Scott-Brown's Otorhinolaryngology Head and Neck Surgery

EIGHTH EDITION

VOLUME 1

Basic Sciences, Head and Neck Endocrine Surgery, Rhinology

VOLUME 2

Paediatrics, The Ear, Skull Base

VOLUME 3

Head and Neck Surgery, Plastic Surgery

Scott-Brown's Otorhinolaryngology Head and Neck Surgery

EIGHTH EDITION

VOLUME 1

Editors

John C Watkinson MSc (Nuclear Medicine; London) MS (London) FRCS (General Surgery) FRCS (ENT) DLO
One-Time Honorary Senior Lecturer and Consultant ENT/Head and Neck and Thyroid Surgeon, Queen Elizabeth Hospital
University of Birmingham NHS Trust and latterly the Royal Marsden and Brompton Hospitals, London, UK
Currently Consultant Head and Neck and Thyroid Surgeon, University Hospital, Coventry and Warwick NHS Trust; and
Honorary Consultant ENT/Head and Neck and Thyroid Surgeon, Great Ormond Street Hospital (GOSH)
Honorary Senior Anatomy Demonstrator, University College London (UCL)
Business Director, Endocrine MDT, The BUPA Cromwell Hospital, London, UK.

Raymond W Clarke BA BSc DCH FRCS FRCS(ORL)
Consultant Paediatric Otolaryngologist, Royal Liverpool Children's Hospital, Liverpool, UK
Senior Lecturer and Associate Dean, University of Liverpool, UK.

Section Editors

Louise Jayne Clark MBChB MD(DIST) FRCS (ORL) FRCS (ENT)
Queen Elizabeth University Hospital, Glasgow, UK.

Adam J Donne PhD FRCS (ORL-HNS)
Consultant Paediatric ENT Surgeon, Alder Hey Children's NHS Foundation Trust, Liverpool,
Honorary Senior Lecturer, Liverpool University, UK.

R James A England FRCS (ORL-HNS)
Consultant Otolaryngologist Head and Neck and Thyroid Surgeon, Honorary Senior Lecturer,
Hull and East Yorkshire NHS Hospitals Trust and Hull University, UK.

Hisham M Mehanna PhD BMedSc (HONS) MBChB (hons) FRCS FRCS (ORL-HNS)
Chair of Head and Neck Surgery and Director of the Institute of Head and Neck Studies and Education,
School of Cancer Sciences, University of Birmingham, UK.

Gerald William McGarry MD MBChB FRCS (ORL-HNS) FFSTed
Consultant Surgeon, Head and Neck and Anterior Skull Base Surgery, Glasgow Royal Infirmary
Greater Glasgow and Clyde NHS, Glasgow, UK
Honorary Clinical Senior Lecturer, University of Glasgow, UK.

Sean Carrie FRCS
Consultant Otolaryngologist, Skull Base Surgeon, Newcastle-upon-Tyne Hospitals NHS Foundation, UK
Honarary Senior Clinical Lecturer, Newcastle University, UK.

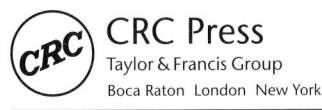

CRC Press
Taylor & Francis Group
Boca Raton London New York

CRC Press is an imprint of the
Taylor & Francis Group, an **informa** business

CRC Press
Taylor & Francis Group
6000 Broken Sound Parkway NW, Suite 300
Boca Raton, FL 33487-2742

© 2019 by Taylor & Francis Group, LLC
CRC Press is an imprint of Taylor & Francis Group, an Informa business

No claim to original U.S. Government works

Printed and bound in India by Replika Press Pvt. Ltd.

Printed on acid-free paper

International Standard Book Number-13: 978-1-138-09461-1 (Hardback; Volume 1)
International Standard Book Number-13: 978-1-138-09463-5 (Hardback; Volume 2)
International Standard Book Number-13: 978-1-138-09464-2 (Hardback; Volume 3)
International Standard Book Number-13: 978-1-4441-7589-9 (Hardback; Set)
International Standard Book Number-13: 978-1-138-19652-0 (Hardback; restricted territorial availability)

This book contains information obtained from authentic and highly regarded sources. While all reasonable efforts have been made to publish reliable data and information, neither the author[s] nor the publisher can accept any legal responsibility or liability for any errors or omissions that may be made. The publishers wish to make clear that any views or opinions expressed in this book by individual editors, authors or contributors are personal to them and do not necessarily reflect the views/opinions of the publishers. The information or guidance contained in this book is intended for use by medical, scientific or healthcare professionals and is provided strictly as a supplement to the medical or other professional's own judgement, their knowledge of the patient's medical history, relevant manufacturer's instructions and the appropriate best practice guidelines. Because of the rapid advances in medical science, any information or advice on dosages, procedures or diagnoses should be independently verified. The reader is strongly urged to consult the relevant national drug formulary and the drug companies' and device or material manufacturers' printed instructions, and their websites, before administering or utilizing any of the drugs, devices or materials mentioned in this book. This book does not indicate whether a particular treatment is appropriate or suitable for a particular individual. Ultimately it is the sole responsibility of the medical professional to make his or her own professional judgements, so as to advise and treat patients appropriately. The authors and publishers have also attempted to trace the copyright holders of all material reproduced in this publication and apologize to copyright holders if permission to publish in this form has not been obtained. If any copyright material has not been acknowledged please write and let us know so we may rectify in any future reprint.

Except as permitted under U.S. Copyright Law, no part of this book may be reprinted, reproduced, transmitted, or utilized in any form by any electronic, mechanical, or other means, now known or hereafter invented, including photocopying, microfilming, and recording, or in any information storage or retrieval system, without written permission from the publishers.

For permission to photocopy or use material electronically from this work, please access www.copyright.com (http://www.copyright.com/) or contact the Copyright Clearance Center, Inc. (CCC), 222 Rosewood Drive, Danvers, MA 01923, 978-750-8400. CCC is a not-for-profit organization that provides licenses and registration for a variety of users. For organizations that have been granted a photocopy license by the CCC, a separate system of payment has been arranged.

Trademark Notice: Product or corporate names may be trademarks or registered trademarks, and are used only for identification and explanation without intent to infringe.

Library of Congress Cataloging-in-Publication Data

Names: Watkinson, John C., editor. | Clarke, Ray (Raymond), editor.
Title: Scott-Brown's otorhinolaryngology and head and neck surgery : basic sciences, endocrine surgery, rhinology / John Watkinson, Ray Clarke.
Other titles: Scott-Brown's otorhinolaryngology, head and neck surgery |Otorhinolaryngology and head and neck surgery.
Description: Eighth edition. | Boca Raton : CRC Press, [2018] | Preceded by Scott-Brown's otorhinolaryngology, head and neck surgery.
7th ed. c2008. | Includes bibliographical references and index.
Identifiers: LCCN 2017032760 (print) | LCCN 2017033968 (ebook) | ISBN 9780203731031 (eBook General) | ISBN 9781351399067 (eBook PDF) | ISBN 9781351399050 (eBook ePub3) | ISBN 9781351399043 (eBook Mobipocket) | ISBN 9781138094611 (hardback : alk. paper).
Subjects: | MESH: Otolaryngology--methods | Otorhinolaryngologic Diseases--surgery | Head--surgery | Neck--surgery | Otorhinolaryngologic Surgical Procedures—methods.
Classification: LCC RF20 (ebook) | LCC RF20 (print) | NLM WV 100 | DDC 617.5/1--dc23
LC record available at https://lccn.loc.gov/2017032760

Visit the Taylor & Francis Web site at
http://www.taylorandfrancis.com

and the CRC Press Web site at
http://www.crcpress.com

Contents

Contributors ix
Foreword xx
Preface xxi
A Tribute to Bill Scott-Brown xxiii
Acknowledgements xxiv
Volume 2 – Table of Contents xxv
Volume 3 – Table of Contents xxix
Abbreviations xxxiii

Section 1 Basic Sciences

Cell biology

1: Molecular biology 3
   Michael Kuo, Richard M. Irving and Eric K. Parkinson

2: Genetics in otology and neurotology 15
   Mohammed-Iqbal Syed

3: Gene therapy 29
   Seiji B. Shibata and Scott M. Graham

4: Mechanisms of anticancer drugs 39
   Sarah Payne and David Miles

5: Radiotherapy and radiosensitizers 51
   Christopher D. Scrase, Stewart G. Martin and
   David A.L. Morgan

6: Apoptosis and cell death 59
   Angela Hague

7: Stem cells 69
   Navin Vig and Ian C. Mackenzie

8: Aetiology and pathogenesis of goitre 75
   Neil Sharma and Kristien Boelaert

9: Genetics of endocrine tumours 83
   Waseem Ahmed, Prata Upasna and Dae Kim

Wound healing

10: Soft and hard tissue repair 93
    Sarah Al-Himdani and Ardeshir Bayat

11: Skin flap physiology 107
    Colin MacIver and Stergios Doumas

12: Biomaterials, tissue engineering and their
    application in the oral and maxillofacial region 119
    Kurt Busuttil Naudi and Ashraf Ayoub

Immunology

13: Defence mechanisms 125
    Ian Todd and Richard J. Powell

14: Allergy: Basic mechanisms and tests 137
    Sai H.K. Murng

15: Evaluation of the immune system 149
    Moira Thomas, Elizabeth Drewe and Richard J. Powell

16: Cancer immunology 157
    Osama Al Hamarneh and John Greenman

17: Human papillomavirus 167
    Mustaffa Junaid and Hisham M. Mehanna

18: Connective tissue diseases: ENT complications 173
    Eileen Baildam

Microbiology

19: Microorganisms 181
    Ursula Altmeyer, Penelope Redding and Nitish Khanna

20: Viruses and antiviral agents 195
    Richard B. Townsley, Camille A. Huser and
    Chris Hansell

21: Fungal infections 205
    Emily Young, Yujay Ramakrishnan, Laura Jackson and
    Shahzada K. Ahmed

22: Antimicrobial therapy 221
    Ursula Altmeyer, Penelope Redding and Nitish Khanna

23: Human immunodeficiency virus 229
    Neil Ritchie and Alasdair Robertson

Haematology

24: Blood groups, blood components and
    alternatives to transfusion 239
    Samah Alimam, Kate Pendry and Michael F. Murphy

25: Haemato-oncology 249
    Robert F. Wynn and Mark Williams

26: Haemostasis: Normal physiology, disorders of
    haemostasis and thrombosis 259
    Elizabeth Jones and Russell David Keenan

Pharmacotherapeutics

27: Drug therapy in otology 275
    Wendy Smith

28: Drug therapy in rhinology 283
    Wendy Smith

29: Drug therapy in laryngology and head and
    neck surgery 293
    Wendy Smith and Rogan Corbridge

Perioperative management

30: Preparation of the patient for surgery 301
    Michael Murray and Urmila Ratnasabapathy

31: Recognition and management of the difficult airway..... 309
    Valerie Cunningham and Alistair McNarry

32: Adult anaesthesia 333
    Daphne A. Varveris and Neil G. Smart

33: Adult critical care 351
    Robert I. Docking and Andrew Mackay

34: Paediatric intensive care 361
    Louise Selby and Robert Ross Russell

Safe and effective practice

35: Training, accreditation and the maintenance of skills 369
    B. Nirmal Kumar, Andrew Robson, Omar Mirza and
    Baskaran Ranganathan

36: Communication and the medical consultation 379
    Uttam Shiralkar

37: Clinical governance and its role in patient safety
    and quality improvement 389
    Samit Majumdar and S. Musheer Hussain

38: Medical ethics 395
    Paul Baines

39a: Medical jurisprudence in otorhinolaryngology 409
    Maurice Hawthorne

39b: Medical negligence in otorhinolaryngology 427
    Maurice Hawthorne

40: Non-technical skills for ENT surgeons 453
    Simon Paterson-Brown and Stephen R. Ell

Interpretation and management of data

41: Epidemiology 465
    Jan H.P. van der Meulen, David A. Lowe and Jonathan
    M. Fishman

42: Outcomes research 483
    Iain R.C. Swan and William Whitmer

43: Evidence-based medicine in medical education
    and clinical practice 495
    Phillip Evans

44: Critical appraisal skills 503
    Paul Nankivell and Christopher Coulson

Advances in technology

45: Electrophysiology and monitoring 525
    Patrick R. Axon and Bruno M.R. Kenway

46: Optical coherence tomography 533
    Jameel Muzaffar and Jonathan M. Fishman

47: Recent advances in technology 541
    Wai Lup Wong and Bal Sanghera

48: Image-guided surgery, 3D planning and
    reconstruction 559
    Ghassan Alusi and Michael Gleeson

49: Interventional techniques 569
    James V. Byrne

50: Laser principles in otolaryngology, head and
    neck surgery 581
    Brian J.G. Bingham

51: Contact endoscopy of the upper
    aerodigestive tract 587
    Mario Andrea and Oscar Dias

Section 2 Head and Neck Endocrine Surgery

Overview

52: History of thyroid and parathyroid surgery 597
    Waraporn Imruetaicharoenchoke, Ashok R. Shaha and
    Neil Sharma

53: Developmental anatomy of the thyroid and
    parathyroid glands 603
    Julian A. McGlashan

54: Developmental anatomy of the pituitary fossa 611
    John Hill and Sean Carrie

55: Physiology of the thyroid and parathyroid glands 619
    Martin O. Weickert

56: Physiology of the pituitary gland 629
    Mária Hérincs, Karen Young and Márta Korbonits

57: Imaging in head and neck endocrine disease 643
    Steve Colley and Sabena Fareedi

58: Thyroid and parathyroid gland pathology 651
    Ram Moorthy, Sonia Kumar and Adrian T. Warfield

Thyroid disease

59: Clinical evaluation of the thyroid patient 705
    Andrew Coatesworth and Sebastian Wallis

60: Investigation of thyroid disease 709
    Anthony P. Weetman

61: Benign thyroid disease 717
    Christopher M. Jones and Kristien Boelaert

62: Management of differentiated thyroid cancer 751
    Hisham M. Mehanna, Kristien Boelaert and Neil Sharma

63: Management of medullary thyroid cancer 757
Barney Harrison

64: Management of anaplastic thyroid cancer/
lymphoma 765
James D. Brierley and Richard W. Tsang

65: Management of locoregionally recurrent
differentiated thyroid cancer 773
Iain J. Nixon and Ashok R. Shaha

66: Non-surgical management of thyroid cancer 779
Laura Moss

Thyroid surgery

67: Thyroidectomy 793
Ricard Simo, Iain J. Nixon and Ralph P. Tufano

68: Surgery for locally advanced and nodal disease 805
Joel Anthony Smith and John C. Watkinson

69: Minimally invasive and robotic thyroid surgery 811
Neil S. Tolley

70: Surgery for the enlarged thyroid 819
Neeraj Sethi, Josh Lodhia and R. James A. England

Parathyroid disease

71: Clinical evaluation of hypercalcaemia 827
Mo Aye and Thozhukat Sathyapalan

72: Investigation of hyperparathyroidism 833
M. Shahed Quraishi

73: Management of hyperparathyroidism 843
Neil J.L. Gittoes and John Ayuk

74: Management of persistent and recurrent
hyperparathyroidism 851
David M. Scott-Coombes

75: Management of parathyroid cancer 857
Pamela Howson and Mark Sywak

Parathyroid surgery

76: Bilateral parathyroid exploration 865
R. James A. England and Nick McIvor

77: Minimally invasive parathyroidectomy 873
Parameswaran Rajeev and Gregory P. Sadler

78: Surgical failure and reoperative surgery 879
Schelto Kruijff and Leigh Delbridge

Thyroid and parathyroid outcomes

79: Complications of thyroid and parathyroid surgery
and how to avoid them 887
*Erin A. Felger, Dipti Kamani and
Gregory W. Randolph*

80: Thyroid and parathyroid surgery: Audit and
outcomes 893
David Chadwick

81: Medicolegal aspects of head and neck
endocrine surgery 899
Barney Harrison

Pituitary disease

82: Clinical evaluation of the pituitary patient 905
Sean Carrie, John Hill and Andrew James

83: Investigation of pituitary disease 915
Thozhukat Sathyapalan and Stephen L. Atkin

84: Primary pituitary disease 923
Christopher M. Jones and John Ayuk

85: Surgical management of recurrent pituitary tumours 941
*Mihir R. Patel, Leo F.S. Ditzel Filho, Daniel M.
Prevedello, Bradley A. Otto and Ricardo L. Carrau*

86: Adjuvant treatment of pituitary disease 951
Andy Levy

Section 3 Rhinology

87: Anatomy of the nose and paranasal sinuses 961
Dustin M. Dalgorf and Richard J. Harvey

88: Outpatient assessment 977
Martyn L. Barnes and Paul S. White

89: Physiology of the nose and paranasal sinuses 983
Tira Galm and Shahzada K. Ahmed

90: Measurement of the nasal airway 991
Ron Eccles

91: Allergic rhinitis 999
Quentin Gardiner

92: Non-allergic perennial rhinitis 1011
Jameel Muzaffar and Shahzada K. Ahmed

93: Occupational rhinitis 1017
Hesham Saleh

94: Rhinosinusitis: Definitions, classification and
diagnosis 1025
Carl Philpott

95: Nasal polyposis 1037
Louise Melia

96: Fungal rhinosinusitis 1047
Eng Cern Gan and Amin R. Javer

97: Medical management for rhinosinusitis 1059
Claire Hopkins

98: Surgical management of rhinosinusitis 1071
A. Simon Carney and Raymond Sacks

99: The frontal sinus 1081
Salil Nair

100: Mucoceles of the paranasal sinuses 1107
Darlene E. Lubbe

101: Complications of rhinosinusitis 1113
Stephen Ball and Sean Carrie

102: The relationship between the upper and lower respiratory tract 1125
Nigel K.F. Koo Ng and Gerald W. McGarry

103: Nasal septum and nasal valve 1135
Shahram Anari and Ravinder Singh Natt

104: Nasal septal perforations 1149
Charles East and Kevin Kulendra

105: Management of enlarged turbinates 1157
Andrew C. Swift and Samuel C. Leong

106: Epistaxis 1169
Gerald W. McGarry

107: Nasal and facial fractures 1183
Dae Kim and Simon Holmes

108: CSF leaks 1203
Scott M. Graham

109: Granulomatous conditions of the nose 1211
Joanne Rimmer and Valerie J. Lund

110: Abnormalities of smell 1227
Richard L. Doty and Steven M. Bromley

111: Disorders of the orbit.. 1243
Nithin D. Adappa and James N. Palmer

112: Diagnosis and management of facial pain 1253
Rajiv K. Bhalla and Timothy J. Woolford

113: Juvenile angiofibroma 1265
Bernhard Schick

114: Endoscopic management of sinonasal tumours 1269
Alkis J. Psaltis and David K. Morrissey

115: Surgical management of pituitary and parasellar diseases 1281
Philip G. Chen and Peter-John Wormald

116: Extended anterior skull base approaches 1289
Carl H. Snyderman, Paul A. Gardner,
Juan C. Fernandez-Miranda and Eric W. Wang

117: Imaging in rhinology 1305
Gregory O'Neill

Index 1319

Contributors

Nithin D Adappa MD
Assistant Professor
Department of Otorhinolaryngology, Head and Neck Surgery
University of Pennsylvania
Philadelphia, USA.

Shahzada K Ahmed BSC(HONS) DLO FRCS (ORL-HNS) PHD
Consultant Rhinologist and Skull Base Surgeon
Queen Elizabeth Hospital
Birmingham, UK.

Waseem Ahmed MBBS BSC FRCS (ORL-HNS)
Clinical Fellow in Otology
Gloucestershire NHS Hospitals Foundation Trust
Gloucester, UK.

Osama Al Hamarneh MBBS MD FRCS (ORL-HNS)
Interface Fellow in Head and Neck Surgical Oncology
Department of Otolaryngology Head and Neck Surgery
Royal Hallamshire Hospital
Sheffield, UK.

Sarah Al-Himdani MBCHB MRCS (ENG)
Plastic Surgery Speciality Registrar
Plastic and Reconstructive Surgery Research
Manchester Institute of Biotechnology
University Hospital of South Manchester NHS Foundation Trust
Institute of Inflammation and Repair, Faculty of Medical and Human Sciences
University of Manchester, Manchester Academic Health Science Centre, Manchester, UK.

Samah Alimam MBCHB MRCP
Haematology Specialty Registrar
Central Manchester Foundation Trust
Manchester, UK.

Ursula Altmeyer MRCP FRCPATH
Consultant Microbiologist
University Hospital Crosshouse
NHS Ayrshire & Arran
Scotland, UK.

Ghassan Alusi PHD FRCS (ORL-HNS)
Consultant Otolaryngologist
ENT Department
Barts and the London NHS Trust
London, UK.

Shahram Anari MD MSC FRCS (ORL-HNS)
Consultant Otorhinolaryngologist/Head & Neck Surgeon
Department of Otolaryngology
Heartlands Hospital
Birmingham, UK.

Mario Andrea MD PHD
Professor of Otolaryngology
Faculty of Medicine
University of Lisbon
Lisbon, Portugal.

Steve L Atkin MBBS PHD
Professor of Medicine
Weill Cornell Medical College Qatar
Qatar Foundation
Education City
Doha, Qatar.

Patrick R Axon MD FRCS (ORL-HNS)
Consultant Otologist and Skull Base Surgeon
Department of Otolaryngology
Cambridge University Hospitals
Cambridge, UK.

Mo Aye MB BS FRCP FRCPE
Consultant Endocrinologist
Centre for Metabolic Bone Disease
Hull Royal Infirmary
Hull, UK.

Ashraf Ayoub PHD BDS MDS FDSRCS FDSRCPS
Professor of Oral and Maxillofacial Surgery
Dental School, School of Medicine
College of Medical, Veterinary and Life Sciences
University of Glasgow
Glasgow, UK.

John Ayuk MD MRCP
Consultant Endocrinologist
Department of Endocrinology
Queen Elizabeth Hospital, Birmingham; and
Honorary Senior Lecturer
University of Birmingham
Birmingham, UK.

Eileen Baildam MBCHB MRCGP DCH FRCP FRCPCH
Consultant Paediatric Rheumatologist
Alder Hey Children's Foundation NHS Trust
Alder Hey, Liverpool; and
Honorary Senior Lecturer
Liverpool University
Liverpool, UK.

Paul Baines MD PHD MRCP FRCA FFICM
Consultant in Paediatric Intensive Care
Alder Hey Children's NHS Foundation Trust
Liverpool, UK.

Stephen Ball MRCS PHD
NIHR Academic Clinical Lecturer & Speciality Registrar in ENT Surgery
Newcastle University & Newcastle Hospitals
Newcastle, UK.

Martyn L Barnes MBBS MD MSC(OXON) FRCS-ORL(EDIN)
Rhinology and Anterior Skullbase Fellow to Dr Richard Douglas, North Shore Hospital, Auckland; and
Honorary Senior Clinical Teacher
University of Dundee; and
Director to SurgTech Ltd
Dundee, UK.

Ardeshir Bayat BSC(HONS) MBBS MRCS(ENG, EDIN) PHD
Clinical Scientist and Associate Professor
Plastic and Reconstructive Surgery Research
Manchester Institute of Biotechnology
University Hospital of South Manchester NHS Foundation Trust
Institute of Inflammation and Repair, Faculty of Medical and Human Sciences
University of Manchester, Manchester Academic Health Science Centre, Manchester, UK.

Rajiv K Bhalla BSC (HONS) FRCS (ORL-HNS) MD PGCERT MED ED
Consultant ENT Surgeon and Rhinologist
Department of Otolaryngology, Head and Neck Surgery
Manchester Royal Infirmary
Manchester, UK.

Brian JG Bingham MBCHB FRCS ED GLAS
Consultant ENT Surgeon
Department of Otolaryngology, New Victoria Hospital & Southern General Hospital; and
Honorary Senior Lecturer in Otorhinolaryngology
University of Glasgow
Glasgow, UK.

Kristien Boelaert MD PHD FRCP
Reader in Endocrinology
Centre for Endocrinology, Diabetes and Metabolism
Institute of Metabolism and Systems Research
College of Medical and Dental Sciences
University of Birmingham; and
Honorary Consultant Endocrinologist
Department of Endocrinology
University Hospital Birmingham NHS Foundation Trust
Birmingham, UK.

James D Brierley MBBS FRCP FRCR FRCSP(C)
Professor
Department of Radiation Oncology
University of Toronto
Princess Margaret Cancer Centre
Toronto, Canada.

Steven M Bromley MD FANN
Director
South Jersey MS Center and Bromley Neurology PC
Audubon
New Jersey, USA.

James V Byrne MD FRCS FRCR
Professor of Neuroradiology
University of Oxford; and
Consultant Neuroradiologist
John Radcliffe Hospital
Oxford, UK.

A Simon Carney BSC (HONS) MBCHB FRCS FRACS MD
Associate Professor and Head of ENT Unit
Flinders University and Flinders Medical Centre
Adelaide, South Australia.

Sean Carrie MB CHB FRCS FRCS (ORL)
Consultant Rhinologist and Hon Senior Lecturer
Newcastle upon Tyne Hospitals NHS Foundation Trust
Newcastle University
Newcastle, UK.

Ricardo L Carrau MD
Professor, Director of the Comprehensive Skull Base Surgery Program
Department of Otolaryngology, Head & Neck Surgery
The Ohio State University Wexner Medical Center
Columbus, Ohio, USA.

David Chadwick BM BCH FRCS(ED) MD
Consultant Endocrine Surgeon
Chesterfield Royal Hospital
Chesterfield, UK.

Philip G Chen MD
Assistant Professor & Program Director
Rhinology & Otolaryngology
Department of Otolaryngology, Head and Neck Surgery
University of Texas Health, San Antonio
Texas, USA.

Andrew Coatesworth FRCS (ORL-HNS)
Consultant ENT Surgeon
York Teaching Hospital NHS Foundation Trust
York Hospital
York, UK.

Steve Colley
Consultant Radiologist
Queen Elizabeth Hospital
Birmingham, UK.

Rogan Corbridge MBBS BSC FRCS FRCS (ORL)
Consultant ENT Surgeon
Oxford Centre for Head and Neck Oncology
John Radcliffe Hospital
Oxford, UK.

Christopher Coulson PHD FRCS (ORL-HNS)
Consultant Otolaryngologist
NIHR Clinical Lecturer, Otolaryngology Head and Neck Surgery
School of Cancer Sciences, University of Birmingham
Queen Elizabeth Hospital
Birmingham, UK.

Valerie Cunningham MBCHB FRCA FFICM
Consultant Anaesthetist
Institute of Neurosciences
Queen Elizabeth University Hospital
Glasgow, UK.

Dustin M Dalgorf MD FRCSC
Clinical Lecturer
Rhinology and Skull Base Surgery
Mount Sinai Hospital and St Joseph's Health Centre
University of Toronto
Toronto, Canada.

Leigh Delbridge MD FRACS
Emeritus Professor of Surgery
University of Sydney
Sydney, Australia.

Oscar Dias MD PHD
Professor of Otolaryngology
Faculty of Medicine
University of Lisbon
Lisbon, Portugal.

Leo FS Ditzel Filho MD
Neurosurgeon
Department of Neurosurgery
Wexner Medical Center at The Ohio State University
Columbus, Ohio, USA.

Robert I Docking MBCHB FRCA
Specialty Registrar, Anaesthesia and
    Intensive Care Medicine
Glasgow Royal Infirmary
Glasgow, UK.

Richard L Doty PHD
Professor and Director
Smell & Taste Center
University of Pennsylvania Medical Center
Philadelphia, USA.

Stergios Doumas MD DDS
Maxillofacial/Head & Neck Fellow
Leeds Teaching Hospitals NHS Trust
Leeds, UK.

Elizabeth Drewe MBBS PHD MRCP MRCPATH
Consultant Clinical Immunologist
Nottingham University Hospitals NHS Trust
Nottingham, UK.

Charles East FRCS
Consultant Surgeon
University College London Hospitals NHS Trust; and
Honorary Senior Lecturer, University College London
London, UK.

Ron Eccles BSC PHD DSC
Professor Emeritus
Common Cold Centre
School of Biosciences
Cardiff University
Cardiff, UK.

Stephen R Ell BSC (HONS) MBBS CERTAVMED MD
    FRCS (EDIN) FRCS (ORL-HNS)
Consultant ENT Surgeon
Hull and East Yorkshire Hospitals NHS Trust; and
Honorary Professor, University of Hull
Hull, UK.

R James A England FRCS (ORL-HNS)
Consultant Otolaryngologist Head and Neck and
    Thyroid Surgeon; and
Honorary Senior Lecturer
Department of Otolaryngology, Head and Neck Surgery
Hull and East Yorkshire Hospitals NHS Trust
Hull, UK.

Phillip Evans BSC(HONS) MSC MED FHEA
Senior University Teacher
College of Medical, Veterinary and Life Science
University of Glasgow
Glasgow, UK.

Sabena Fareedi MBBS BSC MRCP FRCR
Consultant Neuroradiologist
Queen Elizabeth Hospital
Birmingham, UK.

Erin A Felger MD FACS
Associate Program Director of General Surgery
Assistant Professor of Clinical Surgery Georgetown
    University
Endocrine Surgeon
Medstar Washington Hospital Center
Washington DC, USA.

Juan C Fernandez-Miranda MD
Associate Professor of Neurological Surgery
Director of the Complex Brain Surgery Program
Associate Director of the Center for Cranial Base Surgery
Department of Neurological Surgery
University of Pittsburgh School of Medicine
Pittsburgh, USA.

Jonathan M Fishman MA (CANTAB) PHD DOHNS FRCS
    (ORL-HNS)
Clinical Lecturer, Academy of Medical Sciences
University College London
London, UK.

Tira Galm FRCS (ORL-HNS) MBA
Rhinology Fellow
Queen Elizabeth Hospital
Birmingham, UK.

Eng Cern Gan MBBS MRCS (EDIN) MMED (ORL) FAMS
Consultant, Department of Otorhinolaryngology, Head
    & Neck Surgery
Changi General Hospital; and
Senior Clinical Lecturer
Yong Loo Lin School of Medicine
National University of Singapore, Singapore.

Paul A Gardner MD
Neurosurgeon
Department of Neurological Surgery
University of Pittsburgh School of Medicine
Pittsburgh, USA.

Quentin Gardiner MB CHB FRCS (ENG & ED) FRCS (ORL)
Consultant Rhinologist
Ninewells Hospital and Medical School
Dundee, UK.

Neil JL Gittoes PHD FRCP
Consultant Endocrinologist
Department of Endocrinology
Queen Elizabeth Hospital Birmingham; and
Honorary Senior Lecturer
University of Birmingham
Birmingham, UK.

Michael Gleeson MD FRCS
Professor of Otolaryngology and Skull Base Surgery
Institute of Neurology, University College London; and
Consultant
Guy's, Kings and St Thomas' and the National Hospital for Neurology and Neurosurgery; and
Honorary Consultant Skull Base Surgeon
Great Ormond Street Hospital for Sick Children
London, UK.

Scott M Graham MD
Professor of Otolaryngology, Head and Neck Surgery; and
Professor, Department of Neurosurgery
The University of Iowa; and
Director of the Division of Rhinology
University of Iowa Hospital and Clinics
Iowa City, Iowa, USA.

John Greenman PHD
Professor of Tumour Immunology & Scientific Director, Daisy Building
Head, School of Biological, Biomedical and Environmental Sciences
University of Hull
Hull, UK.

Angela Hague BSC PHD
Senior Teaching Fellow
School of Oral and Dental Sciences
University of Bristol
Bristol, UK.

Chris Hansell BSC PHD
Post-Doctoral Research Associate
Institute of Infection, Inflammation and Immunity
University of Glasgow
Glasgow, UK.

Barney Harrison MB BS MS FRCS
Consultant Endocrine Surgeon
Royal Hallamshire Hospital
Sheffield, UK.

Richard J Harvey MD
Program Head and Professor
Rhinology and Skull Base
Applied Medical Research Centre
University of New South Wales
Faculty of Medicine and Health Sciences
Macquarie University
Sydney, Australia.

Maurice Hawthorne FRCS
Consultant Otolaryngologist, Head and Neck Surgeon
James Cook University Hospital
Middlesbrough, UK.

Mária Hérincs MD MBBS
Clinical Fellow
Department of Endocrinology
William Harvey Research Institute
Barts and the London School of Medicine
Queen Mary University of London
London, UK.

John Hill MBBS FRCS FRCSED FCSHK
Consultant Otolaryngologist
Freeman Hospital
Newcastle, UK.

Claire Hopkins FRCS (ORL-HNS) DM
Professor of Rhinology, King's College, London
Consultant ENT Surgeon
Guy's and St Thomas' NHS Trust
London, UK

Simon Holmes BDS MD BS FDS RCS FRCS
Consultant Oral and Maxillofacial Surgeon
Barts and the London NHS Trust
London, UK.

Pamela Howson BMEDSCI MBBS FRACS
Breast, Endocrine and General Surgeon
Concord and Auburn Hospitals
Sydney, Australia.

Camille A Huser BSC MSC PHD
Post-Doctoral Research Associate
MRC University of Glasgow Centre for Virus Research
Glasgow, UK.

S Musheer Hussain MB BS MSC (MANC) FRCS (EDIN) FRCS (ENG) FFST FRCS (ORL)
Consultant Otolaryngologist Head and Neck Surgeon
Honorary Professor of Otolaryngology and Consultant ENT Surgeon
Licenced Teacher of Anatomy
Ninewells Hospital & University of Dundee Medical School
Dundee, UK.

Waraporn Imruetaicharoenchoke MD
Consultant Surgeon
Division of Head Neck and Breast Surgery
Department of Surgery
Faculty of Medicine Siriraj Hospital
Mahidol University
Bangkok, Thailand.

Richard M Irving MD FRCS (ORL-HNS)
Consultant in Neurotology
University Hospital Birmingham NHS Trust and Diana Princess of Wales (Birmingham Children's) Hospital; and
Honorary Senior Lecturer
University of Birmingham
Birmingham, UK.

Laura Jackson BSC PHD MBCHC FRCS(ORL-HNS)
Specialty Registrar ENT
New Cross Hospital
London, UK.

Andrew James BSC MB MCH MD FRCP
Consultant Endocrinologist
Newcastle upon Tyne Hospitals NHS Foundation Trust
Newcastle University
Newcastle, UK.

Amin R Javer BSC MD FRCSC FARS
Clinical Professor of Surgery
University of British Columbia; and
Director, St Paul's Sinus Centre
Vancouver, Canada.

Christopher M Jones BMEDSC(HONS) MB CHB(HONS) MRCP
Wellcome Trust Clinical Research Fellow
Faculties of Biological Sciences, Medicine & Health
University of Leeds
Leeds, UK.

Elizabeth Jones MBCHB BSC (PHARMACOL) MRCPCH FRCPATH
Consultant Haematologist
Wirral University Teaching Hospital Trust
Wirral, UK.

Mustaffa Junaid MBBS BSC (HONS) MRCS DOHNS
Honorary Research Associate
Institute of Head and Neck Studies and Education (InHANSE)
School of Cancer Sciences
University of Birmingham, UK.

Dipti Kamani MD
Harvard Medical School
Research Director Thyroid and Parathyroid Surgical Division
Massachusetts Eye and Ear Infirmary
Boston, Massachusetts, USA.

Russell David Keenan MB CHB FRCP FRCPATH
Consultant Paediatric Haematologist
Alder Hey Children's Hospital
Liverpool, UK.

Bruno MH Kenway BMEDSCI BMBS DOHNS FRCS (ORL-HNS)
Otology Fellow
Department of Otolaryngology
Cambridge University Hospitals
Cambridge, UK.

Nitish Khanna MBCHB BSC DTMH FRCPATH
Consultant Microbiologist
Deputy Director
Scottish MRSA Reference Laboratory & Scottish Salmonella, Shigella and C.difficile Reference Laboratory
Glasgow Royal Infirmary
Glasgow, UK.

Dae Kim MBCHB BDS MSC FRCS PHD
Consultant ENT Surgeon
Queen Alexandra Hospital
Portsmouth, UK.

Márta Korbonits MD PHD FRCP
Professor
Department of Endocrinology
William Harvey Research Institute
Barts and the London School of Medicine
Queen Mary University of London
London, UK.

Schelto Kruijff PHD MD
Consultant Oncology and Endocrine Surgeon
University Medical Center
Groningen, Netherlands.

Kevin Kulendra BSC MBBS DOHNS FRCS (ORL-HNS)
Consultant ENT Surgeon
ENT Department, Oxford University Hospitals NHS Trust
John Radcliffe Hospital
Oxford, UK.

Michael Kuo PHD FRCS (ENG) FRCS (ORL-HNS) DCH
Consultant Otolaryngologist, Head and Neck Surgeon
Birmingham Children's Hospital
Birmingham, UK.

B Nirmal Kumar MPHIL FRCS (ORL-HNS) FACADMED
Consultant Otoloaryngologist Head & Neck Surgeon
Director of Medical Education
Wrightington, Wigan and Leigh NHS Foundation Trust
Wigan, UK.

Sonia Kumar FRCS (ORL-HNS)
Fellow in Paediatric ENT Surgery
Great Ormond St Hospital for Sick Children
London, UK.

Samuel C Leong MPHIL FRCSED (ORL-HNS)
Rhinologist and Anterior Skull Base Surgeon
Aintree University Hospital NHS Foundation Trust
Liverpool, UK.

Andy Levy BMEDSCI MBBS PHD FRCP
Professor of Endocrinology and Honorary Consultant Physician
University of Bristol and University Hospitals
Bristol NHS Foundation Trust
Henry Wellcome Labs
Bristol, UK.

Josh Lodhia MBCHB MRCS
Specialist Trainee
Department of Cardiothoracic Surgery
Hull and East Yorkshire Hospitals NHS Trust
Hull, UK.

David A Lowe BSC FRCSED FRCS
Research Fellow
Clinical Effectiveness Unit
Royal College of Surgeons of England
London, UK.

Darlene E Lubbe MBCHB FCORL(SA)
Principal Specialist
Division of Otorhinolaryngology
University of Cape Town
Cape Town, South Africa.

Valerie J Lund CBE MS FRCS FRCSED
Professor of Rhinology
University College London; and
Honorary Consultant ENT Surgeon
Royal National Throat Nose & Ear Hospital
London, UK.

Andrew Mackay MBCHB FRCA EDIC FFICM
Consultant, Anaesthesia and Intensive Care Medicine
Victoria Infirmary
Glasgow, UK.

Gerald W McGarry MB CHB MD FRCSED FRCS (ORL-HNS) FFSTED
Consultant Surgeon
Department of Otolaryngology and Head and Neck Surgery
Glasgow Royal Infirmary
NHS Greater Glasgow and Clyde
Glasgow, UK.

Julian A McGlashan MBBS FRCS(ORL)
Special Lecturer and Consultant
Department of Otorhinolaryngology
Queen's Medical Centre Campus
Nottingham University Hospitals
Nottingham, UK.

Colin MacIver FRCSS FRD FRCS ED FRCS (OMFS)
Consultant Maxillofacial/Head & Neck Surgeon
Lead Clinician
Maxillofacial Unit
Queen Elizabeth University Hospital
Glasgow, UK.

Nick McIvor MBCHB FRACS
Head and Neck Surgeon
Auckland Regional Head and Neck Service
Auckland District Health Board
New Zealand.

Ian C Mackenzie BDS FDSRCS PHD
Professor of Stem Cell Science
Blizard Institute
Barts and The London Medical School
Queen Mary University of London
London, UK.

Alistair McNarry MA FRCA
Consultant Anaesthetist
Department of Anaesthesia
Western General and St John's Hospitals
NHS Lothian
Edinburgh, UK.

Samit Majumdar MBBS BMEDSCI(HON) FRCS(EDIN) FDS RCPS FRCS(ORL)
Honorary Senior Lecturer and Consultant ENT Surgeon
Fellow, Scottish Patient Safety Programme
Ninewells Hospital & University of Dundee Medical School
Dundee, UK.

Stewart G Martin BSC (HONS) MSC PHD
Associate Professor of Oncology
MSc Course Director and Head of Translational Radiation, Biology Research Group
University of Nottingham
Academic Division of Clinical Oncology
Nottingham University Hospitals
Nottingham, UK.

Louise Melia MBCHB MRCS FRCS ORL-HNS
Specialty Registrar
Department of Otolaryngology
Glasgow Royal Infirmary
Glasgow, UK.

Hisham M Mehanna PHD BMEDSC MBCHB FRCS FRCS (ORL-HNS)
Chair, Head and Neck Surgery; and
Director, Institute of Head and Neck Studies and Education (InHANSE)
Institute of Head and Neck Studies and Education
Institute of Cancer and Genomic Sciences
University of Birmingham
Birmingham, UK.

David Miles FRCP MD
Professor
Medical Oncology Consultant
Mount Vernon Cancer Centre
Northwood, London, UK.

Omar Mirza MBCHB MA MRCS DOHNS
Specialty Registrar in ORL-HNS
Wrightington, Wigan and Leigh NHS Foundation Trust
Health Education North West
Wigan, UK.

Ram Moorthy FRCS (ORL-HNS)
Consultant ENT/Head & Neck Surgeon
Wexham Park Hospital
Frimley Health NHS Foundation Trust
Slough, UK.

David AL Morgan FRCR
Consultant Clinical Oncologist
Department of Clinical Oncology
Nottingham University Hospitals
Nottingham, UK.

David K Morrissey MBBS(HONS) FRACS
Otolaryngology, Head and Neck Surgeon
Department of Otolaryngology, Head and Neck Surgery
The Queen Elizabeth Hospital
Adelaide
School of Medicine
The University of Queensland
St Lucia, Australia.

Laura Moss FRCP FRCR LLM
Consultant Clinical Oncologist
Velindre Hospital
Cardiff, UK.

Sai HK Murng MB BS MRCP(UK) FRCPATH
Consultant Immunologist
Immunology Department
NHS Greater Glasgow and Clyde Glasgow, UK.

Michael F Murphy MD, FRCP, FRCPATH, FFPATH
Professor of Transfusion Medicine
University of Oxford; and
Consultant Haematologist
NHS Blood & Transplant and Oxford University Hospitals NHS Foundation Trust
Oxford, UK.

Michael Murray FRCA FFICM
Consultant Anaesthetist
Department of Anaesthesia
Southern General Hospital
Glasgow, UK.

Jameel Muzaffar BA(HONS) MBBS(HONS) MSC DO-HNS MRCS(ENT)
Specialist Registrar & Honorary Research Fellow
Institute of Head and Neck Studies and Education (InHANSE)
University of Birmingham & University Hospitals Birmingham NHS Foundation Trust
Birmingham, UK.

Salil Nair MD FRCS (ORL-HNS)
Consultant Rhinologist & Honorary Senior Lecturer
Manukau SuperClinic and Auckland University Hospitals
Auckland, New Zealand.

Paul Nankivell PHD FRCS (ORL-HNS)
NIHR Clinical Lecturer, Otolaryngology Head and Neck Surgery
School of Cancer Sciences, University of Birmingham
Queen Elizabeth Hospital
Birmingham, UK.

Ravinder Singh Natt BSC DO-HNS FRCS (ORL-HNS)
Consultant Otorhinolaryngologist/Head & Neck Surgeon
Department of Otolaryngology
Guy's and St Thomas' Hospitals
London, UK.

Kurt Busuttil Naudi DDS MED LTHE BCHD FDS RCSED MFDS RCPS MSURGDENT PGCAP FHEA
Senior Clinical University Teacher / Honoray Consultant in Oral Surgery
Dental School, School of Medicine
College of Medical, Veterinary and Life Sciences
University of Glasgow
Glasgow, UK.

Nigel KF Koo Ng MA BM BCH MFSTED FRCS (ORL-HNS)
Rhinology and Facial Plastic Surgery Fellow
St George's University Hospitals NHS Foundation Trust
London, UK.

Iain J Nixon MBCHB FRCS (ORL-HNS) PHD
Consultant Otorhinolaryngologist Head and Neck Surgeon
University of Edinburgh
NHS Lothian Department of ENT/Head and Neck Surgery
Edinburgh Royal Infirmary
Edinburgh, UK.

Gregory O'Neill BSC(HONS) MBCHB FRCR
Consultant Radiologist
Glasgow Royal Infirmary
Glasgow, UK.

Bradley A Otto MD
Assistant Professor
Director, Division of Rhinology
Department of Otolaryngology, Head & Neck Surgery
Wexner Medical Center at The Ohio State University
Columbus, Ohio, USA.

James N Palmer MD
Associate Professor
Department of Otorhinolaryngology, Head and Neck Surgery
University of Pennsylvania
Philadelphia, USA.

Eric K Parkinson PHD
Professor of Head & Neck Cancer
Centre for Clinical & Diagnostic Oral Sciences
Institute of Dentistry, Barts & The London School of Medicine and Dentistry
Queen Mary University of London
London, UK.

Mihir R Patel MD
Assistant Professor
Department of Otolaryngology, Head & Neck Surgery
Wexner Medical Center at The Ohio State University
Columbus, Ohio, USA.

Simon Paterson-Brown MBBS MPHIL MS FRCS(EDIN) FRCS(ENGL) FCS(HK)
Consultant General and Upper Gastrointestinal Surgeon
Royal Infirmary of Edinburgh; and
Honorary Senior Lecturer
Edinburgh University
Edinburgh, UK.

Sarah Payne MRCP PHD
Medical Manager Oncology, Pfizer UK and Honorary Medical Oncology Consultant
Guy's and St Thomas' NHS Foundation Trust
Medical Oncology
Mount Vernon Hospital
London, UK.

Kate Pendry BSC MBCHB FRCP FRCPATH
Consultant Haematologist
NHS Blood and Transplant
Manchester Blood Centre
Manchester, UK.

Carl Philpott MB CHB DLO FRCS (ORL-HNS) MD PGCME
Professor of Rhinology & Olfactology and Head of Rhinology & ENT Research Group Professionalism Lead
Norwich Medical School; and
Honorary Consultant Rhinologist and ENT Surgeon
James Paget University Hospital
Great Yarmouth, UK.

Richard J Powell MMBS DM FRCP FRCPATH
Consultant and Professor in Clinical Immunology
School of Life Sciences
University of Nottingham
Queen's Medical Centre
Nottingham, UK.

Daniel M Prevedello MD FACS
Professor
Department of Neurological Surgery
The Ohio State University
Columbus, Ohio, USA.

Alkis J Psaltis MBBS(HONS) PHD FRACS
Associate Professor, Division of Surgery, University of Adelaide; and
Head of Department of Otolaryngology, Head and Neck Surgery
The Queen Elizabeth Hospital
Department of Surgery, Division of ENT
The University of Adelaide
Adelaide, Australia.

M Shahed Quraishi OBE FRCS FRCS (ORL-HNS)
Consultant Otolaryngologist, Thyroid and Parathyroid Surgeon
Director, ENT Masterclass®; and
Visiting Professor Capital Medical University, Beijing; and
Honorary Senior Lecturer in Surgical Oncology, University of Sheffield
Doncaster Royal Infirmary
Doncaster, UK.

Parameswaran Rajeev BSC MBBS FRCSI MPHIL FRCS UK
Senior Consultant and Assistant Professor in Endocrine Surgery
National University of Singapore
National University Hospital, Singapore.

Yujay Ramakrishnan MBBCHIR MA CANTAB FRCS (ORL-HNS)
ENT Skull Base Consultant
Queen's Medical Centre
Nottingham, UK.

Gregory W Randolph MD FACS FACE
The Claire and John Bertucci Endowed Chair in Thyroid Surgical Oncology
Harvard Medical School; and
Director General and Thyroid/Parathyroid Surgical Divisions
Massachusetts Eye and Ear Infirmary
Boston, Massachusetts, USA.

Baskaran Ranganathan DOHNS FRCS (ORL-HNS)
Consultant ENT
Manchester University Foundation NHS Trust
Manchester, UK.

Urmila Ratnasabapathy FRCA
Consultant Neuroanaesthetist
Department of Anaesthesia, Southern General Hospital
NHS Greater Glasgow and Clyde Glasgow, UK.

Penelope Redding MB BS FRCPATH
Consultant Microbiologist
Southern General Hospital
NHS Greater Glasgow and Clyde
Glasgow, UK.

Joanne Rimmer FRCS (ORL-HNS)
Specialist Registrar in Otolaryngology
Royal National Throat Nose & Ear Hospital
London, UK.

Neil D Ritchie PHD MBCHB MRCP(UK)(INFECTIOUS DISEASES)
Consultant Physician in Acute Medicine and Infectious Diseases
Queen Elizabeth University Hospital
Glasgow, UK.

Alasdair Robertson FRCS ORL DLO MB CHB
Consultant ENT Surgeon
NHS Greater Glasgow and Clyde
Glasgow, UK.

Andrew Robson FRCS (ORL)
ENT Consultant
North Cumbria University Hospitals NHS Trust
Director of Education ENTUK
Carlisle, UK

Robert Ross Russell MD FRCPCH FHEA
Consultant in Paediatric Respiratory Medicine
Addenbrooke's Hospital
Cambridge, UK.

Raymond Sacks MBBCH FCS(SA)ORL FRACS FARS
Professor and Head of ORL/Head & Neck Surgery
Macquarie University; and
Clinical Professor and Head, ENT Surgery
University of Sydney; and
Past-President Australian and New Zealand Rhinologic Society
Australia.

Gregory P Sadler MD FRCS GEN SURG
Consultant Endocrine Surgeon
Department of Endocrine Surgery
John Radcliffe Hospital
Oxford, UK.

Hesham Saleh FRCS (ORL-HNS)
Consultant Rhinologist/Facial Plastic Surgeon and Honorary Senior Lecturer
Charing Cross and Royal Brompton Hospital
Imperial College
London, UK.

Bal Sanghera PHD MSC
Clinical Scientist
Paul Strickland Scanner Centre Mount Vernon Hospital
Northwood, UK.

Thozhukat Sathyapalan MD FACP FRCP
Reader in Endocrinology and Honorary Consultant
Head of Academic Endocrinology, Diabetes and Metabolism
Hull York Medical School
University of Hull
Hull, UK.

Bernhard Schick MD
Head of Department of ENT
Department of Otorhinolaryngology
Saarland University Medical Center
Hamburg, Germany.

David M Scott-Coombes MS FRCS EBSQ
Consultant Endocrine Surgeon
University Hospital of Wales
Cardiff, UK

Christopher D Scrase MRCP(UK) FRCR
Macmillan Consultant Clinical Oncologist and Honorary Senior Lecturer
The Ipswich Hospital NHS Trust
Ipswich, UK.

Louise Selby BSC MBBS MRCPCH
Paediatric Respiratory Registrar
Royal Brompton Hospital
London, UK.

Neeraj Sethi MBCHB FRCS
Clinical Research Fellow
Leeds Institute of Cancer & Pathology
Leeds, UK.

Ashok R Shaha MD
Professor of Head and Neck Surgery and Oncology
Head and Neck Service
Memorial Sloan Kettering Cancer Center New York
New York, USA.

Neil Sharma MBCHB PHD MRCS DOHNS
NIHR Academic Clinical Lecturer
Centre for Endocrinology, Diabetes and Metabolism
Institute of Metabolism and Systems Research
College of Medical and Dental Sciences
University of Birmingham; and
Specialty Registrar, Otolaryngology
Department of Otolaryngology
University Hospital Birmingham NHS Foundation Trust
Birmingham, UK.

Seiji B Shibata MD PHD
Resident Physician
Department of Otolaryngology, Head and Neck Surgery
University of Iowa
Iowa City, Iowa, USA.

Uttam Shiralkar FRCS MS MRCPSYCH
Consultant Psychiatrist and Psycho-oncologist
Worcestershire Health and Care Trust
and Birmingham University Hospital
Birmingham, UK.

Ricard Simo FRCS (ORL-HNS)
Consultant Otorhinolaryngologist Head and Neck Surgeon
Guy's and St Thomas' Hospital NHS Foundation Trust
Honorary Senior Lecturer
Guy's, King's and St Thomas' Medical and Dental School
London, UK.

Neil G Smart BSC(HONS) MBCHB FFARCSI MBA
Consultant Anaesthetist
Honorary Clinical Senior Lecturer
Department of Anaesthetics
Queen Elizabeth University Hospital
Glasgow, UK.

Joel Anthony Smith MD FRCS MBCHB BMEDSC
Consultant Head Neck and Thyroid Surgeon
Royal Devon and Exeter Hospital
Exeter, UK.

Wendy Smith BPHARM MBBS DLO FRCS (ORL-HNS)
Consultant Otorhinolaryngologist
Department of Otolaryngology
Kettering General Hospital NHS Trust
Kettering, UK.

Carl H Snyderman MD MBA
Professor
Department of Otolaryngology and Neurological Surgery
University of Pittsburgh School of Medicine
Pittsburgh, USA.

Iain RC Swan MD FRCS
Consultant Otologist
Glasgow Royal Infirmary
Glasgow, UK.

Andrew C Swift MB CHB CHM FRCS FRCSED
Consultant Rhinologist and ENT Surgeon
Honorary Senior Lecturer, University of Liverpool; and
Honorary Senior Lecturer, Edge Hill University
Aintree University Hospital
Liverpool, UK.

Mohammed-Iqbal Syed MS DLO FRCS (ORL-HNS)
Consultant Otologist & Skull Base Surgeon and Honorary Senior Lecturer
The Royal Infirmary of Edinburgh
Edinburgh, UK.

Mark Sywak MBBS MMEDSCI(CLIN EPI) FRACS
Associate Professor
Head of Department, Endocrine Surgery and Surgical Oncology
University of Sydney Endocrine Surgical Unit
Royal North Shore Hospital
Sydney, Australia.

Moira Thomas MB CHB MRCP FRCPATH
Consultant Clinical Immunologist
Queen Elizabeth University Hospital
Glasgow, UK.

Ian Todd MA PHD
Associate Professor and Reader in Cellular Immunopathology
Director of Studies for MOL
Faculty of Medicine and Health Sciences
Queen's Medical Centre
Nottingham, UK.

Neil S Tolley MD FRCS DLO
Consultant ENT-Thyroid Surgeon
St Mary's Hospital
London, UK.

Richard B Townsley MBBS BSC MRCS DOHNS
Specialty Registrar, Otolaryngology, Head and Neck Surgery
West of Scotland Deanery
Crosshouse University Hospital
Kilmarnock, UK.

Richard W Tsang MD FRCSP(C)
Professor
Department of Radiation Oncology
University of Toronto
Princess Margaret Cancer Centre
Toronto, Canada.

Ralph P Tufano MD MBA FACS
Charles W Cummings MD Professor
Co-Director of the Johns Hopkins Hospital Multidisciplinary Thyroid Tumor Center; and
Director of the Division of Head and Neck Endocrine Surgery
Department of Otolaryngology, Head and Neck Surgery
The Johns Hopkins University School of Medicine
Baltimore, Maryland, USA.

Jan HP van der Meulen PHD FFPH
Reader in Clinical Epidemiology
Health Services Research Unit, London School of Hygiene and Tropical Medicine
London, UK.

Daphne A Varveris MBCHB FRCA
Consultant Anaesthetist
Department of Anaesthetics
Queen Elizabeth University Hospital
Glasgow, UK.

Navin Vig MBBS BDS MRCS MFDS
Clinical Research Fellow and Specialty Registrar (OMFS)
Blizard Institute
Barts and The London Medical School
Queen Mary University of London
London, UK.

Sebastian Wallis MB CHB FRCS (ORL-HNS)
ENT Consultant
Department of Otolaryngology (Ear, Nose and Throat)
York Hospital
York, UK.

Eric W Wang MD
Associate Professor
Department of Otolaryngology
University of Pittsburgh School of Medicine
Pittsburgh, USA.

Adrian T Warfield FRCPATH
Consultant Histo-Cytopathologist, University Hospital Birmingham NHS Foundation Trust
Honorary Senior Clinical Lecturer, University of Birmingham
Birmingham, UK.

John C Watkinson MSC MS FRCS DLO
One-Time Honorary Senior Lecturer and Consultant ENT/Head and Neck and Thyroid Surgeon, Queen Elizabeth Hospital
University of Birmingham NHS Trust and latterly the Royal Marsden and Brompton Hospitals, London, UK
Currently Consultant Head and Neck and Thyroid Surgeon, University Hospital, Coventry and Warwick NHS Trust; and
Honorary Consultant ENT/Head and Neck and Thyroid Surgeon, Great Ormond Street Hospital (GOSH)
Honorary Senior Anatomy Demonstrator, University College London (UCL)
Business Director, Endocrine MDT, The BUPA Cromwell Hospital, London, UK.

Anthony P Weetman MD DSC
Emeritus Professor of Medicine
Department of Human Metabolism
Faculty of Medicine, Dentistry and Health
University of Sheffield
Sheffield, UK.

Martin O Weickert MD FRCP
Consultant Endocrinology & Diabetes
University Hospitals Coventry & Warwickshire NHS Trust (UHCW)
Warwickshire Institute for the Study of Diabetes, Endocrinology and Metabolism; and
Visiting Professor
Centre for Applied Biological and Exercise Sciences
Coventry University, Coventry, UK; and
Honorary Associate Professor
Division of Metabolic and Vascular Health
Warwick Medical School, University of Warwick
Coventry, UK.

Paul S White MBCHB FRACS FRCS (ED)
Consultant Rhinologist
Ninewells Hospital; and
Honorary Senior Lecturer, University of Dundee
Dundee, UK.

William Whitmer PHD
Senior Investigator Scientist
MRC/CSO Institute of Hearing Research – Scottish Section
Nottingham, UK.

Mark Williams MA MRCP FRCPATH
Senior Registrar in Haematology
Manchester Specialist Registrar Rotation
Manchester, UK.

Wai Lup Wong BA (HONS) LLM FRCP FRCR
Paul Strickland Scanner Centre, Mount Vernon Hospital
Northwood
Honorary Senior Lecturer
University College London
London, UK.

Timothy J Woolford MD FRCS(ORL-HNS)
Consultant ENT Surgeon and Rhinologist
Department of Otolaryngology, Head and Neck Surgery
Manchester Royal Infirmary
Manchester, UK.

Peter-John Wormald MD FRACS FRCS (EDIN) FCS (SA) MBCHB
Chairman and Professor
Department of Surgery, Otolaryngology, Head and
    Neck Surgery; and
Professor of Skull Base Surgery
Adelaide and Flinders Universities
Adelaide, Australia.

Robert F Wynn BA MD MRCP FRCPATH
Consultant Paediatric Haematologist
Director, Blood and Marrow Transplant Unit; and
Honorary Professor of Paediatric Haematology and
    Cellular Therapy
Royal Manchester Children's Hospital and University of
    Manchester
Manchester, UK.

Emily Young MBCHB MPH FRCS (ORL-HNS)
Neurotology Fellow
St Paul's Rotary Hearing Clinic
Vancouver, Canada.

Karen Young MSC FRCS ORL-HNS
Clinical Research Fellow
Department of Endocrinology
William Harvey Research Institute
Barts and the London School of Medicine
Queen Mary University of London
London, UK.

Foreword

The eighth edition of *Scott-Brown* signals the beginning of a new and exciting era for ear, nose and throat surgeons, and also the end of 10 years of very hard work undertaken by John Watkinson and Ray Clarke, the Editors-in-Chief, their team of subeditors and, not least, the publishers. Whatever subspeciality the current generation of trainees decides to follow, they will all have to read and refer to *Scott-Brown* in order to complete their education and gain accreditation. It will be a constant companion and guide throughout their professional lives.

When asked to write the foreword for this edition, I was immediately reminded that I had read John Ballantyne and John Groves's third edition as a trainee, bought the fourth edition as a senior registrar, written chapters for Alan Kerr and Philip Stell in the fifth edition, edited the *Basic science* volume of the fifth edition and was ultimately Editor-in-Chief of the seventh edition. As each edition takes about 10 years to produce, that makes me very old indeed. John and Ray have one final task as Editors-in-Chief: to recommend their successors to the publishers. That was made easy for me as both of them had proved themselves more than capable with the previous edition, and the eighth edition is now their masterpiece. They can enjoy the next 10 years as thousands of surgeons worldwide recognize and thank them for their industry.

This edition reflects the continued expansion of our speciality into fields that Scott-Brown himself could never have imagined. It lays the groundwork for the current generation to make their contribution that will, no doubt, be prompted by technological developments, an evidence base of what is wise and what is not, together with the experience gained by teamwork with other clinicians in today's multidisciplinary approach to patient care.

Simply looking at the table of contents it is clear to see that our role in endocrine surgery has increased dramatically over the last 10 years. The thyroid and parathyroids now account for 30 chapters. How would Scott-Brown have viewed that when the tonsils and adenoids justify just one chapter each, and the sore throat has a mere passing reference? Times have certainly changed and ENT surgery has grown up. We have reflected on our past practices, and the evidence base for our management protocols that was emphasized in the previous edition of *Scott-Brown* has been taken to heart.

I hope that this edition will find its way into every medical library in the world and onto every ENT surgeon's bookshelf. It will serve and guide surgeons throughout the English-speaking world, whether they live in high- or low-income countries. It is said that the tragedy of getting old is that we feel young. Reading these volumes makes me wish that I had my time all over again.

Michael Gleeson

Preface

When we were asked to head up the editorial team for this, the eighth edition of *Scott-Brown*, we were mindful of Michael Gleeson's towering achievement in bringing the seventh edition to fruition. Michael delivered a much-loved text – conceived in the early post-war years when antimicrobials, the operating microscope and the National Health Service were all in their infancy – in an entirely new format that befitted modern surgical scholarship. Authors, editors and readers alike had become acutely conscious of the need to quote high-quality evidence to guide clinical decisions; the concept of grading clinical recommendations – and, by implication, acknowledging gaps in the evidence base of our practice – was born. Recognizing the enormity of Michael's contribution led us into the trap that has befallen every editor who has come before us; we grossly underestimated the task ahead. We had misjudged the pace of change. What began as an 'update' of some outdated chapters became a complete rewrite to reflect the advances that marked the decade between editions, but we were determined to keep the text to a manageable size! In the end, we have 330 chapters, but with a slightly smaller page count than the seventh edition.

The basic science knowledge that underpins our clinical practice is no longer focused just on anatomy and physiology; genetics, molecular biology, new techniques for auditory implantation, information technology, new medical therapies for many old disorders together with seismic changes in endoscopic technology and in medical imaging have transformed our specialty. Today's head and neck surgery would have been unrecognizable to the early authors and editors. Surgical oncologists have recourse to completely different treatment strategies than did their predecessors and now work as part of multidisciplinary teams. They deal with different disease patterns and vastly changed patient expectations. Thyroid and parathyroid surgery has become almost exclusively the domain of the otolaryngologist. Surgery of the pituitary fossa has come within our ambit, as has plastic and reconstructive surgery of the head and neck as well as aesthetic facial surgery. Neurotology, audio-vestibular medicine, rhinology and paediatric otolaryngology are accepted subspecialties, each with its own corpus of knowledge and skills and each warranting a sizeable section of this text. Contemporary otolaryngology is now a collection of subspecialty interests linked by common 'stem' training and a shared passion for looking after patients with disorders of the upper respiratory tract and the head and neck.

There is a view that a single text – even a multivolume tome of this size – cannot cover the entire knowledge base of modern clinical practice. The subspecialist will, of course, need recourse to supplementary reading. The pace of change shows no sign of slowing down, but there is still a need for a comprehensive working text embracing the whole spectrum of our workload. That was the task we set our authors and section editors; we think they have done our specialty proud.

In the new 'digital' editorial world authors create manuscripts on personal computers. They transmit chapters, figures, amendments and revisions across continents and time zones with a few keystrokes. The bulky packages containing grainy photographic prints and the reams of paper with closely-typed and heavily scored text that accumulated on authors' and editors' desks are a distant memory. References, guidelines and systematic reviews are all available online; the editorial 'red pen' has been replaced by a cursor on the screen. This 'new age' has enabled us to look ever further for expertise. We are proud to have enlisted the support of authors from more than 20 countries for this edition. *Scott-Brown* always enjoyed particular affection and respect in Asia, Australia, Africa and the Middle East. It has been a joy to welcome authors in increasing numbers from many of these parts of the world. We are now a truly global specialty and the eighth edition fully reflects this.

What has not changed is the huge time commitment authors and editors need to make. That time now has to be fitted into an increasingly pressurized work environment. Revalidation, mandatory training, more intense regulatory scrutiny, expanding administrative burdens and ever-expanding clinical commitments leave little time for scholarship. Our section editors are all busy clinicians. They have generously given their time, first instructing authors, cajoling them and then editing their chapters, virtually all of which have been completely rewritten since the last edition. Each author was chosen because of his or her specific clinical and scientific expertise and none has disappointed. Authors and section editors receive no reward other than the satisfaction of knowing that they have made a contribution to teaching and learning in a specialty that has given us all so much professional satisfaction. We are profoundly grateful to them and hope that their endeavours spur the next generation of otolaryngologists to carry on this noble tradition. *Scott-Brown* simply wouldn't happen without this generous and dedicated commitment, unstintingly and graciously given.

It is impossible to produce a book like *Scott-Brown* without the contribution of many individuals working behind the scenes. We would like to express our gratitude to our Publishers, Taylor and Francis, and to the staff who have worked on this project from its early days in 2011 to publication in 2018. In particular we would like to mention Cheryl Brandt who with good humour and patience helped to reel in many of the 330 chapters. Miranda Bromage joined the team in 2016 and her publishing experience and enthusiasm for medical education have helped guide this new edition through its final phases to publication. Finally, we are indebted to Nora Naughton who has dedicated so much more than just her extensive publishing skills to this project. Nora's meticulous attention to detail, combined with her warmth and wisdom have encouraged us all at the end of this endeavour.

We are truly 'passing on the torch' of a huge amount of accumulated knowledge and wisdom; it is this that gives us, the Editors-in-Chief, the greatest pleasure.

Read on and enjoy, our thoughts are yours.

RWC
JCW

I wish to acknowledge the love, happiness and inspiration that have been passed on to me by both my parents and grandparents. I recognize and value the friendship of my dear friend Ray Clarke who has been with me all the way on this rewarding and worthwhile endeavour. I would specifically like to thank Esme, Helen and William, without whom none of this would have been achievable. Their love and support has helped guide me through the years leading up to the publication of this tome, and my final thanks go to Angela Roberts and Sally Holden for their typing and editing skills.

JCW 2018

Thanks to my wife Mary for her patience and support. My parents, Emmet and Doreen Clarke, both sadly died during the preparation of this book. They would have been proud to have played a part in such a scholarly enterprise.

RWC 2018

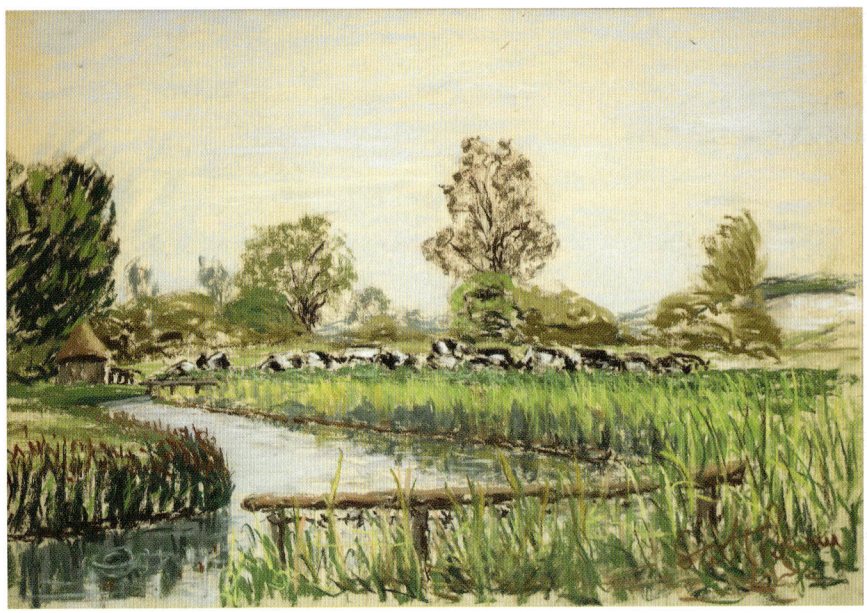

Black Hut on the River Test – Pastel by W G Scott-Brown – circa 1970. Reproduced by kind permission of Mr Neil Weir, who was presented with the original by the artist.

A Tribute to Bill Scott-Brown

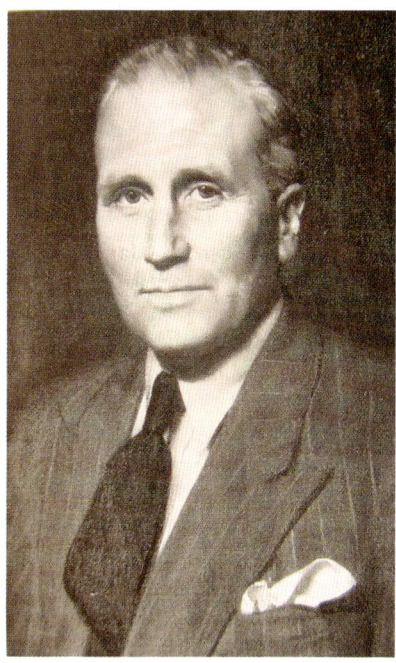

Walter Graham ('Bill') Scott Brown. 1897–1987

Walter Graham ('Bill') Scott-Brown was twenty-three when he arrived at Corpus Christi College Cambridge in 1919. One of the generation of young men whose entry to university and the professions was delayed by their participation in the First World War, he had joined the Gunners in 1915 as an 18-year-old. He considered himself blessed to have survived – although wounded – when so many of his contemporaries never returned from the Front. In those early post-WW1 years the medical school at St Bartholomew's ('Barts') in London was keen to attract 'gentlemen'. To this end a series of scholarships – 'Shuter's scholarships' – was established to lure those with humanities degrees from Oxford and Cambridge into medicine. It was via this scheme that the young Scott-Brown qualified MB, BCh in 1925. By now married to Margaret Bannerman, one of the very few women medical graduates of her generation, the two established a general practice in Sevenoaks, Kent. His work here involved looking after children with poliomyelitis, which was then commonplace, and his MD thesis was on polio-related bulbar palsy. It earned him the Copeman Medal for research from the University of Cambridge. While working in general practice, Bill pursued his interest in the then fledgling specialty of otolaryngology, securing fellowships from London and Edinburgh. Postgraduate training was haphazard; there were no structured programmes or even junior posts, so the young Scott-Brown was fortunate to be awarded a Dorothy Temple Cross Travelling Fellowship. Mrs Florence Temple Cross had set up these awards (now administered by the Medical Research Council) in memory of her daughter, who died in 1927 aged thirty-two.

They were made available to young physicians to help them travel to overseas centres specifically to study tuberculosis, then rampant and one of the commonest causes of death in young adults. The young Scott-Brown visited the leading pioneers of the day in Berlin, Vienna, Budapest, Stockholm, Copenhagen, Madrid and Venice. Here he developed his considerable endoscopy skills. He reported that his first bronchoscopies were done on a Venetian street entertainer who, for a few coins, would inhale sundry objects that the doctors would then dexterously retrieve from his main stem and segmental bronchi – without of course any anaesthesia!

Times were lean on Scott-Brown's return. Margaret ('Peggy') was now a popular and well-established GP who supported him as his private practice developed. Eventually he secured appointments at East Grinstead, the Royal National and Royal Free Hospitals. He had a thriving Harley Street practice and was the favoured otolaryngologist of the aristocracy. His reputation was such that he become laryngologist to the Royal family, was appointed Commander of the Victorian Order and was a particular favourite of the then Princess Royal, HRH Mary the Countess of Harewood.

By 1938 he was wealthy enough to purchase a farm in Buckinghamshire where he bred prize-winning shorthorn cattle. Ironmongery and blacksmith work were hard to come by during the war years, so Scott-Brown prided himself on his ability to make his own agricultural implements, cartwheels and farm wagons in a makeshift forge he himself established on the farm. He would while away endless hours here at weekends following a busy week in London. An accomplished fly fisherman, he was part of the exclusive Houghton Club whose members fished the River Test in Hampshire, where he numbered aristocrats including the Prince of Wales among his circle.

Scott-Brown's celebrated textbook came about in the early 1950s, when he became ill with jaundice and heart trouble. He was advised to rest, and took 6 months off work. Not satisfied with editing what has become the standard UK textbook, he took up painting as well. He became a celebrated artist whose work is still prized in many private collections. One of his pastels is reproduced on the preceding page.

Bill Scott-Brown lived to be 90. He died in July 1987, six weeks after his beloved Peggy and just as the fifth edition of the celebrated textbook that still bears his name was going to press. His legacy lives on in the pages of this book, and we are proud to continue the tradition of scholarship and learning which he established all those years ago.

We would like to thank Martin Scott-Brown for his help in compiling the biography above.

John C. Watkinson and Raymond W. Clarke
London, 2018

Acknowledgements

We acknowledge our debt of gratitude to the many authors who have contributed to previous editions of Scott-Brown's Otorhinolaryngology, and in particular to authors from the seventh edition, published in 2008.

Chapter 1, Molecular biology, contains some material from 'Molecular biology' by Michael Kuo and Richard M Irving. The material has been revised and updated by the current author.

Chapter 3, Gene therapy, contains some material from 'Gene therapy' by Scott M Graham and John H Lee. The material has been revised and updated by the current author.

Chapter 5, Radiotherapy and radiosensitizers, contains some material from 'Radiotherapy and radiosensitizers' by Stewart G Martin and David AL Morgan. The material has been revised and updated by the current author.

Chapter 11, Skin flap physiology, contains some material from 'Skin flap physiology' by A Graeme B Perks. The material has been revised and updated by the current author.

Chapter 15, Evaluation of the immune system, contains some material from 'Evaluation of the immune system' by Elizabeth Drewe and Richard J Powell. The material has been revised and updated by the current author.

Chapter 31, Recognition and management of the difficult airway, contains some material from 'Recognition and management of the difficult airway' by Adrian Pearce. The material has been revised and updated by the current author.

Chapter 34, Paediatric intensive care, contains some material from 'Paediatric intensive care' by Helen Allen and Rob Ross Russell. The material has been revised and updated by the current author.

Chapter 41, Epidemiology, contains some material from 'Epidemiology' by Jan HP van der Meulen and David A Lowe. The material has been revised and updated by the current author.

Chapter 44, Critical appraisal skills, contains some material from 'Critical appraisal skills' by Martin Dawes. The material has been revised and updated by the current author.

Chapter 45, Electrophysiology and monitoring, contains some material from 'Electrophysiology and monitoring' by Patrick R Axon and David M Baguley. The material has been revised and updated by the current author.

Chapter 46, Optical coherence tomography, contains some material from 'Optical coherence tomography' by Mariah Hahn and Brett E Bouma. The material has been revised and updated by the current author.

Chapter 92, Non-allergic rhinitis, contains some material from 'Nonallergic perennial rhinitis' by Claus Bachert. The material has been revised and updated by the current author.

Chapter 107, Nasal and facial fractures, contains some material from 'Nasal fractures' by Brent A McMonagle and Michael Gleeson and 'Fractures of the facial skeleton' by Simon Holmes and Michael Gleeson. The material has been revised and updated by the current author.

Chapter 109, Granulomatous conditions of the nose, contains some material from 'Granulomatous conditions of the nose' by David J Howard and Valerie J Lund. The material has been revised and updated by the current author.

Volume 2 – Table of Contents

Section 1 Paediatrics

1: Introduction to paediatric otorhinolaryngology
   Raymond W. Clarke

2: The paediatric consultation
   Raymond W. Clarke

3: Recognition and management of the sick child
   Julian Gaskin, Raymond W. Clarke and Claire Westrope

4: Anaesthesia for paediatric otorhinolaryngology procedures
   Crispin Best

5: The child with special needs
   Kate Blackmore and Derek Bosman

6: The child with a syndrome
   Thushitha Kunanandam and Haytham Kubba

7: Management of the immunodeficient child
   Fiona Shackley

8: Hearing screening and surveillance
   Sally A. Wood

9: Hearing tests in children
   Glynis Parker

10: Management of the hearing impaired child
    Chris H. Raine, Sue Archbold, Tony Sirimanna and Soumit Dasgoupta

11: Paediatric implantation otology
    James Ramsden and Payal Mukherjee

12: Congenital middle ear abnormalities
    Jonathan P. Harcourt

13: Otitis media with effusion
    Peter J. Robb and Ian Williamson

14: Acute otitis media
    Peter A. Rea and Natalie Ronan

15: Chronic otitis media
    William P.L. Hellier

16: Microtia and external ear abnormalities
    Iain Bruce and Jaya Nichani

17: Disorders of speech and language
    Suzanne Harrigan and Andrew Marshall

18: Cleft lip and palate
    David M. Wynne and Louisa Ferguson

19: Craniofacial anomalies
    Benjamin Robertson, Sujata De, Astrid Webber and Ajay Sinha

20: Balance disorders in children
    Louisa Murdin and Gavin A.J. Morrison

21: Facial paralysis in children
    S. Musher Hussain

22: Epistaxis
    Mary-Louise Montague and Nicola E. Starritt

23: Neonatal nasal obstruction
    Michelle Wyatt

24: Rhinosinusitis and its complications
    Daniel J. Tweedie

25: Lacrimal disorders in children
    Caroline J. MacEwen and Paul S. White

26: The adenoid and adenoidectomy
    Peter J. Robb

27: Paediatric obstructive sleep apnoea
    Steven Powell

28: Stridor
    Kate Stephenson and David Albert

29: Acute laryngeal infections
    Lesley Cochrane

30: Congenital disorders of the larynx, trachea and bronchi
    Chris Jephson

31: Acquired laryngotracheal stenosis
    Michael J. Rutter, Alessandro de Alarcón and Catherine K. Hart

32: Juvenile-onset recurrent respiratory papillomatosis
    Rania Mehanna and Michael Kuo

33: Paediatric voice disorders
    Ben Hartley and David M. Wynne

34: Foreign bodies in the ear, nose and throat
    Adam J. Donne and Katharine Davies

35: Paediatric tracheostomy
    Mike Saunders

36: Perinatal airway management
Pensée Wu, May M.C. Yaneza, Haytham Kubba, W. Andrew Clement and Alan D. Cameron

37: Cervicofacial infections
Nico Jonas and Ben Hartley

38: Diseases of tonsils, tonsillectomy and tonsillotomy
Yogesh Bajaj and Ian Hore

39: Salivary glands
Neil Bateman and Rachael Lawrence

40: Tumours of the head and neck
Fiona McGregor and James Hayden

41: Cysts and sinuses of the head and neck
Keith G. Trimble and Luke McCadden

42: Haemangiomas and vascular malformations
Daniel J. Tweedie and Benjamin E.J. Hartley

43: Drooling and aspiration
Haytham Kubba and Katherine Ong

44: Reflux and eosinophilic oesophagitis
Ravi Thevasagayam

45: Oesophageal disorders
Graham Haddock

Section 2 The ear

Audio-vestibular medicine

46: Anatomy and embryology of the external and middle ear
Peter Valentine and Tony Wright

47: Anatomy of the cochlear and vestibular system: Relating ultrastructure to function
Jonathan Gale and Andrew Forge

48: Physiology of hearing
Soumit Dasgupta and Michael Maslin

49: Physiology of equilibrium
Floris L. Wuyts, Leen K. Maes and An Boudewyns

50: Perception of sounds at the auditory cortex
Frank E. Musiek and Jane A. Baran

51: Psychoacoustic audiometry
Josephine E. Marriage and Marina Salorio-Corbetto

52: Evoked measurement of auditory sensitivity
Jeffrey Weihing and Nicholas Leahy

53: Prevention of hearing loss
Shankar Rangan and Veronica Kennedy

54: Hearing aids
Harvey Dillon

55: Beyond hearing aids: An overview of audiological rehabilitation
Lucy Handscombe

56: Age-related sensorineural hearing impairment
Linnea Cheung, David M. Baguley and Andrew McCombe

57: Noise-induced hearing loss and related conditions
Andrew McCombe and David M Baguley

58: Autosomal dominant non-syndromic SNHL
Polona Le Quesne Stabej and Maria Bitner-Glindzicz

59: Ototoxicity
Andy Forge

60: Idiopathic sudden sensorineural hearing loss
Tony Narula and Catherine Rennie

61: Tinnitus and hyperacusis
Don McFerran and John Phillips

62: Evaluation of balance
Adolfo M. Bronstein

63: Ménière's disease
Vincent W.F.M. van Rompaey

64: Benign paroxysmal positional vertigo
Yougan Saman and Doris-Eva Bamiou

65: Superior semicircular canal dehiscence
Harry R.F. Powell and Shakeel R. Saeed

66: Vestibular neuritis
Charlotte Agrup

67: Vestibular migraine
Louisa Murdin and Lina Luxon

68: Vestibular rehabilitation
Marousa Pavlou

69: Auditory neuropathy spectrum disorder and retrocochlear disorders in adults and children
Rosalyn A. Davies and Raj Nandi

70: Understanding tinnitus: A psychological perspective
Laurence McKenna, Elizabeth Marks and David Scott

71: Auditory processing disorders across the age span
Doris-Eva Bamiou and Cristina Ferraz B. Murphy

72: Neuropsychiatric aspects of vestibular disorders
Julius Bourke, Georgia Jackson and Gerald Libby

Otology

73: Clinical examination of the ears and hearing
George G. Browning and Peter-John Wormald

74: Furunculosis
Malcolm P. Hilton

75: Myringitis
Samuel A.C. MacKeith

76: Keratosis obturans, primary auditory canal cholesteatoma and benign necrotizing otitis externa
Tristram H.J. Lesser

77: Acquired atresia of the external ear
Jonathan P. Harcourt

78: Otitis externa and otomycosis
Simon Carney

79: Periochondritis of the external ear
James W. Loock

80: Exostosis of the external auditory canal
Phillip J. Robinson and Sophie J. Hollis

81: Osteoradionecrosis of the temporal bone
James W. Loock

82: Acute otitis media and otitis media with effusion in adults
Anil Banerjee

83: Chronic otitis media
George G. Browning, Justin Weir, Gerard Kelly and Iain R.C. Swan

84: Myringoplasty
Charlie Huins and Jeremy Lavy

85: Ossiculoplasty
Daniel Moualed, Alison Hunt and Christopher P. Aldren

86: Eustachian tube dysfunction
Holger H. Sudhoff

87: Otoendoscopy
David A. Bowdler, Annabelle C.K. Leong and David D. Pothier

88: Tuberculosis of the temporal bone
Ameet Kishore

89: Otosclerosis
Christopher P. Aldren, Thanos Bibas, Arnold J.N. Bittermann, George G. Browning, Wilko Grolman, Peter A. Rea, Rinze A. Tange and Inge Wegner

90: Otological effects of Paget's disease
Ian D. Bottrill

91: Ear trauma
Stephen C. Toynton

92: Otalgia
Philip D. Yates

Implantation otology

93: Bone-conduction hearing aids
James Ramsden and Chris H. Raine

94: Cochlear implants
Andrew Marshall and Stephen Broomfield

95: Middle ear implants
Maarten J.F. de Wolf and Richard M. Irving

96: Auditory brainstem implants
Shakeel R. Saeed and Harry R.F. Powell

Section 3 Skull base

97: Imaging of the temporal bone
Steve Colley

98: Anatomy of the skull base and infratemporal fossa
Charlie Huins

99: Evaluation of the skull base patient
Jeyanthi Kulasegarah and Richard M. Irving

100: Vascular assessment and management
Joe J. Leyon, Kurdow Nader and Swarupsingh Chavda

101: Natural history of vestibular schwannomas
Mirko Tos, Sven-Eric Stangerup and Per Caye-Thomasen

102: Surgical management of vestibular schwannomas
Shakeel R. Saeed and Christopher J. Skilbeck

103: Stereotactic radiosurgery
Paul Sanghera, Geoffrey Heyes, Helen Howard, Rosemary Simmons and Helen Benghiat

104: Neurofibromatosis 2
Gareth Evans

105: Non-vestibular schwannoma tumours of the cerebellopontine angle
Simon K.W. Lloyd and Scott A. Rutherford

106: Middle fossa surgery
Raghu N.S. Kumar, Sunil N. Dutt and Richard M. Irving

107: Jugular foramen lesions and their management
Rupert Obholzer

108: Petrous apex lesions
Michael Gleeson

109: Approaches to the nasopharynx and Eustachian tube
Gunesh P. Rajan

110: Tumours of the temporal bone
Marcus Atlas, Noweed Ahmad and Peter O'Sullivan

111: Clinical neuroanatomy
John J.P. Patten

112: The facial nerve and its non-neoplastic disorders
Michael Gleeson

113: Tumours of the facial nerve
Patrick R. Axon and Samuel A.C. MacKeith

114: Osteitis of the temporal bone
Cheka R. Spencer and Peter Monksfield

115: Squamous carcinoma of the temporal bone
Liam Masterton and Neil Donnelly

116: Complications of skull base surgery
Abdul Karim Nassimizadeh and Chris Coulson

Volume 3 – Table of Contents

Section 1 Head and Neck

1: History
Patrick J. Bradley

2: Aetiology of head and neck cancer
Pablo H. Montero, Snehal G. Patel and Ian Ganly

3: Epidemiology of head and neck cancer
Kristen B. Pytynia, Kristina R. Dahlstrom and Erich M. Sturgis

4: Staging of head and neck cancer
Nicholas J. Roland

5: The changing face of cancer information
Richard Wight

6: Introducing molecular biology of head and neck cancer
Nikolina Vlatković and Mark T. Boyd

7: Nasal cavity and paranasal sinus malignancy
Cyrus Kerawala, Peter Clarke and Kate Newbold

8: Nasopharyngeal carcinoma
Raymond King-Yin Tsang and Dora Lai-Wan Kwong

9: Benign salivary gland tumours
Jarrod Homer and Andy Robson

10: Malignant tumours of the salivary glands
Vincent Vander Poorten and Patrick J. Bradley

11: Tumours of the parapharyngeal space
Suren Krishnan

12: Oral cavity tumours including lip reconstruction
Tim Martin and Omar A. Ahmed

13: Oropharyngeal tumours
Terry M. Jones with Mererid Evans

14: Tumours of the larynx
Vinidh Paleri, Stuart Winter, Hannah Fox and Nachi Palaniappan

15: Rehabilitation after total laryngectomy
Yvonne Edels and Peter Clarke

16: Management of hypopharyngeal cancer
Prathamesh Pai, Deepa Nair, Sarbani Ghosh Laskar and Kumar Prabhash

17: Neck metastases from an unknown primary
Ricard Simo, Jean-Pierre Jeannon and Maria Teresa Guerrero Urbano

18: Metastatic neck disease
Vinidh Paleri and James O'Hara

19: Principles and practice of radiotherapy in head and neck cancer
Sara Meade and Andrew Hartley

20: Quality of life and survivorship in head and neck cancer
Simon Rogers and Steve Thomas

21: Palliative care for head and neck cancer
Catriona R. Mayland and John E. Ellershaw

22: Transoral laser microsurgery
Mark Sayles, Stephanie L. Koonce, Michael L. Hinni and David G. Grant

23: Anatomy as applied to transoral surgery
Mark Puvanendran and Andrew Harris

24: Chemotherapy
Charles G. Kelly

25: Cysts and tumours of the bony facial skeleton
Julia A. Woolgar and Gillian L. Hall

26: Head and neck pathology
Ram Moorthy, Adrian T. Warfield and Max Robinson

27: Open conservation surgery for laryngeal cancer
Volkert Wreesman, Jatin Shah and Ian Ganly

28: Measures of treatment outcomes
Helen Cocks, Raghav C. Dwivedi and Aoife M. I. Waters

29: Applications of robotics in head and neck practice
Chris Holsinger, Chafeek Tomeh and Eric M. Genden

30: Biologically targeted agents in head and neck cancers
Kevin J. Harrington and Magnus T. Dillon

31: Prosthetic rehabilitation of head and neck defects
Chris Butterworth

32: Multidisciplinary team working
Andrew Davies, Nigel Beasley and David Hamilton

33: Nutritional considerations
Rachael Donnelly, Susannah Penney, Sian Lewis, Lesley Freeman and Pippa Lowe

34: Speech voice and swallow rehabilitation after chemoradiation
Justin W.G. Roe and Katherine A. Hutcheson

35: Surgical anatomy of the neck
Laura Warner, Christopher Jennings and John C. Watkinson

36: Clinical examination of the neck
James O'Hara

37: Imaging of the neck
Ivan Zammit-Maempel

38: Neck trauma
Andrew J. Nicol and Johannes J. Fagan

39: Benign neck disease
Ricard Simo, Jean-Pierre Jeannon and Enyinnaya Ofo

40: Neck space infections
James W. Moor

41: Anatomy and embryology of the mouth and dentition
Barry K.B. Berkovitz

42: Benign oral and dental disease
Konrad S. Staines and Alexander Crighton

43: Salivary gland anatomy
Stuart Winter and Brian Fish

44: Physiology of the salivary glands
Mriganke De and T. Singh

45: Imaging of the salivary glands
Daren Gibson and Steve Colley

46: Non-neoplastic salivary gland diseases
Stephen R. Porter, Stefano Fedele and Valeria Mercadante

47: Anatomy of the pharynx and oesophagus
Joanna Matthan and Vinidh Paleri

48: Physiology of swallowing
Joanne Patterson and Stephen McHanwell

49: Causes and assessment of dysphagia and aspiration
Helen Cocks and Jemy Jose

50: Functional investigations of the upper gastrointestinal tract
Joanne Patterson and Jason Powell

51: Pharyngitis
Sharan Jayaram and Conor Marnane

52: Cricopharyngeal dysphagia
Nimesh N. Patel and T. Singh

53: Oesophageal diseases
Shajahan Wahed and S. Michael Griffin

54: Neurological disease of the pharynx
Kim Ah-See and Miles Bannister

55: Rehabilitation of swallowing disorders
Maggie-Lee Huckabee and Sebastian Doeltgen

56: Chronic aspiration
Guri S. Sandhu and Khalid Ghufoor

57: Temporomandibular joint disorders
Andrew Sidebottom

58: Anatomy of the larynx and tracheobronchial tree
Nimesh N. Patel and Shane Lester

59: Physiology of the larynx
Lesley Mathieson and Paul Carding

60: Voice and speech production
Paul Carding and Lesley Mathieson

61: Assessment and examination of the larynx
Jean-Pierre Jeannon and Enyinnaya Ofo

62: Evaluation of the voice
Julian A. McGlashan

63: Structural disorders of the vocal cords
Yakubu Gadzama Karagama and Julian A. McGlashan

64: Functional disorders of the voice
Paul Carding

65: The professional voice
Declan Costello and Meredydd Harries

66: Speech and language therapy for voice disorders
Marianne E. Bos-Clark and Paul Carding

67: Phonosurgery
Abie Mendelsohn and Marc Remacle

68: Movement disorders of the larynx
Declan Costello and John S. Rubin

69: Acute infections of the larynx
Sanjai Sood, Karan Kapoor and Richard Oakley

70: Chronic laryngitis
Kenneth MacKenzie

71: Contemporary management of laryngotracheal trauma
Carsten E. Palme, Malcolm A. Buchanan, Shruti Jyothi, Faruque Riffat, Ralph W. Gilbert and Patrick Gullane

72: Upper airway obstruction and tracheostomy
Paul Pracy and Peter Conboy

73: Physiology of sleep and sleep disorders
John O'Reilly

74: Obstructive sleep apnoea: Medical management
Dev Banerjee

75: The surgical management of snoring and obstructive sleep apnoea
Bhik Kotecha and Mohammed Reda Elbadawey

76: Laryngotracheal stenosis in adults
Guri S. Sandhu and S.A. Reza Nouraei

77: Reflux disease
Mark G. Watson and Kim Ah-See

78: Paralysis of the larynx
Lucian Sulica and Babak Sadoughi

79: Outpatient laryngeal procedures
Matthew Stephen Broadhurst

Section 2 Plastic Surgery

80: Rhinoplasty following nasal trauma
Charles East

81: Pre-operative assessment for rhinoplasty
Hesham Saleh and Catherine Rennie

82: External rhinoplasty
Santdeep Paun

83: Revision rhinoplasty
Claudia Rudack and Gerhard Rettinger

84: Aesthetic dorsal reduction rhinoplasty
Julian M. Rowe-Jones

85: Nasal reconstruction
Ullas Raghavan

86: Pinnaplasty
Victoria Harries and Simon Watts

87: Blepharoplasty
Brian Leatherbarrow

88: Surgical rejuvenation of the ageing face
Gregory S. Dibelius, John M. Hilinski and Dean M. Toriumi

89: Non-surgical rejuvenation of the ageing face
Lydia Badia, Peter Andrews and Sajjad Rajpar

90: History of reconstructive surgery
Ralph W. Gilbert and John C. Watkinson

91: Grafts and local flaps in head and neck cancer
Kenneth Kok and Nicholas White

92: Pedicled flaps in head and neck reconstruction
Ralph W. Gilbert and John C. Watkinson

93: Reconstructive microsurgery in head and neck surgery
John C. Watkinson and Ralph W. Gilbert

94: Benign and malignant conditions of the skin
Murtaza Khan and Agustin Martin-Clavijo

95: Facial reanimation surgery
Demetrius Evriviades and Nicholas White

96: Partial and total ear construction
Cher Bing Chuo

97: A combined prosthetic and surgical approach
Hitesh Koria, M. Stephen Dover and Steve Worrollo

Abbreviations

1,25-DHCC	1,25 dihydroxycholecalciferol	AEF	auditory-evoked cortical magnetic field
2D	two-dimensional	AERD	aspirin-exacerbated respiratory disease
3D	three-dimensional	AES	assigned educational supervisors
4D CT	four-dimensional computed tomography	AF	atrial fibrillation; or anterior fontanelle
5-FdUMP	5-fluoro-2 deoxyuridine monophosphate	AFAP	attenuated familial adenomatous polyposis
5-FU	5-fluorouracil	AFIP	Armed Forces Institute of Pathology
5-FUMP	5-fluorouridine monophosphate	AFOI	awake fibre-optic intubation
6MP	6-mercaptopurine	AFRS	allergic fungal rhinosinusitis
18-FDG	2-18-fluoro-2-deoxy-D-glucose	AFU	angiofollicular unit
		AGHDA	Assessment of Growth Hormone Deficiency in Adults
A	adenine; or anterior	AH	adenohypophysis
AACE	American Association of Clinical Endocrinologists	AICA	anterior inferior cerebellar artery
AAES	American Association of Endocrine Surgeons	AIDS	acquired immunodeficiency syndrome
AAGBI	Association of Anaesthetists of Great Britain and Ireland	AIFR	acute invasive fungal rhinosinusitis
		AIFS	acute invasive fungal sinusitis
AAOHNS	American Academy of Otolaryngologists/Head and Neck Surgeons	AIH	amiodarone-induced hypothyroidism
		AIP	aryl hydrocarbon receptor-interacting protein
AAV	adeno-associated virus	AIT	amiodarone-induced thyrotoxicosis
ABBA	axillo-bilateral-breast approach	AJCC	American Joint Committee on Cancer
ABG	arterial blood gas	AKT	serine/threonine kinase
ABPA	allergic bronchopulmonary aspergillosis	ALLO	alloimmunization
ABR	auditory brainstem response	ALTB	acute laryngotracheobronchitis
ABRS	acute bacterial rhinosinusitis	ALS	advanced life support; or amyotrophic lateral sclerosis; or acid labile subunit
AC	air conduction; or alternating coupled; or adenylate cyclase		
ACE	angiotensin-converting enzyme	ALSPAC	Avon Longitudinal Study of Parents and Children
ACGME	Accreditation Council for General Medical Education	ALTB	acute laryngotracheobronchitis
		AML	acute myeloid leukaemia
ACh	acetylcholine	AMR	antimicrobial resistance
AchR	acetyl choline receptor	AN	acoustic neuroma; or auditory neuropathy; or audiovestibular nerve
ACR	Americal College of Rheumatology		
ACT	Aid for Children with Tracheostomies	ANA	anti-nuclear antibody
ACTH	adrenocorticotrophic hormone	AN/AD	auditory neuropathy/auditory dyssynchrony
AD	Alzheimer's disease	ANCA	antineutrophil cytoplasmic antibody
ADAM-33	A disintegrin and metalloprotease 33k	ANSD	auditory neuropathy spectrum disorder
ADC	apparent diffusion coefficient	ANTS	anaesthetists' non-technical skills
ADCC	antibody-dependent cellular cytotoxicity	AOM	acute otitis media
ADH	antidiuretic hormone	AON	anterior olfactory nucleus
ADP	adenosine diphosphate	AP	anterior–posterior; or action potential
ADR	adverse drug reaction	APACHE	acute physiology and chronic health evaluation
ADU	avoidable, delayed or undertransfusion		
Ad-VEGF	adenovirus-encoding vascular endothelial growth factor	APC	antigen presenting cell; or activated protein C; or argon plasma coagulation; or adenomatous polyposis coli
AEA	anterior ethmoidal artery		
AED	aerodynamic equivalent diameter		

xxxiii

APIT	activated partial thromboplastic time	BMD	bone mineral density
APOF	aggressive psammomatoid ossifying fibroma	BMI	body mass index
APTT	activated partial thromboplastin time	BMP	bone morphogenetic protein; or bone morphogenic protein
AQP2	aquaporin 2	BOR	brachio-oto-renal; or branchioterenal syndrome
ARIA	allergic rhinitis and its impact on asthma		
ARR	absolute risk reduction	BP	blood pressure
ARS	acute rhinosinusitis	BPE	bilateral parathyroid exploration
ARSAC	Administration of Radioactive Substances Advisory Committee	BSAC	British Society for Antimicrobial Chemotherapy
ART	advanced rotating tomograph; or antiretroviral therapy	BTA	British Thyroid Association
ARIA	allergic rhinitis and its impact on asthma	C	cytosine
ARS	acute rhinosinusitis	CAD	caspase-activated DNase
ASA	aspirin-induced asthma; or aspirin-sensitive asthma; or American Society of Anesthesiologists	CAF	carcinoma-associated fibroblasts
		CAG	curriculum advisory group
		cAMP	3',5'-monophosphate
a-SCC	anterior semicircular canal	CAP	compound action potential; or category of auditory performance; or College of American Pathologists
AT	ataxia telangiectasia; or auditory therapy or training; or autotransplantation		
ATA	American Thyroid Association	CAPS	cryopyrin-associated periodic syndromes
ATC	anaplastic thyroid carcinoma; or air traffic control	CARD	caspase recruitment domain
		CaSR	calcium-sensing receptor
ATD	ascending tract of Deiters; or adult therapeutic dose	CASTLE	carcinoma with thymus-like elements
		CBD	case-based discussion
ATIII	antithrombin III	CBF	ciliary beat frequency
ATP	adenosine triphosphate	CCD	charge-coupled device
ATR	acute transfusion reaction	CCH	C-cell hyperplasia
AVP	arginine vasopressin	CCP	cyclic citrullinated peptide
AW	anterior wall	CCR	chemokine receptor
		CCT	Certificate of Completion of Training
BABA	bilateral axillo-breast approach	CD	cluster of differentiation; or colloid droplets; or compact disk; or Cowden's disease
BAC	bacterial artificial chromosome		
BADS	British Association of Day Surgery	CDA	cold dry air
BAES	British Association of Endocrine Surgeons	CDAD	C. difficile associated diarrhoea
BAETS	British Association of Endocrine and Thyroid Surgeons	CDC	Centers for Disease Control and Prevention
		CDI	C. difficile infection
BAT	basophil activation test	CDK	cyclin-dependent kinase
BCHD	bone conduction hearing device	CEA	carcinoembryonic antigen
BCP	biphasic calcium phosphate	CEFTE	carcinoma of the thyroid with Ewing family tumour elements
BCSH	British Committee for Standards in Haematology		
		CEPOD	Confidential Enquiry into Perioperative Deaths
BD	Behcet's disease		
BDP	beclomethasone dipropionate	CER	control event rate
BFU-E	burst-forming unit erythroid	CESR	Certificate of Eligibility for Specialist Registration
BiPAP	bilevel positive airway pressure		
BIPP	bismuth and iodoform paraffin paste	CEX	clinical evaluation exercises
BIS	bispectoral index	CF	cystic fibrosis; or characteristic frequency
BL	Burkitt's lymphoma	CFD	colour-flow duplex Doppler; or computational fluid dynamics
BMA	British Medical Association; or bone marrow aspirate		
		c-FOS	fos proto-oncogene

CFTR	cystic fibrosis transmembrane conductance regulator
CG	clinical governance
CGD	chronic granulomatous disease
CGH	comparative genomic hybridization
CGIFS	chronic granulomatous invasive fungal sinusitis
CGRP	calcitonin gene-related peptide
CHI	Commission for Healthcare Improvement (UK)
CHOP-R	cyclophosphamide, doxorubicin, vincristine, prednisone and rituximab
CI	cochlear implant; *or* cardiac index; *or* confidence interval; *or* concha inferior
CICV	can't intubate can't ventilate
CIFR	chronic invasive fungal rhinosinusitis
CIFS	chronic invasive fungal sinusitis
CINCA	chronic infantile neurologic cutaneous articular syndrome
CJD	Creutzfeldt–Jakob disease
CK	cytokeratin
CKD-MBD	chronic kidney disease mineral bone disorder
CLL	chronic lymphatic leukaemia; *or* chronic lymphocytic leukaemia
CM	concha media; *or* cochlear microphonic; *or* cricothyroid muscle
CMAP	compound muscle action potential
CML	chronic myeloid leukaemia
CMSO	complementary metal oxide detectors
CMT	Charcot—Marie—Tooth; *or* combined modality therapy
CMV	cytomegalovirus
CN	cranial nerve; *or* cochlear nuclei; *or* cochlear nerve
CNS	central nervous system
CO_2	carbon dioxide
CoAA	coactivator AA
COF	cemento-ossifying fibroma
COMET	Core Outcomes Measures in Effectiveness Trials
CONSORT	Consolidated Standards of Reporting Trials
COPD	chronic obstructive pulmonary disease
COSI	Client Oriented Scale of Improvement
COX-2	cyclo-oxygenase 2
CPA	cerebellopontine angle
CPAP	continuous positive airway pressure
CPD	citrate phosphate dextrose; *or* continuing professional development
CPG	central pattern generator
CRC	colorectal cancer
CRD	component resolved diagnostics
CREB	cAMO binding element
CREST	calcinosis, Raynaud's, oesophageal involvement, sclerodactyly, telangiectasis
CRF	corticotrophin-releasing factor
CRH	corticotrophin-releasing hormone
CRH-R	corticotrophin releasing hormone receptor
CRP	C-reactive protein; *or* canalith repositioning procedure
CRS	chronic rhinosinusitis; *or* congenital rubella syndrome
CRSwNP	chronic rhinosinusitis with nasal polyps
CRSsNP	chronic rhinosinusitis without nasal polyps
CRS	chronic rhinosinusitis; *or* congenital rubella syndrome
CS	corticosteroid; *or* cell salvage and autologous transfusions
CSC	cancer stem cells
CSF	cerebrospinal fluid
CSS	Churg-Strauss syndrome
CST	core surgical training
CT	computed tomography; *or* conventional thyroidectomy
CTA	composite tissue allograft; *or* computed tomography angiography
CTLA	cytotoxic T-lymphocyte-associated antigen
CTM	cricothyroid membrane
Cu-ATSM	Cu(II)-diacetyl-bis-N4-methylthiosemicarbozone
DA	double adenoma
DACH	diaminocyclohexane
DAHANCA	Danish Head and Neck Cancer Study
DAMPs	damage-associated molecular pattern molecules
DAS	Difficult Airway Society
DAT	direct antiglobulin test
DAVF	dural arteriovenous fistulas
dB	decibel
DBM	demineralized bone matrix
DCE MRI	dynamic contrast-enhanced MRI
DCR	dacryocystorhinostomy
DD	death domain
DDAVP	desmopressin
DDE	Doctrine of Double Effect
DED	death effector domain
DFN3	deafness type 3
DFO-H	deferoxamine-hespan
DHI	dizziness handicap inventory
DHTR	delayed haemolytic transfusion reaction
DI	diabetes insipidus
DIC	disseminated intravascular coagulation
DIO	deiodinases

DISC	death inducing signal complex	ECP	eosinophil cationic protein; *or* extra corporeal perfusion
DIT	diiodotyrosine; *or* di-iodothyronine	ECS	extracapsular spread
DLBCL	diffuse large B-cell lymphoma	EDTA	ethylenediaminetetraacetic acid
DM	diabetes mellitus; *or* decision making	EEA	endoscopic endonasal approach
DMARDS	disease-modifying anti-rheumatic drugs	EEG	electroencephalography; *or* electroencephalogram
DMSA	dimercapto succinic acid	EER	experimental event rate
DMSO	dimethylsulfoxide	EFRS	eosinophilic fungal rhinosinusitis
DNA	deoxyribonucleic acid	EFVPTC	encapsulated follicular variant of PTC
DNAR	do not attempt resuscitation	EGF	epidermal growth factor
dNTP	deoxynucleoside triphosphate	eGFR	estimated glomerular filtration rate
DOAC	direct oral anticoagulant	EGFR	epidermal growth factor receptor
DOHNS	Diploma in Otolaryngology – Head and Neck Surgery	ELISA	enzyme-linked immunosorbent assay
DOPS	direct observation of procedural skills	EMG	electromyography
DPA	Data Protection Act (UK)	EMT	epithelial-mesenchymal transition
DPOAE	distortion product otoacoustic emission	EMRS	eosinophilic mucin rhinosinusitis
DR	death receptor; *or* drug resistance	ENA	extractable nuclear antigen
DSA	digital subtraction angiography	ENoG	electroneurography
dsRNA	double-stranded RNA	ENS	empty nose syndrome
DTC	differentiated thyroid cancer	ENT	ear, nose and throat
DTD	DT-diaphorase	EORTC	European Organisation for Research and Treatment of Cancer
dTMP	deoxythymidine monophosphate	EPO	erythropoietin
dUMP	deoxyuridine monophophase	EPOS	European position paper on rhinosinusitis and nasal polyps
DVT	deep vein thrombosis	EQ-5D	EuroQol
DWI	diffusion weighted image	ER	enhancement ratio; *or* endoplasmic reticulum
EAACI	European Academy of Allergology and Clinical Immunology	ERα	oestrogen receptor alpha
EAC	external auditory canal; *or* external acoustic canal	ERAS	enhanced recovery after surgery
EAL	ethmoidal artery ligation	ERK	extracellular signal-regulated kinase
EAT	endoscopic-assisted thyroidectomy	ERS	European Rhinological Society
EBM	evidence-based medicine	ES	embryonic stem; *or* endolymphatic sac
EBNA	Epstein–Barr virus-associated nuclear antigen	ESBL	extended spectrum β-lactamase
EBP	evidence-based practice	ESPAL	endonasal ligation of the sphenopalatine artery
EBRT	external beam radiotherapy	ESR	erythrocyte sedimentation rate
EBSLN	external branch of the superior laryngeal nerve	ESS	endoscopic sinus surgery; *or* Epworth Sleepiness Scale; *or* empty sella syndrome
EBUS	endobronchial ultrasound	ET-1	endothelin-1
EBV	Epstein–Barr virus	ETE	extrathyroidal extension
ECA	external carotid artery	ETT	endotracheal tube
ECAL	external carotid artery ligation	EUA	examination under anaesthesia
ECG	electrocardiogram	EUCAST	European Committee on Antimicrobial Susceptibility Testing
ECM	extracellular matrix	EVAL	ethylene-vinyl alcohol copolymer
ECMO	extracorporeal membrane oxygenation	EWTD	European Working Time Directive
ECochG	electrocochleography		
ECog	electrocochleogram	Fab	fragment antigen binding
ECOG	Eastern Cooperative Oncology Group (USA)	FACT	functional assessment of cancer therapy
		FADD	Fas-associated death domain

Fas-L	Fas ligand	G	guanine
FBC	full blood count	GABA	gamma-aminobutyric acid
Fc	fragment crystallizable	GABHS	group A beta-haemolytic streptococcus
FcεRI	high affinity IgE receptors	GAG	glycosaminoglycan
FD	fibrous dysplasia	GBI	Glasgow Benefit Inventory
FDA	Food and Drug Administration (USA)	GBM	anti-glomerular basement membrane
FDG	fluorodeoxyglucose; or 2-[18F] fluoro-2-deoxy-D-glucose; or F18-fluoro-2-deoxy-D-glucose	GC	glucocorticoid
		G-CSF	granulocyte-colony stimulating factor
		GD	Graves' disease
FD-OCT	fourier domain optical coherence tomography	GERD	gastrooesophageal reflux disease
		GH	growth hormone
FDG-PET	2-[18F] fluoro-2-deoxy-D-glucose positron emission tomography; or fluorine-18-labelled deoxyglucose positron emission tomography	GHABP	Glasgow Hearing Aid Benefit Profile
		GHRH	growth hormone-releasing hormone
		GHRP	growth hormone-releasing peptide
FE	frontal ethmoidal cell	GI	gastrointestinal
FEA	finite element analysis	GMC	ganglion mother cell; or General Medical Council (UK)
FESS	functional endoscopic sinus surgery		
FEIBA	factor VIII inhibitor bypassing agent	GM-CSF	granulocyte-macrophage colony stimulating factor
F-ETNIM	fluorine-18 fluoroerythronitroimidazone		
FFP	fresh frozen plasma	GMS	Gomori's methamine silver stain
FGF	fibroblast growth factor	GnIH	gonadotrophin inhibitory hormone
FHH	familial hypocalciuric hypercalcaemia	GnRH	gonadotrophin-releasing hormone
FIHP	familial isolated hyperparathyroidism	GORD	gastro-oesophageal reflux disease
FiO2	fraction of inspired oxygen	gp	glycoprotein
FIPA	familial isolated pituitary adenomas	GP	general practitioner
FISH	fluorescence in situ hybridization	GPA	granuloma; or granulomatosis with polyangitis
FITS	functional inferior turbinosurgery		
FIV	feline immunodeficiency virus	G protein	guanine nucleotide-binding regulatory protein
FLAIR	fluid attenuated inversion recovery		
FMF	familial Mediterranean fever	GRADE	Grading of Recommendation, Assessment, Development and Evaluation
FMISO	fluorine-18 fluoromisonidazole		
fMRI	functional magnetic resonance imaging	GRB2	growth factor receptor binding protein 2
FMTC	familial medullary thyroid cancer	Gs	G-protein adenylate cyclase stimulator
FN	facial nerve	GSH	glutathione
FNA	fine-needle aspiration/aspirate	GSP	stimulatory G protein
FNAB	fine-needle aspiration biopsy	GTN	nitroglycerin
FNAC	fine-needle aspiration cytology	GTR	guided tissue regeneration
FNHTR	febrile non-haemolytic transfusion reactions	GTV	grow tumour volume
FOI	fibreoptic orotracheal intubation	GvHD	graft-versus-host disease
FRS	fungal rhinosinusitis		
FS	folliculostellate; or frontal sinus	HA	hydroxyapatite
FSH	follicle-stimulating hormone	H&E	haematoxylin and eosin
fT3	free T3	H&N	head and neck
fT4	free T4	H2	histamine receptor type 2
FTC	frequency threshold curve; or follicular thyroid carcinoma	HA	hydroxyapatite
		HAART	highly active antiretroviral therapy
FT-UMP	follicular tumour of uncertain malignant potential	HAI	hospital-acquired infection
		HBME-1	mesothelium-associated antibody
FVPTC	follicular variant of papillary thyroid carcinoma	Hb	haemoglobin
		HbA	adult haemoglobin

HBO	hyperbaric oxygen	HSC	haematopoietic stem cell
HBOT	hyperbaric oxygen therapy	HSCT	haemopoietic stem cell transplant
HCG	human chorionic gonadotrophin	HSD	hydroxysteroid dehydrogenase enzyme
HD	haemodialysis	HSE	handling and storage errors
HDL	high-density lipoprotein	HSV	herpes simplex virus
HDM	house dust mite	HSV-1	herpes simplex virus type 1
HDU	high dependency unit	HSV-2	herpes simplex virus type 2
He-Ne	helium-neon	HSV-TK	herpes simplex thymidine kinase
HEPA	high-efficiency particulate air	HTA	hyalinizing trabecular adenoma; *or* Health Technology Assessment
HES	hospital episode statistics		
HFJV	high-frequency jet ventilation	hTERT	human telomerase reverse transcriptase
HFT	hereditary familial telangiectasia	HTR	haemolytic transfusion reaction
HGF	hepatocyte growth factor	HTT	hyalinizing trabecular tumours
HH	hypogonadotrophic hypogonadism	HU	Hounsfield unit
HHI	Hearing Handicap Inventory; *or* hereditary hearing impairment	HUI	Health Utilities Index
		HVDT	health visitor distraction test
HHIE	Hearing Handicap Inventory for the Elderly	Hz	hertz
		HZV	herpes zoster virus
HHT	hereditary haemorrhagic telangiectasia		
		IAC	internal auditory canal
HHV-6	human herpesvirus 6	IAR	intermittent allergic rhinitis
HHV-8	human herpesvirus 8	IBCT	incorrect blood component transfused
HI	hearing impaired	ICA	internal carotid artery
Hib	*Haemophilus influenzae* b	ICAD	inhibitor caspase-activated DNase
HIDS	hyper-IgD syndrome	ICAM	intercellular adhesion molecule
HIT	heparin-induced thrombocytopenia	ICAM-1	intercellular adhesion molecule 1
HIV	human immunodeficiency virus	ICD	International Classification of Disease
HL	hearing loss; *or* hearing level; *or* hairy leukoplakia	ICF	International Classification of Functioning
HLA	human leukocyte antigen	ICS	intra-operative cell salvage
HLH	haemophagocytic lymphohistiocytosis	ICU	intensive care unit
HM	history of migraine; *or* hemifacial microsomia	IDD	intracellular death domain
		IDT	infant distraction test; *or* intra-dermal test
HMW	high molecular weight	IFN	interferon
HMWC	high molecular weight compound	IFN-α	interferon-alpha
HMWCK	high molecular weight cytokeratin	IFN-β	inteferon-beta
HNSCC	head and neck squamous cell carcinoma	IFN-γ	interferon-gamma
Ho-YAG	holmium yttrium aluminium garnet	IFVPTC	invasive follicular variant of PTC
HPA	hypothalamic–pituitary–adrenal axis	Ig	immunoglobulin
HPC	haemangiopericytoma	IGD	isolated GnRH-deficiency
HPT	hyperparathyroidism	IgE	immunoglobulin E
HPT-JT	hyperparathyroidism-jaw tumour	IGF	insulin-like growth factor
HPV	human papillomavirus; *or* human herpes virus 8	IGF-I	insulin-like growth factor 1
		IGF-II	insulin-like growth factor II
HPZ	herpes zoster	IGFBP	insulin-like growth factor binding protein
HR	hazard ratio	IgG	immunoglobulin G
HRA	Human Rights Act	IgGκC	immunoglobulin G kappa chain
HRQOL	health-related quality of life	IGS	image-guided surgery
HR	heart rate	IHC	immunohistochemistry; *or* inner hair cell
HRT	hormone replacement therapy	IIT	iodide-induced thyrotoxicosis
HRV	rhinoviruses		

IJV	internal jugular vein		K	Kirschner
IL	interleukin		KCCT	kaolin cephalin clotting time
IL-1	interleukin-1		KDOQI	Kidney Disease Quality Outcomes Initiative
IL-2	interleukin-2		keV	kilo electron volt
IL-3	interleukin-3		KOH	potassium hydroxide solution prep test
IL-5	high interleukin		KISS-R	kisspeptin receptor (also known as GR54)
IL-6	interleukin-6		KS	Kaposi's sarcoma
ILMA	intubating laryngeal mask airway		KTP	potassium titanyl phosphate
i.m.	intramuscular			
IMA	internal maxillary artery		LA	lymphangioma
IMAL	internal maxillary artery ligation		LAR	local allergic rhinitis
IMF	intermaxillary fixation		LAT	lateral aberrant thyroid
IMP	importin		LC1	livery cystolic 1
IMRT	intensity-modulated radiation therapy		LCM	laser capture microdissection
iNOS	inducible nitric oxide synthase		LDH	lactate dehydrogenase
INR	international normalized ratio; *or* interventional neuroradiology		LDL	low-density lipoprotein; *or* loudness discomfort level
IOM	institute of Medicine		LED	light-emitting diode
IONM	intra-operative neural/nerve monitoring		LFA	lymphocyte-function associated antigen
IOPTH	intra-operative PTH		LFJV	low-frequency jet ventilation
IOQPTH	intra-operative quick assay of intact parathyroid hormone		LH	luteinizing hormone
			LHB	lateral-head-back
IOUS	intra-operative ultrasound scanning		LH-R	luteinizing hormone receptor
IP	Inverted papilloma		LINAC	linear accelerator
IPD	invasive pneumococcal disease		LKM	liver kidney microsomal
iPSCs	induced pluripotency stem cells		LM	laryngeal mask
IPSS	inferior petrosal sinus sampling		LMA	laryngeal mask airway
IRI	ischaemia-reperfusion injury		LMW	low molecular weight
IRS	insulin receptor substrate; *or* Intergroup Rhabdomyosarcoma Study		LMWC	low molecular weight compound
			LMWH	low molecular weight heparin
ISAAC	International Study of Asthma and Allergies in Childhood		LOCR	lateral opticocarotid recess
			LOD	logarithm to the base 10 of the odds that the markers are linked at a recombination distance of N centimorgans
ISCP	International Surgical Curriculum Programme			
ISL	*in situ* ligation		LOH	loss of heterozygosity
IT	inferior turbinate		LP	lamina papyracea; *or* lichen planus; *or* lymphocyte predominant
ITA	inferior thyroid artery			
ITAM	immunoreceptor tyrosine-based activation motif		LPR	laryngopharyngeal reflux; *or* late phase reactions
ITP	idiopathic thrombocytopenic purpura		LR	likelihood ratio
ITU	intensive therapy unit		LR-OCT	long-range optical coherence tomography
i.v.	intravenous		LTRA	leukotriene receptor antagonists
IVIg	intravenous immunoglobulin		LW	lateral wall
JAK2	Janus kinase 2		M	metastases
JCST	Joint Committee on Surgical Training		M2	Matrix 2 ion channels
JIA	juvenile idiopathic arthritis		MAb	monoclonal antibodies
JLNS1	Jervell and Lange-Nielsen syndrome		MABP	mean arterial blood pressure
JNA	juvenile nasopharyngeal angiofibroma		MAC	membrane attack complex; *or* *Mycobacterium avium* complex
JNK	c-Jun N-terminal kinase			

MAD	mucosal atomization device	MMR	measles, mumps and rubella
MAGE-3	melanoma-associated antigen-3	MNG	multinodular goitre
MALT	mucosa-associated lymphoid tissue	MOCR	medial opticocarotid recess
MAOI	monoamine oxidase inhibitor	MODS	multiple organ dysfunction syndrome
MAP	minimum audible pressure	MOE	malignant otitis externa
MAPK	mitogen-activated protein kinase	MOFT	multiple oxyphil follicular tumour
MAS	mandibular advancement splint; *or* macrophage activation syndromes	MOS	Medical Outcomes Study
MBL	mannose-binding lectin	MPA	microscopic polyangiitis
MC2R	melanocortin 2 receptor	MPTS	Medical Practitioner's Tribunal Service
MCP	monocyte chemotactic protein	MPO	myeloperoxidase
MCS	mental component summary	MPTP	1-methyl-4-phenyl-1,2,3,6-tetrahydropyridine
MCT	medullary thyroid carcinoma	MR	magnetic resonance
MCV	mean corpuscular volume	MRA	magnetic resonance angiography
MDCT	multi-detector row CT	MRC	Medical Research Council (UK)
MDS	myelodysplastic syndrome	MRCS	Member of the Royal College of Surgeons
MDT	multidisciplinary team	MRI	magnetic resonance imaging
ME	middle ear	mRNA	messenger ribonucleic acid
MEG	magnetoencephalography	MRSA	methicillin-resistant *Staphylococcus aureus*
MEK	MAPK/extracellular signal related kinase	MS	multiple sclerosis
MEN	multiple endocrine neoplasia	MSBOS	maximum surgical blood ordering schedule
MeSH	medical subject heading	MSCs	mesenchymal stem cells
MET	middle ear transducer	MSF	multi-source feeback
M-FISH	multifluor FISH	MSSA	methicillin-susceptible strains
MGHD	multiple gland hyperplasia disease	MT	maxilloturbinal; *or* middle turbinate
MGO	methylglyoxal	MTC	medullary thyroid carcinoma
MGUS	monoclonal gammopathy of uncertain significance	mtDNA	mitochondrial DNA
MHC	major histocompatibility complex	mTORC1	mammalian target of rapamycin 1
MHP	massive haemorrhage pack	mTORC2	mammalian target of rapamycin 2
MI	myocardial infarction	MW	medial wall
mIBG	metaiodobenzylguanidine; *or* iodine-123-metaiodobenzylguanidine		
MIBI	sestamibi; *or* technetium-99m	N	nodal
MIC	minimum inhibitory concentration	NADP	nicotinamide adenine dinucleotide phosphate
μOCT	micro-optical coherence tomography	NADPH	reduced form of nicotinamide adenine dinucleotide phosphate
MIFC	minimally invasive follicular carcinoma	NANIPER	non-allergic non-infectious perennial rhinitis
MIP	minimally invasive parathyroidectomy; *or* maximum intensity projection; *or* macrophage inflammatory protein;	NAP4	Fourth National Airway Project
		NARES	non-allergic rhinitis with eosinophilia syndrome
miRNA	micro ribonucleic acid	NBCA	n-butyl-2-cyanoacrylate; *or* N-butylcyanoacrylate
MIST	minimal invasive sinus techniques	NBT	nitro blue tetrazolium
MIT	monoiodotyrosine; *or* mono-iodothyronine; *or* minimally invasive thyroidectomy	NCAS	National Clinical Assessment Service (UK)
		NCEPOD	National Confidential Enquiry into Patient Outcome Death (UK)
MIVAT	minimally invasive video-assisted thyroidectomy	NCIC	National Cancer Institute of Canada
MLKL	mixed lineage kinase domain-like protein	ncRNA	non-coding ribonucleic acid
MLTB	microlaryngotracheobronchoscopy	Nd-YAG	neodymium-yttrium aluminium garnet
MMC	mitomycin C; *or* Modernising Medical Careers	NET	nerve excitability test; *or* neuroendocrine tumour
MMP	mucous membrane pemphigoid; *or* matrixmetalloprotease		

NF1	neurofibromatosis type 1
NF2	neurofibromatosis type 2
NH	normal hearing; *or* neurophypophysis
NHANES	National Health and Nutrition Examination Survey
NHL	non-Hodgkin's lymphoma
NHS	National Health Service (UK)
NHSLA	National Health Service Litigation Authority
NIBP	automatic non-invasive blood pressure
NICE	National Institute for Health and Care Excellence (UK)
NIFTP	non-invasive follicular tumour with papillary-like nuclei
NIH	National Institutes of Health (USA)
NIM	nerve integrity monitor
NIPF	nasal inspiratory peak flow
NIS	Na+/I− symporter
NK	natural killer
nLTP	non-specific lipid transfer protein
NNT	number needed to treat
NO	nitric oxide
NO2	nitric dioxide
NOAC	novel oral anticoagulant
NOE	naso-orbito-ethmoid
NOTSS	non-technical skills for surgeons
NOS	not otherwise specified
NP	nasopharynx; *or* nasopharyngeal
NPC	nasopharyngeal cancer; *or* nasopharyngeal carcinoma
NPSA	National Patient Safety Agency (UK)
NPT	near patient testing
NPV	negative predictive value
NRTIs	nucleoside/nucleotide reverse transcriptase inhibitors
NSAID	non-steroidal anti-inflammatory drug
NSF	national service framework; *or* nasoseptal flap
NSHI	non-syndromic hearing impairment
NTT	near-total thyroidectomy
O3	ozone
OAE	otoacoustic emission
OB	olfactory bulb
OCT	optical coherence tomography
ODP	operating department practitioner
OF	ossifying fibroma
OFDI	optical frequency domain imaging
OIDA	observe; interpret; decide; act
OMC	ostiomeatal complex
OPC	oropharyngeal cancer; *or* oropharyngeal candidiasis
OPCS	Office for Population Censuses and Surveys (UK)
OPF	osteoplastic flap procedure
OR	occupational rhinitis
OREP	olfactory event-related potential
ORL	otorhinolaryngology
OSA	obstructive sleep apnoea
OSATS	obstructive structured assessment of technical skill
OTOF	otoferlin
OXTR	oxytocin receptor
P	phosphate; *or* posterior
PA	pernicious anaemia
PAC	P1 artificial chromosome; *or* pulmonary artery catheter; *or* parathyroid carcinoma
PACS	picture archiving and communication systems
PACU	post-anaesthesia care unit
PAF	platelet-activating factor
PBA	procedure-based assessment
PBP	progressive bulbar palsy
PCA	patient-controlled analgesia
PCC	prothrombin complex concentrate; *or* Professional Conduct Committee (UK); *or* pheochromocytoma
PCD	primary ciliary dyskinesia
PCOS	polycystic ovary syndrome
PCR	polymerase chain reaction
PCS	physical component summary
PD	Parkinson's disease
PDCAT	poorly differentiated carcinoma of the thyroid
PDE	phosphodiesterase
PD1	programmed cell death protein 1
PDGF	platelet-derived growth factor
PDL	pulsed dye laser
PDR	Physicians' Desk Reference
PDS	polydimethylsiloxane
PDT	photodynamic therapy
PE	polyethylene; *or* pulmonary embolism; *or* pharyngo-oesophageal
PEG	percutaneous endoscopic gastrostomy
PER	persistent allergic rhinitis
PET	polyethylene terephthalate; *or* positron emission tomography
PET-CT	positron emission tomography/computed tomography
PET-MRI	positron emission tomography-MRI
PF	posterior fontanelle; *or* cisplatinum/5-fluorouracil

PF4	platelet factor 4
PFAPA	periodic fever, aphthous stomatitis, pharyngitis and cervical adenitis
PFS	progression-free survival
PG	paraganglioma
PGA	polyglycolic acid
PGD2	prostaglandin D2
PGE1	prostaglandin-E1
PGI2	prostacycline; or prostaglandin I2
PGL	persistent generalized lymphadenopathy
PHPT	primary hyperparathyroidism
PI	pulsatility index; or protease inhibitors
PI3K	phosphotidyinositol 3
PICU	paediatric intensive care unit
PIII	parathyroid III
PIP	peak inspiratory pressure
PIV	parainfluenza virus; or parathyroid IV
PKA	protein kinase A
PLAT	paraganglioma-like adenoma of the thyroid
PLD	potentially lethal damage
PM	particulate matter
PNH	paroxysmal nocturnal haemoglobinuria
PNIF	peak nasal inspiratory flow
p.o.	by mouth
POGO	prescription of gain and output
POMC	propiomelanocorticotrophin
PONV	postoperative nausea/vomiting
PP	pyrophosphate
PPD	purified protein derivative; or parathyroid proliferative disease
PPV	positive predictive value
PR3	proteinase 3
PRISMA	Preferred Reporting Items for Systematic Reviews and Meta-Analyses
PRL	polypeptide hormone prolactin
PRP	platelet-rich plasma
PRPP	5-phospho-alpha-D-ribose 1-diphosphate
PSA	prostate-specific antigen; or pleomorphic salivary adenoma; or persistent stapedial artery
PS-OCT	polarization-sensitive OCT
PT	prothrombin time
PTAH	phosphotungstic acid haematoxylin
PTC	papillary thyroid cancer; or psychophysical tuning curve
PTG	parathyroid gland
PTH	parathyroid hormone
PTHrP	parathyroid hormone-related protein; or parathyroid hormone-related peptide
PTMC	papillary thyroid microcarcinoma
pTNM	pathological tumour, nodes, metastases
PTP	post-transfusion purpura
PTU	propylthiouracil
PUOF1	pituitary-specific positive transcription factor 1
PVA	polyvinyl alcohol
PVC	polyvinyl chloride
PW	posterior wall
QALY	quality adjusted life year
QOL	quality of life
RA	retinoic acid
RAE	Ring, Adair, Elwyn
RAF	rapidly accelerated fibrosarcoma signal-regulated kinase
RAI	radioactive iodine
RANKL	regulation of nuclear factor κB ligand
RANTES	regulated on activation, normal T-cell expressed and secreted
RAS	recurrent aphthous stomatitis; or rat sarcoma protein family
RAST	radioallergosorbent test
RAT	rapid antigen testing; or robotic-assisted thyroidectomy
RB	retinoblastoma
RBC	red blood cell
RCC	Rathke cleft cyst; or red cell count
RCoA	Royal College of Anaesthetists
RCT	randomized controlled trial
RET	rearranged during transfection
RF	rheumatoid factor; or radio frequency
RFLP	restriction fragment length polymorphism
RFRP	RFamide-related peptide
RFTVR	radiofrequency tissue volume reduction
rFVIIa	recombinant factor VIIa
rhBMP-7	recombinant human bone morphogenetic protein 7
rhPTH	recombinant human parathyroid hormone
rhTSH	recombinant human TSH
RHD	Reported Hearing Disability
RIG	radiologically inserted gastrostomy
RLN	recurrent laryngeal nerve
RLNP	recurrent laryngeal nerve palsy
RNA	ribonucleic acid
RNP	ribonucleoprotein
ROS	reactive oxygen species
ROSE	rapid on-site evaluation
ROTEM	thromboelastography
RP	rapid prototyping; or relapsing polychondritis
RR	relative risk

RRA	radioiodine remnant ablation	SLE	systemic lupus erythematosus
RRR	relative risk reduction	SLICC	Systemic Lupus International Collaborating Clinics
RSDI	Rhinosinusitis Disability Index		
RSOM	rhinosinusitis outcome measure	SLIT	sublingual immunotherapy; or sublingually in drops or tablets
RSTL	relaxed skin tension line		
RSV	respiratory syncytial virus	SLN	superior laryngeal nerve
RT	radiotherapy	SMAS	superficial or subcutaneous musculoaponeurotic system
RTOG	Radiation Therapy Oncology Group		
rT3	reverse triiodothyronine	SAMD	submucosal diathermy
RTK	receptor tyrosine kinase	SMR	submucosal resection
RUDS	reactive upper airways dysfunction syndrome	SMS	short message service; or indium-111 pentetreotide
		SNHL	sensorineural hearing loss
SA	solitary adenoma; or situational awareness	SNOT	sino-nasal outcome test
SAD	supraglottic airway device	SNUC	sinonasal undifferentiated carcinoma
SAGM	saline-adenine-glucose-mannitol	SO2	sulphur dioxide
SAPS	simplified acute physiology score	SOCS2	suppressors of cytokine signalling 2
SBS	sick building syndrome	SOE	supraorbital ethmoid cells
s.c.	subcutaneous	SOFA	sequential organ failure assessment
SCC	squamous cell carcinoma or cancer; or semicircular canal	SOFT	solitary oxyphil follicular tumour
		SOS	guanine nucleotide exchange factor (son of sevenless)
SCCA	squamous cell carcinoma antigen		
SCCHN	squamous cell carcinoma of the head and neck	SPA	sphenopalatine artery
		SPECT	single photon emission computed tomography
SCID	severe combined immunodeficiency		
SCIT	subcutaneous immunotherapy	SPET	single photon emission tomography
SCL-90	Symptom Checklist-90	SPF	sphenopalatine foramen
SCM	sternocleidomastoid muscle	SPLINTS	scrub practitioners list of intra-operative non-technical skills
SCN	severe congenital neutropenia; or solid cell nests		
		SPT	skin prick test; or station pull through
SEER	Surveillance, Epidemiology, and End Results (program)	SPTX	subtotal parathyroidectomy
		SRS	subacute rhinosinusitis
SERM	selective-oestrogen receptor modifier	SS	somatostatin
SETTLE	spindle cell tumour with thymus-like differentiation	ssDNA	single-stranded DNA
		SSC	superior semicircular canal; or Surviving Sepsis Campaign
SF-36	Medical Outcome Study Short-Form 36-Item Health Survey		
		SSEP	steady-state potential
SFF	speaking fundamental frequency; or solid free form fabrication	SSLP	simple sequence length polymorphism
		SSQ	speech, spatial and qualities
SHC	SH2-containing protein	SSTR1-5	somatostatin receptors 1-5
Shh	sonic hedgehog	SSRI	selective serotonin reuptake inhibitor
SHI	syndromic hearing impairment	ST	superior turbinate; or subtotal thyroidectomy
SHOT	serious hazards of transfusion		
SHPT	secondary hyperparathyroidism	STAT	signal transducer and activator of transcription
SIADH	syndrome of inappropriate antidiuretic hormone		
		STD	standard deviation
sIgE	specific immunoglobulin E	STRP	short tandem repeat polymorphism
SIGN	Scottish Intercollegiate Guidelines Network	SUV	standardized uptake value
SIP	sickness impact profile	SV	stroke volume
siRNA	small interfering ribonucleic acid	SVCO	superior vena caval obstruction
SLD	sublethal damage	SVS	selective venous sampling

SVCO	superior vena cava obstruction		TNM	tumour, node, metastasis
SVR	systemic vascular resistance		TNO	transnasal oesophagosocpy
Syk	signal-propagating kinase		TOE	transoesophageal echocardiography; or *Trichophyton*, *Oidiomycetes* and *Epidermophyton*
T	thymine; or tumour		TOF	tracheo-oesophageal fistula
T1WI	T1-weighted images		TPO	thyroid peroxidase; or thyroperoxidase
T2WI	T2-weighted images		TPP	thyrotoxic periodic paralysis
T3	triiodothyronine		TPTX	total parathyroidectomy
T4	thyroxine		TPZ	tirapazamine
TAA	tumour associated antigens		TRALI	transfusion-related acute lung injury
TACO	transfusion-associated circulatory overload		TRAM	transverse rectus abdominis myocutaneous
TAD	transfusion-associated dysponea		TRH	thyrotrophin-releasing hormone
TAGVHD	transfusion-associated graft-versus-host disease		tRNA	transfer ribonucleic acid
TAM	tumour associated macrophages		TSA	tumour specific antigens
TB	tuberculosis; or *Mycobacterium tuberculosis*		TSH	thyroid-stimulating hormone; or thyrotrophin
TBG	thyroxine-binding globulin		TSHoma	TSH-secreting adenoma
TcT	cytotoxic		TSH-R	TSH receptor
^{99m}Tc	technetium-99m		TT	thrombin time; or total thyroidectomy
Tc-99m (v) DMSA	pentavalent dimercaptosuccinic acid		TTF-1	thyroid transcription factor-1
TC	thyroid cartilage		TTP	thrombotic thrombocytopeniac purpura
TCI	target-controlled infusion		TUNEL	TdT-mediated nick end labelling
TCP	tricalcium phosphate			
TCR	T-cell receptor		U	uracil
t.d.s.	3 times a day		UCT	unclassifiable complications of transfusion
TEG	thromboelastography		UICC	International Union Against Cancer
TFT	thyroid function test		UIC	urinary iodine concentration
TG	thyroglobulin		UKRETS	UK Registry of Endocrine and Thyroid Surgery
TgAb	thyroglobulin antibodies		UMP	uridine monophosphate
TGF	transforming growth factor		UNICEF	United Nations Children's Fund
TGF-α	transforming growth factor alpha		UP	uncinate process
TGF-β	transforming growth factor beta		UPSIT	University of Pennsylvania Smell Identification Test
TGF-β1	transforming growth factor beta 1		URTI	upper respiratory tract infection
Th	T-helper		US	ultrasound; or ultrasonography
Th1	T-helper 1 cell		USH	Usher syndrome
Th2	T-helper 2 cell		USH1B	Usher syndrome type 1B
THST	thyroid hormone suppression therapy		USS	ultrasound scan
THW	thyroid hormone withdrawal		UV	ultraviolet
TI	thyroid isthmusectomy			
TIL	tumour infiltrating lymphocytes		V2R	vasopressin type 2 receptor
TIVA	total intravenous anaesthesia		VA	Veterans' Affairs; or vestibular aqueduct
TKI	tyrosine kinase inhibitor		VAC	vacuum-assisted closure
TL	total lobectomy		VAS	visual analogue scale; or visual analogue score
TME	tumour microenvironment			
TMC1	transmembrane channel-like gene 1		VATS	video-assisted thoracoscopic surgery
TMJ	temporomandibular joint		VC	vocal cord
TNF	tumour necrosis factor			
TNF-α	tumour necrosis factor alpha			

VCAM-1	vascular cell adhesion molecule-1	WDTC	well-differentiated thyroid cancer
vCJD	variant Creutzfeldt—Jakob disease	WDT-UMP	well-differentiated tumour of uncertain malignant potential
VCP	vocal cord paralysis	WHAFFT	worrisome histologic alteration following fine-needle aspiration of the thyroid gland
VDA	vascular disrupting agent		
VEGF	vascular endothelial growth factor		
VEGFR	vascular endothelial growth factor receptor	WHO	World Health Organization
VF	vocal fold	WIFC	widely invasive follicular carcinoma
VHI	Voice Handicap Index	WMD	weighted mean difference
VHI-10	Voice Handicap Index-10	WP	Woodruff's plexus
VHQ	Vertigo Handicap Questionnaire	WPBA	workplace based assessments
VILI	ventilator induced lung injury	WS	Waardenburg syndrome
VN	vestibular nuclei; *or* vagus nerve		
VNO	vomero nasal organ	XLA	X-linked agammaglobulinaemia
VOC	volatile organic compound	XM	crossmatch
VTE	venous thromboembolism		
VTFF	vertex-to-floor	YAC	yeast artificial chromosome
vWD	von Willebrand disease	YAG	yttrium aluminium garnate
vWF	von Willebrand factor		
VZV	varicella zoster virus		
WBS	whole-body scan		
WDC-NOS	well-differentiated carcinoma, not otherwise specified		

Section 1
Basic Sciences

Cell biology
1. Molecular biology 3
2. Genetics in otology and neurotology 15
3. Gene therapy 29
4. Mechanisms of anticancer drugs 39
5. Radiotherapy and radiosensitizers 51
6. Apoptosis and cell death 59
7. Stem cells 69
8. Aetiology and pathogenesis of goitre 75
9. Genetics of endocrine tumours 83

Wound healing
10. Soft and hard tissue repair 93
11. Skin flap physiology 107
12. Biomaterials, tissue engineering and their application in the oral and maxillofacial region 119

Immunology
13. Defence mechanisms 125
14. Allergy: Basic mechanisms and tests 137
15. Evaluation of the immune system 149
16. Cancer immunology 157
17. Human papillomavirus 167
18. Connective tissue disorders: ENT complications 173

Microbiology
19. Microorganisms 181
20. Viruses and antiviral agents 195
21. Fungal infections 205
22. Antimicrobial therapy 221
23. Human immunodeficiency virus 229

Haematology
24. Blood groups, blood components and alternatives to transfusion 239
25. Haemato-oncology 249
26. Haemostasis: Normal physiology, disorders of haemostasis and thrombosis 259

Pharmacotherapeutics
27. Drug therapy in otology 275
28. Drug therapy in rhinology 283
29. Drug therapy in laryngology and head and neck surgery 293

Perioperative management
30. Preparation of the patient for surgery 301
31. Recognition and management of the difficult airway 309
32. Adult anaesthesia 333
33. Adult critical care 351
34. Paediatric intensive care 361

Safe and effective practice
35. Training, accreditation and the maintenance of skills 369
36. Communication and the medical consultation 379
37. Clinical governance and its role in patient safety and quality improvement 389
38. Medical ethics 395
39a. Medical jurisprudence in otorhinolaryngology 409
39b. Medical negligence in otorhinolaryngology 427
40. Non-technical skills for ENT surgeons 453

Interpretation and management of data
41. Epidemiology 465
42. Outcomes research 483
43. Evidence-based medicine in medical education and clinical practice 495
44. Critical appraisal skills 503

Advances in technology
45. Electrophysiology and monitoring 525
46. Optical coherence tomography 533
47. Recent advances in technology 541
48. Image-guided surgery, 3D planning and reconstruction 559
49. Interventional techniques 569
50. Laser principles in otolaryngology, head and neck surgery 581
51. Contact endoscopy of the upper aerodigestive tract 587

Cell biology

CHAPTER 1

MOLECULAR BIOLOGY

Michael Kuo, Richard M. Irving and Eric K. Parkinson

Introduction 3	Molecular aberrations of cellular biology 7
Molecular genetics: DNA structure and function 3	Mapping and identification of genes associated with disease 10
Other regulators of gene expression 4	References 12
Methods in molecular biology 5	Further reading 13

SEARCH STRATEGY

Data in this chapter may be updated by a Medline search using the keywords: molecular biology, genetics and cell biology.

INTRODUCTION

Molecular biology describes the study of the biochemical processes that govern the behaviour of cells. These processes form the fundamental mechanisms by which cell function, cell–cell interactions and cell turnover are regulated. Disruption of this regulation may lead to disease, whilst an understanding of these mechanisms allows the physician to attempt to predict disease behaviour and to explore methods of restoring this regulation at a molecular level. This chapter reviews the principles of molecular genetics and outlines aspects of the molecular biology of the cell in the context of otolaryngological disease processes and describes some of the techniques that form the backbone of current molecular biology. It should give the reader sufficient background knowledge of molecular biology to understand subsequent chapters discussing the molecular biology of specific otolaryngological conditions.

MOLECULAR GENETICS: DNA STRUCTURE AND FUNCTION

Hereditary information in eukaryotes is stored in the form of double-stranded deoxyribonucleic acid (DNA) and is referred to as the genome. DNA forms a double-helix structure as a result of hydrogen bonds between complementary pairs of nucleotides, adenine (A) with thymine (T) and cytosine (C) with guanine (G). The nucleotides on each strand are organized linearly in triplets, known as codons. Each specific sequence determines a single specific amino acid, for example ACU specifies threonine. However, as there are more triplet combinations (64) than commonly encountered amino acids (20), some proteins may be represented by different codons (e.g. lysine by AAA as well as AAG) and some codons (UAA, UGA and UAG) are 'stop' codons, constituting a signal for arrest of translation. The overwhelming majority of this DNA (99.9%) exists in the cell nucleus as the nuclear genome, which, in the human, is estimated to be 3000 megabase pairs in physical size and encodes 30 000–35 000 genes. The remaining DNA (16.6 kilobase pairs) forms the mitochondrial genome, encoding 37 genes. The mitochondrial genome and its potential role in cancer diagnostics will be discussed later.

Each DNA molecule is packaged into a chromosome by complex folding of the DNA around proteins. Diploid human cells contain 22 pairs of autosomes (1 to 22) and a pair of sex chromosomes (XX or XY) that determines the sex of the organism. One of each pair of chromosomes is maternally inherited and the other is paternally inherited. Each chromosome has a distinctive shape, size and banding pattern, but have the common appearance of two arms apparently separated by a constriction. The centromere is microscopically recognizable as the central constriction separating the chromosome into a long arm (q for queue) and a short arm (p for petit), but its biological role lies in anchoring the chromosome to the mitotic spindle for segregation during cell division. The ends of the chromosomes are capped by telomeres, which are specialized structures containing unique simple repetitive sequences. They maintain the structural integrity of the chromosome and provide a solution for complete replication of the extreme ends of the chromosome. The conventional nomenclature for chromosomal locus assignment is given by the chromosome number, followed by the arm and finally the position on the arm, for example, 3p21 indicates position 21(two-one) on the short arm of chromosome three.

During normal cell division, DNA replication is achieved by the separation of the two strands by DNA helicase. Each separated single strand then acts as a template for polymerization, catalyzed by DNA polymerase, of nucleotides forming a new complementary strand and thus double-stranded DNA identical to the original dsDNA. As each daughter DNA consists of one original and one newly synthesized DNA strand, the process is known as semi-conservative replication. The specificity of the complementary relationship between the nucleotides on each strand forms the basis for many techniques of modern molecular biology and molecular cytogenetics.[1] The accuracy with which DNA replication takes place is remarkable with an estimated error rate of less than one in 10^9 nucleotide additions. Such accuracy is of vital importance to the individual as a permanent change in DNA, or mutation may cause inactivation of a gene essential to cell survival or cell cycle control. The high fidelity of DNA sequence replication is achieved by unidirectional 5′-to-3′ direction of DNA replication, a rigorous DNA proofreading mechanism that detects mismatched DNA and efficient DNA repair pathways that excise and repair DNA damage. Failure of these mechanisms, such as is encountered in xeroderma pigmentosum, Fanconi's anaemia and ataxia telangiectasia, leads to accumulation of DNA replication errors and a high incidence of malignancies.

Although the human nuclear genome is 3×10^9 base pairs in size, about 90% of it is non-coding, with all the genes being coded by the remaining 10% of the DNA. Within the non-coding DNA are dispersed short arrays of repeat units of pairs or triplets of nucleotides (di-/trinucleotides). The exact function of these microsatellite repeats is not entirely clear, but their existence and frequency of dispersion throughout the genome have greatly facilitated study of the genetics of tumours and many inherited disorders, which will be discussed later.

A gene is a region of the chromosomal DNA that produces a functional ribonucleic acid molecule (RNA). It comprises regulatory DNA sequences that determine when and in which cell types that gene is expressed, exons that are coding sequences and interspersed introns that are non-coding DNA sequences. These regulatory sequences often consist of CpG islands, short stretches of DNA rich in dinucleotides of cytosine and guanine. The methylation status of these CpG islands determines whether that gene is expressed in a particular cell or tissue, being unmethylated in tissues where the genes are expressed. As will be discussed later, aberration of this control is one of the mechanisms of tumour suppressor gene inactivation. However, these same genes can also be regulated by proteins that recognize methylated sequences called histones[2] and these in turn can be regulated by polycomb genes such as *BMI1*.[3] Transcription is the intra-nuclear process driven by RNA polymerase whereby one of the two DNA strands acts as a template for the synthesis of a single RNA strand which is complementary to the DNA, except that uracil replaces thymine in RNA. This primary RNA transcript then undergoes post-transcriptional processing, or splicing.[4] Traditional dogma held that one gene produces one protein and therefore splicing was considered to occur simply in order to remove the non-coding intronic sequences, producing messenger RNA (mRNA). It is now known that by 'alternative splicing', one gene can result in the production of several different but often related proteins in different tissues.[5]

The mature mRNA then migrates into the cytoplasm where it acts as a template for the synthesis of a polypeptide during translation, a process regulated and catalyzed by cytoplasmic ribosomes. Successive amino acids are added to the polypeptide chain according to the triplet code on the mRNA, which is recognized by the transfer RNA (tRNA), to which each corresponding amino acid is covalently bound. Translation is commenced upon recognition of an initiation codon (usually but not exclusively AUG/methionine) and terminated upon recognition of a stop codon. The polypeptide subsequently undergoes a variable degree of post-translational modification and/or cleavage to produce the mature protein product, which may have an intra-cellular role or may be exported to the endoplasmic reticulum and hence to the extracellular space to execute its function.

The mitochondrial genome is considerably smaller than the nuclear genome, but it deserves mention here because of the increasing recognition of the role of mitochondrial DNA (mtDNA) mutations in human disease. The mitochondrial genome is only 16.6 kb in size, comprising 37 genes, which encode polypeptides that are principally involved in the respiratory chain. mtDNA is double-stranded but does not form a double-helix or chromosomes, but instead takes the form of a circular double-stranded DNA structure with a heavy and a light strand. Unlike the nuclear genome, which is inherited from mother and father, the mitochondrial genome of an individual is entirely maternally inherited.

OTHER REGULATORS OF GENE EXPRESSION

In the last few years it has become apparent that gene expression is 'fine-tuned' by several classes of molecule. Small interfering RNAs (siRNAs) were first discovered in plants and are now widely used as research tools to suppress gene expression. However, natural versions of siRNAs exist (microRNAs- miRNAs) and are thought to be biologically significant regulators of gene expression.[6] miRNAs are small non-coding RNA molecules that function through base-pairing with mRNA, thus preventing their translation into proteins. There may be more than 1000 miRNAs in the human genome[7] and some of them are associated with oral cancer; they are also secreted into body fluids making them candidates for the non-invasive detection of the disease.[8] In addition, long non-coding RNAs (ncRNAs) have been identified that are thought to regulate various aspects of gene expression, including transcription, splicing, translation, siRNA-directed gene regulation and epigenetic regulation.[9] Whilst the study of ncRNAs is still new they have been implicated in a number of diseases, including ageing and cancer.

> **KEY POINTS**
>
> - The double-stranded alpha helical structure of DNA, mainly located in the nucleus, consists of nucleotide triplets called codons which code for specific amino acids and stop signals, and forms the substrate for hereditary information in eukaryotes.
> - The 22 pairs of autosomes and one pair of sex chromosomes, each with their distinctive shape, size and banding pattern, represent a complex folding of DNA around proteins to give the characteristic shape of a central constriction (centromere) separating the chromosome into a long arm (q) and a short arm (p) with a telomere cap at each end to maintain structural integrity.
> - Chromosome locus nomenclature: chromosome number – 3p21 – position on chromosome arm.
> - Semiconservative replication of DNA during normal cell division results in the separation of two strands of DNA by DNA helicase, each strand then acting as a template for polymerization by DNA polymerase. High fidelity is vital to prevent permanent change or mutations.
> - A gene is a region of chromosomal DNA which produces functional RNA consisting of:
>   - regulatory DNA sequences
>   - exons, which are coding sequences
>   - introns, which are non-coding sequences.
> - Transcription is the intra-nuclear process driven by RNA polymerase whereby one of the two DNA strands acts as a template for single-stranded RNA synthesis complementary to the DNA, except that in RNA T is replaced by U. Splicing refers to post-transcriptional processing of RNA.
> - Translation is the cytoplasmic process in which mRNA acts as a template for the synthesis of polypeptide by adding successive amino acids to the polypeptide chain, according to the triplet codon of the mRNA that is recognized by the tRNA to which the corresponding amino acid is covalently bonded. This process is regulated and catalyzed by cytoplasmic ribosomes. Post-translational modification produces mature proteins.
> - Gene expression can be modulated by naturally-occurring miRNAs and ncRNAs.

METHODS IN MOLECULAR BIOLOGY

Basic techniques of DNA fragmentation and identification

Unlike RNA, DNA is extremely stable, which is understandable from the function that each has in the cell. For purposes of studying the DNA and in order to clone specific DNA, the DNA molecule needs to be divided into manageable fragments. Although the ability to cut (and also to join up) DNA molecules now appears to be a

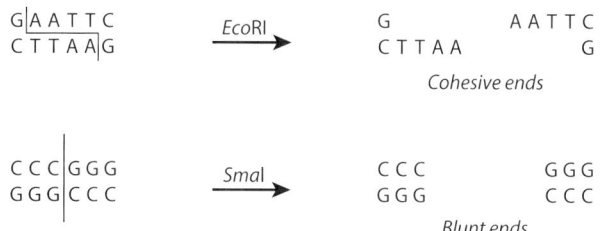

Figure 1.1 **DNA cleavage by restriction endonucleases.** Derived from Ref. 10, with permission.

very straightforward process, it was only 1970 when the first restriction endonuclease was identified in a strain of *Haemophilus influenzae*, hence its name *Hin*dII (pronounced Hin-dee-two). It is believed that this restriction endonuclease acts *in vivo* in bacteria as an immune or host-defence system, recognizing non-self DNA in bacteriophages and cleaving them. By surveying many different bacteria, a wide range of restriction endonucleases is now available, each of which recognizes specific target sites based on sequences of four to eight nucleotides. As a specific, a seven nucleotide sequence (heptanucleotide) will occur less frequently than a four nucleotide sequence (tetranucleotide), statistically, endonucleases recognizing heptanucleotide targets will cut less frequently thereby yielding larger fragments than those recognizing tetranucleotides. As the DNA is double-stranded, the resultant fragments may have blunt ends or cohesive ('sticky') ends (**Figure 1.1**). The nature of the ends of DNA fragments thus generated impact upon the way in which they can be ligated (joined) into recombinant molecules. Ligation of DNA fragments with cohesive ends is more efficient than joining of blunt-ended fragments.

Electrophoresis

Negatively charged phosphate groups on the DNA backbone confer a net negative charge on linear DNA. This allows fragments of different sizes to be resolved within a suitable gel matrix by the application of an electric current across the matrix. The DNA will migrate towards the positive electrode with the smaller fragments travelling faster than the larger fragments.[10] The size of the fragment can be estimated by the use of a graduated DNA ladder containing fragments of known molecular weight. The choice of the particular matrix depends on the fragment sizes that one is trying to resolve. Polyacrylamide gels can resolve differences of just one base pair between fragments of several hundred base pairs in size by virtue of a small pore size in the gel matrix. These gels can be used for DNA sequencing and resolution of alleles varying in only one dinucleotide repeat. Agarose gels can resolve fragment sizes from around 100 bp to 20 kb. Beyond that size, electrophoretic mobility is no longer proportional to fragment size. Resolution of fragments sizes in excess of 50 kb, such as larger bacterial artificial chromosomes (BAC) or yeast artificial chromosomes (YAC) require the use of pulsed field electrophoresis.

Hybridization

Hybridization is the specific annealing of single DNA (or RNA) strands, the probe, to a DNA sample, the target. It serves to detect the presence of a specific sequence of DNA either in the cell or on a hybridization membrane and recognition that hybridization has occurred is achieved either by radioactively labelling the probe and localizing the radioactivity by autoradiography or by labelling the probe with fluorochromes that fluoresce when excited by light of specific wavelengths (**Figure 1.2**). Hybridization on a membrane requires the initial transfer of DNA on to a nitrocellulose membrane from an agarose gel. This elegantly simple process is eponymously known as Southern blotting after the scientist who described the process in 1975. Two other commonly used transfer techniques have their names derived from Southern blotting as jargon terms. Northern blotting is essentially the same process used for transfer of RNA to a membrane. Western blotting is one of the mainstays of protein analysis and involves the transfer of electrophoresed protein bands from a polyacrylamide gel on to a nitrocellulose or nylon membrane to which they bind strongly. Detection of the protein is usually achieved by the use of antibodies to specific antigens presented by the protein with the antibody being labelled radioactively, enzymatically or fluorescently.

Cytogenetics and molecular cytogenetics

Although microscopy had already reached high levels of resolution in the early 1930s, the correct number of human chromosomes was not determined until 1958. The era of classical cytogenetics had thus begun. Cytogenetics is the study of chromosomal abnormalities and rearrangements. It currently has a major role to play in pre-natal diagnosis of Down syndrome and other congenital syndromes characterized by numerical chromosomal abnormalities. In the early part of this century, Theodore Boveri proposed that cancer arose from chromosomal alterations. This hypothesis was not proven until the consistent chromosomal translocation, t(9;22), was demonstrated in chronic myeloid leukaemia. Since that time, cytogenetic analysis has been the mainstay of genetic analysis in reticuloendothelial malignancies, being responsible for the identification of consistent translocations in different leukaemias. Its use in solid tumours has been hampered by the difficulties of establishing short-term primary cultures from head and neck cancers for chromosomal analysis and the erratically acquired chromosomal changes in long-term cell lines, which may have occurred *in vitro*, influenced by culture conditions. Nevertheless, some studies have identified chromosomal areas consistently showing frequent breakpoints suggesting the location of putative tumour suppressor genes (including 3p21, 5p14, 8p11, 17p21, 18q21) and gain or amplification implying the presence of putative protooncogenes at other sites (including 3q, 5p, 8q, 11q13). Although the refinement of karyotyping has been radically enhanced by the introduction of 24-colour combinatorial multifluor FISH (M-FISH), the resolution and therefore utility of solid tumour karyotyping remains limited.[11]

Hybridization to target DNA in cells, using fluorescence detection, is known as fluorescence *in situ* hybridization (FISH). Fluorescence *in situ* hybridization allows the analysis of copy number of a known specific DNA sequence within intact nuclei. In reticuloendothelial malignancies and solid tumour-derived cell lines, the use of both single-copy probes and centromere alpha-satellite repeat probes on metaphase preparations has enhanced and refined classical karyotyping. Interphase FISH has been applied to solid tumour sections to assess the copy number of a known sequence in breast, prostate, bladder, brain, lung and head and neck tumours.

Fluorescence-labelled hybridization has also been combined with cytogenetics to produce the powerful technique of comparative genomic hybridization (CGH).[12] Comparative genomic hybridization permits the rapid medium resolution screening of the entire genome by comparatively hybridizing matched tumour and normal DNA from a patient, which are labelled with different fluorochromes, on to normal metaphase chromosome preparations. Under red-green dual filter fluorescence microscopy and computer-aided image analysis, areas of genetic 'neutrality' appear yellow, under-representation appears green, and over-representation appears red. Areas of genetic under-representation suggest the possibility of a tumour suppressor gene lying within that region while areas of over-representation may indicate the location of a putative oncogene. This technique has been applied to the rapid genetic analysis of many tumour types including squamous cell carcinomas of the head and neck. The advent of molecular cytogenetics has obviated the need for primary short-term cultures and refined the location of chromosomal aberrations in solid tumours.

Polymerase chain reaction

Perhaps the single molecular technique that has had the most dramatic impact on molecular biology has been the polymerase chain reaction (PCR). The original problem lay in obtaining sufficient quantities of a particular DNA sequence such that DNA profiling (e.g. sequencing) and DNA manipulation (e.g. cloning) could be achieved. The only 'requirement' is that the sequences flanking the stretch of DNA of interest is known. With that proviso,

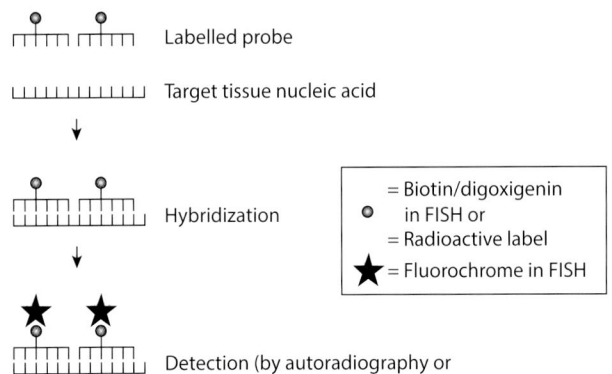

Figure 1.2 *In situ* **hybridization.**

PCR achieves faithful and exponential amplification of a specific sequence of DNA by repeated cycles each consisting of dsDNA denaturation, hybridization of specific oligonucleotides (primers) and extension of the polynucleotide by rapidly altering the reaction temperature between segments of each cycle. dsDNA denaturation is achieved by raising the temperature of the reaction to 94°C for 30 seconds, thus disrupting the hydrogen bonds between the strands and exposing the hydrogen bond donor and acceptor groups to allow base pairing. The oligonucleotide primers are then allowed to hybridize to the denatured DNA (annealing) at around 55–65°C for 90 seconds before the reaction temperature is raised to 72°C to permit extension of the DNA strand by DNA polymerase in the presence of deoxynucleoside triphosphates (dNTPs). With each cycle resulting in the doubling of the copies of the DNA sequence, a 30-cycle PCR taking approximately two hours would amplify a single copy of a DNA sequence 268 million-fold (Figure 1.3). Although the PCR was originally described by Mullis and Faloona in 1987, one practical problem prevented its instant exploitation.[13] The DNA polymerase used in the original reaction was denatured during the DNA denaturation segment and therefore had to be added after each and every cycle. The solution came in 1989 when Lawyer isolated and characterized the DNA polymerase, Taq polymerase, from the thermophilic bacterium *Thermus aquaticus* which normally resided in temperatures above 95°C.[14] This polymerase was therefore 'heat resistant' and did not need to be replenished between cycles.

The PCR holds a central position in many molecular biological techniques as well as clinical diagnostic methods. The fundamental principle of DNA amplification has been adapted to amplify messenger RNA and to amplify areas where the initial flanking oligonucleotide sequences are not known. It is often described as a sensitive and powerful technique, but with great power comes the potential for corruption! In theory, a single copy of DNA can be amplified. Therefore, careless experimental technique may lead to contamination of the DNA sample with other DNA (e.g. from the skin of the investigator) and consequently to an artefactual result. The Taq polymerase originally described in the technique does not have proofreading properties, but newer cloned enzymes such as Pfu polymerase incorporates a proofreading function to increase amplification fidelity for sequencing reactions.

The sensitivity of PCR also presented a problem for the analysis of genetic alterations in certain solid tumours. Squamous cell carcinomas of the head and neck are histologically often characterized by a large stromal element within the tumour. The genetic alterations in the tumour may not be present in the stromal tissue and thus total DNA extracted from the tumour will contain DNA from both benign and malignant tissue. This *in situ* contamination can now be eliminated by the use of laser capture microdissection (LCM) of tumours. LCM involves the placement of a laser-activated film over a tissue specimen. When areas of 'pure' tumour cells are identified, a focal laser pulse lifts the tissue on to the film in specimens down to 30 µm in diameter.[15]

KEY POINTS

- Restriction endonucleases are enzymes that were initially identified in bacteria that can cut and join up DNA. They recognize specific target sites based on sequences of four and eight nucleotides.
- Electrophoresis is a technique for resolving the size of DNA fragments, which carry a negative charge from the phosphate groups on their backbone. Using a gel matrix with an electric current applied across it, the DNA will migrate to the positive electrode at a rate inversely proportional to its size.
- Hybridization is the specific annealing of single DNA or RNA strands (probe) to a DNA sample (target) to detect the presence of a specific sequence of DNA in the cell or hybridization membrane. Variants include the eponymously named Southern, Northern and Western blotting techniques.
- Cytogenetics is the study of chromosomal abnormalities and rearrangements important in the diagnosis of congenital syndromes characterized by numerical chromosomal abnormalities (e.g. Down syndrome and leukaemia types).
- FISH refers to fluorescence *in situ* hybridization which involves hybridization to target DNA cells using fluorescence detection and allows the analysis of copy number of a known specific DNA sequence within intact nuclei.
- PCR achieves faithful and exponential amplification of a specific sequence of DNA by repeated cycles each consisting of:
  - DNA denaturation by heating to 94°C to denature hydrogen bonds between strands
  - annealing (hybridization) of oligonucleotide primers to denatured DNA at 55–65°C
  - extension of DNA strand by DNA polymerase.

MOLECULAR ABERRATIONS OF CELLULAR BIOLOGY

Loss of heterozygosity and the expression of recessive mutant alleles

Retinoblastoma is a childhood cancer, which exhibits both hereditary and sporadic occurrence, with the inherited form transmitted as a highly penetrant autosomal

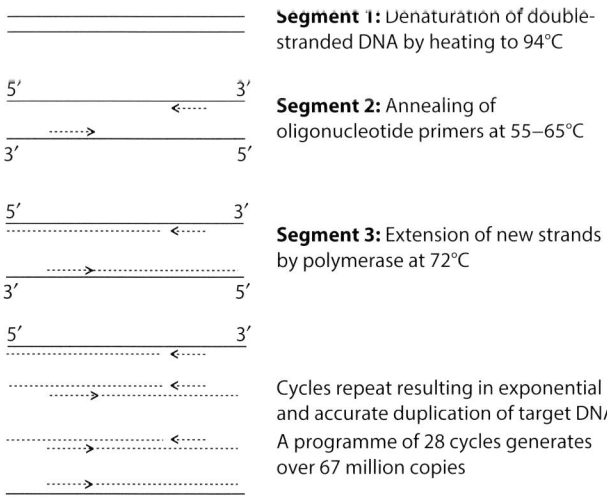

Figure 1.3 The polymerase chain reaction.

dominant trait. The proposition by Alfred Knudson in 1971, based upon a statistical analysis of the occurrence of retinoblastoma in children, that two genetic events were required to inactivate the gene mitigating against development of the cancer, was a major landmark in the understanding of tumour suppressor genetics.[16] In hereditary retinoblastomas, a single additional somatic event in a cell that carried the inherited mutation was sufficient to give rise to the disease while two somatic events were required to produce a sporadic retinoblastoma. This became known as Knudson's 'two-hit' hypothesis. The subsequent study on matched tumour and blood DNA from patients with sporadic retinoblastoma by Webster Cavenee not only proved Knudson's hypothesis but also established the paradigm for all subsequent investigations of tumour suppressor genes.[17] For the first time, the now widely accepted mechanisms of tumourigenesis were reconciled, viz. that neoplasms can arise in a multistep manner, that chromosomal events can lead to tumour formation and that chromosome loss with or without reduplication can lead to expression of recessive mutations. Perhaps even more strikingly, the authors presciently suggested that development of homozygosity for recessive mutant alleles at the *Rb-1* locus may give rise to the development of other tumours and that other additional dominant mutations may be involved in the development of retinoblastoma. Cavenee proposed the various chromosomal mechanisms that could reveal recessive mutations and these are summarized for a putative tumour suppressor gene in **Figure 1.4**, adapted from the figure in his original paper. To these can now be added hypermethylation of the 5′ CpG island resulting in transcriptional inactivation of the gene, discussed below.[18] The simplest way of revealing a recessive mutant allele is by deletion of the wild-type allele, resulting in hemizygosity at the particular locus on the remaining chromosome. It is inferred from this that areas of frequent allelic loss in tumours may represent the location of putative tumour suppressor genes and this hypothesis underpins the commonly employed method of molecular detection of allelic losses, loss of heterozygosity (LOH).

The practical exploitation of the concepts outlined above hinges on the presence of the previously described microsatellites, highly polymorphic non-coding DNA sequences, also referred to as simple sequence length polymorphisms (SSLP) or short tandem repeat polymorphisms (STRP), which are distributed approximately every 100 000 bp throughout the human genome. These microsatellites contain small dinucleotide or trinucleotide repeat units, the number of which may differ between the two alleles in a particular person. Microsatellite markers are now available which map thousands of these sequences to chromosomal loci. When DNA sequences containing these microsatellite markers are amplified by PCR in a person heterozygous for that

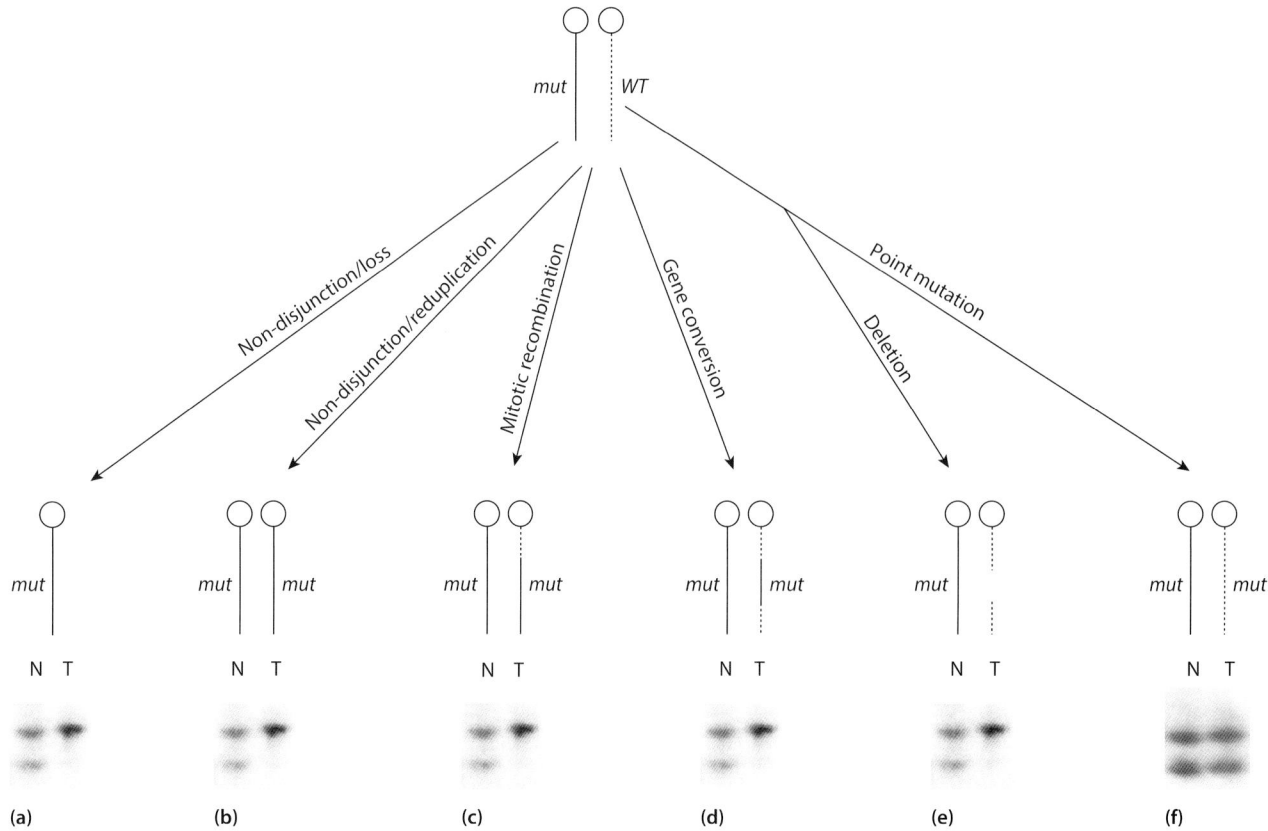

Figure 1.4 Chromosomal mechanisms that could reveal recessive mutations. In this example, before cell division, the tissue concerned carries a mutation in one copy of the hypothetical tumour suppressor gene. In each of the scenarios **(a–f)**, the recessive mutation is revealed. If the individual is heterozygous for a microsatellite marker within or very close to the mutated gene, the hypothetical PCR results are given below each ideotype. The only mechanism that escapes observed loss of heterozygosity is F. *mut*, mutated; N, normal; T, tumour; *WT*, wildtype. After Ref. 17, with permission.

particular microsatellite, the PCR will yield two products of different lengths, which can be resolved on an electrophoretic gel. Where amplification of tumour DNA from such a subject yields only one product, the tumour is said to show LOH, implying allelic loss. Persons who are homozygous for a particular marker are said to be non-informative for that marker. The concept of examining the variation and extent of allelic deletion in tumours was introduced by Vogelstein in an analysis of colorectal carcinomas and termed allelotyping.[19] Allelotypes generated in this fashion have identified several areas of frequent allelic deletion from which some of the responsible tumour suppressor genes have been cloned or identified. The most common areas of loss in HNSCC are at chromosome 9p21, 17p13, 13q14, 4p, 5q21 and several discrete regions on 3p and 8p.[20, 21]

Inactivation of genes and oncogenic transformation

Allelic deletion is only one mechanism by which a copy of a gene can be inactivated. As there are two copies of each gene, inactivation of the gene requires inactivation of both copies of the gene, 'the second hit'. This may occur as a result of a genetic mutation or transcriptional silencing. Conversely, a protooncogene may be converted into an oncogene by a simple increase in the copy number of the gene (gene amplification) resulting in an overproduction of protein or by point mutations that affect the control of protein activity.

Not all mutations result in alteration in function of a gene. DNA mutation may occur as a result of base substitutions, as well as nucleotide insertions and deletions. Insertions and deletions of nucleotides are very rare in coding DNA, but if they occur they may produce a shift in the 'reading frame' that dramatically alters the coding downstream from the mutation. Base substitution is a more common form of mutation in coding DNA, which may have a range of consequences on the function of the gene; a loss of function (e.g. *p53*, *Rb*), a gain in function, often due to stabilization of the active protein (e.g. *c-erbB2*, *K-ras*) or no net functional effect. Since an amino acid may be encoded by different codons with a 'third base wobble' (e.g. GUA, GAC, GUG and GUU all encode valine), a substitution of the third base would result in no change to the amino acid. This is known as a silent substitution. At the other extreme is the nonsense mutation, whereby base substitution results in a stop codon which leads to truncation of the polypeptide and a dramatic reduction in function.

Loss of function in the presence of a normal (wildtype) allele may occur as a result of transcription silencing. The methylation status of CpG islands surrounding the promoter regions of genes determines whether a particular gene is expressed within a cell such that methylation of a CpG island 'switches off' the gene that it is regulating. CpG islands regulating housekeeping genes (i.e. genes encoding proteins essential for cell survival) are unmethylated in all cell types whereas those regulating cell-specific genes (e.g. muscle-specific actin gene in muscle cells), are only unmethylated in the relevant cell. Many tumour suppressor genes (e.g. *CDKN2A* (p16^{INK4A}), *APC*, *RASSF1A*) are now recognized to be inactivated by hypermethylation of the promoter region in malignant tumours.

Gene sequencing

Recently a variety of next generation sequencing methods have been applied to the field. One method is to construct a library of DNA fragments and to use biotinylated RNA baits to capture the exomic sequences using streptavidin coated magnetic beads prior to loading them onto the sequencing machine following digestion of the RNA bait and a few cycles of PCR. This strategy was able to obtain 10 or more sequencing reads for over 90% of the targeted bases and this approach and similar strategies have revealed the mutational landscape of head and neck squamous cell carcinoma, including the frequent mutation of the *NOTCH1* gene, which had not been identified previously.[22–24]

Proteomics and metabolomics

As the Human Genome Mapping Project powers its way towards a high-resolution sequence of the entire genome, the natural progression of research has been towards the elucidation of the repertoire of proteins that control cell signalling and cell growth. Proteomics is the profiling of proteins in cells and serum by two-dimensional gel analysis separating proteins by charge and mass, by X-ray crystallography and by mass spectrometry.[25] Proteomics has the ability to identify post-translational modifications, some of which are cancer cell-specific, which would not be detected by genetic or expression profiling. The power of this approach is particularly evident in cancer studies as it has the ability to compare the entire protein pattern of tumour tissue and normal tissue in a manner analogous to comparative genomic hybridization.

However, the functional consequences of changes to the proteome, especially some enzymes, can only be inferred and a more direct approach is to measure the levels of small molecules, or metabolites. Metabolomics is the global analysis of metabolites but is a relatively new discipline and no single technique is suitable for the analysis of all different types of molecule. Therefore, a mixture of techniques such as gas chromatography, high-pressure liquid chromatography and capillary electrophoresis are used to separate metabolites and the molecules are then identified using methods such as mass spectrometry. Metabolomics has already been applied to the detection of oral cancer in saliva[26] and serum.[27]

Telomerase

Aberration of telomere biology has a now well-recognized role to play in cancer development. The length of the telomere is maintained in germline cells by the enzyme telomerase that is absent in normal somatic cells.[28] This observation led to the theory that progressive shortening of telomeres with each cell division leads to cell senescence and ageing of the organism. Several mechanisms for this have been proposed. A critical shortening of the telomere may leave a non-telomere-free DNA end that signals cell cycle arrest. Telomere loss could also extend to the deletion or inactivation of genes located subtelomerically, again leading to cell cycle arrest. Two important consequences of critical telomere shortening in cells that survive the cell crisis are genomic rearrangements and chromosomal loss, which may in turn lead to malignant transformation. This is particularly relevant to rapidly dividing and regenerating tissues, such as skin and mucosa. Paradoxically, while some of these survivors will subsequently go into cell cycle arrest due to critical telomere length shortening, a proportion will then express telomerase activity. Such activity is capable of cell immortalization by maintaining telomere length indefinitely and its role in cancer is now unquestionable. Telomerase activity has been demonstrated in 80% of oral cancers and around 50% of oral leukoplakia lesions.[29] Even among premalignant lesions, telomerase activity was associated with degree of dysplasia, suggesting that telomerase activation occurs during the late stage of oral premalignancy. The potential for anti-telomerase drugs as a novel treatment remains promising, especially as they are now thought to target cancer stem cells.[30]

> **KEY POINTS**
>
> - Practical techniques based on loss of heterozygosity of tumour DNA are based on Knudson's two-hit hypothesis, which states that two genetic events are required to inactivate the gene that prevents the development of a condition.
> - The number of microsatellite repeats (i.e. non-coding base pairs dispersed throughout the genome) may differ between two alleles in the same person making that person heterozygous for that particular allele. If tumour DNA from such a subject when amplified by PCR yields only one product, the tumour is said to show loss of heterozygosity implying allelic loss.
> - Inactivation of genes can occur by:
>   – allelic deletion
>   – genetic mutation
>   – transcriptional silencing
>   – conversion of protooncogene to oncogene due to gene amplification.
> - Some mutations do not result in change of function. They can be silent or nonsense mutations.
> - Next generation sequencing has produced a mutational landscape of head and neck cancer.
> - Proteomics refers to the profiling of proteins in cells and serum by 2D gel analysis, X-ray crystallography and by examination of protein interactions. This can be used to identify post-translational modifications, some of which are cancer cell specific and are not detected by genetic profiling.
> - Metabolomics can be used to detect small molecules accumulating in the tissues and body fluids of oral cancer patients.
> - Critical telomere shortening or inefficient telomere DNA repair can lead to both cell cycle arrest and cell immortalization due to expression of telomerase, which, for example, has been demonstrated in 80% of oral cancers.

MAPPING AND IDENTIFICATION OF GENES ASSOCIATED WITH DISEASE

The traditional approach to understanding the molecular biology of disease was to look for and characterize the abnormal protein. Diabetes mellitus and sickle cell anaemia are two conditions that were elucidated at the molecular level in this way. Finding the protein when present in minute quantities, in an inaccessible site such as the inner ear, or when nothing is known of its mode of action, is, however, virtually impossible. This is the case with most of the genes involved in cellular growth control and also in inner ear function. Our approach to understanding such conditions relies on determining the chromosomal location, isolating and sequencing the gene so that the structure of the protein can be determined. This is known as the reverse genetic or positional cloning technique.

Strategies employed in determining the sites of these disease genes include cytogenetic analysis, molecular genetic analysis (typically LOH studies) and linkage analysis. Where a clearcut inheritance of a disease can be demonstrated, then linkage analysis can be useful in determining the location of the responsible gene. The key advance that has made this approach increasingly successful has been the construction of a high-resolution linkage map of the entire human genome. This map consists of genetic markers spaced less than 1 centimorgan apart and the process of linkage involves determining which of these the disease gene is close to. Analysis of the coinheritance of the genetic marker and the disease trait in families allows one to determine the probability of their physical proximity or linkage to each other. The statistical probability of linkage is expressed in terms of LOD scores. LOD is short for logarithm to the base 10 of the odds that the markers are linked at a recombination distance of N centimorgans. An LOD score of 3.0 favours linkage while a score of −2.0 effectively rules out linkage.

Successful linkage analysis typically requires large pedigrees with many individuals known to have the disease trait and likewise many confirmed to be free of the disease. The process involves initial family analysis with clinical evaluation and accurate diagnosis. DNA samples are then obtained from each individual and genotyping and linkage analysis can then be carried out. Linkage and molecular deletion analysis generate genetic markers either side of the disease gene location. These genetic markers can be used to identify 'chunks of genomic DNA' cloned into yeast (yeast artificial chromosomes (YAC)) or bacteria (bacterial artificial chromosomes/P1 artificial chromosomes (BAC/PAC)) and organized into libraries. By a number of methods, these 'chunks' of genomic DNA can be directionally organized to produce a physical map of the region of interest from which candidate disease genes can be identified. The Human Genome Mapping Project has, to a great extent, physically mapped the human genome such that in some cases, when the region of interest is sufficiently small, all genes known to be between the markers can be considered positional candidates. The candidates are then analysed in disease families until one is found that demonstrates mutations in affected individuals.

To facilitate the identification of the disease gene from a number of candidates within a particular region, several strategies are available. One such approach exploits our knowledge of animal models of the diseases that parallel human inherited disorders. Another potential source of candidate genes is to identify and characterize genes that are expressed within a particular tissue. Genes expressed within the cochlea, for example, represent the genes critical for cochlear function and thus are excellent candidate genes for hereditary hearing loss.

FUTURE RESEARCH

Although giant strides have already been made in the delineation of molecular events underlying disease processes, the knowledge of these events is far from comprehensive. A clearly identifiable adenoma–carcinoma sequence facilitated the correlation between genetic and histopathological progression models in colorectal cancer.[19] Several similar progression models have been proposed in head and neck squamous cell carcinoma evolution from epithelial dysplasia through to frank carcinoma, but the heterogeneity of carcinomas in different subsites precludes a molecular genetic progression model of equal rigour to that in colorectal cancer. Nevertheless, p16 and p53 inactivation have been identified as the two most frequent and critical events in head and neck carcinogenesis. An understanding of the sequence of genetic aberrations that occur in pathogenesis of tumours can assist in the prediction of progression from premalignant conditions to frank malignancy. An example of this is seen in the accumulation of genetic abnormalities in oral epithelium leading to the progression of oral dysplasia to oral squamous cell carcinoma. By analysing for loss of heterozygosity at 19 microsatellite loci in a series of oral dysplastic lesions and oral malignancies, Rosin et al.[31] showed that LOH at 3p and/or 9p occurred in virtually all cases of oral dysplasia which progressed to frank malignancy implying a 'gatekeeper' role of genes at those loci in the development of oral cancer, in themselves imparting a 3.8-fold increased relative risk of progression to squamous carcinoma. Furthermore, additional LOH at 4q, 8p, 11q or 17p imparted a 33-fold increased relative risk for developing cancer.[31] In certain cases, molecular genetic profiling has added a new dimension to age-old debates. For example, discordant genetic anomalies in inverted sinonasal papillomas and sinonasal carcinomas lend weight to the opinion that the former does not undergo malignant degeneration into the latter.[32]

Traditional methods of allelotyping and mutational analysis remain extremely time-consuming and labour-intensive. Recent years have seen the development of gene arrays (or 'gene chips') that allow the rapid assessment of the genetic profile of tumours or cell lines.[33] cDNA of up to 30 000 genes can be placed in arrays on glass slides on to which DNA and RNA samples can be allowed to hybridize using an automated two-colour fluorescence method for detection.[34] Hybridization with DNA can yield extensive genomic information, while hybridization with RNA takes genetic profiling a step further by semiquantitatively analysing the expression of genes rather than simply the presence or absence of the DNA. As the genetic aberrations and pathways associated with specific tumour development become better dissected, 'designer' chips can be produced that allow for screening for known mutations of those involved genes.[35] Array technology has also been married with molecular cytogenetics to produce array-based comparative genomic hybridization, which obviates the need for metaphase chromosome spreads for CGH.

The clinician might be forgiven for an expression of cynicism regarding the 'molecular revolution', feeling that little has changed despite ambitious predictions. The translation of molecular biology research into clinical practice – 'from laboratory to bedside' – is without doubt the greatest challenge facing the clinician scientist. Progress so far has been largely at the level of disease classification, premorbid diagnosis and patient counselling. However, several discrete arms to translational research have hinted at the future role of genetic analysis determining the likely effectiveness of existing anti-cancer treatments. There are also isolated examples of effective novel therapeutic interventions.

Molecular analysis played a vital role in differentiating neurofibromatosis type I from neurofibromatosis type II, and it now seems difficult to understand how we ever confused the two in the first place. Such clarity of diagnosis is also anticipated for many syndromic and non-syndromic causes of sensorineural hearing loss as the genes are characterized and the clinical features analysed in more detail. This may enable clinicians to determine in which cases hearing loss will be progressive and target monitoring more appropriately. Diagnostic genetic testing will also become increasingly available to families with hereditary hearing loss and clinicians will need to be conversant with the ethical issues of testing and the implications of the results. By characterizing hearing loss at the molecular level we are also developing a greater understanding of inner ear physiology as the critical proteins involved in hearing become elucidated. This may lead to the development of agents able to repair and regenerate the diseased inner ear. The administration of these agents is already being evaluated using miniature infusion pumps.

It is hoped that in the future molecular characterization of tumour tissue will provide for a more accurate diagnosis and prognosis than conventional histopathological analysis. This may lead to a more rational treatment plan based on molecular features. Some genotype–phenotype correlations have already been made, particularly with respect to radio- and chemoresistance in tumours, but confirmation is needed with larger sample sizes as to their applicability into clinical practice. Refinement of the staging of tumours by probing of resection margins and the detection of histological subclinical metastatic disease in regional lymph nodes have been elegantly demonstrated by Brennan et al.[36] at Johns Hopkins. However, the technical complexity of the methodology has precluded its widespread application in the clinical arena. The development of technically simpler but equally sensitive techniques will inevitably render molecular staging routine in oncological practice. Although surveillance for tumour recurrence is less of a problem in the upper aerodigestive tract when compared with intra-abdominal malignancies, the emergence of molecular markers in saliva and serum will have a role in follow-up protocols for head and neck cancers.[37]

A comprehensive understanding of the molecular mechanisms underlying disease processes gives the potential of therapeutic restoration of DNA or protein function, as well as exploitation of the genetic abnormality for targeting of therapy. An example of the latter is the use of ONYX-015. ONYX-015 is an E1B 55-kDa gene-deleted adenovirus engineered to selectively replicate in and lyse p53-deficient cells while sparing normal cells. This tumour-targeting property has led to a successful phase II trial of concomitant ONYX-015 and cisplatin/5-FU in the treatment of recurrent HNSCC, which indicated substantial objective responses as well as a high proportion of complete responses.[38] Post-treatment biopsies of tumour masses confirmed the replication selectivity of the virus *in vivo*.

A consideration of some of the landmarks in molecular biology (e.g. enzymatic DNA cleavage (1970) and PCR (1987)) readily indicates that molecular biology is a relatively young science. However, the rapid development of molecular techniques of such power and diversity as comparative genomic hybridization and gene array technology has permitted the dissection of molecular pathways and the identification of their disruption in disease processes. Some of these processes in specific diseases will be discussed in subsequent chapters. The future in the laboratory lies in the extension of our understanding of these molecular processes and the future in the clinic lies in the exploitation of these molecular techniques in better informing disease classification, staging and treatment:

- Development of a molecular genetic progression model for head and neck squamous cell carcinoma of similar rigour to that for colorectal carcinoma.
- Development of gene arrays or gene chips that allow the rapid assessment of the genetic profile of tumours and can allow semiquantitative analysis of gene expression.
- Designer chips may be produced that allow for screening for unknown mutations of involved genes.
- Potential role for genetic analysis in determining the likely effectiveness of existing anti-cancer treatments.
- Providing more accurate diagnosis and prognosis than conventional histopathological techniques.
- Potential therapeutic restoration of DNA or protein function, as well as exploitation of a genetic abnormality for targeting therapy (e.g. use of ONYX-015).

KEY POINTS

- Strategies employed in determining the sites of disease genes that code for the abnormal proteins include cytogenetic, molecular genetic and linkage analysis.
- Whilst genomics and other omics has generated a large body of data, cancers are complicated tissues. Future research may shift towards understanding the cancer environment and how perhaps to target this in future therapeutic strategies.

REFERENCES

1. Hampson K, Bourn D. Principles of molecular genetics. *J Laryngol Otol* 1998; 112(2): 128–31.
2. Cruickshanks HA, Adams PD. Chromatin: a molecular interface between cancer and aging. *Curr Opin Genet Dev* 2011; 21(1): 100–06.
3. Schwartz YB, Pirrotta V. A new world of polycombs: unexpected partnerships and emerging functions. *Nat Rev Genet* 2013; 14(12): 853–64.
4. Sharp PA. Splicing of messenger RNA precursors. *Science* 1987; 235(4790): 766–71.
5. McKeown M. Alternative mRNA splicing. *Annu Rev Cell Biol* 1992; 8: 133–55.
6. Wu BH, Xiong XP, Jia J, Zhang WF. MicroRNAs: new actors in the oral cancer scene. *Oral Oncol* 2011; 47(5): 314–19.
7. Bentwich I, Avniel A, Karov Y, et al. Identification of hundreds of conserved and nonconserved human microRNAs. *Nat Genet* 2005; 37(7): 766–70.
8. Park NJ, Zhou H, Elashoff D, et al. Salivary microRNA: discovery, characterization, and clinical utility for oral cancer detection. *Clin Cancer Res* 2009; 15(17): 5473–77.
9. Perez P, Jang SI, Alevizos I. Emerging landscape of non-coding RNAs in oral health and disease. *Oral Dis* 2014; 20(3): 226–35.
10. Broomfield A, Bourn D. Basic techniques in molecular genetics. *J Laryngol Otol* 1998; 112(3): 230–34.
11. Speicher MR, Gwyn Ballard S, Ward DC. Karyotyping human chromosomes by combinatorial multi-fluor FISH. *Nat Genet* 1996; 12(4): 368–75.
12. Kallioniemi A, Kallioniemi OP, Sudar D, et al. Comparative genomic hybridization for molecular cytogenetic analysis of solid tumors. *Science* 1992; 258(5083): 818–21.
13. Mullis KB, Faloona FA. Specific synthesis of DNA in vitro via a polymerase-catalyzed chain reaction. *Methods Enzymol* 1987; 155: 335–50.
14. Lawyer FC, Stoffel S, Saiki RK, et al. Isolation, characterization, and expression in Escherichia coli of the DNA polymerase gene from Thermus aquaticus. *J Biol Chem* 1989; 264(11): 6427–37.
15. Emmert-Buck MR, Bonner RF, Smith PD, et al. Laser capture microdissection. *Science* 1996; 274(5289): 998–1001.
16. Knudson Jr AG. Mutation and cancer: statistical study of retinoblastoma. *Proc Natl Acad Sci USA* 1971; 68(4): 820–23.
17. Cavenee WK, Dryja TP, Phillips RA, et al. Expression of recessive alleles by chromosomal mechanisms in retinoblastoma. *Nature* 1983; 305(5937): 779–84.
18. Merlo A, Herman JG, Mao L, et al. 5' CpG island methylation is associated with transcriptional silencing of the tumour suppressor p16/CDKN2/MTS1 in human cancers. *Nat Med* 1995; 1(7): 686–92.
19. Vogelstein B, Fearon ER, Kern SE, et al. Allelotype of colorectal carcinomas. *Science* 1989; 244(4901): 207–11.
20. Ah-See KW, Cooke TG, Pickford IR, et al. An allelotype of squamous carcinoma of the head and neck using microsatellite markers. *Cancer Res* 1994; 54(7): 1617–21.
21. Nawroz H, van der Riet P, Hruban RH, et al. Allelotype of head and neck squamous cell carcinoma. *Cancer Res* 1994; 54(5): 1152–55.
22. India Project Team of the International Cancer Genome Consortium. Mutational landscape of gingivo-buccal oral squamous cell carcinoma reveals new recurrently-mutated genes and molecular subgroups. *Nat Commun* 2013; 4: 2873.
23. Agrawal N, Frederick MJ, Pickering CR, et al. Exome sequencing of head and neck squamous cell carcinoma reveals inactivating mutations in NOTCH1. *Science* 2011; 333(6046): 1154–57.
24. Stransky N, Egloff AM, Tward AD, et al. The mutational landscape of head and neck squamous cell carcinoma. *Science* 2011; 333(6046): 1157–60.
25. Pandey A, Mann M. Proteomics to study genes and genomes. *Nature* 2000; 405(6788): 837–46.
26. Sugimoto M, Wong DT, Hirayama A, et al. Capillary electrophoresis mass spectrometry-based saliva metabolomics identified oral, breast and pancreatic cancer-specific profiles. *Metabolomics* 2010; 6(1): 78–95.
27. Tiziani S, Lopes V, Gunther UL. Early stage diagnosis of oral cancer using 1H NMR-based metabolomics. *Neoplasia* 2009; 11(3): 269–76, 4p following.
28. Greider CW. Telomeres, telomerase and senescence. *Bioessays* 1990; 12(8): 363–69.
29. Mutirangura A, Supiyaphun P, Trirekapan S, et al. Telomerase activity in oral leukoplakia and head and neck squamous cell carcinoma. *Cancer Res* 1996; 56(15): 3530–33.
30. Joseph I, Tressler R, Bassett E, et al. The telomerase inhibitor imetelstat depletes cancer stem cells in breast and pancreatic cancer cell lines. *Cancer Res* 2010; 70(22): 9494–504.
31. Rosin MP, Cheng X, Poh C, et al. Use of allelic loss to predict malignant risk for low-grade oral epithelial dysplasia. *Clin Cancer Res* 2000; 6(2): 357–62.
32. Califano J, Koch W, Sidransky D, Westra WH. Inverted sinonasal papilloma: a molecular genetic appraisal of its putative status as a precursor to squamous cell carcinoma. *Am J Pathol* 2000; 156(1): 333–37.

33. Lakhani SR, Ashworth A. Microarray and histopathological analysis of tumours: the future and the past? *Nat Rev Cancer* 2001; **1**(2): 151–57.
34. Schena M, Shalon D, Davis RW, Brown PO. Quantitative monitoring of gene expression patterns with a complementary DNA microarray. *Science* 1995; **270**(5235): 467–70.
35. Perou CM, Sorlie T, Eisen MB, et al. Molecular portraits of human breast tumours. *Nature* 2000; **406**(6797): 747–52.
36. Brennan JA, Mao L, Hruban RH, et al. Molecular assessment of histopathological staging in squamous-cell carcinoma of the head and neck. *N Engl J Med* 1995; **332**(7): 429–35.
37. Boyle JO, Mao L, Brennan JA, et al. Gene mutations in saliva as molecular markers for head and neck squamous cell carcinomas. *Am J Surg* 1994; **168**(5): 429–32.
38. Khuri FR, Nemunaitis J, Ganly I, et al. A controlled trial of intratumoral ONYX-015, a selectively-replicating adenovirus, in combination with cisplatin and 5-fluorouracil in patients with recurrent head and neck cancer. *Nat Med* 2000; **6**(8): 879–85.

FURTHER READING

Alberts B, Johnson A, Lewis J, et al. *Molecular biology of the cell*. 4th ed. Oxford: Garland Science; 2002.

Latchman D (ed.). *Basic molecular and cell biology*. 3rd ed. London: BMJ Publishing Group; 1997.

Primrose SB, Twyman RM, Old RW. *Principles of gene manipulation*. 6th ed. Oxford: Blackwell Science; 2002.

Strachan T, Read AP. *Human molecular genetics*. 2nd ed. Oxford: BIOS Scientific Publishers; 2001.

CHAPTER 2

GENETICS IN OTOLOGY AND NEUROTOLOGY

Mohammed-Iqbal Syed

Introduction 15	Genetics of neurofibromatosis type 2 21
Molecular genetics of hearing loss 15	Genetics of familial paragangliomas 22
Molecular genetics of non-syndromic hearing impairment (NSHI) ... 16	References 25

SEARCH STRATEGY
Data in this chapter may be updated by a Medline search using a variety of relevant generic keywords, including: DNA, genetics, hereditary hearing loss, connexin 26, neurofibromatosis 2 and familial paragangliomas.

INTRODUCTION

Advances in molecular genetics have helped to identify causative genes and proteins responsible for pathologies; this knowledge is pertinent to molecular target therapy and promises novel therapeutic interventions.

This chapter aims to review the mechanisms and principles of molecular genetics of hearing impairment, vestibular schwannoma, and glomus tumours, and will keep the reader abreast of new developments that may be relevant to identifying and treating these diseases in clinical practice.

MOLECULAR GENETICS OF HEARING LOSS

Hearing loss is the most frequent sensory impairment in humans, with significant social and psychological implications. Permanent childhood hearing impairment of a moderate or greater degree (i.e. detection thresholds 40 decibels hearing level averaged across 0.5, 1, 2 and 4 kHz) is present at birth in about 1.6 per 1000 live births, of which approximately 1.0 in 1000 are bilateral impairments and 0.6 in 1000 are unilateral impairments.[1,2] However, studies have shown that the prevalence of permanent childhood hearing impairment continues to increase through infancy, and by the school entry hearing screen (4–5 years of age) possibly affects 3.5 per 1000 children.[2] It is estimated that at least two thirds of cases of childhood-onset hearing loss have a genetic cause, with the remaining third caused by environmental factors (e.g. cytomegalovirus infection, meningitis, acquired conductive loss, and the impact of extracorporeal membrane oxygenation (ECMO)).[3] Improved clinical knowledge, awareness, and advances in antibiotics and vaccines has led to a decline in hearing loss resulting from environmental factors. Likewise, significant progress in the genetics of hereditary hearing impairment (HHI) has improved our understanding of the causes and early detection of HHI.

Classification

The most useful distinction in hereditary hearing impairment (HHI) is syndromic versus non-syndromic. When SNHL occurs in isolation it is termed non-syndromic and when it is accompanied by other systemic disturbances it is termed syndromic. The majority of hearing impairments are non-syndromic (~70%), whereas a minority are syndromic (~30%).

Non-syndromic HHI is further classified by mode of inheritance:

- Autosomal recessive ~80%
- Autosomal dominant ~18%.[4]

Rare modes of transmission include X-linked and mitochondrial transmission, which account for the remaining 2% of hearing impairment.

MOLECULAR GENETICS OF NON-SYNDROMIC HEARING IMPAIRMENT (NSHI)

Thus far, more than 100 forms of non-syndromic hearing impairment (NSHI) have been discovered (see the Hereditary Hearing Loss website at http://hereditaryhearingloss.org). Most of these are still identified as loci: only the chromosomal location of the defective gene is known.

The different gene loci for non-syndromic deafness are designated DFN (for DeaFNess). Loci are named based on mode of inheritance:

- DFNA: Autosomal dominant
- DFNB: Autosomal recessive
- DFNX: X-linked.

The number following the above designations reflects the order of gene mapping and/or discovery and this information is regularly updated on the Hereditary Hearing Loss website.

Genes for NSHI have been categorized by the function of the proteins each gene encodes. Several superfamilies are represented, including gap junctions, myosins, adhesion proteins and ion channels.

Unlike in some conditions where a common mutation in just one gene is responsible for the majority of cases (e.g. the deltaF508 deletion of three nucleotides in the *CFTR* gene in cystic fibrosis), hearing loss is genetically very heterogeneous involving mutations in many genes.[5] It is therefore not possible to predict the risk of developing hearing loss from assessing a single or even a selection of the genes that have currently been identified.[6]

The most frequent causative genes are discussed below.

Gap junction proteins

Thus far, three connexin genes have been implicated in NSHI: *CX26*, *CX30*, and *CX31*, corresponding to the proteins connexin 26, connexin 30, and connexin 31, which are designated by their molecular mass.

GJB2 (connexin 26) is by far the foremost prominent hearing impairment gene. The discovery that *GJB2*, located at the DFNB1 locus, is a causative gene for hearing impairment[7] led to the unexpected revelation that more than half of the recessive NSHL and approximately 30% to 50% of innate hearing loss are due to *GJB2* mutations.[7, 8] Among the 300 mutations documented worldwide up to now (see The Human Gene Mutation Database at www.hgmd.org), one particular mutation, 35delG, is responsible for 70% of all the *GJB2* mutations.[9] This finding made an enormous impact in the hearing loss field, as it facilitated diagnostic and genetic screening of NSHL patients. Another mutation imperative to note is 167delT, which is most frequent among Ashkenazi Jews and is also present in Palestinians.[10]

The connexion-deafness homepage (http://davinci.crg.es/deafness/) provides a database of all published mutations as well as common polymorphisms in *GJB2* and other connexin genes. More than 100 unique non-syndromic *GJB2* gene variants have already been described. The reported mutations mostly include mutation types that can be detected by sequencing analysis, such as nonsense, missense, splicing and frameshift mutations.

Myosins

Numerous types of unconventional myosins have been identified as NSHI causing genes: *MYO1A*, *MYO3A*, *MYO6*, *MYO7A* and *MYO15A* (encoding myosin I, myosin IIIA, myosin VI, myosin VIIA and myosin XVA proteins, respectively). The term 'unconventional' myosins refers to all non-muscle myosin subclasses (in contrast with the 'conventional' myosins that include only the myosin II subclass). Expression of these unconventional myosins is not limited to the cells and tissues of the inner ear, yet the expression of their dysfunction is largely restricted to hearing impairment.

The myosin VI protein was first implicated in the hearing mechanism when it was found to be mutated in the spontaneously deaf mouse Snell's *waltzer* (*sv*).[11] The role of myosin VI in human deafness remains to be determined.

Myosin VII has been linked to both rodent and human deafness. Mutations in the *MYO7A* human homologue were identified as the genetic cause for Usher syndrome type 1B[12] and Usher syndrome type 2A.[13] Contiguous to this discovery, human *MYO7A* was also linked to NSHL in two distinctive loci: DFNB2[14] and DFNA11.[15]

Myosin XV is the largest of all the myosin heavy chains and mutations in myosin XV have been pathogenically linked to DFNB3 in humans and shaker 2 phenotype in mice. Myosin XV is a critical factor in the evolvement of the hair bundle and in the staircase formation of the bundle[16] and it binds another deafness molecule, whirling at the tip link zone, suggesting that the two molecules might control stereocilia elongation patterning during development and may be implicated in stabilizing connections between stereocilia.[17]

Pendrin

Mutations in the pendrin gene *SLC26A4* are the second most frequent cause of autosomal recessive NSHI, accounting for up to 3.5% of cases.[18] *SLC26A4*, which codes for an anion transport protein, also underlies Pendred syndrome, which is one of the most common forms of syndromic hearing impairment.

Adhesion proteins

Adhesion proteins include a diverse group of distinct protein families including integrins, selectins, members of the immunoglobulin superclass family and cadherins.

Cadherin 23 is a vital member of a specific unit designated for maintaining stereocilia inter-cohesion.[18]

More than 20 mutations in the *CDH23* gene have been identified in people with non-syndromic hearing impairment and more than 30 mutations have been shown to cause the Usher syndrome type 1D. The *USH1D* locus was found to coincide with the recessive NSHI locus *DFNB12*, which is associated with prelingual moderate to profound hearing loss. These data suggested that *DFNB12* and *USH1D* in fact are mutually derived from *CDH23* allelic mutations, both resulting in syndromic and non-syndromic forms of hearing loss.[19, 20]

Autosomal dominant non-syndromic hearing impairment

Unlike autosomal recessive non-syndromic hearing loss, in autosomal dominant non-syndromic hearing loss there is not a single identifiable gene responsible for the majority of cases. The clinical manifestations and molecular genetics of known genes causing autosomal dominant non-syndromic hearing impairment are outlined in **Table 2.1**.

Autosomal recessive non-syndromic hearing impairment

Fifty per cent of people with autosomal recessive non-syndromic hearing impairment have mutations in *GJB2*.[8] The other 50% of cases are attributed to mutations in numerous other genes. The clinical manifestations and molecular genetics of known genes causing autosomal recessive non-syndromic hearing impairment are outlined in **Table 2.2**.

X-linked non-syndromic hearing impairment

DFNX3 is characterized by a mixed conductive-sensorineural hearing loss, the conductive component of

TABLE 2.1 Clinical manifestations and molecular genetics of known genes causing autosomal dominant non-syndromic hearing impairment

Locus name	Gene symbol	Onset/Decade	Audioprofile	Test availability
DFNA1	DIAPH1	Postlingual/1st	Low frequency progressive	Clinical
DFNA2	KCNQ4	Postlingual/2nd	High frequency progressive	Clinical
DFNA2B	GJB3	Postlingual/4th	High frequency progressive	Clinical
DFNA3	GJB2	Prelingual	High frequency progressive	Clinical
	GJB6			Clinical
DFNA4	MYH14	Postlingual	Flat/gently downsloping	Clinical
DFNA5	DFNA5	Postlingual/1st	High frequency progressive	Clinical
DFNA6/14/38	WFS1	Prelingual	Low frequency progressive	Clinical
DFNA8/12	TECTA		Mid-frequency loss	Clinical
DFNA9	COCH	Postlingual/2nd	High frequency progressive	Clinical
DFNA10	EYA4	Postlingual/3rd, 4th	Flat/gently downsloping	Clinical
DFNA11	MYO7A	Postlingual/1st		Clinical
DFNA13	COL11A2	Postlingual/2nd	Mid-frequency loss	Clinical
DFNA15	POU4F3	Postlingual	High frequency progressive	Clinical
DFNA17	MYH9	Postlingual	High frequency progressive	Clinical
DFNA20/26	ACTG1	Postlingual	High frequency progressive	Clinical
DFNA22	MYO6	Postlingual	High frequency progressive	Clinical
DFNA23	SIX1	Prelingual	Downsloping	Clinical
DFNA25	SLC17A8	Postlingual/2nd–6th decades	High frequency progressive	Clinical
DFNA28	TFCP2L3	Postlingual	Flat/gently downsloping	Clinical
DFNA36	TMC1	Postlingual	Flat/gently downsloping	Clinical
DFNA39	DSPP	Postlingual	High frequency progressive	Research only
DFNA44	CCDC50	Postlingual	Low to mid frequencies progressive	Clinical
DFNA48	MYO1A	Postlingual	Progressive	Clinical
DFNA50	MIR96	Postlingual/2nd	Flat progressive	Clinical
DFNA51	TJP2 & FAM189A2	Postlingual/4th	High frequency progressive	Research only

Source: Adapted from Van Camp & Smith [2010] Van Camp G, Smith RJH. The Hereditary Hearing Loss Homepage, 2010, with permission. Available from http://hereditaryhearingloss.org/.

TABLE 2.2 Clinical manifestations and molecular genetics of known genes causing autosomal recessive non-syndromic hearing impairment

Locus name	Gene symbol	Onset	Type	Test availability
DFNB1	GJB2	Prelingual	Usually stable	Clinical
	GJB6			Clinical
DFNB2	MYO7A	Prelingual, postlingual	Unspecified	Clinical
DFNB3	MYO15	Prelingual	Severe to profound; stable	Clinical
DFNB4	SLC26A4	Prelingual, postlingual	Stable, progressive	Clinical
DFNB6	TMIE	Prelingual	Severe to profound; stable	Clinical
DFNB7/11	TMC1			Clinical
DFNB8/10	TMPRSS3	Postlingual, prelingual	Progressive, stable	Clinical
DFNB9	OTOF	Prelingual	Usually severe to profound; stable	Clinical
DFNB12	CDH23	Prelingual	Severe to profound; stable	Clinical
DFNB16	STRC	Prelingual	Severe to profound; stable	Clinical
DFNB18	USH1C	Prelingual	Severe to profound; stable	Clinical
DFNB21	TECTA	Prelingual	Severe to profound; stable	Clinical
DFNB22	OTOA	Prelingual	Severe to profound; stable	Clinical
DFNB23	PCDH15	Prelingual	Severe to profound; stable	Clinical
DFNB24	RDX	Prelingual	Severe to profound; stable	Clinical
DFNB25	GRXCR1	Prelingual	Moderate to profound; progressive	Research only
DFNB28	TRIOBP	Prelingual	Severe to profound; stable	Clinical
DFNB29	CLDN14	Prelingual	Severe to profound; stable	Clinical
DFNB30	MYO3A	Prelingual	Severe to profound; stable	Clinical
DFNB31	DFNB31	Prelingual	—	Clinical
DFNB32/82	GPSM2	Prelingual	Severe to profound; stable	Research only
DFNB35	ESRRB	Unknown	Severe to profound	Clinical
DFNB36	ESPN	Prelingual	—	Clinical
DFNB37	MYO6	Prelingual	—	Clinical
DFNB39	HGF	Prelingual	Severe to profound; downsloping	Clinical
DFNB49	MARVELD2	Prelingual	Moderate to profound; stable	Clinical
DFNB53	COL11A2	Prelingual	Severe to profound; stable	Research only
DFNB59	PJVK	Prelingual	Severe to profound; stable	Clinical
DFNB61	SLC26A5	Prelingual	Severe to profound; stable	Clinical
DFNB63	LRTOMT	Prelingual	Severe to profound; stable	Clinical
DFNB67	LHFPL5	Prelingual	Severe to profound; stable	Clinical
DFNB73	BSND	Prelingual	Severe to profound; stable	Research only
DFNB77	LOXHD1	Postlingual	Moderate to profound; progressive	Clinical
DFNB79	TPRN	Prelingual	Severe to profound; stable	Clinical
DFNB84	PTPRQ	Prelingual	Moderate to profound; progressive	Research only

Source: Adapted from Van Camp & Smith [2010] Van Camp G, Smith RJH. The Hereditary Hearing Loss Homepage, 2010, with permission. Available from http://hereditaryhearingloss.org/.

which is caused by stapedial fixation. In contrast to other types of conductive hearing loss, surgical correction is precluded because an abnormal communication between the cerebrospinal fluid and perilymph results in leakage ('perilymphatic gusher') and complete loss of hearing when the oval window is fenestrated or removed.

Clinical manifestations and molecular genetics of known genes causing X-linked non-syndromic hearing impairment are summarized in **Table 2.3**.

Mitochondrial non-syndromic hearing impairment

The genes and mutations associated with mitochondrial non-syndromic hearing impairment are outlined in **Table 2.4**.

TABLE 2.3 Clinical manifestations and molecular genetics of X-linked non-syndromic hearing impairment

Locus name	Gene	Onset	Type and degree	Frequencies
DFNX1 (DFN2)	PRPS1	Postlingual	Progressive sensorineural; severe to profound	All
DFNX2 (DFN3)	POU3F4	Prelingual	Progressive, mixed; variable, but progresses to profound	All
DFNX4 (DFN6)	SMPX	Postlingual	Progressive sensorineural; mild to profound	All

Source: Adapted from Van Camp & Smith [2010] Van Camp G, Smith RJH. The Hereditary Hearing Loss Homepage, 2010, with permission. Available from http://hereditaryhearingloss.org/.

TABLE 2.4 Mitochondrial Non-syndromic Hearing Impairment

Gene symbol	Mutation	Severity	Penetrance	Test availability
MT-RNR1	961 different mutations	Variable	Highly variable, aminoglycoside induced	Clinical
	1494C>T			
	1555A>G			
MT-TS1	7445A>G		Highly variable	Clinical
	7472insC			
	7510T>C			
	7511T			
MT-CO1	7444G>A	Severe to profound	Complete, aminoglycoside associated; associated with MT-RNR1 1555A>G	Clinical

Source: Adapted from Van Camp & Smith [2010] Van Camp G, Smith RJH. The Hereditary Hearing Loss Homepage, 2010, with permission. Available from http://hereditaryhearingloss.org/.

Molecular genetics of syndromic hearing impairment (SHI)

Hearing impairment is denoted as an integral clinical phenotype in more than 400 genetic syndromes.[21] Syndromic forms of hearing impairment are estimated to be responsible for up to 30% of prelingual deafness, but its contribution to deafness is relatively small reflecting the occurrence and diagnosis of postlingual deafness.

Syndromic hearing loss is discussed further by modes of inheritance.

Autosomal dominant syndromic hearing impairment

WAARDENBURG SYNDROME (WS)

WS is mostly a genetic autosomal dominant disorder, considered to be the most frequent autosomal dominant form of syndromic hearing loss, constituting approximately 2% of all congenital hearing impairment.[22]

The primary phenotypes observed in this syndrome may include variable degrees of sensorineural hearing loss, pigmentation abnormalities (skin, hair, eyes), dystopia canthorum (wide distance between the inner corners of the eyes). Gastrointestinal symptoms like constipation and Hirschsprung disease, neural tube and limb defects may also be observed. Four different types of WS (I to IV) have been described, grouped by distinct physical characteristics. WS I characteristically has the presence and WS II the absence of dystopia canthorum. In WS III there are typically limb abnormalities and in WS IV Hirschsprung disease is present.

All of WS1 and some of WS3 cases are associated with mutations in the PAX3 gene. WS2 is caused by mutations in the transcription factors MITF and SNAI2. WS4 is due to alterations in EDNRB, EDN3 or SOX10 genes.[23]

BRANCHIOOTORENAL SYNDROME

Branchiootorenal (BOR) syndrome is the second most prevalent autosomal dominant syndromic type of hearing loss.[24] The major features of this syndrome are hearing loss (conductive, mixed or sensorineural) in association with branchial cleft cysts or fistulae, deformities of the external, middle or internal ear, and renal malformations.

In approximately 40% of families segregating a BOR phenotype, mutations in EYA1 can be identified; in a few other families mutations have been found in SIX1[25] and SIX5.[26]

STICKLER SYNDROME

Stickler syndrome comprises of progressive sensorineural hearing loss, cleft palate, abnormal development of the epiphysis, vertebral abnormalities and osteoarthritis. Three types are recognized, based on the molecular genetic defect: STL1 (COL2A1), STL2 (COL11A1) and STL3 (COL11A2). STL1 and STL2 are characterized by severe myopia, which predisposes to retinal detachment; this aspect of the phenotype is absent in STL3 because COL11A2 is not expressed in the eye.

NEUROFIBROMATOSIS 2

The hallmark of neurofibromatosis 2 (NF2) is hearing loss caused by bilateral vestibular schwannomas. Approximately 50% of affected patients have no family history of NF2; therefore these patients represent new germ line mutations in the NF2 gene. This is discussed further in the section on NF2 in this chapter.

Autosomal recessive syndromic hearing impairment

USHER SYNDROME

Usher syndrome (USH) is the most frequent autosomal recessive syndromic form of hearing loss. More than 50% of the deaf-blind community in the USA have USH. According to the genotype and phenotype differences, USH has several subtypes:

- Type I: congenital severe-to-profound sensorineural hearing loss, vestibular dysfunction and onset of retinitis pigmentosa in the first decade of life
- Type II: mild-to-severe sensorineural hearing loss, normal vestibular function and onset of retinitis pigmentosa in the first or second decade of life
- Type III: progressive hearing loss, progressive vestibular dysfunction and onset of retinitis pigmentosa is variable.

To date 15 different loci and 12 genes have been reported (http://hereditaryhearingloss.org). One of these identified genes, *MYO7A*, encoding myosin 7A, is a unique molecular motor for hair cells.[27] Cadherin 23, an adhesion molecule, coded by *CDH23* gene may have an important role in cross linking of stereocilia.[28]

PENDRED SYNDROME

This is the second most common type of autosomal recessive syndromic hearing loss. It is usually characterized by severe congenital sensorineural hearing loss and euthyroid goitre that develops in puberty or adulthood. The deafness is also commonly associated with an abnormality of the labyrinth which may be anatomical (Mondini dysplasia or dilated vestibular aqueduct) and/or functional. Almost 50% of the families have *SLC26A4* (PDS) gene mutation on chromosome 7q21-q34. The gene is responsible for sulfate transport. Its protein product, pendrin, is involved in the transport of iodine and chloride ions. *SLC26A4* gene mutation should be investigated in the patients who have progressive hearing loss, Mondini dysplasia or large vestibular aqueduct syndrome. The same mutation can also cause DFNB4.[29]

JERVELL AND LANGE-NIELSEN SYNDROME

This is characterized by a congenital hearing loss and an elongation of the QT interval on electrocardiography. Affected individuals have episodal syncope and may have sudden death. The JLNS1 locus in the *KVLQT1* gene located on chromosome 11p15.5, or the JLNS2 locus in the *KCNE1* (IsK) gene located on chromosome 21q22.1-q22.2 are responsible for the syndrome. These are potassium channel genes.[30]

BIOTINIDASE DEFICIENCY

This condition results from a deficiency of an enzyme required for the normal cycling of the water-soluble vitamin biotin. Clinically it is characterized by a variable sensorineural hearing loss (in 75% of children), with associated neurological, ophthalmological and dermatological abnormalities. Biotinidase deficiency can be prevented with supplementation of biotin.

REFSUM DISEASE

Refsum disease is characterized by severe progressive sensorineural hearing loss and retinitis pigmentosa caused by faulty phytanic acid metabolism.

X-LINKED SYNDROMIC HEARING IMPAIRMENT: ALPORT SYNDROME

Progressive sensorineural hearing loss, renal disorder (glomerulonephritis, haematuria, renal failure) and eye problems (lenticular and macular abnormalities) are observed. Almost 50% develop progressive bilateral hearing loss, which usually begins in the second decade.[30] This syndrome is X-linked in 85%, autosomal recessive in 15% and autosomal dominant in the remainders. In the X-linked form, males are more severely affected than females. The *COL4A5* gene on Xq22 and the *COL4A3* and *COL4A4* genes on chromosome 2q36–q37 are responsible for the syndrome.[30]

Implication of discovery of genes associated with hearing loss

Why has the genetics of hearing loss become such a focus for researchers?

First, from a biological perspective, the amount of information gained about the auditory and vestibular systems has been dramatic. Second, from a diagnostic aspect, clinicians are now able to discern the aetiology of hearing loss of a large number of patients by relatively simple genetic testing. Third, from a genetic counselling aspect, genetic counsellors are able to predict with much greater certainty what the chances are of another child being born with deafness in the family. Fourth, from a therapeutic aspect, the discovery of genes may provide solutions for treatment and therapy for alleviating hearing loss.[22]

Genetics of aminoglycoside toxicity

Aminoglycoside-induced ototoxicity is a potentially preventable form of acquired hearing loss. The mitochondrial 12S rRNA is a hot spot for mutations associated with both aminoglycoside-induced and non-syndromic hearing loss. Of those, the homoplasmic 1555A>G and 1494C>T mutations at the highly conserved decoding region of the 12S rRNA have been associated with hearing loss worldwide.[31] In particular, these two mutations account for a significant number of cases of aminoglycoside ototoxicity. The 1555A>G or 1494C>T mutation is expected to form a novel 1494C–G1555 or 1494U–A1555 base-pair at the highly conserved A-site of 12S rRNA. These transitions make the human mitochondrial ribosomes more bacteria-like and alter binding sites for aminoglycosides. As a result, the exposure to aminoglycosides can induce or worsen hearing loss in individuals carrying one of these mutations.[31]

One of these mutations, 1555A>G, has also been reported in hearing-impaired patients with no history of exposure to aminoglycoside antibiotics, suggesting that in some carriers of this mutation aminoglycoside exposure is sufficient, but not necessary, for hearing loss to occur, and additional environmental and/or genetic risk factors likely exist.[32–34] One way to assess individual risk is by careful evaluation of family history. The other is DNA-based mutation detection technologies, which offer a far more precise method for identification of at-risk individuals, but the appropriateness of screening for these two mutations and the circumstances under which screening should be conducted are not yet clear and perhaps screening only high-risk populations would be a better approach. At-risk populations might be defined as those individuals with increased risk of exposure to aminoglycoside antibiotics because of some other, unrelated condition such as cystic fibrosis or an immunological dysfunction, or individuals in whom the use of aminoglycoside antibiotics is under consideration for treatment of infectious disease.

Data on the prevalence of aminoglycoside use in the population are also needed. Data from such studies will provide information about the clinical utility of testing for genetic susceptibility to aminoglycoside ototoxicity and will support discussions of screening for genetic susceptibility to aminoglycoside ototoxicity by identifying high-risk populations. Data from these types of studies will also help establish guidelines for pretest genetic counselling and informed consent of subjects.

GENETICS OF NEUROFIBROMATOSIS TYPE 2

Neurofibromatosis type 2 (NF 2) is much rarer than NF1, with an incidence estimated to be 1:25 000.[35] Disease prevalence has now risen to 1:60 000 on account of better survival and improved treatment.[36]

Neurofibromatosis type 2 is an autosomal dominant condition with the hallmark of bilateral vestibular schwannomas, but is also associated with meningiomas, ependymomas, and pre-senile cataracts. The mean age of onset of symptoms from vestibular schwannoma is estimated to be 20 years.[37] The majority of vestibular schwannomas are sporadic in occurrence and unilateral, presenting in the fifth decade. The bilateral vestibular schwannomas that occur in patients with NF2 represent 2–4% of all vestibular schwannomas[38, 39] and present in the second and third decades of life.

NF1 and NF2 are recognized as separate genetic and clinical diseases with the localization of the respective genes to chromosomes 17 and 22. The NF2 gene was localized to chromosome 22 through a genetic linkage analysis.[40] Subsequently the NF2 locus was further mapped close to the centre of the long arm of chromosome 22 (22q12).[41] In 1993 the NF2 gene was identified by Rouleau et al.[42] and Trofatter et al.[43] and since then mutations in the NF2 gene have been identified not only in NF2 related vestibular schwannomas, but also in sporadic vestibular schwannomas and meningiomas.

The NF2 gene is spread over approximately 100 000 bases (100kb) on chromosome 22q12.2 and contains 17 exons (or encoding segments). The transcribed mRNA is 1785 base pairs long and produces a protein of 595 amino acids designated as merlin or schwannoma.[42, 43]

The gene product is similar in sequence to a family of proteins including moesin, ezrin, radixin, talin and members of the protein 4.1 superfamily. These proteins are involved in linking cytoskeletal components with the plasma membrane and are located in actin rich surface projections such as microvilli, membrane ruffles, and cell contact regions. The N-terminal region of the merlin protein is thought to interact with components of the plasma membrane and the C-terminal with the cytoskeleton. While the exact function of the NF2 protein is as yet unknown, the evidence available suggests that it is involved in cell–cell or cell–matrix interactions, and that it is important for cell movement, cell shape and communication. There is considerable evidence, in both NF2 knockout mice and *in vitro* schwannoma preparations, that loss of function of the merlin protein results in a loss of contact inhibition and consequently leads to tumourigenesis.[44–46]

NF2 gene defects have been detected in other malignancies including meningiomas, malignant mesotheliomas, melanoma and breast carcinoma.

NF2 mutations and their clinical correlation

The NF2 gene has been postulated to represent a tumour suppressor gene. In approximately 50% of cases, there is no family history of NF2. Therefore, these patients represent new germline mutations in the NF2 gene. To date, more than 200 mutations of the NF2 gene have been identified, including single base substitutions, insertions and deletions.

Mutations were identified in 66% of sporadic cases of vestibular schwannomas, but only in 33% of the NF2 cases; therefore the rate of detection of a mutation in unilateral vestibular schwannomas was significantly higher than that of familial schwannomas.[47] Genotype-to-phenotype correlation studies suggest that the mutations in the NF2 gene that result in protein truncation are associated with a more severe clinical presentation of NF2 (Wishart type) – larger, multiple, faster growing tumours – while missense and splice site mutations are associated with a milder form of the disease (Gardner type) – smaller, few and slow growing tumours. However, this has not been held true in other studies, which showed that some missense mutations associated with a severe phenotype.[47]

Given the heterogeneity of clinical response to various types of mutations, no clear genotype-to-phenotype correlation has been established, and this is further evidenced by the fact that phenotypic variability within the NF2 families with the same mutation has been seen.[48]

Although mutations in the NF2 gene play a dominant role in the biology of vestibular schwannomas, they are not uniformly identified in patients with vestibular schwannomas, which suggests that other genetic loci may contribute to the genesis of vestibular schwannomas and ultimately phenotype of the affected individuals.[49,50]

Genetic testing and antenatal diagnosis

As detection of tumours at an early stage is effective in improving the clinical management of NF2, pre-symptomatic genetic testing is now an integral part of the management of NF2 families.

Once a mutation has been identified in an affected individual, a 100% specific test is available for the family; however, mutation screening may not reveal causative mutation. Predictive diagnosis by linkage analysis using intragenic markers or markers flanking the NF2 gene is also possible in the great majority of families with two or more living affected individuals.[51]

Tumour analysis plays a vital role in providing genetic testing for the offspring of sporadic patients. Indeed analysis should if possible first be carried out on the tumour so that a targeted approach can be used on the blood sample.[51] If both mutational events are identified in the NF2 gene in a tumour and neither is present in the blood the patient must be mosaic for one of these mutations.[52,53] Even if only LOH is identified this still allows exclusion of NF2 in 50% of offspring if they can be shown to have inherited the allele 'lost' in the tumour.[52,53] At-risk individuals who are shown not to have inherited the mutated NF2 gene do not need further follow-up.

Molecular pathophysiology – a link to drug therapy

Recent work on the mechanisms by which the loss of Merlin in the setting of NF2 influences vestibular schwannoma proliferation, has been translated into clinical trials and we are not far away from approved drug therapy for NF2 associated vestibular schwannomas.

The mammalian target of rapamycin (mTOR) is a tyrosine kinase that serves as a hub in the intracellular communication cascade integrating signals from multiple upstream pathways as well as the local intracellular environment. It belongs to two complexes: mTORC1 and mTORC2. mTORC1 is constitutively activated in Merlin-deficient schwannomas.[54] mTORC1 activation in turn leads to phosphorylation of ribosomal S6 kinase (S6K) and the eukaryotic initiation factor 4E binding protein-1 (4EBP-1), ultimately increasing translation, protein production, and cell growth.[55] Subsequent studies have shown decreased phosphorylation of downstream targets with mTOR inhibitors such as rapamycin. This and recent supporting preclinical animal data suggesting mTOR inhibition influences vestibular schwannomas cell proliferation have led to three ongoing clinical trials testing everolimus in patients with radiographic progression of NF2-associated vestibular schwannomas (NCT01345136, NCT01490476, NCT01419639).[56]

The loss of Merlin protein in NF2 has been shown to result in abnormal activation of the epidermal growth factor receptor (EGFR) receptor tyrosine kinases (RTKs) proteins. The proteins implicated include EGFR, ErbB2 and ErbB3. These proteins all span the cell membrane and contribute to feedback loops that regulate both cell death and cell division. When Merlin is inactive, EGFR, ErbB2 and ErbB3 remain constitutively active allowing increased cell proliferation and resistance to cell death.[57] Lapatinib is an oral dual EGFR/ErbB2 inhibitor approved for use in breast cancer. In preclinical studies lapatinib was shown to have substantial inhibition of both cell proliferation and vestibular schwannomas growth.[58,59] Lapatinib is now being investigated in two ongoing clinical studies in patients with NF2.

The contribution of abnormal angiogenesis has recently been recognized in benign tumours and provides a novel therapeutic target for NF2-associated vestibular schwannomas. Vestibular schwannomas and peripheral schwannomas have been shown to express vascular endothelial growth factor (VEGF) in both tumour cells and associated endothelial cells.[60,61] Recent studies indicated that Merlin also regulates angiogenesis via semaphorin 3F (SEMA3F), a protein that inhibits angiogenesis.[62] On these observations, bevacizumab, an angiogenesis inhibitor, is being used in at least two clinical trials.

Ras represents a family of proteins responsible for intracellular communication that are frequently altered in the setting of tumours. Merlin has been shown to regulate the interaction of Ras and various growth factors,[63] and multiple targets in the Ras pathway have been implicated as part of the pathogenesis of NF2-associated tumours. Sorafenib is an oral multitarget inhibitor of several targets downstream from Ras including Raf/Mek/Erk as well as platelet-derived growth factor (PDGF), vascular endothelial growth factor (VEGF) and c-kit. Similar to sorafenib, nilotinib is a RTK inhibitor of breakpoint cluster region-abelson that also targets PDGF receptor and c-kit. It has also shown promising NF2 *in vitro* and is entering a phase 0 trial with a similar design as described for sorafenib.[64]

GENETICS OF FAMILIAL PARAGANGLIOMAS

Paragangliomas (PGs) are tumours of paraganglionic tissue derived from the migration of neural crest cells during foetal development that occur in both sporadic and familial forms. In the head and neck these most commonly arise from the carotid body (carotid body tumours), jugulotympanic region (glomus tympanicum), jugular bulb (glomus jugulare) and vagus nerve (glomus vagale). Another well known but rare paraganglioma is the pheochromocytoma (PCC).

The yearly clinical incidences of paragangliomas and pheochromocytomas are estimated as 1:1 000 000 and 2:1 000 000 respectively.[65]

Familial PG is inherited in an autosomal dominant manner with maternal imprinting. Therefore, when an individual inherits the PG gene from the mother (regardless of whether she herself is affected), that child is unaffected and becomes a silent carrier of the mutated gene. On the other hand, when a child inherits the PG gene from the father, the offspring will have paragangliomas regardless of the affected status of the father. Subsequently, the affected/unaffected child harbouring the abnormal PG gene will be able to pass the gene to his/her children; he/she will have affected children only if the transmitting parent is a father. This unusual form of incomplete genetic penetrance is caused by sex-specific gene modification during gametogenesis.[66]

Because of this unusual form of inheritance, many sporadic PG could in fact be hereditary PG, and the incidence of familial PG could be much higher than the historically quoted rate of 10%. During the last decade mutations in the genes encoding different subunits of the succinate dehydrogenase (SDH) complex have been linked to familial PCC-PG syndrome, and subsequent genetic screenings have revealed that about 30% of PCC and PG are caused by hereditary mutations.[67, 68] Similar to familial PG, sporadic PG also demonstrates loss of heterozygosity at PGL1 and PGL2, and this was demonstrated in 38% sporadic cases of carotid body tumours and glomus tumours by Bikhazi et al.[69] This indirectly tells us that approximately one-third of all sporadic cases of PG may actually be familial.

Currently, four different types of PG are recognized: PGL1, PGL2, PGL3 and PGL4. These are now briefly discussed.

PGL1

PGL1 is caused by germ line mutations of the SDHD gene, located at 11q21.[70] It is the most common PGL.[71, 72]

Multiple head and neck PGs are a key feature of this syndrome and they develop in the majority of patients (60–79%), either synchronous or metachronous.[72–74] There is also a definite risk of developing pheochromocytomas and extra-adrenal PGs (16–21%).[72–74]

In 2012 Van Hulsteijn et al.[75] presented a systematic literature review and meta-analysis on the risk of malignant PG in SDHB and SDHD mutation carriers and found that the prevalence of malignant paraganglial tumours reported in SDHD patients with manifest disease varied widely, ranging from 0% to 23%. The pooled incidence for malignant PG was 8% in SDHD mutation carriers.[75]

Tumour penetrance in SDHD mutation carriers is high. Neumann et al.[76] first published data on age related penetrance in SDHD mutation carriers in 2004. SDHD mutations conferred 50% penetrance by age 31 rising to 86% by the age of 50. In a study by Hensen et al.[77] published in 2010, age related penetrance in SDHD patients was 54% by age 40 and 87% by age 70. The average range of age at diagnosis of SDHD-linked tumours is 25–38 years.[72, 74, 78] As demonstrated by Heesterman et al.[79] there is also a high prevalence of occult paraganglial tumours in asymptomatic SDHD mutation carriers; in their study, MRI detected HNPGs in 28 out of 47 (59.6%) asymptomatic SDHD patients.

Already in 1989, it was observed that PGL1 families exhibit a peculiar inheritance pattern with a distinct 'parent-of-origin-dependent effect'.[80] Whereas SDHD mutations can be inherited both via the maternal and paternal lines, the PGL almost never develops after maternal transmission of the mutation.[72, 76, 80] As maternally derived SDHD mutation carriers will still pass the mutation to their offspring in 50% of cases, PGL1 can appear to skip generations, which may in part explain the occurrence of SDHD germ line mutations in apparently non-familial cases.[72, 74, 76]

This virtually exclusive paternal inheritance of disease is consistent with maternal imprinting of the disease gene.[80] However, imprinting of SDHD has never been established, and the fact that this inheritance pattern is also found in PGL2 families (linked to the SDHAF2 gene, located on 11q13), but not in PGL3 or PGL4 families, suggests that other factors on chromosome 11 explain this phenomenon. It has been found that in SDHD-linked PGs, the whole maternal copy of chromosome 11 is selectively lost.[81] Interestingly, this implies that a second, paternally imprinted tumour suppressor gene located elsewhere on chromosome 11 plays a decisive role in PG tumourigenesis, at least in PGL1 and PGL2.[81] This hypothesis is supported by genetic analysis of the very few 'exceptions to the rule', the reported instances of maternal transmission of disease in PGL1 families. In these rare cases, it was shown that invariably not only the SDHD or SDHAF2 gene but also the 11p15 region was affected.[82, 83] The identity of this secondary tumour suppressor gene remains to be elucidated.[84]

PGL2

PGL2 has a very interesting history, as it was the first PGL to be described.[84] In 1982 Van Baars et al.[85] reported on a large Dutch family (295 living family members) with familial HNPGs. It was not until the year 2009 though, that Hao et al.[86] identified a mutation of the SDHAF2 gene, situated on 11q13, as the underlying cause of PGL2.[86, 87] SDHAF2, also known as SDH5, plays an important role in flavination of SDHA.[86]

Bayley et al.[87] identified a second family with PGL2 in Spain. The authors also looked for SDHAF2 mutations in 443 additional HNPGs and pheochromocytoma patients without finding another case of PGL2, suggesting that SDHAF2 plays a modest role as a causative gene in PGLs. Like PGL1, the PGL2 is strongly associated with the occurrence of multiple HNPGs (70–91%) but so far, no extra-adrenal PGs, pheochromocytomas, or malignant PGs have been described in SDHAF2 mutation carriers.[86–88] As in PGL1, in PGL2 families transmission of the PGL occurs exclusively via the paternal line. Tumour penetrance has been described to be very high in both the Dutch and the Spanish family (88–100%), and the average age at diagnosis is 33–34 years.[86–88]

PGL3

Niemann and Müller[89] first identified a mutation in SDHC, located on 1q21, as the underlying cause of PGL3 in 2000. Until October 2005, only four patients with SDHC mutations had been described.[84] Most authors concluded that SDHC mutations must be exceedingly rare and therefore, HNPG patients were not routinely tested for mutations of the SDHC gene. This only changed when Schiavi et al.[90] reported on a total of 22 SDHC mutation carriers in October 2005.

Nevertheless, SDHC mutations have been detected less frequently than SDHD and SDHB mutations.[72]

In sharp contrast to patients with PGL1 and PGL4, SDHC mutation carriers mostly present with benign, single HNPGs.[72] Multiple HNPGs are found in 19–31%, and pheochromocytomas, extra-adrenal PGs, and malignant PGs are seldom reported in SDHC mutation carriers.[72, 73, 90]

In 2009, Neumann et al.[72] and Burnichon et al.[73] found similar prevalence of 4.3% and 3.6% for SDHC mutations in two large HNPG patient series consisting of 445 and 598 PG patients, respectively. The family history is positive in the minority of SDHC patients (12–25%), suggesting a low tumour penetrance.[72, 73] The average age at diagnosis is higher than for the other PGL (38–46 years).[73, 90]

PGL4

The PGL4 locus is situated on the 1p36 chromosomal band. The first description of the SDHB mutation as the cause of PGL4 dates back to 2001.[91]

In contrast to SDHD mutation carriers, patients with SDHB mutation carriers frequently develop extra-adrenal PGs (in 52–84%) and pheochromocytomas (in 18–28%), and less frequently HNPGs (in 27–31%), while multifocal HNPGs are significantly less frequently found when compared to SDHD patients.[72, 78]

The average age at diagnosis is reported to be between 30 and 37 years.[73, 78]

The most striking clinical feature of PGL4 is the high percentage of malignant pheochromocytomas and malignant HNPGs.[72, 78]

Neumann et al.[72] described malignant paraganglial tumours in 13 out of 63 SDHB mutation carriers (20.6%). Ricketts et al.[78] reported on 40 SDHB patients with malignant PGs and pheochromocytomas in a group of 163 SDHB mutation carriers (25.2%). In a literature review by Pasini and Stratakis,[92] 50 malignant paraganglial tumours were diagnosed in 105 out of 256 SDHB mutation carriers (41%).

As reviewed by Van Hulsteijn et al.[75] prevalence of malignant paraganglial tumours in SDHB patients with manifest disease range from 0% to 54% in the literature. In their systematic literature review and meta-analysis on the risk of malignant PG in SDHB and SDHD mutation carriers, the authors found a pooled incidence of 17% in the SDHB group. The pooled risk in prevalence studies, depending on presence of manifest disease, ranged from 13% to 23% in the SDHB group. The authors concluded that incidence and prevalence of malignant HNPGs and pheochromocytomas are higher in SDHB than in SDHD mutation carriers but lower in the SDHB group than hitherto appreciated.[75]

Identification of an *SDHB* gene mutation is also a factor of poor prognosis.[92] Multivariate analysis of a series of 54 subjects followed in France for PG or malignant pheochromocytoma demonstrated that identification of an *SDHB* mutation was the only risk factor for mortality. The 5-year survival probability was 36% for subjects with an *SDHB* mutation versus 67% for subjects without an *SDHB* mutation with a calculated median survival of 42 months for *SDHB*-mutant patients versus 244 months for wild-type *SDHB* patients.[93]

SDHB mutations follow an autosomal dominant trait of inheritance.[91] Tumour penetrance is somewhat lower than that seen in SDHD mutation carriers. Benn et al.[94] estimated the age related tumour penetrance in SDHB mutation carriers to be at 29% at age 30 rising to 45% at age 40.

KEY POINTS

- Advances in molecular genetics have helped to identify causative genes and proteins responsible for pathologies; this knowledge is pertinent to molecular target therapy and promises novel therapeutic interventions.
- The most useful distinction in hereditary hearing impairment (HHI) is syndromic (majority) and non-syndromic (minority). In autosomal dominant non-syndromic hearing loss there is not a single identifiable gene responsible for the majority of cases whereas in autosomal recessive non-syndromic hearing impairment 50% of people have mutations in the GJB2.
- Waardenburg syndrome, Bronochiootorenal syndrome, Stickler syndrome and NF2 represent the most common causes of syndromic autosomal dominant hearing loss, whereas Pendred syndrome and Jervell and Lange-Neilsen syndrome are the commonest causes of syndromic autosomal recessive hearing loss.
- The mitochondrial 12S rRNA is a hot spot for mutations associated with both aminoglycoside-induced and non-syndromic hearing loss. Of those, 1555A>G and 1494C>T mutations at the 12S rRNA have been associated with hearing loss worldwide and account for a significant number of cases of aminoglycoside ototoxicity.

- The NF2 gene is spread over approximately 100 000 bases on chromosome 22q12.2 and contains 17 exons (or encoding segments). More than 200 mutations of the NF2 gene have been identified, that result in protein truncation are associated with a more severe clinical presentation of NF2 (Wishart type) – larger, multiple, faster growing tumours. While missense and splice site mutations are associated with a milder form of the disease (Gardner type) – smaller, few and slow growing tumours.
- Currently, four different types of PG (tumours of paraganglionic tissue derived from the migration of neural crest cells during fetal development that occur in both sporadic and familial form) are recognized:
  - PGL1- the commonest type caused by germ line mutations of the SDHD gene, located at 11q21
  - PGL2- caused by a mutation of the SDHAF2 gene, situated on 11q13
  - PGL3- caused by a mutation of the SDHC gene located on 1q21
  - PGL4- the locus of which is situated on the 1p36 chromosomal band.

REFERENCES

1. NHS Newborn Hearing Screening Programme 2010–11. *Annual report and 2009–10 data report*.
2. Bamford J, Fortnum H, Bristow K, et al. Current practice, accuracy, effectiveness, and cost effectiveness of the school entry hearing screen. *Health Technol Assess* 2007; **11**(32): 1–168.
3. Linden Phillips L, Bitner-Glindzicz M, Lench N, et al. The future role of genetic screening to detect newborns at risk of childhood-onset hearing loss. *Int J Audiol* 2013; **52**(2): 124–33.
4. Mhatre AN, Lalwani AK. Molecular genetics of deafness. *Otolaryngol Clin North Am* 1996; **29**: 421–35.
5. Van Camp G, Willems PJ, Smith RJ. Non-syndromic hearing impairment: unparalleled heterogeneity. *Am J Hum Genet* 1997; **60**: 758–64.
6. Linden Phillips L, Bitner-Glindzicz M, Lench N, et al. The future role of genetic screening to detect newborns at risk of childhood-onset hearing loss. *Int J Audiol* 2013; **52**(2): 124–33.
7. Kelsell DP, Dunlop J, Stevens HP, et al. Connexin 26 mutations in hereditary non-syndromic sensorineural deafness. *Nature* 1997; **387**: 80–83. (This was the first paper to describe mutations in the GJB2 genes.)
8. Kelley PM, Harris DJ, Comer BC, et al. Novel mutations in the connexin 26 gene (*GJB2*) that cause autosomal recessive (DFNB1) hearing loss. *Am J Hum Genet* 1998; **62**: 792–99.
9. Snoeckx RL, Huygen PL, Feldmann D, et al. *GJB2* mutations and degree of hearing loss: a multicenter study. *Am J Hum Genet* 2005; **77**: 945–57.
10. Shahin H, Walsh T, Sobe T, et al. Genetics of congenital deafness in the Palestinian population: multiple connexin 26 alleles with shared origins in the Middle East. *Hum Genet* 2002; **110**: 284–89.
11. Avraham KB, Hasson T, Steel KP, et al. The mouse Snell's *waltzer* deafness gene encodes an unconventional myosin required for structural integrity of inner ear hair cells. *Nat Genet* 1995; **11**: 369–75.
12. Weil D, Levy G, Sahly I, et al. Human myosin VIIA responsible for the Usher 1B syndrome: a predicted membrane-associated motor protein expressed in developing sensory epithelia. *Proc Natl Acad Sci USA* 1996; **93**: 3232–37.
13. Maubaret C, Griffoin JM, Arnaud B, Hamel C. Novel mutations in *MYO7A* and *USH2A* in Usher syndrome. *Ophthalmic Genet* 2005; **26**: 25–29.
14. Weil D, Kussel P, Blanchard S, et al. The autosomal recessive isolated deafness, DFNB2, and the Usher 1B syndrome are allelic defects of the myosin-VIIA gene. *Nat Genet* 1997; **16**: 191–93.
15. Liu XZ, Walsh J, Mburu P, et al. Mutations in the myosin VIIA gene cause non-syndromic recessive deafness. *Nat Genet* 1997; **16**: 188–90.
16. Belyantseva IA, Boger ET, Friedman TB. Myosin XVa localizes to the tips of inner ear sensory cell stereocilia and is essential for staircase formation of the hair bundle. *Proc Natl Acad Sci USA* 2003; **100**: 13958–63.
17. Delprat B, Michel V, Goodyear R, et al. Myosin XVa and whirlin, two deafness gene products required for hair bundle growth, are located at the stereocilia tips and interact directly. *Hum Mol Genet* 2005; **14**: 401–10.
18. Boeda B, El-Amraoui A, Bahloul A, et al. Myosin VIIa, harmonin and cadherin 23, three Usher I gene products that cooperate to shape the sensory hair cell bundle. *EMBO J* 2002; **21**: 6689–99.
19. Bork JM, Peters LM, Riazuddin S, et al. Usher syndrome 1D and nonsyndromic autosomal recessive deafness DFNB12 are caused by allelic mutations of the novel cadherin-like gene *CDH23*. *Am J Hum Genet* 2001; **68**: 26–37.
20. Astuto LM, Bork JM, Weston MD, et al. *CDH23* mutation and phenotype heterogeneity: a profile of 107 diverse families with Usher syndrome and nonsyndromic deafness. *Am J Hum Genet* 2002; **71**: 762–75.
21. Toriello HV, Reardon W, Gorlin RJ (eds) *Hereditary hearing loss and its syndromes*. New York: Oxford University Press; 2004.
22. Apaydin F, Bereketoglu M, Turan O, et al. Waardenburg syndrome: a heterogenic disorder with variable penetrance. *HNO* 2004; **52**: 533–37.
23. Shalit E, Avraham KB. Genetics of hearing loss. In: Schacht J, Popper AN, Fay RR (eds) *Auditory trauma, protection and repair*. New York: Springer Science+Business Media, LLC; 2008.
24. Steel KP, Kros CJ. A genetic approach to understanding auditory function. *Nat Genet* 2001; **27**: 143–49.
25. Ruf RG, Xu PX, Silvius D, et al. SIX1 mutations cause branchio-oto-renal syndrome by disruption of EYA1-SIX1-DNA complexes. *Proc Natl Acad Sci USA* 2004; **101**: 8090–95.
26. Hoskins BE, Cramer CH, Silvius D, et al. Transcription factor SIX5 is mutated in patients with branchio-oto-renal syndrome. *Am J Hum Genet* 2007; **80**: 800–04.
27. Weil D, Blanchard S, Kaplan J, et al. Defective myosin VIIA gene responsible for Usher syndrome type 1B. *Nature* 1995; **374**(6517): 60–61.
28. Bolz H, von Brederlow B, Ramírez A, et al. Mutation of CDH23, encoding a new member of the cadherin gene family, causes Usher syndrome type 1D. *Nat Genet* 2001; **27**(1): 108–12.
29. Li XC, Everett LA, Lalwani AK, et al. A mutation in PDS causes non-syndromic recessive deafness. *Nat Genet* 1998; **18**: 215–17.
30. Bayazit YA, Yilmaz M. An overview of hereditary hearing loss. *ORL J Otorhinolaryngol Relat Spec* 2006; **68**(2): 57–63.
31. Tang HY, Hutcheson E, Neill S, et al. Genetic susceptibility to aminoglycoside ototoxicity: how many are at risk? *Genet Med* 2002; **4**(5): 336–45.
32. Casano RAMS, Johnson DF, Bykhovskaya Y, et al. Inherited susceptibility to aminoglycoside ototoxicity: genetic heterogeneity and clinical implications. *Am J Otolaryngol* 1999; **20**: 151–56.
33. Fischel-Ghodsian N, Prezant TR, Bu X, Oztas S. Mitochondrial ribosomal RNA gene mutation in a patient with sporadic aminoglycoside ototoxicity. *Am J Otolaryngol* 1993; **14**: 399–403.
34. Gardner JC, Goliath R, Viljoen D, et al. Familial streptomycin ototoxicity in a South African family: a mitochondrial disorder. *J Med Genet* 1997; **34**: 904–06.
35. Evans DG, Moran A, King A, et al. Incidence of vestibular schwannoma and neurofibromatosis 2 in the North West of England over a 10-year period: higher incidence than previously thought. *Otol Neurotol* 2005; **26**(1): 93–97.
36. Evans DG, Howard E, Giblin C, et al. Birth incidence and prevalence of tumor-prone syndromes: estimates from a UK family genetic register service. *Am J Med Genet A* 2010; **152A**(2): 327–32.
37. Kanter WR, Eldridge R, Fabricant R, et al. Central neurofibromatosis with bilateral acoustic neuroma: genetic, clinical and biochemical distinctions from peripheral neurofi-bromatosis. *Neurol* 1980 **30**: 851–59.
38. Lalwani AK, Abaza MM, Makariou EV, Armstrong M. Audiologic presentation of vestibular schwannomas in neurofibromatosis type 2. *Am J Otol* 1998; **19**(3): 352–57.
39. Abaza MM, Makariou E, Armstrong M, Lalwani AK. Growth rate characteristics of acoustic neuromas associated with neurofibromatosis type 2. *Laryngoscope* 1996; **106**(6): 694–99.

40. Rouleau GA, Wertelecki W, Haines JL, et al. Genetic linkage of bilateral acoustic neurofibromatosis to a DNA marker on chromosome 22. *Nature* 1987; **329**(6136): 246–48.
41. Wertelecki W, Rouleau GA, Superneau DW, et al. Neurofibromatosis 2: clinical and DNA linkage studies of a large kindred. *N Engl J Med* 1988; **319**(5): 278–83.
42. Rouleau GA, Merel P, Lutchman M, et al. Alteration in a new gene encoding a putative membrane-organizing protein causes neuro-fibromatosis type 2. *Nature* 1993; **363**: 515–21.
43. Trofatter JA, MacCollin MM, Rutter JL, et al. A novel moesin-, ezrin-, radixin-like gene is a candidate for the neurofibromatosis 2 tumor suppressor. *Cell* 1993; **72**: 791–800.
44. Gutmann DH, Sherman L, Seftor L, et al. Increased expression of the NF2 tumor suppressor gene product, merlin, impairs cell motility, adhesion and spreading. *Hum Mol Genet* 1999; **8**: 267–75.
45. Pelton PD, Sherman LS, Rizvi TA, et al. Ruffling membrane, stress fiber, cell spreading and proliferation abnormalities in human Schwannoma cells. *Oncogene* 1998; **17**: 2195–209.
46. McClatchey AI, Saotome I, Mercer K, et al. Mice heterozygous for a mutation at the Nf2 tumor suppressor locus develop a range of highly metastatic tumors. *Genes Dev* 1998; **12**: 1121–33.
47. Neff BA, Welling DB, Akhmametyeva E, Chang LS. The molecular biology of vestibular schwannomas: dissecting the pathogenic process at the molecular level. *Otol Neurotol* 2006; **27**(2): 197–208.
48. Mautner VF, Baser ME, Kluwe L. Phenotypic variability in two families with novel splice-site and frameshift NF2 mutations. *Hum Genet* 1996; **98**: 203–06.
49. Ruttledge MH, Andermann AA, Phelan CM, et al. Type of mutation in the neurofibromatosis type 2 gene (NF2) frequently determines severity of disease. *Am J Hum Genet* 1996; **59**(2): 331–42.
50. Parry DM, MacCollin MM, Kaiser-Kupfer MI, et al. Germ-line mutations in the neurofibromatosis 2 gene: correlations with disease severity and retinal abnormalities. *Am J Hum Genet* 1996; **59**(3): 529–39.
51. Evans DG. Neurofibromatosis type 2 (NF2): a clinical and molecular review. *Orphanet J Rare Dis* 2009; **4**: 16.
52. Evans DG, Ramsden RT, Shenton A, et al. Mosaicism in NF2 an update of risk based on uni/bilaterality of vestibular schwannoma at presentation and sensitive mutation analysis including MLPA. *J Med Genet* 2007; **44**: 424–28.
53. Kluwe L, Freidrich RE, Tatagiba M, Mautner V. Presymptomatic diagnosis for children of sporadic neurofibromatosis 2 patients, a method based on tumor analysis. *Genet Med* 2002; **4**: 27–30.
54. James MF, Han S, Polizzano C, et al. NF2/merlin is a novel negative regulator of mTOR complex 1, and activation of mTORC1 is associated with meningioma and schwannoma growth. *Mol Cell Biol* 2009; **29**: 4250–61.
55. Acosta-Jaquez HA, Keller JA, Foster KG, et al. Site-specific mTOR phosphorylation promotes mTORC1-mediated signaling and cell growth. *Mol Cell Biol* 2009; **29**: 4308–24.
56. Blakeley J. Development of drug treatments for neurofibromatosis type 2-associated vestibular schwannoma. *Curr Opin Otolaryngol Head Neck Surg* 2012; **20**(5): 372–79.
57. Cole BK, Curto M, Chan AW, McClatchey AI. Localization to the cortical cytoskeleton is necessary for Nf2/merlin-dependent epidermal growth factor receptor silencing. *Mol Cell Biol* 2008; **28**: 1274–84.
58. Ahmad ZK, Brown CM, Cueva RA, et al. ErbB expression, activation, and inhibition with lapatinib and tyrphostin (AG825) in human vestibular schwannomas. *Otol Neurotol* 2011; **32**: 841–47.
59. Ammoun S, Cunliffe CH, Allen JC, et al. ErbB/HER receptor activation and preclinical efficacy of lapatinib in vestibular schwannoma. *Neuro Oncol* 2010; **12**: 834–43.
60. Wong HK, Lahdenranta J, Kamoun WS, et al. Antivascular endothelial growth factor therapies as a novel therapeutic approach to treating neurofibromatosis-related tumors. *Cancer Res* 2010; **70**: 3483–93.
61. Plotkin SR, Stemmer-Rachamimov AO, Barker FG 2nd, et al. Hearing improvement after bevacizumab in patients with neurofibromatosis type 2. *N Engl J Med* 2009; **361**: 358–67.
62. Acevedo LM, Barillas S, Weis SM, et al. Semaphorin 3A suppresses VEGF-mediated angiogenesis yet acts as a vascular permeability factor. *Blood* 2008; **111**: 2674–80.
63. Morrison H, Sperka T, Manent J, et al. Merlin/neurofibromatosis type 2 suppresses growth by inhibiting the activation of Ras and Rac. *Cancer Res* 2007; **67**: 520–27.
64. Ammoun S, Schmid MC, Triner J, et al. Nilotinib alone or in combination with selumetinib is a drug candidate for neurofibromatosis type 2. *Neuro Oncol* 2011; **13**: 759–66.
65. Baysal BE. Hereditary paraganglioma targets diverse paraganglia. *J Med Genet* 2002; **39**(9): 617–22.
66. Hall JG. Genomic imprinting: review and relevance to human diseases. *Am J Hum Genet* 1990; **46**(5): 857–73.
67. Amar L, Bertherat J, Baudin E, et al. Genetic testing in pheochromocytoma or functional paraganglioma. *J Clin Oncol* 2005; **23**(34): 8812–18.
68. Mannelli M, Castellano M, Schiavi F, et al. Italian Pheochromocytoma/Paraganglioma Network. Clinically guided genetic screening in a large cohort of Italian patients with pheochromocytomas and/or functional or nonfunctional paragangliomas. *J Clin Endocrinol Metab* 2009; **94**(5): 1541–47.
69. Bikhazi PH, Messina L, Mhatre AN, et al. Molecular pathogenesis in sporadic head and neck paraganglioma. *Laryngoscope* 2000; **110**(8): 1346–48.
70. Baysal BE, Ferrell RE, Willett-Brozick JE, et al. Mutations in SDHD, a mitochondrial complex II gene, in hereditary paraganglioma. *Science* 2000; **287**: 848–51.
71. Myssiorek D, Ferlito A, Silver CE, et al. Screening for familial paragangliomas. *Oral Oncol* 2008; **44**: 532–37.
72. Neumann HPH, Erlic Z, Boedeker CC, et al. Clinical predictors for germline mutations in head and neck paraganglioma patients: cost reduction strategy in genetic diagnostic process as fall-out. *Cancer Res* 2009; **69**: 3650–56.
73. Burnichon N, Rohmer V, Amar L, et al. The succinate dehydrogenase genetic testing in a large prospective series of patients with paragangliomas. *J Clin Endocrinol Metab* 2009; **94**: 2817–27.
74. Hensen EF, Siemers MD, Jansen JC, et al. Mutations in SDHD are the major determinants of the clinical characteristics of Dutch head and neck paraganglioma patients. *Clin Endocrinol* 2011; **75**: 650–55.
75. Van Hulsteijn LT, Dekkers OM, Hes FJ, et al. Risk of malignant paraganglioma in SDHB-mutation and SDHD-mutation carriers: a systematic review and metaanalysis. *J Med Genet* 2012; **49**: 768–76.
76. Neumann HPH, Pawlu C, Peçzkowska M, et al. Distinct clinical features characterize paraganglioma syndromes associated with SDHB and SDHD gene mutations. *JAMA* 2004; **292**: 943–951.
77. Hensen EF, Jansen JC, Siemers MD, et al. The Dutch founder mutation SDHD. D92Y shows a reduced penetrance for the development of paragangliomas in a large multigenerational family. *Eur J Hum Genet* 2010; **18**: 62–66.
78. Ricketts CJ, Forman JR, Rattenberry E, et al. Tumor risks and genotype-phenotype proteotype analysis in 358 patients with germline mutations in SDHB and SDHD. *Hum Mutat* 2010; **31**: 41–51.
79. Heesterman BL, Bayley JP, Tops CM, et al. High prevalence of occult paragangliomas in asymptomatic carriers of SDHD and SDHB gene mutations. *Eur J Hum Genet* 2013; **21**: 469–70.
80. van der Mey AG, Maaswinkel-Mooy PD, Cornelisse CJ, et al. Genomic imprinting in hereditary glomus tumours: evidence for new genetic theory. *Lancet* 1989; **2**: 1291–94.
81. Hensen EF, Jordanova ES, van Minderhout IJ, et al. Somatic loss of maternal chromosome 11 causes parent-of-origin-dependent inheritance in SDHD-linked paraganglioma and phaeochromocytoma families. *Oncogene* 2004; **23**: 4076–83.
82. Pigny P, Vincent A, Cardot Bauters C, et al. Paraganglioma after maternal transmission of a succinate dehydrogenase gene mutation. *J Clin Endocrinol Metab* 2008; **93**: 1609–15.
83. Yeap PM, Tobias ES, Mavraki F, et al. Molecular analysis of pheochromocytoma after maternal transmission of SDHD mutation elucidates mechanism of parent-of-origin effect. *J Clin Endocrinol Metab* 2011; **96**: E2009–E2013.
84. Boedeker CC, Hensen EF, Neumann HP, et al. Genetics of hereditary head and neck paragangliomas. *Head Neck* 2013; **36**(6): 907–16.
85. van Baars F, Cremers C, van den Broek P, et al. Genetic aspects of nonchromaffin paraganglioma. *Hum Genet* 1982; **60**: 305–09.
86. Hao HX, Khalimonchuk O, Schraders M, et al. SDH5, a gene required for flavination of succinate dehydrogenase, is mutated in paraganglioma. *Science* 2009; **325**: 1139–1142.
87. Bayley JP, Kunst HP, Cascon A, et al. SDHAF2 mutations in familial and sporadic paraganglioma and phaeochromocytoma. *Lancet Oncol* 2010; **11**: 366–72.
88. Kunst HP, Rutten MH, de Mönnink JP, et al. SDHAF2 (PGL2-SDH5) and hereditary head and neck paraganglioma. *Clin Cancer Res* 2011; **17**: 247–54.

89. Niemann S, Müller U. Mutations in SDHC cause autosomal dominant paraganglioma, type 3. *Nat Genet* 2000; **26**: 268–70.
90. Schiavi F, Boedeker CC, Bausch B, et al. Predictors and prevalence of paraganglioma syndrome associated with mutations of the SDHC gene. *JAMA* 2005; **294**: 2057–63.
91. Astuti D, Latif F, Dallol A, et al. Gene mutations in the succinate dehydrogenase subunit SDHB cause susceptibility to familial pheochromocytoma and to familial paraganglioma. *Am J Hum Genet* 2001; **69**: 49–54.
92. Pasini B, Stratakis CA. SDH mutations in tumorigenesis and inherited endocrine tumours: lesson from the phaeochromocytoma-paraganglioma syndromes. *J Intern Med* 2009; **266**: 19–42.
93. Amar L, Baudin E, Burnichon N, et al. Succinate dehydrogenase B gene mutations predict survival in subjects with malignant pheochromocytomas or paragangliomas. *J Clin Endocrinol Metab* 2007; **92**: 3822–28.
94. Benn DE, Gimenez-Roqueplo AP, Reilly JR, et al. Clinical presentation and penetrance of pheochromocytoma/paraganglioma syndromes. *J Clin Endocrinol Metab* 2006; **91**: 827–36.

CHAPTER 3

GENE THERAPY

Seiji B. Shibata and Scott M. Graham

Introduction 29	Head and neck cancer 34
Cystic fibrosis 31	References 36

SEARCH STRATEGY

Data in this chapter may be updated by a Medline and PubMed Central search using the keywords: gene therapy, cystic fibrosis, head and neck cancer, gene transfer, adenoviral vectors, adeno-associated vectors, ballistic gene delivery, chemosensitization and retroviral vectors.

INTRODUCTION

Gene therapy is the means of delivering exogenous genetic material for therapeutic purposes into the host cell target using vectors. This strategy in principle can be utilized in patients who have genetic defects leading to phenotypic impairment. Gene therapy can be restorative, regenerative or protective in nature by replacing/suppressing/enhancing gene expression. Few new treatment protocols reflect the allure of modern science quite as elegantly as gene therapy. The promise of gene therapy in treating a variety of diseases is, simply put, incredible. This promise has captured the hopes and enthusiasm of the scientific and lay communities alike. Notable initial success in treating severe combined immune deficiency (SCID) seemed to herald imminent success in treating a whole variety of other conditions. In reality, however, progress in bringing the allure of the science to a useful clinical application has been quite limited. Even in the group of SCID subjects[1] – an apparent 'cure' – a patient has died from an unusual lymphoproliferative disease.[2] This has led to a reassessment of the risks of retroviral therapy trials. While great strides have been made in understanding the microbiological complexities of disease states and vectors, the barriers to clinical utility continue to be formidable. However in recent years gene therapy has met major milestones in multiple clinical trials for a number of diseases including Leber's congenital amaurosis,[3, 4] X-linked adrenoleukodystrophy[5] and β-thalassemia.[6] In the 10-year follow-up study of aforementioned SCID subjects, 18 out of 20 patients are still alive, including four who had leukemia and 17 who have their immunodifficiency corrected.[7] Additionally the European commission has recently approved alipogene tiparvovec (Glybera®), an AAV viral vector harbouring human lipoprotein lipase, which will be used for the treatment of familial lipoprotein lipase deficiency disease, making it the first commercial available drug using gene therapy technology in Europe.[8] Thus, after experiencing several major setbacks gene therapy is making small but steady steps towards clinical reality.

As of 2012, some 1800 human clinical gene therapy trials (including phase I to IV) exist worldwide.[9] The disease processes involved can be broadly divided into four groups as listed in descending order of number of clinical trials: cancer, monogenetic diseases such as cystic fibrosis (CF) and haemophilia B, cardiovascular disease, and infectious disease trials, which entirely comprise human immunodeficiency virus (HIV). These studies deliver genetic material to target cells via vectors, which act as delivery vehicles to bypass host defences. In the very select circumstances of the skin or eye, a 'gene gun' can be used. The treatment aims to replace or repair the defective gene causing a given disease or to provide a new or altered function in a cell. The most common vectors are a variety of replication-deficient viruses although non-viral vectors, such as liposomes, are also used. The characteristics of commonly used vectors are summarized in **Table 3.1**. We will first review some commonly used gene therapy vectors.

Delivery

The common goal of all gene therapy is to achieve expression of the gene of interest in the targeted cell. To accomplish

TABLE 3.1 The characteristics of commonly used vectors

	Adenovirus	Adeno-associated virus	Retrovirus/lentivirus	Non-viral vectors
Family	*Adenoviridae*	*Parvoviridae*	*Retroviridae*	n/a
Genome	Double-stranded DNA	Single-stranded DNA	Single-stranded DNA	Unlimited size
Infection/tropism	Dividing and non-dividing cells	Dividing and non-dividing cells	Dividing cells	Dividing and non-dividing cells
Host genome interaction	Non-integrating	Non-integrating	Integrating	Non-integrating
Transgene expression	Transient	Potential long lasting	Long lasting	Transient
Packaging capacity	7.5 kb	4.5 kb	8 kb	Unlimited capacity

Source: Adapted and modified from Gene Therapy Net (http://www.genetherapynet.com).

this goal several barriers must be overcome: (i) targeting – ideally only cells which require the gene would be affected; (ii) binding and internalization (transfection) – once a gene reaches the cells it must bind and become internalized; (iii) cellular trafficking to the nucleus (transduction) – most methods of internalization require the gene to escape from endosomal degradation and traffic through the cell to the nucleus; and (iv) nuclear expression – once in the nucleus the quantity of gene expression and stability of expression for a given strategy also need to be determined. Each method of delivering a gene to a cell varies in its ability to overcome these barriers.

Adenovirus

Adenovirus is a human pathogenic, non-encapsulated, DNA virus. It has been extensively studied as a means to deliver transgenes both *in vitro* and in human trials. Adenovirus has several characteristics that make it suitable as a therapeutic vector in gene therapy. Relatively simple amplification methods have been developed to propagate high-titer replication defective vectors.[10] Adenovirus efficiently infects both dividing and non-dividing cells by binding to the cox-adenovirus receptor.[11] Once a cell binds the viral vector, adenovirus is internalized, escapes from the endosome and is trafficked to the nucleus very efficiently. Even if a specific cell is lacking viral receptors, the virus can be combined with complexes to be internalized via non-receptor-mediated mechanisms. In this alternative pathway of entry, the other components of viral gene delivery remain intact, and therefore efficiency is maintained.[12, 13] This relative versatility, its ease of construction, efficiency of infection and the efficient expression of transgene make adenovirus an attractive vector for gene therapy.

Adenovirus does have some drawbacks compared to other viral vectors and non-viral systems. It is immunogenic that which limits its ability to re-infect.[14] Multiple studies have shown that both cell- and humoral-mediated immune systems are activated after viral delivery, especially if greater than 10[10] particles are delivered.[15] This toxicity led to the well-publicized death of a subject in a University of Pennsylvania trial.[1] Besides limiting redelivery, this immune response also results in the clearance of cells expressing the transgene.[16] Several strategies have shown promise in overcoming this immune-stimulatory problem. 'Gutted' vectors, missing almost all of the viral genes, have been shown to be less immunogenic and are expressed for longer periods *in vivo*.[17, 18] Immune modulation at the time of delivery may decrease the initial inflammatory reaction to the virus.[17, 18] A further difficulty with adenovirus is that gene expression is transient. The viral genome does not integrate or persist with cell division and gene expression is lost as the cells divide. As demonstrated by more than 50 current open protocols, the adenoviral vector is a very versatile means of gene delivery. As the obstacles of immune stimulation and persistence are addressed, this vector should only become more useful.

Adeno-associated virus

The AAV vector has more recently emerged as a vector with significant therapeutic promise.[3, 8] AAV is a single-stranded encapsulated virus that belongs to the group of human parvoviruses. Several features of this virus make it attractive as a potential therapeutic tool. First, although it infects human cells this virus has not been associated with a pathologic human disease. It may, therefore, be a safer alternative than other viral vectors. Second, because recombinant AAV vectors do not encode viral proteins, delivery of this vector results in very little immunogenicity.[19, 20] AAV also persists and infects dividing and non-dividing cells. Although the mechanisms are not fully clear, it appears that in quiescent cells AAV integrates into the host chromosome and in rapidly dividing cells it persists as an extrachromosal episome.[21] These factors have made this vector a popular delivery vehicle for many preclinical and human trials. AAV viral vector harbouring human lipoprotein lipase AAV, alipogene tiparvovec (Glybera®) became the first commercially available gene therapy drug in Europe to treat familial lipoprotein lipase deficiency disease in 2012.[8] Disadvantages such as limited loading capacity (up to 4.2 kb), inefficient expression and delayed onset of expression have made AAV less attractive in the past; however, newer generations of recombinant AAV are now becoming available and are proven to have shorter turnover of transcription and enhanced gene expression potencies.

Retrovirus/lentivirus

Retroviral vectors have the substantial advantage of persistent gene expression. A discussion of retroviral vectors requires a basic understanding of the viral genome and replication. Retroviruses are small, encapsulating vectors with a genome composed of two identical single strands of RNA. The virus binds and is internalized into the cell via interactions between the cell membrane and viral capsule. Once internalized the RNA genome is reverse-transcribed and transported to the nucleus where it integrates as a provirus into the host chromosome. In a normal infectious process, this provirus would then produce viral proteins and RNA genomes for viral packaging. In all retroviral gene therapy vectors, the genome of the virus has been made replication-incompetent by removing the components of the viral gene required for packaging. Thus, these vectors integrated and express the desired gene but will not produce infectious particles.

Several retroviral systems for gene therapy are currently available. Murine oncogenic retroviruses have been the most extensively analyzed and used in preclinical studies.[22] Because murine retroviruses only infect dividing cells, the clinical utility of these initial retroviral vectors has been significantly limited.[22] To circumvent this obstacle, newer retroviral systems have been developed based on the lentivirus genus of retroviruses. This group of viral vectors that contains the human immunodeficiency virus offers the advantage of infecting dividing and non-dividing cells. They have shown significant promise in preclinical *in vivo* studies.[5, 6, 23] A further biosafety-related issue of retroviruses is that insertion of the provirus is not controlled. It is possible that insertion of the virus next to a proto-oncogene may lead to therapy-induced cancer. Initial evidence from the first successful therapy in patients with severe combined immune deficiency using retroviral gene replacement suggests that a minority of the patients may have developed a non-typable lymphoproliferative disorder as a result of therapy.[1] In addition to controlling insertion, chromosomal silencing of inserted genes has also been reported. In chromosomal silencing, methylation or acetylation of the promoter leads to significant downregulation of transgene expression.[24, 25] For both of these obstacles, current research has suggested potential solutions. These include controllable chromosomal insertion, chromosomal buffers and methods to controllably excise the provirus.

Non-viral vectors

Naked DNA is one of the most extensively studied methods of gene therapy. This non-viral method of gene therapy has several advantages. These include simplicity, ease of large scale production, minimal immune response and safety.[26] The major obstacle for plasmid gene therapy is efficiency. When DNA is placed in an organism, most of the DNA is not internalized. Even if internalization does occur, endosomal degradation destroys nearly all of the remaining plasmid prior to nuclear membrane transit and expression of the desired gene does not occur. In addition, since plasmid uptake is not receptor-mediated, targeting of the plasmid to a specific cell also remains a major obstacle. In the past 25 years, substantial progress has been made in overcoming these obstacles to non-viral gene transfer. Lastly, plasmid-mediated transfer results in transient expression because the plasmid is lost with cell division. Several methods using site-specific integration or expression of viral proteins have shown promise as a means to overcome this difficulty.[27, 28] Many of the past therapeutic attempts to utilize plasmid-mediated gene transfer have shown only modest potential. However, as all aspects of plasmid efficiency increase, this should directly correlate with the ability to utilize this technology in therapeutic interventions.

In reviewing progress to date in gene therapy, two diseases of interest to otolaryngologists encapsulate the potential and difficulties of this technique. We will review an apparently attractive candidate for gene therapy, a disease caused by a single mutation inherited in an autosomal recessive fashion – cystic fibrosis.[29, 30] We will also review progress in a condition with a variety of causalities and a disparate genetic basis, head and neck cancer[31, 32] – a superficially unattractive candidate for gene therapy. These two diverse diseases serve to illustrate many of the principles, advances and frustrations of gene therapy. In both these examples, human trials remain in nascent stages. Trial sample size is small and results so far do not readily lend themselves to the categorization of levels of evidence, as displayed in other chapters in this text.

CYSTIC FIBROSIS

Cystic fibrosis (CF) represents a seemingly ideal disease for gene therapy. It is the most common lethal genetic disease of one of the wealthiest racial subgroups in the world. There are perhaps 30 000 people with CF in the United States and 70 000 worldwide. It is inherited with an autosomal recessive pattern with carrier rates of 5% in some Caucasian populations.[33, 34] Remarkably, the median survival for CF patients is less than 40 years[35] and unfortunately, the disease remains almost uniformly fatal, invariably from its pulmonary sequelae.[33, 34] Despite dramatic improvements in the understanding of the molecular basis of CF, the pathogenesis of CF remains unclear and there has as yet been no clinically useful breakthrough in its treatment. Clearly, new treatments and novel animal models faithfully mimicking CF are needed. Conceptually, gene therapy offers the promise of a dramatic and new treatment for CF, thereby a majority of gene therapy trials targeting inherited monogenic disorders in Europe and the USA are currently performed in CF patients.[9, 30]

Genetic basis

The discovery of the gene for CF in 1989[36] set in motion a remarkable series of events, often covered by the lay press with the hyperbole of popular culture, which have culminated in attempts at gene therapy. CF is caused by mutations in a cystic fibrosis transmembrane conductance regulator (*CFTR*) gene on the long arm of chromosome 7. This gene encodes a CFTR protein, which has been shown to be a cAMP-dependent chloride channel on the apical surface of the epithelium.[37] Abnormalities of CFTR impairs the chloride channel and dysregulates salt and water transport across a variety of epithelia. This produces the increase of salt in sweat, obstructive pathology of the lung, pancreatic insufficiency, malabsorption of the GI tract and male infertility due to the lack or stenosis of vas deferens.[37] The deletion of three nucleotides results in the deletion of a single phenylalanine residue at position 508 of CFTR, designated ΔF508, is the most common mutation in CF comprising some 70% of cases. Other mutations, now numbering over 1000, are uncommon, occurring in less than 1% of screened populations.

The nasal model for gene transfer in cystic fibrosis

Most interest in CF amongst otolaryngologists has centred on CF sinus disease. Previous reports have claimed benefit from aggressive treatment of CF sinus disease[38] and have also suggested that the rhinologic sequelae of CF are important in production of the eventually life-threatening pulmonary complications. Not as widely reported has been the utility of the nose and sinuses in CF as a model for pulmonary disease.[39] While the eventual goal of CF gene therapy will clearly be intra-pulmonary administration, there are clearly some difficulties using the lungs for routine experimentation.

Chief amongst these concerns is safety. The prospect of an adverse reaction to vector administration in the lungs of a patient with pre-existing pulmonary compromise is real. In a dose-escalating trial reported by Crystal et al.[40] in 1994 of intra-pulmonary adenoviral vector administration, the patient who received the largest dose developed a significant adverse reaction with opacities on chest X-ray. The risk of a significant adverse reaction in a localized area of the nose or sinuses is clearly less.[41] The lungs are also more inaccessible than the nose and the nose and sinuses offer ease of access for vector administration and experimental manipulation. For a variety of reasons, CF clinical trials are performed on adults. These patients invariably have severe pre-existing pulmonary compromise and any incremental benefits in pulmonary function afforded by gene therapy would be difficult to measure.

The nasal potential in CF provides a measurable endpoint for gene transfer experimentation. Nasal mucosa maintains and generates a potential difference across its surface and a characteristic voltage trace can be obtained in normal patients. In CF, the nasal mucosa, like the lung mucosa, exhibits the characteristic chloride transport abnormality. CF patients, because of their abnormal ion transport, produce a nasal potential that is different from normal both in its absolute negativity and in its response to certain pharmacologic influences.[41] This trace is so characteristic for CF that it is referred to as its bio-electric phenotype. This potential can be readily and reproducibly measured, in contrast to a number of bronchopulmonary indices and has been a target of gene therapy strategies in the nose.

In vitro and animal studies

Initially, the feasibility of gene transfer to airway cells was demonstrated *in vitro* and then in a variety of animal experiments. Only one year after the identification of the gene, Rich et al.[42] showed that expression of cDNA for wildtype CFTR corrected the Cl⁻ channel defect in cultured CF airway epithelia. Zabner et al.[43] demonstrated that recombinant adenoviral vectors could deliver CFTR cDNA safely in both cotton rats and rhesus monkeys. Transgenic CF mice provided a means to perform functional testing of CFTR gene expression and have even allowed reversal of the CF phenotype by gene therapy *in utero*.[44] Unfortunately, however, the CF mice do not produce a disease state comparable to the characteristic manifestations of CF on human lungs or other organ systems.[45] Recently Zabner et al.[30, 43, 46] have cloned transgenic CF porcine models that harbour targeted disruption of both CFTR alleles creating an animal model faithfully recapitulating the human phenotype. These transgenic animals also provide the opportunity to study the ion transport defect in the sinuses to further understand the pathogenesis of CF in the nose and sinuses.[47, 48] Innovative advances in basic science are the basis for the development of novel treatments for CF and for the progression to clinical trials to address questions that could only be answered in humans.

The human CF gene therapy trials: Adenovirus vector

Most of the early human cystic fibrosis gene therapy trials in the United States employed adenoviral vectors. Adenovirus has a degree of tropism for respiratory mucosa and a substantial body of knowledge already existed about adenoviruses as respiratory pathogens. Recombinant viruses are produced by replacing the DNA sequence responsible for replication with CFTR cDNA. The viruses are thus replication-deficient, but still remain sufficiently active to transport genetic material into the target cell. In 1993, Zabner et al.[49] reported correction of the CF bioelectric potential in a single-dose study where an escalating dose of vector encoding CFTR was applied to the nasal epithelium of three CF patients. Two CF patients underwent a sham procedure using saline and served as controls. No change was noted in the bioelectric phenotype in these two patients. One year later Crystal et al.[40] published a study in which an adenovirus containing CFTR cDNA was applied to both the upper and lower respiratory tracts of four patients. No statement was made about the nasal potential, but CFTR expression was detected by immunohistochemistry. This report was notable for the widely publicized event of pulmonary toxicity in one of the participants following vector delivery to the lungs. This toxicity was thought to be due to vector-induced inflammation and a reduction of viral vector dose has largely overcome the problem of acute inflammation in subsequent studies. Hay et al.[50] produced a further study revealing partial improvement in the nasal potential in a single escalating-dose protocol the following year.

Knowles et al.[51] found molecular evidence of low efficiency gene transfer, but no correction of the nasal potential in a 1995 report. Their experiment involved administration of logarithmically increasing vector doses to four cohorts of three patients. A further study by Zabner et al.[52] in 1996 addressed the likely need for repeat vector administration. Six patients in two centres in the United States received four or five applications of sequentially escalating concentrations of recombinant adenovirus encoding *CFTR*. In this series, the correction of the nasal potential was more subtle and, importantly, evidence of immunologic response to repeat administration was noted.

Studies involving intra-pulmonary vector administration have scarcely fared better. Zuckerman et al.[53] delivered adenovirus encoding *CFTR* to a segmental bronchus in a dose-escalating study. There was evidence of low-level gene expression, as well as evidence of immune and inflammatory responses. In contrast, a single-escalating dose trial from France revealed gene transfer and no detectable immune or inflammatory response after administration of Ad-*CFTR*.[54]

Adenovirus vectors, while efficient delivery vehicles in the laboratory setting, clearly have difficulties in human trials. The human respiratory tract has evolved to efficiently repel a variety of microbial attacks, including of course adenoviruses. Adenovirus does not integrate into the genome and expression is transient thus repeat administration is required. With repeat administration come concerns of inflammation and immunogenicity. All viral vectors aimed at the epithelial surface suffer from the limitation of the viral receptors being located in the basolateral membrane, away from the cell surface. This may be in part overcome by the use of calcium chelators[55] that briefly disrupt tight epithelial functions, allowing the vector access to the basolateral membrane.

Adeno-associated virus vector

Serotypes 5 and 6 of the adeno-associated virus (AAV) enter airway cells from the apical surface.[45] Furthermore, AAV are thought to have the least cell toxicity and minimal immunoreaction compared to other viral vector counterparts and offer the potential for integration into the host genome. In practical terms, however, AAV are also associated with limited loading capacity, inefficient expression and delayed onset of expression, thereby may not be an ideal vector in treating CF. Indeed using the maxillary sinus model, 10 CF patients who had undergone prior maxillary antrostomy had AAV vector encoding CFTR applied to their maxillary sinus.[56, 57] Molecular evidence of gene transfer was detected as late as 41 days. A functional endpoint of maxillary sinus voltage measurement was also employed, although some evidence of functional improvement was detected at day 14. There appeared to be no effect on maxillary sinusitis, as assessed endoscopically. In summary, although the AAV vector is safe and stable the overall level of CFTR reconstitution has been too low to provide any functional improvement.[57, 58]

Lentivirus vector

Lentiviruses are an apparently attractive addition to the list of possible vectors. They have the ability to integrate into and consequently persist in the host genome. They can transduce non-dividing cells – an advantage in airway epithelium where cell turnover is generally low. While a variety of lentiviral options exists, most work has been carried out with the feline immunodeficiency virus (FIV).[45, 59]

Non-viral vectors

The shortcomings of viral vectors have led to the investigation of non-viral delivery systems. These have included purified or naked DNA in plasmid form or ballistic gene delivery, the so-called gene gun. Only exposed surfaces accessible to a microcarrier coated with DNA are candidates for the gene gun. Although successful in mice lungs this approach is difficult to incorporate in animals with larger lungs due to the lack of equipment design that would match the lung size. Most interest in non-viral gene delivery has centred on liposomes. Liposomes bind to DNA, spontaneously forming complexes that have high affinity for plasma cell membranes. DNA containing liposomes are incorporated into the cell by endocytosis. The advantages of non-viral vectors mainly revolve around safety. They are non-immunogenic and there is no potential for insertion mutagenesis. The main difficulties with non-viral vectors relate to transient expression and less efficient gene transfer as compared to viral vectors.

A 20% correction of nasal potential in nine patients, peaking at three days and disappearing by seven days, was reported by Caplen et al.[60] employing a cationic liposome vector. The vector was applied by a nasal pump spray, a practical method for likely repeat administration should clinical gene therapy become a reality. In 1997, Gill et al.[61] showed functional CFTR gene transfer in six of eight subjects in a further nasal mucosal/liposome study. Alton et al.[62] reported a placebo-controlled study of liposome-mediated CFTR transfer to the lungs and nasal mucosa of CF patients. The treatment group displayed some improvement in airway potential not seen in the liposome-only group. Interestingly, some aspects of toxicity were only seen with pulmonary administration leading the authors to question the value of the nasal model, at least from a safety viewpoint.

> **KEY POINTS**
> - Remarkable progress has been made in understanding the molecular basis of cystic fibrosis.
> - Equally dramatic progress has been made in examining the basic science of vector production and vector interaction with airway cells.
> - The challenge remains to apply this new knowledge and *in vitro* gene therapy success to a clinically relevant and measurable endpoint.

HEAD AND NECK CANCER

In 2000, an estimated 130 000 cases of new head and neck cancer were diagnosed in developed countries.[63] Advances in surgical techniques, radiation treatment strategies and chemotherapy medications have improved the survival and quality of life for many of these patients. Unfortunately, despite these innovations, treatment strategies for advanced stage cancer, squamous cancer and certain other head and neck cancer subtypes have not increased survival over the last 40 years.[64] In order to offer therapy in these advanced cases and to potentially augment current successful therapies, alternative treatment strategies have been examined. Many of these therapies have evolved as a result of our appreciation of the biological basis of oncogenesis. Specifically, this increased understanding has given us gene targets to potentially correct by either replacing or blocking the effect of the mutated gene. The various strategies used in gene therapy fall into four major categories: immune modulation, restorative gene replacement, selective oncolysis and chemosensitization. The following discussion will review both the methods to deliver the genes and the various therapeutic strategies used with these vectors.

Therapy strategies

Gene therapy offers a novel paradigm that leads to the destruction of tumour cells in cancer patients. To date, the approaches to target specific cancer cells fall into four basic categories: (i) chemosensitization; (ii) cytokine gene transfer; (iii) inactivation of protooncogene production; and (iv) selective oncolytic viruses. In the discussion to follow, the rationale and specific results from preliminary gene therapy trials will be presented.

CHEMOSENSITIZATION

Selective sensitization of cancer cells using gene therapy would be an ideal way to kill cancer cells. Using this approach, the expected gene is delivered only to cancer cells and then a second therapy (e.g. radiotherapy or chemotherapy) is used to induce killing in the cells that express the transgene. The best example of this model is delivery of herpes simplex thymidine kinase (HSV-TK).[31, 65] In this strategy, HSV-TK is delivered to cancer cells. Once expressed, this enzyme changes the prodrug gancyclovir to its toxic nucleoside analogue, which induces cell death. Using this system one would expect that 100% infection of the cancer cell would be required in order to be effective. In reality, a phenomenon termed the bystander effect increases the efficiency of such therapies. In the bystander effect, the infected cell spreads the expressed genes to the cells surrounding it via cell–cell contacts. Using mixing experiments, it has been shown that because of this effect, only half of the cells need to initially express the toxic gene to have the desired effect.[65, 66] Transfer of *p53* is another example of chemosensitization, as inclusion of this cellular gene sensitizes a cancer cell to apoptosis after treatment with either radiation therapy or chemotherapy.[67] Initial laboratory studies showed great promise for these types of therapies. Preclinical animal studies, however, showed only modest *in vivo* results.[31, 68] Efficiency and targeting have been shown to be difficult *in vivo*. Methods to increase cancer targeting may make these strategies more amenable for human trials in the future. These strategies include redesigning the adenovirus binding site to increase cancer cell selectivity.[69, 70]

IMMUNE MODULATION

The host immune response has been shown to play a role in cancer eradication. Immune suppression increases the risk of cancer development. In addition to generalized suppression, it has been shown that individuals with head and neck cancer lack an effective local immune response even early in the disease.[71] This immune dysfunction begins at the site of the tumour and progresses systemically with disease progression. This dysfunction occurs as a result of the normal immune system not recognizing the tumour cells. Causes of this include immunological ignorance,[72] downregulation of major histocompatibility complexes and loss of costimulatory receptor and pathways.[73] In some tumours, the cytokine stimulatory pathways (interleukin-2 (IL-2), interferon-gamma and IL-12) that normally upregulate the normal tumour immune response are depressed. One method to break this immune dysregulation is to overexpress the downregulated cytokines. The basis of the first cytokine-based trial for locoregional disease was compelling data from preclinical studies in mice.[74] A subsequent phase I trial using soluble proteins showed three complete responses and three partial responses in 10 patients.[75] All these responses were transient. A subsequent phase II trial showed similar transient responses which did not correlate with dose escalation.[76–78] However, when IL-2 is administered systemically, significant toxicity develops, including capillary leak syndrome. Gene therapy offers the ability to increase local expression and possibly improve tumour response while limiting systemic toxicity. Phase I trials using non-viral plasmids expressing IL-2 have been completed; demonstrating dose escalation safety, subsequent phase II trials are underway.[79] Even if such single agent cytokines do not prove useful, it may be possible to deliver combinations, which activate the immune pathway in a synergistic manner. Many such costimulatory questions are currently being examined in preclinical studies.[80–83] As our understanding of tumour immunity increases, better therapies aimed at reactivating the dysfunctional immune response will develop. Gene therapy may likely play a role in the delivery of such therapies.

RESTORATIVE GENE THERAPY

Restoring the function of a key cellular gene whose dysfunction has resulted in cancer progression can be a major goal of gene therapy. Several strategies to replace dysfunctional genes are currently being tested.[84, 85] The majority of these involve the disrupted apoptotic pathway found in cancer cells. The most common mutations of these genes in squamous cell cancer of the head and neck are *p53* and *p16*. The most extensively studied of these genes in head and neck cancer is suppressor gene *p53*. This gene plays a role in triggering cell death in many different pathways involving apoptosis. Using an adenoviral vector, placed intra-lesionally, this mutated gene was delivered to 33 patients with locally recurrent squamous cell cancer in a phase I trial.[86] The study had two arms, surgical and non-surgical. In the surgical arm, patients received treatment pre-operatively, intra-operatively and post-operatively. Of these patients, four patients were alive and disease-free at one year, nine died of their disease and two died of unrelated causes. In the non-surgical arm, two of 17 had a partial response, six had stable disease and nine had progressive disease. The responses seen were most likely not due to effective replacement of mutated genes because *p53* status did not correlate with response.[86] Gendicine®, a drug with modified adenovirus harbouring *p53* gene was approved by the Chinese State Food and Drug Administration to treat head and neck cancer in China in 2004, becoming the first gene therapy approved for clinical use in humans.[87] However, the western version of Ad-p53 (Advexin®) for the treatment of head and neck cancer was refused for FDA approval in the USA in 2008.[87] The overall efficacy of Ad-p53 therapy in head and neck cancer continues to be closely evaluated.

SELECTIVE ONCOLYTIC VIRUS

Infection with wildtype adenovirus results in viral replication and eventual cell lysis. A therapy that harnesses this virus by only allowing replication in cancer cells would offer a self-propagating treatment that continues to produce virus and lyze cancer cells until a tumour is completely destroyed. Using replication-selective viruses to treat cancer is not entirely new. Initial reports as early as 1912 have used this approach in cancer therapy.[88] With the advent of increased knowledge of the genetic defects in cancer, we have been able to design vectors aimed at only replicating in cancer cells.[89, 90] The ONYX-015 is an adenovirus therapy design to accomplish this goal. ONYX-015 is missing the adenovirus *E1B* gene that normally inhibits the cellular *p53* genes. *p53* cellular expression allows only minimal viral expression. Approximately 60% of squamous cell carcinoma (SCCA) do not express functional *p53*. The ONYX-015 virus will selectively replicate only in SCCA cancers with *p53* mutations. Phase I and II clinical trials have shown significant promise with this strategy.[91–93] The initial phase I trial showed the virus was safe even when given in high doses.[64] Fever and injection site pain were the most common adverse effects. Phase II and III clinical trials are currently underway. In addition to developing this therapy as a single agent treatment, its role in combined therapies is also being examined. Phase II studies have shown this combined approach increases response rates from 33% for chemotherapy (5-fluorouracil (5-FU) and cisplatin) to a 65% response rate when intra-tumoural injections of ONYX-015 are added to the regimen.[93] Another potential advantage of the ONYX-015 vector is that if it is given intravenously it may circulate and offer potential therapy for distant metastasis. The safety of an intravenous delivery approach has been confirmed in phase I trials revealing safe delivery of high titers of viral vectors. The most common side effects were fever, rigours and elevated liver enzymes.[91] To more fully evaluate the potential of this strategy, more work has to be completed in areas of safety and delivery. Overall, however, this self-propagating tumour selective approach offers significant therapeutic promise.

FUTURE RESEARCH

The death of an 10-year-old man in a 1999 adenoviral gene therapy trial in Philadelphia caused scientists around the world to examine more critically the risks of human gene therapy experimentation. Three years later, a three-year-old boy died in France from a leukaemia-like condition, probably as a result of insertional mutagenesis in a retroviral gene therapy trial for SCID. Both of these tragic events have resulted in increased scrutiny for human gene therapy trials. These events have also brought into sharper focus the balance between the risks and the incredible promise of this treatment. However, following these major setbacks, gene therapy seems to have entered a new era with several promising clinical trial results together with recent approval of AAV-based Glybera® as a commercial drug in 2012 in Europe to treat familial lipoprotein lipase deficiency disease. Remarkable progress has been made in the last decade in improving the understanding of the basic science and the complexities of host–vector interaction. The challenge for the next decade continues to be the translation of this new expertise into clinical situations in a safe and effective manner.

KEY POINTS

- Our increased understanding of cellular oncogenesis will lead to the development of novel cancer therapies in the years to come.
- Gene therapy is likely to be a part of these therapies.
- A head and neck oncologist will need to understand both the viral vectors and their strategies of implementation to offer a full range of treatment to the cancer patient.

REFERENCES

1. Check E. A tragic setback. *Nature* 2002; **420**: 116–18.
2. Check E. Regulators split on gene therapy as patient shows signs of cancer. *Nature* 2002; **419**: 545–46.
3. Maguire AM, Simonelli F, Pierce, EA, et al. Safety and efficacy of gene transfer for Leber's congenital amaurosis. *N Engl J Med* 2008; **358**: 2240–48.
4. Cideciyan AV, Hauswirth WW, Aleman TS, et al. Vision 1 year after gene therapy for Leber's congenital amaurosis. *N Engl J Med* 2009; **361**: 725–27.
5. Cartier N, Hacein-Bey-Abina S, Bartholomae CC, et al. Hematopoietic stem cell gene therapy with a lentiviral vector in X-linked adrenoleukodystrophy. *Science* 2009; **326**: 818–23.
6. Cavazzana-Calvo M, Payen E, Negre O, et al. Transfusion independence and HMGA2 activation after gene therapy of human beta-thalassaemia. *Nature* 2010; **467**: 318–22.
7. Hacein-Bey-Abina S, Hauer J, Lim A, et al. Efficacy of gene therapy for X-linked severe combined immunodeficiency. *N Engl J Med* 2010; **363**: 355–64.
8. Bryant LM, Christopher DM, Giles AR, et al. Lessons learned from the clinical development and market authorization of Glybera. *Hum Gene Ther Clin Dev* 2013; **24**: 55–64.
9. Ginn, SL, Alexander IE, Edelstein ML, et al. Gene therapy clinical trials worldwide to 2012: an update. *J Gene Med* 2013; **15**: 65–77.
10. Anderson RD, Haskell RE, Xia H, et al. A simple method for the rapid generation of recombinant adenovirus vectors. *Gene Ther* 2000; **7**: 1034–38.
11. Bergelson JM, Cunningham JA, Droguett G, et al. Isolation of a common receptor for Coxsackie B viruses and adenoviruses 2 and 5. *Science* 1997; **275**: 1320–3.
12. Fasbender A, Lee JH, Walters RW, et al. Incorporation of adenovirus in calcium phosphate precipitates enhances gene transfer to airway epithelia in vitro and in vivo. *J Clin Invest* 1998; **102**: 184–93.
13. Chillon M, Lee JH, Fasbender A, Welsh MJ. Adenovirus complexed with polyethylene glycol and cationic lipid is shielded from neutralizing antibodies in vitro. *Gene Ther* 1998; **5**: 995–1002.
14. Harvey BG, Hackett NR, Ely S, Crystal RG. Host responses and persistence of vector genome following intrabronchial administration of an E1(-)E3(-) adenovirus gene transfer vector to normal individuals. *Mol Ther* 2001; **3**: 206–15.
15. Zaiss AK, Liu Q, Bowen GP, et al. Differential activation of innate immune responses by adenovirus and adeno-associated virus vectors. *J Virol* 2002; **76**: 4580–90.
16. Bristol JA, Gallo-Penn A, Andrews J, et al. Adenovirus-mediated factor VIII gene expression results in attenuated anti-factor VIII-specific immunity in hemophilia A mice compared with factor VIII protein infusion. *Hum Gene Ther* 2001; **12**: 1651–61.
17. Dellorusso C, Scott JM, Hartigan-O'Connor D, et al. Functional correction of adult mdx mouse muscle using gutted adenoviral vectors expressing full-length dystrophin. *Proc Natl Acad Sci USA* 2002; **99**: 12979–84.
18. Hartigan-O'Connor D, Barjot C, Salvatori G, Chamberlain JS. Generation and growth of gutted adenoviral vectors. *Methods Enzymol* 2002; **346**: 224–46.
19. Samulski RJ, Chang LS, Shenk T. Helper-free stocks of recombinant adeno-associated viruses: normal integration does not require viral gene expression. *J Virol* 1989; **63**: 3822–28.
20. Jooss K, Yang Y, Fisher KJ, Wilson JM. Transduction of dendritic cells by DNA viral vectors directs the immune response to transgene products in muscle fibers. *J Virol* 1998; **72**: 4212–23.
21. Ponnazhagan S, Curiel DT, Shaw DR, et al. Adeno-associated virus for cancer gene therapy. *Cancer Res* 2001; **61**: 6313–21.
22. Buchschacher Jr GL, Wong-Staal F. Development of lentiviral vectors for gene therapy for human diseases. *Blood* 2000; **95**: 2499–504.
23. Lewis PF, Emerman M. Passage through mitosis is required for oncoretroviruses but not for the human immunodeficiency virus. *J Virol* 1994; **68**: 510–16.
24. Rosenqvist N, Hard Af Segerstad C, Samuelsson C, et al. Activation of silenced transgene expression in neural precursor cell lines by inhibitors of histone deacetylation. *J Gene Med* 2002; **4**: 248–57.
25. Hanlon L, Barr NI, Blyth K, et al. Long-range effects of retroviral insertion on c-myb: overexpression may be obscured by silencing during tumor growth in vitro. *J Virol* 2003; **77**: 1059–68.
26. Niidome T, Huang L. Gene therapy progress and prospects: nonviral vectors. *Gene Ther* 2002; **9**: 1647–52.
27. Cui FD, Kishida T, Ohashi S, et al. Highly efficient gene transfer into murine liver achieved by intravenous administration of naked Epstein-Barr virus (EBV)-based plasmid vectors. *Gene Ther* 2001; **8**: 1508–13.
28. Stoll SM, Sclimenti CR, Baba EJ, et al. Epstein-Barr virus/human hybrid vector provides high-level, long-term expression of alpha1-antitrypsin in mice. *Mol Ther* 2001; **4**: 122–29.
29. Graham, SM. Gene therapy for cystic fibrosis: perspectives for the otolaryngologist. *Clin Otolaryngol Allied Sci* 1998; **23**: 481–83.
30. Rogers CS, Stoltz DA, Meyerholz DK, et al. Disruption of the CFTR gene produces a model of cystic fibrosis in newborn pigs. *Science* 2008; **321**: 1837–41.
31. Goebel EA, Davidson BL, Graham SM, Kern, JA. Tumor reduction in vivo after adenoviral mediated gene transfer of the herpes simplex virus thymidine kinase gene and ganciclovir treatment in human head and neck squamous cell carcinoma. *Otolaryngol Head Neck Surg* 1998; **119**: 331–36.
32. Goebel EA, Davidson BL, Zabner J, et al. Adenovirus-mediated gene therapy for head and neck squamous cell carcinomas. *Ann Otol Rhinol Laryngol* 1996; **105**: 562–67.
33. Riordan JR, Rommens JM, Kerem B, et al. Identification of the cystic fibrosis gene: cloning and characterization of complementary DNA. *Science* 1989; **245**: 1066–73.
34. Welsh MJ, Ramsay BW, et al. Cystic Fibrosis. In: Scriver CR, Beaudet AL, Sly WS, Valle D (eds). *The metabolic and molecular basis of inherited disease*. 8th ed. New York: McGraw-Hill; 2001, pp. 5121–88.
35. Cystic Fibrosis Foundation. *Patient Registry 2001 Annual Report*. Bethesda, MD: Cystic Fibrosis Foundation; 2002. (Cystic Fibrosis Mutation Database, http://www.genet.sickkids.on.ca/cftr/Home.html)
36. Rommens JM, Iannuzzi MC, Kerem B, et al. Identification of the cystic fibrosis gene: chromosome walking and jumping. *Science* 1989; **245**: 1059–65.
37. Welsh MJ, Anderson MP, Rich DP, et al. Cystic fibrosis transmembrane conductance regulator: a chloride channel with novel regulation. *Neuron* 1992; **8**: 821–29.
38. Davidson TM, Murphy C, Mitchell M, et al. Management of chronic sinusitis in cystic fibrosis. *Laryngoscope* 1995; **105**: 354–58.
39. Graham SM, Launspach JL. Utility of the nasal model in gene transfer studies in cystic fibrosis. *Rhinology* 1997; **35**: 149–53.
40. Crystal RG, McElvaney NG, Rosenfeld MA, et al. Administration of an adenovirus containing the human CFTR cDNA to the respiratory tract of individuals with cystic fibrosis. *Nat Genet* 1994; **8**: 42–51.
41. Welsh MJ, Zabner J, Graham SM, et al. Adenovirus-mediated gene transfer for cystic fibrosis: Part A. Safety of dose and repeat administration in the nasal epithelium. Part B. Clinical efficacy in the maxillary sinus. *Hum Gene Ther* 1995; **6**: 205–18.
42. Rich DP, Anderson MP, Gregory RJ, et al. Expression of cystic fibrosis transmembrane conductance regulator corrects defective chloride channel regulation in cystic fibrosis airway epithelial cells. *Nature* 1990; **347**: 358–63.
43. Zabner J, Petersen DM, Puga AP, et al. Safety and efficacy of repetitive adenovirus-mediated transfer of CFTR cDNA to airway epithelia of primates and cotton rats. *Nat Genet* 1994; **6**: 75–83.
44. Larson JE, Morrow SL, Happel L, et al. Reversal of cystic fibrosis phenotype in mice by gene therapy in utero. *Lancet* 1997; **349**: 619–20.
45. McCray Jr PB. Cystic fibrosis: difficulties of gene therapy. *Lancet* 2001; **358 Suppl**: S19.
46. Rogers CS, Abraham WM, Brogden KA, et al. The porcine lung as a potential model for cystic fibrosis. *Am J Physiol Lung Cell Mol Physiol* 2008; **295**: L240–63.
47. Potash AE, Wallen TJ, Karp PH, et al. Adenoviral gene transfer corrects the ion transport defect in the sinus epithelia of a porcine CF model. *Mol Ther* 2013; **21**: 947–53.
48. Chang GEH, Pezzulo AA, Meyerholz DK, et al. Sinus hypoplasia precedes sinus infection in a porcine model of cystic fibrosis. *Laryngoscope* 2012; **122**: 1898–905.
49. Zabner J. Couture LA, Gregory RJ, et al. Adenovirus-mediated gene transfer transiently corrects the chloride transport defect in nasal epithelia of patients with cystic fibrosis. *Cell* 1993; **75**: 207–16.
50. Hay JG, McElvaney NG, Herena J, Crystal RG. Modification of nasal epithelial potential differences of individuals with cystic fibrosis consequent to local administration of a normal CFTR cDNA adenovirus gene transfer vector. *Hum Gene Ther* 1995; **6**: 1487–96.

51. Knowles MR, Hohneker KW, Zhou Z, et al. A controlled study of adenoviral-vector-mediated gene transfer in the nasal epithelium of patients with cystic fibrosis. *N Engl J Med* 1995; **333**: 823–31.
52. Zabner J, Ramsey BW, Meeker DP, et al. Repeat administration of an adenovirus vector encoding cystic fibrosis transmembrane conductance regulator to the nasal epithelium of patients with cystic fibrosis. *J Clin Invest* 1996; **97**: 1504–11.
53. Zuckerman JB, Robinson CB, McCoy KS, et al. A phase I study of adenovirus-mediated transfer of the human cystic fibrosis transmembrane conductance regulator gene to a lung segment of individuals with cystic fibrosis. *Hum Gene Ther* 1999; **10**: 2973–85.
54. Bellon G, Michel-Calemard L, Thouvenot D, et al. Aerosol administration of a recombinant adenovirus expressing CFTR to cystic fibrosis patients: a phase I clinical trial. *Hum Gene Ther* 1997; **8**: 15–25.
55. Yi SM, Lee JH, Graham S, et al. Adenovirus calcium phosphate coprecipitates enhance squamous cell carcinoma gene transfer. *Laryngoscope* 2001; **111**: 1290–96.
56. Wagner JA, Reynolds T, Moran ML, et al. Efficient and persistent gene transfer of AAV-CFTR in maxillary sinus. *Lancet* 1998; **351**: 1702–03.
57. Wagner JA, Nepomuceno IB, Messner AH, et al. A phase II, double-blind, randomized, placebo-controlled clinical trial of tgAAVCF using maxillary sinus delivery in patients with cystic fibrosis with antrostomies. *Hum Gene Ther* 2002; **13**: 1349–59.
58. Flotte TR, Zeitlin PL, Reynolds TC, et al. Phase I trial of intranasal and endobronchial administration of a recombinant adeno-associated virus serotype 2 (rAAV2)-CFTR vector in adult cystic fibrosis patients: a two-part clinical study. *Hum Gene Ther* 2003; **14**: 1079–88.
59. Sinn PL, Burnight ER, Hickey MA, et al. Persistent gene expression in mouse nasal epithelia following feline immunodeficiency virus-based vector gene transfer. *J Virol* 2005; **79**: 12818–27.
60. Caplen NJ, Alton EW, Middleton PG, et al. Liposome-mediated CFTR gene transfer to the nasal epithelium of patients with cystic fibrosis. *Nat Med* 1995; **1**: 39–46.
61. Gill DR, Southern KW, Mofford KA, et al. A placebo-controlled study of liposome-mediated gene transfer to the nasal epithelium of patients with cystic fibrosis. *Gene Ther* 1997; **4**: 199–209.
62. Alton EW, Stern M, Farley R, et al. Cationic lipid-mediated CFTR gene transfer to the lungs and nose of patients with cystic fibrosis: a double-blind placebo-controlled trial. *Lancet* 1999; **353**: 947–54.
63. Greenlee RT, Hill-Harmon MB, Murray T, Thun M. Cancer statistics, 2001. *CA Cancer J Clin* 2001; **51**: 15–36.
64. Ganly I, Soutar DS, Kaye SB. Current role of gene therapy in head and neck cancer. *Eur J Surg Oncol* 2000; **26**: 338–43.
65. Bi W, Kim YG, Feliciano ES, et al. An HSVtk-mediated local and distant antitumor bystander effect in tumors of head and neck origin in athymic mice. *Cancer Gene Ther* 1997; **4**: 246–52.
66. Frank DK, Frederick MJ, Liu TJ, Clayman GL. Bystander effect in the adenovirus-mediated wild-type p53 gene therapy model of human squamous cell carcinoma of the head and neck. *Clin Cancer Res* 1998; **4**: 2521–28.
67. Thomas SM, Naresh KN, Wagle AS, Mulherkar R. Preclinical studies on suicide gene therapy for head/neck cancer: a novel method for evaluation of treatment efficacy. *Anticancer Res* 1998; **18**: 4393–98.
68. Sewell DA, Li D, Duan L, et al. Safety of in vivo adenovirus-mediated thymidine kinase treatment of oral cancer. *Arch Otolaryngol Head Neck Surg* 1997; **123**: 1298–302.
69. Kasono K, Blackwell JL, Douglas JT, et al. Selective gene delivery to head and neck cancer cells via an integrin targeted adenoviral vector. *Clin Cancer Res* 1999; **5**: 2571–79.
70. Lang S, Zeidler R, Mayer A, et al. Targeting head and neck cancer by GM-CSF-mediated gene therapy in vitro. *Anticancer Res* 1999; **19**: 5335–39.
71. Finke J, Ferrone S, Frey A, et al. Where have all the T cells gone? Mechanisms of immune evasion by tumors. *Immunol Today* 1999; **20**: 158–60.
72. Melero I, Bach N, Chen L. Costimulation, tolerance and ignorance of cytolytic T lymphocytes in immune responses to tumor antigens. *Life Sci* 1997; **60**: 2035–41.
73. Petersson M, Charo J, Salazar-Onfray F, et al. Constitutive IL-10 production accounts for the high NK sensitivity, low MHC class I expression, and poor transporter associated with antigen processing (TAP)-1/2 function in the prototype NK target YAC-1. *J Immunol* 1998; **161**: 2099–105.
74. Forni G, Giovarelli M, Santoni A. Lymphokine-activated tumor inhibition in vivo. I. The local administration of interleukin 2 triggers nonreactive lymphocytes from tumor-bearing mice to inhibit tumor growth. *J Immunol* 1985; **134**: 1305–11.
75. Cortesina G, De Stefani A, Giovarelli M, et al. Treatment of recurrent squamous cell carcinoma of the head and neck with low doses of interleukin-2 injected perilymphatically. *Cancer* 1988; **62**: 2482–85.
76. Cortesina G, De Stefani A, Galeazzi E, et al. Interleukin-2 injected around tumor-draining lymph nodes in head and neck cancer. *Head Neck* 1991; **13**: 125–31.
77. Mattijssen V, De Mulder PH, Schornagel JH, et al. Clinical and immunopathological results of a phase II study of perilymphatically injected recombinant interleukin-2 in locally far advanced, nonpretreated head and neck squamous cell carcinoma. *J Immunother* 1991; **10**: 63–68.
78. Vlock DR, Snyderman CH, Johnson JT, et al. Phase Ib trial of the effect of peritumoral and intranodal injections of interleukin-2 in patients with advanced squamous cell carcinoma of the head and neck: an Eastern Cooperative Oncology Group trial. *J Immunother Emphasis Tumor Immunol* 1994; **15**: 134–39.
79. O'Malley Jr BW, Li D, McQuone SJ, Ralston R. Combination nonviral interleukin-2 gene immunotherapy for head and neck cancer: from bench top to bedside. *Laryngoscope* 2005; **115**: 391–404.
80. Endo S, Zeng Q, Burke NA, He Y, et al. TGF-alpha antisense gene therapy inhibits head and neck squamous cell carcinoma growth in vivo. *Gene Ther* 2000; **7**: 1906–14.
81. Li D, Jiang W, Bishop JS, et al. Combination surgery and nonviral interleukin 2 gene therapy for head and neck cancer. *Clin Cancer Res* 1999; **5**: 1551–56.
82. Day KV, Li D, Liu S, et al. Granulocyte-macrophage colony-stimulating factor in a combination gene therapy strategy for head and neck cancer. *Laryngoscope* 2001; **111**: 801–06.
83. Li S, Ma Z. Nonviral gene therapy. *Curr Gene Ther* 2001; **1**: 201–26.
84. Mobley SR, Liu TJ, Hudson JM, Clayman GL. In vitro growth suppression by adenoviral transduction of p21 and p16 in squamous cell carcinoma of the head and neck: a research model for combination gene therapy. *Arch Otolaryngol Head Neck Surg* 1998; **124**: 88–92.
85. Clayman GL, Frank DK, Bruso PA, Goepfert H. Adenovirus-mediated wild-type p53 gene transfer as a surgical adjuvant in advanced head and neck cancers. *Clin Cancer Res* 1999; **5**: 1715–22.
86. Clayman GL. The current status of gene therapy. *Semin Oncol* 2000; **27**: 39–43.
87. Sheridan C. Gene therapy finds its niche. *Nat Biotechnol* 2011; **29**: 121–28.
88. Ng DP. Case report: cervical cancer regression following rabies vaccination. *Ginnecologia* 1912; **9**: 82.
89. Heise CC, Williams A, Olesch J, Kirn DH. Efficacy of a replication-competent adenovirus (ONYX-015) following intratumoral injection: intratumoral spread and distribution effects. *Cancer Gene Ther* 1999; **6**: 499–504.
90. Heise C, Sampson-Johannes A, Williams A, et al. ONYX-015, an E1B gene-attenuated adenovirus, causes tumor-specific cytolysis and antitumoral efficacy that can be augmented by standard chemotherapeutic agents. *Nat Med* 1997; **3**: 639–45.
91. Nemunaitis J, Cunningham C, Buchanan A, et al. Intravenous infusion of a replication-selective adenovirus (ONYX-015) in cancer patients: safety, feasibility and biological activity. *Gene Ther* 2001; **8**: 746–59.
92. Nemunaitis J, Khuri F, Ganly I, et al. Phase II trial of intratumoral administration of ONYX-015, a replication-selective adenovirus, in patients with refractory head and neck cancer. *J Clin Oncol* 2001; **19**: 289–98.
93. Lamont JP, Nemunaitis J, Kuhn JA, et al. A prospective phase II trial of ONYX-015 adenovirus and chemotherapy in recurrent squamous cell carcinoma of the head and neck (the Baylor experience). *Ann Surg Oncol* 2000; **7**: 588–92.

CHAPTER 4

MECHANISMS OF ANTICANCER DRUGS

Sarah Payne and David Miles

Introduction ... 39	Chemotherapy strategies ... 44
Principles of chemotherapy ... 39	Novel therapies for the future ... 45
Principles of tumour biology ... 39	Immunotherapy ... 48
Classification of chemotherapeutic agents ... 41	Conclusion ... 48
Chemotherapy in head and neck cancer ... 44	References ... 49
Choice of chemotherapy in head and neck cancer ... 44	

SEARCH STRATEGY

Data in this chapter may be updated by a PubMed search using the keywords: mechanisms of chemotherapy; principles of tumour biology, chemotherapy and head and neck cancer; EGFR inhibitors, EGFR monoclonal antibodies; VEGF inhibitors, immunotherapy and head and neck cancer.

INTRODUCTION

Anticancer drugs have been developed and used medically since the 1940s, following the observation that nitrogen mustard gas, a chemical warfare agent used in the Second World War, interfered with haematopoiesis. Since then there have been significant therapeutic advances in the development of anticancer drugs although a cure for all cancer types remains an elusive goal. Alongside trials using more traditional types of chemotherapy, there is also now significant interest in developing more target-directed drug therapies and novel therapies, including immunotherapy.

PRINCIPLES OF CHEMOTHERAPY

Cancer is defined as the uncontrolled growth of cells coupled with malignant behaviour: invasion and metastasis. It arises through a complex interaction between genetic and environmental factors, causing genetic mutations in oncogenes and tumour suppressor genes. Chemotherapy aims to exploit the resulting differences in biological and proliferative characteristics between normal and cancer cells where most cytotoxic drugs preferentially affect dividing cells in tumours.

PRINCIPLES OF TUMOUR BIOLOGY

Cellular kinetics

CELL CYCLE

The cell cycle (**Figure 4.1**) is divided into a number of phases governed by an elaborate set of molecular switches. Normal non-dividing cells are in **G0**. When actively recruited into the cell cycle they then pass through four phases:

1. **G1:** the growth phase in which the cell increases in size and prepares to copy DNA
2. **S (Synthesis):** which allows doubling of the chromosomal material
3. **G2:** a further growth phase before cell division
4. **M (Mitosis):** where the chromosomes separate and the cell divides.

At the end of a cycle the daughter cells can either continue through the cycle, leave and enter the resting phase (**G0**) or become terminally differentiated. Most anticancer agents do not cause cell death during G0.

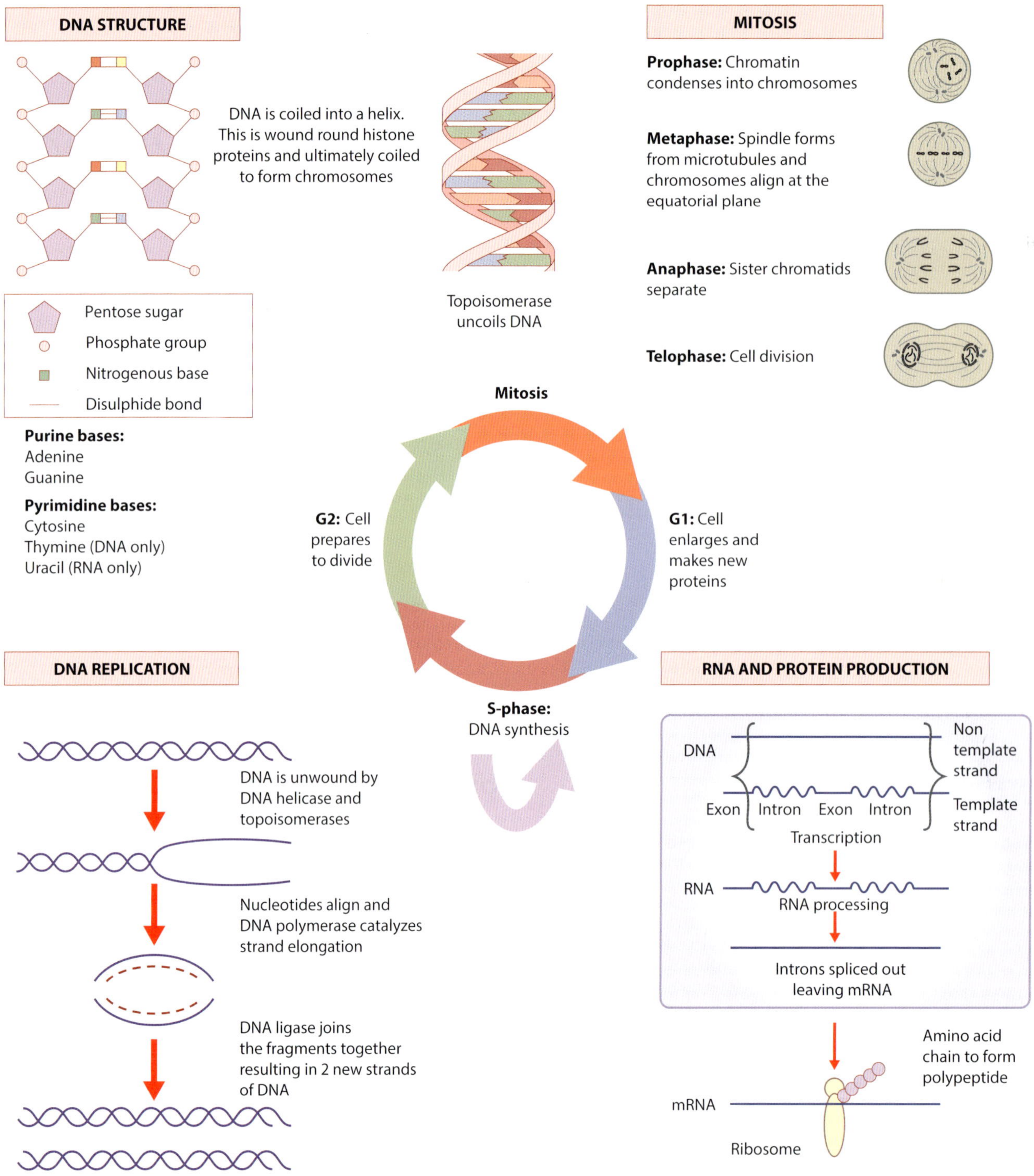

DNA STRUCTURE

DNA is coiled into a helix. This is wound round histone proteins and ultimately coiled to form chromosomes

- Pentose sugar
- Phosphate group
- Nitrogenous base
- Disulphide bond

Purine bases:
Adenine
Guanine

Pyrimidine bases:
Cytosine
Thymine (DNA only)
Uracil (RNA only)

Topoisomerase uncoils DNA

MITOSIS

Prophase: Chromatin condenses into chromosomes

Metaphase: Spindle forms from microtubules and chromosomes align at the equatorial plane

Anaphase: Sister chromatids separate

Telophase: Cell division

Mitosis

G2: Cell prepares to divide

G1: Cell enlarges and makes new proteins

S-phase: DNA synthesis

DNA REPLICATION

DNA is unwound by DNA helicase and topoisomerases

Nucleotides align and DNA polymerase catalyzes strand elongation

DNA ligase joins the fragments together resulting in 2 new strands of DNA

RNA AND PROTEIN PRODUCTION

DNA — Non template strand
Exon | Intron | Exon | Intron — Template strand
Transcription

RNA — RNA processing

Introns spliced out leaving mRNA

mRNA — Ribosome

Amino acid chain to form polypeptide

Figure 4.1 Cell cycle: possible targets for chemotherapy.

TUMOUR GROWTH

The kinetics of any population of tumour cells is regulated by the following:

- **Doubling time:** the cell cycle time, which varies considerably between tissue types
- **Growth fraction:** the percentage of cells passing through the cell cycle at a given point in time, which is greatest in the early stages
- **Cell loss:** which can result from unsuccessful division, death, desquamation, metastasis and migration.

Tumours characteristically follow a sigmoid shaped growth curve, in which tumour doubling size varies with tumour size. Tumours grow most rapidly at small volumes (Gompertzian kinetics). Chemotherapy is therefore more likely to be successful in eradicating a small tumour burden. As they become larger, growth is influenced by the rate of cell death and the availability of blood supply.

Cell signalling

Cells respond to their environment via external signals called growth factors. These interact with cell surface receptors that activate an internal signalling cascade. This ultimately acts at the DNA level through transcription factors that bind to the promoter regions of relevant genes, stimulating the cell cycle and influencing cell division, migration and programmed cell death (apoptosis).

Metastatic spread

A tumour is considered malignant when it has the capacity to spread beyond its original site and invade surrounding tissue. Normally cells are anchored to the extracellular matrix by cell adhesion molecules, including the integrins. Abnormalities of the factors maintaining tissue integrity will allow local invasion and ultimately metastases of the tumour cells.

Mechanism of cell death

There are two main types of cell death: apoptosis and necrosis. Necrotic cell death is caused by gross cell injury, and results in the death of groups of cells within a tissue. Apoptosis is a regulated form of cell death that may be induced or is pre-programmed into the cell (e.g. during development) and is characterized by specific DNA changes and no accompanying inflammatory response. It can be triggered if mistakes in DNA replication are identified. Loss of this protective mechanism would allow mutant cells to continue to divide and grow thereby conserving mutations in subsequent cell divisions. Many cytotoxic anticancer drugs and radiotherapy act by inducing mutations in cancer cells that are not sufficient to cause cell death but that can be recognized by the cell, triggering apoptosis.

FRACTIONAL CELL KILL HYPOTHESIS AND DRUG DOSING

Theoretically the administration of successive doses of chemotherapy will result in a fixed reduction in the number of cancer cells with each cycle.[1] A gap between cycles is necessary to allow normal tissue to recover. Unfortunately these first order dynamics are not observed in clinical practice. Factors such as variation in tumour sensitivity and effective drug delivery with each course result in an unpredictable cell response.

CLASSIFICATION OF CHEMOTHERAPEUTIC AGENTS

Cytotoxic chemotherapy agents have traditionally been classified as phase-specific or non-phase-specific, depending on the effect on the cell cycle. The practical value of this classification is somewhat limited, and as a consequence drugs are more commonly defined by their particular mechanisms of action.

Phase-specific chemotherapy

These drugs (e.g. methotrexate, vinca alkaloids) kill proliferating cells only during a specific part or parts of the cell cycle. Antimetabolites such as methotrexate are more active against cells in the S phase whereas vinca alkaloids are more M-phase-specific. Attempts have been made to time drug administration in such a way that the cells are synchronized into a phase of the cell cycle that renders them especially sensitive to the cytotoxic agent. For example, vinblastine can arrest cells in mitosis. These synchronized cells enter the S phase together and can be killed by a phase-specific agent such as cytosine arabinoside. Most current drug schedules, however, have not been devised on the basis of cell kinetics.

Cell-cycle-specific chemotherapy

Most chemotherapy agents are cell-cycle-specific, meaning that they act predominantly on cells that are actively dividing. They have a dose-related plateau in their cell killing ability because only a subset of proliferating cells remains fully sensitive to drug-induced cytotoxicity at any one time. The way to increase cell kill is therefore to increase the duration of exposure rather than increasing the drug dose.

Some drugs have an equal effect on tumour and normal cells whether they are in the proliferating or resting phase (e.g. alkylating agents, platinum derivatives). They have a linear dose-response curve; that is, the greater the dose of the drug, the greater the fractional cell kill.

According to mechanism

ALKYLATING AGENTS

These include, for example, nitrogen mustards (melphalan and chlorambucil) and oxazaphosphorines (cyclophosphamide and ifosfamide).

These highly reactive compounds produce their effects by covalently linking an alkyl group (R-CH2) to a chemical species in nucleic acids or proteins. The site at which the cross-links are formed and the number of cross-links formed is drug-specific. Most alkylating agents are bipolar (i.e. they contain two groups capable of reacting with DNA). They can thus form bridges between a single strand or two separate strands of DNA, interfering with the action of the enzymes involved in DNA replication. The cell then either dies, or is physically unable to divide or triggers apoptosis. The damage is most serious during the S phase as the cell has less time to remove the damaged fragments.

HEAVY METALS

These include, for example, platinum agents (carboplatin, cisplatin and oxaliplatin).

Cisplatin is an organic heavy metal complex. Chloride ions are lost from the molecule after it diffuses into a cell allowing the compound to cross-link with the DNA strands, mostly to guanine groups. This causes intra- and inter-strand DNA cross-links, resulting in inhibition of DNA, RNA and protein synthesis.

Carboplatin has the same platinum moiety as cisplatin but is bonded to an organic carboxylate group.

Oxaliplatin contains a platinum atom complexed with oxalate and a bulky diaminocyclohexane (DACH) group. It forms reactive platinum complexes that are believed to inhibit DNA synthesis by forming interstrand and intrastrand cross-linking of DNA molecules.

ANTIMETABOLITES

Antimetabolites are compounds that bear a structural similarity to naturally occurring substances such as vitamins, nucleosides or amino acids. They compete with the natural substrate for the active site on an essential enzyme or receptor. Some are incorporated directly into DNA or RNA. Most are phase specific, acting during the S phase of the cell cycle. Their efficacy is usually greater over a prolonged period of time, so they are usually given continuously. There are three main classes: folic acid antagonists, pyrimidine analogues and purine analogues.

Folic acid antagonists

Methotrexate competitively inhibits dihydrofolate reductase, which is responsible for the formation of tetrahydrofolate from dihydrofolate. This is essential for the generation of a variety of coenzymes that are involved in the synthesis of purines, thymidylate, methionine and glycine. A critical influence on cell division also appears to be inhibition of the production of thymidine monophosphate, which is essential for DNA and RNA synthesis. The block in activity of dihydrofolate reductase can be bypassed by supplying an intermediary metabolite, most commonly folinic acid. This is converted to tetrahydrofolate that is required for thymidylate synthetase function (**Figure 4.2**).

Pyrimidine analogues

These drugs resemble pyrimidine molecules and work by either inhibiting the synthesis of nucleic acids (e.g. fluorouracil (**Figure 4.3**)), inhibiting enzymes involved in DNA synthesis (e.g. cytarabine, which inhibits DNA polymerase) or by becoming incorporated into DNA (e.g. gemcitabine), interfering with DNA synthesis and resulting in cell death.

Purine analogues

These are analogues of the natural purine bases and nucleotides. 6 mercaptopurine (6MP) and thioguanine are derivatives of adenine and guanine respectively. A sulphur group replaces the keto group on carbon-6 in these compounds. In many cases, the drugs require initial activation. They are then able to inhibit nucleotide biosynthesis by direct incorporation into DNA.

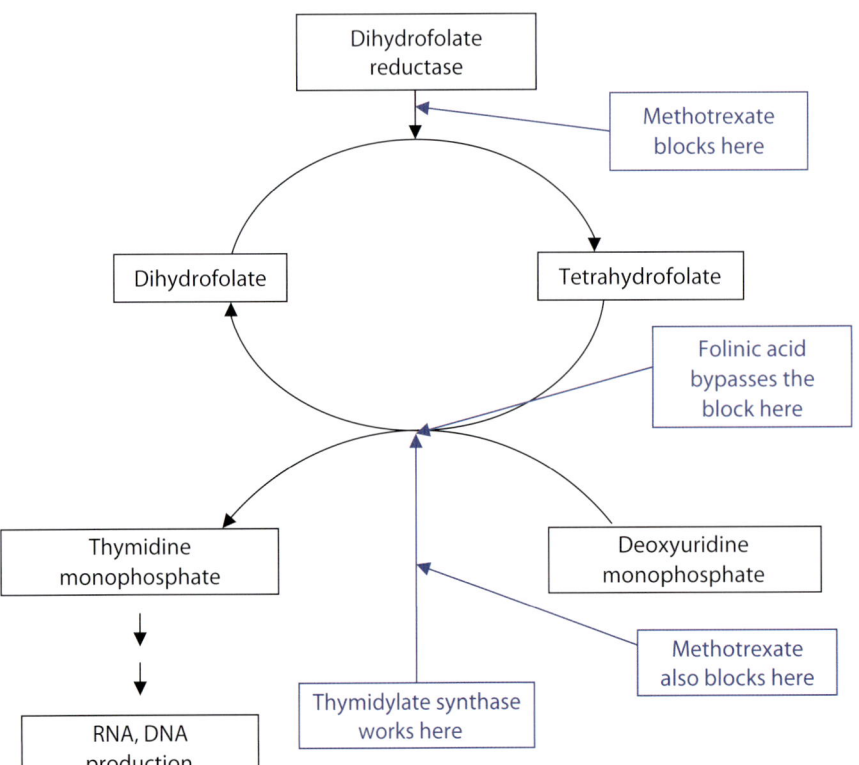

Figure 4.2 Mechanism of action of cytotoxic drugs: methotrexate.

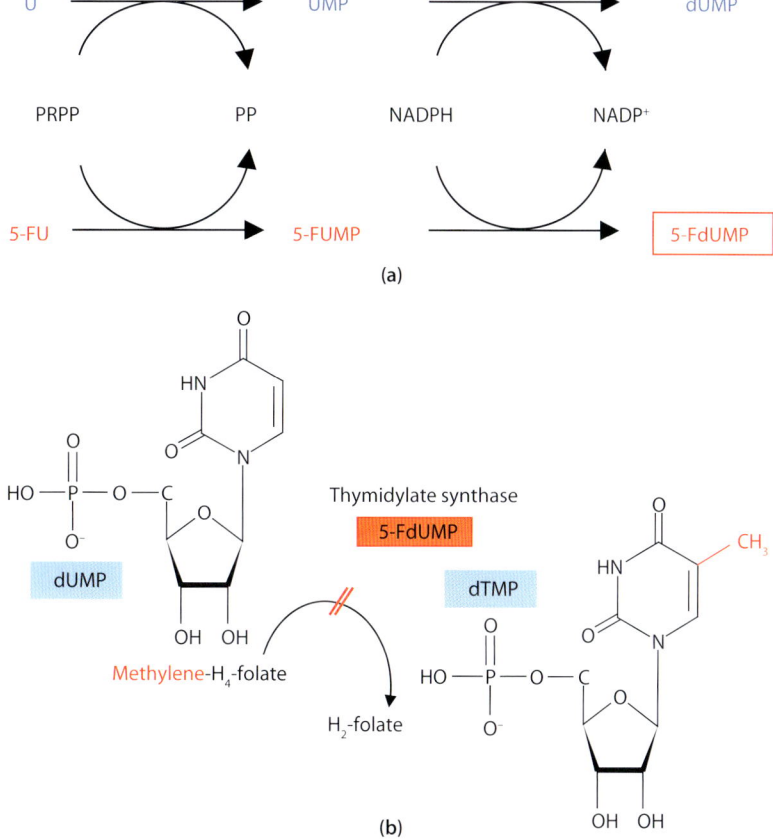

Figure 4.3 Mechanism of action of cytotoxic drugs: fluorouracil. 5-Fluorouracil (5-FU) can participate in many reactions in which uracil would normally be involved. Firstly, it has to be converted to its active form, 5-fluoro-2 deoxyuridine monophosphate (5-FdUMP) **(a)**. This then interferes with DNA synthesis by binding to the enzyme thymidylate synthetase, causing it to be inactivated **(b)**. The binding can be stabilized by the addition of folinic acid. 5-FdUMP, 5-fluorodeoxyuridine monophosphate; 5-FU, 5-fluorouracil; 5-FUMP, binding can be stabilized by the addition of folinic acid. 5-FdUMP, 5-fluorodeoxyuridine monophosphate; 5-FU, 5-fluorouracil; 5-FUMP, 5-fluorouridine monophosphate; dTMP, deoxythymidine monophosphate; dUMP, deoxyuridine monophophase; NADP, nicotinamide adenine dinucleotide phosphate; NADPH, reduced form of nicotinamide adenine dinucleotide phosphate; PP, pyrophosphate; PRPP, 5-phospho-alpha-D-ribose 1-diphosphate; U, uracil; UMP, uridine monophosphate.

CYTOTOXIC ANTIBIOTICS

Most antitumour antibiotics have been produced from bacterial and fungal cultures (often *Streptomyces* species). They affect the function and synthesis of nucleic acids in different ways:

- **Anthracyclines** (e.g. doxorubicin, daunorubicin, epirubicin) intercalate with DNA and affect the topoisomerase II enzyme. This DNA gyrase splits the DNA helix and reconnects it to overcome the torsional forces that would interfere with replication. The anthracyclines stabilize the DNA topoisomerase II complex and thus prevent reconnection of the strands.
- **Actinomycin D** intercalates between guanine and cytosine base pairs. This interferes with the transcription of DNA at high doses. At low doses DNA-directed RNA synthesis is blocked.
- **Bleomycin** consists of a mixture of glycopeptides that cause DNA fragmentation.
- **Mitomycin C** inhibits DNA synthesis by cross-linking DNA, acting like an alkylating agent.

SPINDLE POISONS

Vinca alkaloids

The two prominent agents are vincristine and vinblastine, which act as mitotic spindle poisons. They bind to tubulin, the building block of the microtubules, which inhibits further assembly of the spindle during metaphase, thus inhibiting mitosis. Other examples include vindesine and vinorelbine.

Taxoids

Paclitaxel (Taxol) and docetaxel (Taxotere) promote assembly of microtubules and inhibits their disassembly. Direct activation of apoptotic pathways has also been suggested to be critical to the cytotoxicity of this drug.[2]

TOPOISOMERASE INHIBITORS

Topoisomerases are responsible for altering the 3D structure of DNA by a cleaving/unwinding/rejoining reaction. They are involved in DNA replication, chromatid segregation and transcription. It has previously been considered that the efficacy of topoisomerase inhibitors in the treatment of cancer was based solely on their ability to inhibit DNA replication. It has now been suggested that drug efficacy may also depend on the simultaneous manipulation of other cellular pathways within tumour cells.[3] The drugs are phase-specific and prevent cells from entering mitosis from G2. There are two broad classes:

1. **Topoisomerase I inhibitors (e.g. irinotecan and topetcan).** These bind to the enzyme-DNA complex, stabilizing it and preventing DNA replication.
2. **Topoisomerase II inhibitors (e.g. etoposide).** These stabilize the complex between topoisomerase II and DNA that causes strand breaks and ultimately inhibits DNA replication.

CHEMOTHERAPY IN HEAD AND NECK CANCER

Chemotherapy is regularly employed in the management of head and neck cancer. It has not changed the cure rates of locally advanced head and neck cancer. It has, however, allowed improved organ preservation when combined with radiotherapy and has led to a reduction in rates of distant metastases.

CHOICE OF CHEMOTHERAPY IN HEAD AND NECK CANCER

The single agents active in head and neck cancer, with response rates between 15% and 40%, include methotrexate, cisplatin, carboplatin, fluorouracil, ifosfamide, bleomycin, paclitaxel, and docetaxel. Cisplatin is one of the most active drugs against squamous head and neck cancer.[4] Taxoids and gemcitabine are gaining favour and are being incorporated into many current drug trials.

CHEMOTHERAPY STRATEGIES

Combination chemotherapy

Combinations of cytotoxic agents are widely used for many cancers and may be more effective than single agents. Possible explanations for this include:

- exposure to agents with different mechanisms of action and non-overlapping toxicities
- reduction in the development of drug resistance
- the ability to use combinations of drugs that may be synergistic.

Combination chemotherapy in head and neck cancers usually includes cisplatin.

Adjuvant chemotherapy

This is the administration of chemotherapy after curative surgery or radiotherapy, in patients considered to be at high risk of relapse. The intention is to eradicate micrometastatic disease. Randomized trials assessing the use of adjuvant chemotherapy for the patients with head and neck squamous carcinoma do not suggest a significant survival benefit.[5] [Level 1 evidence]

Neoadjuvant chemotherapy (induction chemotherapy)

Neoadjuvant, or induction chemotherapy, is the use of chemotherapy prior to definitive surgery or radiotherapy in patients with locally advanced disease. The intention is to reduce the tumour bulk before definitive treatment and hence improve local and distant control of the disease. This will also achieve greater organ preservation and overall survival.

Numerous phase III trials have considered the benefit of neoadjuvant chemotherapy. Unfortunately their approaches have been quite heterogeneous, making meta-analysis difficult.[6] VA Laryngeal Cancer Study Group evaluated induction chemotherapy (cisplatin/5-FU) followed by radiotherapy versus surgery and radiotherapy among patients with stage III/IV disease.[7] Chemotherapy responders subsequently received radiotherapy; non-responders underwent laryngectomy. An 85% chemotherapy response rate was documented in this study. No survival differences were noted, but there was the benefit of laryngeal preservation among responders. Subsequent studies have continued to examine the topic of organ preservation. The Radiation Therapy Oncology Group (RTOG) 91-11 trial randomized 547 patients with stage III/IV disease to three treatment arms; induction cisplatin/5-FU followed by radiotherapy, cisplatin-based concurrent chemoradiotherapy, and radiotherapy alone.[8] Concurrent chemoradiation was superior to induction chemotherapy or radiotherapy alone in terms of organ preservation and locoregional control. No differences were observed in relation to overall or disease-free survival comparing induction therapy or concurrent chemoradiation. Taxane-platinum-based combinations have more recently been evaluated and appear superior to cisplatin-5-FU in terms of overall survival, progression free survival, locoregional failure and distant failure for loco-regionally advanced disease.[9, 10] Toxicity, however, can be quite high.

The role of neoadjuvant/induction chemotherapy continues to remain controversial. It is currently considered on a case-by-case basis and further studies are planned. [Level 1 evidence]

Concurrent chemoradiation (CRT)

This involves the synchronous use of chemotherapy and radiotherapy. In the context of head and neck cancer, this is often used after definitive surgery. The rationale is that chemotherapy can sensitize tumours to radiotherapy by inhibiting tumour repopulation, preferentially killing hypoxic cells, inhibiting the repair of sublethal radiation damage, sterilizing micrometastatic disease outside of the radiation fields and decreasing the tumour mass, which leads to improved blood supply and reoxygenation.

Fractionated radiotherapy, in turn, may sensitize tumours to chemotherapy by inhibiting the repair of drug-induced damage and by decreasing the size of the tumour mass, leading to improved blood supply and enhanced drug delivery. Patients with high-risk features (positive lymph nodes, positive margins, extracapsular spread (ECS), perineural/vascular invasion) have been shown to demonstrate an improved 5-year survival by 13%.[11] Two pivotal phase III studies (RTOG 9501 and EORTC 22931) demonstrated improved locoregional control with the addition of chemotherapy in high-risk patients[12, 13] where a post-hoc analysis of the trials confirmed that ECS of tumour and positive margins were the most important indications for adjuvant chemoradiation.[14] At present there is still debate regarding the optimum chemoradiotherapy programme that should become the standard of care.

Local, regional and metastatic recurrence

Patients with localized squamous cell carcinoma of the head and neck are treated with potentially curative therapy. Unfortunately, many patients develop recurrent disease. The recurrence rate in early-stage squamous cell head and neck cancer is approximately 10–20%,[15] whereas the recurrence rate in locally advanced is approximately 50% with a predominance of locoregional failure.[15–18] Patients with recurrent or metastatic squamous cell head and neck cancer have a poor prognosis with median overall survival of under 1 year[19] and is mostly made up of patients who have recurrence after initial treatment for localized disease. A small percentage of patients with localized recurrence can be treated with curative intent, but the vast majority receive palliative treatment with systemic therapy.

Chemotherapy in the first line setting is associated with disappointing opportunities for disease control. Objective response rates to commonly used therapies (including methotrexate, docetaxel, paclitaxel) drop off to well under 20% and median survival in phase 3 trials has been reproducibly reported at approximately 5–6 months.[19–23]

There is clearly a need to explore novel therapies to try to improve disease outcomes. Options being explored include targeted therapies and immunotherapy.

NOVEL THERAPIES FOR THE FUTURE

Despite the introduction of new cytotoxic drugs, the management of advanced head and neck cancer remains challenging. Over the last years interest has focused on the role of novel agents with more targeted mechanisms of action or agents that are able to manipulate the immune system to provide tumour control (immunotherapy).

Targeted therapy

Targeted therapy aims to specifically act on a well-defined target or biologic pathway that, when inactivated, causes regression or destruction of the malignant process.

The main strategies of research have looked at the use of monoclonal antibodies or targeted small molecules.

Monoclonal antibodies

Monoclonal antibodies can be derived from a variety of sources:

- murine – mouse antibodies
- chimeric – part mouse/part human antibodies
- humanized – engineered to be mostly human
- human – fully human antibodies.

Murine monoclonal antibodies may themselves induce an immune response that limits repeated administration. Humanized and, to a lesser extent, chimeric antibodies are less immunogenic and can be given repeatedly.

There are several proposed mechanisms of action of monoclonal antibodies as anticancer agents.[24] These include:

- Direct effects may include:
  - induction of apoptosis
  - blocking of the receptors needed for cell proliferation/function
  - anti-idiotype antibody formation, determinants amplifying an immune response to the tumour cell.
- Indirect effects may include:
  - antibody dependent cellular cytotoxicity (ADCC, conjugating the 'killer cell' to the tumour cell)
  - complement-mediated cellular cytotoxicity (fixation of complement leading to cytotoxicity).

A desirable target for MAbs would have the following properties:

- Wide distribution on tumour cells
- High level of expression
- Bound to tumour, allowing cell lysis
- Absent from normal tissues
- Trigger activation of complement on MAb binding
- Remains unchanged following antibody binding to ensure it remains visible to the immune system (i.e. is not internalized or shredded).

Antibodies have also been used as vectors for the delivery of drugs and radiopharmaceuticals to a target of tumour cells.

Interest in the development of antibodies for solid tumours has become increasingly popular, especially with respect to the epidermal growth factor receptor and the vascular endothelial growth factor receptor.

Epidermal growth factor receptor biology

Epidermal growth factor receptor (EGFR) biology is a 170 kD transmembrane protein composed of an extracellular ligand-binding domain, a transmembrane lipophilic region and an intracellular protein tyrosine kinase domain (**Figure 4.4**). When a substrate binds to the receptor, the

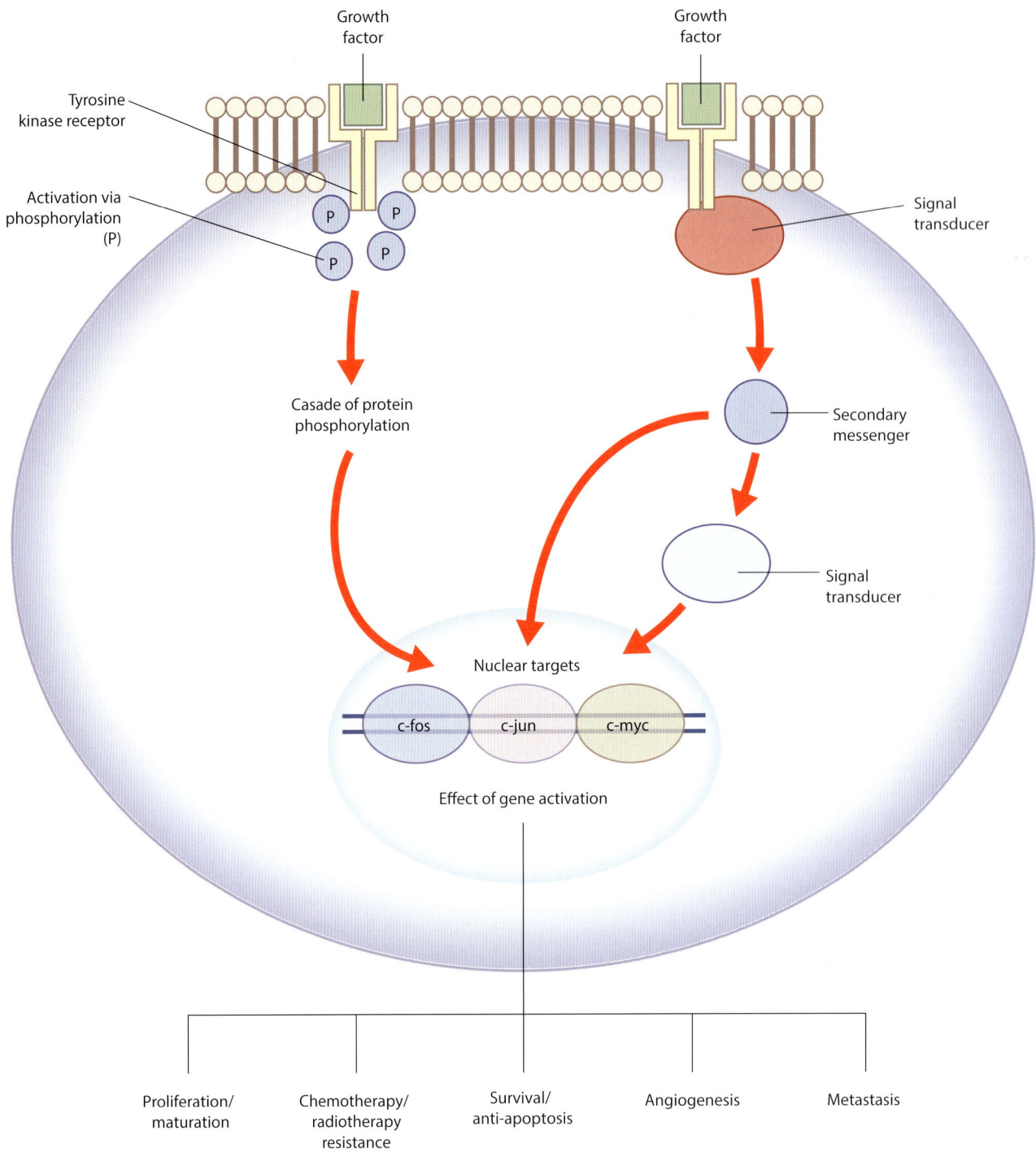

Figure 4.4 Simplified epidermal growth factor receptor signal transduction pathways and opportunities for intervention. GRB2, growth factor receptor binding protein 2; MAPK, mitogen-activated protein kinase; MEK, MAPK/extracellular signal related kinase; SOS, guanine nucleotide exchange factor (son of sevenless); c-fos, c-jun and c-myc, nuclear targets involved in gene transcription/cell cycle progression; P, phosphate; TGFa, transformation growth factor a; PI3-K, phosphotidyinositol 3; AKT, serine/threonine kinase, prosurvival protein; STAT, signal transducing activation of transcription.

ligand-receptor complex dimerizes and is internalized by the host cell. This activates an intracellular protein kinase by autophosphorylation, which in turn activates signal transduction pathways, influencing cell function. This can lead to cell proliferation, as well as invasion and metastasis.

Several investigators have described amplification of the EGFR gene and overexpression of the EGFR surface membrane protein in a large number of human cancers, including squamous cell carcinoma of the head and neck.[25] Overexpression is associated with increased proliferative capacity and metastatic potential and is an independent indicator of poor prognosis.[26] Blockade of the EGFR pathway has been shown to inhibit the proliferation of malignant cells and also appears to influence angiogenesis, cell motility and invasion.[27] Various strategies have been investigated to manipulate EGFR.

Monoclonal antibodies against EGFR

An example of a monoclonal antibody developed against EGFR is the chimeric IgG antibody cetuximab which has the binding affinity equal to that of the natural ligand and can effectively block the effect of epidermal growth factor and transforming growth factor α.[6, 8] It also causes internalization of EGFR and targets the cytotoxic immune effector cells towards EGFR expressing tumour cells.[27]

LOCOREGIONALLY ADVANCED HEAD AND NECK CANCER

The addition of cetuximab to radiotherapy has been shown to improve locoregional control and survival when compared to primary radiotherapy alone for patients with locoregionally advanced head and neck cancer.[28, 29] Randomized controlled trials however have not demonstrated superiority or non-inferiority of cetuximab-radiotherapy compared to concomitant chemoradiotherapy and so cetuximab-radiotherapy is considered an option for treatment in patients who are not candidates for the chemotherapy used with chemo-radiotherapy.[30] [Level 1 evidence]

RECURRENT/METASTATIC HEAD AND NECK CANCER

The addition of cetuximab to platinum-based chemotherapy prolongs median overall survival, progression-free survival, best overall response rate, disease control rate and time to treatment failure in patients with recurrent or metastatic squamous cell carcinoma of the head and neck compared to platinum-based chemotherapy alone and is an option to consider in the first line setting.[31, 32] [Level 1 evidence]

Targeted small molecules against EGFR

Gefitinib (Iressa) and erlotinib (Tarceva) are orally active epidermal growth factor receptor tyrosine kinase inhibitors (EGFR-TKI) that block the EGFR signalling cascade, thereby inhibiting the growth, proliferation and survival of many solid tumours. They have activity as single agents in patients with recurrent or metastatic head and neck cancer, and have an acceptable safety profile compared with conventional chemotherapy.[33, 34] So far, results in locally advanced disease have not demonstrated additional benefit with these drugs.[35, 36]

Inhibitors of angiogenesis

Angiogenesis (**Figure 4.5**) is the process of new blood vessel formation, triggered by hypoxia and regulated by numerous stimulators and inhibitors. It is vital for cancer development.

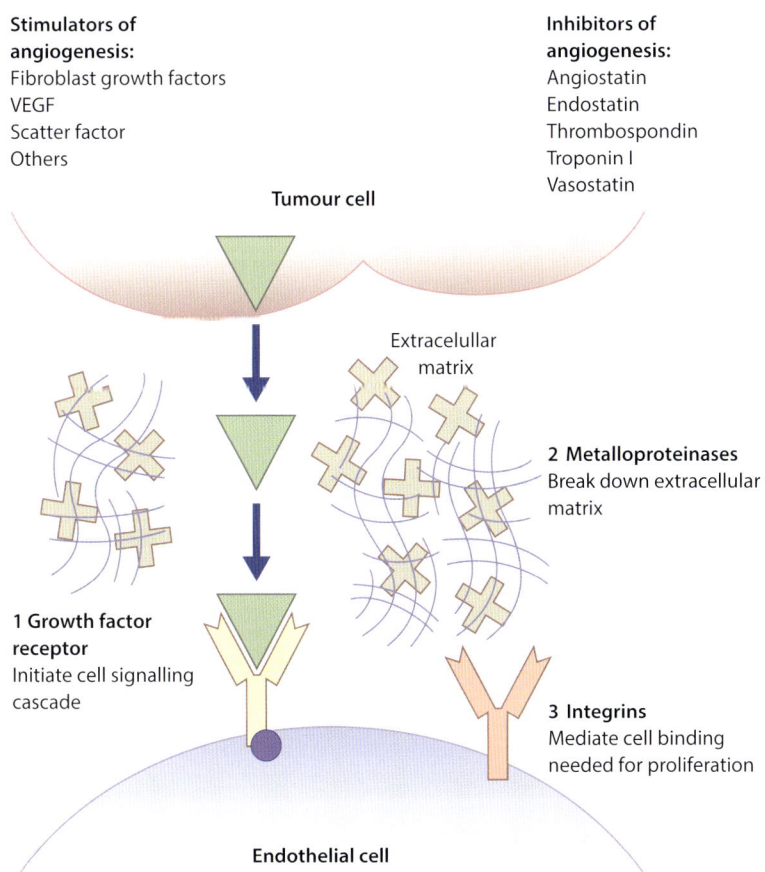

Figure 4.5 Schematic representation of possible anti-angiogenesis targets, including natural stimulators and inhibitors.

A tumour cannot exceed beyond 2–3mm³ without inducing a vascular supply. New vessels develop on the edge of the tumour and then migrate into the tumour. This process relies on degradation of the extracellular matrix surrounding the tumour by matrix metalloproteinases such as collagenase that are expressed at high levels in some tumour and stromal cells. Angiogenesis is then dependent on the migration and proliferation of endothelial cells.

It has been found that anti-angiogenic agents tend to be cytostatic rather than a cytotoxic, hence stabilizing the tumour and preventing spread. As a consequence they may be valuable for use in combination with cytotoxic drugs, as maintenance therapy in early stage cancers or as adjuvant treatment after definitive radiotherapy or surgery. There is evidence to support the fact that suppressing angiogenesis can maintain metastases in a state of dormancy.[34]

Vascular endothelial growth factor receptor

Vascular endothelial growth factor (VEGF) receptor VEGF is a multifunctional cytokine released in response to hypoxia and is an important stimulator of angiogenesis. It binds to two structurally related transmembrane receptors present on endothelial cells. High VEGF protein and receptor expression has been demonstrated in certain head and neck cancers and is associated with a higher tumour proliferation rate and worse survival.[37]

Monoclonal antibodies against VEGFR

Bevacizumab (Avastin) is a humanized murine monoclonal antibody targeting VEGF. It is the first anti-angiogenic drug to have induced a survival advantage in cancer therapy.[38] The use of bevacizumab in head and neck cancer is supported by information derived in preclinical trials.[39] Currently clinical trials are exploring the feasibility and the therapeutic potential of a combination of bevacizumab and EGFR-targeted drugs.[40,41]

IMMUNOTHERAPY

Immune checkpoint inhibitors are a new class of systemic agents being increasingly used in oncology. They function by interrupting the immunosuppressive pathways, called inhibitory checkpoints, which are normally used by tumour cells to prevent detection and elimination by the host immune system.[42,43] Molecular targets of immune checkpoint inhibitors are found on T cells and include cytotoxic T-lymphocyte antigen-4 (CTLA-4) and programmed cell death protein 1 (PD-1) receptor. A third common target is PD-L1, which is found on both tumour and immune cells and is the corresponding ligand to PD-1.[42,43] There is interest in the role of immune checkpoint inhibitors particularly in tumours with high levels of endogenous PD-L1 expression, which include some head and neck squamous cell carcinomas.[42] Current available clinical trial-generated evidence suggests that immune checkpoint inhibitors present a promising new opportunity for a small number of patients with very advanced disease who progress on standard first-line chemotherapy. Objective response rates to immune checkpoint inhibitors are around 20% in patients who have progressed on first-line chemotherapy combinations for recurrent or metastatic squamous head and neck cancer irrespective of PD-L1 expression status.[42] Data suggest that PD-L1 expression correlates with better efficacy to immune-checkpoint inhibitors; however, this correlation is not definitive and no other reliable biomarker has currently been identified for effectively selecting optimally responsive patient subgroups.[42,44] Ongoing studies are investigating the role of immune checkpoint inhibitors in patients with both locally advanced disease and metastatic disease.

CONCLUSION

The majority of conventional chemotherapeutic agents cause cell death by directly inhibiting the synthesis of DNA or interfering with its function. This means that they are often not tumour-specific and are associated with considerable morbidity. Trials have demonstrated that combination chemotherapy regimens can cause dramatic regression of head and neck tumours, especially when used concomitantly with radiotherapy. Unfortunately this has not been associated with an increase in survival rates.

There is now considerable excitement over the development of new target-directed cytotoxic agents. These have been developed to modulate or inhibit specific molecular targets critical to the development of or control of cancer cells. Particular interest has focused on the field of monoclonal antibody development, particularly in relation to the epidermal growth factor. Other drugs affecting signal transduction, programmed cell death, transcription regulation, matrix invasion, angiogenesis and immune modulation are currently involved in clinical trials. The results of these are eagerly awaited and will potentially radically change current therapeutic strategies.

FUTURE RESEARCH

The effect of chemotherapy on non-metastatic head and neck cancers is still being evaluated. The optimum combination of chemotherapeutic agents and the timing of their use in relation to surgery have not been defined, especially in combination with radiotherapy. As this continues to be assessed, significant advances are being made in relation to more specific targeted therapies. The results of clinical trials with these new agents and their incorporation into management regimens are eagerly awaited.

KEY POINTS

- Traditional chemotherapy agents interfere with DNA synthesis and function and are classified according to their mechanism of action.
- Unfortunately they are associated with significant side-effect profiles.
- The role of chemotherapy in head and neck cancer is still being defined but there is increasing popularity of concurrent chemotherapy and radiotherapy regimens.
- Current research, however, is now focusing on more novel approaches including molecular targeted therapy and immunotherapy.
- Strategies recently have particularly looked at the use of monoclonal antibodies.
- There are also drugs being designed that specifically influence signal transduction, cell cycle regulation, apoptosis, matrix invasion and angiogenesis.

REFERENCES

1. Skipper HE, Schabel FM, Jr., Wilcox WS. Experimental evaluation of potential anticancer agents. Xiii. On the criteria and kinetics associated with 'curability' of experimental leukemia. *Cancer Chemother Rep* 1964; **35**: 1–111.
2. Herscher LL, Cook J. Taxanes as radiosensitizers for head and neck cancer. *Curr Opin Oncol* 1999; **11**(3): 183–86.
3. Guichard SM, Danks MK. Topoisomerase enzymes as drug targets. *Curr Opin Oncol* 1999; **11**(6): 482–89.
4. Henk JM. Concomitant chemoradiation for head and neck cancer: saving lives or grays? *Clin Oncol (R Coll Radiol)* 2001; **13**(5): 333–35.
5. Pignon JP, Bourhis J, Domenge C, Designe L. Chemotherapy added to locoregional treatment for head and neck squamous-cell carcinoma: three meta-analyses of updated individual data. MACH-NC Collaborative Group. Meta-analysis of chemotherapy on head and neck cancer. *Lancet* 2000; **355**(9208): 949–55.
6. Forastiere AA, Metch B, Schuller DE, et al. Randomized comparison of cisplatin plus fluorouracil and carboplatin plus fluorouracil versus methotrexate in advanced squamous-cell carcinoma of the head and neck: a Southwest Oncology Group study. *J Clin Oncol* 1992; **10**(8): 1245–51.
7. The Department of Veterans Affairs Laryngeal Cancer Student Group. Induction chemotherapy plus radiation compared with surgery plus radiation in patients with advanced laryngeal cancer. *N Engl J Med* 1991; **324**: 1686–90.
8. Forastiere AA, Goepfert H, Maor M, et al. Concurrent chemotherapy and radiotherapy for organ preservation in advanced laryngeal cancer. *N Engl J Med* 2003; **349**: 2091–98.
9. Lorch JH, Goloubeva O, Haddad RI, et al. Induction chemotherapy with cisplatin and fluorouracil alone or in combination with docetaxel in locally advanced squamous-cell cancer of the head and neck: long-term results of the TAX 324 randomised phase 3 trial. *Lancet Oncol* 2011; **12**(2): 153–59.
10. Blanchard P, Bourhis J, Lacas B, et al. Taxane-cisplatin-fluorouracil as induction chemotherapy in locally advanced head and neck cancers: an individual patient data meta-analysis of the meta-analysis of chemotherapy in head and neck cancer group. *J Clin Oncol* 2013; 31(23): 2854–60.
11. Burchhardt DM, Sukari A. Chemotherapy in head and neck squamous cell cancer. In: Fribley AM, ed. *Targeting Oral Cancer*. New York, NY: Springer International; 2016.
12. Cooper JS, Pajak TF, Forastiere AA, et al. Postoperative concurrent radiotherapy and chemotherapy for high-risk squamous-cell carcinoma of the head and neck. *N Engl J Med* 2004; **350**: 1937–44.
13. Bernier J, Domenge C, Ozsahin M, et al. Postoperative irradiation with or without concomitant chemotherapy for locally advanced head and neck cancer. *N Engl J Med* 2004; **350**: 1945–52.
14. Bernier J, Cooper JS, Pajak TF, et al. Defining risk levels in locally advanced head and neck cancers: a comparative analysis of concurrent postoperative radiation plus chemotherapy trials of the EORTC (22931) and RTOG (9501). *Head Neck* 2005; **27**: 843–50.
15. Zhang X, Yang H, Lee JJ, et al. MicroRNA-related genetic variations as predictors for risk of second primary tumor and/or recurrence in patients with early-stage head and neck cancer. *Carcinogenesis* 2010; **31**(12): 2118–23.
16. Argiris A, Karamouzis MV, Raben D, Ferris RL. Head and neck cancer. *Lancet* 2008; **371**(9625): 1695–709.
17. Baselga J, Trigo JM, Bourhis J, et al. Phase II multicenter study of the antiepidermal growth factor receptor monoclonal antibody cetuximab in combination with platinum-based chemotherapy in patients with platinum-refractory metastatic and/or recurrent squamous cell carcinoma of the head and neck. *J Clin Oncol* 2005; **23**(24): 5568–77.
18. Cho BC, Keum KC, Shin SJ, et al. Weekly docetaxel in patients with platinum refractory metastatic or recurrent squamous cell carcinoma of the head and neck. *Cancer Chemother Pharmacol* 2009; **65**(1): 27–32.
19. Price KA, Cohen EE. Current treatment options for metastatic head and neck cancer. *Curr Treat Options Oncol* 2012; **13**(1): 35–46.
20. Vermorken JB, Trigo J, Hitt R, et al. Open-label, uncontrolled, multicenter phase II study to evaluate the efficacy and toxicity of cetuximab as a single agent in patients with recurrent and/or metastatic squamous cell carcinoma of the head and neck who failed to respond to platinum-based therapy. *J Clin Oncol* 2007; **25**(16): 2171–77.
21. Mehra R, Seiwert TY, Mahipal A, et al. Efficacy and safety of pembrolizumab in recurrent/metastatic head and neck squamous cell carcinoma (R/M HNSCC): pooled analyses after long-term follow-up in KEYNOTE-012. *J Clin Oncol* 2016; **34**(Suppl): 6012.
22. Bauml J, Seiwert TY, Pfister DG, et al. Preliminary results from KEYNOTE-055: pembrolizumab after platinum and cetuximab failure in head and neck squamous cell carcinoma (HNSCC). *J Clin Oncol* 2016; **34**(Suppl): 6011.
23. Machiels JP, Haddad RI, Fayette J, et al. Afatinib versus methotrexate as second-line treatment in patients with recurrent or metastatic squamous-cell carcinoma of the head and neck progressing on or after platinum-based therapy (LUX-head & neck 1): an open-label, randomised phase 3 trial. *Lancet Oncol* 2015; **16**(5): 583–94.
24. Green MC, Murray JL, Hortobagyi GN. Monoclonal antibody therapy for solid tumors. *Cancer Treat Rev* 2000; **26**(4): 269–86.
25. Maurizi M, Almadori G, Ferrandina G, et al. Prognostic significance of epidermal growth factor receptor in laryngeal squamous cell carcinoma. *Br J Cancer* 1996; **74**(8): 1253–57.
26. Perrotte P, Matsumoto T, Inoue K, et al. Anti-epidermal growth factor receptor antibody C225 inhibits angiogenesis in human transitional cell carcinoma growing orthotopically in nude mice. *Clin Cancer Res* 1999; **5**(2): 257–65.
27. Specenier P, Vermorken JB. Cetuximab in the treatment of squamous cell carcinoma of the head and neck. *Expert Rev Anticancer Ther* 2011; **11**(4): 511–24.
28. Bonner JA, Harari PM, Giralt J, et al. Radiotherapy plus cetuximab for squamous cell carcinoma of the head and neck. *N Engl J Med* 2006; **354**(6): 567–78.
29. Bonner JA, Harari PM, Giralt J, et al. Radiotherapy plus cetuximab for locoregionally advanced head and neck cancer: 5-year survival data from a phase 3 randomised trial, and relation between cetuximab-induced rash and survival. *Lancet Oncol* 2010; **11**(1): 21–28.
30. Winquist E, Agbassi C, Meyers BM et al. Head and Neck Disease Site Group. *Current Oncol* 2017; **24**(2): e157–e62.
31. Burtness B, Goldwasser MA, Flood W, et al. Phase III randomized trial of cisplatin plus placebo compared with cisplatin plus cetuximab in metastatic/recurrent head and neck cancer: an Eastern Cooperative Oncology Group study. *J Clin Oncol* 2005; **23**(34): 8646–54.
32. Vermorken JB, Mesia R, Rivera F, et al. Platinum-based chemotherapy plus cetuximab in head and neck cancer. *N Engl J Med* 2008; **359**(11): 1116–27.

33. Cohen EE, Rosen F, Stadler WM, et al. Phase II trial of ZD1839 in recurrent or metastatic squamous cell carcinoma of the head and neck. *J Clin Oncol* 2003; **21**(10): 1980–87.
34. Caponigro F. Rationale and clinical validation of epidermal growth factor receptor as a target in the treatment of head and neck cancer. *Anticancer Drugs* 2004; **15**(4): 311–20.
35. Martins RG, Parvathaneni U, Bauman JE, et al. Cisplatin and radiotherapy with or without erlotinib in locally advanced squamous cell carcinoma of the head and neck: a randomized phase II trial. *J Clin Oncol* 2013; **31**(11): 1415–21.
36. Gregoire V, Hamoir M, Chen C, et al. Gefitinib plus cisplatin and radiotherapy in previously untreated head and neck squamous cell carcinoma: a phase II, randomized, double-blind, placebo-controlled study. *Radiother Oncol* 2011; **100**(1): 62–69.
37. Kyzas PA, Stefanou D, Batistatou A, Agnantis NJ. Potential autocrine function of vascular endothelial growth factor in head and neck cancer via vascular endothelial growth factor receptor-2. *Mod Pathol* 2005; **18**(4): 485–94.
38. Hurwitz H, Fehrenbacher L, Novotny W, et al. Bevacizumab plus irinotecan, fluorouracil, and leucovorin for metastatic colorectal cancer. *N Engl J Med* 2004; **350**(23): 2335–42.
39. Caponigro F, Formato R, Caraglia M, et al. Monoclonal antibodies targeting epidermal growth factor receptor and vascular endothelial growth factor with a focus on head and neck tumors. *Curr Opin Oncol* 2005; **17**(3): 212–17.
40. Caponigro F, Basile M, de Rosa V, Normanno N. New drugs in cancer therapy, National Tumor Institute, Naples, 17–18 June 2004. *Anticancer Drugs* 2005; **16**(2): 211–21.
41. Argiris A, Kotsakis AP, Hoang T, et al. Cetuximab and bevacizumab: preclinical data and phase II trial in recurrent or metastatic squamous cell carcinoma of the head and neck. *Ann Oncol* 2013; **24**(1): 220–25.
42. Schoppy DW, Sunwoo JB. Immunotherapy for head and neck squamous cell carcinoma. *Hematol Oncol Clin North Am* 2015; **29**(6): 1033–43.10.1016/j.hoc.2015.07.009
43. Baksh K, Weber J. Immune checkpoint protein inhibition for cancer: preclinical justification for CTLA-4 and PD-1 blockade and new combinations. *Semin Oncol* 2015; **42**(3): 363–77.10.1053/j.seminoncol.2015.02.015
44. Argiris A, Harrington KJ, Tahara M, et al. Evidence-based treatment options in recurrent and/or metastatic squamous cell carcinoma of the head and neck. *Front Oncol* 2017; 7: 72.

CHAPTER 5

RADIOTHERAPY AND RADIOSENSITIZERS

Christopher D. Scrase, Stewart G. Martin and David A.L. Morgan

Introduction 51	Concurrent chemotherapy.. 55
Fractionation.. 52	Neo-adjuvant chemotherapy 55
Radiosensitizers... 53	Targeted therapies 55
Bioreductive drugs... 54	References 57

SEARCH STRATEGY

Data in this chapter may be updated by a Medline search using the keywords: neoplasms, radiotherapy, fractionation, radiation-sensitizing agents, chemotherapies, hypoxia and immunotherapies.

INTRODUCTION

Radiotherapy is the therapeutic use of ionizing radiation, typically usually high-energy X-rays (photons). Other modalities (e.g. protons) may be used to optimize the therapeutic effect by seeking to optimize the conformality to the target volume. As the name implies, the radiation interacts with matter by ejecting electrons from their orbits, resulting in ionization. The ejected particles interact with further atoms, ejecting further electrons and causing a cascade of ionizations after each initial interaction. In biological material, the free radicals that result, primarily from interactions with water molecules, are highly reactive and are particularly damaging to the cell when they interact with DNA. In total, about 100 distinct lesions have been identified amongst which strand breaks (i.e. sugar-phosphate backbone damage) predominate in terms of importance at the cellular level. Traditionally, the main cause of cell death following radiation was thought to result from direct damage to the DNA. This has gradually been modified over the last few years as an increasing number of studies have shown that ionizing radiation also targets the plasma membrane where it can initiate multiple signal transduction pathways, many of which lead to radiation-induced apoptosis (e.g. hydrolysis of the membrane phospholipid sphingomyelin by the enzyme sphingomyelinase resulting in the generation of ceramide). DNA damage in mammalian cells triggers three pathways: cell cycle arrest, DNA repair and apoptosis. Historically, three types of damage have been recognized: sublethal damage (SLD), potentially lethal damage (PLD) and irreparable or lethal damage. These categories may not reflect different types of damage, but instead reflect the category of repair processes that act to modify the radiation-induced lesions. If the DNA damage is particularly severe then cell death may result, usually when the cell attempts to divide.

The fact that cell death occurs at a time after the actual exposure to irradiation, depending on the time of cell division (and also upon the tissue structure and life span of the mature functional cells), explains one of the most important clinical observations about radiotherapy, that tissues that are dividing rapidly manifest the effects of radiation sooner than those where cell division is slow. Tissues such as bone marrow, skin and the mucosa of the upper aerodigestive tract manifest the effects of radiation within days (i.e. they are classed as 'acute-reacting' tissues). Connective tissue, bone and neural tissue may only show the effect years later, hence being defined as 'late-reacting' tissues. Squamous head and neck cancers, as might be expected, behave as an acute-reacting tissue, like the squamous mucosa from which they originate. In addition to the kinetics (turnover rate) of the population as a whole, the response of tissues and organs is also dependent upon inherent cellular radiosensitivity. The sensitivity of the cell to radiation is determined to some degree by its state of maturity and its functional role. Generally speaking, immature cells are considerably more sensitive to radiation than mature cells and as mitotic activity increases (metabolic activity, proliferation), sensitivity also increases. There is general agreement as to which of the target cells is responsible for acute effects (stem cells of rapidly dividing tissues), but the target cells that determine the late effects have not been defined clearly. In general, if any clonogens from acute responding normal (healthy) tissues survive they can rapidly repopulate and replace lost cells. Late-reacting tissues do not have this ability to repopulate rapidly and therefore whilst most acute reactions heal, most late reactions, if anything, may continue to progress with time. It is the severity of predicted late effects that can limit the delivered dose of radiation. Differentiating between acute and late effects is exploited in the concept of fractionation.

FRACTIONATION

The differences between 'acute-reacting' and 'late-reacting' tissues are thus very important to the science of fractionation in radiotherapy. At low single doses, tumour and early-responding tissues are more sensitive than late-responding tissues (more cells are in cycle). At high doses, the non-dividing late-responding cell response that compensates for tissue loss is slow and therefore organs appear more intrinsically radiosensitive than rapidly dividing tumour and early-responding tissues.

A fraction is the individual dose of radiation delivered at a single session of radiotherapy; in the treatment of head and neck cancer a total course of radiotherapy will take several weeks and consist of numerous fractions. The fraction size, measured in physical dose, is traditionally and almost invariably constant throughout a course of radiotherapy. In conventional radiotherapy, fractions are given once a day, five days per week typically for 4–6 weeks. This accords with normal working practices, rather than being founded on a sound scientific basis, and alternative fractionation schedules have been much studied in recent years.

In general, the relationship between the dose of radiation in a single fraction and the number of cells killed approximates closely to a straight line on a semi-logarithmic graph, conventionally drawing dose arithmetically on the x-axis and surviving fraction of cells on a declining logarithmic scale on the negative y-axis. This is shown in **Figure 5.1**. It should be noted though that while the general relationship is linear, at the lowest doses this is not so, and the line is curved (i.e. it has a 'shoulder'). For most cells, the range in which this shoulder applies is close to most widely used fraction sizes (in other words around 2 Gy) and this has important implications for clinical practice.

The extent of the 'curviness' of the graph varies with many factors. Most importantly for day-to-day routine radiotherapy, late-reacting tissues generally have a more 'curvy' graph than do acute-reacting ones and therefore increasing the fraction size even modestly tends to have a greater effect on late-reacting as opposed to early-reacting tissues: in other words there is more 'late-reacting' tissue damage. The shoulder on the graph is a reflection of the capacity for DNA to repair damaged cells. Thus cells from patients with ataxia-telangiectasia show almost no curve. This is because these patients are deficient in certain mechanisms that act to repair DNA.

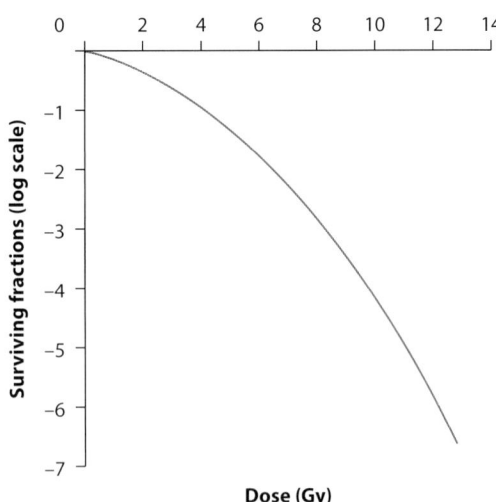

Figure 5.1 Typical radiation dose-response curve following a single radiation exposure. Note that the radiation dose (x-axis) is a linear scale, while surviving fraction (y-axis) is logarithmic. The effect for small doses is relatively 'curvy' compared to that for higher. The consequences of this are explained in the text.

The importance of this shoulder region to radiotherapy relates to the fact that as long as sufficient time elapses between fractions, a subsequent dose of radiation has the same shaped survival curve as an initial dose, including the shoulder (i.e. full repair of the initial damage has occurred). Thus, if the shoulder is considerable, the net effect of two doses is very much less than if the same total physical dose was given as a single fraction. The general shape of the cell survival curves, including the shoulder, is probably best described by the linear quadratic equation:

$$SF = N/No = e^{-(\alpha D + \beta D^2)} \quad \text{or} - \ln SF = \alpha D + \beta D^2$$

In this equation, No is the number of cells in the population originally and N is the number surviving after irradiation with dose D, with N/No representing the surviving fraction (SF). Only two parameters, α (the initial slope) and β (the terminal slope) are required to describe the dose–response curve. Absolute values of α and β are not well known, but the alpha/beta ratio (i.e. the dose at which the contribution to killing from the α component or nonreparable damage, is equal to that of the β component or reparable damage) has been identified with a reasonable degree of approximation for numerous tissues. In general, the α/β ratio tends to be low for late-reacting tissues, and for these the shoulder on the graph is considerable, whereas it is high for acute-reacting tissues, where the shoulder is less marked. When this is translated into practice, the total effect is more fraction size-dependent for late-reacting tissues than for acute-reacting tissues. Thus, for example, the effect achieved with a dose of 70 Gy in 2 Gy fractions given over 7 weeks will differ less from the effect of the same total dose in fractions of 1 Gy for acute-reacting tissues than it will for late-reacting tissues. There will be more 'sparing' of late-reacting tissues by breaking the same total dose up into a greater number of smaller fractions. Having said this, because of the ability of early-reacting tissue to repopulate rapidly, these comparisons are only valid if the overall treatment time is the same for the different schedules. Otherwise the ability of head and neck squamous cell carcinomas (SCC) like acute-reacting normal tissues will negate the intended benefit. This will necessitate a shorter inter-fraction interval for the schedule of many small fractions. This interval still needs to be long enough though for adequate repair of sublethal damage to occur if the full sparing effect on late reactions by reducing factor size is to be seen.

The corollary of this is that by using many small fractions it will be possible to give a higher total dose, but without increasing the amount of late damage, whereas a greater effect will be seen on acute-reacting tissues and thus squamous head and neck cancer cells themselves. This is the theory of 'hyperfractionation'.

The theoretical benefits of hyperfractionation were confirmed in clinical practice in a randomized trial comparing a 'conventional' schedule of 70 Gy in 7 weeks with a hyperfractionated schedule, in which two fractions of 1.15 Gy were given daily, also over 7 weeks, so that the total dose was 80.5 Gy.[1] Better local control was achieved in the experimental hyperfractionation arm, with no observed increase in late side effects. This approach to improve the therapeutic ratio, however, has not gained wide acceptance in the radiotherapy community largely on logistical grounds.

Other ways of modifying radiotherapy fractionation schedules have also been explored in head and neck cancer. The problem of tumour clonogen proliferation during a prolonged course of radiotherapy has already been alluded to. The consequence of this is that if radiotherapy schedules are prolonged for reasons such as holidays, machine breakdowns and so on, tumour control is adversely affected. A number of retrospective series have confirmed this (it cannot, of course, be ethically tested in a prospective randomized trial). The evidence has been strong enough for the Royal College of Radiologists in the UK to publish guidelines on how to minimize the harm done by such interruptions.[2] Of course, if prolongation of schedules is detrimental in terms of control of tumours, it might well be expected that to shorten the overall time ('acceleration') would result in better control. A number of trials have also been conducted to test this hypothesis. The evidence is convincing that shortening overall time is beneficial in terms of tumour control. One problem that all the trials of accelerated treatments have faced is that increasing the effect on the tumour by shortening the overall time also increases the effect on the adjacent normal mucosa, and severe acute reactions are to some extent unavoidable. The problem is compounded by the fact that very severe acute reactions sometimes lead, rather more than might be expected, to an increase in the extent of late reactions, and this has rather limited the extent to which improvements in outcomes can be achieved by shortening radiotherapy schedules. Even so, the many studies published in this area leave little doubt that it is indeed possible to employ the strategy of acceleration without incurring too high a penalty in terms of normal tissue effects, although the optimum strategy in terms of fraction size, interval, number of fractions per day, number of treatment days per week, total dose and overall time, remains elusive.[3] To some extent this debate has been superseded by efforts focussing on systemic agents and their interactions with conventional fractionation.

RADIOSENSITIZERS

As well as modifying the physical parameters of radiotherapy (time and dose through fractionation as well as the modality), other interesting avenues of exploration have involved using various agents to enhance its effects. It is reasonable to refer to all of these as 'radiosensitizers', although the scientific purists may argue about the appropriate use of this term. Numerous types of agent have been used, with varying degrees of success. The rapid advances that are currently occurring in molecular oncology have made and continue to make this an area of fruitful exploration.

The evidence that emerged from laboratory studies that hypoxic cells were relatively radioresistant to X-rays when compared with fully oxygenated ones prompted the earliest attempts at radiosensitization. As the centre of many tumours are necrotic, it was felt that this was evidence that the proliferation of cells within tumours led to growth outstripping blood supply (i.e. the diffusion distance for oxygen is <150–200 μm from an adjacent blood vessel) and that therefore it was logical to assume that there would be many chronically hypoxic cells within tumours (hypoxia can also be acute (momentary) due to the transient opening and closing of tumour blood vessels). It was hypothesized that chronic and acute hypoxia would make the centre of tumours relatively radioresistant. Modern technology has made it possible to precisely measure oxygen levels in tumour and normal tissues, and this hypothesis has indeed been confirmed. If this hypoxic effect could be overcome, radiotherapy would be more likely to be successful. A significant amount of time and effort has been expended over many years testing whether this could be achieved in clinical practice. Many diverse strategies have been employed and new strategies are continually being investigated.

The earliest avenue explored was probably the most direct. In an attempt to ensure greater oxygenation within tumours, patients were placed in hyperbaric oxygen tanks during radiotherapy. Clinical trial results failed to demonstrate that this approach yielded better results than 'standard' radiotherapy. There have been reports that increasing the haemoglobin level could be beneficial as anaemic patients may respond less well to radiotherapy.[4, 5] Initial studies suggested that those patients given transfusions and hyperbaric oxygenation (HBO) did better than those given HBO alone. However, subsequent results from the DAHANCA study group did not support this.[6] Similarly, studies with recombinant erythropoietin (EPO) have discounted the anticipated benefits of using EPO to correct anaemia with such patients actually faring less well.[7]

An alternative approach used the agent nicotinamide, which is thought to dilate small vessels to improve blood flow through the vascularized parts of tumours (i.e. to deal with 'acute' hypoxia), in combination with patients breathing carbogen (a mixture of oxygen and carbon dioxide) during radiotherapy in an attempt to ensure good oxygenization (and thus deal with the 'chronic' hypoxia). Combined with accelerated radiotherapy this approach, called ARCON, was tested in a phase II trial with promising local control.[8] A phase III trial showed locoregional benefits with acceptable toxicity but no gain in overall survival.[9]

A number of pharmaceutical approaches have been used in an attempt to make hypoxic tumour cells more radiosensitive through more direct actions on the cellular structure. True sensitizers have little or no cytotoxic action without radiation, but significantly enhance the efficiency of radiation killing when present during radiation. Apparent sensitizers include a variety of compounds, such as antibiotics, alkylating agents and antimetabolites, that act by diverse mechanisms. In general, sensitizers can be regarded as agents that increase the lethal effects of radiation. They should show a gain between tumours and normal tissues (i.e. to enhance the therapeutic ratio). Such a therapeutic gain could result from selective uptake (concentration), a differential absorption rate or biological half-life. Ideally they should be effective at systemically nontoxic dosages, thereby minimizing side effects.

Halogenated pyrimidines (IUdR, BrdUrd) work by being incorporated into actively dividing tumour cells to a greater degree than slowly dividing (cell maintenance) normal tissues. Appreciable quantities need to accumulate for several generations for them to be incorporated to set up stresses in the DNA and make them more susceptible to radiation damage. They therefore seem to be particularly useful with tumours having a high growth fraction and high labelling index. BrdUrd is also a sensitizer to ultraviolet (UV) radiation, therefore skin may be the limiting tissue. This is less of a problem with IUdR.

Hypoxic cell sensitizers are electron affinic and act to increase the sensitivity of radioresistant hypoxic cells by mimicking O_2. They are not rapidly metabolized and therefore have time to diffuse into poorly vascularized areas.

Cells are more responsive to sensitizers if they are depleted of their natural radioprotector, glutathione (GSH), a radical scavenger that eliminates reactive radicals before they have the opportunity of causing DNA damage. This may be accomplished by incubation with thiol binding agents, such as diamide and diethyl maleate, or inhibition of GSH synthesis with buthionine sulfoximine before delivering the radiation. The effectiveness of hypoxic cell sensitizers is measured in terms of the enhancement ratio (ER).

The nitroimidazoles have been extensively evaluated as potential radiosensitizers. One of the first compounds investigated was metronidazole, a trichomonacide. At 10 mM, an ER of 1.6 was obtained with no effect on aerated cells. The large concentrations required led to investigations for more effective derivatives and other nitroimidazole drugs appeared more promising in this respect.

Although many hypoxic cell sensitizers have been investigated (including misonidazole, metronidazole, benznidazole, desmethylmisonidazole, etanidazole, pimonidazole, nimorazole, ornidazole and doranidazole), controversy exists regarding the role of these agents in conventional radiotherapy. So far only one major randomized trial of the many that have been performed has shown a therapeutic benefit and in this Danish trial, a benefit for nimorazole use during radiotherapy of pharyngeal and supraglottic laryngeal cancers when combined with conventional therapy was shown.[10] Although nimorazole has been shown to be of potential benefit, these sensitizers generally show greater benefit in situations where large, single doses of radiation are given (e.g. intra-operative radiotherapy, interstitial radiotherapy, radiosurgery). As only this one trial out of many has shown a statistically significant benefit, the international clinical community remains unconvinced that there is a true benefit for the use of nitroimidazoles, and they are still not widely used outside Denmark to this day.

BIOREDUCTIVE DRUGS

Adjuncts to radiation, which are not true radiosensitizers, include bioreductive drugs and prodrugs. These agents, which are relatively non-toxic to cells under normal oxygenated conditions, when reduced intracellularly form cytotoxic agents. Bioreduction is favoured under hypoxic conditions due to cytochrome P450 and DT diaphorase reductases. The efficiency of bioreductive drugs may be increased further by inducing increased hypoxia in tumours through the use of vasoactive drugs, such as hydralazine. This induces vasodilation in normal tissues thus diverting blood from the tumour. Bioreductive drugs can be divided into three major groups: the quinones, nitroaromatics and organic nitroxides.

Specific examples of bioreductive drugs include mitomycin C (a quinone) and tirapazamine/SR-4233 (an organic nitroxide). The former is an antitumour antibiotic that is bioreduced to form products that cross-link DNA. It is cell cycle non-specific, is more toxic to hypoxic than aerated cells, is usually administered i.v. and is rapidly cleared from plasma (half-life, 10–15 minutes). The drug does not cross the blood–brain barrier and the major toxicity is myelosuppression. Indoloquinone EO9 is a synthetic analogue of mitomycin C (MMC), which was expected to have similar properties to MMC, but fundamental differences have emerged; for example, EO9 is a much better substrate for DT-diaphorase (DTD) and it has the ability to redox cycle more readily than MMC after reduction by purified DTD. In addition, EO9 has the ability to increase the cytotoxicity to hypoxic cells 49-fold over MMC. The overall capacity of the tumour to metabolize EO9 has been suggested to be the most important determinant for EO9 activity. This, along with the rapid clearance of EO9 in humans, has been suggested as one of the reasons for the disappointing results obtained from phase II clinical trials.[11, 12] Another more efficient quinone, porfiromycin, when assessed in a phase III study showed no benefit over MMC.[13]

A more promising group of bioreductive drugs is the organic nitroxide of which tirapazamine (TPZ) is the most widely known. The benefits, however, in the phase II trials have not been translated into clinical benefits in the phase III setting.[14] It is thought that some of the failure to demonstrate clinical benefit in phase III trials may reflect the need to better identify patient populations with high levels of tumour hypoxia. In addition there is excessive metabolic consumption as it penetrates the extravascular space so that its apparently impressive selectivity for hypoxic cells from 50–300-fold *in vitro* diminishes to a more modest range of 3–5-fold *in vivo*.

To date, as with the hypoxic cell sensitizers mentioned above, there is thus little clinical evidence from large randomized trials of bioreductive agents showing increased efficacy when combined with conventional radiotherapy. There remains a fundamental need to develop drugs that balance small molecule stability against reactivity in a reduction/oxidation equilibrium, so that the intended toxicity is only imparted in tissues that are truly hypoxic. We also need to be mindful that hypoxia is not such a prominent prognostic factor in all forms of head and neck squamous cell carcinomata.[15]

A variety of emerging techniques with more tailored effects on hypoxic tissues are under active investigation:[16]

1. Vascular disrupting agents (VDAs) alter tumour blood flow via activity on the colchicine binding site on tubulin, leading to changes in endothelial cell shape and increased vascular permeability
2. 'New' radiosensitizing agents, e.g. Bevacizumab, a humanized monoclonal antibody specific for vascular endothelial growth factor (VEGF)
3. Drugs that target hypoxia-induced proteins, e.g., Immunomodulating drugs.[17]

CONCURRENT CHEMOTHERAPY

A clinically more successful (therapeutic) strategy than trying to overcome hypoxia thus far has in fact been the rather more empirical approach of simply combining 'conventional' chemotherapy with radiotherapy. Squamous head and neck cancers show a clinical response to a number of chemotherapeutic agents, so the strategy of combining such drugs with radiotherapy seems justifiable.

Many randomized trials have been conducted in which a combination of chemotherapy and radiotherapy have been compared with radiotherapy alone. Although the majority of these trials have been relatively small, when combined there are vast numbers of patients, and the technique of 'meta-analysis' has been applied. This has convincingly shown that the addition of chemotherapy, standardly cisplatin, does give better results than those achieved with radiotherapy alone[18] and confirmed with longer follow-up and later studies.[19, 20] The counterargument has been made that the same could be achieved by simply giving more radiotherapy. However, it is known that beyond a certain level the incidence of complications rises rapidly if additional radiotherapy is given, which is why the doses used in common practice are as they are. It has proved feasible to give chemotherapy in combination with such doses and, to date, there is no strong suggestion that this does lead to an unacceptable increase in damage to normal tissue. The same cannot be said of the proposed strategy of simply giving higher doses of radiotherapy (other than in the context of fractionation trials, particularly hyperfractionation, as discussed previously).[21]

NEO-ADJUVANT CHEMOTHERAPY

Combined chemotherapy and radiotherapy schedules have been tested in randomized controlled trials against a policy of primary surgery for moderately advanced laryngeal and hypopharyngeal cancers. In fact, in these trials the drugs have been given before radiotherapy, so are certainly not acting as 'true' radiosensitizers but are mentioned here for completeness. They have been shown to be no less effective than radical surgery in terms of survival, but confer the advantage of enabling preservation of a functioning larynx in a substantial number of patients.[22, 23] Such 'organ preservation' represents a significant advance in radiotherapy of head and neck cancer, and continues to attract a great deal of attention, with trials of different drug/radiation schedules, and involving other head and neck sites. However there is still no proven benefit in providing chemotherapy prior to definitive chemoradiotherapy for advanced head and neck cancer in terms of improved survival. As such, most consider that further studies are needed to identify potential patient subgroups that may benefit from this treatment intensification.

TARGETED THERAPIES

Our understanding of the molecular mechanisms that drive cancer cells has grown at an accelerating pace within recent years. This has led to the emergence of a range of drugs that act against cancer cells in a more targeted way than the cytotoxic agents that have been the mainstay of chemotherapy in the past. Because of their specificity, such agents hold the promise of being much less toxic than conventional chemotherapy.

Among these new classes of agents there are some interesting suggestions of synergy with radiation. In head and neck cancer, one target has so far attracted significant attention, the epidermal growth factor receptor, EGFR (*erb*B1, HER1). This is one of a family of transmembrane receptor tyrosine kinases, other members being HER2/*neu* (*erb*B2), HER3 (*erb*B3) and HER4 (*erb*B4). Ligand-binding receptor dimerization occurs, which induces a conformational change in the intracellular kinase domain, thereby inducing a cascade of phosphorylation events or activation of signal transduction (e.g. activation of the MAPK or ras signal transduction pathway). As implied by its name and as might be expected in a tumour arising from squamous epithelium, overexpression of this receptor is a very frequent event in head and neck squamous carcinomas and carries with it a worse prognosis.[24] Its overexpression, with or without gene amplification, is often associated with increased production of EGFR ligands, particularly epidermal growth factor (EGF) and transforming growth factor alpha (TGFα). Selective compounds have been developed that target either the extracellular ligand-binding region of the EGFR or the intracellular tyrosine kinase region.

The first of these target the extracellular ligand-binding domain using a monoclonal antibody approach. Cetuximab is a chimeric 'humanized' monoclonal antibody that competitively binds to EGFR (it has a 2-log higher affinity for EGFR than TGFα and EGF). Once bound to the receptor, the complex is internalized and the receptor thereby rendered inactive. Cetuximab has undergone clinical trials in head and neck cancer used both as monotherapy and as combined therapy (radiation, chemotherapy). Results from a large randomized phase III trial were very impressive in that improved locoregional control (24.4 months versus 14.9 months) and improved survival (49 months versus 29.3 months) have been obtained with little increase in toxicity[25] as compared with radiotherapy alone. Cetuximab may, in addition to exerting antiproliferative effects by inhibiting the MAPK signal transduction pathway, act as an antiangiogenic agent and therefore exert radiosensitizing effects via mechanisms described above.[26] Despite these impressive results concurrent chemotherapy using cisplatin remains the gold standard for locally advanced head and neck cancer unless renal function precludes the administration of platinum.

The second approach available to target receptor tyrosine kinases is via the use of small molecules that compete for the ATP binding site of the kinase domain. The low molecular weight of these molecules may allow them to penetrate tumours better and they can be administered orally making them suitable for chronic therapy. Several agents, including gefitinib and erlotinib, showed promise in clinical trials as monotherapy[27, 28] and in combination with standard chemotherapy. Unfortunately these anticipated benefits do not appear to have been translated into studies with radiotherapy.[29]

Another approach to targeted therapies is through the evasion of programmed cell death and immortalization. It is in this area that there is most excitement for new avenues of therapy for treating and improving the outcomes for head and neck squamous cell carcinomata as alluded to earlier.[17] A recently published study in recurrent squamous cell carcinoma of the head and neck has shown the potential for significant activity with anti-PD1 monoclonal antibodies.[30] The question now being evaluated is whether such activity can be translated into the curative setting alongside radiotherapy.

KEY POINTS

- Conventional radiotherapy uses photons that both directly and indirectly damage the DNA, through the production of ions and free radicals. The majority of damage induced by photons is via this 'indirect action'.
- Although the DNA is generally considered to be the most important target for radiation-induced damage, this dogma is gradually being amended to include effects on other cellular constituents, particularly cellular membranes.
- Tissues that are dividing rapidly manifest the effects of radiation sooner than those where cell division is slow. In addition to the kinetics (turnover rate) of the population as a whole, the response of tissues and organs is also dependent upon inherent cellular radiosensitivity. The sensitivity of the cell to radiation is determined to some degree by its state of maturity and its functional role, immature rapidly proliferating cells generally being more radiosensitive than slowly proliferating fully differentiated cells.
- The response of a tumour to radiotherapy is dependent upon inherent radiosensitivity, tumour cell repopulation, redistribution through the cell cycle (G2/M is the most sensitive phase of the cell cycle, late-S phase is the most radioresistant), repair of radiation induced damage and reoxygenation of tumour tissues between fractions. These parameters represent the '5 Rs of radiotherapy'.
- A fraction is the individual dose of radiation delivered at a single session of radiotherapy. In the treatment of head and neck cancer, a total course of radiotherapy will take several weeks and comprise numerous fractions. In conventional radiotherapy, fractions are given once a day, five days per week. The fraction size is, almost invariably, constant throughout a course of radiotherapy. Increasing the fraction size tends to have a greater effect (altered severity) on late-reacting as opposed to early-reacting tissues.
- Hypoxic cells (those under low O_2 tension) are relatively resistant to X-rays when compared with fully oxygenated ones. Chronic and acute hypoxia make tumours relatively radioresistant. If such hypoxia is overcome, radiotherapy is more likely to be successful.
- Many approaches to overcome tumour hypoxia have been evaluated – these include improving blood flow through the vascularized parts of tumours and pharmaceutical approaches to make hypoxic tumour cells more radiosensitive (radiosensitizer drugs).
- The nitroimidazoles have been extensively evaluated as potential radiosensitizers; however, controversy exists regarding the role of these agents in conventional radiotherapy. So far, only one major randomized trial, of the many that have been performed, has shown a therapeutic benefit (with nimorazole).
- Adjuncts to radiation, which are not true radiosensitizers, include bioreductive drugs. These agents are reduced intracellularly to form cytotoxic agents. A number have been evaluated in head and neck cancers.
- Perhaps a clinically more successful (therapeutic) strategy than trying to overcome hypoxia has been the rather more empirical approach of simply combining 'conventional' chemotherapy with radiotherapy. Meta-analyses have not been able to clearly identify which of the various adjuvant chemotherapy options is the best, although a strategy of giving cisplatin concurrently or in rapidly alternating sequences, with radiotherapy (perhaps with other drugs as well) has consistently emerged as the 'front runner'.
- Novel, molecularly targeted, agents hold the promise of being much less toxic than conventional chemotherapy. Of the agents under evaluation, cetuximab, a humanized monoclonclonal antibody that competitively binds to EGFR, has undergone clinical trials in head and neck cancer used both as monotherapy and as combined therapy (radiation, chemotherapy). Results from a large randomized trial were very impressive in that improved locoregional control and reduced mortality have been obtained with little increase in toxicity. Other areas of optimism are in the field of immunotherapy where studies have demonstrated significant gains in the metastatic setting. Whether this will translate into clinical benefit in the curative setting with radiotherapy remains to be seen.

REFERENCES

1. Horiot JC, le Fur R, N'Guyen T, et al. Hyperfractionation versus conventional fractionation in oropharyngeal carcinoma: final result of a randomized trial of the EORTC Cooperative Group of Radiotherapy. *Radiother Oncol* 1992; **25**: 231–41.
2. Board of the Faculty of Clinical Oncology, The Royal College of Radiologists. *The timely delivery of radical radiotherapy: standards and guidelines for the management of unscheduled treatment interruptions.* 3rd ed. 2008.
3. Morgan DAL. Fractionation experiments in head and neck cancer: the lessons so far. *Clin Oncol* 1997; **9**: 302–07.
4. van Acht MJ, Hermans J, Boks DE, Leer JW. The prognostic value of hemoglobin and a decrease in hemoglobin during radiotherapy in laryngeal carcinoma. *Radiother Oncol* 1992; **23**: 229–35.
5. Glaser CM, Millesi W, Kornek GV, et al. Impact of hemoglobin level and use of recombinant erythropoietin on efficacy of preoperative chemoradiation therapy for squamous cell carcinoma of the oral cavity and oropharynx. *Int J Radiat Oncol* 2001; **50**: 705–15.
6. Hoff CM, Lassen P, Eriksen JG, et al. Does transfusion improve the outcome for HNSCC patients treated with radiotherapy? Results from the randomized DAHANCA 5 and 7 trials. *Acta Oncol* 2011; **50**(7): 1006–14.
7. Overgaard J, Hoff C, Hansen HS, et al. Randomized study of Aranesp as modifier of radiotherapy in patients with primary squamous cell carcinoma of the head and neck (HNSCC): final outcome of the DAHANCA 10 trial. *Radiother Oncol* 2010; **96**(Suppl 15 abstract): 197.
8. Kaanders JHAM, Pop LAM, Marres HAM, et al. ARCON: experience in 215 patients with advanced head-and-neck cancer. *Int J Radiat Oncol* 2002; **52**: 769–78.
9. Janssens GO, Rademakers SE, Terhaard CH, et al. Accelerated radiotherapy with carbogen and nicotinamide for laryngeal cancer: results of a phase III randomized trial. *J Clin Oncol* 2012; **30**(15): 1777–83.
10. Overgaard J, Hansen HS, Overgaard M, et al. A randomized double-blind phase III study of nimorazole as a hypoxic radiosensitizer of primary radiotherapy in supraglottic larynx and pharynx carcinoma: results of the Danish Head and Neck Cancer Study (DAHANCA) protocol 5-85. *Radiother Oncol* 1998; **46**: 135–46.
11. Rauth AM, Melo T, Misra V. Bioreductive therapies: an overview of drugs and their mechanisms of action. *Int J Radiat Oncol* 1998; **42**: 755–62.
12. Gutierrez PL. The role of NAD(P)H oxidoreductase (DT-diaphorase) in the bioactivation of quinone-containing antitumor agents: a review. *Free Radical Bio Med* 2000; **29**: 263–75.
13. Haffty BG, Wilson LD, Son YH, et al. Concurrent chemo-radiotherapy with mitomycin C compared with porfiromycin in squamous cell cancer of the head and neck: final results of a randomized clinical trial. *Int J Radiat Oncol* 2005; **61**(1): 119–28.
14. Rischin D, Peters LJ, O'Sullivan B, et al. Tirapazamine, cisplatin, and radiation versus cisplatin and radiation for advanced squamous cell carcinoma of the head and neck (TROG 02.02, HeadSTART): a phase III trial of the Trans-Tasman Radiation Oncology Group. *J Clin Oncol* 2010; **28**: 2989–95.
15. Trinkaus ME, Hicks RJ, Young RJ, et al. Correlation of HPV status and hypoxic imaging using [18F]-misonidazole (FMISO) PET in head and neck squamous cell carcinoma (HNSCC). *J Clin Oncol* 2011; **29**: 5527.
16. Curtis KK, Wong WW, Ross HJ. Past approaches and future directions for targeting tumor hypoxia in squamous cell carcinomas of the head and neck. *Crit Rev Oncol Hemat* 2016: 86–98.
17. Economopoulou P, Perisanidis C, Giotakis EI, Psyrri A. The emerging role of immunotherapy in head and neck squamous cell carcinoma (HNSCC): anti-tumor immunity and clinical applications. *Ann Transl Med* 2016; **4**(9): 173.
18. Pignon JP, Bourhis J, Domenge C, Designe L. Chemotherapy added to locoregional treatment for head and neck squamous-cell carcinoma: three meta-analyses of updated individual data. MACH-NC Collaborative Group. Meta-analysis of chemotherapy on head and neck cancer. *Lancet* 2000; **355**: 949–55.
19. Pignon J-P, le Maître A, Maillard E, Bourhis J. MACH-NC Collaborative Group & Widder, J. Meta-analysis of chemotherapy in head and neck cancer (MACH-NC): an update on 93 randomised trials and 17,346 patients. *Radiother Oncol* 2009; **92**(1): 4–14.
20. Bourhis J, Blanchard P, Landais C, et al. Meta-analysis of chemotherapy in head and neck cancer (MACH-NC): an update on 100 randomized trials and 19,248 patients, on behalf of MACH-NC group. *Ann Oncol* 2016; **27**(6): 328–50.
21. Bourjis J, Overgaard J, Audry H, et al. Meta-analysis of Radiotherapy in Carcinomas of Head and neck (MARCH) Collaborative Group. Hyperfractionated or accelerated radiotherapy in head and neck cancer: a meta-analysis. *Lancet* 2006; **368**(9538): 843–54.
22. Lefebvre JL, Chevalier D, Luboinski B, et al. Larynx preservation in pyriform sinus cancer: preliminary results of a European Organization for Research and Treatment of Cancer phase III trial. EORTC Head and Neck Cancer Cooperative Group. *J Natl Cancer I* 1996; **88**(13): 890–99.
23. The Department of Veterans Affairs Laryngeal Cancer Study Group. Induction chemotherapy plus radiation compared with surgery plus radiation in patients with advanced laryngeal cancer. *New Engl J Med* 1991; **324**(24): 1685–90.
24. Ang KK, Berkey BA, Tu X, et al. Impact of epidermal growth factor receptor expression on survival and pattern of relapse in patients with advanced head and neck carcinoma. *Cancer Res* 2002; **62**(24): 7350–59.
25. Bonner JA, Harari PM, Giralt J, et al. Radiotherapy plus cetuximab for squamous cell carcinoma of the head and neck. *New Engl J Med* 2006; **354**: 567–78.
26. O-charoenrat P, Rhys-Evans P, Modjtahedi H, Eccles S. Vascular endothelial growth factor family members are differentially regulated by c-erbB signalling in head and neck squamous carcinoma cells. *Clin Exp Metastas* 2000; **18**: 155–61.
27. Kirby AM, A'Hern RP, D'Ambrosio C, et al. Gefitinib (ZD1839, Iressa™) as palliative treatment in recurrent or metastatic head and neck cancer. *Brit J Cancer* 2006; **94**: 631–36.
28. Soulieres D, Senzer NN, Vokes EE, et al. Multicenter phase II study of erlotinib, an oral epidermal growth factor receptor tyrosine kinase inhibitor, in patients with recurrent or metastatic squamous cell cancer of the head and neck. *J Clin Oncol* 2004; **22**(1): 77–85.
29. Martins RG, Parvathaneni U, Bauman JE, et al. Cisplatin and radiotherapy with or without erlotinib in locally advanced squamous cell carcinoma of the head and neck: a randomised phase II trial. *J Clin Oncol* 2013; **31**(110): 1415–21.
30. Ferris RL, Blumenschein, Jr G, Fayette J, et al. Nivolumab for recurrent squamous-cell carcinoma of the head and neck. *New Engl J Med* 2016; **375**: 1856–67.

CHAPTER 6

APOPTOSIS AND CELL DEATH

Angela Hague

Introduction 59	Mechanisms of apoptosis regulation 62
Introduction to apoptosis... 59	The PI3K/AKT and MAPK/ERK pathways to cell survival 65
Other types of cell death 61	References 67

SEARCH STRATEGY

Data in this chapter may be updated by searching the following keywords used in PubMed: HNSCC, oropharyngeal, apoptosis, necroptosis, autophagy, senescence, radioresistance, p53, HPV (human papilloma virus), cetuximab and epidermal growth factor receptor (EGFR).

INTRODUCTION

The aim of this chapter is to summarize current understanding of apoptosis and cell death from a clinical perspective, focussing on the head and neck. Reviews cited here have been selected for importance or clear explanations. The basis behind some of the methods to measure cell death is explained to assist in evaluating primary research papers. Emphasis is placed on the role of evasion of apoptosis in head and neck squamous cell carcinoma (HNSCC), although the role of cell death in other processes may be of interest to the specialist clinician, for example: cancers of the head and neck; head and neck development; palatal shelf fusion and cleft palate; autoimmune disease; and hearing loss due to ageing, noise, or exposure to ototoxic agents.

INTRODUCTION TO APOPTOSIS

Apoptosis as a mechanism of programmed cell death regulates cell numbers in tissues and is a key response to cellular damage that cannot be repaired. Resistance to apoptosis is one of the hallmarks of cancer,[1, 2] whereas increased apoptosis contributes to autoimmune and neurodegenerative conditions. In the ear, apoptosis of terminally differentiated sensory hair cells contributes to hearing loss caused by ototoxic agents such as aminoglycoside antibiotics and cisplatin chemotherapy, as well as that caused by excess noise over a prolonged time and general age-related hearing loss.[3] Our understanding of apoptosis regulation provides cancer diagnostic and prognostic markers and is leading to development of cancer therapies specifically targeting cell survival pathways or mimicking pro-apoptotic signalling molecules. Approaches involving sensitization to radiotherapy and chemotherapy are being taken as an alternative to the concept of single agent therapies for cancer. These highlight the need for personalized medicine, such that drugs are given to patients whose cancers, and indeed elusive 'cancer stem cells', can be predicted to respond by undergoing programmed cell death.

There are two signalling pathways that result in apoptosis, the mitochondrial (intrinsic) and the death receptor (extrinsic) pathways. Both involve activation of a family of enzymes called the caspases. Caspases are cysteine proteases that cleave after aspartic acid residues. Caspases are named in the order of their discovery, and while caspases 1, 4 and 5 are involved primarily in the processing of inflammatory mediators, caspases 2, 8, 9 and 10 have roles as initiator caspases for cell death signals, activating downstream effector caspases 3, 6 and 7, which target cellular proteins leading to the condensation of the cell and dissolution of the nuclear membrane. Hundreds of proteins are cleaved by caspases, usually at single sites. Some are cleaved as bystanders, but many structural and regulatory proteins are inactivated by caspases. Some substrates can be activated by cleavage – such as other caspases and Bid (see the section 'Death Receptor Pathway to Apoptosis' below). By cleavage of an inhibitor protein (ICAD), they release a caspase-activated deoxyribonuclease (CAD) that cleaves the DNA of the cell into oligomeric fragments that are integer multiples of 180–200 base pairs. This cleavage pattern can be detected on DNA electrophoresis as a

'DNA ladder'. The cleavage of DNA ensures that the cell is no longer capable of replication, and the destruction of the translational machinery restricts protein synthesis.

In haemotoxylin and eosin stained sections of tissue, apoptotic cells are characterized by condensed chromatin that appears intensely purple stained in smooth shapes. Early stages show chromatin condensed around the periphery of the nuclear membrane, prior to its dissolution, frequently in crescent shapes. As the nuclear membrane disappears, apoptotic cells exhibit single smooth chromatin mass, which subsequently fragments to smaller smooth shaped chromatin masses that can be scattered throughout the cell. Loss of cell–cell and cell–matrix contact, along with shrinkage and rounding up of the cell as the cytoskeletal proteins are cleaved, results in the apoptotic cell appearing isolated among the tissue. The plasma membrane is seen to undergo 'blebbing' and the cell may fragment into apoptotic bodies following invagination of the plasma membrane. Cleavage of poly (ADP-ribose) polymerase (PARP-1) by caspases 3 and 7 gives two fragments of apparent molecular weights of 25 and 85 kDa. These have since been designated as 24 and 89 kD from sequence data. The p85/89 large fragment is a popular marker for identifying apoptosis, either by protein electrophoresis or by using antibodies that specifically recognize this fragment of the cleaved protein for immunostaining of cells or tissues. It is an earlier marker than DNA fragmentation (**Figure 6.1**).[4]

All caspases are produced as inactive zymogens, and are activated by either autocleavage (in the case of initiator caspases) or other upstream caspases. The procaspase is cleaved in two places – a prodomain is removed and two subunits are generated, a large subunit and a small subunit. These are assembled into the active enzyme which is a heterotetramer with head-to-tail alignment of the subunits. As a result of this, protein electrophoresis detection of the small and/or large subunits is indicative of caspase cleavage. *In vivo* detection of apoptosis by immunohistochemistry is facilitated by use of antibodies that recognize only the cleaved, active form (**Figure 6.1**). DNA fragmentation has also been used as a way to detect apoptotic cells. The terminal deoxynucleotide transferase-mediated dUTP-biotin nick end labelling (TUNEL) assay detects both double and single strand breaks by adding labelled dUTP to free 3'-hydroxyl termini of fragmented DNA. The problem with this method is that it picks up DNA fragmentation occurring during necrotic cell death and should therefore be used in conjunction with other methods of apoptosis detection. Alternative *in situ* ligation (ISL) techniques label only 5' double-stranded DNA breaks with either blunt ends or a 3' single base overhang with terminal phosphates, allowing for more specific detection of apoptosis-mediated DNA fragmentation over either necrosis or repairable DNA damage.[5]

The ultimate fate of apoptotic cells *in vivo* is to be phagocytosed by macrophages or neighbouring cells acting as semiprofessional phagocytes. The membrane of apoptotic cells is altered to prevent leakage of intracellular material until phagocytosis, a process involving protein cross-linking by tissue transglutaminase. The lipid components of the membrane are also altered, in that phosphatidyl serine, normally only present on the inner membrane leaflet, is flipped into the outer leaflet and exposed on the cell surface, enabling macrophages to identify and engulf the dying cell. The engulfment of the cell prior to loss of plasma membrane integrity is key to the process of eliminating excess or damaged cells without eliciting an inflammatory response. If this does not occur, the plasma membrane becomes permeable, and the cell is said to undergo 'secondary necrosis', with the leakage of damage-associated molecular pattern molecules (DAMPs) able to elicit a non-infectious immune response. It is exposure of phosphatidyl serine on the outer leaflet that is recognized in the Annexin V assay. Annexin V is an anticoagulant protein from human placenta that binds to phosphatidyl serine lipids.[6] Labelled Annexin V binding in conjunction with propidium iodide staining of unfixed cells distinguishes early apoptosis, as cells that

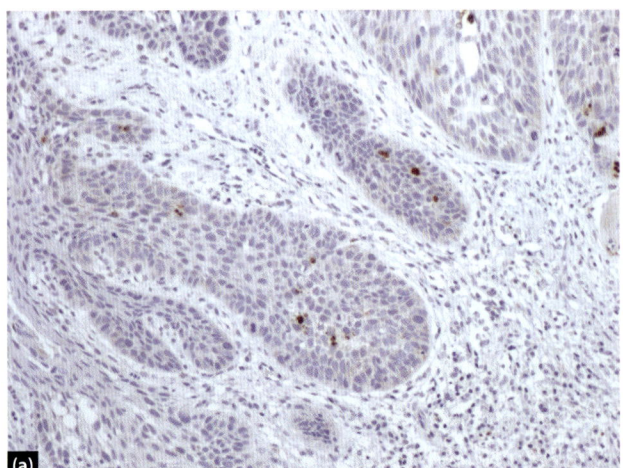
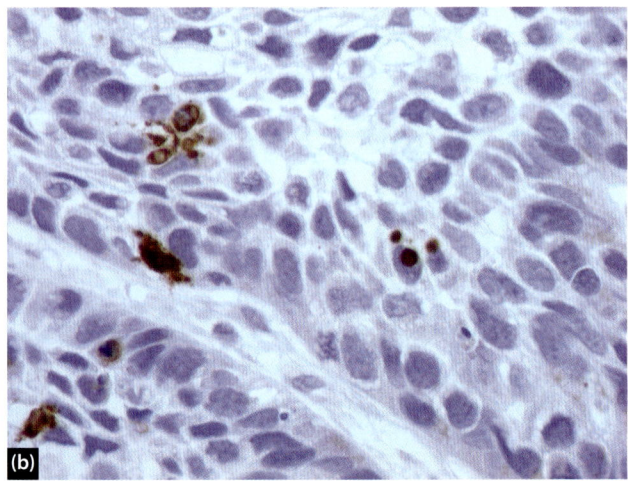

Figure 6.1 Cleaved caspase 3 staining highlights apoptotic cells in human tissue. Staining of apoptotic cells using an antibody that detects active caspase 3 in a human oral squamous cell carcinoma section. **(a)** Low magnification (× 10 objective). **(b)** Higher magnification (× 40 objective).

are not permeable to propidium iodide but are Annexin V positive. However, once the plasma membrane becomes permeable, it can no longer distinguish apoptosis and secondary necrosis, because Annexin V then has access to the inner plasma membrane leaflet. For use in fixed cells or *in vivo*, the cells are labelled before fixation.

OTHER TYPES OF CELL DEATH

Terminal differentiation

Apoptosis is a physiological event that contributes to maintenance of tissues with constant turnover of cells such as the gut epithelium. Tissue homeostasis is maintained by a balance between cell proliferation, differentiation and cell death. However, terminal differentiation in the skin, and indeed oral epithelium, is regulated by a process involving caspase 14. This is a distinct process from apoptosis.[7]

Necrosis

Apoptosis is distinct from necrosis, a pathological, passive process of cellular destruction (**Table 6.1**). Necrosis involves cell swelling and nuclear chromatin 'flocculation' where the swelling nucleus appears more diffuse than normal. Ultimately the cells lyse without detaching from their neighbours and the release of intracellular contents stimulates inflammation.

Necroptosis

Although necrosis is a passive process, a programmed cell death mechanism resulting in necrotic-like death has been identified that is termed 'necroptosis', specifically signalled by receptor-interacting serine/threonine-protein kinases 1 and 3 (RIPK1 and RIPK3) in response to signalling through the tumour necrosis factor receptor (TNFR) family members, toll-like receptors (TLR3 and TLR4) or T-cell receptors (TCR), or in response to DNA damage and viral infection.[9, 10] RIPK3 phosphorylates mixed lineage kinase domain-like protein (MLKL) which homooligomerizes and relocates to the plasma membrane. This appears to be key to the necroptosis signalling pathway, but RIPK1 may or may not be needed.[11]

Necroptosis primarily appears to occur when caspases are inhibited, and one reason why apoptosis normally takes precedence over necroptosis is because active caspase 8 can cleave RIPK1 and RIPK3.[9] Viral infection is a situation that can result in necroptosis because viruses inhibit caspases. Where tumour cells have become apoptosis resistant (perhaps through similar mechanisms to viral infection) necroptosis might be a useful way to eliminate tumour cells, although the consequences of the induction of inflammation to the tumour microenvironment will have to be considered.[12, 13] While microscopically necroptosis appears as a swollen cell with formation of a balloon-like structure, known as oncosis, methods to identify necroptosis currently involve biochemical and fluorogenic assays on lysates or living cells, use of genetically modified mice or cells with RIPK3 or MLKL knockdown, or use of necrostatin and other more specific RIPK1 inhibitors to block the process.[13]

$RIPK3^{-/-}$ and $MLKL^{-/-}$ mice have revealed that necroptosis contributes to ischemia-reperfusion injury and chronic neurodegenerative disorders.[11] Necroptosis is not the only form of 'regulated necrosis' and if multiple pathways lead to cell death with similar morphology, clear understanding of these molecular pathways is needed to devise ways to distinguish these in human tissues as well as to distinguish RIPK3 activation in necroptosis from its role in inflammation.

TABLE 6.1 Summary of differences between apoptosis and necrosis[8]

	Apoptosis	Necrosis
Occurrence	Part of physiological or pathological processes	Always pathological
Initiating factors	Range of extracellular and intracellular factors	Direct result of injury and cellular anoxia
Distribution	Isolated apoptotic cells scattered widely throughout tissues	Occurs in groups/whole areas of tissue
Mechanism	Active process – ATP dependent	Passive
	Regulated mechanism	Regulation lost
Cytoplasmic changes	Cytoplasmic shrinkage	Swelling of cell membrane
	Blebbing of cell membrane into apoptotic bodies	Rupture of cell membrane with loss of contents to extracellular space
	Many organelles preserved and bound into apoptotic bodies	Organelles lost
Nuclear changes	Endonuclease activation, cutting of DNA into oligosomal fragments	Random digestion of DNA
	Chromatin condenses into specific 'crescents' visible on light microscopy	Chromatin flocculates
Effect on surrounding tissue	Little or none	Intense inflammation

Autophagy for survival – or autophagic cell death?

Macroautophagy is a process by which cytoplasm and organelles are engulfed into double membrane bound vesicles called autophagosomes (self-eating), which ultimately fuse with lysosomes for digestion and recycling of contents by lysosomal hydrolases. This process is utilized, for example, in situations of starvation, oxidative stress or hypoxia. Publications frequently specify that it is macroautophagy that is the form of autophagy being referred to (i.e. the use of autophagosomes to transport cargo to the lysosome) and then simply use the term 'autophagy' thereafter. Tumour cells are believed to utilize this process, promoting survival of tumour cells in unfavourable conditions. Autophagy contributes to chemotherapy resistance, for example in esophageal cancer cells treated with cisplatin or 5-fluorouracil.[14] Some agents can induce excessive autophagy leading to cell death, but the consequence of autophagy can be context dependent and the microenvironment can adjust the threshold at which autophagy levels promote cell survival or cell death. There is now believed to be cross-talk between the processes of apoptosis, autophagy and 'regulated/programmed necrosis'.[15]

Measurement of autophagy is difficult, as demonstration of flux of autophagosomes is currently the gold standard method, and this requires living cells in which flux can be blocked at different stages. The autophagy flux reporter mCherry-GFP-LC3 works on the principle that the GFP (green fluorescent protein) signal is sensitive to the acidic and/or proteolytic conditions inside the lysosome, whereas mCherry (red) fluorescence persists. This has been used to show autophagic flux in mouse neurones *in vivo* by adeno-associated virus delivery – autophagosomes appear as yellow dots and autophagolysosomes appear as red dots.[16] A multiprotein class III phosphatidyl inositol-3 kinase (PI3K) complex is needed to produce the isolation membranes that engulf cellular components and pinch off of membranes (usually the endoplasmic reticulum) to form the autophagosomes. Knockdown of active components of this complex can be used to demonstrate if autophagy is important in a particular cellular outcome, for example cell survival or cell death.

> **KEY POINTS**
> - Apoptosis eliminates damaged cells or cells in excess to requirement.
> - Apoptosis involves destruction of the cell by caspases, but the cells are normally engulfed by phagocytes *in vivo*.
> - Excessive apoptosis contributes to autoimmune diseases such as oral lichen planus and degenerative conditions such as apoptosis of the sensory hair cells of the ear, contributing to hearing loss.
> - Resistance to apoptosis is a hallmark of cancer and contributes to therapeutic resistance.
> - Necroptosis involves signalling by RIPK3 and MLKL and is known as 'regulated necrosis or programmed necrosis'.
> - Autophagy involves digestion of cellular material in autophagolysosomes for use as recycled metabolites and is generally a cytoprotective process; it can contribute to resistance to cancer therapy.

MECHANISMS OF APOPTOSIS REGULATION

Mitochondrial pathway to apoptosis

Bcl-2 was originally described as a protooncogene in B-cell lymphomas. In follicular lymphoma the t(8;14) translocation moves Bcl-2 to the immunoglobulin heavy chain locus, leading to its overexpression. Bcl-2 is located in the outer mitochondrial membrane but is also detected in the plasma membrane and endoplasmic reticulum. Its mitochondrial localization allows it to regulate the release of cytochrome c from the intramembrane space into the cytosol and it is this release that is required for the activation of the initiator caspase, caspase 9. Cytochrome c release can be measured as a characteristic marker of a cell's early apoptotic response.[17] A family of Bcl-2 proteins has been identified (**Table 6.2**), some of which are anti-apoptotic like Bcl-2; others are pro-apoptotic.[18] Whereas Bcl-2 is localized constitutively to membranes, the anti-apoptotic Bcl-X_L, Mcl-1 and Bcl-w members of the family are located in the cytoplasm and localize to the mitochondria upon receipt of an apoptotic signal.[19] Bax is a pro-apoptotic protein that was identified as a homologue that bound Bcl-2. When overexpressed, Bax accelerated cell death in response to cytokine deprivation. By contrast, overexpression of Bcl-2 allows cells to tolerate signals to undergo apoptosis. Bcl-2 and other anti-apoptotic family members do this by sequestering pro-apoptotic family members such as Bax and by regulating ion flux to prevent mitochondrial outer membrane depolarization which is required for cytochrome c release.[17] Interestingly, Bax is not always bound to Bcl-2 in viable cells, but cycles on and off mitochondria in a dynamic equilibrium.[20] Bcl-X_L has also been shown to actively transport Bax from the mitochondrial membrane to the cytoplasm.[19] The Bax homologue Bak serves a similar function. Both Bax and Bak function as homooligomeric complexes to release cytochrome c from the mitochondria. Although Bax and Bak mediate responses to different types of cellular stress, the outcome downstream of the mitochondrion is the same, and in fact there is some functional redundancy, as only cells lacking both Bax and Bak molecules fail to undergo apoptosis.[21] By contrast to Bax, which translocates to the

TABLE 6.2 Most commonly studied Bcl-2 family members

Anti-apoptotic	Pro-apoptotic	Pro-apoptotic BH3-only
Bcl-2	Bax	Bad
Bcl-x	Bak	Bim
Bcl-w		Bid
Mcl-1		Puma
Bfl-1/A1		Noxa
		Hrk
		Bik

mitochondrion in response to apoptosis signals, Bak is localized in the outer mitochondrial membrane.

Released cytochrome c binds to the adapter protein Apaf-1, causing a conformational change that allows it to bind dATP. In turn, this triggers oligomerization to a heptomer and exposes the caspase recruitment domain (CARD) of Apaf-1 allowing recruitment of procaspase 9. The heptomeric wheel-like structure carrying procaspase 9 at its hub constitutes an activation platform for caspase 9 and is termed the apoptosome (**Figure 6.2**). Autocleavage of procaspase 9 generates active caspase 9,

the initiator of apoptosis, which subsequently activates further caspases.

While Bcl-2 and most anti-apoptotic proteins of the family have four domains of Bcl-2 homology (BH domains), Bax and Bak have three (BH1-3), which in the folded molecule comprise a hydrophobic groove used for dimerization with the anti-apoptotic proteins. Upstream of the mitochondrion, in addition to Bax translocation, so called 'BH3-only' proteins sense apoptotic signals and transmit these to the mitochondrion. They compete with Bax and Bak for Bcl-2 binding, and displaced Bax is free to

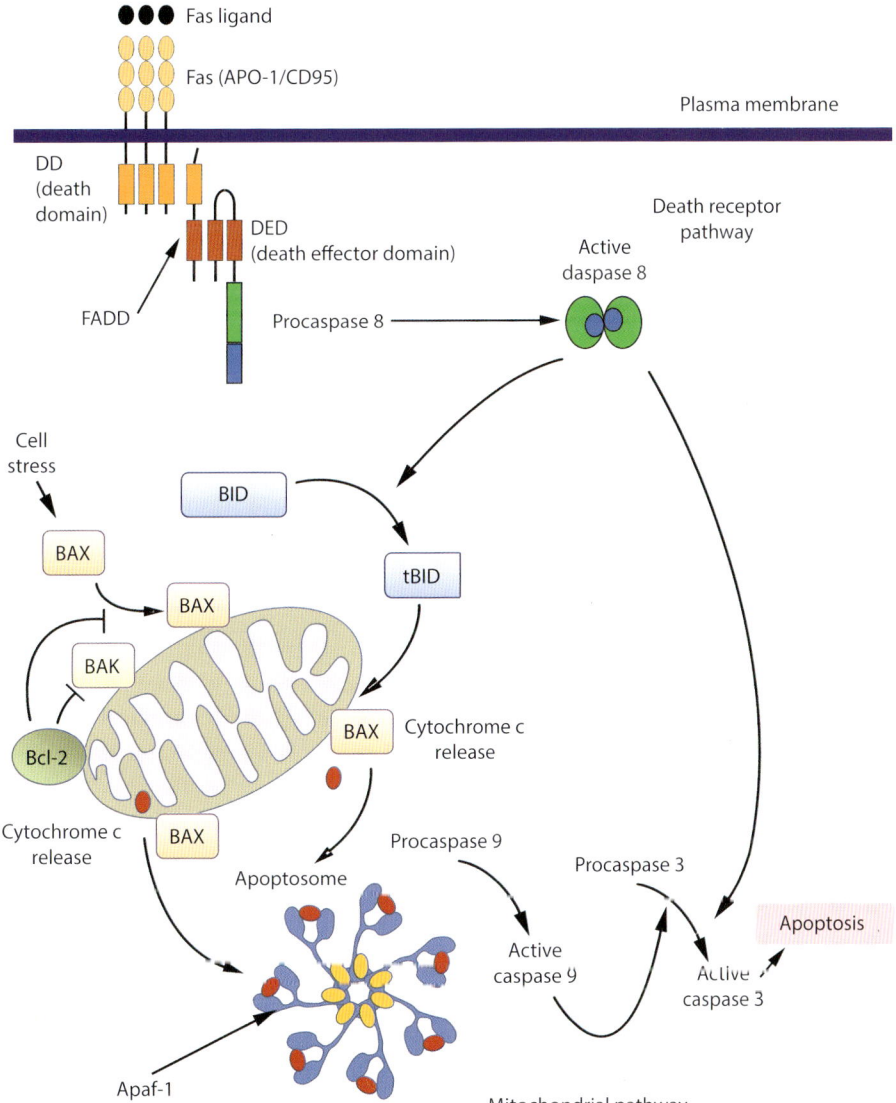

Figure 6.2 Apoptotic signalling. In the mitochondrial cell death signalling pathway, the molecules Bax and Bak can each form homooligomers that release cytochrome c from the inner membrane space of the mitochondrion. These are negatively regulated by anti-apoptotic members of the Bcl-2 family, represented here as Bcl-2. Once released, cytochrome c binds to monomeric Apaf-1, which in the presence of ATP can oligomerize into a heptomer called the apoptosome (blue). Procaspase 9 is recruited to the caspase recruitment domain (CARD) that forms the hub of the apoptosome. Here it autocatalytically cleaves to give rise to a highly active caspase 9 enzyme, which can then activate downstream executioner caspases, represented here by caspase 3. In the death receptor signalling pathway, trimerized receptors recruit the adapter molecule FADD, which recruits procaspase 8, which is autocatalytically processed to form the active enzyme. In type I cells this can result in caspase 3 activation and apoptosis. In type II cells, the BH3-only member of the Bcl-2 family, Bid, is cleaved to a form that can translocate to the mitochondria and interact with Bcl-2 to displace Bax or interact directly with Bax itself and by either of these mechanisms facilitate cytochrome c release, thus engaging the mitochondrial signalling pathway. In type II cells, Bcl-2 overexpression can block death receptor induced apoptosis but in type I cells it does not.

homooligomerize and release cytochrome c. This is the 'sensitizer' function of BH3-only proteins. Some can interact with Bax directly to facilitate conformation change, oligomerization, pore formation and cytochrome c release. This is the 'direct activator' function of BH3-only proteins and a model has been proposed whereby the BH3 protein binds transiently to a rear pocket on Bax distal to the hydrophobic groove.[22] It is likely that Bak does not require this activation because it is already located in the mitochondrial membrane.[19] Whereas Bad is only capable of sensitizer function, Bim, Bid and Puma can serve as direct activators.[23] Different BH3-only proteins mediate different apoptosis signals. In terms of the anti-apoptotic proteins, these may regulate cell life and death during tissue homoeostasis at different stages in cellular differentiation, for example in the colonic crypt, Bcl-2 protects proliferative cells from apoptosis, whereas Bcl-X_L protects the post-mitotic cells in the upper regions of the crypt.[24] The BH3-only proteins also have preferred anti-apoptotic binding partners, for example Bad binds strongly to Bcl-2, Bcl-X_L and Bcl-w, whereas Noxa binds Mcl-1 and Al.[25]

Small molecule drugs have been designed that mimic BH3-only proteins in their action. The most extensively clinically tested of these is ABT-263 (navatoclax; AbbVie), but this does not bind Mcl-1 or Al. Obatoclax (Gemin X) binds both Bad and Noxa targets and is being tested clinically for anti-cancer activity in advanced haematological malignancies. Others are being tested in preclinical models. Interestingly, obatoclax more efficiently induces apoptosis of HNSCC cell lines if autophagy is inhibited by choroquine.[26]

Mitochondrial apoptosis induced by reactive oxygen species is believed to underlie ageing-related deafness and ototoxicity of some pharmaceuticals including aminoglycoside antibiotics such as gentamycin. Resistance to broad spectrum antibiotics and the increase in methicillin-resistant *Staphylococcus aureus* (MRSA) has led to reconsideration of gentamycin. The hair cells are the primary target of ototoxicity but auditory and vestibular ganglion neurons can also undergo cell death.[27] Different *in vitro* and *in vivo* models implicate apoptosis, necrosis or necroptosis as well as cell death subsequent to extrusion from the epithelium. Reactive oxygen species (ROS) generation is believed to induce mitochondrial apoptosis mediated by p53 or c-Jun N-terminal kinase (JNK).[27] Mutations in mitochondrial DNA encoding the 12S ribosomal RNA component of the mitochondrial ribosomes lead to its hypermethylation. Raimundo et al.[28] provided evidence for a model in which A1555G mutation, which confers susceptibility to aminoglycoside-induced deafness, led to enhanced ROS production, and AMP-kinase-dependent induction of the transcription factor, E2F1. E2F1 was expressed at levels high enough to induce pro-apoptotic genes rather than promote cell proliferation. In a mouse model, cleaved caspase 3 positive cells were detected in the stria vascularis and the spiral ganglion neurons, but not in the organ of Corti.[28] A T1095C mutation in the same gene also confers susceptibility to gentamycin mediated apoptosis in an *in vitro* model.[29] Therefore, patients susceptible to gentamycin-induced ototoxicity could be identified by genetic screening. Free radical scavengers have been suggested to protect from aminoglycoside-induced toxicity.[30]

Death receptor pathway to apoptosis

Cells can be induced to undergo apoptosis via engagement of cell surface death receptors (DR) with ligand molecules. These receptors form the tumour necrosis factor receptor family, the other members of which are Fas (APO1/CD95), DR3 (APO3), DR4 (TRAIL-R1) and DR5 (TRAIL-R2). Cell signalling was first elucidated for Fas, which is bound by Fas ligand (Fas-L). The source of Fas ligand may be in membrane-bound form presented on the surface cytotoxic T cells. The Fas ligand-Fas system normally eliminates excess T cells during an immune response, and defects in this signalling can be involved in autoimmune disease. Oral lichen planus involves epithelial apoptosis mediated by Fas ligand due to infiltration of inflammatory cells underneath the oral epithelium. Lichen planus is a condition with a high apoptotic index and is a useful positive control for apoptosis staining.

In apoptosis signalling, receptor trimerization leads to recruitment of FADD (Fas-associated death domain), which binds the intracellular death domain (DD) portion of Fas, and procaspase 8 molecules bind to the death effector domain (DED) of FADD (**Figure 6.2**). Hence, procaspase 8 molecules are clustered and activated by autocleavage on a platform known as the death inducing signal complex (DISC). Trimerized receptors may also cluster into receptor microaggregates. In some cell types (type I cells), caspase 8 activation at the DISC is sufficient for downstream effector procaspase cleavage, but in many cell types (type II cells), the mitochondrial pathway is engaged to amplify the death signal by caspase 8-dependent cleavage of the BH3-only protein Bid, converting it to a form that is able to transmit the apoptotic signal to the mitochondrion. In addition, cytotoxic T cells release perforin, which penetrates the epithelial cell membrane, and granzyme B, a serine protease that can cleave and activate Bid, hence engaging the mitochondrial pathway.

Expression of high levels of Fas ligand by tumour cells can allow them to evade infiltrating T cells that express Fas, so called tumour 'counter-attack'.[31] Tumour-produced Fas may be soluble, as tumour cells may exhibit resistance to Fas-mediated apoptosis. Fas mutations have been found in sporadic myeloma and T-cell leukaemia leading to evasion of apoptosis. FLIP is a molecule that structurally resembles caspase 8 and is able to bind FADD and hence block death receptor signalling. Indeed for death receptors we now know that large complexes can be formed both at the receptors themselves or in complexes that are released into the cytoplasm, and the constitution of these determines downstream signalling consequence. For example, Fas ligand can induce cell survival and contribute to tumour promotion by inducing JNK, ERK (extracellular signal-regulated kinases), NF-κB (nuclear factor kappa-light-chain-enhancer of activated B cells) and PI3K (phosphatidyl inositol 3-kinase) signalling pathways.[32] Tumour necrosis factor-related apoptosis-inducing ligand (TRAIL) induces apoptosis through two of its receptors DR4 (TRAIL-R1) and DR5 (TRAIL-R2). Decoy receptors that bind ligand but do not signal apoptosis can be overexpressed in some cancers. For example, TRAIL-R3 is overexpressed in acute myeloid leukaemia, especially on cancer stem cells.[33] TRAIL-R4 can signal to activate Akt in HeLa cervical carcinoma cells independently of ligand binding, but the mechanism is not yet understood.[34]

Agonistic antibodies that engage death receptors are in trials for various cancers in which the signalling pathway is intact – for example, the TRAIL-R1 antibody Mapatumumab and the TRAIL-R2 antibody Lexatumumab. As single agents these were initially disappointing, in part because TRAIL receptors must trimerize in order to signal effectively, and an antibody can only cross-link two death receptors.[34] However, their combination with other agents is looking more promising, at least *in vitro*. Agents inducing synergistic apoptosis include chemotherapeutic drugs, histone deacetylation inhibitors, proteosome inhibitors, NF-κB inhibitors and BH3 mimetics. Moreover, new TRAIL receptor antibodies that will form higher order complexes are being developed.[35] Other recent strategies use more stable versions of the TRAIL trimer, targeted delivery of TRAIL in nanoparticles, and tumour-targeting of TRAIL constructs.[36]

p53 'guardian of the genome'

Normally wild type p53 protein is rapidly turned over due to its binding to the ubiquitin ligase HDM2 (the human homologue of MDM2), which ubiquitin-tags it for destruction by the proteosome. In recognition of DNA damage, p53 is stabilized and can be detected as nuclear staining. p53 is extensively post-translationally modified and this regulates its binding partners and which gene promoters it engages with. Hence, p53 can activate transcription of either cell cycle arrest and DNA repair genes or genes encoding proteins that promote mitochondrial apoptosis such as Bax, Puma, Noxa and Apaf-1. p53 can also induce Fas, TRAIL, TRAIL-R2, hence modulating death receptor signalling. More recently, p53 has been shown to activate transcription of autophagy regulators under cell stress conditions.[37] p53 knockout mice are developmentally normal, and therefore p53 is thought to play a minimal role in development. However, defects in developmental genes can lead to p53-dependent apoptosis, for example the apoptosis of neural crest cells resulting in craniofacial hypoplasia syndromes such as Treacher Collins.[38]

THE PI3K/AKT AND MAPK/ERK PATHWAYS TO CELL SURVIVAL

In response to engagement of tyrosine kinase receptors, G-coupled protein receptors, integrins, and toll-like receptors, the lipid kinase PI3K phosphorylates phosphatidylinositol 4,5-bisphosphate (PIP2) to generate phosphatidylinositol 3,4,5-triphosphate (PIP3). PTEN antagonizes this pathway by removal of the phosphate at this position of the inositol ring.[39] PIP3 recruits Akt to the plasma membrane ready for activation. Then, upon its activation by phosphorylation, Akt can move to different locations within the cell to phosphorylate many molecular targets, some of which are key regulators of cell survival – for example, Akt-dependent phosphorylation contributes to Bad and caspase 9 inactivation. It also inactivates the Forkhead family of transcription factors that induce expression of pro-apoptotic factors and activates mTOR (mammalian target of rapamycin), a key regulator of autophagy and cell survival in situations of cell stress. The *PIK3CA* gene encodes p110 alpha (p110α) subunit of PI3K and can be mutated in HNSCC.[40]

The mitogen-activated protein kinase MAPK/ERK pathway downstream of Ras activates transcription factors promoting cell survival; however ERK phosphorylation can also lead to phosphorylation, ubiquitination and proteosomal degradation of the 'extra long' isoform of the BH3-only protein, Bim.

Apoptosis and head and neck squamous cell carcinoma

Although resistance to apoptosis is a hallmark of cancer, this does not mean that cancers do not exhibit apoptosis. Apoptosis is uncommon in normal squamous epithelium and eliminates damaged cells rather than contributing to normal tissue homeostasis. The apoptotic index is higher in dysplasia and in HNSCC than corresponding normal tissue.

The genetic changes in head and neck squamous cell carcinoma (HNSCC) have been reviewed by Rothenberg and Ellisen,[41] in particular the exome sequencing results published in *Science* in 2011 by Agrawal et al.[42] and Stransky et al.[43] These include changes that subvert the balance between proliferation, differentiation and apoptosis:

- *CDKN2A* loss (gene encoding tumour suppressor protein and cyclin-dependent kinase inhibitor, p16^{INK4a})
- *CCND1* amplification (gene encoding cyclin D1)
- loss of *TGFBR2* (gene encoding the type II transforming growth factor β receptor) or *SMAD4* (gene encoding the TGFβ signalling molecule), which promote proliferation
- *NOTCH1* loss and/or abnormal expression of *TP63*, both of which deregulate keratinocyte differentiation
- alterations in *CASP8* (gene encoding caspase 8), *EGFR* (gene encoding the epidermal growth factor receptor (EGFR) and *PIK3CA* genes, which promote cell survival.

Loss or mutation of *TP53* is common, leading to defective cell cycle arrest and repair or apoptosis. Mutations in *TP53* can result in stabilized, mutant p53 that lacks function. Alternatively, tumours may lack p53 altogether. Hunter et al.[44] suggested that ~40% of HNSCCs may develop without acquiring immortality and retain wild type p53 and p16. These tumours would likely have better prognosis. Interestingly, cisplatin induces senescence in HNSCC cells with wild type p53.[45]

In development of HNSCC, *TP53* mutations appear early and contribute to 'field cancerization', whereby epithelium that is histologically normal actually carries mutation, and to around half of HNSCC cases. Hence, ways to kill cells harbouring mutant p53 or reconfigure mutant p53 to a transcriptionally active confirmation are being explored. ONYX-015 (dl1520) is an adenovirus modified to only replicate in and kill cells that harbour p53 mutations. Wild type adenoviruses must disable p53 before viral replication can occur and because ONYX-015 has a mutant E1B 55K gene, it cannot neutralize p53, therefore cannot replicate in cells with wild type p53 and does not kill them. Oncolysis of mutant p53-containing tumour cells leads to spread of viral particles and subsequent rounds of tumour-specific replication and cell killing. This virus is in phase III trials for head and neck cancer in the USA. H101, a similar virus to ONYX-015, is licensed in China for treatment of head and neck cancers.[46] An alternative is to use a replication-deficient adenovirus that expresses wild type p53. Phase II/III trials in HNSCC are showing increased patient survival.[43] Small molecules designed to directly reactivate mutant p53 protein are specific to the type of mutation; PRIMA-1(Met) stabilizes unfolded p53 and a 'first in human' study was published in 2012.[47]

Risk factors for HNSCC are primarily smoking and alcohol consumption, with dietary contribution.[48] However, human papilloma virus (HPV) infection, particularly of subtype 16, can increase the risk of oropharyngeal cancer over 4-fold.[49] Unsurprisingly, human papilloma virus positive (HPV+) is genetically distinct from HPV- HNSCC,[50] and patients have longer overall survival and respond better to treatment. Viral proteins E6 and E7 accelerate the degradation of p53 and p16 respectively, resulting in cellular immortalization and reduced ability of cells to repair genetic damage or undergo apoptosis. HPV+ tumours rarely carry p53 mutations, as the E6 protein targets p53 for degradation, yet HPV+ cell lines are generally more radiosensitive than HPV- cell lines, exhibiting a prolonged G2 arrest and increased apoptosis because of residual wild type p53.[50] It should be emphasized that apoptosis can occur by p53-independent mechanisms; for example, HNSCC cells can respond in this way to γ-irradiation.[51]

Since E7 decreases pRb, it frees the transcription factor E2F, normally sequestered by the pRb, permitting cell cycle progresssion. p16 increases in a negative feedback response. Therefore, whereas reduced p16 is common in HPV- HNSCC, in HPV+ cases it tends to be enhanced. Grønhøj Larsen et al.[52] found by systematic review that studies classifying 'p16 positivity' as tumours with a proportion of cells 70% or greater showed strongest correlation with HPV positivity. Using this scoring system, Rietbergen et al.[53] caution that there is also a possibility that p16 positivity may occur independently of HPV involvement, although they analysed HPV DNA and mRNA from formalin fixed paraffin-embedded tumour material and recommended that assays in fresh frozen tissue be conducted. They noted that p16+/HPV- tumours had higher frequency of loss of heterozygosity on chromosomes 3p, 19p and 17p, similar to HPV- tumours.

EGFR activation activates MAPK and PI3K/Akt signalling pathways (**Figure 6.3**). The EGFR and PI3K/Akt/mTOR signalling pathways are of current interest for molecular targeted therapeutics, as they are hyperactivated in HNSCC and contribute to radioresistance.[54] Although the EGFR is rarely mutated in HNSCC, increases in gene copy number do correlate with poor prognosis, and the possibility that EGFR ligands are present in the tumour microenvironment has been suggested.[41] The monoclonal

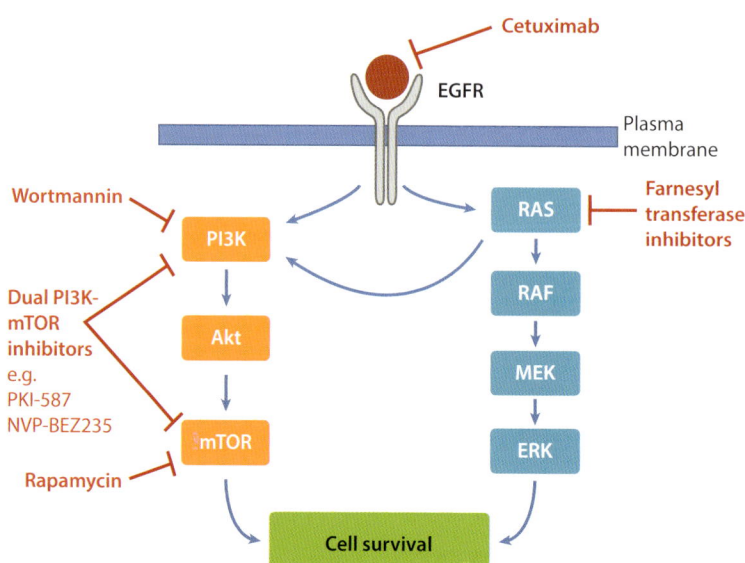

Figure 6.3 Survival signalling and potential targets for cancer therapy. The PI3K and Ras signalling pathways are hyperactivated in HNSCC. There is crosstalk between these two pathways; for example, Ras can potentiate PI3K activity. Targeting a single molecule is ineffective because of development of drug resistance and cells adapt their signalling pathways to overcome the block. Hence strategies are being developed that combine agents with different targets or use drugs with more than one molecular target.

antibody cetuximab targets the EGFR and is now used clinically to significantly enhance patient survival, but resistance remains a problem with downstream activation of PI3K/Akt/mTOR contributing to this. Similarly, resistance to PI3K inhibitors occurs due to the cancer cell's ability to adapt its signalling circuits and to engage feedback mechanisms. Hence, there is a move away from use of single target therapies towards evaluation of combination approaches. Use of PI3K or dual PI3K-mTOR inhibitors in combination with cetuximab is currently being explored.

Cancers with *HRAS* mutation are not likely to respond to EGFR-targeted therapies. Active Ras is needed for Akt activation in HNSCC cells.[55] Farnesyl transferase inhibitors that inhibit activity of Ras and Akt could be an area for research. Cetuximab combined with radiotherapy or chemotherapy is more likely to prolong survival for patients with oropharyngeal carcinomas rather than laryngeal or hypolaryngeal cancers. Although it has been speculated that HPV+ cancers may respond better to cetuximab, this has yet to be investigated.[56]

> **FUTURE RESEARCH**
>
> Molecular targeting approaches are being developed to sensitize tumours to mitochondrial mediated apoptosis (BH3 mimetics at the forefront) and to optimize apoptosis utilizing TRAIL receptor signalling pathways, approaches that may potentially be applicable to HNSCC and nasopharyngeal carcinoma. Frequently, work on cancers of the head and neck lags behind that of other more common cancers. Knowledge can be applied across tumour types, if a full understanding of the molecular basis of the cancer is obtained. Even within HNSCC, subtypes exist that need to be considered when testing agents and drug combinations, and in particular when dealing with the potential for resistance. The potential for inhibiting autophagic cell survival mechanisms could be explored further in these cancers. There is current interest in inhibiting PI3K and mTOR survival pathways. Given the increasing HPV+ HNSCC incidence and low take-up of HPV16 vaccination, targeting HPV DNA or E6 protein in HPV+ cancers to sensitize to p53-mediated apoptosis may be appropriate.

> **KEY POINTS**
>
> - Compromised p53 function leads to resistance to p53-mediated cell cycle arrest and DNA repair as well as apoptosis, leading to accumulation of genetic damage.
> - HPV+ HNSCC is genetically distinct from carcinogen-induced HNSCC and is more likely to respond to traditional therapies; this may be in part because of residual wild type p53 that is not fully degraded in response to E6 binding.
> - Targeting of overexpressed epidermal growth factor receptor (EGFR) using the monoclonal antibody cetuximab is currently used clinically.
> - In HNSCC genetic changes resulting in defects in the PI3K/Akt and Ras/MAPK signalling pathways are common and because tumour cells adapt to single target therapies, a combination approach is being tested.
> - The diversity of HNSCC tumours calls for screening approaches and personalized treatment to maximize cell death and overcome resistance to therapy.

REFERENCES

1. Hanahan D, Weinberg RA. The hallmarks of cancer. *Cell* 2000; **100**: 57–70.
2. Hanahan D, Weinberg RA. Hallmarks of cancer: the next generation. *Cell* 2011; **144**: 646–74.
3. Op de Beeck K, Schacht J, Van Camp G. Apoptosis in acquired and genetic hearing impairment: the programmed death of the hair cell. *Hearing Res* 2011; **281**: 18–27.
4. O'Brien MA, Moravec RA, Riss TL. Poly (ADP-ribose) polymerase cleavage monitored in situ in apoptotic cells. *BioTechniques* 2001; **30**: 886–91.
5. Hornsby PJ, Didenko VV. In situ ligation: a decade and a half of experience. *Methods Mol Biol* 2011; **682**: 49–63.
6. van Engeland M, Nieland LJ, Ramaekers FC, et al. Annexin V-affinity assay: a review on an apoptosis detection system based on phosphatidylserine exposure. *Cytometry* 1998; **31**: 1–9.
7. Candi E, Schmidt R, Melino G. The cornified envelope: a model of cell death in the skin. *Nat Rev Mol Cell Bio* 2005; **6**: 328–40.
8. Saunders, M. Apoptosis and cell death. In: Gleeson M (ed). *Scott-Brown's otorhinolaryngology: head and neck surgery*, 7th edition. Edward Arnold Ltd; 2008, pp. 56–65.
9. Tait SW, Ichim G, Green DR. Die another way: non-apoptotic mechanisms of cell death. *J Cell Sc* 2014; **127**: 2135–44.
10. Vanden Berghe T, Linkermann A, Jouan-Lanhouet S, et al. Regulated necrosis: the expanding network of non-apoptotic cell death pathways. *Nat Rev Mol Cell Bio* 2014; **15**: 135–47.
11. Galluzzi L, Kepp O, Krautwald S, et al. Molecular mechanisms of regulated necrosis. *Semin Cell Dev Biol* 2014; **35**: 24–32.
12. Moriwaki K, Chan FK. RIP3: a molecular switch for necrosis and inflammation. *Gene Dev* 2013; **27**: 1640–49.
13. Sipieter F, Ladik M, Vandenabeele P, Riquet F. Shining light on cell death processes: a novel biosensor for necroptosis, a newly described cell death program. *Biotechnol J* 2014; **9**: 224–40.
14. Sannigrahi M, Singh V, Sharma R, et al. Role of autophagy in head and neck cancer and therapeutic resistance. *Oral Dis* 2014; **21**(3): 283–91.
15. Nikoletopoulou V, Markaki M, Palikaras K, Tavernarakis N. Crosstalk between apoptosis, necrosis and autophagy. *Biochim Biophys Acta* 2013; **1833**: 3448–59.
16. Castillo K, Valenzuela V, Matus S, et al. Measurement of autophagy flux in the nervous system in vivo. *Cell Death Dis* 2013; **4**: e917.
17. Tait SW, Green DR. Mitochondria and cell death: outer membrane permeabilization and beyond. *Nat Rev Mol Cell Bio* 2010; **11**: 621–32.
18. Cory S, Adams JM. The Bcl2 family: regulators of the cellular life-or-death switch. *Nat Rev Cancer* 2002; **2**: 647–56.

19. Chi X, Kale J, Leber B, Andrews DW. Regulating cell death at, on, and in membranes. *Biochim Biophys Acta* 2014; **1843**: 2100–13.
20. Schellenberg B, Wang P, Keeble JA, et al. Bax exists in a dynamic equilibrium between the cytosol and mitochondria to control apoptotic priming. *Mol Cell* 2013; **49**: 959–71.
21. Lindsten T, Roos AJ, King A, et al. The combined functions of proapoptotic Bcl-2 family members bak and bax are essential for normal development of multiple tissues. *Mol Cell* 2000; **6**: 1389–99.
22. Gavathiotis E, Reyna DE, Bellairs JA, et al. Direct and selective small-molecule activation of proapoptotic BAX. *Nat Chem Biol* 2012; **8**: 639–45.
23. Adams JM, Cory S. The Bcl-2 apoptotic switch in cancer development and therapy. *Oncogene* 2007; **26**: 1324–37.
24. Krajewski S, Krajewska M, Shabaik A, et al. Immunohistochemical analysis of in vivo patterns of Bcl-X expression. *Cancer Res* 1994; **54**(21): 5501–7.
25. Chen L, Willis SN, Wei A, et al. Differential targeting of prosurvival Bcl-2 proteins by their BH3-only ligands allows complementary apoptotic function. *Mol Cell* 2005; **17**: 393–403.
26. Yazbeck VY, Li C, Grandis JR, et al. Single-agent obatoclax (GX15-070) potently induces apoptosis and pro-survival autophagy in head and neck squamous cell carcinoma cells. *Oral Oncol* 2014; **50**: 120–27.
27. Sedo-Cabezon L, Boadas-Vaello P, Soler-Martin C, Llorens J. Vestibular damage in chronic ototoxicity: a mini-review. *Neurotoxicology* 2014; **43**: 21–27.
28. Raimundo N, Song L, Shutt TE, et al. Mitochondrial stress engages E2F1 apoptotic signaling to cause deafness. *Cell* 2012; **148**: 716–26.
29. Muyderman H, Sims N, Tanaka M, et al. The mitochondrial T1095C mutation increases gentamicin-mediated apoptosis. *Mitochondrion* 2012; **12**: 465–71.
30. Park MK, Lee DB, Chae SW, et al. Protective effect of NecroX, a novel necroptosis inhibitor, on gentamicin-induced ototoxicity. *Int J Pediatr Otorhinol* 2012; **76**: 1265–69.
31. O'Connell J, Houston A, Bennett MW, et al. Immune privilege or inflammation? Insights into the Fas ligand enigma. *Nat Med* 2001; **7**: 271–74.
32. Villalba M, Rathmore MG, Lopez-Royuela N, et al. From tumor cell metabolism to tumor immune escape. *Int J Biochem Cell B* 2013; **45**: 106–13.
33. Chamuleau MED, Ossenkoppele A, van Rhenen A, et al. High TRAIL-R3 expression on leukemic blasts is associated with poor outcome and induces apoptosis-resistance which can be overcome by targeting TRAIL-R2. *Leukemia Res* 2011; **35**: 741–49.
34. Lalaoui, N, Morlé A, Mérino D, et al. TRAIL-R4 promotes tumor growth and resistance to apoptosis in cervical carcinoma HeLa cells through AKT. *PloS One* 2011; **6**: e19679.
35. Lemke J, von Karstedt S, Zinngrebe J, Walczak H. Getting TRAIL back on track for cancer therapy. *Cell Death Differ* 2014; **21**: 1350–64.
36. de Miguel D, Lemke J, Anel A, et al. Onto better TRAILs for cancer treatment. *Cell Death Differ* **23**(5): 733–47.
37. Napoli M, Flores ER. The family that eats together stays together: new p53 family transcriptional targets in autophagy. *Gene Dev* 2013; **27**: 971–74.
38. Kadakia S, Helman SN, Badhey AK, et al. Treacher Collins syndrome: the genetics of a craniofacial disease. *Int J Paed Otorhinolaryngol* 2014; **78**: 893–8.
39. Chalhoub N, Baker SJ. PTEN and the PI3-kinase pathway in cancer. *Annu Rev Pathol* 2009; **4**: 127–50.
40. Seiwert TY, Zuo Z, Keck MK et al. Integrative and comparative genomic analysis of HPV-positive and HPV-negative head and neck squamous cell carcinomas. *Clin Cancer Res* 2014.
41. Rothenberg SM, Ellisen LW. The molecular pathogenesis of head and neck squamous cell carcinoma. *J Clin Invest* 2012; **122**: 1951–57.
42. Agrawal N, Frederick MJ, Pickering CR, et al. Exome sequencing of head and neck squamous cell carcinoma reveals inactivating mutations in NOTCH1. *Science* 2011; **333**: 1154–57.
43. Stransky N, Egloff AM, Tward AS et al. The mutational landscape of head and neck squamous cell carcinoma. *Science* 2011; **333**: 1157–60.
44. Hunter KD, Thurlow JK, Fleming J, et al. Divergent routes to oral cancer. *Cancer Res* 2006; **66**: 7405–13.
45. Gadhikar MA, Sciuto MR, Alves MVO, et al. Chk1/2 inhibition overcomes the cisplatin resistance of head and neck cancer cells secondary to the loss of functional p53. *Mol Cancer Ther* 2013; **12**: 1860–73.
46. Hallden G, Portella G. Oncolytic virotherapy with modified adenoviruses and novel therapeutic targets. *Expert Opin Ther Tar* 2012; **16**: 945–58.
47. Lehmann S, Bykov VJ, Ali D, et al. Targeting p53 in vivo: a first-in-human study with p53-targeting compound APR-246 in refractory hematologic malignancies and prostate cancer. *J Clin Oncol* 2012; **30**: 3633–39.
48. Bravi F, Bosetti C, Filomeno M, et al. Foods, nutrients and the risk of oral and pharyngeal cancer. *Brit J Cancer* 2013; **109**: 2904–10.
49. Dayyani F, Etzel CJ, Liu M, et al. Meta-analysis of the impact of human papillomavirus (HPV) on cancer risk and overall survival in head and neck squamous cell carcinomas (HNSCC). *Head Neck Oncol* 2010; **2**: 15.
50. Kimple RJ, Smith MA, Blitzer GC, et al. Enhanced radiation sensitivity in HPV-positive head and neck cancer. *Cancer Res* 2013; **73**: 4791–4800.
51. Patel V, Ensley JF, Gutkind JS, Yeudall WA. Induction of apoptosis in head-and-neck squamous carcinoma cells by gamma-irradiation and bleomycin is p53-independent. *Int J Cancer* 2000; **88**: 737–43.
52. Grønhøj Larsen C, Gyldenløve M, Jensen DH, et al. Correlation between human papillomavirus and p16 overexpression in oropharyngeal tumours: a systematic review. *Brit J Cancer* 2014; **110**: 1587–94.
53. Rietbergen MM, Snijders PJF, Beekzada D, et al. Molecular characterization of p16-immunopositive but HPV DNA-negative oropharyngeal carcinomas. *Int J Cancer* 2014; **134**: 2366–72.
54. Perri F, Pacelli R, Della Vittoria Scarpati G, et al. Radioresistance in head and neck squamous cell carcinoma: biological bases and therapeutic implications. *Head Neck* 2015; **37**: 763–70.
55. Rampias T, Giagini A, Siolos S, et al. RAS/PI3K crosstalk and cetuximab resistance in head and neck squamous cell carcinoma. *Clin Cancer Res* 2014; **20**: 2933–46.
56. Yokota T. Is biomarker research advancing in the era of personalized medicine for head and neck cancer? *Int J Clin Oncol* 2014; **19**: 211–19.

CHAPTER 7

STEM CELLS

Navin Vig and Ian C. Mackenzie

Introduction 69	Application of stem cells to clinical problems in otolaryngology 71
General background: Stem cell types and properties 69	Cancer stem cells: Tumour growth, invasion and metastasis 72
Tissue engineering: Methods for generation of tissues and organs from cells 70	References 73

SEARCH STRATEGY

Data in this chapter may be updated by Medline searches based mainly on various combinations of the terms 'stem cells', 'embryonic stem cells', 'tissue regeneration' and 'otolaryngology'. Other sources include published and unpublished information from the author's laboratories.

INTRODUCTION

Tissue abnormalities of the head and neck region, arising from disease, injury or developmental defects, often pose considerable regenerative problems. Historically, the efficacy of surgical reconstruction has been limited by a lack of suitable autologous tissues for reparative or regenerative procedures but the development of methods for *in vitro* and *in vivo* tissue expansion, together with advances in tissue engineering, now provide new therapeutic options.[1] It has become apparent that stem cells, of which there are several varieties, are the cells ultimately responsible for all normal tissue generation and regeneration. Therapeutic regeneration of new tissues therefore also typically depends on direct or indirect manipulation of stem cells and such cells are now a major focus for research. A relatively new aspect of stem cell biology relates to the roles of stem cells in malignancy. This too is of markedly increasing research interest that focuses on their roles in metastasis and the need to target them therapeutically.

Entering the search term 'stem cells' into the PubMed database indicates that more than 20 000 papers relating to stem cells were published in 2015 alone (http://www.ncbi.nlm.nih.gov/pubmed). This brief chapter can only outline some of the aspects of stem cells potentially relevant to otorhinolaryngology and head and neck surgery. The initial aim will be to put stem cells in perspective by outlining the different sorts of stem cells that exist and by describing their common features. The second aim will be to outline current directions of stem cell research related to their potential clinical applications in otolaryngology.

GENERAL BACKGROUND: STEM CELL TYPES AND PROPERTIES

Adult tissue-specific stem cells

It has been known for well over a century that many tissues of the body are continuously renewed by cell division. Detailed studies of cell division in bone marrow, now over 50 years old, indicated that many blood forming cells have some ability to divide but that the ability to divide persistently, the key feature of stem cells, is possessed by only a subset of cells. Subsequent studies indicated that stem cells in the haematopoietic system can be identified by their expression of particular cell surface markers, are clonogenic *in vitro*, and have the ability to completely restore the haematopoietic system in mice whose bone marrow has been destroyed by irradiation.[2] These findings led to the concept of an adult (or 'somatic') stem cell as an immature cell that is capable of dividing indefinitely both to renew itself and produce cells maturing for tissue function. Cells with such properties have now been identified in most normal and malignant tissues.[3]

Although indefinite division is an essential stem cell property, the ability to produce differentiating cells is key to their function of tissue renewal and regeneration.

Some stem cells are able to generate cells entering several different lineages; haematopoietic stem cells, for example, generate cells that differentiate into the diverse range of cell types (e.g. erythrocytes, inflammatory and immune cells) found in blood.[3] Stem cells with the ability to generate many different types of cells are considered 'multipotent'. Other stem cells, for example those of the epidermis, normally produce cells of only a single lineage and are considered 'unipotent'. However, even cells that are normally unipotent may under some conditions, such as wound healing, be capable of generating cells of different lineages.

The advantages of somatic stem cells for clinical use are that they are readily expanded *in vitro*, usually maintain a stable differentiation pattern and, as they can be expanded from autologous tissue, initiate no immune rejection. Examples of established therapeutic uses of somatic stem cells include the transplantation of donor haematopoietic stem cells for the treatment of leukaemia, and the grafting of *in vitro* generated autologous sheets of epithelial cells for the treatment of burns or repair of corneal damage. A large current range of clinical trials of regenerative stem cell procedures include neural stem cell grafting for treatment of spinal cord injuries, embryonic stem (ES) cell-derived retinal cells for treatment of macular degeneration, stem cell-derived β-cells for treatment of Type 1 diabetes, and the use of stem cells to enhance healing after coronary infarction. When somatic stem cells with an appropriate differentiation pattern can be generated from biopsies of autologous tissue this usually forms the simplest approach but, if not, then re-differentiation of a multipotent stem cell of one of the types described below provides an alternative method.

Embryonic stem cells

About 20 years ago, it was discovered that cells of the inner cell mass of mouse blastocysts, the cells that would normally go on to form the embryo, can be isolated, greatly expanded *in vitro* and then differentiated into multiple cell lineages.[4] Such 'embryonic stem cells' (ES cells) were later also derived from human blastocysts. The controlled *in vitro* differentiation of ES cells into a required cell type can be directed using signals that mimic the tissue interactions that guide emergence of regionally appropriate cell lineages during embryonic development. Consequently, ES cells can provide an essentially unlimited source of relevantly differentiated cells.[4] However, ES cells are generated by destruction of living human blastocysts and strong opposition to the use of ES cells has been expressed on ethical grounds. A further major complexity is that tissues produced from ES cells express the histocompatibility antigens genetically determined by the donor embryo and, consequently, their compatibility with recipients is restricted to some immune-privileged sites, requires manipulation of the recipient's immune system, or modification of antigens expressed by the stem cell.

Induced pluripotent stem cells

Studies of ES cells led to the identification of genes associated with the maintenance of 'stemness' and it was found that induced expression of 'stem cell' genes such as *Oct4*, *Sox2*, *cMyc*, and *Klf4* in differentiated cells results in their acquisition of stem cell properties similar to those of ES cells (i.e. the ability to divide indefinitely and the pluripotency that enables differentiation into multiple cell types by *in vitro* manipulation).[5] The generation of such 'induced pluripotency stem cells' (iPSCs) demonstrates a degree of cellular plasticity beyond that previously thought feasible, and iPS cells represent a class of cells able to regenerate a wide range of tissue types. The pluripotency of ES cells, and the possibility of their generation from autologous adult tissues, has greatly stimulated research into their potential clinical use for replacement of tissues that are genetically defective or have been lost to damage or disease.[6] Concerns about potential carcinogenic effects of genetic alterations used to generate iPS cells have been addressed by development of methods for their induction without permanent genetic alteration. In addition to their value for clinical tissue replacement, iPS cells provide *in vitro* models of genetic diseases and for assays of drug effects.

Mesenchymal stem cells

Cells with multipotent stem cell properties can be isolated from various adult and foetal tissues, such as bone marrow, fat, dental pulp and umbilical cord, and it seems likely that similar cells are present in many adult tissues.[7] These mesenchymal stem cells (MSCs) are fibroblast-like, have good expansion and differentiation potentials, and also possess immune-modulatory properties.[8] Typically the cells differentiated from MSCs are osteoblasts or chondrocytes but greater plasticity with an ability to generate cells of non-mesenchymal lineages is suggested by reports of their differentiation into neurons or hepatocytes.[9] The ability to derive MSCs from various tissues and to manipulate their differentiation for use as autologous transplants has generated extensive clinical interest.

TISSUE ENGINEERING: METHODS FOR GENERATION OF TISSUES AND ORGANS FROM CELLS

Methods for the isolation, amplification and differentiation of stem cells can provide the basic cellular materials for tissue reconstruction. However, these biological advances lead to new challenges of how to assemble such cells into functional tissues or organs. Clinical use has so far been largely limited to cells, such as epithelial or chondrocytic stem cells, that are able to self-assemble into an appropriate tissue either *in vitro* or after delivery to an *in vivo* site. The further aim of tissue engineering is to exploit biomaterials and biologically active molecules to facilitate the production of more complex structures. It includes using bioactive substances to control cell behaviour, together with synthetic matrices and engineered scaffolds that both provide physical support for growth and assist with the delivery of constructs. Currently, however, the construction of tissues that are formed of multiple cell types, and of organs that are too large to rely on simple diffusion for the supply of gases and nutrients needed for cell survival provide many technical problems. Biological approaches to overcome problems of construct vascularization have included supporting the growth of cellularized scaffolds by transplantation to surrogate hosts and by complex genetic manipulations that allow implanted human stem cells to form organs during the embryonic development of other species.[10] Rapid advances are, however, being made in three-dimensional cell culture with bio-printing, allowing patterned deposition of cells, and the development of novel perfusion bioreactors providing better support for cell growth.[11, 12] However, the application of these procedures to the regeneration of large organs remains essentially experimental and the cost of such organ production is a significant factor.

APPLICATION OF STEM CELLS TO CLINICAL PROBLEMS IN OTOLARYNGOLOGY

The anatomical area of interest to otolaryngology contains a wide range of tissues but stem cell research has shown the feasibility of generating a range of appropriately differentiated cells for clinical use in regenerating and reconstructing epithelial, cartilaginous, osseous, neural and mucosal tissues.

The ear and nose

Regenerative stem cell properties have been investigated to rectify common structural or functional problems of the ear, nose, tympanic membrane, cochlea, trachea and other structures. Congenital, traumatic, and neoplastic tissue loss, as well as cosmetic reasons, may generate a need to replace or modify the existing structure of the external ear or nose and existing procedures for reconstruction may involve skin expansion, rib harvesting and multistage surgery. An alternative approach is to use autologous stem cells to produce cartilage after seeding onto appropriately shaped scaffolds.[10] If needed, these can be invested in autologous epithelial sheets derived from epidermal stem cells provided by small epidermal biopsies, a well established technique long-employed for skin replacement of burns patients.[13] Such procedures can be expected to provide consistent results that reduce surgical complexity and post-operative morbidity. Small biopsies of ear or rib tissue can provide cartilage stem cells for expansion and aesthetically successful nasal reconstructions have been reported using engineered cartilage grafts generated from cartilage stem cells in biopsies from the nasal septum.[14] The uses of engineered cartilage for various other types of reconstruction are now being assessed. Augmented repair of chronic tympanic membrane perforation has focused mainly on the use of growth factors and biomolecules that have been demonstrated to enhance healing[15] but this appears to be a feasible area for the generation of matrices populated with autologous chondrocytes and epithelial cells.

Cochlea damage or degeneration

Sensorineural hearing loss resulting from inner-ear cochlear dysfunction involves the loss of sensory hair cells and/or spiral ganglion neurons. Loss of inner hair cells is currently irreversible but a range of stem cell procedures that aim to regenerate cochlea structures, such as hair cells and associated peripheral nerves, has been reported.[9] A primary issue is identifying types of stem cells appropriate for differentiation into sensory and neural progenitor cells, but equally challenging secondary issues are the differentiation of stem cells into the desired structures *in situ*, or the delivery of *in vivo* or *in vitro* differentiated stem cells to the right location. Rodent MSCs and some other stem cell types have been shown to differentiate *in vitro* into cells with hair cell properties indicating the feasibility of stem cell use. Of particular interest, a stepwise *in vitro* process that mimics normal developmental interactions, can differentiate murine ES cells into both functional mechano-sensitive hair cells and into sensory neurones that interact to form specialized synapses.[16]

The trachea

Replacement of lost tracheal tissue has been a focus of successful stem cell research. Autologous cartilage has been harvested to replace small defects but malignancy may be associated with more extensive tissue loss that requires more extensive replacement. Larger constructs require the structural strength to withstand collapse due to the negative pressure of inspiration and the need for transplants to clear secretions points to the need for an appropriately differentiated luminal epithelium within a multi-layered functioning trachea.[17] Successful five-year clinical results have been reported using a tissue-engineering strategy of bioreactor growth of a decellularized donor human trachea repopulated with cultured autologous epithelial stem-cells and MSC derived autologous chondrocytes prior to transplantation.[1, 18] Further development that avoids the need for donor tissue has been construction of a bioartificial polymeric scaffold that models tracheobronchial size and morphology and which, after *ex vivo* seeding with autologous bone-marrow mononuclear cells and growth factor-induced mobilization of endogenous stem cells, was successfully transplanted as an airway replacement after cancer surgery.[19]

Larynx and vocal cords

Laryngeal injury and vocal cord (VC) disease can significantly impact upon vocal cord function and thus phonation. Current interventions in the management of vocal fold (VF) dysfunction focus on conservative and surgical approaches. However, the complex structure and precise biomechanical properties of the human VF mean that these strategies have their limitations in clinical practice and may offer inadequate levels of success. Regenerative medicine has the potential to enhance VF recovery beyond that associated with conventional treatments.[20] So far, however, most investigations of the regenerative use of stem cells have been limited to assessment of various types of MSCs in animal models.[21] Cell-free scaffolds of collagen, hyaluronic acid or fibrin enhance laryngeal wound healing and attempts have also been made to activate resident somatic stem cells.[20] MSCs support VC remodelling and reduce scarring when directly injected, either alone or as part of a cell-scaffold composite, and MSCs in hyaluronic acid hydrogels provide both biologically active material and volume allowing for accelerated healing in small animals.[22] However, as VC remodelling can take up to six months in humans, it is uncertain whether MSCs persist long enough to benefit human repair.[22] The non-keratinized epithelium covering the VCs can potentially be replaced by *in vitro* expansion of stem cells from small biopsies of adjacent mucosae but human iPS cells can be differentiated in the presence of matrix molecules and growth factors into an appropriate non-keratinizing epithelium.[23]

Other tissues

Stem cell investigations to assist regeneration of a range of other tissues have been reported. For example, surgery of the head and neck can lead to peripheral nerve damage, with the facial and recurrent laryngeal nerves (RLNs) most commonly affected. Muscle-derived MSCs have been shown to improve outcomes in RLN injuries and work with facial nerve injuries has shown that neural regeneration following axonotomy is enhanced by a combination of neural-induced MSCs and platelet-rich plasma.[24] Interestingly, several regions of the nose act as sources of autologous stem cells, such as olfactory ensheathing cells, which assist neural and other regenerative procedures. Large deficiencies of the maxillofacial skeleton can result from traumatic damage, or resection following malignant invasion, and direct injection of MSCs, together with appropriate materials or scaffolds, can assist regeneration. Stem cells have also been discussed with regard to improvement in scars following surgery or trauma and there is a large body of literature that considers MSCs and scars.

CANCER STEM CELLS: TUMOUR GROWTH, INVASION AND METASTASIS

Many solid tumours respond poorly to current therapies and, on average, only about 50% of HNSCC patients survive longer than five years from diagnosis. Recent work confirms that tumours contain subpopulations of altered stem cells, termed 'cancer stem cells' (CSCs) and that tumour growth is ultimately dependent on these cells.[3, 25] Stem cell patterns have been identified in squamous cell carcinomas and also in the minority glandular tumours.[26, 27] CSCs have unique properties of direct clinical interest including resistance to therapy and the ability to invade locally and metastasize.[25] The mechanisms of the stem cell changes that lead to cancer remain unclear but, despite enhanced stem cell DNA repair,[28] tobacco and alcohol have mutational effects and an increasing number of oropharyngeal tumours result are associated with human papilloma viruses that act to increase the number of SCs and alter their behaviour.[29, 30]

The homeostatic state of renewing tissues such as skin and mucosae is normally maintained by SC divisions that renew the SC population while also producing cells that differentiate. Many signalling pathways that affect division patterns (e.g. Notch, Wnt, Sonic hedgehog) are dysregulated in malignancy leading to a shift of CSC divisions towards greater self-renewal, which leads to an increasing number of CSCs and loss of tumour growth control.[3] Normal stem cells (SCs) have several mechanisms to maintain their integrity and enhancement of these mechanisms in CSCs results in greater resistance when challenged with radiation or chemotherapeutic drugs and provides them with a survival advantage over non-CSCs.[28-31] However, such mechanisms for enhanced tumour growth and resistance do not explain how CSCs escape from a tumour to invade locally or metastasize distantly, the events causing most cancer deaths. Basic research implicates epithelial-mesenchymal transition (EMT) as the process by which tightly cohesive epithelial cells acquire mesenchymal characteristics and lose mutual attachment to gain motility[32] and it is proposed that this mechanism allows CSCs to escape from the tumour and migrate to distant sites where they then revert back to the proliferative epithelial phenotype to produce secondary tumours.[33] The mechanisms of reversion of cells back to the epithelial phenotype are not well understood but the molecular mechanisms of EMT indicate that the level of EMT occurring in a particular tumour depends partly on intrinsic tumour properties and partly on extrinsic stromal factors such as cytokines and hypoxia.[34-36]

CSCs were initially defined by their ability to initiate tumours in immune-deficient mice after their isolation on the basis of their expression of cell surface markers.[3] Such tumour initiating subpopulations of CSC have been identified in both fresh HNSCC and in passaged HNSCC cell lines.[37, 38] Identification was initially achieved using the CD44 marker but a range of other cell surface or enzymatic markers has subsequently been employed. Analyses of CSC behaviour continue to support the conclusion that their elimination is necessary for successful therapy and many different therapeutic mechanisms are being explored to target CSCs.[31] These include using antibodies against particular CSC surface markers to deliver cytolethal agents,[39] development of drugs to inactivate CSC self-renewal pathways,[40] and reducing CSC resistance to radiation or drugs.[41] However, concerning chemotherapeutic drugs, the plasticity of CSCs generates cells that differ in their drug or radiation responses and are also able to switch between phenotypes. Thus elimination of CSCs may require drug combinations and assays to assess drug effects on each of the CSC phenotypic manifestations and these are being developed.[42]

> **KEY POINTS**
>
> - Stem cells are the ultimate origin of the wide variety of cells generated during embryological development and are responsible for all subsequent tissue growth and regeneration.
> - Stem cells are also responsible for the growth and treatment resistance of malignant tissues.
> - Recent research has disclosed many aspects of the control mechanisms underlying stem cell behaviour and has enabled their manipulation.
> - This information is now being used to develop methods for clinical tissue regeneration and for cancer therapy.

REFERENCES

1. Badylak SF, Weiss DJ, Caplan A, et al. Engineered whole organs and complex tissues. *Lancet* 2012; **379**(9819): 943–52.
2. Bonnet D, Dick JE. Human acute myeloid leukemia is organized as a hierarchy that originates from a primitive hematopoietic cell. *Nature Med* 1997; **3**(7): 730–37.
3. Reya T, Morrison SJ, Clarke MF, et al. Stem cells, cancer, and cancer stem cells. *Nature* 2001; **414**(6859): 105–11.
4. Smith AG. Embryo-derived stem cells: of mice and men. *Annu Rev Cell Dev Biol* 2001; **17**: 435–62.
5. Takahashi K, Tanabe K, Ohnuki M, et al. Induction of pluripotent stem cells from adult human fibroblasts by defined factors. *Cell* 2007; **131**(5): 861–72.
6. Nelson TJ, Martinez-Fernandez A, Terzic A. Induced pluripotent stem cells: developmental biology to regenerative medicine. *Nat Rev Cardiol* 2010; **7**(12): 700–10.
7. Zomer HD, Vidane AS, Goncalves NN, et al. Mesenchymal and induced pluripotent stem cells: general insights and clinical perspectives. *Cloning Stem Cells* 2015; **8**: 125–34.
8. Caplan AI. MSCs: the sentinel and safeguards of injury. *J Cell Physiol* 2015; **231**(7) 1413–16.
9. Wormald JC, Fishman JM, Juniat S, et al. Regenerative medicine in otorhinolaryngology. *J Laryngol Otol* 2015; **129**(8): 732–39.
10. Cao Y, Vacanti JP, Paige KT, et al. Transplantation of chondrocytes utilizing a polymer-cell construct to produce tissue-engineered cartilage in the shape of a human ear. *Plast Reconstr Surg* 1997; **100**(2): 297–302; discussion 303–404.
11. Sivayoham E, Saunders R, Derby B, et al. Current concepts and advances in the application of tissue engineering in otorhinolaryngology and head and neck surgery. *J Laryngol Otol* 2013; **127**(2): 114–20.
12. Gjorevski N, Ranga A, Lutolf MP. Bioengineering approaches to guide stem cell-based organogenesis. *Development* 2014; **141**(9): 1794–1804.
13. Green H, Kehinde O, Thomas J. Growth of cultured human epidermal cells into multiple epithelia suitable for grafting. *Proc Natl Acad Sci USA* 1979; **76**(11): 5665–68.
14. Fulco I, Miot S, Haug MD, et al. Engineered autologous cartilage tissue for nasal reconstruction after tumour resection: an observational first-in-human trial. *Lancet* 2014; **384**(9940): 337–46.
15. Hong P, Bance M, Gratzer PF. Repair of tympanic membrane perforation using novel adjuvant therapies: a contemporary review of experimental and tissue engineering studies. *Int J Pediatr Otorhinolaryngol* 2013; **77**(1): 3–12.
16. Koehler KR, Mikosz AM, Molosh AI, et al. Generation of inner ear sensory epithelia from pluripotent stem cells in 3D culture. *Nature* 2013; **500**(7461): 217–21.
17. Naito H, Tojo T, Kimura M, et al. Engineering bioartificial tracheal tissue using hybrid fibroblast-mesenchymal stem cell cultures in collagen hydrogels. *Interact Cardiovasc Thorac Surg* 2011; **12**(2): 156–61.
18. Gonfiotti A, Jaus MO, Barale D, et al. The first tissue-engineered airway transplantation: 5-year follow-up results. *Lancet* 2014; **383**(9913): 238–44.
19. Jungebluth P, Alici E, Baiguera S, et al. Tracheobronchial transplantation with a stem-cell-seeded bioartificial nanocomposite: a proof-of-concept study. *Lancet* 2011; **378**(9808): 1997–2004.
20. Fishman JM, Long J, Gugatschka M, et al. Stem cell approaches for vocal fold regeneration. *Laryngoscope* 2016; **126**(8): 1865–70.
21. Bartlett RS, Gaston JD, Yen TY, et al. Biomechanical screening of cell therapies for vocal fold scar. *Tissue Eng Part A* 2015; **21**(17–18): 2437–47.
22. Svensson B, Nagubothu SR, Cedervall J, et al. Injection of human mesenchymal stem cells improves healing of vocal folds after scar excision: a xenograft analysis. *Laryngoscope* 2011; **121**(10): 2185–90.
23. Imaizumi M, Sato Y, Yang DT, et al. In vitro epithelial differentiation of human induced pluripotent stem cells for vocal fold tissue engineering. *Ann Otol Rhinol Laryngol* 2013; **122**(12): 737–47.
24. Cho HH, Jang S, Lee SC, et al. Effect of neural-induced mesenchymal stem cells and platelet-rich plasma on facial nerve regeneration in an acute nerve injury model. *Laryngoscope* 2010; **120**(5): 907–13.
25. Nguyen LV, Vanner R, Dirks P, et al. Cancer stem cells: an evolving concept. *Nat Rev Cancer* 2012; **12**(2): 133–43.
26. Adams A, Warner K, Nor JE. Salivary gland cancer stem cells. *Oral Oncol* 2013; **49**(9): 845–53.
27. Adams A, Warner K, Pearson AT, et al. ALDH/CD44 identifies uniquely tumorigenic cancer stem cells in salivary gland mucoepidermoid carcinomas. *Oncotarget* 2015; **6**(29): 26633–50.
28. Diehn M, Cho RW, Lobo NA, et al. Association of reactive oxygen species levels and radioresistance in cancer stem cells. *Nature* 2009; **458**(7239): 780–83.
29. Pullos AN, Castilho RM, Squarize CH. HPV infection of the head and neck region and its stem cells. *J Dent Res* 2015; **94**(11): 1532–43.
30. Hufbauer M, Biddle A, Borgogna C, et al. Expression of betapapillomavirus oncogenes increases the number of keratinocytes with stem cell-like properties. *J Virol* 2013; **87**(22): 12158–65.
31. Birkeland AC, Owen JH, Prince ME. Targeting head and neck cancer stem cells: current advances and future challenges. *J Dent Res* 2015; **94**(11): 1516–23.
32. Thiery JP. Epithelial-mesenchymal transitions in development and pathologies. *Curr Opin Cell Biol* 2003; **15**(6): 740–46.
33. Brabletz T, Jung A, Spaderna S, et al. Opinion: migrating cancer stem cells – an integrated concept of malignant tumour progression. *Nat Rev Cancer* 2005; **5**(9): 744–49.
34. Gammon L, Biddle A, Heywood HK, et al. Sub-sets of cancer stem cells differ intrinsically in their patterns of oxygen metabolism. *PLoS One* 2013; **8**(4): e62493.
35. Steinestel K, Eder S, Schrader AJ, et al. Clinical significance of epithelial-mesenchymal transition. *Clin Transl Med* 2014; **3**: 17.
36. Lamouille S, Xu J, Derynck R. Molecular mechanisms of epithelial-mesenchymal transition. *Nat Rev Mol Cell Biol* 2014; **15**(3): 178–96.
37. Locke M, Heywood M, Fawell S, et al. Retention of intrinsic stem cell hierarchies in carcinoma-derived cell lines. *Cancer Res* 2005; **65**(19): 8944–50.
38. Prince ME, Sivanandan R, Kaczorowski A, et al. Identification of a subpopulation of cells with cancer stem cell properties in head and neck squamous cell carcinoma. *Proc Natl Acad Sci USA* 2007; **104**(3): 973–78.
39. Tijink BM, Buter J, de Bree R, et al. A phase I dose escalation study with anti-CD44v6 bivatuzumab mertansine in patients with incurable squamous cell carcinoma of the head and neck or esophagus. *Clin Cancer Res* 2006; **12**(20 Pt 1): 6064–72.
40. Yen WC, Fischer MM, Axelrod F, et al. Targeting Notch signaling with a Notch2/Notch3 antagonist (tarextumab) inhibits tumor growth and decreases tumor-initiating cell frequency. *Clin Cancer Res* 2015; **21**(9): 2084–95.
41. Chang CC, Hsu WH, Wang CC, et al. Connective tissue growth factor activates pluripotency genes and mesenchymal-epithelial transition in head and neck cancer cells. *Cancer Res* 2013; **73**(13): 4147–57.
42. Biddle A, Liang X, Gammon L, et al. Cancer stem cells in squamous cell carcinoma switch between two distinct phenotypes that are preferentially migratory or proliferative. *Cancer Res* 2011; **71**(15): 5317–26.

AETIOLOGY AND PATHOGENESIS OF GOITRE

Neil Sharma and Kristien Boelaert

Introduction 75	Novel therapies 79
Factors influencing goitre formation 76	Summary 79
Pathophysiology 78	References 80
Hormonal factors regulating thyroid growth ... 79	

SEARCH STRATEGY

Data in this chapter may be updated by a Medline search using the keywords: thyroid, goitre, pathogenesis, aetiology, nodular and iodine. Reference lists for selected papers were examined for further sources.

INTRODUCTION

Thyroid enlargement is common, and has been recognized for almost two millennia. The exact definition of goitre has evolved over time, depending on the examination methods available. Based on autopsy studies, a thyroid was initially considered to be enlarged if weighing greater than 35 g, and the use of high-resolution ultrasound has led to the currently accepted definition of >18 mL in women and >25 mL in men.[1,2] Variations in this cut-off globally have meant direct comparison between population studies is often problematic.

Previous autopsy studies reported the prevalence of thyroid nodules to be in excess of 50% in clinically normal thyroids;[3,4] however, these studies were carried out prior to the iodization programs seen in many parts of the world and this is therefore probably an overestimation, with the current incidence lying between 25% and 50%.[1] Goitre can be classified as physiological or pathological – the former is found often in teenage girls and is without clinical significance. The latter comprises both benign and malignant; the focus of this chapter will be the benign multinodular goitre (**Figure 8.1**), with other causes of thyroid enlargement covered in other chapters.

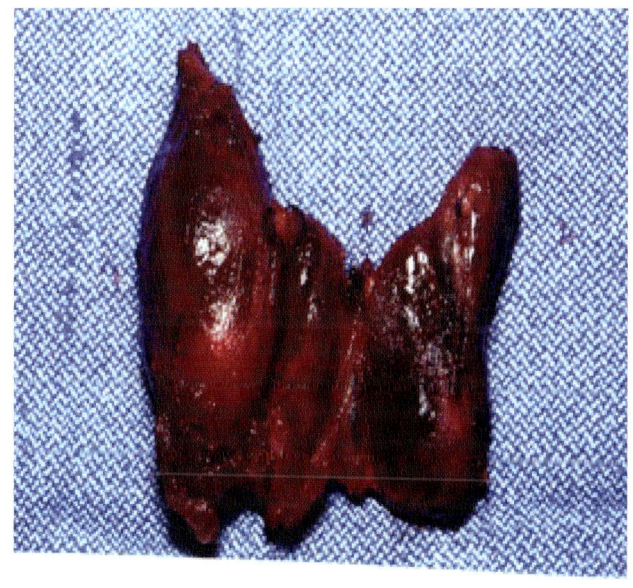

Figure 8.1 A multinodular thyroid following excision.

FACTORS INFLUENCING GOITRE FORMATION

The aetiology of benign pathological goitre can be broadly split into environmental and genetic factors, although these rarely exist in isolation and a thorough understanding of each is therefore essential.

Environmental factors

IODINE DEFICIENCY

Iodine deficiency is the biggest contributor to goitre. In 2004 the World Health Organization estimated that 2 billion people were iodine deficient, including approximately 285 million school-aged children.[5] It is thought around 45% of Europeans are iodine deficient,[6, 7] and in many parts of the world with universal iodine deficiency, goitre is endemic. The most common dietary sources of iodine are fish and dairy products, with a balanced diet being sufficient to maintain an adequate intake of 150 mcg/day for (non-pregnant) adults.[8, 9] Iodine deficiency is measured using the surrogate marker of urinary iodine concentration (UIC), usually corrected for creatinine excretion. Iodine sufficiency is defined as UIC greater than 100 µg/L, moderate deficiency as UIC below 50 µg/L and severe deficiency as UIC below 25 µg/L.[10, 11] Thyroid volume directly correlates to UIC (**Figure 8.2**); in addition, increased UIC also negatively correlates with thyroid nodule prevalence.[1]

Various programs exist across the developed and developing world to improve iodine status, one of the most effective being mandatory iodization of salt. This is not universal, however, and many countries including the UK do not enforce this. In 2006, the World Health Assembly recommended that countries carry out surveys of iodine status using sampling of UIC as a marker.[10] The first national survey in the UK was carried out in 2011 and found that in female schoolchildren between the age of 14 and 15 years, the median UIC was 80.1 µg/L, with 67% of the cohort being iodine deficient (17% moderately or severely so).[12] The consequences of iodine deficiency in relation to prevalence of goitre among school children are shown in **Table 8.1**, and these findings therefore potentially pose a significant public health burden.

The consequences in pregnancy are also potentially severe. A recent study examining mother-child pairs in the UK measured maternal UIC in the first trimester of pregnancy and correlated this with the child's cognitive development at age 8 years. The researchers found that even mild iodine deficiency in early gestation was associated with lower scores for verbal IQ, reading accuracy and reading comprehension (**Figure 8.3**), emphasizing that even in developed countries there is a significant public health risk from iodine deficiency spanning several generations.[13]

Although there are several known environmental goitrogens, all of these must be examined in the context of iodine status of both the individual and the population, as some environmental causes will have significant effects when iodine is deplete, with some or no effect in iodine sufficiency (**Table 8.2**).

POLLUTANTS

Thiocyanate is found in cigarette smoke and also environmentally in cassava, which is a major source of carbohydrate in Africa and associated with an increased incidence of goitre.[19] Nitrate sources include vegetables and drinking water; contamination of water with nitrate from agriculture leads to an odds ratio for goitre of 3 when assessed in iodine-replete Bulgarian school children,[20] although no link was found between urinary nitrite excretion and thyroid volume in a German study.[21]

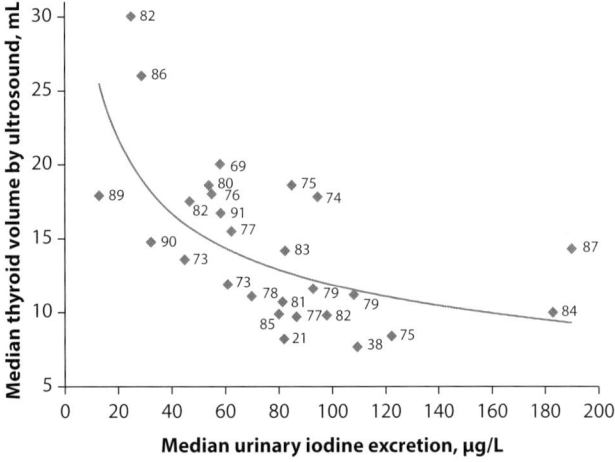

Figure 8.2 Graph demonstrating the fall in thyroid volume as urinary iodine excretion rises. From Carle A, Krejbjerg A, Laurberg P. Epidemiology of nodular goitre. Influence of iodine intake. *Best Pract Res Cl En* 2014; **28**(4): 465–79.[1]

TABLE 8.1 Relationship of iodine status to goitre prevalence in schoolchildren			
Median UIE (µ g/L)	Iodine status	Goitre among schoolchildren	Consequences
<20	Severe ID	>30%	Endemic cretinism, hypothyroidism, endemic nodular goitre
20–49	Moderate ID	20–29.9%	Endemic nodular goitre, low IQ, hyperthyroidism more often than hypothyroidism
50–99	Mild ID	5.9–19.9%	Hyperthyroidism more often than hypothyroidism, nodular goitre
100–199	Iodine sufficiency	<4.9%	Optimal balance between various thyroid disorders

Source: From WHO, UNICEF, ICCIDD. *Assessment of iodine deficiency disorders and monitoring their elimination*. 3rd ed. Geneva: World Health Organization; 2007.

8: AETIOLOGY AND PATHOGENESIS OF GOITRE

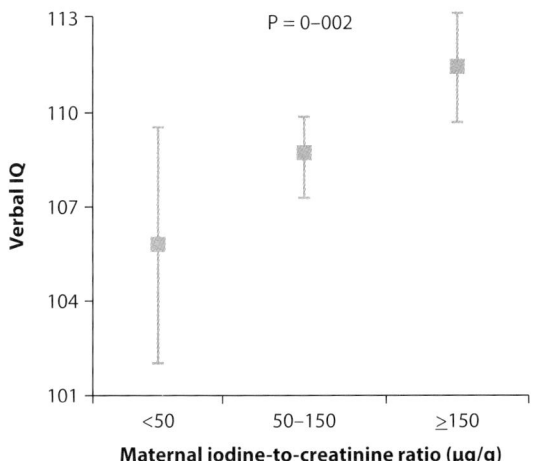

Figure 8.3 A deficient maternal iodine status is associated with poorer performance in a number of cognitive tests in offspring. From Bath SC, Steer CD, Golding J, et al. Effect of inadequate iodine status in UK pregnant women on cognitive outcomes in their children: results from the Avon Longitudinal Study of Parents and Children (ALSPAC). *Lancet* 2013; **382**(9889): 331–37.[13]

Isoflavones are found in soybeans and inhibit thyroid peroxidase; however, population studies give mixed results in terms of goitre formation.[22, 23] In our laboratory, we have used a soybean rich diet in our mouse models of goitre and see an increased thyroid size, a finding that reported by several other researchers.

Organochlorides present in solvents and pesticides have become less prevalent as most of these are now banned. They have, if any, only a mild goitrogenic effect and this should decline as their use tails off.[24]

Perchlorate, a potent inhibitor of iodine uptake, is found in rocket fuel and accelerants, bleach and some fertilizers. It has not been shown to have any effect clinically on thyroid function at the levels encountered though environmental exposure, and it is therefore unlikely to have any effect on thyroid volume.[25] The US Environmental Protection Agency found perchlorate in 4% of drinking water samples tested nationally, and subsequently has issued notice that the perchlorate content of water will be regulated. The cut-off for detectable levels was, however, many orders of magnitude lower than that thought necessary to cause thyroidal effects.

TOBACCO

Tobacco smoking is another major risk factor for goitre development and is most marked in iodine deficient populations. Different studies report an odds ratio of between 1.5 to 3 for goitre in smokers, although variations in background iodine status make meta-analysis challenging.[18] Thiocyanates are a major constituent of tobacco smoke and it is likely that these contribute to the increased risk.

SELENIUM

Selenium, like iodine, is necessary for thyroid hormone synthesis although to a much smaller degree. In addition, selenoproteins are important in the recycling of hydrogen peroxide generated by thyroid peroxidase. It is likely that selenium deficiency plays a cumulative role in nodule formation alongside iodine deficiency.[26]

ORAL CONTRACEPTIVE PILL

While intuitively it may be thought that the OCP would be a risk factor for goitre development, the converse appears to be true. OCP use is associated with a lower thyroid volume (8.5 mL vs. 9.4 mL^2) and low odds ratio (0.6)[27] for the development of goitre compared with no use; the mechanism for this is unexplained, but one theory is that exogenous oestrogens suppress the endogenous, goitrogenic ones. This is an avenue that warrants further exploration.

METABOLIC SYNDROME AND INSULIN RESISTANCE

Insulin resistance is becoming an increasingly studied risk factor given the rise in prevalence of metabolic syndrome across the Western world. Nodules were found in 53% of patients with insulin resistance compared to 19% without, and these results are mirrored in patients with metabolic syndrome, all in areas with a degree of iodine deficiency.[28, 29] Metformin has shown some positive effects in reducing thyroid volume in these patients, although results are not conclusive.[30, 31]

Genetic Factors

In addition to the well-studied environmental factors affecting thyroid growth, the familial clustering of goitres combined with the higher prevalence in females

TABLE 8.2 Relative contribution of genetic and environmental factors to goitre development with varying iodine status

Study	Country	Iodine status	Genetic factors (%)	Environmental factors (%)
Greig et al. 1967[14]	Scotland	Deficient	39	61
Brix et al. 1999[15]	Denmark	Mildly deficient	82	18
Hansen et al. 2004[16]	Denmark	Mildly deficient	71	29
Hansen et al. 2005[17]	Denmark	Mildly deficient	77	23

Source: Adapted from Knudsen N, Brix TH. Genetic and non-iodine-related factors in the aetiology of nodular goitre. *Best Pract Res Cl En* 2014; **28**(4): 495–506.[18]

suggests a genetic component to the disease, and this is becoming increasingly studied. While genetic factors are more significant in iodine deficient areas, families and small groups around the world show increased thyroid volume despite iodine supplementation, adding further evidence to a genetic cause. On a population level, discrete genetic causes are difficult to ascertain and therefore twin studies provide the best direct evidence of a genetic basis to goitre formation. In both endemic and non-endemic areas, monozygotic twins demonstrate a higher concordance for goitre development than dizygotic twins (**Figure 8.4**).

THYROID-SPECIFIC GENES

The identification of specific genes that predispose to goitre formation has mainly focused on those that are known to have a role in the normal physiology of the thyroid gland. Generally speaking, genetic mutations leading to suppression of thyroid hormone production/iodination have been associated with increased thyroid volume (i.e. gene alterations in those coding for the TSH receptor (TSHR), sodium iodide symporter (NIS), pendrin (PDS), thyroid peroxidase (TPO) and thyroglobulin (TG)) (**Table 8.3**).

NON-THYROID-SPECIFIC GENES

A number of putative non-thyroid-specific loci, associated with goitrogenesis, have been identified through genetic linkage analysis. This method uses the rearrangement of known chromosomal markers to identify candidate areas. The specific details are beyond the scope of this chapter but are summarized in **Table 8.4**; for further information see the review by Krohn et al.[32] It remains to be seen whether the increasing use of next-generation whole exome sequencing will elicit more candidate genes; as yet benign goitre has not been a main focus of this research.

Although multiple genes have been identified that predispose to goitre formation, the majority of cases will be polygenic and heavily influenced by the environmental factors discussed above. These factors, inherent and exogenous, all feed into the pathogenic model for goitre formation discussed below.

TABLE 8.3 Thyroid-specific genes with mutations linked to goitre formation

Mutated gene	Thyroid state
TG	Hypothyroid[33, 34]
TPO	Hypothyroid[35] (/euthyroid[36])
TSHR	Euthyroid[37]
PDS	Euthyroid[38]
NIS	Hypo/euthyroid[39, 40]

TABLE 8.4 Non-thyroid-specific genes associated with goitre

Gene candidate	Locus	Reference
MNG-1	14q31	Bignell et al. 1997[41]
MNG-2	Xp22	Capon et al. 2000[42]
MNG-3	3?	Takahashi et al. 2001[43]
N/A	2q, 3p, 7q, 8p	Bayer et al. 2004[44]

PATHOPHYSIOLOGY

Development of a multinodular goitre occurs in two phases: (i) a goitrogenic stimulus leading to global thyrocyte proliferation and increase in overall thyroid size, and (ii) focal increase in proliferation leading to nodules (**Figure 8.5**). Evidence for this is based largely on older animal studies,[45–47] although the same principles do seem applicable to human disease.

Goitrogenic stimulus

Under the influence of (most commonly) iodine deficiency, or another goitrogen, global hyperplasia occurs with increased thyroid hormone synthesis (there is evidence that some patients will adapt to iodine deficiency with hypertrophy without hyperplasia,[48] although the mechanism for this is unclear). This increased production leads to a rise in hydrogen peroxide (H_2O_2) generation and free

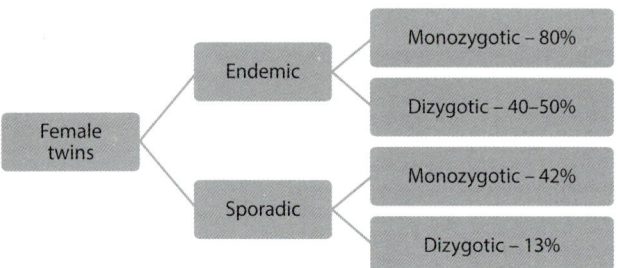

Figure 8.4 Preponderance to goitre in mono- and dizygotic twins. Adapted from Krohn K, Fuhrer D, Bayer Y, et al. Molecular pathogenesis of euthyroid and toxic multinodular goiter. *Endocr Rev* 2005; **26**(4): 504–24.[32]

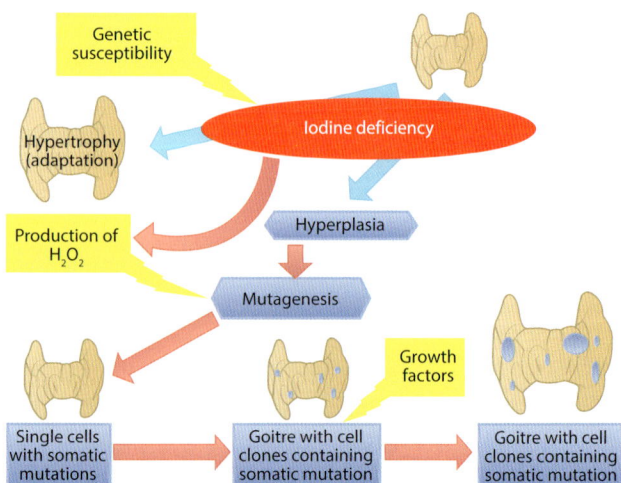

Figure 8.5 The bimodal model for development of goitre. From Krohn K, Fuhrer D, Bayer Y, et al. Molecular pathogenesis of euthyroid and toxic multinodular goiter. *Endocr Rev* 2005; **26**(4): 504–24.[32]

radical formation, resulting in a significant increase in spontaneous mutation rates.

Nodule formation

The combination of high spontaneous mutations coupled with increased cell replication rate results in an increased mutagenic load, and the chances of randomly generated mutations with a growth advantage are therefore significantly increased. The proliferating thyroid will be replete in growth factors (e.g. insulin-like growth factor (IGF), transforming growth factor (TGF), epidermal growth factor (EGF)), which will stimulate the division of all cells, including those with activating mutations. When the goitrogenic stimulus is removed, the proliferation of normal thyrocytes will cease whereas the activated cell clones will continue to proliferate, thus forming nodules. The nature of the mutation will determine whether the nodule is autonomously functioning or 'cold'; for example, an activating mutation of the cyclic AMP cascade will stimulate both growth and function, whereas one in the MAPK pathway will lead to proliferation only and a cold nodule. It follows, therefore, that multinodular goitre is a polyclonal entity, as opposed to a monoclonal one, with different nodules displaying different characteristics, which accounts for their heterogenous appearance on both imaging and pathological studies.

HORMONAL FACTORS REGULATING THYROID GROWTH

Thyroid growth and homeostasis is controlled by a number of factors other than iodine, through endo-, auto- and paracrine pathways. The principal stimulator of growth is TSH, the receptor for which is situated on the basal membrane of thyroid epithelial cells and belongs to the G protein-coupled receptor family. This in turn activates cellular processes including the adenyl cyclase-cAMP system promoting growth. Similar to the Wolff-Chaikoff effect (reduced thyroid function in the presence of very high levels of circulating iodine), high serum TSH concentrations have been shown to have an inhibitory effect on thyroid cell proliferation *in vitro*[49] (**Figure 8.6**).

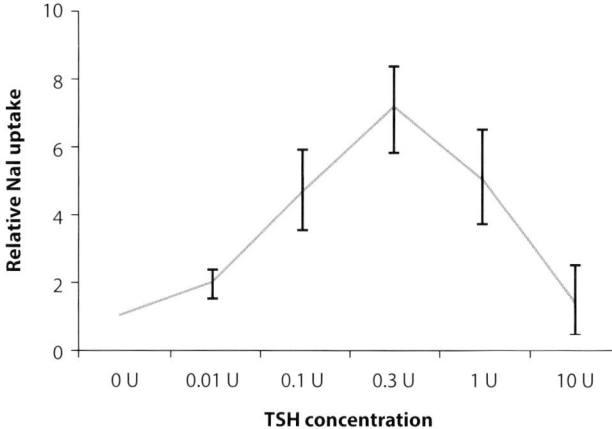

Figure 8.6 Reduction in iodide uptake by primary cultured thyroid cells with high concentrations of TSH.

TABLE 8.5 Growth factors acting on the thyroid gland to promote/inhibit growth

Activation pathway	Factors	Effect
AC-cAMP-PKA	TSH	Stimulatory and inhibitory
	Epinephrine	Stimulatory
Receptor tyrosine kinases	EGF	Stimulatory
	TGF-α	Stimulatory
	FGFs	Stimulatory
	Insulin	Stimulatory
	IGF-I	Stimulatory
	HGF	Stimulatory
	PDGF	Stimulatory
Phosphatidylinositol cascade	TSH	Stimulatory
	Esters	Stimulatory
	TGF-β	Inhibitory
	Iodides	Inhibitory

Source: Adapted from Konturek A. Thyroid growth factors. In: Ward L (ed). *Thyroid and parathyroid diseases*. Intech; 2012.[50]

Other factors that act locally to promote growth and angiogenesis include insulin, EGF, TGF-α/TGF-β, IGFs, fibroblast growth factors (FGFs), hepatocyte growth factor (HGF) and platelet-derived growth factor (PDGF). The particular signalling cascades that involve these mitogenic factors are summarized in **Table 8.5**.[50]

NOVEL THERAPIES

The surgical management of both benign and malignant thyroid disease is covered in depth in other chapters. It is, however, important to remember that globally, for many patients, surgery is not an option, either through patient non-suitability for general anaesthetic or lack of access to the appropriate facilities. Non-surgical treatment modalities are unfortunately lacking, although laboratory studies are ongoing to identify new therapies, usually by targeting specific growth factors receptors such as VEGF-R and FGF-R.[51]

SUMMARY

Goitrogenesis is a complex process reliant on an interplay of environmental and genetic factors, the extent of which is dependent on the underlying iodine status of the individual. While an understanding of these various processes is important, the most important factor to correct globally in order to reduce the prevalence of goitre is iodine deficiency, which continues to be a focus of the WHO – especially in developing countries. The role of iodine deficiency in the developed Western world, however, should not be ignored and continued efforts to ensure populations achieve their required intake should be supported.

FUTURE RESEARCH

➤ The role of iodination programs in the developing world to combat endemic goitre.
➤ Further understanding of the interplay between the metabolic syndrome and goitre formation, especially in view of the worldwide rise in obesity.
➤ Further characterization of the role of non-thyroid-specific genes in goitre formation and progression.
➤ Use of gene targeting therapies/recombinant adenovirus treatments in the non-surgical management of goitre.

KEY POINTS

- Benign thyroid enlargement is common.
- The biggest aetiological factor in the development of goitre is iodine deficiency.
- There is a complex interplay between environmental and genetic factors that determines the nature of the goitre.
- An understanding of the growth factors involved in thyroid hypertrophy and hyperplasia will aid the clinician in determining the likely progression of disease and best treatment options.

REFERENCES

1. Carle A, Krejbjerg A, Laurberg P. Epidemiology of nodular goitre. Influence of iodine intake. *Best Pract Res Cl En* 2014; **28**(4): 465–79.
2. Barrère X, Valeix P, Preziosi P, et al. Determinants of thyroid volume in healthy French adults participating in the SU.VI.MAX cohort. *Clin Endocrinol* 2000; **52**(3): 273–78.
3. Mortensen JD, Woolner LB, Bennett WA. Gross and microscopic findings in clinically normal thyroid glands. *J Clin Endoc Metab* 1955; **15**(10): 1270–80.
4. Ashcraft MW, Van Herle AJ. Management of thyroid nodules. I: History and physical examination, blood tests, X-ray tests, and ultrasonography. *Head Neck Surg* 1981; **3**(3): 216–30.
5. WHO. *Iodine status worldwide*. de Benoist B, Andersson M, Egli I, Takkouche B, Allen H (eds). Geneva: World Health Organization; 2004.
6. Zimmermann MB, Andersson M. Assessment of iodine nutrition in populations: past, present, and future. *Nutr Rev* 2012; **70**(10): 553–70.
7. WHO, UNICEF. *Iodine deficiency in Europe*. de Benoist B, Andersson M (eds). World Health Organization; 2007.
8. WHO, FAO. *Vitamin and mineral requirements in human nutrition*. 2nd ed. World Health Organization; 2004.
9. Andersson M, de Benoist B, Delange F, Zupan J. Prevention and control of iodine deficiency in pregnant and lactating women and in children less than 2-years-old: conclusions and recommendations of the Technical Consultation (vol 10, pg 1606, 2007). *Public Health Nutr* 2008; **11**(3): 327–27.
10. WHO, UNICEF, ICCIDD. *Assessment of iodine deficiency disorders and monitoring their elimination*. 3rd ed. Geneva: World Health Organization; 2007.
11. WHO. *Urinary iodine concentrations for determining iodine status in populations*. Geneva: World Health Organization; 2013.
12. Vanderpump MPJ, Lazarus JH, Smyth PP, et al. Iodine status of UK schoolgirls: a cross-sectional survey. *Lancet* 2011; **377**(9782): 2007–12.
13. Bath SC, Steer CD, Golding J, et al. Effect of inadequate iodine status in UK pregnant women on cognitive outcomes in their children: results from the Avon Longitudinal Study of Parents and Children (ALSPAC). *Lancet* 2013; **382**(9889): 331–37.
14. Greig WR, Boyle JA, Duncan A, et al. Genetic and non-genetic factors in simple goitre formation: evidence from a twin study. *Q J Med* 1967; **36**(142): 175–88.
15. Brix TH, Kyvik KO, Hegedüs L. Major role of genes in the etiology of simple goiter in females: a population-based twin study. *J Clin Endoc Metab* 1999; **84**(9): 3071–75.
16. Hansen PS, Brix TH, Bennedbaek FN, et al. Genetic and environmental causes of individual differences in thyroid size: a study of healthy Danish twins. *J Clin Endoc Metab* 2004; **89**(5): 2071–77.
17. Hansen PS, Brix TH, Bennedbaek FN, et al. The relative importance of genetic and environmental factors in the aetiology of thyroid nodularity: a study of healthy Danish twins. *Clin Endocrinol* 2005; **62**(3): 380–86.
18. Knudsen N, Brix TH. Genetic and non-iodine-related factors in the aetiology of nodular goitre. *Best Pract Res Cl En* 2014; **28**(4): 495–506.
19. Vanderpas J. Nutritional epidemiology and thyroid hormone metabolism. *Annu Rev Nutr* 2006; **26**(1): 293–322.
20. Gatseva PD, Argirova MD. Iodine status and goitre prevalence in nitrate-exposed schoolchildren living in rural Bulgaria. *Public Health* 2008; **122**(5): 458–61.
21. Below H, Zöllner H, Völzke H, Kramer A. Evaluation of nitrate influence on thyroid volume of adults in a previously iodine-deficient area. *Int J Hyg Environ Health* 2008; **211**(1–2):186–91.
22. Elnour A, Hambraeus L, Eltom M, et al. Endemic goiter with iodine sufficiency: a possible role for the consumption of pearl millet in the etiology of endemic goiter. *Am J Clin Nutr* 2000; **71**(1): 59–66.
23. Messina M, Redmond G. Effects of soy protein and soybean isoflavones on thyroid function in healthy adults and hypothyroid patients: a review of the relevant literature. *Thyroid* 2006; **16**(3): 249–58.
24. Pearce EN, Braverman LE. Environmental pollutants and the thyroid. *Best Pract Res Cl En* 2009; **23**(6): 801–13.
25. Tarone RE, Lipworth L, McLaughlin JK. The epidemiology of environmental perchlorate exposure and thyroid function: a comprehensive review. *J Occup Environ Med* 2010; **52**(6): 653–60.
26. Köhrle J. Selenium and the thyroid. *Curr Opin Endocrinol Diabetes Obes* 2013; **20**(5): 441–48.
27. Völzke H, Schwahn C, Kohlmann T, et al. Risk factors for goiter in a previously iodine-deficient region. *Exp Clin Endocrinol Diabetes* 2005; **113**(9): 507–15.
28. Rezzonico J, Rezzonico M, Pusiol E, et al. Introducing the thyroid gland as another victim of the insulin resistance syndrome. *Thyroid* 2008; **18**(4): 461–64.
29. Ayturk S, Gursoy A, Kut A, et al. Metabolic syndrome and its components are associated with increased thyroid volume and nodule prevalence in a mild-to-moderate iodine-deficient area. *Eur J Endocrinol* 2009; **161**(4): 599–605.
30. Rezzonico J, Rezzonico M, Pusiol E, et al. Metformin treatment for small benign thyroid nodules in patients with insulin resistance. *Metab Syndr Relat Disord* 2011; **9**(1): 69–75.
31. Ittermann T, Markus MRP, Schipf S, et al. Metformin inhibits goitrogenous effects of type 2 diabetes. *Eur J Endocrinol* 2013; **169**(1): 9–15.
32. Krohn K, Fuhrer D, Bayer Y, et al. Molecular pathogenesis of euthyroid and toxic multinodular goiter. *Endocr Rev* 2005; **26**(4): 504–24.
33. Medeiros-Neto G, Targovnik H, Knobel M, et al. Qualitative and quantitative defects of thyroglobulin resulting in congenital goiter: absence of gross gene deletion of coding sequences in the TG gene structure. *J Endocrinol Invest* 1989; **12**(11): 805–13.

34. van de Graaf S, Cammenga M, Ponne NJ, et al. The screening for mutations in the thyroglobulin cDNA from six patients with congenital hypothyroidism. *Biochimie* 1999; **81**(5): 425–32.
35. Bakker B, Bikker H, Vulsma T, et al. Two decades of screening for congenital hypothyroidism in the Netherlands: TPO gene mutations in total iodide organification defects (an update). *J Clin Endocrinol Metab* 2000; **85**(10): 3708–12.
36. Hagen Ga, HN, Haibach H, Bigazzi M, et al. Peroxidase deficiency in familial goiter with iodide organification defect. *N Engl J Med* 1971; **285**(25): 1394–98.
37. Peeters RP, van Toor H, Klootwijk W, et al. Polymorphisms in thyroid hormone pathway genes are associated with plasma TSH and iodothyronine levels in healthy subjects. *J Clin Endocrinol Metab* 2003; **88**(6): 2880–88.
38. Reardon W, Trembath RC. Pendred syndrome. *J Med Genet* 1996 Dec; **33**(12): 1037–40.
39. Shen D, Kloos RT, Mazzaferri EL, Jhiang SM. Sodium iodide symporter in health and disease. *Thyroid* 2001; **11**(5): 415–25.
40. Fujiwara H, Tatsumi K, Miki K, et al. Congenital hypothyroidism caused by a mutation in the Na+/I- symporter. *Nat Genet* 1997; **16**(2): 124–25.
41. Bignell GR, Canzian F, Shayeghi M, et al. Familial nontoxic multinodular thyroid goiter locus maps to chromosome 149 but does not account for familial nonmedullary thyroid cancer. *Am J Hum Genet* 1997; **61**(5): 1123–30.
42. Capon F, Tacconelli A, Giardina E, et al. Mapping a dominant form of multinodular goiter to chromosome Xp22. *Am J Hum Genet* 2000; **67**(4): 1004–07.
43. Takahashi T, Nozaki J, Komatsu M, et al. A new locus for a dominant form of multinodular goiter on 3q126.1-q26.3. *Biochem Bioph Res Co* 2001; **284**(3): 648–54.
44. Bayer Y, Neumann S, Meyer B, et al. Genome-wide linkage analysis reveals evidence for four new susceptibility loci for familial euthyroid goiter. *J Clin Endoc Metab* 2004; **89**(8): 4044–52.
45. Many MC, Denef JF, Hamudi S, et al. Effects of iodide and thyroxine on iodine-deficient mouse thyroid: a morphological and functional study. *J Endocrinol* 1986 Aug; **110**(2): 203–10.
46. Denef JF, Haumont S, Cornette C, Beckers C. Correlated functional and morphometric study of thyroid hyperplasia induced by iodine deficiency. *Endocrinology* 1981; **108**(6): 2352–58.
47. Van Middlesworth L. T-2 mycotoxin intensifies iodine deficiency in mice fed low iodine diet. *Endocrinology* 1986; **118**(2): 583–86.
48. Dumont JE, Ermans AM, Maenhaut C, et al. Large goitre as a maladaptation to iodine deficiency. *Clin Endocrinol* 1995; **43**(1): 1–10.
49. Sharma N. Novel binding partners of PBF in thyroid tumourigenesis. PhD Thesis: University of Birmingham; 2013. Available from http://etheses.bham.ac.uk/4766/1/Sharma14PhD.pdf
50. Konturek A. Thyroid growth factors. In: Ward L (ed). *Thyroid and parathyroid diseases*. Intech; 2012.
51. Ramsden JD, Buchanan MA, Egginton S, et al. Complete inhibition of goiter in mice requires combined gene therapy modification of angiopoietin, vascular endothelial growth factor, and fibroblast growth factor signaling. *Endocrinology* 2005; **146**(7): 2895–902.

CHAPTER 9

GENETICS OF ENDOCRINE TUMOURS

Waseem Ahmed, Prata Upasna and Dae Kim

| Genetics of thyroid tumours .... 83 | Inherited cancer syndromes and genetic testing .... 87 |
| Genetics of parathyroid tumours .... 86 | References .... 89 |

SEARCH STRATEGY

Data in this chapter may be updated by a PubMed search using the keywords: thyroid cancer, molecular biology, parathyroid cancer, parathyroid adenoma and molecular genetics.

GENETICS OF THYROID TUMOURS

Introduction

Thyroid malignancy is the most common cancer of the endocrine organs. Most thyroid cancers originate from thyroid follicular cells and can be subdivided into well differentiated papillary and follicular carcinoma, poorly differentiated carcinoma and anaplastic carcinoma.[1] Medullary thyroid cancer (MTC) accounts for a small proportion of thyroid cancers.[2]

Understanding of the molecular pathogenesis of thyroid cancer has progressed rapidly in the last decade. The genetic aberrations and alterations in signalling pathways have helped reshape our insights into thyroid cancer aetiology and management of patients with thyroid nodules.

Oncogenes and tumour suppressor genes in thyroid cancer

Cancer is a complex, multistep process. However, recent years have seen major advances in understanding the role of two classes of genes that are of particular importance in carcinogenesis that provide a more comprehensive picture: oncogenes and tumour suppressor genes. Several of the known oncogenes have been consistently detected in differentiated thyroid neoplasms. Some are more strongly associated than others and, interestingly, few are limited to specific forms of thyroid tumours.

GENE MUTATIONS

B-RAF (BRAF) mutation

BRAF is a serine/threonine kinase and is a member of the mitogen-activated protein kinase (MAPK) pathway, involved in the transduction of mitogenic signals from the cell membrane to the nucleus within. *BRAF* gene mutations have been shown to be common in many different human cancers.[3] Several studies have recently identified the most common *BRAF (V600E)* mutation, T1796A transverse mutation, in 29–69% of papillary thyroid cancers.[4–8] *BRAFV600E* mutation has been demonstrated to be a novel prognostic biomarker that predicts poor clinic-pathological outcomes such as extra-thyroidal invasion, advanced pathological stage invasion, metastasis and relapse of PTC.[8–9] *BRAF* mutation has also been associated with loss of radioiodine avidity and treatment failures.[10]

In contrast to classical genetic mutations in thyroid cancers such as *RET-PTC* and *RAS* mutations, which are also apparent in some benign thyroid lesions, this mutation has consistently been reported to be 100% specific for PTC. Consequently, *BRAF* mutation has been proposed as a specific molecular marker with high sensitivity for the diagnosis of PTC and represents a useful diagnostic adjunctive technique in the evaluation of thyroid nodules with indeterminate cytological findings.

RAS

The *RAS* proto-oncogene codes for a G-protein, p21, which is found within cell membranes. p21 plays a critical intermediate role in connecting the stimulatory signal from tyrosine kinases such as EGF receptor and via Raf-1 to a mitogenic cascade involving the MAP kinases.[11] *RAS* mutations are found in 30% of human cancers, making this the most widely mutated human proto-oncogene. Activated *RAS* has been detected previously in 20% of papillary carcinomas and 53% of follicular carcinomas.[12] Three families of *RAS* oncogenes have been identified (*K-RAS*, *H-RAS* and *N-RAS*), each located in separate chromosomal locations. Although downstream targets of *RAS* mutations include MAPK and P13K signalling, there appears to be preferential activation of the P13K-AKT pathway.[13]

The prevailing view is that *RAS*-activation probably represents an early event in thyroid tumourigenesis and is itself not sufficient for malignant transformation. Studies have shown *RAS* to be present in a high proportion of the earliest forms of thyroid tumours. Others have noted normal cells immediately adjacent to *RAS*-containing tumour cells also to harbour *RAS*.[14]

C-Myc, c-Fos, c-Met

Mutations of several other proto-oncogenes such as *c-Myc* (nuclear transcriptional factor family), *c-Fos* and *c-Met* have also been demonstrated in differentiated thyroid cancers (see Reviews).[15–16]

The *c-Myc* proto-oncogene encodes a nuclear protein that binds to DNA and acts as a transcriptional factor for genes involved in growth and differentiation. *c-Fos* is an immediate/early gene that regulates the expression of specific target genes by binding to their regulatory sequence of DNA. Aberrant activation of this transcriptional regulator has been demonstrated in thyroid tumours.[17]

Met protein is a transmembrane receptor with tyrosine kinase activity. Oncogene activation is associated with mitogenesis as well as motogenesis and has been suggested to contribute to tumour aggressive and metastatic behaviour.[18] *Met* oncogene is seen in various cancer human types, including up to 70% of papillary and 25% of follicular carcinomas, although it is not detected either in MTC or in normal thyroid tissues.[19]

GENE TRANSLOCATIONS

RET-PTC gene rearrangements

The thyroid carcinoma gene, *PTC*, is an oncogene found in 25% of papillary thyroid cancers, which was initially described by Fusco et al.[20] Subsequently, it was discovered to be a fusion between a gene of unknown function (*D10S170*) and the TK domain of the *RET* proto-oncogene as a result of a chromosomal rearrangement.[21] The *RET* proto-oncogene codes for a transmembrane protein with tyrosine kinase activity, the activity of which is normally restricted to a subset of cells derived from embryonic neural crest cells.[22]

Although the *RET* proto-oncogene is not expressed in normal thyroid follicular cells, the rearranged *RET/PTC* oncogene is highly expressed in some papillary thyroid cancer cells.[23] *PTC/RET* rearrangements are generally specific for papillary carcinomas and have been found in 5–40% of papillary thyroid cancers (PTC) in adults and are more common in paediatric PTC, as well as in cancers from children exposed to ionizing radiation.[24, 25–28]

There are more than 10 types of translocation, the most common being *RET/PTC1* and *RET/PTC3*.[29–30] The oncogenic capabilities of *RET/PTC* are achieved through activation of both MAPK and P13K-AKT pathways.

PAX8/PPARG rearrangement

The paired box 8 (*PAX8*)–peroxisome proliferator-activated receptor-γ (*PPARG*) fusion gene (*PAX8/PPARG*) rearrangement occurs as a genetic translocation between chromosomes two and three. This inhibits the tumour suppressor activity of *PPARG* and also transactivates certain *PAX8*-responsive genes.[31] The rearrangement occurs in up to 60% of follicular thyroid carcinoma (FTC) and follicular variant of papillary thyroid carcinoma (FVPTC).[32]

TUMOUR SUPPRESSOR GENES

P53

The tumour suppressor p53 regulates cell response to DNA damage and allows for repair or apoptosis when cells are severely damaged. Inactivating mutations of p53 gene are common in human cancers; however, they are only present in 10% of thyroid malignancies.[33] The majority of such mutations are found in poorly differentiated and aggressive histotypes.[34] This suggests p53 plays a minor role in thyroid malignant transformation and in early stages of thyroid cancer, unlike many other human malignancies. However, evidence suggests that although p53 mutations may not occur in thyroid tumours, its activity may be inhibited by other mechanisms,[35] especially in early stage thyroid cancer.[36]

SIGNALLING PATHWAYS

There are several important signalling pathways involved in the development and propagation of thyroid cancer. The common mutations described above are key genes in these signalling pathways.

The MAPK signalling pathway

The mitogen-activated protein kinase (MAPK) pathway plays a major role in the regulation of cell proliferation and survival and in human tumourigenesis. Activation is often due to mutated *RAS*, *BRAF* or by *RET-PTC* reported widely in papillary thyroid cancer.[37] Secondary molecular events amplifying this pathway such as hypomethylation and genome-wide hypermethylation, and upregulation of various oncogenic proteins can also occur. These include chemokines, nuclear factor kB (NF-kB), vascular endothelial growth factor A (VEGFA), matrix metalloproteinases (MMPs), and transforming growth factor-β1 (TGFβ1).[38]

The PI3K-AKT signalling pathway

The role of P13K-AKT pathway in thyroid tumourigenesis became apparent when the association of follicular thyroid adenoma and carcinoma was noted with Cowden's syndrome (caused by germline mutations of *PTEN*),[39] and high levels of AKT expression established in the latter (when compared to PTC or normal thyroid tissue).[40] Furthermore, evidence of AKT mutations and their occurrence in metastatic thyroid cancer[41] has validated the central role of PI3K-AKT pathway in the invasive and metastatic capabilities of FTC. Aberration of the PI3K/AKT pathway appears to play a pivotal role in tumourogenesis in both FTC and ATC, promoting progression of adenoma to FTC, and subsequently ATC.

The NF-κB signalling pathway

It has been suggested that activation of NF-κB may promote dedifferentiation of PTCs and FTCs.[42] Studies have demonstrated the NF-κB pathway's role in anti-apoptotic and proliferative signalling pathways in thyroid cancer.[43] Emerging evidence of deregulated NF-κB activity in ATC helps provide further insight into the molecular biology of thyroid cancer and identify it as a potential target to inhibit the pro-survival signalling in thyroid malignancy.[43]

The WNT-β-catenin signalling pathway

The pathway plays a role in regulating cell proliferation and differentiation. Abnormal signalling and its role in thyroid tumourogenesis has been established. Activation of WNT-β-catenin pathway is secondary to mutations of CTNNB1 (which encodes β-catenin),[44] a likely late event not evident in well differentiated carcinomas. Expression of β-catenin, a cytoplasmic protein regulating the coordination of cell–cell adhesion and gene transcription, is more prominent in ATC compared to DTC.[45]

ABERRANT GENE METHYLATION

Epigenetic silencing through aberrant gene methylation are hallmarks of cancers including thyroid malignancy. Methylation of thyrotropin receptor (TSHR), E-cadherin (ECAD), sodium iodide symporter protein (NIS-L) are frequent in PTC.[46] The BRAFV600E mutation has been associated with a combination of hypermethylation and hypomethylation of genes involved in important metabolic and cellular functions in PTC.[47] Hypermethylation of several tumour suppressor genes are also associated with increased PTC aggressiveness.[48] Evidence shows down-regulation of PTEN tumour suppressor due to changes in methylation is associated with increased activity of the PI3K-AKT pathway, in thyroid cancer.[49]

Genetic alterations in medullary thyroid cancer

Medullary thyroid cancer (MTC) is an aggressive form of thyroid cancer, accounting for less than 5% of thyroid malignancies.[50] It is a neuroendocrine carcinoma arising from the parafollicular C-cells and associated with secretion of calcitonin and various other hormones such as carcinoembryonic antigen (CEA). Sporadic MTC accounts for 75% of cases, with inherited MTC accounting for the remainder. The majority of the latter occurs in association with multiple endocrine neoplasia (MEN) type 2A, MEN2B, and familial medullary thyroid carcinoma syndrome (FMTC) syndromes.

RET GENE

The various forms of hereditary MTC are caused by germline RET mutations and are all autosomal dominant with high penetrance. Somatic RET mutations are responsible for a subset of sporadic MTC.[51] The RET oncogene plays a major role in MTC tumourogenesis, with RET mutations being identified in 98% of MEN2A patients, 95% of MEN2B patients, and 88% of those with FMTC.[52] As noted previously, RET signalling activates both MAPK and PI3K-AKT pathways, playing a key role in cell growth, differentiation and survival.

ABERRANT GENE METHYLATION

Hypermethylation of RASSF1A (RASSF1), a known tumour suppressor gene within the PI3K-AKT pathway, has been noted in the majority of FTCs and less frequently in benign adenomas and PTC.[53] Due to its high prevalence in MTC (85%), it may indicate a role in MTC tumourogenesis.[54]

MICRORNAS

MicroRNAs are small non-coding RNA genes (containing about 22 nucleotides) that function in RNA silencing and post-translational regulation of gene expression. MicroRNAs deregulation in MTC is thought to be an early event in parafollicular C-cell carcinogenesis.[55]

Genetic alterations in anaplastic thyroid cancer

Anaplastic thyroid carcinoma remains a devastating disease. ATC constitutes 5% of all thyroid cancer and yet accounted for 50% of all thyroid cancer deaths in the United States in 2006.[56] Molecular research in anaplastic carcinoma has been limited due to its rarity and aggressiveness, relying mainly on in vivo cell line studies. Experimental models involving xenografts in athymic mice has allowed further study of this aggressive endocrine disease. Despite our limited understanding, it is generally accepted that anaplastic cancer does not arise de novo, but is likely to evolve from established well-differentiated thyroid cancer (PTC or FTC).[57]

There are two groups of mutations evident in the ATC tumourogenesis. The first set of mutations is abundant within well differentiated thyroid cancer (WDTC) and ATC. Examples include BRAF and RAS point mutations and are likely to represent early changes.[58] The second group are found largely in ATC and are noted for their absence in WDTC. These are likely to represent late changes and are involved in dedifferentiation; p53 and β-catenin.

Mutations in p53 impairing transcriptional activity are found in 55% of ATCs[58] enabling accelerated genomic instability, growth, angiogenesis and dedifferentiation. Redifferentiation of ATC tissue has been demonstrated with reintroduction of wild type p53 and the restoration of cellular responsiveness to physiologic stimuli (thyroid stimulating hormone) and re-expression of thyroid peroxidase.[59] E-cadherin and β-catenin are epithelial adhesion molecules in normal epithelium. There is reduced expression of both in ATCs when compared to the originating WDTC from which they evolve, suggesting the E-cadherin/β-catenin complex plays a role in this transformation process.[60]

> **KEY POINTS**
>
> - Several gene mutations and alterations in signalling pathways are now recognized as important events in the development and progression of thyroid cancer.
> - RAS mutations appear to be an early event, as they are common to benign and malignant tumours. The subsequent pathways leading to follicular or papillary carcinoma are divergent.
> - Mutational activation of BRAF and RET/PTC oncogenes are specific to papillary carcinomas. Conversely, loss of function of a gene on chromosome 11q13, possibly MEN1 gene, may direct the tumour clone towards a follicular phenotype.
> - Mutations of p53 are highly prevalent in anaplastic thyroid carcinomas, and together with mutations in the RB gene, may represent the critical transitional step in the progression of well-differentiated tumours into these aggressive thyroid cancers.

GENETICS OF PARATHYROID TUMOURS

Introduction

Primary hyperparathyroidism is a commonly detected endocrine disorder having a prevalence of 1–3:1000 in the general European population.[61] The most common cause of primary hyperparathyroidism is a parathyroid adenoma accounting for ~85% of cases. Parathyroid adenomas are more commonly sporadic, or inherited as part of multiple endocrine neoplasia (MEN) syndromes, familial hyperparathyroidism or hereditary hyperparathyroidism with jaw tumours (HPT-JT). Parathyroid carcinomas are rare and account for less than 1% of cases of hyperparathyroidism.[62]

Parathyroid adenomas

Previous investigations of the molecular pathogenesis of parathyroid tumours have only yielded mutations accounting for the minority of tumours. Investigations of the PTH gene, which is located on chromosome 11q15, detected restriction fragment length polymorphism (RFLP) abnormalities in sporadic parathyroid adenomas.[63] Further analysis demonstrated the rearrangement of part of the PTH gene onto chromosome location 11q13. The protein that was overexpressed as a result of this rearrangement was designated PRAD 1 (parathyroid adenoma 1), and encodes a novel member of the cyclin-D family of cell-cycle regulatory proteins. Up to 20–40% of sporadic parathyroid adenomas have been shown to overexpress cyclin D1.[64-65]

There has also been interest in the role of cyclin dependent kinase inhibitors (CDK1) genes conferring low-penetrance predisposition to hyperparathyroidism by providing a selective growth advantage to parathyroid cells.[66] Another genetic abnormality that appears to be important in the aetiology of parathyroid adenoma is the tumour suppressor gene associated with MEN type 1; 12–20% of patients with sporadic parathyroid adenomas have been shown to harbour bi-allelic defects in the MEN1 gene.[67] Parathyroid adenomas are also associated with MEN syndrome type 2a. Although C-RET mutations are responsible for MEN2a, a search for the most common mutation at codon 634 has proved to be negative, suggesting a different mechanism responsible for the development of sporadic and inherited parathyroid adenomas.

Whole exome and direct sequencing of parathyroid adenomas has lead to mutations being identified in the ZFX gene, a gene believed to have a role in the regulation of stem cell renewal. The identified mutations did not overlap with somatic mutations in the MEN1 gene. Also implicated in other cancers such as that of the larynx, lung and prostate, the ZFX gene may as an oncogene provide gain of function in parathyroid tumour cells, possibly linked to cyclin D1.[68]

Parathyroid hyperplasia

Comparison of genes between parathyroid hyperplasia and adenomas does demonstrate greater genetic heterogeneity and more complex expression of genetic mutations in hyperplasia, which is consistent with its polyclonal nature. Examples include the CDH1 gene, which is not exclusive to but more highly expressed in hyperplasia versus adenoma (but not in carcinoma).[69]

Parathyroid carcinoma

Although rare, parathyroid carcinoma is clinically aggressive. Whether it arises pre-existing adenomas or *de novo* remains controversial. As noted previously, cyclin D1 gene expression is overexpressed in parathyroid adenomas compared to normal parathyroid tissue. Recently, Zhao et al. examined seven parathyroid carcinomas and noted expression of CCND1 (a gene encoding for cyclin D1) was significantly overexpressed in carcinomas when compared with adenomas.[62]

The RB tumour suppressor gene responsible for the pathogenesis of retinoblastomas is involved in the pathogenesis of various other human tumours. Allelic deletion of RB gene was demonstrated in all parathyroid carcinomas in one study, with abnormal histological staining patterns for Rb protein in 50% of carcinomas but none in the adenomas.[70] Together, these observations suggests an important role for RB gene in the development of parathyroid carcinomas, and may help in the histological diagnosis of parathyroid carcinoma.[61]

Shattuck et al. directly sequenced the *HRPT2* gene (associated with hyperparathyroidism-jaw tumour syndrome) in 21 parathyroid carcinomas from 15 patients who had no known family history of primary hyperparathyroidism or the HPT-JT syndrome at presentation.[71] Parathyroid carcinomas from 10 of the 15 patients had *HRPT2* mutations. In contrast, mutations of *HRPT2* are not evident in benign parathyroid tumours. Some have suggested that all patients with parathyroid carcinoma should be considered for germline testing for *HRPT2* mutations as up to 20% of them may have unrecognized HPT-JT.[66]

INHERITED CANCER SYNDROMES AND GENETIC TESTING

In about 5–10% of individuals predisposition to a specific group of cancers is the result of a heritable mutation in a cancer predisposing gene, so-called germline mutation. The at-risk individuals tend to develop tumours at an earlier age than usual and are at risk of developing more than one primary tumour. In addition, the siblings and offspring of an affected individual each have a 50% chance of inheriting the cancer predisposing mutation, consistent with autosomal dominant inheritance.

Multiple endocrine neoplasia type 1 (MEN1)

MEN1, also known as Wermer's syndrome, represents the combination of more than 20 different endocrine and non-endocrine tumours. A practical definition is a case with two or three main MEN1-related endocrine tumours: parathyroid adenoma, entero-pancreatic endocrine tumour and pituitary tumour. MEN1 syndrome is usually an autosomal, dominantly inherited condition, although in 10% of cases arise *de novo*. The prevalence of MEN in the UK is estimated to be ~10 per 100 000 with equal sex distribution.[72]

Parathyroid tumours occur in 95% of MEN1 patients and is the most common endocrinopathy with a typical age of onset of 20–25 years (reaching nearly 100% penetrance by the age of 50 years).[73] In contrast, MEN1 is rare and represents only 2–4% of all cases of primary HPT. Patients with MEN1 generally have parathyroid tumours in three or all four parathyroid glands. These tumours are asymmetric in size and are regarded as independent clonal adenomas. The issue of which operation is optimal remains controversial.[72–74]

The gene causing MEN1 was localized to chromosome 11q13 by genetic mapping studies. Further studies defined the *MEN1* gene in 1997, consisting of 10 exons that codes a novel 610 amino acid protein named MENIN.[67] MENIN is a ubiquitously expressed nuclear protein that has been demonstrated to have roles in transcriptional regulation, genome stability, cellular proliferation, cell cycle control and apoptosis.[67, 75]

More than 1000 germline mutations of the *MEN1* gene have been described and the majority (>80%) of these are inactivating, and are consistent with its role as a tumour suppressor gene.[72] More than 10% of the *MEN1* gene germline mutations arise *de novo* and may be transmitted to subsequent generations.[76] Importantly, 5–10% of MEN1 patients do not harbour mutations in the coding region of the *MEN1* gene, and these individuals may have mutations in the promoter and untranslated regions, which remains to be clarified. Correlations between *MEN1* mutations and the clinical manifestations are absent, and this contrasts with the situation in MEN2 and the *RET* gene.

MEN1 GENETIC TESTING FOR FAMILIAL MEN1 SYNDROME

The first step in the analysis is to identify the specific *MEN1* mutation in the germline DNA derived from a peripheral blood sample from the affected index case using direct DNA sequencing strategies. In most index cases of familial MEN1, a germline mutation of *MEN1* will be identified. However, many large studies have failed to find a *MEN1* germline mutation in 10–20% of index cases for familial MEN1.[77] Such failures are believed to be due to mutations in untested parts of the *MEN1* gene or large deletions that are transparent to PCR methods. Current recommendations suggest genetic testing should be performed in index cases with two or more MEN1 tumours, and first-degree relatives of a known mutation carrier. All individuals who are offered genetic testing should receive appropriate genetic counselling.[78]

Multiple endocrine neoplasia type 2 (MEN2)

The MEN2 syndrome describes the association of medullary thyroid carcinoma (MTC), pheochromocytoma, and parathyroid tumours. MEN2 is an autosomal dominant syndrome caused by mutations in the *RET* proto-oncogene with variations in the penetrance resulting in three variants: MEN2a; MEN2b; and familial medullary thyroid cancer (FMTC). All variants show a high penetrance for medullary thyroid cancer; 90% of MEN2 carriers will eventually show evidence for MTC. MEN2a is the most common variant (95%), and the development of multicentric MTC (almost 100%) is associated with pheochromocytoma (50%) and parathyroid adenomas (20%). MEN2b, which represents 5% of all MEN2 cases, is characterized by the occurrence of MTC, pheochromocytoma in association with Marfanoid habitus and mucosal neuromas. Parathyroid tumours do not usually occur in MEN2b. FMTC is a variant in which only MTC is the sole manifestation and is the mildest subtype. MTC is the first neoplastic manifestation in most MEN2 patients because of its earlier and overall higher penetrance. Earlier studies reported mortality of 15–20% when treatment was initiated after identification of a thyroid nodule.[79] However, carrier diagnosis before adulthood allowing early thyroidectomy has lowered the mortality from hereditary MTC to less than 5%.[80]

The *c-ret* proto-oncogene encodes a transmembrane tyrosine kinase receptor and is located on chromosome 10q11.2.[81] The RET protein is involved in cellular signalling pathways that regulate cell proliferation, differentiation, survival and regeneration (ref10). Specific activating mutations of C-RET have been described for each of the three MEN2 variants. The aggressiveness of MTC correlates with the MEN2 variant syndrome and with the mutated RET codon.[82] Prevention or cure of inevitable MTC is by surgery, and should be performed before the age of possible malignant progress.

The presence of somatic RET mutations (which occur in up to 75% of sporadic MTC patients) confers a more aggressive clinical course when compared to RET-negative sporadic patients. The absence of RET mutations in some patients suggests that other loci may predispose to MEN1 and sporadic MTC.

MEN2 GENETIC TESTING

In 1997, a consensus was reached that the decision to perform prophylactic thyroidectomy in MEN2 should be based predominantly on the result of ret mutation testing, rather than CT testing.[83] Genetic testing for MEN2 has enabled detection of nearly 100% of carriers and is one of the few examples of a genetic test that mandates a highly effective clinical intervention. Sequencing DNA for RET mutation is effective and widely available. The likelihood of a ret germline mutation in a patient with apparently sporadic MTC is 1–7%.[84] Despite the modest mutation yield, all cases of sporadic MTC should be tested for germline ret mutation because the critical clinical implications of finding a ret mutation. A germline ret mutation is more likely if the sporadic MTC is of early age onset or there is multiplicity in the thyroid gland. Further, the specific ret codon mutation correlates well with the MEN2 variant and with clinical behaviour. Genetic information allows stratification of MTC risk and provides a basis for a 3-level stratified thyroid management (Table 9.1).[85]

Hyperparathyroidism-jaw tumour (HPT-JT) syndrome

The HPT-JT syndrome is an autosomal dominant disorder characterized by the development of parathyroid adenomas and carcinomas and fibro-osseous jaw tumours. In HPT-JT, patients usually have single adenoma or a carcinoma, whilst MEN1 patients will often have multigland disease.

The gene causing HPT-JT, HRPT2, is located on chromosome 1q25 and encodes for an ubiquitously expressed 531 amino acid protein PARAFIBROMIN.[87] To date,

TABLE 9.1 Genotype-phenotype correlations, risk levels for MTC and recommended interventions based on ATA risk level of genotype 2015[86]

ATA group	RET genotype		MEN2 classification	Recommended start interventions			
	Exon	Codon mutation		PE/US/Ctn	TTX	Screening PHEO	Screening HPT
HST	16	M918T	MEN2B	1 month	Before the first year of life	11 years	NA
H	11	C634F/G/R/S/W/Y	Classical MEN2A / MEN2A + CL	3 years	At or before 5 years of age	11 years	11 years
	15	A883F	MEN2B				NA
MOD	10	C609F/G/R/S/W/Y C611R/S/W/Y C618F/G/R/S/W/Y C620F/G/R/S/W/Y	Classical MEN2A	5 years	Childhood or young adulthood	16 years	16 years
		C611F	FMTC			NA	NA
		C609G C611S C618/R/S C620/R/S/W	MEN2A + HD				
	11	C630R/Y D631Y S649L K666E	Classical MEN2A			16 years	16 years
	13	E768D	FMTC			NA	NA
		L790F Y791F	Classical MEN2A			16 years	16 years
	14	V804L/M	Classical MEN2A / MEN2A + CL			16 years / NA	16 years / NA
	15	S891A	Classical MEN2A			16 years	16 years
	16	R912P	FMTC			NA	NA

13 different heterozygous mutations translating truncated forms of parafibromin, have been reported in HPT-JT families. Although no consensus clinical guideline exists for *HRPT2* genetic testing, testing for germline HRPT2 mutations are available commercially.[88]

Cowden's disease

Cowden's disease (CD), also known as multiple hamartoma syndrome, is a rare autosomal dominantly inherited disease. Multiple trichilemmomas of the skin are common diagnostic features found in >90% of affected individuals. Patients with CD have an increased risk for carcinomas of the breast and thyroid; up to a 10% lifetime risk of follicular or papillary thyroid cancer. Approximately 70% of people with Cowden syndrome will have benign thyroid abnormalities, including multinodular goitre, adenomatous nodules and follicular adenomas. Marsh et al. identified *PTEN* mutations in 30 of 37 (81%) Cowden disease families.[89] The *PTEN* gene is involved in the previously PI3/AKT or PI3-AKT intracellular signalling pathway. Although no consensus clinical guideline exists testing for germline *PTEN* mutations are available commercially.

Other inherited syndromes

Mutations in the *APC* gene cause FAP and attenuated familial adenomatous polyposis (AFAP). FAP is inherited as autosomal dominant and is characterized by multiple adenomatous polyps in the colon and rectum with a natural history of progression to colorectal carcinoma in nearly 100% of cases, usually by the age of 40. People with FAP have up to a 2% lifetime risk of developing papillary thyroid cancer (PTC). Women with FAP appear to be at greater risk than men (80:1) and develop a particular histological variant of PTC (cribriform morular variant of PTC) that demonstrates more indolent behaviour than the sporadic type.[90]

Gardner syndrome (colonic polyposis, osteomas, and characteristic retinal lesion) is now known to be a phenotypic variant of FAP, caused by mutation in the *APC* gene. Herve et al. estimated that the incidence of thyroid carcinoma in patients with Gardner syndrome approached 100 times that of the general population. Genetic testing for mutations in the *APC* gene is available.[91]

KEY POINTS

- Our understanding of parathyroid tumour biology is less developed than thyroid; however, advancements in genetic testing have demonstrated areas of potential. Several genes have been studied (*MEN1*, *PTH*, *HRPT2*, *ZFX*) and have been postulated to play an important role in the development of parathyroid tumours.
- PCR and immunohistochemistry techniques based on products of specific genetic mutations may aid in differentiation of adenomas, hyperplasia and carcinoma.
- Genetic testing in endocrine disease relates to the MEN syndromes. Genetic testing plays a key role in the management of MEN type 2 and less prominent role in MEN type 1.
- *RET* mutational analysis is a key investigation in the management of patients with MEN type 2. *RET* analysis offers a risk stratification based on the codons mutated and guides clinical management.
- Further identification of genes may allow targeted anti-neoplastic agents in the age of targeted molecular therapeutics.

REFERENCES

1. Nikiforov YE. Thyroid tumors: classification and general considerations. In: Nikiforov YE, Biddinger PW, Thompson LDR (eds). *Diagnostic pathology and molecular genetics of the thyroid*. Baltimore: Lippincott Williams & Wilkins; 2009, pp. 94–102.
2. Howlader N, Noone AM, Krapcho M, et al. SEER Cancer Statistics Review 1975–2009 (Vintage 2009 Populations) National Cancer Institute. 2012 [online], http://seer.cancer.gov/csr/1975_2009_pops09.
3. Davies H, Bignell GR, Cox C, et al. Mutations of the BRAF gene in human cancer. *Nature* 2002; **417**: 949–54.
4. Kimura ET, Nikiforova MN, Zhu Z, et al. High prevalence of BRAF mutations in thyroid cancer: genetic evidence for constitutive activation of the RET/PTC-RAS-BRAF signaling pathway in papillary thyroid carcinoma. *Cancer Res* 2003; **63**(7): 1454–57.
5. Cohen Y, Xing M, Mambo E, et al. BRAF mutation in papillary thyroid carcinoma. *J Natl Cancer Inst* 2003; **95**(8): 625–27.
6. Soares P, Trovisco V, Rocha AS, et al. BRAF mutations and RET/PTC rearrangements are alternative events in the etiopathogenesis of PTC. *Oncogene* 2003; **22**(29): 4578–80.
7. Namba H, Nakashima M, Hayashi T, et al. Clinical implication of hot spot BRAF mutation, V599E, in papillary thyroid cancers. *J Clin Endocrinol Metab* 2003; **88**(9): 4393–97.
8. Nikiforov YE, Nikiforova MN. Molecular genetics and diagnosis of thyroid cancer. *Nature* 2011; **7**: 569–80.
9. Nikiforova MN, Kimura ET, Gandhi M, et al. BRAF mutations in thyroid tumors are restricted to papillary carcinomas and anaplastic or poorly differentiated carcinomas arising from papillary carcinomas. *J Clin Endocrinol Metab* 2003; **88**(11): 5399–404.
10. Xing M, Westra WH, Tufano RP, et al. BRAF mutation predicts a poorer clinical prognosis for papillary thyroid cancer. *J Clin Endocrinol Metab* 2005; **90**: 6373–79.
11. Marshall CJ. Ras effectors. *Curr Opin Cell Biol* 1996; **8**: 197–204.
12. Wright PA, Lemoine NR, Mayall ES, et al. Papillary and follicular thyroid carcinomas show a different pattern of ras oncogene mutation. *Br J Cancer* 1989; **60**: 576–7.
13. Abubaker J, Jehan, Z, Bavi, P, et al. Clinicopathological analysis of papillary thyroid cancer with PIK3CA alterations in a Middle Eastern population. *J Clin Endocrinol Metab* 2008; **93**: 611–18.
14. Schark C, Fulton N, Kaplan EL, et al. N-ras 61 oncogene mutations in Hürthle cell tumours. *Surgery* 1990; **108**: 994–99.
15. Kim DS, McCabe CJ, Buchanan MA, Watkinson JC. Oncogenes in thyroid cancer. *Clin Otolaryngol* 2003; **28**(5): 386–95.
16. Farid NR, Shi Y, Zou M. Molecular basis of thyroid cancer. *Endocr Rev* 1994; **15**(2): 202–32.
17. Curran T. *The fos oncogene*. New York: Elsevier; 1988.
18. Matsumato K, Nakamura J. Hepatocyte growth factor: molecular structure, roles in liver regeneration and other biological functions. *Crit Rev Oncog* 1992; **3**: 27–54.
19. Di Renzo MF, Narsimhan RP, Comoglio PM, et al. Expression of the Met/HGF receptor in normal and neoplastic human tissues. *Oncogene* 1991; **6**: 1977–2003.
20. Fusco A, Grieco M, Vecchio G, et al. A new oncogene in human papillary thyroid carcinomas and their lymph-nodal metastases. *Nature* 1987; **328**: 170–72.
21. Pierotti MA, Santoro M, Vecchio G. Characterization of an inversion on the long arm of chromosome 10 juxtaposing D10S170 and Ret and creating the oncogene sequence ret/PTC. *Proc Natl Acad Sci USA* 1992; **89**: 1616–20.

22. Santoro M, Carlomagno F, Hay ID, et al. Ret oncogene activation in human thyroid neoplasms is restricted to the papillary cancer subtype. *J Clin Invest* 1992; **89**(5): 1517–22.
23. Grieco M, Santoro M, Vecchio G, et al. PTC is a novel rearranged form of the ret proto-oncogene and is frequently detected in vivo in human thyroid papillary carcinomas. *Cell* 1990; **60**: 557–63.
24. Fagin JA. Minireview: branded from the start-distinct oncogenic initiating events may determine tumor fate in the thyroid. *Mol Endocrinol* 2002; **16**(5): 903–11.
25. Santoro M, Melillo RM, Carlomagno F, et al. Molecular mechanisms of RET activation in human cancer. *Ann NY Acad Sci* 2002; **963**: 116–21.
26. Nikiforov YE, Rowland JM, Bove KE, et al. Distinct pattern of ret oncogene rearrangements in morphological variants of radiation-induced and sporadic thyroid papillary carcinomas in children. *Cancer Res* 1997; **57**(9): 1690–94.
27. Fugazzola L, Pilotti S, Pinchera A, et al. Oncogenic rearrangements of the RET proto-oncogene in papillary thyroid carcinomas from children exposed to the Chernobyl nuclear accident. *Cancer Res* 1995; **55**(23): 5617–20.
28. Bongarzone I, Fugazzola L, Vigneri P, et al. Age-related activation of the tyrosine kinase receptor protooncogenes RET and NTRK1 in papillary thyroid carcinoma. *J Clin Endocrinol Metab* 1996; **81**(5): 2006–09.
29. Rabes HM, Demidchik EP, Sidorow JD, et al. Pattern of radiation-induced RET and NTRK1 rearrangements in 191 post-chernobyl papillary thyroid carcinomas: biological, phenotypic, and clinical implications. *Clin Cancer Res* 2000; **6**: 1093–103.
30. Santoro M, Thomas GA, Vecchio G, et al. Gene rearrangement and Chernobyl related thyroid cancers. *Br J Cancer* 2000; **82**: 315–22.
31. Placzkowski KA, Reddi HV, Grebe SK, et al. The role of the PAX8/PPARr fusion oncogene in thyroid cancer. *PPAR Res* 2008; **2008**:672829.
32. Kroll TG, Sarraf P, Pecciarini L, et al. PAX8-PPARi fusion oncogene in human thyroid carcinoma. *Science* 2000; **289**: 1357–60.
33. Olivier M, Eeles R, Hollstein M, et al. The IARC TP53 database: new online mutation analysis and recommendations to users. *Hum Mutat* 2002; **19**: 607–14.
34. Faggin JA, Matsuo K, Karmakar A, et al. High prevalence of mutations of the p53 gene in poorly differentiated human thyroid carcinoma. *J Clin Invest* 1993; **91**(1): 179–84.
35. Malaguarnera R, Vella V, Vigneri R, Frasca F. p53 family proteins in thyroid cancer. *Endocr Relat Cancer* 2007; **14**: 43–60.
36. Fagin, JA, Tang SH, Zeki K, et al. Reexpression of thyroid peroxidase in a derivative of an undifferentiated thyroid carcinoma cell line by introduction of wild-type p53. *Cancer Res* 1996; **56**(4): 765–71.
37. Xing M. Recent advances in molecular biology of thyroid cancer and their clinical implications. *Otolaryngol Clin North Am* 2008; **41**: 1135–46.
38. Omur O, Baran Y. An update on molecular biology of thyroid cancers. *Crit Rev Oncol Hematol* 2014; **90**: 233–52.
39. Liaw D, Marsh DJ, Li J, et al. Germline mutations of the PTEN gene in Cowden disease, an inherited breast and thyroid cancer syndrome. *Nat Genet* 1997; **16**(1): 64–67.
40. Ringel MD, Hayre N, Saito J, et al. Overexpression and overactivation of Akt in thyroid carcinoma. *Cancer Res* 2001; **61**: 6105–11.
41. Ricarte-Filho JC, Ryder M, Chitale DA, et al. Mutational profile of advanced primary and metastatic radioactive iodine-refractory thyroid cancers reveals distinct pathogenetic roles for BRAF, PIK3CA, and AKT1. *Cancer Res* 2009; **69**(11): 4885–93.
42. Li X, Abdel-Mageed AB, Mondal D, Kandil E. The nuclear factor kappa-B signaling pathway as a therapeutic target against thyroid cancers. *Thyroid* 2013; **23**(2): 209–18.
43. Pacifico F, Leonardi A. Role of NF-kappaB in thyroid cancer. *Mol Cell Endocrinol* 2010; **321**(1): 29–35.
44. Garcia-Rostan G, Tallini G, Herrero A, et al. Frequent mutation and nuclear localization of β G. et a in anaplastic thyroid carcinoma. *Cancer Res* 1999; **59**: 1811–15.
45. Wiseman SM, Griffith OL, Gown A, et al. Immunophenotyping of thyroid tumors identifies molecular markers altered during transformation of differentiated into anaplastic carcinoma. *Am J Surg* 2011; **201**: 580–86.
46. Smith JA, Fan CY, Zou C, et al. Methylation status of genes in papillary thyroid carcinoma. *Arch. Otolaryngol Head Neck Surg* 2007; **133**: 1006–11.
47. Hou P, Liu D, Xing M. Genome-wide alterations in gene methylation by the BRAF V600E mutation in papillary thyroid cancer cells. *Endocr Relat Cancer* 2011; **18**: 687–97.
48. Xing M. Gene methylation in thyroid tumorigenesis. *Endocrinology* 2007; **148**: 948–53.
49. Hou P, Ji M, Xing M. Association of PTEN gene methylation with genetic alterations in the phosphatidylinositol 3-kinase/AKT signaling pathway in thyroid tumors. *Cancer* 2008; **113**: 2440–47.
50. Hundahl S, Fleming I, Fremgen A, et al. A national cancer data base report of 53,856 cases of thyroid carcinoma treated in the U.S., 1985–1995. *Cancer* 1998; **83**: 2638–48.
51. Drosten M, Pützer BM. Mechanisms of disease: cancer targeting and the impact of oncogenic RET for medullary thyroid carcinoma therapy. *Nat Clin Pract Oncol* 2006; **3**: 564–74.
52. Figlioli G, Landi S, Romei C, et al. Medullary thyroid carcinoma (MTC) and RET proto-oncogene: mutation spectrum in the familial cases and a meta-analysis of studies on the sporadic form. *Mutat Res* 2013; **752**: 36–44.
53. Xing M, Cohen Y, Mambo E, et al. Early occurrence of rassf1a hypermethylation and its mutual exclusion with braf mutation in thyroid tumorigenesis. *Cancer Res* 2004; **64**: 1664–68.
54. Schagdarsurengin U, Gimm O, Hoang-Vu C, et al. Frequent epigenetic silencing of the CpG island promoter of RASSF1A in thyroid carcinoma. *Cancer Research* 2002; **62**: 3698–701.
55. Abraham D, Jackson N, Gundara JS, et al. MicroRNA profiling of sporadic and hereditary medullary thyroid cancer identifies predictors of nodal metastasis, prognosis, and potential therapeutic targets. *Clin Cancer Res* 2011; **17**: 4772–81.
56. Are C, Shaha AR. Anaplastic thyroid carcinoma: biology, pathogenesis, prognostic factors, and treatment approaches. *Ann Surg Oncol* 2006; **13**: 453–64.
57. Wiseman SM, Loree TR, Rigual NR, et al. Anaplastic transformation of thyroid cancer: review of clinical, pathologic, and molecular evidence provides new insights into disease biology and future therapy. *Head Neck* 2003; **25**: 662–70.
58. Nikiforov YE. Genetic alterations involved in the transition from well-differentiated to poorly differentiated and anaplastic thyroid carcinomas. *Endocr Path* 2004; **15**: 319–27.
59. Moretti F, Nanni S, Farsetti A, et al. Effects of exogenous p53 transduction in thyroid tumor cells with different p53 status. *J Clin Endocrinol Metab* 2000; **85**: 302–08.
60. Wiseman SM, Masoudi H, Niblock P, et al. Derangement of the E-cadherin/catenin complex is involved in transformation of differentiated to anaplastic thyroid carcinoma. *Am J Surg* 2006; **191**: 581–87.
61. Árvai K, Nagy K, Barti-Juhász H, et al. Molecular profiling of parathyroid hyperplasia, adenoma and carcinoma. *Pathol Oncol* 2012; **18**: 607–14.
62. Zhao L, Sun L, Liu D, et al. Copy number variation in CCND1 gene is implicated in the pathogenesis of sporadic parathyroid carcinoma. *World J Surg* 2014; **38**: 1730–37.
63. Arnold A, Kim H, Gaz R, et al. Molecular cloning and chromosomal mapping of DNA rearranged with the parathyroid hormone gene in a parathyroid adenoma. *J Clin Invest* 1989; **83**: 2034–40.
64. Hsi E, Zukerberg L, Yang WI W, Arnold A. Cyclin D1/PRAD1 expression in parathyroid adenomas: an immunohistochemical study. *J Clin Endocrinol Metab* 1996; **81**: 1736–39.
65. Agarwal A, Pradhan R, Kumari N, et al. Molecular characteristics of arge parathyroid adenomas. *World J Surg* 2016; **40**: 607–14.
66. Costa-Guda J, Soong C, Parekh V, et al. Germline and somatic mutations in cyclin-dependent kinase inhibitor genes CDKN1A, CDKN2B and CDKN2C in sporadic parathyroid adenomas. *Horm Canc* 2013; **4**: 301–07.
67. Chandrasekharappa S, Guru S, Manickam P, et al. Positional cloning of the gene for multiple endocrine neoplasia-type 1. *Science* 1997; **276**(5311): 404–07.
68. Soong C, Arnold, A. Recurrent ZFX mutations in human sporadic parathyroid adenomas. *Oncoscience* 2014; **1**(5): 360–66.
69. Velazquez-Fernandez D, Laurell C, Saqui-Salces M, et al. Differential RNA expression profile by cDNA microarray in sporadic primary hyperparathyroidism (pHPT): primary parathyroid hyperplasia versus adenoma. *World J Surg* 2006; **30**: 705–13.
70. Cryns V, Thor A, Xu H, et al. Loss of the retinoblastoma tumorsuppressor gene in parathyroid carcinoma. *New Engl J Med* 1994; **330**: 757–61.
71. Shattuck T, Valimaki S, Obara T, et al. Somatic and germ-line mutations of the HRPT2 gene in sporadic parathyroid carcinoma. *New Eng J Med* 2003; **349**: 1722–29.
72. Walls G. Multiple endocrine neoplasia (MEN) syndromes. *Semin Pediatr Surg* 2014; **23**: 96–101.

73. Marx, S. *Multiple endocrine neoplasia type 1*. 8th ed. New York: McGraw-Hill; 2001.
74. Uchino S, Noguchi S, Sato M, et al. Screening of the MEN1 gene and discovery of germ-line and somatic mutations in apparently sporadic parathyroid tumors. *Cancer Res* 2000; **60**: 5553–57.
75. Lemos M, Thakker R. Multiple endocrine neoplasia type 1 (MEN1): analysis of 1336 mutations reported in the first decade following identification of the gene. *Hum Mutat* 2008; **29**(1): 22–32.
76. Thakker R. Genetics of endocrine and metabolic disorders: parathyroid. *Rev Endocr Metab Disord* 2004; **5**: 37–51.
77. Basset JH, Forbes SA, Pannett AA, et al. Characterization of mutations in patients with multiple endocrine neoplasia type I. *Am J Hum Genet* 1988; **62**: 232–44.
78. Thakker R, Newey P, Walls G, et al. Clinical practice guidelines for multiple endocrine neoplasia type 1 (MEN1). *J Clin Endocrinol Metab* 2012; **97**(9): 2990–3011.
79. Kakudo K, Carney J, Sizemore G. Medullary carcinoma of thyroid: biologic behavior of the sporadic and familial neoplasm. *Cancer* 1985; **55**: 2818–21.
80. Gagel R, Tashjian Jr A, Cummings T, et al. The clinical outcome of prospective screening for multiple endocrine neoplasia type 2a: an 18-year experience. *N Engl J Med* 1988; **318**: 478–84.
81. Hofstra R, Landsvater R, Ceccherini I, et al. A mutation in the RET proto-oncogene associated with multiple endocrine neoplasia type 2B and sporadic medullary thyroid carcinoma. *Nature* 1994; **367**(6461): 375–76.
82. Eng C, Clayton D, Schuffenecker L, et al. The relationship between specific RET proto-oncogene mutations and disease phenotype in multiple endocrine neoplasia type 2I. International RET mutation consortium analysis. *JAMA* 1996; **276**: 1575–79.
83. Lips C. Clinical management of the multiple endocrine neoplasia syndromes: results of a computerized opinion poll at the Sixth International Workshop on Multiple Endocrine Neoplasia and von-Hippel-Lindau disease. *J Intern Med* 1998; **243**: 589–94.
84. Eng C, Mulligan L, Smith D, et al. Low frequency of germline mutations in the RET proto-oncogene in patients with apparently sporadic medullary thyroid carcinoma. *Clin Endocrinol (Oxf)* 1995; **43**: 123–27.
85. Brandi M, Gagel R, Angeli A, et al. Guidelines for diagnosis and therapy of MEN type 1 and type 2. *J Clin Endocrinol Metab* 2001; **86**: 5658–71.
86. Wells S, Asa S, Dralle H, et al. Revised American Thyroid Association guidelines for the management of medullary thyroid carcinoma. *Thyroid* 2015; **6**: 567–610.
87. Carpten J, Robbins C, Villablanca A, et al. HRPT2, encoding parafibromin, is mutated in hyperparathyroidism-jaw tumor syndrome. *Nat Genet* 2002; **32**: 676–80.
88. Howell V, Cardinal J, Richardson A, et al. Rapid mutation screening for HRPT2 and MEN1 mutations associated with familial and sporadic primary hyperparathyroidism. *J Mol Diagn* 2006; **8**(5): 559–66.
89. Marsh D, Coulon V, Lunetta, K, et al. Mutation spectrum and genotype-phenotype analyses in Cowden disease and Bannayan-Zonana syndrome, two hamartoma syndromes with germline PTEN mutation. *Hum Mol Genet* 1998; **7**: 507–15.
90. Cetta F, Montalto G, Gori M, et al. Germline mutations of the APC gene in patients with familial adenomatous polyposis-associated thyroid carcinoma: results from a European cooperative study. *J Clin Endocrinol Metab* 2000; **1**: 286–92.
91. Herve R, Farret O, Mayaudon H, et al. Association of Gardner syndrome and thyroid carcinoma. *Presse Med* 1995; **24**: 415.

Wound healing

CHAPTER 10

SOFT AND HARD TISSUE REPAIR

Sarah Al-Himdani and Ardeshir Bayat

Introduction 93	Wound assessment 101
Types of wound healing 93	Excessive wound healing 102
Phases of wound healing 94	Wound dressings 102
Repair of hard tissue/bone 97	Management of specific wounds 103
Linking basic knowledge to practice – key questions 98	References 105
Classification of wounds 99	

SEARCH STRATEGY

Data in this chapter may be updated by Medline and Embase searches using the key words: wound healing, tissue repair, tissue regeneration, chronic wounds and wound dressings. Information from these resources was critiqued and the information included is from levels of evidence 1 and 2.

INTRODUCTION

A wound is defined as a break in the integrity of the skin epithelium, often accompanied by concurrent disruption of the underlying dermis.[1] Having a clear understanding of wound healing is fundamental in all aspects of surgery. Whether small or large, acute or chronic, all wounds heal by a complex, dynamic, highly orchestrated biological process and a surgeon's success is largely dependent upon the uncomplicated successful procession through the different phases of normal wound healing.[2] In order to be able to both prevent wound formation and treat pathologic wounds, one must first appreciate the normal process of wound healing.

Wound healing has been divided into four overlapping stages: haemostasis, inflammation, proliferation and remodelling. However, this complex process is by no means constant, with genetics (susceptibility to abnormal scarring), age, site, tension, nutrition and disease all very important influencing factors. A wound is 'healed' when:

- connective tissue repair and complete re-epithelialization have occurred
- skin cover has been resorted with scar tissue without the necessity of drains or dressings.

When the process of wound healing fails to occur in an orderly and timely fashion, wounds become chronic and non-healing, requiring continued management by drainage and dressing.[1]

On the other hand, aberrant healing (excessive scar formation) may also result in the formation of abnormal scarring, such as in hypertrophic scarring or keloid disease.

TYPES OF WOUND HEALING

Primary healing (healing by first intention)

Healing by first intention is characterized by closure of a wound within 12–24 hours of its formation. These wounds are clean and well perfused, for example following surgical excision or a clean laceration. Wound edges are approximated using sutures, skin glue, steri-strips or other mechanical devices/instruments.[1] Apposition of wound edges reduces the distance for epidermal proliferation and wound closure (**Figure 10.1**).

Secondary healing (healing by secondary intention)

Healing by secondary intention usually occurs in large wounds where it is not possible to appose the edges or in wounds that are complicated by infection. Wounds may be

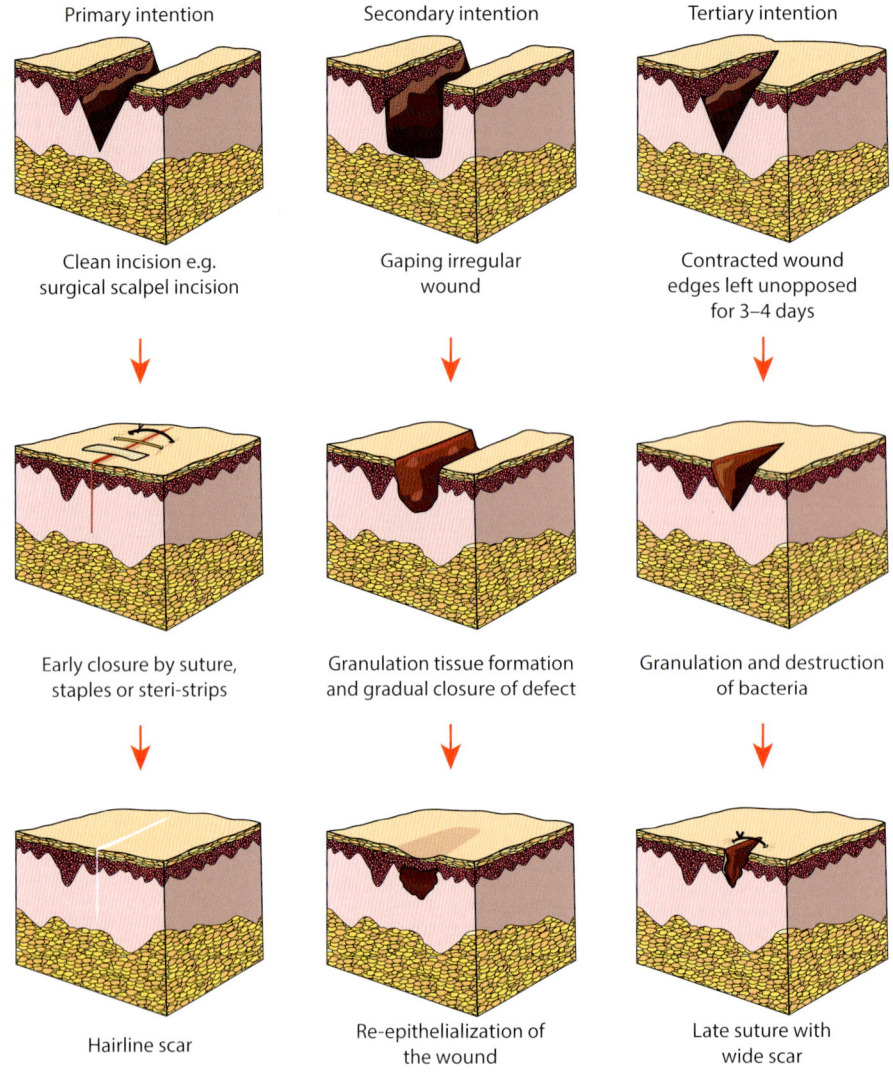

Figure 10.1 Diagrammatic representation of healing by primary, secondary and tertiary intention.

gaping and the edges lacerated. In these situations, sealing of the epithelium across the wound bed does not occur rapidly. Epithelial cells must grow both downwards and across the wound bed, with granulation tissue filling the defect. Healing of these wounds is achieved by wound contraction and subsequent epithelialization. Myofibroblasts play a key role in this process, usually appearing around 3 days following wound formation. Compared to healing by first intention, wound healing by secondary intention is a much slower process and may lead to subsequent contracture formation potentially resulting in functional impairment.[1]

Delayed primary healing (healing by tertiary intention)

This process mainly occurs in contaminated wounds, for example following bites and in abdominal wounds after peritoneal soiling. The wound edges are left unopposed in order for host defences to aid in debridement of the wound. The wound edges are usually approximated after 3–4 days, during which host phagocytes are recruited and inflammatory cells destroy the contaminating bacteria.[1]

Healing of superficial (partial-thickness) wounds

This process occurs following partial-thickness burns, split-thickness skin grafts and following abrasions, can extend through the epidermis and to the papillary dermis. The basal cell layer of the epidermis often remains intact and dermal regeneration can occur from epithelial cells within dermal appendages (hair follicles and sebaceous glands) and from the basal cell layer that replicate and migrate to the wound. The healing process occurs by re-epithelialization and is usually complete.[1]

PHASES OF WOUND HEALING

The complex, co-ordinated cascade of wound healing (as occurs in primary wound healing) is characterized by a number of cellular activities, including phagocytosis, cytokine release, chemotaxis, inflammation and synthesis of the extracellular matrix (ECM).[1] Following tissue

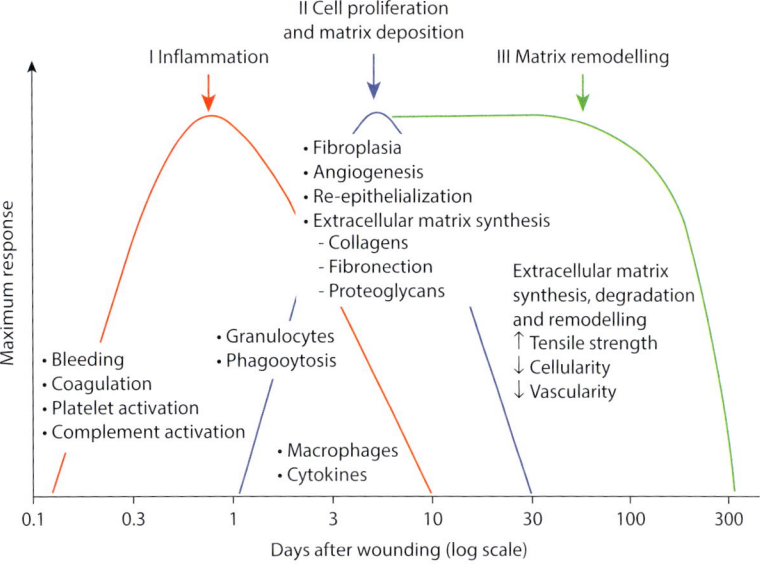

Figure 10.2 Phases of wound healing. Adapted from Greaves et al., 2013.[1]

injury, these processes have been described to occur in four phases: haemostasis, inflammation, proliferation and remodelling (**Figure 10.2**). Growth factors and cytokines are essential throughout the whole process of wound healing (**Tables 10.1** and **10.2**).

Haemostasis

Tissue injury results in disruption of the vascular endothelium, extravasation of blood constituents and exposure of the basal lamina. Constriction of endothelial cells and platelet activation then ensues. As well as initiating the coagulation cascade, aggregation, activation and degranulation of platelets leads to the release of several important growth factors that play important roles in chemotaxis (platelet-derived growth factor), deposition of the extracellular matrix (transforming growth factor-β), epithelialization (epidermal growth factor) and angiogenesis (vascular endothelial growth factor).[2–3]

TABLE 10.1 Major cell types and their roles in wound healing

Cell type	Role in wound healing
Platelets	• Clot formation • Release cytokines through degranulation (TGF-β, PDGF, platelet factor-4, β-thromboglobulin)
Neutrophils	• First cells attracted to wound site • Phagocytosis and intracellular destruction of bacteria
Macrophages/monocytes	• Phagocytosis of bacteria • Remove debris and necrotic tissue • Release important cytokines • Essential for fibroblast division, synthesis of collagen and angiogenesis
Lymphocytes	• Role unclear • May release some cytokines
Fibroblasts	• Produce most of the ECM • Form granulation tissue • Reorganize and structure the ECM • Wound contracture through formation of myofibroblasts
Keratinocytes	• Identification and destruction of foreign microorganisms • Wound re-epithelialization

TABLE 10.2 Major cytokines/growth factors, their sources and roles in wound healing

Cytokine/Growth factor	Sources	Role in wound healing
TGF-α	Macrophages, platelets, epithelial cells	• Stimulates epithelial cells and fibroblasts • Forms granulation tissue
TGF-β	Platelets, macrophages, fibroblasts, neutrophils, keratinocytes	• Stimulates fibroblast and smooth muscle proliferation • Chemotactic for macrophages
VEGF	Platelets, neutrophils	• Stimulates angiogenesis and collateral blood vessel formation in peripheral vascular disease
PDGF	Platelets, macrophages, endothelial cells	• Stimulates proliferation of fibroblasts • Stimulates angiogenesis • Stimulates wound contracture
FGFs	Fibroblasts, endothelial cells, smooth muscle cells, macrophages	• Chemotactic and mitogenic for fibroblasts and keratinocytes • Stimulates angiogenesis
IL-1	Macrophages, lymphocytes	• Activates granulocytes and endothelial cells • Stimulates haematopoiesis

Growth factors attract and activate fibroblasts, macrophages and endothelial cells. Four processes, essential to wound healing, are initiated following these events:

- Clotting cascade
- Complement cascade
- Kinin cascade
- Plasmin generation

The clot that forms acts as a matrix for subsequent cell migration. Vasoactive mediators released from the platelets lead to vasodilatation and increased vascular permeability.

Inflammation

This process usually lasts up to 4 days and can be divided into early and late phases. The cell type and response differ in these phases.

EARLY INFLAMMATION (DAYS 1–2)

Activation of the classical and alternative complement cascades leads to neutrophil infiltration of the wound usually within 24–48 hours of injury. These chemoattractants include:[1]

- transforming growth factor-β
- complement constituents
- bacterial peptide products
- fragments of extracellular matrix proteins.

Neutrophils adhere to endothelial cells of the surrounding blood vessels (margination) and move through the vessel wall (diapedesis). Further neutrophils are attracted to the site and release proteolytic enzymes, which digest the bacteria and debris. Neutrophils also form oxygen-free radicals (through a myeloperoxidase pathway), which sterilize the wound of bacteria.[4]

Throughout this period, basal cells exhibit increased mitotic activity and epithelial cell migration and proliferation occurs across the dermis. Neutrophil activity usually stops within a few days of tissue injury, once the contaminating bacteria and debris have been removed. Macrophages also aid in this process by phagocytosing redundant cells. The main function of the neutrophil is to remove bacterial contamination and debris from the wound and thus prevent infection.

LATE INFLAMMATION (DAYS 2–3)

Monocytes are attracted to the wound by chemoattractants including cytokines, complement components and breakdown products of collagen and elastin. At the wound site, they differentiate into macrophages, which are the most important cell type of the late inflammation stage (48–72 hours). In addition to phagocytosis of bacteria and cell debris, macrophages play a key role in granulation tissue formation and proliferation by releasing important cytokines: PDGF (platelet derived growth factor), TGF-β (transforming growth factor beta), TGF-α (transforming growth factor alpha), FGF (fibroblast growth factor) and IL-1 (interleukin one).[5] Macrophages also play important roles in:

- formation of the ECM by fibroblasts
- proliferation of smooth muscle cells
- endothelial cell proliferation and subsequent angiogenesis
- phagocytosis and enzyme release in the early inflammatory phase.

Macrophage or monocyte depletion leads to poor wound healing with poor debridement, delayed proliferation of fibroblasts, delayed ECM synthesis, inadequate angiogenesis and poor fibrosis.[6] During the late inflammatory stage, collagen fibres become evident at the incision margins of the wound but do not bridge the incision. A thickened epidermal covering layer is produced by continued epithelial proliferation.

Proliferation (day 3 to week 2)

This process, starting around day 3 and which can last up to 4 weeks, encompasses re-epithelialization and granulation tissue formation.

RE-EPITHELIALIZATION

This process involves replication and movement of the epidermal cells from the wound edges in order to reconstitute an organized, keratinized, stratified squamous epithelium. Increased mitotic activity within the basal cells of the wound edges occurs within 12 hours of wounding. Initially, migration of epidermal cells creates a delicate covering over the raw area, a process also known as 'epiboly'. These cells then migrate, usually as a sheet, by extending lamellipodia (from the Latin *lamina* – thin sheet, *pod* – foot) from the free edge of the cut epidermis, across the defect. This process of migration is dependent on the oxygen tension present in the wound and is most rapid in hyperbaric conditions.[7] 'Contact inhibition' prevents movement when epithelial sheets meet. Gradually, a continuous squamous cell epithelium is restored.

In partial-thickness wounds, the skin appendages (hair follicles and sebaceous glands) act as a source of epithelial cells for regeneration of the epidermis. During the process of migration, keratinocytes play an important role in bacteriological control. Foreign particles, once detected are phagocytosed and non-viable tissue is sloughed off.

Migration ceases once the sheets of epidermal cells meet. Re-epithelialization is complete and epidermal cells return to their normal morphology. Through this process, the barrier properties of the skin are restored, preventing the development of complications such as infection.

GRANULATION TISSUE FORMATION

Granulation tissue formation is composed of three important steps: fibroplasia, wound contraction and angiogenesis.

Fibroplasia

This process comprises of recruitment and proliferation of fibroblasts, which are essential in production of the ECM and the organization of components of the granulation tissue.[8] Fibroblasts are attracted to the wound 2–4 days after injury by growth factors including PDGF and TGF-β. Once at the wound site, fibroblasts proliferate and produce a number of important proteins (fibronectin, hyaluronin, collagen and proteoglycans) used to construct the new ECM. After wounding, fibroblasts undergo phenotypic alterations with altered expression of fibronectin.[9] These cells, called myofibroblasts, have capacity for contraction and increased motility and play an essential role in contraction during both normal and pathological wounding.[9] Mechanical tension and PDGF are important factors reported in myofibroblast formation.[9]

Fibroblasts secrete the ECM matrix, composed of fibrous structural proteins (collagen, elastin) and an interstitial matrix (glycoproteins in a proteoglycan and glycosaminoglycan gel). The interstitial matrix becomes organized around the epithelial cells, smooth muscle cells and endothelial cells and forms a new basement membrane. Fibronectin is a glycoprotein secreted in the ECM that aids adhesion of fibroblasts to the ECM, stimulates fibroblast migration, provides support for collagen deposition and mediates wound contraction.

Structural proteins (collagen and elastin) are vital for providing structure and strength. Several growth factors stimulate collagen synthesis during both the proliferative and remodelling phases, including: PDGF, basic fibroblast growth factor, TGF-β, IL-1, and TNF (tissue necrosis factor). Around 18 different types of collagen exist. Collagen type III is secreted maximally within 5–7 days of wounding.

Wound contraction

This begins 7 days after wounding and peaks at 2 weeks. This process reduces the size of the defect and the need for scar tissue, usually occurring at a rate of 0.6–0.7 mm per day.[10] The degree of contraction varies with depth. However, in humans, in whom the skin is relatively immobile, contraction alone rarely completely closes a wound. Contraction must be closely regulated; when there is limited contraction, this can lead to delayed wound closure, bleeding and infection whilst excessive contracture can cause contractures.

Angiogenesis

This is the process of new blood vessel formation, commencing 2–3 days after wounding. This is essential to healing, as metabolic activity in a healing wound cannot occur without a specific blood supply. Granulation is composed of proliferating fibroblasts and loops of capillaries in a loose ECM. Important steps required for angiogenesis include: degradation of the basement membrane of the parent vessel, endothelial cell migration towards the angiogenic stimuli, endothelial cell proliferation with subsequent maturation into capillary tubes.[1]

Important factors inducing angiogenesis include: VEGF, PDGF, TGF-β and basic fibroblast growth factor. Invasion of the wound by capillaries creates a microvascular network within the wound. Chronic wounds, characterized by delayed healing, may occur when vascular supply to the wound is insufficient.[11]

Remodelling and scar maturation (from week 1 to several weeks)

The ECM and collagen fibres are continually synthesized and remodelled throughout the process of wound healing (this occurs simultaneously with granulation tissue formation). As collagen is formed, it is also degraded. Metalloproteinases (collagenases, gelatinases and stromelysins) are proteolytic enzymes synthesized by fibroblasts, neutrophils and macrophages responsible for this process. Regulation of metalloproteinase activity is necessary to ensure that collagen degradation, which in excess may impair wound healing, is closely controlled. Typically, these enzymes are initially inactive and activation is necessary before they can act. Tissue inhibitors of metalloproteinases also prevent their action and allow for control of collagen breakdown. Around 21 days following injury, equilibrium is reached between collagen formation and degradation. Continued remodelling leads to eventual reduced activity of metalloproteinases, reduced macrophages and fibroblasts, reduced capillary outgrowth and reduced size of contractile connective tissue.

Scar maturation results in the breakdown of fibronectin and hyaluronan as well as a larger diameter of collagen bundles. Though increasing in strength through the process of remodelling, the collagen will never reach the same strength as that of unwounded skin and usually a maximum of 80% of the strength in unwounded skin is reached.

REPAIR OF HARD TISSUE/BONE

Repair of bone is similar to that of soft tissue, with an added osteogenic component. Following injury, haemorrhage occurs with clot formation. Neutrophils, macrophages and mast cells move into the injury site and release growth factors and cytokines, stimulating the process of healing. Cytokines of importance in bone formation include:

- TGF-β, which is a potent chemotactic cytokine for osteoprogenitor cells and macrophages. This also stimulates proliferation of mesenchymal and osteoprogenitor cells, osteoblasts and chondrocytes.
- TNF-α, which promotes recruitment of mesenchymal stem cells. Absence of TNF-α prohibits bone formation.
- Bone morphogenic proteins, which regulate the transcription of target genes, in particular playing a critical role in regulation of growth, differentiation and apoptosis of osteoblasts, chondroblasts, neural cells and epithelial cells.

Osteoclasts and macrophages remove wound debris and gradually granulation tissue is formed and replaces the clot. This process usually takes several days, but the duration is also dependent on the site and the severity of the injury.

Vascular endothelial cells and perivascular mesenchymal cells provide osteoprogenitor cells, which become osteoblasts. Several cytokines stimulate osteoblast activation including PDGF, TGF-β, FGFs and bone morphogenetic proteins (BMPs).[12] Chondroblasts may also become activated, particularly when oxygen levels are low. Within the new matrix, mainly at the site of the periosteum, cartilage cells begin to develop. Osteoblasts also release calcium, which is deposited into the new matrix and on to the cartilage. At this stage, the bone is flexible and is called soft callus.

Once the soft callus is formed, subperiosteal and endochondral ossification occurs continually. Hard callus is formed once the ends of the bone become united, after approximately 2 months. Once formed, the remodelling process continues leading to the formation of mature lamellar bone. This process requires osteoblasts and osteoclasts. Through further remodelling, the marrow cavity and the contour of the bone are restored. External forces applied to the bone can alter the remodelling process.

LINKING BASIC KNOWLEDGE TO PRACTICE – KEY QUESTIONS

A number of different pathological processes may lead to abnormal wound healing. Prompt diagnosis and appropriate treatment is key. When incorrectly diagnosed, delayed wound healing followed by other morbid complications may ensue.

1. What are the causes of abnormal wound healing?
2. Which local and systemic factors impede wound healing?
3. How do we assess wounds?
4. How do we manage wounds?

What are the causes of abnormal wound healing?

Several local and systemic factors may impede wound healing (**Figure 10.3**). This section will review some of these important factors in more detail.

PATIENT AGE

Local and systemic factors affecting wound healing are more common in elderly patients. Failure of wound healing can become a chronic disabling condition and may incur significant social and medical costs to the elderly population affected. Ageing has a number of effects on the different stages of wound healing including:[13–15]

- delayed epithelialization
- altered inflammatory and cell adhesion molecule profile

LOCAL FACTORS
- Poor blood supply
- Infection
- Increased skin tension
- Presence of foreign body
- Underlying osteomyelitis
- Poor venous drainage
- Malignant transformation

SYSTEMIC FACTORS
- Obesity
- Increasing age
- Systemic diseases e.g. diabetes mellitus
- Protein deficiency
- Chemo/radiotherapy
- Immunosuppressant therapy
- Disorders of neutrophils or macrophages
- Lymphoedema or venous oedema
- Peripheral vascular disease

Figure 10.3 Local and systemic factors contributing to impaired wound healing.

- reduced collagen content and 'fragmented' appearing elastic fibres leading to reduced tensile strength
- reduced number of inflammatory cells
- impaired granulation tissue formation
- impaired angiogenesis.

NUTRITIONAL STATUS

Malnutrition adversely affects wound healing. In particular, dramatic degrees of protein calorie malnutrition delays the wound healing response.[16] Additionally, several 'pro-healing' nutrients have been identified including: arginine, vitamins A and C and zinc.

Markers of nutrition identified in previous studies include:[17, 18]

- serum albumin (<30 g/l), shown to predict delayed wound healing; however, albumin levels can be affected by other conditions such as fluid retention and distribution. It also has a long half-life
- pre-albumin (<10 mg/dl), an indicator of malnutrition and poor wound healing with a shorter half-life than albumin
- serum transferrin (<1.5 g/l) also shown to predict delayed wound healing; however, transferrin levels are also dependent upon body iron status.

Assessment of nutritional needs and supplementation is essential in those with or at risk of malnutrition. Dieticians play a vital role in the assessment and management of these patients.

Important screening questions when assessing nutritional intake include[17] height, weight, recent unintentional weight loss, and change in food intake. It is also important to find out how physically active patients are and whether they have had any additional gastrointestinal symptoms such as chronic diarrhoea or vomiting.

Several formal screening tools have also been developed, such as 'MUST'. This categorizes patients into low,

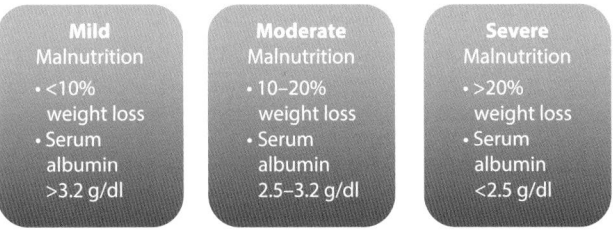

Figure 10.4 Mild, moderate and severe categories of malnutrition.

medium and high-risk groups according to their score. Those at high risk should be assessed by a dietician and receive nutritional support.[19] Pre-operative nutritional support is recommended for patients with moderate to severe malnutrition (**Figure 10.4**).

UNDERLYING CHRONIC CONDITION

Diabetes mellitus, atherosclerosis, hypothyroidism, chronic venous insufficiency and obesity can all delay wound healing. The effect of increased serum glucose, in diabetic patients, on wound healing is multifactorial. Some of these effects include:[20–23]

- increased vascular permeability leading to pericapillary albumin deposition and impaired diffusion of oxygen and nutrients
- inhibition of function of structural and enzymatic proteins due to non-enzymatic glycolization
- glycosylated collagen resistance to enzymatic degradation.

Animal and human models have shown that as a result of these effects, diabetic wounds demonstrate decreased granulation tissue, decreased collagen, slow wound maturation and decreased numbers of fibroblasts.

Animal studies have also demonstrated that reduced thyroid hormone levels can adversely affect fibroblast function and subsequent wound strength. In addition to the specific effects of absent thyroid hormone, systemic complications of the disease such as heart failure can also compound these effects.[20] Treating the underlying condition is an essential step in wound management in patients with both diabetes mellitus and hypothyroidism.

INFECTION

Local wound infection and foreign bodies delay wound healing by prolonging the inflammatory phase. When the bacterial count is greater than 10^5/g of tissue or beta-haemolytic streptococcus is present, the wound will not heal. Bacteria prolong the inflammatory phase of wound healing and also deleteriously affect rate of epithelialization, contraction and collagen deposition.[20]

MEDICATIONS

Patients with chronic wounds often suffer from chronic diseases for which they may take several medications. These medications may contribute to delayed wound healing. It is thus vital to review a patient's list of medications. The following medications may contribute to delayed wound healing:[24]

- steroids,[25] which arrest inflammation by interfering with wound macrophages, angiogenesis and wound contraction
- NSAIDs,[26] which reduce collagen synthesis, thought to be related to impaired prostaglandin metabolism
- chemotherapeutic agents,[24] which reduce wound contraction and fibroblasts proliferation.

CLASSIFICATION OF WOUNDS

Wounds can be categorized in a number of different ways. In this section we will describe some of the important classifications.

Acute vs. Chronic

Acute wounds most often occur secondary to trauma. These wounds generally heal very well.

Chronic wounds usually occur in patients with an underlying condition, for example diabetes mellitus, malignancy and chronic venous insufficiency. These wounds may start from an initial trauma and persist beyond 6 weeks, due to an abnormal underlying physiology affecting the process of wound repair, such as diabetes, or peripheral vascular disease. In addition, these wounds have the potential for malignant transformation, also known as Marjolin's ulcer.

ACUTE WOUNDS

Examples of acute wounds include:

- thermal wounds
- surgical wounds
- traumatic wounds.

Thermal Wounds

Both extremes of temperature and radiation may lead to thermal wounds. Radiotherapy is often used treat head and neck cancers and leads to permanent damage to the skin's microvasculature. These wounds often heal poorly and can become infected.

Burns are the commonest type of thermal injury and exact assessment of the degree/level of depth of burn is critical. Most commonly burns are classified as:

1 Superficial:
   - Wound appears erythematous.
   - This affects the upper layer of the epidermis. Generally no intervention is necessary.
2 Partial-thickness:
   - Appear blistered.
   - Further subdivided into **superficial partial-thickness**, **mid-dermal** and **deep-dermal**.

- This affects the epidermis and part of the dermis. Generally minimal intervention may be required if only the most superficial part of the epidermis is affected, the so-called superficial partial-thickness wounds. Mid-dermal and deep-dermal should be closely observed as skin grafting may be necessary, particularly if these wounds extend.
3. Full-thickness:
   - Appear charred/white and insensate
   - These wounds affect the epidermis, dermis and can extend into the subcutis. Skin grafts are always required in these wounds.

Surgical Wounds

There are many types of surgical wounds and examples include incisions, excisions, skin grafting (involving split-thickness skin grafts or full-thickness skin grafts), amputations and skin biopsies:

- **Incisions/excisions:** A scalpel is the most common device used to make these wounds. This extends through the whole thickness of the skin to the underlying tissues. If the incision involves removal of tissue, this will be considered an excision. Post-operatively the wound is sutured closed (healing by primary intention) or in the case of excision, this may require skin grafting or use of skin flaps.
- **Skin grafts:** These are commonly used following deep (full-thickness) burn injuries. The grafts can be either split-thickness or full-thickness depending on the depth of the harvest. Split-thickness includes the epidermis and the papillary dermis.
- **Amputations:** This type of wound is created following surgical removal of a limb, either as a result of disease, trauma or infection. Healing of these wounds is usually by either primary or secondary intention depending on the initial indication for the amputation.
- **Skin biopsies:** These wounds usually involved surgical excisional removal of a full-thickness area of skin for histological assessment. These wounds are normally left to heal and close by secondary intention although the larger wounds are closed directly using sutures following the biopsy and healing by primary intention.

Surgical wounds have also been classified according to the level of contamination during the operation from I–IV (**Table 10.3**).

Traumatic Wounds

These are other acute injuries, which usually result from a physical force. They may result from small, common cutaneous injuries to life-threatening limb/head/trunk injuries. Examples include:

- abrasions
- puncture
- laceration
- bruises
- gunshots
- blisters
- bites
- stab
- crush.

CHRONIC WOUNDS

The vast majority of chronic wounds can be classified into the following categories:

- diabetic ulcers
- pressure ulcers
- venous ulcers
- arterial ulcers.

Diabetic Ulcers

The effect of diabetes on wound healing was described previously. Diabetics have a 15% greater risk of amputations compared to the general population, due to chronic lower limb ulcers.[27] Wounds often form secondary to diabetic neuropathy. Loss of pain perception results and patients often develop wounds from repeated injury that they fail to notice.

Pressure Ulcers

These wounds typically occur over bony prominences where skin is subject to excessive pressure forces. Chronic conditions such as diabetes mellitus may also predispose patients to developing pressure sores. Common sites affected include the heels, shoulder blades and sacrum. Pressure ulcers can be classified according to the depth of the wound:

1. Stage I:
   - Non-blanching erythema
   - Skin temperature, tissue consistency or sensation may be altered

TABLE 10.3 Classification of surgical wounds

Class and type of wound	Description of wound	Wound closure
Class I Clean	• Wound made aseptically • No contact made with respiratory, alimentary or urinary tract	• Closed by primary intention
Class II Clean-contaminated	• Wound made aseptically • Enters respiratory, alimentary or urinary tract	• Closed by primary intention
Class III Contaminated	• Wound is open or involves major breaks in sterile technique or gross spillage from gastrointestinal tract	• Closed by primary or secondary intention. • Requires significant washing before closure
Class IV Dirty	• Dirty infected wounds • This retains devitalized tissue or involves pre-operative existing infection or perforated viscera	• These wounds are often left open for drainage

2. Stage II:
   - Partial-thickness skin loss
   - Involves epidermis and dermis
   - Appears as an abrasion, blister or shallow crater
3. Stage III:
   - Full-thickness skin loss
   - Extends to but not through the underlying fascia
   - Presents as a deep crater
4. Stage IV:
   - Full-thickness tissue loss
   - Extends to muscle, bone, or supporting structures (e.g. tendon or joint capsule)

Venous Ulcers

These are the most commonly occurring ulcers and result from venous insufficiency. Venous drainage and blood supply are reduced in the affected tissue, leading to extensive ulceration following a minor injury.

Characteristics of these ulcers include:

- often located around medial malleolus
- shallow depth
- large in size
- irregular edges
- sloughy base with pink granulation tissue.

Arterial Ulcers

These are caused by a lack of blood flow to the lower limbs. This leads to tissue hypoxia and ischemia. These ulcers occur more commonly in diabetics and smokers.

Characteristics of these ulcers include:

- often sited around the lateral malleolus
- small in size
- regular shape
- deep, often to bone
- no granulation tissue.

Types of wound tissue

GRANULATION TISSUE

This appears red, moist, shiny and granular. On biopsy, an abundance of capillaries, macrophages and fibroblasts may be seen.

EPITHELIAL TISSUE

Once wounds are filled with granulation tissue, a new epithelial layer grows from the edges of the wound moving towards the centre. This tissue appears pink/white in colour. As well as from the edges of the wound, epithelial cells may also be derived from skin appendages, producing islands of skin in the middle of the granulation tissue.

NECROTIC TISSUE

There are two types of necrotic tissue that may appear in a wound: slough and eschar. Slough is dead devitalized tissue that appears moist, loose and stringy. It is typically yellow and found on the wound bed. It is commonly present in chronic or infected wounds. Eschar commonly occurs after burns and appears as dry, thick, leathery tissue. It may be black and should be promptly excised.

INFECTED TISSUE

A number of classical features can be used to identify infected tissue:

- Pyrexia
- Pus
- Erythema (particularly when spreading)
- Malodour
- Wound dehiscence
- Poor healing
- Increased pain
- Sinus formation

When a wound infection is suspected, the following steps should be taken:

1. Wound swab: Traditionally 10^5 bacteria per gram has been used as the cut-off point at which it is thought that bacteria inhibit wound healing. Wounds with this level or greater of bacteria are classed as being infected.
2. Sensitivities: From the wound swab, the sensitivities of the organisms to antibiotic treatment can be determined.

WOUND ASSESSMENT

Size of the wound

The wound size should be assessed on first presentation and regularly thereafter. The outline of the wound can be traced onto transparent acetate sheets. The surface area may be calculated by multiplying the longest diameter in one plane by the longest diameter in the plane at right angles (in a circular shaped wound).[28]

Edges of a wound

Examination of the edges of a wound is useful in identifying the aetiology of the wound. Venous ulcers often have sloping edges whilst arterial appear well demarcated or 'punched out'. When rolled or everted edges are observed, malignancy must be excluded by biopsy.

Location of the wound

The site of a wound also aids in the diagnosis. Venous ulcers most commonly occur in the gaiter region, around the medial malleolus. Diabetic foot ulcers commonly occur over pressure areas such as under the hallux, under the first and fifth metatarsal heads and under the heel.

Wound bed

The appearance of the wound bed gives an indication of the type of wound. Healthy granulation tissue appears pink. Dark red and bleeding granulation tissue

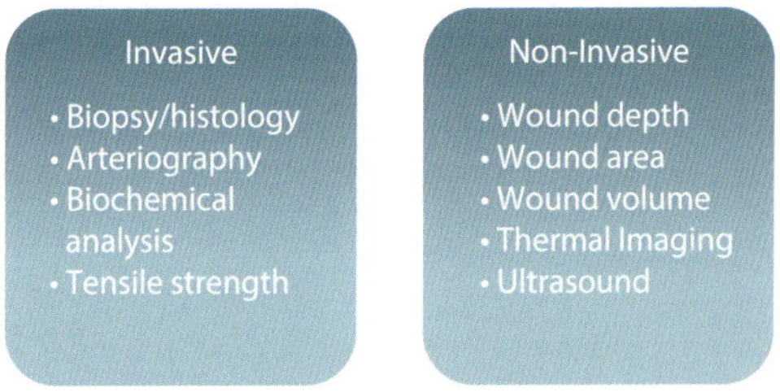

Figure 10.5 Invasive and non-invasive techniques for assessing wounds.

- Invasive
  - Biopsy/histology
  - Arteriography
  - Biochemical analysis
  - Tensile strength
- Non-Invasive
  - Wound depth
  - Wound area
  - Wound volume
  - Thermal Imaging
  - Ultrasound

may indicate infection. Excess granulation tissue may be present in chronic poorly healing wounds. This excess tissue must be debrided to aid wound healing. Techniques for assessing wounds may be either invasive or non-invasive (**Figure 10.5**).

EXCESSIVE WOUND HEALING

Hypertrophic scars and keloids occur as a consequence of excessive wound healing leading to abnormal fibrotic scar formation. These result from overproduction of fibroblasts, collagen, elastin and proteoglycans. These occur in up to 5–15% of all wounds, with rates much higher in the non-Caucasian population with pigmented skin.[1]

Hypertrophic scars

These scars are more common in:[1]

- wounds that are under tension
- deep dermal burns
- wounds healing by secondary intention.

Keloid

This is a benign fibroproliferative scar that continues to grow beyond the confines of the original wound, invading into healthy surrounding tissue.[29] No specific cause has been elucidated, although it is known that keloids have a strong genetic predisposition.[30] In most instances, the magnitude of the injury does not correlate with the size of the keloid scar, although in every case, a form of dermal injury has been associated with development of a keloid scar.

WOUND DRESSINGS

Ideal wound dressings sustain a moist wound environment for optimal wound healing. Dressings can be comprised of synthetic polymers (formed into fibres, wafers or membranes).[31] These membranes are considered to be semipermeable to gases (oxygen, CO_2 and moisture) and usually impermeable to liquids. These dressings are also named occlusive dressings. There are five types of such dressings:

1. Hydrogels
2. Hydrocolloids
3. Foams
4. Films
5. Alginates.

The principle reasons for applying a dressing include:

- to produce rapid and cosmetically acceptable healing
- to reduce pain
- to remove odour
- to treat or prevent infection
- to cover a cosmetically unpleasant wound.

Several factors should be considered when choosing a dressing including:

- wound-related factors:
  - size
  - depth
  - amount and characteristics of exudate
  - necrotic/viable
  - surrounding tissue appearance (pigmented, scarred or cellulitic)
- product factors
- patient factors.

Dressings for acute wounds

Several dressings may be used for acute wounds. These include:

- low-adherence dressings (e.g. Mepore®, Mölnlycke Healthcare), for example for skin tears
- transparent film (e.g. OpSite™, Smith & Nephew), which is used in clean, dry wounds.

Dressings for chronic wounds

NECROTIC WOUNDS

The aim with these wounds is to rehydrate the skin so that the dead skin/scab will separate from the normal skin. Options include:

- wet dressings using saline or hypochlorite
- hydrocolloid when wounds are dry and necrotic
- hydrogel (e.g. Aquasorb™) when wounds are dry and necrotic
- surgical/mechanical debridement
- biological debridement (e.g. larvae)
- enzymatic debridement (e.g. collagenase).

SLOUGHY WOUNDS

These should be debrided in order to remove the abnormal matrix of slough (inflammatory cells and exudate). This can be done surgically or using an agent which soaks up the debris forming a moist gel. Dressing options include:

- hydrofibres
- hydrogels
- hydrocolloids
- polysaccharide dressings (beads or paste)
- alginate dressings
- mechanical debridement.

GRANULATING WOUNDS

Granulation tissue is highly vascular. It contains collagen and proteoglycans. The dressing choice depends on depth and exudate from the wound.

For light-medium exudative wounds consider:

- hydrocolloids
- thin foam dressings
- hydrogel, sheets or gels.

For shallow exuding ulcers:

- alginate dressings
- hydrophilic foam materials
- hydrocolloids.

For deep cavity wounds:

- alginate fibre ribbons
- foams
- silicone foam dressings
- hydrofibers (e.g. Aquacel®)
- vacuum-assisted closure (VAC) therapy.

EPITHELIALIZING WOUNDS

These are superficial wounds. Dressing choice depends on whether the wounds are dry or exude fluid. For dry superficial wounds, the following dressings are recommended:

- hydrocolloids
- film dressings
- perforated plastic film dressings
- knitted viscose non-adherent dressings.

For exudative wounds (e.g. burns and graft donor sites) dressing options include:

- paraffin gauze covered with gauze and cotton (Gamgee)
- hydrocolloids
- alginates
- hydrofibers (e.g Aquacel®).

For very exudative wounds:

- impregnated gauze dressings may be used. Twice daily dressing changes may be required.

INFECTED WOUNDS

These wounds can have an unpleasant odour. For this reason and in order to prevent spread of infection, they should be covered. Antibacterial agents are included in a number of the dressings:

- framycetin
- fusidic acid
- chlorhexidene
- iodine
- honey dressings
- silver sulfadiazine dressings (e.g. Silvadene) or an ionic silver hydrofiber dressings (e.g. Aquacel-AG).

MANAGEMENT OF SPECIFIC WOUNDS

Over/hypergranulation tissue occurs when the inflammatory phase is prolonged unnecessarily. The most frequent dressing options include:

- change from occlusive to non-occlusive dressings
- light pressure application to wound bed with bandaging
- short-term topical steroid application.

For pressure wounds:

- comfortable dressing, for example an extra-thin hydrocolloid
- off-loading devices such as comfort boots in heel ulcers
- securing dressings in a very moist area such as the sacrum is challenging. A wafer hydrocolloid is a comfortable and highly adherent dressing.

For venous ulcers:

- the dressing type should be according to the tissue type in the ulcer bed
- compression bandages.

For diabetic foot ulcers:

- optimal blood sugar control
- appropriate comfortable footwear
- daily saline dressing to provide a moist wound environment
- debridement if necessary
- antibiotics if soft tissue infection or osteomyelitis present.

For burns or scalds:

- cold running water
- cling film prior to assessment.

For superficial burns:

- semipermeable films
- hydrocolloids
- Aquacel®
- Mepitel®
- foams.

For partial thickness burns:

- Flamazine®
- alginates
- Mepitel®
- Aquacel®.

For full-thickness burns:

- assessment at a specialist burn centre for need for skin grafting
- Flamazine®
- hydrogels
- Mepitel®.

Care of the surrounding skin:

- To secure a dressing when surrounding skin is fragile, hydrogel sheets and non-adhesive foams are useful.
- Topical creams such as Diprobase may be used to rehydrate the skin.

BEST CLINICAL PRACTICE

- ✓ Ensure a relevant history and careful examination is undertaken in order to elicit factors contributing to poor wound healing:
    - ✓ age: delayed wound healing with increasing age
    - ✓ nutritional status: malnutrition impairs wound healing
    - ✓ chronic disease: diabetes, peripheral vascular disease and chronic venous insufficiency all predispose to ulceration and poor wound healing
    - ✓ several medications impair wound healing, in particular: steroids, non-steroidal anti-inflammatory drugs, cytotoxic agents and immunosuppressants
    - ✓ pressure-prone anatomical areas can lead to ulcer formation
    - ✓ infection impairs wound healing.
- ✓ Wounds can be classified in a number of ways:
    - ✓ acute vs. chronic: (i) acute: thermal wounds, surgical wounds and traumatic wounds; (ii) chronic: diabetic ulcers, pressure ulcers, venous ulcers, arterial ulcers and mixed ulcers.
    - ✓ according to the type of wound tissue: granulation tissue, epithelial tissue, necrotic tissue or infected tissue.
- ✓ Wound assessment involves evaluation of: wound size, edges, and location (anatomical site) and status of wound bed and tissue. Invasive as well as a number of non-invasive techniques can be utilized in wound assessment.
- ✓ Five main types of wound dressing are used: hydrogels, hydrocolloids, foams, films and alginates.
- ✓ The following factors should be considered in order to choose the optimal dressing:
    - ✓ type of wound/ulcer
    - ✓ wound size
    - ✓ wound site
    - ✓ depth
    - ✓ amount and characteristics of exudate
    - ✓ necrotic/viable tissue
    - ✓ surrounding tissue appearance (pigmented, scarred or cellulitic).

FUTURE RESEARCH

Pre-clinical studies have demonstrated the potential benefit in the application of topical growth factors onto wounds.[32] Future treatments may include gene therapy with insertion of human growth factors genes direction into wound cells using vectors.[33] Additionally research has demonstrated benefit in utilizing mesenchymal stem cells to promote wound healing.[34]

In addition, the role of electrical stimulation (ES) in acceleration of cutaneous repair has gained recent scientific and clinical interest. A number of recent studies have shown that application of ES can enhance tissue repair not only by increasing angiogenesis but also by reducing inflammation.[35-36]

KEY POINTS

- Wounds may heal by primary, secondary or tertiary intention.
- Healing by primary intention involves:
    - clean wound edges closed within 24 hours
    - surgical incision/laceration
    - approximation using sutures, skin glue or steri-strips
    - hairline scar.
- Healing by secondary intention involves:
    - large gaping or infected wounds
    - epithelial cells grow downwards and across the wound bed
    - contraction and epithelialization occurs
    - slower than healing by primary intention and may lead to contracture formation.
- Healing by tertiary intention involves:
    - contaminated wounds
    - wound edges left unopposed for up to 4 days for phagocytosis to occur
    - wound edges then approximated, often loosely.
- Cutaneous wound healing may be divided into four stages:
    1. Haemostasis
    2. Inflammation
    3. Proliferation
    4. Remodelling.
- The following steps occur in the haemostasis phase:
    - disruption of the vascular endothelium
    - blood extravasation and clot formation
    - endothelial cell constriction and platelet activation
    - release of growth factors and cytokines by platelets.
- The inflammation phase comprises of early and late phases:
    - The early phase (days 1–2) comprises neutrophil infiltration within 24–48 hours of injury. These digest bacteria and debris.
    - The late phase (days 2–3) involves monocyte/macrophage attraction to the wound. Macrophages phagocytose bacteria and release essential cytokines including PDGF, TGF-β, TGF-α, FGF and IL-1.

- The proliferative phase:
  - Occurs from day 3 up to week 2.
  - Encompasses: re-epithelialization and granulation tissue formation (fibroplasia, wound contraction and angiogenesis).
  - Re-epithelialization starts within 12 hours of wounding and is the replication and reconstitution of the organized, keratinized, stratified squamous epithelium.
  - Fibroplasia is recruitment and proliferation of fibroblasts, which produce the extracellular matrix that acts as a scaffold for the healing tissue.
  - Fibroblasts, as well as releasing important cytokines and growth factors also produce important structural proteins (collagen, hyaluronin and proteoglycans). Phenotypic alterations in fibroblasts after wounding (day 7 to week 2) lead to myofibroblast formation. These contract and aid in wound closure.
  - Angiogenesis (day 2–3) is the process of new blood vessel formation and this is essential for the metabolic activity of the wound during healing. Several cytokines induce angiogenesis: VEGF, PDGF, TGF-β and basic fibroblast growth factor. A poor vascular supply leads to poor wound healing.
- Remodelling and scar maturation:
  - Occurs from week 1 to several weeks following tissue injury.
  - Involves collagen formation that is balanced closely with its degradation by metalloproteinases.
  - Continued remodelling eventually leads to scar formation.
  - Scar collagen is usually a maximum of 80% of the strength of unwounded skin.
- Healing of hard tissue/bone involves:
  - A similar process to that of soft tissue, with an added osteogenic component.
  - Important cytokines include: TGF-β, TNF-α and Bone morphogenic proteins.
  - Osteoclasts and macrophages remove wound debris and gradually granulation tissue is formed.
  - Chondroblasts and osteoblasts create a soft callus.

REFERENCES

1. Greaves NS, Ashcroft KJ, Baguneid M, Bayat A. Current understanding of molecular and cellular mechanisms in fibroplasia and angiogenesis during acute wound healing. *J Dermatyol Sci* 2013; **72**(3): 206–17.
2. Janis JE, Harrison B. Wound healing: part I. Basic science. *Plast Reconstr Surg* 2014; **133**(2): 199e–207e.
3. Barrientos S, Stojadinovic O, Golinko MS, et al. Perspective article: Growth factors and cytokines in wound healing. *Wound Repair Regen* 2008; **16**(5): 585–601.
4. Yager DR, Nwomeh BC. The proteolytic environment of chronic wounds. *Wound Repair Regen* 1999; **7**(6): 433–41.
5. DiPietro LA. Wound healing: the role of the macrophage and other immune cells. *Shock* 1995; **4**(4): 233–40.
6. Leibovich SJ, Ross R. The role of the macrophage in wound repair: a study with hydrocortisone and antimacrophage serum. *Am J Pathol* 1975; **78**(1): 71–100.
7. LaVan FB, Hunt TK. Oxygen and wound healing. *Clin Plas Surg* 1990; **17**(3): 463–72.
8. Stephens P, Davies KJ, Al-Khateeb T, et al. A comparison of the ability of intra-oral and extra-oral fibroblasts to stimulate extracellular matrix reorganization in a model of wound contraction. *J Dent Res* 1996; **75**(6): 1358–64.
9. Tomasek JJ, Gabbiani G, Hinz B, et al. Myofibroblasts and mechano-regulation of connective tissue remodelling. *Nat Rev Mol Cell Biol* 2002; **3**: 349–63.
10. Winter GD. Formation of the scab and the rate of epithelization of superficial wounds in the skin of the young domestic pig. *Nature* 1962; **193**: 293–94.
11. Witte MB, Barbul A. General principles of wound healing. *Surg Clin N Am* 1997; **77**(3): 509–28.
12. Dimitriou R, Tsiridis E, Giannoudis PV. Current concepts of molecular aspects of bone healing. *Injury* 2005; **36**(12): 1392–404.
13. Holt DR, Kirk SJ, Regan MC, et al. Effect of age on wound healing in healthy human beings. *Surgery* 1992; **112**(2): 293–97; discussion 7–8.
14. Van De Kerkhof PMC, Van Bergen B, Spruijt K, Kuiper JP. Age-related changes in wound healing. *Clin Exp Dermatol* 1994; **19**(5): 369–74.
15. Ashcroft GS, Horan MA, Ferguson MW. Aging alters the inflammatory and endothelial cell adhesion molecule profiles during human cutaneous wound healing. *Lab Invest* 1998; **78**(1): 47–58.
16. Albina JE. Nutrition and wound healing. *Jpen-Parenter Enter* 1994; **18**(4): 367–76.
17. Lennard-Jones JE, Arrowsmith H, Davison C, et al. Screening by nurses and junior doctors to detect malnutrition when patients are first assessed in hospital. *Clin Nutr* 1995; **14**(6): 336–40.
18. Casey J, Flinn WR, Yao JS, et al. Correlation of immune and nutritional status with wound complications in patients undergoing vascular operations. *Surgery* 1983; **93**(6): 822–27.
19. Stratton RJ, Hackston A, Longmore D, et al. Malnutrition in hospital outpatients and inpatients: prevalence, concurrent validity and ease of use of the malnutrition universal screening tool, (MUST) for adults. *Brit J Nutr* 2004; **92**(5): 799–808.
20. Broughton G, Janis JE, Attinger CE. Wound healing: an overview. *Plast Reconstr Surg* 2006; **117**(7S): 1e–S–32e–S 10.1097/01.prs.0000222562.60260.f9.
21. Bucalo B, Eaglstein WH, Falanga V. Inhibition of cell proliferation by chronic wound fluid. *Wound Repair Regen* 1993; **1**(3): 181–86.
22. He Z, King GL. Microvascular complications of diabetes. *Endocrin Metab Clin* 2004; **33**(1): 215–38.
23. Chow LWC, Loo WYT, Yuen KY, Cheng C. The study of cytokine dynamics at the operation site after mastectomy. *Wound Repair Regen* 2003; **11**(5): 326–30.
24. Stadelmann WK, Digenis AG, Tobin GR. Impediments to wound healing. *Am J Surg* 1998; **176**(2, Supplement 1): 39S–47S.
25. Stephens FO, Dunphy JE, Hunt TK. Effect of delayed administration of corticosteroids on wound contraction. *Ann Surg* 1971; **173**(2): 214–18.
26. Kulick MI, Smith S, Hadler K. Oral ibuprofen: evaluation of its effect on peritendinous adhesions and the breaking strength of a tenorrhaphy. *J Hand Surg* 1986; **11**(1): 110–20.
27. Snyder RJ. Treatment of nonhealing ulcers with allografts. *Clin Dermatol* 2005; **23**(4): 388–95.
28. Grey JE, Enoch S, Harding KG. Wound assessment. *BMJ* 2006; **332**(7536): 285–88.
29. Shih B, Bayat A. Genetics of keloid scarring. *Arch Dermatol Res* 2010; **302**(5): 319–39.
30. Bayat A, Bock O, Mrowietz U, et al. Genetic susceptibility to keloid disease and hypertrophic scarring: transforming growth factor beta1 common polymorphisms and plasma levels. *Plast Reconstr Surg* 2003; **111**(2): 535–43; discussion 544–46.
31. Chaby G, Senet P, Vaneau M, et al. Dressings for acute and chronic wounds: a systematic review. *Arch Dermatol* 2007; **143**(10): 1297–304.
32. Goldman R. Growth factors and chronic wound healing: past, present, and future. *Adv Skin Wound Care* 2004; **17**(1): 24–35.
33. Liechty KW, Nesbit M, Herlyn M, et al. Adenoviral-mediated overexpression of platelet-derived growth factor-B corrects ischemic impaired wound healing. *J Invest Dermatol* 1999; **113**(3): 375–83.
34. Wu Y, Chen L, Scott PG, Tredget EE. Mesenchymal stem cells enhance wound healing through differentiation and angiogenesis. *Stem Cells* 2007; **25**(10): 2648–59.
35. Ud-Din S, Sebastian A, Giddings P, et al. Angiogenesis is induced and wound size is reduced by electrical stimulation in an acute wound healing model in human skin. *PLoS One* 2015; **10**(4): e0124502.
36. Sebastian A, Syed F, Perry D, et al. Acceleration of cutaneous healing by electrical stimulation: degenerate electrical waveform down-regulates inflammation, up-regulates angiogenesis and advances remodeling in temporal punch biopsies in a human volunteer study. *Wound Repair Regen* 2011; **19**(6): 693–708.

CHAPTER 11

SKIN FLAP PHYSIOLOGY

Colin MacIver and Stergios Doumas

Definition 107	Skin biomechanics 112
History 107	The compromised flap 113
Flap design 108	Physical interventions 116
Applied anatomy and physiology 108	References 117
Skin vessel biomechanics 111	

SEARCH STRATEGY

Data in this chapter may be updated by a Medline search using the keywords: skin flap, tissue transfer, free flap, physiology, biomechanics, vessel and skin.

Make a plan and a pattern for this plan.

Sir Harold Gillies (1882–1960)

DEFINITION

A skin flap is a block of tissue transferred from the donor site and inserted to the recipient site while maintaining a continuous attachment to the body (the pedicle). The flap may consist of skin and subcutaneous fat but could also include mucosa, fascia, muscle, bone, nerve or combinations thereof.

Traditionally, the term free flap refers to autologous tissue transfer from a distant donor site to reconstruct a defect after the pedicle has been completely detached. Blood supply is reinstated by means of microsurgical anastomoses of donor artery and vein(s) to the recipient artery and vein(s).

Flap viability is initially dependent on its robust blood supply via the pedicle so that metabolic demands of the mobilized tissue are met. Multiple anatomical and physiological factors that hamper adequate perfusion, before the collateral capillary network develops, can be detrimental for the flap survival.

Flaps currently represent the workhorses for head and neck reconstruction. However, allotransplantation holds promise for non-oncological reconstruction. Also, tissue engineering is another fast growing field in head and neck reconstruction.

HISTORY

The term 'flap' is alleged to originate from the Dutch *Flappe*, meaning something broad and loose that hangs attached only at one side.[1]

Reconstructive skin flap surgery owes a great deal to the work of the Indian Ayurvedic medical practice of nasal reconstruction. *Sushruta Samhita*, the classical surgery textbook written around 600 BCE, describes the first cheek flaps utilized for nose repair.[2] The English surgeon Joseph Carpue (1764–1840) is given credit for introducing the Indian forehead rhinoplasty technique into the English language, based on a letter to the editor in 1794 relating the nasal reconstruction of a bullock driver called Cowasjee. An extremely well-referenced discussion of the history of this flap reconstructive technique is given by Nichter et al.[3]

Seminal studies in anatomical description of blood supply, pharmacological manipulation of the circulation and the advent of anaesthesia and aseptic techniques in surgery led to a better understanding of skin flaps. In this context, in 1889 Manchot published on many of the distinct cutaneous vascular territories served by identified named arteries.[4] Spalteholz described the fasciocutaneous vessels, as well as those passing through muscle, and provided the origin of the concept of the musculocutaneous blood supply to flaps.[5] In France, Salmon added to these ideas by performing radiographs on cadaver skin following intraarterial contrast injection.[6]

In 1921, Carl-Olof Siggesson Nylen, a Swedish ear, nose and throat (ENT) surgeon, built the first microscope. However, its use was confined to ENT and neurosurgical procedures. The first modern microscope is credited to Zeiss in the 1950s, and the first diploscope, operated by two surgeons simultaneously, was produced in 1961.[7]

Two years later, McGregor and Morgan described how skin flaps could be considered axial or random and therefore the length-to-width ratio was given an anatomical basis (drawing of random and axial flap). Having studied intra-arterial fluorescine injections in 14 patients, McGregor and Morgan deduced that an axial pattern flap could be safely raised beyond the standard dimensions of a random pattern flap of 1:1 length-to-width ratio and introduced the paramedian forehead flap.[8] They went on to postulate that changes in pressure between one territory and an adjacent territory could create the effect of reverse flow in the adjacent axial vessels. This was further developed by Taylor and Palmer who postulated that each of the composite blocks (angiosomes) were connected by true anastomoses or reduced calibre 'choke vessels'.[9] These choke vessels are analogous with the description by Salmon of 'retiform anastomoses' and as such are the defining limits of the vascular territories. They name the accompanying veins 'oscillating veins' in which flow could occur in any direction. In 1970, Milton reported that 'the surviving length of flaps made under similar conditions of blood supply is constant regardless of width. The only effect of decreasing width is to reduce the chance of the pedicle containing a large vessel'.[10]

The first attempts at free flaps without any magnification assistance were made in the late 1950s. Seidenberg et al. pioneered this by using a free jejunal autograft anastomosed to the superior thyroid artery and anterior facial vein via a stapling method, following a pharyngo-esophagectomy for squamous cell carcinoma in 1959. The patient survived for 8 days post-op, apparently dying of an unrelated cerebrovascular accident, with the jejunal graft found to be completely viable on autopsy.[11]

Nevertheless, the first reports of free flaps as we understand them today appeared in the early 1970s. Harry Buncke and Donald McLean used omentum, in 1972, to restore a large scalp defect following squamous cell carcinoma resection with exposed bone.[12]

As microsurgery field research advanced, it became evident that any clinically relevant perforator has the potential to be harvested as either a pedicle perforator flap or a free flap, depending on the diameter and length of the source artery and vein. The perforator flap era began in 1989, when Koshima and Soeda first described an inferior epigastric artery skin flap with the rectusabdominis muscle for reconstruction of floor-of-mouth and groin defects. Recently, Saint-Cyr et al. introduced the term 'perforasome' after conducting a three-dimensional (static) and four-dimensional (dynamic) computed tomographic angiography (CTA) in 40 fresh cadavers.[13] Another breakthrough in the field of free-tissue transfer has been achieved by means of extracorporeal tissue perfusion. This method potentially opens avenues in cases of vessel depleted neck and severed limbs.[14]

FLAP DESIGN

In general, flaps are divided into two main categories, based on whether the pedicle remains attached to the donor site or not; pedicled and free flaps, respectively. The former are further subdivided based on the pattern of blood supply and tissue composition into random, arterial cutaneous (axial), fasciocutaneous, musculocutaneous and venous flaps. Similarly, free flaps are divided into fasciocutaneous, musculocutaneous, osteocutaneous, muscular or combinations thereof (chimeric free flaps). The latter allow for three-dimensional reconstruction of massive defects.

APPLIED ANATOMY AND PHYSIOLOGY

The skin is the outermost human organ in direct contact with the environment. It weighs approximately 3.8 kg and measures about 1.7 m² in surface area.[15] The superficial part known as the epidermis is an impermeable, renewing, metabolically active, multi-layered, keratinizing, squamous epithelium. The epidermis consists of keratinocytes, melanocytes, Langerhans cells and Merkel cells. Hence, it serves as a sensory organ as well as a protective organ against insult and infection. Skin appendages, namely hair follicles, sebaceous glands, and eccrine and apocrine sweat glands derive from the epidermis. The epidermis and its appendages are all of ectodermic origin. Epidermis renewal is achieved by the so-called asymmetric division of the interfollicullar stem cells located in the basal layer.[16]

The dermis, derived from mesoderm, is primarily a connective tissue layer between the epidermis and the subcutaneous (subdermal) fat and muscle. Being 15–40 times thicker than the epidermis, it invariably accounts for the skin bulk. It accommodates nerve and vascular networks, epidermal appendages, fibroblasts, macrophages and others. Collagen type I and type III to a lesser extent abound in the extracellular matrix. Elastin fibres and the ground substance (proteoglycans, glycosaminoglycans and filamentous proteins) are also found in dermis. All fibres and the ground substance are synthesized by fibroblasts and confer skin pliability, elasticity and tensile strength.

The superficial layer of dermis has a waveform pattern in proximity to the rete pegs, which is known as the papillary layer. The deeper counterpart is known as the reticular dermis. The papillary dermis has an enriched capillary network that is 10–20 microns in diameter. Deeper to it, there are several arteriovenous shunts (diameter of 10–30 microns), most notable in the reticular dermis. The capillary plexus provides nutritional support to the epidermis, whereas the arteriovenous shunt contributes to the thermoregulation and systemic blood pressure of the body. They are both connected with the deep subdermal plexus. Under normal skin conditions blood flow though the skin amounts to approximately 9 mL/min per 100 g of tissue, 10 times above the rate fulfilling the skin's metabolic needs. In extremely hot climates blood flow can increase up to 20 times with maximal vasodilation.

11: SKIN FLAP PHYSIOLOGY   109

In contrast, when the body is exposed to cold, blood flow can reduce to levels that are marginal for skin nutrition.[17]

Two sphincter types regulate skin blood flow. The capillary system is controlled by a ring of smooth muscle, the pre-capillary muscle, located at the point where capillaries originate from metarteriole. It is mainly responsible for controlling nutritional support to the skin. Hence, skin hypoxia and metabolic by-products released into the microcirculation result in local vasodilation. However, blood flow can bypass by virtue of the arteriovenous shunts. The so-called pre-shunt sphincters are the main regulators of this system. Low blood pressure and extreme cold lead to pre-shunt sphincter contraction via norepinephrine released by the post-ganglionic sympathetic fibres. A similar effect is achieved by catecholamines released into the blood stream, as skin is perceived as a 'non-vital' organ in generalized hypoperfusion states.[18]

As mentioned above, Taylor and Palmer coined the term 'angiosome' in order to describe the spatial pattern of blood supply in various parts of the integument. Houseman et al. describe 13 angiosomes in the head and neck region mostly supplied from the external carotid, internal carotid and subclavian arteries. All 13 but the lingual, vertebral and ascending pharyngeal angiosomes contribute to the abundant subdermal vascular network (**Figure 11.1**). In the face and scalp, major contributing vessels radiate from fixed points, either from bony foramina or from sites where the deep fascia is attached to the bone. These arteries further arborize into smaller perforators that feed the subdermal plexus by penetrating the underlying muscle or bypassing through its fascia, hence are called musculocutaneous and fasciocutaneous perforators, respectively. Multiple arterial arches are encountered

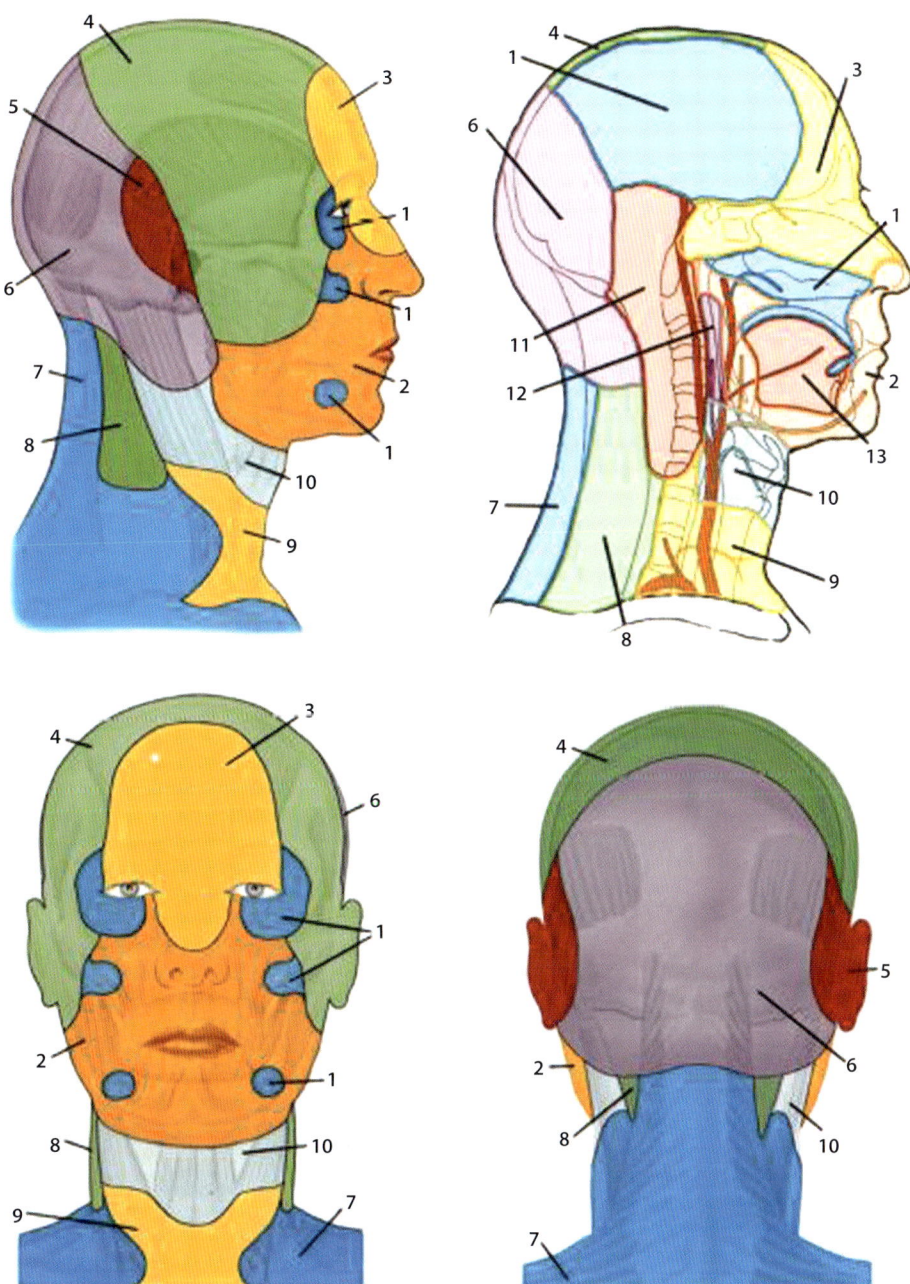

Figure 11.1 The angiosomes of the head and neck coloured and numbered. The additional territories defined in the neck are the transverse cervical (7), deep cervical (8), inferior thyroid (9) and superior thyroid (10) (above, right). Sagittal section showing the three angiosomes, vertebral (11), ascending pharyngeal (12) and lingual (13), which do not reach the skin surface.

in midline by connection of paired arteries. The head and neck region is the smallest one with approximately 25 perforators greater than 0.5 mm in diameter. The average diameter and area of irrigation by a single perforator are 0.9 mm and 32 cm², respectively.[19]

In analogy to 'angiosomes', Saint-Cyr et al. recently introduced the term 'perforasomes' as well defined vascular territories nourished by a single perforator. They carried out static and dynamic CTA in order to study detailed vascular anatomy, flow characteristics, and the contribution of both the subdermal plexus and fascia to flap perfusion after raising 247 flaps in 40 fresh cadavers. Perforator flaps on the anterior trunk, posterior trunk, and extremities were studied. They concluded that:

- Each perforasome carries a multidirectional flow pattern that is highly variable and complex. These perforasomes are linked to one another by both direct and indirect linking vessels, which themselves are linked by communicating branches (**Figure 11.2**). These numerous vascular connections confer further protection from ischemia and vascular injury in case of trauma or flap raising. Linking vessels allow communication with adjacent perforasomes and follow a direction that is parallel to the direction of perforator flow. Therefore, perforator flap skin paddles should be parallel to the linking vessel orientation whenever possible. These linking vessels make it possible to harvest large perforator flaps based on a single perforator, such as the extended anterolateral thigh flap.
- When a perforator flap is harvested, all muscle and cutaneous branches from the source artery are ligated, which results in hyperperfusion of the selected perforator. Increased vascular filling pressures clinically dilate the perforator itself and allow extensive inter-perforator flow by means of opening and recruitment of additional linking vessels. These linking vessels, both direct and indirect, are subject to higher than normal filling pressures and are able to capture additional adjacent perforator vascular territories (perforasomes) (**Figure 11.3**).

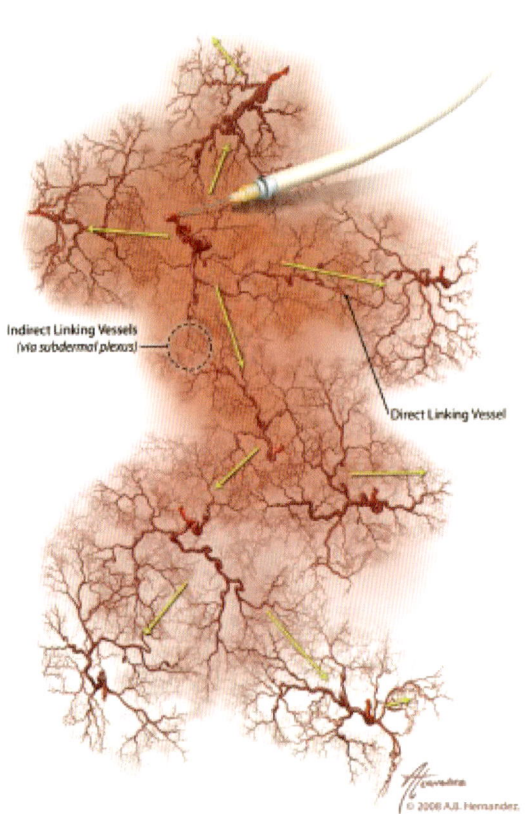

Figure 11.2 Interperforator flow occurs from the selected main perforator to multiple adjacent perforators by means of direct linking vessels and indirect linking vessels (recurrent flow from subdermal plexus). High perfusion pressures through the main perforator opens multiple direct and indirect linking vessels and allows perfusion of multiple other perforasomes. In this way, large flaps such as the anterolateral thigh flap can be harvested based on a single perforator. (Adapted from Saint-Cyr M, Wong C, Schaverien M, et al. The perforasome theory: vascular anatomy and clinical implications. *Plast Reconstr Surg* 2009; **124**: 1529–44. © American Society of Plastic Surgeons.)

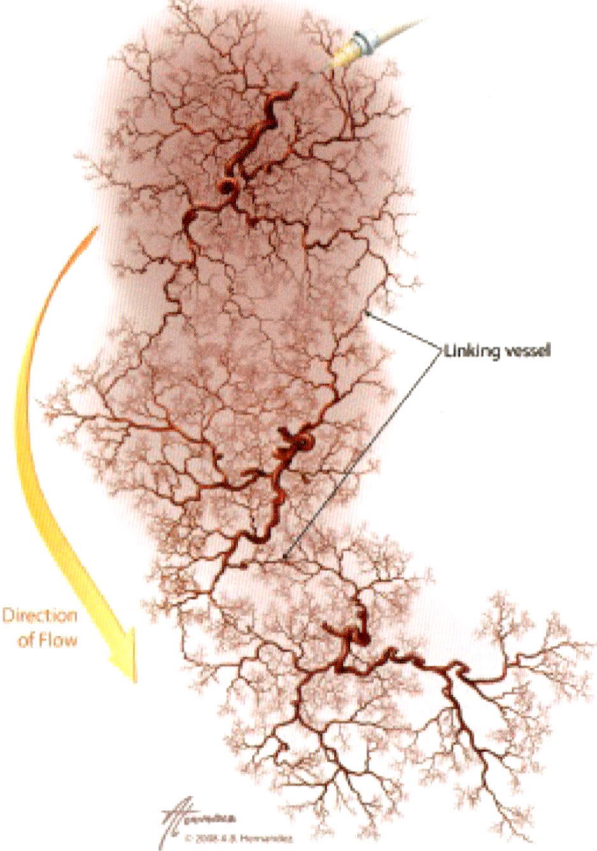

Figure 11.3 Perfusion in multiple perforasomes via linking vessels. Vascular density is maximal within the cannulated perforator and its corresponding perforasome and decreases distally away from the midline of the trunk or an articulation. The orientation of linking vessels determines the orientation of vascular flow within the flap. Direction of flow is predominantly perpendicular to the trunk midline and parallel to the vertical axis of the limbs. (Adapted from Saint-Cyr M, Wong C, Schaverien M, et al. The perforasome theory: vascular anatomy and clinical implications. *Plast Reconstr Surg* 2009; **124**: 1529–44. © American Society of Plastic Surgeons.)

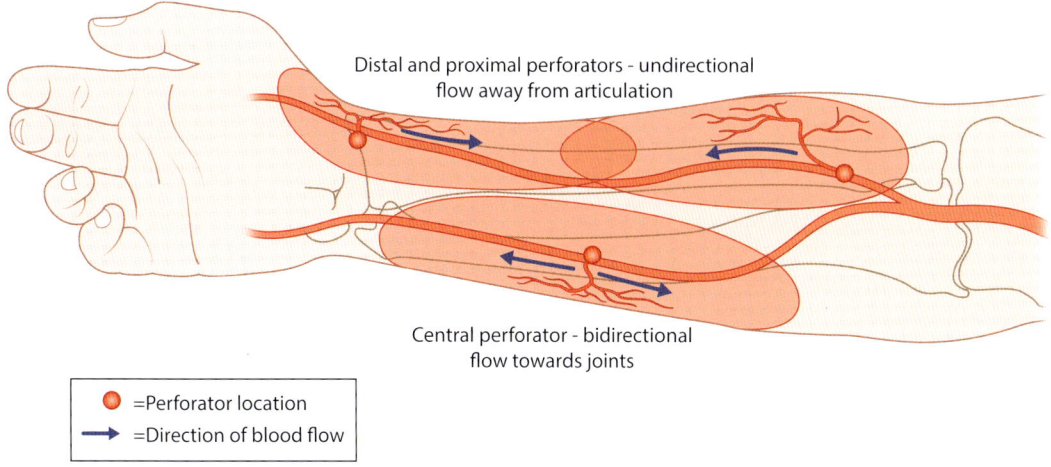

Figure 11.4 Direction of perforator flow between articulations. Perforators in the extremities that are found close to an articulation will have preferential flow away from that articulation, whereas midpoint perforators will have bidirectional flow. (Adapted from Saint-Cyr M, Wong C, Schaverien M, et al. The perforasome theory: vascular anatomy and clinical implications. *Plast Reconstr Surg* 2009; **124**: 1529–44. © American Society of Plastic Surgeons.)

- Perforator flaps designed at a midpoint between two articulations can be designed in multiple fashions because of the multidirectional perforator flow distribution. However, perforators located in proximity to one articulation seem to have unidirectional flow, i.e. distally located forearm perforators (wrist joint) course towards the proximal forearm (elbow joint), and vice versa (**Figure 11.4**).[13]

SKIN VESSEL BIOMECHANICS

Blood flow

Flap survival depends on flow though the pedicle of the flap.[20] Although the fluid mechanics of blood flow are complex, certain factors applicable to the small vessels supplying the flap are well established. Vessel blood flow (Q) is determined by:

- pressure difference (ΔP) between the two ends of the vessel
- the resistance to flow (R) produced in the vessel.

The mathematical expression of this blood flow is:

$$Q = \Delta P/R$$

where the letters are defined above.

The flow of blood through a smooth, straight vessel behaves as if there are concentric laminae, with the fastest flow in the centre creating a paraboloid wave front. The smaller the vessel becomes, the closer the central lamina becomes to the vessel wall. While this formula and lamina flow hold true for a straight, smooth vessel, any deformity such as vessel angulation, branching, obstruction or intraluminal irregularity will interfere with lamina flow. Disturbance in lamina flow is known as turbulence. Because all the flow is no longer in the same concentric laminae, fluid flowing across the direction of flow down the vessel will increase resistance to the flow. Resistance to lamina blood flow in a vessel is created by marginal adherence of molecules to the vessel wall.

The smaller the vessel diameter, the closer the fastest flowing central lamina becomes to the margin. Therefore, these molecules become closer to the slow moving marginal molecules, which increases the resistance to flow. The effect of reducing the vessel diameter can be expressed as mean velocity (ι) and described in the formula:

$$\iota = \Delta P r^2 / 8 \varsigma L$$

where ι is velocity in cm/s; ΔP is pressure gradient (dynes)/cm^2; r is the radius of the vessel in cm; ς is the viscosity in poises; and L is the length of vessel in cm.

The rate of blood flow through a vessel (Q) is related to the velocity of flow (ι) multiplied by the cross-sectional area:

$$Q = \delta \Delta P r^4 / 8 \varsigma L.$$

Thus it can be seen that if $Q = \Delta P/R$ and $Q = \delta \Delta P r^4 / 8 \varsigma L$ such that:

- the resistance of a blood vessel (R) is directly proportional to the viscosity of the fluid and the length of the vessel
- the resistance is inversely proportional to the fourth power of the radius. Therefore the smaller the vessel (r), the greater the resistance of the flow. Thus, any interference with the resting tone in the blood vessel, which reduces the vessel radius, will have a detrimental effect on blood flow.

$$R = 8 \varsigma L / \delta r^4.$$

In general, radius (r) plays a major role in larger vessels, whereas viscosity (ς) seems to determine blow flow in smaller vessels. Viscosity varies with the speed of blood flow; the faster the flow, the lower the viscosity because Poiseuille's law does not apply fully *in vivo*. The Fahraeus-Lindqvist effect appears with reducing vessel diameter below 1.5 mm. The viscosity of blood in vessels narrower than 1.5 mm is so much smaller that viscosity in the capillaries is half that of large-calibre vessels. In a 100-micron arteriole, red blood cells randomly orientated whilst in a 15-micron vessel more regular orientation of the red cells occurs. Bloch postulated that the vessel flow has a marginal layer with few cells and red cells congregate in the centre of the stream, which reduces the viscosity of the layer in contact with the vessel wall. In the 10-micron capillary, the red cells travel in single file paraboloids, rather then the usual bioconcave shape.[21]

Vessel wall tension

From Laplace's law, the tangential vessel wall tension (T) is proportional to the vessel diameter (D) and the pressure exerted across the vessel wall (P) such that:

$$T \, \alpha \, DP.$$

This has critical importance in a small vessel in which vessel diameter reduces, as does the pressure within the vessel. The vessel will collapse at the point elastic tension in the vessel wall exceeds the transmural pressure (P). This is known as critical closure pressure. Any increase in the resting tone in the blood vessel (spasm in clinical setting) that reduces the vessel radius, will thus have a deleterious effect on blood. Equally, any interstitial pressure increase (e.g. severe flap oedema) above the critical closure pressure can compromise the flap. As flap edges distal to the perforator are nourished by smaller calibre vessels they are more vulnerable to ischaemic necrosis. Laplace's law also applies to Milton's theory that 'the surviving length of flaps made under similar conditions of blood supply is constant regardless of width'. This is notably known as fallacy of the length-to-width ratio (**Figure 11.5**).[18]

SKIN BIOMECHANICS

As mentioned earlier, skin is a composite material consisting of a collagen-rich fibrous network embedded in a ground substance matrix. The proteoglycan-rich matrix provides skin its viscous nature at low loads, whereas collagen and elastin provide structural stiffness and elasticity to the skin. Skin exhibits anisotropic, non-linear, viscoelastic properties, in which the direction of minimal extensibility correlates with the fibrous network's principal direction. Skin is also a dynamic tissue, changing with age and influenced by gender.[22]

Recently, finite element analysis (FEA) has been used in order to understand skin flap dynamics. It is a computerized technique that can determine the stresses, strains and displacements in solid body given the geometry, material behaviour and load/displacement boundary

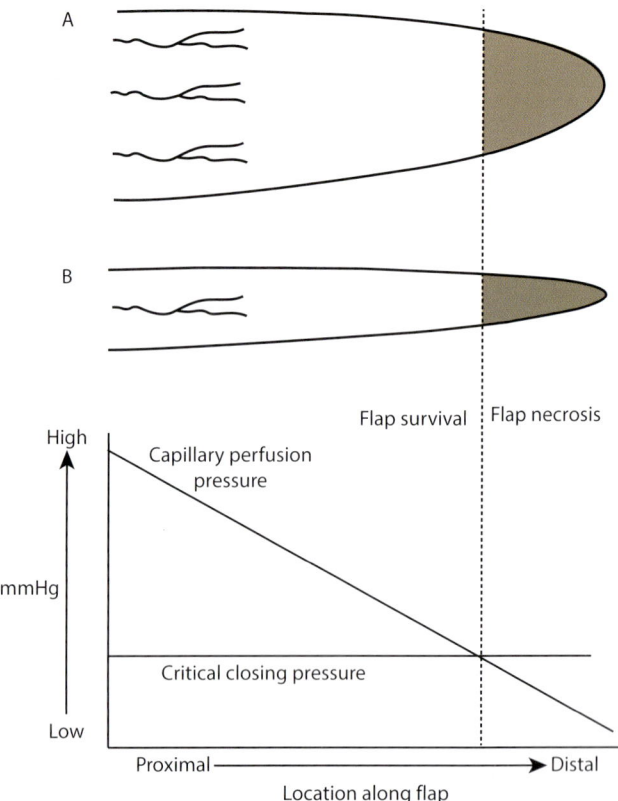

Figure 11.5 Fallacy of the length-to-width ratio. Slope of decreasing perfusion pressure versus flap length does not change with incorporation of additional vessels (flap A versus flap B) with some perfusion pressure. Flap necrosis occurs when perfusion pressure falls below critical closing pressure of the capillary bed. (Adapted from Hom DB, Goding GS. Skin flap physiology. In: Baker SR (ed). *Local flaps in facial reconstruction*. 2nd ed. Philadelphia: Mosby Elsevier; 2007, pp. 15–30.)

conditions acting on that body. In this context, Lovald et al. performed FEA on a monopedicle (advancement) skin flap model concluding that the length of the flap should not exceed 3 times the size of the defect as benefit in reducing deformation is diminished beyond that point. Nevertheless, authors admitted that not all skin mechanical or local anatomical properties were studied. Although simulation models are useful instruments for a better understanding of skin flap biomechanics, success is dependent on the surgeon's ability to choose the best flap pattern on a given patient.[23]

Non-linearity

This property refers to the limited lengthening of the skin when it is acutely stretched. It is ascribed to collagen, elastin, ground substance, capillaries, nerve fibres and lymphatics. Moreover, the relationship between the applied force (stress) exerted on a given skin length and its ensuing length increase (strain) is non-linear. Skin is initially resilient to the forced applied as fibres recruited along the lines of the stress have little resistance. However, in the intermediate stage, further deformation requires much more stress as more collagen fibres are recruited into a load-carrying role. The final portion demonstrates almost complete rigidity of the skin regardless of the force applied as all of the collagen fibres are deployed in the direction of the stress. The rationale of skin non-linearity is to preserve its structural integrity especially under excessive stress. As eloquently shown in the stress-strain curve diagram, there are age dependent changes in skin deformation. Aged skin is less 'malleable' at initial stages due to the paucity of elastic fibres. However, young and aged skin stress-strain curves coincide in phase 3 alluding to the same degree of refractoriness at higher forces.

Although non-linearity confers protection to skin, lack of further deformation at high forces has a deleterious effect on blood flow. As mentioned above, peripheral (small caliber) vessels are more prone to occlusion due to their decreased diameter. Hence, increasing the amount of flap tension can hamper circulation, leading to necrosis of the distal part of any flap (**Figure 11.6**).[24]

Anisotropy

Anisotropy refers to the directional qualities of the skin. In most regions of skin, there is tension in every direction, being greatest along the relaxed skin tension line (RSTL). Hence, an incision placed perpendicular to the RSTL will result in a wide gaping wound. Increased tension will also affect scarring and flap survival.

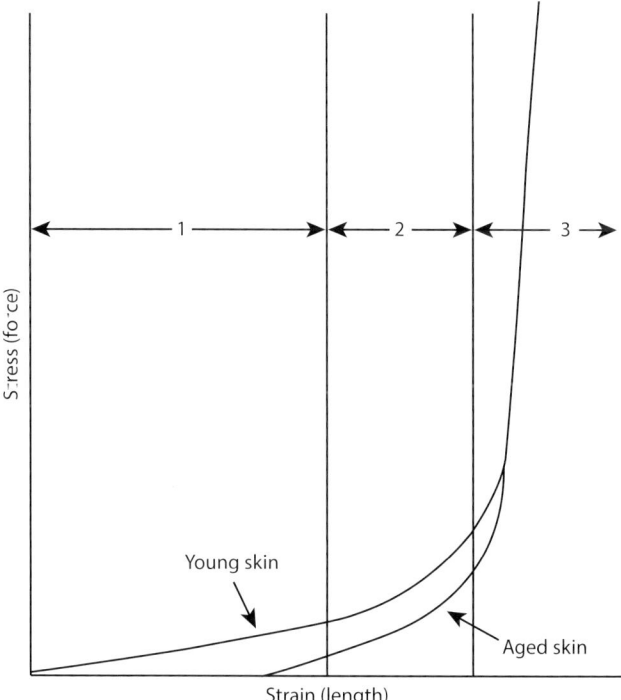

Figure 11.6 Stress-strain curve for isolated skin can be divided into three separate regions. Aged skin deforms under its own weight, shifting apparent origin of the curve along the x axis. (Adapted from Larrabee WF Jr. Immediate repair of facial defects. *Dermatol Clin* 1989; **7**: 661–76.)

Viscoelasticity

Viscoelastic properties of the skin are better understood by the terms *creep* and *stress relaxation*. Creep refers to the increase in strain seen after a sudden constant load applied to the skin. Stress relaxation refers to a decrease in stress by means of stretching when a constant stress is applied to the skin. Viscoelasticity seems to be the background of the tissue expansion and serial sections.[18]

THE COMPROMISED FLAP

'The after care is as important as the planning' is the 15th principle postulated by Sir Harold Gillies.[25] His principle reads, 'How futile it is to lose flap or graft for the lack of a little postoperative care. If in any doubt about the progress slip your hands out of your pockets and get down to the haematoma.' This advice holds as true today as it did when it was published, the most common cause for the flap failure being failure to recognize a compromised circulation.

Indeed, Pohlenz et al. recently conducted a single-centre retrospective study looking at complications and outcomes of 1000 microvascular free flaps transplanted in the head and neck region for the interim between 1987 and 2010. Vascular occlusion (thrombosis) of one of the vessels was the primary (4.5% arterial, 6.8% venous) reason for flap loss, with venous thrombosis being more common than arterial occlusion. The majority of flap failures occurred within the first 36 hours. The main reasons for flap failure were the use of compression bandages, tapes around the neck or tracheal strips with extrinsic compression of the vascular pedicle (n = 7). Tight wound closure or wound haematoma may also compromise the flap by obstructing venous outflow. Major bleeding (4.9%) was a common cause of failure in microvascular free tissue.[26]

Factors affecting flap survival can be considered as either extrinsic or intrinsic.

Extrinsic factors

External compression of the circulation to the flap is either due to a tight dressing, tension in the skin wound closure, which more commonly occurs if the flap is angulated over an underlying rigid bony surface, or soft tissue swelling; this can be due to oedema or a post-operative haematoma. The flap is usually blue and engorged, indicative of venous congestion. Haematomas seem to cause tissue injury even in absence of a pressure effect or pedicle thrombosis by a complex sequence of inter-related biochemical and cellular processes merging on a common pathway of local tissue ischaemia, which the overlying tissue is unable to regulate. In 2012, Glass et al. reviewed the literature relating haematoma to tissue compromise including free transferred tissue, vascularized flap models and brain injury. The authors acknowledged that all experimental data of this study were done in rat or pig modes. They postulated that degraded platelets release cytokines, which attract neutrophils. The latter release reactive oxygen species (ROS) causing direct tissue damage. Additionally, the complement cascade is triggered by thrombin. Ferrous ions, freed by complement-mediated lysis of erythrocytes and degradation of haemoglobin, also promote generation of ROS. Reactive oxygen species, complement and activated neutrophils cause endothelial cell disruption, leading to activation of pro-thrombotic mechanisms and small vessel occlusion, with consequent tissue ischaemia, which in turn generates further ROS.[27]

The prompt release of thigh bandages, dressings and removal of wound sutures and heamatoma drainage may salvage the situation. If the free flap blood blow is compromised, urgent exploration of pedicle vessels is warranted. In general, earlier intervention confers better outcome in flap survival. In the case of a local flap, repositioning back on to the donor site should be considered if there is concern that the pedicle has been kinked, thus following the old adage, 'It is better to have a live flap out of position than a dead flap in position'.

Intrinsic factors

Reconstructive surgery for the head and neck is mainly aimed at elderly cancer patients with a long history of excessive smoking and drinking. These patients also suffer from other comorbidities (myocardial ischaemia, atherosclerosis/peripheral vascular disease, pulmonary diseases, diabetes mellitus (DM), cachexia, anaemia of chronic disease), hence are more vulnerable to flap-related as well as generalized complications.

Age per se should not be considered as an aggravating factor in terms of free-flap survival. Yang et al. conducted a retrospective cohort study on 53 head and neck cancer patients, aged >80 years, who underwent a free-flap reconstruction from 1996 to 2011 at an academic medical centre. There were zero flap failures or peri-operative deaths. Similar encouraging results were published by others.[28–29]

Rosado et al. performed a systematic review and meta-analysis to determine whether diabetic patients have an increased rate of post-operative complications compared to non-diabetic patients after head and neck free-flap reconstruction. They reported that the prevalence of DM in patients with failed free flaps for head and neck reconstruction is 15%. The incidence of diabetes mellitus in these patients with failed free flaps is 2.3 times higher than in the general population.[30]

Vasospasm in the flap following raising of the flap is a normal physiological response to reduce blood loss. Under normal circumstances, this vasospasm resolves without intra-vascular thrombosis because the spasm empties the lumen of the vessel. In addition, vessel lumen irrigation with heparin can resolve potential clots during anastomosis. In the presence of intact endothelium, the coagulation cascade is not activated. Hence, endothelial cell integrity plays a vital role in the maintenance of blood flow. Where flow to the flap is not established (or is compromised for a prolonged period of time) it has been shown experimentally in rabbits that 'no flow' occurs after a period of several hours of ischaemia. This has become known as

'no reflow phenomenon' coined by Ames et al. in 1968 and studied first in flap reperfusion in 1978.[31–32] In the no reflow phenomenon, reperfusion of the ischaemic tissue results in the formation of oxygen-derived free radicals. Furthermore, it has been shown that the vasodilator effect of acetyl choline is mediated through endothelial production of nitric oxide.[33] The net effect of acetyl choline following reperfusion is the presence of damaged endothelial cells in vasoconstriction.

Nitric oxide is produced by nitric oxide synthase from the amino-acid L-arginine. Elegant experimental research in mice with targeted disruption of the inducible nitric oxide synthase (iNOS) gene (iNOS knockout mice) has shown pharmacological and genetic evidence that iNOS activity promoted survival of ischaemic tissue. The administration of nitro-L-arginine methyl ester (a constitutive NOS, endothelia NOS and neuronal NOS inhibitor) significantly increased flap survival in these mice.

In a pig ischaemia-reperfusion injury flap model, there was a disruption of constitutive nitric oxide synthase expression and activity, which may have led to decreased nitric oxide production.

A great deal of laboratory research has been undertaken to reduce flap failure by pharmacological means. Much attention has been paid to drugs that could act as 'free radical scavengers'. Superoxide dismutase has been shown to improve flap survival in animals[34–35] but not in humans. Angel et al.[36–37] have been at the forefront of superoxide radical scavenger therapy, publishing work on the beneficial effects of the iron chelator deferoxamine. These benefits, however, occur with significant toxicity that can be ameliorated (in pigs) by the conjugated form, deferoxamine-hespan (DFO-H). DFO-H has a longer half-life, but with reduced efficacy in augmenting flap survival. This was postulated to decrease its ability to reach the intracellular oxygen free radicals.[38]

It has also been shown that allopurinol can augment flap survival.[39–40] Allopurinol is a xanthine oxidase inhibitor, although elevated levels of xanthine oxidase and malonylodialdehyde have been noted to be elevated in ischaemic flap tissue in animals.[41] A beneficial effect has yet to be shown in humans. Innumerable other animal experiments have been performed on such things as anti-adrenergic drugs[42] and magnesium-ATP (a supply of high energy phosphometabolites),[43] both approaches being to increase the levels of ATP in the tissues.

Others researchers have looked at prostacycline (PGI2) and prostaglandin-E1 (PGE1). Both cause peripheral vasodilatation and inhibition of platelet aggregation.[44–47]

Endothelin-1 (ET-1) is an endogenous vasoactive (vasoconstrictor) peptide, produced in ischaemic flap tissues. In human microvascular breast reconstruction flaps, a statistically significant increase in (skin biopsy) tissue levels of endothelin-1 after clamping of the flap pedicle has been demonstrated. The authors concluded that endothelin-1 levels were elevated in free flaps following reperfusion.[48]

Recent studies have shown that this detrimental effect can be blocked in experimental porcine transverse rectus abdominis myocutaneous (TRAM) flaps by tezosentan, a endothelin receptor blocker. The authors suggest that tezosentan improves oxygenation and metabolism in the jeopardized contralateral flap tissue, probably as a result of a decrease in venous vascular resistance and fluid extravasation.[49]

This beneficial effect on the venous outflow would fit with observations on the sensitivity of the human musculocutaneous perforator vessels to vasoconstrictors and vasodilatators *in vitro*. The vasoconstrictor potency of norepinephrine, endothelin-1 and thromboxane-A2 mimetic were shown to be significantly higher in the vein than in the artery, hence the maximal venous effect of ET-1 blockade.[50] The severity of tissue necrosis correlated well with tissue levels of ET-1 in rat skin flaps, whilst topical nifedipine antagonized the vasoconstrictive effects of ET-1.

Topical nitroglycerin (GTN) has also been shown to exert a greater vasodilatator effect on the venous circulation than on arterial vessels. Rohrich et al.[51] reported improved survival of axial flaps in pigs and rats treated with nitroglycerin ointment. Topical GTN paste is used in clinical practice but with variable success. On the contrary, recent meta-analyses have shown that intra-operative use of vasopressors in free flap surgery is safe (hNJ).

Direct smooth muscle relaxants nifedipine and verapamil increased flap survival in rats.[52-54] These are calcium-channel blockers that act on the vascular smooth muscles to cause vasodilatation but are restricted in clinical practice to topical application on to microvascular anastomoses, as there is no trial evidence to support their systemic use.

Surgically induced neutrophil recruitment in skin flaps has been shown to impair flap survival experimentally in the rat.[55] Myeloperoxidase (a marker for neutrophil recruitment) was significantly reduced by low-intraperitoneal calcitonin gene-related peptide (CGRP) without affecting the circulating neutrophil count, with improved random pattern flap survival.

One Japanese group[56] have studied sulphatide which binds to L-selectin and P-selectin, important in the initiation of neutrophil–endothelial interactions. Pre-treated experimental skin flaps showed little histological evidence of leukocyte invasion compared to that in the dermal layer of control flaps 48 hours after elevation. They went on to show augmented protection against ischaemia-reperfusion in rat skin flaps when combining sulphatide with anti-rat ICAM-1 and anti-rat LFA-1 antibodies.

The monoclonal antibody to the primary neutrophil adherence-mediating glycoprotein CD18 improves the survival length of the random pattern flap. Histological examination 24 hours after reperfusion in the treated group demonstrated only slight leukocyte invasion into the flap, and myeloperoxidase activity 24 hours after reperfusion was significantly reduced. This study indicated that sulphatide and monoclonal antibodies combined protect rat skin flaps from ischaemia-reperfusion injury.[57]

The platelet glycoprotein IIb/IIIa receptor antagonist Abciximab promoted experimental skin flap survival secondary to blocked platelet activation/aggregation and decreased activated-platelet deposition on the vascular endothelium in the rat.[58] Thus, administration may save the skin flap from reperfusion injury after a long period of ischaemia.

Dimethylsulfoxide (DMSO) is the only substance that has been shown experimentally to improve flap survival in animals and then been supported in a randomized control trial of mastectomy skin flap survival by Rand-Luby et al.[59] This is one of only two controlled trials referenced by the Cochrane database. The authors concluded that the topical application of DMSO safely reduced human mastectomy skin flap ischaemia.

The other clinical trial on the Cochrane database reported a selective phosphodiesterase III inhibitor (Amrinone), which prevents breakdown of cyclic adenosine monoposphate.[60] Statistically proven to improve positively the microcirculatory blood flow of transferred flaps, the authors proposed that this occurred by relief of intra-operative vasospasm.

Another work in rats by Pang et al. concluded that the administration of exogenous vascular endothelial factor (VEGF) 'could protect flaps from ischaemia-reperfusion injury through the regulation of pro-inflammatory cytokines and the inhibition of cytotoxic nitric oxide production'.[61]

Adenovirus-mediated gene therapy with vascular endothelial growth factor delivered into the subdermal space of compromised epigastric skin flaps in a rat model has improved skin flap survival.[62] Viral transfection with subdermal injections of adenovirus-encoding VEGF (Ad-VEGF) was performed two days before flap elevation. Compared with controls, a significant reduction in the area of necrotic and hypoxic zones of the flap was demonstrated following both local and midline subdermal injections of Ad-VEGF.

Others have reported that the survival of flaps treated with VEGF A165 or B167 cDNA was significantly greater than controls.[63] However, neither study could produce evidence that the mechanism was due to angiogenesis using light microscopy, microvessel count or angiography on the treated flap. This is in contrast with histologically demonstrated angiogenesis at the skin paddle-recipient bed interface following the subcutaneous administration of VEGF into the recipient bed of a skin tube flap.[64]

Further support for VEGF therapy comes from Kryger et al., who showed that all routes of administration (systemic, subdermal into the flap, subfascial into the recipient bed) improved survival of a full thickness random pattern flap in the rat compared with controls.[65]

By contrast, Rinsch et al. demonstrated that FGF-2, was more efficacious than either VEGF(121) or VEGF(165) in treating acute skin ischaemia and improving skin flap survival when delivered from encapsulated cells positioned under distal flap.[66]

Thus, with improved delivery strategies, VEGF and FGF-2 may have a role in the management of surgical ischaemia. However, novel gene therapies to improve flap survival have not yet translated into clinical flap surgery.

Dextran and heparin have been shown to improve flap survival in experimental studies of microvascular anastomoses, but not in improving survival of a failing flap.[67-68]

PHYSICAL INTERVENTIONS

Surgical delay

The only well-established technique to improve skin flap survival is by the 'delay procedure' with which all surgeons should be familiar. 'Delay' is a surgical procedure that renders a flap partially ischaemic several days prior to its transfer in order to increase its viability at transfer. Though much debate exists regarding the actual mechanism of vascular delay, most agree that changes in the microcirculation play a key role.

The latest work by Dhar and Taylor showed that when a flap is delayed, there is a dilation of existing vessels within the flap, not ingrowth of new vessels. The maximal anatomic effect on the arterial tree occurs at the level of the reduced-caliber 'choke' (or linking) anastomotic vessels that link adjacent adjacent vascular territories.

They describe 'an active process associated with both an increase (hyperplasia) and enlargement (hyper trophy) of the cells in all layers of the choke artery wall and a resultant increase in calibre of these vessels'.[69]

Tissue expansion can be considered a form of skin flap delay, where expanded porcine flaps showed 150% greater length survival compared with acute non-delayed flap.[70] The expanded flaps had 50% greater length survival compared with the delayed flaps. Angiography showed increased axial vessel calibre in the tissue expanded flaps, subsequently confirmed by Taylor's work. A controlled clinical trial of TRAM flap breast reconstruction confirmed by colour flow Doppler showed an increase in the diameter of flap vessels in which surgical delay was performed one month prior to transfer.[71] A lower flap necrosis rate was found using a delayed TRAM (7.1%) compare with a standard TRAM (30%).

Conditioning

This term describes an endogenous phenomenon in which the application of one or more brief cycles of sublethal ischaemia and reperfusion to an organ or tissue to protect itself or another one distant to it (remote ischaemic conditioning) from the detrimental effect of ischaemia-reperfusion injury (IRI). Depending on the timing of application in relevance to the actual IRI it is classified as ischaemic pre-, post- or conditioning.

Ischaemic preconditioning was first described in 1986 by Murry et al. in canine myocardiac infract models.[72] In 2003, Zhao et al.[73, 74] introduced ischaemic post-conditioning as a procedure to minimize acute myocardial infarction (MI) after applying alternate cycles of ischaemia and reperfusion. Both procedures require direct intervention on the tissue or organ. In contrast, remote ischaemic conditioning achieves a protective effect by applying the sublethal cycles to an easily accessed tissue or organ (i.e. arm).[74]

Kraemer et al. studied the microcirculatory benefits of remote ischaemic preconditioning in 27 healthy individuals. The baseline cutaneous microcirculation of the left thigh (corresponding to ALT flap) was tested using combined Laser-Doppler and photospectrometry. Similar tests in the same skin region were performed after three 5-minute ischaemic cycles on the contralateral arm. Statistically significant increase in tissue oxygen saturation and capillary blow flow (29%, 35%, p = 0.001) was noted.[75]

Extracorporeal perfusion

Recently, there have been attempts to revascularize severed limbs or free flaps in vessel-depleted necks both in animal models and humans via extracorporeal perfusion (ECP). This technique refers to a pump-assisted perfusion of the tissues in order to obviate the deleterious effects of prolonged ischaemia. In 2005, Newsome et al. presented a case report of a boy with chondroblastic osteosarcoma of the right hemipelvis with involvement of the common, internal, and external iliac vessels on the right side. The patient underwent hemipelvectomy and high above-knee amputation of the ipsilateral leg. The amputated extremity was placed on extracorporeal bypass using an extracorporeal machine oxygenation (ECMO) circuit connected to the femoral vessels for 162 min. at 32°C. While maintaining extracorporeal circulation, an anterior thigh free flap was created and later used for soft-tissue reconstruction.

In 2016, Wolff et al. reported successful free flap transfer using ECP in three consecutive cases with vessel-depleted neck.[76, 77]

Lasers

Low energy helium-neon (He-Ne) laser irradiation has been shown to improve the viability of skin flaps in rats and in clinical flap repair after avulsion injury.[78, 79] In rat capillaries and fibroblasts, proliferation was demonstrated histologically while clinical improvement was attributed to improved superoxide dismutate activity.

Leeches

Hirudo medicinalis, the medicinal leech, exerts its effect by injecting hirudin, a naturally occurring anticoagulant, into the affected part. In addition, leeches secrete hyalurodinase into the tissues, as well as a vasodilator, which contributes to prolonged bleeding. The main use for leeches is in the congested microvascular flap when there is no other way of improving venous outflow.[80] Useful in selected cases, there is nonetheless a serious risk of secondary infection with the leech enteric organism *Aeromonas hydrophila*, which can kill the skin flap. Antibiotic cover should be provided when using leeches.

KEY POINTS

- Skin is the largest organ of the human body and confers protection against mechanical and bacterial insults as well as thermoregulation.
- Better understanding of the pertinent anatomy and skin and vessel biomechanics can minimize mistakes and improve outcomes in reconstructive surgery.
- Several intrinsic and extrinsic factors may compromise flap viability.
- Conditioning, surgical delay and/or extracorporeal perfusion may optimize flap survival.

REFERENCES

1. Cormack GC, Lamberty BGH. *The arterial anatomy of skin flaps*. London: Churchill Livingstone; 1986, pp. 2–4.
2. Sushruta: Sushruta Sahmita. In: Bhishagratna, K. (ed.) *An English translation of the Sushruta Sahmita, based on original Sanskrit text*. Calcutta: Bose, 1907. Quoted in Nichter LS, Morgan RF, Nichter MA (eds). The impact of Indian methods for total nasal reconstruction (historical perspectives of plastic surgery). *Clin Plast Surg* 1983; **10**: 637–38.
3. Nichter LS, Morgan RF, Nichter MA. The impact of Indian methods for total nasal reconstruction (historical perspectives of plastic surgery). *Clin Plast Surg* 1983; **10**: 635–47.
4. Manchot C. *Die Hautarletien des menschlichen Kotpers*. Leipzig: Vogel.
5. Spalteholz W. Die Verteilung der Blutgefasse in der Haut. *Archives d'Anatomie Physiologie* 1983; **1**: 1–4.
6. Salmon N. *Arteres de la peau*. Paris: Masson; 1936. Quoted in Taylor GI, Razzaboni RM (eds). *Michel Salmon anatomic studies*. St Louis, MI: Quality Medical Press; 1994, pp. 13–17.
7. Steel BJ, Cope MR. A brief history of vascularized free flaps in the oral and maxillofacial region. *J Oral Maxillofac Surg* 2015; **73**(4): 786. e1–11.
8. McGregor IA, Morgan G. Axial and random pattern flaps. *Brit J Plast Surg* 1973; **26**: 202–13.
9. Taylor GI, Palmer JH. The vascular territories (angiosomes) of the body: experimental date and clinical applications. *Brit J Plast Surg* 1987; **40**: 113–41.
10. Milton SH. Pedicle to skin flap: the fallacy of the length:width ratio. *Brit J Plast Surg* 57: 502–8.
11. Seidenberg B. Immediate reconstruction of the cervical esophagus by a revascularized isolated jejunal segment. *Ann Surg* 1959; **149**(2)162–7.
12. McLean DH, Buncke HJ Jr. Autotransplant of omentum to a large scalp defect, with microsurgical revascularization. *Plast Reconstr Surg* 1972; **49**: 268–74.
13. Saint-Cyr M, Wong C, Schaverien M, et al. The perforasome theory: vascular anatomy and clinical implications. *Plast Reconstr Surg* 2009; **124**: 1529–44.
14. Fichter AM, Ritschl LM, Rau A, et al. Free flap rescue using an extracorporeal perfusion device. *J Craniomaxillofac Surg* 2016; **44**(12): 1889–95.
15. Goldsmith LA. My organ is bigger than your organ. *Arch Dermatol* 1990; **126**: 301–2.
16. Hsu YC, Li L, Fuchs E. Emerging interactions between skin stem cells and their niches. *Nat Med*. 2014; **20**: 847–56.
17. Honrado CP, Murakami CS. Wound healing and physiology of skin flaps. *Facial Plast Surg Clin North Am*. 2005; **13**: 203–14.
18. Hom DB, Goding GS. Skin flap physiology In: Baker SR (ed). *Local flaps in facial reconstruction*. 2nd ed. Philadephia: Mosby Elsevier; 2007, pp. 15–30.
19. Houseman ND, Taylor GI, Pan WR. The angiosomes of the head and neck: anatomic study and clinical applications. *Plast Reconstr Surg* 2000; **105**: 2287–313.
20. Gumley GJ. Chapter 7. In: O'Brien B McC, Morrison WA (eds). *Reconstructive microsurgery*. London: Churchill Livingstone; 1987, pp. 65–73.
21. Bloch EH. A quantitate study of the haemodynamics in the living microvascular system. *Am J Anat* 1962; **11**: 125–53.
22. Corr DT, Hart DA. Biomechanics of scar tissue and uninjured skin. *Adv Wound Care (New Rochelle)* 2013; **2**: 37–43.
23. Lovald ST, Topp SG, Ochoa JA, Gaball CW. Biomechanics of the monopedicle skin flap. *Otolaryngol Head Neck Surg* 2013; **149**: 858–64.
24. Larrabee WF Jr. Immediate repair of facial defects. *Dermatol Clin*. 1989; **7**: 661–76.
25. Gillies H, Millard DR. *The principles and art of plastic surgery*. Vol 1. London: Butterworths; 1957, pp. 15–20.
26. Pohlenz P, Klatt J, Schön G, et al. Microvascular free flaps in head and neck surgery: complications and outcome of 1000 flaps. *Int J Oral Maxillofac Surg* 2012; **41**: 739–43.
27. Glass GE, Nanchahal J. Why haematomas cause flap failure: an evidence-based paradigm. *J Plast Reconstr Aesthet Surg* 2012; **65**: 903–10.
28. Yang R, Lubek JE, Dyalram D, et al. Head and neck cancer surgery in an elderly patient population: a retrospective review. *Int J Oral Maxillofac Surg* 2014; **43**: 1413–17.
29. Saçak B, Akdeniz ZD, Certel F, et al. Risk assessment for free tissue transfers: is old age a determining factor? *J Craniofac Surg* 2015; **26**: 856–59.
30. Rosado P, Cheng HT, Wu CM, Wei FC. Influence of diabetes mellitus on postoperative complications and failure in head and neck free flap reconstruction: a systematic review and meta-analysis. *Head Neck* 2015; **37**: 615–18.
31. Ames A III, Wright LR, Kowada M, et al. Cerebral ischaemia II. No reflow phenomenon. *Am J Pathol* 1968; **52**: 437–45.
32. May JW Jr., Chait LA, O'Brien BM, Hurley JV. The no-reflow phenomenon in experimental free free flaps. *Plast Reconstr Surg* 1978; **61**: 256–67.
33. Furchgott RF, Zawadzki JV. The obligatory role of endothelial cells in the relaxation of arterial smooth muscle by acetylcholine. *Nature* 1980; **288**: 373–76.
34. Im MJ, Manson PN, Burkley GB, Hoopes JE. Effects of superoxide dismutase and allopurinol on the survival of acute island skin flap. *Ann Surg* 1985; **201**: 357–59.
35. Manson PN, Narayan KK, Im MJ, et al. Improved survival in free skin flap transfers in rats. *Surgery* 1986; **99**: 211–15.
36. Angel MF, Narayanan K, Swartz WM, et al. Deferoxamine increases skin flap survival: additional evidence of free radical involvement in ischaemic flap surgery. *Brit J Plast Surg* 1986; **39**: 469–72.
37. Angel MF, Mellow CG, Knight KR, et al. A biochemical study of acute ischaemia in rodent skin free flaps with and without prior elevation. *Ann Plas Surg* 1991; **26**: 419–24.
38. Hom DB, Golding Jr. GS, Price JA, et al. The effects of conjugated deferoxamine in porcine skin flaps. *Head Neck* 2000; **22**; 579–84.
39. Im MJ, Shen WH, Pak CJ, et al. Effects of allopurinol on the survival of hyperemic islands skin flaps. *Plast Reconstr Surg* 1984; **73**: 276–78.
40. Angel MF, Ramasastry SS, Swartz WM, et al. Augmentation of skin flap survival with allopurinol. *Ann Plas Surg* 1987; **18**: 494–98.
41. Angel MF, Ramasastry SS, Swartz WM, et al. The critical relationship between free radicals and degrees of ischemia: evidence for tissue tolerance of marginal perfusion. *Plast Reconstr Surg* 1988; **81**: 233–39.
42. Jurell G, Hjemdahl P, Fredholm BB, On the mechanism by which antiadrenergic drugs increase survival of critical skin flaps. *Plast Reconstr Surg* 1983; **72**; 518–25.
43. Zimmerman TJ, Sasaki GH, Khattab S. Imroved ischaemic island skin flap survival with continuous intra-arterial infusion of adenosine triphosphate-magnesium chloride and superoxide dismutase: a rat model. *Ann Plas Surg* 1987; **18**: 218–23.
44. Emerson DJM, Sykes PJ. The effect of prostacyclin on experimental random pattern flaps in the rat. *Brit J Plast Surg* 1981; **34**: 264–66.
45. Zachary LS. Effects of exogenous prostacyclin on flap survival. *Surg Forum* 1982; **33**: 588.
46. Suzuki S, Isshiki N, Ogawa Y, et al. Effect of intravenous proglandidn E1 on experimental flaps. *Ann Plas Surg* 1987; **19**: 49–53.
47. Sasaki GH, Pang CY. Experimental evidence for involvement of prostaglandins in viability and acute skin flaps: effects on viability and mode of function. *Plast Reconstr Surg* 1981; **67**: 335–40.

48. Lantieri LA, Carayon A, Maistre O, et al. Tissue and plasma levels of endothelin in free flaps. *Plast Reconstr Surg* 2003; **111**: 85–91.
49. Erni D, Wessendorf R, Wettstein R, et al. Endothelin receptor blockade improves oxygenation in contralateral TRAM flap tissue in pigs. *Brit J Plast Surg* 2001; **54**: 412–18.
50. Zhang J, Lipa JE, Black CE, et al. Pharmacological characterization of vasomotor activity of human musculocutaneous perforator artery and vein. *J Applied Physiol* 2000; **89**: 2268–75.
51. Rohrich R, Cherry GW, Spira M. Enhancement of skin-flap survival using nitroglycerin ointment. *Plast Reconstr Surg* 1984; **73**: 943–48.
52. Hira M, Tajima S, Sano S. Increased survival length of experimental flap by calcium channel antagonist nifedipine. *Ann Plas Surg* 1990; **24**: 45–48.
53. Pal S, Khazanchi RK, Moudgil K. An experimental study on the effect of nifedipine on ischaemic skin flap survival in rats. *Brit J Plast Surg* 1991; **44**: 299–301.
54. Carpenter RJ, Angel MF, Amiss LR. Verapamil enhances the survival of primary ischemic venous obstructed rodent skin flaps. *Archiv Otolaryngol* 1993; **119**: 1015–17.
55. Jansen GB, Torkvist L, Lofgren O, et al. Effects of calcitonin gene-related peptide on tissue survival, blood flow, and neutrophil recruitment in experimental skin flaps. *Brit J Plast Surg* 1999; **52**: 299–303.
56. Akamatsu J, Ueda K, Tajima S, Nozawa M. Suplhatide elongates dorsal skin flap survival in rats. *J Surg Res* 2000; **92**: 36–39.
57. Ueda K, Nozawa M, Nakao M, et al. Sulfatide and monoclonal antibodies prevent reperfusion injury in skin flaps. *J Surg Res* 2000; **88**: 125–29.
58. Kuo YR, Jeng SF, Wang FS, et al. Platelet glycoprotein IIb/IIIa receptor antagonist (abciximab) inhibited platelet activation and promoted skin flap survival after ischemia/reperfusion injury. *J Surg Res* 2002; **107**: 50–55.
59. Rand-Luby L, Pommier RF, Williams ST, et al. Improved outcome of surgical flaps treated with topical dimethylsulfoxide. *Ann Surg* 1996; **224**: 583–89.
60. Ichioka S, Nakatsuka T, Ohura N, et al. Clinical use of amrinine (a selective phosphodiesterase II inhibitor) in reconstructive surgery. *Plast Reconstr Surg* 2001; **108**: 1931–37.
61. Pang Y, Lineweaver WC, Lei MP, et al. Evaluation of the mechanism of vascular endothelial growth factor improvement of ischemic flap survival in rats. *Plast Reconstr Surg* 2003; **112**: 556–64.
62. Lubiatowski P, Goldman CK, Guruluoglu R, et al. Enhancement of epigastric skin flap survival by adenovirus-mediated VEGF gene therapy. *Plast Reconstr Surg* 2002; **109**: 1986–93.
63. O'Toole G, MacKenzie D, Lindeman B, et al. Vascular endothelial growth factor gene therapy in ischaemic rat skin flaps. *Brit J Plast Surg* 2002; **55**: 55–58.
64. Zhang F, Richards L, Angel MF, et al. Acceleration flap maturation by vascular endothelial growth factor in a rat tube flap model. *Brit J Plast Surg* 2002; **55**: 59–63.
65. Kryger Z, Zhang F, Dogan T, et al. The effects of VEGF on survival of a random flap in the rat: examination of various routes of administration. *Brit J Plast Surg* 2000; **53**: 234–39.
66. Rinsch C, Quinodoz P, Pitter B, et al. Delivery of FGF-2 but not VEGF by encapsulated genetically engineered myoblasts improves survival and vascularization in a model of acute skin flap ischemia. *Gene Ther* 2001; **8**: 523–33.
67. Salemark L, Knudsen F, Dougan P. The effects of dextran 40 on patency following severe trauma in small arteries and veins. *Brit J Plast Surg* 1995; **48**: 121–26.
68. Cox GW, Runnels S, Hsu HSH, Das SK. A comparison of heparinised saline irrigation solutions in a model of microvascular thrombosis. *Brit J Plast Surg* 1992; **45**: 345–48.
69. Dhar SC, Taylor GI. The delay phenomenon: the story unfolds. *Plast Reconstr Surg* 1999; **104**: 2079–91.
70. Saxby PJ. Survival of axial pattern flaps after tissue expansion: a pig model. *Plast Reconstr Surg* 1988; **81**: 30–34.
71. Ribuffo D, Muratori l, Antoniadou K, et al. A hemodynamic approach to clinical results in the TRAM flap after selective delay. *Plast Reconstr Surg* 1997; **99**: 1706–14.
72. Murry CE, Jennings RB, Reimer KA. Preconditioning with ischemia: a delay of lethal cell injury in ischemic myocardium. *Circulation* 1986; **74**: 1124–36.
73. Zhao ZQ, Corvera JS, Halkos ME, et al. Inhibition of myocardial injury by ischemic postconditioning during reperfusion: comparison with ischemic preconditioning. *Am J Physiol Heart Circ Physiol* 2003; **285**: 579–88.
74. Lim SY, Hausenloy DJ. Remote ischemic conditioning: from bench to bedside. *Front Physiol* 2012; **3**: 27.
75. Kraemer R, Lorenzen J, Kabbani M, et al. Acute effects of remote ischemic preconditioning on cutaneous microcirculation: a controlled prospective cohort study. *BMC Surg* 2011; **23**: 32.
76. Newsome RE, Warner MA, Wilson SC, et al. Extracorporeal bypass preserved composite anterior thigh free flap (periosteo-musculo-fascio-cutaneous) for hemipelvectomy reconstruction: utilizing the periosteal component for abdominal wall fascial reconstruction. *Ann Plast Surg* 2005; **54**: 318–22.
77. Wolff KD, Mücke T, von Bomhard A, et al. Free flap transplantation using an extracorporeal perfusion device: first three cases. *J Craniomaxillofac Surg* 2016; **2**: 148–54.
78. Amir A, Solomon AS, Giler S, et al. The influence of helium-neon laser irradiation on the viability of skin flaps in the rat. *Brit J Plast Surg* 2000; **53**; 58–62.
79. Luo Q, Xiong MG, Gu H. Effect of intravascular low level laser irradiation used in avulsion injury. *Chinese Journal of Reparative and Reconstructive Surgery* 2000; **14**: 7–9.
80. Batchelor AGG, Davison P, Sully L. The salvage of congested skin flaps by the application of leeches. *Brit J Plast Surg* 1984; **37**: 358–60.

BIOMATERIALS, TISSUE ENGINEERING AND THEIR APPLICATION IN THE ORAL AND MAXILLOFACIAL REGION

Kurt Busuttil Naudi and Ashraf Ayoub

Introduction 119	Tissue engineering 122
Biomaterials 119	References 123

SEARCH STRATEGY

Data in this chapter may be updated by a Medline and Embase search using the keywords: biomaterials, tissue engineering, head and neck, and focussing on gold standard tissue engineering techniques as well as new developments. Clinical applications are limited due to the novelty of the subject; most of the published research is based on the preclinical applications of biomaterials.

INTRODUCTION

The reconstruction of large defects, particularly bony defects, in the head and neck region continues to be an area of significant debate. These defects are usually created after the surgical removal of cancer lesions or as a result of bone loss following major trauma. The critical size of the created surgical defect, combined with the detrimental effect of post-surgical radiation therapy on the blood supply of the surrounding tissues contribute to the limited healing capabilities of the surgical site and the challenging reconstructions. Most of the available data on the management of such defects are based on expert opinion; the comprehensive studies provide limited objective guidelines for successful treatment.[1]

Bone provides the support and foundation for the overlying soft tissues so its replacement is essential for successful reconstruction. Various bone graft materials have been used for the restoration of head and neck bone defects. An ideal bone graft needs to promote osteogenesis, osteoinduction and osteoconduction.[2] *Graft osteogenesis* is provided by the cellular elements within a donor graft that survive the transplantation and synthesize new bone at the recipient site, an example of which would be mesenchymal stem cell-derived osteoblasts. *Graft osteoinduction* is new bone formation through the active recruitment of host mesenchymal stem cells from the surrounding tissue, which then differentiate into bone-forming osteoblasts. This is a property held by various cytokines including bone morphogenetic proteins (BMP). *Graft osteoconduction* is achieved by new bone formation into a defined supporting scaffold (matrix) that can be the non-vascularized bone itself or with the application of allografts or synthetic substitute. Other important graft properties include biocompatibility, bioactivity, biodegradability and the ability to attain adequate mechanical properties. Because autogenous bone grafts possess all of the aforementioned properties they continue to be the gold standard for the repair of such defects but the morbidity associated with harvesting such grafts inspired the development of substitutes.[3]

This chapter looks at the main types of biomaterials that have been applied for the reconstruction of the oral and maxillofacial region and looks at the various bioengineering methods that have been developed to try and replicate as well as promote the body's natural healing capabilities.

BIOMATERIALS

The biomaterials that will be discussed in this section were developed to support the concepts described previously. The materials described will possess one or more of the three fundamental properties of osteoconduction, osteoinduction and osteogenesis.

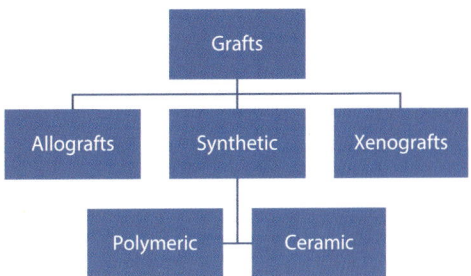

Figure 12.1 The main types of alternative grafts available for use in the head and neck region. Hybrids of these different types are also available.

Scaffold biomaterials used for tissue engineering vary in porosity, composition and biodegradability to best mimic the requirements of the tissue to be replaced. For this reason a vast array of scaffold materials (available as powders, granules, dense blocks, putties, injectable pastes, gels and porous scaffolds) have been developed as they are able to provide osteoconduction and in some cases (e.g. porous block scaffolds) help restore the shape of the critical-sized defect.

Scaffolds can be broadly divided into three main types: allogenic, xenogenic and synthetic graft materials. Allogenic grafts are derived from donors of the same species as the recipient, xenografts are derived from donors that are from a species different to that of the recipient and synthetic grafts, as their name implies, are manufactured in a laboratory. These synthetic grafts are then further subdivided into ceramics and polymeric materials (**Figure 12.1**). Several hybrids (composites) of all the above scaffolds have also been developed. Most of these grafts only have osteoconductive properties providing a foundation for cells to migrate from the wound edges. Because of this limitation they are usually combined with osteoinductive materials.

Allografts

Allografts are grafts obtained from donors that are of the same species as the recipient. Demineralized bone matrix (DBM) is derived from human cadaveric bone that has been demineralized, processed and sterilized, leaving a denatured form of the protein matrix. This process is required to remove the risk of disease transmission to or an immunological response in the recipient. However, heavy processing can also result in the denaturing of the cytokines in the graft so that it loses its osteoinductive properties and remains only osteoconductive. It has been shown that DBM, when placed in sites where bone is not normally produced, can induce ectopic bone formation.[4]

Xenografts

Xenograft usage in the head and neck region is mostly limited to the use of bone minerals derived from the bones of pigs, cows and horses. The preparation of the materials results in the removal of all organic components leaving a granular, porous material with good osteoinductive properties. Collagen xenografts are also commercially available where the collagen is extracted from porcine small intestine submucosa. Bio-oss is an example of a xenograft derived from bovine bone that is routinely used for augmentation of the jaw bones. The main barriers to the usage of these materials in the past have been the risk of disease transmission; this is now unlikely due to the processing methods. However, the ethical issues related to xenograft usage remain, so detailed informed consent is essential prior to their clinical use.

Synthetic grafts

The most researched synthetic grafts are the ceramics, of which hydroxyapatite (HA), tricalcium phosphate (TCP) or a mixture of the two (biphasic calcium phosphate, BCP) are most widely used (**Table 12.1**). Ceramics are brittle materials with limited tensile strength but are available in the form of blocks with more extensive interconnected porosity permitting faster bony ingrowth; the ideal pore size is thought to be between 150 and 500 microns.[5] So as to overcome their inherent brittleness, ceramics are also available as composite materials where they have been combined with either polymers or allograft materials such as DBM.[6]

Cytokines

Cytokines are important low molecular weight, soluble cell signalling proteins that are released by cells to stimulate, 'induce', other cells through specific receptors. Usually cytokines act only over a short distance and for short periods of time and must therefore be newly produced. This has to be repeated frequently, usually in response to a stimulus. They are pleiotropic (can influence various cell types) as well as redundant (can share similar functions). Cytokines promote and control immune responses against

TABLE 12.1 Types of scaffolding materials used in tissue engineering

Natural	Synthetic
Collagen: • Gels, nanofibers, porous scaffolds, films Fibrin: • Injectable adhesive gels Alginate: • Hydrogels Silk: • Nanofibers, films Hyaluronan: • Gels, sponges, pads Chitosan: • Sponges, porous scaffolds, nanofibers Agarose: • Hydrogels	Ceramics: • Calcium phosphate cements: • Low-temperature calcium orthophosphate cements • Bioactive glasses • Hydroxyapatite • β-tricalcium phosphate Titanium Polymeric materials: • Poly(α-hydroxy esters): • Poly(L-lactic acid) • poly(glycolic acid) • Poly(lactic-co-glycolic acid) • Poly(propylene fumarate) • polyethylene glycol Ceramic reinforced polymers

inflammation, infections and cancer, with the malignant transformation process being associated with an altered response to cytokine stimulation.[7]

Cytokines such as interleukins (IL-1, IL-3, IL-6, IL-11), tumour necrosis factor (TNF), platelet-derived growth factor (PDGF), fibroblast growth factors (FGF) and vascular endothelial growth factor (VEGF) have been linked with functions that range from further cytokine release, angiogenesis, metastasis and osteoblast/osteoclast development.

There is a complex interaction that takes place between the various bone modelling cells (osteoblasts and osteoclasts) and their haematopoietic precursors as well as the cytokines themselves that results in bone formation or deposition. Cytokines also play an important role in cell activation leading to chemotaxis and release of inflammatory mediators, help in vascular remodelling (neoangiogenesis) and promote the synthesis of matrix enzymes required for the remodelling of cartilage and bone.

BONE MORPHOGENETIC PROTEINS

Bone morphogenetic proteins (BMP) are probably the most effective cytokines in relation to bone formation and healing. There are more than 20 subtypes, all forming part of the transforming growth factor β (TGF-β) superfamily.[8] BMPs induce stem and mesenchymal cell differentiation into osteogenic cells capable of producing bone. BMPs are secreted as signalling molecules that activate intracellular cascades by binding to cell surface receptors. The BMP signalling pathway has been shown to be involved in a number of developmental processes and is critical for the formation of the majority of the craniofacial elements including the cranial neural crest, the facial primordia, teeth, lips and palate.

With the use of recombinant gene technology, large quantities of recombinant human BMPs (rhBMPs) have become readily available. BMP-2 and BMP-7 (also known as Osteogenic Protein-1) are recognized to be the most effective cytokines in the maxillofacial region, inducing osteoprogenitor cells to produce bone, and resulting in chemo-attraction of mesenchymal stem cells to the defect area.[9] They are both approved for clinical use and have been used for spinal fusion, the repair of long bone fractures and non-unions as well as the repair of craniomaxillofacial defects.[9]

Due to their nature cytokines need to be placed in a scaffold, such as the ones mentioned above, to control the shape of the regenerate. Even though they are widely available and appear to be very effective at inducing bone formation, cytokines continue to be very expensive. This is due to the very time-consuming purification and concentration steps before the produced dimer protein can be refolded into its functional form. This currently significantly limits their widespread use.

Mesenchymal stromal cells

The last important bone regeneration property is osteogenesis; this is a property potentially held by pluripotent cells such a mesenchymal stromal cells (MSC). These cells are capable of differentiation into three main cell lineages – osteogenic, chondrogenic and adipogenic – as well as potentially into myogenic, neurogenic and tenogenic lineages. These cells, by their very nature, can therefore be *induced* to transform into bone forming cells if given the right stimulus and microenvironment.[10] This microenvironment is implicated in both the support and maintenance of the MSCs. There are different elements that could affect the cells; these are oxygen tension, glucose concentration, growth factors, the physiochemical nature of the environment including the pH and ionic strength (e.g. Ca^{2+} concentration). Their roles are critical for the maintenance of stem cell properties and the possibility of reprogramming their commitment prior to application in the surgical defect. MSCs can be obtained from the bone marrow, spleen and thymus as well as several other sites including adipose tissue.[11]

Autogenous bone marrow aspirate (BMA) is readily obtainable from the bone marrow of, for example, the anterior iliac crest. The aspirate is highly cellular containing osteoprogenitor cells (osteogenic) and provides a concentration of protein factors (cytokines) that stimulate bone growth (osteoinductive). For this reason it has become a cost effective alternative to the recombinant osteoinductive cytokines mentioned above.[6]

Platelet-rich plasma

Platelet-rich plasma (PRP) is blood that is taken from the patient, centrifuged, ultra-concentrated and then reimplanted after processing. It contains a mixture of platelets and growth factors such as platelet derived growth factors (PDGF), transforming growth factor-β (TGF-β), as well as insulin-like growth factor-I (IGF-I). These growth factors (cytokines) can stimulate mitogenesis of marrow stem cells and angiogenesis.[12] The expensive processing methods for the production of PRP limit its clinical use; for this reason, second generation platelet-rich fibrin (PRF), which requires no biochemical handling, has been developed.[13]

Bioreactors

In tissue engineering a bioreactor is a device that simulates the natural environment of a tissue so as to promote its growth. It is usually a perfusion chamber connected to a pump system that allows peristaltic pumping of fresh medium, and is kept at a controlled oxygen level. This allows the maintenance of ideal physiologic conditions that promote development of the required tissue. This helps to recreate the microenvironment that was described above. Other parameters that can be controlled include the application of forces or stresses to the tissues in both two or three dimensions, thus simulating the environment in which, for example, bone develops.[14] These devices are becoming increasingly popular for the development of grafts for use in the head and neck region as they are able to overcome one of the main problems in tissue engineering, which is the maintenance of a good oxygen supply and removal of cellular waste products. They also allow the maturation of the graft in the laboratory prior to its placement into the surgical recipient site.

TISSUE ENGINEERING

Bone is a complex tissue with highly porous central spongy bone and solid compact outer cortical bone. Therefore bone tissue engineering requires the design of three-dimensional (3D) scaffolds that closely mimic this anatomical organization of bone. Changes in scaffold geometry can impact on the flow of media across the scaffold and thus affect the supply of gases and nutrients and the removal of metabolites. An increase in pore number and size in various scaffolds is associated with increased vascularization and osseointegration *in vivo*, but the increased pore volume reduces the mechanical stability of the scaffold.[15]

A sufficient blood supply is required to achieve successful tissue regeneration. This remains a significant barrier to the effective reconstruction of large defects in the head and neck region. The stimulation of angiogenesis from endothelial precursors is therefore essential. The best-known angiogenic factor is vascular endothelial growth factor (VEGF), which creates an environment that promotes endothelial cell migration and proliferation.[16]

Clinical trials

The clinical application of the above mentioned novel materials is still in its early stages but some successful outcomes have been reported.

Fibroblast growth factors (FGFs) have been successfully applied for the repair of tympanic membrane perforations[17] as well as the treatment of the ageing vocal folds,[18] due possibly to the effect that this cytokine has on the key extracellular matrix components in the lamina propria.[17]

Recombinant human bone morphogenetic protein 7 (rhBMP-7) in a type I collagen carrier was used for the reconstruction of unilateral and bilateral alveolar cleft defects. The patients were followed up for an average of 6.5 years and objective radiographic evaluation demonstrated very good bone regeneration in the defects.[19]

Cultured bone marrow cells that were exposed to an osteogenic environment and placed in a mineral base of β-tricalcium phosphate and hydroxyapatite were used to treat three clinical cases. These cases had osteoradionecrosis of the maxilla and mandible with pathological fracture; a non-healed fracture with bone loss, and bilateral paraesthesia; and a very large maxillary bone deficiency. All showed signs of osteogenesis, nerve reinnervation and skin regeneration.[20]

Thirteen consecutive cases of cranio-maxillofacial hard-tissue defects in the frontal sinus (three cases), cranial bone (five cases), mandible (three cases) and nasal septum (two cases) were treated with autologous adipose stem cells derived from adipose tissue obtained from the abdominal wall. The cells were seeded onto bioactive glass or β-tricalcium phosphate scaffolds together with recombinant human bone morphogenetic protein 2. Ten out of the thirteen cases had successful outcomes.[21]

A large mandibular discontinuity defect was repaired with a custom bone transplant grown inside the latissimus dorsi muscle of an adult male patient. This was achieved using computed tomography scanning and computer-aided design techniques to produce a virtual replacement (in the form of a titanium mesh) for the mandibular defect. This was filled with bone mineral blocks, recombinant human bone morphogenetic protein 7 and the patient's bone marrow. Seven weeks after placement in the latissimus dorsi muscle the graft was successfully transplanted as a free bone-muscle flap to repair the mandibular defect.[22]

FUTURE RESEARCH

Molecular therapy in bone bioengineering

Modification of the properties of cells at the molecular level can have significant potentially useful effects within tissue engineering. Liposome-mediated and adenovirus cell-mediated BMP-2 gene transfer into MSCs in preclinical studies has resulted in cells that are able to repair critical-size bony defects.[23] Gene-modified cells could potentially be given all the properties required for tissue regeneration and they could be then implanted into the surgical defect. Alternatively these cells could be place in a bioreactor and allowed to create the required tissue 'bone' *ex vivo* after which it would be implanted into the surgical recipient site.

Biomimetic scaffolds

Scaffolds currently used for tissue engineering are either granular or manufactured in predetermined shapes. With the use of computer-based solid free form fabrication (SFF) using 3D printers it is possible to create custom-made scaffolds designed to specifically fit the defect that is being treated. Also the nano-topography and nano-chemistry of the scaffold can be structured in detail to try and reproduce the natural tissue that it is designed to replace, even at the cellular level. This would help promote the growth of all the required cellular elements for tissue regeneration (e.g. blood vessels and bone).

Improved vascularity

New methods that can improve the vascularity of the donor sites/grafts will significantly enhance the regenerative abilities. The bioreactors mentioned earlier can help in this respect but specific methods of inducing controlled vascular proliferation within the surgical site still need to be developed, possibly using synthetic polymers.

KEY POINTS

- The reconstruction of large defects, particularly bony defects, in the oral and maxillofacial region continues to be an area of significant development.
- An ideal bone graft should promote osteogenesis, osteoinduction and osteoconduction, as well as be biocompatible, bioactive, biodegradable and possess adequate mechanical properties.
- The harvesting of the autogenous bone graft 'gold standard' is associated with donor site morbidity; this is the main drive force for the search for synthetic substitutes and further investigation in tissue bioengineering.
- Biomaterial scaffolds can be broadly divided into three main types; allogic, xenogenic and synthetic graft materials.
- Most synthetic scaffolds have only osteoconductive properties and are combined with osteoinductive materials.
- The ethical issues related to xenograft usage remain, so patient informed consent is essential prior to their clinical use.
- The most researched synthetic grafts are hydroxyapatite (HA), tricalcium phosphate (TCP) or a mixture of the two (biphasic calcium phosphate, BCP).
- Cytokines are important low molecular weight, soluble cell signalling proteins that have an effect on other cells through specific receptors affecting several processes that include tumour growth and bone remodelling.
- Mesenchymal stromal cells, which can be obtained from the bone marrow, spleen, thymus and adipose tissue, are capable of differentiation into the three main cell lineages; osteogenic, chondrogenic and adipogenic.
- The cytokine bone morphogenetic protein induces mesenchymal cell differentiation into osteogenic cells capable of producing bone.
- A bioreactor is a device that simulates the natural environment of a tissue so as to promote its growth.

REFERENCES

1. Assael LA. Mandibular reconstruction: expert opinion and outcome studies remain a fragile guide to treatment. *J Oral Maxil Surg* 2009; 67: 2557–58.
2. Perciaccante V, Jeffery J. Oral and maxillofacial reconstruction. In: AbuBake O, Benson K. *Oral and maxillofacial secrets.* 2nd ed. Philadephia: Elsevier; 2007, pp. 389–403.
3. Younger EM, Chapman MW. Morbidity at bone graft donor sites. *J Orthop Trauma* 1989; 3: 192–95.
4. Urist MR. Bone: formation by autoinduction. *Clin Orthop Relat Res* 1965; 4–10.
5. Tanner KE. Bioactive composites for bone tissue engineering. *P I Mech Eng H* 2010; 224: 1359–72.
6. Ilan DI, Ladd AL. Bone graft substitutes. *Oper Tech Plast Reconstr Surg* 2002; 9: 151–60.
7. Pries R, Wollenberg B. Cytokines in head and neck cancer. *Cytokine Growth F R* 2006 17: 141–46.
8. Matthews SJ. Biological activity of bone morphogenetic proteins (BMPs). *Injury* 2005; 36(Suppl.3): S34–S37.
9. Herford AS, Stoffella E, Tandon R. Reconstruction of mandibular defects using bone morphogenic protein: can growth factors replace the need for autologous bone grafts? A systematic review of the literature. *Plast Surg Int* 2011, 165824.
10. Bianchi G, Muraglia A, Daga A, et al. Microenvironment and stem properties of bone marrow-derived mesenchymal cells. *Wound Repair Regen* 2001; 9: 460–66.
11. Dicker A, Le Blanc K, Astrom G, et al. Functional studies of mesenchymal stem cells derived from adult human adipose tissue. *Exp Cell Res* 2005; 308: 283–90.
12. Lieberman JR, Daluiski A, Einhorn TA. The role of growth factors in the repair of bone: biology and clinical applications. *J Bone Joint Surg Am* 2002; 84A: 1032–44.
13. Martínez CE, Smith PC, Palma Alvarado VA. The influence of platelet-derived products on angiogenesis and tissue repair: a concise update. *Front Physiol* 2015; 6: 290.
14. Griffith LG, Swartz MA. Capturing complex 3D tissue physiology in vitro. *Nat Rev Mol Cell Biol* 2006; 7: 211–24.
15. Karageorgiou V, Kaplan D. Porosity of 3D biomaterial scaffolds and osteogenesis. *Biomaterials* 2005; 26: 5474–91.
16. Hughes GC, Biswas SS, Yin BL, et al. Therapeutic angiogenesis in chronically ischemic porcine myocardium: comparative effects of bFGF and VEGF. *Ann Thorac Surg* 2004; 77: 812–18.
17. Ohno T, Hirano S. Treatment of aging vocal folds: novel approaches. *Curr Opin Otolaryngol Head Neck Surg* 2014; 22: 472–76.
18. Teh BM, Marano RJ, Shen Y, et al. Tissue engineering of the tympanic membrane. *Tissue Eng Part B Rev* 2013; 19: 116–32.
19. Ayoub A, Roshan CP, Gillgrass T, et al. The clinical application of rhBMP-7 for the reconstruction of alveolar cleft. *J Plast Reconstr Aesthet Surg* 2015; S1748-6815(15)00437-4. [Epub]
20. Mendonça JJ, Juiz-Lopez P. Regenerative facial reconstruction of terminal stage osteoradionecrosis and other advanced craniofacial diseases with adult cultured stem and progenitor cells. *Plast Reconstr Surg* 2010; 126: 1699–709.
21. Sándor GK, Numminen J, Wolff J, et al. Adipose stem cells used to reconstruct 13 cases with cranio-maxillofacial hard-tissue defects. *Stem Cells Transl Med* 2014; 3: 530–40.
22. Warnke PH, Springer IN, Wiltfang J, et al. Growth and transplantation of a custom vascularised bone graft in a man. *Lancet* 2004; 364: 766–70.
23. Park J, Ries J, Gelse K, et al. Bone regeneration in critical size defects by cell mediated BMP-2 gene transfer: a comparison of adenoviral vectors and liposomes. *Gene Ther* 2003; 10: 1089–98.

Immunology

CHAPTER 13

DEFENCE MECHANISMS

Ian Todd and Richard J. Powell

Innate and adaptive immunity 125	Immunity to cytosolic infectious agents 132
Antigen recognition 126	Inflammation and hypersensitivity 132
Immunity to extra-cellular and vesicular infectious agents 129	Further reading 135

SEARCH STRATEGY

Data in this chapter may be updated by a PubMed search using the keywords: innate immunity, adaptive immunity, antigen, B lymphocyte, T lymphocyte, antibody, immunoglobulin, antigen presentation, cytokine, complement, inflammation, hypersensitivity, allergy and autoimmunity.

INNATE AND ADAPTIVE IMMUNITY

The immune system has evolved for protection against infectious agents that invade the body. In order to achieve this, the immune system has recognition properties to locate and identify the invader, and to activate defence processes to repel or destroy the invader. There are an enormous number and variety of infectious agents within the main categories of viruses, bacteria, fungi, protozoa and parasitic worms. In order to provide effective immunity against each of these agents, the immune system has to be able to meet the challenges they pose: this is achieved by a diverse range of molecular and cellular components in the body that cooperate with each other in order to maximize their defensive activities. Some of these components generate innate immunity, whereas others provide adaptive (or acquired) immunity. The main cell types of the immune system are the leucocytes that develop from stem cells in the bone marrow.

The innate immune system is evolutionarily older than the adaptive system and provides generic defence against categories of microbes. It is composed of a range of cells and proteins found in the circulation and in tissues: these include macrophages (and their monocyte precursors), granulocytes (i.e. neutrophils, eosinophils, basophils), and mast cells, natural killer cells, complement proteins, regulatory proteins called cytokines. The innate system employs an inherited repertoire of receptor proteins (known as pattern-recognition molecules) that recognize characteristic structures that are commonly expressed by microbes, and changes to cells induced by infection. The advantage of this innate system is that it is rapidly activated by infectious agents that penetrate tissues. However, it is only moderately efficient; hence, an adaptive immune response is also required to enhance the elimination of many pathogens.

Adaptive immunity is mediated by T lymphocytes and B lymphocytes (also known as T cells and B cells). Similar to the leucocytes involved in the innate system, lymphocytes develop from bone marrow stem cells. The precursors of T cells migrate to the thymus to complete their maturation. Each T or B cell expresses receptors that specifically recognize one particular chemical structure of a microbial molecule (known, in this context, as an antigen). Activated B cells also secrete a soluble form of their antigen receptors, known as antibodies or immunoglobulins (Ig). An enormously diverse repertoire of antigen receptors is somatically generated by recombination events involving the receptor genes during the development of lymphocytes, resulting in the potential to recognize millions of different antigens. The recruitment, activation and proliferation of resting lymphocytes specific for the antigens of an invading microbe takes time (possibly several days), but the lymphocytes generate a highly efficient defence. In addition, some of the lymphocytes activated by specific antigens are maintained in the body as resting cells after the elimination of the infection and constitute a memory population of cells that are able to generate a bigger and faster response upon subsequent exposure to the same antigens: this demonstrates the adaptive properties of lymphocytes.

The innate and adaptive systems interact and synergize to generate optimal immunity. Specifically, lymphocyte activation is dependent not only on antigen recognition, but also on co-stimulatory signals provided by cells and molecules of the innate system. Furthermore, the antibodies produced by B cells and the cytokines secreted primarily by T cells enhance the defensive activities of the innate system.

Stages of an immune response

The immediate response to an invading pathogen is mounted by innate components resident within the infected tissues (**Figure 13.1a**). In particular, tissue macrophages (and other cells with innate immune functions) express a range of pattern recognition receptors for microbial structures, including mannose receptor, scavenger receptors and Toll-like receptors, whose ligands include various microbial polysaccharides, lipids and nucleic acids. Complement proteins are also directly activated by microbes via the alternative pathway (see 'The Complement System' below). Inflammatory products of macrophages and complement, together with those released by tissue mast cells activated by the complement peptides C3a and C5a (known as anaphylatoxins), induce the migration of granulocytes, natural killer cells and more complement proteins from the blood stream into the infected tissues (**Figure 13.1b**).

Whilst these innate processes are providing early defence to limit growth and spread of the infection within the body, other processes are set in train to generate the antigen-specific adaptive response (**Figure 13.1c**). The activation of lymphocytes does not initially take place within the infected tissues themselves, but in specialized collections of lymphoid tissues such as lymph nodes, the spleen and mucosa-associated lymphoid tissues (MALT) that includes Waldeyer's ring. Antigens therefore have to be transported from the infected tissues to local lymphoid tissues. Some antigens may be passively carried in the tissue fluid forming the lymph that drains into regional lymph nodes. However, a significant role is played by dendritic cells found in most tissues. These, like the macrophages described above, express pattern-recognition receptors for microbial structures and actively engulf microbial material. This induces maturation of the dendritic cells, which then migrate from the site of infection and carry the microbial antigens to the local lymphoid tissues where T and B lymphocytes have the opportunity to interact with the antigens leading to their activation. Only a very small proportion of the millions of lymphocytes in a particular lymphoid organ will have receptors that specifically recognize the antigens associated with a particular microbe. It is the antigen-activated lymphocytes that proliferate and mature into effector cells contributing to defence against the pathogen. These effector lymphocytes leave the lymphoid tissues and recirculate via the blood stream to the site of infection in order to enhance the destruction and elimination of the pathogen in cooperation with the innate components described above.

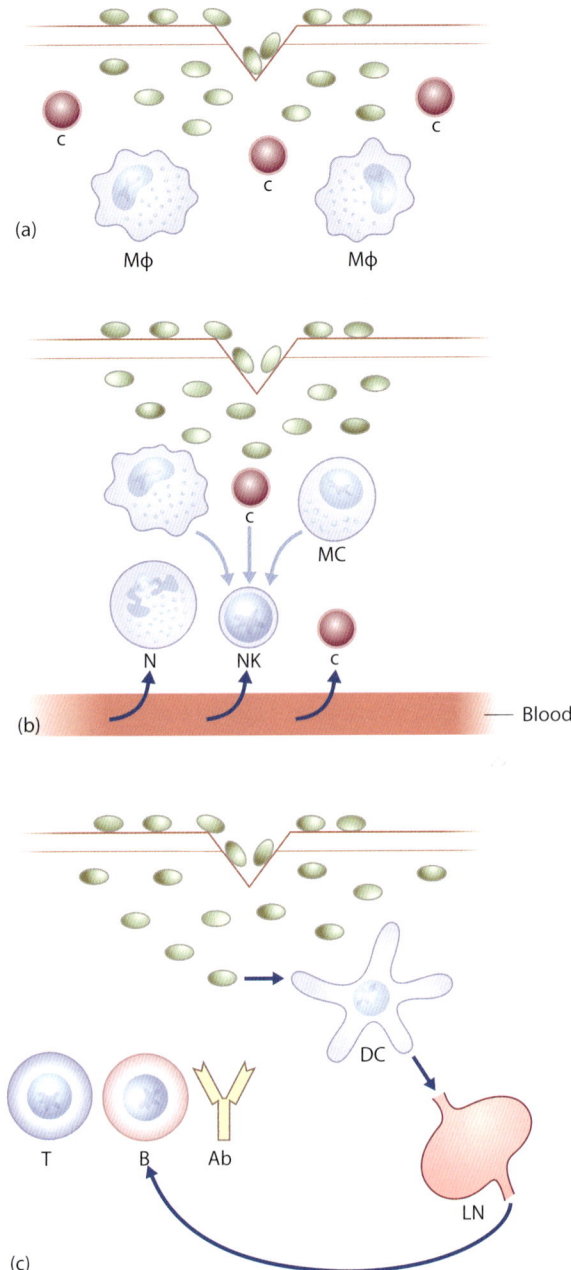

Figure 13.1 Stages of an immune response. (See text for details.) a) Immediate local innate response; b) Early induced response (innate/inflammatory); c) Later adaptive response. Ab, antibody; B, B lymphocyte; C, complement; DC, dendritic cell; LN, lymph node; MC, mast cell; MΦ, macrophage; N, neutrophil; NK, natural killer cell; T, T lymphocyte.

ANTIGEN RECOGNITION

Antigen recognition involves a high affinity interaction between an antigen and the specialized antigen combining site of a lymphocyte's antigen receptor protein (or of an antibody molecule). The binding involves non-covalent intermolecular attractive forces that require the interacting surfaces to have complementary shapes that fit snugly together (rather like a lock and a key), allowing interactions to occur between complementary chemical groups of the antigen and the combining site. Each lymphocyte clone (i.e. group of cells derived from a single parent lymphocyte) expresses antigen receptors with a single type of combining site that is unique in shape and amino acid composition to that clone contrasting with the millions of other lymphocyte clones in the body: this is why millions of differing antigens can be recognized by the adaptive immune system. Furthermore, the specificity of the adaptive response arises because those lymphocytes whose receptors have the highest affinity for an antigen that enters the body are the ones most likely to bind it and hence be activated by it: this is termed clonal selection.

B cells and antibodies (immunoglobulins)

The B cell's receptor is essentially a membrane bound form of the antibody that a particular B cell secretes, and is called surface immunoglobulin (sIg) (**Figure 13.2**). It is made up of two identical large polypeptides (heavy chains) and two identical smaller light chains (which can be one of two types called κ and λ light chains). Each chain is composed of a series of homologous globular regions called Ig domains: two in the light chains and four or five in the heavy chains.

The receptor has two identical antigen combining sites, each of which is composed of the amino terminal domains of a heavy and a light chain: these are called variable domains because they vary in structure between different B cell clones, thereby conferring the differences in antigenic specificity between B cells. Different types of chemicals can serve as antigens for direct interaction with different B cell receptors and antibodies, including proteins, carbohydrates, lipids and even nucleic acids.

The combining site constitutes only a small part of a whole Ig molecule and can accommodate approximately four to six amino acids of a protein antigen: the precise region of an antigen molecule that interacts with a combining site is termed the antigenic determinant or epitope. Each variable domain contains three hypervariable loops, so called because they differ most in amino acid sequence between different clones of B cells; they are also known as complementarity determining regions, being complementary to the epitope and forming the main interactions with it. Following B cell activation, modifications can occur to the variable domains by somatic mutation. This involves nucleotide changes to the variable domain genes during B cell replication that affect the amino acid sequence (particularly of the complementarity determining regions) and therefore affect the antigenic specificity of the antigen combining sites. This can generate combining sites that fit even more tightly with the epitope, improving further the affinity for the antigen.

The other domains are called constant domains because they have the same structure in the sIg of different B cells. Human B cells can express one of nine different forms or isotypes of Ig (both surface and secreted) that differ in the structure and number of their heavy chain constant region domains, and constitute five immunoglobulin classes. These are called IgM, IgG (with subclasses IgG1, IgG2, IgG3 and IgG4), IgA (with subclasses IgA1 and IgA2), IgE and IgD. All B cells are initially programmed to express IgM (with IgD), but can undergo Ig class switching to produce one of the other isotypes following stimulation by antigen, without changing their antigenic specificity. They do this by changing the heavy chain constant region domains that they express, but maintain expression of the same variable domain on the heavy chain and the same light chain variable and constant domains.

The sIg is anchored in the surface membrane of a B cell by a transmembrane amino acid sequence at the carboxy terminus of the heavy chains. When a resting B cell is activated by an antigen, it can differentiate into a plasma cell that produces large numbers of Ig molecules that lack the transmembrane sequence. These are secreted from the cell as antibodies with the same antigenic specificity and isotype as the B cell's sIg. Because B cells initially express sIgM, the first antibodies produced during an immune response (i.e. on first exposure to a particular antigen) are also IgM (there is little, if any, secretion of IgD systemically), but IgG, IgA and IgE antibodies appear later in the response as activated B cells undergo class switching. Furthermore, the memory population is derived from B cells that have undergone class switching, so that IgG, IgA and IgE are produced at the start of a secondary response on repeated exposure to the same antigen. The advantages of producing a range of antibody isotypes are that they have different physiological and defensive activities.

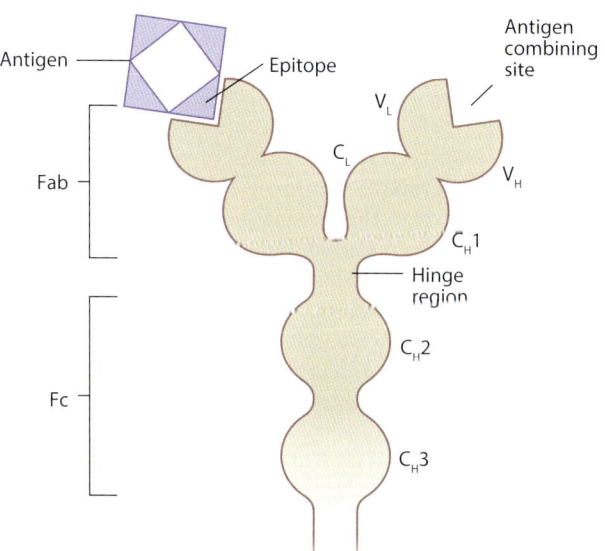

Figure 13.2 A schematic structure of a generic immunoglobulin (surface or secreted). (See text for details.) The variable domains of the heavy and light chains are labelled V_H and V_L, respectively. Similarly, the constant domains are labelled C_H1-3 and C_L. The pale region below C_H3 indicates the transmembrane region and cytoplasmic tail present in sIg, but not in secreted antibodies.

T cells and antigen presentation

The T-cell receptor (TCR) for an antigen shows both similarities and differences to B cell sIg (**Figure 13.3**). The TCR is a much smaller molecule, being made up of two

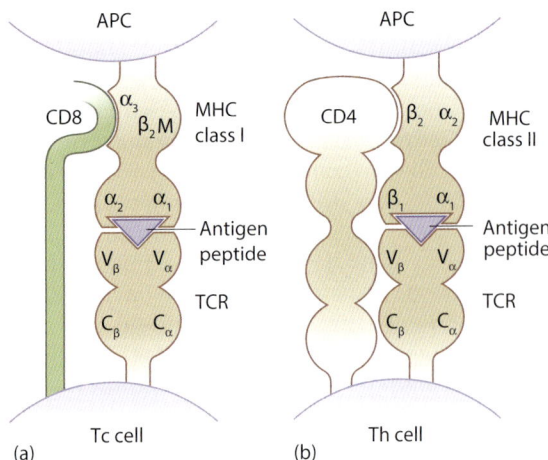

Figure 13.3 Antigen recognition by T cells. (See text for details.) APC, antigen presenting cell; β2M, β2-microglobulin; C, constant domain; MHC, major histocompatibility complex; Tc, cytotoxic T cell; TCR, T cell receptor; Th, helper T cell; V, variable domain.

polypeptide chains each of which is about the same size as an Ig light chain, with both expressing a transmembrane sequence. However, T cells do not produce a secreted form of the TCR (i.e. they do not release proteins equivalent to antibodies). The TCR polypeptides expressed by the majority of T cells are called α and β chains, whereas a minority express γ and δ chains. Each chain is composed of two domains that show strong structural homologies with those of the immunoglobulins. Similar Ig-like domains are found in many other surface molecules of lymphocytes and other cells: this indicates evolutionary genetic relationships between these molecules, constituting the immunoglobulin superfamily. The two amino terminal, membrane-distal domains of the TCR chains are variable between T cells and constitute the single antigen combining site. The membrane-proximal domains are constant in structure.

Unlike B cell immunoglobulins, conventional TCR cannot interact directly with antigenic epitopes of proteins; rather, they only bind to short peptides that are derived from protein antigens, and are expressed on the surface of other cells of the body that are known, in this context, as antigen presenting cells (APC). This is because the main function of T cells is to interact with other cells within the context of an immune response: binding to antigenic peptides held on the surface of a cell thereby directs a T cell to exert effects on that particular APC. There are two main functional types of T cell: helper T cells (Th) regulate the activity of other cells of the immune system, whereas cytotoxic T cells (Tc) kill cells that are infected. In order for this to happen, protein antigens that enter the cytoplasm of an APC are processed (i.e. degraded) into peptides, some of which associate with proteins of the major histocompatibility complex (MHC), known in humans as HLA (human leucocyte antigens). The MHC molecule/peptide complexes are then expressed on the surface of the APC where they can interact with T cells whose TCR have combining sites specific for the particular antigenic peptides presented, much in the same way as an Ig combining site interacts with an antigen epitope. This interaction binds the T cell to the surface of the APC, enabling these cells to exert effects on each other.

There are two types of MHC molecule, called MHC class I and MHC class II (**Figure 13.3**). They have similar three-dimensional structures, but are made up of different types of polypeptide chains. The MHC class I protein is composed of a large α-chain non-covalently associated with the smaller $β_2$-microglobulin, whereas MHC class II is composed of similarly sized α and β chains. Both class I and class II have two Ig-like domains adjacent to the cell membrane (i.e. they are members of the Ig superfamily), whereas distal to the membrane is the antigen peptide binding cleft. Two α-helices form the walls of the cleft and sit on a platform of β-pleated sheet; antigen peptide is held within the cleft in a linear conformation (rather like a hotdog sausage in a bun!) with its exposed surface available for interaction with a TCR. Peptides eight or nine amino acids in length can be accommodated within the cleft of MHC class I molecules, whereas the peptides that associate with MHC class II molecules can be between 12 and 20 amino acids in length because they can extend beyond the ends of the peptide binding cleft.

MHC class I molecules present antigens primarily to Tc cells because these cells express a protein called CD8 that binds to the side of the class I α-chain when the TCR interacts with the peptide and binding cleft (**Figure 13.3a**). Most tissue cells of the body express MHC class I molecules on their surfaces and thus have the potential to be targets for Tc cells if they become infected by microbes that enter the cytosol, such as viruses. The processing pathway for cytosolic proteins delivers the peptides to MHC class I molecules for binding and presentation. Tc cell clones that specifically bind to these peptides have various ways of killing infected cells by inducing them to undergo apoptosis (programmed cell death):

- The Tc cells secrete two types of proteins stored in cytoplasmic granules: perforins that polymerize to create pores through the plasma membranes of the target cells, and granzymes that enter the target cells through the perforin pores, inducing apoptosis.
- Fas-ligand expressed on the surface of Tc cells, or tumour necrosis factor (TNF alpha) secreted by Tc cells can induce apoptosis when they bind to their receptors on infected target cells (Fas and TNFR1, respectively).

MHC class II molecules present peptides mainly to Th cells because these cells express the CD4 protein that binds to the side of the MHC class II β-chain (**Figure 13.3b**). The expression of MHC class II molecules is mainly restricted to cells of the immune system whose functions are to activate, and be activated by, Th cells: these are dendritic cells, macrophages and B cells. These cells deliberately engulf exogenous antigens that, for example, bind to Toll-like receptors expressed on macrophages and dendritic cells, or specifically bind to the sIg of selected B cell clones. In either case, the surface-bound

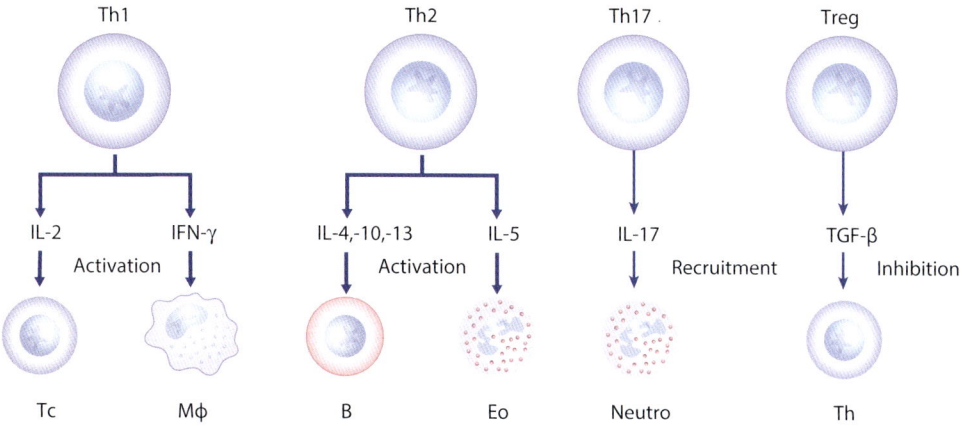

Figure 13.4 Cytokine-mediated regulation by Th1, Th2, Th17 and Treg cells. B, B lymphocyte; Eo, eosinophil; IFN-γ, interferon-γ; IL, interleukin; MΦ, macrophage; Neutro, neutrophil; Tc, cytotoxic T cell; TGF-β, transforming growth factor β; Th1, T helper 1 cell; Th2, T helper 2 cell; Th17, T helper 17 cell; Treg, regulatory T cell.

antigens are endocytosed into membrane-bound vesicles within the cytoplasm. The processing pathway for these vesicular proteins delivers peptides to MHC class II molecules for binding and presentation. Th cell clones that specifically bind to these peptides can then be triggered by the APC to exert their regulatory activities. A range of cell surface and secreted molecules mediate the mutual effects of Th cells and APC. First, there are the interactions of TCR and CD4 with the peptide/MHC class II complex, with the signal resulting from TCR binding being delivered to the interior of T cells by the CD3 protein. Second, a number of other membrane proteins interact between the surfaces of the T cells and APC to deliver co-stimulatory signals: particularly important are interactions of CD28 with B7, and CD40-ligand with CD40, but others include the interactions of CD2 with LFA-3, and LFA-1 with ICAM (in each case on the T cells and APC, respectively). Third, both the APC and the T cells secrete cytokines as soluble regulatory proteins that bind to specific cell surface receptors. For example, interleukin-1 (IL-1) and IL-12 are important T cell activators secreted by dendritic cells.

When activated, different Th cells preferentially secrete differing combinations of cytokines (**Figure 13.4**). Th1 cells produce interferon-γ (IFN-γ), which is an important macrophage activator, and IL-2, which stimulates T cells (including Tc cells); hence, Th1 cells induce primarily cell-mediated immunity, although they do also stimulate B cells to produce IgG antibodies (subclasses 1-3). In contrast Th2 cells produce IL-4, IL-10 and IL-13, which stimulate B cells to produce antibodies, and particularly induce Ig class switching to production of IgG (subclasses 1-4), IgE and IgA; they also secrete IL-5, which stimulates eosinophils. Th1 and Th2 cells can in fact inhibit each other's activities via the cytokines they release. These patterns of type 1 and type 2 cytokine secretion are observed with other cell types, including Tc cells and B cells. Other subpopulations of T cells have been defined and include Th17 cells, which secrete IL-17, recruit neutrophils to infected tissues and induce the production of inflammatory cytokines and chemokines. Regulatory T cells (Treg cells) inhibit the activity of T helper cells, thereby controlling adaptive immunity; they do this partly by secreting suppressive cytokines, a key example of which is transforming growth factor-beta (TGF-β).

There are several subpopulations of lymphocytes that display properties of both innate and adaptive immunity. These include NKT cells and γδT cells, whose antigen receptors show limited diversity and interact with ligands that differ from the peptide-MHC complexes recognized by 'conventional' T cells. Additional 'innate lymphoid cells' include the well-characterized natural killer (NK) cells and more recently identified lymphoid cells that lack antigen-specific receptors and rapidly produce cytokines when activated.

IMMUNITY TO EXTRA-CELLULAR AND VESICULAR INFECTIOUS AGENTS

Differing defence mechanisms are required to deal with infectious agents that occupy different compartments within the body. A major distinction is whether an infectious agent is in an extra-cellular environment or has entered the cytoplasm of cells, joining the intra-cellular environment (**Figure 13.5**). This distinction is important because extra-cellular organisms are directly accessible to defensive molecules secreted by cells of the immune system, whereas intra-cellular ones are not. Consequently, antibodies play a major role in the adaptive immune response to extra-cellular pathogens (**Figure 13.5a**).

Antibody effector functions

Antibodies are bifunctional molecules with one end having the antigen binding properties while the other end triggers the defensive activities. These functional regions are separated by a relatively flexible amino acid sequence between the first and second heavy chain constant

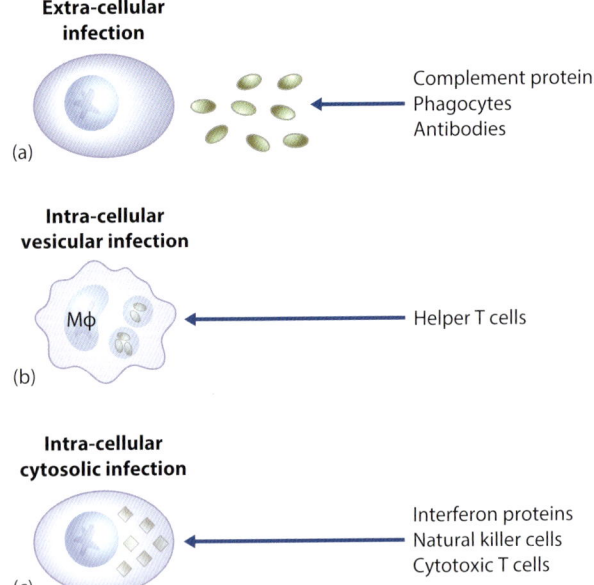

Figure 13.5 Immune responses to different types of infections.

domains called the hinge region (**Figure 13.2**). The two arms containing the antigen combining sites are called the fragment antigen binding (Fab) regions: each is composed of a light chain and the variable and first constant domain of a heavy chain. The other constant domains of the two heavy chains constitute the Fragment crystallizable (Fc) region (because it can form crystals when isolated experimentally).

As described under Antigen recognition above, there are five classes of Ig molecules expressed as B cell sIg, four of which are also secreted as antibodies (i.e. IgM, IgG, IgA and IgE, but not IgD). The classes have different heavy chain constant domains, and thus differ primarily in their Fc regions (**Table 13.1**). The heavy chains of IgG, IgA and IgD each have two constant domains in the Fc region, whereas IgM and IgE have three.

In addition, IgM forms pentamers (five Ig monomers) held together by a J (joining) chain polypeptide, whereas IgA can similarly form dimers. The large size of IgM results in it being predominantly restricted to the blood stream (except at sites of inflammation), whereas the other classes can more readily diffuse into tissues. IgG is the most abundant antibody class in the blood, and also is transported across the placenta from the maternal to the fetal circulation during the last three months of pregnancy. This maternal IgG in the newborn baby provides the protection against infection until the baby's immune system produces significant levels of antibodies. Very premature babies have limited maternal antibody. IgA in its dimeric form is transported across mucosal epithelia in large quantities and thus constitutes the main antibody class conferring protection in secretions and at mucosal surfaces. Part of the mucosal receptor that binds and transports IgA across the epithelium remains associated with it as the secretory piece. IgA is also secreted into milk and thus confers protection in the gastro-intestinal tract of suckling babies. In humans, IgD is present in secretions of the upper respiratory and digestive tracts where it may play important roles in neutralization of pathogenic microbes and exclusion of commensals.

Antibodies can neutralize microbes and their toxins simply by binding to them, hence inhibiting their functions and infectivity. However, antibodies can also contribute to the destruction of infectious agents by interacting with other defensive components, as described below.

The complement system

(See **Figure 13.6**.) The complement proteins found in the circulation and tissue fluids constitute an important defensive system that can be activated by the Fc regions of IgM and IgG antibodies in what is termed

TABLE 13.1 Functional properties of antibody classes and subclasses

	IgM	IgG1	IgG2	IgG3	IgG4	IgA1	IgE	IgD
Molecular weight (kDa)	970 (pentamer)	146	146	165	146	160 (monomer)	188	184
Adult serum level (mg/ml)	1.5	9	3	1	0.5	3	5×10^{-5}	0.04
Serum half-life (days)	10	21	20	7	21	6	2	3
Extra-vascular diffusion	±	+++	+++	+++	+++	++ (monomer)	+	+
Transport across epithelium	+	−	−	−	−	+++ (dimer)	−	++
Transport across placenta	−	+++	+	++	±	−	−	−
Neutralization	+	++	++	++	++	++	−	++
Binding to phagocytes	−	+++	±	++	+	+	−	+
Binding to NK cells	−	++	−	++	−	−	−	−
Binding to mast cells and basophils	−	−	−	−	−	−	+++	+
Classical complement pathway activation	+++	++	+	+++	−	−	−	−
Alternative complement pathway activation	−	−	−	−	−	+	−	−

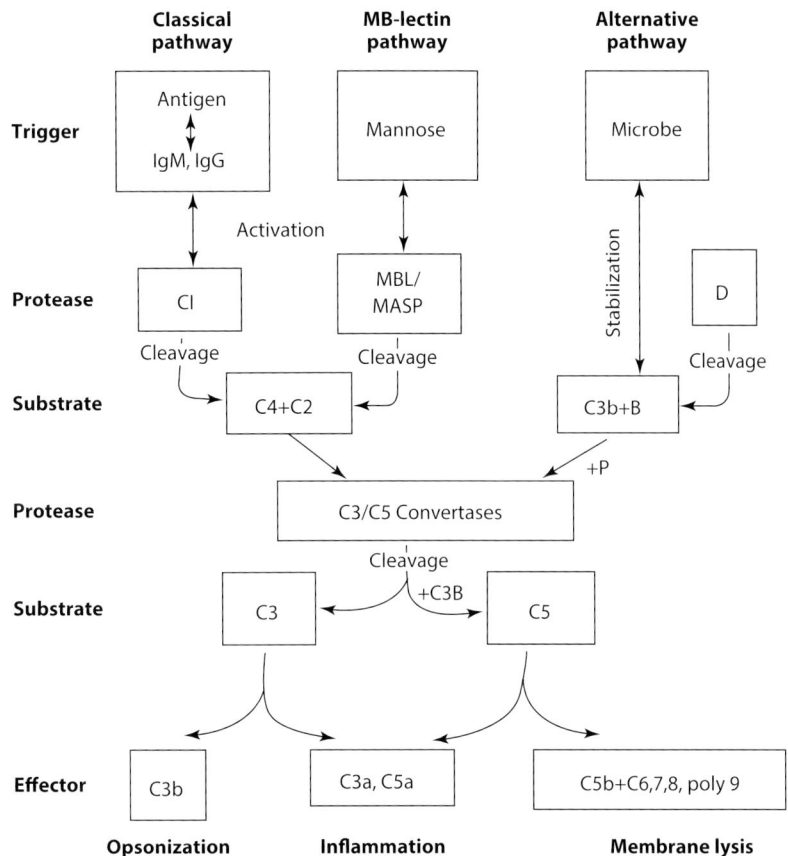

Figure 13.6 Complement activation pathways and effector functions. Ig, immunoglobulin; MASP, MBL-associated serine protease; MBL, mannan-binding lectin.

the classical pathway of complement activation. This is triggered when IgM or several IgG antibodies that are bound to antigen, interact with the complement C1 protein complex, resulting in the formation of a C3 convertase enzyme from C4 and C2 (C4b2a). This same C3 convertase can be generated when the pattern recognition molecule mannan-binding lectin (MBL) interacts with mannose residues of microbial surfaces. (MBL is a member of a family of secreted carbohydrate-binding collagenous defensive proteins called collectins.) A different C3 convertase is produced when certain complement proteins directly form a stable complex (C3bBbP) on microbial surfaces in what is termed the alternative pathway of complement activation. IgA can also activate the alternative pathway.

The conversion, or splitting, of complement protein C3 by the C3 convertase enzymes into fragments C3a and C3b is the central and crucial event during complement activation and generates a range of biological effects. Some of the C3b can be used to generate more of the alternative pathway C3 convertase; it also modifies the activity of the C3 convertase enzymes to split C5 into C5a and C5b. As mentioned in 'Innate and adaptive immunity' above, C3a and C5a activate mast cells and thus promote inflammation: they also attract and activate neutrophils (particularly C5a). The C5b fragment forms the membrane attack complex (MAC) with C6, C7, C8 and several molecules of C9: this last complement protein has structural and functional similarities to perforin and forms pores through lipid bilayers. Thus, the MAC has direct anti-microbial effects by disrupting microbial membranes. Finally, in addition to its other activities, C3b opsonizes (i.e. coats) infectious agents, which facilitates their interaction with leucocytes, as described below.

Digestive and inflammatory leucocytes

Some leucocytes have surface receptor proteins that bind to the Fc regions of antibodies (FcR), and others that bind to complement C3b (CR). As described above, the phagocytes (macrophages and neutrophils) express pattern-recognition molecules that enable them to bind microbes directly. However, they also possess FcR specific for IgG or IgA and CR that have particularly high affinities for their respective ligands. Thus, microbes such as bacteria can be firmly bound to the surface of phagocytes when opsonized by antibodies and C3b. This facilitates and activates phagocytosis (i.e. engulfing) of the microbes into membrane-bound cytoplasmic vesicles. The microbes can then be destroyed by lysosomal enzymes and reactive oxygen molecules.

Some microbes, such as the mycobacteria that cause tuberculosis and leprosy, are relatively resistant to the digestive activities of phagocytes and are able to survive and multiply within the cytoplasmic vesicles of macrophages. In this environment the microbes are protected from the activities of extra-cellular antibodies and complement proteins. The effective control of such infections is then dependent on the activity of Th1 cells that, as described in 'T cells and antigen presentation' above, produce the potent macrophage activating cytokine IFN-γ: this promotes macrophage digestive activity against microbes in intra-cellular vesicles (**Figure 13.5b**).

Other infective agents, particularly parasitic worms like schistosomes and helminths, are much too large to be engulfed for intra-cellular digestion by phagocytes. In such circumstances, eosinophils are recruited to undertake extra-cellular digestion by releasing their digestive proteins (e.g. major basic protein) onto the surface of the parasites. Eosinophils possess FcR (specific for IgG or IgE) and CR, and so again will bind most avidly to opsonized targets.

The other main cells that express FcR for IgE are the tissue mast cell and blood basophils, whose defensive roles are to promote inflammation, rather than directly destroying pathogens. These cells are activated when an antigen binds and cross-links several FcR-bound surface IgE molecules. This induces the immediate release of pre-formed inflammatory mediators, particularly histamine, that are stored in cytoplasmic granules. It also induces the *de novo* synthesis and later release of leukotrienes. (As mentioned above, mast cells are also activated by the complement peptides C3a and C5a.) Furthermore, IgD produced in the upper aerodigestive tract can bind to receptors expressed by basophils, mast cells, monocytes and neutrophils. Cross-linking of IgD antibodies on the surface of basophils by the antigens to which they bind promotes basophil activity in promoting both innate and adaptive immunity.

IMMUNITY TO CYTOSOLIC INFECTIOUS AGENTS

(See **Figure 13.5c**) Some infectious agents, such as viruses, actively infect cells by entering the fluid cytosol. Viruses are obliged to infect cells in order to use the machinery of the cells they enter in order to replicate themselves. Although antibodies and complement can neutralize viruses whilst they are outside cells, other immune mechanisms are required to interact with intra-cellular viruses.

An innate mechanism of anti-viral defence is the production and secretion of IFN-α and/or IFN-β by the infected cells. These type 1 interferons are structurally unrelated to the IFN-γ (type 2 interferon) that is produced by activated T cells and natural killer (NK) cells. Both types derive their name from their ability to *interfere* with viral replication. Type 1 interferons secreted by virally infected cells induce an anti-viral state in neighbouring non-infected cells by stimulating these cells to produce enzymes that block viral replication. In addition, type 1 interferons enhance MHC class I expression, which is necessary for Tc cell recognition of target cells, and they activate NK cells. Both these types of killer cells are important in the immune response to intra-cellular viruses as killing the infected cells inhibits viral replication and hence spread within the body. NK cells are the first killer cells to be activated, and they employ the same mechanisms of cytotoxicity as those described for Tc cells under the 'T cells and antigen presentation' above. However, unlike Tc, NK cells do not possess antigen-specific receptors; rather, they detect abnormalities in the expression of a cell's own surface molecules that may be indicative of the cell being virally infected. NK cells possess two types of receptors that interact with potential target cells: killer activating receptors; and killer inhibitory receptors, with the latter providing a dominant inhibitory signal that prevents NK cells from killing normal (uninfected) cells. The ligands for killer inhibitory receptors are often MHC class I molecules, whose expression may be reduced by viral infection of a cell: this makes the cell susceptible to the activity of NK cells because they then bind predominantly via their killer activating receptors. The ligands for some of the killer activating receptors are MHC class I-like molecules whose expression on target cells can be induced by infection, malignant transformation or other forms of cellular stress, thereby increasing the susceptibility of these cells to killing by NK cells.

NK cells also express FcR specific for IgG and so can interact with, and kill, target cells via antibodies that have bound to antigens expressed in the surface membranes of the target cells, as may happen during the process of budding by viruses. This is termed antibody-dependent cellular cytotoxicity (ADCC).

Interferons and NK cells are very important in limiting the replication and spread of a virus during the early stages of an infection, but may not be able to eliminate the infection. The adaptive Tc cells will take longer to be activated, as described under 'Stages of an immune response' above, but can then specifically and efficiently target the infected cells, as described under 'T cells and antigen presentation' above.

INFLAMMATION AND HYPERSENSITIVITY

Inflammatory processes are necessary to recruit components of the immune system to sites of infection. The importance of tissue mast cells as a source of inflammatory mediators has been discussed in previous sections, but many cell types can produce a range of inflammatory mediators, including cytokines and other proteins as well as other types of chemicals (e.g. prostaglandins and leukotrienes). A number of these have particular effects on the vessels that supply blood to infected tissues, promoting vasodilatation and increased vascular permeability, and enhancing endothelial expression of adhesion molecules (particularly selectins and integrins). The interaction of circulating leucocytes with the adhesion molecules facilitates their migration across the blood vessel walls and into the infected tissues in response to chemotactic factors.

In addition to localized inflammatory events within infected tissues, systemic effects are induced by cytokines that enter the blood stream, particularly IL-1, IL-6 and tumour necrosis factor (TNF). These have effects on the hypothalamus to induce fever, on the bone marrow to promote leucocyte release, and on the liver leading to the release of acute phase proteins: in particular the liver-derived pentraxins called C-reactive protein and serum amyloid P possess innate anti-microbial activities.

The enormous destructive potential of the immune system that is unleashed against invading microbes can be equally damaging to the body's own tissues. Thus, during every immune and inflammatory response, a balance must be struck between beneficial and tissue damaging effects. The immune system has evolved regulatory processes to limit the latter but, in some instances, immunological tissue damage becomes the main clinical feature, generating the problems of hypersensitivity.

Allergy and autoimmunity

Tissue damaging adaptive immune mechanisms can be triggered by foreign antigens or the body's own components. The former can be microbes, inducing the immune-mediated tissue damage associated with infective diseases, or can be inert (non-infective) materials that cause allergies. Up to 30% of the population is affected by allergies in developed countries, with a host of different allergens affecting different individuals (e.g. pollen, house dust mite, insect venom, food proteins, latex). Conversely, reactivity to self-components can lead to autoimmune diseases. Collectively, these affect over 3% of the population, with a much higher incidence of sub-clinical autoimmunity. In organ-specific autoimmunity, the stimulating autoantigens are restricted to particular tissues or organs, such as thyroid peroxidase and thyroglobulin in autoimmune thyroiditis, insulin and glutamate decarboxylase in type 1 diabetes mellitus. By contrast, systemic autoimmunity involves reactivity against widely spread tissue components, such as DNA, histones and ribonucleoproteins in systemic lupus erythematosus and IgG and citrullinated proteins in rheumatoid arthritis.

Mechanisms of hypersensitivity

Although allergic and autoimmune disorders differ in the nature of the stimulating antigens, they involve similar mechanisms of tissue damage, referred to as the four mechanisms of hypersensitivity (**Figure 13.7**).

> **Type I (immediate or reaginic) hypersensitivity** occurs in a variety of atopic allergies (**Figure 13.7**). It involves activation of tissue mast cells when an inducing allergen specifically binds to at least two IgE antibodies on the surface of mast cells. The IgE cross-linking induces the release of inflammatory mediators, as described under 'Digestive and inflammatory leucocytes' above, which induce vasodilatation, increased vascular permeability and smooth muscle contraction. For example, inhaled allergens that induce immediate mast cell activation commonly cause allergic rhinitis and extrinsic asthma. These conditions may be seasonal (eg. hay fever), or perennial in allergies to house dust mite and cat, for example. Severe systemic acute forms of type 1 hypersensitivity are seen in anaphylaxis (e.g. to nuts, insect stings, drugs).

> **Type II (cell or membrane reactive) hypersensitivity** involves antibodies of the IgG, IgA or IgM classes that bind to antigens associated with cell surface membranes or basement membranes (**Figure 13.7**). The antigen-bound antibodies then activate complement, which may damage the membranes directly via the membrane attack complex, but also attract and activate neutrophils via the actions of C5a and C3a. The release of digestive enzymes and reactive oxygen species by the neutrophils can then exacerbate the membrane damage. Bullous pemphigoid is an example of a disease involving antibodies to basement membrane antigens. By contrast, in pemphigus, autoantibodies bind to desmoglein in the epidermal intra-cellular cement, and clearly correlate with tissue damage. Goodpasture's syndrome is a further example of a disease where autoantibodies bind to basement membranes; in this case, the autoantigen is type IV collagen in alveolar and glomerular basement membranes, causing the typical haemoptysis and haematuria. The muscle weakness of myasthenia gravis is induced by autoantibodies to the acetylcholine receptors in the post-synaptic membranes of muscles: these antibodies induce complement-mediated damage, receptor internalization and blockade, leading to inhibition of neurotransmission by acetylcholine.

> **Type III (immune complex mediated) hypersensitivity,** like type II hypersensitivity, involves IgG, IgA and IgM antibodies, but in this case reacting with soluble antigens to form cross-linked molecular lattices containing multiple antibody and antigen molecules known as immune complexes (**Figure 13.7**). These complexes can become too large to remain soluble and so precipitate within tissues where they can activate complement and neutrophils, leading to tissue damage. Allergic immune complex disease is exemplified by extrinsic allergic alveolitis that is triggered by inhalation of allergens that form immune complexes in the alveolar walls leading to tissue damage and fibrosis. Common allergens are fungal spores (e.g. in farmer's lung) and avian plasma proteins (e.g. in bird fancier's lung). In systemic lupus erythematosus immune complex deposition can occur in various tissues, including the skin, joints, lungs, brain and kidneys: these complexes are frequently composed of DNA and anti-DNA antibodies, with contributions from other nuclear and cytoplasmic autoantigens.

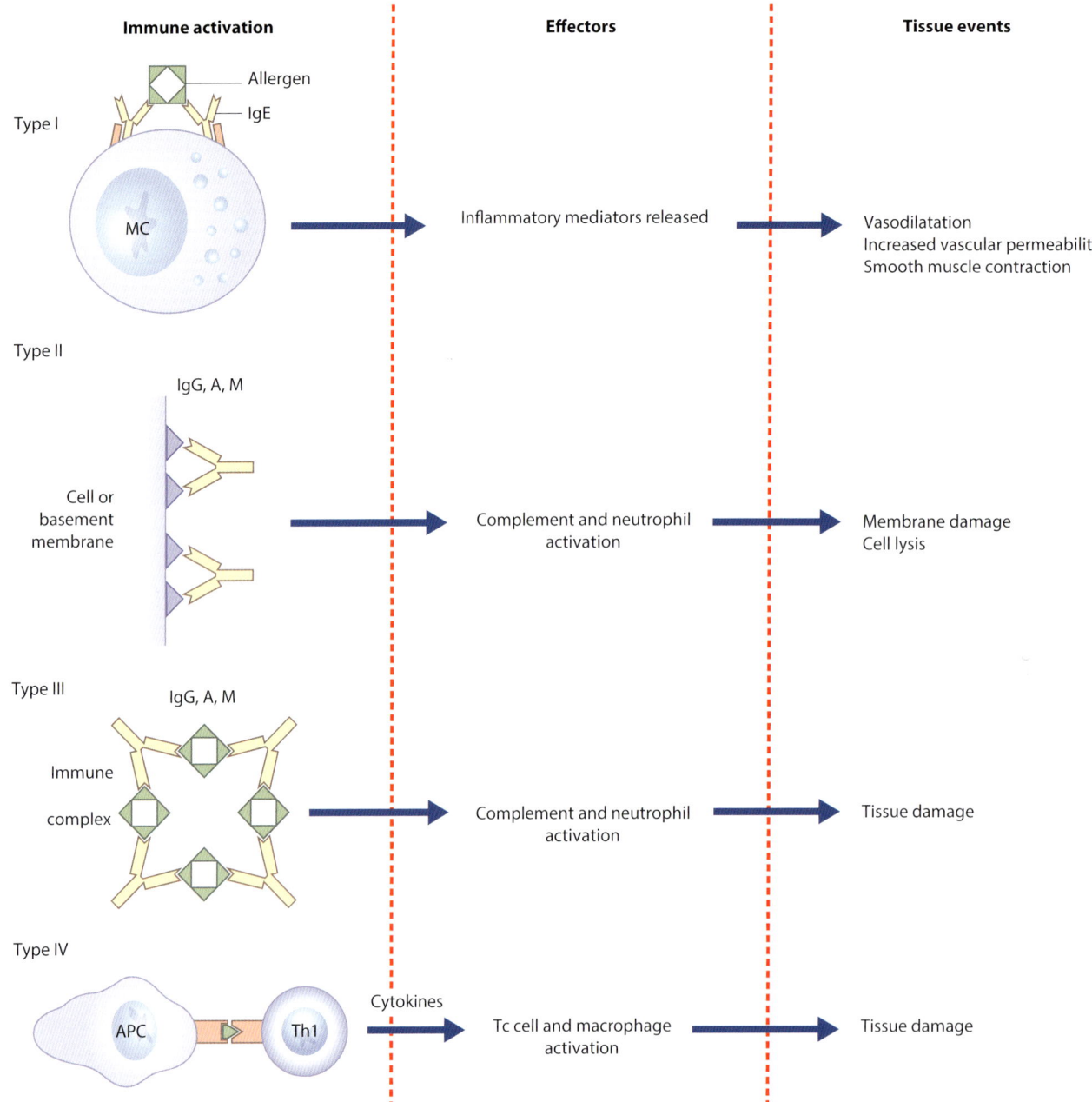

Figure 13.7 **Mechanisms of hypersensitivity.** (See text for details.) APC, antigen presenting cell; Ig, immunoglobulin; MC, mast cell; Th1, T helper 1 cell.

Type IV (cell-mediated) hypersensitivity is distinguished from the other three types by not involving antibodies. It is principally dependent on the activities of T cell and macrophages with Th1 cells producing cytokines like IL-2 and IFN-γ that activate cytotoxic T cells and macrophages, respectively (Figure 13.7). Much of the tissue damage in autoimmune diseases is brought about by cell-mediated mechanisms, although autoantibodies are also present (e.g. thyroiditis in the autoimmune thyroid diseases, insulitis in type 1 diabetes and synovitis in rheumatoid arthritis). Sjogren's syndrome is characterized by lymphocytic destruction of exocrine tissues, particularly the lacrimal and salivary glands, resulting in dry eyes and mouth. Much of the pathology associated with certain infectious diseases is also due to immune-mediated tissue damage. For example, in tuberculosis, infection of lung macrophages by *Mycobacterium tuberculosis* – which is resistant to intra-cellular digestion – leads to chronic T cell activation and cytokine production.

Despite the clinical problems of hypersensitivity diseases, the severe, persistent, unusual and recurrent infection problems associated with immunodeficiency disorders highlight the vital defensive role of the immune system.

KEY POINTS

- Immunity provides protection against pathogenic organisms, and the functions of the immune system are recognition of these foreign pathogens and defence of the body against them.
- Innate and adaptive immunity constitute the two main arms of the immune system which differ in their recognition and activation properties. Adaptive immunity improves with repeated exposure to the same antigens.
- The early innate response to infection stimulates an inflammatory response and initiates the processes that result in the adaptive lymphocyte response.
- Adaptive immunity involves the specific recognition of antigens by B and T lymphocytes.
- B-cell antigen receptors and antibodies can bind antigen in its native, unmodified form, recognizing accessible surface epitopes. In contrast, T-cell receptors recognize antigenic peptides bound to HLA molecules expressed on the surface of antigen-presenting cells or target cells; this requires processing (fragmentation) of the antigen, and epitopes may be derived from any part of the antigen.
- A typical immunoglobulin/antibody is composed of two identical heavy chains and two identical light chains. The amino-terminal variable domains of a heavy and a light chain form an antigen-combining site within one of the two Fab portions of the molecule. The Fc portion is composed of the heavy chain constant regions on the carboxy-terminal side of the hinge region.
- Cytotoxic function is associated with CD8+ T cells and HLA class I-associated antigen recognition. This facilitates T-cell recognition and killing of abnormal tissue cells.
- Helper function is associated with CD4+ T cells and HLA class II-associated antigen recognition. This facilitates T cell help by interaction with cells such as interdigitating dendritic cells, macrophages and B cells.
- Th1 and Th2 cells secrete cytokines that promote principally cell-mediated immunity and antibody-mediated immunity, respectively. Th17 cells promote inflammatory responses, whereas various types of Treg cells suppress Th cell-driven responses.
- Immunoglobulin isotypes (i.e. classes and subclasses) are defined by differences in their heavy chain constant regions. These determine their biological characteristics, e.g. complement activation, cellular association via Fc receptors and tissue distribution.
- Complement consists of several plasma proteins that operate as an enzyme cascade giving rise to various biological activities, including immune adherence, inflammation and membrane lysis.
- Macrophages and neutrophils are called phagocytes because of their ability to ingest and destroy microbes.
- Mast cells and basophils are activated by multivalent antigens cross-linking surface-bound IgE molecules; this induces the release of inflammatory mediators. Certain mast cell and basophil mediators are preformed and stored in granules (e.g. histamine) and are released immediately upon activation, whereas other mediators are synthesized *de novo* (e.g. leukotrienes and prostaglandins).
- There are two types of killer lymphocytes: cytotoxic T cells (Tc cells) and natural killer cells (NK cells). They are cytotoxic to target cells that have become infected or malignant.
- The immune system can cause inflammatory damage to the body's own tissues that may be triggered by infection, non-infective foreign antigens (in allergies), or the body's own autoantigens (in autoimmune disease).
- The mechanisms of immunologically mediated tissue damage are classified into four main types: Type I, IgE-mediated immediate hypersensitivity; Type II, antibody-mediated; Type III, immune complex-mediated, Type IV: T cell-mediated, DTH. More than one mechanism may operate in an inflammatory process.

FURTHER READING

Chapel H, Haeney M, Misbah S, Snowden N. *Essentials of clinical immunology*. 6th ed. Oxford: Wiley-Blackwell, 2014.

Male D, Brostoff J, Roth D, Roitt I. *Immunology*. 8th ed. Oxford: Elsevier; 2012.

Murphy K, Weaver C. *Janeway's immunobiology*. 9th ed. New York: Garland Science; 2016.

Todd I, Spickett G, Fairclough L. *Lecture notes: immunology*. 7th ed. Chichester: Wiley-Blackwell; 2014.

CHAPTER 14

ALLERGY: BASIC MECHANISMS AND TESTS

Sai H.K. Murng

Introduction 137
Aetiology of sensitization 137
Basic mechanisms 138
Tests in allergy diagnosis 143
References 148

SEARCH STRATEGY

Data in this chapter may be updated by PubMed and Ovidsp Medline searches using the keywords: allergy basic mechanisms, allergic rhinitis, anaphylaxis, skin prick tests, specific IgE, allergen component, basophil activation test, immunotherapy, mast cell signalling. The references of relevant articles were also checked. In addition, major immunology and allergy journals, and immunology textbooks were scanned. The evidence in this chapter is mainly levels 2/3 with some level 1 evidence. The clinical and laboratory recommendations are based on guidance from the UK and international professional associations, grade A and B.

INTRODUCTION

Allergy is defined as a hypersensitivity reaction initiated by specific immunologic mechanisms.[1] By a specific definition, it describes objectively reproducible symptoms or signs initiated by an exposure to a defined stimulus at a dose tolerated by normal persons.[1] *Hypersensitivity* is an altered immune response to an antigen that can cause damage. Immunologically four types of hypersensitivity reactions are generally recognized (**Table 14.1**).

An *allergen* is an antigen (usually protein) that causes allergic diseases. Allergic airway diseases including rhinitis are due to inhaled allergens (**Table 14.2**). *Atopy* is a tendency to become sensitized and produce allergen-specific immunoglobulin E (sIgE) in response to ordinary exposures to allergens. Clinically this is demonstrated by positive skin prick tests and/or increased serum sIgE concentration to one or more allergens. Not all sensitized individuals are symptomatic. Therefore allergy is a disease manifestation of sensitization.

We will consider the basic mechanism of allergy initially in which an individual is predisposed to allergy by sensitization to allergens. Then we will consider the immunological process involved in some allergic diseases and the effect of treatment including current understanding of specific allergen immunotherapy. Finally the principles of diagnostic tests will be considered.

AETIOLOGY OF SENSITIZATION

Type 1 immunoglobulin E (IgE) mediated immediate hypersensitivity occurs only in a sensitized individual. Immune responses to innocuous antigens leading to sensitization are multi-factorial. In general these include host factors such as genetic predisposition and environmental factors such as pollution.

Up to 40% of the population in the industrialized countries have been reported to have a tendency to atopy. An atopic person usually has a high total IgE level, a strong familial tendency and increased susceptibility to allergic diseases such as allergic rhinitis and atopic dermatitis. Many genetic loci have been shown to be associated with allergic diseases. These include chromosome 11q12-13 (encodes β subunit of high-affinity IgE receptor) and chromosome 5 (encodes Th2 promoting cytokines such as IL4, TIM gene family that regulates Th1/Th2 balance, p40 subunit of IL12, β2 adrenergic receptor). Polymorphism in these genes altered disease susceptibility of a person to allergic diseases. Another inherited variation seen in IgE response to specific antigen is human major histocompatibility complex (MHC) class II region (e.g. HLA DRB1*1501 in ragweed pollen sensitization). Therefore an allergic individual can be associated with both general tendency and allergen-specific predisposition to develop a stronger Th2 response than their normal counterpart.

TABLE 14.1 Types of hypersensitivity (adapted from Coombs and Gell Classification)

Features	Type I	Type II	Type III	Type IV
Mechanism	Immediate hypersensitivity	Cytotoxic hypersensitivity	Immune complex reaction	Cell-mediated hypersensitivity
Immune reactant	IgE	IgG	IgG	T cell
Effectors	Mast cells, basophils, eosinophils	Complement, phagocytes	Complement, phagocytes	Macrophages
Disease examples	Allergic rhinitis	Haemolytic anaemia	Serum sickness, SLE	Contact dermatitis

TABLE 14.2 Inhaled allergens

Seasonal	Perennial	Occupational
Grass, trees	House dust mites	Laboratory animals, flour, latex
Weeds	Cats, dogs	Colophony, isocyanates
Moulds	Horses	Acid anhydrides

Environmental factors such as exposure to infectious diseases in early childhood, environmental pollution and dietary changes also contribute to allergic diseases. *Hygiene hypothesis* has been one of the well-known discussions since 1989. Early life exposure to infectious diseases has been shown in mice models as being associated with promoting Th1 rather than Th2 response. Th1 response is proinflammatory and responsible for killing intracellular pathogens and for perpetuating autoimmune responses. Th2 response is not only essential in defence against pathogens such as helminths (e.g. hookworm) but also promotes allergic conditions. Therefore the prevalence of allergic diseases is higher in children who grew up in a hygienic environment (e.g. industrialized Western countries) than in less hygienic regions where infectious diseases are more common.

A *counter-regulation hypothesis* has proposed that regulatory cytokines (e.g. IL10, TGF-β) are upregulated in the presence of infection. As a result atopy is less common despite Th2 response being predominant in infections. In addition proinflammatory cytokines (e.g. interferon-γ) resulting from infection also stimulate dendritic cells (DC) to suppress Th2 inflammation and promote regulatory cytokines.

Regulatory T cells are also considered to have an important role in allergic diseases. This has been supported by a FoxP3 deficient mice model that develops manifestations seen in allergic conditions such as eosinophilia, increased IgE level and allergic airway inflammation suggesting Treg (CD4+CD25+) cell deficiency can predispose to this phenotype.

BASIC MECHANISMS

Mast cells and basophils are the principle effector cells that produce mediators (**Table 14.3**) responsible for allergic diseases. IgE mediated immediate allergy can be associated with early and late responses. The early phase is due to preformed mediators release (e.g. anaphylaxis). The late phase is due to newly synthesized mediators and infiltration of other leucocytes that can be followed by a chronic allergic inflammation in some conditions (e.g. allergic asthma). Late phase response involves Th2 cytokines resulting in activation of eosinophils and other leucocytes. Chronic allergic inflammation is characterized by tissue destruction and remodelling and is essentially type IV hypersensitivity in nature.

Effectors of allergic diseases

The essential effector cells of immediate hypersensitivity are cells expressing high affinity IgE receptors (FcεRI) such as mast cells, basophils and eosinophils. Other effectors include antigen presenting cells (e.g. dendritic cells) and Th2 cells that promote allergen-specific IgE synthesis by B cells.

MAST CELLS

Mast cells are haemopoietic stem cell derivatives and mature locally. They reside near the surface where our body is exposed to pathogens and allergens. Based on the distribution they are known as either mucosal mast cells or tissue mast cells. They are often found in close proximity to blood vessels. FcεRI is capable of being tightly bound to sIgE even in the presence of a very low serum concentration. On exposure to their specific allergens, cross-linking of the receptor and signalling follow to produce clinical phenomena (**Figure 14.1**). FcεRII is a low affinity IgE receptor (CD23). It is present in many cells including B cells, activated T cells, monocytes, eosinophils, platelet and follicular dendritic cells. The role of FcεRII in an allergic reaction is not fully understood.

Mast cells granules contain preformed mediators that are responsible for the immediate symptoms of allergic reactions. Mast cells also produce other mediators upon FcεRI signalling. Mediators that are rapidly synthesized are involved in the immediate symptoms of allergic reactions. Other mediators may lead to late phase responses and chronic allergic inflammation (**Table 14.4**).

BASOPHILS

Basophils develop from bone marrow granulocyte-monocyte progenitor. There is increasing evidence that basophils involve significantly in allergic diseases. They respond to many stimuli including cytokines, antibodies, proteases and antigens. Cross-linking of IgE bound FcεRI receptors on basophils have been shown to produce mediators (**Table 14.4**). Basophils have been identified in nasal washes of patients with allergic rhinitis.

TABLE 14.3 Physiologic actions of mediators	
Types of mediator	Effects
Enzymes: • tryptase, chymase, carboxypeptidase A • eosinophil peroxidase • eosinophil collagenase • matrix proteinase	– tissue destruction – toxic to target, histamine release from mast cells – connective tissue remodelling – matrix protein degradation
Eosinophil major basic protein	– toxic to parasite, histamine release form mast cells
Proteoglycans - histamine, heparin	– increase vascular permeability, smooth muscle contraction
Cytokines: • TNF-α • IL4, IL13 • IL3, IL5 • TGF-α, TGF-β	– promote inflammation – amplify Th2 response – activate eosinophil – epithelial proliferation and myofibroblast formation
Chemokines: CCL3, CXCL8	– influx of leucocytes
Platelet-activating factor (PAF)	– attracts leucocytes and increases lipid mediators production
Arachidonic acid metabolites: • prostaglandins D2 (PgD2), leucotrienes C4 (LtC4)	– smooth muscle contraction and increase vascular permeability

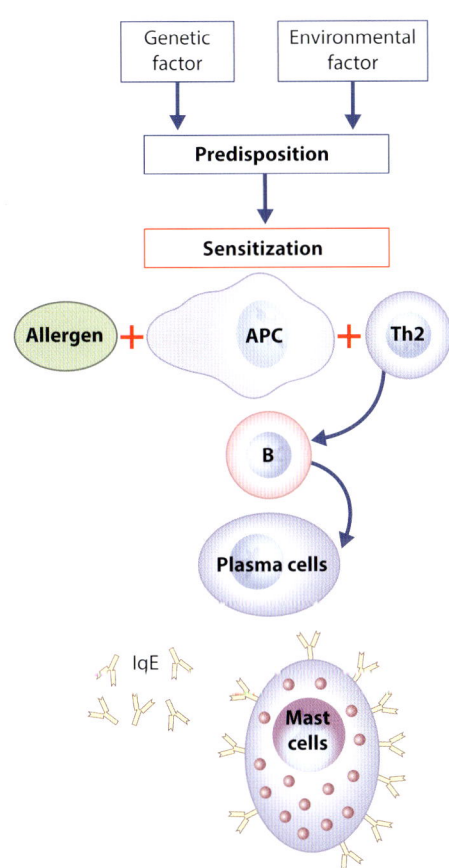

Figure 14.1 Development of sensitization.

EOSINOPHILS

Eosinophils are granular leucocytes that mainly reside in submucosal connective tissue in respiratory, gastrointestinal and urogenital tracts. They play an essential role in defence against helminths. Eosinophils also express FcεRI receptors and are capable of releasing mediators (Table 14.4).

T LYMPHOCYTES

T cells are central to the pathogenesis of allergic diseases since they are the only cells capable of recognizing antigens presented by antigen presenting cells. Maturation of a naive T cell takes place on activation by signals including specific peptide-MHC via T cell receptor and costimulatory signal via CD28. T helper cells (CD3+CD4+) differentiated into many types depending upon the type of immune response taking place and cytokine environment. Th1 cells differentiate in the presence of interferon gamma (IFN-γ) and IL-12, and produce predominantly IFN-γ and interleukin 2 (IL-2). Th2 cells differentiate in the presence of IL-4 and produce IL-4, IL-5 and IL-13 cytokines preferentially. Recruitment of Th2 cells, their activation in tissues and generation of Th2 cytokines are main features of both allergic rhinitis and asthma. Low dose antigen exposure via mucosal surface with inhaled allergen is typical of Th2 response in allergic rhinitis, where as high dose allergen delivered by injection favour Th1 response.

DENDRITIC CELLS

Dendritic cells are professional antigen presenting cells (APC), which are abundant in the epithelium and submucosa of both upper and lower respiratory mucosa in patients with allergic diseases. Traditionally dendritic cells have been classified as myeloid derived DC1 cells (derived from human blood monocytes) or DC2, plasmacytoid cells (derived from lymphoid cells). DC1 cells produce a high level of IL-12 and favour Th1 development. DC2 cells are low IL-12 producers and support preferential Th2 differentiation. However, in dendritic cells subpopulations, differential function may depend on their location, their degree of maturation and local cytokines milieu.

Immature cells express high levels of immunoglobulin receptors and are highly endocytic in keeping with

TABLE 14.4 Mediators of effector cells			
Types of mediator	Mast cells	Basophils	Eosinophils
Preformed mediators	tryptase, chymase, carboxypeptidase A, histamine, heparin, TNF-α	histamine, TNF-α	eosinophil peroxidase, eosinophil collagenase, matrix proteinase, eosinophilic cationic protein
Newly synthesized cytokines and lipid mediators	IL4, IL13, TNF-α, IL3, IL5, PAF, PgD2, LtC4	IL4, IL13, PAF, LtC4	IL3, IL5, TGF-α, TGF-β, LtC4, PAF

efficient antigen capture. In contrast, mature cells express high levels of MHC class II and have upregulated CD86 expression and produce abundant cytokines, features consistent with their role in allergen presentation and immune modulation. Rapid maturation (within 2 hours) was observed in dendritic cells within the bronchial wall and not peripheral lung. Rapid dendritic cells recruitment to the bronchial mucosa in atopic asthmatic patients has also been observed within the time frame of late asthmatic responses following local segmental allergen challenge. Plasmacytoid dendritic cells (CD123) IL-3R α-chain+CD45RA+ cells increase dramatically in number following local allergen challenge repeatedly for 7 days. This is of particular interest since plasmacytoid dendritic cells matured *in vitro* can induce preferential Th2 development.

IMMUNOGLOBULIN E (IGE)

IgE concentration is the lowest immunoglobulin isotype (approximately 100–400 ng/mL) in human serum. The majority of IgE is tissue-bound with a half-life of approximately 2 days. FcεRI is a high affinity receptor for IgE, which is mainly present on mast cells, basophils and eosinophils. But low-level expressions are detected in dendritic cells, monocytes, and macrophages that are in different molecular structures. Their significance remains uncertain. IgE also bind to a low affinity receptor FcεRII (CD23) on B cells, monocytes and macrophages.

IgE is developed from isotype switching of IgM. B cells secrete IgM following antigen recognition (**Figure 14.2**). Isotype switching is influenced by specific Th2 cells and the cytokine environment. IgE production is favoured by IL-4 and Il-13 derived from Th2 cells. It is also perpetuated by IL-4 and IL-13 from mediator release as a result of degranulation in allergic reaction. IgE production generally occurs in the bone marrow and the draining regional lymph nodes. But local IgE production has been reported in local forms of allergic conditions (e.g. allergic rhinitis). Local IgE synthesis has been considered as the cause in some situations – allergic symptoms without sensitization on skin prick test and increased sIgE; some atopic individuals develop rhinitis whereas other develop asthma or eczema, and others may have sensitization without any clinical manifestation.

HISTAMINE

Histamine is generated from histidine decarboxylase and stored in granules of mast cells and basophils. Elevated

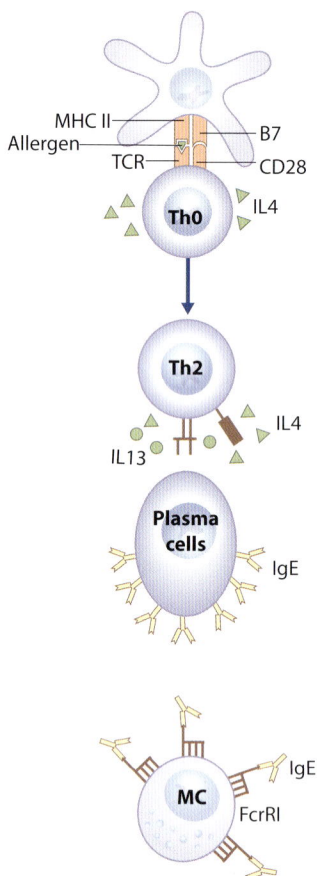

Figure 14.2 Th2 development and IgE production. APC, antigen presenting cell; MC, mast cell.

histamine levels correlate well and indicate higher sensitivity than tryptase in anaphylaxis. Tryptase level is elevated in 60% whereas histamine and PAF are elevated in 70% and 100% respectively in anaphylaxis.[2] However, histamine is highly soluble and rapidly diffuses away after the release. The majority of histamine is metabolized within minutes of release by many enzymes such as histamine N-methyl transferase, monoamine oxidase and diamine oxidase. The short plasma half-life and sample handling issue are major limiting factors for histamine measurement in routine laboratory use. Urinary metabolites (N-methyl histamine) can be detected several hours after anaphylaxis. But there are potential confounding factors for this measurement such as the effect of histamine producing bacteria, histamine containing foods and so on. In scombroidosis, the urinary histamine level can be increased despite a normal serum tryptase level.

SERUM TRYPTASE

Tryptase is produced by mast cells and basophils. In humans, tryptase exists in two isotypes (alpha and beta), which are in two forms – mature and immature. Beta tryptase is the predominant isotype in mast cells. Protryptase is the immature form and is spontaneously secreted by unstimulated mast cells. Mature tryptase is stored in the intracellular granules and released on degranulation. Therefore it is normally undetectable. The normal reference range of total tryptase is 1–13 ng/mL in our laboratory. The total tryptase levels peak 30–60 minutes after the onset of symptoms due to degranulation, and reduce afterwards with a half-life of about 2 hours. Tryptase levels can be measured in both serum and plasma but in a sample left at room temperature for more than 1–2 days may give falsely low values.

Normal tryptase levels do not exclude anaphylaxis. Other causes of increase tryptase levels include mastocytosis, acute myelocytic leukaemia, myelodysplastic syndrome and the myeloid varaints of hypereosinophilic syndrome. Elevated total tryptase has also been reported in some conditions such as onchocerciasis treatment and administration of recombinant stem cell factor.

There are two mechanisms leading to mediators release in mast cells and basophils. The FcɛRI signalling as a result of the sIgE-antigen complex is the underlying mechanism in the IgE mediated hypersensitivity. However, mediator release can also occur by other factors that are capable of IgE independent direct stimulation. These include viral proteins (e.g. HIV gp120), bacterail proteins (e.g. LPS), drugs (e.g. opiate), chemical and physical stimuli, complement activation and neuropeptides, cytokines and so on.

High affinity receptor (FcɛRI) signalling in allergic reaction

Allergic reactions are overlapping and synergistic physiological effects resulting from mediators release due to the activation of mast cells and basophils through a mechanism generally understood to involve FcɛRI signalling. This signalling has been extensively investigated using passive cutaneous and passive systemic anaphylaxis models.[3]

Unlike other immunoglobulin isotypes, the majority of IgE is tightly bound to FcɛRI. There is no signalling until these receptors are cross-linked by their specific antigens. The high level of IgE has potential to enhance IgE dependent effector function. FcɛRI is a tetrameric receptor consisting of three subunits: a IgE binding unit (α chain); a signal transducing unit (β chain); and two signal regulator units (γ chain).

Allergen–sIgE binding is followed by early signalling events including phophorylation of cytosolic domains of the receptor known as immunoreceptor tyrosine-based activation motif (ITAM). This phophorylation is mediated by Src family proteins. There are two types of Src family protein in these events, namely signal-initiating kinase (Lyn) and signal-propagating kinase (Syk). This is followed by the recruitment of many signalling proteins to form multi-molecular signalling complexes. The downstream effect of this signalling results in an activation of protein kinase C and liberation of intracellular calcium. These lead to degranulation within minutes. In addition eicosanoid generation and activation of transcription factors for the production of cytokines and other mediators of allergic reaction follow within hours (**Figure 14.2**).

ROLES OF SENSORY NERVES

Activation of sensory nerves is an important mechanism in rhinitis in many ways. These include generation of acute rhinitis symptoms, nasal hyper-reactivity to non-specific triggers, release of neuropeptides such as substance 'p' and neurokinin from inflamed sensory nerves. Neurogenic inflammation is self-perpetuating and represents an important component of the allergen-IgE interaction. Nerve growth factor can be detected in nasal fluids in chronic allergic rhinitis. It is increased after allergen challenge. Therefore immediate response is due to a complex interaction between mediators release and target organs such as the sensory nerve, the vasculature and mucus secreting glands. Hyper-responsiveness of target organs associated with late response and day-to-day allergic disease is likely to relate to a combination of both inflammation and increased sensory nerve activation. The contribution of these components varies in different individuals.

Clinical features of IgE mediated hypersensitivity[4-6]

The American College of Allergy, Asthma and Immunology Epidemiology of Anaphylaxis Working Group has estimated that a lifetime prevalence of anaphylaxis is 0.05–2.0%. The clinical features of allergic reactions are the effects of mediator release and may involve many systems. Most commonly, these include cutaneous, respiratory, cardiac and gastrointestinal systems (**Table 14.5**).

The onset of immediate allergy depends on the route of exposure to an allergen but it is usually within minutes. An anaphylaxis due to intravenous allergen (e.g. drug) occurs within seconds. Electrocardiographic abnormalities such as T inversion, supraventricular arrhythmias and bundle branch blocks have been reported in anaphylactic reactions during anaesthesia. In general an immediate allergy develops within 60 minutes of allergen challenge. Myocardial infarctions following anaphylaxis have also been reported. The late-phase reactions (LPR) have been described in respiratory and cutaneous allergy. Biphasic reaction patterns have been reported when both immediate and LPR have occurred.

Post-mortem finding of fatal anaphylaxis often shows few pathologic changes but may reveal oedematous obstruction of the airways, laryngeal oedema, pulmonary hyperinflation, pulmonary oedema, eosinophilic infiltration around the bronchi, and swelling of liver, spleen and intestine.

LOCAL ALLERGIC RHINITIS[8]

Local allergic rhinitis (LAR) has been described as a localized nasal allergic response. In contrast to generally

TABLE 14.5 Clinical features of immediate allergy (adapted from Ring and Messmer[7])

System	Manifestations
Prodromal	– feeling of anxiety, paresthetic sensations on palms and soles
Cutaneous	– pruritus, flush, urticaria, or angioedema
Respiratory	– sneezing, rhinorrhea, dyspnoea due to laryngeal obstruction or bronchospasm, hoarseness, feeling of 'tight throat', cough or wheezing, cyanosis and respiratory arrest
Cardiac	– early tachycardia, changes in blood pressure (sometimes an initial rise, followed by hypotension), arrhythmia, shock, cardiac arrest
Gastrointestinal	– nausea and cramping (uterine cramps may also occur), vomiting, diarrhoea, urination
Non-specific	– sweating, headache and disorientation

Severity grading of an allergic reaction

Severity	Cutaneous	Cardiac	Respiratory	Abdominal
Grade 1	Urticaria, flushing, angioedema			
Grade 2	Urticaria, flushing, angioedema	Tachycardia, blood pressure change (>20 mmHg systolic)	Rhinorrhoea, hoarseness, breathlessness	Nausea
Grade 3	Urticaria, flushing, angioedema	Shock	Laryngeal oedema, wheezing, cyanosis	Nausea, vomiting, diarrhoea
Grade 4	Urticaria, flushing, angioedema	Cardiac arrest	Respiratory arrest	Nausea, vomiting, diarrhoea

known allergic rhinitis (AR), allergic sensitizations are not detectable by serum-specific IgE or skin testing in LAR. LAR is usually diagnosed by a positive nasal allergen provocation test (NAPT). Many patients previously diagnosed with non-allergic rhinitis are now being classified as having LAR. In one of the Spanish cohort, LAR accounts for 15% of all cases of rhinitis.

A local specific IgE production in the nasal mucosa with a TH2 inflammatory pattern response has been considered as a pathophysiologic mechanism in LAR. A proportion of patients with LAR have detectable basal aeroallergen sIgE (e.g. house dust mite, cat, dog, grass etc.) in their nasal secretion. These sIgE levels rapidly increase after NAPT in 22% of LAR with perennial symptoms and 35% of those with seasonal symptoms. Measurement of nasal sIgE in LAR has a high specificity but low sensitivity (up to 40%). Clinically patients with LAR often present with typical symptoms of AR including ocular symptoms and good response to oral antihistamine and nasal corticosteroid.

RHINITIS AND ASTHMA LINK

The link between rhinitis and asthma has been highlighted in a World Health Organization report, *Allergic rhinitis and its impact on asthma* (ARIA).[9] Approximately 30% of patients with rhinitis develop asthma and up to 80% of patients with perennial asthma have rhinitis. However, the causal link between these conditions is not fully understood (Table 14.6).

It is important to recognize and treat asthma in patients presenting with allergic rhinitis. Airflow obstruction should be assessed in an ENT clinic including using peak expiratory flow, spirometry and reversibility testing. If these are unavailable, patients should be referred to a respiratory physician.

Basic mechanisms of treatment of allergic diseases

The majority of current drug treatments for allergic diseases are symptomatic therapies targeting the mediators (e.g. antihistamines and adrenaline) or general immunosuppressive drugs (e.g. corticosteroids). New approaches are now developing to modify the pathogenesis of allergy. The most promising is specific allergen immunotherapy such as pollen desensitization for seasonal allergic rhinitis.

Antihistamines act through histamine H1 receptors. They are effective in the partial suppression of immediate allergic responses in the skin and respiratory tract in AR. However, they have little or no effect in late response in allergic asthma and bronchial asthma.

Corticosteroids bind to intracellular receptors, leading to an anti-inflammatory effect due to alteration in transcription factors. Allergen-induced Th2 proliferation and cytokines secretion are exquisitely sensitive to corticosteroids in low 10^{-10} to 10^{-8} molar concentration. They also act on membrane receptors that lead to non-genetic mechanism, resulting in more rapid action. Corticosteroid has no effect on immediate response but is highly effective in inhibiting allergen-induced late response and bronchial asthma. The topical steroid effects of corticosteroid have been extensively studied in AR. These can be summarized as follows:

- Reduction of inflammatory mediators such as cytokines, prostaglandins, nitric oxide
- Inhibition of inflammatory cells migration by inhibiting the expression of adhesion molecules
- Promotion of apoptosis of leucocytes due to upregulation of endonucleases.

TABLE 14.6 Features of allergic rhinitis and asthma		
Features	Similarities	Differences
Anatomical features	Pseudostratified epithelium	• Prominent erectile venous sinusoids and submucosal glands in the nose • Disruption of epithelium with thickening of the sub-basement membrane zone in asthma but intact epithelium with normal basement membrane zone in rhinitis • Airway smooth muscles are present in bronchi and increase in asthma
Pathogenesis	Th2 driven inflammation	Airway remodelling in chronic asthma
Treatment response	Corticosteroid, antileukotriene, anticholinergic	Selective effectiveness of antihistamine in rhinitis and β2 agonists in asthma

Allergen-specific immunotherapy is the only curative approach for allergic rhinitis, allergic asthma and venom allergy. This involves a step-wise administration of increasing doses of an allergen, in order to suppress symptoms on subsequent re-exposure to that allergen. Allergen-specific immunotherapy has been reported to be highly effective in allergic rhinitis in a Cochrane systematic review.[10]

Subcutaneous immunotherapy (SCIT) has an earlier onset of the therapeutic effect than sublingual immunotherapy (SLIT) in seasonal allergic rhinitis. Both have been shown to give long-lasting benefit after stopping treatment. Alternative methods of administration of allergen have been used in smaller cohort to improve the uptake and reduce the side effects. These include nasal immunotherapy, epicutaneous immunotherapy, intra-lymphatic immunotherapy and oral immunotherapy.

The precise mechanism of allergen-specific immunotherapy is being elucidated. Current understanding is based on evaluating benefits and immunological changes following the immunotherapy.[11–13] These can be summarized as follows:

- Inhibition of mediators release due to rapid desensitization of mast cells and basophils by allergens. The exact molecular pathway is not well understood. However, the susceptibility of these cells to degranulation decreases but the subsequent threshold for activation increases. Upregulation of histamine receptor expression on basophils were observed in venom immunotherapy. Rapid upregulation of histamine receptor strongly suppresses FcεRI induced activation of basophils
- Upregulation of blocking specific IgG4 antibodies that reduce the antigen presentation by the relevant cell types as a result of binding to epitopes on the surface of the allergen
- Inhibition of IgE-facilitated antigen presentation due to immunotherapy-induced specific IgG antibodies and subsequent reduction in the activation and proliferation of allergen-specific T-cells that are responsible for the production of cytokines (IL-4, IL-13) and further IgE synthesis
- Skewing effector cells towards regulatory phenotypes due to induction of T-reg and B-reg cells. Numbers of tissue mast cells and eosinophils, and subsequent mediators release decrease.

The clinical effects of immunotherapy have been shown in many studies. It induces an early and further reduction in symptoms/need for medication and reduction in hyper-responsiveness that persist after the end of the treatment period. It has been proposed as a prevention of new sensitivities and progression of disease (e.g. rhinitis into asthma). Therefore immunotherapy has been considered as a potentially curative treatment in allergic rhinitis due to its immunomodulatory effect.

A subcutaneous anti-IgE antibody (omalizumab) has been shown to be effective in a proportion of patients with severe perennial allergic asthma and in seasonal allergic rhinitis. Other therapies such as anti-CD23 monoclonal antibody (IDEC-152) and CCR3 targeted therapy have not been proved with clinical significance so far.

New knowledge arises for more targeted strategies in AR that inhibits Th2 cytokines IL4 and IL5 to prevent the activation of B cells from producing IgE. IL4 induces B cell class switching, upregulates IgE receptors on mast cells, increases VCAM-1 expression on vascular endothelium, induces mucus secretion and promotes Th2 polarization. In a small study, using an inhaled soluble IL-4 receptor during the withdrawal of inhaled corticosteroids has been shown to be effective in preventing relapse in moderately severe atopic asthma.

IL5 is a major factor responsible for terminal differentiation of eosinophils. Inhaled IL5 induces airway hyper-responsiveness and sputum eosinophila. Anti-IL5 blocking monoclonal antibody was effective in reducing allergen-induced eosinophila and deposition of extracellular matrix proteins in the bronchial subepithelial basement membrane zone in patients with mild asthma.

TESTS IN ALLERGY DIAGNOSIS

Allergy diagnosis includes an assessment of clinical presentations followed by *in vivo* and/or *in vitro* tests to identify the culprit allergen responsible for the immunologic mechanism of immediate hypersensitivity. Demonstration of sensitization to a suspected allergen (i.e. the presence of allergen-specific IgE) is required for the diagnosis. But not all sensitized individuals are clinically allergic. Therefore confirmation of allergy diagnosis requires either a convincing relevant history or a reproducible allergic phenomenon by a 'controlled challenge test' (provocation test). Hence, 'challenge test' is accepted as the gold standard test in allergy diagnosis.

Skin testing

Skin testing is a bioassay. When specific allergens are introduced into the skin, cross-linking of the FcεRI occurs if allergen-specific IgEs are present in sufficient quantities on the cutaneous mast cells. Transient wheal and flare responses develop as a result of mast cell activation and mediators release. These represent the immediate phase of the allergic reaction. However, the size of the wheal does not directly correlate with the amount of histamine released. In some individuals deep tissue swellings with warmth, pruritus and erythema at skin test sites may develop 1 to 2 hours after testing and resolve in 24 to 48 hours (late phase responses). But they are not used in allergy diagnosis.

Skin testing is widely used in the diagnosis of a variety of IgE-mediated allergies (Table 14.7). The performance of skin testing in allergy diagnosis is influenced by many factors (Table 14.8). Skin testing and interpretation require specific training and knowledge. The diagnostic utility of skin testing depends on the pre-test probability. It should be performed by an allergy expert, because there is a small but definite risk of a systemic allergic reaction.

The two major methods of skin testing currently in use are the skin prick test (SPT) and the intra-dermal test (IDT). SPT is the most appropriate initial test with overall positive predictive value (PPV) of less than 50% for all allergens but negative predictive value (NPV) is very high (≥95%) (Table 14.9). IDT has much higher sensitivity (100–1000 folds) but lower specificity with a greater risk of a systemic reaction. IDT should only be performed after a negative SPT.

Skin prick test

After cleaning with a 70% alcohol solution, 1:10 or 1:20 weight/volume allergen extract solutions are placed at least 2 cm apart on the volar surface of the forearm or upper back. A separate commercially available test device (lancet) is used to prick through each droplet of allergen.

TABLE 14.7 Indications, cautions and contraindications of skin testing

Indications	Notes
1. Aeroallergy (e.g. rhinitis, allergic asthma)	Well validated
2. Food allergy (e.g. nut, milk, egg)	Well validated
3. Drug allergy (e.g. penicillin)	Often used in the evaluation of many other drugs including antibiotics, chemotherapeutic agents and anaesthetic drugs but the significance of results are less well defined
4. Venom allergy (e.g. wasp, bee)	The diagnostic test of choice; well-validated
5. Latex allergy	The diagnostic test of choice when using standardized test preparations
Cautions and contraindications	**Notes**
1. High risk patients	Poorly controlled asthma, clinical histories of severe reactions to minute amounts of allergen, significant cardiovascular diseases such as coronary heart disease, cardiac arrhythmias
2. Recent anaphylaxis	The skin can render temporarily non-reactive after anaphylaxis for 2 to 4 weeks
3. Interfering medications	Recent antihistamine use
4. Unsuitable skin conditions	Dermatographism, urticaria, dermatitis, cutaneous mastocytosis

TABLE 14.8 Factors affecting results of skin testing

Factors	Notes
Medications	Many drugs can interfere with skin testing and should be stopped prior to skin testing: • Antihistamine – stop 3 days for non-selective short acting, 7 days for long acting (e.g. Cetirizine) • H2 receptor antagonists – stop 48 hours • chronic and relatively high dose systemic corticosteroids (>20 mg/day) may partially suppress skin testing • omalizumab may depress skin reactivity for up to 6 months or longer • tricyclic antidepressants, phenothiazines may decrease skin reactivity for up to 2 weeks • other drugs may affect skin testing – some muscle relaxants and antiemetic drugs with antihistamine action.
Physiologic factors	Extreme age may reduce skin reactivity. Forearms produce smaller wheals than the skin of the back.
Technical factors	The quality of allergenic extracts, testing devices, and techniques: • the major inhalant allergens are well characterized and standardized, except for moulds • although extracts of milk, eggs, peanuts, soy, fish, shellfish, and tree nuts are reliable, most commercially available food extracts are not standardized (e.g. commercial extracts of fruits and vegetables).
Allergen preparation	Allergen extracts used in current clinical practice are obtained mainly from natural sources. There is immense variability in the commercial preparation of these products – season, growth conditions, genetic differences between geographic regions, etc.

TABLE 14.9 Reported diagnostic values of SPT[14]		
Preparation	Wheal mm	PPV %
HDM	≥3	95
Peanut	≥8	95
Egg	≥4	95
Grass	≥3	80
Hazel	≥4	80
Dog	≥10	80
Cat	≥7	80
Birch	≥3	80
Cladosporium	≥7	80
Alternaria	≥8	80

PPV = positive predictive value.

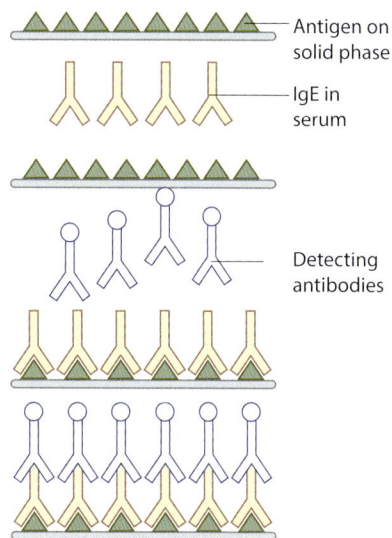

Figure 14.3 Enzyme immunoassay diagram of serum sIgE measurement.

Prick by prick testing is a skin prick test (SPT) when a fresh food is used as a source of the allergen. The test device is used to prick the food initially and then the patient's skin. A positive prick prick test (PPT) should be confirmed on a non-allergic individual, to exclude an irritant effect.

Histamine dichloride (10 mg/mL) and a negative control of diluent identical to that of the allergen extracts (usually glycerinated saline) should always be included in the test.idt

A wheal ≥3 mm with flare after 15 to 20 minutes is considered positive – the presence of sensitization. For research purposes, a more precise measurement is usually used – the mean of the longest wheal diameter (D) and the diameter perpendicular to D (d) expressed as (D+d)/2.

Potential systemic reactions are reported to be about 33:100,000 (SPT) and 0.5% of PPT using fresh food in infants. One fatality due to SPT has been reported in a large survey (American Academy of Allergy Asthma & Immunology).[15] Appropriate training and full emergency equipment and medications are essential when skin testing is used.

End-point dilution technique (a variant of IDT) to identify the concentration of an extract that produces a reaction of a defined size is not routinely used in the clinical practice. Potential systematic reactions (0.5%) and fatalities (6) have been reported with IDT without prior SPT.

Serum-specific IgE measurement

Allergen-specific IgE (sIgE) measurement is an *in vitro* test to demonstrate sensitization.[16] Serum sIgE can be measured by sensitive immunoassays such as radioimmunoassay, enzyme immunoassay or fluorescent immunoassay. In these assays a serum is incubated with an allergen of interest bound solid phase. IgEs with the specificity to the allergen of interest will remain on the solid phase, which is then detected by a labelled anti-IgE antibody (**Figure 14.3**). The level of signal is proportionate to the concentration of sIgE. SIgE can be falsely elevated if total IgE > 1000 kU/L due to non-specific binding. Solid phase varies in different assay systems – the ImmunoCAP by Phadia (cellulose sponge matrix in the form of a small cap), the Immulite System (avidin solid phase) and the HYTEC-288 system (cellulose wafer). Similarly reagents used in the different systems vary. Therefore sIgE results from different systems are not interchangeable. The ImmunoCAP system is currently most widely used for sIgE measurement in the UK.

SIgE measurement is indicated in the following situations: high risk for anaphylaxis; use of medications that can cause interference in SPT; skin lesions unsuitable for SPT; small children; and so on. The level of sIgE is not directly correlated with the severity of allergy.

Until recently allergen sources have usually been based on the conventional extract. Allergen extract is a mixture of proteins (components) from the allergen source. More recently component resolved diagnostics (CRD) are used in detecting sIgE to allergen components. CRD has improved our knowledge in risk assessment and treatment such as allergen-specific immunotherapy.

Multiple component-specific IgEs can be detected using microarray techniques (e.g. ImmunoCAP ISAC). This can be useful by providing a sensitization profile for risk assessment. Allergen components can be categorized into species-specific and cross-reactive component. Cross-reactive components labile proteins (e.g. profilin) can be associated with multiple sensitivities and symptoms but are less likely to cause systemic symptoms. In contrast, cross-reactive stable proteins such as non-specific lipid transfer protein (nLTP) are often associated with more systemic symptoms. This knowledge is increasingly being applied in the management of multiple fruit/food allergy (**Table 14.10**).

Basophil activation test (BAT)

The Basophil Activation Test (BAT) (**Figure 14.4**) is an *in vitro* study of peripheral basophils responses to stimuli.[18–20] BAT can use whole blood and therefore is more accessible than mast cells to study IgE mediated

TABLE 14.10 Allergen components and clinical relevance[17]

Component	Allergen source	Protein nature	Clinical relevance
Ara h 2	Peanut	Species-specific	Severe peanut allergy
Ves v 1	Wasp	Species-specific	Wasp allergy
Api m 1	Bee	Species-specific	Honey bee allergy
Gal d 1	Egg	Species-specific	Persistent egg allergy
Tri a 19 (O5g)	Wheat	Species-specific	Food dependent exercise induced anaphylaxis
Phl p 1	Timothy grass pollen	Cross-reactive (profilin)	Seasonal allergic rhinitis
Ara h 8	Peanut	Cross-reactive (PR-10)	Oral allergy syndrome
Pru p 3	Peach	nsLTP	Peach allergy/oral allergy syndrome

responses in allergic reaction. These can be assessed mainly by two methods: measurement of mediator release (e.g. histamine); or detecting the increase in cell surface molecules or newly expressed cell surface molecules (e.g. CD63, CD69, CD203c).

The whole blood of the patient is incubated with the allergen of interest. Basophils are stimulated due to the cross-linking of the specific IgE-FcεRI on basophil. Degranulation of basophils leads to the expression of molecules (e.g. CD63) on the basophil cell surface. In an unstimulated phase these molecules are anchored on the membrane of intracellular basophil granules, which contain histamine. CD63 expression closely correlates with histamine release in the degranulation. These can be detected by the flow cytometry method.

The assay performance from many studies and reports indicates BAT is comparable to serum sIgE in allergy diagnoses. For house dust mite sensitivity, BAT has claimed to have sensitivity of 85% (allergic rhinitis) and 50% (local allergic rhinitis), specificity of 93%, positive predictive value of 0.92 (allergic rhinitis) and 0.89 (local allergic rhinitis), and negative predictive value of 0.87 (allergic rhinitis) and 0.62 (local allergic rhinitis). BAT has been used to assess allergic response for allergens that are not commercially available for sIgE measurement. These include aeroallergens, drugs, venom and food allergens.

There are limitations in BAT. It is not well standardized (e.g. allergen concentration). It requires a fresh sample and highly skilled technicians. Interpretation of the test demands a highly trained immunologist/allergist given there is a concern about false positive related CD63 expressing platelet. Therefore BAT is currently available in limited numbers of diagnostic laboratories.

Non-validated tests

The following tests have not been validated to be used in allergy diagnosis:

- vega test
- kinesiology
- hair analysis
- provocation-neutralization
- iridology
- leucocytotoxic testing
- auriculo-cardiac reflex.

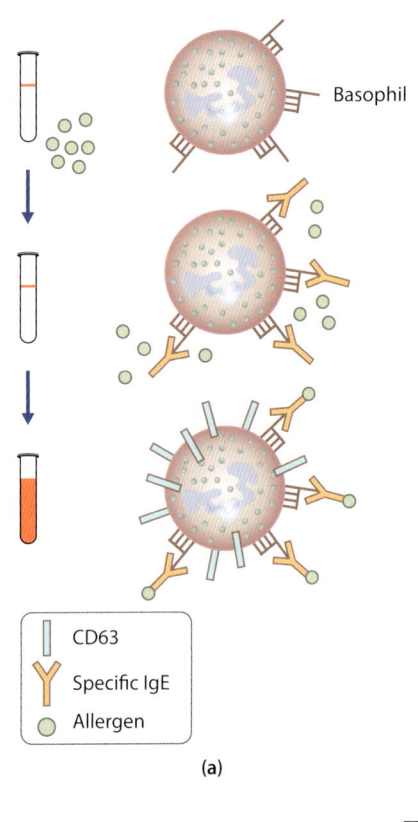

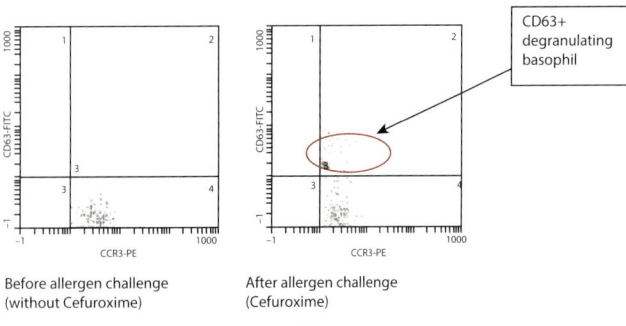

Figure 14.4 (a) Assay principle diagram of basophil activation test. (b) BAT histogram from flow cytometry using activating markers CD63. This patient has a history of anaphylaxis following intravenous cefuroxime. SPT, strongly positive to cefuroxime.

BEST CLINICAL PRACTICE

- ✓ Diagnosis of allergic disease is principally on a careful clinical history. An approach to allergy diagnosis is outlined in **Figure 14.5**.
- ✓ Allergic rhinitis can cause significant morbidities, and the impact of the disease upon the patient's work and leisure activities should be considered. Respiratory symptoms may indicate the presence of associated asthma.
- ✓ The examination of allergic rhinitis should include nasoendoscopy to exclude other conditions or exacerbating factors (nasal polyps, septal deflection or chronic rhinosinusitis).
- ✓ The presence of sensitization can be demonstrated by *in vivo* or *in vitro* tests, which must be interpreted with the clinical history.
- ✓ The routine panel of skin prick testing to demonstrate atopy includes house dust mite, animal danders (cat fur, dog hair, horse hair), moulds (*Aspergillus, Alternaria, Cladosporium*) and pollens (birch, timothy grass, weeds), positive control (histamine 10 mg/L) and negative control (allergen diluent).
- ✓ Serum sIgE measurement is preferred when SPT is likely to be equivocal in certain conditions such as severe eczema or use of medications that may interfere with the SPT (**Table 14.6**). Serum sIgE has a wider spectrum of allergens than SPT.
- ✓ Pharmacotherapy is the mainstay of treatment for allergic rhinitis. Most medications are designed to target mediators.
- ✓ Antihistamines are H1 receptor antagonists that are effective in early symptoms of allergic rhinitis.
- ✓ Intra-nasal corticosteroids are considered first-line treatment for more severe allergic rhinitis and are highly effective provided they are administered correctly. Training and health education of patients regarding the timing, technique and adequate dosing are essential in order to achieve the maximal benefit.
- ✓ A short course of prednisolone (e.g. 20 mg daily for 5 days) may be prescribed and is highly effective at relieving all nasal symptoms including nasal obstruction in the majority of patients.
- ✓ Sodium cromoglycate is a mast cell membrane stabilizer. It reduces nasal discharge and congestion but is less effective than topical corticosteroids. The eye drop preparations are useful for allergic ocular symptoms.
- ✓ Intra-nasal cholinergic relieves rhinorrhoea but is less effective for other symptoms of allergic rhinitis.
- ✓ Leucotriene receptor antagonists (e.g. montelukast) have beneficial effects in asthma but are less effective in rhinitis.

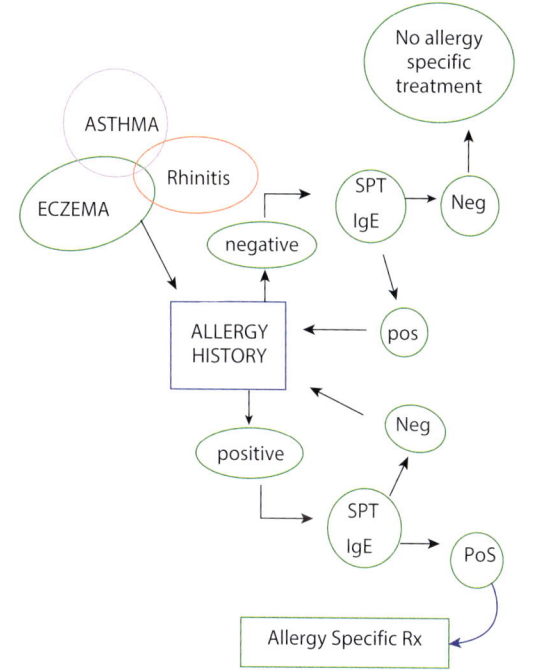

Figure 14.5 An approach to allergy diagnosis.

- ✓ Allergen avoidance is possible and essential for some allergens (e.g. peanut, cat fur, latex) but less effective in allergic rhinitis due to ubiquitous allergen (e.g. grass, house dust mite).
- ✓ House dust mite avoidance is often recommended. However, trials to date have been small and of suboptimal methodology.
- ✓ Allergen-specific immunotherapy is an effective intervention that can modify the disease process and long-lasting benefit has been reported. There are potential side effects including anaphylaxis, especially in patients with concomitant asthma. Efficacy can be limited in patients with multisensitivities. Therefore allergen-specific immunotherapy should be delivered in specialist centres and comply with the clinical guidelines (e.g. British Society for Allergy and Clinical Immunology).

FUTURE RESEARCH

- ➤ Improve understanding of mechanism of different methods of specific immunotherapy
- ➤ Multicentre studies for better application of component resolved diagnostics (CRD) in risk assessment
- ➤ External quality assurance of tests – CRD, BAT
- ➤ Multicentre studies for translation of new biomarkers, use of specific immunotherapy other than SCIT and SLIT
- ➤ Prevention of allergic diseases development

KEY POINTS

- Genetic and environmental factors interact as causes of allergic disease.
- Type 1 IgE mediated immediate hypersensitivity occurs only in a sensitized individual.
- Allergic inflammation is characterized by IgE dependent activation of mast cells and tissue eosinophils infiltration. These events are under the regulation of Th2 cells.
- Biomarkers are useful in allergy diagnosis. Normal levels of tryptase do not exclude anaphylaxis.
- The majority of IgE is tightly bound to FcεRI. There is no signalling until these receptors are cross-linked by their specific antigens.
- Skin testing and sIgE indicate sensitization only and must be interpreted in the context of the clinical history.

- Allergic rhinitis and asthma are commonly associated.
- Corticosteroids are general immunosuppressive agents.
- Allergen-specific immunotherapy is the only curative approach for allergic rhinitis, allergic asthma and venom allergy.
- Of the new novel therapeutic targets in clinical trials only anti-IgE therapy has been successful.

REFERENCES

1. Johansson SG, Bieber T, Dahl R, et al. Revised nomenclature for allergy for global use: report of the Nomenclature Review Committee of the World Allergy Organization, October 2003. *J Allergy Clin Immunol* 2004; **113**: 832–36.
2. Vadas P, Perelman B, Liss G. Platelet-activating factor, histamine, and tryptase levels in human anaphylaxis. *J Allergy Clin Immunol* 2013; **131**: 144–49.
3. Metcalfe DD, Peavy RD, Gilfillan AM. Mechanisms of mast cell signaling in anaphylaxis. *J Allergy Clin Immunol* 2009; **124**: 639–46; quiz 47–48.
4. Simons FE. Anaphylaxis: recent advances in assessment and treatment. *J Allergy Clin Immunol* 2009; **124**: 625–36; quiz 37–8.
5. Tejedor Alonso MA, Sastre DJ, Sanchez-Hernandez JJ, et al. Idiopathic anaphylaxis: a descriptive study of 81 patients in Spain. *Ann Allergy Asthma Immunol* 2002; **88**: 313–18.
6. Ring J, Darsow U. Idiopathic anaphylaxis. *Curr Allergy Asthma Rep* 2002; **2**: 40–45.
7. Ring J, Messmer K. Incidence and severity of anaphylactoid reactions to colloid volume substitutes. *Lancet* 1977; **1**: 466–69.
8. Rondon C, Campo P, Togias A, et al. Local allergic rhinitis: concept, pathophysiology, and management. *J Allergy Clin Immunol* 2012; **129**: 1460–67.
9. Bousquet J, Hellings PW, Agache I, et al. ARIA 2016: Care pathways implementing emerging technologies for predictive medicine in rhinitis and asthma across the life cycle. *Clin Trans Allergy* 2016 **6**: 47.
10. Cochrane Systematic Review. 10.1002/14651858.CD0001936.pub2/enhanced/exportCitation/
11. Akdis M, Akdis CA. Mechanisms of allergen-specific immunotherapy: multiple suppressor factors at work in immune tolerance to allergens. *J Allergy Clin Immunol* 2014; **133**: 621–31.
12. Casale TB, Stokes JR. Immunotherapy: what lies beyond. *J Allergy Clin Immunol* 2014; **133**: 612–19.
13. Jacobsen L, Wahn U, Bilo MB. Allergen-specific immunotherapy provides immediate, long-term and preventive clinical effects in children and adults: the effects of immunotherapy can be categorised by level of benefit -the centenary of allergen specific subcutaneous immunotherapy. *Clin Transl Allergy* 2012; **2**: 8.
14. Haahtela T, Burbach GJ, Bachert C, et al. Clinical relevance is associated with allergen-specific wheal size in skin prick testing. *Clin Exp Allergy* 2013; **44**: 407–16.
15. Bernstein DI, Wanner M, Borish L, et al. Twelve-year survey of fatal reactions to allergen injections and skin testing; 1990-2001. *J Allergy Clin Immunol* 2004; **113**: 1129.
16. Hamilton RG. Clinical laboratory assessment of immediate-type hypersensitivity. *J Allergy Clin Immunol* 2010; **125**: S284–96.
17. Treudler R, Simon JC. Overview of component resolved diagnostics. *Curr Allergy Asthma Rep* 2013; **13**:110–17.
18. MacGlashan DW, Jr. Basophil activation testing. *J Allergy Clin Immunol* 2013; **132**: 777–87.
19. Korosec P, Silar M, Erzen R, et al. Clinical routine utility of basophil activation testing for diagnosis of hymenoptera-allergic patients with emphasis on individuals with negative venom-specific IgE antibodies. *Int Arch Allergy Immunol* 2013; **161**: 363–68.
20. Gomez E, Campo P, Rondon C, et al. Role of the basophil activation test in the diagnosis of local allergic rhinitis. *J Allergy Clin Immunol* 2013; **132**: 975-6 e1-5.

CHAPTER 15

EVALUATION OF THE IMMUNE SYSTEM

Moira Thomas, Elizabeth Drewe and Richard J. Powell

Introduction to evaluation of the immune system 149
Immunological tests 149
References 155

SEARCH STRATEGY

Data in this chapter are taken from standard UK immunology laboratory practice. They reflect expert opinion (level 4 evidence) with regards to immunology tests currently performed in the UK.

INTRODUCTION TO EVALUATION OF THE IMMUNE SYSTEM

Evaluation of the immune system broadly encompasses the investigation of immunodeficiency, autoimmune disease including vasculitis, allergy and lymphoproliferative disease. Diagnosis results from studying the combination of clinical presentation and investigations including immunological, haematological, microbiological and histopathological, with increasing recognition of the place of genetic and molecular biological approaches. However, immunology tests in isolation are rarely diagnostic. Some understanding of the sensitivity (proportion of true positives correctly identified), specificity (proportion of true negatives correctly identified), positive predictive value (likelihood an individual has a disease given a positive result) and negative predictive value (likelihood an individual does not have the disease given a negative result) for each test is required.

Interpretation of results is dependent upon the age of the patient. This is particularly important for the investigation of childhood immunodeficiency when, for example, a lymphocyte count that would be normal for an adult could be well below the age-related normal range and may signify an underlying immunodeficiency in an infant. Similarly, a weak positive anti-nuclear antibody (ANA) titre may be a common incidental finding in a middle-aged female whereas may signify an autoimmune process in a child.

The choice of investigations will ultimately depend on the clinical presentation and may be guided through discussion with a clinical immunologist. Whilst rare immunological diseases will only be recognized by the appropriate investigation, consideration must also be given to commoner diseases with a similar presentation, for example, cystic fibrosis.

IMMUNOLOGICAL TESTS

Immunodeficiency

Immunodeficiency should be considered in any patient with persistent or recurrent infections not responding to antibiotics, or patients with unusual or opportunistic infections.[1] Immunodeficiency may be either primary or secondary to therapies such as immunosuppressive drugs or chemotherapy or secondary to diseases such haematological malignancies, diabetes or HIV infection; in many patients the secondary cause will be clearly apparent but in others, infection will be the presenting feature. Primary immune deficiency can arise from defects in any part of the immune system so may manifest in a myriad of ways across a wide age range but with the common hallmark of increased susceptibility to infection. Sinopulmonary infections are a common feature of primary antibody deficiency and ENT clinical staff should look out for these individuals and initiate the appropriate investigations. It is estimated that half of the patients with primary antibody deficiency in the UK remain undiagnosed.[2] Remember that early diagnosis of primary immunodeficiency does lead to an improved outcome, emphasizing the need to consider this diagnosis.

When considering immunodeficiency, the type of pathogen may provide a clue to the underlying disease and appropriate tests required (**Tables 15.1** and **15.2**). Certain tests, especially those involving functional assays, require rapid transport of samples and prior laboratory preparation. Accordingly early discussion with the local laboratory is recommended.

TABLE 15.1 Outline of associations between pathogens and specific immunodeficiencies

Pathology	Immunodeficiency
Bacterial infections	Antibody deficiency
	T cell deficiency
	Complement
	Neutrophil disorders
Viral infections	T cells
	Antibody deficiency
Fungal infections	Neutrophil disorders
	T cells
Neisserial infections	Complement
Abscess formation	Neutrophil disorders
Mycobacterial infection	T cells
	Macrophage/cytokines

TABLE 15.2 Outline of immunological tests for primary immunodeficiency

Deficiency	Tests
T lymphocytes	HIV serology
	Lymphocyte subsets - numbers of CD4 and CD8 T cells, B and NK cells
	Lymphocyte proliferation studies
Antibody deficiency	Immunoglobulins (IgG, IgA and IgM) and serum electrophoresis
	Specific antibodies and responses to immunization
	Lymphocyte subsets
Phagocyte disorders	Differential white cell count (neutrophil numbers)
	Neutrophil respiratory burst analysis
	Neutrophil adhesion markers
Complement disorders	Functional complement assays
	Assay individual complement components

C-REACTIVE PROTEIN

C-reactive protein (CRP) levels reflect the acute phase response and are particularly elevated in bacterial infections and active vasculitis. An elevated CRP may indicate intercurrent infection in immunodeficiency and individuals on high dose steroids. Rarely the lack of an appropriate acute phase response in the face of invasive bacterial infection can be a feature of certain rare immune deficiencies such as Hyper IgE Syndrome.

IMMUNOGLOBULINS

Serum immunoglobulins (IgG, IgA and IgM) are a useful first line test for investigation of immunodeficiency although normal or even high levels do not exclude all forms of immune deficiency. Very low levels of all immunoglobulins are typical in boys with X-linked agammaglobulinaemia (XLA). IgG and IgA levels are typically low in children and adults with common variable immunodeficiency, although, as the name suggests, the pattern can vary and in some patients immunoglobulin levels may only be slightly below the normal range. Other types of immune deficiency such as HIV infection and defects of neutrophil function such as chronic granulomatous disease are characterized by raised immunoglobulin levels. Other indications for immunoglobulin testing include infective and inflammatory diseases in which polyclonal increases in immunoglobulins are often seen and the evaluation of lymphoproliferative disease when serum and urine electrophoresis should also be requested to identify any paraproteinaemia.

SPECIFIC ANTIBODIES (ALSO TERMED FUNCTIONAL ANTIBODIES)

Assessment of dynamic antibody responses to immunization plays an important part in the assessment of antibody deficiency especially in patients with borderline or normal immunoglobulin levels. Specific antibody levels are measured before and 4–6 weeks after immunization with tetanus toxoid, pneumococcal, Haemophilus influenza b or other non-live vaccines depending upon local immunization schedules and availability of specific antibody tests. Failure to mount an adequate response is a pointer to an underlying immunodeficiency. Of course, live vaccines must not be given to any patient with a suspected immunodeficiency.

IMMUNOGLOBULIN G SUBCLASSES

IgG subclasses are sometimes useful in the investigation of possible antibody deficiency where IgG subclass deficiency may be associated with selective IgA deficiency and/or failure to respond to pneumococcal immunization. However, isolated low IgG2 levels may be found in asymptomatic individuals especially in childhood. Increasingly the main indication for the measurement of IgG subclasses is now suspected autoimmune pancreatitis and other IgG4-related diseases. This group of inflammatory disorders, which may affect a wide range of organs including sinuses, salivary glands and thyroid, is characterized by an infiltrate of IgG4 positive plasma cells, fibrosis and raised IgG4 levels.

LYMPHOCYTE PHENOTYPING (ALSO TERMED LYMPHOCYTE SUBSETS)

A reduced lymphocyte count in the full blood count may provide an early clue to the presence of immune deficiency; indeed in infants a persistent unexplained lymphocyte count of $<2.8 \times 10^9/l$ should prompt consideration of severe combined immune deficiency. Lymphocyte phenotyping by flow cytometry allows accurate measurements of the different lymphocyte subsets by detection of cell surface markers. The two main T cell subsets are evaluated by assessing $CD3^+CD4^+$ and $CD3^+CD8^+$ numbers whilst $CD19^+$ cells identify B cells and $CD3^-CD16/56^+$ cells represent NK cells. Very low T cells are characteristic of severe combined immunodeficiency whereas absence of B cells is a feature of X-linked agammaglobulinaemia. However, these findings are not diagnostic and may be affected by drugs or intercurrent infection.

Low CD3+CD4+ cell numbers are characteristic of human immunodeficiency virus (HIV) infection. However, a normal CD4 count does not exclude HIV nor should it be used as a covert screening test. A wide range of additional cell surface markers and lymphocyte subsets can be measured and so close dialogue with the laboratory is advised in order to select the most appropriate panels for individual patients and also to interpret the results. Lymphocyte phenotyping is also valuable in the diagnosis of lymphoproliferative disease.

LYMPHOCYTE PROLIFERATION AND OTHER FUNCTIONAL ASSAYS

These specialized tests are reserved for the investigation of suspected cellular immunodeficiency usually following discussion with an immunologist. The proliferation of lymphocytes can be measured following *in vitro* stimulation by mitogens such as phytohaemagglutinin, or antigens such as tetanus, to which the patient has previously been exposed. Additional more specialized functional tests are possible, for example to assess production and function of cytokines in the gamma interferon and interleukin 12 pathways in patients with recurrent atypical mycobacterial infections.

COMPLEMENT PATHWAY LEVELS (C3-, C4-, C1-INHIBITOR)

Measurement of C3 and C4 levels is helpful in the assessment of patients with systemic inflammatory disorders. As complement components are acute phase proteins, levels of both C3 and C4 are typically raised in systemic vasculitides, sepsis and other inflammatory disorders. However, complement is consumed in systemic immune complex disorders so levels of both C3 and C4 are typically low in active systemic lupus erythematosus (SLE) and levels may vary with disease activity. Isolated low C3 levels with normal C4 levels are a feature of certain glomerulopathies including post-streptococcal nephritis. Complement levels also play a vital role in the investigation of angioedema. Patients with C1-inhibitor deficiency (hereditary angioedema) have low C4 levels (but normal C3 levels) due to uncontrolled turnover of the classical complement pathway; a normal C4 level during an attack of angioedema essentially excludes this diagnosis. C1-inhibitor levels are low in the majority of hereditary angioedema patients but a small proportion have type 2 C1-inhibitor deficiency whereby they have normal levels of a dysfunctional C1-inhibitor. Functional C1-inhibitor assays can be undertaken in those patients with angioedema without urticaria and a low C4 level. Appropriate care must be taken in handling and transport of the sample to avoid in vitro degradation of C1-inhibitor function.

HAEMOLYTIC COMPLEMENT ACTIVITY

Deficiencies in the classical complement pathway typically present with early onset atypical or severe lupus-like illness or invasive bacterial infection with encapsulated organisms such as pneumococcus. Deficiencies in the alternate and terminal pathways predispose to meningococcal infection especially with unusual serotypes. The CH100 (or CH50) haemolytic complement test assesses activity of the classical and terminal complement pathways and the AP100 (or AP50) haemolytic complement test assesses activity of the alternate and terminal pathways. Thus the combination of these tests can identify the presence and likely location of any deficiency that can be followed up by measurement of the appropriate individual complement components. As haemolytic complement tests rely upon complement function, samples should be taken when patients are clinically stable and blood samples must be separated and frozen within a short time of venepuncture to avoid *in vitro* depletion of complement causing false positive results.

NEUTROPHIL FUNCTION

Patients with chronic granulomatous disease (CGD) have deficient neutrophil respiratory burst and their neutrophils are unable to kill ingested organisms, especially catalase positive organisms such as staphylococcus aureus, serratia and also fungi such as aspergillus. Therefore assessment of neutrophil respiratory burst is indicated in patients presenting with recurrent abscesses and lymphadenitis, deep seated abscesses or recurrent bacterial infections. The traditional nitro blue tetrazolium (NBT) test, which assessed the ability of patient neutrophils to oxidize pale yellow NBT into a dark blue precipitate, has now mainly been superceded by flow cytometric assays. Female carriers of the X-linked form of CGD may also be identified using the flow cytometric test. Neutrophils have a short life span so analysis needs to be carried out within a short period of time after venepuncture whilst cells are still viable, so prior discussion with local laboratory is recommended.

MOLECULAR AND GENETIC STUDIES

Mutations in more than 300 genes are now known to cause primary immune deficiency with the number of causative genes increasing each year. Genetic testing for primary immune deficiency by means of Sanger sequencing of the suspected faulty gene is now routinely available for many disorders and also allows carrier detection and prenatal diagnosis where appropriate. However, with this new genetic knowledge has come the recognition that many primary immune deficiencies have overlapping and wider clinical phenotypes than were initially described. The advent of next generation sequencing technologies is paving the way for new approaches to genetic investigation of suspected immune deficiency by enabling large panels of immunological genes to be examined simultaneously. As well as providing a means to identify lesions in multiple genes known to cause immune deficiency, this approach can also enable the discovery of new genetic conditions.

Allergy

A brief discussion of allergy tests follows, although this subject is discussed further in Chapter 14, Allergy: basic mechanisms and tests. When diagnosing allergy, a clear and detailed history is paramount. Evidence of sensitization to specific allergens can be detected *in vivo* by skin prick tests or *in vitro* on serum by measuring allergen-specific IgE levels.

SKIN PRICK TESTS

Drops of aqueous solutions of relevant allergens, negative (allergen buffer) and positive controls (histamine) are applied to the skin. A pinprick is made through the drop placed on the epidermis and excess solution removed with tissue. The size of any localized skin reaction is measured at 15 minutes, and results > 2–3 mm diameter larger than the negative control are considered positive. Antihistamines should be stopped before testing, to prevent false negative results. Positive results indicate sensitization but do not necessarily indicate clinical allergy, emphasizing the need to correlate with the patient's history.

IgE

Total IgE levels may be raised in allergic diseases, particularly eczema, and also with certain parasitic infections, immunodeficiencies and lymphomas. Therefore a raised total IgE level does not necessarily imply allergic disease and a normal level does not exclude allergic disease. Very high total IgE levels such as those found in severe eczema can result in many weak false positive allergen-specific IgE levels.

ALLERGEN-SPECIFIC IgE

These are now measured by enzyme-linked immunoassay rather than radioallergosorbent assay test (RAST) although the latter term remains in common usage. A wide range of aeroallergens, food and other allergens is available. Choice of appropriate allergens should be based on the clinical history, for example in patients with seasonal allergic rhinitis the most useful allergens will be the pollens in season at the time of the patient's symptoms; in patients with perennial rhinitis allergens such as house dust mite or household pets are more likely to be informative. The presence of specific IgE indicates sensitization but does not necessarily indicate clinical allergy, emphasizing the importance of correlation with the patient's history. Results also depend upon the sensitivity and specificity of the tests which does vary between individual allergens. *In vitro* tests are especially useful if patients are unable to undergo skin testing (e.g. because they are unable to stop antihistamine therapy, have widespread skin disease or are dermatographic).

ANAESTHETIC REACTION TESTING

Anaphylaxis occurring during surgery may be difficult to differentiate from other simultaneous haemodynamic events. Tryptase is released from mast cells during anaphylaxis and can be measured by laboratories and may be helpful in this setting. Serum tryptase levels typically peak 1–2 hours after onset of an anaphylactic event with levels falling towards normal within 24 hours. Accordingly a series of timed and clearly labelled samples for tryptase is required. However a rise in tryptase is only seen in approximately 60% of anaphylactic events so normal results do not completely exclude anaphylaxis. Allergen-specific IgE can be measured to a limited range of anaesthetic drugs, antibiotics, chlorhexidine and latex but there is an increased risk of false negative results within the first 6 weeks after the acute event. Further specialist assessment and skin testing is often required to identify the most likely culprit allergen.

Autoimmune disease including vasculitis

The detection of serum autoantibodies is a helpful aid in the investigation of autoimmune diseases and vasculitis and should be considered in the light of the clinical history and the outcome of appropriate tissue biopsies.[4] Some autoantibodies such as anti-glomerular basement membrane (GBM) and acetyl choline receptor antibodies play a direct role in disease pathogenesis; these antibodies generally have very high sensitivity and specificity for the disease in question. In contrast, other autoantibodies such as anti-nuclear antibodies (ANA) are thought to be secondary to tissue damage or represent epiphenomona but are nevertheless useful disease markers; these antibodies are often less specific. Autoantibodies may be useful for diagnosis, assessment of prognosis and disease monitoring, and in some cases may be detected prior to the development of disease.

ANCA AND VASCULITIS

The investigation of suspected vasculitis requires integration of clinical, laboratory and biopsy information. Antineutrophil cytoplasmic antibodies (ANCA) play a critical role in identifying ANCA-associated vasculitis (AAV). ANCA is detected by indirect immunofluorescence on human neutrophils. Two main patterns of fluorescence may be seen; cytoplasmic staining denotes a C-ANCA and is usually due to reactivity against proteinase 3 (PR3) and are associated with polyangiitis with granulomatosis (formally called Wegener's granulomatosis). Perinuclear staining denotes a P-ANCA which is usually due to myeloperoxidase (MPO) antibodies and associated with microscopic polyangiitis, rapidly progressive glomerulonephritis or Churg–Strauss syndrome. Other atypical staining patterns of ANCA may be seen but these are usually due to reactivity against other antigens and are rarely associated with systemic vasculitis. Care is needed in interpreting ANCA results. Negative results can be found in AAV, especially localized polyangiitis with granulomatosis, and false positive results can be found in a range of conditions including HIV infection, infective endocarditis and atrial myxoma, which may mimic vasculitis (**Table 15.3**). Other tests are also useful in the investigation of suspected vasculitis. Complement levels may be useful. For example, if both C3 and C4 are low, SLE, subacute bacterial endocarditis and hypocomplementaemic vasculitis should be considered; if C4 alone is low cryoglobulinaemia should be considered; and if C3 alone is low, then post-streptococcal nephritis should be considered in the differential diagnosis. Other autoantibodies may be useful, for example, anti-nuclear, anti-glomerular basement membrane and anti-phospholipid antibodies, depending upon the clinical picture and organ involvement.

TABLE 15.3 Guide to interpretation of ANCA

Result	Guide to interpretation
Positive C-ANCA with PR3 antibodies	Polyangiitis with granulomatosis
Positive P-ANCA with MPO antibodies	Microscopic polyangiitis
	Churg–Strauss syndrome
Positive C-ANCA without PR3 antibodies	Inflammatory bowel disease
	Infection, malignancy
Positive P-ANCA without MPO antibodies	Vasculitis, connective tissue disease

ANTI-NUCLEAR ANTIBODIES (ANA), DOUBLE-STRANDED DNA ANTIBODIES AND ANTIBODIES TO EXTRACTABLE NUCLEAR ANTIGENS (ENA)

Anti-nuclear antibodies (ANA) are found in systemic lupus erythematosus (SLE). ANA is a useful screening test, as a negative ANA makes SLE very unlikely. However, positive ANAs are also found in other connective tissue disorders and autoimmune hepatitis, as well as a wide range of other autoimmune, inflammatory and infective disorders. ANAs are also found in healthy individuals especially older females. Different patterns of ANA are seen and reflect reactivity against different nuclear antigens including centromere, dsDNA and ENA (Ro, La, Sm, ribonucleoprotein, Scl70 and others) and may help categorize the connective tissue disease present. Whilst antibodies against centromere, dsDNA and ENA are much more specific for individual connective tissue disorders, they are less sensitive. Table 15.4 shows the main disease associations. Advances in technology mean that many multiplex assays are now readily available and often termed 'connective tissue disease screens'. These typically comprise a mixture of the main ENA and dsDNA antigens enabling patient samples to be screened more rapidly with detection of only the more disease-specific autoantibodies. However, there may be a loss of sensitivity and some patients with clinically relevant positive ANA but negative ENA and dsDNA abs may be missed. Clinicians are encouraged to become familiar with the details of the tests offered by their local laboratory as the different methods may differ significantly in sensitivity, specificity and range of autoantibodies included in the screen.

RHEUMATOID FACTOR (RF) AND CYCLIC CITRULLINATED PEPTIDE (CCP) ANTIBODIES

RF and CCP antibodies may both be found in a proportion of patients with rheumatoid arthritis. CCP antibodies are more specific than rheumatoid factor, which is also found in many healthy individuals. Rheumatoid factor is also found in Sjogren's syndrome and cryoglobulinaemia.

CARDIOLIPIN ANTIBODIES AND ANTIPHOSPHOLIPID SYNDROME

Anti-phospholipid syndrome presents with features including recurrent venous and arterial thrombosis, recurrent pregnancy loss, thrombocytopaenia and neurological

TABLE 15.4 Interpretation of ANA, centromere, dsDNA and ENA antibodies

Autoantibodies	Interpretation
Anti-nuclear antibody (ANA)	SLE Other connective tissue diseases – Sjogren's syndrome, scleroderma, undifferentiated connective tissue disease Autoimmune hepatitis Other autoimmune, inflammatory and infective disorders, malignancy Healthy individuals – incidence increases with age, females > males
dsDNA antibodies	SLE Autoimmune hepatitis
Ro (SSA)	SLE, Sjogren's syndrome, neonatal heart block in the fetus of a Ro positive mother
La (SSB)	SLE, Sjogren's syndrome
Sm	SLE
Ribonucleoprotein (RNP)	SLE, overlap syndromes eg mixed connective tissue disease
Scl70	Systemic sclerosis
CENP-B	CREST syndrome (calcinosis, Raynaud's, oesophageal dysmotility, scleroderma, telangiectasia)

disease due to both small and large vessel occlusion plus the presence of phospholipid antibodies. These consist of a group of related autoantibodies – anti-cardiolipin antibodies, anti-β-2 glycoprotein 1 antibodies and lupus anticoagulant. Patients may have one or more of these autoantibodies. Repeat testing may be indicated to exclude transient autoantibody production (e.g. secondary to infection).

CRYOGLOBULINAEMIA

Cryoglobulins are immunoglobulins that form gels or precipitates on cooling. Clinical features include purpura, Raynaud's syndrome, thrombosis, neuropathy and vasculitis. They are associated with infections, connective tissue disease and lymphoproliferative disease. Detection relies on the appropriate collection into a prewarmed blood tube in a waterbath/vacuum flask. Cold agglutinins are autoantibodies that reversibly agglutinate erythrocytes in the cold and should not be confused with cryoglobulins.

COELIAC DISEASE

Coeliac disease is characterized by malabsorption and weight loss but can present with oral ulceration, anaemia and malaise. The presence of villous atrophy on duodenal biopsy remains the gold standard for diagnosis but serological tests are an invaluable screen. Over 95% of patients with Coeliac disease have positive IgA tissue transglutaminase or IgA endomysial antibodies; these are essentially the same autoantibodies, the different terminology reflecting the different test methodology. Serology typically becomes negative on a gluten-free diet so it is important to ensure that the patient has been consuming gluten regularly (typically at least twice a day for at least 6 weeks) prior to testing to avoid obtaining a false negative result. Paradoxically individuals with IgA deficiency (defined as IgA < 0.06 g/l) have an increased incidence of Coeliac disease but of course the usual IgA based serology is of no value. IgG tissue transglutaminase or IgG endomysial antibodies can be measured instead but sensitivity and specificity may be less than that of the IgA based serology.

BULLOUS PEMPHIGOID AND PEMPHIGUS

Bullous pemphigoid and pemphigus are blistering disorders associated with autoantibodies to desmoglein in the basement membrane zone or intercellular type VII collagen respectively. These may be detected in blood or in tissue biopsies using direct immunofluorescence.

LIVER AUTOANTIBODIES

Several autoantibodies are associated with autoimmune liver disease. Typical screens based on indirect immunofluorescence on rodent liver/kidney/stomach multi-block can detect mitochondrial, smooth muscle, liver kidney microsomal (LKM), liver cytosolic 1 (LC1) and anti-nuclear antibodies. M2 mitochondrial antibodies are associated with primary biliary cirrhosis, ANA and smooth muscle antibodies are associated with autoimmune hepatitis, LC1 and LKM antibodies may be associated with more aggressive forms of autoimmune hepatitis. However, overlapping serology and clinical pictures may be seen.

GASTRIC PARIETAL CELL AND INTRINSIC FACTOR ANTIBODIES

Gastric parietal cell antibodies are present in the majority of patients with pernicious anaemia and may pre-date onset of disease. They are also found in up to 15% of the healthy elderly. Intrinsic factor antibodies are much more specific but less sensitive for pernicious anaemia. In the past, recent B12 treatment could interfere with the intrinsic factor antibody assays but this is much less of a problem with modern methodologies.

ACETYL CHOLINE RECEPTOR ANTIBODIES, MYASTHAENIA GRAVIS AND THYMOMA

Myasthaenia gravis is characterized by increased skeletal muscle fatiguability. Facial and bulbar muscle involvement may cause nasal speech, ptosis, diplopia and difficulty in swallowing. Generalized weakness occurs in approximately 85% of patients. Autoantibodies to the acetyl choline receptor (AchR) at the neuromuscular junction are detectable in 90% of patients. Myasthenia gravis is associated with thymoma and other autoimmune diseases.

Lymphoproliferative disease

Many of the immunological tests required to investigate lymphoproliferative disease have already been mentioned and are used in combination with bone marrow and lymph node biopsies.

IMMUNOGLOBULINS, SERUM AND URINE ELECTROPHORESIS AND SERUM-FREE LIGHT CHAINS

Multiple myeloma is a malignancy of plasma cells that produce monoclonal immunoglobulin (paraprotein). Paraproteins may be detectable in both serum and/or urine. Twenty percent of myelomas only produce monoclonal light chains, which may only be detectable in urine as Bence Jones protein or in serum using a serum-free light chain assay. Therefore a full myeloma screen requires both blood for immunoglobulins and electrophoresis plus either serum-free light chains or urine for electrophoresis. This combination of tests will detect all but the very rare non-secretory myelomas. These tests are also required for the investigation of possible AL amyloid. As paraprotein levels may be relatively low and difficult to detect in AL amyloid, close liaison with the laboratory is recommended as more sensitive detection methods such as immunofixation may be required. Although paraproteins are the hallmark of myeloma, Waldenstrom's macroglobulinaemia and AL amyloid, the majority of paraproteins detected in routine clinical practice are not associated with any identifiable lymphoproliferative disorder and are termed monoclonal gammopathy of uncertain significance (MGUS). Some MGUS may progress to lymphoproliferative disease with an overall rate of 1–2% per annum.

BEST CLINICAL PRACTICE

✓ Immunological tests always need to be interpreted in the context of the clinical case.

FUTURE RESEARCH

➤ The majority of current tests are performed on peripheral blood due to its accessibility. Tests that reflect activity at local surfaces, for example defensins, and tests that are more reflective of *in vivo* pathology, such as intracellular cytokine analysis, may enter clinical practice.
➤ Many patients have severe, persistent, unusual and recurrent infections yet no immunological cause is identified. Advancing knowledge, particularly regarding the innate immune system (e.g. toll receptors), may account for such disease and diagnostic tests will subsequently follow.
➤ Increasing use of molecular diagnosis and development of tests looking at functional pathways will occur. It is becoming increasingly apparent that individuals with the same genetic mutation may have diverse disease phenotypes, e.g. btk mutation associated with complete absence of B cells or IgG subclass defect. Identification of genetic polymorphisms may predict patients at risk of severe disease requiring a more aggressive management strategy.

KEY POINTS

- Immunodeficiency may present to ENT specialists with severe, persistent, unusual or recurrent infection. Early diagnosis may reduce morbidity and mortality.
- Immunological tests may help in diagnosis and monitoring of disease but must always be considered in association with clinical presentation and biopsy findings.
- Liaise with your clinical immunologist/immunology laboratory to ensure the appropriate tests are being requested. If clinical history is particularly suggestive of a disease, further tests may be required even in the presence of initial negative investigations.

REFERENCES

1. Picard C et al. Primary immunodeficiency diseases: an update on the Classification from the International Union of Immunological Societies Expert Committee for Primary Immunodeficiency 2015. *J Clin Immunol* 2015; **35**: 696–726.
2. Spickett GP, Misbah SA, Chapel HM. Primary antibody deficiency in adults. *Lancet* 1991; **337**: 281–84.
3. Rusznak C, Davis RJ. ABC of allergies. *Brit Med J* 1998; **316**: 686–89.
4. Jury EC, D'Cruz D, Morrow WJW. Autoantibodies and overlap syndromes in autoimmune rheumatic disease. *J Clin Pathol* 2002; **54**: 340–47.

CHAPTER 16

CANCER IMMUNOLOGY

Osama Al Hamarneh and John Greenman

Introduction 157	Immunotherapy 161
Tumour microenvironment (TME) 157	Conclusions 162
Tumour escape mechanisms 160	References 163
Tumour biomarkers 161	

SEARCH STRATEGY

This chapter provides an overview of the main concepts involved in the immunology of head and neck tumours, including disease progression, monitoring and immunotherapy. Data in this chapter may be updated by a PubMed search using the keywords: head and neck cancer, tumour microenvironment and Immunotherapy.

INTRODUCTION

Major technical and conceptual advances in immunology and cancer immunology in particular over the last two decades has led to a better, although by no means as yet complete, understanding of the complex relationship between the immune system, tumour initiation and progression, and immunotherapy. Specifically much attention has focused on changes in individual immune profiles of patients treated with conventional, biological or combination therapies; such work is underpinned by high-throughput proteomic and genomic platforms. This has led to a huge amount of interest in using immune biomarkers to both diagnose and monitor tumour response to therapy, as well as acting as a potential therapeutic option alone or in combination with chemo- or radiotherapy.

In this chapter, we endeavour to explore the fundamentals of the complex interactions within the tumour microenvironment and how malignancies effectively 'escape' immune detection. The roles of key immune cells and proteins will be discussed with a focus on tumour biomarkers and the application of anti-tumour immunity knowledge that underpins recent immunotherapeutic trials.

This chapter will discuss concepts of tumour immunebiology that will be of help to clinicians and their patients, focusing on head and neck squamous cell carcinomas (HNSCC), as tumours head and neck originating from squamous epithelia are the most prevalent tumour type within the head and neck region.

TUMOUR MICROENVIRONMENT (TME)

In general, cancers arise from the accumulation of genetic and epigenetic changes, together with abnormalities in the cancer-associated signalling pathways causing the acquisition of cancer-related phenotypes. These changes include limitless replicative potential of tumours, self-sufficiency in growth signals and insensitivity to anti-growth signals, ability to evade apoptosis, increased angiogenesis, invasion and metastasis.[1] However, tumours are complex tissues that not only contain malignant cells but surrounding stroma, which comprises various types of mesenchymal cells, extracellular matrix and immune cells. Collectively, these tissues are referred to as the tumour microenvironment (TME).[2]

As tumours progress, the surrounding microenvironment co-evolves into an activated state through continuous tumour–host interactions.[1] The TME contains many different cell types including normal fibroblasts, carcinoma-associated fibroblasts (CAFs), myofibroblasts, smooth muscle cells, endothelial cells and their precursors, pericytes, neutrophils, eosinophils, basophils, mast cells, T and B lymphocytes, natural killer cells, macrophages and dendritic cells.[2] Many components of the immune system contribute to the rejection of tumours; however, under the influence of the malignancy, they can actually act to promote tumour growth and invasion (**Figure 16.1**). Several studies have shown that tumour stroma contains growth factors and

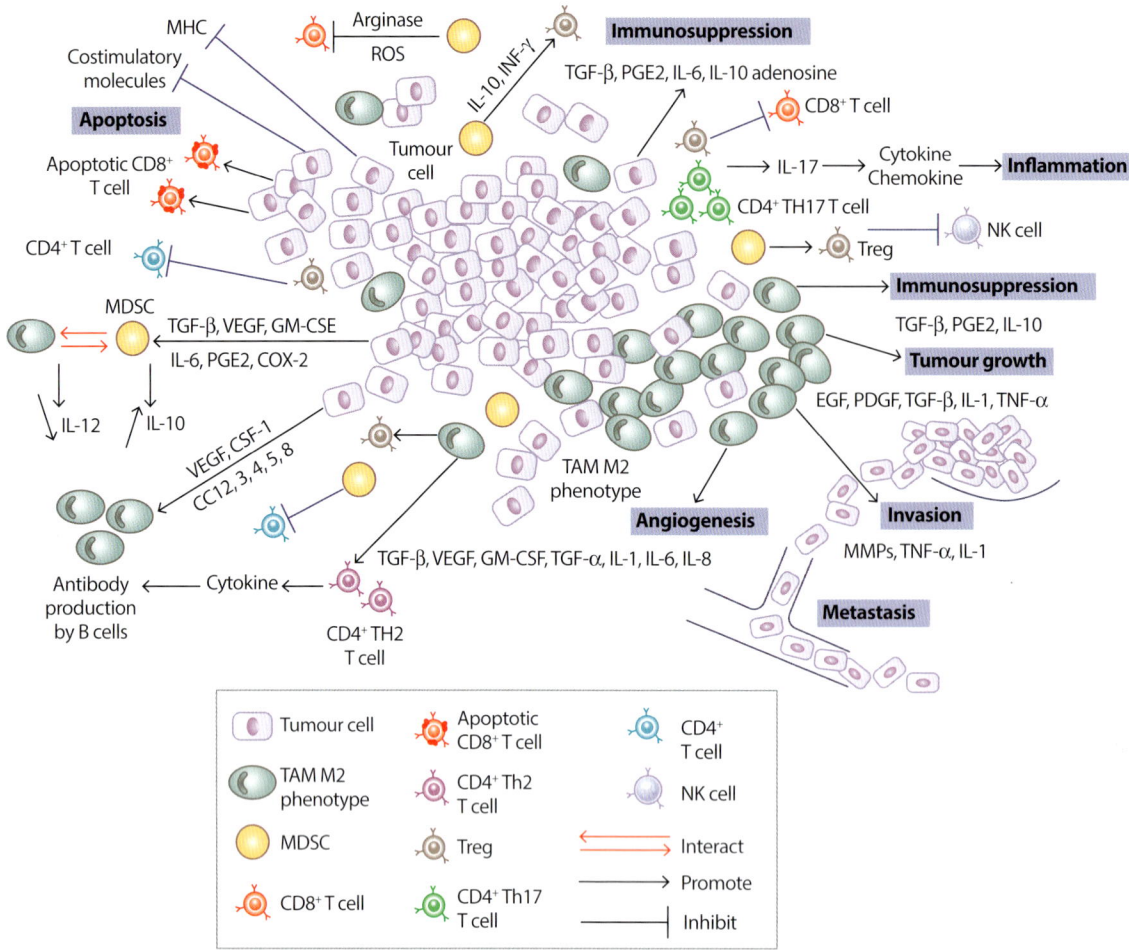

Figure 16.1 Immunosuppressive mechanisms in the tumour microenvironment.

cytokines that can promote angiogenesis, tissue invasion and metastasis. In addition, it has become evident that the stroma provides a chemoresistant capability to the tumour, most likely due to the presence and function of CAF and tumour associated macrophages (TAM) that promote resistance to oncological therapies.[3–5]

The cellular component of TME

T lymphocytes are considered an essential component of anti-tumour immunity. *In vitro*, malignant cells presenting 'altered self' peptides (molecules that have undergone mutations or are aberrantly expressed in the tumour cell) in association with major histocompatibility complex (MHC) class I molecules, can be recognized by CD8+ T cells causing tumour cell-lysis and/or apoptosis through the release of toxic molecules such as perforin and granzymes. Conversely, CD4+ T cells are programmed to release cytokines and may differentiate into one of an ever growing type of T helper cells (i.e. Th1, Th2, Th17) or regulatory T cells (Treg cells), which differ in the cytokine repertoire they produce and therefore their function[6] when interacting with antigen-presenting cells such as dendritic cells or macrophages expressing altered self peptides by host MHC II molecules. In general the CD4+ Th1 cells serve to 'help' and enhance the magnitude and duration of the anti-tumour response.[7] However, CD4+ Th2 cells and CD4+ Treg cells are capable of suppressing effective CD8+ anti-tumour responses.[5] *In vivo* studies by several groups have found dysfunctional circulating and tumour-infiltrating T cells in HNSCC patients, with functional assays identifying multiple defects in T-cell activation and effector functions, suggesting that the tumour has successfully suppressed an otherwise robust lymphocytic response.[8–11]

The TME can become dominated by CD4+ Treg cells that suppress anti-tumour effector T cells by the production of suppressive cytokines such as TGF-β, interleukin-10 (IL-10), prostaglandin E2 (PGE2) and adenosine.[5] Although the full relevance of different subsets of Treg cells is not yet known one subtype, inducible Treg cells (iTreg cells or Tr1 cells), have been shown to very effectively suppress cytotoxic T cell activity both in the TME of several cancers and the peripheral circulation.[12–13] It is becoming increasingly clear that the balance between inflammatory effector cells and Treg cells is critical in producing an effective immune response. A relatively crude measure of the effectiveness is to determine the ratio between cytotoxic CD8+ T cells and Treg cells within the tumour microenvironment. Higher CD8+/Treg cell ratios have been shown to be associated with a favourable prognosis in a range of human cancers including ovarian,[14] hepatocellular,[15] breast,[16] lung[17] and HNSCC.[13]

Tumour infiltrating lymphocytes (TIL) have been shown to promote angiogenesis and therefore tumour progression and metastasis. Cells with such activity in HNSCC include mast cells,[18] CD34 progenitor cells,[19] Th17 cells[20] and TAM.[21] A high level of infiltration of TAM within HNSCC defined by the overexpression of macrophage content, monocyte chemoattractant protein 1 (MCP1) and macrophage inflammatory protein (MIP)-3alpha levels was also found to be a strong predictor of lymph node metastasis, extracapsular spread and advanced stages of the disease; all considered as poor prognostic markers.[22-23] Stromal cells have been shown to secrete cytokines and growth factors including vascular endothelial growth factor (VEGF), platelet derived growth factor (PDGF) and IL-8, which are strong inducers of angiogenesis and tumour progression.[24-26] VEGF expression, which is responsible for facilitating proliferation of endothelial cells and neo-vascularization, correlated significantly with adverse prognosis in HNSCC patients.[27] VEGF-C, a member of the VEGF family, plays an important role in tumour lymphangiogenesis; raised tumour-tissue levels of VEGF-C are associated with a worse prognosis due to increased tumour lymphatic vessel density that correlates with lymph node metastasis in HNSCC.[28]

Carcinoma-associated fibroblasts are the major cell population in the tumour stroma.[2, 29] Within the TME, there is evidence suggesting that CAF use protease and mechanical remodelling of the extracellular membrane to lay tracks along which HNSCC tumour cells invade.[30] When compared with normal oral cavity fibroblasts, CAF were found to exhibit rapid growth, increased proliferation and viability and produce α-smooth muscle actin (α-SMA) and membrane metalloproteinase 2 (MMP-2), which represent markers of chronic inflammation that normal tissue fibroblasts do not produce.[31]

Cytokines and chemokines in TME

Cytokines are small molecular weight molecules that regulate all aspects of the immune response (e.g. inflammation, immunity and haematopoiesis). This group of molecules is divided into subfamilies according to their structure or function and includes: interleukins (IL), interferons (IFN), cytokines, tumour necrosis factors (TNF) and other cell-specific growth factors.[7] Chemokines are a superfamily of small proteins with chemoattractant and activation properties for different cell types involved in inflammatory reactions and are considered the main facilitators of cell trafficking.[32] Cytokines and chemokines are key in controlling communication within and between individual cells in the TME.

Tumours produce cytokines in a dysregulated manner that contributes to an ineffective host immune response.[33-34] One such cytokine is tumour growth factor beta (TGF-β), which acts broadly to suppress cell-mediated immunity and is released by tumour cells and Treg cells conferring inhibitory action.[35] Further observations in HNSCC, as well as in many other cancers, have shown that tumour development can significantly alter serum levels of key Th1 and Th2 type cytokines in the body. Commonly there appears to be an imbalance, towards a Th2 cell cytokine profile that becomes more pronounced at later stages of tumour growth.[36-37] The Th2 cell profile is characterized by the production of IL-4, IL-5, IL-6, IL-10, IL-13 and granulocyte-macrophage colony stimulating factor (GM-CSF) whilst Th1 responses are characterized by the production of interferon gamma (IFN-γ), IL-2, IL-12 and IL-18. Some of the Th2 cell cytokines, particularly IL-10, have been clearly shown to suppress the cellular immune response effectively, thus permitting tumour growth.[38]

Immune suppressive cytokines, whether produced by tumour cells or by stromal cells, seem to control the crosstalk between cells within the TME during tumour progression (Figure 16.1). Furthermore the release of such cytokines induces ECM remodelling, basement membrane degradation, tumour cell proliferation and angiogenesis, and hence favours tumour progression and metastasis. In studies on HNSCC cell lines, fibroblasts and stromal endothelial cells have been shown to express a suppressive cytokine/chemokine milieu when co-cultured with HNSCC cells.[39] CAF showed an increase in the expression of a number of pro-inflammatory cytokines and chemokines including CCL7, CXCL1, CXCL2, CXCL3 and CXCL8 when compared with CAF cultured alone.[40] Similarly, type I collagen was found to markedly stimulate immune-suppressive cytokine expression such as IL-1α, IL-1β, IL-6, TNF-α, TGF-β and MMP-2 in metastatic HNSCC cell lines compared with that of the primary cancer cell lines.[41]

Chemokines co-ordinate the trafficking, migration and organization of cells to various tissue compartments.[42-43] Thus understanding alterations in chemokine levels within HNSCC is likely to offer useful prognostic information. Initial work by Muller and colleagues demonstrated that upregulation and activation of CXCR4 and CCR7, facilitate leukocyte migration to regional lymph nodes; in breast cancer this is capable of inducing actin polymerization, migration and invasion both *in vitro* and *in vivo* studies.[44] Upregulation of CXCR4 and CCR7 expression has been observed in tumour tissue and lymph nodes of HNSCC patients.[45-48] Overexpression of CXCR4 was shown to be a significant prognostic indicator for poor survival in patients with oral squamous cell carcinoma[46] while upregulation of CCR7 was also found to correlate with poorer survival in patients with HNSCC.[49] Furthermore, it was reported that hypoxia, a major stimulator of tumour progression, enhances CXCR4 expression by activating hypoxia inducible factor 1 alpha (HIF-1α) in tissue from oral squamous cell carcinoma patients.[50]

A recent systematic review of cytokine/chemokine profiles and their clinical significance in various cancers has shown that, despite tumour heterogeneity, patients with advanced-stage cancer seem to experience a simultaneous immune-stimulation and immune-suppression, with increased concentrations of cytokines Macrophage Inhibitory Factor (MIF), TNF-α, IL-18, IL-8, IL-6, TGF-β, and IL-10. The result of the described cytokine pattern is local immunostimulation and inflammation with synchronous functional immune-suppression and attraction of immune cells that are then tolerized, thus protecting tumour cells locally from detection and destruction. The review concluded that, independent of tumour histological changes, the immune-suppressive cytokine cascade links the functional status of the immune system with the extent of cancer disease and patients prognosis and ultimately is an expression of the systemic disease in cancer.[51]

Inflammation in TME

A chronic inflammatory environment is associated with neoplastic transformation and progression in many malignancies including HNSCC.[52–54] Oncogenes that are activated early in the development of tumours can incite strong inflammatory responses. For example, lung tumours that are initiated by a mutation in the K-ras oncogene produce chemokines that attract immune cells to the TME;[55] or the RET–PTC protein, that causes constitutive activation of the RET tyrosine kinase domains in thyroid tumours, modulates nuclear factor-κB, a transcription factor that controls the production of immune-regulatory cytokines. The RET–PTC protein increases the production of GM-CSF and monocyte chemotactic protein 1, that contribute to a pro-inflammatory microenvironment.[56] Products of dying tumour cells (e.g. heat-shock proteins and monosodium urate) are some of the many inflammatory substances that further exacerbate immune responses in a relatively non-specific manner.[57]

The pro-inflammatory conditions within the TME have also been shown to contribute to tumour progression, proliferation and metastasis. Cyclooxygenase (COX)-2 and 5-lipoxygenase (5-LOX) pathways, which both produce derivatives from arachidonic acid, are activated during HNSCC development.[58] The COX-2 enzymes specifically catalyze the production of prostaglandins (PG). PG are increased in HNSCC (e.g. raised PGE2 in HNSCC is known to promote tumour growth and inhibit apoptosis by upregulating Bcl-2 expression). PGE2 is also known to increase the production of angiogenic factors such as VEGF and MMP, resulting in the promotion of invasion and tumour metastasis. Higher expression of COX-2 in tumour cells is seen in parallel with an increased PGE2 expression in HNSCC.[59–60]

TUMOUR ESCAPE MECHANISMS

In order for the immune system to identify and eliminate tumours, it needs to recognize the malignant growth in some way. Some antigens are solely presented by tumour cells and never by normal cells, thus are called tumour-specific antigens (TSA); for example, MAGE-1, a melanoma-specific antigen,[61] or NY-ESO-1 antigen, a molecule that belongs to a family of cancer–testis antigens.[62] Other antigens are presented by tumour cells but at raised levels when compared with normal cells; these are termed tumour-associated antigens (TAA).[63] Examples of TAA in HNSCC include the epidermal growth factor receptor (EGFR)[64] and wild-type p53.[65] Tumours associated with viral infection display viral antigens that can serve as tumour markers. Good examples are the products of the E6 and E7 genes of the human papilloma virus, the causative agent of both cervical[66–67] and oropharyngeal carcinoma,[68] and EBNA-1, the Epstein–Barr virus nuclear antigen expressed by Burkitt's lymphoma and nasopharyngeal carcinoma cells.[69]

The discovery and identification of tumour antigens has helped scientists begin to understand the key steps in an anti-tumour immune response. In animal models, the encounter between the immune system and tumours initiates a process termed 'immunoediting'.[70] This process can bring about three outcomes: elimination of the tumour; tumour equilibrium, in which there is immune selection of less immunogenic tumours during an anti-tumour immune response;[71] and tumour escape, the growth of tumour variants that resist immune destruction.

Tumour escape mechanisms have been broadly divided into two main groups. Either the tumour cells are poor stimulators of immune cells and hence are simply not recognized, and/or they actively interfere with immune function and survival of the immune cells.[72–73] Tumour-escape from immune-surveillance in HNSCC is due to a combination of multiple mechanisms involving tumour cells, cytokines and immune cells (Table 16.1). The most common mechanism is the loss of MHC class 1 molecules that reduces/prevents TAA expression, which, coupled with deficient antigen-presenting and processing mechanisms by immature dendritic cells and overexpression of Treg cell, all contribute to avoidance of the immune system. Major regulators behind dysregulated cytokine and chemokine function include imbalanced STAT1/STAT3 signalling within tumour cells,[74] hepatocyte growth factor (HGF) production by tumour-associated fibroblasts,[75, 76] and production of immunosuppressive molecules by TAM such as VEGF, IL-10 and TGF-β.[77, 78] Finally, effector cell dysfunction allows tumour escape through an increased level of spontaneous apoptosis and anergy, as well as signalling defects in the T cell receptor signalling complex (Table 16.1).

TABLE 16.1 Immune-suppressive tumour-escape mechanisms in HNSCC

- Spontaneous apoptosis/anergy of tumour infiltrating and circulatory T cells[10, 105, 106]
- Imbalanced and decreased absolute counts of T cell subsets[107, 108]
- Signalling defects in effector cells[109, 110]
- Cytokine imbalance favouring immunosuppression[51, 111, 112]
- Poor expression of co-stimulatory molecules and high expression of co-inhibitory receptors on tumour cells[106, 113, 114]
- Deficient antigen-presenting and processing mechanisms[115–117]
- Loss of HLA class I molecules by HNSCC cells[118, 119]
- Inhibition of NK cell activity[73, 120, 121]
- Overexpression of Treg cells both in the circulation and intra-tumourally[6, 122]

HLA: human leukocyte antigen; NK cells: natural killer cells; Treg cells: regulatory T cells; HNSCC: Head and neck squamous cell carcinoma.

TUMOUR BIOMARKERS

As our knowledge of the anti-tumour response increases the idea of using biomarkers as surrogate endpoints of clinical response is becoming a reality.[2]

Tumour biomarkers can be divided into either disease-related ones (i.e. at the time of diagnosis prior to any therapy) or therapy-related ones (i.e. prior to, during and after therapy).[79]

Seminal work in colorectal cancer (CRC) by Golan and colleagues,[80–83] reporting on TIL using modern techniques of systems biology, and an objective scoring system based on image analysis data, showed that the type, density and location of immune cells within tumours predicted clinical outcome. T cell infiltrates emerged as the strongest independent prognostic factor, more significant than the conventional clinicopathological criteria such as tumour size, depth of infiltration, differentiation, or the nodal status. Based on these results, a proposal has been drafted for a routine evaluation of the tumour microenvironment for the density, location, phenotype and function of T cells in order to define an 'immune score' for each tumour as a part of the standard pathological examination. Although not yet incorporated in routine pathological practice, this approach represents the first serious immunological marker of risk in cancer with a potential to be incorporated into prognostically relevant immune classification of human CRC equal to or better than the conventional TNM classification.[81] In HNSCC, the value of tumour-infiltrating CD4+ T cell subpopulations is under evaluation as a prognostic marker; however, this too has not yet been incorporated into clinical practice.[84–85]

One of the other validated biomarkers is the B cell signature, which has emerged as the most robust prognostic factor in breast cancer.[86–87] A multicentred trial has identified the immunoglobulin G kappa chain (IgGκC) as an immunological biomarker of prognosis and response to chemotherapy breast cancer, ovarian cancer, non-small cell lung cancer, and CRC. The IgGκC was microscopically identified as a product of plasma cells present in the tumour stroma and was validated as a prognostic biomarker by RNA and protein-based expression studies independently performed in thousands of formalin-fixed, paraffin-embedded specimens at 20 different centres.[87] However, the most important finding was that IgGκC predicted responses to neo-adjuvant therapy in breast cancer and thus qualifies it as the first immune marker of response to cancer treatment. Supporting the key role of the B cell signature in HNSCC is a study by Pretscher et al. where intra-tumoural CD20+ B cells were significantly more frequent in metastatic lesions than in primary tumours when 193 tissue cores from 33 patients were examined. Further, large numbers of peri-tumoural B cells together with increased numbers of intra-epithelial CD8+ T cells in metastatic tumours were associated with favourable outcome in patients with oro- and hypopharyngeal carcinoma.[88]

Recent evidence has suggested that the total white blood count and especially the elevated neutrophil count compared with a depressed lymphocyte count (i.e. high neutrophil-to-lymphocyte ratio (NLR)) measured prior to oncological therapies predicts adverse clinical outcome in patients with lung, breast, renal, ovarian and HNSCC. Further, high NLR was found to be a significant but not yet validated marker of poor response to chemotherapy in these cancers.[89] These observations are in agreement with previous studies that reported low lymphocyte counts in patients with HNSCC, for example spontaneous apoptosis of circulating CD8+ antigen-responding effector T cells, leading to rapid lymphocyte turnover and depressed absolute numbers of T cell subsets tested prior to any form of treatment, have been reported.[4]

Multiple other biomarkers have been identified in various cancers including HNSCC, but are not yet validated. Examples include the frequency and function of circulating Treg cells,[13, 90] markers of CD8+ T cell apoptosis such as Fas L+ microvesicles and their immunosuppressive cytokines PDL-1 &TGF-β,[91] the frequency of circulating CD8+ CCR7+ cells,[92] and the functional status of tumour peptide-specific CD8+ T cells.[93] A recent review summarizes the biomarkers measured by immunohistochemistry in the different anatomical subgroups of HNSCC and their clinical relevance;[94] as yet no marker is sufficiently robust to become a routine test in HNSCC.

IMMUNOTHERAPY

Early clinical trials of immunotherapy in the majority of cancers were troubled by systemic toxicity or difficulties in local administration. Now, interest in immunotherapy has been revitalized by mechanistic insights into immune evasion, coupled to ongoing developments of novel immunotherapies.[95]

Any form of immune-based therapy must overcome the main factors hindering an effective immune response; a representative selection of ongoing trials is detailed in **Table 16.2**. Multiple components of the immune system, such as immunization with tumour antigens, cytokines and T cells, have all been studied in multiple immune-based therapies. The aim of these therapies is to cause the tumour to be targeted in a specific fashion by the host immune defences.

Immune-based therapies are classified according to their target cell or molecule. Targeting specific elements of the immune system such as tumour antigens with antibodies and therapeutic cancer vaccines have all shown promising results.[96] Some of the most promising immune-based therapies involve the administration of monoclonal antibodies against tumour antigens (e.g. Trastuzumab, an antibody against the HER2 receptor expressed on 15–25% of breast cancers;[97] rituximab that binds CD20 expressed on 90% of Non-Hodgkin B-cell lymphomas;[97] or cetuximab, that binds to EGFR that is upregulated in HNSCC, lung and colorectal cancer);[98–100] these have all been shown to be clinically effective and are already incorporated into mainstream treatment modalities.

TABLE 16.2 Key areas and promising immunotherapies in HNSCC		
Key area	Example of drug mechanisms	Phase of development
TA-specific monoclonal antibodies	**Cetuximab**: Anti-EGFR chimeric IgG1 mAb[98] blocks growth factor signalling	NICE and FDA approved
	Nimotuzumab: Anti-EGFR IgG1 humanized mAb[123] blocks growth factor signalling	II
Targeting cytokines	**IL 12**: Cytokine agonist causes NK cell activation[95]	II
	Bevacizumab: Anti-VEGF IgG1 humanized mAb[123] a drug that inhibits angiogenesis	III
	IRX-2: various cytokines including IL-1b, IL-2, IL-6, IL-8, GM-CSF, IFNγ and TNFα, to enhance anti-tumour immune responses[125]	I/II
Targeting T cell checkpoint inhibitors	**Ipilimumab**: Anti-CTLA4 IgG1 humanized mAb[95] that prevents co-stimulatory signals	I
Therapeutic cancer vaccines	**MAGE-3 and HPV-16 vaccine**: Trojan construct peptide vaccine[126]	I
	HPV pNGVL4a-CRT/E7 (Detox) DNA vaccine: Detoxified E7 DNA in a pNGVL4a plasmid backbone[127]	I
	Multi-epitope p53 vaccine: Wild type peptide/autologous dendritic cell vaccine[95]	I

Examples of key areas during anti-tumour immune responses, where immunotherapeutic agents are being utilized and trialled. TA: tumour associated; EGFR: epidermal growth factor receptor; IgG: immunoglobulin G; mAb: monoclonal antibody; IL: interleukin; NK cells: natural killer cells; VEGF: vascular endothelial growth factor; GM-CSF: granulocyte macrophage-colony stimulating factor; IFNγ: interferon gamma; TNFα: tumour necrosis factor alpha; CTLA4: cytotoxic T-lymphocyte antigen 4; MAGE-3: melanoma-associated antigen-3; HPV: human papilloma virus. (For a current list of immunotherapy-based trials, please refer to clinicaltrials.gov.)

Several mechanisms are developed by cancerous cells to escape the immune system such as a loss or a reduction of the expression of MHC class 1 molecules and co-stimulatory molecules, the expression of FasL to induce apoptosis of tumour-infiltrating lymphocytes and the production of immunosuppressive molecules such as TGF-β, PGE2, IL-6, IL-10 and adenosine. Among the subpopulations of naïve CD4+ T cells, CD4+ Th17 T cells promote inflammation by secreting IL-17 whereas CD4+ Th2 T cells promote antibody production by B cells. Tregs promote tumour progression by inhibiting the functions of CD4+ and CD8+ T cells and NK cells. TAMsM2 phenotype induce the expression of CD4+ Th2 T cell and Tregs. Moreover, M2 phenotype promotes growth tumour (EGF, PDGF, TGF-β, IL-6, IL-1 and TNF-α), angiogenesis (TGF-β, VEGF, GM-CSF, TGF-α, IL-1, IL-6 and IL-8), invasion (MMPs, TNF-α, IL-1), immunosuppression (TGF-β, PGE2 and IL-10) and metastasis. MDSCs induce Treg cells, secrete IL-10, and inhibit CD4+ and CD8+ T cells. (Adapted from Duray et al.[128])

Seminal work by Bonner et al. reported that the administration of cetuximab with radiotherapy, when compared to radiotherapy alone, has significantly prolonged progression free survival without increasing the common toxic effects associated with radiotherapy to the head and neck in a multicentred phase III clinical trial.[98] So far, cetuximab is the only approved antibody by FDA and NICE for use in patients with locally advanced HNSCC. In addition, a variety of other anti-EGFR agents such as the small molecule tyrosine kinase inhibitors (TKI) lapatinib, dacomitinib and afatinib and the anti-EGFR mAbzalutumumab, nimotuzumab and panitumumab, are currently under investigation in phase II and III clinical trials in different HNSCC therapeutic settings. The EGFR-targeting TKI erlotinib is currently in phase III development for oral cancer prevention (NLM Identifer NCT00402779), while bevacizumab, an anti VEGF monoclonal antibody, has been shown to produce favourable efficacy when combined with chemoradiotherapy for locally advanced HNSCC.[101] Numerous other biological agents are in early stages of development for HNSCC treatment, including novel anti-EGFR mAb such as necitumumab, small-molecule TKIs (vandetanib, icotinib and dasatinib), and drugs (temsirolimus and everolimus). Overall, a wealth of clinical trial data are expected in the coming years, with the potential to modify significantly the approach to anti-EGFR therapy for HNSCC.[102]

The key areas for targeting the immune system through immune-based therapies with promising results in HNSCC are summarized in Table 16.2. It is worth noting that in HNSCC the degree of immune-suppressive cross-talk suggests that single immunotherapies will be inadequate. Thus, integration of immune therapies with standard treatments for cancer is seen as the best avenue and revealing promising results.[95]

CONCLUSIONS

It is evident now that cancer creates an immunosuppressive environment locally and systemically. This tumour microenvironment interferes with maturation and activation of antigen-presenting cells and naïve cytotoxic T cells,[103] hence creating immune-suppressive conditions that favour tumour proliferation and progression. As our understanding of the TME grows, specific key areas and immune end points can be explored with the ultimate goal that they may act as potential targets for tumour detection, prognosis and ultimately therapy.

In HNSCC, several reports have shown that immune cells within the peripheral circulation, associated lymph nodes and tumour tissue are responsible for supressing effective CD8+ anti-tumour responses and are associated with poorer prognosis in patients. Such cells include CD4+ Th2 cells, TD4+ Treg cells, TAM and CAF. Products of these cells in the form of cytokines and chemokines have also been linked to immune suppression and poor prognosis in HNSCC patients, for example IL-10, TGF-β, CXCR4 and CCR7.

Most tumour biomarkers, whether reflecting cancer presence, progression or response to therapy, have a potential to serve as intermediate biomarkers of outcome.

However only a few, including T-cell and B-cell immune signatures or the NLR, have been validated in independent clinical studies encompassing sufficiently large cohorts of patients with different tumour types to give statistically valid data. In HNSCC, a histopathological 'immune score' of TIL as a robust clinical prognostic marker is under evaluation based on work in colorectal cancer that has been reported recently. HPV p16 status in HPV-associated head and neck tumours is the only validated biomarker in HNSCC to date. Treatment protocols of HNSCC, especially oropharyngeal tumours, have now fully incorporated HPV p16 status in their guidelines.[104]

Precise clinicopathological analysis and clinical follow-up in well-defined, relatively uniform cohorts of patients in each subunit of the head and neck offers the best option for confirming immune endpoints as biomarkers of outcome. This is particularly important in tumours of the head and neck as multiple anatomical subsites with different molecular biology and immune reactions are usually studied and reported together. This point has clearly been shown to be relevant in oropharyngeal tumours, and more precisely tonsillar and tongue base tumours that are HPV related, and nasopharyngeal tumours that are EBV related.[104] Much work remains to confirm the reliable association of immune biomarkers with clinical endpoints and to validate each of these potentially promising biomarkers in a series of prospective clinical trials appropriately powered to determine effects on each head and neck subsite.

Much has been learned about the potential of the immune system to control cancer and the various ways that immunotherapy can boost the potential of the immune system for the benefit of the patient. This knowledge has stimulated the invention of many new therapeutic antibodies, cell-based treatments, and vaccines, which are starting to be used in clinical practice, either alone or in various combinations. Cetuximab, the only immune-based therapy incorporated in the treatment of advanced HNSCC so far, has paved the way for a wealth of ongoing and future trials exploring multiple agents in key areas during tumour progression and spread. Future immune-based therapies in HNSCC specifically, and solid tumours generally, are expected to result in improved cancer treatment.

KEY POINTS

- The tumour microenvironment strongly influences tumour development and outcome through a combination of cell activities; Tumour Associated Macrophages and Treg cell populations appear to play prominent roles.
- Currently, no biomarkers have been identified which possess prognostic or diagnostic value above TMN classification, but it is likely that tumour subtype-specific molecules will be identified in the future.
- The number of trials involving immunotherapies in HNSCC continues to increase; the use of novel checkpoint inhibitors has shown positive preliminary data.

REFERENCES

1. Hanahan D, Weinberg RA. Hallmarks of cancer: the next generation. *Cell* 2011; **144**(5): 646–74.
2. Koontongkaew S. The tumor microenvironment contribution to development, growth, invasion and metastasis of head and neck squamous cell carcinomas. *J Cancer* 2013; **4**(1): 66–83.
3. Albini A, Sporn MB. The tumour microenvironment as a target for chemoprevention. *Nat Rev Cancer* 2007; **7**(2): 139–47.
4. Whiteside TL. Immune responses to cancer: are they potential biomarkers of prognosis? *Front Oncol* 2013; **3**: 107.
5. Whiteside TL. What are regulatory T cells (Treg) regulating in cancer and why? *Semin Cancer Biol* 2012; **22**(4): 327–34.
6. Zou W. Regulatory T cells, tumour immunity and immunotherapy. *Nat Rev Immunol* 2006; **6**(4): 295–307.
7. Topping KP, Fletcher LM, Agada FO, et al. Head and neck tumour immunology: basic concepts and new clinical implications. *J Laryngol Otol* 2009; **123**(1): 9–18.
8. Albers AE, Schaefer C, Visus C, et al. Spontaneous apoptosis of tumor-specific tetramer+ CD8+ T lymphocytes in the peripheral circulation of patients with head and neck cancer. *Head Neck* 2009; **31**(6): 773–81.
9. Prado-Garcia H, Romero-Garcia S, Aguilar-Cazares D, et al. Tumor-induced CD8+ T-cell dysfunction in lung cancer patients. *Clin Dev Immunol* 2012; 741741.
10. Hoffmann TK, Dworacki G, Tsukihiro T, et al. Spontaneous apoptosis of circulating T lymphocytes in patients with head and neck cancer and its clinical importance. *Clin Cancer Res* 2002; **8**(8): 2553–62.
11. Reichert TE, Strauss L, Wagner EM, et al. Signaling abnormalities, apoptosis, and reduced proliferation of circulating and tumor-infiltrating lymphocytes in patients with oral carcinoma. *Clin Cancer Res* 2002; **8**(10): 3137–45.
12. Alhamarneh O, Amarnath SM, Stafford ND, Greenman J. Regulatory T cells: what role do they play in antitumor immunity in patients with head and neck cancer? *Head Neck* 2008; **30**(2): 251–61.
13. Drennan S, Stafford ND, Greenman J, Green VL. Increased frequency and suppressive activity of CD127(low/-) regulatory T cells in the peripheral circulation of patients with head and neck squamous cell carcinoma are associated with advanced stage and nodal involvement. *Immunology* 2013; **140**(3): 335–43.
14. Leffers N, Gooden MJ, de Jong RA, et al. Prognostic significance of tumor-infiltrating T-lymphocytes in primary and metastatic lesions of advanced stage ovarian cancer. *Cancer Immunol Immunother* 2009; **58**(3): 449–59.
15. Gao Q, Qiu SJ, Fan J, et al. Intratumoral balance of regulatory and cytotoxic T cells is associated with prognosis of hepatocellular carcinoma after resection. *J Clin Oncol* 2007; **25**(18): 2586–93.
16. Ladoire S, Mignot G, Dabakuyo S, et al. In situ immune response after neoadjuvant chemotherapy for breast cancer predicts survival. *J Pathol* 2011; **224**(3): 389–400.
17. Petersen RP, Campa MJ, Sperlazza J, et al. Tumor infiltrating Foxp3+ regulatory T-cells are associated with recurrence in pathologic stage I NSCLC patients. *Cancer* 2006; **107**(12): 2866–72.
18. Iamaroon A, Pongsiriwet S, Jittidecharaks S, et al. Increase of mast cells and tumor angiogenesis in oral squamous cell carcinoma. *J Oral Pathol Med* 2003; **32**(4): 195–99.
19. Grote K, Salguero G, Ballmaier M, et al. The angiogenic factor CCN1 promotes adhesion and migration of circulating CD34+ progenitor cells: potential role in angiogenesis and endothelial regeneration. *Blood* 2007; **110**(3): 877–85.
20. Kesselring R, Thiel A, Pries R, et al. Human Th17 cells can be induced through head and neck cancer and have a functional impact on HNSCC development. *Brit J Cancer* 2010; **103**(8): 1245–54.
21. El-Rouby DH. Association of macrophages with angiogenesis in oral verrucous and squamous cell carcinomas. *J Oral Pathol Med* 2010; **39**(7):559–64.
22. Marcus B, Arenberg D, Lee J, et al. Prognostic factors in oral cavity and oropharyngeal squamous cell carcinoma. *Cancer* 2004; **101**(12): 2779–87.

23. Chang KP, Kao HK, Yen TC, et al. Overexpression of macrophage inflammatory protein-3alpha in oral cavity squamous cell carcinoma is associated with nodal metastasis. *Oral Oncol* 2011; **47**(2): 108–13.
24. Sawatsubashi M, Yamada T, Fukushima N, et al. Association of vascular endothelial growth factor and mast cells with angiogenesis in laryngeal squamous cell carcinoma. *Virchows Arch* 2000; **436**(3): 243–48.
25. Bran B, Bran G, Hormann K, Riedel F. The platelet-derived growth factor receptor as a target for vascular endothelial growth factor-mediated anti-angiogenetic therapy in head and neck cancer. *Int J Oncol* 2009; **34**(1): 255–61.
26. Li C, Shintani S, Terakado N, et al. Microvessel density and expression of vascular endothelial growth factor, basic fibroblast growth factor, and platelet-derived endothelial growth factor in oral squamous cell carcinomas. *Int J Oral Max Surg* 2005; **34**(5): 559–65.
27. Kyzas PA, Stefanou D, Batistatou A, Agnantis NJ. Hypoxia-induced tumor angiogenic pathway in head and neck cancer: an in vivo study. *Cancer Lett* 2005 **225**(2): 297–304.
28. Sedivy R, Beck-Mannagetta J, Haverkampf C, et al. Expression of vascular endothelial growth factor-C correlates with the lymphatic microvessel density and the nodal status in oral squamous cell cancer. *J Oral Pathol Med* 2003; **32**(8): 455–60.
29. Xouri G, Christian S. Origin and function of tumor stroma fibroblasts. *Semin Cell Dev Biol* 2010; **21**(1): 40–46.
30. Gaggioli C, Hooper S, Hidalgo-Carcedo C, et al. Fibroblast-led collective invasion of carcinoma cells with differing roles for RhoGTPases in leading and following cells. *Nat Cell Biol* 2007; **9**(12): 1392–400.
31. Liu Y, Hu T, Shen J, et al. Separation, cultivation and biological characteristics of oral carcinoma-associated fibroblasts. *Oral Dis* 2006; **12**(4): 375–80.
32. Sarvaiya PJ, Guo D, Ulasov I, et al. Chemokines in tumor progression and metastasis. *Oncotarget* 2013; **4**(12): 2171–85.
33. Sparano A, Lathers DM, Achille N, et al. Modulation of Th1 and Th2 cytokine profiles and their association with advanced head and neck squamous cell carcinoma. *Otolaryng Head Neck* 2004; **131**(5): 573–76.
34. Inagaki A, Ishida T, Ishii T, et al. Clinical significance of serum Th1-, Th2- and regulatory T cells-associated cytokines in adult T-cell leukemia/lymphoma: high interleukin-5 and -10 levels are significant unfavorable prognostic factors. *Int J Cancer* 2006; **118**(12): 3054–61.
35. Drabsch Y, ten Dijke P. TGF-beta signalling and its role in cancer progression and metastasis. *Cancer Metast Rev* 2012; **31**(3–4): 553–68.
36. Neuner A, Schindel M, Wildenberg U, et al. Prognostic significance of cytokine modulation in non-small cell lung cancer. *Int J Cancer* 2002; **101**(3): 287–92.
37. Kumar R, Kamdar D, Madden L, et al. Th1/Th2 cytokine imbalance in meningioma, anaplastic astrocytoma and glioblastoma multiforme patients. *Oncol Rep* 2006; **15**(6): 1513–16.
38. Pries R, Wollenberg B. Cytokines in head and neck cancer. *Cytokine Growth F R* 2006; **17**(3): 141–46.
39. Sweeny L, Liu Z, Lancaster W, et al. Inhibition of fibroblasts reduced head and neck cancer growth by targeting fibroblast growth factor receptor. *Laryngoscope* 2012; **122**(7): 1539–44.
40. Jung DW, Che ZM, Kim J, et al. Tumor-stromal crosstalk in invasion of oral squamous cell carcinoma: a pivotal role of CCL7. *Int J Cancer* 2010; **127**(2): 332–44.
41. Koontongkaew S, Amornphimoltham P, Yapong B. Tumor-stroma interactions influence cytokine expression and matrix metalloproteinase activities in paired primary and metastatic head and neck cancer cells. *Biol Int* 2009; **33**(2): 165–73.
42. Strieter RM, Belperio JA, Phillips RJ, Keane MP. Chemokines: angiogenesis and metastases in lung cancer. *Novart Fdn Symp* 2004; **256**: 173–84; discussion 84–8, 259–69.
43. Zlotnik A. Chemokines in neoplastic progression. *Semin Cancer Biol* 2004; **14**(3): 181–85.
44. Muller A, Homey B, Soto H, et al. Involvement of chemokine receptors in breast cancer metastasis. *Nature* 2001; **410**(6824): 50–56.
45. Delilbasi CB, Okura M, Iida S, Kogo M. Investigation of CXCR4 in squamous cell carcinoma of the tongue. *Oral Oncol* 2004; **40**(2): 154–57.
46. Lee JI, Jin BH, Kim MA, et al. Prognostic significance of CXCR-4 expression in oral squamous cell carcinoma. *Oral Surg Oral Med O* 2009; **107**(5): 678–84.
47. Tan CT, Chu CY, Lu YC, et al. CXCL12/CXCR4 promotes laryngeal and hypopharyngeal squamous cell carcinoma metastasis through MMP-13-dependent invasion via the ERK1/2/AP-1 pathway. *Carcinogenesis* 2008; **29**(8): 1519–27.
48. Wang J, Xi L, Hunt JL, et al. Expression pattern of chemokine receptor 6 (CCR6) and CCR7 in squamous cell carcinoma of the head and neck identifies a novel metastatic phenotype. *Cancer Res* 2004; **64**(5): 1861–66.
49. Mburu YK, Egloff AM, Walker WH, et al. Chemokine receptor 7 (CCR7) gene expression is regulated by NF-kappaB and activator protein 1 (AP1) in metastatic squamous cell carcinoma of head and neck (SCCHN). *J Biol Chem* 2012; **287**(5): 3581–90.
50. Ishikawa T, Nakashiro K, Klosek SK, et al. Hypoxia enhances CXCR4 expression by activating HIF-1 in oral squamous cell carcinoma. *Oncol Rep* 2009; **21**(3): 707–12.
51. Lippitz BE. Cytokine patterns in patients with cancer: a systematic review. *Lancet Oncol* 2013; **14**(6): e218–28.
52. Le Bitoux MA, Stamenkovic I. Tumor-host interactions: the role of inflammation. *Histochem Cell Biol* 2008; **130**(6): 1079–90.
53. Grivennikov SI, Greten FR, Karin M. Immunity, inflammation, and cancer. *Cell* 2010; **140**(6): 883–99.
54. Del Prete A, Allavena P, Santoro G, et al. Molecular pathways in cancer-related inflammation. *Biochem Medica* 2011; **21**(3): 264–75.
55. Ji H, Houghton AM, Mariani TJ, et al. K-ras activation generates an inflammatory response in lung tumors. *Oncogene* 2006; **25**(14): 2105–12.
56. Russell JP, Engiles JB, Rothstein JL. Proinflammatory mediators and genetic background in oncogene mediated tumor progression. *J Immunol* 2004; **172**(7): 4059–67.
57. Rock KL, Hearn A, Chen CJ, Shi Y. Natural endogenous adjuvants. *Springer Semin Immun* 2005; **26**(3): 231–46.
58. Ondrey FG. Arachidonic acid metabolism: a primer for head and neck surgeons. *Head Neck* 1998; **20**(4): 334–49.
59. Camacho M, Leon X, Fernandez-Figueras MT, et al. Prostaglandin E(2) pathway in head and neck squamous cell carcinoma. *Head Neck* 2008; **30**(9): 1175–81.
60. Mauro A, Lipari L, Leone A, et al. Expression of cyclooxygenase-1 and cyclooxygenase-2 in normal and pathological human oral mucosa. *Folia Histochem Cyto* 2010; **48**(4): 555–63.
61. van der Bruggen P, Traversari C, Chomez P, et al. A gene encoding an antigen recognized by cytolytic T lymphocytes on a human melanoma. *Science* 1991; **254**(5038): 1643–47.
62. Chen YT, Scanlan MJ, Sahin U, et al. A testicular antigen aberrantly expressed in human cancers detected by autologous antibody screening. *P Natl Acad Sci USA* 1997; **94**(5): 1914–18.
63. Renkvist N, Castelli C, Robbins PF, Parmiani G. A listing of human tumor antigens recognized by T cells. *Cancer Immunol Immunother* 2001; **50**(1): 3–15.
64. Schuler PJ, Boeckers P, Engers R, et al. EGFR-specific T cell frequencies correlate with EGFR expression in head and neck squamous cell carcinoma. *J Transl Med* 2011; **9**: 168.
65. Albers AE, Ferris RL, Kim GG, et al. Immune responses to p53 in patients with cancer: enrichment in tetramer+ p53 peptide-specific T cells and regulatory T cells at tumor sites. *Cancer Immunol Immunother* 2005; **54**(11): 1072–81.
66. Albers A, Abe K, Hunt J, et al. Antitumor activity of human papillomavirus type 16 E7-specific T cells against virally infected squamous cell carcinoma of the head and neck. *Cancer Res* 2005; **65**(23): 11146–55.
67. Melief CJ, Vasmel WL, Offringa R, et al. Immunosurveillance of virus-induced tumors. *Cold Spring Harb Sym* 1989; **54**(Pt 1): 597–603.
68. Ringstrom E, Peters E, Hasegawa M, et al. Human papillomavirus type 16 and squamous cell carcinoma of the head and neck. *Clin Cancer Res* 2002; **8**(10): 3187–92.
69. Hislop AD, Taylor GS, Sauce D, Rickinson AB. Cellular responses to viral infection in humans: lessons from Epstein-Barr virus. *Annu Rev Immunol* 2007; **25**: 587–617.
70. Dunn GP, Old LJ, Schreiber RD. The three Es of cancer immunoediting. *Annu Rev Immunol* 2004; **22**: 329–60.
71. Koebel CM, Vermi W, Swann JB, et al. Adaptive immunity maintains occult cancer in an equilibrium state. *Nature* 2007; **450**(7171): 903–07.
72. Young MR. Protective mechanisms of head and neck squamous cell carcinomas from immune assault. *Head Neck* 2006; **28**(5): 462–70.
73. Whiteside TL. The tumor microenvironment and its role in promoting tumor growth. *Oncogene* 2008; **27**(45): 5904–12.

74. Leibowitz MS, Srivastava RM, Andrade Filho PA, et al. SHP2 is overexpressed and inhibits pSTAT1-mediated APM component expression, T-cell attracting chemokine secretion, and CTL recognition in head and neck cancer cells. *Clin Cancer Res* 2013; **19**(4): 798–808.
75. Leef G, Thomas SM. Molecular communication between tumor-associated fibroblasts and head and neck squamous cell carcinoma. *Oral Oncol* 2013; **49**(5): 381–86.
76. Singhal E, Sen P. Hepatocyte growth factor-induced c-Src-phosphatidylinositol 3-kinase-AKT-mammalian target of rapamycin pathway inhibits dendritic cell activation by blocking IkappaB kinase activity. *Int J Biochem Cell B* 2011; **43**(8): 1134–46.
77. Siveen KS, Kuttan G. Role of macrophages in tumour progression. *Immunol Lett* 2009; **123**(2): 97–102.
78. Galdiero MR, Bonavita E, Barajon I, et al. Tumor associated macrophages and neutrophils in cancer. *Immunobiology* 2013; **218**(11): 1402–10.
79. Butterfield LH, Palucka AK, Britten CM, et al. Recommendations from the iSBTc-SITC/FDA/NCI Workshop on Immunotherapy Biomarkers. *Clin Cancer Res* 2011; **17**(10): 3064–76.
80. Galon J, Costes A, Sanchez-Cabo F, et al. Type, density, and location of immune cells within human colorectal tumors predict clinical outcome. *Science* 2006; **313**(5795): 1960–64.
81. Galon J, Pages F, Marincola FM, et al. The immune score as a new possible approach for the classification of cancer. *J Transl Med* 2012; **10**: 1.
82. Fridman WH, Pages F, Sautes-Fridman C, Galon J. The immune contexture in human tumours: impact on clinical outcome. *Nat Rev Cancer* 2012; **12**(4): 298–306.
83. Fridman WH, Galon J, Pages F, et al. Prognostic and predictive impact of intra- and peritumoral immune infiltrates. *Cancer Res* 2011; **71**(17): 5601–05.
84. Badoual C, Hans S, Rodriguez J, et al. Prognostic value of tumor-infiltrating CD4+ T-cell subpopulations in head and neck cancers. *Clin Cancer Res* 2006; **12**(2): 465–72.
85. Fridman WH, Galon J, Dieu-Nosjean MC, et al. Immune infiltration in human cancer: prognostic significance and disease control. *Curr Top Microbiol* 2011; **344**: 1–24.
86. Schmidt M, Bohm D, von Torne C, et al. The humoral immune system has a key prognostic impact in node-negative breast cancer. *Cancer Res* 2008; **68**(13): 5405–13.
87. Schmidt M, Hellwig B, Hammad S, et al. A comprehensive analysis of human gene expression profiles identifies stromal immunoglobulin kappa C as a compatible prognostic marker in human solid tumors. *Clin Cancer Res* 2012; **18**(9): 2695–703.
88. Pretscher D, Distel LV, Grabenbauer GG, et al. Distribution of immune cells in head and neck cancer: CD8+ T-cells and CD20+ B-cells in metastatic lymph nodes are associated with favourable outcome in patients with oro- and hypopharyngeal carcinoma. *BMC Cancer* 2009; **9**: 292.
89. Perisanidis C, Kornek G, Poschl PW, et al. High neutrophil-to-lymphocyte ratio is an independent marker of poor disease-specific survival in patients with oral cancer. *Med Oncol* 2013; **30**(1): 334.
90. Britten CM, Janetzki S, van der Burg SH, et al. Minimal information about T cell assays: the process of reaching the community of T cell immunologists in cancer and beyond. *Cancer Immunol Immunother* 2011; **60**(1): 15–22.
91. Whiteside TL. Immune modulation of T-cell and NK (natural killer) cell activities by TEXs (tumour-derived exosomes). *Biochem Soc T* 2013; **41**(1): 245–51.
92. Czystowska M, Gooding W, Szczepanski MJ, et al. The immune signature of CD8(+)CCR7(+) T cells in the peripheral circulation associates with disease recurrence in patients with HNSCC. *Clin Cancer Res* 2013; **19**(4): 889–99.
93. Schaefer C, Butterfield LH, Lee S, et al. Function but not phenotype of melanoma peptide-specific CD8(+) T cells correlate with survival in a multiepitope peptide vaccine trial (ECOG 1696). *Int J Cancer* 2012; **131**(4): 874–84.
94. Wallis SPL, Stafford ND, Greenman J. Clinical relevance of immune parameters in the tumor microenvironment of head and neck cancers. *Head Neck* 2015; **37**(3): 449–59.
95. Gildener-Leapman N, Ferris RL, Bauman JE. Promising systemic immunotherapies in head and neck squamous cell carcinoma. *Oral Oncol* 2013; **49**(12): 1089–96.
96. Agada FO, Alhamarneh O, Stafford ND, Greenman J. Immunotherapy in head and neck cancer: current practice and future possibilities. *J Laryngol Otol* 2009; **123**(1): 19–28.
97. Piccart-Gebhart MJ, Procter M, Leyland-Jones B, et al. Trastuzumab after adjuvant chemotherapy in HER2-positive breast cancer. *New Engl J Med* 2005; **353**(16): 1659–72.
98. Bonner JA, Harari PM, Giralt J, et al. Radiotherapy plus cetuximab for squamous-cell carcinoma of the head and neck. *New Engl J Med* 2006; **354**(6): 567–78.
99. Giaccone G. Epidermal growth factor receptor inhibitors in the treatment of non-small-cell lung cancer. *J Clin Oncol* 2005; **23**(14): 3235–42.
100. Marechal R, De Schutter J, Nagy N, et al. Putative contribution of CD56 positive cells in cetuximab treatment efficacy in first-line metastatic colorectal cancer patients. *BMC Cancer* 2010; **10**: 340.
101. Yoo DS, Kirkpatrick JP, Craciunescu O, et al. Prospective trial of synchronous bevacizumab, erlotinib, and concurrent chemoradiation in locally advanced head and neck cancer. *Clin Cancer Res* 2012; **18**(5): 1404–14.
102. Cohen RB. Current challenges and clinical investigations of epidermal growth factor receptor (EGFR)- and ErbB family-targeted agents in the treatment of head and neck squamous cell carcinoma (HNSCC). *Cancer Treat Rev* 2014; **40**(4) 567–77.
103. Kareva I, Hahnfeldt P. The emerging 'hallmarks' of metabolic reprogramming and immune evasion: distinct or linked? *Cancer Res* 2013; **73**(9): 2737–42.
104. Bonilla-Velez J, Mroz EA, Hammon RJ, Rocco JW. Impact of human papillomavirus on oropharyngeal cancer biology and response to therapy: implications for treatment. *Otolaryng Clin N Am* 2013; **46**(4): 521–43.
105. Saito T, Dworacki G, Gooding W, et al. Spontaneous apoptosis of CD8+ T lymphocytes in peripheral blood of patients with advanced melanoma. *Clin Cancer Res* 2000; **6**(4): 1351–64.
106. Badoual C, Hans S, Merillon N, et al. PD-1-expressing tumor-infiltrating T cells are a favorable prognostic biomarker in HPV-associated head and neck cancer. *Cancer Res* 2013; **73**(1): 128–38.
107. Kuss I, Hathaway B, Ferris RL, et al. Decreased absolute counts of T lymphocyte subsets and their relation to disease in squamous cell carcinoma of the head and neck. *Clin Cancer Res* 2004; **10**(11): 3755–62.
108. Kuss I, Hathaway B, Ferris RL, et al. Imbalance in absolute counts of T lymphocyte subsets in patients with head and neck cancer and its relation to disease. *Adv Otorhinolaryngol* 2005; **62**: 161–72.
109. Reichert TE, Scheuer C, Day R, et al. The number of intratumoral dendritic cells and zeta-chain expression in T cells as prognostic and survival biomarkers in patients with oral carcinoma. *Cancer* 2001; **91**(11): 2136–47.
110. Kuss I, Donnenberg AD, Gooding W, Whiteside TL. Effector CD8+CD45RO-CD27-T cells have signalling defects in patients with squamous cell carcinoma of the head and neck. *Br J Cancer* 2003; **88**(2): 223–30.
111. Akhurst RJ. TGF beta signaling in health and disease. *Nat Genet* 2004; **36**(8): 790–92.
112. Jebreel A, Mistry D, Loke D, et al. Investigation of interleukin 10, 12 and 18 levels in patients with head and neck cancer. *J Laryngol Otol* 2007; **121**(3): 246–52.
113. Wang S, Chen L. Co-signaling molecules of the B7-CD28 family in positive and negative regulation of T lymphocyte responses. *Microbes Infect* 2004; **6**(8): 759–66.
114. Baruah P, Lee M, Odutoye T, et al. Decreased levels of alternative co-stimulatory receptors OX40 and 4-1BB characterise T cells from head and neck cancer patients. *Immunobiology* 2012; **217**(7): 66975.
115. Lopez-Albaitero A, Nayak JV, Ogino T, et al. Role of antigen-processing machinery in the in vitro resistance of squamous cell carcinoma of the head and neck cells to recognition by CTL. *J Immunol* 2006; **176**(6): 3402–09.
116. Ferris RL, Whiteside TL, Ferrone S. Immune escape associated with functional defects in antigen processing machinery in head and neck cancer. *Clin Cancer Res* 2006; **12**(13): 3890–95.
117. Leibowitz MS, Andrade Filho PA, Ferrone S, Ferris RL. Deficiency of activated STAT1 in head and neck cancer cells mediates TAP1-dependent escape from cytotoxic T lymphocytes. *Cancer Immunol Immunother* 2011; **60**(4): 525–35.
118. Campoli M, Chang CC, Ferrone S. HLA class I antigen loss, tumor immune escape and immune selection. *Vaccine* 2002; **20**(Suppl 4): A40-5.
119. Ferris RL, Hunt JL, Ferrone S. Human leukocyte antigen (HLA) class I defects in head and neck cancer: molecular mechanisms and clinical significance. *Immunol Res* 2005; **33**(2): 113–33.

120. Bauernhofer T, Kuss I, Henderson B, et al. Preferential apoptosis of CD56dim natural killer cell subset in patients with cancer. *Eur J Immunol* 2003; **33**(1): 119–24.
121. Dasgupta S, Bhattacharya-Chatterjee M, O'Malley BW, Jr., Chatterjee SK. Inhibition of NK cell activity through TGF-beta 1 by down-regulation of NKG2D in a murine model of head and neck cancer. *J Immunol* 2005; **175**(8): 5541–50.
122. Whiteside TL, Schuler P, Schilling B. Induced and natural regulatory T cells in human cancer. *Expert Opin Biol Ther* 2012; **12**(10): 1383–97.
123. Rojo F, Gracias E, Villena N, et al. Pharmacodynamic trial of nimotuzumab in unresectable squamous cell carcinoma of the head and neck: a SENDO Foundation study. *Clin Cancer Res* 2010; **16**(8): 2474–82.
124. Lionello M, Staffieri A, Marioni G. Potential prognostic and therapeutic role for angiogenesis markers in laryngeal carcinoma. *Acta Oto-Laryngol* 2012; **132**(6): 574–82.
125. Freeman SM, Franco JL, Kenady DE, et al. A phase 1 safety study of an IRX-2 regimen in patients with squamous cell carcinoma of the head and neck. *Am J Clin Oncol* 2011; **34**(2): 173–78.
126. Voskens CJ, Sewell D, Hertzano R, et al. Induction of MAGE-A3 and HPV-16 immunity by Trojan vaccines in patients with head and neck carcinoma. *Head Neck* 2012; **34**(12): 1734–46.
127. Peng S, Lyford-Pike S, Akpeng B, et al. Low-dose cyclophosphamide administered as daily or single dose enhances the antitumor effects of a therapeutic HPV vaccine. *Cancer Immunol Immunother* 2013; **62**(1): 171–82.
128. Duray A, Demoulin S, Hubert P, et al. Immune suppression in head and neck cancers: a review. *Clin Dev Immunol* 2010; 701657.

HUMAN PAPILLOMAVIRUS

Mustaffa Junaid and Hisham M. Mehanna

Introduction 167	HPV life cycle 167
HPV genotypes 167	HPV and cancer 169
HPV genome and proteins 167	References 171

SEARCH STRATEGY

Data in this chapter may be updated by a PubMed searches using keywords related to human papillomavirus, molecular biology, cancer pathogenesis and epidemiology.

INTRODUCTION

In recent years there has been increasing evidence related to head and neck cancer pathogenesis and viral infections, particularly human papillomavirus (HPV). In 1907 Giuseppe Ciuffo was able to demonstrate the viral origin of common warts, with the potential for human–human transmission.[1] Subsequently in 1976 Harald zur Hausen was the first to suggest a link between HPV infection and cervical cancers,[2] with HPV now considered a sexually transmitted disease. Our current knowledge of HPV and disease pathogenesis is based mainly on cervical cancer models. This chapter will review the molecular biology of HPV and related cancer pathogenesis.

HPV belongs to the papovaviridae family of viruses, which also includes the polymaviruses. The HPV virion is composed of an 8 kb double-stranded DNA genome contained within a protein capsid, and forms a non-enveloped icosahedral structure measuring 55 nm in diameter. The virus only infects epidermal cells, such as skin or mucosa.

HPV GENOTYPES

To date, more than 120 HPV types have been identified.[3] These can be divided into mucosal or cutaneous genotypes, with approximately one-third causing mucosal infections. Furthermore the HPV types can be classified into low- or high-risk, depending upon their malignant potential. Low-risk HPV includes types 6 and 11, which are traditionally associated with genital warts but are also related to laryngeal papillomatosis. The high-risk HPV types 16 and 18 have been implicated in head and neck squamous cell carcinomas (HNSCC), such as laryngeal and oropharyngeal cancers. Reported HPV prevalence in HNSCC varies between studies, and is dependent on anatomical subsite. For example, the RTOG 0129 randomized controlled study reported 63.8% HPV prevalence among patients diagnosed with oropharyngeal cancer, of whom 96% were HPV 16 positive.[4]

HPV GENOME AND PROTEINS

The HPV genome is composed of approximately 8000 base pairs coding for eight main viral genes, which are subdivided into early and late gene products (**Figure 17.1**). The LCR (long control region) contains *cis*-regulatory elements, which control and regulate viral DNA replication. The functions of the early and late genes are summarized in **Table 17.1**. The key viral proteins involved in cancer pathogenesis are E6 and E7.

HPV LIFE CYCLE

Transmission

HPV is transmitted between individuals by direct contact of skin or mucosa. While HPV can be considered a sexually transmitted disease this is by no means the only mode of transmission. Studies have demonstrated HPV infection in children, which is likely caused by vertical transmission from the mother during birth. Indeed there is evidence that risk of HPV transmission from mother to infant is

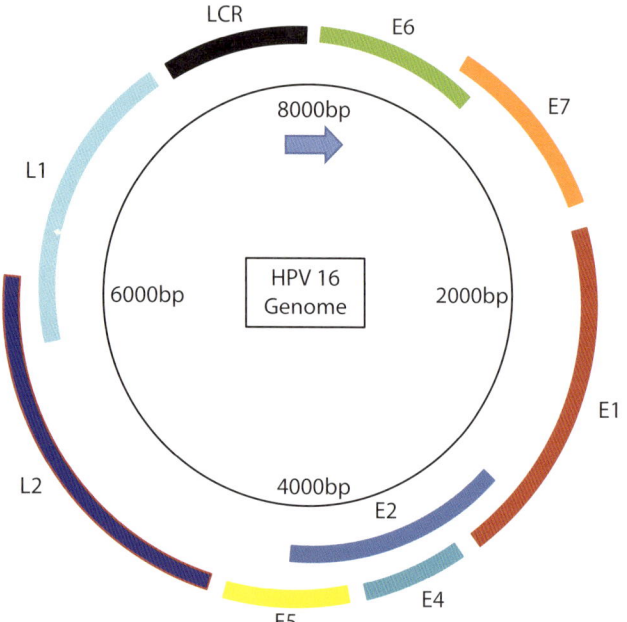

Figure 17.1 Schematic diagram of the HPV 16 genome.

TABLE 17.1 HPV gene products and functions[5, 6]

Viral protein	Functions
E1	Initiates viral DNA replication via ATP-dependent helicase activity
E2	Combined activity with E1 to initiate viral replication Regulates viral transcription Suppresses E6 and E7 activity
E4	Disrupts host cell keratin structure Supports viral amplification and maturation
E5	Enhances E6 and E7 activity Role in evading host immune response
E6	Binds to p53 and causes its degradation by proteolysis, leading to inhibition of apoptosis
E7	Binds to and inactivates pRb, causing loss of cell cycle regulation
L1	Major capsid protein
L2	Minor capsid protein

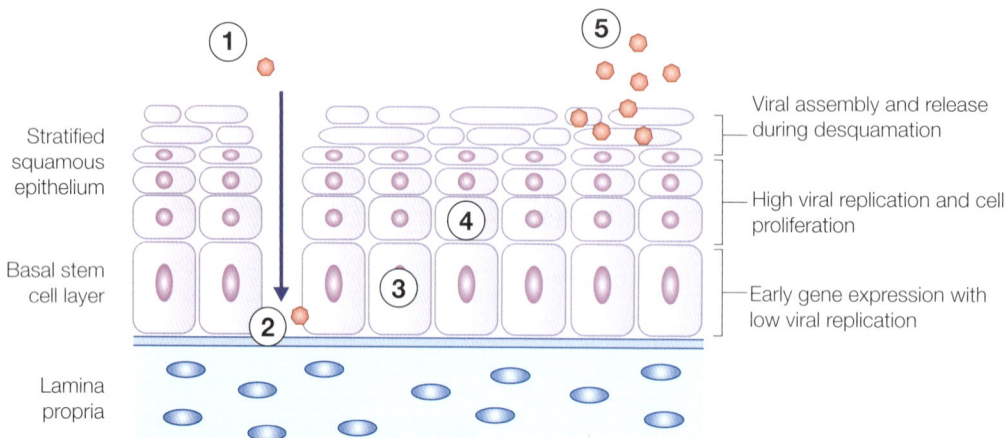

Figure 17.2 Life cycle of HPV. 1) HPV gains access to basal stem cells through areas of micro-trauma in the epithelial cell layer, 2) Entry into basal cells via endocytosis, 3) Maintenance phase with low viral replication, 4) Differentiation-dependent phase with high viral replication, 5) Complete HPV particles are released during normal epithelial desquamation.

reduced in caesarean sections.[7] Transmission may also occur by autoinoculation or indirectly via fomites.[8] The HPV particles are shed by the outermost epithelial layer of skin or mucosa, and are highly infectious. The life cycle of HPV (**Figure 17.2**) is ideally adapted to the host cell cycle, ensuring evasion from the immune system.

Epithelial exposure

The HPV particle has a tropism to epithelial surfaces but must first acquire access to the dividing basal stem cell layer. This can occur via micro-trauma to the epithelial layer, for example during sexual contact. As the normal host cell response to injury is recruitment of dividing epithelial cells, this enhances the infectious ability of the virus.[9] However, the exact mechanism of establishing HPV infection is not clearly understood, particularly in head and neck sites.

Attachment and entry

In order to gain access into the basal stem cells the virus requires attachment to surface receptors, the L1 and L2 viral capsid proteins are believed to be involved in this process. Initially the L1 capsid protein binds to exposed heparin sulfate proteoglycans and causes a conformational change leading to cleavage of L2 capsid protein by furin.[10] Further interaction with host cell receptors occurs, with α6 integrin proposed as one of the main target receptors.

Entry into the host cells then occurs via endocytosis utilizing various pathways. These include clathrin-mediated and caveolar endocytosis.[10–11] Once internalized the viral particle migrates to the host cell nucleus. The incubation period of the virus can last for weeks, months or even years after initial exposure.

Replication

The replication stage can be subdivided into the maintenance and differentiation-dependent phases.[12] The HPV particle utilizes the host cellular mechanisms to initiate DNA replication within the host cell nucleus and cause persisting infection. During the maintenance phase there are a low number of episomal viral copies produced within the basal stem cells, between 50–100 copies per cell.[13] The E1 and E2 viral proteins function together to maintain viral DNA replication. Dividing stem cells produce daughter cells that either remain within the basal layer or move towards the suprabasal layer. The low number of viral copies within the basal layer ensures evasion from the host immunity. Within the suprabasal layer the cells begin to differentiate, with E6 and E7 viral proteins encouraging further cell proliferation. Cells moving into the suprabasal layer lose their ability to divide and therefore undergo terminal differentiation, with HPV replication entering the differentiation-dependent phase. Activation of late viral promoters during this phase causes a dramatic increase in viral copies to several thousand per cell.[14] The E1, E4 and E5 viral proteins function to support viral amplification and maturation at this stage. While E6 and E7 function to promote cell proliferation the E2 viral protein suppresses their activity to allow cell differentiation and completion of the HPV life cycle. The delayed expression of large viral numbers within terminally differentiated cells prevents an immune reaction and ensures long-term persistence of the virus.

Shedding

Expression of L1 and L2 capsid proteins is the final step prior to release of the viral particles from the host cells. Maturation of HPV occurs in the most superficial layer of the epithelium. Release of complete viral particles occurs during normal epithelial shedding. Unlike other viruses, which lyse the host cells for viral release, the papillomavirus has adapted to utilize the normal epithelial cell cycle. Release of viral particles by this method prevents host cell immune recognition and ensures no abnormal inflammatory response.[12]

Persistence and clearance

Following initial infection the majority of individuals will clear the virus, although the period of active infection is unknown in head and neck sites. Cell-mediated immune response and activation of Langerhans cells play a role in viral clearance from the host cells.[13] However, considering the life cycle of HPV, undetectable infection may persist for an extended period with possible reactivation. Several factors, such as host cell immune status and hormonal levels, are likely to contribute to persistence and future reactivation.

HPV AND CANCER

Pathogenesis

Infection with HPV, particularly high-risk types, increases the risk of developing cancer. Failure to clear

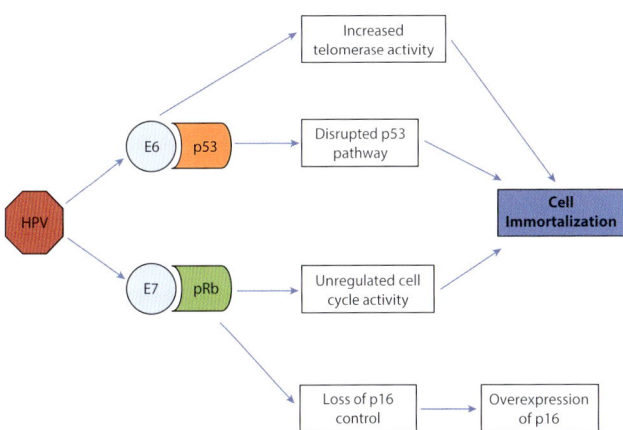

Figure 17.3 Illustration of HPV E6 and E7 interactions with host cell pathways.

the virus is likely to result in unregulated cell proliferation, accumulation of mutations and cancer formation. While the various HPV proteins contribute to viral replication, the E6 and E7 viral oncoproteins are critical in malignant transformation (**Figure 17.3**). Working together they can lead to epithelial cell immortalization. E6 binds to p53 and promotes its degradation via ubiquitin-dependent protease pathways.[15] The wild-type p53 is normally activated by DNA damage or cellular stress, and acts as a tumour suppressor. P53 functions include modulation of cell cycle, regulation of apoptosis and cell senescence.[16] E6 also activates the hTERT promoter to induce telomerase activity, which also leads to cell immortalization.[17]

The E7 viral protein binds to and inactivates pRb (retinoblastoma protein). The pRb is also an important tumour suppressor. The normal function of pRb is to block cell cycle progression by binding to E2F transcription factor and therefore blocking progression from G1 to S-phase.[18] Disruption of pRb-E2F complex therefore leads to unregulated cell cycle entry into S-phase causing increased cell proliferation. Interestingly unregulated S-phase activity would normally cause apoptosis via the p53 pathway. However, suppression of p53 activity by E6 interrupts this pathway and prevents cell death. Consequently immortalized cells lose the ability to repair DNA damage and therefore accumulate mutations and chromosomal instability. This can eventually lead to cancer formation.

During the complex interactions between E6 and E7 and the host cell pathways numerous cellular proteins can be disrupted, including p16. The p16 gene was first discovered in 1993 and codes for a cyclin-dependent kinase (CDK) inhibitor.[19] The CDK family plays an important role in cell cycle control. The p16 protein acts to prevent G1 to S-phase cell cycle progression, and also interacts with the pRb pathway.[20] The pRb function varies according to its phosphorylated state, which is controlled by the cyclin D-CDK4/6 complex. The p16 protein inhibits CDK4/6 and prevents phosphorylation of pRb. Hypo-phosphorylated pRb binds to and inactivates E2F transcription factors, leading to cell cycle arrest as described. Activity of p16 is controlled by functional pRb via a negative feedback mechanism.[21] Considering the effect of E6 on pRb function, an overexpression of p16 is expected in HPV active infections.

Epidemiology and risk factors

Among the head and neck cancers there appears to be a significant increase in the incidence of oropharyngeal cancer (OPC). In a large retrospective study examining incidence rates of OPC within 23 countries between 1983 and 2002, increasing incidence was observed mainly in developed countries such USA, UK and France.[22] In England the incidence rate of OPC more than doubled between 1990 and 2006,[23] with similar trends observed in Sweden and Scotland.[24-25]

Traditional risk factors of HNSCC include smoking and alcohol. However, increasing evidence has implicated HPV in cancer pathogenesis. The majority of HPV-related head and neck cancers occur within the oropharynx. In one systematic review there was a 26% overall prevalence of HPV infection within HNSCC cases, with the greatest proportion in the oropharyngeal cohort with a prevalence of 36%.[26] Other studies have also shown a strong association between HPV positivity and the oropharynx.[27] Recent evidence also appears to show prevalence of HPV infection in oropharyngeal cancer is increasing, whilst prevalence in non-oropharyngeal sites has remained static.[28]

Recently a geographic variation in prevalence has been demonstrated, with high prevalence in oropharyngeal cancers demonstrated in Western Europe (37%) compared with Eastern Europe (6%) and Asia (2%).[29] The increasing prevalence of HPV-related cancers can be attributed to changes in sexual practices. Risk factors for high-risk HPV infection in oropharyngeal cancer include younger age group (< 55 years), higher number of sexual partners, early sexual contact, oral-genital and oral-anal sex.[30-31]

Prognostic markers

There has been increasing interest in the role of HPV in HNSCC and the prognostic significance of HPV-related tumours. Various studies have correlated improved overall survival and disease-specific survival in HPV positive cancers.[27, 32, 33] In a retrospective study of the RTOG 0129 data, 3-year overall survival was 82.4% in HPV positive OPC cases compared to 57.1% in HPV negative cases.[4] Further analysis of the data showed HPV status was the most important determinant of survival, followed by number of smoking pack years. Recently a number of systematic reviews and meta-analyses have confirmed the improved prognostic outcomes in HPV positive HNSCC.[34-36]

Other prognostic markers proposed for HPV infection include p16 overexpression. The use of p16 testing as a surrogate marker for HPV-related OPC is now commonplace.[37] Overexpression of p16 is considered an independent prognostic marker, with improved overall survival and disease-free survival.[38]

Diagnosis

HPV detection can involve several methods including direct and indirect assays. Direct methods include polymerase chain reaction (PCR), in-situ hybridization (ISH), Southern blot analysis and HPV antibody detection. The common detection methods included PCR and ISH. The PCR assay is highly sensitive but not specific, requiring only a low level of viral DNA. However, traditional PCR is time and resource intensive and is unable to distinguish between episomal and integrated HPV infection.

In contrast to PCR, the ISH assay is highly specific but not sensitive. An estimated 10 viral copies per cell are required for a positive reaction.[39] The advantages of ISH are the ability to differentiate between episomal and integrated HPV infection, and it can be a fully automated process.

Indirect HPV testing includes p16 detection, which utilizes monoclonal antibodies against p16. Staining patterns and cut-off values vary between studies and are observer-dependent. HPV testing algorithms incorporating these various methods have been proposed.[40]

> **FUTURE RESEARCH**
>
> ▶ Current knowledge of HPV infection and cancer pathogenesis is based on cervical cancer studies. Further studies are required to determine the exact life cycle and natural history of HPV in head and neck sites.
> ▶ Initial infection mechanisms in the upper aerodigestive tract remain unknown.
> ▶ Receptors involved in HPV epithelial cell attachment and exact cell entry pathways are yet to be identified.
> ▶ Further studies are needed to determine the incubation and latency period of HPV infection in head and neck sites.
> ▶ Epidemiological studies into incidence and prevalence rates of HPV infection in the healthy population are required.
> ▶ Exact mechanisms of malignant transformation are yet to be elucidated.
> ▶ The interaction between host immune system and HPV is not fully understood, particularly the reasons why infection can persist in some individuals.
> ▶ Accurate biomarkers are required to determine a causal link between HPV infection and cancer pathogenesis. Ideal assays should be highly sensitive, specific and cost effective.
> ▶ The best methods of HPV detection have not been determined, particularly a consensus on accurate p16 testing among researchers.
> ▶ Models of risk stratification based on HPV status can have the potential for personalized prognosis and treatments.

KEY POINTS

- The HPV virion is a small, non-enveloped virus composed of an 8 kb double-stranded DNA contained within a protein capsid.
- HPV only infects skin or mucosal epidermal cells.
- Human papillomavirus is considered a sexually-transmitted disease, although transmission can occur by other methods such as vertical transmission between mother and infant.
- More than 120 HPV types have been described and divided into low-risk (e.g. 6 and 11) and high-risk (e.g. 16 and 18).
- The majority of HPV positive oropharyngeal cancers are caused by HPV 16.
- HPV proteins are classified into early and late gene products.
- E6 binds and degrades p53, E7 binds and inactivates pRb. Both E6 and E7 contribute to cell immortalization.
- Persisting HPV infection is likely to cause accumulated mutations and chromosomal instability, leading to cancer pathogenesis.
- p16 overexpression occurs via pRb inactivation, and is considered a surrogate marker of HPV infection.
- Recent evidence suggests improved prognosis for HPV positive HNSCC, particularly oropharyngeal cancer.
- Risk factors for HPV-related OPC include younger age group, increased sexual partners and oral-related sex.

REFERENCES

1. Javier RT, Butel JS. The history of tumor virology. *Cancer Res* 2008; **68**(19): 7693–706.
2. zur Hausen H. Condylomata acuminata and human genital cancer. *Cancer Res* 1976; **36**(2 pt 2): 794.
3. Bernard HU, Burk RD, Chen Z, et al. Classification of papillomaviruses (PVs) based on 189 PV types and proposal of taxonomic amendments. *Virology* 2010; **401**(1): 70–79.
4. Ang KK, Harris J, Wheeler R, et al. Human papillomavirus and survival of patients with oropharyngeal cancer. *New Engl J Med* 2010; **363**(1): 24–35.
5. Lace MJ, Anson JR, Turek LP, Haugen TH. Functional mapping of the human papillomavirus Type 16 E1 Cistron. *J Virol* 2008; **82**(21): 10724–34.
6. Morshed K, Polz-Gruszka D, Szymański M, Polz-Dacewicz M. Human papillomavirus (HPV): structure, epidemiology and pathogenesis. *Otolaryngologia Polska* 2014; **68**(5): 213–19.
7. Tseng CJ, Liang CC, Soong YK, Pao CC. Perinatal transmission of human papillomavirus in infants: relationship between infection rate and mode of delivery. *Obstet Gynec* 1998; **91**(1): 92–96.
8. Syrjanen S, Puranen M. Human papillomavirus infections in children: the potential role of maternal transmission. *Crit Rev Oral Biol M* 2000; **11**(2): 259–74.
9. Miller DL, Puricelli MD, Stack MS. Virology and molecular pathogenesis of human papillomavirus (HPV): associated oropharyngeal squamous cell carcinoma. *Biochem J* 2012; **443**(2): 339–53.
10. Letian T, Tianyu Z. Cellular receptor binding and entry of human papillomavirus. *Virol J* 2010; **7**: 2.
11. Horvath CA, Boulet GA, Renoux VM, et al. Mechanisms of cell entry by human papillomaviruses: an overview. *Virol J* 2010; **7**: 11.
12. Bodily J, Laimins LA. Persistence of human papillomavirus infections: keys to malignant progression. *Trends Microbiol* 2011; **19**(1): 33–39.
13. Doorbar J, Quint W, Banks L, et al. The biology and life-cycle of human papillomaviruses. *Vaccine* 2012; **30**(Suppl 5): F55–70.
14. Bedell MA, Hudson JB, Golub TR, et al. Amplification of human papillomavirus genomes in vitro is dependent on epithelial differentiation. *J Virol* 1991; **65**(5): 2254–60.
15. Scheffner M, Werness BA, Huibregtse JM, et al. The E6 oncoprotein encoded by human papillomavirus types 16 and 18 promotes the degradation of p53. *Cell* 1990; **63**(6): 1129–36.
16. Zilfou JT, Lowe SW. Tumor suppressive functions of p53. *CSH Perspect Biol* 2009; **1**(5): a001883.
17. Liu X, Dakic A, Zhang Y, et al. HPV E6 protein interacts physically and functionally with the cellular telomerase complex. *P Natl Acad Sci USA* 2009; **106**(44): 18780–85.
18. Giacinti C, Giordano A. RB and cell cycle progression. *Oncogene* 2006; **25**(38): 5220–27.
19. Serrano M, Hannon GJ, Beach D. A new regulatory motif in cell-cycle control causing specific inhibition of cyclin D/CDK4. *Nature* 1993; **366**(6456): 704–07.
20. Romagosa C, Simonetti S, Lopez-Vicente L, et al. p16(Ink4a) overexpression in cancer: a tumor suppressor gene associated with senescence and high-grade tumors. *Oncogene* 2011; **30**(18): 2087–97.
21. Hara E, Smith R, Parry D, et al. Regulation of p16CDKN2 expression and its implications for cell immortalization and senescence. *Mol Cell Biol* 1996; **16**(3): 859–67.
22. Chaturvedi AK, Anderson WF, Lortet-Tieulent J, et al. Worldwide trends in incidence rates for oral cavity and oropharyngeal cancers. *J Clin Oncol* 2013; **31**(36): 4550–59.
23. Oxford Cancer Intelligence Unit. *Profile of head and neck cancers in England: incidence, mortality and survival.* Oxford: Oxford Cancer Intelligence Unit; 2010.
24. Robinson KL, Macfarlane GJ. Oropharyngeal cancer incidence and mortality in Scotland: are rates still increasing? *Oral Oncol* 2003; **39**(1): 31–36.
25. Hammarstedt L, Dahlstrand H, Lindquist D, et al. The incidence of tonsillar cancer in Sweden is increasing. *Acta Oto-Laryngol* 2007; **127**(9): 988–92.
26. Kreimer AR, Clifford GM, Boyle P, Franceschi S. Human papillomavirus types in head and neck squamous cell carcinomas worldwide: a systematic review. *Cancer Epidem Biomar* 2005; **14**(2): 467–75.
27. Gillison ML, Koch WM, Capone RB, et al. Evidence for a causal association between human papillomavirus and a subset of head and neck cancers. *J Natl Cancer I* 2000; **92**(9): 709–20.
28. Mehanna H, Beech T, Nicholson T, et al. Prevalence of human papillomavirus in oropharyngeal and nonoropharyngeal head and neck cancer: systematic review and meta-analysis of trends by time and region. *Head Neck* 2013; **35**(5): 747–55.
29. Mehanna H, Franklin N, Compton N, et al. Geographic variation in human papillomavirus-related oropharyngeal cancer: data from four multinational randomized trials. *Head Neck* 2016 [Epub ahead of print].
30. Smith EM, Ritchie JM, Summersgill KF, et al. Age, sexual behavior and human papillomavirus infection in oral cavity and oropharyngeal cancers. *Int J Cancer* 2004; **108**(5): 766–72.
31. Heck JE, Berthiller J, Vaccarella S, et al. Sexual behaviours and the risk of head and neck cancers: a pooled analysis in the International Head and Neck Cancer Epidemiology (INHANCE) consortium. *Int J Epidemiol* 2010; **39**(1): 166–81.
32. Mellin H, Friesland S, Lewensohn R, et al. Human papillomavirus (HPV) DNA in tonsillar cancer: clinical correlates, risk of relapse, and survival. *Int J Cancer* 2000; **89**(3): 300–04.
33. Klozar J, Kratochvil V, Salakova M, et al. HPV status and regional metastasis in the prognosis of oral and oropharyngeal cancer. *Eur Arch Oto-Rhino-Laryngol* 2008; **265**(Suppl 1): S75–82.
34. Dayyani F, Etzel CJ, Liu M, et al. Meta-analysis of the impact of human papillomavirus (HPV) on cancer risk and overall survival in head and neck squamous cell carcinomas (HNSCC). *Head Neck Oncol* 2010; **2**: 15.
35. O'Rorke MA, Ellison MV, Murray LJ, et al. Human papillomavirus related head and neck cancer survival: a systematic review and meta-analysis. *Oral Oncol* 2012; **48**(12): 1191–201.
36. Ragin CC, Taioli E. Survival of squamous cell carcinoma of the head and neck in relation to human papillomavirus infection: review and meta-analysis. *Int J Cancer* 2007; **121**(8): 1813–20.
37. El-Naggar AK, Westra WH. p16 expression as a surrogate marker for HPV-related oropharyngeal carcinoma: a guide for interpretative relevance and consistency. *Head Neck* 2012; **34**(4): 459–61.
38. Weinberger PM, Yu Z, Haffty BG, et al. Prognostic significance of p16 protein levels in oropharyngeal squamous cell cancer. *Clin Cancer Res* 2004; **10**(17): 5684–91.
39. Venuti A, Paolini F. HPV detection methods in head and neck cancer. *Head Neck Path* 2012; **6**(Suppl 1): S63–74.
40. Smeets SJ, Hesselink AT, Speel EJ, et al. A novel algorithm for reliable detection of human papillomavirus in paraffin embedded head and neck cancer specimen. *Int J Cancer* 2007; **121**(11): 2465–72.

CHAPTER 18

CONNECTIVE TISSUE DISEASES: ENT COMPLICATIONS

Eileen Baildam

Introduction 173	Notes on specific vasculitides with ENT implications.................. 175
ENT presentations in autoimmune rheumatic disease 173	Effects of immunosuppression from disease or treatment.......... 179
Systemic symptoms and signs that are red flags of autoimmune rheumatic diseases 174	Treatments including disease-modifying anti-rheumatic drugs (DMARDS) and biologic therapies... 179
Laboratory features of specific rheumatological disease 175	References 180
Rheumatological conditions with ENT features or complications .. 175	

SEARCH STRATEGY

Data in this chapter may be updated by a Medline search using the keywords: ENT complications of autoimmune rheumatic disease, rheumatoid arthritis, spondylarthropathy, sarcoidosis, SLE, Sjögren's syndrome, juvenile idiopathic arthritis, scleroderma, systemic sclerosis, Behçet's disease, dermatomyositis, polymyositis, periodic fever syndromes, PFAPA, mouth ulcers, TMJ arthritis, jaw growth, vasculitis, Wegener's granulomatosis, Churg-Strauss syndrome, microscopic polyangiitis, Kawasaki vasculitis, relapsing polychondritis, lymphadenopathy and polychondritis.

INTRODUCTION

Many rheumatological disorders are multi-system in nature where ENT symptoms and signs may provide a fundamental diagnostic clue to the overall condition, for example, mouth ulcers and lymphadenopathy often seen in systemic lupus erythematosus (SLE). On the other hand, ENT complications may constitute a life-threatening emergency, as in arthritis of the crico-arytenoid with associated vocal cord dysfunction. Long-term secondary damage may occur in under-treated granulomatosis with polyangiitis (GWP), the old Wegener's granulomatosis, where late tracheal stenosis or collapse of the nasal bridge are pathognomic. Sudden onset deafness, trigeminal nerve or facial nerve dysfunction can be seen in many autoimmune and chronic inflammatory rheumatological conditions.

The key to assessment is a whole patient screening review of systems and general examination by the ENT specialist, as well as good ENT assessment by the physician or paediatrician. This ensures that a second or multiple presentation is noticed enabling an early, accurate diagnosis without delay of definitive treatment.[1]

Constitutional symptoms of general malaise, tiredness, weight loss, unexplained fevers, rashes, hair loss, photosensitivity, arthralgia, arthritis, myalgias or muscle weakness, neurological features such as neuropathies, hypertension or unexplained haematuria or proteinuria, mouth ulcers, lymphenopathy, hepatosplenomegaly, shortness of breath, chronic cough, crepitations on chest auscultation, heart murmurs and absent pulses all occur in rheumatic disorders such as in SLE, the vasculitides, complicated rheumatoid arthritis, and in overlap connective tissue disorders.

Localized arthritis of the temporomandibular joints, cervical vertebrae and the cricoarytenoid can present with local and referred pain, or specific signs. Erosion or collapse of vertebrae from arthritis or secondary osteoporosis can present with torticollis (more often in childhood) or loss of movement and/or neurological signs.

ENT PRESENTATIONS IN AUTOIMMUNE RHEUMATIC DISEASE

The clinical symptoms and signs of many conditions may overlap and appear similar so that it is the patterns and combinations of symptoms, signs and subsequent investigations that will lead to the most likely diagnosis. However, as these diagnoses are made by clinical pattern recognition it is important that the expert opinion of a rheumatologist is sought as early as possible to avoid any dangerous delays in making an accurate diagnosis.

ENT management needs to be in conjunction with an expert specialist rheumatology or paediatric rheumatology team depending on the age of the patient.

1. Mouth ulcers and nasal ulcers may be found in Behçet's disease, systemic lupus erythematosus (SLE).
2. Sore throat may be the presenting symptom in:
   a. Acute rheumatic fever
   b. Systemic onset juvenile idiopathic arthritis (JIA)
   c. Macrophage activation syndromes (MAS)/haemophagocytic lymphohistiocytosis (HLH), either primary or secondary to other autoimmune inflammatory states
   d. Periodic fever syndromes including periodic fever, aphthous stomatitis, pharyngitis and adenitis (PFAPA) syndrome.
3. Lymphadenopathy may be associated with many rheumatological disorders:
   a. SLE
   b. Systemic onset JIA, with or without MAS/HLH
   c. Sarcoidosis or Blaus syndrome
   d. Kawasaki disease
   e. Rosai-Dorfman disease
   f. Kikuchi syndrome.
4. Nasal disorders: GWP, eosinophilic granulomatosis with polyangiitis (Churg-Strauss syndrome), relapsing polychondritis and sarcoidosis.
5. Sinusitis: GWP, eosinophilic granulomatosis with polyangiitis, relapsing polychondritis and sarcoidosis.
6. Vasculitic lesions: petechial lesions, ulcerated non-healing lesions (e.g. in pinna, on the palate, nasal mucosa, perforated nasal septum).
7. Hearing disturbances (either through autoimmune neuropathy or with vasculitic damage to small vasa-nervorum). Seen in SLE, GWP, relapsing polychondritis, polyarteritis nodosa, Cogan's syndrome, Sjögren's syndrome, and less frequently in eosinophilic granulomatosis with polyangiitis and Behçet's disease.
8. Stridor:
   a. Arthritis of the synovial joints of the cricoarytenoid joint with an emergency presentation of vocal cord dysfunction. Occurs in rheumatoid arthritis, ankylosing spondylitis, juvenile idiopathic arthritis and gout. Osteoarthritic changes have also been described.
   b. Mucosal inflammation and swelling in GWP, Churg-Strauss vasculitis, rheumatoid arthritis, SLE, extranodal mucosal disease with lymphoid hyperplasia as in lymphomas.
   c. Myaesthenia gravis including neonatal disease with transplacental transfer of anti-Musk antibodies.
9. Dysphonia and vocal cord paralysis is found in association:
   a. Cervical cord changes due to osteophyte
   b. Cervical cord damage associated with cervical vertebral erosion with JIA
   c. Hoarseness from anatomical and functional problems.
10. Sjögren's syndrome. Xerostomia or a dry mouth is a common feature of primary and secondary Sjögren's syndrome (occurring with most autoimmune rheumatological disorders). Salivary gland enlargement may be also seen in these patients, as well as in patients with sarcoidosis. In childhood parotid gland enlargement is the most frequent presentation of Sjögren's syndrome. People with Sjögren's are at increased risk of developing non-Hodgkin lymphoma.
11. Trigeminal nerve dysfunction may occur in patients with Sjögren's syndrome, systemic sclerosis, SLE and mixed connective tissue disease.
12. Peripheral facial nerve palsy may complicate Sjögren's syndrome and sarcoidosis.
13. Motility disorders of upper and/or lower portions of the oesophagus have been reported in patients with dermatomyositis/polymyositis, systemic sclerosis and SLE.
14. Chondritis of the pinna in relapsing polychondritis.
15. Skin thickening, dyspigmentary changes, hemi-facial hypertrophy (Parry Romberg syndrome), gum retraction, tympanic membrane involvement in localized scleroderma.
16. Swallowing difficulties:
    a. Due to weakness in dermatomyositis, myasthenia gravis
    b. Due to oesophageal constriction in scleroderma.

SYSTEMIC SYMPTOMS AND SIGNS THAT ARE RED FLAGS OF AUTOIMMUNE RHEUMATIC DISEASES

- Joint pain, stiffness especially early morning stiffness and joint swelling seen in inflammatory arthritis
- Fevers
- Malaise, tiredness, weakness, weight loss
- Mouth ulcers, nasal ulcers, genital and perianal ulceration
- Rashes:
  ○ psoriasis
  ○ photosensitive, malar erythema in SLE
  ○ salmon pink, urticarial in systemic onset juvenile idiopathic arthritis
  ○ purple/black ulcerated vasculitic rashes
  ○ scalp rash or ulceration
  ○ skin thickening or hardening with dyspigmentary changes in localized scleroderma
  ○ erythema nodosum in sarcoidosis and streptococcal infection
- Alopecia either with or without scalp rashes in SLE
- Sclerodactyly, sclerodermatous facial pinching with decreased mouth opening in systemic sclerosis
- Puffy eyelids, heliotrope violaceous look around eyelids in diabetes mellitus (DM)
- Skin ulceration in vasculitis
- Nail fold capillary changes in systemic sclerosis, DM, SLE
- Lymphadenopathy (e.g. Kikuchi syndrome, massive lymphadenopathy with histiocytosis)
- Cardio-vascular features in SLE, vasculitis:
  ○ Raynaud's phenomenon
  ○ hypertension

- peripheral vascular pulses loss of diminished, or peripheral aneurysms
- pericarditis, endocarditis, myocarditis
- Thromboembolic phenomenon from primary or secondary anti-phospholipid syndrome
- Respiratory symptoms (e.g. shortness of breath, chronic cough, interstitial pneumonitis, pulmonary arterial hypertension in SLE, scleroderma, DM)
- Nephritis with haematuria, proteinuria, renal impairment, hypertension in SLE or vasculitis
- Gastrointestinal abdominal pain, dysphagia, altered bowel habit, bloody diarrhoea SLE or vasculitis
- Neurological features of neuropathies, myopathies, CNS direct involvement with various presentations including headaches, reduction in intellectual function, loss of memory in SLE or vasculitis
- Opthalmological disease of uveitis, retinal vasculitis, retinal vein thrombosis
- Laboratory features: raised ESR and or CRP, thrombocytosis, cytopenias, haemolytic anaemia, raised ferritin, abnormal U and Es, LFTs, raised CK, LDH. Abnormal thyroid function tests and thyroid antibodies, raised immunoglobulins, abnormal antibodies antithyroid peroxisomal, antinuclear factor, positive extractable nuclear antibodies, anti-ds DNA, positive p and c ANCA, positive anti-MPO and anti-proteinase 3 (PR3) antibodies, anti-centromere antibodies, anti-scl 70 antibodies.

LABORATORY FEATURES OF SPECIFIC RHEUMATOLOGICAL DISEASE

SLE features include positive antinuclear antibodies (ANA), positive extractable nuclear antibodies (ENA) especially anti-Ro and anti-La, anti-Smith, anti-dsDNA, abnormal thyroid tests, raised immunoglobulins, abnormal antibodies (i.e. antithyroid peroxisomal, raised ESR and/or CRP), thrombocytosis, cytopenias (e.g. lymphopenia, Coombs positive haemolytic anaemia), systemic sclerosis positive ANA, positive anti-centromere antibodies, positive anti-scl 70 (topisomerase antibodies).

Vasculitic suggestive features include raised inflammatory markers, positive ANCA. Raised serum angiotensin converting enzyme may be seen in sarcoidosis. Sjögren's syndrome positive ANA, positive extractable nuclear antibodies, especially anti-Ro and La. Other causes of raised ACE include Hodgkin disease, diabetes, alcoholic hepatitis and hyperthyroidism.

RHEUMATOLOGICAL CONDITIONS WITH ENT FEATURES OR COMPLICATIONS

Vasculitides

There are many ways of classifying vasculitis including the size of the blood vessel involved, whether there is a granulomatous histology, whether there is ANCA positivity, immune complex deposition. **Table 18.1** lists most named types of vasculitis. Presentation is often specific with low-grade fever, tiredness, malaise with rashes, arthritis and multi-organ disease.

TABLE 18.1 Classification of vasculitis

I	Predominantly large vessel vasculitis	a) Takayasu arteritis b) Giant cell arteritis
II	Predominantly medium sized vessel vasculitis	a) Childhood polyarteritis nodosa b) Cutaneous polyarteritis c) Kawasaki disease
III	Predominantly small vessel vasculitis	Granulomatous: a) Granulomatosis with polyangiitis (Wegener's granulomatosis); eosinophilic granulomatosis with polyangiitis (Churg-Strauss syndrome) b) Microscopic polyangiitis Non-granulomatous: a) Microscopic polyangiitis b) Henoch-Schonlein purpura/IgA vasculitis c) Isolated cutaneous leucocytoclastic vasculitis d) Hypocomplementic urticarial vasculitis (possibly drug induced) e) Cryoglobulinaemic vasculitis associated with RA, SLE, Sjögren's syndrome f) Anti-GBM disease
IV	Variable	Cogan's syndrome Behçet's disease
V	Other vasculitides	a) Behçet's disease b) Vasculitis secondary to infection (including polyarteritis nodosa associated with hepatitis B or streptococcal infections), malignancies, drugs (including hypersensitivity vasculitis) c) Vasculitis associated with connective tissue disease (systemic lupus erythematosus, dermatomyositis, rheumatoid arthritis d) Isolated vasculitis of the central nervous system e) Unclassified

NOTES ON SPECIFIC VASCULITIDES WITH ENT IMPLICATIONS

Kawasaki disease

Kawasaki disease is the most common vasculitis seen in childhood. Typical features of Kawasaki disease are fever persisting for at least 5 days (mandatory criterion) plus four of the following five features:

- changes in peripheral extremities or perineal area
- polymorphous exanthema
- bilateral conjunctival injection
- changes of lips and oral cavity: injection of oral and pharyngeal mucosa
- cervical lymphadenopathy.

In the presence of coronary artery involvement (detected on echocardiography) and fever, fewer than five additional features are required to be certain of the diagnosis. Note that atypical cases occur that do not fulfill all criteria.

In terms of ENT features, the mucosal inflammation may present with swollen red tongue and lips, cracked lips, and angular stomatitis enough to make swallowing impossible. Clinically this can look similar to Stevens Johnson syndrome

The eyes may be red with aseptic conjunctivitis. Peripheral oedema of the dorsum of hands and feet may occur with or without rashes. The most frequent feature not in the diagnostic criteria is irritability and may signify cerebral irritation. The illness can be life-threatening acutely from myocarditis or later from coronary artery aneurysms. Treatment is evidence-based with intravenous immunoglobulin and aspirin, although steroids and immunosuppressants may be needed in non-responsive and severe cases. Coronary artery aneurysms can occur in atypical cases with incomplete diagnostic criteria where treatment is still needed.

Granulomatosis with polyangiitis (Wegener's granulomatosis)

Necrotizing granulomatous inflammation usually involves the upper and lower respiratory tracts with rhinosinusitis leading to bloody discharge, chronic nasal ulceration, nasal chondritis (**Figure 18.1**) leading to a saddle nose, laryngeal stenosis, chronic destructive sinusitis, proptosis, orbital wall damage leading to orbitonasal fistulas. Conductive hearing loss caused by middle ear inflammation, or eustachian tube dysfunction, pulmonary granulomata, necrotizing glomerulonephritis, skin rashes, arthritis, neuropathies, CNS, heart and GI involvement can all occur. In the localized phase of the disease 50% are ANCA negative whereas when generalized disease is present 90% are positive for PR3 ANCA.

The disease has a high mortality and requires urgent intensive treatment with high dose steroids, cyclophosphamide, plasma exchange for severe cases with methotrexate and/or rituximab in milder cases.

Eosinophilic granulomatosis with polyangiitis (Churg-Strauss syndrome)

This is a vasculitis characterized by asthma, hypereosinophilia, pulmonary infiltrates with eosinophilia rich granulomatous inflammation in the respiratory tract. Sinuses are affected with allergic rhinitis, sinusitis and polyps. Myocarditis, neuropathies, arthritis, skin purpura, renal and gut disease can occur. ANCA, usually with anti-MPO specificity, is detected in 40% of patients.

ENT manifestations of Behçet's disease

Behçet's disease (BD) is a multi-system vasculitis characterized by recurrent oral and genital ulceration, skin lesions and ocular inflammation. Diagnostic criteria are based on recurrent oral ulcers occurring three times in 12 months plus two of the following: scarring recurrent genital ulcers, ocular involvement (uveitis or retinal vasculitis), skin lesions (such as erythema nodosum, pseudofolliculitis/pustolosis) and positive pathergy test (skin reaction to needle insertion). Other observed manifestations are arthritis, neurological disease and ENT involvement.

Audiovestibular involvement is frequent with sensorineural hearing loss in 23–32% of patients.[2] This is usually bilateral, affecting high frequencies and may be due

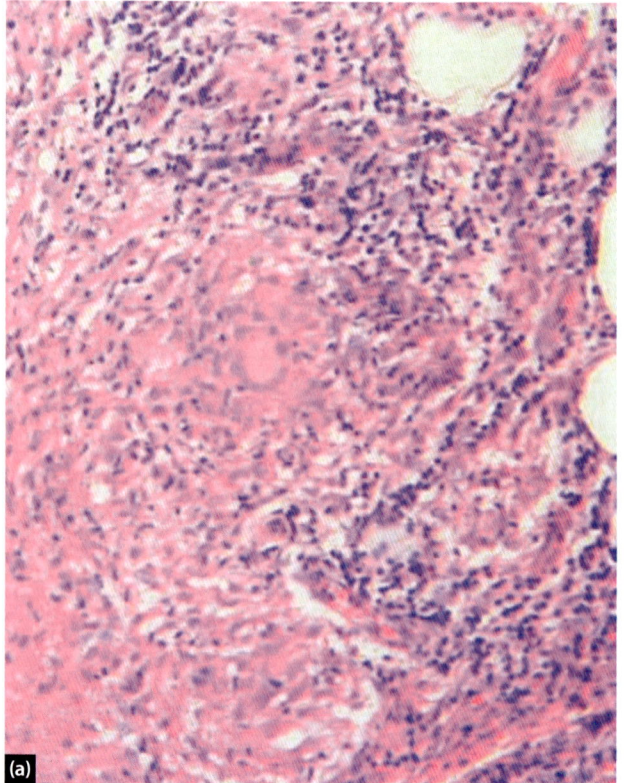

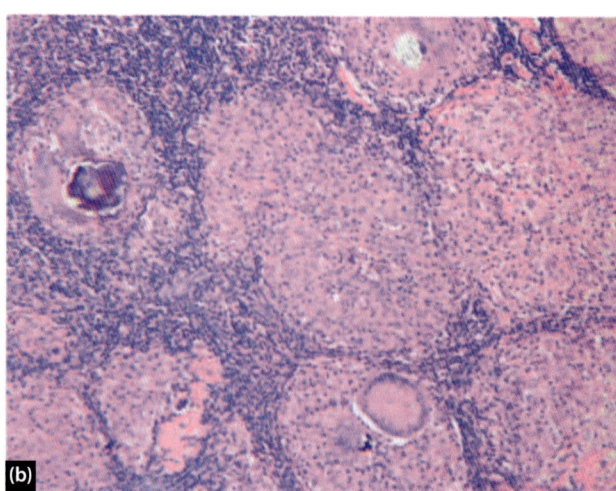

Figure 18.1 The changes in crusting found inside the nose from a patient with active granulomatosis with polyangiitis: (a) shows early changes with an angry mucosa and mucous hypersecretion; **(b)** demonstrates the end result of gross activity.

to vasculitis of vessels supplying the cochlea. Recurrent vertigo, bilateral vestibular hypofunction causing instability and bilateral Meniere's syndrome can occur. Neuro-Behçet's may present with vestibular neuronitis. Although CNS involvement is infrequently seen, peripheral nerve involvement with isolated case reports of facial paralysis and vocal cord paralysis are reported.

Ulceration of the oral cavity is common but oropharyngeal ulceration may be misdiagnosed as tonsillitis or pharyngitis. Rarely, laryngeal or oesophageal ulceration can lead to pharyngolaryngeal stenosis. Infrequently nasal symptoms such as nasal ulceration, dysosmia, obstruction and pain are experienced.

MAGIC syndrome

There is an association of autoimmune disorders such as Behçet's disease with relapsing polychondritis and inflammation of the auricular cartilages seen as part of the MAGIC syndrome (mouth and genital ulcers with inflamed cartilage).

Cogan syndrome

This is an autoimmune disorder of young people characterized by[3]:

- ocular symptoms with non-syphilitic interstitial keratitis
- audio-vestibular symptoms similar to those of Meniere's syndrome (sudden onset of tinnitus and vertigo accompanied by gradual hearing loss)
- an interval between the onset of the ocular and audio-vestibular features of less than 2 years.

Atypical cases occur without any inflammatory ocular manifestations, with interstitial keratitis and with delays of more than 2 years between the eye and ear symptoms. There are often neurological or systemic features of vasculitis with possible infectious or autoimmune triggers. Anti HSP 70 antibodies may be a marker for the autoimmune nature of the hearing loss. ANCA positivity may occur. Treatment is with corticosteroids followed by immunosuppressive therapy with cyclophosphamide, methotrexate, azathioprine, cyclosporine or anti-TNF blockers such as etanercept and infliximab. Rituximab is also used.

Relapsing polychondritis (RP)

RP is a rare autoimmune disease with episodic flares of progressive inflammatory destruction of cartilage either as a primary condition or overlapping with rheumatoid arthritis, spondylarthropathies, vasculitis or as a paraneoplastic condition. Acute phase reactants are raised and biopsy of affected tissues is characteristic. Elastic cartilage of the ear, hyaline cartilage of the tracheobronchial tree and joints, and fibrocartilage of the axial skeleton are involved. Because of significant morbidity and mortality systemic immunosuppression is required.

Systemic lupus erythematosus (SLE)

SLE is truly a multi-system inflammatory disorder affecting every organ with multiple presentations, a true masquerading condition where diagnosis can be difficult requiring specialist advice. Recently the Systemic Lupus International Collaborating Clinics (SLICC) classification 2012 has been proposed in addition to the 1997 American College of Rheumatology (ACR) diagnostic criteria (**Tables 18.2** and **18.3**). Both include a glossary of detailed definitions of component parts but are a start in making sense of a multifaceted disorder.

From an ENT perspective mucosal presentations occur in up to 45% of cases. In the mouth these include irregular raised white plaques with areas of erythema, silvery white scarred lesions, actual ulcers with surrounding redness occurring on soft or hard palates or on the buccal mucosa. These have a wide differential diagnosis including lichen planus, candidiasis, aphthous stomatitis, intra-oral herpes, Behçet's disease, bite induced lesions, leukoplakia and malignancy.

Oral and nasal ulcers occur. These are usually painless and may be the first presentation of the SLE. Discoid lesions may occur on the lips with erythema, swelling or atrophy and depigmented areas. Lymphadenopathy occurs in around 40% of cases with soft, non-tender discrete glands in the cervical, axillary or inguinal regions. These may warrant a biopsy to exclude other causes.

TABLE 18.2 Systemic Lupus International Collaborating Clinics (SLICC) classification criteria for systemic lupus erythematosus[4]

Clinical criteria	Immunologic criteria
Requirements; 4 or more criteria (at least 1 clinical and 1 laboratory criteria) OR biopsy-proven lupus nephritis with positive ANA or Anti-DNA.	
1. Acute cutaneous lupus	1. ANA
2. Chronic cutaneous lupus	2. Anti-DNA
3. Oral or nasal ulcers	3. Anti-Sm
4. Non-scarring alopecia	4. Antiphospholipid Ab
5. Arthritis	5. Low complement (C3, C4, CH50)
6. Serositis	6. Direct Coombs test (do not count in the presence of haemolytic anaemia)
7. Renal	
8. Neurologic	
9. Haemolytic anaemia	
10. Leukopenia	
11. Thrombocytopenia (100,000/mm³)	

From Petri et al., 2012[4]

TABLE 18.3 American College of Rheumatology revised criteria for diagnosis of systemic lupus erythematosus 1997

Criteria	Definition
Malar rash	Fixed erythema, flat or raised, over the malar eminences, tending to spare the nasolabial folds
Discoid rash	Erythematous raised patches with adherent keratotic scaling and follicular plugging: atrophic scarring occurs in older lesions
Photosensitivity	Skin rash as a result of unusual reaction to sunlight, by patient history or physician observation
Oral ulcers	Oral or nasopharyngeal ulceration, usually painless, observed by a physician
Arthritis	Non-erosive arthritis involving two or more peripheral joints, characterized by tenderness, swelling or effusion
Serositis	a. Pleuritis: convincing history of pleuritic pain or rub heard by a physician or evidence of pleural effusion, or b. Pericarditis: documented by ECG or rub or evidence of pericardial effusion
Renal disorder	a. Persistent proteinuria >0.5g per day or 3+ if quantification is not performed or b. Cellular casts: may be red cell, haemoglobin, granular, tubular or mixed
Neurological disorder	a. Seizures: in the absence of offending drugs or known metabolic derangements (eg. uraemia, acidosis, or electrolyte imbalance) b. Psychosis: in the absence of offending drugs or known metabolic derangements (eg uraemia, acidosis, or electrolyte imbalance)
Haematological disorder	a. Haemolytic anaemia with reticulocytosis, or b. Leucopenia <4000/mm^3, or c. Lymphopenia <1500 mm^3, or d. Thrombocytopenia <100 000 mm^3 in the absence of offending drugs
Immunological disorder	a. Anti-DNA antibody to native DNA in abnormal titre, or b. Anti-Sm, presence of antibody to Sm nuclear antigen, or c. Positive finding of antiphospholipid antibodies based on: (1) an abnormal serum concentration of IgG or IgM anticardiolipin antibodies, (2) a positive test result for lupus anticoagulant using a standard method, or (3) a false positive test for syphilis known to be positive for at least 6 months and confirmed by Treponema pallidum immobilization or fluorescent treponemal antibody absorption test
Antinuclear antibody	An abnormal titre of antinuclear antibody by immunofluorescence or an equivalent assay at any point in time and in the absence of drugs known to be associated with 'drug-induced lupus' syndrome

Autoinflammatory diseases/hereditary periodic fever syndromes (HPFSs)

These rare genetic conditions are characterized by short and recurrent attacks including fever, often with a sore throat, tonsillitis, lymphadenopathy and general debility, with a severe inflammatory reaction (with raised leucocytosis, ESR, CRP, fibrinogen, serum amyloid A protein) with the patient well between attacks. Infection has to be excluded as it is clinically indistinguishable in an individual attack and often it is only after multiple courses of antibiotics that the pattern of the disorders is clear. Genetic testing needs to be through specialist clinics and specialist laboratories. Clinical clues are in recurrent or continuous symptoms, especially fever, rash, joint pain or arthritis, accompanied by very high acute phase reactant with a wide differential diagnosis. If attacks recur for longer than a year and especially if there is a family history, HPFS should be considered. Some may present very late into adult life.

They are disorders of the inflammasome with triggers including emotional and physical stress, the menstrual cycle and pregnancy, vaccination reactions in hyper-IgD syndrome (HIDS), local mucosal trauma (e.g. in PFAFA), cold as in some cryopyrin-associated periodic syndromes (CAPS) syndromes:

- **Familial Mediterranean fever (FMF)** is due to a gene mutation *MEFV*, location 16p13.3 proteins affected pyrin and marenostrin. FMF may cause sensorineural hearing loss.
- Hyperimmunoglobulinemia D (or hyper IgD syndrome) with periodic fever syndrome (HIDS) gene mutation *MVK* located at 12q24, proteins affected mevalonate kinase deficiency. Most cases have marked reactions to immunizations. Febrile episodes with lymphadenopathy, rashes sometimes with hepatosplenomegaly, arthralgia, abdominal pain, irritability.
- **Tumour necrosis factor (TNF) receptor–associated periodic syndrome (TRAPS)** gene *TNFRSF1A* located 12p13, proteins affected TNF-receptor Type 1

Cryopyrin-associated periodic syndromes (CAPS):

- This is a group of hereditary periodic fever syndromes with the same gene mutations but with very different phenotypes. The gene *NLRP3 (CIAS1) mutation* at 1q44 affects the protein cryopyrin (NALP3/PYPAF1).
- Muckle-Wells syndrome (MWS) gene *NLRP3 (CIAS1)* at 1q44 inheritance protein affected cryopyrin (NALP3/PYPAF1). Clinical presentation with conjunctivitis in 44%, hearing loss in 32% with recurrent urticaria and uveitis.
- **Familial cold autoinflammatory syndrome (FCAS)** *NLRP3 (CIAS1)*, 1q44 protein affected Cryopyrin (NALP3/ PYPAF1). Symptoms such as lip swelling after cold contact.
- **Chronic infantile neurologic cutaneous articular syndrome (CINCA)**, also known as neonatal-onset multi-system inflammatory disease (NOMID) *NLRP3 (CIAS1)*, 1q44 protein affected, Cryopyrin (NALP3/PYPAF1). Although onset is from the

neonatal period, diagnoses may not be made until adult. Features include daily fever, a measles-like macular rash (very like that in systemic onset arthritis), lymphadenopathy, splenomegaly and sensorineural deafness with ocular optic neuritis papillitis, intermittent oligoarticular arthritis with pathognomic patellar overgrowth and learning difficulties preventable with treatment. Treatment is with daily anakinra injections or with canakinumab, both IL1 receptor antagonists.

- **Shnitzlers syndrome** is like CAPS but late onset with no family history. Diagnosed only in adults. Consisting of an IgM gammopathy, chronic urticarial rashes, acute phase reactants, intermittent fever, arthralgia and arthritis, splenomegaly, lymphadenopathy, some deafness. There is a long-term risk of Waldenstrom's macroglobulinemia. It is interleukin-1 (IL-1) driven with 100% of cases responding to anakinra.
- **PFAPA syndrome** (periodic fever, aphthous stomatitis, pharyngitis and adenitis syndrome). The most frequent disorder in childhood accounting for around 50% of recurrent fever syndromes. There is no identifiable gene associated with this so the diagnosis is clinical. This disorder often responds to tonsillectomy; however, PFAPA may recover spontaneously. The evidence for adenoidectomy in addition to tonsillectomy is not established.[7] Short courses of oral corticosteroids may help this condition. Although PFAPA is usually self-limiting attacks can occur frequently throughout childhood from a median age of 2.5 years and can last for a decade.
- **Blau syndrome and sarcoidosis:** sarcoidosis is a systemic disorder characterized by non-caseating granulomata affecting the lungs, skin, joints with arthritis, bony changes of osteitis, eyes with uveitis, calcium metabolism causing hypercalcaemia, muscle, and heart with skin lesions of lupus pernio, papules, nodules in infiltrated scars and erythema nodosum. Neurosarcoid can result in cranial nerve palsy and obstructive sleep apnea. Lymphadenopathy occurs in 15%. Salivary gland involvement (e.g. solitary parotid enlargement) occurs. Other ENT presentations include nasal perforation, sinonasal disease (where the nasal mucosa resembles apple jelly; (Figure 18.2)), laryngeal disease, and vocal cord deposits, trigeminal nerve or facial nerve mediated pain. Chest X-ray to look for perhilar lymphadenopathy or pulmonary infiltrates, and urinalysis for proteinuria or haematuria suggestive of a nephritis as the rare renal involvement should always be done. Patients should be sent for ophthalmological review for signs of uveitis that may be subclinical. In childhood, chest and kidney involvement is rare. Blau syndrome is associated with CARD15/NOD 2 mutations and is very like young onset sarcoidosis. Most patients develop polyarticular arthritis, with cutaneous and eye manifestations.

Systemic sclerosis

This condition is caused by a combination of low-grade inflammation with increased fibrosis in soft tissues and in blood vessels. As well as Raynaud's phenomenon, the skin becomes stiff and vascular insufficiency can lead to finger-tip ulcers. The antinuclear factor is usually positive. Lung and renal disease and pulmonary hypertension are significant causes of death. From an ENT perspective the soft tissues of the mouth can become stiff with decreased mouth opening.

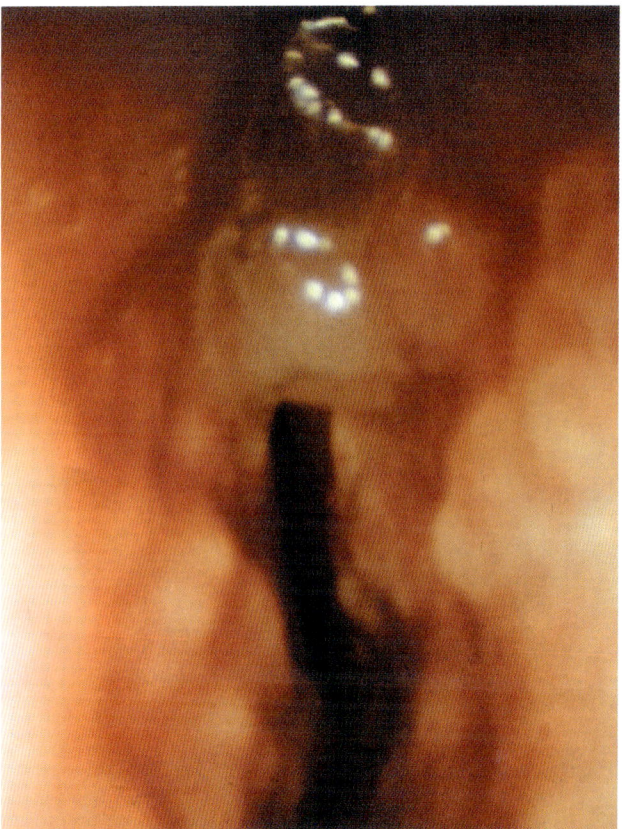

Figure 18.2 Examination of the nasal mucosa from a patient with sarcoidosis reveals apple jelly nodules.

EFFECTS OF IMMUNOSUPPRESSION FROM DISEASE OR TREATMENT

Many of the rheumatological conditions are immune-suppressive in themselves, as are the drugs, including steroids, used to treat the conditions. ENT infections may be increased in these situations. Immunizations against winter flu, pneumococcus and any killed vaccines are safe and are important to reduce infection risk although the efficacy may vary according to the time between vaccination and drug treatments.

TREATMENTS INCLUDING DISEASE-MODIFYING ANTI-RHEUMATIC DRUGS (DMARDS) AND BIOLOGIC THERAPIES

Treatments of the rheumatic disorders include steroids, disease-modifying anti-rheumatic drugs (DMARDS – methotrexate, ciclosporin, azathioprine, leflunamide) cyclophosphamide and biologic drugs against specific cytokines (e.g. anti-TNF blockers – etanercept, infliximab, adalimumab), anti-IL6 blocker (tocilizumab), anti-IL1 blockers (anakinra or canakinumab and rilonocept), anti-B cell drugs such as rituximab and belimumab and the anti-costimulatory molecule blocker abatacept. Immunomodulatory doses of intravenous immunoglobulin may be used. Colchicine may be used. Several drugs in combination are often required.

> **FUTURE RESEARCH**
>
> ➤ Long-term outcome studies of childhood ENT diseases such as GWP with laryngeal stenosis
> ➤ Trials of early aggressive treatment of isolated ENT auto-immune disease

> **KEY POINTS**
>
> - Airway and anaesthetic risks occur:
>   - arthritis of the TMJ and decreased jaw growth
>   - arthritis of the cricoarytenoid joint
>   - arthritis of the cervical spine
>   - disorders with tracheal stenosis.
> - Patients with systemic sclerosis with tight soft tissues and decreased mouth opening.
> - Many rheumatological disorders have a relatively high mortality rate and high morbidity rates if treatment is delayed.
> - Multi-system disorders may have ENT features as the clue to diagnosis.
> - Lymphomas and leukaemias can be associated with autoimmune presentations with raised auto-antibodies occurring as an epi-phenomenon and unless tissue diagnosis is sought misdiagnoses can occur.

REFERENCES

1. Papadimitraki ED, Kyrmizakis DE, Kritikos I, Boumpas DT. Ear-nose-throat manifestations of autoimmune rheumatic diseases. *Clin Exp Rheumatol* 2004; **22**(4): 485–94.
2. Webb CJ, Moots RJ, Swift AC. Ear, nose and throat manifestations of Behçet's disease: a review. *J Laryngol Otol* 2008; **122**(12): 1279–83.
3. Greco A, Gallo A, Fusconi M, et al. Cogan's syndrome: an autoimmune inner ear disease. *Autoimmun Rev* 2013; **12**: 396–400.
4. Petri M, Orbi AM, Alarcón GS, et al. Derivation and validation of the Systemic Lupus International Collaborating Clinics classification criteria for systemic lupus erythematosus. *Arthritis Rheum* 2012; **64**(8): 2677–86.
5. Hochberg MC. Updating the American College of Rheumatology revised criteria for the classification of systemic lupus erythematosus. *Arthritis Rheum* 1997; **40**(9): 1725.
6. Greco A, Gallo A, Fusconi G, et al. Cogan's syndrome: an autoimmune inner ear disease. In: Watts R (ed). *Oxford Textbook of Rheumatology*. 4th ed.
7. Burton MJ, Pollard AJ, Ramsden JD, et al. Tonsillectomy for periodic fever, aphthous stomatitis, pharyngitis and cervical adenitis syndrome (PFAPA). *Cochrane Database Syst Rev* 2014; **9**: CD008669.

Microbiology

CHAPTER 19

MICROORGANISMS

Ursula Altmeyer, Penelope Redding and Nitish Khanna

Introduction 181	Classification of bacterial organisms 183
Basic concepts in microbiology 181	References 193

SEARCH STRATEGY

This chapter collates basic consensus knowledge of bacteriology. Laboratory practices described are based on Public Health England's Standards for Microbiology Investigations (SMI). Data in this chapter may be updated by a PubMed search using the keywords: basic concepts in microbiology; classification of bacteria based on gram staining; gram positive; gram negative; staphylococci, streptococci, enterobacteriaceae, anaerobes; mycobacteriae; spirochetes.

INTRODUCTION

The human body is a habitat that supports single-cell microorganisms in numbers that by far exceed the number of its own cells. Most of these organisms have evolved over millions of years in close association with our own species, forming what is referred to as the human microbiome.

Contained in their ecological niche, these bacteria can be essential for the survival of the host body, although if given the opportunity to leave their niche, for example through injury or surgery, their presence may equally lead to disease. Some of these beneficial, or at least harmless, tenants also have the potential to cause opportunistic infections in host organisms that are particularly susceptible, whether that be due to overall poor health, extremes of age, or constitutional or iatrogenic immunosuppression.

In comparison, the number of pathogens whose presence is always abnormal and will always lead to disease is relatively small.

The advent of antimicrobials in the first half of the 20th century has been one of the most transformative developments in medicine for both good and bad.

The emergence of antimicrobial resistance and the increasing number of resistant strains in circulation together with a lack of new antimicrobial agents means that modern healthcare is under pressure to reassess its attitude towards infection and develop alternative diagnostic and therapeutic approaches.

BASIC CONCEPTS IN MICROBIOLOGY

The human body is colonized with a wide range of microorganisms and different body sites will have a very characteristic normal or resident flora (**Table 19.1**).

A few sites are considered sterile (**Table 19.2**) and recovery of any bacterial growth from such a site should merit consideration of systemic treatment if infection is clinically suspected. In this context it is important to be able to differentiate between possible contamination and infection; this becomes easier if multiple samples can be submitted and examined (**Table 19.3**).

Most organisms commonly recovered from clinical specimens can be identified on the basis of few simple tests:

- Gram staining and light microscopy
- growth requirements (e.g. aerobic or anaerobic growth)
- metabolic properties.

The best known of these techniques is the Gram stain, which was developed by the Danish microbiologist Hans-Christian Gram (1853–1938) as a stain that is able to differentiate between human and bacterial tissue more readily than the histological stains in use at the time. The presence or absence of an outer membrane leads to differences in uptake of methylene blue, and has coined the terms 'Gram positive' and 'Gram negative' (**Figure 19.1**).

This technique is still in daily use and is performed on any positive blood culture and any sterile site sample submitted for bacterial culture.

TABLE 19.1 Resident flora of selected body sites

Site	Examples of resident flora
Skin	Predominantly Gram positive organisms: • staphylococci • streptococci • corynebacteriae Gram negatives may be present on lower body half
Oral cavity	Mixed flora: • staphylococci • streptococci • anaerobic organisms • bacillus species • yeasts Consider cover of oral flora in both human and animal bite wounds.
Upper respiratory tract	Predominantly Gram positives: • staphylococci • streptococci, incl S. pneumoniae and S. pyogenes Some Gram negative organisms, e.g.: • Haemophilus influenzae • Moraxella catharrhalis • Neisseria meningitis
Digestive tract, especially colon	Mixed flora: • anaerobic organisms • Gram negatives – 'coliforms' • some Gram positive organisms – enterococcus species • yeasts

TABLE 19.2 Sterile sites

Sterile body sites
Blood stream
Central nervous system
Pleural space
Peritoneal cavity
Bones and joints
Deep muscle tissue
Bladder and upper urinary tract
Healthy lower respiratory tract

TABLE 19.3 Contaminant versus infection

More likely contaminant	More likely to represent infection
Few organisms present on microscopic examination	Large number of organisms present on microscopic examination
Lack of white blood cells on microscopic examination	White blood cells present on microscopic examination
Growth absent from routine culture, present in enrichment only	Abundant growth in routine culture
No clinical signs of infection	Patient displays clinical signs of infection

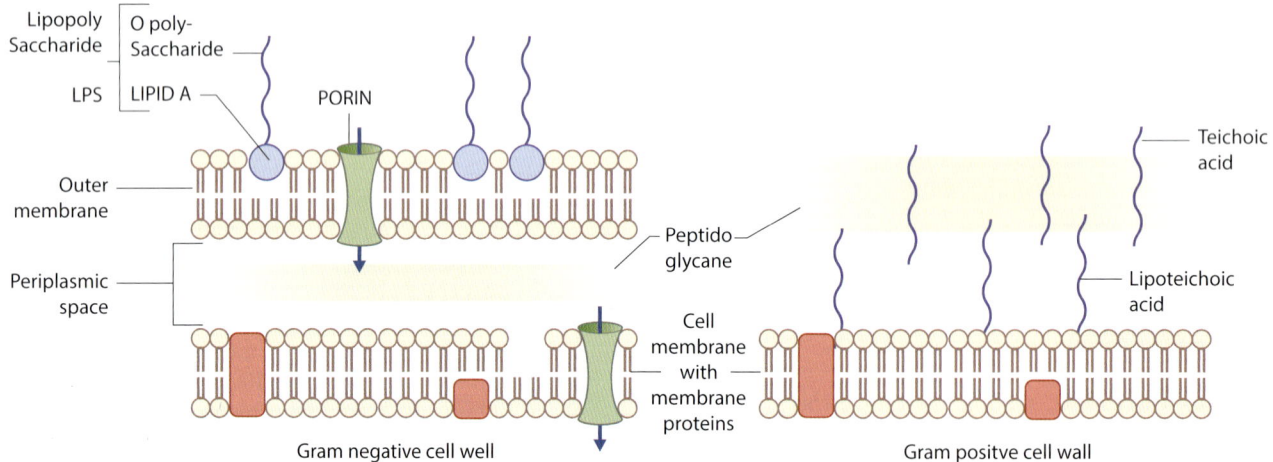

Figure 19.1 Gram positive and Gram negative cell wall structure in comparison.

Depending on the sample site and its resident flora, different sets of bacterial culture media are inoculated and incubated overnight. By careful choice of medium and incubation environment (e.g. CO_2, anaerobic, different incubation temperatures) it is possible to encourage growth of a wide range of potential pathogens.

Clinical information often provides clues about potential pathogens and may therefore play a crucial role in selection of appropriate media, for example selective media for mycobacteria or Actinomyces (Table 19.4).

For some organisms (e.g. *Staphylococcus aureus* or *Streptococcus pyogenes*), a formal identification is possible by performing very simple tests on the first day a growth is observed on the culture medium.

The majority of Gram negative organisms, however, will look very similar in culture and require further differentiation on the basis of their metabolic profiles. This is usually done by automated or semi-automated systems that are able to perform an entire range of different reactions in one step and often also carry out antibiotic susceptibility testing at the same time.

Some tests, especially susceptibility testing, whether performed manually as disc testing or by automation, require the organism to be grown in pure culture and can,

TABLE 19.4 Different types of media used for bacterial culture

Medium type	Use	Example
Enrichment medium	Improves recovery of organisms from sterile sites when only few organisms may be present in the sample and there is no resident flora	Robertson's Cooked Meat Broth Blood culture medium
Nutrient medium	Improves recovery of fastidious organisms	Chocolated blood agar
Selective medium	Selectively allows growth of organisms of interest while suppressing growth of normal flora	Hoyle's tellurite medium for recovery of corynebacterium species

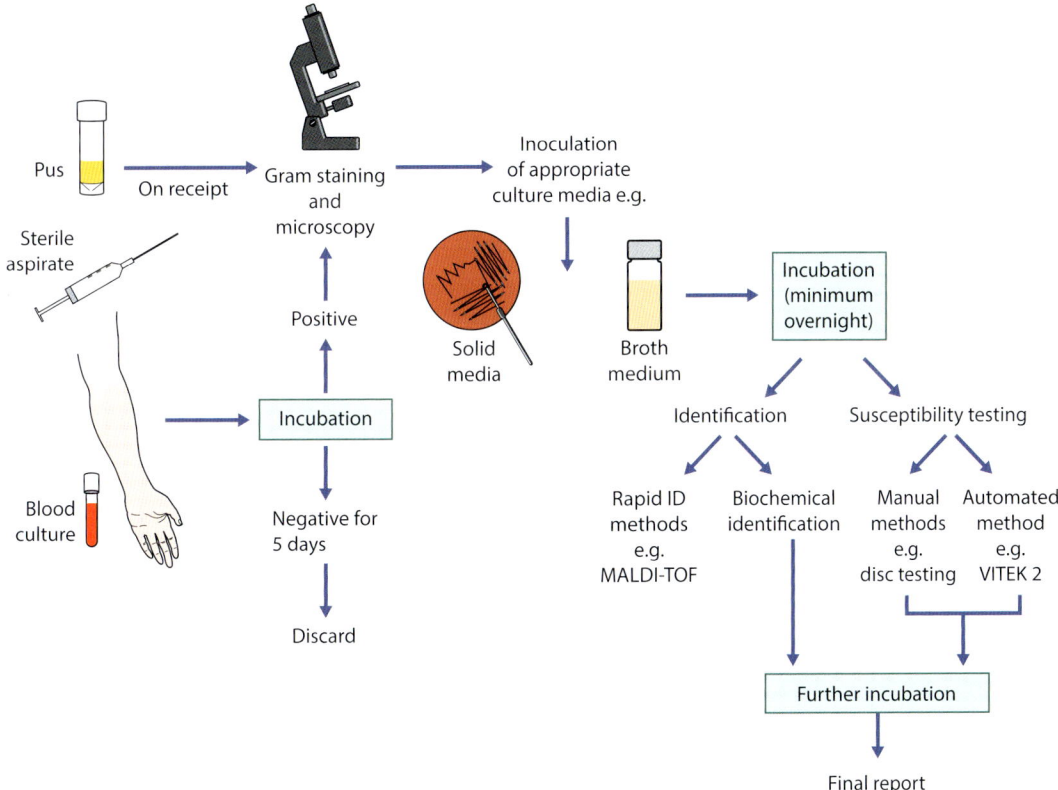

Figure 19.2 Processing of sterile site samples involves several overnight incubation steps. If organisms are not present in pure culture in the original sample a further step of subculture and incubation may be required in order to be able to perform formal identification and susceptibility testing. On average 48 hours are required to produce a final report on a sterile site sample.

at the earliest, be performed after overnight incubation of a sample (Figure 19.2).

Polymerase chain reaction (PCR) has been a mainstay technique in virology for some time and is also available for bacteriological diagnosis. It is widely employed in reference laboratories for typing purposes and CSF is often tested for presence of genomic material from *Streptococcus pneumoniae*, *Haemophilus influenzae* and *Neisseria menigitidis*.

Another more rapid diagnostic technique that has recently come into routine use in many laboratories is matrix-assisted laser desorption/ionization and time of flight analysis, or MALDI-TOF, which uses mass spectrometry to measure species-specific profiles of biomolecules, such as peptides and sugars, and larger organic molecules following laser ionization of a sample absorbed onto a specific test matrix. This is currently only possible from a pure culture, but may become available as a technique usable directly on clinical samples.

In the future, whole genome sequencing may come to supersede conventional culture techniques entirely, as it is able to not only identify bacterial species directly from clinical samples, but is also able to deliver a full profile of antimicrobial resistance. This has the benefit of identifying genes responsible for resistance (genotype) as opposed to current conventional susceptibility testing that detects phenotypic resistance.

CLASSIFICATION OF BACTERIAL ORGANISMS

The Gram stain continues to be one of the most frequently used and simple tests performed in clinical microbiology laboratory practice, and gram staining of pus and tissue samples can provide vital early information on possible causative organisms in an infective process. **Figure 19.3** provides an overview of gram positive organisms and gram negative organisms (**Figure 19.5**) commonly encountered in clinical practice.

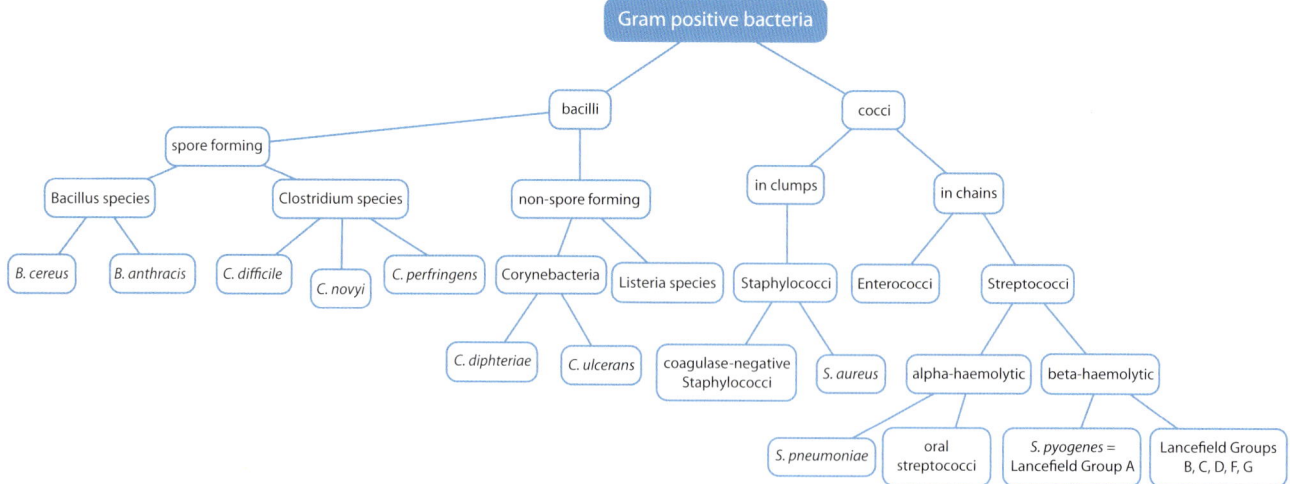

Figure 19.3 Overview of medically important Gram positive organisms.

Gram positive organisms

STAPHYLOCOCCI

Staphylococci are Gram positive, catalase positive organisms that on microscopy after Gram staining lie together in clusters, reflecting the fact that they are able to divide in more than one geometrical plane. Staphylococcal species form part of the normal skin flora.

There are several species of coagulase negative staphylococci. Most are skin commensals with low pathogenic potential, although they are able to cause indolent infections of intravascular devices and implants. An exception to this is *Staphylococcus lugdunensis*, which although coagulase negative, produces infections which present clinically much like infections with *Staphylococcus aureus*.

S. aureus is the major human pathogen in this group and it can be distinguished from other staphylococci by presence of a coagulase, which clots plasma.

This allows the organism to become coated in plasma and evade detection by phagocytes. It also plays a role in the formation of abscesses, which sequester the organism from access by the host immune system. *S. aureus* also produces a hyaluronidase, which facilitates spreading of the organism through host connective tissue.

Some strains are capable of producing exotoxins, among which are several enterotoxins, an exfoliative toxin and a toxin capable of producing staphylococcal toxic shock. Another important exotoxin is the Panton-Valentine leukocidin (PVL) toxin, which is associated with an increased ability to cause disease, usually in the form of skin and soft tissue infection with recurrent abscesses. In the UK, about 2% of all *S. aureus* isolated from clinical samples are PVL positive.[1]

Rarely, strains carrying this exotoxin can cause severe necrotizing pneumonia with a high mortality rate. Specific infection control measures should be adhered to if a patient carries a PVL positive strain and guidance regarding this is available from public health authorities.

S. aureus most commonly colonizes the anterior nares; about 20% of the population are permanent carriers and 60% carry it intermittently; the remaining 20% are non-carriers which are almost never colonized.[2]

The main manifestations of community-acquired disease caused by *S. aureus* are superficial skin and soft tissue infections, purulent infections in the form of folliculitis and deep tissue abscesses. Enterotoxin carrying strains are a cause of food poisoning.

In the hospital environment, the organism plays a major role in hospital-acquired infection, most commonly in surgical site infection, infection of surgical implants and intravascular device infection.

S. aureus bacteraemia (SAB) is a severe complication of *S. aureus* infection, which has a mortality rate of up to 30% and frequently involves secondary deep foci of infection, such as solid organ abscesses, spondylodiscitis and endocarditis. Even if treated adequately with intravenous antibiotics and removal of the focus of infection, a significant number of cases will experience a relapse or develop metastatic infection.

The majority of strains of *S. aureus* currently in circulation produce a penicillinase that renders them resistant to benzyl-penicillin, making penicillinase-stable penicillins, such as flucloxacillin, the first-line treatment. Unless the patient is penicillin allergic, intravenous treatment with one of these agents is the gold standard treatment of invasive *S. aureus* infection.

For penicillin allergic individuals, or if the isolate is methicillin-resistant (MRSA), vancomycin is the agent of choice for invasive infection.

If the infection is clinically severe or likely to involve a biofilm, as in prosthetic joint or intravascular device infections, a second anti-staphylococcal agent is sometimes added. The choice of this second agent will depend on the antibiotic susceptibility profile, but may include agents such as gentamicin, rifampicin, fusidic acid, trimethoprim, and clindamycin. However, there is scant clinical evidence that dual therapy for SAB is any more efficacious than single agent therapy.[3]

Methicillin-resistant *S. aureus* (MRSA) first emerged in the 1960s, but since has become widespread, both within the hospital environment as well as in the community and causes the same range of infections as the methicillin-susceptible strains (MSSA).

All strains of MRSA are resistant to penicillinase-stable β-lactams such as flucloxacillin; this is mediated by carriage of a resistance gene cassette, *mecA*, which codes for altered cell wall components which the β-lactam agents are unable to bind to.

Susceptibility to other anti-staphylococcal agents varies, but in contrast to initial concerns, vancomycin resistant strains are extremely rare (case reports only from the United States, Japan and most recently Portugal)[4] and the agent remains the intravenous treatment of choice for MRSA infection.

Biofilms

Like many other organisms, *S. aureus* is capable of forming a biofilm, in which the organisms form an aggregate within a slime-like extracellular matrix.

These are well known to form on non-biological surfaces which are immersed in a liquid, such as a intravascular devices immersed in the blood stream, but may also exist on mucosal surfaces within the body, such as the tonsils or the mucosa of the sinuses and the middle ear.[5]

The importance of biofilms is becoming recognized in a range of fields, from treatment of intravascular device infections, in marine engineering and shipbuilding, to use of biofilms for removal of oil spills from marine environments (**Table 19.5**).

The formation of a biofilm initially involves a stage of reversible attachment of the planctonic (free-living) form of the organism to a surface. As the biofilm develops, this attachment becomes irreversible and the bacterial community becomes covered in an extracellular matrix slime. Within this matrix the individual cells communicate with each other via a process called quorum sensing, which allows regulation of gene expression throughout the colony. A fully mature biofilm is able to release planktonic organisms back into the environment. Biofilms may involve more than one bacterial species.

Treatment of infections involving a biofilm are complicated by both the presence of the extracellular slime, which makes penetration of antimicrobials difficult, and the fact that the bacteria themselves will exhibit reduced metabolic activity and divide less frequently than as their free-living planktonic forms. This renders many antimicrobials ineffective. Agents that act on the ribosome, such as rifampicin or macrolide agents, remain effective in these organisms, unless a resistance mechanism is present. Successful treatment of infections involving a biofilm may require mechanical debridement of the biofilm and if a device is involved, this may ultimately require removal. Development of improved device surfaces that do not allow attachment of the organisms to initiate biofilm formation is a focus of research that may in the future prevent device-related infections.[7]

Research into treatment strategies involving disruption of the biofilm by mechanical measures and eradication of the biofilm with topical agents such a mupirocin or manuka honey may also result in more effective new treatments of biofilm infection.[8]

STREPTOCOCCI

Streptococci form the second group of medically important Gram positive cocci. On microscopy, they appear to lie in chains, the length of which can vary. In the laboratory, they are initially classified by examining growth on a blood agar plate for the presence and type of haemolysis (**Figure 19.4** and **Table 19.6**).

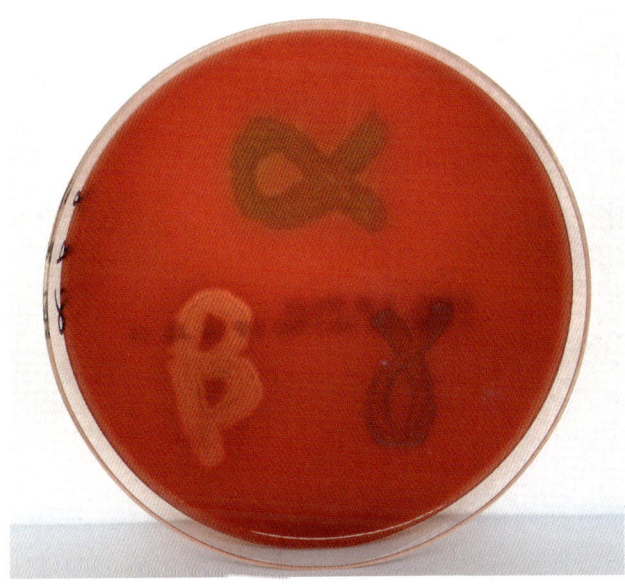

Figure 19.4 Alpha, beta and gamma haemolysis on blood agar. Courtesy of Jasminder Karde and Margaret Woods, Department of Microbiology, Golden Jubilee National Hospital, Clydebank, UK.

TABLE 19.5 Examples of biofilms[6]
Biofilms in medicine
• Dental plaque • Otitis media • Chronic rhinosinusitis • Colonization of the lung in chronic respiratory disease, e.g. cystic fibrosis • Colonization of chronic wounds • Osteomyelitis • Intestinal microbiome • Endocarditis • Device-related infections

TABLE 19.6 Streptococci by type of haemolysis	
Type of haemolysis	**Examples**
α-haemolysis	S. pneumoniae Oral streptococci - 'viridans' group Some *enterococci*
β-haemolysis	S. pyogenes S. agalactiae S. anginosus/milleri Some *enterococci*
γ-haemolysis	Denotes a lack of haemolytic activity

β-haemolytic streptococci

The β-haemolytic streptococci are usually further classified by using a latex agglutination test to determine their Lancefield group.

Medically relevant streptococci usually belong to Lancefield groups A–D, F and G (Table 19.7).

Of the β-haemolytic streptococci, *Streptococcus pyogenes* is particularly worth noting, partly due to the range of clinical presentations caused by this organism, but also due to its particular virulence (Table 19.8). It not only expresses a wide range of proteins which enable it to evade host defence mechanisms, but certain strains also produce an exotoxin capable of acting as a superantigen, leading to streptococcal toxic shock syndrome. This represents a true medical emergency with a high mortality and a substantial number of patients with this presentation require transfer to an intensive care facility as they frequently require circulatory and ventilatory support as well as renal replacement therapy.[9]

S. pyogenes causes a range of suppurative infections from tonsillitis to skin and soft tissue infections, but is also capable of eliciting a number of non-suppurative immunological complications (Table 19.9), with certain M-protein type strains showing association with specific presentations.

S. pyogenes remains sensitive to penicillins and is usually also sensitive to macrolide antibiotics and clindamycin. Clindamycin has a particular role in the treatment of severe infection with *S. pyogenes*, as it reduces toxin production by interrupting protein synthesis at the bacterial ribosome.

Streptococci of the Lancefield groups C and G are also capable of causing severe skin and soft tissue sepsis that is clinically indistinguishable from infections with *S. pyogenes*.

Group F streptococci, also commonly referred to as the *Streptococcus milleri* group, are part of the normal flora of the gut and occasionally the oral cavity. They have a particular propensity to cause deep-seated abscesses and infection should be treated by drainage of the abscess, followed by a prolonged course of antibiotics to minimize the rate of recurrence.

α-haemolytic streptococci

Streptococcus pneumoniae is the clinically most important organism amongst the α-haemolytic streptococci. It colonizes the healthy upper respiratory tract, more often in children (carriage rate up to 53%) than in adults (carriage rate 4%).[10]

S. pneumoniae can be more difficult to grow in culture than other streptococci, but when it does it can readily be identified in the laboratory by a characteristic 'draughtsman' shape of the individual colonies, alpha-haemolysis on blood agar and an inhibitory zone to a disc containing optochin, which disrupts the fragile cell wall.

Prior to introduction of the heptavalent pneumococcal vaccine into paediatric vaccination schedules, *S. pneumoniae* was the most common bacterial cause of otitis media in children. It has now been replaced by *Haemophilus influenzae*, but still remains the second most common bacterial cause.[11]

Overall, the introduction of the vaccine has led to a shift of circulating strains from those included in the vaccine to previously less common strains.

In the adult population, *S. pneumoniae* is most commonly found in the classic lobar pneumonia, but also plays a role as a causative agent of bacterial meningitis which may arise from an infected mastoid or sinus cavity and has a high rate of neurological sequelae, especially permanent hearing loss.

Contiguous infection from the mastoid or sinuses may also result in formation of intra-cerebral abscesses. These are a radiological diagnosis, and ideally drainage and sampling should precede initiation of antimicrobial treatment. Drainage itself is mandatory to achieve cure of disease and intravenous treatment with an agent that penetrates well into the brain tissue should be extended to at least 6 weeks.

TABLE 19.7 β-haemolytic streptococci by Lancefield group

Lancefield group	Species
A	S. pyogenes
B	S. agalactiae
C	S. dysgalactiae, S equisimilis, S equi, S zooepidemicus
D	S. bovis, enterococci
F	S. anginosus/milleri
G	S. canis

TABLE 19.8 Virulence factors of *S. pyogenes*

Virulence factor	Function
Capsule hyaluronidane	Mimics host connective tissue
Hyaluronidase	Spread through connective tissue
M protein	Adhesion to epithelium and evasion of complement
Protein F	Adhesion
Streptolysin O and S	Evasion, haemolysis
C5a peptidase	Evasion; cleaves complement factor C5a, a potent chemotactic stimulant of neutrophils
Streptococcal pyrogenic antitoxins	Superantigens, responsible for manifestations of scarlet fever and toxic shock syndrome

TABLE 19.9 Clinical syndromes caused by *S. pyogenes*

Suppurative	Non-suppurative complications
Pharyngitis, tonsillitis	Rheumatic fever
Impetigo	Carditis
Cellulitis	Glomerulonephritis
Necrotizing fasciitis	Sydenham's chorea
Surgical site infection	
Puerperal sepsis	

Invasive strains of *S. pneumoniae* are usually capsulated, rendering asplenic individuals particularly vulnerable to infection and therefore available vaccines against capsulated organisms (i.e. against *S. pneumoniae*, *H. influenzae* and *N. meninigitidis*) should be administered to any patient undergoing splenectomy.

High dose intravenous benzyl-penicillin is the treatment of choice of pneumococcal sepsis, but in some countries, especially in southern Europe, strains with a raised minimum inhibitory concentration for penicillin (MIC) are in circulation, which display intermediate susceptibility or resistance to benzyl-penicillin. Invasive infection with these strains should be discussed with an infection specialist, who may recommend treatment with a third generation cephalosporin, vancomycin and rifampicin or a fluoroquinolone with activity against *S. pneumoniae*, such as levofloxacin or moxifloxacin.

Ciprofloxacin has little useful activity against *S. pneumoniae* and should be avoided.

Other α-haemolytic streptococci, often referred to as viridans streptococci alluding to the green tinge of the blood agar caused by the α-haemolysis, mainly play a role in medicine as causative agents of sub-acute bacterial endocarditis.

ENTEROCOCCI

Enterococci are relatives of the streptococci most commonly found as gut commensals. They are indistinguishable from streptococci on Gram stain and haemolysis on blood agar can be variable. They frequently react with the reagent for the Lancefield group D.

In clinical samples, they often represent colonization rather than infection, especially in samples from chronic wounds or the nasopharynx of patients currently on antimicrobial treatment. They can contribute to intra-abdominal infections and cause urinary tract infections. Enterococcal bacteraemias may lead to infective endocarditis and merit further investigation with an echocardiogram; they should be treated with an appropriate course of intravenous antimicrobials.

Enterococci are commonly sensitive to amoxicillin or vancomycin, but can carry multiple resistance genes, including resistance to glycopeptides (i.e. vancomycin), making treatment difficult.

Gram positive bacilli

The main distinction between the different Gram positive bacilli lies in the presence or absence of spore formation.

Bacillus species, such as *Bacillus anthracis* and *Bacillus cereus* and *Clostridium* species, like *Clostridium tetani*, *Clostridium perfringens* and *Clostridium difficile*, all form spores, which preserve the organism in unfavourable conditions and can remain viable for considerable amounts of time. This has implications for both treatment and infection control aspects – treatment may have to be prolonged, taking into account that spores may reactivate after antimicrobials have been discontinued (e.g. post-exposure prophylaxis of inhalatory anthrax) and any disinfecting agents have to be active against the spore form (e.g. lack of activity of alcohol hand gels against spores of *C. difficile*).

CLOSTRIDIUM DIFFICILE

Toxin-producing strains of this spore forming anaerobic Gram positive rods are the causative agent of a form of toxin-mediated bacterial diarrhoea (now called *C. difficile* infection (CDI), previously referred to as *C. difficile* associated diarrhoea (CDAD)), which may lead to the development of potentially lethal pseudomembranous colitis.

Carriage rates of *C. difficile* vary in different age groups – in infants the carriage rate can be as high as 70%, in healthy adults it is usually < 3%.[12]

The use of certain antimicrobial classes is associated with an increased risk of CDI (**Table 19.10**), although other risk factors, such as use of proton pump inhibitors, presence of naso-gastric tubes, abdominal surgery or length of hospital stay also play a role. One possible control strategy of CDI is therefore restricting the use of these agents.

If CDI is suspected, the patient should be isolated and faecal samples tested for the presence of *C. difficile* toxin. Any contributing factors, such as proton pump inhibitors and antimicrobials should be removed, if possible.

Clinical severity of disease should be assessed and treatment strategies appropriate for the severity of the disease should be chosen. This may include oral metronidazole or vancomycin, but may also include intravenous immunoglobulins or colectomy in life-threatening cases.

Fidaxomycin is a recently licensed macrocyclic antibiotic that targets clostridium species specifically. The agent has recently been approved for restricted use in NHS Scotland, but guidance on its use in English NHS trusts is still outstanding.

As the concept of treating an infection caused by antimicrobials with another antimicrobial is somewhat illogical, non-antimicrobial methods of treating CDI are being investigated. A novel approach to the treatment of recurrent CDI that is becoming increasingly popular is the use of faecal transplantation to replace the abnormal gut flora with organisms that prevent overgrowth of *C. difficile*. This method of enhancing 'colonization resistance' has shown promising results in a number of studies.[13, 14]

Local protocols for treatment and infection control procedures are available in most hospitals.

TABLE 19.10 Antibiotics and CDI

Antibiotic classes most frequently associated with CDI
• Clindamycin
• Quinolones
• Broad-spectrum penicillin – β-lactamase inhibitor combinations
• Cephalosporins

CORYNEBACTERIA

The *corynebacteria* and *listeria* are non-sporeforming Gram positive bacilli.

On Gram staining, both appear as pleomorphic Gram positive rods, often lying together in formations resembling Chinese lettering.

The different species of *corynebacteria* are indistinguishable on Gram stain, and in blood cultures they are frequently found as the result of contamination with skin commensals. These species may be involved in intravascular device associated infection.

Corynebacterium diphtheriae is the most important human pathogen. Diphtheria classically presents as a severe pharyngitis with pathognomonic formation of pseudomembranes. The organism can be grown on selective media containing tellurite and produces characteristic black colonies with a 'daisy head' edge.

There are four subspecies of *C. diphtheriae*, all of which are able to produce diphtheria toxin, the gene for which is integrated into bacterial genome by a lysogenic phage.

This toxin is made up of two protein subunits. Subunit B mediates entry of the toxin into the cell, where subunit A interrupts protein synthesis by inhibiting the elongation factor EF-2.

Mortality may arise from upper airway obstruction as a result of severe soft tissue swelling, but toxin-mediated myocarditis and polyneuritis are important contributing factors and anti-toxin should be administered to prevent death as well as significant neurological sequelae.

As the diphtheria toxoid vaccine is part of the routine childhood vaccination programme and has a good uptake (>94%), diphtheria is rare in the British population. The last case of respiratory diphtheria in Britain occurred in 1997, with only eight cases all in all since 1986. The patients in all cases had travelled to endemic areas (figures from Public Health England).[15]

Arcanobacterium haemolyticum is a Gram positive bacillus that produces haemolysis on blood agar. It is a cause of bacterial pharyngitis associated with a maculopapular rash in young adults, which clinically is similar to pharyngitis caused by Group A streptococci.

Gram negative organisms

As mentioned earlier, **Figure 19.5** provides an overview of gram negative organisms commonly encountered in clinical practice.

The Gram negatives are distinguished from Gram positive organisms by a different cell wall structure.

In Gram negatives, the teichoic acid component that stains blue in Gram staining is much thinner and surrounded by an outer bi-layer membrane.

This membrane contains lipopolysaccharides that can act as superantigens and are responsible for triggering cytokine cascades that cause the systemic effects seen in Gram negative sepsis. This is sometimes referred to as the Gram negative endotoxin.

The periplasmic space between the outer membrane and the cell wall is where a number of Gram negative antibiotic resistance mechanisms are located (see also **Figure 19.1**).

GRAM NEGATIVE COCCI

Neisseria

Neisseria are the medically most important Gram negative cocci.

A number on non-pathogenic *Neisseria* spp. are commensals in the upper respiratory tract, but even the potentially highly pathogenic *N. meningitis* is carried asymptomatically by almost 24% of 19-year-olds; the carriage rates in young children and adults are generally lower than this.[16]

On Gram staining, neisseriae appear as small Gram negative diplococci. They will usually grow readily on a nutrient rich medium, such as chocolate blood agar, but selective media are available.

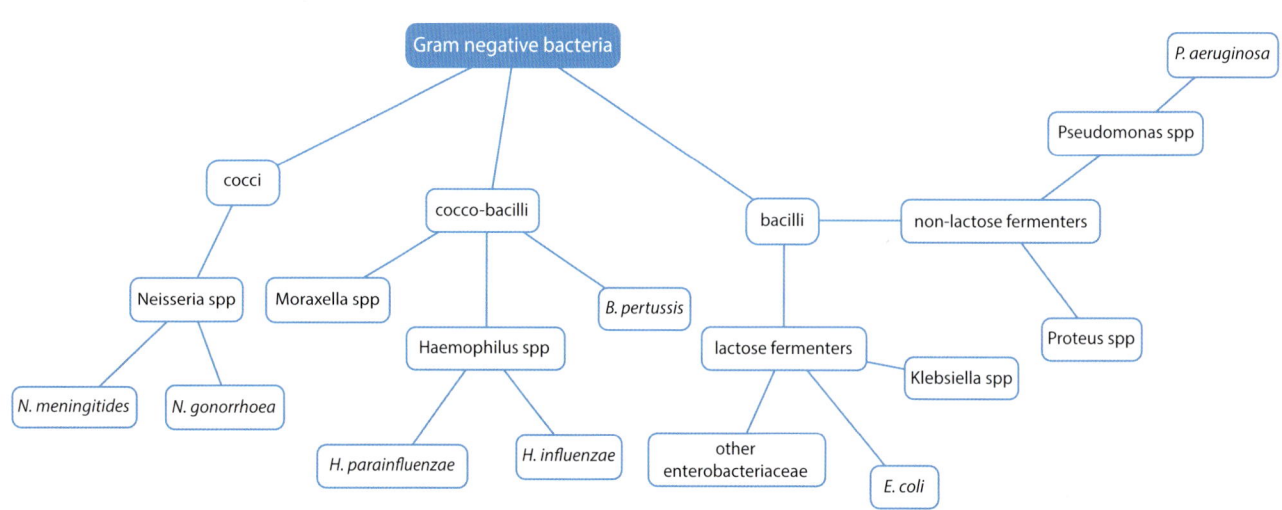

Figure 19.5 Overview of medically important Gram negative organisms.

Clinically *N. meningitis* can present with three distinct clinical syndromes: meningococcal meningitis, meningococcal septicaemia and meningococcal septic arthritis.

The first line treatment for suspected infection with *N. meningitis* is high dose ceftriaxone (i.e. 2g IV twice daily). In patients with anaphylaxis to penicillins or cephalosporins, therapy should be discussed urgently with an infection specialist.

The infection is a notifiable disease and referral to public health should be made in order to allow early contact tracing and, where indicated, offer post-exposure prophylaxis to household contacts and healthcare workers.

Vaccines targeting specific surface lipopolysaccharides are available for all major serogroups of *N. meningitidis*, but at present only the vaccine against serogroup C forms part of the UK vaccination schedule.

Neisseria gonorrhoea is indistinguishable from *N. meningitidis* on both Gram staining and appearance in culture, but they differ in their capability to metabolize glucose and maltose, which is used in the laboratory to identify them biochemically.

N. gonorrhoea can be carried asymptomatically in the upper airway as well as in the genito-urinary tract; infection may present as bacterial pharyngitis and it is not uncommon to isolate them from throat swabs.

Haemophilus influenzae

Haemophilus influenzae appears on microscopy as a Gram negative very short rod or cocco-bacillus. It has specific growth requirements in form of haemin and nicotinamide adenide dinucleotide and therefore grows more readily on a nutrient agar like chocolate blood agar.

Some strains are encapsulated, and six capsular serogroups (a–f) have been described.

Encapsulated strains, particularly strains of serogroup b, are associated with invasive disease. Asymptomatic carriage is common.

Infection can present as otitis, sinusitis or mastoiditis, acute bacterial meningitis and epiglottitis, but the most frequent presentation is as a lower respiratory tract infection.

Similarly to *S. pneumoniae*, *H. influenzae* may also be a causative agent in intra-cerebral abscess formation.

Moraxella catarrhalis is a Gram negative cocco-bacillus which is very similar to *Haemophilus* in that it forms part of the normal flora of the respiratory tract, but can play a role in otitis, sinusitis and infections of the lower respiratory tract, such as bronchitis and exacerbations of chronic obstructive pulmonary disease.

Some strains of *Moraxella* and *Haemophilus* produce a β-lactamase that renders them resistant to amoxicillin, but these strains will usually be sensitive to a penicillin with a β-lactamase inhibitor, such as amoxicillin with clavulanic acid and cephalosporins; other treatment options may include macrolides, quinolones or a tetracycline.

Bordetella pertussis

Bordetella pertussis, the causative agent of whooping cough, is a Gram negative organism of the upper respiratory tract that is exceedingly fastidious and conventional culture of this organism for diagnostic purposes has now been entirely abandoned in favour of PCR and serology.

Whooping cough is characterized by a bi-phasic clinical course. The early stage presents relatively non-specific with malaise and fever and is followed by a lengthy toxin-mediated phase of severe paroxysmal coughing, which may be accompanied by post-tussive emesis and is followed by a rapid intake of breath, the characteristic whooping.

In infants, the paroxysmal coughing can lead to significant hypoxia and be potentially fatal. Other risk groups include the elderly, immunosuppressed individuals and patients with chronic respiratory disease

Whooping cough is notifiable and contacts, especially if small children are among them, should be offered post-exposure prophylaxis.

Cases of pertussis have been increasing in the past few years. The vaccine is included in the vaccination schedule, but it is unclear for how long the vaccination actually protects against the effects of pertussis toxin. Due to this a pertussis booster vaccination is offered to women in the third trimester of pregnancy, as immunity of the mother will minimize the risk of the infant becoming infected.

Gram negative bacilli

As appearances in Gram staining and often also in culture are very similar between different species of this group, identification is usually performed on the basis of biochemical properties.

One of these is dependence on the presence of oxygen; although most organisms are facultative anaerobes that are capable of anaerobic metabolism if required, dependence on oxygen or strictly anaerobic growth can be a useful pointer towards a putative identification of a Gram negative organism.

Another useful reaction is the ability to metabolize lactose, and on the basis of this they can be split into lactose fermenters and non-fermenters. A number of commonly used media for the culture of Gram negative organisms, such as the MacConkey agar, contain a colour indicator and if the organism ferments lactose the resulting change in pH will lead to a colour change (**Figure 19.6**), allowing for a categorization of the organism on the first day that growth is observed.

The third bench procedure that may aid in early identification of certain Gram negative bacilli is the test for the presence of cytochrome oxidase.

Further identification is usually undertaken by means of semi-automated methods.

Overall, there is a large number of Gram negative bacillus species, but of these only a few are commonly found in human disease.

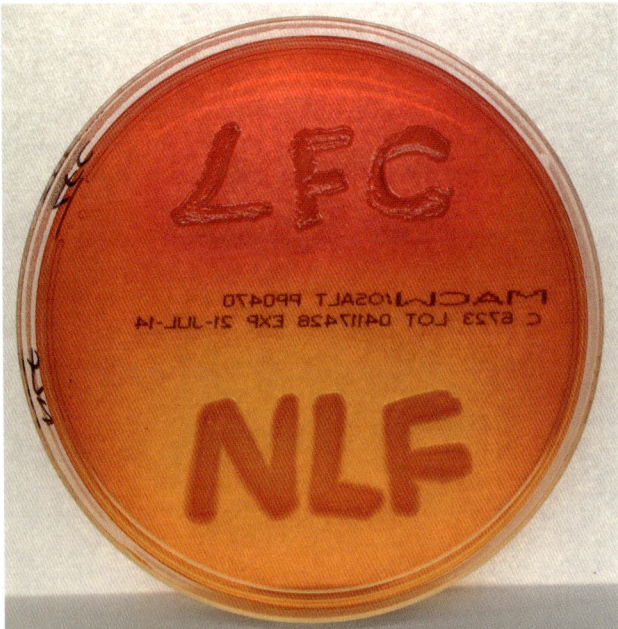

Figure 19.6 Non-lactose-fermenting (NLF) and lactose-fermenting (LFC) enterobacteriaceae on MacConkey agar. Courtesy of Jasminder Karde and Margaret Woods, Department of Microbiology, Golden Jubilee National Hospital, Clydebank, UK.

ENTEROBACTERIACEAE

The enterobacteriaceae are a group of Gram negative bacilli that are part of the resident flora of the human gut. They are facultatively anaerobic and many of these organisms are common in clinical isolates, although only few of them are invariably pathogenic (**Table 19.11**).

Enterobacteriaceae usually possess one or more flagellae and are therefore mobile – an extreme example of these are *Proteus* spp., which are capable of swarming across an entire agar plate and overgrow other organisms that may be present in the sample.

Clinically, infections with enterobacteriaceae most commonly present as urinary tract or intra-abdominal infections and they play an important in hospital-acquired infection. Most commonly, it will be the patient's own resident Gram negative flora that is involved in these infections.

Gram negative bacilli are frequent colonizers of the skin below waist level, chronic wounds and the mouth and respiratory tract, most frequently in individuals who are undergoing antimicrobial therapy and it can be difficult to judge the relevance of these organisms without careful clinical assessment.

If thought to be clinically relevant, a number of antimicrobial agents are available for treatment, but the choice of agent will usually be based on antimicrobial susceptibilities, as resistance patterns and mechanisms are manifold, widespread and difficult to predict.

Gram negative bacilli that display resistance against broad spectrum penicillins and third-generation cephalosporins via production of extended spectrum β-lactamases as well as the current emergence of carbapenem-resistant Gram negatives are developments that are likely to evolve into a major healthcare challenge.

PSEUDOMONAS

Pseudomonas spp. are aerobic oxidase positive Gram negative bacilli. They are widespread in the environment, but commonly present as opportunistic pathogens in a clinical context.

The best known species is *Pseudomonas aeruginosa*, which is easily recognized in culture due to a characteristic fruity smell and green pigment production by some strains (**Figure 16.7**).

It is a common causative agent of acute otitis externa, but also a frequent isolate from the respiratory tract or chronic wounds.

In the healthcare setting it also plays an important role in infections of venous access lines, as well as catheter-related urinary tract infections and hospital-acquired pneumonia and can cause bacteraemia secondary to these.

Treatment of pseudomonas infection is complicated by the fact that *Pseudomonas* spp. are carriers of a number of antimicrobial resistance genes, which may restrict options for antimicrobial treatment significantly. Severe infection (e.g. bacteraemia) is often treated with dual antimicrobial therapy (e.g. with an anti-pseudomonal penicillin or cephalosporin together with an aminoglycoside), as resistance has been shown

TABLE 19.11 Examples of species of enterobacteriaceae	
Opportunistic enterobacteriaceae	Pathogenic enterobacteriaceae
Escheria coli Klebsiella spp. Serratia spp. Citrobacter spp. Enterobacter spp. Morganella spp. Proteus spp.	Salmonella spp. Shigella spp.

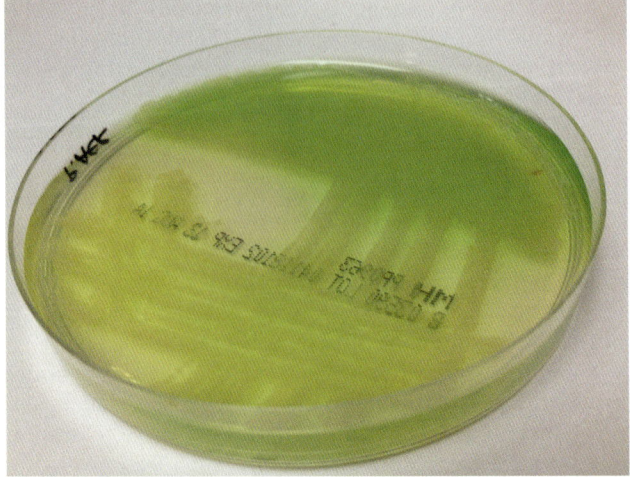

Figure 19.7 A pigment-producing strain of *P. aeruginosa*. Courtesy of Jasminder Karde and Margaret Woods, Department of Microbiology, Golden Jubilee National Hospital, Clydebank, UK.

to develop rapidly using a single agent; however, there is little evidence linking combination therapy with improved outcomes.[17]

Anaerobes

The anaerobes are a phyllogenetically heterogeneous group of organisms that are united by two characteristics – they grow in culture under strict anaerobic conditions and are sensitive to metronidazole (Table 19.12).

Their strictly anaerobic lifestyle makes isolation of these organisms from clinical samples a challenge. It is very difficult to grow them from swabs and recovery from a volume of pus sent in a container or capped syringe with all air expelled is usually more successful. In order to maximize the chances of isolating anaerobes, selective media are incubated in specific anaerobic cabinets for an extended period of time.

Anaerobic organisms form the majority of the resident flora of the gut and are commonly found in the oral cavity and as colonizers in wounds.

Most commonly, anaerobes cause pathology in the context of polymicrobial infections and an anaerobic organism being responsible for significant morbidity and mortality on its own is rare (Table 19.13).

One of these rare exceptions is *Fusobacterium necrophorum*. The name, literally translated, means 'the spindle-shaped bringer of death'. The organism is an anaerobic Gram negative rod, the shape of which is similar to a cigar or spindle.

The organism is classically the causative agent of Lemièrre's syndrome, although other *Fusobacterium* spp. are also able to produce the same presentation.

Lemièrre's syndrome usually affects young healthy individuals who initially develop bacterial pharyngitis with a peritonsillar abscess. In the anaerobic conditions of the abscess fusobacteria are able to multiply rapidly, invade the circulation and go on to cause severe systemic sepsis associated with septic embolic phenomena, classically in the form of lung abscesses arising from a septic thrombus of the internal jugular vein.

As the name suggests the condition is associated with a significant mortality rate.

Common to all anaerobic organisms is the susceptibility to metronidazole, although other antimicrobials such as clindamycin and rifampicin as well as β-lactam-β-lactamase-inhibitor combinations such as amoxicillin with clavulanic acid or piperacillin-tazobactam are also active against anaerobes.

Mycobacteria

The cell wall architecture of mycobacteria is characterized by the presence of mycolic acid, which is found in high concentrations in the waxy hydrophobic outer layer of the cell wall. Arabinogalactan connects this outer layer with an inner peptidoglycan layer. This makes the entire cell wall significantly thicker than that of either Gram negative or Gram positive organisms and conveys its typical staining properties of 'acid and alcohol fastness'.

If subjected to Gram staining, mycobacteria will typically present as slender, Gram positive rods, but the stain is only taken up very poorly, resulting in an irregular or beaded appearance. If a sample is examined for mycobacteria, specific stains such as the Ziehl-Neelsen method or an auramine stain will be performed.

In the laboratory, mycobacteria are subject to specific restrictions in terms of processing and handling in order to minimize the risk of laboratory acquired infection.

If mycobacterial infection is clinically suspected, this should therefore be indicated on the sample request form.

Growth requirements for *Mycobacterium* spp. also differ significantly from most other bacterial organisms. The organisms divide only slowly, which means that incubation times of up to 6 weeks are not unusual. An exception is the atypical or fast-growing mycobacteria, but even those will still grow much less readily that other bacteria. Due to this, PCR methods play currently play an important role in the diagnosis of mycobacterial infection.

Speed of growth is one characteristic by which mycobacteria can be categorized, but nowadays more common is the distinction between tuberculous mycobacteria or *M. tuberculosis* complex, which all cause a clinical presentation of tuberculosis and the non-tuberculous mycobacteria, which are able to cause a pulmonary disease resembling tuberculosis, but also

TABLE 19.12 Anaerobic organisms

Examples of anaerobic organisms
Clostridium spp.
Bacteroides spp.
Finegoldia spp.
Peptostreptococcus spp.

TABLE 19.13 Polymicrobial Infections

Type of infection	Common organisms
Bites	Animal: • *Pasteurella multocida* • *Capnocytophaga canimorsus* • Gram negative organisms • Anaerobes Human: • Oral streptococci • Gram negatives • Anaerobes • Nocardia • Actinomyces • Blood-borne viruses
Brain abscesses	• S. pneumoniae • H. influenzae • Oral streptococci • S. aureus • Anaerobes
Necrotizing fasciitis	• S. pyogenes • S. aureus • Gram negatives • Anaerobes

TABLE 19.14 Examples of mycobacteria	
Non-tuberculous mycobacteria	***M. tuberculosis* complex**
M. avium intracellulare complex	M. tuberculosis
M. kansasii	M. bovis
M. chelonae	M. africanum
M. fortuitum	M. microti
M. marinum	
M. abscessus	
M. gordonae	
M. ulcerans	

cause cervical lymphadenitis in children, skin infections and may cause disseminated disease in immunosuppressed individuals (Table 19.14).

Mycobacterium leprae is characterized by extremely slow growth and is the causative agent of lepra, which is still endemic in areas of the developing world.

Three agents form the mainstay of anti-tuberculous therapy: rifampicin, ethambutol and isoniazid, and most anti-tuberculous regimens will include some or all of these agents. Other agents may include aminoglycosides, such as amikacin or kanamycin.

The aminoglycoside streptomycin was the first available agent for the treatment of tuberculosis, but it has somewhat fallen out of favour due to high resistance rates.

The treatment regimen should be determined on the basis of a susceptibility profile and treatment regimens should be discussed with an infection or respiratory specialist.

It is worthwhile noting that some commonly used antimicrobials like macrolides and quinolones have anti-tuberculous properties and therapy with these in a patient with suspected mycobacterial disease may prevent microbiological diagnosis.

Due to the slow-growing nature of the organism, anti-tuberculous therapy is usually lengthy, often between 6 months and up to a year and in order to minimize resistance development patient concordance with therapy can be monitored.

Spirochaetes

Spirochaetes have a characteristic spiral shape, which is supported by an axial filament that is fixed to either end of the organism, but located outside the cytoplasm. The organisms wrap around this filament, which leads to a tumbling, rotating motion. This can be observed directly in dark field microscopy.

They cannot be grown in routine culture and PCR and serology are the investigations of choice for diagnosis.

There are many non-pathogenic species, but a few cause disease in humans.

Treponema pallidum is the causative agent of syphilis, which is a sexually transmitted disease which, if untreated, follows a multi-phasic course of initial painless ulcers at the site of entry which may be genital, anal or oral (primary syphilis) followed by early systemic symptoms such as a rash involving palms and soles (secondary syphilis), a period of latency and later systemic manifestations, including tabes dorsalis, dementia, polyneuropathy and mesaortitis (tertiary syphilis).

Borellia burgdorferi is transmitted via tick bites and causes Lyme disease, which initially causes a characteristic skin rash, the erythema migrans, and may be followed by a number of systemic effects, such as arthritis, cardiac conduction abnormalities and neuropathy, which may present as facial nerve palsy.

Actinomycetes

Actinomyces spp. are a group of Gram positive bacilli that are strictly speaking facultative anaerobes, but generally grow best under anaerobic conditions.

They are part of the normal oral and gut flora.

On Gram film, individual rod-shaped organisms form a structure that looks like fungal hyphen, giving the organism its Greek name that translates as 'ray fungus'.

The organism is slow growing and usually requires specific culture media for optimum recovery.

Infection with actinomycetes usually presents as a deep soft tissue or intra-abdominal abscess and is usually the result of penetrating trauma into the oral cavity or viscus.

Pus drained from actinomycotic collections characteristically contains the organism in distinct granula, often called sulphur granules due to their colour.

Treatment of tissue actinomycosis is usually with penicillins; alternatives are clindamycin, tetracyclines or cephalosporins. Depending on the site of infection and its accessibility for drainage, treatment is continued for anything between 6 months and life-long.

> **KEY POINTS**
> - A large variety of bacterial organisms can be involved in clinical infection. Some of these form part of the human normal bacterial flora and it may be difficult to distinguish between colonizing and infecting agents.
> - Most organisms display characteristic virulence factors, such as formation of biofilms or toxin production, which will influence a therapeutic approach to infection with a specific organism.
> - Processing of clinical specimens in the laboratory involves several steps that require overnight incubation. The average time from receipt of a sample to formal identification and sensitivities in a sterile site sample is 48 hours.
> - Bacterial culture results need to be interpreted in the context of the clinical assessment in order to identify significant results.

REFERENCES

1. Holmes A, Ganner M, McGuane S, et al. Staphylococcus aureus isolates carrying Panton-Valentine leucocidin genes in England and Wales: frequency, characterization, and association with clinical disease. *J Clin Microbiol* 2005; **43**: 2384–90.
2. Kluytmans J, van Belkum A, Verbrugh, H. Nasal carriage of Staphylococcus aureus: epidemiology, underlying mechanisms, and associated risks. *Clin Microbiol Rev* 1997; **10**(3): 505–20.
3. Thwaites GE, Edgeworth JD, Gkrania-Klotsas E, et al., for the UK Clinical Infection Research Group. Clinical management of *Staphylococcus aureus* bacteraemia. *Lancet Infect Dis* 2011; **11**: 208–22.
4. Melo-Cristino J, Resina C, Manuel V, et al. First case of infection with vancomycin-resistant Staphylococcus aureus in Europe. *Lancet* 2013; **382**(9888): 205.
5. Tonnaer EL, Mylanus EA, Mulder JJ, et al. Detection of bacteria in healthy middle ears during cochlear implantation. *Arch Otolaryngol Head Neck Surg* 2009; **135**: 232–37.
6. Bjarnsholt T. The role of bacterial biofilms in chronic infections. *APMIS* 2013; **121** (Suppl. 136): 1–54.
7. Vlastarakos PV, Nikolopoulos TP, Maragoudakis P, et al. Biofilms in ear, nose, and throat infections: how important are they? *Laryngoscope* 2007; **117**(4): 668–73.
8. Smith A, Buchinsky FJ, Post JC. Eradicating chronic ear, nose, and throat infections: a systematically conducted literature review of advances in biofilm treatment. *Otolaryngol Head Neck Surg* 2011; **144**(3): 338–47.
9. Stevens DL. Streptococcal toxic-shock syndrome: spectrum of disease, pathogenesis, and new concepts in treatment. *Emerg Infect Dis* 1995; **1**(3): 69–78.
10. Regev-Yochay G, Raz M, Dagan R, et al. Nasopharyngeal carriage of Streptococcus pneumoniae by adults and children in community and family settings. *Clin Infect Dis* 2004; **38**(5): 632–39.
11. Coker TR, Chan LS, Newberry SJ, et al. Diagnosis, microbial epidemiology, and antibiotic treatment of acute otitis media in children. *JAMA* 2010; **304**(19): 2161–69.
12. Barbut F, Petit J-C. Epidemiology of clostridium difficile-associated infections. *Clin Microbiol Infection* 2001; 7(8): 405–10.
13. van Nood E, Vrieze A, Nieuwdorp M, et al, Duodenal infusion of donor feces for recurrent Clostridium difficile. *N Engl J Med* 2013; **368**: 407–15.
14. Bakken JS. Fecal bacteriotherapy for recurrent Clostridium difficile infection. *Anaerobe* 2009; **15**: 285–89.
15. Public health control and management of diphtheria (in England and Wales): 2015 guidelines, via: https://www.gov.uk/government/uploads/system/uploads/attachment_data/file/416108/Diphtheria_Guidelines_Final.pdf
16. Christensen H, May M, Bowen L, et al. Meningococcal carriage by age: a systematic review and meta-analysis. *Lancet Infect Dis* 2010; **10**(12): 853–61.
17. Peña C, Suarez C, Ocampo-Sosa A, et al. Spanish Network for Research in Infectious Diseases (REIPI). Effect of adequate single-drug vs combination antimicrobial therapy on mortality in *Pseudomonas aeruginosa* bloodstream infections: a post hoc analysis of a prospective cohort. *Clin Infect Dis* 2013; **57**(2): 208–16.

CHAPTER 20

VIRUSES AND ANTIVIRAL AGENTS

Richard B. Townsley, Camille A. Huser and Chris Hansell

Introduction 195	Rubivirus 199
Viral proteins 195	Human papilloma virus 199
Viral genomes 196	Conditions with a viral aetiology 200
The virus life cycle 196	Viruses and malignancy 201
Detection of viruses in clinical samples 196	Vaccines 202
Respiratory viruses 197	Antivirals 202
Herpes viruses 199	References 204
Retroviruses 199	

SEARCH STRATEGY

Data in this chapter may be updated by a PubMed/Google Scholar search using the keywords: virus, head and neck, and specific virus names.

INTRODUCTION

Viruses are small acellular infectious agents that can only replicate within cells. They characteristically comprise of genetic material made of nucleic acids (DNA or RNA) encased in a protective capsule of proteins, the nucleoprotein or nucleocapsid (**Figure 20.1**). Some also contain lipid envelopes. Envelopes originate from the cells in which the virus particle was made (through a process called budding), and are essentially lipid bi-layer vesicles enclosing the virus particle. During budding, the cell's membrane proteins are replaced with viral proteins, which are important for the virus's entry into a new host cell. Although they vary in size and shape enormously (range 20 nm to 500 nm), at a mode of around 100 nm in diameter, they are approximately 10 times smaller than bacteria. Viruses are therefore not normally visible by light microscopy. Classifying viruses is done according to three parameters: type of nucleic acid; shape and size of capsid; and presence of a lipid envelope.

VIRAL PROTEINS

The virus genome codes for viral proteins, which usually fall into two categories: structural proteins, such as those

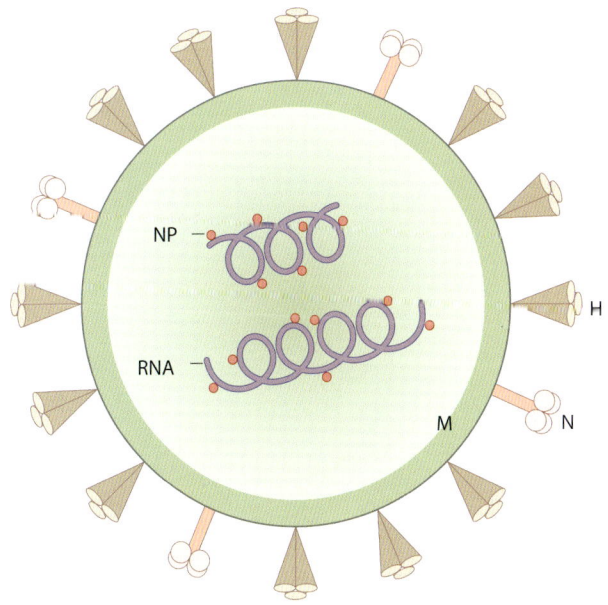

Figure 20.1 Diagram of influenza virus. H, haemaglutinin; M, matrix protein; N, neuraminidase; NP, nucleoprotein; RNA, ribonucleic acid.

comprising the capsid (including haemagglutinin, neuraminidase and matrix protein); and non-structural proteins such as viral enzymes (including integrase and reverse transcriptase), usually essential for viral replication.

VIRAL GENOMES

There are four main categories of viral genome: double-stranded DNA (dsDNA), single-stranded DNA (ssDNA), double-stranded RNA (dsRNA) and single-stranded RNA (ssRNA) viruses. The genomes of dsDNA viruses exist as a single DNA molecule, and usually contain a small amount of genetic information. On the other hand, the genome of dsRNA viruses is usually split into several fragments. ssRNA viruses are the most common type of virus. The RNA is termed either positive strand (if it can be used directly as a template for mRNA) or negative strand (if it must first be made into complementary RNA).

THE VIRUS LIFE CYCLE

There are as many life cycles as there are viruses, but there are some shared or common aspects (**Figure 20.2**). Firstly, viruses attach to the cells they will infect. The attachment is usually dependent on binding between proteins on the virus's surface and receptors on the cell membrane. This allows specificity of viruses for particular species and cell types: the virus can only infect cells that express the appropriate receptor on their surface. Following attachment, the virus enters the cell, usually through endocytosis. Once inside the cell, the viral capsid is removed in a process called uncoating, which involves proteases from either viral or cellular origin. Once the virus has uncoated and the genetic material is exposed, viral proteins are expressed and replication of the genetic material occurs, using both viral and cellular proteins and enzymes. Finally, new virus particles are assembled and released through host cell lysis or budding for viruses with envelopes.

DETECTION OF VIRUSES IN CLINICAL SAMPLES

Diagnostic virology has now become part of mainstream medicine for several reasons. Firstly, novel antiviral therapies, which are expensive and have side effects, have generated a need to precisely identify virus infections in order to treat patients appropriately. Secondly, novel technologies allow precise and rapid identification of a wide range of viruses. Thirdly, viral identification plays a greater role in the clinical management of chronic diseases such as HIV and hepatitis C. Finally, specific viral diagnosis is important for public health to track and control potential epidemics. There are several methods used to identify viruses: viral culture, antigen detection, nucleic acid detection and serology.[1] Viral culture is the more traditional method, and is slow and expensive. It involves growing the virus in cultured cells, and looking for characteristic phenotypic changes. Although it is slowly being phased out by molecular methods, it is the only method capable of maintaining a viable isolate for further tests. Antigen detection involves the use of specific tagged antibodies (usually to a fluorescent molecule) to detect specific viral proteins in clinical samples. Antigen detection using techniques such as enzyme-linked immunosorbent assay (ELISA) is of particular use for viruses that grow very slowly in culture, but is not suitable for certain viruses with wide antigenic heterogeneity, such as rhinoviruses. Serology, the detection of virus specific antibodies, is limited to cases in which

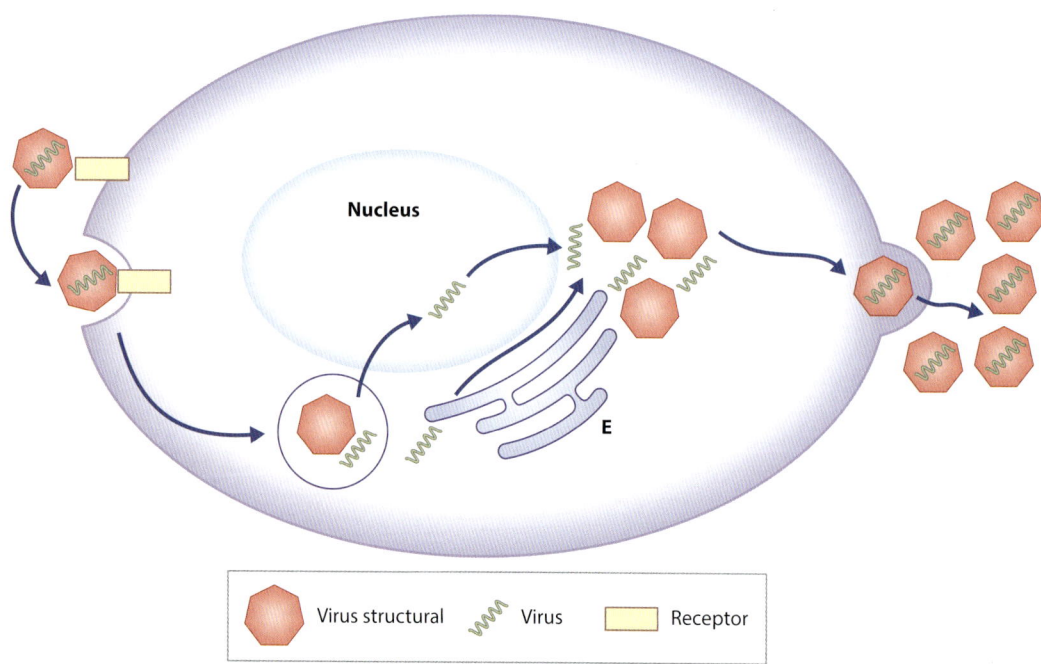

Figure 20.2 Schematic of a virus life cycle.

differentiation between acute and convalescent infection is essential. Differentiation is established by analysing levels of IgM (acute disease) and IgG (convalescent infection). Many diagnostic laboratories are adopting polymerase chain reaction (PCR) to identify viruses and virus strains. PCR is a technique used to specifically detect nucleic acid sequences, and can potentially detect the presence of any virus for which at least part of the genomic sequence is known. PCRs are sensitive and specific. Furthermore, viral RNA can be measured, giving an indication of viral load as well as strain using quantitative real-time reverse transcription PCR. Multiplex PCRs allow for the detection of a number of different viruses within one test, and can even detect viruses and other pathogens within a single test. Viral diagnostic tests can be performed on respiratory, cutaneous or blood specimens, depending on virus location.

RESPIRATORY VIRUSES

Respiratory viruses are the most common cause of illness in humans, and cause around 30% of child deaths in the developing world.[2]

Rhinoviruses (HRV)

Rhinoviruses (**Figure 20.3**) are a group of ssRNA viruses, which cause approximately half of all upper respiratory tract infections, otherwise known as the common cold.[3] The ssRNA genome of Rhinoviruses consists of a single gene, which is then cleaved to produce message for 11 proteins. Most rhinoviruses use the receptor ICAM-1 to enter cells and others use the low density lipoprotein receptor (LDLR). A new species of rhinoviruses was recently identified (HRV-C), whose mechanism of entry remains to be identified. Rhinoviruses are transmitted through contact or aerosol, via the intra-nasal or conjunctival routes. Rhinoviruses generally do not cause much pathology in the upper respiratory tract, but do disrupt the epithelial cell barrier, allowing transmigration of bacteria and exposure of toll-like receptors. In addition, it is now understood that rhinoviruses can exacerbate asthma, chronic obstructive pulmonary disease (COPD) and cystic fibrosis.

Corona viruses (HCoV)

Corona viruses are enveloped positive strand ssRNA viruses. They cause around 15% of upper respiratory infections otherwise known as common colds. There are two serotypes of corona viruses that were identified in the 1960s: group I or 229E, and group II or OC43. A third strain, SARS-CoV was discovered in 2003, followed by a fourth strain, HCoV-NL63. There are no vaccines available and immunity following infection wanes after a year or two.

Adenoviruses (HAdV)

These dsDNA viruses (**Figure 20.4**) cause acute respiratory disease, epidemic keratoconjunctivitis, as well as pharyngitis and pharyngeal-conjunctival fever in infants.[4] At the latest count, there were 67 different serotypes that are known to infect humans, and new serotypes are still being discovered. The large number of serotypes is due to frequent homologous recombination of viral genomes, and the detection and classification is greatly aided by improved methodologies such as rapid whole genome sequencing and bioinformatic analysis. In epithelial cells, HAdV infection causes the lysis of the cell when new viral particles are released. In lymphoid cells, fewer virus particles are released and the cell remains intact. HAdV have been linked to oncogenic transformation by two mechanisms: viral proteins such as E1A and E1B can transform human cells and the adenoviral DNA can integrate within the host cell DNA to cause oncogenic transformation.

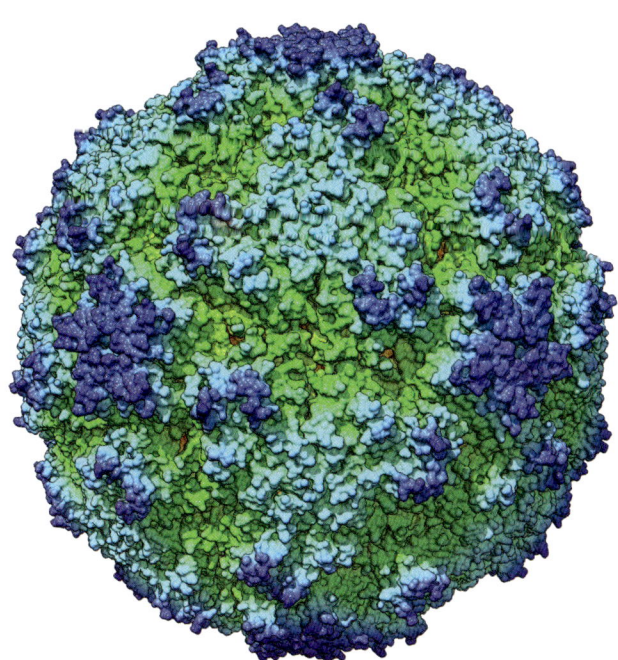

Figure 20.3 Rhinovirus. Courtesy of Dr. D. Bhella, MRC-University of Glasgow Virus Research Centre.

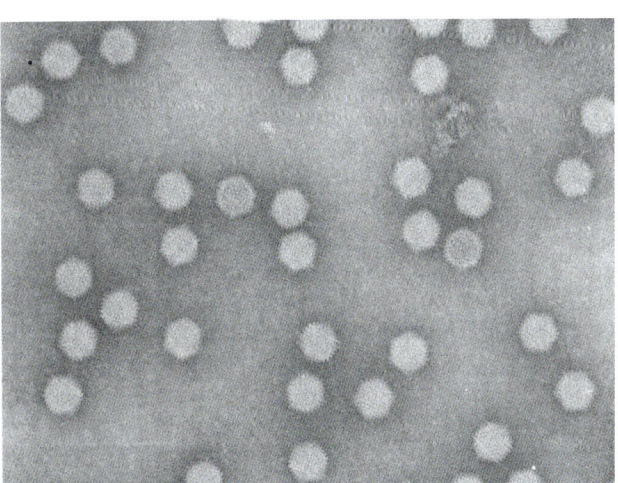

Figure 20.4 Electron micrograph of adenovirus. Courtesy of Dr D. Bhella, MRC-University of Glasgow Virus Research Centre.

Influenza

Enveloped and containing negative sense ssRNA, influenza viruses (**Figures 20.5** and **20.6**) are responsible for both seasonal endemic infections and occasional pandemics.[5] They cause respiratory disease with significant morbidity and mortality. Complications such as pneumonia, haemorrhagic bronchitis or laryngotracheitis (croup) can arise in patients with co-morbidities such as chronic pulmonary or cardiac disease, or diabetes mellitus. There are three subtypes of influenza virus: A, B and C. Types B and C are almost exclusive to humans while type A infects a very wide range of species. Influenza A viruses are further divided according to the antigenic subtype of their surface proteins haemagluttinin (H) and neuroaminidase (N). There are 16 H variants and 9 N. Currently, H3N2 and H1N1 ('swine flu') are the dominant circulating types, and H5N1 is the 'avian flu' type. Vaccination and antiviral drugs are used for prophylaxis. However, influenza viruses display continuous antigenic drift (i.e. they continuously acquire mutations which allow them to escape established immunity) so the vaccines are not effective for long. For this reason, the World Health Organization continuously monitors influenza infections in order to predict which specific vaccine will be required. Furthermore, the RNA genome of influenza viruses is segmented, and can recombine between two viruses of different subtypes if co-infection occurs in the same patient or animal. This allows antigenic shift and is how new subtypes such as H5N1 arise.

Paramixoviridae

The paramixoviruses are a family of enveloped negative strand ssRNA viruses (**Figure 20.7**), responsible for a number of significant human diseases including those listed below.

RESPIRATORY SYNCYTIAL VIRUS (RSV)

RSV is the most common cause of respiratory tract infection in humans. In 1–2% of cases, complications such as broncholitis can occur, and are especially dangerous in infants and the elderly. Furthermore, it can exacerbate asthma and COPD. Despite ongoing research, no vaccine has yet been licensed for RSV, and the use of the neutralizing monoclonal antibodies palivizumab and motavizumab has at best, mild effects.[6]

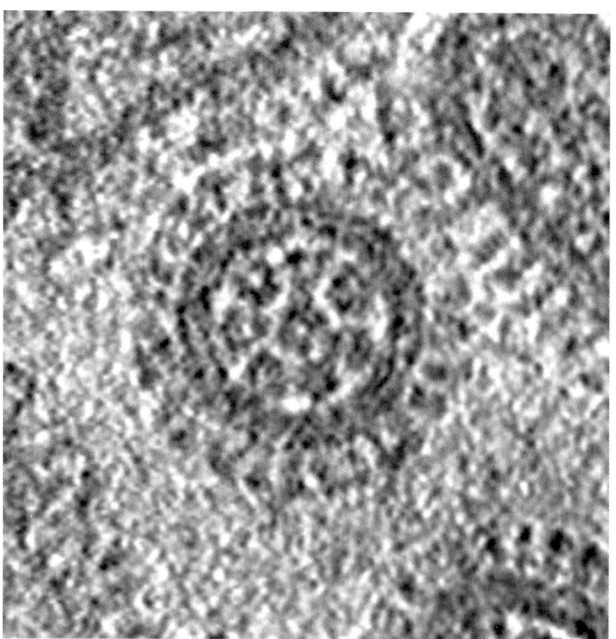

Figure 20.5 Electron micrograph of influenza virus. Courtesy of Dr D. Bhella, MRC-University of Glasgow Virus Research Centre.

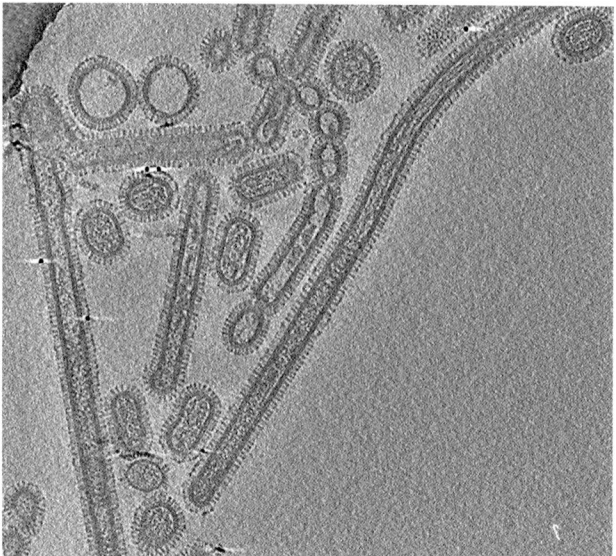

Figure 20.6 Tomogram slice of influenza-A virus. Courtesy of Dr D. Bhella, MRC-University of Glasgow Virus Research Centre.

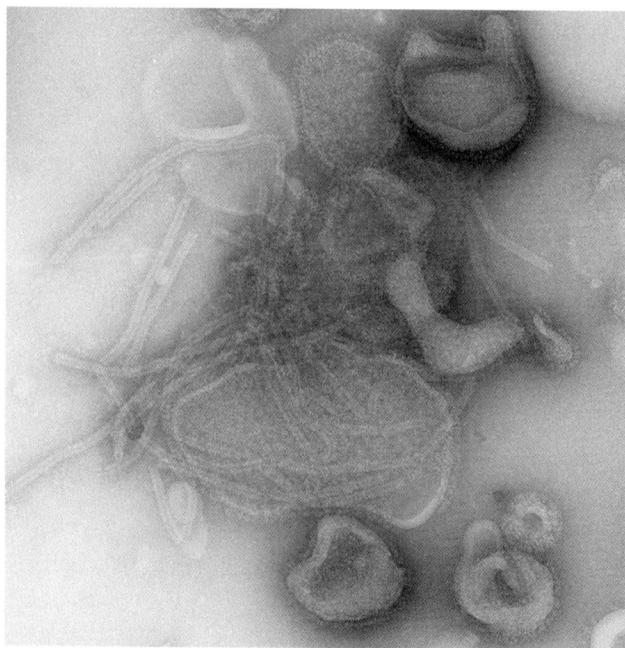

Figure 20.7 Electron micrograph of a paramixoviridae. Courtesy of Dr D. Bhella, MRC-University of Glasgow Virus Research Centre.

PARAINFLUENXA (hPIV)

This group of viruses is the second most common cause of child hospitalization for respiratory illness after RSV. There are four subtypes, which cause diseases such as croup (laryngotracheobronchitis, hPIV-1 and -2), bronchiolitis and pneumonia (hPIV-3). hPIV-4 causes asymptomatic or mild disease. There are also rare associations with viral meningitis and Guillain-Barré syndrome.

MUMPS

Mumps (Parotitis) is highly infectious and spreads through saliva. The virus probably penetrates the body via the mouth and can be detected in the oral cavity 1–6 days prior to the appearance of swollen salivary glands (especially parotid glands), a symptom that typifies the disease.[7] Other symptoms include fever and complications include oophoritis, orchitis, pancreatitis and viral meningitis. Transient hearing loss is a common symptom (approximately 1 in 20), but in extremely rare cases (1 in 20000) can become permanent. Although the illness can occur at any age, most cases present in children between the ages of 5 and 10. The disease is self-limiting and in most children the symptoms are generally not severe. There is no cure for mumps and therefore treatment is restricted to symptom relief. Clearance of the virus leads to lifelong immunity and immunization with the live virus MMR vaccine between the ages of 12 to 15 months provides a similar level of immunity and protection from subsequent infection.

MEASLES

Measles is extremely contagious, and causes coryza, conjunctivitis, fever, and a typical maculopapular rash that appears 1–3 days after the onset of other symptoms. The infective stage extends from around 2–4 days prior to the appearance of a rash to 2–5 days after. In the early phase of the disease the infection is primarily spread via contact with nasal or oral excretions, and in the later stages via contact with the rash itself. Measles infection is associated with a number of serious complications including encephalitis and pneumonia, leading to death in approximately 1 in 5000 cases.[8] The group most at risk of developing such complications are infants less than 12 months old. In around 1 in 1000 cases, measles causes permanent bilateral deafness. Like mumps there is no cure for measles, and treatment is focused on ameliorating symptoms. However, the MMR vaccine given to children between the ages of 12 and 15 months elicits a highly effective and lifelong protection.

HERPES VIRUSES

Herpes viruses (HHVs) are a class of enveloped double-stranded DNA viruses that most commonly cause oral mucosal infections. They affect patients of all ages, and can cause significant pain and dysfunction.

Herpes simplex virus

Herpes simplex virus Type-1 (HSV-1) is the most common HSV affecting the mouth and is usually the cause of blisters in the skin and mucosal membrane called 'cold sores', although in rare cases, HSV-2 (which normally causes genital herpes) may be involved.[9] Lesions heal with a characteristic scab. HSV chronically but latently infects cells of the nervous system, hiding in the cell bodies. HSVs are spread through contact with saliva. The initial infection is resolved by the innate immune system, while the adaptive immune system clears the remaining active infection. The latent infection cannot be treated at present, but general antivirals are used to treat active infections.

Epstein-Barr virus

Epstein-Barr virus (EBV) is also called human herpes virus 4 (HHV4), and is the cause of infectious mononucleosis or 'glandular fever'. It is transmitted through contact with saliva. Viral entry into cells occurs through binding to CD21 (entry into B cells) and β1 integrin (entry into epithelial cells). Similarly to HSV, after the primary infection, the infection enters a chronic latent phase that at the moment cannot be cured. As further detailed below, EBV is associated with several malignancies.

RETROVIRUSES

One large class of single-stranded RNA viruses are the Retroviridae, or retroviruses, which contain the enzyme reverse transcriptase, allowing them to synthesize double-stranded DNA from their RNA genome. One such virus is the human immunodeficiency virus (HIV), which is discussed in Chapter 23.

RUBIVIRUS

Rubella, also known as German measles, is a positive sense ssRNA virus with a lipoprotein envelope. Viral replication occurs in cells of the respiratory system. It is a purely human virus, with no animal reservoir, so could theoretically be eliminated with global vaccination strategies. In developed countries, vaccination has reduced the incidence of rubella to non-endemic levels. If contracted during pregnancy, rubella can cause congenital rubella syndrome in the foetus, with profound and serious consequences including ocular and neurological abnormalities and deafness.[8]

HUMAN PAPILLOMA VIRUS

Human papilloma virus (HPV) is a family of DNA viruses. There are at least 70 subtypes of HPV so far identified. Many of these are thought to be asymptomatic; however, a subset of HPV subtypes is associated with human disease (**Table 20.1**).

CONDITIONS WITH A VIRAL AETIOLOGY

Viruses are responsible for a wide range of pathologies involving the head and neck (see Table 20.2 for a non-exhaustive list), and some of the most common ones are briefly described below.

Laryngeal papillomatosis

HPV6, 11 and more rarely HPV 16 are specifically associated with laryngeal papillomas. Treatment requires repeated laryngoscopy and bronchoscopy to facilitate surgical ablation of forming papillomas and avoid airway obstruction. Although malignant transformation can occur it is rare and typically associated with patients with additional risk factors such as smoking or long-term illness.

TABLE 20.1 Conditions associated with particular HPV types

Condition	Usual HPV type	Less common HPV type
Oral papilloma	6, 7, 11, 16, 32	
Common warts	2, 7, 22	
Plantar wart	1, 2, 4, 63	
Anogenital warts	6, 11, 42, 44	
Heck's disease	13, 32	
Multiple papillomatosis	6, 11	67
Laryngeal papillomatosis	6, 11	16
Oropharyngeal carcinoma	16, 18	6, 11, 30
Inverted papilloma	6, 11	18
Genital cancers	16, 18, 31, 45	various

TABLE 20.2 Pathologies and associated viruses

Pathology	Virus(es)
Acute otitis media (AOM), and miringitis bullosa	Parainfluenza viruses, influenza viruses, rhinovirus, RSV, adenovirus
Asthma exacerbation	HRV, RSV, influenza, hPIV, adenovirus
Cold sores	HSV-1
Bronchiolitis	RSV, hPIV-3, influenza, adenovirus
COPD exacerbation	HRV, RSV, influenza, hPIV, adenovirus
Conjunctivitis	Adenovirus, HSV, VZV, HIV, poxvirus, picornavirus, measles
Typical maculopapular rash	Measles, rubella, parvovirus B19, HHV 6,7, EBV
Encephalitis	HSV-1,2, VZV, CMV, EBV, HHV6, adenovirus, influenza, measles, mumps, rubella, arboviruses
Cystic fibrosis exacerbation	HRV
Keratoconjunctivitis (epidemic)	Adenoviruses
Facial paralysis	Herpes zoster
Guillain-Barré syndrome	hPIV, EBV, HIV
Hearing Loss	Mumps, measles virus, VSV, cytomegalovirus, rubella virus, herpes zoster, parainfluenza viruses, influenza viruses
Infectious mononucleosis (glandular fever)	EBV
Labyrinth disease	HSV, varicella zoster, rubella, cytomegalovirus
Laryngeal papillomas	HPV-6, -11, -16
Laryngotracheitis (croup)	hPIV-1, hPIV-2, influenza viruses
Oophoritis	Mumps
Orchitis	Mumps
Parotitis	Mumps, HIV
Pharyngitis	Adenovirus, Coxsackie A, parainfluenza viruses, enterovirus-echo, HSV, EBV, VRS, influenza viruses, cytomegalovirus
Pneumonia	Influenza, hPIV-3, measles
Rhinitis	Adenovirus, coronavirus, parainfluenza viruses, rhinoviruses
Rhinosinusitis (predisposing to bacterial infection)	hPIV, influenza viruses, adenovirus, rhinoviruses
Stomatitis	EBV, HSV
Tonsillitis	Adenovirus, parainfluenza viruses, EBV, other viruses (42%)
Viral meningitis	Enteroviruses, hPIV, mumps, EBV, HSV, VZV, measles

Bell's palsy

Bell's palsy is an acute, idiopathic mononeuropathy affecting the facial nerve. The annual incidence is approximately 11–40/100 000 with a lifetime risk of 1 in 60. The course is usually benign with complete resolution in 71% of untreated cases.[10] Although the aetiology remains unknown, one theory that has gained popularity is that the reactivation of latent varicella-zoster virus or herpes simplex causes inflammation and entrapment of the facial nerve in the narrow labyrinthine segment. This theory gained popularity after detection of the HSV-1 genome in endoneurial fluid in patients with Bell's palsy. However, a recent Cochrane review has shown antivirals against HSV are no more effective than placebo treatment in producing complete recovery.[11] This casts doubt on HSV being the causative agent for Bell's palsy. More recently, HPV-6 has been suggested as a possible causative agent after detection of significantly higher DNA copies in the saliva of Bell's palsy patients in comparison to healthy donors.[12]

Sensorineural hearing loss

Many viruses, including those that cause the common cold, have been implicated in sensorineural hearing loss (SNHL).[13]

In congenital hearing loss, cytomegalovirus (CMV) and rubella are the implicated viruses. CMV is the most common cause of non-hereditary congenital SNHL. In infants with congenital CMV infection, 33% of symptomatic and 21% of asymptomatic infants were found to have SNHL. The hearing loss progresses in 11% and fluctuates in 16% of cases.[14] A histological study of inner ear lesions in congenitally CMV infected foetuses identified the structures within the inner ear infected with the virus. These structures were all involved in endolymph secretion and potassium homeostasis and the authors therefore postulated that the mechanism of damage to the inner ear may be related to potassium dysregulation, which causes secondary degeneration of the sensory structures.[15]

Idiopathic sudden SNHL is often attributed to viral aetiology. Potential viruses involved include measles, mumps, rubella, CMV, HSV, varicella zoster virus (VZV), EBV, HHV, adenoviruses and arenaviruses. The viral hypothesis postulates two potential direct mechanisms, the first being cochleitis or neuritis, in which the virus invades the fluid and soft tissues of the cochlea or the cochlear nerve, respectively. The second mechanism involves reactivation of a latent virus in inner ear tissues. A third, indirect, viral mechanism has been hypothesized, which implicates a systemic or distant viral infection that either elucidates an antibody response which cross-reacts with an antigen in the inner ear, or that triggers a circulating ligand that in turn produces a pathologic activation of the cellular stress pathways in the cochlea.[16]

Acute otitis media

Acute otitis media (AOM) is a polymicrobial disease that in many cases occurs following a viral upper respiratory tract infection (URTI). One third of children with viral URTI develop AOM within four weeks of its onset.[17] Viral URTI plays a pivotal role in the pathogenesis of AOM by causing nasopharyngeal inflammation, alteration of mucous properties, reduction of the normal mucociliary clearance of the epithelial cells in the nasopharynx, middle ear and Eustachian tube. This causes changes in bacterial adherence properties and Eustachian tube dysfunction.

In viral AOM, rhinovirus and RSV are most commonly detected and adenovirus, coronavirus and PIV are found less frequently.[18] Furthermore, viral-bacterial interactions are thought to play a significant role in the pathogenesis of AOM.

VIRUSES AND MALIGNANCY

A virus that can cause cancer is called an oncovirus. In 2008, of the estimated 12.7 million new cases of cancer worldwide, 1.9 million were attributable to hepatitis B and C virus, human papilloma virus and helicobacter pylori infections.[19] With regard to primary head and neck malignancies, the International Agency for Research on Cancer has identified Epstein-Barr virus and human papilloma virus as causative oncoviruses for nasopharyngeal cancer and oropharyngeal cancer respectively.[20]

Epstein-Barr virus

Epstein-Barr virus (EBV), the first identified human oncovirus, was isolated from Burkitt Lymphoma (BL) cells in 1964[21] and its association with nasopharyngeal cancer was first recognized in 1966.[22] It has been implicated in a number of malignant diseases including nasopharyngeal carcinoma, Burkitt's lymphoma (BL) and B-cell lymphoma.

BL is a B-cell tumour typically involving the mandibular area and occurs in children aged 4–12 years. Malaria is considered a cofactor as BL is endemic in certain areas of Africa where malaria is hyperendemic. EBV can be detected in 95% of BL tumours.[23] Cyclophosphamide is the treatment of choice.

Nasopharyngeal carcinoma has a high incidence in south China, Indonesia and Vietnam. As well as racial predisposition and genetic factors, environmental factors have also been identified, in particular the consumption of salted fish and other processed foods containing volatile nitrosamines. In addition, EBV is widely accepted as a cofactor in the development of nasopharyngeal carcinoma. Higher EBV antibody titres are observed in most nasopharyngeal patients. Latent EBV infection is identified in cancer cells of virtually all cases of nasopharyngeal cancer in endemic regions. The clonal EBV genome is consistently detected in invasive carcinomas and high-grade dysplastic lesions.[24]

Hairy oral leukoplakia is considered a pre-malignant condition consisting of painless, white, raised lesions on the lateral aspect of the tongue. The condition occurs in

HIV infection and other causes of immunosuppression. Squamous epithelial cells have been demonstrated to contain large amounts of actively replicating EBV. Acyclovir inhibits EBV replication but only allows transient lesion regression.

Lymphomas occur more commonly in immunocompromised and HIV-infected individuals. In Hodgkin's and oral T-cell lymphoma, EBV proteins are expressed by tumour cells. Persistent EBV infection becomes uncontrolled in the immunosuppressed and there is an increase in viral replication and the numbers of virus-carrying B lymphocytes. Although this condition can remain 'silent', loss of immune control can lead to EBV-associated lymphomas.[25]

Human papilloma virus

Human papilloma virus (HPV) is a double-stranded DNA papovavirus with a predilection for human epithelial cells. It is causally associated with benign and malignant diseases of the upper airway. Multiple studies and reviews have collected sufficient evidence to link infection with HPV-16 to the development of oropharyngeal cancer.[26,27] The association is strongest between HPV16 and tonsil cancer.[28] However, recent research has indicated that HPV positive head and neck squamous cell cancer is associated with improved prognosis over those which are HPV negative.[29]

VACCINES

Vaccination has been highly effective in controlling measles, mumps, rubella and influenza viruses. They are however ineffective against viruses which have multiple serotypes, such as rhinovirus.

Vaccines can be produced in a number of ways.

Live attenuated vaccines, such as the measles, mumps and rubella vaccines, use a weakened version of the live virus. This can be created by passaging the virus through a series of cell cultures or animal embryos. In this way, the virus loses its ability to replicate in human cells, creating a virus that can be recognized by the immune system and elicits an immune response, but cannot replicate well enough to cause disease.

Inactivated viruses, such as the polio and hepatitis A vaccines, are created by inactivating the virus using heat or chemicals. This renders the virus unable to replicate yet allows recognition of the virus by the immune system.

Subunit vaccines, such as the HPV vaccine, contain only elements of the virus. The HPV vaccines are created by the isolation of a single viral protein from each strain. These particles contain no genetic material from the virus but prompt an immune response that confers future protection against HPV infection.

ANTIVIRALS

Antivirals are a large class of drugs used to treat or prevent viral infections. Antivirals do not 'kill' the virus, but impede its replication or function. For this reason, specific antivirals are required for each virus type.

Matrix 2 ion channel blockers

The Matrix 2 ion channels (M2) are part of the influenza virus envelope, and play a crucial role in viral infection and replication. M2 blockers such as amantadine and rimantadine are effective for treatment of influenza A infections, but resistance is an increasing problem. For this reason, and as they are not well tolerated, these compounds are not recommended to treat influenza.[30]

Interferon

Interferons (IFN) were the first cytokines that demonstrated efficacy in the treatment of viral infections. They are a group of naturally occurring cytokines with important immunomodulatory and antiviral activities. Clinically, they have uses in the treatment of certain malignancies and also as antiviral agents. IFNs exert their therapeutic action both by direct cellular effects, via action on cell surface receptors leading to activation of signalling pathways, and by indirect mechanisms involving induction of host anti-tumour responses.[31] Interferon as a therapeutic agent is less effective *in vivo* than hoped. Unpleasant adverse effects such as 'flu-like' symptoms and haematological complications limit its use. However, alpha-interferon is used with success in chronic hepatitis B and C infection, often in conjunction with lamivudine and ribavirin, respectively.

Acyclovir

Acyclovir, a pro-drug, is phosphorylated by the thymidine kinase of the herpes virus. The active monophosphate inhibits herpes DNA replication. Acyclovir is used in the treatment of HSV and herpes zoster (HZV) infections and given as prolonged courses in those with recurrent HSV-1 and -2 infections. It is used as prophylaxis in bone marrow and organ transplant patients. High doses are given for varicella zoster virus (VZV) or HSV in the immunocompromised and HSV encephalitis.

Ganciclovir is a related compound with more activity against cytomegalovirus (CMV) than acyclovir. It is also more toxic and usually reserved to treat conditions such as CMV oesophagitis and retinitis in the immunocompromised.

Influenza neuraminidase inhibitors

Neuraminidase is a protein found on the surface of the influenza virion. Its function is to enable the release of progeny virions from the cell surface and prevent their self-aggregation. These antiviral agents prevent release and spread of progeny virions by blocking neuraminidase function.[32] Zanamivir is an influenza A and B neuraminidase inhibitor administered by powder inhalation. A Cochrane review of the use of zanamivir and oseltamivir in healthy adults found that both drugs shortened the duration of symptoms of influenza-like illness by less than a day and that oseltamivir did not affect the number of hospitalizations. Prophylaxis trials showed that oseltamivir and zanamivir reduced the risk of symptomatic influenza in individuals and households. Oseltamivir was associated with side-effects, but zanamivir showed no increased risk of reported adverse events in adults.[33] Current guidance is that oseltamivir and zanamivir should only be used prophylactically for 'at risk adults' who have not been effectively protected by vaccination[34] and that use of these drugs in the treatment of influenza should also only be used for 'at risk' patients when national surveillance schemes indicate that influenza A or B is circulating.[30]

Ribavirin

Ribavirin is a synthetic analogue of guanosine. *In vitro* it has good activity against a range of viruses including RSV, measles, influenza A and B, hepatitis A, B and C as well as HIV. However, *in vivo* it has dose-limiting toxic effects and few clinical indications. It is used in hepatitis C infection and is administered by aerosol inhalation in paediatric cases of severe RSV infection. Its efficacy is controversial with many studies failing to show significant benefit.[35]

BEST CLINICAL PRACTICE

- ✓ Influenza immunization is recommended for at risk groups including those over 65, patients with chronic liver, cardiac, respiratory and renal disease, diabetes, immunosuppression and those in institutions.
- ✓ Influenza neuraminidase inhibitors are recommended only for 'at risk' patients.
- ✓ Although acyclovir is not always necessary in the immunocompetent patient, it is recommended in the immunocompromised, and at high dose in serious infection.
- ✓ In recurrent HSV infection, famciclovir or valacyclovir should be taken immediately upon the appearance of symptoms.
- ✓ There is no significant benefit in the use of anti-HSV antivirals in the treatment of Bell's palsy.

FUTURE RESEARCH

- ➤ **Virotherapy:** In recent years, research into the use of viruses for disease treatment has been re-energized by the ability to genetically engineer viruses. One category showing promise are oncolytic viruses, which kill cancer cells. For example, reovirus, a natural cancer cell-targeting virus that does not otherwise cause disease in humans is currently in Phase III trials for head and neck squamous carcinoma, in conjunction with chemotherapy. Viruses are also being engineered for their use in gene therapy, as a method of delivering therapeutic genes specifically to cancer cells. However, caution remains with integrating viruses, as inadvertent insertional mutagenesis and hence cancer development can result, as was seen in the trials for *Il2rg* gene therapy. To date, only one gene therapy treatment, Gendicide, is licensed for head and neck squamous cell cancers in China, but many clinical trials are ongoing internationally.
- ➤ Bacteriophages, a sub-group of viruses that infect bacteria are used to treat some bacterial infections. Future research may allow them to play a greater role in antibacterial treatment.
- ➤ **Novel antivirals:** Some specific novel small molecule compounds are showing promise as antivirals for influenza A and B by either interfering with the polymerase complex or with the RNA promoter. Other small molecules have been shown to interrupt protein interactions in a range of virus processes. It is possible that in the future, the emergence of specific small molecule antiviral therapeutics will improve treatment of viral diseases, but will require improved diagnostics due to their specificities for virus species and strains.
- ➤ **Vaccines:** Vaccine research is ongoing. Clinical trials and studies are underway to ascertain the impact of polyvalent HPV vaccines in the treatment of recurrent respiratory papillomatosis and in the prevention of head and neck cancers.

KEY POINTS

- Respiratory viruses are very common and cause significant morbidity and mortality.
- EBV and HPV are associated with a variety of malignant and pre-malignant conditions in the head and neck.
- Vaccination is highly effective in certain viral diseases. In others the characteristics of the virus have prevented effective vaccine development.
- Some antivirals, such as acyclovir, are highly effective while others have a limited role in controlling illness.

REFERENCES

1. Storch G. Diagnostic virology. *Clin Infect Dis* 2000; **31**(3): 739–51.
2. Hinman AR. Global progress in infectious disease control. *Vaccine* 1998; **16**: 1116–21.
3. Jacobs SE, Lamson DM, St George K, Walsha TJ. Human rhinoviruses. *Clin Microbiol Rev* 2013; **26**(1): 135–62.
4. Ghebremedhin B. Human adenovirus: viral pathogen with increasing importance. *Eur J Microbiol Immunol (Bp)* 2014; **4**(1): 26–33.
5. Taubenberger JK, Morens DM. The pathology of influenza virus infections. *Annu Rev Pathol-Mech* 2008; **3**: 499–522.
6. Andabaka T, Nickerson JW, Rojas-Reyes MX, et al. Monoclonal antibody for reducing the risk of respiratory syncytial virus infection in children. *Cochrane DB Syst Rev* 2013; (4): CD006602.
7. Hviid A, Rubin S, Mühlemann K. Mumps. *Lancet* 2008; **371**(9616): 932–44.
8. White SJ, Boldt KL, Holditch SJ, et al. Measles, mumps, and rubella. *Vlin Obstet Gynecol* 2012; **55**(2): 550–59.
9. Egan KP, Wu S, Wigdahl B, Jennings SR. Immunological control of herpes simplex virus infections. *J Neurovirol* 2013; **19**(4): 328–45.
10. McCaul JA, Cascarini L, Godden D, et al. Evidence based management of Bell's palsy. *Brit J Oral Max Surg* 2014; **52**(5): 387–91.
11. Lockhart P, Daly F, Pitkethly M, et al. Antiviral treatment for Bell's palsy (idiopathic facial paralysis). *Cochrane DB Syst Rev* 2009; (4): CD001869.
12. Turriziani O, Falasca F, Maida P, et al. Early collection of saliva specimens from Bell's palsy patients: quantitative analysis of HHV-6, HSV-1 and VZV. *J Med Virol* 2014.
13. Linthicum Jr FH. Viral causes of sensory-neural hearing loss. *Otolaryng Clin N Am* 1978; **11**: 29–33.
14. Foulon I, Naessens A, Foulon W, et al. A 10-year prospective study of sensorineural hearing loss in children with congenital cytomegalovirus infection. *J Pediatr* 2008; **153**: 84–88.
15. Teissier N, Delezoide AL, Mas AE, et al. Inner ear lesions in congenital; cytomegalovirus infection of human foetuses. *Acta Neuropathol* 2011; **122**: 763–74.
16. Merchant SN, Durand ML, Adams JC. Sudden deafness: is it viral? *ORL J Oto-Rhino-Laryngol* 2008; **70**: 52–60.
17. Chonmaitree T, Revai K, Grady JJ, et al. Viral upper respiratory tract infection and otitis media complication in young children. *Clin Infect Dis* 2008; **46**: 815–23.
18. Arola M, Ruuskanen O, Ziegler T, et al. Clinical role of respiratory virus infection in acute otitis media. *Pediatrics* 1990; **86**: 848–55.
19. De Martel C, Ferlay J, Franceschi S, et al. Global burden of cancers attributable to infections in 2008: a review and synthetic analysis. *Lancet Oncol* 2012; **13**(6): 607–15.
20. IARC. *A review of carcinogen-Part B: biological agents*. Monographs on the evaluation of carcinogenic risks to humans. Volume 100. Lyon: International Agency for Research on Cancer; 2011.
21. Epstein MA, Achong BG, Barr YM. Virus particles in cultured lymphoblasts from Burkitt's lymphoma. *Lancet* 1964; 1(7335): 702–03.
22. Old LJ, Boyse EA, Oettgen HF, et al. Precipitating antibody in human serum to an antigen present in cultured Burkitt's lymphoma cells. *P Natl Acad Sci USA* 1966; **56**: 1699–704.
23. Collier L, Oxford J. Viruses and cancer. In: Collier L, Oxford J (eds). *Human virology*. Oxford: Oxford University Press; 2000, pp. 49–56.
24. Raab-Traub N. Epstein Barr virus in the pathogenesis of NPC. *Semin Cancer Biol* 2002; **12**(6): 431–41.
25. Epstein MA, Crawford DH. The Epstein-Barr virus. In: Ledingham JGG, Warrell DA (eds). *Concise Oxford textbook of medicine*. Oxford: Oxford University Press; 2000, pp. 1505–08.
26. Gillison ML, Alemany L, Snijders PJF, et al. Human papillomavirus and disease of the upper airway: head and neck cancer and respiratory papillomatosis. *Vaccine* 2012; **30**(Suppl 5): F34–F54.
27. Sudhoff HH, Schwarze HP, Winder D, et al. Evidence for a causal association for HPV in head and neck cancers. *Eur Arch Oto-Rhino-Laryngol* 2011; **268**: 1541–47.
28. Hobbs CGL, Sterne JAC, Bailey M, et al. Human papillomavirus and head and neck cancer: a systematic review and meta analysis. *Clin Otolaryngol* 2006; **3**: 259–66.
29. Fakhry C, Westra WH, Li S, et al. Improved survival of patients with human papilloma virus positive head and neck squamous cell carcinoma in a prospective clinical trial. *J Natl Cancer I* 2008: **100**: 261–69.
30. National Institute for Clinical Excellence. *Guidance on the use of amantadine, oseltamivir and zanamivir for the treatment of influenza*. Technology appraisal guidance, TA168; February 2009.
31. Parmer S, Platanias LC. Interferons: mechanism of action and clinical applications. *Curr Opin Oncol* 2003; **15**(6): 431–39.
32. McKimm-Breschkin JL. Influenza neuraminidase inhibitors: antiviral action and mechanism of resistance. *Influenza Other Resp* 2013; 7 (Suppl 1): 25–36.
33. Jefferson T, Jones M.A, Doshi P, et al. Neuraminidase inhibitors for preventing and treating influenza in healthy adults and children. *Cochrane DB Syst Rev* 2014.
34. National Institute for Clinical Excellence. *Guidance on use of Oseltamivir, amantadine and zanamivir for the prophylaxis of influenza*. Technology appraisal guidance, TA158; September 2008.
35. DeVincenzo J. Prevention and treatment of respiratory syncytial virus infections (for advances in paediatric infectious diseases). *Adv Paediatr Infect Dis* 1997; **13**: 1–47.

CHAPTER 21

FUNGAL INFECTIONS

Emily Young, Yujay Ramakrishnan, Laura Jackson and Shahzada K. Ahmed

Introduction 205	Conidiobolus 208
Fungal taxonomy 205	Cryptococcus 208
Fungal tissue diagnosis 206	Rhinosporidiosis 208
Aspergillus species 206	Fungi in ENT clinical practice 208
Candida species 207	References 218
Trichophyton 207	

SEARCH STRATEGY

Data in this chapter may be updated by a Medline search using the keywords: fungal infections in ENT, fungal infections in otolaryngology, fungal sinusitis, fungal rhinosinusitis, invasive fungal sinusitis, acute invasive fungal sinusitis, chronic invasive fungal sinusitis, chronic invasive granulomatous fungal sinusitis, fungal ball, allergic fungal sinusitis, oropharyngeal candida, otomycosis and speech valves fungal infection.

INTRODUCTION

Many thousands of species of fungi have been identified and these organisms are extremely diverse in terms of morphology and habitat. Only a small proportion of these organisms, however, are medically important pathogens, and even fewer of these are commonly encountered in otolaryngology practice.

In this chapter, we aim to expand upon previous editions by providing an introduction into the basic science of fungal infections, and their laboratory identification, as well as providing a concise update on the subject of fungal infections in ENT. This is presented in a subsite specific manner, and is based upon a comprehensive review of the literature on the subject. The basic science material has been obtained from salient texts[1–3] along with online resources aimed at scientists and medical professionals, and governed by the national mycological associations of Britain, America and Australia.

FUNGAL TAXONOMY

Fungi are one of four major groups of microorganisms (bacteria, viruses, parasites and fungi). They are eukaryotic organisms that reproduce through spore formation, and are distinct from both plants and animals. Based on the case or sac in which the spores are produced, fungi are classified into four divisions: Ascomycota (sac fungi), Basidiomycota (club fungi), Zygomycota (zygote forming fungi) and Deuteromycota (imperfect fungi).

Fungi exist in nature in one of two forms: as unicellular yeasts or as branching filamentous moulds. Some fungi are dimorphic – they change from one form to another depending on their environment. While yeasts cannot be seen with the naked eye, moulds can be seen as growths on ageing foods, or as mildew in damp bathrooms. Of the vast array of fungi in the environment, less than 200 species are associated with human disease and of these, only 20 to 25 species are common causes of infection.[1, 2]

Fungi with importance in otolaryngology typically belong to the divisions Ascomycota and Deuteromycota, divisions to which *Aspergillus* species and *Candida* species belong respectively. Whilst Candidiasis and Aspergillosis account for the majority of fungal infections, Zygomycetes also contribute to a significant proportion.[4] Pathogens in the Zygomycota phylum, including Mucor, Apophysomyces, Rhizomucor, Rhizopus and Absidia, more frequently cause infections in immunosuppressed patients with underlying conditions, such as diabetes and malignancy.[5]

FUNGAL TISSUE DIAGNOSIS

Specific tests are used to determine the causative agent of a fungal infection, and to guide the clinician towards appropriate treatment. For many superficial skin and yeast infections, a clinical examination of the patient and microscopic examination of the sample may be sufficient to determine that a fungal infection is present. Identification of the specific organism is not always necessary as several topical and oral antifungal treatment options are available for clinicians to prescribe empirically based on best practice guidelines and personal experience.

Fungi do not stain well with routine stains and special silver-impregnated fungal stains are required. The latter is not species specific. Other fungal tests including potassium hydroxide solution (KOH) prep test also detect fungi but are not species specific. This is a rapid test, which dissolves non-fungal elements in a sample. It is widely used on skin scrapings, tissue, body fluids and sputum. After the non-fungal elements of the sample are dissolved, yeast cells and fungal hyphae can be visualized directly on a microscope slide.

Similarly, the Calcofluor white stain (**Figure 21.1**) detects fungi rapidly in a non-specific manner from a similar range of samples to the KOH prep test. The stain binds to fungal elements in a sample and fluoresces under ultraviolet light allowing direct visualization on a microscope slide.

Fungal cultures are used to identify the specific fungi present in persistent fungal infections and in those that penetrate into deeper tissues or cause systemic infections. Fungi are typically slow-growing and must be isolated in specific fungal enrichment media that inhibit bacterial growth. Fungal culture can take several weeks depending upon the species isolated. Susceptibility testing performed on fungi isolated from a culture is used to determine which antifungal is best to use for treatment

When a fungal infection is persistent, involves deep tissues or there is systemic upset, more extensive testing may be required. As a minimum, susceptibility testing following fungal culture determines the most effective antifungal agents to use. This can take days to weeks after primary culture.

Serology for fungal antigens and antibodies may be used to determine if a patient has a specific fungal infection. They are more rapid than fungal cultures but only test for a specific fungal species, so are limited by the index of suspicion for a specific organism that the requesting clinician has. Fungal antibodies can also be present from a prior exposure to the organism so a single antibody test cannot always confirm the presence of a current infection in isolation. If antibody tests are requested to see if antibody titres are changing, results may take several weeks.

Molecular tests for nucleic acids are also available that detect genetic material of certain specific fungi. These are performed on samples of fungus isolated in culture and are not yet widely available (https://labtestsonline.org). The results of these tests may take days to weeks from the sample reaching the lab.

ASPERGILLUS SPECIES

The genus *Aspergillus* includes over 185 species. Around 20 species have so far been reported as causative agents of infections in humans. They are ubiquitous fungi found in the environment and are commonly isolated from soil and plant debris. The most commonly isolated species are *Aspergillus fumigatus* (**Figure 21.2**), *Aspergillus flavus* and *Aspergillus niger* (**Figure 21.3**). All three of these species are implicated in otomycosis, a superficial fungal infection of the ear canal, although in general *Aspergillus niger* is the most commonly isolated; this can be population dependent.[6]

Aspergillus species (*Aspergillus* spp.) are implicated in opportunistic infections, allergic states and toxicoses. Immunosuppression is the major factor predisposing to development of opportunistic infections. These can present as minor local infections or disseminated aspergillosis. Almost any organ or system in the human body may be involved. In ENT practice, *Aspergillus* spp. most

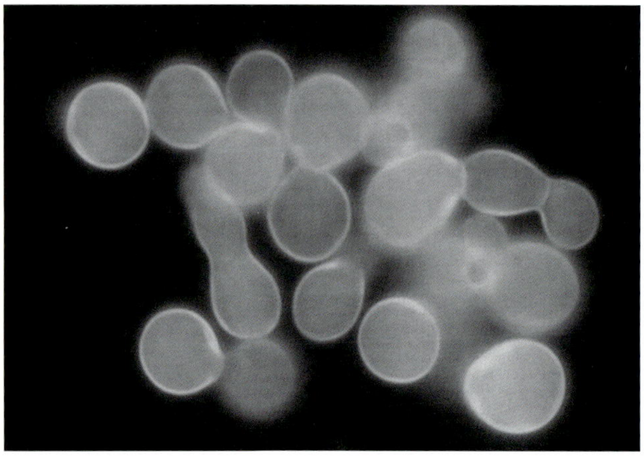

Figure 21.1 Blastomycosis-Calcofluor white stain of yeast phase growth at 30°C (1000x magnification). Courtesy of http://www.mycology.adelaide.edu.au/gallery/dimorphic_fungi/

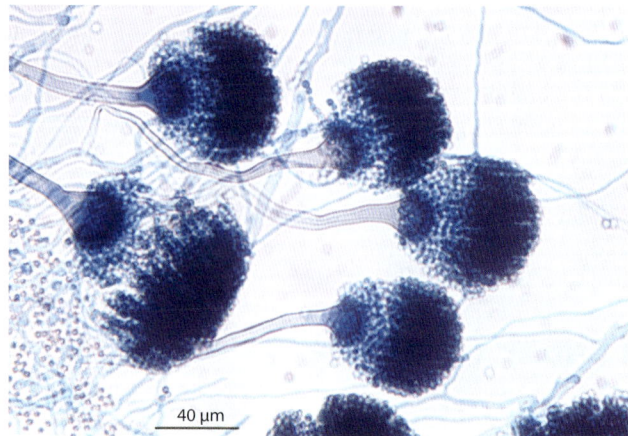

Figure 21.2 *Aspergillus fumigatus* colony growth on Czapek dox agar showing atypical blue-green surface pigmentation. Courtesy of http://www.mycology.adelaide.edu.au/gallery/hyaline_moulds/

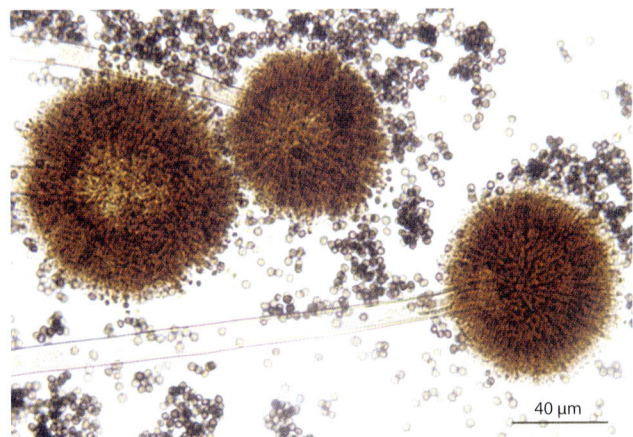

Figure 21.3 *Aspergillus niger* – **microscopic morphology.**
Courtesy of http://www.mycology.adelaide.edu.au/gallery/hyaline_moulds/

commonly infect the sinuses, which can rarely result in meningitis or cerebral aspergillosis, and the external ear canals, resulting in otomycosis. Construction in hospital environments poses a major risk for development of aspergillosis by unearthing spores from the environment. This is particularly risky in immunosuppressed, or neutropenic patients.

It is important to note, however, that since *Aspergillus* spp. are found in the natural environment, they are also common laboratory contaminants and therefore an awareness of the clinical features of their infections is paramount to allow for accurate clinical correlation of laboratory reports.

Within the Aspergilli, the major macroscopic features remarkable in species identification are the growth rate, colour of the colony, and thermotolerance. For the otolaryngologist, these finer details are something to be aware of, but will not be considered further in the context of this chapter.

CANDIDA SPECIES

Candida species (*Candida* spp.) are yeasts and the most common cause of opportunistic mycoses worldwide. *Candida* spp. are frequent colonizers of human skin and mucous membranes lining the mouth, vagina and gastrointestinal tract. As well as being a colonizer and opportunistic pathogen, it is found in the environment, on leaves, flowers, water and soil.

The genus *Candida* includes around 154 species, the majority of which are not frequently isolated in human infections. While *Candida albicans* is the most abundant and significant species, there has been a recent increase in infections due to non-albicans *Candida* spp. Patients who receive fluconazole prophylaxis, for example head and neck oncology patients, are at risk of infections with fluconazole-resistant *Candida krusei* and *Candida glabrata* strains. The diversity of pathogenic *Candida* spp. is expanding and the emergence of other species is a real possibility.

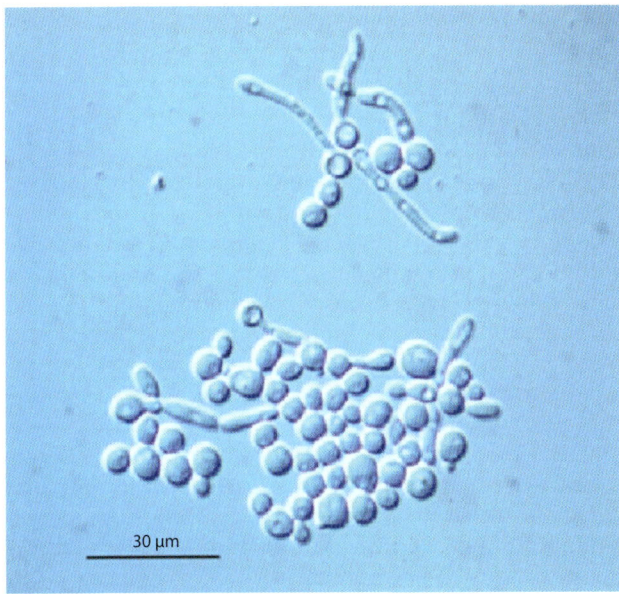

Figure 21.4 *Candida albicans* – **microscopic morphology.**
Courtesy of http://www.mycology.adelaide.edu.au/gallery/yeast-like_fungi/

Infections caused by *Candida* spp. are in general referred to as candidiasis. The clinical spectrum of candidiasis is extremely diverse. In otolaryngology, the most frequently encountered candida infections are of the oropharynx, larynx and external ear canal, although almost any organ or system in the body can be affected. Infection can be superficial and local or deep-seated and disseminated. Disseminated infections tend to arise via haematogenous spread from the primary infection site. *Candida albicans* (**Figure 21.4**) is the most pathogenic and most commonly encountered species. Its ability to adhere to host tissues, produce secretory aspartyl proteases and phospholipase enzymes, and transform from yeast to hyphal phase are the major determinants of its pathogenicity. Several host factors predispose to candidiasis including pregnancy, extremes of age, trauma, immunosuppression (including steroid use), endocrine disease and antibiotic use.

Candidiasis is mostly an endogenous infection, arising from overgrowth of the fungus inhabiting in the normal flora. However, it may occasionally be isolated from exogenous sources (such as catheters or prosthetic devices such as speech valves in laryngectomy patients) or by person-to-person transmission, such as oral candidiasis in neonates of mothers with vaginal candidiasis.

TRICHOPHYTON

Trichophyton is a dermatophyte that ordinarily inhabits soil. It is a leading cause of hair, skin and nail infections in humans and is most commonly encountered by the otolaryngologist as a causative agent of pinna dermatosis. There are several species of Tricophyton, most commonly being *Trichphyton mentagrophytes*, *Trichophyton rubrum* and *Trichophyton schoenleinii*. Trichophyton is a keratinophilic filamentous fungus with the ability to invade keratinized tissues. It produces enzymes such as proteinases, elastase, and keratinases, which are the major virulence factors of these fungi.

CONIDIOBOLUS

The genus Conidiobolus contains several species. The most common ones are *Conidiobolus coronatus*, *Conidiobolus incongruus* and *Conidiobolus lamprauges*. Conidiobolus is a mould most commonly found in soil and decaying plant debris. It is mostly distributed in tropical areas and particularly in Central America, equatorial Africa and India (www.mycology.adelaide.edu.au). The most common clinical picture caused by *Conidiobolus* spp. is a subcutaneous infection involving nasal mucosa and maxillofacial tissues. This chronic inflammatory granulomatous disease is also referred to as entomophthoromycosis conidiobolae.[7] It involves facial subcutaneous tissues and paranasal sinuses, leading to formation of firm, subcutaneous nodules or polyps. The infection may be acquired via inhalation of spores or a minor trauma such as an insect bite. The infected host is frequently an otherwise healthy individual working outdoors in tropical areas. However, the infection may also develop in patients with underlying pathologies, such as neutropenia or Burkitt's lymphoma.

On potato dextrose agar and following incubation at 25° *Conidiobolus* spp. produce rapidly growing colonies which are glabrous and waxy initially and become powdery after development of aerial hyphae. The colonies mature in about 5 days. (mycosesstudygroup.org)

In vitro data on the activity of antifungal agents against Conidiobolus isolates are very limited.

There is as yet no standard regimen for treatment of Conidiobolus infections. Potassium iodide, trimethoprim sulfamethoxazole, and azole derivatives have been used.

CRYPTOCOCCUS

Cryptococcus is an encapsulated yeast. Following its first identification in nature from peach juice samples, the major environmental sources of *Cryptococcus neoformans* have been shown to be either soil contaminated with pigeon droppings (*Cryptococcus neoformans* var. *neoformans*) or eucalyptus trees and decaying wood forming hollows in living trees. The genus Cryptococcus includes around 37 species. Among these, *Cryptococcus neoformans* is the only species that is pathogenic. It has four serotypes, A to D. *Cryptococcus neoformans* was generally accepted to include two varieties; var. *gattii* and var. *neoformans*.

The definitive identification of *neoformans* and *gattii* varieties is possible by biochemical tests, such as resistance to canavanine and EDTA.

Cryptococcus neoformans is the causative agent of cryptococcosis. Given the neurotropic nature of the fungus, the most common clinical form of cryptococcosis is meningoencephalitis. The course of the infection is usually subacute or chronic.

The polysaccharide capsule and phenol oxidase enzyme of *Cryptococcus neoformans*, as well as its ability to grow at 37°C, are its major virulence factors. The infection commonly starts following inhalation of the yeasts.

Colonies of *Cryptococcus neoformans* are fast growing, although the growth rate is slower than *Candida* and usually takes 48 to 72 h. It grows well at 25°C as well as 37°C. Ability to grow at 37°C is one of the features that differentiates *Cryptococcus neoformans* from other *Cryptococcus* spp.

RHINOSPORIDIOSIS

Rhinosporidiosis is an infectious disease caused by an aquatic protozoan previously considered to be a fungus. The aetiologic agent of rhinosporidiosis, *Rhinosporidium seeberi*, is closely related to several proctoctistiae fish pathogens. The infection affects nasal mucous membranes and ocular conjunctivae of humans and animals, producing slowly growing masses that degenerate into polyps. As this is no longer considered to be a fungal pathogen it will be considered no further in this chapter.

FUNGI IN ENT CLINICAL PRACTICE

Otomycosis

Otomycosis is a fungal infection of the external ear canal that can also affect mastoid cavities and in complicated cases, the middle ear. It is more common in hot, humid climates compared to temperate ones. Approximately 9% of cases of otitis externa are due to otomycosis.[8] Other studies have reported a prevalence of up to 30% in patients presenting with inflammatory conditions of the ear.[9] There is no preponderance of either gender, and it can affect any age, although it is rare in young children.

PREDISPOSING FACTORS

The most common causal fungal organisms are *Aspergillus niger*, *Candida albicans*, *Actinomyces*, *Trichophyton*, *Aspergillus fumigatus* and *Candida tropicalis*. Common predisposing factors include prolonged treatment with topical antibiotics, hearing aid use, regular swimming in contaminated water, trauma to the ear canal and immunosuppression.[10]

CLINICAL FEATURES

The symptoms of otomycosis are non-specific and include itching, otalgia, otorrhoea, aural fullness, hearing loss and tinnitus. Furthermore, although the classic sign of otomycosis is the presence of waving conidiophores, this is not universally present. Yeasts, such as *Candida* species, do not form the closely woven mass of hyphae that are formed by moulds, such as *Aspergillus* (**Figure 21.5**).[8]

More common is the finding of generalized inflammatory changes of the external canal (oedema, hyperaemia, granulomatous myringitis and aural discharge of variable colour.[11]

COMPLICATIONS

Fungal malignant otitis externa is a skull base osteomyelitis and occurs when inadequately treated fungal infection spreads through small gaps in the cartilaginous floor of the external ear canal, and spreads medially to the skull base. From here, bony destruction continues, with cranial nerve palsies occurring, particularly affecting the facial nerve. Other lower cranial nerves including IX, X, XI and XII can also be affected. Malignant otitis externa should be suspected in a patient with severe otalgia, which interrupts sleep, and often occurs in immunocompromised patients. In a review of all reported cases of fungal malignant otitis externa, 84% of patients had conditions causing immunocompromise, including diabetes, AIDS and acute myeloid leukaemia.[12] Forty-four per cent had an associated cranial nerve palsy. Amphotericin B is traditionally used as a treatment for fungal malignant otitis externa, although more recently voriconazole has become more popular, due to its more favourable side effect profile.[13]

MANAGEMENT

The treatment for otomycosis includes elimination of predisposing factors, thorough aural cleaning and antifungal agents. Topical antifungals can be specific (clotrimazole, miconazole, econazole, nystatin, tolnaftate, potassium sorbate) or non-specific (acetic acid, alcohol, boric acid, m-cresyl acetate, and gentian).[14]

Overall, there are four main classes of antifungal treatments: azoles, polyenes, nucleoside analogues and echinocandins. Azoles are synthetic agents that block the synthesis of ergosterol, an essential component of fungal plasma membranes. Clotrimazole is one of the most widely used azoles in otomycosis and is highly effective, with efficacy rates of between 95% and 100%.[15] Other azoles that are widely used include fluconazole, ketoconazole and miconazole. Polyenes, such as nystatin, are thought to interact with sterols in the fungal plasma membrane, causing pores to form within the membrane, thus causing altered permeability and fungal death.[16] Although nystatin is not available as an otic preparation it can be prepared as a solution or suspension, or applied as a cream, ointment or powder. Amphotericin B, another polyene antifungal agent, is used in severe, life-threatening infections, such as fungal malignant otitis externa. Nucleoside analogues, such as flucytosine, interfere with fungal DNA, RNA and protein synthesis. Flucytosine has a reported efficacy of 90% and is available as an ointment.

Other agents less commonly used include Gentian Violet, boric acid and cyclopiroxolamine. Boric acid is a keratolytic non-specific agent, more commonly used in countries with less availability of specific antifungal agents.

Fungal disease of the paranasal sinuses

Fungi can affect the paranasal sinuses through inhalation of spores. Fungi are ubiquitous within the environment, but can rarely cause disease within the paranasal sinuses, often but not always in the presence of predisposing factors. The spectrum of disease is largely dependent on the immunological competence of the host.

Fungal disease affecting the sinuses can be defined as acute or chronic (lasting over 4 weeks) or as invasive or non-invasive. Invasive fungal disease is defined as the presence of fungal hyphae within mucosa, submucosa, bone, blood vessels and nerves of the paranasal sinuses. Non-invasive fungal disease implies colonization of the surface of epithelial tissues, rather than invasion. Currently, fungal rhinosinusitis is classified into three invasive (acute necrotizing, chronic invasive, and granulomatous invasive) and two non-invasive (fungal ball and allergic fungal) subgroups (**Table 21.1**).

Acute invasive fungal rhinosinusitis (AIFR)

AIFR is a rare but rapidly progressive disease process that can result in fatality within days. It is the most lethal form of fungal sinusitis with mortality rates of at least 50%.[17] *Aspergillus* and *Zygomycetes* (particularly *Mucor* and *Rhizopus*) are the causative fungi in most cases. A high degree of clinical suspicion is required in order to correctly and promptly diagnose and manage this condition.

Following inhalation of spores, the fungi grow and invade neural and vascular structures, leading to vessel thrombosis and resultant mucosal necrosis. The fungi then extend beyond the affected sinus through a combination of bony destruction, perineural and perivascular spread.

PREDISPOSING FACTORS

Two main groups of patients are thought to be at risk of AIFR: diabetics, particularly with ketoacidosis, and patients who are immunocompromised (severe neutropenia, haematologic malignancy, systemic chemotherapy, steroid therapy, bone marrow transplantation, AIDS). Diabetic patients are particularly at risk from

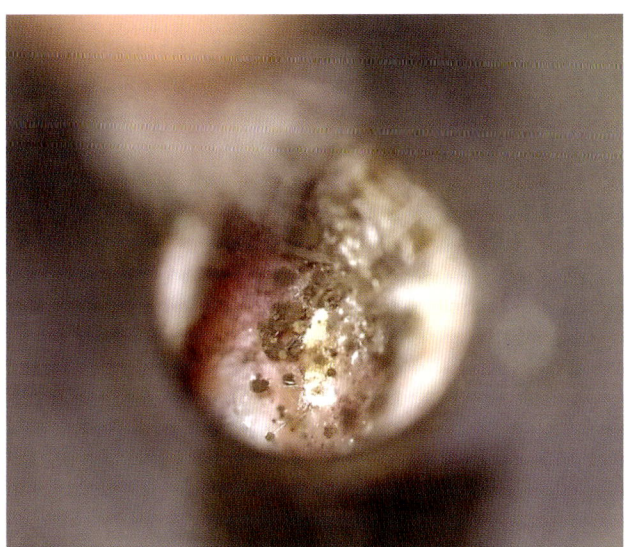

Figure 21.5 *Aspergillus niger* causing otitis externa.

TABLE 21.1 Definitions of fungal disease affecting the paranasal sinuses

	Non-invasive		Invasive		
	Fungal ball (mycetoma)	**Allergic fungal sinusitis**	**Acute invasive fungal; sinusitis**	**Chronic invasive fungal sinusitis**	**Chronic granulomatous invasive fungal sinusitis**
Pathogen	*Aspergillus* species; *Pseudallescheriaboydii*	Primarily dematiaceous species: *Bipolaris, Alternaria, Curvularia*; also *Aspergillus* species and multiple other moulds	Mucormycosis (Diabetics); *Aspergillus Fumigatus* (immunocompromised), *Candida* species, *Fusarium*	*Aspergillus flavum, A. fumigatus*	*Aspergillus flavum*
Immune status of host	Immunocompetent	Atopic	Immunocompromised	Immunocompetent or mildly immunocompromised	Immunocompetent
Geographical distribution	Humid area	Humid area	Non-specific	Non-specific	North Africa
Radiological findings	Hyperdense on CT, especially maxillary and sphenoid sinus	CT-heterogenous sinus opacification, bony remodelling +/− erosion MRI – signal void on T2 depending on metal concentration within mucin	CT-sinus opacification, bony erosion and tissue infiltration	CT-sinus opacification, bony erosion and tissue infiltration	CT-sinus opacification, bony erosion and tissue infiltration
Treatment	Surgical	Surgical + medical	Reversal of underlying Immunocompromise, surgical + antifungal therapy	Surgical + medical	Surgical + medical

Zygomycetes (*Rhizopus*, *Mucor*) as these organisms have an active ketone reductase system and thrive in high glucose acidotic conditions. *Aspergillus* species commonly affect immunosuppressed patients.[18] Iron-overload is also thought to be a predisposing factor, particularly after treatment with deferoxamine, an iron chelator, for iron overload due to multiple blood transfusions. *Rhizopus* binds to deferoxamine and uses it to bind iron, which it requires for growth.[19]

CLINICAL FEATURES

The clinical hallmark of AIFR is febrile neutropenia and facial pain with or without nasal congestion and orbital signs.

Symptoms and signs occur rapidly, often within hours, depending on the pattern of invasion into nearby structures. Nasal features include discolouration of nasal mucosa, granulation, ulceration and crusting. Later, spread to the orbit and intra-cranially can result in proptosis, diplopia, visual loss and neurological deficit. Infection can extend to the cavernous sinus via the orbital apex, causing palsies of cranial nerves III, IV and VI resulting in opthalmoplegia and orbital pain (ophthalmic division of trigeminal nerve). Orbital signs and symptoms are common presentations, occurring in around half of patients in a recent systematic review by Turner et al. examining survival outcomes in AIFR.[20] Thrombosis of the cavernous section of the carotid artery can extend to other branches at the circle of Willis. As a result once disease has spread to the cavernous sinus, cerebral or brainstem infarction is almost inevitable. Intra-cranial extension presents as headaches, neurological deficit, seizures and coma. Around a fifth of patients in Turner's systematic review presented with altered mental status.

Interestingly, patients can present with advanced AIFR with orbital and cerebral complications with few signs or symptoms of rhinosinusitis and nasoendoscopy may be essentially normal.[21] This reinforces the need to have a high degree of suspicion in patients with immunocompromise presenting with orbital or cerebral signs, with or without symptoms of sinus disease.

DIAGNOSIS

Changes in mucosal appearance and/or sensation (anaesthesia) are typical on endoscopic examination. In the early stages, the mucosa may appear pale. Necrosis resulting from angioinvasion results in black crusts and sloughing of the mucosal surface of the nose and septum; septal perforation may be present. Biopsies should be taken from multiple sites, particularly the middle turbinate and septum in order to confirm the diagnosis and the causal fungal organism. The gold standard of diagnosis is pathological examination of permanent sections, prepared in potassium hydroxide. This allows the identification of invasive features, and can often distinguish *Mucorales* from *Aspergillus* fungi. However, this process is time consuming and may delay the diagnosis and institution of treatment. Frozen section is a technique that is useful in order to provide rapid evidence of invasion, and has been found to have a sensitivity of 84% and a specificity of 100% for the diagnosis of AIFR compared to gold standard permanent sections.[22] Culture should also be undertaken in order to confirm the species of fungus responsible and sensitivity to antifungal agents, although culture has been found only to have a sensitivity of 54%.

Both CT and MRI are invaluable in the diagnosis of AIFR. CT allows detection of bony destruction while MRI is better at detecting mucosal, skin invasion, orbital or intra-cranial involvement. Non-contrast CT may show hypoattenuating mucosal thickening in the affected sinuses, bony erosion and/or thickening of periantral fat planes. MRI is superior at evaluating extra-sinus disease, such as intra-cerebral and intra-orbital spread. Early orbital changes include inflammatory changes in orbital fat and extra-ocular muscles and resulting proptosis. There may be subtle obliteration of periantral fat. Early changes in the cerebrum include leptomeningeal enhancement, which may preclude the development of frank abscesses or granulomas. There may be evidence of cerebral infarction or subarachnoid haemorrhage due to either thrombosis of the carotid artery and branches or mycotic aneurysm.[23]

MANAGEMENT

The mainstay of treatment is reversing the underlying immunosuppression (e.g. ketoacidosis or neutropenia) aggressive surgical debridement and broad spectrum antifungal therapy. Hyperglycaemia should be reversed and blood glucose levels should be tightly controlled. Reversal of neutropenia, if possible, improves survival, and there may be a role for granulocyte-colony stimulating factor in these patients.[18, 24]

Surgical treatment (endoscopic or open) aims to confirm the diagnosis and remove non-viable tissue. Debridement is carried out until clear, bleeding margins are observed. There is little evidence that radical resection, including orbital exenteration and radical maxillectomy, improves survival. In fact, in the systematic review carried out by Turner et al.,[20] patients who underwent endoscopic resection had significantly improved survival compared to those who underwent open surgery, although this may partly be due to the fact that patients undergoing open surgery had far more advanced disease. There is little consensus as to the role of orbital exenteration, although most agree that it should be reserved for those with a completely non-functioning eye.[25] A multidisciplinary approach utilizing ophthalmology, maxillofacial and neurosurgical expertise is paramount.

Broad-spectrum antifungal therapy should be started as soon as a diagnosis of AIFR is suspected. Fungal cultures are essential in determining sensitivity to anti-fungal agents. Amphotericin B is a polyene antifungal with activity against both *Mucorales* and *Aspergillus*. Amphotericin B deoxycholate is used as the mainstay of treatment prior to identification of the causal fungus, usually at doses of 1–1.5 mg/kg per day. However, the toxicity of amphotericin B has led to the development of safer lipid-formulations of the drugs such as amphotericin B lipid complex and liposomal amphotericin B. These formulations are less nephrotoxic and can be used at higher concentrations for longer. Liposomal amphotericin B is used at doses of 5–10 mg/kg per day, and although expensive is safer and may be more effective than amphotericin B deoxycholate, particularly in cancer patients with mucormycosis.[26]

Once mucormycosis is ruled out, treatment may be changed to a less toxic azole that is more effective against *Aspergillus* but has less reliable activity against mucormycosis. A randomized unblinded trial showed that voriconazole led to improved survival and fewer side effects in patients with invasive aspergillosis compared to amphotericin B.[27] Voriconazole is used at an initial dose of 6 mg/kg iv for two doses, followed by 4 mg/kg iv every 12 hours. It is now recommended as first line treatment for invasive aspergillosis of the sinuses by the Infectious Disease Society of America. An alternative azole, posaconazole may be used as a step-down to oral treatment when clinical improvement is seen, to enable long-term treatment.

Hyperbaric oxygen therapy (HBOT) has been proposed an adjunct to treatment of AIFR.[28] HBOT acts directly via increased production of oxygen-based free radicals and indirectly by reversing growth-promoting lactic acidosis and restoration of phagocytosis.[29] To date there is no clear evidence of the efficacy of HBOT in the treatment of AIFR.

PROGNOSIS

In the recent systematic review by Turner et al.,[20] diabetic patients were found to have better prognosis, despite often more aggressive disease, possibly due to the fact that their underlying condition was more easily reversed than other conditions. Patients who have intra-cranial involvement, or who do not receive surgery as part of their therapy, have a poor prognosis.

Chronic invasive fungal rhinosinusitis

Chronic invasive fungal rhinosinusitis (CIFR) has a similar clinical appearance to AIFS but a slower progressive course, occurring over months to years. It also tends to occur in immunocompetent individuals.

Aspergillus spp. (*flavus* or *fumigatus*) or *Mucor* spp. are the most common causative organisms.[30] In the initial stages of disease symptoms may be subtle and non-specific and include unilateral bloody nasal discharge, nasal obstruction, headache, cacosmia and purulent nasal discharge. Patients may present with advanced disease with proptosis, orbital apex syndrome and cranial nerve deficits reflecting invasion into the orbit. Destruction of the bony walls of the maxillary sinus causes palatal erosion and soft tissue swelling of the cheek. Disease invading into the cribriform plate and anterior cranial fossa may cause chronic headache, seizures and focal neurological deficit.

DIAGNOSIS

CT imaging may mimic the features of malignancy, which is the primary differential in most cases. CT shows a hyperattenuating mass in one or more of the sinuses with destruction of the sinus bony walls. MRI typically shows decreased signal intensity on both T1- and T2-weighted images.[23] Invasion into anterior cranial fossa may result in meningitis seen as meningeal enhancement on contrast enhanced MRI. Cavernous sinus thrombosis typically results in a swollen non-enhancing sinus with compression of the carotid artery on coronal post-contrast T1-weighted MRI.

Biopsies should be obtained to assess for mucosal invasion. Microsopically, there are few inflammatory cells (unlike AIFS) and CIFS lacks granulomas often witnessed in granulomatous invasive fungal sinusitis.

MANAGEMENT

The treatment of CIFS is similar to AIFS, that is, a combination of surgical and antifungal treatments. Surgical resection should be carried out until clear, bleeding margins are observed. Systemic and topical amphotericin B should be started until cultures exclude *Mucor* species. Amphotericin B has proven efficacy against invasive Aspergillosis, although its side effect profile may limit the length of treatment and the optimal dose.[27] Whilst newer lipid-formulations are safer they are also more expensive and can only be given in the intravenous route. Azole drugs such as voriconazole and itraconazole are promising alternatives as they are effective via the oral route and are therefore easier and cheaper to administer for longer term treatment but are less effective against *Mucor* spp. A prospective randomized unblinded study compared amphotericin B (conventional or liposomal) and itraconazole in the management of CIFR and found that both were equally efficacious.[31]

Chronic granulomatous invasive fungal sinusitis

Chronic granulomatous invasive fungal sinusitis is distinguished from CIFS by the geographical distribution of the disease, type of pathogen and microscopic findings. It is rarely seen in the West and is more common in North Africa, the Middle East and Asia. *Aspergillus flavus* is the most common causative fungi. It is defined by the presence of non-caseating granulomas with Langhan's type giant cells and fungal hyphae, although it may coexist with other types of fungal sinusitis.[32] Similar to CIFR, it follows an indolent cause and may be found in both immunocompetent and immunodeficient patients.

It is treated by surgery (resection of involved tissues to bleeding margins) followed by antifungals. Antifungals like voriconazole instead of amphoteracin may be used as the disease is caused by *Aspergillus flavus*. Rupa et al.[32] recommend post-operative treatment with either oral itraconazole or voriconazole for disease with limited extension and oral voriconazole for advanced disease extending to the brain. Amphotericin B was not recommended as first-line therapy for CGFS.

Allergic fungal rhinosinusitis

Allergic fungal rhinosinusitis (AFRS) is a non-invasive fungal disease, first reported by Safirstein[33] in 1976 in a patient with allergic bronchopulmonary aspergillosis (ABPA). This condition shares similar histopathologic features with ABPA. Unlike other forms of sinusitis, it has distinct clinical, histopathological and prognostic findings. Debate concerning the underlying pathogenesis and optimal treatment strategy is ongoing.

AFRS is more common in younger individuals (mean age 21–33 years) compared to CRS. It is also more frequent in warm, humid environments and lower socio-economic status.[34] Atopic individuals tend to suffer from AFRS.

DIAGNOSTIC CRITERIA

Allergic fungal rhinosinusitis is often misdiagnosed, and there are many controversies surrounding its diagnosis and even its very existence. However, most experts use Bent and Kuhn criteria[35] for diagnosis (Table 21.2). These consist of both major and minor criteria, and all five major criteria must be met in order for a diagnosis to be made. The presence of minor criteria supports the diagnosis of AFR.

De Shazo et al.[36] proposed a slightly revised set of criteria, reflecting the controversy surrounding the role of atopy in AFRS, and suggested the following: (1) sinusitis confirmed on CT scanning; (2) the presence of allergic mucin; (3) demonstration of fungal hyphae within the allergic mucin; (4) the absence of fungal invasion; and (5) the absence of diabetes or immunodeficiency states. In 2004 a panel of experts redefined AFRS as 'histological confirmation of eosinophilic mucin and the presence of type 1 hypersensitivity to fungi in CRS patients'.[37]

PATHOGENESIS

The pathogenesis of AFRS is not completely understood and subject to controversy. The most common pathogens in AFRS are the dematiaceous species (*Curvularia, Bipolaris, Alternaria*). Due to the histopathological similarity of AFRS to ABPA, a common pathophysiological mechanism was attributed. In ABPA, both elevated IgE and IgG to either *Aspergillus fumigatus* or *A. flavus* are present. Both Type I (specific IgE antibody-antigen interaction) and Type III (IgG antibody-antigen complex) reactions have been postulated in the pathogenesis of ABPA. The immune pathogenesis of AFRS is supported

TABLE 21.2 Bent and Kuhn diagnostic criteria

Major	Minor criteria
Type I hypersensitivity (history, skin test or *in vitro* testing)	Asthma
Nasal polyposis	Unilateral disease
Characteristic CT findings	Radiological bone erosion
Eosinophilic mucin without invasion	Fungal cultures
Positive fungal stain	Serum eosinophilia
	Charcot-Leyden crystals

by Manning and Holman;[38] eight AFRS patients with culture-positive Bipolaris showed skin test positivity to Bipolaris as well as RAST IgE to Bipolaris and ELISA IgG antibodies for Bipolaris. In contrast, only 1 in 10 controls had a positive skin test for Bipolaris, as well as IgE and IgG antibodies to Bipolaris. On examination of mucosal specimens from AFRS patients, eosinophilic mediators predominated over neutrophil-derived mediators compared to control patients with unrecognized AFS.

In AFRS, a Type I (and possibly Type III hypersensitivity reaction) to inhaled airborne fungi is believed to result in tissue inflammation, oedema and production of an 'eosinophilic mucin'. This consists of eosinophilic inflammator cells and Charcot-Leyden crystals (breakdown of cells by eosinophilic enzymes).

Interestingly, some patients with a clinical picture of AFRS did not display signs of systemic allergy. Collins et al[39] proposed a theory that AFRS is the result of a local Type I hypersensitivity rather than a systemic response. His study demonstrated fungal-specific IgE in sinus mucin in AFRS patients and may explain why the response was confined to the nose and paranasal sinuses without systemic involvement.

However, controversy exists about whether a Type 1 sensitivity reaction is central to the pathogenesis of AFRS. Ponikau et al.[40] prospectively studied 210 patients with CRS, with or without nasal polyps, and used rigorous methods to collect and culture fungus from nasal mucin. Cultures were positive for fungus in a surprising 96% of patients with CRS. Furthermore, all healthy control patients, with no history of sinonasal disease, had fungal-positive cultures, suggesting that fungi are ubiquitous within the sinuses and nasal passages. When using deShazo's criteria for a diagnosis of AFRS, 93% of CRS patients undergoing surgery (thereby providing samples for histological examination), had AFRS. Of patients diagnosed with AFRS, less than a third had elevated fungus specific IgE level by RAST. Ponikau's study has been criticized for a number of reasons. Furthermore, Ponikau states that 'allergic mucin' (required for a diagnosis of AFRS) was found in the vast majority of patients with CRS, whilst multiple studies have estimated the prevalence of allergic mucin to be much lower in patients requiring surgery for CRS.[41] AFRS is usually associated with the production of copious amounts of allergic mucin, whereas the patients in Ponikau's study often only produced small pockets of mucin.

There is strong evidence that patients with 'simple' CRS show abnormal immunological responses to fungal elements within the nose and sinuses. Shin et al.[42] demonstrated that patients with simple CRS showed exaggerated humoral and cellular responses to commonly found airborne fungi compared to healthy controls. However, it is important to recognize that whilst fungal allergy may play a role in the pathogenesis of simple CRS, AFRS is a distinct entity with very strict criteria for diagnosis, and more is needed for diagnosis over and above merely the existence of allergy to fungal elements in a patient with sinusitis.

CLINICAL FEATURES

Typically patients presenting with AFRS are young, immunocompetent individuals, with a history of atopy or asthma. They present often with unilateral, but sometimes bilateral, symptoms of nasal congestion, post-nasal drip, and a thick dark nasal discharge. There is often a history of recurrent symptoms following previous treatment or surgery and typically patients show an excellent response to oral corticosteroids, but not antibiotics. Patients may also present with signs and symptoms of bony erosion and involvement of the orbit, including proptosis and telecanthus.

On examination, there is usually gross nasal polyposis with thick, highly viscous mucin, classically described as the consistency of peanut butter. Green or black casts consisting of allergic mucin may be present. Microscopic examination of the fungal mucin with haematoxylin and eosin (H&E) staining typically shows the presence of Charcot-Leyden crystals and eosinophilic breakdown products, and often the eosinophils themselves form sheets. Fungi do not stain with H&E staining, but can be seen on special stains. Culture of the mucin may or may not be positive for fungus; however, this does not rule out AFRS as the yield of culture is typically fairly low. The fungi most commonly identified in the eosinophilic mucin include *Alternaria*, *Bipolaris*, *Cladosporium*, *Curvularia*, *Drechslera* and *Helminthosporium* from the dematiaceous family and *Aspergillus* species.[43]

IMAGING

CT imaging typically shows characteristic pansinusitis, hyperattenuation of the intrasinus contents (representing thick allergic mucin) surrounded by lower attenuation hyperplastic mucosa. The 'double density' sign may be seen in affected sinuses (i.e. heterogeneous signal intensity due to the deposition of heavy metals within the mucin) (**Figure 21.6**). The affected sinus is often expanded and there may be erosion of the sinus walls (**Figure 21.7**). This erosion is not due to invasion by fungal elements, but due to local inflammation and the expansive nature of mucin, which differentiates it from invasive fungal sinusitis.[44] MRI, if interpreted in the absence of CT, can be misleading; on T2-weighted images, the high metal concentration within proteinaceous allergic fungal mucin may show up as a signal void, mimicking the appearance of a normally aerated sinus. On T1-weighted images the material is hypointense to isointense.[23] Both T1- and T2-weighted images shows peripheral enhancement (**Figure 21.8**).

MANAGEMENT

The mainstay of AFRS treatment remains surgery although adjunctive medical management is critical for optimal outcomes. The aim of functional endoscopic sinus surgery (FESS) is to remove all antigenic fungal elements, and to re-establish drainage of the affected sinuses. During the endoscopic procedure, all specimens including polyps and allergic mucin should be sent for microscopic examination

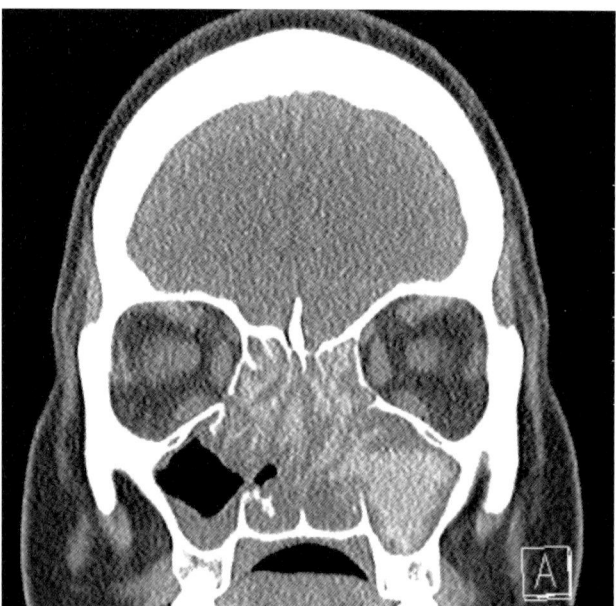

Figure 21.6 Coronal CT sinus showing classic 'double density' sign seen in AFRS.

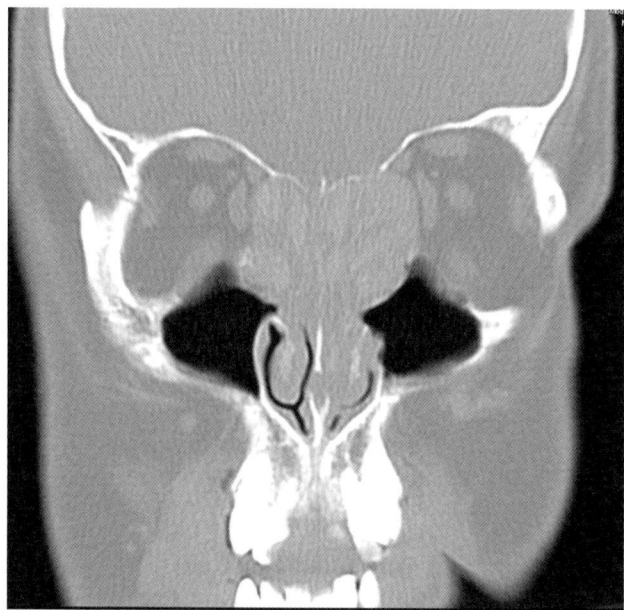

Figure 21.7 Coronal CT sinus demonstrating erosion of lamina papyracea and skull base.

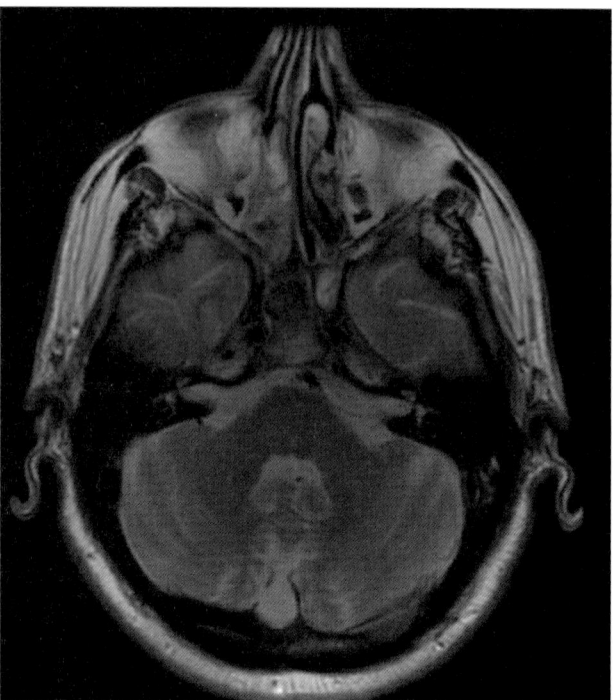
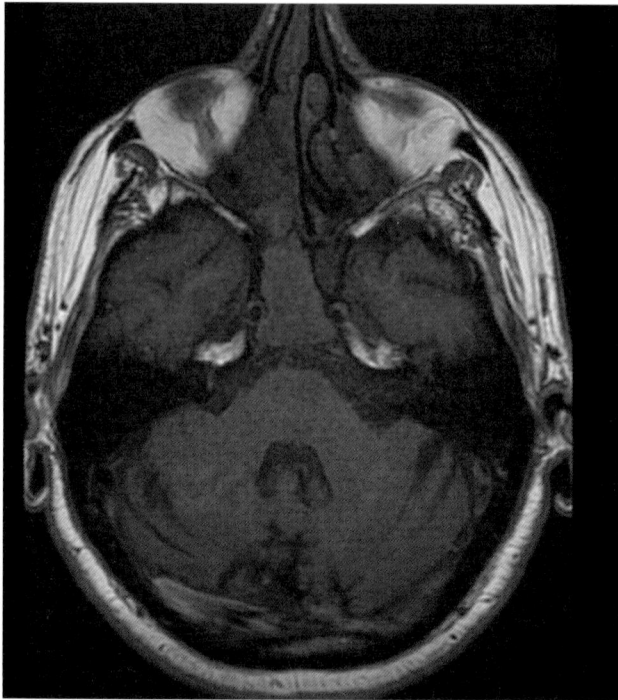

Figure 21.8 Axial MRI sinus showing near signal void in sphenoid sinus on T2-weighted (left) compared to T1-weighted images (right).

and staining for fungi, and all should be sent for culture. In particular, invasion of vasculature or mucosa should be excluded.

In 2014 Gan et al.[45] published an evidence-based approach for the post-operative medical management of AFRS. The review concluded that post-operative systemic and standard topical nasal steroids are recommended; oral antifungals, and immunotherapy are options in cases of refractory AFRS; and did not provide recommendations for topical antifungals and leukotriene modulators due to lack of evidence. Recently, AFRS which is refractory to surgery and conventional medical treatment has been shown to be responsive to anti-IgE antibody, omalizumab.[46]

Oral steroids

Gan et al.[45] recommend the use of oral steroids in the post-operative period, using grade B evidence from four studies (level 2b: 2 studies, level 4: 2 studies), and report a reduction in post-operative mucosal disease and inflammatory markers. The four studies included a total of 76 patients fulfilling the Bent and Kuhn criteria for AFRS, although two were case series lacking comparison with control. In 2010, Rupa et al.[47] published a prospective, randomized, placebo-controlled trial of post-operative oral steroids in AFRS comparing the use of oral prednisolone (n = 12) and placebo (n = 12). They concluded that post-operative oral steroid in a tapering dose produces significant subjective and objective improvement of patients with AFRS.

Topical nasal steroids

Topical nasal steroids achieve effective drug concentration at the sinonasal mucosa with few systemic side effects. There is little evidence for the use of topical steroids post-operatively in AFRS. A randomized controlled trial examined the use of post-operative topical nasal steroids and nasal douching in patients with AFRS compared with nasal douching alone, and nasal douching plus itraconazole. This study showed no significant benefit at 6 months for topical nasal steroids, although there were limitations to the study.[48]

Oral antifungals

The use of oral antifungals in AFRS should theoretically reduce fungal sinus load and therefore reduce the type 1 hypersensitivity reaction. However, there are numerous side effects associated with oral antifungals, and therefore they should be used with caution. Three level 4 studies (all case series) were included in Gan's review[45] and their use was restricted to patients with a poor post-operative response to oral or topical steroids. These studies show a reduction in symptoms, prevention of disease recurrence and reduced dependence on oral steroids (level C evidence). Itraconazole was used at a dose of 200 mg to 400 mg daily in divided doses for up to 6 months.

Topical antifungals

Topical antifungals may be used to reduce the risk of side effects associated with oral antifungals. However, to date there is no high quality evidence regarding the use of topical antifungals in AFRS.

Immunotherapy

There is level C evidence (two case-control studies and three prospective case series) that allergen immunotherapy shows improvement with reduced reliance of post-operative steroids, post-operative exacerbations and revision surgery.[45] Double-blind placebo controlled trials are lacking, and therefore conclusive evidence of efficacy is not yet available.

Bassichis et al.[49] studied a database of 82 patients and compared patients with AFRS who had been treated with post-operative immunotherapy against those who had not (36 versus 24 patients). They found a re-operation rate of 33% in those who did not receive immunotherapy compared to 11.1% in those who did. Folker et al.[50] published a case-control study comparing 11 patients who received IT for at least 12 months with those who did not and found improvements in mucosal endoscopic staging, quality of life and reliance on oral and systemic steroids. It is less clear if immunotherapy leads to significant reduction in recurrence of disease in the long term.[51]

To date, there remains no evidence of unusual side effects or immune complex formation in AFRS patients receiving immunotherapy.

Leukotriene modulators

To date there is no evidence that leukotriene modulators, such as montelukast, have a role in the treatment of AFRS. Only one case study has reported a benefit from using 10 mg oral montelukast in a patient with recalcitrant AFRS, with recurrent symptoms following three previous attempts at sinus surgery.[52]

Fungal ball

A fungal ball consists of sequestered fungal hyphal elements within a sinus without invasive or granulomatous changes. It is distinct from saprophytic fungal infestation, which corresponds to fungal spores found on crusts and mucus in the nose. Fungal balls are typically found in immunocompetent individuals and may coexist with other forms of fungal sinusitis.

DEFINITION

DeShazo[53] developed a clear definition for the diagnosis of fungal ball of the paranasal sinuses. A dense mass of hyphae is found in the affected sinus, which separates easily from the sinus mucosa, and macroscopically resembles a clay-like or cheesy material. Microscopically there is no evidence of invasion of the mucosa, vessels or bone. There are typical radiological changes (see below) and non-specific inflammatory changes of the mucosa, with no predominance of eosinophils, no granuloma and no allergic mucin.

PREDISPOSING FACTORS

There is little evidence that the presence of pre-existing medical conditions predispose to fungal balls, and furthermore, no evidence that pre-existing sinus disease or anatomical abnormalities does so either. An association between previous dental treatment, particularly fillings, and fungal balls has been suggested with reports showing that between 56% and 84% of patients found to have fungal balls have had previous dental treatment.[54]

PATHOGENESIS

Two theories as to the pathogenesis of fungal balls have been proposed. The first proposes that a large amount of inhaled fungal spores enter the sinuses through the natural ostium (the aerogenic pathway). The second suggests that fungal colonization of the sinuses occurs via an iatrogenic pathway when an oro-antral fistula is created during endodontic treatment with overfilling of the dental canal. Commonly used endodontic sealers may promote the growth of fungus, as demonstrated by experimental work, which showed that zinc oxide found in sealers promotes the growth of *Aspergillus*, whereas the second component, a liquid called eugenol, may inhibit its growth. Over time, however, the inhibitory effect of eugenol fades, allowing the promotion of fungal growth many years after the initial dental treatment. This would explain why the maxillary sinus is the most commonly affected sinus, and why many patients with fungal balls have a history of previous endodontic treatment.

CLINICAL FEATURES

Fungal balls most often affect one sinus, most commonly the maxillary sinus (94%), followed by the sphenoid sinus. Symptoms are non-specific, and the patient may be completely asymptomatic, hence the reason why patients are often diagnosed late. Other symptoms include headache or facial pain, post-nasal drip and cacosmia. Fungal balls affecting the sphenoid sinus may present with retro-orbital pain at the vertex. Symptoms may be recurrent, coinciding with superimposed bacterial sinus infection, with relatively symptom-free periods between episodes.

Examination findings may be unremarkable, but careful examination with a flexible or rigid endoscope may reveal localized inflammatory changes at the natural ostium of the affected sinus, including the presence of small polyps or purulent mucopus (**Figure 21.9**).

Macroscopically the fungal ball consists of cheesy like material, which is green, yellow, brown or black. The underlying mucosa may be normal or hypertrophic. Microscopically at low power the ball is seen to consist of densely packed hyphae, and may have an onion-skin-like appearance, due to the alternating zones of dense and less-dense growth. The mucosa may show non-specific inflammation, but in particular there is an absence of invasion by fungal elements, or granulomatous reaction.

Aspergillus is the most commonly identified fungus in fungal balls, and can often be seen on haematoxylin-eosin slides. However, all samples, including mucosa and fungal samples should be stained with silver impregnation stains in order to identify the presence of fungi. Whilst stains may be able to identify their presence, only culture will confirm the species of fungus. However, culture typically has a low yield of up to 50%.[54]

IMAGING

CT scanning is the imaging of choice for suspected fungal balls. Five CT features are commonly found on CT imaging of fungal balls, including a heterogenous soft tissue density in a single unilateral sinus, absence of an air-fluid level, erosion of the inner wall of the sinus, sclerosis of the lateral sinus wall and the presence of calcification. In particular, the presence of erosion of the inner wall of the sinus and the presence of calcification have a positive predictive value in the diagnosis of fungal balls of 94.6% and 93.2% respectively.[55] The presence of calcification is thought to be due to the deposition of calcium salts within the fungal ball.

MRI scanning is not usually necessary, but may be used as an adjunct to CT imaging to differentiate mucosal swelling or mucous retention from a fungal ball. On T2-weighted MR imaging fungal balls are often hypointense compared to mucous or mucosal swelling, which is hyperintense.

MANAGEMENT

The treatment of fungal balls is surgical with no adjunctive medical treatment usually necessary. Functional endoscopic sinus surgery (FESS) is employed to create a wide opening of the affecting sinus ostium. All fungal material should be removed, and biopsies taken from the underlying mucosa to rule out invasion. Any dental filling material present in the sinus should also be removed. In immunocompetent patients there is no role for the use of systemic antifungal agents.

Oropharyngeal candidiasis

Fungal infection of the oral cavity and pharynx is most often caused by fungi belonging to the genus *Candida* (*Candidiasis*). There are three subtypes of oropharyngeal candidiasis (OPC) that are recognized: pseudomembranous, atrophic and hyperplastic candidiasis. Whilst candidiasis of the oral cavity is not uncommon, and is in most cases easily treated, in this section we consider oropharyngeal candidiasis in two populations: patients with HIV and head and neck cancer patients.

OROPHARYNGEAL CANDIDIASIS IN HIV PATIENTS

Candida albicans is found as part of the normal skin, genitourinary and gastrointestinal microflora, and may be isolated in up to 65% of healthy individuals. Prior to the development of antiretroviral therapy (ART) for treatment of HIV, OPC was seen in up to 90% of patients with

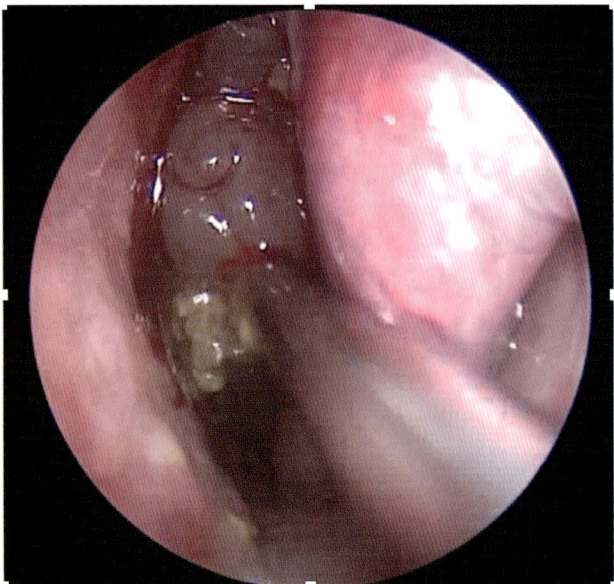

Figure 21.9 Endoscopic findings of AFRS showing nasal polyposis and thick mucinous secretions.

HIV, reflecting their underlying immunosuppression.[56] Since the introduction of ART, the incidence of OPC has declined, although it remains a problem for patients with limited access to ART, those with a poor response to ART and those with infections resistant to conventional antifungal treatment. In one study of 122 patients with advanced HIV, 81% were colonized by oral candida, and of these 33% had symptomatic infection.[56] *Candida albicans* was the most common candida species isolated in 54% of samples, with *C. dublinensis* and *C. glabrata* next most common. Rarer species of *Candida* may often be resistant to fluconazole and are important causes of recalcitrant oropharyngeal candidiasis.

HIV patients are at greater risk of OPC once their immunity drops to a certain level, normally taken to be an absolute CD4+ T-lymphocyte count of less than 200 cells/µL. Viral load is also found to be a contributing factor for the development of OPC, and the risk of OPC increases as HIV viral load surpasses 10,000 copies/mL.

Pseudomembranous candidiasis is the most common subtype of OPC in HIV patients. Painless, often asymptomatic plaques appear on the tongue, buccal mucosa and oropharynx, and can typically be wiped away leaving an erythematous base, which may bleed (**Figure 21.10**). Patients may complain of altered taste or pain if ulceration occurs. Distal spread to the larynx or oesophagus causes dysphonia, odynophagia and dysphagia. Erythematous OPC may also be seen in the HIV patient and clinically appears as flat, red lesions anywhere in the oral cavity, but often the dorsal tongue or palate. Hyperplastic candidiasis presents as firm, white plaques of varying sizes, which, in contrast to pseudomembranous OPC cannot be removed. These are important lesions to recognize as whilst they are rare in all populations, they have malignant potential.

Mild disease can be treated with topical nystatin suspensions, whilst more severe disease will require a 14-day course of fluconazole 200mg daily.[57] However, there is increasing recognition of *Candida* species that are resistant to fluconazole, estimated to cause up to 5% of OPC. A multicentre randomized trial evaluating posaconazole as an alternative to fluconazole has shown posaconazole to be as effective and even better at sustaining clinical remission and is an alternative for fluconazole-resistant disease. Posaconazole suspension is given at a dosage of 400mg twice daily for 3 days, followed by 400mg daily for up to 28 days. Other alternatives include voriconazole, itraconazole or amphotericin B oral suspension. Refractory candidiasis may require parenteral treatment with amphotericin B or caspofungin.[57]

OROPHARYNGEAL CANDIDIASIS IN HEAD AND NECK CANCER PATIENTS

Pseudomembranous and erythematous OPC are the most common variants of candidiasis in head and neck cancer patients.[58] The prevalence of OPC in patients receiving either radiotherapy or chemotherapy for head and neck cancer is approximately 38%.[58] *Candida albicans* is the most frequent species isolated, but other species are recognized including *C. tropicalis* and *C. glabrata*. The increased risk of OPC in these populations is likely related to salivary hypofunction. Amisfostine, an agent that acts to preserve salivary gland function, has been shown to reduce the risk of clinical OPC in patients receiving radiotherapy.[59] OPC in cancer patients is important to treat and recognize early as maintenance of oral intake and nutritional status is vital in patients receiving chemotherapy and radiotherapy. In addition, patients receiving such treatment are vulnerable to systemic dissemination of fungal infection via lesions associated with oral mucositis; this can be fatal. Non-albicans species are more likely to spread into the systemic circulation.

Treatment of OPC in head and neck patients is similar to the treatment of OPC in other populations; however, topical treatment may be uncomfortable in patients with significant mucositis. Oral fluconazole is the recommended first-line treatment for moderate or severe OPC. The use of fluconazole as a prophylactic measure should be used with caution, in view of the emergence of fluconazole resistant strains of OPC and should be restricted to frequent and disabling infection.

Laryngectomy patients with silicone trachea-oesophageal voice prostheses may develop the formation of *Candida* biofilms, which can invade the silicone, causing deterioration of the valve. Valves deteriorate fairly rapidly after placement and normally need replacing after between 3 and 5 months. The main reason for replacement is leakage of fluid into the trachea via an incompetent valve, which is thought to be related to biofilm formation. In 100 Provox2 voice prostheses that were analysed following removal due to leakage of fluid, the most common isolate from the biofilm was *Candida albicans* (53% of isolated fungi), followed by *C. krusei* and *C. tropicalis*.[60] Eighty three per cent of the valves were found to have biofilms of fungi and bacteria. A promising area has been the development of a nontoxic deoxyribonuclease that has been shown to be effective *in vitro* at dispersing biofilms from discarded voice prostheses contaminated with mixed biofilms.

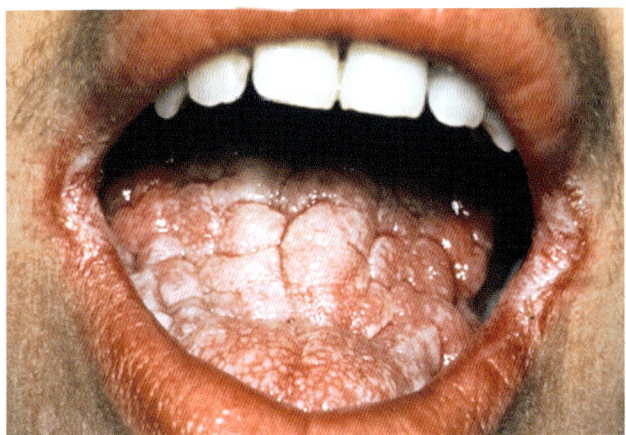

Figure 21.10 Chronic oral candidiasis of the tongue and mouth corners (angular chelitis) in an adult with an underlying immune deficiency. Courtesy of http://www.mycology.adelaide.edu.au/gallery/yeast-like_fungi/

KEY POINTS

- Fungi exist in nature as yeasts or branching moulds; of the thousands of fungi present naturally in the environment, only around 30 species are commonly associated with human disease.
- Fungal infection within the ear canal results in otomycosis, most commonly caused by *Aspergillus niger* and *Candida albicans*. Rarely, in immunocompromised hosts, fungal otomycosis can result in malignant otitis externa.
- Fungal infection affecting the sinuses can be divided into five main groups: acute invasive fungal sinusitis, chronic invasive fungal sinusitis, chronic granulomatous invasive fungal sinusitis, allergic fungal sinusitis and fungal ball.
- Oropharyngeal candidiasis can be a significant issue in patients with immunocompromise, particularly patients receiving treatment for HIV or head and neck cancer.

REFERENCES

1. Larone DH. *Medically important fungi: a guide to identification*. ASM Press: 2011.
2. Ellis DH, Davis S, Alexiou H, et al. *Descriptions of medical fungi*. Adelaide Medical Centre for Women & Children: 2007.
3. Rippon J. *Medical mycology: the pathogenic fungi and the pathogenic actinomycetes*. Philadelphia: Saunders 1988.
4. Neofytos D, Horn D, Anaissie E, et al. Epidemiology and outcome of invasive fungal infection in adult hematopoietic stem cell transplant recipients: analysis of Multicenter Prospective Antifungal Therapy (PATH) Alliance registry. *Clin Infect Dis Off Publ Infect Dis Soc Am* 2009; **48**: 265–73.
5. Roden MM, Zaoutis TE, Buchanan WL, et al. Epidemiology and outcome of zygomycosis: a review of 929 reported cases. *Clin Infect Dis Off Publ Infect Dis Soc Am* 2005; **41**: 634–53.
6. Abdelazeem M, Gamea A, Mubarak H, Elzawawy N. Epidemiology, causative agents, and risk factors affecting human otomycosis infections. *Turk J Med Sci* 2015; **45**: 820–26.
7. Isa-Isa R, Arenas R, Fernández RF, Isa M. Rhinofacial conidiobolomycosis (entomophthoramycosis). *Clin Dermatol* 2012; **30**: 409–12.
8. Mugliston T, O'Donoghue G. Otomycosis: a continuing problem. *J Laryngol Otol* 1985; **99**: 327–33.
9. Kurnatowski P, Filipiak A. Otomycosis: prevalence, clinical symptoms, therapeutic procedure. *Mycoses* 2001; **44**: 472–79.
10. Jia X, Liang Q, Chi F, Cao W. Otomycosis in Shanghai: aetiology, clinical features and therapy. *Mycoses* 2012; **55**: 404–09.
11. Paulose KO, Al Khalifa S, Shenoy P, Sharma RK. Mycotic infection of the ear (otomycosis): a prospective study. *J Laryngol Otol* 1989; **103**: 30–35.
12. Walton J, Coulson C. Fungal malignant otitis externa with facial nerve palsy: tissue biopsy AIDS diagnosis. *Case Rep Otolaryngol* **2014**: 192318.
13. Tarazi AE, Al-Tawfiq JA, Abdi RF. Fungal malignant otitis externa: pitfalls, diagnosis, and treatment. *Otol Neurotol Off Publ Am Otol Soc Am Neurotol Soc Eur Acad Otol Neurotol* 2012; **33**: 769–73.
14. Khan F, Muhammad R, Khan MR, et al. Efficacy of topical clotrimazole in treatment of otomycosis. *J Ayub Med Coll Abbottabad JAMC* 2013; **25**: 78–80.
15. Munguia R, Daniel SJ. Ototopical antifungals and otomycosis: a review. *Int J Pediatr Otorhinolaryngol* 2008; **72**: 453–59.
16. Ghannoum MA, Rice LB. Antifungal agents: mode of action, mechanisms of resistance, and correlation of these mechanisms with bacterial resistance. *Clin Microbiol Rev* 1999; **12**: 501–17.
17. Waitzman AA, Birt BD. Fungal sinusitis. *J Otolaryngol* 1994; **23**: 244–49.
18. Gillespie MB, O'Malley BW, Francis HW. An approach to fulminant invasive fungal rhinosinusitis in the immunocompromised host. *Arch Otolaryngol Head Neck Surg* 1998; **124**: 520–26.
19. Larcher G, Dias M, Razafimandimby B, et al. Siderophore production by pathogenic mucorales and uptake of deferoxamine B. *Mycopathologia* 2013; **176**: 319–28.
20. Turner JH, Soudry E, Nayak JV, Hwang PH. Survival outcomes in acute invasive fungal sinusitis: a systematic review and quantitative synthesis of published evidence. *Laryngoscope* 2013; **123**: 1112–18.
21. Thurtell MJ, Chiu ALS, Goold LA, et al. Neuro-ophthalmology of invasive fungal sinusitis: 14 consecutive patients and a review of the literature. *Clin Experiment Ophthalmol* 2013; **41**: 567–76.
22. Ghadiali MT, Deckard NA, Farooq U, et al. Frozen-section biopsy analysis for acute invasive fungal rhinosinusitis. *Otolaryngol Head Neck Surg* 2007; **136**: 714–19.
23. Aribandi M, McCoy VA, Bazan C. Imaging features of invasive and noninvasive fungal sinusitis: a review. *Radiogr Rev Publ Radiol Soc N Am Inc* 2007; **27**: 1283–96.
24. Abzug MJ, Walsh TJ. Interferon-gamma and colony-stimulating factors as adjuvant therapy for refractory fungal infections in children. *Pediatr Infect Dis J* 2004; **23**: 769–73.
25. Zuniga MG, Turner JH. Treatment outcomes in acute invasive fungal rhinosinusitis. *Curr Opin Otolaryngol Head Neck Surg* 2014; **22**: 242–48.
26. Spellberg B, Walsh TJ, Kontoyiannis DP, et al. Recent advances in the management of mucormycosis: from bench to bedside. *Clin Infect Dis Off Publ Infect Dis Soc Am* 2009; **48**: 1743–51.
27. Herbrecht R, Denning DW, Patterson TF, et al. Voriconazole versus amphotericin B for primary therapy of invasive aspergillosis. *N Engl J Med* 2002; **347**: 408–15.
28. Kajs-Wyllie M. Hyperbaric oxygen therapy for rhinocerebral fungal infection. *J Neurosci Nurs J Am Assoc Neurosci Nurses* 1995; **27**: 174–81.
29. Tragiannidis A, Groll AH. Hyperbaric oxygen therapy and other adjunctive treatments for zygomycosis. *Clin Microbiol Infect Off Publ Eur Soc Clin Microbiol Infect Dis* 2009; **15**(Suppl 5): 82–86.
30. Li Y, Li Y, Li P, Zhang G. Diagnosis and endoscopic surgery of chronic invasive fungal rhinosinusitis. *Am J Rhinol Allergy* 2009; **23**: 622–25.
31. Mehta R, Panda NK, Mohindra S, et al. Comparison of efficacy of amphotericin B and itraconazole in chronic invasive fungal sinusitis. *Indian J Otolaryngol Head Neck Surg* 2013; **65**: 288–94.
32. Rupa V, Maheswaran S, Ebenezer J, Mathews SS. Current therapeutic protocols for chronic granulomatous fungal sinusitis. *Rhinology* 2015; **53**: 181–86.
33. Safirstein BH. Allergic bronchopulmonary aspergillosis with obstruction of the upper respiratory tract. *Chest* 1976; **70**: 788–90.
34. Wise SK, Ghegan MD, Gorham E, Schlosser RJ. Socioeconomic factors in the diagnosis of allergic fungal rhinosinusitis. *Otolaryngol Head Neck Surg* 2008; **138**: 38–42.
35. Bent JP, Kuhn FA. Diagnosis of allergic fungal sinusitis. *Otolaryngol Head Neck Surg* 1994; **111**: 580–88.
36. deShazo RD, Swain RE. Diagnostic criteria for allergic fungal sinusitis. *J Allergy Clin Immunol* 1995; **96**: 24–35.
37. Meltzer EO, Hamilos DL, Hadley JA, et al. Rhinosinusitis: establishing definitions for clinical research and patient care. *Otolaryngol Head Neck Surg* 2004; **131**(6 Suppl): S1–62.
38. Manning SC, Holman M. Further evidence for allergic pathophysiology in allergic fungal sinusitis. *Laryngoscope* 1998; **108**: 1485–96.
39. Collins M, Nair S, Smith W, et al. Role of local immunoglobulin E production in the pathophysiology of noninvasive fungal sinusitis. *Laryngoscope* 2004; **114**: 1242–46.
40. Ponikau JU, Sherris DA, Kern EB, et al. The diagnosis and incidence of allergic fungal sinusitis. *Mayo Clin Proc* 1999; **74**: 877–84.
41. Heffner DK. Allergic fungal sinusitis is a histopathologic diagnosis; paranasal mucocele is not. *Ann Diagn Pathol* 2004; **8**: 316–23.
42. Shin S-H, Ponikau JU, Sherris DA, et al. Chronic rhinosinusitis: an enhanced immune response to ubiquitous airborne fungi. *J Allergy Clin Immunol* 2004; **114**: 1369–75.

43. Pant H, Schembri MA, Wormald PJ, Macardle PJ. IgE-mediated fungal allergy in allergic fungal sinusitis. *Laryngoscope* 2009; **119**: 1046–52.
44. Ghegan MD, Lee F-S, Schlosser RJ. Incidence of skull base and orbital erosion in allergic fungal rhinosinusitis (AFRS) and non-AFRS. *Otolaryngol Head Neck Surg* 2006; **134**: 592–95.
45. Gan EC, Thamboo A, Rudmik L, et al. Medical management of allergic fungal rhinosinusitis following endoscopic sinus surgery: an evidence-based review and recommendations. *Int Forum Allergy Rhinol* 2014; **4**: 702–15.
46. Evans MO, Coop CA. Novel treatment of allergic fungal sinusitis using omalizumab. *Allergy Rhinol Provid RI* 2014; **5**: 172–74.
47. Rupa V, Jacob M, Mathews MS, Seshadri MS. A prospective, randomised, placebo-controlled trial of postoperative oral steroid in allergic fungal sinusitis. *Eur Arch Otorhinolaryngol* 2010; **267**: 233–38.
48. Gupta RP, Bahadur S, Thakar A, et al. Management protocols of allergic fungal sinusitis. *Indian J Otolaryngol Head Neck Surg* 2007; **59**: 35–40.
49. Bassichis BA, Marple BF, Mabry RL, et al. Use of immunotherapy in previously treated patients with allergic fungal sinusitis. *Otolaryngol Head Neck Surg* 2001; **125**: 487–90.
50. Folker RJ, Marple BF, Mabry RL, Mabry CS. Treatment of allergic fungal sinusitis: a comparison trial of postoperative immunotherapy with specific fungal antigens. *Laryngoscope* 1998; **108**: 1623–27.
51. Marple B, Newcomer M, Schwade N, Mabry R. Natural history of allergic fungal rhinosinusitis: a 4- to 10-year follow-up. *Otolaryngol Head Neck Surg* 2002; **127**: 361–66.
52. Schubert MS. Antileukotriene therapy for allergic fungal sinusitis. *J Allergy Clin Immunol* 2001; **108**: 466–67.
53. deShazo RD, O'Brien M, Chapin K, et al. Criteria for the diagnosis of sinus mycetoma. *J Allergy Clin Immunol* 1997; **99**: 475–85.
54. Grosjean P, Weber R. Fungus balls of the paranasal sinuses: a review. *Eur Arch Otorhinolaryngol* 2007; **264**: 461–70.
55. Chen J-C, Ho C-Y. The significance of computed tomographic findings in the diagnosis of fungus ball in the paranasal sinuses. *Am J Rhinol Allergy* 2012; **26**: 117–19.
56. Thompson III GR, Patel PK, Kirkpatrick WR, et al. Oropharyngeal candidiasis in the era of antiretroviral therapy. *Oral Surg Oral Med Oral Pathol Oral Radiol Endod* 2010; **109**: 488–95.
57. Pappas PG, Kauffman CA, Andes D, et al. Clinical practice guidelines for the management of candidiasis: 2009 update by the Infectious Diseases Society of America. *Clin Infect Dis* 2009; **48**: 503–35.
58. Lalla RV, Latortue MC, Hong CH, et al. A systematic review of oral fungal infections in patients receiving cancer therapy. *Support Care Cancer* 2010; **18**: 985–92.
59. Nicolatou-Galitis O, Sotiropoulou A, Velegraki A, et al. Oral candidiasis in head and neck cancer patients receiving radiotherapy with amifostine cytoprotection. *Oral Oncol* 2003; **39**: 397–401.
60. Tićac B, Tićac R, Rukavina T, et al. Microbial colonization of tracheo-esophageal voice prostheses (Provox2) following total laryngectomy. *Eur Arch Otorhinolaryngol* 2010; **267**: 1579–86.

CHAPTER 22

ANTIMICROBIAL THERAPY

Ursula Altmeyer, Penelope Redding and Nitish Khanna

Introduction 221	Mechanisms of resistance 225
Classification of antimicrobial agents 222	Controlling antimicrobial resistance 226
Susceptibility testing 222	Principles of antimicrobial treatment............................226
Antimicrobial resistance (AMR) 224	References 227

SEARCH STRATEGY

The information in this chapter is based on standard clinical microbiology practice in the UK; evidence level 4 (Expert opinion). Laboratory practices described are based on Public Health England's Standards for Microbiology Investigations (SMI). Data in this chapter may be updated by a PubMed search using the keywords: classification of antimicrobials; antimicrobial spectrum; susceptibility testing; antimicrobial resistance and principles of antimicrobial treatment.

INTRODUCTION

Historically, the prevention and treatment of infection had been one of the most pressing problems medicine was trying to solve. Following the introduction of anti-infective agents in the first half of the 20th century, it seemed as if infection had in all but the most severe cases become a manageable event, rather than a potentially life-threatening catastrophe.

The advances afforded by effective antimicrobial treatments in terms of both surgical and medical interventions have saved millions of lives.

However, shortly after introduction of antimicrobials into clinical practice, resistant organisms developed and began to spread.

When penicillin was first introduced in 1942, all strains of *S. aureus* were susceptible to it and its use during the Second World War contributed to a significant drop in infection associated mortality among wounded soldiers. Already by the mid-1940s, though, the first penicillin resistant strains had developed; they now dominate the circulating strains of *S. aureus* entirely.

Bacterial generation times are short (only 10 minutes for a division of *Escherischia coli*) and their inaccurate genetic replication mechanisms favour random point mutation. Any of these mutations has the potential to result in a new antimicrobial resistance mechanism.

Initially, the development of new antimicrobial compounds was rapid (**Table 22.1**) and able to keep at least apace with emerging resistances, but since the early 1990s there has been a decline in production of novel agents.

In short: this is a competition in which we're unlikely ever to retain the upper hand.

The threat posed by antimicrobial resistance is now widely recognized (**Table 22.2**). In March 2013 the Chief Medical Officer, Dame Sally Davies, highlighted the emergence of antimicrobial resistance as a major challenge in her annual report, stating:

The supply of new replacement antimicrobial agents has slowed dramatically and we face the prospect of a future where we have far fewer options in the treatment of infectious disease and infections that, previously easy to control, will become much more significant threats to health. Standard surgical procedures, such as hip replacements, could become riskier with widespread antimicrobial resistance, as would treatments that result in immunosuppression, such as chemotherapy or organ transplant, which rely on the ability to treat infections that occur in this very vulnerable group of patients.

TABLE 22.1 Historical overview of antimicrobial development

Year	Antimicrobial
1935	Protonsil - sulphonamide pro-drug
1942	Benzyl-penicillin
1944	Streptomycin – first aminoglycoside
1948	Chlortetracycline
1949	Chloramphenicol
1952	Erythromycin – first macrolide
1955	Vancomycin – first glycopeptides
1960	Metronidazole
1964	Cephalotin – first cephalosporin
1967	Rifampicin
1968	Clindamycin
1971	Gentamicin
1972	Amoxicillin
1980	Amoxicillin-clavulanic acid
1982	Ceftriaxone – 3rd generation cephalosporin
1987	Ciprofloxacin
1990	Clarithromycin
1992	Piperacillin-tazobactam
1996	Meropenem
2000	Linezolid
2011	Fidaxomycin

TABLE 22.2 Current and emerging problem resistances

- Methicillin resistant *S. aureus* (MRSA)
- Vancomycin resistant enterococci (VRE), also known as glycopeptide resistant enterococci (GRE)
- Penicillin-intermediate or resistant *S. pneumoniae*
- Extended spectrum β-lactamase (ESBL) producing enterobacteriaceae
- Carbapenemase-producing enterobacteriaceae

CLASSIFICATION OF ANTIMICROBIAL AGENTS

Antimicrobial agents can be classified according to several characteristics:

- chemical structure (e.g. β-lactams, quinolones)
- site of action (e.g. cell wall or ribosome)
- mode of action (i.e. bactericidal or bacteriostatic).

A summary of the properties of the most frequently used classes of antibacterial agents can be found in **Table 22.3**. Tables 22.4–22.7 list important antibacterial agents with their expected spectrum of activity. Please note that the information in these tables should be correlated with local resistance data, and cannot replace local empirical antimicrobial guidance.

SUSCEPTIBILITY TESTING

Once the identity of an organism is known, typical susceptibility patterns can be predicted for some organisms, for example penicillin susceptibility in strains of *S. pyogenes*.

These expected susceptibility patterns form the basis of empirical antibiotic choices.

The majority of resistance patterns are however highly variable and any isolate thought to be clinically significant will be tested formally against panels of antibiotics for their susceptibilities and resistances.

The panels in use may vary from laboratory to laboratory, depending on prevailing patterns of susceptibilities and local antimicrobial policies.

Several different methods for antimicrobial susceptibility testing exist.

Which method will be used may differ between certain organisms, but ultimately all methods demonstrate in vitro presence or inhibition of growth of the organism when exposed to a defined concentration of the tested antimicrobial.

The most accurate method for determining this is the broth dilution method (**Figure 22.1**), in which test tubes containing a broth medium are spiked with serial dilutions of the tested antimicrobial. A standardized inoculum of the organism of interest is then added and the tubes are observed for the presence of bacterial growth after a period of incubation. The first dilution with which no growth is observed represents the minimum inhibitory concentration (MIC) of the tested antibiotic.

While this process will yield very accurate information, it is time and labour intensive and routine use in a diagnostic lab is impractical; however, it forms the basis of most automated methods of susceptibility testing.

An alternative method that is in widespread use is antimicrobial disc diffusion testing (**Figure 22.2**).

In this, a specific testing medium is inoculated evenly with a standardized suspension of the test organism and a selection of paper discs containing defined amounts of antimicrobials is placed on the medium.

The antibiotic will diffuse from the disc into the medium, leading to a gradient of concentration with the highest concentration just around the disc.

A check for growth patterns takes place after a defined period of incubation and the zone of inhibited growth is measured. In order to be classified as susceptible, this zone must be equal or greater than a certain diameter, which varies between different organisms and different antimicrobials.

The interpretation of these results relies on extensive databases of susceptibility break points (i.e. zone diameters that are deemed to represent clinical susceptibility or resistance). Such databases are compiled by external agencies, such as the British Society for Antimicrobial Chemotherapy (BSAC) or the European Committee on Antimicrobial Susceptibility Testing (EUCAST).

A third method, known as the E-test, uses plastic strips that are coated with the tested antimicrobial forming a concentration gradient along the strip. This is placed on a testing medium inoculated with the test organism and

TABLE 22.3 Commonly used classes of antimicrobials

Chemical class	Site of action	Mode of action	Comments
β-lactams: • Penicillins • Cephalosporins	Cell wall	Bactericidal	• Short plasma half lives requiring frequent dosage intervals • Optimum action on actively dividing organisms • Cephalosporins have good penetration through the blood–brain barrier
Carbapenems	Cell wall	Bactericidal	• Very broad spectrum • Cautious use, ideally only if confirmed resistances • Once daily dosing possible with some agents • Good penetration through blood–brain barrier
Glycopeptides: • Vancomycin	Cell wall	Bactericidal	• Large molecules • Not absorbed from GI tract • Penetration into tissues variable • Potential nephrotoxicity • Require therapeutic drug monitoring
Aminoglycosides: • Gentamicin • Amikacin	Ribosome	Bactericidal	• Rapidly bactericidal • Nephrotoxic • Ototoxic • Require therapeutic drug monitoring
Macrolides	Ribosome	Bacteriostatic	• Good oral absorption • Gastro-intestinal side effects, but less pronounced with newer agents
Trimethoprim	Di-hydrofolate reductase	Bacteriostatic	• Contra-indicated in pregnancy, especially 1st trimester
Sulfamethoxazole	Di-hydropteroate synthetase	Bacteriostatic	• Given with trimethoprim as Cotrimoxazole • Inhibits earlier step in tetrahydrofolate synthesis • Contra-indicated in pregnancy, especially 1st trimester
Quinolones	DNA topoisomerase II, gyrase	Bacteriostatic	• Good oral bioavailability • Good tissue penetration
Lincosamides: • Clindamycin	Ribosome	Bacteriostatic	• Good tissue penetration
Oxazolinidones: • Linezolid	Ribosome	Bacteriostatic	• Excellent tissue penetration • Bone marrow toxicity
Nitroimidazoles: • Metronidazole	Directly damages DNA and proteins through formation of radicals	Bactriocidal	• Exclusively anaerobic cover • Excellent tissue penetration

TABLE 22.4 Commonly used penicillins

Agent	Expected spectrum of activity
Penicillin V Benzyl-penicillin	Alpha-haemolytic streptococci S. pneumoniae S. pyogenes
Amoxicillin	Streptococci, enterococci Some Gram-negative cover
Flucloxacillin	Methicillin-sensitive S. aureus
Amoxicillin with clavulanic acid Piperacillin with tazobactam	Broad spectrum Gram-positive, Gram-negative and anaerobic cover, but not MRSA

TABLE 22.5 Commonly used cephalosporins and carbapenems

Commonly used cephalosporins	Expected spectrum of activity
Cefuroxime (2nd generation) Cefotaxime (3rd generation) Ceftriaxone (3rd generation)	Broad spectrum Gram-positive and Gram-negative cover, but not MRSA
Commonly used carbapenems	
Meropenem Ertapenem	

TABLE 22.6 Commonly used macrolides

Commonly used macrolides	Expected spectrum of activity
Erythromycin Clarithromycin	S. pyogenes S. pneumoniae S. aureus, including some strains of MRSA

TABLE 22.7 Commonly used quinolones

Commonly used quinolones	Expected spectrum of activity
Ciprofloxacin Levofloxacin Moxifloxacin	Broad spectrum Gram-negative cover S. aureus Levofloxacin and moxifloxacin have enhanced Gram-positive cover especially against S. pneumoniae

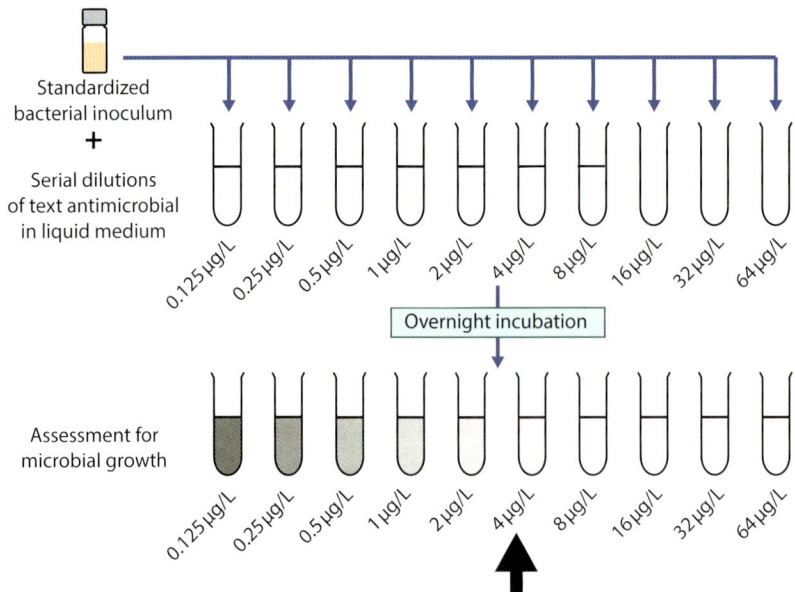

Figure 22.1 Determination of minimum inhibitory concentration by broth dilution method.

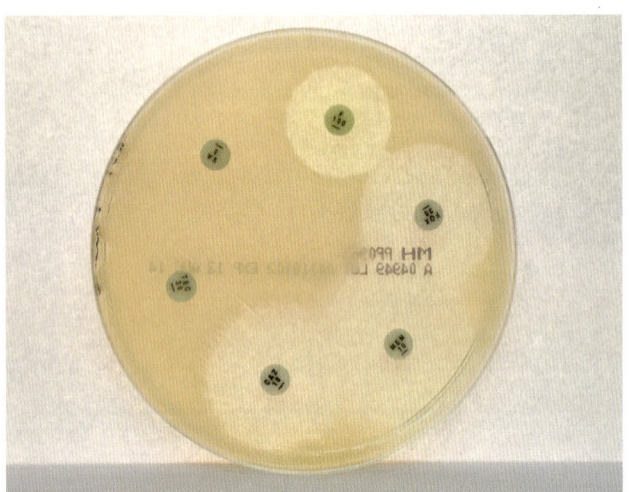

Figure 22.2 Disc diffusion method of susceptibility testing. Courtesy of Jasminder Karde and Margaret Woods, Department of Microbiology, Golden Jubilee National Hospital, Clydebank, UK.

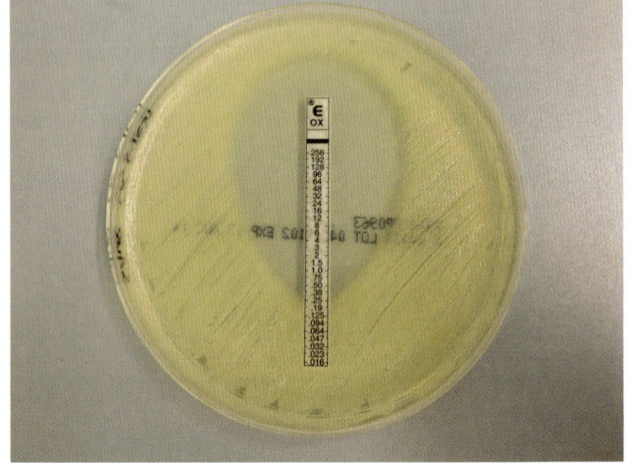

Figure 22.3 Determination of MIC by E-test. The MIC is read where the inhibition zone intersects the test strip. Courtesy of Jasminder Karde and Margaret Woods, Department of Microbiology, Golden Jubilee National Hospital, Clydebank, UK.

again read after a period of incubation. An elliptical zone of inhibition is visible around the test strip, which intersects it at the measured MIC (**Figure 22.3**).

This test combines aspects of both the above methods – it yields information regarding the minimal inhibitory concentration, while retaining the ease of use of the disc diffusion method.

ANTIMICROBIAL RESISTANCE (AMR)

Broadly speaking, there are two principal types of antimicrobial resistance: intrinsic resistance and acquired resistance.

Intrinsic resistance

In 1984 the bodies of two members of an Arctic expedition led by the British explorer Captain Sir John Franklin in 1845 were exhumed on Beechey Island and autopsied. *Clostridium* spp. were isolated from their guts which were resistant to clindamycin and the second-generation cephalosporin cefoxitin, although they could not have been exposed to any modern antimicrobial.[1]

This is an example of intrinsic resistance, which has its basis on traits common to all strains of an organism, such as characteristics of the cell wall or the metabolism, which render them impervious to the effects of an antimicrobial (**Table 22.8**).

TABLE 22.8 Examples of intrinsic resistance

Organism	Intrinsic antimicrobial resistances	Mechanism
Gram-negative organisms	Vancomycin	Agent unable to penetrate outer membrane of cell wall
Aerobic bacteria	Metronidazole	Aerobic metabolism unable to reduce the agent to its active form
Anaerobic bacteria	Aminoglycosides	Active uptake of agent dependent on oxidative metabolism

TABLE 22.9 Mechanisms of horizontal gene transfer

Mechanism	Genetic element transfer	Method of transfer
Transformation	Free genetic material from lysed organisms	Uptake of exogenous DNA from the environment
Conjugation	Mobile genetic elements, e.g. plasmids or transposons	Via direct cell-to-cell contact or through specific cell bridges (pili)
Transduction	Mobile genetic elements, e.g. plasmids or transposons	Introduction of foreign genetic material via viral (phage) vector

Acquired resistance

If a bacterial organism becomes resistant to an antimicrobial agent or class to which it was previously susceptible, it is said to have developed an acquired resistance.

This may be the result of a new mutation or the transfer of resistances from other organisms.

Chromosomal resistance is the result of a randomly occurring spontaneous mutation, resulting in resistance to an antimicrobial agent. If the host is exposed to the antimicrobial in question, organisms carrying the mutation will have a survival advantage and replace the susceptible isolates. The mutation will be passed on to the progeny of this organism with every cell division; this is referred to as vertical transfer and may lead to treatment failures, but the resistance is unlikely to spread to other strains or types of organisms.

The second, and more worrying, way of acquiring resistance is via mobile genetic elements, which can spread easily between different strains of the same organism, but also between different types of organisms.

This is called horizontal transfer and there are several ways this transfer can occur (Table 22.9).

MECHANISMS OF RESISTANCE

While there are many resistance genes, the effects of them fall broadly into three categories.

Alteration or removal of the antimicrobial's target

Resistance to flucloxacillin in *S. aureus* is the result of the alteration of the binding site of penicillin in the organism's cell wall components.

Usually, penicillin disrupts cell wall synthesis by attaching to a part of the peptidoglycan component known as the penicillin binding protein (PBP) and prevents cross linking of the components into a normal cell wall structure.

The *mecA* gene of methicillin-resistant strains of *S. aureus* (MRSA) encodes for an altered penicillin binding protein called PBP2a, which does not allow attachment of any β-lactam agent and therefore renders the organism resistant to this class of antibiotic.

Alteration of the drug leading to loss of activity

Many Gram-negative organisms produce enzymes called β-lactamases that are able to cleave the β-lactam ring of penicillins, rendering them resistant to their effects. They are usually located in the peri-plasmic space between the outer membrane and the peptidoglycan cell wall.

This enzyme can be inhibited, and several penicillin-β-lactamase inhibitor combination agents are available, such as amoxicillin with clavulanic acid or piperacillin with tazobactam.

If the enzyme is able to cleave not only the β-lactam ring of penicillins, but also that of third-generation cephalosporins, this enzyme would be classed as an extended spectrum β-lactamase (ESBL).

If the enzyme in question cleaves not only the β-lactam ring of penicillins and third-generation cephalosporins but also the carbapenem ring, it is classed as a carbapenemase.

Gram-negative organisms carrying various β-lactam resistance mechanisms are endemic in many parts of the world and frequently carry resistance mechanisms conferring resistance to additional classes of antimicrobials, rendering the organisms difficult to treat.

Alteration of the drug's access to its target

The easiest way of preventing a drug from acting on its target is by removing the drug before it even reaches the target.

Many bacteria have incorporated efflux pumps that share some molecular components with the flagellar apparatus into their cell walls. This comes at a price – while many of these efflux pumps are able to remove more than one type of antibiotic, the transport of the drug across the membrane is an active process that uses significant amounts of energy.

Resistance to tetracyclines in Gram-positives is the result of such an efflux pump.

Resistance to an agent may be mediated via different mechanisms in different organisms and different mechanisms conferring resistance to multiple antimicrobial classes may coexist in the same organism; listing all possible combinations of organisms and resistance mechanisms would be beyond the scope of this chapter.

CONTROLLING ANTIMICROBIAL RESISTANCE

The rise of resistant organisms has been recognized as a major healthcare challenge on a national and international level and the World Health Organization and the British Department of Health have both recently published guidance documents on AMR control.

The issue is a complex one, as antimicrobials in the form of antibacterial, antifungal, antiviral and antiparasitic chemotherapy are used not only in a human healthcare setting, but also in veterinary medicine and agriculture.

In addition to this, resources, prescribing practice and surveillance programmes differ markedly between countries, making it difficult to develop an approach that is suitable for global application.

In the UK, the following key factors have been identified by the Department of Health:[2]

- Enhanced surveillance in order to identify existing and novel resistance patterns quickly
- Optimizing prescribing practice and antimicrobial stewardship, ensuring that antibiotics are only prescribed when needed and the correct agent is given for the correct amount of time
- Improving infection prevention and control
- Encouraging the development of new antibiotics, diagnostic strategies and novel therapies

PRINCIPLES OF ANTIMICROBIAL TREATMENT

Antimicrobials are amongst the most commonly prescribed medication in both primary and secondary care. Approximately one-third of all inpatients at any given time are receiving some form of antimicrobial treatment.[3]

In order to ensure that unnecessary prescribing is minimized, it is good practice to adhere to some basic principles when considering antimicrobial treatment.

Identification of the source of infection

Ideally, antibiotics should only be prescribed when a clear clinical source has been identified. This relies heavily on careful clinical examination and consideration whether or not a bacterial infection is likely.

In suspected deep-seated infections, such as intracranial abscesses, imaging forms an integral part of the diagnostic process.

Appropriate sampling

Clinical samples from the suspected focus of infection should be collected before any antimicrobial therapy is commenced.

If the patient is septic (i.e. fulfils the criteria of systemic inflammatory response with a suspected infective focus), at least one set of blood cultures should be taken peripherally, and from any vascular access devices if present.

If a deep infection is present and the patient is stable, it may in some cases be possible to delay antimicrobial therapy until a diagnostic tap or drainage can be performed in order to maximize the chances of recovering the causative organism.

Source control

If the source of infection is identified as an abscess or collection, this should be drained wherever possible, as abscesses are not vascularized and penetration of antimicrobials into the cavity is very poor, even if given intravenously.

Recovery of organisms is more likely to be successful if a volume of pus in a sterile container is sent to the laboratory as opposed to a swab.

If the infection involves prosthetic material or a device, treatment success may depend on removal of the foreign material as this is obviously not perfused and may harbour bacteria in a sticky polysaccharide matrix known as a biofilm.

Choice of initial antimicrobial agent

Empirical antimicrobial therapy targets the most likely causative agents of a clinical syndrome, and local policies should be adhered to as they will take into account local resistance patterns.

Ideally, empirical broad-spectrum cover should be avoided as it will disrupt the normal protective gut flora and may also prevent a microbiological diagnosis. In a patient assumed to be bacteraemic, inclusion of a rapidly bactericidal agent in the regimen should be considered.

Appropriate dosing

Giving an appropriate dose of the correct antimicrobial maximizes the chance for cure of disease and may prevent development of resistance due to exposure to subtherapeutic levels of antimicrobials.

A variety of reasons may prompt dose adjustments in antimicrobial treatment.

Patients with renal disease and low creatinine clearance require dose adjustments for many classes of antimicrobials.

The dosing of aminoglycosides and glycopeptides is usually adjusted to the patient's body weight and creatinine clearance. Local guidelines for dose calculation should be adhered to.

A special case is the dosing of antimicrobials in the morbidly obese, where standard dosing may not result in achievement of therapeutic serum or tissue levels.

These cases should be discussed with a pharmacist to ensure that appropriate doses are prescribed and serious side effects are avoided.

Route of administration

Many uncomplicated infections, especially in the primary care setting, will only require oral antimicrobial treatment. Indeed, depending on the source of infection, topical antimicrobials alone may be indicated, for example in the treatment of mild otitis externa.

However, if the infection is accompanied by signs of systemic upset and sepsis is suspected, the patient may well be bacteraemic and antimicrobial treatment should be given intravenously initially.

Bacteraemia should always be treated with an appropriate intravenous antimicrobial; the duration of intravenous treatment may depend on the organism involved and the underlying source of infection.

In deep-seated infections or infections in poorly vascularized tissue, intravenous treatment is likely to continue for a prolonged course.

De-escalation and switch to oral administration of treatment

Once culture results are available, antimicrobial therapy should be adjusted according to the susceptibility of the organism in order to allow targeted treatment with a narrow spectrum agent.

If treatment has commenced via the intravenous route and clinical improvement is observed, the administration route should be reviewed after 48 hours by the latest and a switch to oral antimicrobials considered, provided blood cultures remained negative and oral treatment is appropriate for the source of infection.

Completing a course of treatment

Giving an antimicrobial for an appropriate amount of time maximizes the rate of cure of disease and reduces the risk of relapse and need for further courses of likely broader spectrum antimicrobials.

The duration of the course will differ between different foci and also partly depend on the organism involved. Generally speaking, deep-seated infections and infections in poorly vascularized tissue such as cartilage and bone will require extended courses of treatment with agents that are able to penetrate into these tissues to reach therapeutic levels.

KEY POINTS

- Antimicrobials may be classified by chemical class and mechanism of action.
- Organisms can display intrinsic resistance to certain agents.
- Acquired resistance may arise as a direct consequence of exposure to antimicrobial agents. There are a number of resistance mechanisms, some of which can spread within bacterial populations and between different bacterial species via mobile genetic elements.
- The control of antimicrobial resistance is a major public health challenge.
- Any decision to commence antimicrobial therapy should comply with best practice principles.

REFERENCES

1. Notman D, Beattie O. The palaeoimaging and forensic anthropology of frozen sailors from the Franklin Arctic expedition mass disaster (1845–1848): a detailed presentation of two radiological surveys. *New Scientist*, 11 Feb 1989, p. 34.

2. Department of Health. *UK five year antimicrobial resistance strategy 2013 to 2018*. London: Department of Health; 2013. Available from https://www.gov.uk/government/uploads/system/uploads/attachment_data/file/238872/20130902_UK_5_year_AMR_strategy_FINAL.pdf

3. Health Protection Scotland. *Healthcare Associated Infection Annual Report 2014*. Glasgow: Health Protection Scotland; 2015. Available from http://www.hps.scot.nhs.uk/haiic/sshaip/publications.aspx and also via this link: http://www.hps.scot.nhs.uk/haiic/sshaip/resourcedetail.aspx?id=1718

CHAPTER 23

HUMAN IMMUNODEFICIENCY VIRUS

Neil Ritchie and Alasdair Robertson

Introduction 229	Kaposi's sarcoma 231
Human immunodeficiency virus 229	Otologic 232
HIV testing 230	Nose and paranasal sinuses 233
Therapy 230	Oral cavity 233
Otorhinolaryngological manifestations 231	Pharynx, larynx and oesophagus 235
Acute HIV infection 231	Salivary glands 235
Cervical lymphadenopathy 231	References 236

SEARCH STRATEGY

Data in this chapter may be updated by a PubMed search using the keywords: acquired immunodeficiency syndrome, antiretroviral therapy, highly active, HIV, HIV infections, lymphadenopathy, otolaryngology, otorhinolaryngologic diseases, sarcoma and kaposi.

INTRODUCTION

Human immunodeficiency virus (HIV) has had a profound impact on global healthcare in the 30 years since its discovery. In 1981 healthy young men in America started to become gravely ill with atypical infections and tumours, previously only seen in the severely immunocompromised; the term acquired immuno-deficiency syndrome (AIDS) was coined. In 1983, HIV was isolated and identified as the causal agent. HIV is now a worldwide epidemic that affects individuals of every age, sex and socioeconomic group, with 34 million people infected.[1]

Sub-Saharan Africa continues to bear the brunt of the epidemic, and accounted for 69% of all people living with HIV and 72% of new cases in 2011. Since 1998 more than 1 million people a year have died from HIV infection in Sub-Saharan Africa. South Africa alone has 5.6 million infected people, compared to 1 million in Western and Central Europe and 1.3 million in North America. The number of people infected with HIV continues to increase; however, the number of new cases per year and the number of deaths per year have been falling since the peak of the disease in 1997. Eastern Europe and Central Asia (particularly the Russian Federation and Ukraine) are bucking the trend for HIV control, with a 250% increase in HIV infection from 2001 to 2010. Changing health policies and new treatments are responsible for the relative decline of the HIV epidemic. Public health campaigns have helped to change behaviour with an increase in condom use and a decrease in the number of sexual partners. Antiretroviral therapy for pregnant HIV-infected women has reduced mother-to-child spread. Targeting of high-risk groups such as sex workers (free condoms) and intravenous drug users (needle exchange programmes) has been effective. The effectiveness of these interventions is impeded by the number of people living with HIV who are unaware of their infected status; 84% of HIV-infected adults in Kenya were unaware of their infection[2] and in the UK the figure is 24%.[3]

Head and neck manifestations of the disease are prevalent and up to 100% of HIV patients will have some head and neck presentation of the disease during the course of their illness.

HUMAN IMMUNODEFICIENCY VIRUS

HIV is a retrovirus, of the lentivirus genus. There are two strains of the virus: HIV-1 and HIV-2. HIV-1 is the global epidemic strain, while HIV-2 is largely limited to West Africa and is less virulent. The HIV genetic material is a diploid, single-stranded ribonucleic acid (RNA) that uses the enzyme reverse transcriptase to convert its single-stranded RNA into double-stranded deoxyribonucleic acid (DNA). The viral RNA encodes three virus specific genes: *pol*, *gag* and *env*. *Pol* encodes the enzymes for viral replication (polymerase, integrase and protease) while *gag* encodes the inner structural proteins. *Env* encodes the glycoproteins responsible for the viral envelope; this envelope contains two glycoproteins, gp41 and gp120, which form a complex essential for viral proliferation. gp120 binds to the glycoprotein receptor CD4 on the host-cell membrane. CD4 is found in highest concentrations on T helper lymphocytes and it is through these cells that HIV primarily proliferates. Once gp120 and CD4 are bound, the viral and host cell membranes fuse. This allows the viral contents to be injected into the host cell. Reverse transcriptase then catalyses the synthesis of viral DNA from RNA. The viral DNA then migrates into the host nucleus and is incorporated into the host cell genome through the action of integrase. This means that the viral genome is replicated along with the host cell DNA and passed onto progeny cells. Once activated, the provirus begins to synthesize new virus particles using host cell transcription machinery. Cells of the monocyte/macrophage lineage also express CD4 and thus can be infected by HIV and act as reservoirs.[4,5]

HIV infection is characterized by three distinct phases: seroconversion, asymptomatic infection and AIDS. Seroconversion starts within 2 weeks of inoculation; viraemia occurs with widespread dissemination of the virus throughout the body. Reservoirs of infection are created in macrophages. The viral load is high and a sharp decline in the number of CD4+ cells occurs. The individual is very infectious at this stage. Eventually the immune system attains a degree of control and this leads to a reduction in the viral load and a recovery of the peripheral CD4 cell count but infection is not eradicated. Half of seroconverting patients experience symptoms, typically a 'flu-like' illness with fever malaise and generalized rash. The next phase of HIV infection lasts for several years, during which the patient is asymptomatic. During this latency period viral replication and CD4 lymphocyte destruction continues; however, the body's immune response keeps the viral load in check. Circulating CD4 counts are generally high during this period. Once the CD4 count starts to decrease, symptomatology may resume, beginning with fatigue and generalized lymphadenopathy. Further decreases in CD4 count produce more constitutional symptoms including fever, sweats, chills, weight loss, night sweats and diarrhoea. Eventually the CD4 cells reach a level where an effective immune response can no longer be mounted (less than 200 cells per microlitre). At this stage, the incidence of opportunistic infections and AIDS associated neoplasms greatly increases. T helper cells are important in the immune response against viruses and fungi, hence these infections are the most commonly encountered. Conditions such as *Pneumocystis carinii* pneumonia and Kaposi's sarcoma are diagnostic for AIDS. Untreated AIDS is universally fatal.

HIV TESTING

With prompt treatment, HIV morbidity and mortality can be minimized. One of the most important factors in poor prognosis is late presentation.[6] Furthermore, undiagnosed individuals pose a significant risk of further transmission. Detection of HIV infection is therefore an essential pillar of HIV interventions. There are two main misconceptions regarding HIV testing: it requires extensive pre-test counselling and it will have an impact on future insurance polices for the patient. Where an HIV test is clinically indicated, extensive pre-test counselling is not required. Informed consent should be taken including discussion of the benefit of testing and how the results will be given. It is recommended that if a test is positive the clinician should have identified the appropriate local treatment providers and established a clear plan for onward referral prior to the consultation.[7]

Testing for HIV, by an otolaryngologist, should be carried out whenever HIV infection enters the differential diagnosis. In particular otolaryngologists should test patients with the following conditions: unexplained oral candidiasis, hairy leukoplakia of the tongue, atypical head and neck cancers, parotid cysts, cervical lymphadenopathy, chronic parotitis and pyrexia of unknown origin. High-risk groups should also be offered testing. In the UK all patients who attend antenatal, genito-urinary medicine clinics and drug dependency services are offered HIV testing. In the United States, the Preventative Services Task Force has recommended screening for all individuals aged between 15 and 65.[8]

THERAPY

Over the past 15 years significant progress has been made in the treatment of HIV-infected individuals. Highly active antiretroviral therapy (HAART) has transformed the prognosis for people living with HIV, turning the disease from a fatal affliction into a manageable chronic condition. HAART is a treatment consisting of various regimens of multiple pharmaceutical agents. Each drug in a HAART regimen inhibits a different part of the viral lifecycle. By inhibiting the virus at multiple stages effective viral suppression can be obtained. The commonly used drugs inhibit one of the three main viral enzymes for replication: reverse transcriptase, protease and integrase.

Two classes of drugs inhibit reverse transcriptase; nucleoside/nucleotide reverse transcriptase inhibitors (NRTIs) and non-nucleoside reverse transcriptase inhibitors (NNRTIs). NRTIs are the oldest antiretroviral drugs and still have a central role in antiretroviral therapy. NRTIs are structurally similar to DNA nucleosides. Since reverse transcriptase lacks error correction, when it incorporates NRTIs into the proviral DNA, the replication process is terminated. NNRTIs inhibit reverse transcriptase by binding directly to its active site.

HIV protease catalyses the maturation of viral particles by cleaving polypeptides responsible for capsule formation. Protease inhibitors (PIs) are highly robust antiretrovirals but their complex absorption kinetics require complex regimes and lack patient acceptability. However, the use of the PI ritonavir as a pharmacological booster has revolutionized their use by allowing once or twice daily regimes without difficult dietary restrictions.

Other classes of antiretrovirals include integrase inhibitors, entry inhibitors and fusion inhibitors but these are usually reserved for patients intolerant of first-line therapy or with resistant infection.

When used as monotherapy, antiretroviral resistance rapidly develops through the accumulation of mutations in viral genome caused by the relatively imprecise action of reverse transcriptase. This means that antiretroviral therapy must be delivered as combinations, usually of three drugs. The most common first-line regimes consist of two NRTIs (the backbone) with either a NNRTI or PI. With current HAART regimes, up to 95% of patients can achieve viral suppression with an undetectable viral load.

Not all people living with HIV need HAART. Current UK guidelines suggest healthy patients in the asymptomatic phase with a high CD4 count only require monitoring. Current British HIV Association guidelines suggest a CD4 threshold of 350 cells/ul. Development of serious HIV related infections or malignancies are other indications for initiation of HAART.

OTORHINOLARYNGOLOGICAL MANIFESTATIONS

The relative sparing of the humoral immune response in HIV-infected patients means that the incidence of most bacterial infections is similar to non-HIV-infected patients. Conditions such as bacterial otitis externa, bacterial sinusitis and tonsillitis have generally the same infective agents and treatments in HIV and non-HIV patients. This chapter will concentrate on the more challenging and unusual conditions that HIV patients encounter.

ACUTE HIV INFECTION

Patients recently infected with HIV can present to the otolaryngologist with the symptoms of their initial infection. Detection of infection at this stage is important both for the patients and from the perspective of public health. Patients with acute infection usually have a very high viral load and are therefore highly infectious. Early diagnosis gives an opportunity to intervene before further infections occur. Acute infection usually presents non-specifically; however, common symptoms include fever, pharyngitis, lymphadenopathy, oropharyngeal ulceration and rash. Heterophile antibody testing is usually negative but there are reports of positive tests in acute HIV.

UK testing guidelines recommend all patients with a mononucleosis-like illness should be offered an HIV test.

CERVICAL LYMPHADENOPATHY

The presence of peripheral lymphadenopathy is common in patients infected with HIV. In the era of HAART, AIDS-associated malignancies have become less common and it has become clear that patients with HIV are also at increased risk of non-AIDS malignancies including head and neck, lung and upper-gastrointestinal cancers with an overall odds-ratio of around 2–4.

Persistent generalized lymphadenopathy is a common feature of early symptomatic HIV infection, with cervical nodes the most commonly involved. Lymph nodes are usually small, symmetrical and non-tender. Biopsy is not required unless an alternative diagnosis is suspected and is usually prompted by continued enlargement or asymmetry. When biopsy is conducted, it reveals follicular hyperplasia and no treatment is required.

Other causes of lymphadenopathy common in patients with HIV include non-Hodgkin's lymphoma, Hodgkin's lymphoma, tuberculosis, syphilis, Kaposi's sarcoma (KS) and metastatic solid organ malignancies. Less common causes include infections such as mycobacterium avium complex, syphilis, dimorphic fungi and toxoplasmosis.

Castleman disease is a rare lymphoproliferative disorder. In most immunocompetent patients it is a localized disorder that rarely causes systemic symptoms. However, in HIV associated disease most patients present with constitutional symptoms associated with organ involvement (multicentric disease). The disorder is associated with human herpes virus-8 (HHV-8) infection, which is also the viral cause of KS.[9] Patients with multicentric Castleman disease present with fever, weight loss and lymphadenopathy. Diagnosis is made with excision biopsy.

KAPOSI'S SARCOMA

Kaposi's sarcoma (KS) is a malignant spindle cell tumour. Initially it was a rare condition seen in elderly Mediterranean men (classical KS); however, it is now mostly associated with HIV infection. KS is an AIDS-defining condition and is the most common HIV related tumour. KS is caused by the co-infection of HIV and HHV-8. Untreated HIV KS is an aggressive tumour; however, the advent of HAART has lead to a decrease in the incidence and severity of KS.

KS presents with cutaneous or mucosal lesions, most commonly in the head and neck. Visceral organs and lymph nodes can also be involved. Cutaneous lesions are variable in nature; the colour varies from purple to dark brown, the size is from a few millimetres to several centimetres, there may be multiple lesions or a single lesion, and the lesions may be flat, raised or nodular. Oral mucosa lesions are classically raised and red and may ulcerate. Patients with suspected KS should have an HIV test and CD4 count; a biopsy will confirm the diagnosis.

HAART is the mainstay of KS treatment; as the immune system recovers the condition regresses. In advanced cases HAART may not be sufficient and local treatment is required. Localized radiotherapy to cutaneous or oral lesions provides good control of the disease although HIV patients are more prone to radiation side effects.[10] Surgical excision also provides local control; however, recurrence is common even with clear margins of excision. Other treatment modalites include topical retinoids, intra-lesional chemotherapy, laser coagulation and cryotherapy.

Bacillary angiomatosis is a condition that mimics KS and should be considered in the differential diagnosis. Bacillary angiomatosis is a bartonella infection in HIV patients that causes a vascular proliferation. The resulting lesions have an angiomatous appearance very similar to KS. Biopsy and microbiological studies will differentiate from KS. Bacillary angiomatosis resolves with antibiotics; erythromycin is the drug of choice.

OTOLOGIC

External ear

Malignant otitis externa (MOE) has a higher incidence in HIV patients. Osteomyelitis of the skull base causes facial nerve or cranial nerve dysfunction. Diagnosis can be confirmed using a computerized tomography (CT) scan of the temporal bone or a technetium 99m bone scan. The causative agent for malignant otitis externa is usually *Pseudomonas aeriuginosa*, although in patients with very low CD4 count *Aspergillus* is common and can be very invasive.[11, 12] In *Pseudomonas aeriuginosa*, the treatment is 6–8 weeks of antibiotics. A combination of an antipseudomonal third-generation cephalosporin with either ciprofloxacin or aminoglycoside is appropriate.[13] Invasive *Aspergillus* should be treated with intravenous antifungals such as amphoteracin B. Surgical debridement may be necessary in more severe cases.

Pneumocystis jiroveci (previously known as *Pneumocystis carinii*) can infect the extenal auditory canal but may also involve the middle ear and mastoid bone. It may present as either a cyst or polyp, and the cyst if allowed to grow can occlude the external auditory canal or spread to the middle ear cleft and middle cranial fossa. The diagnosis is made by biopsy. Treatment with trimethoprim/sulphamethoxazole and/or dapsone[14] usually results in resolution of infection.

Middle ear

The most common otologic entities seen in HIV-positive individuals are serous and recurrent otitis media. There are a variety of aetiologies that includes Eustachian tube dysfunction, nasopharyngeal neoplasms, adenoid hypertrophy and sinusitis/allergies. Nasopharyngeal neoplasms should be ruled out in HIV-infected individuals, particularly with unilateral otitis media. Myringotomy and tympanostomy tube placement can offer symptomatic relief easily and quickly. Treatment of associated sinusitis or allergies should be instituted. Adenoidectomy may be indicated when more conservative measures fail.

Mycobacterium tuberculosis (TB) is a common infective agent in HIV. *Mycobacterium tuberculosis* should be considered in patients with an otitis media unresponsive to conventional therapy. The classical TB otitis media signs of multiple tympanic membrane perforations, granulations, painless otorrhoea and bone necrosis may not be evident in HIV patients. Tissue biopsies and microbiology cultures may be diagnostic; however, false negatives are common. Antituberculous chemotherapy should be continued for a minimum of 6 months. Surgery to remove sequestrum may speed up recovery; however, a conservative approach has also been shown to be effective.[15, 16] Atypical mycobacteria such as *Mycobacterium avium* complex are also reported to cause otitis media in patients with HIV.[17]

Inner ear

Vestibular and cochlear symptoms are common in HIV-infected individuals. Sensorineural hearing loss is reported to be more common than in uninfected patients and to correlate with stage of disease.[18] Sudden sensorineural hearing loss is also reported to be more than twice as common in this patient population.[19] Identified causes of hearing loss include direct HIV central nervous system involvement, opportunistic infection, immune-reconstitution and drug induced ototoxicity.

Opportunistic infections associated with hearing loss include cytomegalovirus, herpes simplex virus, varicella zoster virus, Cryptococcus neoformans and syphilis. The role of antiretrovirals in sensorineural hearing loss is unclear; a cohort study suggested an association with NRTIs but this was not confirmed prospectively. Other drugs commonly used in patients with HIV associated with hearing loss include macrolides, aminoglycosides and isoniazid. There is some evidence that patients with HIV are more susceptible to aminoglycoside ototoxicity.

Otosyphilis is a rare but important cause of hearing loss in HIV. Patients with HIV can have an abbreviated course of syphilis with features of neurological involvement occurring early. Otosyphilis classically presents with hearing loss sparing the mid-range frequencies, tinnitus and vertigo mimicking Meniere's disease. Diagnosis is with serological testing. Treatment is with high dose procaine penicillin in combination with probenecid. The role of corticosteroids is controversial and evidence is limited but some experts recommend their addition.

Facial nerve palsy can occur in up to 7.2% of HIV patients and is referable to direct infection by the HIV, neoplasms, opportunistic infections, AIDS encephalopathy and toxoplasmosis. Bell's palsy is the most frequent diagnosis given for CN VII paralysis. It is postulated to be caused by HSV and is a diagnosis of exclusion. Complete recovery usually occurs within 3 weeks to 3 months.

Ramsay Hunt syndrome (herpes zoster oticus) usually occurs later in HIV infection and is more prevalent in AIDS patients. Symptoms include peripheral facial nerve palsy, herpetic vesicles along the seventh nerve dermatome and in the conchal bowl, and severe herpetic pain. Treatment is with high-dose acyclovir and high-dose steroids when not contraindicated.

Bilateral facial nerve palsies have been reported[20] and usually represent a systemic disease. Serology tests for syphilis, cytomegalovirus, herpes simplex, herpes zoster and Epstein Barr virus should be carried out. MRI of the brain and CSF analysis will aid the diagnosis.

Patients with a low CD4 count may present with central nervous system disease with few or ambiguous clinical signs. There should be a low threshold for neuroimaging and lumbar puncture. Investigation and management should be undertaken in consultation with a physician with expertise in the management of HIV.

NOSE AND PARANASAL SINUSES

Thirty to sixty-eight per cent of HIV-positive patients will manifest some form of nasal and/or sinus symptom.[21] Nasal obstruction secondary to a variety of aetiologies is a complaint that commonly causes these patients to see an otolaryngologist. Adenoidal hypertrophy can present as nasal obstruction, as can hypertrophy of any of the tissues in Waldeyer's ring. Any non-paediatric patient with adenoid hypertrophy should be tested for HIV.

Neoplasms such as KS or non-Hodgkin's lymphoma can also cause nasal obstruction. Both lesions can arise from the nasal cavity or nasopharynx. Kaposi's sarcoma can also arise from the nasal septum. Non-Hodgkin's lymphoma can also arise from the sinuses.

Sinusitis in HIV-positive individuals is similar to that in non-infected persons with *S. pneumonia*, *M. catarrhalis* and *H. influenzae* the main infective agents. In HIV-positive persons with fever of unknown origin, the sinuses should always be investigated for possible infection. The bacteriology of chronic sinusitis differs from that of acute sinusitis. In patients with CD4 counts less than 200/mL, *S. aureus*, *P. aeruginosa* and anaerobes become more prominent, and antibiotic therapy should be broadened to include these organisms. As the CD4 count decreases below 50/mL, fungal infection of the sinuses can occur (**Figure 23.1**), with the majority of fungal infections caused by *Aspergillus*. Other pathogens reported in the literature include CMV, *Microsporidia*, *Acanthamoeba castellani* and *Legionella pneumophila*.

Evaluation of sinusitis in HIV involves bacteriology culture, nasal endoscopy and CT scanning. The mainstays of medical management of sinusitis are antibiotics and decongestants. First-line antibiotics include amoxicillin, co-amoxiclav, cephalosporins and co-trimoxazole. Topical nasal steroids may also be considered as an adjunctive therapy. There is also evidence suggesting a role for guaifensin therapy for these patients.[22]

Surgery is advocated in patients with persistent symptoms despite medical therapy, or in any patient at any time with extra-sinus symptoms (mental status changes, cranial nerve dysfunction, intra-cranial extension, abscess, etc.). Endoscopic sinus surgery is safe and effective. The goal of surgery should be symptomatic relief, as well as optimizing nasal anatomy to facilitate drainage of the sinuses. However, as HIV disease progression continues and CD4 counts decrease, the physician can expect recurrent sinus infections that become more difficult to treat.

ORAL CAVITY

Oral cavity manifestations of HIV are extremely common and have been reported in up to 100% of AIDS patients. Oral manifestations are also common in patients with relatively high CD4 counts and are often the first manifestation of HIV in otherwise asymptomatic patients. Oral manifestations are also common in patients on HAART, despite the generally low incidence of manifestations of immunosuppression in this group.

Recurrent apthous ulcers are common in immunocompromised patients and are generally larger than those in non-immunocompromised patients. On examination, the lesions are solitary or multiple, have an erythematous halo that is well circumscribed, and may have an exudate or pseudomembrane. The lesions are tender to palpation, and in giant apthous ulcers can cause severe odynophagia and pain. In severe cases, the pain may accentuate the anorexia and dehydration common in advanced HIV. Treatment is primarily to provide symptomatic relief. Topical anaesthetics or steroids are often effective in less severe cases. Topical tetracycline or systemic clindamycin are effective agents when superimposed infection is present. An intralesional steroid injection with triamcinolone acetonide has been shown to have analgesic effects within 24–48 hours after injection, and has very few side effects.[23] Oral thalidomide has been shown in some studies to heal ulcers completely in 55% of patients and partially in 90% of patients, but is only recommended to be used for 2–4 weeks at a time secondary to increased HIV viral load. Thalidomide also has teratogenic effects limiting its use in women. Ulcers that do not respond to local treatment should be biopsied for pathological examination.

Oral candidiasis is a common infection in HIV patients. The most prevalent form is pseudomembraneous candidiasis (thrush) and is characterized by a tender white plaque atop an erythematous and erosive mucosal surface. In the

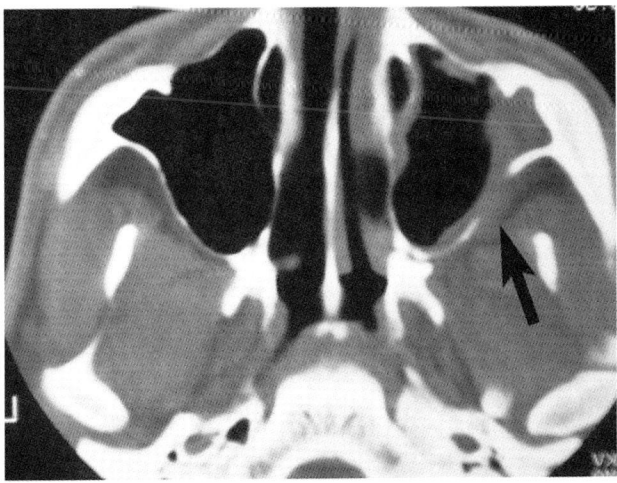

Figure 23.1 In advanced HIV disease, invasive fungal infection of the paranasal sinuses must be considered. As seen in this axial CT scan, subtle bony erosion with extension into the infratemporal fossa (arrow) indicates an invasive fungal process.

chronic hypertrophic form, the plaques are heaped up and not easily removed with scraping. As with recurrent apthous ulcers, the lesions can be extremely painful, leading to malnutrition, dehydration and wasting if not effectively treated. Oesophageal candidiasis can coexist with oropharyngeal lesions and patients should be questioned about oesophageal symptoms since oesophageal involvement will require systemic therapy. Treatment of mild disease consists of Nystatin mouthwash. Clotrimazole or amphotericin lozenges are also effective. Systemic therapy is indicated in patients with worsening immunocompromise or thrush unresponsive to topical agents. Fluconazole is the most commonly used agent – failure to respond can indicate resistance and samples for culture should be sent for sensitivity testing. A minority of cases require intravenous therapy with amphotericin or echinocandins.

Hairy leukoplakia is unique to HIV-positive individuals and typically arises on the lateral border of the tongue as a white, raised, corrugated or filiform lesion. It can also arise on the dorsal tongue, buccal and labial mucosa, floor of mouth or soft palate. It requires no treatment and is usually asymptomatic (**Figure 23.2**).

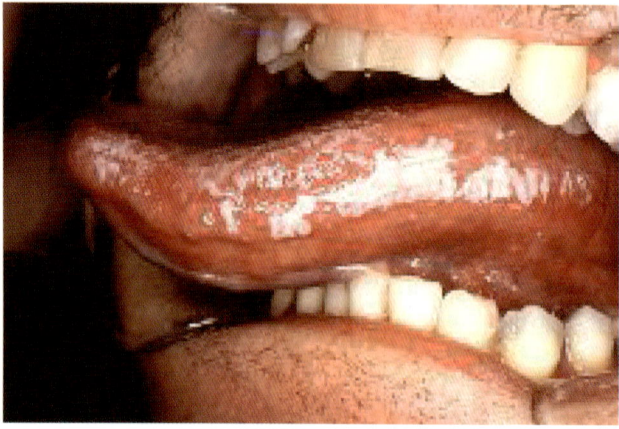

Figure 23.2 Hairy leukoplakia of the tongue.

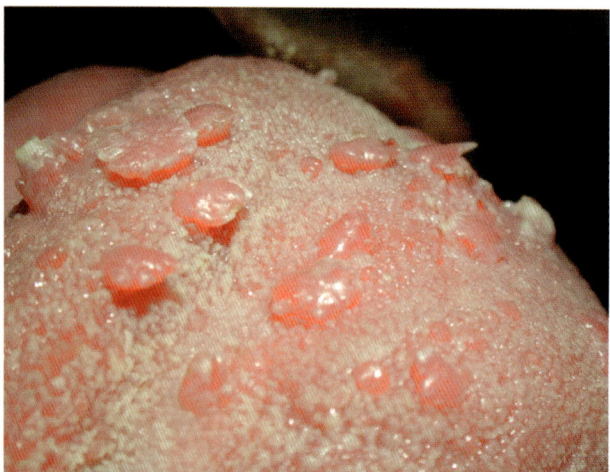

Figure 23.3 While often presenting as solitary lesions, oral papillomas can be widespread covering much of the oral and oropharyngeal mucosa. This patient has multiple papillomas of the dorsal tongue, which predictably recurred following surgical management.

Oral herpes simplex commonly presents as herpes labialis (fever blisters, cold sores). The lesions frequently present as small bullae that form ulcerations after they rupture. These lesions are painful and are generally larger in HIV patients than in immunocompetent individuals. Treatment consists of oral acyclovir; long-term secondary prophylaxis may be required for frequent recurrence.

Gingivitis in HIV patients tends to be more severe than in non-infected patients. Bleeding from the gums can occur with minimal or no trauma. Periodontitis presents as loosening of periodontal attachments. It can progress to acute necrotizing ulcerative gingivitis, which is an ulcerative process along the gingival margin leading to destruction of the periodontal soft tissues. Treatment consists of antibiotics aimed at anaerobic organisms and topical irrigations with chlorhexidine gluconate. If available, a referral to a dentist or oral surgeon should be made early in the process.[24]

Human papilloma virus can present as a verrucous, flat or spiky lesion in the oral cavity. It appears similar to venereal warts and usually appears in synchrony with anal or genital lesions. While often solitary lesions, these can occur as widespread involvement of the entire oral cavity and oropharyngeal mucosa (**Figure 23.3**). Treatment consists of surgical excision, but recurrence is likely.

Xerostomia secondary to chronic inflammation of the major and minor salivary glands is frequently seen in HIV patients. The treatment is for symptomatic relief and consists of oral irrigations, saline rinses, salivary substitutes and sialogogues.

KS is the most common HIV-related oral malignancy, with the majority arising on the palate. This tumour can also appear on the gingiva (**Figure 23.4**) or oropharynx.

Non-Hodgkin's lymphoma (NHL) may also arise in the oral cavity. In AIDS patients, NHL is usually a poor prognostic indicator of disease progression. Recurrences are common despite chemotherapy and radiation. The lesions may present as ulcerative lesions, but typically appear red and exophytic. They usually involve the gingiva and alveolar ridges and may arise from Waldeyer's ring.[25]

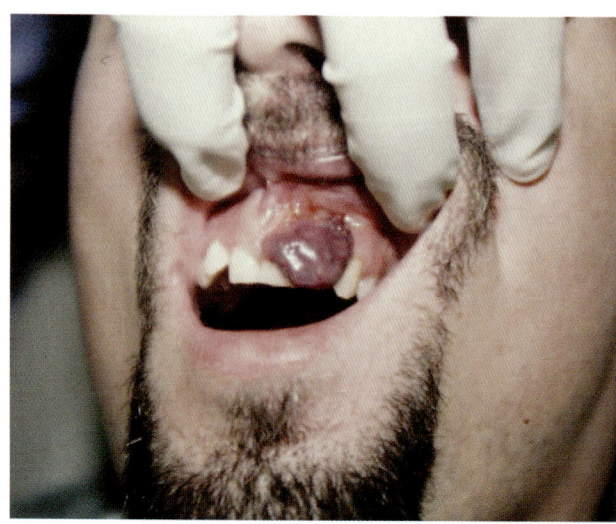

Figure 23.4 The gingival is a common site for presentation of Kaposi's sarcoma.

TABLE 23.1 Characteristics and treatment of the most common oral manifestations of HIV

Disease		Management	Comment
Gingival disease	Can develop gingival tissue loss, tooth loosening/loss, bone exposure	Best treatment is frequent dental cleanings, flossing, etc. Aggressive antibiotics and/or surgical management when advanced	Common in HIV. Requires close dental evaluations and frequent management
Oral thrush	Pseudomembranous candidiasis: • Typical plaque-like lesions • Atrophic form with erythematous lesions on palate, buccal mucosa, tongue • Angular cheilitis	Topical agents such as clotrimazole. Systemic agents (e.g. fluconazole) for refractory cases in patients with advanced disease	Prolonged or frequent use of fluconazole increases risk of azole-resistance candidiasis
Oral aphthous ulcers	Lesions may be large. Biopsy confirms non-neoplastic, non-viral aetiology	Topical steroid therapy. Intra-lesional or systemic steroids. Thalidomide. Antiretroviral therapy	Are usually difficult to treat. Produce severe pain, odynophagia. Often cause substantial morbidity
Kaposi's sarcoma	Typically on hard, soft palate. Occasionally on gingival, buccal mucosa	Symptomatic relief. When functionally problematic, low-dose radiotherapy or intra-lesional vinblastine or systemic chemotherapy	
Radiation mucositis	Side effect of treatment for other oral lesions	Topical therapy (steroids, antifungals, etc.) Supportive care – nutrition, pain management, hydration	Can result even from low doses of radiation
Hairy leukoplakia	Usually occurs on side of tongue. Probably Epstein-Barr virus related	No treatment necessary if asymptomatic	Must be differentiated from other more serious oral disorders

Table 23.1 reviews the characteristics and treatment of many of the most common oral manifestations of HIV disease.

PHARYNX, LARYNX AND OESOPHAGUS

Many of the same processes that affect the oral cavity can also affect the larynx and pharynx. Many of these processes present with similar symptoms: odynophagia, dysphagia and in some cases, chest pain. Correctly identifying and treating these processes can not only provide symptomatic relief but also in many cases help in dealing with the wasting and malnutrition that can occur.

Candidiasis of the oesophagus and pharynx can cause severe dysphagia, odynophagia and weight loss. Laryngeal infection presents as hoarseness and in severe cases stridor and shortness of breath. Barium swallow will show an irregular cobblestone surface to the mucosa. Direct visualization can be obtained with panendoscopy and biopsy will exclude KS. Treatment is with systemic fluconazole.

Cytomegalovirus is the second most common infectious ulcerative condition of the upper aerodigestive tract. Of patients who fail empirical antifungal therapy, approximately one-third will have CMV ulcerations.[26, 27] These ulcers tend to occur more commonly in the distal oesophagus with a raised indurated border and necrotic base. While occasionally occurring as solitary ulcers, CMV can also form multiple or diffuse ulcerations and lacking any defined pathognomonic appearance. Unfortunately, other than biopsy and culture, there are also no disease specific clinical characteristics that differentiate this from other forms of ulcerative oesophagitis. Once the diagnosis has been established, treatment can be instituted using intravenous ganciclovir or foscarnet.

Herpes simplex viral infection in the pharynx, larynx or oesophagus can present with similar symptoms as oesophageal and laryngeal candidiasis. Examination reveals discrete vesicles with mucosal ulceration. Biopsy and viral culture of lesions confirm diagnosis. The occurrence of HSV is usually associated with significant immune dysfunction, usually occurring only when the CD4 level is well below 100/mm[28] Treatment usually starts with intravenous acyclovir followed by oral agents.

Idiopathic oesophageal ulcer arises with the same frequency as CMV oesophagitis. Its aetiology is unclear and there is usually no associated specific infectious aetiology. These lesions also usually occur with severe immunocompromise. The endoscopic appearance is similar to CMV lesions, often with solitary, large ulcerations with raised indurated margins. Treatment has been effective using systemic steroids.[29] Successful treatment has also been described with thalidomide.[30]

Kaposi's sarcoma can present primarily in the pharynx and/or larynx or extend to adjacent areas including the oral cavity. Oesophageal KS may present with dysphagia or odynophagia. Laryngeal lesions may present as shortness of breath, hoarseness or severe airway compromise.

SALIVARY GLANDS

Both major and minor salivary glands can be involved in disease processes in the HIV-infected individual. The most common complaint is xerostomia.

Lymphoepithelial cysts is a disease process that is almost diagnostic of HIV infection. Lymphoepithelial cysts present as progressive parotid swellings, which are usually multiple, bilateral and non-tender (**Figures 23.5** and **23.6**).

Facial nerve dysfunction should lead the physician to suspect a malignant neoplasm. Fine-needle aspiration

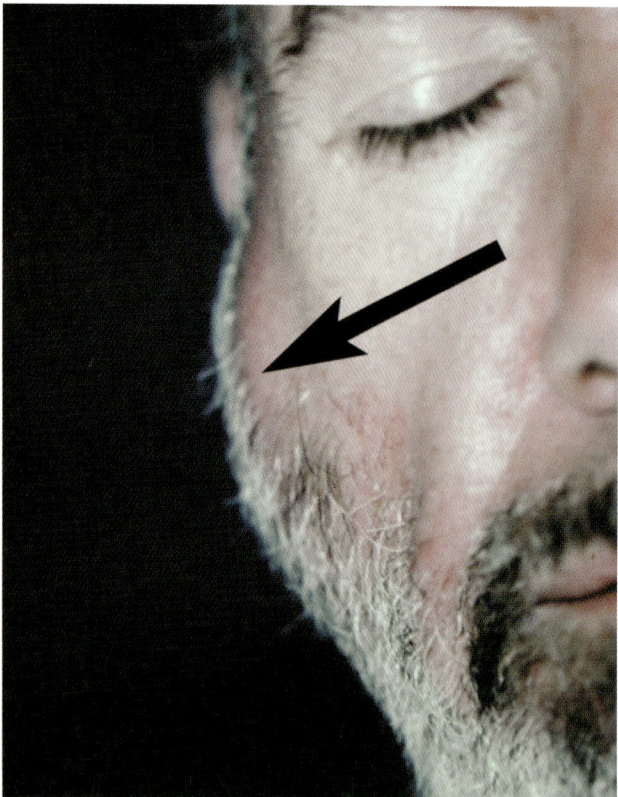

Figure 23.5 The most common etiology of an asymptomatic parotid mass in the HIV-infected patient is the lymphoepithelial cyst (arrow).

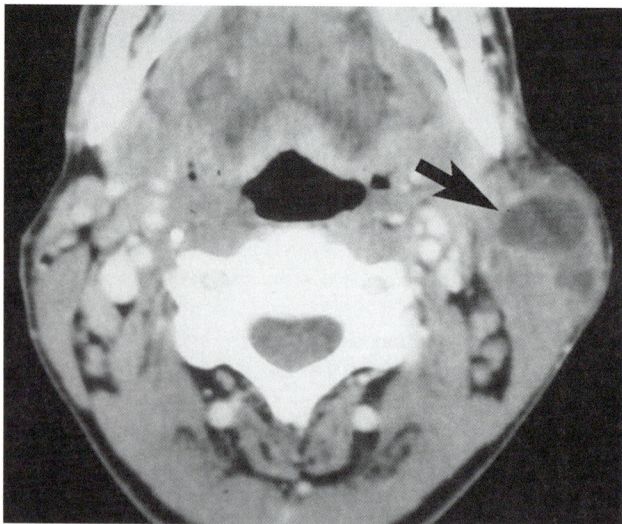

Figure 23.6 This axial CT scan demonstrates the typical findings (arrow) of a benign parotid lymphoepithelial cyst.

reveals fluid with lymphocytes and squamous epithelial cells. Computed tomography or ultrasound imaging will show multiple thin walled cysts in the parotid gland. With fine-needle aspiration biopsy (FNAB) and imaging, open biopsies or surgical excision for diagnosis is rarely indicated. The cysts usually resolve with HAART and surgery is only necessary for enlarged lesions that are a cosmetic challenge or where the diagnosis is equivocal. Needle aspiration of cyst contents is ineffective for long-term cure as recurrence almost always happens.[31] In patients not receiving HAART, slerotherapy with alcohol or sodium morrhuate can be effective.[32,33]

> **KEY POINTS**
>
> - HIV infection continues to be a global health problem.
> - Infection with the Human Immunodeficiency Virus leads to immunosuppression, opportunistic infections and Acquired Immunodeficiency Syndrome.
> - Highly active anti-retroviral therapy (a combination of various anti-retroviral agents) is an effective treatment for HIV infection.
> - Otolaryngologists should test for HIV infection whenever it enters the differential diagnosis.
> - ENT manifestations of HIV infection are very common.
> - Kaposi's sarcoma is a malignant tumour caused by the co-infection of HIV and Human Herpes Virus 8.

REFERENCES

1. Joint United Nations Programme on HIV/AIDS (UNAIDS). *Global Report: UNAIDS report on the global AIDS epidemic 2012*. ISBN 9789291739967 (Printed version).
2. *Kenya AIDS Indicator Survey (KAIS) 2007*. Available from http://www.prb.org/pdf09/kaiskenyadatasheet.pdf
3. Health Protection Agency. *HIV in the UK: 2012 report*. London: Health Protection Services. Available from http://www.medfash.org.uk/uploads/images/file/HIV%20annual%20report%202012.pdf
4. McElrath MJ, Pruett JE, Cohn ZA. Mononuclear phagocytes of blood and bone marrow: comparative roles as viral reservoirs in human immunodeficiency virus type 1 infections. *P Natl Acad Sci USA* 1989; **86**: 675–79.
5. Witiak DG, Tami TA. AIDS and otolaryngology. In: English GM (ed). *Otolaryngology*. Philadelphia: Lippincott, Williams and Wilkins; Chapter 63.
6. Health Protection Agency (HPA), Centre for Infections. The UK Collaborative Group for HIV and STI Surveillance. *Testing times. HIV and other sexually transmitted infections in the United Kingdom: 2007*. Available from http://webarchive.nationalarchives.gov.uk/20140714084352/http://www.hpa.org.uk/web/HPAweb&HPAwebStandard/HPAweb_C/1203084355941
7. British HIV Association. *UK National Guidelines for HIV Testing 2008*. Available from http://www.bhiva.org/HIV-testing-guidelines.aspx
8. Moyer VA. Screening for HIV: US Preventative Services Task Force recommendation statement. *Ann Intern Med* 2013; **159**: 51–60.
9. Chang Y, Cesarman E, Pessin, et al. Identification of herpesvirus-like DNA sequences in AIDS-associated Kaposi's sarcoma. *Science* 1994; **266**: 1865–9.
10. Nobler MP, Leddy ME, Huh SH. The impact of palliative irradiation on the management of patients with acquired immune deficiency syndrome. *J Clin Oncol* 1987; **5**(1): 107–12.
11. Munoz A, Martinez-Chamorro E. Necrotizing external otitis caused by Aspergillus fumigatus: computed tomography and high resolution magnetic resonance imaging in an AIDS patient. *J Laryngol Otol* 1998; **112**: 98–102.
12. Dropulic LK, Leslie JM, Eldred LJ, et al. Clinical manifestations and risk factors of Pseudomonas aeriginosa infection in patients with AIDS. *J Infect Dis* 1995; **171**: 930–37.
13. Weinroth SE, Schessel D, Tuazon CU. Malignant otitis externa in AIDS patients: case report and review of literature. *Ear Nose Throat J* 1994; **73**: 772–74, 777–78.

14. Rinaldo A, Brandwein MS, Devaney KO, Ferlito A. AIDS related otological lesions. *Acta Otolaryngol* 2003; **123**: 672–74.
15. Cho YS, Lee HS, Kim SW, et al. Tuberculous otitis media: a clinical and radiologic analysis of 52 patients. *Laryngoscope* 2006; **116**: 921–27.
16. Singh B. Role of surgery in tuberculous mastoiditis. *J Laryngol Otol* 1991; **105**: 907–15.
17. Viehman JA, Khalil DM, Barhoma C, Hanna RM. Mycobacterium avium-intracellulare otomastoiditis in a young AIDS patient: case report and review of the literature. *HIV AIDS* 2013; **5**: 61–66.
18. Van der Westhuizen Y, Swanepoel de W, Heinze B, Hofmeyr LM. Auditory and otological manifestations in adults with HIV/AIDS. *Int J Audiol* 2013; **52**: 37–43.
19. Lin C, Lin SW, Weng SF, Lin YS. Increased risk of sudden sensorineural hearing loss in patients with human immunodeficiency virus aged 18 to 35 years: a population-based cohort study. *JAMA Otolaryngol Head Neck Surg* 2013; **139**: 251–55.
20. Abboud O, Saliba I. Isolated bilateral facial paralysis revealing AIDS: a unique presentation. *Laryngoscope* 2008; **118**: 580–84.
21. Tami TA, Wawrose S. Diseases of the nose and paranasal sinus in the human immunodeficiency virus-infected population. *Otolaryng Clin N Am* 1992; **25**: 1199–210.
22. Wawrose SF, Tami TA, Amoils CP. The role of guaifenesin in the treatment of sinonasal disease in patients infected with the human immunodeficiency virus (HIV). *Laryngoscope* 1992; **102**: 1225–28.
23. Friedman M, Brenski A, Taylor L. Treatment of aphthous ulcers in AIDS patients. *Laryngoscope* 1994; **104**: 566–70.
24. Dichtel WJ. Oral manifestations of human immunodeficiency virus infection. *Otolaryng Clin N Am* 1992; **25**: 1211–24.
25. Finn DG. Lymphoma of the head and neck and acquired immunodeficiency syndrome: clinical investigation and immunohistological study. *Laryngoscope* 1995; **105**: 1–18.
26. Parente F, Cernuschi M, Rizzardini G. Opportunistic infections of the esophagus not responding to oral systemic antifungals in patients with AIDS: their frequency and treatment. *Am J Gastroenterol* 1991; **86**: 1729–34.
27. Wilcox CM, Straub RF, Schwartz DA. Prospective endoscopic characterization of cytomegalovirus esophagitis in AIDS. *Gastrointest Endosc* 1994; **40**: 481–84.
28. Genereau T, Lortholary O, Bouchaud O, et al. Herpes simplex esophagitis in patients with AIDS: report of 34 cases. The Cooperative Study Group on Herpetic Esophagitis in HIV Infection. *Clin Infect Dis* 1996; **22**: 926–31.
29. Kotler DP, Reka S, Orenstein JM, Fox CH. Chronic idiopathic esophageal ulceration in the acquired immunodeficiency syndrome: characterization and treatment with corticosteroids. *J Clin Gastroenterol* 1992; **15**: 284–90.
30. Jacobson JM, Spritzler J, Fox L, et al. Thalidomide for the treatment of esophageal aphthous ulcers in patients with human immunodeficiency virus infection. National Institute of Allergy and Infectious Disease AIDS Clinical Trials Group. *J Infect Dis* 1999; **180**: 61–67.
31. Echavez MI, Lee KC, Sooy CD. Tetracycline sclerosis for treatment of benign lymphoepithelial cysts of the parotid gland in patients infected with human immunodeficiency virus. *Laryngoscope* 1994; **104**: 1499–502.
32. Meyer E, Lubbe DE, Fagan JJ. Alcohol sclerotherapy of human immunodeficiency virus related parotid lymphoepithelial cysts. *J Laryngol Otol* 2009; **123**: 422–25.
33. Marcus A, Moore CE. Sodium morrhuate sclerotherapy for the treatment of benign lymphoepithelial cysts of the parotid gland in the HIV patient. *Laryngoscope* 2005; **115**: 746–49.

Haematology

CHAPTER 24

BLOOD GROUPS, BLOOD COMPONENTS AND ALTERNATIVES TO TRANSFUSION

Samah Alimam, Kate Pendry and Michael F. Murphy

Introduction 239
Blood donation 240
Blood groups 240
Blood grouping and crossmatch process 241
Planning for surgery 241
Emergencies 242
Blood components 243
Transfusion reactions 244
Reversal of anticoagulation 246
Alternatives to blood transfusions 246
Jehovah's witnesses 247
References 248
Further reading 248

SEARCH STRATEGY

Data in this chapter may be updated by a Medline search using the keywords: transfusion, components, alternatives, blood sparing and adverse events.

INTRODUCTION

Surgical specialties are responsible for the transfusion of up to 40% of blood and blood components in the UK. It is therefore imperative for those in surgical practice to have a sound understanding of the principles of safe transfusion, the appropriate use of blood and measures for blood avoidance (**Box 24.1**).

The UK has been successful at improving the safety of blood and blood component transfusion over the last 25 years. The risk of death has dropped to under 3 in 1 000 000 per blood components issued, since the serious hazards of transfusion (SHOT) scheme started in 1996.

BOX 24.1 Principles of safe and appropriate transfusion

1. Do not just act on numbers. Not all anaemic patients need transfusing – consider the patient's symptoms, comorbidities and possible treatable underlying cause.
2. Transfuse based on clinical assessment and evidence-guided practice.
3. Involve the patient in the decision to transfuse (or not) and obtain consent.
4. Ensure the right blood is transfused to the right patient at the right time in the right place and for the right indication.

This reduction has been largely due to increased awareness of the hazards of transfusion, better screening of donors and improvements in the processing of blood and its components. A frequently encountered error in blood transfusion remains that of ABO incompatibility as a consequence of clerical error. Examples of this and other transfusion complications will be covered later in the chapter.

Blood is used in the management of anaemia, in surgical blood loss and in patients with acute massive haemorrhage. However, blood and its components are a scarce resource both within the UK and worldwide. Only 5% of eligible adults in the UK are blood donors, and this valuable resource needs to be used in a responsible and safe manner.

In relation to ENT surgery, a retrospective review of transfusion in patients undergoing sinus surgery in Germany found that only 0.46% of these patients actually needed a transfusion; this likely represents excellence in surgical techniques and patient management to avoid blood transfusion.[1] A study in the United States concluded that transfusion is no longer necessary during routine bimaxillary orthognathic surgery. Patients requiring double-jaw procedures are often the ENT patients most likely to require a blood transfusion.[2]

BLOOD DONATION

Extensive screening of altruistic, unpaid volunteers has been a major factor in the provision of safe blood in the UK. First-time donors in the UK have to be between the ages of 17 and 65 years, minimum weight of 50 kg, in good health and undergo a thorough health questionnaire and screening programme to exclude high-risk donors. There is no upper age limit for donors but after the age of 66 years, donors are required to undergo an annual review. Male donors can donate blood every 12 weeks up to a maximum of four donations in 12 months. Female donors can donate every 16 weeks up to three times a year. The minimum haemoglobin concentration (Hb) required for donation is 125 g/L for female and 135 g/l for male donors (for full eligibility criteria consult https://www.blood.co.uk).

Following thorough cleaning of the skin at the needle entry point, blood is collected into a sterile bag containing anticoagulant and preservative. It is labelled with the donor details and transported to a blood centre where it is processed. Whole blood is filtered and then separated into its blood components. Filtration eliminates leucocytes, which are associated with several complications of transfusion including febrile (non-haemolytic) transfusion reactions, human leukocyte antigen (HLA) alloimmunization and transmission of cytomegalovirus (CMV). Leucocyte depletion was introduced as a variant Creutzfeldt–Jakob disease (vCJD) risk reduction measure and the other effects were a useful by-product of this decision. From each unit of blood donated, red cells, platelets, fresh frozen plasma and cryoprecipitate can be obtained.

A sample from the donor on each occasion is tested for blood-borne viruses and syphilis (Table 24.1). Platelets undergo bacteriological testing requiring incubation for 36 hours to exclude any significant bacteria before release.

Due to concerns regarding the transmission of vCJD by blood transfusion, universal leucocyte-reduction of blood components was implemented in the UK in 1999. In addition, a number of restrictions on blood donors were put in place to reduce the risk of transmission. Individuals are restricted from donating if they have:

- previously received a blood transfusion after 1980
- received human pituitary-derived hormones, graft of human dura mater, cornea, sclera or other ocular tissue
- come from a family at risk of inherited prion disease
- been notified that they are at risk of vCJD due to exposure to infected individual via blood transfusion, transplanted tissue or surgical instruments
- been notified they are at risk because a recipient of their blood or tissue has developed a prion-related disease

Additionally, individuals born after 1996 who require plasma products are only transfused with non-UK plasma.

BLOOD GROUPS

There are more than 300 blood groups with around 23 being clinically significant. The most important are the ABO and RhD groups because of their association with haemolytic transfusion reactions and haemolytic disease of the newborn. However, some patients especially those who are multi-transfused may develop antibodies against other blood group antigens and thus it is important to look beyond the ABO and RhD in patients requiring transfusion.

ABO group

The ABO grouping of blood was first recognized in 1901 by Landsteiner. The ABO system is the most important because of the presence of naturally occurring anti-A and anti-B antibodies, which develop in the first months of life. The ABO system consists of three allelic genes – A, B and O – and each of these is responsible for production of antigens on the surface of red blood cells (Table 24.2). ABO incompatible transfusions are very serious because anti-A and anti-B are IgM antibodies causing intravascular haemolysis activation of coagulation and cytokines resulting in major morbidity and mortality. In the UK, blood group O is commonest, found in 47% of the population. Historically, blood group O individuals were considered to be universal donors and AB universal recipients. As a result, Group O, RhD negative blood is often used in emergency situations. Group O RhD negative blood is in short supply, consequently except in true emergencies it is desirable to establish the ABO and RhD group of emergency patients to ensure group specific blood is issued. Group AB is the rarest group in the UK and due to lack of donors they are often given group A or B blood.

TABLE 24.1 Screening for infectious agents

Routine screening of donor blood	Further screening may include (depending on travel history):
• Hepatitis B • Hepatitis C • Human immunodeficiency virus • Human T cell lymphotropic virus • Syphilis	• Malaria • West Nile virus • Trypanosoma cruzi

TABLE 24.2 ABO groups

Blood group	Antigen	Antibody	UK frequency %
O	None	Anti A, Anti B	47
A	A	Anti B	42
B	B	Anti A	8
AB	AB	None	3

Rh antigens

The Rh system was discovered later by Landsteiner and Weiner in 1940. The RhD antigen is the most important, although others do also exist (Cc and Ee). The RhD gene maybe either absent or present (i.e. RhD+ or RhD−); 85% of the UK population is RhD+. Rh antibodies are IgG antibodies causing extra-vascular haemolysis. They do not occur naturally but as a result of sensitization secondary to transfusion or pregnancy. The commonest significant event is that of a RhD− mother, developing an antibody as a result of carrying a RhD+ foetus. If not addressed, this can result in the fatal haemolytic disease of the newborn or hydrops fetalis. The UK programme of antenatal administration of anti-D for the prevention of RhD immunization in pregnancy and postpartum has reduced its incidence. However, it is imperative that all RhD− women of childbearing age only receive RhD− blood components.

BLOOD GROUPING AND CROSSMATCH PROCESS

Compatibility testing is carried out in accredited hospital blood transfusion laboratories by trained biomedical scientists. There is now increasing use of automated processes but there is still an important role for the clinical scientist.

As previously mentioned, the first step is determination of the ABO and RhD groups of the recipient: 'blood grouping'. This is rapid and can be done in less than 15 minutes. Once a patient is grouped an antibody screen is performed to identify any clinically significant red cell antibodies; this process takes up to 45 minutes in total. If the antibody screen is positive, the blood group specificity of the antibodies should be identified by testing the patient's plasma against panels of red cells with a wide range of known blood group antigens.

The full crossmatch takes up to 60 minutes and involves testing the patient's plasma against a sample of the donor red cells to be transfused. In many hospitals this serological crossmatch has been omitted as a negative antibody screen makes it highly unlikely that there will be any incompatibility with the donor units. A greater risk is that of a transfusion error involving the collection of the patient sample or a mix-up of samples in the laboratory. Laboratories can use their information system to check the records of the patient and authorize the release of the donor units (computer or electronic crossmatching/issue).

Electronic blood issue, as described above, can be extended to issue previously unallocated blood at blood fridges remote from the main laboratory ('remote blood issue'). This is possible using blood fridges electronically linked to the blood transfusion laboratory information system. The printing of compatibility labels for the blood and its collection are under electronic control using the same rules as electronic issue from the main laboratory. Issue of blood using this process reduces the time it takes to provide blood for patients needing it urgently, particularly at hospitals without a blood transfusion laboratory because transport of blood from the central laboratory is not required.

In an emergency it is possible to provide group specific blood (same ABO and RhD groups as the patient) within a few minutes and follow this up with a full crossmatch. If time is short it is possible to administer group O blood, and for women of childbearing age this must also be RhD negative.

In elective surgical patients, blood grouping and antibody screening can be done weeks in advance of surgery. The British Committee for Standards in Haematology (BCSH) guidelines[3] recommend a second sample be tested for confirmation of ABO group for all patients undergoing transfusion for the first time. With regards to the timing of pre-transfusion compatibility testing the following is recommended:

1. Samples should not be more than 3 days old in those who have been transfused or pregnant within last 3 months.
2. An extension to 7 days can be considered for those regularly transfused or pregnant women with no significant alloantibodies.

PLANNING FOR SURGERY

Many operations can take place without the need for transfusions. Blood transfusion laboratories can issue blood and blood components rapidly if there is unexpectedly large bleeding, and there is rarely a need to provide large numbers of units in advance.

It is important in elective surgical procedures to optimize the patient's Hb prior to surgery to minimize the need for transfusion. If there is evidence of anaemia this should be investigated and treated pre-operatively. Thirty per cent of patients found to be anaemic pre-operatively are iron deficient; this can be corrected with oral iron or, in patients who are intolerant to oral iron or those that have a short pre-operative period, intravenous iron can be used.

Maximum surgical blood ordering system (MSBOS)

In surgical procedures that have a high probability of requiring transfusion, an MSBOS should be agreed between the surgical team and transfusion laboratory. This must specify the number of units of each blood component that should be reserved routinely guided by evidenced based practice (Table 24.3). The recommended aim is to have a crossmatched to transfused ratio of <2:1 with regular review and audit of actual blood use.

TABLE 24.3 Examples of MSBOS

Surgical procedure	MSBOS
Tumour of palate	Group and Save only
Laryngectomy	2 units
Radical neck dissection	2 units
Commando	4 units

EMERGENCIES

Emergency requests for blood require clear communication between the clinical team and laboratory staff. If there is a massive haemorrhage (i.e. blood loss greater than 50% of patients' blood volume in 3 hours or more than one total blood volume within 24 hours or greater than 150ml per minute associated with shock), the 'massive haemorrhage protocol' must be activated. **Figure 24.1** gives an example of such a protocol. Early recognition and intervention to stop bleeding is vital for patient survival. It is important for the clinical team to liaise closely with the

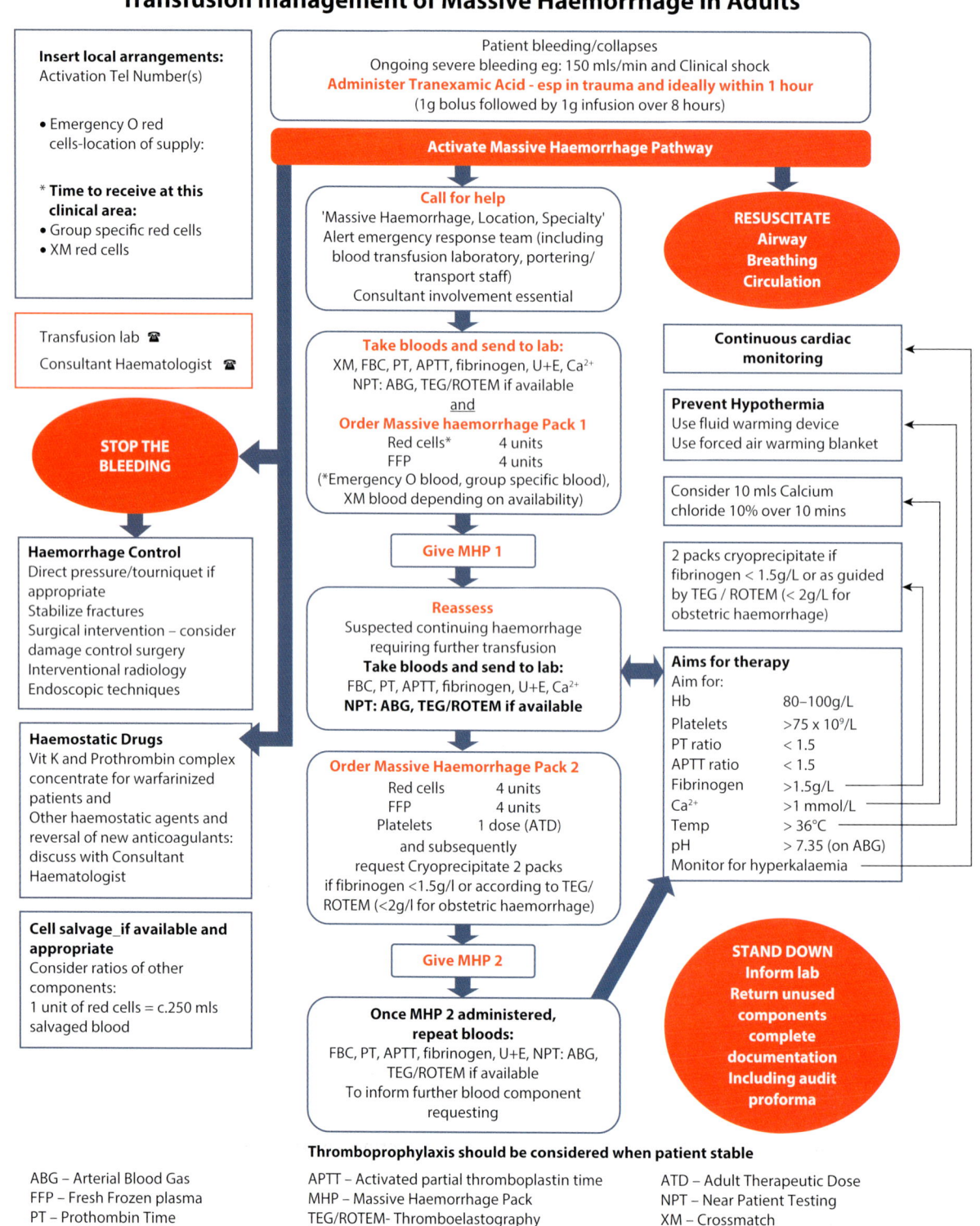

Figure 24.1 Suggested algorithm for management of massive haemorrhage. (Adapted from the North West Massive Hemorrhage tool kit with permission from Dr Kate Pendry.)

blood transfusion laboratory and ensure the appropriate products are requested, issued and administered rapidly. Close monitoring of haemostasis is essential as a massive transfusion can result in platelet and coagulation factor depletion especially of fibrinogen, which will require replacement.

BLOOD COMPONENTS

Whole blood is composed of a number of components that are separated during blood processing in transfusion centres. Whole blood is not used in modern clinical practice and use of individual components makes for more efficient and safer therapy. Figure 24.2 outlines the different components of blood and their preparation.

Red blood cells (RBC)

Red blood cells are responsible for the transport of oxygen. Transfusion of RBC is indicated in massive haemorrhage, symptomatic anaemia, after chemotherapy and in chronic haematological conditions. ABO and RhD compatibility are essential for safe transfusion as described above. RBC are stored at 2–6 °C for up to 35 days. Irradiated blood, which is required for immunocompromised individuals at risk of transfusion-associated graft versus host disease (TA-GVHD), has a shorter shelf life of 14 days. It is important for the clinical team to inform the transfusion laboratory of this requirement. TA-GVHD is explained in more detail later in this chapter.

There is no universal agreed trigger for the transfusion of RBC, and it is important to be aware of local guidelines. Patients must be assessed clinically for symptoms of anaemia or bleeding. Emphasis must be on clinical evaluation over correction based purely on numbers. A Cochrane review has recommended evaluated transfusion triggers and recommended target haemoglobin of 70 to 80 g/L and the transfusion of 1 unit followed by assessment of the patient's response. This current trend in practice favours restrictive rather than liberal transfusion; the groundbreaking TRICC study[4] reported no significant difference in 30-day mortality in critically ill patients who were randomized to either a restrictive or liberal transfusion strategy. Additionally the group was able to demonstrate a benefit in outcomes in younger patients who received the restrictive transfusions.[4] The recommendation that followed from this trial changed critical care practice, as now unless contraindicated the recommended policy is not to transfuse until haemoglobin has fallen below 70 g/L aiming for a target haemoglobin of 70 to 90 g/L. This restrictive transfusion practice has received support from other randomized controlled trials in cardiac surgery and acute upper gastrointestinal haemorrhage and is now widely adopted throughout clinical practice. The only exceptions to this are patients with acute cardiac ischaemia and those on long-term transfusion programmes, for example thalassaemia and myelodysplastic syndrome, who may have a trigger haemoglobin of 80 g/L or greater to maintain a good quality of life (this should be discussed with the haematologist).

Platelets

Platelets are central to haemostasis. Platelet transfusions may be needed in patients with thrombocytopenia or platelet function disorders. Platelet concentrates are prepared either by centrifuging whole blood or from a single donor via plateletpheresis using a cell separator. Platelets are stored at 22 °C in an incubator that is constantly agitated for optimal platelet storage. Platelets have a shelf life of 7 days following the recent introduction of bacterial screening in the UK.

Platelets have ABO antigens on their surface and ideally should be ABO compatible. Although adverse reactions are rare, the survival time may be reduced if there is an ABO mismatch. As with RBC, only RhD negative platelets should be given to women of childbearing age. Irradiated platelets should be administered to those at risk of transfusion-associated graft-versus-host disease TA-GVHD. Platelets express HLA antigens and some patients with HLA antibodies fail to increase their platelet counts with platelets from random donors and require HLA-matched platelets. If HLA-matched platelets are required, early recognition is necessary as advance notice is required to identify compatible donors.

It is important to investigate the cause of thrombocytopenia to determine if it is autoimmune, secondary to bone marrow failure, drug-induced or secondary to platelet sequestration in the spleen or consumption, for example, in disseminated intra-vascular coagulation (DIC). In a haemodynamically stable patient with ear, nose or throat bleed with bleeding associated with thrombocytopenia or a platelet function disorder, it is important to consider

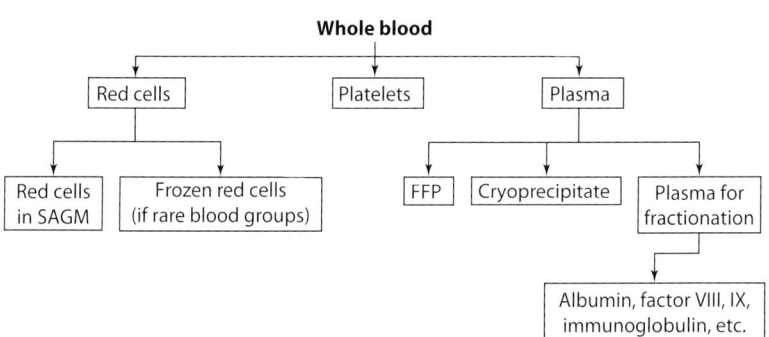

Figure 24.2 Blood components and products derived from whole blood.

Procedure where platelet threshold is greater than 50	Procedures where platelet threshold is greater than 100
• Lumbar puncture • Gastroscopy and biopsy • Insertion of indwelling lines • Transbronchial biopsy • Liver biopsy • Laparotomy or similar procedures	• Ocular region • Neurosurgery *Spinal anaesthesia requires platelet count >80*

TABLE 24.4 Examples of platelet thresholds

measures such as tranexamic acid or surgical repair of bleed as well as a platelet transfusion.

The BCSH guidelines (2003)[5] suggest the thresholds for platelets in surgical and medical procedures as outlined in **Table 24.4**. However, transfusion of platelets must be assessed on an individual basis taking into consideration clinical factors and the presence or absence of other disorders of haemostasis. After a platelet transfusion it is important to assess whether it has been effective in stopping bleeding (if it was administered to a patient with thrombocytopenic bleeding) and perform a repeat sample 15–30 minutes later to determine its effect on the platelet count.

Platelets are relatively contraindicated in patients with thrombotic thrombocytopenic purpura and heparin-induced thrombocytopenia due to increased thrombotic risk. However, in bleeding patients with these conditions, it is advised to discuss the patients with a haematologist.

Fresh frozen plasma (FFP)

Fresh frozen plasma is derived from whole blood through centrifugation; it is rich in coagulation factors. FFP must be ABO compatible because of the presence of anti-A and anti-B in the plasma. FFP is indicated for the treatment of coagulation factor deficiency where a suitable factor concentrate is not available, coagulopathy associated with liver disease, massive haemorrhage and DIC. The usual dose is 12–15 ml/kg. FFP is no longer recommended for the reversal of warfarin. Reversal of warfarin and the newer anticoagulants will be covered later in the chapter. The response to FFP can be monitored by measuring the patient's prothrombin time and activated partial thromboplastin time.

FFP is frozen at −25 °C to maintain the activity of the coagulation factors and can be stored for up to 36 months. When requested it must be thawed, which can take up to 30 minutes. Once thawed it can be stored at 4 °C for 24 hours. In the UK, children born after 1 January 1996 should receive FFP from countries with a low risk of vCJD; the preparation provided in the UK is also treated with methylene blue, which inactivates bacteria and viruses.

Solvent detergent plasma, which is prepared from more than 1000 donation pools of plasma, undergoes pathogen inactivation including bacteria and viruses such as hepatitis B and C and HIV. Donations are sourced from countries at low risk of vCJD. As it is pooled, the concentration of coagulation factors is more standardized.

It is recommended for patients who have thrombotic thrombocytopenic purpura.

Cryoprecipitate

Cryoprecipitate is made from thawing FFP at 4 °C. It is rich in fibrinogen, factor VIII and von Willebrand factor. It is used as source of fibrinogen, especially in massive haemorrhage where fibrinogen concentration is less than 1.5 g/l. The recommended dose is two pools of 5 units (1 unit per 5–10 kg body weight). Cryoprecipitate is stored at −25 °C and has a shelf life of 36 months. Once thawed, it must be used within 4 hours.

TRANSFUSION REACTIONS

All transfusion-associated reactions and errors should be reported to the transfusion laboratory and/or hospital transfusion committee, who report them to the national haemovigilance scheme, serious hazards of transfusion (SHOT). SHOT produces an annual report with recommendations about transfusion safety, which is accessible online. In 2012, 62% of the errors reported to SHOT were secondary to preventable mistakes in the transfusion process, highlighting the scale of the problem (**Figure 24.3**).[6] Blood sampling errors resulting in 'wrong blood in tube' continue to be a major preventable problem that can result in ABO-incompatible red cell transfusions with severe consequences.

Although not a drug, blood and its components should be treated as such. Blood products should be prescribed and administered by trained individuals. Patients should be transfused in areas where they can be directly monitored; observations should be performed and documented before transfusion, after 15 minutes to detect any immediate transfusion reaction, and at the end of transfusion. Transfusions should generally be avoided overnight unless they are urgently needed.

Acute transfusion reactions

These present within 24 hours of the transfusion and vary in severity. The diagnosis of an acute transfusion reaction can be challenging especially in the acutely unwell patient. As acute transfusion reactions can have profound morbidity, it is essential for the clinical staff to recognize them and respond promptly. **Box 24.2** summarizes a suggested approach to acute transfusion reactions:

SEVERE ACUTE TRANSFUSION REACTIONS

Immediate haemolytic transfusion reaction

Immediate haemolytic transfusion reactions are the most severe transfusion reactions caused by acute haemolysis secondary to destruction of donor red blood cells by IgM complement-fixing antibodies present in the recipient's serum, usually anti-A and/or anti-B. These antibodies can result in rapid intravascular destruction of donor red blood cells. It can also result in activation of coagulation and

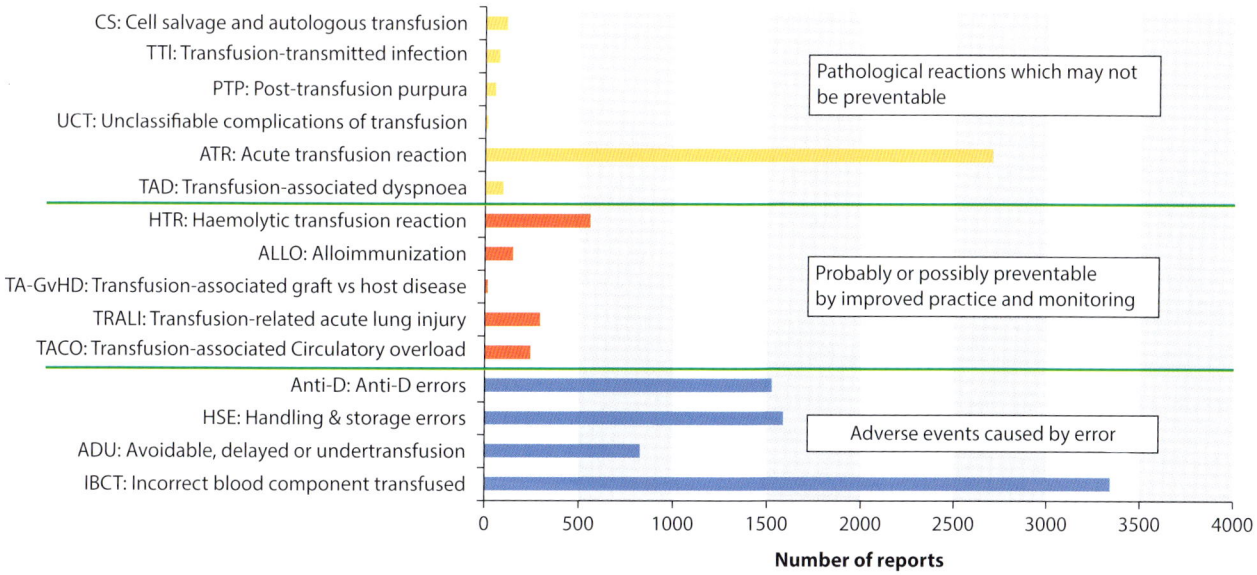

Figure 24.3 Cumulative data from SHOT reports 1996–2012.

BOX 24.2 Approach to management of an acute transfusion reaction

1. Stop the transfusion.
2. Assess patient: Airway, Breathing and Circulation.
3. Maintain venous access with physiological saline.
4. Check the identification of the patient and compatibility of the blood component.
5. Inspect the component for clumps or discolorations (important in platelets).
6. Assess for evidence of blood loss.
7. Unless mild allergic or febrile reaction, perform full blood count, renal and liver screen, blood culture if temperature rise, direct Coombs test, repeat group and screen urine for haemoglobinuria.
8. Inform the transfusion laboratory.
9. Unless mild allergic or febrile reaction, return the blood components to the transfusion laboratory.
10. Report to SHOT.

release of cytokines and cause renal failure and disseminated intravascular coagulation. It is commonly caused by human clerical error and occurs in around 1 in 180 000 red cells transfused. Features include pain at infusion site, chest and back pain, hypotension and haemoglobinuria. Mortality can be as high as 10%.

Bacterial contamination

Although a rare complication of transfusion, it may be fatal. The patient becomes acutely unwell, pyrexial, hypotensive and may develop septic shock. The actions that should be taken when a bacterial contamination of blood is suspected include checking the appearance of the contents of the transfused component; there may be clots or purple discoloration of red cells, platelets may have clumps or green discoloration. Blood cultures should be taken immediately and the patient commenced on broad spectrum antibiotics. The component should be returned to the transfusion laboratory for microbiological testing and the transfusion service should be informed so that other components from the same donor can be recalled.

Anaphylaxis

Severe anaphylaxis following transfusion is very rare but can be fatal. Symptoms may include wheeze, stridor and angioedema. Flushing and urticaria may occur in less severe reactions. Immediate resuscitation is imperative with administration of intramuscular adrenaline, intravenous chlorpheniramine and intravenous hydrocortisone. If further transfusions are needed, management should be discussed with the immunologist and haematologist.

Transfusion-related acute lung injury (TRALI)

TRALI typically occurs after transfusion of platelets or FFP. It has been the commonest cause of severe morbidity and mortality after transfusion. It is due to anti-leucocyte antibodies in the donor plasma reacting with the recipient's neutrophils, monocytes and pulmonary endothelium. Severe hypoxia may develop immediately or at the latest within 6 hours of the transfusion and be associated with hypotension and bilateral lung infiltrates. It is important to differentiate TRALI from acute respiratory distress syndrome and pulmonary oedema. Treatment is supportive with high flow oxygen and ventilator support if required.

Transfusion-associated circulatory overload (TACO)

This is a common adverse effect of transfusion in older patients and those with history of cardiac disease. It is often not diagnosed in a timely manner. It is defined as acute or worsening pulmonary oedema within 6 hours of transfusion.

Features include dyspnoea, tachycardia, hypertension and a positive fluid balance. Treatment involves stopping transfusion, administering oxygen and diuretics. TACO can be avoided by careful assessment of its risk factors and appropriate measures for its avoidance such as co-administration of diuretics and the use of single unit transfusions in small frail adults.

LESS SEVERE ACUTE TRANSFUSION REACTIONS

Febrile non-haemolytic transfusion reactions (FNHTR)

This is a very common transfusion-associated reaction. However, as it is associated with the recipient's anti-leucocytes antibodies, its incidence has reduced since the implementation of universal leucocyte-reduction of blood components in the UK. Features include pyrexia accompanied by rigours, nausea and muscle pain. Mild reactions, where temperature is greater than 38 °C but less than 2 °C above starting temperature can be managed by slowing the transfusion and/or giving anti-pyretic agents such as paracetamol. If the temperature rise is greater than 39 °C or greater than a 2 °C rise, the transfusion should be discontinued. When fever is associated with transfusion, immediate haemolytic transfusion reactions and bacterial contamination should be excluded.

Mild allergic reactions

Urticarial reactions to donor plasma proteins can be treated by slowing the transfusion rate and using antihistamines whilst the patient is monitored carefully. If repeated reactions occur and do not respond to antihistamines, washed red blood cell or platelet transfusions (washed in saline to remove plasma proteins) may be appropriate management for future transfusions.

DELAYED TRANSFUSION REACTIONS

Delayed haemolytic transfusion reaction (DHTR)

Delayed haemolytic transfusion reactions can occur in those who have had previous transfusions or have had a previous pregnancy and result from alloantibodies (e.g. Rh, Kell, and Duffy) that have fallen to low levels so they are undetectable in compatibility testing. Re-exposure to the antigen results in a secondary immune response with production of IgG antibodies and consequent extravascular haemolysis of the transfused red cells, usually a few days after the transfusion has taken place. Typical features include jaundice, haemoglobinuria, fever and fatigue. Investigations reveal a drop in haemoglobin, a positive direct Coombs test and rise in bilirubin. Renal failure may also be a feature. It is important to perform a repeat group and screen on the pre-transfusion and post-transfusion blood samples of the patient.

Post-transfusion purpura

In this condition, there is severe thrombocytopenia usually with a platelet count $< 10 \times 10^9/l$ 7–12 days post-transfusion. There may be severe bleeding. It usually occurs in previously pregnant and/or transfused females who are HPA-1a antigen negative and who develop high levels of anti-HPA-1a after the transfusion. It has become rare since leucocyte-reduction of blood components. The condition responds well to administration of high-dose intravenous immunoglobulin.

Transfusion-associated graft versus host disease (TA-GVHD)

This is a rare and usually fatal complication of blood transfusion caused by donor lymphocytes engrafting in the recipient and mounting an immune response against the transfusion recipient. Initial symptoms of TA-GVHD include fever, rash, diarrhoea, jaundice and bone marrow failure. It can occur up to 30 days post-transfusion.

Immunocompromised patients at risk of TA-GVHD include those with inherited immunodeficiency, HIV, recipients of certain chemotherapy agents such as fludarabine and post bone marrow transplant. It is important to identify at-risk patients and provide gamma irradiated blood components that prevent TA-GVHD.

REVERSAL OF ANTICOAGULATION

FFP is no longer first-line recommended management for the reversal of warfarin therapy. The BCSH guidelines (2012)[7] recommend the use of Vitamin K (oral or IV in emergencies) and prothrombin complex concentrate (PCC). FFP should only be used if PCC is not available. PCC contains factors II, VII, IX and X. It is used for the reversal of warfarin in patients with a raised INR and significant bleeding. It has also been used in treating coagulopathy associated with liver disease. There is a small thrombotic risk associated with its use but this has to be weighed up in light of bleeding risk. It is given intravenously and the recommended dose is 25 to 50 units/kg based on the INR.

There is increasing use of the new oral anticoagulants such as the direct thrombin inhibitor Dabigatran and the anti Xa inhibitor Rivaroxaban, which are increasingly prescribed for the treatment of atrial fibrillation and deep vein thrombosis. There is no licensed antidote to these agents. However, if severe bleeding occurs, it is recommended to consider the use of PCC or recombinant factor VIIa and contacting the haematology team for further guidance.

ALTERNATIVES TO BLOOD TRANSFUSIONS

There have been many recent developments in the use of alternatives to blood and the avoidance of transfusion. The use of these alternative measures requires organization and a multidisciplinary approach to the patient, which is now often described as 'patient blood management'.

Pre-operative anaemia management

Surgical patients who are anaemic are more likely to require blood transfusion, have post-operative infection and a prolonged hospital stay, and so patients who have a low Hb should be identified prior to surgery. In collaboration with the pre-operative team these patients should be investigated and managed to optimize the Hb before surgery. It is important to identify if there is any iron or haematinic deficiency and also exclude any underlying causes such as an undiagnosed malignancy.

Where iron deficiency is identified, it should be treated with oral iron, but if it is not tolerated or there is no response after 4–6 weeks, or if surgery is urgent, then intravenous iron can be used. In patients who have anaemia on a background of chronic renal failure, malignant diseases or haematological conditions such as myelodysplasia, recombinant erythropoietin can be used with good effect to improve the Hb before surgery. Erythropoietin is not widely employed due to the considerable health economic costs associated with its use.

Any drugs known to increase risk of bleeding, such as aspirin and clopidogrel, should be withdrawn in advance of surgery; advice should be sought from the prescribing physician if necessary. Post-operatively, non-steroidal anti-inflammatory drugs should be avoided as they may contribute to bleeding.

Acute normovolaemic haemodilution

Blood is removed immediately prior to surgery, often post-anaesthesia, and returned post-operatively or if significant bleeding occurs. The patient's blood volume is maintained by the infusion by crystalloid or colloid fluids. There is little evidence for its effectiveness and thus this technique is rarely employed outside of cardiac surgery.

Cell salvage

Cell salvage can be used intra-operative or post-operatively.

INTRA-OPERATIVE CELL SALVAGE (ICS)

A number of devices are available and are widely in use. Blood lost during surgery is aspirated into a collection reservoir and filtered to remove any debris. Blood is treated with heparin and citrate to prevent clot formation. If adequate blood is collected and the patient meets requirements for transfusion, the collected blood is centrifuged, washed and re-infused via a leucocyte-reduction filter in a closed and automated system within 4 hours. ICS is indicated in surgery where anticipated blood loss is greater than 20% of the patient's blood volume, greater than 1l in an adult (e.g. major orthopaedic, cardiac, vascular and cancer surgery).

POST-OPERATIVE CELL SALVAGE

This has very little role in ENT surgery. Blood is collected from wound drains and filtered or washed before it is re-infused via a closed automated system.

Tissue sealants

These are biological agents derived from human or animal clotting products such as thrombin, fibrinogen and calcium. They are applied directly to the bleeding point and fibrin clot formation occurs, impeding blood loss. Tissue sealants are commonly used in accident and emergency departments and minor injury clinics for minor cutaneous bleeds.

Tranexamic acid

Tranexamic acid is an antifibrinolytic drug that inhibits the conversion of plasminogen to plasmin and hence hinders fibrinolysis. It is inexpensive and can be given orally, topically or intravenously. It has a recognized role in the management of massive haemorrhage and reducing bleeding post-operatively. There is also a mouthwash preparation that can be helpful in managing minor oral cavity bleeds.

JEHOVAH'S WITNESSES

Jehovah's Witnesses have contributed considerably to the understanding of minimum blood requirements. JWs do not accept red cell transfusions, whether donor blood or their own pre-donated blood, although most patients will accept the use of cell-salvaged blood provided the blood is returned to them without a break in the circuit. When treating patients, it is important to take an individualized approach and discuss all options for blood avoidance. Most hospitals will have a Jehovah's Witness liaison committee that can be consulted.

KEY EVIDENCE

- The use of blood in surgery is in decline.
- There is increasing recognition that surgical patients can avoid transfusion through the application of patient blood management practices and more restrictive thresholds for transfusion.
- An organized approach to massive haemorrhage is key for improved survival.
- There is no role for FFP in the reversal of warfarin. Prothrombin complex concentrates should be used.

FUTURE RESEARCH

Patient blood management is integral to modern transfusion practice, with increasing evidence favouring restrictive blood transfusion. Ongoing trials are evaluating the expansion of restrictive transfusion to patient groups other than those undergoing critical care. Further research is needed to determine the optimal use of alternatives to transfusion.

KEY POINTS

- Before requesting a blood transfusion, assess the patient clinically, evaluate laboratory investigations and consider whether it is necessary.
- Patient identification is essential: ensure the right blood is transfused to the right patient at the right time in the right place.
- Early recognition of transfusion reactions is essential. Stop the transfusion, maintain intravenous access and assess the patient. Follow local protocols and inform the transfusion laboratory.
- Correction of pre-operative anaemia is fundamental in minimizing transfusion requirements.
- Surgical planning is key. A group and screen should be done a minimum of 24 hours pre-operatively. Where a large volume of blood is anticipated, agree with the transfusion laboratory how much blood should be provided.
- Early recognition of massive haemorrhage is imperative; activate local protocols and ensure a coordinated process takes place.
- There are many alternatives to blood transfusion that should be considered and discussed with patients.

REFERENCES

1. Maunes, Jeckstrom W, Thomsen H, Rudert H. Indication, incidence and management of blood transfusion during sinus surgery: a review over 12 years. *Rhinology* 1997; **35**: 2–5.
2. Gong SG, Krishnan V, Waack D. Blood transfusions in bimaxillary or orthognathic surgery: are they necessary? *Int J Adult Orthodon Orthognath Surg* 2002; **17**: 314–17.
3. Milkins C, Berryman J, Cantwell C, et al. Guidelines for pre-transfusion compatibility procedures in blood transfusion laboratories. British Committee for Standards in Haematology. *Transfusion Med* 2013; **23**: 3–35. Available from http://www.bcshguidelines.com
4. Hebert PC. The TRICC trial: a focus on the sub-group analysis. *Int J Transfus Med* 2002; **83**(S1): 387–96.
5. BCSH Transfusion Task Force. Guidelines for the use of platelet transfusions. *Brit J Haematol* 2003; **122**: 10–23. Available from http://www.bcshguidelines.com
6. Serious Hazards of Transfusion (SHOT). *Annual Shot Report 2012*. Available from www.shotuk.org
7. Makris, M, Ven Veen J, Tait C, et al. Guidelines on the management of bleeding in patients on antithrombotic agents. *Br J Haematol* 2012; **160**: 135–46. Available from http://www.bcshguidelines.com

FURTHER READING

Baskett PJF. Management of hypovolaemic shock. *Brit Med J* 1990; **300**: 1453–57.

British Committee for Standards in Haematology, Blood Transfusion Task Force (2004). Guidelines for the use of fresh-frozen plasma, cryoprecipitate and cryosupernatant. *Brit J Haematol* **126**: 11–28. Available from http://www.bcshguidelines.com

Goodnough LT, Levy JH, Murphy MF. Concepts of blood transfusion in adults. *Lancet* 2013; **381**: 1845–54.

Kotze, A, Carter LA, Scally AJ. Effects of a patient blood management programme on preoperative anaemia, transfusion rate and outcome after primary hip or knee arthroplasty: a quality improvement cycle. *Brit J Anaesth* 2012; **108**(6): 943–52.

Murphy MF, Pamphilon DH, Heddle NM. *Practical transfusion medicine*. 4th ed. Hoboken, NJ: Wiley Blackwell.

Murphy MF, Waters JH, Wood EM, Yazer MH. Transfusing blood safely and appropriately. *Brit Med J* 2013; **347**: f4303.

Norfolk, D. *Handbook of transfusion medicine*. 5th ed. Norwich: TSO.

Tinegate H, Birchall J, Gray A, et al. Guideline on the investigation and management of acute transfusion reactions. Prepared by the British Committee for Standards in Haematology blood transfusion task force. *Brit J Haematol* 2012; **159**: 143–53. Available from http://www.bcshguidelines.com

Treleaven J, Gennery A, Marsh J, et al. Guidelines on the use of irradiated blood components. Prepared by the British Committee for Standards in Haematology blood transfusion task force. *Brit J Haematol* 2010; **152**: 35–51. Available from http://www.bcshguidelines.com

CHAPTER 25

HAEMATO-ONCOLOGY

Robert F. Wynn and Mark Williams

Introduction 249	Laboratory haematology and the ENT surgeon 254
Overview of basic haematology 249	Special considerations in chronic haematological diseases 256
Haematological disorders presenting to ENT 251	References 257
ENT complications of haematological therapies 253	

SEARCH STRATEGY

Data in this chapter may be updated by a PubMed search using the keywords: haemostasis, erythropoiesis, leukaemia, lymphoma, myeloma, sickle cell disease, otolaryngology, fungal rhinosinusitis and ototoxicity.

INTRODUCTION

Many patients with haematological malignancies will present initially to an ENT surgeon, for example with nodal disease of the head and neck. Patients with known haematological disease can also develop numerous problems of the ear, nose and throat as a result of either their disease or its treatment. Similarly many of the therapies used for primary ENT disorders can have important haematological effects.

The aim of this chapter is to provide clinically relevant information that enables practicing ENT surgeons and trainees to interpret basic haematological laboratory parameters, recognize the haematological disorders that present to their services and facilitate appropriate timely referral, manage the haematological complications of ENT disorders and interventions, understand potential ENT complications of haematological therapies and appreciate special considerations in the management of ENT conditions in patients with chronic haematological disorders.

OVERVIEW OF BASIC HAEMATOLOGY

Components of blood: their function and production

Blood is a liquid tissue whose cellular compartment consists of red cells (erythrocytes), white cells (leukocytes) and platelets. Erythrocytes, the most numerous blood cells, are bi-concave discs that contain an abundance of haemoglobin, the protein responsible for oxygen transportation in vertebrates.[1] They have a lifespan of approximately 120 days after which they are removed by the spleen.[2] Leukocytes are a diverse group of cell types that are capable of migration into tissues where they have vital roles in the processes of immunity, inflammation and wound healing. Neutrophils are the most common white cell in adult peripheral blood and are a key component of innate immunity, providing defence against bacteria, which they are able to ingest and kill. Lymphocytes are the cellular effectors of the adaptive immune system and are capable of producing antibodies or recognizing and killing virally infected cells; some are long-lived, permitting anamnestic immune responses.[3] Platelets are the cellular element of the haemostatic system but they also have functions in tissue repair and cytokine signalling. Their life span is 8–9 days.[4] The liquid phase of blood is plasma, which contains a wide range of hormones, electrolytes and proteins; including albumin, immunoglobulins, fibrinogen, clotting factors and complement.

All of the cellular components of blood are derived from a common progenitor, the haematopoietic stem cell (HSC), which is capable of self-renewal as well as giving rise to a variety of progenitors and from there all cells of the blood (**Figure 25.1**).[5] The presence of various combinations of haematopoietic growth factors, such as erythropoietin (EPO) and granulocyte-colony stimulating factor (G-CSF), will determine which progenitors successfully proliferate and differentiate, thus ensuring homeostatic

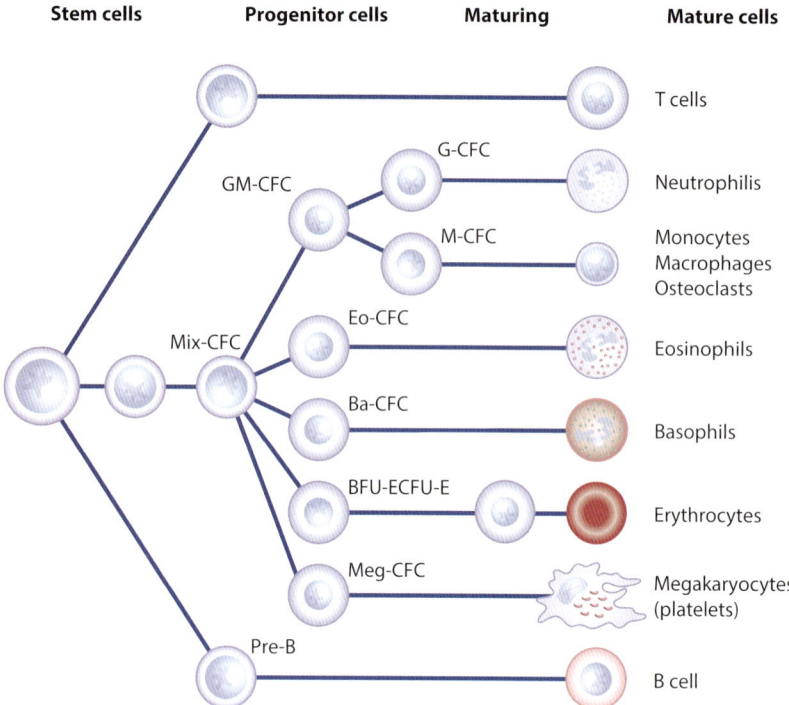

Figure 25.1 Schematic representation of haemopoiesis.

control over mature cell numbers.[6] For example, in response to tissue hypoxia the kidney secretes EPO, which increases red cell production and restores oxygen delivery.[7] Understanding the haematopoietic hierarchy helps to predict the behaviour of haematological malignancies (see below) and the effects of commercially available recombinant growth factors (G-CSF and EPO).

Haematopoiesis initially occurs in the yolk sac of the embryo, followed by the foetal liver and spleen. During the third trimester HSCs migrate to the bone marrow, which becomes the dominant site of haematopoiesis by term. Whilst the majority of the infant bone marrow is active, by adulthood only the axial skeleton and the proximal ends of the long bones are haematopoietic.[8] However, if increased cell production is required then haematopoiesis can expand back down the long bones, resume activity in the liver and spleen and can even occur in soft tissue deposits outside these organs. This is seen in several haematological disorders such as thalassaemia major and myelofibrosis and it also explains the propensity for many haematological malignancies to involve the liver and spleen.[9]

Lymphatics and the mononuclear phagocyte system

The lymphatic system consists of a network of vessels that drain extracellular tissue fluid through a series of nodes and back to the venous circulation.[3] This organization ensures that foreign material passes through lymph nodes where lymphocytes can compete for survival on the basis of their affinity for the antigen, allowing the selective expansion and activation of cells that are capable of producing an effective antibody. The architecture of lymph nodes reflects these complex processes and the pattern of its disruption gives vital clues as to the nature of lymphoid malignancies (see below).[10]

Monocytes are produced by the bone marrow but migrate into tissues where they develop specialized functions, often involving the phagocytosis of debris. Examples include the Kupffer cells of the liver, lymph node dendritic cells, alveolar macrophages and the microglia of the central nervous system.[11] Collectively these cells are known as the mononuclear phagocyte system; the spleen is the largest component and has multiple functions, including the removal of senescent blood cells, recycling of iron and the phagocytosis of antibody coated bacteria.

Haematological malignancy: Principles of diagnosis and management

The cells of the bone marrow are actively dividing throughout life, predisposing them to the acquisition of genetic mutations. Lymphocytes also perform somatic recombination to produce their immunoglobulin, which involves breaking DNA and risks chromosomal translocation; with the result that translocations are commonly found in lymphoid tumours and frequently involve the immunoglobulin loci.[12] Haematological malignancies are the result of cells that have acquired defects in their apoptotic and/or proliferative pathways giving them a survival advantage that allows their uncontrolled expansion; leading to tissue disruption, organ damage and, ultimately, death. Whilst exposure to radiation and certain chemotherapeutic agents certainly increases the risk of myeloid malignancy, in practice this accounts for a small number of patients and the majority of cases of haematological malignancy are sporadic relating to the accumulation of somatic mutation. Notable exceptions include endemic Burkitt's lymphoma, believed to be caused by EBV infection in the context of chronic malaria, and adult T-cell leukaemia/lymphoma, which is caused by the virus HTLV-1.[13]

Oncogenesis can occur at any stage in the haematopoietic hierarchy (Figure 25.1), resulting in a diverse spectrum of malignancies. Diagnosis is frequently dependant on the demonstration that a population of cells are 'clonal', meaning that they are all related to a common ancestor. Clonality can be confirmed by unique patterns of expression of cell surface antigens (immunophenotype), the presence of a shared genetic aberration (cytogenetics, molecular genetics) or by expression of the same immunoreceptor (immunoglobulin/TCR rearrangement studies).[14] Whilst the concept that a malignant population consists of many identical cells remains clinically useful there has been increasing evidence in recent years that these cancers are genetically diverse disorders with multiple clones often populating the same patient.[15] For example, acute myeloid leukaemia (AML) was shown to consist of 2–5 distinct clones in just over half of patients studied. It is likely that such studies significantly underestimate the number of clones present as current methods can only detect clones of a certain size (> 5–10% of cells).[16] The prognostic significance of the clonal structure remains unclear at this time.

Haematological malignancies will generally involve predominantly the blood and bone marrow (leukaemias) or the lymph nodes (lymphomas), but there is often considerable overlap. Many of these cancers are 'liquid', insofar as they are widely circulating at presentation and conventional notions of anatomical staging do not apply (e.g. acute leukaemia); others behave as solid tumours with orderly spread to contiguous lymphatic regions (e.g. Hodgkin's lymphoma). Bone marrow involvement frequently presents with pancytopenia causing fatigue, breathlessness, infection and bleeding. Whereas nodal disease presents with visible enlargement, the effects of local compression, or constitutional symptoms such as weight loss and night sweats.

The nature of the presenting symptoms will guide the diagnostic process; pancytopenia requires prompt assessment of the bone marrow by aspiration, trephine biopsy, flow cytometric evaluation and cytogenetic analysis. Nodal disease will require imaging to assess the extent of the disease followed by biopsy.

Treatment usually involves combination chemotherapy, the principles of which are similar to that of solid tumour regimes.[17] Most haematological malignancies are radiosensitive but the widespread nature of these conditions restricts the use of radiotherapy to the control of troublesome deposits or the treatment of localized lymphomas. Increasingly monoclonal antibodies and small molecule inhibitors are used to target and disrupt disease-specific processes. The most striking example is the tyrosine kinase inhibitor (TKI), imatinib, which has transformed the management of chronic myeloid leukaemia (CML) from an often-fatal disease to one that is held in remission by oral medication.[18] In the era before TKIs CML would invariably transform into an acute leukaemia that was usually fatal. The only patients who survived were a proportion of those who were fit enough to undergo a stem cell transplant. With current therapies > 90% of patients remit and contemporary trials are exploring the possibility of stopping treatment in those who appear to be cured.

Whilst some haematological cancers can be cured with conventional therapy many have high rates of relapse and patients with responsive diseases who can tolerate the procedure are offered haematopoietic stem cell transplantation (HSCT). Allogeneic HSCT is an extreme form of immunotherapy that involves conditioning the recipient with immunosuppressive chemotherapy to allow engraftment of infused haematopoietic stem cells from a matched donor.[19] The donor stem cells form a new immune system that is capable of engaging the recipient's neoplasm, but the price of this graft-versus-disease effect is graft-versus-host disease (GvHD). Acutely GvHD typically presents with diarrhoea, rash and liver dysfunction, whereas chronic GvHD is a truly protean disorder, with inflammation and scarring affecting any tissue.[20] GvHD is one of the major complications of HSCT, causing considerable morbidity and mortality and the management can be very challenging. To reduce the incidence of GvHD patients are given immunosuppressive therapy (typically Ciclosporin) for a period after transplantation, but in contrast to solid organ transplantation where lifelong immunosuppression is mandated, stem cell transplant recipients will typically stop these medications 3–9 months post-HSCT.

HAEMATOLOGICAL DISORDERS PRESENTING TO ENT

Head and neck lymphadenopathy

The most common presentation of a haematological malignancy to an ENT surgeon is that of a 'neck lump'; most lumps are cervical lymphadenopathy and a significant proportion of these will be lymphoma.[21] It is important that lymphoma is considered early in the diagnostic process as an appropriately focused history and examination can save the patient time, stress and unnecessary investigations.

Symptoms of unexplained fever, drenching night sweats and weight loss (> 10% in 6 months) are highly suspicious of lymphoma; in this context they are termed 'B-symptoms' and are also of prognostic significance, typically predicting an inferior outcome.[22] However, these symptoms also occur in a range of infections and chronic inflammatory disorders, especially tuberculosis (TB); careful attention to any history of TB exposure should help to make this distinction. Generalized pruritus or alcohol-induced lymph node pain suggest Hodgkin's lymphoma (HL), which is the lymphoma most commonly associated with localized cervical disease, especially in younger patients, and usually has an excellent prognosis. Attention should also be paid to the time course of the symptoms as these give an indication of the pace of the disease and important clues as to the likely diagnosis. Indolent lymphomas can cause stable lymphadenopathy over many years, the nodes of HL often fluctuate in size with observation, whilst the most aggressive lymphomas can enlarge over the course of days and may require admission for urgent therapy.

Examination should be used to describe the neck lump and its relationship to surrounding structures, as well as establishing the extent of nodal involvement elsewhere; this must include examination of the liver and spleen, enlargement of the latter being highly suggestive of lymphoid malignancy. The oropharynx should be inspected for involvement of Waldeyer's ring, which is infiltrated in 5–10% of non-Hodgkin's lymphoma (NHL) but rarely in HL. The nodes of lymphoma are usually painless, often rubbery to palpate and can be mobile or fixed depending on whether the capsule has been infiltrated. In the absence of symptoms asymmetric palatine tonsils carry a low risk of malignancy. A review of 792 patients undergoing tonsillectomy identified 53 patients with asymptomatic asymmetric tonsils, all of whom had normal histology.[23] However, the presence of pain, dysphagia, ulceration, progressive enlargement or B-symptoms should prompt biopsy/removal. A more recent meta-analysis has suggested that whilst there is an association between tonsil asymmetry and lymphoma the risk is dramatically increased by the presence of other signs of malignancy.[24]

Distended neck veins and facial oedema suggest superior vena cava obstruction (SVCO) by mediastinal disease, most commonly bronchogenic carcinoma but also HL or lymphoblastic lymphoma.[25] SVCO is a medical emergency that mandates urgent imaging and immediate referral to oncology/haematology, thoracic surgery and radiology.[26] In the case of lymphoid malignancy high dose dexamethasone can provide rapid relief. However, the tumour response to steroids can be so impressive that the diagnostic yield of subsequent biopsy is significantly reduced (see 'Airway obstruction' below). Careful consideration must therefore be given to the timing of biopsy and early involvement of oncology/haematology and thoracic surgery is vital in this regard.

A full blood count should be performed as pancytopenia suggests bone marrow infiltration and lymphocytosis raises the possibility of circulating disease. Chronic lymphocytic leukaemia (CLL – synonymous with small lymphocytic lymphoma) is the most common leukaemia in adults, has typical blood film appearances and can usually be diagnosed by performing flow cytometry on peripheral blood, without recourse to lymph node biopsy.[27] Renal and liver biochemistry should also be taken as derangement can suggest infiltration or compression and organ function is an important consideration when planning chemotherapy.

If malignancy is suspected then computed tomography (CT) of the chest, abdomen and pelvis should be performed to stage the disease. Early involvement of haematology or oncology at this point is helpful so that the most appropriate type and site of biopsy can be planned. The diagnosis of a specific lymphoma usually requires an extended immunohistochemical panel to be performed and an appreciation of the growth pattern within the node is often useful; as such whole node biopsies are preferred.[10] Core biopsy can be useful when the tumour is inaccessible (e.g. retroperitoneal), but contains little information regarding architecture making the diagnosis of certain low-grade NHLs challenging.

Fine-needle aspiration (FNA) is commonly used in the initial investigation of neck lumps because it is quick, safe and diagnostic of many malignancies; but its role in lymphoma diagnosis has been controversial. Some lymphomas (especially HL) consist of small numbers of malignant cells within a reactive cellular background; in this situation FNA may yield only reactive cells and wrongly suggest an infective or inflammatory aetiology. This has led many organizations to advise against the use of FNA for suspected lymphoma, to avoid diagnostic delay or false negative results. However, increasing use of flow cytometry and immunocytochemistry has enabled many lymphomas to be accurately defined cytologically and the ability of this technique to provide fresh samples for DNA microarray analysis suggests that there may be an increasing role for FNA in the future.[28] Centres with sufficient expertise in these techniques are able to use FNA for preliminary diagnosis, although excision biopsy is often performed for confirmation and uncertainty can still arise with certain low grade B-cell malignancies, such as marginal zone lymphoma, where the markers themselves are not specific and an appreciation of tissue architecture is needed.[29] Overall we would still advocate proceeding directly to whole node biopsy when symptoms are highly suggestive of lymphoma, and using FNA only when there are several possible diagnoses and there is sufficient local expertise for cytology to be discriminatory.

Airway obstruction

On occasion lymphomas of the oropharynx, larynx or neck can cause intrinsic occlusion or extrinsic compression of the airway. In this context ENT surgeons can be asked to provide direct visualization with fibre-optic laryngoscopy and to advise regarding the security of the airway. Where a malignant condition is suspected then consideration must be given to both the immediate stabilization of the patient and the need for urgent diagnosis. Dexamethasone can be used to shrink tumours and rapidly relieve compressive symptoms, but the effect on certain lymphomas can be so dramatic that the diagnosis cannot be ascertained unless tissue is sampled prior to the administration of steroids. Clearly the priority in a situation of life-threatening airway compromise is to secure the airway, but where the presentation is less acute then priority must be given to urgently obtaining tissue for diagnosis, as this will allow definitive treatment to be started. Regular (daily) assessment will allow surgery that is both safe and likely to yield diagnostic tissue.[30]

Extranodal and extramedullary disease

A quarter of NHL patients will present with extranodal disease, which commonly involves the CNS or GI tract, but can occur anywhere. Extranodal sites of head and neck lymphomas include salivary glands (marginal zone lymphoma – especially in patients with Sjögren's syndrome,[31] sinuses (usually diffuse large B-cell lymphoma) and the nasal cavity (NK/T nasal type lymphoma). Bone marrow malignancies such as acute myeloid leukaemia and myeloma are also capable of forming extramedullary deposits, referred to as chloromas and plasmacytomas respectively. The latter commonly involve the head and neck and frequently present diagnostic difficulties. Whilst most occur in the context of systemic myeloma a minority are solitary and potentially cured with radiotherapy.[32-33] Deposits of extramedullary haematopoiesis can also occur at any site and often mimic the appearance of tumours; these should be considered when a paranasal lesion is found in a patient with chronic anaemia, especially a child with thalassaemia major or sickle cell disease.[9]

Hyperviscosity and leucostasis

Both myeloma and lymphoplasmacytoid lymphoma are capable of secreting large amounts of immunoglobulin; if the concentration of this paraprotein is sufficiently high it will thicken the blood and cause impairment of the microcirculation, a condition known as hyperviscosity syndrome. Leucostasis refers to a similar situation that results from very high white cell counts (typically > 100×10^9/L), usually at initial presentation of acute myeloid leukaemia or CML. Impairment of blood flow causes a constellation of symptoms and signs that may include blurring or loss of vision, headache, hearing loss, vertigo, nystagmus, tinnitus, diplopia and ataxia. Untreated these conditions can progress to seizures, stroke, coma and death.[26] Plasmapheresis or leucopheresis can be used to rapidly remove the excess immunoglobulin or malignant cells (respectively), but the essence of successful management is the prompt instigation of disease directed therapy (e.g. chemotherapy). Although rare there have also been several case reports of sudden-onset bilateral deafness as the initial presenting feature of CML.[34]

Bony disease

Multiple myeloma can affect any bone and cases of temporal bone involvement causing otitis media, hearing loss and mastoid effusions have been reported. Whilst this would be a rare presentation, myeloma is a common malignancy and should be considered whenever lytic bone lesions are identified.[35-36]

ENT COMPLICATIONS OF HAEMATOLOGICAL THERAPIES

Infections

Patients with haematological malignancies are often severely immunocompromised as a result of both their disease and the effects of treatment, making them susceptible to infection from a wide range of common organisms and opportunistic pathogens, including bacteria, viruses, fungi and protozoa. Whilst patients are often taking a variety of prophylactic antimicrobials these offer incomplete protection.

Certain congenital (constitutional) haematological disorders are associated with either neutropenia or disordered neutrophil function and similarly increase the risk of bacterial or fungal infection. These disorders not infrequently present with discharging ears or lymphadenitis.[37]

These infections can be of unexpected severity or duration and can occur at unusual sites; clinical signs can be subtle or misleading as the inflammatory response that usually produces symptoms is often attenuated or absent. Fungal rhinosinusitis can be fatal.[38]

Bacterial infections are most frequent in patients with neutropenia (post-chemotherapy, acute leukaemia, aplastic anaemia etc.) or impaired neutrophil function (myelodysplasia). Otitis media and sinusitis are common acute infections that can become chronic and problematic for patients with persistent neutrophil defects.[39]

Viral infections are common in patients rendered hypogammaglobulinaemic by CLL, HSCT or myeloma; they are usually upper respiratory tract infections or rhinosinusitis and tend to last longer than in an immunocompetent host, sometimes persisting for several weeks. More profoundly suppressed patients can experience reactivation of latent CMV, VZV or HSV 1+2; the latter is often associated with severe ulceration of the oropharynx and even abscess formation.[40]

Fungal spores are ubiquitous in the environment and are continuously inhaled, often leading to colonization of the respiratory tract. Invasive infection is less common but occurs in the context of prolonged neutropenia or patients with GvHD, who have impaired immune reconstitution and are often taking multiple immunosuppressive agents.[41-42] Acute fungal rhinosinusitis is an invasive infection with a high mortality usually caused by *aspergillus* species or pin moulds (mucorales).[38] The initial symptoms include fever, nasal congestion, facial pain and epistaxis; examination of the oral cavity and nasal passages may reveal mucosal thickening or areas of necrotic tissue. Invasion of the palate, orbit, cavernous sinus, cranial nerves and brain can occur within hours, days or weeks depending on the specific organism and the depth of immunosuppression.[43] Some patients have extension beyond the sinuses at presentation leading to visual disturbance, diplopia, facial numbness, altered cognition or seizures.

Rapid diagnosis is essential for survival so a high index of suspicion is required when immunocompromised patients develop sinus symptoms; early input from radiology, ENT and pathology is vital in this regard. Multiple sinuses are usually involved and can be recognized using CT by the presence of opacification, mucosal thickening and bony erosions; the maxillary and ethmoid sinuses are the most commonly affected.[44] If invasion of surrounding structures is suspected then magnetic resonance imaging (MRI) is needed to characterize intra-cranial involvement.[45] Whilst imaging is not diagnostic of fungal infection, it is important to define the extent of the disease and identify extension into the brain or orbit, so that surgical intervention can be planned. Early nasal endoscopy is crucial to look for necrosis, which can appear as sloughing or perforation of the nasal septum, or palatal eschars;[46] biopsy of the affected area should be performed and sent for both culture and histopathology. Diagnosis depends on histological demonstration of fungal hyphae penetrating surrounding tissue and blood vessels, to distinguish invasive infection from colonization. Culture of the specimen permits identification of the fungus, which has important consequences for the choice of antifungal therapy.

When fungal infection is first suspected empirical therapy with intravenous amphotericin B should be commenced. The mucorales are resistant to voriconazole and this agent should only be considered if mucormycosis has been excluded.[47] Other species of fungus have varying sensitivities, highlighting the importance of early identification of the organism and discussion with microbiology. Where immunosuppression can be withdrawn then this should be considered, although in the context of haematological malignancy and HSCT it is often a case of buying time with antifungal therapy whilst immune reconstitution occurs. The surgical management of fungal rhinosinusitis can be challenging and is discussed in detail in Chapter 96 (Fungal Rhinosinusitis).

Mucormycosis of the palate and middle ear have also been described in the context of haematological disease and HSCT, emphasizing the need to keep an open mind when assessing ENT problems in this population.[47–49]

Ototoxicity

Cisplatin and carboplatin are platinum-containing chemotherapy agents that are used for the treatment of relapsed lymphomas and numerous non-haematological malignancies. They are potent neurotoxins that are capable of damaging the outer hair cells and the epithelium of the lateral wall of the cochlea. Cisplatin is the most ototoxic of this class, typically causing high-frequency sensorineural hearing loss with tinnitus in 15–20% of patients; audiometric changes can be demonstrated in many more, up to 75% in some studies.[50] Onset is variable with some patients suffering severe hearing loss after a single dose, whilst others develop symptoms several months after the last dose. The toxicity is dose dependant but there is considerable variation between individuals, suggesting significant polymorphism in the pathways responsible for the drugs metabolism. Risk is increased by the presence of renal failure and the concomitant use of other ototoxic therapies, especially radiotherapy (RT), which has a synergistic effect and also causes serous otitis media, potentially complicating assessment. Children are particularly susceptible, partly because of age but also the regimes that they receive are commonly high dose, combined with RT or contain two platinum based compounds. Avoiding ototoxicity is particularly important in children as it has profound consequences for speech and language development.[51] Extended high-frequency audiometry is recommended to allow early detection of hearing loss before the frequencies required for hearing speech are affected.[52] Distortion product otoacoustic emissions (DPOAEs) are also more sensitive than conventional audiometry and can be used in children under 5 years of age. Damage is typically irreversible and management should focus on prevention through early recognition and dose reduction or cessation where possible.[53] Sodium thiosulphate has been trialed as a protective agent but the development of this and similar agents has been hampered by a lack of consensus regarding ototoxicity assessment criteria.

The ototoxicity of the aminoglycosides is well documented and gentamicin is commonly used in combination with extended spectrum penicillin for the treatment of neutropenic sepsis. Other ototoxic agents used in the management of haematological disorders include desferrioxamine (used to prevent iron overload in the chronically transfused), loop diuretics, vancomycin, amphotericin B, cytarabine, methotrexate and the vinca alkaloids.[54]

Stridor during treatment of haematological malignancy

The ENT surgeon may be called to the haematology ward to see patients with respiratory compromise due to airway obstruction. Several causes should be considered:

- There may be mucosal inflammation of the mouth and pharynx secondary to intensive chemotherapy. This is known as mucositis and is related to the intensity of chemotherapy. It occurs in the weeks after such therapy and is self-limiting. There is evident inflammation of the mucosa with thick secretions that might contribute to airway compromise.[55]
- Stridor secondary to vocal cord paralysis is rarely recorded secondary to vincristine chemotherapy, which is usually part of the treatment of childhood leukaemia.[56] The paralysis may be of long-standing duration.

LABORATORY HAEMATOLOGY AND THE ENT SURGEON

The full (complete) blood count

All basic laboratory haematology is fully automated. The full (or complete) blood count (FBC) will give the requesting clinician the following:[57]

- The number of red cells (red cell count, RCC), their size (mean corpuscular volume, MCV) and the haemoglobin concentration within them (mean corpuscular haemoglobin, MCH or mean corpuscular haemoglobin concentration, MCHC).[58] It will also measure the haemoglobin concentration (Hb) within whole blood. The haemoglobin can be low and the red cell count high if those red cells don't contain much haemoglobin within them (as in certain haemoglobinopathies). Most analysers will also offer a reticulocyte count. Reticulocytes are simply young red cells recently made in the marrow and if the reticulocyte count is high then the marrow is making lots of red cells.
- The total white cell count; and usually a 5-part differential giving the number of neutrophils, monocytes, lymphocytes, eosinophils and basophils. The counters discriminate these cells on the basis of size and staining.
- The platelet count.

The analysers are good but abnormalities may be confirmed after examination of the blood smear. Samples that are clotted or diluted give erroneous results and should be repeated. Similarly samples that are not freshly analysed may give inaccurate results.

Cytopenia indicates reduction of a blood cell number and pancytopenia is a reduction in the blood of all cell types – red cells, white cells and platelets. Any cytopenia is either caused by diminished production of the cell in the marrow or by increased peripheral consumption. The causes of pancytopenia are given in **Box 25.1**.

BOX 25.1 Causes of pancytopenia

- Decreased bone marrow function
- Aplasia
- Acute leukaemia, myelodysplasia, myeloma
- Infiltration with lymphoma, solid tumours, tuberculosis
- Megaloblastic anaemia
- Paroxysmal nocturnal haemoglobinuria
- Myelofibrosis
- Haemophagocytic syndrome
- Increased peripheral destruction
- Splenomegaly

Anaemia

The haemoglobin (Hb) is low on the analyser FBC. The practising ENT surgeon should be readily able to discriminate the likely causes for any anaemia from the clinical situation of the patient and the details of both the red cell parameters and the reticulocyte count:

- **Bleeding.** This might be obvious from the history of the patient. The red cells are usually normal in size and shape (unless the bleeding has been chronic and associated with iron deficiency) and there should be a raised reticulocyte count as the marrow compensates for the blood that has been lost with increased production. Note that reticulocytes are larger than normal cells and a reticulocytosis might be associated with a raised MCV and note also that the platelet count maybe increased by bleeding.
- **Iron deficiency.** Iron is needed to make haemoglobin and when there is iron deficiency then the Hb will be low. The red cells will be small (low MCV) without much haemoglobin within them (low MCH and MCHC). The diagnosis can be confirmed by measuring the serum iron or the ferritin. Iron deficiency may be associated with a poor diet or with chronic blood loss. If the patient is female then take a history of menstrual bleeding and consider the gut as a source of bleeding – this might be asymptomatic and referral to the gastroenterology team might be indicated.
- **Haemolytic anaemia.** Haemolysis is shortened red cell survival so that they are surviving for fewer than their usual 120 days. The marrow should compensate for the shortened survival with a reticulocytosis (perhaps with a raised MCV). Red cell breakdown will result in unconjugated hyperbilirubinaemia. The cause might be immune mediated with antibody on the red cell surface, which will manifest as a positive Coombs test (direct antiglobulin test, DAT).
- **Anaemia of chronic disease.** Sick patients will often be anaemic. This will include those with cancer and those with chronic infection or autoimmune disease. The anaemia is usually normochromic and normocytic (normal red cell parameters) or slightly microcytic.
- **Anaemia associated with haematological diseases.** Patients known to haematology services may have anaemia associated with their primary disease or its treatment.

Polycythaemia

This is a raised Hb with a raised red cell count. It may be secondary to hypoxia, which itself is most commonly associated with chronic cardiopulmonary disease and the arterial oxygen saturation is low. Such patients simply need more red cells to deliver oxygen to the tissues since each red cell delivers less since it picks up less in the lung. Sometimes polycythaemia might be part of a myeloproliferative condition where there is an endogenous and primary overproduction of red cells by the bone marrow.

Disorders of platelet number

An increase in the platelet count is known as thrombocytosis. Just as with polycythaemia it might be secondary or part of a myeloproliferative condition. Primary causes include bleeding and surgery. The count may also be raised in chronic inflammatory disease including infection.

Thrombocytopenia is a reduced platelet count. It may present with bleeding including bleeding from the nose and into the mouth. Causes that the surgeon should consider must include:

- Immune thrombocytopenic purpura (ITP). In this condition then there are autoantibodies directed at the platelet. The platelet count may be dramatically low (into single figures). In children it may resolve spontaneously. Steroids and other immunosuppressant drugs are used to improve the count, especially in adult patients.[59] Referral to haematology services is indicated.
- As part of a coagulopathy including disseminated intravascular coagulation (DIC). In DIC there is activation and consumption of clotting factors and platelets in association with severe illness such as severe bacterial infection or widespread metastatic malignancy. Where there is thrombocytopenia the coagulation profile should be checked and the hallmarks of DIC are prolongation of the prothrombin time (PT) and activated partial thromboplastin time (APTT) with reduction in fibrinogen and elevation of fibrin degradation products (expressed as FDP or D-Dimers).[4]
- Heparin can cause thrombocytopenia and there may be paradoxical thrombosis, which can be severe in heparin-induced thrombocytopenia (HIT). If HIT is suspected then an urgent referral to haematology is

indicated as there are specific investigations to detect the culpable antibodies and specific intervention will be initiated.
- Thrombocytopenia might be associated with primary haematological illness.

Disorders of neutrophil number

Neutrophil leucocytosis – an increase in the neutrophil count – is usually secondary to bacterial infection. It may be secondary to other inflammatory illness, to malignancy and it will frequently be raised post-operatively. Sometimes it may be part of a primary haematological process including myeloproliferative disease and leukaemia.

Neutropenia may also be associated with infection including viral infections and significant bacterial infection. As with ITP there may be immune mediated neutropenia. It may be associated with primary haematological disease and its treatment.

Abnormalities of lymphocyte appearance and number

The practising surgeon should recognize that lymphocytes deal with viruses and may be altered in number or appearance in viral infection or primary haematological disease. Certain conditions are worthy of specific mention:

- The lymphocyte may appear differently – often referred to as 'atypical mononuclear cells' or 'atypical lymphocytes' – in certain viral infections and particularly in the EBV infection know as infectious mononucleosis. In this illness there maybe be fever, lassitude, sore throat, with atypical lymphocytes seen on the blood smear.[60] Diagnosis is with EBV serology. Note that this illness may be indistinguishable from other virus infection such as CMV.
- There may be a lymphocytosis in other viral infections. It may be elevated in bacterial infection especially in children and classically with pertussis infection (whooping cough).
- The lymphocyte count may be chronically elevated in chronic lymphocytic leukaemia (CLL). There will often be associated lymph node enlargement as the malignant cells infiltrate nodes. The diagnosis can easily be made from peripheral blood investigations (starting with blood smear and then flow cytometry) and biopsy of an enlarged node might therefore be avoidable.

Monocytes, eosinophils and basophils

Monocytosis is seen in chronic infection and in primary haematological disease. Where it is part of a reactive picture there is usually an associated neutrophil leucocytosis.[60]

Eosinophila is seen in allergic conditions (asthma, eczema), in parasitic infections and in association with certain drugs. It is classically also seen in Hodgkin's lymphoma and the association of lymphadenopathy with eosinophilia should alert the clinician to this potential diagnosis.[61]

Basophils are infrequently found in the peripheral blood. They may be increased in chronic myeloid leukaemia where the total white cell count is usually typically greatly elevated.

SPECIAL CONSIDERATIONS IN CHRONIC HAEMATOLOGICAL DISEASES

Sickle cell disease

Sickle cell disease is a common haemoglobinopathy, which is encountered worldwide, although usually in patients of Afro-Caribbean, Middle Eastern or Asian ancestry. There is a single base pair substitution leading to a single amino acid change in the β-globin chain of the haemoglobin molecule.[62] It can be considered as two diseases:

- There is a haemolytic anaemia with shortened red cell survival and anaemia with the generic features of haemolysis including reticulocytosis and jaundice.
- There is also a vaso-occlusive illness. The red cells occlude blood vessels during crises and either affect the oxygen delivery to that organ (stroke, painful crisis) or affect blood flow from that organ (sequestration crisis).

There are several points that the ENT surgeon should note.[63] All children with a possible diagnosis of sickle cell anaemia should be screened prior to surgery since there is an increased risk associated with anaesthesia. Safe surgery requires the meticulous avoidance of dehydration, hypoxia or hypothermia as these may trigger sickling.[64]

In some countries including the UK there will have been implemented a national neonatal screening strategy. Otherwise it is easy to screen rapidly by testing for sickling in the lab (the sickledex test) and by looking at the blood film. Haemoglobin electrophoresis will detect haemoglobin S and distinguish it from normal adult haemoglobin A.

There is an increased risk of sensorineural deafness in children with sickle cell disease presumably as a consequence of the vasculopathy of sickle cell. Affected children have an increased incidence of obstructive sleep apnoea caused by adeno-tonsillar hypertrophy and surgical correction might reduce the risk of painful crises. Priapism of the nasal turbinates is a cause of nasal obstruction and partial turbinectomy might be indicated.[63]

Bone marrow (stem cell) transplant

During stem cell transplant the recipient receives a stem cell donation from either a relative or an unrelated individual as part of their treatment of a primary haematological malignant or non-malignant disease. The stem cell donation follows a period of 'conditioning' high dose chemotherapy or radiotherapy that gets rid of both the patient's immune system so that the donation is not rejected and the patient's own bone marrow so that there is 'space' for the donated stem cells to engraft into.

The conditioning therapy will regularly and reliably generate mucositis (see 'Stridor during treatment of haematological malignancy' above). There will be the risk of infection including fungal infection that is discussed in 'Infections' above and in the management of which the ENT team will be not infrequently involved.

The transplant may involve immunological rejection of host tissue by the engrafted, regenerating donor immune system. This is the process of graft versus host disease (GvHD) and is the opposite of graft rejection. GvHD in the early months after transplant will involve attack on the skin (presenting as rash), the gut (presenting as diarrhoea) and the liver (presenting as jaundice). However there may be involvement of any organ in the months that follow. During this chronic GvHD phase there may be immunological destruction of the salivary gland and xerostomia.[65]

Management is supportive and symptom-directed but also immunosuppressive.

Splenectomy

The spleen protects against infection with encapsulated organisms including *pneumococcus* and *haemophilus* species.[3] Hyposplenism is rarely constitutional but usually follows surgical splenectomy, which may be done following trauma or as part of treatment of a haematological condition. The patient will usually receive protection against such infection with prophylactic antibiotics and with regular vaccination against *pneumococcus*, *meningococcus* and *haemophilus*. Malaria prophylaxis in endemic areas is also important. The FBC may be abnormal in the splenectomized individual with leucocytosis and thrombocytosis. The smear will show Howell-Jolly bodies in the red cells – these are nuclear fragments that the spleen will usually remove from the mature, circulating red cell.[60]

KEY POINTS

- Haematological malignancies often present to the otolaryngologist as nodal disease in the neck.
- Patients with haematological malignancies may have severely compromised immune systems due both to the disease process and the treatment. This leads to increased risk of severe upper respiratory infections including rhinosinusitis, mastoiditis, supraglottitis and neck space infections.
- Invasive fungal rhinosinusitis can complicate haematological disorders.
- Lymphomas of the head and neck can progress rapidly in size, leading to airway obstruction.
- Severe mucositis of the aerodigestive tract can complicate the treatment of haematological malignancies.
- Vincristine is an uncommon but important cause of vocal cord palsy.

REFERENCES

1. Hoffbrand AV, Moss PAH, Pettit JE. *Essential haematology*. 6th ed. Malden, MA: Wiley-Blackwell; 2011.
2. Kruse A, Uehlinger DE, Gotch F, et al. Red blood cell lifespan, erythropoiesis and hemoglobin control. *Contrib Nephrol* 2008; **161**: 247–54.
3. Delves PJ, Roitt IM, Ebook Library. *Roitt's essential immunology*. Chichester, West Sussex: Wiley-Blackwell; 2011.
4. Marder VJ. *Hemostasis and thrombosis basic principles and clinical practice*. 6th ed. Philadelphia: Wolters Kluwer/Lippincott Williams & Wilkins Health; 2013.
5. Wintrobe MM, Greer JP. *Wintrobe's clinical hematology*. 12th ed. Philadelphia: Wolters Kluwer Health/Lippincott Williams & Wilkins; 2009.
6. Borghesi L. Hematopoiesis in steady-state versus stress: self-renewal, lineage fate choice, and the conversion of danger signals into cytokine signals in hematopoietic stem cells. *J Immunol* 2014; **193**(5): 2053–58.
7. Koulnis M, Porpiglia E, Hidalgo D, Socolovsky M. Erythropoiesis: from molecular pathways to system properties. *Adv Exp Med Biol* 2014; **844**: 37–58.
8. Ciau-Uitz A, Monteiro R, Kirmizitas A, Patient R. Developmental hematopoiesis: ontogeny, genetic programming and conservation. *Exp Hematol* 2014; **42**(8): 669–83.
9. Rivella S. Ineffective erythropoiesis and thalassemias. *Curr Opin Hematol* 2009; **16**(3): 187–94.
10. Ioachim HL, Medeiros LJ, Ovid Technologies Inc. *Ioachim's lymph node pathology*. Philadelphia, PA: Lippincott Williams & Wilkins; 2009.
11. Davies LC, Taylor PR. Tissue-resident macrophages: then and now. *Immunology* 2015; **144**(4): 541–48.
12. Chiarle R. Translocations in normal B cells and cancers: insights from new technical approaches. *Adv Immunol* 2013; **117**: 39–71.
13. Kimura H, Kawada J, Ito Y. Epstein-Barr virus-associated lymphoid malignancies: the expanding spectrum of hematopoietic neoplasms. *Nagoya J Med Sci* 2013; **75**(3–4): 169–79.
14. Bain BJ. *Leukaemia diagnosis*. 2nd ed. Oxford: Blackwell Science; 1999.
15. Notta F, Mullighan CG, Wang JC, et al. Evolution of human BCR-ABL1 lymphoblastic leukaemia-initiating cells. *Nature* 2011; **469**(7330): 362–67.
16. Genomic and epigenomic landscapes of adult de novo acute myeloid leukemia. *New Engl J Med* 2013; **368**(22): 2059–74.
17. Chabner B. *Cancer chemotherapy and biotherapy: principles and practice*. 5th edn. Philadelphia: Walter Klowers, 2010
18. Iqbal N, Iqbal N. Imatinib: a breakthrough of targeted therapy in cancer. *Chemother Res Pract* 2014; (2014): 357027.
19. Bishop MR. *Hematopoietic stem cell transplantation*. New York: Springer; 2009.
20. Socie G, Ritz J. Current issues in chronic graft-versus-host disease. *Blood* 2014; **124**(3): 374–84.
21. Moor JW, Murray P, Inwood J, et al. Diagnostic biopsy of lymph nodes of the neck, axilla and groin: rhyme, reason or chance? *Ann Roy Coll Surg* 2008; **90**(3): 221–25.
22. Crnkovich MJ, Leopold K, Hoppe RT, Mauch PM. Stage I to IIB Hodgkin's disease: the combined experience at Stanford University and the Joint Center for Radiation Therapy. *J Clin Oncol* 1987; **5**(7): 1041–49.
23. Cinar F. Significance of asymptomatic tonsil asymmetry. *Otolaryngol Head Neck* 2004; **131**(1): 101–03.

24. Guimaraes AC, de Carvalho GM, Correa CR, Gusmao RJ. Association between unilateral tonsillar enlargement and lymphoma in children: a systematic review and meta-analysis. *Crit Rev Oncol Hemat* 2015; **93**(3): 304–11.
25. Dubashi B, Cyriac S, Tenali SG. Clinicopathological analysis and outcome of primary mediastinal malignancies: a report of 91 cases from a single institute. *Ann Thorac Med* 2009; **4**(3): 140–42.
26. Khan UA, Shanholtz CB, McCurdy MT. Oncologic mechanical emergencies. *Emerg Med Clin N Am* 2014; **32**(3): 495–508.
27. DiGiuseppe JA, Borowitz MJ. Clinical utility of flow cytometry in the chronic lymphoid leukemias. *Semin Oncol* 1998; **25**(1): 6–10.
28. Skoog L, Tani E. Immunocytochemistry: an indispensable technique in routine cytology. *Cytopathology* 2011; **22**(4): 215–29.
29. Chen YH, Gong Y. Cytopathology in the diagnosis of lymphoma. *Canc Treat* 2014; **160**: 211–40.
30. Hack HA, Wright NB, Wynn RF. The anaesthetic management of children with anterior mediastinal masses. *Anaesthesia* 2008; **63**(8): 837–46.
31. Thieblemont C, Bertoni F, Copie-Bergman C, et al. Chronic inflammation and extra-nodal marginal-zone lymphomas of MALT-type. *Semin Cancer Biol* 2014; **24**: 33–42.
32. Straetmans J, Stokroos R. Extramedullary plasmacytomas in the head and neck region. *Eur Arch Otorhinolaryngol* 2008; **265**(11): 1417–23.
33. Sasaki R, Yasuda K, Abe E, et al. Multi-institutional analysis of solitary extramedullary plasmacytoma of the head and neck treated with curative radiotherapy. *Int J Radiat Oncol* 2012; **82**(2): 626–34.
34. Resende LS, Coradazzi AL, Rocha-Junior C, Zanini JM, et al. Sudden bilateral deafness from hyperleukocytosis in chronic myeloid leukemia. *Acta Haematol* 2000; **104**(1): 46–49.
35. Li W, Schachern PA, Morizono T, Paparella MM. The temporal bone in multiple myeloma. *Laryngoscope* 1994; **104** (6 Pt 1): 675–80.
36. Jun HJ, Choi J, Kim KM, Chae SW. Multiple myeloma with isolated plasmacytoma in temporal bone. *Otol Neurotol* 2013; **34**(7): e107–08.
37. Fuchs HA, Tanner SB. Granulomatous disorders of the nose and paranasal sinuses. *Curr Opin Otolaryngol Head Neck Surg* 2009; **17**(1): 23–27.
38. Zuniga MG, Turner JH. Treatment outcomes in acute invasive fungal rhinosinusitis. *Curr Opin Otolaryngolo* 2014; **22**(3): 242–48.
39. Pagano L, Caira M. Risks for infection in patients with myelodysplasia and acute leukemia. *Curr Opin Infect Dis* 2012; **25**(6): 612–18.
40. Gonen C, Uner A, Cetinkaya Y, et al. Tonsillar abscess formation due to herpes simplex type-1 in a severely immunocompromised stem cell transplant patient with chronic myeloid leukemia. *Transpl Infect Dis* 2006; **8**(3):166–70.
41. Walsh TJ, Gamaletsou MN. Treatment of fungal disease in the setting of neutropenia. *Hematology* 2013; (**2013**): 423–27.
42. Epstein VA, Kern RC. Invasive fungal sinusitis and complications of rhinosinusitis. *Otolaryngol Clin N Am* 2008; **41**(3): 497–524.
43. Thompson GR 3rd, Patterson TF. Fungal disease of the nose and paranasal sinuses. *J Allergy Clin Immun* 2012; **129**(2): 321–26.
44. Middlebrooks EH, Frost CJ, De Jesus RO. Acute invasive fungal rhinosinusitis: a comprehensive update of CT findings and design of an effective diagnostic imaging model. *AJNR Am J Neuroradiol* 2015; **36**(8) 1529–35.
45. Kim JH, Kang BC, Lee JH, et al. The prognostic value of gadolinium-enhanced magnetic resonance imaging in acute invasive fungal rhinosinusitis. *J Infect* 2015; **70**(1): 88–95.
46. Idris N, Lim LH. Nasal eschar: a warning sign of potentially fatal invasive fungal sinusitis in immunocompromised children. *J Pediatr Hematol Oncol* 2012; **34**(4): e134–36.
47. Al Akhrass F, Debiane L, Abdallah L, et al. Palatal mucormycosis in patients with hematologic malignancy and stem cell transplantation. *Med Mycol* 2011; **49**(4): 400–05.
48. Olalla I, Ortin M, Hermida G, et al. Autologous peripheral blood stem cell transplantation in a patient with previous invasive middle ear mucormycosis. *Bone Marrow Transpl* 1996; **18**(6): 1183–84.
49. Caira M, Trecarichi EM, Mancinelli M, et al. Uncommon mold infections in hematological patients: epidemiology, diagnosis and treatment. *Expert Rev Anti-Infect Ther* 2011; **9**(7): 881–92.
50. Rademaker-Lakhai JM, Crul M, Zuur L, et al. Relationship between cisplatin administration and the development of ototoxicity. *J Clin Oncol* 2006; **24**(6): 918–24.
51. Knight KRG, Kraemer DF, Neuwelt EA. Ototoxicity in children receiving platinum chemotherapy: underestimating a commonly occurring toxicity that may influence academic and social development. *J Clin Oncol* 2005; **23**(34): 8588–96.
52. Knight KR, Kraemer DF, Winter C, Neuwelt EA. Early changes in auditory function as a result of platinum chemotherapy: use of extended high-frequency audiometry and evoked distortion product otoacoustic emissions. *J Clin Oncol* 2007; **25**(10): 1190–95.
53. Brock PR, Knight KR, Freyer DR, et al. Platinum-induced ototoxicity in children: a consensus review on mechanisms, predisposition, and protection, including a new International Society of Pediatric Oncology Boston ototoxicity scale. *J Clin Oncol* 2012; **30**(19): 2408–17.
54. Chiodo AA, Alberti PW, Sher GD, et al. Desferrioxamine ototoxicity in an adult transfusion-dependent population. *J Otolaryngol* 1997; **26**(2): 116–22.
55. Chaimberg KH, Cravero JP. Mucositis and airway obstruction in a pediatric patient. *Anesth Analg* 2004; **99**(1): 59–61.
56. Latiff ZA, Kamal NA, Jahendran J, et al. Vincristine-induced vocal cord palsy: case report and review of the literature. *J Pediatr Hematol Oncol* 2010; **32**(5): 407–10.
57. Bain BJ, Dacie JV, Lewis SM. *Dacie and Lewis practical haematology*. Edinburgh: Elsevier Churchill Livingstone; 2012.
58. Minetti G, Egee S, Morsdorf D, et al. Red cell investigations: art and artefacts. *Blood Rev* 2013; **27**(2): 91–101.
59. Provan D, Stasi R, Newland AC, et al. International consensus report on the investigation and management of primary immune thrombocytopenia. *Blood* 2010; **115**(2): 168–86.
60. Bain BJ. *A beginner's guide to blood cells*. Hoboken: Wiley; 2008.
61. Roufosse F, Garaud S, de Leval L. Lymphoproliferative disorders associated with hypereosinophilia. *Semin Hematol* 2012; **49**(2): 138–48.
62. Bain BJ, WRLC EBSCO E-books. *Haemoglobinopathy diagnosis*. Malden, MA: Blackwell Pub; 2006.
63. Abou-Elhamd KE. Otorhinolaryngological manifestations of sickle cell disease. *Int J Pediatr Otorhinolaryngol* 2012; **76**(1): 1–4.
64. Stanley AC, Christian JM. Sickle cell disease and perioperative considerations: review and retrospective report. *J Oral Maxil Surg* 2013; **71**(6): 1027–33.
65. Imanguli MM, Alevizos I, Brown R, et al. Oral graft-versus-host disease. *Oral Dis* 2008; **14**(5): 396–412.

CHAPTER 26

HAEMOSTASIS: NORMAL PHYSIOLOGY, DISORDERS OF HAEMOSTASIS AND THROMBOSIS

Elizabeth Jones and Russell David Keenan

Introduction 259	Platelet disorders 267
Clotting cascade 259	Thrombotic disorders 269
Interpretation of coagulation screening tests 263	Blood products and factor replacement in bleeding disorders 272
Bleeding disorders 264	How to get the best from your local haematologist 273
Coagulation factor disorders 265	References 274

SEARCH STRATEGY

Data in this chapter may be updated by a PubMed search using the keywords: haemostasis and thrombosis.

INTRODUCTION

It is common for surgeons to come across disorders of haemostasis. The three main scenarios are: i) peri-operative severe and potentially life-threatening bleeding; ii) pre-operative assessment that identifies or suggests a patient may be at increased risk of bleeding; and iii) post-operative thrombosis. The aim of this chapter is to provide the physiological and practical knowledge to manage these scenarios together with your haematology team.

In order to interpret laboratory tests and manage patients' safely it is important to have a working understanding of blood clotting. Blood clotting is somewhat confusing as clotting factors are numbered according to when they were discovered and this is not related to where they are in the clotting cascade. They are labelled in Roman numerals. Factors III, IV and VI are not referred to because, following their discovery, it became clear that they were already known substances (i.e. thromboplastin, calcium and factor Va).

While the traditional cascade model of clotting is not exactly what happens in the body it is still useful and important to understand in order to interpret laboratory tests and safely manage patients. In the body, blood clotting is a much more dynamic process also involving other blood cells and the blood vessel walls. It involves a fine balance between excessive bleeding and clotting, either of which is pathological.

CLOTTING CASCADE

Blood clotting is the conversion of soluble fibrinogen (coagulation factor I), which is present as small monomers, to insoluble long chains of fibrin. Long strands of fibrin are insoluble; however, they are not strongly bound together until the long fibrin strands are cross-linked. This cross-linked fibrin is very strong and stable and the principal structure of the blood clot.

Thrombin is the only factor able to cause fibrinogen to generate fibrin, so thrombin generation is therefore essential for clot formation. Thrombin also controls many other parts of the blood clotting system including forming the cross-linked bonds through activation of factor XIII (**Figure 26.1**).

Common pathway

Prothrombin (factor II) is cleaved to form thrombin and itself can only be activated by activated factor X (Xa). This involves a complex reaction with factor V as a cofactor. Calcium and phospholipid are also required for this to occur.

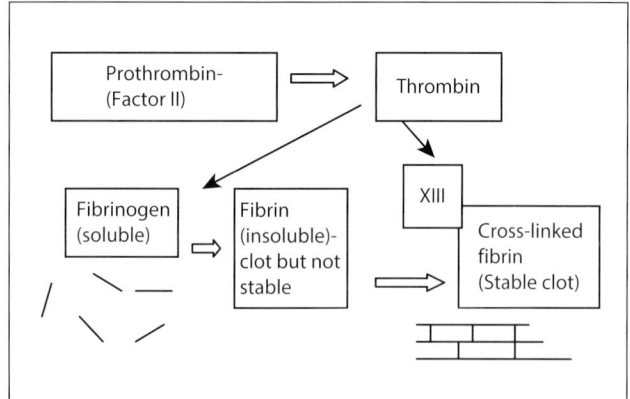

Figure 26.1 The action of thrombin to form cross-linked fibrin.

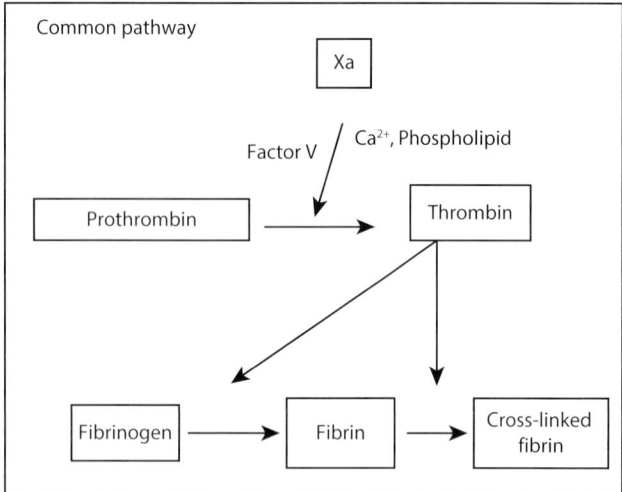

Figure 26.2 The common pathway of blood coagulation.

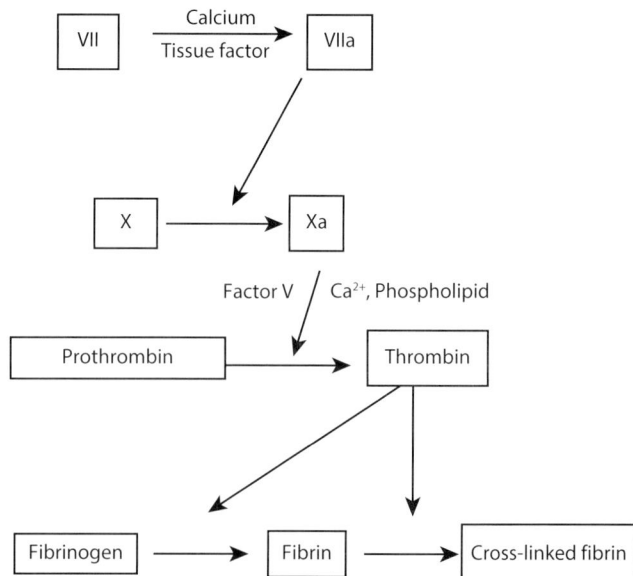

Figure 26.3 The extrinsic and common pathway of blood coagulation.

This section of the process is referred to as the common pathway (**Figure 26.2**). Descriptions of the clotting cascade are traditionally referred to as the common pathway, the intrinsic pathway and the extrinsic pathway. These will be discussed shortly.

Factor Xa can be formed in the laboratory in two different ways. In the prothrombin time (PT) test an **external** factor called 'tissue factor' is required; hence this is called the **extrinsic** pathway. In the partial thromboplastin time (PTT) – also known as activated partial thromboplastin time (APTT) or Kaolin cephalin clotting time (KCCT) – there is no additional biological factor so all the factors are already present **in** the plasma so it is called the **intrinsic** pathway.

Extrinsic pathway (Figure 26.2)

The PT is the time, in seconds, for a clot to form once tissue factor (made from rabbit's brain) and calcium are added to the patient's plasma. During this time factor VII is activated by tissue factor and calcium to become factor VIIa, which in turn directly activates factor X to become Xa, and so on through to the formation of fibrin (**Figure 26.3**).

Note that the PT includes all of the cascade from factor VII through to fibrin formation, but does *not* include cross-linked fibrin (so the PT is normal in factor XIII deficiency).

Intrinsic pathway

The PTT measures the time in seconds for a clot to form once calcium is added to the patient's plasma after a pre-incubation with kaolin which acts as a catalyst (required within laboratory testing to allow the reaction to occur). This covers the time from the conversion of factor XII to XIIa, which then drives activation of factor XI to XIa. Factor XIa in turn activates IX to IXa, which leads to the activation of X to Xa. Factor VIII is a cofactor required for the action of IXa (**Figure 26.4**).

The physical structures of cofactors VIII and V (in the common pathway) are very similar to each other and they participate in similar ways in the reactions. The PTT measures the time for the process from Factor XII through to formation of fibrin, but again *not* to cross-linked fibrin so again this is also normal in factor XIII deficiency.

While the above pathways do not precisely represent what occurs in the body it is a useful working understanding of clotting in laboratory testing that can be used to identify deficiencies in specific factors. The above screening tests allow a measure of the presence and function of the patient's factor levels. However, the differences that occur within the human body include thrombin, also providing positive feedback towards the formation of factors IX, X, XI and VII. Within the body factor VII also activates primarily factor IX, factor IX then activates factor VII in a positive feedback. These extra levels of positive feedback accelerate the process, and create a powerful amplification of the cascade. At each stage of the reaction the amplification is such that one molecule of a particular

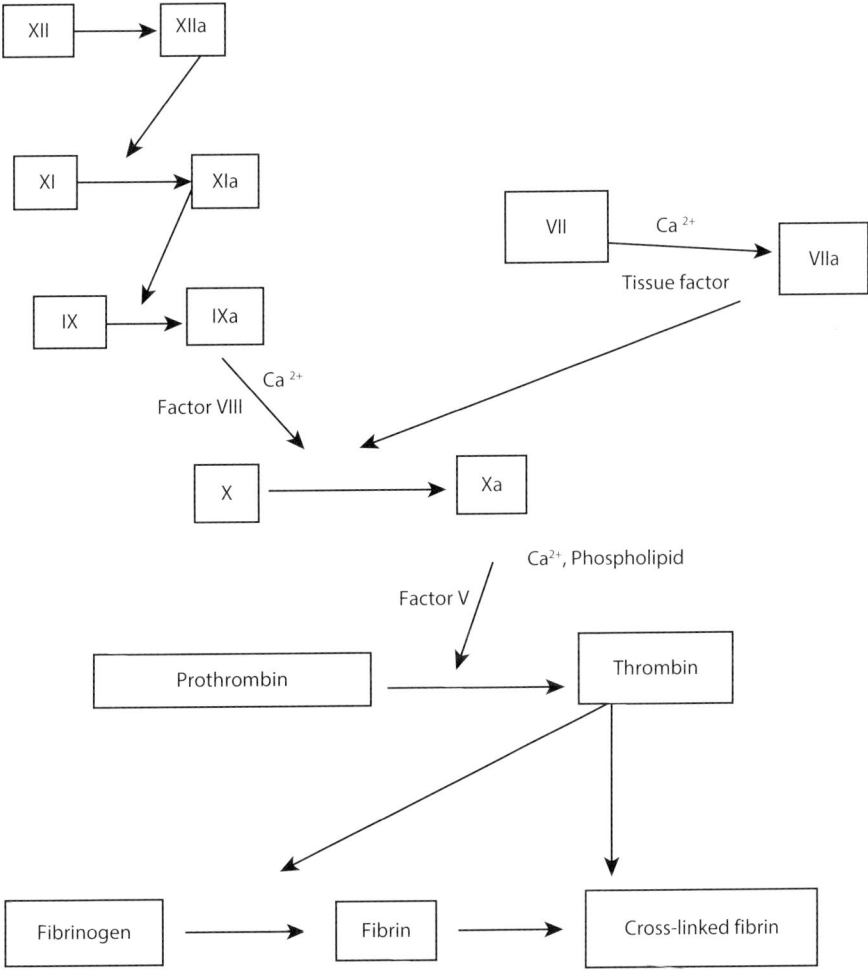

Figure 26.4 The intrinsic, extrinsic and common pathways of blood coagulation.

factor activates 100 molecules of the next factor in line. This allows rapid clot formation from a small initial stimulus. This speed is obviously essential when somebody is bleeding and differs from other much slower enzymatic reactions in the body.

Inhibitory systems

Inhibitory systems are in place to prevent clotting continuing extensively where it is not required. There are two main inhibitory systems; 1) antithrombin (previously referred to as antithrombin III) and 2) protein C with protein S.

Antithrombin's main action is, as the name suggests, inhibition of thrombin. Antithrombin also inhibits at multiple other levels within the cascade, the serine proteases, factors X, IX, XI and XIIa, which share some molecular features.

Factors V and VIII are structurally similar to each other but very different from the other factors. Not surprisingly, therefore, they have a different inhibition system, protein C and its cofactor protein S.

Deficiencies in any of these inhibitory proteins are a risk factor for the generation of clots in patients. An abnormality of the blood clotting system that predisposes to clots is called thrombophilia ('clot loving').

The role of platelets

Platelets are the smallest cell in the body and are fragments of cytoplasm formed from megakaryocytes in the bone marrow. Platelets contain 'packages' (granules) of various elements needed for coagulation, including clotting factors, ADP, serotonin, von Willebrand factor (vWF) and fibrinogen. They have two main receptors on their surface allowing them to stick to exposed collagen on a damaged blood vessel wall and allowing them to stick to each other directly and via vWF.

The steps in platelet function include:

- adherence – sticking to collagen exposed by damaged endothelium
- activation – secreting a range of chemicals to induce clot formation, vasoconstriction and start the healing process
- aggregation – sticking together (stimulated by ADP and thromboxane) (**Figure 26.5**).

ADHERENCE

This is the platelets sticking to exposed collagen underlying the damaged endothelium. There are two main

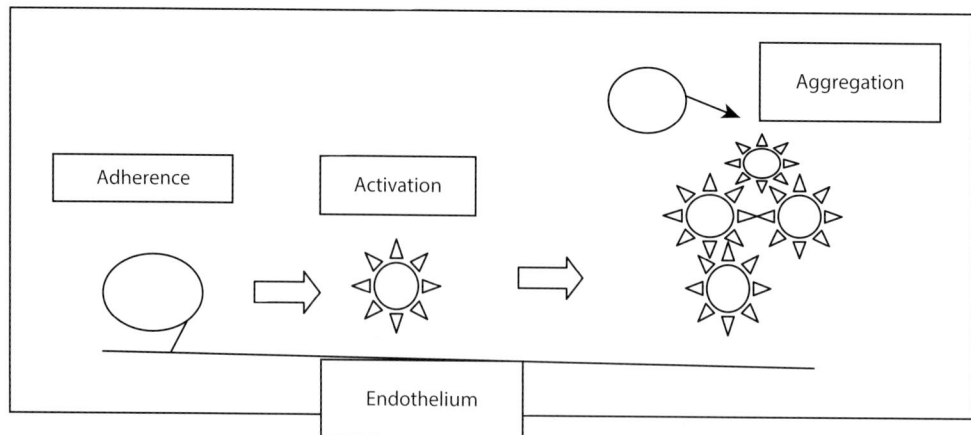

Figure 26.5 Platelet adherence, activation and aggregation.

membrane bound sticky molecular complexes that have this function:

1. Glycoprotein IIb/IIIa complex, which sticks to collagen directly. If this glycoprotein is missing it causes a severe bleeding disorder called Glanzmann's thrombasthenia.
2. Glycoprotein Ib/V/IX complex, which sticks to collagen indirectly via von Willebrand factor. If this glycoprotein is missing it causes a severe bleeding disorder called Bernard Soulier disease.

ACTIVATION

This is the process of locally secreting factors that promote blood clot formation, platelet aggregation, vasoconstriction and the start of tissue healing. One critical process is the 'arachidonic acid pathway'. Arachidonic acid is freed from cell membrane phospholipid molecules and converted to prostaglandin by cyclo-oxygenase (COX) enzymes. In turn the prostaglandin then forms thromboxane (via thromboxane synthetase present in platelets) and prostacyclin (via prostacyclin synthetase in endothelial cells). The thromboxane is a vasoconstrictor that stimulates further platelet aggregation and activation (aspirin irreversibly blocks this process, rendering the platelet function reduced for the rest of its 12-day life span), whereas prostacyclin has opposite effects, causing vasodilation and platelet inhibition.

Aggregation

This is when the activated platelets recruit other platelets to an enlarging 'platelet aggregate'. Much of this is by the release of ADP from dense granules and also through generation of thromboxane.

The role of von Willebrand factor

Von Willebrand factor (vWF) is in plasma and platelets. It is also released from the special storage granules in the endothelium called Weibel Palade bodies.

vWF has two main functions:

1. It makes platelets stick to each other and to damaged blood vessel walls. This can only occur when the vWF sticks to itself in ultra large high molecular weight multimers. These multimer molecules can be huge (from 500 to 20 000 kDa)
2. It chaperones circulating factor VIII – this stabilizes factor VIII to prolong the half-life.

Interpreting laboratory results and diagnosing von Willebrand disease is not straightforward and is beyond the scope of this chapter. Difficulties arise firstly in that vWF is a highly labile protein that goes up with stress (which could include surgery) and also in pregnancy. In addition, the laboratory tests are difficult and results are not always robust, commonly giving falsely low levels.

The role of the vessel wall

The formation of a clot usually starts when there is damage to the endothelial wall. The endothelial wall in its healthy state is active in inhibiting platelet adhesion by the production of substances such as nitric oxide and prostacyclin. It therefore functions as a 'non-stick' surface. When collagen is exposed, allowing platelets to come into contact, they then become active. The two main anticoagulant systems discussed earlier (i.e. antithrombin and proteins C and S) are potentiated by normal endothelium. Antithrombin is bound on the endothelial cell surface by 'heparin like' glycosaminoglycans and is made much more powerful. Another molecule on the endothelial surface called thrombomodulin binds thrombin. Thrombin, instead of being the critical promoter of coagulation, then stops all procoagulant function and potentiates protein C. In effect thrombin becomes an anticoagulant in the presence of normal endothelium and limits the clot to the damaged surface (**Figure 26.6**).

When a platelet plug has formed, the larger blood vessels in particular need cross-linked fibrin to stabilize it. In smaller vessels this is not always a vital step and this partly explains the difference in bleeding manifestations in different disease states.

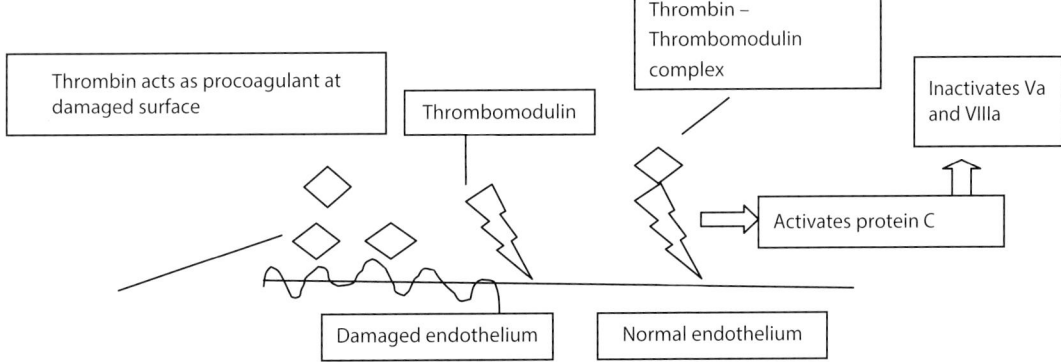

Figure 26.6 Natural anticoagulation via thrombomodulin, protein C and protein S pathway.

The flow of blood within the blood vessel can also affect the type of clot formed. Red clot, mostly erythrocyte (red cell) and fibrin, is formed where flow is reduced with no blood vessel damage (i.e. cases of DVT); they are generally treated best with anticoagulants. White clot is platelet and fibrin, forming where blood vessel damage has occurred and characteristically occurs in faster flow vessels/arteries (i.e. myocardial infarction), which is best treated with antiplatelets. Of course clots may be both white and red, especially where white clots are initially formed leading to alteration of flow and additional formation of red clot.

Blood clot breakdown (fibrinolysis)

As soon as a clot is formed the process of clot breakdown called fibrinolysis starts and is mediated via plasmin. Plasmin is generated from plasminogen, which is bound by fibrin. It is then converted to its active form by plasminogen activators. There are inhibitors to this process, which prevent the degradation occurring too quickly (e.g. plasminogen activator inhibitor PAI-1 and activated protein C) (**Figure 26.7**). All of the products of this breakdown are call fibrin degradation products. D-dimer is the specific product formed only by breakdown of cross-linked fibrin and can be used as an indicator of thrombus formation; however it will also be raised in other states of inflammation/infection.

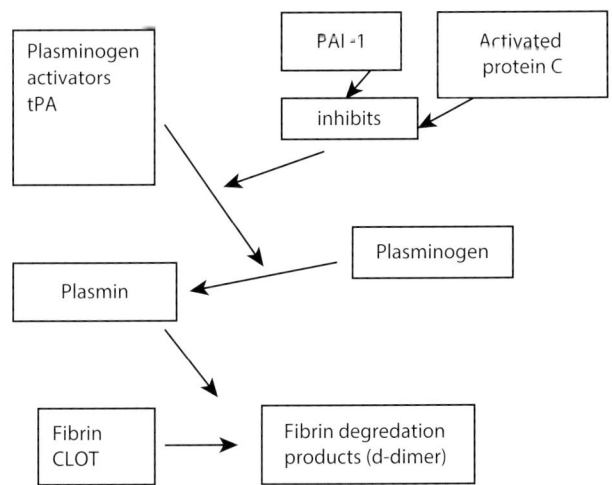

Figure 26.7 Fibrinolysis.

INTERPRETATION OF COAGULATION SCREENING TESTS

(See **Table 26.1**)

International normalized ratio

Technically, an international normalized ratio (INR) should only be used for monitoring of warfarin as this is the setting validated for its use. In all other instances the PT should be requested. The INR is purely the PT ratio multiplied by a 'fiddle factor' specific to the laboratory to allow comparison between laboratories. Therefore there is no additional information in an INR compared with a PT.

With suspected Vitamin K deficiency (if time allows) the usual practice would be to treat with Vitamin K, either oral or IV, depending on concerns regarding gastrointestinal absorption (i.e. 10 mg for 3 to 5 days with a repeat test following this as a 'proof of suspicion') rather than checking Vitamin K levels.

Thromboelastography/rotational thromboelastography

In many settings there is now increasing use of thromboelastography (TEG) and rotational thromboelastography (ROTEM). This technology gives a quick guide as to the global coagulation functioning indicating the patient's current status. It produces a trace providing information of time to formation of clot, and its stability, enabling a more 'real time' guide to product use (**Figure 26.8**). It has particularly been employed in setting with major blood loss (i.e. trauma, vascular surgery).

The trace has a variety of measurements that help in interpreting (**Figure 26.8**):

- **R time** – time until clot first detected (prolonged if on anticoagulants or factor deficiency)
- **K time** – time to clot formation (time from initiation of clot to maximum amplitude/strength)
- **alpha angle** – helps guide if the patient is in a hypercoagulable state.

TABLE 26.1 Interpretation of abnormal laboratory tests

Test	Causes	Further laboratory investigations to consider
Prolonged PT only (with other tests normal). Can only be caused by factor VII deficiency, which in turn may be related to a variety of causes	• Vitamin K deficiency • Antagonists, e.g. warfarin • Dietary. Vitamin K in green vegetables • Early liver disease • Congenital deficiency (very rare)	• LFTs • FVII assay • If dietary deficiency is considered, giving oral Vitamin K and repeating the PT is a simple way of excluding other serious causes.
Prolonged APTT only (deficiency of one or more of: factor VIII, IX, XI, XII)	• Heparin • Lupus anticoagulant or other inhibitor • Congenital deficiency (haemophilias)	• Thrombin time • Reptilase time, which neutralizes heparin
Prolonged PT and APTT	• DIC (also may have low platelets and low fibrinogen) • Liver failure • Vitamin K deficiency • Warfarin • Factor X or V or II deficiency	• LFT • Fibrinogen, factors V, X, II
Low fibrinogen	• DIC • Afibrinogenaemia/dysfibrinogenaemia	• Fibrinogen assay (In routine coagulation testing the result is often a derived value rather than direct testing).
Low platelets	• Clumping/artefact • ITP • Bone marrow failure (many causes) • Drug cause • Infection/DIC	• If a single low count that is unexpected, repeat sample • Blood film • Further investigation depends on the history
Normal tests but abnormal bleeding	• **Consider surgical causes**; it may be obvious but surgery is the commonest cause of bleeding post-operatively • LMWH • Abnormal platelet function • Von Willebrand disease • Factor XIII deficiency • Mild factor deficiency	• Von Willebrand screen • Factor XIII assay • Platelet aggregation studies

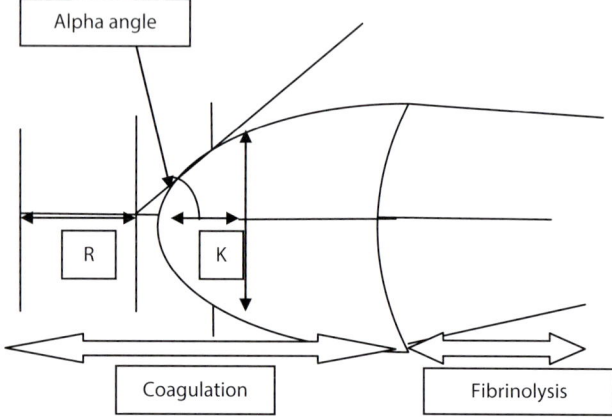

Figure 26.8 Thromboelastography.

The shape of the trace produced gives a lot of information on the coagulation and fibrinolysis and very typical traces can be seen in pathological states such as disseminated intravascular coagulation (DIC) when a patient is hypercoagulable with reduced R and K times and secondary fibrinolysis.

Specific factor assays

These are performed to quantify the levels of specific coagulation factors in a patient. They are needed for initial diagnosis and then for guiding response treatment and further management. Using a plasma known to be deficient in a specific factor (which are now manufactured, although can be plasma from patients known to have haemophilia) and normal plasma, either the PT or PTT test can be performed, depending on which factor is to be assayed. By mixing the 100% normal plasma and 0% deficient plasma in different proportions to create a standard curve, the patient's plasma can then be tested and a specific factor level deduced from this curve. This is the basis of testing for all factor levels in the extrinsic and intrinsic pathways.

BLEEDING DISORDERS

It is vital to identify any underlying bleeding disorder prior to surgery. Patients with severe bleeding disorders can have life-threatening bleeding even with minor procedures. Patients with bleeding disorders should always be managed jointly with the haematology team.

Different bleeding disorders present with different bleeding symptoms, for example joint bleeds in haemophilia and mucocutaneous bleeding (i.e. bruising, bleeding from the nose, mouth and menorrhagia) with von Willebrand disease and platelet disorders. This is because the defect in the clotting system affects different aspects of function. Bleeding disorders may be genetic/congenital or acquired. The history is crucial to guide further investigation and it is not always possible to fully interpret the laboratory investigations without the history.

It is useful to know that bleeding symptoms are common in the normal population. In a survey of normal controls, up to 25% of males and 46% of females with normal haemostasis are likely to have at least one bleeding manifestation (including menorrhagia, post-operative bleeding, bleeding post dental extraction).[1] Almost all of us will get a nose bleed at some point and 25% of younger children have recurrent nose bleeds. Most children experience fewer nose bleeds by the time they are teenagers. In some studies 65% of normal women in the control population would describe themselves as having menorrhagia. Bruising is normal with an active childhood lifestyle and if easy bruising is a symptom then objective questioning on the location, frequency, size and trauma associated with the bruising is essential. Bleeding scores have been developed to aid decisions on how significant the history is, but they are not necessarily in widespread use.

COAGULATION FACTOR DISORDERS

Haemophilia

One of the better known bleeding disorders is haemophilia. The genetic forms of this are grouped as haemophilia A (deficiency of factor VIII) or haemophilia B – Christmas disease (deficiency of factor IX). These are then classified as mild, moderate or severe depending on the patient's baseline factor level (mild is factor level <30%, moderate <5% and severe <1%). In most haemophilias the genetic defect 'runs true' within the family, therefore the severity of haemophilia also runs true within families.

Haemophilia A and B are X-linked genetic disorders and as such classically affect males. However, there are rare instances of female carriers presenting with increased bleeding tendency related to a low factor level (i.e. carriers of severe haemophilia). There are also instances of affected females with very low factor levels due to other complicated inheritance genetics (extreme X chromosome lyonization and mosaicism). Lastly it should be remembered that there are rare families who have two completely separate bleeding disorders, which can lead to some individuals having a much more severe bleeding phenotype than would be normally expected because they have inherited both. This means the patient's personal history and bleeding manifestations are of vital importance in treatment decision-making.

Severe and moderate haemophilias are usually diagnosed in childhood with many cases having been suspected antenatally when family history is known. Milder cases may present in adulthood. Spontaneous new mutations occur in approximately 20% of cases (therefore there is no family history). People with severe haemophilias have increased bruising but this does not usually cause a problem. The main issues for these patients are spontaneous joint and muscle bleeds and excessive bleeding following even minor procedures. All patients with a diagnosis of or suspected haemophilia should have surgery managed in a centre with specialist haematology experience.

Patients with haemophilia A or B would be expected to have a significantly prolonged APTT on screening tests. Further assays can then be performed to ascertain specific factor levels.

Management of haemophilia

The management of patients ideally revolves around appropriate intravenous recombinant or plasma derived factor replacement. This can be 'on-demand' treatment for bleeds or 'prophylaxis' given regularly (usually 2–3 times weekly and often taken when sports or activities dictate). No oral factor replacement therapy is available as yet. Many patients who are newly diagnosed are now given primary prophylaxis and may not have experienced significant bleeds. Patients (particularly older ones) are generally very knowledgeable about symptoms of joint bleeds and most will self-treat at home, only attending hospital for review by the medical team if significant bleeding is experienced or if it is not settling. Acute bleeds require increased factor administration (i.e. often at least twice a day) with rest initially being advised followed by appropriate physiotherapy.

In developing countries expensive recombinant factor is often not available. Plasma derived factor is often cheaper but can carry the risk of blood-borne infection transmission. Simple measures of bleed management should always be considered in addition to factor replacement including RICE (rest, ice, compression and elevation) along with use of the relatively inexpensive tranexamic acid (an antifibrinolytic agent).

Management of any bleeding condition is a partnership between patient and multidisciplinary team. Perioperative management and dosing of factor replacement will usually be guided by exact levels and review of bleeding symptoms. The administered factor will be consumed more quickly in the face of bleeding and close monitoring of bloods may be required for a week or more post-operatively in the event of major surgery. Treatment options include bolus and continuous infusion of factor.

The management of haemophilia (and other bleeding disorders) may be complicated further by the development of inhibitors. This is an immune response with neutralizing antibodies against the factor treatment, which is viewed by the body as a foreign protein. The development of an inhibitor would be suspected in cases where there is an inadequate clinical response to treatment. Inhibitors are also usually monitored via laboratory testing as part of routine follow-up care. As the factor therapy is rendered ineffective, patients with inhibitors are very difficult to treat and can suffer life-threatening bleeding. Surgery should be avoided where possible until the inhibitor is controlled. Acute bleeds in these situations require administration of factor VIII inhibitor bypassing agent (FEIBA), which is a plasma derived concentration of a number of other factors or high dose recombinant factor VIIa (rFVIIa) to gain control. Patients with significant problems with inhibitors generally require treatment aimed at eradicating the inhibitor; however, this usually takes many months to be an effective strategy.

Acquired haemophilia

Acquired haemophilia is very rare but is important to mention as it can present to surgeons and has disastrous consequences if not identified. This usually occurs in older adults but can also occur in pregnancy. It is a type of autoimmune disease where patients develop (auto)antibodies to a coagulation factor (their own endogenous factor). This is most commonly FVIII or von Willebrand factor. It can present with no past history of bleeding manifestation. On presentation their bleeding, manifestations tend to be very different to those with congenital haemophilia and may consist of very extensive bruising and prolonged surgical bleeding. It does not usually lead to joint bleeds. From a laboratory point of view they will have a similar finding of markedly prolonged APTT, which would of course require further investigation. There will be a very low factor level. A 50:50 mix of patient plasma and normal plasma is a quick and easy test that all laboratories can perform even out of hours. The prolonged APTT does not correct as the inhibitor also destroys the factor in the normal plasma that is added (whereas it would normally correct in a congenital deficiency as enough factor is added with the 'normal plasma' and it is not destroyed by antibody). There may be an underlying condition driving the formation of the antibodies (i.e. malignancy, pregnancy). Patients with acquired haemophilia are complex and unbelievably expensive to manage and require two aspects of treatment: i) management of acute bleeding, which is similar to the management of a patient with congenital haemophilia who has an inhibitor; and ii) immunosuppression in an attempt to control the antibody, often with agents such as steroid, ciclosporin or Rituximab (a monoclonal antibody directed against CD20 cell marker that destroys mature B lymphocytes). Patients may spontaneously remit depending on whether an underlying driver can be treated but may have further episodes of relapse.

Von Willebrand disease

Von Willebrand disease is an inherited bleeding disorder. It can be seen with autosomal dominant or recessive inheritance. It is categorized into three types. The most common is type 1. This is usually a relatively mild partial quantitative deficiency, that is, a reduced amount of a normal von Willebrand factor (vWF). Type 2 is split into further groups but all involve abnormal vWF, usually with reduced function. Type 3 is near absence of vWF that leads to a severe bleeding phenotype very similar to severe haemophilia A.

It is often quoted that von Willebrand disease is very common at around 1% of the population.[2] This is false. The 'rumour' followed an Italian study that identified nine normal school children with low vWF levels out of 1000 tested. This in reality was just validating the reference range, which if set at 2 standard deviations from the mean will exclude 5% of the normal population (2.5% below and above). This paper is still repeatedly quoted today in literature but what is rarely quoted is the follow-up paper on the nine children, most of whom had surgery and none of whom had any clinically relevant bleeding problems. In 2004–2005, UK international diagnostic guidelines were published that were much more restrictive.[3] This is important as it will not be uncommon for someone to present with a historical diagnosis of von Willebrand disease and when you contact your haematologist to review they may retract the diagnosis.[4] It is also recognized that as people get older their levels often improve, which may be another reason for altered management.[5]

Surgeons will frequently encounter patients with a personal or family member with a historical diagnosis. The international diagnostic guidelines have minor differences but essentially the diagnosis relies upon clinical significant bleeding symptoms and a vWF antigen (or activity level of vWF) of 40 iu/dL or less on repeat occasions. A patient's blood group is also related to vWF levels, with group O patients having 30% lower levels then group A and B. This may well be the reason why blood group O patients are less likely to have thrombotic problems such as ischaemic stroke.

MANAGEMENT OF VON WILLEBRAND DISEASE

Management of vWD in most cases is by use of DDAVP (which leads to release of endogenous stores of vWF and factor VIII) or plasma derived product containing vWF and FVIII. There is as yet no recombinant product available. DDAVP is not effective in all cases so for routine surgery patients would normally have a trial of DDAVP prior to the procedure to assess response. Of course levels would still need to be checked prior to surgery even if a previous good response has been demonstrated. DDAVP leads to a rise in plasma level of FVIII and vWF, caused by increase release from Weibel Palade granules in endothelial cells. Once these storage granules release their contents there is a latency period before the treatment will be effective again. DDAVP should be avoided in patients with evidence of atherosclerosis. Fluid retention can be a problem post-administration, often leading to headaches, so patients should be fluid restricted following it. DDAVP also cannot be used in very young children who are prone to life-threatening sodium toxicity. It should be noted that different strengths of DDAVP are available depending on the indication so it is vital to ensure the correct formulation is used.

Other rare congenital factor deficiencies

Patients can present with deficiency of any coagulation factor. The next most common factor deficiency is factor XI. This is a very variable cohort of patients and the factor level does not necessarily correlate with bleeding manifestations. It can be treated with factor concentrate but levels should not be increased to above 70% as the risk of thrombosis becomes high. Tranexamic acid (an antifibrinolytic agent) should not be used at the same time as factor replacement in this group but could be an alternative strategy. As only small amounts of factor XI are required in mild factor XI deficiency adequate haemostasis can often be achieved with FFP.

Dys- or afibrinogenaemia may be a qualitative or quantitative defect of fibrinogen. It may manifest as abnormal bleeding following trauma or surgery. The severity depends on the exact defect. It is managed by replacement with fibrinogen concentrate; often twice weekly is sufficient.

Factor VII plays a vital role in initiating coagulation but only a small amount is required. However, a severe deficiency causes a similar bleeding phenotype to haemophilia with spontaneous bleeds occurring. Factor VII has the shortest half-life and therefore replacement during a bleed is required 3–4 times per 24 hours. There is a recombinant product available.

Factor II, V and X deficiency are all exceedingly rare. There are also cases of deficiencies seen in combination that can lead to diagnostic confusion.

Factor XIII is important in fibrin stabilization, so has a typical delayed bleeding after surgery. The classical presentation is in neonates with prolonged umbilical stump bleeding. It has a long half-life and in deficient patients treatment once a month with concentrate is adequate prophylaxis. Plasma derived concentrate has been used for many years but a recombinant factor XIII is available in some countries.

Factor XII deficiency leads to a prolonged PTT but it does not lead to clinical bleeding or symptoms, so is only relevant in relation to its effect on the laboratory parameter.

Disseminated intravascular coagulation (DIC)

Disseminated intravascular coagulation (DIC) can be a confusing condition with both bleeding and clotting problems being present. There is widespread over-activation of the coagulation system leading to significant, usually arterial, thrombosis. The extensive formation of tiny blood clots throughout the body can lead to consumption of coagulation factors. These deficiencies can then lead to bleeding. It is usually bleeding that causes the life-threatening problems (Table 26.2).

TABLE 26.2 The causes of disseminated intravascular coagulation (DIC)

Infection
Trauma: • bleeding post-surgery • shock/hypotension
Tissue necrosis (e.g. organ destruction, e.g pancreatitis)
Malignancy-solid tumours, leukaemia
Obstetric-amniotic fluid embolism, placental abruption, pre-eclampsia
Vascular abnormalities – haemangioma and vascular aneurysm
Severe liver failure
Toxic and immunological insults-snake bites, drugs, ABO incompatible transfusion

The management revolves around 'treating the underlying cause' (Table 26.2) and supportive care (either by transfusion and other organ support, with or without anticoagulation dependent on the most problematic symptom). From a laboratory perspective it is usually diagnosed when an abnormal clotting screen is present with low platelets. The trend of blood counts should be monitored[6] and would include a rising PT and APTT, reducing fibrinogen and platelets with a raised D-dimer. The decision to use FFP and/or cryoprecipitate depends on the relative PT, PTT and fibrinogen, and the clinical problem. Again it is wise to involve a haematologist if this condition is suspected to guide on what is likely to be the most effective product and to ensure that the laboratory is expecting and turning around samples and provision of blood products quickly.

PLATELET DISORDERS

Immune thrombocytopenic purpura

Immune thrombocytopenic purpura (ITP) is a relatively common cause of an isolated low platelet count. Platelets are usually produced normally but are destroyed by the immune system so it is an auto-immune phenomenon. In the paediatric setting it is usually a condition that spontaneously resolves often not requiring specific treatment. However in the adult setting, and occasionally in children, it can be a chronic condition. In either case patients generally do not respond well to platelet transfusion, only getting poor transient increments due to rapid destruction. Patients who have a low platelet count should be discussed with the haematology team whether they have a specific diagnosis already or not. When a patient newly presents, other causes of thrombocytopenia would need to be ruled out. A repeat full blood count (FBC) is always essential as clumping of platelets can give a falsely low result on automated counters. A blood film can confirm if it is a consistent result and look for other abnormalities. Advice on management would depend on the clinical presentation, mainly if the patient has haemorrhagic manifestations. The platelet count does not always correlate with the level of bleeding or bruising and in ITP patients often tolerate very low counts without symptoms.

If an immediate rise in platelet count is needed, advice is likely to include administration of intravenous immunoglobulin (IVIg) to gain a quick response, high dose steroid (IV or oral), which takes longer to act, and platelet transfusions.[7] Despite a likely poor response, platelets are usually advisable in an emergency setting. IVIg is also often employed in an elective perioperative management plan. If a patient has previously been diagnosed they may well be on treatment which could include oral steroid or immunosuppression (i.e. azathioprine, ciclosporin, etc). Another treatment becoming more commonly used is Rituximab. Splenectomy can be very effective in some patients, but this leads to increased risk of sepsis, particularly from encapsulated organisms. Lastly the thrombopoetin (TPO) agonists are a newer treatment option with oral and subcutaneous administration routes that stimulate increased platelet production.

Thrombocytosis

Very high platelet counts (> 1000) can also lead to thrombosis or bleeding as the platelets are dysfunctional and also absorb increased amounts of von Willebrand factor, which then becomes depleted, contributing to the problems. The most common scenarios that cause this are myeloproliferative disorders, usually essential thrombocythaemia in older adults. The platelet count in this situation needs to be controlled because of both the bleeding risk and the risk of stroke or other thromboembolic events. Thrombocytosis in children is very rarely due to a primary blood disorder and is usually in response to infection or inflammation. This reactive picture is also seen in adults and in this situation no specific action is required other than monitoring.

Heparin-induced thrombocytopenia (HIT)

Many patients on prolonged heparin can develop a mild thrombocytopenias. This is not usually a clinical problem and heparin can often be continued. However, a rare drug reaction can be a severe thrombocytopenia that paradoxically also causes thrombosis as well as bleeding. This is a complication whereby a patient forms antibodies to heparin and the antibodies form immune complexes with heparin and PF4, which bind to platelet Fc receptors and lead to aggregation and thrombocytopenia. It may be suspected when a platelet count falls when on heparin (usually to between 20 and 50 or a drop of 50% compared with the baseline, with no other explanation) and when new thrombosis occurs. There are scoring systems to assess the likelihood, and testing for causative PF4 antibodies can be undertaken.[8] Heparin should be stopped and treatment should be given with an alternative anticoagulant (i.e. danaparoid, argatroban, bivilarudin, Fondaparinux). The platelet count should increase over the next 2–5 days. Patients should not be re-exposed to heparin (or low molecular weight heparin) as recurrence is common.

Thrombotic thrombocytopenic purpura

Thrombotic thrombocytopenic purpura (TTP) is a rare life-threatening condition that requires urgent treatment when recognized. It is a haematological emergency. Patients present haematologically with low platelets and anaemia (due to haemolysis) with fragments of red cells (schistocytes) seen on blood film, a microangiopathic haemolysis. Patients can have clinical symptoms of fever and neurological features (confusion, seizures) along with renal failure. In TTP the low platelets are caused by thrombosis in small blood vessels. The fibrin strands act as a 'cheese wire' leading to the red cell fragments. The underlying pathology is a reduction in a protein called ADAMTS13, which is normally involved in controlling vWF. With reduced ADAMTS13 vWF builds up into even bigger multimers than normal. The molecules can even get to the size of cells. Treatment is aimed at the underlying cause, reducing the abnormal vWF molecules and also replacing ADAMTS13. At the moment this is most effectively done by plasma exchange. Steroids and further immunosuppressive agents are also needed to gain control of the underlying drivers in the acquired form (there is a congenital variant of the condition with deficiency of ADAMTS13 and replacement by plasma infusion is sufficient treatment). When the platelet count rises thromboprophylaxis should be instigated as thrombosis is common in recovery.

Bone marrow failure syndromes

Myelodysplastic syndrome (MDS) is a collection of conditions where blood cell production in the bone marrow is abnormal and can affect one or all blood cell lines. Patients may therefore have features of anaemia, low platelets or low white cells. In most surgical situations patients will be managed with platelet transfusions if there is a bleeding risk. They may also need antibiotics to cover infection.

Other causes of bone marrow failure include conditions such as leukaemia and aplastic anaemia. Again the mainstay of bleeding management involves platelet transfusion. It may be appropriate to check a 'platelet increment', that is, repeat an FBC either 1 hour after the transfusion or 24 hours after. This may be particularly relevant if the patient has had previous transfusions and therefore a greater possibility of antibodies adversely affecting response to transfusion, or if a major procedure is planned to determine if further treatment is required.

Abnormalities of platelet function

Platelet function abnormalities generally present with post-surgical bleeding, mucocutaneous bleeding and/or menorrhagia. Platelet function abnormalities are most usually seen secondary to medication but there are very severe inherited disorders worth discussing here. Investigation of platelet function disorders will depend on a significant bleeding history usually with normal coagulation tests. A prolonged bleeding time is characteristic of platelet function disorders. A bleeding time is a very simple test where a cut of defined length, thickness and depth is made on the medial anterior aspect of the forearm and the time is measured in seconds until the bleeding stops. The bleeding time is rarely used as it is difficult to control and there is significant observer variability as well as the risk of scarring. Other platelet tests available include a screening test called the PFA-100 and more formal platelet aggregation studies. Platelet aggregation studies take a senior coagulation scientist a few hours and must be performed on fresh platelets. Therefore, this is an assay that must be booked with your laboratory in advance. In addition, intracellular platelet nucleotides can also be measured to aid diagnosis. Lastly, confirmation of some disorders may be sought by use of flow cytometry with monoclonal antibodies directed against absent receptors.

Platelet storage pool disorder is a term that covers abnormalities of the granules in the platelet cytoplasm. It includes deficiency of either alpha granules (grey platelet syndrome) or dense granules (MYH9 anomalies, Hermansky-Pudlak etc.) or both.

Platelet receptor anomalies include Glanzmann's thrombasthenia, where there is absent or abnormal glycoprotein IIb/IIIa (a receptor for fibrinogen and vWF), and Bernard Soulier disease with absent or abnormal glycoprotein Ib/V/IX complex (a receptor for vWF).

Management of bleeding problems in these structural platelet disorders will usually include platelet transfusions. However, these patients often need repeated platelet transfusions throughout their lives and frequently develop antibodies to the platelet antigen in the transfused platelets that they are missing. For this reason when planning minor procedures, where possible, the use of platelets is avoided. Other treatment options may include use of an antifibrinolytic such as tranexamic acid (mouthwash/PO or IV), avoiding antiplatelet agents and on occasion recombinant factor VIIa. Surgical technique should also be considered to minimize bleeding problems. To reduce the chance of developing antibodies any transfused platelets should be HLA matched irradiated and leucodepleted.

Medical problems

RENAL DISEASE

Renal disease and uraemia mostly affects platelet function, although anaemia also contributes to bleeding manifestations. The platelets, as the smallest constituent in blood, normally flow and travel along next to the endothelium so they are closest to the site where they will function. In anaemia they are not pushed out to the side as much, therefore increasing bleeding when injury occurs. Correcting the anaemia and the use of agents such as tranexamic acid or DDAVP are useful strategies to improve haemostasis in these patients when bleeding.

LIVER DISEASE

Liver disease has a potentially large impact on coagulation due to its role in the production of coagulation factors, particularly the Vitamin K-dependent ones (II, VII, IX, X and protein C and S) along with fibrinogen and the other coagulation factors. Portal hypertension can also lead to splenomegaly, which in turn can lead to a thrombocytopenia due to increased destruction of platelets.

THROMBOTIC DISORDERS

When a patient presents with thrombosis (the pathological formation of blood clot) an assessment should be undertaken as to the potential drivers behind clot formation. According to Virchow's Triad, three broad categories of factor contribute to thrombus formation: i) hypercoaguability (i.e. problems within the blood); ii) haemodynamic/blood flow changes; and lastly, iii) endothelial injury or dysfunction. Within this framework it is easier to see how certain states contribute towards a hypercoagulability by one or more mechanism (i.e. surgery, inflammatory conditions, infection, pregnancy, dehydration, immobility). Most hospital inpatients are assessed on admission and a decision made regarding prophylaxis for venous thromboembolism (VTE), most commonly with low molecular weight heparin (LMWH).

Investigation of thrombosis may include a thrombophilia screen, although this is done much less frequently now, as usually the results do not change the management of the patient. However, where it would alter management it should be taken into account.[9] Thrombophilia tests are best delayed until after the acute thrombus setting, ideally being done around 6 weeks after discontinuing anticoagulation treatment. Some patients will be tested because of their own history (e.g. VTE at a young age); however, some may be tested because of their relatives and family history. For the purposes of this chapter we will concentrate on the haematological abnormalities that lead to clots rather than the acquired non-haematological ones, of which there is a long list (i.e. dehydration, malignancy, advanced age, obesity, vascular malformation).

Table 26.3 gives an idea of comparable relative risks for various states in a large retrospective study.[10] It is worth noting that a prospective study found much lower risks for both heterozygosity (3.7) and homozygosity (24) for factor V Leiden.[11]

Thrombophilia screen

This includes:

- deficiency of natural anticoagulants (antithrombin; protein C; protein S)
- other genetic thrombophilias (factor V Leiden, an abnormal form of factor V protein which is resistant to protein C inactivation; prothrombin gene mutation (causing increased production of thrombin).

Deficiencies in protein C, protein S and ATIII mostly occur as a genetically inherited phenomenon. Heterozygous inheritance (one abnormal gene copy) of factor V Leiden or prothrombin gene mutation leads to only a small increase

TABLE 26.3 Relative risk factors for thrombosis

Risk factor	Relative risk
Antithrombin deficiency (Heterozygous)	5
Factor V Leiden	8.1
Factor V Leiden homozygous	80
Hospitalization	11.1
Immobilization	8.9
Oral contraceptive	3.8
Pregnancy	4.2
Protein C deficiency	3.1
PT gene mutation	2.8
Puerperium	14.1
Surgery	5.9

in risk of thrombosis compared to the normal population and, depending on the clinical scenario, would not require any specific treatment. However, where there is homozygous expression, or co-inheritance with other defects the risk increases significantly and patients would often be on long-term anticoagulation, particularly if there is a personal history of blood clot (**Table 26.3**).

Patients with a deficiency of antithrombin, protein C or S generally have a more severe clotting phenotype and each case should be assessed on an individual basis with regards to anticoagulation.

Hyperhomocysteinaemia, which can be inherited or acquired, can also lead to increased propensity to clot, this raised level of homocysteine affects collagen and causes damage to the endothelial wall. It is managed by vitamin B6, B12 and folic acid (B9) supplementation as this reduces the concentration of homocysteine in the blood. This is not necessarily included as part of the basic screen.

Acquired causes of thrombosis

Antiphospholipid syndrome is an acquired condition and has strict criteria for diagnosis requiring both clinical (thrombotic events, unexplained miscarriage or premature labour) and laboratory findings (two out of; anticardiolipin antibodies, anti beta-2 glycoprotein or a lupus anticoagulant found persistently over a period of 3 months). Again with these patients anticoagulant decisions should be made upon consideration of their clinical history. It is important to mention that a lupus anticoagulant is a relatively common cause of a prolonged APTT and when found without other features mainly causes 'diagnostic issues' rather than clinical problems.

Rarities

There are also other haematological conditions such as paroxysmal nocturnal haemoglobinuria (PNH) and myeloproliferative disorders that can lead to an increased propensity to form clots. These should also be considered if investigating for thrombophilia, particularly where rare or unusual thrombus occurs (i.e. intra-abdominal) but they would commonly have an associated abnormality on the full blood count.

Treatment of venous thrombosis

When a patient presents with venous thrombosis, initial treatment is usually with low molecular weight heparin (LMWH) followed by warfarin or a direct oral anticoagulant (DOAC). Apixiban, Dabigatran, Edoxaban and Rivaroxaban are all licensed DOACs and are in increasing use. Decisions need to be taken regarding the length of treatment based on an assessment of risk factors, depending on whether it was provoked, the family history, whether hereditary thrombophilia is present, whether symptoms have resolved and if the risk factors present are modifiable or are going to resolve.

Post-operative deep vein thrombosis (DVT) without other suspected predisposition can usually be treated for 3 months, previously treatment for pulmonary embolus (PE) was given for 6 months, although there are more recent suggestions that 3 months may be adequate for PE if long-term anticoagulation is not indicated. When considering the risks of repeat events it is worth bearing in mind that it is most common to have the same type of event again, so if a patient has a PE they are more likely to have a further PE rather than DVT. There is evidence now to suggest that a raised d-dimer following the completion of treatment can be predictive of a repeat clot and this may be taken into account and a discussion between patient and medical team about the risks of recurrent clot versus the risks of side effects/bleeding on the anticoagulant is needed to decide if long-term anticoagulation should be continued. Decisions on anticoagulation need to be reviewed and the risk benefit balance needs to be reassessed if there is a change in the patients' situation.

Managing a patient on anticoagulation who needs surgery

Managing a patient on anticoagulation in an emergency requires consideration of how best to reverse it (if possible). For an elective procedure 'bridging' anticoagulation should be considered, depending on whether the patient is low or high risk for clotting (i.e. atrial fibrillation (AF) is low risk, compared with metallic heart valve or recent clot-high risk) and whether surgery is low or high risk for serious bleeding (tonsillectomy would be considered a high risk procedure in terms of bleeding, dental extraction of tooth low risk). If the patient is low risk and the surgery high risk, discontinuation of anticoagulation may be required. However if the patient is high risk and the surgery low risk it may be reasonable to continue as normal. In the middle of these extremes it may be necessary to switch onto an alternative, such as from warfarin to LMWH, which can be discontinued 24 hours before the procedure and restarted when haemostasis is secured post-operatively (24–48 hours). With NOACs generally, their half-life allows discontinuation 24–48 hours prior to an operation depending on renal function (although up to 5 days may be advisable in some cases). Where a clot has occurred recently (within 6 weeks to 3 months) an IVC (inferior vena cava) filter may be considered to add a level of protection from PE on the discontinuation of anticoagulation for theatre. Filters should be removed as soon as possible post-procedure otherwise they become permanent and have potential long-term complications. Again, discussion with the anticoagulation team or haematologist should be helpful in managing these situations

Medication affecting haemostasis
WARFARIN/COUMARINS

Warfarin is often described as a Vitamin K antagonist. It does not actually antagonize Vitamin K but it inhibits the enzyme that recycles Vitamin K (Vitamin K epoxide reductase) and therefore active Vitamin K will run out, which usually takes 2–3 days. The Vitamin K dependent clotting factors are depleted (II, VII, IX and X), leading to increased bleeding tendency and the intended benefit of reducing clot formation. However, when it is first initiated patients are rendered prothrombotic because protein C and S are also dependent on Vitamin K and their levels can reduce before the other factors. When patients present with an acute clot it is advisable to overlap initial treatment with LMWH and warfarin until therapeutic. All coumarins have a narrow therapeutic window and, due to various polymorphisms, are metabolized with a lot of inter-individual variation. Warfarin needs to be monitored by the international normalized ratio (INR). The INR is a PT ratio of the patients compared to normal, to the power of an adjustment factor called the ISI that is specific for the laboratory. This gives a result that is comparable amongst laboratories internationally. The indications for coumarins include: treatment of VTE; prevention of VTE; anticoagulation for prosthetic heart valves; and reduction of stroke risk in AF. Patients may be on them for a period of a few months, or may be on lifelong treatment. The most common side effect is bleeding.

REVERSING A RAISED INR DUE TO WARFARIN

The availability of product needs to be taken into consideration if the patient is bleeding and also how quickly reversal is required. In reversing a patient's anticoagulation there should always be discussion with your haematologist. The need for reinstating anticoagulation also needs to be considered.

HEPARIN AND LOW MOLECULAR WEIGHT HEPARIN

Unfractionated heparin (UFH, administered by intravenous infusion) acts by binding to antithrombin and causing a conformational change. The antithrombin then inactivates thrombin, along with the other proteases, mostly factor Xa. Low molecular weight heparins (LMWH, administered by subcutaneous injection) are much smaller molecules so their mechanism of action is mediated more predominantly through anti factor Xa action. The main indications for these drugs are acute VTE or coronary thrombotic event. Some patients remain on LMWH long term, particularly those with malignancy. Unfractionated heparin (UFH) is monitored by APTT ratio and LMWH by anti-factor Xa levels. Most patients do not require monitoring of LMWH (the exceptions where it is useful include children, pregnancy, renal impairment, obesity and when in long-term use).

There is no specific reversal treatment, although protamine sulphate can have some neutralizing effect if given soon after administration, particularly when IV unfractionated heparin has been used. It is much less predictable in subcutaneous LMWH reversal and can act as a weak anticoagulant in its own right in high dose. Prior to surgery, UFH will be fully reversed if stopped 6 hours before with normal renal function; LMWH prophylaxis dose should be last given 12 hours before procedures and treatment doses 24 hours before.

OTHER PARENTERAL ANTICOAGULANTS

These are rarely used. Danaparoid is a heparinoid with mostly anti-Xa action and a little anti-IIa activity. It is renally excreted with no specific antidote. Fondaparinux is a pentasaccharide (synthetic) that acts indirectly through its anti-Xa activity. Again, it is renally excreted with no specific antidote. Bivalirudin is a direct thrombin inhibitor and has a short half-life but IV infusion is required for ongoing anticoagulation, so stopping it and general haemostatic measures are usually adequate.

DIRECT ORAL ANTICOAGULANT AGENTS (DOACS)

Dabigatran is an oral direct thrombin inhibitor. It has a half-life of 13 hours and is mostly excreted by the kidney. There is a specific antidote available called Idarucizumab for use in an emergency setting.

Rivaroxaban, Apixaban and Edoxaban are direct anti-Xa inhibitors. Both are 75% metabolized by the liver with 25% excreted unchanged by the kidney. They are both used as prophylaxis or treatment in VTE or used in stroke prevention in atrial fibrillation. Emergency management of bleeding consists of general haemostatic measures and use of prothrombin complex concentrate (PCC), activated PCC, also known as factor eight bypassing agent (FEIBA) or rFVIIa as there are no specific antidotes currently available,[12] although reversal agents have been developed and are likely to be available shortly

ANTIPLATELET AGENTS

Antiplatelet agents (i.e. aspirin, clopidogrel, dypirimdamole, ticagrelor, abciximab, other NSAIDs, prasugel)

TABLE 26.4 Reversing a raised INR			
Product/drug	Dose	Advantages	Disadvantages
Vitamin K	0.5–10 mg	Cheap	Slow, takes over 7 hours for detectable effect and takes up to 24 hours for complete reversal
FFP	15 mls/kg	Cheap	Plasma product, not very effective as doesn't replace some of the factors enough
Prothrombin complex concentrate (ideally 4 factor)	25–50 units/kg	Quick to act	Plasma product with more of factors II, IX and X
rVIIa	90 mcg/kg	Quick to act	Expensive, prothrombotic; not viewed as first line treatment

generally have a short half-life although the length of effect depends on whether the effects are irreversible or not. There are no specific reversal agents. If they have irreversible binding (like aspirin) the action lasts as long as the life of the platelets, and in many cases they need to be discontinued 7–14 days before procedures where possible. The mechanism of action of most of the agents is as P2Y12 antagonists or as GP IIb/IIIa inhibitors.

Aspirin acts by irreversibly inhibiting cyclo-oxygenase (COX) 1 and 2 (in contrast to some NSAIDs that reversibly act). Aspirin in low dose blocks the formation of thromboxane A2 in platelets for the life of the platelet; however, there is little effect on prostacyclin (because endothelial cells have a nucleus to produce further enzyme to produce more prostacyclin). The balance of increasing prostacyclin and reducing thromboxane A2 inhibits platelet aggregation. Platelet transfusion is the only way to reverse the effects of antiplatelet agents and only really helps if the drug has not been taken recently (otherwise the transfused platelets will also be affected).

FIBRINOLYTIC AGENTS

Fibrinolytic agents (i.e. streptokinase, tenecteplase, urokinas) all act by promoting plasmin indirectly and thus mediating clot breakdown. They are short acting and all potentially give a high bleeding risk. They are most commonly used in the acute management of stroke and myocardial infarction. In the event of serious bleeding, use of tranexamic acid and FFP or fibrinogen concentrates is indicated with other treatment guided by coagulation tests.

BLOOD PRODUCTS AND FACTOR REPLACEMENT IN BLEEDING DISORDERS

Included in this section is a brief summary of products.[13,14] Most of the coagulation factor therapies are either very expensive or extremely expensive. When available, recombinant factor concentrates are preferred as there is almost zero risk of infection transmission. In the 1980s, plasma derived coagulation factors caused tremendous (unintentional) suffering in a generation of patients with transmission of HIV/AIDS, and hepatitis B and C. Concerns over transmission of prion (specifically vCJD) have led to the UK government abandoning all UK sourced blood donors as sources for plasma factor concentrates. In an era of significantly improved safety of product and increased knowledge regarding use of prophylactic treatment the younger generations of patients have a good chance of not developing such disabling chronic joint problems that previous generations have suffered.

Platelets

Platelets are suspended in patient plasma, either apheresis units from one donor or pooled units from a few donors. Each unit is approximately 250 ml and they are stored at 22 °C. They are therefore a higher risk for bacterial transfusion transmitted infection. Usually used as one adult dose, more may be required in order to gain an appropriate increment for surgery. They are useful in major haemorrhage, platelet dysfunction and bone marrow failure; but are generally not indicated in ITP or TTP, except with life-threatening bleeding. They are generally administered over 15–30 minutes.

Fresh frozen plasma

Plasma is the 'liquid' part of the blood, therefore it contains coagulation factors. It is indicated for bleeding where there are abnormal coagulation results. Fresh frozen plasma (FFP) is used to correct multiple coagulation factor defects and in major haemorrhage. It is also beneficial as replacement of congenital factor deficiency where a specific concentrate is not available.

Dosing is usually 15 mls/kg (approximately 4 units in a 70 kg adult). Each unit is given over around 15–30 minutes. They must be defrosted prior to being issued and made from human plasma.

Cryoprecipitate

Cryoprecipitate is made by the controlled thawing of FFP to produce a cryolobulin concentrate, which is rich in fibrinogen, FVIII and von Willebrand factor. It is administered over 15–30 minutes and a dose of 2 pooled units would be expected to give a rise of 1 g/L in fibrinogen. It is mainly used as a more concentrated form of fibrinogen compared to FFP (see also fibrinogen concentrate).

Prothrombin complex concentrate

Prothrombin complex concentrate (PCC) can be 3 or, ideally, 4 factors (II, VII, IX and X but also contains protein C and S). It is made from human plasma. Dosing is usually 25–50 units per kg. It is indicated for reversal of warfarin and can be used in liver disease, especially where volume overload is a problem or in bleeding with DOACs.

Recombinant factor

This is available following discovery of the genes used in production of factor (first used in FVIII). It is produced by recombinant DNA technology, whereby a cell line (usually animal-based) is modified to express the gene that produces the factor protein. Therefore no exposure to human plasma occurs and a high purity, safe product is formed. They have no risk of transmission of blood-borne virus or prion. Currently there are recombinant products for FVIII, FIX and rVIIa. Other factors are becoming available including Factor XIII.

Plasma derived factor concentrate

There are specific factor concentrates available for FVIII, IX, X, XIII and von Willebrand disease (containing

VIII and vWF). They are treated to reduce risks associated with administration of human plasma but still carry a possibility of infection transmission. They are rarely used where a recombinant factor is available and affordable.

Fibrinogen concentrate

Fibrinogen concentrate is currently licensed for congenital fibrinogen disorders, although some centres are using it in acquired states of low fibrinogen. It is made from donor plasma, but again has had viral inactivation treatment.

Intravenous immunoglobulin

This product is made from large pools of donor plasma. It is used in the treatment of autoimmune phenomena (i.e. ITP). In other settings it is also used as replacement therapy in hypogammaglobulinaemia and targeted against specific infection in the immunocompromised.

HOW TO GET THE BEST FROM YOUR LOCAL HAEMATOLOGIST

Most patients with a significant bleeding or thrombotic disorder should be managed in conjunction with the clinical and laboratory haematology team so that a perioperative treatment plan can be agreed upon. Discussion is needed to weigh up the risk factors for bleeding and thrombosis. It is important the patient is aware of the management plan, particularly as many are experts in their own condition.

This section gives some guidance on how to get the best advice.

Information to communicate to a haematologist about a bleeding patient

- The patient's personal history regarding bleeding (previous procedures and obstetric history; severity of bleeds, i.e. requiring transfusion; type of bleeds i.e. mucocutaneous).
- Whether the patient has ever had treatment for bleeding or thrombosis.
- Their family history, especially regarding siblings, parents, children, grandparents, aunts/uncles' bleeding and how their condition was managed.
- Medication the patient is currently on or has previously used, especially anything that could lead to bleeding and, if they have a diagnosis, what product they usually have (i.e. factor brand, as it is usual to try and continue with the same one).
- Do they have an alert/ information card with diagnosis details and baseline factor levels?
- Ensure FBC, PT, APTT and fibrinogen results are available. Where possible if an elective procedure is planned results should be reviewed with time to carry out further investigations or the procedure should be delayed.
- What surgery is planned, with an idea of what bleeding would be expected in a haemostatically normal patient. Do not assume a haematologist will know a lot about procedures, particularly if new or complex.

For significant bleeding disorders it is usually advisable to carry out surgery at a centre of haemostasis expertise so the medical and laboratory advice is easily accessible. Usually, NSAIDs would be avoided, along with intramuscular injections. It is important to remember that patients on treatment may have a similar (or even higher) risk of thrombosis so VTE prophylaxis may still be indicated. In planning surgery patients may require admission even if the procedure is usually done as a day case for closer observation. Post-operatively they will require both clinical and laboratory assessment to guide further use of factor replacement.

Information to communicate to a haematologist about a clotting patient

- The patient's personal history regarding thrombosis including the type of clot, when it occurred and precipitants (i.e. hormones, perioperative, related to malignancy and treatment).
- Whether they have ever had treatment for bleeding or thrombosis.
- Their family history, especially regarding siblings, parents, children, grandparents, aunts/uncles' thrombosis and how it was managed.
- Medication they are currently on or have previously used, particularly anticoagulants and antiplatelets, and the indication.
- What surgery is planned. Do not assume a haematologist will know a lot about procedures, particularly if new or complex.

For advice on management of anticoagulation in an emergency (e.g. warfarin reversal in a patient who has attended A&E with significant bleeding) it is important to have information about why they are on the drug and how quickly reversal is required.

For warfarin, a weight is helpful so that dosing of PCC can be discussed. For LMWH, antiplatelets and DOACs it is important to know renal function and when the last dose was taken. Other comorbidities should be also taken into account to aid management.

The commonest cause of post-surgical bleeding is surgery

Post-surgical bleeding does not always equal a problem with the clotting system. Surgical causes and the need for a return to theatre should always be considered.

FUTURE RESEARCH

➤ More experience in direct oral anticoagulation agents (DOACs) and specifically in their reversal
➤ Further work on global coagulation testing and its applications
➤ Gene therapy as treatment and other novel therapies for haemophilia and other bleeding disorders

KEY POINTS

- Patients with bleeding disorders should be managed with close liaison between the haematology, laboratory and surgical teams.
- Pre-operative assessment should include bleeding history and medication. Where possible when screening coagulation tests are performed they should be reviewed with time for further investigation prior to procedures when needed.
- Bridging of anticoagulation therapy needs consideration for elective procedures.

REFERENCES

1. Sadler JE. Von Willebrand Type I: a diagnosis in search of a disease. *Blood* 2003; **101**: 2089–93.
2. Rodeghiero F, Castaman G, Dini, E. Epidemiological investigation of the prevalence of von Willebrand's disease. *Blood* 1987; **69**(2): 454–59.
3. Laffan M, Brown SA, Collins PW, et al. The diagnosis of Von Willebrand disease: a guideline from the UK Haemophilia Doctors Organisation. *Haemophilia* 2004; **10**(3): 199–217.
4. Dutt T, Burns S, Mackett N, Keenan, R. Application of UKHCDO 2004 guidelines in type 1 von Willebrand Disease: a single centre paediatric experience of the implications of altered or removed diagnosis. *Haemophilia* 2011; **17**(3): 522–26.
5. Kadir RA, Economides DL, Sabin CA, et al. Variations in coagulation factors in women: effects of age, ethnicity, menstrual cycle and combined oral contraceptive. *Thromb Haemost* 1999; **82**(5): 1456–61.
6. Levi M, Toh CH, Thachil J, Watson HG. Guidelines for the diagnosis and management of disseminated intravascular coagulation. *Br J Haematol* 2009; **145**(1): 24–33.
7. Provan D, Stasi R, Newland AC, et al. International consensus report on the investigation and management of primary immune thrombocytopenia as published in Blood Journal. *Blood* 2009; **115**: 168–86.
8. Watson H, Davidson S, Keeling D. Guidelines on the diagnosis and management of heparin-induced thrombocytopenia: second edition. *Br J Haematol* 2012; **159**(5): 528–40.
9. Baglin T, Gray E, Greaves M, et al. Clinical guidelines for testing for heritable thrombophilia. *Br J Haematol* 2010; **149**: 209–20.
10. Van der Meer FJ, Koster T, Vandenbroucke JP, et al. The Leiden Trombophilia Study (LETS). *Thromb Haemost* 1997; **78**(1): 631–5.
11. Cushman M, Tsai AW, White RH, et al. Deep vein thrombosis and pulmonary embolism in two cohorts; the longitudinal investigation of thromboembolism etiology. *Am J Med* 2004; **117**: 19–25.
12. Makris M, Van Veen JJ, Mumford AD, et al. Guideline on the management of bleeding in patients on antithrombotic agents. *Br J Haematol* 2012; **160**: 35–46.
13. Keeling D, Tait C, Makris M. Guideline on the selection and use of therapeutic products to treat haemophilia and other hereditary bleeding disorders. *Haemophilia* 2008; **14**: 671–84.
14. Norfolk D (ed). *Handbook of transfusion medicine*. 5th ed. Norwich: TSO; 2013.

Pharmacotherapeutics

CHAPTER 27

DRUG THERAPY IN OTOLOGY

Wendy Smith

Introduction 275
Topical ear preparations 275
Preparations used in the management of vertigo 279
Drugs used in sudden sensorineural hearing loss 280
Sodium fluoride treatment in otosclerosis 280
Acknowledgements 281
References 281

SEARCH STRATEGY
Data in this chapter may be updated by a Medline search using the keywords: otitis externa, ear drops, antibiotics, betahistine, gentamicin, Menières, acyclovir and sodium fluoride.

INTRODUCTION

Medicines are commonly prescribed in the management of otological diseases. Whilst the efficacy of some treatments may be uncertain, it is important to understand how these drugs act, their indications, contraindications and side effects. This chapter discusses these factors in relation to a number of specific types of otological medications.

TOPICAL EAR PREPARATIONS

Ear drops are solutions or suspensions of medicaments in water, glycerol, diluted alcohol, propylene glycol or other suitable solvent for instillation into the ear. A solution comprises a solute (drug) dissolved in the solvent, whereas a suspension consists of an insoluble drug distributed in a liquid. Some preparations used in otology are also used as eye or nose drops. Since these drops are in multiple-application containers, the vehicle contains a bactericidal and fungicidal agent such as benzalkonium chloride (0.01%). Other adjuvants in ear and eye drops include buffers such as sodium metabisulphite and disodium edetate. The buffers are used to maintain the pH to minimize breakdown of the active constituents or to increase comfort for the patient. Both sodium metabisulphite and disodium edetate are effective at retarding oxidation reactions and the latter can enhance the bactericidal activity of benzalkonium chloride and chlorhexidine acetate. Information on excipients contained in drops is found in the British National Formulary or its equivalent. This information is useful since some patients may be allergic to topical ear medication and this allergy may not be to the primary constituent but to the excipients.

Ear drops are dispensed in coloured fluted glass bottles with a plastic screw cap incorporating a glass dropper tube and rubber teat, or, more commonly, in plastic squeeze bottles fitted with a plastic cap incorporating a dropper device. Such containers are designed to prevent light degradation of the contents.

Some ear preparations are available as creams or ointments where the antimicrobial and/or anti-inflammatory substance is prepared in a suitable base such as liquid paraffin, wool fat and yellow soft paraffin. Both are semi-solid preparations but in a cream the base is absorbed into the skin, whereas in an ointment only the medication is absorbed from the greasy base. In general, ointments are useful in dry scaly conditions whereas creams can also be used in weeping skin conditions.

Again, warnings that the preparation contains lanolin (wool fat) are useful since some patients are allergic to lanolin.

Topical ear preparations for inflammatory and infective conditions

INDICATIONS
A number of topical ear preparations in the form of drops or ointments are available for the treatment of otitis

externa and discharging mastoid cavities. Many are also used in discharging ears with a perforated tympanic membrane or ears with a grommet *in situ*. In this latter situation this is an unlicensed indication for the use of many of these preparations. Manufacturers' data sheets continue to state that even plain steroid drops are contra-indicated in the presence of a perforation. In chronic suppurative otitis media, it has been shown that aural toilet and topical antibiotics, especially a quinolone, is effective in resolving otorrhoea and eradicating bacteria from the middle ear. This treatment used by specialists is now recognised in the BNF.[1] Topical antibiotic preparations are more effective than oral preparations and the addition of oral therapy to topical antibiotics confers no greater benefit than the latter used alone.[2]

SPECIFIC PREPARATIONS

Acetic acid 2% has antifungal and antibacterial properties and can be used to treat mild otitis externa. Aluminium acetate is an astringent that can be applied as drops or onto a gauze wick. An astringent is an agent that causes shrinkage or constriction and is usually applied topically. The hydroscopic effect reduces oedema in the inflamed ear canal, opening the meatus. Aluminium acetate has a tendency to form crystals in the ear. Regular aural toilet is required to remove both the crystals that form as well as the debris produced by the inflammatory process. This treatment can be safely used in pregnancy. Boric acid has been used in the past for its weak fungistatic and bacteriostatic activity and is used as a mild disinfectant in lotions, ointments and powders in concentrations of up to 5%. It is absorbed through damaged skin and may cause systemic toxicity. Acute and chronic toxicity can occur, presenting with gastrointestinal disturbance, rash, central nervous system and renal involvement that may result in death. Slow excretion of boric acid can lead to cumulative toxicity during repeated use.

Some preparations contain only a steroid and are used in eczematous otitis externa. The steroid reduces inflammatory swelling and helps control irritation. The steroid stimulates the synthesis of lipocortin in leukocytes. This protein inhibits phospholipase A_2 that reduces the formation of arachidonic acid, the precursor of many inflammatory mediators. Betamethasone sodium phosphate (Betnesol®) and prednisolone sodium phosphate (Predsol®) are steroids available as ear drops. These steroids are combined with anti-infective agents for use in the management of infected otitis externa. Other steroids found in combination with anti-infective drugs include dexamethasone (Otomize® – with neomycin and glacial acetic acid; Sofradex® – with framycetin sulphate and gramicidin), flumetasone pivalate (Locorten-Vioform® – with flumetasone pivalate and clioquinol), hydrocortisone acetate (Gentisone HC® – with gentamicin; Neo-Cortef® – with neomycin sulphate) and triamcinolone acetonide (Audicort® – with neomycin undecanoate and Tri-Adcortyl Otic® – with gramicidin, neomycin and nystatin). Clioquinol (found in Locorten-Vioform) is an 8-hydroxyquinolone with both antibacterial and antifungal properties and is useful when a mixed infection is suspected. Its use is contra-indicated in patients with iodine sensitivity. The other antibiotics included in ear preparations are framycetin sulphate, gentamicin and neomycin sulphate which are all aminoglycosides. They are bactericidal, inhibiting microbial protein synthesis and are effective against aerobic Gram-negative bacteria. Bacteria may acquire resistance via plasmids against one aminoglycoside but these bacteria rarely exhibit resistance to other aminoglycosides. This accounts for the benefit in changing the ear drops if the otitis externa fails to respond to one preparation.

Some of these preparations are available as ear sprays (Otomize), and there is some evidence that these cover the external meatus more effectively than traditional ear drops[3] and are easier for the elderly to apply. However, in some clinical situations, drops are more likely to reach the infected and inflamed parts of the external ear, middle ear or mastoid cavity at which treatment is aimed. Prolonged use of antibiotic/steroid preparations may sensitize the skin and may lead to fungal infections.

Clotrimazole is an azole derivative with a broad-spectrum antifungal activity that acts by inhibiting ergosterol synthesis in the fungal cell membrane. At lower concentrations, clotrimazole merely inhibits fungal growth but at higher concentrations, fungi are killed by clotrimazole action causing direct membrane damage. Clotrimazole should be continued for at least 2 weeks after apparent resolution of the infection. Increasingly, ciprofloxacin eye drops are used as ear drops in the management of *Pseudomonas* spp. ear infections. This is an unlicensed use in the UK where licensed ciprofloxacin ear drops are unavailable. Ciprofloxacin drops have been used widely in the rest of Europe, North America and beyond.

CONTRAINDICATIONS

The use of preparations containing only a steroid is contraindicated in untreated infections since the immunosuppressive effect of corticosteroids may exacerbate the infection. More controversial is the use of preparations with anti-infective agents in the presence of a perforated tympanic membrane because of the potential for ototoxicity.

SIDE EFFECTS

The most common side effects with these preparations are hypersensitivity reactions and local irritation, burning and itching.

The use of anti-infective ear drops in the presence of a tympanic membrane perforation

The product licences do not permit the use of anti-infective ear drops in ears with perforated tympanic membranes as a result of cochlear damage that occurred when such drops were instilled into guinea pig ears.[4,5] These authors recognize that the round window niche in humans is relatively deep and often protected by a pseudomembrane whilst in the guinea pig the round window is completely exposed. In patients with active chronic suppurative otitis media there is no evidence that the use of these ear drops causes sensorineural deafness.[6-8]

Topical ear preparations for removal of ear wax

Many cerumenolytics, including oils and aqueous preparations, are available to soften wax prior to syringing or to disintegrate or disperse the wax, to avoid the need for syringing altogether. Burton and Dorée[9] undertook a systematic review and found nine clinical trials. All had a small number of participants, and most were of poor methodological quality. The review concluded that there is insufficient evidence to favour any one particular cerumenolytic. Water and sodium chloride 0.9% seem to be as effective as any proprietary agent. Sodium bicarbonate 5% ear drops, olive or almond oil ear drops are also safe and inexpensive although their effectiveness has not been evaluated in randomized controlled trials. These findings were supported by Clegg et al. in a more recent systematic review.[10] If the wax is impacted, these drops can be used twice a day for a few days prior to syringing. Some proprietary preparations contain organic solvents (chlorbutanol, paradichlorobenzene) that may cause irritation to the meatal skin. The rational for inclusion of these ingredients in the preparations is not clear and the vehicle alone is often effective.

SYSTEMIC ANTIBIOTICS

Indications

Systemic antibiotics are prescribed in the otological conditions of acute otitis media (AOM), cellulitis associated with furunculosis, otitis externa and perichondritis.

In AOM, the use of antibiotics is controversial. Venekamp et al.[11] found that antibiotic usage in AOM in children varied from 31% in the Netherlands to 98% in the USA and Australia. Their Cochrane review concluded that antibiotics provide a small benefit; however, since most cases resolve spontaneously, this benefit must be weighed against possible adverse reactions. Twenty children must be treated to prevent one child from having pain after 2 days. Antibiotic treatment did however produce a statistically significant reduction in tympanic membrane perforations and contralateral AOM episodes. Antibiotic treatment may play an important role in reducing the risk of mastoiditis in populations where it is more common. It is recommended that in children without systemic features, antibacterial treatment may be started after 72 hours if no improvement or earlier if systemically unwell or if at a high risk of serious complications (patients who are immunocompromised, the presence of mastoiditis or in children under 2 years with bilateral otitis media). If antibiotics are used, amoxicillin appears to be the first-line treatment, with clarithromycin in those who are penicillin sensitive. Should treatment fail, second-line agents include co-amoxiclav and cephalosporins. Usually 5 days treatment is required but may be longer if severely ill.

Conservative management of acute mastoiditis (without subperiosteal abscess) has been adopted since a third of patients will settle in 24–48 hours with intravenous antibiotics.[12-14]

Flucloxacillin is the antibiotic of choice in treating cellulitis due to staphylococcus. Penicillin V is used in erysipelas due to streptococcus.

Ciprofloxacin is the drug of choice in malignant otitis externa and is also used in treating perichondritis due to *Pseudomonas aeruginosa*.

Mechanisms of actions

The penicillins have a bactericidal action, inhibiting cell wall synthesis by preventing the formation of peptidoglycan cross-bridges. The penicillinase-resistant penicillins, flucloxacillin, cloxacillin and methicillin, are semisynthetic penicillins, resistant to penicillinase by virtue of an isoxazolyl group on R_1. Many bacterial β-lactamases are inhibited by clavulanic acid, and a mixture of this inhibitor with amoxicillin (co-amoxiclav) is available. The cephalosporins are also bactericidal. They contain a β-lactam ring and their mechanism of action is similar to the penicillins.

The macrolides, for example erythromycin, act by inhibiting bacterial protein synthesis. It binds to the 50s bacterial ribosome subunit inhibiting translocation.

Metronidazole was initially used in protozoal infections but was found to be very effective against anaerobic bacteria. The drug is reduced to active metabolites that interfere with nucleic acid function. Ciprofloxacin is a fluoroquinolone and acts on both stationary and dividing bacteria by inhibiting DNA gyrase, an enzyme that compresses the bacterial DNA into supercoils. Cell death is thought to occur as a result of the unwinding of the supercoils.

Antibacterial spectrum

Table 27.1 demonstrates the antibacterial spectrum of the various antibiotics. The penicillinase-sensitive penicillins have a greater spectrum of activity than the β-lactamase resistant drugs, but the combination of clavulanic acid with amoxicillin enables protection of the β-lactam ring, allowing this essential part of the penicillin molecule to remain active.

Dosage

Specific dosage recommendations can be found in the British National Formulary.[1] Phenoxypenicillin, amoxicillin and flucloxacillin have better oral absorption than ampicillin but all should be taken at least 30 minutes before food since they are destroyed, to some extent, by gastric acid. The penicillins have good penetration to most tissues but poor entry to CSF (overcome by giving higher doses intravenously). Dosage modification is required in patients with severe renal failure.

TABLE 27.1 The antibacterial spectrum of antibiotics

Penicillins	Antibacterial spectrum
Benzylpenicillin and phenoxymethylpenicillin	Streptococcal, non β-lactamase producing staphylococcal, pneumococcal, clostridial infection, meningococcal, gonococcal, spirochaetes (syphilis), anthrax, actinomycosis
Ampicillin and amoxicillin	As above and *Strep. faecalis*, most *Haemophilus influenzae* and many coliforms
Methicillin, cloxacillin, flucloxacillin	Similar to penicillin but less active. Stable to staphylococcal β-lactamase
Carbenicillin and ticarcillin	Similar to amoxicillin and in addition activity to *Ps. aeruginosa*, most *Proteus* spp. and against bacteroides
Mezlocillin, azlocillin, piperacillin	Similar to ticarcillin and in addition to *Klebsiella* spp. and greater activity against pseudomonads
Mecillinam	Coliforms, little activity against Gram-positive bacteria
Cephalosporins	**Antibacterial spectrum**
First generation: cephaloridine, cephalothin, cephalexin, cefradine and cephazolin	Broad spectrum except against *Strep. faecalis*, *Ps. aeruginosa*, *H. influenzae* and *Bacteroides* spp. Staphylococcus is sensitive, except for MRSA
Second generation: cefaclor, cefuroxime, cefamandole, cefoxitin	Broad spectrum with stability against β-lactamases. Active against *H. influenzae* and *Bacteroides* spp. but less activity against staphylococcus
Third generation: cefotaxime, latamoxef, ceftazidime, cefsulodin, ceftriaxone, cefixime, cefpodoxime proxetil Fifth generation: ceftaroline fosamil	As for second generation but also active against *Ps. Aeruginosa* Similar to cefotaxime but also against Gram-positive bacteria including methicillin-resistant *Staphylococcus aureus* and multidrug-resistant *Streptococcus pneumonia*.
Macrolides: erythromycin, azithromycin, clarithromycin	See penicillins but also active against *H. influenzae*, *Bord. Pertussis*, *Bacteroides* spp., *Campylobacter* spp. *Legionella pneumophilia*, *Mycoplasma pneumoniae* and *Chlamydiae*
Sulphonamides and trimethoprim: co-trimoxazole	Broad, active against Gram-positive and Gram-negative bacteria except *Ps. aeruginosa*
Aminoglycosides: gentamicin, tobramycin, netilmicin, amikacin, kanamycin and neomycin Carbapenems: imipenem, meropenem, doripenem and ertapenem	Coliforms, *Ps. aeruginosa* and staphylococci; streptomycin; mycobacteria Broad spectrum of activity including many Gram-positive and Gram-negative bacteria and anaesrobes. Good activity against *Pseudomonas aeruginosa* except ertapenem
Vancomycin	Staphylococci including MRSA, streptococci and clostridia
Tetracyclines: tetracycline, chlortetracycline, oxytetracycline, doxycycline, minocycline	Broad; Gram-positive and -negative bacteria, brucellae, *M. pneumoniae*, rickettsia, *Coxiella burneti* and *Chlamydiae*. Some resistance to *Strep. pyogenes*, pneumococci and *H. influenzae*. *Ps. aeruginosa* and *Proteus* spp. resistant
Metronidazole	Anaerobic bacteria and protozoa
Ciprofloxacin	Broad; Gram-negative bacteria including *Ps. aeruginosa*, staphylococci including MRSA, streptococci less sensitive
Monobactams: aztreonam	Narrow, active against aerobic Gram-negative bacteria (less sensitive to *Ps. aeruginosa*)

Ciprofloxacin can achieve high concentrations in bone and soft tissue, even after oral administration. A dosage of 1.5 g daily over a period of 6–12 weeks has been recommended in the treatment of malignant otitis externa.[15,16]

Contraindications

In all cases the prescribing of these drugs is contraindicated when the patient is known to be allergic to the ingredients or related compounds. Immediate hypersensitivity to penicillins occurs in 0.05% of patients, the severity of which ranges from urticaria or wheezing to a life-threatening anaphylactic response. Less than 5% of patients may develop a delayed hypersensitivity response to penicillins, usually a rash. Occasionally, haemolytic anaemia, leukopenia and interstitial nephritis may occur. There is a 10% hypersensitivity crossover with cephalosporins.

Precautions

The prolonged use of antibiotics may result in superinfection with unsusceptible organisms. There is no evidence that the penicillins, cephalosporins or erythromycin are hazardous in pregnancy but metronidazole should be avoided in high dosages and ciprofloxacin must be avoided in all trimesters of pregnancy. Antibiotics are secreted into breast milk and ciprofloxacin should be avoided in lactation. Other antibiotics, such as the penicillins and cephalosporins, are secreted into breast milk but may not be harmful to the infant. Antibiotics, such as the cephalosporins and ciprofloxacin, cleared by the kidneys may require dosage adjustments in patients with renal impairment. Similarly, antibiotics metabolized by the liver, for example erythromycin, may require dosage adjustments or to be avoided in patients with liver failure.

Interactions

Before prescribing a specific medication, the reader is advised to check for interactions in, for example, The British National Formulary.[1] Antibiotics may lead to oral contraceptive failure, probably because of diminished enterohepatic circulation. The anticoagulant effect of warfarin is affected by the penicillins, macrolides, metronidazole and quinolones.

Erythromycin interacts with some antihistamines and cisapride, resulting in cardiac arrhythmias. It also increases the plasma level of a number of drugs.

Metronidazole produces a disulfiram-like reaction with alcohol. Acetaldehyde accumulates in the body producing facial flushing, headaches, palpitations, nausea and vomiting.

Indigestion, iron or zinc therapies must not be taken within 2 hours of ciprofloxacin since absorption of this antibiotic is significantly affected.

Side effects

Most antibiotics may produce diarrhoea, rashes, blood disorders, nausea and vomiting. Ampicillin and amoxicillin have a unique adverse effect, comprising a rash, in up to 90% of patients with mononucleosis or chronic lymphocytic leukaemia. Reversible hearing loss has been reported with erythromycin. Angioneurotic oedema and anaphylaxis are, fortunately, relatively rare.

PREPARATIONS USED IN THE MANAGEMENT OF VERTIGO

Betahistine

Betahistine hydrochloride is commonly prescribed in the management of vertigo, usually when associated with Menière's disease or syndrome.

Betahistine is thought to reduce the endolymphatic pressure through improved microvascular circulation in the stria vascularis of the cochlear[17] or by inhibiting activity of the vestibular nuclei.[18]

There is insufficient evidence from high quality randomized trials to say whether or not betahistine has any effect on Menières.[19] It may reduce vertigo, and possibly tinnitus, but does not seem to influence the hearing loss.

Betahistine should be used with caution in patients with asthma, a history of peptic ulcer disease, in pregnancy and breastfeeding. It is contraindicated in patients with phaeochromocytoma. The side effects include gastrointestinal disturbance, headaches, rashes and pruritis; however, these are uncommon. Betahistine is prescribed initially at 16 mg three times a day; a maintenance daily dose of 24–48 mg has been recommended.

Dopamine antagonists

Prochlorperazine (Stemetil®) is a dopamine antagonist and acts centrally by blocking the chemoreceptor trigger zone and thereby blocking the vomiting centre. The vomiting centre also has afferent input from the vestibular apparatus. This region has a high concentration of muscarinic receptors and histamine H_1-receptors.

Prochlorperazine belongs to group three of the phenothiazines. This means it has less sedative effects, fewer antimuscarinic effects but more pronounced extra-pyramidal side effects when compared to the other phenothiazine groups.

Prochlorperazine is available as tablets, syrup, effervescent sachets, injection, suppositories and as a buccal preparation (Buccastem®). These last two preparations are useful because patients using prochlorperazine often vomit and fail to absorb the orally ingested form. The oral dosage varies from 5 mg three times a day increasing to 30 mg daily.

Antihistamines

The antihistamines are competitive antagonists of histamine at H_1-receptors, and their main action is on the vomiting centre rather than on the chemoreceptor trigger zone. They have weak anticholinergic effects and may occasionally produce a dry mouth and blurred vision. Drowsiness, occasional insomnia and euphoria are side effects that have been reported. These central effects are accentuated with alcohol. Cinnarazine (Stugeron®) and cyclizine (Valoid®) are less sedating than promethazine teoclate (Avomine®). Cinnarizine has been used in the prophylaxis and treatment of Menière's at a dosage of 30 mg three times a day. Cyclizine may be given in the acute attack orally or parentally at a dosage of 50 mg three times a day.

Gentamicin therapy in Menière's disease

Intra-tympanic gentamicin therapy was described by Beck and Schmidt[20] in 1978 and has been used both in Canada and the UK. Since its introduction, a variety of gentamicin dosage regimens and methods of administration have been developed and remain in clinical practice. These range from injection through the tympanic membrane, through a grommet or via intra-tympanic or round window catheters.

Other medical treatment for Menières disease

The use of salt restriction and diuretic therapy (hydrochlorothiazide, acetazolamide and co-triamterzide 50/25 (Dyazide®) are aimed at reducing the accumulation of endolymph. Although a study with Dyazide showed a reduction in vestibular symptoms, there was no effect on hearing loss or tinnitus. Acetazolamide may initially increase the hydrops and Brookes and Booth[21] concluded that this drug has no place in treating Menière's disease. Steroids and immunological therapy have also been proposed by those who believe that a disorder of the immune system underlies Menière's disease or syndrome.

DRUGS USED IN SUDDEN SENSORINEURAL HEARING LOSS

Corticosteroids

Steroids are commonly used in patients with sudden sensorineural hearing loss (SSNHL), but evidence for their effectiveness is lacking. There are several alternative dosage regimes when a 'short reducing course' of steroids is required. One such consists of enteric-coated prednisolone, 60 mg on the first day, 50 mg on the second day, 40 mg daily for 3 days, 30 mg daily for 3 days and a further reduction so that therapy is discontinued after 3 weeks.

Antiviral agents

Aciclovir (acycloguanosine) is an antiviral agent active against herpesviruses and is prescribed in patients with Ramsay Hunt syndrome (herpes zoster oticus). It acts by inhibiting nucleic acid synthesis. Herpes simplex and varicella zoster contain a thymidine kinase that converts the aciclovir to a monophosphate that is then phosphorylated by the host cell enzymes of acycloguanosine triphosphate that inhibits viral DNA polymerase and viral DNA syntheses. Selectivity for infected cells is achieved since the DNA polymerase of herpesvirus has a much greater affinity for the activated drug than the cellular DNA polymerase.

Aciclovir may be administered orally at a dosage of 800 mg five times a day for 5 days. If treatment is commenced prior to 72 hours after the onset of the rash, acyclovir may shorten the rash duration and acute symptoms and reduce the incidence of post-herpetic neuralgia.[22] Aciclovir should be used with caution in patients with renal impairment or who are pregnant or breastfeeding. Side effects include nausea, vomiting, gastrointestinal disturbances, rash, photosensitivity and, rarely, hepatitis, acute renal failure and neurological reactions. Two newer antiviral agents are famiclovir (a prodrug of penciclovir) and valaciclovir (an ester of aciclovir), which, depending on indication and co-morbidities, are administered up to three times a day (see British National Formulary[1] for further details).

SODIUM FLUORIDE TREATMENT IN OTOSCLEROSIS

Sodium fluoride has been used for 35 years in an attempt to slow down or arrest sensorineural hearing loss in patients with stapedial otosclerosis or after stapedectomy. It has also been used in patients with 'pure' cochlear otosclerosis.

Sodium fluoride is an enzyme inhibitor and reduces osteoclastic bone resorption. The clinical benefit of sodium fluoride is controversial. Causse et al.[23] found that in 'otospongiosis-otosclerosis', sodium fluoride influenced the underlying bony changes in the labyrinth so as to arrest or prevent the onset of hearing loss. In their prospective clinical double-blind, placebo-controlled study of 95 patients, Bretlau et al.[24] found that there was a statistically worse deterioration of hearing loss in the placebo group than in the active treated (40 mg sodium fluoride daily) group. Further work by Colletti[25] showed benefit in 50% of patients 5 years after a 2-year treatment with sodium fluoride (dosages up to 16 mg/day). Cruise et al. in a review of the literature 1966 to 2009 concluded that there is low evidence suggesting sodium fluoride may be of benefit to preserve hearing and reduce vestibular symptoms in patients with otosclerosis.[26] Treatment doses used vary greatly and the optimum treatment time has yet to be determined. Deka et al.[27] suggested the use of Florical at a dosage of two capsules three times a day in active cochlear otospongiosis. Their study showed that variation in absorption occurs with the use of different preparations and also amongst individuals.

The side effects of sodium fluoride need to be considered. In a prospective case-controlled study of ten patients with otosclerosis receiving sodium fluoride 30 mg/day and matched healthy volunteers, Das et al.[28] found a high incidence (70%) of dyspeptic symptoms in those taking sodium fluoride, as well as histological and electron microscopic abnormalities.

BEST CLINICAL PRACTICE

✓ Before prescribing, ensure that the patient is not known to be allergic to the medicine or adjuvants (such as the preservatives).
✓ Ensure medication does not interact with patient's established medication or medical conditions.
✓ Prescribe medicines at the lowest dose for the shortest time that is effective.
✓ Review whether medication is still required.

FUTURE RESEARCH

➤ There is insufficient evidence to favour any one particular cerumenolytic and a randomized controlled trial may be useful to determine the most clinically and cost-effective preparations for this purpose.
➤ There is insufficient evidence from high-quality randomized trials to determine whether betahistine, diuretics, steroids and immune therapy have any effect in Menière's disease.

KEY POINTS

- Topical ear preparations can be used for a limited period in discharging ears with a perforated tympanic membrane or a grommet *in situ*.
- The use of topical ear preparations containing a steroid only is contraindicated in untreated infections since the immuno-suppressive action of the corticosteroid may exacerbate the infection.
- Flucloxacillin is the antibiotic of choice in cellulitis due to staphyloccus. Penicillin V is used in erysipelas due to streptococcus. Ciprofloxacin is the antibiotic of choice in malignant otitis externa.

ACKNOWLEDGEMENTS

Acknowledgement is made for Martin J. Burton's contribution to this chapter in the previous edition of Scott-Brown.

REFERENCES

1. British Medical Association, Royal Pharmaceutical Society of Great Britain. *British National Formulary 65*. London: Pharmaceutical Press; 2013.
2. Macfadyen CA, Acuin J, Gamble C. Systemic antibiotics versus topical treatments for chronically discharging ears with underlying eardrum perforations. *Cochrane Database Syst Rev* 2006; **25**(1).
3. Mcgarry GW, Swan IRC. Endoscopic photographic comparison of drug delivery by ear drops and by aerosol spray. *Clin Otolaryngol* 1992; **17**: 359–60.
4. Kohonen A, Tarkanen J. Cochlea damage by ototoxic antibiotics by intratympanic application. *Acta Otolaryngol* 1969; **68**: 90–97.
5. Brummett RE, Harris RF, Lindgren JA. Detection of ototoxicity from drugs applied topically to the middle ear space. *Laryngoscope* 1976; **86**: 1177–87.
6. Browning GG, Gatehouse S, Calder IT. Medical management of active chronic otitis media: a control study. *J Laryngol Otol* 1988; **102**: 491–95.
7. Fairbanks DNF. Antimicrobial therapy for chronic suppurative otitis media. *Ann Otol Rhinol Larynol Suppl* 1981; **90**: 58–62.
8. Phillips JS, Yung MW, Burton M, Swan IRC for the Clinical Audit and Practice Advisory Group, British Association of Otolaryngologists – Head and Neck Surgeons (ENT-UK). *Use of aminoglyco-side-containing ear drops in the presence of a perforation: evidence review and ENT-UK consensus statement* (in press).
9. Burton MJ, Dorée CJ. Ear drops for the removal of ear wax. *Cochrane Database Syst Rev* 2009.
10. Clegg AJ, Loveman E, Gospodrevskay E, et al. The safety and effectiveness of different methods of earwax removal: a systematic review and economic evaluation. *Health Technol Assess* 2010; **14**(28): 1–192.
11. Venekamp RP, Sanders S, Galsziou PP, et al. Antibiotics for acute otitis media in children. *Cochrane Database Syst Rev* 2013.
12. Rubin JS, Wei WI. Acute mastoiditis: a review of 34 patients. *Laryngoscope* 1985; **95**: 963–65.
13. Ogle JW, Lauer BA. Acute mastoiditis: diagnosis and complications. *Am J Dis Child* 1986; **140**: 1178–82.
14. Nadal S, Herrmann P, Baumann A, Fanconi A. Acute mastoiditis: clinical, microbiological, and therapeutic aspects. *Eur J Pediatr* 1990; **149**: 560–64.
15. Brody T, Pasak ML. The fluoroquinolones. *Am J Otol* 1991; **17**: 902–04.
16. Levenson MJ, Parisier SC, Dolitsky J, Bindra G. Ciprofloxacin: drug of choice in the treatment of malignant external otitis. *Laryngoscope* 1991; **101**: 821–84.
17. Martinez DM. The effect of Serc on the circulation of the inner ear in experimental animals. *Acta Otolaryngol* 1972; **Suppl 305**: 29–46.
18. Timmerman H. Pharmacotherapy of vertigo: any news to be expected? *Acta Otolaryngol* 1994; **Suppl 573**: 28–32.
19. James A, Burton MJ. Betahistine for Menieres disease or syndrome. *Cochrane Database Syst Rev* 2001.
20. Beck C, Schmidt CL. 10 years experience with intratympanally applied streptomycin (gentamicin) in the therapy of Morbus Meniere. *Arch Otorhinolaryngol* 1978; **221**: 149–52.
21. Brookes GB, Booth JB. Oral acetazolamide in Menieres disease. *J Laryngol Otol* 1984; **98**: 1087–95.
22. Collier J. Acyclovir in general practice. *Drug Ther Bull* 1992; **30**: 101–04.
23. Causse JR, Causse JB, Uriel J, et al. Sodium fluoride therapy. *Am J Otol* 1993; **14**: 482–90.
24. Bretlau P, Causse J, Causse JB, et al. Otospongiosis and sodium fluoride: a blind experimental and clinical evaluation of the effect of sodium fluoride treatment in patients with otospongiosis. *Ann Otol Rhinol Laryngol* 1985; **94**: 103–07.
25. Colletti V, Fiorino FG. Effect of sodium fluoride on early stages of otosclerosis. *Am J Otol* 1991; **12**: 195–98.
26. Cruise AS, Singh A, Quiney RE. Sodium fluoride in otosclerosis treatment: review. *J Laryngol Otol* 2010; **124**(6); 583–86.
27. Deka RC, Kacker SK, Shambaugh Jr GE. Intestinal absorption of fluoride preparations. *Laryngoscope* 1978; **88**: 1918–21.
28. Das TK, Susheela AK, Gupta IP, et al. Toxic effects of chronic fluoride ingestion on the upper gastrointestinal tract. *J Clin Gastroenterol* 1994; **18**: 194–99.

CHAPTER 28

DRUG THERAPY IN RHINOLOGY

Wendy Smith

Introduction 283	Agents used to block the parasympathetic nervous system 289
Treatment of rhinosinusitis with corticosteroids 283	Vaccination 289
Treatment of rhinosinusitis with antibiotics 285	Related topics 289
Treatment of rhinosinusitis with other medicines 286	Acknowledgements 290
Medication that may improve the immune response 288	References 291
Nasal and antral irrigation with saline 288	Further reading 292
Antileukotrienes 288	

SEARCH STRATEGY

Data in this chapter may be updated by a Medline search using the keywords: acute rhinosinusitis, chronic rhinosinusitis, nasal polyposis, fungal rhinosinusitis and medical treatment. The chapter has also relied on a review produced by the European Rhinological Society and the European Academy of Allergology and Clinical Immunology (EAACI) that was published as a supplement by *Rhinology* in March 2012, and their abbreviations are used in this chapter.

INTRODUCTION

This chapter covers the medical treatment, in particular the use of corticosteroids and antibiotics, in managing the various types of rhinosinusitis. A separate section is devoted to other medicines that are used in the management of rhinosinusitis. Finally, other medical treatments used in rhinology are discussed under related topics.

Rhinosinusitis is a significant health problem that reduces the quality of life for individuals and places a large financial burden on society. The evidence for the effectiveness of medical treatment of rhinosinusitis has been reviewed by the European Rhinological Society (ERS) and the European Academy of Allergology and Clinical Immunology (EAACI), and the authors of this chapter have relied on the ERS/EAACI review.[1]

Rhinosinusitis is an inflammatory process involving the mucosa of the nose and one or more of the sinuses. Factors contributing to the inflammation include mucociliary impairment, bacterial infection, allergy, swelling of the mucosa for other reasons and mechanical obstruction. Inflammation around the osteomeatal complex is of particular importance and treatment is aimed at reducing the factors causing inflammation and ensuring adequate ventilation in this area. The classification of rhinosinusitis includes: acute rhinosinusitis (ARS) (viral or post-viral; a few of these having acute bacterial rhinosinusitis (ABRS)), and then chronic rhinosinusitis with (CRSwNP) or without (CRSsNP) nasal polyps.[1]

TREATMENT OF RHINOSINUSITIS WITH CORTICOSTEROIDS

Topical corticosteroids have improved the treatment of rhinosinusitis and asthma. Their efficacy may partly depend on their ability to reduce the viability and activation of eosinophils and to reduce the secretion of chemotactic cytokines by the nasal mucosa. This is mediated through activation of intracellular glucocorticoid receptors that are expressed in many tissues and cells. Other beneficial effects of steroids include: change of vascular permeability, reduction of mast cell degranulation and reduction of squamous metaplasia of allergic nasal polyps.

Acute rhinosinusitis (ARS)

In published studies, where either a placebo or a topical steroid has been added to antibiotic treatment for ARS, the results generally show that the patients who were treated with a topical corticosteroid improved more rapidly than when the antibiotic was combined with a placebo. A representative study by Meltzer et al.[2] found Mometasone furoate 400 μg a day improved the symptom score more than placebo in patients with ARS also treated with amoxicillin clavulanate potassium for 21 days. Recently a double-blind, double-dummy, placebo-controlled trial found topical corticosteroid given twice daily as monotherapy to be more effective than amoxicillin twice daily in ARS[3] and has been supported by others[4,5] as well as a Cochrane review.[6]

Gehanno et al.[7] looked at the effectiveness of systemic steroids in the treatment of ARS. Eight milligrams of methylprednisolone was given three times a day for 5 days as an adjunct to 10 days' treatment with amoxicillin clavulanate potassium in patients with ARS. The diagnostic criteria consisted of facial pain, purulent nasal discharge and purulent secretions from the middle meatus, together with opacities on CT scan. The conclusion was that there was no difference in the therapeutic outcome at day 14 between the steroid group and the placebo group, although 4 days after initiating treatment, the headache and facial pain was significantly less in the steroid group. A Cochrane review suggests systemic steroids may be a useful adjunctive therapy to oral antibiotics in the short-term relief of symptoms of ARS.[8]

There is very low evidence for a prophylactic effect of nasal corticosteroids in preventing recurrence of acute rhinosinusitis.[1]

Chronic rhinosinusitis without nasal polyps (CRSsNP)

Most studies compare topical steroid versus placebo as an adjunctive treatment to antibiotics. Two large trials of 407 and 967 patients, respectively, found that mometasone furoate produced a significant improvement in symptom score over the placebo. In one study topical steroid did not help the symptom of post-nasal drip[9] but it did in the second study.[10] There was no statistical difference in the CT findings of the treatment group compared with placebo.

A systematic review of level 1 or randomized controlled trials (RCTs) failed to demonstrate a universal benefit of local intra-nasal corticosteroids in CRSsNP. The method of delivery and post-surgical improved access were significant but the type of corticosteroid was not.[1] Epistaxis, dry nose, nasal burning and nasal irritation may occur as side effects to topical corticosteroid use but these are usually mild, the benefit outweighing the risk. There is a lack of clinical data to support the use of systemic corticosteroids in patients with CRSsNP.

Chronic rhinosinusitis with nasal polyps (CRSwNP): Topical steroids

In patients with CRSwNP the studies have tended to consider the effectiveness of the treatment on the rhinitic symptoms and then, as a separate outcome measure, the effect of the treatment on the size of the polyps.

In a landmark paper published in 1979, Mygind et al.[11] showed that beclomethasone dipropionate (BDP) was more effective than placebo at reducing nasal symptoms in CRSwNP but no reduction in the size of the polyps occurred in 3 weeks.

A systematic review found 34 studies in which a topical steroid has been compared to placebo. Three compared two agents and three compared topical steroid against no intervention in patients with CRSwNP. Topical steroid is more effective than placebo in reducing symptoms, particularly nasal blockage. About half report improvement in sense of smell and reduction in polyp size. The response was greater in post-surgical patients; however, their improvement in symptoms and nasal flow was not statistically significant.[1]

A comprehensive study compared fluticasone propionate 400 μg daily, with BDP 400 μg daily and with topical placebo over a 12-week period in a double-blind randomized parallel group that was conducted in a single centre study.[12] The symptom score was significantly improved in the fluticasone group and the nasal cavity volume improved in both active treatment groups when measured with acoustic rhinometry. The peak nasal and inspiratory flow also improved in both active groups but the improvement was quicker in the fluticasone propionate group. After 12 weeks there was no difference statistically in the symptoms between the two active groups.

In conclusion, therefore, there is good evidence that topical corticosteroids improve the symptoms associated with nasal polyps, in particular nasal blockage, nasal secretions and sneezing, and in some patients they are effective at improving the sense of smell. In the majority of patients, topical corticosteroids also appeared to reduce the size of the nasal polyps, provided they were used for several weeks.

Chronic rhinosinusitis with nasal polyps (CRSwNP): Systemic steroids

A Cochrane review updated in 2010 identified three level 1 studies supporting the use of systemic steroids in CRSwNP. In one study, oral prednisolone was given in doses of 60 mg daily to 25 patients with severe nasal polyposis for 4 days and, for each of the following 12 days, the dose was reduced by 5 mg daily. Antibiotics and antacids were also given. Seventy-two per cent of patients experienced a symptom improvement due to the involution of polyps and in 52% of patients an improvement was seen on the CT. Nasal obstruction reduced and sense of smell improved. This study supports the general clinical impression that systemic steroids are highly effective in treating patients' symptoms whilst taking the systemic steroid but the beneficial effects seem to be lost once the steroid is stopped.[13] The chronic nature of CRSwNP has to be considered along with the short-lived benefits of systemic corticosteroids. Local corticosteroid treatment appears to be useful so long as it can be administered effectively.

The post-operative treatment of patients with chronic rhinosinusitis and nasal polyps (CRSwNP) with steroids

Six studies have found topical steroids do reduce the recurrence rate of nasal polyps after nasal polyp surgery. To quote from two of the representative studies, Karlsson and Rundcrantz[14] treated 20 patients with BDP and 20 were followed with no treatment after polyp surgery. The follow-up period was for 30 months. After 6 months, there was a statistically significant difference between the groups in favour of BDP and its effect increased during the study period over the next 30 months.

Hartwig et al.[15] used budesonide 6 months after polypectomy in a double-blind parallel group on 73 patients. In the budesonide group, 'polyp' scores were significantly lower than in the controls after 3 and 6 months. Interestingly, this difference was only significant for patients with recurrent nasal polyposis and not those who had had a polypectomy operation for the first time.

TREATMENT OF RHINOSINUSITIS WITH ANTIBIOTICS

The exact incidence of rhinosinusitis within populations is not known but it is a common condition for which antibiotics are frequently prescribed. According to the National Ambulatory Medical Care Survey in the USA, rhinosinusitis is the fifth most common diagnosis for which antibiotics are prescribed, accounting for 9% of all paediatric antibiotic prescriptions and 21% of all adult antibiotic prescriptions written in 2002.[16]

Recurrent acute rhinosinusitis

A recent Cochrane review compared antibiotics against placebo or between antibiotics of different classes in the management of acute maxillary sinusitis in adults.[17] Fifty-nine studies met the appropriate criteria for inclusion in this review and included six placebo-controlled studies and 53 comparing different classes or dose regimens of antibiotics. Compared to placebo only a slight statistical difference in favour of antibiotics was found although the clinical significance was equivocal with cure or improvement being high in both the placebo (80%) and antibiotic group (90%).

A previous Cochrane review in which comparisons were made between the newer non-penicillins (cephalosporins, macrolides, minocycline) versus penicillins (amoxicillin and penicillin V), no significant differences were shown. The rates of cure or improvement appeared to be 84% for both antibiotic classes. Adverse effects were infrequent with no significant difference between the two groups of antibiotics. Sixteen trials (4818 patients) compared newer non-penicillin antibiotics (macrolide or cephalosporin) to amoxicillin/clavulanate with similar cure or improvement rates (72%) but less adverse effects occurred with cephalosporin antibiotics. Relapse rates within one month of successful therapy did not differ between the groups.[18] Six trials, of which three were double-blinded (1067 patients), compared a tetracycline (doxycycline, tetracycline, minocycline) to a heterogeneous group of antibiotics (folate, cephalosporin, macrolide, amoxicillin) and no relevant differences were found.

The Cochrane reviewers[18] concluded that for recurrent ARS, confirmed radiologically, current evidence is limited but supports the use of penicillin or amoxicillin for 14–17 days. In the Cochrane review, local differences in susceptibility of microorganisms to antibiotics used were not acknowledged, although it is known that resistance patterns of predominant pathogens, such as *Streptococcus pneumoniae*, *Haemophilus influenzae* and *Moraxella catarrhalis*, vary considerably.[19] The prevalence and degree of antibacterial resistance in common respiratory pathogens is also increasing worldwide, presumably because of the increase in antibiotic consumption. The choice of which antibiotic is used may depend on local resistance patterns and disease aetiology.

Antibiotic treatment for chronic rhinosinusitis

It is significantly more difficult to evaluate the efficacy of antibiotic treatment in chronic compared to intermittent ARS because of the difficulties of defining the clinical diagnosis of CRS in the literature. In many studies there is no radiological diagnosis and, therefore, data supporting the use of antibiotics in CRS are limited; however, a number of open studies using macrolides have shown a response rate of 60–80%.

In a double-blind prospective study by Legent et al.,[20] 251 adult patients with CRSsNP were treated with ciprofloxacin or amoxicillin/clavulanic acid for 9 days. Only 141 of the 251 patients had positive bacterial cultures from the middle meatus at the beginning of the study. At the end of the treatment period, the nasal discharge disappeared in 60% of the patients in the ciprofloxacin group and 56% of those in the amoxicillin/clavulanic acid group. The clinical cure and bacteriological eradication rates were 59% and 89% for ciprofloxacin versus 51% and 91% for amoxicillin/clavulanic acid, respectively. The differences were not significant. In 2002 Namyslowski reported the results of an open parallel randomized clinical trial of 206 adults with exacerbation of CRS had either amoxicillin/clavulanic acid or cefuroxime axetil. The clinical response was similar (95% and 88% respectively) as was the bacterial cure rate (65% and 68% respectively).[21] Short-term treatment of CRSsNP may be considered in exacerbations with a positive culture. In patients with CRSwNP one RCT has shown that doxycycline for 3 weeks had a small effect on polyp size and post-nasal discharge but no effect on other symptoms compared to placebo.[22]

There is some evidence that long-term treatment with low-dose macrolide antibiotics may be effective in treating patients with CRSsNP that has not been cured by surgery or corticosteroid treatment. In animal studies, macrolides have been shown to increase mucociliary transport and reduce goblet cell secretion. There is evidence *in vitro*, as well as clinical experience, that macrolides reduce the virulence and tissue damage caused by chronic bacterial colonization without actually eradicating the bacteria, that is their action is immune-modulatory rather than anti-bacterial.

Clinical studies have shown that long-term treatment with macrolide antibiotics increases ciliary function.[23] In a prospective RCT, 90 patients with CRSwNP and CRSsNP were randomized to erythromycin for 3 months, or endoscopic sinus surgery, and followed up over a year. The outcome measures included a symptom score, the SNOT 22, the SF 36, nitrous oxide levels, acoustic rhinometry, saccharine clearance times and nasal endoscopy. Both the medical and surgical treatment of CRS significantly improved almost all the subjective and objective parameters with no significant difference between the two groups, or between CRSwNP and CRSsNP, except for the increase in total nasal volume, which was greater following surgery.[23] Further studies are necessary to determine the effect of long-term treatment with antibiotics in CRSwNP.

There are two placebo-controlled studies on the effectiveness of long-term antibiotic treatment. One using roxithromycin showed efficacy in patients with CRSsNP. The other study included CRSwNP as well and although more responded in the treatment group this was not significant. Data suggest patients with high IgE levels are less likely to respond to macrolide treatment than patients with normal IgE levels.[24] Studies comparing different antibiotics did not show any significant difference between ciprofloxacin versus amoxicillin/clavulanic acid. The few available prospective studies showed a positive effect on the patient's symptoms in 56–95% of patients.

Long-term low-dose macrolide treatment may be of use if surgery and/or steroids and saline irrigation have failed. Further placebo-controlled studies should be performed to establish the efficacy of macrolides if this treatment is to be accepted in the future. There is also an urgent need for randomized placebo-controlled studies to investigate the effectiveness of antibiotics in general for CRS.

There are three placebo-controlled trials with topical antibiotics in CRSsNP. None showed any additive effect compared to saline.[25–27] There are no data on the effect of topical antibiotics in CRSwNP.

TREATMENT OF RHINOSINUSITIS WITH OTHER MEDICINES

Decongestants

After corticosteroids and antibiotics, the medications that are perceived to be most useful for treating rhinosinusitis are decongestants. The rationale behind the use of decongestants is to improve sinus ventilation and drainage. Radiological studies using CT and MRI scanning show that topical decongestants markedly reduce the size of the inferior and middle turbinates and improve osteomeatal complex patency but have no effect on ethmoidal and maxillary sinus mucosa.[28, 29]

Experimental studies suggest that topical decongestants (xylometazoline and oxymetazoline) have a beneficial anti-inflammatory action that is caused by decreasing nitric oxide synthetase.[30] A controlled clinical trial showed improved mucociliary clearance *in vivo* after 2 weeks of oxymetazoline for ABRS when compared to fluticasone and hypertonic saline and saline. The clinical course of the disease between the three groups, however, was not significantly different.[31] This, together with another study using decongestants in addition to a penicillin treatment in acute maxillary sinusitis, suggests that decongestion of the sinus ostia is not of primary importance during the healing of ARS.[32]

Topical decongestants are also recommended for individuals who have problems clearing their ears while flying or diving. The decongestants are all alpha adrenergic agonists and act on the two types of alpha receptor, one of which controls the venous capacitance vessels of the nasal tissues, which are responsible for erectile function, and the other alpha receptors, which mediate contraction of arterioles that supply the mucosa.

Ephedrine nasal drops (0.5% and 1%) are weak sympathomimetics whilst oxymetazoline and xylometazoline are more potent causing intense vasoconstriction. The rebound effect that occurs after the vasoconstriction wears off is more with the potent decongestants and patients should be advised not to use topical decongestant for more than 10 days. In patients who become addicted to decongestant drops or sprays, there is a risk of developing rhinitis medicamentosa where the nasal mucosa becomes permanently damaged.

One preparation combines the steroid dexamethasone isonicotinate with the sympathomimetic tramazoline hydrochloride (Dexa-Rhinaspray Duo). The spray is promoted for the treatment of allergic rhinitis. The suggestion is that the decongestant allows better mucosal access for the steroid. Clinical experience suggests that this is a useful spray. The use of all sympathomimetic preparations is contraindicated in patients on monoamine oxidase inhibitors (MAOIs) and they should be used with caution in patients with hypertension, hyperthyroidism, cardiovascular disease, diabetes mellitus and closed angle glaucoma, and in infants of less than 3 months of age.

The use of decongestants for CRS has not been evaluated in any RCTs. There are no controlled trials to test the efficacy of decongestants for the treatment of nasal polyps.

Systemic decongestants appear to be less effective than local preparations but rebound nasal congestion on withdrawal of the drug does not arise. Pseudo-ephedrine is available over the counter in the UK, both in tablet form and as a linctus. Little evidence supports the use of systemic decongestants in the treatment of rhinosinusitis.

Mucolytics

The rationale for using mucolytics in the treatment of rhinosinusitis is to reduce the viscosity of the nasal secretions. There is minimal evidence to support the use of mucolytics in the treatment of rhinosinusitis. One RCT study (report in Italian) suggests bromhexine is superior to placebo in acute rhinosinusitis.[33] In one paediatric study, an RCT did not prove bromhexine to be superior to saline inhalation for children with CRS.[34]

Antihistamines

These can be used orally and as a nasal spray. Clinical experience suggests that they reduce rhinorrhoea, sneezing and itching, but have little effect on nasal obstruction. There is no evidence that antihistamines reduce or abolish the symptoms of the common cold. The non-sedating antihistamines acrivastine (Semprex), cetirizine hydrochloride (Zirtek), desloratadine (Neoclarityn) and fexofenadine hydrochloride (Telfast) cause less sedation and psychomotor impairment because they penetrate the blood–brain barrier to a lesser degree than the older type of antihistamines. Side effects of antihistamines include hypotension, hypersensitivity reactions, extrapyramidal effect, dizziness, blood disorders and liver dysfunction.

In the treatment of ARS, the beneficial effect of loratadine (the predecessor of desloratadine) for patients with allergic rhinitis was confirmed in a multicentre randomized double-blind placebo-controlled trial. Patients receiving loratadine as an adjunct to antibiotic treatment suffered significantly less sneezing and obstruction on daily visual analogue scale (VAS) scores.[35]

In CRS there is little evidence that antihistamines are effective. However, they are often prescribed for patients with CRS, particularly in the USA. One randomized placebo-controlled trial on patients with residual or recurrent nasal polyps was identified using cetirizine 20 mg twice a day or placebo for 3 months. Inhaled steroids for asthma was allowed. The end point was poorly defined and no significant improvement in symptoms found using cetirizine over placebo.[36] The use of antihistamines may be useful in patients with CRSwNP with concomitant nasal allergies. No RCTs are identified for treatment of CRSsNP or CRSwNP with antihistamines without previous sinus surgery.

Sprays such as azelastine hydrochloride (Rhinolast) and levocabastine (Livostin) are topical antihistamines that are promoted for use in allergic rhinitis. Topical antihistamines are considered less effective than topical steroids and good evidence to support their use is lacking.

Sodium cromoglicate

Sodium cromoglicate is available as a 4% aqueous nasal spray (Rynacrom) and a 2% nasal spray (Vividrin), and it is also combined with xylometazoline (Rynacrom) and is promoted for prophylactic use in allergic rhinitis. Depending on the preparation, it needs to be taken either four or six times a day. Its mechanism of action is debatable; it was originally thought to act by preventing mediator release from mast cells. However, agents subsequently developed with this property do not demonstrate the same anti-asthmatic affects as cromoglicate. There is some evidence that cromoglicate depresses the exaggerated neuronal reflexes generated by irritant receptor stimulation.

Side effects are few and include local irritation and transient bronchospasm. It may have a role in the treatment of allergic rhinitis in children but the fact that it needs to be taken several times a day means that compliance is low.

Antifungal agents used in rhinology

Fungal infections may be superficial or systemic. Antifungal agents can be classified into polyenes, flucytosine, imidazoles and triazoles. The polyenes, amphotericin and nystatin interact with ergosterol in the fungal cell membrane. Pores are formed through which the fungal cell contents are lost. Selectivity is obtained since the human cell membrane contains mostly cholesterol rather than ergosterol.

Amphotericin has a wide spectrum of activity and is used parentally in severe systemic infections since oral absorption is poor. Side effects are common and include nausea and fevers. Renal impairment can occur but is reversible if detected early. Liposomal amphotericin is significantly less toxic but is more expensive. It is likely that it will become the agent of choice. Nystatin is used principally for *Candida albicans* infections of the skin and mucosal membranes.

Flucytosine is given orally or intravenously to treat systemic candidiasis or cryptococcal infections, often in combination with amphotericin to prevent resistance. Flucytosine is converted in fungal cells to flurouracil which inhibits DNA synthesis.

The imidazoles, miconazole, ketoconazole and clotrimazole, are mostly used to treat topical infections. They are broad-spectrum antifungals that prevent ergosterol synthesis. Ketoconazole is better absorbed by mouth than the other imidazoles but it has been associated with fatal hepatotoxicity.

The triazoles include fluconazole and itraconazole and both can be given orally and parentally. Itraconazole is active against Aspergillus but has been associated with heptatoxicity.

There has been interest in the role of fungi as a possible cause for the various types of rhinosinusitis. Antimycotics have been used topically and systemically and as an adjunct to sinus surgery in the treatment of allergic fungal rhinosinusitis, invasive fungal rhinosinusitis and conventional recurrent ARS.

Surgery is considered the first-line treatment for allergic fungal rhinosinusitis,[37] and surgery and systemic antimycotics are used in the treatment of invasive fungal rhinosinusitis.[38] Although the use of antimycotics in the treatment of allergic fungal rhinosinusitis has not been tested in controlled trials, a high dose of post-operative itraconazole, combined with oral and topical steroids in a cohort of 139 patients with allergic fungal rhinosinusitis, reduced the need for revision surgery.[39] The antifungal prophylaxis in immunocompromised patients did not prevent the development of invasive zygomycosis but treatment with liposomal amphotericin B resulted in improved response and survival rates with early detection being as important as the surgical and antifungal treatments.[40]

Researchers from the Mayo Clinic proposed that CRS may arise because of a local immune response to fungi that are present in nasal and sinus secretions.[41] Given the correct equipment, fungi can be detected in nasal secretions in virtually all patients with CRSwNP, but also in a controlled disease-free population. There is no definitive proof that fungi are involved in the aetiology of the inflammatory response in some patients. One double-blind randomized placebo-controlled trial in 60 patients with CRSwNP, comparing topical treatment with amphotericin B with saline douching,[42] found radiological and subjective scores were actually worse in the treatment group. One trial with nasal amphoteracin B treatment significantly reduced symptoms at 2 but not 4 weeks and endoscopy scores and fungal culture rates did not significantly differ. This treatment is not recommended in CRSsNP.[43]

MEDICATION THAT MAY IMPROVE THE IMMUNE RESPONSE

Since an altered immune response to bacterial infection or fungal infection may be responsible for some of the episodes of recurrent rhinosinusitis, there is interest in medications that may alter the immune response.

Bacterial lysate preparations

Bacterial lysate preparations (e.g. ribosomal fractions of *Klebsiella pneumoniae*, *Streptococcus pneumoniae*, *Streptococcus pyogenes* and *Haemophilus influenzae*) have been tested against placebo in three multicentre placebo-controlled trials and the evidence from these studies suggested that this type of therapy may reduce the need for antibiotics in the treatment of chronic rhinosinusitis.[44-46] Based on the results of one RCT oral OM-85 BV treatment may be considered as an adjunct to standard medical treatment in adults with CRSsNP.[1]

Treatment with more expensive agents that either stimulate or modulate the immune system (e.g. recombinant human granulocyte colony stimulating factor) have been tested in a randomized controlled trial in a group of patients with CRS that were refractory to other types of treatment. The studies showed there was no significant improvement with this expensive treatment.

A pilot study has looked at treatment with gamma interferon and it suggested that this treatment may be beneficial in treating resistant CRS; but the number of patients was small.[47]

NASAL AND ANTRAL IRRIGATION WITH SALINE

Saline irrigation

A number of RCTs have tested nasal irrigation with isotonic or hypertonic saline in the treatment of ARS and CRS comparing modalities of application. There was limited evidence of benefit with nasal saline irrigation in adults with ARS.[48] The evidence is that nasal washout with isotonic or hypertonic saline is beneficial in alleviating symptoms and improves endoscopic findings in patients with CRS. Irrigation with saline has also shown to significantly improve nasal mucociliary clearance, as measured by saccharine tests in healthy volunteers.[49]

ANTILEUKOTRIENES

The role of leukotrienes in the pathogenesis of bronchial asthma has been well documented and increased levels of these mediators have been detected in patients with rhinosinusitis and nasal polyps. Antileukotrienes have been evaluated in the treatment of asthmatics, especially in those with the aspirin-induced asthma (ASA) triad.

When seasonal allergic rhinitis was considered, antileukotrienes were not found to be superior to placebo in reducing symptom scores in a randomized controlled trial.[50]

For patients with CRSwNP, one study looked at antileukotriene treatment in 36 patients and found that when antileukotrienes were added to standard treatment regimes, there was a significant reduction in symptom score.[51]

Two other studies support the use of antileukotriene treatment as an adjunct to standard treatment in patients with nasal polyps, asthma and aspirin intolerance.[52, 53]

Leukotriene antagonists can cause skin rash, mood changes, tremors or shaking and occasionally can worsen the symptoms of sinus symptoms and asthma. Currently data do not support the use of antileukotriene antagonist in CRSwNP.

Aspirin desensitization

This treatment has been used in patients with aspirin-exacerbated respiratory disease (AERD) having CRSwNP, bronchial asthma and hypersensitivity to Cox-1 inhibitors (including aspirin). It was observed that following exposure to aspirin, these patients became refractory to the effects of aspirin for 24 to 72 hours. Several case series suggest a weak clinical benefit from oral aspirin desensitization.[54, 55] There is no randomized placebo-controlled trial on oral aspirin in AERD patients. In one trial, 14 patients who reacted to an aspirin provocation test were allocated to 100 mg or 300 mg aspirin daily for 1 year. It was found that all patients on 100 mg aspirin had recurrence of nasal polyps but no polyps were found in patients on 300 mg aspirin daily.[56]

Nasal administration of lysine-aspirin may reduce the risk of severe hypersensitivity reactions as well as gastrointestinal side effects. In a randomized, double-blind placebo-controlled trial patients with AERD were given either 16 mg lysine-aspirin or placebo every 48 hours for 6 months but no significant clinical benefit was found in the treatment group compared to the placebo group.[57]

Based on current data, the benefit of oral or nasal aspirin desensitization in patients with AERD has yet to be determined.

AGENTS USED TO BLOCK THE PARASYMPATHETIC NERVOUS SYSTEM

Ipratropium bromide (Rinatec) is a muscarinic receptor antagonist blocking the parasympathetic nervous system. It should be effective in anyone with a wet dripping nose due to parasympathetic overactivity. In practice, it is effective for some elderly men with a dripping nose! Side effects include a dry mouth, epistaxis and dryness of the nose. A Cochrane review identified seven studies and concluded that ipratropium bromide is effective in reducing the rhinorrhoea with no effect on congestion experienced by those with the common cold.[58]

VACCINATION

Although vaccination does not have a direct effect in the treatment of ARS, a study showed that in the 5-year period following the introduction of 7-valent pneumococcal vaccination when compared to the previous 5-year period, the cause of acute maxillary sinusitis by *Streptococci pneumonae* decreased by 18% but *Haemophilus influenza* increased by 8%.[59]

RELATED TOPICS

Preparation of the nasal mucosa prior to surgery

Cocaine solution (5% or 10%) or cocaine paste (25%) has been used to prepare the nose prior to surgery for more than 100 years. The majority of rhinologists believe it to be the most effective way of ensuring good operating conditions providing sufficient time for the drug to work is allowed. The application of Moffat's solution by a spray (**Figure 28.1**) is one method of preparing the nose and it is sensible to do this immediately after the induction of anaesthesia.

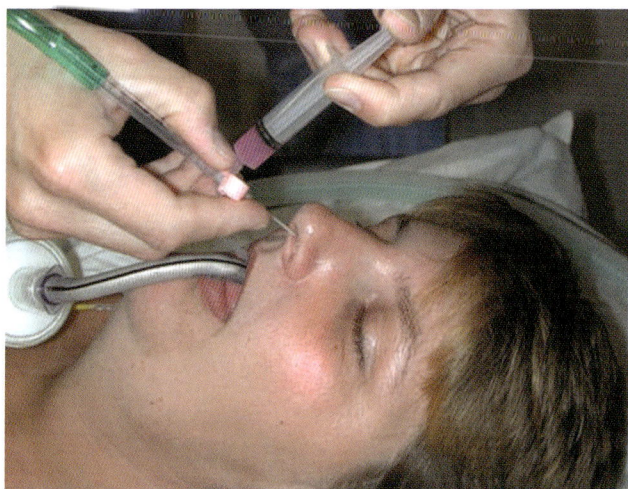

Figure 28.1 The application of Moffat's solution by a spray.

Moffat's solution consists of 2 mL of 5% cocaine, 1 mL of 1:1000 adrenaline and a small amount of bicarbonate solution. In order to avoid systemic effects, the maximum dose recommended for application to the nasal mucosa in fit adults is 1.5 mg/kg. The solution is dyed pink reducing the risk of it being mistaken for other drugs in the anaesthetic room.

Vestibulitis

Non-infective vestibulitis may be treated by applying vaseline or a mild topical corticosteroid to the vestibule. In the presence of infection an antibiotic ointment active against *Staphylococcus aureus* is required. A combination of chlorhexidine and neomycin (Naseptin) or mupirocin (Bactroban nasal) are available. The latter is used as a second-line agent for the eradication of methicillin-resistant *Staphylococcus aureus* (MRSA). The ointment is applied three times a day for 5 days and a swab is taken 2 days later to determine whether MRSA has been successfully eradicated. Naseptin includes arachis (peanut) oil and should not be used in patients with peanut allergy. Naseptin is contraindicated in pregnancy.

Hereditary familial telangiectasia

The epistaxis associated with hereditary familial telangiectasia (HFT) is difficult to treat and a variety of medical and surgical treatments have been tried. Systemic and topical oestrogen provoke squamous metaplasia of the epithelium and in this way provide a protective coat over the blood vessels. Ethinyloestradiol may be used under supervision for the treatment of HFT in women. The side effects include nausea, fluid retention and thrombosis. It is not popular in men because of the gynaecomastia it induces.

Atrophic rhinitis

Steam inhalation, humidification and saline nasal douching are useful in atrophic rhinitis. A 25% glucose in glycerine solution restores moisture to the nasal mucosa: 25 g of glucose is dissolved in 75 g glycerine (gently warmed). Once bottled the drops have a 3-month life span. The drops can be used several times a day and provide some relief to this distressing condition.

METHODS OF ADMINISTERING TOPICAL NASAL PREPARATIONS

If two nasal sprays are to be administered to each nostril, one spray should be directed upwards and the other backwards whilst the patient does not breathe or breathes in gently.

The best position for administering nasal drops is head-down, as in **Figure 28.2**.

Fluticasone propionate nasules (400 μg) can be used to increase the topical dose of steroid. One nasule is shared between each nostril once daily; thus the dose given is precisely known.

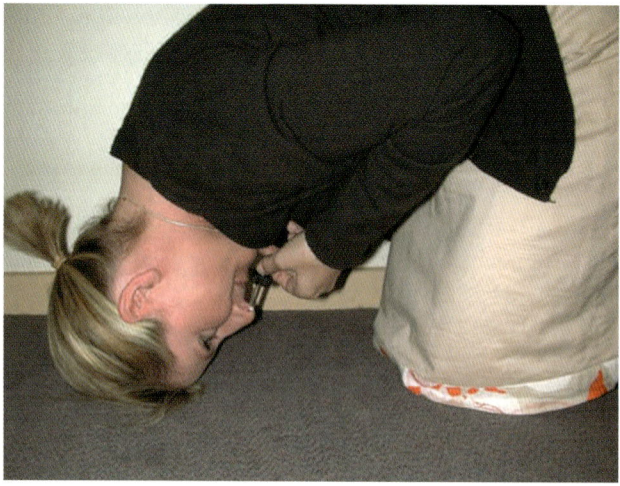

Figure 28.2 The best position for administering steroid drops.

BEST CLINICAL PRACTICE

- ✓ Topical steroids improve the symptoms associated with nasal polyps and reduce the recurrence rate of nasal polyps after surgery.
- ✓ The best position for administering steroid drops is head-down (**Figure 28.2**).
- ✓ One way of introducing cocaine into the nose is by spraying Moffat's solution into the nose immediately after induction of anaesthesia, increasing the chances of obtaining a 'bloodless surgical field'.
- ✓ Before prescribing naseptin, ensure the patient is not allergic to peanuts and is not pregnant.

FUTURE RESEARCH

- ➤ Topical steroids reduce the recurrence rate of nasal polyps following surgery but there is yet to be an effective long-lasting medical polypectomy.
- ➤ The optimum length of treatment with topical steroids is yet to be established with the different clinical scenarios.
- ➤ A large prospective study is required to determine the role of antibiotics in preventing acute complications.
- ➤ The aetiology of polyps is yet to be identified.

KEY POINTS

- Rhinosinusitis is one of the most common healthcare problems. It diminishes patients' quality of life and consumes resources.
- Corticosteroids are useful topically in post-viral ARS, CRSsNP and CRSwNP (in both adults and children). Oral steroids are useful in adults with CRSwNP.
- Antibiotics with oral corticosteroids in adults and topical corticosteroids in children are effective treatments for acute bacterial rhinosinusitis.
- Oral antibiotic therapy (< 4 weeks) may be useful in CRS during exacerbations.
- Topical decongestants are a useful adjunct to analgesia and antihistamines in viral ARS in adults.
- Antihistamines reduce rhinorrhoea, sneezing and itching but not nasal obstruction and may be useful in patients with CRSwNP in allergic patients.
- Saline irrigation of the nose is an effective treatment for rhinosinusitis.

ACKNOWLEDGEMENTS

Acknowledgement is made to the late Grant Bates, a valuable co-author to this chapter published in the previous edition of Scott-Brown.

REFERENCES

1. Fokkens W, Lund VJ, Mullol J, et al. European position paper on rhinosinusitis and nasal polyps. *Rhinology* 2012; 50(supplement 23): 1–329.
2. Meltzer EO, Orgel HA, Backhaus JW, et al. Intranasal flunisolide spray as an adjunct to oral antibiotic therapy for sinusitis. *J Allergy Clin Immun* 1993; **92**: 812–23.
3. Meltzer EO, Bachert C, Staudinger H. Treating acute rhinosinusitis: comparing efficacy and safety of mometasone furoate nasal spray, amoxicillin, and placebo. *J Allergy Clin Immun* 2005; **116**(6): 1289–95.
4. Bachert C, Meltzer EO. Effect of mometasone furoate nasal spray on quality of life of patients with acute rhinosinusitis. *Rhinology* 2007; **45**(3): 190–96.
5. Keith PK, Dymek A, Pfaar O, et al. Fluticasone furoate nasal spray reduces symptoms of uncomplicated acute rhinosinusitis: a randomised placebo-controlled study. *Prim Care Resp J* 2012; **21**(3): 267–75.
6. Zalmanovici A, Yaphe J. Intranasal steroids for acute sinusitis. *Cochrane Database Syst Rev (Online)* 2009; (4): CD005149.
7. Gehanno P, Beauvillain C, Bobin S, et al. Short therapy with amoxicillin-clavulanate and corticosteroids in acute sinusitis: results of a multicentre study in adults. *Scand J Infect Dis* 2000; **32**: 679–84.
8. Venekamp RP, Thompson MJ, Hayward G, et al. Systemic corticosteroids for acute sinusitis. *Cochrane Database Syst Rev (Online)* 2011; **12**: CD008115.
9. Meltzer EO, Charous BL, Busse WW, et al. Added relief in the treatment of acute recurrent sinusitis with adjunctive Mometasone furoate nasal spray. The Nasonex Sinusitis Group. *J Allergy Immun* 2000; **106**: 630–37.
10. Nayak AS, Settipane GA, Pedinoff A, et al. Effective dose range of Mometasone furoate nasal spray in the treatment of acute rhinosinusitis. *Ann Allerg Asthma Immunol* 2002; **89**: 271–78.
11. Mygind N, Pedersen CB, Prytz S, Sorensen H. Treatment of nasal polyps with intranasal Beclomethasone dipropionate aerosol. *Clin Allergy* 1975; **5**: 159–64.
12. Keith P, Nieminen J, Hollingworth K, Dolovich J. Efficacy and tolerability of Fluticasone propionate nasal drops 400 microgram once daily compared with placebo for the treatment of bilateral polyposis in adults. *Clin Exp Allergy* 2000; **39**: 1460–68.
13. van Camp C, Clement PA. Results of oral steroid treatment in nasal polyposis. *Rhinology* 1994; **32**: 5–9.
14. Karlsson G, Rundcrantz H. A randomized trial of intranasal Beclomethasone dipropionate after polypectomy. *Rhinology* 1982; **20**: 144–48.
15. Hartwig S, Linden M, Laurent C, et al. Budesonide nasal spray as prophylactic treatment after polypectomy (a double blind clinical trial). *J Laryngol Otol* 1988; **102**: 148–51.
16. Anon JB, Jacobs MR, Poole MD, et al. Antimicrobial treatment guidelines for acute bacterial rhinosinusitis. *Otolaryngol Head Neck* 2004; **130**: 1–45.
17. Ahovuo-Saloranta A, Borisenko OV, Kovanen N, et al. Antibiotics for acute maxillary sinusitis. *Cochrane Database Syst Rev (Online)* 2008; **16**(2): CD000243.
18. Williams Jr. JW, Aguilar C, Cornell J, et al. Antibiotics for acute maxillary sinusitis (Cochrane review). *Cochrane Database Syst Rev* 2003; (4).
19. Hoban D, Felmingham D. The PROTEKT surveillance study: antimicrobial susceptibility of Haemophilus influenzae and Moraxella catarrhalis from community-acquired respiratory tract infections. *J Antimicrob Chemoth* 2002; **59**: 49–59.
20. Legent F, Bordure P, Beauvillain C, Berche P. A double-blind comparison of ciprofloxacin and amoxycillin/clavulanic acid in the treatment of chronic sinusitis. *Chemotherapy* 1994; **40**: 8–15.
21. Namyslowski G, Misiolek M, Czecior E, et al. Comparison of the efficacy and tolerability of amoxycillin/clavulanic acid 875 mg b.i.d. with cefuroxime 500 mg b.i.d. in the treatment of chronic and acute exacerbation of chronic sinusitis in adults. *J Chemother* 2002; **14**(5): 508–17.
22. Van Zele T, Gevaert P, Holtappels G, et al. Oral steroids and doxycycline: two different approaches to treat nasal polyps. *J Allergy Clin Immunol* 2010; **125**(5): 1069–76. e4.
23. Ragab SM, Lund VJ, Scadding G. Evaluation of the medical and surgical treatment of chronic rhinosinusitis: a prospective, randomised, controlled trial. *Laryngoscope* 2004; **114**: 923–30.
24. Haruna S, Shimada C, Ozawa M, et al. A study of poor responders for long-term, low-dose macrolide administration for chronic sinusitis. *Rhinology* 2009; **47**(1): 66–71.
25. Gysin C, Alothman GA, Papsin BC. Sinonasal disease in cystic fibrosis: clinical characteristics, diagnosis, and management. *Pediatr Pulmonol* 2000; **30**(6): 481–89.
26. Desrosiers MY, Salas-Prato M. Treatment of chronic rhinosinusitis refractory to other treatments with topical antibiotic therapy delivered by means of a large-particle nebulizer: results of a controlled trial. *Otolaryngol Head Neck Surg* 2001; **125**(3): 265–69.
27. Videler WJ, van Drunen CM, Reitsma JB, Fokkens WJ. Nebulized bacitracin/colimycin: a treatment option in recalcitrant chronic rhinosinusitis with Staphylococcus aureus? A doubleblind, randomized, placebo-controlled, cross-over pilot study. *Rhinology* 2008; **46**(2): 92–98.
28. Stringer SP, Mancuso AA, Avino AJ. Effect of a topical vasoconstrictor on computed tomography of paranasal sinus disease. *Laryngoscope* 1993; **103**: 6–9.
29. Benammar-Englmaier M, Hallermeier JK, Englmaier B. Alphamimetic effects on nasal mucosa in magnetic resonance tomography. *Digitale Bilddiagn* 1990; **10**(2): 46–50.
30. Westerveld GJ, Voss HP, van der Hee RM, et al. Inhibition of nitric oxide synthase by nasal decongestants. *Eur Respir J* 2000; **16**: 437–44.
31. Inanli S, Ozturk O, Korkmaz M, et al. The effects of topical agents of fluticasone propionate, oxymetazoline, and 3% and 0.9% sodium chloride solutions on mucociliary clearance in the therapy of acute bacterial rhinosinusitis in vivo. *Laryngoscope* 2002; **112**: 320–25.
32. Wiklund L, Stierna P, Berglund R, et al. The efficacy of oxymetazoline administered with a nasal bellows container and combined with oral phenoxymethyl-penicillin in the treatment of acute maxillary sinusitis. *Acta Otolaryngol Suppl* 1994; **515**: 57–64.
33. Tarantino V, Stura MG, Leproux GB, Cremonesi G. Advantages of treatment with bromhexine in acute sinus inflammation in children: randomized double-blind study versus placebo. *Minerva Pediatr* 1988; **40**(11): 649–52.
34. Van Bever HP, Bosmans J, Stevens WJ. Nebulization treatment with saline compared to bromhexine in treating chronic sinusitis in asthmatic children. *Allergy* 1987; **42**: 33–36.
35. Braun JJ, Alabert JP, Michel FB, et al. Adjunct effect of loratadine in the treatment of acute sinusitis in patients with allergic rhinitis. *Allergy* 1997; **52**: 650–55.
36. Haye R, Aanesen JP, Burtin B, et al. The effect of cetirizine on symptoms and signs of nasal polyposis. *J Laryngol Otol* 1998; **112**(11): 1042–46.
37. Schubert MS. Medical treatment of allergic fungal sinusitis. *Ann Allerg Asthma Immunol* 2000; **85**: 90–97; quiz 97–101.
38. Kuhn FA, Javer AR. Allergic fungal rhinosinusitis: perioperative management, prevention of recurrence, and role of steroids and antifungal agents. *Otolaryng Clin N Am* 2000; **33**: 419–33.
39. Rains BM 3rd, Mineck CW. Treatment of allergic fungal sinusitis with high-dose itraconazole. *Am J Rhinol* 2003; **17**: 1–8.
40. DelGaudio JM, Clemson LA. An early detection protocol for invasive fungal sinusitis in neutropenic patients successfully reduces extent of disease at presentation and long term morbidity. *Laryngoscope* 2009; **119**(1): 180–83.
41. Ponikau JU, Sherris DA, Kern EB, et al. The diagnosis and incidence of allergic fungal sinusitis. *Mayo Clin Proc* 1999; **74**: 877–84.
42. Weschta M, Rimek D, Formanek M, et al. Topical antifungal treatment of chronic rhinosinusitis with nasal polyps: a randomized, double-blind clinical trial. *J Allergy Clin Immunol* 2004; **113**: 1122–28.
43. Liang KL, Su MC, Shiao JY, et al. Amphotericin B irrigation for the treatment of chronic rhinosinusitis without nasal polyps: a randomized, placebo-controlled, double-blind study. *Am J Rhinol* 2008; **22**(1): 52–58.
44. Habermann W, Zimmermann K, Skarabis H,. [Reduction of acute recurrence in patients with chronic recurrent hypertrophic sinusitis by treatment with a bacterial immunostimulant (Enterococcus faecalis Bacteriae of human origin]. *Arzneimittelforschung* 2002; **52**: 622–27.
45. Serrano E, Demanez JP, Morgon A, et al. Effectiveness of ribosomal fractions of Klebsiella pneumoniae, Streptococcus pneumoniae, Streptococcus pyogenes, Haemophilus influenzae and the membrane fraction of Kp (Ribomunyl) in the prevention of clinical recurrences of infectious rhinitis: results of a multicenter double-blind placebo-controlled study. *Eur Arch Otorhinolaryngol* 1997; **254**: 372–75.

46. Heintz B, Schlenter WW, Kirsten R, Nelson K. Clinical efficacy of Broncho-Vaxom in adult patients with chronic purulent sinusitis: a multi-centric, placebo-controlled, double-blind study. *Int J Clin Pharm Ther Toxicol* 1989; **27**: 530–34.
47. Jyonouchi H, Sun S, Kelly A, Rimell FL. Effects of exogenous interferon gamma on patients with treatment-resistant chronic rhinosinusitis and dysregulated interferon gamma production: a pilot study. *Arch Otolaryngol* 2003; **129**: 563–69.
48. Hildenbrand T, Weber R, Heubach C, Mosges R. Nasal douching in acute rhinosinusitis (Article in German). *Laryngorhinootologie* 2011; **90**(6): 346–51.
49. Talbot AR, Herr TM, Parsons DS. Mucociliary clearance and buffered hypertonic saline solution. *Laryngoscope* 1997; **107**: 500–03.
50. Pullerits T, Praks L, Skoogh BE, et al. Randomized placebo-controlled study comparing a leukotriene receptor antagonist and a nasal glucocorticoid in seasonal allergic rhinitis. *Am J Resp Crit Care* 1999; **159**: 1814–18.
51. Parnes SM, Chuma AV. Acute effects of antileukotrienes on sinonasal polyposis and sinusitis. *Ear Nose Throat J* 2000; **79**: 18–20, 24–25.
52. Ulualp SO, Sterman BM, Toohill RJ. Antileukotriene therapy for the relief of sinus symptoms in aspirin triad disease. *Ear Nose Throat J* 1999; **78**: 604–06, 613, passim.
53. Ragab S, Parikh A, Darby YC, Scadding GK. An open audit of montelukast, a leukotriene receptor antagonist, in nasal polyposis associated with asthma. *Clin Exp Allergy* 2001; **31**: 1385–91.
54. Forer B, Kivity S, Sade J, Landsberg R. Aspirin desensitization for ASA triad patients: prospective study of the rhinologist's perspective. *Rhinology* 2011; **49**(1): 95–99.
55. Kamani T, Sama A. Management of nasal polyps in 'aspirin sensitive asthma' triad. *Curr Opin Otolaryngol* 2011; **19**(1): 6–10.
56. Rozsasi A, Polzehl D, Deutschle T, et al. Long-term treatment with aspirin desensitization: a prospective clinical trial comparing 100 and 300 mg aspirin daily. *Allergy* 2008; **63**(9): 1228–34.
57. Parikh AA, Scadding GK. Intranasal lysine-aspirin in aspirin-sensitive nasal polyposis: a controlled trial. *Laryngoscope* 2005; **115**(8): 1385–90.
58. Albalawi ZH, Othman SS, Alfaleh K. Intranasal ipratropium bromide for the common cold. *Cochrane Database Syst Rev (Online)* 2011; (7): CD008231.
59. Brook I, Gober AE. Frequency of recovery of pathogens from the nasopharynx of children with acute maxillary sinusitis before and after the introduction of vaccination with the 7-valent pneumococcal vaccine. *Int J Pediatr Otorhinolaryngol* 2007; **71**(4): 575–79.

FURTHER READING

British Society for Allergy and Clinical Immunology, ENT Sub-Committee. *Rhinitis Management Guidelines*. 3rd ed. London: Martin Dunitz.

CHAPTER 29

DRUG THERAPY IN LARYNGOLOGY AND HEAD AND NECK SURGERY

Wendy Smith and Rogan Corbridge

Introduction	293
Antiplatelet drugs	293
Anticoagulants	293
Antibiotics	295
Preparations used to irrigate wounds	295
Local anaesthetic sprays and lozenges	295
Mouthwashes	295
Throat lozenges and pastilles	295
Solutions, suspensions and syrups	295
Treatment of dry mouth	296
Cough medicines	296
Management of stridor	296
Drug therapy in angioneurotic oedema	296
Use of botulinum toxins in spasmodic dystonia	296
Collagen injection of paralyzed vocal cords	297
Drugs used in thyroid disease including the management of hypocalcaemia	297
Treatment of reflux oesophagitis and laryngopharyngeal reflux	298
Chemotherapeutic agents	299
Management of fungating wounds	300
References	300
Further reading	300

SEARCH STRATEGY

Data in this chapter may be updated by a Medline search using the keywords: antiplatelet, anticoagulant, antibiotic prophylaxis, and head and neck surgery. This chapter relied on the medicines listed in the *British National Formulary*.[1]

INTRODUCTION

The laryngologist and head and neck surgeon prescribes medicines for prophylactic purposes, for example antibiotics and anticoagulants, as well as for therapeutic use in the management of infections, immune conditions and voice/throat problems. An appreciation of the pharmacology, preparations available, side effects and contraindications is required for appropriate and safe prescribing. This chapter addresses these matters.

ANTIPLATELET DRUGS

These reduce platelet aggregation and thereby thrombus formation in the arterial circulation where thrombi are primarily composed of platelets with little fibrin. Aspirin, clopidogrel and dipyridamole are often encountered in ENT patients with comorbidities to prevent atherosclerotic and thromboembolic events (see NICE guidelines[2]). The decision to stop these preparations prior to surgery is based on the balance of risk of bleeding versus the risk of thrombus formation. Sylvester and Coatesworth[3] found that there is a significant morbidity and mortality associated with early cessation of antiplatelet agents but evidence from cardiac surgery suggests that the operative blood loss is only marginally greater in patients on aspirin and clopidogrel. They, like others,[4] suggest the management of these patients in the perioperative period should be made after multidisciplinary consultation.

ANTICOAGULANTS

The perioperative management of patients taking anticoagulants may be complex and should be considered on an individual patient basis, taking into account the increased risk of haemorrhagic complications in that procedure with the risk of thromboembolism if the anticoagulation therapy is stopped. Where necessary, involvement of the haematology/medical teams is advised.

The anticoagulant drugs heparin and warfarin are widely used in the prevention and treatment of venous thrombosis and embolism perioperatively. Anticoagulants should not be used where there is a history of haemorrhagic disorders, peptic ulcer disease, severe hypertension and severe liver disease. **Figure 29.1** illustrates the clotting pathway and the action of heparin and oral anticoagulants.

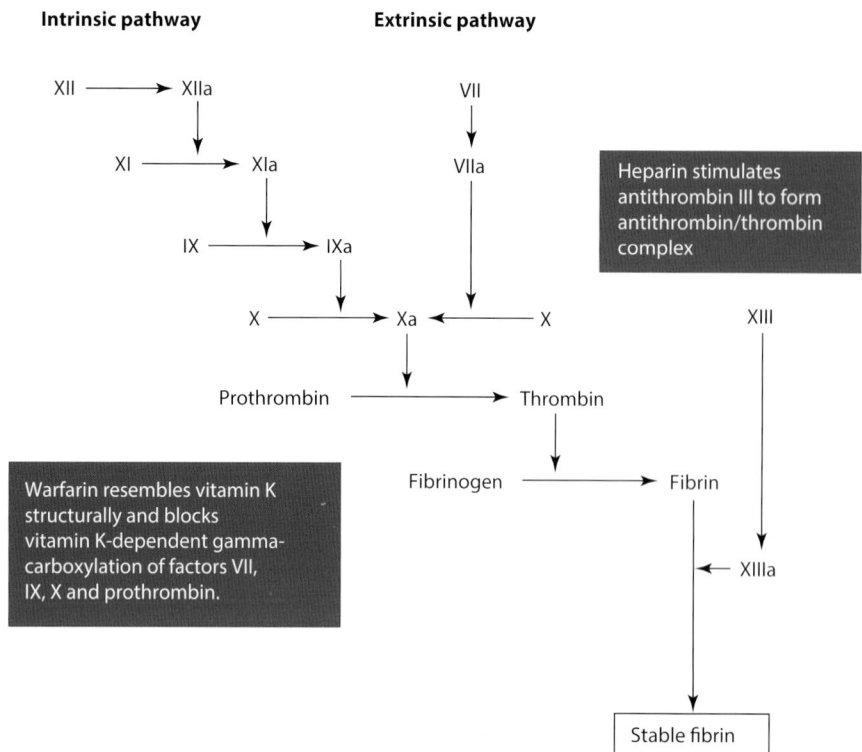

Figure 29.1 The clotting pathway and the mechanism of action of heparin and oral anticoagulants.

Heparin is a family of mucopolysaccharides with a molecular weight of 4000–30 000. The molecules are attached to a protein backbone consisting entirely of serine and glycine residues. Heparin is found in mast cells, in plasma and in the endothelial cell layer of blood vessels. This highly acidic substance is extracted from beef lung or hog intestinal mucosa for therapeutic use. Heparin's main action is preventing fibrin formation by interacting with the protease inhibitor antithrombin III enhancing (by 1000-fold) the binding of antithrombin III with thrombin. In addition, the heparin–antithrombin III complex has inhibitory effects on factors IXa, Xa, XIa and XIIa.

Heparin is not absorbed from the gastrointestinal mucosa because of its charge and large molecular weight; therefore it must be given intravenously or by subcutaneous injection. Intramuscular injection is avoided to prevent haematoma formation. The onset of action of heparin is immediate and it has a half-life of 40–90 minutes. It is inactivated by heparinase in the liver and platelet factor IV released from activated platelets may also have a role.

When used for prophylaxis of deep vein thrombosis in surgery, 5000 units of heparin should be given 2 hours before surgery, then 8–12-hourly for 7 days or until the patient is ambulant. Monitoring is not required in this situation but when used to treat a thrombosis, a regime of 5000 units intravenously followed by 15–25 units/kg/hour intravenous infusion or 15 000 units 12-hourly necessitates monitoring of the thrombin time, which should be increased by a factor of 2 to 3.

Low molecular weight heparins (certoparin, dalteparin, enoxaparin, reviparin and tinzaparin) are also effective in the prophylaxis of venous thromboembolism and their once daily subcutaneous administration is more convenient. These can also be used to treat deep vein thrombosis and monitoring is not required.

Platelet counts should be measured in patients receiving heparin since thrombocytopenia (an immune reaction) may occur but this does not usually happen until 6 to 10 days after the start of treatment. Should thrombocytopenia, or a 50% reduction of the platelet count occur, and further anticoagulation is required, patients should be given the heparinoid, danaparoid, or the hirudin, lepirudin.

Heparin inhibits aldosterone and may result in hyperkalaemia, especially in patients with diabetes mellitus, chronic renal failure, acidosis, raised plasma potassium or those taking potassium-sparing drugs.

The oral anticoagulants prevent the reduction of vitamin K that is required as an active cofactor of carboxylase in factors II, VII, IX and X. The effect on fibrin formation depends upon the balance between the decreased rate of carboxylation and the unaltered rate of degradation of factors already carboxylated. Warfarin has a half-life of 40 hours and a duration of action between 2 and 6 days. It takes at least 48–72 hours for the anticoagulant effect to develop fully and so heparin is also used initially when an immediate anticoagulant effect is required. Warfarin is the most commonly prescribed oral anticoagulant; nicoumalone and phenindione are rarely used. The drugs are metabolized by the mixed function oxidases in the liver.

Monitoring of the prothrombin time (usually reported as the international normalized ratio, INR) is required and dose adjustments made accordingly. Target INR values (usually between 2 and 4) are detailed in the

British National Formulary. The INR can be dramatically altered by coprescribing other medication and the reader is again directed to the British National Formulary[1] prior to coprescribing.

ANTIBIOTICS

Antibiotics are commonly prescribed prophylactically, even in so-called clean operations.[5, 6] The use of antibiotics post-tonsillectomy has failed to show a reduction in the secondary haemorrhage rate but may reduce pain at day 5 post-operatively.[7, 8] Where there is no violation of mucosa, no pre-operative inflammation and no drain, the incidence of wound infection in the head and neck is 2%. In surgery such as laryngectomy, prophylactic antibiotics with a broad spectrum are used to prevent wound infections. A pre-operative dose (given to allow a high tissue level at the time of surgery) and three post-operative doses of a cephalosporin and metronidazole are suitable. Violaris and Bridger, using a cephalosporin at 8 hours pre-operatively with the premedication and three doses 8-hourly post-operatively, reduced the development of pharyngocutaneous fistulae.[9] Johansen et al.[10] found prophylactic metronidazole resulted in a highly significant decrease in the frequency of post-operative fistulae.

Antibiotic prophylaxis is also necessary in patients with artificial heart valves or cardiac valve disease. Local policies may vary but amoxicillin 3 g orally or 1 g intramuscularly can be given 1 hour before surgery and 6 hours post-operatively.

The choice of antibiotic to treat an established infection is initially on a 'best guess' policy based on the probable pathogen until swab results and sensitivities become available.

PREPARATIONS USED TO IRRIGATE WOUNDS

Before closing a wound following tumour excision it has been recommended that it should first be washed out well. Stell and Maran[11] describe the use of Savlon, hydrogen peroxide and sterile water as suitable solutions since it appears that the mechanical process of washing rather than the lytic action on the cells is important. They recommend the use of at least 1 L of solution. In a xenograft model of tumour-cell wound contamination, Allegretto et al.[12] found that irrigation with water, saline or gemcitabine delayed tumour development: the latter two improved rates of long-term disease control.

LOCAL ANAESTHETIC SPRAYS AND LOZENGES

These preparations are used to desensitize the mouth and pharynx prior to examination, investigation or treatment. Lidocaine (lignocaine) is effectively absorbed from mucous membranes and is available as a pump spray as a 10% solution (maximum dose is 20 sprays in pharynx, larynx or trachea) and more commonly as a topical 4% solution (maximum dose is 7.5 mL). Benzocaine is a neutral, water-insoluble local anaesthetic of low potency and is only used for surface anaesthesia in non-inflamed tissue in the mouth and pharynx. It is available in lozenges and sprays, sometimes combined with antiseptics. Sensitization may occur and there is little evidence for the benefit in using these combined preparations. Patients should be advised not to eat or drink until the numbness has worn off. Lidocaine belongs to the amide class, benzocaine to the ester class of local anaesthetics. Both bind to a receptor on the sodium channel in the axon preventing the opening of the channels, thereby preventing depolarization of the nerve. In over dosage, cardiac toxicity can occur.

MOUTHWASHES

Mouthwashes are usually aqueous solutions in a concentrated form of substances with deodorant, antiseptic, local anaesthetic or astringent properties. Sometimes they should be diluted before use. They have a mechanical cleansing action. Hydrogen peroxide mouthwash is a 6% solution and 15 mL should be diluted in half a cup of warm water two to three times daily. It contains an oxidizing agent and is useful in the treatment of acute ulcerative gingivitis. It froths in contact with oral debris, thereby having a mechanical cleansing effect, hence its use in the management of secondary tonsillectomy haemorrhages. Chlorhexidine gluconate, used when tooth-brushing is not possible or in combating oral infection, inhibits plaque formation on teeth but has the side effect of causing reversible brown staining of the teeth. Since chlorhexidine gluconate can interact with some of the ingredients in toothpaste, a 30-minute interval is advised between using this mouthwash and toothpaste.[1]

THROAT LOZENGES AND PASTILLES

Lozenges and pastilles are both used to deliver medicaments for local effect, either to soothe or treat infections. Lozenges consist of medicaments incorporated into a flavoured base that dissolves or disintegrates slowly in the mouth. They are prepared either by moulding and cutting or by compression. Colours, flavours and sweetening agents may be incorporated. Heavy compression is used to ensure slow disintegration in the mouth.

Pastilles consist of medicaments in a base containing gelatin and glycerol or a mixture of acacia and sucrose. Sodium benzoate and citric acid monohydrate may be used as a preservative and antioxidant, respectively. Flavourings such as lemon oil may be incorporated.

SOLUTIONS, SUSPENSIONS AND SYRUPS

Solutions are liquid preparations containing one or more soluble ingredients, usually dissolved in water. They may be used internally, externally or for instilling into body cavities and may be sterile or unsterilized depending on the application. Solutions given orally usually result in rapid absorption. Problems with solubility, taste and stability may prevent this formulation being available for a particular drug.

Suspensions are formulations in which the drug does not dissolve in the solvent but is distributed within it. It usually provides a more rapid dispersion and dissolution of the drug when compared to tablets and capsules so long as the drug has a suitable particle size and does not settle or cake on storage. The primary particle size may grow due to the action of surfactants, emulsifiers and other adjuvants.

Syrups are concentrated aqueous solutions of sucrose or other sugars to which medicaments or flavourings are added. Glycerol, sorbitol and polyhydric alcohols may be added to reduce the rate of crystallization of sucrose and to increase the solubility of other ingredients. Growth of microorganisms is usually retarded by sucrose concentrations greater than 65% w/w.

TREATMENT OF DRY MOUTH

Artificial saliva can be useful to relieve dry mouth resulting from radiotherapy or diseases affecting the salivary glands. These preparations should be of neutral pH and contain electrolytes approximating to the composition of saliva. These preparations are available as oral sprays, lozenges and pastilles. Pilocarpine (Salagen) is a muscarinic and can stimulate any residual salivary gland function. Side effects relate to the muscarinic action and its use is contraindicated in those with significant respiratory and cardiovascular disease, angle-closure glaucoma, pregnancy and breastfeeding.

COUGH MEDICINES

These are divided into cough suppressants and the expectorant and demulcent cough preparations. After excluding an underlying cause of a cough, such as asthma and gastro-oesophageal reflux, cough suppressants may be used. It is thought that these drugs act by an ill-defined central action in the nervous system and may depress the 'cough centre' in the brain stem. The narcotic analgesics are effective as antitussives in subanalgesic doses. Codeine phosphate is useful for dry or painful coughs but it also inhibits the secretion and mucociliary clearance of sputum, is constipating and dependence can develop. Pholcodine (related to codeine) and dextromethorphan (a non-narcotic, nonanalgesic) have lesser side effects. Over the counter preparations include sedating antihistamines, such as diphenhydramine, and may work by causing drowsiness.

There is no evidence that expectorants (ammonium chloride, ipecacuanha and squill) are effective at promoting expulsion of bronchial secretions. Their action is more placebo. Demulcent cough preparations may relieve a dry irritating cough by virtue of the fact that they contain a syrup or glycerol that has a soothing effect. Simple linctus (a sugar-free preparation is also available) is harmless and inexpensive.

MANAGEMENT OF STRIDOR

The treatment required depends upon the cause and severity of the stridor. Heliox is useful in an acute situation but antibiotics, adrenaline, steroids and antihistamines may be required, as may surgery.

Helium is a colourless, odourless, tasteless gas that when mixed, one volume of helium to two volumes of air, diffuses more rapidly than air itself. Breathing such a mixture requires less effort due to the lower density. An air–helium mixture or a mixture of 21 volumes of oxygen and 79 volumes of helium (Heliox) has been used in the management of stridor.

DRUG THERAPY IN ANGIONEUROTIC OEDEMA

Swelling of the face and lips, and occasionally of the larynx, occurs in angioneurotic oedema of allergic origin. Antihistamines and corticosteroids are prescribed and, if life-threatening, 1 mL/1 : 1000 adrenaline can be administered subcutaneously. The non-allergic type results from a serum deficiency of the C1 esterase inhibitor protein. An acute attack is treated with an intravenous injection of 1000 units of C1 esterase inhibitor protein (derived from human plasma). This can also be given prior to surgery for prophylaxis. Conestat alfa (contraindicated if allergic to rabbits) and icatibant are also licenced in treating acute attacks of hereditary angioedema in adults with C1 esterase inhibition.[1] Long-term prophylaxis is achieved with epsilon aminocaproic acid or its derivative tranexamic acid or with androgen methyltestosterone or its derivative danazol. These stimulate the production of C1 esterase inhibitor protein.

USE OF BOTULINUM TOXINS IN SPASMODIC DYSTOMIA

Botulinum is available as botulinum A toxin–haemagglutinin complex (Botox, Dysport) and botulinum B toxin (NeuroBloc). The dosage is specific to each individual preparation and therefore the product literature must be consulted prior to use. In laryngeal dystonia, localization of the involved muscles and confirmation of correct needle position can be achieved by electromyographic guidance. The effect of botulinum toxin is observed within a few days. Patients may initially have worsening of their voice, dysphagia with the potential for aspiration and occasionally airway compromise. Improvement is seen 2 weeks post-injections and the effects of treatment may last for 3 to 6 months.

Botulinum toxin is contraindicated in patients known to be hypersensitive to ingredients, bleeding disorders, pregnancy and lactation, concurrent or potential aminoglycoside or spectinomycin administration (neuromuscular blockade is enhanced). It should not be used in patients with generalized muscle disorders such as myasthenia gravis. No information is available on its use in patients with renal or hepatic impairment. Adrenaline should be available in case anaphylaxis occurs.

COLLAGEN INJECTION OF PARALYZED VOCAL CORDS

As a result of Teflon injection being unavailable in the UK, collagen (Contigen) is now used to medialize paralyzed vocal cords. It is a purified bovine dermal gluteraldehyde cross-linked collagen and has been used in genuine stress incontinence. A skin test (0.1 mL collagen and lignocaine, injected intra-dermally into the volar surface of the forearm) should be carried out 4 weeks prior to the treatment. Many patients requiring this treatment have a short life expectancy and so a compromise with the skin test performed only a week prior to vocal cord injection is practised. A positive response is defined as erythema, induration, tenderness or swelling with or without purities, persisting for more than 6 hours or first appearing more than 24 hours after the injection.

The use of collagen injection is contraindicated in patients hypersensitive to the ingredients, with a positive skin test, in pregnancy and lactation and in patients with autoimmune disease or a history of multiple severe allergies.

DRUGS USED IN THYROID DISEASE INCLUDING THE MANAGEMENT OF HYPOCALCAEMIA

Thyroid hormones

The two preparations levothyroxine sodium/thyroxine sodium (Eltroxin) and liothyronine sodium (Tertroxin) are available for use in the management of hypothyroidism, diffuse non-toxic goitre, Hashimoto's thyroiditis and thyroid carcinoma. Levothyroxine sodium (thyroxine sodium) is used for maintenance therapy, usually as a single dose before breakfast. The initial dose is 50–100 μg daily increasing at 2- to 3-week intervals by 25–50 μg increments until normal metabolism is obtained. In the elderly, patients with cardiac insufficiency or severe hypothyroidism, the initial dose is 25 μg, increased by 25 μg every 4 weeks until normal metabolism is achieved. The usual maintenance dose is 100–200 μg, the higher dose is used to suppress T4 in thyroid carcinoma.

Liothyronine has a shorter half-life with a more rapid onset of action and shorter duration of action. Twenty micrograms of liothyronine is equivalent to 100 μg of thyroxine sodium. It can also be given intravenously. A pre-therapy ECG should be performed since hypothyroidism can produce changes resembling ischaemia. The starting dose is 10–20 μg every 8 hours. The usual maintenance dose is 60 μg daily in three divided doses. Sometimes it is coadministered with carbimazole to treat thyrotoxicosis. It may be used in severe hypothyroid states when a rapid response is required and is used in patients awaiting radioactive iodine scan following thyroid surgery. The latter enables patients to remain euthyroid in this interval period and patients need to stop liothyronine only 2 days prior to the scan.

These thyroid hormones must be used with caution in patients with hypertension, diabetes mellitus and insipidus, cardiovascular disorders, angina, the elderly, lactation, pregnancy (especially the first trimester) and in adrenal insufficiency. Interactions include sucralfate, phenylbutazone, warfarin, carbamazepine, phenytoin, rifampicin, barbiturates and propranolol. The side effects of arrythmias, insomnia, tremor, palpitations, sweating, weight loss, thyroid crisis, vomiting, diarrhoea and headache have been reported.

Drugs used in hyperthyroidism

Antithyroid drugs are used for hyperthyroidism either pre-operatively or for long-term management. Carbimazole (Neo-Mercazole) is the most commonly used in the UK; propyluracil is used in patients sensitive to carbimazole. Both are thionamides containing a thiocarbamide group ($S=C-N$) that is essential for their activity. Carbimazole is rapidly converted to methimazole *in vivo*. Methimazole is available in the USA. Thioamides prevent the synthesis of thyroid hormones by competitive inhibition of I^- to I^2 by peroxidase and also block the coupling of the iodotyrosine, especially in forming diiodothyronine. More controversial is the possibility that the thionamides have immunosuppressive properties. These drugs are administered orally and accumulate within the thyroid gland. Their delayed onset of action of 3 to 4 weeks results from the need of preformed hormones to be depleted first.

The main concern with thionamides is the development of neutropenia and agranulocytosis. Carbimazole has an incidence of causing agranulocytosis in 0.1% of patients; propylthiouracil has an incidence of four times this (explaining the preference for carbimazole in the UK).

The Committee on Safety of Medicines recommends that:

- patients should be asked to report symptoms and signs suggestive of infection, especially sore throat
- a white blood count should be performed if there is any clinical evidence of infection
- the drug should be stopped promptly if there is clinical or laboratory evidence of neutropenia.

Iodine is used as an adjunct to antithyroid drugs in the pre-operative management of thyrotoxicosis. An aqueous iodine oral solution (Lugol's solution) is given at a dose of 0.1–0.3 mL three times a day, taken well diluted with water or milk. Patients may develop flu-like symptoms, headache, rashes, insomnia, lacrimation, conjunctivitis, laryngitis and bronchitis. It must be used with caution in pregnancy and be avoided in lactation.

Drugs used in hypocalcaemia

Following thyroid or parathyroid surgery, patients may develop hypoparathyroidism either temporarily or permanently. Parathormone (PTH) is the most important regulator of the extracellular calcium concentration. Hypocalcaemic tetany is first managed by an initial intravenous injection of 10 mL 10% calcium gluconate followed by a continuous infusion of 40 mL daily or oral calcium with careful monitoring of the plasma calcium concentration. Bradycardia, arrhythmias and irritation after intravenous injection may occur as can gastrointestinal disturbances after oral administration. Failure to obtain and maintain a corrected calcium concentration within the normal range with calcium supplements alone necessitates the additional administration of a vitamin D preparation. **Figure 29.2** demonstrates the control of calcium plasma concentration by vitamin D. Vitamin D is a prohormone, metabolized to hormones that increase intestinal absorption of calcium, mobilize calcium from bone and inhibit renal excretion. The hypocalcaemia of hypoparathyroidism often requires doses of up to 2.5 mg (1 000 000 units) calciferol daily. Calcifediol is the main derivative of liver hydroxylation and this is further hydroxylated in the kidney to the potent calcitriol. The latter step is regulated by PTH. A synthetic derivative of vitamin D commonly prescribed in hypoparathyroidism is alfacalcidiol.

TREATMENT OF REFLUX OESOPHAGITIS AND LARYNGOPHARYNGEAL REFLUX

Initial treatment depends on the severity of the symptoms and treatment response. Changes to lifestyle (avoid excess alcohol and fatty foods), weight reduction, stopping smoking and raising the head of the bed may be advised. Antacids and alginates alone may be used for mild symptoms. The alginates are said to form a raft on the surface of the stomach's contents to reduce reflux and protect the oesophageal mucosa. McGlashan et al. in a prospective randomized controlled trial demonstrated a significant improvement in symptom scores and clinical findings with liquid alginate suspension compared to the control group in patients with laryngopharyngeal reflux.[13]

Histamine H_2 receptor antagonists (cimetidine, famotidine, nizatidine and ranitidine) block the action of histamine on the parietal cells and reduce acid secretion. They should be used with caution in patients with liver or renal disease, in pregnancy and breastfeeding. Side effects include diarrhoea, altered liver function tests, rashes and, more rarely, hypersensitivity reactions, AV block and blood dyscrasias. Cimetidine has been reported to cause gynaecomastia and it binds to cytochrome P-450 reducing the hepatic metabolism of drugs such as warfarin.

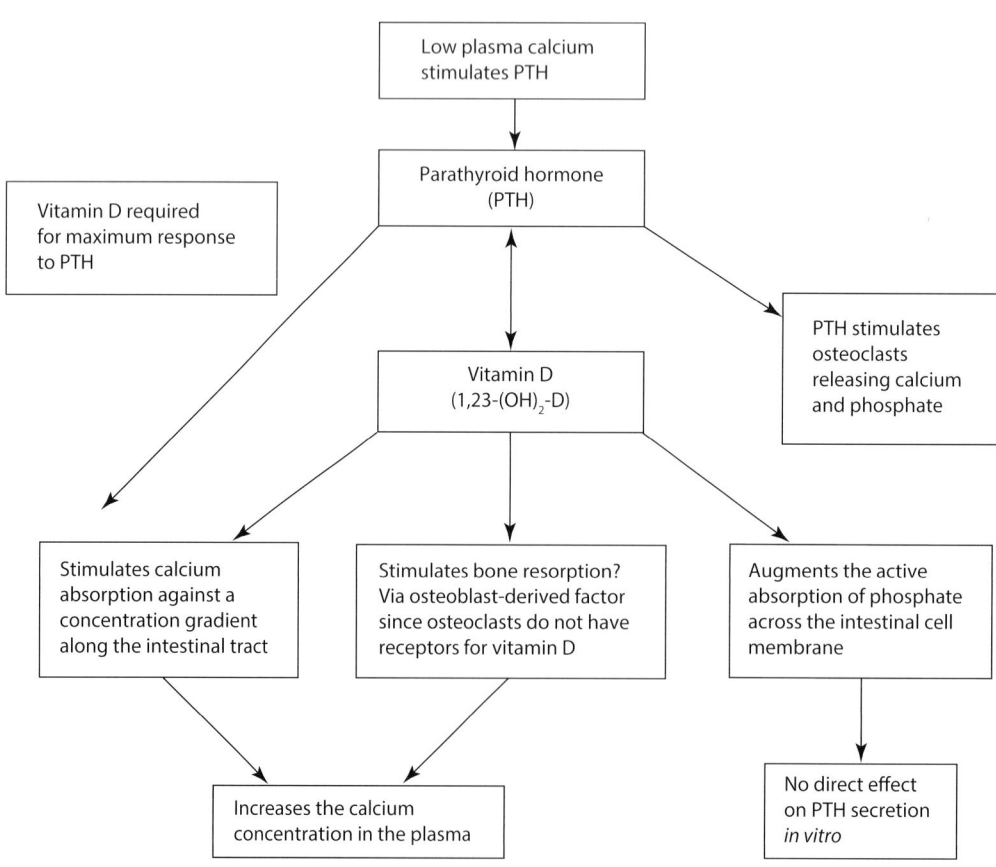

Figure 29.2 Calcium homeostasis and the role of Vitamin D.

The proton pump inhibitors (omeprazole, esomeprazole, lansoprazole, pantoprazole and rabeprazole sodium) react with sulphydryl groups in the H+/K+ ATPase (proton pump) responsible for the transportation of H+ ions out of the parietal cells. Although their use is well established in the treatment of reflux oesophagitis, their use in larygopharyngeal reflux is based on poor levels of evidence from uncontrolled studies. The few randomized controlled trials failed to show any benefit over placebo in this condition.[14]

CHEMOTHERAPEUTIC AGENTS

These drugs are used either alone or in combination with surgery and/or radiotherapy with the aim to cure or palliate a cancer. They inhibit the mechanisms of cell proliferation and rely upon malignant tumours having a greater proportion of cells undergoing division than in normal proliferating cells, especially in the bone marrow, gastrointestinal mucosa and in hair follicles. Chemotherapeutic agents are classified with respect to their site of action, as demonstrated in **Figure 29.3**.

Alkylating agents (mustine, cyclophosphamide, chlorambucil, cisplatin and busulphan) cross-link the two strands of the double helix of DNA. The antibiotics actinomycin D, doxorubicin, mitomycin, mithramycin and bleomycin interact with the DNA preventing RNA production. DNA synthesis is prevented by a group of antimetabolites (methotrexate, flurouracil, mercaptopurine and thioguanine) that prevent purine or pyrimidine synthesis. The vinca alkaloids (vincristine and vinblastine) bind to the microtubular proteins inhibiting mitosis. Glucocorticoids are included in regimes since they inhibit cell division by interfering with DNA synthesis.

Side effects such as nausea and vomiting, intestinal ulceration, diarrhoea, alopecia and bone marrow suppression are common but may become life-threatening.

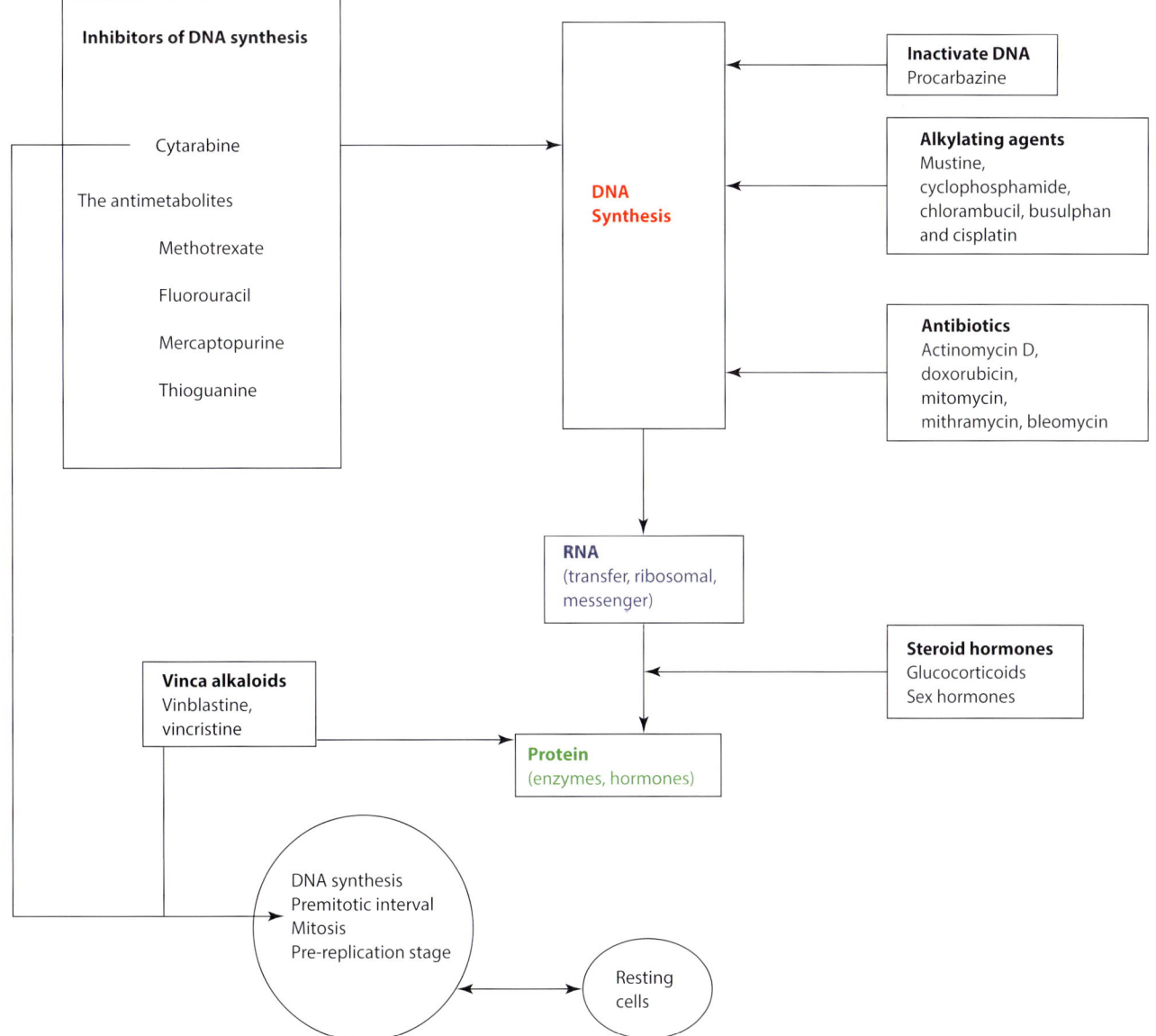

Figure 29.3 Site of action of chemotherapy.

MANAGEMENT OF FUNGATING WOUNDS

Charcoal dressings have been used to help combat malodorous fungating tumours. When this fails, topical metronidazole gel (Anabact or Metrotop) can be applied to the cleaned wound once or twice a day and covered with a non-adherent dressing. The metronidazole has antimicrobial activity against the anaerobes likely to be responsible for the odour.

Alginate dressings may stop bleeding from fungating wounds and, if moistened prior to a dressing change, the risk of bleeding at this time can be reduced.

> **BEST CLINICAL PRACTICE**
>
> ✓ The starting or stopping of antiplatelet drugs and anticoagulants should be in accordance with guidance from the haematologist and medical colleagues, taking into account other prescribed medications that may interact.
> ✓ Platelet counts should be monitored in patients on heparin to detect any thrombocytopenia.
> ✓ Cefuroxime and metronidazole should be given at induction and for at least three post-operative doses in head and neck procedures where the mucosa is breached.
> ✓ Heliox is easier to breathe than air and buys useful time in patients with stridor; however, it is important to take additional steps to treat the underlying cause and to secure the airway.
> ✓ First-line treatment of angioneurotic oedema consists of intravenous antihistamines and steroids with nebulized or subcutaneous adrenaline but C1 esterase inhibitor protein is the first-line treatment of hereditary angioedema.
> ✓ In order to avoid severe hypersensitivity reactions, preoperative test injections of collagen are necessary where this is used to perform vocal cord medialization.

> **KEY POINTS**
>
> - Perioperative antibiotics have not been shown to reduce bleeding rates after tonsillectomy but may reduce pain.
> - The use of perioperative cephalosporins and metronidazole reduce the rates of fistula formation in head and neck operations.
> - Pilocarpine (used in the treatment of dry mouth) is contraindicated in patients with significant respiratory/cardiovascular disease, glaucoma, pregnancy or breastfeeding.
> - Rarely, carbimazole can cause agranulocytosis.
> - Botulinum is available as botulinum A toxin–haemogglutinin complex and botulinum B toxin. It is important to realize that the dosage is specific to each preparation.

REFERENCES

1. British Medical Association, Royal Pharmaceutical Society of Great Britain. *British National Formulary 65*. London: Pharmaceutical Press; 2013.
2. NICE guidelines. Available from www.nice.org.uk
3. Sylvester JR, Coatesworth AP. Antiplatelet therapy in ENT surgery: a review. *J Laryngol Otol* 2012; **126**: 331–36.
4. Savage JR, Parmar A, Robinson PJ. Antiplatelet drugs in elective ENT surgery. *J Laryngol Otol* 2012; **126**: 886–92.
5. Fennessy BG, Harney M, O'Sullivan MJ, Timon C. Antimicrobial prophylaxis in otorhinolaryngology/head and neck surgery *Clin Otolaryngol* 2007; **32**: 204–07.
6. Verschuur HP, de Wever WW, Van Benthen PP. Antibiotic prophylaxis in clean and clean-contaminated ear surgery. *Cochrane Database Syst Rev* 2004 (3).
7. Lee WC, Duignan MC, Walsh RM, McRae-Moore JR. An audit of prophylactic antibiotic treatment following tonsillectomy in children. *J Laryngol Otol* 1996; **110**: 357–59.
8. Telian SA, Handler SD, Fleisher GR, et al. The effect of antibiotic therapy on recovery after tonsillectomy in children: a controlled study. *Arch Otolaryngol* 1986; **112**: 610–15.
9. Violaris N, Bridger M. Prophylactic antibiotics and post laryngectomy pharyngocutaneous fistulae. *J Laryngol Otol* 1990; **104**: 225–28.
10. Johansen LV, Overgaard J, Elbrønd O. Pharyngo-cutaneous fistulae after laryngectomy: influence of previous radiotherapy and prophylactic metronidazole. *Cancer* 1988; **61**: 673–78.
11. Watkinson JC, Gaze MN, Wilson JA (eds). *Stell and Maran's head and neck surgery*. 4th ed. London: Arnold; 2000, pp. 55–56.
12. Allegretto M, Selkaly H, Mackay JR. Intraoperative saline and gemcitabine irrigation improves tumour control in human squamous cell carcinoma-contaminated surgical wounds. *J Otolaryngol* 2001; **30**: 121–25.
13. McGlashan JA, Johnstone LM, Sykes J, et al. The value of a liquid alginate suspension (Gaviscon Advance) in the management of laryngopharyngeal reflux. *Eur Arch Otorhinolaryngol* 2009; **266**: 243–57.
14. Karkos PD, Wilson JA. Empirical treatment of laryngopharyngeal reflux with proton pump inhibitors: a systematic review. *Laryngoscope* 2006; **116**: 144–48.

FURTHER READING

bnf.nice.org.uk and bnfc.nice.org.uk

Hardman JG, Limbird LE, Molinoff PB, et al. (eds). *The pharmacological basis of therapeutics*. 9th ed. New York: McGraw-Hill; 1996.

Johnson JT, Myers EN, Thearle PB, et al. Antimicrobial prophylaxis for contaminated head and neck surgery. *Laryngoscope* 1984; **94**: 46–51. PMID: 6361430.

Lambert HP, O'Grady FW (eds). *Antibiotic and chemotherapy*. 6th ed. London: Churchill Livingstone; 1992.

Lund W (ed). *Pharmaceutical codex principles and practice of pharmaceutics*. 12th ed. London: Pharmaceutical Press; 1994.

Rang HP, Dale MM. *Pharmacology*. London: Churchill Livingstone; 1990.

Perioperative management

CHAPTER 30

PREPARATION OF THE PATIENT FOR SURGERY

Michael Murray and Urmila Ratnasabapathy

Patient pathway 301	Consideration of special requirements 306
Pre-operative assessment 302	Planning and scheduling of theatre time and post-operative care 306
Pre-operative investigations...................................... 303	Preparation on the day of surgery 306
Obtaining patient consent for planned surgery 304	Enhanced recovery after surgery 307
Consideration of venous thromboembolism (VTE) prophylaxis 305	References 308

SEARCH STRATEGY

This included recent publications in scientific journals, from professional bodies and the UK Department of Health. Data may be updated using keywords such as consent, enhanced recovery, suitability for day surgery, pre-operative assessment, pain, anti-coagulation, pre-operative preparation and venous thromboembolism prevention.

PATIENT PATHWAY

The patient pathway describes the 'route' taken by a patient from initial referral to regaining health. A pathway includes processes and documentation, and should be amenable to audit and external review. Generally, the surgeon makes a broad judgement at the time of seeing the patient as to whether or not the patient is fit for surgery. The in-hospital segment of the pathway begins here and, within the confines of a busy clinic, the patient requiring surgery should be placed into one of five routes:

- day surgery
- inpatient, scheduled admission within a few weeks
- inpatient, elective surgery, fit patient
- planned inpatient but requiring prior medical/anaesthetic review
- immediate admission.

Suitability for day surgery

There are guidelines[1] about which patients are suitable for day surgery in a particular hospital. There are three main criteria for the selection of patients as being suitable for same day surgery: social, medical and surgical.

Social factors

- The patient must understand the planned procedure, post-operative care and have consented to day surgery.
- Following most procedures under general anaesthesia, a responsible adult should escort the patient home and provide support for the first 24 hours.
- The patient's domestic circumstances should be appropriate for post-operative care.

Medical factors

- Fitness for a procedure should relate to the patient's health as determined at pre-operative assessment and not be limited by arbitrary limits such as ASA status (**Table 30.1**), age or body mass index (BMI).
- Patients with stable chronic disease such as diabetes, asthma or epilepsy are often better managed as day cases because of minimal disruption to their daily routine.
- Obesity per se is not a contraindication to day surgery as even morbidly obese patients can be safely managed in expert hands, with appropriate resources. The incidence of complications during the operation or in the early recovery phase increases with increasing BMI. However, these problems would still occur with

TABLE 30.1 Physical status grading of American Society of Anesthesiologists	
Grade	Physical status
Grade 1	Normal healthy patient without any clinically important comorbidity
Grade 2	Patient with a mild systemic disease
Grade 3	Patient with one (or more) severe systemic disease which does not present a constant threat to life
Grade 4	Patient with systemic disease processes which present a constant threat to life
Grade 5	Patient not expected to survive more than 24 hours

inpatient care and have usually resolved or been successfully treated by the time a day case patient would be discharged. In addition, obese patients benefit from the short-duration anaesthetic techniques and early mobilization associated with day surgery.

Surgical factors

- The procedure should not carry a significant risk of serious complications requiring immediate medical attention (e.g. haemorrhage, cardiovascular instability).

Pre-operative assessment is an essential part of perioperative management in order to determine primarily if the patient is a suitable patient for day surgery. It is part of the UK governmental strategy to have 75% of all elective surgical cases carried out as day case surgery as it confers significant cost savings. The NHS Institute for Innovation and Improvement, Delivering for Health[1] suggests a fundamental shift in patient and NHS culture so that day surgery is regarded as the norm for elective surgery. Expansion of day surgery as an anaesthetic speciality in its own right and interest therein has grown vastly in recent times.

The following statements are from the consensus document[1] produced by expert members of a working party established by the Association of Anaesthetists of Great Britain and Ireland (AAGBI) and British Association of Day Surgery (BADS):

- Day surgery is a continually evolving speciality performed in a range of ways across different units.
- In recent years, the complexity of procedures has increased with a wider range of patients now considered suitable for day surgery.
- Effective pre-operative preparation and protocol-driven, nurse-led discharge are fundamental to safe and effective day and short stay surgery.
- Patients presenting with acute conditions requiring urgent surgery can be efficiently and effectively treated as day cases via a semi-elective pathway.
- Central neuraxial blockade and a range of regional anaesthetic techniques, including brachial plexus and paravertebral blocks, can be used effectively for day surgery.

- Each anaesthetist should develop techniques that permit the patient to undergo the surgical procedure with minimum stress and maximum comfort, and optimize his/her chance of early discharge.
- Every day surgery unit must have a clinical lead with specific interest in day surgery and whose remit includes the development of local policies, guidelines and clinical governance.
- Good quality advice leaflets, assessment forms and protocols are in use in many centres and are available to other units.
- Effective audit is an essential component of good care in all aspects of day and short stay surgery.
- Enhanced recovery is based on established day surgery principles and is aimed at improving the quality of recovery after inpatient surgery such that the patient is well enough to go home earlier and healthier.

PRE-OPERATIVE ASSESSMENT

Pre-operative assessment is often carried out by specialist nursing staff in the outpatient setting using pre-agreed screening forms. Significant issues detected are referred to an anaesthetist who can make recommendations for optimization or review the patient in a pre-admission clinic. The anaesthetic assessment includes review of:

- patient and family history of anaesthetic and/or surgical problems
- cardiorespiratory system including blood pressure measurement
- significant other medical conditions
- coagulation disorders (i.e. bleeding tendency or thromboembolic risk)
- assessment of difficulty with airway management or presence of airway aspiration risk
- likelihood of post-operative nausea and/or vomiting (PONV)
- difficulties with pain control
- medications, allergies, weight
- smoking, alcohol and illicit drug use
- home/family circumstances for post-operative discharge.

Cardiovascular disease

The pattern of presentation of cardiovascular disease and recommendations for assessment has changed markedly over the last 20 years with the advent of earlier detection and better management of these conditions.

In pre-operative assessment, the main considerations are as follows.

DETECTING PREVIOUSLY UNDIAGNOSED DISEASE BY MEANS OF CAREFUL HISTORY-TAKING AND RELEVANT INVESTIGATIONS

If a patient can manage two flights of stairs then this is a good indicator of cardiac ability and is generally used as an assessment of functional capacity. Investigations for a patient with moderate or severe dyspnoea on mild exertion or at rest may include chest X-ray and echocardiography. As a screening test for left ventricular dysfunction a normal ECG corresponds with around a 95% chance of having a normal echocardiogram.[2] All patients should get blood pressure recorded. Uncontrolled hypertension should be controlled before elective surgery. ECG (electrocardiogram) is undertaken for selected patients (see preoperative investigations below). Note that dysrhythmias are uncommon but can be detected by examination or ECG.

ASSESSMENT OF EXISTING CARDIOVASCULAR DISEASE

Deteriorating pathology, exhibited by increasing symptoms (e.g worsening angina) or decreasing exercise capacity, are indications for further investigation and management. Heart failure may present with limited exercise tolerance, dyspnoea, orthopnoea, paroxysmal nocturnal dyspnoea and ankle oedema. Echocardiography will demonstrate size of chambers, wall thickness, wall motion, valve function and allow an estimate of ejection fraction.

MANAGEMENT OF SPECIFIC CONCERNS

Antiplatelet therapy for coronary stenting

There is considerable variation regarding the use of aspirin in the perioperative period. In a recent study, it had no impact on myocardial infarction or pulmonary embolus but was associated with an increase in bleeding.[3] There is still uncertainty regarding definitive treatment and large trials are necessary to determine optimal management.[4] In patients with coronary arterial stents the situation is complex and advice should be sought from a cardiologist.

There is considerable variation in risk for transient ischaemic attack and stroke in atrial fibrillation ranging between 1% and 18% depending on risk factors.[5]

Discontinuation of aspirin or other thrombo-prophylactic therapy is calculated on the individual risk benefit ratio for the patient (i.e. the risk of bleeding vs the time of discontinuation of therapy). Aspirin is usually discontinued 5 to 7 days before an operation as it affects platelet function irreversibly. Patients who are on warfarin usually need inpatient management with discontinuation approximately 3 days prior to surgery and use of either low molecular weight heparin or an intravenous heparin infusion. Direct thrombin inhibitors such as dabigatran should be managed in a similar way as warfarin. These drugs are however of greater concern in emergency surgery as no reversal agent is currently available.

Cardiac medications

Cardiac medications may need to be considered perioperatively and the anaesthetist will usually advise on this.

Pacemakers

Pacemakers should be checked for correct functioning, preferably by a pacemaker clinic, and implantable defibrillators should be turned off immediately before surgery and on again post-operatively. Patients with valvular disease, prosthetic valves or cardiomyopathy are at risk of bacterial endocarditis and should receive antibiotic prophylaxis at surgery.

Review by a cardiologist may sometimes be required pre-operatively to review patients with new onset, severe or increasing frequency angina. The cardiologist may arrange additional testing (e.g. exercise stress testing or coronary angiography) and optimize cardiac medication.

Risk indices[6] have been developed over the years and, generally, coronary artery disease, heart failure, cerebrovascular disease, elevated creatinine, insulin-dependent diabetes and high-risk surgery have all been associated with increased perioperative cardiac morbidity. Age is another risk factor[7] with the overall 30-day mortality associated with surgery and anaesthesia rising from 2.2% (age 60–69 years) to 8.4% (age >90 years).

Respiratory disease

Common conditions are chronic bronchitis, emphysema, chronic obstructive airways disease and asthma. Generally, a patient with known, mild, stable disease under review by the GP or respiratory department will not need special pre-operative assessment. Accurate assessment of disease severity is important. In the absence of clinical signs, chest X-ray is generally unhelpful. Asthmatic patients often know their normal peak flow measurement and this is a simple test to carry out. An assessment of functional exercise capacity, clinical examination and pulse oximetry are generally more helpful than pulmonary function tests. A respiratory physician and/or anaesthetic review should be sought for patients with severe respiratory disease. All patients should be advised to stop smoking.

Acute respiratory tract infection is an indication for postponement of elective surgery until resolution because of an increased risk of intra-operative bronchospasm and post-operative chest infection.

PRE-OPERATIVE INVESTIGATIONS

The National Institute for Clinical Excellence (NICE)[8] produced recommendations for the use of routine preoperative tests for elective surgery which were updated in April 2016. Specific recommendations are made according to grade of surgery (minor, intermediate, major, complex), ASA status, presence of diabetes, obesity, cardiovascular, respiratory or renal comorbidities and consideration of existing medication (NG45). Pre-operative tests may be ordered on a selective basis for purposes of guiding or optimizing perioperative management, but should not be ordered routinely. The Association of Anaesthetists of Great Britain and Ireland[9] states that 'blanket routine preoperative investigations are inefficient, expensive and unnecessary'.

Written guidelines are, therefore, hospital or department-based and should be discussed during induction of new department members. Reasonable guidelines for pre-operative tests in adult patients undergoing head and neck surgery are:

- dipstick urinalysis
- haemoglobin in all females, males aged over 40 years and any patient in whom blood grouping will be undertaken
- urea and electrolytes in all patients over 40 years or when indicated by disease process or medication
- clotting studies when indicated by history
- sickle cell testing in all patients of African or Afro-Caribbean origin
- pregnancy testing when pregnancy is possible
- blood grouping (group and save) in patients with a normal pre-operative haemoglobin and an anticipated blood loss of 10–15% blood volume (blood volume 70 mL/kg in adult), and all patients who have had a previous blood transfusion in case of the presence of antibodies
- blood grouping and cross-matching in all patients with an expected blood loss in excess of 15% blood volume (>750 mL in the average adult) or at significant risk of sudden severe haemorrhage. The number of blood units requested for a particular surgical procedure should follow written guidelines drawn up in consultation with the hospital transfusion committee
- electrocardiography (ECG) in any patient with cardiovascular disease or in asymptomatic patients aged over 60 years.

Audiometry should be undertaken on all patients undergoing surgery on the middle ear, and vocal cord function visualized when surgery might damage the recurrent laryngeal nerve.

Failure of the initial broad screening will direct the patient into the wrong pathway and may lead to substantial delays or frustration and patient harm. It is the pathway of medical/anaesthetic review prior to surgery that is particularly testing since it involves initial detection of problem patients, sending them for review, initiating treatment as required and waiting for optimal response before admission for surgery. It is clear that perioperative mortality is reduced by pre-operative optimization, particularly of cardiac and respiratory disease.[10]

OBTAINING PATIENT CONSENT FOR PLANNED SURGERY

Currently, in the UK, the process of obtaining informed consent for planned surgery is carried out by a member of the surgical team and, ideally, by the surgeon who will be performing the operation. In taking consent, it is important that full information is provided to the patient including indications for the proposed treatment including its implications and significant as well as common risks. Some ENT departments (e.g. Cambridge University Hospital) have consent forms for specific surgeries (e.g. tonsillectomy, tympanoplasty), which detail surgical risks relevant to the specific operations.[11] The process of consent should be seen as a stimulus for active discussion with patients about treatment options and decision-making following that discussion. ENT UK have produced 22 patient information leaflets which cover some common operations but also conditions.

Patients who have consented to surgery are considered to have implied consent to anaesthesia as specific written consent for anaesthesia is not required in the UK. However, as anaesthesia is associated with its own specific risks that are quite distinct and separate from those associated with the surgery, anaesthetists are advised to obtain specific consent for anaesthesia.[12] Ideally, each patient should receive a general leaflet about anaesthesia in the outpatient clinic.[13] This allows the patient time to consider relevant anaesthetic issues. Discussion between the anaesthetist and patient should include:

- previous medical/surgical/anaesthetic history including problems (e.g. latex allergy, anaphylaxis, difficult or failed intubation, pulmonary aspiration, post-operative nausea or vomiting, awareness, suxamethonium apnoea, malignant hyperpyrexia or unexpected admission to a high dependency or intensive care unit)
- likely difficulties in provision of anaesthesia for the planned surgery (e.g. possibility of fibreoptic tracheal intubation/tracheostomy under local anaesthesia/alternative method of securing the airway)
- local anaesthesia options (either as an adjunct to analgesia or as an alternative to general anaesthesia)
- general conduct of general anaesthesia to include fasting advice, pre-medication, administration of intravenous fluids, blood transfusion, pain relief, control of nausea/vomiting, urinary catheterization, nasogastric tube insertion, placement of arterial and central venous lines
- immediate recovery period and post-operative destination (e.g. HDU/ITU/ward/day case discharge)
- complications related to anaesthesia (e.g. dental damage, cardiovascular complications).

Patient anxieties in relation to anaesthesia are predominantly around the issues of death, brain damage, intra-operative awareness, loss of control, memory loss, pain control, nausea or vomiting and needle insertion.[14] Deaths caused by anaesthesia are very rare. A collection of 14 articles about specific risks associated with having an anaesthetic has been developed to be used with the patient information leaflets. The risk articles are available on the website www.rcoa.ac.uk/patientinfo

In the UK, the pre-operative anaesthetic visit often occurs only minutes before planned surgery. Ideally, all patients should be seen in an outpatient anaesthetic clinic before surgery. This gives time for proper pre-operative assessment, pre-operative preparation and discussion of anaesthetic options and this is what UK services should strive for as it allows for better patient satisfaction, same day admissions (therefore better use of resources) and a smaller likelihood of short notice cancellation due to poor patient preparation.

Patients should have adequate time to consider the indications and implications of any potential operation.[15] The process of informed consent for surgery is a continuous process and rushing a patient to give consent has ethical as well as medico-legal consequences. The UK General Medical Council (GMC) code of Good Medical Practice was updated in 2008 and comprehensively covers consent issues.[16] Ideally, consent for elective procedures should be taken well in advance of the proposed surgery (e.g. at a pre-assessment clinic). This gives the patient time to assimilate the information, discuss with family members if they wish and make appropriate choices. There have been successful cases of litigation when consent has been taken on the day of surgery.[17]

There is a specific consent form in the UK both for parents consenting for children and for those adults that are unable to consent (incapacity form). For those adults that lack capacity, the clinician has to record on this form how they have come to the conclusion that the patient lacks capacity to make this particular healthcare decision and why the proposed treatment would be in the patient's best interests.

Acute pain management plans

Acute pain management plans are made after discussion with the patient in the pre-operative period. Modifications to the WHO analgesic ladder[18] may be useful when considering prescribing post-operative analgesia for patients. Some patients may already be on analgesics pre-operatively. Those patients who are on larger doses of opioids pre-operatively will require larger amounts of analgesia intra- and post-operatively to treat pain. Early liaison with the acute pain team should be made for patients in whom acute pain is anticipated to be difficult to manage.

Simple analgesics include paracetamol and ibuprofen/diclofenac. The vast majority of patients undergoing surgery will receive some intravenous opioid intra-operatively (e.g. fentanyl, alfentanil or morphine). Some patients may require continuing opioids (e.g. codeine or morphine) for a period post-operatively. Tramadol is another analgesic that may be considered.

Drugs should be given orally as far as possible. If they cannot be taken orally then other routes to be considered include sublingual, parenteral (including patient controlled analgesia (PCA)), rectal suppository, nasogastric/percutaneous endoscopic gastrostomy (PEG)/radiologically inserted gastrostomy (RIG) tube and transdermal patch. It is important to know doses, duration of action, contraindications and side effects of analgesics prescribed. The British National Formulary can be a useful guide if there are no local prescription procedures in place.

The correct dose of analgesic for the individual patient should be given at regular intervals to achieve adequate pain relief with minimal side effects and titrated according to pain intensity using regularly measured pain severity scores. It is important to ensure that the patient understands and is involved in their pain management.

As part of multi-modal analgesic delivery, surgeons can infiltrate wound sites with chirocaine (Levo-Bupivacaine) 0.5% (maximum dose 2 mg/kg) at the end of surgery. Elastomeric pumps that can deliver local anaesthetic infusions into wounds are also used particularly in free tissue transfer surgery. By providing a continuous infusion, the pumps have the potential to provide continuous analgesia, eliminating the peaks and troughs in analgesic effect that occur with intermittent local or systemic analgesics. Unlike simple incisional infiltration with local anaesthetics, evidence for the efficacy of local anaesthetic wound catheters is abundant.[19] In a recent systematic review[20] it was concluded that continuous local anaesthetic wound infiltration resulted in a consistently reduced requirement for post-operative opioids, a subsequent reduction in post-operative nausea and vomiting, quicker return to normal bodily function and ambulation and a reduced length of hospital stay, especially in cardiothoracic and orthopaedic populations. Despite the cost of the equipment, the reduction in complications may lead to overall cost savings.

Local anaesthetic infiltration and infusions have recently been incorporated into enhanced recovery programmes.

CONSIDERATION OF VENOUS THROMBOEMBOLISM (VTE) PROPHYLAXIS

VTE is a recognized complication in hospital inpatients. It is associated with significant morbidity and mortality hence the importance in assessment and regular reassessment in patients with a view to the need for anticoagulation. Approximately 25 000 patients in England die each year from preventable hospital acquired VTE.[21] The cost of treating non-fatal symptomatic VTE and associated long-term disability is around £640 million per year. It is not surprising therefore that efforts should be focused on prevention.

In the UK the DoH,[22] the National Institute of Clinical Excellence (NICE)[23] and the Scottish Intercollegiate Guidelines Network (SIGN)[24] have stated that risk assessment and preventative measures for VTE are major patient safety interventions that must be made to save lives. Government policy states that every adult patient should undergo an individual risk assessment for VTE on admission to hospital and this should be a systematic and auditable process.[25]

Therefore, medical and surgical patients who are expected to be in hospital for more than 24 hours are assessed for risk (of both VTE and bleeding) and risk stratified based on various factors including age, period of immobility, obesity and malignancy so that appropriate VTE preventative measures may be instituted (unless contraindicated or refused by the patient). Assessment outcomes must be documented. All patients (or carers) should receive written guidance and verbal information on VTE.

Methods of prophylaxis to be considered include general measures (mobilization, hydration), mechanical techniques (anti-embolic stockings, pneumatic compression boots) and pharmacological agents. Haematology opinion should be sought if hypercoagulable states are present (e.g. protein C or S deficiency) or if patients are on long term anti-coagulation for other medical conditions.

Reassessment must be carried out every 24–48 hours and after any major clinical change. Appropriate discharge VTE prophylaxis should be prescribed.

CONSIDERATION OF SPECIAL REQUIREMENTS

Patients undergoing surgery in the head and neck region may lose, temporarily or permanently, sensation or motor activity in the distribution of the cranial nerves. Particularly important from a patient's perspective are the loss of communication arising from impairment of hearing, speech or vision, disabling sensation such as vertigo through vestibular dysfunction or alteration to normal activity such as eating, drinking or breathing. Patients who will be unable to speak post-operatively require a plan for communication, such as a bell to attract attention, prepared cards indicating common needs, pen and paper or the use of hand-signals. For those patients undergoing laryngectomy, the pre-operative period is the appropriate time to discuss voice reconstruction options and for the patient to meet the speech therapist and another patient who has undergone, and recovered from, similar surgery.

The disease process or nature of surgery may interfere with nutrition. Failure of adequate nutrition may lead to morbidity and mortality through infection, failure of wound healing and gross catabolism. Nutrition may be provided orally, through a nasogastric tube, via a percutaneous or open gastrostomy, via an open feeding jejunostomy or intravenously. The enteral route is superior in all regards to the intravenous route and should be used whenever possible. Poorly nourished patients require pre-operative supplementation and there is some evidence that a week of enteral (but not parenteral) nutrition improves outcome. A feeding gastrostomy or jejunostomy can be placed in a planned manner at the time of extensive surgery to cover post-operative feeding.

Patients in whom the small or large bowel is required for surgical reconstruction of the upper gastrointestinal (GI) tract may require bowel preparation with a low residue diet or intravenous fluids and laxatives.

PLANNING AND SCHEDULING OF THEATRE TIME AND POST-OPERATIVE CARE

The Confidential Enquiry into Postoperative Deaths (CEPOD) process identifies patients as being **elective** when the surgery can be planned for the convenience of the patient and surgeon, **scheduled** when admission will be prioritized within a few weeks of initial referral, **urgent** indicating an unplanned admission where resuscitation can be achieved before theatre and **emergency** in which surgery is required coexistent with resuscitation. A better scheme starts by indicating whether the patient is listed or unlisted, since the classification of CEPOD urgent or emergency is not always understood or useful.

The operating theatre list should be presented to theatre reception in the manner required within that hospital. Generally, a theatre list should contain the patient's name, hospital number, date of birth or age and planned surgery. The side of surgery should be recorded as left or right. Some hospitals use the Office for Population Censuses and Surveys (OPCS) or Read codes. The first patients on a list are generally children in ascending age, or shorter operations before longer ones or patients with diseases such as diabetes. Patients with latex allergy must be scheduled first to allow correct preparation of the operating theatre. Similarly, the anaesthetist and senior charge nurse in theatre should be informed regarding patients who are either MRSA positive or have other infections as far in advance as possible. These patients should be placed last on the list wherever possible to allow the theatre to be cleaned adequately after the procedure. Scheduling problems should be resolved by discussion between the surgeon, anaesthetist and theatre sister. Some patients will require a planned extended stay in recovery, or admission to a high dependency unit (HDU) or intensive therapy unit (ITU). Generally, this will be for longer, major procedures, when ventilation is required post-operatively, when the airway is at risk or if extended patient monitoring is required for cardiorespiratory disease. Patients should know about the plans for the immediate recovery period (which may change) and may benefit from seeing the HDU/ITU pre-operatively or talking to a nurse from the unit.

PREPARATION ON THE DAY OF SURGERY

It should be possible to estimate a provisional time of surgery and preparation aims to make certain that the patient is ready when the theatre calls for the patient. Most units use a form with tick boxes to cover the areas of baseline blood pressure, heart rate, weight, allergies, false or capped teeth, patient's wrist band present, consent form signed, notes and X-rays present, investigations present, blood cross-matched, time of last oral intake and details of pre-medication. The side and site of surgery should be indicated with an indelible marker by the surgeon who reviews the patient on the day.

Oral intake on the day of surgery

Fasting guidelines are in existence for planned surgery to minimize the risk of regurgitation and aspiration pneumonitis at induction of anaesthesia.

Historically, surgical patients were fasted routinely from food and drink for unnecessarily prolonged periods sometimes exceeding 12 hours before anaesthesia. Recent studies have shown that reduced pre-operative fasting time without increasing risk of harm from adverse events[26] is beneficial in terms of patients' well-being to include increased patient comfort and hydration. Shortening the fluid fast may also lead to less anxiety pre-operatively[27] and less nausea and vomiting post-operatively.[28] The volume of administered fluids does not appear to have an impact on patients' residual gastric volume and gastric pH when compared to a standard fasting regimen.[29]

The Royal College of Nursing has produced fasting guidelines[30] for elective surgery. There is a '2–6' rule for adults, which advises that patients may have unlimited amounts of water and other clear fluid up to 2 hours before induction of anaesthesia and solids including milk containing drinks up to 6 hours before surgery. For children, there is a '2–4–6 rule' which recommends that water/clear fluids are advised up to 2 hours, breast milk at 4 hours and formula milk, cows' milk or solids 6 hours before induction of anaesthesia. As an advance to these guidelines the AAGBI guidance[31] allows chewing gum as long as it is not swallowed, for up to 2 hours before induction of anaesthesia.

Regular medication taken orally should be continued pre-operatively unless there is anaesthetist/surgeon advice to the contrary. Diabetic medication needs to be specifically addressed by the anaesthetist. Up to 30 ml water may be given orally to help patients take their medication. If an elective operation is delayed, consideration should be given to giving the patient a drink of water to prevent excessive thirst and dehydration.

ENHANCED RECOVERY AFTER SURGERY

Enhanced Recovery After Surgery (ERAS) is a multimodal perioperative care pathway designed to achieve early recovery for patients undergoing major surgery. ERAS reviews traditional practices and replaces them with evidence-based best practices if applicable. It encompasses all areas of the patient's journey throughout the surgical process.[32] Use of the ERAS pathway has been shown to result in a significant reduction in both length of hospital stay and post-operative complications.[33]

ERAS has mainly been studied in colorectal surgery,[34] vascular surgery,[35] thoracic surgery[36] and radical cystectomy.[37] The rationale behind these programs is to try to modify the physiological and psychological responses to major surgery.

The key principles of the ERAS protocol[38–40] include:

- pre-operative patient counselling
- pre-operative nutrition, avoiding use of bowel preparation, carbohydrate loading* up to 2 hours pre-operatively, early commencement of feeding post-operatively
- goal directed fluid therapy and a standardized anaesthetic
- avoiding opioid analgesia
- early mobilization
- maintaining intra-operative normothermia.

There has been a recent publication with consensus recommendation[40] from the ERAS Society for Peri-operative Care in major Head and Neck surgery free flap reconstruction. In the OMFS Regional Centre in Glasgow, an Enhanced Recovery after Head and Neck Cancer Surgery (ERAHNCS) protocol for major free flap reconstructive surgery for OMFS/ENT oncology patients was introduced in 2013. The multimodule integrated care pathway focuses on multidisciplinary team involvement to achieve early recovery for patients undergoing head and neck oncology surgery.

There is a drive to introduce early enteral feeding to patients particularly as a component of part of the ERAS programme. Nutritional status is assessed (e.g. Malnutrition Universal Screening Tool (MUST) score in Greater Glasgow and Clyde) pre-operatively and regularly reassessed. There should be a critical care/ward policy in place for introduction of enteral feed for those who require it.

At the Glasgow Centre referred to above, carbohydrate-containing oral drinks are consumed the night before surgery and 2 hours before induction of anaesthesia. This has been shown to reduce hospital stay.[40] If the patient is unable to take oral intake or swallow then the drinks are administered via an enteral feeding tube. Currently, patients with delayed gastric emptying, galactosaemia and diabetes are excluded from the carbohydrate loading aspect of the ERAHNCS programme.

---

* The stress response to surgery results in a catabolic state and insulin resistance, which is a known risk factor for post-operative complications. Aggressive insulin therapy post-operatively has been shown to reduce morbidity and mortality. Similar results can be achieved when insulin resistance is attenuated and protein losses minimized by the use of pre-operative carbohydrate loading.

BEST CLINICAL PRACTICE

- ✓ The patient should be directed into the correct pathway as soon as surgery is contemplated, and sufficient oral and written information given to inform the patient and initiate the consent process.
- ✓ Attendance at a pre-admission clinic a few weeks before surgery allows a full history and examination to be taken, leading to the identification of any medical, anaesthetic or personal problems. This is particularly important when the interval between scheduling and admission for surgery is more than a few months.
- ✓ The requirement for specific pre-operative blood tests, investigations and blood cross-matching should be agreed by the whole team and produced in a written form which is available to doctors and nurses involved in pre-operative preparation.
- ✓ Pre-operative assessment of the problem patient by an anaesthetist, preferably the one who will be involved, is valuable and ideally should be arranged.
- ✓ Pre-operative tests taken at pre-admission should be reviewed before the admission for surgery so that abnormalities can either be treated in time or the patient rescheduled.

> **KEY POINTS**
>
> - Consider day surgery where possible.
> - Assess the risk balance of operation/anaesthesia.
> - Moderate or severe cardiorespiratory disease requires medical/anaesthetic review.
> - Routine pre-operative tests are expensive and unnecessary.
> - Valid, written consent is required for most surgery.
> - Consider venous thromboembolism prevention.
> - Consider the need for an HDU/ITU bed post-operatively.

REFERENCES

1. Verma R, Alladi R, Jackson I, et al. Day case and short stay surgery: 2. *Anaesthesia* 2011; **66**: 417–34.
2. Davie AP, Francis CM, Love MP, et al. Value of the electrocardiogram in identifying heart failure due to left ventricular systolic dysfunction. *BMJ* 1996; 312(7025): 222.
3. Devereaux PJ, Mrkobrada M, Sessler DI. Aspirin in patients undergoing non cardiac surgery. *N Engl J Med* 2014; 370: 1494–503.
4. Burger W, Chemnitius JM, Kneissl GD, Rucker G. Low-dose aspirin for secondary cardiovascular prevention: cardiovascular risks after its perioperative withdrawal versus bleeding risks with its continuation – review and meta-analysis. *J Intern Med* 2005; **257**: 399–414.
5. National Institute for Clinical Excellence. *Atrial fibrillation: The management of atrial fibrillation*. NICE guidelines [CG36]. 2006.
6. Goldman L, Caldera DL, Nussbaum SR. Multifactorial index of cardiac risk in non-cardiac surgical procedures. *N Engl J Med* 1977; **297**: 845–50. PMID: 904659.
7. Jin F, Chung F. Minimizing perioperative adverse events in the elderly. *Brit J Anaesth* 2001; **87**: 608–24. PMID: 11878732.
8. National Institute for Clinical Excellence, or www.nice.org.uk
9. The Association of Anaesthetists of Great Britain and Ireland. *Preoperative assessment: the role of the anaesthetist*. London: The Association of Anaesthetists of Great Britain and Ireland; 2001.
10. Prause G, Ratzenhofer-Komenda B, Smolle-Juettner F, et al. Operations on patients deemed 'unfit for operation and anaesthesia': what are the consequences? *Acta Anaesth Scand* 1998; **42**: 316–22. PMID: 9542559.
11. Cambridge University Hospitals ENT procedure specific consent forms. Available from http://www.cuh.org.uk/addenbrookes-hospital/for-patients/patient-information-and-consent-forms/consent-forms
12. White SM. Consent for Anaesthesia. *J Med Ethics* 2004; **30**: 286–90.
13. The Association of Anaesthetists of Great Britain and Ireland. Consent for Anaesthesia 2. London: The Association of Anaesthetists of Great Britain and Ireland; 2006. Available from www.aagbi.org/sites/default/files/consent06.pdf
14. Matthey P, Finucane BT, Finegan BA. The attitude of the general public towards preoperative assessment and risks associated with general anaesthesia. *Can J Anaesth* 2001; **48**: 333–39. PMID: 11339773.
15. Department of Health. *Good practice in consent implementation guide: consent to examination or treatment*. London: Department of Health, 2001. Available from http://webarchive.nationalarchives.gov.uk/20040419095927/http://www.dh.gov.uk/asset-Root/04/01/90/61/04019061.pdf
16. General Medical Council. *Consent: patients and doctors making decisions together*. London: GMC; 2008. Available from http://www.gmc-uk.org/guidance/ethical_guidance/consent_guidance_index.asp
17. Berry NH, Phillips JS, Salam MA. Written consent: a prospective audit of practices for ENT patients. *Ann R Coll Surg Engl* 2008; **90**(2): 150–52.
18. Grisell Vargas-Schaffer. Is the WHO analgesic ladder still valid? 24 years of experience. *Can Fam Physician* 2010; 56(6): 514–17. PMCID: PMC2902929.
19. Whiteman A, Bajaj S, Hasan M. Novel techniques of local anaesthetic infiltration. *Contin Educ Anaesth Crit Care Pain* 2011; 11(5): 167–71.
20. Liu SS, Richman JM, Thirlby RC, Wu CL. Efficacy of continuous wound catheters delivering local anaesthetic for postoperative analgesia: a quantitative and qualitative systematic review of randomised controlled trials. *J Am Coll Surg* 2006; **203**(6): 914–32.
21. House of Commons Health Committee. *The prevention of venous thromboembolism in hospitalised patients*. Publication HC99, 2005. Available from http://www.publications.parliament.uk/pa/cm200405/cmselect/cmhealth/99/9902.htm
22. Arya, R (ed). *Venous thromboembolism prevention: a patient safety priority*. London: Department of Health; 2009. Available from http://webarchive.nationalarchives.gov.uk/20130123200125/http://www.dh.gov.uk/en/Publicationsandstatistics/Publications/PublicationsPolicyAndGuidance/DH_101398
23. National Institute for Health and Clinical Excellence. *Venous thromboembolism: reducing the risk of venous thromboembolism (deep vein thrombosis and pulmonary embolism) in patients admitted to hospital*. London: NICE; 2010. Available from http://www.nice.org.uk/guidance/CG92
24. SIGN. 122: *prevention and management of venous thromboembolism: a national clinical guideline*. Edinburgh: Scottish Intercollegiate Guidelines Network, 2010. Available from http://www.sign.ac.uk/assets/sign122.pdf
25. Department of Health. *Report of the independent expert working group on the prevention of venous thromboembolism in hospitalised patients*. London: Department of Health; 2007. Available from http://www.dh.gov.uk/prod_consum_dh/groups/dh_digitalassets/documents/digitalasset/dh_073950.pdf
26. Corbett MC, Mortimer AJ (1997) Pre-operative fasting: how long is necessary? *Eur J Anaesth* 1997; **14**: 555–57.
27. Read MS, Vaughan RS. Allowing pre-operative patients to drink: effects on patients' safety and comfort of unlimited oral water until 2 hours before anaesthesia. *Acta Anaesthesiol Scand* 1991; **35**: 591–95.
28. Smith AF, Vallance H, Slater RM. Shorter preoperative fluid fasts reduce postoperative emesis. *BMJ* 1997; **314**: 1486.
29. Brady M, Kinn S, Stuart P, Preoperative fasting for adults to prevent perioperative complications. *Cochrane DB Syst Rev* 2003; **4**: CD004423.
30. Royal College of Nursing. *Peri-operative fasting in adults and children. AN RCN guideline for the multidisciplinary team*. London: RCN; 2005. Available from http://www.rcn.org.uk/__data/assets/pdf_file/0009/78678/002800.pdf
31. Association of Anaesthetists of Great Britain. *AAGBI safety guideline. Pre-operative assessment and patient preparation: the role of the anaesthetist 2*. London: AAGBI; 2010. Available from http://www.aagbi.org/sites/default/files/preop2010.pdf
32. ERAS Society (http://www.erassociety.org).
33. Varandhan KK, Neal KR, Dejong CH, et al. The enhanced recovery after surgery (ERAS) pathway for patients undergoing major elective open colorectal surgery: a meta-analysis of randomized trials. *Clin Nutr* 2010; **29**(4): 434–40.
34. Wind J, Polle SW, FungKon Jin PH, et al. Systematic review of enhanced recovery programmes in colonic surgery. *Br J Surg* 2006; **93**: 800–09.
35. Podore PC, Throop EB. Infrarenal aortic surgery with a 3-day hospital stay: a report on success with a clinical pathway. *J Vasc Surg* 1999; **29**: 787–92.
36. Tovar EA, Roethe RA, Weissig MD, et al. One-day admission for lung lobectomy: an incidental result of a clinical pathway. *Ann Thorac Surg* 1998; **6**(3)5: 803–06.
37. Koupparis A, Dunn J, Gillatt D, et al. Improvement of an enhanced recovery protocol for radical cystectomy. *Brit J Med Surg Urol* 2010; **3**: 237–40.
38. Wilmore DW, Kehlet H. Management of patients in fast track surgery. *BMJ* 2001; **322**: 473–76.
39. Kehlet H, Wilmore DW. Multimodal strategies to improve surgical outcome. *Am J Surg* 2002; **183**(6): 630–41.
40. Dort JC, Farwell DG, Findlay M, et al. Optimal peri-operative care in major head and neck cancer surgery with free flap reconstruction. A consensus recommendation from the ERAS society. *JAMA Otolaryngol Head Neck Surg* 2017; **143**(3): 292–303.

CHAPTER 31

RECOGNITION AND MANAGEMENT OF THE DIFFICULT AIRWAY

Valerie Cunningham and Alistair McNarry

Definitions 309	Laryngeal mask airways 317
Prevalence 310	Failed ventilation and emergency cricothyrotomy 319
Evaluation 310	Obstructed airway 321
Prediction of difficulty 313	Extubation and recovery 328
Strategy 314	Follow-up 329
Alternative techniques to Macintosh laryngoscopy blades 315	References 330

SEARCH STRATEGY

Data in this chapter may be updated by a PubMed search using the keywords: difficult intubation, difficult airway, obstructed airway.

DEFINITIONS

The difficult airway is the clinical situation in which a practitioner experiences difficulty with adequate maintenance and/or protection of the airway. The most commonly used adjunct airway devices that help maintain a patent airway are the face mask, with or without a guedel airway, the laryngeal mask, and the tracheal tube. These devices are designed to maintain the patency of an airway and hence reduce impedance to ventilation. A cuffed tracheal tube offers the airway the highest level of security from obstructions or contaminations as the other devices are 'supraglottic'. Tracheal tubes are often the adjunct of choice in head and neck surgeries.

Two broad categories of airway problems can be defined: difficult ventilation and difficult intubation. Difficult mask ventilation is defined by the American Society of Anesthesiologists (ASA)[1] as the 'inability to maintain the oxygen saturations above 90% by face-mask inflation with 100% inspired oxygen or to reverse signs of inadequate ventilation'. Oxygen stores in the body are exhausted within a few minutes and difficulty or failure to ventilate will rapidly result in morbidity or mortality from hypoxaemia. Maintenance of oxygenation but inability to ventilate effectively (we will discuss this later) may still be associated with significant morbidity and mortality related to hypercarbia.

Difficulty or failure to intubate is defined by the ASA as 'the inability to establish tracheal intubation within three attempts at direct laryngoscopy or within ten minutes'. In the UK, the Difficult Airway Society (DAS) guidelines for failed intubation also recommend no more than three attempts at direct laryngoscopy before accepting that intubation by this method has failed.[2] Provided that face-mask ventilation is possible, failed tracheal intubation by itself should not result in hypoxaemia unless the failure of airway protection leads to gross airway soiling from gastric contents, blood, pus or debris. Failure to recognize that tracheal intubation has been unsuccessful is associated with morbidity and mortality. This may occur in cases of unrecognized oesophageal intubation or dislodgement of endotracheal tubes. Continuous capnography from induction to extubation of the patient in the perioperative period is now a basic recommended standard of practice.

Cormack and Lehane[3] described the commonly used classification of the best view of laryngeal structures seen at direct laryngoscopy. Grade I is visualization of the entire laryngeal aperture, grade II is visualization of the posterior portion of the laryngeal aperture, grade III is visualization of the epiglottis only and grade IV is no view of any laryngeal structures. Difficulty with intubation of the trachea is more likely in laryngoscopy grades III/IV and in cases where multiple attempts at conventional direct laryngoscopy in these grades have failed to improve the direct view of the larynx.[4] Classification of laryngeal view has also been described as a percentage of glottic opening or POGO scoring. This method is reported to have good inter- and intra-physician reliability when grading the laryngeal view; however, there is limited evidence for this and in general it is the Cormack and Lehane system that is most commonly used.[5,6] If there has been a requirement to use a specialized aid or device to aid direction of the endotracheal tube when intubating, this also would indicate that there has been a level of difficulty to intubate. Specialized devices such as tube stylets or gum elastic bougies are used to direct endotracheal tubes towards the glottis opening in cases of difficult laryngeal view. In addition different blades used with the direct laryngoscope, for example the Millar or Henderson straight blades, can be used to improve laryngeal view in 'poor grades' III and IV. The recognition of the need for additional adjuncts or devices has led to theatre suites ensuring specifically stocked carts or trolleys are available for use in cases of difficult or failed intubation. Difficult direct laryngoscopy is only one cause of difficulty with intubation. It may be easy to visualize the larynx but intubation is unsuccessful because the larynx, subglottis or trachea are abnormally narrowed or distorted.

PREVALENCE

Both difficult intubation and difficult ventilation are uncommon. The prevalence of Cormack and Lehane laryngoscopic grade III is 1.5% in the general population. Requiring more than three attempts at direct laryngoscopy occurs in approximately 0.4% of patients and the average anaesthetist will abandon intubation in approximately 1:2500 of general surgical patients. In 1200 consecutive ENT and general surgical patients the overall prevalence of difficult intubation (defined as requiring specialist equipment) was 4.2%.[7] The highest prevalence was 12.3% in ENT cancer surgery, 3.5% in ENT non-cancer surgery and 2.0% in general surgical patients. This confirms the clinical impression that difficult intubation is more common in patients undergoing head and neck surgery, particularly in those patients following extensive surgery, flap reconstruction and post-operative radiotherapy or with an obstructed airway.

It is difficult to know the precise prevalence of difficult face-mask ventilation.[8] Catastrophic failure leading to serious morbidity or mortality is generally quoted as 1:10000–1:100000. However, in any large series, a number of problem patients are identified pre-operatively and these patients may not receive a general anaesthetic. A North American study that involved 18 500 patients of whom 18 200 were intubated under general anaesthesia quoted that only 1.8% of patients required more than two attempts at direct laryngoscopy and no patient was impossible to mask ventilate.[9] Approximately 300 patients underwent awake intubation and it is this group of patients that is likely to contain those who would have proved difficult to ventilate if anaesthetized. Another study of 1502 patients determined a prevalence of difficult mask ventilation of 5% but the definition used was that the anaesthetist considered the difficulty was clinically relevant and could have led to potential problems if mask ventilation had to be maintained for a longer period.[8] More recent data from the Fourth National Airway Project (NAP4) run by the Royal College of Anaesthetists (RCoA) of Great Britain and Ireland in 2012 reported an incidence of adverse airway events as 1:22 000 and an incidence of death related to an airway event as 1:180 000. More than 3 million anaesthetics were audited in this data collection.[10]

EVALUATION

The aim of perioperative airway management is to adequately maintain and protect the airway throughout this period. Adequate assessment and evaluation of each individual patient is paramount to make the most appropriate management strategy. Face-mask anaesthesia is impractical and provides no airway protection for head and neck surgery patients and so has limited application. The appropriate use of either a supraglottic airway or a tracheal tube is dependent on multiple factors such as patient comorbidity and pathology, the length of surgery and the level surgical access to the head and neck structures needed. The need for positive pressure ventilation during the procedure and minimizing the risk of airway soiling from blood, pus, cerebrospinal fluid or gastric contents are also of major importance.

The airway may be evaluated according to the scheme outlined in **Table 31.1**.

History

The anaesthetic or hospital notes may indicate previously encountered difficulty with airway management. The patient may pass on verbal or written information from a previous anaesthetist that they are difficult, or difficulty may be inferred from a history of displaced front teeth, bruised lips, excessive sore throat or an unexpected stay in ITU. Past surgery or radiotherapy, or the current surgical condition, may be relevant if it affects the head, neck or mediastinum. A number of medical conditions, such as rheumatoid arthritis, obstructive sleep apnoea and acromegaly, have some association with difficult airway management. For example, the incidence of Cormack and Lehan grade III larynx, which is associated with difficult intubation, is reported as 10% in acromegalics. This is six to eight times higher than in the general population.[11] In this group there is also an association with difficulty with

TABLE 31.1 Scheme for evaluation of the airway

Evaluation	
History	Previous airway difficulty Previous surgery Current surgical condition Current medical condition
Examination	General Specific predictive tests
Investigations	MR imaging CT imaging Flow-volume loop Flexible nasendoscopy

bag valve mask ventilation due to the soft tissue hypertrophy of the tongue. Rheumatoid arthritis patients may have reduced neck mobility or have had surgery for fusion of cervical vertebrae and therefore the optimum position for intubation or the 'sniffing the morning air' cannot be achieved. There are a number of congenital conditions, such as Treacher-Collins and Pierre-Robin, in which airway management, particularly intubation, is often difficult. Anatomical hypoplasia of the mandible in these conditions is often associated with poor laryngeal view.

Figure 31.1 illustrates a patient with Hunter's syndrome, in which abnormal mucopolysaccharide is deposited in the tissues. Characteristically, he was difficult to intubate for a tonsillectomy to alleviate obstructive sleep apnoea and required an emergency tracheostomy in the recovery period. He is pictured in his late teens when his original standard tracheostomy tube had been replaced by one designed to circumvent lower tracheal and carinal deposits. This T-Y silastic stent passes from just below the vocal cords into each main bronchus (an inverted Y shape) with a limb passing out through the tracheostomy (the T component).

Examination

General examination is aimed at identifying individual physical findings that may be associated with difficult intubation:

- trauma, burn, swelling, infection, scarring, haematoma of the mouth, tongue, larynx, trachea or neck
- large tongue, receding jaw, high-arched palate, prominent upper incisors, short thick neck, large breasts, microstomia, fixed larynx, impalpable cricothyroid membrane, limited mouth opening, limited head/neck movements
- voice change, shortness of breath, stridor, inability to lie down.

A number of these factors, such as the appreciation of a short neck or receding jaw (**Figure 31.2**), are subjective. This does not diminish their importance since professional judgements may often be subjective.

A number of subjective tests are used as predictors of difficult intubation. The five tests most commonly used are gape, jaw slide, thyromental distance, Mallampati and atlanto-occipital movement.

GAPE

Patients with small mouths, large teeth, previous surgeries or obvious physical deformity, among other things, may have reduced mouth opening.

Gape is the measurement of maximal mouth opening and is usually expressed as inter-incisor distance in fingerbreadths (fb) or centimetres. Normal values are 3 fb or 5 cm. A mouth opening of 2 fb is limited and 1 fb is severely limited, making direct laryngoscopy very difficult. It is difficult to insert a laryngeal mask when the gape is less than 2 cm (**Figure 31.3**). Relatively long upper incisors may also contribute to difficulty.

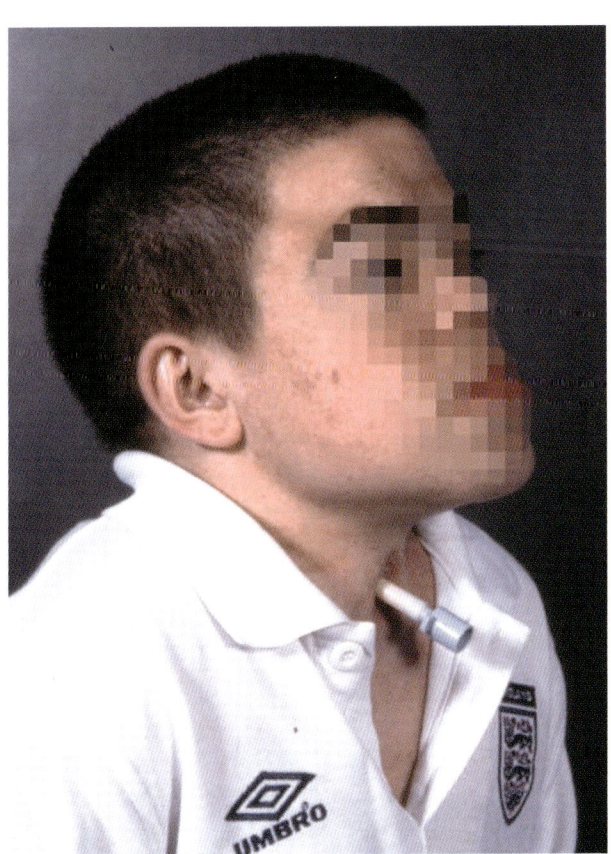

Figure 31.1 Mucopolysaccharidosis (Hunter's syndrome).

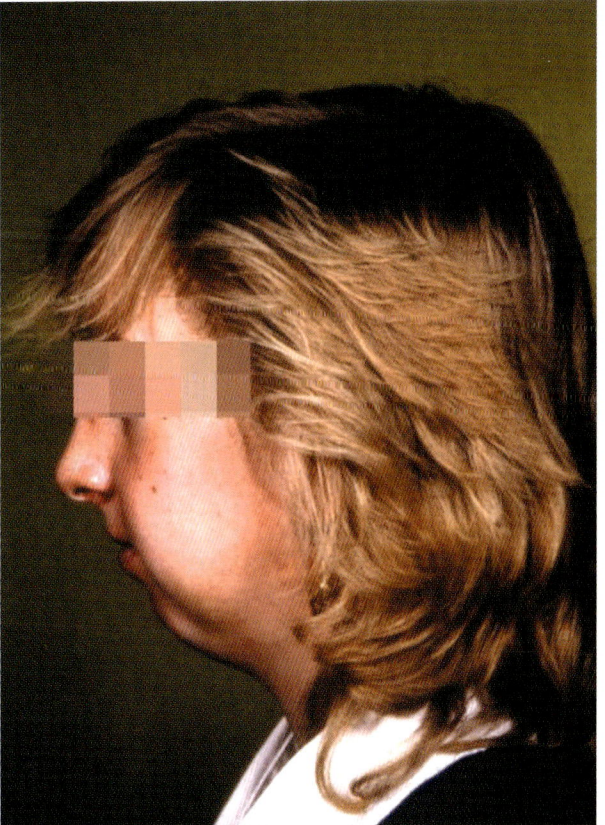

Figure 31.2 Receding jaw.

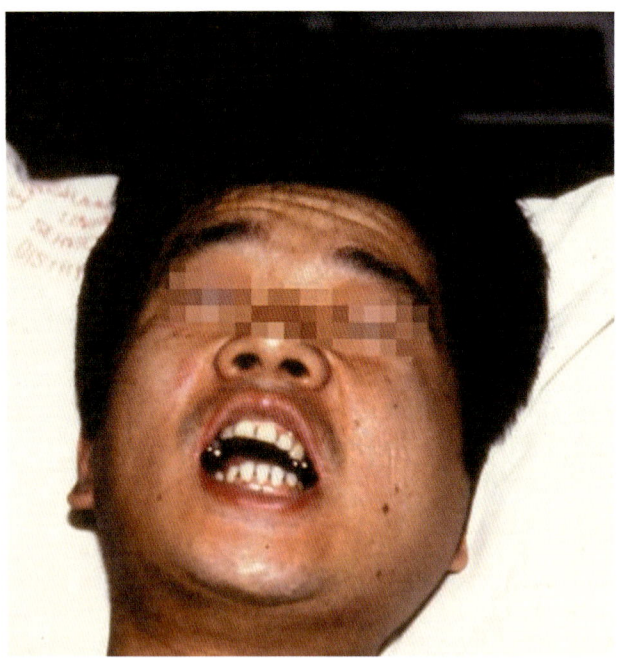

Figure 31.3 Limited mouth opening due to dental abscess.

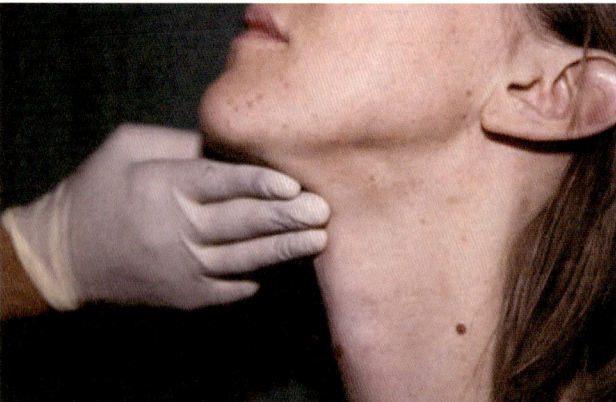

Figure 31.4 A normal thyromental distance.

This measurement, described by Patil,[13] is from the mentum to thyroid notch in full neck extension. The normal measurement is 6–7 cm or 3 fb (Figure 31.4). A short distance (2 fb) indicates a 'high' larynx and difficult direct laryngoscopy.

MALLAMPATI

Mallampati scoring is a commonly used scoring system for anaesthetists. While the scoring system may not be highly sensitive it is an easy bedside test that is generally regarded as useful in prediction of difficulty with intubation. Mallampati grading is commonly recorded on anaesthetic records.

Mallampati's contribution was a test to assess oropharyngeal space. The test asks a seated patient to open their mouth fully and extend the tongue maximally. The practitioner notes which posterior pharyngeal structures are visible. Mallampati described only three grades:

- class 1 indicates that the posterior pharyngeal wall, fauces and uvula are visible
- class 2 indicates that only a part of the fauces, posterior wall and uvula are visible
- class 3 indicates that the tongue meets the palate; the uvula is not visible.

Samsoon and Young[14] arbitrarily introduced a subdivision of class 3 (tongue against soft palate) and class 4 (tongue meets hard palate).

ATLANTO-OCCIPITAL MOVEMENT

Optimal head and neck positioning for direct laryngoscopy requires cervical spine flexion and almost maximal extension of the head on the spine. A simple clinical test to look at atlanto-occipital movement is for the clinician to ask the patient to flex their neck maximally and then nod; the observer's hand placed posteriorly on the neck makes certain that the nodding motion is at the level of the cranium on the upper cervical vertebrae. Atlanto-occipital extension may be clinically graded as normal or reduced or measured and the normal value is 35°. Connective tissue conditions such as ankylosing spondylitis and

JAW SLIDE OR MANDIBULAR PROTUSION

Patients with a prominent overbite may be considered more likely to be an intubation challenge, as are patients who are unable to bring their mandibular incisors anterior to their maxillary incisors. The relationship between the maxillary and mandibular incisors during normal jaw closure and voluntary protrusion of the mandible have been graded in an attempt to predict significance to difficulty with intubation.

Functions are graded as follows:

- class A if the lower jaw can be protruded beyond the top teeth
- class B if the lower teeth can only reach the top teeth
- class C if the lower teeth will not reach the top teeth

The value of testing this function is that, in intubation by direct laryngoscopy, the lower jaw must slide forward. In some scoring systems, mouth opening and jaw slide are combined, the greatest difficulty indicated by a gape of < 3.5 cm and class C jaw slide. Another method of testing mandibular protrusion is the upper lip bite test[12] in which the patient demonstrates how much of the upper lip may be covered by the lower incisors. Class 1 indicates 'biting' above the vermilion line, class 2 below the vermilion line and class 3 an inability to bite the upper lip.

THYROMENTAL DISTANCE

Patients who physically have short, fat, thick necks or reduced compliance of the submandibular space (e.g. radiotherapy, induration) may also be difficult to intubate. Many of these patients could have reduced thyromental distances.

rheumatoid arthritis are associated with pronounced reduction in atlanto occipital movement. Instability of the cervical spine may render movement of the spine impossible due to the presence of a collar, traction or halo frame.

Investigations

Plain X-rays may demonstrate abnormalities, such as enlargement of the retropharyngeal space (**Figure 31.5**), a swollen epiglottis, tracheal deviation or narrowing, a radio-opaque foreign body or obstructive emphysema suggesting a ball-valve obstruction in the relevant bronchus. However, imaging of the whole airway by CT or MR scan is better and will show narrowing or distortion and allow planning of airway instrumentation. Flexible nasendoscopy under topical anaesthesia is extremely useful in delineating supra- or glottic pathology, and a longer flexible fibrescope can inspect the whole respiratory tract although generally this requires sedation.

Another useful test is the flow-volume loop. This expresses flow during expiration and inspiration as a function of lung volume. Airflow is measured during inhalation from residual volume to total lung capacity and exhalation back to residual volume. Extrathoracic obstruction causes limitation of inspiratory flow whilst intrathoracic obstruction causes limitation in expiratory flow. Limitation in expiratory flow is particularly noticeable because the highest flow-rates are usually present in peak expiration.

PREDICTION OF DIFFICULTY

The practitioner forms a professional judgement as to whether airway management plans need to be altered from that carried out normally based on information gathered from the history and examination of the patient, the nature of the pathological process and surgeries planned and investigations and imagine undertaken. Key predictors of difficulty as previously discussed would be a known history of failed intubation, presentation with breathing difficulty or stridor, absent mouth opening or previous head and neck reconstructive surgery. In pathological processes of the laryngopharynx supraglottic tumour is highly predictive of difficulty with intubation,[15] as is the presence of tracheal compression, the presence of dyspnoea and cancerous pathology in patients with a goitre undergoing thyroid surgery.[16]

However, when there are no abnormalities in the anaesthetic, medical or surgical history, the presenting disease process does not affect the head, neck or mediastinum and the patient does not 'look' difficult, then it is not possible to predict difficulty accurately.

Most attention has been on predicting difficult direct laryngoscopy using various specific or predictive tests (described above), combination of tests and scoring systems. All are imperfect and the reason is partly the low prevalence of difficult intubation. Test sensitivity indicates the ability of the test to label a difficult patient as difficult, test specificity the ability to label a normal patient as normal and the positive predictive value (PPV) is the proportion of patients found to be difficult out of all patients predicted by that test to be difficult. **Table 31.2** shows values of test sensitivity, specificity and PPV for the various tests. It can be seen that an individual test, such as Mallampati, has a low PPV indicating that most patients predicted to be difficult will, in fact, be normal.

It is likely that the upper lip bite test and the Mallampati are both poor predictors as single screening tests;[17] however, the more tests that are abnormal in one patient, the increased likelihood that the patient will be difficult to intubate.

Another approach may be to produce a score from consideration of various predictive tests, with appropriate weighting. This may provide a system with higher

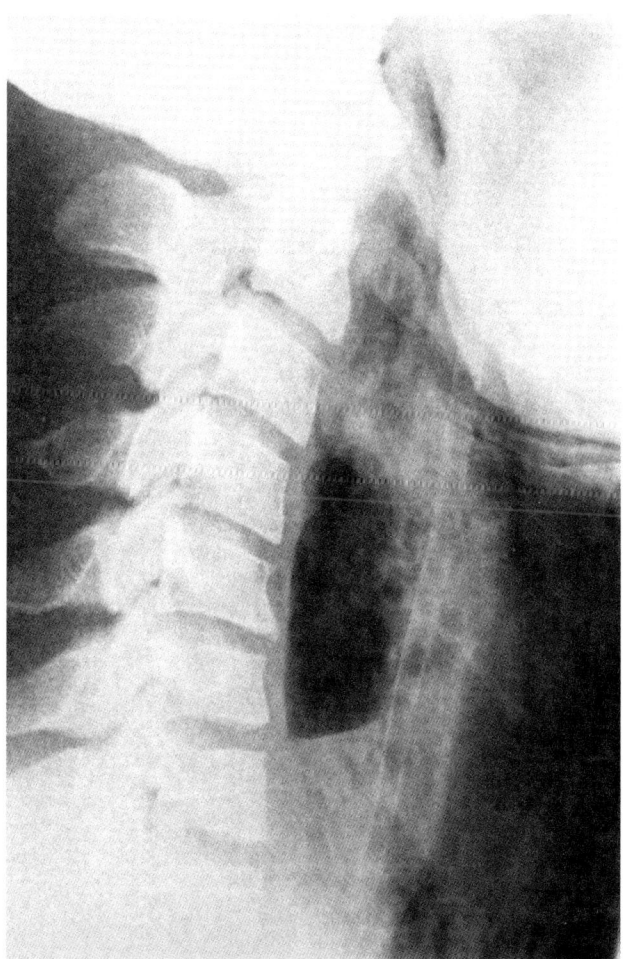

Figure 31.5 Retropharyngeal abscess.

TABLE 31.2 Test sensitivity, specificity and positive predictive value from the literature and reference[19]

Test	Sensitivity %	Specificity %	PPV %
Thyromental	65–91	81–82	8–15
Mallampati	42–56	81–84	4–21
Wilson risk sum	42–55	86–92	6–9
Mouth opening	26–47	94–95	7–25
Neck movement	10–17	98	8–30

sensitivities and specificities; however, the subject of prediction of difficulty is fraught with difficulties arising from studies with small numbers of patients, definitions, curious mathematics and inappropriate conclusions.[7, 18, 19] Some meta-analysis data of bedside screening tests for predicting difficult intubation in apparently normal patients propose that they have limited value.[20]

Objective tests aim only to predict difficult direct laryngoscopy when the tongue has a normal compliance and the respiratory tract is normal. Viewing the larynx using direct laryngoscopy with a standard Macintosh blade is reliant on anterior elevation of the mandible and sweeping the tongue to the left while at the same time lifting the epiglottis to open the laryngopharyngeal space and view the glottis. Restriction of tongue movement due to poor tissue compliance may result because of multiple pathologies including tumour, infection, post-radiotherapy or scarring and oedema. Fixation or restricted movement of the tongue is known to cause difficulty.[21] Unexpected difficulty with intubation occurs in cases such as a vallecular cyst and lingual tonsillar hypertrophy, which may be symptomless but will not be predicted, but also in cases with no physical pathology who have anatomically high and anterior larynx which are poor Cormack and Lehane views.[3, 22, 23]

Airway evaluation is an essential part of pre-operative assessment. It may be rewarded by the detection of severe or obvious problems that necessitate a strategy different to 'normal' management. When there are no obvious problems, evaluation is imperfect and safe airway management in all circumstances depends on the adoption of an airway strategy that is able to respond to unexpected difficulty with intubation or oxygenation.

STRATEGY

The recommendations of the ASA on management of the airway[1, 4] promoted the five-step linear model of evaluation of the airway, preparation for difficulty, strategy at intubation, strategy at extubation and follow-up. The ASA difficult airway algorithm presents an overall scheme of planning airway management (**Figure 31.6**).[24]

In September 2004 the Difficult Airway Society Guidelines were published in the United Kingdom. Similarly to the ASA guidelines, they were aimed at providing a standardized logical series of steps following a failed intubation in particular circumstances. The guidance was issued for unanticipated difficult intubation during routine induction of anaesthesia and following rapid sequence induction in the non-obstetric adult patient. They are widely accepted in the UK as a gold standard of care in airway management and they are based on a series of consecutive plans from A to D (**Table 31.3**).

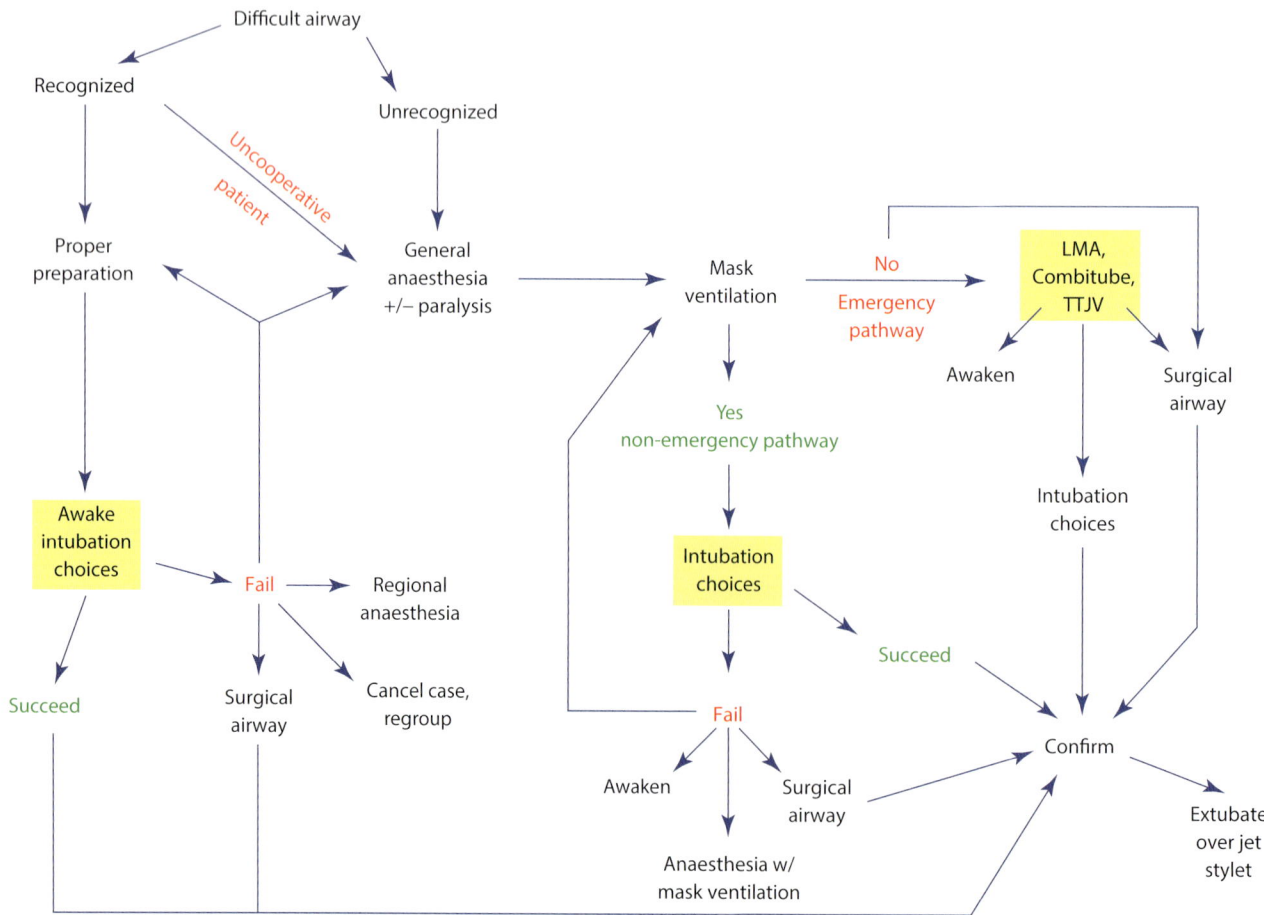

Figure 31.6 ASA difficult airway algorithm. Redrawn from ref. 20, with permission.

TABLE 31.3 Plans A–D in the failed intubation flowchart

Plan	Step following direct laryngoscopy, any issues arising and immediate call for help
A	Initial tracheal intubation plan; no more than four attempts at intubation while maintaining oxygenation with face mask
B	Secondary tracheal intubation plan following failure to intubate; supraglottic airway (LMA) not more than two insertions plus or minus fibre-optic/Aintree catheter guided assistance
C	Maintenance of oxygenation ventilation, postponement of surgery and awakening
D	Rescue techniques in the can't intubate can't ventilate scenario/proceed to needle or surgical cricothroidotomy

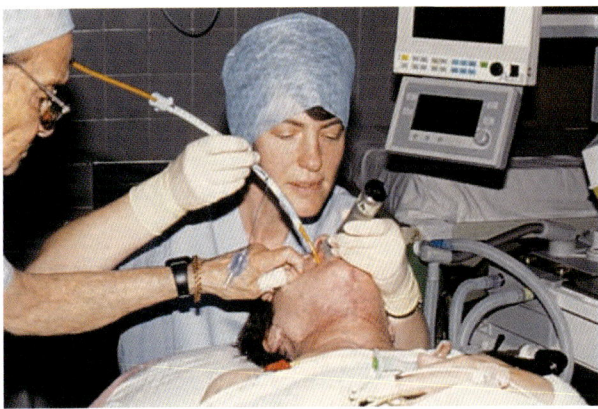

Figure 31.7 The gum-elastic bougie is an effective aid to intubation.

Forming a 'management strategy' rather than one isolated plan is the underlying principle of both societies' guidelines. The practitioner is encouraged to plan in advance the steps they will take based upon the success or failure of the first-line plan or 'plan A' that they make following assessment of the patient. Following the publication by the RCoA of the NAP4 study data, it was concluded that this 'strategy' is fundamental to improving outcome from problems resulting from airway difficulties. This conclusion was consolidated by analysis of the reasons that problems arose during airway management. Such problems were shown to be potentiated by poor forward planning, preparation, training and communication. In 2011, the DAS published guidelines on extubation. This followed the recognition that although complications at intubation have been decreasing since the turn of the century, the incidence of complications at extubation has not improved.[25] Extubation scenarios will be discussed later.

Management strategies may not necessarily mean the initial plan A will employ the technique of direct laryngoscopy or the standard curved Macintosh blade to intubate the trachea; however, this is by far the commonest first-line approach. Recommendations when this approach fails are first to attempt to perform basic manoeuvres. Reposition the patient, maximize jaw thrust and neck extension, possibly in combination with backward upward pressure on the larynx by external manipulation to improve the view. During rapid sequence induction relaxation of cricoid force may be needed. Introduction of the tube may be aided by low-tech devices such as a tube stylet, bougie or Magills forceps.

The bougie is a useful 'low-tech' device (**Figure 31.7**) with proven success rates.[26] Its correct use during attempted direct laryngoscopy is by placement through the glottis, either blindly or by educated guess. Correct placement is confirmed by feeling the tracheal rings and hold-up at 25 cm when the bougie contacts the carina. This is followed by railroading the tracheal tube with the laryngoscope still *in situ*. There are traumatic complications to bougie use, epithelial damage or placement into the bronchus resulting in trauma. Caution should be exerted when railroading the tube not to further advance the bougie towards the smaller airways as the tracheal tube is passed over it.

It is widely accepted that generally no more than three or four attempts should be made at direct laryngoscopy, including a change from a Macintosh blade to a straight or alternative blade, and there is some evidence to suggest morbidity with more than two attempts.[27] The correct decision is to acknowledge early a 'failed intubation' and abandon plan A. Defaulting to plan B, both failed ventilation and failed intubation are addressed by using alternative techniques to direct laryngoscopy with a standard Macintosh blade.[2]

ALTERNATIVE TECHNIQUES TO MACINTOSH LARYNGOSCOPY BLADES

Although the Macintosh curved design is the blade most commonly used by anaesthetists, there are a variety of blades that have proven their worth. Straight blades (for example, the Millar and Henderson blades) are used by a slightly different technique to the paraglossal approach with the Macintosh and they have been reported to provide superior views in some cases of lingual tonsillar hypertrophy.[28] It is a similar technique to the rigid laryngoscopy that is employed by head and neck surgeons. Another blade, originally invented by McCoy, employs a lever to increase markedly the angulation of the tip (**Figure 31.8**). A number of direct laryngoscopy blades have been introduced over the years incorporating prisms or mirrors to try and provide an indirect view of the larynx but these have not become mainstream devices.

Videolaryngoscopes

Rigid fibrescopes like the Upsherscope and Bullard, which incorporated fibre-optic viewing bundles into rigid curved blades, have been superceded by new generation videolaryngoscopes (**Figure 31.9**).[29] These devices, designed as aids to intubation, provide an indirect view of the larynx on a small LCD screen on a handheld device or a satellite screen and they have been shown to improve the view at laryngoscopy.[30, 31] There is evidence suggesting that they have a shorter learning curve than direct laryngoscopy, may improve the learning of direct laryngoscopy and require less mouth opening.[32] The LCD camera on these

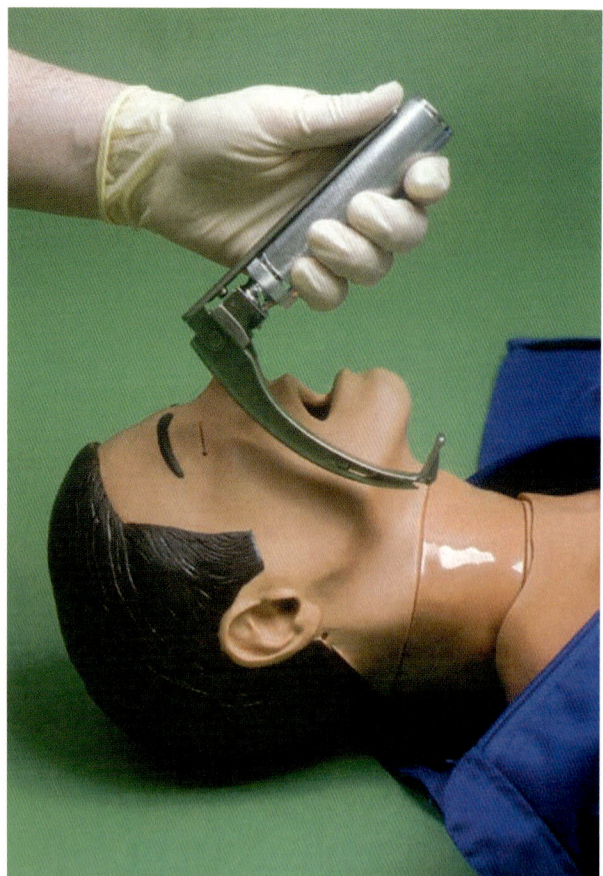

Figure 31.8 McCoy blade with a hinged tip.

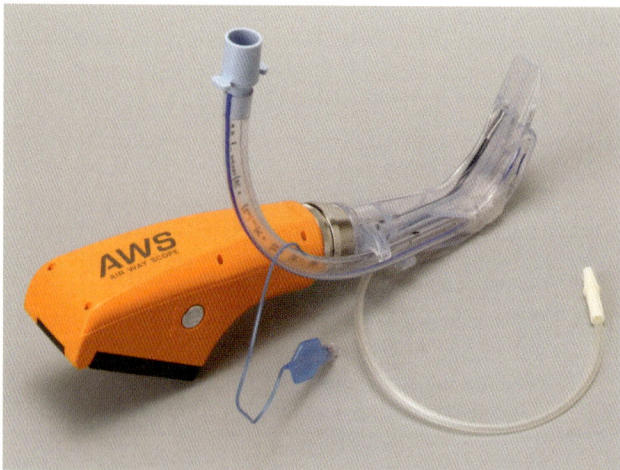

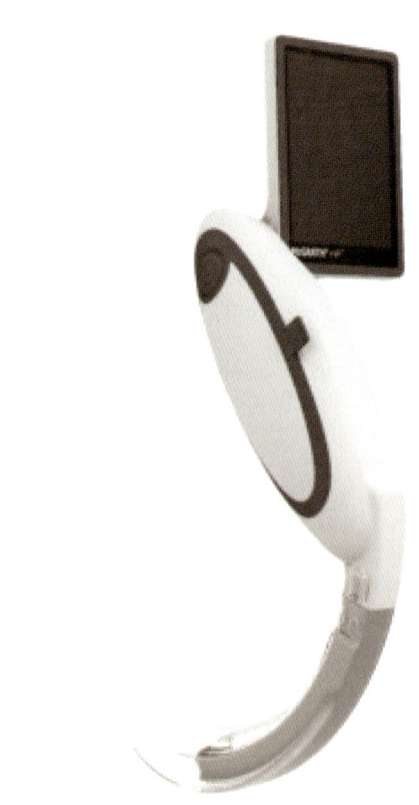

Figure 31.9 (a) Pentax AWS videolaryngoscope side mounted channel; difficult airway blade. **(b)** McGrath MAC videolaryngoscope with a Macintosh style blade.

handheld devices was developed from CMSO (complementary metal oxide detectors) technology and provides high fidelity small screens similar to those on current phones such as the iPhone 4 and HTC. Videolaryngoscopes can be divided into two large categories: those with Macintosh style blades (direct and indirect view of the larynx is possible); and those with difficult airway blades (indirect view possible only).

Some videolaryngoscopic devices, such as the McGrath MAC and Stortz CMAC, have both types of blade attachment. Some devices have a guide channel for side mounting endotracheal tubes to help direct the tip through the laryngeal inlet, while others require the use of a stylet or bougie to mould the tube to the correct hockey stick shape or guide the tube through the inlet. Although scientific evidence suggests that videolaryngoscopes will consistently improve the view of the larynx there is little evidence to support one particular device over the other.[33] Currently videolaryngoscopes are in widespread use and are gaining in popularity. It can be assumed that successful use of the technique is dependent not only on adequate training but also on operator dexterity and skill, judgement and patient selection. The technique of videolaryngoscopy involves four stages: introduction of the device under direct vision into the mouth, followed by obtaining the best view indirectly by using the LCD screen, followed by introduction of the tracheal tube into the mouth or nose under direct vision. Ultimately the tube is advanced while observing indirectly on the screen. Within a management strategy these devices would be used within one of the four attempts at intubation in plan A.

Flexible fibre-optic scopes

Tracheal intubation using the flexible fibrescope was first described in 1967 by Peter Murphy,[34] an anaesthetic senior registrar working at the National Hospital, Queen Square, London, and flexible intubating fibrescopes have been commercially available for over 20 years. Several textbooks[35, 36] are concerned solely with the technique. A standard adult intubating fibrescope has a length of 60 cm and a nominal external diameter of 4 mm. Its narrow diameter allows it to pass through the nose or mouth, its flexibility allows it to conform to the anatomy of the patient, the working channel can be used to instil local anaesthesia, oxygen or to pass wires in the antero- or retrograde direction to aid intubation, the technique is visual and can be used to confirm correct positioning of the tube in the trachea. It is fairly easy to use anaesthetic breathing system connectors or attachments that allow concurrent ventilation of the patient during intubation, or specially adapted airways to make oral intubation easier. It is not surprising that such an instrument has become the safest and most successful technique of intubation. A failed intubation rate of 0.045% is reported in one study and a success rate of 98.4% in another.[37, 38] The complication rate is extremely low.

Fibre-endoscopic skills appear in the core competencies for trainee anaesthetists and include visual inspection of the respiratory tract for diagnostic purposes and placement of double lumen tracheal tubes. The problems associated with the intubating fibrescope are that it is a skilled technique requiring training and practice, the devices are expensive and require careful handling, and disinfection requires chemical agents. There has been particular concern over the inability of cold sterilizing agents to destroy prions. The recommendation from the Department of Health is that a register should be maintained such that all patients treated with an individual fibrescope can be traced easily. Fibre-optic intubation may be part of a practitioners initial plan A strategy or part of a plan B, possibly an asleep fibre-optic intubation or in conjunction with an intubating laryngeal mask airway or supraglottic airway device–Aintree catheter technique.

Intubating laryngeal mask airway

The intubating laryngeal mask was devised by Brain and introduced in 1999. The intubating laryngeal mask airway (ILMA) kit (**Figure 31.10**) differs from the classic laryngeal mask (LM) in several ways. The stem is a rigid highly curved metal tube with a handle, there is an epiglottic elevator bar, a ramp at the junction of the stem and bowl directs the tube appropriately and it is supplied with a special wire-spiral tracheal tube with novel bevel. Single use systems are now widely available. The described technique of intubation in the anaesthetized, paralyzed patient is for the mask to be placed and the patient ventilated through it. Mask placement appears to be easy provided the mouth opening is more than 2 cm. The tracheal tube is inserted through the stem and advanced slowly without force. As the tip of the tube emerges from the stem, it lifts the epiglottic elevator bar and the route is now clear for the tube to be advanced into the trachea. This blind intubation has a success rate of 95% or so if two to three manipulations of mask position and tube advancement are allowed. A fibre-optic modification is recommended that allows a visually guided technique and would seem to

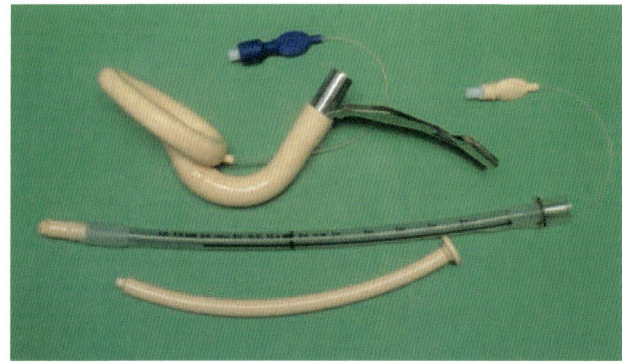

Figure 31.10 Components of the intubating laryngeal mask airway.

be preferable. Published figures suggest a successful intubation rate of 96.5% with a blind technique and 100% when used with the fibrescope[37, 38] although a small North American study[39] compared intubation by the ILMA in anaesthetized patients with awake fibre-optic intubation with suspected difficult intubation and found them both to be 100% successful.

Lighted stylets

The technique of transillumination of the neck to guide oro- or nasotracheal intubation was described first in 1959. A lighted stylet[40] uses the principle of trans illumination and takes advantage of the anterior or superficial location of the trachea. A number of commercially available devices have been produced over the years and the most recent, the Trachlight, appears to be the most successful. The tracheal tube is loaded onto the stylet, which has a distal bulb, and the stylet is shaped into a hockey-stick. The lighted stylet is introduced into the oropharynx from the side and brought into the midline. The tip of the light wand is passed around the tongue and a bright, well-circumscribed circle of light seen externally at the level of the hyoid indicates that the tip lies in the vallecula. The tube is advanced into the trachea without resistance. In skilled hands it has been shown to be an effective and rapid technique although it has not gained widespread popularity in the UK. Concerns over heat damage to the mucosa from the lighted stylet Trachlight™ during prolonged attempts have led the manufacturers to design the bulb to flash on and off every 20 seconds.

LARYNGEAL MASK AIRWAYS

The Classic laryngeal mask (LM) has proven itself highly successful among supraglottic airway devices for maintenance of the airway. The classic laryngeal mask airway (LMA™) is the original design of the mask, which consisted of an elliptical high volume low pressure silicone cuff, a breathing tube and connector piece for connection to a breathing circuit or bag. Large study data put the incidence of failed placement as 1:600 patients. They were designed and marketed from the late 1980s for maintenance of the airway in planned, elective surgery and within three years of launch had been used in over 2 million anaesthetics. There are now many different companies marketing their own disposable version of the device. LMA use has the advantages, when compared with tracheal intubation, of easier placement, no requirement for muscle relaxation and is tolerated *in situ* by the awakening patient. The major disadvantages are that it does not offer the same level of airway protection as a cuffed tracheal tube against gross gastric regurgitation and it does not traverse the larynx, so is no protection against airway occlusion by glottic or infraglottic pathology. LMA design has evolved in recent years with second-generation laryngeal masks (proseal LMA, LMA supreme) having the proposed benefit of a better pharyngeal seals allowing for more efficient controlled ventilation.

They also aim to provide an oesophageal seal or protection reducing the likelihood of aspiration of gastric contents and some (for example the LMA Supreme™ Teleflex®) have integral bite blocks. They have the advantage of having a drainage channel that, when positioned correctly, lies over the oesophageal opening and can be used to assist placement of the mask or pass a gastric tube. The NAP4 study executive summary now recommends the use of a second generation LMA in cases where there is a small but increased concern about regurgitation in preference to first-generation LMAs. There is also a recommendation that all hospitals should have second-generation LMA with an integral bite block available for use. LMAs in general have proved themselves to be a very useful device in difficult airway management and appear in several places in airway algorithms (**Box 31.1**).

BOX 31.1 Role of the classic LM in difficult airway management

- As the desired airway device
- Instead of a tracheal tube
- Rescue device in failed ventilation
- Conduit during emergence
- Conduit for fibre-endoscopy of the airway
- Conduit for intubation:
    - blind
    - bougie
    - fibre-optic-guided bougie
    - fibre-optic
    - Aintree catheter

Intubation via the LM

In normal use, the LM should be seated in close proximity to the vocal cords and it is not surprising that it can provide a route for passage of a tracheal tube. There are five methods for this (**Box 31.1**). A size 6.0 mm will pass through the stem/connector of a size three or four Classic LMA™ and a size 7.0 mm tube will pass through the size five Classic LMA™. This may not be the case for different brand disposable LMAs and should be checked in advance by any practitioner who would use the technique of intubating through these devices as part of a management strategy. Blind placement, in which the tube is lubricated and advanced blindly, has a success rate of only 50–90% and passing a bougie through the LM first has an even lower success rate. Techniques under vision have appreciably higher success rates and flexible fibre-optic techniques are particular useful. It is now not recommended that blind placement of the tube is attempted where fibre-optic equipment is available.

Fibre-optic-assisted techniques are useful because they are visually guided (**Figure 31.11**). The core technique is to insert the LM, load a 6.0 mm tube onto the fibrescope, pass the fibrescope into the trachea through the stem of the LM and slide the well-lubricated tube into the trachea. It is also possible to ventilate an anaesthetized patient through the LM whilst intubation is in progress. This introduces the concept of the laryngeal mask as a dedicated airway,[41] a device used for maintenance of the airway whilst other airway interventions (e.g. intubation) are in progress. Development of this concept led to the design of the Aintree catheter,[42] a hollow bougie that may be placed over the fibrescope and inserted through the LM into the trachea (**Figure 31.12**). Effectively, the technique places a hollow bougie under vision into the airway, over which a tracheal tube is railroaded.

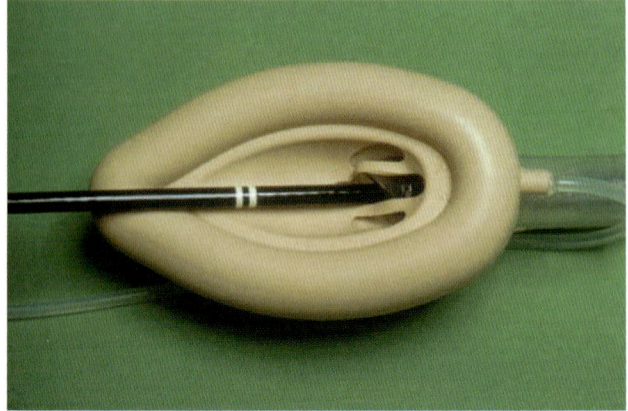

Figure 31.11 The laryngeal mask is a good conduit for fibre-optic intubation.

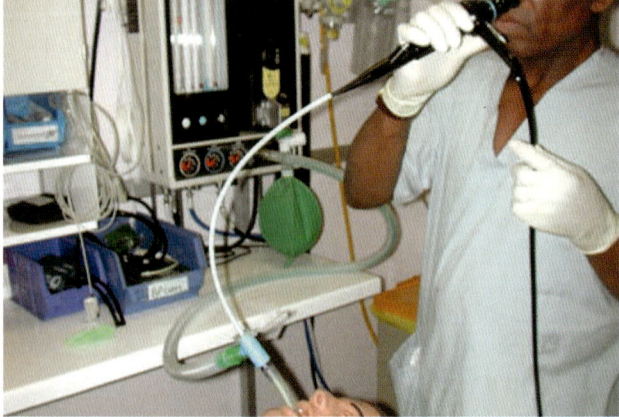

Figure 31.12 Aintree catheter – a hollow bougie inserted over a fibrescope.

FAILED VENTILATION AND EMERGENCY CRICOTHYROTOMY

Failed ventilation refers to the situation where a patient has been anaesthetized and muscle relaxants administered but it is not possible to provide positive pressure ventilation by use of the face mask and oral airway. A prepared sequence of steps (for example, DAS guidelines steps plan A–C) should commence to provide rescue oxygenation as quickly as possible. Bag/mask ventilation in which two hands are used to try to maintain airway patency and another hand squeezes the anaesthetic reservoir bag should be followed by insertion of an LMA. This may prove life-saving and must always be considered. If oxygenation cannot be achieved by face mask or LM, it may be worthwhile attempting intubation by direct laryngoscopy. This must be a brief attempt only and must not delay oxygenation by the next step.

In a can't intubate and can't ventilate scenario (CICV), and if it is known that the patient has normal airway anatomy or no airway pathology, it may be a consideration to follow the 'awaken patient' limb of the algorithm. If a non-depolarizing muscle relaxant has been given Sugammadex, a modern reversal agent should be administered and anaesthesia discontinued. Sugammadex is a synthetic modified gamma-cyclodextrin. It is the only selective binding agent that provides rapid reversal of the neuromuscular blockers rocuronium and vecuronium. It should be given in a dose of 16 mg/kg for reversal of neuromuscular blockade within approximately 7 minutes of administration of vecuronium or rocuronium. Careful consideration may be given to reversal of benzodiazepines or opiates to increase the speed of emergence.

Airway deaths, unfortunately, often involve prolonged fruitless attempts to intubate when oxygenation is the immediate necessity. Prolonged attempts to intubate patients who initially may have been low risk and appropriate to attempt wakening up may lead to a situation where this cannot be performed due to airway trauma or unconsciousness as a result of hypoxia and hypercarbia. The CICV accounts for 25% of all anaesthetic deaths.

When the anaesthetized patient cannot be oxygenated by face mask or LM, and tracheal intubation is not possible, the practitioner should proceed with emergency oxygenation attempts directly into the respiratory tract below the level of the vocal cords. When attempting emergency front-of-neck access, routing via the cricothyroid membrane (CTM) has a number of desirable properties:

- superficial
- easy landmarks to locate
- present in most patients
- rarely calcifies
- relatively avascular
- wide enough to accept 6.0 mm tube
- inferior to vocal cords
- cricoid ring holds airway open
- posterior lamina protects back wall.

There are three types of cricothyrotomy as detailed in the following sections.[43]

Needle or small bore cannula cricothyrotomy

A narrow-calibre rigid needle or flexible cannula is inserted through the CTM in a caudad direction. In adults, an appropriate size is 14 G with an internal diameter of 2 mm (Figure 31.13). Anatomically bevelled kink resistant cannulas specifically designed for cricothyroid puncture are commercially available. The old-fashioned technique of using a venous cannula has become obsolete. The resistance to flow through such a small calibre needle is high and this has implications for inspiration and expiration. In inspiration, adequate gas flows cannot be obtained by the pressures generated within a standard anaesthetic breathing system and exhalation of 500 mL takes >30 seconds. Inspiratory gas flows of 500 mL/s require oxygen at a pressure of 2–4 bar supplied by a jet injector (Figure 31.14). Traditionally the Sanders injector has been described for jet injection via a cricothyroidotomy cannula. It attaches to the 4 bar (400 kPa, 4 atmospheres) oxygen pipeline and has a hand-operated lever to control gas flow during inspiration and historically has been the common injector available in head and neck surgery for jet injection during rigid bronchoscopy. More recently the

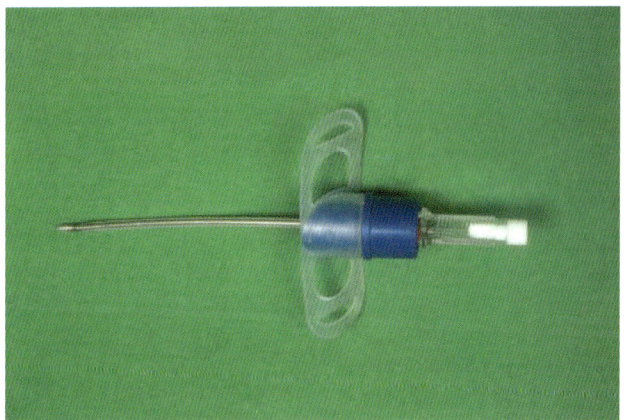

Figure 31.13 Ravussin style cricothyrotomy cannula.

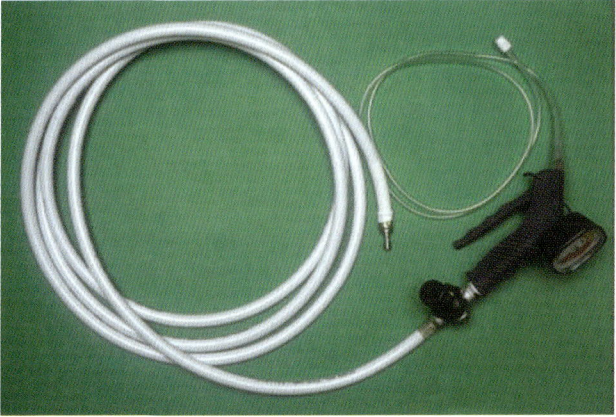

Figure 31.14 Sanders injector.

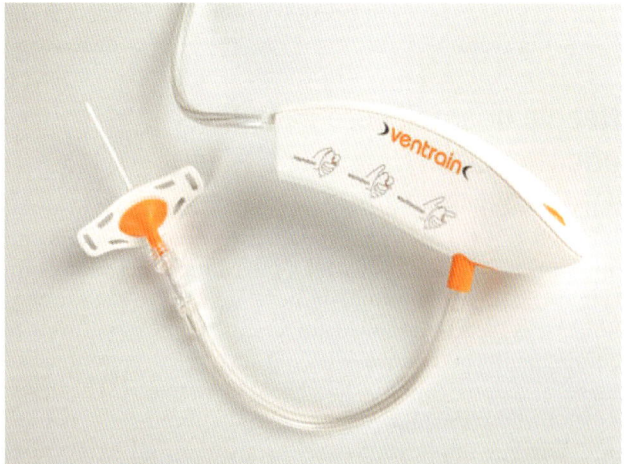

Figure 31.15 Ventrain device.

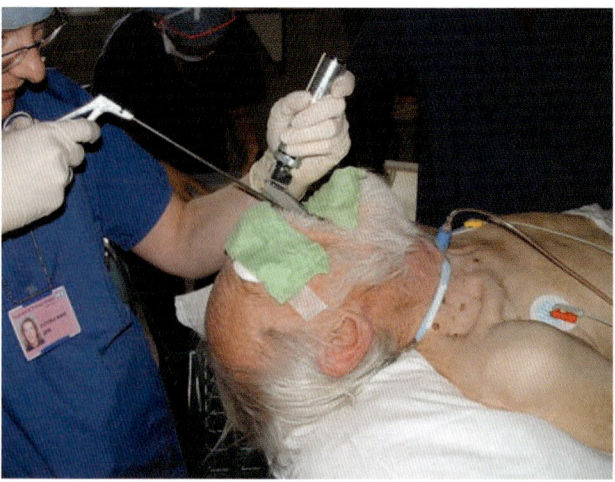

Figure 31.16 Planned use of transtracheal jet ventilation.

Manujet (VBM Medizintechnik GmbH, Sulz, Germany) has been widely used. It has the advantage of an adjustable pressure gauge to tailor inspiratory pressures between 0.5 and 4 bars. Other disposable devices for jet injection are available, such as the ENK flow modulator (Cook) and the Ventrain device (Dolphys medical; **Figure 31.15**), which can actively assist expiration. It is recommended that the pressure that should be used need be only the minimum required to raise the chest wall for inspiration (individual considerations would have to be accounted for if the patient had poor chest wall or lung compliance).

Exhalation occurs through the upper airway and particular attention must be taken to ensure that this happens, otherwise airway pressures rise and pulmonary barotrauma develops, as do haemodynamic consequences. A needle cricothyrotomy is a temporary measure; it will provide for oxygenation and so will give some time. However, it does not allow for adequate gas exchange and fatal hypercarbia can ensue. Consideration must be given to creation of a tracheostomy or competent airway allowing for adequate ventilation in relevant circumstances. It is possible for ventilation via needle cricothyrotomy to be used in the planned elective or urgent case. **Figure 31.16** shows a patient whose partial denture had fallen into the pharynx in such a position that the larynx was obscured. The cricothyrotomy needle was placed in the awake patient and its correct position in the trachea confirmed by aspiration of free air and attachment of the capnograph to show an appropriate trace. Following intravenous anaesthesia and muscle relaxation, the Sanders technique of intermittent application of high-pressure oxygen provided adequate oxygenation and ventilation. Exhalation through the upper airway was unobstructed.

Large cannula cricothyrotomy

A purpose-built cannula with an internal diameter of >4 mm allows adequate inspiratory gas flows with the pressures generated by the standard breathing system and exhalation of 500 mL takes approximately 5–6 seconds. This is an advantage because there is no requirement for high-pressure oxygen. It is easy to attach the capnograph

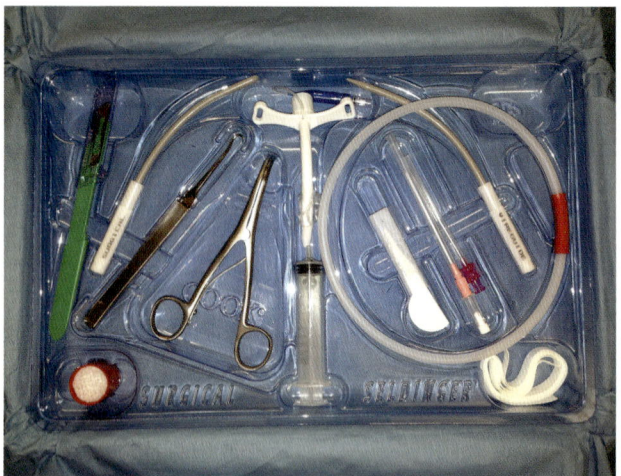

Figure 31.17 Combined Melker cricothyroidotomy set.

to the circuit for confirmation of correct positioning within the trachea, and to suction the respiratory tract. Exhalation occurs through the cannula, even in the presence of complete upper airway obstruction. The cannula may be a cannula-over-needle or a Seldinger-type dilatational device. Cannula-over-needle devices place an uncuffed tube whereas the Melker Seldinger device allows positioning of a 6.0 mm cuffed tube (**Figure 31.17**). There are advantages in placing a cuffed tube in allowing controlled positive pressure ventilation and protecting the airway.

Surgical cricothyrotomy

The technique is to make a 3 cm midline incision in the skin followed by a horizontal stab incision in the inferior part of the cricothyroid membrane. The incision is spread horizontally and vertically and a 6 mm tube is inserted. The complication rate was 40% in one series of 38 emergency surgical cricothyrotomies. Misplacement and bleeding requiring ligation of vessels were the most common problem. A more rapid four-step technique has been described[44] in which a single horizontal incision is made through the skin and cricothyroid membrane together. In a cadaver study, emergency physicians compared the standard and rapid technique. The rapid technique was faster than the standard 43 versus 134 seconds, but the complication rate was higher. The horizontal incison through the skin may cause more haemorrhage. A cricothyrotomy tube should not be left in place for more than a few days and conversion to tracheostomy prevents the complications of dysphonia and subglottic stenosis.

OBSTRUCTED AIRWAY

The obstructed airway[45] is one in which the primary symptoms or signs are due to narrowing or distortion of the airway. There are two broad clinical presentations. In acute obstruction (**Figure 31.18**), a previously normal person develops problems over a matter of minutes or hours. The aetiology is usually one of inhaled foreign body or abnormal fluid accumulation, such as blood, pus or oedema. Typical clinical scenarios are infections in the head and neck, post-operative haematoma, and airway swelling secondary to anaphylaxis or angiotensin-converting enzyme inhibitors. The rapidity of onset produces prominent signs of difficulty with breathing and the patients may present in extremis. Imaging of the airway by X-ray, CT or MR scan is desirable but often inappropriate because the patient may be unable to adopt the necessary position to complete the procedure and the radiology suite is not an appropriate location for a patient with a deteriorating airway. The management of acute obstruction includes 100% oxygen by face mask and continuous positive airway pressure (CPAP), adrenaline (epinephrine) if oedema is prominent, steroids intravenously and a trial of administration of heliox. This is known as CASH management, with the rapid institution of these measures in a stridulous patient aimed at buying time until pus is drained and tracheal intubation, emergency cricothyrotomy or tracheostomy is performed and the airway secure. Heliox is a combination of oxygen 21% and helium 79% and is three times less dense than air because of the low atomic weight of helium (4) compared with nitrogen (14). In airway obstruction, turbulent gas flow is inversely proportional to the square root of density and the use of heliox improves gas flow in turbulent conditions and also promotes laminar flow (**Figure 31.19**). It is suggested also that carbon dioxide molecules diffuse four to five times faster through heliox than an equivalent oxygen–nitrogen mixture and this may enhance carbon dioxide excretion in the airway.

In chronic obstruction, the airway pathology has developed over a period of weeks or months and is usually due to growth of tissue or to scarring. The slow onset allows development of enlarged intercostal muscle mass and patients can tolerate a very significantly narrowed airway without symptoms. Generally, a patient will not be dyspnoeic at rest until the airway is narrowed to <5 mm diameter, although they are likely to be short of breath on exercise. The slower time course of obstruction allows complete imaging of the airway and controlled intervention. Appropriate imaging in the stable, chronic condition is through flexible nasendoscopy and CT or MR imaging of the entire airway. Flow-volume loops may be helpful in detecting that a patient's problem is large airway narrowing and not truly pulmonary, or assessing the degree of tracheal narrowing before planning surgery.

Evaluation of the obstructed airway seeks to define the degree of obstruction, likely site, rapidity of onset and likely time course of deterioration by history, examination and special investigations. The history from the relative or patient usually indicates whether this is acute, chronic

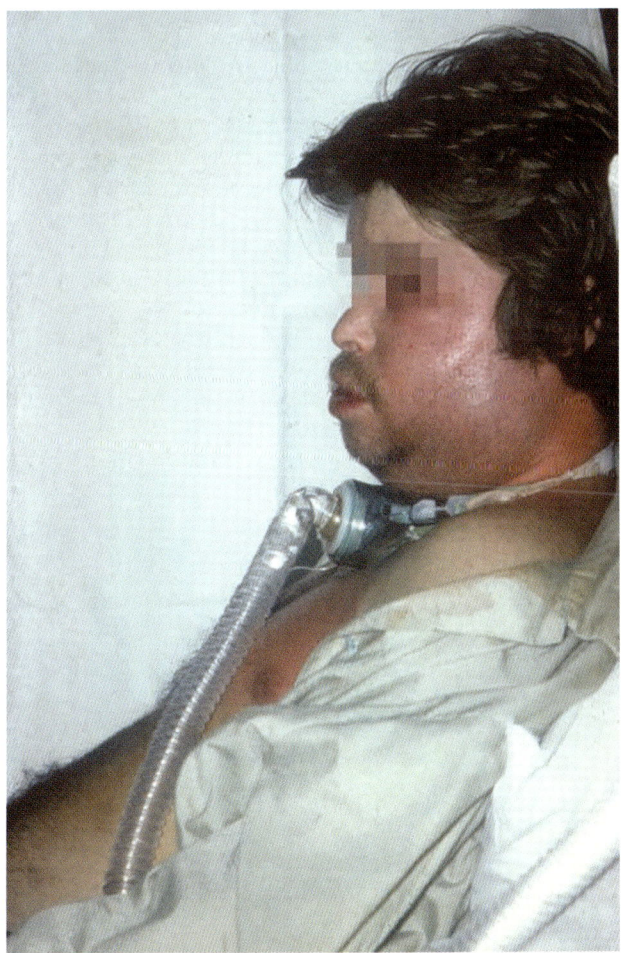

Figure 31.18 Patient with Ludwig's angina.

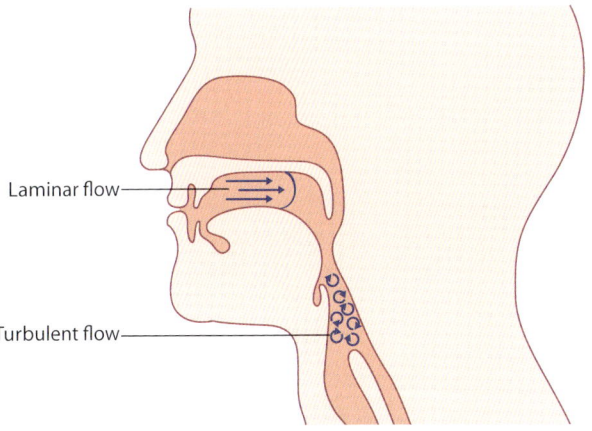

Figure 31.19 Laminar to turbulent flow.

or acute-on-chronic. Specific symptoms/signs in airway obstruction are degree of difficulty with breathing, stridor (noisy breathing) and phase of respiration of any stridor. Stridor indicates that the airway is narrowed to < 50% of normal diameter, but this degree of airway narrowing is not always accompanied by stridor. Expiratory stridor indicates an infraglottic problem and inspiratory stridor a supra or glottic aetiology. There may be a positional aspect to the difficulty with breathing and patients may be more comfortable in the sitting or lateral position. Voice change and difficulty with swallowing may indicate the site or extent of disease, and pyrexia or sepsis indicates an infective component. Unilateral reduction in breath sounds indicate specific bronchial obstruction. With progressive obstruction, signs of ineffective ventilation and poor gas exchange are present. These include agitation, anxiety, confusion, restlessness and depressed level of consciousness. Increased work of breathing is indicated by a high respiratory rate, use of accessory muscles of respiration, flaring nostrils, sweating and tachycardia. Oximetry is not a good monitor of work of breathing and normal oxygen saturation does not indicate that all is well. In severe acute obstruction with untrained respiratory muscles, exhaustion occurs relatively quickly with a resulting decrease in effective minute ventilation, hypoxaemia, bradycardia and death.

Management strategy in the obstructed airway

Deaths resulting from an airway that is obstructed due to a pathological process are usually due to the underlying disease process. However, cases with these pathologies where the airway has been difficult to maintain in the theatre or recover unit have led to deaths.[46] In the NAP4 study 70% of adverse events reported in patients having head and neck surgeries were in patients with an obstructed airway. This includes patients with stridor but also those without. Patients with friable necrotic tumours may be made much worse by attempts at intubation causing swelling, oedema and bleeding and progressive difficulty in face-mask ventilation and this was reflected in the case studies that were reported. In addition, gas induction with the maintenance of spontaneous respiration in patients with obstruction is difficult, the airway liable to deterioration as anaesthesia deepens and airway tone is lost. Those patients with painful faces or necks associated with obstruction are liable to laryngospasm when the chin is lifted and pressure is placed on painful tissues by a face mask. This is explored in more depth later.

Patients should be seen by a senior surgeon and anaesthetist who consider carefully the plan for securing the airway and a backup strategy. Imaging of the airway should be obtained, if possible, to allow delineation of whether the airway is narrowed at supraglottic, glottic or infraglottic level. There should be coherence between the individual plans A–D. For example if a long-acting muscle relaxant is used in plan A, plan B cannot rely on a patient 'waking-up'. If a surgical tracheostomy is the back-up plan, anaesthesia should start in the operating theatre with the equipment, surgeon and theatre team immediately ready – it is foolish to start anaesthesia in the anaesthetic room and scramble into theatre when plan A fails. There has been much discussion in the anaesthetic literature about provision of anaesthesia in the presence of the abnormal airway but general agreement that classification according to the site of obstruction is helpful. Currently, the terms used by anaesthetists are not as precise as the ones used by surgeons to localize tumours.

'SUPRAGLOTTIC' OBSTRUCTION

In 'supraglottic' obstruction the obstruction is above or superior to the glottis and the glottic aperture is of normal dimensions. An example would be a base of tongue tumour (**Figure 31.20**), although clearly this is not truly a supraglottic structure in disease terminology. Direct laryngoscopy is likely to prove difficult and may cause bleeding if the blade contacts the tumour. It may also prove difficult to ventilate by face mask following induction of general anaesthesia. In this circumstance it is helpful to retain spontaneous respiration and to use an alternative means of intubation. Awake fibre-optic intubation (**Figure 31.21**) by the nasal or oral route has much to recommend it.[47] It is used successfully in adult patients with deep neck infections including classical Ludwig's angina.[48]

Awake intubation is a misnomer because it is very difficult to intubate a truly awake patient. The more correct term is tracheal intubation under topical anaesthesia with conscious sedation. It has a very good record of safety in airway management because the patient maintains his or her own airway and continues with spontaneous respiration until the airway is secure. It is possible for the patient to adopt a change in position, such as sitting up, and to aid intubation by protruding their tongue, vocalizing or taking deep breaths. There are a number of intubation techniques in an awake patient, such as oral direct laryngoscopy, blind intubation through the nose, through the classic or intubating laryngeal masks or a retrograde wire technique, although none of these are commonly practised.

Awake fibre-optic intubation (AFOI) appears to be the best technique, combining awake intubation with a

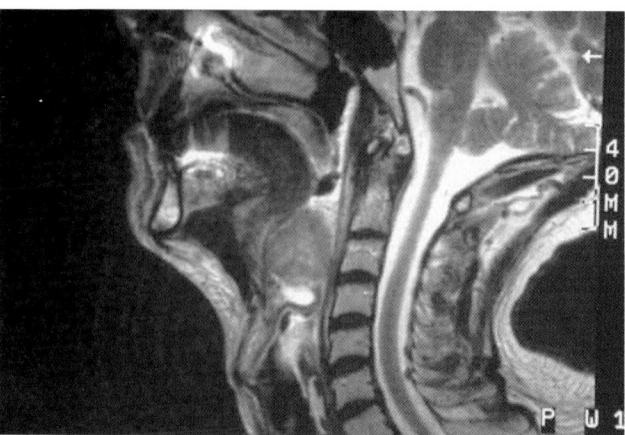

Figure 31.20 Magnetic resonance image of tongue base tumour.

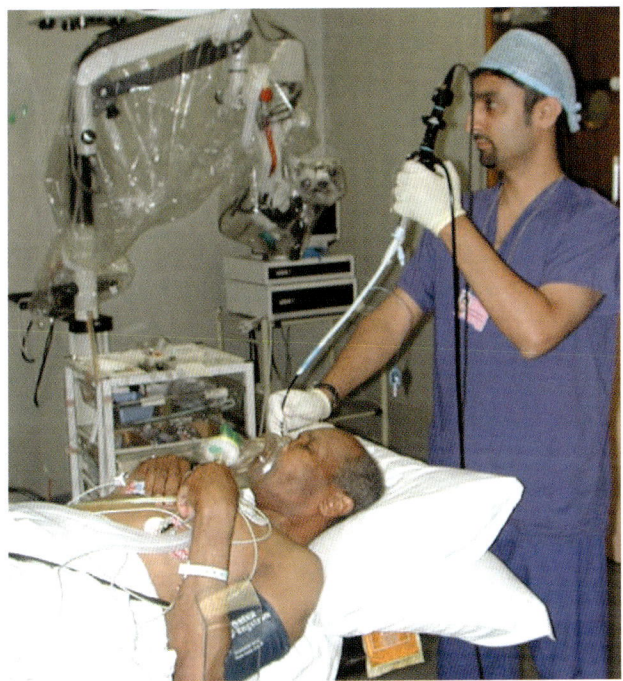

Figure 31.21 Awake fibre-optic intubation.

visually guided method of both inspecting and intubating the airway, applying local anaesthesia to the airway and confirming correct positioning of the tube within the trachea. Fibre-optic intubation is generally easier in the awake rather than anaesthetized, paralysed patient because airway patency is maintained, the airway opens and closes with respiration and the flow of gas indicates the route to the larynx.

There are a number of specific practical steps and attention to detail is required. Premedication may be employed if there is no airway embarrassment, but should be avoided if there are symptoms or signs of airway obstruction. An antisialogogue is important and absence of secretions allows earlier and more profound topical anaesthesia, and easier fibre-endoscopy. Pre-operative intramuscular atropine 0.6 mg, hyoscine 0.4 mg or glycopyrrolate 0.4 mg are suitable. Although it is common to administer glycopyrrolate 0.2–0.4 mg intravenously as soon as the patient arrives in the operating room, the antisialogogue effect when used this way is limited and patients may develop tachycardia.

Sedation aims to provide a comfortable patient who maintains spontaneous respiration, airway patency and verbal contact.

Remifentanil is an ultra-short-acting opioid that is commonly used nowadays by target-controlled infusion (TCI) or in micrograms per kilogram per minute for conscious sedation. It has a profound effect on airway reflexes and the cough response that is desirable during AFOI. It is often used as the sole sedative technique for AFOI.[49]

Small incremental doses of a benzodiazepine and opioid may administered, taking care not to produce over sedation. Typical total doses are midazolam 1–5 mg and fentanyl 25–100 μg. Both drugs have a peak onset of 5 minutes and a specific antagonist (flumazenil and naloxone, respectively).

Benzodiazepines cause relaxation of genioglossus and destabilization of the airway and opioids are associated with central respiratory depression so neither drug is benign. However, appropriate doses produce a compliant patient who is not unduly upset by airway topicalization or instrumentation, and is usually amnesic.

Propofol, an anaesthetic agent, provides sedation at subhypnotic concentrations and is used by some anaesthetists for conscious sedation by target-controlled infusion. TCI devices are sophisticated syringe pumps that incorporate a pharmacokinetic model of the relevant drug. The operator enters the age and weight of the patient and the desired blood level. The TCI pump calculates and delivers the appropriate bolus dose to reach the required blood level and the subsequent infusion required to maintain it. Appropriate starting blood levels for propofol are 0.5–1.0 μg/mL.

There are a variety of ways of topicalizing the airway with lignocaine, most practitioners having their 'own way' of administering the local to the mucosa. There is no evidence reporting one technique being better than the other; however, it is important to keep in mind the that local anaesthetic effect will be reduced if tissues are acidotic and that local anaesthetic toxicity is a small risk when using larger doses that are then followed by infiltration of tissues as part of a surgical procedure. The majority of lignocaine administered by topicalization will be swallowed and metabolized by first pass metabolism and so will contribute little to plasma concentrations. However, that fraction that reaches the larynx trachea and bronchial tree will raise blood levels.

If the nasal route is chosen for intubation, a topical vasoconstrictor should be applied. This may be xylometazoline or phenylephrine spray, ephedrine 0.5% drops or cocaine (3 mL 5%), which produces both vasoconstriction and topical anaesthesia. The use of cocaine as a vasoconstrictor for AFOI has reduced in popularity in the last 10 years.

Topical anaesthesia with lignocaine may be provided by:

- nebulization
- translaryngeal administration
- specific nerve blocks
- transendoscopic administration.

Nebulization sounds attractive but use of the technology that provides particles for alveolar deposition of drug (e.g. salbutamol nebulizer) may lead to disappointing results, partly because the particles are too small but also because a large amount of the drug escapes to the atmosphere. High drug concentrations may be effective and nebulized lignocaine 10% in a dose of 6 mg/kg has been described as effective.

A useful variant is the production of a larger droplet size produced during inspiration. This manual spray-and-inhale technique historically employed a 22g Venflon attached to a constant oxygen flow rate of 1–2 L/min. Specific mucosal atomizer devices are now widely available for this purpose. Small increments of lignocaine 4%

are injected and coordinated with inspiration. One spray-and-inhale regime is to use 3 mL lignocaine 4% with ephedrine 15 mg to the nose, wait 3 minutes and apply the second 3 mL lignocaine 4%, asking the patient to inspire deeply and slowly through the nose. The droplets are inhaled and deposited onto the larynx and trachea. After a 3-minute wait, a further 3 mL lignocaine 4% is nebulized during slow forced inspiration. Maximum lignocaine dosage should be 9 mg/kg.

Translaryngeal administration has a long history of safe use.[50] A 22 G cannula or needle is passed through the cricothyroid membrane or trachea and 3–4 mL lignocaine 4% is injected preferably at end-expiration. The injection provokes a short period of intense coughing, which distributes the drug to the glottis and above. The experimental addition of methylene blue to the local anaesthetic shows staining of the superior aspect of the vocal cords in 95% of patients.

Appropriate specific nerve blocks are of the superior laryngeal and glossopharyngeal nerves and are uncommonly used for AFOI. The internal branch of the superior laryngeal nerve supplies sensation to the under surface of the epiglottis and the superior surface of the vocal cords. It may be blocked on each side as it traverses the thyrohyoid membrane. Extension of the head and neck aids identification of the hyoid and thyroid cartilages. A 22 G needle is placed inferiorly to the greater horn of the hyoid, passed into the membrane and 2 mL lignocaine 2% is injected. The glossopharyngeal nerve supplies sensation to the posterior third of the tongue, superior part of the epiglottis, lateral pharyngeal wall and inferior surface of the soft palate. The nerve may be blocked behind the anterior pillar of the tonsillar fossa. With full mouth opening the tongue is grasped and pulled to the contralateral side. A 20 G spinal needle is inserted to a depth of 5 mm into the base of the anterior tonsillar pillar at the level of the reflection onto the tongue, and 2 mL lignocaine 2% injected. Bilateral glossopharyngeal nerve blocks will abolish the gag reflex and allow greater manipulation in the oropharynx or direct laryngoscopy, perhaps when placing a large double lumen tube. These specific nerve blocks are not performed routinely.

Transendoscopic administration of lignocaine 4% through the working channel of the intubating fibrescope is an extremely effective means of applying local anaesthetic to the airway under vision. This spray-as-you-go technique is highly favoured and non-invasive. The intubating fibrescopes have connectors for injection but an easier alternative is to place an epidural catheter, cut to produce one terminal hole, substantially into the working channel (**Figure 31.22**). Aliquots of lignocaine 4% to a maximum dose of 9 mg/kg are administered.

It is helpful for the fibrescope to be attached to a CCTV system, particularly for training. An appropriate size tracheal tube is loaded onto the fibrescope and the scope is introduced under vision into the mouth or more patent nostril. The fibrescope is advanced without touching the mucosa until the vocal cords are seen. Additional local anaesthetic may be applied before the fibrescope is advanced to the carina. The tube is advanced or railroaded over the fibrescope. This may be difficult because the bevel impinges on the larynx. Use of a small diameter tube and rotation of the tube minimize this problem.

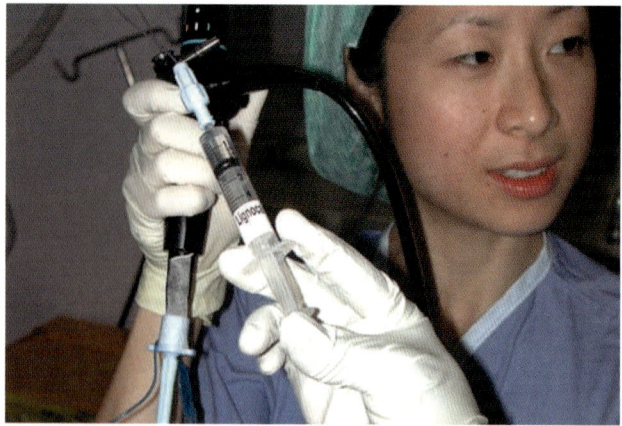

Figure 31.22 Injection of lignocaine through an epidural catheter inserted into working channel of fibrescope.

Awake fibre-optic intubation may be difficult when the airway anatomy is abnormal and when there is blood or secretions in the airway. An illustrative case scenario indicates some of the pitfalls in management. An adult patient underwent removal of a fishbone impacted in the lower pharynx/upper oesophagus. Three days later the patient was pyrexial, with a sore throat, unable to swallow and with limited mouth opening. A lateral X-ray of the neck showed a retropharyngeal abscess. The patient was seen by two anaesthetic trainees, who did not inform the consultant on call. They decided on an awake fibre-optic intubation but administered too much sedation. In a deteriorating situation with a semi-rousable patient they attempted nasal fibre-optic orotracheal intubation (FOI) with the patient supine. They were unsuccessful and were moved aside by the consultant surgeon who managed to intubate the patient fibre-optically with the patient sitting, leaning forward on the edge of the operating table. Mistakes made here include failure to appreciate the seriousness of the condition and to inform a consultant, failure to realize that awake nasal FOI in the supine position would be difficult in the presence of retropharyngeal swelling and failure to realize that airway patency would be compromised by any sedation.

PERIGLOTTIC/GLOTTIC OBSTRUCTION

In these situations it may be difficult to visualize the vocal cords by direct laryngoscopy and the glottic aperture may be significantly narrowed or distorted. Much lively discussion is evident over the correct anaesthetic technique. When awake fibre-optic intubation is used, it allows visualization of the airway but becomes less useful in the patient with stridor due to glottic narrowing. The fibrescope has little rigidity to 'push' through a narrow hole and attempts to do this may precipitate bleeding and oedema. If the scope is passed through a small hole, the airway is completely obstructed for a short time and patients feel uncomfortable at this stage. Panic and ongoing obstruction with this 'corking the bottle' effect can lead to airway catastrophe. There have been a few reports[51, 52] of destabilization of the airway by applying anaesthetic agent to the airway and this is a reminder of the need to work at all times in the correct environment for immediate activation of the pre-formulated back-up plan. Awake fibre-optic intubation is, therefore, a technique that should always be considered but may not be suitable. It is not appropriate when adequate operator skill is not present, in children and uncooperative adults and in the opinion of some anaesthetists when stridor is present.

Mason and Fielder[53] argue that the correct anaesthetic technique in the presence of stridor due to periglottic/glottic pathology is inhalational induction of general anaesthesia. This permits a gradual onset of anaesthesia and maintains spontaneous respiration, even at a depth of anaesthesia appropriate for direct laryngoscopy and intubation. The maintenance of spontaneous respiration is viewed as highly desirable with supraglottic airway obstruction. A typical case scenario would be a child with epiglottitis and, in a survey of college tutors in the UK, 98% of anaesthetists would choose this form of anaesthesia. The face mask is applied to the patient who is in the most comfortable position (sitting if necessary) and 100% oxygen administered for a few minutes. The volatile agent is administered in increasing concentrations until a surgical level of anaesthesia is obtained. The agent commonly used initially is either halothane or sevoflurane and both drugs are non-irritant so do not provoke coughing. The speed of onset of anaesthesia is inversely proportional to the blood–gas solubility and is therefore faster with sevoflurane (0.6) than halothane (2.4). However, it is more difficult to establish sufficient depth of anaesthesia to instrument the airway with sevoflurane and it has a more rapid offset than halothane. Halothane may be associated with increased cardiac rhythm irritability and is now difficult to obtain in the UK. It is usual, therefore, to start with sevoflurane and consider a change over to isoflurane which does permit adequate levels of anaesthesia.

It is not an easy anaesthetic to administer in the presence of stridor and requires a sanguine anaesthetist. There may be periods of increasing obstruction due to glottic irritability or change in position. Generally, there should be no change in the position of the anaesthetist's hands or the face mask and no attempt in light planes of anaesthesia to provide positive pressure ventilation. Insertion of an oral airway is risky but there may be benefit in a nasopharyngeal airway, although it is perhaps useful to have applied a vasoconstrictor to the nasal mucosa first. Glottic irritability is confined to light planes of anaesthesia and should resolve, although induction may take much longer than normal because of the reduced alveolar ventilation. When an adequate depth of anaesthesia is reached, which may take 20 minutes, direct laryngoscopy is undertaken. The view may be quite abnormal and it may be necessary to press on the chest and observe the egress of bubbles to detect the glottis. A small tube will be needed and the use of a bougie should be considered. If intubation is not possible, the face mask is reapplied and a tracheostomy undertaken. Plan B must be formulated and ready so that anaesthesia is induced in the operating theatre with the surgeon scrubbed and ready to undertake tracheostomy.

It is apparent that the safety of any approach is the combination of plans and the close cooperative working of the surgeon, anaesthetist and theatre team. In the common scenario of a known obstructing glottic tumour that requires initial histology and debulking, it is possible to construct a primary plan of (in the operating theatre) preoxygenation, followed by intravenous induction and rapid muscle relaxation. Direct laryngoscopy using a bougie and size 5.0 mm microlaryngeal tube is attempted. If it is unsuccessful, the surgeon is in the best situation to undertake tracheostomy – the patient is as well oxygenated as possible, unconscious and remains still. This technique is logical and popular but appears 'heretical' since it abolishes spontaneous respiration. However, it illustrates that safety lies in the combination of plans rather than any particular plan A. It also demonstrates that the site of obstruction requires plans that are specific for that level of obstruction and the safety that arises from the close working of experienced surgeon and anaesthetist.

There is an increasing evidence-base to the practice of planned prior placement of a transtracheal ventilation catheter under local anaesthesia and using this as a route for oxygenation and ventilation during intubation attempts under general anaesthesia.[54]

TRACHEOSTOMY UNDER LOCAL ANAESTHESIA

This should be considered in any patient with an obstructed airway. It is particularly appropriate as the primary plan when the disease process is a large friable mass or abscess in the supraglottis or glottis and intubation attempts may destabilize or compromise the airway. There are differences between countries and between surgeon–anaesthetist pairs as to when the patient undergoes traditional intubation in the awake or anaesthetized state or awake tracheostomy. Elements within the decision-making are the availability of a skilled fibre-endoscopist, the ability of the patient to cooperate with the procedure and adopt a suitable position, the pretracheal anatomy and the likely time for resolution of the disease process. It may be a very difficult procedure in patients with short stocky necks, a previous tracheostomy or post-radiotherapy with respiratory distress. Considerations may be complicated by front-of-neck pathology or the patient's inability to lie flat.

Tracheostomy under local anaesthesia is undertaken in the operating theatre with the patient breathing oxygen or heliox, monitored by non-invasive blood pressure, ECG and pulse oximetry with intravenous access. CASH management can be continued throughout the procedure in the semi-sitting position with a roll under the shoulders and neck extension is ideal. Generally, reassurance is given to the patient but intravenous sedation is not required and should be used cautiously. Restlessness during the procedure may be due to hypoxia, hypercarbia or an inability to breathe in that position. Sedation may destabilize the airway leading to sudden hypoxia and loss of consciousness. Consideration may be given to conscious sedation with remifentanil with the primary aim of obtunding the airway reflexes and improving the distress of the patient; however, caution is highly advisable. The anaesthetist must be prepared for the back-up plan if the patient deteriorates. Placement of a cricothyrotomy needle at the outset may be useful when it is known that the pathology is supraglottic. The cricothyrotomy needle does not interfere with a surgical tracheostomy and can be used to provide oxygenation. If the patient becomes so restless that the surgeon is unable to operate, consideration should be given to providing general anaesthesia and oxygenation through the needle.

Another option in the distressed patient is to provide sedation/anaesthesia by addition of a volatile anaesthetic agent, such as sevoflurane, to the breathing system with 100% oxygen. At best, the airway proves to be adequate enough to allow a surgical plane of anaesthesia to be reached and the tracheostomy is undertaken in a relatively unhurried fashion on 100% oxygen/sevoflurane by face mask. At worst, the airway deteriorates with the onset of sedation/anaesthesia but the patient stops moving and a rapid emergency tracheostomy can be undertaken. In a rapid tracheostomy, the surgeon enters the airway with one or two incisions and a small cuffed microlaryngeal or armoured tube size 5.0–6.0 mm is inserted. Once the patient has been stabilized, a more measured exploration of the neck and fashioning of a formal tracheostomy may be undertaken.

It is important to verify that the tube is within the trachea before ventilation starts, otherwise gas may be forced into the mediastinal tissues. Signs of correct placement when undertaking a tracheostomy under local anaesthesia (with the patient breathing spontaneously) are firstly regular respiratory movement of the reservoir bag of the anaesthetic breathing system connected to the tracheostomy tube, and the presence of six successive breath-related carbon dioxide traces on the capnograph. If no carbon dioxide is detected in the breathing system, inflation of the cuff of the tracheal tube or tracheostomy and connection of the capnograph to the breathing system should be checked first. If both are correct, failure to detect carbon dioxide indicates that the tube is not in the airway. When an emergency tracheostomy is undertaken in an apnoeic patient, the confirmatory signs of anaesthetic bag movement and capnography can be obtained only by applying a number of positive pressure breaths. If the tube is not within the trachea, these positive pressure breaths into the mediastinum may prove deleterious. An alternative confirmatory device in these circumstances, although not widely used, is the oesophageal detector device. The principle is simple and takes advantage of the structural differences between the oesophagus and trachea. In the original version described by Wee in 1988,[55] an empty 60 mL syringe is attached to the 15 mm connector of the inserted tracheal tube and aspiration attempted. Aspiration of air is not possible if the tube is in the oesophagus because the mucosa is 'sucked' over the end of the tube, whereas the more rigid cartilaginous structure of the trachea allows free aspiration of air. The syringe can be replaced by a self-inflating bulb with a volume of approximately 75 mL and in this version the bulb is squeezed flat before being attached to the inserted tube. If the bulb re-inflates immediately, the tube is in the trachea and if the bulb does not re-inflate the tube is in a false passage or the oesophagus.

SUBGLOTTIC AND MIDTRACHEAL OBSTRUCTION

Imaging is particularly useful in delineating the length of narrowing, the diameter of the airway at its narrowest and that sufficient distance is present inferiorly to the obstruction to permit the cuff of a tracheal tube to be positioned above the carina. The obstruction may arise from external pressure, such as a retrosternal goitre or other mediastinal mass, from a mass arising from the trachea, from an inflammatory condition such as Wegener's granulomatosis, from previous surgery or from damage due to prolonged intubation. The type of narrowing may range from a short subglottic stenosis due to previous prolonged intubation to a narrowing of several centimetres in the midtrachea due to tumour. In the presence of stridor, the principles of management vary according to whether it can be bypassed by tracheostomy. This will be true for subglottic disease but the Confidential Enquiry into Patient Outcome and Death (CEPOD) assessors noted that in two patients it had been difficult to bypass a mid/low tracheal lesion with a standard length tracheostomy tube. Awake fibre-optic intubation has a role in management of trachea narrowing, allowing inspection of the airway and confirmation that the tip of the tracheal tube has passed beyond the obstruction. Rigid bronchoscopy is an extremely effective means of managing these patients.

LOW TRACHEAL OBSTRUCTION

Narrowing of the lower trachea or carina presents great difficulty. The anaesthetic literature contains case reports of failed airway maintenance leading to death.[56] This characteristically occurs after induction of general anaesthesia or muscle relaxation when, presumably due to loss of muscle tone, airway patency is lost. Tracheal intubation may not provide an adequate airway because the obstruction is beyond the tip of the tube. Occasionally, the presence of carinal obstruction is not known and anaesthetic induction, intubation or indeed extubation may result in unexpected disaster. When imaging has provided good pre-operative localization of obstruction, a number of options may be used. Rigid bronchoscopy is invaluable and will often provide a route for ventilation (**Figure 31.23**). The rigid bronchoscope may also act as a guide to therapy, such as lasering of a tumour or introduction of a tracheobronchial stent. Surgical resection of carinal lesions requires specialist anaesthetic techniques including jet ventilation and undertaking surgery during cardiopulmonary bypass.

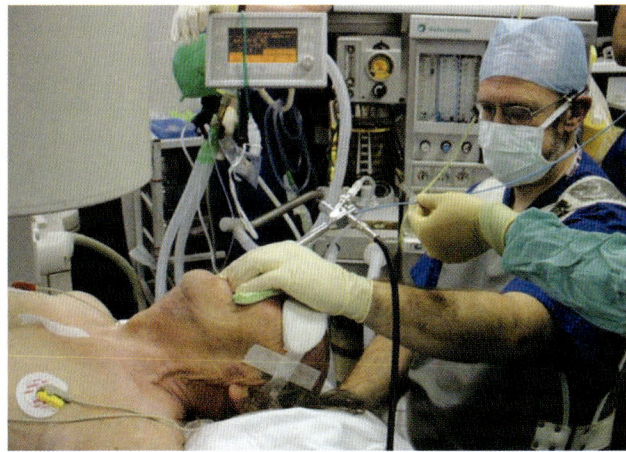

Figure 31.23 Rigid bronchoscopy used for ventilation and conduit for tracheal stent.

JET VENTILATION

Jet ventilation as an in-theatre technique is associated with allowing access in Head and Neck/ENT surgery and also as an airway rescue technique. It has also been described as a technique for facilitating thoracic radiology procedures and rigid bronchoscopy, and was first described as such over 40 years ago.[57–59] This chapter does not consider its use as a mode of ventilation on critical care.

It is best considered by its nature (high- or low-frequency) and by its position (supraglottic, subglottic or transtracheal). Delivery of each of these has advantages and disadvantages. High-frequency jet ventilation is defined as a respiratory rate of between 1 and 10 Hz and requires the use of a specific device. Low-frequency jet ventilation can be delivered by a Manujet (VBM) at a lower rate (**Figure 31.24**). More complex modes of jet ventilation are described. Superimposed High-Frequency Jet Ventilation combines HFJV with LFJV and has been shown to be effective in patients and offers potential benefits in terms of end-expiratory volumes.[60, 61]

Mechanism: The most common mistake made about jet ventilation is in its mechanism of action. It does not work by the Venturi effect; it works by friction. There are actually six postulated mechanisms as to how it might function:

1. Convective or Bulk flow.
2. Laminar flow in the small airways.
3. Pendelluft.
4. Cardiogenic mixing.
5. Molecular Diffusion.
6. Taylor type dispersion.

Describing jet ventilation

Jet ventilation can be defined in terms of the Driving Pressure (up to 4 bar), the pressure generated by the ventilator, the frequency (or cycles per second) of jet ventilation (between 60 and 600 Hz) and the pause pressure. Pause pressure is sensed in the last 10 milliseconds of the expiratory pause. If the pause pressure alarm value is

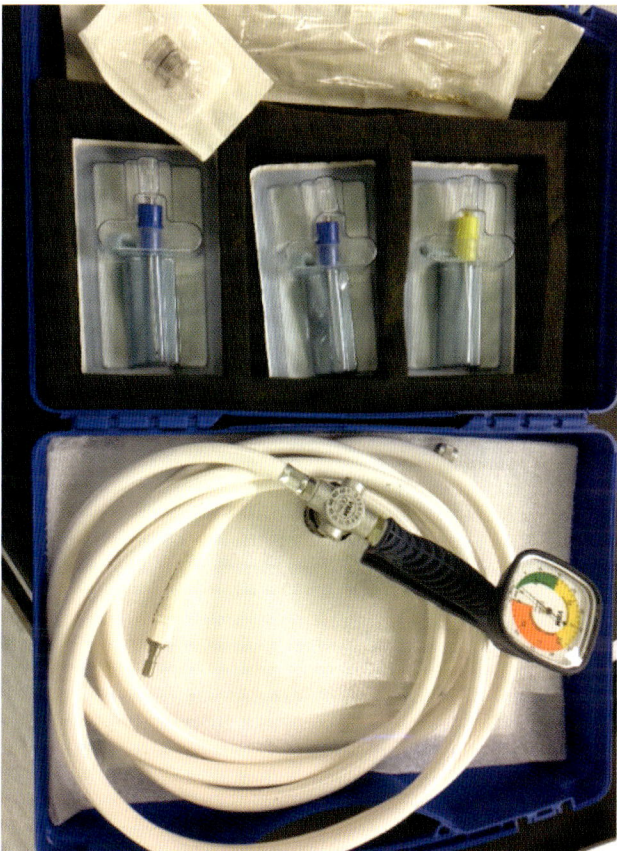

Figure 31.24 A low-frequency jet ventilation system. Simple to use, however lacking the safeguards of a more complex high-frequency jet ventilator.

exceeded then cycling is stopped preventing breath stacking. This is well described by Wiedemann and Mannle.[62]

Various articles have looked at the complications of jet ventilation. Hu et al reported a series of 839 cases using the Hunsaker tube.[63] They reported a complication rate of 5.8%, although 47 of the 58 complications were cited as hypoxia (Spo2 < 90%) or hypercarbia (CO2 > 60 mmHg). There were 2 cases of barotrauma and 4 cases of airway obstruction. They cited risk factors for complication as being a higher BMI, ASA class 3 or 4, history of heart disease, history of previous laryngeal surgery, longer case duration, and use of a laser. Patel and Rubin have reported 2 series; 142 cases who were grade I laryngoscopy with a complication rate of 0.7% (Rubin JS 2005) and a difficult airway series looking at 89 cases where they reported no anaesthetic or surgical complications, but noted that higher BMI patients required an increased driving pressure.[64, 65] Jaquet et al. reported a series of 734 jetted patients with 24 minor complications and 4 major ones.[66] Transtracheal jet ventilation was associated with a significantly higher complication rate than transglottal jet ventilation. Serious complications occurred when jetting took place in the presence of airway outflow obstruction. They concluded that the use of a transtracheal jet ventilation catheter was the major independent risk factor. Bougain et al. provide different evidence of transtracheal jet ventilation.[67] In their series of 643 episodes of transtracheal high-frequency jet ventilation they reported a 1% pneumothorax rate (57% required drainage) and an 8.4% rate of surgical emphysema. They concluded that transtracheal ventilation from an automatic ventilator with a cut-off alarm was safe for experienced users.[67] In their survey in 2008 Cook and Alexander noted that complications over a 5 year period were evenly spread between subglottic, supraglottic and transtracheal techniques although deaths all occurred in departments using low-frequency jet ventilation (no pressure alarms).[68] The three centres performing more than 100 cases of transtracheal jet ventilation did not report any serious complications.

The future

In 1990, Smith suggested that high frequency ventilation was here to stay.[69] However, in recent years, there have been innovations that may offer an alternative technique. The ventrain was designed by Enk, as an alarm-free manually operated device that permits transtracheal ventilation.[70] Driven by a conventional wall oxygen flowmeter it can generate a driving pressure for inspiration of 2.3 bar (pressure). However, crucially it can also generate a suction pressure to facilitate expiration (EVA-expiratory ventilation assistance) and avoid air trapping. Unfortunately, clinical trials of the device are limited at present. Unlike other forms of jet ventilation the Ventrain works by the Bernoulli principle.

High-flow oxygen therapy may also an alternative to jet ventilation; however this technique is yet to be evaluated in patients under general anaesthesia.[71]

EXTUBATION AND RECOVERY

At the end of surgery a decision is made as to where and when the airway device should be removed. There is little problem with removal of a laryngeal mask. This is usually tolerated well by a patient until they are awake. Tracheal intubation is common in head and neck surgery due to the constraints of providing clear operative fields for the surgeon and maintaining a secure airway to the distal trachea. Extubation requires as much thought, and gives rise to as much difficulty, as intubation. Transient difficulties with oxygen saturations are common due to coughing, breath-holding and laryngospasm, particularly in children. Extubation problems may arise in those patients who were difficult to intubate and those who were not difficult to intubate but in whom surgery has affected the airway. Of the NAP4 reports, 28% of airway complications were reported at emergence or during recovery from anaesthesia and in all cases airway obstruction was the problem.

Default strategy at extubation when no difficulty is expected is for the anaesthetist to remove any pharyngeal packs, suction the pharynx under direct vision, administer 100% oxygen, antagonize residual neuromuscular blockade and consider whether to remove the tube in the anaesthetized or awake state. After extubation, 100% oxygen is administered by face mask and the patient observed by the anaesthetist until it is clear that the patient is safe to go to the post-anaesthetic care unit (Recovery).

In the patient with a normal airway who was difficult to intubate, it is prudent to make certain that oxygen stores are maximal and to extubate in the awake state. Lung oxygen stores can be considered maximal when the end-tidal (i.e. alveolar) oxygen is 91%. This may take at least 5 minutes of breathing 100% oxygen or longer if nitrous oxide has been used. Awake extubation refers to removal of the tracheal tube when the person has opened their eyes and is able to obey commands. An additional option is to assess the leak around the tube before removal. This may be carried out by applying positive pressure to the tube, deflating the cuff and listening for egress of gas around the tube, or alternatively occluding the tube in spontaneous respiration and making certain that inspiration can occur around the tube. Failure of a leak test indicates that the tube is a very tight fit within the airway and an inadequate air passage may be left after extubation.

In the patient with an abnormal airway, either present pre-operatively or due to surgery, consideration should be given to keeping the tracheal tube in situ for 24–48 hours until any airway oedema subsides. The patient should be nursed in a high-dependency unit with an appropriate level of sedation to avoid inadvertent removal of the tube. In some circumstances it is appropriate to perform a tracheostomy to provide a secure airway in the first few post-operative days.

Extubation of the high-risk airway requires a strategy. Anticipation of complications may be possible, for example long complicated head down surgeries may be accompanied by laryngeal oedema. Awake extubation after maximal oxygenation in the presence of an anaesthetist in a well-equipped environment may be a good plan A, but what happens if it fails? The situation rapidly becomes critical with a struggling, hypoxic patient possibly with blood in the oropharynx. One possibility is to extubate over a thin bougie and to leave the bougie in the airway for a period until it is certain that the patient is coping satisfactorily. The bougie acts as a guide if reintubation is required and, if it is hollow, may be used for emergency oxygenation.

Problems may arise in the Recovery unit or post-operatively on the ward. Of most concern is post-operative bleeding following carotid endarterectomy or removal of a parapharyngeal mass. The physical presence of a mass of blood may compress the airway itself but also induces mucosal oedema, perhaps by impairment of lymphatic drainage. The deterioration of the airway may be very dramatic and necessitate emergency cricothyrotomy or tracheostomy as part of resuscitation. In a dire situation it is always worth fitting an LM. It is helpful to open the wound and evacuate the blood clot and this may provide temporary improvement. The patient is returned to theatre for surgical exploration. Intubation should take place with the patient breathing spontaneously, if possible. This may be by awake intubation or with inhalational anaesthesia. Blood in the pharynx may impair the view and the first response

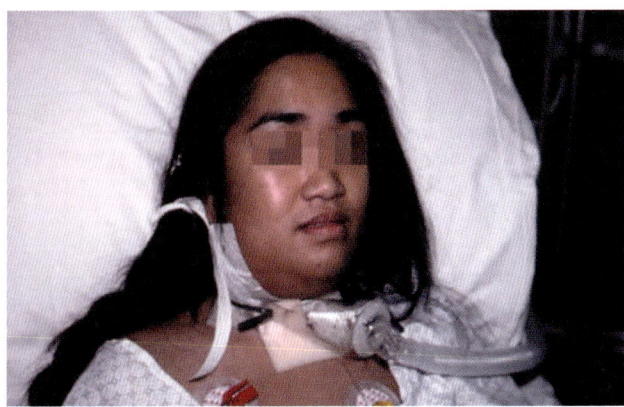

Figure 31.25 Post-extubation emergency tracheostomy.

is to try suctioning. An LM may cover the larynx and provide some respite before being used as a conduit for intubation. Emergency tracheostomy may be required. In the patient in **Figure 31.25**, drainage of a peritonsillar abscess had been undertaken with intubation by awake fibre-optic intubation. The patient had been extubated and returned to Recovery. Approximately 45 minutes later, the patient developed severe breathing difficulties and was returned immediately to the operating theatre. Awake intubation was not possible due to soiling of the airway, the patient was too restless to adopt a position suitable for formal tracheostomy and, in a deteriorating situation, the surgeon managed to carry out a rapid emergency tracheostomy.

The Difficult Airway Society have recently seen published extubation guidelines in an effort to reduce complications at extubation.[23]

FOLLOW-UP

Following difficulties with airway management, a certain scheme should be followed. An account of the problem and management should be written in the anaesthetic record and in the hospital notes. The patient needs to be reviewed clinically to detect and treat any morbidity, an explanation is required for the patient with details of the problem encountered and management, and a written account should be sent to the patient with a copy to their general practitioner.[72] If the problem with airway management is likely to be recurrent with subsequent anaesthetics, consideration should be given to the patient registering with Medic Alert and wearing a bracelet or to registering the patient with the difficult airway database supported by the Difficult Airway Society.

Immediate morbidity or mortality from difficult airway management arise from the effects of severe hypoxia, hypercarbia or cardiovascular responses, from failure to adequately protect the airway leading to aspiration and from physical trauma to the airway during attempts at intubation or resuscitation. Airway damage may occur even when airway management has not been notably difficult. Valuable information can be obtained from detailed analysis of the medical information contained in insurance reports, once claims for negligence have been settled or closed. In an analysis of such closed claims in North America,[73] 6% of 4460 claims were for airway injury. The most frequent sites of injury were the larynx (33%), pharynx (19%) and oesophagus (18%). Approximately 20% of laryngeal injuries were associated with difficult intubation and included granuloma formation, arytenoid dislocation and hoarseness. Injuries to the pharynx and oesophagus had a much stronger association with difficult airway management. Half of all pharyngeal injuries and 68% of pharyngeal perforations were associated with difficult intubation.

There were five deaths in the pharyngeal injury claims and all involved perforation and the development of mediastinitis. The oesophageal injuries involved a significantly greater proportion of females and patients older than 60 years than the other sites and oesophageal perforation involved difficult intubation in 67% of claims. Oesophageal injuries were the most severe and were associated with a poor outcome with 19% mortality. Pharyngo-oesophageal perforation is a serious condition (overall mortality 25%) and risk factors include difficult intubation, emergency intubation and intubation by inexperienced personnel. Perforation may also be caused by passage of a nasogastric tube. The triad of surgical emphysema, chest pain and pyrexia should be sought and treatment with antibiotics, limitation of oral intake and surgical review initiated as soon as possible. In the closed claims study, surgical emphysema was only evident in 56% of patients and the diagnosis was sometimes delayed. It is suggested that treatment within 24 hours improves outcome.

BEST CLINICAL PRACTICE

- ✓ All patients should undergo airway evaluation as part of pre-operative assessment.
- ✓ Strategy must cover unexpected failed intubation and failed ventilation.
- ✓ The LM is a versatile airway device and should always be available.
- ✓ Decisions about management of the obstructed airway are made by senior anaesthetists and surgeons.
- ✓ Awake fibre-optic intubation and tracheostomy under local anaesthesia should be considered in the obstructed airway.
- ✓ Maintenance of spontaneous respiration is recommended when general anaesthesia is employed in the presence of upper airway obstruction.
- ✓ Consider placement of a transtracheal ventilation catheter prior to inducing general anaesthesia in the difficult upper airway.
- ✓ Always confirm correct placement of the tube in the trachea.
- ✓ A strategy is required for extubation.
- ✓ Follow-up is important to detect and treat morbidity caused by airway management.

FUTURE RESEARCH

➤ Unified surgical and anaesthetic terms describing the location of disease pathology in the airway.
➤ Randomized comparative studies of anaesthetic techniques in management of the obstructed airway.
➤ National collection of serious adverse incidents resulting from airway management in head and neck disease.
➤ National audit of attempts at emergency cricothyrotomy.
➤ Annual publication of circumstances of death within 28 days of surgery for the obstructed airway.

KEY POINTS

- The difficult airway is an important feature in head and neck surgery.
- Difficult intubation and difficult mask ventilation are different entities.
- Evaluation of the airway is imperfect and may fail to predict difficulty.
- Airway obstruction may be acute or chronic.
- Imaging of the airway is essential, when possible, to delineate the level of obstruction.
- Airway strategy means a primary plan A and back-up plan B.
- The anaesthetic room is an inappropriate location for plan A if plan B is a surgical tracheostomy.
- Pharyngo-oesophageal perforation due to intubation attempts has a high mortality and needs early detection and treatment.

REFERENCES

1. Caplan RA, Benumof JL, Berry FA, et al. A practice guideline for management of the difficult airway. *Anesthesiology* 1993; **78**: 597–602.
2. Henderson JJ, Popat MT, Latto IP, Pearce AC. Difficult Airway Society guidelines for management of the unanticipated difficult intubation. *Anaesthesia* 2004; **59**: 675–94.
3. Cormack RS, Lehane J. Difficult tracheal intubation in obstetrics. *Anaesthesia* 1984; **39**: 1105–11.
4. American Society of Anesthesiologists Task Force on Management of the Difficult Airway. Practice guidelines for management of the difficult airway: an updated report by the American Society of Anesthesiologists Task Force on Management of the Difficult Airway. *Anesthesiology* 2003; **98**: 1269–77.
5. Levitan RM, Ochroch EA, Kush S, et al. Assessment of airway visualisation: validation of the percentage of glottis opening POGO score. *Acad Emerg Med* 1998; **5**(9): 919–23.
6. Ochroch EA, Hollander JE, Kush S, et al. Assessment of laryngeal view:percentage of glottis opening score vs Cormack and Lehane grading. *Can J Anaesth* 1999; **46**(10): 987–90.
7. Arne J, Descoins P, Fusciardi J, et al. Preoperative assessment for difficult intubation in general and ENT surgery: predictive value of a clinical multivariate risk index. *Brit J Anaesth* 1998; **80**: 140–6.
8. Langeron O, Masso E, Huraux C, et al. Prediction of difficult mask ventilation. *Anesthesiology* 2000; **92**: 1229–36.
9. Rose DK, Cohen MM. The airway: problems and prediction in 18 500 patients. *Can J Anaesth* 1994; **41**: 372–83.
10. Cook TM, Woodall N, Frerk C, and on behalf of the Fourth National Audit Project. Major complications of airway management in the UK: results of the Fourth National Audit Project of the Royal College of Anaesthetists and the Difficult Airway Society. Part 1: Anaesthesia. *Br J Anaesth* 2011; **106**(5): 617–31.
11. Schmitt H, Buchfelder M, Radespiel-Troger M, Fahlbusch R. Difficult intubation in acromegalic patients. *Anesthesiology* 2000; **93**: 110–14.
12. Khan ZH, Kashfi A, Ebrahimkhani E. A comparison of the upper lip bite test (a simple new technique) with modified Mallampati classification in predicting difficulty in endotracheal intubation: a prospective blinded study. *Anesth Analg* 2003; **96**: 595–99.
13. Patil VU, Stehling LC, Zauder HL. Predicting the difficulty of intubation utilizing an intubation gauge. *Anesthesiol Rev* 1983; **X**: 32–3.
14. Samsoon GL, Young JR. Difficult tracheal intubation: a retrospective study. *Anaesthesia* 1987; **42**: 487–90.
15. Ayuso MA, Sala X, Luis M, Carbo JM. Predicting difficult orotracheal intubation in pharyngo-laryngeal disease: preliminary results of a composite index. *Can J Anaesth* 2003; **50**: 81–85.
16. Bouaggad A, Nejmi SE, Bouderka MA, Abbassi O. Prediction of difficult tracheal intubation in thyroid surgery. *Anesth Analg* 2004; **99**: 603–06.
17. Eberhart LH, Arndt C, Cierpka T, et al. The reliability and validity of the upper lip bite test compared with the Mallampati classification to predict difficult laryngoscopy: an external prospective evaluation. *Anesth Analg* 2005; **101**: 284–89.
18. Wilson ME, Spiegelhalter D, Robertson JA, Lesser P. Predicting difficult intubation. *Brit J Anaesth* 1988; **61**: 211–16.
19. Yentis SM. Predicting difficult intubation: worthwhile exercise or pointless ritual? *Anaesthesia* 2002; **57**: 105–09.
20. Shiga T, Wajima Z, Inoue T, Sakamato A. Predicting difficult intubation in apparently normal patients: a meta-analysis of bedside screening test performance. *Anesthesiology* 2005; **103**: 429–37.
21. Rosenstock C, Kristensen MS. Decreased tongue mobility: an explanation for difficult endotracheal intubation? *Acta Anaesth Scand* 2005; **49**: 92–94.
22. Kamble VA, Lilly RB, Gross JB. Unanticipated difficult intubation as a result of an asymptomatic vallecular cyst. *Anesthesiology* 1999; **91**: 872–73.
23. Ovassapian A, Glassenberg R, Randel GI, et al. The unexpected difficult airway and lingual tonsillar hyperplasia: a case series and review of the literature. *Anesthesiology* 2002; **97**: 124–32.
24. Benumof JL. Laryngeal mask airway and the ASA difficult airway algorithm. *Anesthesiology* 1996; **84**: 686–99.
25. Popat M, Mitchell V, Dravid R, et al. Difficult Airway Society guidelines for the management of tracheal extubation. *Anaesthesia* 2012; **67**(3): 318–40.
26. Combes X, Le Roux B, Suen P, et al. Unanticipated difficult airway in anesthetized patients: prospective validation of a management algorithm. *Anesthesiology* 2004; **100**: 1146–50.
27. Mort TC. Emergency tracheal intubation: complications associated with repeated laryngoscopic attempts. *Anesth Analg* 2004; **99**: 607–13.
28. Henderson JJ. The use of paraglossal straight blade laryngoscopy in difficult tracheal intubation. *Anaesthesia* 1997; **52**: 552–60.
29. Crosby ET, Cooper RM, Douglas MJ, et al. The unanticipated difficult airway with recommendations for management. *Can J Anaesth* 1998; **45**: 757–76.
30. Stroumpoulis K, Pagoulatou A, Violari M, et al. Videolaryngoscopy in the management of the difficult airway: a comparison with the Macintosh blade. *Eur J Anaesthesiol* 2009; **26**(3): 218–22.
31. Niforopoulou P, Pantazazopoulos P, Demestiha T, et al. Video-laryngoscopes in the adult airway management: a topical review of the literature. *Acta Anaesth Scand* 2010; **54**(9): 1050–61.
32. Butchart AG, Young P. The learning curve for videolaryngoscopy. *Anaesthesia* 2010: **65**: 1145–46.

33. Minhai R, Blair E, Kay H, Cook TM. A quantitative review and meta-analysis of performance of non-standard laryngoscopes and rigid fibreoptic intubation aids. *Anaesthesia* 2008; **63**: 745–60.
34. Murphy P. A fibre-optic endoscope used for nasal intubation. *Anaesthesia* 1967; **22**: 489–91.
35. Popat M. *Practical fibreoptic intubation*. Oxford: Butterworth Heinemann; 2001.
36. Hawkins N. *Fibreoptic intubation*. London: Greenwich Medical Media; 2000.
37. Heidegger T, Gerig HJ, Ulrich B, Kreienbuhl G. Validation of a simple algorithm for tracheal intubation: daily practice is the key to success in emergencies – an analysis of 13 248 intubations. *Anesth Analg* 2001; **92**: 517–22.
38. Ovassapian A. *Fiberoptic endoscopy and the difficult airway*. Philadelphia: Lippincott-Raven; 1996.
39. Joo HS, Kapoor S, Rose K, Naik VN. The intubating laryngeal mask airway after induction of general anesthesia versus awake fiberoptic intubation in patients with difficult airways. *Anesth Analg* 2001; **92**: 1342–46.
40. Davis L, Cook-Sather SD, Schreiner MS. Lighted stylet tracheal intubation: a review. *Anesth Analg* 2000; **90**: 745–56.
41. Charters P, O'Sullivan E. The dedicated airway: a review of the concept and an update of current practice. *Anaesthesia* 1999; **54**: 778–86.
42. Atherton DP, O'Sullivan E, Lowe D, Charters P. A ventilation-exchange bougie for fibreoptic intubations with the laryngeal mask airway. *Anaesthesia* 1996; **51**: 1123–26.
43. Vanner R. Emergency cricothyrotomy. *Curr Anaesth Crit Care* 2001; **12**: 238–43.
44. Brofeldt BT, Panacek EA, Richards JR. An easy cricothyrotomy approach: the rapid four-step technique. *Acad Emerg Med* 1996; **3**: 1060–03.
45. Popat M, Dudnikov S. Management of the obstructed upper airway. *Curr Anaesth Crit Care* 2001; **12**: 225–30.
46. National Confidential Enquiry into Patient Outcome and Death. 1996/97 Report. London: NCEPOD, cited April 2007. Available from: http://www.ncepod.org.uk/sum96.htm 32
47. Woodall N. Awake intubation. *Curr Anaesth Crit Care* 2001; 12: 218–24
48. Ovassapian A, Tuncbilek M, Weitzel EK, Joshi CW. Airway management in adult patients with deep neck infections: a case series and review of the literature. *Anesth Analg* 2005; **100**: 585–89.
49. Rai MR, Parry TM, Dombrovskis A, Warner OJ. Remifentanil target controlled infusions vs propofol target controlled infusions for conscious sedation for awake fibre optic intubation: a double blind randomised controlled trial. *Br J Anaesth* 2007; **100**(1): 125–30.
50. Gold MI, Buechel DR. Translaryngeal anesthesia: a review. *Anesthesiology* 1959; **20**: 181–85.
51. Shaw IC, Welchew EA, Harrison BJ, Michael S. Complete airway obstruction during awake fibreoptic intubation. *Anaesthesia* 1997; **52**: 582–85.
52. Ho AM, Chung DC, To EW, Karmakar MK. Total airway obstruction during local anesthesia in a non-sedated patient with a compromised airway. *Can J Anaesth* 2004; **51**: 838–41.
53. Mason RA, Fielder CP. The obstructed airway in head and neck surgery. *Anaesthesia* 1999; **54**: 625–28.
54. Gerig HJ, Schnider T, Heidegger T. Prophylactic percutaneous transtracheal catheterisation in the management of patients with anticipated difficult airways: a case series. *Anaesthesia* 2005; **60**: 801–05.
55. Wee MYK. Assessment of a new method to distinguish oesophageal from tracheal intubation. *Anaesthesia* 1988; **43**(1): 27–29.
56. Goh MH, Liu XY, Goh YS. Anterior mediastinal masses: an anaesthetic challenge. *Anaesthesia* 1999; **54**: 670–74.
57. Chung DY, Tse DM, Boardman P, et al. High-Frequency Jet Ventilation under General Anesthesia Facilitates CT-Guided Lung Tumor Thermal Ablation Compared with Normal Respiration under Conscious Analgesic Sedation. *J Vasc Interv Radiol* 2014; **25**: 1463–9.
58. Pathak V, Welsby I, Mahmood K et al. Ventilation and Anesthetic Approaches for Rigid Bronchoscopy. *Ann Am Thor Soc* 2014; **11**: 628–34.
59. Sanders RD. Two ventilating attachments for bronchoscopes. *Delaware Med J* **39**; 170–76.
60. Rezaie-Majd A, Bigenzahn W, Denk D-M, et al. Superimposed high-frequency jet ventilation (SHFJV) for endoscopic laryngotracheal surgery in more than 1500 patients, *Br J Anaesth* 2006; **96**: 650–9.
61. Sütterlin R, Priori R, Larsson A, et al. Frequency dependence of lung volume changes during superimposed high-frequency jet ventilation and high-frequency jet ventilation. *Br J Anaesth* 2014; **112**: 141–9.
62. Wiedemann K, Männle C. Anesthesia and gas exchange in tracheal surgery. *Thorac Surg Clin* 2014; **24**: 13–25.
63. Hu A, Weissbrod PA, Maronian NC, et al. (2012), Hunsaker mon-jet tube ventilation: A 15-year experience. *Laryngoscope* 2012; **122**: 2234–39.
64. Rubin JS, Patel A, Lennox P. Subglottic jet ventilation for suspension microlaryngoscopy. *J Voice* 2005; **19**: 146–50.
65. Patel A, Rubin JS. The difficult airway: the use of subglottic jet ventilation for laryngeal surgery. *Logoped Phoniatr Vocol* 2008; **33**: 22–24.
66. Jaquet Y, Monnier P, Van Melle G, et al. Complications of different ventilation strategies in endoscopic laryngeal surgery: a 10-year review. *Anesthesiology* 2006; **104**: 52–9.
67. Bourgain JL, Desruennes E, Fischler M, Ravussin P. Transtracheal high frequency jet ventilation for endoscopic airway surgery: a multicentre study. *Br J Anaesth* 2001; **87**: 870–5.
68. Cook TM, Alexander R. Major complications during anaesthesia for elective laryngeal surgery in the UK: a national survey of the use of high-pressure source ventilation. *Br J Anaesth* 2008; **101**: 266–72.
69. Smith BE. High frequency ventilation: past, present and future? *Br J Anaesth* 1990; **65**: 130–8.
70. Hamaekers AE, Borg PA, Enk D. Ventrain: an ejector ventilator for emergency use. *Br J Anaesth* 2012; **108**(6): 1017–21.
71. Dysart K, Miller TL, Wolfson MR, Shaffer TH. Research in high flow therapy: mechanisms of action. *Respir Med* 2009; **103**: 1400–5.
72. Barron FA, Ball DR, Jefferson P, Norrie J. Airway alerts: how UK anaesthetists organise, document and communicate difficult airway management. *Anaesthesia* 2003; **58**: 73–77.
73. Domino KB, Posner KL, Caplan RA, Cheney FW. Airway injury during anesthesia. *Anesthesiology* 1999; **91**: 1703–11.

CHAPTER 32

ADULT ANAESTHESIA

Daphne A. Varveris and Neil G. Smart

Principles of general anaesthesia 333
Premedication 334
Anaesthetic agents 334
Devices used in airway management 336
Factors influencing choice of device in airway management 339
Conduct of anaesthesia: Principles guiding induction of anaesthesia 340
Monitoring in anaesthesia 341
Basic intra-operative monitoring 341
Anaesthetic technique: Principles for specific ENT operations 343
References 349

SEARCH STRATEGY

Data in this chapter may be updated by a Medline search using the keywords: anaesthesia, ear, nose, throat and maxillofacial, and combinations of the words. Reference lists of retrieved papers were searched manually as were reference lists of standard text (listed in the reference list at the end of the chapter).

As is the case with anaesthesia in general the evidence levels are largely from observational, non-experimental, non-controlled studies or expert opinion (i.e. levels 3 and 4), or in the case of clinical evidence from low-quality case-controlled/cohort studies or clinical series and expert opinion (i.e. grades C and D). This arises purely due to the paucity of randomized controlled trials or meta-analyses of the common questions covered in this chapter.

PRINCIPLES OF GENERAL ANAESTHESIA

Derived from the Greek 'an aesthesis' meaning 'without sensation', anaesthesia is a relatively modern speciality. In 1846, Dr William Morton publicly demonstrated the use of ether to facilitate successful ENT surgery (the removal of a neck tumour). By the early twentieth century, the importance of pain relief and reduction of the stress response in reducing mortality had been recognized. Anaesthesia has continued to evolve not only to enable surgery but also to provide organ support, patient stabilization and long-term pain relief. Based on perioperative mortality statistics, anaesthetic care is often cited as a model for its improvements with regard to patient safety.[1] High quality, low morbidity anaesthesia is tailored to individual patients and their concurrent illnesses and begins with meticulous pre-operative assessment. The role of the anaesthetist as perioperative physician continues to develop.

To facilitate surgery, modern practice seeks to deliver the 'triad' of anaesthesia:

1. Hypnosis – loss of consciousness, implicit and explicit memory
2. Akinesia – prevention of movement
3. Analgesia – obtundation of subconscious response to pain, stress and trauma.

At first a single agent such as ether or chloroform was used to achieve these aims but at perilously high doses. In contrast, modern anaesthesia tackles the triad of anaesthesia using a combination of drugs or agents to satisfy each of the aims separately. This has become known as 'balanced anaesthesia'.

In balanced anaesthesia, the 'anaesthetic vapour' (isoflurane, sevoflurane or desflurane) is used to depress cognitive function and provide the element of 'hypnosis'. This is achieved at relatively low concentrations far below

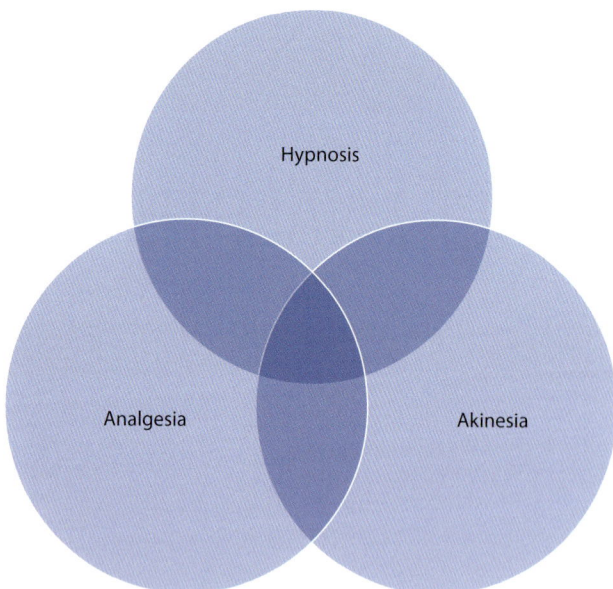

Figure 32.1 Triad of anaesthesia.

those required to achieve akinesia and analgesia and far below concentrations associated with respiratory depression and cardiovascular collapse.

Analgesia is provided by specific drugs such as the opioid fentanyl or the opiate morphine, or by supplemental use of regional or local anaesthetic blocks.

The combination of hypnotic and analgesic drugs may also be sufficient to provide akinesia and abolish movement in response to stimulus yet the patient may still breathe spontaneously. However, it may be desirable to abolish all movement and to relax the tone in all skeletal muscle, for example to facilitate endotracheal intubation or to provide good conditions for laser surgery. This can be achieved by specific drugs such as rocuronium or atracurium, which block the neuromuscular junction and paralyse skeletal muscle. When the element of akinesia is provided in this way, it is possible to reduce the doses of hypnotic and analgesic drugs yet further. So by judicious use of hypnotics, analgesics and muscle relaxants, a state of balanced anaesthesia can be achieved in which the dose of anaesthetic agent is a fraction of that which would be required if it were used as a sole agent (**Figure 32.1**).

PREMEDICATION

Premedication was originally introduced in the nineteenth century to reduce the amount of chloroform required and thereby speed the onset of surgical anaesthesia. Morphine and its derivatives were often combined with an anticholinergic antisialagogue such as atropine and this reduced patient anxiety and facilitated anaesthesia. Although now uncommon, the combination of an antisialagogue with or without an opiate can still find use prior to an anticipated fibre-optic or difficult intubation.

With the advent of quicker acting anaesthetics and the move to day surgery and same-day admission, sedative premedicant drugs have fallen out of favour. In very anxious patients, an anxiolytic may still be indicated and oral short-acting benzodiazepines such as temazepam are most commonly used in such circumstances. These need to be given approximately one hour prior to surgery.

Other premedication drugs are still commonly administered to improve patient safety and facilitate anaesthesia. For example, pulmonary aspiration of gastric contents can cause a severe pneumonitis. In at-risk patients such as those with diabetes, renal impairment, obesity or gastro-oesophageal reflux disease (GORD), H2 blockers (ranitidine), proton pump inhibitors (omeprazole), gastric alkalinizers (sodium citrate) or prokinetic agents (metoclopramide) may be used.

Paracetamol and non-steroidal anti-inflammatory agents can also be administered orally prior to surgery. These are well absorbed from the stomach and oral administration is cost-effective. Evidence that this is better in preventing pain in the early post-operative period than a similar analgesic treatment initiated after surgery, so called pre-emptive analgesia, is weak. Although widely used, care must be taken with non-steroidal anti-inflammatory drugs (NSAIDS), particularly in the elderly and in patients with dyspeptic symptoms or renal impairment. Altered platelet function and coagulation is an additional consideration in some types of surgery.

> **KEY POINTS**
>
> - Sedative premedication is seldom used in modern anaesthetic practice, especially as day-case surgery is increasing.
> - Antiemetic and antacid prophylaxis should be given pre-operatively to high-risk patients.
> - Pre-operative oral administration of simple analgesics is cost-effective but NSAIDS must be prescribed with caution in some patient groups.

ANAESTHETIC AGENTS

Intravenous agents

Intravenous (i.v.) anaesthetic agents are most commonly used to induce anaesthesia although they can also be used for maintenance. Their rapid onset of action relates to their high lipid solubility, which allows them to diffuse rapidly into the lipid-rich brain. The brain has a high blood flow and so the drug is delivered quickly to its site of action. After a single induction dose, plasma levels rise and then fall rapidly. This is not due to metabolism, but rather redistribution to other lipid-rich tissues with lower blood flows. Metabolic clearance mostly occurs after hepatic metabolism but this accounts for a much slower 'background' elimination of drug and in most clinical situations plays no part in emergence from anaesthesia.

For many years, the thiobarbiturate thiopentone dominated this class of drugs. However, by far the most commonly used i.v. induction agent in the Western world is propofol, which is a derivative of phenol. This white emulsion mixture has a rapid onset and offset as a consequence of its short context-sensitive half time so patients wake up quickly. The quality of recovery is good with a low incidence of post-operative nausea and vomiting and a quick return to street fitness. Further benefits include bronchodilation, safety in porphyria and in malignant hyperpyrexia patients, and a lack of active metabolites.

Like most anaesthetic agents, thiopentone and propofol are associated with a fall in blood pressure mediated by a number of mechanisms, including a reduction in central sympathetic vasomotor tone and cardiac contractility. These features are particularly marked in the elderly and patients who are dehydrated or hypovolaemic.

Propofol, unlike thiopentone, can also be used to maintain anaesthesia. This relates to its favourable pharmacokinetics. With a large volume of distribution (Vd), recovery occurs quickly even after prolonged infusions due to drug redistribution. Again the quality of recovery is good with a low incidence of post-operative nausea and vomiting.

Algorithms using population-based pharmacokinetic models (Marsh or Schneider) allow the delivery of propofol by target-controlled infusion and this makes administration safe and predictable.

Propofol is often used in combination with remifentanil, an ultra short-acting synthetic opioid, as part of a total intravenous anaesthesia (TIVA) technique. Remifentanil is metabolized by non-specific plasma esterases and with a context sensitive half-time of 3 minutes and elimination half-time of 6 minutes, it has minimal active metabolites. Used by infusion including target control with the Minto pharmacokinetic model, remifentanil has a short, predictable duration of action with no accumulating effect. Deep intra-operative analgesia can be achieved quickly and yet reversed rapidly. This can contribute to improved intraoperative cardiovascular stability and may also be used to negate the need for neuromuscular blocking drugs, useful when nerve monitoring is required. At the end of surgery, faster recovery and less respiratory depression are achieved in comparison with other opioids but the short duration of action means that alternative post-operative analgesia is required.[2] Remifentanil can also be used to provide sedation during awake fibre-optic intubation. By suppressing airway reflexes, it facilitates excellent intubating conditions (**Figure 32.2**).[3]

> **KEY POINTS**
> - Intravenous induction agents owe their rapid onset and offset of action to rapid diffusion across the blood–brain barrier due to their high lipid solubility.
> - Hepatic clearance is moderately slow, and does not play a significant part in the return of consciousness after a bolus dose of intravenous agent.
> - Propofol by target-controlled infusion can be used to maintain anaesthesia.
> - Remifentanil is a short-acting synthetic opioid often administered intravenously along with propofol as part of a total intravenous anaesthesia technique.

Inhalational agents

Inhalational or 'volatile' agents may be used for induction and/or maintenance of anaesthesia, although they are more commonly used for maintenance alone. The historical

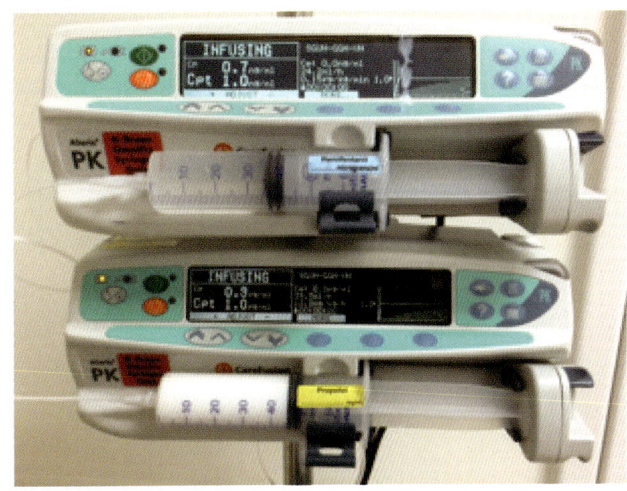

Figure 32.2 Target controlled infusion pumps for propofol and remifentanil. Pharmacokinetic algorithms calculate drug delivery taking into account patient age, weight and, for remifentanil, height.

archetype is 'ether' (actually diethyl ether), now replaced with less flammable and toxic modern agents such as isoflurane, desflurane (halogenated methyl-ethyl ethers) and sevoflurane (isopropyl ether). Like the intravenous agents, the volatile agents are lipid soluble; the higher the lipid solubility, the higher the potency. Modern agents are extremely lipid soluble and so their potency is sufficiently high to require only an inspired concentration of a few percent to induce anaesthesia. The depth of anaesthesia is determined by the partial pressure (i.e. the effective concentration) of the volatile agent in the brain. Since the brain is in equilibrium with the arterial blood, and the latter is in equilibrium with the alveolar gas, then the depth of anaesthesia should be determined by the partial pressure (or concentration) of volatile agent in the alveoli. Given that the concentration of the anaesthetic vapour in the alveoli (i.e. in the expired breath) can be measured easily, the anaesthetic depth can therefore be estimated reliably. In contrast, there is no means of doing this for intravenous agents.

Volatile agents can also be used to induce anaesthesia, and some do so more quickly than others. The rate of onset (and offset) of a volatile agent is determined by its blood solubility. It has already been stated that the depth of anaesthesia is determined by the partial pressure of the agent in the alveoli/blood/brain. In the blood, only molecules that are not in solution contribute to the partial pressure. For more soluble agents such as halothane, the rate of rise of alveolar partial pressure is comparatively slow because some of the agent is able to enter the blood in solution rather than remaining in the alveolus to contribute to the rise in partial pressure. In contrast, modern agents such as sevoflurane and desflurane have a high lipid solubility and so low blood solubility. This results in a rapid rate of rise in partial pressure in the alveolus and in the blood and brain in turn and so induction is quick. Likewise, when volatile administration is discontinued, elimination is rapid and recovery quick with an early return of airway reflexes.

Sevoflurane is preferred to desflurane for inhalational induction because of its lack of airway irritation. Desflurane has a rapid rate of recovery in prolonged cases and has an important place in some ENT procedures of long duration.

> **KEY POINTS**
> - Older agents (ether, halothane) have high solubility in blood and therefore a slow onset and offset of action.
> - Modern agents (sevoflurane, desflurane) have low solubility in blood and therefore rapid onset and offset of action.
> - Because vapour concentrations can be measured in the expired breath, adequate depth of anaesthesia can be determined with confidence.

DEVICES USED IN AIRWAY MANAGEMENT

The sections above outline the drugs that can be used to induce and maintain anaesthesia. This section examines the devices used in airway management during anaesthesia. One of the hallmarks of anaesthesia for ENT surgery is the concept of the 'shared airway'. The surgeon operates in the same anatomical region as the anaesthetic devices used to maintain the airway. Therefore, the detailed properties of the airway device selected and precise conduct of anaesthesia are particularly important to ENT surgery as compared with many other types of surgery.

The simple face mask

The upper airway is composed of a wide array of soft tissues, muscles and bony structures that modulate its patency. Induction of anaesthesia invariably causes a degree of collapse and the oropharynx behaves as a Starling resistor with airflow critically dependent on pharyngeal tone and transmural pressure.

Pharyngeal collapse is governed by a complex interplay of mechanical and neuromuscular factors but reduction in the tone of the pharyngeal dilator muscles and genioglossus is key. These muscles are innervated by the efferent outflow of the 'respiratory centre', and tone varies cyclically in much the same way as does the diaphragm under the command of the phrenic nerve. Drugs that depress the respiratory centre and have a tendency to produce a 'central' apnoea, also by this mechanism have a tendency to produce an 'obstructive' apnoea. Central and obstructive apnoeas are therefore inextricably linked and cannot adequately be categorized as separate entities.[4]

If neuromuscular blocking drugs are used, then spontaneous ventilation is abolished completely. All these factors require the use of devices that both give anatomical support to the upper airway and facilitate ventilation. Perhaps the simplest means of achieving these aims is a face mask that, when connected to a suitable supply of oxygen and anaesthetic gas, may be used to support the airway manually or (if spontaneous ventilation is absent) allow hand-ventilation of the patient's lungs. Problems with the face-mask technique include poor surgical access to the face, head or airway; it requires that one or both of the anaesthetist's hands are occupied in airway maintenance; and active ventilation of the patient's lungs can often be inefficient as not all the tidal volume administered enters the patients lungs, some being lost as a 'leak'.

Supraglottic airway devices

A range of supraglottic airway devices (SADs) have been developed which reduce some of these problems. First introduced into clinical practice as the classic LMA (cLMA), these are tubes with a distal component, often inflatable, to 'hold' the airway in place. They lie in the oropharynx, above the level of the glottis. SADs allow spontaneous breathing and, similar to the face-mask techniques, facilitate active ventilation. However, since SADs lie above the glottic opening and so do not seal it, there is a risk that positive pressure ventilation of the lungs may not always be possible with leakage of ventilating gas into the oesophagus and stomach. If gastric fluid should then regurgitate, SADs will not completely protect the airway from lung soiling. Second generation SADs such as the ProSeal, LMA Supreme and i-gel, seek to improve on the classic laryngeal mask airway to improve efficacy (airway seal) and safety (gastric access and protection from aspiratiob). These are modified with an oesophageal drain tube and structures to improve the seal with positive pressure ventilation. They have significant use in modern airway management and resuscitation; however, their value in ENT is more restricted when a 'shared' airway is required (Figure 32.3).[5]

Tracheal tubes

Tracheal tubes maintain airway patency and protect against aspiration of gastric contents. In adult anaesthesia

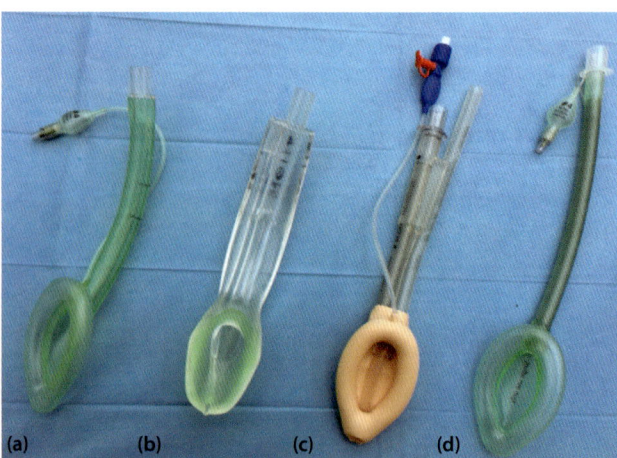

Figure 32.3 SADs (a) standard disposable; **(b)** i-gel (intersurgical) – a second generation mask with non-inflatable cuff, improved seal pressure over cLMA, and gastric vent; **(c)** Proseal – has additional posterior cuff and deeper mask. Drain tube acts as vent if regurgitation occurs; **(d)** flexible wire reinforced SAD allows tube to be moved out of surgical field without cuff displacement and is resistant to compression.

cuffed tracheal tubes are most commonly used and these are sited so that the tip lies in the trachea above the carina. To minimize the risk of late onset tracheal stenosis, high volume low-pressure cuffs are preferred and these are inflated with air (saline or methylene blue in laser surgery). The cuff improves the efficiency of ventilation by minimizing leaks and helps maintain the tube in the centre of the trachea. In addition, the airway is protected from soiling by blood coming from above in mouth, nose or laryngopharyngeal surgery and from regurgitated gastric contents.

Since tracheal tubes form a sealed conduit into the trachea, they are primarily used when the patient is paralysed and requires positive pressure ventilation (there is no risk of blowing air into the stomach). It is indeed possible to allow the patient to breathe spontaneously through a tracheal tube, but since the glottis and trachea are richly innervated, deep anaesthesia is required to prevent the patient from reflex coughing. The dose required to achieve this may lead to dose-related side effects (as described below). Whereas most SAD devices can be used effectively after relatively short periods of training, the techniques used by the anaesthetist to insert a tracheal tube are more specialized and are described in more detail in Chapter 31, 'Recognition and management of the difficult airway'.

Tracheal tubes may be passed either orally or nasally and choice of route can depend upon the type of surgery performed. For example, a nasotracheal tube better facilitates surgical access for oral surgery, but is clearly a hindrance during operations of the nose.

The shape, size and material used in manufacture are important in relation to the intended use. Preformed endotracheal tubes (ETTs), such as the Ring, Adair, Elwyn (RAE) tube, direct anaesthetic circuits away from the surgical field to improve access whilst wire-reinforced ETTs also prevent obstruction from kinking. Microlaryngoscopy ETTs are small diameter, large cuff tubes of long length (e.g. 31 cm long, 4–6 mm internal diameter) designed to optimize the surgical view on direct laryngoscopy (**Figure 32.4**).

In thyroid and parathyroid surgery the Nerve Integrity Monitor (NIM) electromyography (EMG) ETT can be used to identify and monitor the recurrent laryngeal and vagus nerves. With two integrated bipolar stainless steel electrodes on each side of the low-pressure cuffed silicone tube, it is placed in close contact with the vocal cords to allow monitoring of the EMG activity of the intrinsic laryngeal musculature. Electrode contact with the true vocal cords is important to ensure adequate response. Nerve stimulation is carried out using a sterile monopolar or bipolar probe. Both electrodes and nerve stimulators require grounding electrodes, usually placed on the sternum or shoulder. These are then attached to the NIM monitor, which produces an audible and visual electromyographic signal whenever the recurrent laryngeal nerve or vagus nerve is stimulated (**Figure 32.5**).[6]

Endotracheal tubes designed for airway laser surgery are constructed to minimize the potential damage to surrounding tissues from heat and toxins. These are further discussed below.

Regardless of which airway device is selected, it is vital that there is constant communication between surgeon and anaesthetist regarding the other's needs during surgery. The airway device must not hinder the surgical process because of its size or shape; it must be properly secured in place to prevent dislodgement during head movement by the surgeon and the direction of the airway device shaft must be appropriate to the operation. Use of surgical gags and props may compress the airway device, so the anaesthetist must be vigilant about the patency of the airway. Even with the presence of a cuffed tube, throat packs are commonly used to protect the airway from blood soiling in nasal surgery and careful removal of these prior to extubation must be ensured. Airway obstruction may occur not only during induction of anaesthesia, but also after extubation and in some circumstances it is important that the surgeon is present at extubation.

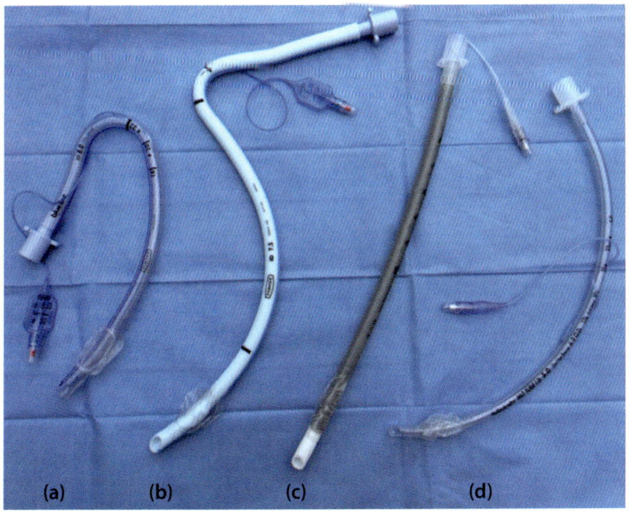

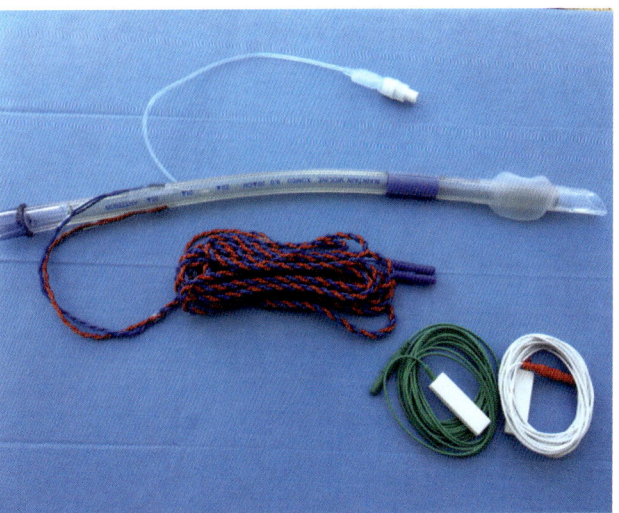

Figure 32.4 Different types of endotracheal tube. **(a)** RAE oral south; **(b)** RAE nasal north; **(c)** reinforced; **(d)** microlaryngoscopy (MLT).

Figure 32.5 Medtronic Xomed NIM tube. Two of the four exposed wire electrodes can be seen in the blue area. These come into contact with the mucosa of the vocal cords.

Jet ventilation techniques and tubeless surgery

Jet ventilation was first described in 1967 by Douglas Sanders as a technique to allow patient ventilation during rigid bronchoscopy. It improves access to the airway, particularly in laryngeal surgery, and avoids the need for an endotracheal tube. Low (LFJV) and high frequency jet ventilation (HFJV) systems are available. Both systems work on the premise that high pressure jets of gas are delivered intermittently either manually or automatically. This generates a tidal volume supplemented by the entrainment of gases at the jet nozzle. Expiration is a passive process. No volatile agents can be administered by jet and total intravenous anaesthesia is required.

In LFJV, gas exchange is achieved by direct alveolar ventilation or bulk flow. Most commonly, a hand-triggered manual jet ventilator (e.g. Sanders injector /Manujet III) is used and the lungs insufflated at a frequency of 8–10 breaths per minute to allow adequate expiration. The gas source (usually oxygen piped at 4 bar) is passed through pressure reducing valves, which can be further adjusted via a regulator to a pressure that produces the desired chest-wall movement and maintains oxygenation. It is important for the injector cannula to be aligned with the airway to improve ventilation and prevent gastric distension, particularly when placed in the supraglottic position. Ventilation may be difficult in patients with poor lung or chest wall compliance (**Figure 32.6**). End-tidal CO_2 ($ETCO_2$) is not usually monitored except when a Hunsaker tube is used.

In high frequency jet ventilation, tidal volumes smaller than anatomical dead space are delivered at supraphysiological frequencies of 1–10 Hz. Gas exchange takes place by Pendelluft, Taylor dispersion and cardiogenic mixing.

HFJ ventilators such as the Mistral or Monsoon jet ventilator (Acutronic Medical Systems) humidify and warm gas jets to minimize heat loss and reduce the likelihood of complications arising from the airway drying out. Peak airway pressures are limited by an automatic cut-out device and are lower than with LFJV but barotrauma remains a risk. Surgical conditions are very good with minimal movement of the surgical field (**Figure 32.7**).

Jet ventilation can be applied above or below the vocal cords or in emergencies via the cricothyroid membrane. The supraglottic approach allows a completely tubeless surgical field although there is greater vocal cord movement than with other techniques and a risk of blowing debris including tumour into the distal airway. It is not possible to monitor end-tidal CO_2 ($ETCO_2$) or airway pressures and there is a risk of gas trapping and barotrauma. The inspired oxygen concentration is unknown as significant entrainment occurs. The airway is maintained during the procedure by the surgeon and the quality of ventilation can be impaired by misalignment of the jet with the airway during attempts to access the operative site. Good communication between surgeon and anaesthetist is thus required to ensure adequate ventilation.

In comparison, the subglottic approach requires a narrow catheter or tube such as a Hunsaker and this may limit surgical access posteriorly. However, vocal cord movement is minimal. Furthermore, $ETCO_2$ can be monitored and with minimal entrainment of air, inspired oxygen delivery is more consistent (**Figure 32.8**).[7] Transtracheal jet ventilation can be used as a rescue technique.

> **KEY POINTS**
>
> - Anaesthesia and loss of consciousness result in reduced tone in the pharyngeal dilators and posterior displacement of the tongue.
> - The oropharynx behaves as a Starling resistor: airflow is critically dependent on pharyngeal tone and transmural pressure.
> - A variety of devices and techniques can be used to maintain the airway during anaesthesia and include the simple face mask, supraglottic airway device and tracheal tube, as well as jet ventilation.
> - Jet ventilation is useful in airway surgery to improve the surgical field but TIVA is required and high driving pressures increase the risk of barotrauma.

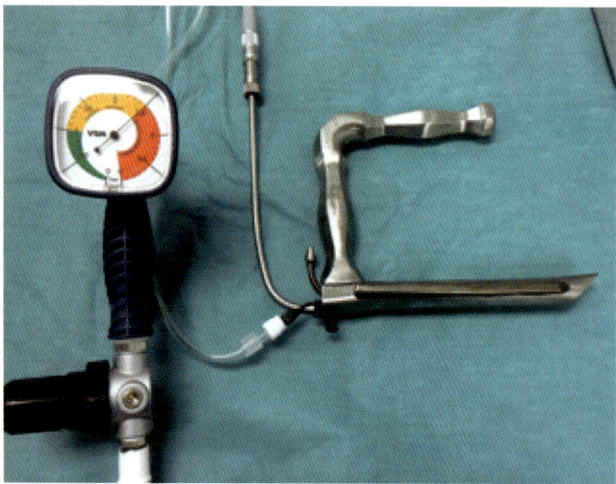

Figure 32.6 Manujet LFJV directly attached to surgical laryngoscope for supraglottic ventilation.

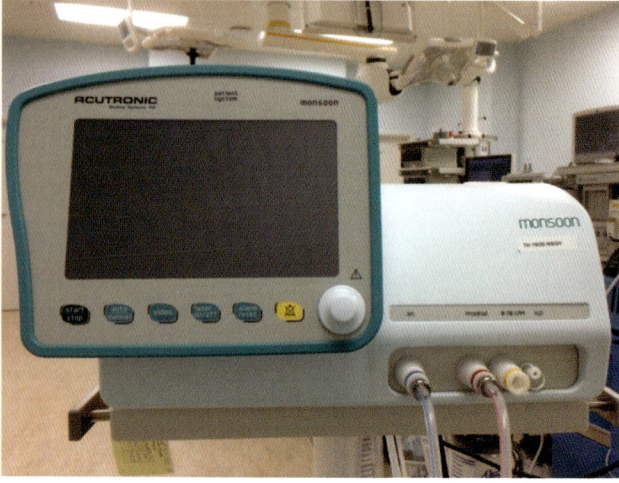

Figure 32.7 Monsoon jet ventilator Acutronic Medical Switzerland.

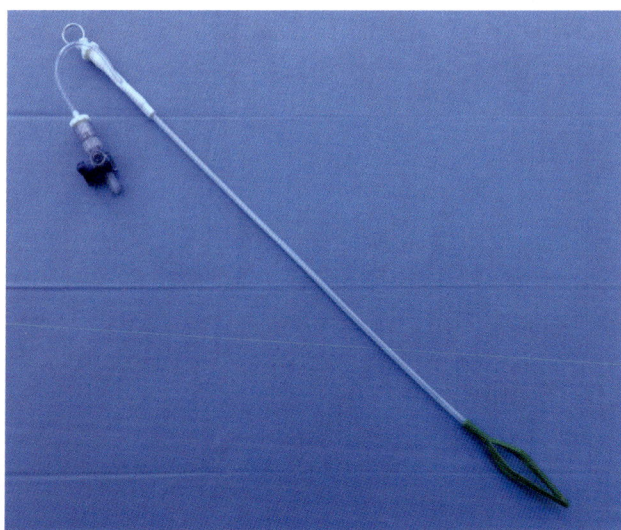

Figure 32.8 Laser safe Hunsaker tube provides self-centring, subglottic ventilation with both manual and automated jet ventilation. The jet ventilator is attached via the luer lock and there is a gas sampling lumen.

FACTORS INFLUENCING CHOICE OF DEVICE IN AIRWAY MANAGEMENT

The selection of airway device in individual patients is influenced by several considerations. In general terms, these can be divided into patient factors and surgical requirements.

Patient factors influencing choice of airway device

Of the many patient factors determining choice between an SAD or endotracheal tube, preventing aspiration, maintaining airway patency and facilitating ventilation are the most important.

GASTRO-OESOPHAGEAL REFLUX

Hiatus hernia, symptomatic reflux, pregnancy, abdominal sepsis or injury and recent ingestion of solids or particulate liquids all predispose to regurgitation of gastric contents. Endotracheal intubation minimizes the risk of subsequent aspiration and lung soiling. In high-risk cases, rapid sequence induction with cricothyroid pressure is employed to reduce the time between loss of protective airway reflexes and lung protection by inflation of the tracheal cuff.

OBESITY

Obese patients do not always find it easy to breathe when lying supine, even when awake. This results from both a reduction in lung volume and a restrictive defect. When anaesthetized, this difficulty is exacerbated and tracheal intubation is often necessary to facilitate positive pressure ventilation.

OBSTRUCTIVE SLEEP APNOEA

Closely correlated with morbid obesity, although other ENT related abnormalities of the nose, pharynx and larynx can also be the cause, obstructive sleep apnoea (OSA) is characterized by repetitive intermittent pharyngeal airway collapse during sleep. This results in obstruction of the airway, apnoea and desaturation. Anaesthesia exacerbates OSA and an airway secured with an endotracheal tube is preferred. Potential difficulties with intubation require identification pre-operatively and formulation of an appropriate management plan. Risk extends into the post-operative period following extubation.

PATIENTS WITH KNOWN OR ANTICIPATED DIFFICULT AIRWAY

In cases of known or anticipated difficult intubation where general anaesthesia is the sole option, it can be argued that it is prudent to intubate the trachea electively and so achieve a definitive 'secured airway' before surgery begins. While it is also acceptable to use a SAD device (and sometimes necessary should tracheal intubation fail), the risk remains that, should urgent tracheal intubation be necessary during the course of surgery, this might be difficult or impossible to achieve in a short space of time.

Surgical factors influencing choice of airway device

A number of surgical requirements reasonably influence the choice of airway device.

FACTORS RELATED TO THE 'SHARED AIRWAY'

As a result of the large distal cuff, most SAD devices do not permit a good view of structures distal to the oropharynx. Thus, for almost all periglottic, laryngeal and subglottic operations in which an unobstructed view of the relevant anatomy is required, a tracheal tube is preferred. A tracheal tube is also less likely to be dislodged by excessive movements of the head and neck.

SAD devices may, however, be used for operations related to the tonsils, anterior tongue, nose, teeth and ears without obstructing the surgical field. There may be reduced incidence of coughing and gagging at emergence but care must be taken to ensure the orophaynx is clear of blood to prevent soiling of the airway.

LASER SURGERY

Standard (polyvinyl chloride) tracheal tubes can ignite if struck by a laser beam and manufacturers discourage the use of unprotected PVC tracheal tubes in such airway operations. Wrapping conventional tubes with metallic tape or other materials to shield the flammable material from laser contact has also been described and this reduces the risk of combustion.

More effective protection is provided by specialized laser resistant endotracheal tubes. A number have been developed and these are manufactured from a variety of materials including metals, ceramics and Teflon. Double cuffs

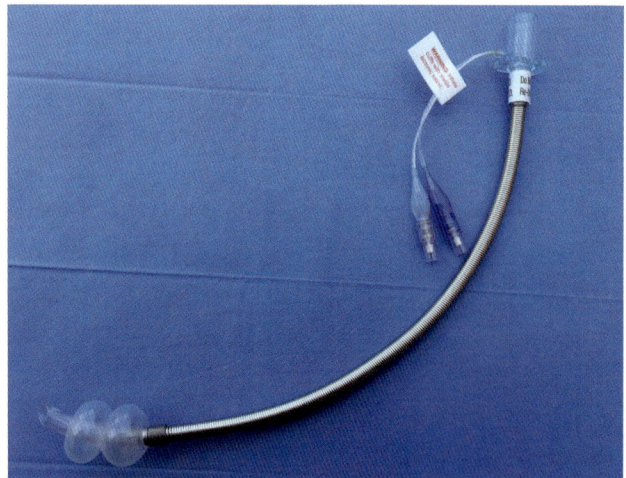

Figure 32.9 Metal spiral armoured laser tube. Note the twin cuffs, which are inflated with saline or methylene blue.

reduce the leak risk resulting from cuff damage and so minimize the fire risk resulting from an oxygen leak. None are completely laser-proof and may combust in certain circumstances (**Figure 32.9**).

The flexible wire reinforced laryngeal mask airway has also been shown to have some laser-resistance but is not used routinely. Anaesthesia for laser surgery is further discussed below.

REQUIREMENT FOR NEUROMUSCULAR BLOCKADE

Neuromuscular blockade is a reliable way of preventing patient movement, coughing and swallowing and this is particularly important for certain operations such as skull base, laryngopharyngeal, and laser surgery. With paralysis, positive pressure mechanical ventilation is required and an endotracheal tube is most commonly used to facilitate this. Rocuronium, a short acting non-depolarizing aminosteroid neuromuscular blocker, has the advantage that it can be reversed quickly and reliably with sugammadex, a cyclodextrin that encapsulates and binds the active drug. Profound muscle relaxation can thus be used for short procedures including panendoscopy.

POST-OPERATIVE PLAN

After some major operations of the head and neck the risk of post-operative swelling and subsequent obstruction is best mitigated by admission to an intensive care unit with an endotracheal tube *in situ*. Post-operative ventilation might also be necessary in the presence of certain medical conditions such as poor lung function.

> **KEY POINTS**
> - In ENT, shared airway surgery is common; a variety of airway devices exist and appropriate selection is particularly important.
> - Choice of airway device is influenced by a variety of medical and surgical factors.
> - Communication between surgeon and anaesthetist is vital.

Conduct of anaesthesia: Principles guiding induction of anaesthesia

Anaesthesia is planned taking into consideration the requirements of the surgical procedure and the comorbidities of the patient that may impact on safety. Both intravenous and inhalational induction can result in haemodynamic instability, loss of airway tone, apnoea and desaturation. Risk can be reduced with preoxygenation and appropriate monitoring.

Preoxygenation

Before induction of anaesthesia, it is common to preoxygenate by administering 100% oxygen via a tight fitting face mask for two to three minutes. Perhaps counter-intuitively, breathing 100% oxygen in this way may not increase the oxygen content of the blood. This is because for most patients, the arterial blood is almost fully saturated with oxygen even when breathing room air, so breathing oxygen cannot really improve on this. Rather, the purpose of this manoeuvre is to wash out the nitrogen-rich air within the lungs and thereby increase the mass of oxygen within the alveolar compartment. A reservoir of oxygen is created that serves to delay the rate of desaturation during a subsequent apnoea. As an alternative, four successive vital capacity breaths of 100% oxygen over 30 seconds can provide effective preoxygenation.

Intravenous induction

The commonest method of induction of anaesthesia is by intravenous administration of one of the drugs listed above but most commonly propofol. Surgical anaesthesia is rapidly induced in one 'arm–brain circulation time' and Guedel's stage 2 anaesthesia, first described using ether and associated with coughing, vomiting, struggling and laryngospasm, is avoided.

The dose of intravenous agent is guided by patient weight but should be titrated slowly according to the observed effect. Injudicious dosing can result in cardiovascular compromise and loss of spontaneous ventilation.

If there is any doubt that ventilation can be maintained post-induction, then the safety of the technique should be questioned and alternative management plans considered. The details and nature of these doubts (i.e. the ability to predict a patient who is difficult to intubate or ventilate) are discussed in Chapter 31, 'Recognition and management of the difficult airway'.

Prior to neuromuscular blockade it is not uncommon to 'check' the ability to ventilate by face mask. This precaution is predicated in the belief that if for some reason the trachea cannot be intubated, then ventilation can at least be achieved and oxygenation preserved. This practice is not universal and in the 'can't intubate, can't ventilate' group of patients neuromuscular blockade with short acting muscle relaxants such as suxamethonium or rocuronium has been advocated as a rescue route to improve mask ventilation.[8]

The Fourth National Airway Project (NAP4) recognizes the importance of a rescue plan in all patients but highlights the importance in head and neck patients, in whom 40% of the serious airway complications occurred.[9]

Rapid sequence induction

Rapid sequence induction seeks to protect the airway from soiling by minimizing the time between loss of protective reflexes and inflation of the ETT cuff. It is particularly indicated in emergency surgery where a patient may have a full stomach or in hiatus hernia with active reflux. It may also be considered where there is airway or gastrointestinal haemorrhage.

Following preoxygenation, a bolus of intravenous induction agent is administered and quickly followed with a neuromuscular blocker. Either suxamethonium or rocuronium (1 mg/kg) are used. No attempt is made to confirm that the lungs can be ventilated by face mask prior to administration of neuromuscular blocker.

As soon as consciousness is lost, the anaesthetic assistant applies 'cricoid pressure' to the larynx. A force of 40 N (4 kg weight) applied to the cricoid cartilage using the finger and thumb compresses the oesophagus posteriorly against the C6 cervical vertebral body and so prevents passive spillage of gastric contents. Laryngoscopy and intubation are now undertaken in the usual manner.

Inhalation induction

Inhalational induction is now relatively uncommon but still remains relevant in ENT practice, particularly in the management of the difficult airway. One advantage of the technique is that spontaneous ventilation is maintained. If the upper airway collapses as anaesthesia deepens and breathing becomes obstructed, then no further anaesthetic vapour can enter the lungs. The anaesthetic is redistributed during apnoea and the patient begins to wake up, thereby restoring upper airway tone and breathing. For this reason, inhalational induction has been advocated as a safe option for patients with perilaryngeal tumours and stridor. In contrast to intravenous induction, therefore, inhalational induction may be used even when there are doubts about the ability to intubate the trachea or maintain ventilation.

Inhalational induction may also be the technique of choice in patients with little cardiovascular reserve and relatively stable conditions can be provided in patients at risk from hypotension, hypertension and tachycardia.

However, there are some practical disadvantages. First, because induction is slow, there is a danger that the stage of excitability is prolonged. Second, should collapse of the upper airway occur during inhalational induction then not only anaesthetic vapour but also oxygen is prevented from reaching the lungs. Thus, inhalational induction may not be as safe or controlled as may be claimed.

In clinical practice, sevoflurane has now largely supplanted halothane for inhalational induction, its rapid onset and offset being accompanied by a pleasant smell and minimal airway irritation.

Induction after securing the airway

Certain conditions require techniques that achieve tracheal intubation with the patient awake or sedated, anaesthetic induction occurring only after the airway is secured. These methods are discussed further in Chapter 31, 'Recognition and management of the difficult airway'. Planned awake tracheostomy under local anaesthesia is an additional option.

MONITORING IN ANAESTHESIA

Derived from the Latin *monere*, to warn, monitoring is used to describe measurements whose prime purpose is to 'warn' of imminent (possibly injurious) events, and allow action to be taken to avoid them, or moderate their effect. The Association of Anaesthetists of Great Britain and Ireland publishes guidelines for minimum monitoring standards, and these are reviewed from time to time (**Figure 32.10**). Both at induction and throughout the operation, the most important 'monitor' is undoubtedly the anaesthetist who can synthesize information derived from clinical observation and specialized devices and take appropriate action.

BASIC INTRA-OPERATIVE MONITORING

ECG

Continuous ECG recording is universally used, its purpose being to detect the development of dysrhythmias and myocardial ischaemia.

The lead II configuration best displays rhythm disturbances (atrial fibrillation, heart block, asystole, ventricular tachycardia, ventricular fibrillation) while the CM5 placement best detects myocardial ischaemia (ST depression, T wave inversion).

The ECG gives no information about pump function and circulation.

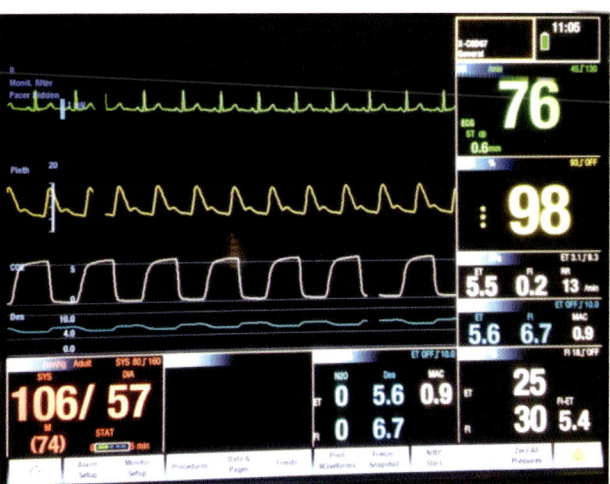

Figure 32.10 Minimal standards of monitoring; ECG, pulse oximetry, $ETCO_2$, NIBP.

Pulse oximetry

Pulse oximetry provides safe, non-invasive monitoring of arterial oxygen saturation. Based on spectrophotometry and the different light absorption characteristics of oxygenated and deoxygenated blood, these devices shine two different wavelengths of red light through an extremity (usually a finger) and measure the absorbance of transmitted light. A number of substances absorb or scatter this light, including arterial haemoglobin, venous haemoglobin, skin, bone and nail-bed. However, in addition to the background absorbance, there is a component that varies throughout the cardiac cycle, and this pulsatile absorbance is due to the added volume of arterial blood that enters during or shortly after systole. If this pulsatile signal is subtracted from the background, the resulting absorbance signal is wholly accounted for by the composition of arterial blood. The proportions of oxygenated and deoxygenated haemoglobin can then be identified and SpO_2 calculated.

The pulsatile waveform displayed on the oximeter screen also gives a beat-to-beat indication of circulation, the electronic equivalent of keeping one's finger on the pulse.

Most accurate above 90% saturation, reliability decreases at lower saturations below 70%. Accuracy is also affected by poor peripheral perfusion, electrical interference, and the use of dyes such as methylene blue.

Oxygenation rather than ventilation is measured. Hence patients breathing supplemental oxygen may still be well saturated, despite being virtually apnoeic and at risk of imminent respiratory arrest. In high-risk patients at risk of respiratory depression or obstruction post-operatively, pulse oximetry must not be relied upon to monitor the adequacy of ventilation.

Automatic non-invasive blood pressure

Automatic non-invasive blood pressure (NIBP) monitoring uses the principle of oscillotonometry applied to an inflatable cuff around the arm. These devices record blood pressure intermittently and have gained widespread acceptance because they are safe and easy to use but they do have limitations.

While the mean blood pressure measurement is reasonably accurate, the systolic and particularly the diastolic values are less so and low pressures tend to be overestimated and high pressures underestimated. Readings may be inaccurate or difficult to record in the presence of an irregular cardiac cycle resulting from a rhythm disturbance such as atrial fibrillation, or in patients who are shocked or peripherally shut down.

As blood pressure measurement is not continuous, detection of sudden changes including cardiovascular collapse may be delayed.

Invasive monitoring of blood pressure

Blood pressure can be measured invasively through a cannula sited in a suitable artery, usually the radial. This allows beat-to-beat measurement and the detection of rapid changes in real time. The morphology of the arterial 'waveform' including the rate of upstroke, pulse pressure and the presence of 'pulsus paradoxus' provides useful information on circulatory and vasotonic status. Blood gas sampling via the arterial cannula is also facilitated. Unlike non-invasive blood pressure measurement, invasive monitoring is reliable and accurate in both high and low pressure states. Disadvantages are few, but include the fact that siting such cannulae can be difficult, and the disposables are relatively expensive. There is a very small risk of unrecognized disconnection and bleeding, drug injection error, thrombosis, distal ischaemia and infection.

Oxygen analysis

It is axiomatic that oxygen is vital for safe anaesthesia. Since it is odourless and colourless, the use of an oxygen analyzer with audible alarm is vital to monitor the composition of gases leaving the anaesthetic machine and entering the patient airway. Gas is continuously sampled from the airway and a rapid gas analyzer displays the concentration of inspired and expired oxygen breath-by-breath. Most analyzers are also capable of monitoring other gases including CO_2 and anaesthetic vapours.

Inspired and expired CO_2

Inspiration of CO_2 raises $PaCO_2$ and severe hypercapnia may be life threatening, hence inspired CO_2 should be zero or near zero. Rising inspired CO_2 concentrations indicate that the patient is rebreathing exhaled breath and this usually results from a faulty breathing circuit, inadequate gas supply from the anaesthetic machine, or exhaustion of the CO_2 absorber.

The capnograph measures end-tidal CO_2 ($ETCO_2$) and is one of the most important monitors in anaesthesia. It provides robust evidence of tracheal intubation; expired CO_2 confirms endotracheal placement while the absence of an alveolar waveform is strongly suggestive of oesophageal intubation.

'End-tidal' refers to the concentration at the very end of expiration and is taken to be representative of alveolar gas. The $ETCO_2$ is therefore useful to confirm the adequacy of alveolar ventilation and identify hypoventilation and hyperventilation.

In metabolic states such as malignant hyperpyrexia and thyroid storm, a rising $ETCO_2$ on capnography can assist in diagnosis.

Capnography can also play a part in the identification of a number of cardiorespiratory abnormalities including a falling cardiac output, pulmonary embolus, and V/Q mismatch.

Inspired/end-tidal anaesthetic agent concentration

By sampling the concentration (or partial pressure) of anaesthetic vapours in the expired breath, the anaesthetic partial pressure in the alveolar gas and hence the arterial blood and brain can be estimated. This is a reliable way of monitoring anaesthetic depth because the dose-response curves (or more accurately the partial pressure-response curves) for these agents show very little inter-individual variation.

Airway pressure and tidal volume

Measurement of airway pressure and expired volume is important, particularly during mechanical ventilation. Airway pressure is influenced by the compliance (or elastance) of the lung and chest wall and by the resistance to airflow. Compliance is influenced by muscle paralysis, surgical manipulation and pneumothorax. Sudden changes in airway pressure resulting from increased resistance to airflow may result from bronchospasm, endotracheal tube displacement or compression by a Boyle Davis gag.

Temperature

Patients tend to cool during anaesthesia and inadvertent hypothermia is associated with adverse effects which include delayed wound healing, depressed immunity, increased risk of pressure sores and impaired coagulation.

Defined as a core temperature below 36°C, hypothermia develops as a consequence of:

- heat loss to the environment (cold theatre, exposed body surface/cavities, vasodilation caused by anaesthetic drugs)
- altered thermoregulation under anaesthesia
- loss of the behavioural response to cold.

Effective temperature management begins with accurate measurement. The thermistor probe is the most commonly used type of measurement device. Common sites for placement include oro/nasopharynx, tympanic membrane, rectum and bladder. Several different types of patient warming device are available for prevention and treatment and the National Institute for Health and Clinical Excellence (NICE) recommends forced air convection warming (e.g. Bair-Hugger) and the Inditherm warming mattress. Fluid warmers are of value should the administration of cold products such as blood or blood products be required.

Monitoring of neuromuscular function

Neuromuscular blockade is measured by means of a peripheral nerve stimulator, now considered essential when using muscle relaxants. Four successive supramaximal stimuli are delivered at 2 Hz, 50 mA by two adhesive electrodes placed on the skin over a convenient peripheral nerve (usually the ulnar, facial or common peroneal). With increasing degrees of block, the twitches in the train of four progressively fade. The only reliable guarantee of return of safe motor function is a train of four ratio > 0.9.

This differs from the facial nerve monitor used by the ENT surgeon, which detects microvolts of EMG activity, rather than gross movement. It is possible for patients to be moderately but adequately blocked from the anaesthetic perspective but sufficiently unblocked for safe facial nerve monitoring. The important point here is that if this approach is used, the surgeon needs to be aware of it.

The problems of neuromuscular blockade in the context of facial nerve monitoring in middle ear and parotid surgery are discussed below.

Central venous pressure/pulmonary artery wedge pressure/cardiac output/transoesophageal echocardiography

This is **not** routine monitoring, but is used where indicated by:

- the patient's pre-operative medical condition (e.g. left ventricular failure, sepsis)
- surgery that is likely to produce significant deviations in these parameters (e.g. large blood loss or compression of the mediastinum and great vessels).

The aim is to detect and correct changes in left and/or right ventricular preload, afterload or contractility indicated by changes in venous and pulmonary pressures, arterial pressure and cardiac output.

Transoesophageal echocardiography (TOE) has grown in popularity as it provides information on ventricular volume rather than pressure. Initially used mainly as a monitor of left ventricular ischaemia, it now provides real-time dynamic information about heart physiology and can be used to guide therapy in haemodynamically unstable patients

Depth of anaesthesia monitors: EEG/AEP/BIS

A number of devices that measure and process EEG signals are available for estimating anaesthetic depth during surgery. Such monitors are recommended in patients at greater risk of awareness and in patients receiving TIVA. However, data on effectiveness remains mixed and such devices should be used along with clinical observation. For patients breathing spontaneously and unparalyzed, 'awareness' under anaesthesia has an incidence of 1 : 136 000. In contrast, the incidence rises to 1 : 8000 when muscle relaxants are used. This likely reflects difficulty in detecting the early warning signs of awareness such as movement and coughing in this group.

ANAESTHETIC TECHNIQUE: PRINCIPLES FOR SPECIFIC ENT OPERATIONS

The above sections indicate broad principles used to determine choice of anaesthetic drugs, airway device, mode of induction and monitoring. We now turn to some specific operations in ENT surgery and the particular

TABLE 32.1 Considerations for anaesthesia in ENT	
Shared airway	• Communication • Surgical access • Inaccessible airway intra-operatively (head position distant to anaesthetist) • Disconnection/displacement/compression potential • Airway soiling • Hidden blood loss
Positioning	• Reverse Trendelenburg to reduce bleeding, neck extension and complications
Dental trauma	• From anaesthetic or surgical access
Laser	• Airway fire prevention
Nerve monitoring	• E.g. facial/recurrent laryngeal nerve
Post-operative	• PONV • Airway soiling • Tracheostomy care • Airway irritation (coughing) • Post-operative airway oedema

challenges posed. In general terms, anaesthesia for ENT has many unique considerations and these are summarized in **Table 32.1**.

Tonsillectomy and adenoidectomy

In adults, the most common indication for adenotonsillectomy is chronic or recurrent infection. Although tonsillitis is less common in adults than in children, it tends to be more severe and in some cases is complicated by peritonsillar abscess (quinsy). Obstructive sleep apnoea syndrome (OSA), snoring resulting from upper airway obstruction secondary to tonsillar hypertrophy and excision biopsy for suspected malignancy are also strong indications.

PERIOPERATIVE MANAGEMENT

Tonsillectomy in adults is associated with an increased risk of post-operative bleeding and pain when compared with the paediatric population.

Pre-operative consideration should include identification and assessment of OSA.

Either intravenous or inhalational induction with sevoflurane can be employed but the intravenous route is preferred in adults because hypertrophied adenotonsils can be associated with early airway obstruction and a more challenging induction.

In management of the shared airway, an endotracheal tube or reinforced laryngeal mask can be placed. A preformed south-facing RAE endotracheal tube is commonly used to protect the airway from soiling by blood and to facilitate ventilation. Secured in the midline, it is designed to point 'south' (or caudad) thereby facilitating surgical access by allowing placement in the split blade tongue depressor of the Boyle-Davis gag. A careful check of ventilation and airway pressures should be made when the gag is deployed to exclude obstruction or displacement of the tube. Alternatively, a reinforced tube with an integral metallic spiral in the shaft provides protection from external compression and kinking.

The flexible, reinforced version of the LMA is also kink resistant and with a narrower shaft than the standard LMA, provides good surgical access. In adenotonsillar hypertrophy, initial placement may be problematic but dislodgement on neck extension is rare. The inflated cuff sits around the outside of the laryngeal inlet and acts as an effective barrier to lung soiling with blood. There is no requirement for neuromuscular blockade and the device is well tolerated at emergence with a low incidence of coughing. Complications include laryngospasm and, as with an endotracheal tube, airway obstruction from the throat gag.

Neck extension is necessary to facilitate surgical access and is most commonly achieved with a pad under the shoulders. Care should be taken to ensure that the ETT or LMA has not been displaced by movement.

Opioid analgesia is the mainstay of perioperative analgesia but non-steroidal anti-inflammatory drugs and paracetamol also have an important part to play. A Cochrane database review suggests that the use of NSAIDs in tonsillectomy does not increase the incidence of bleeding but that nausea and vomiting may be reduced. Paracetamol administered orally (pre-operatively), rectally (in children) or intravenously (intra-operatively) reduces the opioid requirement. Local anaesthetic administration into the tonsillar bed has not been shown to reduce post-operative pain.

The incidence of post-operative nausea and vomiting is high without antiemetic prophylaxis and may be a cause of prolonged stay. High dose dexamethasone decreases the incidence of nausea and vomiting and may also reduce pain, although higher doses may be associated with an increase in haemorrhage.

Ketamine and dexmedetomidine have been used as analgesics but as yet their benefit is unclear and they are not in routine use.

EXTUBATION/RECOVERY

At the end of the case, the laryngeal inlet is examined under direct vision to confirm haemostasis and the oro/nasopharynx judiciously suctioned. In intubated adult patients, extubation is most commonly performed awake after the return of protective reflexes. Deep extubation reduces the risk of immediate haemorrhage by reducing coughing but is associated with a higher risk of laryngospasm. During this time, the risk of blood or secretions soiling the airway can be reduced if the patient is placed in the left lateral/head down 'tonsil position' and this should be maintained until laryngeal reflexes return.

In the post-anaesthesia care unit (PACU), oxygen should be administered until the patient is fully recovered. Opiates may be required and regular paracetamol and ibuprofen should be prescribed if appropriate. Routine observations should include pulse and blood pressure for evidence of post-operative bleeding, and respiratory rate and pain scores should also be recorded.

Variant Creutzfeldt-Jakob disease may be transmitted between patients undergoing tonsillectomy due to the presence of prions in lymphoid tissue. Single use ETTs, LMAs and either sheathed or single use laryngoscope blades are recommended to reduce the risk of cross-contamination.

The post-operative bleeding tonsil

This is a serious complication. Bleeding can occur in the first 24 hours following the operation (primary), or later (secondary). Patients with secondary bleeds frequently present between 5 and 9 days after their procedure. Management is based on **fluid resuscitation, airway protection and haemostasis at the bleeding site.** Most of the blood may have been swallowed so blood loss cannot be measured and fluid resuscitation may be required prior to theatre. Induction poses special problems for the anaesthetist due to the probability of a full stomach and a high risk of regurgitation and aspiration. A rapid sequence induction minimizes the risk. At the same time the trachea may be difficult to intubate due to the presence of blood in the oropharynx and oedema from the recent surgery. There must be good communication between the teams and the surgeon must be prepared to establish an emergency surgical airway or tracheostomy should tracheal intubation fail. At the end of the procedure, extubation should be performed awake. A prolonged stay in PACU is advisable to ensure that the bleeding has stopped.

Thyroid and parathyroid surgery

THYROIDECTOMY

Thyroid surgery is the most common endocrine surgery and is almost always elective. Indications include thyroid cancer, symptomatic goitre or failure of medical treatment in hyperthyroidism. Patients with uncontrolled myxoedema or hyperthyroidism are at considerable risk and pre-operative management seeks to achieve a euthyroid state.

In hyperthyroidism, a thyroid storm is life-threatening and function can be normalized pre-operatively with radioactive iodine ablation, antithyroid drugs such as propythiouracil, and Lugol's solution, which may help reduce iodine uptake and the vascularity of the gland. In the presence of uncontrolled hyperthyroidism, additional treatment with beta blockers in addition to steroid may be required. Increased risk extends into the post-operative period and care should continue in a high dependency unit (HDU) setting.

From an anaesthetic perspective, it is important to define the size and location of the thyroid in relation to the trachea and vascular structures. Laryngeal deviation, tracheal compression, vocal cord changes or previous thyroid or neck surgery raise the possibility of difficulties with airway management. Assessment should include diagnostic indirect laryngoscopy and CT scanning.

The vast majority of thyroidectomies are carried out under general anaesthesia using a reinforced ETT to maintain airway patency. The more recent use of intra-operative nerve monitoring requires optimal placement of a specialist silicone wired reinforced endotracheal tube with embedded or surface electrodes in contact with the vocal cords (Nerve Integrity Monitor EMG ETT – see above). This allows monitoring of the recurrent laryngeal nerve directly or indirectly via vagal stimulation. Muscle relaxation is contraindicated.

Alternatively, a laryngeal mask and spontaneous breathing allows endoscopic evaluation of vocal cord movement. Total intravenous anaesthesia may be of benefit by reducing the incidence of coughing and improving the quality of recovery.[10] However, the risk of mask displacement is high and careful team work is required.

Local anaesthesia with deep and superficial cervical plexus blocks used in combination with sedation or general anaesthesia has also been described but remains uncommon.

Post-operatively, surgical infiltration with local anaesthetic, simple analgesics such as non-steroidal anti-inflammatories and paracetamol, or weak opioids are usually sufficient to provide good post-operative analgesia.

PARATHYROID SURGERY

Primary hyperparathyroidism (PHPT) is most commonly caused by a benign parathyroid adenoma and surgery is the only curative treatment. Secondary hyperparathyroidism is a compensatory response to hypocalcaemia from another disease process and the majority of patients are managed with medical therapy, although in around 25% this is unsuccessful. Pre-operatively, symptomatic patients or those with significantly raised calcium levels require medical control with adequate hydration, diuretics and biphosphonates. Cardiac arrhythmias resulting from hypercalcaemia should be excluded.

With improved identification of the parathyroid gland, minimally invasive surgery can be performed under local anaesthesia in some patients. In more challenging cases or those with concomitant thyroid disease a general anaesthetic is required, the considerations being similar to those described above for thyroid surgery.

Hypocalcaemia is a common problem after parathyroidectomy but is usually mild and transient. In 'hungry bone syndrome' hypocalcaemia is rapid in onset and severe with associated hypophosphataemia and hypomagnesaemia. It results from sudden removal of the effect of high circulating levels of parathyroid hormone (PTH) in patients with severe PHPT and pre-operative high bone turnover. Plasma calcium levels should be monitored post-operatively to allow early detection and prompt management.

Salivary gland surgery

Salivary gland excision may be performed for tumour, stone or chronic infection. The most common procedure is complete or superficial parotidectomy and carries with it the risk of facial nerve injury. EMG monitoring may minimize this by identifying the facial nerve and its branches. Needle electrodes are placed in the orbicularis oculi and oris muscles and these detect EMG potentials generated as a result of surgical or electrical stimulation of the facial nerve. The electrical activity is converted into an audible signal, which warns of the proximity of the nerve. A functioning neuromuscular junction is a prerequisite and muscle relaxants should be avoided or used with caution. Long-acting neuromuscular blockers should be avoided altogether but it is possible to use a short-acting alternative to facilitate intubation on the premise that the effect will have worn off by the time monitoring is required. Offset of muscle relaxation should be confirmed with a peripheral nerve stimulator. Partial neuromuscular blockade does not significantly interfere with the facial EMG but the information derived may be unreliable.

Alternatively, intubation may be accomplished without muscle relaxants by administration of high doses of opioids or volatile anaesthetic agents. An infusion of remifentanil often produces good conditions for intubation and allows stable levels of anaesthesia during surgery.

The facial nerve monitor can be tested before surgery by using the peripheral nerve stimulator. A short burst of tetanic stimulation applied in front of the ear over the facial nerve produces visible muscle contractions and both visual and audible alerts from the monitor.

Laryngeal microsurgery

Direct laryngoscopy is performed for diagnostic or therapeutic purposes and may be combined with an examination of the pharynx, oesophagus or bronchial tree. Rigid instruments are used requiring the atlantoaxial joint to be fully extended and so underlying pathology should be excluded. Often, lasers are used to treat isolated lesions of the larynx.

Competition for space within the airway necessitates the use of a small size (6 mm or less) microlaryngeal tube that is sufficiently flexible and long that it does not interfere with the surgical field. If lasers are to be used an appropriate laser-resistant type is required. Alternatively, a tubeless technique using jet ventilation can be used (see above).

The operation is usually relatively short, but a severe sympathetic-mediated stress response may be provoked with up to 4% of patients showing signs of cardiovascular ischaemia post-operatively.

Laryngospasm, bleeding or post-operative airway obstruction due to oedema of the vocal cords may occur. The risk of oedema may be minimized if steroid (for example dexamethasone 8 mg intravenously) is used perioperatively.

Laser surgery

The use of laser has become widespread, especially for laryngeal microsurgery. Also used for stapedectomy, tympanoplasty, turbinate surgery and oropharyngeal surgery, there are various types of laser (CO_2, Nd:Yag, KTP) all named after the source of substrate for the laser beam and producing light at different wavelengths. Most commonly used in ENT surgery is the CO_2 laser, which can be used as a precision cutting tool or to vaporize tissue.

The neodymium-doped yttrium-aluminium-garnet (Nd:Yag) laser was introduced in the 1980s and penetrates tissue more deeply than the CO_2 laser. It can also be delivered by means of a flexible fibre-optic light cable that can be used in conjunction with a fibre-optic bronchoscope to treat lesions in the trachea and bronchi. The potassium titanyl phosphate (KTP) laser is a variant of the Nd:Yag, in which the laser beam is passed through a potassium titanyl phosphate crystal.

Airway management in laser surgery can be challenging. Aside from the underlying pathology and its impact on safe airway management, the greatest concern is the possibility of uncontrolled combustion of either tissues or extraneous materials including airway devices and surgical drapes. A fire in the airway is always serious and often fatal. Oxygen and nitrous oxide both support combustion; nitrous oxide should be replaced by air as the carrier gas and the lowest inspired oxygen concentration which maintains oxygen saturation should be used. In practice, inspired oxygen concentration is usually between 21% and 30%. A number of special laser-resistant endotracheal tubes are available.[11] These diminish but do not abolish the risk of tube fire and reflection damage to adjacent tissue. The cuffs of tracheal and SAD devices are more vulnerable to laser strike than are the shafts. Therefore, the cuffs should be filled with saline (or water coloured with methylene blue) rather than air. This protects them, to some extent, from combustion with laser strike; it slows any deflation of the cuff after strike; it aids, to some extent, in preventing spread of any fire; and the leak of fluid allows the surgeon to see that the cuff has been ruptured.

Surgical access can be improved by use of a 'tubeless' technique employing jet ventilation. This may reduce the fire risk because there is no endotracheal tube as a source of ignition. However, not every patient can be successfully ventilated by jet, and there is a risk of barotrauma including pneumothorax and pneumomediastinum. A TIVA technique is required.

Post-operatively, airway obstruction can arise from tissue oedema. This may be delayed following Nd:YAG use. Again intra-operative dexamethasone can reduce oedema as well as acting as an antiemetic.

BEST PRACTICE IN LASER SURGERY

- ✓ Direct laser strikes to the airway device should be avoided. This risk might be minimized during oral surgery if a Boyle Davis gag without the Doughty modification is used, thus protecting the shaft of most airway devices. If the Doughty modification is used, then the shaft of the airway device might be protected using damp gauze or swabs.
- ✓ The minimum power output of the laser should be used and the duration of laser strike limited. The risk of combustion increases with duration of strike at the same power.
- ✓ Eye protection for both patient and staff is important as CO_2 lasers are associated with corneal injuries and Nd:YAG with retinal damage. For patients, taping the eyes shut and then covering them with saline soaked gauze provides protection. For staff, protective goggles matched to the wavelength of light emitted by the laser are used.
- ✓ A smoke evacuator and appropriate face masks should be used especially if virus particles are present to reduce the potential risk of cross-infection.

Laryngectomy

Usually performed for tumour of the larynx, a total laryngectomy involves removal of all the tissues from the vallecula (and sometimes base of tongue) to the second or third tracheal rings. Occasionally, the thyroid gland also needs to be removed. The pharynx is closed in a T-shape, and the trachea is brought out to the skin as a stoma (so no special tube is required long term to maintain airway patency). There are variations of this operation. A supraglottic laryngectomy involves resection of all tissue from the base of tongue to the vocal cords (which are left intact). The strap muscles are also preserved. A temporary tracheostomy is required post-operatively. A hemilaryngectomy involves removal of the epiglottis and just one half of the larynx (including one true and false vocal cord).

Areas of consideration for anaesthesia include:

- pre-operative comorbidities
- tracheal intubation at induction
- change of airway device during surgery.

PRE-OPERATIVE PATIENT STATE

Laryngeal tumours most commonly occur in elderly smokers, often with coexistent cardiovascular and respiratory disease. Where possible, coexistent medical conditions should be optimized pre-operatively with particular attention to nutritional status. Intra-operatively, invasive arterial pressure, and less commonly central venous monitoring placed distant to the site of surgery, may be necessary. If lung function is poor, a period of elective post-operative ventilation in intensive care may be required.

TRACHEAL INTUBATION

The presence of a laryngeal tumour may make tracheal intubation difficult. Previous radiotherapy is also a risk factor and may make bag and mask ventilation difficult. Imaging, which may include nasendoscopy, in combination with good communication between surgeon and anaesthetist, is essential in formulating a management plan.

Specialized techniques such as awake fibre-optic intubation may be necessary and these are further discussed in Chapter 31, 'Recognition and management of the difficult airway'.

THE AIRWAY DURING SURGERY

To facilitate access as surgery proceeds, the oro/nasotracheal tube is exchanged for a tracheal tube inserted percutaneously into the trachea and shaped to lie against the neck, pointing caudally. Examples include the Montandon tube, RAE tube or reinforced flexible tube. Then when the permanent end-tracheostomy is fashioned the tracheal tube is removed. Thus, the anaesthetist needs to have ready a number of sterile airway devices, sterile connectors and tubing, which often need to be sited directly by the surgeon. Close communication is clearly necessary.

Tracheo-oesophageal puncture allows the placement of a voice prosthesis between the trachea and the oesophagus. The voice prosthesis is a one-way valve that allows air to pass from the trachea to the pharynx when the tracheal stoma is occluded, thus preserving voice, but preventing contamination of the trachea from above.

> **KEY POINTS**
>
> - Anaesthesia for head and neck surgery epitomizes the quintessential anaesthetic 'art' of airway mastery.
> - It requires a unique dialogue between surgeon and anaesthetist who share the same territory. As such it requires, perhaps more than any other branch of surgery, an understanding of, and respect for each other's contribution towards a common end.

Nasal and sinus surgery

Nasal surgery is performed for cosmetic or functional restoration of the nasal airway, and includes operations such as septoplasty (operation to the nasal septum), rhinoplasty (operation to move the nasal contour), turbinectomy or these combined. Sinus surgery is performed to eliminate infection, polyps or neoplastic conditions of the sinuses, and the goal is to provide aeration of the sinuses so that secretions can drain adequately into the nasopharynx.

Anaesthetic considerations for all these operations are similar. An oral rather than nasal airway device is necessary, usually an ETT in combination with a throat pack to collect any debris from the nose. Topical cocaine mixtures have long been used to shrink the nasal mucosa, reduce bleeding and so improve the surgical field. The intense vasoconstriction is accompanied by a local anaesthetic action that contributes to post-operative analgesia. However, mucosal surface uptake is rapid and large doses are associated with severe hypertension and dysrhythmias. Cophenylcaine (Phenylephrine 0.5% and Lidocaine 5%) may be a safer alternative,[12] but again the maximum safe dose should not be exceeded.

At the end of surgery, coughing and straining can exacerbate bleeding and smooth extubation may be challenging. The nose is usually packed so a good oral airway is essential. Swallowed blood can be an irritant and antiemetic prophylaxis should be given intra-operatively.

Ear surgery

Surgery on the external ear is performed for a variety of reconstructive or cosmetic indications.

Middle ear surgery is performed to restore hearing, eliminate infection, treat cholesteatoma and rarely for neoplasm. Outcomes have been improved by advances in technology including high magnification microscopes, enhanced imaging and improved nerve monitoring. Surgery tends to be complex, long and delicate. The principle aim of anaesthesia is to obtain a clear dry operative field by minimizing even small amounts of bleeding that could obscure the view. This can be achieved by maintaining a stable depth of anaesthesia, having a moderate degree of hypotension (without compromising vital organ perfusion particularly in the elderly) and restricting or preventing extrinsic movement caused by monitoring or patient movement.

Blood in the surgical field may arise from arterial, capillary or venous bleeding. Arterial bleeding is directly proportional to mean arterial blood pressure (MABP). Moderate controlled hypotension to achieve a MABP of 60–70 mmHg provides optimal operating conditions. Techniques to reduce the blood pressure using hypotensive agents such as beta blockers (esmolol or labetalol), sodium nitroprusside or calcium channel blockers have in general been superseded by the use of short acting opioid agents. Remifentanil is an effective and titratable hypotensive agent during ear surgery.[13]

Capillary bleeding depends on local flow in the capillary bed, which in turn is dependent on upstream arterial pressure and downstream venous tone, in addition to local metabolic factors. Capillary bleeding can be moderated by the use of locally infiltrated adrenaline (although the systemic effects of this will transiently confound the anaesthetist's attempts to control blood pressure) and by reduction in arterial and venous partial pressure of carbon dioxide (PCO_2) by hyperventilation.

A reduction in venous tone and backpressure will reduce both capillary and venous bleeding. Venous tone can be moderated by the use of intravenous nitrates, and a 25° head uptilt can reduce the hydrostatic venous pressure.

The surgical approach is often a post-auricular route through the mastoid. The head must be turned so that the ear on which the operation occurs is uppermost. Unlike most other ENT procedures, the airway is not 'shared' and so anaesthetic rather than surgical considerations predominate in choice of airway. Access may be difficult intra-operatively and so tracheal intubation using a south facing ETT and IPPV ventilation is commonly employed. A flexible SAD is an alternative and may reduce coughing at emergence. However, there is a greater risk of displacement, particularly if controlled ventilation is required to prevent hypoventilation.

Facial or cranial nerve monitoring may be required and the use of muscle relaxants is best avoided post-induction. Smooth emergence and prevention of post-operative nausea and vomiting are important to prevent graft failure.[13]

Where tympanoplasty, tympanomeatal flaps, stapedotomy or stapedectomy is performed it is advisable to avoid nitrous oxide. Due to its relative solubility, nitrous oxide enters the middle ear cavity at a rate faster than nitrogen (the ambient gas in the air) leaves the space. Consequently, there is a rise in middle ear pressure that can displace the structures being operated on. Care must be taken to prevent extensive head turning and to protect the eyes from corneal abrasions.

Myringoplasty, mastoidectomy and stapedectomy are increasingly carried out as day surgery procedures and TIVA is commonly used. Advantages include improved cardiovascular stability, decreased post-operative nausea and vomiting and a short recovery time. Post-operative pain is relatively low and is well managed with paracetamol and NSAIDs except in the mastoidectomy group when opioid analgesia is required. Routine use of antiemetic prophylaxis with dexamethasone and a 5HT3 antagonist is advisable.

KEY POINTS

- Care should be taken when positioning patients for ear surgery.
- Moderate hypotension may help to reduce bleeding in the surgical field.
- Short acting opioids such as remifentanil allow greater control of cardiovascular stability and facilitate moderate hypotension.
- Hypotension should be limited in patients with uncontrolled hypertension, cerebrovascular or ischaemic disease.

FUTURE RESEARCH

Looking into the future, several new issues are emerging.

The imperatives of improving quality of care, reducing length of stay and limiting the physiological impact of surgery so that return to 'normal' is rapidly achieved provide significant drivers for change.

Current IV anaesthetic agents have limitations. To address the broadening agenda, new drugs based on etomidate, benzodiazepines and propofol are under development

In the search for a hypnotic agent with pharmacokinetic properties similar to remifentanil, methoxycarbonyl etomidate showed initial promise. This has an ester moiety which is very rapidly hydrolyzed by plasma esterases but potency is low and therefore large amounts are required. To overcome these limitations, other spacer linked etomidate esters are under development and these are more potent and metabolized more slowly.

Remimazolam is a benzodiazepine that acts on gamma-aminobutyric acid (GABA) receptors but has organ dependent metabolism similar to remifentanil. Following prolonged infusions, residual effects are minimal. Preliminary data suggest that it has potential for sedation in theatre and ITU.

Fospropofol is a prodrug of propofol. Unlike propofol, it is water-soluble and benefits include less pain at the site of intravenous administration, less potential for hyperlipidemia with prolonged administration, and a reduction in the incidence of bacteraemia. Slower in onset than propofol, further research is needed to establish an appropriate role for fospropofol in sedation, anaesthesia and the management of the critically ill.

The search for new drugs that minimize or treat post-operative nausea and vomiting (PONV) is also important. PONV is a significant cause of patient distress and effective management not only improves quality of life but also reduces costs by reducing delayed discharge from hospital. Neurokinin-1 receptor antagonists such as aprepitant were originally developed for chemotherapy-induced nausea and vomiting. When used in surgery, aprepitant may decrease the incidence of vomiting by 70–80% and has similar efficacy against nausea and greater efficacy against vomiting compared with other commonly used antiemetics. Administered orally, its expense currently limits its use to high-risk patients. An intravenous preparation is also available.

Outwith the development of novel drugs in anaesthesia, recent advances in airway management have seen the introduction of videoscopes such as Airtrach and McGrath. These have reduced the requirement for expensive fibre-optic techniques, which also require considerable training and expertise. Further development of equipment for the management of the difficult airway in head and neck surgery that is low-cost and requires minimal expertise remains desirable. However, developing such devices or techniques will require far more understanding of the reasons underlying the concept of the 'difficult airway' than we have at present.

Beyond the more technical aspects of anaesthesia described above, attention is turning towards the dramatic variation in patient outcomes for major surgery between different centres. Although harm directly attributable to the conduct of anaesthesia is rare (less than 1 : 50 000 mortality), these differences have spurred interest in the role of the anaesthetist as perioperative physician. Stretching across the care pathway, from pre-operative optimization to intra-operative management, which includes measures to reduce post-operative side effects and into the post-operative management of pain and identification and treatment of early complications, the changing contribution of the anaesthetist may well be an important driver of future improvement.

KEY POINTS

- Anaesthesia for ENT surgery requires constant communication and cooperation between anaesthetist and surgeon. The pre-operative surgical brief is particularly important in planning management to achieve a satisfactory outcome.
- Anaesthetic technique must balance safe airway management with surgical requirements such as nerve integrity monitoring, difficult access requiring a tubeless field or laser surgery.
- In patients undergoing head and neck surgery, the complications associated with a 'shared airway', positioning of the patient to facilitate surgery and the high risk of dental trauma should be considered.

Tonsillectomy and adenoidectomy

- Evidence supports the use of either endotracheal tube or laryngeal mask airway and the choice is one of operator preference.

- The post-operative bleeding tonsil is a serious complication which poses special problems for the anaesthetist due to the probability of a full stomach and obscured laryngoscopy.

Ear surgery

- A stable depth of anaesthesia, moderate hypotension without compromising vital organs perfusion particularly in the elderly may help to reduce bleeding in the surgical field.
- Best practice during laser surgery should be maintained at all times to ensure patient and staff safety.

REFERENCES

1. Bainbridge D, Martin J, Arango M, Cheng D. Evidence-based Peri-operative Clinical Outcomes Research (EPiCOR) Perioperative and anaesthetic-related mortality in developed and developing countries: a systematic review and meta-analysis. *Lancet* 2012; **380**(9847): 1075–81.
2. Komatsu R, Turan AM, Orhan-Sungur M, et al. Remifentanil for general anaesthesia: a systematic review. *Anaesthesia* 2007; **62**(2): 266–80.
3. Vennila R, Hall A, Ali M, et al. Remifentanil as single agent to facilitate awake fibreoptic intubation in the absence of premedication. *Anaesthesia* 2011; **66**(5): 368–72.
4. Farmery AD. Physics and physiology. In: Calder I, Pearce A (eds). *Core topics in airway management*. Cambridge: Cambridge University Press; 2011, pp. 19–27.
5. Cook TM, Howes B. Supraglottic airway devices: recent advances. *Contin Educ Anaesth Crit Care Pain* 2011; **11** (2): 56–61.
6. Julien N, Mosnier I, Bozorg Grayeli A, et al. Intraoperative laryngeal nerve monitoring during thyroidectomy and parathyroidectomy: a prospective study. *Eur Ann Otorhinolary* 2012; **129**(2): 69–76.
7. Evans E, Biro P, Bedforth N. Jet ventilation. *Contin Educ Anaesth Crit Care Pain* 2007; **7** (1): 2–5.
8. Broomhead RH, Marks RJ, Ayton P. Confirmation of the ability to ventilate by facemask before administration of neuromuscular blocker: a non-instrumental piece of information? *Br J Anaes* 2010; **104**; 313–17.
9. Cook T, Woodall N, Frerk C. Major complications of airway management in the UK: results of the Fourth National Audit Project of the Royal College of Anaesthetists and the Difficult Airway Society. Part 1: Anaesthesia. *Br J Anaes* 2011; **106** (5): 617–31.
10. Lee W, Kim M, Kang S, et al. Type of anaesthesia and patient quality of recovery: a randomized trial comparing propofol–remifentanil total i.v. anaesthesia with desflurane anaesthesia. *Br J Anaes* 2015; **114** (4): 663–68.
11. Lai HC, Juang SE, Liu TJ, Ho WM. Fires of endotracheal tubes of three different materials during carbon dioxide laser surgery. *Acta Anaesthesiol Sin* 2002; **40**(1); 47–51.
12. Smart NG, Hickey S, Nimmo A. Head neck and airway blocks. In: McLeod G, McCartney JA, Wildsmith JAW (eds). *Wildsmith and Armitage's principles and practice of regional anaesthesia*. 4th ed. Oxford: Oxford University Press; 2013, pp. 201–08.
13. Degoute CS, Ray MJ, Manchon M, et al. Remifentanil and controlled hypotension; comparison with nitroprusside or esmolol during tympanoplasty. *Can J Anaesth* 2001; **48**(1): 20–27.

CHAPTER 33

ADULT CRITICAL CARE

Robert I. Docking and Andrew Mackay

Introduction 351	Death and dying in ICU 358
Organ support 352	References 359
The interface between critical care and ENT 356	

SEARCH STRATEGY

Data in this chapter may be updated by a PubMed search using the keywords: critical care, sepsis, ventilation and organ support.

INTRODUCTION

The development of modern critical care started during the polio epidemic of the 1950s, when the need to deliver positive pressure ventilation on a widespread scale encouraged the design and production of ventilators that allowed the continuation of ventilation into the post-operative period. This facility allowed surgeons to undertake more invasive and complicated procedures that would be impossible without an option for extending recovery (ruptured aneurysms, cardiothoracic surgery), and the experience gained was then used to improve the support of critically ill medical patients.

Modern critical care units are now essential to the function of any acute hospital, with resources including equipment, medical and nursing staff as well as ancillary support including physiotherapy and outreach teams. Traditionally in the UK, medical staffing has originated from anaesthesia, but the recent establishment of the Faculty of Intensive Care Medicine has led to creation of an independent specialty that allows doctors from a wide range of disciplines to complete training as critical care specialists.

Normally a high dependency unit (HDU) would care for Level 1 and Level 2 patients (**Box 33.1**), whereas an intensive care unit (ICU) would take in Level 2 and Level 3 patients. A national trend towards specialization and centralization of specialist and tertiary services has led to consolidated critical care areas, based on the premise that caring for higher volumes of patients leads to improved outcomes through refinement of processes and more rapid cycling of quality improvement measures. This has led to larger units with a broader spread of intensity from patients with simple post-operative analgesia requirements such as an epidural catheter to patients receiving multiple modes of organ support. Having units with such diverse intensity, or a geographically close HDU/ICU setup means that 'stepping up' and 'stepping down' as the clinical case evolves is easier and more efficiently done.

Critical care is truly a multidisciplinary specialty. The medical and nursing teams should be trained specifically in critical care, and be supported by the referring teams for specific issues. Critical care units will also have

---

BOX 33.1 Definitions

In 2000 the United Kingdom Department of Health authored a document, *Comprehensive Critical Care*, which sought to classify critical care as to the intensity of care delivered:

- **Level 0:** Patients whose needs can be met through normal ward
- **Level 1:** Patients at risk of their condition deteriorating or with higher levels of care whose needs can be met on advice and support from the critical care team
- **Level 2:** Patients requiring more detailed observation or intervention, single failing organ system or post-operative care, and higher levels of care
- **Level 3:** Patients requiring advanced respiratory support alone or basic respiratory support together with support of at least two organ systems. This level includes all complex patients requiring support for multi-organ failure

significant requirements for physiotherapy, nutrition, microbiological and laboratory input. The medical staff should have no competing commitments during their time working in the unit, and should be easily accessible both to referring teams and the nursing staff. The lead clinician should spend the majority of their time in the critical care environment, and be able to take an overview of the issues confronting the unit. In terms of physical environment, the unit should have the space to safely look after patients, with suitable distance between beds to minimize cross-infection rates and facilitate patient care and procedures.

The management of critical care has been subject to several models. To illustrate differing approaches one may look at 'open' versus 'closed' models of care. The open model allows all admission and treatment decisions to be made by the referring specialties, with the critical care team providing only the procedural and nursing input as outlined by the referrer. This is difficult to support as continuity of care is hard to maintain, and treatment decisions can be delayed and potential harm incurred. The closed model sees all decisions made by the critical care team, often without reference to the originating parent team. While this aids continuity and speeds decision-making time, it can lead to professional friction and barriers and removes the valuable knowledge resource of the referring team when it comes to specialist input. A more cohesive approach aims to involve referring teams in the ongoing care of their patients, but with clear boundaries regarding the decision-making process.

The decision to admit a patient to critical care is often a challenging one, made after consultation with the patient, their family and their parent team. However, the nature of critical illness is such that often many of the discussions that would be useful are impossible to pursue in the available time period. Admission to critical care should only be made when there is a potential for reversal of pathology/organ failure, and with an assessment as to whether the burden of treatment is acceptable for the patient. A stay in critical care carries with it substantial physical and psychological ramifications, with recovery to a similar pre-morbid level often taking a year or more following hospital discharge. This must therefore inform part of the decision-making process prior to and during an admission to critical care.

Scoring systems

Illness severity scores are widely used in the critical care environment to predict outcome, assess organ dysfunction and analyse use of resources. The multitude of scoring systems that have been developed support the fact that there is no single gold standard; each system will have individual merits and a composite of these scores is likely to be most useful. Scoring systems in ICU can be broadly divided into:

- scores that assess disease severity at point of admission in an attempt to predict outcome (Acute Physiology and Chronic Health Evaluation (APACHE), Simplified Acute Physiology Score (SAPS), Mortality Probability Model (MPM))
- scores that assess the presence and severity of organ dysfunction (Multiple Organ Dysfunction Score (MODS), Sequential Organ Failure Assessment (SOFA))
- scores that assess nursing workload use (Therapeutic Intervention Scoring System (TISS)).

The most commonly used system is APACHE-II. The original APACHE score was described in 1981 and scored both physiological derangement of the acute illness and an assessment of chronic health. APACHE-II was a refinement of the original with fewer physiological variables, each scored on the most deranged value in the first 24 hours, combined with age and chronic health evaluation to give a score of up to 71, which is then combined with admission diagnosis to give a predicted mortality.[1] Although on an individual basis scoring systems have little value, as ICU survival is a binary outcome, the score permits population studies and objective comparison of outcomes between patient groups or even different units.

ORGAN SUPPORT

The fundamental approach of critical care is diagnosing the cause of illness, and direct efforts to treat the underlying cause while providing appropriate organ support until such point that the patient's intrinsic organ function returns. Multiple negative trials of 'magic bullet' interventions (Activated Protein C, TNF-alpha antagonists, steroid use for septic shock) have reinforced the need for reliable and safe implementation of relatively uncomplicated modes of support, and the introduction of 'bundle' approaches to help clinicians achieve the reliability that is required in the high-risk critical care environment.

At all times the progress of the patient should be considered, and if improvement is either slow or absent then alternative diagnoses should be investigated. A failure to improve at an expected time course is often a sign that either the wrong diagnosis has been made, or that the severity of the illness has been underestimated. Complications often have differing implications depending upon the diagnosis. For example, atrial fibrillation in the setting of pneumonia is a sign of disease severity whereas following an oesophagectomy it may suggest an anastomotic leak with mediastinitis and therefore the investigation and treatment of the same arrhythmia will differ significantly.

Respiratory support

For many, the provision of respiratory support is the defining element of critical care. There has been a rapid increase in the range, variety and nomenclature of modes of both non-invasive and invasive ventilation in the last decade, but the fundamental aim remains the same: to augment oxygenation and to clear carbon dioxide while limiting iatrogenic harm.

The provision of intensive ratios of nursing care means that critical care units are the only places outwith theatre where prescribed oxygen therapy can be reliably and accurately provided. Humidification of delivered gases reduce the toxic drying effects of high flow gas, and allied to regular physiotherapy help mobilization of secretions and reversal of atelectasis.

The classification of respiratory support suffers from a variety of differing nomenclature, driven by both clinicians and manufacturers. Table 33.1 separates those that require tracheal intubation, and those that do not:

Institution of invasive respiratory support carries with it both benefits and risks. It reduces or eliminates the work of breathing, which reduces patient discomfort and oxygen consumption, and allows access to the lower respiratory tree for clearance, suction and reinflation. However, it usually requires sedation, bypasses the usual defence mechanisms of the upper airways and equally opens the lower respiratory tree up to damage by excesses of pressure, volume and infection – so-termed ventilator induced lung injury (VILI).

Weaning off respiratory support is the process whereby support is gradually reduced to the point where the patient can breathe unaided. There is little to support one way of doing this over another, but it generally takes the form of establishing a spontaneous mode of ventilation then reducing the support until extubation can occur. For any weaning process to be successful, several things need to have occurred:

- The underlying diagnosis needs to have been appropriately treated.
- The patient needs an adequate respiratory drive.
- Any source of pain needs to be identified and controlled.
- The patient needs a reasonable cough and swallow mechanism.

Predicting successful extubation is not an exact science, but reintubation is associated with poorer outcomes in critical care. Whether this is associative or causative is more difficult to ascertain. The use of non-invasive ventilation as a treatment for failed extubation is difficult to support, unless there is strong evidence of chronic obstructive pulmonary disease in which case extubating straight to non-invasive ventilation is an option. In all but this subset there seems to be an excess mortality associated with non-invasive 'rescue', most probably due to delaying reintubation and loss of reserve.

Acute respiratory distress syndrome (ARDS) is a clinical and pathological diagnosis that is the common final pathway of many disparate pulmonary and extra-pulmonary conditions, typified by bilateral diffuse airspace oedema, without overt ventricular failure, and resultant hypoxaemia. The current consensus criteria[2] are:

- acute onset, <1 week after insult
- bilateral widespread radiological infiltrates unexplained by other pathology
- no clinical signs of LV failure or fluid overload
- hypoxaemia, with a PaO_2/FiO_2 ratio of <40 for mild ARDS, <27 for moderate ARDS and <13 for severe ARDS.

The treatment of ARDS can exacerbate the underlying disease process by using harmful techniques to try and 'normalize' physiological parameters. Many therapies have been tried, but the best evidence supports relatively simple interventions including 'lung protective ventilation', a strict attention to management of fluid balance and early treatment of infection. The best evidence for ventilation comes from the ARDSnet RCT from 2000,[3] which compared a ventilatory strategy that aimed to normalize blood gas values with high tidal volumes and pressures (12 ml/kg tidal volume and plateau airway pressures of <50 cmH$_2$O) and a low volume strategy (6 ml/kg tidal volume and pressures of <30 cmH$_2$O). This large RCT was stopped early due to a mortality reduction of 8.8% in the low volume group, and this has formed the central tenet of modern ventilatory strategy for ARDS.

The realization that ventilation can exacerbate, prolong and worsen the pathophysiological effects of critical illness has led to a renewed interest in alternative treatment strategies, particularly extracorporeal membrane oxygenation (ECMO). This approach of using an extracorporeal circuit to oxygenate and remove carbon dioxide from blood has evolved from cardiopulmonary bypass techniques, and has been well established in the neonatal and paediatric critical care environment. A protagonist-driven RCT from the UK,[4] randomizing patients with severe ARDS to management in their hospital of origin, or transfer to a centre for consideration of ECMO showed a small but significant reduction in mortality or disability.

TABLE 33.1 Classification of respiratory support

Non-invasive		Invasive
Variable performance devices (concentration depends on effort/rate)	• Nasal cannulae • Hudson masks • Non-rebreathing 'trauma' masks	• Spontaneous modes (CPAP, ASB, APRV) • Mandatory modes (VCV, PCV) • Mixed modes (SIMV, BIPAP, ASV)
Fixed performance devices (concentration is independent of effort/rate)	• Venturi masks • High-flow nasal oxygen	
Pressure delivery devices	• Continuous pressure airway pressure masks (CPAP) • Bilevel airway pressure masks (NIV, NIPPV, BiPAP)	

This was published during an H1N1 influenza pandemic that resulted in a large number of young critically hypoxic patients presenting to critical care, and encouraged the formation of regional specialist centres where ECMO can be used to reduce iatrogenic lung damage. The circuits require the use of significant anticoagulation and there are appreciable complications involving spontaneous bleeding, albeit in a patient group with a high predicted mortality.

Cardiovascular support

The primary function of the heart is to deliver oxygen to tissues, which requires a flow from the lungs, through the left heart and on to the peripheral tissues. At that point uptake can be blocked on a cellular or mitochondrial level, but generally the aim of critical care cardiorespiratory support is to increase tissue oxygen delivery.

As can be seen from the equations in **Box 33.2**, increasing oxygen delivery can be achieved in a number of ways, including using fluid challenges, vasoactive drugs, transfusion of blood and optimizing oxygenation. Choosing which of these methods to use, and how to assess the efficacy of the chosen intervention is an ongoing source of debate in the critical care community.

Commonly used ways of assessing both inadequate oxygen delivery and the response to treatment include: trends in serum lactate as a marker of anaerobic metabolism; central venous oxygen saturation as an index of oxygen extraction; and more basic methods like peripheral warmth and capillary refill time.

In the past extrapolation of the use of pulmonary artery catheters (PACs) in high-risk surgical patients led to the widespread use of PAC as cardiac output monitoring in the majority of critical care patients.[4] Following a prospective trial,[5] and large retrospective database analyses, no evidence for benefit was found and significant numbers of procedure-related complications have resulted in far lower rates of use. Less invasive cardiac output monitors have been introduced to the market with reasonable concordance with PAC-derived values, but there remains a lack of evidence that their use improves outcome. The modes vary in their alleged benefits as detailed below, but can give trending values of most haemodynamic variables. Some of these are directly measured but many are calculated using a variety of assumptions based on normative data that may or may not be true in the critically ill patient. A summary of the available cardiac monitors can be seen in **Table 33.2**.

In terms of the drugs used to aid the cardiovascular system during critical illness, the majority are related to the catecholamine family and increase sympathetic tone. Unlike in theatre where intermittent boluses are given, most patients receiving vasoactive drugs will receive them as continuous infusions with nursing staff adjusting dosage in response to monitored variables. Alpha agonists like noradrenaline predominantly produce increased vascular tone and therefore raise blood pressure, while beta agonists like dobutamine or adrenaline increase myocardial contractility and heart rate and thus increase cardiac output directly. Catecholamines all increase myocardial oxygen consumption, and have diverse effects including modulation of the immune response, glycaemic metabolism and gut blood flow.

BOX 33.2 Increasing oxygen delivery

$DO_2 = CO \times CaO_2$

$CO = HR \times SV$

$CaO_2 = (Hb \times 1.34 \times SaO_2) + (0.003 \times PaO_2)$

Abbreviations: DO_2 = oxygen delivery; CO = cardiac output; CaO_2 = arterial oxygen content; HR = heart rate; SV = stroke volume; Hb = haemoglobin; SaO_2 = arterial oxygen saturation; PaO_2 = dissolved arterial oxygen tension

---

TABLE 33.2 Cardiac output monitors

	Mode of action	Strengths	Weaknesses
Pulmonary artery catheter	Inserted as a central line, measures thermodilution in pulmonary circulation, Fick principle	• 'Gold standard' • Direct measurements of flow and pressure	• Invasive • Potential complications include PA rupture • Infections
Oesophageal Doppler	Nasal Doppler probe that measures blood flow in thoracic aorta	• Easy to insert • Few complications	• Prone to movement and measurement artefact • Poorly tolerated unless deeply sedated
LiDCO	Pulse contour analysis of arterial line, calibrated with transpulmonary lithium dilution	• Easy to use • Does not require central access	• May not respond accurately to interventions • Inaccurate with dysrhythmias
PiCCO	Pulse contour analysis of arterial line, calibrated with transpulmonary thermodilution	• Relatively easy to use • Large number of displayed variables	• Requires central access and modified arterial line • Inaccurate with dysrhythmias
Echocardiography	Ultrasound examination of heart and great vessels, either trans-thoracic or trans-oesophageal	• Direct visualization • Able to diagnose cause of low/high cardiac output	• User dependent • Interpretation variable • Intermittent observation

Fluids

In the early stages of a critical care admission there is often the need for large volume fluid resuscitation, either to correct overt hypovolaemia or relative underfilling in vasodilated states like sepsis. The debate as to what is the ideal replacement fluid is ongoing, as is the debate as to how to assess response to therapy.

In terms of fluid type, both crystalloid and colloids are available for use. Crystalloids have a better safety profile in terms of anaphylaxis and cost less, but larger volumes may be required to produce an equivalent response. The disparity between the two is probably far less than the previously quoted 3:1 ratio, and crystalloids seem to have less of a deleterious effect upon the glycocalyx of the basement membrane than colloids. Use of balanced 'physiological' solutions is on the rise, as non-physiological solutions like 0.9% NaCl being linked to hyperchloraemic acidosis and impaired renal function.

Colloids are solutions with polymers suspended within them. Examples include gelatins like Gelofusin, starches like Voluven and non-synthetic colloids like human albumin solution. Many fluid optimization papers have used colloids for their bolus regimes, but concerns over safety have led to the decline of colloid use and withdrawal of starches from the European market.

After the initial resuscitation period fluid requirements revert to basal needs. These needs can be met by intravenous fluid, gastric feed and drugs. Patients on multiple antibiotics and drug infusions can receive over 2 L of fluid a day from drugs alone, and without a watchful eye on fluid balance can become cumulatively overloaded. Positive fluid balance during a critical care stay has a strong association with poorer outcomes and although causation is harder to prove, avoiding fluid overload in the post-resuscitation phase is a worthwhile aim. In the case of ARDS, a restrictive fluid therapy regime improved gas exchange, shortened duration of ventilation and had no harmful effects on renal function.[6] Conversely, positive fluid balance has been shown to worsen outcomes in acute kidney injury although this again may well be indicative of disease severity.

Renal support

The development of renal failure in critical care is usually multifactorial, with sepsis as the most common aetiology. The degree of failure can be quantified by looking at changes in serum creatinine or urine output with the RIFLE or AKIN criteria.[7] Support focuses on treating the underlying condition, ensuring adequate hydration and lack of urinary tract obstruction and if complications supervene then providing renal replacement therapy (RRT).

Generally accepted indications for RRT include:

- hyperkalaemia
- acidosis
- uraemia – urea >30
- fluid overload/pulmonary oedema
- toxic drug accumulation

RRT can be achieved using either dialysis or haemofiltration,[8] with the latter being the most common modality used in critical care. A dedicated large bore central line is used to pump blood through a membrane lined filter, which utilizes a concept called 'solute drag', whereby water that passes out of the filter pores draws solutes like urea and creatinine alongside it. This results in a large amount of ultrafiltrate that needs to be replaced and therefore commercially manufactured replacement fluids containing physiological concentrations of solutes are added to the 'return' limb of the renal line. This extracorporeal circuit normally requires a degree of anticoagulation to reduce the likelihood of clot formation, and most units use an unfractionated heparin infusion for this purpose.

The optimum dose of renal replacement therapy is another area of contention. More intense sessions, either judged by frequency of dialysis or volume of replacement in haemofiltration, have a physiological rationale for providing better clearance of waste products. This was examined in a single centre trial[9] where three separate effluent doses were targeted for patients receiving haemofiltration. This trial showed a significantly increased mortality in the low dose group, and no significant complications in the higher dose groups. This work was replicated in the field of intermittent haemodialysis,[10] comparing three times a week dialysis with six times a week, showing a significant mortality benefit in the more frequent group. This concept of intensity has been re-examined by two much larger studies,[11,12] which were unable to replicate the mortality benefit. There is likely to be a complex dose-response curve with renal replacement, and while under-dosing should be avoided there is insufficient evidence to support higher dose intervention.

Nutritional support

In order to survive critical illness, nutrition must be maintained and supported. For short stays of <48 hours there is no rush to institute feeding, but for stays longer than this an assessment of how to feed must be made. There is little firm evidence that enteral nutrition is necessarily better than parenteral nutrition other than the risk of central line associated infection, but most units will pursue the enteral route as first line. If the enteral route fails, or is contraindicated, then parenteral nutrition should be used through a dedicated feeding line if possible.

Feeding can be difficult to establish due to slow gastric emptying, impaired hormonal flux and altered enteral circulation. Methods of encouraging successful enteral nutrition include gradually increasing feeding rate, prokinetic drugs and insertion of postpyloric feeding tubes rather than the standard nasogastric placement. The standard approach is to target an energy intake of 25 kcal/kg/24 hrs, with a mix of protein, fat, carbohydrate and essential vitamins. Enthusiasm has waxed and waned for 'immuno-nutrition' with supplementation of substances purported to boost immune function, but there is not enough evidence to support this when subjected to meta-analysis.

Poor glycaemic control is linked to increasing infection rates, poorer wound healing and worse outcomes in a variety of disease states. Critically ill patients tend to develop hyperglycaemia in response to a number of factors including the stress response, relative insulin resistance, increased circulating levels of cortisol, catecholamines as well as exogenous administration of drugs including steroids and additional catecholamines as part of their support. Interest was raised when a 2001 RCT[13] comparing a 'tight' glycaemic control protocol targeting blood glucose values of 4.4 to 6.1 mmol/L against a 'conventional' protocol target of 10 to 12 mmol/L was published and showed a raft of positive effects including reduction in all-cause mortality, incidence of AKI needing RRT, bloodstream infections and critical care acquired weakness. Many centres adopted this so-called 'intensive insulin therapy' approach, but a subsequent trial by the same group[14] looking at a wider range of patients (as opposed to the original cardiac surgery cohort) failed to support the same findings. A more recent 2009 RCT,[15] far larger than the previous cohorts, compared the intensive target to a conventional target of < 10 mmol/L and showed an increased all-cause mortality in the intensive group, seemingly independent of the effects of hypoglycaemia. Certainly hyperglycaemia should be avoided and treated if it occurs, but intensive control cannot be supported.

Sedation

The majority of patients in critical care will require some form of sedation or analgesia to help provide their care. The presence of an endotracheal tube is intensely stimulating, so the use of opioids for their anti-tussive effects is key. Acute pain related to operations, critical care related procedures and positioning is extremely common and critical illness interrupts the sleep-wake cycle meaning that sedation is also often required.

The most commonly used regime involves the short-acting anaesthetic agent propofol, alongside an opioid (morphine, alfentanil, remifentanil). Benzodiazepines, such as midazolam, have lost favour due to the implication of increasing the incidence of delirium. Stopping sedation on a regular basis may help to shorten stay, and allows for more accurate assessment of neurological function.[16]

Delirium, an acute alteration in consciousness and alertness associated with many disease states, has recently become far more readily recognized in critical care. Up to 70% of critical care patients will experience an episode of delirium, and it is associated with longer stays, longer duration of ventilation, increased mortality and long-term cognitive decline. There are no proven interventions to treat delirium, but generally non-pharmacological measures (sedation breaks, orientation aids like clocks and natural light) have fewer side effects than the pharmacological measures like haloperidol and atypical antipsychotics.

THE INTERFACE BETWEEN CRITICAL CARE AND ENT

Post-operative care

Like all other surgical specialties, patients undergoing ENT operations may be admitted to critical care either in a planned or unplanned fashion. The type of admission can be generalized into one of three categories as follows:

1. Caused by the acute illness (e.g. the ongoing management of shock following post-tonsillectomy haemorrhage)
2. Caused by the nature of the surgery (e.g. major head and neck operations where it is anticipated that airway swelling or compromise may persist for several days after the operation)
3. Caused by pre-existing disease processes (e.g. severe left ventricular dysfunction in someone undergoing an unrelated ENT procedure)

Early discussion with critical care allows for potential pre-operative optimization, or modification of intra-operative management to aid post-operative recovery. Depending on developments in the post-operative period these admissions may be brief, or unexpectedly protracted. Regular communication between the ENT and critical care team allows for both sides to improve decision-making processes and support the patient and family during what is an emotionally fraught time.

Sepsis

ENT can be involved in the management of sepsis in critical care either in ENT patients who have developed perioperative sepsis either as a primary or secondary infection, or in the investigation of occult sepsis in non-ENT patients. Most critical care patients have indwelling tubes through the nasal passages, and as such are at increased risk of sinusitis that may be difficult to diagnose. In such cases ENT may be asked to help investigate, or provide washouts to remove a potential source of sepsis.

Although the terminology has been well defined, various phrases are used interchangeably, which can lead to diagnostic confusion. Initial consensus definitions derived three states of sepsis, increasing in severity: sepsis; severe sepsis; and septic shock. The most recent iteration of the Surviving Sepsis Campaign (SSC) guidelines[17] classes these as shown in **Table 33.3**.

The underlying pathophysiology of sepsis is that of an uncontrolled physiological response to infection leading to systemic vasodilation produced by a host of cytokines including, but not limited to, Il-6, Il-18, TNF-α, inducible nitric oxide synthase and arginine. The 'classic' septic patient will display a hyperdynamic circulatory pattern with low filling pressures, maintained or increased cardiac output and microcirculatory dysfunction. This textbook presentation is often not seen, with a wide range of patients from those with a maintained blood pressure but

TABLE 33.3 Three states of sepsis		
Sepsis	Severe sepsis	Septic shock
Documented or suspected infection with the presence of systemic manifestations of infection	Sepsis with signs of organ hypoperfusion (hypotension, raised creatinine, raised bilirubin, prolonged INR, hypoxia, thrombocytopaenia, lactataemia)	Severe sepsis with hypotension refractory to initial resuscitation – classed as a MAP <70mmHg or systolic <90mmHg after 30ml/kg fluid resuscitation and initial vasopressor use

organ dysfunction, to those with marked sepsis-induced myocardial dysfunction who are far from hyperdynamic.

The early and aggressive management of sepsis has been a focus of recent media attention with campaigns including Surviving Sepsis and the UK-based Sepsis Six, based on work that suggests that both early administration of antibiotics[18] and resuscitation targeted to endpoints[19] reduced mortality and morbidity in sepsis. Management hinges on having a high suspicion of the diagnosis, investigating the potential sources using microbiology, radiology and surgery early, restoring tissue oxygen delivery by resuscitation and administering appropriate broad-spectrum antibiotics tailored to the most likely source of sepsis. The following list summarizes the Sepsis Six approaches that are recommended to be implemented within this first hour of a patient being diagnosed with sepsis:

1. Administer high flow oxygen.
2. Take blood cultures.
3. Give broad spectrum antibiotics.
4. Give intravenous fluid challenges.
5. Measure serum lactate.
6. Measure hourly urine output.

This bundle approach aims to make the early diagnosis and management of sepsis more reliably achieved within a short timeframe by junior staff, but does require ongoing senior input including making the escalation to critical care if appropriate.

Improving tissue oxygen delivery relies upon the restoration of both an appropriate circulating volume, and perfusing pressure. As previously mentioned, the SSC guidelines advocate the use of a 30ml/kg crystalloid resuscitation approach, with early use of noradrenaline as the first-line vasopressor alongside fluid resuscitation to restore organ autoregulatory flow. Suggested endpoints for resuscitation include trends in lactate, venous oxygen saturations, or urine output. In cases of reduced cardiac output suggested by findings such as low venous oxygen saturations, echocardiography or lack of response to vasoconstrictor therapy, predominantly inotropic agents like dobutamine or adrenaline are indicated.

Airway management

The involvement of ENT with airway management in critical care falls into two main groups. The first is the management of difficult or potentially difficult airways in critical care, while the second is the provision of tracheostomies for patients with an ongoing need for ventilatory support.

DIFFICULT AIRWAYS

Difficult airways can be known, suspected or not recognized. The experience of the clinician assessing the airway is key, as is access to previous documentation if available. A national UK survey of airway complications[20] showed that 20% of all reported complications occurred in the critical care unit, and that the degree of harm that occurred to these patients was far higher than those that happened in theatre or the emergency department. The majority of complications were related to tracheostomies, both new and existing, but securing *de novo* airways also featured heavily. Common reasons identified for complications included lack of training, lack of equipment and lack of preparation. Reasons for increased complication rates include the above, but also the rapid need for intubation in the critically ill, the lack of cardiorespiratory physiological reserve, and the regular lack of an escape option where abandoning the need for ventilation is not possible.

The difficult airway can be due to obstruction or distortion at any level, and the potential management options will vary due to aetiology:

- supralaryngeal – tumour, infection, anaphylaxis
- laryngeal – infections, tumours, surgery, anaphylaxis
- infralaryngeal – tumour, infection, tracheomalacia, subglottic stenosis.

Where possible, the most senior staff available should be present, with full monitoring as would occur in theatre, and with trained skilled assistance. If predicted to be difficult there is a strong case for attempting the intubation in a theatre setting.

TRACHEOSTOMY

For patients who have an ongoing need for ventilation, there are several potential benefits for exchanging a translaryngeal tube for a tracheostomy tube. These include:

- reduced sedation needs due to lack of glottic stimulation
- reduced deadspace (probably less important than previously thought)
- reduced tube resistance and work of breathing
- improved mouth care
- ongoing bronchial toilet when weaned.

These benefits need to be balanced against the complications of tracheostomy insertion, the patient specific factors like coagulopathy or body habitus and the predicted duration of ventilation need. There is little evidence to support the optimal timing of tracheostomy insertion, with a recent UK trial[21] comparing early (before day 4) and late (after day 10) tracheostomy insertion. This trial stopped early due to difficulties in recruitment, but with 900 of 1200 planned recruited patients failed to show a benefit in mortality with early tracheostomy insertion with similar lengths of stay, ventilation and antibiotic use.

The method of tracheostomy insertion is essentially between a percutaneous dilational technique, most often performed by critical care staff under bronchoscopic control, and traditional open surgical tracheostomies. Meta-analysis[22] has shown equivalence of the techniques, with a percutaneous approach leading to less wound infections and a similar complication rate. The percutaneous techniques involve partial withdrawal of the endotracheal tube under general anaesthesia and neuromuscular blockade, then a Seldinger based technique of needle insertion, guidewire pass and dilation using a serial dilator, graduated dilator or blunt forcep dilation before placing the tracheostomy tube over the wire.

There are situations where surgical techniques are more appropriate and these include:

- obesity, more for the availability of suitable percutaneous kit
- anatomical variance including previous surgery and goitres
- coagulopathy or bleeding diatheses.

ASSESSING VOCAL CORDS

This may be asked for in patients who have failed extubation, who have impaired cough mechanisms or suspected recurrent aspiration. Cord dysfunction may be due to mechanical issues after long-term intubation, surgical complications especially after thyroid or parathyroid surgery, or some apical lung tumours. Other nerve dysfunction should be sought, including bulbar or pseudobulbar dysfunction that may suggest alternative diagnoses. Assessment can be performed at the bedside using either rigid or flexible bronchoscopy methods, ideally without neuromuscular blockade.

DEATH AND DYING IN ICU

Mortality in critical care is steadily decreasing, despite dealing with ageing populations with increasing comorbidity. Figures vary between countries and case mix, but in a mixed medical and surgical ICU in a first world country, one would expect a unit mortality of around 20% and a hospital mortality of 35%. While improvements in mortality are encouraging, this still means that around one in five patients admitted will die and therefore medical and nursing staff need to be familiar with the caring of the dying patient and the support of their family.

Communication

Communication with both the patient and their family is a key part of the critical care workload. Often critically ill patients are unable to communicate or retain information, and the bulk of the communication given is to the family. This carries with it issues surrounding confidentiality and it is always best to have the patient give their permission prior to such conversations. This is not always possible, and the situation must be approached with tact and careful judgement. It should be remembered that having a relative who is critically ill is a heavy emotional burden for any family, and that even simple messages may have to be repeated at each conversation to ensure understanding.

Identification of the next-of-kin is a useful approach, allowing for clarity of communication and the reduction of misinterpretation. It is a laudable aim for a senior clinician to meet with a family within the first day following admission, and to have continuity of communication throughout the stay especially if prolonged.

Regardless of communication content, a few key points are universal:

- Time for communication must be made, ideally free from interference, in a dedicated relatives' area.
- Introductions should be clear, outlining roles and responsibilities and ensuring that you know who you are addressing.
- It is valuable to spend time at the beginning of each conversation investigating what has previously been said, and what has been understood – this can help to reduce 'mixed messages'.
- Be familiar with the case, including dates of admission and significant events.
- Always aim to summarize your conversation aims at the end, and allow time for questions.

Care of the dying in critical care

Every day in a large critical care unit there will be a patient who has their focus of care changed from a curative intent to the provision of palliation. This change in focus can happen quickly, or follow a more indolent course. It is usually due to a patient worsening, or a recognition that the patient would not wish to survive with such a marked reduction in functional outcome or quality of life. The latter is a particularly difficult decision to make, and needs to be carefully approached given the inherently subjective nature of such judgements.

Such decisions should be made in conjunction with the patient if their condition allows it, the family, and the referring team.[23] Concordance in the decision is the most desirable outcome, and if there is dissent then the best approach is to address this openly and to continue ongoing support until an agreement is reached.[24] As the emotional element of such decisions is so high, the process can often be reached over a longer period of time allowing time for grieving and acceptance of the situation at hand. Pursuing a decision in the face of unease or unhappiness is a common finding in complaints.

In critical care, the change of focus to palliation often encompasses either limitation of therapy or withdrawal of organ support. From an ethical standpoint the two are identical, but some will struggle with withdrawal of support more than non-institution. Regardless of the mode of palliation, the comfort and the dignity of the patient are paramount, and only interventions that will increase patient comfort should be pursued. This may include starting or increasing analgesic infusions, extubation if appropriate, and cessation of blood sampling whilst continuing to ensure good oral cleaning, regular position changes and good nursing care. Communication should continue with the family, and addressing any concerns they may have during the process.

'Do not attempt resuscitation' (DNAR) orders are ways of communicating advance decisions regarding the appropriateness of undertaking cardiopulmonary resuscitation. The forms themselves are not legally mandated in the UK, but are seen as good clinical practice as they prompt medical teams to discuss decisions about resuscitation with patients and their families. Controversies surrounding DNAR decisions mainly stem from lack of communication, and misunderstanding of the role and realistic outcomes of cardiopulmonary resuscitation.

FUTURE RESEARCH

One of the major problems facing research in critical care is the application of single interventions to heterogeneous disease states. A desire to classify and compartmentalize broadly similar presentations has lead to umbrella terms, such as ARDS or sepsis. While these approaches make sense in terms of broadly similar pathophysiology or clinical presentation, the application of targeted treatments to clustered disease states does lead to potentially missing true treatment effects.

A common theme in modern critical care developments has been the early identification of organ dysfunction. A promising area of research is the development of reliable biomarkers of organ dysfunction that could allow early intervention and prevention of further deterioration. For example, serum lactate has been identified as a marker of tissue hypoxaemia that can be used to guide resuscitation and monitor progress in sepsis; and development of point-of-care tests could allow for quicker detection of the critically ill patient. This and other potential biomarkers would all have to be validated and suitable levels of sensitivity and specificity agreed upon.

As mentioned earlier in the chapter, an admission to critical care carries with it a substantial morbidity and the effect this has on future quality of life in survivors forms a key research priority. There is emerging evidence that an episode of acute inflammation such as a critical illness can lead to a chronic low-grade pattern of inflammation. This can have effects upon an individual's ability to recover from their acute event, and upon the potential for future accelerated organ deterioration. Both qualitative and quantitative research in this area is needed to help inform clinicians about the burden of admission on patients.

KEY POINTS

- Critical care has evolved to occupy a central role in the modern acute hospital.
- The most important interventions in critical care are the assiduous application of good basic medical and nursing care.
- Critical care admission is a multifactorial decision incorporating acute and chronic medical, social and ethical considerations.
- Advanced organ support is crucial to optimize the physiological state and permit time for definitive interventions to take effect.
- The majority of interactions between ENT and critical care will be for the provision of elective and emergency post-operative care and for advanced airway intervention, including difficult airway management and tracheostomy.
- Due to the high mortality rate among ICU patients, management of death and the dying patient is of paramount importance, as is recognizing that effective and empathetic communication assists this process.

REFERENCES

1. Knaus WA, Draper EA, Wagner DP, Zimmerman JE. APACHE II: a severity of disease classification system. *Crit Care Med* 1985; **13**(10): 818–29.
2. Ranieri VM, Rubenfeld GD, Thompson BT, et al. Acute respiratory distress syndrome: the Berlin Definition. *JAMA* 2012; **307**(23): 2526–33.
3. The Acute Respiratory Distress Syndrome Network. Ventilation with lower tidal volumes as compared with traditional tidal volumes for acute lung injury and the acute respiratory distress syndrome. *N Engl J Med* 2000; **342**(18): 1301–08.
4. Peek GJ, Elbourne D, Mugford M, et al. Efficacy and economic assessment of conventional ventilatory support versus extracorporeal membrane oxygenation for severe adult respiratory failure (CESAR): a multicentre randomised controlled trial. *Lancet* 2009; **374**(9698): 1351–63.
5. Harvey S, Harrison DA, Singer M, et al., Assessment of the clinical effectiveness of pulmonary artery catheters in management of patients in intensive care (PAC-Man): a randomised controlled trial. *Lancet* 2005; **366**(9484): 472–77.
6. The National Heart, Lung, and Blood Institute Acute Respiratory Distress Syndrome (ARDS) Clinical Trials Network. Comparison of two fluid-management strategies in acute lung injury. *N Engl J Med* 2006; **354**(24): 2564–75.
7. Van Biesen W, Vanholder R, Lameire N. Defining acute renal failure: RIFLE and beyond. *Clin J Am Soc Nephrol* 2006; **1**(6): 1314–19.
8. Bagshaw SM, Berthiaume LR, Delaney A, Bellomo R. Continuous versus intermittent renal replacement therapy for critically ill patients with acute kidney injury: a meta-analysis. *Crit Care Med* 2008; **36**(2): 610–17.
9. Ronco C, Bellomo R, Homel P, et al. Effects of different doses in continuous veno-venous haemofiltration on outcomes of acute renal failure: a prospective randomised trial. *Lancet* 2000; **356**(9223): 26–30.
10. Schiffl H, Lang SM, Fischer, R. Daily hemodialysis and the outcome of acute renal failure. *N Engl J Med* 2002; **346**(5): 305–10.
11. The VA/NIH Acute Renal Failure Trial Network. Intensity of renal support in critically ill patients with acute kidney injury. *N Engl J Med* 2008; **359**(1): 7–20.

12. Bellomo R, Cass A, Cole L, et al. Intensity of continuous renal-replacement therapy in critically ill patients. *N Engl J Med* 2009; **361**(17): 1627–38.
13. Van den Berghe G, Wouters P, Weekers F, et al. Intensive insulin therapy in critically ill patients. *N Engl J Med* 2001; **345**(19): 1359–67.
14. Van den Berghe G, Wilmer A, Hermans G, et al. Intensive insulin therapy in the medical ICU. *N Engl J Med* 2006; **354**(5): 449–61.
15. The NICE-SUGAR Study Investigators. Intensive versus conventional glucose control in critically ill patients. *N Engl J Med* 2009; **360**(13): 1283–97.
16. Kress JP, Pohlman AS, O'Connor MF, Hall JB. Daily interruption of sedative infusions in critically ill patients undergoing mechanical ventilation. *N Engl J Med* 2000; **342**(20): 1471–77.
17. Dellinger RP, Levy MM, Rhodes A, et al. Surviving Sepsis Campaign: international guidelines for management of severe sepsis and septic shock: 2012. *Crit Care Med* 2013; **41**(2): 580–637.
18. Kumar A, Roberts D, Wood KE, et al. Duration of hypotension before initiation of effective antimicrobial therapy is the critical determinant of survival in human septic shock. *Crit Care Med* 2006; **34**(6): 1589–96.
19. Rivers E, Nyugen B, Havstad S, et al. Early goal-directed therapy in the treatment of severe sepsis and septic shock. *N Engl J Med* 2001; **345**(19): 1368–77.
20. Cook TM, Woodall N, Harper J, Benger J. Major complications of airway management in the UK: results of the Fourth National Audit Project of the Royal College of Anaesthetists and the Difficult Airway Society. Part 2: intensive care and emergency departments. *Br J Anaesth* 2011; **106**(5): 632–42.
21. Young D, Harrison DA, Cuthbertson BH, et al. Effect of early vs late tracheostomy placement on survival in patients receiving mechanical ventilation: the TracMan randomized trial. *JAMA* 2013; **309**(20): 2121–29.
22. Higgins KM, Punthakee X. Meta-analysis comparison of open versus percutaneous tracheostomy. *Laryngoscope* 2007; **117**(3): 447–54.
23. Sjökvist P, Nilstun T, Svantesson M, Nerggren L. Withdrawal of life support – who should decide? Differences in attitudes among the general public, nurses and physicians. *Intensive Care Med* 1999; **25**(9): 949–54.
24. Levack P. Live and let die? A structured approach to decision-making about resuscitation. *Br J Anaesth* 2002; **89**(5): 683–86.

CHAPTER 34

PAEDIATRIC INTENSIVE CARE

Louise Selby and Robert Ross Russell

Introduction	361	Major surgery	365
General principles	361	Summary	366
ENT emergencies in PICU	363	References	367

SEARCH STRATEGY

Data for this chapter are mostly generic management strategies for children in intensive care. The target audience is ENT surgeons involved in caring for children, rather than paediatric intensivists who are looking after ENT patients. The material is relevant to both groups within the chapter.

The data were gathered through reference to standard texts on paediatric intensive care, notably Rogers and Nichols' *Textbook of Paediatric Intensive Care*.[1] Specific information on ENT trauma in children was obtained through PubMed using the keywords: 'laryngeal trauma and laryngeal injury', limiting the search to children aged 0–18 years. This revealed 90 review articles of which 7 were found relevant and scrutinized. Information on bronchoscopy was located on PubMed using the keywords: 'fibreoptic bronchoscopy and intensive care', limiting the search to children aged 0–18 years. This yielded five papers, but by looking at related citations we were able to find two relevant articles.[2, 3]

INTRODUCTION

Children are liable to present acutely with ENT pathologies, many of which are specific to the paediatric population and may require intensive care management. Those children undergoing major ENT surgery also frequently require admission to a paediatric intensive care unit in the post-operative period. This chapter aims to outline the general management principles of ENT patients within the paediatric intensive care setting. Important differences in the anatomy and physiology of children compared to adults are reviewed. A systematic approach to evaluation of children admitted to the paediatric intensive care unit (PICU) is outlined, together with general principles of fluid and analgesia management in children. Specific issues relating to the care of the major paediatric emergencies, as well as the post-operative management of patients undergoing major ENT surgical procedures are discussed. Finally, indications for performing flexible and rigid bronchoscopy are outlined.

GENERAL PRINCIPLES

Anatomical and physiological considerations

The paediatric airway differs from the adult airway in many aspects. Understanding these differences in structure is essential in order to manage the paediatric airway successfully. The head of the infant and small child is proportionately larger, accounting for nearly 10% of body surface area compared to 3.5% in adults. Infants and young children have a more prominent occiput with a shorter neck and these factors in combination increase neck flexion. Children also have a relatively large tongue and a small mandible, potentially making airway access difficult.[4]

In all young children the epiglottis is a 'horseshoe shape' and the larynx sits high (opposite the third cervical vertebrae, compared to the fifth or sixth in an adult) and anterior. The larynx itself is conical, unlike the cylindrical

TABLE 34.1 Physiological parameters at different ages			
Age	Heart rate (bpm)	Respiratory rate (bpm)	Mean BP (mmHg)
Newborn	110–140	50–60	50–60
1 year	90–110	30–40	70–90
2–5 years	75–90	25–30	80–100
5–12 years	60–90	20–25	90–110
>12 years	50–80	15–20	100–120

TABLE 34.2 Issues to be considered on admission of a child to PICU	
	Issues to consider
Airway	Clear? ETT position? ETT secured properly?
Breathing	Air entry? Adequate ventilation?
Circulation	Peripheral perfusion? Adequate access?
Fluids	Drug infusions? Blood sugar? Urine output?
Analgesia/sedation	Pain control and sedation adequate? Muscle relaxant needed?
Tests	Blood gas? Electrolytes? Full blood count?

adult larynx and the narrowest part lies at the cricoid cartilage. Finally the tracheal cartilage is often less rigid than in adults, and may compress if the neck is overextended.[5]

Infants up to the age of 6 months are obligate nasal breathers.[5] When this is combined with the relatively small airways and risk of mucus obstruction, airway compromise is common. Between 3 and 6 years of age, tonsillar and adenoidal hypertrophy further contribute to airway obstruction.

Physiologically, there are also substantial and important differences. Respiratory muscle function is affected by the position of the ribs in infants, which lie perpendicular to the spine rather than running caudally as in adults. This makes the diaphragm the only effective inspiratory muscle. Infants and children have a faster respiratory rate than adults (Table 34.1), which is partly related to an increased metabolic rate. In infants, increased chest wall compliance can increase the work of breathing substantially.

In the cardiovascular system, a limited stroke volume necessitates a faster heart rate in children and they also display a lower mean blood pressure. Their response to cardiovascular stress is limited and cardiac output can only be increased significantly by increasing the heart rate, therefore tachycardia is common.

Evaluation

Admission of a child into the PICU is a difficult and important moment in the child's care. The care of the child is transferred to a new team of doctors and nurses and the family are moved to a new and stressful environment. It is essential that handover of the child is structured and complete. Ideally there should be a face-to-face handover between medical and nursing teams involved in the care of the child. The background history, current problems and care plan should be clearly documented.

The family of the child need to be included in this handover. When the admission is planned, for example post-operatively, families should be offered the chance to visit the intensive care unit prior to the surgery so they have met some of the staff and seen the environment. There should be an area for them to stay whilst procedures are being carried out and regular progress updates from medical and nursing staff.

The doctors admitting the child also need to evaluate the child carefully on admission. This should follow a standard 'ABC' assessment, assessing the airway, breathing and circulation. Issues regarding fluid balance, medications and results of investigations should also be clarified (Table 34.2).

Fluid management

The principles of fluid balance in children are the same as in adults but there are complicating factors. Any fluids that need to be given are based on a child's weight or occasionally body surface area (tables for which are found in the British National Formulary for Children). The distribution of fluids between compartments is different for adults and children. Total body water is distributed between the intracellular, interstitial and intra-vascular spaces, moving from one compartment to another. At birth approximately 80% of a baby's body weight is water, with this percentage falling gradually to 60% in adulthood. The infant has approximately one third of their body weight as interstitial fluid – twice as much as in an adult.[1]

Normally fluid balance is tightly controlled by thirst, hormonal responses and renal function. In illness and injury there may be rapid fluid shifts with clinical consequences.

THE NEWBORN INFANT

The full term infant requires approximately 150 ml/kg per day of fluid from day 5 of life (less in the first few days). Of this, approximately 30 ml/kg will be accounted for by insensible losses. Normal fluid intake is entirely as milk, which provides fluid and nutrition for approximately the first 6 months of life. Fluid requirements (per kg) gradually reduce thereafter as shown in Table 34.3; however, these requirements may require adjustment in disease.[5]

Electrolyte requirements also vary with age, though not as dramatically as fluid volume. In the infant, immature renal function increases the salt requirements and 3 mmol/kg of sodium and 2 mmol/kg of potassium are required daily. In older children this falls to approximately 2 mmol/kg per day of each ion. Calcium, magnesium and other ions are broadly in the same dose (per kg) as adults.

Glucose requirements are critical, especially in young children. The daily calorie requirement of infants is approximately 100 kcal/kg, more than double that in adults.

TABLE 34.3 Fluid and electrolyte requirements at different ages

Age	Daily fluid requirements	Sodium/potassium requirements
1 day	60 ml/kg	2–3 mmol/kg/day
5 days	150 ml/kg	2 mmol/kg/day
1 month	120 ml/kg	1–2 mmol/kg/day
6 months	110 ml/kg	
1 year	100 ml/kg	
>1 year	1000 ml for the first 10 kg, 500 ml for the next 10 kg, then 20 ml/kg for the rest of body weight	

Maintenance of adequate glucose levels in infants is critically important and hypoglycaemia can cause brain damage. In infants and small children, enough glucose must be given to maintain blood glucose levels.

THE UNWELL CHILD

Fluid requirements following surgery can be quite variable. In most units, children are started on a regime restricting their input to approximately two-thirds of normal requirements. This is especially true if oral feeds are not to be used and fluids are being given intravenously. Intravenous fluids should be chosen with care. A National Patient Safety Agency (NPSA) alert in 2007 prompted the removal of hypotonic fluids (0.18% saline) from paediatric wards following incidences of mortality secondary to hyponatraemia.[6] Solutions containing adequate sodium (such as 0.9% saline, or 0.45% saline and 5% dextrose) are therefore recommended. Whatever regime is used, it needs to be remembered that children are prone to becoming dehydrated or fluid-overloaded quite rapidly (particularly during illness) and need to be monitored carefully. In infants especially, blood glucose levels need to be measured up to every 4 hours.

Analgesia

Appropriate analgesia needs to balance the sedative and respiratory suppressive effects of opiates against the need for good pain control. Oral paracetamol and other non-steroidal anti-inflammatory drugs (NSAIDs) may be adequate, but opiates (e.g. morphine) may be needed. A morphine infusion of 10–30 mcg/kg/hour can be given or as a patient-controlled analgesia pump for older children. Infusions can be set up to give background rates of 10 mcg/kg/hour with additional boluses for breakthrough pain but should be discussed with an anaesthetist. Midazolam is a sedative and amnesic drug and may be needed for patients in the PICU, especially if they are ventilated or undergoing painful procedures. Midazolam can be given as bolus doses of 0.1 mg/kg up to every 4 hours or as an infusion (50–250 mcg/kg/hour). Patients need close observation of physiological parameters with either bolus dosing or intravenous infusions.[5]

ENT EMERGENCIES IN PICU

Trauma

All trauma cases, including those who have sustained craniofacial trauma should be managed acutely according to paediatric life support guidelines, with immediate evaluation of airway, breathing and circulation.[5] Laryngeal trauma consists of a rare but precarious set of injuries, often requiring a high index of suspicion to promptly diagnose and appropriately treat. Cases of blunt laryngeal trauma are rare. Laryngeal trauma is seen less frequently in infants and children because of their involvement in fewer car crashes and cases of 'interpersonal conflict'.[7] They may occur if a child is unrestrained in a car involved in a road traffic accident if they hit the dashboard when the head and neck are in a hyperextended position. In the child presenting with laryngotracheal injuries in the absence of such a history, the possibility of non-accidental injury with a direct blow to the anterior neck should be considered as a possible aetiology.

Children surviving a near strangulation event are at risk for significant airway compromise. Studies looking at near hanging events between 2001 and 2010 found four cases with documented laryngeal injury and one child requiring a tracheostomy.[8] 'Near hanging' or 'choking games' are reported in the teenage population.[9]

Management of laryngeal trauma must begin by evaluating the adequacy and patency of the airway. If airway obstruction is a concern, a surgical airway in the form of emergency tracheostomy should be established urgently. The preferred management in children consists of gas anaesthesia with rigid bronchoscopy to evaluate the injuries as well as securing the airway so tracheostomy can be performed over the rigid bronchoscope.[8] Orotracheal intubation must be undertaken with caution to avoid extending damage or losing the airway.

In patients with moderate injuries, the degree of damage can be further assessed using CT scanning once the airway has been protected. Open exploration is recommended where the injuries are severe, and laryngeal trauma is commonly associated with other injuries to the neck or chest.[8]

Upper airway obstruction

The small cross sectional area and conical shape of the paediatric airway renders children particularly susceptible to upper airway obstruction. Airway resistance is inversely proportional to the fourth power of the radius of the airway. Therefore a relatively small reduction in the radius of the airway through mucosal oedema, secretions or a foreign body results in a significant increase in airway resistance.[5]

Stridor on inspiration is indicative of upper airway obstruction. In children where severe upper airway obstruction is suspected as a diagnosis it is imperative to avoid all invasive procedures and aspects of the examination that may distress the child as this may cause complete upper airway occlusion. Children should be kept warm and calm while experienced anaesthetic and surgical staff are assembled. Examination can then be undertaken in a controlled manner. A full examination of the child is also needed at a convenient point. Birthmarks and haemangiomas should be recorded as this may indicate there is a vascular laryngeal lesion. If a child is dysmorphic, a genetic opinion may help identify a syndrome that may have airway implications. Patients with micrognathia as seen in Pierre Robin syndrome, Robin sequence and Treacher Collins syndrome, and those with the mucopolysaccharidoses where progressive dermatan sulphate accumulation in body tissues including the oropharynx and airway, can make airway management challenging.[4]

The patient recovering from burns presents additional challenges. Contractures of the face, neck and chest may result in microstomia, granuloma formation, subglottic stenosis, tracheomalacia and fixed flexion of the neck.[10]

EPIGLOTTITIS

The vaccine included in childhood immunization schedules should protect against *Haemophilus Influenzae B* (Hib) infections and has led to a marked decline in the incidence of epiglottitis such that it is a rare condition. Occasional cases do occur in unimmunized children or in those in whom the vaccine has failed.

The clinical presentation is a child usually aged between 2 and 7 years who is toxic, stridulous and drooling. Immediate management is to secure the airway either by endotracheal intubation by experienced personnel or by emergency tracheostomy. The child will remain ventilated in intensive care whilst receiving intravenous antibiotics (third generation cephalosporins) until the swelling of the epiglottis has reduced, usually within 24–36 hours.[11]

CROUP

Acute viral laryngotracheobronchitis (viral croup) is a common cause of upper airway obstruction in children characterized by hoarseness, barking cough and inspiratory stridor. *Parainfluenzae* virus type 1 is the agent most commonly identified in cases of croup. Only severe cases require admission to the PICU.

Localized inflammation and oedema of the upper airway caused by a virus can increase airway resistance and significantly increase the work of breathing in young children. Glucocorticoids in the form of nebulized budesonide or systemic dexamethasone are believed to reduce the degree of upper airway inflammation and swelling leading to decreased effort in breathing. A recent Cochrane review found when corticosteroids were compared to placebo in treatment for croup, dexamethasone and budesonide were effective in relieving symptoms as early as 6 hours after treatment, resulting in reduced hospital stay and fewer hospital re-admissions.[12] Some clinical improvement can occur within 30 minutes of glucocorticoid dose.[5]

If airway obstruction is severe, short-term relief can be achieved by nebulizing adrenaline (1 ml/kg of 1 : 1000 up to a maximum dose of 5 ml) with oxygen. A small number of children with croup (<5%) will require intubation. However glucocorticoids and nebulized adrenaline have both been shown to reduce length of hospital stay in management of croup.[12,13] A comparison of the clinical features of croup and epiglottitis are included in Table 34.4.

TABLE 34.4 Features of croup vs epiglottitis

	Croup	Epiglottitis
Age	1–3 years	2–7 years
Cause	Parainfluenza viruses	Hib
Prodrome	1–2 days coryza	Hours, sore throat, dysphagia, drooling.
Fever	<38°C	>38°C
Appearance	Lethargic	Pale and toxic, drooling and dysphagia, sitting with neck extended
Stridor	Barking cough, loud stridor	Muffled stridor
Hypoxia	Unusual	Frequent
Severity	<5% hospitalized cases require intubation	All require intubation

Bacterial tracheitis

Bacterial tracheitis, or pseudomembranous croup, is much less common than viral croup but it is potentially life threatening. The majority of patients (over 80%) will require intubation to secure their airway whilst receiving treatment with intravenous antibiotics. The responsible pathogens are usually *staphylococcus aureus, streptococci* or *Haemophilus influenzae B*, which infect the tracheal mucosa causing necrosis and the production of purulent secretions that may occlude the upper and lower airway. Clinically, a child with bacterial tracheitis is septic with a high fever, barking cough and signs of progressive upper airway obstruction. Coughing without drooling can help to distinguish it from epiglottitis.[5]

Foreign body inhalation and ingestion

Foreign body inhalation most commonly occurs in children aged 1 to 3 years and should be suspected if there is sudden onset of stridor and upper airway obstruction with no preceding fever or illness (please see Chapter 31 for more details). Without early treatment it is a cause of morbidity in children, sometimes resulting in a fatal outcome.[14] Foreign body injuries can be described by anatomical site. Upper airway involvement varies from complete obstruction with hypoxia and cardiorespiratory compromise to partial obstruction with cough, stridor, and respiratory distress. Lower airway involvement can lead to pulmonary changes depending on the site of the impaction including collapse and consolidation of the bronchopulmonary segment seen on chest X-ray.[15] Foods, particularly nuts and seeds, are the usual cause. However, small magnets or other metallic parts found within some toys can become lodged in the hypopharynx or oesophagus and rapidly cause pressure necrosis of mucosal tissues.[16]

If a child presents with increasing dyspnoea, apnoea or loss of consciousness that has not responded to simple airway manoeuvres then advanced paediatric life support guidelines for managing a choking child should be followed. Blind finger sweeps of the mouth are not recommended as these can push the object tighter into the larynx. In the older child the Heimlich manoeuvre can be safely attempted, or if the child is unconscious and supine then abdominal thrusts may be as effective.[5]

On clinical examination there may be unilateral wheeze and reduced breath sounds. A chest X-ray may show air trapping possibly with (mediastinal shift), atelectasis, pneumothorax or have a normal appearance.[15] Patients require general anaesthetic for rigid bronchoscopic removal and may require admission to the PICU post procedure. Complications of delayed diagnosis of inhaled foreign body can include tracheal lacerations, inflammation, oedema, atelectasis and bronchopneumonia[12,13] contributing to prolonged hospital stay. There can also be bleeding with manipulation of the object and it can be difficult to dislodge and retrieve.[16]

Laryngopharyngeal injury can also occur following accidental ingestion, particularly of liquid detergent capsules. These contain irritant cleansing ingredients that can cause rapid onset of mucosal oedema. Consequences can be severe, with possible oesophageal perforation and necrotic extension to the tracheobronchial tree requiring endotracheal intubation or tracheostomy.[17]

MAJOR SURGERY

Craniofacial surgery and cleft lip and palate

Children who undergo craniofacial surgery or a cleft lip or palate repair may require admission to the PICU or high dependency unit (HDU), particularly if there is a risk of the airway becoming compromised by post-operative swelling. If the child returns from theatre ventilated, sedation and analgesia need to be maintained for the duration of ventilation. A partially sedated child may struggle against an endotracheal tube (ETT) and this may damage a palatal or laryngeal repair. It may be necessary to muscle relax a child once they are adequately sedated, usually by using short acting anaesthetic agents, so if extubation is planned the child can be woken quickly. Using longer-acting drugs can lead to accumulation of the drug within the tissues and a period of suboptimal wakefulness as it is metabolized.

Other important considerations include the use of an orogastric rather than nasogastric tube best sited intra-operatively (nasogastric tubes can traumatize a palate repair). Nursing staff should be aware to use a soft wide-bore flexible suction catheter to remove visible oral secretions. Patients should not be nursed close to other children who may be infectious if at all possible.

Surgery of the nose and upper airway

Patients who have nasal surgery rarely require admission to the PICU in the post-operative period; however, infants requiring surgery for choanal atresia or stenosis may require a nasal stent and close observation for the first few days post-operatively.

Those undergoing surgery to the upper airway are frequently admitted to the PICU for a period post-operatively due to the high risk of developing upper airway obstruction as oedema evolves around the surgical site. This includes operations for laryngeal reconstruction but also for more minor procedures such as ary-epiglottoplasty and those children who have undergone adenotonsillectomy for severe sleep apnoea. It is therefore important to ensure a PICU/HDU bed is available before proceeding with surgery. Children who have major upper airway surgery, such as laryngotracheal reconstruction, are electively ventilated for a period of 5 to 7 days post-operatively to allow the oedema to resolve before the ETT is removed. In these patients, sedation and analgesia are critical (see 'Craniofacial surgery and cleft lip and palate', above). Muscle relaxants are used in this patient group to prevent trauma to the surgical site and exacerbation of upper airway oedema due to movement of the ETT whilst *in situ*. Close observation of cardiovascular parameters in muscle-relaxed patients will detect tachycardia and hypertension suggestive of inadequate sedation or pain. It is important that if a significant leak is allowed to develop around the ETT before extubation is attempted this may signify that the post-operative oedema is resolving and that extubation is more likely to be successful.

Laryngeal surgery and tracheostomy

Managing a tracheostomy in the PICU involves the management of the newly formed stoma, care of an established tracheostomy and training requirements for families looking after long-term tracheostomies. In children, tracheostomy is most frequently performed in the first year of life as a result of premature infants requiring prolonged ventilation.[18]

In the first week after a tracheostomy is formed the airway is dependent on the tracheostomy stent (i.e. the tube) to maintain airway patency. Loss of the stent over this period can allow the airway to close, and reinsertion of a tube through an immature tracheostomy can be difficult, as the tracheal opening can be obscured and the tube can easily be passed into the wrong place causing airway obstruction and ventilation of the neck tissues. This complication, known as accidental tube dislodgement, is minimized in a fresh tracheostomy when stay sutures are used. These are attached to the edges of the trachea at surgery and allow the trachea to be brought to the surface of the neck in an emergency, facilitating tube reinsertion. Additionally, maturation sutures attach skin directly to the edge of the trachea to reduce creation of a false passage during the first tracheostomy tube change. Velcro tracheostomy tube ties can also be used if available.[18]

However, many departments prefer to use ties rather than Velcro in the early post-operative phase.

If a tracheostomy tube does become dislodged in this period and cannot easily be reinserted, then (in a child with an adequate upper airway), a conventional ETT should be inserted to secure the airway. This allows planned replacement of the tracheostomy tube at a later stage.

Following the first tracheostomy tube change (usually at 7 days post-operatively), the tracheostomy is more secure. Care of an established stoma involves the establishment of routine tube changes, tape care and training for care givers. The development of difficulties with tube insertion or bleeding should raise the possibility of obstructive granuloma formation.[18]

Bronchoscopy in PICU

FIBREOPTIC BRONCHOSCOPY

Fibreoptic bronchoscopy is a safe and effective method of investigating airway problems when used in a planned and controlled manner.[2] It is a useful technique to directly visualize the lung by passing a fibreoptic scope through an ETT. The scope can visualize all lobes of the lung and identify static (e.g. mucus plugging) and dynamic (e.g. bronchomalacia) problems. The general difficulties with bronchoscopy include hypoxia and hypercapnia as a result of an inability to effectively ventilate through the scope and a narrow suction channel that blocks easily. The scope can be passed through a rubber valve in the ETT allowing continued ventilation around the scope, but this is difficult if the scope diameter is close to that of the ETT. Ventilation may also be worsened for hours after the procedure due to removal of endogenous lung surfactant and atelectasis. The main contraindication to bronchoscopy is that it may provide no useful information.[2,3]

Bronchoscopy can be classed as 'diagnostic' to assess airway patency and anatomy or obtain lavage specimens to aid diagnosis or 'therapeutic' to aid secretion clearance for example.[19]

RIGID BRONCHOSCOPY

This technique is much more effective at removing debris from the airway, and may be easier to use in the very unstable patient as ventilation can be continued through the scope during the procedure.

There are several indications for either fibreoptic or rigid bronchoscopy in PICU:

- **Persistent collapse of lobe/lung:** Ventilated children may develop complete collapse of a lung, usually secondary to blockage of the major airways with secretions and mucus plugs (secondary to severe pneumonia). This can lead to major ventilatory problems with shunting. Fibreoptic bronchoscopy down the ETT can often identify the degree of blockage but a rigid bronchoscope may be needed to clear thick secretions. Intra-tracheal recombinant human DNAase (rhDNase) has been reported to be of benefit in segmental collapse.[18]
- **Assessment of malacia:** Clinical tracheo or bronchomalacia may be difficult to confirm. Flexible bronchoscopy may help locate the site and degree of weakness, but needs to be carried out with the patient self-ventilating as positive pressure ventilation can stent the airway open artificially.
- **Assisted intubation:** This is a rare indication as conventional intubation is usually relatively easily accomplished. However if a child has a craniofacial syndrome that may make this particularly difficult and bronchoscopic intubation may be indicated. The bronchoscope is threaded through an appropriately sized ETT and the endotracheal tube is advanced over the fibreoptic bronchoscope into position.
- **Collection of broncho-alveolar lavage:** The diagnosis of lung pathogens can be difficult, particularly in patients who are immunosuppressed. Many probable pathogens for pneumonia in these patients are not tracheal commensals. Broncho-alveolar lavage may be very useful in this situation. It can be carried out 'blind' by passing a nasogastric tube into the lungs, washing in 0.9% saline then aspirating or using a fibreoptic scope to direct the lavage to a particular part of the lung. If a good quality lavage is negative then an open lung biopsy maybe necessary.

SUMMARY

Principles of care for children are similar to those of adults, but physiological responses seen in children vary with age. Some ENT procedures are also specific to the younger age group, and in units that are not undertaking paediatric surgery frequently, well maintained guidelines for the care of these children is essential.

BEST CLINICAL PRACTICE

- ✓ General principles:
    - ✓ Anatomical and physiological differences between adults and children need to be recognized.
    - ✓ Fluid and electrolyte administration must be age and weight appropriate.
    - ✓ Appreciation of family carers and their involvement is essential.
- ✓ ENT emergencies in PICU:
    - ✓ Laryngeal trauma in children may require a tracheostomy.
    - ✓ Epiglottitis is now rare in the UK because of the Hib vaccination.
    - ✓ Foreign body inhalation is an important, if uncommon, cause of acute respiratory distress in young children.

- ✓ Major surgery:
    - ✓ Muscle relaxation may be needed following palatal and tracheal surgery to avoid damage from a struggling child.
    - ✓ Infection is a major cause of palatal breakdown in children following surgery.
- ✓ Flexible bronchoscopy in children can clear secretions, but the size of the bronchoscope limits its suctioning ability.
- ✓ Suspected foreign bodies should be removed through a rigid bronchoscope.

FUTURE RESEARCH

Many of the clinical practices on PICU have evolved through sharing of experience rather than being substantiated by medical evidence or clinical trials and the potential for research projects aimed at providing evidence to support or refute current practices is huge. However there are significant practical limitations to undertaking such research, for example the ethics of research in children, difficulties obtaining parental consent for entry into trials and recruiting sufficient numbers of patients to achieve adequate power.

KEY POINTS

- Paediatric anatomy and physiology differs significantly to that of an adult.
- Foreign body inhalation (or ingestion) should be suspected in any child with unexplained stridor or respiratory problems.
- Fluid and electrolyte prescriptions for children individually according to body weight.
- All patients with suspected epiglottitis require intubation.
- Trauma and infection are threats to palatal repairs.
- Good evidence to support clinical practice in PICU is limited.

REFERENCES

1. Rogers MC, Nichols DG (eds). *Textbook of paediatric intensive care*. 4th ed. Baltimore, MD: Lippincott Williams and Wilkins; 2008.
2. Davidson M, Coutts J, Bell G. Flexible bronchoscopy in paediatric intensive care. *Pediatr Pulm* 2008; 43: 1188–92.
3. Bush A. Bronchoscopy in paediatric intensive care. *Paediatr Respir Rev* 2003; 4: 67–73.
4. Levy R, Helfaer M. Pediatric airway issues. *Crit Care Clin* 2000; 16(3): 489–504.
5. Advanced Life Support Group. *Advanced paediatric life support*. London: BMJ Publishing Group; 2005.
6. National Patient Safety Agency. *Patient safety alert 22 reducing the risk of hyponatraemia when administering intravenous fluids in children*. London: NHS; 2007.
7. Atkins B, Abbate S, Fisher S, et al. Current management of laryngotracheal trauma: case report and literature review. *J Trauma* 2004; 56: 185–90.
8. Hackett A, Kitsko D. Evaluation and management of pediatric near-hanging injury. *Int J Pediatr Otorhl* 2013; 77: 1899–901.
9. Davies D, Lang M, Watts R. Paediatric hanging and strangulation injuries: a 10 year retrospective description of clinical factors and outcomes. *Paediatr Child Health* 2011; 16: e78–e81.
10. Caruso T, Janik L, Fuzaylov G. Airway management of recovered paediatric patients with severe head and neck burns: a review. *Pediatr Anesth* 2012; 22: 462–68.
11. Damm M, Eckel HE, Jungehulsing M, et al. Management of acute inflammatory childhood stridor. *Otolaryngol Head Neck Surg* 1999; 121: 633–38.
12. Russell K, Liang Y, O'Gorman K, et al. Glucocorticoids for croup. *Cochrane Database Syst Rev* 2011. John Wiley and Sons Ltd.
13. Bjornson C, Russell K, Vandermeer B, et al. Nebulised epinephrine for croup (in children). *Cochrane Database Syst Rev* 2013 John Wiley and Sons Ltd.
14. Gregori D, Salerni L, Scarinzi C, et al. Foreign bodies in the upper airways causing complications and requiring hospitalisation in children aged 0–14 years: results from the ESFBI study. *Eur Arch Otorhinolaryngol* 2008; 265: 971–78.
15. Foltran F, Ballali S, Rodriguez H, et al. Inhaled foreign bodies in children: a global perspective on their epidemiological, clinical and preventive aspects. *Pediatr Pulm* 2013; 48: 344–51.
16. Brown J, Baik F, Ou H, et al. Upper aerodigestive magnetic foreign bodies in children. *Laryngoscope* 2014; 124(6): 1481–85.
17. Fraser L, Wynne D, Clement W, et al. Liquid detergent capsule ingestion in children: an increasing trend. *Arch Dis Child* 2012; 97(11): 1007.
18. Mitchell R, Hussey H, Setzen G, et al. Clinical Consensus statement tracheostomy care. *Otolaryngol Head Neck Surg* 2013; 148(1): 6–20.

Safe and effective practice

CHAPTER 35

TRAINING, ACCREDITATION AND THE MAINTENANCE OF SKILLS

B. Nirmal Kumar, Andrew Robson, Omar Mirza and Baskaran Ranganathan

Principles of training	369
GMC standards of assessment	371
Evolution of surgical training	371
Structure of UK postgraduate and ENT specialty training	373
Delivery of training	373

Maintenance of skills	375
Appraisal and revalidation for surgeons: Specialty-specific guidelines	375
Future of training in ENT	376
References	377

SEARCH STRATEGY

Data in this chapter may be updated by a PubMed search using the keywords: otolaryngology, training, surgical education, educational models, clinical competence, academic legislation & jurisprudence, European Union and United Kingdom.

PRINCIPLES OF TRAINING

A training programme in any postgraduate medical specialty, which includes otorhinolaryngology (ORL), is designed to ensure that a doctor progressing through that programme is competent to perform as an independent specialist within the healthcare system in which they work. It follows that the first goal to agree upon, when designing a programme, is the level at which competence should be set and what the scope of the competencies should be. A curriculum will then be written, agreed upon by stakeholders and published. A curriculum has the following areas of content:

- aims and objectives
- content or syllabus
- resources
- assessment strategy
- evaluation.

Aims and objectives

A clearly stated aim of a curriculum is required to ensure that it has the right content and assessment strategy. In the UK in 2016 the aim of the curriculum in ORL for postgraduate training is to train a surgeon who is emergency safe and has the ability to develop an area of special interest. Being emergency safe requires a high degree of knowledge as well as technical and clinical skills, not least because of the need to manage a wide range of unselected patients with a variety of conditions. To demonstrate safe management of emergencies the curriculum can identify elective procedures that may be used as proxy for the less common emergency procedures. For example, competence in a (relatively common) selective neck dissection can, in conjunction with clinical, non-operative experience, be used as a proxy for competence in managing neck trauma and deep neck abscesses. This requirement for a high level of technical expertise in managing emergencies has the consequence of lengthening training time compared to a programme where competence in emergency care is not a prerequisite for completion of training. Shorter specific fellowship programmes should also have a curriculum with specific aims so that one can assess competence against curriculum objectives. So, for example, an advanced otology fellowship programme may state that an aim of the programme is 'competence in cochlear implant surgery'.

The aim of a curriculum should take into account a variety of stakeholders. Indeed, one motivation could be political, whereby a particular programme is designed with a public health policy in mind that needs to be implemented. A specialist needs to be 'fit for purpose' and capable of working effectively within a healthcare system. Therefore, when designing a curriculum, it is imperative to consult patient groups, employers, commissioners, trainee representatives and, importantly, those responsible for delivering training (e.g. in England these are the Local Education and Training Boards (LETBs)) to ensure that a specialist is in the best position to deliver care to those who receive it (the patients) and those who commission it (ultimately the government). With increasing input from lay people and non-specialists in the design of surgical curricula, there has been a greater emphasis on professional and leadership skills where the importance of effective communication, leadership, teaching and keeping up to date is made, as well as assessed.

In the UK, the General Medical Council (GMC), along with specialty input, is responsible for the design and delivery of curricula. The process of curriculum approval by the GMC is governed through the Curriculum Advisory Group (CAG), where medical royal colleges, faculties and specialty associations are held accountable to the standards and requirements for curricula and assessment systems in accordance with the Medical Act 1983.[1,2]

Syllabus

Once the primary aim of a curriculum is established, a syllabus then needs to be formulated that allows the delivery of curriculum objectives in a clear, unambiguous way. A syllabus will define in a variable amount of detail the areas that need to be learnt and the requirements needed to demonstrate competence to ensure the aim is realized. A syllabus will usually be written in sections or topics where the knowledge, clinical and technical skills required are defined against the level of competence necessary. A syllabus is defined by a specialty curriculum group which takes into account the breadth of skills required, the caseload available for training, as well as the level of expertise at which those who are awarded a Certificate of Completion of Training (CCT) should expect to be competent. The concept of 'desirability' of inclusion of topics, with the understandable aspiration for expertise in all areas, must be balanced with 'deliverability' whereby a pragmatic approach to setting competence levels should be adopted so that competence can be achieved by all. For example, it is unnecessary in the UK programme for all trainees to be expected to be competent in stapedectomy and neither is it realistic to be able to deliver this training opportunity to all. A syllabus indicates the supreme aims of a programme through ensuring that trainees understand what is required to achieve competence, and in what areas they will be assessed to demonstrate competence, prior to certification.

Resources

Once an aim of a programme is agreed and a syllabus written, the resources required to deliver it need to be established. If appropriate resources are not available, then the curriculum may need to be reviewed and modified, as it is a *sine qua non* that a curriculum can only be achieved if the resources required to fulfil it are available to all. The following resources are required for curriculum delivery:

- **Caseload:** Enough cases are needed to enable *all* trainees to have equitable access sufficient to meet training needs. With healthcare delivery evolving this requires regular evaluation. For example, over the next few years exposure to transnasal oesophagoscopy (TNO) is likely to increase in the UK, whilst with the changing management of head and neck oncology, exposure to total laryngectomy is likely to reduce.
- **Faculty:** There should be adequate access to expert faculty to train those going through the programme. In surgical programmes faculty is represented by consultant surgeons who have competing interests for their professional responsibilities. Faculty need to be trained and accredited for their role within a teaching programme.
- **'Off the job' training:** Increasingly there is an emphasis on simulated or technology enhanced learning, which has the principle of providing a safe environment to hone essential technical and non-technical skills before exposure to real patients (e.g. in human factors training).[3] There is some evidence that simulation training improves the rate of acquisition of skills, but this has to be balanced with the increased cost of equipment, time away from patient care and requirements for trained faculty to supervise learning in this environment. There is a move in the UK towards mandatory simulated surgical training in order to satisfy some aspects of the curriculum.
- **Time for training:** A purely supernumerary trainee is aspirational, with the tradition for service delivery as a means of acquiring competence embedded in UK training. Training lists and clinics take longer than pure service lists, and the balance needs to be struck between the two. Skilful supervision will mitigate the time lost to training whilst developing a trainee's skills and this is one of the aims of courses in educational supervision.
- **Pastoral support:** Support for those experiencing difficulties in achieving outcomes is necessary to ensure all trainees have the opportunity to achieve the aims of the curriculum of the programme they are training in.

Assessment

Trainees within programmes need to be assessed to ensure they are on track in their development and to prove that they have achieved the aims of the programme. Assessments may be formative (assessment for learning), which tend to use workplace-based assessments (WPBA) on a regular basis, or summative (assessment of learning), which are high stakes assessments (i.e. a pass/fail exam). Each is complementary, but a continuous cycle of low stakes 'on the job' assessments will, when used correctly, encourage reflective learning and steady development in clinical, technical and professional skills. Summative assessments need to be developed and assured that they are assessing the whole curriculum and assessing trainees at the correct level in their training.

In the UK this is overseen by the GMC as part of its role in quality assuring all aspects of postgraduate training.

Evaluation

Programmes also need to be evaluated to ensure that they are fit for purpose, that is, delivering a surgeon capable of achieving the aim of the programme. This can be achieved by 'triangulation' of feedback from trainees, faculty and users of the service. Analysis of assessments can also demonstrate that a programme is delivering a properly trained surgeon. Evaluation should feed into the review of a curriculum so that it can be modified appropriately to best reflect the requirements of service users, whilst also ensuring trainees are being treated fairly and receiving support and opportunities to accomplish their aims. In the UK the annual GMC and Joint Committee on Surgical Training (JCST) trainee survey is producing increasingly meaningful data capable of evaluating programmes and helping to identify areas for development. Analysis of data from workplace-based assessments within trainee portfolios are being used to demonstrate the validity and utility of such tools.[4]

GMC STANDARDS OF ASSESSMENT

The GMC supervises the standards that medical royal colleges, faculties and specialty associations must apply in developing, monitoring and assessing curricula. The GMC defines an assessment system as an integrated set of assessments that is in place for the entire postgraduate training programme and that is blueprinted against and supports the approved curriculum. The importance of a robust assessment system is to:[5]

- determine whether trainees are meeting the standards of competence and performance specified at various stages in the curriculum for surgical training
- provide systematic and comprehensive feedback as part of the learning cycle
- determine whether trainees have acquired the common and specialty-based knowledge, clinical judgement, operative and technical skills, and generic professional behaviour and leadership skills required to practise at the level of CCT in the designated surgical specialty
- address all the domains of *Good Medical Practice* and conform to the principles laid down by the GMC.[6]

In order to be included in an assessment system, the assessment methods selected must meet the following criteria:[5]

- **Validity:** To ensure face validity, WPBAs comprise of direct observations of workplace tasks. The complexity of the tasks increases in line with progression through the training programme. To ensure content validity all the assessment instruments have been blueprinted against all standards of *Good Medical Practice*.
- **Reliability:** In order to increase reliability, there will be multiple measures of outcomes. Intercollegiate Surgical Curriculum Programme (ISCP) assessments make use of several observers' judgements, multiple assessment methods (triangulation) and take place frequently. The planned, systematic and permanent programme of assessor training for trainers and assigned educational supervisors (AES) through the Deaneries/LETBs is intended to gain maximum reliability of placement reports.
- **Feasibility:** The practicality of the assessments in the training and working environment has been taken into account. The assessment should not add a significant amount of time to the workplace task being assessed and assessors should be able to complete the scoring and feedback part of the assessment in 5–10 minutes.
- **Cost-effectiveness:** Once staff have been trained in the assessment process and are familiar with the online ISCP portfolio, the only significant additional costs should be the extra time taken for assessments and feedback and the induction of a new AES. The most substantial extra time investment will be in the regular appraisal process for units that did not previously have such a system.
- **Opportunities for feedback:** All the assessments, both those for learning and of learning, include a feedback element. Structured feedback is a fundamental component of high-quality assessment and should be incorporated throughout workplace-based assessments.
- **Impact on learning:** The workplace-based assessments are all designed to include immediate feedback as part of the process. A minimum number of three appraisals with the AES per clinical placement is built into the training system. The formal examinations all provide limited feedback as part of the summative process. The assessment process thus has a continuous developmental impact on learning, a process enriched further with emphasis on reflective practice within the portfolio.

EVOLUTION OF SURGICAL TRAINING

Postgraduate surgical training has undergone significant change over recent decades. Historically surgical training in the UK was considered to be an apprenticeship, taking several years to learn the theoretical background and cultivate operative competence to achieve expertise.[7] Although there were advantages to the conventional time-based apprenticeship model of training and it did successfully produce competent consultant surgeons over many years, several limitations did exist and it gradually became outdated. Training was considered unstructured, occurring over an undefined period of time, and often consisted of unsupervised service rather than training. This was associated with an inherent difficulty in measuring trainee competence and was criticized for lacking transparency, reliability and validity. This not only failed to meet training needs, but also did not satisfy the changing expectations and demands of both patients and an evolving

National Health Service requiring a greater number of consultants to deliver care and train the next generation of surgeons, due to both the mounting demands of patient safety and the ever increasing medico-legal unacceptability of complications due to inexperience.

The Calman Report in 1993 outlined the future direction of training and this was reinforced further in the chief medical officer's report, *Unfinished Business*, in 2002, in which recommendations were made for the establishment of a national benchmark for training, comprehensive specialty curriculums and regular assessment of trainee competence, as well as consultant-delivered, rather than consultant-led, patient care.[8,9] As a result, Modernising Medical Careers (MMC) was initiated in 2003 and this was followed by the implementation of a shortened, restructured continuous pathway of specialty training based on a model of proficiency in developing trainee competence according to predetermined approved standards.[10] A shift to a more competency-based form of training has assured the provision of a high standard of training with less importance placed on service delivery and a greater emphasis on formal supervision from consultant trainers appropriately qualified to train, assess and give feedback. Following satisfactory completion of training, having developed the required competencies to practice independently and having reached a definite educational end point after a predetermined period of time, a trainee is awarded a certificate of completion of training (CCT) and is able to practice as a consultant.

A further challenge has been the delivery of a shortened and reorganized training paradigm within the restrictions imposed by the compulsory implementation of the European Working Time Directive (EWTD).[11,12] The significant reduction in the time available to train has had a dramatic impact, especially on surgical specialties, where developing and achieving expertise relies heavily on operative experience and exposure. The concept of experiential learning suggests that to truly understand something a learner must experience it first-hand.[13] With a traditional time-based model of training, trainees would have had an estimated 25–30,000 hours of training before reaching consultant level, allowing deliberate practice so that replication of events leads to a full understanding and the development of subconscious pattern recognition. The current competency-based training is thought to only offer around 6000 hours.[14] To attain a level of expertise in a certain field subconscious pattern recognition is vital, and it has been suggested that at least 10,000 hours of training is necessary for this to occur.[15]

As such, a greater need has been identified in order to maximize learning, develop acquired competences, accelerate skills acquisition and reduce learning curves in order to meet the educational needs of surgical trainees within the confines of a 48-hour working week. Accordingly, higher surgical training curricula have also evolved to incorporate alternate educational modalities, such as simulation, in order to bridge this gap and compensate for the significant reduction in the time available for training (**Figure 35.1**). Simulation provides a realistic exposure equivalent environment that allows deliberate practice in order to achieve expertise in a non-threatening environment without risk to patients.[15] Behavioural models have shown high fidelity controlled environments akin to real life can show correct practice and through accumulative experience cement learning.[16] Objective assessment is also possible, enhancing the learning process by facilitating reflection and reinforcing positive behaviours and identifying negative actions.

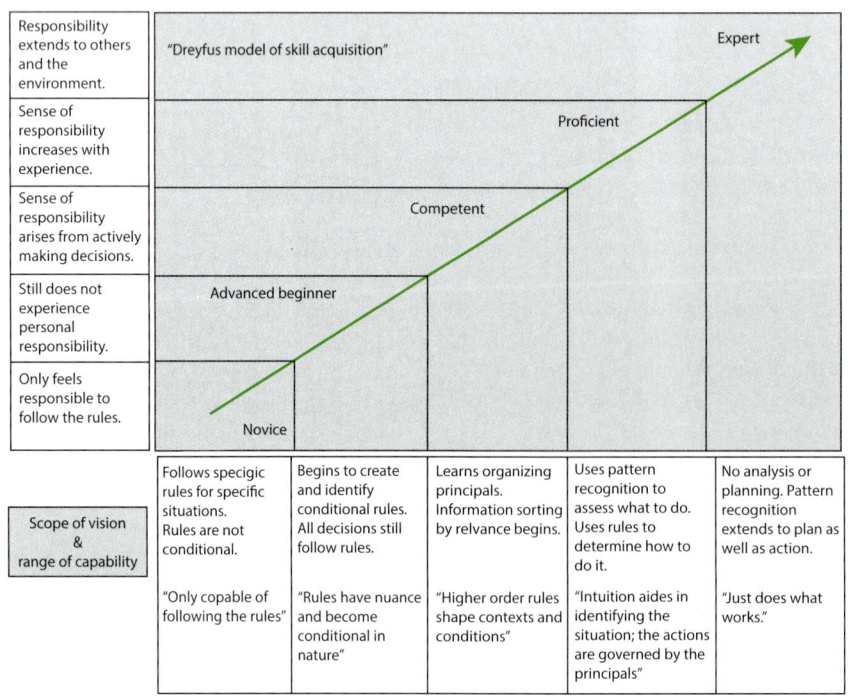

Figure 35.1 Dreyfus model of skills acquisitions. Learning through simulation hopes to alter the trajectory to quicken the learning curve passing from novice to attaining expertise.[17]

STRUCTURE OF UK POSTGRADUATE AND ENT SPECIALTY TRAINING

Trainees begin their postgraduate medical education by entering the foundation training programme, which was implemented in 2005 as part of MMC. This has replaced the traditional house officer and senior house officer grades, and allows junior doctors to rotate through core disciplines in order to develop the generic skill set required to practice safely in their onward specialties. Those wishing to pursue a career in surgery then apply to a generic 2-year Core Surgical Training (CST) programme, themed to their chosen surgical discipline (**Figure 35.2**). The CST programme is a broad-based initial training in surgery that enables trainees to establish the necessary competences, fundamental skills and breadth of experience required for progress on to higher specialty training (HST). Membership of the Royal College of Surgeons (MRCS) and Diploma in Otolaryngology – Head and Neck Surgery (DOHNS), or alternatively the MRCS (ENT) examinations are sat at this stage, and are, along with other defined mandatory criteria, an essential component of satisfactory completion of CST, before being eligible to apply to an HST programme. Recruitment to both CST and HST is through competitive national selection.

ORL HST is a 6-year programme that allows trainees to develop the necessary competencies in order to achieve a CCT. During this period a trainee can embark on additional out of programme activities (OOPA) in addition to conventional training, such as alternative training or experiences (OOPT/OOPE), research (OOPR) or fellowships. Towards the end of HST, the Fellowship of the Royal College of Surgeons (FRCS(ORL-HNS)) exit exam is sat.

Subspecialization in ENT surgery has been well established for many years and trainees are encouraged to show a special interest in a particular subspecialty during their training period. Fellowship programmes offer this additional training opportunity to pre- and post-CCT trainees and are available both in the UK and abroad. The JCST interface group, in conjunction with allied surgical specialties, offer interface fellowship programmes for UK trainees in ORL, plastics and maxillofacial surgery.[18] These fellowship programmes are accredited and have a structured, defined syllabus, and are monitored regularly for quality assurance. Alternative UK, European and international fellowships in other subspecialties also exist.

The Certificate of Eligibility for Specialist Registration (CESR) is a route to entry onto the specialist register for those doctors who have not entered through HST but are able to demonstrate experience, skills and knowledge equivalent to CCT. The application process is arbitrated by the GMC, and the JCST has issued specialty-specific guidelines for applicants applying through this process that outline the relevant supporting evidence, mapped to the four domains of *Good Medical Practice*, which are required.[18] Applications should also be supported by six consultant referees who are able to give a structured report regarding a candidate's clinical and non-clinical performance. The submitted documents are assessed against these requirements, as well as against the current ORL HST curriculum, by a GMC-approved assessor before CESR is awarded.

DELIVERY OF TRAINING

The aim of a competency-based surgical curriculum is to provide an assured, high quality of surgical training to ensure it produces proficient trainees able to deliver a high standard of surgical care, safely to patients. A competency model of training satisfies the need for an objective measurement of surgeon competence and performance. This delivers reassurances to the public that surgeons are being trained to an appropriate standard, whilst providing evidence to educational peers that trainees are demonstrating

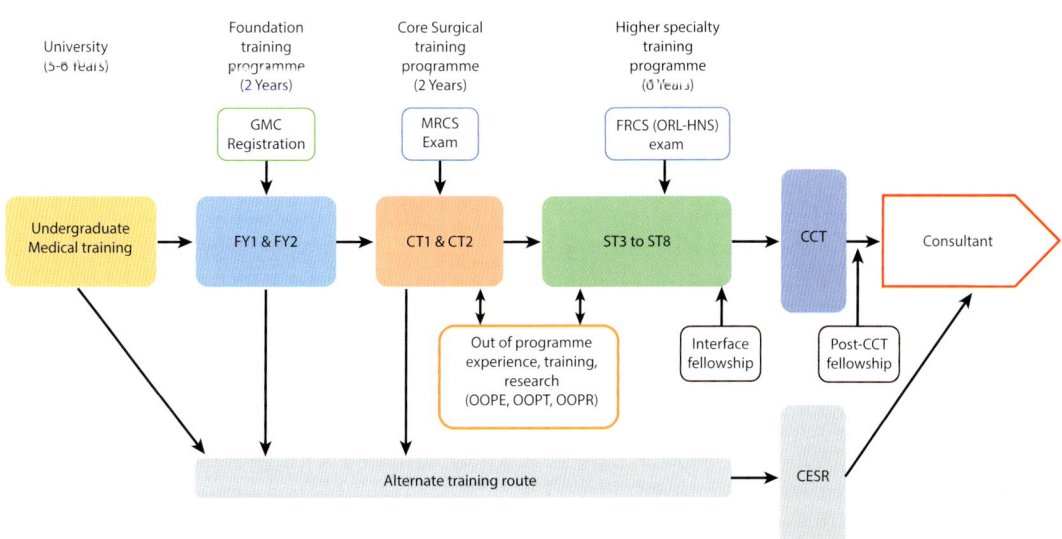

Figure 35.2 Current typical UK postgraduate training pathway for a career in ORL.

continuous development commensurate with their stage of training. The ISCP, a real time, online web portfolio (https://www.iscp.ac.uk), allowing an interface between trainer and trainee, has become a central component in supporting this process.[5] It has a clearly defined competency-based syllabus to which trainees are able to integrate their completed WPBA and additional educational achievements and map them to the curriculum as evidence of progress through training. Summative records of formal educational meetings and annual appraisal are also recorded to form a comprehensive record of training.

During their 6 years, ENT specialty trainees will expect to rotate to at least three different training units within their Deanery/LETB in order gain exposure to all the ENT subspecialties and to develop the required skill set and competences to satisfy curriculum standards. Rotation to a particular unit may be decided by trainee preference, individual educational requirements and stage of training. Each training placement is expected to be able to provide:

- at least three or more consultant supervised outpatient clinics per week, including a combination of routine, emergency and special interest clinics, limited to 10–14 new and follow-up patients
- four (or more) supervised operating sessions per week with a suitable elective and emergency case mix in a unit with a minimum output of 500 cases per year per trainee
- opportunities to manage patients presenting acutely at least once a week
- weekly formal local teaching, as well as regular regional teaching
- exposure to audit, research and other educational activities to develop teaching, management and leadership skills.

For each placement a trainee will have an AES with an overall educational and supervisory responsibility for the trainee, along with other departmental consultant trainers, or clinical supervisors (CS), who will also deliver teaching, train and have involvement in the assessment process. Traditionally, it may have been assumed that all consultants were good trainers. However, it is increasingly apparent that this is not true, and the skills required to teach, train and give feedback may not necessarily be inherent, but instead need to be learned and developed. The key to an effectively deployed competency-based curriculum are suitably qualified trainers able to reliably assess and give constructive feedback. As such, there is an increasing expectation that consultant trainers, and even trainees during their higher specialty training, undergo formal training or gain a higher qualification in teaching principles and methodology before they assume a formal role as a trainer.

Although consultant trainers do have a facilitatory role, the responsibility of training remains primarily with the trainee. At the start of each placement a 'learning agreement' (LA) is set by the trainee with their AES, agreeing on the educational objectives for the forthcoming placement. This is recorded on the ISCP and is revisited with the trainee during interval formative and summative appraisals typically in the middle and at the end of the placement. Throughout the placement trainees are expected to complete a set number and a variety of WBAs assessing knowledge, clinical judgement, procedural and technical competences, as well as professional behaviour and attitudes such as communication, team working and management skills. These include:

- case-based discussion (CBD)
- clinical evaluation exercises (CEX)
- direct observation of procedural skills (DOPS)
- procedure-based assessment (PBA)
- multi-source feedback (MSF).

Assessment is made to determine whether a trainee is meeting curriculum standards of competence and performance expected for their stage of training. Each completed WPBA can be linked to the ISCP syllabus as evidence and can be used to demonstrate evolving progression up to demonstrating fully competent, independent practice as a trainee progresses through specialty training. As training is no longer time-defined, assimilating acquired competences may vary according to trainee exposure and ability. In addition, WPBAs can also effectively be used as a formative tool at the time of completion. The process of reflection and feedback helps consolidate the learning process by reinforcing positive practice, but also enables the trainee to identify specific learning points for onward development. Learning through objective feedback is an essential component of enhancing the educational process by directing learning towards desired outcomes. WPBAs can, however, be incorrectly used and seen as a time-consuming 'tick-box' exercise, which can have a negative impact on the reliability and validity of the assessment. In order for these assessments to retain their educational value, they must be used correctly, as a continuous, formative tool to provide constructive feedback to trainees.

Collectively, WPBAs, in addition to the end of placement AES and CS reports, and additional recorded evidence of educational activity (including involvement in audit, research, publications, attendance at courses and conferences), are evaluated in an annual review of competence progression (ARCP). This summative face-to-face appraisal is to assess whether a trainee is developing satisfactorily and has achieved the necessary competencies in order to progress to the next stage of training. Equally, if a trainee is underperforming, this can be identified and additional support given to meet their specific educational needs.

Towards the end of specialty training, and provided a trainee is meeting their educational requirements of training, they are able to sit the FRCS(ORL-HNS) exit exam. This traditional summative assessment complements competency-based training positively by formally assessing what has been learnt throughout specialty training. In order for recommendation to be made to the GMC for an award of the CCT, a trainee should have gained all required curricula competencies, passed the FRCS(ORL-HNS), and completed a pre-defined number of 'index' operative procedures (elective and emergency) to a specified level of competence, in addition to the total number of defined major operations required to be completed in the generality of ORL so as to cover the fundamental subspecialties (head and neck, rhinology, otology and paediatric ORL).

MAINTENANCE OF SKILLS

Continuing professional development (CPD) is the engagement in lifelong self-directed learning outside formal postgraduate training. It is the duty of all doctors to keep up to date, and maintain and improve their knowledge and skills in order to provide a high standard of care to patients and the public throughout their career. The obligations of doctors are specified in *Good Medical Practice* and *Good Surgical Practice*.[6, 19] The key points addressed are:

1. The essence of CPD is to be competent and up to date across all clinical and non-clinical aspects of the practice.
2. CPD should be a combination of formal and informal teaching and should include the activities within the local institution as well as at regional, national and international levels. Surgeons should aim for a mix of at least three activities including clinical, academic and professional (including managerial).
3. The minimum requirement for CPD in the UK is 50 credits per annum. One credit represents one hour of activity. To encourage a range of activities, normally no more than 20 of the minimum 50 hours per year should come from a single activity.[20]
4. Surgeons are encouraged to record the activities electronically, such as in the 'surgeons portfolio' developed by the Royal College of Surgeons (RCS), which helps to record the activities securely and assists surgeons with the appraisal and revalidation process (**Table 35.1**).[20]
5. There is a range of organizations that accredit the CPD activities including the medical royal colleges, specialty associations and LETBs. The RCS has established criteria and standards for accreditation of CPD activities.[21] ENT-UK accredits educational activities relevant to the specialty. The organization seeking accreditation must demonstrate compliance to the academic and competence standards:
    - CPD is awarded on the basis of course content and delegates' feedback.
    - The activity should have clear scientific and educational purpose and should address the learning needs of the participants.
    - The course organizers and faculties should have a proven relevant expertise, and appropriate skills and knowledge.
    - Robust quality assurance is required with course inspection and evaluation.
    - Attendance records should be maintained.
    - Feedback forms should be submitted for further accreditations of the event.

APPRAISAL AND REVALIDATION FOR SURGEONS: SPECIALTY-SPECIFIC GUIDELINES

Appraisal and revalidation is based on the principles of *Good Medical Practice*. Doctors practising in the UK must participate in an annual appraisal process to reflect on their practice and performance based on which the responsible officer (RO) makes recommendation to the GMC to renew their licence to practice every 5 years. The GMC and RCS have provided a number of documents to describe the supporting information required for appraisal and revalidation.[23] The surgeons are expected to collect and maintain a portfolio of supporting information to demonstrate that they are continuing to meet the principles and values set out in *Good Medical Practice*, which consists of four domains as follows:[6]

1. Knowledge, skills and performance
2. Safety and quality
3. Communication, partnership and teamwork
4. Maintaining trust.

Checklists are available to guide the surgeon through the suggested components of the revalidation process (**Table 35.2**).

Individual surgeon and departmental outcome measures are playing an increasing role in the surgical appraisal

TABLE 35.1 Examples of activities that will qualify for CPD[18]

	Internal	External	Personal
Clinical	Courses, workshops and meetings	Courses, workshops and meetings	Self directed learning, e.g. reading journals
Academic	Audit, research	Participating in national audits, research trials and presentations	Publications and peer-reviewing articles
Professional	Teaching, training and mentoring activities	Examiner, e.g. undergraduates, MRCS, FRCS Standard setting for exams	Courses on management, leadership and teaching/training

Note: The list in this table is not exhaustive and individuals should discuss with their appraiser to plan the activities that will address individual educational needs.

TABLE 35.2 Supporting information for revalidation checklist based on the Academy of Medical Royal Colleges and Faculties' Core Guidance[22]

General information	Personal information Scope of work Record of annual appraisal Personal development plan (PDP) Probity Health	Current job plan Description of clinical and non-clinical activities Appraisal portfolio Agreed objectives from previous PDP Self declaration of Probity and health
Keeping up to date	CPD	Evidence of CPD activities
Review of current practice	Clinical audit Review of clinical outcome Case review or discussion Clinical incidents	Details of participation in local/national audits Details of outcome data Participation mortality and morbidity meeting Records of clinical incidents and reflection
Feedback on your practice	Patients' feedback Colleagues' feedback Complaints and compliments	Multisource feedback from colleagues and patients Details of complaints and compliments

and revalidation process. This supports best practice and ultimately improves patient care. ENT-UK supports the participation in national clinical audit and, for example, has previously jointly collaborated with RCS of England to conduct and publish outcomes of the national prospective tonsillectomy audit. Currently ENT-UK is managing surgeon activity data for laryngeal surgery and airway intervention registry for paediatric balloon dilatation procedures for airway stenosis. It is important to also mention that some recorded individual surgeon's outcome data can be published and subsequently accessed by the public, a development aiming for greater transparency and accountability. For example, members of the British Association of Endocrine and Thyroid Surgeons (BAETS) are required to participate in the UK Registry of Endocrine and Thyroid Surgery (UKRETS), which is an electronic audit of endocrine operations. All thyroid surgeries must be recorded in UKRETS, which is the published openly via the surgeon specific outcomes report for endocrine surgery.

FUTURE OF TRAINING IN ENT

The specialty of ORL has evolved significantly over the last four decades with expanding subspecialization, introduction of new technologies and as a result of the development of new surgical techniques. Furthermore, the move in the UK to the provision of full '7-day working' and an anticipated shift of the provision of ORL services to both community outpatient-based and super-specialized tertiary centres will have a dramatic impact on the provision of training and the expectations of the ENT surgeon. This will inevitably need to be matched by constant review and subsequent modifications of learning curricula in future ORL surgical training. The challenge is to address new advancements and potential changes in training within a safe timeframe in order to continue to create a surgical workforce that is able to deliver competent, safe and high quality patient care.

KEY POINTS

- The objective of the curriculum for higher surgical training in ENT is to train a surgeon who is emergency safe and competent to practice independently in the healthcare system.
- In the UK, the General Medical Council (GMC) supervises the standards of the curriculum developed by the Royal colleges, faculties, and specialty associations.
- The syllabus is written in sections where the knowledge, clinical and technical skills required are defined against the level of competence necessary. The trainees are expected to achieve those set competencies in order to progress in their training to obtain completion of certification of training.
- In the UK, post-graduation training begins with two years of foundation training and a further two years core surgical training in a chosen specialty to gain broad-based initial training prior to progressing on to higher surgical training which is six years for ENT.
- Throughout the placement, trainees are expected to complete a set number of work-based assessments to assess the knowledge, clinical and procedural skills, professional behavior and attitudes. To gain CCT, trainees are expected to achieve all competencies outlined in the curriculum, completion of FRCS (ORL-HNS) and performance of a defined number of 'Index' procedures.
- Doctors practising in the UK must participate in an annual appraisal process and revalidation once in every five years to renew their license to practice by the GMC. The above process is to ensure doctors are up to date, maintain their skills and knowledge to provide a high standard of care to the patients.
- ENT specialty is evolving rapidly with expanding subspecialization and introduction of new diagnostic and surgical techniques. There is a need for constant review and modification in the surgical curriculum and training in future to match the changes.

REFERENCES

1. http://www.gmc-uk.org/education/approval_curricula_and_assessment_system.asp
2. http://www.gmc-uk.org/about/legislation/medical_act.asp
3. Department of Health. *A framework for technology enhanced learning.* London: Department of Health; 2011. Available from https://www.gov.uk/government/uploads/system/uploads/attachment_data/file/215316/dh_131061.pdf
4. Awad Z, Hayden L, Muthuswamy K, et al. Utilisation and outcomes of case based discussion in otolaryngology training. *Clin Otolaryngol All Sci* 2015; **40**: 86–92.
5. https://www.iscp.ac.uk
6. General Medical Council. *Good medical practice.* London: General Medical Council; 2014.
7. Halsted W. The training of the surgeon. *Bull Johns Hopkins Hosp* 1904; **15**: 267–76.
8. Department of Health. *A guide to specialist training.* London: Department of Health; 1993.
9. Department of Health. *Unfinished business: proposals for the reform of the SHO grade.* London: Department of Health; 2002.
10. Department of Health. *Modernising medical careers.* London: Department of Health; 2003.
11. Council of the European Union. European Working Time Directive, No. 93/104/EC.
12. Department of Health. *New deal for junior doctors.* London: Department for Health; 1991.
13. Kolb DA. *Experiential learning: experience as the source of learning and development.* Englewood, NJ: Prentice Hall; 1984.
14. Chalmer C, Joshi S, Bentley P, et al. The lost generation: impact of the 56 working hour week on current surgical training. *B Roy Coll Surg Eng* 2010; **92**(3): 102–06.
15. Ericsson K, Prietula M, Cokely E. The making of an expert. *Harv Bus Rev* 2007; **85**(7–8): 114–21.
16. Watson JB, Skinner BF, cited in Rachlin H. *Introduction to modern behaviorism.* New York: Freeman; 1991.
17. Dreyfus HL, Dreyfus SE. *Mind over machine: the power of human intuition and expertise in the age of the computer.* Oxford: Basil Blackwell; 1986.
18. Joint Committee on Surgical Training. *Training interface groups.* Available from http://www.jcst.org/training-interface-groups
19. General Medical Council. *Specialty specific guidance for otolaryngology.* Available from http://www.gmc-uk.org/SGPC___SSG___Otolaryngology___DC2320.pdf_48455281.pdf
20. The Royal College of Surgeons of England. *Good surgical practice.* London: The Royal College of Surgeons of England; 2014.
21. Directors of CPD Subcommittee of the Academy of Medical Royal Colleges. *Continuing professional development scheme for surgery.* London: Academy of Medical Royal Colleges; 2014
22. Joint Committee on Surgical Training. *Training interface groups.* Available from http://www.jcst.org/training-interface-groups
23. Federation of Surgical Specialty Associations, The Royal College of Surgeons of Edinburgh, The Royal College of Surgeons of England, The Royal College of Physicians and Surgeons of Glasgow. *Revalidation guide for surgery Jan 2014.* Available from http://www.baps.org.uk/content/uploads/2017/03/Revalidation-Guide-for-Surgery-2014.pdfA

CHAPTER 36

COMMUNICATION AND THE MEDICAL CONSULTATION

Uttam Shiralkar

Introduction 379	Non-verbal communication 383
Why communication skills are important for doctors 380	Communicating adverse incidents 384
Why communication skills are important for surgeons ... 380	Addressing issues around loss 385
Why communication skills are important for ENT surgeons ... 380	Discussing medical errors 385
Literature 381	Conclusion 386
Learning communication skills 381	References 386
Communication models 381	

SEARCH STRATEGY

Data in this chapter may be updated by Medline, Embase and PsychINFO searches using the keywords: communication skills, doctor-patient communication, communication skills and surgeons, training communication for health professionals, communication and clinical outcome.

INTRODUCTION

How important is it for a surgeon to have good communication skills? Not many people would think this to be of 'life-and-death' importance. Unfortunately, this was exactly the case for one plastic surgeon in Madrid, who was killed by one of his dissatisfied patients. That was not a unique incident. Between 1995 and 2005, five surgeons were killed by disgruntled patients in the USA.[1] Although these extreme acts of violence are rare, many surgeons face abuse, complaints or legal actions due to communication problems between them and patients. Every day of our working lives we rely upon communication skills to build up relationships with our patients. These skills are vital in establishing trust with those who come to us with problems. This chapter explores the communication issues related to outpatient visits. Since practical communication training is available in various formats such as written material, workshops, videos and online training, this chapter will focus on the fundamentals to deliver a broader perspective.

As a doctor, consultation is the most common clinical procedure we employ. Our communication with a patient has a therapeutic effect. Compared to other therapeutic modalities, communication has an immediate palliative effect as it can reduce a patient's distress instantly. Comparatively, it has a wider therapeutic index since this treatment-related morbidity and mortality has never occurred! The most common problem observed regarding its use is suboptimal dosing.[2] Good communication is not just 'being nice' or having a 'touchy-feely' talk. It is a specific task and observable behaviour that includes interviewing a patient to obtain clinical information, explaining diagnosis or prognosis, and giving treatment advice and information needed for an informed consent to undergo procedures. It also involves providing counselling to patients to motivate participation in the management.[3] Conventionally our management tends to focus only on bio-medical aspects of the treatment since we adopt a 'disease perspective'.[4] Lately there has been a realization of the limitation of a narrow 'disease perspective' and the need to treat the patient from an 'illness perspective'. When doctors interact with the patient through the 'illness perspective' the impact of a disease on the patient from a personal aspect is taken into account so that the care becomes 'patient-centred'. Patient-centred care entails involving the patient in decision-making and activating their sense of responsibility.[5] Without appropriate communication skills the surgeon will not be able to deliver patient-centred care.

WHY COMMUNICATION SKILLS ARE IMPORTANT FOR DOCTORS

There are various advantages of taking the skill of communication seriously:

- A skilful interview improves diagnostic accuracy by gathering a superior quantity and quality of information.[6]
- Doctors with excellent communication skills establish good understanding with their patients and consequentially improve the patients' compliance and outcomes.[7]
- In contrast, poor communication seems to be correlated with patient dissatisfaction.[8] Studies have shown that communication skills are the single most important factor in patients' satisfaction. Practising surgeons will be interested to know that a satisfied patient will tell, on average, three other patients about their positive experience. On the other hand, patients who are dissatisfied with their encounter will tell, on average, 19 other individuals about their unpleasant experience.[9]

WHY COMMUNICATION SKILLS ARE IMPORTANT FOR SURGEONS

Communication between surgeons and their patients is particularly important. A randomized trial specific to surgical communication showed that patients undergoing surgery had better pain scores and lower analgesic use postoperatively when the pre-operative communication with the patient was appropriately conducted.[7] Patients visiting surgeons, in comparison to visiting other specialists, may be more anxious due to the concerns of undergoing invasive procedures. Surgeons need to conduct conversations about complicated medical issues, treatment choices and complexities of surgical options, and they have to address patients' anxieties.[10]

A study that analysed surgeons' communication behaviours identified that failure to adequately explain the medical condition, failure to show interest in the patient, failure to ask whether they had any questions and failure to answer their questions were the main factors for patients not recommending the surgeon.[11] There is evidence showing that very few patients or their families are able to absorb what the surgeon has explained to them before surgery. Six months after surgery, patients may be unable to recall what kind of information the surgeon gave to them during the informed consent process. Additionally, some patients may even deny that this process occurred despite the existence of objective evidence.[12]

A stereotypical image of a surgeon is someone who is not a very good communicator.[13] Studies have found disparities between surgeons' self-assessments and patient's perceptions about the surgeons' communication skills.[14] There is a need to acknowledge these gaps and to make efforts to reduce them. It has been observed that when surgeons improve their communication skills, it is not just patients but the surgeons themselves who are beneficiaries. Good communication makes working in a specialty more enjoyable and acts as a preventative factor to burnout.[15, 16] After an untoward incidence in surgical practice, the possibility of the matter ending up in court is greater if the communication with the patient is not handled satisfactorily. Sometimes malpractice suits are the results of differences in expectations between a patient and the surgeon. Good communication helps the surgeon to understand patient expectations, thereby reducing liability exposure.[17]

WHY COMMUNICATION SKILLS ARE IMPORTANT FOR ENT SURGEONS

For ENT surgeons there is a need to take a particular interest in communication for various reasons. Otorhinolaryngology is a unique surgical specialty dealing with clinical problems that have a wide range of psychological implications for the patient. Otolaryngologists perform procedures like rhinoplasty purely for cosmetic improvement but also head and neck cancer surgery to improving a patient's survival. We perform emergency procedures, such as the removal of a foreign body, that give immediate relief, and we perform surgical interventions in rhinosinusitis where the patient may continue to experience some symptoms despite surgery. Some patients with sensorineural deafness may not be offered a cure but with a successful stapedectomy, hearing improvement is instant. Thus we need to prepare the patient, as well as ourselves, for the anticipated outcome, whatever that may be.

Patients visiting otolaryngologists experience symptoms that have an emotional contribution. Significant percentages of patients who experience symptoms such as dysphonia, vertigo or facial pain have underlying psychological problems.[18] Unless these psychological factors are addressed, symptom resolution will not be achieved. Chronic pain anywhere in the body invokes emotional reactions and pain in the facial region carries far more emotional reaction. An otolaryngologist with good communication skills will be able to pick up psychological cues, thereby avoiding delay in symptomatic relief.

Otolaryngologists come across patients (e.g. those with allergic rhinosinusitis) for whom curative surgery is not possible or for whom surgery will offer only partial relief. Appropriate consultation will help the patient to accept the best possible treatment. In some cases, like inoperable malignancy, the surgeon will be not be able to offer the patient anything apart from empathetic conversation, the efficacy of which is directly proportional to the surgeon's communication skills.

Otolaryngologists deal with patients who have difficulties with important sensory organs (i.e. hearing). There is a special responsibility to be sensitive to the sensory loss and at the same time not to underestimate the patient's ability to adapt.[19] This can be understood only with the help of efficient communication.

In the era of technological development and implementation of new techniques, adequate communication between otolaryngologist and patient is very important. This is especially relevant if the procedure is not very well established. In the event of a complication after the use of an uncommon or novel technique, the surgeon may be accused of not adequately explaining the consequences.[20]

LITERATURE

Despite the importance of effective communication to surgeons, the vast majority of literature in the field of medical communication has focused on primary care interactions. There have been relatively few studies describing communication between surgeons and patients.[21] The first ever study on communication between surgeon and patient was published in 1999.[4] This study underscored the differences in both the content and process of routine surgical visits compared with primary care visits. The study concluded that unlike other medical specialties, surgical consultations had a narrow biomedical focus with little consideration of the psychosocial problems the patient might experience due to the disease.

A systematic review on directly observed surgeon–patient communication was recently published.[22] The reviewers evaluated 2794 citations, 74 full-text articles, 21 studies and 13 companion reports. This systematic review highlighted the gaps that need to be addressed by training both trainee and practicing surgeons. The studies confirmed that surgeons spend the majority of consultation time in educating patients and discussing treatment options.[4, 23] Thus, surgeons use the communication mostly for the purpose of informed decision-making. Studies found that surgeons are good in providing information about the surgical conditions.[10, 24] However, they are lacking in areas such as assessing patients' understanding of therapeutic options and discussing risks. Since these elements are important for patients to make good informed choices, there is a need to improve the quality of informed decision-making conversations in surgery. It is also felt that surgeons need to focus greater attention on the emotional aspects of consultation.

LEARNING COMMUNICATION SKILLS

Although the clinical value of these skills has been known for the last few years, it has traditionally been difficult for many to accept the idea that something as supposedly intuitive as communication could or should be influenced by teaching. It was a commonly held belief that communication skills could not be taught; they were natural talents – inborn attributes of the 'good doctor' – and a young doctor was either endowed with them or not. It was debated whether these techniques could be learned, and whether anything could be done to bring the awkward communicator to a reasonable level. Mounting evidence has clearly shown that these goals are achievable and that these skills can be taught, do change patient satisfaction and can be retained over time.[25]

Surgeons receive limited formal education in the communication skills necessary for patient-centred care, although they perform more than 100 000 consultations during their careers.[26] In one study researchers developed an innovative empathy-relational skills training protocol focusing on the underlying neurobiological mechanisms of empathy and the interpersonal processes that positively affect the patient–doctor relationship. The authors tested the effectiveness of this protocol with ENT trainees. The results showed that a brief series of three empathy-training sessions significantly improved the surgeon's knowledge of the neurobiology and physiology of empathy, as well as their self-reported capacity to empathize with patients. As a result of improved empathetic consultation, improvement in patient satisfaction was observed.

From a practical perspective, improving communication skills is similar to improving operating skills. It involves seeking information, implementing the techniques and evaluating the outcome. The efforts that are put into improving clinical communication do make an indelible impression on patients. If done poorly, the patient may never forgive the surgeon; if done well, they may never forget the surgeon![27]

COMMUNICATION MODELS

There have been various attempts to describe the overall structure of a doctor–patient relationship and to create a standard model of conversation between the two that aims to facilitate training and the learning of communication skills.[27] The Calgary-Cambridge model is one model that describes a sequence of tasks to aid an effective consultation.[28]

There is no single way that a consultation plays out. Every interaction is unique, as it depends on how the surgeon and the patient contribute and react to the interactions. However, if a surgeon is aware of the basic tenets of an ideal consultation, it will provide a useful framework to build upon (**Figure 36.1**).

Engagement

Engaging the patient requires making a personal connection with him/her. This can be achieved by appropriate body language and introductory conversation. Initial questions like 'How can I help you?' will initiate the engagement. It is strongly recommended that you listen to the response to this question patiently. Patients usually disclose most of the useful information within the first two minutes; however, it is observed that a surgeon often interrupts a patient in less than half a minute and starts asking specific or closed questions.[6] Closed questions at this stage of the conversation are unlikely to reveal what is of greatest concern to the patient. Instead of closed questions, comments like 'tell me more about that' or 'what concerns do you have about that' will allow the patient to give their own view and initiate the engagement.

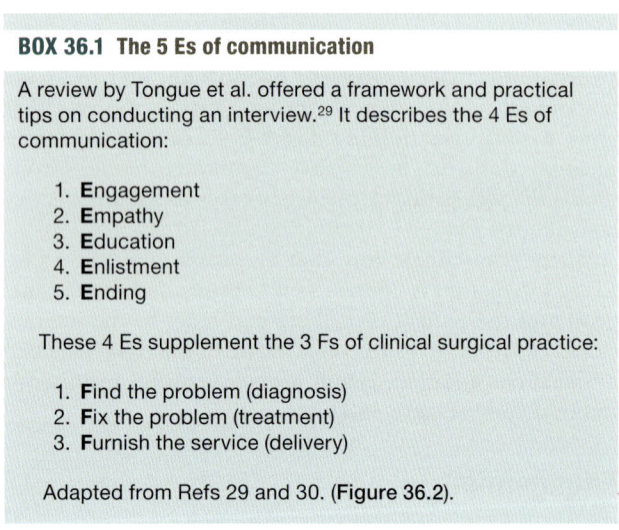

Figure 36.1 Expanded framework.

BOX 36.1 The 5 Es of communication

A review by Tongue et al. offered a framework and practical tips on conducting an interview.[29] It describes the 4 Es of communication:

1. **E**ngagement
2. **E**mpathy
3. **E**ducation
4. **E**nlistment
5. **E**nding

These 4 Es supplement the 3 Fs of clinical surgical practice:

1. **F**ind the problem (diagnosis)
2. **F**ix the problem (treatment)
3. **F**urnish the service (delivery)

Adapted from Refs 29 and 30. (**Figure 36.2**).

Empathy

'The patient will never care how much you know until they know how much you care.'[31]

Unfortunately, the most common weakness in communication with patients is a failure to demonstrate an empathic response. Studies show that surgeons often miss opportunities to express empathy.[32] The potential effect of this is that patients may feel that their surgeons have not addressed their concerns. The gaps between the patient's expectations and the surgeon's approach leads to patient dissatisfaction.[33,34]

Empathetic conversation reveals the surgeon's understanding of and concern about the patient's thoughts. It involves acknowledging the emotional content of the communication, without necessarily sharing the emotion itself. It is necessary to clarify the difference between

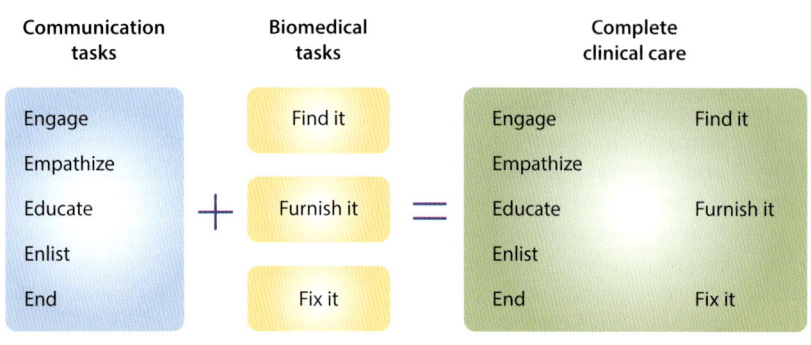

Figure 36.2 The five Es and three Fs of communication. From Tongue JR, Epps HR, Forese L. Communication skills for patient-centered care: Research-based, easily learned techniques for medical interviews that benefit orthopaedic surgeons and their patients. *J Bone Joint Surg* 2005; **87**(3): 652–58.

empathy and sympathy. Sharing the emotion fully would be sympathy and, although we may be sympathetic with some emotions, we generally do not share the emotions of most of our patients. It is not expected – in fact, it may be unhelpful for a surgeon to experience what the patient is feeling. As the saying goes, you don't need to have pain in your own right iliac fossa in order to diagnose a patient's appendicitis.

However, good communicators are expected to reflect a patient's emotion in the conversation, for example: 'It must be frightening to lose your hearing suddenly. Many people would feel that way.'

The process of acknowledging emotions is not too complex. The empathic response consists of three steps:

1. Identifying the emotion
2. Identifying the source of the emotion
3. Responding in a way that shows you have made the connection between the first two steps.

Surgeons may run short of time during consultations; hence they may be reluctant to address emotional issues, thinking that it may lengthen the consultation. However, several studies have uncovered a positive relationship between addressing the emotions and the length of the visit. Levinson et al. found that visits in which the surgeon directly addressed a patient's clue about a concern or worries were shorter than visits in which the clue was ignored.[35] This observation could be explained as the patients whose worry was addressed were able to put the concern to rest more quickly than those whose concern was unaddressed. Similarly, Braddock et al. found that visits with more complete, informed, decision-making conversations were only modestly longer than those that were less complete.[36]

Education

Educating the patient involves providing the diagnosis, the prognosis and the options for treatment in a language that the patient understands. It is necessary to be aware that the amount of information the patient requires will vary. It may be helpful to ask, 'Does that match what you have been thinking about this problem?' That will allow the patient to bring up other outstanding issues. In the later part of the consultation it is a good idea to check that important details have been understood. Providing supplementary written material – especially about important pre-operative or post-operative instructions – should be considered.

Enlistment

Enlisting or enrolling extends an offer to the patient to actively participate in decision-making. Enlistment acknowledges that the patient controls much of what can happen in his or her healthcare treatment plan.[37] Different surgeons and patients will vary in their preferences about the degree of patient involvement. Orienting patients to the process of care and discussing risks frankly but positively will help to empower patients facing surgery.

Ending

The last E that needs to be considered is Ending the consultation on a positive note, with an expectation of a satisfactory outcome, phrased accordingly. Closing in a manner that gives patients hope is an effective strategy. It is worth reiterating that after leaving the consulting room, patients normally forget a significant part of what has been said during the consultation. Written material can supplement, but not replace, effective communication.

NON-VERBAL COMMUNICATION

Patients are particularly sensitive to non-verbal cues from their doctors, although many doctors are unaware of their influence in this respect. It is said that in a consultation less than 35% of contact is established through verbal means, while 65% is conveyed through non-verbal cues including facial expression and eye contact.[38] It is important to recognize the importance of subtle behavioural cues that are highly influential in determining the direction of consultation and the subsequent outcome.

Some consideration of how some non-verbal factors are effective through the clinic set-up arrangements is necessary. These factors include the layout of furniture, the relative positions of doctor and patient and the distance between them. A relaxed interaction is likely when both chairs are positioned at the same height to ensure good eye contact. The ideal positioning between a surgeon and the patient is approximately 2–4 ft (0.6–1.2 m). It is advisable for the surgeon not to stand while the patient is seated during the medical interview.

A desk represents a potential barrier between the doctor and patient and may be an important factor limiting the free flow of conversation. In one interesting experiment, the influence of the desk was analysed during consultations between a cardiologist and his patient. On alternate days the cardiologist removed the desk from his consulting room to assess the impact upon non-verbal cues and body language. When the desk was absent, more than half of all patients sat back and relaxed, but when the doctor was positioned behind the desk fewer than 1 in 10 assumed a relaxed body posture and this corresponded with a drop in the level of meaningful interaction between the two.[38]

Knapp looked into the importance of seating arrangement. He identified four sitting positions for any interaction: the corner position, the cooperative position and the competitive-defensive position (**Figure 36.3**). In the corner position, the individuals are positioned in such a way that the corner of the desk intervenes. It usually results in casual friendly conversation. It allows unlimited eye contact and a full appreciation of gesture. The corner of the desk behaves as a partial barrier but does not intrude as a territorial division.[39]

The cooperative position differs from the corner position in the absence of any barrier and a straight face-to-face sitting posture. While this favours a mutualistic

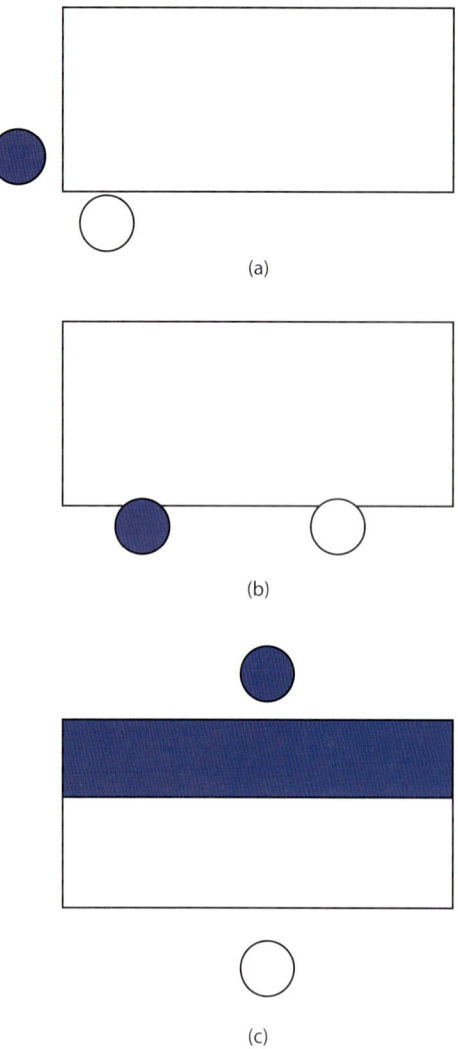

Figure 36.3 Examples of seat and desk arrangements. (a) The corner position; **(b)** The cooperative position; **(c)** The competitive-defensive position (the territorial line); Redrawn from Ref. 39, with permission.

relationship, a number of individuals feel threatened by the lack of a firm boundary. In the competitive-defensive position, the desk constitutes a firm physical barrier. Not only does this prevent intimacy, but it may also create competition for control of the consultation.

BOX 36.2 Optimizing communication

Behaviours in Western culture that can communicate to the patient that the surgeon is making an effort to optimize the personal aspect of the communication experience include:[40]

- shaking hands
- maintaining eye contact
- welcoming the patient
- thanking the patient for coming
- apologizing for being late
- appearing relaxed
- appearing genuinely interested
- acknowledging emotions
- not writing and listening at the same time.

COMMUNICATING ADVERSE INCIDENTS

Bad news is a routine part of many surgical practices. A good surgeon will offer the appropriate words and actions in the setting of a dangerous operation or devastating diagnosis. Patients need to be able to absorb bad news, and they need to be able to prepare for the worst while hoping for a cure. This requires careful, balanced communication. Learning the skills to break bad news can prevent interactions in which it is delivered insensitively or too bluntly. Such 'hit and run' delivery of bad news may result from a surgeon's own emotional discomfort.

Sharing bad news with patients is difficult to do well. A number of simple techniques may help you to undertake this more sensitively. Some techniques may appear obvious, like planning the consultation in advance, checking the facts and avoiding interruptions to ensure privacy. Breaking bad news can take a significant amount of time and it is important to avoid being rushed. The use of simple straightforward language and avoiding jargon is helpful. Many patients value an invitation to bring a relative or close friend for support, and it is necessary to establish the nature of their relationship in order to understand how the news will impact upon them also.

As mentioned earlier, non-verbal messages are as important as verbal ones. Patients need to be given sufficient time for silence, tears or anger. Even when the future looks bleak, we need to be careful in using the phrase 'nothing can be done'. There are always ways of encouraging hope in any dire situation. However, it is equally important to admit when we do not know the answers to difficult questions, such as life expectancy after a diagnosis of terminal disease. Most patients value the offer of ongoing support, and follow-up is especially valuable.

BOX 36.3 SPIKES

Oncologist Robert Buckman has suggested a framework called SPIKES when breaking bad news, standing for setup, perception, invitation, knowledge, emotions, summarize and strategy.[41]

- **S**etup refers to finding an appropriate time and place for a discussion, somewhere quiet, private, seated, at eye level and free of distractions.
- **P**erception indicates the technique of asking the patient what he/she knows about the situation. This is a good starting point for the discussion as they may already know the bad news or have guessed it. However, they still want further clarification.
- **I**nvitation means asking the patient what else they would like to know or whether they would like to know more.
- **K**nowledge implies offering information. Many patients want to know all that the doctor knows or understands.
- **E**motions are commonly expressed when facing loss of health or loss of life. These emotions should be acknowledged and empathized with. Sometimes silence on behalf of the surgeon may constitute effective communication. 'I wish' statements can be used to convey empathy.
- **S**ummarize and strategy.

ADDRESSING ISSUES AROUND LOSS

Patients may experience concern about potential disfigurement and loss of function as a result of surgery. The surgeon has a duty to address these issues in appropriate depth. Within otolaryngology, patients undergo loss of speech, swallowing, balance or hearing. Perhaps not surprisingly, those who cope less well with the loss of body function are those with a history of pre-morbid anxiety or depression, and these are factors that are easy to overlook in a busy consultation. Consequently, a professional assessment of mental health may be useful part of pre-operative planning for some patients prior to surgery.[42]

The effect of hearing loss depends greatly on the age of onset and the extent of any residual function. The distinction between truly deaf individuals and those who become deafened later in life is important. Properly nurtured, the congenitally deaf individual is able to develop normal communication skills within the deaf community without any requirement for the spoken word. However, the individual who encounters hearing loss after normal development suffers an immeasurable handicap without augmentation or alternative aids.

For patients with acquired hearing loss there are a number of simple methods for improving communication within the consultation. Slow, deliberate speech of adequate volume in a room with low ambient noise will assist those with a modest hearing loss. A face-to-face position and clear enunciation of words enables lip-reading in those with long-standing loss. Other simple measures include diagrams and picture boards.

DISCUSSING MEDICAL ERRORS

Surgical error seems pervasive today, mostly because it is increasingly sought and increasingly recognized. Surgeons face a difficult dilemma when deciding whether and how to disclose a harmful error to a patient. When a patient has had an adverse outcome and if the surgeon's reaction is defensive, it results in the patient not being fully informed. However, it is recommended to follow appropriate disclosure. A study found that patients who had received full disclosure after an error were less likely to change doctor and had greater satisfaction[43] than patients who did not receive full disclosure. In some cases, disclosure decreased the risk of legal action, although a positive response was not guaranteed since it was dependent on the clinical outcome and the details and severity of the error.[44] In another study, investigators assessed the attitudes of 149 randomly chosen adults about medical errors. Patients were more likely to commence litigation following moderate and severe errors if there had been no disclosure.[45]

A study, the first to assess how surgeons currently disclose errors, revealed that surgeons vary widely in their approach and in many cases, surgeons fail to use recommended error disclosure skills.[46] After a harmful error patients expect reliable information: an explicit statement that an error occurred, what the error was, why the error happened, how the error will impact their health and an apology. They want someone to take responsibility. Many surgeons struggle with these aspects. A surgeon's reluctance to state explicitly that an error has occurred might in part reflect the advice they receive that the disclosure of an error should not include any statements that could constitute an admission of liability. However, a surgeon's failure to communicate clearly about errors can make patients feel angry and misled, feelings that frequently contribute to the decision to file a malpractice claim.[47, 48]

While communicating errors, direct, clear statements are important, as are their delivery, particularly the tone of voice. One interesting study analysed the quality of surgeons' speech and malpractice history.[49] They observed that surgeons who were judged to be more dominant in their tone were more likely to have been sued than those who sounded less dominant. These findings indicate that even brief exposure to a surgeon's speech may be perceived by patients as expressing dominance and lacking concern. Dominance in the voice may imply a surgeon's indifference and lead a patient to launch a malpractice suit when poor outcomes occur.

Empathetic communication is especially important when discussing difficult issues like error. However, some aspects of errors, such as a surgeon's discomfiture about an error or concerns about liability, may make it difficult for them to discuss empathetically. Validating patients' views may also conflict with the surgeon's desire to persuade the patient that the error was not as serious as it may appear to them. However, failing to communicate empathetically with patients may give an impression that the surgeon is not concerned about what happened.[50, 51]

There are some techniques that are useful in communicating adverse error events. The conversation may start with, 'I am afraid I have some bad news'. It is advised to communicate in a manner that is open as well as acknowledging emotional responses. Complex reactions of fear, anger and mistrust can be expected. An apology without assigning blame is acceptable and does not denote an admission of liability. Statements like 'I am sorry this has happened to you' will go some way in that regard. Many patients also want to know that steps are being taken to continue their care or rectify the error, and that steps are being taken to minimize a similar error happening in future. Thus, at the end of the discussion it will be effective if the patient is given an explicit plan of the support to be provided.

Communication is of significant importance with a somatizing patient. These are patients for whom no organic cause for their symptoms can be found and they fail to respond to the standard treatment. In interacting with these patients, surgeons experience a sense of frustration or irritation; some identify them as 'heart-sink' patients. These patients need to be managed by improved communication strategies including the identification of underlying situations that cause the stress that is responsible for the lack of therapeutic response. A number of special skills exist to combat the heart-sink encounter including a 'holding strategy' for listening and understanding the patient's problem without feeling the need to tackle all issues in that consultation.

BOX 36.4 Compliance

Research has shown that compliance depends on three factors:

1. Good understanding of advice
2. High level of satisfaction
3. An ability to recall information given by the doctor.

Evidence suggests that following the end of the consultation the patient retains surprisingly little factual information. For example, in one study over a third of patients failed to recall the name of their prescription medicine and a quarter failed to appreciate the duration of the course of their medication. Simple and effective techniques for increasing compliance include provision of written information, keeping explanations simple and repeating important points.[52]

CONCLUSION

As clinicians, consultation is the most common clinical procedure we employ. Our communication with patients has a therapeutic effect, and can be positive as well as negative. A stereotypical image of a surgeon is someone who is not a very good communicator. It has been observed that when surgeons improve their communication skills, it is not just patients but surgeons themselves who are beneficiaries. Mounting evidence has shown that improvement in communication skills is achievable and that these skills can be taught, do change patient satisfaction, and can be retained over time. Improving communication skills is similar to improving operating skills. It involves seeking information, implementing the techniques and evaluating the outcome.

KEY POINTS

- Communication is the most commonly used therapeutic tool in ENT practice.
- The surgeon needs to be mindful of verbal as well as non-verbal communication.
- Like operative skill, good communication is a skill that needs to be developed. It involves seeking information, applying appropriate techniques and monitoring outcome.
- There are various models of doctor-patient communication. One needs to choose appropriate model according to the situation and personalities.
- Special consideration is advisable in communicating undesired.

REFERENCES

1. Terino E. Psychology of the aesthetic patient: the value of personality profile testing. *Facial Plast Surg Clin Am* 2008; 16: 165–71.
2. Buckman R. Communications and emotions: skills and effort are key. *BMJ* 2002; 325: 672.
3. Coulehan JL, Block MR. *The medical interview: mastering skills for clinical practice*. 4th ed. Philadelphia: F.A. Davis Company; 2001.
4. Levinson W, Chaumeton N. Communication between surgeons and patients in routine office visits. *Surgery* 1993; 125: 127–34.
5. Stewart M, Brown JB, Weston WW, et al. *Patient-centered medicine: transforming the clinical method*. Thousand Oaks, CA: Sage Publications; 1995.
6. Beckman H, Frankel R. The effect of physician behavior on the collection of data. *Ann Intern Med* 1984; 101: 692–96.
7. Stewart MA. Effective physician-patient communication and health outcomes: a review. *Can Med Assoc J* 1995; 152: 1423–33.
8. Levinson W, Roter DL, Mullooly JP, et al. Physician–patient communication: the relationship with malpractice claims among primary care physicians and surgeons. *J Amer Med Assoc* 1997; 277: 553–59.
9. Baily BJ. Physician communication skills: an essential competency. In Bailey BJ, Johnson JT, Newlands, SD (eds). *Head and neck surgery: otolaryngology*. Philadelphia: Wolters Kluwer/Lippincott Williams & Wilkins; 2013, vol 1, 2819 –26.
10. Braddock C, Hudak PL, Feldman JJ, et al. Surgery is certainly one good option: quality and time-efficiency of informed decision-making in surgery. *J Bone Joint Surg Am* 2008; 90: 1830–38.
11. McLafferty RB, Williams RG, Lambert AD, Dunnington, GL. Surgeon communication behaviours that lead patients to not recommend the surgeon to family members and friends: analysis and impact. *Surgery* 2006; 140(4): 616–24.
12. Fischer JE. The effect of litigation on surgical practice in the USA. *Brit J Surg* 2000; 87: 833–34.
13. Herndon JH, Pollick KJ. Continuing concerns, new challenges, and next steps in physician-patient communication. *J Bone Joint Surg Am* 2002; 84: 309–15.
14. Canale ST. How the orthopaedist believes he is perceived by the public and how the public actually perceives the orthopaedist. AAOS Symposium, Patient-Physician Communication. Presented at the Annual Meeting of the American Association of Orthopaedic Surgeons; 15–18 Mar 2000; Orlando, FL.
15. DiMatteo M. The physician-patient relationship: effects on the quality of health care. *Clin Obstet Gynecol* 1994; 37: 149–61.
16. Krasner MS, Epstein RM, Beckman H, et al. Association of an educational program in mindful communication with burnout, empathy, and attitudes among primary care physicians. *J Amer Med Assoc* 2009; 302: 1284–93.
17. Beckman H, Markakis K, Suchman A, Frankel R. The doctor-patient relationship and malpractice: lessons from plaintiff depositions. *Arch Intern Med* 1994; 154: 1365–70.
18. Bridger MWM, Epstein R. Functional voice disorder: a series of 109 patients. *J Laryngol Otol* 1993, 97: 1145–48.
19. Fitzgerald RG, Parkes M. Coping with loss: blindness and loss of other sensory and cognitive function. *BMJ* 1998; 316: 1160–63.
20. Mavroforou A, Giannoukas AD, Katsamouris A, Michalodimitrakis E. The importance of communication between physician and patients. *Int Angiol* 2002; 21(1): 99–102.
21. Rao JK, Anderson LA, Inui TS, Frankel RM. Communication interventions make a difference in conversations between physicians and patients: a systematic review of the evidence. *Med Care* 2007; 45: 340–49.
22. Levinson W, Hudak P, Tricco AC. A systematic review of surgeon–patient communication: atrengths and opportunities for improvement *Patient Educ Couns* 2013; 93: 3–17.
23. van Dulmen AM. Communication during gynecological out-patient encounters. *J Psychosom Obst Gyn* 1999; 20: 119–26.
24. Braddock 3rd CH, Edwards KA, Hasenberg NM, et al. Informed decision making in outpatient practice: time to get back to basics. *J Am Med Assoc* 1999; 282: 2313–20.

25. Maguire P, Fairbairn S, Fletcher C. Consultation skills of young doctors: benefits of feedback training in interviewing as students persist. *BMJ* 1986; **292**: 1573–76.
26. Ramirez AJ, Graham J, Richards MA, et al. Mental health of hospital consultants: the effects of stress and satisfaction at work. *Lancet* 1996; **347**: 724–28.
27. Riess H, Kelley JM, Bailey R, et al. Improving empathy and relational skills in otolaryngology residents: a pilot study. *Otolaryng Head Neck* 2011; **144**: 120–22.
28. Silverman J, Kurtz S, Draper J. *Skills for communicating with patients*. 2nd ed. Oxford: Radcliffe Publishing; 2005.
29. Tongue JR, Epps HR, Forese LL. Communication skills. *Instr Course Lect* 2005; **54**: 3–9.
30. Howard A. Communication skills for surgeons. *Surgery in Africa Review* July 2012.
31. Canale ST. Falling in love again. *J Bone Joint Surg Am* 2000; **82**: 739–42.
32. Kain ZN, MacLaren JE, Hammell C, et al. Healthcare provider-child-parent communication in the preoperative surgical setting. *Paediatr Anaesth* 2009; **19**: 376–84.
33. Hickson GB, Clayton EW, Entman SS, et al. Obstetricians' prior malpractice experience and patients' satisfaction with care. *J Amer Med Assoc* 1994; **272**: 1583–87.
34. Larson EB, Yao X. Clinical empathy as emotional labor in the patient–physician relationship. *J Amer Med Assoc* 2005; **293**: 1100–06.
35. Levinson W, Gorawara-Bhat R, Lamb J. A study of patient clues and physician responses in primary care and surgical settings. *J Amer Med Assoc* 2000; **284**: 1021–27.
36. Braddock CH, Fihn SD, Levinson W, et al. How doctors and patients discuss routine clinical decisions: informed decision making in the outpatient setting. *J Gen Intern Med.* 1997; **12**(6): 339–45.
37. Makoul G. Essential elements of communication in medical encounters: the Kalamazoo consensus statement. *Acad Med* 2001; **76**: 390–93.
38. Pietroni P. Language and communication in general practice. In: Tanner B (ed). *Communication in general practice surgery*. London: Hodder and Stoughton; 1976.
39. Knapp M. *Non-verbal communication in human interaction*. 2nd ed. New York: Holt, Rinehart and Winston; 1978.
40. Leach DC. Building and assessing competence: the potential for evidence-based graduate medical education. *Qual Manag Health Ca* 2002; **11**: 39–44.
41. Bradley CT, Brasel KJ. Core competencies in palliative care for surgeons: interpersonal and communication skills. *Am J Hosp Palliat Care* 2007; **24**: 499–507.
42. Maguire P, Parkes CM. Coping with loss: surgery and loss of body parts. *BMJ* 1998; **316**: 1086–88.
43. Mazor K, Simon S, Yood R. Health plan members' views about disclosure of medical errors. *Ann Intern Med* 2004; **140**: 409–18.
44. Witman A, Park D, Hardin S. How do patients want physicians to handle mistakes? A survey of internal medicine patients in an academic setting. *Arch Intern Med* 1996; **156**: 2565–69.
45. Wu AW, Cavanaugh TA, McPhee SJ, et al. To tell the truth: ethical and practical issues in disclosing medical mistakes to patients. *J Gen Intern Med* 1997; **12**: 770–75.
46. Chan D, Gallagher T, Reznick R, Levinson W. How surgeons disclose medical errors to patients: a study using standardised patients. *Surgery* 2005; **138**: 851–58.
47. Huycke LI, Huycke MM. Characteristics of potential plaintiffs in malpractice litigation. *Ann Intern Med* 1994; **120**: 792–98.
48. Shapiro R, Simpson DE, Lawrence SL, et al. A survey of sued and non-sued physicians and suing patients. *Arch Intern Med* 1989; **149**: 2190–96.
49. Ambady N, LaPlante D, Nguyen T, et al. Surgeons' tone of voice: a clue to malpractice history. *Surgery* 2002; **132**: 5–9.
50. Bosk CL. *Forgive and remember: managing medical failure*. Chicago: University of Chicago Press; 1979.
51. Fallowfield L, Jenkins V. Communicating sad bad and difficult news in medicine. *Lancet* 2004; **363**: 312–19.
52. Ley P. Improving patients' understanding, recall satisfaction and compliance. In: Broom AK (ed). *Health psychology: processes and applications*. London: Chapman and Hall; 1989, pp. 74–102.

CHAPTER 37

CLINICAL GOVERNANCE AND ITS ROLE IN PATIENT SAFETY AND QUALITY IMPROVEMENT

Samit Majumdar and S. Musheer Hussain

Historical background 389	Francis, Keogh and Berwick reports 393
Definition 390	Current issues 393
The 7 pillars of clinical governance 391	Role of CEO, NHS board and senior management 393
Relationship between clinical governance, patient safety and quality improvement 392	Conclusions 393
	References 394

SEARCH STRATEGY

Data in this chapter may be updated by a Medline search as well as reports for the Department of Health and website Institute of Health Improvement (IHI) using the keywords: clinical governance, patient safety, quality improvement and adverse events.

HISTORICAL BACKGROUND

'The only way to be sure that they do the right thing is to keep an eye on them, to challenge them, to hold them to account and, above all, to take part in them.'

The Nolan Committee[1]

The last decade of the twentieth century saw some colossal tragedies in our practice of medicine in the UK, including the cases of Beverly Allit,[2] Harold Shipman[3] and Bristol Paediatric Cardiology practice.[4] While we were coming to terms with these tragedies, trying to make sense of and learn from them, on the other side of the Atlantic the Institute of Medicine (IOM) published a report that sent shock waves around the world. *To Err Is Human: Building a safer health system*[5] made a conservative estimate that 98 000 people die in hospitals in the United States every year due to medical errors while they are receiving some form of healthcare intervention. The US Department of Health and IOM set out robust steps to reduce the mortality by 50% in the 5 subsequent years. The patient safety revolution crossed many geographical and political boundaries and the World Health Organization set up the World Alliance for Patient Safety in response.

To Err Is Human helped us to understand that medical errors are often the result of multifactorial problems within a healthcare delivery system – it is rarely the fault of a single individual. The importance of teamwork in patient safety and quality improvement emerged as a more fundamental need. The focus shifted from the healthcare professional to the structural clarity and robustness of the operating system, that is, the organization (microsystem, mesosystem, macrosystem).

Dealing with the serious public repercussions of a number of significant tragedies in the National Health Service, the then Labour government came up with a new plan to reform the health service with a new philosophical concept of practice: clinical governance. In December 1997, the new Labour government published a White Paper,[6] *The New NHS*. In July 1998, the Chief Medical Officer, Liam Donaldson, co-authored a paper in the *British Medical Journal* titled 'Clinical governance and the drive for quality improvement in the new NHS in England'.[7] We saw the birth of clinical governance – an eclectic concept that was strangely alien to most of the frontline workers in the NHS. As a new cognitive structure, it incorporated **clinical audit, risk management, incident reporting** and **continuous professional development (CPD)**. It was described as a package that housed all the disparate and fragmented practice of quality improvement.

DEFINITION

'Clinical governance is a system through which NHS organizations are accountable for continuously improving the quality of their services and safeguarding high standards of care by creating an environment in which excellence in clinical care will flourish.'[8]

A robust framework of a high-performance system was proposed where healthcare professionals and managers would be working together towards a common goal of delivering safe and high quality care to our patients. This vision of a healthcare system was described based on an integrated intelligent matrix of communication pathways connecting all its parts and people. The capability of preserving and learning from our experience (memory) of individuals and groups on the front line was described. This new phrase clinical governance was partly harvested from the Cadbury report (1992)[9] on the financial aspects of corporate governance with some intrinsic support from the NHS constitution. For the first time, quality improvement was put at the heart of medical practice in the NHS. The chief executive officers of the NHS hospital and primary care trusts were made accountable for the quality of care provided by their organization. The attention was expected to shift from the traditional target- and performance-driven, management-led organizational culture, to a refreshingly appropriate practice of medicine within an established framework of patient safety and quality improvement, led by senior clinicians. Safe, effective, patient-centred care with efficient utilization of resources and focused practice of risk management became the essence of good quality service. In 1997, the Department of Health introduced a 10-year programme to improve the quality of clinical care provided by NHS organizations and positively change the public perception. The National Institute for Clinical Excellence (NICE) was created to establish clear national standards through National Services Frameworks. The Clinical Governance Support Team, National Patient Safety Agency and National Clinical Assessment Authority were also established to support the development and good practice of clinical governance. The Commission for Health Improvement (CHI) was founded in 2000 by the Health Act 1999, as an external body to review the performance of each healthcare provider.[10]

Scally and Donaldson[7] described the integrated approach to the practice of clinical governance under six interconnected domains:

1. Culture:
   - good leadership
   - ethos of teamwork
   - patient partnership
   - education and research valued
   - open and participative

2. Coherence:
   - goals of individuals, teams, organizations aligned
   - excellent communication
   - external partnership forged

3. Infrastructure:
   - access to evidence
   - time allowed to plan
   - training and development strategies
   - information technology supports practice

4. Risk avoidance:
   - well trained staff
   - safe environment
   - clear procedures

5. Quality methods:
   - good practice spread
   - clinical policies evidence based
   - lessons learned from failures
   - improvement process integrated

6. Poor performance:
   - early recognition
   - decisive intervention
   - effective self-regulation
   - feedback on performance.

It is important to note the World Health Organization has used the term clinical governance in relation to building high quality healthcare service. WHO had described it as four dimensions of quality:

1. Patient satisfaction
2. Professional performance
3. Risk management
4. Resource allocation.

In essence, clinical governance is a framework of safety with a whole system integrated approach to care and continuous quality improvement.

The main principles of clinical governance are:

- clear lines of responsibility and accountability for the overall care
- a comprehensive programme of quality improvement
- education and training
- clear policies for risk management
- managing poor performance.

In 1999, the Secretary of State for Health stipulated proposals for professional regulations of staff in the consultation document, *Supporting doctors, protecting patients*. Professional regulation of individuals working at the frontline of the NHS was considered necessary and plans were unveiled. *An organisation with a memory*[11] was published in the year 2000. This report of an expert group on learning from adverse events in the NHS highlighted the extent of the harm patients could face when under the care

> **BOX 37.1 The 7 pillars of clinical governance**
>
> 1. Patient and public involvement
> 2. Risk management
> 3. Clinical audit
> 4. Staffing and staff management
> 5. Education and training
> 6. Clinical effectiveness
> 7. Use of information

of our NHS hospitals. It stated that adverse events resulting in patient harm occur in around 10% of all admissions to NHS hospitals. This is equivalent to an incidence in excess of 850 000 patients per year. The estimated cost of managing this is £2 billion a year in additional hospital stays alone. The establishment of NICE in 1999 and CHI in 2000 aimed to safeguard patient care through evidence-based support and regulation. CHI described clinical governance as a platform held up by the 7 pillars of clinical governance (**Box 37.1**). It was widely perceived that changing organizational culture and creating a robust, well-connected system with clarity of structure and function was the essential key to successful clinical governance and the survival of the NHS beyond its 50th birthday.

THE 7 PILLARS OF CLINICAL GOVERNANCE

Patient and public involvement

The National Health Service belongs to the citizens of the UK and is run on public funding. The voices of patients and the public are essential to maintain its integrity, growth and evolution. Feedback from patients and the public should be dealt with carefully so as not to miss any learning opportunity that may come with it. The creation of clear structures for handling such feedback ensures the generation of functional memory and creates a learning environment that allows us to improve our provision of care every day.

Risk management

DEFINITION OF RISK

Risk can be defined as any potential for the occurrence of an unwanted effect because of an intended action.

RISK TO PATIENTS

The practice of medicine is a high-risk business. Every healthcare intervention must be risk assessed and continuously monitored to reduce any risk to patients. All incidents and near misses must be reported, recorded in the organizational memory and carefully analyzed. Knowledge gained from these and through significant clinical event analysis should change behaviours of clinical practice with resultant reduction of both non-human factors and human factor-related risk and incidents. All critical events must be audited. The introduction of surgical checklists has led to a reduction of risk and adverse incidents in surgical patients. Statutory regulatory bodies (i.e. Medicine Control Agency, Data Protection Act, etc.) can help in the reduction of risks and incidents. The use of software (e.g. DATIX) can facilitate all aspects of risk management and the successful use of these has been reported by some health organizations. Regular training of staff and routine and random checks of systems and practices are essential for maintenance of the highest standards of safety.

RISK TO THE PRACTITIONER

Protecting healthcare professionals from occupational hazards by immunization, improving and creating a safe work environment, assessing and reducing human factor-related incidents are recommended good practice.

RISK TO THE NHS ORGANIZATION

Any incidence of poor practice has the potential to damage the professional reputation of an organization. Significant events of poor practice are usually the reflection of poor organizational culture and serious lack of leadership across all parts of the system. Examples of such tragedies are plentiful in our recent history (i.e. Bristol, Mid-Staffordshire, Lanarkshire, Blackpool, etc.). The Francis, Keogh and Berwick reports will speak of the risk associated with poor organizational culture for decades to come. We must not miss the opportunity to learn from these situations.

Aligning the individual, team and organizational values creates resonance and avoids conflicts of interest. This is essential for the success of clinical governance.

Clinical audit

Clinical audit is a quality improvement process that seeks to improve patient care and outcomes through systematic review of care against explicit criteria and implementation of change.[12,13]

In 1989, medical audit was introduced in the NHS by the Department of Health,[14] with clear instructions for all hospital doctors to take part in audit by 1991. This had been duly endorsed by the General Medical Council in its advice to all doctors. In 1997, clinical audit was integrated into clinical governance. Clinical audit comprises the essential core of clinical governance. It is the most appropriate way to check for the safety, effectiveness and quality of all healthcare interventions, both processes and outcomes. When applied carefully and methodically, clinical audit is excellent in its ability to monitor healthcare delivery services in its entirety. The recommendations from the Report of the Public Inquiry into Children's Heart Surgery at Bristol Royal Infirmary (1984–95) strongly supported audit to be the tool for monitoring clinical performance. It also stressed that clinical audit should be thoroughly supported by all healthcare organizations and all healthcare professionals should be contractually bound to take part in local audits. The recent introduction of the revalidation process for renewal of doctors' licence to practise by the General Medical Council requires all doctors to perform clinical audits.

Factors contributing to the success of any audit are:[15]

- organizational support
- evidence-based guidelines
- participation of patients
- good relationship with patient support groups
- improved record-keeping
- good use of information technology
- professional help and support in designing and application.

Lack of ring-fenced time within doctors' job plans, lack of resources, poor microsystems and organizational culture and deficient managerial support in efforts towards clinical quality improvement can all be significant deterrents to effective clinical audit. Johnston et al. reviewed 93 publications to explore the barriers and facilitating factors for effective clinical audit. They have highlighted professional attitudes and presence of coherent strategies as significant variables influencing outcomes of clinical audits.[16]

The tragedies of Bristol Royal Infirmary should deter anyone from dismissing the significant role of clinical audit in achieving patient safety and quality improvement.[12]

Staffing and staff management

Recruiting highly trained staff with a passion for working in the NHS is fundamental to providing excellent patient care. Of equal importance in the provision of safe, effective and patient-centred care is ensuring the optimum skill mix of well supported staff in every clinical area. Tired, harassed, psychologically disengaged staff cannot provide good quality care.[17]

Education and training

Continuous professional development through well supported in-house and national courses is essential to keep all NHS staff up to date with the rapid pace of progress of modern medicine. The reduction of junior doctors' training hours to comply with European working time directives has certainly caused difficulties in terms of the training of doctors because of the significant lack of the most important resource – time. The introduction of consultant contracts with 90% of time spent in direct patient care, with a paucity of time and funding for study leave time, has a serious detrimental effect on the education and training of senior doctors.

The education and training of all healthcare professionals, throughout their career, must be supported and guarded as sacrosanct in order to allow safe and best quality practice to thrive. It is a duty of all employers to safeguard this. A very good example of this is the work of NHS Education for Scotland.[18]

Clinical effectiveness

Ensuring that each and every patient gets safe and effective healthcare is the core function of clinical effectiveness. Standards of safety and quality of care must not fluctuate across timelines or postcodes. All aspects of healthcare should be based on the current body of evidence and be patient centred. Clinical effectiveness is all about doing the right intervention, for the right patient, at the right time, in the right way. Eradicating wastage, minimizing harm and variations of practice should be at the heart of the practice of clinical effectiveness. In essence, clinical effectiveness measures how good an intervention is at achieving what it is intended for and is weighed up by the hierarchy of evidence. This has been derived from the evidence-based medicine movement of the 1990s.

The development of CHI, NICE and the Scottish Intercollegiate Guidelines Network (SIGN) have been at the heart of the promotion of good practice based on the best evidence. It has also been established that safe and effective practice is also more cost-effective.

Use of information

Effective and efficient management of information is the key to the ultimate success of an operational system, that is, the NHS organization (macrosystem). This involves understanding data protection, methods of collection, evaluation, interpretation and application of all relevant data to improve processes and, therefore, the outcomes of a system. A good example of this is the improvement of clinical performance based on monthly or annual outcome data of one or many interventions. Data are extremely powerful tools to show the quality of any practice (i.e. patient feedback information allows us to improve our care pathways). Data handling is hugely labour intensive. Every NHS organization needs to ensure modern technology and appropriately trained staff are in place to harvest and make good use of data. This is a key infrastructure requirement for the success of clinical governance.

RELATIONSHIP BETWEEN CLINICAL GOVERNANCE, PATIENT SAFETY AND QUALITY IMPROVEMENT

The concept of clinical governance was introduced by the Department of Health in 1997 as an integrated framework within the NHS to safeguard patient safety and continuous quality improvement. For clinical governance to be successful it is imperative that an organization will have safe, effective and patient centred care in day-to-day practice. Patient safety and continuous quality improvement are at the heart of clinical governance and should not be separated. However, NHS organizations often show separation and conflicts between clinical and managerial approaches to patient safety and quality improvement.

Realignment of organizational goals with the goals of the frontline healthcare professionals will ensure that patient safety remains at the heart of the practice of clinical governance.

FRANCIS, KEOGH AND BERWICK REPORTS

Hope is not a plan and a plan is not always a good strategy that can survive the test of time. 2013 saw the publication of several landmark government-funded reports into failures of healthcare delivery systems. Many devastating high-profile failures of provision of care, mishaps and deplorable quality of practice plagued us throughout the early twenty-first century. The second cycle of the Francis report made 290 recommendations over 1782 pages.[19] The essential recommendations were: openness, transparency and candour throughout the healthcare system (including a statutory duty of candour); fundamental standards for healthcare providers; improved support for compassionate caring; committed nursing; and stronger healthcare leadership.

Bereaved and angered patients' families and friends had questions. Many of these questions sadly still remain unanswered. A review of mortality figures in 14 hospitals in England was the next revelation to hit the medical profession. Keogh summarized his recommendations as eight ambitions.[20] Listening to the frontline staff (i.e. the nurses and junior doctors) is one of the most highlighted areas, along with the need for the creation of a climate of safety and positive organizational culture.

Don Berwick, founder and past president of the IHI, a physician, philosopher and a passionate believer of robust systems, individual accountability and the human touch in patient care, was the third leader invited by the government to analyze and report on the problems affecting patient safety in NHS hospitals. Berwick expressed his thoughts succinctly in the form of four eloquent letters in a document, *A promise to learn – a commitment to act: improving the safety of patients in England*.[21] The summary of his recommendations is simple, clear, extremely powerful and poignant (**Box 37.2**).

BOX 37.2 Four recommendations by Don Berwick

1. Engage, empower, and hear patients and carers throughout the entire system, and at all times.
2. Foster wholeheartedly the growth and development of all staff, especially with regard to their ability and opportunity to improve the processes within which they work.
3. Insist upon, and model in your own work, thorough and unequivocal transparency, in the service of accountability, trust and the growth of knowledge.
4. Embrace transparency unequivocally and everywhere, in the service of accountability, trust and the growth of knowledge.

CURRENT ISSUES

There are a number of issues that can be highlighted to show why clinical governance has not thrived:

- lack of defined input, structure and process for clinical governance
- poor organizational culture
- poor and deficient leadership
- disengaged, disillusioned staff
- historical glass walls of poor culture or practice separating clinicians and managers
- financial targets and misaligned performance indicators
- disconnected microsystems
- confines and silos of good practice
- poor, cumbersome feedback system
- lack of patient involvement and regular public scrutiny.

ROLE OF CEO, NHS BOARD AND SENIOR MANAGEMENT

In 1998, chief executives of all NHS primary and secondary care organizations were made directly accountable for the quality of the service provided by their organizations. In the absence of a clear, defined framework of safety, clinical governance will fail to meet any of its lofty goals. The chief executive officer with the senior management team and board members need to ensure there is an environment where good practice thrives. The lines of accountability and responsibility for overall patient safety and quality improvement must be clearly identified. Organizational goals aligned with those of individual healthcare professionals dedicated to value-based practice will create an environment in which clinical governance will thrive.

CONCLUSIONS

Primum non nocere, the Hippocratic Oath of first doing no harm in our every endeavour, has been at the core of our medical practice for centuries. Patient safety and quality improvement is everyone's business. Without willing contribution from the majority of NHS staff, the goals of patient safety and quality improvement will never be realized. However, we urgently need some effective measures to engage our disillusioned staff in value-based patient care. This will not be possible until the clinical priorities are met.

It should be our goal to see that all staff are well connected, well informed, well supported and working in resonance towards their common goal of delivering safe, effective and patient-centred care to every patient every time, 365 days a year. Financial, political and performance related goals should not override the goals for patient safety and quality improvement.

The National Health Service[22] was born on 5 July 1948. It did not have any intrinsic or extrinsic system for safety or quality improvement for the first four decades of its existence. The 10 years leading to its 50th birthday saw some major failures, with consequent public scrutiny. This triggered a deluge of white papers, reforms and introduction of laws. Despite the implementation of all these measures, British citizens have seen repetitions of many mistakes in the NHS. Sadly its recent history has demonstrated that the NHS as an organization does not have a functional memory and has failed to learn from its major mistakes. We cannot solve a problem with the same level of intelligence that created it – a paradigm shift in organizational culture is required to ensure that patient safety and continuous quality improvement are at the heart of the practice of medicine throughout the NHS.[23] This will only be possible with strong leadership from front-line clinicians in partnership with excellent senior managers.

> **KEY POINTS**
>
> - Clinical governance is a system through which NHS organizations are accountable for continuously improving the quality of their services and safeguarding higher standards of care by creating an environment in which excellence in clinical care will flourish.
> - Clinical audit comprises the essential core of clinical governance.
> - Data are a key infrastructure requirement for the success of clinical governance.
> - Medical errors are often the result of multifactorial problems within a healthcare delivery system – it is rarely the fault of a single individual.
> - Feedback from patients is the most valuable resource. It should be actively encouraged at all parts of a patients' journey.
> - Risk can be defined as any potential for the occurrence of an unwanted effect because of an intended action.
> - Tired, harassed, psychologically disengaged staff cannot provide a decent quality of care.

REFERENCES

1. The Nolan Committee. *The first Nolan report on standards in public life*. 1995.
2. Vincent M, Richmond C. Beverly Allitt: the nurse who killed babies. *J R Soc Med* 2008; **101**: 110–15.
3. Baker R. Implications of Harold Shipman for general practice. *Postgrad Med J* 2004; **80**: 303–06.
4. Savulescu J. Beyond Bristol: taking responsibility. *J Med Ethics* 2002; **28**: 281–82.
5. Kohn LT, Corrigan JM, Donaldson MS. *To err is human: building a safer health system*. Washington, DC: National Academy Press; 2000. Available from: http://www.nap.edu/openbook.php?isbn=0309068371
6. Department of Health. *The new NHS*. White paper, 1997. Available from: https://www.gov.uk/government/publications/the-new-nhs
7. Scally G, Donaldson LJ. Clinical governance and the drive for quality improvement in the new NHS in England. *BMJ* 1998; **317**: 61–65.
8. Scally G, Donaldson LJ. Clinical governance and the drive for quality improvement in the new NHS in England. *BMJ* 1998; **317**(7150): 61–65.
9. The Committee on the Financial Aspects of Corporate Governance and Gee and Co Ltd. *Report of the Committee on the Financial Aspects of Corporate Governance. (The Cadbury Report)*. London: Gee; 1992. Available from: http://www.ecgi.org/codes/documents/cadbury.pdf
10. Health Act 1999. Available from: http://www.legislation.gov.uk/ukpga/1999/8/pdfs/ukpga_19990008_en.pdf
11. Department of Health. *An organisation with a memory: report of an expert group on learning from adverse events in the NHS*. London: Stationery Office; 2000.
12. Available from: http://www.hqip.org.uk/resources/hqip-local-clinical-audit-handbook-for-physicians/download [accessed 4 Oct 2017].
13. National Institute for Clinical Excellence. *Principles for best practice in clinical audit*. Abingdon: Radcliffe Medical Press, 2002. Available from: http://www.nice.org.uk/media/796/23/BestPracticeClinicalAudit.pdf
14. www.hqip.org.uk/public/cms/253/625/19/186/HQIP-Criteria
15. Shaw CD, Costain DW. Guidelines for medical audit: seven principles. *Br Med J* 1989; **299**: 498–99.
16. Johnston G, Crombie I, Davies H, et al. Barriers and facilitating factors for effective clinical audit. *Qual Health Care* 2000; **9**: 23–36.
17. National Advisory Group on the Safety of Patients in England. *A promise to learn – a commitment to act*. London: TSO; 2013. Available from: https://www.gov.uk/government/uploads/system/uploads/attachment_data/file/226703/Berwick_Report.pdf
18. NHS Education for Scotland. *Education and training*. Available from: http://www.nes.scot.nhs.uk/education-and-training
19. *Final report of the Mid Staffordshire NHS Foundation Trust Public Inquiry*. 2013. Available from: http://www.midstaffspublicinquiry.com/
20. NHS England. *NHS England's Sir Bruce Keogh sets out plan to drive seven-day services across the NHS*. 15 December 2013. Available from: http://www.nhs.uk/NHSEngland/bruce-keogh-review/Pages/published-reports.aspx
21. Department of Health. *Independent report: Berwick review into patient safety*. 2013. Available from: https://www.gov.uk/government/publications/berwick-review-into-patient-safety
22. *The history of the NHS in England*. Available from: http://www.nhs.uk/NHSEngland/thenhs/nhshistory/Pages/NHShistory1948.aspx
23. https://www.good-governance.org.uk/wp-content/uploads/2017/04/Good-Governance-Handbook.pdf

CHAPTER 38

MEDICAL ETHICS

Paul Baines

What is ethics?..395	Some practical matters in medical ethics....................401
Methods in ethics...396	Conclusions..406
Important concepts in ethics...................................397	References..406

SEARCH STRATEGY

Data in this chapter may be updated by a PubMed search using the keywords: ethics, methods, autonomy, interests, welfare, principles, consequentialism, deontology, reasons, informed consent, children, relativism, research ethics, resource allocation, truth-telling and confidentiality.

WHAT IS ETHICS?

'The purpose of ethical reflection is to help us to decide how to act in the real world, all things considered. This means ethical reflection must take into account all aspects of a proposed course of action, it must rely on good factual evidence and on an understanding of the social and legal contexts in which action has to take place.'[1]

Sometimes decisions in medical ethics are presented as though they are separate from mainstream medical decisions, but this is not so. Succinctly, good medicine demands good ethics and this requires correct facts: ethics necessarily cannot be divorced from the real world.

Two broad academic approaches can be distinguished in ethics. The first, empirical ethics, describes ethical interactions through the methods of social sciences, using questionnaires, interviews and focus groups (amongst others) in studying what happens, or how people approach situations that involve ethics. The methods are both quantitative and qualitative and often come from psychology or sociology.[2] The other broad approach (adopted in this chapter) is philosophical, or analytic, ethics. This is the study of what *ought* to be done and includes questions such as what ethics is and how doctors should behave towards patients and each other. Ethical questions in this tradition are about what *should* happen, not about what does happen. Within this approach to ethics, some consider more abstract questions, such as whether there are moral facts or whether moral truths are relative to society. This discipline is called meta-ethics. These questions are not immediately relevant to clinical practice. Others ask more down to earth questions, such as: What is needed for research to be ethical? Is abortion acceptable? This discipline is called normative ethics. Meta-ethics and normative ethics are not independent, as answers to meta-ethical questions may inform normative conceptions and vice versa. The important difference between these disciplines and empirical ethics is that these studies describe the world, recounting how things are, whereas philosophical ethics concentrates on what would be *right* or how things *should* be. As an example of the distinction, empirical ethics can report on whether or not abortion is carried out and the reasons that people offer for their involvement (or non-participation) in abortion, but philosophical ethics attempts to answer the question of whether or not abortion should be performed. That abortion is (or is not) performed does not indicate whether it ought to be performed.

The distinction between how things are and how they should be, or between what people do and what they should do is one manifestation of the 'is-ought gap'. Hume argued, 'In every system of morality which I have hitherto met with, I have always remarked, that the author proceeds for some time in the ordinary way of reasoning, and establishes the being of a God, or makes some observations concerning human affairs; when of a sudden I am surprised to find that instead of the usual copulations of propositions, *is*, and *is not*, I meet with no proposition that is not connected with an *ought*, or an *ought not* ... a reason should be given, for what seems altogether inconceivable, how this new relation can be a deduction from others, which are entirely different from it'.[3] This distinction is important: clinicians are educated in biomedical scientific methodology, but the methods, and knowledge, of ethics are different from those that they are used to.

Most pressingly, ethics asks the question: What should *I* do? As Singer argues in criticising relativism, 'Anyone who has thought about a difficult ethical decision knows that being told what our society thinks we ought to do does not settle the quandary. We have to reach our own decision.'[4] When a clinician is confronted by an ethical decision, particularly one that is disputed or troubling, the choice that must be made seems deeply personal, and in that way is different from technical questions in medicine (such as the choice of antibiotic to treat sinusitis in a previously well 20-year-old). Although colleagues or confidantes can offer advice and guidance, there is much less sense that an expert can know the right decision when it comes to matters of ethics than in matters of technical medicine (indeed, the notion of whether or not there are ethics experts is contested).[5,6] However, what I want to emphasize is the strong sense that what I do in ethics matters personally.

At different times different questions have concerned those interested in medical ethics. Partly this has been driven by advances in biomedical knowledge and expertise (an example is the advances in reproductive techniques) and partly this has been driven by a change in the focus of ethical interest to different aspects of medical practice. In the recent past medical ethics was more concerned with the professional behaviour of doctors (for example, the acceptability of advertising, and in relationships between doctors); then focus turned to the relationship between the individual clinician and the patient. More recently attention has turned more towards public health ethics and the ethics of the distribution of the social determinants of health.

Some people believe that it is unlikely that there will be progress in ethics because ethics have been studied for several thousand years, so there is nothing new to say, but others are more optimistic: 'Some people believe that there cannot be progress in Ethics, since everything has already been said ... I believe the opposite. How many people have made Non-Religious Ethics their life's work? ... Non-Religious Ethics has been systematically studied, by many people, only since the 1960s. Compared with the other sciences, Non-Religious Ethics is the youngest and least advanced.'[7]

In this chapter I will briefly consider the methods that are used in ethics, then continue to consider some important concepts that are used in ethics and conclude by considering some topics of relevance to practising otolaryngologists. Although I will review the ethics of clinical research there are topics that I will not consider (including, for example, the concerns around stem cell therapies).

METHODS IN ETHICS

The emphasis, in clinical medicine, is on the evidence-base that justifies the performance of diagnostic tests and the effectiveness of medical interventions. Medical decisions that are not supported by a high standard of empirical evidence are taken to be suspect. But this approach will not work in ethics as the questions are different. Ethics involves claims about what *should* be done and what *ought* to happen. These normative questions are different from the questions of evidence-based medicine. To answer these different questions, different methods are needed.

The methods of ethics are essentially those of philosophy or critical thinking and include the critical evaluation of concepts and the use and evaluation of rational arguments in a logical and consistent fashion. The techniques are many and varied but a sense of them can be found in books such as *The Philosopher's Toolkit*[8] and *Thinking from A to Z*[9] and can often be found in introductory textbooks such as *Medical Ethics and Law: The Core Curriculum*.[10] However, as well as philosophy, a broad range of disciplines contribute to medical ethics including, amongst others, legal scholars and lawyers, theologians and historians alongside practising clinicians and other healthcare professionals.

Reasoning and rational justification is at the heart of ethics. In ethics it is important that the conclusions are justified by reasons (though it is important to acknowledge the position that emotion may have in ethics). An important commitment in ethics is that judgements are universalizable. This means that is that there is a requirement to treat all similar cases in the same way. There can be no special pleading along the lines of 'she's my daughter': a reason for your daughter is a reason for all daughters, for all girls, for all children. This means that significant weight is placed on deciding whether two cases are morally similar, or alternatively morally different. One approach in ethics that has achieved prominence in recent times is reflective equilibrium.[11] In this approach all of a person's beliefs and theories are involved when making a decision. Neither the facts of the situation, nor any high level abstract principles take priority over other beliefs, there is a to-and-fro examination of the complete set of a person's beliefs in an attempt to develop a coherent approach. Should there be disagreement or inconsistency, then all of the person's beliefs may be revisited in order to achieve a coherent and consistent set of thoughts. Importantly, all beliefs are subject to revision. Abstract principles do not necessarily trump more down-to-earth concerns.

Within the discipline of normative ethics several different approaches are used to analyze the ethics of medical interventions. These methods include principlism, the claim that principles guide moral action. The most popular principlist approach is the four principles advocated by Beauchamp and Childress,[12] but this is only one form of principlism. Another approach is casuistry, which objects to the 'top-down' approach that starts with abstract principles, insisting that we should attend to the particular circumstances of individual cases. Virtue ethics, another approach, characterizes ethical actions as those in which the virtuous person will 'assess each situation individually, searching for action guidance in considering what a characteristically virtuous person would do'.[13] And yet another is the ethics of care, originating in the work of

Carol Gilligan, emphasizing empathy and compassion, describing ethics in terms of relationships. Gilligan found (in empirical work) that women took the care ethics approach, whereas men appealed more to abstract principles (such as 'justice') in ethical analysis. This is not an exhaustive list of the approaches to ethical analysis.

Importantly, although ethics and law are related, the two are separate disciplines. Some laws neither have nor need an ethical underpinning (the legal requirement to drive on one side of the road for example). Other laws may have some ethical justification, but even in these cases the relationship between ethics and law is not straightforward: some actions are legal but unethical (some would want to describe abortion – legal in many countries – in this way). Some actions are ethical but illegal (some would want to describe assisted suicide, which is illegal in the UK, as an example). And even if there were clear agreement over which actions were ethical and which were not, it is a separate question whether an action that is unethical should be illegal: 'it is one thing to show what a woman ought to do in relation to her unborn child and quite another thing to say that this obligation ought to be enforced'.[14] One way in which it is clear that there is not a direct relation between the law and ethics is the differences in laws between adjacent, but similar, countries. For example, abortion is illegal in Ireland, but legal, in certain circumstances, a 30-minute flight away in the UK. Furthermore, although there is some moral obligation to obey the law, there are also circumstances in which there may be a moral obligation to disobey a bad law. The civil disobedience campaigns in the United States are examples of this.

Similarly the relation between religion and ethics is troubled. Important contributions have been made to ethical thought by religious scholars (amongst other examples in the analysis of the doctrine of double effect), but the foundations of religious ethics – that they are the revealed word of God, or some equivalent, and so their authority is unquestioned – are not accepted by all. And this is compounded by the several different competing religions in pluralistic societies (alongside the arguments of militant atheism). No one dominant religious approach is able to claim a secure knowledge of the good.

Many different institutions and agencies develop and have developed prescriptive guidance on matters of ethics. For example, in the UK, the body responsible for licensing doctors, the General Medical Council (GMC), produces guidance[15] in the form of pamphlets guiding medical practice in general, and pamphlets that also address specific areas of practice such as dealing with children, or research. In law, the GMC's guidance is often taken to indicate the correct approach. As well as GMC guidance, professional bodies such as the British Medical Association and the Royal Colleges (responsible for postgraduate medical education in the UK) produce ethical guidance. Although the guidance may be useful in practice, it requires interpretation by the practitioner to be applied. As well as this, even with clear guidance, there may be conflict between different components of the guidance. Again, interpretation and ethical wisdom is needed in the clinical application of advice.

IMPORTANT CONCEPTS IN ETHICS

Relativism

Relativism is the claim that ethical judgments are made relative to a particular society and time. If this is true, there is no single correct ethical judgement for all and 'when in Rome, do as the Romans do' is true. One support for relativism is the presence of differences between societies in their approaches to ethics. This evidence then leads to the claim that there are no right answers in ethics, just different right answers in different contexts. But this need not be the response; in some circumstances disagreement just indicates that one side is wrong. If we disagree about the distance from Paris to London it doesn't mean that there isn't a right answer, just that one (or both) of us is wrong.

With the prominence of respect for autonomy, relativism can seem the correct response to the challenge 'who are you to judge?' Amongst the advantages of relativism is that it is sensitive to the criticism of ethical imperialism and, in avoiding the claim that a person is wrong, may encourage negotiation instead of confrontation. Confrontation is likely to entrench disagreement whereas negotiation may lead to reasoned agreement.

However, there are significant problems with relativism. Firstly, relativism implies that there is no progress in ethics. If ethical relativism is true, then in slave-owning societies slavery is not wrong. The recognition of the wrongs of slavery and the moral progress in banning slavery is not acknowledged. A second problem for relativism is that ethical disagreement becomes a matter of fact. So again, the claim that slavery is wrong is just a factual claim about a society. But the wrong of slavery is not something that anthropology can judge. Ethical wrongs are not anthropological disagreement.

Importantly, there are different ways that a person can be a 'relativist', and so two relativists can disagree with one another. This brief review only skims the complexity of relativism.[16]

Principles

Principles are laws or truths that offer guidance in ethics. The dominant approach in medical ethics is the four principles approach of Beauchamp and Childress.[12] There are several different principled approaches (see Veatch[17] for a summary of some of these), all with competing justifications. The justification that is often offered is that the chosen principles best condense moral intuitions, or best reflect common-sense morality. Perhaps the most famous principle-based approach is that of Kant[18] with his single categorical imperative (see below).

Not all ethical approaches depend on principles. Some reject a principled approach. Moral particularism claims that 'moral judgment can get along perfectly well without any appeal to principles ... abandoning the mistaken link between morality and principles is if anything a defence of morality rather than an attack on it'.[19] As well as this, other approaches, such as virtue ethics, do not depend on principles.

Autonomy

Respect for autonomy has become the pre-eminent value of our times, and not just in medical ethics: 'to be autonomous is to be one's own person, to be directed by considerations, desires, conditions, and characteristics that are not simply imposed externally upon one, but are part of … one's authentic self'.[20] Although autonomy may seem straightforward, it is highly contested. It includes, at least, freedom from external manipulation (neither physical nor emotional control by others) as well as an internal ability to control oneself (a person does not choose unwisely, driven by impassioned urges or addiction).[20, 21] As rational, morally responsible people, we should adopt our own long-term commitments, goals and values and make our own important decisions about how to live our own lives. Only in this way are we truly human, living a genuine life as a rational person.

Respect for autonomy replaced a more paternalistic model of medicine, where because the technical expertise of the doctor in medicine was respected and accepted, the clinician chose what was best for the patient. However, requirements of autonomy are such that although the clinician has technical expertise, the person with the medical problem knows better the effects of the disease and the therapies on their own life and life goals. In this way it is only the person, guided by the clinician, who is able to make the right decisions about medical interventions.

Kant's morality grounds autonomy in the demands of pure reason. Kant distinguished a hypothetical imperative from the moral categorical imperative. A hypothetical imperative recognizes that one should act in a certain way to achieve a specific goal: consult the map *if* you want the quickest route to the next town. The categorical imperative (the rational demand of morality) is universal, and (in one construction) states, 'Act as if the maxim of your action were to become through your will a universal law of nature' [Kant, 1948; 84].[18] An autonomous decision then is not just simply an individual's choice, it is a supremely rational decision, devoid of misinformation and faulty reasoning, standing for all people for all time: it is the right action. Amongst the criticisms is that such a choice is an impossibly demanding standard. Importantly, many choices do not approach this stringency and so are not (in this sense) autonomous. A different justification that personal choice should be respected comes from libertarianism – such as Mill's. Mill set out the harm principle, 'the only purpose for which power can be rightfully exercised over any member of a civilized community, against his will, is to prevent harm to others. His own good, either physical or moral, is not a sufficient warrant.'[22] This is because when another person chooses they are 'quite as likely to be wrong as right'.[22] Even so, Mill recognizes some limits. He gives the example of a person crossing an unsafe bridge who may be 'seized and turned back' if unaware of the danger. A Millian justification of respect for choice is less demanding than a Kantian justification.

An autonomous decision is one that affects only the individual involved. So preventing smoking in public based on the risks of passive smoking does not conflict with the respect that is due to autonomous choices (it is not paternalistic). One criticism is that very few, if any, decisions have repercussions only for the individual concerned. Almost all of us have family and friends: we are not atomic individuals bound by rights. The Nelsons argued that the locus for medical decisions should be the family and not the individual.[23] Feminist criticism of autonomy draws attention to the fiction of the lone 'autonomous' individual free of ties, drawing attention to the relational nature of autonomy. A further criticism of autonomy is that pervasive discrimination can impoverish a person's self-esteem and so desires. If so, the choices a person makes are not truly autonomous: 'our desires are shaped by our expectations which are shaped by our circumstances'.[24]

Sometimes autonomous individuals can choose a course that seems (at least to others) not to be good for the individual (even the individual themself may come to recognize their choice was mistaken). Some deny this, arguing that an autonomous individual is always the best judge of their welfare (for example, 'Competent adults are allowed to define their own concept of "best interests"…'[25]). That an individual makes the correct choice about their welfare depends on the individual being informed and reasoning correctly. We can all recognize episodes when we have been mistaken about what would be good for us as individuals, in which our choices have not been to our benefit. In this way there is a tension between autonomous choices and an individual's welfare. Bosk observed that 'the dark side of patient autonomy is abandonment'.[26]

An ethics based on respect for autonomy does not account for public health commitments (to water fluoridation or to clean water and air as examples). These cannot be a matter of autonomous choice for individuals, as it is unlikely that all individuals will choose (or refuse) them.

Some people are not autonomous, lacking some – or all – of the abilities needed to be autonomous. Young children are one group. They will be considered later on. Another is incompetent adults. When dealing with incompetent adults, all attempts should be made to maximize the person's capacity. Incompetence may be temporary (perhaps while ill or intoxicated) or permanent (in severe dementia). Sometimes a person's capacity, and so their competence, fluctuates. The broad approach to those who lack autonomy (if they were previously competent) is to choose as the individual would have chosen. Medical decisions can be guided by written instructions that the individual has left (an advance directive). Alternatively, the now incompetent person may have chosen someone to make decisions on their behalf (in the UK this is named a Lasting Power of Attorney). In the absence of these, evidence of the incompetent person's preferences (from family and friends) guides medical decisions, in order to choose as the person would have chosen (a substituted judgement). As well as this, the views of the not competent individual should be sought so that their views may be included. In the absence of all of these, the decision for an incompetent person will be based on some objective or impersonal sense of the individual's best interests.[27]

Welfare, well-being, 'good for', in a person's (best) interests, beneficence

Often the role of medicine is taken to be to make people better, specifically to improve their health, but there can be disagreement about what this means. One problem is that there is not a clear boundary between health and disease, nor is there a clear boundary between treating disease, preventing disease and improving health. Some believe that although doctors treat disease caused by smoking, clinicians overreach their role in campaigning against smoking or advocating restrictions on smoking. Importantly non-healthcare interventions can improve health. Literacy campaigns reduce overall mortality and neonatal mortality,[28] but would not usually be taken to be a healthcare intervention. Some seek to define the role of medicine as the treatment of physiological disorders, appealing to the role of disturbances to what is 'scientifically' normal function. There are many difficulties with these approaches. One example is in reproduction. Medical roles encompass both abortion, in terminating pregnancy, and assisted reproductive techniques in initiating and maintaining pregnancy. A physiological definition of medical goals is unhelpful here. Importantly, as well as benefits for physical health, mental well-being is also important.

Medicine is not limited to the treatment of disease (an example is the importance of health promotion exemplified by vaccination programmes) but how far into the promotion of health medicine should go is controversial. The WHO defines health as 'a state of complete physical, mental and social well-being and not merely the absence of disease or infirmity'.[29] Daniels responds, 'Health is not all there is to well-being or happiness, contrary to the famous World Health Definition (WHO) definition … The WHO definition risks turning all of social philosophy and social policy into health care.'[30] In general in medicine, clinicians act in a way that is 'good for' their patients, though their actions are limited both by the law and by the consent of the patient.

This aim can be expressed in several different ways: that clinicians should do good for their patients; that they should act in their patients' interests; or best interests; or with attention to their patients' welfare or well-being or for their good. In this sense, a person's interests are at the core of ethics. Or, describing it another way, when acting or choosing between actions, a significant (although perhaps not the only) factor in ethics is the effect the action will have on people's interests.

However, in modern pluralist societies there are often different senses of what would be good for someone. In a well-rehearsed example, Jehovah's Witnesses believe that the voluntary acceptance of blood transfusion leads to damnation, so a blood transfusion, even when life-saving, is not in their interests. Others would see that a blood transfusion is clearly beneficial. Can we resolve these dilemmas? Philosophers disagree about how best to conceptualize a person's interests, some (utilitarians) arguing that what is best is what makes most people most 'happy' (though they may disagree about what is meant by happiness). Others argue that what is best is where more of a person's desires are fulfilled and fewer desires are left unfulfilled (desire-satisfaction theories). A further approach is that some things are just good for people (sufficient food) and some things are just bad for people (pain). To be healthy is just good. This is called an objective list account. There is insufficient space in this chapter to take this further (but see Degrazia's[31] paper or Griffin's book *Wellbeing*[24]), but we should recognize that not only do we not have a clear grasp of a person's interests but we also do not have a clear way to go about working out what a person's interests are. These concerns led the House of Lords to claim '"best interests" is probably the most abused and misunderstood phrase in health and social care. It has too often been the vehicle for poor decision-making'.[32]

It is rare that any medical intervention is a source of unmitigated benefit; all interventions have some adverse effects in terms of pain or unpleasantness, or even (for the most trivial of interventions) the time that the intervention requires could have been spent more profitably. So in considering the benefit to an individual, the severity and the likelihood of harm (maleficence) must be considered alongside the extent and likelihood of benefit in coming to a conclusion about the benefits of medical intervention. For example, in the Belmont Report (considering the ethics of research), harm is included in the calculation of beneficence which is described as '(1) do not harm and (2) maximize possible benefits and minimize possible harms.'[33] Beauchamp and Childress,[12] in their influential four principles, separate beneficence from non-maleficence.

Non-maleficence

Avoidance of harm is sometimes prioritized as a first principle, often phrased in the Latin *primum non nocere* – above all do no harm. I have argued already that it is usually necessary to balance benefits and harms each against the other in judging the overall advantage (or disadvantage) of medical interventions. If the first, overriding, responsibility is taken to be to do no harm, then it is likely to rule out all medical interventions as none can be guaranteed to be without adverse effects.

A reason to separate non-maleficence from beneficence is that a person may have a broader responsibility to avoid harm to others, than to do good to them. A clinician has a responsibility to benefit her patients, but she need not help others. The clinician, though, does have a more general responsibility to avoid harm even to those who are not her patients.

Paternalism

Paternalism describes an intervention that is done solely to benefit a person, but which that person has not chosen, or perhaps would not choose (there are different forms of paternalism). This sort of intervention is excluded by Mill's harm principle. Failing to intervene (refusing to refer for abortion for example) can also be paternalistic. Because of the importance of the principle of respect for autonomy the objection 'you're being paternalistic' is generally taken to knock down a proposed action. The only justification for intervention should be that an autonomous individual has consented to it. However, paternalism is manifest in different forms and there is some sense of appropriate paternalism: '"paternalistic" in an innocent, non-pejorative sense, namely that of "protective in a manner characteristic of parents"'.[34] Others resist this claim, arguing that paternalism is always wrong.

Paternalism has been characterized further, to distinguish when paternalism may be appropriate, though the terms used are used inconsistently (see for example Dworkin[35] and Childress[36]). Amongst other distinctions, some interventions involve autonomous persons, others non-autonomous persons, and sometimes the person's autonomy is uncertain. Another distinction lies in separating pure paternalism (the intervention solely benefits the person involved) from impure paternalism (justified by benefits both to the person involved and to others – such as laws restricting smoking that benefit both the smoker and those around her). A further distinction is found when the intervention helps a person to achieve values they hold (soft paternalism) contrasted with hard paternalism where the person does not accept the goals of the intervention. Accepting these distinctions, it is clear that paternalistic interventions need not be wrong and the important point lies in deciding when paternalism is unjustified. The waters have been muddied still further by the inclusion of 'maternalism'[1] and nudging, efforts to guide people in the right direction.

Rights

Rights are commonly, and increasing commonly, used in moral discourse. Codes or declarations of rights, having started with the UN Declaration of Human Rights in 1948 (provoked by the outrages of the Second World War) are increasing in number. Legal rights must be distinguished from moral or natural rights. Legal rights are ensconced in law, and are a matter for legal debate, for lawyers to resolve, and so are not the concern here. I will consider natural or moral rights that are independent of and go beyond the law, so that a person in a country where there is no right to free speech (for example) can say, 'I have a right to speak'. This is an appeal to a human right, not a legal right. Some dispute the existence of human rights at all, most famously Bentham: 'right with me is the child of the law ... a natural right is a son that never had a father'.[37]

How could we know whether a claim is a human right or just a matter of convention, politeness or good manners? One response is to look to the codes or declarations of rights, but problematically the codes differ in their content. Furthermore, this response just pushes the question back one step: why are *those* rights in the declaration?

Regardless of these concerns, rights-based claims are common. The power of rights-based claims is in demanding access to healthcare for individuals and groups who are ignored or discriminated against. They are less useful in clinical problems where conflicting rights may not clearly be resolvable. Diane Pretty (afflicted by multiple sclerosis) used the European Convention of Human Rights (her right to life, a prohibition from torture, and a right to private and family life alongside a prohibition of discrimination) to ask that her husband would not be prosecuted should he assist her in ending her life. The UK government argued successfully against her claimed rights.[38] Often, when rights come into conflict there is no clear way to decide which right should triumph and which will be vanquished.

Justice

The concept of justice used in medical ethics is that of distributive justice. A formal statement of justice is that equals should be treated equally, but the presence of significant morally relevant differences indicates individuals should be treated differently.

The weight then is placed on deciding which differences are morally relevant. Most would want to agree that age or gender are not relevant differences in determining medical interventions. Some diseases are a consequence of personal choice (for example, smoking-inflicted diseases, such as coronary artery disease). If we agree that people are responsible for the consequences of the choices that they make, and if we agree that personal choices are an important cause of some diseases, then (the argument runs) treatment for smokers should be assigned a lower priority, than treatment for (the same conditions) for non-smokers. And the reason for the lower priority is that smokers deserve a lower priority because they are at least partly responsible for their disease. There are several concerns with this argument. One response is that smokers are addicted to smoking: smoking is not the free, uncoerced 'autonomous' choice that people should be held responsible for. Furthermore, many smokers started smoking when they were young (often when they were less than 16 years old), at the age when children should be protected from unwise choices. Similar arguments run for other diseases that may be self-inflicted (such as those provoked by alcohol or obesity). These arguments for responsibility are less often used for other self-inflicted diseases (the orthopaedic injury of the sportsman) and the concern here is that we are then imposing our choice of values on individuals who should be free to make their own choices. Be this as it may, the concept of justice is that if people are to be treated differently then there should be clear reasons why this is justified.

Consequentialism

Consequentialist approaches to ethics distinguish the ethically correct course as that which produces the best outcomes. Consequentialists differ in the outcomes that they value. Utilitarianism is one form of consequentialism in which the outcome that matters is 'utility' taken as the balance between pleasure and pain. Utilitarians seek to maximize overall utility.

Consequentialism is implicitly appealing to many healthcare practitioners, in seeking the best outcome: when choosing between two treatments, it seems obvious to choose the intervention, which has the least mortality or highest function or whatever, both for an individual patient and for populations. In fact it is a puzzle to many why anything other than the best outcome should be sought (I will consider a contrasting approach – deontology – in the next section). A consequentialist approach underlies the use of quality adjusted life years (QALYs) in the allocation of limited healthcare resources. There are often ethical decisions to be made about what is the 'best' outcome.

Consequentialist approaches can differ in what is taken to be the best outcome. One difference lies in the outcome that is taken to be best. As an example, a longer life is usually taken to be a better outcome, but some would choose a life of 60 years of full health with a sudden end in contrast to a life of 65 years, the last 10 years of which are blighted by unremitting pain. Another difference lies in the way that outcomes are amalgamated. In maximizing consequentialism, the best outcome is sought with no attention to the distribution of the outcomes. Often in health promotion programmes those who are most likely to suffer from the disease are least likely to take advantage of the programme. If so the intervention with the greatest efficiency in reducing disease increases inequality.[39] Most would agree that inequality matters and that it should not be exacerbated by healthcare interventions. I do not intend to resolve the debate here, just to note that even if consequentialism is taken to be a preferred approach, there are important questions about which form of consequentialism should be adopted.

Deontological

Consequentialism is often contrasted with deontological approaches. Deontology has its origin in the Greek work *deon*, meaning duty. Deontological theories are those that characterize ethics in terms of duty: actions are obligatory, permissible or forbidden. The paradigmatic deontological approach (though not by any means the only one) is the well-worked out ethics of the Roman Catholic Church.

Deontological approaches can be seen in contrast to consequentialist theories. One criticism of consequentialist theories is that they are too demanding. In consequentialist approaches, an individual is obliged always to choose the action that will maximize the good. Consequentialists may recognize no distinction between acts and omissions. A person then should act in the best way for the overall outcome. If so a person may have no time for their own projects, indeed they almost cease to be a person (with characteristics and individual values) becoming a machine to produce the best outcome. In contrast a deontological approach is characterized by permissible and forbidden actions. Some actions are required (for example those of a parent in relation to their child), but the required actions are much less frequent than the forbidden actions. Because of this, the deontologist does not face the overwhelming demands of a consequentialist (see, for example, Singer[4]).

Another distinction between deontology and consequentialist theories is that consequentialism permits too much. If only consequences matter, then any action may be acceptable in pursuing the outcomes. An example of these fears is the well-worked transplant example. Imagine that a surgeon has two dying patients, whose lives could be saved by organ transplantation. Some consequentialists would allow (or even demand) the sacrifice of a randomly chosen individual whose organs could save the two (or more) lives.[40] Deontological approaches, in which some actions are impermissible, forbid the taking of an innocent life, whatever the potential gains.

Medical practice, in which doctors are guided or constrained by the guidance provided by the various official bodies, often seems to have a deontological underpinning.

The four principles approach (Beauchamp and Childress)

Beauchamp and Childress[12] developed and popularized the four principles approach, which has become the dominant paradigm in Western medical ethics. The four principles are: respect for autonomy; beneficence; non-maleficence; and justice. These have been considered individually. Although used to the greatest extent in medical ethics these four principles are claimed to underlie a common approach to ethics. As Gillon has it, 'the four principles approach to ethics will be recognized to have far wider moral relevance than its application to health care ethics. Indeed I predict its increasing acceptance as the basis for a global ethics, compatible with and acceptable across the range of the world's moral cultures, sensitively negotiating the delicate path between moral relativism and moral imperialism.'[41]

There are many other approaches that are advocated by their supporters; several have been mentioned already. There is insufficient space to discuss the other approaches in any detail. The important point is that although the four principles may seem to be the only approach, there are other approaches used to analyze the ethics of medicine. Introductions to the other approaches can be found in *Principles of Health Care Ethics*[42] or in the Festschrift edition of the *Journal of Medical Ethics*[43] devoted to methods in ethics.

SOME PRACTICAL MATTERS IN MEDICAL ETHICS

Informed consent

Given the importance of autonomous choice, consent becomes crucial for medical interventions. In an early medico-legal case Cardozo stated, 'Every human being of adult years and sound mind has a right to determine what shall be done with his own body; and a surgeon who performs an operation without his patient's consent, commits an assault'.[44] For significant interventions, consent is usually written, giving proof that a consent discussion took place (and perhaps in giving a signature the person recognizes a greater significance to the consent discussion) but what is important is the consent of the person – not the signature. Should someone withdraw consent, the document is no longer evidence of consent.

Consent requires a persistent sense of self with personal values, an understanding and knowledge of the available choices, and an ability to reflect on (and judge between) the options, and having done this, to communicate the decision. The person must have sufficient information about the available options. What counts as 'sufficient' information is disputed, but broadly it is the information that would affect the person's choice, recognizing that different factors may be important to different individuals. There is a tension between an attempt to limit the information needed to make decisions easier for those on the boundaries of competence (to prevent people being overwhelmed by information), but also to provide more information (so that people are more fully informed). Consent suggests that the patient agrees to one of the options put forward by the clinician; true respect for autonomy requires negotiation and agreement and is perhaps better described as concordance.

Consent may be modified in various ways. Implied consent is not explicit. An example is when a patient pulls their sleeve up when informed a blood test is needed, though no formal consent discussion has taken place. Another form of consent is assumed consent, where interventions are assumed to have consent. Patients may have been informed by posters or by mailed information. Examples of assumed consent are to the use of data collected for other purposes, and to patients being examined by students. Here assumed consent is often not consent at all, but a lack of resistance or lack of dissent. A further modification of consent is deferred consent. In emergencies, the research subject may be unconscious and so unable to consent, or the intervention may need to be administered quickly allowing no opportunity for an informed consent discussion. Here deferred consent may be used. The question here is: what is the person consenting too when asked later on? Not to the intervention (which has already taken place) but to the use of their information, or to continuing participation in the research, if the intervention is continuing. And if so, then the justification for the research intervention at the time it starts is different from the justification offered by 'true' consent.

Consent is important in medical ethics, but some adults are unable to consent. They will be considered in the next section.

The incompetent adult

Some adults are not competent to make decisions about their own healthcare. The presumption is that adults are competent to make their own choices, but some adults are temporarily (perhaps through drugs or disease), and others permanently incompetent to make their own decisions. All attempts should be made to ensure that a person is most able to make decisions for themselves, perhaps by delaying decisions if there is a prospect that competence may return. If not, decisions are made in a variety of ways, which have been discussed above.

The fact that a patient disagrees with a clinician's proposed treatment does not in itself indicate that the patient is incompetent; a competent patient may disagree with a clinician. However, if disagreement over treatment is likely to harm a patient, then the patient's competence may come into question (though it may not were he to agree with proposed treatment).

Children

Children range from a newly born baby, totally dependent on others, to adolescents on the cusp of competence who may fare perfectly well on their own and so have varied abilities. All are described as children. Not all children are incompetent to make their own medical decisions (in England and Wales this is established as the concept of Gillick Competence[45] and in the United States there is the concept of mature minors).

Children differ from others who are incompetent for a variety of reasons. Children grow towards personhood and the most important achievements of their lives, whereas most adult incompetents fall away from moral personhood: their achievements lie behind them. As well as this, parents play a particularly important role in their child's life that is not matched by the role of relatives of grown adults. Importantly, the way that children are treated will affect, sometimes determining, the adult that the child becomes. Parents are offered broad latitude, though not complete freedom, in the way that they bring up their children.

Young children cannot be taken to be competent. The mainstream approach is that parents consent for treatment that is in their child's interests, and the only treatment that should be offered is treatment that is in the child's interests. But it is not so simple. Firstly there may be dispute about what treatment is in a child's interests (an example is male circumcision, which some will claim is in a child's interests though others deny this). Secondly, sometimes parental authority extends to the refusal of treatment that is unequivocally in a child's interests (the requirement for parental consent for vaccination is an example of this). As children grow older, the approach to medical decisions changes so that the child's views should be taken into account when decisions are taken, but medical decisions are still made by the child's parents. And as children approach maturity, they may be recognized to be competent to make their own medical decisions.

I have already described problems with knowing a person's interests, and because children have the potential to develop in many different ways, one response to this is to claim a 'right to an open future' for children:[34] children should mature with as many life choices as possible. One practical application is that interventions with momentous consequences should (when possible) be delayed until the child is able to make their own decision. But this is not always possible. Cochlear implantation provides an example. Two broad approaches can be adopted for deaf children. Conventionally, deafness is taken to be a disability. Oralism encourages the use of spoken language. Hearing aids (and now cochlear implants) maximize the child's ability to hear, and are combined with intensive speech therapy. Sign language is banned in some cases, to encourage children to interact with spoken language. Some deaf children, particularly those with some hearing, achieve success with this route, but others, especially those with profound deafness, don't. The second strategy embraces Deaf culture and the Deaf World (with a capital 'D'), encouraging signing and rejecting spoken language. Deaf culture is celebrated. Communication is fundamentally different: imagine poetry in sign language. As a result there are two separate paths for deaf children: oralism or Deaf culture. The earlier a person starts to sign, the better their signing becomes and vice versa. Compounding this, those who have some hearing or use verbal communication may not be taken to be 'properly' deaf and so are excluded from the Deaf community. The reverse may also be true. In deciding how to rear their deaf child, Deaf parents are at some advantage. They have their own experiences, and they may have considered the possibility of a deaf child (and indeed some have chosen a deaf child*). A compounding problem is that the Deaf community may have expectations of the choices that Deaf parents should make (to preserve the Deaf community). Parents of deaf children have important choices to make at an early stage in their child's lives: 'Deaf people in the hearing world are always going to be at a disadvantage. So the question is whether people prefer to be marginal in a mainstream world, or mainstream in a marginal world and many people quite understandably prefer the latter.'[47] And the question must be answered when the child is young. An attempt to keep both options open – a right to an open future – is unlikely to lead to success in either option.

Research

Research is vital to maintain and advance scientific medical practice. Whereas interventions by clinicians are intended to benefit the patient in front of them, the aim of research is to further knowledge. Although research may benefit patients in the future, the advantage may not accrue to individual research participants. There are many examples in medical research, where the new 'better' intervention has worse outcomes than the traditional 'control' therapy (and indeed the point of therapeutic research is to determine which of the tested treatments is better).

Appropriate ethical standards in research are protected by the requirement that research should only take place with the consent of the research participant, and through an extensive system of research governance, policed by the healthcare practitioners' professional bodies (the GMC and the World Medical Association as examples), and the academic journals and universities and hospitals, and (in many countries) by the law. An important principle is that research depends on the consent of the research participant. An influential statement dates from the Nuernberg War Crimes Trial: 'the voluntary consent of the human subject is absolutely essential'.[48] Since then it has generally been accepted that all research should be preceded by consent. Any variation to this requirement requires good reasons (for example, deferred consent may be acceptable in emergency situations where prior consent is impossible). This statement could be taken to exclude research participation by children, but an equivalent for children's participation is generally taken to be the consent of the child's parents and (if appropriate) the assent of the child.

As well as this, there are extensive systems of research governance, professional standards are often reinforced by the law. The Nuernberg standards for research were updated in the World Medical Association's Declaration of Helsinki (and are kept up to date by further revisions). The requirements are broad and include that research is reviewed before it starts, that the research is performed to standards to ensure the scientific validity of the findings, and that research participants are protected (as best they can be) from harm. As part of the review, the risks and benefits of the project to participants are assessed and minimized, and must be proportionate to the benefits of the research. An important part of the review is that patients should be involved in determining research priorities and designing trials.

There are different sorts of research, some involving medical interventions, perhaps with random allocation, some involving patients, but with more trivial interventions and some involving only identifiable information about patients. Different standards may be required for these different forms of research.

Sometimes the boundary between research and audit is unclear. Some projects are clearly research – for example, the random allocation of children to different fluid resuscitation regimes – but some projects are clearly audit – for example, monitoring post-operative mortality or infection rates. The distinction between research and audit is taken to be important because of the rigour of research governance. However, this may not be the important distinction. Merely because an activity is taken to be audit does not mean that it is ethically unproblematic, as audit may produce the same sort of ethical concerns (confidentiality, for example) as research. And the correct response is to recognize that research and audit should be carried out to the same standards.

The distinction between acts and omissions

A common view is that we are more responsible for the consequences of our acts than we are for our omissions. This may be why some believe that it is acceptable not to intervene towards the end of life ('passive' euthanasia) whereas an act to shorten life ('active' euthanasia) is often taken to be wrong. Others do not recognize the distinction between acts and omissions. Consequentialists judge actions by their outcomes, and so hold a person as

---

* 'A deaf lesbian couple in the United States deliberately created a deaf child. Sharon Duchesneau and Candy McCullough used their own sperm donor, a deaf friend with five generations of deafness in his family, to ensure that their child would be deaf.'[46]

responsible for the consequences that follow from a failure to act as they do for those that result from actions. Rachels seeks to undermine what some see as the clear difference between acts and omissions. He asks us to imagine two uncles. Smith deliberately drowns his cousin in the bath in order to benefit from a large inheritance. In another family, Jones enters the bathroom to drown his cousin (to benefit from an inheritance) to see that his cousin has slipped, is submerged unconscious, and will drown if unaided. Jones merely stands by while his cousin drowns. Rachels asks, 'Smith killed the child, whereas Jones "merely" let the child die ... Did either man behave better from a moral point of view?'[49]

Despite Rachels' arguments, there is a strong intuition that we are more responsible for our acts than our omissions. Why is this? It may be that there are other aspects that often go along with the distinction between acts and omissions, but that are separable from it. These include the fact that causation is often stronger for actions. Another difference between acts and omissions is the intention of the person involved. But the moral importance of intention can be questioned and our ability to know another's intention must be questioned.

Perhaps the solution is that the distinction between acts and omissions is blurred. Ethics depends on many overlapping considerations and the distinction between acts and omissions is one, but only one, amongst many factors that need to be evaluated in assessing the morality of an action.

The doctrine of double effect

The doctrine of double effect (DDE) is sometimes invoked towards the end of life, allowing that interventions that may have adverse effects (and so that by deontology's values are *always* forbidden) may be used if the bad results are *foreseen* but not *intended*. The paradigm case is the use of opiates towards the end of life to alleviate pain, whilst accepting that opiates may shorten life (a bad effect is foreseen but not intended). The origins of the DDE lie in Aquinas' justification of murder in self-defence. For the DDE to be applicable, several conditions must be fulfilled: the act itself must be morally good or indifferent; the agent must not intend (but merely foresee) the bad effect; the benefit must not be obtained *by* the bad effect (DDE could not be invoked for euthanasia for a patient in severe pain, as the benefit occurs through the bad effect); and the final condition is that there is proportionality between the bad effect and good effect.

Although these may seem clear conditions, there are several problems with the DDE. How can the outcomes that are 'intended' be distinguished from those that are merely 'foreseen'? The criticism is that the DDE is just sophistry: wordplay allows an unacceptable action to become acceptable.

Rationing and resource allocation

Rationing, or resource allocation decisions, recognizes that there are situations where treatment is not determined solely by the autonomous choice of the patient (or the welfare of an incompetent patient) but that – at times – limited resources must be distributed in some way that is fair.

Resource allocation decisions need to be made at different levels. The highest (macro) level decisions involve decisions at governmental level regarding the total spending on health, and how much allocation within the whole of the health budget should be on geriatrics and how much on paediatrics, amongst many other decisions. The micro-allocation level involves direct clinical decisions at the level of individual patients. So an example would be the decision in a flu epidemic of which of two patients who need intensive care should be admitted to the single remaining critical care bed. There are other resource allocation decisions that must be made between these two levels.

Sometimes these decisions are made by default, or on the basis of historical priorities. In the UK, the National Institute for Health and Care Excellence (NICE) was established so that decisions about NHS resource allocation are made in a consistent and structured way. These decisions may be less pressing when healthcare is purchased and so distributed to those who are able to pay, but even in these systems during periods of limited resources, or excessive demand (such as a flu epidemic), decisions about resource allocation may be needed. There are a variety of ways in which these decisions can be made, none of which are agreed.

Truth-telling, deception, and disclosure of errors

Until recent times, medicine was practised paternalistically: clinicians often deliberately concealed diagnoses and treatments and were certainly less likely to inform patients. There was greater respect for expertise and alongside the power imbalance between doctor and patients, the expectations that patients would be fully informed and (on occasion) even told the truth were lower. But with acknowledgement of the importance of autonomous choice, truth-telling is fundamental to respect for people and consent. Consent is essentially meaningless if it is uninformed.

What then are the circumstances under which a commitment to truth-telling may be undermined? A relatively straightforward justification is when the context is entirely inappropriate. For example, if a clinician is in the supermarket and encounters a patient who asks, 'My tests were okay, weren't they Doc?', the clinician may justifiably dissemble if they weren't, and arrange an early appointment.

Another threat to honest communications comes from patient's relationships. A patient may require that relatives are not informed of a diagnosis, sometimes to 'protect' them. Parents may sometimes not fully inform their children (of the risks of death or the unpleasantness of therapies) and may ask that the clinical team join in their deception. As parents play a fundamental role in the care of a child their requirements may seem reasonable in some circumstances (perhaps with younger children) but may seem wrong in other circumstances (with older children).

With deception, there is always the possibility of inadvertent disclosure by staff who are used to dealing with fully informed patients. The child themself may see they are admitted to the oncology ward and ask what oncology is. Some clinicians may accept a passive role in failing to inform the child but cannot condone a direct lie. The relationship with the child will be destroyed if the clinician isn't honest and the lie is discovered, but the therapeutic relationship with the parents may be destroyed if clinicians refuse to join in the deception. In these situations it is sensible to explore the parent's reasons for withholding information from their child in order that any misunderstandings can be corrected. Many children understand more than their parents believe. Often both parents and child will benefit from the opportunity for a frank discussion with acknowledgement of the reality of the situation.

In a discussion of truthfulness, it is important to acknowledge that there are many steps between complete truth and a deliberate lie. It may be acceptable to fail to mention a complication (if it is rare or of minor importance) but a direct question about the same complication deserves an honest response. Although there is a fundamental commitment to full and honest disclosure, at times, as Higgs (a strong proponent of truth-telling) argues, 'unwavering honesty can seem as pathological as paternalistic concealment'.[50] In these situations a deviation from truthfulness demands explicit reasons.

An important part of truth-telling is that errors should be disclosed to patients when they have happened. This is for several reasons. Firstly, we should treat patients with respect, and this means that they deserve full information. This is how we would choose to be dealt with ourselves. A further reason is that, following medical accidents or an adverse outcome, many patients give their reasons for suing as the fact that no one would tell them what had happened. It is likely that giving patients full information at the time would prevent at least some of the malpractice lawsuits.

Confidentiality/privacy

Confidentiality is the requirement that the information that is disclosed in the course of healthcare consultations should remain confidential to the treating clinical team. This is justified by respect for the patient's autonomy and by the doctor's professional responsibilities and duties. There are also pragmatic justifications that if it were known that clinical teams did not keep information confidential then people would be cautious in disclosing information to clinicians that could be embarrassing or harmful. Without complete clinical information, diagnosis and treatment become more difficult.

Healthcare has become more dependent on technology, which has provided many challenges to confidentiality, with the development of computerized records adding the problems of loss or deliberate hacking of electronically stored information to concerns in confidentiality. As well as this, as healthcare is more often delivered by large teams and as healthcare governance teams extend the number of those who need (or believe that they need) information, the demands in maintaining confidentiality are not as simple as they were in the past.

The right to confidentiality is not absolute and, if there are good reasons, confidentiality may be broken. Situations where it may be appropriate to breach confidentiality include those where there is a threat of harm to the patient or to others. If confidentiality is to be broken, it may be appropriate to negotiate the disclosure with the patient. Where the individual lacks capacity and is incompetent to make choices about their own healthcare, it is likely to be appropriate to disclose information in the patient's interests, but again the disclosure should be negotiated with the patient. The disclosed information should be limited to that which is necessary and no more, and should be to the appropriate authorities.

The threat of harm to a competent individual (and harm only to that person) is unlikely to justify disclosure of confidential information. However, disclosure of confidential information can be justified if there is the prospect of harm to another individual. Again there should be an attempt to negotiate disclosure with the person: they may agree. However, there may be situations where disclosure is justified, even when the person does not agree. Indeed, disclosure of confidential information is sometimes required by law; for example, the Abortion Act (1991) in the UK requires that the name and address of the woman is notified to the appropriate authorities. There are several other statutory obligations in the UK (listed by the GMC).[51]

Clinical ethics committees and consultation

In some situations, clinicians may be concerned about the ethics of a particularly complex clinical situation, or a novel clinical scenario. When ethical concerns appear, what can clinicians do? A first response is to discuss the circumstances and the focus of the concern with colleagues. Even just laying out the problem to another may lead to a solution, but if not, talking through the problem with clinical colleagues may provide a solution to the ethical concerns. Another approach is to consult official guidance and policy. In the UK these include sources such as the Royal Colleges, who oversee education, or the institutions responsible for licensing doctors (in the UK the GMC offers useful advice in pamphlets that are available on its website) and the medical societies (the British Medical Association in the UK, for example, has an ethics department, and the specialist societies often have written guidance and policies). However, the guidance is rarely directly applicable to individual situations and needs to be interpreted in application to clinical problems.

More recently the importance of clinical ethics advice has been acknowledged and clinical ethics has developed as a specialism. Many hospitals have appointed clinical ethics specialists and have established clinical ethics committees.[52] These are often distinct from the longer-established research ethics committees. The committees may have several roles, but one important role is to advise on clinical case consultations. Other roles may involve policy development, education and the organizational ethics of the hospital. Usually there is a broad representation of healthcare staff on the committee, alongside members from those outside the organization. Specific disciplines that are often included are lawyers and religious representatives such as chaplains or leaders of other faiths. Some committees encourage the participation of patients and their families when considering ethical problems, and indeed it would seem wrong to fail to canvass the opinion of the patients and those close to them.

CONCLUSIONS

In this chapter I have given a brief introduction to medical ethics. Medical ethics is a large and developing field, in which some of the more outlandish claims made by some who are remote from clinical practice may cause clinicians to dismiss medical ethics as irrelevant to clinical practice. This is the wrong response. The correct response when challenged by conclusions that seem to be incorrect is to engage with the arguments that are given, to work out the flaws in the arguments, and so demonstrate the weaknesses of the mistaken claim. It is also useful to rehearse the arguments of one's own position, making sure that these are sufficiently strong. Good arguments for one's own position are insufficient in their own right: if each side has good arguments to support their position, but neither can demonstrate a flaw in the opposing arguments, there is insufficient reason to come to a conclusion. Often it is through the conflict of two claims that a third, more defensible solution is found.

Should the reader wish to study ethics further, several useful texts are given in the reference list. *Medical Ethics and Law: The Core Curriculum*[10] is a sound introductory text. Beauchamp and Childress'[12] book is almost the bible of medical ethics, but advocates strongly for only one approach – the four principles. The second edition of the *Principles of Health Care Ethics*[42] is intimidatingly large, but magisterial and comprehensive. There are several short courses in ethics and many universities have developed Master's level degrees in medical ethics, often combined with law, for further study.

KEY POINTS

- The methods used in ethics generally – and so in medical ethics – are different from the methods of evidence-based medicine.
- Respect for the informed autonomous choice of a patient is a dominant approach in western medical ethics.
- The patient's (and patients') welfare, well-being or interests are an important factor in medical decisions for incompetent patients, children and populations.

REFERENCES

1. Holm S. Obesity interventions and ethics. *Obes Rev* 2007; s1, **8**: 207–10.
2. Sugarman J, Pearlman RA, Taylor HA. Empirical approaches to health care ethics. In Ashcroft RE, Dawson A, Draper H, McMillan, JR (eds). *Principles of health care ethics*. 2nd ed. Chichester: John Wiley & Sons, Ltd; 2007.
3. Hume D. *A treatise of human nature*. Book III, part i, section i. Available from http://www.davidhume.org/search.html?T1=on&T2=on&T3=on&A=on&L=on&ad=on&es=on&E=on&M=on&P=on&N=on&D=on&q=%22is%2C+and+is+not%22
4. Singer P. *Practical ethics*. 3rd ed. Cambridge: Cambridge University Press; 2011, p. 6.
5. Archard D. Why moral philosophers are not and should not be moral experts. *Bioethics* 2011; **25**(3): 119–27.
6. Vogelstein R. The nature and value of bioethics expertise. *Bioethics* 2015; **29**(5): 324–33.
7. Parfit D. *Reasons and persons*. Oxford: Clarendon Press; 1984, p. 453.
8. Baggini J, Fosl PS. *The philosopher's toolkit*. 2nd ed. Oxford: Wiley-Blackwell; 2010.
9. Warburton N. *Thinking from A to Z*. 3rd ed. London: Routledge; 2007.
10. Hope T, Savulescu J, Hendrick J. *Medical ethics and law: the core curriculum*. Edinburgh: Churchill Livingstone Elsevier; 2008.
11. Daniels N. Reflective equilibrium. In Zalta, EN (ed). *The Stanford encyclopedia of philosophy*. Winter 2013. Available from http://plato.stanford.edu/archives/win2013/entries/reflective-equilibrium
12. Beauchamp TL, Childress JF. *Principles of biomedical ethics*. 6th ed. Oxford: Oxford University Press; 2009.
13. Gardiner P. A virtue ethics approach to moral dilemmas in medicine. *J Med Ethics* 2003; **29**: 297–302.
14. Draper H. *Women, forced caesareans and antenatal responsibilities*, vol. 1 (Working Paper no. 1). University of Liverpool: Feminist Legal Research Unit; 1992.
15. GMC. *Good Medical Practice*. 2013. Available from http://www.gmc-uk.org/guidance/index.asp
16. Sheehan M. Relativism in principles. In Ashcroft RE, Dawson A, Draper H, McMillan, JR (eds). *Principles of health care ethics*. 2nd ed. Chichester: John Wiley & Sons, Ltd; 2007.
17. Veatch RM. How many principles for bioethics? In Ashcroft RE, Dawson A, Draper H, McMillan, JR (eds). *Principles of health care ethics*. 2nd ed. Chichester: John Wiley & Sons, Ltd; 2007, pp. 43–47.
18. Kant I. *The fundamental principles of the groundwork of morality*. Trans. HJ Paton. London: Routledge; 1948.
19. Dancy J. *Ethics without principles*. Oxford: Clarendon Press; 2004, p. 1
20. Christman J. Autonomy in moral and political philosophy. In Zalta, EN (ed). *The Stanford encyclopedia of philosophy*. Spring 2011. Available from http://plato.stanford.edu/archives/spr2011/entries/autonomy-moral
21. Dworkin R. *The theory and practice of autonomy*. Cambridge: Cambridge University Press; 1988.
22. Mill JS. *On liberty*. Project Gutenberg ebook 2011. Available from http://www.gutenberg.org/files/34901/34901-h/34901-h.htm
23. Nelson HL, Nelson JL. *The patient in the family: an ethics of medicine and families*. London: Routledge. 1995.
24. Griffin J. *Well-being: its meaning measurement and moral importance*. Oxford: Oxford University Press; 1986, p. 47.
25. Ethics Department BMA. *Medical ethics today: the BMA's handbook of ethics and law*. 2nd ed. London: BMJ Publishing Group; 2004, p. 136.
26. Bosk CL. *All God's mistakes: genetic counselling in a paediatric hospital*. Chicago: University of Chicago; 1992, p. 158.
27. Buchanan AE, Brock DW. *Deciding for others: the ethics of surrogate decision making*. Cambridge: Cambridge University Press; 1990.
28. Grosse RN. Literacy and health status in developing countries. *Annu Rev Publ Health* 1989; **10**: 281–97.
29. Constitution of the World Health Organization as adopted by the International Health Conference, New York, 19–22 June, 1946; signed on 22 July 1946 by the representatives of 61 States (Official Records of the World Health Organization, no. 2, p. 100) and entered into force on 7 April 1948. Available from http://www.who.int/about/mission/en/

30. Daniels N. *Just health: meeting health needs fairly.* Cambridge: Cambridge University Press; 2008, p. 37.
31. Degrazia D. Value theory and the best interests standard. *Bioethics* 1995; **9**(1): 50–61.
32. House of Lords Select Committee on the Mental Capacity Act 2005. *Mental Capacity Act 2005: Post-legislative Scrutiny*, p. 45. London: House of Lords; 2014 Available from http://www.publications.parliament.uk/pa/ld201314/ldselect/ldmentalcap/139/139.pdf
33. The National Commission for the Protection of Human Subjects of Biomedical and Behavioral Research. *The Belmont report: ethical principles and guidelines for the protection of human subjects of research.* Department of Health Education and Welfare Publication No. (OS) 78-0012. 1978.
34. Feinberg J. The child's right to an open future. In Aiken W, LaFollette H (eds). *Whose child? Children's rights, parental authority and state power.* Totowa, NJ: Rowman and Littlefield; 1980, pp. 141–2.
35. Dworkin G. Paternalism. In Zalta, EN (ed). *The Stanford encyclopedia of philosophy.* Summer 2014. Available from http://plato.stanford.edu/archives/sum2014/entries/paternalism
36. Childress JF. Paternalism in health care and health policy. In Ashcroft RE, Dawson A, Draper H, McMillan, JR (eds). *Principles of health care ethics.* 2nd ed. Chichester: John Wiley & Sons, Ltd; 2007.
37. Waldron J (ed). *Theories of rights.* Oxford: Oxford University Press; 1984, p. 4.
38. *Pretty v. Director of Public Prosecutions and Secretary of State for the Home Department* [2001] UKHL 61 (29 November, 2001).
39. Reading R, Colver A, Openshaw S, Jarvis S. Do interventions that improve immunisation uptake also reduce social inequalities in uptake? *BMJ* 1994; **308**: 1142.
40. Harris J. The survival lottery. *Philosophy* 1975; **50**: 81–87.
41. Gillon R. Ethics needs principles – four can encompass the rest – and respect for autonomy should be 'first among equals'. *J Med Ethics* 2003; **29**: 307–12.
42. Ashcroft RE, Dawson A, Draper H, McMillan, JR (eds). *Principles of health care ethics.* 2nd ed. Chichester: John Wiley & Sons, Ltd; 2007, p. 312.
43. *J Med Ethics* 2003; **29**(5).
44. *Schloendorff, Appellant, v. The Society of the New York Hospital, Respondent Court of Appeals of New York* 211 N.Y. 125; 105 N.E. 9.
45. *Gillick v. West Norfolk and Wisbech Area Health Authority and Another* [1986] 1 AC 112.
46. Savulescu J. Deaf lesbians, 'designer disability' and the future of medicine. *BMJ* 2002; **325**: 771.
47. Solomon A. *Far from the tree: a dozen kinds of love.* London: Vintage; 2013, p. 107.
48. Nuernberg Military Tribunals. *Trials of war criminals before the Nuernberg military tribunals. Volume II: The medical case*, p. 181. 1946–49. Available from https://www.loc.gov/rr/frd/Military_Law/pdf/NT_war-criminals_Vol-III.pdf
49. Rachels J. Active and passive euthanasia. *NEJM* 1975; **292**: 78–80.
50. Higgs R. Truth telling, lying and the doctor-patient relationship. In Ashcroft RE, Dawson A, Draper H, McMillan, JR (eds). *Principles of health care ethics.* 2nd ed. Chichester: John Wiley & Sons, Ltd; 2007, p. 336.
51. GMC. *Confidentiality.* Manchester: GMC; 2009. Available from http://www.gmc-uk.org/Confidentiality___English_1015.pdf_48902982.pdf
52. RCP Working Party on Clinical Ethics. *Ethics in practice: background and recommendations for enhanced support.* London: Royal College of Physicians; 2005.

CHAPTER 39a

MEDICAL JURISPRUDENCE IN OTORHINOLARYNGOLOGY

Maurice Hawthorne

Introduction 409	The role of the expert 418
Tort 410	Performance and complaints 420
Negligence 410	The Human Rights Act 421
Duty of candour 414	The criminal law 421
Consent 415	Guidelines 423
Confidentiality 417	Hospital administration 423
The coroner 417	References 425

SEARCH STRATEGY
Data in this chapter are based largely on the author's long experience as an expert witness and on landmark legal judgements, some of which are alluded to in the text.

INTRODUCTION

The last two decades have seen some changes in how claims of clinical negligence are decided but the developments in other fields such as consent, confidentiality and clinical performance have been much more significant. The medical profession in general has been put in the spotlight by very major events that were subject to intense media interest. The Bristol Royal Infirmary Inquiry into unacceptable complication rates in the paediatric cardiac surgery unit and the events following the trial of Harold Shipman, who was convicted of murdering an unknown number of his patients, have changed the way that the public views the medical profession. The response from politicians has been to try to tighten the legal framework in which doctors practise so that the public can be reassured that such events can never happen again.

The law differs in different jurisdictions, even within the UK, but most of the principles are the same. The first major subdivision is into criminal law and civil law. In criminal law, the state prosecutes an individual or an organization (the defendant) alleging breach of a law or statute. If the case is proven, the individual or organization is subject to a sentence, often a fine or a custodial term of some kind. In civil law, one individual or organization (now known as the claimant) brings a suit for damages against a defendant and seeks redress from that defendant. Ideally, the damages would exactly redress the loss suffered by the claimant. For instance, a claimant proved to have been swindled out of his car by a defendant might be happy merely to have his car back. In medical negligence cases, it is manifestly impossible to restore negligently caused losses so the damages are monetary. There are three important forms of monetary damages in clinical negligence: general; special; and punitive or exemplary.

General damages are those awarded to compensate the successful claimant for pain and suffering. Special damages are those awarded to take account of loss of income, special nursing needs and so on, arising from the negligence. Punitive damages are exactly what they say they are: damages awarded to the claimant to punish the negligent defendant. These are similar in a way to a fine in criminal cases but are not awarded in clinical negligence cases in the UK where most defendants have insurance to cover any damages awarded against them.

Civil and criminal processes differ in two other important ways: in the standard of proof required and in the influence of statutes. In criminal cases, the standard of proof is 'beyond reasonable doubt', which is often taken to imply a probability of guilt of at least 95%. In civil cases the standard of proof is 'on the balance of probabilities' which means greater than 50% probability. The source of the criminal law is founded in the common law and on statutes passed by Parliament and European law.

Statutes, precedent and European legislation state what actions constitute criminal behaviour. In the course of a criminal trial, counsel may well cite a precedent of what has been said and what decisions were made by courts in the past in similar cases. In a civil trial, there may be no statute that has any relevance to the questions to be decided so the decisions are based almost entirely on what happened in previous cases. This is referred to as the common law. The common law is in a state of continuous development as civil cases are tried by high courts, such as the Court of Appeal and the House of Lords, which can introduce subtle changes in decisions that then become the common law. Much argument may then occur as to what exactly their Lordships meant. Was what they said in a previous case relevant to the one currently being tried? Even more debatable is whether or not the important remark was part of a judgement or some sort of subjunctive aside to the judgement in the form of 'if this case had been similar to case A then I would have decided as follows'. The next section of the chapter (see 'Causation', below) illustrates exactly how one word in a judgement can be important when the case referred to as Bolitho[1] is considered.

Besides major sections devoted to clinical negligence and the duties of an expert medical witness, this chapter examines the two most common issues raised via a medical indemnity organization's helpline: consent and the doctor's duty of confidentiality. The criminal law and the role of the coroner as they are likely to apply to surgeons in their professional activities are discussed. The duties of a consultant surgeon as a doctor and the mechanisms that are or shortly will be in place to ensure that these are complied with are described and the additional duties of that consultant as a trainer are also mentioned.

TORT

Before discussing clinical negligence and consent issues, it is relevant to review the legal principle on which these are largely based. This is the law of tort or wrong done by one party to another. The two forms of tort that are relevant to surgeons are negligence, and assault and battery.

There are four essential elements of the legal tort of negligence:

- there must be a duty of care
- there must be a breach of that duty
- harm must have occurred
- the breach must have caused the harm.

Negligence occurs when party A is considered to owe a duty of care to party B, to have breached that duty and, as a result, harm has come to B. It must be shown that A could reasonably have foreseen that the breach might cause the harm. For instance, a driver travelling quickly on a country road should have it in mind that there might be a cyclist just around the corner. A second important aspect of negligence on which many clinical negligence cases fail is causation. This works on the so-called 'but for' test. It must be proved that, 'but for' the breach of duty by the defendant, the damage suffered by the claimant would not have occurred.

Assault is the threat of physical violence, and battery is any unlawful touching or physical contact of one person by another. Only with consent does a medical examination become lawful. Without consent, approaching a patient with a shining Lack's tongue depressor at the ready is an assault and using it to depress the tongue is a battery. Although the act of opening the mouth probably implies consent, the patient has the option of lodging a civil claim alleging battery or even of reporting a possible criminal battery to the police. It is important to note that civil actions for battery, unlike those for negligence, do not require that there has been any harm. Patients seeking damages for lack of adequate consent can sue either in negligence (where the 'but for' test applies but consent must be truly informed) or in battery (where causation is not an issue but a much less rigorous consent is enough to refute the allegations).

NEGLIGENCE

Standard of skill and care

In deciding negligence the claimant must establish first the four essential elements of tort.

To establish a duty it is necessary for a doctor/patient relationship to be in existence. There is no Good Samaritan law in the UK, and doctors only have a legal responsibility to people they have agreed to treat. In general practice the agreement arises by virtue of accepting a patient onto one's list. In a hospital setting, the agreement arises either out of the doctor's terms and conditions of employment or, with private patients, as a result of contract.

Patients tend to be seen by several different doctors and, therefore, the question 'who owes the duty of care?' may be a pertinent one. In the National Health Service (NHS), the employing authority will usually be named as first defendant as it would be liable to pay damages arising from any successful action by virtue of the principle of vicarious liability. Individual doctors may then be named as subsequent defendants.

An unresolved issue is who should be sued if a patient is placed on a waiting list but suffers additional damage in the time it takes to receive a first appointment. Is the defendant the referring GP, or the authority, or the NHS Trust at whose clinic the patient is awaiting an appointment?

The standard of care is that of the reasonably skilled and experienced doctor. The appropriate test, known as the Bolam (*Bolam v. Friern Hospital Management Committee*) test,[2] states that it is:

> the standard of the ordinary skilled man exercising and professing to have that special skill. A man need not possess the highest expert skill; it is well-established law that it is sufficient if he exercises the ordinary skill of an ordinary competent man exercising that particular art.

The standard of care relates to the specialty in which the doctor practises. A GP will not be required to possess the skills of a specialist. An inexperienced doctor cannot rely on his lack of experience as a defence to alleged negligence (*Wilsher v. Essex Area Health Authority*).[3] However, a junior doctor may discharge his duty by seeking the help of a superior.

While a doctor is under a duty to keep him- or herself appraised of developments in his area, this is subject to the bounds of reasonableness. Failure to read one article, which might have prevented the negligent act, could be excusable, while failure to be aware of new techniques that have become widespread may be inexcusable (*Crawford v. Board of Governors of the Charing Cross Hospital*).[4]

A doctor will not be negligent simply because he acted in a way that another doctor would not have done. The Bolam test establishes that a man is not negligent if he is acting in accordance with a practice merely because there is a body of medical opinion that would take a contrary view, provided there is a responsible body of opinion that supports the practice. A body of opinion must consist of at least two people. This statement has recently been qualified by the case referred to as Bolitho (*Bolitho v. City and Hackney Health Authority*).[1]

Causation

In Bolitho, a registrar in paediatrics was accepted to be in breach of her duty of care by failing to visit an infant with breathing difficulties. Her defence was that, given the clinical circumstances at the time she should have visited, she would not have intubated the infant. The Court of Appeal had found that the failure to attend the infant constituted negligence. The House of Lords heard opposite expert opinions, one asserting that there was a body of opinion that would undoubtedly have intubated in those circumstances and the other that there was also a responsible body of opinion that would not have intubated. Their Lordships then reversed the judgement saying that the defendant's assertion that she would not have intubated, a practice supported by a reasonable body of opinion, meant that on the balance of probabilities the brain damage would have occurred even if the registrar had visited. The causal link from the failure to discharge her duty of care by visiting the patient to the harm suffered was therefore broken so no negligence could be proved.

Bolitho is important because it clearly brings Bolam into the field of causation and also because of the dissenting judgement of Lord Browne-Wilkinson. Referring to the reasonable body of medical opinion that would allow a Bolam-based defence, Lord Browne-Wilkinson said, 'The use of these adjectives – responsible, reasonable and respectable – all show that the court has to be satisfied that the exponents of the body of opinion relied on can demonstrate that such opinion has a **logical** basis' (our emphasis). Later in judgement he qualified this by saying, 'it will very seldom be right for a judge to reach the conclusion that views genuinely held by a competent medical expert are unreasonable'. It is not yet clear how these comments will be used as precedents for future cases but they certainly will be. An example might be the practice of stripping all the mucosa from a vocal cord in Reinke's oedema. There may still be a body of expert opinion that would condone the practice but, in view of our knowledge of the physiology of the superficial lamina propria, is it logical to operate in this way and can that body of expert opinion be considered responsible?

Proof of medical negligence

The onus lies upon the claimant to prove that the surgeon's negligent treatment caused the injury. It is not sufficient simply to prove that the surgeon's actions were reprehensible or even reckless if the claimant cannot go on to show that their injury is directly attributable to the surgeon's poor performance. Hence, while it was clear that a casualty officer was in breach of his duty of care when he failed to examine a patient attending his department with the obvious signs of poisoning, there was a complete defence (*Barnett v. Chelsea & Kensington Hospital*)[5] when it was shown that there was no antidote to the poison taken by the patient. This is similar to the reasoning in Bolitho above, although that case was much more complicated than Barnett. In Barnett, it was a straightforward and uncontested statement that the workmen who had accidentally ingested arsenic in their tea were doomed whether or not they received medical attention. In Bolitho the courts had to decide whether or not, on balance of probabilities, the hypoxic brain damage would have occurred even if the registrar had visited the child.

The standard to which the claimant must prove his case is on the balance of probabilities. This means that the claimant must show that his version of events and expert analysis are more likely to be true than those put forward by the defence. If the case for each side is evenly balanced then the claimant will fail. Hence, where a patient suffers a nerve palsy that could equally have been due to negligence, or could have occurred as an inherent risk of the operation even when performed with proper skill and care, the claimant's case will fail in the absence of some item of evidence to tip the scales in favour of negligence (*Ashcroft v. Mersey Regional Health Authority*).[6]

An apparent reversal of the burden of proof can occur where the likelihood of negligence is so obvious that it 'speaks for itself' (*res ipsa loquitur*). In other words, a defendant may find that he is obliged at least to provide an explanation of the patient's injury that is consistent with reasonable care having been taken, even where the claimant has no positive evidence of negligence, where:

- there is no evidence as to how or why the accident occurred
- the accident is such that it would not occur without negligence
- the defendant is proved to have been in control of the situation in which the accident occurred.[7]

The doctrine first evolved in simple personal injury cases concerning falling objects (*Scott v. London & St Katherine's Docks*,[8] *Byrne v. Boadle*[9] and *Pope v. St Helen's Theatre*[10]), but has obvious attractions to a claimant in a medical case, where there may well be very real uncertainty as to how an injury came about, and where the often unconscious patient is entirely under the control of the medical team. Despite the fact that it is often pleaded, in England the doctrine has more often been conceded than litigated in medical cases, and so its ambit is unclear.[11] In practice the courts are reluctant to apply a doctrine derived from the relatively simple 'bumps and thumps' of stevedoring to the complex issues of causation found in medical litigation. It has been said (*Girard v. Royal Columbian Hospital*[12]):

> *The human body is not a container filled with a material whose performance can be predictably charted. ... because of this medical science has not yet reached the stage where the law ought to presume that a patient must come out of an operation as well or better than when he went into it.*[12]

Thus, as a matter of law, the onus of proving negligence will almost always fall on the claimant, although in cases where there is a strong and obvious inference of negligence from the very facts themselves (e.g. a retained swab (*Mahon v. Osborne*)[13] or where the claimant woke from his anaesthetic with the septic finger still attached and an adjacent one in the bucket[14]) the defence may well find that onus discharged unless they are able to provide some alternative theory, not involving negligence, to answer the claimant's case.

Damages

A claimant having established negligence, and having proved injury as a consequence, the question turns to the assessment of the compensation to be paid. The court must award a sum of money that will, as nearly as possible, put the injured person in the same position as he would have been had he not been injured (*Livingstone v. Rawyards Coal Company*).[15] In some jurisdictions (notably the United States) an element of punitive damages may be awarded. Such an approach has been rejected in England and Wales (*Kralj v. McGrath*)[16] and the rest of the UK for mere inadvertent negligence.

Damages are broadly classified into two categories: general damages and special damages.

GENERAL DAMAGES

These include damages for pain, suffering and loss of amenity. This is the aspect of the claimant's loss that is not ascertainable by a mathematical calculation of economic loss and, in the past, was determined by a jury (*Ward v. James*).[17] Juries were effectively abolished in personal injury trials in the mid-1960s. While the level of general damages will depend on the claimant's circumstances, and the suffering which the particular injury has caused the individual, a general bracket for a particular injury will be determined with reference to awards (adjusted for inflation) from previously decided cases. Obviously, it is impossible to 'compensate' someone for loss of a limb or for a life of continual pain so the awards are essentially conventional figures. As a guide, the current conventional figure for injuries of the utmost severity is between £150 000 and £170 000, and so injuries of lesser significance will be a proportion of that 'maximum'.

SPECIAL DAMAGES

These are the specific 'out-of-pocket' monetary expenses and losses the claimant has incurred up until the date of the trial. These will include loss of earnings, medical expenses, travel costs and the cost of any special equipment consequent upon the injury. Often there will be a claim for losses expected in the future. (Future loss is technically an item of general damages as its assessment is uncertain and it was formerly a matter for the jury to determine. As a matter of practice, the calculation of future loss is inseparable from that of past loss, many of the same arguments rehearsed in both, and one flows naturally to the other.) The amount of money at issue will depend almost exclusively on the particular circumstances of the claimant (*Lim v. Camden Health Authority*),[18] guided by the principle that a claimant should only recover what he has lost as a result of the injury. He must prove that his expenditure was (or will be) reasonably necessary, and that his needs cannot be met more cheaply by other reasonable means.

As a rule, English law seeks to compensate a claimant by way of a single lump sum award. This creates obvious problems where a claimant is likely to remain unemployed or requires continuing care for many years in the future. The only certain result is that the claimant will be either under- or overcompensated, depending on how circumstances unfold. This problem has not been solved, but ameliorated in certain cases. Where a claimant suffers a condition that may deteriorate significantly in the future, rather than receive a small sum to represent the risk, they can apply for an order for 'provisional damages', which leaves it open to the claimant to come back to court at a later date.[19]

In very large claims where the claimant's life expectancy will determine the level of the award, the risk can be borne by an insurance company by the purchase of an annuity. This is known as a 'structured settlement'.

Dealing with medical negligence claims

What happens when a surgeon is sued?[20] The 86th update of The Civil Procedure Rules 1998[21] came into effect on 3 October 2016. They require that, in cases of clinical disputes, a pre-action protocol be followed. This sets procedures and time limits for various stages of the process of being sued. There are also recommendations for Trusts about how they should respond to a claim and what processes should be in place to ensure that they are able to respond in an appropriate and timely way. In effect, the pre-action protocol will penalize a Trust that has such a poor clinical governance structure that it is unable to respond to a claim in a relatively short time.

What the individual consultant surgeon will experience if his patient sues him alleging negligence will differ in some ways, depending whether the patient was a private patient or an NHS patient. The first stage of the proceedings is the same: the patient, having found some means of financial support for his or her claim against the healthcare provider (a matter outside the remit of this chapter but considerably more difficult than formerly) will request, via a solicitor, release of notes. In private practice, the consultant will need to release these notes himself and is wise to check with his anaesthetist, the private hospital and other doctors involved in the secondary care that they will do the same. The consultant would be most unwise at this stage if he did not inform his medical indemnity organization and seek their help and advice. If the case is an NHS one, the matter must be referred to the Trust's legal department immediately. If the clinical governance system in the Trust is working well, there is a good chance that the events have already been reported to the legal section via an incident form and that contemporaneous statements have already been taken and filed in preparation for a potential claim. Alternatively, the claimant may already have used the NHS complaints procedure so all the statements from that will be available. A Trust is vicariously liable for the actions of its employees and so the legal department should take over all further responses to solicitors and communication with the defendant legal team. Both Trusts and independent practitioners have 40 days to provide the copy medical records and failure to meet this deadline will prejudice any defence.

The potential claimant's solicitors will now obtain an expert report on the medical records with examination of their client, if appropriate, and can decide whether or not the claim has merit. If it has, they will serve a letter of claim on the healthcare provider setting out a summary of facts, the main allegations of negligence, description of injuries and an outline of losses. This may include an offer to settle. The defendant organization or individual must provide a reasoned answer within three months of receipt.

In addition, the defendant's solicitors will be concerned to obtain guidance from experts swiftly and, once received, be able to form an initial view about whether or not the claim is defensible. The assessment of a claim at this stage will be facilitated by recent rule changes that have been made concerning the conduct of personal injury actions, including medical negligence litigation. These changes require that at the time of service of a writ, a claimant must also submit a medical report setting out the claimant's condition and prognosis, together with a Schedule of Special Damages said to result from any alleged negligence. Traditionally, such information was not available until much later in the litigation process. The change has resulted in a defendant's solicitors being able to assess the potential value of a claimant's claim at an early stage. Accordingly, following that initial expert opinion, a settlement can be proposed early in the proceedings on behalf of the otolaryngologist, if appropriate.

If settlement is desired but cannot be negotiated between the solicitors, then the solicitors acting for the otolaryngologist may try to settle the claim by what is known as a 'payment into court'. In making a payment into court, the defendant can make an assessment of the damages that might be awarded in due course at trial, if negligence is established. If the trial judge awards a sum higher than the level of the payment in, the claimant will receive his or her costs in the usual way. If, however, the sum awarded is the same or a lesser sum then, as a general rule, all costs of the action, including the defendant's costs after the payment into court, must be borne by the claimant. The claimant has 21 days to decide whether or not to accept the payment in. Thereafter the costs conservancies will operate. In cases where the claimant is legally aided, this device is of more limited assistance to a defendant. In other circumstances, there may well be a strong incentive to a claimant to accept a payment into court through fear of being prejudiced on costs in this way.

Following the service of a defence, in response to allegations contained in the statement of claim, both parties may raise requests for further information about their respective pleadings, and the claimant may choose to file a reply to the defence.

Directions concerning the conduct of a claim will be given by the court, usually after the pleadings are completed. In the High Court, a formal hearing will take place to consider these directions, but in personal injury actions brought in the County Court, a series of so-called automatic directions is given by the court. These are rarely, if ever, appropriate in medical negligence cases and it is therefore usual for the parties to apply to the court for specific directions to be given. These directions will provide for, among other things, the disclosure of witness statements as to fact and expert reports. It is usual for witness statements to be disclosed, followed shortly thereafter by expert reports, in order that experts can consider this information available from the other side in preparing the report. The exchange of both statements and reports gives a further opportunity for review of the case, both by claimant and medical defendant. At this stage the claimant may realize that the claim is weak and the case may be discontinued. Equally, the defence may feel that the case is not defensible and settlement negotiations or a payment into court may follow.

TRIAL AND PREPARATION FOR TRIAL

If the exchange of witness statements and expert reports does not promote the settlement of a claim, then the case proceeds towards trial. In medical negligence actions, a fixed date for trial will usually be given by the court because of the significant number of clinicians who may have to make themselves available, either as experts or as witnesses of fact.

By way of preparation for trial, both parties should arrange conferences with counsel in order to review the case in detail, and ensure all preparations are complete. If the defence considers that the case should be settled, or there are certain aspects of the case where a defendant may be vulnerable, a payment into court may be made. The payment in may be limited to those aspects of the claim where the defendant could be found liable. The claimant has 21 days within which to accept the payment in before the penalty of costs starts to run. As a significant proportion of the costs of an action result from the trial itself, the defendants are usually anxious to make any payment into court before 21 days in advance of the trial. Thereafter bundles of documents must be prepared for use in the court by all parties, which will include the pleadings, medical records, witness statements and expert reports.

A proportion of cases are settled literally at the doors of the court, the last opportunity for compromise before further significant costs of trial are incurred.

If no compromise can be reached, the trial will commence with an explanation of the case to the judge by counsel for the claimant, setting out the relevant events and the nature of the allegations. The claimant's counsel will then call witnesses of fact, usually followed then by expert witnesses. Each witness will be cross-examined in turn by the defence, and then re-examined by claimant's counsel if necessary. When the claimant's evidence has been called, the defence case is then put in the same way, and usually in the same order.

The trial judge may allow variation in this order of evidence, particularly in complex cases, so that witnesses for both sides are called first, to be followed then by experts. This will allow experts to hear all the evidence of fact before giving a final opinion. However, the present arrangements for disclosure of witness statements make such variation rare.

At the conclusion of the case, the judge will usually hear submissions from counsel on the law to be applied and the appropriate level of damages to be awarded if the claimant is successful. It is usual then for the judge to reserve judgement, to be delivered at a later date, as most negligence cases are complex and will require some consideration. Once judgement is given, and if the claimant is successful, the judge will indicate the level of damages to be awarded. Only at that stage is the judge informed about any payment into court that may have been made, and the costs to be awarded can then be considered.

FUNDING OF NEGLIGENCE CLAIMS

Otolaryngologists may well have been concerned at the possibility that medical negligence actions in England and Wales will follow the pattern of the United States, and that the perceived increase in the number of actions here may continue. However, with the reduction in the eligibility for legal aid, many actions that would have been funded by legal aid in the past will now have to be funded privately. The introduction of contingency or conditional fees is unlikely to assist all those who are no longer eligible for legal aid. As an incentive for the claimant's solicitor, the conditional fee system[22] will allow the solicitor to claim twice the rate of fees they might have otherwise obtained in a successful action. There is a risk that the solicitor might receive no payment at all if the case is unsuccessful. As suggested above, solicitors acting for patients are therefore likely to take on fewer claims,[23] concentrating on those where liability is obvious and can be quickly established. The result is likely to be that there will be no significant increase in the number of medical negligence actions in the short term. Indeed, it is possible that there will be a reduction at the expense of patients who might otherwise have had successful claims for compensation.

The *NHS Litigation Authority 2015/2016 Annual Report*[24] stated that the number of new clinical negligence claims received that year had fallen by 4.6% from 11 497 to 10 965. Damages paid out that year to patients rose from £774.4 million to £950.4 million. That is an average pay out to patients of £86 675 per claim. The provision set aside to pay agreed and estimated future damages is £56.4 billion with 75% of it due to be paid in 2021 and beyond.

DUTY OF CANDOUR

The Health and Social Care Act 2008 (Regulated Activities) (Amendment) Regulations 2015[25] extend the fit and proper person requirement for directors and the duty of candour to all providers from 1 April 2015. Regulation 20 defines what constitutes a notifiable safety incident for health service bodies and all other providers (such as primary medical and dental practices, adult social care and independent healthcare providers). Specifically, paragraph 8 defines the harm thresholds that trigger the duty of candour for health service bodies. Paragraph 9 defines the thresholds for all other providers.

The introduction of Regulation 20 is a direct response to recommendation 181 of the Francis Inquiry report into Mid Staffordshire NHS Foundation Trust,[26] which recommended that a statutory duty of candour be introduced for health and care providers. This is further to the contractual requirement for candour for NHS bodies in the standard contract, and professional requirements for candour in the practice of a regulated activity. In interpreting the regulation on the duty of candour we use the definitions of openness, transparency and candour used by Robert Francis in his report:

- Openness – enabling concerns and complaints to be raised freely without fear and questions asked to be answered
- Transparency – allowing information about the truth about performance and outcomes to be shared with staff, patients, the public and regulators
- Candour – any patient harmed by the provision of a healthcare service is informed of the fact and an appropriate remedy offered, regardless of whether a complaint has been made or a question asked about it.

This does not mean that a consultant should immediately give his version of an adverse event to a patient or relative. It does mean that the consultant should report the adverse event using standard reporting facilities within his Trust. This then allows the adverse event to be thoroughly investigated, after which the truth can be shared with the patient and their relatives. There is an inherent risk in relatives getting only a partial truth or inaccurate information should there be an immediate 'knee-jerk reaction' to tell the patient what has gone wrong. This does not mean, though, that the patient should not be told that an adverse event has occurred and is being investigated.

CONSENT

Much medical litigation is caused by the practitioner's failure to disclose adequate information about the risks inherent in a given procedure. Common law recognizes the principle that every person has the right to have his or her bodily integrity respected. There is a presumption that a person should not be exposed to risk unless he has voluntarily accepted that risk, based on adequate information and adequate comprehension.

Obtaining consent to carry out an operation is necessary to avoid three sorts of legal jeopardy. The first and second arise because any touching of another person is a potential battery. (Assault is the threat of causing physical injury. An unconscious person can be battered but cannot be assaulted.) This means that, in very exceptional circumstances, a surgeon performing an operation without consent may be prosecuted in the criminal courts for alleged criminal battery. A more likely outcome of such surgery is a civil case seeking damages for the tort (or wrong) of battery. There is no need to show that anything went wrong with the surgery, merely that it was carried out without valid consent. The third, and much the most likely legal outcome regarding consent, is that the claimant tries to show that he was not warned of the risks of a proposed therapy that resulted in harm and that, had he been warned of those risks, he would have refused the treatment. An example might be a patient with a dead ear after a competently performed stapedotomy who was not warned of that risk before surgery. He may well be able to claim damages from the surgeon because he can say that 'but for' the surgeon's failure to warn of the risk, he would not have undergone the surgery. It is immediately obvious that any careful surgeon must record what potential adverse outcomes of a proposed operation have been discussed with a patient. If it is not recorded in the notes, courts have become sceptical of a statement such as 'it is my usual practice to warn of these risks'.

The question of how much information must be given to the patient would vary from situation to situation, but was generally set by the professional standard according to the Bolam test, with doctors being arbiters of how much information should be given. This meant that, in the example above, if the defendant surgeon could assemble a responsible body of opinion whose practice would not be to warn of the risk of dead ear, his conduct did not breach a duty of care.

This was modified to a degree by the case of Sidaway (*Sidaway v. Board of Governors of the Bethlem Royal Hospital*)[27] in which the House of Lords held that where the proposed treatment involved a substantial risk of grave or adverse consequences such that, notwithstanding any practice to the contrary, a patient's right to decide whether to consent to the treatment was so obvious that no prudent medical man could fail to warn of the risk (save in emergency or some other sound clinical reason for nondisclosure), then it would be negligent not to warn. To continue the example above, the claimant could argue that total deafness in one ear is such a disability that any reasonable patient would wish to be told about it pre-operatively.

Accordingly, the right of the doctor (acting in accordance with a reasonable body of medical opinion) to decide what the individual patient should be told remained enshrined in English case law. Such medical paternalism, which may be in the best interest of some of our patients, is currently and repeatedly being questioned. The doctor should realize that in Sidaway when the question 'Is informed consent a part of English law?' was put to the five law lords, the answer was not unanimous. Scarman said 'yes'; Diplock said 'no'; and Bridge, Keith and Templeman said 'yes with reservations'.

In assessing which material risks should be mentioned, doctors should consider the degree of probability of the risk materializing and seriousness of possible injury if it does. A risk, even if it is a mere possibility, should be disclosed if its occurrence would cause serious circumstances (*Hopp v. Lepp*).[28] Medical evidence will be necessary for the court to assess the degree of probability and the seriousness. A further medical factor upon which expert evidence will also be required is to assess the character of the risk; that is, is this risk common to all surgery or is it specific to the particular operation? Special risks inherent in a recommended operation are more likely to be material.

The legal standard of disclosure required in response to direct questions is also set by the professional standard (*Blyth v. Bloomsbury Health Authority*).[29] Although the amount of information given must depend upon the circumstances, as a general proposition it was governed by the Bolam test (supra).

In Australia, the doctrine of informed consent went one stage further from Sidaway where the reasonable patient was considered the arbiter of what risks should or should not be disclosed pre-operatively. In *Rogers v. Whittaker*,[30] it is clear that the risks that must be disclosed are those that affect that one patient and not the generality of reasonable patients. To take the stapedotomy analogy one last stage further, few surgeons would warn of a dead ear risk of 1 in 2000 operations and probably the reasonable patient would be unlikely to want to know that this was a complication as it is so unlikely. The question arises of whether the patient having that operation on an only hearing ear might view the risk differently and want to be aware of it in making a decision.

In 2004, the issue of consent moved further in the patient's favour in the case of *Chester v. Afshar*.[31] In this case whilst the injury occurred despite a competent surgical technique, the claimant argued that had she known about the risk she would have taken time to consider the risk that would have resulted in the surgery occurring at a different time and therefore the adverse outcome would not have occurred in this spinal surgery case.

Montgomery v. Lanarkshire Health Board[32] heard in the Supreme Court in Scotland in 2016 has now shifted the requirements of what a patient should be told to 'what a reasonable person would expect to be told'. The claimant alleged that had she been told that there was a significant risk of shoulder dystocia resulting from a vaginal birth that occurred in 1999 she would have elected for a caesarean section. The law lords found unanimously in favour of the claimant, effectively ending the era of

Bolam applying to consent. This has now enshrined in law the principles laid down in the 2008 GMC guidance, *Consent: Patients and Doctors Making Decisions Together*.[33]

Who can give consent?

There are three categories of patient described in the Department of Health's reference guide to consent for examination or treatment: the adult with capacity to consent; the adult without capacity to consent; and children and young people.

CHILDREN

Section 8(1) of the Family Law Reform Act 1969 provides that a person over 16 may give a valid consent to medical treatment as though he was an adult. As regards children under 16, the general principle is that laid down in the Gillick (*Gillick v. West Norfolk and Wisbech Area Health Authority*) case,[34] that the parental right to determine whether or not a child under 16 should have medical treatment terminates when the child achieves a significant understanding and intelligence to enable him or her to understand fully what is proposed. Until such time, the parents, or others acting *in loco parentis*, may give their consent or refusal to medical treatment. Recent case law suggests that it may still be possible to treat a seemingly competent child who is refusing to give consent, providing someone else with the capacity to consent provides consent on the child's behalf (in Re R, and in Re W).[35, 36]

MENTALLY INCOMPETENT PATIENTS

Where a patient is unable to provide consent on his or her own behalf by reason of mental incapacity, no one else, including a court, may give consent on that person's behalf. The doctrine of necessity, however, permits a doctor to lawfully operate on or give other treatment to adult incompetent patients, provided that the treatment is in their best interest, either to save their lives or to ensure improvement in their physical or mental health (Re F).[37] However, mental illness does not mean mental incompetence as was tested in the case of Re C (1994),[38] a paranoid schizophrenic held at Broadmoor, when he refused consent to have a gangrenous leg amputated despite the wishes of his managing medical team.

The Mental Capacity Act 2005 sets out five principles on which the legal requirements are based. The principles are:

1. A person must be assumed to have capacity unless it is established that they lack capacity.
2. A person is not to be treated as unable to make a decision unless all practicable steps to help him or her do so have been taken without success.
3. A person is not to be treated as unable to make a decision merely because he or she makes an unwise decision.
4. An act done or decision made, under this Act for or on behalf of a person who lacks capacity must be done, or made in his or her best interests.
5. Before the act is done, or the decision is made, regard must be had to whether the purpose for which it is needed can be as effectively achieved in a way that is less restrictive of the person's rights and freedom of action.

That a person has been judged to lack capacity in relation to a previous decision regarding their care does not mean that they lack capacity to make decisions in all situations. Capacity of an individual to make decisions should be made on a situation-by-situation basis. Capacity can vary with the nature of the decision and may change over time.

Understanding what constitutes acting in the best interests of a patient who lacks capacity can present challenges as to what the person's best interests are. Section 5 of the Mental Capacity Act 2005 states that 'An act done or decision made, under this Act for or on behalf of a person who lacks capacity must be done, or made in his best interests'; and that 'As long as these acts or decisions are in the best interests of the person who lacks capacity to make the decision for themselves, or to consent to acts concerned with their care or treatment, then the decision-maker or carer will be protected from liability'.

In deciding the best interests of a person lacking in capacity the ENT surgeon should:

- encourage the patient to take part in the decision-making process and take all reasonable steps to improve their ability to be involved in making the decision
- identify, as far as possible, all factors that patients lacking capacity would consider, were they to decide for themselves
- make all reasonable efforts to establish the patient's views including past wishes, beliefs, behaviour, decisions and values (e.g. religious, moral, political cultural or personal) and any other relevant factors that may have a bearing on their best interests; reasonable efforts include talking to family members and, where appropriate, seeking the support of an individual mental capacity advocate
- avoid making assumptions on a person's interests based solely on factors such as age, race, gender or condition
- decide whether the person may regain capacity at a later time and, if so, whether the decision can be safely delayed till this is possible
- never be motivated in any way by a desire to bring about the death of the person without capacity in decisions concerning life-sustaining treatment
- remember that the person who lacks capacity has a right to privacy and dignity and so it may not be appropriate to share all information with everyone involved in their care or those related to them through family ties.

JEHOVAH'S WITNESSES

Certain groups of patients, including Jehovah's Witnesses, may refuse to receive blood transfusions or other life-saving therapies. The Court of Appeal has affirmed patients' rights to refuse medical treatment, even if this will result in their death; nevertheless, for such a refusal to be effective, the court must be satisfied that at the time of refusal the patient's capacity is not diminished by illness or medication or given on the basis of false assumptions or misinformation. In the case of Re T,[39] Lord Donaldson said:

> An adult patient who suffers from no mental incapacity has an absolute right to choose whether to consent to medical treatment, to refuse it or to choose one rather than another of the treatments being offered.

A decision to refuse medical treatment does not have to be sensible, obviously rational or well considered, and in the case of a competent patient, the doctor cannot override the patient's wishes because he believes it to be in the patient's best interests.

OTHER SPECIAL GROUPS

Pregnant women, patients who are human immunodeficiency virus positive or suffering from acquired immunodeficiency syndrome and the elderly do not represent special categories for the purposes of consent. Although the amount of information that has to be given to a patient varies from case to case, a decision to withhold information solely on paternalistic grounds that it may deter the patient from accepting the therapy is not justified in law.

CONFIDENTIALITY

Doctors are well aware of their duty of confidentiality, originally stated in the Hippocratic oath. What is often not appreciated is the common law and statutory basis of this duty and the circumstances in which confidential information may legally be revealed. There is a common law duty placed upon professionals to guard confidential information. A patient may sue a doctor through the civil courts if there is alleged to have been damage as a result of breach of confidentiality. The Data Protection Act (1997) places a statutory duty on anyone who holds patient identifiable data (in any form) to guard and release that information under strict controls. Any surgeon who keeps any sort of patient identifiable information at his residence (where his employer's blanket registration under the act will probably not apply) and who is not registered with the data commissioner breaches the provisions of the Act. It is particularly important to note in this context that, if disclosure is properly requested, it is an offence to fail to disclose all of the records, both computerized and manual.

The second statute that obliges surgeons to care for information appropriately is the Human Rights Act (1998). This enshrines in UK law the sixth clause of the European Convention on Human Rights granting citizens an absolute right to privacy and to family life.

There are a number of instances in which confidential information can be released. The first is with the consent of the patient. This is sometimes implied consent such as applies when a GP releases confidential information in a referral to a consultant (and so to both secretaries).

On other occasions, there needs to be expressed consent, for instance in release of information to insurers when a holiday must be cancelled. Sometimes a doctor is obliged to release information. The statutory examples concern the Terrorism Act 2000 and its successors such as the Terrorism Act 2006, the Counter-Terrorism Act 2008, the Abortion Act 1967 and the infectious diseases regulations. A court has power to require disclosure of records and there are several cases where disclosure is appropriate in the public interest. These are to protect the rights of others, such as reporting to prevent or detect serious crime or to prevent suspected child abuse and in reports to the Driver and Vehicle Licensing Authority. In all cases of this nature where the disclosure is not governed by the Data Protection Act, the information released must be no more than that necessary to comply with the public duty. A surgeon with any doubt as to how to resolve the conflict between duties of confidentiality and the public interest is well advised to consult his or her medical indemnity organization and to ensure that the final decision is one with which a responsible body of medical opinion would concur (Bolam).

The situation after the death of the patient is different. Doctors have a duty to disclose on death certificates and to national confidential enquiries as well as to the police and courts, especially the coroner. Data protection no longer applies and the relevant statute is the Access to Health Records Act 1990. This clarifies that executors or, failing them, next of kin can consent to release of medical records. It appears that anyone with a legitimate claim to view the record can see that part of the record that is relevant.

THE CORONER

The Coroners and Justice Act 2009 was implemented in 2013 and saw a change in the coroner service in the UK. Going forward, newly appointed coroners now have to be legally qualified. The Act also created the post of the Chief Coroner. The coroners' service remains a local service funded by the local authority and provides a service to the local community. There has been a dramatic reduction in the number of inquests still open after a year and it has been proposed that a system of medical examiners be introduced, which is likely to reduce the number of deaths reported to the coroner's office.

When the coroner is mentioned, most doctors ask three questions: What deaths must be reported to the coroner? What verdicts can be brought and will these criticize the doctor? And what must I do if required to write a report for or appear before the coroner?

The following must be reported to the coroner:

- violent or unnatural death
- death in custody (even if the prisoner was licensed on leave to attend the hospital)
- death where no doctor is able to issue a death certificate.

Most jurisdictions also have local agreements about the reporting of deaths within a certain period after hospital admission and after surgical procedures. Coroners usually wish to know about deaths from notifiable diseases and industrial diseases, and deaths of those in receipt of war pensions.

The range of verdicts that the coroner can return is limited. The coroner's court (in theory at least) is not adversarial and no finger of blame should be pointed by the court. The coroner's remit is to establish the identity of the deceased, the time and place of death and the mode of death. Although death due to gross neglect is an acceptable verdict, death due to negligence is not. In practice, of course, the family of the deceased and their lawyers may use the proceedings of the coroner's court to assess whether or not an action in negligence is likely to succeed.

What about the surgeon called upon to provide a report to the coroner? The first piece of advice would be for the surgeon to contact his or her defence organization for support. The report itself should be factual, full and directed to a non-medical audience. The report should not contain opinion but just facts. In particular, a report to a coroner should never contain the words 'negligent' or 'negligence'. Not only are these a matter of opinion and not fact, but they also have special well-defined meanings for lawyers that may not be apparent to doctors.

In most cases, the report will be all that the coroner needs and the doctor will not be required to appear. If the coroner feels that the evidence that the doctor can give may be crucial to his investigations, then he will summon the doctor to the inquest. Sometimes the family of the deceased will see this as their opportunity to confront the doctor, who they see as the source of their grief. To be fair, sometimes the process works well, the family see that the doctor is not some kind of ogre and the resentment fades. Even if this does not occur, the coroner should ensure that the family do not persecute the doctor and that the proceedings remain directed towards establishing the who, when, where and how but not why the deceased perished.

If the doctor anticipates a difficult inquest, he may be accompanied by legal assistance but the solicitor may not answer for him and there is no cross-examination of the other side. Defence organizations can advise the doctor but there is always a risk that the presence of a legal advisor will make the family (and the coroner) suspect that some sort of cover-up is being attempted.

Doctors summoned to the coroner's court need to follow the usual rules of court appearances – dress smartly but conservatively and do show appropriate respect to the coroner. Bring the notes or fair copies and copies of the reports already supplied and read them through before the case opens. Remember that the doctor is a witness and not an advocate or defendant and so there is no problem in asking for a question to be repeated or for a pause while the notes are consulted before answering.

THE ROLE OF THE EXPERT

An expert medical witness is instructed by either the defence or the claimant to give his or her opinion on the medical matters pertinent to the case to the court. This evidence is different from that of a material witness who is asked for the facts. The expert's job is to interpret the facts for the court. In simple terms, it is 'to give impartial advice and opinion'. Many otolaryngologists will be called upon to give expert opinion on personal injury cases where neither the claimant nor the defendant is a clinician. The many reports on noise-induced hearing loss that have been written by otolaryngologists are a form of written expert testimony in just such personal injury cases. A few otolaryngologists will be asked to prepare reports that assist courts in deciding clinical negligence claims and the special circumstances that pertain to these are discussed below.

Until the Civil Procedure Rules 1998 came into force, experts were retained by either the claimant or defendant's side and to some extent this remains the case. In theory, an expert's report would be the same whether he was instructed by the solicitors of the claimant or those of the defendant. The 1998 Rules have made it clear that the duty of an expert, whether he is expecting to be paid by the defendant or by the claimant, is to produce for the court an unbiased opinion. The 1998 Rules encourage a court, where practical, to appoint a single joint expert to produce such an opinion. They also give direction about exchange of reports, communication between and with experts and the expert's right to ask the court for directions.

In practice, the expert's evidence is usually contained in a report and it is rare for an expert to have to appear in court. The form and content of an expert report were previously based upon a well-known civil case.

In the Ikarian Reefer (*National Justice Compania Naviesa SA v. Prudential Assurance Company Ltd, The Ikarian Reefer*),[40] Mr Justice Cresswell stated that he considered that a misunderstanding on the part of some of the expert witnesses had taken place concerning their duties and responsibilities which had contributed to the length of the trial. Although this was a shipping case, the seven duties and responsibilities laid down have equal validity for medical experts:

1. Expert evidence presented to the court should be, and should be seen to be, the independent product of the expert uninfluenced as to form or content by the exigencies of litigation.
2. Independent assistance should be provided to the court by way of objective unbiased opinion regarding matters within the expertise of the expert witness. (An expert witness should never assume the role of advocate.)
3. Facts or assumptions upon which the opinion was based should be stated together with material facts that could detract from the concluded opinion.
4. An expert witness should make it clear when a question or issue fell outside his expertise.
5. If the opinion was not properly researched because it was considered that insufficient data were available then that had to be stated with an indication that the opinion was provisional. If the witness could not assert that the report contained the truth, the whole truth and nothing but the truth, then that qualification should be stated on the report.

6. If after exchange of reports an expert witness changed his mind on a material matter then the change of view should be communicated to the other side through legal representatives without delay and when appropriate to the court.
7. Photographs, plans, survey reports and other documents referred to in the expert evidence had to be provided to the other side at the same time as exchange of reports.

More recently, the Civil Procedure Rules have modified these directions. The expert should obtain the Civil Procedure Rules Chapter 35 and read sections 1.1 to 1.6, which is too extensive to reproduce here.

Before writing a report the expert should be aware of what the solicitor requires. Reports usually refer to one or more of the following six areas:

1. An initial statement on the possible merits of an allegation for a claimant before notes and other evidence are obtained
2. Liability
3. Causation
4. Current condition
5. Prognosis
6. Expert opinion on an area of medicine.

A quote should be given on the cost of the report in advance. Lawyers may have no concept of the cost in time and research to answer what to them may be the simplest of questions. The solicitor will not be pleased to receive a report of 100 pages with detailed bibliography costing £2000 when the damages sought are only £500 for a relatively minor event.

The report should be double spaced and typed on A4 paper. Each sheet should have the name of the claimant or defendant typed in the top right-hand corner and be separately numbered. It is also helpful to number the paragraphs. The names of the parties should be stated, as should the requesting solicitor or insurance company. It is inadvisable to use the word 'negligent' in the report. Negligence may be implied by using phrases such as 'falling below an acceptable standard' or 'followed a course of action that could not be supported by any body of medical opinion'. Phrases such as 'reckless action' or 'flagrant disregard' may have a special meaning and lead to criminal charges rather than a civil case.

There is always the possibility that the credentials of the expert will be tested in court. It is extremely unwise for the expert to step outside his field. Should he be forced to comment outside his field of expertise he should add the rider that he is speaking only as an average medical practitioner. The expert will need to be *au fait* with up-to-date research in his own field.

The medical expert in clinical negligence

The medical expert retained in a case of medical negligence is usually asked to elucidate the areas of medical contention within a case. He needs to be aware of the various views on current practice, even if these views are held by a minority of doctors, provided always that the minority is a reasonable one and that the practices supported are logical (Bolitho). Although the temptation is to be an arbitrator of medical colleagues, in court, this is the province of the judge. Nevertheless, the expert will be asked to comment as to whether the claimant's complaint has merit. When acting for the defence the expert will inevitably come across cases where defence is impossible. Here it is the expert's duty to advise that a speedy settlement be made to the aggrieved patient. This will have the secondary benefit of avoiding a colleague's professional shortcomings being exposed to public criticism in court. Rarely, some doctors expect their colleagues to defend them whatever the circumstances. Hence, being an expert can lead to criticism or alienation by colleagues.

Medical negligence cases can take an inordinate amount of time. Not only may the expert have to inspect all the records, examine the claimant and prepare reports, he will have to do research, attend meetings with solicitors and counsel and attend court. A single case may, in unusual circumstances, take up to 100 hours of time or more. The expert should never take on a case if he cannot afford the time.

Subsection 1.6 of the practice direction requires that experts comply with the relevant approved expert's protocol. As might be expected, there is a detailed pre-action protocol for the resolution of clinical disputes. Although this is aimed primarily at the legal profession, it is required reading for any doctors involved in providing expert testimony in clinical negligence cases. In particular, the times allowed by the court for the completion of various stages of the claim and the defence are clearly stated.

The doctor as an expert witness in court

The purpose of expert opinion given in court is to persuade the judge that one side of a case has greater merit than the other. This does not mean that he should ignore inconvenient facts which mitigate against his argument. In persuading the judge, the expert should be seen to weigh up all the facts both in favour of his view and those in favour of an alternative view. Then he should give the reasons why the judge should favour one interpretation of the facts over another. It is the judge who will decide between the two sides of the argument. The expert should not be tempted to usurp the role of the judge for this may do untold damage to his own side or at the very least earn a rebuke which may undermine his confidence.

In court, the expert should wear conservative clothes. Evidence should be given in a straightforward, unequivocal manner. A personal view may be represented especially in response to a direct question but should always be tempered with information about acceptable alternative practice and opinion. He should always be prepared to concede points if it is appropriate to do so, and not to adhere rigidly to one view when that cannot be sustained. The expert often has difficult concepts to convey to the judge. The expert should not hesitate to use pictures, models or even video to illustrate a point but should avoid being seen as a flamboyant 'show off' lest he discredits himself by not giving due respect to the court.

The usual course of examining a witness in court is that the barrister for the side calling the witness will examine that witness and try to anticipate and pre-empt difficult questions from the other side. Counsel for the opposing side will then cross-examine the witness and may attempt to undermine the evidence given by the expert or the standing of the expert in his profession. Above all, the expert must not see this as a personal insult lest he should lose his temper and hence his dignity. After this potentially hostile cross-examination, the first barrister is permitted to re-examine the witness and try, if necessary, to restore the faith of the judge in that witness.

PERFORMANCE AND COMPLAINTS

Besides using the legal system to sue a surgeon in tort, patients have recourse to a number of mechanisms to resolve concerns about how they have been treated or managed. Some of these mechanisms have the potential to involve doctors in disciplinary or performance investigations so the two elements are considered together. A patient or a family unhappy with the outcome of a surgical process can of course sue in the tort of negligence but this is expensive and will succeed in only a few cases. Another option is a complaint to the Trust employing the surgeon. Trusts are obliged to have a complaints procedure and the patient is entitled to a prompt reply from the chief executive. In practice, the time limits are so tight that, especially when the complaint is a complex clinical one (rather than the more usual gripes about hospital food or parking for visitors), the first reply is a letter of acknowledgement. Following this the complaint should be answered point by point with an apology if appropriate. The chief executive must report to the complainant what action has been taken. Among the possible actions are Trust disciplinary procedures or referral of staff to their regulatory body. If this is rejected by the patient then the patient may request that the Health Service Commissioner investigate the complaint. This officer, also referred to as the ombudsman, can review the decisions made by the Trust. There may also be grounds for appeal to the ombudsman if there are problems with the terms of reference or the conduct of an independent review.

If the investigation of a complaint leads to further investigation of the conduct or performance of a doctor, there are a number of forms that this can take. One is an internal investigation by the doctor's Trust. Although there are regulations that govern the conduct of such investigations, there is such a variety of approaches that this chapter cannot be dogmatic. It is clear that a Trust must not unjustifiably suspend a doctor pending investigation and then drag its heels in the investigation. There may well be a case against the trust under the Human Rights Act (1998) and the doctor is probably best advised to consult his or her defence organization.

Two NHS organizations may put a doctor's reputation or right to practise in jeopardy. These are the National Clinical Assessment Service (NCAS) and the Care Quality Commission (CQC). The NCAS, which has been part of the NHS Litigation Authority since 2013, will deal with concerns about the performance of individual doctors by investigating problems and arranging performance assessments where necessary. Memoranda of understanding have been agreed between the NCAS and both CQC and the GMC as well as some of the medical Royal Colleges so it is clear that a suggestion of deficient performance or conduct uncovered by one of the three organizations may well be reported to the other two.

The organization that these newer groups feed to and that has disciplinary control over doctors in the UK is the General Medical Council (GMC). This organization has a statutory duty to maintain standards and ensure that doctors registered with the GMC do not endanger the public. The GMC is bedevilled by lots of committees with similar acronyms but there are basically three routes through the system. The first stage is usually the reporting to the GMC by a Trust, by a member of the public, by another doctor or the NCAS.

Increasingly, the GMC is looking at reports in the media that suggest poor performance or conduct, and is initiating proceedings on the basis of these. The complaint is screened and the decision made to reject it at this stage or to refer it on for investigation. The screener decides which of the three routes – health, conduct or performance – is the most appropriate. More than one route may be pursued.

In 2012 the adjudication process was split off from the GMC and delegated to the Medical Practitioner's Tribunal Service (MPTS). If the screener at the GMC feels that the allegations against a doctor are serious or pose a threat to patient safety the doctor's case can be brought before the Interim Orders Tribunal, which can temporarily suspend or restrict a doctor's registration whilst the allegations are investigated or a performance assessment undertaken.

Health procedures are aimed at rehabilitating a doctor whose illness is affecting his or her work. The four stages of the process are: initial assessment; medical examination; then decision by two case examiners, one medical and one lay.

The performance procedures apply where there is 'a departure from good professional practice ... sufficiently serious to call into question a doctor's registration'. Referrals are examined and the doctor is likely to be asked to have a performance assessment. If he or she refuses, the Interim Orders Committee of the MPTS may order an assessment. Two case examiners consider the outcome of the assessment process.

After an investigation of a doctor's conduct, health or performance assessment the case examiners will: decide that no further action is required; agree undertakings with the doctor such as counselling, training, or that restriction of practice are required; issue a warning; or decide that the case is so serious that referral to the MPTS is required (this is also the case if the doctor has refused assessment). A Medical Practitioner's Tribunal can leave a doctor's registration intact, impose conditions, suspend or erase. A Medical Practitioner's Tribunal hearing is, to all intents and purposes, a court of law with a panel, advised by a legal assessor, sitting in judgement. The GMC and the doctor can be represented by barristers if necessary and, unlike the health process, the tone is adversarial. Formerly, outcomes of all three processes could be appealed to the judicial committee of the Privy Council but now appeals are heard by the High Court.

Recently, the government has established the Professional Standards Authority. If it is felt that a decision of the GMC or the MPTS has been too lenient then the decision can be appealed through the courts by this commission in the interests of protecting the public.

THE HUMAN RIGHTS ACT

Perhaps the two most potentially influential recent statutes affecting surgeons are the Data Protection Act (DPA) (1998) and the Human Rights Act (HRA) (1998). The first of these is discussed under the heading of confidentiality, where its effects, although far-reaching, are relatively easy to predict. The HRA formally enshrines in UK legislation, the European Convention on Human Rights.

The European Convention on Human Rights

Many people understand this convention to be a product of the European Community and compliance with it to be a condition of membership. In reality it is a convention to which the UK government signed up in the 1950s. The requirement until the HRA became law was that national legislation should be interpreted in accordance with the convention. The HRA enshrines the rights defined in the convention in UK law, allowing UK citizens to claim in UK courts that their rights have been breached and seek damages or perhaps a stay of criminal proceedings.

A number of rights are described in the HRA and these are divided into qualified and absolute rights. The ones of most relevance to otolaryngologists are Articles 2, 3, 6 and 8.

Article 2 states the right to life. There are a number of ways in which this is relevant. Perhaps this is another route by which the family of a dead patient may seek redress if there is the suggestion that the death occurred due to corporate or individual error. The verdicts that are open to a coroner are discussed under the criminal law below, but, as described, this important field is changing. The coroner is a public body under the terms of the HRA and so must ensure that verdicts are in line with that act. Will we soon see a verdict of death in contravention of Article 2 of the European Convention on Human Rights returned as a halfway house between death by misadventure and unlawful killing? What would be the consequences for a subsequent negligence claim? If the strong lobby seeking to legalize assisted suicide in certain circumstances is successful, how will this sit with the right to life? It is not clear in the legislation how a patient can personally renounce his or her rights under Article 2.

Article 3 is the right not to be subject to torture or to inhumane or degrading treatment or punishment. This appears to influence the facilities that must be made available by hospitals for the care of patients as well as powerful implications for the whole consent process. Surely it will not be long before a Trust is sued by a patient alleging that the wait on a trolley for 24 hours in casualty constituted inhumane or degrading treatment. There is also a suggestion that the coroner will have to pay regard to Article 3 as well if, in his view, there was inhumane and degrading treatment leading to a death.

There are two other Articles with relevance to otolaryngologists: Articles 6 and 8. These two interact with each other when the question of GMC and other legal and paralegal proceedings are considered. Article 6 affirms the right of all citizens to a fair and timely trial. A magistrate in the UK has already stayed a prosecution because he judged that the prosecution had taken an unreasonably long time to bring the case to trial. As the defendant was a doctor and now leaves the criminal court without even having been tried, let alone convicted, it is possible that this judgement will profoundly affect his treatment by the GMC.

Since GMC committees are trials within the meaning of the HRA, they are subject to exactly the same legal liabilities as courts and coroners. It is here that Article 6 may begin to conflict with Article 8, which grants the right to respect for private and family life. Consider the position of a surgeon seeking to refute at the GMC committee on professional performance an allegation that there is a consistent pattern of poor professional competence. In order to defend himself and to liaise with his professional advisers (solicitors and counsel), he would surely need access to the notes of the patients that he cared for and to whom he may have given substandard care. Also, the GMC might wish to call the patients as material witnesses to the substandard care. At present, there is no obligation on a patient, unwittingly a witness at a GMC committee, to grant consent to release of his or her confidential information to either the doctor or the GMC. The patient has rights under the DPA to know what is being done with his or her data and, except in certain circumstances, to withhold consent for release of that information. The exceptions do not seem to apply to GMC proceedings. Surely a patient who found out that a Trust had divulged notes to a surgeon and his legal advisors or to the GMC, in pursuit of a fair trial, could bring action under both the HRA and the DPA. Perhaps also, a patient or even a doctor other than the one being investigated, obliged by subpoena to attend a GMC hearing as a witness and subsequently hounded by the press, can argue that no respect has been shown to his or her privacy.

The whole question of how the HRA (1998) will affect surgeons is under active consideration at present. The only guarantee in this field is that lawyers will continue to use the act to push the common law in new and unusual directions.

THE CRIMINAL LAW

Otolaryngologists rarely face criminal proceedings in connection with medical practice, but mention should be made concerning two types of criminal offence that may flow from medical treatment.

INVOLUNTARY MANSLAUGHTER

In recent years, an increasing number of doctors have faced the prospect of prosecution following the deaths of their patients, allegedly as the result of medical malpractice. The English law relating to involuntary manslaughter has been in a confused state, and clarification has only very recently been provided by the Court of Appeal. Traditionally, the test for involuntary manslaughter has been one of gross negligence. In the words of the then Lord Chief Justice, Lord Hewart, in the case of *R v. Bateman*,[41] in order to establish criminal liability the facts must be such that 'the negligence of the accused went beyond a mere matter of compensation between subjects and showed such a disregard for life and safety of others as to amount to a crime against the state and conduct deserving of punishment'. Adjectives such as 'gross', 'wicked' and 'criminal' were used to describe the degree of negligence required. This is effectively something of a 'gut reaction' test for the jury. In a crime of this nature, it is arguably best left open to the jury to make the determination of criminality.

An attempt was made to further define gross negligence by the House of Lords in the case of *Andrews v. DPP*.[42] In that instance, 'reckless' was considered to be the *adjective* that most closely described the concept. In this way, the House of Lords was endeavouring to ascribe as guilty states of mind the appreciation of risk, coupled with a determination to run it, or the wilful indifference to the question of whether such a risk existed. However, 'mere inadvertence' was not considered to merit criminal responsibility.

The test was thrown into confusion in 1981 as a result of decisions in two cases (*R v. Caldwell*[43] and *R v. Lawrence*[44]) by the House of Lords, which redefined the concept of 'recklessness'. The cases concerned the offences of criminal damage and causing death by reckless driving. It was determined that the defendant would be reckless if his action created an obvious and serious risk (to a victim in the case of manslaughter) and the defendant either appreciated the risk but went on to run it or failed to appreciate the risk. This test has been criticized as being unduly harsh. It allows no realistic explanation of the defendant's state of mind to be put forward. Thus, a doctor under pressure, perhaps through overwork and being asked to perform tasks which he or she should not otherwise have been required to do, would have no opportunity to explain those circumstances as part of defence. The mere fact that an obvious and serious risk had been created to the patient, as a result of which the patient had died, would be sufficient to secure a conviction.

The test was applied in a case of motor manslaughter (*R v. Seymour*)[45] by the House of Lords in 1983. Thereafter, however, there was significant confusion as to whether the case should extend to all cases as an involuntary manslaughter. As a result, in some cases involving doctors charged with involuntary manslaughter the traditional test of gross negligence was applied; in others the new harsh formulation for recklessness was considered appropriate. In yet other cases, attempts were made to combine the two tests.

This unsatisfactory situation has been resolved to a degree by the case of *R v. Prentice and Sulliman*.[46] The case involved two junior doctors, Dr Prentice being a pre-registration house officer who, as part of the chemotherapy treatment, injected vincristine intra-thecally in error. As the Court of Appeal observed, the mitigating circumstances in relation to both doctors were many, but a version of the recklessness test was put to the jury, resulting in their convictions. These were quashed by the Court of Appeal (*R v. Prentice and Sulliman*)[47] on the basis that the test of recklessness was not appropriate for cases of involuntary manslaughter where a breach of duty is concerned, particularly for cases involving doctors, where the court observed: 'Often there is a high degree of danger to the deceased's health, not created by the defendant, and pre-existing risks to the patient's health is what causes the defendant to assume the duty of care with consent. His intervention will often be in situations of emergency.' The traditional test for gross negligence was preferred.

The court set out the matters that need to be established for a prosecution of manslaughter, namely the existence of a duty of care, the breach of the duty causing death, and gross negligence which the jury considers justifies criminal conviction. The Court of Appeal went on to set out various states of mind that it considered could probably lead the jury to making a finding of gross negligence:

- indifference to an obvious risk of injury to health
- actual foresight of a risk coupled with the determination nevertheless to run it
- an appreciation of the risk, coupled with an intention to avoid it but also coupled with such a high degree of negligence in the attempted avoidance as the jury considers justifies conviction
- inattention to or failure to avert a serious risk that goes beyond mere inadvertence in respect of an obvious and important matter that the defendant's duty demanded he should address.

The first three are not unduly onerous. The fourth, however, may present particular problems to medical practitioners. Medical treatment generally may be considered to amount to an obvious and important matter. Further, many serious risks are inherent in treating patients and, accordingly, medical practitioners remain in danger of falling foul of the criminal law relating to manslaughter. At the conclusion of the judgement of the Court of Appeal in the case of Drs Prentice and Sulliman, the court expressed the view that the Law Commissioners should look at the law in relation to involuntary manslaughter as a matter of urgency.

In Canada,[48] manslaughter may be committed where a doctor causes the death of a patient by, among other things, criminal negligence that may be committed where someone under a duty shows a wanton or reckless disregard for the lives or safety of others. The precise meaning of 'wanton or reckless disregard' is in doubt. In a recent case (*R v. Tutton and Tutton*)[49] the Supreme Court of Canada was divided between those who considered that a defendant should have an intention to run a prohibited risk, or a wilful blindness to the risk, and those who considered that a marked and substantial departure from a standard of behaviour expected of a reasonably prudent individual would suffice. This dilemma is similar to that recently addressed by the Court of Appeal in this jurisdiction in the case of Drs Prentice and Sulliman.

In the Court of Appeal in the matter of *R v. Sellu*,[50] the conviction of Mr Sellu was quashed as being unsafe following the finding that the instructions to the jury of the trial judge on the meaning of gross negligence manslaughter were inadequate. In the judgement their Lordships made the point that 'mistakes even very serious mistakes, errors of judgment even very serious errors of judgement, and the like, are not enough for a crime as serious as manslaughter to be committed. You must go on to consider the nature of the carelessness.' They go on to say that 'the key is that the breach of duty must be gross. It must have been so bad, so obviously wrong, that, having regard of the risk of death involved in it, it can be properly condemned as criminal.'

In New Zealand (*R v. Yogasakaran*),[51] the test for manslaughter is that of mere negligence, and a breach of the civil standard of care resulting in the death of a patient is all that is required. Similarly in Greece, the offence under the Greek Criminal Code[52] is of causing death by negligence, mere civil negligence being sufficient. The charge is often seen as a precursor to civil proceedings, where a victim's family may make complaint to prosecuting authorities, effectively as part of the bargaining process for compensation.

ASSAULT, BATTERY AND BODILY HARM

Charges of assault and battery are considered very infrequently by the prosecuting authorities in this jurisdiction in relation to medical practitioners. Courts are reluctant to consider actions in tort for battery arising out of a failure to obtain consent, let alone criminal charges. Very few doctors will intend to inflict harm on a patient, the overall aim being to provide some form of therapeutic benefit. However, where the clinician performs a procedure that goes substantially beyond that to which the patient has consented and that is known to the clinician, or the clinician is reckless as to whether or not the patient's consent will authorize the procedure actually performed, then such an offence may be made out, even if it is of therapeutic benefit. In circumstances where surgical intervention takes place, an offence of greater seriousness than mere assault may result, for example, assault occasioning grievous bodily harm.

Punitive damages

Punitive (exemplary) damages are not normally awarded in jurisdictions of the UK and Australasia but in 2002 the Privy Council heard the case of *A v. Botrill*[53] from New Zealand. This case involved the wholesale misreading of cervical smears by a private pathologist in Gisborne, New Zealand. Between 1990 and 1994 he examined four smears from Mrs A. After Mrs A had a radical hysterectomy for invasive cancer the smears were reviewed and all four slides had been misread or misreported. Mrs A made a successful claim for accident compensation. Disciplinary proceedings against Dr Botrill found him guilty of conduct unbecoming of a medical practitioner. Mrs A then brought court proceedings claiming exemplary damages. Justice Young dismissed the action, applying the principle 'exemplary damages may be awarded, but only if the level of negligence is so high that it amounts to outrageous and flagrant disregard for the plaintiff's safety, meriting condemnation and punishment'.

Two events then occurred: Mrs A found another 10 women whose slides had been misread, and there was public concern about smear reporting in the Gisborne area. This led to a review of Dr Botrill's slides, which showed that Dr Botrill's false reporting rate was 50% or higher. In the light of the new evidence Mrs A applied for a retrial, which was granted. Dr Botrill then appealed this decision and his appeal was successful. Mrs A sought leave to appeal to the Privy Council, which was granted. The argument for Mrs A was that cases of reprehensible wrongdoing that are totally unacceptable to the community but arise from inadvertent negligence should not be put beyond the reach of exemplary damages. Dr Botrill's argument was that there was no conscious, outrageous and flagrant disregard for the plaintiff's safety. The Privy Council agreed with Mrs A and allowed her appeal on a majority decision.

Although this is a New Zealand case it now brings the possibility of punitive damages for reprehensible wrongdoing even if there was no flagrant disregard of risk. It seems that now inadvertent negligence may lead to exemplary damages in selected cases of the worst kind of professional practice.

GUIDELINES

Nowadays, many treatments are the subject of guidelines or protocols, drawn up locally or nationally from organizations such as the National Institute for Health and Clinical Excellence (NICE). These documents purport to set proper standards. Although from a litigation viewpoint they are best considered to be indicative of an accepted course of practice rather than the final arbiter of professional standards, contravention of them without good reason may make defence of a claim very difficult. Where guidelines are departed from the wise practitioner will take particular care to record the reasons in the patient records.

HOSPITAL ADMINISTRATION

A claim may arise where a patient has been lost to follow-up and only represents with an extensive recurrence of a cancer or a complication of a chronic disease such as chronic suppurative otitis media or a systemic condition such as sarcoid. Such cases may have a prospect of being successful where the patient can establish that had there been a regular examination advancing disease would have been easily identified at an early stage.

It is therefore important that health trusts have a robust system of tracking down those patients who fail to attend for their expected appointment. Trusts should be seen to communicate with the GP in order to establish whether the address that they have is correct, and furthermore to inform the GP that the patient has not attended and request the GP to investigate the reasons why. Failure to do so may be difficult to defend, unless the trust can establish that they have emphasized to the patient the importance of regular follow-up and examination following treatment for the tumour. There is considerable merit in a letter being sent to the patient, giving details of the diagnosis, treatment and the planned follow-up care, for the purposes of identifying early recurrence of disease. It is not uncommon for an expert to examine a claimant's notes and identify frequent non-attendance in outpatient departments of various specialties. However, the claimant usually alleges that they failed to receive the appointment in the mail. Although the treating physician may have a healthy scepticism of such allegations, it must be borne in mind that many people live in multiple occupancy dwellings in which security of mail may indeed be in doubt. As such, where follow-up is important, it is advisable that the GP is asked to investigate for repeated failures to attend.

BEST CLINICAL PRACTICE

- ✓ Where there is evidence of a flagrant disregard for safety or recklessness in performing a surgical technique, then the public may need to be protected by requesting the General Medical Council for a competency assessment.
- ✓ Where an adverse outcome of treatment has occurred, prompt offer of transfer to another department and another surgeon may assuage the patient's anger.
- ✓ Trusts should have a robust system of tracking down those patients who fail to attend for their expected appointment.
- ✓ It will be increasingly difficult to justify a single surgeon operating in excess of four hours without having a short rest.

KEY POINTS

- Clinical negligence is a matter for civil law.
- Damages awarded are general and special.
- The standard or proof is 'on the balance of probabilities'.
- There are four essential elements of the legal tort of negligence:
  - there must be a duty of care
  - there must be a breach of that duty
  - harm must have occurred
  - the breach must have caused the harm.
- The standard of care is that of the reasonably skilled and experienced doctor.
- 'It will very seldom be right for a judge to reach the conclusion that views genuinely held by a competent medical expert are unreasonable.'
- If the case for each side is evenly balanced then the claimant will fail.
- The court must award a sum of money that will, as nearly as possible, put the injured person in the same position as she would have been had she not been injured.
- The result of the introduction of contingency fees is likely to be that there will be no significant increase in the number of medical negligence actions in the short term.
- Where a proposed treatment involves a substantial risk of grave or adverse consequences such that, notwithstanding any practice to the contrary, a patient's right to decide whether to consent to the treatment was so obvious that no prudent medical man or woman could fail to warn of the risk, then it would be negligent not to warn.
- The parental right to determine whether or not a child under the age of 16 should have medical treatment terminates when the child achieves a significant understanding and intelligence to enable him or her to understand fully what is proposed.
- 'An adult patient who suffers from no mental incapacity has an absolute right to choose whether to consent to medical treatment, to refuse it or to choose one rather than another of the treatments being offered.'
- Any surgeon who keeps any sort of patient identifiable information at his or her residence and who is not registered with the data commissioner breaches the provisions of the DPA.
- The coroner's remit is to establish the identity of the deceased, the time and place of death and the mode of death.
- Articles 2, 3, 6 and 8 of the HRA are those most relevant to surgeons.
- Modifications to the law on involuntary manslaughter are awaited; currently the traditional description of gross negligence resulting in death usually applies.
- Just because a recognized complication occurs, it does not automatically mean that surgical technique has been below a satisfactory standard.

REFERENCES

1. *Bolitho v. City and Hackney Health Authority* [1997] Weekly Law Report 151.
2. *Bolam v. Friern Hospital Management Committee* [1957] 1 Weekly Law Reports 582.
3. *Wilsher v. Essex Area Health Authority* [1988] 1 All England Reports 871, House of Lords.
4. *Crawford v. Board of Governors of Charing Cross Hospital* [1953] Times Law Reports, 8 December 1953, Court of Appeal.
5. *Barnett v. Chelsea & Kensington Hospital* [1968] 1 All England Reports 1068.
6. *Ashcroft v. Mersey Regional Health Authority* [1985] 2 All England Reports 96.
7. Picard E. Legal liability of doctors and hospitals in Canada. In: Kennedy I, Grubb A (eds). *Medical law: text and materials.* London: Butterworths; 1989, p. 423.
8. *Scott v. London & St. Katherine's Docks* [1865] 3 Hurlstone & Coltman's Exchequer Reports 596 ExCh (sugar bags).
9. *Byrne v. Boadle* [1863] 2 Hurlstone & Coltman's Exchequer Reports 722 (a barrel of flour).
10. *Pope v. St. Helen's Theatre* [1947] Kings Bench 30 (the ceiling of a theatre).
11. M.A.M.S. Leigh. Res ipse Loquitur: What does it mean? *Medical Defence Union Journal* 1993; 9: 66.
12. *Girard v. Royal Columbian Hospital* [1976] 6 Dominion Law Reports (3d) 676.
13. *Mahon v. Osborne* [1939] 2 Kings Bench 1450.
14. Personal correspondence.
15. *Livingston v. Rawyards Coal Company* [1880] 5 Appeal Cases 25 @ 39, House of Lords per Lord Blackburn.
16. *Kralj v. McGrath* [1986] All England Law Reports 54.
17. *Ward v. James* [1965] 2 All England Reports 563, Court of Appeal.
18. *Lim v. Camden Health Authority* [1979] 2 All England Reports 910, House of Lords, per Lord Scarman.
19. Rules of the Supreme Court: Order 37 Rules 7–10.
20. See generally the Rules of the Supreme Court and the County Court Practice for Procedure.
21. Civil Procedure Rules 1998.
22. S.58 Courts and Legal Services Act 1990.
23. Preliminary results of the Law Society Survey of Personal Injury Specialists. *LS Gaz* 29 September 1993: 3.
24. *NHS Litigation Authority Annual Report 2015/2016.* London: HMSO; 2016.
25. The Health and Social Care Act 2008 (Regulated Activities) (Amendment) Regulations 2015. HMSO; 2015.
26. *Report of the Mid Staffordshire NHS Foundation Trust Public Enquiry.* London: HMSO; February 2013.
27. *Sidaway v. Board of Governors of the Bethlem Royal Hospital* [1985] Appeal Cases 871, House of Lords.
28. *Hopp v. Lepp* [1979] 112 Dominion Law Reports 3d 67.
29. *Blyth v. Bloomsbury Health Authority* [1993] 4 Medical Law Reports, Court of Appeal.
30. *Rogers v. Whitaker* [1993] 4 Medical Law Reports 79, High Court of Australia.
31. *Chester v. Afshar* [2004] Appeal Cases 41, House of Lords.
32. *Montgomery v. Lanarkshire Health Board.* Available from: www.supremecourt.uk/decided-cases/docs/UKSC_2013_0136_Judgment.pdf
33. *Consent: patients and doctors making decisions together.* London: The General Medical Council; 2008.
34. *Gillick v. West Norfolk and Wisbech Area Health Authority* [1986] Appeal Cases 112, [1985] 3 All England Reports 402, House of Lords.
35. In Re R [1991] 4 All England Reports 177, Court of Appeal.
36. In Re W [1992] 3 Weekly Law Reports 758.
37. Re F [1990] 2 Appeal Cases 1, House of Lords.
38. Re C [1994] 1 Weekly Law Reports 290, [1994] 1 All England Reports 819.
39. In Re T (Adult: Refusal of treatment) [1992] 3 Weekly Law Reports 783.
40. *National Justice Compania Naviera SA v. Prudential Assurance Company Ltd. (Ikarian Reefer)* [1993] Times Law Reports, 3rd March 1993.
41. *R v. Bateman* [1925] 19 Criminal Appeal Reports 8, Court of Appeal.
42. *Andrews v. DPP* [1937] Appeal Cases 576, PC.
43. *R v. Caldwell* [1982] Appeal Cases 341, House of Lords.
44. *R v. Lawrence* [1982] Appeal Cases 510, House of Lords.
45. *R v. Seymour* [1983] 2 Appeal Cases 493, House of Lords.
46. *R v. Prentice and Sulliman* (unreported 1 November 1991, Owen J).
47. *R v. Prentice and Sulliman* [1993] 4 All England Reports 935, Court of Appeal.
48. *The Annotated Tremear's Criminal Code* 1992, Sections 219, 220, 222.
49. *R v. Tutton and Tutton* [1989] 48 Canadian Criminal Cases (3d) 129, Canadian Supreme Court.
50. *R v. Sellu* [2016] EWCA Crim 1716, Court of Appeal.
51. *R v. Yogasakaran* [1990] 1 New Zealand Law Reports 399, New Zealand Court of Appeal.
52. Article 302 Greek Penal Code.
53. *A v. Botrill* [2002] UKPC 44.

CHAPTER 39b

MEDICAL NEGLIGENCE IN OTORHINOLARYNGOLOGY

Maurice Hawthorne

Introduction 427	Specific conditions and procedures..................................430
Interpretation of images.......................................427	Rhinology and facial plastic surgery..................................430
Interpretation of histological investigations 428	Otology and neuro-otology..439
Failure to consider conservative treatment.....................428	Paediatric otolaryngology...445
Patient selection 428	Head and neck surgery...448
Consent to surgery 429	References..451
Tumour recurrence 430	

SEARCH STRATEGY

Data in this chapter are based largely on the author's long experience as an expert witness and on landmark legal judgements, some of which are alluded to in the text.

INTRODUCTION

Chapter 39a dealt with the general principles that govern legal aspects of medical practice in otorhinolaryngology. This chapter explores recurrent themes to guide safe practice and then focuses on specific scenarios that give rise to claims of negligence in general otolaryngological practice and within the subspecialties.

INTERPRETATION OF IMAGES

In many hospitals, there is no radiologist with a special interest in ENT. Consequently, the experienced consultant ENT surgeon may be just as competent at reading radiological films as the specialist radiologist. In all departments it is wise that both the clinician and the radiologist assess the radiological films within the clinical context of the patient's disease. From time to time, a difference of opinion may arise, and a failure to address this difference of opinion can lead to a delay in diagnosis, with a significant impact on prognosis for the patient. Where films have been discussed, and a difference of opinion continues, then it is advisable that a further opinion is sought from a radiologist with a special interest in the field. Nowadays, films can be easily transferred electronically and the vagaries of the postal system do not have to be endured. Where there is a difference of opinion between the clinician and the radiologist, most patients would expect the radiological investigation to be repeated after some weeks. Although the radiologist, and indeed the clinician, may have some concerns about the increased dosage of X-rays necessitated by repeat films, where there is a possibility of malignancy, the patient will see this risk as being trivial, and would be much more concerned about obtaining peace of mind about what they see as a real and existing problem, compared to some theoretical risk of developing a malignancy in the future. Therefore, the wise clinician should argue for a repeat investigation or discuss with his radiological colleague using another imaging modality.

In the field of endoscopic sinus surgery, whether it is functional, diagnostic or treating an iatrogenic complication, it is essential to have a complete demonstration of the radiological anatomy by computed tomography (CT) scan. The nose should be scanned from its rostral extremity as far back as the basilar artery. In addition, it is essential that the window setting is such as to maximize the bony detail and also a second series should be saved with window settings to give some soft tissue information. Litigation may arise when the clinician either has not viewed the imaging or ignores a report demanding that action should be taken. For example, it is normal practice that immediate post-operative plain films of cochlear implants are taken. In two cases, settlement had to be explored where an electrode had partially slipped out immediately following surgery, and was shown on the post-operative films but only detected by the team when the films were reviewed some months later as the patient was not doing as well as expected.

INTERPRETATION OF HISTOLOGICAL INVESTIGATIONS

Much of what has been said above on radiological investigations also applies to histopathological investigations. The wise otolaryngologist will be well aware of the pitfalls that can arise. These are especially true in salivary gland and nasal neoplasia. Also, fine-needle aspiration cytology needs to be carefully considered in the light of the clinical picture and if a lesion deemed benign on cytological examination does not appear to be behaving clinically as such, rebiopsy should be undertaken speedily.

FAILURE TO CONSIDER CONSERVATIVE TREATMENT

This issue appears to arise more commonly in private practice. It is not uncommon for the patient who has had a mishap following sinus surgery to state that conservative options for treatment, such as oral steroids and antibiotics in the case of nasal polyposis, had never been discussed, but that an immediate recommendation for surgery had been made by the practitioner. In the case of simple, benign, nasal polyposis in a fit individual, there is rarely any defence for not discussing the possibility of a course of oral steroids, with or without antibiotics. If there is doubt as to the nature of the polyps, a simple biopsy can be undertaken, followed by conservative treatment, rather than an attempt to radically clear the disease, as first-line treatment.

In those patients with nasal obstruction due to enlarged inferior turbinates, first-line treatment should normally be conservative. Adequate investigation to identify the presence of any allergy and then treatment either by allergen avoidance or topical steroid treatment would usually be first-line treatment. If the general practitioner has already undertaken this in an adequate and thorough manner, it may be reasonable to proceed with an offer of surgery. However, a significant complication occurring following turbinate surgery in the patient who has not been offered an initial trial of conservative treatment can be very difficult to defend.

PATIENT SELECTION

When a patient attends with trauma or cancer, the surgeon has little choice but to either provide the treatment that is necessary or refer on to a specialist who is more fitted to handle the case. Ultimately, the patient is going to require treatment and a failure to provide prompt treatment after diagnosis may in itself lead to litigation.

However, in the non-urgent situation, there is time for the patient to choose his surgeon and also for the surgeon to choose his patient. The wise surgeon will pay heed to features that suggest an increased risk of dissatisfaction, and will attempt to manage these before undertaking any surgical treatment. Only once the surgeon is convinced that a patient understands what the experience and the result of surgery is likely to be should the planned surgery proceed. This is especially so where there is a cosmetic element to the proposed treatment.

Beware the patient with no physical abnormality. A patient who has a physical abnormality visible to the surgeon and a clear understanding of what he or she wishes to be achieved is more likely to be satisfied with the result of cosmetic surgery than a patient with no visible abnormality. If a patient's nose is too long or too wide, the tip too bulbous or deviated, and is obviously outwith the norm, then successful surgery is possible. A patient who refuses to accept that the nose is within the range of normality and clearly believes it to be too large may be suffering from dysmorphophobia. These patients will be dissatisfied with surgery and should be referred to a psychiatrist with experience in the field for assessment and possible treatment.

Beware the patient whose appearance is at either end of the normal spectrum, obsessively neat and tidy or dishevelled and unkempt. Both types may prove difficult for the surgeon to achieve a result that satisfies the patient. The immaculate patient may be seeking a result beyond the capability of surgery, and may also find the normal scar maturation process too slow. The patient who does not care about his or her appearance may not comply postoperatively, compromising the result. If such a patient is looking for an improvement in social life, attention to personal hygiene may be more appropriate than changing facial appearance. In particular, it requires considerable tact to explain this, but undertaking a cosmetic surgical procedure on his or her face is unwise.

Beware the patient who is dissatisfied with other surgeons or the results of previous surgery. The surgeon who has refused a patient elsewhere is likely to have had good reasons for not proceeding. Furthermore, the patient's perception of these reasons will almost certainly be given with a bias that the wise would recognize. If the patient has had an unacceptable result from surgery and yet in your evaluation the result is well within the range of results produced by most competent practitioners, then dissatisfaction from further surgery is likely. However, there are those who see plastic surgery as an adjunct to all the other means of enhancing appearance, and a patient seeking another plastic surgical operation on a part of the body that has not been enhanced before should not necessarily be seen as a potentially problematical patient, particularly if the patient expresses satisfaction at previous operative procedures.

Beware the patient with the bizarre request. Occasionally, patients may present with a request that is so bizarre, the surgeon is unlikely to have come across it before. For example, a patient may believe that he or she is part-snake, part-human, and consequently requests splitting of the tongue to give it a forked appearance. Underlying such requests may be a psychotic delusion and, whenever the surgeon is in doubt, an opinion from a psychiatrist should be sought before offering surgery.

Beware the aggressive and violent patient. Individuals who express their dissatisfaction or who fail to solve their daily problems by the spoken word and consequently resort to violence may hide an underlying personality disorder. Such people may have problems with interpersonal relationships that they have focused onto one aspect of their appearance. If this aspect is changed and their interpersonal relationship problems do not improve, they may seek retribution from the surgeon. Surgeons have been murdered by dissatisfied patients.

CONSENT TO SURGERY

Issues of consent on their own are rare in relation to sinus surgery and they are much more common when coupled with allegations of incompetent surgical technique. However, it is in the field of turbinectomy, particularly in the adolescent and young adult, that issues of consent arise. Torrential haemorrhage following inferior turbinectomy is not uncommon, probably happening in most surgeons' practice, with an incidence of between 1 in 60 and 1 in 200 cases. It does appear to be more common where a posterior turbinectomy has been undertaken, rather than removal of the anterior end of the interior turbinates. Nevertheless, torrential haemorrhage can happen in any form of turbinate surgery. When this occurs, and the patient has undergone the usual treatment to arrest the haemorrhage and correct the blood loss, an allegation of permanent psychological damage may arise, accompanied by the allegation that the patient was not warned of the risk and had they been, then they would have refused consent for the surgery. In taking consent, the wise surgeon must assess the personality of the patient and ask himself whether they would have the mental fortitude to withstand the psychological trauma that can accompany a severe nasal haemorrhage, particularly as it may appear life-threatening to the patient and their family. If the patient, despite warning of such haemorrhage, still wishes to proceed with the surgery, then it should be carefully annotated in the notes that the warning has been given and understood.

Since the introduction of functional endoscopic sinus surgery on a wide basis, between 1988 and 1992, consent for these procedures seems, on the whole, to be well annotated in the case-notes, particularly from the point of view of the risks of injury to orbital contents and breach of the dura. However, where contention may arise, it is not that the patient was warned of these anatomical risks, but that they did not understand the consequences of these risks on their day-to-day life or that, should such risks occur, secondary complications may supervene. One patient, an intelligent banker, freely admitted that he had been warned of the risk of cerebrospinal fluid leaking from his nose, but was adamant that he had been given no warning that this could lead to meningitis and subsequent intellectual impairment, which had occurred in his particular circumstances.

However, the claimant may find it difficult to establish in court that, had they been fully warned, they would not have gone on to subject themselves to the surgical procedure.

The landmark Australian case, *Rogers v. Whitaker*,[1] in which it was felt the risk of sympathetic ophthalmitis, with a risk of approximately 1 in 30 000, should have been explained to a patient, has not found favour in the English courts. The risk of blindness as the result of submucosal diathermy, or the use of adrenalin-containing local anaesthetic in rhinological surgery, is somewhat similar. In one case, a young woman woke up following a general anaesthetic for a submucosal diathermy to the inferior turbinates and had totally lost sight in one eye. Thorough investigation did not reveal any evidence of direct trauma to orbital or retro-orbital structures, and a literature search revealed that this can happen despite competent surgical technique. On the Bolam principle, as virtually no ear, nose and throat surgeon practising in the UK would warn of this risk, her case would fail and therefore her solicitor advised that she should not pursue the issue. A Legal Aid Certificate was not granted to test the principle that such a loss was so catastrophic that, despite its rarity, it should have been warned of and that any reasonable patient would expect that this issue be mentioned. Now in the post-Montgomery era it is likely that such a complication would meet the reasonable patient test and so the issue may be tested in the courts in the future. A major point of debate will be around just what really rare complications the consenting surgeon should actually be aware of.

Time should be spent carefully outlining: the common complications; the likelihood of them occurring; what the effects of them would be; what treatment may be necessary to correct matters should such complications arise; and, most importantly, whether such extra treatment will be charged for. Providing this free of charge goes a long way to having a satisfied patient and reduces the chance of litigation. Carefully worded patient information leaflets are helpful, either sent to the patient to read before the consultation or given for reading afterwards, but they are not a substitute for proper discussion and informed consent. The surgeon should take care to ensure that such leaflets are directly applicable to the patient's problem and to the way in which the surgeon plans to treat the patient, both at the operation and post-operatively. Some commercial leaflets are too vague or, worse, impart information that does not apply to your practice or the patient concerned. This may cause litigation problems later.

Patients should not make a final, irrevocable decision about surgery at the initial consultation. A period of time, perhaps two weeks, for the patient to reflect upon what has been said is invaluable. Many patients will undertake their own research, often using the internet or discussing matters with friends or relatives during this period. Although the surgeon may be inconvenienced or disappointed if a patient changes his or her mind and decides not to undergo a procedure, the wise surgeon will realize that she or he has probably been saved a considerable amount of time and inconvenience by not performing the operation discussed.

TUMOUR RECURRENCE

An allegation of inadequate primary resection of a tumour, either malignant or benign, usually follows the unexpected diagnosis of a recurrence. This may seem surprising to the profession, but sadly a combination of belief in modern surgical techniques, plus the confident statement from the operating surgeon that 'all the tumour has been removed', can lead to an accusation of incompetent technique. Clearly, a confident statement on tumour resection is meant to reassure the patient and improve their psychological well-being. However, there is no excuse to take on a patronizing role, supported by frank lies. It is important that the patient is told the exact situation, as best as can be determined, and if the outcome for the future appears to be bleak, then such bad news needs to be adequately supported with appropriate psychological therapy. It is possible that any psychological damage may be looked upon seriously by the courts, and appropriately rewarded, especially when the major defence to the bulk of the claim is that 'the patient would have died anyway'.

In circumstances where resection margins are being monitored by frozen section examination during the surgery, it is vital that all specimens are sent. Thus, when a report says that the tumour is at the margin of resection, on one specimen it is useful to have a subsequent specimen indicating that there is a clearance. Obviously, where the tumour is up to, but not invading, a nerve sheath, the surgeon may have to exercise clinical judgement and decide whether to resect such a nerve sheath or not. These points should be carefully noted in the records. Thus, a histological report that indicates that the margin of resection is up to the edge of the tumour can be seen to have been acted upon appropriately.

SPECIFIC CONDITIONS AND PROCEDURES

Just because a recognized complication happens, it does not automatically mean that surgical technique has been below a satisfactory standard. A complication such as damage to the medial rectus muscle in endoscopic sinus surgery may occur, despite all care being taken by the surgeon. On the other hand, it may occur as a result of a 'gung ho' or slapdash technique, in which due respect and identification of the relevant surgical landmarks has not been attempted. For the claimant, it can be difficult, if not impossible, to prove that the damage has occurred because of the latter surgical technique, rather than the former. It would indeed be rare for a claimant to successfully identify a witness, present at the time of the surgery, who was willing to testify in court as to incompetent technique practised by the surgeon.

Increasingly, video is used in theatre and, in the case of endoscopic sinus surgery, operating via camera is a common technique. If the surgery is recorded and the tapes kept until it is established there is no significant post-operative complication, the recording may be available to both parties in which an adverse outcome to the surgery has developed.

In a recent MPTS case, examination of recordings kept on DVD by an expert was key evidence that led to the erasure from the medical register of the surgeon.

For example, in one case, a trainee undertook a difficult nasal polypectomy endoscopically. The procedure was recorded and a breach of the anterior cranial fossa, and how it was acquired, could clearly be seen on the video. In this particular instance there was a dehiscence of the cribriform plate, with absence of bone in the anterior cranial fossa. The repair was also filmed. An explanation was given to the patient, who was quite satisfied. However, his children, who lived some distance away, attended the hospital some days later. One daughter, a nurse in a maxillofacial surgical department, clearly felt that causing a cerebrospinal fluid (CSF) leak had to be negligent. Fortunately the video material was available, which was immediately shown to the family and carefully explained. This diffused the aggression and was successful in preventing litigation.

Occasionally, massive injury can be sustained in which the degree of damage is so gross that basic surgical technique has to have been ignored, or not understood. For example, in one case a patient failed to regain consciousness from the anaesthetic following intra-nasal surgery. On arrival at the intensive care unit, a 2 × 1 × 1 cm piece of cerebral cortex was retrieved from the oropharynx; subsequently an extensive resection of the anterior cranial fossa was identified, and the nose contained a huge herniation of the brain. The neuroradiological expert in the case felt that there was clear evidence of instrument tracks within the substance of the frontal lobes of the brain, suggesting that instruments had been passed repeatedly into this brain substance. In this particular case, pre-operative CT scans did not reveal any evidence of a congenital abnormality of the anterior skull base. Not surprisingly the surgeon's insurers sought a settlement early on in the process of the case.

Where the evidence is strong that the lack of standard of care would suggest a flagrant disregard for safety, or recklessness in performing the surgical technique, then the public may need to be protected by requesting a competency assessment by the General Medical Council.

RHINOLOGY AND FACIAL PLASTIC SURGERY

Negligence in general practice in relation to rhinological disease is unusual. It appears to occur mainly due to a failure in recognizing the significance of certain symptoms or signs.

One of the most common areas is in failure to arrange timely treatment for a nasal fracture. In most practices, the best opportunity in effectively manipulating a nasal fracture is within the first 21 days of the injury. Failure to undertake timely treatment may lead to the necessity of performing a formal septorhinoplasty. The consequence of this is a longer period off work than would otherwise be necessary, as well as additional pain and suffering such as periorbital bruising. A delayed referral can rarely be defended and usually the best outcome is to seek a speedy settlement. There are exceptions and one of the most important is the cartilaginous injury of the nasal tip or septum when simple manipulation does not give the best results and a septorhinoplasty is indicated as first-line treatment.

A delay in referral of sinusitis is also a common area that leads to litigation. The general practitioner (GP) usually fails to realize when a sinus infection has spread beyond the sinus and is involving the orbit, bone, meninges or soft tissues. The most common examples of this are orbital and forehead swelling. It is only the onset of symptoms in relation to brain abscess, meningitis, blindness or severe orbital swelling that leads to a speedy referral.

The significance of unilateral nasal symptoms, such as discharge, may be ignored by the GP and so a delay in diagnosis of a tumour or foreign body occurs.

Sadly, it is not just the GP who may fall into the situation of delaying a diagnosis. Inexperienced trainees within the specialty, accident and emergency doctors, and occasionally other specialists within hospital practice, may all find themselves at the centre of litigation arising from these relatively common areas of negligence.

Inadequate pre-surgical management

Failure to investigate significant symptoms arises from time to time. Wegener's granulomatosis is a condition that regularly goes unrecognized. Often it may be mistaken for atrophic rhinitis or even industrial rhinitis, and the patient treated symptomatically, without adequate investigation. It is only when other systems are involved, such as the renal or respiratory system, that adequate investigations are triggered and the condition identified. Clearly if the condition has progressed to frank renal failure requiring dialysis before diagnosis has been made, then the patient may have a strong claim. It is common to find that other conditions, such as scleritis, flitting arthropathy or skin lesions, have not been not linked to the nasal symptoms.

Circumstances arise in which the investigations for this condition, such as a raised plasma viscosity or erythrocyte sedimentation rate (ESR), which are usually raised, are within the normal range. Occasionally even the antineutrophil cytoplasmic antibody (ANCA) test is negative, and where adequate investigations have been undertaken but the diagnosis has been delayed, a reasonable defence can be mounted.

From time to time, a post-nasal space carcinoma may present as a neck lump to another specialist. Although the malignant nature of the neck lump is identified, occasionally the primary site is missed. The ear, nose and throat (ENT) expert may be asked to comment on such a delay. It is of course inappropriate for him to deal with issues of liability concerning delay in diagnosis by another specialist, but it would be expected for him to comment on how the delay may affect the prognosis of the patient.

Similarly, a restriction in eye movement may indicate early involvement of orbital contents or a cranial nerve by a sinus malignancy. Clinical examination may not reveal an obvious restriction in movement, due to the partial nature of the malignant process. Sudden onset of double vision, without an obvious cause such as head injury, or orbital displacement should never be ignored, and requires thorough investigation to exclude a pathological cause requiring treatment.

External drainage of the frontal sinus

Frontal sinus trephine may lead to supratrochlear nerve damage and indeed supraorbital nerve damage. Where there is significant oedema in the surgical area, most surgeons could understand how the supraorbital nerve might be stretched by retractors, or indeed cut. However, in a simple drainage procedure, there can be no excuse for extending the incision so far laterally as to divide the supraorbital nerve. The Lynch–Howarth procedure gives wider access to the frontal and ethmoid sinuses. In extensive disease it may be necessary to sacrifice the supraorbital and the supratrochlear nerve. This should be anticipated before the surgery and the patient warned. In addition, the patient should be warned of the possibility of double vision post-operatively due to the detachment of the trochlea.

Caldwell-Luc procedure

Caldwell-Luc surgery is now rarely undertaken. Resting cheek retractors against the supraorbital rim in a Caldwell-Luc procedure, or similar surgery, can lead to a neuropraxia of the supraorbital nerve. This usually recovers; however, it is a well-recognized risk and adequate precautions can usually be taken to prevent it happening. On the other hand, infraorbital nerve neuropraxia in Caldwell-Luc surgery can be inflicted despite all care being taken, and does not indicate *de facto* substandard technique.

Septal surgery

A major saddle deformity of the supra tip area, following septal surgery, causes such a deformity that it can be difficult to prevent the angry and embittered patient from seeking redress. If the complication has occurred as the result of a post-operative septal abscess, and the patient has been warned of the possibility when consent was taken, then sympathetic handling can usually prevent the patient seeking redress through the court. A careful explanation that infection had destroyed the septal cartilage may suffice. Rarely the saddle could be due to a failure to recognize and diagnose disorders such as Wegener's granulomatosis, sarcoidosis or relapsing polychondritis. The wise surgeon, when presented with such an unexpected outcome, should take the appropriate tests to exclude such disorders. Clearly the presence of an alternative explanation for a septal collapse or perforation may present an opportunity for a defence.

Septal perforation is another common complication, especially in submucous resection of the nasal septum that causes such symptoms that a patient may seek compensation. It should always be mentioned when septal surgery is being offered. The presence of a perforation does not automatically imply a substandard technique; it is more likely to be an indicator of a severely fractured nasal septum or the presence of another disease, such as atrophic rhinitis or a granulomatous disease.

The circumstances of a submucosal resection, in which the surgeon has made an error of judgement and resected too much cartilage, are likely to be much more difficult for the patient to accept. Once more, recognition of the patient's concern is the key to good management. In addition to offering surgery to correct the deformity, it is important to recognize that the patient may no longer have confidence in the surgeon, or indeed even in the hospital in which they have been treated, and so a prompt offer of transfer to another department and another surgeon may assuage the patient's anger.

In the last few years the author has seen a rise in claims in which there has been a subtle change in the appearance of the nose following septoplasty. In these cases the surgery has clearly been performed competently but the patient claims that they were reassured that the operation would not alter their appearance.

Examination under anaesthesia and diagnostic sinus lavage

Prior to the 1980s, it was very common practice to undertake a 'proof puncture' of the maxillary antra. This would often be done at the time of a tonsillectomy or adenotonsillectomy, in older children and young adults. It was considered a legitimate investigation to detect the possibility of chronic sinus infection. Many surgeons advocated its routine use, even in the absence of any sinus or nasal symptoms. Such an invasive procedure, which carries the risk of damage to unerupted secondary dentition, the inferior orbital nerve and the orbital contents, in the absence of sinus symptoms, can no longer be justified without taking a formal consent for the procedure and offering alternative methods of investigation. In addition, several cases have arisen due to misunderstanding of the term 'examination under anaesthesia'. Some claimants who have sustained complications as a result of such procedures have asserted that they only gave consent for the surgeon to look, but not to biopsy. A typical examination would be obtaining consent for examination of the post-nasal space in a child or adult with glue ear, and then proceeding to perform an adenoidectomy having identified a significant pad of lymphoid tissue in the post-nasal space, the damage occurring usually being a secondary haemorrhage. It is important therefore, in taking consent, to include the potential risks that may arise for any additional procedure, usually a biopsy of an excisional or incisional nature.

Intra-operative monitoring

This term usually invokes thoughts of nerve monitoring in the context of ENT surgery, but it is still particularly important in rhinological surgery, although the monitoring may be purely visual in nature. In endoscopic sinus surgery, it is the orbital contents that are at risk. Clues to a significant intra-orbital incursion can be obtained by careful observation of both eyes during the procedure. This may not be possible by the operating surgeon, as it is likely that he or she will be observing the operating field either indirectly through a camera or directly through an eye-piece. However, an operating assistant, such as a scrub nurse or other colleague, should be in a position to observe both orbits and watch for the tell-tale signs of a complication arising. These may include a sudden movement of the globe of the eye, the development of proptosis or subconjunctival haemorrhage. Although in the early parts of the procedure it is important to protect the cornea from damage, at points in the surgery in which the eye may be in a critical, or vulnerable state, it is permissible for the eyelid to be opened and the globe observed for brief periods. Early identification of an incursion into the orbit is essential to reduce the risk of damage. Equally, in the recovery area, post-operative observation of the orbits and eyes is essential, particularly if a significant retrobulbar haemorrhage is to be identified, monitored and, if necessary, treated before permanent damage to the eyesight occurs.

Post-operative monitoring

Even though frontal sinus infection has been adequately drained at surgery, the patient still has the potential of developing an intra-cranial complication, though this is now much less. It is likely that the infection has spread through the venous system prior to the actual drainage of the sinuses and so the intra-cranial symptoms usually commence 24–48 hours after surgery. Complaint of severe headache that is progressive, along with drowsiness, confusion or disinhibition, should alert the wary to the onset of a frontal lobe infection. Usually the patient should be on an antibiotic with a high ability to cross the blood–brain barrier, but if this is not the case, then with the onset of these symptoms the antibiotic will need to be changed. Inadequate monitoring in the post-operative period may also lead to delay in detection of a cerebrospinal fluid leak. Although these may be blatantly obvious when there is a striking flow of clear fluid from the nose and the patient has an accompanying headache, the occasional case may be intermittent. In one case, the patient re-attended the hospital on three occasions complaining of watery nasal discharge, which was ignored. No investigations were undertaken, other than admission and observation on the ward, on one occasion only for 48 hours. On the final attendance at hospital the patient presented with a small bottle containing a sample of the CSF and symptoms of frank meningitis. The confusing issue is that nasal discharge that may be watery in nature is not uncommon following sinus surgery, or indeed may be related to the underlying sinus disorder. It is quite likely that minor CSF leaks are probably more common than is actually realized, but fortunately they close spontaneously without any secondary damage.

Benign skin lesions

Patients often believe that small skin lesions can be removed without leaving a scar. It is very important that the inevitability of a scar, its length and width, the duration of the scar maturation process and the risk of scar hypertrophy and/or keloid formation is explained to the patient as part of the informed consent procedure.

When excising a skin lesion as an ellipse, the length of the scar will be two or three times the diameter of the lesion. Once the sutures have been removed, the scar will initially be a relatively fine line. As the proliferative phase of wound healing progresses, the vascularity increases, making the scar red and noticeable. This appearance may last for between two weeks and two months after injury.

With entry into the collagen maturation phase the appearance of the scar improves, but full maturation may take up to two years in some patients. Those with a heavy, sebaceous skin, or ginger colouring, may have a noticeable scar for longer than average. Overexposure of an immature scar to ultraviolet light from bright sunshine or from a sun bed will cause burning more easily than in normal skin or a mature scar. Patients should be advised to avoid or protect the skin from such overexposure by applying high protection factor sun cream and by keeping out of the direct rays of the sun.

The patient dissatisfied with the early appearance of a scar should be advised that early revision is rarely indicated as many scars settle without surgery being necessary. Regular communication with the patient whilst the scar matures is the keystone of treatment, as brushing off the patient or disregarding the patient's perception that there is a problem may lead to litigation. Although the scar may well settle whilst the complaint proceeds, the problems of having an ongoing case are not to be dismissed lightly. Regular outpatient consultations, encouragement that the scar is likely to settle in time and sympathy with the patient will minimize the risk of litigation.

Patients with factors known to adversely affect the final appearance of scars must be counselled about this. Adolescents with spotty, pubertal skin are best not operated on until their skin has calmed down unless there is a suspicion of malignancy. Patients with previous hypertrophic scarring, patients with coloured skin and those with lesions on areas of the face more likely to make a hypertrophic scar, such as along the line of the mandible, must be warned appropriately. In some parts of the face, particularly the tip of the nose, it is difficult to achieve a fine scar even with no adverse factors.

In trauma, the method of injury influences the final appearance of a scar. Dirty or infected wounds, traumatic tattooing, closure under tension, non-perpendicular wound edges and wounds crossing skin tension lines will lead to poor quality scars. Trapdoor scarring is a particular problem in traumatic wounds: a flap of skin is raised, often tangentially and thus with bevelled edges, and the scar heals with contraction and localized lymphoedema within the confines of the scar. Simple excision and resuture is unlikely to resolve the problem and a patient must be advised clearly of the limited improvement that may be achieved by scar revision.

Suture marks are not acceptable and, if they occur, litigation will be difficult to defend. Careful choice of suture material and its thickness, accurate placement of the sutures and their tightness, and timing of removal are critical. It has been suggested that scar stretching can be minimized using subcuticular sutures left in place for weeks or months, but clinical experience does not generally support this.

All lesions excised should be submitted for histological examination, however benign the lesion looks, unless the patient specifically instructs that this is not to be done. In such a situation, this instruction must be recorded in the notes.

Keloid and hypertrophic scars

Both hypertrophic and keloid scars contain excess collagen. In a hypertrophic scar, the collagen remains within the borders of the scar, but in a keloid scar it extends into the surrounding undamaged skin. Hypertrophic scars usually settle spontaneously, although they may take a few years and leave unsightly scars, but keloid scars persist. Hypertrophic scarring is more common in young people, can occur on any part of the body and is more common if there has been wound infection and breakdown or healing by secondary intention. Keloid scarring may be familial, is much more common in Afro-Caribbeans than in Caucasians and has a predilection for certain parts of the body, such as in the head and neck, the ear lobes and more rarely the post-auricular skin.

Treatment of keloid scarring is difficult and often unsuccessful. Patients find it difficult to believe that simple excision will not solve the problem and that keloid recurrence is not only inevitable but may be worse. Triamcinolone injections are the mainstay of treatment, although great care must be taken that the steroid is of the correct strength (10 mg/mL and not 40 mg/mL) as the concentration of steroid used for intra-articular injections rapidly causes localized fat atrophy which takes two or more years to recover. Steroid impregnated tape and topical application of hydrocortisone can also help, as can pressure garment therapy.

Patients should be warned pre-operatively of the risk of keloid scarring occurring with an indication of the degree of risk for the site or procedure. For example, keloid scars developing after a pinnaplasty are rare but when they occur it is a cosmetic disaster and frequently the cause of a claim. It can be difficult when the effect of the complication is so great to defend such a claim on the grounds simply that the complication is rare and that the patient therefore did not need a warning.

Nasal trauma

DELAYED TREATMENT

Nasal fractures with bony deformity should ideally be reduced within at most 10 days following the injury to avoid callus formation and rigid bony union. Delayed treatment may lead to permanent osseocartilaginous deformity, which can only be corrected by septorhinoplasty. This may lead to a successful claim for negligence. It is essential to have a referral mechanism between accident and emergency departments and otolaryngology departments so that early assessment can take place and arrangements can be made for manipulation of a nasal fracture under anaesthesia. The decision to manipulate a nasal fracture is clinical. Plain X-rays have little to offer.

SEPTAL HAEMATOMA

Failure to recognize acute septal haematoma can lead to a permanent deformity if a septal abscess subsequently develops. In most instances of septal abscess, a doctor has not previously examined the child but occasionally a haematoma is missed or is diagnosed but not drained. The saddle nose deformity that results can be difficult to correct and as such the compensation can be relatively expensive to cover the pain and suffering of additional surgery and the cosmetic deformity.

Rhinoplasty and septorhinoplasty

The importance of proper selection of the patient and the procedure appropriate to that patient in connection with a rhinoplasty cannot be overemphasized as it is an area in which expectations are very high. It is particularly important to identify those patients who are being unrealistic. Those bringing cuttings from magazines showing the nose that they want and those with concerns about a deformity that the surgeon cannot see should make the surgeon wary of proceeding.

Pre-operative photographs must be taken and studied carefully as they may show abnormalities that the surgeon has missed on examination, or which the patient may be unaware of, such as an asymmetry that might otherwise be blamed later on the operation.

In most rhinoplasties, osteotomies are performed which narrow the nasal airway. This may cause obstructive symptoms, and assessment of the airway pre-operatively is important if nasal obstruction is to be avoided.

Patients who have a congenitally wide nose may require alar base reduction at the same time as a rhinoplasty. This will leave a permanent scar at each nostril base and patients must be warned of this.

There is a recognized revision rate following rhinoplasty, which ranges from 5% to 15% in published series. Patients must be advised that this may be required and should be regarded as normal. It is wise to include the cost of this surgery in the price quoted for the initial rhinoplasty, or to agree the cost before the first operation, as additional unexpected charges can turn a patient from accepting a less-than-perfect outcome to starting litigation.

Elderly patients with thin, fine skin are particularly difficult to manage. Any material left under the skin, such as bone dust or fragments, can easily show through once the healing process is complete. Furthermore, if the osteotomies are not carefully positioned and the bone fragments align in an unsatisfactory position, the edges of the bone or the osteotomies themselves may show through the skin. Occasionally, it may even be wise to advise a patient with such skin not to undergo a rhinoplasty procedure. Elderly skin will have lost its elasticity and will not retract satisfactorily when it is re-draped over the bony and cartilaginous framework at the end of the procedure, so resection, particularly of a bony hump, must be very conservative to avoid unsightly, redundant skin.

Tight application of a plaster-of-Paris splint against the unyielding bed when osteotomies have not been performed can lead to skin necrosis. Paper splints, such as self-adhesive dressing strips, are best used instead to prevent subdermal haematomas. Many surgeons overlap these strips and care needs to be taken that they overlap adequately otherwise a bleb of skin can herniate between them, become strangulated and lead to an ulcer and subsequently a permanent external scar.

The occurrence of unacceptable deformities, such as the pollybeak and the columella retraction deformity, do not always indicate a substandard technique and may arise from tissue loss as the result, for example, of infection. Infections must be treated promptly and with the appropriate antibiotics, either by the operating surgeon or by the patient's GP. It is important to record the treatment in the patient's records, if only to rebut a later legal claim.

The surgical technique is vitally important, not only to achieve a patient's aspirations but also to avoid complaints and litigation. A successful rhinoplasty is a balance between resection and preservation of cartilage. As the nasal skin is simply redraped over the modified cartilage framework, the cartilage left behind is at least as important as what is resected. Excision should generally err on the conservative side as a small excision can result in a significant and adequate change but a large excision can cause an unacceptable deformity, such as excessive bony hump removal.

Many changes that patients may express concern about are normal post-operative appearances and are not the result of negligent surgery. Patients will need reassurance about these changes and regular follow-up. Discharging a dissatisfied patient even though the surgeon knows that the complication is likely to resolve spontaneously may well lead to a complaint, and once this has happened the patient will be much more difficult to satisfy. These complications include particularly those occurring within the first six months after surgery, such as discolouration, loss of tip sensation and oedema. As post-operative oedema settles, irregularities of shape may appear. These may settle spontaneously but may be those that occur in the 10–15% of patients who require revision surgery. This sort of irregularity tends to be minor in size, such as a small ridge or lump on the bridge line, but a patient can become so focused on it that they feel that the deformity is noticeable to every casual observer. In most cases, any revision rhinoplasty should be delayed until at least one year to allow the tissues to mature and soften, giving time for any resolution to occur, making the surgery easier, and giving the surgeon the best chance of rectifying the problem.

More major abnormalities, such as a saddle nose or ski-slope deformity, alar retraction, pollybeak deformity, tip and alar-columella deformities, and pinching of the lateral alar walls, are likely to be due to surgical failure. With any revisional surgery, the patient must be warned that post-operative settling takes much longer after a second operation. The final result may not be seen until a year afterwards.

A saddle nose or ski-slope deformity usually results from over-resection of dorsal bone and cartilage, but can arise after post-operative trauma leading to a septal haematoma or following an abscess, causing loss of septal support. Rarely, a granulomatous or autoimmune disease can be the cause. The treatment requires augmentation, ideally with a cartilaginous autograft. Alloplastic materials may be used as an alternative, but patients must be warned pre-operatively of the risks of infection and rejection.

Alar retraction is usually caused by excessive excision of cartilage and vestibular skin. The combination of lack of support and contraction causes retraction of the ala. These patients sometimes also get nasal obstruction due to loss of the external valve. Treatment should follow the basic plastic surgical principle of replacement of all parts of the missing tissue, and thus both cartilage and skin will be required. A composite graft, such as from the concha, will be needed and support from the graft will help to keep the external valve patent.

Causes of the pollybeak deformity, or supratip fullness, include both inadequate and excessive resection of dorsal septal cartilage, and excessive lower lateral cartilage excision, leading to loss of tip support. Despite careful surgery, however, some patients still develop a pollybeak deformity. This is commonest in patients with thick skin. Treatment is by correction of the cause with further resection or augmentation with cartilage grafts.

Tip and alar-columella deformities include bossa formation (knob-like protuberances in the region of the domes), pinching of the nasal tip, columella retraction and alar retraction. A bossa occurs after extensive lower lateral cartilage surgery or by leaving sharp or rough edges after cartilage resection. Typically, it is not evident in the early post-operative period but shows up as the swelling settles. It usually requires revision as it is unsightly. Pinching of the lateral alar walls results from over-excision of the lower lateral cartilage. It may be accompanied by collapse of the external nasal valve, causing obstructive symptoms. Cartilage grafting is needed.

Columella retraction is usually due to over-excision and is treated by a composite graft or a cartilage graft.

In a septoplasty, one particular complication is supratip depression. A careful septoplasty technique should avoid this complication but this cosmetic disaster can still occur if a septal abscess develops or the nose sustains significant trauma in the immediate post-operative period. Commonly, however, supratip depression presents because a submucous resection technique has been used and excessive cartilage removed.

A subdermal haematoma can also occur after a septorhinoplasty, collecting underneath the dressings. Such a haematoma may go unnoticed until the external plaster or dressings are removed a week later. If this has occurred then evacuation of the haematoma is required promptly in order to try and ameliorate any adverse cosmetic result.

Pinnaplasty

There are two commonly used techniques in this surgery. One is the anterior cartilage scoring technique as described by Stenstrom. The other is the placing of permanent nonabsorbable sutures to hold the pinna back as described by Mustardé. Whichever technique is used, the patient, and the patient's parents if the patient is a child as is often the case, must be warned of the risk of recurrence of the deformity, what surgery if any will be required to correct such a recurrence, the presence of a post-auricular scar, and the rare but cosmetically disastrous risk of keloid scarring behind the ear.

In both techniques the skin and cartilage are marked with ink. It is important not to use Indian ink as this can leave permanent tattoo marks. Methylene blue is the ink of choice, but Bonney's blue and gentian violet are alternatives.

In the cartilage scoring technique the skin is elevated off the cartilage of the pinna. This can lead to haematoma collection and, subsequently, cauliflower ear deformity. Great care needs to be taken in haemostasis and the application of the dressings to prevent haematoma formation and also to ensure that the dressings do not come off prematurely in the active child. Haemostasis must, however, be achieved carefully as it is very easy to cause a full-thickness burn of the anterior pinna skin with diathermy, causing a permanent and visible scar.

Patients and parents must be warned that constant pain post-operatively, particularly if unilateral, must be reported to the surgeon who will need to remove the dressings to see if a haematoma has developed. If so, the haematoma must be drained to minimize the risk of cartilage necrosis. Once a haematoma has formed and revision surgery has been required, antibiotics should be prescribed as there is the additional risk of infection and this also may lead to permanent deformity of the pinna. Excessively tight bandages or knots from ribbon gauze placed to pull the bandages away from the eyes may cause skin ulceration and are indicative of substandard care.

In the Mustardé technique, there is a significant risk of the sutures either cutting out or becoming undone, leading to a recurrence of the bat ear deformity. In young children the cartilage may be particularly soft and so the Mustardé technique may be unsuitable. The surgeon needs to evaluate each case and decide a technique appropriate to the child.

The advantage of the Stenstrom technique is that it generally gives a good result and the ear is less likely to unfold with a return of the original deformity than in the

Mustardé technique where the recurrence rate is of the order of 15%.

Skin cancer, flaps and grafts

DELAY IN DIAGNOSIS

Despite head and neck skin cancer being one of the most common cancers in this country, cases of delay in diagnosis are unusual. The condition is more common in the elderly and occasionally diagnosis may be delayed in those that suffer from dementia, who live alone and fail to attend their GP. If there has been an administrative error within the NHS and an appointment has not been received, such patients may not seek clarification of the situation about their outpatient appointment until many months have passed.

Occasionally, an amelanotic melanoma is not recognized. It can be thought to be a benign skin lesion and may be excised in a minor surgery procedure by the family doctor or otolaryngologist. This is not a problem if the specimen is sent for histology but occasionally the excised lesion may be discarded and the true nature of the disease not picked up until a recurrence or distant metastasis develops at a later date.

In dealing with skin lesions it has been suggested that a failure to use Mohs technique for surgical excision amounts to substandard care *de facto*. However this is not the case. It is but one technique for treatment of skin cancers. Many hard-pressed histopathology departments are unable to offer the service due to shortages of staff or lack of training. In addition, in many parts of the country the histopathology department is on a different site to where the surgery is undertaken. In these circumstances it is not practicable to rush specimens by taxi from one hospital to another. Finally, there are certain parts of the face in which the technique would be inappropriate, such as the inner surface of the nasal vestibule.

Excision of the lesion with frozen section monitoring of the margins of excision is a widely used technique that is an acceptable alternative to Mohs surgery. If this is not available then excision with clinically adequate margins and repair with a skin graft rather than a flap can be carried out, the graft being removed and replaced by a flap at a later stage once histological clearance has been given and if the graft is unlikely to give an acceptable cosmetic appearance.

SKIN GRAFTS

If a patient requires a skin graft to repair a defect after trauma or excision of a lesion, appropriate pre-operative warnings must be given. Patients generally think that a skin graft looks the same as normal skin (i.e. there is an invisible mend) but it should be emphasized that this is not the case, that there may be a significant colour, texture or contour mismatch, and that other complications such as hyper- or hypopigmentation and hypertrophy may occur.

Ideally there should be 100% take of a graft. The commonest causes of graft failure are haematoma or seroma formation, infection and shearing of the graft on its bed. Small areas of graft loss should be managed conservatively but large areas may need regrafting. In both situations the scarring is likely to be worse than if there had been normal healing.

Patients should be warned of the slight risk of graft loss and that grafts look very unsightly for several weeks after surgery. Crusting of grafts is extremely common and requires application of moisturising cream. Grafts may change colour as they heal: split grafts from the abdomen, buttocks and thighs may become yellowish, and full thickness grafts may look redder than the surrounding skin.

Split skin graft donor sites should heal within two to three weeks. If when harvesting the graft, too deep a graft is taken, healing will be longer and the eventual scarring more noticeable, particularly as it may become hypertrophic. If a full thickness cut is made whilst taking the graft this should be sutured immediately and the patient told. A linear scar which heals well will leave a scar but when the scar is fully mature 6–12 months after surgery its appearance is not likely to be as bad as might seem initially.

Full thickness grafts should be taken from an area where a good colour match is more likely, such as the postauricular or supraclavicular regions. Unfortunately, even grafts from these areas may not match well or develop hyperpigmentation, a troublesome problem that is very hard to treat. Full thickness donor sites appear as linear scars and can undergo hypertrophy, remain narrow or stretch, all of which a patient should be warned about.

Split thickness skin grafts donor sites also become crusty for the first few months and require moisturizing cream. Milia may appear initially but these stop within a few months. Most donor sites become pale within 6–12 months but occasionally pigmentation or hypopigmentation occurs, particularly in coloured skin. Immature donor sites should be protected from excessive ultraviolet light or else they may pigment or burn.

SKIN FLAPS

A flap is needed rather than a skin graft when repairing an avascular wound, such as in an irradiated area, or to restore more tissue than can be achieved by a graft. The disadvantages of a flap are that an additional wound is made, the secondary defect, with additional scarring, that designing and raising a flap safely is technically demanding and may be got wrong, that flaps can necrose and that a flap can be too bulky, needing revision. Like grafts, the colour of a flap may not match the surrounding skin, but pigmentary changes do not usually occur.

Facelift

There are many potential problems with facelift surgery, ranging from physical complications, such as facial nerve injury and unsatisfactory scarring, to more generalized problems, such as disappointment with the rejuvenating effect of the procedure. The latter may be caused by unrealistic expectations.

The surgeon should ask why a patient wants a facelift, and look for initiating factors that might indicate the potential for dissatisfaction, such as recent occupational or marital stresses. Surgery will not alter a patient's lifestyle and will not cure failing relationships or difficulties at work. The surgical goal should be reasonable. The ideal patient will have been thinking about a facelift for some time and not just for a very short period, will have specific signs of ageing that can be seen, such as jowls or excess baggy skin under the chin, and will understand that surgery will refresh the face rather than make them look younger, particularly not taking 10 years off the appearance. Patients falling outside these groups run a high risk of being disappointed with the result of a facelift and may need to be advised against proceeding.

Patients who are dissatisfied with previous facial rejuvenation surgery, who have fallen out with other surgeons, who have a history of litigation, and who have seen several other surgeons, are very high risk medicolegally. Careful consideration should be given before accepting them for surgery.

As with other forms of facial plastic surgery, the preoperative assessment of the patient is very important. Clinical photographs should be reviewed with the patient so that he or she has a clear indication of what might and, perhaps more importantly, might not be achieved by the proposed surgery. The patient's hairstyle and use of make-up should be noted as these may alter the placement of the incisions.

With increasing age, damage from excessive sun exposure and previous irradiation therapy, the elasticity of the skin, the flap vascularity and the skin's healing ability lessen. This will affect the result of a facelift and may increase the complication rate.

Dark-skinned patients may develop hyperpigmentation post-operatively. Specific questions should be asked about: any previous facial surgery as this will affect the site of incisions; any history of alopecia as this may herald post-operative hair loss; and whether there has been a previous Bell's palsy as this might recur. Generalized medical problems should also be enquired about, such as hypertension or other cardiovascular problems, chronic obstructive airways disease, diabetes and coagulation disorders, including anticoagulant therapy and the taking of aspirin or similar drugs that can lead to post-operative bleeding. Cigarette smoking is a relative contraindication for surgery because of the high risk of flap necrosis, particularly in the post-auricular region, and smokers should stop for at least two weeks pre-operatively.

Each part of a facelift operation has its own risks and these must be explained to the patient. Care must be taken over the amount of local anaesthetic that is infiltrated to reduce bleeding, particularly if extensive neck procedures are being performed. The maximum dose of lignocaine and/or adrenaline must not be exceeded, and care must be taken for the injections to be in the right plane to avoid injury to the frontal and marginal mandibular nerves.

Correct placement of the incision is important as incorrect siting may lead to a complaint about unsightly or particularly visible scarring, pulling forward of the tragus to expose the external auditory meatus, or an abnormal shape of the earlobes. The incisions should be hidden within the hair as far as possible and must be made parallel to the direction of the hair follicles to prevent post-operative hair loss.

Flap elevation is in the superficial subcutaneous plane to achieve a thin flap but to retain the viability of the sub-dermal-dermal plexus. Haemostasis must be meticulous to prevent haematoma formation. The flap must be a consistent thickness or else post-operative irregularities in the contour will be visible. Special care when elevating the flap is needed to protect the frontal and mandibular branches of the facial nerve and the greater auricular nerve, the latter causing permanent numbness of the pinna. Dissection of the superficial musculo-aponeurotic system (SMAS) puts the facial nerve at risk, and SMAS plication may injure the buccal nerve or the parotid gland with the risk of a parotid fistula.

Draping of the skin flap after SMAS plication must be carried out with care as excessive posterior tension or failure to rotate the flap will give an unsatisfactory appearance. Excess tension near the tragus may pull it forward.

If liposuction is performed at the same time as a facelift, it is important to achieve a smooth result. The port of the liposuction tube should be held with the port away from the dermis to avoid 'buttonholing' the skin and excessive fat removal.

As with any operation, post-operative complications can occur after a facelift. Prompt and adequate treatment is required to avoid permanent unwanted effects. Haematoma is the commonest early complication. Some are minor and can be aspirated or milked after removal of some sutures but many require drainage. If untreated, at best an inflammatory response occurs leading to soft tissue irregularities, and at worst skin necrosis and infection.

Skin flap necrosis is not common, except in smokers or if the dressings are applied too tightly. It is best managed expectantly initially, but a large area will require skin grafting when the wound is clean. Careful wound care and, when appropriate, antibiotic therapy is vital. The patient will need much reassurance about the prolonged healing time and the resultant scars.

Facial nerve paralysis occurs in 0.5–3% of patients, most commonly involving the frontal and marginal mandibular branches. Most paralyses resolve spontaneously. Unless an injury is noted at the time of surgery, in which case it should be repaired, nerve injuries should be managed conservatively. Permanent paralysis may require additional surgery, such as an eyebrow lift. Sensory changes, such as hypoaesthesia of the facial skin, are common for several weeks. The greater auricular nerve may be injured. If it is noticed at surgery that the nerve has been divided it should be sutured, but otherwise treatment should be conservative. Permanent numbness will occur and a troublesome neuroma may develop.

Later complications include: hypertrophic scarring, often post-auricular and made worse by haematoma; infection and skin flap necrosis; earlobe distortion from excessive tension, a permanent deformity possibly needing further surgery such as a V-Y plasty; unfavourable hairline changes, alopecia, permanent hair loss occurring in approximately 2–3% of patients, temporary loss with thinning more frequently but with hair regrowth within several weeks; bald scars due to incorrect bevelling of incisions; and hyperpigmentation from bruising or just spontaneous.

Mentoplasty

This is indicated as part of a rhinoplasty or as a separate procedure. A slight increase in projection of the chin is usually carried out with an alloplastic implant, usually Silastic. Projection of more than 1 cm may require a sliding genioplasty. Choosing the correct size and shape to match the shape of the patient's chin is important, particularly the curve of the implant and the length of it as it wraps round the mandible. Excessively long implants may result in the prosthesis being visible or palpable.

The surgical approach can be intra-oral or submental. The intra-oral incision is made in the labial sulcus. In a submental approach the incision must be posterior to the submental crease or else it will become visible as it is pulled forward by the implant. In both approaches a subperiosteal pocket for the implant is then created. Failure to match the size and shape of the implant exactly may lead to movement of the implant later, and great care must be taken not to damage the mental nerves. Other complications include haematoma, seroma and infection. In the long term, implants tend to give rise to some bone resorption.

Malar augmentation

Malar implants can be inserted through an intra-oral, a subciliary or a conjunctival approach. In the intra-oral route, care must be taken to avoid Stensen's duct. In the subciliary incision, a submuscular approach reduces the risk of eyelid retraction. The infraorbital nerve must be preserved. The implant is placed subperiosteally through a periosteal incision placed anterior to the orbital rim to minimize adhesions that might cause ectropion and lower lid contracture. The implant can be sutured in place to minimize the risk of movement out of place.

Eyelid surgery

A full pre-operative assessment for eyelid reduction surgery is very important. This should include assessment of the lid margin for ptosis, differences in the level of and ptosis of the eyebrows, the level of the lid creases, the degree of excess skin and the location and extent of fat pads. Lid laxity should be assessed with the snap test and the pinch test.

Pre-operative photographs are necessary in case there are minor degrees of asymmetry more visible photographically rather than clinically. These may be the cause of a complaint post-operatively if not detected.

Eliciting any pre-operative history of dry eye is very important and lacrimal secretion should be assessed by the Schirmer test if there is doubt. Patients with dry eyes can have a blepharoplasty but artificial tears and ophthalmic lubricants will be needed. Care must be taken to limit the degree of skin excision in both upper and lower eyelids to minimize the risk of intractable dryness.

Patients should be warned pre-operatively about the recognized complications of blepharoplasty, dry eyes, haematoma, globe injury, infection, lagophthalmos and ectropion, the possibility of visual loss, irregularities in healing and the need for secondary surgery in a small percentage of cases.

A post-operative haematoma may be a cause of visual loss. It also delays resolution of periorbital oedema and can lead to subcutaneous haemosiderin deposits that cause pigmentation.

Injuries to the cornea and globe should not occur in blepharoplasty and cannot be defended. Swabs are very abrasive and easily cause corneal abrasions. Instruments should not be passed over the eyes during surgery. Corneal protectors may be used for added security but may distort the shape of the lid. The inadvertent injection of local anaesthetic into the globe can occur. This can cause a selective parasympathetic palsy with a fixed dilated pupil.

Under- or over-resection of the fat pads, particularly on the lower lids, may give a poor cosmetic appearance. Rarely, the lacrimal gland may be injured or even resected, causing dry eye symptoms.

Poor placement of lid scars is difficult to correct. If the upper lid incision goes too far medially, an epicanthal web may develop needing a Z-plasty to correct it. If the upper lid incision is too close to the lid margin or too high, the scar will be visible. Correction is difficult. In the lower lid, the incision should be made close to but not involving the eyelashes or else permanent loss of the lashes will result.

Great care must be taken over the amount of skin that is excised. Lagophthalmos, incomplete upper eyelid closure, is a normal occurrence in the first 48 hours after surgery. It usually resolves spontaneously but a large lagophthalmos (greater than approximately 3 mm), or if it persists, indicates overexcision of upper eyelid skin. If left untreated, dry eye symptoms and corneal exposure occur. The best treatment is replacement of the excised skin, providing that this has been stored in a refrigerator at the time of the operation, as this provides the best match. Ectropion is often due to excessive removal of skin but may be due to other causes such as scar contracture or a lax lid margin. Taping of the lower lid, and if necessary a support stitch, for a few weeks may resolve the problem but permanent ectropion will require skin grafting that will leave additional scars.

Loss of vision is the most feared complication following blepharoplasty. It is very rare but, because it is such a serious complication, all patients considering a blepharoplasty should be warned of the risk of it happening. The mechanism of action is not clear but it may be due to acute elevation of intra-ocular and intra-orbital pressures due to retrobulbar haemorrhage from a bleeding artery retracting into the retrobulbar space. The elevated intra-orbital pressure leads to optic nerve head ischaemia and central retinal artery occlusion. Meticulous haemostasis is the best prevention.

Laser skin resurfacing

Lasers are commonly used for reducing wrinkles around the mouth and eyes, ablating areas of actinic damage and generally 'tightening up' the skin due to elastosis. The two lasers used are the pulsed carbon dioxide (CO_2) and the erbium:yttrium-aluminium-garnet (Er:YAG). The CO_2 laser removes 50–100 µm of tissue with each pass of the laser, whereas the Er:YAG laser removes only 25–30 µm of tissue. There is less collateral dermal energy with the latter and adverse effects, such as the risk of scarring, may therefore be less. Pre-operative assessment must include careful assessment of the skin, including photographs. Contraindications to surgery include active acne, recent retinoid treatment and an active herpes lesion.

Post-operative infection, including fungal and viral infections, will cause scarring and must be treated early. Post-operative pigmentation problems are most likely to be troublesome in patients with type IV and type V skin. Patients with black skin should not be treated because of the likelihood of hypopigmentation. All patients will experience some erythema after treatment but more unwelcome complications are persistent hypopigmentation and hyperpigmentation. Hypopigmentation may respond to topical treatment. For several weeks after treatment, exposure to bright sunshine may cause hyperpigmentation.

Rhinophyma

Rhinophyma is a bulbous enlargement of the nose and is caused by hypertrophy of the sebaceous glands, soft tissues and blood vessels of the nasal tip. If large, it can lead to obstruction of the nares. Misdiagnosis by assuming that the bulbousness is due to the underlying nasal cartilage may make the surgeon excise nasal cartilage instead of the soft tissues, leading to an abnormal shape of the nasal tip. Rhinophyma is usually treated by direct excision with a scalpel or by dermabrasion, but laser excision or cryotherapy can be used. Great care must be taken not to excise or dermabrade too deeply or else the area will heal slowly and by secondary intention, leading to unsightly scarring. If the patient develops an infection in the excised area, deepening of the skin loss may occur, leading to additional scarring which the patient may find unacceptable. Full thickness excision of all the rhinophymatous tissue followed by skin grafting has been advocated in the past but this is not considered now to be an acceptable procedure because of the extensive resultant scarring.

OTOLOGY AND NEURO-OTOLOGY

Hearing disorders

DELAYED DIAGNOSIS

Although parents may be convinced that there has been a significant delay in the diagnosis of a child with profound hearing loss, it is often difficult for them to prove this. Often the child will have passed the health visitor screening tests early in life; the claimant may find it difficult to establish that these were improperly undertaken and led to the wrong conclusion. A child may be born with a mild to moderate hearing impairment, which gradually deteriorates.

A delay in diagnosis of meningitis may also account for a claim for profound hearing impairment. In the case of pneumococcal or meningococcal meningitis this may amount to only a matter of hours, and there is often dispute as to whether the signs and symptoms of meningitis were evident at the time when the first doctor missed the diagnosis at the onset of the illness. This is especially so in babies. If not, a case can be defended successfully as there is evidence that the onset of profound deafness is early in the course of the disease, especially in pneumococcal cases. In one case, tuberculous meningitis was misdiagnosed as a viral infection, despite the fact that at the same time the child's mother had just been diagnosed with open tuberculosis. Nobody had linked the presence of the tubercular cough as being a likely source of infection and cause of the baby's ill health.

ESTABLISHING DAMAGES

Even if there is clear evidence from GP records that a child's mother attended on frequent occasions complaining about the child's ability to hear, the mother may have grave difficulties in establishing that the child has been damaged by any delay that may have occurred. The problem becomes more difficult if the child has other developmental abnormalities, particularly if they affect language development. A child in whom the diagnosis is delayed until the age of, say, two-and-a-half years may then be fitted with hearing aids and it is uncertain what deleterious effect the delay brought about. If the child is older and the optimum time for fitting a cochlear implant has been missed, then the prospect of the child developing the ability to understand spoken language and to communicate orally may have been lost. With a trend towards earlier implantation it has become more difficult to argue that diagnostic delay did not bring about adverse consequences.

NEGLIGENT CAUSATION

Profound deafness at birth may arise from a negligent act in the antenatal period. For example, in one case a mother was established as lacking immunity to rubella following the birth of her first child. The hospital failed to arrange a rubella vaccination, as did the GP. A year later the mother attended at nine weeks gestation with her second pregnancy, having just contracted rubella. The GP reassured her that, as it was coming to the end of her first trimester, there was no risk to the foetus of damage from the maternal rubella infection. As a result of this advice, the mother decided not to pursue a termination of the pregnancy, which had been her original intention. The child was born profoundly deaf. Judgement was in the claimant's favour.

DEAFNESS WRONGLY DIAGNOSED

Litigation may also arise due to decisions made on the false assumption that the child has a profound hearing impairment. In the young infant and toddler, a detected hearing loss assessed by brain stem evoked response audiometry may give thresholds in the region of 80 dB. The child may be fitted with hearing aids, and educational decisions based on a hearing difficulty may lead the child to be placed in a school for children with special needs. Such a child may also have a fluctuating conductive hearing loss, due to otitis media with effusion, and the true sensorineural thresholds may only become established when the child reaches the age of 5 or 6. At this point, it may become clear that the hearing impairment is only in the order of 30–40 dB, and that placement in a mainstream school can be considered. The parents of such a child often feel aggrieved.

They may feel that their child is being disadvantaged educationally and attempt to seek compensation. Although the diagnosis in such circumstances of the degree of hearing loss may have been incorrect, it is a challenge for the claimant to establish that alternative management would firstly have been instituted, and secondly would have led to a materially different and improved outcome.

Congenital fixation of the stapes

Rarely, a child may present with a conductive hearing loss and no middle ear effusion or significant past history of middle ear suppuration. This may be misdiagnosed in the older child as otosclerosis and surgery recommended. In these circumstances a range of congenital abnormalities can be present and not be recognized by the inexperienced. When a stapedotomy is attempted, the result is frequently a dead ear secondary to a perilymph 'gusher'. Problems may also arise from attempting to perforate a mobile thin footplate. This happens when the anterior crus is attached to the promontory rather than to the footplate. This abnormality, rather than a fixed footplate, accounts for the conductive loss. Correct management is to either divide the anterior crus alone or else close the ear. It is rare that poor outcomes from stapes surgery in children can be defended. Not only do surgical errors occur, but also often the consent has been inadequate, not taking into account the special problems of such surgery in children. Where a stapedectomy is planned in a child under 10, most experts in the field would expect that high definition CT scans of the cochlear and vestibular aqueducts had been obtained beforehand. Congenital abnormalities of the inner ear are a specific contraindication to such surgery.

Matters become more complex in the case of the adult with congenital fixation of the stapes, as not surprisingly there are often no records from childhood. The past history of childhood hearing loss can be then erroneously ascribed to otitis media with effusion.

Ear syringing

Nearly all of the cases of negligent ear syringing take place in general practice.[2] The first common failure is failure to take an adequate history, asking in particular for previous ear surgery or ear infections with perforation of the eardrum as contraindications to undertaking the procedure.

The advent of the pulsed jet of water produced by a device connected to a simple pump has, in recent times, reduced the number of injuries sustained as a result of faulty bulb or barrel ear syringes disassembling during syringing.

Occasionally, irrigation fluid at the wrong temperature can cause the patient to move suddenly. This can happen either because excessively hot or cold liquid surprises the patient or, more commonly, a marked caloric effect with dizziness causes the patient to become stressed. Rarely, a sudden movement may lead to trauma of the external auditory canal.

Failure to ensure that all the wax has been removed can lead to a soggy mass of wax and dead skin left in the external auditory canal. This almost inevitably leads to an external ear infection and a dissatisfied customer. If the eardrum is perforated through trauma then it is probably wise to give a short course of prophylactic antibiotics to reduce the risks of otitis media. The presence of a perforation of a traumatic type following ear syringing does not automatically imply negligence: a perforation of the eardrum can still happen even if an adequate history has been taken and the procedure was performed competently. This usually happens in those patients who have had a previous perforation in the past, which has healed by a thin two-layer repair. The patient may not be aware that this has happened in the past and consequently have failed to declare the problem. However, a defence is unlikely to be successful if there is clear evidence in the GP's records of a previous acute otitis media that settled following an episode of aural discharge.

Otosclerosis

It should always be remembered that a bilateral conductive audiogram is a common finding in assessing a patient for surgery in otosclerosis. This presents the dilemma of wondering whether it is a true bilateral conductive hearing impairment or whether the phenomenon of central masking has led to the failure to detect a dead ear on one side.[3] In the patient who has had no previous surgery and appears to derive benefit from a single hearing aid worn in either ear, it is reasonable to assume that the patient does have a bilateral conductive hearing impairment. The problem arises in those patients who have had a stapedectomy on one side that has been unsuccessful, in that the hearing has not improved and the audiogram is showing a bilateral conductive hearing impairment. These patients would usually confirm that wearing a hearing aid in the operated ear provides no benefit. However, the only reliable way of determining whether there is inner ear function in both ears is to undertake pre-operative electrocochleography. In one case in which the patient had had several procedures on one ear it was decided that a stapedectomy should be undertaken on the ear that had never had any previous operations because his audiogram showed a bilateral conductive hearing loss. When the patient awoke following this surgery he had no hearing left whatsoever and subsequently had to be managed with a cochlear implant (unpublished data*). Electrocochleography should be seriously considered in those patients, who detect no improvement in hearing from a hearing aid worn in one ear, or where a previous stapes operation has been performed without apparent benefit.

Having established that the patient has a true bilateral conductive hearing impairment then the process of consent for surgery commences. It is important that the patient clearly understands that a hearing aid is a valid and relevant treatment. Once the patient has been counselled of the risks of stapedectomy including loss of hearing, balance dysfunction and tinnitus, the patient should be asked once again whether they are absolutely sure that they do not wish to consider at least a trial of wearing a hearing aid. It should be clearly documented in the notes that the patient has refused to either continue using a hearing aid or is absolutely refusing a hearing aid trial despite counselling.

Stapedotomy is the preferred operation in managing otosclerosis for more than 35 years. Stapedectomy is rarely indicated and is probably only appropriate as a management in certain complications of the stapedotomy operation. There are two basic techniques in stapedotomy: the first is where the fenestra is closed with a vein graft prior to positioning the prosthesis; and the second is where the fenestra is closed directly by the prosthesis itself. Both techniques are still widely practised and, despite the arguments put forward by the proponents of each, both techniques are still acceptable practice.

Complications may arise directly relating to the prosthesis itself. In the type of prosthesis in which the barrel is made of Teflon attached to a piece of wire, there have been incidences of the Teflon barrel becoming detached from the wire during the operation. In one case the Teflon barrel fell through the fenestra into the inner ear. In these circumstances probably the wisest thing to do is to close the fenestra with a vein graft but sadly, in this case, the surgeon attempted to remove the Teflon barrel and the patient subsequently developed a total loss of hearing (unpublished data*).

Litigation may arise post-operatively where a dead ear is the result of either a perilymph fistula or granuloma formation. Prompt diagnosis of a suspected stapedectomy granuloma with urgent exploration of the ear does have a reasonable chance of saving some inner ear function. This can also occur in sudden significant perilymph fistula. However, the patient with the suspected minor perilymph leak that is being treated conservatively is a much more difficult management problem from the point of view of choosing the optimum time for surgery. In many instances it can be reasonably demonstrated that even if surgery had taken place promptly there was still a likelihood that a total loss of hearing would occur. If conservative management is advocated with bed rest then it is essential to monitor the hearing daily and if the sensory thresholds are falling exploration and sealing any perilymph leak is required.

Iatrogenic facial nerve damage

This is a rare complication and is probably sustained as a result of negligence in about 1 in 600–1500 major ear operations. In the author's hospital there have been only two cases of permanent inadvertent iatrogenic facial nerve damage in middle ear surgery over a 20-year period, which gives an approximate incidence of 1 in 2000 cases of middle ear surgery excluding minor procedures, such as ventilation tube insertion and procedures on the external auditory canal (in which there were no palsies). In 1982, Wiet[4] estimated the risk of iatrogenic damage as being 0.6–3.6% in the USA, which is considerably higher than in the UK, but not all cases of iatrogenic damage are due to negligence. It has been reported in operations such as stapedotomy, but is so rare that it was doubtful that even despite the devastating effect that a palsy has, it was not a requirement to warn patients as part of the consenting process. This may no longer be the case in this post-Montgomery era. In the UK in 2016 the patient should be advised about the risks to the facial nerve from cholesteatoma surgery even if the surgeon has evidence from personal audit that it is not a common risk in their hands.

The occurrence of a facial palsy following an ear operation does not *de facto* indicate that a negligent surgical technique has been employed. In cases where the disease has exposed the nerve or where the nerve is covered in granulation tissue as a response to infection, facial palsy can occur despite the fact that all care has been taken. Also in cases where the nerve is found in a congenitally abnormal position[5] and is injured as a result then often a defence can be mounted. However, in these rare situations it is advisable to make detailed records supplemented by verification by another surgeon or photography if at all possible.

There are several common errors made in ear surgery that account for a facial palsy that are usually impossible to defend:[6]

- thermal injury as a result of drilling with inadequate irrigation
- failing to find the nerve in an area of normal anatomy and following it into the area where the pathology lies
- inexperience in recognizing the cardinal anatomical landmarks in a normal temporal bone.

This final situation is most common in trainees and usually occurs when undertaking a cortical mastoidectomy and the descending portion of the nerve is injured.

Injury to the facial nerve is much more common in parotid surgery and also joint replacement surgery on the temporomandibular joint.

Sadly, although the cause of the injury may be defensible, it is all too often that the management of the injury is substandard. The unexpected facial palsy that does not recover in a few hours goes unexplored, even though it is clear from the notes that the surgeon has no idea how the nerve has been injured. When an unexpected facial nerve injury occurs, the wise surgeon seeks guidance from a colleague and the patient is reassured that the injury is being taken seriously. Where neuronography indicates that a serious injury has been sustained, then urgent exploration of the facial nerve with repair is required.[7]

Settlements in the United States for facial nerve damage are much higher than in the UK. Wiet[8] quotes settlements of between US$200 000 and US$1.6m, whereas the largest settlement excluding loss of earnings in the UK is £40 000 (US$62 000). Dr Yeager of the Medical Inter-Insurance Exchange of New Jersey reported that in the 10 years from 1977 to 1987 they settled a total of 79 cases (four were iatrogenic facial palsies) arising from ear surgery.[9]

Nerve monitoring has now become widely available. Facial nerve monitoring has the ability to give the surgeon warning of proximity to the nerve in those cases where the nerve is dehiscent or in an abnormal position. However, such cases are usually defensible anyway. As yet, it is not standard practice to use a nerve monitor in major ear surgery, such as for cholesteatoma. In all the cases of iatrogenic facial nerve palsy that I have opined upon, only one case was the result of surgery by a consultant, with the rest due to operations performed by various grades of trainee or non-consultant career grade doctors. Usually the injury was gross with complete transection of the nerve and one of the circumstances indicated in the records is a failure to identify the major landmarks that indicate the position of the nerve. In the case of a trainee, there was usually no direct supervision. In all cases that are indefensible, adherence to the cardinal rules of mastoid surgery and adequate supervision by a trainer would have prevented the accident. It is debatable that these cases can be prevented by the use of facial nerve monitoring. A large prospective series of monitored mastoid procedures undertaken by trainees would probably be enough to convince the profession or, even better, a randomized controlled trial, but this is unlikely to happen for some time given the UK's track record on multicentre studies of otological surgery. Interestingly the last six cases of iatrogenic facial nerve injury that I have opined upon were all fitted with a facial nerve monitor.

Cholesteatoma

DIAGNOSTIC OR TREATMENT DELAY

Delay in diagnosis usually occurs due to a failure of the GP to refer a patient with a chronic aural discharge. Occasionally, particularly in those cases of congenital cholesteatoma with an intact eardrum, a mother may have attended either the GP, and/or the hospital, complaining that their child has a unilateral hearing impairment. It is quite permissible in those children under the age of 8, particularly if the tympanogram is abnormal, to wait the usual three months for a middle ear effusion to resolve. If the condition has not resolved, then serious consideration should be given to an examination of the ear under anaesthesia, and if there is any doubt, a CT scan. Plain radiography often gives a clue in these cases, due to the loss of the septae in the air cell system, as well as the cloudiness due to the presence of the cholesteatoma.

Although parents may be aggrieved by the delay in diagnosis, they are usually unable to establish that any additional damage has occurred as a result of the delay, unless there has been an intra-cranial complication.

If patients have been referred and diagnosed and placed on the waiting list for excision of a cholesteatoma, complications such as facial nerve paralysis, meningitis or other intra-cranial sepsis may occur whilst the patient is on the waiting list. In these cases it is rarely possible to prove negligence, as it is difficult for the claimant to establish that the waiting list has been managed such as to amount to providing substandard care. However, whether increased delays to some patient's treatment caused by prioritizing 'long waiting' patients amounts to negligence has not been tried in the courts. Cholesteatomas are often large in children despite a relatively short history and consequently it is probably only a matter of time until there is a challenge to waiting list management arguing that a child with a cholesteatoma should be given priority over an adult who may have waited longer. This may be especially so today as waiting list management is increasingly being taken out of the hands of consultants who know the patients and is being controlled more by hospital managers. As such managers are not medically qualified, there is an argument that the Bolam principle should not apply.

The cornerstone of the argument that is usually advanced in cases that develop intra-cranial complications while on the waiting list is that the patient should have been given priority over routine mastoid surgery. For example, in one case a patient lost all hearing in their only hearing ear while waiting for excision of cholesteatoma in that ear and the consultant and defence argued that all cholesteatomas were potentially life-threatening and as such should be treated in the order that they presented. The claimant argued that the fact he had such poor hearing in the other ear meant that should he lose all hearing in the diseased ear then he was going to have a greater loss than the other patients on the waiting list. The defence also was on Bolam. The case settled out of court in favour of the claimant (unpublished data*).

NEGLIGENT MANAGEMENT

As yet no litigation has arisen as a result of creation of an open cavity. However, patients are becoming increasingly sophisticated in their expectations and demanding of being involved in choices concerning their health, which has been upheld by the Montgomery case.[10] Having an open cavity effectively bars the patient from many jobs and, in particular, from joining the armed forces. In areas where the armed forces are major employers of young men who have little prospect of any other employment, choice of ear operation to eradicate cholesteatoma is important. Patients have been angry to discover that there was a choice of either canal wall up surgery or canal wall down surgery, and had a canal wall up procedure been undertaken there would have been a prospect of passing an army medical. They were angry that an open cavity had been created and as such there was now a considerable restriction on job opportunities. It is only a matter of time until this point is litigated.

Technical errors in performing mastoid surgery are still all too common. In one case, an aural polypectomy was performed that revealed cholesteatoma. Several months later, an atticotomy for cholesteatoma was undertaken on the same ear. Five days following surgery the child was admitted to another hospital with meningism and cerebritis. An exploration of the ear was undertaken by an experienced ear surgeon who found that extensive cholesteatoma still remained. This was despite the operation note for the atticotomy indicating that all cholesteatoma was removed. The case was settled for an interim payment of £15 000 as fortunately, the child had made a full recovery from the brain infection, but should epilepsy subsequently develop then further compensation would be paid.

Ossiculoplasty

Ossicular reconstruction appears to attract remarkably little litigation. This suggests that in everyday practice not that many cases of ossicular reconstruction are being undertaken, or else those that are doing them are not making errors. The key to a satisfied patient is to manage their expectations. The patient with normal hearing in the other ear needs particularly careful handling. In these circumstances, for the patient to appreciate a significant improvement, the operated ear will need to reach within about 20 dB in the important speech frequencies of the other ear for the patient to notice a benefit. Consequently, if there is a significant sensorineural component on the side with the conductive loss, it may be impossible to give the patient a noticeable hearing benefit. To offer ossicular surgery in these circumstances would generally be considered substandard care. Fortunately, litigation in these circumstances is rare as even if the operation is successful all the patient feels is that the operation did not work. It usually requires a loss of amenity for the patient to seek redress, such as the development of chronic discharge, pain, tinnitus or altered taste sensation.

Rarely, serious damage can occur during ossicular surgery. This has included gluing an instrument to the stapes with histoacryl glue with accidental removal of the stapes on removal of the instrument.

Recently two cases have occurred where a prosthesis with a shoe that rests on the footplate has given trouble. In this design there is a central wire core to the prosthesis. This wire has gone through the shoe and penetrated the footplate causing a perilymph leak.

Sudden sensorineural deafness

From time to time, a patient will attempt to litigate following a sudden loss of hearing. This usually arises when the patient presents to a specialty other than ENT, such as general practice or orthopaedics. Examples include patients told by their GPs that they had colds with middle ear effusion, although they had no cold symptoms, and patients awaking from non-otological surgery with total hearing loss in one ear. Cases that subsequently litigate have usually been told to consult their GP. There can be trouble if they are subsequently told that prompt treatment with a vasodilator or steroids would have restored their hearing. These cases can usually be defended as there is no evidence that any therapy is effective in acute sudden sensorineural deafness apart from acyclovir in herpetic infection and perhaps steroids in acute autoimmune cochleitis and tertiary syphilis.

Dizziness

Failure to diagnose a cause of dizziness can lead to litigation, but the likelihood of success usually depends on the final diagnosis. Vestibular schwannoma appears to be the number one disorder for which the public will attempt litigation if diagnosis has been delayed. However, cases are rarely successful due to the slow growth rates of the tumour and difficulties in establishing that any damage has been caused by the delay. It is in those disorders where there is an effective, reliable treatment that litigation is likely to be successful.

A good example is provided by the failure in one case to diagnose bilateral labyrinthine failure in a young professional. The patient attended her GP with acute rotatory vertigo and was seen by her local ENT surgeon. Following a history, and a brief clinical examination with audiometry and a magnetic resonance scan, the surgeon diagnosed acute vestibular neuronitis and reassured the patient that she would get better. Six months later the patient was still off work despite having seen her local physiotherapist. The patient then went privately to see another ENT surgeon with a special interest in balance dysfunction. By the end of a half-hour consultation that impressed the patient, the surgeon diagnosed bilateral vestibular failure, which was confirmed by caloric tests, and instituted Herdman exercises. The patient was back to work within six weeks and felt considerably better. She litigated for the six months' loss of salary and brought a complaint against the original specialist through the NHS complaints procedure (unpublished data*).

Benign paroxysmal positional vertigo is another disorder that if missed may lead to a prolonged period off work but there has not yet been litigation for failure to diagnose and treat this condition as far as I am aware.

Dizziness can be the presenting symptom for a number of serious conditions. Failing to be suspicious of cardiac causes and undertaking a basic examination in a patient presenting with dizziness can lead to allegations of negligence. Checking someone's pulse will detect arrhythmia and heart block. Failing to identify such serious disorders will depend on the circumstances and the symptoms complained of but could lead to litigation. Similarly, failing to diagnose and act on severe untreated hypertension or marked hypotension can lead to a successful claim.

Menière's disease

Failure to diagnose Menière's disease is unlikely to succeed as the patient would have to establish that they would have been successfully treated within the time frame of the delay. Litigation therefore tends to arise because of side effects of the treatment that the patient was not expecting.

SACCUS DECOMPRESSION SURGERY

The structures that are at risk of damage in this procedure are the facial nerve, posterior semicircular canal, the dura and the lateral venous sinus. Damage to the facial nerve or the posterior semicircular canal is usually indefensible unless the nerve is in a congenitally abnormal position. Opening the dura with cerebrospinal fluid leak is an inherent risk of many of the advocated procedures on the sac, such as excision, insertion of a valve, and so on, and so a defence can often be mounted. In one case the lateral sinus was injured and led to major complications. During the procedure a cutting burr opened the sinus. The surgeon chose not to repair the sinus but to pack it. Before doing this he chose not to refer to the scans that had been done to exclude a vestibular schwannoma. Following the procedure, the patient developed bilateral VI nerve palsies and chronic headache due to packing of the only lateral sinus, as there was a congenital absence on the other side. This may be seen as incredibly bad luck, but it is a complication that could have been foreseen and prevented by the simple measure of having the scans in the theatre and checking them before deciding on how to manage the complication (unpublished data*).

The unusual

Occasionally the bizarre turns up. The following are some of those cases that have occurred that could not be foreseen by most experts in the field of otology.

HYPERSALIVATION

The patient complained of having excessive mucus and saliva at the back of the throat. She was a senior executive in a stressful occupation with an introspective personality. Despite normal sinus radiology the surgeon undertook a range of sinus procedures including washouts and intranasal antrostomies, none of which produced any long-term resolution of her symptoms, which she was beginning to dwell on. He then diagnosed 'hypersalivation', even though the patient was not on any medication known to cause this, and advocated a tympanic neurectomy, which was duly carried out and produced no benefit. He then persuaded her to have a tympanic neurectomy on the other side, which did not help either. At this point, the patient sought a second opinion.

SHAM SURGERY

A patient with Menière's disease attended an otologist privately and after a consultation and discussion it was agreed that a saccus decompression should take place. After the operation the patient was no better and thus sought a second opinion. On this occasion, a computed tomography scan was undertaken as part of the investigations, which revealed that no saccus decompression operation could have taken place as the mastoid air cell system was present and normal. The patient had not received the operation for which she had paid and, as such, had been defrauded. The patient chose to treat this as a criminal matter and reported it to the police who subsequently took action against the doctor concerned. It is essential when billing a patient that they are billed for exactly what they received.

Causation of loss of hearing

From time to time, expert opinion is sought on the matter of causation of deafness, where the alleged injury has been perpetrated by a doctor from another specialty. There are some areas of practice in which this happens again and again.

FAILURE TO DIAGNOSE MENINGITIS

Usually the doctor involved is a paediatrician, accident and emergency specialist or GP. In most circumstances, the date and time when the disease should have been diagnosed can be established with some certainty. It is usually easier to express an opinion if the infecting organism is known. Placing the hearing loss in the context of other neurological damage is much more difficult. In other words, it may be possible to state with some conviction that hearing would have been saved, but it is much more difficult in some cases to assert that the interpretation of sound would have been normal, especially if it is likely that other central neurological damage would have occurred. In expressing an opinion on such matters, it is useful to discuss the hearing loss and neurological damage with a neurologist. This is particularly important if requested to give an opinion on the management of the claimant's current condition with a cochlear implant and the claimant also has a severe neurological deficit.

OTOTOXICITY

It is unusual for the claimant to allege that the negligence occurred at the hands of an otolaryngologist, but from time to time indiscriminate use of ototoxic ear drops are accused of causing deafness. Establishing causation can be difficult. First, it may be claimed that the deafness has occurred because of chronic suppuration. Second, there is nothing in the medical literature that establishes beyond doubt that topical ear drops are ototoxic when used in short courses. Third, it may be argued that when used to treat Menière's disease, buffered gentamicin does cause deafness and the literature gives many accounts of this; however, the counter-argument is that topical gentamicin ear drops are not buffered and therefore do not act in the same way as buffered gentamicin. Nevertheless, where a patient has been using ototoxic ear drops in the presence of a perforation or mastoid cavity on a daily basis for many months or years contrary to the advice in standard texts, it is a real possibility that having heard the scientific argument a judge will give the benefit of the doubt to the claimant.

Ototoxicity is much more common where the drug has been administered parenterally. Consequently, where the drug is an aminoglycoside, knowledge of renal function and inspection of the drug charts and any blood levels usually makes it clear at what point the ototoxic deafness occurred. Rarely, the doses and drug levels appear to be within the therapeutic range, yet there appears to be no other explanation for the deafness occurring other than ototoxicity. In these circumstances the possibility of synergy between drugs causing an ototoxic effect has to be considered. Common synergistic combinations are furosemide and/or vancomycin with an aminoglycoside. Also a rare genetic predisposition to ototoxic effects of aminoglycosides could explain deafness where drugs have been used within recognized therapeutic parameters. Opinion from a clinical pharmacologist may be valuable in trying to determine the possible cause of the claimant's deafness.

Dermatological products containing steroid and aminoglycoside may cause sensorineural deafness after prolonged usage on inflamed skin. Any patient presenting with symmetrical deafness should be asked about usage of skin preparations. A typical situation may be prolonged usage of Betnovate® with neomycin to manage generalized eczema. The patient should be advised of the possible cause and, after excluding other causes, it is reasonable to attribute the hearing loss to the obvious. As usage has been prolonged, often over many years, it is much more difficult to advise the court at what point the hearing loss started as opposed to when the claimant noticed a problem. The easiest way may be to quantify the hearing loss and then divide it by the number of years over which the product was used. However, this may not be fair as the history of usage of the product is not likely to indicate even consumption but variation as the underlying skin disorder waxes and wanes.

The court, however, needs a practical solution, which may often be reached following discussion with the expert for the other side. Both experts need to demonstrate that they have considered all reasonable ways of calculating the onset of the hearing loss and why they have discarded some methods in favour of another.

POST-SURGICAL LOSS OF HEARING

Very rarely, sudden sensorineural deafness can occur as a result of surgery in the posterior cranial fossa. The otologist may be asked to give an opinion as to the likely cause. This may be a 'fishing expedition' on behalf of the claimant by their lawyers. Any operation in the posterior cranial fossa can cause deafness. The cause may be obvious, such as vestibular schwannoma surgery or a meningioma involving the VIIth and VIIIth nerve. On the other hand, it may be something unrelated to the VIIIth nerve such as a microvascular decompression of the Vth nerve for trigeminal neuralgia or VIIth nerve for hemifacial spasm. The cause of the deafness is frequently not clear. Each case has to be considered individually but in most cases the answer comes down to vasospasm, embolism, thrombosis, dividing the blood supply or venous drainage surgically, or cutting the VIIIth nerve.

Embolism causing deafness is rare but it occurs most commonly on heart bypass surgery and following major limb injury when it is believed to be fat embolism in the presence of a right to left cardiac shunt, say through an atrial septal defect.

PAEDIATRIC OTOLARYNGOLOGY

Tonsillectomy and adenoidectomy

DENTAL DAMAGE

Most anaesthetists will advise that loose milk teeth are removed prior to surgery and consequently inhalation of a milk tooth is unusual. Occasionally, secondary dentition can get chipped in the older child or adult. Many hospitals now have speedy internal access to dental services to effect a repair, which often forestalls litigation.

CONSENT AND BLEEDING

One of the commonest sources of complaint revolves around post-operative haemorrhage. Many parents when they are giving consent do not grasp that a haemorrhage can be large, require a blood transfusion and even become life-threatening. Most parents will acknowledge that they were warned that bleeding could occur, but most do not have in their mind a collapsed, shocked child with a young doctor desperately trying to get venous access – or even worse, medical and nursing staff showing signs of panic as they realize they are losing control of the situation. Parents who have come through this scenario with their child almost all say that they would not have consented had they known of this risk. Actual haemorrhage rates are between 5% and 10% with severe bleeds happening in approximately 1–2%. A landmark case in October 2004 in the House of Lords[11] now means that it is no longer necessary for the claimant to establish that had they known of the risk they would not have had the surgery; it is just necessary to establish that they would have delayed surgery whilst they sought further advice. This effectively means that it is now essential that every parent be warned of the risk of major haemorrhage and blood transfusion.

Occasionally, the haemorrhage can go unrecognized by nursing staff. This can happen when nursing staff do not follow post-operative instructions on monitoring or, worse, carefully chart a rising pulse in a restless child up to the point that the child has a massive haematemesis or even loses consciousness.

Errors in the resuscitation of the shocked child may be less common now with the introduction of paediatric life support and advanced paediatric life support training courses.

POOR SURGICAL TECHNIQUE

Diathermy burns in the mouth and on the lips are still produced. Considerable care needs to be taken especially if using diathermy dissecting instruments or scissors as these can cause large burns, particularly on the tongue. It is generally impossible to mount a defence.

Perforation of the palate – deemed to be due to negligent surgery – has been reported with diathermy dissection.

Excessive resection of the soft palate leading to velopharyngeal incompetence can occur. Where these changes in speech and swallowing reverse within a few weeks a defence can usually be mounted. However if the changes due to nasal escape persist beyond two years the loss of soft palate tissue is usually so excessive that a defence is impossible.

Acute epiglottitis

Since the introduction of haemophilus influenzae B (HiB) vaccination, epiglottitis is on the decrease. No child died from epiglottitis in England and Wales in 2013 while there were nine adult deaths, all aged over 45. In the recent past it was failure to diagnose or suspect the condition that would lead to a patient being sent home only to return hours later with grave breathing problems or even to die at home. Not only may it be a failure to recognize clinical symptoms and signs, but also the classical radiographic appearance can go unrecognized, thus leading to an indefensible claim.

Acute airway obstruction is more commonly due to acute laryngotracheobronchitis (ALTB or croup), especially in infants. If an artificial airway is needed this is now best managed by intubation. The anaesthetist may wish to have an ENT surgeon standing by to undertake a tracheotomy should intubation be impossible and the airway become compromised. Emergency tracheotomy in this situation is nowadays extremely rare. If the airway is not quickly secured, brain damage ensues. Whether substandard care is deemed to have occurred will depend on each individual case.

Tracheotomy

Problems with the operation being undertaken as a planned procedure are unusual. Rarely, in very young children a pneumothorax can develop as can injury to the brachiocephalic vein. In the immediate post-operative period, should the tracheostomy tube become dislodged then there can be problems with maintaining the airway. This is why the tube may be sutured to the skin or stay sutures placed on either side of the tracheal incision to help find the opening should the tube be dislodged.

Most litigation relating to tracheotomy surgery can be attributed to complications arising from poor nursing care. Many patients who have tracheotomies have been long-stay patients on intensive care. These patients frequently have chest infections with production of thick secretions. The secretions leading to acute airway obstruction can block the tracheostomy tube. Speedy identification of the problem by close monitoring of the patient usually results in aggressive suction of the airway with saline lavage or bronchoscopy with lavage if necessary. If this does not cause a rapid relief of the problem, the tracheostomy tube can be removed altogether. Unfortunately problems arise on general wards where the nursing staff may have many patients to look after and are unfamiliar with tracheostomy care. Ward nurses on ENT and neurosurgery wards are often experienced in nursing tracheotomies patients but this cannot be said for the other wards. The timid nurse is often frightened to introduce a suction catheter deep into the lungs. In fact it is failing to pass the catheter right through the tube into the trachea that leads to the deep part of the tube obstructing with dried secretions. Also, these nurses may not have been trained to undertake bronchial lavage to loosen secretions and so bronchial plugging happens, which reduces the patient's oxygenation.

When the patient's airway obstructs, speedy removal of the 'inner' tube and aggressive suction is required. If there is no inner tube then rapid removal of the whole tracheostomy tube and insertion of a clean tube is required. The tracheotomy tube is then connected to an Ambu-bag for inflation of the lungs. Despite the obvious fact that the tracheotomy was undertaken for obstruction to the airway above the stoma, there have been cases where the nursing staff attempted ventilation via the mouth with a facemask and ignored the tracheostomy. It was only when the cardiac arrest team arrived that the blocked tracheostomy was dealt with, but by then severe brain damage had been sustained.

Foreign bodies

THE EAR

The safest way to deal with a foreign body in the ear of a small child is under a general anaesthetic. Attempts to remove a foreign body from the ear without a general anaesthetic by syringing or the use of a strong electromagnet are often successful and carry a low risk of injury. However, instrumentation of the ear in a fractious child can lead to serious injury; such an action can only rarely be defended. Fortunately the injury is usually just limited to laceration of meatal skin, but perforation of the eardrum, ossicular injury and even complete avulsion of the stapes has occurred.

THE NOSE

Failure to diagnose a foreign body is a common cause of complaint and even litigation. The presence of a unilateral or even bilateral foul nasal discharge, which does not settle, should alert the otolaryngologist to the possibility of a foreign body in the nose in a child. In most cases the mother has attended on several occasions at the GP, the accident and emergency department and the ear, nose and throat department where a junior doctor has failed to realize the significance of the problem.

It is a common practice to wrap the small child in a blanket, then to remove the foreign body. However, if this method is employed, it is vital that all care is taken to avoid injury and the practice should not be used on those at risk of atlanto-axial subluxation. Injury occurring in these circumstances is difficult to defend when it could be argued that a general anaesthetic carries less risk.

THE OESOPHAGUS

Problems usually only arise with sharp foreign bodies. The main risk is of perforation but often this can be defended with a sharp foreign body. However, litigation is more likely to arise when there is a delay in recognizing the perforation or inappropriate management once recognized.

THE AIRWAY

Occasionally an inert foreign body can be present for some time before it is recognized. Complaint usually only arises when a significant symptom such as stridor is ignored and then subsequently it is found to have been due to a foreign body.

An unjustifiable delay in undertaking an examination where a foreign body has been inhaled may lead to problems. Any history of a suspected inhaled foreign body accompanied by a severe bout of coughing or noisy breathing mandates an examination of the airway and bronchoscopy. This is especially so when the foreign body is of a vegetable material such as a peanut. The delay can lead to swelling of the peanut with subsequent obstruction to that lung segment and bronchiectasis or lung abscess.

It should always be remembered that a normal chest radiograph does not exclude a foreign body and is not a defence against neglecting to undertake a bronchoscopy.

BUTTON BATTERIES

These modern foreign bodies can cause considerable damage if left in place for any length of time. If they are left in place in the nose or oesophagus they cause caustic burns with marked swelling and a risk of subsequent stenosis. Litigation may arise if a child is not treated as an emergency but is left until the next available routine list.

IATROGENIC FOREIGN BODIES

My experience of this includes a nasal splint retained for 17 years, a guidewire left in the airway for several weeks after a percutaneous tracheotomy and swabs left in the airway after adenoidectomy.

Cervical lymphadenopathy

Once a patient presents with a neck lump, delay in referral is rare. When it occurs it is nearly always in young adults or children.

Once a patient is referred there can be a preoccupation with investigating for cancer rather than on some of the more esoteric conditions such as infections, for example tuberculosis and cat scratch fever. History taking may be inadequate so that exposure to an infection is missed and investigations are not considered. Fortunately, investigating for cancer does usually bring to light the alternative diagnosis.

Surgery may be considered to establish a histological diagnosis in persistent cervical adenopathy. Trauma to the accessory nerve with resultant shoulder drop can arise as a result of dissection in the posterior triangle. Patients need to be explicitly warned of this risk and its consequences prior to surgery. Ultrasound imaging may avoid the need for surgery in some neck masses. Proper surgical technique will avoid injury to the accessory nerve. Firstly it is usually best to undertake the open biopsy under a general anaesthetic without muscle relaxant or infiltration of local anaesthetic. The accessory nerve should be found in an area of normal anatomy and traced towards the node that is being biopsied. Traction should be used judiciously and use of the diathermy kept to a minimum and always where the tissue being cauterized is seen. On completion of the surgery it is well worthwhile assessing accessory nerve function and recording it.

If an injury to the nerve is identified then it should be thoroughly assessed. If neuronography suggests a major lesion then exploration of the nerve should be undertaken and a repair effected if necessary. If a lesion is detected after some months then EMG evaluation can be useful to predict likely recovery or to indicate a major lesion. Discussion can then take place on the pros can cons of late exploration of the injured nerve.

Salivary gland tumours and congenital anomalies in children

This is a complex group of disorders. Claims usually arise because of delay in diagnosis or facial paralysis. Adverse outcomes occur especially where a surgeon is persuaded to manage a condition that he has little or no experience of rather than insisting the child is seen in a tertiary referral centre.

Epistaxis

In children, the commonest site for repeated epistaxis is the nasal septum. Cautery with silver nitrate is still commonly practised. This rarely causes a problem, but excessive use on both sides of the nasal septum at the same time can lead to a septal perforation. This can also occur when hot wire cautery is used. In occasional circumstances, a severe vestibulitis following the cautery may be a significant contributory factor. Usually, such a complication cannot be defended.

Trichloroacetic acid is rarely used nowadays in the UK to cauterize the nasal septum. However it is now more commonly seen being used as a chemical peel agent in facial plastic surgery. This needs to be handled very carefully as if too much or the wrong concentration is applied it can run on to the upper lip and cause a permanent scar.

Complicated sinusitis

The usual practice is to treat the frontal and ethmoidal sinusitis with decongestants and antibiotics, which is often successful. However, if there is a failure to respond or there is evidence of infection spread beyond the sinus, then drainage of the sinus is required. Failure to recognize that the infection beyond the sinus can lead to orbital abscess and intra-cranial infection. Within the hospital setting, spread of the infection should be recognized within 24 hours of the first signs or symptoms of this complication developing.

If the infection spreads beyond the frontal sinus, then infection of the bony walls of the sinus can be inferred, as well as thrombosis of the venous channels through the bone. This infection is difficult to eradicate and requires prolonged use of antibiotics in the order of 8–12 weeks. When a patient presents with marked swelling of the soft tissues of the forehead, perhaps with a subperiosteal abscess, there may be an initial settling of the symptoms with a two-week course of antibiotics. The dramatic improvement in the patient's condition may lull either doctor and/or patient into a false sense of security and the antibiotic course is terminated as a result. Then, weeks later, the features of chronic osteomyelitis develop or even secondary intra-cranial sepsis. It is indefensible not to give a prolonged course of antibiotics where there is a significant risk of osteomyelitis.[12]

Atlanto-axial instability

Children with trisomy 21 (Down syndrome) have a high risk of atlanto-axial instability. This can result in excessive movement of the odontoid process during anaesthesia, such as to cause pressure on the spinal cord and neurological dysfunction, including permanent tetraplegia. It is often the anaesthetist who is blamed, especially if the induction has been fraught and the parent was present. However, it is more likely that it is the surgeon and the theatre team who cause this event by over-vigorous movement of the head while the child is hypotonic under the anaesthetic, often with muscle relaxants. High-risk children should be assumed to have the disorder. The practice of ordering routine plain radiographs of the cervical spine prior to surgery on Down syndrome children is outdated and no longer appropriate. It is more important to ensure that all theatre personnel move the child's head with extreme care. There is a salutary lesson to be learned with reference to this: a case was brought after a myringoplasty from which the child awoke with a partial tetraparesis. Post-operative radiology indicated that it was a rotational injury probably caused by the surgeon pushing the head away from himself to get a view of the anterior margin of the perforation whilst trying to position the graft. The mother dropped the case when she learned that it was more likely that the surgeon rather than the anaesthetist had caused the injury, as she liked the surgeon and thought he was a kind and caring doctor.

HEAD AND NECK SURGERY

Thyroid surgery

In times gone by it was standard practice to leave a clip remover attached to the end of the bed of any patient that had thyroid surgery so that, should a haemorrhage arise, rather than the patient having an airway obstruction with death or brain damage, they just got a bad scare. I was surprised only this year to have two cases where no clip remover was present. In one the patient died; in the other, by the time the sutures were released the patient had sustained a major brain injury. This should not happen and I would suggest that this misadventure would be a good candidate to join the list of never events.

Recurrent laryngeal nerve injury remains the mainstay of clinical negligence in thyroid surgery. The key to preventing litigation is to ensure that training covers the techniques of finding the recurrent and superior laryngeal nerves; the key to defending litigation is a good operation note that details how the recurrent laryngeal nerves were identified and protected during the surgery. Monitoring can also be used and can be especially helpful where the gland is grossly enlarged and in supervising trainees. It is extremely unusual to find a claimant who alleges they had no warning of recurrent laryngeal nerve injury and the risk of change of voice; however there appear to be occasions when the risk of bilateral recurrent nerve palsy and its consequences has not been mentioned. It is such a devastating injury that a claimant having surgery for a benign condition has a good chance of persuading the court that they would have postponed surgery or considered an alternative treatment such as radio iodine. In operative cases where the vagus nerves and/or the recurrent laryngeal nerves are at risk it is wise to record vocal cord function found at a pre-operative laryngeal examination as occasionally a patient will be found to have an unrecognized cord palsy.

It is essential that all thyroid specimens are subject to histology. This also goes for thyroglossal cysts as rarely a malignancy may be found.

Acute loss of parathyroid function can occur. In some cases it can even be predicted, such as the risk occurring after removing a functioning parathyroid tumour or after a total thyroidectomy for cancer. It is the unsuspected case that catches out the unwary. As a general rule if both lobes of the thyroid have been disturbed and not necessarily at the same operation then it is wise to monitor calcium function and blood levels at least once in the post-operative period. The same holds true in laryngectomy surgery even if a thyroid lobe with its parathyroids has been preserved.

Submandibular gland surgery

STONES

The main issue with stones is failing to warn of the risk of leaving a stone behind when opening the duct in the floor of the mouth to extract stones. Usually there is a floor of mouth radiograph to compare the extracted stones with. It is also wise to lavage the duct after removing the stones just to wash out any grit that might be present. However, despite these steps, occasionally a stone will be encountered that will not come out easily. If the patient has been duly warned there is rarely a problem. However, if there is a post-operative infection secondary to a retained stone litigation can follow.

SUBMANDIBULECTOMY

If a discrete lump can be felt within the gland then it is malignant until proven otherwise. Fine-needle aspiration cytology can be of particular help when it confirms a malignancy but if it is equivocal or even if a report of a benign condition comes back, the wise surgeon should still treat the gland as potentially containing a cancer. Stones and sialectasis can usually be confirmed radiologically.

It is essential to warn of the risks of marginal mandibular branch of the facial nerve palsy, lingual, and hypoglossal nerve injuries. Anaesthesia of the skin over the gland post-operatively is common.

Some series quote as many as 30% of excisions as being accompanied by a nerve injury with mandibular branch of the facial leading the way with an external excision technique and the lingual with an intra-oral approach.

There are two techniques for managing the marginal mandibular branch of the facial and the technique used should be recorded. In the first technique the lower border of the gland is identified and the capsule incised. The capsule of the gland is left attached to the skin and subcutaneous tissues, in which will be the nerve. The dissection is performed in the subcapsular plane. This is also the quickest technique. The other way is to actually find the retromandibular vein and follow it superiorly to locate the nerve and then dissect the nerve. In this way the nerve is always kept in view and the risks of injury reduced. Care has to be taken to dissect close to the gland in benign cases to reduce the risk of injury to the hypoglossal and lingual nerves on the deep aspect of the gland. Injury to the nerve is not *de facto* evidence of poor surgical technique but to convince a court that the operation was done competently, a good note dealing with how these nerves were protected is important.

Parotid disease

Management of chronic sialadenitis leads to litigation as it is often underestimated by both surgeon and patient. Problems arise when the patient has unrealistic expectations of the surgery. The risk to the facial nerve is extremely high when attempting a total resection of the gland. Opinion is divided as to whether total excision is required of the whole gland. As a general rule if any glandular tissue is left behind there is a risk of further active infection but radical excision of the gland carries high risk of facial nerve injury. The golden rule is always to try and treat conservatively. If a point comes where there is no choice but to operate then it is essential that the patient accepts that they will probably have some degree of loss of facial movement.

Salivary gland fistulae if persistent can lead to allegations of substandard care. It is generally accepted that botulinum toxin injected into the remaining gland is first line treatment. Should this fail, ligation of the fistulous tract is worth a try. In recent times histoacryl glue has been used to block the fistula and the National Institute for Health and Clinical Excellence (NICE) has produced guidance on this technique. Once again litigation can be avoided by managing patient expectations from the outset. It is a risk that should be mentioned at consent and when it occurs the patient needs to understand that they can be troublesome to stop. However, leaving the patient to leak saliva from the incision with only reassurance is unacceptable care.

PAROTID TUMOURS

If the histology of a tumour has not been revealed by a fine-needle aspiration cytology then the lump needs to be excised with a substantial cuff of tissue around it. This is because, should the tumour be malignant or a pleomorphic adenoma, then local recurrence is a real risk and will be difficult to defend. Occasionally a GP will remove a parotid lump, often expecting it to be a benign skin lesion such as a sebaceous cyst, and get a surprise when the histology of a pleomorphic adenoma comes back. If such a patient is referred, the hospital consultant has a choice as to what to recommend to the patient. The choices are radiotherapy, revision superficial parotidectomy or watch and wait. There is no right thing to do and each case has to be weighed up, taking into consideration the size of the specimen removed and the age of the patient. Should the tumour be a low-grade malignancy then total parotidectomy with facial nerve preservation is usually the treatment of choice but all such cases now should be managed through a multidisciplinary team (MDT).

Where a tumour is located hard up against the skull base at the stylomastoid foramen it is substandard to try and locate the main trunk of the facial, as the tumour will for sure have moved the nerve to an abnormal anatomical position. The nerve should always be located in an area of normal anatomy. If the tumour is known to be benign then it best to identify a peripheral branch such as the marginal mandibular branch of the facial nerve and trace it back towards the main trunk and the tumour. This will usually effect a successful excision without a nerve palsy. Where the tumour is malignant then it is best to open the mastoid and identify the descending facial nerve and follow it towards the tumour. This has the advantage that in a low-grade malignancy the nerve can usually be kept intact but if that is not possible grafting is permitted.

With an increasing interest in patient outcomes it is wise for the ENT surgeon to keep a record of all his salivary gland surgery and the outcomes and complications so that he can defend his position if there is any argument about his competency.

Chronic laryngitis

Poor outcomes of surgery lead to litigation especially in the professional voice user. One of the commonest allegations is lack of conservative management in the early course of the condition and going for a surgical option without trying alternatives. In some instances this can be defended, especially where the patient abuses tobacco and alcohol and cancer is suspected. Nevertheless the wise surgeon should explain his reasons for recommending biopsies in the larynx and counsel on any long-term risk to the voice.

The main reason for a poor result is post-operative tethering of the mucosa, often as a consequence of stripping away too much tissue and damaging the underlying vocal ligament.

Another reason for litigation is misdiagnosis or failure to make a diagnosis at all of rare neurological conditions that can affect the voice and larynx. Such conditions include Shy Drager syndrome, laryngeal dystonia, motor neurone disease, neuroferritinopathy and neuroacanthocytosis. These conditions usually present with such a range of symptoms that affect other parts of the body as well as the larynx that they rarely present in an ENT department and when they do the systemic nature of the disorder is usually spotted. In the early stages they can just present with voice and laryngeal symptoms or the ENT surgeon fails to ask about any general symptoms. I have seen a case of delayed diagnosis of Shy Drager syndrome in which the ENT surgeon completely failed to appreciate the significance of the patient's fainting episodes and chronic diarrhoea. She went into a crisis requiring an emergency tracheotomy after six months of progressing problems and subsequently successfully litigated.

DELAY IN DIAGNOSIS

Delays in diagnosing cancer rarely occur in general practice these days. Prompt referral of patients with a greater than six-week history of voice change to the two-week wait clinic is the norm, meaning that more than 90% of patients in the two-week wait clinic do not have cancer. Problems arise when biopsies come back showing dysplasia or just chronic inflammation. Discharge of patients back to the GP or on to speech and language therapy for a course of treatment can only be justified if there are no 'red flag' symptoms suggesting cancer, such as persistent unilateral earache in a normal ear or intractable pain in the throat. A good rule for patients who smoke and/or drink who have symptoms of cancer but a negative biopsy is that they have cancer but just require more in-depth urgent investigation. A three-month wait in a smoker with intractable earache and evidence of laryngitis cannot be justified. Rebiopsy, PET scanning or CT scanning should be seriously considered on receipt of a negative biopsy and tests ordered even before discussion at an MDT.

Rare tumours or common cancers with unusual presentation can be diagnosed late. Examples of these include sarcomas, malignant tumours of blood vessels and locally destructive tumours such as ameloblastoma. There is no doubt that if the patient sees someone inexperienced, such as a young consultant or trainee, then there is an increased risk of delay. In the cases where litigation is successful there has usually been a reluctance on behalf of the managing practitioner to bring the case to a more experienced colleague or to discuss the case at an MDT. In addition there is often a series of errors. Another common error is in the management of the case with an unusual presentation. In such cases, it is important to go back to first principles taught at medical school and take a thorough history followed by detailed examination. If the surgeon does not go back to first principles, important steps that may give key clues to the diagnosis may get missed. Examples include failure to palpate the tongue, transilluminate or auscultate a lump.

Delays in diagnosis have differing consequences. The commonest allegation is that a resection would have been smaller, which may lead to allegations that a different less disfiguring reconstruction would have been used, a prosthesis would have been avoided or neurological deficits would not have occurred.

The next allegation is that surgery would have been avoided and another treatment modality would have been used such as radiotherapy in cancer of the larynx.

Conversely, allegations may include that chemotherapy and side effects such as ototoxicity would have been avoided or that radiotherapy with consequent scarring, stricture formation or xerostomia would have been avoided.

SURGICAL INFECTION

Allegations of substandard surgical technique in the management of head and neck cancer are unusual and mainly revolve around salivary gland and thyroid surgery. Where allegations occur is in the ward management of the post-operative patient. These usually revolve around the management of infection. MRSA (methicillin resistant *Staphylococcal aureus*) infection can lead to the claimant alleging failure to adhere to Trust policies on infection control. Nowadays with the emergence of resistant strains of bacteria there is wisely an increasing reluctance to use antibiotics, especially where wounds are dirty or contaminated, but there is little indication of systemic or spreading infection. Not surprisingly, getting such wounds to heal especially if there are salivary fistulae can take many weeks. Claimants can make allegations that but for the failure of prescribing antibiotics they would have been discharged earlier and with less scarring.

Conversely, allegations arise in the case of hospital-acquired infections (HAI) such as *C. difficile* and their consequences, which would not have occurred but for the injudicious use of antibiotics in the post-operative period. This can be difficult to repudiate if the claimant has been on an antibiotic for weeks with no evidence of review.

BEST CLINICAL PRACTICE

✓ Sudden onset of double vision should never be ignored.
✓ It is wise that both the clinician and the radiologist assess the radiological films, within the clinical context of the patient's disease.
✓ In the field of endoscopic sinus surgery, it is essential to have a complete demonstration of the radiological anatomy by CT scan.
✓ If a lesion deemed benign on cytology does not appear to be behaving clinically as such, rebiopsy should be undertaken speedily.
✓ In the case of simple, benign, nasal polyposis, there is rarely any defence for not discussing the possibility of a course of oral steroids, with or without antibiotics.
✓ A post-operative saddle nose deformity could, rarely, be due to a failure to recognize and diagnose disorders such as Wegener's granulomatosis or sarcoidosis. In such an event, the appropriate tests to exclude such disorders should be taken.

KEY POINTS

- Ear syringing and stapes surgery are the commonest procedures leading to litigation in otology.
- The only reliable way of determining whether there is inner ear function in both ears is to undertake pre-operative electrocochleography.
- The argument that is usually advanced in cases that develop intra-cranial complications while on the waiting list is that the patient should have been given priority over routine mastoid surgery. Disease in the other ear with hearing loss is usually given as the reason for priority.
- Cases of failure to treat sudden deafness can usually be defended as there is no evidence that any therapy is effective except acyclovir in herpetic infection.
- Establishing that sensorineural deafness is caused by ototoxic ear drops can be difficult.
- Wegener's granulomatosis is a condition that regularly goes unrecognized.
- Issues of consent on their own are rare in relation to sinus surgery.
- Where contention may arise is not that the patient was warned of anatomical risks, but that they did not understand the consequences of these risks on their day-to-day life, or that, should such risks occur, secondary complications may supervene.
- Infraorbital nerve neuropraxia in Caldwell-Luc surgery can occur despite all care being taken and does not indicate de facto substandard technique
- A decision not to investigate is probably only best confined to those patients who have such gross comorbidity that no surgeon or anaesthetist would consider them for surgical management.
- Unless progressive sensorineural deafness in a young adult is investigated, cases of treatable disease such as neurofibromatosis will be missed.
- Failure to act on a unilateral sensory neural deafness is rarely defensible.
- Misinterpretation of brainstem-evoked responses can lead to a failure of instigating radiological tests and subsequently a delay in diagnosis of a vestibular schwannoma.
- Failure to diagnose an olfactory groove meningioma usually occurs when there is another plausible explanation for the loss of smell.
- Meningitis is such a devastating disease when it occurs that clearly a degree of risk has to be considered acceptable when undertaking the investigations for a suspected CSF leak.
- In lateral skull base surgery, every surgeon should now give careful consideration as to which lower motor cranial nerves should be monitored.

REFERENCES

1. *Rogers v. Whitaker* [1993] 4 Medical Law Reports 79, High Court of Australia.
2. Hawthorne M, Dingle AF. In: Varian JPW (ed). *Handbook of medicolegal practice*. Oxford: Butterworth Heineman; 1991, p. 166.
3. Rose RM, Rosenblum J. Medicolegal otology. *Am J Otol* 1983; 4: 251–54.
4. Wiet RJ. Iatrogenic facial paralysis. *Otolaryngol Clin N Am* 1982; 15: 773–80.
5. Dew LA, Shelton C. Iatrogenic facial nerve injury: prevalence and predisposing factors. *Ear Nose Throat J* 1996; 75: 724–28.
6. Harner SG, Leonetti JP. Iatrogenic facial paralysis prevention. *Ear Nose Throat J* 1996; 75: 715–19.
7. House J. Iatrogenic facial paralysis. *Ear Nose Throat J* 1996; 75: 720–23.
8. Wiet RJ. The legal aspects of surgical facial nerve injury. *Ear Nose Throat J* 1996; 75: 737–38.
9. Yeager HP, Kuehm SL. Ten year experience in otolaryngology medical malpractice claims in New Jersey. *New Jers Med* 1988; 10: 819–23.
10. *Montgomery v. Lanarkshire Health Board*. Available from: www.supremecourt.uk/decided-cases/docs/UKSC_2013_0136_Judgement.pdf
11. *Chester v. Afshar* [2004] Appeal Cases 41, House of Lords.
12. Hawthorne M. Clinical negligence in rhinological surgery. *Clinical Risk* 2003; 9: 44–48.

*This refers to case reports written by the author and court cases attended by and involving the author.

CHAPTER 40

NON-TECHNICAL SKILLS FOR ENT SURGEONS

Simon Paterson-Brown and Stephen R. Ell

Introduction 453	Leadership 460
Behavioural markers 454	The surgical checklist and NOTSS 463
The non-technical skills for surgeons (NOTSS) system 454	Summary 463
Situational awareness (SA) 454	Acknowledgements 463
Decision-making (DM) 457	References 463
Communication and teamwork (C&T) 459	

SEARCH STRATEGY

The information described in this chapter comes directly from the NOTSS project, with details in the reference section. Further details can be found at www.rcsed.ac.uk/professional-support-development-resources/learning-resources.

All tables provided in this chapter are based on those developed in the NOTSS project but adapted for use by ENT surgeons.

INTRODUCTION

Technical skills in ENT surgery relate to the hand-eye coordination that enables the surgeon to move the scalpel or drill exactly, to cut with the correct pressure to a precise depth without injuring adjacent structures; to hold the tissues gently; to create the space to work and to diathermy only the bleeding vessel, keeping collateral damage to a minimum. Technical skills are the craftsmanship of surgery.

Non-technical skills relate to those additional abilities of situational awareness, decision-making, communication and teamwork, and leadership that allow the technical work to proceed efficiently, safely and calmly, and are equivalent, in aviation, to crew resource management skills, which are part of the human factors well known in aviation circles. The influence of these skills in healthcare on both good and poor performance is now well recognized. Surgery is particularly susceptible to complications and these adverse events are much more likely to follow failures in non-technical rather than technical skills.[1] It has been estimated that adverse events, not directly related to the underlying condition, occur in 10–15% of hospital admissions. Half of these occur in surgical patients and around half are avoidable.[2]

Despite the introduction of the World Health Organization (WHO) peri-operative surgical checklist, which reported significant reduction in morbidity and mortality,[3,4] there remains an alarming rate of 'never events'.[5] The problem, until recently, was that the surgical fraternity did not know much about these so-called 'non-technical' skills,[6] what they were and how they could be observed, taught or even assessed. These skills are not new or mysterious behaviours; they represent what the safest and most efficient surgeons do on a consistent basis. In ENT, training in 'theatre behaviour' was given only by example, both good and bad, was incomplete, was random and depended on the awareness and perspective of the training consultant. It is now clear that these skills underpin everything surgeons do, supporting technical and clinical excellence, reducing errors and improving outcomes. In a reply to an anonymous postal survey in South East Scotland, 68 consultant surgeons from all specialties identified 70 skills that they considered important to be a successful surgeon.[7] Only 19 (27%) of these were technical and 22 (31%) clinical; 29 (41%) related to communication, teamwork and the application of knowledge. Problems with decision-making, communication and teamwork have been shown to be related to surgical failure.[8–10]

Following the example of civil aviation and other high risk industries (e.g. offshore oil exploration and nuclear power generation) that have developed training and assessment of non-technical skills,[11] surgery has developed its own 'non-technical skills for surgeons' (NOTSS) that are required in the intra-operative environment to support the surgeon's technical expertise. These were identified in a joint project between

Aberdeen University and the Royal College of Surgeons of Edinburgh,[12] and an associated classification was developed along with good and poor behavioural markers, which can be used to assess surgeons. Several studies have now demonstrated that these are usable, reliable and reproducible, and can be informative for trainee feedback.[12–14]

BEHAVIOURAL MARKERS

Observational methods for identifying and rating non-technical skills in medicine were first developed for anaesthetists,[15] now called anaesthetists' non-technical skills (ANTS). Other studies have explored team factors, which support good surgical performance.[16–18] NOTSS is a system designed 'by surgeons for surgeons' to observe and rate individual surgeons. Subsequent phases of the NOTSS project have used the classification for debriefing trainees after surgery,[12] in surgical simulation, and as a central part of a master-class to train surgeons to observe and rate non-technical skills.[19] NOTSS has also been subject to an independent trial of workplace assessment systems along with procedure-based assessment (PBA) and objective structured assessment of technical skill (OSATS),[20] with encouraging results in the operating room.[21] NOTSS has been adopted by the Royal Australasian College of Surgeons as part of their competence assessment and recommended by the Accreditation Council for General Medical Education (ACGME).[22] A large-scale trial in Japanese hospitals is also underway.[23] A similar system has subsequently been developed for theatre scrub practitioners: scrub practitioners list of intra-operative non-technical skills (SPLINTS).[24]

THE NON-TECHNICAL SKILLS FOR SURGEONS (NOTSS) SYSTEM

The aim of the NOTSS project was to develop a non-technical skills classification, with associated behavioural markers, which could be used in the training and assessment of surgeons during the intra-operative phase of surgery. The resulting NOTSS classification is made up of four main skills categories, each with three levels of associated elements as shown in Table 40.1.

TABLE 40.1 Non-technical surgical skills classification

Skill category	Level	Element
Situational awareness	I	Gathering information
	II	Understanding information
	III	Projecting and anticipating future state
Decision-making	I	Considering options
	II	Selecting and communicating options
	III	Implementing and reviewing decisions
Communication and teamwork	I	Exchanging information
	II	Establishing a shared understanding
	III	Coordinating team activities
Leadership	I	Setting and maintaining standards
	II	Supporting others
	III	Coping with pressure

It is important to understand that this is not about personality, but about observable characteristics within the operative environment. For training purposes, to provide feedback, and to assess surgeons, behaviours associated with each element may be scored as follows:

- **Good** (score 4): Performance of a consistently high standard, enhancing patient safety, which could be used as a positive example for others
- **Acceptable** (score 3): Performance of a satisfactory standard, but could be improved
- **Marginal** (score 2): Performance indicated a cause for concern, considerable improvement is needed
- **Poor** (score 1): Performance endangered, or potentially endangered, patient safety; serious remediation is required.

Sometimes a particular behaviour is not required, or not relevant, in a particular situation. In this case 'Not Applicable' or 'N/A' is recorded. This is not to be used if the behavioural skill is lacking. If the skill is lacking then a score of Poor (score 1) or Marginal (score 2) is recorded.

Although these elements appear distinct, several of the elements may occur at the same time during a particular event. For example, gathering information about a developing, urgent, life-threatening situation, such as worsening stridor, will require good communication, exchanging information about all possible options and potential outcomes, establishing a shared understanding, and leading to a balanced decision on the next best step to take to maintain standards and safety, all the time coping with the stress. Although NOTSS relates to the intra-operative environment, these skills are also important in all aspects of surgical care, on the wards, in the clinics, and when dealing with managerial and secretarial staff. For each category, shown in **Tables 40.2–40.13**, a selection of 'good' and 'poor' behaviours associated with each of the three elements within that category, relevant to ENT surgeons, will be discussed, though the broader picture may be applied to all surgeons. Examples from aviation and industry may be used for comparison or illustration.

SITUATIONAL AWARENESS (SA)

Situational awareness is the ability to develop and maintain a dynamic awareness of the present situation based on fitting together environmental information, understanding its meaning and thinking ahead to what might happen next. Good SA in the operating theatre is essential for all the other non-technical skills and comprises three distinct levels, which may be inferred from the above definition: Level I – gathering information; Level II – interpreting the information, which requires understanding; and Level III – projecting and anticipating future states based on this information.[25]

Level I – gathering information

The information gathered relates to ensuring the safety of both patients (clinical information) and staff (non-clinical information), and forms the foundation of forward

TABLE 40.2 Situational awareness Level I. Gathering information – examples of good and poor behaviours

Good behaviours	Poor behaviours
• Has reviewed patient in the clinic and explained relevance of investigations to surgery: begins consent process • Carries out pre-operative checks of patient notes, especially previous surgery • Ensures that all relevant imaging/investigations are available and have been reviewed in detail, e.g. CT sinuses before FESS • Identifies hazardous anatomy on CT, e.g. sloping skull base (Keros I), Onodi cells; exposed ant. ethmoid artery and optic nerve • Liaises with anaesthetist about comorbidities affecting anaesthetic plan, e.g. hypotension and tolerable blood loss • Monitors staff well-being • Asks anaesthetist for regular updates on e.g. blood loss	• Has not seen the patient before the day of surgery • Doesn't see the patient pre-operatively, but expects the trainee to have done so • Reviews results superficially at the last minute, or does not review them at all • Is unaware of the pressures on the operating theatre staff, e.g. numbers, skill mix, impending urgent cases • Does not listen to the concerns of the anaesthetic team, e.g. about using hypotension during FESS or ear surgery to reduce bleeding in a patient with cardio-vascular disease • Asks theatre staff to read from patient notes during procedure because surgeon has not read notes pre-op. • Fails to review pertinent information collected by the operating theatre team • Ignores the assistant/nurse who may be struggling to assist, or standing for long periods of time, for reasons unknown to the surgeon • Ignores anaesthetic or theatre alarms • Is unaware of patient's allergies

planning to make the surgical procedure as efficient and free of complications as possible. If information is poor or absent, all future planning will suffer. This information may be obvious, or subtle. Obvious information should be noted by all but the most obtuse; subtle information may be observed only by the experienced (e.g. a past history of significant peri-operative bleeding, despite all blood and clotting parameters being normal, may indicate a rare platelet malfunction under certain surgical conditions).

In order to gather information the surgeon needs to be able to manage mental focus. Focus, or level of concentration, may be classified as broad or narrow, external or internal, and the agility to move observational abilities from broad to narrow focus, and vary the intensity of the focus, as the situation demands, is an important skill for situational awareness and other non-technical skills. Managing focus is important in managing fatigue.

A broad external focus, which may be thought of as a relaxed focus with reduced concentration, would best be used when all appears to be going well. This may be thought of as 'scanning the horizon' for signs of trouble, for gathering less critical information, such as the number of medical and nursing staff available and their skill mix with respect to the complexity of an oncoming difficult procedure, and observing any staff health issues, both emotional and physical, that may reduce their resilience under pressure. A narrow external focus, which may be thought of as intense focus, would best be used when absolute concentration is needed for the moment, such as decompressing a facial or an optic nerve, or placing a stapes prosthesis, or carving an incus for a transposition ossiculoplasty. The operating theatre is often a busy and noisy place, but during these moments of intense focus, distractions must be reduced to a minimum, since all the surgeon's senses will be heightened, especially hearing. Background conversation, or music, or both, must be stopped, no doors allowed to slam and telephones switched to silent. All this must be communicated to the surgical team at the WHO pre-op team briefing as a 'critical step', so that all who are present in the operating theatre are prepared for 'silent running' (a maritime term used to describe submarines in stealth mode), and the surgeon is freed from distraction and able to concentrate wholly on the critical task. In aviation this 'silent running' is called 'sterile cockpit', used during take-off and landing, or in an emergency, when non-essential communication or distractions cease, and messages are confirmed by repeating the message back.[26]

Equally, due to the intense concentration of narrow external focus, which is tiring, the surgeon may either miss other information, or miss its importance. This is termed 'inattentional or perceptual blindness'.[27] It is important to recognize the psychological draining effect of prolonged intense concentration and a mid-procedure break is wise, especially during long cases using the microscope. A 5-minute break in a 2–3-hour operation speeds up the procedure significantly. It gives time to review progress, to plan the rest of the operation, to relieve the nurses and to have a hot drink. This broadens the focus, de-stresses the mind and facilitates 'coping with pressure' (*vide infra*), and is why all craftsmen have a tea break. Clearly, the surgeon must focus on the task in hand, but must also realize constantly, perhaps at a subconscious level, that important information might be missed. The most perfectly placed stapes prosthesis would be to no avail if the patient was arresting under the hypotensive anaesthetic. During such an event, even when locked within the high concentration of narrow focus, the surgeon must listen to the theatre environment and secure the operating field as quickly as possible, get away from the patient and hand over control to the anaesthetic team. Even in less dramatic circumstances, such as a disconnected monitor lead, stopping the procedure to reassess the situation and discuss progress with colleagues will help regain Level I situational awareness. In these examples, decision-making and communication and teamwork also play a large part in the NOTSS.

Level II – understanding information

After all the relevant information has been received, the surgeon must understand its significance, which requires training and experience. Inexperienced surgeons may

TABLE 40.3 Situational awareness Level II. Understanding information – examples of good and poor behaviours

Good behaviours	Poor behaviours
• Changes surgical plan in proportion to the patient's condition, when appropriate • Acts according to information gathered from previous investigations • Studies the CT scan and points out important features • Reflects and discusses significance of information with team, e.g. links stridor and tracheomalacia in a child with a trachea-oesophageal fistula (TOF) • Discusses surgical priorities	• Overlooks or ignores important results until hazard encountered peri-op, e.g. history of bleeding • Asks questions that demonstrate a lack of understanding or preparation • Poorly coordinates investigation: essential blood tests done in theatre • Flicks through the CT scan and misses hazardous anatomy • Fails to prepare, e.g. a ventilating bronchoscope for MLTB in a patient with a TOF and tracheomalacia • Reads the summary of the radiologist's report, not the report detail • Discards rather than discusses results that don't 'fit the picture'

be unaware of the significance of certain facts and may not respond, or respond differently, from more experienced surgeons. This process is dynamic, since new information will require processing within the context of established information, and different interpretations may lead to different actions. When interpreting information, it is important that the surgeon avoids 'confirmation bias', whereby ill-fitting information is filtered out, since it does not fit with the surgeon's established view. Yet ill-fitting information may suggest an alternative path and require an unpleasant course of action, which must be faced. This error may be avoided by analyzing all the available information (co-morbidities, blood results and imaging) with the anaesthetic, radiological and surgical teams in their turn, and discussing what actions or precautions are required (e.g. an unusually low or perhaps dehiscent skull base, unreported on the scan, may indicate a surgical hazard).

Level III – projecting and anticipating future state

After receiving and understanding the information available, the surgeon must then anticipate what might happen next and this will help to decide on the best plan of action. Incorrect anticipation can be avoided by discussing possible future situations with colleagues and reviewing alternative strategies. A good example of this would be management of a difficult airway problem in theatre, depending on the urgency. The team briefing would extend the 'critical steps' discussion and include various 'what if' events, such as a failure to intubate, tracheal bleeding after removal of a foreign body or tracheal biopsy, or a peanut splitting in two and blocking each main bronchus. For each potential situation, the surgeon rehearses what they would do and tells the team. Each member of the team can then rehearse what they would do for each situation and three levels of situational awareness repeated until all are content. Although this process improves situational awareness, it relies on good communication and teamwork (see below). In this example, the anaesthetist would plan, with the operating department practitioner (ODP), which methods she might use to intubate and the equipment needed, and define what parameters determine failed intubation, so the surgeon knows when to act. The surgeon would go through, step by step, what facilities need to be ready and in place for a swift tracheostomy: position of the patient, surgical instruments and suction ready and working before intubation is attempted. This rehearsal is especially important when transferring responsibility of the airway between the anaesthetist and the surgeon in paediatric cases using the ventilating bronchoscope, or for peanut recovery, or to prevent both lungs filling with blood after a tracheal biopsy. In aviation, and in the film industry, this process is called 'pre-visualization' and improves situational awareness by predicting difficult or unexpected circumstances. Pre-visualization enables all in the team to plan and to know their role, so the team can act swiftly in a coordinated fashion, should such disasters occur. Making 'pre-visualization' a habit helps prepare for complications with routine surgery too (e.g. excessive bleeding from adeno-tonsillectomy).

TABLE 40.4 Situational awareness Level III. Projecting and anticipating future state – examples of good and poor behaviours

Good behaviours	Poor behaviours
• Has contingency plans for peri-operative complications: requesting required equipment to be available: cerebrospinal fluid (CSF) repair kit, fibrin glue, Floseal® • Keeps anaesthetist informed about procedure progress, e.g. exposed dura or venous sinus, and estimated finish • Verbalizes what may be required later in operation • Anticipates post-op problems: a tracheostomy tube placed in the TOF	• Overconfident attitude and continues with no regard for what may go wrong • Does not discuss potential problems with team • Tells the anaesthetist about excessive bleeding late, or not at all • Fails to anticipate a predictable problem and responds late • Does not plan ahead, assuming 'all will go well', rather than 'all will go ill' • Fails to tell the anaesthetist about potential problems in recovery; tracheomalacia in the presence of a TOF which may require an ITU bed post-operatively • Failing to plan (= planning to fail)

Projecting and anticipating the future state is fluid and dynamic and will change many times during the course of an operation. Surgeons with good situational awareness will regularly stop what they are doing (even if only mentally) to avoid 'inattentional blindness' and reassess how the operation is progressing, asking themselves the question: are we where we expect to be at this time? If not, what needs to be done to get the operation back on track? This will undoubtedly require the ability to collect all the relevant information including non-verbal clues (anaesthetic activity, scrub nurse concerns and monitor warnings), understanding what they all mean and what is likely to occur later. Non-operating observers with a broad focus can often see a problem developing, which operating surgeons would recognize if they were not locked within intense concentration. In this situation, the scrub nurse should be informed and she would look for a safe opportunity to alert the surgeon, allowing action to be taken well before the inevitable 'event' occurs.

DECISION-MAKING (DM)

Decision-making may be defined as the thought process of selecting the best logical choice of an appropriate course of action from the available options. This means considering all the alternatives and weighing the positives and negatives of each option. To be effective, the surgeon must also be able to forecast the outcome of each option and determine which would be best for a particular situation. This skill requires thinking time, which is dependent on the understanding gained through surgical experience and the urgency of the situation. Although experience helps, it does not create expertise, and expertise is not infallible: sometimes the decision made, on the information available at the time, is not the best when viewed leisurely with hindsight.

Although the various types of decision-making have been much studied and written about, the simplest model is that described by Daniel Kahneman[28] in his book *Thinking Fast and Slow*. Fast thinking, also known as *System 1* thinking, is quick, automatic, requires little or no effort, and has no sense of voluntary control. *System 1* decisions, often made in stressful situations, reduce threats and can be both instinctive, such as fear of blood loss, and learned through prolonged practice and experience, such as recognizing the subtle change in pitch of the drill when it touches the *tegmen tympani*: the sound moving away from the rumble and towards the scream as the thin plate of bone vibrates under the touch of the burr; or the glimpse of the whiter bone of the skull base; or the yellow tinge of the *lamina papyracea* during endoscopic sinus surgery. *System 1* thinking may be thought of as intuitive, and instantly tells the experienced surgeon to hold back and proceed cautiously, and is used when the risk is high and time is short; however, it is not always correct. The pallor of the skull base, seen in the distance, may be a simple mucous retention cyst, yet it could be a meningocele, or an encephalocele. In these situations the main consideration is safety; danger is recognized and disaster averted. Fast, *System 1* thinking can also be called *recognition-primed* DM (RPD) and is a type of pattern recognition that experts use to make satisfactory decisions under times of high stress or time-pressure.[29]

Slow thinking, or *System 2* thinking, also termed *analytical* DM, is more familiar and is the type of thinking used to check the validity of a complex logical argument. *System 2* thinking allocates mental processing capacity or focused attention to the effortful analysis of a situation; assessing options, weighing up the pros and cons and deciding on a course of action. Often this produces a better course of action than *System 1* thinking and is used when risk is low and time is available. Clinically, *System 2* thinking would be used to diagnose and treat, for example, a patient with complex balance problems. In theatre, *System 2* thinking would be used to plan the next few steps of an operation, with diversion options in mind if the plan fails, and alternative reconstruction methods if the pathology is not as expected, as used in head and neck surgery, or in otology, for example following a cholesteatoma avoiding dehiscent structures while considering primary or staged hearing reconstruction possibilities.

Analytical DM requires more focused concentration than recognition-primed DM. In times of stress, when an individual's working or short-term memory is overloaded, 'freezing' can occur, which is the inability to make any decision at all. In this situation, someone else can help by taking on some of the mental workload, freeing up working memory and allowing the individual to think about what to do next (see below). One recent study demonstrated that during the intra-operative phase of surgery, surgeons use analytical DM in around 50% of cases.[30]

There is another main form of decision-making, which is *rule-based*, and is somewhere between fast and slow thinking in terms of the working memory required. It is particularly useful in times of stress when 'thinking' is more difficult. It is used by both trainee and expert surgeons and follows the algorithmic process of 'if X occurs then I'll do Y'. This is usually based on well-known guidelines and protocols; for example, when a cerebrospinal fluid leak occurs during sinus surgery, while the fibrin glue is defrosted, the bleeding is stopped, the area is cleaned, fat is harvested and mucosal flaps lifted in preparation for repair. An injured dural sinus during mastoid surgery is covered immediately with a damp swab, the head lowered to prevent air embolus, followed by a muscle graft, or haemostatic gelatin (Floseal®), or occlusive BIPP packing: all these critical events having been discussed at the WHO pre-op team briefing.

For completion, DM that relies on creating brand new solutions in theatre should only be a last resort when the above three methods fail, and, in general, it requires an inordinate amount of time and does not work well. Pre-visualization works better.

There are three elements of decision-making: Level I – considering options; Level II – selecting and communicating options; and Level III – implementing and reviewing decisions.

Level I – Considering options

When the situation is urgent and high risk, and a decision is needed swiftly, there may be only one option. When there is more time and less risk, alternative options may be weighed in the balance.

Level II – Selecting and communicating options

This should progress naturally from considering alternative options, but one option can only be selected if the surgeon appreciates the alternatives. Ignoring valid alternatives ensures an easy decision, but which sometimes is wrong. Telling the team which option has been selected is a 'sense check' and strengthens the team's cohesion.

Level III – Implementing and reviewing decisions

Once a decision has been made and acted upon, reviewing progress should run in parallel to monitor if all is going well, or badly, so that alternative choices can be made in a timely manner; for example, the decision to carve an incus remnant, for a transposition ossiculoplasty, may be abandoned in favour of a prosthesis or a bone chip, if the incus remnant proves to be too small or too crumbly. In this situation the three levels of decision-making are repeated, but this can be done only if the original decision is reviewed.

Situational awareness and decision-making represent the two cognitive non-technical skills in the NOTSS classification: the skills that require 'brain power'. In aviation, these are reduced to the more rapid process of observe; interpret; decide; act (OIDA) and this pattern is followed repeatedly, so the pilot's mind flies 'in front of the aircraft'. Surgeons work in the same way when concerned with patient care, thinking ahead to the next step. The next two non-technical skills are the social skills of communication and teamwork, and leadership.

TABLE 40.5 Decision-making Level I. Considering options – examples of good and poor behaviours

Good behaviours	Poor behaviours
• Weighs the chances of success of primary or staged reconstruction • Considers changing list order for clinical need • Considers autograft versus prosthetic ossicular reconstruction with respect to comorbidities • Considers asking for help if in difficulty • Considers early start to list to prevent late finish • Considers an alternative instrument to do the same manoeuvre • Is open to new options suggested by others	• Reconstructs the same way regardless of the clinical situation • Reconstructs in suboptimal conditions, e.g. myringoplasty in presence of *pseudomonas* infection • Fails to consider changes to list order, e.g. for diabetics, young children, anaesthetist's request • Considers it a failure to request help with a procedure/list • Fails to consider alternatives when new information becomes known • Does not consider any alternative • Insists on a particular instrument when another would work almost as well, e.g. periosteal elevators • Ignores alternative suggestions made by others

TABLE 40.6 Decision-making Level II. Selecting and communicating options – examples of good and poor behaviours

Good behaviours	Poor behaviours
• Tells the team the decision in an urgent situation (*System 1* thinking) • Requests a moment to think when decision is complex (*System 2* thinking) • Verbalizes options, with associated pros and cons • Absorbs information provided by others to refine selected option	• Selects an option but does not tell the team, e.g. decides on an ossicular prosthesis but gives no prior warning • Is unable to make a selection of a technique, an instrument set, or tool, so requests everything • Does not select an option when there are clear alternatives and ignores resources: skill of a colleague, nurse/anaesthetist. • Uses information unrelated to patient care to select an option

TABLE 40.7 Decision-making Level III. Implementing and reviewing decisions – examples of good and poor behaviours

Good behaviours	Poor behaviours
• Makes a decision and sets a timescale for review of progress, e.g. estimates duration of operation and updates anaesthetist peri-operatively • Checks a decision is acceptable, e.g. changes in list order • Reviews the quality of the decisions/work in progress; is flexible	• Does not make a clear decision and continues with no clear direction • Makes a decision and carries on regardless of new information • Ignores poor progress, or the poor outcome of a decision made, when re-evaluation may improve matters • Assumes repair is satisfactory when it could be tested peri-operatively, e.g. ossicular reconstruction or a repaired CSF leak (with an anaesthetic Valsalva)

COMMUNICATION AND TEAMWORK (C&T)

Communication skills, and working as part of a team, are important skills for the surgeon that underpin and link the other non-technical skills of situational awareness, decision-making and leadership. Being able to communicate clearly and succinctly, and hear others' perspectives, ensures the team has a shared understanding of the situation, of the challenge to be faced and the overall objective, so that individuals can complete their tasks by working together effectively. These skills are important throughout the peri-operative period, but particularly so during the WHO pre-op team briefing. Knowing each team member by name improves prompt information exchange and efficient working when under pressure. Communication and teamwork may be divided into three levels: Level I – exchanging information; Level II – establishing a shared understanding; and Level III – coordinating team activities.

Level I – Exchanging information

This is the free exchange of information pertinent to the situation, from all members of the team, and a complete picture is best gained if the atmosphere is easy and unstrained. This is not the didactic surgeon telling the team how it is and who should do what in a bombastic way, brooking no argument. Each member of the team brings a personal understanding of what might be required of them, but not how that might fit in with other members of the team; therefore, individuals tell the rest of the team their thoughts, concerns and impressions, that they feel are important to their role in the team. Clarity is achieved by questions and answers; however, reticent members of the team may need to be 'drawn out' and asked directly if there is anything they would like to say, or ask. Information given by one member of the team may trigger further information or questions from another and sufficient time needs to be allocated for this. All relevant concerns should be shared. Holding back information, or minor concerns, because these are thought to be unimportant, may not be helpful, since a situation may arise when these concerns become highly important. Experienced professionals develop a 'sixth sense' when something is about to go wrong and sensing this may initiate checking emergency equipment, such as additional means of intubation, or that the crash trolley is well stocked and has serviceable defibrillators. This process of exchanging information is necessary to develop a 'shared mental model' of the situation.

The exchange of information is not confined to the WHO pre-op team briefing. It is also a crucial part of the communication between the scrub nurse and the surgeon to avoid misunderstanding and increase efficiency, especially during critical phases of the operation. In aviation, during critical phases of the flight, instructions from Air Traffic Control (ATC) are repeated back to ATC by the pilot, for example take-off and landing. This confirms to ATC that the pilot has received the message correctly. If the pilot makes an error, the word 'correction' is used and the process is repeated. Although this sounds like practising to be a parrot, and seems to be a waste of time, it is the most efficient way to communicate when misunderstanding could be fatal. In surgery, this method is used, especially for critical moments of the procedure, for example, the surgeon requests an instrument by name: 'micro-scissors'. The scrub nurse hands over the instrument and repeats back the name: 'micro-scissors'. If the surgeon initially asks for the wrong instrument, for example, the surgeon says: 'Knife, correction, Beaver Blade', the nurse diverts to the correct instrument and passes this to the surgeon and repeats back: 'Beaver Blade'. This discipline reduces the chances of a wrong instrument being used at a critical moment and is good practice at all times when using sharp instruments.

Level II – Establishing a shared understanding

Once there has been a full exchange of information, each individual has a greater appreciation of the whole situation, its challenges and objectives, and how they, as individuals, might contribute to achieving the objectives by working with other members of the team; how they might help others, and in turn, be helped by others to ensure the work progresses in a coordinated fashion. This is especially important for the surgeon, anaesthetist, scrub nurse and ODP, for example, in the case of an airway emergency when time is of the essence. Prior practice and pre-visualization promotes performance. Once a shared

TABLE 40.8 Communication and teamwork Level I. Exchanging information – examples of good and poor behaviours

Good behaviours	Poor behaviours
• Has a relaxed attitude allowing individuals to speak	• Overconfident attitude and disregards others' concerns
• Asks if anyone has any questions/concerns at the end of the WHO team briefing	• Does not communicate with, or consider the pressures on, the operating theatre staff, e.g. numbers, skill mix.
• Explains need for 'silent running' during times of intense concentration at briefing	• Intimidates colleagues/juniors, allowing no-one else to raise concerns about clinical safety
• Encourages scrub nurse to repeat back instrument names, especially sharp instruments	• Shouts/speaks harshly to theatre staff to be quiet during the procedure
• Is clear about when the operation is paused and control is handed over to the anaesthetic team, e.g. during a cardiac arrest	• Shouts/speaks harshly to scrub nurse because she misheard the name of the instrument requested

TABLE 40.9 Communication and teamwork Level II. Establishing a shared understanding – examples of good and poor behaviours

Good behaviours	Poor behaviours
• Checks everyone understands what needs to be done • Checks that objectives are clear • Pre-visualizes alternative situations and rehearses what each person would do, e.g. in an airway emergency • Communicates clearly to all when the situation has changed, so all understand an alternative route is underway • Re-explains patiently if someone in the team is unsure	• Does not communicate with anaesthetist, especially, e.g. over a shared airway during a laryngeal procedure, or blood pressure control during FESS or ear surgery • Does not ensure all team members are clear what needs to be done if things do not go as planned • Assumes all can tell when things are not going well and ignores the resources and help of the anaesthetic and nursing team • Is intolerant of inexperience

TABLE 40.10 Communication and teamwork Level III. Coordinating the team – examples of good and poor behaviours

Good behaviours	Poor behaviours
• Fits in when other team members lead when appropriate • Coordinates with scrub nurse when setting up, each doing separate things for efficiency, e.g. surgeon sets the endoscope demister, nurse sets the diathermy • Tells the nurse when 'silent running' is needed peri-operatively • An unscrubbed surgeon follows theatre communication etiquette when another surgeon is operating	• Insists on being in command at all times • Positions the patient after towelling up, when it would have been easier to coordinate before • Fails to warn staff of the procedure duration, so staff are unprepared for the next case • A visiting surgeon speaks directly to an operating surgeon without waiting for the scrub nurse to indicate a good time to speak

understanding has been established, potential changes to that situation, causing diversions from the plan, are readily apparent to all and the team can change direction as one with little disturbance to the smooth running of the case.

Level III – Coordinating the team

This is more likely to be successful once Levels I and II have been followed, but coordinating the team does not fall to one person at all times. There will be times when the anaesthetist and ODP coordinate activity, such as transfer of the patient to and from the operating table when the surgeon may act as a helper. During patient positioning, the anaesthetist and ODP help the surgeon. During towelling up, the surgeon and the scrub nurse work together with the anaesthetist to ready the patient for surgery. During times of 'silent running', when the surgeon is in intense concentration and fully occupied, the scrub nurse coordinates the (silent) theatre, but in a medical emergency, such as a cardiac arrest, the anaesthetist takes command. This flexibility of hierarchy, like the Knights of the Round Table, uses the skill mix of the team to maximum effect and is most efficient when teams work together regularly.

Not surprisingly, problems with communication are usually associated with the most adverse events.[8, 10, 31] When communication improves between members of the team, the shared mental model will undoubtedly be better and overall teamwork and performance will benefit.

LEADERSHIP

There are many industrial definitions of leadership, but in the operating theatre the skill of leadership may be considered as: 'a social process of influence that ensures the best work of the theatre team to achieve the objective of safe, high quality patient care', in other words, a successful operation. Leadership skills are essential for the efficient and safe performance of the surgical team and require emotional intelligence.

Leadership is not an inherent part of seniority, associated with fancy titles or domineering or charismatic personal attributes, and it is much more than the ability to command or to realize a vision: it incorporates the ability to earn respect and trust. Respect and trust may be earned by maintaining high standards of clinical care, being considerate to others and being calm under pressure.

During the NOTSS development process, the leadership behaviours were grouped into three elements: Level I – setting and maintaining standards; Level II – supporting others; and Level III – coping with pressure. These social leadership skills were more reliably rated than the cognitive skills in NOTSS.[32] Leadership skills may be divided into those related directly to the *team* and those related to the *task*.[33] There is a degree of overlap between these three levels. For example, by reviewing blood results and scans, and setting up the microscope before an otological procedure in good time, the surgeon sets an example for trainee surgeons, supports the nursing staff by being ready and eases the stress of last minute or peri-operative microscope adjustments.

Level I – Setting and maintaining standards

In theatre, this includes adhering to theatre protocols of sterility, communication and etiquette, and respecting the high standard of care given by the anaesthetist, the nurses

TABLE 40.11 Leadership Level I. Setting and maintaining standards – examples of good and poor behaviours

Good behaviours	Poor behaviours
• Endorses the WHO checklist • Changes gloves/gown when advised sterility has been compromised • Follows theatre etiquette • Allows for inexperienced team members • Respects seniority	• Arrives late, or has to be searched out by theatre staff • Does no pre-op planning, delegates the briefing to a junior • Disregards theatre protocols • Is impatient with inexperienced staff • Does not use facial nerve monitor appropriately when it is available

TABLE 40.12 Leadership Level II. Supporting others – examples of good and poor behaviours

Good behaviours	Poor behaviours
• Supports trainees appropriately for their surgical skill level • Liaises with the anaesthetist and accepts constraints associated with comorbidities • Is approachable, takes heed of staff well-being • Is tactful and discreet when supporting those having a tough time.	• Leaves trainee to 'go solo' with an operation beyond their skill level • Intolerant of anaesthetic constraints, fails to suggest requesting more senior help, if appropriate • Is bullish, unapproachable and intolerant of staff 'excuses' • Is tactless and indiscreet, so is denied knowledge useful for the smooth running of the operating list.

and the ODP. Although the most important person in the theatre is the patient, the surgeon and anaesthetist are close behind: the operating surgeon holding the knife or drill, and the anaesthetist for keeping the patient alive despite, on occasion, the activities of the surgeon. Theatre personnel rely on the surgeon to set an example and also for guidance, for doing the right thing and upholding the culture of safety, for example endorsing the WHO checklist as an important method of preventing errors and maintaining standard of care.

Checklists have been used in aviation for decades and have been honed and refined to prevent basic errors of omission, manage complex technology and free up mental processing capacity (working memory) to focus on the current task. Once the checklist is complete, the surgeon (and pilot) can relax, knowing nothing has been missed, and can concentrate on operative planning.

In the UK, personal attributes of politeness and good manners are respected and rudeness and bad manners are not; however, what is polite in one culture may be considered rude in another and, in certain company, it would be respectful to be culturally aware.

Level II – Supporting others

A team works well because the strength of one team member makes up for the weakness of another. In the operating theatre, all are trained, or are being trained, to the high standards essential for safe patient care. In those being trained, technical and knowledge deficiencies are expected, and they are supported by further training and study to improve deficiencies until the trainee can 'go solo'. Supporting anaesthetic and surgical colleagues in theatre, by being receptive to the anaesthetic constraints of comorbidities, and to the skill needs of trainees, has been written into the traditions of operating theatre culture since surgery began; however, not all traditional surgeons have been receptive, approachable and willing to help secure patient safety by supporting others.

Supporting others in non-technical terms is a social skill, which, for some, can be difficult to master in the cut and thrust of the operating theatre. Not all members of the team are strong at all times, and most will not complain if they are feeling unwell, or are dealing with stressful issues away from the operating theatre. Most people do not allow personal difficulties to interfere with their professional work; they 'keep calm and carry on'. To support those going through a tough time, it is a social skill to be aware that all is not well, yet not to enquire too deeply into personal matters.

An approachable surgeon is more likely to be advised of such a situation, since it is likely that he will adjust his mental model of the team's strengths and weaknesses and ensure the team is able to make allowances and cope with the pressures of the operating list. This becomes important when the team is under pressure and good judgement is required to know how far someone can be pushed without buckling, or if that person needs some time out, or even time off work.

An unapproachable surgeon, insensitive to the needs of others, bullish in manner or both, is unlikely to listen to any excuse for poor work and is likely to be intolerant in the operating theatre, which puts the rest of the team under greater pressure. The work must go on, the operation takes priority and supporting others can be a delicate business and difficult to get right every time. It is also linked with how well the surgeon can cope with the pressure of operating (see below) when she depends on the strength of the team supporting her.

Level III – Coping with stress

Potential stressful situations can be countered before they escalate by making a practice of assessing situational awareness, decision-making, communication and teamwork; however, coping with stress can be difficult and depends on the degree of stress. Forward planning and training can mitigate most stressful situations by having the resources and the ability to deal with the situation.

TABLE 40.13 Leadership Level III. Coping with pressure – examples of good and poor behaviours	
Good behaviours	**Poor behaviours**
• Has pre-assessed the situation and is aware of potential difficulties • Carries out a 'stress assessment' and raises concerns pre-operatively (WHO checklist) • Rehearses dealing with potential complications (pre-visualization) • Forward-plans equipment needs • Calls for help appropriately • Mentally checks I'M SAFE and makes adjustments	• Is unaware of potential difficulties • Is unprepared for the operation and unaware of potential complications • Tackles an operation outside comfort zone without asking for help from a colleague • Is unprepared for an operative complication • Is unable to remain calm under pressure • Blames others for personal failings

Confidence in your technical ability to complete the surgery to a high standard reduces the stress of complex procedures and is learned through focused training. In most theatre lists this is the normal situation. There are, however, technical and non-technical factors that increase the stress, which vary in number and severity. Many small stressors may be equivalent to one big stressor. As a general rule, more than two big stressors are too many and steps need to be taken to reduce the number and severity of the stressors. In the same way that risk is assessed by a risk assessment, it is wise for the operating surgeon to do a 'stress assessment' pre-operatively, even if this is just mentally rehearsing the procedure and dealing with potential peroperative complications. This surgical pre-visualization may be done whist scrubbing up and uses a narrow internal focus (see above). Often this will bring to mind the need for additional equipment, for example, fibrin glue and the Rhoton® neurosurgical micro-dissectors to facilitate the repair of a cerebrospinal fluid (CSF) leak occurring during FESS, which may have been forgotten during the WHO pre-op team briefing.

If a procedure is outside your comfort zone because you supra-specialized (e.g. an otologist tackling a neck stabbing), then swallowing your pride and calling for help from a friendly colleague reduces stress. Your colleague provides more than technical know-how; they also provide support that is emotional, practical, informative (advice) and provides companionship (EPIC), and all these ease the stress significantly.

Sometimes a case is especially tricky and having the support of a well trained, familiar theatre team is essential. Confidence in the nurse's ability to provide the exact instruments in a timely manner ensures a flowing, relaxed procedure, and knowing the anaesthetist and ODP will keep the patient safe, and asleep, during surgery is quite calming. Unfortunately, this is not always so. If the case is complex and high risk, such as a third revision mastoid exploration in an only hearing ear, in which the lateral semi-circular canal, facial nerve and dura are exposed, and the nurse is new to the procedure and has not memorized the instruments, some of which may be missing or damaged, and you are expected to train an inexperienced registrar, and explain the procedure to medical students, and your new anti-hypertensive medication is associated with postural hypotension, there are too many stressors, especially when a peri-operative complication occurs and you are being handed the wrong instruments.

It would be wise to explain, at the team briefing, that this case is complex, delicate and requires your full concentration. Politely request the help of an experienced scrub nurse; ask the registrar or the anaesthetist, or both, to teach the students quietly, outside theatre if possible; request more instruments and a comfortable chair to sit on during the procedure. Warn the theatre staff that there will be episodes of 'silent running' (i.e. when dissecting matrix off the lateral semi-circular canal, facial nerve and dura).

It would be unwise to get deep into the procedure before requesting these things; it would be even wiser to arrange all this before surgery after your assessment of the situation is complete (situational awareness), and perhaps quietly tell a friendly colleague of the situation so your mind benefits from EPIC support, even if this is remote.

A surgeon's ability to cope with stress is also proportional to his well-being and this was alluded to above when mentioning the surgeon's hypertension. A surgeon who is hydrated, fed and rested is more likely to operate more skilfully (and be less stressed and less grumpy) than a dehydrated, hypoglycaemic and tired surgeon. In aviation safety, to check if a pilot is fit to fly, the well-known personal mnemonic: I'M SAFE is used and we can use this in surgery to check if we are fit to operate. This is a quick check-list to cover:

- Illness (Am I well? Is my angina under control?)
- Medication (Are there side effects?)
- Stress (Feuds and performance targets?)
- Alcohol (No alcohol in the bloodstream is the only safe option)
- Fatigue (Enough sleep, well rested?)
- Eating (Had something suitable and nutritious to eat before operating?)

This self-assessment would be an example of broad internal focus (see above).

A responsible surgeon with such insight will know when he is unsafe and, if unsure, will discuss with a trusted colleague. Better this than the patient coming round to discover he is being intubated by the anaesthetist while the ODP bounces on his chest underneath an arc of spurting blood coming from his carotid.

THE SURGICAL CHECKLIST AND NOTSS

As discussed throughout this chapter, the WHO introduced the concept of the 'surgical checklist' in order to provide a final error trap before surgery.[3] In addition to providing a final 'check' before surgery, it has undoubtedly contributed to the improvement of the various non-technical skills required for better team-working in the operating room. *Situational awareness* around the diagnosis and procedure, along with the instruments/equipment required and possible difficulties that may be encountered (projection/anticipation), are all discussed. *Decision-making* is improved by early identification of possible difficulties and *communication* throughout the team is expressed out loud and acknowledged. *Teamwork* has to be improved by the knowledge of all the names of people in the operating room. Good *leadership* can be observed by completing the checklist in the appropriate manner, demonstrating a commitment to patient safety and both recognizing the roles, and supporting other members, of the operating team.

Practising these skills in the day to day running of the operating theatre will ensure they become habitual and instinctive, so that during an urgent surgical emergency the pre-visualized processes can be followed swiftly and smoothly, reducing the likelihood of error.

SUMMARY

This chapter has described those non-technical skills that have been identified by experienced surgeons as being important for safe and successful surgery, recognizing that technical proficiency alone is not enough. These skills are both cognitive and social and can be observed by the demonstration of good and bad behaviours, as outlined in each section of the chapter. As surgeons strive to improve their operative performance, they will need the support of the whole operating team. Only with good non-technical skills will errors and adverse events be reduced and outcomes improved. Now that these skills have been recognized the challenge in the future is to incorporate them into undergraduate teaching as well as post-graduate training and assessment.

KEY POINTS

- Good surgeons have good 'non-technical skills' which support good operative performance and better outcomes for patients.
- These non-technical skills for surgeons (NOTSS) have now been identified as Situational awareness, Decision-making, Communication & Teamwork and Leadership
- Using the NOTSS taxonomy these skills can be observed, assessed, rated and taught.
- Better understanding of these skills will improve overall clinical performance and outcomes for patients with reduced adverse events.

ACKNOWLEDGEMENTS

The authors recognize the enormous work carried out by Dr. Stephen Yule and Prof. Rhona Flin on the NOTSS project along with the support of Aberdeen University, NHS Education Scotland (NES) and the Royal College of Surgeons of Edinburgh.

Further information can be found at: www.rcsed.ac.uk/professional-support-development-resources/learning-resources

REFERENCES

1. Flin R, Mitchell L. *Safer surgery: analysing behaviour in the operating theatre.* Ashgate: Aldershot; 2009.
2. Vincent C, Neale G, Woloshynowych M. Adverse events in British hospitals: preliminary retrospective record review. *BMJ* 2001; **322**: 517–19.
3. Haynes AB, Weiser TG, Berry WR, et al. A surgical safety checklist to reduce morbidity and mortality in a global population. *NEJM* 2009; **360**: 491–99.
4. De Vries EN, Prins HA, Crolla RMPH, et al. Effect of a comprehensive surgical safety system on patient outcomes. *NEJM* 2010; **363**: 1928–37.
5. Stahel PF, Sabel AL, Victoroff MS, et al. Wrong-site and wrong-patient procedures in the universal protocol era (analysis of a prospective database of physician self-reported occurrences). *Arch Surg* 2010; **145**: 978–84.
6. Yule S, Flin R, Paterson-Brown S, Maran N. Non-technical skills for surgeons: a review of the literature. *Surgery* 2006; **139**: 140–49.
7. Baldwin PJ, Paisley AM, Paterson-Brown S. Consultant surgeons' opinions of the skills required of basic surgical trainees. *Brit J Surg* 1999; **86**: 1078–82.
8. Gawande AA, Zinner MJ, Studdert DM, Brennan TA. Analysis of errors reported by surgeons at three teaching hospitals. *Surgery* 2003; **133**: 614–21.
9. Christian CK, Gustafson ML, Roth EM, et al. A prospective study of patient safety in the operating room. *Surgery* 2006; **139**: 159–76.
10. Greenberg CC, Regenbogen SE, Studdert DM. Patterns of communication breakdowns resulting in injury to patients. *J Am Coll Surg* 2007; **204**: 533–40.
11. Flin R, Martin L, Goeters K, et al. The development of the NOTECHS system for evaluating pilots' CRM skills. *Human Factors and Aerospace Safety* 2003; **3**: 95–117.
12. Yule S, Flin R, Paterson-Brown S, et al. Development of a rating system for surgeons' non-technical skills. *Med Educ* 2006; **40**:1098–104.
13. Yule S, Flin R, Maran N, et al. Surgeons' non-technical skills in the operating room: reliability testing of the NOTSS behaviour rating system. *World J Surg* 2006; **32**: 548–56.
14. Yule S, Flin R, Rowley D, et al. Debriefing surgical trainees on non-technical skills (NOTSS). *Cogn Technol Work* 2008; **10**: 265–74.
15. Fletcher GCL, McGeorge P, Flin RH, et al. The role of non-technical skills in anaesthesia: a review of current literature. *Br J Anaes* 2002; **88**: 418–29.
16. Undre S, Sevdalis N, Healey AN, Vincent CA. The Observational Teamwork Assessment for Surgery (OTAS): refinement and application in urological surgery. *World J Surg* 2007; **31**: 1373–81.
17. Dickinson TL, McIntyre RM. A conceptual framework for teamwork measurement. In: Brannick MT, Salas E, Prince C (eds). *Team performance assessment and measurement: theory, methods, and applications*. Series in applied psychology. Mahwah, NJ: Erlbaum Associates Inc; 1997.

18. Mishra A, Catchpole K, McCulloch P. The Oxford NOTECHS system: reliability and validity of a tool for measuring teamwork behaviour in the operating theatre. *QSHC* 2009; **18**: 104–08.
19. Royal College of Surgeons of Edinburgh – see 'courses' at www.rcsed.ac.uk
20. Martin JA, Regehr G, Reznick R, et al. Objective structured assessment of technical skill (OSATS) for surgical residents. *Br J Surg* 1997; **84**: 273–78.
21. Crossley J, Marriott J, Purdie H, Beard J. Prospective observational study to evaluate NOTSS (Non-Technical Skills for Surgeons) for assessing trainees' non-technical performance in the operating theatre. *Br J Surg* 2011; **98**: 1010–20.
22. Swing SR, Clyman SG, Holmboe ES, Williams RG. Advancing resident assessment in graduate medical education. *J Grad Med Educ* 2009; **December**: 278–86.
23. Yule S, Wilkinson G. Test of cultures. *Surgeons News* October 2009.
24. Mitchell L, Flin R, Yule S, et al. Thinking ahead of the surgeon: an interview study to identify scrub practitioners' non-technical skills. *Int J Nurs Stud* 2011; **48**: 818–28.
25. Endsley M, Garland D. *Situation awareness: analysis and measurement*. Mahwah, NJ: LEA; 2000.
26. Wadhera R, Henrickson Parker S, Burkhart H, et al. Is the 'sterile cockpit' concept applicable to cardiovascular surgery critical intervals or critical events? The impact of protocol-driven communication during cardiopulmonary bypass. *J Thorac Cardiovasc Surg* 2010; **139**: 312–19.
27. Simons DJ & Chabris CF. Gorillas in our midst: sustained inattentional blindness for dynamic events. *Perception* 1999; **28**: 1059–74.
28. Kahneman D. *Thinking fast and slow*. London: Penguin; 2011.
29. Klein G. A recognition-primed decision (RPD) model of rapid decision making. In: Klein G, Orasanu J, Calderwood R, Zsambok C (eds). *Decision making in action*. New York: Ablex; 1993.
30. Flin R, Youngson GG, Yule S. How do surgeons make intraoperative decisions? *QSHC* 2007; **16**: 235–39.
31. Lorelei Lingard S, Espin S, Whyte G, et al. Communication failures in the operating room: an observational classification of recurrent types and effects. *QSHC* 2004; **13**: 330–34.
32. Yule S, Rowley D, Flin R, et al. Experience matters: comparing novice and expert ratings of non-technical skills using the NOTSS system. *ANZ J S* 2009; **79**: 154–60.
33. Henrickson Parker S, Yule S, Flin R, McKinley A. Towards a model of surgeons' leadership in the operating room. *BMJ Qual Saf* 2011; **20**: 7, 570–79.

Interpretation and management of data

CHAPTER 41

EPIDEMIOLOGY

Jan H.P. van der Meulen, David A. Lowe and Jonathan M. Fishman

Introduction 465	Choosing the design study 474
What is epidemiology? 466	Concluding remarks 480
'Streams' of epidemiology 466	Acknowledgements 481
The 'anatomy' and 'physiology' of epidemiological research 468	References 481

SEARCH STRATEGY

Data in this chapter may be updated by a PubMed search using the keywords: epidemiology; public health; clinical trials; research; research design; patient outcome assessment; statistics; epidemiological studies; methods; data interpretation; sample size; evidence-based medicine; bias (epidemiology) and confounding factors (epidemiology).

INTRODUCTION

This chapter presents epidemiology as a methodological discipline that provides important principles for clinical and health services research. It introduces the 'determinant-occurrence relationship' as a key epidemiological concept. On the basis of this concept, we will demonstrate how epidemiological methods and techniques can be used to address a wide range of questions. This chapter is intended to inform those who want to read the medical literature and evaluate research evidence. In other words, it has been written especially with the needs of the 'consumers' of research in mind.

We will concentrate on the choice of a study design for different types of research questions with the ultimate aim of developing a study that produces results that are relatively precise (free of random error) and accurate (free of systematic error or bias). An additional consideration is that the study needs to be efficient (affordable in terms of time and money). Strengths and weaknesses of study designs will be discussed as much as possible on the basis of examples related to diseases of the ear, nose and throat.

This chapter is not based on a specific literature search strategy. It amalgamates information and points of view as can be found in major textbooks and reviews of epidemiology, methods of health services research and evidence-based clinical practice.

Example: The indication for tonsillectomy

Simple, but well-designed, epidemiological research can be of great importance for clinical practice. A recent systematic review indicated that the effectiveness of tonsillectomy in adults is uncertain (although modest in children)[1] and in turn, that the indications for tonsillectomy are controversial. Nevertheless, tonsillectomy is one of the commonest surgical procedures carried out in children as well as in adults.

In the 1930s, an estimated 200 000 tonsillectomies were performed annually in England and Wales, a huge number compared to an annual number of approximately 40 000 in the year 2000. In the pre-war period, tonsillectomy had become popular to the point of being fashionable, and there was marked variation in its frequency according to geographical location, social class and sex.[2] It was estimated that at least 85 children lost their lives each year as a direct result of tonsillectomy.

Another study, carried out in the 1940s, demonstrated that there was great uncertainty about effectiveness and indications,[3] as cited in a book by Sackett and co-workers.[4] Among 389 11-year-old schoolchildren with intact tonsils examined by a group of clinicians, tonsillectomy was recommended in 174 (45%). A second opinion was requested in the 215 schoolchildren for whom tonsillectomy was not recommended, and tonsillectomy was recommended for 99 (46%). The remaining 116 children, in whom on the two previous occasions tonsillectomy was not recommended, were then examined for the third time, and tonsillectomy was recommended in 51 (44%) of them. The most remarkable finding is that tonsillectomy was recommended in each of the three cycles for approximately 45% of the children.

These historical examples illustrate that uncertainty about diagnostic and management decisions can lead to overtreatment, which may have serious consequences for patients. Given the fact that there is still no high-quality evidence on the effectiveness of tonsillectomy more than 50 years later, the same problem may still exist, albeit to a lesser extent. The only published study on the effectiveness of tonsillectomy that could be included in one systematic review studied 91 children and was affected by important baseline differences in the characteristics of the surgical and the control group.[1] It is obvious that this kind of clinical uncertainty can only be solved by epidemiological evidence of high quality.

WHAT IS EPIDEMIOLOGY?

Epidemiology is a relative young discipline, but during its short life many definitions of epidemiology have emerged.[5] Many of these describe epidemiology in terms of its subject matter. The perhaps most frequently cited definition in this context states that epidemiology is the study of the distribution and determinants of disease frequency in human populations.[6] These three closely related components – distribution, determinants and frequency – encompass many epidemiological principles and methods.[7] For example, an epidemiological study that would fit perfectly within this definition is that of the frequency of head and neck cancer in a certain geographical area. This study could also consider the distribution of the disease among different subgroups. The determinants of disease occurrence would then derive from these two.

Although this definition has its merits in that it covers many epidemiological studies, some of which attracted large media attention (for example, smoking and lung cancer, cholesterol and heart disease, effect of diethylstilbestrol on offspring, unprotected sex and the acquired immune deficiency syndrome), a growing number of epidemiologists feel that the above-cited definition does not cover their work. The reason is that the subject matter of what can be considered epidemiological studies has become rather heterogeneous. Attempts to produce a definition of epidemiology based upon its subject matter therefore produce confusion rather than clarity.

The concept of the determinant-occurrence relationship

In the last two decades, an alternative definition has arisen that defines epidemiology as a discipline that studies the functional relationship between the occurrence of disease (or related health outcomes) and its determinants.[8] This may seem a trivial step, but this focus on the concept of the 'determinant-occurrence relationship' rather than the subject matter has considerably broadened the scope of epidemiology in medicine.

One of the major reasons why epidemiology has gained such far-reaching importance lies in the nature of medical knowledge. Medical knowledge is, to a large extent, derived from the experience obtained in groups of similar patients. Medicine is therefore an empirical science, and many of the empirical relationships in medicine can be considered as determinant-occurrence relationships. It is especially this realization on the basis of which epidemiology has become a basic science in medicine.

Epidemiology as a methodological discipline

An alternative approach to clarify the definition of epidemiology is to consider it as a methodological discipline. From this perspective, the subject of epidemiological inquiry is not so much the determinants of the occurrence of disease and other health outcomes, but the principles and methods for the study of determinant-occurrence relationships.

As a methodological discipline, epidemiology allows a large number of different questions to be answered. As explained earlier, it may play a role in describing the distribution of health and disease in a population. Who is affected? Where and when does this health problem occur? Why does it occur in a particular population?

However, other questions can be considered as well. Once a health problem occurs, epidemiology also provides methods for monitoring the course and outcome of a health problem. What is the outcome of the health problem? It may answer questions regarding the outcomes of interventions. Is intervention A more effective than intervention B? How well does a diagnostic test distinguish between people with and without the target disorder?

Epidemiological research is also essential for the assessment of the burden of disease and the need for health services and evaluation of the access to services. How much suffering does this health problem cause in a population? How many people need a certain intervention? Who uses the intervention? What factors explain differences in healthcare use?

'STREAMS' OF EPIDEMIOLOGY

Given the extension of the boundaries of epidemiology – based on the introduction of the determinant-occurrence relationship as the key epidemiological concept and the realization that epidemiological principles provide the methodological underpinning for the study of a wide range of questions – one can recognize several 'streams' of epidemiological research. These streams differ largely according to the types of questions they address, but they share most of the methodological concepts and principles.

Classical epidemiology

The first stream of research is 'classical epidemiology', sometimes referred to as 'aetiological epidemiology' or 'risk factor epidemiology', of which the ultimate goal is 'the elaboration of causes that can explain patterns of disease occurrence'.[5] The geographical distribution of a disease, the variations in its frequency over time, and the special characteristics of people affected by it, are typical objects of study.

There is often a natural progression in this type of epidemiological research.[7] First, there is a concern about the possible influence of a particular factor on the occurrence of disease. This suspicion can have many origins – clinical practice, laboratory research, theoretical speculation – but it often arises from examination of disease distributions, and leads to the formulation of a specific hypothesis about its causes. It can then be further explored in studies of individuals that include an appropriate comparison group. A systematic collection and analysis of data may reveal that a statistical association exists. It is then essential to assess whether random errors or systematic errors might be responsible for the findings. Finally, a judgement needs to be made about whether an observed association represents a cause-effect relationship.

An otolaryngological example of this type of epidemiological research is the study of the distribution of head and neck cancers and the association of the occurrence of this disease with traditional risk factors such as diet, smoking and drinking habits or socioeconomic status. Another more specific example is the testing of the hypothesis that there is a link between human papillomavirus and the occurrence of a subset of these cancers. The result of aetiological research may guide the first steps towards the development of primary prevention that keeps disease from occurring at all.

However, the reductionist nature of classical epidemiology has been criticized. It has been argued that epidemiological studies often ignore 'the interdependence of multiple agents and how human populations become exposed and susceptible to them'.[9] Epidemiological research that focuses on the effect of risk factors measurable at the level of the individual neglects the population context and the social and cultural determinants that act at population level.

Clinical epidemiology

The second stream of research is 'clinical epidemiology'. The adjective 'clinical' is added because clinical epidemiology 'seeks to answer clinical questions and to guide clinical decision making with the best available evidence'.[10] Clinicians are mainly concerned with problems of individual patients. It may seem paradoxical that results of epidemiological studies that are derived from groups of patients should be applicable to the problems of individual patients. It is obvious, however, that this is because the best evidence to solve a clinical problem is derived from the experience of a large number of similar patients.

Advocates of evidence-based medicine have addressed this paradox directly. They state that clinicians need to carry out 'the particularization, to the individual patient, of our prior experiences (both as individual clinicians and collectively) with groups of similar patients'.[4] A good clinician should therefore use the best available external evidence together with his own unsystematic clinical experience and intuition – based on a blend of knowledge derived from anatomy, physiology and other basic sciences.[11] Evidence alone is never sufficient to make a clinical decision. Decision-makers always trade the benefits and risks, inconvenience and costs associated with alternative management strategies, and in doing so should especially consider the patients' values and preferences.

The significance of the definition of epidemiology as a methodological discipline that addresses determinant-occurrence relationships is based on the reach of the concept of determinant-occurrence relationships in itself. If one considers the presence of disease as the outcome and the diagnostic information as the determinant, then this represents a diagnostic problem. The object of study is, in this case, the functional relationship between diagnostic information and the presence of disease. If one considers the occurrence of a disease or a health-related event in the future as the outcome and the presence of certain patient characteristics as the determinants, then this represents a prognostic problem. One of these patient characteristics can be the use of a specific therapy, and in that case, this represents a therapeutic problem. In the latter case however, to achieve accurate results the '*ceteris paribus* principle' – the condition that all other determinants are equal – is a fundamental notion that we will explicitly address in the section 'Randomized controlled trials' below.

A study of the diagnostic accuracy of fine-needle aspiration as a test for malignant disease in patients with nodular thyroid disease is an otolaryngological example of diagnostic research. The influence of the age of patients with an oropharyngeal carcinoma on long-term survival constitutes a prognostic research question. The effect that early surgery compared with watchful waiting for glue-ear has on language development in pre-school children represents a therapeutic research question.

It is useful at this point to distinguish between the epidemiological terms, 'incidence' and 'prevalence'. Incidence is defined as the number of new cases that occur in a specific time period. Prevalence is defined as the proportion of the population that actually has a disease, or condition, at a specific point in time. Unlike prevalence, incidence is a true rate because it includes a measure of time. Prevalence on the other hand is a 'snapshot' of a situation at a single point in time and for this reason is sometimes also called the 'point' prevalence.

Epidemiology and health services and public health research

Epidemiology is also one of the core disciplines of health services research and public health. Whereas classical epidemiology and clinical epidemiology focus largely on determinants of health and disease and related conditions in individuals, health services research is more directed towards questions addressing the quality and organization of healthcare systems and public health research towards the health and healthcare problems in communities. One could consider this as a third stream of epidemiological research.

Important questions for health services research are those that address the variations in processes and outcomes of healthcare services, as well as the determinants of these variations. Research in public health may be concerned with the influence of environmental factors, socioeconomic conditions and health services on health in the community. It will be clear by now that many of these questions take the form of determinant-occurrence relationships, which again confirms the crucial role of an epidemiological approach.

A study comparing the outcome of thyroid surgery performed by experienced surgeons and surgeons in training is an example of an epidemiological study directly addressing a determinant of the quality of otolaryngological care.[12] Another example is a study of the impact that the publication of a guideline on the treatment of persistent glue-ear in children had on the rate of surgery.[13] A systematic review of studies addressing the effectiveness of screening young children to undergo early treatment for glue-ear is a third example of public health research.[14]

THE 'ANATOMY' AND 'PHYSIOLOGY' OF EPIDEMIOLOGICAL RESEARCH

We cannot discuss the different study designs before we have examined what epidemiological research is made up of and how it works. The easiest way to do this is to describe the components of a study protocol and the way results are used to draw inferences from the study results about the truth in the universe. The following sections are based largely on the introductory chapters of a recent book by Hulley and colleagues about designing clinical research.[15]

Essential components of a protocol for an epidemiological study

A research protocol is a document that provides all essential details of a study. A protocol is necessary for guiding all the decisions that need to be made in the course of the study. The process of writing a protocol itself helps the investigator to enhance the scientific rigour and efficiency of the project. Most research involves teamwork and a written document ensures that all members know how the study should be implemented and what they are expected to contribute. A good protocol provides answers to a number of essential questions.

WHAT QUESTION WILL THE STUDY ADDRESS?

The research question defines what you want to achieve. Many experienced researchers will agree that formulating a question that can be translated into a feasible and valid study can be surprisingly hard. What often happens is that instead of a 'research question', a 'topic' is formulated. 'Framing' the research question is the first step for every new project, of which the importance cannot be overestimated. Conversely, many studies fail not so much because the study design is flawed or the execution of study is poor, but because the question was not formulated adequately in the first place.

An otolaryngological example of such a 'topic' that needs further research is the concern about the rising complication rate after tonsillectomy in the UK. It is clear that we need to provide more detail and structure before we are able to formulate a relevant and answerable 'research question'. The concept of the determinant-occurrence relationship may provide some guidance in this context. In other words, we need to be specific about what outcomes we want to study as well as what determinants we want to consider. Finally, we need to specify the target population, the kind of people for whom the study should provide answers.

In epidemiological research, a good research question therefore has four components, which can be summarized by the acronym PICO:

1. the target population or participants (P);
2. the intervention (I);
3. the comparison or control group (C), at least if there is any;
4. the outcome(s) of interest (O).

An example of a 'good' research question for a study addressing the complication rates after tonsillectomy could be: 'In patients undergoing tonsillectomy for recurrent tonsillitis, does the use of the bipolar diathermy forceps increase the occurrence of tonsil bleeds severe enough to require return to theatre in the first 28 days after surgery, compared to other tonsillectomy dissection types?' Admittedly, this is a rather convoluted sentence, and is only given here to illustrate how the four components of a research question can be covered in one question. In practice, the question will be shortened to 'Does bipolar diathermy increase the haemorrhage rate after tonsillectomy', but in that case the details that define the target population, intervention, comparison and outcome of interest need to be provided separately.

WHY IS THE STUDY QUESTION IMPORTANT?

Good epidemiological research should also pass the 'so what' test. In the Introduction or Background section of a protocol, it should be argued that answering the research question will provide a significant contribution to our state of knowledge or, in other words, add to what is already known about the problem. It is therefore important to be on top of the published literature before developing a study. It should also be clear that the results of the proposed study will help to resolve current uncertainties, which may lead to new scientific understanding and influence clinical and public health policies.

It is often 'scholarship' that will identify the gaps in the current knowledge and how these can be addressed in an optimal way by learning from the work of others. For example, a recent systematic review of the literature on the effect of tonsillectomy in patients with chronic or recurrent tonsillitis concluded a lack of evidence to guide decision-making for this surgical intervention in adults or children.[1] More importantly in this context, the authors of the systematic review also concluded on the basis of the results of their review that future trials should address the effectiveness of tonsillectomy in subgroups according to age, severity and disease frequency, and that patients should be followed up for at least one year to assess outcomes such as general well-being, behaviour, growth, sleep and eating patterns in addition to severity and frequency of infections. These conclusions based upon a systematic review provide powerful arguments for the direction of future research.

HOW IS THE STUDY STRUCTURED?

Choosing the study design is a complex issue. The actual choice depends strongly on the research question. The study should be designed in such a way that it produces results that are relatively precise (free of random error) and accurate (free of systematic error or bias). An additional consideration is that the study needs to be efficient (affordable in terms of time and money).

A simplistic 'taxonomy' of study designs, presented in **Figure 41.1**, shows that two fundamental decisions have to be made. First, the investigators have to decide whether they want to assign the determinants themselves in an 'experimental study', or whether they want to examine events as nature takes its course in an 'observational study'. Second, if an observational study design is chosen, the next step is to decide whether the study needs a comparison or control group. If so, the study is often called 'analytical'. If not, it is a 'descriptive' study. Descriptive studies are often used as a first step into a new area of study – the scientific 'toe in the water',[15] and followed by analytical studies to answer questions that can address determinant-occurrence relationships.

A more detailed presentation of study designs follows under the section 'Choosing the study design' below.

WHO ARE THE STUDY SUBJECTS AND HOW WILL THEY BE SELECTED AND RECRUITED?

A good choice of the study subjects ensures that the results of the study will accurately represent what is going on in the population of interest, the target population, the set of people best suited to the research question (for example, patients with early laryngeal squamous cell carcinoma for a study comparing radiotherapy and surgery for laryngeal cancer). The protocol must also specify the study sample, which is the subset of the target population available for study (for example, all consecutive patients with this disease condition referred to a regional head and neck cancer centre in a defined period of time). The study sample should be a subset of the target population that can be studied at an acceptable cost and is large enough to control random error and representative enough to control systematic error.

In many cases, controlling both random error and systematic error sets conflicting demands, which is sometimes referred to as the 'precision–bias' dilemma. For example, a study that aims to evaluate the usefulness of the endoscope compared to the headlamp for sinonasal surgery should carefully consider which patients to include.

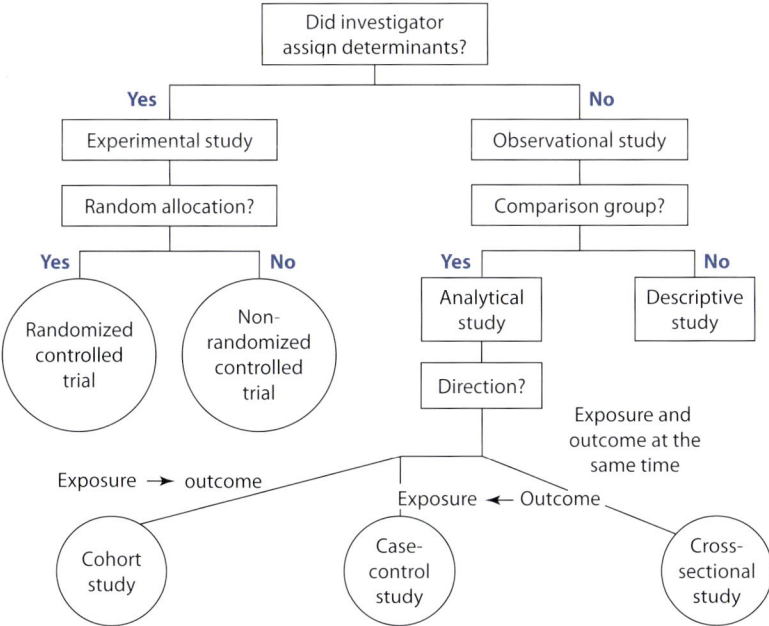

Figure 41.1 Algorithm for classification of types of clinical research. Reproduced from Grimes and Schulz, 2002,[16] with permission from Elsevier.

It is highly likely that the results of the study will differ according to the extent of the surgery. The comparison might be most relevant for patients who undergo surgery for procedures around the middle meatus and the anterior ethmoid. Including patients who undergo only simple polypectomy, who comprise approximately 50% of the total number of patients who undergo a form of sinonasal surgery, may seem an attractive option because it will double the size of the study. However, including these patients will diminish the extent to which the study sample represents the population for which the research question is of interest.

In an ideal world without practical and financial limitations, we would study the entire target population. Often, if not always, the target population is too large and the study will be carried out in a sample. Earlier, we gave as an example the study comparing radiotherapy and surgery for early laryngeal carcinoma that was carried out in consecutive patients visiting a regional centre in a defined period of time. This type of sampling, including patients that are easily accessible to the investigator, is called 'convenience sampling'. It is very frequently used in clinical research. It has obvious advantages in terms of costs and logistics, but its drawback is that it might not sufficiently represent the target population. Consecutive sampling, including without interruption all accessible people, is especially useful in this context given that it reduces the possibility that selection either by the investigators or self-selection by the subjects influences the results. Probability sampling is the gold standard for ensuring that the study sample is representative of the target population, except for the effect of chance variation. There are several probability-sampling methods. With simple random sampling, every individual in a population has the same chance of being included. However, in some cases, a form of stratified sampling (random sampling with a known sample size within subgroups) is desirable. For a study of patient satisfaction of patients visiting an otolaryngology outpatient clinic, for example, the investigators may wish to divide patients in 'strata' according to their diagnosis or the procedure that was being carried out, and then sample specified numbers from each stratum.

The choices made about the selection of the study subjects (the intended sample) are important as they have an impact on the extent to which the study findings can be generalized. The sampling procedures can affect the generalizability of the results in a number of ways. First, the actual sample might be different from the intended sample. For example, people who were eligible for the study might have refused, and people who participated might be different (more or less healthy, dependent on the study context) from those who did not. Second, the study sample should be sufficiently similar to the target population. For example, the 'spectrum' of disease in patients with laryngeal squamous cell cancer might differ from one centre to the next, and in turn the effects of radiotherapy and cancer might differ as well. Third, the investigator must form an opinion about whether the results can be generalized to people outside the target population. In terms of our example, do radiotherapy and surgery have similar effects in other countries, in patients with more advanced disease, or in patients who are on average older or younger? This will always be a subjective judgement that depends on findings in other studies, more general scientific knowledge, and what is sometimes called 'a feeling for the organism'. It is not a yes-or-no decision, and may trigger debate among experts. This debate may be informed by the study itself if the study population is diverse enough to explore the constancy of effects in different subgroups within the study.

WHAT MEASUREMENTS WILL BE MADE?

The quality of a study depends on how well the variables measured in the study represent the phenomena of interest. Another concern is how the variables of interest can be measured as precisely (free of random error) and accurately (free of systematic error) as possible without making the study unreasonably expensive.

It is important to have some understanding about the types of variables that are encountered in epidemiological research, and how they can be measured. Any variable can be considered to be of one of two basic types: continuous variables and categorical variables. This distinction determines the way in which these variables should be measured as well as analyzed. As a general rule, with categorical variables, the analysis will involve a description or comparison of the proportion of subjects falling into the various categories. With continuous variables, the descriptions or comparisons are most often presented in terms of average values or medians if the sample is small and the average value is considered to be inappropriate to describe the 'midpoint' of the variable's distribution.

Theoretically, continuous variables can take all possible values on a continuum along a specific range. Many clinical parameters are continuous. Variables, such as blood pressure, body weight, body temperature, are not restricted to particular values and are only limited by the accuracy and precision of the measuring procedures. The units in which a continuous variable is expressed specify a uniform difference along the entire length of the scale. A difference in blood pressure of 10 mmHg has the same interpretation irrespective of whether it occurs at the lower or the upper end of the blood pressure scale.

Discrete variables can only take certain numerical values – in most cases only integers (whole numbers). If discrete variables have a considerable number of possible values, they can often be treated as if they were continuous. Examples of these 'quasi-continuous' variables are counts (such as the number of cigarettes smoked, number of episodes of acute tonsillitis in last year, or number of days spent in hospital) or scores on 'clinimetric scales' (such as the 20-item Sino-Nasal Outcome Test) that measures symptom severity of sinonasal conditions on a scale with discrete values ranging from 0 (no symptoms) to 100 (very severe symptoms)[17] or the Epworth Sleepiness Scales, used in patients with obstructive sleep apnoea, that can take discrete values from 0 (no daytime sleepiness) to 24 (very severe daytime sleepiness).[18] Strictly speaking, considering scores on a clinimetric scale as continuous is somewhat problematic, as the interpretation of a difference of one unit may vary along the length of the scale. For example, does an increase from 5 to 10 on the Epworth Sleepiness Score correspond to an increase from 15 to 20?

Phenomena that cannot be measured quantitatively can often be measured by classifying them into categories, and then counting the number of subjects that fall within the defined categories. In its simplest form, there are only two categories (such as man/woman, or dead/alive), and these variables are called dichotomous or binary variables. When there are more than two possible categories, the variables are termed poly- or multichotomous variables. Polychotomous variables can be further classified into those that are ordered, called ordinal variables, and those that are not, called nominal variables. Socioeconomic status, ASA grades describing fitness to undergo surgery,[19] and degree of pain are examples of the former, and race, marital status and blood type are examples of the latter.

As a general rule, continuous variables are more 'informative' than categorical variables. It is therefore advisable to use continuous variables as much as possible. For example, 'body temperature' as a continuous variable should be preferred to a categorical variable dividing patients into those with a temperature below and above a certain threshold.

Good measurements are precise and accurate. There are largely three sources of random and systematic error: (i) variability due to the observer; (ii) variability due to the subject; and (iii) variability due to the instrument used.

A number of strategies can be followed to increase simultaneously both precision and accuracy of the measurements. First, the measurement procedures should be standardized and clearly described in the study protocol. Second, those who are involved in taking the measurements should be trained and their performance monitored in the course of the study. Third, the measurements should be carefully chosen in terms of what is known about their performance. Fourth, calibration procedures should be carried out against a 'gold standard'. This is especially essential for mechanical devices such as weighing scales, thermometers and blood pressure measuring devices. Furthermore, a simple and rather effective approach to increase measurement precision is to repeat the measurements and to use the mean of two or more observations. The latter approach is commonly used in studies measuring blood pressure. An important approach to reduce systematic error is blinding, which conceals information about determinants, or in some cases outcomes, to the observers and/or subjects. This reduces the possibility that the observers or the study subjects distort the overall accuracy of the measurements, consciously or unconsciously. Blinding, however, does not ensure overall accuracy of the measurements, but it may eliminate 'differential bias' that affects one study group more than another. Blinding is especially relevant for measurements that incorporate some subjective judgement. For example, a study comparing early surgery with watchful waiting for glue-ear in pre-school children used a tester of language development who was unaware of what treatment the children had received.[20]

HOW WILL THE RESULTS BE ANALYZED?

The main statistical methods that are going to be used to analyze the results should be defined in the study protocol. Choosing the statistical methods after the results have become available will increase the likelihood of finding associations between determinants and outcome on the basis of chance alone.

An important element of the analysis plan is the description of how the outcome variable is going to be analyzed. For example, a trial on early surgery for glue-ear that measured language development with the Reynell development language scales (a test of expressive language and verbal comprehension abilities in children aged 6 months to 6 years) could analyze the Reynell data as a continuous variable.[20] Conversely, it could define groups with normal language development and with delayed language development by dichotomizing the Reynell data, and use this categorical variable as the main outcome measure.

If a categorical variable is used as the outcome measure, the 'denominator problem' should be considered. **Figure 41.2** summarizes the questions that have to be answered in this respect. The first question asks whether the numerator is going to be included in the denominator. If the answer is yes, the next question is whether time is included in the denominator or not.

Let us first consider the case when the numerator is included in the denominator, but time is not. A first example of this would be a measure of the occurrence of sensorineural hearing loss in neonates. One could simply report the proportion of neonates with hearing loss: the numerator would be the number of neonates with hearing loss and the denominator would be the total number of

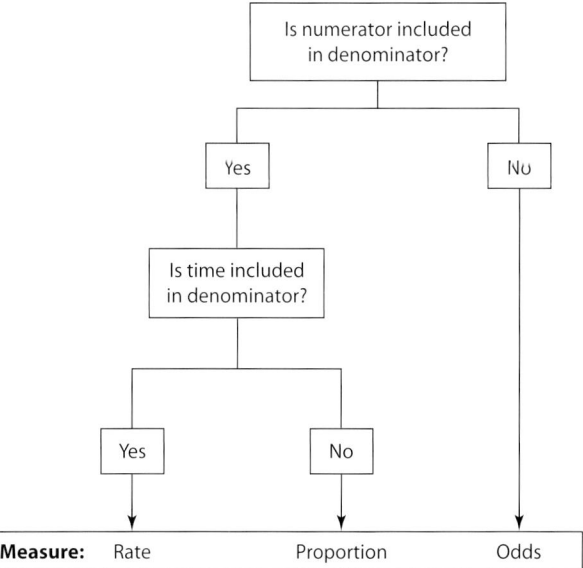

Figure 41.2 Algorithm for distinguishing rates, proportions and odds. Adapted from Grimes and Schulz, 2002,[16] with permission from Elsevier.

neonates included in the study. This proportion is often referred to as *prevalence*. A second example would be a measure of the occurrence of head and neck cancer in people, initially free of the disease, who developed the disease within a specified time period. The numerator would be the number of subjects who developed the disease during follow-up and the denominator would be the total number of subjects at the beginning of the study. This proportion is often referred to as *cumulative incidence*. Suppose that 1000 smokers are followed up during 5 years and that 15 develop head and neck cancer, the cumulative incidence would be 1.5%.

The calculation of a proportion as an estimate of disease occurrence, as described above, assumes that the entire study sample has been followed up for the specified time period. This is often not the case. Some subjects might enter the study later, and others might be lost to follow-up. An alternative way of measuring outcomes that takes these varying follow-up time periods into account is to include time in the denominator. The numerator would be exactly the same as for proportions, but the sum of the time that each individual was followed up and at risk of becoming a case would be used as the denominator. In this case, an incidence rate (also called incidence density, force of morbidity/mortality, hazard) could be calculated that is equal to the number of people who develop cancer divided by the total person-time at risk during follow-up. For example, on the basis of the previous example of the occurrence of head and neck cancer in smokers, one could have expressed the incidence rate of cancer as approximately 3 cases per 1000 people per year (or 15 divided by approximately 5×1000 years of person-time at risk). Because the incidence is very low, a simple relationship holds: cumulative incidence ≈ incidence × average follow-up time.

Many epidemiological studies report, in some form or other, outcomes expressed as 'odds'. It is important to distinguish odds from probability. A probability can be estimated as the proportion of people in whom a particular characteristic, such as the presence of disease, is present. The larger the group of people under study, the better the observed proportion of people with the disease reflects the 'true' probability. Odds, on the other hand, represents the ratio of two complementary probabilities. For example, if the probability of disease is 0.20, then the odds are $0.20/0.80 = 1:4 = 0.25$. Another way of calculating the odds is by dividing the number of subjects with the characteristic by the number without it. In other words, the numerator is not included in the denominator (**Figure 41.2**).

Most frequently, it is not the odds itself that is reported in epidemiological studies, but the odds ratio – the ratio of odds in different groups. This can be the 'outcome odds ratio', or the ratio of the odds of the outcome of interest in the group with the determinant to the odds of the outcome in the group without the determinant. Conversely, this can also be the 'determinant odds ratio', or the odds of the determinant in the group with the outcome compared to the odds of the determinant in the group without the outcome of interest. One reason why epidemiologists find odds ratios so attractive is that 'outcome odds ratios' are equivalent to 'determinant odds ratios', which is a fact used in the analysis of case-control studies (see 'Case-control studies' below). For example, **Table 41.1** presents fictitious findings of a study on risk factors for post-operative complications after tonsillectomy. The outcome odds ratio is the same as the determinant odds ratio, which can be easily understood as both odds ratios simplify to the 'cross product' of the cell frequencies of a 2 × 2 table. The 'outcome odds ratio' can be calculated as

TABLE 41.1 'Outcome odds ratios' and 'determinant odds ratios' – fictitious example of complication rates after tonsillectomy

Dissection instruments used	Post-operative complication					
	Yes		No		Total	
Bipolar diathermy	36	a	264	b	300	a+b
Other	24	c	676	d	700	c+d
Total	60	a+c	940	b+d	1000	

$$\frac{\dfrac{a}{a+b}\Big/\dfrac{b}{a+b}}{\dfrac{c}{c+d}\Big/\dfrac{d}{c+d}} = \frac{a/b}{c/d} = \frac{a \times d}{b \times c} = \frac{36 \times 676}{24 \times 264} = 3.8.$$

Similarly, the 'determinant odds ratio' can be calculated as

$$\frac{\dfrac{a}{a+c}\Big/\dfrac{c}{a+c}}{\dfrac{b}{b+d}\Big/\dfrac{d}{b+d}} = \frac{a/c}{b/d} = \frac{a \times d}{b \times c} = 3.8.$$

When a dichotomous outcome variable is used (for example, alive/dead, or disease present/absent) 'risk differences' and 'risk ratios' are commonly used as 'measures of effect'.[10] The 'risk' in this circumstance can represent 'prevalence', 'cumulative incidence', 'incidence' or even 'odds', as described above. One might ask, 'What is the additional risk of head and neck cancer in people who smoke, over and above that in people who do not?' The answer to this question is obviously a risk difference. In a previous fictitious example, we supposed that we followed up 1000 smokers for a period of 5 years and that we found that 15 of them developed head and neck cancer. The cumulative incidence of cancer in this group is therefore 1.5%. We can also suppose that we did the same in 1000 non-smokers and that we found cancer in 7 of them. The cumulative incidence in non-smokers is 0.7%. The risk difference attributable to smoking is therefore 0.8% (= 1.5–0.7%). On the other hand, one might ask, 'How many times are smokers more likely to get head and neck cancer compared to non-smokers?' Following our example, we could calculate the risk ratio as 2.1 (= 1.5%/0.7%). In other words, smokers are approximately twice as likely to develop head and neck cancer over a 5-year period as non-smokers. This risk ratio does not tell us anything about the magnitude of the risk difference. Even for large risk ratios, the risk difference might be quite small if the outcome is uncommon. As a rule of thumb, risk differences are more meaningful as a measure of effect in clinical situations, because it represents the actual additional probability in those exposed. On the other hand, relative risks are more meaningful as effect measures of a causal relationship in aetiological studies.

HOW LARGE IS THE STUDY GOING TO BE?

A major problem of many studies is that the study size is too small. Small studies lead to imprecise results. Small studies often increase, rather than reduce, the scientific and clinical uncertainty in a specific area. Although one might argue that small studies have a value of their own because they might be included in a systematic review and meta-analysis, which would mimic the results of a larger study, it should be the goal of every study to include a number of subjects that would in itself produce 'meaningful' results. A considerably less frequent problem is that of a study that is larger than necessary to be meaningful. Larger studies are more difficult to carry out and may be more costly than necessary. The most important issue in this context is of course to determine what can be considered meaningful.

How can the appropriate size of a study be determined? This question is most commonly answered on the basis of a statistical 'sample size calculation'. Although the answer of a sample size calculation is exact (for example, the number of subjects to be included in a study), in many cases it depends on a number of rather subjective choices. The way that the sample size of study is to be calculated depends on whether it is an analytical study (study with a comparison or control group) or a descriptive study.

For analytical studies, a research hypothesis should be formulated that further refines the study question. This hypothesis sets out the basis for statistical significance testing. Because this hypothesis guides the statistical analysis, it should be simple (addressing one determinant or comparison and the occurrence of one outcome) and specific (defining unambiguously the target population, the control and comparison group, and the outcome of interest). For the purpose of statistical significance testing, this hypothesis should be given in the form of a 'null hypothesis' that states that there is no association between the determinant and the outcome. A statistical test helps to estimate the probability that an association observed in a study is due to chance (the 'p-value'). The 'alternative hypothesis' states that there is such an association. Sometimes, a distinction is made between one-sided and two-sided hypotheses. Two-sided hypotheses state only that an association exists between determinant and outcome, whereas one-sided hypotheses specify the direction of the association. For example, the null hypothesis of a study comparing early surgery with watchful waiting for glue-ear in pre-school children could be that there is no difference in the language development in the two treatment groups. The one-sided null hypothesis would state that language development with early surgery is poorer than with watchful waiting. One-sided p-values are appropriate in selected circumstances, when only one direction of the association is important. One-sided p-values may seem attractive as, generally speaking, with a one-sided significance test the p-value would be half the size of that with a two-sided test, but, on the other hand, if the results of the study would suggest that the language development is indeed poorer with surgery, then this would produce a large p-value as it is likely to observe a result like that given that the null hypothesis (language development with surgery is poorer) is true. For this reason, it is convention to use two-sided hypotheses when planning the size of a study as well as two-sided p-values when analyzing the results, unless there are well-argued reasons for the contrary.

When developing a study protocol for an analytical study, the investigator does not know the size of the effect that the determinant of interest has on the outcome, as one of the objectives of the study is to estimate it. For example, the investigators of the study of the effect that early surgery has on language development in children with glue-ear had to decide the smallest effect of surgery that in their view would be of clinical importance. This quantity is often called effect size or target difference. Determining this effect size is the most arbitrary step in a sample size calculation. The smaller the effect size, the larger the study needs to be, other things being equal. Previous studies could help to make a guess about what can be expected, but they do not provide any guidance about what is an important difference and what is not.

Before a sample size can be calculated, two further arbitrary choices need to be made. First, the 'alpha level' or 'significance level' has to be chosen that defines the cut-off point for the p-value – conventionally 0.05 – to classify a result either as 'significant' (if p-value $\leq$ cut-off), in which case the null hypothesis is rejected, or as 'not significant' (if p-value $>$ cut-off), in which case the null hypothesis is not rejected. Second, the 'power' of the significance test has to be chosen – commonly used values are 0.80 or 0.90 – that defines the probability to obtain a significant result if we assume that the defined effect size or target difference would be the 'true effect' or 'true difference'.

Finally, and only if a continuous outcome variable is going to be analyzed, a measure of the variability (spread) of that outcome – standard deviation or variance – is needed. The greater the variability in the outcome variable among the subjects, the more difficult it will be to demonstrate a difference between two groups, and the larger the study needs to be.

The required sample size can be obtained on the basis of the above-described ingredients either by using the formulae presented in statistical textbooks, from published tables or by using commonly available statistical software packages. The ingredients and the formulae for study size are purely technical. They do not take into account the value of the information obtained in the study. The most important decision is to determine the 'right balance' between the value of greater precision in study results against the greater costs. Essentially, this decision boils down to a cost-benefit analysis in which the benefits are more difficult to quantify than the costs.

For descriptive studies, concepts such as null hypothesis, effect size, alpha level and power do not apply. Instead, descriptive statistics, such as means and proportions, are presented. The sample size of descriptive studies depends on how precise the investigator wants these descriptive statistics to be. Confidence intervals, such as 95% or 99% confidence intervals, are commonly used to represent the precision of the estimates. For example, a study of the 5-year survival after surgical treatment in 228 patients with hypopharynx carcinoma found that the survival was 27.2% with a 95% confidence interval ranging from 21.5% to 33.5%.[21] This interval indicates that we can be 95% confident (which can be considered more or less the same as saying that there is 95% chance) that the 'true' 5-year survival probability lies within this interval. When estimating the sample size for descriptive studies, the investigator specifies the desired width of the confidence interval, and the sample size derives from that and can be read from tables or obtained from statistical software packages. This approach can be followed for any type of descriptive variable for which confidence intervals can be calculated.

TABLE 41.2 Oxford Centre for Evidence-Based Medicine – classification of levels of evidence

Level	Evidence
1a	Systematic review of RCTs; meta-analyses
1b	Individual RCT
2a	Systematic review of cohort studies
2b	Individual cohort study
2c	'Outcomes' research
3a	Systematic review of case-control studies
3b	Individual case-control study
4	Case-series (and poor quality cohort and case-control studies)
5	Expert opinion, anecdotal evidence, case reports or based on physiology, bench research or 'first principles'

Modified from http://www.cebm.net/oxford-centre-evidence-based-medicine-levels-evidence-march-2009

CHOOSING THE DESIGN STUDY

The taxonomy of study designs presented in **Figure 41.1** provides a simple decision aid for choosing the most appropriate design. A number of questions have to be answered with the ultimate goal being to create an affordable study that provides results that are relatively precise (free of random error) and accurate (free of systematic error or bias). A first distinction that has to be made is that between studies in which the investigator actively assigns the determinants (experimental studies) or those in which this is not the case (observational studies). A second distinction that has to be made is that between observational studies that do or do not have a comparison or control group. If so, the study is called analytical, if not, descriptive.

The following sections are largely based on a series of short essays on clinical research published in the Lancet,[16] and chapters of recent books about designing clinical research by Hulley and colleagues[15] and clinical epidemiology.[10] We start this section by describing observational studies and will end with the description of experimental studies (randomized controlled trials).

Levels of evidence

Individual studies are frequently graded according to a hierarchy whereby those at the top are considered to provide stronger evidence than those lower down the scale. The Oxford Centre for Evidence-Based Medicine has provided one such framework as shown in **Table 41.2**.

Caution, however, is recommended in exercising such a rigid hierarchical approach to all studies. Thus, randomized controlled trials (RCTs) for a particular intervention are not always available and not all interventions can be evaluated in RCTs; a lack of RCT evidence does not equate to a lack of evidence. In addition, although guidelines are based on the best available published evidence, not all evidence makes it into the literature. Finally, this approach fails to take into consideration the quality of individual studies. A well-designed and properly conducted cohort or case-control study may provide better evidence than a small or poorly conducted RCT.

An alternative approach is to classify studies not only by their *design* but also according to the *quality of evidence* they provide. For example, The Grading of Recommendation, Assessment, Development and Evaluation Working Group (GRADE Working Group) has developed a system for grading the quality of evidence.[22]

Minimizing bias and confounding

We indicated earlier that the precision of study results depends mainly on two factors: the size of the study design and the methods used to obtain the measurements. Furthermore, a study should be designed in such a way that it avoids systematic error or bias. A great number of different types of bias have been documented but it is not a major simplification to consider all these types of biases in three categories: selection bias, information bias and confounding.

To examine whether selection bias would introduce systematic error in the study results, two questions need to be answered: 'Do the sample of study subjects sufficiently represent the population of interest?' and 'Are the groups that are going to be compared similar in all important respects apart from the determinant(s) of interest?' The first question is especially relevant when designing a randomized controlled trial, because trials usually enrol patients who tend to be different (often healthier) from the target population and the results tend to overestimate the effects compared to what they would be in routine practice. This contributes to the differences between the efficacy of a therapy observed in the highly controlled circumstances in selected clinical settings and the effectiveness of a treatment in actual practice. The second question refers directly to the comparability of the groups. In other words, do the groups differ importantly aside from the comparison that is being studied?

Information bias results from incorrect information about the determinant or the outcome or both. The important question that has to be answered is: 'Has information been gathered in the same way?' In cohort studies (see 'Cohort studies' below), information about the outcome should be obtained in the same way for those with and without the determinants under consideration. Also, those who collect the information about the outcome should be unaware of ('blind to') the determinant status of the subjects as much as possible. In case-control studies (see below), information about the determinant status should be collected in the same way for cases and controls.

Confounding occurs when two determinants or risk factors are associated with each other. In that case, the effect of one is confounded with, or distorted by, the effect of the other. Confounding can occur because of selection bias, by chance, or because the two determinants are really associated in nature. Selection bias and confounding are not mutually exclusive, but they are often presented differently as they represent problems at different stages in a study. Selection bias is an issue when the sampling procedures for patients are determined during the design phase of a study, whereas confounding is an issue to consider during the analysis phase.

Often in the same study more than one bias operates, as in the following example. Imagine a study that compared the effect that surgical and non-surgical management had on speech and language development in children with persistent otitis media with effusion. In this example, selection bias could have been present if the children who received surgical treatment came from a different background and had parents who were on average of higher socioeconomic status, or if they had a family history of chronic ear infection. Information bias could have occurred because the assessment of language development might have been influenced by the fact that those who were applying and interpreting the speech and language tests knew the treatment the children had received. Finally, the conclusion that surgical treatment improved speech and language development might have been the result of confounding if the children who received surgical treatment had had more serious or more frequent ear infections. The latter bias is often referred to as 'confounding by clinical indication'.

When designing studies, investigators should try as much as possible to rule out bias. The concerns about bias need to be thought through very carefully. This relates directly to the three components of a good research question, and these components should be represented adequately in the study design. First, the study sample should adequately represent the target population. Second, the measurement of the determinants should adequately represent the comparison of interest. Third, the measurements of the outcomes should adequately represent the outcome(s) of interest.

When confounding is anticipated, the investigator should consider design and analysis strategies to control its influence on the outcomes. The simplest approach in the design phase is restriction or specification. For example, investigators could decide to include only non-smokers in a study on the effect of human papillomavirus and oropharyngeal cancer. The disadvantage of this strategy is that it reduces recruitment and prohibits generalization of the results to smokers. Another potential approach in the design phase is matching, which means that subjects with matching values for the confounding variables are included. This can be done individually (pair wise matching) or in groups (frequency matching). However, the use of matching has many disadvantages. The recruitment process can become rather cumbersome. Special analytical techniques are required that represent the fact that the subjects are not sampled independently. There is also the danger of overmatching – matching on the basis of a variable that is not a confounder, which would reduce the study's power. Given these disadvantages, matching should be avoided if other strategies could provide sufficient control for confounding.

In the analysis phase, the investigator can use either stratification or adjustment. Stratification ensures that the analysis compares like with like, first by comparing subjects within a group (or stratum) of subjects with similar values of one or more confounding variables and then, in a second step, by calculating an overall estimate by pooling the stratum-specific results. The most important disadvantage of this approach is the limited number of variables that can be controlled for. Adjustment on the basis of a statistical multivariate model does not suffer from this limitation, but its effects depend on the adequacy of the model fit. Both approaches depend on the completeness, precision and accuracy of the measurements of the confounders.

Observational studies

DESCRIPTIVE STUDIES

Descriptive studies can describe the experience in only one individual, a case report, or a report on a series of individual cases, the case-series report. Case series are the most frequently published studies in surgery. An important function of descriptive studies is that they can describe the distribution of diseases or disease-related conditions and events in a specified population.

Good descriptive research should address the five 'W' questions – who, what, why, when and where – although as soon as these questions are addressed on the basis of the data, the distinction between descriptive studies (no comparison) and analytical studies (comparison between groups essential) starts to disappear; but a distinctive characteristic of descriptive studies is that they cannot directly quantify the risk that can be attributed to a specific determinant. For example, a series of three cases was published recently of perichondritis of the pinna as a result of 'high' ear piercing, and was used to focus attention on the risks of body piercing.[23] The study also presented the increasing trend in the number of hospital admissions for perichondritis of the pinna in the UK and Wales from approximately 600 in 1990–91 to approximately 1200 in 1997–98. The latter is an example of a surveillance study, which is another important type of descriptive study. A surveillance study is an ongoing and systematic collection, analysis and interpretation of health data essential to the planning, implementation and evaluation of health services and public health practice. The fact that this particular descriptive study cannot quantify the attributable risk might not be a weakness as most cases of perichondritis of the pinna may be due to piercing practices in the first place.

The strength of descriptive studies is that they often use existing data and thus are inexpensive and efficient to carry out. Furthermore, few ethical limitations exist. The disadvantages are that there is a danger of over-interpretation. For example, in early 2001 the UK government recommended that single-use instruments should be used for adenotonsillectomy to minimize the risk of transmission of variant Creutzfeldt-Jacob disease (vCJD). In the course of the same year, suspicion was raised about the post-operative haemorrhage rate. It was thought that the increase in the haemorrhage rate was due to the poor quality of the single-use instruments and, in late 2001, the UK government recommended the reintroduction of reusable instruments. The need to consider alternative explanations arose later as more detailed analyses of hospital admission data revealed that there also had been a gradual increase in the post-tonsillectomy complication rate from 3.9% in 1995–96 to 7.3% in 2000–01.[24]

Analytical studies

An important distinction that is often made with respect to observational studies that are analytical is whether the determinants and outcomes relate to phenomena that occur at the same time. If so, it is called a cross-sectional study. If not, it is either a cohort study (looking forward in time from determinant to outcome) or a case-control study (looking backward from outcome to determinant).

CROSS-SECTIONAL STUDIES

The single most important characteristic of cross-sectional studies is that the determinant(s) as well as the outcome(s) measured occur at the same time, and that there is no follow-up period. Cross-sectional designs are very well suited to describe the prevalence of health and disease-related conditions and their distribution patterns. For example, a study was carried out in 864 school children in the UK to investigate the effect of parental smoking on middle ear disease.[25] Data on parental smoking were collected with a questionnaire and glue-ear was considered to be present in children with a flat tympanogram. The study identified 82 cases in total, 45 in the 407 households with at least one smoker and 37 in the 457 households with no smokers, and a risk ratio of 1.4 (=11.0%/8.1%, with a 95% confidence interval ranging from 0.9 to 2.1) could be calculated.

The major strength of cross-sectional studies is that they examine the presence or absence of an outcome and determinant at the same time. Cross-sectional studies are therefore fast, relatively cheap, and there is no 'loss to follow-up'. A major disadvantage of cross-sectional studies is that they provide only a snapshot of complicated temporal relationships between determinant and outcome. Parental smoking, for example, is likely to be persistent, but chronic middle ear infection in children is an intermittent disease. As a consequence, causal relationships are difficult to establish with cross-sectional studies. For the same reasons, they are not suitable for producing information on prognosis or the natural history of a condition.

Studies of the accuracy of diagnostic tests are a special case of cross-sectional studies. A key feature of such studies is that the diagnostic test results and 'gold standard information' or reference test results about the presence or absence of the conditions of interest are collected at the same time. The subjects should have both undergone the diagnostic test in question (for example, ultrasound-guided fine-needle aspiration to diagnose malignant disease in patients with nodular thyroid disease), as well as the reference test (histology after surgical resection). The results of one test should not be available to those who are carrying out the other. In terms of the example, the pathologist examining the surgical specimen should be 'blind' to the results of the fine needle aspiration. Another important criterion for a valid evaluation of the diagnostic accuracy is that the diagnostic test is evaluated in 'an appropriate spectrum of patients' (such as those in whom we would use it in practice).

The accuracy of a diagnostic test, a measure of how well the test results help to distinguish between individuals with and individuals without the disease or target disorder, is often expressed in terms of sensitivity and specificity. However, it is important to realize that this is, in most cases, a simplified representation of the diagnostic accuracy. Sensitivity and specificity can only be calculated for a test with dichotomous results, often called 'positive' if the result suggests that the disease is present and 'negative' if it suggests that disease is absent. The sensitivity is estimated as the proportion of individuals with the disease who have a positive test result. The specificity corresponds to the proportion of individuals without the disease who have a negative test result. The sensitivity and specificity of a 'perfect' test are 100%. The sum of the sensitivity and specificity is sometimes used as a single measure of the diagnostic accuracy. The sum of the sensitivity and specificity for a 'worthless' test, a test that would perform no better than tossing a coin, is expected to be 100% and for a perfect test 200%.

In many cases, however, relying on sensitivity and specificity as measures of diagnostic accuracy is too simplistic. For example, many tests, if not all, have more than two possible outcomes, and dichotomizing the results in a positive and a negative test result reduces the amount of diagnostic information that a test can provide. Furthermore, if one would like to dichotomize the test results, it is not immediately obvious what the cut-off value between positive and negative results should be. Lastly, the actual aim of performing a diagnostic test is not to distinguish between individuals with and without the disease, but to identify those individuals for whom the expected benefit of treatment outweighs the expected harm. This indicates that the classic diagnostic 'stepping-stone approach', jumping from signs and symptoms to diagnosis and then from diagnosis to treatment, is rather artificial in many cases. This should be reflected in studies assessing diagnostic tests. They should focus on clinical effectiveness (effect on patient outcomes) rather than on diagnostic accuracy alone (for a comprehensive review of methods for the evaluation of diagnostic technologies, see Knottnerus).[26]

COHORT STUDIES

Cohort studies follow groups of individuals over time. The word 'cohort' originates from the Latin word for a group of 300 to 600 soldiers in a Roman legion. This is appropriate as the same rule applies for epidemiological cohorts as once for Roman cohorts: if a person joins a cohort, he will be a member of that cohort forever, which emphasizes the need for the completeness of follow-up. Most follow-up studies are analytical (comparing the occurrence of outcomes according to presence or absence of certain determinants), but they can be descriptive as well.

The design of many cohort studies is relatively straightforward. A group of people is assembled, none of whom have experienced the outcome of interest, but all of whom could experience it. On study entry, people may be classified according to the determinants of interest. These people are then observed over time to see in which of them the outcome of interest occurs. Despite this simple design, the terminology used to describe these studies can be confusing. For example, terms such as 'longitudinal study', 'prospective study' or 'incidence study' are often used interchangeably. The only real problematic issues in this respect is the use of the term 'prospective study', as cohort studies can consider data that are collected prospectively as well as retrospectively.

The terms 'retrospective' and 'prospective' refer to the way that the data have been collected rather than to the study design. The essential characteristic of prospective data collection is that data are being collected on determinants and outcomes that manifest themselves after the establishment of a study protocol. In all other situations, the data collection should be considered to be retrospective. Retrospective data collection can be based on data recorded in the past for other purposes or on the memory of the study subjects, investigators or other parties. It is obvious that the precision and accuracy of prospectively collected data can be expected to be better than retrospectively collected data. Cohort studies can be based entirely on retrospective data (using retrospective data on both the determinants and the outcome), based entirely on prospective data (using prospective data on both the determinants and the outcome), or based on a mix of retrospective data on determinants and prospective data on the outcome.

Cohort studies have many attractive features. They are the best way of ascertaining the incidence of a disease or health-related event or condition, as well as the natural history of a disorder. They also provide insight into the temporal order of determinants and outcome, which strengthens the inferences that can be made about whether an observed risk factor is a cause of the outcome. Furthermore, multiple outcomes can be considered, which is especially relevant if cohort studies are compared with case-control studies (see 'Case-control studies' below). However, the dangers of considering multiple outcomes are also obvious since testing many hypotheses may lead to misleading results. Lastly, prospective cohort studies are especially valuable for the study of fatal diseases, or more general studies of the occurrence of disease-related conditions with a short duration. When these kinds of conditions are studied retrospectively, the observed occurrences may be an under-representation of all occurrences.

The major drawback of cohort studies is that they are relatively expensive and therefore an inefficient way to study rare outcomes. Cohort studies become more efficient as the outcomes become more common. Another disadvantage for cohort studies that collect outcome prospectively is that the results may not be available for a long time. A prospective study of the effect of passive smoking on the head and neck cancer incidence may take more than 10 years to come up with relevant results.

However, not all prospective cohort studies need to take a very long time to complete. A cohort study could be used, for example, to study the risk factors for complications after tonsillectomy. Such a study could prospectively collect patient characteristics as well as data on surgical technique, instruments used and experience of the surgeons. Every patient could be followed up for a certain period, say one month, and the occurrence of complications could be registered. Such a study would provide insight into the incidence of complications – it might even distinguish between primary haemorrhage, secondary haemorrhage as well as infection, and also in the way this incidence depends on relevant risk factors.

CASE-CONTROL STUDIES

Case-control studies can be considered as 'research in reverse'.[16] Many epidemiologists consider them as one of the most important tools in their armamentarium. The design of case-control studies can be appreciated by again considering the example of the study on risk factors for complications after tonsillectomy. For this study, we could also use a case-control design. All the patients who experience a complication in the first month after surgery could be considered as 'cases', and patients without postoperative complications as 'controls'. The investigators then have to look back in time to find data on the patient's risk factors that were present at the time of surgery.

The essential feature of a case-control study is that not all controls need to be included but that a selection would suffice. Many case-control studies include only one control for each case, whereas others included more but hardly ever more than four or five. The reason that the number of included controls per case is seldom higher is that including more controls will have only a small effect on the power of the study and on the precision of the estimates ('law of diminishing returns'). The fact that only information has to be collected for a selection of the controls makes that, in many circumstances, case-control studies are the most efficient design in terms of time, effort and therefore money. Hence, case-control studies are especially relevant if the occurrence of the outcome of interest is low. However, if the frequency of the determinant of interest is low, case-control studies might become inefficient. For example, if the frequency of a certain risk factor of post-tonsillectomy complications is low, investigators have to examine many cases and controls to find some who have been exposed. Some have advocated a 'rule of thumb' stating that cohorts are more efficient than case-control studies if the occurrence of the outcome is more frequent than that of the determinant and vice versa.

Unlike cohort studies, case-control studies cannot produce an estimate of the occurrence of the outcome of interest since we lack information about the denominator. A case-control study of post-tonsillectomy complications will neither provide information on how many patients underwent the operation nor on what their risk factors were. The relevant effect measure that a case-control study can provide is the odds ratio for a determinant, derived from the proportions in cases and in controls (more precisely, the odds) in whom the determinant is present. Earlier, we referred to this odds ratio as the 'determinant odds ratio'. This determinant odds ratio is equivalent to the 'outcome odds ratio' and the odds ratio obtained from a case-control study can therefore be used as a measure of relative risk.

The advantage of case-control studies (efficiency in time, effort and money) comes at a price, however, because two methodological issues may introduce major systematic errors: selecting the control group and obtaining information about the determinants. The selection of cases is relatively straightforward provided that the definition of the outcome being studied (the 'case definition') is clear. The selection of the control group is more problematic. Two criteria need to be met. First, controls should be representative of the population at risk of becoming cases. In other words, the controls should have been selected as cases had they developed the disease or outcome of interest themselves. Second, selection of the cases should be independent of the determinant(s) being investigated. Therefore, a case-control study of risk factors for post-tonsillectomy haemorrhage should include as controls only patients who underwent a tonsillectomy themselves. Furthermore, it seems inappropriate to select as controls all patients who underwent a tonsillectomy immediately after patients who developed complications. If that were the case, it would be very likely that the same surgeon using the same technique and the same type of instruments treated these patients. It is left as an exercise for the reader to decide what an appropriate strategy to select controls would be.

RANDOMIZED CONTROLLED TRIALS

Randomized controlled trials are cohort studies with prospective data collection. Their distinctive feature is that they use a random allocation scheme to assign the determinant. With randomization, you can expect that the prognostic characteristics of the randomized groups or 'arms' of the trial are similar except for differences due to chance variation. Randomization eliminates the influence of both known and unknown confounders that are present at the time of randomization. Without randomized treatment allocation, it cannot be excluded and is in practice very likely that imbalances in prognostic factors between the groups occur that are the result of selection bias – a type of bias often called 'confounding by clinical indication'.

The ethical argument in favour of a random process deciding what intervention patients receive is that there is equipoise, or a state of genuine uncertainty on the part of the clinical investigator regarding the comparative merits of each intervention. If there is genuine uncertainty about which treatment is best, it is not possible to recommend one over the other, which justifies that a random process decides. The problem, however, is that equipoise depends on subjective judgements and that therefore experts may disagree. Furthermore, preferences of patients or those who are candidates to receive the intervention have to be taken into account. The process of informed consent should address all these issues to ensure that patients can evaluate the potential risks and benefits of the study from their own perspective before they agree to participate.

It is important that the randomization process is 'concealed' from the investigators who include the participants into the trial. Proper allocation concealment requires that the investigators do not know the arm to which a participant will be allocated until the participant has definitively been recruited and included in the study. Concealment of the randomization is the only way to prevent the investigators influencing the balance of the prognostic characteristics between the groups that are being compared. For example, prior knowledge of the next allocation may allow investigators to exclude certain candidate participants from the trial because they are perceived to be allocated to an inappropriate group. More directly, the investigators may try to influence the order of inclusion. Concealment of treatment allocation is so important that with inadequate concealment a randomized controlled trial should be considered non-randomized. Empirical studies have shown that trials with inadequate concealment overestimate the treatment effect by as much as 40% on average.

Another important feature of many randomized controlled trials is the use of a form of blinding, which prevents the participants and the investigators who are in contact with the participants from being aware of which treatment has been offered. Blinding can help to prevent bias in a number of ways. First, if participants do not know what treatment they are receiving, it is less likely that their perceptions and expectations of the treatment that they receive can influence their compliance and the physical and psychological response to the intervention. For example, most patients expect that a new treatment is better than an existing one. Second, blinding investigators is important, as this would prevent them consciously or unconsciously managing the participants in the trials differently. Also, their attitude towards the treatment can influence how patients respond to the treatment. Third, blinding participants and investigators will prevent outcomes from being assessed differently. The terms 'single-blind' and 'double-blind' are often used to indicate trials in which only the participants or both the participants and the investigators are blinded.

Double blinding is impossible in almost all surgical trials. To avoid biased management, the investigators should then try to standardize other potential treatments as much as possible. Approaches to minimize biased assessment of outcomes could include the use of a third party who is unaware of the treatment originally given. When blinded assessment is not possible, one should try as much as possible to use 'hard outcomes' (based on measurements resistant to bias). Another alternative includes the use of standardized outcome measurement scales that can be completed by the participant. This approach is likely to produce less biased outcomes than the judgement of an investigator.

Many people also consider the use of a placebo treatment as an essential feature of a randomized controlled trial. Placebo treatment is a form of treatment indistinguishable from the 'active treatment' under study, but it does not have a specific known mechanism to influence a patient's health. Blinding often requires the use of placebo treatment. Apart from that, the choice whether to use placebo treatment depends on the question that the trial tries to answer. First, if the question is whether intervention A is better than intervention B, then it is obvious that one should compare the effects of A and B with each other and not against placebo treatment. Second, if the question is whether intervention A is better than no treatment at all, the answers may be different for researchers and clinicians. Researchers are likely to be more interested in the specific effects – effects that can be attributed to the 'active component' of an intervention. Clinicians are likely to be more interested in the combined effects of the active and placebo components. On the other hand, it is always useful to know what part of the total effect is due to the active component and what part to the placebo when balancing the potential benefits against potential harms and costs, which are likely to differ between the active and placebo components. It is obvious that placebo treatment is rarely an option for randomized controlled trials in surgery. For example, in a trial comparing tonsillectomy with non-surgical management, it would require a form of 'sham surgery' to provide a placebo treatment. It is left to the reader to decide what the advantages and disadvantages of using such a form of placebo treatment in this context would be.

If a substantial number of participants do not receive the study interventions, do not comply with the study protocol or are lost to follow-up, the trial is likely to be underpowered and its results biased. Strategies to maximize compliance and follow-up should therefore be an integral part of every trial protocol. An obvious strategy is to make participation in a trial as convenient, painless and enjoyable as possible. Some trials have a 'run-in period' that can be used to 'screen out' patients who may not adhere to the study protocol and the follow-up procedures. It is essential to ascertain that compliance and completeness of follow-up do not differ between the trial arms as this could lead to biased estimates of the effects of the interventions.

The results of trials can be analyzed in two ways. First, the comparison of the intervention can be carried out according to the intervention to which the patients were randomized ('intention-to-treat' analysis) or according to the treatment they actually received ('per protocol' analysis). The advantage of an intention-to-treat analysis is that the question that is being addressed corresponds exactly with the one clinicians and patients try to answer in clinical practice. The disadvantage is that if many patients do not receive the treatment they were randomized to, this would obscure the difference between the trial arms. Per protocol analysis, on the other hand, addresses which intervention is better more directly. With this form of analysis, the treatments are being compared according to the treatments that the patients actually received. The problem with this approach is that if many patients do not receive the treatment to which they were randomized, the study no longer represents an experimental study.

The analysis should focus on a single outcome – often referred to as the 'primary endpoint' – to avoid the problems of interpreting the outcome of multiple hypothesis tests. This primary endpoint should also be used for the power calculation in the design phase of the trial. It is often desirable to consider a number of secondary endpoints – outcomes that represent different aspects of the outcome of interest – to provide a more detailed picture of the effects of the interventions under study. For example, a randomized controlled trial of tonsillectomy and non-surgical management could consider the reduction in the number of episodes of tonsillitis or sore throat as primary endpoint, but could also collect information on postoperative complications, reduction in time off work and reduction in the use of certain drugs, such as analgesics and antibiotics.

Subgroup analyses are comparisons between randomized groups in a subset of the patients with specific characteristics. The most important question that subgroup analyses try to answer is whether the effect measure is different in different subgroups by carrying out a statistical test for interaction (or 'effect modification'). For example, one could investigate – when analyzing the results of the trial on tonsillectomy – whether the effects of tonsillectomy on recurrence of tonsillitis are different in children younger than 5 years compared to children of 5 years and older.

Subgroup analyses can be dangerous and misleading, but they can also provide an important extra insight into the generalizability of the results. One danger arises from the fact that multiple comparisons are carried out, which increases the risk of producing false-positive results. To avoid this risk, only a limited number of subgroup analyses should be carried out and they should be specified in the study protocol, in other words, before the results of the trial are known and on the basis of patients characteristics that are measured before randomization.

Furthermore, the actual number of subgroup analyses carried out should be reported. Another approach to minimize the risk of false-positive results is to reduce the significance level of the statistical tests for interaction (for example, from the conventional 0.05 to 0.05 divided by the number of tests carried out as specified by the Bonferroni method). A further danger is the limited power of the subgroup analyses, because the group size is, by definition, smaller than that of the original trial population.

An important problem of randomized controlled trials is that of generalizability. Most trials are carried out in highly controlled conditions in a selected group of patients. Their results therefore provide evidence about the efficacy of an intervention (does the treatment work under ideal circumstances?) and not about the effectiveness (does the treatment work in actual practice?). It depends on the question that needs to be answered as to what extent the design of a trial should focus on efficacy or on effectiveness. An explanatory trial (addressing the efficacy question) is needed in the early stage of a new intervention. However, a pragmatic trial (addressing the effectiveness question that aims to create study conditions that reflect as much as possible actual practice when effectiveness is more important) is more appropriate to answer whether an intervention should be included in the 'repertoire' of available services.

The Consolidated Standards of Reporting Trials (CONSORT) statement has been developed to alleviate the problems arising from inadequate reporting of randomized controlled trials.[27] The CONSORT statement is an evidence-based, minimum set of recommendations for reporting randomized trials and offers a standard way for authors to prepare reports of trial findings, facilitating their complete and transparent reporting, and aiding their critical appraisal and interpretation.

It is obvious that not all questions about the effectiveness of surgical procedures can be addressed with a randomized controlled trial.[28] A number of obstacles have been identified that make randomized controlled trials inappropriate (outcome of interest relatively rare, relevant outcomes far in the future, or randomization affecting the effectiveness of a procedure), impossible (refusal of clinicians or patients to participate, ethical obstacles) or inadequate (low generalizability of experimental studies).[29] As an example, the EaStER trial (Early Stage glottic cancer: Endoscopic excision or Radiotherapy) was closed early with recruitment of only 17 patients. Four principle reasons were found to contribute to poor recruitment into the trial: (i) surgeons and nurses involved in the trial were not in equipoise between the two trial arms and did not fully agree with the trial protocol; (ii) surgeons differed about primary outcome measures; (iii) recruiters focused on the treatment process rather than treatment per se; (iv) logistical issues in some centres made trial participation difficult.[30] If the obstacles are insurmountable, carefully designed observational studies should be considered.

Studying surgical innovation

Innovations are essential to the advancement of otolaryngology. However, the overall number of RCTs in surgical innovation remains small compared with the number of RCTs evaluating medical interventions. On this backdrop, The IDEAL Collaboration was set up in Oxford, UK. They concluded that innovation in surgery follows a different pathway to that of pharmacological developments and that a different approach was needed. The collaboration proposed a framework for the stages in surgical innovation (idea, development, exploration, assessment, and long-term study) and developed a set of recommendations on how evaluation should be conducted at each stage.[31]

Schwartz described three categories of surgical innovation: practice variation (minor changes to routine surgical practice); experimental research (formal trials); and a 'transition zone' between the two.[32] She outlined the ETHICAL model for studies in this 'transition zone' (expertise, technical skill, hazard awareness, informed consent, conflict of interest avoidance, analysis of results, and literature publication). This seeks to protect patients and surgeons, guides decision-making and assists in the generation of scientific hypotheses, without unduly hampering surgical progress.

CONCLUDING REMARKS

This chapter introduces the 'determinant-occurrence relationship' as a key concept for medical research, and epidemiology as a methodological discipline with immediate relevance for otolaryngological research. A basic understanding of epidemiological principles is therefore essential for all people who are involved in clinical research and desirable for all clinicians who want to read the medical literature critically.

We have only presented a broad picture of epidemiological concepts and principles, but it will be clear to the reader that studies vary according to the likelihood that their results are accurate (free of systematic error) and precise (random error). For this reason, a 'hierarchy of evidence' has been suggested.[11] For therapeutic issues, this hierarchy ranges from well-conducted randomized controlled trials at the top – preferably summarized in a systematic review and meta-analysis – to case-reports and expert opinion at the bottom (used throughout this book). For diagnostic and prognostic issues, very different hierarchies are necessary. These hierarchies of evidence are not absolute. If the therapeutic effects are very large in comparison to the potential effects of bias – for example, effects of insulin in ketoacidosis – a description of a series of cases may already provide compelling evidence. Nevertheless, it should be a leading principle that users of research try to look for the best available evidence from this hierarchy.

KEY POINTS

- Epidemiology is a methodological discipline. Epidemiological concepts and principles will help to design empirical studies that are relatively precise (free of random error), accurate (free of systematic error or bias) and efficient (affordable in terms of time and money).
- The 'determinant-occurrence relationship' is a key epidemiological concept, and many clinical research questions can be 'framed' as determinant-occurrence relationships.
- Epidemiological studies can be distinguished into experimental studies (investigators assign the determinants themselves, e.g. randomized controlled trial) and observational studies (investigators examine events as nature takes its course). Observational studies without a comparison or control group are called descriptive studies.
- A research protocol is a document that provides all essential details of a study. It should contain information on:
  - research question
  - study design
  - selection and recruitment of the subjects
  - measurements
  - statistical analysis
  - sample size calculation.
- A 'hierarchy of evidence' has been suggested on the basis of the likelihood that results are accurate and precise. For therapeutic issues, this hierarchy ranges from well-conducted randomized controlled trials at the top – preferably summarized in a systematic review and meta-analysis – to case-reports at the bottom.

ACKNOWLEDGEMENTS

Jan van der Meulen is supported by a National Public Health Career Scientific Award, Department of Health, NHS R&D, UK. David Lowe was supported by a project grant from the Department of Health, UK. Jonathan Fishman is supported by a research grant from The Academy of Medical Sciences, UK.

REFERENCES

1. Burton MJ, Glasziou P, Chong LY, Venekamp RP. Tonsillectomy or adenotonsillectomy versus non-surgical treatment for chronic/recurrent acute tonsillitis (Cochrane Review). *Cochrane DB Syst Rev* 2014: CD001802.
2. Glover JA. The incidence of tonsillectomy in school children. *Proc Roy Soc Med* 1938; **21**: 1219–36.
3. Bakwin H. Pseudodoxia pediatrica. *New Engl J Med* 1945; **232**: 691–97.
4. Sackett DL, Haynes RB, Guyatt GH, Tugwell P. *Clinical epidemiology: a basic science for clinical medicine*. Boston: Little Brown; 1985.
5. Rothman KJ, Greenland S. *Modern epidemiology*. Philadelphia: Lippincott Williams & Wilkins, 1998.
6. MacMahon B, Pugh TF. *Epidemiology: principles and methods*. Boston: Little Brown; 1970.
7. Hennekens CH, Buring JE. *Epidemiology in medicine*. Philadelphia: Lippincott Williams and Wilkins; 1987.
8. Miettinen OS. *Theoretical epidemiology: principles of occurrence research in medicine*. New York: John Wiley and Sons; 1985.
9. Loomis D, Wing S. Is molecular epidemiology a germ theory for the end of the twentieth century? *Int J Epidemiol* 1990; **19**: 1–3.
10. Fletcher RH, Fletcher S, Wagner EH. *Clinical epidemiology: the essentials*. Philadelphia: Lippincott Williams & Wilkins; 1996.
11. Guyatt G, Haynes B, Jaeschke R, et al. Introduction: the philosophy of evidence-based medicine. In: Guyatt G, Rennie D (eds). *Users' guides to the medical literature: essentials of evidence-based clinical practice*. Chicago: AMA Press; 2002.
12. Manolidis S, Takashima M, Kirby M, Scarlett M. Thyroid surgery: a comparison of outcomes between experts and surgeons in training. *Otolaryngol Head Neck Surg* 2001; **125**: 30–33.
13. Mason J, Freemantle N, Browning G. Impact of effective health care bulletin on treatment of persistent glue ear in children: time series analysis. *BMJ* 2001; **323**: 1096–97.
14. Simpson SA, Thomas CL, van der Linden MK, et al. Identification of children in the first four years of life for early treatment for otitis media with effusion (Cochrane Review). *Cochrane Database Syst Rev* 2007: CD004163.
15. Hulley SB, Cummings SR, Browner WS, et al. *Designing clinical research*. Philadelphia: Lippincott Williams & Wilkins; 2001.
16. Grimes DA, Schulz KE. An overview of clinical research: the lay of the land. *Lancet* 2002; **359**: 57–61.
17. Piccirillo JF, Merritt Jr MG, Richards ML. Psychometric and clinimetric validity of the 20-Item Sino-Nasal Outcome Test (SNOT-20). *Otolaryngol Head Neck Surg* 2002; **126**: 41–47.
18. Johns MW. A new method for measuring daytime sleepiness: the Epworth Sleepiness Scale. *Sleep* 1991; **14**: 540–45.
19. https://www.asahq.org/resources/clinical-information/asa-physical-status-classification-system
20. Maw R, Wilks J, Harvey I, et al. Early surgery compared with watchful waiting for glue ear and effect on language development in preschool children: a randomised trial. *Lancet* 1999; **353**: 960–63.
21. Eckel HE, Staar S, Volling P, et al. Surgical treatment for hypopharynx carcinoma: feasibility, mortality, and results. *Otolaryngol Head Neck Surg* 2001; **124**: 561–69.
22. Guyatt GH, Oxman AD, Vist GE, et al. GRADE: an emerging consensus on rating quality of evidence and strength of recommendations. *BMJ* 2008; **336**: 924–26.
23. Hanif J, Frosh A, Marnane C, et al. Lesson of the week: 'high' ear piercing and the rising incidence of perichondritis of the pinna. *BMJ* 2001; **322**: 906–07.
24. Unpublished data. Van der Meulen JHP, 2003.
25. Strachan DP. Impedance tympanometry and the home environment in seven-year-old children. *J Laryngol Otol* 1990; **104**: 4–8.
26. Knottnerus JA (ed.). *The evidence base of clinical diagnosis*. London: BMJ Books; 2002.
27. Schulz KF, Altman DG, Moher D; CONSORT Group. CONSORT 2010 statement: updated guidelines for reporting parallel group randomised trials. *BMJ* 2010; **340**: c332.
28. McCulloch P, Taylor I, Sasako M, et al. Randomised trials in surgery: problems and possible solutions. *BMJ* 2002; **324**: 1448–51.
29. Black N. Why we need observational studies to evaluate the effectiveness of health care. *BMJ* 1996; **312**: 1215–18.
30. Hamilton DW, de Salis I, Donovan JL, Birchall M. The recruitment of patients to trials in head and neck cancer: a qualitative study of the EaStER trial of treatments for early laryngeal cancer. *Eur Arch Otorhinolaryngol* 2013; **270**: 2333–37.
31. McCulloch P, Cook JA, Altman DG, et al. IDEAL framework for surgical innovation 1: the idea and development stages. *BMJ* 2013; **346**: f3012.
32. Schwartz JA. Innovation in pediatric surgery: the surgical innovation continuum and the ETHICAL model. *J Pediatr Surg* 2014; **49**: 639–45.

CHAPTER 42

OUTCOMES RESEARCH

Iain R.C. Swan and William Whitmer

Aim of chapter 483	Specific instruments 489
Introduction 483	How to choose a patient-based outcome measure 491
What are patient-based outcome measures? 483	Which generic instrument? 491
Why use patient-based outcome measures in research? .. 484	The future 492
Assessment of patient-based outcome measures 484	References 492
Types of patient-based outcome measure 487	Further reading 494
Generic instruments 487	

SEARCH STRATEGY

There is a vast literature on this subject, so there was no formal literature search.

AIM OF CHAPTER

The aim of this chapter is to explain the background to patient-based outcomes research. The emphasis is on instruments relevant to otolaryngology. The instruments described are simply examples for the reader. The authors do not suggest that these are the best instruments in their subject area. A list of recommended reading is included for readers who wish further information.

INTRODUCTION

Clinical outcomes research examines the outcomes of treatment or of disease. Traditionally outcomes of medical care are based on clinical observations or laboratory measurements. While these measures provide useful information for the clinician, they are often of limited interest to patients. There is often poor correlation between clinical outcomes and functional capacity and well-being, which are the areas of most interest to the patient. There has been increasing recognition that traditional measures need to be complemented by some measure reflecting the impact of the intervention on the patient in terms of health status and health-related quality of life. These terms refer to experiences of illness such as pain, fatigue, disability and broader aspects of the individual's physical, emotional and social well-being. Medicine, in particular surgery, formerly had the principal objective of reducing mortality and morbidity. These objectives are usually straightforward to assess. Nowadays, a large proportion of clinical practice is either cancer or chronic disease. There has been little improvement for some time in survival in cancer while treatments often have associated side effects and functional impairment that significantly affect the patient's quality of life. There is an increasing prevalence of chronic diseases with an ageing society and here the aims of treatment are to arrest or reverse decline in function.[1] These factors have led to an increased interest in patient-based outcome measures.

At the same time, increased attention is being given to patients' opinions and wishes in relation to their health. Patients should be involved in decisions about their treatment. To contribute usefully, they need information about the outcomes of treatment, not just in terms of surgical results but in terms of the possible effects on their quality of life. Financial resources limit healthcare around the world, and increasingly the distribution of these resources is influenced by the benefits perceived by patients, their carers and society as a whole.

WHAT ARE PATIENT-BASED OUTCOME MEASURES?

Patient-based outcome measures are, in general, questionnaires that ask patients about their perception of their health. Usually these instruments are made up of a number of items or questions. These items are linked in a number of domains or dimensions. A domain refers to an area of behaviour or experience, such as mobility, self-care, depression, pain, social functioning and general well-being. Many questionnaires focus on physical function, such as the patient's ability to walk, climb stairs, wash and dress themselves. Others ask about the impact of health on various areas of an individual's life, such as ability to socialize with members of their family and friends. These are aspects of health-related quality of life (HRQoL). Overall quality of life is influenced by many factors other than health, such as social, financial and physical factors. Patient-based outcome measures assess only one aspect of quality of life and are not measures of overall quality of life.

Patient-based outcome measures assess some aspect of the patient's subjective experience of health and the consequences of illness – and of treatment. As these experiences are those of an individual patient with an individual personality and lifestyle, they cannot be objectively verified. This point is sometimes raised as a criticism of patient-based outcome measures, but it should be borne in mind that many clinician-based outcomes are the subjective opinion of the clinician.

WHY USE PATIENT-BASED OUTCOME MEASURES IN RESEARCH?

In the early days of research, few if any studies included assessment of health-related quality of life. It is increasingly argued now that clinical trials should include patient-based outcome measures except where it is clear that these are not relevant outcomes. The UK Medical Research Council (MRC), the European Organisation for Research and Treatment of Cancer (EORTC) and the National Cancer Institute of Canada (NCIC) all have policies stating that the likely impact on quality of life should be assessed, or justification provided for not doing so.[2] Patient-based outcome measures have been used as the primary outcome measure in randomized controlled trials in many areas including cancer and heart disease. They are also useful in providing evidence of the overall value of a treatment in a way that allows comparison with other treatments in the same area or in other areas.

Patient-based outcome measures are particularly relevant in otolaryngology. Head and neck cancer forms a small proportion of our patients, though a much larger proportion of our clinical workload. The majority of our patients do not have a life-threatening condition and the morbidity is small. Most of our patients simply want us to make them feel better. In many cases we do not have reliable, objective clinical measures to assess the outcome of treatment. To justify our treatment we need patient-based outcome measures to demonstrate the efficacy of treatment – improvement in HRQoL. We also need patient-based outcome measures to demonstrate the effects of these non-life-threatening conditions on HRQoL.

Even when we have objective measures (e.g. closure of a tympanic membrane in myringoplasty), we often know little about the effects on HRQoL. There are also occasions where there is disagreement between clinical measures of success and HRQoL outcomes (e.g. septal surgery for deviated nasal septums). It is likely that the results from one of the measures are unreliable or that they are measuring different things – the validity of both measures should be questioned.

ASSESSMENT OF PATIENT-BASED OUTCOME MEASURES

There are eight criteria that should be applied to patient-based outcome measures: appropriateness, validity, reliability, responsiveness, precision, interpretability, acceptability and feasibility (Table 42.1).[3] There are few patient-based outcome measures for which there is sufficient evidence to allow judgement on all of these criteria.

Appropriateness

The first and most fundamental question when selecting a patient-based outcome measure is how to identify one that is appropriate to the aims of the particular trial. The aims of the trial, the patient group being studied, the type of treatment and the relevant quality of life questions should be carefully considered. The instrument should measure aspects of patients' lives that patients consider important, and should not omit aspects of HRQoL that are important to the patients in the trial.[4] Clinicians often think that they know what aspects of HRQoL are important to patients. Many studies have demonstrated, however, that patients' views often differ from those of clinicians. The most effective way of establishing the importance to patients is asking patients their views. A list of aspects of HRQoL can be drawn up by clinicians and patients. A group of

TABLE 42.1 Assessment of patient-based outcome measures

Criterion	Meaning
Appropriateness	Does the content of the instrument match the intended purpose of the trial?
Validity	Does the instrument measure what it claims to measure?
Reliability	Does the instrument produce the same results when repeated in the same population?
Responsiveness	Does the measure detect clinically meaningful changes in the patient condition?
Precision	Can the instrument detect small differences between patient groups?
Interpretability	Can results from the measure be interpreted clinically and are they relevant?
Acceptability	Are the format of the instrument and the questions acceptable to the planned subjects?
Feasibility	Is it feasible to use this instrument in this setting with these subjects?

patients can then be asked which of these items are problems for them and how important these items are. This is the method commonly used in creating the patient-based outcome measures that are widely used, such as the SF-36 (see 'Generic instruments' below).

The purpose of the trial must be specified precisely in order to select an instrument that fits that purpose. In many studies, the rationale for selection of outcome measures is not clear. Careful consideration of content and relevance of a questionnaire to the purpose of the trial should be given. The instrument selected must be as relevant to the health problem and the proposed intervention as possible.

It is often recommended that one generic and one disease-specific instrument be used in a trial to increase the likelihood of appropriate assessment of outcomes.

Validity

The validity of a measure is an assessment of the extent to which it measures what it claims to measure. Validity is not a fixed property of a measure but is assessed in relation to a specific purpose and setting.[5] It is, therefore, meaningless to refer to a validated outcome measure, as many reports do. Evidence of validity of an outcome measure in one situation does not mean that there will be adequate validity in another research setting.

This apparently simple property depends on a range of different types of evidence including how the content was chosen and its relationship to other variables. There are several different ways of assessing validity of a patient-based outcome measure. No single set of observations is likely to determine validity, so assessment of validity in relation to a specific trial is not straightforward.

CRITERION VALIDITY

Criterion validity is the correlation of a measure with an objective or 'gold standard' measure. As gold-standard measures rarely exist in assessment of quality of life, criterion validity is rarely relevant in patient-based outcome measures, and validity is judged by more indirect assessment of content and construct validity. It can be assessed when a shorter version of an instrument is used to predict the results of a full-length version.

FACE AND CONTENT VALIDITY

Face and content validity are among the most relevant issues for the use of patient-based outcome measures in clinical trials. They address whether items clearly address the intended subject matter and whether the range of aspects is adequately covered. They are explained by Guyatt et al.:[6] 'Face validity examines whether an instrument appears to be measuring what it is intended to measure, and content validity examines the extent to which the domain of interest is comprehensively sampled by the items or questions in the instrument.' In other words, does the questionnaire look right and does it cover the right things? Face and content validity are mainly based on careful examination of the content of the instrument and qualitative judgement rather than statistical criteria. Evidence of how the questionnaire was initially developed is useful. Questionnaires with good validity are constructed in phases with involvement of patients with experience of the particular health problem. The content of poor-validity questionnaires is chosen without consultation.

CONSTRUCT VALIDITY

Construct validity is also very relevant but is a quantitative assessment of the relationship of a construct to other variables. A construct is a theoretical idea about the domain to be measured. For example, patients with hearing disability should have poorer audiometric thresholds. Many patient-based outcome measures are multidimensional: they assess, for example, physical, psychological and social aspects of an illness. Those questions related to psychological aspects should correlate with each other much more than with questions assessing physical function. The internal structure of such instruments is established by construct validation, most commonly factor analysis. For a detailed discussion of assessment of construct validity, the reader is referred to Fitzpatrick et al.[3]

Reliability

Reliability is the reproducibility and internal consistency of an instrument. It assesses the extent to which the instrument is free from random error. It is essential to establish that any changes observed in a trial are due to the treatment and not to problems in the measuring instrument. As the random error increases, the size of the sample required to produce an accurate result increases.

REPRODUCIBILITY

Reproducibility is the degree to which an instrument gives the same results on repeated applications with the same subjects, and is also known as the test-retest reliability. An instrument should produce the same or very similar results on two or more administrations. This should be relatively straightforward to assess but care must be taken with the time interval between tests. Repeat measurements should be far enough apart in time for the subject to forget their earlier answers but not so far apart that their health status might have changed. This is commonly reported as a correlation coefficient. However, a correlation coefficient measures the strength of association between two measures and not the extent of agreement. Bland and Altman recommend plotting the scores from the two tests graphically, which is certainly a simpler method than a statistical comparison of repeated scores.[7]

INTERNAL CONSISTENCY

More than one question is usually used to measure one domain in a questionnaire because several related observations will produce a more reliable estimate than one. Individual questions in a domain should correlate highly with each other and with the total score for questions in that domain. This is the internal consistency of a patient-based outcome measure. The correlation is often measured using Cronbach's alpha.[8, 9] If all the questions in a domain are the same, Cronbach's alpha will be 1, while if there is no relationship Cronbach's alpha will be 0. If the correlation is too high, it is likely that the questions are addressing a very narrow aspect of an attribute and some items may be redundant, which then reduces the content validity. It is therefore suggested that Cronbach's alpha should be between 0.7 and 0.9.[10]

Responsiveness to change

Responsiveness is the ability of an instrument to detect clinically important change, even if that change is small.[11] This is sometimes called sensitivity to change but the term sensitivity has other, more general uses. It is particularly important in clinical trials when changes might correspond to therapeutic effects of treatment. An instrument can be both reliable and valid but not responsive to change.

There are several statistical methods of assessing responsiveness. The simplest method is to compare change scores for an instrument over time with changes in another variable or variables. The other variable preferably should be an objective indicator, such as a physiological measurement, or a clinician-based outcome measure.

An alternative method of assessing responsiveness is calculation of the effect size in a given clinical situation. This is the size of change in a measure between assessments, for example before and after treatment, compared with the variability of scores for that measure on one assessment. The effect size is defined as the mean change in a variable divided by the standard deviation of that variable.[12] The effect size can then be expressed in standardized units that allow comparisons with other outcome measures. It has been suggested that effect sizes can be used to assess the size of change in a study arm: an effect size of 0.2 is small, 0.5 is medium and 0.8 or greater is a large change.[12]

Other more complex statistical measures of responsiveness are described by Fitzpatrick et al.[3]

One of the main limitations on the responsiveness of an instrument is when the wording of questions does not allow reporting of very good or very poor health states: ceiling and floor effects. Subjects with initial high scores may not show any improvement following effective treatment and those with initial poor scores may not show any deterioration when their clinical situation deteriorates.

As with validity, evidence of responsiveness in one situation does not mean that there will be adequate responsiveness in another research setting.

Precision or sensitivity

The preferred term is precision as sensitivity has a number of other uses in research. Precision is the ability of the instrument to reflect true differences in health states. As clinical trials often aim to detect small differences between patient groups, precision is a desirable capability.

One of the main influences on the precision of an instrument is the format of the answers. The simplest answers are 'yes' or 'no' but they do not allow any assessment of difficulty or severity. The most commonly used graded response is a Likert scale, such as:

- very satisfied
- satisfied
- neither satisfied or dissatisfied
- dissatisfied
- very dissatisfied.

There is some evidence that using seven response categories rather than five increases precision, though this is rarely used.

The main alternative to a Likert scale is a visual analogue scale, where patients can mark any point on a line to represent their answer. Though this would appear to offer more precision, comparison studies of Likert scales and visual analogue scales have found no advantage of visual analogue scales. In addition, it appears that visual analogue scales are less acceptable to many patients, who find it difficult to translate their feelings into numbers. It is important to note that the questions should be worded as to potentially elicit all points along whichever scale is used (i.e. avoid wording that elicits only yes or no responses).

Patients' responses in patient-based outcome measures are generally converted into numerical values for statistical analysis. Most instruments use simple ordinal values, for example 1 to 5 (or 7) for a Likert scale, which are capable of less precision. However, the majority of published reports of health status measures use parametric statistical analysis that is appropriate for interval scales,[13] though the interval between 1 and 2 (very satisfied and satisfied) may not be the same as between 4 and 5 (dissatisfied and very dissatisfied).

Some patient-based outcome measures use an explicitly derived weighting system for responses. The weights can be assigned by a panel of patients and health professionals, for example the Nottingham Health Profile,[14] or be based on preference measurements obtained from a random sample of the general population, such as the Health Utilities Index.[15, 16] The fact that weighted scoring systems appear to be much more exact with their scoring suggests that they might be more precise but this may well be deceptive. Several studies have compared weighted and ordinal scoring systems and have not shown any significant difference in precision between these two methods of scoring.

Ceiling and floor effects may influence scores of instruments. Some patient-based outcome measures do not include questions that would identify very poor levels of health, so all patients with poor health have similar scores and further deterioration will not be identified. Sometimes patients with minor health problems will be scored as having excellent health so treatment of their problem will not result in any improvement in score.

One other important factor in precision is bias. This can be reduced by general aspects of study design, such as making assessments blind to intervention. In many cases it is not possible to keep the patient blind to which treatment arm of a trial he is in, so his judgement of outcomes may be influenced.

Patient-based outcome measures may therefore vary in how precisely their scores relate to underlying distributions of patients' health status. Researchers need to carefully consider factors that might influence precision. The degree of precision required of a patient-based outcome measure will depend on other aspects of trial design such as sample size and the expected differences between arms of the trial.

Interpretability

Can results from the measure be interpreted clinically and are they relevant? The interpretability of an instrument is concerned with how meaningful are the baseline scores or a change in scores. Clinically important changes in scores can be estimated by comparison with clinical or laboratory tests in the same patient group. Representative data are available from the general population for some widely used instruments such as the Health Utilities Index (see 'Utility measures' below) and the SF-36. The scores from the trial patients can be compared with the means and standard deviations for the general population. A significant change in the score in the trial could be set at one-and-a-half standard deviations from the population mean.[10] Normative data can be key to interpreting both state and change questionnaires, as assumptions of no treatment resulting in no change in outcome can be erroneous. For example, in a study of hearing-aid interventions, those who were not given hearing aids exhibited participant acquiescence: a statistically significant increase in benefit without intervention.[17]

Acceptability

Clearly it is essential that the format of the instrument and the questions are acceptable to patients. An instrument should not cause distress to patients or be difficult to understand. In general, shorter instruments are more acceptable to patients. The instructions to patients should make it very clear that their answers will not influence their treatment. Acceptability is also important in order to obtain high response rates to questionnaires to make results of trials easier to interpret, more generalizable and less prone to bias due to non-response. When choosing an instrument, it is useful to know if the instrument has been used in similar settings before.

Ideally acceptability of an instrument should be directly tested at the design stage by seeking the views of patients. Subsequently, evidence of acceptability can be found in patient response rates.

Feasibility

The feasibility of an instrument is dependent on the time available for its completion and the staff available to help with its completion, either by interviewing patients or explaining the instrument to patients. The data collected have to be entered onto a computer and the time required and ease of entering has to be considered. The measure must be short enough to be completed or administered in the intended setting and with the types of patients and families involved in the trial. This is one of the criteria of patient-based outcome measures that can usually be easily judged by investigators in the research setting. If in doubt, feasibility can be assessed by piloting the study methods.

TYPES OF PATIENT-BASED OUTCOME MEASURE

There are two basic types of patient-based outcome measure: generic and specific. Generic instruments access multidimensional health profiles, overall medical condition and personal function. Specific instruments focus on the problems found in individual diseases, disabilities and patient groups.[11] Within each of these categories there are different types of instruments (Table 42.2).

TABLE 42.2 Types of patient-based outcome measure

Category	Type	Example
Generic	Health profile	SF-36, Sickness Impact Profile, Nottingham Health Profile, Glasgow Benefit Inventory.
	Utility	Health Utilities Index (HUI), EQ-5D
Specific	Disease-specific	Dizziness Handicap Inventory (DHI)
	Site-specific	Sino-Nasal Outcome Test (SNOT-20)
	Dimension-specific	McGill Pain Questionnaire

GENERIC INSTRUMENTS

Generic instruments are designed to access a broad range of aspects of health status and the consequences of illness and therefore to be relevant to a wide range of patient groups and conditions. The advantage of generic instruments is that they can be used for a broad range of health problems and this enables comparisons across different groups of patients with diverse conditions. Because of their broad range of content and general applicability, such instruments have been used to assess the health of samples from the general population. Such data have been used to generate normative values across populations with which other groups of patients with specific health problems can be compared. Since generic instruments are used more often than specific instruments, there are usually more data available about their reliability and validity.

As generic questionnaires cover a broad range of aspects of health status, many items may be irrelevant to a particular condition. These items result in a wide range of scores that are not relevant to the condition being studied. As there are few questions relevant to a specific condition, the instrument may be insensitive to changes that might occur as a result of treatment for that condition.

Health profile

SF-36

The most commonly used health profile instrument is the Medical Outcome Study Short-Form 36-Item Health Survey (SF-36).[18, 19] The SF-36 is a 36 item, self-completed questionnaire that measures health status in eight dimensions: physical functioning; role limitations due to physical problems; role limitations due to emotional problems; social functioning; mental health; energy and vitality; pain; and general perceptions of health. It can be completed by the patient in less than 10 minutes. Responses are summed to give a score for each dimension: physical component summary (PCS) and mental component summary (MCS).[20] It has been used in a wide variety of patient groups and conditions, including many otorhinolaryngological conditions (Table 42.3). Data from trial subjects can be compared with normative data for the population.[21] Garratt et al.[22] identified 408 papers that included aspects of development and evaluation of the SF-36 over a 10-year period (1990–99). It can also be used in a reduced 12-item version that is a subset of the original SF-36.[23] However, the larger instrument gives more reliable estimates of individual levels of health and is therefore the better choice of instrument in small studies.

Recently, Brazier et al.[24] derived from the SF-36 a preference-based single index measure, the SF-6D, to make the instrument more useful in evaluations of cost-effectiveness (see 'Utility measures' below). This weighted scoring model could potentially be applied to any SF-36 data set. However, initial validation studies demonstrated some inconsistencies and further assessment of the scoring model is required.[25]

WORLD HEALTH ORGANIZATION DISABILITY ASSESSMENT SCHEDULE 2.0

The World Health Organization's Disability Assessment Schedule 2.0 (WHO-DAS 2) was designed to measure domains coincident with the definitions of the WHO's International Classification of Functioning (ICF), a replacement for the stigmatized labels of impairment, disability and handicap. It is very similar to the SF-36 except that its six domains – cognition, mobility, self-care, interaction, life activities (e.g. leisure and work limitations) and 'social participation' (e.g. emotional and social burden) – fit the ICF framework. To date, it has only been applied in otorhinolaryngology with regard to hearing aids, where it was found to be sensitive to intervention, but the effect size was modest compared to hearing-specific questionnaires.[17]

SICKNESS IMPACT PROFILE

The Sickness Impact Profile (SIP) is a general health-status questionnaire comprising 136 questions answered as either 'yes' or 'no'.[34] They are grouped into 12 categories: walking; body care and movement; mobility; social interaction; alertness behaviour; emotional behaviour; communication; sleep and rest; eating; home management; recreational activities; and work. Each item is weighted, and the scores of all answered questions are combined. There are 12 category scores, 2 summary scores (physical and psychosocial) and a total score. The scores are standardized and range from 0 to 100 points, with 100 indicating the poorest function. The test-retest reliability and internal consistency are high and it has good content and construct validity.[34] It is, however, a long questionnaire and is usually administered by interview. Its acceptability and feasibility in a trial must be carefully considered.

NOTTINGHAM HEALTH PROFILE

The Nottingham Health Profile is a generic, self-administered questionnaire designed to measure perceived physical, social and emotional health problems.[14, 35] An initial pool of statements was collected from patients at interview, and from this pool 38 items were chosen relating to six dimensions: physical mobility, pain, social isolation, emotional reaction, energy and sleep. The scores can be compared with the average scores in a population matched for gender and age.

GLASGOW BENEFIT INVENTORY

As other generic instruments are often insensitive to the non-acute disorders generally seen in an ORL clinic, the Glasgow Benefit Inventory (GBI) was developed for use in patients with otolaryngological conditions.[36] The GBI is a post-intervention questionnaire that assesses the effects of interventions on the health status of patients, rather than the actual health status. The GBI has 18 items in three domains: psychological, social and physical well-being. Rather than attempt to assess the difference between before and after treatment measures, it asks directly about the change in health status resulting from treatment. It is likely, therefore, to be more sensitive to such change than two separate instruments before and after intervention. In addition, compliance will be significantly higher because patients are only required to complete one questionnaire. The response to each question is based on a five-point Likert scale, for example: 'Since your *operation/intervention*, have you found it easier or harder to deal with company?' The words in italics (*operation/intervention*) in each question are replaced by words appropriate to the intervention of interest. Responses are scored using

TABLE 42.3 Examples of the use of the SF-36 in otolaryngology

ORL condition	Reference
Chronic rhinosinusitis	van Agthoven et al.,[26] Gliklich and Metson,[27] Piccirillo et al.[28]
Chronic otitis media	Nadol et al.[29]
Dysphonia	MacKenzie et al.[30]
Laryngeal cancer	Stewart et al.[31]
Meniere's disease	Lopez-Escamez et al.[32]
Rhinoplasty and otoplasty	Klassen et al.[33]

TABLE 42.4 Examples of the use of the GBI

ORL intervention	Reference
Bone-anchored hearing aids	Dutt et al.[38]
Hearing aids	Swan et al.[39]
Cochlear implants	UK Cochlear Implant Study Group[40]
Treatment of acoustic neuroma	Brooker et al.[41]
Speech therapy for dysphonia	Wilson et al.[42]
Rhinoplasty	McKiernan et al.[43]
Tonsillectomy	Bhattacharyya et al.[44]
Surgery for snoring	Uppal et al.[45]

a weighted scale from a population sample to give a score between −100 and +100.

The GBI has been used to assess the benefit experienced by patients following various treatments (**Table 42.4**). Details of the questionnaire and its use can be found at www.ihr.gla.ac.uk. Hendry et al.[37] wrote a comprehensive review of the use of the GBI.

Utility measures

Multi-attribute utility measures access a broad range of aspects of health status, like other generic instruments, but have a particular form of numerical weighting or valuation of health states. Utility measures have been developed from economics and decision theory in order to provide an estimate of individual patients' overall preferences for different health states. They are scored as a single number between 1 (full health) and 0 (death). The weighted scoring method is based on preference measurements obtained from samples of a general population. They are asked to value different aspects of health as defined by the instrument using one of a number of valuation techniques, most commonly standard gamble, time trade-off and visual analogue scales (see Brazier et al.[46] for explanation).

Utility scores reflect the health status and value of that health status to the patient. As utility measures are scored as a single value, they do not define individual dimensions of health that contribute to the individual's overall sense of well-being. They are relatively insensitive to small but relevant changes in health and are therefore more suited to studies of large populations.

There are several health utility measures that have been widely used. Brazier et al.[46] carried out an extensive review of these and recommended the Health Utilities Index (HUI) and the EuroQol (EQ-5D) as the instruments of choice.

HEALTH UTILITIES INDEX

The Health Utilities Index (HUI-I) evolved from studies in neonatal intensive care.[47] A second version (HUI-II) was developed to assess outcomes in long-term survivors of childhood cancer but is suitable for use in a wider range of children.[16] Though it is claimed to be a generic instrument, its content is explicitly aimed at children with questions specifically aimed at developmental age.

The HUI-II was revised to make it more relevant to an adult population. The HUI-III assesses eight aspects of health status: vision, hearing, speech, ambulation, dexterity, emotion, cognition, self-care and pain.[48] It has 15 questions with 4 to 6 available responses for each and is easy for patients to complete. The HUI-III has been used in a wide variety of clinical studies and has been shown to be reliable and responsive.[49] It is one of the few generic patient-based outcome measures that specifically assesses hearing and speech and is therefore potentially useful in many areas of otolaryngology. Normative data have been collected from large populations and from these data weighted scoring scales have been devised.[16] It has been used in a cost-utility study of cochlear implants[50] and in the UK cochlear implant study.[51]

EQ-5D

The EQ-5D is a self-completed questionnaire with five dimensions: mobility, self-care, usual activities, pain/discomfort and anxiety/depression.[52] It is easy to complete and is very acceptable to patients. Responses can be scored using a weighted scale from a large general population sample.[53] It is very brief with only five questions and three levels of response for each.[54] It was compared with the Euroquol and the SF-36 in a survey of 1980 adults and the Euroquol was found to be less sensitive.[54] However, it was originally intended to complement other forms of health-related quality of life measures. It has been widely used and its test-retest reliability is good.[55]

SPECIFIC INSTRUMENTS

Disease- or condition-specific instruments

The aim of these instruments is to provide the patient's perception of the problems related to a specific disease or condition. It should be remembered that disease may have a broad impact on the patient's life. To make these instruments comprehensive, a detailed survey of patients suffering from the condition should be conducted when developing the instrument. They may also not detect problems associated with a disease and its treatment that have not been anticipated by the developers if patients have not been involved in the planning. As all of the questions are developed specifically to assess a particular health problem, the content should be very relevant for use in studies of that condition: high validity. They are more likely to detect changes that occur in that particular condition as there should be few if any irrelevant questions: high responsiveness. They are also more acceptable to patients as the relevance of the questions to their condition is obvious so completion rates should be high.

The major disadvantage of disease-specific instruments is that they do not allow comparison to be made with other patient groups with other diseases or conditions.

Such comparisons require generic instruments designed for use with any health problem, and for this reason it is often useful to combine a specific instrument with a generic one.

VERTIGO

The Dizziness Handicap Inventory (DHI) is a 25-item questionnaire designed to measure the self-perceived disability and handicap caused by dizziness or imbalance.[56] They reported good internal consistency and test-retest repeatability. The questions were grouped in three domains of functional, emotional and physical aspects of dizziness with three possible answers to each question: yes, sometimes and no. The questions were selected from an initial bank of 37 questions chosen from the case histories of patients. They take a clinical perspective of disability and handicap in daily activities and therefore content validity should be carefully inspected before choosing this instrument for use in a trial. It is preferable to have more input from patients in the selection of items to include in a questionnaire (see 'Face and content validity' above. This instrument has been widely used in studies of imbalance in general. It has been shown to have a moderate correlation with balance performance measures.[57]

The Vertigo Handicap Questionnaire (VHQ) was developed from patients' accounts of the problems that they experienced with vertigo.[58] It has 25 questions about restriction of physical and social activities and emotional distress, each scored on a 5-point Likert scale. It has good reliability and validity but has not been widely used.

HEARING

There are many instruments that have been developed for use in audiology. Assessing hearing disability has one major difference from assessing most other disabilities in otolaryngology – there is a gold standard, at least for audibility – pure-tone audiometry. One of the most widely used measures is the Hearing Handicap Inventory for the Elderly (HHIE).[59] This instrument has been shown to have good face and content validity.[60] Further, it has good sensitivity and specificity when used properly in tandem with an audioscope.[61] A more in-depth instrument is the Speech, Spatial and Qualities of Hearing questionnaire (SSQ),[62] which asks situation-specific questions on understanding speech, locating sound sources, and various qualities of sounds (e.g. detection, naturalness), resulting in an overall score and the three subscales of its title. It has shown good validity and reliability, and has been translated into many languages. Details of the SSQ and its use can be found at www.ihr.gla.ac.uk.

While there are reliable tools for measuring hearing, assessment of the efficacy of hearing aid provision and comparison of benefits from different prescription strategies are heavily reliant on patient-based outcome measures. The HHIE has been used for this purpose[63] but it has been shown to have poor precision when changes in the HHIE were compared with changes in the Speech Intelligibility Index when using a hearing aid.[64] This is probably because the HHIE assesses predominantly the emotional and psychological response to hearing impairment. There are many self-report hearing-aid tools available, to such an extent that a good guide for how to choose one already exists.[65] Two of the more popular hearing-aid questionnaires that deserve additional mention are the Glasgow Hearing Aid Benefit Profile (GHABP)[66] and the Client-Oriented Scale of Improvement (COSI).[67] The GHABP was developed as a measure of hearing disability and the benefit obtained from use of a hearing aid.[66] It assesses unaided disability, handicap, benefit from a hearing aid, residual disability and patient satisfaction in eight listening situations – four specified and up to four chosen by the patient. It has been used as one of the primary outcome measures in the NHS programme of modernizing hearing-aid services in England. Details of the questionnaire and its use can be found at www.ihr.gla.ac.uk. The COSI asks the patient to provide (up to) five specific situations that are important to them. Communication ease is then rated before and after fitting (or change in fitting) for those specific situations, and benefit derived from the pre/post-fitting difference in ease. The 'open-set' approach of the COSI is notable in avoiding the assumption of experience with the hypothetical situations proposed by many questionnaires.

OTITIS MEDIA

The Otitis Media-6 (OM6) was developed for use in children with recurrent acute otitis media and otitis media with effusion.[68] Six domains (physical suffering, hearing loss, speech impairment, emotional distress, activity limitation, caregiver concerns) are each addressed by a single question. Test-retest repeatability was high, and responsiveness was demonstrated by significant change in scores after surgery for ventilation tube insertion.[69] The criterion validity has been questioned, however, in that it does not correlate well with other markers of disease severity, such as audiometry and severity of symptoms of recurrent acute otitis media.[70] Kubba also suggested that the instrument lacks precision as it does not differentiate between children with otitis media and others with sore throats.[70]

CANCER

The European Organization for Research and Treatment of Cancer Quality of Life Study Group developed the EORTC QLQ-C30 as an instrument of 30 items for use in international trials in cancer.[71] Further modules have been developed which can be added to the core instrument to provide assessment of specific cancers, for example head and neck cancer.[72] This allows collection of data for comparison across cancer groups and additional data that are particularly relevant to specific cancers. The questionnaire has been translated into more than 60 languages and is widely used around Europe and the rest of the world.[73]

Site-specific instruments

These instruments contain items that are particularly relevant to patients having treatment for a specific region of the body and should be sensitive to changes experienced by patients following treatment in that region. They are particularly useful in otolaryngology and have the advantage that patient groups are not limited to a specific disease classification. They thus allow comparison of patients with similar symptoms but different pathology. Because they have a narrow focus, they are unlikely to detect any change in broader aspects of health or quality of life following intervention.

SINONASAL DISEASE

Many patient-based outcome measures have been designed for use in sinonasal disease. The 20-item Sino-Nasal Outcome Test (SNOT-20)[74] is a modification of the previously used 31-item Rhinosinusitis Outcome Measure (RSOM-31).[28] The 20 questions refer to specific sinonasal symptoms and some general health questions. It has good internal consistency (Cronbach's alpha 0.9), and showed good responsiveness to change. Face and content validity seemed good and the construct validity was high when compared with clinical assessment of disease. Test-retest scores were highly correlated (r = 0.9) though this measures the association between tests rather than repeatability (see 'Reproducibility' above). Piccirillo et al.[74] report the SNOT-20 to be a valid outcome measure in their particular research setting. The questionnaire is easily completed by the patient and acceptability is high. It has since been modified with the addition of two further questions (the SNOT-22);[75] its validity and ease of use were confirmed in a study of more than 2000 patients.

VOICE

There is no generally accepted objective test to serve as a 'gold standard' for the assessment of voice disorders. Various questionnaires have been developed for evaluation of the consequences of dysphonia. The Voice Handicap Index (VHI) was designed to assess the self-perceived effect on quality of life of voice disorders.[76] It is a 30-item questionnaire divided into 3 subscales: functional handicap, emotional handicap and physical handicap. The questions use a 5-point Likert scale. It has been used to assess the impact of a number of voice disorders, including vocal cord polyps, cord palsy, spasmodic dysphonia and functional disorders. Its construct validity has been confirmed by comparing its subscales with appropriate subscales of the SF-36 in assessment of the health-related quality of life in patients after treatment for laryngeal cancer.[31] A shortened version, the Voice Handicap Index-10, has been proposed as an equally effective alternative.[77] Carding et al.[78] wrote a review of measures of voice outcomes.

Dimension-specific instruments

These instruments assess one specific aspect of health status. The most commonly assessed dimension is psychological well-being. Another common dimension, more relevant to otolaryngology, is pain. The McGill Pain Questionnaire is one of the most widely used measures of pain severity for both clinical and research purposes.[79] It comprises 20 subclasses of pain descriptors that provide pain severity scores across sensory–discriminative, motivational–affective and cognitive–evaluative dimensions. It has been found to have good short-term repeatability in chronic pain conditions, and it discriminates well between different types of pain syndromes. A short form of the McGill Pain Questionnaire has been developed.[80] It is highly correlated with the original longer version and has comparable sensitivity. It may be a useful instrument in situations in which the standard questionnaire takes too long to administer.

The advantage of dimension-specific instruments is that they provide a more detailed assessment in the area of concern than is possible in more general instruments. They are perhaps most useful in a study where they are used in combination with another instrument (e.g. van Agthoven).[26]

HOW TO CHOOSE A PATIENT-BASED OUTCOME MEASURE

The choice of patient-based outcome measure depends on the purpose of the study. To assess the effects on health-related quality of life of a disease or condition, a generic instrument is required. Specific instruments are of little value as they do not allow comparison with other conditions. A specific instrument may provide additional information by assessing the severity of the disease if no objective measure is available, for example in tinnitus. Comparison of the scores from the specific instrument with the generic instrument may be valuable.

If the aim of the study is to assess the efficacy of treatment, it is usually recommended that two instruments be combined, a generic and a specific instrument. The two different measures are likely to produce complementary evidence. A disease-specific measure will be more responsive to the main effects of intervention, and therefore produce the evidence most relevant to the clinician. A generic measure may allow comparisons across interventions and disease groups, but is likely to be relatively insensitive to the effects of the intervention. It is possible, however, that the additional burden on the patient may reduce overall compliance, especially if there is overlap between questions in the two instruments.

WHICH GENERIC INSTRUMENT?

Acceptability to the patient and feasibility of completing the questionnaires are obviously important. The time required to complete the commonly used instruments varies. The Health Utilities Index (HUI) Mark II takes 3 minutes, the SF-36 10 minutes and the Sickness Impact Profile 20 minutes.[81]

Appropriateness depends on the study. Utility measures are, in general, only appropriate for studies with large numbers of subjects. Small studies would probably be better to choose a generic health status questionnaire. Some generic instruments have been shown to be better than others in assessing patients with particular problems. Edelman et al.[81] reported that the HUI was better used for evaluating relatively healthy populations because of some floor effects, while the SIP was better for more severely ill populations as their study patients were grouped at the healthy end of the scale. Other authors have similarly reported that the SIP has ceiling effects.[82–84]

A careful evaluation of reports of the use of these instruments in similar patient groups and study settings should be carried out before making a final choice. In the absence of this, the SF-36 appears to be the safest choice. The HUI Mark III is suitable for large studies and has the advantage for otolaryngology research of including items about hearing and speech.

THE FUTURE

Development of a valid and acceptable patient-based outcome measure takes a lot of time and effort. Large numbers of subjects are needed as development requires several stages. Patient involvement in the selection of items is essential. There have been many patient-based outcome measures that have been reported once and never used again. On the other hand, the currently available and widely used patient-based outcome measures are not ideal. We need better ones.

KEY POINTS

- Patient-reported outcome measures assess the patient's subjective experience of illness and of treatment.
- Generic instruments access a broad range of aspects of health status, enabling comparisons across different patient groups with diverse conditions, but may not be sensitive to particular illnesses or treatments.
- Specific instruments are more sensitive to the effects of specific diseases or conditions, but do not allow comparison to be made with other patient groups with other diseases or conditions.
- The best assessment is usually achieved by using both a generic and a specific outcome measure.

REFERENCES

1. van den Bos GAM, Limburg LCM. Public health and chronic diseases. *Eur J Public Health* 1995; **5**: 1–2.
2. Fayers PM, Hopwood P, Harvey A, et al. Quality of life assessment in clinical trials – guidelines and a checklist for protocol writers: the UK Medical Research Council experience. MRC Cancer Trials Office. *Eur J Cancer* 1997; **33**: 20–28. UI: 9071894.
3. Fitzpatrick R, Davey C, Buxton MJ, Jones DR. Evaluating patient-based outcome measures for use in clinical trials. *Health Technol Assess* 1998; **2**(14): i–iv, 1–74. UI: 9812244
4. Guyatt GH, Cook DJ. Health status, quality of life, and the individual. *JAMA* 1994; **272**: 630–31. UI: 8057520.
5. Jenkinson C. Evaluating the efficacy of medical treatment: possibilities and limitations. *Soc Sci Med* 1995; **41**: 1395–401. UI: 8560307.
6. Guyatt GH, Feeny DH, Patrick DL. Measuring health-related quality of life. *Ann Int Med* 1993; **118**: 622–29. UI: 8452328
7. Bland JM, Altman DG. Statistical methods for assessing agreement between two methods of clinical measurement. *Lancet* 1986; **1**: 307–10. UI: 2868172.
8. Cronbach LJ. Coefficient alpha and the internal structure of tests. *Psychometrika* 1951; **16**: 297–334.
9. Bland JM, Altman DG. Cronbach's alpha. *BMJ* 1997; **314**: 572. UI: 9055718.
10. Streiner DL, Norman GR. *Health measurement scales: a practical guide to their development and use*. Oxford: OUP; 1995.
11. Guyatt GH, Veldhuyzen van Zanten≈SJO, Feeny DH, Patrick DL. Measuring quality-of-life in clinical trials: a taxonomy and review. *Can Med Assoc J* 1989; **140**: 1441–48. UI: 2655856.
12. Kazis LE, Anderson JJ, Meenan RF. Effect sizes for interpreting changes in health status. *Med Care* 1989; **27**(Suppl): S178–89. UI: 2646488.
13. Coste J, Fermanian J, Venot A. Methodological and statistical problems in the construction of composite measurement scales: a survey of six medical and epidemiological journals. *Stat Med* 1995; **14**: 331–45. UI: 7746975.
14. Hunt SM, McEwen J, McKenna SP. Measuring health status: a new tool for clinicians and epidemiologists. *Brit J Gen Pract* 1985; **35**: 185–88. UI: 3989783.
15. Feeny D, Furlong W, Boyle M, Torrance GW. Multi-attribute health status classification systems. Health Utilities Index. *Pharmacoeconomics* 1995; **7**: 490–502. UI: 10155335.
16. Feeny D, Furlong W, Torrance GW, et al. Multi-attribute and single-attribute utility functions for the Health Utilities Index Mark 3 system. *Med Care* 2002; **40**: 113–28. UI: 11802084.
17. McArdle R, Chisolm T, Abrams H, et al. The WHO-DAS II: Measuring outcomes of hearing intervention for adults. *Trends in Amplif* 2005; **9**: 127–43.
18. Ware JE Jr, Sherbourne CD. The MOS 36-item short-form health survey (SF-36). I. Conceptual framework and item selection. *Med Care* 1992; **30**: 473–83. UI: 1593914.
19. McHorney CA, Ware JE Jr, Raczek AE. The MOS 36-Item Short-Form Health Survey (SF-36): II. Psychometric and clinical tests of validity in measuring physical and mental health constructs. *Med Care* 1993; **31**: 247–63. UI: 8450681.
20. Ware JE. *SF-36 Physical and mental health summary scales: a user's manual*. Boston: Health Assessment Lab, New England Medical Center, 1994.
21. Jenkinson C, Coulter A, Wright L. Short form 36 (SF36) health survey questionnaire: normative data for adults of working age. *BMJ* 1993; **306**: 1437–40. UI: 8518639.
22. Garratt A, Schmidt L, Mackintosh A, Fitzpatrick R. Quality of life measurement: bibliographic study of patient assessed health outcome measures. *BMJ* 2002; **324**: 1417. UI: 12065262.
23. Ware J Jr, Kosinski M, Keller SD. A 12-item short-form health survey: construction of scales and preliminary tests of reliability and validity. *Med Care* 1996; **34**: 220–33. UI: 8628042.
24. Brazier J, Usherwood T, Harper R, Thomas K. Deriving a preference-based single index from the UK SF-36 Health Survey. *J Clin Epidemiol* 1998; **51**: 1115–28. UI: 9817129.
25. Brazier J, Roberts J, Deverill M. The estimation of a preference-based measure of health from the SF-36. *J Health Econ* 2002; **21**: 271–92. UI: 11939242.
26. van Agthoven M, Fokkens WJ, van de Merwe JP, et al. Quality of life of patients with refractory chronic rhinosinusitis: effects of filgrastim treatment. *Am J Rhinol* 2001; **15**: 231–37. UI: 11554654.
27. Gliklich RE, Metson R. Techniques for outcomes research in chronic sinusitis. *Laryngoscope* 1995; **105**: 387–90. UI: 7715384.
28. Piccirillo JF, Edwards D, Haiduk A, et al. Psychometric and clinimetric validity of the 31-item Rhinosinusitis Outcome Measure (RSOM-31). *Am J Rhinol* 1995; **9**: 297–306.
29. Nadol JB Jr, Staecker H, Gliklich RE. Outcomes assessment for chronic otitis media: the Chronic Ear Survey. *Laryngoscope* 2000; **110**: 32–35. UI: 10718413.

30. MacKenzie K, Millar A, Wilson JA, et al. Is voice therapy an effective treatment for dysphonia? A randomised controlled trial. *BMJ* 2001; **323**: 658–61. UI: 11566828.
31. Stewart MG, Chen AY, Stach CB. Outcomes analysis of voice and quality of life in patients with laryngeal cancer. *Arch Otolaryngol* 1998; **124**: 143–48. UI: 9485104.
32. Lopez-Escamez JA, Viciana D, Garrido-Fernandez P. Impact of bilaterality and headache on health-related quality of life in Meniere's disease. *Ann Otol Rhinol Laryngol* 2009; **118**: 409–16.
33. Klassen A, Jenkinson C, Fitzpatrick R, Goodacre T. Patients' health related quality of life before and after aesthetic surgery. *Brit J Plast Surg* 1996; **49**: 433–38. UI: 8983542.
34. Bergner M, Bobbitt RA, Carter WB, Gilson BS. The Sickness Impact Profile: development and final revision of a health status measure. *Med Care* 1981; **19**: 787–805. UI 7278416.
35. Hunt SM, McKenna SP, McEwen J, et al. A quantitative approach to perceived health status: a validation study. *J Epidemiol Community Health* 1980; **34**: 281–86. UI: 7241028.
36. Robinson K, Gatehouse S, Browning GG. Measuring patient benefit from otorhinolaryngological surgery and therapy. *Ann Otol Rhinol Laryngol* 1996; **105**: 415–22. UI: 8638891.
37. Hendry J, Chin A, Swan IRC, et al. The Glasgow Benefit Inventory: A systematic review of the use and value of an otorhinolaryngological generic Patient Recorded Outcome Measure [PROM]. *Clin Otolaryngol* 2016; **41**(3): 259–75.
38. Dutt SN, McDermott AL, Jelbert A, et al. The Glasgow Benefit Inventory in the evaluation of patient satisfaction with the bone-anchored hearing aid: quality of life issues. *J Laryngol Otol* 2002; Suppl (28): 7–14. UI: 12138792.
39. Swan IRC, Guy FH, Akeroyd MA. Health-related quality of life before and after management in adults referred to otolaryngology: a prospective national study. *Clin Otolaryngol* 2012; **37**: 35–43.
40. UK Cochlear Implant Study Group. Criteria of candidacy for unilateral cochlear implantation in postlingually deafened adults 1: theory and measures of effectiveness. *Ear Hearing* 2004; **25**: 310–35.
41. Brooker JE, Fletcher JM, Dally MJ, et al. Quality of life among acoustic neuroma patients managed by microsurgery, radiation, or observation. *Otol Neurotol* 2010; **31**: 977–84.
42. Wilson JA, Deary IJ, Millar A, Mackenzie K. The quality of life impact of dysphonia. *Clin Otolaryngol Allied Sci* 2002; **27**: 179–82. UI: 12071993.
43. McKiernan DC, Banfield G, Kumar R, Hinton AE. Patient benefit from functional and cosmetic rhinoplasty. *Clin Otolaryngol Allied Sci* 2001; **26**: 50–52. UI: 11298168.
44. Bhattacharyya N, Kepnes LJ, Shapiro J. Efficacy and quality-of-life impact of adult tonsillectomy. *Arch Otolaryngol* 2001; **127**: 1347–50. UI: 11701072.
45. Uppal S, Nadig S, Jones C, et al. A prospective single-blind randomized-controlled trial comparing two surgical techniques for the treatment of snoring: laser palatoplasty versus uvulectomy with punctuate palatal diathermy. *Clin Otolaryngol* 2004; **29**: 254–63.
46. Brazier J, Deverill M, Green C, et al. A review of the use of health status measures in economic evaluation. *Health Technol Assess* (Winchester, England) 1999; **3**(9): i–iv, 1–164. UI: 10392311.
47. Torrance GW, Boyle MH, Horwood SP. Application of multi-attribute utility theory to measure social preferences for health states. *Oper Res* 1982; **30**: 1043–69. UI: 10259643.
48. Torrance GW, Furlong W, Feeny D, Boyle M. Multi-attribute preference functions. Health Utilities Index. *Pharmacoeconomics* 1995; **7**: 503–20. UI: 10155336.
49. Furlong WJ, Feeny DH, Torrance GW, Barr RD. The Health Utilities Index (HUI) system for assessing health-related quality of life in clinical studies. *Ann Med* 2001; **33**: 375–84. UI: 11491197.
50. Palmer CS, Niparko JK, Wyatt JR, et al. A prospective study of the cost-utility of the multichannel cochlear implant. *Arch Otolaryngol* 1999; **125**: 1221–28. UI: 10555693.
51. Barton GR, Summerfield AQ, Marshall DH, Bloor KE, on behalf of the POCIA Collaboration. *Choice of instrument for measuring the gain in utility from cochlear implantation*. Oxford: Health Economics Study Group; 2001.
52. EuroQol Group. EuroQol: a new facility for the measurement of health-related quality of life. *Health Policy* 1990; **16**: 199–208. UI: 10109801.
53. MVH Group. The measurement and valuation of health: final report on the modelling of valuation tariffs. York: Centre for Health Economics, University of York; 1995.
54. Brazier J, Jones N, Kind P. Testing the validity of the Euroqol and comparing it with the SF-36 health survey questionnaire. *Qual Life Res* 1993; **2**: 169–80.
55. Brooks R. EuroQol: the current state of play. *Health Policy* 1996; **37**: 53–72. UI: 10158943.
56. Jacobson GP, Newman CW. The development of the Dizziness Handicap Inventory. *Arch Otolaryngol* 1990; **116**: 424–27. UI: 2317323.
57. Vereeck L, Truijen S, Wuyts FL, Van de Heyning PH. The Dizziness Handicap Inventory and its relationship with functional balance performance. *Otol Neurotol* 2006; **28**: 87–93.
58. Yardley L, Putman J. Quantitative analysis of factors contributing to handicap and distress in vertiginous patients: a questionnaire study. *Clin Otolaryngol Allied Sci* 1992; **17**: 231–36. UI: 1387052.
59. Ventry IM, Weinstein BE. The Hearing Handicap Inventory for the Elderly: a new tool. *Ear Hearing* 1982; **3**: 128–34. UI: 7095321.
60. Weinstein BE, Spitzer JB, Ventry IM. Test-retest reliability of the Hearing Handicap Inventory for the Elderly. *Ear Hearing* 1986; **7**: 295–99. UI: 3770324.
61. Lichtenstein MJ, Bess FH, Logan SA. Validation of screening tools for identifying hearing-impaired elderly in primary care. *JAMA* 1988; **259**: 2875–78.
62. Gatehouse S, Noble W. The Speech, Spatial and Qualities of Hearing Scale (SSQ). *Int J Audiol* 2004; **43**: 85–99.
63. Newman CW, Weinstein BE. The Hearing Handicap Inventory for the Elderly as a measure of hearing aid benefit. *Ear Hearing* 1988; **9**: 81–85. UI: 3366309.
64. Gatehouse S. *Outcome measures for the evaluation of adult hearing aid fittings and services. Scientific and Technical Report to the Department of Health*. Glasgow: MRC Institute of Hearing Research; 1997.
65. Cox R. Choosing a self-report measure for hearing aid fitting outcomes. *Semin Hear* 2005; **26**: 149–56.
66. Gatehouse S. Glasgow Hearing Aid Benefit Profile: derivation and validation of a client-centred outcome measure for hearing aid services. *J Am Acad Audiol* 1999; **10**: 80–103.
67. Dillon H, James A, Ginis J. Client Oriented Scale of Improvement (COSI) and its relationship to several other measures of benefit and satisfaction provided by hearing aids. *J Am Acad Audiol* 1997; **8**: 27–43.
68. Rosenfeld RM, Goldsmith AJ, Tetlus L, Balzano A. Quality of life for children with otitis media. *Arch Otolaryngol* 1997; **123**: 1049–54. UI: 9339979.
69. Rosenfeld RM, Bhaya MH, Bower CM, et al. Impact of tympanostomy tubes on child quality of life. *Arch Otolaryngol* 2000; **126**: 585–92. UI: 10807325.
70. Kubba H, Swan IRC, Gatehouse S. How appropriate is OM6 as an instrument to assess the impact of otitis media? *Arch Otolaryngol* 2004; **130**: 705–09.
71. Aaronson NK, Ahmedzai S, Bergman B, et al. The European Organization for Research and Treatment of Cancer QLQ-C30: a quality-of-life instrument for use in international clinical trials in oncology. *J Nat Cancer Inst* 1993; **85**: 365–76. UI: 8433390.
72. Bjordal K, Ahlner-Elmqvist M, Tollesson E, et al. Development of a European Organization for Research and Treatment of Cancer (EORTC) questionnaire module to be used in quality of life assessments in head and neck cancer patients. EORTC Quality of Life Study Group. *Acta Oncologica* 1994; **33**: 879–85. UI: 7818919.
73. Koller M, Aaronson NK, Blazeby J, et al. on behalf of the EORTC Quality of Life Group. Translation procedures for standardised quality of life questionnaires: The European Organisation for Research and Treatment of Cancer (EORTC) approach. *Eur J Cancer* 2007; **43**: 1810–20.
74. Piccirillo JF, Merritt MG Jr, Richards ML. Psychometric and clinimetric validity of the 20-Item Sino-Nasal Outcome Test (SNOT-20). *Otolaryngol* 2002; **126**: 41–47. UI: 11821764.
75. Hopkins C, Gillett S, Slack R, et al. Psychometric validity of the 22-item Sinonasal Outcome Test. *Clin Otolaryngol* 2009; **34**: 447–54.
76. Jacobson BH, Johnson A, Grywalski C, et al. The Voice Handicap Index (VHI): development and validation. *Am J Speech Lang Path* 1997; **6**: 66–70.
77. Rosen CA, Lees AS, Osborne J, et al. Development and validation of the Voice Handicap Index-10. *Laryngoscope* 2004; **9**: 1549–46.
78. Carding PN, Wilson JA, MacKenzie K, Deary IJ. Measuring voice outcomes: state of the science review. *J Laryngol Otol* 2009; **123**: 823–29.

79. Melzack R. The McGill Pain Questionnaire: major properties and scoring methods. *Pain* 1975; **1**: 277–99. UI: 1235985.
80. Melzack R. The short-form McGill Pain Questionnaire. *Pain* 1987; **30**: 191–97. UI: 3670870.
81. Edelman D, Williams GR, Rothman M, Samsa GP. A comparison of three health status measures in primary care outpatients. *J Gen Int Med* 1999; **14**: 759–62. UI: 10632822.
82. Andresen EM, Rothenberg BM, Panzer R, et al. Selecting a generic measure of health-related quality of life for use among older adults: a comparison of candidate instruments. *Eval Health Prof* 1998; **21**: 244–64. UI 10183346.
83. Coons SJ, Rao S, Keininger DL, Hays RD. A comparative review of generic quality-of-life instruments. *Pharmacoeconomics* 2000; **17**: 13–35. UI: 10747763.
84. De Korte J, Mombers FM, Sprangers MA, Bos JD. The suitability of quality-of-life questionnaires for psoriasis research: a systematic literature review. *Arch Dermatol* 2002; **138**: 1221–27. UI: 12224984.

FURTHER READING

Streiner DL, Norman GR. *Health Measurement Scales: a practical guide to their development and use*, 5th edn. Oxford: OUP, 1995.

An invaluable practical guide for those who wish to develop a new patient-based outcome measure. Very good and readable explanation of theory behind these instruments.

Fitzpatrick R, Davey C, Buxton MJ, Jones DR. Evaluating patient-based outcome measures for use in clinical trials. *HTA* 1998; **2**(14): i–iv, 1–74.

Extensive review of the literature to describe the range of patient-based outcome measures available and the criteria for selecting an instrument for use in a trial.

Fayers PM, Hopwood P, Harvey A, et al. Quality of life assessment in clinical trials – guidelines and a checklist for protocol writers: the UK Medical Research Council experience. *Euro J Cancer* 1997; **33**: 20–28.

Good advice from authors with experience of reviewing grant applications submitted to the MRC.

Coons SJ, Rao S, Keininger DL, Hays RD. A comparative review of generic quality-of-life instruments. *Pharmacoeconomics* 2000; **17**: 13–35.

De Korte J, Mombers FM, Sprangers MA, Bos JD. The suitability of quality-of-life questionnaires for psoriasis research: a systematic literature review. *Arch Dermatol* 2002; **138**: 1221–7.

These two papers provide good reviews of the three most widely used generic instruments: the SF-36, the Nottingham Health Profile and the Sickness Impact Profile.

Whitmer WM, Wright-Whyte KF, Holman JA, Akeroyd MA. Hearing Aid Validation. In: Popelka G., Moore B., Fay R., Popper A. (eds). *Hearing Aids*, 2016. Springer Handbook of Auditory Research, vol 56. New York: Springer.

Extensive look at hearing-aid specific outcome measures, including an examination of the repetition of domains, followed by a discussion of the different perspectives on the measuring of benefit.

CHAPTER 43

EVIDENCE-BASED MEDICINE IN MEDICAL EDUCATION AND CLINICAL PRACTICE

Phillip Evans

Introduction 495	Gathering the evidence 498
Begin with the patient 495	Critical evaluation 498
Ask the right questions 497	Preparing the evidence 498
Structuring the search 497	Conclusion 500
Conducting the search 497	References 501
Setting the scope 498	

SEARCH STRATEGY

Data in this chapter may be updated by a PubMed search using the keywords: evidence-based medicine and EBM.

INTRODUCTION

Professor David Sackett's definition of evidence-based medical (EBM) practice still holds true: 'the conscientious, explicit and judicious use of current best evidence in making decisions about the care of individual patients'.[1] The principles are now considered to be 'core' in professional practice and praxis, across the four main phases of training, in the UK (**Figure 43.1**). Furthermore, endorsement by the World Federation of Medical Education and the World Health Organization secures it as an international characteristic of the medical profession, and therefore one that should be promoted globally.

EBM may be described as a patient-centred cycle with three linked phases: the clinical phase, the search phase and the evidence review phase (**Figure 43.2**). Taken together, this becomes a framework for teaching, learning and curriculum delivery in the continuum of professional training.

BEGIN WITH THE PATIENT

In addition to being at the heart of the ethos of care, the patient has a central role in medical education.

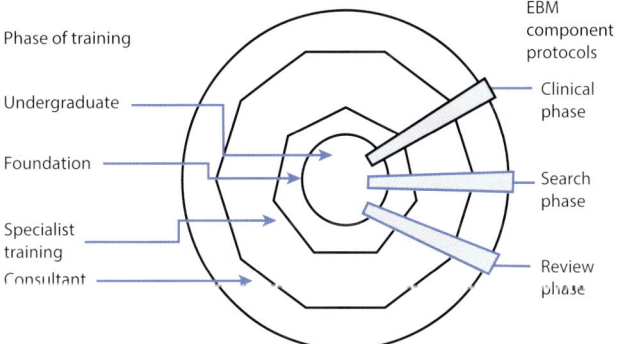

Figure 43.1 Evidence-based medicine is core to all four professional phases.

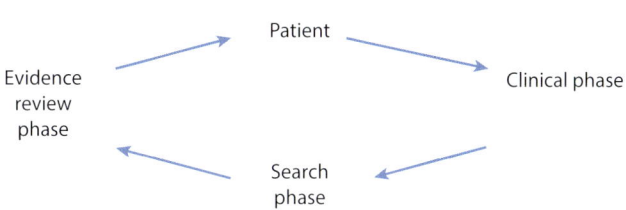

Figure 43.2 Patient-centred evidence-based cycle.

The patient may be actual, or described as a theoretical case, or the two may be used in combination. As actual cases for teaching and learning, real patients are frequently 'opportunistic', and therefore theoretical cases are normally constructed by clinicians as a vehicle for teaching and learning. The topics for the cases are chosen because they are common or frequent or, if rare, because they are important in understanding the fundamental principles or concepts of a particular condition. One such example is the autoimmune condition known as Wegener's disease. A portfolio of cases in otolaryngology will include examples from the following areas:

- plastic surgery
- oral and maxillofacial surgery
- general upper GI surgery
- neurosurgery
- paediatric surgery
- cardiothoracic surgery
- ophthalmology
- accident and emergency medicine.

Well-structured cases may be prepared using a systematic framework (Figure 43.3), which is intended to encourage students and trainees to explore the bio-medical spectrum of relevance to that particular condition.

The cases themselves normally relate to the learning outcomes that are relevant and appropriate to the particular professional stage (Table 43.1). In the UK, these may be sourced from Tomorrow's Doctors, The Foundation Programme,[3] and the college documentation.[4]

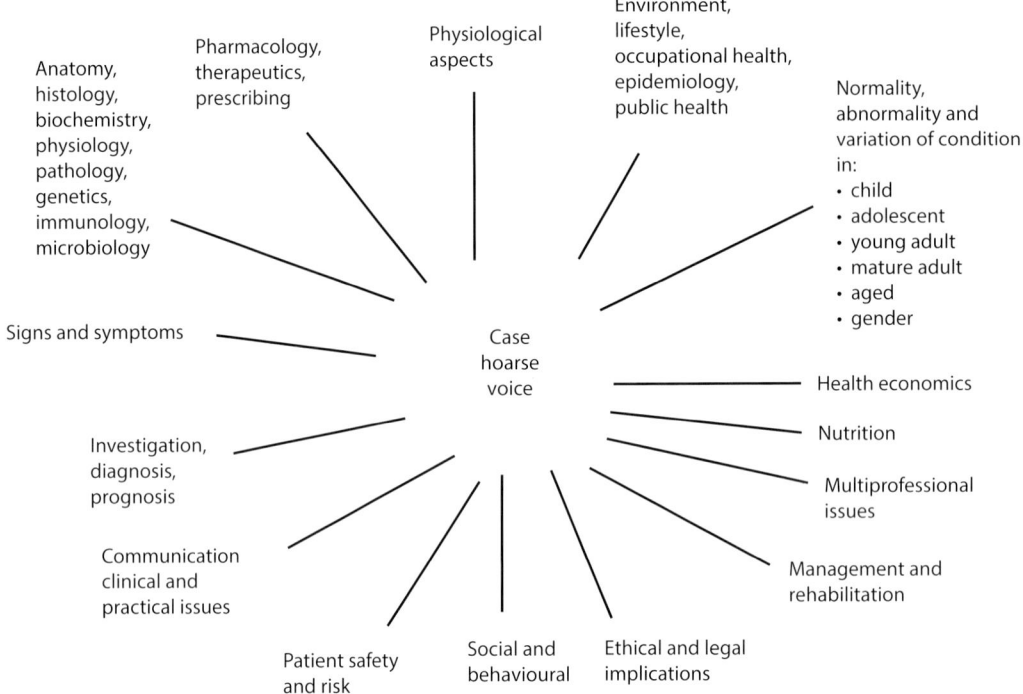

Figure 43.3 Factors to consider in writing and analyzing a case.

TABLE 43.1 A matrix for developing cases appropriate to the stage of expertise			
	Outcomes relevant to the stage of the student		
Core case from	Undergraduate	Foundation	Specialist training
Plastic surgery			
Oral and maxillofacial surgery			
General upper GI surgery			
Neurosurgery			
Paediatric surgery			
Cardiothoracic surgery			
Ophthalmology			
Accident and emergency medicine			

Outcomes are entered by the teacher in the relevant column.

Whilst it is suggested that EBM is used routinely for keeping up to date, clinical supervisors and other teachers should offer their students or trainees selected cases as part of the training process. The supervisor should give one case at the beginning of the week, with the expectation of it being presented as the basis for discussion with the supervisor towards the end of the week, together with a report summarizing the key points and a reasoned evidence-based appraisal of the critical points of the case. This might be included in the student's reflective portfolio. There may be an advantage for the student or trainee to work with a partner (peer-assisted learning) or in a small group (case-based learning). The case itself is part of the normal spectrum of activities in the student's or trainee's normal experience of workplace learning and assessment, and may be linked to a DOPS, MiniCex or video-based discussion. The cases should be central to the curriculum, should form a structured framework for the student's or trainee's self-directed learning, and should be part of the normal provision of teaching and learning activities (blended learning). The case presentation at the end of the week confirms and tests the professional judgement of the student or trainee, and provides an opportunity for extending their understanding.

The student or trainee will undertake the following steps to prepare and present the case thoroughly:

1. Appraise the patient and the condition
2. Identify and ask the questions, in an appropriate way
3. Establish the evidence
4. Critique the evidence
5. Present the conclusions and discuss the case.

ASK THE RIGHT QUESTIONS

At all stages, the trainee should think ahead, and form a judgement as to how best to proceed, and this normally requires asking two categories of questions:

1. What do I need to know to understand the case?
2. What do I need to know to form a clinical judgement?

The nature and quality of the questions posed will vary according to the age and stage of the student or trainee. Clearly an undergraduate student will be expected to read more widely about the basic and clinical science related to the case. In addition, they will also require more guidance about appropriate communication skills, performing the clinical and practical skills, and interpretation of tests. Trainees with more experience will consolidate their knowledge and extend their understanding of diagnosis and management of the condition.

Questions related to the 'best' clinical judgement require greater thought and refinement, and a higher level of skill with respect to searching the literature and interpreting the available evidence. A suitable search strategy should take into consideration the following aspects:

- an overall structure for the search
- anticipation of the nature of papers found in the search
- forethought about conducting the search itself
- a strategy for reading the literature.

STRUCTURING THE SEARCH

PICO is the acronym commonly used as a strategy when searching the bibliographic databases:

P = **Patient/Population:** Who was the subject of the investigation?
I = **Intervention:** What was done?
C = **Comparison:** What are the alternatives and appropriate options?
O = **Outcome:** What are you trying to accomplish or achieve with this case?

The search structure should seek the best evidence for diagnosis, therapy, prognosis, and harm or aetiology, and at this stage it is also useful to anticipate the nature of the papers present in the literature. The most common categories are:

- **Cases.** Reports of individual patients, groups of patients or cohort studies, which may be retrospective or prospective, are highly valid and authentic, but have low reliability.
- **Randomized controlled clinical trial.** An RCT is a carefully structured prospective study, in which bias and influence have been carefully controlled. These are highly specific.
- **Systematic reviews and synopses.** The author has undertaken an extensive literature search and review of a particular clinical topic, and has prepared our systematic analysis of the quality of the evidence. Such papers are beneficial as they save the individual a great deal of time, but the assumption is that the review is up to date. Therefore it is wise to search for the most recent evidence.
- **Meta-analysis.** This combines the results of valid studies in that field, and uses statistical analysis to combine the results in a way that expresses the conclusions as if the collected reports were a single study.
- **Qualitative or humanistic enquiries.** These explore questions and issues related to psycho-social and attitudinal aspects that cannot be measured in a prospective randomized controlled trial.

CONDUCTING THE SEARCH

The search should be organized and planned[5] by focusing on the purpose of the search, and identifying the characteristics that are sought (**Table 43.2**).

TABLE 43.2 The purpose of the search

Focus	Outcomes sought
Goal	Establish the recommendations
Perspective	Establish the clinical evidence
Coverage	Selective and relevant
Organization	That the scientific style is robust
Audience	What type of clinician?

TABLE 43.3 Establishing alternative terms

Question component	Subject or MeSH term	Synonyms
Patient	Patient Inpatient Outpatient	Person Case
Cause		Reasons
Sudden hearing loss (SHL)	Hearing loss, sudden	Deafness

A search of the literature is essentially a text-matching exercise between the search question and the text in the databases. The first step is to clarify one key question,[6] for example, 'What is the cause of sudden hearing loss?'.

Due to the complexity and ambiguity of the English language, it is necessary to establish alternative words (refer to a thesaurus), keywords or medical subject headings (MeSH terms) used by other authors. These are identified and written down at the start of the search, and may be augmented with experience from the search (**Table 43.3**).

The search terms will be used, with truncations (if appropriate) and use 'variant spelling' if possible, singly and then in combination, using the Boolean operational commands, AND, OR, NOT and AND & OR.

SETTING THE SCOPE

It is desirable to establish the scope of the search by establishing the inclusion and exclusion criteria of the paper. Examples of inclusion criteria are:

- meta-analyses
- systematic reviews of randomized trials
- physiological studies
- English language only
- time-frame (last 5 years).

Examples of exclusion criteria are:

- studies that do not cover clinical evidence
- studies published prior to the 5-year cut-off, except key papers or definitive studies.

GATHERING THE EVIDENCE

Searching the literature in otolaryngology may be relatively straightforward. The options are to conduct an electronic search of NICE, the Cochrane Collaboration (Embase) and databases such as Medline (PubMed), and to complete a 'hand-search' of specific journals. Google Scholar may be an unattractive alternative because it can throw up an enormous number of results, though there may be benefits if it highlights 'grey literature', such as book reviews and web pages. Reference manager software, such as Mendeley or Zotero, is an aid in managing the papers found in the literature.

A pathway for completing the exercise is given in **Figure 43.4**.[7]

CRITICAL EVALUATION

A critical evaluation of the significant papers is necessary at this stage. The first step is to review the type of paper. Categories are as follows:

- randomized controlled trial (RCT)
- systematic review of RCTs
- methods that are not RCTs
- systematic review of papers that are not RCTs
- basic science paper (physiology, microbiology, genetics)
- other (clinical observation or case study, synopsis, guideline).

A critique of each paper entails a systematic evaluation of the following points:

- The title: is it relevant?
- The method: is it valid?
- The results: what are they?
- The conclusions: in what way are they useful?

The summary in **Table 43.4** is an example of a useful, but not definitive, framework for the process.

Evidence for each phase of the case report should be set out and considered using questions that are appropriate for the information available. The framework in **Table 43.5** might be used as an example.

The papers may also be categorized using the PICO approach. Dividing the papers into these categories allows a systematic analysis of the evidence about diagnosis, therapy, prognosis and risk of harm. It is necessary to establish that the validity and significance of the evidence has been demonstrated in the paper. If it has not, then the necessary data may be extracted and analyzed by an appropriate statistical instrument to establish the level of confidence.

PREPARING THE EVIDENCE

The final case discussion should provide an overview of each stage in the process, setting out the evidence used in determining the conclusions. The correct answer is not arriving at the diagnosis, but understanding the basis on which the clinical judgement is made, and declaring the evidence (**Table 43.6**).

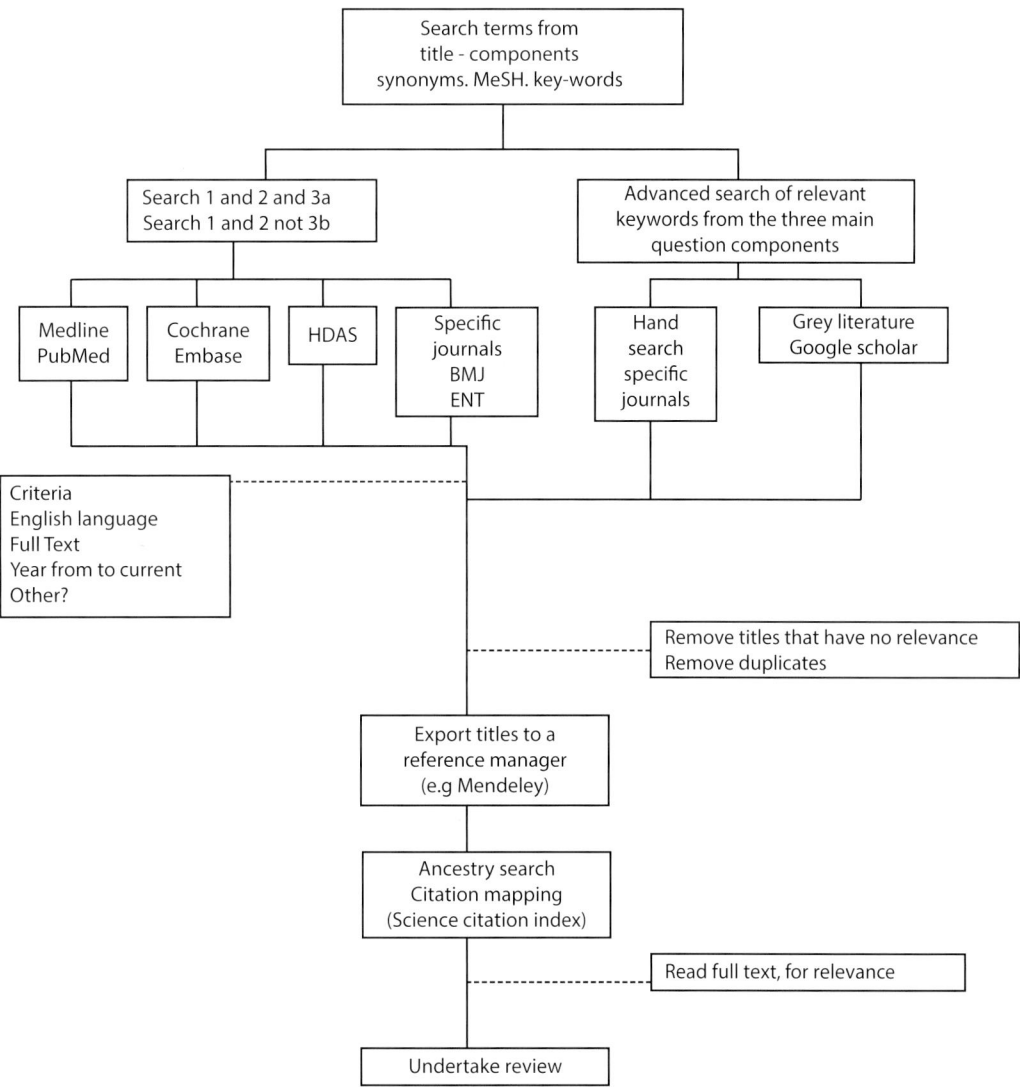

Figure 43.4 Flow chart of search strategy.

TABLE 43.4 Example framework			
	Paper		
	1. Author/ Year	**2. Author/ Year**	**3. Author/ Year**
Type of study			
Participants: • cohort • cross-sectional • purposive selection			
Method: • how was the evidence gathered? • instruments for analysis			
Results • do they answer the question? • significance			
Conclusions • relevance			
Limitations, bias			
Other points and your conclusions			

Adapted from Sackett et al.[8]
Information to be entered in Table 43.4 from the papers found in the literature search.

TABLE 43.5 Framework for considering evidence

	Evidence from the literature	Relevance to patient (information to be completed by the user, with reference to the patient.)
History and examination	Were these controlled and confirmed?	
Aetiology	Were these reported and recorded?	
Test results	Confirmed by replication? Levels of probability? Results presented in sufficient detail? Was the index test compared to a gold standard?	
Diagnosis	Based on a blind trial? Representative sample? Reference standard? Specificity? Sensitivity? Predictive validity?	
Therapy	Was it a 'blind' trial? Did the sample change? Assigned or randomized? Were other variables controlled? Size and nature of impact?	
Prognosis	Was it a 'blind' trial? Was the sample declared and described? Was the follow-up sufficient?	
Risks	Placebo rate (control)? Absolute risk? Relative risk? Numbers needed to treat?	
Care and compliance	Were all variables considered and controlled? What was the sample size?	

Adapted from Sackett et al.[8]

TABLE 43.6 Providing an overview and setting out the evidence

	PICO component (information to be added by the student with relevance to the patient)			
	Problem	Intervention	Comparison	Outcomes
History				
Examination				
Aetiology				
Possible diagnosis				
Differential diagnosis				
Tests				
Management options				
Care and compliance				

CONCLUSION

The exponential increase in scientific papers, and expansion of 'what is known' makes it almost impossible not to make clinical judgements without some reference to the evidence in the literature. It may be argued that the expansion of the literature has surpassed our capacity to maintain a comprehensive review of all the information available. However, as the flexibility of modern information technology allows convenient access to a wide range of resource materials, this is less problematic now than in times past. Indeed, web-based information is a commonly used platform for learning and keeping up to date. Therefore, acquiring a rational and systematic competence in finding and using valid, reliable and appropriate information is a fundamental part of clinical praxis. However, this is not to dismiss the values of professional judgement based on experience and often 'gut reaction'. Indeed, it has been acknowledged that the capability of forming a professional judgement is a greater order of magnitude than mere technical competence.[9] Yet it is certainly the case that, in this digital age, evidence in the literature does provide a significant input into informing the *best* clinical judgement.

KEY POINTS

- EBM is fundamental to clinical practice, globally.
- It has a series of skills that require mastery
- It contributes to an informed clinical judgement.

REFERENCES

1. Sackett D. Evidence based medicine: what it is and what it isn't . *BMJ* 1996; **312**: 71–72.
2. General Medical Council. Available from http://www.gmc-uk.org/education/under-graduate/tomorrows_doctors_2009.asp
3. General Medical Council. Available from http://www.gmc-uk.org/4___Foundation_Programme_curriculum_final.pdf_29557735.pdf
4. Royal College of Surgeons. Available from https://www.rcseng.ac.uk/media/media-background-briefings-and-statistics/the-surgical-specialties-3-2013-ear-nose-throat-ent
5. Cook D. Narrowing the focus and broadening horizons: complementary roles for systematic and nonsystematic reviews. *Adv Health Sci Educ* 2008; **13**: 391–95.
6. Haig A, Dozier M. BEME Guide no. 3: Systematic searching for evidence in medical education, part 2. *Med Teach* 2003; **25**(4): 463–84.
7. César Orsini. Personal communication, 2013.
8. Sackett D, Straus SE, Richardson WS, et.al. *Evidence-based medicine: how to practice and teach EBM*. Edinburgh: Churchill Livingstone; 2000.
9. Eraut M. *Developing professional knowledge and competence*. London: Falmer; 2002.

CHAPTER 44

CRITICAL APPRAISAL SKILLS

Paul Nankivell and Christopher Coulson

Why do we need critical appraisal?...........503	Appraising therapy articles........................512
Tips for practising evidence-based healthcare...........504	Appraising systematic reviews...................515
Basics of critical appraisal 505	Worksheets..521
Forming answerable questions 506	References...521
Appraising diagnostic articles 508	

SEARCH STRATEGY

Data in this chapter may be updated by a PubMed search using the keywords: critical appraisal, evidence-based care, evidence-based healthcare, systematic reviews. As this chapter is essentially a 'How I do it,' there was no formal strategy used.

WHY DO WE NEED CRITICAL APPRAISAL?

Evidence-based practice (EBP) begins and ends with patients. We can harm patients by giving inaccurate information about prognosis, make assumptions about diagnostic test results that are false, give therapy that is ineffective or harmful, or fail to give effective therapy. The only way to prevent this happening is to ensure that we have the most up-to-date knowledge available so that we can share that information with patients.

There were 26 randomized control trials regarding otitis media alone published in the last two years. Therefore, even with maintaining a diligent approach to reading journals during continuing professional development (CPD) time and attending postgraduate seminars, it is becoming increasingly difficult for clinicians to keep up to date with everything that is important affecting their patients. EBP starts with the clinician accepting that there is uncertainty about what we do and that sometimes (when that uncertainty occurs frequently or when it is important) we should search for the latest knowledge. Pragmatically, what we do at present is ask colleagues. The inherent flaw here is the inability to assess the quality of the evidence presented to you by your colleague. Does this matter? If the question is important or frequent then yes, it does matter.

Research evidence can be approached from two angles. The first is the clinician who wants to undertake research and the second is the clinician who wants an answer to a clinical question. The latter wants to know what to believe. Is it the randomized trial, or the case series or case-control trial? What papers should they look for to answer their question?

Levels of evidence have been proposed to help clinicians identify trials most likely to yield the 'truth' and associated with these are grades of recommendation. For questions about the efficacy of a therapy, these state that a systematic review of homogenous trials is likely to be the most believable evidence.

The process of EBP therefore requires that one searches for the best evidence. For therapeutic decisions, this is usually going to be a systematic review, where data from relevant randomized control trials on the topic of interest have been identified and screened according to pre-defined inclusion criteria. Data may potentially be combined together in the form of a meta-analysis. Systematic reviews should include the data from all up-to-date trials with this completeness being one of the significant advantages of this method of review. Yet, it is not an approach to be underestimated. A search for papers to be included in the review might often generate a list of more than a thousand papers, with all the titles and abstracts being read to select relevant articles. The full text of these relevant articles must then be obtained (in itself a time-consuming and expensive task) and read to ensure they meet the selection criteria. The data then have to be independently abstracted from the selected articles. Undertaking a valid, well carried out systematic review is no easy task, but is essential for clinicians to determine the latest evidence.

Once a trial or trials have been found that seems to answer your question, you have to check three things. Is the study valid? What are the results? Can these be applied to my patients?

The need to check for validity seems, on the surface, to be bizarre. Surely this is what journals should be doing. That assumption is correct but in reality the job of a journal is primarily to make a profit. Therefore you will find articles with flawed trials in even the most highly cited journals.[1]

Journals started as the diaries of researchers. These were then passed around colleagues so that the information could be shared. The development of trials and the assessment of bias are subsequent to that descriptive era. What we are now faced with are seemingly complex long papers with obscure statistical analyses. The scenario is no different to a medical student facing their first anatomy class. By reading around the subject and by practice, will be able to quickly identify key anatomical structures. The same is true of reading scientific articles. You can learn certain aspects of trial design very quickly to be able to assess whether an appropriate design was used for a certain research question. The journal *Evidence-Based Medicine* critically appraises the literature from over 100 journals. However, it only includes a few that are likely to change the way you think about a problem or change the way you practise. Sadly for the other articles, we must appraise them ourselves.

The need to assess the methodology of individual trials is extremely important. In large systematic reviews of the same clinical outcome with the same therapy, researchers have compared the results of those trials that were randomized and those that were not randomized. There are some large differences in certain studies that are more than one would expect by chance. One cannot always say that randomized trials show less effect than non-randomized trials.[2]

However, it is not enough to accept that a trial is believable at face value. There is now overwhelming evidence that trial methodology has a major influence on the results of therapeutic trials.[2, 3] Concealment of randomization, masking and randomization itself are three main components of randomized trial design. The numbers of patients involved in the study and their follow-up are the other key features.

Inadequate concealment of randomization may exaggerate the efficacy of a treatment compared to trials where adequate concealment has occurred. The size of this effect may be considerable, over 40% in some studies although it should be noted that it is not possible to quantify the size or direction of such bias on effect size from study to study.[4, 5] Surprisingly, perhaps of lesser importance is blinding (masking) – the doctor looking after the patient, or the patient themselves, knowing whether they are giving (being given) the experimental or placebo treatment. If there is no blinding, the results may exaggerate the effectiveness of the treatment by 15%. If less than 80% of patients are followed up, one cannot tell what is happening and the results become meaningless.

To assess a study there are checklists some of which have now been incorporated into computer programmes such as that found at the Centre for Evidence-Based Medicine website (www.cebm.net) that enable health professionals to appraise the quality of the evidence for themselves.

Systematic reviews therefore need to assess the individual validity of the trials that are included. If they do not assess whether there was concealed randomization, for example, then you, the reader, may be given incorrect information. The assessment of methodological quality – now better termed risk of bias – of a randomized controlled trial may be carried out using a variety of available systems. The Cochrane Collaboration has recently updated their tool for assessing risk of bias in randomized trials.[6] Furthermore, systematic reviews should be conducted using the Preferred Reporting Items for Systematic Reviews and Meta-Analyses (PRISMA) guidelines, an evidence-based minimum set of items for reporting in systematic reviews and meta-analyses.[7] The PRISMA guidelines have replaced the previously used Quorum statement.[8]

For systematic reviews, effective transparent searches and defined inclusion and exclusion criteria are important. The homogeneity (similarity) of the studies is also critical in determining whether a meta-analysis of the data is appropriate. The meta-analysis (combination of the results of the individual trials) is usually only appropriate when there is clinical and methodological homogeneity (that is, the methods and clinical outcomes and starting points are similar). In addition, the results must be put into context of present formats of care.

The need to understand how trials may come to the 'wrong' conclusion is as important as understating the treatment itself. Clearly, all this may be daunting to a busy clinician so there are sensible short cuts. Always start by looking at evidence that has already been appraised such as that in *Evidence-Based Medicine* and *Clinical Evidence*. The essential part of effective clinical practice is to continue to ask questions.

We need to make sure that what we do is based on the soundest evidence possible. If the only evidence is experiential and anecdotal then that is perfectly satisfactory. However, if there is a systematic review of randomized control trials that all point to an alternative treatment being more effective then that should only be ignored at your patients' peril.

TIPS FOR PRACTISING EVIDENCE-BASED HEALTHCARE

Tip 1: Ask questions

Try making one question per clinic. Select one question because:

- There is likely to be an answer.
- The question has arisen more than once or is important:
  - record briefly the problem, for example, 'Sudden onset hearing loss'

○ write down the question, for example, 'are steroids an effective treatment (efficacy and morbidity)?'
○ put time aside each week to research the answer to the question.

Tip 2: Searching

- Search one question regularly: every two weeks, every month or every quarter!
- Conduct your search in a logical order:
  ○ clinical evidence
  ○ journal EBM
  ○ Cochrane
  ○ PubMed.

Keeping up to date with literature searches can be facilitated by developing highly specific search strategies (for example using PubMed). These searches are set up to deliver regular alerts directly via email. Any new articles relevant to the topic of interest will then be sent through on a regular basis without the need to specifically perform a search each time.

Often you will find too few articles, or that the articles you do find are not in your library or will take a long time to obtain. Sometimes you will find too many articles and a systematic review is needed. Unless you have time and the question is desperately important, pass and move on to the next question – let someone else answer this one!

Appraise only the article(s) that answer your question, have the highest level of evidence and are readily available.

Tip 3: Appraisal

- Look for letters about the article in subsequent issues of the journal.
- Appraise with others until confident.
- Appraise using worksheets or using software, for example CATmaker.
- Mark (highlight) on the printed article where you found the important data.
- Get someone else to check it for you.
- Appraise the article as part of a departmental journal club.

Tip 4: Share your knowledge

- Try sharing uncertainty with your colleagues.
- Discuss your questions with colleagues (maybe they have already answered them).
- Find fault with the article(s) rather than your colleagues.

BASICS OF CRITICAL APPRAISAL

Read the abstract

Assuming you have three or four articles to appraise, how should you start? First read the abstract. Read it briefly trying to gain an overview firstly of the methods used and secondly the results. For example, a parent brings in a child referred by their GP for recurrent epistaxis but is worried about surgery (describing cautery in dramatic terms) and wonders whether a cream used by a friend's child might help (Naseptin). You make a note of this and later formulate the question 'In children with recurrent epistaxis, is Naseptin effective, compared with placebo, at reducing attacks of epistaxis?' and find this paper.[9] The abstract is available online. It takes a minute or two to read through the abstract:

> *Epistaxis is common in children. Trials show antiseptic cream is as effective as cautery, but it is not known whether either is better than no treatment. We wished to know the efficacy of cream in children with recurrent epistaxis. The design was a single-blind, prospective, randomized controlled trial set in the otolaryngology clinic in a children's hospital.*
>
> *The participants were 103 children referred by their general practitioner for recurrent epistaxis. Excluded were those with suspected tumours, bleeding disorders or allergies to constituents of the cream. Referral letters were randomized to treatment and no treatment groups.*
>
> *Treatment was antiseptic cream to the nose twice daily for four weeks, which was prescribed by the general practitioner before clinic attendance. All children were given an appointment for eight weeks after randomization.*
>
> *The main outcome measures were the proportion of children in each group with no epistaxis in the four weeks preceding clinic review. Complete data were available for 88 (85%) of the children. Of the treatment group, 26/47 (55%) had no epistaxis in the four weeks before the clinic appointment. Of the controls, 12/41 (29%) had no epistaxis over the four weeks. This is a relative risk reduction of 47% for persistent bleeding (95% CI 9–69%) and an absolute risk reduction of 26% (95% CI 12–40%), giving a number needed to treat of 3.8 (95% CI 2.5–8.5).*
>
> *We conclude that antiseptic cream is an effective treatment for recurrent epistaxis in children.*

The format of any abstract should be similar to this. If there is a complex description of the trial that is confusing, ask yourself why. Is it because the authors are hiding an overall negative result or is it really a necessary peculiar design?

So, in this study there were 103 patients with epistaxis in a single blind randomized controlled trial with various outcomes described and a promising result overall.

Does the paper answer the question you are asking?

This is a qualitative judgement that you must make on reading the abstract. Unless the paper is the highest level of evidence (systematic review) and deals specifically with the question you have posed it will be necessary to next look for individual randomized controlled trials that address the specific outcomes relevant to your patient.

Find answers to the validity questions using a checklist for the relevant study

It is very much easier to read an article when you know what you are looking for. The same occurs when an experienced doctor finds it easier to filter the enormous number of questions and signs they can ask or examine for, and homes in on specific areas they think are relevant. This ability to put the patient's symptoms quickly into context is the key to skilful practice. In exactly the same way, learning what to look for in a research article is key. When teaching medical students, we give them exactly the same list of questions that are shown below. This gives them focus and they will work through an article in 10 minutes answering all the validity questions.

The first place to check for validity questions about the methods employed is, not surprisingly, in the methods section of the paper. However, you will frequently find that certain elements of the methodology may be mentioned in the introduction, results or even the discussion. So if you cannot find out, for example, the rate of follow-up in the methods, then scan the rest of the text for the answer.

What sort of research design is the trial?

You may have to resort to checking the methods section of the paper to obtain this. The trial under discussion was a randomized control trial with single blinding.[9]

Assess the level of bias

At this stage, you have all the methodology neatly summarized. For example, in the paper under discussion there were some problems with follow-up. They had data available on 88 of the 103 patients randomized, but 15 of these were assessed by telephone. This introduces an element of bias that may reduce the validity. If this was less than 80% then really the trial is so severely compromised that you cannot make any interpretation of the result. If there is not concealed randomization (see 'Concealed randomization' below) then the results *may* overestimate the effectiveness of the treatment. So, assessing bias is the art of appraisal. In the end you have to decide whether the effect of the treatment demonstrated is likely, taking into consideration the level of bias, to translate into benefit in your patient.

Translate the results into something clinically meaningful

If the article describes analysis data with quoted figures for risk reduction, how does that apply to an individual patient? A frequent term used now is numbers needed to treat. This puts the effect into the context of the patient and lets them decide whether the benefit is worth the trouble or potential side effect(s).

How can I implement this?

Does this help my practice, either by reinforcing what I know and making me more confident, or does it change my practice? If it is the latter, how am I going to go about implementing that change?

The numbers

The most frequent fear expressed is that of the statistics. How can I tell whether these were the correct statistics to be used? This can initially be tackled obliquely. First, ask what is likely to represent a clinically beneficial outcome for your patients. Is a reduction in mortality of 1% enough for an invasive procedure, or should it be 5%? This is by far the most important feature of the results. If the trial was designed to establish a benefit that you regard as clinically insignificant then no further examination of the study is necessary.

Following this example a little further, assume a 5% reduction in mortality is considered a clinically meaningful difference, and the results of the trial demonstrate that this was achieved. The statistical test is there to show you that this difference was very unlikely to have occurred by chance in two ways. First, that the difference observed in this trial was unlikely to have happened by chance (p value) and, second, if this trial were repeated 100 times, 95% of the trials would have shown a similar result (confidence interval). How they determine the p value (i.e. with a student t test or a chi-square) is beyond the scope of this article but a quick tip is to check the letters written in response to the article because, if the article is in a major journal, statisticians will be quick to point out the incorrect use of statistics. In our experience, there is much less use of incorrect statistical tests than there is of poor trial methodology.

To summarize, check that the difference is clinically significant and did not occur by chance.

Summary

Critical appraisal is a logical way of assessing the likely truth of a piece of research, evaluating the results in terms of individual patient care, and then assessing the whole and determining whether it is useful for your practice. It combines some knowledge of trial design, a small amount of basic arithmetic and some qualitative judgements.

FORMING ANSWERABLE QUESTIONS

The reason we do not usually ask questions is they are so difficult to answer. This was clearly illustrated in the *Hitchhiker's Guide to the Galaxy* when the super computer gave the answer '42' to the Ultimate Question of Life, the Universe, and Everything.[10] The people asking the question were horrified and angry. The computer calmly suggested that, instead of panicking, they should go back and consider the question and that he would of course help them do this. Clearly, this is an extreme example of where the question has been so badly formed that the answer is meaningless.

Imagine a patient with diabetes. Their control has been haphazard and they have had repeated haemoglobin A1C (HbA1C) tests performed over the last year. Their control seems better now but the HbA1c test is expensive to perform. How effective is blood glucose at monitoring diabetes? A search for 'blood glucose' and 'diabetes mellitus' identifies 25 000 articles.

Two mistakes were made here. The search was unstructured, the terms so vague that a manageable list of relevant items unable to be generated. This arose partly because of the unfocused nature of the question. The goal was to discover how 'effective' the test is. What is meant by that? If it is negative does that rule out poor control – or if it is positive (high) does that mean they have poor control? In this case it is the former that really is of interest.

You could start with a textbook and read thoroughly about diabetes. For a broad overview of the topic area textbooks may be ideal; however, they are often many years out of date. For understanding more about therapy in general, a resource such as *Clinical Evidence*[11] is extremely valuable (*Clinical Evidence* cites all the evidence from which therapeutic recommendations are made). This form of enquiry is termed a 'background question' or one that helps the person understand the problem in general. This in contrast to what is being discussed here, which are termed 'foreground questions' or decision-making questions. As a student, you ask mainly background questions but as your experience with a condition increases and the clinical need for decision-making increases, the proportion of background questions fall as the foreground questions rise (**Figure 44.1**).

Incorporating this, the question now becomes: In diabetics, is fasting blood glucose (compared with HbA1c) effective at excluding poor diabetic control?[12] (A fasting blood glucose < 7.8 rules out poor glycaemic control.)

The query is becoming better but the first part is still vague. Including something about non-insulin-dependent diabetics would further refine the question. By structuring a question, the answer may be found more efficiently.[13] It is therefore important to try to break the question down into several parts, the most common approach being to use the PICO format:

- **p**atient and problem
- **i**ntervention (or diagnostic test)
- **c**omparison intervention (optional)
- **o**utcomes.

Patient and problem

The first part is to identify the problem or the patient. Some healthcare problems are not always about patients! For example, an administrator may want to know whether having acute medical beds in a temporary holding ward next to the accident and emergency department is any better than having conventional acute medical wards in the hospital. Make sure at this stage in the question you are describing the problem or patients that you see. However, if you are too specific at this stage you may miss some important evidence and there is a balance to be struck between obtaining evidence about exactly your group of patients and obtaining all the evidence about all groups of patients.

Intervention

The intervention is equally important. It may in fact be a postponement of an action, such as an operation. In patients with abdominal pain lasting less than 12 hours, does an additional 24-hour delay before referral to hospital alter outcome? Most interventions are more straightforward, such as types of dressings, drug therapies or counselling. Alternatively, they can be about the provision of differing environmental factors, such as the décor of waiting rooms or dealing with the way in which information is given to patients, i.e. positively or negatively.[14]

The intervention can be a diagnostic test. However, specify whether you are trying to detect or exclude a disease.

Comparison intervention

Sometimes, there is a comparison of the intervention. For example, you might seek papers comparing the use of an active compound compared with either a placebo or another active drug. Considering whether you are looking for comparative studies will help when searching for that evidence. You may be comparing one diagnostic test against another.

Outcomes

Outcome measures are particularly important when considering the question. It is worth spending some time working out exactly what it is you want. In serious diseases it is often easy to concentrate on the mortality and miss the important aspects of morbidity. For example, the use of toxic chemotherapies for cancer may affect both aspects.

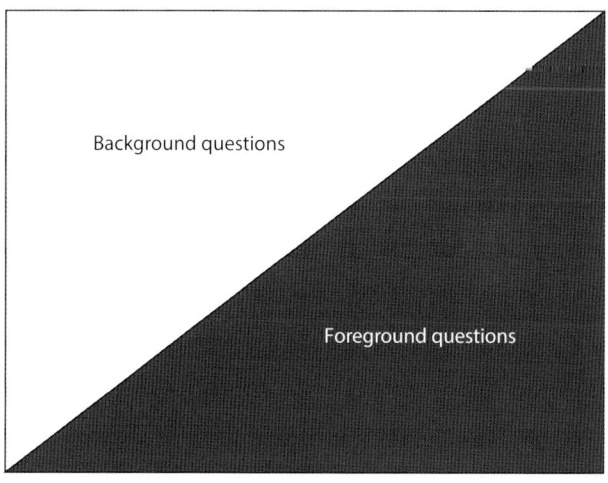

Figure 44.1 Foreground and background questions.

This is also the time when it is important to know what outcome is relevant to the patient. In Menière's, deafness and tinnitus may occur but the patient may only really be interested in controlling one problem as a priority. The search should primarily focus on that outcome. The Core Outcome Measures in Effectiveness Trials (COMET) initiative aims to develop and encourage application of agreed standardized sets of outcomes, known as 'core outcome sets'. These can be applied to both controlled and non-controlled trials. The intention is not to limit the range of outcomes measured but to ensure a minimum core set is included in all studies of a particular condition such that pooling or comparison of trial data can be more meaningful.[15]

Type of question

Once we have created a question, it is helpful to think about what type of question you are asking, as this will affect where you look for the answer and what type of research you can expect to provide the answer. For example, although randomized controlled trials (RCTs) are a very valid type of study, it would be unethical to perform an RCT on harm. (Would you volunteer for the exposure arm of such a study?) Questions about harm should look for different types of research, such as case-control studies or cohort studies.

APPRAISING DIAGNOSTIC ARTICLES

Diagnoses are usually made through interpreting and combining information from a combination of the clinical history, examination findings and the results of investigations, such as blood tests and X-rays. An important component of evidence-based healthcare is working out how useful these different pieces of information are in making a diagnosis. For example, if you test a patient's urine and find protein in it, how likely is it that this represents kidney disease? A test result needs to be interpreted in the light of how accurate you think the test is, and what you already know about the patient.

In making a diagnosis you are consciously (or subconsciously) weighing up probabilities. Each question you ask or each observation changes those probabilities. For example, if a patient limps in then there is a probability of arthritis being the cause of the limp. If the patient is 70 years of age, the probability is higher than if the patient is 30. The age of the patient is a diagnostic test, either increasing or decreasing the probability. It is essential, when contemplating a test, that the person requesting the test has some idea of the probability of the diagnosis. They will also need to decide whether the test is helping them exclude or include the diagnosis. Finally, they need to know what is the likely probability of the diagnosis after a positive or a negative result.

What is meant by test accuracy? Accuracy is a description of how well the test diagnoses and excludes the disease when the result is positive or negative (see 'What are the results?' below).

Sensitivity reflects the ability of a test to identify people who have disease and specificity reflects the ability of the test to identify 'normality', or people who do not have disease. So this means that tests with very high sensitivities and specificities can be extremely useful at either excluding or including a diagnosis. It is not uncommon to spend time seeing the worried well. These are patients who present with symptoms caused by a mild or self-limiting disease but are naturally worried that it may be something more serious. In these cases what is required are tests that mainly exclude disease. In hospital, where patients are potentially significantly unwell, what is required is to be able to make a diagnosis (including disease).

To see an example of how high sensitivity and specificity values of a test can be used in clinical practice, let us consider how general practitioners deal with patients with a sore throat. This is a common presenting complaint in general practice and it would be useful to know whether a new 'rapid test' could be useful in helping diagnose bacterial sore throats.[16] This particular paper is selected for illustrative purposes rather than it being the 'best' level of evidence.

In the paper four patient features were determined:

- fever ≥ 38°C
- lack of cough
- tonsillar exudates
- anterior cervical lymphadenopathy.

Five hundred and fifty-eight patients older than 11 years presenting with sore throat were swabbed and examined for these features. They all also had a rapid streptococcal antigen detection test for detecting group-A B-haemolytic streptococcus (GABHS).

The next step was to go through the paper checking for validity.

Is the study valid?

- **Did the authors answer the question?** The question is often found at the end of the introduction section of the paper. Some authors leave you guessing as to what the original question might have been. If the paper does not have a clear question, it cannot give any clear answer, so you can save yourself time by moving on to the next paper. You should also consider whether the research question is relevant to your clinical question.
- **What were the characteristics of the groups?** This would contain some description about the numbers of patients, their race and gender, age and any other features that are pertinent to the study. This would also include any characteristics that are known or likely confounders (i.e. factors that might introduce bias if highly represented in one group compared to the other).
- **Is it clear how the test was carried out?** To be able to apply the results of the study to your own clinical practice, you need to be confident that the test is performed in the same way in your setting, as it was in the study.

What was the test undertaken? How was it done and by whom? Was it a multi-level test (i.e. a serum level) with different thresholds?

- **Is the test result reproducible?** This is essentially asking whether you obtain the same result if different people carry out the test, or if the test is carried out at different times on the same person. One thing to consider here of course is the distinction between reproducibility and validity. It is perfectly possible for a study to generate a series of results that are reproducibly wrong.
- **Was the reference standard (gold standard) appropriate?** To start with, we need to find out how the study found out what the 'truth' really was about patients. That is to say, how did the investigators know whether or not someone really had a disease? To do this, they will have needed some reference standard test (or series of tests) which they know 'always' tells the truth.
- **Were the reference standard and the diagnostic test interpreted blind and independently of each other?** If the study investigators know the result of the reference standard test, this might influence their interpretation of the diagnostic test and vice versa. The potential effect of non-blinding of investigators has already discussed.
- **Was the reference standard applied to all patients?** Ideally, both the test being evaluated and the reference standard should be carried out on all patients in the study. There may be a temptation, for example, if the test under investigation proves positive, not to bother administering the reference standard test. In many cases, the reference standard test may be invasive and may expose the patient to some risk and/or discomfort. While it would usually be ethical to use such a test on a patient in whom you had grounds to suspect that it might be positive, it would not be ethical if you thought that the test would be negative (i.e. if the diagnostic test being evaluated had been negative). Therefore, when reading the paper, you need to find out whether the reference standard was applied to all patients, and if it was not look at what steps the investigators took to find out what the 'truth' was in patients who did not have the reference test.
- **Was the test evaluated on an appropriate spectrum of patients?** Another complication is that a test may perform differently depending upon the sort of patients on whom it is carried out. For example, the more severe a disease is, the easier it tends to be to detect. Thus, you might find that testing for bacterial sore throats might be 'better' at detecting infection when evaluated in patients who attend an ENT clinic, than in those attending family practice. This may be because people with chronic disease who attend an ENT clinic will be more symptomatic and have more bacteria in general, making it easier to detect. This problem is referred to as spectrum bias. A test is going to perform better in terms of detecting people with disease if it is used to identify it in people in whom the disease is more severe, or advanced. Similarly, the test will produce more false-positive results if it is carried out on patients with other diseases that might mimic the disease that is being tested for.

The issue to consider when appraising a paper is whether the test was evaluated on the typical sort of patients in whom the test would be carried out in real life.

The optimal study method for the assessment of a diagnostic test is a cohort study evaluating the test in a group of patients thought to be at risk of having the disease. A less valid alternative method that has been used is a case-control study. The latter method studies patients known to have the disease and control patients without the disease. The performance of the test in the two groups is compared. This sort of study has been shown to overestimate the effectiveness of the diagnostic tests.[17]

What are the results?

In an ideal world, a positive test would mean that someone has disease, and a negative test would mean they do not have disease. Unfortunately, this is rarely the case. When a test is carried out, there are four possible outcomes:

1. The test can correctly detect disease that is present (a true positive result).
2. The test can detect disease when it is really absent (a false-positive result).
3. The test can correctly identify that a disease is not present (a true negative result).
4. The test identifies someone as free of a disease when it is really present (a false-negative result).

These possible outcomes are illustrated in **Table 44.1**.

Given that a test may potentially mislead us if we obtain a false-positive or a false-negative result, we need to have some way of characterizing how accurate the test really is (**Table 44.2**). What does this mean? The high specificity means that there is a high true negative rate (359 out of 375). Or put another way, only a few (16) falsely positive test results were found out of the 375 people who did not have GABHS. So that means (using some reverse logic) that if the rapid test was positive (going across the row), by inference they almost certainly have the disease.

We can simplify this to say that in tests with high **specificities**, where the result is **positive**, it rules the diagnosis **in**. The mnemonic for this is **SpPIn**.

TABLE 44.1 Possible outcomes of a diagnostic test

Test result	'True condition status'		
	Condition present	Condition absent	Totals
Positive	a True positive	b False positive	a+b
Negative	c False negative	d True negative	c+d
Totals	a+c	b+d	a+b+c+d

Sensitivity = a/(a+c) Positive predictive value = a/(a+b).
Specificity = d/(b+d) Negative predictive value = d/(c+d).
Prevalence = (a+c)/(a+b+c+d).
Accuracy = a+d/a+b+c+d.

TABLE 44.2 Results of rapid test screening for group-A β-haemolytic streptococcus (GABHS) in patients with a sore throat

Test result	'True condition status'		
	GABHS+ve	GABHS–ve	Totals
Positive	119	16	135
Negative	64	359	423
Totals	211	375	558

Sensitivity = 119/211 = 65%.
Specificity = 359/375 = 96%.
Positive predictive value = 119/135 = 88%.
Negative predictive value = 359/423 = 85%.
Prevalence = 211/558 = 33%.
Accuracy = 478/558 = 85%.

In tests with high **sensitivities** and the test is **negative** then it rules **out** the disease. So the mnemonic for this is **SnNOut**. Clearly it is not 100% accurate at excluding (that would only happen if the sensitivity was 100%). How you take that finding and put it into practice depends on the severity of the disease as well as the other symptoms and signs that indicate the pretest probability of the disease.

In reality, patients who are well where you are trying to exclude disease need tests with high sensitivities (primary care). Patients who are ill need tests with high specificities to determine the cause of the illness. This is an oversimplification of the process of diagnosis but is helpful in terms of remembering what tests do.

Often, of course, we are faced with tests whose sensitivity and specificity are not so high that we can use the test to rule in or rule out a disorder. For such cases, we need a measure of a particular test result's ability to predict the presence or absence of disease.

We might think that this is provided by the positive and negative predictive values (for positive and negative results, respectively). However, in practice we find that these values can change depending on the prevalence of the target disorder amongst the test population: if the disorder is more common, the positive predictive value will be higher and the negative predictive value lower.

For example, if the results show a much lower prevalence (Table 44.3), the sensitivity remains similar and the specificity is the same but the positive predictive value

TABLE 44.3 Potential results of a rapid test screening for GABHS in patients with sore throat in an imaginary low prevalence setting

Test result	'Truth'		
	GABHS+ve	GABHS–ve	Totals
Positive	12	16	28
Negative	6	359	365
Totals	18	375	393

Sensitivity = 67%.
Specificity = 96%.
Positive predictive value = 43%.
Negative predictive value = 98%.
Prevalence = 4.5%.

drops considerably. Now the test only has a 50:50 chance of detecting someone with disease. You can see how the prevalence will sometimes significantly alter the effectiveness of a test. It is important always to consider the setting before recommending tests that perform well in an alternative healthcare setting.

However, since sensitivity and specificity are not affected by disease prevalence, we can combine them to create a combined measure of the efficacy of a particular test result. This can be thought of as, for a given test result, the likelihood that a patient with the disorder would yield that test result compared to the likelihood that a patient without the disorder would yield that same test result. This is the likelihood ratio (LR). As a rule of thumb, for positive test results, an LR of 10 or above shows that the test result is good at ruling in disease; for negative test results, an LR of 0.1 or less shows that the test result is good at ruling out disease.

Two additional benefits of the LR are that they can be used to generate specific post-test probabilities for your patient and that, where we have multiple independent tests, the LRs can be multiplied together to yield a much more powerful test.

The prevalence of GABHS was 33%. If the test is positive it is very likely they have GABHS, but what about if it is negative?

What you can do is work out the likelihood ratios: Figure 44.2 shows the nomogram for likelihood ratios. To use the nomogram a line is drawn from the pre-test probability of 33% through 16 (on the likelihood ratio line) to obtain a post-test probability of approximately 90% if the result is positive and through 0.36 (roughly) to obtain a post-test probability of approximately 12% if the result is negative.

But what if our patient has a lower pre-test probability? For example, this might be a patient with only a 20% pre-test probability. Using a ruler, see what their post-test probability would be. The nomogram lets you quickly see the implications of a positive or negative result in terms of post-test probability.

Will the results help my patient?

ARE THE RESULTS RELEVANT TO YOUR PATIENT?

So far, we have considered how to interpret results of tests for your patients. However, it may be that you feel that the results of studies carried out to assess the accuracy of the test are not generalizable (or relevant) to your setting, or you may consider that it would not be helpful to your patient to perform the test.

GENERALIZABILITY TO YOUR SETTING

One aspect to consider is whether the assessment(s) of test validity that have been carried out are applicable to your setting. We have already seen how predictive value is dependent upon prevalence, so the predictive value of a test in one setting is usually not the same in another setting.

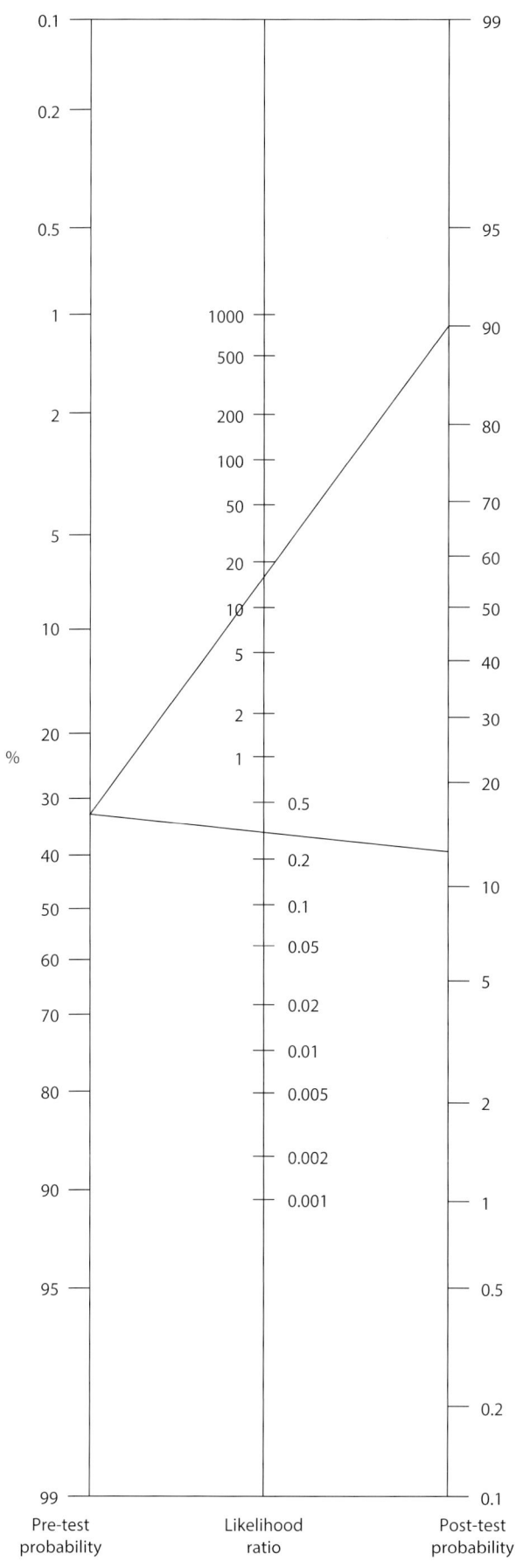

Figure 44.2 Nomogram for likelihood ratios.

Sensitivity and specificity (and likelihood ratios) are not dependent on prevalence, but they can vary according to the type of patients on which the test is carried out. The sensitivity of a test will depend upon the severity of disease in the population being tested. The more advanced or severe the disease, the more likely the test is to identify it.

The specificity of a test will depend upon the prevalence of other diseases in the population that might lead to false-positive results. The more that other diseases are present, the more likely a false-positive result.

A second aspect to consider is whether the test is carried out the same way in your setting as it was in the study. Some diagnostic tests depend upon the skill of the person carrying out the test, and the skill of the people interpreting the test result. Tests may be carried out in different ways, and it is important to know that it is carried out the same way in your local hospital or laboratory as it was in the study which evaluated the test.

WILL IT HELP YOUR PATIENT?

One way to think about whether or not to perform the test is whether it will influence the management of the patient or groups of patients you are likely to see. If you think that a disease is unlikely in a particular patient, it may be that if you carried out the test and it was positive, you would still think that the disease was unlikely, so it would not influence your management. Conversely, if you think that a disease is likely in a given patient, it may be that a negative test result would not stop you treating the patient, since you would still think that the disease is likely whatever the test result. Putting this in terms of pre- and post-test probabilities, in the first instance the pre-test probability of disease is so low, that even with a positive test result, the post-test probability will be less than 50%. In the second instance, the pre-test probability of disease is so high that even with a negative test result, the post-test probability will be more than 50%.

In practice, knowledge about the accuracy of diagnostic tests will perhaps be most useful when planning protocols or guidelines to manage particular groups of patients.

Summary

An evidence-based approach to deciding whether a test is effective for your patient involves the following steps:

- Frame the clinical question.
- Search for evidence concerning the accuracy of the test.
- Assess the methods used to determine the accuracy of the test.
- Find out the likelihood ratios for the test.
- Estimate the pre-test probability of disease in your patient.
- Apply the likelihood ratios to this pre-test probability using the nomogram to determine what the post-test probability would be for different possible test results.
- Decide whether or not to perform the test on the basis of your assessment of whether it will influence the care of the patient, and the patient's attitude to different possible outcomes.

APPRAISING THERAPY ARTICLES

When we are required to answer a question about therapy, the identification of information from an article is not straightforward. The layout is frequently different depending on the journal you are reading. One is often relying on the editorial board of the journal, as well as the people who reviewed the article, to have ensured the quality of the article. There may be confusing statistics that make interpretation of the data seem difficult. These problems seem to be very daunting when one is trying to identify information that may affect the care of a patient. These following questions will help you identify the real validity of the therapy article.

- **Is the study valid?** Did the authors answer the question? For this example I shall be using the Kubba paper[9] on Naseptin and epistaxis. The abstract of this article is shown under 'Read the abstract' above. Kubba et al.[9] have answered their question about the effectiveness of Naseptin in epistaxis. They state clearly how they did this and what they used to determine 'effective'.
- **What were the characteristics of the groups?** This would contain some description about the numbers of patients, their race and gender, age and any other features that are pertinent to the study. This is usually found in Table 1 in most papers but in this case is described in the protocol part of the subjects and methods section.
- **Are the comparison groups similar?** To determine whether bias has occurred in the selection procedure, certain potentially relevant characteristics of the two populations should be displayed in tabular form. Usually these include age, sex, duration of illness and other demographic and functional characteristics. This is covered in the first paragraph of the results section of the paper being considered here. There were more boys than girls, but the age and duration of history were the same in both groups. Is it likely that girls and boys would differ in response? The aim is not to find whether there are statistical differences between the two groups but to find whether there are clinically significant differences. You as a clinician reader should judge whether you think the differences are clinically significant.
- **What was the treatment?** In this case it was either Naseptin or nothing. The authors describe clearly the reasons for not using a placebo.

Equal treatment

The groups in the trial were treated equally throughout apart from the experimental intervention. It should be clear from the article that, for example, there were no co-interventions that were applied to one group but not the other, or more frequent or detailed assessments on one group compared to the other.

Placebo control

Patients do better if they think they are receiving a treatment than if they do not, even if the treatment is an inactive substance: the placebo effect is a widely accepted potential bias in trials. A placebo is an inactive treatment that is given so that the patient does not know whether he or she has been given the active treatment; the control group in a trial will often receive a placebo treatment so that this effect is equal in both groups. Patients in both groups of the trial should not know whether or not they are receiving the active therapy. However there is a twist in the tail – one can have a placebo-controlled trial where the patients are having active treatments in both arms of the study in addition to the new treatment or the placebo. So the term 'placebo-controlled trial' does not exclude the use of active treatments (as long as both groups get the same).

Follow-up

There are three major aspects to assessing the follow-up of trials:

- Did so many patients drop out of the trial that its results are in doubt?
- Was the study long enough to allow outcomes to become manifest?
- Were patients analyzed in the groups to which they were originally assigned (intention-to-treat)?

Drop-out rates

A good clinical trial requires the complete follow-up of patients in both the control and experimental groups. If less than 80% of patients are adequately followed up then the results may be invalid. In this study they had problems and had to phone subjects as they did not attend the outpatient clinic. This weakness of the study was evaluated in the discussion.

Length of study

The length of the study is critical in determining the clinical significance of the results. For a disease of short duration, such as an acute infectious disease, the period of the study need only be long enough to cover the course of that infection. Where the disease is more progressive and lengthy then the duration of the study needs to reflect that. The question that the research is trying to answer will also be helpful in deciding the appropriate length of the study.

Intention-to-treat

Because anything that happens after randomization can affect the chances that a patient in a trial has an event, it is important that all patients are analyzed in the groups to which they were randomized. This is an essential prerequisite for valid evidence about therapy. For example, it has been repeatedly shown that patients who do and do not take their study medicine have very different outcomes, even when the study medicine they have been prescribed is a placebo. The correct form of analysis, in which patients are analyzed in the groups to which they were assigned, is called 'intention-to-treat' analysis.

Were the groups randomized?

The major reason for randomization is to prevent bias. The largest potential cause of bias in research about effectiveness of an intervention is if the patients allocated to the treatment group are different from those allocated to the control group in a way that might influence outcome. To reduce this bias as much as possible, the decision as to which treatment a patient receives should be determined by random allocation. Why is this important?

There could be any number of confounding variables that affect a given situation, some of which we know about, but also others that our knowledge of human physiology has not yet uncovered. Randomization is important because it spreads all confounding variables evenly amongst the study groups, even the ones we do not know about. Occasionally, simple randomization may not ensure that there is an equal balance between treatment groups of known confounding variables. Where there are important confounders known and a need to be sure these are balanced between two groups, a process of stratified randomization can be employed.

CONCEALED RANDOMIZATION

As a supplementary point, clinicians who are recruiting patients into a trial may consciously or unconsciously distort the balance between groups if they know the treatments that will be given to patients. For this reason, it is preferable that the randomization list be concealed from the clinicians. The amount of impact the lack of concealment may have is larger than if the trial was not blinded. If there is inadequate concealment, the size of the effect may be overemphasized by as much as 30%.

BLINDING

It is also important that, if possible, both clinician and patient be 'blind' to whether or not they are receiving treatment. Lack of blinding may lead to exaggeration of the effectiveness of the therapy by as much as 20%.[3]

Outcome measures

To determine the impact of an intervention on patient health, one needs to define clearly the outcome that needs to be measured. This sounds straightforward enough but it can take up a larger amount of the preparation time of the research. An outcome measure is any feature that is recorded to determine the progression of the disease or problem being studied. In this paper a comprehensive questionnaire was used to determine outcomes.

What are the results?

- How large is the treatment effect?
- How precise is the estimate of the treatment effect?

In any clinical therapeutic study there are three explanations for the observed effect:

- the effect of the treatment
- chance variation between the two groups
- bias.

Good research will explicitly endeavour to reduce the effects of chance and bias by using special designs, as we have seen.

NUMBERS NEEDED TO TREAT

The most common approach is to describe the effect of a drug in terms of the risk reduction. The risk is usually of continuing to have, for example, pain or an event. When evaluating a paper on a therapeutic manoeuvre, it is possible to establish its clinical effectiveness by determining the proportion of patients receiving treatment who gain benefit.

Table 44.4 shows the results drawn from the paper.

From the paper the following results are drawn:

The simple statement above obscures the fact that identifying the correct table in the paper and then obtaining the correct figures from it is often not as easy as it sounds. This is one of the parts of appraisal that it is often useful to share with others to ensure you have the correct data.

From **Table 44.4** it can be seen that 47 patients were assigned to the active treatment (or experimental) group and 41 to the watchful waiting (or control) group. There were a total of 50 children with epistaxis; 21 occurred in the experimental group and 29 in the control group.

EVENT RATES

It is important to set some standard methods of describing these data. In therapy, we start by converting the numbers of patients into event rates. In the control group, 29 out of 41 patients had epistaxis. This may be presented as an event rate of $(29/41) = 0.71$. So the control event rate (CER) is 0.71 (this number is also the risk of epistaxis in the control group, and corresponds to a percentage risk of 71%).

In the experimental treatment group there were 21 children with epistaxis out of 47 children. The experimental

TABLE 44.4 Results of a trial of Naseptin against watchful waiting in stopping epistaxis in children

	Epistaxis	No epistaxis for four weeks	Total
Active treatment (Naseptin)	21	26	47
Watchful waiting	29	12	41
Total	50	38	88

event rate (EER) was therefore 0.44 (44%). Now that we have these numbers we can start working with them.

RELATIVE RISK

One way of combining the event rates is to use relative risk (RR). Here, we make a ratio of the two risks to show which group has a higher or lower risk. The relative risk is calculated by dividing the risk of having epistaxis in the treatment group by the risk of the control group = 0.44/0.71 = 0.62. This means that the risk of epistaxis continuing with Naseptin was 0.62 (or 62%) of the risk without Naspetin.

Relative risk reduction

It is also possible to show the extent of the benefit compared to the original risk by calculating the relative risk reduction (RRR). This is similar to relative risk, except that we take the difference in risk between the two groups and divide that by the control group's risk: RRRs are often presented as percentages.

The RRR means that the treatment reduced the risk of continued nosebleeds by 38% relative to that occurring in this control population (the RRR given by the authors is for persistent bleeding whereas I have calculated for cessation of bleeding). This is a large risk reduction in a population that are all bleeding. But what if it was an RRR for primary stroke reduction where the events are far fewer? So the RRR has to be judged against the prevalence of the outcome we want to prevent.

Absolute risk reduction

The absolute risk is that 71% of individuals in the placebo group had nosebleeds and that 44% of the treatment group had nosebleeds. The difference (absolute risk reduction (ARR)) between these gives us another view of the effectiveness of the treatment. The ARR of this therapy is 0.27 (CER − EER = 0.71−0.44).

ARR = CER − EER

Consider 100 people given this treatment. We would expect 27 fewer children to have epistaxis if this group were given Naseptin than if they were not. We can convert this into how many people we would need to treat to prevent one child continuing to have epistaxis. This number is the reciprocal of the ARR. In this example 1/0.27 = 3.7. Therefore, to prevent a child continuing to have epistaxis we need to treat four people. This is the number needed to treat (NNT). It is more useful than relative measures because, as well as measuring the benefit of a therapy, it also represents the baseline risk and the absolute benefit you can expect from the therapy.

NNT = 1/ARR

Sometimes, papers will present their results in the form of NNTs, as in this one, which is very helpful, but often they do not, and prefer to present risk ratios (perhaps not surprisingly, since these tend to make beneficial results look more spectacular) or similar measures. You will often be required to calculate NNTs from the data in the study. Fortunately, the arithmetic is fairly straightforward. Some other examples of NNTs are included in Bandolier (http://www.bandolier.org.uk/band59/NNTcalc.html).

This is a small study and like the relative risk there is a confidence interval around the NNT. To calculate this[18] it is easier to use software (www.ebm.net). Also, there is the 'believability' issue of a relatively small trial. This is where the clinical judgement comes in – would you use this treatment based on 100 patients?

Will the results help my patient?

- Can the results be applied to my patient?
- Were all clinically relevant outcomes considered?
- Are the benefits worth the harms and costs?

Given that your patient was not in the trial and may not even have been eligible for it (due to age, sex, comorbidity, disease severity or for a host of other sociodemographic, biologic or clinical reasons), how can you extrapolate from the external evidence to your individual patient? (We use the term 'extrapolate' here, although this might more accurately be described as 'particularizing' the results of a trial (which looks at a generic population) to your particular patient.) This requires that you apply some of your knowledge of human biology and clinical experience to answer the question: 'Is my patient so different from those in the trial that its results cannot help me make my treatment decision?'

When analyzing the results of a trial it is important therefore to identify whether the trial has been designed to be explanatory or pragmatic in its approach. The former is often used to test whether the intervention works under ideal conditions – often in a highly selected cohort. This design may also be able to quantify the magnitude of any effect. A pragmatic design on the other hand often has much less strict inclusion criteria and consequently much more closely represents a 'real world' scenario. The results of a pragmatic trial may be more easily translated into a likely benefit for your particular patient.

HOW MUCH BENEFIT CAN YOU EXPECT FOR YOUR PATIENT?

Given that you have decided that your patient is sufficiently similar to those in the study for the effect to be applicable, the next questions is how much? Here is one way of going about this.

f method

First estimate, as a decimal fraction, your patient's risk compared to the control group from the study. Thus, if your patient is twice as susceptible as those in the trial, $f = 2$; if half as susceptible, $f = 0.5$. As long as the treatment produces a constant RRR across a range of susceptibilities, the NNT for your patient is simply the trial's reported NNT divided by f. (This is a big assumption and we are only beginning to learn when assuming a constant RRR is appropriate (for numerous medical treatments such as antihypertensive drugs) and inappropriate (for some operations such as carotid endarterectomy, where the RRR rises with increasing susceptibility). So, in the above example, we might assign an f of 0.7 (70% chance of having epistaxis to the control group of subjects), which would yield an NNT of $(3.7/0.7) = 5$.

INCORPORATING YOUR PATIENT'S VALUES AND PREFERENCES

What does your patient think? Have you talked to them about their personal preferences, concerns and expectations? Here, we must try to determine whether the outcome of the therapy actually serves the values and preferences of the patient. Many factors can come into play, not least the difficulty of representing them. Sometimes, the situation may be very clear-cut or demand immediate action. For example, in a patient having a heart attack, the value of survival and the preference for a simple, low-risk intervention such as aspirin, given the efficacy of this regimen, usually makes this decision quickly agreed and acted upon. In other cases, the answer may take weeks and several visits to sort out, such as in choosing between radiation and adjuvant chemotherapy for stage II carcinoma of the breast.

These questions are perhaps the most important, yet have the least written about them in this chapter. That is because they are also the most complex and depend to a great extent on the clinical situation.

Summary

An evidence-based approach to deciding whether a therapy is effective for your patient involves the following steps:

- Frame the clinical question.
- Search for evidence concerning the accuracy of the test.
- Assess the methods used to carry out the trial of the therapy.
- Determine the NNT of the therapy.
- Decide whether the NNT can apply to your patient, and estimate a particularized NNT.
- Incorporate your patient's values and preferences in to deciding on a course of action.

APPRAISING SYSTEMATIC REVIEWS

What happens when there is more than one randomized control trial on the same treatment or diagnostic test? In this case you want to look for a paper that has combined these trials together.

What you need here is a systematic review, a publication that collects all of the evidence in a particular area and summarizes it. More formally, a systematic review is 'a review of a clearly formulated question that uses systematic and explicit methods to identify, select and critically appraise relevant research, and to collect and analyze data from studies that are included in the review. Statistical methods may or may not be used to analyze and summarize the results of the included studies.'

This section will look at how you appraise studies that search for all research on a specific question and in some way combine it.

You may be familiar with the narrative reviews traditionally found in many journals. Normally someone, usually an expert, looks at the evidence in a certain area. Mulrow[19] argues that traditional reviews do not routinely use systematic methods to identify, assess and synthesize information. Thus, normally there is no methods section for the actual conduct of the review. The reader then has no way of knowing whether the review is based on a systematic review of the evidence, or on a collection of papers that the author has found in a less systematic way and thus the evidence presented may not be complete. There is a need for systematic reviews of the evidence. This needs to be undertaken in just as rigorous a way as any primary piece of research, with a clear question and explicit methods for all stages of the process, such that another person could replicate the review. Three key features of such a review are:

- a strenuous effort to locate all original reports on the topic of interest
- critical evaluation of the reports
- conclusions drawn based on a synthesis of studies that meet preset quality criteria.

When synthesizing results, a meta-analysis may be undertaken. This is 'the use of statistical techniques in a systematic review to integrate the results of the included studies', which means that the authors have attempted to synthesize the different results into one overall statistic.

Where can you find systematic reviews?

Systematic reviews have been published in a variety of journals, and in addition the Cochrane Collaboration provides an important resource in this area. The Cochrane Collaboration is an international collaboration that is committed to 'preparing, maintaining and disseminating systematic reviews of the effects of health care'. It promotes and publishes the Cochrane Library (www.cochrane.org). This contains the Cochrane Database of Systematic Reviews. These reviews have a prespecified protocol, where every stage of the process of undertaking the review is made explicit.

Sections covered in a protocol include background, objectives, criteria for considering studies for the review (including types of participants, types of interventions, types of outcome measure, types of study), search strategy for identification of studies, study selection, methodological quality assessment, data extraction, meta-analysis, the comparisons to be made, subgroup analysis and sensitivity analysis to be undertaken. The point to note here is that all these aspects of the protocol are set out before the review is undertaken. The PRISMA guidelines are freely available online (www.prisma-statement.org) and contain a checklist to assist when performing a systematic review.

Many journals now require adherence to these guidelines and will ask for the article to be peer reviewed against them.

Many of the systematic reviews so far completed are based on evidence of effectiveness of an intervention from RCTs.

Is the review valid?

In this section we will focus on systematic reviews of therapy. Of course, systematic reviews exist for other types of research.[20]

- **What databases and other sources did the authors of this review search?** The paper should give a comprehensive account of the sources consulted in the search for relevant papers, and the search strategy used to find them. Since standard databases fail to correctly index up to half of published trials, and negative trials are less likely to be published in the first place, the search strategy should include hand searching of journals and searching for unpublished literature. Other questions to ask yourself about the search strategy are: Have any obvious databases been missed? Did the authors check the reference lists of articles and of textbooks? Did they contact experts (to obtain their list of references checked for completeness and to attempt to find out about ongoing or unpublished research)? Search terms used are also important – has an obvious medical subject heading (MeSH) (a standard thesaurus for medical indexing) term been missed or is there another term they have not used? For example, when searching for papers looking at care of the elderly, use of the term 'senior' in the North American literature may be overlooked. Searching should include languages other than English. Unpublished data are useful to include because studies with significant results are more likely to be published than studies without significant results, known as publication bias. For example, research that is carried out by non-English language teams is more likely to be published in English if it shows a strong result in favour of an intervention than if it shows a negative or indifferent result.
- **How were the studies selected – eligibility criteria?** You should look for a statement of how the trial's validity was assessed, using criteria such as those in the therapy guides. It is particularly reassuring when two or more investigators applied these criteria independently and achieved good agreement in their results. You need to know what criteria were used to select the research. This should include who the study participants were, what was done and what outcomes were assessed. A point to consider is that the narrower the inclusion criteria, the less generalizable are the results. However, this needs to be balanced with using very broad inclusion criteria, when heterogeneity becomes an issue. Such studies may cover a wide range of patients and/or interventions and/or outcomes and the justification for then combining these differing groups comes into question. The importance of a clear statement of inclusion criteria is that studies should be selected on the basis of these criteria (that is, any study that matches these criteria is included) rather than selecting the study on the basis of the results.
- **How were the data abstracted?** Data are usually obtained by two individuals working separately (independently) and then compared later. Where consensus between reviewers cannot be reached it is customary for a third reviewer to act as arbiter. Often the data are not available within the paper and there may be a statement about obtaining the raw data from the authors.
- **Is there a description of the quality of each trial?** A table of the studies meeting the inclusion criteria should include some data on the validity checks itemized in the section on randomized control trials.[4]
- **Were the results consistent from study to study?** Although we might expect some variation from study to study, we would be concerned if some trials confidently concluded a beneficial effect of the therapy, while others confidently concluded harmful or no effects. Unless this heterogeneity can be explained to your satisfaction (such as by differences in patients, dosage or duration of treatment), this should lead you to be very cautious about believing any overall conclusion about efficacy from the review.

Statistical heterogeneity exists when there is greater variation between the results than is likely due to chance. The chi-square statistic on which they are based has on average a value equal to its degrees of freedom. Values much larger than the degrees of freedom suggest a smaller p value and thus significant statistical heterogeneity. This means greater variation exists between the studies than is likely by chance alone. One might then conclude that the studies are so different that it makes no sense to combine them. Since this test of heterogeneity is described as having a low power, a non-significant test cannot be interpreted as evidence of homogeneity. The aim of the authors should be to clearly describe the influences of specific clinical differences between the studies, rather than purely relying on an overall statistical test of heterogeneity.

Clinical and statistical heterogeneity need to be distinguished. Clinical heterogeneity refers to differences between settings, patients, techniques and outcomes, which might lead you to suggest it does not make sense to combine the data.

What are the results?

Terms that you will probably come across when looking at systematic reviews include odds ratios, relative risks, weighted mean differences and fixed and random effects, amongst others.

BINARY OR CONTINUOUS DATA

The type of data will dictate what you see when you look at a meta-analysis:

- binary data (for example, an event rate: something that happens or it does not, such as myocardial infarction, stroke, improved/not improved) is usually combined using odds ratios

- continuous data (for example, numbers of days, peak expiratory flow rate) are combined using differences in mean values for treatment and control groups (weighted mean differences (WMDs)) when units of measurement are the same (for example, all using the same anxiety scale), or standardized mean differences when units of measurement differ (for example, using a variety of anxiety scales, where one numerical value could mean very different things, depending on the scale used). Here, the difference in means is divided by the pooled standard deviation.

Thus when you look at a meta-analysis, you will see odds ratios or relative risks and/or weighted mean differences or standardized mean differences, depending on the outcomes measures that have been used in the included studies.

ODDS RATIO

Odds are another way of describing risk. The odds of an event are the probability of it occurring compared to the probability of it not occurring. We cannot do a randomized control trial to assess whether gastrooesophageal reflux disease (GERD) may be associated with laryngeal neoplasm. However, we can do a case-control study looking at people with and without cancer.[21]

We do not know the incidence of laryngeal cancer in the population from this study as they took cases with cancer and compared them to controls, but we can work out the odds (Table 44.5). For GERD, the odds of having cancer is 731/1315 = 0.555. This clearly is not the risk in the general population! The odds of having laryngeal cancer in non-GERD patients was 0.237. The odds ratio was 0.555/0.237 = 2.3. So patients with GERD in this study had 2.3 times the odds of having laryngeal carcinoma. This was unadjusted for the other major risk factor of smoking. In large studies, odds ratios approximate risk ratio.

Clearly, as in randomized controlled trials with risk reduction, unless we know the baseline risk it is impossible to put odds ratios into context. A number needed to treat can be derived from an odds ratio but remember that many assumptions have been made in that process and treat them with some caution.

Many systematic reviews use odds ratios to represent differences between treatment and control groups. Relative risk and absolute risk reduction may also be used to express these sorts of differences, as we have already seen.

TABLE 44.5 Prevalence of gastrooesophageal reflux disease (GERD) in a case control study of patients with and without laryngeal cancer

	GERD	No GERD
Laryngeal cancer	731	7497
No laryngeal cancer	1315	31,597
Total	2046	39,094

WHAT DO ODDS RATIOS USED IN A META-ANALYSIS LOOK LIKE?

The square box on the Forrest Plot (Figure 44.3) is the individual study effect (technically referred to as the point estimate), with its associated confidence interval as lines either side of that box (technically known as the interval estimate). Sometimes the size of the box may vary to reflect the weight that particular study is given, with larger boxes representing higher weighting. Lower weighted studies are usually those with smaller samples and large confidence intervals. The overall or summary effect (from combining or pooling the studies) is usually depicted as a diamond. Since patients may respond differently to treatment, this pooling may need to be supplanted by summarizing evidence along multiple covariates of interest. Thus, although one overall number is appealing in its simplicity, it may oversimplify a more complex situation.

An odds ratio of 1 on a linear scale means there is no difference between the experimental and control group. This value of 1 is the line down the middle of the figure (sometimes with the wording 'favours treatment' on one side and 'favours control' on the other). If the confidence interval does *not* cross the line, it means that there is a 95% chance that there is a true difference between the groups. That is, that there is a significant difference on that particular outcome between the intervention and control groups. If the confidence interval does cross this vertical line labelled '1' it means that any difference in that outcome between the treatments could have occurred by chance (that is, there are no statistically significant differences). It may be that a very wide confidence interval is due to a very small sample size, and it would reduce with more people in the study. A 95% confidence interval covers likely results from a set of similar studies. It therefore provides a more realistic view of what will happen in practice than a point estimate, because it takes potential variability into account.

It is worth noting that a lack of evidence for an intervention is not the same as evidence of a lack of effect.

HOW PRECISE ARE THE RESULTS?

This is asking whether there are any confidence intervals used, so the reader can see the range of values around the effect size, where one has 95% confidence that the 'true' effect would lie. The *Cochrane Handbook* (2011)[22] defines precision as 'a measure of the likelihood of random errors. It is reflected in the confidence interval around the estimate of effect from each study … more precise results are given more weight'. Thus the more precise the results, the narrower (smaller) the confidence interval. NNTs can be calculated from the odds ratios. However, these should be treated with caution as they can oversimplify.

WILL THE RESULTS HELP ME IN CARING FOR MY PATIENTS?

- **Can the results be applied to my patient care?** How similar are the patients you care for to those included in the review? The wider the type of patients included

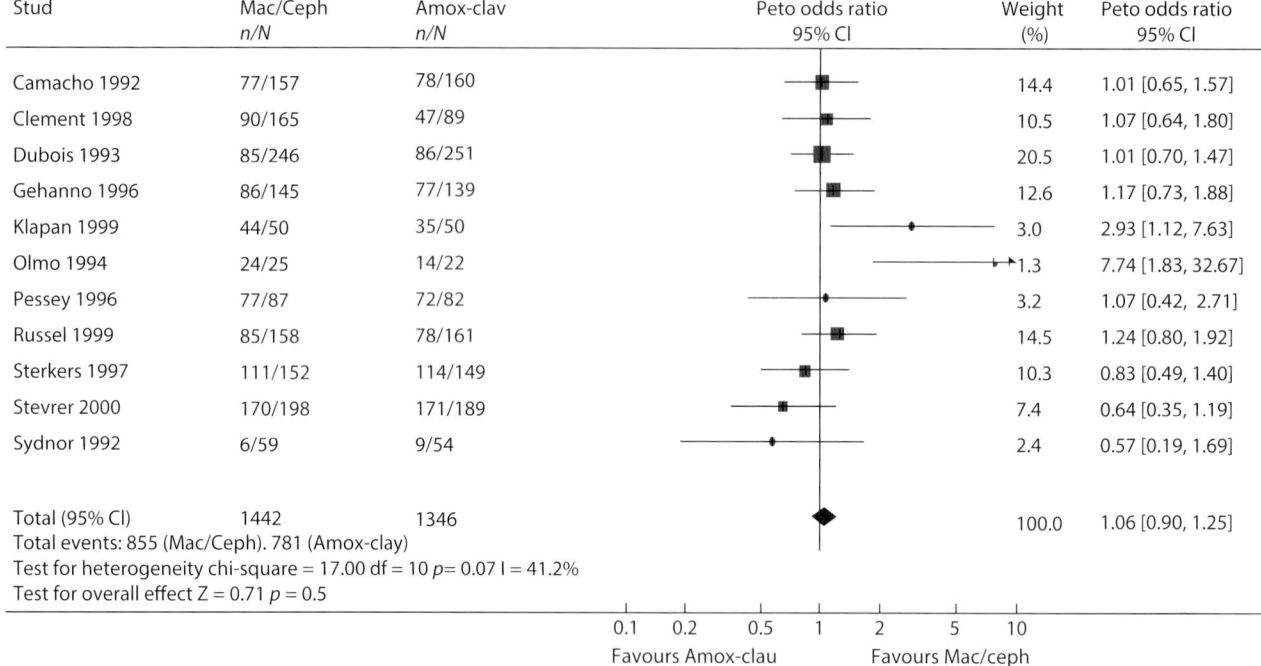

Figure 44.3 A Forrest plot. Redrawn from Ref. 23, with permission.

in the review, the more likely you are to feel the results may apply across a range of different patients. However, it is sometimes a difficult decision to know whether, for example, something that works on men will be equally effective on women, or something that works in younger people will work in the same way in older people. Subgroup analysis may be one way of addressing this, although there are concerns with this approach.
- Were all clinically important outcomes considered? What is clinically important can depend on your perspective. Sometimes, whilst factors such as bone density may be included in a review to assess the effectiveness of certain orthopaedic procedures, it may be some other outcome, such as ability to get to the shops, that needs to be considered as this sort of outcome may be crucial from the patient's perspective.
- Are the benefits worth the harms and costs? This may cover a range of factors, such as benefit of early treatment following a positive cervical smear versus the harms of high anxiety. Or it may be the benefits of a chemotherapeutic agent versus its unpleasant side effects. An economic evaluation may be included.

What is sometimes difficult using a set of criteria like this, is that you end up with a variety of 'no's' or 'can't tell's' in answer to the questions you pose. It is sometimes difficult to decide when a review is 'too bad' to give you any confidence in the findings. Perhaps one pragmatic approach would be that when you have several 'no's' or 'can't tell's' you are more wary about the validity and robustness of the review's findings. What this does illustrate is that,

like undertaking a systematic review, critically appraising these reviews is not an exact science, but there are many subjective decisions along the way. Just like undertaking a systematic review, making explicit your decisions in the critical appraisal is therefore very important.

Although a systematic review can provide you with high quality evidence, clinical experience and patient preferences are an important part of evidence-based medicine. It may be that even high quality evidence does not apply to a particular patient. Similarly, Cochrane reviews do not include recommendations, as reviewers cannot know the local situation or the patient, and this is the province of the health professional caring for the patient.

Levels of evidence

Table 44.6 provides a breakdown of the types of research that answers questions on therapy, prognosis, diagnosis, differential diagnosis or prevalence and economic studies. For each type of research a level of evidence is shown. This helps the reader identify the likely validity of the research. It does not mean that all systematic reviews are 'better' than randomized controlled trials. It should be used more as a pointer for searching and then a guide to the likely level of evidence. If one has a therapeutic question then looking for a systematic review first is logical. If there is no review then one next looks for a randomized controlled trial, etc.

If there is no trial evidence then consensus statements becomes the highest level of evidence answering that question. This just makes the grade of recommendation D rather than A if there was a systematic review. The grades

TABLE 44.6 Levels of evidence

Level	Therapy/prevention, aetiology/harm	Prognosis	Diagnosis	Differential diagnosis/ symptom prevalence study	Economic and decision analyses
1a	SR (with homogeneity)[a] of RCTs	SR (with homogeneity)[a] of inception cohort studies; CDR[b] validated in different populations	SR (with homogeneity)[a] of Level 1 diagnostic studies; CDR[b] with 1b studies from different clinical centres	SR (with homogeneity)[a] of prospective cohort studies	SR (with homogeneity)[a] of level 1 economic studies
1b	Individual RCT (with narrow Confidence interval)[c]	Individual inception cohort study with >80% follow-up; CDR[b] validated in a single population	Validating[k] cohort study with good[h] reference standards; or CDR[b] tested within one clinical centre	Prospective cohort study with good follow-up[c]	Analysis based on clinically sensible costs or alternatives; systematic review(s) of the evidence; and including multi-way sensitivity analyses
1c	All or none[d]	All or none case-series	Absolute SpPins and SnNouts[g]	All or none case-series	Absolute better-value or worse-value analyses[j]
2a	SR (with homogeneity)[a] of cohort studies	SR (with homogeneity)[a] of either retrospective cohort studies or untreated control groups in RCTs	SR (with homogeneity)[a] of Level >2 diagnostic studies	SR (with homogeneity)[a] of 2b and better studies	SR (with homogeneity)[a] of level >2 economic studies
2b	Individual cohort study (including low quality RCT; e.g., <80% follow-up)	Retrospective cohort study or follow-up of untreated control patients in an RCT; Derivation of CDR[b] or validated on split-sample[f] only	Exploratory[k] cohort study with good[h] reference standards; CDR[b] after derivation, or validated only on split-sample[f] or databases	Retrospective cohort study, or poor follow-up	Analysis based on clinically sensible costs or alternatives; limited review(s) of the evidence, or single studies; and including multi-way sensitivity analyses
2c	'Outcomes' research; Ecological studies	'Outcomes' research		Ecological studies	Audit or outcomes research
3a	SR (with homogeneity)[a] of case-control studies		SR (with homogeneity)[a] of 3b and better studies	SR (with homogeneity)[a] of 3b and better studies	SR (with homogeneity)[a] of 3b and better studies
3b	Individual case-control study		Non-consecutive study; or without consistently applied reference standards	Non-consecutive cohort study, or very limited population	Analysis based on limited alternatives or costs, poor quality estimates of data, but including sensitivity analyses incorporating clinically sensible variations
4	Case-series (and poor quality cohort and case-control studies)[e]	Case-series (and poor quality prognostic cohort studies)[i]	Case-control study, poor or non-independent reference standard	Case-series or superseded reference standards	Analysis with no sensitivity analysis
5	Expert opinion without explicit critical appraisal, or based on physiology, bench research or 'first principles'	Expert opinion without explicit critical appraisal, or based on physiology, bench research or 'first principles'	Expert opinion without explicit critical appraisal, or based on physiology, bench research or 'first principles'	Expert opinion without explicit critical appraisal, or based on physiology, bench research or 'first principles'	Expert opinion without explicit critical appraisal, or based on economic theory or 'first principles'

The levels of evidence used throughout this book are as stated in the prelims on the How to use this book page. These are very similar to the five levels given in this table, except that Levels 3 and 4 of the system described in this table are equivalent to Level 3, and Level 5 (expert opinion) is equivalent to Level 4 in the system used in this book.

Produced by Bob Phillips, Chris Ball, Dave Sackett, Doug Badenoch, Sharon Straus, Brian Haynes and Martin Dawes since November 1998.

Users can add a minus sign '−' to denote the level of that fails to provide a conclusive answer because of:

- EITHER a single result with a wide confidence interval (such that, for example, an ARR in an RCT is not statistically significant but whose confidence intervals fail to exclude clinically important benefit or harm).
- OR a systematic review with troublesome (and statistically significant) heterogeneity.
- Such evidence is inconclusive, and therefore can only generate Grade D recommendations.

a   By homogeneity we mean a systematic review that is free of worrisome variations (heterogeneity) in the directions and degrees of results between individual studies. Not all systematic reviews with statistically significant heterogeneity need be worrisome, and not all worrisome heterogeneity need be statistically significant. As noted above, studies displaying worrisome heterogeneity should be tagged with a '−' at the end of their designated level.
b   Clinical decision rule. (These are algorithms or scoring systems which lead to a prognostic estimation or a diagnostic category.)
c   Good follow-up in a differential diagnosis study is >80%, with adequate time for alternative diagnoses to emerge (e.g. 1 to 6 months acute, 1 to 5 years chronic).
d   Met when *all* patients died before the Rx became available, but some now survive on it; or when some patients died before the Rx became available, but *none* now die on it.
e   By poor quality *cohort* study we mean one that failed to clearly define comparison groups and/or failed to measure exposures and outcomes in the same (preferably blinded), objective way in both exposed and non-exposed individuals and/or failed to identify or appropriately control known confounders and/or failed to carry out a sufficiently long and complete follow-up of patients. By poor quality *case–control* study we mean one that failed to clearly define comparison groups and/or failed to measure exposures and outcomes in the same (preferably blinded), objective way in both cases and controls and/or failed to identify or appropriately control known confounders.
f   Split-sample validation is achieved by collecting all the information in a single tranche, then artificially dividing this into 'derivation' and 'validation' samples.
g   An 'Absolute SpPin' is a diagnostic finding whose Specificity is so high that a Positive result rules-*in* the diagnosis. An 'Absolute SnNout' is a diagnostic finding whose Sensitivity is so high that a *Negative* result rules out the diagnosis.
h   Good, better, bad and worse refer to the comparisons between treatments in terms of their clinical risks and benefits.
i   Good reference standards are independent of the test, and applied blindly or objectively to applied to all patients. *Poor* reference standards are haphazardly applied, but still independent of the test. Use of a non-independent reference standard (where the 'test' is included in the 'reference', or where the 'testing' affects the 'reference') implies a level 4 study.
j   Better-value treatments are clearly as good but cheaper, or better at the same or reduced cost. Worse-value treatments are as good and more expensive, or worse and the equally or more expensive.
k   Validating studies test the quality of a specific diagnostic test, based on prior evidence. An exploratory study collects information and trawls the data (e.g. using a regression analysis) to find which factors are 'significant'.
l   By poor quality prognostic cohort study we mean one in which sampling was biased in favour of patients who already had the target outcome, or the measurement of outcomes was accomplished in <80% of study patients, or outcomes were determined in an unblinded, non-objective way, or there was no correction for confounding factors.

TABLE 44.7	Grades of recommendation
A	Consistent level 1 studies
B	Consistent level 2 or 3 studies **or** extrapolations from level 1 studies
C	Level 4 studies **or** extrapolations from level 2 or 3 studies
D	Level 5 evidence **or** troublingly inconsistent or inconclusive studies of any level

'Extrapolations' are where data are used in a situation that has potentially clinically important differences than the original study situation.

of recommendations vary from country to country and organization to organization and should only be considered as a guide (**Table 44.7**).

WORKSHEETS

The worksheets shown in **Figures 44.4, 44.5** and **44.6** can be used to appraise a randomized controlled trial, a diagnostic study or a systematic review. They are aide memoirs about the items to look for in a paper when appraising the validity, identifying the results and assessing the applicability.

They can be used in journal clubs or in other settings when an important new paper is being discussed. The data from these checklists can be entered into software to make your own electronic database of critical appraisals and saved as web pages or text documents.

KEY POINTS

Appraising diagnostic articles

- Criteria for validity of diagnosis trials: was there a reference standard, was it appropriate and was it applied blind, independently and to all patients?
- Appropriate spectrum of patients; clear and reproducible description of test, follow-up, intention-to-treat.
- Outcome measures.
- Measures of the accuracy of diagnostic tests: sensitivity, specificity, positive predictive value negative predictive value, likelihood ratios.
- Applying the results to your patient: pre- and post-test probability, SpPin and SnNOut.

Appraising therapy articles

- Criteria for validity of therapy trials: randomization, blinding, placebo control, equal treatment, follow up, intention-to-treat, outcome measures.
- Measures of the importance of the results of therapy trials: risk, event rates, NNTs.

Appraising systematic reviews

- Criteria for validity of systematic reviews: search for relevant trials, assessment of included trials' quality, heterogeneity.
- Measures of the importance of the results: risk, event rates, NNTs, odd ratios.

REFERENCES

1. Kraaijenhagen RA, Haverkamp D, Koopman MM, et al. Travel and risk of venous thrombosis. *Lancet* 2000; **356**: 1492–93.
2. Ioannidis JP, Haidich AB, Pappa M, et al. Comparison of evidence of treatment effects in randomized and nonrandomized studies. *J Am Med Assoc* 2001; **286**: 821–30.
3. Juni P, Altman DG, Egger M. Systematic reviews in health care: assessing the quality of controlled clinical trials. *BMJ* 2001; **323**: 42–46.
4. Schulz KF, Chalmers I, Hayes RJ, Altman DG. Empirical evidence of bias. Dimensions of methodological quality associated with estimates of treatment effects in controlled trials. *JAMA* 1995; **273**: 408–12.
5. Odgaard-Jensen J, Vist GE, Timmer A, et al. Randomisation to protect against selection bias in healthcare trials. *Cochrane DB Syst Rev* 2011 (4). Art No. MR000012.
6. Higgins JP, Altman DG, Gøtzsche PC, et al. The Cochrane Collaboration's tool for assessing risk of bias in randomised trials. *BMJ* 2011; **343**: d5928.
7. Moher D, Liberati A, Tetzlaff J, et al. Preferred Reporting Items for Systematic Reviews and Meta-Analyses: The PRISMA Statement. *BMJ* 2009; **339**: b2535.
8. Moher D, Cook DJ, Eastood S, et al. Improving the quality of reports of meta analyses of randomised controlled trials: the QUORUM statement. *Onkoligie* 2000; **23**: 597–602.
9. Kubba H, MacAndie C, Botma M, et al. A prospective, single-blind, randomized controlled trial of antiseptic cream for recurrent epistaxis in childhood. *Clin Otolaryngol* 2001; **26**: 465–68.
10. Adams D. *Life, the universe, and everything: The hitchhiker's guide to the galaxy.* London: Millenium (Orion); 1994, vol. 3.
11. www.clinicalevidence.com
12. Bouma M, Dekker JH, van Eijk JT, et al. Metabolic control and morbidity of type 2 diabetic patients in a general practice network. *Fam Pract* 1999; **16**: 402–06.
13. Booth A, O'Rourke AJ, Ford NJ. Structuring the pre-search reference interview: a useful technique for handling clinical questions. *Bull Med Libr Assoc* 2000; **88**: 239–46.
14. Thomas KB. General practice consultations: is there any point in being positive? *BMJ (Clin Res Ed)* 1987; **294**: 1200–02.
15. www.comet-initiative.org
16. Dagnelie CF, Bartelink ML, van der Graaf Y, et al. Towards a better diagnosis of throat infections (with group A beta-haemolytic streptococcus) in general practice. *Brit J Gen Pract* 1998; **48**: 959–62.
17. Lijmer JG, Mol BW, Heisterkamp S, et al. Empirical evidence of design-related bias in studies of diagnostic tests. *J Am Med Assoc* 1999; **282**: 1061–66.
18. Bender R. Calculating confidence intervals for the number needed to treat. *Control Clin Trials* 2001; **22**: 102–10.
19. Mulrow CD. The medical review article: state of the science. *Ann Intern Med* 1987; **106**: 485–88.
20. Oxman AD, Cook DJ, Guyatt GH. Users' guides to the medical literature. VI. How to use an overview. Evidence-Based Medicine Working Group. *J Am Med Assoc* 1994; **272**: 1367–71.
21. El-Serag HB, Hepworth EJ, Lee P, Sonnenberg A. Gastroesophageal reflux disease is a risk factor for laryngeal and pharyngeal cancer. *Am J Gastroenterol* 2001; **96**: 2013–18.
22. Higgens JPT, Green S, (eds). *Cochrane Handbook for Systematic Reviews of Interventions.* Version 5.1.0 [updated March 2011]. The Cochrane Collaboration, 2011. Available from http://handbook.cochrane.org
23. Williams Jr. JW, Aguilar C, Cornell J, et al. Antibiotics for acute maxillary sinusitis. *Cochrane DB Syst Rev* 2003; **2**: CD000243.

522 Section 1: Basic Sciences

The answer:	

Are the results of this single preventive or therapeutic trial valid?

PICO QUESTION	
Search terms used	
Databases searched to find this article	
Citation of article	
Why did you select this article(s)?	
Did the authors answer the question?	
1. What were the characteristics of the patients?	
2. Were the groups similar at the start of the trial?	
3. Aside from the experimental treatment, were the groups treated equally?	
4. What was the treatment and what was it compared against (placebo)?	
5a. Was the assignment of patients to treatments randomized? 5b. and was the randomization list concealed?	
6a. Were all patients who entered the trial followed up at its conclusion? 6b. and were they analyzed in the groups to which they were randomized (Intention to treat)?	
7. Were patients and clinicians kept 'blind' to which treatment was being received?	
8. Was the length of study appropriate?	

Are the valid results of this randomized trial important?

YOUR CALCULATIONS:

		Absolute risk reduction (ARR)	Number needed to treat (NNT)	Relative risk reduction (RRR)
Control group rate (CER)	Experimental Group Rate (EER)	CER-EER	1/ARR	ARR/CER

95% Confidence Interval (CI) on an NNT = 1/(limits on the CI of its ARR) =

$$\pm 1.96 \sqrt{\frac{CER \times (1-CER)}{\text{No. of control pts.}} + \frac{EER \times (1-EER)}{\text{No. of exp. pts.}}} =$$

Can you apply this valid, important evidence about a treatment in caring for your patient?

Do these results apply to your patient?	
Is your patient so different from those in the trial that its results cannot help you?	
How great would the potential benefit of therapy actually be for your individual patient?	
Method I: f	Risk of the outcome in your patient, relative to patients in the trial. expressed as a decimal: _____ NNT/F = _____ / _____ = _____ (NNT for patients like yours)

Are your patient's values and preferences satisfied by the regimen and its consequences?	
Do your patient and you have a clear assessment of their values and preferences?	
Are they met by this regimen and its consequences?	

Figure 44.4 Randomized control trial worksheet.

The Answer:	

Are the results of this diagnostic study valid?

PICO QUESTION	
Search terms used	
Databases searched to find this article	
Citation of article	
Why did you select this article(s)	
Did the authors answer the question?	
1. What were the characteristics of the patients?	
2a. New diagnostic test description. Is it clear how the test was carried out? 2b. Is the test reproducible in your setting?	
3a. Gold standard description. 3b. Was there an independent, blind comparison with a reference ('gold') standard of diagnosis?	
4. Was the reference standard applied regardless of the diagnostic test result?	
6. Was the diagnostic test evaluated in an appropriate spectrum of patients (like those in whom it would be used in practice)?	

YOUR CALCULATIONS:

		Target disorder		Totals
		Present	Absent	
Diagnostic test result	Positive	a	b	a + b
	Negative	c	d	c + d
	Totals	a + c	b + d1770	a + b + c + d

Sensitivity = a/(a + c) =
Specificity = d/(b + d) =
Likelihood ratio for a positive test result = LR+ = sens/(1−spec) =
Likelihood ratio for a negative test result = LR−= (1−sens)/spec =
Positive predictive value = a/(a + b) =
Negative predictive value = d/(c + d) =
Pre-test probability (prevalence) = (a + c)/(a + b + c + d) =
Pre-test-odds = prevalence/(1−prevalence) =
Post-test odds = Pre-test odds x likelihood ratio =
Post-test probability = post-test odds/(post-test odds + 1) =

Can you apply this valid, important evidence about a diagnostic test in caring for your patient?

Is the diagnostic test available, affordable, accurate and precise in your setting?	
Can you generate a clinically sensible estimate of your patient's pre-test probability (from practice data, from personal experience, from the report itself or from clinical speculation)	
Will the resulting post-test probabilities affect your management and help your patient? (Could it move you across a test-treatment threshold?; Would your patient be a willing partner in carrying it out?)	
Would the consequences of the test help your patient?	

Additional notes:

Figure 44.5 Diagnosis worksheet.

The Answer:

Are the results of this systematic review of therapy valid?

PICO QUESTION	
Search terms used	
Databases searched to find this article	
Citation of article	
Why did you select this article(s)?	
Did the authors answer the question?	
1. What databases and other sources did the authors of this review search?	
2. What were their eligibility criteria (inclusion and exclusion) for papers in this study? Do these seem appropriate?	
3. Was their independent data extraction of the results by the reviewers (then compared later)?	
4. Is there a description of the quality of each trial included?	
5. Were the results consistent from study to study (Homogeneous)?	

Are the valid results of this systematic review important?

What was the odds ratio?	
What was the control group rate (PEER)	

Can you apply this valid, important evidence from a systematic review in caring for your patient?

Do these results apply to your patient?	
Is your patient so different from those in the overview that its results cannot help you?	
How great would the potential benefit of therapy actually be for your individual patient?	
To calculate the NNT for any OR and PEER $$NNT = \frac{1 - (PEER^* (1 - OR))}{(1 - PEER) * PEER^* (1 - OR)}$$ Or use calculator from www.cebm.net	

Are your patient's values and preferences satisfied by the regimen and its consequences?

Do your patient and you have a clear assessment of their values and preferences?
Are they met by this regimen and its consequences?
Should you believe apparent qualitative differences in the efficacy of therapy in some subgroups of patients? Only if you can say 'yes' to all of the following:
Do they really make biologic and clinical sense?
Is the qualitative difference both clinically (beneficial for some but useless or harmful for others) and statistically significant?
Was this difference hypothesized before the study began (rather than the product of dredging the data), and has it been confirmed in other, independent studies?
Was this one of just a few subgroup analyses carried out in this study?

Additional notes:

Figure 44.6 Systematic review (of therapy) worksheet.

Advances in technology

CHAPTER 45

ELECTROPHYSIOLOGY AND MONITORING

Patrick R. Axon and Bruno M.R. Kenway

Development of facial nerve monitoring 525
Technique for continuous facial nerve monitoring 526
Predicting post-operative facial function 527
Difficulties of monitoring facial function 527
Monitoring facial function for non-otological procedures 527
Monitoring auditory function 527
Techniques 528
Evidence of the efficacy of monitoring auditory function 529
References 529

SEARCH STRATEGY

Data in this chapter may be updated by a Medline search using the keywords: intra-operative monitoring, facial nerve, cranial nerve and auditory evoked potentials.

DEVELOPMENT OF FACIAL NERVE MONITORING

The first description of intra-operative cranial nerve stimulation was by Fedor Krause in 1898.[1] During cochlear nerve section for tinnitus, he noted 'unipolar faradic stimulation of the (facial) nerve-trunk with the weakest possible current of the induction apparatus resulted in contractions of the right facial region, especially of the orbicularis oculi, as well as the branches supplying the nose and mouth'. Over the next three-quarters of a century, a series of articles refined the technique, all relying on observing movement of the face in order to confirm the functional integrity of the facial nerve.[2–7] The evoked facial twitch was observed by either the anaesthetist or ancillary staff under the drapes using a flashlight or mirror. These techniques lacked both quantitative control of the stimulus and objective recording of the evoked responses.

In 1979, Delgado and colleagues first described the use of evoked compound muscle action potentials (CMAP) to monitor facial nerve function in response to stimulating the intra-cranial portion of the facial nerve.[8] The introduction of facial electromyography (EMG) enabled not only facial nerve identification either by electrical stimulation or inadvertent manipulation, but also the possibility of mapping its course through the temporal bone and assessing changes in function during surgical resection of tumour from the nerve's surface.[9] Facial nerve monitoring has proved an invaluable aid during vestibular schwannoma surgery.[10–12] The introduction of an auditory signal enabled instantaneous real-time auditory feedback to the surgeon during tumour dissection without information passing through an intermediary.[13, 14]

Three trials tested the hypothesis that facial nerve outcome improved when using intra-operative facial nerve monitoring. Harner and colleagues[12] demonstrated the usefulness of facial nerve monitoring in 91 consecutive cases of vestibular schwannoma resection via the suboccipital route. At 1 year, 78% of those patients who were monitored demonstrated facial function, compared with 65% in an unmonitored group, these data were not studied statistically. Niparko and colleagues[15] described the results of 29 patients who underwent translabyrinthine removal of vestibular schwannoma and compared them with a similar group of 75 unmonitored patients. They demonstrated that monitoring was associated with a significant improvement of facial function at 1 year for tumours over 2 cm intra-cranial diameter. Kwartler and colleagues[16] demonstrated that monitored patients with tumours over 2.5 cm had a significant improvement of facial function when compared with a matched unmonitored group.

The benefit of facial nerve monitoring during surgery for chronic middle ear disease is less certain. Facial nerve injury after otological surgery is rare in experienced hands and there are no randomized controlled trials examining its efficacy. Silverstein and others recommend that the facial nerve should be monitored during all general anaesthetic cases where the facial nerve is at risk.[17, 18] This view is in contrast to most American otolaryngologists, although those who trained in the 1990s, those in an academic setting and those who perform more otology than other types of surgery are more likely to use monitoring techniques.[19, 20] Hu et al. reported a survey that showed an increase in the number of surgeons who felt that facial nerve monitoring should be used as a standard of care from 32% in a similar study performed 10 years previously, to 49% in their more recent survey group.[21] This proportion is thought to be higher in the UK and Australia, however.[22]

Increasing usage of nerve monitors has implications for litigation cases. In general such cases question whether a reasonable body of practitioners would employ a nerve monitor during surgery (Bolam test). If any such body is likely to recommend use of monitoring, then failure to use a monitor would likely become indefensible, as breach of duty could be established. The principle remains, however, that if any adverse outcome would have occurred regardless of the lack of nerve monitoring, then the claim would fail. The claimant must therefore establish causation. At the time of writing, a freedom of information request from the NHS litigation authority had identified 15 claims for facial nerve injury during otological surgery from 2003 to 2013, 9 of which had been successful with total damages claimed of £488,571.

Facial nerve injury often occurs when there is an unexpected change to normal middle ear anatomy, precisely the time when monitoring is so valuable. The senior surgeon must take responsibility to ensure that the equipment is functioning normally. A simple technique for confirming equipment function is described under 'Technique for continuous facial nerve monitoring' below. Intra-operative facial nerve monitoring is no substitute for experience in the otological setting and should not replace good surgical practice, but if the operating team adopt the approach that all patients are monitored, the set-up technique becomes routine and more reliable. With developments in robotic surgery, investigators have evaluated facial nerve monitoring systems that have been integrated into the drill system, to determine whether such systems could reliably warn of impending facial nerve contact during robot-assisted direct cochlear access procedures. At present, however, such systems lack sensitivity and repeatability.[23]

TECHNIQUE FOR CONTINUOUS FACIAL NERVE MONITORING

The operating theatre is filled with electrical interference generated by the equipment surrounding the anaesthetized patient. Monitoring techniques have developed to minimize this interference and amplify only relevant information. Two sets of subdermal platinum or stainless steel needle recording electrodes are inserted into the upper and lower face. The electromyographic electrical response is biphasic (as electrical potential moves past one electrode it becomes negatively charged compared to its paired neighbour, until it reaches that electrode and the situation reverses). The amplifiers amplify the difference between the potentials recorded at each electrode. This arrangement has the advantage of common mode rejection; electrical interference from other sources is recorded by both electrodes equally and therefore does not create a potential difference between the two closely aligned electrodes. A number of commercial EMG cranial nerve monitoring systems are now available including the NIM-2 (Xomed Treace, Jacksonville, FL, USA) and the Neurosign (Magstim, Whitland, UK). They rely on recording facial muscle activity and delivering the information as a visual and audible representation of the CMAP response. The audible response is presented as either raw EMG activity or a characteristic sound when EMG activity reaches a set threshold.

All systems are isolated and self-contained electrical nerve stimulator and monitoring units. The electrodes are connected to a preamplifier pod, which is attached to the operating table. The recorded electrical signal is filtered through high- and low-pass filters and either rectified and displayed on a logarithmic bar chart or presented as a CMAP waveform. Different systems use different methods of presenting the same information to the surgeon. The logarithmic bar chart has a delayed response decay to enable calculation of rectified CMAP amplitude. Systems that present a CMAP waveform present it as visual and audible real-time information or utilize image capture strategies that also give waveform amplitude information. This allows the surgeon time to examine the waveform and size of the CMAP. So-called 'repetitive responses' occur as a result of repetitive depolarizations after surgical manipulation has ended. They can be used as a measure of nerve irritability as a result of early damage (e.g. from thermal injury). Compare this with non-repetitive responses that are indicative of direct mechanical stimulation of the nerve.

Familiarity with the set up and function of a chosen monitoring system is essential. The senior surgeon must take responsibility and should check that the equipment is functioning normally. Tapping the skin overlying the two sets of subdermal electrodes will generate a recorded response on the monitor. This confirms that electrodes are connected to the preamplifier pod and in turn the preamplifier pod is connected to the monitor, which is switched on. The volume should be checked so that a response is audible over background theatre noise.

Facial nerve stimulation is delivered as a short (0.1 ms) electrical pulse. This is the default setting for most monitors. The stimulating electrode is either monopolar or bipolar. The monopolar electrode is favoured because it is simple to use, but has the disadvantage of stimulating a larger area. The bipolar electrode requires careful positioning of both electrode tips on to the tissue surface; this can prove difficult in the tight confines of the temporal bone. The use of constant voltage stimuli has an advantage over constant current stimuli because it delivers a relatively reliable current to the nerve whatever the medium that surrounds the nerve. In 2013 the American Society of Neurophysiological Monitoring established a position statement on intra-operative motor evoked potential monitoring, based upon best available evidence,[24] which included guidelines on proper usage, interpretation and general anaesthesia use in a variety of clinical settings including facial nerve monitoring. Regarding general anaesthesia, Choe et al. also concluded that induction of total intravenous anaesthesia with propofol and remifentanil provided reliable conditions for facial nerve monitoring during complex ear surgery.[25]

PREDICTING POST-OPERATIVE FACIAL FUNCTION

A number of studies have described an objective technique that correlates parameters of the evoked CMAP to eventual facial outcome.[15, 26–29] The test gives non-dichotomous results and therefore a retrospective cut-off point is used to predict those patients who have a good prognosis. Results indicate that a low stimulation threshold, across the site of tumour dissection, is a valuable prognostic indicator of good long-term facial function. The technique, which is simple to perform, assesses the minimum current required to evoke a muscle response after tumour resection. The drawback to the described technique is that the majority of patients have some degree of facial function immediately after surgery. This group will almost certainly have good long-term outcome.[30] It is the small group of patients with poor facial function immediately after surgery that will benefit most from a sensitive and specific predictive test. Axon and Ramsden compared post-dissection minimal stimulation thresholds with immediate post-operative facial function for predicting long-term facial function in 184 patients undergoing vestibular schwannoma surgery.[30] Post-dissection stimulation thresholds demonstrated only a moderate relation to eventual outcome, which was of limited clinical value. The test criteria were then applied to patients with poor immediate post-operative facial function for predicting long-term outcome; the predictive accuracy fell, further reducing test validity.

Some studies compared the supramaximal CMAP to either facial nerve stimulation proximal and distal to tumour dissection or before and after tumour dissection. These techniques have been advocated as more accurate methods of analysing data, because they remove absolute amplitude comparisons and rely on comparison of ratios.[31, 32]

DIFFICULTIES OF MONITORING FACIAL FUNCTION

All otological procedures rely on a facial muscle response, warning the surgeon that the facial nerve is near. A simple audible noise is all that is required. Recent monitoring systems have increased the amount of information available to the surgeon, stimulating the desire to expand monitoring techniques and so improve patient outcome. This information is superfluous to most procedures and of benefit to only a few. Facial CMAPs represent a complicated interplay between groups of muscle fibres depolarizing in response to facial nerve stimulation. The muscles of the face are very different to those found in the limbs. The facial motor units are small, often having only 25 muscle fibres supplied by each motor neuron compared with many thousands in more peripheral muscles. As a consequence, each muscle has a wide, ill defined motor end-plate zone. The muscles are also arranged in an almost haphazard arrangement, overlying each other and aligned in different directions. This makes meaningful electrophysiological recording difficult. Intra-subject variability (test-retest variability) is high and intersubject comparison almost impossible. The CMAP waveform is usually multiphasic instead of the well-recognized biphasic responses recorded from peripheral muscles, a consequence of phase cancellation. Calculation of maximum amplitude or area under the waveform bears little relation to the number of motor neurons innervating the muscle fibres that create the response.

MONITORING FACIAL FUNCTION FOR NON-OTOLOGICAL PROCEDURES

The facial nerve is at risk of iatrogenic injury in the cerebellopontine angle and parotid. Intra-operative facial nerve monitoring has been advocated during microvascular decompression and superficial parotidectomy.[33, 34] Arguments for adopting its use for all surgical procedures are the same as those for otological surgery.

MONITORING AUDITORY FUNCTION

The aim of monitoring the status of the auditory pathway during cerebellopontine angle (CPA) surgery is the prevention of avoidable post-operative hearing deficit. The achievement of this laudable aim is fraught with difficulty and hearing preservation rates in comparison with facial nerve outcomes remain poor.[35] The cochlear nerve is sensitive to mechanical manipulation and easily damaged, as the intra-cranial section of the nerve is sheathed in central myelin and has no perineurium.[36] Additionally, the cochlear nerve is intimately involved with pathologies, such as vestibular schwannoma, and hence at very considerable risk during the surgical removal of such lesions, even when every care is taken to preserve the nerve anatomically. The basic principle of intra-operative monitoring is that changes in recordable neuroelectric potentials occur whilst the injury is still reversible and before permanent deficits result.[37] Recent research[38] has demonstrated that this principle holds for changes in auditory brainstem responses (ABR) wave V amplitude (and to a lesser extent latency) in rat auditory nerves manipulated in a fashion analogous to that undergone in humans during vestibular schwannoma removal. It is therefore theoretically feasible that monitoring auditory function may inform the surgeon of reversible injury to the cochlear nerve.

One prerequisite of monitoring auditory function during surgery is that sufficient pre-operative hearing must remain such that meaningful recordings may be made in the operating theatre and change observed if and when it occurs. If ABR or electrocochleography (ECochG) are the monitoring techniques of choice, a further prerequisite is for pre-operative recordings with that technique. Monitoring with ABR is not possible if waveforms are absent or of grossly abnormal morphology.

Whilst the techniques and equipment utilized for auditory monitoring may seem familiar from the outpatient clinic, their use in monitoring is significantly different. Rather than comparing an individual's data with group data, in monitoring, one is comparing a sequence of waveforms over time and evaluating for change. The time allowed for eliciting each recording is limited and this will influence the choice of recording parameters. The decision whether to inform the surgeon of a change in recorded activity is both urgent and crucial. As such, the person undertaking monitoring should be familiar with the operating theatre environment and team, and be able to interpret and communicate observed and measured change to the surgeon confidently and concisely.[39] Such skills are rare and this may prove to be a hindrance to the widespread adoption of these techniques.

Lloyd et al.[40] have shown that patients benefit from cochlear implantation after a translabyrinthine approach for acoustic neuroma excision with cochlear nerve preservation. Such findings highlight the clinical relevance of being able to monitor the eighth nerve intra-operatively in order to reliably predict who might benefit from such strategies.

TECHNIQUES

Otoacoustic emissions

Cane et al.[41] undertook a feasibility study of the use of otoacoustic emissions (OAE) as a technique for monitoring the auditory pathway during surgical removal of a vestibular schwannoma. The experience was that OAE recordings were feasible despite the noise within the surgical environment, but the study did not indicate that OAE would be a useful indicator of early, reversible injury. Theoretically, OAE recording may furnish evidence of cochlear function, but as the site of surgery is the internal auditory canal (IAC), one would not be measuring activity deriving from the point of possible injury. OAE monitoring might therefore give information about ischaemic or noise injury to the cochlea, but it has not yet been demonstrated that this would be at a point where the injury was reversible. At the present time, however, the use of OAE in monitoring auditory function during surgery is rare.

Electrocochleography

Similarly, electrocochleography records activity associated with cochlear function and the distal portion of the cochlear nerve, rather than the intra-cranial portion of the cochlear nerve, which is acutely at risk during surgery. As such, even strong advocates of ECochG in monitoring have seen it as adjunct to ABR, and not providing the surgeon with the required information when used alone. There is research evidence that responses to auditory stimulation recorded by ECochG persist after complete transection of the eighth nerve in the rat,[42] and so this technique has the potential to mislead if used in isolation.

One potential advantage of the use of ECochG is the large amplitude of the activity recorded.[43] This allows interpretation of the elicited waveform after fewer averages, so that decision-making may be more rapid.[44] As with ECochG in the outpatient context, there is debate about the optimal site of the recording electrode, with advocates for extratympanic intra-meatal placement[36] and transtympanic placement.[45] A further advantage is that ECochG recordings are less compromised by acoustic noise or by electrical artefact as may occur during cautery, and may serve some purpose whilst these are present.[46]

Auditory brainstem responses

Auditory brainstem responses have a theoretical advantage over other techniques in that certain peaks within the waveform derive from anatomical structures at risk of injury during surgery. The generator of wave I is considered to be the distal portion of the cochlear nerve, the site also held to be the generator of the N1 component of the compound action potential recorded by ECochG.[36] Wave II is associated with the proximal section of the cochlear nerve,[37] wave III with the lower pons (specifically the superior olivary complex)[47] and wave V with the inferior colliculus.[47] The generators of waves III and V are, therefore, unlikely to be directly challenged by surgical manipulation during hearing preservation surgery for space occupying lesions of the CPA, but the latencies of these easily identifiable waves are used during monitoring as change reflects latency change of waves I and II.

Specific methodologies and parameters utilized in intra-operative ABR have been described in detail. The reader who intends to perform this procedure is directed to the comprehensive reviews by Moller[37] and Martin and Mishler.[36] Several points should be noted. There is considerable variability in the methods advocated and clinical trial evidence is not apparent. Second, this variability may account in part for the lack of a strong evidence base for the benefits of auditory monitoring. Further, the reviews cited underline the difference between utilizing ABR in the outpatient clinic and the operating theatre, the need for the technique not to inconvenience surgical techniques and the utility of clear and timely interpretation and communication of change in recordings to the surgeon. In more recent work the importance of obtaining pre-operative ABR has been highlighted.[48] The authors concluded that knowledge of the ABR before surgery helps to solve problems such as choosing to monitor the interaural latency difference of wave V, cochlear nerve action potential or alternative sound-evoked ABR.

Direct recordings from the cochlear nerve

The need for rapid acquisition of responses may be met by recording directly from the cochlear nerve, the large amplitude of the elicited activity obviating the need for lengthy averaging.[49] This technique was first developed to monitor cochlear nerve function during microvascular decompression surgery, but has been adapted for use during surgical removal of space occupying lesions of the CPA.[44] The site of recording is usually the root entry zone, and both monopolar and bipolar electrodes have their advocates.[50] Click stimuli similar to those used in ABR are used to elicit the response, which comprises a compound action potential. Changes in latency, amplitude and morphology should all be reported to the surgical team.[37] Ehrmann-Müller et al.[51] compared direct cochlear recordings using a ball electrode, to ABR results, to evaluate its effectiveness in predicting hearing outcomes after acoustic neuroma excision. They found that such direct recordings gave a sensitivity of 100% and specificity of 70%, and it was possible even in cases where they were unable to obtain reliable ABR results.

Combining techniques

Given that each of the techniques described above has technical challenges and shortcomings, many teams choose to utilize more than one, the most common combination being direct cochlear nerve recording and ABR.[52]

EVIDENCE OF THE EFFICACY OF MONITORING AUDITORY FUNCTION

Authors have reported hearing preservation rates following vestibular schwannoma excision, but the heterogeneity of pathological status, surgical technique, surgical experience and criteria for reporting of hearing preservation combine to frustrate analysis of the clinical utility of auditory monitoring. Observational evidence in this area abounds.[53],[55] The need for well-designed, hypothesis-driven clinical trials in this field is paramount.

A similar dearth of evidence is found when determining the relative efficacy of techniques or combinations of techniques. Several studies have reported that direct cochlear nerve recordings are more effective in the maintenance of hearing function than ABR, to an extent that is statistically significant.[56],[57] This effect is said to be due to the immediacy of direct recordings.[58]

Despite the lack of evidence, a consensus is building that monitoring auditory function during CPA surgery is best practice,[50] and that a combination of ABR and direct cochlear nerve recording is optimal,[43] with the adjunctive use of ECochG if desired.[45]

BEST CLINICAL PRACTICE

- ✓ Regarding monitoring of facial nerve function, there is evidence that these techniques offer benefit in improving facial nerve outcomes in surgery that may challenge the facial nerve. As such it is strongly indicated.
- ✓ The evidence base for monitoring auditory nerve function is less robust, but it should be regarded as best clinical practice.

FUTURE RESEARCH

- ▶ Further work is required to develop an intra-operative technique that enables accurate assessment of clinical facial nerve function at any point during skull base procedures. Only accurate estimation of motor neuron function will give the surgeon a true representation of immediate facial function and hopefully then enable development of a valid predictive technique.
- ▶ The specialty as a whole requires a good evidence base to support the use of intra-operative facial nerve monitoring as the standard for all otological procedures that place the facial nerve at risk.

KEY POINTS

- Monitoring facial nerve function is straightforward and neither hampers nor impedes surgery.
- There is good evidence that monitoring facial nerve function improves outcomes of facial function.
- A consensus has not yet been reached on techniques for monitoring auditory function, but it looks likely that a combination of techniques will be optimal.

REFERENCES

1. Krause F (ed). *Surgery of the brain and spinal cord*. New York: Rebman Company; 1912.
2. Frazier CH. Intracranial division of the auditory nerve for persistent aural vertigo. *Surg Gynaecol Obstet* 1912; **15**: 524–29.
3. Olivecrona H. Acoustic tumors. *J Neurol Neurosur PS* 1940; **3**: 141–46.
4. Hullay J, Tomits GH. Experiences with total removal of tumours of the acoustic nerve. *J Neurosurg* 1965; **22**: 127–35.
5. Rand RW, Kurze TL. Facial nerve preservation by posterior fossa transmeatal microdissection in total removal of acoustic tumors. *J Neurol Neurosur PS* 1965; **28**: 311–16.
6. Poole JL. Suboccipital surgery for acoustic neurinomas: advantages and disadvantages. *J Neurosurg* 1966; **24**: 483–92.
7. Albin MS, Babinski M, Maroon JC. Anesthetic management of posterior fossa surgery in the sitting position. *Acta Anaesth Scand* 1976; **20**: 117–28.
8. Delgado TE, Buchheit WA, Rosenholtz HR. Intraoperative monitoring of facial muscle evoked responses obtained by intracranial stimulation of the facial nerve: a more accurate technique for facial nerve dissection. *Neurosurgery* 1979; **4**: 418–21.
9. Silverstein H, Willcox Jr TO, Rosenberg SI, Seidman MD. Prediction of facial nerve function following acoustic neuroma resection using intraoperative facial nerve stimulation. *Laryngoscope* 1994; **104**: 539–44.

10. Moller AR, Janetta PJ. Preservation of facial function during removal of acoustic neuromas: use of monopolar constant voltage stimulation and EMG. *J Neurosurg* 1984; **61**: 757–60.
11. Benecke JE, Calder HB, Chadwick G. Facial nerve monitoring during acoustic neuroma removal. *Laryngoscope* 1987; **97**: 697–700.
12. Harner SG, Daube JR, Beatty CW, Ebersold M. Intraoperative monitoring of the facial nerve. *Laryngoscope* 1988; **98**: 209–12.
13. Prass RL, Luders H. Acoustic (loudspeaker) facial electromyography (EMG) monitoring: I. Evoked electromyographic (EMG) activity during acoustic neuroma resection. *Neurosurgery* 1986; **19**: 392–400.
14. Prass RL, Kenney SE, Hardy RW, et al. Acoustic (loudspeaker) facial EMG monitoring: II. Use of evoked EMG activity during acoustic neuroma resection. *Otolaryng Head Neck* 1987; **97**: 541–51.
15. Niparko JK, Kileny PR, Kemink JL. Neurophysiologic intraoperative monitoring: II. Facial nerve function. *Am J Otol* 1989; **10**: 55–61.
16. Kwartler JA, Luxford WM, Atkins J, Shelton C. Facial nerve monitoring in acoustic tumor surgery. *Otolaryng Head Neck* 1991; **104**: 814–17.
17. Silverstein H, Smouha EE, Jones R. Routine intraoperative facial nerve monitoring during otologic surgery. *Am J Otol* 1988; **9**: 269–75.
18. Noss RS, Lalwani AK, Yingling CD. Facial nerve monitoring in middle ear surgery. *Laryngoscope* 2001; **111**: 831–36.
19. Greenberg JS, Manolidis S, Stewart MG, Kahn JB. Facial nerve monitoring in chronic ear surgery: US practice patterns. *Otolaryng Head Neck* 2002; **126**: 108–14.
20. Pensak ML, Willging JP, Keith RW. Intraoperative facial nerve monitoring in chronic ear surgery: a resident training program. *Am J Otol* 1994; **15**: 108–10.
21. Hu J, Fleck TR, Xu J, et al. Contemporary changes with the use of facial nerve monitoring in chronic ear surgery. *Otolaryng Head Neck* 2014; **151**(3): 473–77.
22. Flukes, S, Ling SS, Leahy T, Sader C. Intraoperative nerve monitoring in otolaryngology: a survey of clinical practice patterns. *Int J Otolaryngol Head Neck* 2013; **2**: 21–26.
23. Ansó J, Stahl C, Gerber N, et al. Feasibility of using EMG for early detection of the facial nerve during robotic direct cochlear access. *Otol Neurotol* 2014; **35**(3): 545–54.
24. Macdonald DB, Skinner S, Shils J, et al. Intraoperative motor evoked potential monitoring: a position statement by the American Society of Neurophysiological Monitoring. *Clin Neurophysiol* 2013; **124**(12): 2291–316.
25. Choe WJ, Kim JH, Park SY, Kim J. Electromyographic response of facial nerve stimulation under different levels of neuromuscular blockade during middle-ear surgery. *J Int Med Res* 2013; **41**(3): 762–70.
26. Selesnick SH, Carew JF, Victor JD, et al. Predictive value of facial nerve electrophysiologic stimulation thresholds in cerebellopontine-angle surgery. *Laryngoscope* 1996; **106**: 633–38.
27. Prasad S, Hirsch BE, Kamerer DB, et al. Facial nerve function following cerebellopontine angle surgery: prognostic value of intraoperative thresholds. *Am J Otol* 1993; **14**: 330–33.
28. Silverstein H, Willcox TO, Rosenberg SI, Seidman MD. Prediction of facial nerve function following acoustic neuroma resection using intraoperative facial nerve stimulation. *Laryngoscope* 1994; **104**: 539–44.
29. Nissen AJ, Sikand A, Curto FS, et al. Value of intraoperative threshold stimulus in predicting postoperative facial nerve function after acoustic tumor resection. *Am J Otol* 1997; **18**: 249–51.
30. Axon PR, Ramsden RT. Intraoperative EMG for predicting facial function in vestibular Schwannoma surgery. *Laryngoscope* 1999; **109**: 922–26.
31. Axon PR, Ramsden RT. Assessment of real-time clinical facial function during vestibular Schwannoma surgery. *Laryngoscope* 2000; **110**: 1911–15.
32. Goldbrunner RH, Schlake HP, Milewski C, et al. Quantitative parameters of intraoperative electromyography predict facial nerve outcomes for vestibular schwannoma surgery. *Neurosurgery* 2000; **46**: 1140–46; discussion 1146–48.
33. Mooj JJ, Mustafa MK, van Weerden TW. Hemifacial spasm: intraoperative electromyographic monitoring as a guide for microvascular decompression. *Neurosurgery* 2001; **49**: 1365–70; discussion 1370–71.
34. Lopez M, Ouer M, Leon X, et al. Usefulness of facial nerve monitoring during parotidectomy. *Acta Otorrinolaringol Esp* 2001; **52**: 418–21.
35. Oh T, Nagasawa DT, Fong BM, et al. Intraoperative neuromonitoring techniques in the surgical management of acoustic neuromas. *Neurosurg Focus* 2012; **33**(3): E6.
36. Martin WH, Mishler ET. Intraoperative monitoring of auditory evoked potentials and facial nerve electromyography. In: Katz J (ed). *Handbook of clinical audiology*. Philadelphia: Lippincott Williams and Wilkins; 2001, pp. 323–48.
37. Moller AR. Intraoperative neurophysiological monitoring. In: Roeser RJ, Valente M, Hosford-Dunn H (eds). *Audiology diagnosis*. New York: Thieme; 2000, pp. 545–70.
38. Sekiya T, Shimamura N, Yagihashi A, Suzuki S. Axonal injury in auditory nerve observed in reversible latency changes of brainstem auditory evoked potentials (BAEP) during cerebellopontine angle manipulations in rats. *Hearing Res* 2002; **173**: 91–99.
39. Fisher RS, Raudzens P, Nunemacher M. Efficacy of intraoperative neurophysiological monitoring. *J Clin Neurophysiol* 1995; **12**: 97–109.
40. Lloyd SK, Glynn FJ, Rutherford SA, et al. Ipsilateral cochlear implantation after cochlear nerve preserving vestibular schwannoma surgery in patients with neurofibromatosis type 2. *Otol Neurotol* 2014; **35**(1): 43–51.
41. Cane MA, O'Donoghue GM, Lutman ME. The feasibility of using oto-acoustic emissions to monitor cochlear function during acoustic neuroma surgery. *Scand Audiol* 1992; **21**: 173–76.
42. Rosahl SK, Tatagiba M, Gharabaghi A, et al. Acoustic evoked response following transection of the eighth nerve in the rat. *Acta Neurochir* 2000; **142**: 1037–45.
43. Mullatti N, Coakham HB, Maw AR, et al. Intraoperative monitoring during surgery for acoustic neuroma: benefits of an extratympanic intrameatal electrode. *J Neurol Neurosur PS* 1999; **66**: 591–99.
44. Yingling CD. Intraoperative monitoring of cranial nerves in neurotologic surgery. In: Cummings CW, Fredickson JM, Harker LA, et al. (eds). *Otolaryngology head and neck surgery*. 3rd ed. St Louis: Mosby; 1998, pp. 3331–55.
45. Schlake HP, Goldbrunner R, Milewski C, et al. Technical developments in intraoperative monitoring for the preservation of cranial motor nerves and hearing in skull base surgery. *Neurol Res* 1999; **21**: 11–24.
46. Schlake HP, Milewski C, Goldbrunner RH, et al. Combined intra-operative monitoring of hearing by means of auditory brainstem responses (ABR) and transtympanic electrocochleography (EcochG) during surgery of intra and extrameatal acoustic neurinomas. *Acta Neurochir* 2001; **143**: 985–95.
47. Legatt AD. Mechanisms of intraoperative brainstem auditory evoked potential changes. *J Clin Neurophysiol* 2002; **19**: 396–408.
48. Aihara N1, Murakami S, Takahashi M, Yamada K. Preoperative characteristics of auditory brainstem response in acoustic neuroma with useful hearing: importance as a preliminary investigation for intraoperative monitoring. *Neurol Med Chir (Tokyo)* 2014; **54**(4): 267–71. Epub 27 Dec 2013.
49. Moller AR. Intraoperative neurophysiologic monitoring. In: Brackmann DE, Shelton C, Arriaga MA (eds). *Otologic surgery*. Philadelphia: WB Saunders; 2001, pp. 645–61.
50. Nguyen BH, Javel E, Levine SC. Physiologic identification of eighth nerve subdivisions: direct recordings with bipolar and monopolar electrodes. *Am J Otol* 1999; **20**: 522–34.
51. Ehrmann-Müller D, Mlynski R, Ginzkey C, et al. Direct recording from cochlear nerve via a ball-electrode in transtemporal acoustic neuroma surgery. *Laryngorhinootologie* 2012; **91**(1): 22–27.
52. Mann WJ, Maurer J, Marangos N. Neural conservation in skull base surgery. *Otolaryngol Clin N Am* 2002; **35**: 411–24.
53. Radtke RA, Erwin CW, Wilkins RH. Intraoperative brainstem auditory evoked potentials: significant decrease in postoperative morbidity. *Neurology* 1989; **39**: 187–91.
54. Harper CM, Harner SG, Slavit DH, et al. Effect of BAEP monitoring on hearing preservation during acoustic neuroma resection. *Neurology* 1992; **42**: 1551–53.
55. Fischer G, Fischer C, Remond J. Hearing preservation in acoustic neurinoma surgery. *J Neurosurg* 1992; **76**: 910–17.

56. Colletti V, Fiorino FG, Mocella S, Policante Z. EcochG, CNAP and ABR monitoring during vestibular schwannoma surgery. *Audiology* 1998; **37**: 27–37.

57. Jackson LE, Roberson Jr. JB. Acoustic neuroma surgery: use of cochlear nerve action potential monitoring for hearing preservation. *Am J Otol* 2000; **21**: 249–59.

58. Colletti V, Fiorino FG. Advances in monitoring of seventh and eighth cranial nerve function during posterior fossa surgery. *Am J Otol* 1998; **19**: 503–12.

CHAPTER 46

OPTICAL COHERENCE TOMOGRAPHY

Jameel Muzaffar and Jonathan M. Fishman

Introduction 533	Clinical studies utilizing OCT 536
OCT: System operation..534	Summary...537
OCT imaging of the larynx...535	Acknowledgements 538
Polarization-sensitive OCT 536	References 538

SEARCH STRATEGY

Data in this chapter may be updated by PubMed, Embase and the Cochrane Library performed by an information specialist librarian. Searches used the following keywords: optical coherence tomography, needle biopsy, surgical guidance, nasal, vocal cord and/or otology. Levels of evidence are not really applicable to the scientific principles of this area, but the human studies that underlie the discussion of optical coherence tomography as applied to otorhinolaryngology are observational, or at best non-randomized.

INTRODUCTION

Medical imaging technology has advanced rapidly over the past 25 years, providing physicians with essential information on the macroscopic anatomy of patients. Techniques capable of imaging subepithelial structure *in situ*, such as conventional X-ray radiography, magnetic resonance imaging (MRI), computed tomography (CT) and ultrasonography have allowed the non-invasive investigation of relatively large-scale structures in the human body, with resolutions ranging from 100 μm to 1 mm. Resolution on this scale, however, is insufficient to detect the subtle changes in tissue microstructure characteristic of many ear, nose and throat (ENT) pathologies.

In the field of laryngology, light endoscopy currently forms the cornerstone of clinical imaging and biopsy guidance, yet conventional light endoscopic techniques are unable to reveal information concerning subepithelial tissue. Since many laryngeal pathologies originate near the boundary between the epithelium and the underlying mucosa, or within the mucosa itself, the inability to image subepithelial tissue represents a serious limitation of conventional light endoscopy. Even as a method for guiding biopsy, conventional light endoscopy gives only a relatively coarse indication of prospective biopsy locations. Frequently, a large number of biopsies are required to achieve high diagnostic accuracy, a situation that is often undesirable or unfeasible given the fragility of adjacent structures. This is particularly true for the vocal folds, which have a specialized and delicate microstructure that is highly intolerant of trauma. These limitations restrict the effectiveness of light endoscopy for the diagnosis, monitoring and treatment of many laryngeal pathologies. Clinical laryngology would thus greatly benefit from a non-invasive imaging technology capable of resolving subepithelial tissue microstructure in the range of conventional biopsy.

Optical coherence tomography (OCT) is a relatively new optical imaging modality that allows high-resolution, cross-sectional imaging of tissue microstructure. OCT can image with an axial resolution of 1–15 μm and has an imaging depth of 2–3 mm in non-transparent tissue. OCT was first applied in 1991 to imaging optically transparent structures, such as the anterior eye and retina.[1, 2] Subsequent technological advances have enabled high-resolution imaging of non-transparent tissue in the cardiovascular system[3] and the gastrointestinal,[4] urinary[5] and female reproductive tracts.[6] In addition, the application of OCT to surgical guidance[7] and carcinoma detection[6, 8] has been explored.

The aforementioned imaging studies have demonstrated that OCT is particularly informative in tissues in which non-keratinized epithelium is separated from the underlying stroma by a smooth basement membrane zone, suggesting that OCT may have a strong clinical relevance in laryngology. This indication is further strengthened by several features of the OCT system itself:

- OCT imaging can be performed *in situ* and non-destructively, enabling the imaging of tissue for which biopsy should be avoided or is impossible.
- OCT gives images of high resolution, 10–100 times that of conventional MRI or ultrasound.
- Imaging can be performed in real time, without the need to process a specimen, as in conventional biopsy, and without the need for a transducing medium, as in ultrasound imaging.
- OCT is fibre-optically based and can thus be interfaced to a wide range of instruments including catheters, endoscopes, laparoscopes and surgical probes.
- OCT systems can be engineered to be compact, portable and low cost, depending on the desired system specifications.

Although now entering human trials in a variety of areas within otolaryngology, early research focused on the potential applications of OCT to laryngeal tissue, imaging of the middle ear[9] and of rat cochlea[10] *ex vivo* and nasal tissues[11] with promising results. Before presenting and discussing OCT images of larynges *ex vivo*, it is useful to briefly describe the basis by which OCT systems form subepithelial images.

OCT: SYSTEM OPERATION

Optical coherence tomography performs high-resolution tomographic imaging by measuring light backscattered, or backreflected, from internal tissue structures. OCT imaging is analogous to ultrasound B-mode imaging, but is based on the detection of infrared light waves, instead of sound. Like acoustic waves, light is characterized by its propagation direction. Light is distinct, however, in that it has an additional vector characteristic known as polarization. The polarization direction is orthogonal to the propagation direction and can be influenced by the medium in which the light propagates. This is known as 'birefringence'. Polarization measurements can be used to provide additional insights into the microscopic structure and integrity of tissues. An adjunct to conventional OCT, polarization-sensitive OCT (PS-OCT), exploits birefringence as an additional contrast mechanism for imaging tissue. PS-OCT will be discussed in further detail under 'Polarization-sensitive OCT' below.

The analogy with ultrasound is a useful starting point for understanding the basics of OCT. In ultrasound, a high frequency acoustic pulse travels into the tissue and is reflected, or backscattered, from internal structures having different acoustic properties. The magnitude and the delay time of the echoes are electronically detected, and the structural properties of the internal tissues are determined from the measured signals. In OCT, imaging is performed by measuring the echo delay time and magnitude of light backreflected, or backscattered, from internal structures with distinct optical properties. Unlike in ultrasound, though, the speed of light is very high, rendering electronic measurement of the echo delay time of the reflected light impossible. OCT systems circumvent this limitation by using low coherence interferometry, also known as white light interferometry, to characterize optical echoes.

The most common OCT echo detection scheme is based on a Michelson interferometer set up with a scanning reference delay arm, shown in **Figure 46.1**. Within the interferometer, the beam leaving the optical light source is split into two parts, termed the reference and sample beams, at the beam splitter. The reference beam then travels to a mirror, located at a known distance from the detector and subsequently returns to the beam splitter. The sample beam travels to the tissue sample and is reflected back towards the detector by scattering sites within the tissue. Light reflecting from deeper tissue layers has traversed a greater optical pathlength (optical distance) and therefore arrives at the detector at a later time. In addition, the various backreflected parts of the sample beam will have different amplitudes based on the differing strengths of the scattering sites. The reflected portions of the sample beam then return to the beam splitter where they interact with the reflected reference beam and are directed towards the detector.

When two waves from the same source recombine in this manner, an interference pattern will result if the optical path length travelled by the two waves is identical. The output detector measures the intensity of this interference pattern and thus only measures information contained in the portion of the sample beam that has travelled the same optical distance as the light in the reference arm. Information about the remaining tissue layers can be extracted by moving the mirror in the reference arm, which changes the optical path length travelled by the reference beam. Two- or three-dimensional images are produced by scanning the beam across the sample and

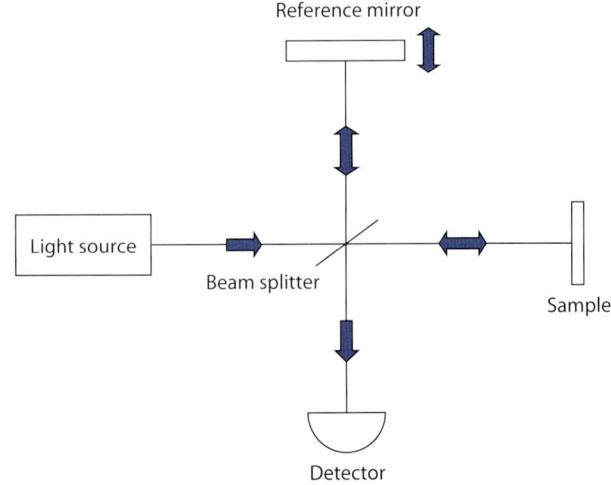

Figure 46.1 Schematic of an optical coherence tomography system using a Michelson interferometer with scanning reference delay arm.

recording the optical backscattering versus depth at different transverse positions. The resulting data is a two- or three-dimensional representation of the optical backscattering of the sample on a micron scale.

OCT IMAGING OF THE LARYNX

To assess the potential value of OCT imaging technology in improving visualization and pathology, as well as the diagnosis and treatment of a given organ system, it is essential to first image normal tissue from that particular organ and then reference the resulting OCT images to parallel histology.

Initial studies of the laryngeal imaging using OCT[12, 13] have focused on the following structures due to clinical relevance:

- the laryngeal surface of the epiglottis
- the false folds
- the inferior surface of the true folds.

The images presented are based on a similar focus. It should be noted, however, that since OCT can be readily adapted to fibre optic-based probes, other areas of traditionally poor visibility in light endoscopy, such as the anterior commissure, the subglottis and the laryngeal ventricle, could also be readily imaged using this technology.

In **Figure 46.2**, an OCT image of the laryngeal surface of an ovine (sheep) epiglottis and the associated histological section are shown. Several different layers of the epiglottic tissue are visible, with epithelium, lamina propria and cartilage being clearly demarcated. Glandular structures and vessels are also frequently visible.

Figure 46.3 presents an OCT image taken along the inferior portion of a porcine true fold, as evidenced by the transition from free-edge non-glandular mucosa to subglottal glandular mucosa observed in the OCT image and corresponding histological section. This image illustrates the ability of OCT to allow visualization of the epithelium, basement membrane and lamina propria of the true fold, as well as of certain structural features, such as glands and vessels. Note in particular that local epithelial thickness and transparency of the true fold can be readily deduced from these images, implying that OCT may prove useful for the diagnosis of hyperplasia, early-stage keratosis and papillomas, and other pathologies resulting in epithelial abnormalities not normally visible by conventional light endoscopy until an advanced stage. Since many laryngeal pathologies originate at the border between the mucosa and the epithelium, the ability to observe the integrity

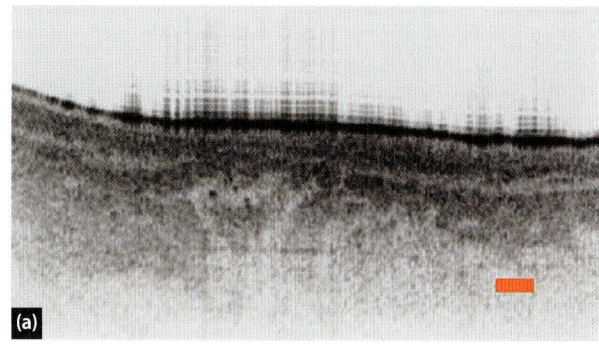

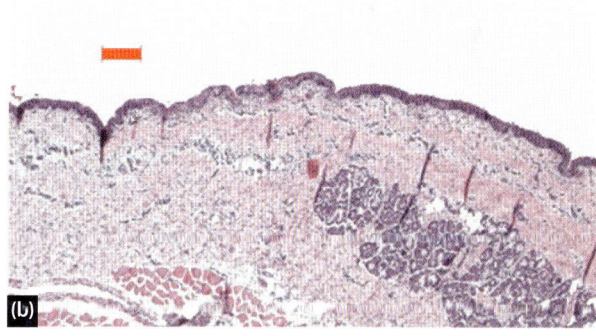

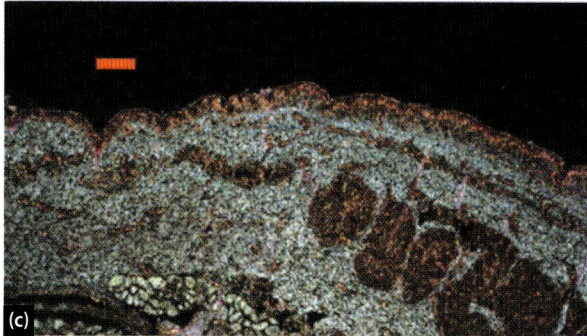

Figure 46.3 (a) OCT image of the inferior surface of a porcine true fold; **(b)** corresponding haematoxylin and eosin histology section; **(c)** phase-contrast viewing of the stained histology section. Scale bars represent 150 μm.

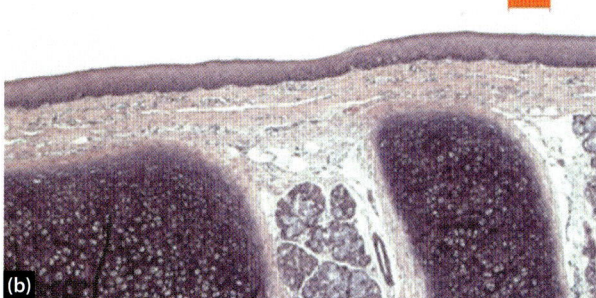

Figure 46.2 (a) OCT image of an ovine epiglottis; **(b)** corresponding haematoxylin and eosin histology section. Scale bars represent 150 μm.

of the basement membrane via OCT imaging may have important implications for the use of this technology in aiding the diagnosis and monitoring of such laryngeal disorders, possibly including early stage carcinoma.

POLARIZATION-SENSITIVE OCT

A monochromatic light wave carries three potential sources of information contained in the amplitude, phase and polarization state of its electrical field vector. Conventional OCT, by detecting only the intensity of the interference pattern resulting from interaction of the sample and reference optical beams, fails to quantify the effects of tissue on the polarization state of the sample light beam. An adjunct to conventional OCT, known as polarization-sensitive OCT, therefore has focused on exploiting the information contained in the polarization state of the light backreflected, or backscattered, from the sample relative to that of the reference beam to obtain information about the tissue microstructure.

In order to appreciate the power of PS-OCT and its potential applications, it is helpful to describe briefly the main mechanisms by which tissue alters the polarization state of light. Two mechanisms dominate the changes in the polarization state of light propagating through biological tissue: scattering and birefringence. Scattering changes the polarization of light mainly in a random manner, so it is generally not useful in mapping tissue structure. Organized linear structures, on the other hand, such as collagen fibre bundles with a clear orientation, can exhibit birefringence, resulting in a predictable change in polarization state. Many biological tissues exhibit birefringence, such as tendons, muscle, nerve, bone, cartilage and teeth.[14] Since changes in birefringence may, for instance, indicate changes in functionality, structure or viability of tissues, PS-OCT images may contain information that can be used to evaluate tissue microstructure and health beyond the level possible with the use of OCT alone.[15]

The potential implications for clinical laryngology of the sensitivity of PS-OCT to organized linear structures, such as oriented collagen fibre bundles, are numerous. To illustrate, the human vocal fold lamina propria is generally subdivided into the superficial, intermediate and deep layers, with each layer having a characteristic composition and functionality. The relative thickness and integrity of these various layers appear to have a profound impact on voice. This idea is supported by the fact that the average adult will experience marked thinning of the superficial lamina propria relative to the intermediate and deep layers with increasing age,[16] with a concomitant reduction in voice quality.

Histological studies of normal adult human vocal fold tissue have repeatedly noted increased density and longitudinal orientation of collagen fibres as one progresses from more superficial to deeper lamina propria layers.[16] PS-OCT, due to its sensitivity to oriented collagen fibre bundles, may thus allow indirect detection of these lamina propria layers in situ and hence monitoring and possibly improving treatment of voice ageing. In the case of vocal fold scarring, the biomechanical integrity of the lamina propria is disrupted, resulting in reduced vocal fold pliability and thus decreased vocal range and quality. Scar tissue has collagen fibre orientation and density that is generally distinct from that of normal tissue and therefore PS-OCT may also prove useful in visualizing, localizing and treating vocal fold scars within the lamina propria. These capabilities could have a profound impact in the area of voice management.

Figure 46.4 compares a PS-OCT image of the inferior surface of a human true fold with the corresponding OCT image and histological section. Note the banding pattern apparent in the PS-OCT image of the vocal fold. A transition from white to black banding indicates a change in the polarization state of light. In particular, observe the marked increase in the thickness of the initial subepithelial white band in the leftmost portion of the PS-OCT image (corresponding to the true fold free edge) relative to that in the more subglottic tissue. The spatial location of this thickened initial band corresponds closely with the increased prominence of the superficial lamina propria in this region. Since collagen in normal superficial lamina propria is sparse and relatively randomly oriented, a net change in the polarization state of light will be slow to occur in this region. Hence, the thickness of the superficial lamina propria can potentially be inferred from the thickness of the initial subepithelial PS-OCT band. The true fold superficial lamina propria features critically in vocal health and disease. Although the presented results are not definitive, the potential of PS-OCT to detect changes in the superficial lamina propria thickness and collagen alignment is an exciting area for future study.

Again, it must be stressed that further studies must be carried out to determine what the observed vocal fold polarization patterns truly indicate. In the case that these studies show that the relative thickness and/or health of the lamina propria layers can indeed be indirectly assessed by this imaging adjunct, PS-OCT could prove very useful to the study of lamina propria health and in the development of targeted scar treatment strategies.

CLINICAL STUDIES UTILIZING OCT

A number of studies have explored OCT use *in vivo*. Whilst these studies are predominantly non-randomized pilot or proof of concept studies they illustrate potential clinical applications for widespread clinical practice.

The most studied area of interest in otolaryngology has been for imaging of the larynx. A number of studies have utilized OCT in conjunction with microlaryngoscopy, with or without histology for a range of benign and malignancy pathologies.[17, 18] Initial experience is promising, with good correlation between OCT and histological diagnosis. However, the exact role of OCT remains unclear and we currently lack large-scale studies to justify replacement of histological confirmation.

Furthermore, OCT may be helpful to evaluate cartilage in the lower trachea or bronchi. Congenital absence of cartilaginous tracheal rings associated with esophageal atresia and trifurcated carina: a novel anomaly?[21] Again whilst these avenues show promise there remains some distance from definitive trials likely to change routine practice.

In head and neck surgery, one study has demonstrated the feasibility of using two newer generation OCT systems – optical frequency domain imaging (OFDI) and micro-optical coherence tomography (µOCT) imaging – to identify parathyroid tissue with histology-like levels of certainty, without the need for frozen section.[22] It is not too much of a leap to imagine a handheld probe used in a similar manner to a nerve stimulator for intraoperative localization, though this is not currently available. Another study reported two cases where OCT was combined with endobronchial ultrasound (EBUS) for the potential identification of residual hypertrophic and persistent inflammatory tissue (known contributors to stricture recurrence) following laryngotracheal dilation of post-intubation laryngotracheal stenosis, with some promising results, although the sample size was small.[23]

Within Otology OCT imaging has been demonstrated in combination with robotic surgery for localization and electrode placement for cochlear implantation has been demonstrated on dry-fixed human temporal bones.[24] Further small case series advocate the use of OCT to identify the stapes footplate in revision stapes surgery[25] and as an adjunct to otomicroscopy for the identification of myringitis and potential biofilm formation.[26]

SUMMARY

OCT and OCT adjuncts have enormous potential for improving the diagnosis, monitoring and both surgical and non-surgical management of diseased ENT tissues. Conventional OCT provides objective information concerning the structure of tissue elements with distinct optical backscattering and backreflection properties. With regard to the larynx, conventional OCT studies of healthy laryngeal tissues *ex vivo* have demonstrated that OCT can detect spatial changes in the thickness and transparency of the epithelium, the content of the connective tissues in terms of glands and vessels, as well as pronounced transitions in connective tissue type and the architecture of the basement membrane.[27] PS-OCT holds promise for permitting indirect visualization of the layers of the true fold lamina propria, as well as of vocal fold scar beds. In addition, a number of other OCT adjuncts, such as spectroscopic OCT[28] and phase dispersion tomography[29] exist, or are currently in development, each with distinct imaging advantages and capabilities over conventional OCT imaging. Whilst not yet in widespread use in clinical practice, OCT has the potential to significantly alter the diagnostic and treatment pathway across the range of otolarygology. The next few years provide the opportunity for future research and discovery in this fascinating field.

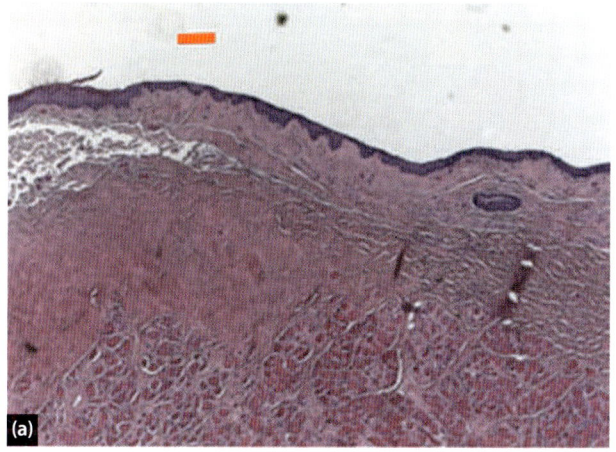
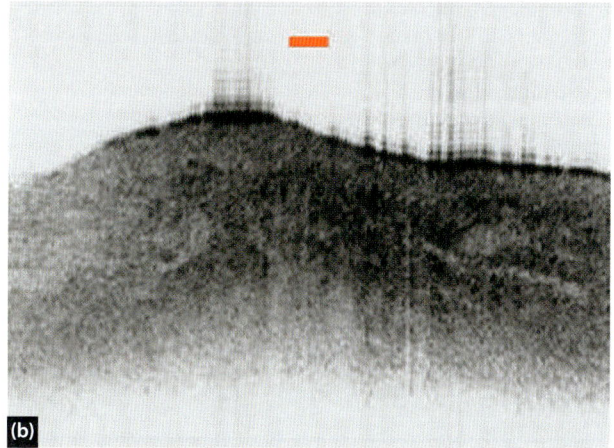
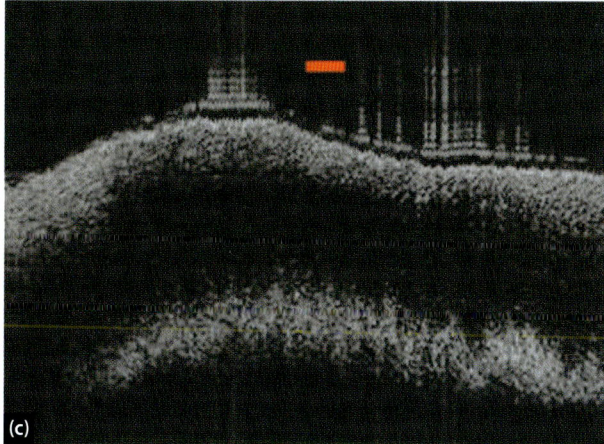

Figure 46.4 (a) Haematoxylin and eosin histology section of the inferior surface of a human true fold; **(b)** corresponding OCT image; **(c)** corresponding PS-OCT image. Scale bars represent 150 µm.

In paediatric otolaryngology studies have explored the use of fourier domain optical coherence tomography (FD-OCT) and long-range optical coherence tomography (LR-OCT) for the development of computerized airway models for predicting neonatal subglottic stenosis following intubation[19] and localizing the site of upper airway obstruction in children with sleep disordered breathing.[20]

FUTURE RESEARCH

Although OCT and OCT adjuncts hold substantial promise for improved visualization of ENT-related tissues, OCT/OCT-adjunct feasibility studies for most of these tissues are either extremely limited or entirely lacking. For those ENT tissues that have been imaged with OCT, the primary focus of the imaging studies has been the necessary, but insufficient, first step of assessing the degree to which normal tissue microstructure can be accurately identified from OCT images. Before the OCT imaging modality can be regarded as a diagnostic tool in ENT, rigorous correlation of OCT/OCT-adjunct images of diseased tissue with parallel histology must be carried out to demonstrate that a given disease state can be accurately and reliably identified from OCT image structures. In the case of the larynx, although conventional OCT images of pathological laryngeal structures *in vivo* have been recorded,[12] the corresponding histology necessary to guide OCT image interpretation has most often been lacking. Thus, whether OCT/OCT-adjuncts can reproducibly and accurately identify laryngeal pathology or other ENT pathologies remains to be determined and constitutes an exciting and vital area of future work.

In addition to pathology identification, OCT or certain OCT adjuncts may prove useful in guiding laser and non-laser-based microsurgery of ENT tissues. In laser microsurgery, PS-OCT may be particularly applicable, since laser damage of collagenous tissue has been shown to alter the tissue's effect on the polarization state of incoming light.[30] This is yet another exciting avenue for future research.

In brief, the following are a few of the many vital areas for current and future investigation:

- correlation of histology with OCT images of pathologic laryngeal specimens
- further investigation of the potential use of OCT in laryngology and correlation of PS-OCT images to laryngeal microstructure
- investigation of other OCT adjuncts, such as spectroscopic OCT, to laryngeal imaging
- further exploration of the possible applications of OCT/OCT adjuncts to ear-related imaging and a feasibility study of OCT applied to nasal tissue
- exploration of the use of OCT in conjunction with image guidance and/or robotic systems.

KEY POINTS

- The diagnosis and treatment of many ENT pathologies would benefit from the ability to image subepithelially and with high resolution *in situ*.
- Optical coherence tomography enables subepithelial imaging of tissue with a resolution ranging from 1 to 15 µm and is fibre-optically based, allowing OCT systems to be interfaced with a wide range of instruments, including catheters and endoscopes.
- Conventional OCT appears to be able to detect spatial changes in the thickness and transparency of laryngeal epithelium; the content of the connective tissue, including the presence of glands and vessels; and the integrity of the basement membrane.
- Polarization-sensitive OCT, with its sensitivity to organized linear structures, such as oriented collagen fibre bundles, may prove useful for vocal fold visualization and health assessment.
- OCT and OCT adjuncts hold substantial promise for improved diagnosis and treatment of many ENT disorders, a potential that remains largely untapped and constitutes an exciting avenue for future research, development and discovery.

ACKNOWLEDGEMENTS

The authors acknowledge the work on the previous iteration of this chapter by Dr Mariah Hahn of Texas A&M University and Dr Brett Bouma of Harvard Medical School. Their work was funded in part by the Advisory Board Foundation, Eugene B Casey Foundation and the National Science Foundation Graduate Fellowships. Mr Jonathan Fishman is supported by a research grant from The Academy of Medical Sciences, UK.

REFERENCES

1. Hee MR, Izatt JA, Swanson EA, et al. Optical coherence tomography of the human retina. *Arch Ophthal – Chicago* 1995; **113**: 325–32.
2. Swanson EA, Izatt JA, Hee MR, et al. *In vivo* retinal imaging by optical coherence tomography. *Optics Letters* 1993; **18**: 1864–66.
3. Jang IK, Bouma BE, Kang DH, et al. Visualization of coronary atherosclerotic plaques in patients using optical coherence tomography: comparison with intravascular ultrasound. *J Am Coll Cardiol* 2002; **39**: 604–09.
4. Bouma BE, Tearney GJ, Compton CC, Nishioka NS. Endoscopic optical coherence tomography of the gastrointestinal tract. *Gastroint Endosc* 1999; **49**: 390, Part 2.
5. Tearney GJ, Brezinski ME, Southern JF, et al. Optical biopsy in human urologic tissue using optical coherence tomography. *J Urology* 1997; **157**: 1915–19.
6. Pitris C, Goodman A, Boppart SA, et al. High-resolution imaging of gynecologic neoplasms using optical coherence tomography. *Obstet Gynecol* 1999; **93**: 135–39.
7. Boppart SA, Bouma BE, Pitris C, et al. Intraoperative assessment of microsurgery with three-dimensional optical coherence tomography. *Radiology* 1998; **208**: 81–86.
8. Jesser CA, Boppart SA, Pitris C, et al. High resolution imaging of transitional cell carcinoma with optical coherence tomography: feasibility for the evaluation of bladder pathology. *Brit J Radiol* 1999; **72**: 1170–76.
9. Pitris C, Saunders KT, Fujimoto JG, Brezinski ME. High-resolution imaging of the middle ear with optical coherence tomography: a feasibility study. *Arch Otolaryngol* 2001; **127**: 637–42.
10. Wong BJF, de Boer JF, Park BH, et al. Optical coherence tomography of the rat cochlea. *J Biomed Opt* 2000; **5**: 367–70.
11. Mahmood U, Ridgway J, Jackson R, et al. In vivo optical coherence tomography of the nasal mucosa. *Am J Rhinol* 2006; **20**: 155–59.
12. Gladkova ND, Shakhov AV, Feldstein F. Capabilities of optical coherence tomography in laryngology. In: Bouma B, Tearney G (eds). *Handbook of optical coherence tomography*. Basel: Marcel Dekkar; 2002, pp. 705–24.

13. Pitris C, Brezinski ME, Bouma BE, et al. High resolution imaging of the upper respiratory tract with optical coherence tomography: a feasibility study. *Am J Resp Crit Care* 1998; **157**: 1640–44.
14. de Boer JF, Srinivas SM, Nelson JS. Polarization sensitive OCT. In: Bouma B, Tearney G (eds). *Handbook of optical coherence tomography*. Basel: Marcel Dekkar; 2002, pp. 237–74.
15. Drexler W, Stamper D, Jesser C, et al. Correlation of collagen organization with polarization sensitive imaging of *in vitro* cartilage: implications for osteoarthritis. *J Rheumatol* 2001; **28**: 1311–18.
16. Hammond TH, Gray SD, Butler JE. Age- and gender-related collagen distribution in human vocal folds. *Ann Otol Rhinol Laryngol* 2000; **109**: 913–20, Part 1.
17. Volgger V, Stepp H, Ihrler S, et al. Evaluation of optical coherence tomography to discriminate lesions of the upper aerodigestive tract. *Head Neck* 2013; **35**(11): 1558–66.
18. Burns JA, Kim KH, deBoer JF, et al. Polarization-sensitive optical coherence tomography imaging of benign and malignant laryngeal lesions: an in vivo study. *Otolaryng Head Neck Surg* 2011; **145**(1): 91–99.
19. Volgger V, Sharma GK, Jing JC, et al. Long-range Fourier domain optical coherence tomography of the pediatric subglottis. *Int J Pediatr Otorhinol* 2015; **79**(2): 119–26.
20. Lazarow FB, Ahuja GS, Loy AC, et al. Intraoperative long range optical coherence tomography as a novel method of imaging the pediatric upper airway before and after adenotonsillectomy. *Int J Pediatr Otorhinol* 2015; **79**(1): 63–70.
21. Torre M, Speggiorin S, Roebuck DJ, et al. Congenital absence of cartilaginous tracheal rings associated with esophageal atresia and trifurcated carina: a novel anomaly? *J Pediatr Surg* 2012; **47**(5): 1008–11.
22. Freitas LC, Phelan E, Liu L, et al. Optical coherence tomography imaging during thyroid and parathyroid surgery: a novel system of tissue identification and differentiation to obviate tissue resection and frozen section. *Head Neck* 2014; **36**(9): 1329–34.
23. Murgu SD, Colt HG. Combined optical coherence tomography and endobronchial ultrasonography for laser-assisted treatment of postintubation laryngotracheal stenosis. *Ann Oto Rhinol Laryngol* 2013; **122**(5): 299–307.
24. Pau HW, Lankenau E, Just T, Hüttmann G. Imaging of cochlear structures by optical coherence tomography (OCT): temporal bone experiments for an OCT-guided cochleostomy technique. *Laryngol Rhinol Otol* 2008; **87**(9): 641–46.
25. Just T, Lankenau E, Hüttmann G, Pau HW. Optical coherence tomography of the oval window niche. *J Laryngol Otol* 2009; **123**(6): 603–08.
26. Guder E, Lankenau E, Fleischhauer F, et al. Microanatomy of the tympanic membrane in chronic myringitis obtained with optical coherence tomography. *Eur Arch Oto-Rhino-Laryngol* 2015; **272**(11): 3217–23.
27. Burns JA, Zeitels SM, Anderson RR, et al. Imaging the mucosa of the human vocal fold with optical coherence tomography. *Ann Oto Rhinol Laryngol* 2005; **114**: 671–76.
28. Morgner U, Drexler W, Kartner FX, et al. Spectroscopic optical coherence tomography. *Opt Lett* 2000; **25**: 111–13.
29. Yang CH, Wax A, Dasari RR, Feld MS. Phase-dispersion optical tomography. *Opt Lett* 2001; **26**: 686–88.
30. de Boer JF, Milner TE, vanGemert MJC, Nelson JS. Two-dimensional birefringence imaging in biological tissue by polarization-sensitive optical coherence tomography. *Opt Lett* 1997; **22**: 934–36.

CHAPTER 47

RECENT ADVANCES IN TECHNOLOGY

Wai Lup Wong and Bal Sanghera

Positron emission tomography (PET) – computed tomography (CT)...541	Non-squamous cell carcinoma..................................549
Squamous cell carcinoma...544	Other malignant tumours..550
Recurrent disease...546	Limitations/pitfalls..551
Emerging applications..549	Radiotracers other than FDG....................................552
	References..556

SEARCH STRATEGY

This chapter is based on literature obtained by electronic searches of four biomedical databases (Medline, Embase, Cochrane Library, PubMed) using combinations of keywords including PET, PET-CT, FDG, positron emission tomography, tomography emission computed, FDG, head and neck, cancer, neoplasm, squamous cell cancer, thyroid cancer, neck, staging, nodal metastases, occult primary, recurrence, surveillance, MR . Studies were also sought from hand searches of H&N surgery and other relevant journals, and scanning the reference lists of relevant articles. No beginning date limit was used and the search was updated on November 2, 2016.

PET-CT has replaced PET. Notwithstanding, there is good justification for continuing to take into account the FDG PET evidence when considering FDG PET-CT as both assess the same aspects of tissue metabolism . Also, the whole body is routinely scanned in both techniques. Furthermore, there is evidence that PET-CT is more accurate as a diagnostic test compared with PET because PET-CT can more sensitively detect radiotracer emitted from the body and more accurate anatomical localization of the radiotracer emitted.[1] In other words, PET studies set a baseline for performance which is likely to be improved by PET-CT.[2]

POSITRON EMISSION TOMOGRAPHY (PET) – COMPUTED TOMOGRAPHY (CT)

The main role of PET-CT in head and neck surgery is in the assessment of people with head and neck (H&N) cancer using the radiotracer 2-[^{18}F] fluoro-2-deoxy-D-glucose (FDG). So the focus of the chapter, after consideration of the principles of PET-CT, is on FDG PET-CT in people with H&N squamous cell cancer (SqCC). Separate short commentaries are provided on the role of FDG PET-CT for other tumours and on the evolving role of radio-tracers beyond FDG. In addition, brief observations are made on the current status of PET-MR.

Computed tomography (CT), magnetic resonance (MR) and ultrasound predominantly produce anatomical images, whereas positron emission tomography (PET) identifies pathology based on altered tissue metabolism. Modern whole-body PET scanners are physically integrated with standard CT scanners enabling the creation of accurately computed combined [registered] fused PET-CT scans.

CT component of PET-CT

The CT component of PET-CT has two important functions. Firstly, it contributes directly to more accurate diagnosis. It does this by facilitating precise anatomical location of radiotracer activity which leads to more exact anatomical localization of pathology and more accurate distinction between pathology and normal appearances. Secondly, the CT component corrects for the reduction in PET signal [attenuation] as it travels through the patient's body; the deeper the site the signal arises in the body the greater the attenuation. The correction results in more accurate measurement of radiotracer uptake.

CT is usually performed with a lower radiation dose than conventional diagnostic CT. Also, unlike conventional diagnostic CT, PET-CT is commonly performed without intravenous contrast. This is because there is

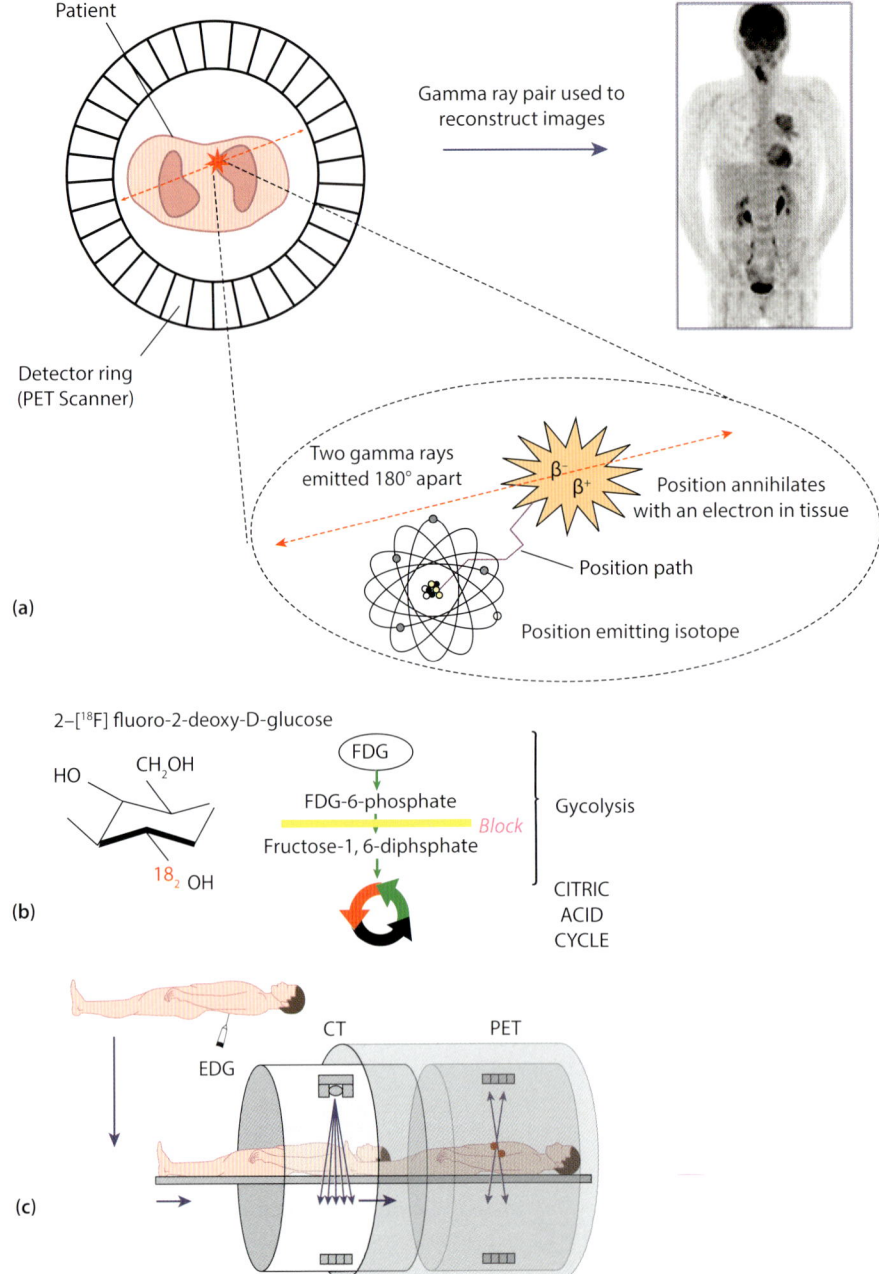

FIGURE 47.1 (a) Projection FDG-PET shows a patient with a primary bronchogenic carcinoma with extensive bony and cutaneous deposits. (b) Schematic representation of FDG metabolism. (c) Schematic representation of scanning with integrated PET/CT. The radiation burden is equivalent to two whole body diagnostic CTs. The CT is usually obtained using a low-voltage technique with no intravenous contrast given, but it provides diagnostic information.

some evidence to suggest that intravenous contrast results in PET artefacts. That said, the actual impact intravenous contrast makes to interpretation of clinical PET-CT scans is debatable. This has prompted some centres to carry out PET-CT scanning with intravenous contrast in an effort to reduce the number of investigations for patients. More typically, however, if a contrast-enhanced CT is required it is performed following low dose attenuation CT.

Recently, similar to CT, manufacturers have introduced continuous bed motion PET acquisition systems with potential for less artefacts and increased sensitivity.

This is in contrast to conventional whole-body PET-CT scans which comprises a series of overlapping static 'step and shoot' bed acquisitions taking approximately 30 mins in total to perform.[3]

PET component of PET-CT

PET is a functional imaging technique which relies on a radioactive molecule (radiotracer) that decays with positron emission. The radiotracer is given intravenously to the patient and is taken into cells. The cell recognizes it as being 'foreign' and as a consequence it is trapped early in its metabolic pathway. Malignant cells trap more radiotracer compared with non-malignant cells. The local radiotracer concentration can be measured *in vivo* since these unstable radiotracers decay by positron emission. Positrons travel a short distance in tissue before colliding with electrons. When they collide, the annihilation reaction results in two photons also known as gamma rays of 511 kilo electron volts (keV) each emitted at approximately 180° to each other. The photons are detected by opposing detectors. A computer reassembles these signals into images that represent radiotracer uptake in the part of the body scanned.

One of the main strengths of PET is the ability to perform quantitative studies. Absolute quantification is not often carried out in clinical practice as it is complicated to obtain and can demand direct arterial blood sampling. The standardized uptake value (SUV), which provides a semi-quantitative index of radiotracer uptake is widely used in clinical PET:

$$\frac{\text{Tracer uptake (MBq/mL)}}{\text{Administered activity (MBq)/(patient weight (kg)} \times 1000)}$$

Depending on the radiotracer used, different aspects of tissue metabolism can be studied, such as distribution of blood flow, oxygen utilization and protein synthesis. The overwhelming majority of clinical studies are in conjunction with an analogue of glucose, 2-[^{18}F] fluoro-2-deoxy-D-glucose (FDG), which reflects glucose metabolism. Cancer cells have a greater avidity for glucose than normal cells. Otto Warburg and colleagues made this observation in the 1920s.[4] FDG can be used to exploit the differences in glucose metabolism between cancer cells and normal cells.

FDG-PET has been used effectively for imaging of a variety of malignancies including breast, lung, colorectal, oesophageal cancer, brain tumours, malignant melanoma and lymphoma.[45] Seifert and others demonstrated that H&N cancers take up FDG, an observation which was subsequently confirmed by other studies.[6]

Occult primary tumours

The cornerstone for investigating people with malignant nodes and no primary site on usual assessment is biopsy of suspicious sites and sites likely to harbour the primary site at examination under anaesthesia (EUA). There is universal agreement that FDG PET-CT should be included prior to EUA.[7] Applied in this context, FDG PET-CT influences the management plan in three main ways. Firstly, and primarily, FDG PET-CT detects an unexpected primary site, and with FDG PET-CT superior to FDG PET. A National Institute of Care and Health Excellence (NICE) review, based on the combined results of 5 FDG PET-CT studies and 198 patients, provided an estimated sensitivity of 0.89 and specificity 0.73.[8] In addition, one meta-analysis of eight studies which included 430 people, FDG PET-CT detected 31.4% more primary sites not diagnosed at usual assessment.[9] This compares favourably with FDG PET where in a meta-analysis of 16 studies with 302 patients FDG PET detected 24.5% more primary sites not apparent after conventional work-up.[10] However, the exact likelihood of detecting an unexpected primary site will depend on the investigations prior to FDG PET-CT, and the more investigations the less likely the value of FDG PET-CT.

Secondly, FDG PET-CT improves diagnosis by contributing directly to detecting unexpected nodal and unexpected distant metastases, albeit infrequently.

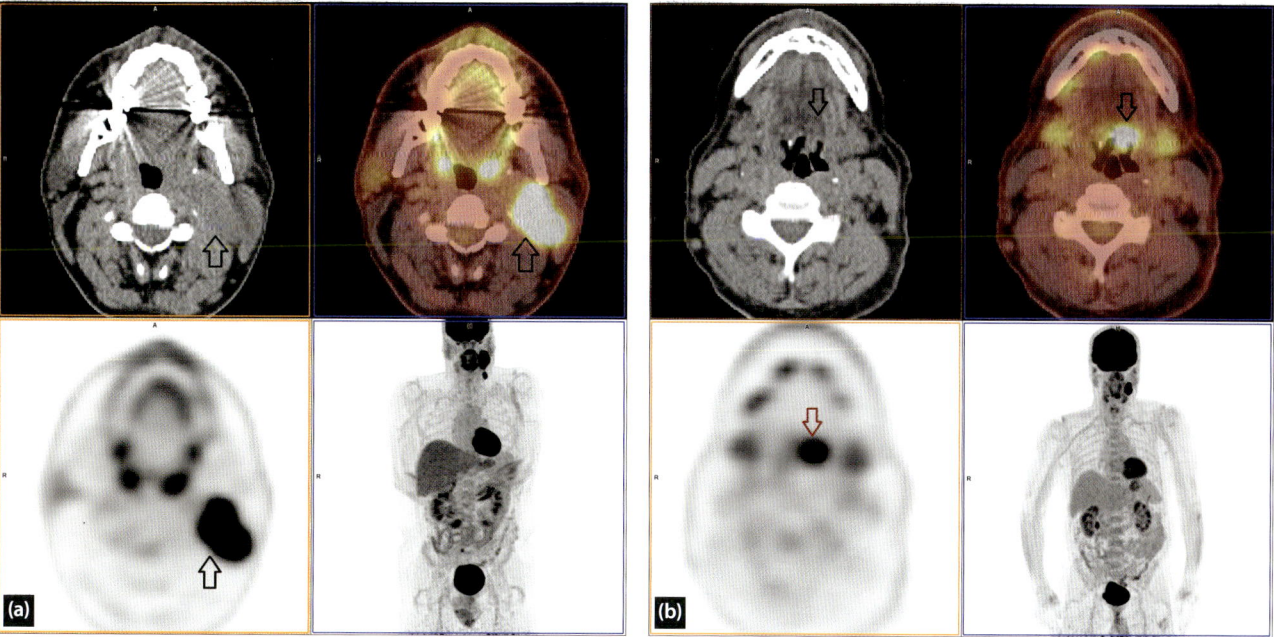

Figure 47.2 A 55-year-old man presented with a left neck lump due to an enlarged neck node infiltrated with SqCC. No primary site on clinical assessment and usual assessment including indirect laryngoscopy and MRI. FDG PET-CT (a) shows the left neck node (hollow arrows), and (b) the subtle base of tongue primary site (hollow arrow), confirmed at subsequent EUA and biopsy.

In a retrospective cohort study of 78 people, one of the largest studies in this area, FDG PET-CT detected primary tumours in 30 people not identified on usual assessment which included flexible fibre-optic nasoendoscopy and CT/MR or both; unexpected contralateral neck nodal disease in two, mediastinal nodal disease in one, and liver metastases in one.[11] Finally, occasionally, but importantly, FDG PET-CT detects occult synchronous cancers, most often silent lung and colorectal cancers.[9, 10] The former because of the linked causes between H&N and lung cancer and the later because colorectal cancer is a common cancer and is often initially asymptomatic.

Currently, many centres offer FDG PET-CT only after clinical assessment and CT/MR shows no primary site, and prior to EUA and biopsy. Increasing confidence in the use of FDG PET-CT and the wider availability of PET-CT scanners is leading to a growing view that FDG PET-CT should be considered as the initial investigation, reserving CT/MR only if necessary for treatment planning.[12] This approach is justified on the grounds that it will improve patient experience by reducing the number of investigations prior to EUA and without overall compromise to detection of occult primary sites.

That said, the diagnostic pathway requires critical consideration. Firstly, it does not take into account the complementary potential of emerging MR techniques, and specifically diffusion MR.[13, 14] In addition, one study showed FDG PET-CT was cost effective in N1 and N2 occult H&N primaries but questioned the cost effectiveness of FDG PET-CT for N3 occult H&N primaries.[15] Finally, given that in HPV-positive people the occult primary site is almost invariably in the tongue base and palatine tonsil the question arises whether a different approach should be taken in HPV-positive people from those who are HPV negative; specifically, as to whether FDG PET-CT should be only for the HPV-negative group. While for those who are HPV-positive, advancing those patients directly to surgical diagnostic assessment, including consideration of emerging techniques such as narrow-band imaging and tongue-base mucosectomy, if no primary site is identified on CT/MR.[16]

SQUAMOUS CELL CARCINOMA

Primary disease

STAGING

FDG PET-CT has a limited use in the staging of the primary site and for assessment of nodal disease in the neck. FDG PET-CT can detect the majority of clinically visible primary tumours. This capability is of limited clinical value in the main, but can occasionally be utilized to more precisely delineate the primary tumour where submucosal extension of disease is a feature, such as in post-cricoid carcinoma and tracheal carcinoma.

With regard to the neck, FDG PET-CT is also of limited clinical value. It is clear from the literature that FDG-PET cannot consistently detect subclinical disease and that reactive nodes can be FDG avid.[14–20] So FDG PET-CT cannot obviate elective neck treatment. However, it can have a role in those with equivocal nodal disease following conventional assessment. In those with a moderate to high risk of neck metastases, a positive FDG PET-CT scan will be highly indicative of neck nodal disease and this can be particularly useful for highlighting possible contralateral or bilateral nodal disease. Conversely, in those with a low risk of nodal metastases, a negative FDG PET-CT is highly indicative of no nodal disease. In other words, FDG PET-CT can highlight possible additional

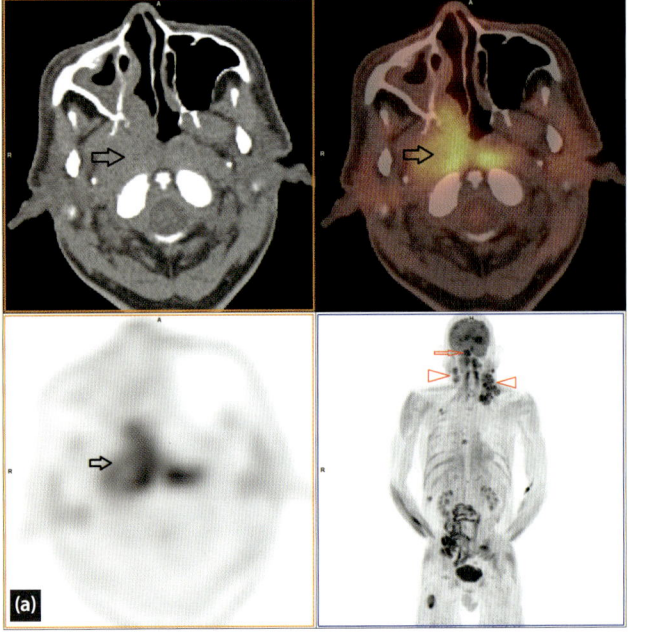 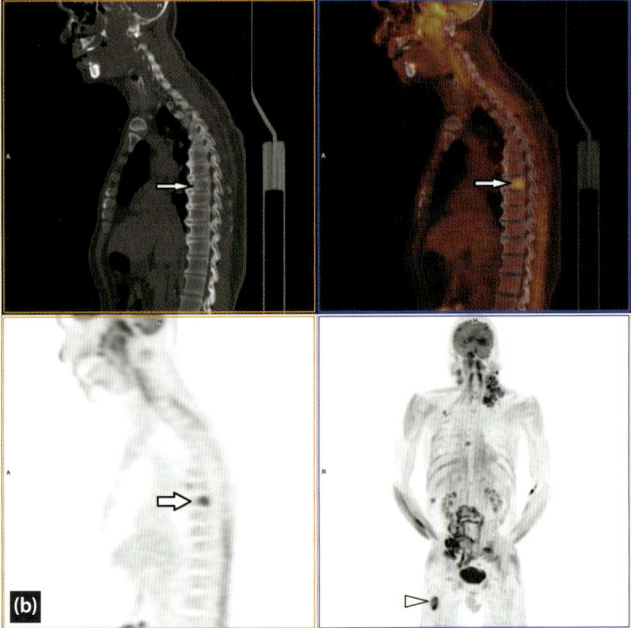

Figure 47.3 A 49-year-old man with nasopharyngeal cancer (NPC). Staging FDG PET-CT **(a)** shows the primary NPC (red hollow arrow), bilateral neck nodes (red arrowhead), and **(b)** two bone metastases, one in a vertebral body (arrow), corresponding to a lucent lesion on CT component (arrow) and one in the RT femur (hollow arrowhead).

unexpected nodal disease which may have a direct and immediate impact. In some it will justify further neck assessment; this is most often initially ultrasound with fine-needle aspiration cytology. In others, treatment may be modified to include the suspicious node or nodes. Determining which nodes are potentially significant is largely influenced by the probability of nodal disease at the location and this will influence the interpretation of nodes that are potentially significant. If the node lies in the nodal drainage area for the primary site and there is a moderate to high probability for nodal disease at this site then the node, notwithstanding its relatively small size and mild FDG uptake, requires consideration. On the other hand, if a node lies outside the drainage area and there is low probability for disease at this site then it is unlikely that the node contains tumour. For example, a right level II node, 8 mm, mildly FDG avid, SUVmax 3.0, in a person with nasopharyngeal cancer must be viewed with much more suspicion than that of a node in a person with a left maxillary antral cancer.

The main role of FDG PET-CT in the assessment of people with primary disease is in the detection of distant metastases. In a significant number, FDG PET-CT detects metastases not diagnosed on usual assessment.[21–23] In a meta-analysis, including 1147 patients from eight studies, FDG PET-CT had a pooled sensitivity and specificity for detecting distant metastases of 0.83 and 0.96 respectively, compared with usual assessment, 0.44 and 0.96, respectively. In addition, the superiority of FDG PET-CT applied to both nasopharyngeal cancer and non-nasopharyngeal head and neck cancers.[24] Specifically with regard to bone metastases, in a meta-analysis which included 1184 patients from five comparative studies, which compared FDG PET CT to bone scanning, FDG PET-CT was more sensitive, with a pooled sensitivity of 0.85 compared with 0.55.[25]

There is divergence in guidance as to whom should be offered FDG PET-CT. Taking cost-effectiveness considerations into account, recent NICE guidelines recommend offering FDG PET-CT only to people with T4 nasopharyngeal and hypopharyngeal cancer and to people with advanced neck disease (N3).[8] Other guidelines recommend FDG PET-CT more extensively.[7] This divergence highlights the many factors that come into play with complex decision-making processes, beyond guideline development process and methodology, and they include the value beliefs and value systems of the individual on the panel making the decisions.[7]

Post-treatment assessment

FDG PET-CT has a high negative predictive value, greater than 90%, 8 weeks or more after chemo-radiotherapy (CRT).[26, 27] Stratification for neck dissection with FDG PET-CT after chemo-radiotherapy results in fewer neck dissections and a reduced incidence of complications.[28] In a prospective study of 564 people with H&N SqCC and advanced neck nodal disease following CRT, 282 were recruited into the neck dissection arm, 282 had FDG PET-CT 8–12 weeks following CRT and neck dissection only if FDG PET-CT showed residual disease. Fifty-four neck dissections were performed in the surveillance arm with 22 surgical complications; 221 neck dissections in the neck arm with 85 complications. FDG PET-CT surveillance was cost-effective compared to planned neck dissection with a £1,415 per person saving and an additional gain of 0.07 quality added life years (QALY).[28]

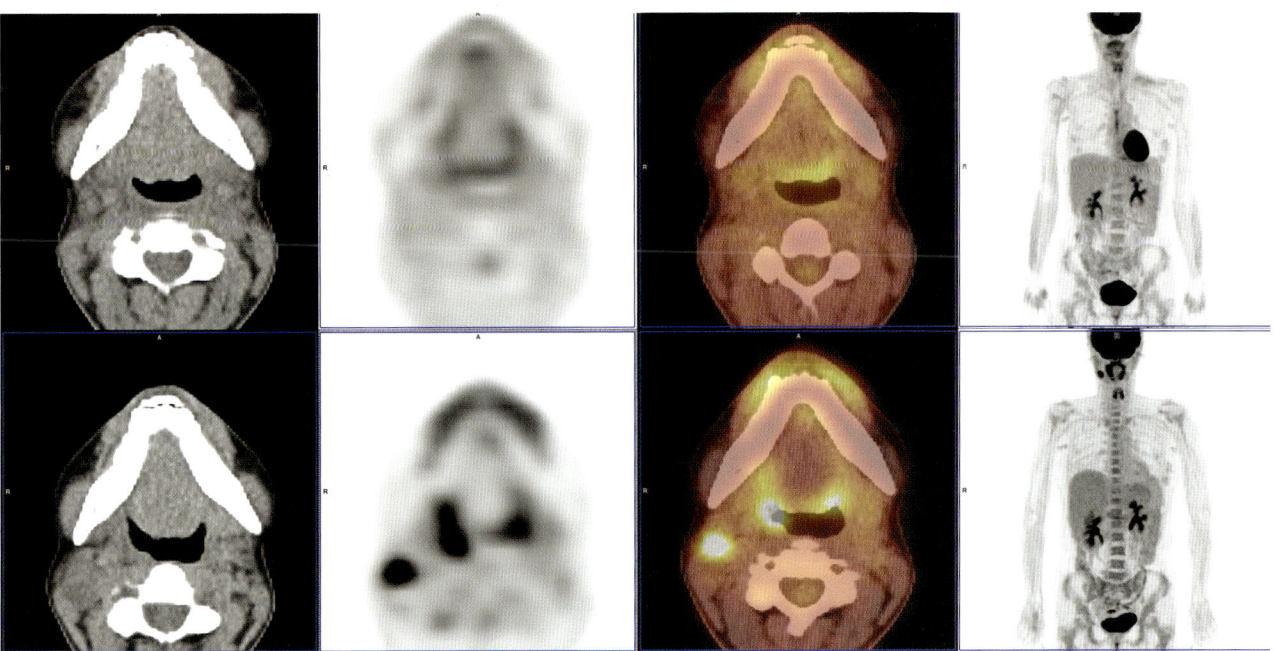

Figure 47.4 FDG PET-CT (bottom row) shows intense FDG avidity of the right glosso-tonsillar fossa SqCC and right neck nodal disease. FDG PET-CT 12 weeks post chemo-radiotherapy (top row) there is resolution of FDG uptake at the primary site and no FDG uptake in the residual right neck node on CT.

Of current interest is the influence of HPV status on FDG PET-CT in the assessment of residual nodal disease following CRT.[29] HPV-positive nodal disease can take longer to involute.[30] So enlarged nodes with no residual disease occur at the 12-week assessment following CRT. Several studies have shown that FDG PET-CT is more accurate than CT for distinguishing nodes with residual disease from those with no disease.[31, 32] In one study, FDG PET and PET-CT at a mean of 12 weeks following treatment, with a range of between 8 and 16 weeks, was significantly more accurate at predicting complete response compared to contrasted CT assessment, 90% compared with 46%, and especially for the HPV-positive group, 93% compared with 50%.[31] In one of the largest studies to date which specifically considered FDG PET-CT response in HPV-positive oropharyngeal cancer, FDG PET-CT at 12 weeks post-CRT demonstrated high-negative predictive value for loco-regional failure though the positive predictive value and sensitivity was disappointing.[32] However, Pryor et al. demonstrated that surveillance strategies including FDG PET-CT was more cost effective than CT-guided surveillance alone, regardless of HPV status. Furthermore, that study showed that combined strategies using CT followed by FDG PET-CT in non-responders were only marginally more cost effective than FDG PET-CT alone, and were highly sensitive to changes in circumstances.[33] Therefore, some advocate that HPV-positive people with enlarged nodes but with no FDG avidity after 12 weeks post-CRT may be considered for close surveillance with serial scanning, with limiting neck dissection for those with FDG avid enlarged nodes, especially if HPV-negative or at high risk and HPV-positive.

This approach however is challenged. In one prospective study, FDG PET-CT had no advantage over CT in low-risk non-smokers with HPV-positive oropharyngeal primaries. In addition, in that study, FDG PET-CT was only better than CT in high-risk patients who have HPV-negative disease, non-oropharyngeal primaries or who have a smoking or alcohol history.[34] The authors acknowledge that the study is limited for several reasons. Firstly, it was performed in a high-throughput cancer institution where the proportion of high-risk patients and radiotherapy non-responders may be greater than in other treatment settings. Secondly, FDG PET-CT nodal response was assessed at a mean of 8 weeks, with a range of between 5 to 12 weeks following treatment, which may not be the optimal timing for FDG PET-CT after radiotherapy.[30, 31] Finally, histopathology of post-CRT neck dissection was used as evidence of persistent disease, which is known to overestimate persistence.[27, 33]

As yet, independent validation of CT scan-driven response systems or comparison with PET-CT-driven systems in multicentre, randomized settings have not been published. As a final comment, even if further studies establish that FDG PET-CT is of limited value in HPV-positive patients, in many countries, HPV-positive patients constitute only a minority, and FDG PET-CT would still have an important role in the majority of patients.

RECURRENT DISEASE

FDG PET-CT is accurate at detecting recurrent disease. A survey of the literature identified 23 studies which

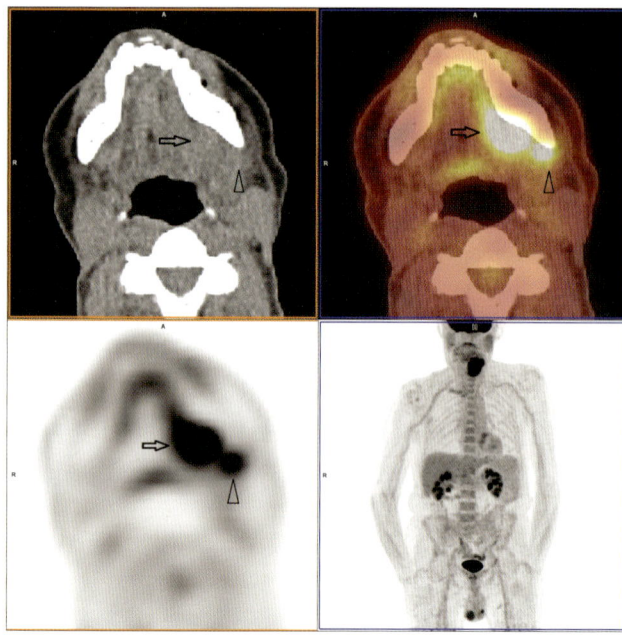

Figure 47.5 A 73-year-old man with clinical suspicion of floor of mouth SqCC recurrence. FDG PET-CT shows the left floor of mouth recurrence (arrow) and a metastatic ipsilateral level IB node (arrowhead).

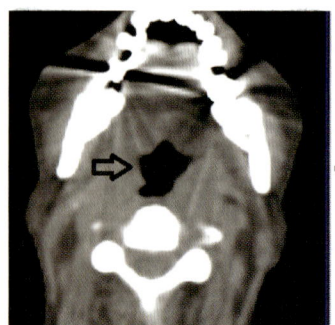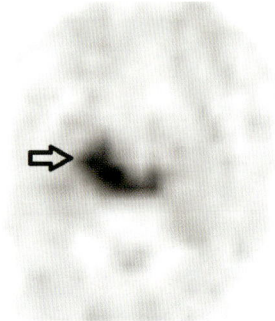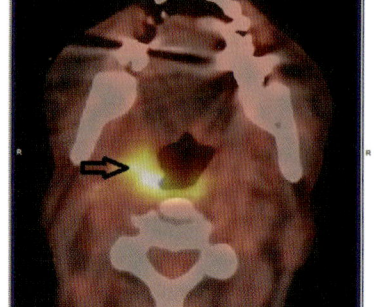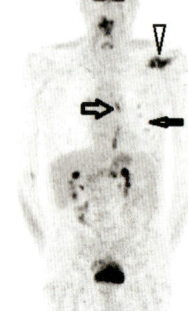

Figure 47.6 FDG PET-CT shows the right poster-lateral oropharyngeal wall recurrence (arrow). It also shows metastases in the lungs (narrow arrow) and within subcutaneous tissue around the left shoulder (arrowhead). It also shows incidental linear FDG in the chest due to oesophagitis (broad arrow).

considered the accuracy of FDG PET-CT done at least 4 months after therapy for detecting active disease at the primary site, within neck nodes and distant metastases.[35] Drawing on the pooled data of 2247 patients from 12 FDG PET and 11 FDG PET-CT studies, the pooled sensitivity and specificity for detection of disease were 0.92 and 0.87, respectively. The pooled sensitivity and specificity performed 4 to 12 months after treatment were 0.95 and 0.78, respectively, and for scans performed at or more than 12 months after treatment, 0.92 and 0.91 respectively. These results concur with a meta-analysis which reported a sensitivity and specificity for the primary site of 0.92 and 0.87, respectively, and for neck nodes 0.90 and 0.94, respectively.[36] Another meta-analysis which included 10 studies reported a sensitivity of 0.92 and specificity of 0.95 for detecting distant metastases in people with suspected head and neck cancer.[36] Individual studies show varying results and this is a reflection not only on the small number of patients in each study, but also on the various clinical situations where FDG PET was used.[35-37]

Compared with other imaging, prospective studies provide evidence that FDG PET is effective and superior to CT and MR for distinguishing active disease from treatment sequelae in people who develop symptoms during follow-up.[38-45] In a study of 38 people, FDG PET differentiated between post-irradiation laryngeal recurrent cancer from laryngeal oedema with an accuracy of 79% and was superior to CT (61%) and clinical assessment (43%).[44]

In addition, a recent study evaluated the accuracy of FDG PET-CT with intravenous contrast for suspected recurrent H&N SqCC in 170 people who underwent FDG PET-CT, which consisted of non-contrast-enhanced and contrast-enhanced CT, to investigate suspected recurrence. Diagnostic performance of FDG PET-CT / contrast enhanced CT (FDG PET-CT/ceCT), FDG PET-CT / non-contrast-enhanced CT (FDG PET-CT/ncCT) and contrast-enhanced CT (ceCT) for local or regional recurrence, distant metastasis, overall recurrence and second primary cancer was evaluated. FDG PET CT was a more accurate restaging tool than ceCT. The added value of ceCT to FDG PET-CT is minimal.[46] The study supports the conclusion from a previous retrospective study which compared FDG PET-CT to that of contrast-enhanced CT and to standard-of-care follow-up, physical examination and endoscopy, in detecting locally recurrent H&N cancer. FDG PET-CT had higher accuracy than contrast-enhanced CT alone and increases the sensitivity and negative predictive value of physical examination and endoscopy.[47]

The value of FDG-PET as a surveillance tool for patients with high risk of relapse remains unclear. A survey of the literature extending to March 2012 found a lack of evidence to support FDG PET-CT surveillance of people with H&N cancer.[2] There have subsequently been several further published studies. These studies show FDG PET-CT can detect disease before it is clinically evident. One retrospective review included 512 patients who underwent surveillance FDG PET-CT. FDG PET-CT was performed at 3-month intervals, starting 2 months after the conclusion of therapy with scans routinely obtained at 2, 5, 8 and 14 months after therapy. Patients were assessed clinically and radiographically for at least 12 months from their last FDG PET-CT (mean, 26 months; median, 28 months; range, 12–89 months) to determine recurrence rates. All suspected recurrences underwent biopsy for confirmation. A single FDG PET-CT with negative findings carried a NPV of 91%, which is not adequate to defer further radiological surveillance. Two consecutive FDG PET-CT examinations with negative findings within a 6-month period, however, resulted in a NPV of 98%, which could obviate further radiological imaging in the absence of clinical signs of recurrence.[48]

One single institution prospective study performed FDG PET-CT at 6 months after the end of treatment in all 116 patients treated for histologically proven H&N cancer from April 2009 to May 2012 who did not show any findings suggestive of recurrence at 6 months of their usual follow-up. FDG PET-CT findings were correlated with histopathology or imaging follow-up. Results from the study included 116 patients. Of the 82 FDG PET-CT considered as negative, only one had a recurrence. Among the 34 positive FDG PET-CT, 22 relapsed whereas 12 did not show evidence of recurrence. The sensitivity and specificity of FDG PET-CT were 96% (22/23) and 87 % (81/93), respectively. The positive predictive value was 65% (22/34). The negative predictive value was 99% (81/82). The overall accuracy was 89% (103/116). Of the 116 patients, FDG PET-CT highlighted 22 (19%) subclinical recurrences. These results confirmed that FDG PET-CT is more accurate than conventional follow-up physical examination alone in the assessment of recurrence after previous curative treatment for H&N SqCC.[49] One retrospective review was performed on a series of H&N patients at a single institution who had undergone FDG PET-CT as an integral part of follow-up after definitive treatment. Of the 123 patients, 24 (20%) had asymptomatic lesions (either recurrent or new primaries) on FDG PET-CT (8% of surveillance scans) at an average interval of 35.7 weeks post treatment. Asymptomatic lesions were detected most frequently at distant sites, with 50% being thoracic, but also included were primary (9%), regional (9%), and other distant (32%) sites. At last follow-up of the 24 patients in whom an asymptomatic lesion was detected, 14 have died of disease; 10 remain alive, 4 with disease; and 1 patient had a subsequent recurrence treated and is currently disease-free. The authors concluded that FDG PET-CT is an effective tool for detecting asymptomatic disease in people previously treated for H&N cancer. Disappointingly, they found that even with early detection of recurrent disease, the mortality rate remains high.[50] In a 10-year retrospective analysis of H&N cancer patients with long-term serial imaging, those with negative 3-month imaging appear to derive limited benefit from subsequent FDG PET-CT surveillance. Furthermore, no survival differences were observed between PET/CT-detected and clinically detected recurrence.[51] So even if results substantiate the ability to predict recurrence earlier than conventional assessment, there remains the question of whether earlier detection afforded by FDG PET-CT results in an improved clinical outcome.

Other comments

CHARACTERIZATION OF INDETERMINATE LESIONS

In common with other cancers, FDG PET-CT is a key investigation for the assessment of lesions indeterminate on usual assessment when improved characterization can change the treatment plan. These indeterminate lesions are usually in the lung, liver and adrenal glands, with the lung being the most common site. FDG PET has been shown to be an accurate non-invasive test for the diagnosis of pulmonary lesions. In a meta-analysis limited to pulmonary nodules including 13 studies with a total of 450 nodules, FDG PET had a sensitivity of 93.9% and specificity of 85.8% respectively.[52] Another meta-analytic comparison of the cross-sectional imaging modalities for the diagnosis of malignancy in SPNs (up to 3 cm diameter) from a pooled analysis of 1008 nodules from 22 eligible studies reported a similar sensitivity and specificity of FDG PET, 95% and 82%, respectively.[53] Abscesses and granulomas including those due to sarcoid, tuberculosis (TB), anthracite and fungus (asperilloma, blastomycosis, coccidiomycosis, cryptococcosis, histoplasmosis) can mimic malignant lesions.[54,55] False-negative FDG PET-CT results are unusual, although mucinous carcinomas such as those arising from the stomach, highly-differentiated neuroendocrine carcinoma and adenocarcinoma, especially within a scar, can cause confusion.[54,55] Lesions smaller than 1 cm across can be detected by FDG PET-CT, as detection is influenced not only on size but also FDG avidity of the lesion. That said, with lesions less than 1 cm false-negative results occur and so a negative FDG PET-CT must be interpreted with caution and cannot reliably exclude malignancy.[55] Recent British Thoracic Society Guidelines recommend FDG PET-CT as the preferred investigation in the further evaluation of pulmonary nodules, partly because it is widely available and partly because no alternative investigation shows superiority.[56]

In detection of synchronous and metachronous malignancies (**Figures 47.7** and **47.8**) FDG PET-CT will detect synchronous other H&N cancers and lung cancers, linked by their common aetiologies. In addition, FDG PET-CT will also diagnose unexpected other cancers. The cumulative incidence of a second malignancy following H&N cancer is up to 18%.[57] Fewer than half will have a detectable synchronous primary malignancy and almost half will be detected by a thorough clinical assessment and a further number by chest CT. So the expected pick-up rate of FDG PET-CT at the time of primary diagnosis is likely to be in the order of 2–3%. This is substantiated by one South Korean study of 349 patients. FDG PET-CT detected second primary H&N cancer over 2 years in 14 people, 10 (2.8%) at initial staging and 4 (1.2%) during the follow-up, with a mean duration of 15 months; H&N cancer arising from the

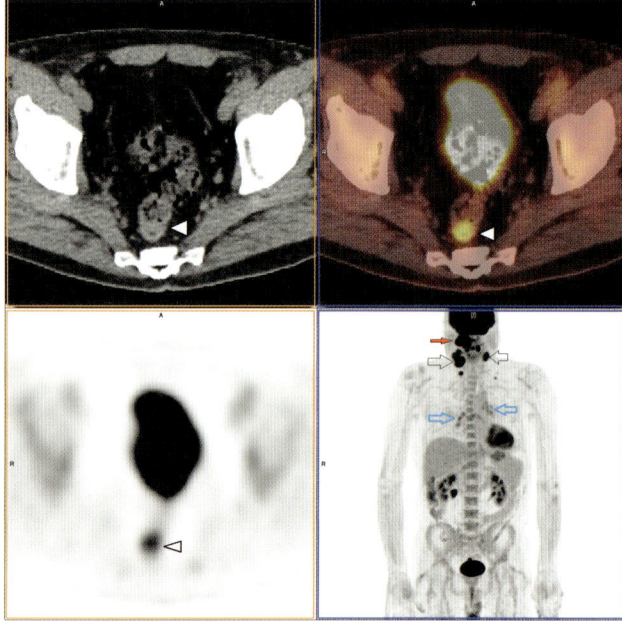

Figure 47.7 A 45-year-old man with nasopharygeal cancer. FDG PET-CT shows incidental focal intense FDG uptake in the pelvis (arrowhead). Excision biopsy confirms a small rectal cancer. The maximum intense projection (MIP) image shows the nasopharyngeal cancer (red arrow) and bilateral neck nodal disease (hollow arrow). It also shows FDG avid nodes in the chest due to a sarcoid like reaction (blue arrow).

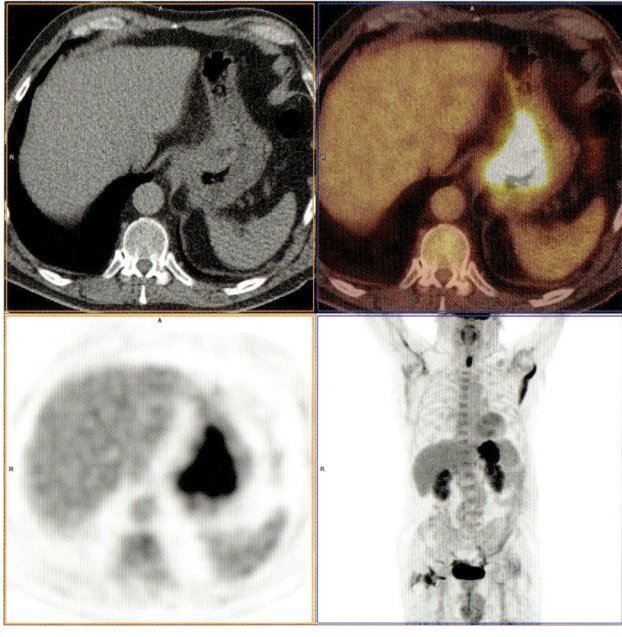

Figure 47.8 FDG PET-CT shows the primary laryngeal cancer. It also shows a silent synchronous stomach cancer. FDG uptake in the stomach is usually due to Helicobacter Difficile infection, which can be focal or diffuse and FDG PET-CT cannot reliably distinguish between the two conditions.

nasal cavity: one, lung cancers: seven, colorectal cancer: two, thyroid: two, upper GI tract: two.[57] The low rate of synchronous malignancy perhaps does not justify routine screening. However, when FDG PET-CT is indicated for other reasons, detection of an unexpected second cancer may influence the plan of treatment. The main dilemma is that both malignant and benign incidental lesions are FDG avid and often only biopsy or excision of the lesion can distinguish between the two. This may lead, in some people, to unnecessary investigations and in some the additional unnecessary tests may contribute to delayed initiation of treatment.

FDG uptake and outcomes

There is increasingly strong evidence that pre-treatment FDG PET-CT uptake at the primary site and within involved nodes is an independent predictor of subsequent prognosis. Two meta-analyses concluded that there was a correlation between SUVmax and outcome in people with H&N cancer.[58, 59] Most studies included in the meta-analyses, however, report either univariate or relatedly small multivariate analyses. More recently, one single-centre study which included 287 people confirmed FDG uptake retains statistical significance in multivariate analysis and has a clinically relevant prognostic impact.[60] The contribution of FDG uptake to personalized treatment of H&N cancer has yet to be formally assessed.

EMERGING APPLICATIONS

Response assessment

The role of FDG PET/CT in this area is evolving. With revived enthusiasm in chemotherapy for H&N SqCC, there is interest in non-invasive imaging which can distinguish responders from non-responders early during treatment. FDG PET-CT has been shown to predict early-on response to neo-adjuvant chemotherapy in a variety of solid tumours including oesophageal carcinoma. There is currently one published study for H&N SqCC. In 15 patients, an FDG response after two cycles of chemotherapy predicted event-free survival.[61]

Radiotherapy (RT) planning

FDG PET-CT is increasingly used for radiotherapy target volume delineation.[62] Benefits include inter-observer variability in gross tumour volume (GTV) delineation reduction, GTV size reduction and identification of tumour that would not otherwise have been treated but for PET-CT, reducing geographical misses. However, two major challenges prevail. Firstly, inflammation leads to tumour margin over-estimation. Secondly, there is presently no reliable, universally accepted, standardized method of identifying tumour margins. Notwithstanding, two small retrospective studies show significantly better overall survival and event-free survival applying FDG PET-CT-based intensity modulated radiotherapy (IMRT), compared with the control group.[63, 64] More studies are needed to clarify the benefits of FDG PET-CT in this area.

NON-SQUAMOUS CELL CARCINOMA

Thyroid cancer

FDG PET-CT is of limited value for the pre-operative assessment of thyroid nodules as both malignant and benign thyroid lesions can be equally avid for FDG.[65] However, it has an important role in the assessment of differentiated thyroid cancer, which includes papillary and follicular histological types, following treatment.[66] In this group, metastases have an alternating pattern of uptake with 131-iodine and FDG where either some 131-iodine uptake combined with low FDG trapping or no 131-iodine uptake combined with high FDG trapping.[67] The hypothesis was that persistent iodine metabolism is consistent with better cell differentiation, while the loss of this ability together with increased glucose metabolism is consistent with dedifferentiation.[67] A meta-analysis of 958 patients from 20 studies which

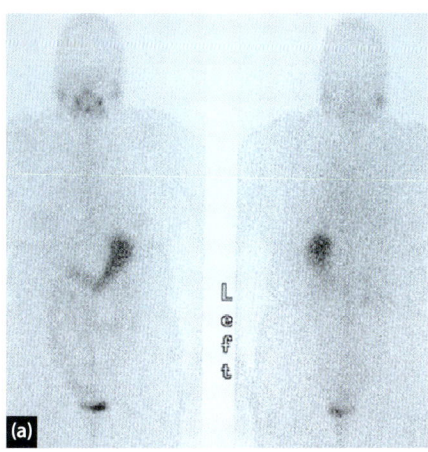
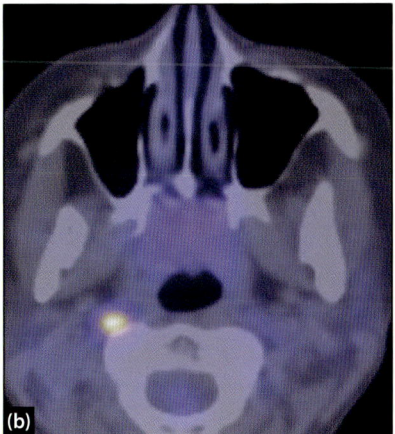
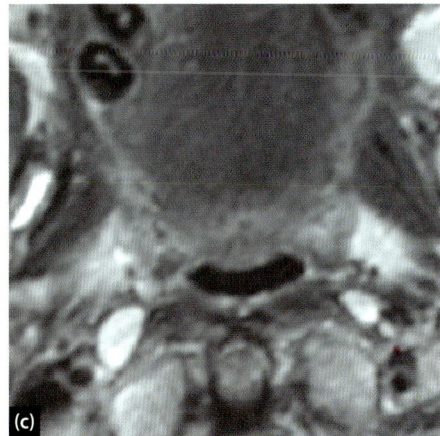

Figure 47.9 A 48-year-old woman following treated for follicular thyroid cancer with elevated and raising serum thyroglobulin levels.
(a) No unaccountable uptake on 131 I-iodine scan (b) FDG PET-CT shows a left prevertebral node in keeping with active disease at this site. It also shows no other suspicious areas. (c) The node corresponded to an indeterminate node on MRI. Subsequent surgery confirmed the FDG PET-CT; subsequent fall in serum thyroglobulin level following surgery.

included 11 studies that used FDG PET only, 7 FDG PET-CT only and 2 studies which used both FDG PET and FDG PET-CT, confirmed the value of FDG PET-CT in treated papillary and follicular thyroid cancer patients who have suspected recurrent disease and negative 131-iodine scan, with a pooled sensitivity of 95%, and specificity 81%, respectively, and compared favourably with FDG PET, sensitivity and specificity 84%.[66]

With regard to other histological types of thyroid cancer, FDG PET-CT can detect Hurthle cell carcinoma and anaplastic carcinoma.[68, 69] However, the clinical role of FDG PET-CT in these tumours is currently unclear. Concerning medullary thyroid cancer, preliminary results suggest FDG PET to be an accurate technique for detecting metastases and recurrent disease. The largest study in the literature, a German multicentre retrospective survey, reviewed 100 FDG PET studies performed on 85 patients.[70] The results of the FDG PET were compared with 46 indium-111 pentetreotide (SMS) studies, 33 Pentavalent technetium dimercaptosuccinate acid (DMSA) scans, 8 hexakis (2 Methoxyisobutyl isonitirile) technetium-99m (MIBI) scans, 64 CT and 37 MR. One hundred and eighty-one lesions were identified by at least one technique; FDG PET detected the majority of lesions with a lesion detection probability of 68% compared with 25% for SMS, 29% for DMSA, 6% for MIBI, 53% for CT and 58% for MR. In the 55 lesions confirmed histologically, FDG PET had the highest overall accuracy with a sensitivity of 78% and specificity of 79%; MR had a slightly higher sensitivity of 82%, but a specificity of 67% and MIBI had a specificity of 100%, but a sensitivity of only 25%.

OTHER MALIGNANT TUMOURS

There is limited evidenced guidance for the use of FDG PET-CT here, beyond anecdotal reports, as these tumours are extremely rare. Notwithstanding, FDG PET/CT is often done prior to treatment and for several reasons. Firstly, to demonstrate that the tumour is FDG avid. And if so, FDG PET-CT is considered for pre-treatment staging, and subsequently to detect residual/ recurrent disease.

In one published report of post-operative parathyroid carcinoma, FDG PET provided more accurate information compared with other imaging.[71] FDG PET-CT cannot reliably distinguish between malignant and benign major salivary gland tumours as both can be equally FDG avid.[72] It can, however, be useful for distinguishing active disease from sequelae of treatment.[73] Caveat, muco-epidermoid and adenoid cystic cancers may not be FDG and particularly following treatment.[74] FDG PET-CT is effective for detecting lymphoma except low-grade non-Hodgkin's lymphoma and extra-nodal marginal zone B-cell lymphoma, which are not consistently FDG avid.[75, 76] H&N malignant melanomas, sarcomas and paraganglionomas have been shown to be FDG avid.[77, 78]

Normal variants and artefacts

Brown adipose-tissue FDG uptake can be difficult to distinguish from adjacent small FDG avid nodes, especially when there is slight mis-registration of PET to CT.

Skeletal muscle FDG uptake is usually linear and symmetrical and does not pose a diagnostic quandary. Occasionally, pre-vertebral muscle FDG uptake and

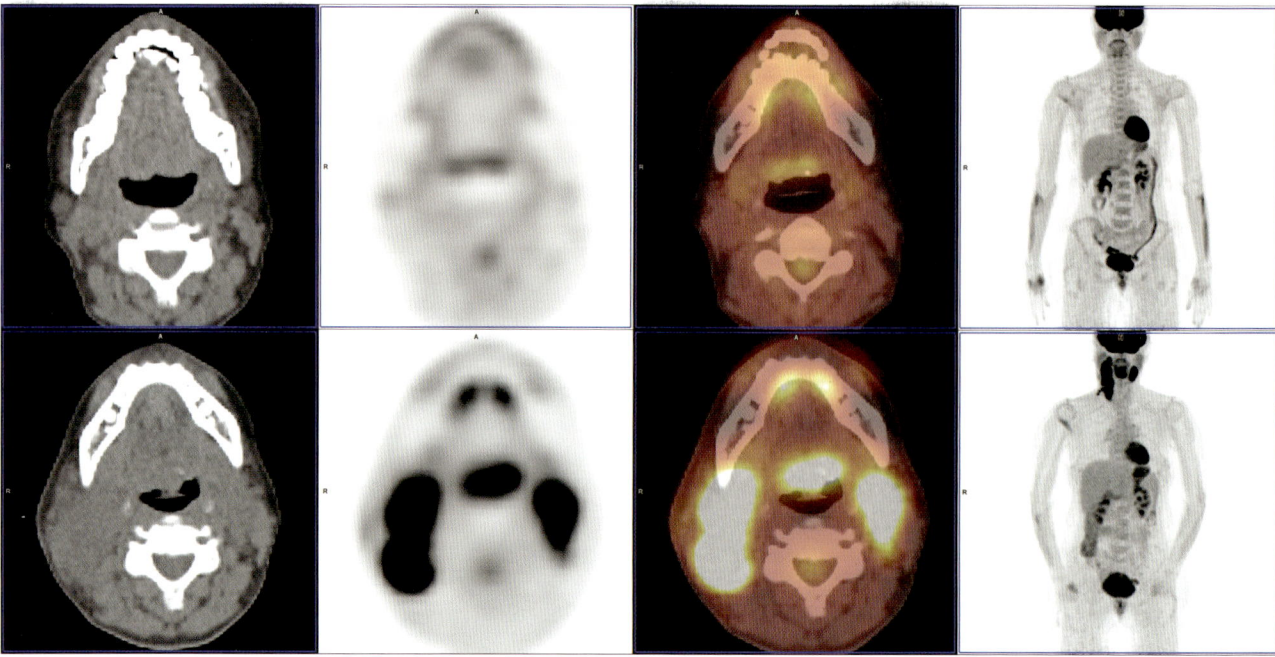

Figure 47.10 A 36-year-old woman with non-Hodgkin's lymphoma. FDG PET-CT shows (bottom row) intense FDG uptake in enlarged nodes in the neck on both sides and within Waldeyer's ring lymphoid tissue in the tongue base, (top row) following completion of chemotherapy, there is resolution of FDG activity in the tongue base and neck nodes; all that remains are indeterminate non FDG avid nodes in the neck.

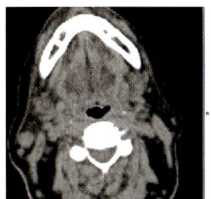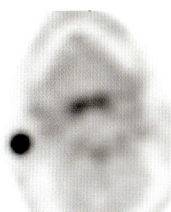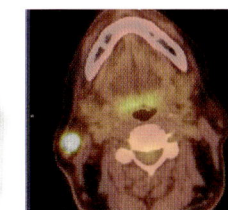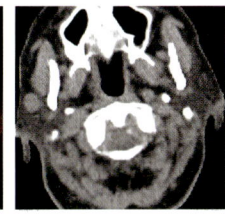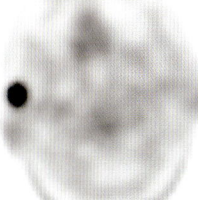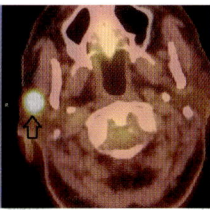

Figure 47.11 A 25-year-old woman who presented with a neck node due to malignant melanoma. FDG PET-CT shows (top row) intense FDG uptake in the involved right neck node. It also shows (bottom row) an intensely FDG avid nodule within the right parotid gland. Malignant and benign parotid lesions are FDG avid and so fine-needle aspiration cytology was required to confirm the diagnosis. Both lesions were resected and provided histological confirmation of the FDG PET-CT diagnosis. Importantly, FDG PET-CT demonstrated that there was no disease beyond the head and neck.

especially when asymmetrical, needs separating from pre-vertebral nodal FDG uptake, and this may not be possible without resorting to correlation with MR or post-intravenous contrast CT.

Waldeyer's ring normal lymphoid tissue FDG uptake in the nasopharynx, tongue base (lingual tonsil) and palatine tonsils needs careful distinction from FDG uptake from an occult primary tumour arising at these sites, these being common sites for an occult primary tumour. That said, the role of FDG PET-CT is not to make the diagnosis but to increase the number of malignancies diagnosed at EUA and biopsy. In this setting, a low threshold for diagnosing abnormality should be adopted and any asymmetrical FDG uptake at these sites reported. SUV measurement is of limited use because of the overlap of values between tumour and normal lymphoid tissue.[79]

Dental amalgam causes FDG uptake in the anterior two thirds of the mouth. In practice, this rarely poses a clinical dilemma. If there is doubt as to the cause, direct inspection and palpation will almost invariably provide reassurance.

LIMITATIONS/PITFALLS

As on CT/MR, branchial cysts can be challenging to distinguish from necrotic nodes. No FDG uptake in the wall of the lesion favours the diagnosis of a branchial cyst. On the other hand, presence of FDG uptake in the lesion wall does not assist, as both pathologies can show this appearance, the necrotic node due to tumour and inflammation and the branchial cyst due to inflammation.

Granulomatous disease mimicking metastases deserve comment. Firstly, sarcoid and sarcoid-like reaction. With FDG uptake in chest nodes careful distinction needs to be made between those due to sarcoid-like reaction and cancerous nodes. Sarcoid-like reaction is not rare in H&N cancer. There is also an increased likelihood in recurrent disease. The pattern of FDG uptake assists. FDG uptake in normal-sized nodes which include those in paratrachea, both hila and subcarina would favour sarcoidosis, especially if there are no FDG avid neck nodes, but even when there is neck nodal disease.[80] In addition, sarcoid can mimic disease beyond chest nodes including in the lung, liver and bone.[81] Secondly, TB needs distinction from malignancy, and especially from lung metastases and synchronous lung malignancy.

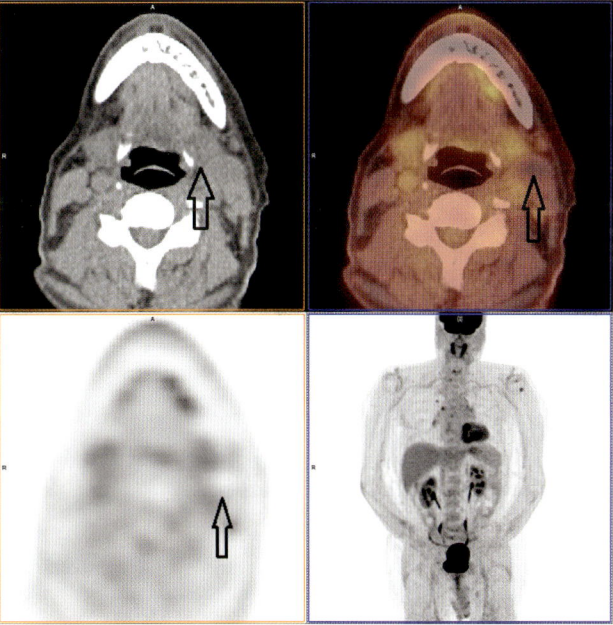

Figure 47.12 Branchial cyst. FDG PET-CT shows a left level IIA cystic lesion with no FDG uptake (hollow arrow).

Lung metastases and synchronous lung cancers can pose a challenge to diagnosis. Adeno-carcinoma may not be FDG avid. Also small sub-centimetre lung metastases may not be FDG avid.

Post-treatment, before making the diagnosis of residual or recurrent disease FDG uptake due to treatment sequelae needs careful consideration (**Table 47.1**). In clinical practice, taking a pragmatic approach, and drawing from experience, a definitively positive FDG PET-CT should be taken as highly suspicious of disease as long as there is no infection. A negative scan is highly likely to represent absence of active disease, but still demands careful surveillance as microscopic foci of active disease cannot be excluded. An equivocal scan requires biopsy of areas of FDG activity or an early repeat FDG PET-CT. False-positive and false-negative results occur and so FDG PET-CT findings must be interpreted, not in isolation but in the context of the overall assessment.[35–37, 38–45] This is especially pertinent as determination of definitely positive, definitely negative and equivocal FDG uptake is still relatively subjective as, notwithstanding efforts, there is

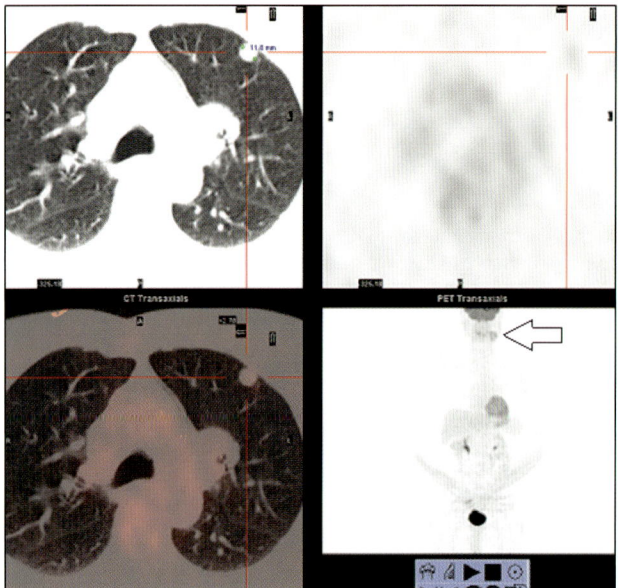

Figure 47.13 A 61-year old-man with SqCC recurrence in the left post-treatment neck FDG PET-CT shows the neck recurrence (arrow) and a left upper lobe lung adenocarcinoma, which shows no FDG uptake (centre of red cross-hairs).

currently no universal consensus agreement on the meaning of these terms.[82]

There is a commonly held view that recent biopsies cause focal FDG uptake in the H&N. This concern is probably overestimated as biopsies are usually tiny and limited to the mucosa.

RADIOTRACERS OTHER THAN FDG

Thymidine 3-Deoxy-3-^{18}F-fluorothymidine [FLT]

Currently, its only potential role is for more accurately distinguishing lung metastases and from benign lesions, compared with FDG.[83–85] However, if confirmed that FLT is only taken up by malignant cells, then this may be of value on the rare occasion when more information on the extent of disease at the primary site is required following usual assessment for treatment planning. Also, FLT may be effective for detecting residual disease following RT and chemotherapy and to predict the outcome to RT and chemo-RT.[86–88]

TABLE 47.1 Sequelae of interventions that mimic active disease following surgery

Residual tongue mimicking recurrent disease Asymmetrical FDG uptake in the oral cavity and oro-pharynx following partial resection of the tongue and hypertrophy of the normal residual tongue. Such an appearance also occurs following radiotherapy to the tongue.	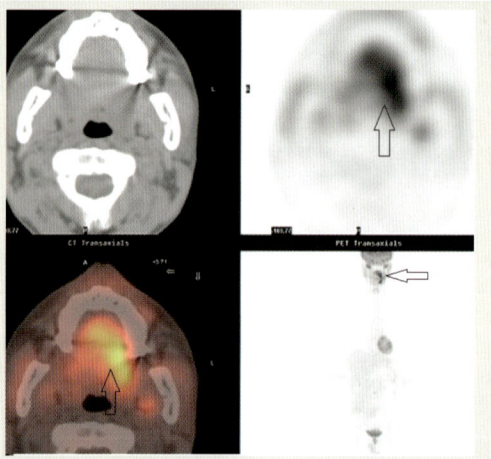 FDG PET-CT shows intense FDG uptake in the left oral cavity and oro-pharynx following radiotherapy which included the right side of the oral cavity and oropharynx [hollow arrow].
Post-tonsillectomy The normal palatine tonsil mimics a palatine tonsil lesion, particularly relevant when looking for an occult primary site or assessing for recurrent disease.	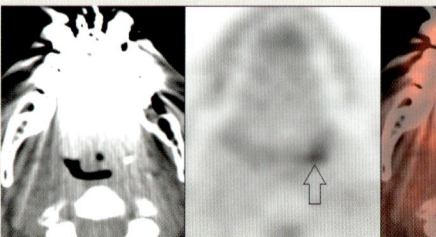 The normal left palatine tonsil mimics a palatine tonsil lesion. [hollow arrow], following a previous right tonsillectomy,

(Continued)

TABLE 47.1 *(Continued)* Sequelae of interventions that mimic active disease following surgery

Osteonecrosis following surgery
This can also occur following radiotherapy. FDG PET-CT cannot reliably distinguish osteonecrosis from infection and recurrence.

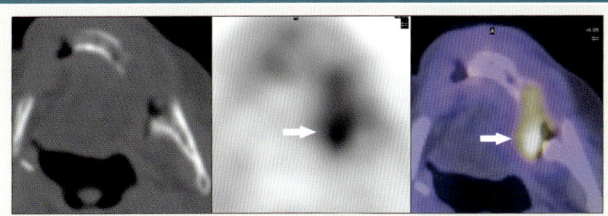

FDG PET-CT shows intense FDG uptake due to osteonecrosis following surgery to the left mandible (arrow).

Following recent neck dissection
FDG uptake occurs directly related to inflammation post-surgery. Cylous collections also cause FDG uptake.

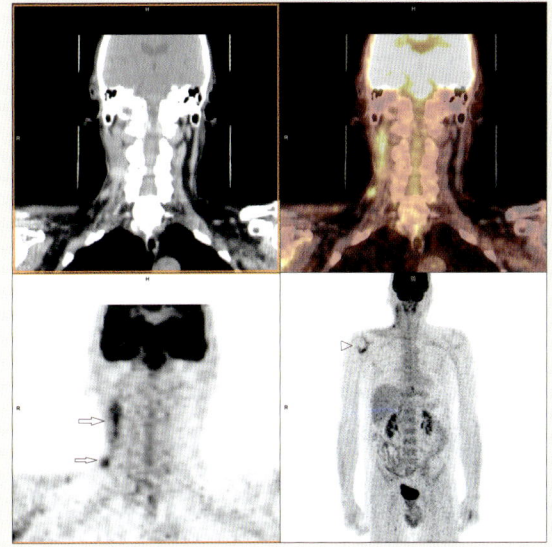

FDG PET-CT shows intense FDG uptake in the right neck 6 weeks following neck dissection (arrow). Right gleno-humeral joint synovitis due to osteoarthritis causing incidental FDG uptake (arrowhead).

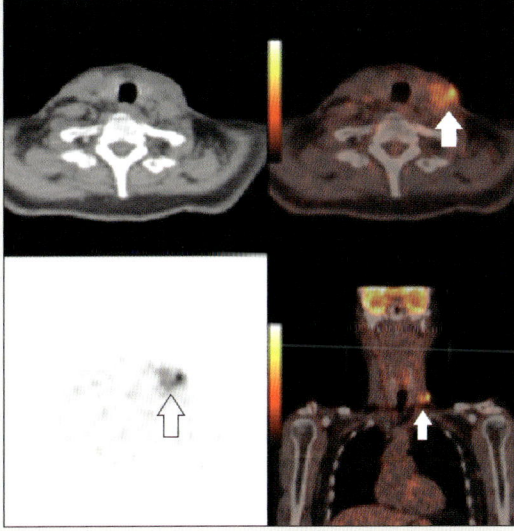

FDG PET-CT shows intense FDG uptake related to a cylous collection complicating neck dissection.

(Continued)

TABLE 47.1 *(Continued)* Sequelae of interventions that mimic active disease following surgery	
Granulomas Specifically, vocal cord injection with Teflon and collagen needs distinction from a primary vocal cord cancer. Stitch granuloma following neck dissection also very rarely causes increased FDG uptake and needs distinction from a neck node containing disease.	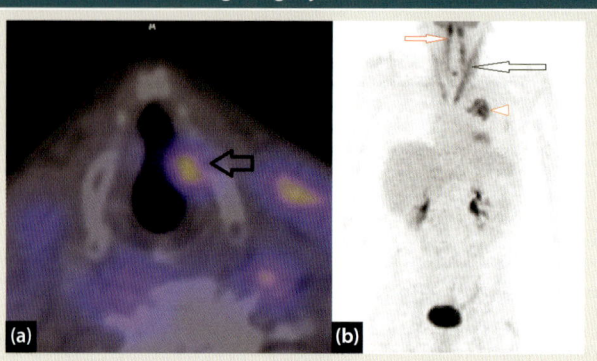 **(a)** FDG PET CT shows intense FDG uptake related to a granuloma post vocal cord injection (hollow black arrow). **(b)** FDG PET-CT also shows the cause of the left vocal cord palsy, namely a left upper lobe non-small cell cancer invading the mediastinum and causing left recurrent laryngeal nerve paralysis (arrowhead). There is also FDG uptake in normal prevertebral (hollow red arrow) and steno-mastoid muscles (hollow black arrow).
Following other interventions	
Radiation myelitis A very rare complication with modern radiotherapy techniques.	
Around stoma sites FDG uptake due to inflammation needs consideration as an alternative to recurrence around the tracheostomy stoma site and tract. FDG uptake is also present around gastrostomy stoma sites.	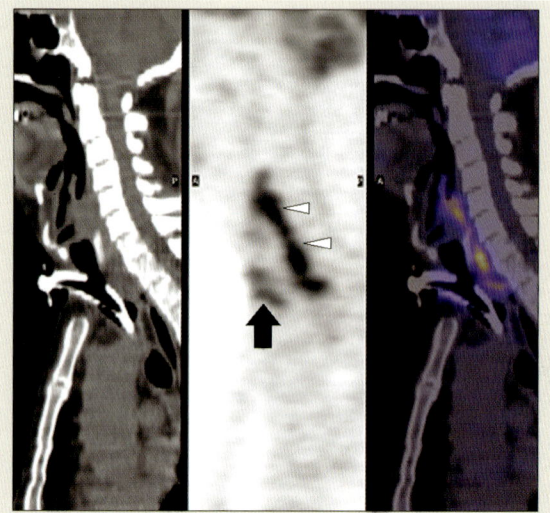 Increased FDG uptake around the tracheostomy stoma site and tract (arrow). There is also FDG uptake related post cricoid SqCC (arrowhead).
Gastrostomy stoma site	
Post-chemo-radiotherapy neck Especially in HPV-positive people mild FDG uptake can persist in post-treatment neck nodes beyond 8 weeks.	

Radiotracers for detecting hypoxia

There has been considerable interest in PET tracers which can detect hypoxia in H&N SqCC, because inadequate treatment of hypoxic cells is one of the main causes of failure to effectively treat the primary site. Hypoxic cells require three times more radiation to kill compared with non-hypoxic cells; often it is not possible to deliver the required dose because of the damage it will cause to surrounding normal tissue. Imaging of hypoxia would provide the opportunity to apply RT to the subvolume of hypoxic cells only.[89, 90]

Fluorinated nitromidazole compounds, including 1-[2-nitro-1-imidazolyl-3[^{18}F]fluoro-2-propanol [[^{18}F]FMISO], have been used for imaging hypoxia in H&N SqCC*. Copper isotopes of varying half-life, including ^{60}Cu, ^{61}Cu, ^{62}Cu and ^{62}Cu labelled to copper-diacetyl-bis(N^4-methyl-thiosemicabazone) [Cu-ATSM] and copper-pyruvaldehyde-bis(N^4-methylthiosemicarbazone [Cu-PTSM] have also

---

* Other florinated nitromidazole compounds that have been studied include 1-(5-[^{18}F]fluoro-5-deoxy-α-D-arabinofuranosyl)-2-nitro-imidazole [[^{18}F]FAZA], ^{18}F-2-(2-Nitro-imidazol-1-yl)-N-(3,3,3-trifluropropyl)-Acetamide [^{18}F-EF3] and ^{18}F-Fluoroerythronitromidazole [^{18}F-FETNIM]

been studied. There is as yet no one clear front runner. [18F]FMISO is the most commonly used and best validated tracer and most studies have shown correlation between hypoxia and [18F]FMISO uptake.[91] But it is only slowly cleared from the blood compartment and the radiotracer passively diffuses into the cell which takes a relatively long time. This means that for imaging to be effective it has to be done between 2 to 3 hours post-injection.[92] There are as yet inadequate data to recommend the other tracers as superior.

11C-choline PET/CT

In a pilot study 11C-choline improved the delineation of orbital and skull involvement compared with FDG PET/CT in people with nasopharyngeal cancer.[93] This is because physiological 11C-choline uptake in the brain and extra-ocular eye muscles is minimal compared with FDG. The advantage of 11C-coline beyond this specific scenario has been questioned.[94]

PET-MRI [magnetic resonance imaging]

Integrated PET-MRI is an emerging technology, a development of registering PET with MRI obtained from different scanners.[95] Combining PET with MRI for assessment of H&N cancer is an area of considerable interest because MRI is often performed as a complement to PET-CT in the assessment of H&N cancer. The added value of PET-MRI compared with separate PET-CT and MRI scanning has yet to be fully evaluated. Beyond a significantly lower dose of ionizing radiation, the advantage of PET-MRI as an alternative to PET-CT is unclear. A pilot study of 25 patients designed to evaluate the accuracy of FDG PET-MR for loco-regional tumour evaluation compared to FDG PET-CT and MRI in initial tumour and recurrence diagnosis in histo-pathologically confirmed H&N SqCC found no significant differences were observed in T and N staging among the three modalities. In 13 patients undergoing hybrid imaging for cancer recurrence diagnosis, diagnostic accuracy was 57% with MRI and 72% with FDG PET-CT and FDG PET-MRI, respectively.[96] In a study designed to evaluate and compare the diagnostic potential of FDG PET-MRI to FDG PET-CT for people with cancer of unknown primary a total of 20 patients underwent a dedicated head and neck and whole-body FDG PET-CT and subsequent simultaneous FDG PET-MRI. Both hybrid imaging techniques provide a comparable diagnostic ability for detection of primary cancer and metastases, with comparably high-lesion conspicuity and diagnostic confidence, offering superior assessment of cervical lesions in PET-MRI and potentially of pulmonary lesions in PET-CT.[97]

BEST CLINICAL PRACTICE

FDG PET-CT is not necessary for all people with Head and Neck cancer. For many, clinical assessment complemented by conventional imaging will give all the necessary information for providing the person with H&N cancer with enough information to make an informed choice of treatment and for the planning treatment. However, with the current evidence:
In SqCC:

✓ Offer FDG PET-CT in T3, T4 nasopharyngeal and hypopharyngeal cancer and N3 nodal disease; consider FDG PET-CT in others with a moderate and high risk of disseminated disease.
✓ Consider FDG PET CT where staging is difficult clinically; for example, where there is uncertainty on other imaging or equivocal findings that would preclude radical treatment.
✓ Offer FDG PET-CT following completion of chemoradiotherapy in advanced neck nodal disease to inform the need for neck dissection.

✓ Consider FDG PET CT when there is suspicion of recurrent disease and equivocal on radiological assessment.

Consider FDG PET-CT in occult primary tumours prior to EUA.
Offer FDG PET-CT in papillary and follicular thyroid cancer post-treatment with suspected recurrence.
Consider FDG PET-CT in treated medullary thyroid carcinoma associated with elevated calcitonin levels with equivocal or normal cross-sectional imaging, bone and octreotide scintigraphy.
Consider FDG PET-CT pre-treatment in rare cancers to confirm that the tumour is FDG avid, and especially if there is a reasonable chance that subsequently FDG PET-CT may be considered for detection of residual / recurrent disease.
Consider FDG PET-CT in indeterminate lesions which are not accessible to biopsy or where a biopsy would be particularly hazardous.

FUTURE RESEARCH

► Large prospective studies evaluating FDG PET-CT as an early predictor of response to neo-adjuvant treatment in Head and Neck SqCC.
► Large prospective studies evaluating the value of FDG PET-CT as a surveillance tool in Head and Neck SqCC with high risk of recurrence.

► PET-CT studies with hypoxic and cell proliferation markers for evaluating the biology of malignant Head and Neck tumours.

> **KEY POINTS**
>
> - The use of FDG PET-CT in Head and Neck cancer is supported mainly by data from observational and non-randomized studies. There are limited randomized controlled trials available.
> - The body of evidence shows that FDG PET-CT appropriately used can contribute to more accurate assessment of Head and Neck cancer, including more accurate staging, earlier and more accurate detection of residual and recurrent disease, improved detection of the occult primary and earlier detection of occult disease in treated differentiated thyroid cancer.

REFERENCES

1. Schroder H, Yeung HWD, Gonen M, et al. Head and neck: clinical usefulness and accuracy of PET CT image fusion. *Radiol* 2004; **231**(1): 65–72.
2. Patel K, Hadar N, Lee, J et al. The lack of evidence for PET or PET/CT surveillance of patients with treated lymphoma, colorectal cancer, and head and neck cancer: a systematic review. *J Nucl Med* 2013; **54**: 1518–27.
3. Acuff SN, Osborne D. Clinical workflow considerations for implementation of continuous-bed-motion PET/CT. *J Nucl Med Technol* 2016; **44**(2): 55–8.
4. Warburg O, Wind F, Negelein G. Uber den Stoffwechsel von Tumoren im Korper. *Klinische Wochenschrift*. 1926; **5**: 829–32.
5. Hustinx R, Benard F, Alavi A. Whole body FDG-PET imaging in the management of patients with cancer. *Semin Nucl Med* 2002; **32**: 35–46.
6. Seifert E, Schadel A, Haberkorn U, Strauss LG. Evaluating the effectiveness of chemotherapy in patients with head and neck tumours using positron emission tomography. *HNO* 1992; **40**: 90–3.
7. Wong WL, Ross P, Corcoran M. Evidence based guidelines recommendations on the use of PET CT imaging in head and neck cancer from Ontario and guidelines in general: some observations. *Clin Oncol* 2013; **25**: 242–5.
8. Cancer of the upper aero-digestive tract tumours: assessment and management in people aged 16 and over. NICE guideline 36. February 2016.
9. Dong MJ, Zhao K, Lin XT, et al. Role of fluorodeoxyglucose-PET versus fluorodeoxyglucose-PET/computed tomography in detection of unknown primary tumor: a meta-analysis of the literature. *Nucl Med Commun* 2008; **29**(9): 791–8.
10. Rusthoven KE, Koshy M, Paulino AC. The role of fluorodeoxyglucose positron emission tomography in cervical lymph node metastases from an unknown primary tumor. *Cancer* 2004; **101**(11): 2641–49.
11. Wong WL, Sonoda LI, Gharpurhy A, et al. 18F-fluorodeoxyglucose positron emission tomography/computed tomography in the assessment of occult primary head and neck cancers: an audit and review of published studies. *Clin Oncol* 2012; **24**: 190–19.
12. Thoeny HC, Kweyzer FD, King AD. Diffusion-weighted MR imaging in the head and neck. *Radiol* 2012; **263**(1): 19–32.
13. Bhatia KSS, King AD, Yeung DKW, et al. Can diffusion weighted imaging distinguish between normal and squamous cell carcinoma of the palatine tonsil? *BJR* 2010; **83**(993): 753–8.
14. Smith KA, Dort JC, Hall SF, Rudmik L. Cost effectiveness of PET-CT in the evaluation of cancer of the unknown primary. *Head Neck* 2015; **37**(12): 1781–7.
15. Koivunan P, Black L, Laranne J, Irjala H. Unknown primary: diagnostic issues in the biological endoscopy and PET scan era. *Otolaryngol* 2015 **23**: 121–6.
16. Braams JW, Pruim J, Freling NJM, et al. Detection of lymph node metastases of squamous cell cancer of the head and neck with FDG-PET and MR. *J Nucl Med* 1995; **36**: 211–16.
17. Laubenbacher C, Saumweber D, Wagner-Manslau C, et al. Comparison of fluorine-18-fluorodeoxyglucose PET, MR and endoscopy for head and neck squamous cell carcinoma. *J Nucl Med* 1995; **36**: 1747–57.
18. Myers LL, Wax MK, Nabi H, et al. Positron emission tomography in the evaluation of the N0 neck. *Laryngoscope* 1998; **108**: 232–6.
19. Stoeckli SJ, Steinert H, Pflaltz M, Schmid S. Is there a role for positron emission tomography with 18F-fluorodeoxyglucose in the initial staging of nodal negative oral and oropharyngeal squamous cell carcinoma. *Head Neck* 2002; **24**: 345–9.
20. Nowak B, Di Martino E, Janicke S, et al. Diagnostik maligner Kopf-Hals-Tumouren durch F-18-FDG PET im vergleich zu CT/MRT. *Nuklearmedizin*. 1999; **38**: 312–18.
21. Haerle SK, Schmidt DT, Ahmad N, et al. The value of f-18-FDG PET/CT for the detection of distant metastases in high risk patients with head and neck squamous cell carcinoma. *Oral Oncol* 2011; **47**(7): 653–9.
22. Ng SH, Chan SC, Liao CT, et al. Distant metastases and synchronous second primary tumours in patients with newly diagnosed oropharyngeal and hypopharyngeal carcinomas: evaluation of (18) F-FDG and extended field multi-detector row CT. *Neuroradiology* 2008; **50**(11): 969–79.
23. Liu FY, Lin CY, Chang JT, et al. [18]-F FDG PET can replace conventional workup in primary M staging of non-keratinizing nasopharyngeal carcinoma. *J Nucl Med* 2007; **48**: 1614–19.
24. Xu G, Li J, Zou X, Li C. Comparison of whole body positron emission tomography (PET)/PET-computed tomography and conventional anatomic imaging for detecting distant malignancies in patients with head and neck cancer: a meta-analysis. *Laryngoscope* 2012; **122**: 1974–8.
25. Yi X, Fan M, Liu Y, et al. 18FDG PET and PET-CT for the detection of bone metastases in patients with head and neck cancer: a meta-analysis. *J Med Imag Radiat Oncol* 2013; **57**: 674–9.
26. Gupta T, Master Z, Kannan S, et al. Diagnostic performance of post-treatment FDG PET or FDG PET/CT imaging in head and neck cancer: a systematic review and meta-analysis. *Eur J Nucl Med Mol Imaging* 2011; **38**(11): 2083–95.
27. Porceddu SV, Pryor DI, Burmeister E, et al. Results of a prospective study of positron emission tomography-directed management of residual nodal abnormalities in node-positive head and neck cancer after definitive radiotherapy with or without systemic therapy. *Head Neck* 2011; **33**(12): 1675–82.
28. Mehanna H, Wong W, McConkey CC, et al. PET-CT surveillance versus neck dissection in advanced head and neck cancer. *N Engl J Med* 2016; **374**: 1444–54.
29. Mehanna H, Wong WL, Dunn J. Management of advanced nodal disease in patients treated with primary chemoradiotherapy. *Curr Opin Oncol* 2016: **28**(3): 201–4.
30. Huang SH, O'Sullivan B, Zhao H, et al. Temporal nodal regression and regional control after primary radiation therapy for N2-N3 head and neck cancer stratified by HPV status. *Int J Radiation Oncol Biol Phys* 2013; **87**(5): 1078–85.
31. Mak D, Hicks, RJ , Rischin D, et al. Treatment response in the neck: p16+ versus p16- oropharyngeal cancer. *J Med Imaging Radiat Oncol* 2013; **57**(3): 364–72.
32. Vainshtein JM, Spector ME, Stenmark MH, et al. Reliability of post chemotherapy F-18-FDG PET/CT for prediction of locoregional failure in human papillomavirus-associated oropharyngeal cancer. *Oral Oncol* 2014; **50**(3): 234–9.
33. Pryor DI, Porceddu SA, Scuffman PA, et al. Economic analysis of FDG PET CT guided management of the neck after primary chemoradiotherapy for node positive head and neck squamous cell carcinoma. *Head Neck* 2013; **35**: 1287–94.
34. Moeller BJ, Rana V, Cannon BA, et al. Prospective risk adjusted [18F]FDG PET and CT assessment of radiation response in head and neck cancer. *J Clin Oncol* 2009; **27**(15): 2509–15.
35. Sheikhbahaei S, Taghipour M, Ahmad R, et al. Diagnostic accuracy of follow-up FDG PET or PET/CT in patients with head and neck cancer after definitive treatment: a systemic review and meta-analysis. *Am J Radiol* 2015; **205**: 629–39.
36. Gupta T, Master Z, Kannan S, et al. Diagnostic performance of post-treatment FDG PET or FDG PET/CT imaging in head and neck cancer: a systematic review and meta-analysis. *Eur J Nucl Med Mol Imaging* 2011; **38**: 2083–95.

37. Shuichao G, Shisheng L, Xinming Y, Qinglai T. 18FDG PET-CT for distant metastases in patients with recurrent head and neck cancer after definitive treatment: a meta-analysis. *Oral Oncol* 2014; **50**: 163–7.
38. Anzai Y, Carroll WR, Quint DJ, et al. Recurrence of head and neck cancer after surgery or irradiation: prospective comparison of 2-deoxy-2-(F-18)fluoro-d-glucose PET and MR imaging diagnoses. *Radiol* 1996; **200**: 135–41.
39. Bailet JW, Sercarz JA, Abemayor E, et al. The use of positron emission tomography for early detection of recurrent head and neck squamous cell carcinoma in postradiotherapy patients. *Laryngoscope* 1995; **105**: 135–9.
40. Fischbein NJ, Aassar OS, Caputo GR, et al. Clinical utility of positron emission tomography with 18F-fluorodeoxyglucose in detecting residual/recurrent squamous cell carcinoma of the head and neck. *Am J Neuroradiol* 1998; **19**: 1189–96.
41. Hanasono MM, Kunda LD, Segall GM, et al. Uses and limitations of FDG positron emission tomography in patients with head and neck cancer. *Laryngoscope* 1999; **109**: 880–5.
42. Kim HJ, Boyd J, Dunphy F, Lowe AV. F-18 FDG PET scan after radiotherapy for early-stage larynx cancer. *Clin Nucl Med* 1998; **23**(11): 750–2.
43. Lapela M, Grenman R, Kurki T, et al. Head and neck cancer: detection of recurrence with PET and 2-(F-18) fluoro-2-deoxy-D-glucose. *Radiology* 1995; **197**: 205–11.
44. McGuirt WF, Greven KM, Keyes JW, et al. Laryngeal radionecrosis versus recurrent cancer: a clinical approach. *Ann Otol Rhinol, Laryngol* 1998; **107**: 293–6.
45. Li P, Shuang H, Mozley PD, et al. Evaluation of recurrent squamous cell carcinoma of the head and neck with FDG positron emission tomography. *Clin Nucl Med* 2001; **26**: 131–5.
46. Suenaga Y, Kitajima K, Ishihara T, et al. FDG-PET/contrast-enhanced CT as a post-treatment tool in head and neck squamous cell carcinoma: comparison with FDG-PET/non-contrast-enhanced CT and contrast-enhanced CT. *European Radiol* 2016; **26**: 1018–30.
47. Rangaswamy B, Fardanesh MR, Genden EM, et al. Improvement in the detection of locoregional recurrence in head and neck malignancies: F-18 fluorodeoxyglucose-positron emission tomography/computed tomography compared to high-resolution contrast-enhanced computed tomography and endoscopic examination. *Laryngoscope* 2013; **123**(1): 2664–9.
48. McDermott M, Hughes M, Rath T, et al. Negative predictive value of surveillance PET/CT in head and neck squamous cell cancer. *Am J Neuroradiol* 2013; **34**: 1632–6.
49. Robin P, Abgral R, Valette G, et al. Diagnostic performance of FDG PET/CT to detect subclinical HNSCC recurrence 6 months after the end of treatment. *Eur J Nucl Med Mol Imaging* 2015; **42**: 72–8.
50. Medhat M, Osman MD, Brandon M, et al. PET-CT and the detection of the asymptomatic recurrence or second primary lesions in the treated head and neck cancer patient. *Laryngoscope* 2013; **123**: 2161–4.
51. Ho AS, Tsao GJ, Chen FW, et al. Impact of positron emission tomography/computed tomography surveillance at 12 and 24 months for detecting head and neck cancer recurrence. *Cancer* 2013; **119**: 1349–56.
52. Gould MK, Maclean CC, Kushner WG, et al. Accuracy of positron emission tomography for the diagnosis of pulmonary nodules and mass lesions: a meta-analysis. *JAMA* 2001; **285**(7): 914–24.
53. Cronin P, Dwamena BA, Kelly AM, et al. Solitary pulmonary nodules: meta-analytic comparison of cross-sectional imaging modalities for diagnosis of malignancy. *Radiol* 2008; **246**: 772–82.
54. Wong WL, Campbell H, Saunders M. Positron emission tomography (PET) evaluation of indeterminate pulmonary lesions. *Clin Oncol* 2002; **14**: 123–8.
55. Lin EC, Alavi A. (eds) *Thoracic neoplasms in PET and PET CT: a clinical guide.* New York: Thieme; 2005.
56. Callister MEJ, Baldwin DR, Akram AR, et al. British Thoracic Society guidelines for the investigation and management of pulmonary nodules. *Thorax* 2015; **70**: ii1–ii54.
57. Kim SY, Roh J-L, Yeo N-K, et al. Combined 18F-fluorodeoxyglucose-positron emission tomography and computed tomography as a primary screening method for detecting second primary cancers and distant metastases in patients with head and neck cancer. *Ann Oncol* 2007; **18**: 1698–1703.
58. Xi P, Li M, Zhao H, et al. 18F-FDG PET or PET CT to evaluate prognosis for head and neck cancer: a metaanalysis. *J Cancer Res Clin Oncol* 2011; **137**: 1085–109.
59. Zhang B, Li X, Lu X. Standardised uptake value is of prognostic for outcome in head and neck squamous cell cancer. *Acta Otolaryngol* 2010; **130**: 756–62.
60. Rasmussen JH, Vogelius IR, Fishcher BM, et al. Prognostic value of 18-F uptake in 287 patients with head and neck squamous cell cancer. *Head Neck* 2015; 37:1274–81.
61. Abgal R, Le Roux P-Y, Keromnes N, et al. Early prediction of survival following induction chemotherapy with DCF using FDG PET/CT imaging in patients with locally advanced head and neck cancer. *Eur J Nucl Med Mol Imaging* 2012; **39**: 1839–47.
62. Troost EGC, Schinagl DAX, Bussinka J, et al. Clinical evidence on PET CT for radiation planning in head and neck tumours. *Radiother Oncol* 2010; 96: 328–34.
63. Vernon MV, Maheshwari M, Schultz CJ, et al. Clinical outcomes of patients receiving integrated PET CT radiotherapy for head and neck carcinoma. *Int J Radiat Oncol Biol Phys* 2008; **70**: 678–84.
64. Rothschild S, Studer G, Seifert B, et al. PET/CT staging in IMRT improves treatment outcome of locally advanced pharyngeal cancer: a matched pair comparison. *Radiat Oncol* 2007; **2**: 22.
65. Lin EC, Alavi A. Thyroid cancer. In: *PET and PET CT: a clinical guide*. Lin EC, Alavi A. (eds). New York: Thieme; 2005.
66. Caetano R, Basto CRG, Olivera IAG de, et al. Accuracy of PET and PET CT in the detection of differentiated thyroid cancer recurrence with negative 131-I whole body scan results: a meta-analysis 2016. *Head Neck* 2016; **38**: 316–27.
67. Feine U, Lietzenmayer R, Hanke JP, et al. 18FDG-Ganzkorper-PET bei differenzierten Schilddrusenkarzinomen. *Nucl Med* 1995; **34**: 127–34.
68. Wang W, Macapinlac H, Larson SM, et al. (18F)-2-Fluoro-2-deoxy-D-glucose positron emission tomography localizes residual thyroid cancer in patients with negative diagnostic 131I whole body scans and elevated serum thyroglobulin levels. *J Clin Endocrinol Metab* 1999; **84**: 2291–302.
69. Lind P, Kumnig G, Matschnig S, et al. The role of F-18FDG PET in thyroid cancer. *Acta Med Austriaca* 2000; **27**: 38–41.
70. Diehl M, Risse JH, Brandt-Mainz K, et al. Fluorine-18 fluorodeoxyglucose positron emission tomography in medullary thyroid cancer: results of a multicentre study. *Euro J Nucl Med* 2001; **28**: 1671–6.
71. Neumann DR, Esselstyn CB, Kim EY. Recurrent post operative parathyroid carcinoma: FDG PET and sestamibi SPECT findings. *J Nucl Med* 1996; **37**: 2000–1.
72. Rassekh CH, Cost JL, Hurst MK, et al. PET in Wartin's tumour mimicking malignancy impacts the evaluation of head and neck patients. *Am J Otolaryngol* 2015; **36**: 259–63.
73. Lin EC, Alavi A. Head and Neck cancer. In *PET and PET CT a clinical guide* eds. Lin EC, Alavi A. Publ. Thieme New York Stuttgart. 2005.
74. Hadiprodjo D, Ryan T, Truong MT, et al. Parotid gland tumours: preliminary data for value of FDG diagnostic performance. *AJR* 2012; **198**:185–190.
75. Walsh RM, Wong WL, Chevretton EB, Beaney RP. The use of PET-18FDG imaging in the clinical evaluation of head and neck lymphoma. *Clin Oncol* 1996; **8**: 51–4.
76. Hoffman M, Kletter K, Becherer A, et al. 18F-fluorodeoxyglucose positron emission tomography (18F FDG PET) for staging and follow-up of marginal zone B-cell lymphoma. *Oncol* 2003; **64**: 336–40.
77. Goerres GW, Stoeckli SJ, von Schulthess GK. FDG PET for mucosal malignant melanoma of the head and neck. *Laryngoscope* 2002; **112**: 381–5.
78. Wittekindt C, Theissen P, Jungehulsing M, Brochhagen HG. FDG-PET imaging of malignant paraganglioma of the neck. *Ann Otol Rhino Laryngol* 1999; **108**: 909–12.
79. Wong WL, Gibson D, Sanghera B, et al. Evaluation of normal FDG uptake in palatine tonsil and its potential value for detecting occult head and neck cancers: a PET CT study. *Nucl Med Comm* 2007; **28**(9): 675–80.
80. Abdel-Galiil K, Anand R, Sharma S, Brennan PA. Incidence of sarcoidosis in head and neck cancer. *Br J Maxillofac Surg* 2008; **46**: 58–60.
81. Chowdhury U, Sheerin F, Bradley, KM, Gleeson FV. Sarcoid-like reaction to malignancy on whole body integrated 18F-FDG PET/CT: prevalence and disease pattern *Clin Radiol* 2009; **75**: 675–81.
82. de Bree R, Hoekstra OS. Evaluation of neck node response after radiotherapy minimizing equivocal results. *Euro J Nucl Med Mol Imaging* 2016; **43**: 605–8.
83. Hoshikawa H, Nishiyama Y, Kishino T, et al. Comparison of FLT-PET and FDG-PET for visualization of head and neck squamous cell cancers. *Mol Imaging Biol* 2011; **13**: 1172–7.

84. Troost EG, Vogel WV, Merkx MA, et al. 18F-FLT PET does not discriminate between reactive and metastatic lymph nodes in primary head and neck cancer patients. *J Nucl Med* 2007; **48**: 726–35.
85. Hoshikawa H, Kishino T, Morit T, et al. The value of 18F-FLT for detecting second primary cancers and distant metastases in head and neck cancer. *Clin Nucl Med* 2013; **38**: 318–24.
86. Troost EG, Bussink J, Hoffmann AL, et al. 18F-FLT PET/CT for early response monitoring and dose escalation in oropharyngeal tumors. *J Nucl Med* 2010; **51**: 866–74.
87. Hoeben BA, Troost EG, Span PN, et al. 18F-FLT PET during radiotherapy or chemoradiotherapy in head and neck squamous cell carcinoma is an early predictor of outcome. *J Nucl Med* 2013; **54**: 532–40.
88. Kishino T, Hoshikawa H, Nishiyama Y, et al. Usefulness of 3'-deoxy-3'-18F-fluorothymidine PET for predicting early response to chemoradiotherapy in head and neck cancer. *J Nucl Med* 2012; **53**: 1521–7.
89. Chang JH, Wada M, Anderson NJ, et al. Hypoxia-targeted radiotherapy dose painting for head and neck cancer using (18)F-FMISO PET: a biological modeling study. *Acta Oncol* 2013; **52**(8): 1723–9.
90. Bollineni VR, Koole MJ, Pruim J, et al. Dynamics of tumor hypoxia assessed by (18)F-FAZA PET/CT in head and neck and lung cancer patients during chemoradiation: possible implications for radiotherapy treatment planning strategies. *Radiother Oncol* 2014; **113**(2): 198–203.
91. Horsman MR, Motensen LS, Peterson JB, et al. Imaging hypoxia to improve RT outcomes. *Nat Rev Clin Oncol* 2012; **9**(12): 674–87.
92. Carlin S, Humm JL. PET of hypoxia: current and future perspectives. *J Nucl Med* 2012; **53**: 1171–4.
93. Wu HB, Wang QS, Wang MF, et al. Preliminary study of ^{11}C-choline PET/CT for T staging of locally advanced nasopharyngeal carcinoma: comparison with ^{18}F-FDGH PET/CT. *J Nucl Med* 2011; **52**: 341–6.
94. Ito K, Kubota K, Morooka, M, Yokoyama J. Comparison of PET CT with F18-FDG and with C11-choline for the detection of recurrence of head and neck cancer after radiotherapy. *J Nucl Med* 2009; **50**: (suppl 2) 1780.
95. Wong WL, Hussain K, Chevretton EB, et al. Validation and clinical application of computer combined CT and PET with FDG head and neck images. *Am J Surg* 1996; **172**: 628–32.
96. Schaarschmidt BM, Heusch P, Buchbender C, et al. Locoregional tumour evaluation of squamous cell carcinoma in the head and neck area: a comparison between MRI, PET/CT and integrated PET/MRI. *Euro J Nucl Med Mol Imaging* 2016; **43**(1): 92–102.
97. Ruhlmann V, Ruhlmann M, Bellendorf A, et al. Hybrid imaging for detection of carcinoma of unknown primary: a preliminary comparison trial of whole-body PET/MRI versus *J Nucl Med* PET/CT. *Eur J Radiol* 1016; **85**(11): 1941–7.

CHAPTER 48

IMAGE-GUIDED SURGERY, 3D PLANNING AND RECONSTRUCTION

Ghassan Alusi and Michael Gleeson

Introduction 559	Visualization of image data 561
Background and overview 559	Image-guided surgery 565
Image reconstruction 560	References 566

SEARCH STRATEGY
Data in this chapter may be updated by a Medline search using the keywords: image-guided surgery, endoscopic sinus surgery and skull base surgery.

INTRODUCTION

The use of X-ray images to guide a surgeon dates back to the middle of the 20th century. Pioneering attempts to use Cartesian coordinates to determine locations of target points in the brain in three-dimensional space predated the development of computers. The limitations of radiographic images did not stop scientists from developing over 40 stereotactic apparatus by the 1950s.[1]

The development of both computers and digital imaging opened up the field of computer-aided surgery to include their use in diagnosis, pre-operative planning, surgical simulation, intra-operative image guidance, robotics, telemedicine and, no doubt, numerous other applications yet to come.

The term computer-aided surgery is used to describe computer-aided surgical planning, surgical simulation, intra-operative image guidance, robotics and prosthetics design and manufacture. Computer-aided surgery has become an integral part of modern surgical practice and training in all surgical specialties including neurosurgery, otorhinolaryngology, maxillo-facial, general and orthopaedic surgery.

BACKGROUND AND OVERVIEW

A CT or MRI scan produces a stack of digital images to create a 3D volume.[2] The data within this volume can be extracted and used as an accurate representation of the patient anatomy. Anatomical structures can be displayed in a variety of ways to show skin, bone, muscles, tumour and other structures, including vessels, nerves and so on.[3] The data can then be made to be transparent/semi-transparent, opaque and even colour coded. Multiple data sets can be superimposed to show different tissues and structures. An MRI could be fused to a CT 3D volume and displayed simultaneously to show accurately bone and soft tissues.

A CT scan contains an extremely accurate coordinate system of the patient data. This can be used to generate 3D models of every structure including a whole head (using skin coordinates), bones, blood vessels, lesions and bone defects. These 3D models can then be used (on screen) to make measurements, and drive numerically controlled milling machines and 3D printers to create physical models representing the patients anatomy. In maxillo-facial surgery, this is extensively used to produce prostheses for reconstruction of defects in the skull.[4]

Digital image processing algorithms have been developed to segment (extract), enhance and suppress the display of any structure contained within the 3D volume.

The 3D volume of data as well as virtual surgical tools can be aligned (registered) with the patient's real world coordinates such that the surgeon would be able to navigate surgical tools and these be displayed on a computer screen to indicate their position in relationship to patient anatomy.

The display of the data to the surgeon may be presented as three orthogonal 2D images or as a 3D volume. Augmented reality displays present the real-world patient with 3D structures or even vectors superimposed to guide the surgeon. These images may be displayed through the operating microscope as overlays on the surgical field.[5]

Alternatively, part of the 3D data set can be superimposed on the patient's anatomy, thus providing the surgeon with an extraordinary 'X-ray' type vision[6] (**Figure 48.1**).

As the normal anatomy is often distorted by disease, trauma or previous surgery, and as minimally invasive surgical techniques have been developed, intra-operative image guidance has become became an invaluable tool.[7]

These 3D virtual models can be used to simulate surgery. Using appropriate devices, the surgeon is able to practice surgical techniques using a virtual model and virtual tools. These virtual tools may be used to simulate different actions including cutting, suturing, manipulation and drilling. Exercises can be designed to improve hand–eye coordination and to monitor and measure a trainee's progress and development. Some of these surgical simulators include a haptic feedback mechanism that produces a realistic 'feel' to the tool that is being used. Haptic feedback allows mistakes to be made that are essential to understanding limitations as the exercises can be repeated over and over until the trainee develops the confidence needed to perform surgery on real patients.

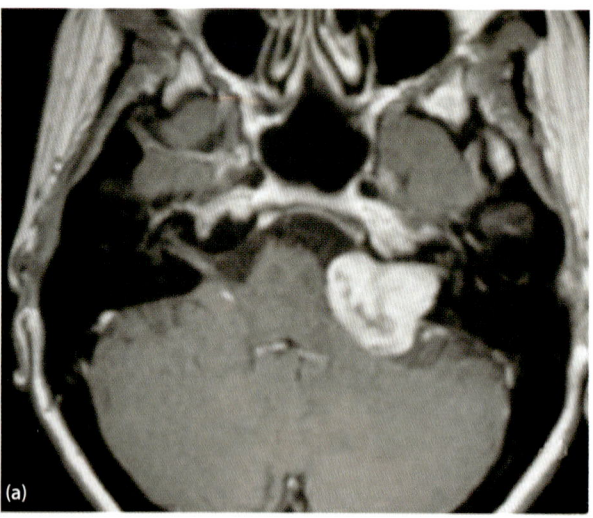

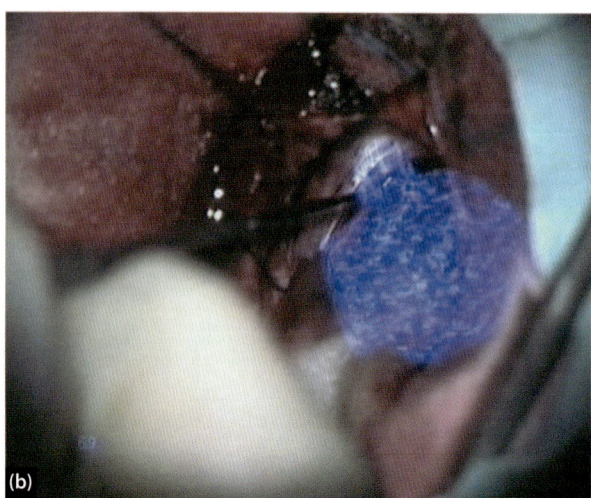

Figure 48.1 Vestibular schwannoma. (a) MR scan; **(b)** intra-operative view through the microscope with the segmented image data overlain on the operative scene.

Trainers are able to monitor progress by reviewing technical data produced by the simulator to enable them to decide whether to progress the trainee on to the next step in their surgical training.

Today's doctors are relaxed and comfortable with using computers in all aspects of their lives and this extends to their surgical practice. The use of 3D models and reconstructions as well as image processing algorithms to enhance images extends to diagnosis and pre-operative surgical planning. It is difficult to imagine a surgeon performing endoscopic sinus surgery without first reviewing a CT scan (with a bone window) of the patient's individual anatomy. The surgeon still has to reconstruct a 3D model, in his or her mind, using these 2D images and their learned and prior knowledge of anatomy. 3D reconstruction removes the guesswork and utilizes all the information to make surgery safer and to provide better training of future surgeons.

Robots have, for some time now, been used by orthopaedic surgeons to perform accurate drilling of the femur and tibia during hip and knee replacement surgery. Urologists now routinely use robots to perform prostatectomy surgery and indeed general surgeons have started to use these robots when performing minimally invasive laparoscopic surgery. ENT as a specialty has now started to use robots in transoral resection of tumours as well as thyroid surgery. The size of the robotic arms prohibits them from being used as an aid in endoscopic sinus surgery, yet it is only a matter of time before these arms are made smaller to facilitate their use as an aid to endoscopic sinus and skull base surgery.

Robots offer several advantages that enable accurate, safer and ultimately better surgery for the patient. They are extremely accurate and, when operated by a surgeon, eliminate tremor. They provide a higher degree of freedom, which enables the surgeons to perform manoeuvres that are not normally possible. The surgeon's hand movement can be magnified or miniaturized to enable extremely small and delicate movements in a small or confined space.[8, 9]

The geometric accuracy of these robots and of the image guidance devices depends, not only on the precision of these instruments, but also the accuracy of the 3D data that are input to represent the patient coordinates. It is also dependent on the accuracy of registration of the data to real-world coordinates, image reconstruction and segmentation, tracking devices and the displays. In the next section we will discuss these components to enable a better understanding of the principles of computer-aided surgery, image navigation and guidance.

IMAGE RECONSTRUCTION

CT and MRI data are acquired on a 2D plane. Sequential 2D images are then stacked to create a 3D volume. The geometric accuracy of the 2D slices is extremely high and in the case of CT is even higher to a resolution as high as 0.2 mm per pixel on a 512 × 512 matrix. The 2D slices can be as thin as 0.5 mm and this, along with slice separation, will affect the resolution in the Z (longitudinal) direction and therefore affect the resolution of the coronal and axial reconstructions. This is also applicable to multislice spiral CT scanners that acquire images in a contiguous manner. These scanners are faster, have a better resolution and expose the patient to less radiation.

Pixels and voxels

Two-dimensional slice sections are composed of pixels, which are the smallest picture elements. The more pixels, the better the resolution. Currently, the highest resolution available for both CT and MRI is 512×512 pixels per image. In a field that is 30×30 cm, this gives a high definition picture, whereas in a larger field this gives a low resolution. By convention, the image resolution is stated by the number of pixels in the x and y axis.

Each pixel has a value ranging, in the case of the CT scan, from −1000 to 3096. This is referred to as Hounsfield units (HU). CT scans are calibrated such that the value of 0 equates to the density of water. By convention, high pixel values are displayed as white. The lower the value, the lower the density of the tissue (X-ray absorption) and the darker the pixel would appear. Pixels are two-dimensional, but it is possible to convert these picture elements into a 3D block. This 3D block is referred to as a voxel or a volumetric picture element. Voxels can be a cube or cuboid depending on the inter-slice distance.

Volume averaging

If a structure falls partially within a pixel, the true value of that structure will then be assigned a value less than the normal value of the structure. In the case of bone, which has a value of say 1000 HU, the value of a pixel that includes a part of that part of the bone will be much less, perhaps 500 HU. This is referred to as partial volume averaging and is a major problem in delineating where the edge of a structure should lie within a given image. Higher resolution images would overcome that problem to some extent. This is not always possible as higher X-ray dosages would be required and an order of magnitude increase in the complexity of the hardware. Algorithms have been developed to overcome this problem and define the edge of a structure with a greater degree of confidence. Each one has its own unique problems and for clinical use in the area of neurosurgery and otorhinolaryngology the accuracy difference is submillimetric and can be ignored.

VISUALIZATION OF IMAGE DATA

Many factors have to be considered when deciding which visualization technique to use. The clinical purpose for which the data are to be used is the most significant and the image data are rendered for that purpose. *Rendering* is the process of generating computer images that represent the three-dimensional anatomy with varying degrees of tissue transparency.[10]

Surface rendering

Optical surface scanners produce structured 3D coordinate point sets that relate to an anatomical surface.[9] Triplets of data points are generally grouped as the vertices of adjacent triangles that interconnect to make up the entire surface. These triangular surface patches are known as facets or polygons.

The rendering of surfaces from volume data requires pre-processing. The properties of voxels containing anatomical surfaces must first be decided and voxels with these properties can then be processed. Usually voxels are considered to lie on a surface if they are connected and all have the same associated property within a given range of values. The derived surfaces are called isosurfaces and are selected to correspond to the surfaces of anatomical structures or to surfaces of equal functional activity.

Geometric primitives are also derived from volumetric data by processes such as contour tracing, surface extraction or boundary following. Alternatively, voxels belonging to anatomical parts may be isolated from the full data set by applying thresholds to the data values associated with them. This extraction of tissue topology has become known as 'segmentation'. The derived geometric primitives (such as polygon meshes or contours) are rendered for display using conventional computer graphics techniques.

Figure 48.2b shows the rendering of a facial surface that is made up of a large set of triangular facets that are also shown in **Figure 48.2a**. This type of image can be produced using data from an optical scan of the face.

Volume rendering can be undertaken for notional surfaces between distinct tissue types. The surface normals are derived directly from the voxel values neighbouring the boundary. These derived surface normals are used for calculating the final image using algorithms. A technique of this sort was used to produce the image depicted in **Figure 48.2c**.

Volume rendering

Volume rendering has become the most commonly used method with which to visualize 3D medical image data. The basic idea is that 3D volumes are composed of voxels and that these are analogues of their 2D counterparts, the pixels. Fine details throughout a volume of interest are displayed, enabling a more direct understanding of visualized data with fewer artefacts.

This visualization technique works by projecting each voxel on to a viewing plane with a value related to the physical property represented in the voxel array. For example, a voxel containing bone with a high X-ray absorption coefficient might be projected with a high value. The most advanced systems allow the operator to construct a look-up table that relates the physical value associated with the voxel to the value it contributes to the image at the chosen viewing plane. A pixel in the viewing plane usually receives contributions from many voxels and the operator may control the manner in which these contributions are composed. For example, the operator may choose to

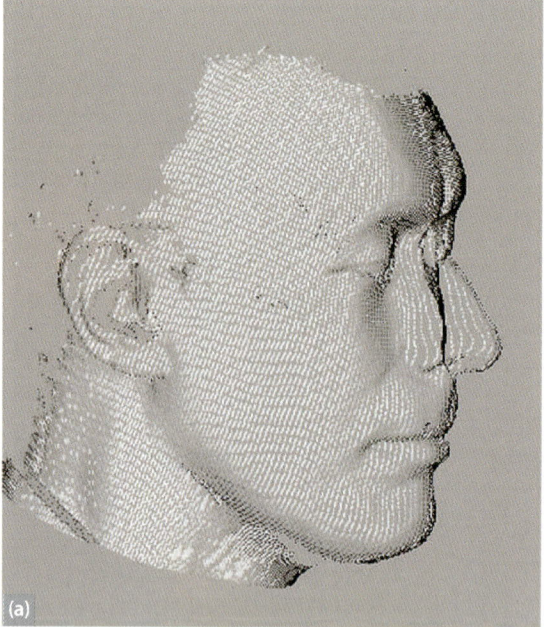
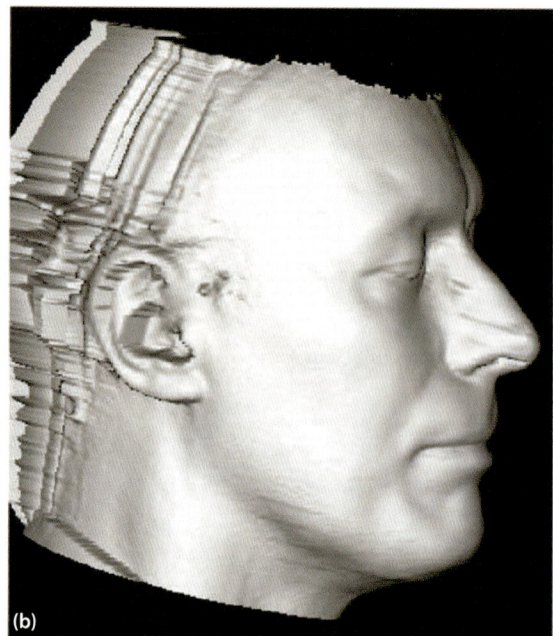
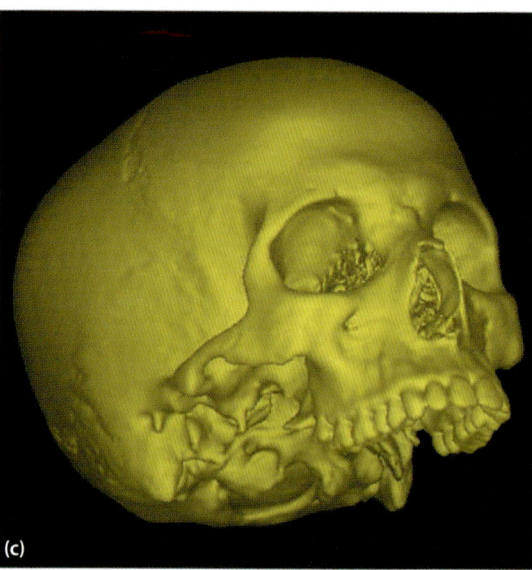

Figure 48.2 **(a)** Wire mesh; **(b)** polygon-rendered; and **(c)** volume surface.

display only the maximum contribution from any voxel along a ray. This produces an image known as the maximum intensity projection (MIP). On the other hand, any individual voxel-associated value may be assigned a maximum opacity value to produce the same images as would be produced by surface rendering.

Figure 48.3 shows two volume-rendered images with different look-up tables. These demonstrate how different anatomical structures may be made visible through others that are being rendered transparent. Major blood vessels, for example, may be effectively rendered visible within the anatomical data set.

Generally, a volume-rendered image appears different from that of a surface-rendered image in that anatomical structures are presented as having some degree of transparency. For some clinical procedures, such as image-guided biopsy or transcutaneous thermal ablation, transparency may greatly enhance depth perception and thus increase the accuracy of the procedure. It is apparent that surfaces are not explicitly rendered, but human perception reconstructs images that are perceived to be in the correct spatial relationship. The transparency that volume rendering offers also enables the placement of surgical instruments within 3D structures with great accuracy.[10]

Registration

Once the patient is secured on the operating table, registration of the Cartesian coordinates of the CT scan to that patient in the theatre is achieved by one of two methods. The first is by locating anatomical landmarks visible both on the patient and image data using a probe that is visible to the tracking device. For example, using navigation

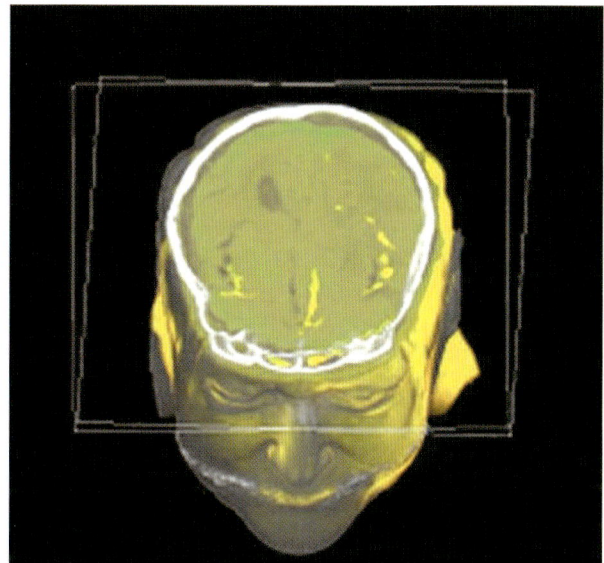

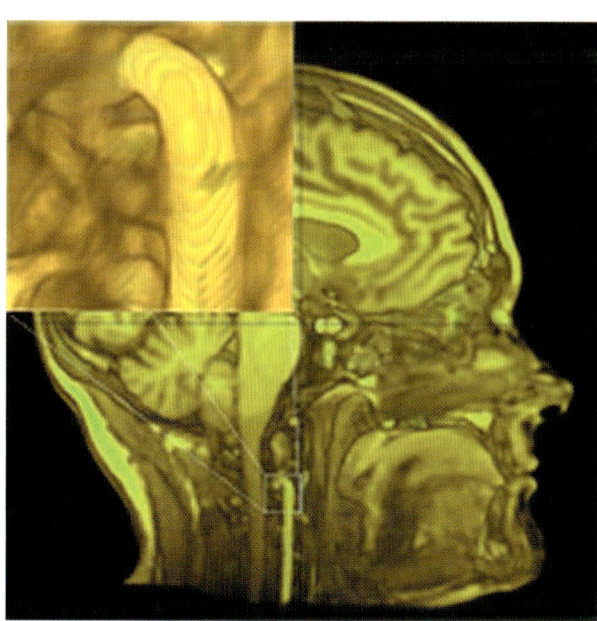

Figure 48.3 Volume-rendered data with different look-up tables.

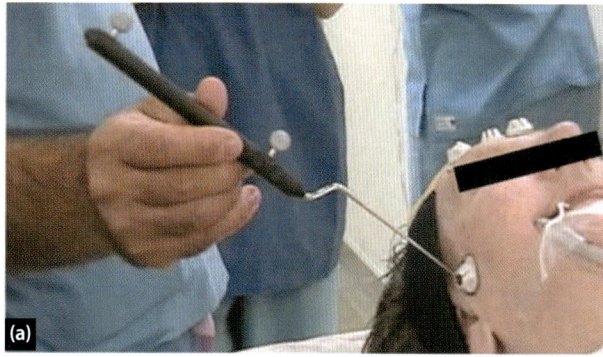

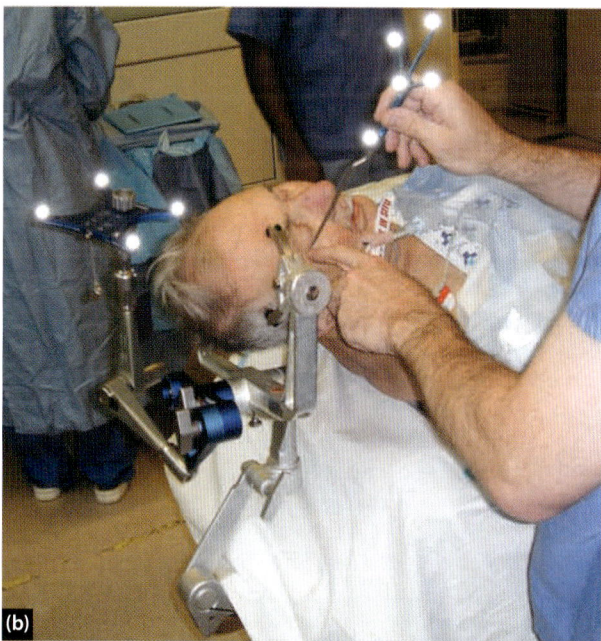

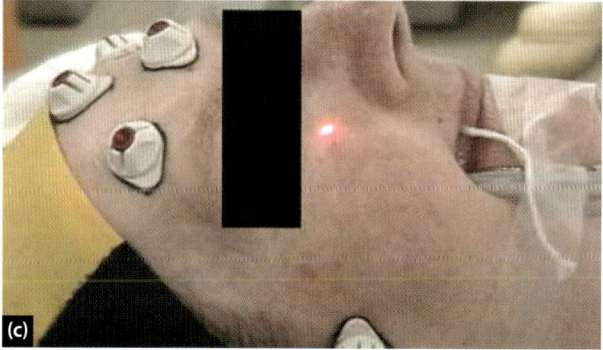

Figure 48.4 **(a)** A laser registration being undertaken before endoscopic sinus surgery; **(b)** the laser beam is shone on to the skin around the operative site; **(c)** a band onto which fiducial balls have been mounted is attached to the patient's head.

software, the surgeon would point to pre-specified landmarks, such as the tragus, outer canthus and nasion. This is usually sufficient to achieve a registration accuracy or error of 3–4 mm. This can then be improved by entering a random sample of points from around the operative region (typically 40–100 points) using the probe. The position of the tip of the probe is identified by the tracking device and the coordinates are fed back to the navigation software. In this way, accuracy/errors of 2–3 mm can be achieved.

Other methods of registration use masks[11] and laser scanning tools (**Figure 48.4**)[12] that speed up the acquisition of surface points. With all these methods, calculations made in real time indicate the point accuracy. It is then up to the surgeon to reject or accept that point in order to improve the overall registration accuracy. Some types of image guided systems make use of fiducial markers that are applied to the patient before scanning on the day of surgery. These markers are clearly visible in both MR and CT data sets and, of course, on the patient when in theatre. They help to improve the accuracy of registration.

No matter whether skin fiducials or anatomical landmarks are used for registration, these reference points should describe or be immediately adjacent to the surgical field. Failure to pay attention to this results in navigational inaccuracies. It is important to realize that the registration error is only a measure of the accuracy of correlation between selected points in the virtual data set and the fiducial markers or anatomical landmarks identified on the patient. It is not synonymous with target error, which is the error that could be expected if a probe was placed on a random point of interest within the surgical field. The target error is influenced by the registration error and is unlikely to be much worse if the target is within the volume described by the fiducial markers. However, if the point is outside that volume, the target error will be proportionately greater.

Tracking

Sensors that provide dynamic positional information are known as 'tracking devices'. They are employed in a multitude of everyday situations that range from virtual reality games, GPS systems, to missile guidance and electronic tagging of prisoners.[13] Although these measurement acquisition systems may be similar, each has different tracking properties that are optimal for a particular application. Without some form of tracking device, it would not be possible to move the patient once they had been registered. In surgical practice, tracking systems must be very precise, consistently accurate, fast enough to provide more than 25 readings per second, and be insensitive to changes in air temperature, unaffected by metal objects and able to track at least two objects simultaneously.

Several tracking systems have been employed over the years. Some of the earliest devices were mechanical arms fitted with potentiometers at every joint. These were fast and accurate but were cumbersome, had a restricted range of movement and hindered the movement of the tracked object to which they had to be attached. Systems based on magnetic field distribution are effective and relatively cheap. However, their disadvantage is that tracking accuracy can be both easily and significantly affected by the presence of metal objects. The quality and accuracy of these types of tracking devices is constantly improving and because there are no line-of-site issues, these are ideal for ENT applications. The latest types of electro-magnetic tracking devices are flexible, again making them ideal for areas that are difficult to reach such as the frontal sinus.

Infrared light sensors are the most commonly used image-guided surgical systems. They are referred to as either active or passive devices. Active devices sense infrared light from light-emitting diodes (LED) attached to the patient or location probe. Passive tracking devices detect infrared light reflected from metallic balls attached to the patient or probe. In the latter case, the infrared light source is situated on the sensing device itself (**Figures 48.5** and **48.6**). In order to detect changes in the patient's head position, haloes or arches with light-emitting diodes or reflective spheres can be fitted to a Mayfield clamp or the patient's head. Systems based on light-emitting diodes are reliable if the light path is not impeded.[14] Within the operating theatre an accuracy of 2–5 mm can usually be achieved.[4] In general, optical tracking systems are expensive. Cheaper variations do exist, but they lack high degrees of accuracy.

Inertial trackers have also been developed that are small and accurate enough for virtual reality applications. These devices generally provide one rate of change of rotational measurement only; hence, a number would be required. They are also not accurate for slow position changes. Systems based on standard ultrasound signals have the potential to achieve much greater accuracy, but are susceptible to changes in temperature and air currents. Other drawbacks include long lag times and interference from echoes and other noises in the environment.

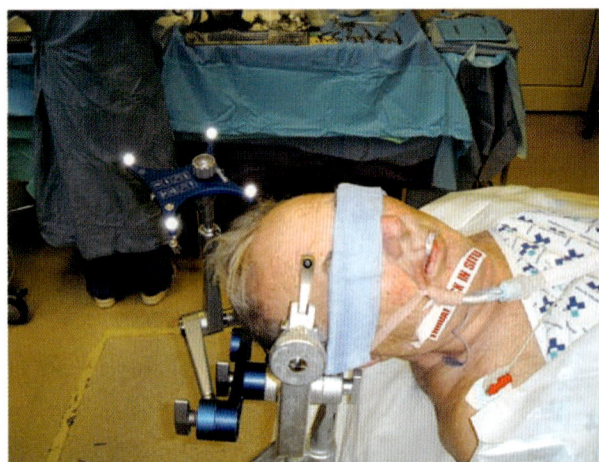

Figure 48.5 A patient with their head held in a Mayfield clamp being prepared for image-guided surgery. An arc with metallic ball fiducials has been attached to the clamp. The arc describes the operative volume. A laser light is being centred on the field to find the optimal position for the tracking device.

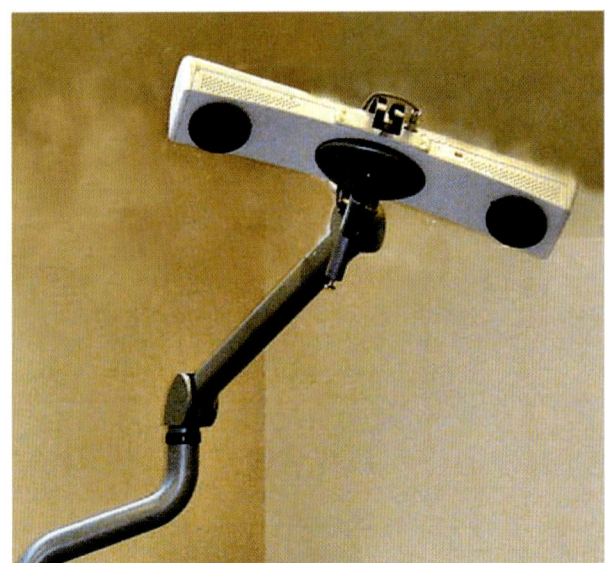

Figure 48.6 An infrared optical tracking system. In the centre of the gantry is a laser light that is used to position the arm during the set-up procedure.

Clinical applications

Image-guided surgery (IGS) offers most promise in the areas of skull base and endoscopic sinus surgery. Skull base surgeons have found this technology particularly useful for pre-operative surgical planning, design of bone flaps, identification of important structures and for finding small tumours in obscure parts. This takes on additional importance when normal anatomy is distorted by disease or anatomical variations.

In rhinology, IGS systems are already in use in difficult revision endoscopic sinus surgery where there are no recognizable anatomical landmarks (**Figure 48.7**).[15] In particular, surgeons have found the guidance systems useful to localize the frontal recess during Draf type 2 and 3 procedures, where the floor of the frontal sinus is to be opened.[16] With the help of these systems, the need to perform open, external procedures will become less. Extended applications of endoscopic sinus surgery include trans-sphenoidal, trans-nasal endoscopic hypophysectomy where conventionally X-ray image intensifiers have been used to localize the sella.[17–19]

In the field of otology, IGS has been used to aid the surgeon in locating the facial nerve, identifying and localizing lesions of the petrous apex[20] and tumours, particularly in the internal auditory meatus. These include meningiomas and vestibular schwannomas.[21, 22] It is possible that when these systems gain in acceptance, are more accurate and involve shorter set-up times, they may become mainstream intra-operative equipment in all types of mastoid surgery. Their role then would be to aid the surgeon in localizing important anatomical structures such as the facial nerve, dura, brain and jugular bulb, as well as diseases such as cholesteatoma and acoustic schwannoma.

Surgical planning

Surgical planning is usually carried out in the surgeon's mind, drawing on past experience, knowledge of anatomy and anatomical variation. Some individuals are able to do this very well, others are not. In endoscopic sinus surgery, the surgeon must have the ability to think in 3D, having studied the information available from 2D CT slices.

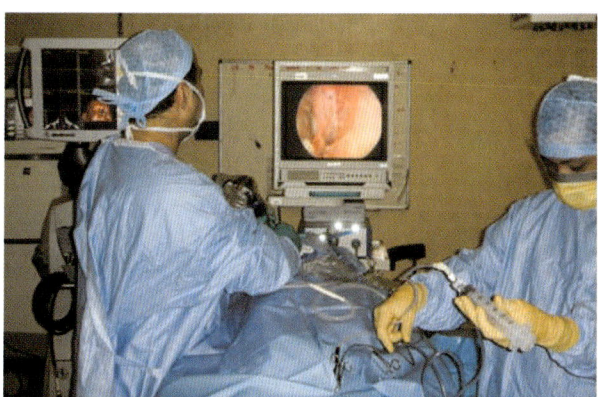

Figure 48.7 Functional endoscopic surgery being undertaken using image guidance.

Surgeons may or may not be able to communicate their impressions to other surgeons. Furthermore, their mental image cannot be reviewed, audited or measured by other surgeons or indeed by the surgeon themselves when assessing patients at a later date. Planning using reconstructed 3D data enables the surgeon to assess the patient's anatomy objectively, to communicate this with other surgeons and to review these films at a later date. The data can be segmented and manipulated to familiarize the surgeon with specific features pertinent to that patient and the procedure to be performed.

Surgical simulation

The major driving force behind the development of surgical simulators was the morbidity that accompanied the introduction of new techniques such as endoscopic 'keyhole' surgery. These techniques were conceptually different from traditional surgery. Surgeons had to operate using a 2D image on a television monitor and had to develop new hand–eye coordination skills not previously required for open surgery. Training surgeons in these new skills and the assessment of their competence was entirely different from the 'apprentice–master' approach that had been the mainstay of traditional surgical teaching. Three-dimensional reconstructions of image data can be used for surgical simulation. Simulators that create a virtual surgical environment or a set of tasks that enhance hand–eye coordination skills seem to be the answer.[23, 24]

Surgical simulators are now being developed and employed in other surgical specialties, for example skull base surgery. They are being used by trainees and experienced surgeons who might find it useful to practise a specific difficult surgical technique before performing the actual operation. Surgeons are able to 'virtually' manipulate, move and drill the mastoid process, to perform laparoscopic or endoscopic sinus procedures. The sensations and resistance encountered during real surgery may be simulated using positive feedback mechanisms in the form of a passive robotic arm.

IMAGE-GUIDED SURGERY

A thorough knowledge of anatomy is essential for all types of surgery, particularly those using microscopes and endoscopes. Pre-operative imaging alerts the surgeon to variations of anatomy that are either inherent in the patient or caused by a disease process or previous surgery. As stated before, image guidance offers the surgeon the ability to use the patient's image data intra-operatively to determine position, distance to vital organs and other anatomical features that might be hidden from direct vision. Structures in the vicinity of the skull base are either embedded or closely adherent to bone, making this region ideal for image guidance as CT has great spatial accuracy.

Two fundamental processes are required for intra-operative image guidance, registration and tracking. Registration is the process that relates the patient in the operating theatre to pre-operatively acquired image data sets. Tracking is the mechanism of following the position of the patient or an instrument within the operative field. Both processes are potentially subject to significant mathematical error and it is vital that how this might happen is fully appreciated.

> **FUTURE RESEARCH**
>
> - Image-guided and augmented reality surgery relies heavily on technology research in the areas of computer hardware (processors, graphics and tracking) and software for segmentation and registration. Developments in these fields are driven by a variety of customer-driven demands. It is vital that clinicians make these demands and provide ideas for the computer scientists.
> - The most important requirements are for accurate, robust, fail-safe systems that will give clinicians greater confidence. These systems must be user-friendly and ergonomically efficient. Computer user interface remains the biggest deterrent to regular use of these systems. These need to be simplified and easy to operate. Surgeons will eventually develop trust in the accuracy of these systems.
> - In the future, we are likely to see more developments in the areas of surgical simulation and planning. Surgical training should benefit from simulators that will enable the trainee to develop their hand–eye coordination skills prior to applying them in clinical practice.
> - At present, augmented reality still has to prove its position in surgical practice. Several research groups are producing encouraging results and future reliance on these types of systems is likely to replace traditional IGS systems.
> - Robots are already being used for drilling in the field of orthopaedics and to manoeuvre and control cameras in laparoscopic surgery. These are far more accurate than humans and are likely to enter other fields of surgery where there is a reliance on power instrumentation, including drills and debriders.
> - In the future, we are likely to use IGS systems to audit surgical procedures as they already have the inherent capacity to store all information relating to intra-operative navigation. This will be an invaluable and auditable operative record.

> **KEY POINTS**
>
> - IGS aids the surgeon in diagnosing the extent of disease, planning surgery and providing intra-operative positional information.
> - Image-guided surgical techniques may reduce complications in endoscopic sinus surgery.
> - IGS techniques offer greater accuracy and confidence in structure and disease localization.
> - Major applications are skull base and revision nasal surgery where there is complex or distorted anatomy.

REFERENCES

1. Guildenberg PL. General concepts of stereotactic surgery. In: Guildenberg PL (ed.) *Modern stereotactic neurosurgery*. Boston: Martinus Nijhof; 1988.
2. Herman GT, Liu HK. Three-dimensional display of human organs from computed tomograms. *Comput Vision Graph* 1979; **9**: 1–21.
3. Linney AD, Tan AC, Richards R, et al. The use of three dimension data on human body for diagnosis and surgical planning. *Rec Neuroradiol* 1992; **5**: 483–88.
4. Vannier MW, Marsh JL, Warren JO. Three-dimensional computer graphics for craniofacial surgical planning and evaluation. *ACM SIGGRAPH Comp Graph Quart* 1983; **17**: 263–73.
5. Edwards PJ, Hawkes DJ, Hill DL, et al. Augmentation of reality using an operating microscope for otolaryngology and neurosurgical guidance. *J Image Guided Surg* 1995; **1**: 172–78.
6. Lapeer RJ, Tan AC, Alusi G, Linney AD. Computer-assisted surgery and planning using augmented reality (CASSPAR): visualisation and calibration. In: *2003 IEEE/ACM International Symposium on Mixed and Augmented Reality*. Washington: IEEE Computer Society; 2005, pp. 272–73.
7. Olson G, Citardi MJ. Image-guided functional endoscopic sinus surgery. *Otolaryng Head Neck* 2000; **123**: 188–94.
8. Davies B. Jakopec M, Harris SJ, et al. Active-constraint robotics for surgery. *Proc IEEE* 2006; **94**(9): 1696–1704.
9. Kienzle III TC, Stulberg SD, Peshkin MA, et al. A computer-assisted total knee replacement surgical system using a calibrated robot. In: Taylor RH, Lavallée S, Burdea GS, Mösges R (eds). *Computer integrated surgery*. Cambridge, MA: MIT Press; 1996, pp. 409–16.
10. Linney AD, Alusi GH. Clinical applications of computer aided visualization. *J Visual* 1998; **1**(1): 95–109.
11. Albritton FD, Kingdom TT, DelGaudio JM. Malleable registration mask: application of a novel registration method in image guided sinus surgery. *Am J Rhinol* 2001; **15**: 219–24.
12. Raabe A, Krishnan R, Wolff R, et al. Laser surface scanning for patient registration in intracranial image-guided surgery. *Neurosurgery* 2002; **50**: 797–801; discussion 802–03.
13. Watanabe K, Kobayashi K, Munekata F. Multiple sensor fusion for navigation systems vehicle navigation and information systems. In: *Vehicle navigation and information systems conference, 1994 proceedings*. Washington: IEEE Computer Society; 1994, pp. 575–78.
14. Azuma R, Bishop G. Improving static and dynamic registration in an optical see-through HMD. In: *Proceedings of the 21st annual conference on computer graphics and interactive techniques*. New York: ACM Press; 1994, pp. 197–204.
15. Metson R. Image-guided sinus surgery: lessons learned from the first 1000 cases. *Otolaryng Head Neck* 2003; **128**: 8–13.
16. Neumann Jr AM, Pasquale-Niebles K, Bhuta T, Sillers MJ. Image-guided transnasal endoscopic surgery of the paranasal sinuses and anterior skull base. *Am J Rhinol* 1999; **13**: 449–54.
17. Otori N, Haruna S, Yoshiyuki M, Moriyama H. Endoscopic endonasal surgery with image-guidance. *Nippon Jibiinkoka Gakkai Kaiho* 2000; **103**: 1–6.
18. Kajiwara K, Nishizaki T, Ohmoto Y, et al. Image-guided transsphenoidal surgery for pituitary lesions using Mehrkoordinaten Manipulator (MKM) navigation system. *Minim Invas Neurosur* 2003; **46**: 78–81.
19. Sandeman D, Moufid A. Interactive image-guided pituitary surgery: an experience of 101 procedures. *Neurochirurgie* 1998; **44**: 331–38.

20. Van-Havenbergh T, Koekelkoren E, De-Ridder D, et al. Image guided surgery for petrous apex lesions. *Acta Neurochir* 2003; **145**: 737–42; discussion 742.
21. Sargent EW, Bucholz RD. Middle cranial fossa surgery with image-guided instrumentation. *Otolaryng Head Neck* 1997; **117**: 131–34.
22. Klimek L, Mosges R, Schlondorff G, Mann W. Development of computer-aided surgery for otorhinolaryngology. *Comput Aided Surg* 1998; **3**: 194–201.
23. Caversaccio M, Eichenberger A, Hausler R. Virtual simulator as a training tool for endonasal surgery. *Am J Rhinol* 2003; **17**: 283–90.
24. Bockholt U, Muller W, Voss G, et al. Real-time simulation of tissue deformation for the nasal endoscopy simulator (NES). *Comput Aided Surg* 1999; **4**: 281–85.

CHAPTER 49

INTERVENTIONAL TECHNIQUES

James V. Byrne

Introduction 569	Embolization for specific tumours 572
Indications 569	Embolization for epistaxis 576
Tools and techniques 570	References 578
Application of embolization techniques 571	

SEARCH STRATEGY

Data in this chapter may be updated by a Medline search using the keywords: interventional neuroradiology, endovascular therapy, embolization, meningioma, paraganglioma, epistaxis, tumour embolization.

INTRODUCTION

This chapter reviews the role of interventional neuroradiology (INR) in the management of patients with pathologies of the head and neck and describes common techniques. Endovascular embolization originated in surgery when Brooks[1] closed a cavernous-carotid fistula with a muscle embolus introduced by arteriotomy in 1930. The need for vascular imaging to monitor embolization was obvious, but the capacity developed slowly after the first description of cerebral angiography by Egas Moniz in 1927.[2] As a result, embolization for head and neck pathologies is generally performed in Neuroradiology departments.

Endovascular embolization is the most common technique. It is used to treat arterio-venous shunts, devascularize tumours and close large arteries prior to surgical resections. But also included in the INR repertoire are percutaneous techniques for embolization of vascular malformations and tumours, image guided biopsy and focused endovascular delivery of chemotherapy agents. The technologically driven evolution of the discipline will almost certainly produce new methods and applications to replace more invasive surgery in the future.

INDICATIONS

MR or CT scanning is usually adequate for diagnosis and pre-operative assessment of head and neck lesions so digital subtraction angiography (DSA) is rarely needed unless there is a possible role for INR. Combining embolization using DSA means that the indications for INR techniques should be considered early in treatment planning. This process involves considering a lesion's blood supply as well as its extent and relationship to normal structures. Pre-operative embolization may be indicated and information about adjacent major vessels may be vital, either because of tumour proximity or because their sacrifice may be a necessary component of the surgical approach or resection.

Embolization of vascular tumours is indicated prior to surgical resection to reduce intra-operative blood loss, operation times and facilitate complete resection. It can be considered as the definitive intervention in patients with minimal symptoms in whom surgery is contraindicated. It may also be indicated as palliative treatment to relieve pain for patients when surgery, radiotherapy or chemotherapy are unsuitable or to manage haemorrhage or increasing neurological symptoms. It is most effective in tumours with high blood flows. In most instances this can be inferred from the degree of contrast enhancement evident on CT or MR scanning but it should be remembered that the uptake of radiographic contrast within a tissue reflects the degree of extravascular leakage of these agents and not necessarily the blood supply. So occasionally tumours showing pronounced enhancement are not suitable for embolization.

Embolization is targeted to occlude the smaller arteries of the tumour vascular bed since the proximal occlusion of arteries is a relatively ineffective method of causing tumour necrosis and/or regression.

Large artery occlusions are sometimes indicated as pre-operative manoeuvres and rarely for tumour palliation. Emergency embolization may be required to manage tumour haemorrhage.

Functional testing by temporary vessel occlusion is indicated prior to endovascular ligations and may be useful when surgical resections are likely to require the ligation of a large artery or vein. Blood flow in the target vessel is occluded by inflating a balloon with the patient awake so that neurological examination can be performed and collateral blood flows can be assessed by DSA. Permanant occlusion by endovascular ligation is performed after a satisfactory test. The potential of INR to access lesions under imaging control, either using highly flexible endovascular microcatheters or by direct puncture, can also be exploited for the selective delivery of drugs for sclerotherapy, chemotherapy or functional tests of nerve function using sedative agents, such as barbituates (in brain) or lignocaine (in spine).

The decision to perform an INR procedure depends on clinical and anatomical factors. These should be reviewed in multidisciplinary consultations between the treating otolaryngologist (or other specialist) and interventional neuroradiologist. For pre-operative embolization, the guiding principle is that an additional INR procedure should not add to the management's overall risk. This risk/benefit analysis may require information that can only be obtained at the time of DSA. Therefore close cooperation and a team approach is needed, to ensure that the risks of complications caused by embolization or pre-operative invasive functional tests are acceptable and are justified because they are likely to improve the outcome of subsequent surgery. These issues, as they apply to specific tumour types, and the use of embolization in the management of epistaxis, will be discussed below. The purpose and potential benefits of INR techniques are summarized in **Table 49.1**.

TOOLS AND TECHNIQUES

Endovascular catheters

The catheters used for transarterial or transvenous catheterization are available in a range of sizes and shapes. They are used to select and inject radiographic contrast media in cranial vessels for angiography or as guiding catheters for smaller catheters used for the selection of small vessels (i.e. microcatheters). Microcatheters are generally 0.02 inches (0.5 mm) or smaller in diameter and are used to inject embolization materials. They are constructed with flexible distal ends for navigation through tortuous vessels and stiffer proximal sections to allow the operator to advance them by pushing.

Two basic types of microcatheter are used: flow directed and over-the-wire catheters. The former have extremely light and supple distal ends so that they are carried by antegrade blood flow to the target position. The latter are pushed over a guide wire to the objective. Flow directed catheters work best when blood flow is increased and are therefore used to treat arteriovenous shunts. Their size limits their use to the injection of liquids or very small particles. Over-the-wire catheters are used when blood flow is slower. The combination of guide wire and a stiffer catheter makes navigation easier and their larger lumen allows the delivery of liquids and both particles or coils. They are usually used in the treatment of head and neck tumours.

Materials used for embolization

PARTICLES

Embolic agents can be categorized on various criteria. Traditionally, they are divided according to whether the resulting devascularization is permanent or temporary. Examples of temporary agents are autologous blood clot, gelfoam powder and microfibrillar collagen, which are biodegradable, whilst particles manufactured from non-degradable materials are considered permanent agents (**Table 49.2**). However, the effectiveness of embolization using non-degradable particles is liable to be temporary because small vessel occlusions may be circumvented by the development of new collateral vessels.[3, 4] In practice, the development of a new blood supply is likely given time but is less likely if particles can be deposited in small vessels within the tumour bed rather than in proximal arteries. To ensure the deep penetration of injected particles, they are engineered to mix well with radiographic contrast so that they can be injected as an even suspension. Non-degradable particles in current use are made of polyvinyl alcohol (PVA),[5] trisacryl gelatin[6] or cellulose porous beads,[7] which are coated or mixed with radiographic contrast material to make them radioopaque and visible on X-ray fluoroscopy. They are available in sizes varying between 40–800 microns in diameter. The choice

TABLE 49.1 Interventional neuroradiology techniques and their uses		
Procedure	Technique	Purpose/benefit
Biopsy	Percutaneous needle	Histology and treatment selection
Functional testing	Temporary balloon occlusion	Assessment of collateral blood supply prior to surgical or endovascular ligations
Embolization of small vessels	Particle, liquid embolics, sclerosants	Devascularization of tumour to reduce operative blood loss, palliation or cure
Embolization of large vessels	Balloon, coils, plug devices, liquid embolics, sclerosants	To aid surgical exposure/dissection, palliation or cure
Chemotherapy	Endovascular or intra-lesion injection	To maximize drug delivery to the lesion

TABLE 49.2 Embolic agents

Agent	Embolization	Target vessels
Autologous blood clot	Temporary	Afferent arteries
Gelfoam	Temporary	Afferent arteries
Polyvinyl alcohol particles	Permanent	Tumour vessels
Trisacryl gelatin particles	Permanent	Tumour vessels
Coils	Permanent	Large arteries/veins
Balloons	Permanent	Large arteries
Alcohol (ethanol)	Permanent	Malformations or tumour vessels
Sodium tetradecyl sulphate	Permanent	Malformations or tumour vessels
Cyanoacrylate adhesives (NBCA)	Permanent	Malformations or tumour vessels
Ethylene vinyl alcohol copolymer (Onyx)	Permanent	Malformations or tumour vessels

of particle size is important because, though smaller particles will penetrate to smaller vessels, they are more likely to pass through arteriovenous shunts and reach the lungs. They are also more likely to cause ischaemic damage to normal tissues. On the other hand larger particles occlude proximal arteries and achieve less reliable tumour devascularization.[8]

The effect of PVA or gelatin particles on tissues is to cause an initial acute inflammatory response, which is followed by a chronic foreign body reaction within weeks.[4,9] Devascularization causes ischaemia and necrosis within hours, which in turn causes tumours to swell (exacerbating symptoms and causing pain) or haemorrhage. For this reason pre-operative embolization is often performed immediately prior to operation.

COILS AND BALLOONS

Embolization coils are made from steel, tungsten or platinum. Because of problems of corrosion, tungsten is generally no longer used and platinum, though expensive, is preferred because it is inert and not liable to magnetization effects during MRI. A new development is to enhance their effect by adding a thrombogenic coating. The materials used include collagen, bioabsorbable polymers and dacron fibres.[10] Originally coils were simply pushed through a delivery catheter and could not be retrieved or repositioned. Retrievable coils with controlled delivery are now standard. There are various methods for controlling their detachment from a delivery wire. These include couplings released by mechanical or hydrostatic pressure, electrolysis or thermal heating.[11]

Balloons are made of latex or silicone.[12] They are either fixed to a catheter tip for temporary test occlusions or can be detached for vessel occlusion. They are inflated by injecting fluid; usually radiographic contrast media. Detachable balloons are released mechanically from a delivery microcatheter but their detachment is less reliable than the newer methods developed for coils. In many centres they have been superseded by coils.

Coils or balloons are used for large artery occlusion (i.e. endovascular ligations), usually after a satisfactory temporary balloon occlusion test. High blood flow fistulas are occluded with coils or balloons positioned at the point of transition between artery and vein. The delivery of coils is easier to control than balloons and they can be positioned more accurately. They are used to embolize large veins or dural sinuses in order to close dural arteriovenous fistulas (DAVF) and less often for tumour embolizations.

LIQUID EMBOLIC AGENTS

Various liquids are used for embolization including sclerosants, adhesives and soluble plastics. They have the advantage over coils and particles of being injectable via smaller lumen catheters or needles. Most commonly used are quick-setting adhesives and polymers. Examples of liquid agents are the tissue adhesive N-butyl-2-cyanoacrylate (NBCA) and ethylene-vinyl alcohol copolymer (EVAL). There are various commercial formulations available (e.g. NBCA marketed as Histoacryl and Glubran, and EVAL marketed as Onyx).[13,14] NBCA thickens and sets on exposure to blood and copolymers set after injection as the solvent (e.g. dimethyl sulfoxide) in which they are dissolved disperses. Both agents are liable to embed the delivery catheter within vessels and require considerable expertise to deliver safely, but they are generally regarded as producing the most permanent form of embolization. They are therefore preferentially used for definitive or palliative treatments as well as for pre-operative embolization. Sclerosants such as ethanol or sodium tetradecyl sulphate are used to treat facial vascular malformations, bleomycin is effective in certain types of low flow vascular malformations[15] and mannitol has been used to embolize meningiomas.[16]

APPLICATION OF EMBOLIZATION TECHNIQUES

Tumour embolization

TRANSARTERIAL

Embolization of tumours of the head and neck is most often performed to reduce blood loss and facilitate surgical resection or for palliation. It is rarely curative. Pre-operative embolization is performed for vascular tumours such as meningioma,[9,11,17] haemangioblastoma, juvenile nasopharyngeal angiofibroma,[18] schwannoma and paraganglioma[19] (Table 49.3). Pre-operative functional evaluations by temporary balloon occlusion of at-risk major arteries can also be performed. Pre-operative embolization is largely reserved for extra-axial intra-cranial tumours and only rarely are highly vascular intra-axial CNS tumours, such as haemangioblastoma, treated.

Pre-operative transarterial embolization is usually performed with PVA particles (sized to occlude the pathological circulation) or liquid agents (e.g. NBCA or Onyx).[20]

TABLE 49.3 Head, neck and skull base tumours treated by embolization

Commonly treated tumours	Less frequently treated tumours
Meningioma	Schwannoma
Paraganglioma	Carcinoid
Juvenile angiofibroma	Alveolar sarcoma
Haemangiopericytoma	Thyroid carcinoma
	Granular cell myoblastoma
	Capillary haemangioma
	Esthesioneuroblastoma
	Neurinoma

Liquid agents can also be injected directly into tumours (see below). Serious procedural complications occur in about 4% of patients and these include cranial nerve palsies (including blindness), stroke due to unrecognized spread of emboli and induced bleeding due to vessel perforation or secondary to tissue necrosis.[21] Complicating cranial nerve palsies are more common when very small particles or NBCA are used.[22] Though technically relatively straightforward, safe embolization of skull base lesions should only be undertaken after adequate training. Safe embolization demands a sound knowledge of vascular anatomy and the potential sites of spontaneous external to internal carotid artery or vertebral artery anastomoses, if cerebral or spinal migration of emboli is to be avoided.[23]

PERCUTANEOUS EMBOLIZATION

This technique involves the injection of a liquid embolic or sclerosant directly into tumour vessels. The objective is to devascularize tumours before surgical resection or for palliation of symptoms by causing tumour involution. Pre-operative embolization is usually performed following percutaneous puncture but perioperative needling can be performed. The technique was first used to devascularize hypervascular juvenile angiofibromas[24] but has also been used to treat haemangiopericytoma and paraganglioma.[25,26] The technique is particularly attractive for the management of recurrent lesions and has been reported to achieve total or near-total tumour devascularization.[27]

Delivery of chemotherapy agents

Selective catheterization allows endovascular delivery of chemotherapy drugs directly into tumours to maximize the local dose. Direct puncture of tumour vessels under X-ray or ultrasound imaging is an alternative. The objective is to deliver higher doses in the target tumour whilst avoiding systemic toxic symptoms. The amount of drug delivered to a tumour is proportional to its rate of plasma clearance within the tissue and inversely related to tumour plasma flow.[28] Selective catheterization allows the delivery rate to be fine-tuned to the prevailing rate of blood flow. This benefit has been used in studies of local chemotherapy for cancers of the head and neck, specifically advanced squamous cell carcinomas.[29] Combination therapies with radiotherapy, for example RADPLAT, have been effective at inducing remission and Kumar and Robbins[30] recently reviewed their use. The systemic toxic effects of Cisplatin can be mitigated by the simultaneous intravenous administration of its competitive antagonist thiosulphate. Despite logistical problems associated with catheterization and long infusion times, preliminary trials have shown the technique to be effective at causing tumour shrinkage.[31]

Temporary and permanent large artery occlusions

Temporary endovascular occlusion of large arteries prior to head and neck surgery allows neurological testing of the awake patient and angiographic assessment of the consequences of vessel sacrifice.

There are many described protocols for temporary artery occlusion and dynamic testing. Only two elements are common to all: that the procedure is performed under local anaesthesia so that the patient is accessible for neurological examination; and that anticoagulants are given. Test occlusion involves inflating a balloon in the target artery for 20–30 minutes and assessing the effect on cerebral blood flow. The adequacy of collateral blood flow to the territory of the occluded vessel can be demonstrated by angiography, Doppler ultrasound, xenon CT, single photon emission computed tomography (SPECT) and positron emission tomography (PET) scanning. Additional provocative testing can be performed by simultaneously lowering the systemic blood pressure or administering a vasodilator drug such as acetazolamide.[32] All these techniques are designed to improve the reliability of the test but the lack of a consensus protocol testifies to the fact that there remains a risk of the collateral blood flow being inadequate, despite normal test data.

It is generally accepted that preliminary testing reduces the risk of delayed stroke, but its value depends on risk posed by the test. Reported rates of morbidity come largely from audits of its use in aneurysm patients.[33, 34] Amongst patients undergoing ligation for skull base tumours, rates for complications range between 5% and 20%.[35] The additional risks faced by cancer patients was documented in a single institution report, which found the complication rate to be 10% whilst that of aneurysm patients was only 3%.[36] Following a satisfactory period of temporary occlusion, the artery is permanently occluded by detaching the balloon or replacing it with embolization coils. Some practitioners prefer the latter because the detachment systems for coils are more reliable. It is obviously important that permanent occlusion is performed at the same arterial level (i.e. at the same place) as the test occlusion.

EMBOLIZATION FOR SPECIFIC TUMOURS

The commonly treated tumour types will be described in detail to illustrate the goals of INR in the management of patients with tumours of the skull base and neck.

Meningioma

These typically benign tumours originate from arachnoid cap cells found in arachnoid granulations. They therefore arise in continuity with dura. Though generally intracranial they are found at extra-cranial sites by extension from a dural origin or rarely occur entirely extra-cranially (presumably from ectopic dural rests). Thus tumours may involve the skull base, orbit and cervical spine or the upper neck. They occur in middle age, affect women twice as commonly as men and are linked to a genetic deficit on chromosome 22. Multiple lesions occur in patients with neurofibromatosis II and meningiomatosis.[37,38] Associations have been reported with exposure to ionizing radiation[39] and hormonal influences due to the presence of androgen and other hormone receptors.[38] They may be locally invasive and the WHO classification of histological findings recognizes three grades (grade 1 – benign, grade 2 – atypical and grade 3 – anaplastic), which are independent of the traditional histopathological descriptions of meningothelial, fibrous, transitional, syncytial and psammomatous subtypes. They are usually highly vascular tumours with the transitional subtype being most vascular and the psammomatous subtype least vascular.

Clinical presentation varies according to location and imaging by CT scan or MRI is usually adequate for diagnosis and pre-operative assessment. Tumour calcification and skull hyperostosis is easier to recognize on CT than MRI and suggests a less vascular subtype. Enlarged vessels within or adjacent to more vascular tumour are easier to see on MRI. Tumour enhancement after intravenous contrast media administration is typical and is more avid in vascular tumours, but such enhancement does not imply that a particular lesion is suitable for embolization.

Treatment is by resection, and radiotherapy is reserved for more aggressive histological types. Pre-operative embolization in indicated for vascular tumours and for the palliation of inoperable newly diagnosed or recurrent tumours. Intra-arterial angiography is required to assess the extent of tumour vascularity and therefore the potential of embolization. In a minority of tumours, dense calcification on CT or lack of enhancement after contrast media administration, imply a less vascular tumour and that embolization will not contribute to management but the majority warrant angiography to select tumours likely to benefit from embolization.

The vascular supply to meningioma seen on DSA is typically arranged in a radial pattern of dilated feeding arteries of decreasing size with a delayed venous phase of contrast passage (often termed a 'blush') through the tumour bed. Arterial supply may be from external carotid artery branches or from dural or trans-pial branches of the internal carotid artery or a mixture of the two (**Figure 49.1**). The endovascular therapist therefore needs a detailed pre-embolization DSA to evaluate the feasibility (and risks) associated with superselective catheterization and embolization. In practice treatment and diagnostic DSA are usually combined in the same session and scheduled as part of the patient's overall treatment plan.

A universal need for pre-resection embolization is controversial and patients are usually selected on a case-by-case basis after multidisciplinary review. The goal is to reduce operative blood loss and facilitate complete resection. It may be performed using particles (e.g. PVA), or liquid embolic agents (e.g. NBCA or Onyx). Since the typical blood supply is by arteries and arterioles of gradually reducing size, small particles (for example, 150 microns) are used first to obstruct intra-tumour vessels and larger particles injected subsequently to obstruct larger afferent arteries (**Figure 49.1**). Effective embolization will cause acute tumour infarction and swelling. The optimum timing of subsequent operation is debatable; the argument for early operation is that symptoms due to swelling or haemorrhage are avoided whilst for delayed surgery that operative blood loss is lessened and surgery facilitated.[40] If operation is delayed then steps must be taken to ensure that worsening neurological symptoms or signs are quickly detected and treated. Rarely, tumour necrosis causes bleeding and life threatening expansion of tumours. Prolonged delay risks revascularization, due to growth of vessels and new blood supply to the meningioma, which can occur within as short a period as 3–4 weeks after particulate embolization.

Another indication for meningioma embolization is to arrest or impede tumour growth when lesions are inoperable and radiotherapy inappropriate.[41] In theory, particles delivered into the tumour bed only, will cause tissue ischaemia/necrosis without stimulating growth of collateral blood vessels. In this situation, very small particles (50 microns) are injected slowly and no attempt is made to obstruct larger feeding arteries. Tumour devascularization and shrinkage is monitored by MRI enhanced by intravenous gadolinium administration. Areas of non-enhancement imply devascularization (**Figure 49.3f**).

The efficacy of pre-operative embolization is difficult to objectively evaluate. Criteria used in reported studies include comparisons of blood transfusion volumes between tumour resection operations performed with or without pre-operative embolization, surgery times, lengths of hospital stay, extent of tumour necrosis and clinical outcomes. A reduced need for blood transfusion was reported by Teasdale et al.[42] and Oka et al.,[43] shorter lengths of hospital admission by Dean et al.[44] and Oka et al.,[43] and improved clinical results by Oka et al.[43] when adjuvant embolization was performed. A reduction in neurological complications after surgery was reported by Oka et al.[43] but this benefit was only evident for patients with large tumours (greater than 6 cm in diameter). Delaying surgery until 7 days or more after embolization is associated with lower blood transfusion volumes[45] and greater induced tumour necrosis.[46] The conduct and evaluation of such studies is difficult because of the variations in size and site of the tumours studied.

Several specific complications have been reported after meningioma embolization due to inadvertant occlusion of vessels supplying normal tissues, the effects of tumour swelling and haemorrhage. Intra-tumoural haemorrhage resulting from devascularization may occur 24–36 hours after embolization. In the author's practice, this complication has occurred once in 40 treatments over the

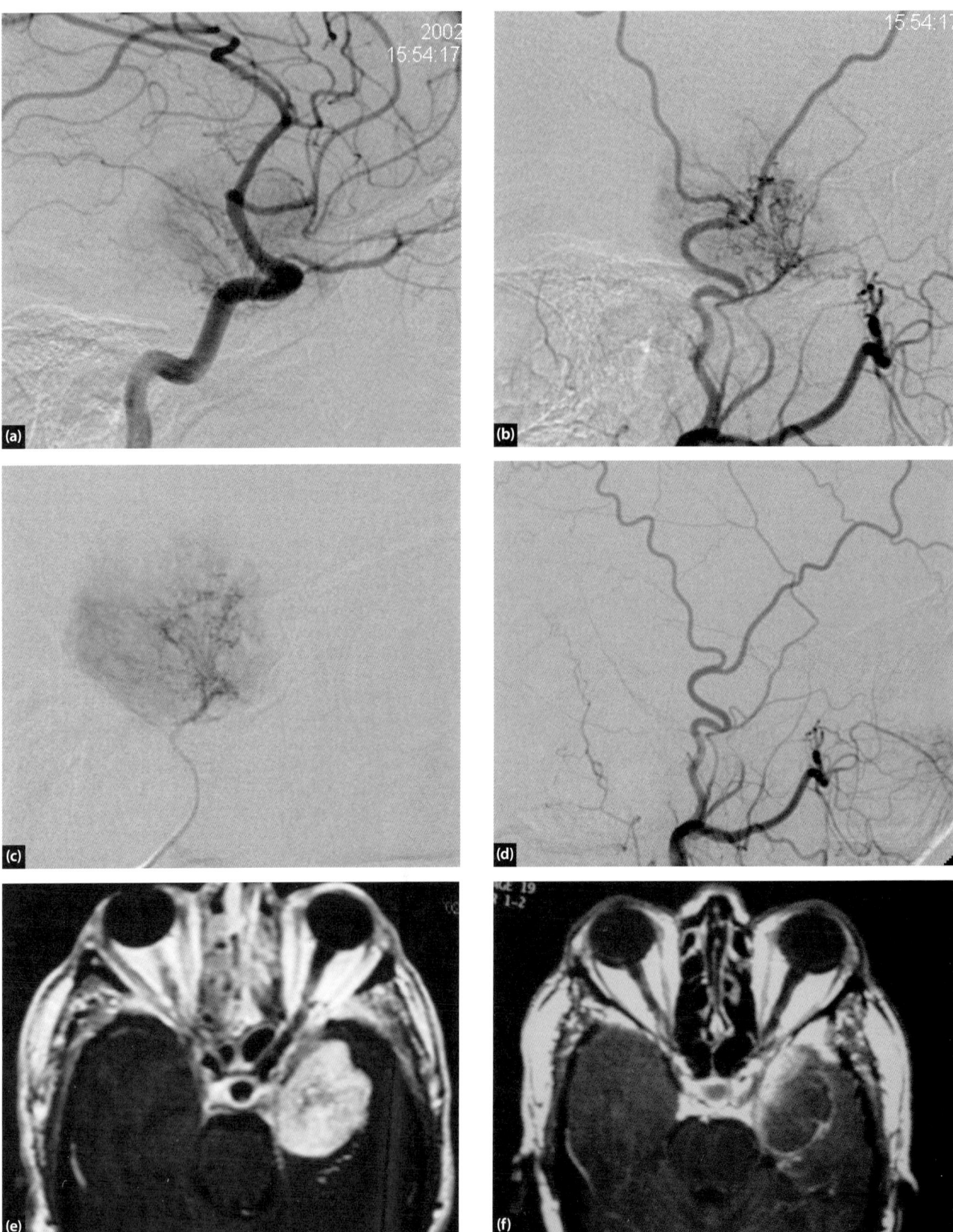

Figure 49.1 Parasellar meningioma. This tumour is supplied by meningeal branches arising from both internal and external carotid arteries. Figures **(a)** and **(b)** are lateral views from internal and external carotid injections respectively. Pre-operative embolization of the external carotid supply only was performed after selective catheterization of the accessory meningeal artery **(c)**. The effect of embolization is seen in **(d)**; compare this DSA with **(b)**. Figures **(e) (f)** are axial T1W gadolinium enhanced MRI of the tumour before and after embolization of the external carotid blood supply. Note that enhancement occurs in only the medial portion of the tumour on **(f)**.

last 5 years. Selective catheterization risks causing vessel damage, perforation and rupture. The last is more likely to occur at sharp bends in vessels. Such bends occur in the course of the middle meningeal artery (a common route for meningioma embolization) and rupture of this artery has been reported to cause bleeding or delayed arteriovenous shunting.[32, 33] The incidence of complications related to pre-operative embolization ranges from 3% to 6% with about half due to haemorrhage.[20, 21] Gruber et al.[47] reported morbidity of 6.4% and mortality of 6.2% in a small series of patients treated with combined surgery and embolization.

Paraganglioma

These benign but locally invasive tumours arise from paraganglionic chemoreceptor cells of neural crest origin. About 50% occur in the temporal bone, arising from either the cochlear promontory (i.e. typanicum) or the jugular blub (i.e. jugulare), 35% in the carotid body, 12% in the region of the high cervical vagus and the rest at various other sites in the head and neck.[48]

Though relatively rare tumours they are usually targets for embolization because of their highly vascular nature. Most occur sporadically though familial cases occur with autosomal dominant inheritance. In approximately 10% of patients tumours are multifocal and up to 5% of tumours secrete catecholamines. Symptoms are related to tumour location and typically are due to compression of adjacent structures, tinnitus (tympanicum) cranial nerve palsy (jugulare, vagale) and pain. The role of imaging by plannar scanning is to support the clinical diagnosis and usually includes both CT and MRI. The former (performed with high resolution parameters) will best demonstrate bony involvement and MRI will best demonstrate the soft tissue character of tumours.

Tumour vascularity and extent can be assessed from scans performed after intravenous contrast administration and evidence of involvement of the carotid artery or intracranial invasion should be sought. Intra-arterial angiography is usually undertaken as part of a pre-embolization evaluation rather than diagnosis.[49] Though the typical angioarchitecture of this tumour type makes angiography a very specific diagnostic test and it should be considered prior to biopsy.

On intra-arterial angiography feeding arteries are found to be enlarged and there is an early and intense blush in the tumour bed. The intra-tumoural angioarchitecture comprises centripetally orientated arterioles estimated to be 90 microns in diameter at the periphery and 300–600 microns in the centre of the tumour with arteriovenous shunts (**Figure 49.2**).[50] To further complicate embolization, the majority of tumours show a multi-compartment pattern of blood supply with arterial and venous supply confined to haemodynamic unit so that separate injections of embolic agent have to be made into each feeding artery. The technique for embolization has evolved with the development of embolization particles small enough to penetrate the smaller peripheral arteries (**Figure 49.3**). The presence of intra-tumour shunts may justify the use of the percutaneous (or intra-operative) direct puncture technique with injections of a liquid embolic agent[26] since spread of emboli to the lungs is less likely; however, AV shunting is rarer in paraganglioma than within the vascular bed of some other tumour types (e.g. nasopharyngeal angiofibroma, see below).[51]

Embolization is usually performed as an adjuvant to surgical resection. When surgery and/or radiotherapy are considered inappropriate, embolization may alone provide symptomatic relief by stabilizing tumour growth.[52] The benefits of pre-operative embolization have been demonstrated in several single institution reports.[53, 54]

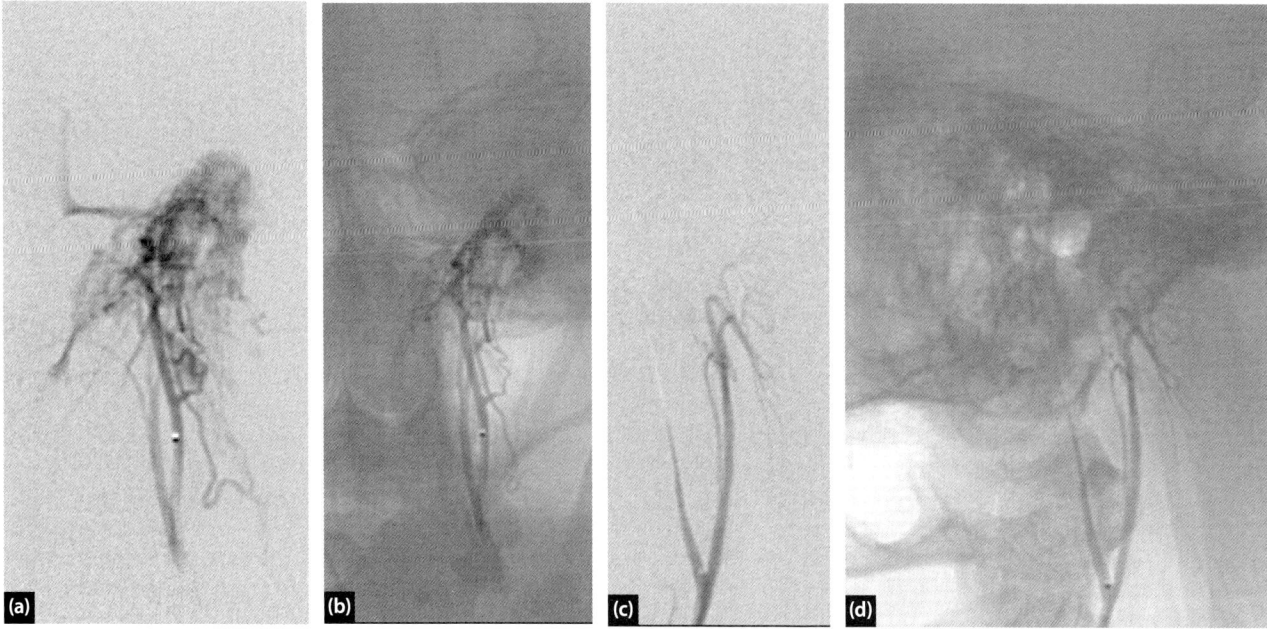

Figure 49.2 Temporal paraganglioma. Lateral subtracted **(a) (c)** and unsubtracted **(b) (d)** angiograms following selective injections into the ascending pharyngeal artery before **(a) (b)** and after **(c) (d)** embolization with particles.

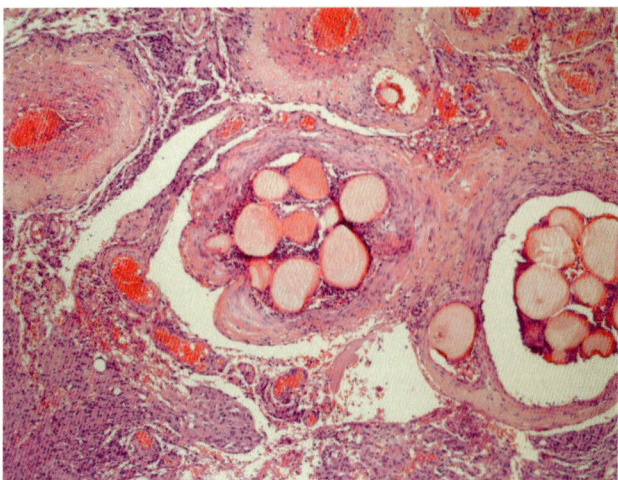

Figure 49.3 Histological section showing embolization particles (trisacryl gelatin microspheres) within tumour vessels.

Murphy and Brackmann assessed the effects of per-operative embolization in a cohort of 35 glomus jugulare tumour patients, and found pre-operative embolization reduced the volume of operative blood loss and the duration of procedures but not the length of bed stay.[55] Tikkakoski et al. reported that pre-operative embolization improved operating conditions with subjective benefits to surgical results if performed by superselective catheterization with effective devascularization of the tumour vascular bed.[56]

Juvenile nasopharyngeal angiofibroma

These benign locally invasive tumours of the nasopharynx are also commonly embolized prior to surgical resection. The histological features include the presence of vascular cavities with an endothelial layer but no muscle layer which are mixed with a more conventional arteriocapillary tree with muscle layers. There are similarities between the appearance of cells of the nasal mucosa, genital erectile tissue and vascular spaces of this tumour type. The target cells of the nasal mucosa are assumed to develop into muscularized vascular channels secondary to testosterone stimulation and oestrogen hypersensitivity at pubery.

Patients present with epistaxis and symptoms due to nasal obstruction. Epistaxis may lead to anaemia and require embolization for control though embolization is usually performed as part of planned resection procedures.

CT and MRI performed with contrast enhancement should define the extent of the tumour and be able to differentiate tumour extension into adjacent paranasal sinuses from sinusitis due to retained secretions. Diffuse or patchy enhancement with bone expansion suggests tumour invasion, and dural enhancement may suggest intra-cranial extension. The blood supply arises from branches of the external carotid artery and the internal carotid artery if local spread has occurred. DSA typically shows enlarged intra-tumoural vessels mixed with more regular arterioles (**Figure 49.4**). In the venous phase there is an intense inhomogenious blush which shows the full extent of tumour.

Complete surgical removal is the optimum treatment. Pre-operative embolization is a well established surgical adjuct to induce tumour shrinkage, improve surgical access and reduce blood loss.[51] Originally embolization was performed transarterially with particles (i.e. PVA) or liquids (i.e. NBCA) and since most tumours are supplied by branches of the external carotid artery it is relatively straightforward with a low risk of complications.[57] Intra-cranial tumour spread and supply by branches of the internal carotid arteries increase the risk of embolization causing neurological deficit and limits the potential for complete devascularization.[58] For this reason a direct tumour puncture technique with injections of liquid embolic agents (i.e. NBCA or Onyx) was introduced.[59] The goal is to facilitate surgery and reduce operative blood loss since pre-resection embolization does not appear to improve long-term outcomes.[60]

The introduction of the direct puncture technique with Onyx injection has been shown to improve the extent of devascularization after embolization[61] but the transarterial method still has its advocates.[62] Similarly the introduction and success of endoscopic surgical resection has changed some surgeons' opinion on the need for pre-operative embolization for smaller tumours (i.e. without spread) with some now considering pre-operative embolization unnecessary.[63]

Pre-operative embolization commonly causes a facial dull ache. Other reported effects are generally mild. These include transient facial numbness and hemiparesis.[59, 64] But there have been case reports describing blindness and permanant disability.[65]

EMBOLIZATION FOR EPISTAXIS

Transarterial embolization using particles, coils or balloons has been used to control intractable idiopathic epistaxis. For effective embolization, superselective catheterization of the sphenopalatine artery is performed after locating the bleeding site. This goal is hampered if prior surgical ligation of the internal maxillary artery has been performed or if the site of bleeding cannot be established. In these situations, particles may need to be injected via both internal maxillary and facial arteries.

There is no consensus on the most effective timing of embolization after the onset of spontaneous epistaxis and different definitions of intractable epistaxis make it difficult to compare published reports. The vast majority of patients admitted to hospital with epistaxis respond to packing, balloon tamponade or local cautery and only a small minority will need embolization.[66] Whether embolization is substantially safer or more effective than internal maxillary artery (IMA) ligation is also debated. In a recent review of the literature comparing embolization with IMA ligation, Cullen and Tami[67] found that embolization was generally reported to be more reliable, but this was not the case in their institution, where outcomes were similar but the procedural complication rate was

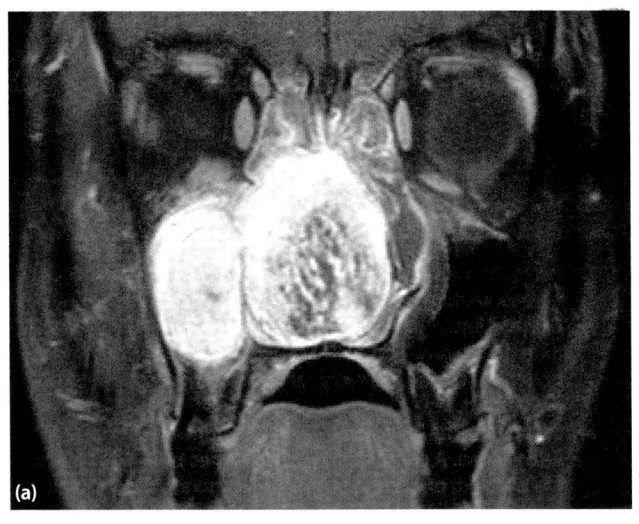
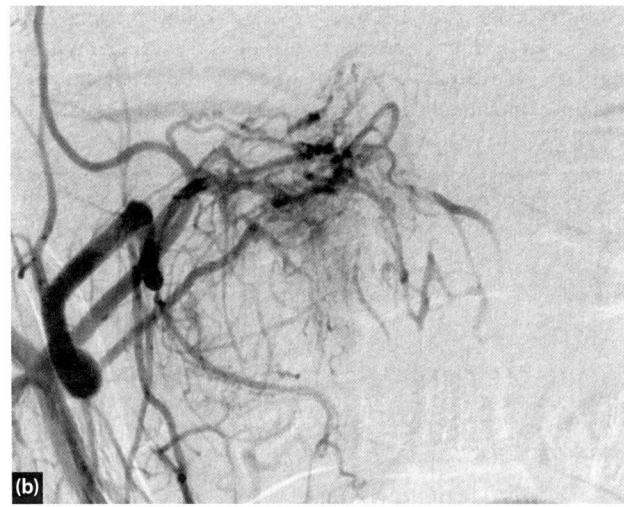
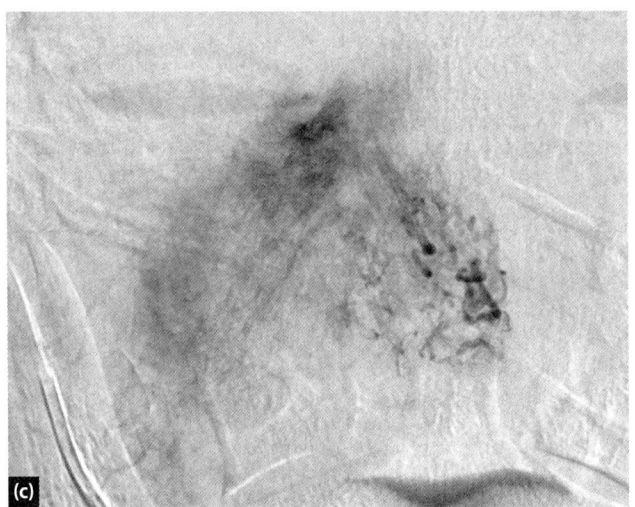
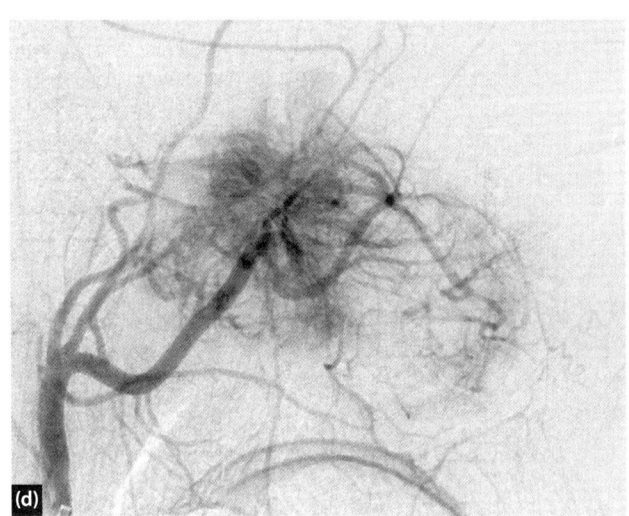
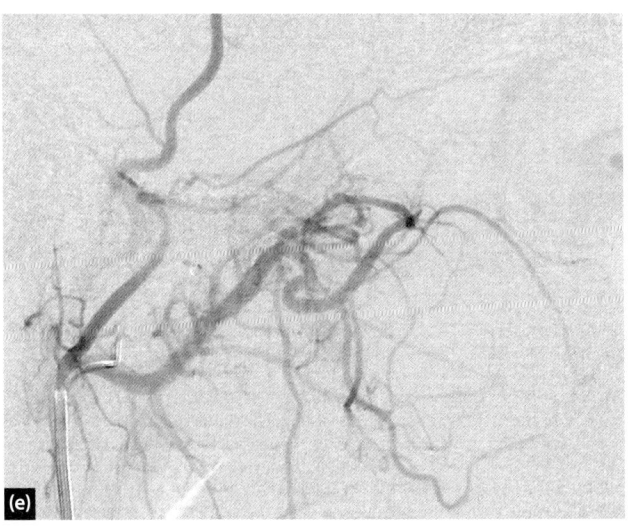

Figure 49.4 Juvenile angiofibroma. MRI **(a)** after gadolinium administration shows enhancement of tumour in the nose and right maxillary sinus. Lateral DSA performed by selective injection in the distal right external carotid artery shows mixed sized arteries and vascular spaces within the tumour **(b)** and a venous 'blush' in the late phase **(c)**. The effect of embolization with particles is shown on lateral DSA before **(d)** and after **(e)** embolization.

higher after IMA ligation. Even if the risks are no greater, it is logical to perform embolization before IMA ligation because ligation limits the effectiveness of subsequent embolization.

For patients with epistaxis secondary to a vascular malformation or nasal tumour, particulate embolization is indicated to stop acute haemorrhage. In patients with Osler-Weber-Rendu disease, multiple sessions may be required to induce remission and embolization is rarely curative.[10] In patients with epistaxis due to the rare internal carotid aneurysm or pseudoaneurysm that erodes the sphenoid bone and bleeds intra-nasally, emergency embolization can be life saving. Embolization also has a small but important role in the management of patients' bleeding as a result of head and neck cancers. Haemorrhage may occur from large or small vessels and may be associated with radiation induced tissue necrosis. A variety of embolization techniques using particles, coils, stents and balloons may be needed to control such bleeding.[68]

FUTURE RESEARCH

The evidence-base for most INR treatments is lacking. Research has largely involved reports of single institute case audits. Large-scale trials are difficult because relatively small patient numbers are treated at each hospital and multicentre cooperation is needed. This problem is being addressed by various specialist interest groups who organize case registries and multicentre trials to study the efficacy of embolization in different situations.

Areas for future research include:

➤ **Technical:**
  ➤ Development of non-X-ray imaging. Fluoroscopy using magnetic resonance imaging is now feasible. This avoids the potential hazards of ionizing radiation but requires the development of new catheters and embolic agents. Attempts to develop liquid agents that remain stable in high strength magnetic fields are proving difficult. A great deal of investment is being made to develop ways of monitoring minimally invasive surgical techniques without X-ray fluoroscopy.
  ➤ Current liquid embolic agents are to a greater or lesser extent adhesive and non-adhesive materials that remain coherent during delivery and permanent need to be developed.
  ➤ Improvements in reliability of data from functional tests are needed. A great deal of research has been directed at the problem of falsely reassuring temporary vessel occlusion tests. A completely reliable protocol is still needed.

➤ **Biological:**
  ➤ The evolution of embolized tissue has been studied but we do not know much about the mechanisms that cause secondary haemorrhage in some tumours.
  ➤ The potential benefits of local delivery for gene therapy and future chemotherapy agents will probably open new areas of research. The *in vivo* response of lesions will need further study.

KEY POINTS

- Pre-operative embolization should be considered for all vascular tumours.
- Tumour vascularity can only be inferred from CT and MR scans. Intra-arterial angiography is still required to identify tumours suitable for embolization.
- Functional testing of vessels 'at risk' during surgery is performed under local anaesthesia by temporary inflation of an endovascular balloon.
- Most embolizations are performed transarterially but direct percutaneous injections of tumour or vascular malformation vessels, or transvenous injections are also possible.
- Occasionally embolization alone is used for palliation and management of inoperable tumours.
- Embolization should be considered early rather than late in the management of intractable epistaxis

---

REFERENCES

1. Brooks B. The treatment of traumatic arteriovenous fistula. *South Med J* 1930; **23**(2): 100–06.
2. Moniz E, Lima A, Caldas P. Angiographie en serie de la circulation de la tete. *Revue Neurol (Paris)*; 1934.
3. Quisling R, Mickle J, Ballinger W. Small particle polyvinyl alcohol embolization of cranial lesions with minimal arteriolar-capillary barriers. *Surg Neurol* 1986; **25**(3): 243–52.
4. Hamada J-i, Kai Y, Nagahiro S, et al. Embolization with cellulose porous beads, II: Clinical trial. *Am J Neuroradiol* 1996; **17**(10): 1901–06.
5. Derdeyn CP, Moran CJ, Cross D, et al. Polyvinyl alcohol particle size and suspension characteristics. *Am J Neuroradiol* 1995; **16**(6): 1335–43.
6. Laurent A, Beaujeux R, Wassef M, et al. Trisacryl gelatin microspheres for therapeutic embolization, I: Development and in vitro evaluation. *Am J Neuroradiol* 1996; **17**(3): 533–40.
7. Kai Y, Hamada J-i, Morioka M, et al. Clinical evaluation of cellulose porous beads for the therapeutic embolization of meningiomas. *Am J Neuroradiol* 2006; **27**(5): 1146–50.
8. Latchaw R. Preoperative intracranial meningioma embolization: technical considerations affecting the risk-to-benefit ratio. *Am J Neuroradiol* 1993; **14**(3): 583–86.
9. Kerber C, Bank W, Horton J. Polyvinyl alcohol foam: prepackaged emboli for therapeutic embolization. *Am J Roentgenol* 1978; **130**(6): 1193–94.
10. Byrne JV. *Interventional neuroradiology: theory and practice*. Oxford: Oxford University Press; 2002.
11. Guglielmi G, Vinuela F, Dion J, et al. Electrothrombosis of saccular aneurysms via endovascular approach: Part 2: Preliminary clinical experience. *J Neurosurg* 1991; **75**(1): 8–14.
12. Serbinenko F. Balloon catheterization and occlusion of major cerebral vessels. *J Neurosurg* 1974; **41**(2): 125–45.
13. Raffi L, Simonetti L, Cenni P, et al. Use of Glubran 2 acrylic glue in interventional neuroradiology. *Neuroradiology* 2007; **49**(10): 829–36.
14. Gore P, Theodore N, Brasiliense L, et al. The utility of onyx for preoperative embolization of cranial and spinal tumors. *Neurosurgery* 2008; **62**(6): 1204–12.
15. Sainsbury DC, Kessell G, Fall AJ, et al. Intralesional bleomycin injection treatment for vascular Birthmarks: a 5-year experience at a single United Kingdom Unit. *Plast Reconstruct Surg* 2011; **127**(5): 2031–44.
16. Feng L, Kienitz BA, Matsumoto C, et al. Feasibility of using hyperosmolar mannitol as a liquid tumor embolization agent. *Am J Neuroradiol* 2005; **26**(6): 1405–12.
17. Manelfe C, Lasjaunias P, Ruscalleda J. Preoperative embolization of intracranial meningiomas. *Am J Neuroradiol* 1986; **7**(5): 963–72.
18. Davis KR, Debrun GM (eds). Embolization of juvenile nasopharyngeal angiofibromas. *Semin Intervent Radiol* 1987; **4**: 309–20.

19. Lacour P, Doyon D, Manelfe C, et al. Treatment of chemodectomas by arterial embolization (glomus tumors). *J Neuroradiol* 1975; **2**: 275–87.
20. Borg A, Ekanayake J, Mair R, et al. Preoperative particle and flue embolization of meningiomas: indications, results and lessons learned from 117 consecutive patients. *Neurosurgery* 2013; **73**(2): 244–51.
21. Carli D, Sluzewski M, Beute G, Van Rooij W. Complications of particle embolization of meningiomas: frequency, risk factors, and outcome. *Am J Neuroradiol* 2010; **31**(1): 152–54.
22. Lasjaunias PL, Berenstein A. *Endovascular treatment of craniofacial lesions.* Berlin: Springer-Verlag; 1987.
23. Valavanis A. Preoperative embolization of the head and neck: indications, patient selection, goals, and precautions. *Am J Neuroradiol* 1986; **7**(5): 943–52.
24. Tranbahuy P, Borsik M, Herman P, et al. Direct intratumoral embolization of juvenile angiofibroma. *Am J Otolaryngol* 1994; **15**(6): 429–35.
25. George B, Casasco A, Deffrennes D, Houdart E. Intratumoral embolization of intracranial and extracranial tumors: technical note. *Neurosurgery* 1994; **35**(4): 771–74.
26. Wanke I, Jackel M, Goericke S, et al. Percutaneous embolization of carotid paragangliomas using solely Onyx. *Am J Neuroradiol* 2009; **30**(8): 1594–97.
27. Chaloupka JC, Mangla S, Huddle DC, et al. Evolving experience with direct puncture therapeutic embolization for adjunctive and palliative management of head and neck hypervascular neoplasms. *Laryngoscope* 1999; **109**(11): 1864–72.
28. Howell S. Pharmacokinetic principles of regional chemotherapy. *Contr Oncol* 1988; **29**: 1–8.
29. Lee Y-Y, Dimery IW, Van Tassel P, et al. Superselective intra-arterial chemotherapy of advanced paranasal sinus tumors. *Arch Otolaryngol* 1989; **115**(4): 503–11.
30. Kumar P, Robbins T. Treatment of advanced head and neck cancer with intra-arterial cisplatin and concurrent radiation therapy: the 'RADPLAT' protocol. *Curr Oncol Rep* 2001; **3**(1): 59–65.
31. Kerber C, Wong H, Howell S, et al. An organ-preserving selective arterial chemotherapy strategy for head and neck cancer. *Am J Neuroradiol* 1998; **19**(5): 935–41.
32. Rogg J, Rutigliano M, Yonas H, et al. The acetazolamide challenge: imaging techniques designed to evaluate cerebral blood flow reserve. *Am J Roentgenol* 1989; **153**(3): 605–12.
33. Byrne JV, Guglielmi G. Results of endovascular treatment. In: *Endovascular Treatment of Intracranial Aneurysms.* Berlin: Springer; 1998. pp. 207–33.
34. Sudhakar K, Sawlani V, Phadke R, et al. Temporary balloon occlusion of internal carotid artery: a simple and reliable clinical test. *Neurol India* 2000; **48**(2): 140–43.
35. Standard SC, Ahuja A, Guterman LR, et al. Balloon test occlusion of the internal carotid artery with hypotensive challenge. *Am J Neuroradiol* 1995; **16**(7): 1453–58.
36. Gonzalez C, Moret J. Balloon occlusion of the carotid artery prior to surgery for neck tumors. *Am J Neuroradiol* 1990; **11**(4): 649–52.
37. Langford LA. Pathology of meningiomas. *J Neurooncol* 1996; **29**(3): 217–21.
38. Black PM. Meningiomas. *Neurosurgery* 1993; **32**(4): 643–57.
39. Bondy M, Ligon BL. Epidemiology and etiology of intracranial meningiomas: a review. *J Neurooncol* 1996; **29**(3): 197–205.
40. Chun JY, McDermott MW, Lamborn KR, et al. Delayed surgical resection reduces intraoperative blood loss for embolized meningiomas. *Neurosurgery* 2002; **50**(6): 1231–37.
41. Lazzaro MA, Badruddin A, Zaidat OO, et al. Endovascular embolization of head and neck tumors. *Front Neurol* 2011; **2**: 64.
42. Teasdale E, Patterson J, McLellan D, Macpherson P. Subselective preoperative embolization for meningiomas: a radiological and pathological assessment. *J Neurosurg* 1984; **60**(3): 506–11.
43. Oka H, Kawano N, Tanaka T, et al. Long-term functional outcome of suprasellar germinomas: usefulness and limitations of radiotherapy. *J Neurooncol* 1998; **40**(2): 185–90.
44. Dean B, Flom R, Wallace R, et al. Efficacy of endovascular treatment of meningiomas: evaluation with matched samples. *Am J Neuroradiol* 1994; **15**(9): 1675–80.
45. Kai Y, Hamada J-i, Morioka M, et al. Appropriate interval between embolization and surgery in patients with meningioma. *Am J Neuroradiol* 2002; **23**(1): 139–42.
46. Nania A, Granata F, Vinci S, et al. Necrosis score, surgical time, and transfused blood volume in patients treated with preoperative embolization of intracranial meningiomas: analysis of a single-centre experience and a review of literature. *Clin Neuroradiol* 2014; **24**(1) 29–36.
47. Gruber A, Bavinzski G, Killer M, Richling B. Preoperative embolization of hypervascular skull base tumors. *Minim Invasive Neurosurg* 2000; **43**(2): 62–71.
48. Zak FG, Lawson W. *The paraganglionic chemoreceptor system: physiology, pathology, and clinical medicine.* New York: Springer-Verlag; 1982.
49. Phelps PD, Cheesman AD. Imaging jugulotympanic glomus tumors. *Arch Otolaryngol* 1990; **116**(8): 940.
50. Willis A, Birrell J. The structure of a carotid body tumor. *Cell Tissues Org* 1955; **25**(2–4): 220–65.
51. Schroth G, Haldemann AR, Mariani L, et al. Preoperative embolization of paragangliomas and angiofibromas: measurement of intratumoral arterio-venous shunts. *Arch Otolaryngol* 1996; **122**(12): 1320–25.
52. Maier W, Marangos N, Laszig R. Paraganglioma as a systemic syndrome: pitfalls and strategies. *J Laryngol Otol* 1999; **113**(11): 978–82.
53. Ogura J, Spector G, Gado M. Glomus jugulare and vagale. *Ann Otol Rhinol Laryngol* 1978; **87**(5 Pt 1): 622.
54. Simpson GT, Konrad HR, Takahashi M, House J. Immediate postembolization excision of glomus jugulare tumors: advantages of new combined techniques. *Arch Otolaryngol* 1979; **105**(11): 639.
55. Murphy TP, Brackmann DE. Effects of preoperative embolization on glomus jugulare tumors. *Laryngoscope* 1989; **99**(12): 1244–47.
56. Tikkakoski T, Luotonen J, Leinonen S, et al. Preoperative embolization in the management of neck paragangliomas. *Laryngoscope* 1997; **107**(6): 821–26.
57. Ballah D, Rabinowitz D, Vossough A, et al. Preoperative angiography and external carotid artery embolization of juvenile nasopharyngeal angiofibromas in a tertiary referral paediatric centre. *Clin Radiol* 2013; **68**(11): 1097–106.
58. Valavanis A, Christoforidis G (eds). Applications of interventional neuroradiology in the head and neck. *Sem Roentgenol* 2000; **35**(1): 72–83.
59. Herman B, Bublik M, Ruiz J, Younis R. Endoscopic embolization with onyx prior to resection of JNA: a new approach. *Int J Pediatr Otorhinolaryngol* 2011; **75**(1): 53–56.
60. Petruson K, Rodriguez-Catarino M, Petruson B, Finizia C. Juvenile nasopharyngeal angiofibroma: long-term results in preoperative embolized and non-embolized patients. *Acta Otolaryngol* 2002; **122**(1): 96–100.
61. Gemmete J, Patel S, Pandey A, et al. Preliminary experience with the percutaneous embolization of juvenile angiofibromas using only ethylene-vinyl alcohol copolymer (Onyx) for preoperative devascularization prior to surgical resection. *Am J Neuroradiol* 2012; **33**(9): 1669–75.
62. Elhammady MS, Johnson JN, Peterson EC, Aziz-Sultan MA. Preoperative embolization of juvenile nasopharyngeal angiofibromas: transarterial versus direct tumoral puncture. *World Neurosurg* 2011; **76**(3): 328–34.
63. Khoueir N, Nicolas N, Rohayem Z, et al. Exclusive endoscopic resection of juvenile nasopharyngeal angiofibroma: a systemic review of the literature. *Otolaryngol Head Neck Surg* 2014; **150**(3): 350–8.
64. Itar Ogawa A, Aurelio Fornazieri M, Da Silva LV, et al. Juvenile angiofibroma: major and minor complications of preoperative embolization. *Rhinology* 2012; **50**(2): 199–202.
65. Casasco A, Houdart E, Biondi A, et al. Major complications of percutaneous embolization of skull-base tumors. *Am J Neuroradiol* 1999; **20**(1): 179–81.
66. Pollice PA, Yoder MG. Epistaxis: a retrospective review of hospitalized patients. *Otolaryngol Head Neck Surg* 1997; **117**(1): 49–53.
67. Cullen MM, Tami TA. Comparison of internal maxillary artery ligation versus embolization for refractory posterior epistaxis. *Otolaryngol Head Neck Surg* 1998; **118**(5): 636–42.
68. Morrissey DD, Andersen PE, Nesbit GM, et al. Endovascular management of hemorrhage in patients with head and neck cancer. *Arch Otolaryngol Head Neck Surg* 1997; **123**(1): 15–19.

CHAPTER 50

LASER PRINCIPLES IN OTOLARYNGOLOGY, HEAD AND NECK SURGERY

Brian J.G. Bingham

Introduction 581	Laser applications in otolaryngology 584
History 581	Laser safety 584
Principles of laser action 581	Photodynamic therapy in otorhinolaryngology 584
Laser light delivery devices 582	References 585
Laser–tissue interaction 583	

SEARCH STRATEGY

Data in this chapter may be updated by a Medline search using the keywords: head and neck cancer and photodynamic therapy.

INTRODUCTION

Laser is the acronym for light amplification by stimulated emission of radiation. Surgical lasers are devices that amplify light and create coherent light beams ranging from the infrared to the ultraviolet parts of the spectrum.

HISTORY

In 1917, Albert Einstein described the theory of stimulated emission that is the underlying process for laser action. The American physicists, Arthur Schawlow and Charles Townes, described the working principles of lasers in 1958.[1] In 1960 Theodore Maiman demonstrated the first laser action in solid ruby[2] and a year later Ali Javan built the first helium-neon gas laser.[3] C Kumar N Patel introduced the carbon dioxide (CO_2) gas laser in 1962. In 1972, in Boston, USA, Jako and Strong were the first to pioneer the use of the CO_2 laser in otolaryngology, head and neck surgery.[4–6]

PRINCIPLES OF LASER ACTION

A laser empowers atoms to store and emit light in a coherent form. The electrons in the atoms of a laser medium are first pumped or energized to an excited state by an external energy source. These electrons are then stimulated by external photons to emit their stored energy in the form of photons. This process is 'stimulated emission'.

The photons emitted have a frequency characteristic to their atoms and travel in step with the stimulating photons. These photons now strike other excited atoms to release even more photons. These photons move back and forth between two parallel mirrors triggering further stimulated emission. This part of the process is known as 'light amplification'. One mirror in the laser tube is partially silvered and it allows the exit or leak of the intense, collimated, monochromatic and coherent laser light.

Nature of laser light

A beam of laser light is:

- **coherent**: the photons or waves travel in step, or in phase with one another
- **collimated**: the laser light travels in one direction
- **monochromatic**: one wavelength or colour (if the energy is in the visible spectrum).

Types of lasers

Depending on the type of laser medium used, lasers can be classified as solid state, gas, semiconductor, liquid or free electron.

A pioneering example of a solid-state laser is the ruby laser. The neodymium yttrium aluminium garnate (YAG) laser and the related (frequency doubled) potassium titanyl phosphate (KTP) are examples of solid-state lasers in surgical practice.

The carbon dioxide laser (CO_2) is a very efficient gas laser that delivers laser light as an invisible continuous wave beam. The carbon dioxide surgical laser has been the most widely applied laser in oral and laryngological practice. The helium-neon laser is a gas laser with high frequency stability, good colour stability (red) and minimal beam spread. The helium-neon gas laser is often superimposed on an invisible laser beam, such as the CO_2, to facilitate surgical targeting. Activation of chemicals in photodynamic therapy can be achieved with the helium-neon laser.

The gallium arsenide laser is the most commonly used semiconductor laser. This laser is used in CD players and laser printers and has some surgical applications.

The most common medium for a liquid laser is an inorganic dye contained in a glass vessel. This laser is pumped or energized by intense flash lamps or by a gas laser in a continuous wave mode. The frequency of a tuneable dye laser can be altered with the aid of a prism inside the laser cavity. Tuneable dye lasers can be well suited for treating pigmented cutaneous lesions.

Lasers that utilize beams of electrons unattached to atoms and spiralling around magnetic field lines were initially developed in 1977 and are important research instruments. Free-electron lasers are tuneable and, in theory, could cover the electromagnetic spectrum from infrared to X-rays. Free-electron lasers could be capable of producing very high power radiation and may have medical applications in the future.

Patterns of laser output

The configuration of the resonator cavity and the method in which an energy source is applied to the 'active laser medium' will determine the pattern of a laser output. The output may be continuous wave or pulsed. A continuous wave laser operates with a constant intensity. A laser that operates with a continuous output for longer than 0.1 seconds is considered a continuous wave laser. A pulsed laser produces a single or train of pulses with each individual pulse less than 0.1 seconds. A Q-switch is an electro-optical component that facilitates the production of a very short (less than 1 microsecond) but high intensity pulse of laser energy.

Basic laser tissue interaction

The reaction of laser energy with living tissue can be photoablative, photochemical, photomechanical or photothermal. Most lasers react with a combination of all these mechanisms although for a specific wavelength and delivery system one form of tissue reaction may predominate:

- **Photoablative** reactions occur when molecular bonds are divided. The ruby laser, for example, can split the molecular bonds of tattoo ink with minimal local thermal damage. Macrophages remove the tattoo ink after the molecular bonds are broken.
- **Photochemical** reactions occur when infrared, visible or ultraviolet laser light interacts with photosensitizers to produce chemical and physical reactions. This forms the basis for photodynamic therapy that is discussed later in this chapter.
- A **photomechanical** effect occurs when the laser energy is pulsed to disrupt tissue or stones by the mechanism of shock waves. An example of this mechanism would be the use of the Holmium YAG laser to shatter ureteric and renal calculi.
- The conversion of absorbed laser light into heat is a **photothermal** reaction. The tissue effect can be cutting, coagulation or vaporization depending on the laser wavelength and the laser delivery device. The photothermal mechanism is predominant in laser use in otolaryngology and examples include CO_2 microlaryngoscopy and the argon laser for stapedotomy.

LASER LIGHT DELIVERY DEVICES

Many delivery devices are available to deliver laser energy to tissue in a safe and efficient manner. Most delivery devices are suited specifically for the wavelength that they transmit. Examples of delivery systems would be an articulated arm, a mirror lens system, micromanipulator, fibre optic fibre, shaped tip fibre optic fibres and robotized scanners.

An articulated arm uses a system of hollow tubes and mirrors to direct the laser beam to the target area. Most articulated arms have a lens system to focus the emerging beam on the target tissue. The carbon dioxide laser wavelength is absorbed in fibre optic material and hence this laser energy is delivered with an articulated arm system.

Micromanipulators and other focusing devices can be connected to microscopes. Micromanipulators and focusing devices will create an accurate and reproducible spot on target tissue. This facilitates very accurate and multiple laser strikes, which suits surgical techniques in otology and laryngology.

Laser energy exits from a micromanipulator or focusing device in a similar style to the 'laser beam weapon' of science fiction. This means that inadvertent strikes beyond the target tissue or misdirection from a reflective surface are a significant operative risk. This also means that a mirror can deliberately redirect a 'laser beam'. An example of this would be to use a mirror to redirect CO_2 laser energy on to adenoid tissue or on to lymphoid tissue on the base of the tongue.

The bare fibre optic fibre is the most common technique for delivering laser energy to tissue. The flexibility and diameter of fibre optic fibre facilitates their use with both rigid and flexible endoscopes. This means that laser energy can be delivered to almost any tissue that can be seen with an endoscope.

Laser light exits the tip of the fibre optic fibre in what is called the 'angle of divergence'. The light exiting from the tip of the fibre projects in a similar manner to water projecting from the nozzle of a hosepipe. The smallest light spot and, consequently, the highest concentration of energy is found very close to the fibre tip and as the distance from the fibre to tissue increases, the projected area of light decreases and the energy intensity reduces. Consequently, the tissue response to laser energy exiting from the tip of a fibre can be controlled by altering the distance of the fibre from the tissue. Changing the distance between the fibre and the tissue can produce all the tissue photothermal effects of coagulation, incision and vaporization. A fibre 'in contact' with tissue will create an incision. The cut is similar to a saw rather than a knife. This means that some tissue is removed like the kerf of a saw as compared to being split with a scalpel. There is a degree of tactile control with a laser fibre 'in contact' mode. As the fibre is retracted and hovers above the tissue (2–4 mm), it is in the 'near contact' position and vaporizes tissue. As the laser fibre is retracted even further from tissue into the 'non-contact' mode, then the tissue effect is coagulation.

A fibre optic laser cable can be inserted through the biopsy channel of a fibre optic endoscope. The end of the laser fibre must protrude beyond the end of the endoscope or heat damage to the endoscope can occur when the laser is fired. To simplify this problem one can perform a preliminary check of the length of fibre required to achieve a satisfactory distal position and then mark the laser fibre with a 'steristrip' at the entry port.

A fibre optic laser fibre can be inserted through a narrow metal tube to help direct the laser energy. In otology, for example, the laser fibre can be presented through a hollowed out needle. An aspiration channel can be added to the hollow metal fibre carrier to remove smoke from the surgical site. **Figure 50.1** shows a modified ear suction tube and fibre holder that is used for endoscopic intra-nasal surgery. In the design of these instruments, the curves of the fibre carrier should create sufficient resistance that when combined with the torque of the laser fibre it results in a fibre that is 'held' in position without any additional mechanism. In **Figure 50.2**, the 0.6-micron laser fibre can be set at the position of choice for the surgeon and will not move unless the surgeon applies additional pressure. The indent of the finger shows the pressure to overcome the self-retaining torque.

A shaped tip laser is a laser fibre with a tip constructed of another material, such as metal or synthetic sapphire. The laser energy heats the tip and it is the conduction of heat from the tip that produces the tissue interaction. Different materials and shapes of tip will create different tissue reactions. Some tips become so hot that a secondary cooling mechanism is required. An example of this type of device in head and neck practice would be a sapphire tipped neodynium YAG fibre used to ablate tracheobronchial tumours.

Robotized scanners can facilitate laser treatment by reproduction of previous instrument settings or by being able to control precisely the distance a laser is placed or 'hovered above' the target tissue. A robotized scanner can 'trace' an area of treatment before delivery of laser energy to ensure accuracy or can apply a pattern to the area of laser treatment. At present, the greatest use for

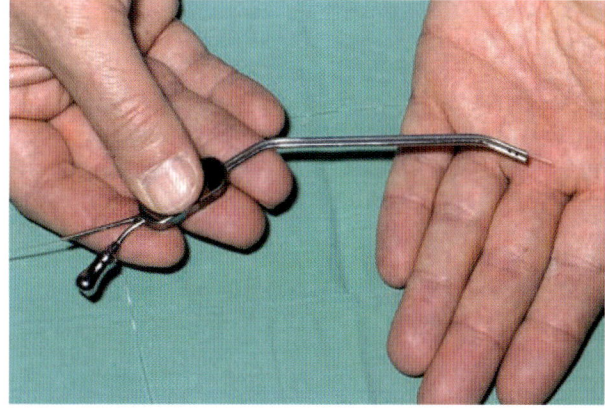

Figure 50.1 A 0.6-micron laser fibre inserted through a modified aural suction tube to create a laser delivery device. The natural torque of the fibre holds the laser fibre in place.

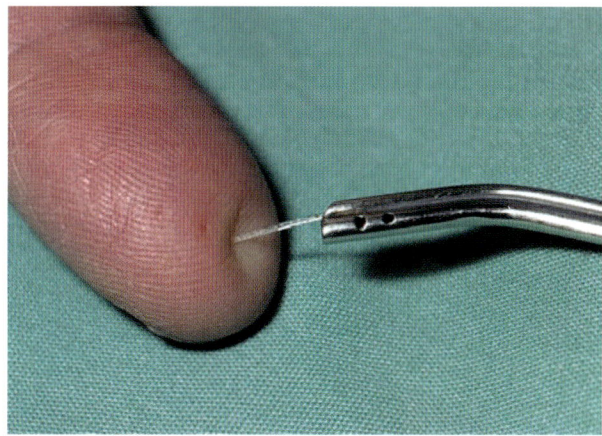

Figure 50.2 The pressure required to move or regress the laser fibre tip into the delivery device.

robotized scanners is in the cutaneous treatment of pigmented lesions and for skin resurfacing or recontouring.

LASER–TISSUE INTERACTION

When laser light strikes tissue, it scatters until all the laser energy is either absorbed or reflected. The absorption of laser energy heats tissue. The volume of tissue affected is larger than the area shown by the laser spot size. The depth of penetration by a given wavelength of laser light is determined by the absorption and scattering of the type of tissue and the wavelength of the laser.

The strength of the tissue effect is altered by changing the fluence. Fluence is defined as the laser power in watts, multiplied by the length of exposure in seconds, divided by the area (mm^2) of the target tissue. This implies that when the distance between a fibre optic tip and the tissue varies, the spot sizes become bigger or smaller and the fluence will accordingly increase or decrease.

The heat in the tissue produces a series of changes in the tissue as the temperature rises. The changes are denaturation, coagulation, vaporization, carbonization and incandescence. Cutting with a laser is narrow controlled vaporization! The heat produced by the absorption of laser light is partly dissipated into air but also produces a secondary thermal effect in surrounding tissue. This lateral thermal effect produces haemostasis by coagulation. The lateral haemostasis effect varies with wavelength of laser, the rate at which the energy is applied, fluence and the nature of the tissue.

LASER APPLICATIONS IN OTOLARYNGOLOGY

The specific clinical applications of lasers are not described in this chapter, but the following list identifies particular lasers for disease-specific regions:

- stapedectomy and tympanomastoid surgery: CO_2 laser, KTP laser, argon laser
- endonasal dacrocystorhinostomy: Holmium YAG laser, KTP laser, 810 nm laser
- nasal and sinus surgery, including tumour surgery, telangectasia destruction, antrostomy creation and turbinate reduction: Holmium YAG laser, KTP laser, Nd YAG laser, argon laser, 810 nm
- nasal polyp reduction: CO_2 laser 'swiftlase' (oscillating device)
- microlaryngeal surgery: CO_2 laser
- laryngopharyngeal tumour resection/ablation: CO_2 laser.

LASER SAFETY

Throughout the world each country applies different safety regulations. Usually the Medical Devices Agency of a country or state will produce guidance for clinicians and hospitals. In the UK, the local Medical Physics Department will produce local laser rules (based on national guidance) and ensure training of all staff involved in the use of the laser. Training for medical and nursing staff should be mandatory. A laser company will typically provide a safety manual on their particular wavelength of laser. Staff should read the laser safety manual and in many countries produce signed documentation that the manual has been read.

The principles of safety are as follows:

- A laser beam may hit or damage objects outside the target area and cause a fire, tissue damage or eye/visual damage.
- The patient should be shielded by wet gauze or fireproof material from accidental strikes.
- The anaesthetic tube and airway should be protected from accidental strikes that could produce a fire.
- All personnel in the operating room should wear correct eye protection appropriate to the wavelength of the laser.
- A warning sign plus locked doors should prevent unprotected and unprepared individuals from walking into the operating room when the laser is in use.
- The key to switch on the laser should be held by a senior member of the operating team to ensure only properly qualified individuals use the laser.
- The operating room and windows should be laser protected.
- Endoscopic equipment should be blackened to reduce accidental reflective strikes of the laser.

PHOTODYNAMIC THERAPY IN OTORHINOLARYNGOLOGY

Principles of photodynamic therapy

Phototherapy is the use of light in the treatment of disease. An example would be the treatment of neonatal hyperbilirubinaemia with visible light.

Photochemotherapy is a subset of phototherapy where a treatment requires the administration of a drug in addition to the application of light. An example would be treatment of a skin condition such as psoriasis with the combination of a furocoumarin sensitizer drug and UV-A (320–400 nm) light.

Photodynamic therapy (PDT) is a subset of photochemotherapy where, in addition to an administered drug and the application of light, oxygen is required to complete the process. The administered drug is known as a 'photosensitizer'. This type of drug accumulates within a cell and reacts with light and oxygen to form 'singlet' oxygen. The 'singlet' oxygen damages the cell membranes and produces cell death.

One of the attractions of PDT for oncology is that the photosensitizer drug is, typically, retained in tumour tissue for a longer period than in normal tissue. This improves the therapeutic effect while reducing toxicity to normal tissue. The use of PDT is not affected by prior radiotherapy, chemotherapy or surgery. To date, the principle shortcomings of PDT have been the limited depth of tissue penetration and extensive skin phototoxicity. This skin phototoxicity requires that the patient is not exposed to daylight during treatment or they develop extensive and painful skin reactions.

In photodynamic therapy for head and neck cancer the photosensitizer is usually administered by intravenous infusion. The perfect photosensitizer drug would be absorbed selectively only by tumour tissue in the drug uptake period (also called the drug–light interval). The drug uptake period may last between 3 and 96 hours. The tumour is then irradiated with a measured light dose. Singlet oxygen is released to kill only tumour cells and thus destroy the target tumour.

The tumour targeting arises firstly from the structure of the photosensitizer that leads to the selective uptake by a tumour and secondarily by the accurate application of an appropriate light wave.

There are many potential applications for PDT but few, currently, in routine practice. The diseases in which trials of photodynamic therapy have taken place include malignant tumours, such as squamous carcinoma of the oral cavity, squamous carcinoma of the nasopharynx, oesophageal carcinoma and metastatic squamous carcinoma of the neck. Non-malignant disease such as inverted papilloma of the sinonasal cavity has also been targeted.

Photodynamic clinical reports in otorhinolaryngology

Both palliative and curative therapy has been reported for oesophageal cancer. The patients receive a photosensitizer followed by light delivered via optical fibres through a flexible endoscope. A phase II trial[7] randomized 218 patients to receive palliative oesophageal PDT (porfimer sodium sensitizer) versus Nd:YAG laser ablative therapy. Each arm gave an equivalent improvement in dysphagia but with fewer perforations in the PDT group (1 versus 7%, $p < 0.05$).

Overholt and Panjehpour[8] reported the results of 55 patients with dysplasia or early carcinoma in Barrett's mucosa of the lower end of the oesophagus treated with PDT. The patients received porfimer sensitizer followed at 48 hours with red light therapy. There was a good response at the 6-month follow-up. Forty-three patients with high-grade dysplasia/adenocarcinoma had endoscopic-proved ablation of their problem. Eleven of the 12 patients with low-grade dysplasia had no dysplasia on endoscopic review. Oesophageal stricture, however, developed in 53% of the patients.

There has been hope for PDT in the treatment of head and neck tumours. The endoscopic access to squamous tumours of the upper aerodigestive tract combined with the tendency to develop 'field cancerization' make these tumours good candidates for PDT. Gluckman[9] treated a mixture of carcinoma *in situ*, early and advanced squamous cell carcinoma of the head and neck. Dihaematoporphyrin ether and light at 630 nm were used to treat these patients. The best results were obtained in the oral cavity and oropharynx where 11 out of 13 patients had a complete response and 2 out of 13 a partial response. Four of these tumours had recurrence within 1 year of treatment. Eight patients with advanced tumours were treated palliatively, but the results were no better that with standard regimes of the time.

Karakullukcu et al.[10] analyzed the outcomes of photodynamic therapy in 170 patients with early stage oral cavity and oropharynx neoplasms giving results of a 90% response rate and a 70% complete response (cure) rate.

Biel[11] treated 25 patients with early squamous cell tumours of the larynx, obtaining a complete response in patients despite the fact that radiation therapy had previously been unsuccessful in 17 of them.

Biel[12] also reported a summary of the results of a collection of studies on the treatment of early squamous cell carcinoma of the head and neck with PDT. There were a total of 217 patients. One hundred and ninety-four (89%) showed a complete response to treatment, 23 (10.6%) showed a partial response and no patient failed to show any response to the therapy.

Dilkes et al.[13] had considerable experience with the use of PDT using the sensitizers m-TPHC, photofrin II and ALA for squamous carcinoma at multiple sites in the head and neck during the mid-1990s. The patients they treated included palliative, primary and adjunctive forms of treatment and, in nearly all cases, the authors identified a visible response to the effects of PDT. Their complications included local pain at the photosensitizer injection site and, in some patients where appropriate precautions had not occurred, post-treatment skin photosensitivity.

Lofgren et al.[14] used PDT in 5 patients with circumscribed nasopharyngeal carcinoma. The drug was activated with laser light under topical anaesthesia and after 4 years, 3 of the patients has no evidence of disease.

> **FUTURE RESEARCH**
>
> All of the papers on photodynamic therapy for head and neck cancer suggest that photodynamic therapy has a significant place in the future management of this disease. The problem is in determining the exact type of photodynamic therapy associated with which photosensitizer and whether primary therapy, adjunctive therapy or palliation is the optimum course.

> **KEY POINTS**
>
> - Laser light amplification by stimulated emission of radiation.
> - Laser light – collimated, coherent and monochromatic.
> - Laser tissue action – photoablative, photochemical and photomechanical.
> - Laser 'star wars' beam of micromanipulator – hosepipe type jet of fibre optic laser delivery.
> - Read and follow the safety regulations for your laser and operating room.
> - PDT requires administered drug, light and oxygen.
> - Skin phototoxicity and limited tissue penetration are the current PDT shortcomings.
> - PDT has a future place in head and neck cancer management.

REFERENCES

1. Schawlow AL, Townes CH. Infrared and optical lasers. *Phys Rev* 1958; **112**: 1940–49.
2. Maiman TH. Stimulated optical radiation in ruby. *Nature* 1960; **187**: 493–94.
3. Javan A, Bennett WR, Harriott DR. Population inversion and continuous laser oscillation in a gas discharge containing He-Ne mixtures. *Phys Rev Lett* 1961; **6**: 106.
4. Jako GJ. Laser surgery of the vocal cords: an experimental study with carbon dioxide lasers on dogs. *Laryngoscope* 1972; **82**: 2204–16. PMID: 4675172.

5. Strong MS, Jako GJ. Laser surgery in the larynx: early clinical experience with continuous CO2 laser. *Ann Oto Rhinol Laryn* 1972; **81**: 791–98. PMID: 4636137.
6. Strong MS, Jako GJ, Vaughan CW, et al. The use of C02 laser in otolaryngology: a progress report. *T Am Acad Opthalmol* 1976; **82**: 595–602. PMID: 1035443.
7. Lightdale CJ, Heier SK, Marcon NE, et al. Photodynamic therapy with porfimer sodium versus thermal ablation therapy with Nd:YAG laser for palliation of esophageal cancer: a multicenter trial. *Gastrointest Endosc* 1995; **42**: 507–12. PMID: 8674919.
8. Overholt BF, Panjehpour M, Halberg D, et al. Photodynamic therapy for Barret's oesophagus with dysplasia and/or early stage carcinoma: long-term results. *Gastrointest Endosc* 2003; **58**: 183–8.
9. Gluckman JL. Hematoporphyrin photodynamic therapy: is there truly a future in head and neck oncology? Reflections on a 5 year experience. *Laryngoscope* 1991; **101**: 36–42. PMID: 1701843.
10. Karakullukcu B, van Oudenaarde K, Copper MP, et al. Photodynamic therapy of early stage oral cavity and oropharynx neoplasms: an outcome analysis of 170 patients *Eur Arch Otorhinolaryngol* 2011; **268**(2): 281–88.
11. Biel MA. Photodynamic therapy and the treatment of neoplastic diseases of the larynx. *Laryngoscope* 1994; **104**: 399–403. PMID: 8164476.
12. Biel MA. Photodynamic therapy and the treatment of head and neck neoplasia. *Laryngoscope* 1998; **108**: 1259–68. PMID: 9738739.
13. Dilkes MG, Alusi G, Djaezeri BJ. Treatment of head and neck cancer with PDT: clinical experience. *Rev Contemp Pharmaco* 1999; **10**: 47–57.
14. Lofgren LA, Hallgren S, Nilsson E, et al. Photodynamic therapy for recurrent nasopharyngeal cancer. *Arch Otolaryngol* 1995; **121**: 997–1002. PMID: 7646870.

CHAPTER 51

CONTACT ENDOSCOPY OF THE UPPER AERODIGESTIVE TRACT

Mario Andrea and Oscar Dias

Introduction 587	Normal and pathological patterns 589
Technique 588	Conclusion 593
Cellular and microvascular structure of the mucosa of the upper aerodigestive tract 588	References 594

SEARCH STRATEGY

Data in this chapter may be updated by a PubMed search using the keywords: contact endoscopy, mucosal vascular network, narrow band imaging and Methylene blue.

INTRODUCTION

The investigation of blood vessels and their microcirculation has been an area of interest to surgeons for many years. In 1970, surgeons[1] started research on the arterial vascularization of the larynx. Over the years, anatomical and clinical research on the pathways of extension of laryngeal tumours has been published.[2-5] The systematic evaluation of operated specimens allowed for a better understanding of the progression and invasion of the laryngeal tumours.

In order to enhance the evaluation of the operative specimens, nasal endoscopes and endoscopes of other territories and specialities were used. It soon became obvious that the endoscopes offered a superior view compared the operative microscope alone.[6] With the microscope the assessment is limited by a straight line of vision.

A group of endoscopes were produced by Karl Storz (1995)[7] that were specifically designed for the intraoperative evaluation of the larynx. This technique is called contact endoscopy and typically involves examination of the superficial epithelium of the larynx. Rigid endoscopy associated with microlaryngoscopy[8-9] allowed the direct observation of the vascular networks and alterations. This led to the the next phase in which contact endoscopy was used to visualize the microvascular networks.[10]

The first description of contact endoscopy is atributed to Desormaux in 1865,[11] who observed the vascular network of the bladder mucosa. The development of this technique was only possible due to technological progress. In 1955, Jaupitre[12] promoted contact cystoscopy associated to photography and cinematography and in 1983, Hamou[13] developed the microcolpohysteroscopy used in gynaecology. This technique allowed for the better comprehension of the pathology of the uterine cervix, but due to its complexity and difficulty, its use remained only within a limited number of centres.

The contact microlaryngoscope was developed in 1995[14] and the study of the larynx using contact endoscopy was initiated.

Contact endoscopy, using amplifications of 60x and 150x, allows for the *in vivo* and *in situ* observation of the mucosal vessels. By staining the mucosa with methylene blue, it is possible to visualize the cells of the superficial layer of the mucosa of the larynx, which allows diagnosis, the evaluation of the extension of the lesions and, when tumour is present, defining the safety margins. The advantages of this technique led to it being used daily in clinical practice.[15–22]

Contact endoscopy was further developed and systematized for the other areas of the aerodigestive tract. Confronted with the richness of the microcirculatory and cellular images obtained with contact endoscopy, new endoscopes were designed and produced by Karl Storz, for use in the nasal fossa, in the nasopharynx, mouth, oropharynx, hypopharynx and trachea.[23–26]

In 2007, observation of the mucosal vascular network was enhanced by combining contact endoscopy with an Olympus system of illumination called 'narrow band imaging'.[27] This produces a specific wavelength, which is selectively captured by haemoglobin and allows a better contrast of the vessels relative to the neighbouring tissues. This enhances the visualization of the deeper vessels.

With contact endoscopy, anatomical-pathological concepts of mucosal illnesses are evaluated clinically in multiple sites and stages, at times associated with aetio-pathological factors. With this technique vascular and cellular alterations of the mucosa can be observed both in the outpatient clinic and in the operating theatre.

With contact endoscopy, the notion of illness has surpassed the classic concept of the macroscopic lesion that was biopsied.

With these techniques, the non-invasive pathological evaluation can be made during an endoscopic examination. This allows, in many cases, for the diagnosis to be made at the time of observation, having a direct implication on the planning and method of treatment that is chosen. Contact endoscopy may deliver further information on the subclinical staging and improve understanding of the physiopathology of the diagnosed condition.

The objective of contact endoscopy is not to visualize at the surface what is expected to be observed from histological sections and it should not be considered a substitute for biopsy. Instead it is a clinical method that adds to the information available during an endoscopic examination. It is an anatomical-pathological examination that supports the cytology.

The development of contact endoscopy of the upper aerodigestive tract has led to establishing parallels with other areas such as gynaecology, gastroenterology, pulmonology and opthalmology, as we further converge at the pathological and cytological level.

Contact endoscopy is now used in centres with benefits for patients around the world. The same principles are being used in other specialties, as can be seen through work published in the medical literature.[28–49] Technological evolution and collaboration between centres will contribute to the further development of this technique.

TECHNIQUE

The contact microlaryngoscope (Karl Storz 8715 AA) is an endoscope with a diameter of 5.8 mm, and 24 cm in length. Another contact endoscope with an angulation of 30° (Karl Storz 8715 BA) was manufactured in order to improve the access to certain locations of the larynx. Later, shorter contact endoscopes (18 cm) with a smaller diameter (4 mm) for the observation of the nasal cavity, the oral cavity, the oro- and the nasopharynx (Karl Storz 7215 AA e 7215 BA) have also been designed.

At the level of the larynx and hypopharynx contact endoscopy is performed under general anaesthesia with endotracheal intubation. The nasal mucosa, nasopharynx, mouth and oropharynx can be observed, in many cases, without the need for any anaesthetic.

For the observation of the vessels the contact endoscope is applied directly on the mucosa without any staining. The microcirculation is visible with illumination from a regular endoscopy light source. However when the illumination is changed for the Olympus 'narrow band imaging', the emitted light is absorbed by the haemoglobin of the erythrocytes, improving substantially the visibility of the vascular network allowing the identification of deeper vessels.

To observe the cells of the epithelum the mucosa is stained with methylene blue. The contact endoscope is gently applied to the mucosal surface. The colouration lasts for 4 to 5 minutes.

The contact endoscope has a round control near the proximal ocular end that allows a change of magnification (60× to 150×) and controls focus. Sliding the contact endoscope over the mucosa, it is possible to visualize the cells and their alterations at the level of the lesion and of the neighbouring areas. Furthermore, it allows mapping of the disease or the various diseases that can occur in distinct sites and stages.

Contact endoscopy must always be performed with video recording and if possible in high definition. The image is immediately shared and the recording can be reviewed and analyzed later by the otolaryngologist and pathologist or cytologist.

CELLULAR AND MICROVASCULAR STRUCTURE OF THE MUCOSA OF THE UPPER AERODIGESTIVE TRACT

The mucosa that covers the upper aerodigestive tract is constituted by ciliated epithelium and by squamous stratified epithelium in accordance with the function of the different regions. Acting as an interface with the external environment, this mucosa is subjected to frequent stimuli and insults that may cause clinical and subclinical alterations at different tissue levels. Alterations of one part of the aerodigestive tract may cause consequences of other anatomical territories within the aerodigestive tract.

Contact endoscopy in otolaryngology reinforces clinical evaluation through the concept of the anatomical and functional units, as it allows a non-invasive method to identify alterations at various anatomical territories that would not be perceived in other ways.

NORMAL AND PATHOLOGICAL PATTERNS

The systematic observation of the various organs and territories of the upper aerodigestive tract with contact endoscopy allows a better understanding of how the mucosa reacts to the conditions and insults to which it is subjected. In each of the territories the pathology acquires specific characteristics; however, the overall behaviour of the mucosa, in general, is very similar.

Normal pattern

When observed by contact endoscopy the cells of normal squamous epithelium have a polyhedric shape, being in continuity with each other. The nuclei are round and dark. The cytoplasm has a light blue colouration. The nucleus:cytoplasm ratio is regular and the general morphological pattern is homogeneous (**Figure 51.1**).

The ciliated epithelium observed with contact endoscopy has a distinct appearance. The nuclei are round and dark but the cytoplasm limits are difficult to define. The nuclei are very close to each other creating a higher density of nuclei per optic field (**Figure 51.2**). The filamentous structures displaced by the endoscope are due to bundles of cillia. These bundles of cillia may have variable size, being very exhuberant at the level of the nasal and nasopharyngeal mucosa.

The transition of squamous to ciliated epithelium is easily observed with contact endoscopy. In some cases there is a very sharp line of separation (**Figure 51.3**). In other cases the transition is less well defined. Occasionally islands of squamous epithelium are found in the middle of the ciliated epithelium.

Glandular orifices are observed scattered through the mucosa of the upper aerodigestive tract.

The mucosa undergoes a process of metaplasia with age and particularly when submitted to damaging factors. For example, the ciliated epithelium of the larynx changes into squamous epithelium in chronic smokers. The same happens with the trauma of reflux at the posterior commissure of the larynx. The same phenomena occur at the nasal and nasopharyngeal sites when exposed to traumatic factors.

Contact endoscopy allows a detailed observation of the mucosal vessels. The most superficial microvascular network is situated immediately below the basal membrane. The morphology of the vascular network is conditioned by the topography and function of the mucosa. In most of the mucosa of the upper aerodigestive tract the vessels have a course parallel to the surface and are connected by many anastomoses constituting a plexus. In specific sites, vessels with a perendicular course to the surface are identified in gums, hard palate, cheek mucosa, superior surface of the tongue and in the papillae of the nasal mucosa. At the level of the vocal cords the blood vessels are parallel to each other (**Figure 51.4**) and are connected by transverse anastomotic vessels. This arrangement favours the vibratory movements of the vocal mucosa.

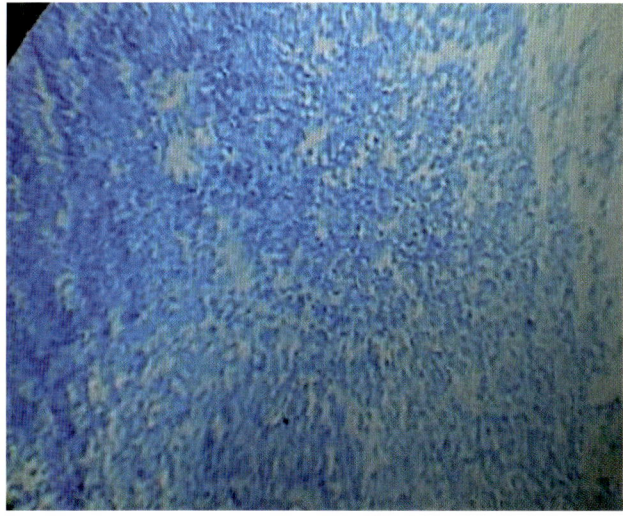

Figure 51.2 Normal ciliated epithelium of the vocal cord, 60X.

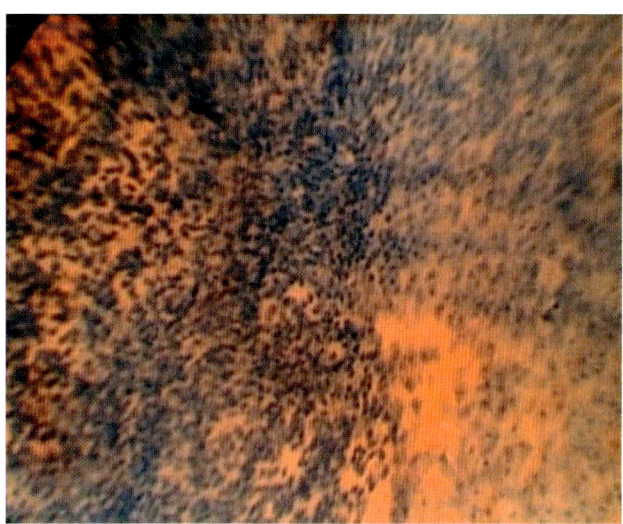

Figure 51.3 Transition of the ciliated epithelium to squamous epithelium of the vocal cord, 60X.

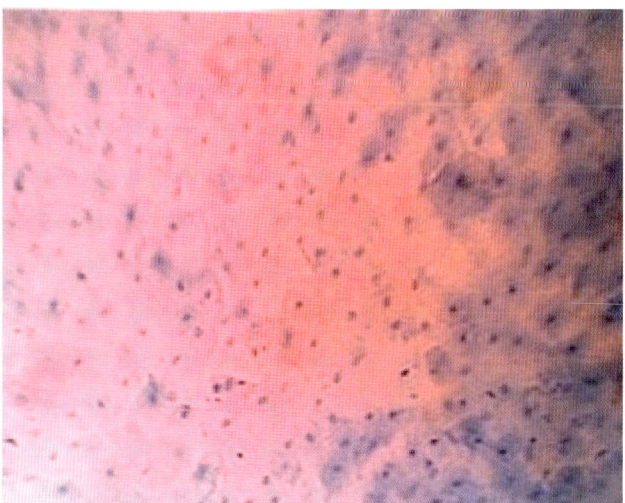

Figure 51.1 Normal squamous epithelium of the vocal cord. The nuclei are regular and homogeneous, 60X.

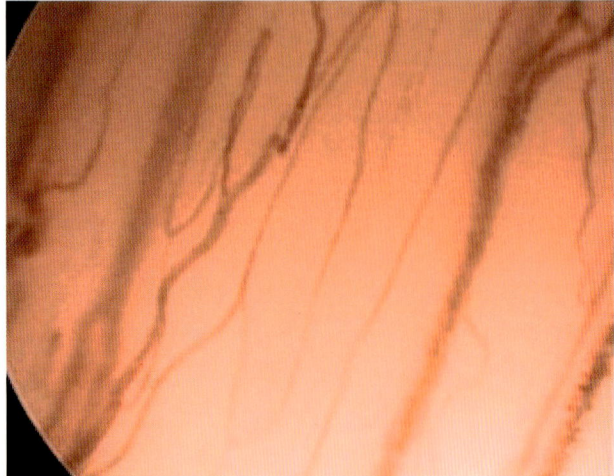

Figure 51.4 Normal vessels of the vocal cord. The vessels are thin and parallel, 60X.

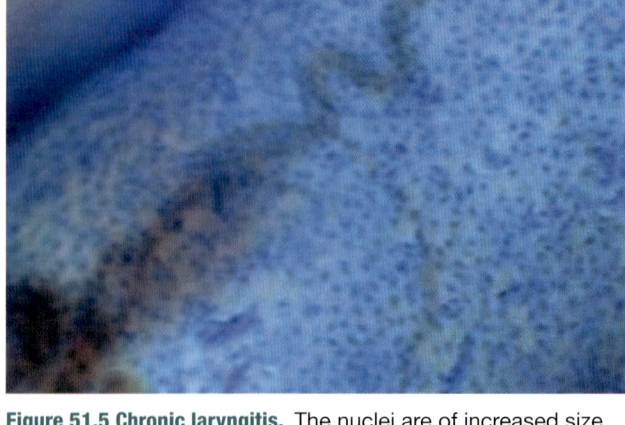

Figure 51.5 Chronic laryngitis. The nuclei are of increased size with a homogeneous pattern, 60X.

The more superficial microvascular network drains to venules that go to collecting vessels of larger calibre at the deeper planes. The angioarchitecture of this deeper plane depends on the thickness of the mucosa and the neighbouring structures. Contact endoscopy offers a fascinating image of the blood flow. The red cells circulate to the rhythm of the heartbeat and travel in several directions, and sometimes change direction with the pressure of the contact endoscope on the mucosa.

Chronic inflammation

When chronic inflamed mucosa is observed through contact endoscopy, the general aspect of the squamous epithelium is homogeneous, but the size of the nuclei is larger with an increased nucleus/cytoplasm ratio (**Figure 51.5**). As the cellular turnover is accelerated due to the inflammation, more immature cells become visible at the surface, similar to those that are observed at the intermediate layers of the normal epithelium.

The mucosa of chronic inflammation has a higher vascular density due to the increased number of vessels and vessel enlargement. However, the pattern of distribution remains organized.

FUNGAL INFECTION

In some cases of chronic inflammation, in addition to the typical pattern of increased diameter of the nuclei, it is possible to identify with contact endoscopy small dark dots that seem to spoil the image. These correspond to fungal spores (**Figure 51.6**). Hyphae and miceliums can also be observed as well as filamentous structures.

Contact endoscopy has identified that fungal infections are in many cases associated with chronic inflammatory changes, and dysplastic or neoplastic lesions in different anatomical sites. In general the fungal infection does not disturb the microcirculation more than inflammation due to other aetiologies. However, in more

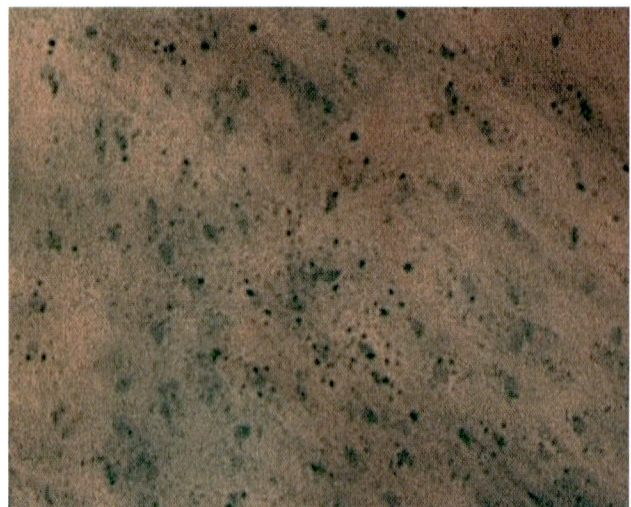

Figure 51.6 Laryngeal fungal infection and dysplasia, 60X.

aggressive forms of disease there are profound vascular changes, including aberrant shaped vessels causing thrombosis and tissue necrosis.

KERATOSIS

In the same patient, and even within the same lesion, different degrees of keratinization can be observed by contact endoscopy. Initially isolated cells without nuclei are identified. Unfortunately, it is not possible to identify individual cells in areas of amorphous or laminar structure (**Figure 51.7**). Keratosis is present in different clinical entities. In some cases keratinization is very discrete while in others it is pronounced. Occasionally keratosis is not suspected and its finding with contact endoscopy is a surprise.

With leukoplakias, in addition to keratosis, other types and degrees of cellular alterations can be observed by contact endoscopy, including heterogeneity of the cellular population. The variety of the cellular images can be accounted for as different pathological alterations such as

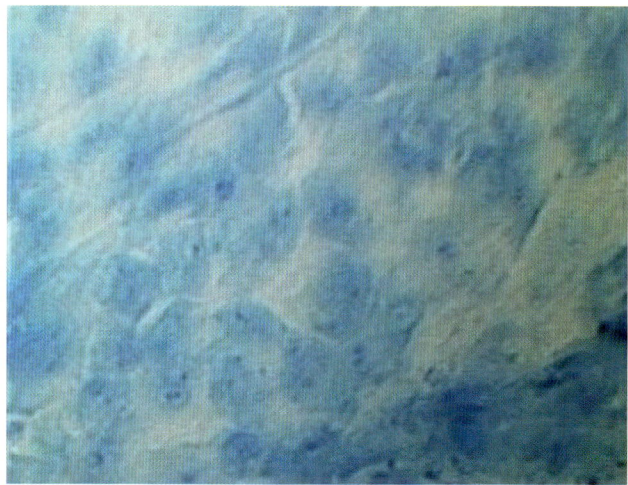

Figure 51.7 Keratosis of the vocal cord, 60X.

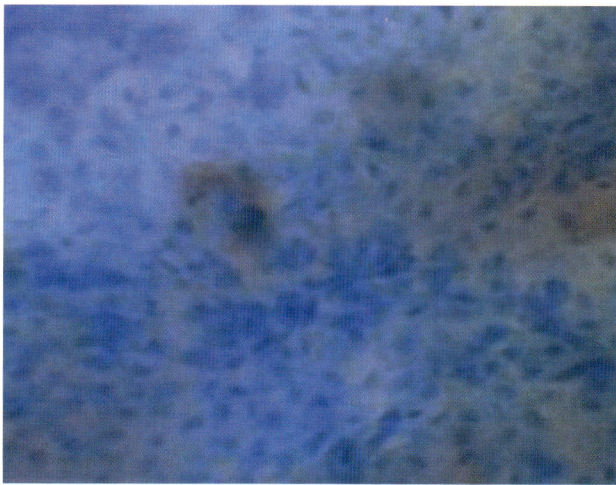

Figure 51.8 Dysplasia, 60X.

hyperkeratosis and dysplasia can occur simultaneously. In other clinical entities such as chronic inflammation, papillomas and tumours, keratosis can also exist in different degrees.

While in some cases the vessels pass below the area containing keratosis they may sometimes surround the leukoplastic lesion.

DYSPLASIA

In the majority of the cases of dysplasia, there are alterations at the superficial layers, making it accessible to contact endoscopy. Most tissue alterations that are necessary for the diagnosis of dysplasia by a pathologist are also identifiable by contact endoscopy, specifically alterations in size, shape and colouration of nuclei, altered nucleus:cytoplasm ratio (dyskaryosis and anisokaryosis) and keratosis (**Figure 51.8**). The more pronounced the changes observed by contact endoscopy the more severe is the dysplasia.

The microvascular alterations that accompany the dysplastic lesion are fundamental to the understanding of the pathology hence its treatment. The normal microvasculature is substituted by vessels with different degrees of alteration.

When the vascular network becomes disorganized and the vessels are irregular it can be interpreted that the pathology of the epithelium has passed the boundary of the basal membrane, which may be damaged, thus allowing the vessels to penetrate the epithelium. The mobility of the contact endoscope allows assessment of the regions neighbouring the lesion. This information benefits an understanding of the main lesion.

TUMOUR

In carcinoma, contact endoscopy identifies the marked cellular irregularity and heterogeneity. The nuclei have different sizes, shapes and colouration. The nucleus:cytoplasm ratio is very irregular (**Figure 51.9**). Sometimes nuclear inclusions, prominent nucleoli and mitosis are identified.

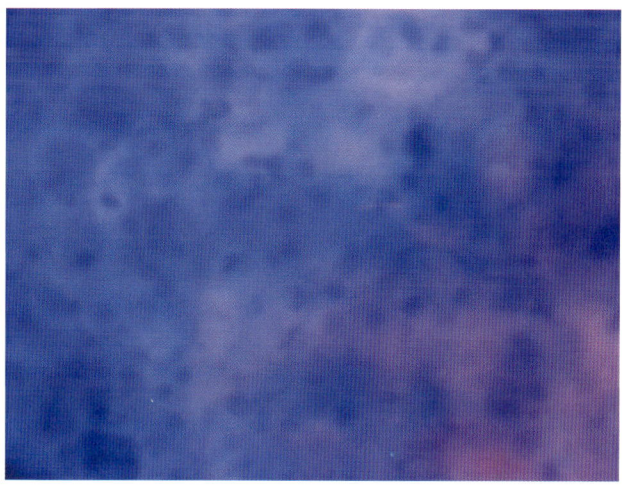

Figure 51.9 Tumour of the larynx observed by contact endoscopy. Nuclei are irregular in size, shape and colouration.

The angioarchitecture is also very disturbed. The blood vessels are atypical with differences in size and shape, but also ectasias, haemorrhages and reduced blood flow, which results in thrombosis (**Figure 51.10**).

Depending on the anatomical region of the tumour, distinct images can be observed. In places where the tumour growth infiltrates the deep planes but does not reach the surface, vascular alterations can be identified with normal superficial epithelial cells.

The direct demonstration *in vivo* and *in situ* of a tumoural pattern in the operating room and in the outpatient clinic is a reality. Contact endoscopy also allows the assessment of transition areas, the identification of early stages of disease, guidance of biopsies, guidance of sample collections for cytology, establishment of safe margins and demonstration of different diseases.

PAPILLOMA

Contact endoscopy contributes to the assessment of the papilloma, allowing the identification of its extent, offering

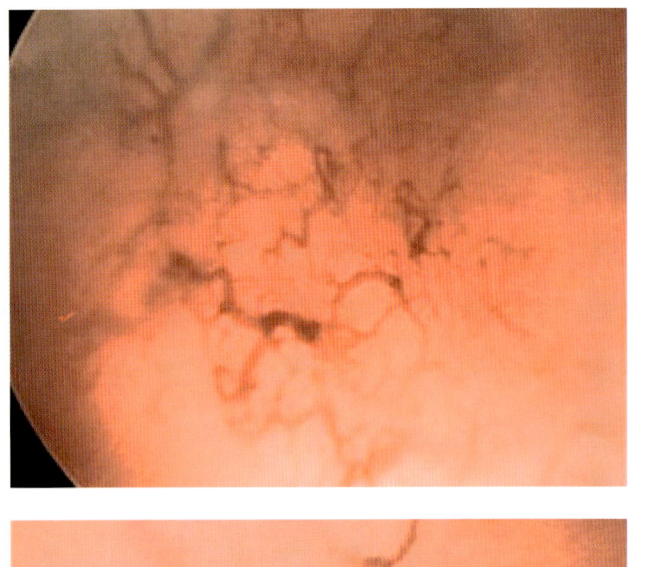
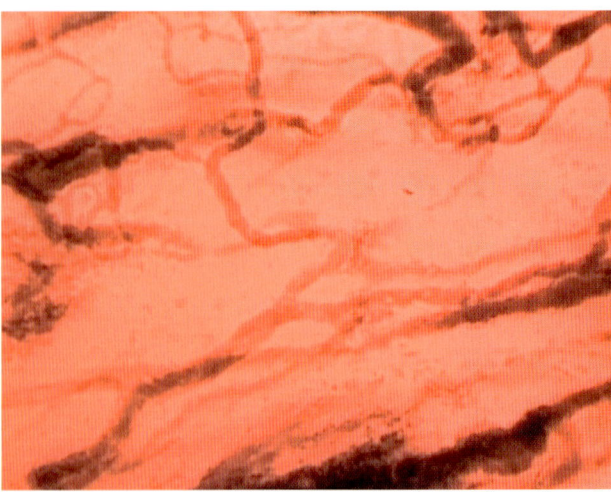
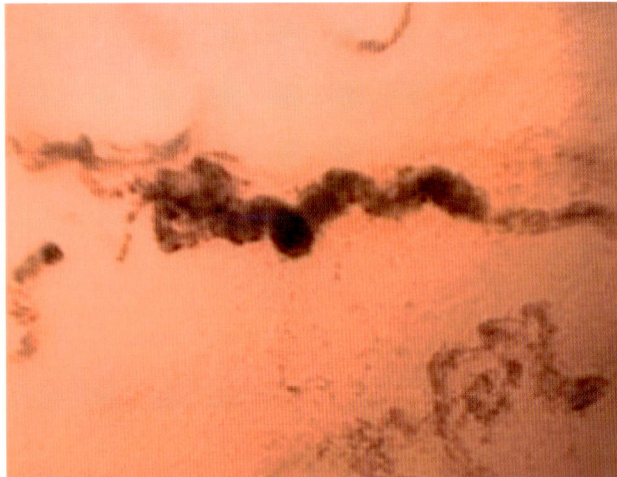
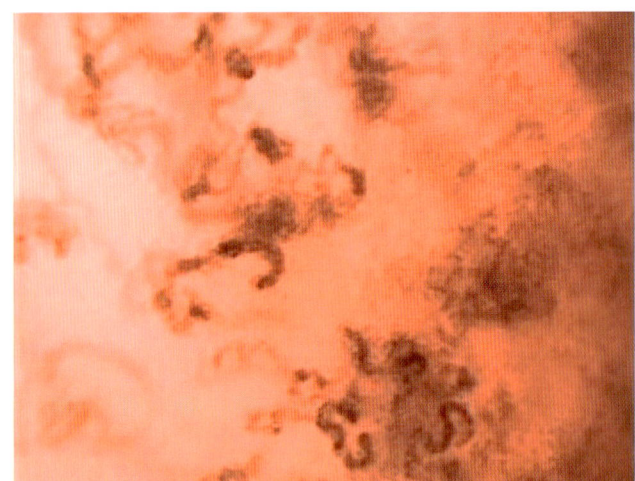

Figure 51.10 Tumoural vessels.

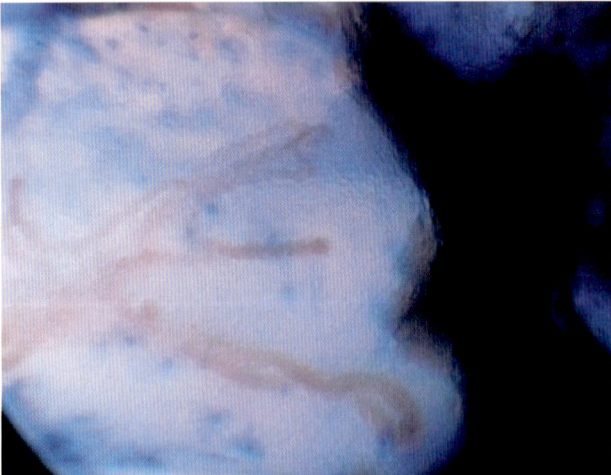
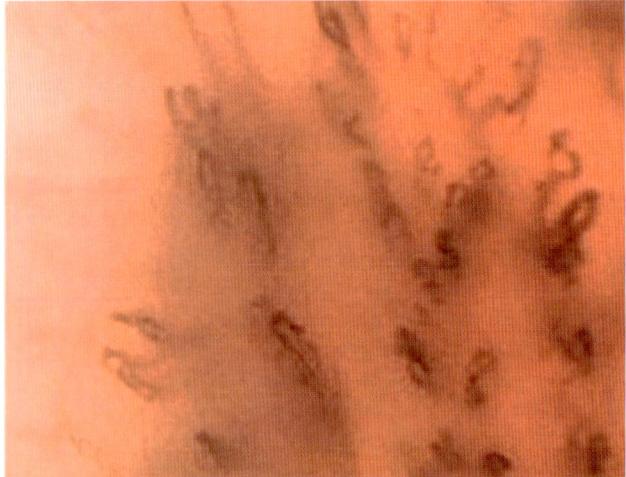

Figure 51.11 Papilloma of the larynx. Vascular axis of the papillas, 60X.

Figure 51.12 Papilloma of the larynx. Vascular axis of the papillas observed with NBI, 60X.

better conditions for removal and potentially reducing the risks of residual disease.

The direct application of the contact endoscope allows the identification of the typical vascular loops (**Figures 51.11, 51.12**). The degree of visualization of the vascular structure depends on the density of the keratosis that is associated with the disease in some cases.

With the vital stain, in some cases it is possible to identify the typical koilocytes (ballooned cells) (**Figure 51.13**) and inflammatory infiltrates. Koilocytes are typical of human papillomavirus infected cells.

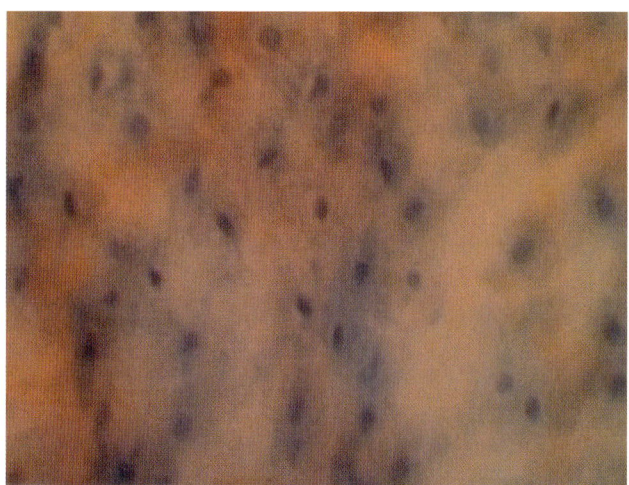

Figure 51.13 Papilloma of the larynx. Koilocytes are identified, 150X.

Beyond the characterization of the lesions, contact endoscopy allows the assessment of neighbouring areas, and sometimes it is possible to identify subclinical stages of the disease.

CONCLUSION

Contact endoscopy is a non-invasive clinical technique and is currently the only technique that allows an *in vivo* and *in situ* assessment based on the observation of the microvascular networks and of the cells of the superficial layers of the epithelium.

In some cases, the cellular alterations precede or are more evident than the vascular alterations. In other cases the modifications of the vascular networks and the course of the vessels that are present occur before the identification of cellular changes.

Contact endoscopy allows not only the observation of vessels and cells of the lesion or of a suspected area identified macroscopically, but also of all the anatomical territory. The application of the contact endoscope to several anatomical sites allows an assessment of the extent of pathology and importantly the transition of a normal to pathological tissue.

The information that is obtained (vascular and cellular alterations of a pathological entity) is obtained in real time. These alterations are not limited to the macroscopic lesion and become integrated in a much wider concept – the concept of disease. This occurs in the subclinical stages that become associated with the main lesion.

The visualization of vascular network alterations simultaneously with the observation of the cells of the superficial layers of the mucosa opens an enormous window for the understanding of the physiopathology allowing a more correct and precise diagnosis, with repercussions in the therapeutic planning, in the follow-up and prognosis.

Contact endoscopy of the upper aerodigestive tract, with the exception of the larynx and trachea, can be performed in the outpatient setting. Beyond being minimally invasive, it does not cause pain to the patient, typically does not even require local anaesthesia and the image recording of the image allows a single endoscopy. The high definition video technology allows a more detailed analysis.

The association of contact endoscopy with the 'narrow band imaging' is currently the most detailed way (in clinical practice) of studying the microvasculature of the mucosa of a patient with upper aerodigestive pathology.

Combining the conventional endoscopic techniques with contact endoscopy and analyzing the patterns with the cellular and vascular changes, it is possible to aid diagnose in a more precise way for chronic inflammation, fungal infections, some viral infections, mechanical trauma, metaplasia, keratosis, dysplasia and tumours, hence improving the mapping of alterations of the disease.

Having access to all this information can modify the therapeutic approach, medical as well as surgical, and in some cases changing both simultaneously.

Whatever the developments of new therapies, there is little doubt that a more detailed and profound knowledge of a disease with the *in vivo* and *in situ* observation of the vascular networks combined with the alterations at the cellular level will create a new way of thinking.

Contact endoscopy represents a new phase of the development of endoscopy. With experience from different centers and technological progress, new ideas, concepts and instruments will occur. If all this progress facilitates a more thorough examination it will also require a more detailed knowledge and understanding of each organ and anatomical territory of the upper aerodigestive tract.

Images obtained by contact endoscopy promote intense and fruitful interdisciplinary work. This will continue to be fundamental to the development of the technique.

KEY POINTS

- Contact endoscopy allows non-invasive evaluation of micovasculature and cells.
- Contact endoscopy allows appreciation of cellular differences at transition zones.
- Most upper aerodigestive mucosa has vessels which run parallel to the surface mucosa.
- Contact endoscopy may assist the identification of safe margins during surgery.

REFERENCES

1. Andrea M. *Vascularização arterial da laringe, distribuição macro e microvascular*. Tese de Doutoramento: Faculdade de Medicina de Lisboa; 1975.
2. Andrea M, Guerrier Y. L'Epiglotte et ses amarrages. *Cahiers d'ORL Chir Cervicofac* 1979; **14**: 793–803.
3. Andrea M, Guerrier Y. Microvascularization de la muqueuse laryngée et trachéale: introduction à la physiopathologie des lésions sténosantes. *Ann Oto-laryngol Chir Cervicofac (Paris)* 1980; **97**: 409–21.
4. Andrea M, Guerrier Y. The anterior commissure of the larynx. *Clin Otolaryngol* 1981; **6**: 259–64.
5. Andrea M. Vasculature of the anterior commissure. *Ann Otol Rhinol Laryngol* 1981; **90**: 18–20.
6. Andrea M, Dias O, Paço J, Santos A. Endoscopia rígida associada a microcirurgia endolaríngea, contribuição para o estudo da patologia benigna, pré-maligna e maligna das cordas vocais. *J Ciências Médicas* 1993; **157**: 15–35.
7. Andrea M, Dias O. *Rigid endoscopy associated with microlaryngeal surgery (REMS)*. Endo World – ORL 25E, Karl Storz; 1995.
8. Andrea M, Dias O, Paço J, et al. Anatomical borders in staging: rigid endoscopy associated to microlaryngeal surgery. In: Smee R, Bridger G (eds). *Laryngeal cancer*. Sidney, Australia: Elsevier Science BV; 1994, pp. 233–35.
9. Andrea M, Dias O, Paço J. Endoscopic anatomy of the larynx. In: Fabian R and Gluckman J (eds). *Current review of otolaryngology & head and neck surgery*. London: Churchill Livingstone, 1995.
10. Andrea M, Dias O, Santos A. Contact endoscopy during microlaryngeal surgery: a new technique for endoscopic examination of the larynx. *Ann Otol Rhinol Laryngol* 1995; **104**: 333–39.
11. Desormaux A. *De l'endoscope et de ses applications au diagnostique et au traitement des affections de l'uréthre et de la vessie*. Paris, 1865.
12. Jaupitre M. La cystocinématographie en couleur. *Communication au Congrés Français d'Urologie* 1955; 128.
13. Hamou J. *Hysteroscopy and microcolpohysteroscopy, text and atlas*. Norwalk, CT: Appleton & Lange, 1991.
14. Andrea M, Dias O. *Contact endoscopy associated to microlaryngeal surgery (CEMS)*. Endo World – ORL 30E, Karl Storz, 1996.
15. Andrea M, Dias O. *Atlas of rigid and contact endoscopy in microlaryngeal surgery*. Philadelphia: Lippincott-Raven Publishers, 1995.
16. Andrea M, Dias O, Santos A. Contact endoscopy of the vocal cord. Normal and pathological patterns. *Acta Otolaryngol (Stock)* 1995; **115**: 314–16.
17. Andrea M, Dias O. Rigid and contact endoscopy associated to microlaryngeal surgery. In: Fried M (ed) *The larynx: a multidisciplinary approach*. 2nd ed. St Louis: Mosby Year Book; 1996.
18. Andrea M, Dias O. Rigid and contact endoscopy during microsurgery. In: Yanagisawa E (ed). *Color atlas of diagnostic endoscopy in otorhinolaryngology*. Tokyo: Igaku Shoin; 1996.
19. Andrea M, Dias O. Endoscopic assessment of early vocal cord cancer. In: *Proceedings of IV International Conference of Head and Neck Tumors*. Toronto, 1996.
20. Andrea M, Dias O. Newer techniques of laryngeal assessment. In: Cummings C, Frederikson J, Harker L, et al. (eds). *Otolaryngology head and neck surgery*. 3rd ed. St Louis: Mosby; 1998.
21. Andrea M, Dias O. La Endoscopia rígida y de contacto en la evaluación de las lesiones premalignas de la laringe. In: Suarez Nieto C (ed). *Tratado de Otolaringologia y Cirugia de Cabeza y Cuello*. Madrid: Proyectos Médicos; 1999.
22. Andrea M, Dias O. Rigid and contact endoscopy of the larynx. In: Ferlito A (ed). *Diseases of the larynx*. London: Arnold/Oxford University Press; 2000, pp. 1001–11.
23. Andrea M, Dias O, Macor C, et al. Contact endoscopy of the nasal mucosa. *Acta Otolaryngol (Stock)* 1997; **117**: 307–11.
24. Andrea M, Dias O. *Contact endoscopy of the nasal mucosa*. Endo World – ORL 40E, 1998.
25. Andrea M, Dias O. *Contact endoscopy*. Tutlingen: Endo-Press; 1999.
26. Andrea M, Dias O. Contact endoscopy. In: Gleeson M, Jones N, Burton M, et al. (eds). *Scott-Brown's otorhinolaryngology head and neck surgery*. 7th ed. New York: Hodder Arnold; 2008.
27. Piazza C, Cocco D, De Benedetto L, et al. Narrow band imaging and high definition television in the assessment of laryngeal cancer: a prospective study on 279 patients. *Eur Arch Oto-Rhino-Laryngol* 2010; **267**: 409–14.
28. Arens C, Malzahn K, Dias O, et al. Endoskopische bildegebende Verfahren in der Diagnostik des Kehlkopfkarzinoms und seiner Vorstufen. *Laryngorhinootologie* 1999; **78**: 685–91.
29. Arens C, Glanz H, Dreyer T, Malzahn K. Compact endoscopy of the larynx. *Ann Otol Rhinol Laryngol* 2003; **112**: 113–19.
30. Carriero E, Galli J, Fadda G, et al. Preliminary experiences with contact endoscopy of the larynx. *Eur Arch Otorhinolaryngol* 2000; **257**: 68–71.
31. Cikojević D, Gluncić I, Pesutić-Pisac V. Comparison of contact endoscopy and frozen section histopathology in the intra-operative diagnosis of laryngeal pathology. *J Laryngol Otol* 2008; **122**: 836–39.
32. D'Avila J. Estudo comparativo da microvascularização das cordas vocais humanas acometidas por cisto e reação nodular contra-lateral 'in vivo', através das endoscopias rígida e de contato da laringe. PhD thesis. Universidade de S. Paulo, 2002.
33. Dedivitis R, Pfuetzenreiter E, Guimarães A. Contact endoscopy of the larynx as an auxiliary method to the surgical margins in frontolateral laryngectomy. *Acta Otorhinolaryngol Ital* 2009; **29**: 16–20.
34. Guimarães A, Brandão L, Dedivitis R. Contact endoscopy for identifying the parathyroid glands during thyroidectomy. *Acta Otorhinolaryngol Ital* 2010; **30**(1): 20–26.
35. Just T, Pau H, Witt M, Hummel T. Contact endoscopic comparison of morphology of human fungiform papillae of healthy subjects and patients with transected chorda tympani nerve. *Laryngoscope* 2006; **116**: 1216–21.
36. Konstantinidis I, Chatziavramidis A, Printza A, et al. Effects of smoking on taste: assessment with contact endoscopy and taste strips. *Laryngoscope* 2010; **120**(10): 1958–63.
37. Pak M, To K, Leung S, Van Hasselt C. In vivo diagnosis of nasopharyngeal carcinoma using contact rhinoscopy. *Laryngoscope* 2001; **11**: 1453–58.
38. Pak M. The use of office-based contact rhinoscopy for in vivo real time diagnosis of nasopharyngeal carcinoma. PhD thesis. The Chinese University of Hong Kong, 2008.
39. Pau H, Dommerich S, Just T, Beust M. Cholesteatoma recurrences caused by intraoperative cell seeding? Contact endoscopic and cytologic studies. *Laryngo Rhino Otol* 2001; **80**: 499–502.
40. Pelucchi S, Bianchini C, Travagli M, Pastore A. Contact endoscopy of the oral mucosa: preliminary results. *Acta Otorhinolaryngol Ital* 2007; **27**: 59–61.
41. Prado F, Weber R, Romano F, Voegels R. Evaluation of inverted papilloma and squamous cell carcinoma by nasal contact endoscopy. *Am J Rhinol Allergy* 2010; **24**(3): 210–14.
42. Richtsmeier W, Huang P, Scher R. In situ identification of normal visceral tissues using contact telescopic microscopy. *Laryngoscope* 1999; **109**: 216–20.
43. Saeki N, Tsuzuki K, Negoro A, et al. Utility of real-time diagnosis using contact endoscopy for oral and lingual diseases. *Auris Nasus Larynx* 2011; **38**: 233–39.
44. Sone M, Sato E, Hayashi H, et al. Vascular evaluation in laryngeal diseases: comparison between contact endoscopy and laser doppler flowmetry. *Arch Otolaryngol Head Neck Surg* 2006; **132**: 1371–74.
45. Szeto C, Wehrli B, Whelan F, et al. Contact endoscopy as a novel technique in the detection and diagnosis of mucosal lesions in the head and neck: a brief review. *J Oncol* 2011. article ID 196302, 6 pages.
46. Tarnawski W, Fraczek M, Jelen M, et al. The role of computer assisted analysis in the evaluation of nuclear characteristics for the diagnosis of precancerous and cancerous lesions by contact laryngoscopy. *Adv Med Sci, Poland* 2008; **53**: 221–27.
47. Wardrop PJ, Sim S, Mclaren K. Contact endoscopy of the larynx: a quantitative study. *J Laryngol and Otol* 2000; **114**: 437–40.
48. Warnecke A, Averbeck T, Leinung M, et al. Contact endoscopy for the evaluation of the pharyngeal and laryngeal mucosa. *Laryngoscope* 2010; **120**: 253–56.
49. Xiaoming H, Haiqiang M, Manquan D, et al. Examination of nasopharyngeal epithelium with contact endoscopy. *Acta Otolaryngol (Stock)* 2001; **121**: 98–102.

Section 2
Head and Neck Endocrine Surgery

Overview

52 History of thyroid and parathyroid surgery............... 597
53 Developmental anatomy of the thyroid and parathyroid glands 603
54 Developmental anatomy of the pituitary fossa 611
55 Physiology of the thyroid and parathyroid glands.... 619
56 Physiology of the pituitary gland.............................. 629
57 Imaging in head and neck endocrine disease 643
58 Thyroid and parathyroid gland pathology 651

Thyroid disease

59 Clinical evaluation of the thyroid patient 705
60 Investigation of thyroid disease 709
61 Benign thyroid disease... 717
62 Management of differentiated thyroid cancer 751
63 Management of medullary thyroid cancer 757
64 Management of anaplastic thyroid cancer/lymphoma 765
65 Management of locoregionally recurrent differentiated thyroid cancer 773
66 Non-surgical management of thyroid cancer 779

Thyroid surgery

67 Thyroidectomy 793
68 Surgery for locally advanced and nodal disease 805
69 Minimally invasive and robotic thyroid surgery 811
70 Surgery for the enlarged thyroid.............................. 819

Parathyroid disease

71 Clinical evaluation of hypercalcaemia...................... 827
72 Investigation of hyperparathyroidism....................... 833
73 Management of hyperparathyroidism 843
74 Management of persistent and recurrent hyperparathyroidism 851
75 Management of parathyroid cancer......................... 857
76 Bilateral parathyroid exploration 865

Parathyroid surgery

77 Minimally invasive parathyroidectomy 873
78 Surgical failure and reoperative surgery.................. 879

Thyroid and parathyroid outcomes

79 Complications of thyroid and parathyroid surgery and how to avoid them................................ 887
80 Thyroid and parathyroid surgery: Audit and outcomes 893
81 Medicolegal aspects of head and neck endocrine surgery 899

Pituitary disease

82 Clinical evaluation of the pituitary patient 905
83 Investigation of pituitary disease.............................. 915
84 Primary pituitary disease.. 923
85 Surgical management of recurrent pituitary tumours... 941
86 Adjuvant treatment of pituitary disease 951

Overview

CHAPTER 52

HISTORY OF THYROID AND PARATHYROID SURGERY

Waraporn Imruetaicharoenchoke, Ashok R. Shaha and Neil Sharma

Thyroid surgery 597	Summary 601
Parathyroid surgery 600	References 601

SEARCH STRATEGY

Data in this chapter may be updated by a Medline search using the keywords: thyroid, goitre, history, endocrine, surgery. Key historical texts were consulted in print where possible, or via online access if not. Reference lists were examined for further sources of evidence.

THYROID SURGERY

The dark ages: Shoe laces, seaweed and the King's touch

Thyroid surgery has its roots over one millennium ago, with goitre being recognized well before that. Pliny the Elder (AD 23–73) in his work *Naturalis Historia* mentions hernia gutteres, as does Aëtius of Amida (c.5th–6th century) in his compilation the *Tetrabiblion*. In this time, the thyroid gland was not recognized as a normal structure and these enlargements were considered new formations. In time, the thyroid was seen as a normal organ, although its function was still unknown. In 1511, during the Italian Renaissance, Leonardo Da Vinci was the first person to draw the anatomical shape of the thyroid gland correctly, but he misinterpreted its function as only filling up empty space in neck. In the 16th century, Andreas Vesalius described the thyroid structure, considering it a laryngeal gland, while Bartholomeus Eustachius correctly noticed that this gland had two lobes conjoined by isthmus; Aelius Galemus reported its role was lubrication of the larynx. In 1656 Thomas Wharton named it the 'glandulae thyroidea' or 'thyroid' because of the juxtaposition to the thyroid cartilage, which is shield-shaped.[1,2]

Treatment of thyroid goitre was first described in 2700 BC in Chinese literary works; this involved administering seaweed and burnt sea sponge (we now know this is due to their high iodine content). The earliest recorded operation on the thyroid was performed by Albucasis (Abu al-Qasim al-Zahrawi, AD 936–1013), a Moorish physician, using simple ligatures and hot cautery irons; however, his works seemed to be forgotten. Indeed, Ruggiero Frugadi (pre AD 1140–1195) of the Salerno School of Surgery is often credited as performing the first goitre surgery in 1170, using bootlaces as setons to ligate and transfix a pedunculated goitre, allowing it then to slough off.[3] King Henry IV of France (1553–1610) practised the 'King's touch', akin to the laying on of hands, in the 16th century. This technique was famous in Europe between 1100 and 1600 with many thousands of people reportedly 'cured' of different ailments.

The true beginnings: Foolhardy performances and horrid butchery

Despite these early attempts, thyroid surgery did not progress for several centuries. Early attempts by Benjamin Gooch (1708–1776) resulted in fatal haemorrhage and the thyroid's adherence to the trachea meant that for many years it was considered impossible to safely separate the two structures. During the French Revolution, Pierre-Joseph Desault (1744–1795) performed a successful thyroidectomy on a 20-year-old woman.[4] He demonstrated that careful dissection coupled with ligation of the key vessels would allow the surgeon to remove the thyroid gland and for the patient to survive through the postoperative period. For many years, Desault's technique was the accepted standard, but mortality in 1850 was still in the region of 41%.[5] Most patients suffered with both primary or secondary haemorrhage and an almost inevitable sepsis.

The unacceptably high mortality and morbidity rates, both short- and long-term, led to the French Academy of Medicine banning thyroid surgery. It was described as 'breathtaking heroics fraught with danger to the patient and almost certain bereavement for the family'.[6] Johann Dieffenbach (1792–1847), a German surgeon who reportedly tried every method known to treat vesicovaginal fistula, thought of thyroid operations as 'foolhardy performances' and 'one of the most thankless, most perilous undertakings which, if not altogether prohibited, should at least be restricted'.[7] Even the great American surgeon Samuel Gross (1805–1884) wrote that 'every step he takes will be environed with difficulty, every stroke of his knife will be followed by a torrent of blood, and lucky will it be for him if his victim lives long enough to enable him to finish his horrid butchery' and 'also no honest and sensible surgeon will ever engage in it'.[8] However, as the 19th century progressed, the practice of thyroid surgery was revolutionized by three advances that took it from the realms of a last-ditch approach for the rapidly succumbing patient to a recognized, valid treatment for goitre.

The new dawn: Three great advances and the fathers of thyroid surgery

During the mid 1800s, three important discoveries changed the evolution of thyroid surgery.[5] In 1842 Crawford Williamson Long (1815–1878), an American surgeon, was the first doctor to administer inhaled ether as an anaesthetic agent, although at the time the credit was given to the dentist Horace Wells (1815–1848) and the surgeon John C. Warren (1778–1856) for an operation in 1846. The first thyroidectomy under ether anaesthesia took place in St Petersburg under Nikolay Pirogoft (1810–1881) in 1849.[9] Secondly, and a few years later in 1867, Joseph Lister's (1827–1912) theories of antisepsis using carbolic acid, followed shortly after by asepsis, dramatically reduced the infection and sepsis rates after surgery and did a great deal to reduce mortality.[4] The last development was of haemostatic forceps, used in central Europe in 1870 by Thomas Spencer Wells (1818–1897)[10] and redesigned as the operative haemostat in 1874 by Jules-Emile Péan (1830–1898).[6] These led to improved haemorrhage control over the traditional methods such as the artery hook, mass ligature, crushing forceps and crude cautery.

These three developments prepared the way for Christian Albert Theodor Billroth (1829–1894) (**Figure 52.1a**), arguably the most famous surgeon of his day. Billroth trained at the University of Berlin before becoming the chair of surgery at the University of Zurich at the age of 31. In his first year at Zurich, he performed 20 thyroidectomies, but his mortality rate was around 40%, mostly from sepsis. Despite becoming disheartened and abandoning thyroid surgery for almost 10 years, he returned to it when he moved to the chair of surgery at the University of Vienna. He embraced anaesthesia and initiated the use of antisepsis and haemostats. He was also the first surgeon to wear gloves, albeit cotton, when operating, and his mortality rate fell from nearly 40% to 8%, making him the most well-known thyroid surgeon at that time. Despite this, he was still troubled by post-operative tetany and damage to the recurrent laryngeal nerve.

Billroth's most valuable contribution to thyroid surgery is arguably the students he taught, many of whom went on to become outstanding surgeons in their own right. Anton Wölfler (1850–1917), Anton von Eiselsberg (1860–1939), Jan von Mikulicz-Radecki (1850–1905) and Hans von Haberer (1875–1958) all contributed not only to thyroid surgery but to surgery in general. However, Billroth's greatest student, and the surgeon who can be truly considered the 'Father of thyroid surgery', was Emil Theodor Kocher (1841–1917) (**Figure 52.1b**).

Having trained with Lucke, Billroth and Langenbeck, Kocher studied and acted on the successes and failures of those around him, constantly updating his technique to give better results. His knowledge of anatomy and circulation aided his meticulous dissection technique, and he adopted the now standard collar incision that bears his name in 1890.

Kocher was also one of the first surgeons to audit his own results. In a review of his 101 cases in the mid 1880s, he found that most of his unilateral excision patients were well, but all of the total resections were suffering with symptoms we would now recognize as hypothyroidism. This had also been described by Jacques-Louis Reverdin, with patients who underwent total thyroidectomy experiencing

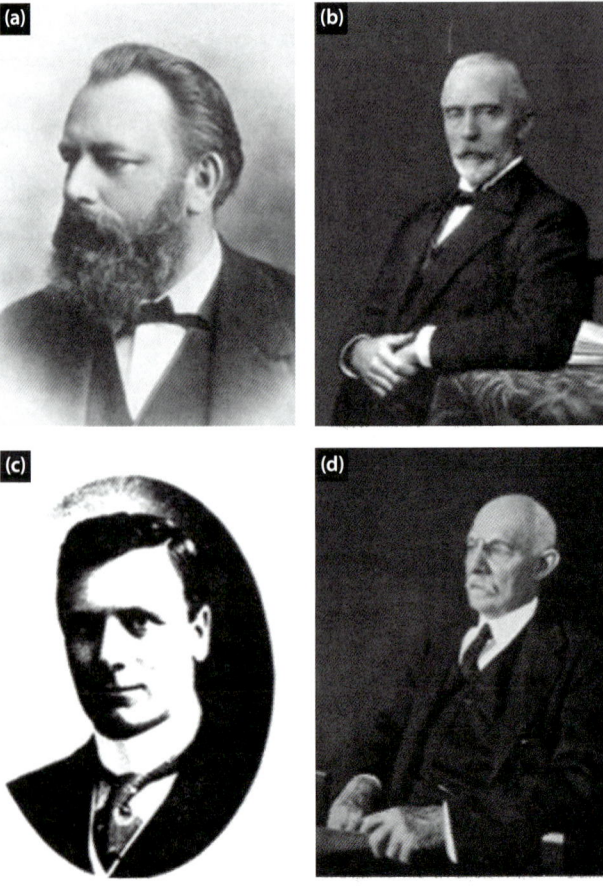

Figure 52.1 The fathers of thyroid surgery. (a) Theodor Billroth, **(b)** Theodor Kocher, **(c)** William Halsted, **(d)** Thomas Dunhill.

personality change and distressed physical features named 'myxoed me operatoire'.[11] Kocher realized that this adverse condition was caused by deprivation of thyroid hormone, and then called it 'cachexia thyreopriva', acknowledging that the thyroid gland had a function. Subsequently, Kocher prohibited total thyroidectomy except in the treatment of thyroid cancer, to avoid this condition. His method of preventing damage to the recurrent laryngeal nerve was to switch from extracapsular to intracapsular dissection, leaving thyroid tissue behind posteriorly. He was also an early proponent of iodinizing drinking water to prevent goitrogenesis. Kocher kept detailed outcome records and it is a testament to his ability as a surgeon and innovator that, when he presented his surgical experience to the Swiss Surgical Congress in 1917, his mortality was 0.2% for ordinary goitre and 2% for what we now consider hyperthyroid goitre, all in an era before antithyroid drugs and radioactive iodine.[12] His work in physiology, pathology and surgery on thyroid gland led to the award of the Nobel Prize in Medicine in 1909.[13]

Kocher went on to train William Halsted (1794–1878, **Figure 52.1c**), an American surgeon who studied in Vienna. On his return to America, Halsted popularized the use of haemostatic forceps and his work on parathyroid preservation and post-operative calcium/parathyroid extract supplementation to prevent hypocalcaemia did much to improve thyroid surgery. Halsted also swapped Billroth's cotton gloves for ones made from rubber. He later concluded that: 'The extirpation of the thyroid gland for goiter typifies perhaps better than any other operations the supreme triumph of the surgeon's art'.[9]

Another difficulty that thyroid surgeons were encountering was that of the patient with exophthalmic goitre. First described by Caleb Hillier Parry (1755–1822) in a posthumous publication in 1825,[1] the condition we now know as Graves' disease linked thyrocardiac symptoms, such as palpitations and tachycardia, with exophthalmos, extreme nervousness, and goitre. Surgery in these patients was reserved for those in extremis as the operation was fraught with difficulty, and mortality was very high. Nevertheless, in 1884 Ludwig Rehn (1849–1930) reported the full recovery of patients from thyrotoxic symptoms following thyroid surgery due to compressive goitres. In 1887, Theodor Kocher demonstrated increased vascularization of the thyroid gland in a patient diagnosed with Graves' disease and recommended that the thyrotoxic symptoms originated by an increase in thyroid hormone level. Thereafter, he practised staged thyroidectomy, first ligating the main feeding vessels to the gland and then removing one lobe at a second operation.

Over the following decade, the mortality rate for surgery for Graves' disease improved to around 6%; however, 25% patients developed recurrent disease requiring a second operation.[14] In 1905 Frank Hartley advocated that the cure rate of thyroidectomy for Graves' disease relied on removing a sufficient amount of the thyroid gland, and he recommended resecting one thyroid lobe and some portions of the opposite lobe for treatment of hyperthyroid patients.[15] Thomas Dunhill (1876–1957) (**Figure 52.1d**) followed Hartley's theory and in 1912 published the outcomes of 380 thyrotoxic patients who underwent surgery, with a mortality of around 1% and a minimal recurrence rate.[16] Over the next two decades, Dunhill gradually moved to carrying out bilateral subtotal thyroidectomy, as Jan Mikulicz-Radecki (1850–1905) did for the treatment of simple goitre.[17]

The pre-operative preparation of hyperthyroid patients became more widely recognized as key to reducing complications. Charles Mayo (1865–1939) and George Crile (1864–1943) worked closely with the endocrinologist Henry Plummer (1874–1936), pioneering this cross-specialty collaboration in the United States.

Plummer began treating hyperthyroid patients with iodine before passing them on to Mayo for surgery; this approach decreased the incidence of thyroid storm and also mortality rate.[18] Consequently, the staged thyroid operation could be abandoned and the whole gland removed in one sitting. The improved survival and cure rate moved thyroidectomy for Graves' disease from an operation reserved for moribund patients to a curative procedure for those with much milder disease. The introduction of radioiodine in Boston and Berkley for the treatment of thyroid cancer and Graves' disease in 1942[19, 20] did much to improve outcomes further, as did the use of the antithyroid drugs thiourea and thiouracil created and advocated by Edwin Bennett Astwood (1909–1976) in Boston.[21]

The modern age

The history of thyroid surgery belongs to general surgery, but over the past three decades we have seen a shift towards otolaryngologists and head and neck surgeons working together with endocrine surgeons. Endocrine surgery has now come of age and, from a thyroid and parathyroid point of view, multidisciplinary and collaborative specialist work began when Dick Welbourn founded the British Association of Endocrine Surgeons (BAES) in 1983 (later to become the British Association of Endocrine and Thyroid Surgeons (BAETS)). This organization focused on specialist endocrine multidisciplinary working to include education and research and welcomed the ear, nose and throat (ENT) surgeon into its fold. It was much more recently that the American Association of Endocrine Surgeons (AAES) included otolaryngology in their membership.

Modern-day greats of endocrine/head and neck surgery reflect the shared responsibility between general surgery and otolaryngology. In the United States, general surgeons Jatin Shah, Ashok Shaha, Keith Heller and Joseph Attie (New York) and Orlo Clark from San Francisco as well as Samuel Wells from Duke have led the way in both surgical techniques and education. Significant contributions from otolaryngology in the USA have come from David Terris (Augusta), Greg Randolph (Massachusetts), and David Eisele and Ralph Tufano (both Baltimore). In Australia, Leigh Delbridge and Tom Reeve (Sydney) did much to advance endocrine surgery, in particular the creation and maintenance of prospective surgical databases.

In Europe, Charles Proye from Lille and Jean Françoise Henri from Marseilles (both general surgeons) led the way; in the United Kingdom, much is owed to Professor Malcolm Wheeler (general and endocrine surgery) from Cardiff and Omar Shaheen (otolaryngology) from Guy's Hospital; the link between general surgery and otolaryngology in the UK and the USA was cemented when John Watkinson (Birmingham) was the first ENT surgeon to be elected President of the BAETS (2011–13) and recently Greg Randolph has become the first otolaryngologist member of the AAES.

With the advent of thyroid specialists, the operative technique has undergone significant refinement and subsequent changes in the extent of surgery performed. While initially total thyroidectomy/lobectomy were the procedures of choice, concerns over preservation of the parathyroid glands and recurrent laryngeal nerves, as well as maintaining some functioning thyroid tissue, led to a move towards sub-total thyroidectomy. This has been largely abandoned now, however, and the current recommendations are for either total lobectomy or total thyroidectomy as the only valid operations, with near-total acceptable to preserve a nerve at risk. These changes have resulted from the era of evidence-based medicine and subsequent focus on outcomes. The prognostic factors and risk group analyses in thyroid cancer were very well defined by Hay from the Mayo Clinic[22] and Cady from the Lahey Clinic,[23] as well as Shaha from Memorial Sloane Kettering.[24] The American Thyroid Association (ATA) has now incorporated these risk groups into the third edition of their thyroid cancer guidelines, published in 2015, which is a landmark document for the management of thyroid cancer.[25] For medullary thyroid cancer, Sam Wells defined the implications of RET mutation and the role of prophylactic thyroidectomy in these patients,[26] and recent guidelines have further detailed the timing of surgery.[27]

While other chapters will cover the latest technological advances that relate to thyroid surgery, a review of their development is appropriate here. The first major change has been the approach to the gland itself. While Kocher's classic 8–10 cm transverse incision was the standard for almost a century, the move towards minimally invasive approaches has resulted in scars commonly of 3–6 cm in length being usual for both thyroid and parathyroid surgery.[28] As well as smaller scars for access, the use of the endoscope has found its way into the thyroid surgeon's armamentarium. First described in 1997 by Paulo Mucozi,[29] this has evolved into minimally invasive video-assisted thyroidectomy (MIVAT) with access from the neck,[30] the axilla[31] or lateral approaches.[32,33] Thus far, complication rates are comparable to open surgery[34] and although operation time is longer, cosmesis and recovery appear improved over open. An almost inevitable extension from endoscopic thyroid surgery has been robot-assisted operations as pioneered by Chung at Yonsei University, South Korea. Designed to address the limitations of two-dimensional visualization and basic endoscopic instruments, a number of centres are now performing robotic thyroidectomy more often. The advantage of absent neck scar is currently countered by the extra dissection needed to reach the thyroid bed, longer operation time, learning curve and significant cost associated with the procedure. Whether this technique represents the future of thyroid surgery remains unclear.

The tools available to the surgeon have also advanced greatly, although their uptake has been variable. The intraoperative nerve monitor epitomizes this, with surgeons divided across the world as to its benefits versus disadvantages. As litigious medicine becomes more universal, the requirement for both real-time monitoring and assessment following surgery will surely increase. Dissection tools such as the harmonic scalpel and Ligasure™ are most widespread, and proponents herald the associated reduced operating time and improved haemostasis. Again, cost is a factor that rules these out for many units.

Surgical outcomes are now routinely measured in some manner by all hospitals, whether this be a personal or national audit. With the increased demand for transparency from the public, the requirement to participate in a national audit will become mandatory, as will the need for multidisciplinary meetings for suspected cancer cases.

The medical treatment of thyroid disease has also seen great leaps over the past half-century. In the post-war period, radioiodine treatment, antithyroid drugs and the technology surrounding thyroid surgery have advanced significantly. For thyrotoxic patients, medical treatment now carries high remission rates and reduces the number of patients requiring surgical treatment. Those who do progress or choose to have an operation are usually rendered euthyroid pre-operatively to decrease peri- and post-operative morbidity and mortality.

What is without doubt is that, in the modern era, the thyroid surgeon must act as a 'thyroidologist', capable of understanding the complexities of medical care as well as the nuances of surgery, and be willing to adapt their techniques and methods as modern technologies continue to gain ground.

PARATHYROID SURGERY

What we now know as the parathyroid glands were first identified by Sir Richard Owen, Hunterian Professor and Conservator of the Museum at the Royal College of Surgeons of England, in 1862 when he was asked to perform an autopsy on a Great Indian Rhinoceros. Owen described 'a small compact yellow glandular body attached to the thyroid at the point where the vein emerged',[35] resulting in the occasional use of the name 'Owen's glands'. However, the naming and description of the parathyroid glands is credited in 1880 to the Swedish medical student Ivan Viktor Sandstrom (1852–1889). Sandstrom's finding was unrecognized for more than 10 years until in 1891 Eugene Gley (1857–1930) repeated his discovery and also found that removal of these glands in animals resulted in tetany.[36] William George MacCallum (1874–1944) and Carl Voegtlin (1879–1960) subsequently discovered that the tetany produced by parathyroidectomy could be treated with a calcium infusion.[37] In parallel to these findings, Friedrich von Recklinghausen (1833–1910), a pathologist in Strasbourg, described the characteristics of a specific bone disease which correlated with parathyroid lesion in 1891,[38] followed by the report in 1904 by Max Askanazy (1865–1940) of a female patient with a severe bone condition and a tumour lateral to her thyroid gland. Askanazy incorrectly interpreted that the parathyroid lesion was secondary to the bone disease rather than being the primary lesion itself.[39] In 1915, Friedrich Schlagenhaufer (1866–1930) suggested that parathyroid tumours themselves are the primary lesions affecting severe skeletal changes.[40] Nearly a decade later, Felix Mandl (1892–1957) treated a patient suffering from osteitis fibrosa cystica of the femur who had failed treatment with thyroid and parathyroid extract. Mandl planned to perform a parathyroid transplantation, but on exploring the neck he discovered a parathyroid tumour, which he proceeded to excise. The patient's post-operative serum calcium levels returned to normal and their bone disease recovered, supporting Schagenhaufer's hypothesis.

In 1926, Edward Delos Churchill (1895–1972) set out to explore the neck in a patient with primary hyperparathyroidism but failed to find a parathyroid tumour.[1] Just 3 years later, however, David Barr and Harold Bulger carried out the first successful parathyroidectomy for a patient with parathyroid disease, and they originated the term 'hyperparathyroidism'.[41] More surgeons began to perform the procedure, although there were still patients in whom no tumour was found.

One such patient was Captain Martell, treated by Oliver Cope (1902–1994). Cope, a student of Churchill who went on to become a leader in parathyroid surgery in his own right, performed numerous unsuccessful neck explorations before asking Churchill's opinion. Churchill proceeded to find the adenoma in the anterior mediastinum via a partial sternotomy, becoming the first surgeon to describe this.[42] As well as the anatomical variants of the parathyroid glands, advances in the understanding of the physiology of parathyroid hormone (PTH) continued throughout the early to middle 20th century. PTH was first isolated in 1923 by Adolph Hanson (1888–1959) and successfully extracted by James Collip (1892–1965).[43]

It was Gerald Aurbach (1927–1991), however, who first purified the hormone in 1959.[44] In 1963, Solomon Aaron Berson (1918–1972) and Rosalyn Yalow (1921–2011) developed a radioimmunoassay to quantify PTH levels in the bloodstream, which greatly aided the diagnostic process.[45] After that period, determination of parathyroid disease and parathyroid surgery were greatly advancing.

From then to the present day, as for thyroid surgery, the management of parathyroid disease has been improved through previously described multidisciplinary working and advances in imaging, medical therapies and surgical techniques. Key among these advances is the use of localization studies (ultrasound, sestamibi and computed tomography (CT), specifically SPECT-CT scans and 4D CT with venous sampling) to identify the site of a diseased gland, thus greatly reducing the need for multigland exploration, and the risks inherent to operating in the central compartment on both sides of the neck – all of this facilitates minimally invasive techniques and targeted approaches. Intra-operative PTH measurement has allowed the surgeon to check for a fall in the PTH minutes after removing a suspect adenoma, again to determine whether further exploration in needed.

However, despite all the advances, the key to parathyroid surgery remains as it was when Edward Churchill described it: 'the success of parathyroid surgery must lie in the ability of the surgeon to know a parathyroid gland when he saw it, to know the distribution of glands, where they hide, and also be delicate enough in technique to be able to use this knowledge'.[42]

SUMMARY

The history of thyroid and parathyroid surgery is rich in the names of famous surgeons who advanced the practice from butchery to art form. With technological advances being made regularly, we can expect to see further changes over the coming years, although it will be some time before the original operation, described by Kocher over a century ago, ceases to be the gold standard.

KEY POINTS

- Thyroid surgery has a rich history stretching back a thousand years, and it is replete with the names of the most famous surgeons of the day.
- While technology has leapt forward over the past 50 years, thyroidectomy is still based on Kocher's original description.
- More recent advances have led to both thyroid and parathyroid surgery becoming increasingly specialized.

REFERENCES

1. Welbourn RB. *The history of endocrine surgery*. New York: Praeger; 1990.
2. Medvei VC. *The history of clinical endocrinology*, 2nd ed. New York: Parthenon; 1993.
3. Corner G. *The rise of medicine at Salerno in the twelfth century*. New York: P.B. Hoeber; 1931.
4. Zimmerman LM, Veith I. *Great ideas in the history of surgery*. Baltimore: Williams & Wilkins; 1961.
5. Becker WF. Pioneers in thyroid surgery. *Ann Surg* 1977; **185**(5): 493–504.
6. Tapscott WJ. A brief history of thyroid surgery. *Curr Surg* 2001; **58**(5): 464–6.
7. Diffenbach JF. *Die Operative Chirurgie*. Leipzig: F.A. Brockhaus; 1848.
8. Gross S. *A system of surgery*. Philadelphia: H.C. Lea; 1866.
9. Halsted W. *The operative story of goitre: the author's operation*. Baltimore: Johns Hopkins Press; 1919.

10. Wells S. The use of torsion in surgical operations. *BMJ* 1874; **1**(680): 47.
11. Welbourn RB. Highlights from endocrine surgical history. *World J Surg* 1996; **20**(5): 603–12.
12. McGreevy PS, Miller FA. Biography of Theodor Kocher. *Surgery* 1969; **65**(6): 990–9.
13. Choong C, Kaye AH. Emil Theodor Kocher (1841-1917). *J Clin Neurosci* 2009; **16**(12): 1552–4.
14. Kocher E. The surgical treatment of exophthalmic goiter. *J Am Med Assoc* 1907; **49**(15): 1240–4.
15. Hartley F. II. Thyroidectomy for exophthalmic goitre. *Ann Surg* 1905; **42**(1): 33–48.
16. Dunhill TP. A discussion on partial thyroidectomy under local anaesthesia, with special reference to exophthalmic goitre: an address introductory to a discussion on the subject. *Proc R Soc Med* 1912; **5**(Surg sect): 61–9.
17. Cope O, Welch CE. The care of patients requiring thyroidectomy. *N Engl J Med* 1942; **227**(23): 870–4.
18. Plummer HS, Boothby WM. The value of iodine in exophthalmic goiter. *Ill Med J* 1924; **46**: 401–7.
19. Hertz S, Roberts A. Radioactive iodine in the study of thyroid physiology: the use of radioactive iodine therapy in hyperthyroidism. *J Am Med Assoc* 1946; **131**: 81–6.
20. Hamilton J, Lawrence J. Recent clinical developments in the therapeutic application of radio-phosphorus and radio-iodine. *J Clin Invest* 1942; **21**: 624.
21. Astwood EB. Treatment of hyperthyroidism with thiourea and thiouracil. *J Am Med Assoc* 1943; **122**: 78–81.
22. Hay ID, Bergstralh EJ, Goellner JR, et al. Predicting outcome in papillary thyroid-carcinoma: development of a reliable prognostic scoring system in a cohort of 1779 patients surgically treated at one institution during 1940 through 1989. *Surgery* 1993; **114**(6): 1050–8.
23. Cady B, Rossi R, Silverman M, Wool M. Further evidence of the validity of risk group definition in differentiated thyroid-carcinoma. *Surgery* 1985; **98**(6): 1171–8.
24. Shaha AR, Shah JP, Loree TR. Risk group stratification and prognostic factors in papillary carcinoma of thyroid. *Ann Surg Oncol* 1996; **3**(6): 534–8.
25. Haugen BR, Alexander EK, Bible KC, et al. 2015 American Thyroid Association management guidelines for adult patients with thyroid nodules and differentiated thyroid cancer. *Thyroid* 2016; **26**(1): 1–133.
26. Wells SA, Skinner MA. Prophylactic thyroidectomy, based on direct genetic testing, in patients at risk for the multiple endocrine neoplasia type 2 syndromes. *Exp Clin Endocrinol Diabetes* 1998; **106**(1): 29–34.
27. Lairmore TC, Diesen D, Goldfarb M, et al. American Association of Clinical Endocrinologists and American College of Endocrinology disease state clinical review: timing of multiple endocrine neoplasia thyroidectomy and extent of central neck lymphadenectomy. *Endocr Pract* 2015; **21**(7): 839–47.
28. Brunaud L, Zarnegar R, Wada N, et al. Incision length for standard thyroidectomy and parathyroidectomy: when is it minimally invasive? *Arch Surg* 2003; **138**(10): 1140–3.
29. Huscher CS, Chiodini S, Napolitano C, Recher A. Endoscopic right thyroid lobectomy. *Surg Endosc* 1997; **11**(8): 877.
30. Inabnet WB, Chu CA. Transcervical endoscopic-assisted mediastinal parathyroidectomy with intraoperative parathyroid hormone monitoring. *Surg Endosc* 2003; **17**(10): 1678.
31. Ikeda Y, Takami H, Sasaki Y, et al. Endoscopic neck surgery by the axillary approach. *J Am Coll Surg* 2000; **191**(3): 336–40.
32. Sebag F, Palazzo FF, Harding J, et al. Endoscopic lateral approach thyroid lobectomy: safe evolution from endoscopic parathyroidectomy. *World J Surg* 2006; **30**(5): 802–5.
33. Palazzo FF, Sebag F, Henry JF. Endocrine surgical technique: endoscopic thyroidectomy via the lateral approach. *Surg Endosc* 2006; **20**(2): 339–42.
34. Miccoli P, Berti P, Frustaci GL, et al. Video-assisted thyroidectomy: indications and results. *Langenbecks Arch Surg* 2006; **391**(2): 68–71.
35. Felger EA, Zeiger MA. The death of an Indian rhinoceros. *World J Surg* 2010; **34**(8): 1805–10.
36. Carney JA. The glandulae parathyroideae of Ivar Sandström: contributions from two continents. *Am J Surg Pathol* 1996; **20**(9): 1123–44.
37. Maccallum WG, Voegtlin C. On the relation of tetany to the parathyroid glands and to calcium metabolism. *J Exp Med* 1909; **11**(1): 118–51.
38. Councilman W. Friedrich Daniel Von Recklinghausen (1833-1910). *Proc Am Acad Arts Sci* 1918; **53**: 872–4.
39. Vermeulen AH. The birth of endocrine pathology: how Erdheim misunderstood parathyroids. *Virchows Arch* 2010; **457**(3): 283–90.
40. Lew JI, Solorzano CC. Surgical management of primary hyperparathyroidism: state of the art. *Surg Clin North Am* 2009; **89**(5): 1205–25.
41. Bulger HA, Dixon HH, Barr DP. The functional pathology of hyperparathyroidism. *J Clin Invest* 1930; **9**(1): 143–90.
42. Churchill ED, Cope O. The surgical treatment of hyperparathyroidism: based on 30 cases confirmed by operation. *Ann Surg* 1936; **104**(1): 9–35.
43. Li AJB, Collip AM. Hanson and the isolation of the parathyroid hormone, or endocrines and enterprise. *J Hist Med Allied Sci* 1992; **47**(4): 405–38.
44. Aurbach GD. Isolation of parathyroid hormone after extraction with phenol. *J Biol Chem* 1959; **234**(12): 3179–81.
45. Berson SA, Yalow RS, Aurbach GD, Potts JT. Immunoassay of bovine and human parathyroid hormone. *Proc Natl Acad Sci USA* 1963; **49**(5): 613–17.

CHAPTER 53

DEVELOPMENTAL ANATOMY OF THE THYROID AND PARATHYROID GLANDS

Julian A. McGlashan

Introduction	603	Parathyroid glands	607
The thyroid gland	603	References	609

SEARCH STRATEGY AND EVIDENCE BASE

Much of the evidence for this topic is well documented in standard tomes on this subject such as *Werner and Ingbar's The thyroid*[1] and Bilezikian's *The parathyroids – Basic and clinical concepts*.[2] Medline, Embase and Google Scholar searches were performed for the years 1993–2013 to review new evidence pertinent to the topic using the keywords: thyroid gland, parathyroid gland, developmental anatomy, embryology, histopathology, and microstructure.

INTRODUCTION

Study of the developmental anatomy of the thyroid and parathyroid glands helps in the understanding of the normal and abnormal variations in anatomy seen at surgery and the related pathology of these organs. Although the main steps in the developmental anatomy have been known for over half a century, it is only in the last decade that the morphogenesis, control of cell growth and cellular differentiation of these organs have begun to be unravelled.[3] This has followed significant advances in our understanding of the molecular biology[4, 5] and genetic[3, 6–8] basis of thyroid and parathyroid function in health and disease in the last 20 years. There is now increasing knowledge of the role of the cellular aspects of thyroid stem cell biology[9] and pathogenesis of many thyroid and parathyroid diseases.[6, 10] Much of the information has been obtained from limited human studies and more extensive investigations in rodents and sheep. The events of thyroid development are roughly comparable to humans except for the timing.[11] Detailed discussion is beyond the scope of this chapter, which will focus on summarizing the key anatomical features and stages in the development of the thyroid and parathyroid glands relevant to surgical practice. There is also an emphasis on the link between developmental abnormalities and some of the more common clinical presentations. Further information on the physiology of the thyroid and parathyroid glands can be found in Chapter 55. For details of cellular development and their abnormalities, see Chapter 9, Genetics of endocrine tumours.

THE THYROID GLAND

Macroscopic anatomy

The thyroid gland is situated in the lower anterior neck straddling the upper trachea. It is the largest endocrine organ in the body. It weighs 15–20 g in adulthood.[12, 13] It is a highly vascular, reddish-brown, bi-lobed structure with each lobe joined together by a narrow isthmus (**Figure 53.1**). Each lobe is pear-shaped, measuring approximately 5 cm in length, 3 cm in width and 1.5 cm in depth. The apex of each lobe is narrow and extends beneath the sternothyroid muscle up to its insertion on the oblique line of the thyroid cartilage. The more rounded lower pole extends down to the level of the fourth or fifth tracheal ring. It lies lateral to the trachea and oesophagus and medial to the carotid sheath. The isthmus overlies the second to fourth tracheal rings.

The thyroid gland, together with the oesophagus and trachea, is invested in a visceral layer of deep fascia known as the pretracheal fascia.[1] It is attached superiorly to the hyoid bone and extends inferiorly into the mediastinum, fusing with the fascia surrounding the aorta, pericardium and parietal pleura at the level of the carina. Laterally the fascia blends with the carotid sheath. Anteriorly the fascia forms a distinct layer separating the thyroid from the strap muscles and posteriorly it merges with the prevertebral fascia. On the posterior aspect of the isthmus the fascia is sometimes known as the anterior tracheal ligament and is perforated by small

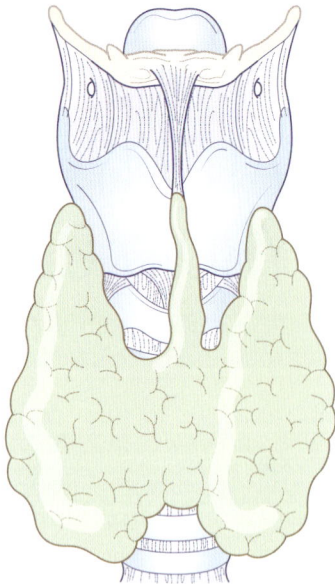

Figure 53.1 Relationship between thyroid gland, larynx and trachea. A pyramidal lobe +/– a fibrous or fibromuscular band is a common finding, particularly on the left side. It may arise from the isthmus or upper poles of the thyroid and extend a variable distance up to the body of the hyoid.

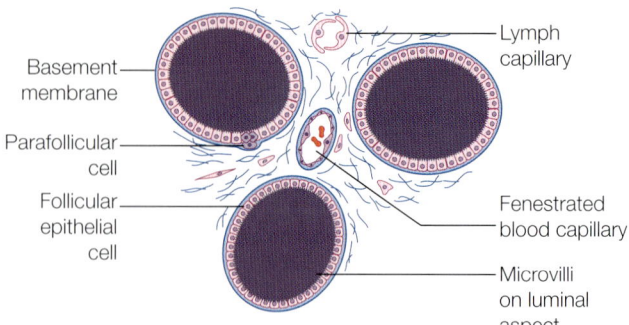

Figure 53.2 Angiofollicular unit and relationship between thyroid follicles and parafollicular cells.

tracheal vessels, but at the upper part on each side it is much thicker and binds the gland firmly to the sides of the cricoid cartilage and first tracheal ring. This condensation is known as the lateral ligament of the thyroid or the 'suspensory ligament of Berry'. Its fixation to the trachea causes the thyroid gland to move up and down on swallowing. During thyroid surgery it must be divided with care and by sharp dissection as the recurrent laryngeal nerve may lie lateral, medial or within the ligament just before it enters the larynx.

Microscopic anatomy

The thyroid gland is made up of multiple lobules supplied by a lobular artery.[14] A thyroid lobule consists of 20 to 40 follicles which are spherical in shape and 0.02–0.9 mm in diameter.[15] Each follicle is an aggregate of follicular cells which are one cell thick surrounding a central pool of viscous colloid (**Figure 53.2**). When the gland is relatively inactive, the cells are flattened and the colloid is abundant, dense and homogenous in appearance. On prolonged and excessive thyroid-stimulating hormone (TSH) stimulation the follicular cells become hypertrophied and hyperplastic and they adopt a more columnar shape.

The follicular cells have the characteristic cytoplasmic features of an endocrine gland in that they have long segments of rough endoplasmic reticulum and a large Golgi apparatus for synthesizing and packaging protein and prominent electron-dense lysosomal bodies. The plasma membranes of the apical and basal layers have separate functions and are kept separate by tight junctions which bind adjacent cells together. This allows the cell to control the storage of the thyroid hormones in the colloid and their release into the circulation. When stimulated by TSH, the intracellular organelles become more prominent and microvilli develop on their apical surfaces.[16] The microvilli enable the colloid to be absorbed by endocytosis. This is associated with the development of 'reabsorption lacunae' and a reduction in the size of the follicular lumen. The process is also associated with an overall increase in vascularity of the gland. The thyroid hormones released into the circulation ensure that the metabolic demands of the tissues of the body are met by stimulating oxygen consumption and regulating carbohydrate and lipid metabolism. They are also essential for embryonic development, normal growth and especially for brain maturation.

Each follicle is invested and interlaced with loose connective tissue (stroma) containing a close-meshed plexus of fenestrated capillaries forming morphological and functional angiofollicular units (AFUs).[17, 18] The inter-follicle connective tissue spaces are relatively large and contain a collagenous matrix, fibroblasts, unmyelinated nerve fibres with Schwann cells, and fat cells, plasma cells, macrophages, expanded lymphatics and lymphocytes.[14, 16, 19] The fibroblasts form a highly organized 'neuro-reticular network' by linking their long, thin, branching cytoplasmic processes. These processes are surrounded by autonomic nerve endings in a similar manner to that found in bone marrow and in the submandibular gland. The presence of CD34-positive antigen on the fibroblasts may mean they play an important role in immune surveillance.[19]

Scattered in the stroma are some embryologically distinct cells known as parafollicular cells or C cells (**Figure 53.2**). They are found either singly or in small clumps and are characterized by their polygonal or spindle shape, their relatively large size and their 'light' cytoplasm.[14, 20] They secrete calcitonin in response to elevated serum levels of calcium or gastrin. A total thyroidectomy does not always abolish calcitonin secretion as it can be produced by other organs such as the brain, gastrointestinal tract, urinary bladder, thymus and lungs.[21] Calcitonin lowers serum calcium and phosphate levels by inhibiting the osteoclastic resorption of bone and enhancing the excretion of calcium by the kidneys. Its physiological importance is debatable as parathyroid hormone and vitamin D are thought to be more important in calcium haemostasis.[22]

Developmental anatomy

The thyroid gland is the earliest endocrine organ to appear in mammalian development. It is formed from both the endodermal cells of the primitive pharynx, known as the median anlage, and from neural crest cells from the lateral anlagen or ultimobranchial bodies.[3, 23–25]

MEDIAN ANLAGE

The median anlage (**Figure 53.3**) develops from a midline thickening of the ventral surface of the endodermal epithelium of the primitive pharynx between the first and second branchial arches adjacent to the developing myocardium. A diverticulum forms from this thickening at about the sixteenth or seventeenth gestational day. This out-pouching expands laterally at its distal tip to form a rudimentary bilobed structure. It is pulled into position by the descent of the heart and reaches its final location, immediately anterior to the trachea, in the seventh gestational week. Initially the descending thyroid remains attached to the pharyngeal floor by a tubular stalk. During the seventh to tenth week the lumen of the stalk becomes filled with cords of thyroid progenitor cells but eventually fragments and disappears before birth. The residuum of the attachment of the stalk forms the foramen caecum in the midline at the junction of the posterior third and anterior two-thirds of the tongue.[25]

LATERAL ANLAGEN (ULTIMOBRANCHIAL BODIES)

The two lateral anlagen (**Figure 53.3**), also known as the ultimobranchial bodies, are thought to develop as evaginations of the fourth pharyngeal pouches.[25, 26] They become separated from them by attenuation and rupture from the common pharyngobranchial duct. The ultimobranchial bodies fuse with the median thyroid anlage by the sixth week of development, contributing approximately 10% of the mass of the thyroid gland.[25, 27] It is thought that rarely the ultimobranchial bodies can fail to fuse resulting in a true 'lateral thyroid lobe', although this has been disputed.[28] The ultimobranchial bodies also contribute the calcitonin-producing parafollicular cells (C cells). The exact origin of these cells in humans remains controversial although they are thought to migrate from the neural crest.[23–25]

HISTOGENESIS OF THE THYROID FOLLICLE

Histological differentiation of follicular cells can be seen to pass through three stages, defined by their production of colloid.[23]

1. The 'precolloid stage' (7–13 weeks) is from the first appearance of immature follicular cells to the beginning of differentiation into cells that are capable of producing colloid.
2. In the second stage (13–14 weeks) an intracellular structure known as the canaliculus begins to dilate. This structure is thought to be an extension of the smooth endoplasmic reticulum and is associated with the accumulation of increasingly electron-dense material. This material is then discharged into the extracellular space where it is retained by the intracellular connections to form a central colloid space.
3. In the third stage there is an increase in colloid production and storage with a consequent increase in size of the follicles. The follicular cells also show an increase in the number of lysosomes representing endocytosis of the colloid in preparation for storage and release of the thyroid hormones into the circulation.

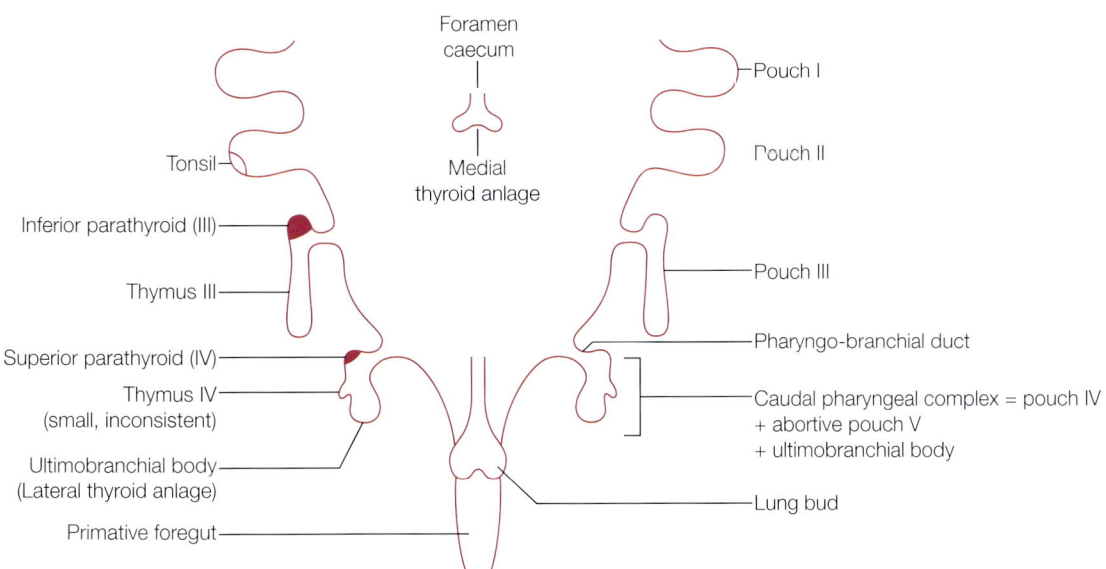

Figure 53.3 Schematic representation of the early development of the median and lateral analagen of the thyroid gland and the parathyroid glands.

TABLE 53.1 Timeline of development of thyroid gland in humans	
Gestational age	**Development**
Embryonic day 10	Endodermal thickening seen
Embryonic day 16–17	Median and lateral anlagen discernible
Embryonic day 24	Median anlage has developed a thin, flask-like diverticulum, extending from the floor of the buccal cavity down to the fourth branchial arch
Embryonic day 30	Formation of bi-lobulated structure
Embryonic day 40	Median and lateral anlagen have fused Degeneration of thyroglossal duct into fibrous stalk
Embryonic day 50	Lateral expansion Descent of the heart and thyroid reaches its final location, immediately anterior to the trachea Precolloid phase starts
Embryonic day 60	Definite shape Follicle formation Onset of thyroglobulin expression
Gestational week 10	Colloid phase Thyroid hormone receptors detectable in brain Fibrous thyroglossal stalk disappears
Gestational week 11	Histogenesis of the thyroid is virtually complete Foetal thyroid is capable of trapping and oxidizing iodide Thyroglobulin present in foetal thyroid Thyroxine can be detected in foetal serum
Gestational week 16	Increasing TSH secretion the principal regulator of thyroid hormone biosynthesis and secretion Significant increase of thyroid hormone receptors in foetal brain
Gestational week 17.5	Structural maturity of thyroid gland
Gestational week 20	Increasing organification of iodide and foetal T4 secretion
Gestational week 24	T3 detectable
Birth	Gland weight 1.5 g

Thyroxine can be detected in foetal serum at 11 weeks.[29] Structural maturity of the foetal thyroid gland is achieved at 17.5 weeks (**Table 53.1**).[30]

Anatomical variations and pathological conditions resulting from developmental abnormalities of the thyroid gland

ASYMMETRIES AND COMMON NORMAL VARIANTS

Asymmetries of the gland are frequently found with the right side being larger than the left.[12] A third conical protrusion known as the **pyramidal lobe** is present in 12–81% of cases. The prevalence depends on the method of identification, i.e. autopsy, ultrasonography, CT, scintigraphy, intra-operative finding, the presence of pathology and possibly the population studied.[31–33] Most authors report the pyramidal lobe to originate more commonly on the left side, from either the medial aspect of the upper poles or the isthmus (40–60%),[34] but it can also arise from the midline of the isthmus or the right lateral lobe. Reported as being between 3 mm and 63 mm in length,[34] it can extend superiorly as a short stump or a long process that can reach the upper border of the thyroid cartilage or even the hyoid bone[32, 34, 35] (**Figure 53.1**). Its high prevalence indicates that this is a normal variant and represents the persistence of the distal part of the embryonic thyroid and thyroglossal duct.[34, 36] Its apex may be replaced by fibrous or fibromuscular tissue when it is then known as the 'levator of the thyroid gland'.[36]

> **KEY POINT**
>
> The prevalence of the pyramidal lobe is high enough to warrant exploration in every case of thyroid surgery. If a pyramidal lobe is present on the side of surgery, it should be removed with the main lobe to avoid leaving behind functioning thyroid tissue.[34]

The **tubercle of Zuckerkandl** is a lateral or posterior projection of the thyroid lobe which can be identified in up to 60% of surgical dissections.[14, 37, 38] It is thought to represent the point of embryological fusion of the ultimobranchial body and median anlage.

> **KEY POINT**
>
> The surgical importance of the tubercle of Zuckerkandl is threefold:
>
> - the recurrent laryngeal nerve most often runs medial to it
> - the superior parathyroid gland is usually attached to its cranial aspect
> - when enlarged as part of the goitre, a significant portion of thyroid tissue may be inadvertently left behind if subtotal thyroidectomy is performed.

ABNORMAL DESCENT AND DEVELOPMENT OF THE THYROID GLAND

Rarely the migration of the thyroid may become arrested anywhere along the descent pathway from the foramen caecum to low in the neck.[39] The most common abnormality is a lingual thyroid. Ectopic thyroid tissue may also be found in the sublingual, high cervical and mediastinal regions or within the cardiac endothelium.[39] Hemiagenesis with absence of a lobe or lobe and isthmus can be rarely encountered.[40, 41] The left lobe is more commonly absent (5:1) than the right.[41]

More commonly the descending thyroid stalk can persist anywhere between the foramen caecum and thyroid isthmus. Subsequent infection of adjacent lymphoid tissue to the tract is thought to stimulate the epithelial remnants so that they undergo cystic change.[42] Typically thyroglossal duct cysts are midline with 25% being paramedian; 60–80% are found below the hyoid bone.[28, 43-45] The tract is in close proximity to the hyoid bone, lying within the periosteum or even passing through the bony substance. During development, the point of origin of the embryonic thyroid is situated anteriorly to the second branchial arch so the thyroglossal tract ends up running ventrally to the developing hyoid bone. As the hyoid matures it rotates to assume its adult position. During this rotation the thyroglossal tract is drawn posteriorly and cranially around the inferior edge of the bone. It then continues descending downward and anteriorly to thyroid membrane.[42] A persisting thyroglossal tract may become entrapped in the midline mesenchymal condensation that is now thought to form the body of the hyoid bone in the midline.[46, 47]

Lateral aberrant thyroid rests

Normally the ultimobranchial bodies fuse with the expanding lateral lobes of the median thyroid and differentiate into thyroid tissue, which is usually indistinguishable from the rest of the thyroid gland. Aberrant follicular thyroid tissue or gland has been identified lateral to the main body of the thyroid gland and situated lateral to the internal jugular vein and not associated with any lymphoid tissue. The majority of these deposits or nodules are likely to represent metastatic follicular or follicular variant papillary thyroid carcinoma and perhaps should be managed as such.[48] On rare occasions a few follicles of normal thyroid tissue can also be found within the capsule of cervical lymph nodes situated in the central compartment of the neck. Again, the majority are likely to represent metastatic deposits but on rare occasions with no evidence of a carcinoma in the thyroid gland on painstaking histological examination they have to be attributed to ectopic tissue.[48]

Solid cell nests

These are irregularly shaped clusters of inter-follicular cells delineated by basal lamina within the thyroid gland. The dominant cell component comprises polygonal to fusiform cells with an epidermoid appearance.[49] Less commonly they show glandular morphology and may be microcystic, micropapillary and/or mucinous.[49] They may be found in approximately 25% of resected thyroid glands and are thought to represent remnants of the ultimobranchial apparatus.[9, 31, 50] They are more prevalent in the thyroid of infants and children and gradually decline with advancing age. Their biological significance remains controversial but there is some evidence that they harbour stem cells with capacity for self-renewal and end differentiation. They can be a source of confusion in thyroid pathology as they can mimic a number of pathological conditions.[51]

Medullary carcinoma

Normally the calcitonin-producing parafollicular cells (C cells) migrate to become distributed throughout the thyroid gland. However, they often remain more numerous near the point of fusion between the two anlagen.[52, 53] There is therefore a tendency for medullary carcinomas to develop in the central portions of the middle and upper thirds of the thyroid lobes.[53]

Struma ovarii (thyroid tissue within the ovary)

This is not a developmental anomaly of the thyroid but a germ-cell tumour, i.e. a monodermal teratoma. It accounts for approximately 5% of ovarian teratomas and the teratoma must comprise more than 50% of thyroid tissue to be classed as Struma ovarii. The thyroid tissue in this condition rarely functions but there have been rare instances of thyrotoxicosis (5–8%)[54] and malignancy with peritoneal and distant metastases.[55-57]

PARATHYROID GLANDS

Macroscopic and microscopic anatomy

The parathyroid glands are generally found in close proximity to the posterior surface of the thyroid gland. They are small, yellowish-brown, oval or bean-shaped and their colour often darkens with age. In most cases (84%) there are four parathyroid glands.[58] The size of each gland can vary but on average they are 6 mm in craniocaudal dimension and 3–4 mm in transverse diameter. They are usually paired and named superior and inferior glands. Around 85% of superior glands are within a 2 cm diameter of a point 1 cm above the crossing of the inferior thyroid artery and recurrent laryngeal nerve.[58-60] The inferior glands are frequently situated below the artery level or within 1 cm of the lower pole of the thyroid gland.

The parathyroid glands are enveloped by a thin fibrous capsule which extends into the parenchyma partitioning the gland into lobules. The parenchymal cells are arranged in clusters or cords nourished by a rich capillary network. Within the fibrovascular stroma there are other cells including adipocytes, macrophages and mast cells. They are likely to be involved in parathyroid hormone (PTH) secretion, signalling functions and as a detoxification storage site for lipophilic agents such as Vitamin A. The amount of stromal fibroadipose tissue increases with age, eventually comprising 50% of the gland substance in the elderly.[61]

The dominant cell type within the parathyroid glands are known as chief cells or principal cells. They produce PTH and together with calcitonin and an active metabolite of vitamin D, 1.25-dihydroxyvitamin D3, play an essential role in calcium homeostasis. Tight regulation of serum calcium levels is essential for neural transmission, muscle contraction and relaxation, exocrine secretion, blood clotting and cellular adhesion. Chief cells undergo morphological changes corresponding to different stages of the secretory cycle. They range from being cuboidal in shape in the inactive phase to oval or polygonal in the active phase.[4] They are characterized by their rather scant, slightly eosinophilic cytoplasm. This is in contrast to the other main cell type, the oxyphil cells. Oxyphil cells are much less prevalent and are found singly or in small clusters. They can be identified by their larger size, eosinophilic cytoplasm due to their high mitochondrial content, prominent nucleoli and randomly enlarged nuclei.[2] Oxyphil cells are thought to be derived from chief cells and their numbers increase with age or after excessive functional stress (e.g. long-term stimulation of the parathyroid glands or chronic kidney disease).[4] Their function is not fully understood but they have the potential to produce PTH, PTH-related protein (PTHrP) and calcitriol. They may also have autocrine and paracrine functions.[62] A further cell type known as parathyroid water-clear cells can occasionally be found in normal parathyroid glands. They are much more prevalent in hyperfunctional parathyroid states associated with hyperplasia and parathyroid adenomas.[63]

Developmental anatomy

In humans the parathyroid primordia first appear at about 32 days of embryonic development.[59] Each superior parathyroid gland is derived from the endoderm of the dorsal part of the fourth pharyngeal pouch together with the ultimobranchial body.[4] It is commonly referred to as Parathyroid IV (PIV) in the embryological literature to indicate its site of origin. Each inferior parathyroid gland (Parathyroid III (PIII)) develops from endodermal cells from a common parathyroid/thymus primordium found in the third pharyngeal pouch (**Figure 53.3**). The dorsal/anterior part of the common primordium contributes the parathyroid component while the ventral/distal part contributes to the thymus component. PIII migrates with the thymus and PIV migrates together with the ultimobranchial bodies respectively at about 44 days (**Figure 53.4**).

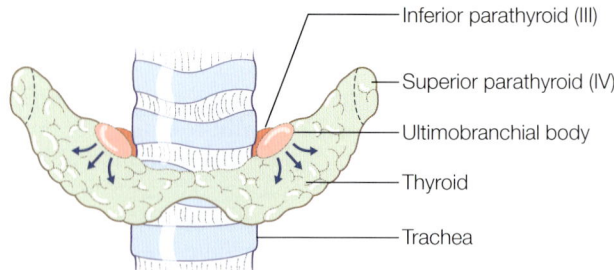

Figure 53.4 Schematic representation during development of relative positioning of the parathyroids and ultimobranchial body during fusion.

Later in development the inferior glands separate from the thymus and come to lie caudal to the superior parathyroids.

Anatomical variations and pathological conditions resulting from developmental abnormalities of the parathyroid glands

GLAND NUMBERS, SIZE AND POSITION

Although four parathyroid glands is the commonest number present, the number can range from two to six with some authors reporting as many as twelve glands.[64] Each gland weighs 30–40 mg, giving a combined weight of the glands in adults of 120 ± 3.5 mg in men and 142 ± 5.2 mg in women.[65] If a single gland's weight is greater than 60 mg, it is considered pathological.

As the thymus has a longer course of descent into the superior mediastinum, the accompanying inferior parathyroids have a more variable location, and a higher chance of ectopic location. They are responsible for supernumerary glands most commonly found in the cervical thymus (39%) or within the mediastinal thymus itself (6%).[60] Normal superior parathyroids can occasionally be found in the posterior neck, retropharyngeal–oesophageal space, carotid sheath and posterior mediastinum (1–4%). Parathyroid adenomas are found in posterior locations in 40% of cases. Most 'intrathyroidal' parathyroids reported on histological resections are located within indentations of the thyroid gland surrounded by perithyroidal fat.[2] Intravagal parathyroid tissue has been documented in 6% of cases in autopsy reports.[66]

KEY POINTS

- In most cases (84%) there are four parathyroid glands but the number can vary between two and six.
- 85% of superior parathyroid glands are within a 2 cm diameter of a point 1 cm above the crossing of the inferior thyroid artery and recurrent laryngeal nerve.
- The inferior glands have a more variable position but are frequently situated below the artery, level or within 1 cm of the lower pole of the thyroid gland.
- Ectopic or supernumerary glands can be found in the thymus gland, posterior neck, retropharyngeal – oesophageal space, carotid sheath and posterior mediastinum.

REFERENCES

1. Braverman LE, Utiger RD (eds). *Werner and Ingbar's The thyroid*, 8th ed. Philadelphia: Lippincott William & Wilkins; 2000.
2. Bilezikian JP (ed.). *The parathyroids: basic and clinical concepts*. 3rd ed. New York: Elsevier Sciences; 2015.
3. Gillam MP, Kopp P. Genetic regulation of thyroid development. *Curr Opin Pediatr* 2001; **13**: 358–63.
4. Chen H, Senda T, Emura S, Kubo K-Y. An update of the structure of the parathyroid glands. *Open Anat J* 2013; **5**: 1–9.
5. Ozaki T, Nagashima K, Kusakabe T, et al. Development of thyroid gland and ultimobranchial body cyst is independent of p63. *Lab Invest* 2011; **91**(1): 138–46.
6. Van Vliet G. Development of the thyroid gland: lessons from congenitally hypothyroid mice and men. *Clin Genet* 2003; **63**: 445–55.
7. Xu P-X, Zheng W, Laclef C, et al. *Eya1* is required for the morphogenesis of mammalian thymus, parathyroid and thyroid. *Development* 2002; **129**(13): 3033–44.
8. Carre A, Rachdi L, Tron E, et al. Hes1 is required for appropriate morphogenesis and differentiation during mouse thyroid gland development. *PloS One* 2011; **6**(2): e16752.
9. Thomas D, Friedman S, Lin R-Y. Thyroid stem cells: lessons from normal development and thyroid cancer. *Endocr Relat Cancer* 2008; **15**: 51–8.
10. Kondo T, Ezzat S, Asa SL. Pathogenetic mechanisms in thyroid follicular-cell neoplasia. *Nat Rev Cancer* 2006; **6**(4): 294.
11. Fisher DA, Brown RS. Thyroid physiology in the perinatal period and during childhood. In: Braverman LE, Utiger RD (eds). *Werner and Ingbar's The thyroid*. 8th ed. Philadelphia: Lippincott William & Wilkins; 2000, pp. 960–72.
12. Clark OH. Surgical anatomy. In: Braverman LE, Utiger RD (eds). *Werner and Ingbar's The thyroid*. 8th ed. Philadelphia: Lippincott William & Wilkins; 2000, pp. 455–61.
13. Langer P. Minireview: discussion about the limit between normal thyroid goiter. *Endocr Regul* 1999; **33**(1): 39–45.
14. Klinck GH. Structure of the thyroid. In: Hazard JB, Smith DE (eds). *The thyroid*. Baltimore: Williams & Wilkins; 1964.
15. Williams PL, Warwick R. Endocrine glands: the thyroid gland. *Gray's Anatomy*. Edinburgh: Churchill-Livingstone; 1984, pp. 1449–53.
16. Sobrinho-Simoes M, Johannessen JV. Scanning electron microscopy of the normal human thyroid. *J Submicrosc Cytol* 1981; **13**(2): 209–22.
17. Colin IM, Gerard AC. The thyroid angiofollicular units, a biological model of functional and morphological integration. *Bull Mem Acad R Med Bel* 2010; **165**(5–6): 218–30.
18. Colin IM, Denef JF, Lengelé B, et al. Recent insights into the cell biology of thyroid angiofollicular units. *Endocr Rev* 2013; **34**(2): 209–38.
19. Yamazaki K, Eyden BP. Interfollicular fibroblasts in the human thyroid gland: recognition of a CD34 positive stromal cell network communicated by gap junctions and terminated by autonomic nerve endings. *J Submicrosc Cytol Pathol* 1997; **29**(4): 461–76.
20. LiVolsi VA. Pathology of thyroid diseases. In: Braverman LE, Utiger RD (eds). *Werner and Ingbar's The thyroid*. 8th ed. Philadelphia: Lippincott William & Wilkins; 2000, pp. 488–511.
21. Becker KL, Snider RH, Moore CF, et al. Calcitonin in extrathyroidal tissues of man. *Acta Endocrinol (Copenh)* 1979; **92**(4): 746–51.
22. Baran DT. The skeletal system in thyrotoxicosis. In: Braverman LE, Utiger RD (eds). *Werner and Ingbar's The thyroid*. 8th ed. Philadelphia: Lippincott Williams & Wilkins; 2000, pp. 658–66.
23. Pintar JE. Normal development of the hypothalamic-pituitary-thyroid axis. In: Braverman LE, Utiger RD (eds.). *Werner and Ingbar's The thyroid*. 8th ed. Philadelphia: Lippincott William & Wilkins; 2000, pp. 7–43.
24. Fuse Y. Development of the hypothalamic–pituitary–thyroid axis in humans. *Reprod Fertil Dev* 1996; **8**: 1–21.
25. Di Lauro R, De Felice M. Anatomy and development. In: De Groot LJ, Jameson LJ (eds). *Endocrinology*. 4th ed. Philadelphia: W.B. Saunders; 2001, pp. 1268–77.
26. Ohri AK, Ohri SK, Singh MP. Evidence of thyroid development from the fourth branchial pouch. *J Laryngol Otol* 1994; **108**: 71–3.
27. Mérida-Velasco JA, García-García JD, Espín-Ferra J, Linares J. Origin of the ultimobranchial body and its colonizing cells in human embryos. *Acta Anatomica* 1989; **136**(4): 325–30.
28. Haller JR, Davis RK. Ectopic thyroid and thyroglossal duct cysts. In: Randolph GW (ed.). *Surgery of the thyroid and parathyroid glands*. London: Saunders, Elsevier Sciences; 2003, pp. 56–60.
29. Ballabio M, Nicolini U, Jowett T, et al. Maturation of thyroid function in normal human foetuses. *Clin Endocrinol* 1989; **31**(5): 565–71.
30. Bocian-Sobkowskal J, Malendowicz LK, Woíniakl W. Morphometric studies on the development of human thyroid gland in early fetal life. *Histol Histopath* 1992; **7**: 415–20.
31. Kim DW, Jung SL, Baek JH, et al. The prevalence and features of thyroid pyramidal lobe, accessory thyroid, and ectopic thyroid as assessed by computed tomography: a multicenter study. *Thyroid* 2013; **23**(1): 84–91.
32. Harjeet A, Shani D, Jit I, Aggarwal AK. Shape, measurements and weight of the thyroid gland in northwest Indians. *Surg Radiol Anat* 2004; **26**: 91–5.
33. Geraci G, Pisello F, Li Volsi F, et al. The importance of pyramidal lobe in thyroid surgery. *G Chir* 2008; **29**(11–12): 479–82.
34. Zivic R, Radovanovic D, Vekic B, et al. Surgical anatomy of the pyramidal lobe and its significance in thyroid surgery. *S Afr J Surg* 2011; **49**(3): 110, 112, 114.
35. Capan CC. Anatomy. In: Braverman LE, Utiger RD (eds). *Werner and Ingbar's The thyroid*. 8th ed. Philadelphia: Lippincott William & Wilkins; 2000, pp. 20–51.
36. Milojevic B, Tosevski J, Milisavljevic M, et al. Pyramidal lobe of the human thyroid gland: an anatomical study with clinical implications. *Rom J Morphol Embryol* 2013; **54**(2): 285–9.
37. Gauger PG, Delbridge LW, Thompson NW, et al. Incidence and importance of the tubercle of Zuckerkandl in thyroid surgery. *Eur J Surg* 2001; **167**(4): 249–54.
38. Gurleyik E, Gurleyik G. Incidence and surgical importance of Zuckerkandl's tubercle of the thyroid and its relations with recurrent laryngeal nerve. *ISRN Surg* 2012 Article ID 450589, 5 pages http://dx.doi.org/10.5402/2012/450589.
39. Guerra G, Cinelli M, et al. Morphological, diagnostic and surgical features of ectopic thyroid gland: a review of literature. *Int J Surg* 2014; **12**: S3–S11.
40. McDougall IR, Cavalieri RR. In vivo radionuclide tests and imaging. In: Braverman LE, Utiger RD (eds). *Werner and Ingbar's The thyroid*. 8th ed. Philadelphia: Lippincott Williams & Wilkins; 2000, pp. 355–75.
41. Wu YH, Wein RO, Carter B. Thyroid hemiagenesis: a case series and review of the literature. *Am J Otolaryngol* 2012; **33**(3): 299–302.
42. Allard RHB. The thyroglossal cyst. *Head Neck Surg* 1982; **5**: 134–46.
43. Rincon S, Caruso P, Curtin H. Imaging of the thyroid gland. In: Randolph GW (ed.). *Surgery of the thyroid and parathyroid glands*. London: Saunders, Elsevier Sciences; 2003, pp. 163–75.
44. Josephson GD, Spencer WR, Josephson JS. Thyroglossal duct cyst: the New York Eye and Ear Infirmary experience and a literature review. *Ear Nose Throat J* 1998; **77**(8): 642–4.
45. Ewing CA, Kornblut A, Greeley C, Manz H. Presentations of thyroglossal duct cysts in adults. *Eur Arch Otorhinolaryngol* 1999; **256**(3): 136–8.
46. Rodríguez-Vázquez JF, Kim JH, Verdugo-López S, et al. Human fetal hyoid body origin revisited. *J Anat* 2011; **219**(2): 143–9.
47. Inoue K, Bando Y, Sakiyama K, et al. Development and regression of the thyroglossal duct in mice. *Ann Anat* 2015; **200**: 54–65.
48. LiVolsi VA. Pathology of thyroid diseases. In: Braverman LE, Utiger RD (eds). *Werner and Ingbar's The thyroid*. 8th ed. Philadelphia: Lippincott-Williams & Wilkins; 2000, pp. 488–511.
49. Cameselle-Teijeiro J, Varela-Duran J, Sambade C, et al. Solid cell nests of the thyroid: light microscopy and immunohistochemical profile. *Hum Pathol* 1994; **25**(7): 684–93.
50. Akhtar M, Scognamiglio T. Solid cell nests: role in thyroid disease. *Adv Anat Path* 2007; **14**(2): 141–2.
51. Ríos Moreno MJ, Galera-Ruiz H, De Miguel M, et al. Inmunohistochemical profile of solid cell nest of thyroid gland. *Endocr Pathol* 2011; **22**(1): 35–9.
52. Gibson W, Croker B, Cox C. C cell populations in normal children and young adults. *Lab Invest* 1989; **42**: 119.
53. Ball DW, Baylin SB, De Bustros AC. Medullary thyroid carcinoma. In: Braverman LE, Utiger RD (eds). *Werner and Ingbar's The thyroid*. 8th ed, Philadelphia: Lippincott Williams & Wilkins; 2000, pp. 930–43.
54. Yoo SC, Chang KH, Lyu MO, et al. Clinical characteristics of struma ovarii. *J Gynecol Oncol* 2008; **19**: 135.

55. Devaney K, Snyder R, Norris HJ, Tavassoli FA. Proliferative and histologically malignant struma ovarii: a clinicopathologic study of 54 cases. *Int J Gynecol Pathol* 1993; **12**: 333–43.
56. Leite I, Margarida Cunha T, Pinto Figueiredo J, Félix A. Papillary carcinoma arising in struma ovarii versus ovarian metastasis from primary thyroid carcinoma: a case report and review of the literature. *J Radiol Case Rep* 2013; 7(10): 24–33.
57. Billan S, Abdah-Bortnyak R, Cohen H, et al. Metastatic malignant struma ovarii. *IMAJ* 2011; **13**: 247–8.
58. Åkerström G, Malmaeus J, Bergström R. Surgical anatomy of human parathyroid glands. *Surgery* 1984; **95**(1): 14–21.
59. Gilmour JR. The gross anatomy of the parathyroid glands. *J Pathol* 1938; **46**: 133–48.
60. Wang CA. The anatomic basis of parathyroid surgery. *Ann Surg* 1976; **183**: 271–5.
61. Johnson SJ. Changing clinicopathological practice in parathyroid disease. *Histopathol* 2010; **56**: 835–51.
62. Ritter CS, Haughey BH, Miller B, Brown AJ. Differential gene expression by oxyphil and chief cells of human parathyroid glands. *J Clin Endocrinol Metab* 2012; **97**: E1499–505.
63. Roth SI. The ultrastructure of primary water-clear cell hyperplasia of the parathyroid glands. *Am J Pathol* 1970; **61**: 233–4.
64. Seethala RR, Virji MA, Ogilvie JB. Pathology of the parathyroid glands. In: Barnes L (ed.). *Surgical pathology of the head and neck*, vol. III. New York, NY: Informa Health Care; 2009, pp. 1429–72.
65. Grimelius L, Åkerström G, Johansson H, Bergström R. Anatomy and histopathology of human parathyroid glands. *Pathol Annu* 1981; **16**(Pt 2):1–24.
66. Pawlik TM, Richards M, Giordano TJ, et al. Identification and management of intravagal parathyroid adenoma. *World J Surg* 2001; **25**(4): 419–23.

DEVELOPMENTAL ANATOMY OF THE PITUITARY FOSSA

John Hill and Sean Carrie

Embryology 611	Cavernous sinuses 616
Endoscopic anatomy of the sphenoid and anterior sella wall 612	Endoscopic anatomy of cavernous sinuses 617
Pituitary gland anatomy 613	References 618
Sella turcica 614	Further reading 618
Endoscopic anatomy of the pituitary fossa 616	

SEARCH STRATEGY AND EVIDENCE BASE

This chapter was prepared from anatomy and physiology texts and supported by a Medline search using the keywords anatomy, endoscopic, pituitary and cavernous sinus. The anatomical studies quoted constitute level 3 evidence.

EMBRYOLOGY

The adenohypophysis is derived from the placodal ectoderm of the stomodeum roof. The neurohypophysis is derived from an evagination of the floor of the forebrain and the third ventricle.

There is a saccular depression in the roof of the stomodeum immediately in front of the oropharyngeal membrane. This saccular depression evaginates to form the pouch of Rathke. This area remains in close contact with the ventral surface of the forebrain. The pouch of Rathke develops into the adenohypophysis. The anterior part becomes the pars anterior and the posterior part, in contact with the forebrain, becomes the pars intermedia. The section of the forebrain in close contact with the pars intermedia becomes the neurohypophysis (**Figure 54.1**). In foetal life and childhood the vestige of Rathke's pouch remains as the hypophyseal cleft separating the pars anterior and pars intermedia. The pars intermedia is rudimentary in humans and is of little functional significance. Remnants of Rathke's pouch may persist below the sphenoid in the roof of the nasopharynx forming a pharyngeal pituitary. The clivus and the dorsum sellae of the future sphenoid bone are formed from mesenchymal condensations surrounding the hypophysis.[1] The cavernous sinus is derived from the primary head vein (**Figure 54.1**).

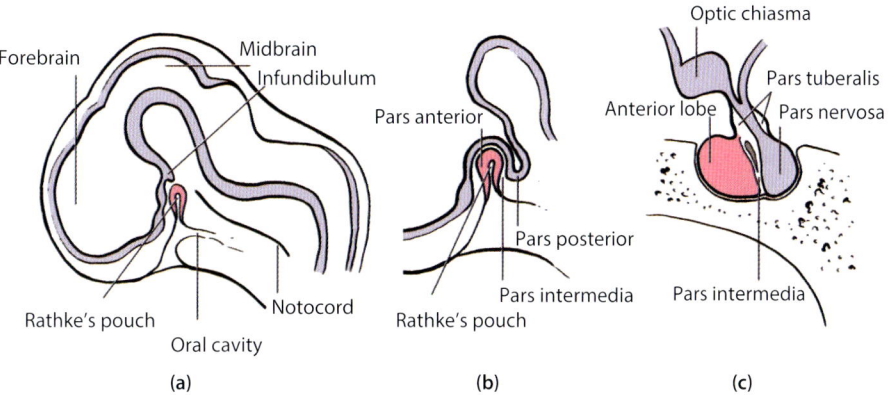

Figure 54.1 Embryological development of the hypophysis.

ENDOSCOPIC ANATOMY OF THE SPHENOID AND ANTERIOR SELLA WALL

The anatomical considerations for the endoscopic pituitary surgeon are:

- the degree of pneumatization of the sphenoid and the localization of the anterior sella wall
- the position of the intra-sphenoid sinus septae
- the positioning of the carotid arteries and optic nerves in the posterior sphenoid wall.

The degree of pneumatization of the sphenoid was originally described by Hammer and Radberg in 1961.[2] They divided the sphenoid sinus into three types: sellar, pre-sellar and conchal. In the sellar type the sphenoid is well pneumatized and the floor of the pituitary fossa (sella) performs an easily identifiable bulge in the posterosuperior aspect of the sphenoid sinus. In most series this arrangement is found in approximately 80% of sinuses. The posterior wall of the sphenoid sinus is in the same plane as the midpoint of the pituitary fossa or more posteriorly placed. In a small subgroup the pneumatization can be described as 'post-sella' whereby the entire sella floor protrudes down from the roof of the sphenoid sinus. In 'pre-sella' pneumatization (approximately 20%), the posterior wall of the sphenoid sinus is in the same plane as the anterior wall of the sella. In these cases it may be difficult to delineate the anterior bulge of the anterior sphenoid wall and intra-operative radiology or navigation systems may be needed to help the endoscopic surgeons. In 2% of cases there is no pneumatization of the sphenoid. This arrangement is much more common in Asian populations where it may occur in up to 28% of cases.[3]

Intra-sphenoid sinus septae

The arrangement of the septae is highly variable. The standard textbook depiction of a single septum running in the midline from the rostrum of the sphenoid back to the anterior pituitary fossa wall is found in only 14% of individuals. Almost any arrangement of septae can be encountered by the surgeon. The commoner arrangements are of a single septum (48%) or two septae (48%) rather than multiple septations. The septae may be incomplete or complete whereby they extend from the anterior to the posterior wall of the septum. Anteriorly, a complete septum is usually inserted in the midline, but its posterior attachment is variable. Midline posterior attachment occurs in only 14% of individuals and more commonly the arrangement is that the posterior attachment is laterally placed close to the paraclival carotid eminence. In 87% of cases at least one septum will be inserted posteriorly close to the carotid.[4] Care is therefore needed when drilling down these septae to gain surgical access (**Figure 54.2**).

Transverse septations as well as vertical septations are also encountered. Where there are horizontal sphenoid

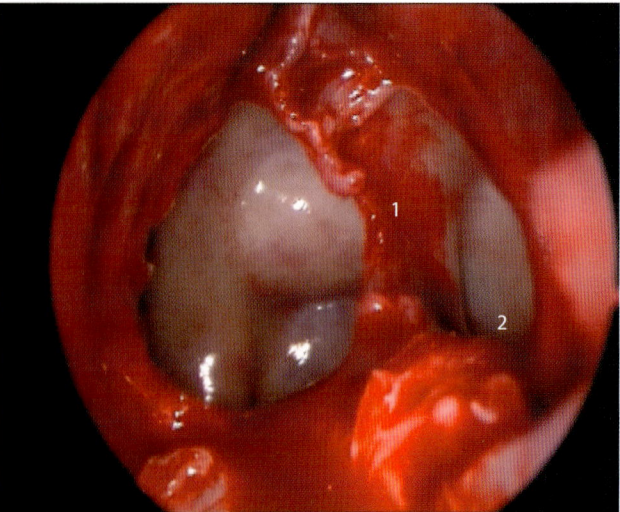

Figure 54.2 Endoscopic view of sphenoid. Single intra-sphenoid septum (1) inserting into the left carotid artery eminence (2).

septae, this is due to posterior ethmoids pneumatizing over the top of sphenoid sinuses. This can be surgically relevant: if they are not opened, the surgeon may not be able to visualize and reach all of the anterior wall of the pituitary fossa.

Carotid arteries and optic nerves

In a well-pneumatized sphenoid the pituitary fossa will form a bulge in the midline in the posterosuperior aspect of the sinus. **Figure 54.3** shows that inferolateral to the fossa is the paraclival carotid (a). Lateral to the fossa is the bulge formed by the carotid as it curves anteriorly then posteriorly as it ascends in the cavernous sinus (b). Superolateral to the fossa is the position of the optic nerve (c), although this is visible in only a small proportion of the sphenoid sinuses. The small fossa bounded by the

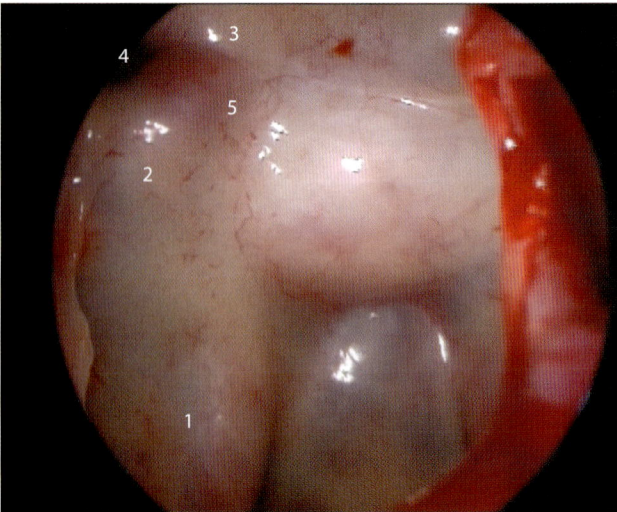

Figure 54.3 Endoscopic view of posterior wall of sphenoid. Indentations caused by the internal carotid artery (1,2) and optic nerve (3), lateral opticocarotid recess (4) and medial opticocarotid recess (5).

optic nerve superomedially and the carotid artery inferomedially is termed the lateral opticocarotid recess (LOCR) and it corresponds to the anterior clinoid process intra-cranially. The triangular depression bounded by the optic nerve superolaterally, the carotid inferomedially and the the pituitary fossa medially is termed the medial opticocarotid recess (MOCR) and that corresponds to the medial clinoid intra-cranially.

The bony covering over the sella is thin, usually less than 0.5 mm. In cases where an adenoma is present, the bony covering may be absent. The carotico-optic recess is triangular in shape and is limited by the optic nerve superiorly, the carotid artery inferomedially and the oculomotor nerve laterally. The carotid protuberance or C shape of the carotid artery is immediately lateral to the pituitary fossa and is formed by the serpentine carotid artery as it bends forwards in the cavernous sinus before curving backwards as it ascends before entering the anterior cranial fossa medial to the anterior clinoid process.

The optic nerves and the carvernous sinuses are usually covered by bone, although a dehiscence over the carotid artery is present in up to 5% of cases.[5]

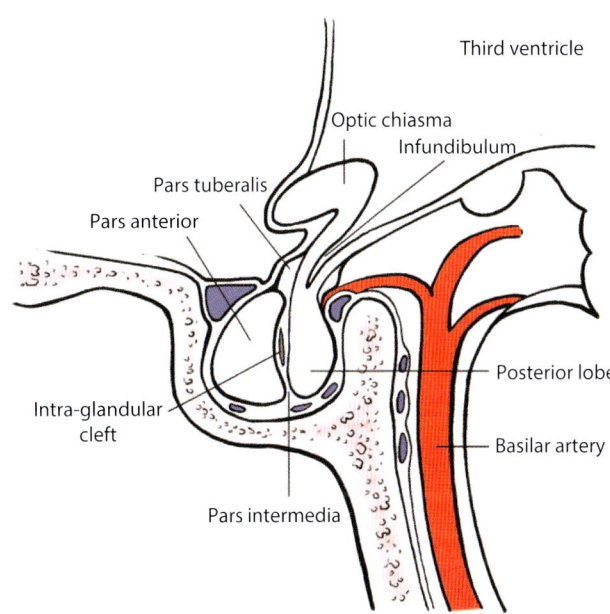

Figure 54.4 **Lateral view of the hypophysis in the sella turcica.** The intercavernous venous sinuses are indicated in blue.

PITUITARY GLAND ANATOMY

The pituitary gland or hypophysis cerebri is an ovoid body measuring approximately 8 mm in the anteroposterior diameter by 12 mm transversely by 4 mm high. By the age of puberty it weighs approximately 100–500 mg. It doubles in size during pregnancy and usually remains larger in females. The adenohypophysis constitutes two-thirds of the volume.

There are two major parts to the hypophysis:[6]

- **adenohypophysis:** includes the pars anterior, pars intermedia and pars tuberalis
- **neurohypophysis:** includes the pars posterior, infundibular stem and median eminence.

Both these parts include parts of the infundibulum and are preferred to the old terms anterior and posterior lobes (**Figure 54.4**).

Adenohypophysis

This structure is highly vascular and consists of epithelial cells arranged in follicles and cords between which lie thin-walled, vascular sinuses. This arrangement is supported by a delicate skeleton of reticular tissue.

Traditionally, cell types of the adenohypophysis have been divided up by their staining characteristics into chromophil (acidophilic, basophilic) and chromophobe cells. Modern immunohistochemical techniques allow us to identify cells by the hormones that they produce, as follows.

- **Somatotrophs:** (acidophilic), the largest and most abundant chromaphil cells, these secrete the protein somatotrophin or growth hormone (GH).
- **Mammotrophs:** (acidophilic), secrete the polypeptide hormone prolactin (PRL). They become the dominant cell during pregnancy and lactation.
- **Mammosomatotrophs:** (acidophilic) secrete growth hormone and prolactin simultaneously.
- **Corticotrophs:** (basophilic), produce the precursor molecule pro-opiomelanocorticotropin (POMC), which is broken down into adrenocorticotropin (ACTH), beta-lipotropin and beta-endorphin.
- **Thyrotrophs:** (basophilic), secrete thyroid-stimulating hormone (TSH).
- **Gonadotrophs:** (basophilic) secrete follicle-stimulating hormone (FSH) and luteinizing hormone (LH).
- **Chromophobe cells:** these small cells constitute the majority of the cells in the adenohypophysis. They include stem cells and degranulated secretory cells.
- **Folliculostellate (FS) cells:** these are the supporting cells of the adenohypophysis, with growth factor and cytokine activity. Their expression of cytokeratins supports the theory that the adenohypophysis is derived from Rathke's pouch.[7]
- **Pars tuberalis:** this contains large number of blood vessels as well as the secreting cells listed above. In some species this area is rich in receptors for the pineal hormone melatonin.

Neurohypophysis

Axons with their cell bodies in the supraoptic and paraventricular nuclei of the hypothalamus run to the neurohypophysis. Some terminate in the median eminence from where they can influence the action of the adenohypophysis (see below); others run down through the stalk of the hypophysis to the main mass of the neurohypophysis where they terminate close to the sinusoids. The latter transport polypeptide hormones in conjunction with a glycoprotein (neurophysin) to the neurohypophysis where they are stored prior to release. The two hormones secreted in this way are:

- anti-diuretic hormone (ADH) or vasopressin
- oxytocin.

Blood supply of the hypophysis

The arterial supply of the hypophysis is from single inferior hypophyseal arteries and several superior hypophyseal arteries on each side, all of which are branches of the internal carotid. The superior hypophyseal arteries supply the median eminence and the infundibulum. The inferior hypophyseal arteries anastamose to form an arterial ring around the infundibulum, which gives fine branches supplying the capillary bed of the neurohypophysis. The adenohypophysis does not have a direct arterial supply but is supplied by long and short portal vessels, which run from the median eminence and the lower infundibulum respectively to the capillary bed of the adenohypophysis (Figure 54.5).

The hormones of the adenohypophysis are secreted by exocytosis into the nearby sinusoids. The major signal for this secretion involves the release of specific releasing factors from neurones in the median eminence, which are then transported to the adenohypophysis by the portal system.[8]

The venous drainage of the hypophysis is less clear but has important implications in understanding the control of pituitary hormone secretion. Possible drainage is via:

- long and short portal vessels to the infundibulum
- large inferior hypophyseal veins into the dural venous sinuses
- the median eminence to the hypothalamus
- reversible flow between the adenohypophysis and neurohypophysis.

Pituitary gland capsule

The gland has a capsule made up of soft fibrous tissue that is in continuity with the fibrous connective tissue of the gland. The gland appears to be loosely attached to the surrounding connective tissue, which forms a smooth nest for the hypophysis. Bridging veins, capsular arteries and fibrous bundles cross this space.[9]

SELLA TURCICA

The sella turcica or Turkish saddle is the deep depression in the body of the sphenoid bone. It contains the hypophysis cerebri, dural layers and the intercavernous sinuses. The hypophysis fills 50–85% of the fossa.

The bony landmarks around the fossa are as follows (Figure 54.6):

- The **optic canal** lies between the roots of the lesser wing and the body of the sphenoid medially. It descends slightly anterolaterally, and it contains the optic nerve, ophthalmic artery and meninges.
- The **anterior clinoid process** is the posterior projection from the lesser wing of the sphenoid.
- The **tuberculum sellae** is a midline ridge in the anterior slope of the sella turcica.
- The **dorsum sellae** is the posterior wall of the sella turcica. The superolateral projections of the dorsum form the posterior clinoid processes.
- The **groove** for the internal carotid artery is formed as the artery turns anteriorly from the foramen lacerum. The groove can be seen on the sphenoid lateral to the sella turcica.
- The **middle clinoid process** is a small elevation in the median edge of the groove. In approximately 10% of skulls the middle and anterior clinoid processes are joined to form a continuous ring called the caroticoclinoid foramen.[10]

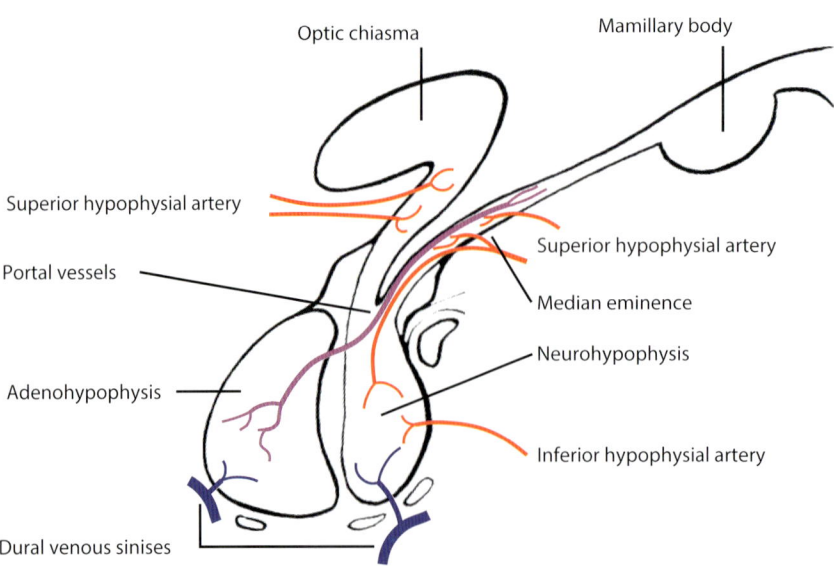

Figure 54.5 Vasculature of the hypophysis.

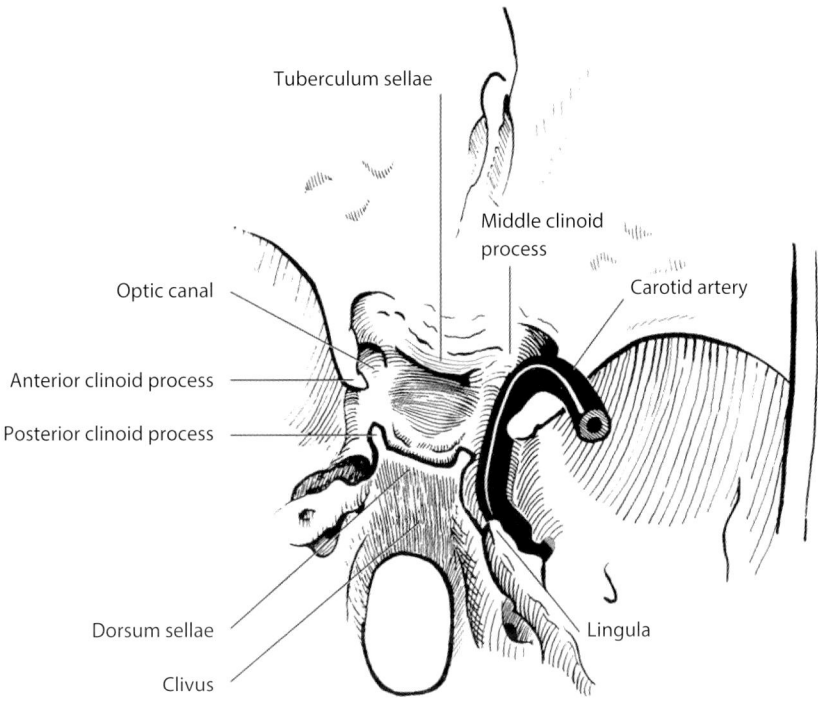

Figure 54.6 **Posterosuperior view of the sella turcica of a skull.** The position of the right internal carotid is demonstrated.

- The **lingula** is a small projection arising on the posterolateral aspect of the carotid groove.
- The **clivus** is made up of the body of the sphenoid bone behind the dorsum sellae and the basioccipital bone. The upper part of the pons lies adjacent to the clivus.

In approximately 2% of skulls there is a bony bridge joining the anterior clinoid and posterior clinoid processes called the tinea interclinoidea. In approximately 1% of skulls there is a bony projection in the floor of the sella called the sella spine. It is a bony spicule that projects from the junction of the anterior and inferior walls of the sella towards the middle of the hypophyseal fossa and it is usually 1mm in diameter and 2–5mm in length. It probably represents an ossified remnant of the notochord.[11]

Dural reflections

The diaphragmatica sella is a sheet of dura mater that forms the roof of the sella turcica. This small, flat, horizontal circular sheet covers over the fossa between the clinoid processes and is continuous with the roof of the cavernous sinus. There is a central defect in the diaphragm called the foramen diaphragmatis to allow through the pituitary stalk or infundibulum. It is of variable diameter up to 5mm.[12] In the region of the foramen of the dura, arachnoid and pia mater fuse with each other and with the capsule of the pituitary gland to form one fibrous layer that lines the hypophyseal fossa. In the fossa it is not possible to differentiate the fibrous layers and there are no subdural or subarachnoid spaces. Therefore there is no cerebrospinal fluid (CSF) in the normal pituitary fossa. The diaphragmatica sella separates the contents of the pituitary fossa from the CSF in the region of the foramen. The barrier may be very thin and consist of only arachnoid mater.[13]

The tentorium cerebelli is the main dural sheet that loops around the brain stem and separates the cerebral hemispheres from the cerebellum, forming the floor of the middle cranial fossa. It arises from the anterior clinoid processes and has a U-shaped free border looping posteriorly. The peripheral attachments of the tentorium run from the anterior clinoid process backwards as a ridge of dura mater to the apex of the petrous temple bone. This ridge is at the junction of the roof and the lateral part of the cavernous sinus. From here the attachment runs backwards to the posterior clinoid process, forming the roof of the cavernous sinus, and is continuous with the diaphragmatica sella. The remainder of the peripheral attachment of the tentorium is to the superior surface of the petrous temporal bone in the region of the superior petrosal sinus and to the occipital bone in the region of the transverse sinuses.

Intercavernous venous sinuses

The two cavernous sinuses are connected across the floor of the pituitary fossa by the intercavernous venous sinuses. Some texts indicate that there is a single anterior and single posterior vein in the floor of the fossa, hence the old term 'inferior circular sinus of Winslow'. Cast studies have shown, however, that the arrangement is much more variable, with multiple interconnections across the floor possible. The superior and inferior connections may be found behind the anterior wall of the fossa and the connections may widen out laterally as they enter the cavernous sinuses (**Figure 54.4**).[14]

Relations of the pituitary fossa

Superior:

- The diaphragmatica sella
- The pituitary stalk and infundibulum
- The optic chiasm anterior to the infundibulum; 5–10 mm above the diaphragm
- Anterior cerebral artery and anterior communicating artery anterior to the optic chiasm
- Internal carotid artery/middle cerebral artery lateral to the infundibulum
- CSF surrounds the above structures above the diaphragmatica sella
- The third ventricle lies above the infundibulum

Posterior:

- Lamellar bone of the dorsum sella
- Dura mater of the poster fossa, behind the lamellar bone
- Basilar artery, behind the dura mater
- CSF

Lateral:

- Upper part of the cavernous sinus containing:
  - horizontal portion of the internal carotid artery
  - oculomotor, trochlear and abducens nerves

Anterior and inferior:

- Sphenoid sinus
- Intra-sphenoid sinus septum

ENDOSCOPIC ANATOMY OF THE PITUITARY FOSSA

There is a thin layer of bone (<0.5 mm) over the anterior surface of the pituitary fossa. In pathological cases where a macro-adenoma is present the bone may be dehiscent or thinned.

In a cadaver study, the average dimensions of the anterior sella wall were measured.[15] The distance between the medial margins of the optic nerves at the level of the carotico-optic recess was found to be 12 mm; the width of the pituitary fossa between the carotid prominences was 21 mm; and the height of the anterior sella wall was 8 mm. Inside the pituitary fossa the height of the pituitary gland was 7 mm and the average separation of the superior aspect of the gland from the optic chiasm was 5 mm. There is, however, great variation in the normal anatomy of this region and the inter-carotid distance can be much narrower (**Figure 54.7**). The pathological processes will also distort the anatomy and macroadenomas can result in the intra-carotid distance being increased to up to 3 cm.[16]

During the endoscopic surgical approach to the fossa the first layer encountered will be the bony covering of the anterior sella wall, followed by a layer of dura lining the fossa. This is a single layer of dura except where it splits to accommodate the intercavernous sphenoid

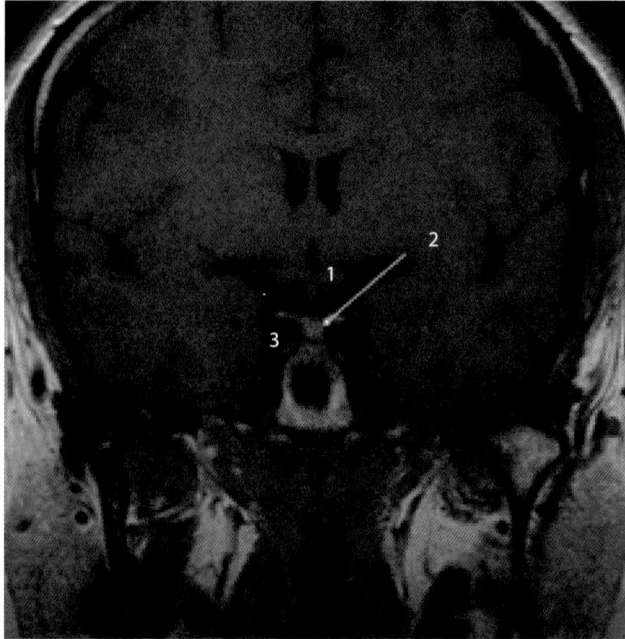

Figure 54.7 Coronal MR scan. The optic chiasm (1) and the pituitary gland (2) between medially placed carotid arteries (3).

sinuses (see above). Inside the dural layer is the substance of the gland itself. *In vivo* normal healthy pituitary gland tissue is slightly yellowish in appearance. There is a clear plane of dissection between the substance of the gland and its soft fibrous capsules. If the pituitary gland is removed *in vivo*, it is possible to see the diaphragm bulging down from above. The diaphragm is an easily identifiable sheet of fibrous tissue. Laterally the soft fibrous tissue of the medial wall of the cavernous sinuses is visible.

CAVERNOUS SINUSES

These sinuses lie on the lateral aspect of the sphenoid body and are the lateral relations of the sella turcica. The term 'cavernous' was adopted when it was thought that these sinuses were a single cavern with a few trabeculae. Work using corrosion casts has established that these sinuses are plexiform in nature, i.e. they are made up of an intertwined network of thin-walled venous channels of varying sizes that divide and coalesce and incompletely surround the carotid arteries.[17]

The sinuses are approximately 1 cm wide and 2 cm long and are wider at the roof than at the base. They extend forwards from the apex of the petrous temporal bone to the superior orbital fissure. The carotid arteries have a variable course inside the sinuses. They enter posteroinferiorly, having passed through the carotid canal, and then turn anteriorly, passing horizontally through the sinus before turning superiorly to enter the anterior cranial fossa medial to the anterior clinoid processes. The horizontal portion of the artery is usually the lateral relation of the hypophysis. There is significant individual variation and the artery may be up to 7 mm away from the gland with the intervening space filled with venous plexus or it may be as close as 1 mm with little intervening venous tissue. The lateral wall of the cavernous sinus is a thick sheet of dura mater; the medial wall is much thinner. There is no thick dural sheet and the capsule of the pituitary is the only barrier to spread of adenoma from the pituitary fossa.

The oculomotor nerve, trochlear nerve and ophthalmic division of the trigeminal nerve are closely related to, but not in, the lateral wall of the sinus as they pass anteriorly towards the superior orbital fissure.[18] The abducens nerve runs inferolaterally to the carotid artery in its horizontal portion. The sympathetic plexus runs with the carotid artery.

The sinus receives tributaries from the superficial middle cerebral vein, inferior cerebral vein, sphenoparietal sinus, inferior ophthalmic vein and sometimes the central retinal vein and frontal tributaries of the middle meningeal vein. The sinus then drains into the internal jugular vein via the inferior petrosal sinus, to the transverse sinus via the superior petrosal sinus, and small emissary veins drain through the foreman lacerum and foramen ovale to the pterygoid plexus.

ENDOSCOPIC ANATOMY OF CAVERNOUS SINUSES

If the bone of the posterior sphenoid sinus is taken down laterally to the anterior sella wall, the anterior aspect of the cavernous sinus is exposed. The prominent anatomical feature is the bulge of the C-shaped curve of the intra-cavernous portion of the internal carotid artery (**Figure 54.8a**). The nerves in the cavernous sinus are all placed laterally to the carotid artery and the carotid artery needs to be displaced medially in order to identify these (**Figure 54.8b**). Along the lateral wall of the cavernous sinus the oculomotor, trochlear and abducens nerves may be seen. In addition, the ophthalmic and occasionally the maxillary divisions of the trigeminal nerves may be visible. The oculomotor nerve is large and easily recognizable. It is located superiorly closest to the optic nerve, the trochlear nerve is smaller and is found just below the oculomotor nerve, and the abducens nerve is located more medially and inferior to the carotid artery.[19]

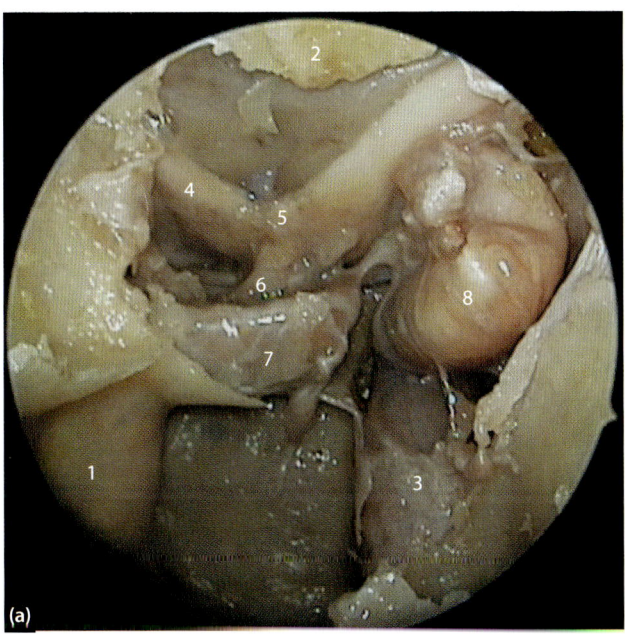 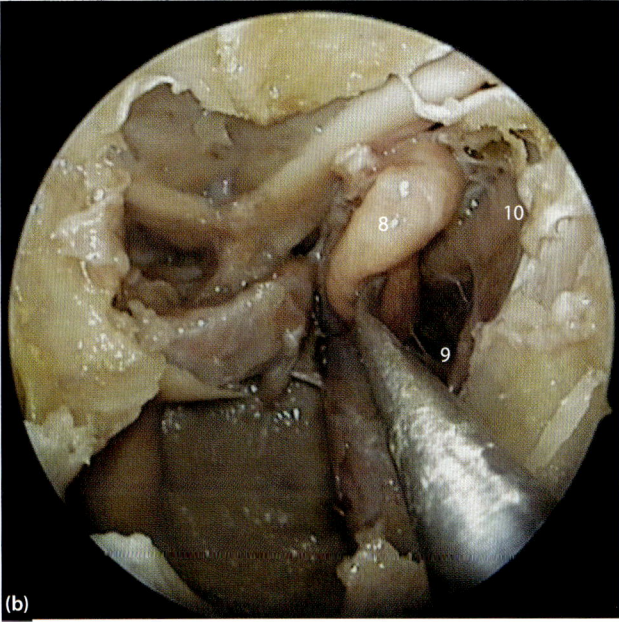

Figure 54.8 Endoscopic view of the sella and cavernous sinus in a frozen cadaver. (a) The right ascending carotid (1) is behind its bony covering. Bone, dura and the diaphragm have been removed over the pituitary fossa and left cavernous sinus up to the roof of the sphenoid (2). The left ascending carotid (3), optic nerves (4), chiasm (5), pituitary stalk (6) and the pituitary gland (7) are exposed. The anterior bulge of the left carotid artery (8) is seen in the cavernous sinus. **(b)** The left carotid artery (8) is displaced medially to show the cavernous sinus (9) and the oculomotor nerve (10) in its lateral wall.

> **KEY POINTS**
>
> - Intra-sphenoid septae are highly variable and often inserted close to the carotid artery on the posterior sphenoid wall.
> - Endoscopic view allows good visualization of the posterior sphenoid wall and the landmarks of the carotid arteries and optic nerves are often visible.
> - The lateral optico-carotid recess corresponds to the anterior clinoid process intracranially.
> - Understanding the variable, tortuous course of the carotid artery in the sphenoid and cavernous sinus is the key to performing safe pituitary surgery.
> - The pituitary fossa does not normally contain CSF but does contain small inter-cavernous venous sinuses.

REFERENCES

1. Langman J. *Medical embryology.* 4th ed. Philadelphia: Williams & Wilkins; 1981.
2. Hammer G, Radberg C. The sphenoid sinus: an anatomical and roentgenologic study with reference to transsphenoid hypophysectomy. *Acta Radiol* 1961; **56**: 401–22.
3. Tan HKK, Ong YK. Sphenoid sinus: an anatomic and endoscopic study in Asian cadavers. *Clin Anat* 2007; **20**: 745–75.
4. Fernandez-Miranda JC, Prevedello DM, Madhok R, et al. Sphenoid septations and their relationship with internal carotid arteries: anatomical and radiological study. *Laryngoscope* 2009; **119**: 1893–6.
5. Sareen D, Agarwal A, Kaul JM, et al. Study of sphenoid sinus anatomy in relation to endoscopic surgery. *Int J Morphol* 2005; **23**(3): 261–6.
6. Williams PL (ed.). *Gray's anatomy.* 38th ed. Edinburgh: Churchill Livingstone; 1995.
7. Tsudchida T, Hruban RH, Carson BS, Philips PC. Folliculostellate cells in the human anterior pituitary express cytokeratins. *Pathol Res Pract* 1993; **189**: 184–8.
8. Page RB, Bergland RM. Pituitary vasculature. In: Allen MB, Makesh VB (eds). *The pituitary: a current review.* New York: Academic Press; 1977, pp. 9–17.
9. Dietemann JL, Lang J, Francke JP, et al. Anatomy and radiology of the sella spine. *Neuroradiol* 1981; **21**(1): 5–7.
10. Lang J. Structure and postnatal organisation of the heretofore uninvestigated and infrequent ossifications of the sella turcica region. *Acta Anat* 1977; **99**: 121–30.
11. Dietemann JL, Kehrli P, Maillot C, et al. Is there a dural wall between the cavernous sinus and the pituitary fossa? Anatomical and MRI findings. *Neuroradiol* 1998; **40**: 627–30.
12. Hempel KJ. Zur Pathologie der Sellaregion. *Radiologe* 1970; **10**: 425–9.
13. Sheahy CN, Jackson CCR, Pearson O, Kaufman B. Submucosal infranasal transphenoid hypophysectomy. *Bull Los Angeles Neurol Soc* 1968; **33**: 564–73.
14. Kaplan HA, Browder J, Krieger AJ. Intercavernous connections of the cavernous sinuses: the superior and inferior circular sinuses. *J Neurosurg* 1976; **45**: 166–8.
15. Unlu A, Meco C, Uqur HC, et al. Endoscopic anatomy of sphenoid sinus for pituitary surgery. *Clin Anat* 2008; **21**(7): 627–32.
16. Hamid O, El Fiky L, Hassan O, et al. Anatomic variations of the sphenoid sinus and their impact on trans-sphenoid pituitary surgery. *Skull Base* 2007; **18**(1): 9–15.
17. Parkinson D. Carotid cavernous fistula: direct repair with preservation of the carotid artery. Technical note. *J Neurosurg* 1973; **38**: 99–106.
18. McGrath P. The cavernous sinus: anatomical survey. *Aust NZ J Surg* 1977; **47**: 601–13.
19. Bassim MK, Senior BA. Endoscopic anatomy of the parasellar region. *Am J Rhinol* 2007; **21**: 27–31.

FURTHER READING

Cappabianca P, Alfieri A, De Divitis E, Tschabitscher M. *Atlas of endoscopic anatomy for endonasal intracranial surgery.* New York: Springer-Verlag; 2001.

Schwartz TH, Anand VK. *Endoscopic pituitary surgery. Endocrine, neuro-opthalmologic and surgical management.* New York: Thieme; 2012.

Cushing HJB. *Pituitary body and its disorders.* Philadelphia: Lippincott Co.; 1912.

CHAPTER 55

PHYSIOLOGY OF THE THYROID AND PARATHYROID GLANDS

Martin O. Weickert

Introduction 619	Summary of considerations of patients with disorders of the
Physiology of the thyroid gland 619	thyroid or parathyroids... 626
Physiology of the parathyroid glands 623	References 627

SEARCH STRATEGY

Data in this chapter may be updated by a Medline search using the keywords: thyroid, parathyroid glands, hypothyroidism, thyrotoxicosis, thyroid-stimulating hormone (TSH), thyroglobulin, thionamides, neutropenia, osteoporosis, vitamin D.

The information in this chapter summarizes the physiology of the thyroid and the parathyroid glands, with a focus on aspects that are important for the endocrine surgeon.

INTRODUCTION

The thyroid is the largest endocrine organ, weighing 10–25 g. The highly vascular gland is located in front of the trachea in the anterior neck and consists of a left and a right lobe, connected by the isthmus. The parathyroid glands can vary in number and location, but in over 80% of humans there are four glands which are most commonly located posterior to the thyroid, although the location especially of the inferior glands can be more variable. Importantly, apart from sharing anatomical neighbourhood and part of the name, thyroid and parathyroid glands are independent endocrine organs that share no obvious functional similarities. However, due to the close anatomical location, surgery of the thyroid can impair parathyroid function transiently or permanently.

At the beginning of modern thyroid surgery in the 1860s, the mortality associated with thyroidectomy was high,[1,2] mainly related to thyroid storm in thyrotoxic patients, as well as post-surgical hypothyroidism and hypocalcaemia. 'Cachexia strumipriva' in patients after total thyroidectomy, as described by Kocher in 1883,[3] was later causally linked to surgical hypothyroidism. Tetany was thought to be caused by 'hysteria'. The parathyroid glands in humans were discovered in 1880 by Sandstrom,[4] but the fact that hypocalcemia was the definitive cause of tetany was not accepted until decades later.[2]

Improved insights in the physiology of thyroid and parathyroid glands have made a major contribution to transforming surgery of these organs to relatively low-risk routine procedures. The aim of this chapter is to provide a brief overview of the physiology of the thyroid and parathyroid glands, with a focus on aspects that are relevant to the ENT surgeon.

PHYSIOLOGY OF THE THYROID GLAND

Hormones secreted by the thyroid are critical for the development of the foetus and newborn, with key influences on the development of the brain and normal growth. In adults, major roles of the thyroid include involvement in the regulation of energy homoeostasis.[5] Thyroid hormones influence the function of various target organs, primarily by stimulating cell metabolism and activity. Both over- and under-function of the thyroid influence the well-being of the patient, with major dysfunction in both directions being potentially life-threatening.

Key controlling factors of thyroid hormone synthesis include the availability of external iodine; and regulation by the hypothalamic–pituitary axis (HPA).

The thyroid produces and releases tetraiodothyronine (T4) and triiodothyronine (T3), which are essential hormones for the regulation of metabolic processes. Iodine from dietary sources is absorbed and carried to the thyroid as iodide, where it is actively concentrated via the natrium (sodium) iodide symporter (NIS) and transported

TABLE 55.1 Effects and key functions of thyrotoxic or hypothyroid states in adults

	Thyrotoxicosis	Hypothyroidism
Energy metabolism	Increased basal metabolic rate Heat intolerance Weight loss*	Decreased basal metabolic rate Cold intolerance Weight gain
Carbohydrate metabolism	Stimulation of carbohydrate metabolism	
Lipid metabolism	Stimulation of lipolysis, T3 mediated down regulation of SREBP1c mRNA;47 reduction in body fat mass[1]	Reduced lipolysis, increase in body fat mass
Protein metabolism	Protein degradation, reduction of body lean mass	Decreased protein synthesis, increased body mass
Cardiovascular	Increased efficacy of catecholamines, tachycardia, tremor, peripheral vasoconstriction (skin) with increased central blood flow	Decreased efficacy of catecholamines, bradycardia, reduced exercise tolerance and myocardial contractility, exacerbated heart failure
Central nervous system	Enhanced catecholamine activity	Impairment of intellectual activity, movement and speech, impaired memory, delayed tendon reflexes, muscle weakness
Bone	Increased bone turnover, osteopaenia, osteoporosis¶	Decreased bone turnover
Various	Turnover of vitamins, increased gut motility, erythropoiesis, involvement in the regulation of the menstrual cycle	Dry/coarse skin, hair loss, breathlessness, oligomenorrhea/amenorrhea, menorrhagia, normocytic anaemia

* In some 10% of patients, weight loss can be observed in the thyrotoxic state, related to increased appetite which may override the catabolic metabolic state.
¶ Related to activation of osteoclasts.

into thyroid follicles. The endoplasmic reticulum of the thyrocyte produces thyroglobulin (Tg) and thyroid peroxidase (TPO). Iodide is then attached to Tg via TPO, resulting in the production of mono-iodothyronine (MIT) and di-iodothyronine (DIT), with subsequent production of T3 and T4 via enzymatic coupling.

Thyroid hormone release is a complex process, involving endocytosis of Tg-containing vesicles and fusion with follicular epithelial phagolysosomes, proteolytic digestion and cleavage of Tg, intra-cellular deiodination of MIT and DIT and reuse of iodide, and finally release of T3 and T4 from the basolateral membrane into the circulation.[5,6] Almost all of these steps are influenced by thyroid-stimulating hormone (TSH).[7] Table 55.1 summarizes some of the key functions of thyroid hormones in adults.

Hormones secreted by the thyroid

The thyroid produces thyroid hormones T4 and T3 and releases them into the circulating blood. Approximately 80% of thyroid hormone is secreted as T4 and peripherally converted via deiodination into T3, which shows around fivefold more potency. The half-life of circulating T3 is ≅1.5 days, as compared with ≅7 days of T4. Combined, this results in ≅40-fold higher plasma concentrations of T4 versus T3.[5] T3 production is reduced in acute illness and starvation. Locally produced T3 plays important roles in several fundamental mechanisms, including thyroid homeostasis, energy balance and glucose metabolism.[8]

Thyroid hormones are bound to binding proteins in the peripheral blood. In circulating blood, only the free hormones (fT3 and fT4) exert relevant physiological actions. To assess the function of the thyroid, it is usually sufficient to measure plasma fT4, along with TSH. However, the measurement of plasma fT3 can be valuable in situations where there is suspected excess production and release of T3, i.e. in patients with a toxic thyroid adenoma.

Synthesis of thyroid hormones

Iodine is a crucial component of thyroid hormones, which are iodothyronines. By weight, iodine comprises 65% of T4 and 58% of T3. Ingested iodine is absorbed in the small intestine and transported via the plasma to the thyroid follicular cells, where it is concentrated. Thereafter, iodine is rapidly oxidized and bound to tyrosyl residues in Tg. This is followed by intra-colloidal modification of Tg, which comprises iodination of tyrosine residues; formation of iodothyronines by oxidative coupling of two iodotyrosines; and storage of iodinated Tg as colloid. The next steps include endocytosis of iodinated Tg, merging with lysosomes and finally, mediated via TPO, conversion of the respective iodinated tyrosine residues MIT and DIT to the thyroid hormones T3 (from MIT + DIT) and T4 (from DIT + DIT) (**Figure 55.1**).[6,9]

Selenium is another essential element for thyroid hormone synthesis. It is involved in synthesis of various enzymes, especially glutathione peroxidase.[10]

Antithyroid drugs interfere with the synthesis of thyroid hormones. The most important inhibitory drugs of thyroid hormone synthesis are the thionamides: methimazole and, more widely used in the UK, its prodrug carbimazole; and propylthiouracil. Propylthiouracil shows a less favourable side-effect profile compared with the thiamazoles in terms of possible agranulocytosis (not dose-dependent) and hepatic reactions, but it is preferred during the first trimester of pregnancy, due to the extremely rare possible side effect of aplasia cutis of the scalp in the foetus that has been observed with treatment with carbimazole.

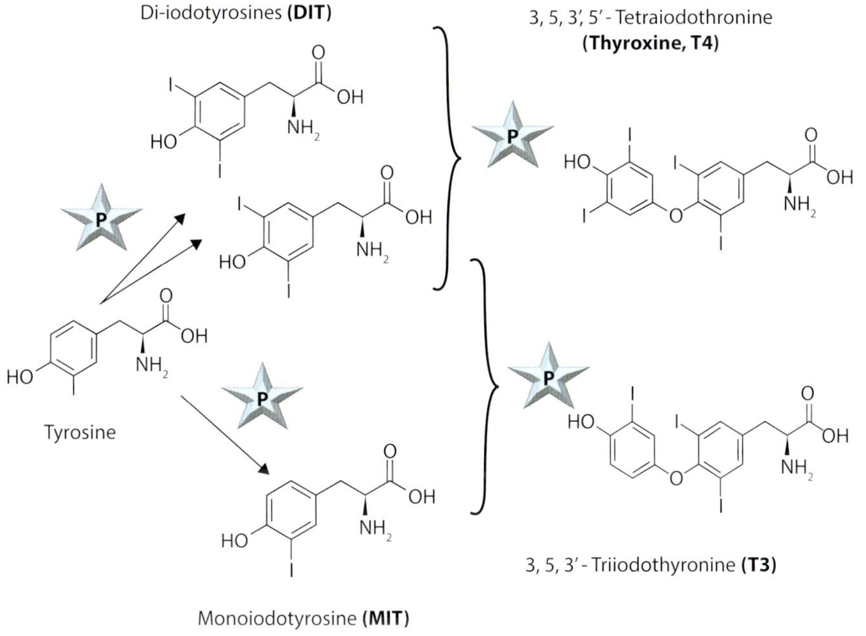

Figure 55.1 Thyroid hormone synthesis. Following the uptake of iodide into the follicular thyroid cell, thyroid peroxidase drives the iodination of tyrosine residues within the thyroglobulin matrix. Iodothyronines are formed by peroxidase coupling of iodothyrosyl residues, with 2 di-iodotyrosines (DIT) forming T4 and 1 MIT + 1 DIT forming T3. P, thyroid peroxidise.

Control of thyroid hormone synthesis

Release of thyroid hormones into the circulating blood involves the negative feedback system of the HPA.[11] A decrease in circulating T3 concentrations or a low metabolic rate signal the hypothalamus to secrete thyrotropin-releasing hormone (TRH), which in turn stimulates the secretion of TSH from the anterior pituitary gland. On the contrary, elevated circulating T3 concentrations inhibit the release of TRH and TSH directly.[7] T4 plays an indirect role, exerting inhibitory roles mainly after conversion to T3 within the pituitary or hypothalamus. **Figure 55.2** depicts the feedback inhibition of thyroid hormones on the release of TRH and TSH.[6]

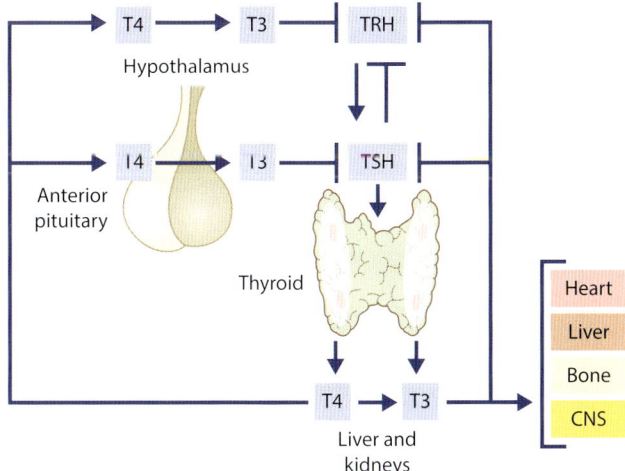

Figure 55.2 Feedback inhibition of thyroid hormones. The anterior pituitary gland increases the secretion of thyroid-stimulating hormone (TSH) when stimulated by hypothalamic thyrotropin-releasing hormone (TRH). The action of TRH is inhibited either directly by circulating T3, or indirectly, after conversion of T4 to T3, by the hypothalamus and pituitary.

TSH is a glycoprotein hormone from the anterior pituitary that influences almost all steps in both the synthesis and the release of thyroid hormones. The α-subunit is similar to that of luteinizing hormone, follicle-stimulating hormone and human chorionic gonadotropin, whereas the β-subunit is unique to TSH. It stimulates the TSH receptor (TSH-R) on thyroid follicular cells. The effects on thyroid hormone secretion appear to be mediated through the cAMP cascade, whereas the effects on synthesis are mediated by the Gq/phospholipase C cascade.[7] TSH stimulates the expression of NIS, TPO and Tg, the generation of hydrogen peroxide (H_2O_2), and the formation of T3.[7] Further functions of TSH involve altering the priority of iodination and hormonogenesis among tyrosyls and promoting the rapid internalization of Tg by thyrocytes. These steps are interrelated and have the net effect of increasing available iodine to the cells and finally of producing and releasing an increased amount of biologically active T3.[7]

Stimulation of TSH-R also increases the vascularity of the thyroid, an effect that is mediated via vascular endothelial growth factor (VEGF) secretion by the follicular cells. Presence of stimulating TSH R antibodies explains that patients with Graves' disease can show excessive vascular flow in the thyroid. Although TSH is the primary regulator of thyroid function, there is evidence for additional autoregulation of the thyroid, mainly related to iodine transport and organification.

Normal range for TSH

Expert opinion on the normal range for TSH varies widely. Some assays give excessively wide 'normal ranges' from 0.35–6 mU/L, which is in part related to the use of not well-characterized cohorts from cross-sectional studies, including assumed healthy individuals with occult thyroid disease.[12, 13] The American Association of Clinical Endocrinologists (AACE) defines a normal range for TSH of 0.3–3.0 mU/L and the National Academy of Clinical Biochemistry of 0.4–2.5 mU/L.[14] Notably, the population mean for TSH in various ethnicities appears to be lower, at 1–2 mU/L.[15–18] Even higher normal TSH levels (>2.5 mU/L) may be related to adverse outcomes, which include associations with parameters of metabolic risk.[19] After thyroidectomy, it appears reasonable titrating TSH within the ideal range in most patients. In subjects with moderate or high risk differentiated thyroid carcinomas, where TSH suppression is indicated, fT4 should be titrated towards the upper normal range. Importantly, TSH suppression is sufficient, whereas over-treatment resulting in excess fT4 levels is unnecessary and should be avoided due to risks of palpitations, atrial fibrillation and depletion of bone mass.

Iodine

Iodine is an essential mineral and the main substrate involved in thyrocyte metabolism. Potassium iodide is a man-made salt compound of iodine with increased absorption in the intestine. The normal human thyroid maintains a concentration of iodide that is 20–50 times higher than plasma concentrations, depending on the amount of available iodine and the activity of the gland.[20]

The thyroid concentrates iodide from the extracellular fluid by an active, energy-dependent and saturable process via NIS, which is located at the basolateral membrane of the acinar cell.[6] Iodide then diffuses via pendrin channels from the cell to the lumen at the apical membrane. Several types of control have been identified, which involve rapid and transient TSH-mediated stimulation of iodide efflux, TSH-induced blunted capacity of the active iodide transport, and transient inhibition of thyroid blood flow by iodide.[9] The rate of uptake of iodide by the thyroid normally exceeds the rate of its incorporation into amino acids (organification) and diffusion back to the extracellular fluids, which ensures high intra-thyroidal iodide concentrations.

Adequate dietary intake of iodine is essential for thyroid hormone synthesis. The daily iodine intake of adult humans varies from less than 10 μg in areas of extreme deficiency to several hundred milligrams. In the United States, urine iodine concentrations indicate generally sufficient intake of iodine[21], but intake in most of Europe appears to be lower. The Institute of Medicine has set the Recommended Dietary Allowance (RDA) for iodine in adults at 150 mcg/day. The minimum daily requirement to prevent goitre from iodine deficiency is thought to be 50–75 mcg/day. Both under- and over-supply of iodine influence thyroid function. Low supply with iodine is common and leads to impaired production of thyroid hormones, causing increased TSH secretion and possibly goitre in an compensatory attempt.[7] Various other iodine deficiency disorders of the thyroid have been reported.[22]

Excess iodide acutely inhibits the synthesis of thyroid hormones, the Wolff–Chaikoff effect.[23] Possible mechanisms include inhibiting the production of H_2O_2 and thus blocking the iodination of TG.[24] Importantly, this effect is typically short-lived, often lasting for several days only (escape from the Wolff–Chaikoff effect). Thereafter, in patients with pre-existing goitre, excess iodine can cause severe thionamide-resistant thyrotoxicosis. Blocking an overactive thyroid with high-dose iodine before surgery is therefore not encouraged by all centres; if this procedure is chosen, thyroid surgery should be performed within the next few days. Thyrotoxic effects of excess iodine can also be observed in thyrotoxicosis type-1 induced by amiodarone (an antiarrhythmic drug that contains 75 000 μg of iodine per tablet) and in patients with goitre following the use of iodine-containing contrast medium when performing computer tomographic (CT) scans.

Thyroglobulin

Tg is the most abundant protein in the thyroid gland, with up to 200-300 g/L being stored in the follicular lumen. The main function of Tg is to provide the polypeptide backbone for the synthesis and storage of thyroid hormones.[7] Further functions include depot capacity for the storage of iodine, thereby compensating for fluctuations in the supply of external food derived iodine. Thyroid hormones that are bound to Tg are biologically inactive.

Given that Tg is exclusively produced in thyroid, it can serve as a tumour marker after complete removal of the thyroid (total thyroidectomy followed by radioiodine treatment in patients with differentiated thyroid cancer). However, the presence of anti-Tg antibodies needs to be excluded. Interference of these antibodies with various assays can lead to either false positive and false negative results, possibly delaying the detection of a relapse, or resulting in unnecessarily repeated investigations involving radiation.

Thyroid peroxidase

TPO is produced in the endoplasmic reticulum of the thyrocytes. TPO oxidizes iodine, thereby facilitating the formation of T3 and T4 (**Figure 55.1**). The presence of TPO antibodies increases the risk of developing autoimmune thyroiditis.

Release of thyroid hormones

Unlike most other endocrine organs, which do not store relevant amounts of hormone, the thyroid contains the supply of Tg-bound thyroid hormones for several weeks.[6] Upon stimulation by TSH, iodothyronines are released from Tg due to effects of lysosomal proteases, with fT4 and fT3 diffusing from the thyroid cell into the bloodstream. Both iodide and TG normally remain in the thyroid cells and are reused for hormone resynthesis.[6] After variable periods of storage in thyroid follicles, Tg is proteolysed and the released hormones are secreted into the circulation, where specific binding proteins, most notably thyroxine-binding globulin (TBG), transport them to their respective target tissues.

Thyroxine-binding globulin in plasma (TBG)

In circulating blood ≅80% of T4 and T3 are bound to TBG and other binding proteins, which help maintain

TABLE 55.2 Effects of various factors on circulating thyroxine-binding globulin (TBG)	
Circulating TBG	**Causal factors**
Increased TBG	Pregnancy Hepatitis Acute intermittent porphyria Drugs (i.e. oestrogen, tamoxifen, opiates, etc.) Hereditary TBG excess
Decreased TBG	Genetic reasons Chronic liver disease Nephrotic syndrome Malnutrition Cushing's disease Drugs (i.e. androgens, steroids, etc.) Acromegaly

FUTURE RESEARCH

- To develop uniform evidence-based recommendations for the follow-up of patients with differentiated thyroid cancers, with respect to risk assessment (low, medium or high risk)
- Advanced strategies to avoid inadvertent damage to the parathyroids in patients requiring total thyroidectomy
- Potential differences between thyroid hormone action in circulating blood, as compared to cellular and tissue levels
- Influence of age and developmental status on thyroid function
- Further defining risk assessment in patients with thyroid nodules
- Molecular treatment approaches for different histotypes of thyroid cancer

serum free T3 and T4 concentrations within a tight range. Only unbound thyroid hormone is available to the tissues and therefore biologically active. T3 is less strongly bound than T4 and has a more rapid onset of action.

Oestrogens stimulate the expression of TBG in the liver. Therefore, from about 20 weeks of gestation, pregnant women with hypothyroidism need their L-thyroxine replacement doses to be increased to avoid hypothyroidism (**Table 55.2**).

Action of thyroid hormones at the tissue level

At the tissue level, the biological activity of thyroid hormone is regulated by deiodinases (DIO). DIO-1 and DIO-2 are responsible for the generation of T3 from T4, whereas DIO 3-is the major inactivating enzyme, leading to an increase of reverse T3 (rT3).[25] The ratio between T3 and rT3 (T3/rT3-ratio) is a sensitive indicator of peripheral thyroid hormone metabolism. The ratio is positively influenced by DIO-1 and DIO-2 and negatively by DIO-3. The T3/rT3-ratio is relatively independent of both thyroidal T4 production and thyroid hormone-binding protein variation in serum.[25]

Calcitonin

Calcitonin is produced by the neural crest cell-derived parafollicular C-cells. The role of calcitonin in humans is not completely understood.

Calcitonin (and, less specific, carcinoembryonic antigen – CEA) can be used as tumour markers in medullary thyroid carcinoma (MCT), a rare ($\cong$4% of all thyroid cancers) and frequently aggressive cancer that is often located in the upper central lobe of the thyroid gland. C-cell hyperplasia defines a MTC *in situ*, with better prognostic features. Around 80% of MCT occur sporadically. The remaining 20% are inherited syndromes such as multiple endocrine neoplasia (MEN) types 2A, 2B, or MTC only. Catecholamine-producing pheochromocytomas are a concern in MEN-2, with important implications when preparing for safe thyroid surgery.

KEY POINTS

- TSH is the best overall parameter for assessing thyroid function and for monitoring replacement therapy.
- In medium- to high-risk thyroid cancer, TSH suppression with high normal fT4 is the aim.
- Replacement with L-thyroxine (T4) is standard. Replacement with Liothyronine (T3) is more likely to result in fluctuations of thyroid function tests and side effects, but it may be needed in rare conditions with impaired conversion of T4 to T3 or for preparation of radioiodine treatment if recombinant TSH is not available.
- Thyroid hormones should be taken at least 30 min before breakfast and isolated from caffeine-containing beverages and other tablets to facilitate more reliable absorption.
- TSH can react slowly to changes in hormone supply, especially after longer term dysfunction. Here, monitoring of fT4 (or fT3, if appropriate) gives more timely information.
- Thionamides are the treatment of choice to control thyrotoxicosis prior to surgery.
- Replacement of vitamin D before total thyroidectomy reduces the risk of severe hypocalcaemia related to inadvertent damage to the parathyroid glands.
- Screening for catecholamine-producing tumours is mandatory before performing surgery for MCT.

PHYSIOLOGY OF THE PARATHYROID GLANDS

The main function of the parathyroids is the regulation of calcium homoeostasis via the secretion of PTH. There are usually four (40 mg each) parathyroid glands. Five per cent of the population have only three glands and an additional fifth gland can be found in 12–15%, with six or more glands being occasional findings.[26] The secretion of PTH is under negative feedback regulation by ionized calcium in the extracellular fluid. However, PTH remains detectable even when serum calcium is excessively raised, indicating that further factors contribute to the regulation of PTH secretion.

Calcium homoeostasis

Calcium homeostasis is a complex process, involving serum calcium, phosphate, 1,25-dihydroxyvitamin D3 (synonyms: 1,25(OH)$_2$ vitamin D3, 'active' vitamin D, or calcitriol) and PTH. The main involved organs are the parathyroid glands, bones, kidneys and the intestine; the skin, kidneys and liver regulate vitamin D metabolism.

More than 99% of the human calcium reserve ($\cong$1.1 kg) is stored in the bones and teeth. 'Free' ionized calcium, comprising $\cong$50% of body calcium, has crucial physiological roles including cell signalling, the functioning of the heart and the nervous system, the contraction of muscles and the clotting of blood.[6] The remainder of the calcium pool is protein-bound (40%) or forms soluble complexes with phosphate and citrate (10%). Most protein-bound calcium is attached to albumin and influenced by the pH, with acidosis increasing and alkalosis decreasing ionized calcium levels.[5]

Serum calcium concentrations are tightly regulated (normal range 2.14–2.6 mmol/L, assay-dependent). Even relatively mild acute changes can be symptomatic. Major changes in both directions can be life-threatening.

Parathyroid hormone (PTH)

The parathyroid glands secrete parathyroid hormone (PTH) after cleavage from pre-pro-PTH (115 amino acids) to pro-PTH (90 amino acids) and finally the active peptide hormone (84 amino acids). PTH is released when calcium sensors on the surface of the parathyroid glands detect low circulating serum calcium concentrations, and rapidly increases serum calcium levels. The release of PTH is inversely proportional to serum calcium, with small calcium fluctuations producing large changes in PTH secretion.[26] PTH blocks the renal reabsorption of phosphate in the proximal tubule and facilitates the reabsorption in the ascending loops of Henle, distal tubules and collecting tubules. In addition, PTH activates the enzyme 1-hydroxylase in the proximal renal tubules, thereby converting 25-OH vitamin D to its active metabolite, calcitriol.

In the bone, PTH promotes the absorption of calcium via a rapid and a slow phase.[27] The rapid phase appears to be mediated at the level of the bone cells. In response to hypocalcaemia, PTH concentrations change within 1 min, peak in 4–10 min and decline again within 60 min. The half-life of PTH is approximately 3 min. The slow phase of bone resorption is regulated via activation and proliferation of osteoclasts, with effects taking several days. These actions appear to be mediated by the differentiation of osteoclast precursors which, unlike mature osteoclasts, possess vitamin D and PTH receptors; or via cytokines that are released by activated osteocytes and osteoblasts.[27] Feedback inhibition of PTH release occurs primarily by direct effects of circulating calcium at the level of the parathyroid gland.

In humans, PTH fluctuates episodically at a frequency of 6–7 bursts per hour. Non-pulsatile secretion accounts for $\cong$70% of total PTH secretion. Patients with excess PTH secretion (i.e. primary hyperparathyroidism, PHPT) show both pulsatile and tonic excess secretion but unchanged pulse frequency. Constantly elevated PTH has detrimental effects on bone mass density and bone structure,[28] primarily due to up-regulation of nuclear factor κB ligand (RANKL) and inhibition of osteoprotegerin expression, leading to an increase in osteoclast formation and activity.[29] In contrast, intermittent administration of recombinant PTH stimulates bone formation, explaining its pharmacological use for the treatment of osteoporosis.[30] In hypercalcaemic states, measurement of PTH is the most important measure to distinguish between PHPT and other causes of hypercalcaemia where circulating PTH is typically low, i.e. in patients with Vitamin D intoxication or malignancy (where hypercalcaemia can result from PTH related peptide (PTHrp) excess; osteolytic bones metastases; immobilization or dehydration. Importantly, patients with raised PTH together with low or lower end of normal adjusted calcium concentrations have secondary hyperparathyroidism (frequently caused by vitamin D deficiency or insufficiency), which is a physiological reaction of the parathyroids to increased serum calcium levels. Here, imaging of the parathyroids or surgical intervention would be inappropriate.

Vitamin D

Vitamin D3 (colecalciferol, previously cholecalciferol) is formed in the skin when a cholesterol precursor, 7-dehydroxycholesterol, is exposed to ultraviolet light (UV-B). 'Active' vitamin D (1, 25-(OH)$_2$ vitamin D3) occurs after (i) 25-hydroxylation in the liver and (ii) 1-hydroxylation in the kidney (**Figure 55.3**), with major effects on calcium homoeostasis. Compared with PTH, vitamin D exerts much slower but long-acting regulatory effects on calcium balance.

Active vitamin D is calciotropic, raising serum calcium by several mechanisms. These include promoting the absorption of calcium in the intestine and stimulating the formation of calcium-binding protein in the intestinal epithelial cells. Further functions include increasing bone resorption and renal calcium reabsorption, actions that are in part shared with those of PTH. Vitamin D also promotes intestinal absorption of phosphate. In bone, vitamin D may play a synergistic role with PTH in stimulating osteoclast proliferation and bone resorption, with high PTH and low phosphate levels as stimulating and with low PTH and high phosphate as inhibiting factors.[6]

Recent research also links calcitriol precursors to various physiological functions. The exact mechanisms of how increased vitamin D3 intake intake inhibits PTH secretion need further investigation but are unlikely to be exclusively dependent on circulating calcitriol.[31–34] Local mRNA and protein expression of 1-alpha hydroxylase has been described in human parathyroid glands, and this expression appears to be altered in various disorders of the parathyroids.[33, 35, 36] Further proposed mechanisms include non-1,25(OH)$_2$ vitamin D-mediated effects of colecalciferol or other vitamin D metabolites on PTH production, or stimulation of parathyroid tissue vitamin D receptors.[32–34] Further actions may include vitamin D-mediated regulation of the expression of the calcium-sensing receptor (CaSR).[31, 37, 38] Treatment of

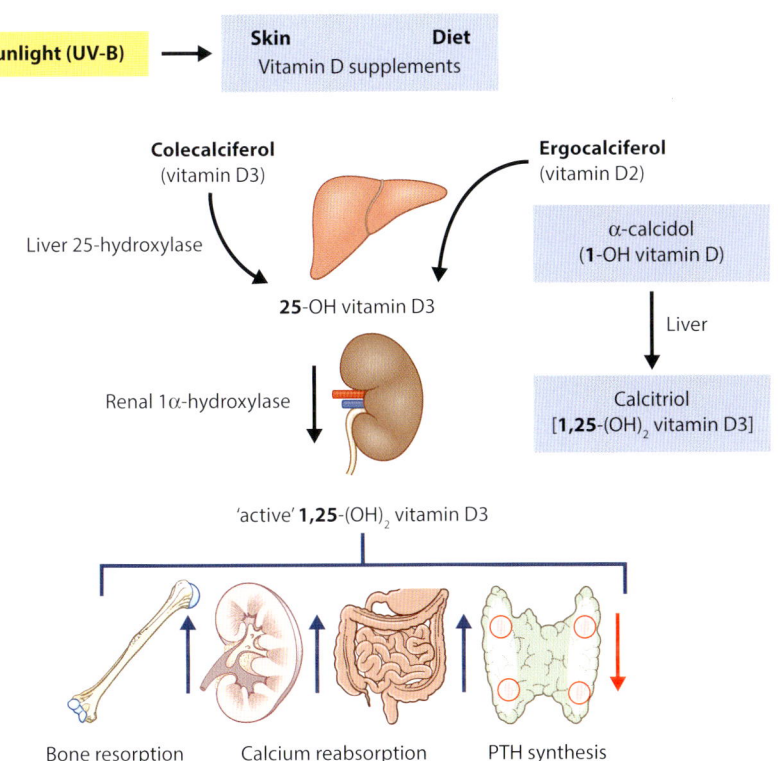

Figure 55.3 Vitamin D metabolism and replacement drugs. Unlike calcitriol, alfacalcidol is a prodrug that is inactive prior to hydroxylation in the liver. This process can be impaired in patients with liver disorders.

vitamin D deficiency appears to reduce circulating PTH in patients with PHPT, without adverse effects on serum calcium concentrations.[31] Various factors support the replacement of vitamin D deficiency in patients with PHPT: suboptimal dietary intake of vitamin D stimulates parathyroid adenoma growth and reduces the calcaemic response to PTH.[31] Apart from elevated markers of increased bone turnover,[39, 40] patients with coexisting PHPT and vitamin D deficiency are more likely to have a larger parathyroid adenoma and higher PTH levels.[34, 41] Recent guidelines encourage vitamin D replacement to serum 25-OH vitamin D concentrations above 50 nmol/L in all monitored patients with pHPT.[42]

Post-operative hypoparathyroidism

Post-operative hypoparathyroidism can result in severe hypocalcaemia. Early symptoms may include anxiety, tingling of the fingers and toes, or peri-oral numbness. Acute and severe hypocalcaemia may result in papilledema, tetany, seizures and even death. In patients with MEN type 1, all parathyroids should be removed, although autotransplantation of half a gland into the sternocleidomastoid muscle or forearm is advised to avoid severe hypocalcaemia and often major fluctuations in serum calcium levels despite replacement with active vitamin D. Post-operative hypoparathyroidism happens accidentally, for example during total thyroidectomy for thyroid cancer, Graves' disease, or surgery for multinodular goitre. It is more often temporary but can be permanent. Frequency of this complication is usually reported as 5%, but could be as high as 20% after combined thyroidectomy and radical neck dissection.[2, 43] Treatment with radioiodine may play a role as well, but is considered to be a rare cause of symptomatic hypocalcaemia.

Post-operative hypoparathyroidism is most frequently caused by disruption of the fine vessels that supply the parathyroids, rather than by accidental removal of all parathyroid glands.[2] The risk of accidental devascularization can be reduced by dissecting close to the thyroid capsule and by ligating the branches of the inferior thyroid artery on the thyroid capsule distal to their supply of the parathyroid glands, rather than by ligating the inferior thyroid artery as a single trunk.[2]

There is an increased risk of severe and potentially life-threatening hypocalcaemia in patients with combined PHPT and vitamin D deficiency following parathyroidectomy.[41] Correcting vitamin D deficiency has been shown to reduce both the incidence of post-operative hypocalcaemia and the length of stay in hospital.[44]

Calcium-sensing receptor

The calcium-sensing receptor (CaSR) is a class C G-protein coupled receptor which senses extracellular levels of calcium ions. In the parathyroid gland CaSR controls calcium homeostasis by regulating the release of PTH. Mutations that inactivate the CaSR gene cause familial hypocalciuric hypercalcemia (FHH), which generally is asymptomatic and does not require treatment. Therefore, it is important to distinguish this benign disorder from PHPT. Not all patients with PHPT require surgical treatment, and there is consensus that asymptomatic patients with adjusted calcium concentrations below 3 mmol/L and absence of end-organ damage related to longer-term PTH excess such as osteoporosis can be safely observed. Calcimimetics are a class of drugs with calcium-sensing receptor agonist properties that act directly on the parathyroid gland and decrease PTH release and serum calcium levels, and may also beneficially influence parathyroid tumour growth. Calcimimetics can be useful in patients with PHPT who are not eligible for surgical intervention.

Calcitonin

Calcitonin counteracts many of the functions of PTH in various species. However, in humans the biological role of calcitonin is not well defined, with both lack of calcitonin after thyroidectomy and excess of calcitonin in medullary thyroid carcinoma exerting no obvious effects on serum calcium or bone mass. Calcitonin of some other species (e.g. that of salmon, which is >15-fold more potent) is used pharmacologically for the treatment of osteoporosis and malignant hypercalcaemia.[6] Calcitonin acts in response to acute changes in serum calcium concentrations by inhibiting calcium resorption from the bones and tubular reabsorption in the kidneys.[5] Physiological stimuli of calcitonin secretion include hypercalcaemia and high circulating levels of gastrin.

SUMMARY OF CONSIDERATIONS OF PATIENTS WITH DISORDERS OF THE THYROID OR PARATHYROIDS

Patients undergoing surgery of the thyroid should be euthyroid. Correction of thyrotoxicosis is assessed by measurement of serum fT3 (and more slowly reacting fT4, due to longer plasma half-life; note that fT4 will show delayed decrease when the conversion of fT4 to fT3 is pharmacologically blocked), whereas a suppressed TSH alone does not define risk and may need weeks to normalize. Hypothyroidism should be treated before surgery, if possible. In emergency situations, intravenous treatment with thyroid hormones for patients with severe hypothyroidism can be provided during surgery. In patients with thyrotoxicosis and contraindications against thionamides drugs (i.e. due to carbimazole-induced agranulocytosis, with known cross-reactivity of at least 50% with all other drugs in this class), urgent surgery is mandatory to save the patient's life. Measures to reduce risk in this situation may include high-dose treatment with propranolol (>140 mg/day are needed to block conversion T4 to T3), high-dose hydrocortisone, low-dose lithium (400–500 mg daily) (unlicensed use; with various inhibiting effects on thyroid hormone synthesis and release;[45] higher doses are discouraged and increase the rate of side effects only); or iodine, although with the latter the situation may worsen in patients with multinodular goitre related to pre-existing iodine deficiency; and surgery must be performed within the next few days.

Following total thyroidectomy, the replacement dose of L-thyroxine is usually ≅1.6 µg/kg body weight, to be taken first thing in the morning and at least 30 minutes before food, caffeine-containing beverages and any other tablets or supplements to facilitate more reliable absorption. Initially smaller doses with stepwise increases are advised, especially in geriatric patients and patients with risk factors such as atrial fibrillation. When TSH needs to be raised transiently (typically to >30 mU/L) prior to radioiodine treatment, the preferred choice is administration of recombinant TSH over 2 days. Alternatively, L-thyroxine can be paused and replaced by Liothyronine (T3; 20% of the dose of L-thyroxine), which is eliminated more rapidly after withdrawal. Although more cost-efficient, this method results in significant morbidity related to overt hypothyroidism, which can include severe weight gain and clinically relevant depression.

Measurement of serum-adjusted calcium, 25-OH vitamin D and PTH concentrations, and pre-operative replacement of vitamin D are recommended in patients undergoing total thyroidectomy or surgery of the parathyroid glands. Endoscopic or indirect laryngoscopy should be performed to exclude potentially asymptomatic pre-existent lesions of the vocal cords. In patients following removal of parathyroid gland(s) or in patients who underwent total thyroidectomy, close monitoring of serum calcium levels and appropriate replacement with active vitamin D preparations is crucial to avoid significant morbidity.

In patients with PHPT due to MEN 1, all parathyroid glands need to be explored and thymectomy considered, particularly when fewer than four parathyroid glands are identified.[46] Leaving a viable remnant or performing autotransplantation is recommended to avoid major swings in serum calcium levels following surgery. Patients with MTC require pre-surgical assessment (and treatment, if appropriate) for possible coexisting catecholamine excess.

> **FUTURE RESEARCH**
>
> ► Additional strategies for preserving parathyroid function in patients undergoing total thyroidectomy; and improved strategies for the long-term treatment of patients with permanent hypoparathyroidism and hypocalcaemia
> ► Improved methods for the pre-operative identification of small parathyroid adenomata
> ► Further improvement of decision pathways for performing surgery vs. an observational approach in patients with PHPT
> ► Improved diagnostic and therapeutic strategies for patients with parathyroid carcinoma

KEY POINTS

- PTH concentrations are altered within 1 min, peak in 4–10 min and decline in 60 min. Absence of PTH (e.g. after inadvertent damage to the parathyroids) can result in major problems including life-threatening hypocalcaemia.
- Additional vitamin D deficiency in patients with PHPT may introduce additional (secondary) stimulation to the parathyroid glands, with further negative effects on bone mass.
- Correcting vitamin D deficiency before parathyroid surgery and total thyroidectomy can reduce both the incidence of postoperative hypocalcaemia and the length of stay in hospital.
- Alfacalcidol is a prodrug and may not work effectively in hypoparathyroid patients with impaired liver function.
- Patients with MEN 1 generally have tumours in several or all four parathyroid glands and may have additional ectopic glands (e.g. in the thymus). Minimally invasive parathyroidectomy is not recommended. Leaving a viable remnant or performing autotransplantation is recommended to avoid major swings in serum calcium levels following surgery.

REFERENCES

1. Hasselgren PO. Surgery in Sweden at the time of Halsted. *Arch Surg* 2004; **139**(1): 100–12.
2. Kaplan E, Angelos P, Applewhite M, et al. Surgery of the thyroid. In: *Thyroid disease manager*. Available from: http://www.thyroidmanager.org/chapter/chapter-21surgery-of-the-thyroid/ [Accessed June 09, 2017]; 2012.
3. Trohler U. Towards endocrinology: Theodor Kocher's 1883 account of the unexpected effects of total ablation of the thyroid. *J R Soc Med* 2011; **104**(3): 129–32.
4. Thompson NW. The history of hyperparathyroidism. *Acta Chir Scand* 1990; **156**(1): 5–21.
5. Molina PE. *Endocrine physiology*. New York: McGraw-Hill; 2004; Lange Physiology Series.
6. Kovacs WJ, Ojeda SR. *Textbook of endocrine physiology*. Oxford: Oxford University Press; 2012.
7. Miot F, Dupuy C, Dumont JE, Rousset B. Thyroid hormone synthesis and secretion. In: *Thyroid disease manager*. Available from: http://www.thyroidmanager.org/chapter/chapter-2-thyroid-hormone-synthesis-and-secretion/ [Accessed June 09, 2017]; 2012.
8. Salvatore D. Thyroid endocrinology: the future is now. *Front Endocrinol* 2010; **1**: 7.
9. Dumont JE, Opitz R, Christophe D, et al. Ontogeny, anatomy, metabolism and physiology of the thyroid. In: *Thyroid disease manager*. Available from: http://www.thyroidmanager.org/chapter/ontogeny-anatomy-metabolism-and-physiology-of-the-thyroid/ [Accessed June 09, 2017]; 2011.
10. Brown KM, Arthur JR. Selenium, selenoproteins and human health: a review. *Public Health Nutr* 2001; **4**(2B): 593–9.
11. Wartofsky L. Diseases of the thyroid. In: Isselbacher KJ, Braunwald E, Wilson JD, et al (eds). *Harrison's principles of internal medicine*. 17th ed. New York: McGraw-Hill; 1994, pp. 1930–53.
12. Wartofsky L, Dickey RA. The evidence for a narrower thyrotropin reference range is compelling. *J Clin Endocrinol Metab* 2005; **90**(9): 5483–8.
13. Wier FA, Farley CL. Clinical controversies in screening women for thyroid disorders during pregnancy. *J Midwifery Womens Health* 2006; **51**(3): 152–8.
14. Spencer CA. Assay of thyroid hormones and related substances. In: *Thyroid disease manager*. Available from: http://www.thyroidmanager.org/chapter/assay-of-thyroid-hormones-and-related-substances3/ [Accessed June 09, 2017]. 2013.
15. Andersen S, Pedersen KM, Bruun NH, Laurberg P. Narrow individual variations in serum T(4) and T(3) in normal subjects: a clue to the understanding of subclinical thyroid disease. *J Clin Endocrinol Metab* 2002; **87**(3): 1068–72.
16. Baloch Z, Carayon P, Conte-Devolx B, et al. Laboratory medicine practice guidelines: laboratory support for the diagnosis and monitoring of thyroid disease. *Thyroid* 2003; **13**(1): 3–126.
17. Hollowell JG, Staehling NW, Flanders WD, et al. Serum TSH, T(4), and thyroid antibodies in the United States population (1988 to 1994): National Health and Nutrition Examination Survey (NHANES III). *J Clin Endocrinol Metab* 2002; **87**(2): 489–99.
18. Vanderpump MP, Tunbridge WM, French JM, et al. The incidence of thyroid disorders in the community: a twenty-year follow-up of the Whickham Survey. *Clin Endocrinol* 1995; **43**(1): 55–68.
19. Ruhla S, Weickert MO, Arafat AM, et al. A high normal TSH is associated with the metabolic syndrome. *Clin Endocrinol* 2010; **72**(5): 696–701.
20. Berson SA, Yalow RS. The iodide trapping and binding functions of the thyroid. *J Clin Invest* 1955; **34**(2): 186–204.
21. Soldin OP, Soldin SJ, Pezzullo JC. Urinary iodine percentile ranges in the United States. *Clin Chim Acta* 2003; **328**(1–2): 185–90.
22. Dunn JT. What's happening to our iodine? *J Clin Endocrinol Metab* 1998; **83**(10): 3398–400.
23. Wolff J, Chaikoff IL. The inhibitory action of iodide upon organic binding of iodine by the normal thyroid gland. *J Biol Chem* 1948; **172**(2): 855.
24. Corvilain B, Van Sande J, Dumont JE. Inhibition by iodide of iodide binding to proteins: the "Wolff-Chaikoff" effect is caused by inhibition of H_2O_2 generation. *Biochem Biophys Res Commun* 1988; **154**(3): 1287–92.
25. Ruhla S, Arafat AM, Weickert MO, et al. T3/rT3-ratio is associated with insulin resistance independent of TSH. *Horm Metab Res* 2011; **43**(2): 130–4.
26. Bruder JM, Guide TA, Mundy GR. Mineral metabolism. In: Felig P, Frohman LA (eds). *Endocrinology and metabolism*. 5th ed. New York: McGraw-Hill; 2001, pp. 1079–177.
27. Essig GF, Jameson MJ, Carter WB, Carron JD. *Parathyroid physiology*. Medscape; 2012.
28. Feldman D. Vitamin D, parathyroid hormone, and calcium: a complex regulatory network. *Am J Med* 1999; **107**(6): 637–9.
29. Silva BC, Costa AG, Cusano NE, et al. Catabolic and anabolic actions of parathyroid hormone on the skeleton. *J Endocrinol Invest* 2011; **34**(10): 801–10.
30. Schmitt CP, Homme M, Schaefer F. Structural organization and biological relevance of oscillatory parathyroid hormone secretion. *Pediatr Nephrol* 2005; **20**(3): 346–51.
31. Rao RR, Randeva HS, Sankaranarayanan S, et al. Prolonged treatment with vitamin D in postmenopausal women with primary hyperparathyroidism. *Endocr Connect* 2012; **1**(1): 13–21.
32. Carling T, Rastad J, Szabo E, et al. Reduced parathyroid vitamin D receptor messenger ribonucleic acid levels in primary and secondary hyperparathyroidism. *J Clin Endocrinol Metab* 2000; **85**(5): 2000–3.
33. Grey A, Lucas J, Horne A, et al. Vitamin D repletion in patients with primary hyperparathyroidism and coexistent vitamin D insufficiency. *J Clin Endocrinol Metab* 2005; **90**(4): 2122–6.
34. Rao DS, Honasoge M, Divine GW, et al. Effect of vitamin D nutrition on parathyroid adenoma weight: pathogenetic and clinical implications. *J Clin Endocrinol Metab* 2000; **85**(3): 1054–8.
35. Correa P, Segersten U, Hellman P, et al. Increased 25-hydroxyvitamin D3 1alpha-hydroxylase and reduced 25-hydroxyvitamin D3 24-hydroxylase expression in parathyroid tumors: new prospects for treatment of hyperparathyroidism with vitamin D. *J Clin Endocrinol Metab* 2002; **87**(12): 5826–9.
36. Segersten U, Correa P, Hewison M, et al. 25-hydroxyvitamin D(3)-1alpha-hydroxylase expression in normal and pathological parathyroid glands. *J Clin Endocrinol Metab* 2002; **87**(6): 2967–72.
37. Brown AJ, Zhong M, Finch J, et al. Rat calcium-sensing receptor is regulated by vitamin D but not by calcium. *Am J Physiol* 1996; **270**(3 Pt 2): F454–60.
38. Chakrabarty S, Wang H, Canaff L, et al. Calcium sensing receptor in human colon carcinoma: interaction with Ca(2+) and 1,25-dihydroxyvitamin D(3). *Cancer Res* 2005; **65**(2): 493–8.

39. Moosgaard B, Christensen SE, Vestergaard P, et al. Vitamin D metabolites and skeletal consequences in primary hyperparathyroidism. *Clin Endocrinol* 2008; **68**(5): 707–15.
40. Stein EM, Dempster DW, Udesky J, et al. Vitamin D deficiency influences histomorphometric features of bone in primary hyperparathyroidism. *Bone* 2011; **48**(3): 557–61.
41. Silverberg SJ. Vitamin D deficiency and primary hyperparathyroidism. *J Bone Miner Res* 2007; **22** Suppl 2: V100–4.
42. Bilezikian JP, Khan AA, Potts JT Jr. Third International Workshop on the Management of Asymptomatic Primary H. Guidelines for the management of asymptomatic primary hyperparathyroidism: summary statement from the third international workshop. *J Clin Endocrinol Metab* 2009; **94**(2): 335–9.
43. Pattou F, Combemale F, Fabre S, et al. Hypocalcemia following thyroid surgery: incidence and prediction of outcome. *World J Surg* 1998; **22**(7): 718–24.
44. Brasier AR, Nussbaum SR. Hungry bone syndrome: clinical and biochemical predictors of its occurrence after parathyroid surgery. *Am J Med* 1988; **84**(4): 654–60.
45. Temple R, Berman M, Robbins J, Wolff J. The use of lithium in the treatment of thyrotoxicosis. *J Clin Invest* 1972; **51**(10): 2746–56.
46. Powell AC, Alexander HR, Pingpank JF, et al. The utility of routine transcervical thymectomy for multiple endocrine neoplasia 1-related hyperparathyroidism. *Surgery* 2008; **144**(6): 878–83; discussion 883–74.
47. Viguerie N, Millet L, Avizou S, et al. Regulation of human adipocyte gene expression by thyroid hormone. *J Clin Endocrinol Metab* 2002; **87**(2): 630–4.

CHAPTER 56

PHYSIOLOGY OF THE PITUITARY GLAND

Mária Hérincs, Karen Young and Márta Korbonits

Introduction 629	Conclusion 640
Anterior lobe of the pituitary gland 630	References 641
Posterior lobe of the pituitary gland 638	

SEARCH STRATEGY

Data in this chapter may be updated by a PubMed search using the keywords: pituitary hormones, growth hormone (GH), prolactin (PRL), adrenocorticotrophic hormone (ACTH), thyroid stimulating hormone (TSH), luteinising hormone (LH), follicle stimulating hormone (FSH), argenine vasopressin (AVP) and oxytocin.

INTRODUCTION

The existence of the pituitary gland (also referred to as hypophysis cerebri, derived from the Greek words *hypo*, meaning under, and *physis*, meaning growth) was known before the time of Aristotle, but its role in physiology puzzled scientists for many centuries. In AD 150, the Greek physician and philosopher Galen described the pituitary gland in detail, proposing that its role was to drain the phlegm from the brain to the nasopharynx. The gland was named with this in mind – from the Greek *ptuo* (to spit) and the Latin *pituita* (mucous) and *pituitarius* (mucous-secreting). The pituitary gland's true functions emerged over the 19th and 20th centuries, when its function as an endocrine organ was finally recognized.[1]

The pituitary gland is usually less than 8 mm in length when measured in the craniocaudal plane. However in certain physiological conditions, such as puberty and pregnancy, it can be enlarged (reaching 10–12 mm). It is quite remarkable that such a small organ controls diverse and complex functions of the whole body. Although the pituitary gland is often referred to as the 'master gland' of the body (since many other endocrine glands depend on hypophyseal stimulation), the hypothalamus is the true superior regulator of the hormonal system.[1] The hypothalamus (forming the most ventral part of the diencephalon or 'midbrain') is a key regulator of homeostasis, controlling not only the release of pituitary hormones but also a range of autonomic and behavioural functions including temperature regulation, food and water intake, sleep, circadian rhythms and mediation of emotion. The various nuclei located within the hypothalamus allow signals to pass between the nervous and endocrine system, via the pituitary gland. The hypothalamus receives both hormonal and neural input from the periphery and the brain, and it exerts its action via neural as well as humoral pathways. There are extensive vascular (long portal vessels) and neural (axons in the pituitary stalk) connections between the hypothalamus and the anterior and posterior lobe of the pituitary, as well as a vascular connection between the anterior and posterior lobe via the short portal vessels.[2]

Control of the endocrine system is primarily achieved by negative feedback loops, which not only act as the main form of regulation but are also important in fine-tuning the functions of the hypothalamic–pituitary–peripheral organ axis. The interplay of stimulatory and inhibitory hormones from the hypothalamus and the pituitary hormones is influenced by negative feedback loops between the periphery and central organs, as well as between the pituitary and the hypothalamus (**Figure 56.1**). Positive feedback also exists, primarily in the gonadal axis at the time of puberty and ovulation.[3]

Diagnosing pituitary tumours is often challenging, as symptoms can initially be rather non-specific. In later stages the pituitary mass may lead to local tumour effects,

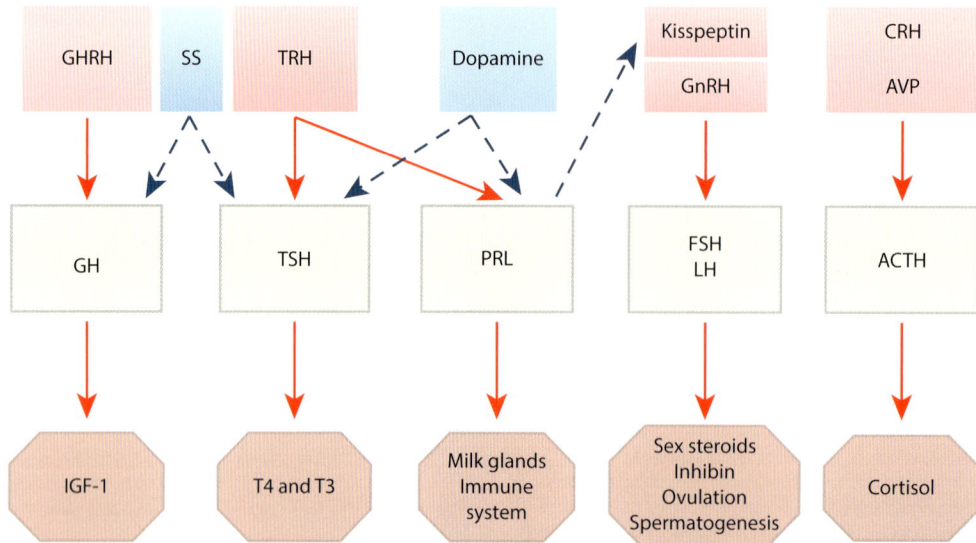

Figure 56.1 Interplay of stimulatory and inhibitory hormones from the hypothalamus and the pituitary hormones. Primary hormone deficiency results from the damage of the peripheral gland or its function, which usually leads to elevated pituitary stimulatory hormone levels. For example, primary hypothyroidism results in high TSH, adrenal failure leads to high ACTH levels, etc. Secondary hormone deficiency is due to damage to the pituitary, such as a pituitary lesion destroying the gland. Tertiary deficiency is due to damage to the hypothalamus. Blue arrows show inhibition; red arrows show stimulatory effects.

Abbreviations: GHRH: growth hormone-releasing hormone; SS: somatostatin; TRH: thyrotrophin-releasing hormone; GnRH: gonadotrophin-releasing hormone; CRH: corticotropin-releasing hormone; AVP: arginine vasopressin; GH: growth hormone; TSH: thyroid-stimulating hormone; PRL: prolactin; FSH: follicle-stimulating hormone; LH: luteinizing hormone; ACTH: adrenocorticotropic hormone; IGF-1: insulin-like growth factor 1; T3: triiodothyronine; T4: thyroxine.

such as headaches and characteristic visual field defects if the tumour is large enough to compress nearby tissues, particularly the optic chiasm.

ANTERIOR LOBE OF THE PITUITARY GLAND

The anterior lobe of the pituitary, the adenohypophysis, comprises approximately 75% of the total pituitary volume. It is functionally linked to the hypothalamus by blood vessels in the pituitary stalk which transmit regulatory hypothalamic hormones to the pituitary. These stimulate or inhibit the synthesis and release of pituitary hormones. The anterior pituitary consists of five major cell types (each secreting specific hormones), organized into cords of cells located around venous sinusoids. The six major hormone products of the anterior pituitary (**Table 56.1**) are secreted into the sinusoids from which they enter the circulation.

Other less common cells in this area include somatomammotrophs, a rare cell type that secretes both growth hormone (GH) and prolactin (PRL) and a unique starshaped, non-endocrine cell type, the so-called folliculostellate cell. These cells have been shown to be important for cell-to-cell interaction and regulation within the pituitary.[4] More recently, a few stem cell-like cells have also been discovered in the adult pituitary located mostly at the border of the anterior and posterior lobe ('marginal zone') and their role in pituitary tumorigenesis is currently under investigation.[5, 6]

The growth hormone axis

The existence of a hormone responsible for growth was first proposed by Cushing in the early 1910s but the hormone itself was not isolated until 1956.[7] Growth hormone (GH) is a 191-amino acid polypeptide synthesized by the somatotroph cells, which make up 40–50% of anterior pituitary cells. The main functions of GH are to stimulate growth and regulate cell turnover and repair. At a cellular level, this results in enhanced protein synthesis, facilitating amino-acid transport, mobilizing free fatty acids from adipose tissues, decreasing glucose uptake and increasing gluconeogenesis. The most notable targets of GH are the growth plates of long bones leading to the characteristic increases in bone length seen during childhood, but GH also regulates soft-tissue growth. GH excess in childhood results in overly increased linear bone length and gigantism, while in adults (in whom the epiphyseal plates are now fused, preventing further elongation of the long bones) increases in bone width occur instead, resulting in the characteristic facial and hand/foot changes associated with the diagnosis of acromegaly. Other clinical features of acromegaly include prominent soft-tissue swelling of internal organs, such as the heart, bowels and liver. Cartilaginous enlargement also occurs, leading to rheumatological problems and altered laryngeal anatomy, with resultant deepening of the voice. Finally, as the skull enlarges, the paranasal sinuses also increase in size, particularly the frontal sinuses, and the jaw enlarges with resultant malocclusion and prognathism.

GH acts via the GH receptor (GHR), which belongs to the type I cytokine receptor family. GH binding to the dimerized GHR activates Janus kinase 2 (JAK2) and signal transducer and activator of transcription (STAT) (**Figure 56.2**). While

TABLE 56.1 Main cell types of the anterior pituitary gland

Cell type	Percentage of total pituitary cells (%)	Hypothalamic regulatory hormone	Hormone secreted	Main target organs
Somatotrophs	45–50	Stimulation: growth hormone releasing hormone (GNRH) and ghrelin Inhibition: somatostain (SST)	Growth hormone (GH)	Liver, muscle, bone, cartilage, adipose tissue
Thyrotrophs	5	Stimulation: thyrotrophin releasing hormone (TRH)	Thyroid-stimulating hormone (TSH)	Thyroid gland
Lactotrophs	10–30	Stimulation: TRH Inhibition: dopamine	Prolactin (PRL)	Mammary gland
Gonadotrophs	10–15	Stimulation: gonadotrohin releasing hormone (GnRH)	Follicle-stimulating hormone (FSH) Luteinizing hormone (LH)	Ovary and testis
Corticotrophs	10–20	Stimulation: corticotrophin releasing hormone (CRH), argenine vasopressin (AVP)	Adrenocorticotrophic hormone (ACTH)	Adrenal gland (cortex)

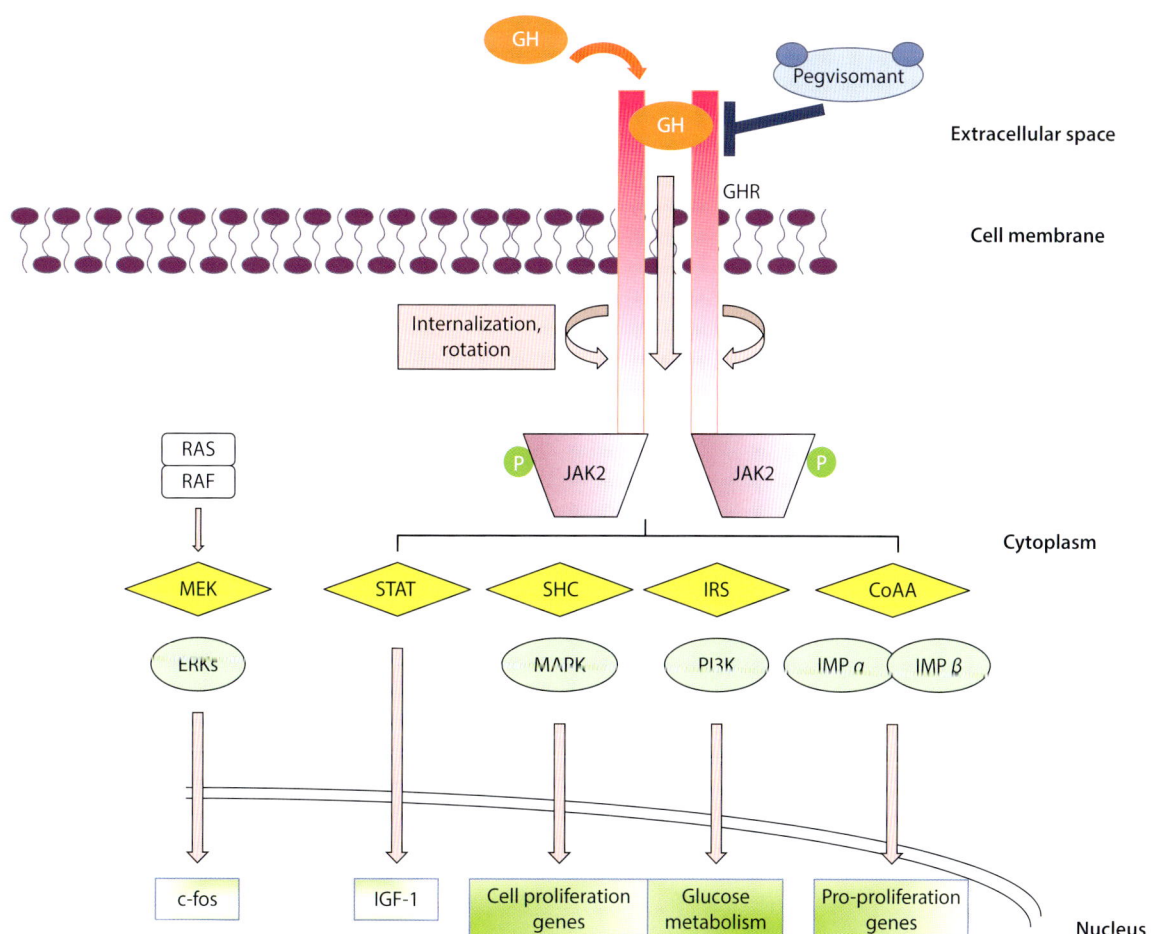

Figure 56.2 GH action. Ligand binding to the pre-formed GHR dimer results in internalization and relative rotation of the subunits in the homodimer, subsequently causing JAK2 phosphorylation (P) and signal transduction. GH signalling may be mediated by JAK2-independent signalling (Src/ERK) pathways. GH targets include IGF-I, c-fos, genes involved in cell proliferation, glucose metabolism and cytoskeletal proteins. IGF-I may also block GHR internalization, acting in a feedback loop. The GHR antagonist pegvisomant used in the treatment of acromegaly, blocks GHR signalling via inhibitory rotation.

Abbreviations: GH: growth hormone; GHR: growth hormone receptor JAK2: Janus kinase 2; P: phosphor group; STAT: signal transducer and activator of transcription; SHC: SH2-containing protein; IRS: insulin receptor substrate; CoAA: nuclear receptor coactivator AA; IMP α/β: importin α/β; MAPK: mitogen-activated protein kinases; PI3K: phosphatidylinositide 3-kinase; ERK: extracellular signal-regulated kinase; MEK: MAP kinase kinase; RAS: rat sarcoma protein family; RAF: rapidly accelerated fibrosarcoma protein kinase family; c-fos: Fos Proto-Oncogene; AP-1: Transcription Factor Subunit; IGF-1: insulin-like growth factor 1.

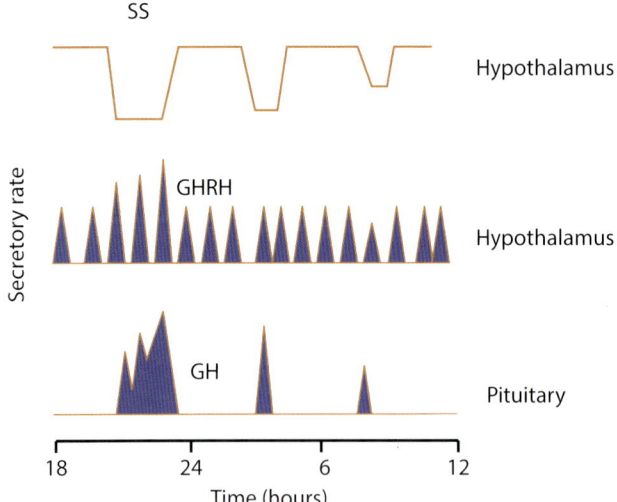

Figure 56.3 Secretion of growth hormone. A simplified schematic representation of pulsatile secretion of growth hormone (GH) in response to growth hormone-releasing hormone (GHRH) and growth hormone inhibitory hormone (SS, somatostatin) impulses. (Adapted from Hartman et al. Temporal structure of *in vivo* growth hormone secretory events in humans. Redrawn from ref.)[9]

GH exerts its direct metabolic effects via this pathway, other effects are exerted through insulin-like growth factor type 1 (IGF-1), synthesized not only in the liver but in all local tissues, and responsible for the growth effects of the hormone. IGF-1 binds to the type 1 IGF receptor, which belongs to the membrane-bound tyrosine kinase receptor family.[8]

GH is secreted in a pulsatile manner (**Figure 56.3**)[9] in response to an interplay of hypothalamic hormones. GH release is stimulated by both growth hormone-releasing hormone (GHRH) and ghrelin (the brain-gut peptide, mainly synthesized by neuroendocrine cells in the gastric mucosa) while somatostatin (SS) is inhibitory in action. Animal data suggest that ghrelin-induced GH release has a role in maintaining glucose levels during fasting.[10] GHRH, SS and ghrelin act by binding G-protein coupled receptors: the GHRH receptor, five major subtypes of SS receptors and the type 1a growth hormone secretagogue receptor (also called ghrelin receptor). Animal data suggest that a tightly regulated network of somatotroph cells, known as 'clusters', allows rapid, large increases in circulating GH levels.

GHRH has a complex regulatory function on GH:

- It causes immediate release via activation of cAMP and Ca^{2+} in somatotrophs.
- GHRH triggers GH synthesis by stimulating the transcription factor POU class 1 homeobox 1 (PUOF1, previously called Pit1).
- It increases GH cell number.
- It stimulates the formation of GH cell clusters.

An understanding of the second messenger pathway of the GHRH receptor is important, since several genetic defects involving this pathway can result in excess GH secretion and its associated complications (**Figure 56.4**). The stimulatory subtype of the alpha subunit of the G protein (Gsalpha) activates adenylyl cyclase, following which

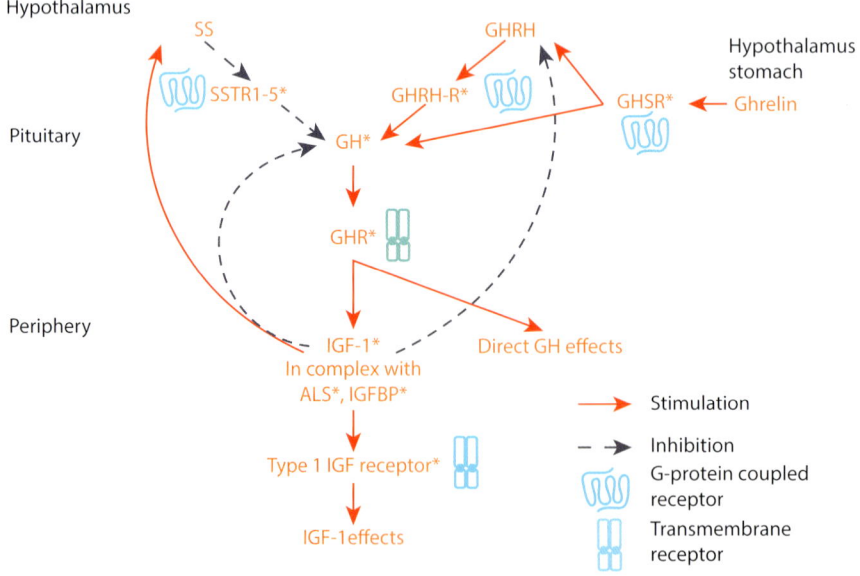

Figure 56.4 Growth hormone axis. A simplified scheme of the growth hormone (GH) axis. Inhibitory somatostatin (SS) and stimulatory growth hormone-releasing hormone (GHRH) impulses coming from the hypothalamus regulate GH release from the pituitary. GH exerts its effects either directly or via IGF-1. GH stimulates IGF-1 synthesis in all peripheral tissues. Circulating IGF-1 primarily represents liver IGF-1 synthesis. Ghrelin is also a potent GH-releasing hormone. IGF-1 regulates GH release via negative feedback to the hypothalamus and the pituitary.

Abbreviations: GH: growth hormone; GHRH: growth hormone releasing hormone; GHRH-R: growth hormone releasing hormone receptor; SS: somatostatin; SSTR1-5: somatostatin receptors 1-5; IGF-1: insulin-like growth factor 1; IGFBP: insulin-like growth factor binding protein; ALS: acid labile subunit.

*Mutations in these components of the pathway have been described in patients presenting with short stature.

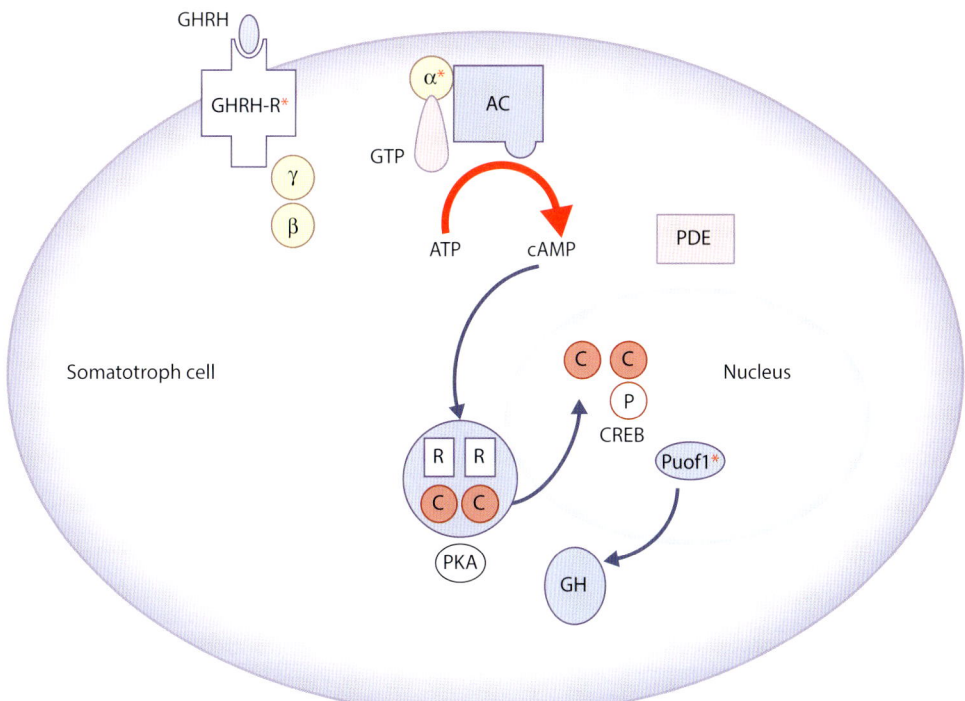

Figure 56.5 Signal transduction in the growth hormone cell. Following ligand binding, the alpha subunit of the Gs protein dissociates from the beta and gamma subunits and activates AC. cAMP is synthesized, and this binds to and inhibits the regulatory subunit (R) of protein kinase A (PKA). The catalytic subunit (C) is now free to enter the nucleus and phosphorylate the CREB, which upregulates GH synthesis. A gain of function mosaic (McCune-Albright syndrome) or somatic mutation (seen in 40% of sporadic acromegaly adenomas) in the Gs alpha subunit (GSP) leads to GHRH-independent upregulation of the pathway. In Carney complex there is a loss of function in the regulatory subunit of PKA, or gain of function of the catalytic subunit leading to cAMP-independent activation of PKA. Alterations are marked with yellow leading to different disease conditions.

Abbreviations: Gs: G-protein adenylate cyclase stimulator; AC: adenylate cyclase; cAMP: cyclic adenosine monophosphate; PDE: phosphodiesterase; PKA: protein kinase A; CREB: cAMO binding element; GH: growth hormone; GHRH: growth hormone releasing hormone; GHRH-R: growth hormone releasing hormone receptor; ATP: adenosine triphosphate; Puof1: pituitary-specific positive transcription factor 1; GSP: stimulatory G protein.

*Mutations in these components of the pathway have been described in patients presenting with short stature.

synthesized cAMP binds and inhibits the regulatory subunit of protein kinase A. The catalytic subunit of protein kinase A phosphorylates the cAMP response element binding protein which in turn upregulates PUOF1 and GH synthesis (**Figure 56.5**).[11]

GH levels change throughout life. The highest levels occur during puberty, after which there is a gradual decline (**Figure 56.6**).[12] GH levels also show circadian variation with the highest levels occurring during the night, and low, often undetectable levels during the day. We clinically utilize this circadian rhythm when serial GH samples are taken in the diagnostic workup of GH-excess or GH-deficient patients.[13] IGF-1 circulates in a complex with IGF-binding proteins (mostly IGFBP3). The acid labile subunit and IGF-1 levels are steady during the day and a gradual decline is seen with age, therefore age-specific normal ranges should be used to assess circulating hormone levels.

The regulation of growth and the GH axis is a complex process. It is influenced by various activities such as sleep (GH levels are high during the night), calorie intake (GH levels increase at fasting), exercise (increases GH release) and inflammation (chronic inflammation reduces the activity of the growth axis). Oestrogen stimulates GH release both via the hypothalamus and by direct action on the pituitary gland but it inhibits GH effects via upregulating an inhibitor of GH receptor signalling pathway SOCS2 (suppressors of cytokine signalling 2).[14] Overall, females need higher GH levels to achieve the same IGF-1 level.

The thyroid axis

Thyroid-stimulating hormone (TSH) is synthesized in the thyrotroph cells and its release is triggered by binding of thyrotrophin-releasing hormone (TRH) to the TRH receptor (**Figure 56.7**). TRH is synthesized in the paraventricular nucleus of the hypothalamus. TSH secretion is inhibited by somatostatin.[3] Interestingly, TRH also stimulates prolactin release from the pituitary. This is clinically relevant since in untreated primary hypothyroidism the high TRH level stimulates prolactin release, leading to hyperprolactinaemia and hypogonadism, which could pose a diagnostic problem if the link were not appreciated.[3] The glycoprotein hormone TSH is a heterodimer comprising two subunits. The alpha subunit, a protein made up from 89 amino acids, is common to TSH, LH, FSH and human choriogonadotrophin (HCG), while the beta subunit (112 amino acids) is specific to TSH. TSH is produced by the thyrotroph cells of

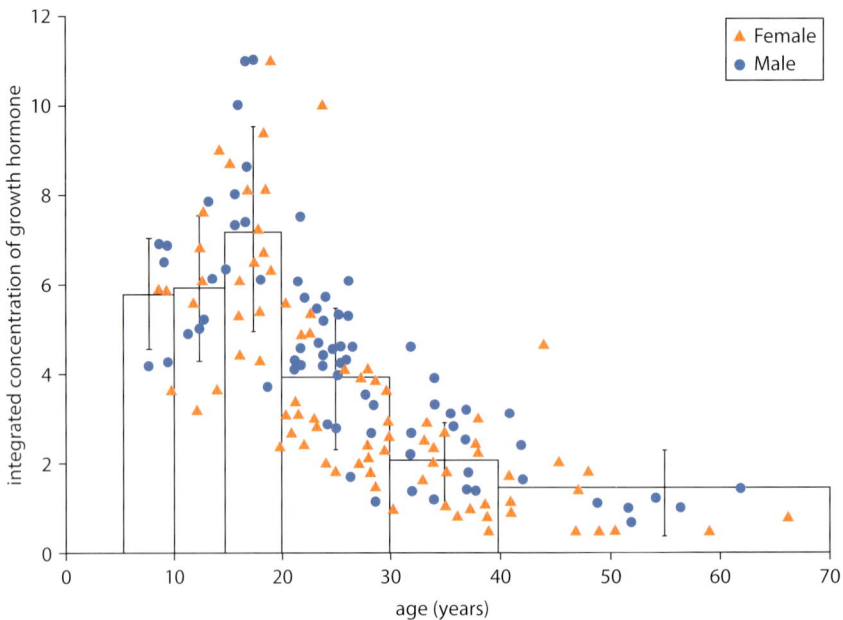

Figure 56.6 The 24-hour integrated concentration of GH. The mean 24-h concentration of growth hormone, designated the integrated concentration levels change throughout life, reaching a peak level during puberty then decreasing by age. Figure adapted from Zadik et al.[12]

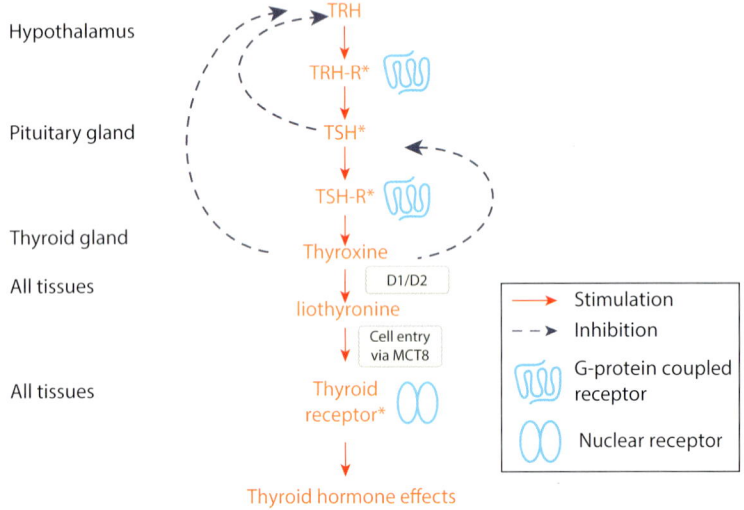

Figure 56.7 Thyroid axis. A simplified scheme of the hypothalamo–pituitary–thyroid gland axis. Hypothalamic hormone TRH stimulates TSH release from the pituitary. TSH binds to the TSH-receptor on the thyroid gland and activates thyroid cells, which results in increased iodine uptake, thyroglobulin synthesis, thyroid peroxidase activity and thyroxine release.

Abbreviations: TRH: thyroid releasing hormone; TRH-R: thyroid releasing hormone receptor; TSH: thyroid stimulating hormone; TSH-R: thyroid stimulating hormone receptor.

* Mutations in these components of the pathway have been described in patients presenting with abnormal thyroid function.

the anterior pituitary and is essential for regulating the thyroid gland and consequently the metabolic activity of the body.[2,3] TSH activates thyroid cells by binding to the TSH receptor, thus stimulating the cAMP pathway, leading to increased iodine uptake, thyroglobulin synthesis, thyroid peroxidase activity and thyroxine release.[15] Iodine is a crucial component of both thyroxine and triiodothyronine, and lack of iodine in the diet can lead to reduced thyroid hormone synthesis, therefore elevated TSH due to negative feedback and significant thyroid enlargement (endemic goitre). Recently, 'thyrostimulin', an alternative TSH receptor ligand, has been identified, but its precise physiological role is yet to be elucidated.[16]

Circulating TSH is known to exhibit a circadian rhythm with higher levels during the night and its pulsatile secretion is synchronized with hypothalamic PRL pulses, as TRH has a stimulatory effect on the release of both PRL and TSH.[3] The availability of sensitive TSH assays allows us to diagnose subclinical hypo- or hyperthyroidism. Screening for congenital hypothyroidism using the Guthrie-devised heel-prick blood test relies on sensitive TSH measurements to identify hypothyroidism in neonates 2–3 days old. Recent data suggest that women planning pregnancies should have strictly normal TSH levels for the optimal central nervous system development of the foetus. Patients with pre-existing thyroid hormone replacement need usually increase the dose of hormone replacement during early stages of pregnancy.

Thyroid cells synthesize thyroxine (T4) and in smaller amounts its active derivative triiodothyronine (T3), which has a much shorter half-life. Thyroid hormones circulate in the bloodstream in a ratio of approximately 20:1 T4:T3, bound to thyroglobulin (Tg), which is synthesized by the follicular cells of the thyroid gland. Thyroglobulin levels can be used as tumour markers in patients with papillary or follicular thyroid cancers, hence regular Tg level monitoring may facilitate detection of early recurrence. Sex steroids can alter thyroglobulin synthesis, so measurement of free thyroid hormones (fT4 and fT3) is a better reflection of thyroid status.[17] T4 is converted to the active T3 form in peripheral tissues; T3 is inactivated by conversion to reverse T3 (under the influence of D3 deionidase enzyme). Deiodinase enzymes contain selenium, therefore dietary selenium insufficiency can result in low T3 levels and there is now evidence that selenium supplements are beneficial for patients with Graves' ophthalmopathy.

Thyroid disease is one of the most common endocrine diseases. A wide range of congenital and acquired aetiologies underlie thyroid disease including: euthyroid goitre (due to mild iodine deficiency), thyroid nodules, thyroid cancer, autoimmune hypothyroiditis (Hashimoto's thyroiditis) or hyperthyroidism (Graves disease), contrast agent- or amiodarone-induced abnormalities, TSH-secreting pituitary tumours and a range of genetic syndromes affecting pituitary transcription factors. Less common causes include sick euthyroid syndrome, where the patient's blood tests demonstrate a pattern of thyroid hormone alterations during non-thyroidal illness with normal TSH, low total T4, fT3 and elevated reverse T3 levels,[18] and Pendred syndrome, a congenital autosomal recessive disease which results from a mutation in the iodine/chloride transmembrane transporter pendrin. In thyroid cells, pendrin transports iodine from the cytoplasm to the colloid, where it is organized into thyroglobulin during thyroid hormone synthesis. Mutations in this transporter cause progressive bilateral high-frequency sensorineural hearing loss (often secondary to minor head trauma) possible vestibular dysfunction and abnormal thyroid hormone synthesis with goitre developing in early puberty/young adulthood.[18] This condition is often associated with Mondini malformation of the cochlea and enlarged vestibular aqueducts.

Prolactin

The lactotroph hormone prolactin (PRL) was discovered in the early 1930s and was named for its effect on lactation and mammary gland development.[19] Both PRL (198 amino acid protein) and its receptor share similarities with GH. Primarily synthesized and secreted by the lactotroph pituitary cells,[20] PRL is also secreted by extrapituitary sites such as the mammary gland, placenta, uterus and T lymphocytes.[21] The most prominent effects of prolactin are the effect on milk production, inhibition of the gonadal axis and regulation of immune function. Its hypothalamic control is different from other pituitary hormones. The hypothalamus has a primary inhibitory input on prolactin synthesis and release, therefore any damage to the hypothalamus or pituitary stalk can result in hyperprolactinaemia.[19]

Prolactin levels in maternal blood rise from the fifth week of pregnancy and peak at parturition. Loss of placental oestrogen and progesterone disinhibits the milk ejection response to suckling.[2, 20] Basal prolactin level typically returns to normal within a couple of weeks after the delivery, but each nursing episode results in temporarily increased PRL secretion.[2] Prolactin exerts its inhibitory action on the gonadal axis via inhibiting kisspeptin release from the kisspeptin neurons.[23] Furthermore, it has been shown to counteract the effects of dopamine on sexual arousal (dopamine rises during intercourse and decreases rapidly afterwards), which may explain the decreased libido frequently reported by patients suffering from hyperprolactinaemia. TRH stimulates prolactin release and this is of clinical importance in primary hypothyroidism, since mild hyperprolactinaemia frequently accompanies primary hypothyroidism.[19–21]

Although high prolactin is a typical sign of a prolactin-secreting pituitary adenoma (prolactinoma), the differential diagnosis of hyperprolactinaemia is broad. High prolactin levels occur physiologically during pregnancy, stress and exercise. PRL can be elevated by administering dopamine antagonist drugs including psychotropic drugs (used to treat depression and schizophrenia), as well as verapamil, metoclopramide, opiates, cocaine and protein inhibitors, even after short-term use. It is also affected by some medicinal herbs, such as star anise, fenugreek, fennel seeds and red clover.[2] Other causes of raised prolactin levels include polycystic ovary syndrome (PCOS), herpes zoster infection of the chest, thoracic surgery, renal failure and liver cirrhosis.[24, 25] PRL levels can double due to stress, increase to 5 times the upper limit of normal due to stalk effect (pituitary stalk compression), increase 5–10 times due to small microadenomas or drugs, and 10–100+ times due to larger adenomas. Pituitary-dependent hyperprolactinaemia can result from a prolactinoma or an adenoma (endocrinologically active or inactive) compressing the pituitary stalk, preventing dopamine (prolactin release inhibiting hormone) reaching lactotrophs.[26, 27] Prolactin-secreting tumours lead to inhibition of the gonadal axis and can induce galactorrhoea and cause local tumour effects. Small adenomas (microprolactinomas, <1 cm) are more commonly identified in females, while males usually harbour macroprolactinomas (>1 cm) at presentation. In the majority of the cases dopamine agonist drugs (cabergoline or bromocriptine) have an excellent effect both on hormone reduction and on tumour shrinkage.[24, 25] Prolactinomas can be part of multiple endocrine neoplasia type 1 syndrome (MEN1) which is associated with hyperparathyroidism and pancreatic adenomas.

The gonadal axis

Luteinizing hormone (LH) and follicle-stimulating hormone (FSH) are glycoprotein hormones. Although they are both synthesized in the gonadotroph cells and regulated by the same stimulatory hypothalamic hormone gonadotroph-releasing hormone (GnRH), their levels vary considerably during the female cycle. The frequency of GnRH pulses is the main determinant of this differential regulation with slow pulses leading to FSH release and rapid pulses to LH release.[3] Numerous further factors regulate the system (**Figure 56.8**). Pulsatile GnRH secretion is an important hallmark of gonadal regulation. If continuous GnRH secretion is present, the GnRH receptors in the

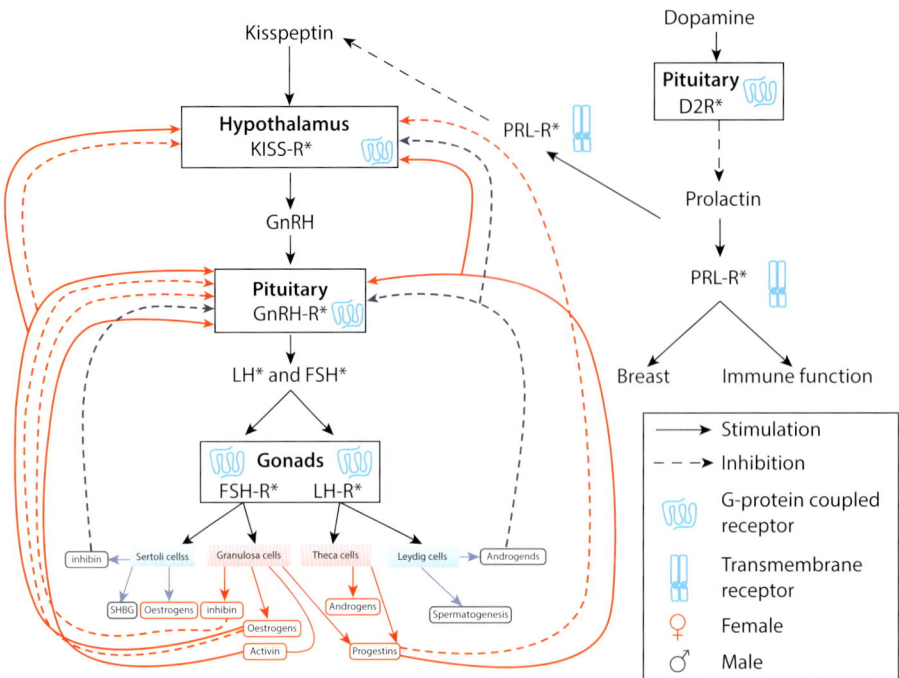

Figure 56.8 Gonadal axis. A simplified scheme of the gonadal axis. Hypothalamic hormone GnRH stimulates LH and FSH release from the pituitary gland. Prolactin inhibits the gonadal axis by inhibiting kisspeptin release from the kisspeptin neurons in the hypothalamus. As shown in the diagram, there are differences between male (blue lines) and female (red lines) with respect to signalling and feedback loops. SHBG (in the testis, also called androgen binding protein).

Abbreviations: KISS-R: kisspeptin receptor (also known as GPR54); GnRH: gonadotrophin releasing hormone; LH: luteinising hormone; LH-R: luteinising hormone receptor; FSH: follicle stimulating hormone receptor; SHBG: sex hormone binding globulin; D2R: dopamine receptor 2; PRL-R: prolactin receptor.

*Mutations in these components of the pathway have been identified in patients with abnormal gonadal hormone synthesis.

pituitary desensitize and the gonadal axis is turned off. This phenomenon is utilized in treatment of some diseases where gonadal steroids need to be inactivated, such as prostate cancer, breast cancer and endometriosis, or when premature puberty needs to be delayed.[28] Patients with tertiary hypogonadism (hypogonadotrophic hypogonadism) can be treated with pulsatile GnRH treatment using a pump device.[28]

Secretion of GnRH is primarily regulated by 17β-oestradiol (E_2) acting via oestrogen receptor alpha (ERα). However, as GnRH neurons do not express ERα, regulation of hypothalamic function by oestradiol is mediated by kisspeptin neurons, which do express this receptor and are thought to relay information regarding oestrogen levels directly to the GnRH neurons.[29] In addition, the inhibitory feedback of prolactin on the gonadal axis occurs via kisspeptin, as GnRH neurons do not express prolactin receptors either, therefore rendering them insensitive to circulating prolactin levels.[30] Kisspeptin and its receptor KISS-R (G-protein-coupled receptor 54, GPR54) are recently identified members of the gonadotroph axis. Kisspeptin is synthesized in several hypothalamic nuclei including the arcuate nucleus and the preoptic area. More recently, a gonadotrophin inhibitory hormone (GnIH) has been described in birds.[31] The role of its mammalian counterpart RFamide-related peptide (RFRP) and its putative G-protein coupled receptor OT7T022 (also known as neuropeptide FF receptor type 1) is currently under investigation.

There is an interesting interface between the gonadal axis and the olfactory system. During embryogenesis, GnRH cells are located at the top of the nasal cavity together with cells of the olfactory system. GnRH cells then migrate to the hypothalamus. Patients with loss-of-function mutations in peptides involved in this migration develop hypothalamic hypogonadism. When this condition occurs in combination with decreased sense of smell, either partial (hyposmia) or total (anosmia), the underlying condition is referred to as Kallmann syndrome.[32] From an ENT perspective, the condition is associated with craniofacial defects such as cleft palate and sensorineural hearing loss.

LH

In females, LH is responsible for follicular development, ovulation and development of the corpus luteum, while in the male it acts on Leydig cells within the testis, stimulating testosterone production.[2] Binding to the G-protein-coupled transmembrane receptor, the luteinizing hormone receptor (LH-R) exerts its effects on the ovarian theca cells to enhance oestrogen production of the granulosa cells. At the beginning of the cycle, FSH stimulates these granulosa cells, leading to elevated oestrogen levels and follicular maturation. Elevated oestrogen levels may lead to ovulation by a positive feedback effect on arcuate kisspeptin neurons that stimulate GnRH, thus leading to sudden LH release. This 'LH surge' acts as the trigger for ovulation, resulting in the egg leaving the follicle and the follicle beginning to become the corpus luteum, secreting progesterone to make the endometrium ready for implantation.[2]

Slightly elevated LH levels are observed in polycystic ovary syndrome and precocious puberty. Marked elevation is typically due to the lack of gonadal negative feedback, which results in excessive production of LH and FSH in the anterior pituitary, such as in primary ovarian failure and the menopause. Low LH levels are associated with hyperprolactinaemia, eating disorders and certain congenital conditions where patients present with infertility. Synthetic LH-analogues (such as human chorionic gonadotropin – better known as HCG) are commonly used for ovulation induction and managing male infertility.

FSH

FSH stimulates follicular growth. Its level drops after the follicle has reached full maturation but rises slightly again at the end of the menstrual cycle, contributing towards the initiation of the next cycle. In males, FSH stimulates the gonadal Sertoli cells to produce spermatozoa as well as inhibin, which in both females and males inhibits FSH production. Low FSH secretion can be observed in conditions resulting in infertility and loss of gonadal functions.[2] High FSH is an early sign of the menopause or primary gonadal damage (e.g. autoimmune or cytostatic-induced). Synthetic FSH is available for ovulation induction or induction of spermatogenesis.

The hypothalamic–pituitary–adrenal axis

Adrenocorticotropic hormone (ACTH), secreted by corticotroph cells, is derived from the pro-hormone pro-opiomelanocortin (POMC). Typically produced in response to stress, ACTH functions to increase production and release of corticosteroids. It stimulates cortisol synthesis and release from the adrenal cortex (but it also has some effect on aldosterone and androgen secretion) (**Figure 56.9**).[2] ACTH release from the pituitary is regulated by corticotrophin-releasing hormone (CRH) and arginine vasopressin (AVP), both synthesized in the paraventricular nucleus. The latter hormone reaches the anterior pituitary gland via the short portal vessels.[2]

Nearly all types of stress, physical or emotional, and food intake lead to immediate and significant increase in ACTH and cortisol secretion.[2] There is a prominent circadian rhythm operating in the HPA axis, with high hormone levels in the early morning hours. This is followed by a gradual reduction in hormone levels through the day such that cortisol levels during the night are undetectable.[2]

In addition, ACTH secretion has a superimposed pulsatile release pattern. The increase in cortisol is crucial for the appropriate stress response of the body and, if the hypothalamic–pituitary–adrenal (HPA) axis is compromised, cortisol treatment is life-saving in stress situations such as infection or surgery. Since ACTH is derived from POMC, conditions that lead to synthesis of large amounts of ACTH will also result in accumulation of other POMC-derived peptides. Raised levels of the alpha melanocyte-stimulating hormone lead to characteristic

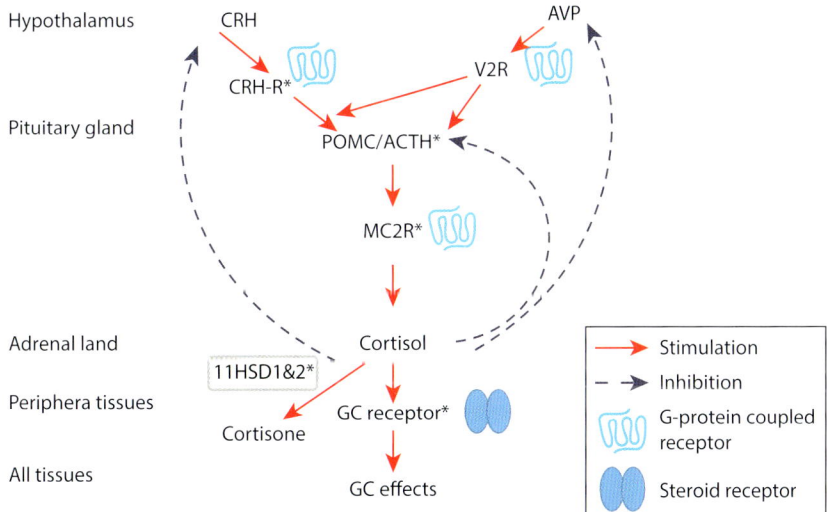

Figure 56.9 Hypothalamic–pituitary–adrenal (HPA) axis. A simplified scheme of the hypothalamic–pituitary–adrenal (HPA) axis. The hypothalamic hormone CRH stimulates ACTH release. Arginine vasopressin (AVP), which is also a hormone of the posterior pituitary and has a role in regulating water balance, is another significant stimulator of ACTH. Its main effect is acting synergistically with CRH, but it also has a direct effect on the pituitary. It has been suggested recently that CRH is the basis of constant basal release of ACTH, while AVP adds peaks in stress situations. ACTH binds to its receptor MC2R and stimulates cortisol release. Cortisol may undergo alteration via the 11 beta hydroxysteroid dehydrogenase type 1 and 2 (11HSD1&2) before binding the glucocorticoid receptor.

Abbreviations: CRH: corticotrophin releasing hormone; CRH-R: corticotrophin releasing hormone receptor; POMC: pro-opiomelanocortin; ACTH: adrenocorticotropic hormone; MC2R: melanocortin 2 receptor; GC: glucocorticoid; HSD: hydroxysteroid dehydrogenase enzymes.

* Mutations in these components of the pathway have been identified in patients with abnormal HPA axis hormone synthesis.

darkening of the skin. This phenomenon is seen in adrenal insufficiency, ectopic ACTH-secreting tumours and Nelson syndrome.

Abnormalities can occur in the HPA axis at several levels. Depression can cause chronic central stimulation of the HPA axis. ACTH-secreting adenomas, ectopic ACTH-secreting tumours and adrenal cortisol-secreting tumours lead to Cushing's syndrome. Cushing's syndrome is a hormone disorder that results from high levels of cortisol in the blood, while Cushing's disease refers to one specific cause of Cushing's syndrome, a corticotroph adenoma in the pituitary gland that produces large amounts of ACTH. POMC mutations lead to glucocorticoid deficiency together with altered skin colouring and obesity due to the lack of ACTH and alpha melanocyte-stimulating hormone. Damage to the adrenal gland (causes include autoimmune and infective, e.g. tuberculosis) results in Addison's disease (primary adrenal insufficiency). Familial glucocorticoid deficiency arises secondary to mutations in the *MC2R* or its accessory protein MRAP (*MC2R* accessory protein), and further genes have been recently identified in the steroidogenic pathway. Abnormalities in the steroid synthesis pathway (as seen in congenital adrenal hyperplasia) may lead to glucocorticoid deficiency in some cases. Finally, abnormalities in the pre-receptor metabolism of cortisol or mutations in the glucocorticoid receptor itself will also lead to abnormalities in the HPA axis.

The most common and clinically relevant situation regarding the HPA axis occurs in patients receiving exogenous glucocorticoid treatment, usually in the form of prednisolone or dexamethasone. In these patients the endogenous HPA axis is suppressed and they do not exhibit a normal stress hormone response. For infections, doubling the standard glucocorticoid replacement dose is advisable; for surgery, intra-muscular 100 mg hydrocortisone every 8 hours for 24 hours and then oral treatment in gradually decreasing doses is recommended.

POSTERIOR LOBE OF THE PITUITARY GLAND

The posterior lobe of the pituitary gland, the neurohypophysis, consists of nerve fibres originating from the supraoptic and paraventricular nuclei of the hypothalamus. The supraoptic and paraventricular nuclei synthesize two cyclic nonapeptides. The resulting hormones are known as arginine vasopressin (AVP, previously known as antidiuretic hormone, ADH) and oxytocin, respectively (**Figure 56.10**). The hormones are transported to the posterior lobe of the pituitary gland via the pituitary stalk, loosely bound to their carrier protein neurophysin. Within the posterior lobe of the pituitary, nerve axon terminals are located close to blood vessels. Upon activation, the secretory granules rapidly release the hormones by a calcium-dependent exocytic process,[2] allowing them to diffuse into the local capillary network. The role of AVP in rapid ACTH release has been well described.[2]

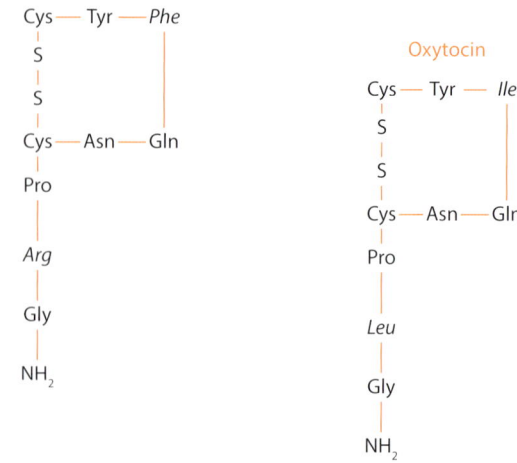

Figure 56.10 The chemical structure of arginine vasopressin (AVP) and oxytocin. Both AVP and oxytocin are nine amino acid peptide hormones (nonapeptides) released from the posterior lobe of the pituitary gland. Their structural similarity (they have all but one amino acid in common) may be the reason behind their functional similarities.

Arginine vasopressin

Arginine vasopressin (AVP) is primarily produced in response to reductions in plasma volume and/or increased plasma osmolality.[2] The plasma half-life of AVP is relatively short (15–30 minutes) therefore plasma levels can vary greatly over short periods of time.[33] AVP regulates renal excretion of water and is the primary determinant of urine concentration. Very small amounts of AVP can have a significant inhibitory action on water excretion in the kidneys, an effect known as antidiuresis. AVP is released from the posterior hypothalamus in response to increases in plasma osmolality (**Figure 56.11**). As more water is reabsorbed, the urine becomes more concentrated. Certain drugs can modify AVP plasma levels: for example, ethanol, mineralocorticoids and glucocorticoids decrease AVP level, while selective serotonin reuptake inhibitors (SSRIs), nicotine and carbamazepine can increase its level in peripheral blood.

The precise mechanism by which increased plasma osmolality triggers AVP release is yet to be elucidated; however, it is suggested that osmoreceptor cells release water upon higher fluid concentration via osmosis, ultimately leading to increased AVP production and secretion in the hypothalamus and neurohypophysis.[2] In addition to increasing osmolality, carotid, aortic and pulmonary baroreceptors detect the resulting hypotension, which stimulates vasopressin release (**Figure 56.12**).[2]

In patients with complete absence of AVP, the collecting tubules and ducts are almost impermeable to water resulting in daily fluid loss of up to 20 litres via the urinary tract.[2, 34]

Insufficient AVP or reduced AVP action results in production of excessive amounts of inappropriately dilute urine, a hallmark of diabetes insipidus (DI). This disease can be either central (hypothalamic) or nephrogenic. In central DI there is a defect in AVP synthesis or secretion, typically due to pituitary stalk damage, head trauma,

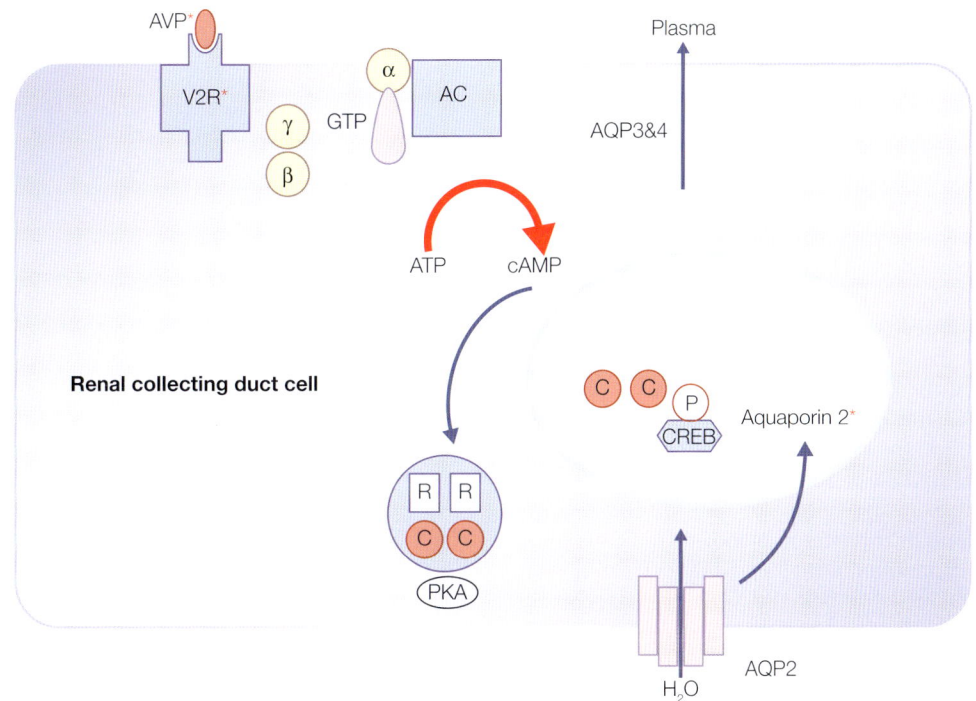

Figure 56.11 Signal transduction in the renal collecting duct cell. Following the binding of AVP by the V2R, the alpha subunit of the Gs protein dissociates from the beta and gamma subunits and activates adenylyl cyclase. cAMP is synthesized, which binds to and inhibits the regulatory subunit (R) of protein kinase A (PKA). The catalytic subunit (C) can enter the nucleus and phosphorylate the cAMP binding element (CREB), which upregulates aquaporin 2 synthesis. Four AQP2 molecules assemble to create a water channel at the luminal border, allowing water to be reabsorbed from the collecting duct back to the cell, and then via AQP3 and AQP4, from the cell back to the plasma.

Abbreviations: AVP: argenine vasopression; V2R: vasopressing type 2 receptor; AC: adenylate cyclase; GTP: guanosine triphosphate; ATP: adenosine triphosphate; cAMP: cyclic adenosine monophsphate; PKA: protein kinase A; CREB: cAMP binding element; AQP2: aquaporin 2.

*Mutations in these components of the pathway have been identified with abnormal function.

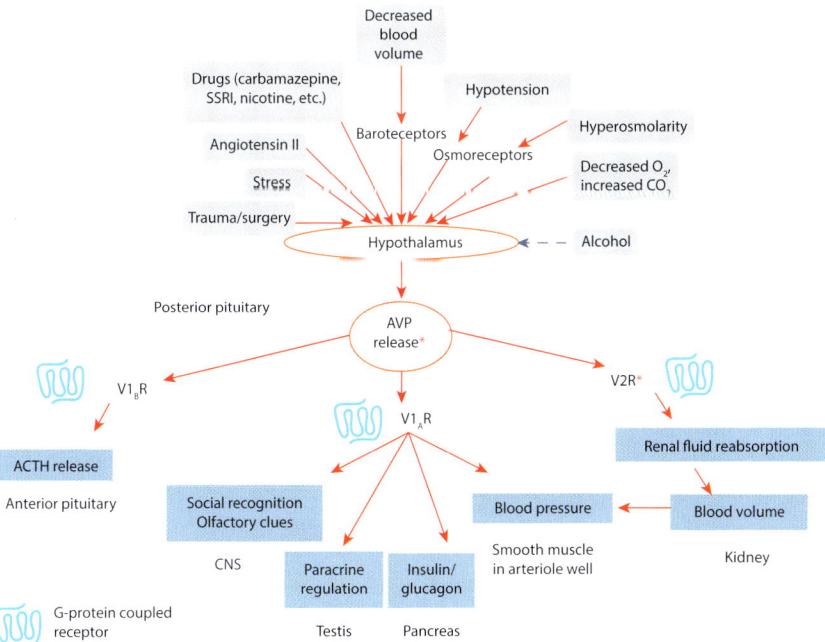

Figure 56.12 Regulation of AVP release. AVP release stimulators increase AVP release from the posterior pituitary. AVP then acts via three receptor subtypes: V1AR, V1BR and V2R. V1AR and V1BR are responsible for the vasoconstrictive effect, and V2R for the antidiuretic effect.

Abbreviations: AVP: argenine vasopressin; VR: vasopressin receptors 1A, 1B and 2; CNS: central nervous sytem; ACTH: adrenocorticotrophic hormone.

*Mutations in these components of the pathway have been identified with abnormal function.

infection or tumour or mutation in the AVP gene; in nephrogenic DI the kidneys are unable to respond to AVP because of renal disease or a mutation in the vasopressin type 2 receptor (V2R) or in aquaporin 2 (AQP2).

Central DI is managed by administering an exogenous AVP analogue. The analogue used in clinical practice is desmopressin, which, with its strong antidiuretic but relatively low vasopressive effect, is a good therapeutic option not only in central DI but also as treatment for enuresis in children. In nephrogenic DI, thiazide diuretics can be beneficial (inhibiting reabsorption of sodium (Na+) and chloride (Cl-) ions from the distal convoluted tubules in the kidneys by blocking the thiazide-sensitive Na+-Cl- symporter as well as increasing calcium reabsorption at the distal tubule). In contrast, the syndrome of inappropriate antidiuretic hormone (SIADH or Schwartz-Bartter syndrome) is characterized by excessive release of AVP from the posterior pituitary gland or from neuroendocrine tumours, typically small-cell carcinoma of the lung. This is treated using V2R antagonists, which block the V2R receptors in the collecting duct and therefore result in aquaresis (excretion of water that is free of electrolytes). V2R blockers must be used cautiously since rapid reversal of hyponatraemia carries a risk of severe central nervous system complications.

Oxytocin

Oxytocin was first discovered by British pharmacologist Sir Henry Dale in 1906.[35] The name (derived from the Greek words meaning 'quick birth') refers to its well-known role in stimulation of uterine-contraction during delivery.[35] Oxytocin acts via receptors which activate the phospholipase signalling pathway.[36–38] Plasma oxytocin levels are markedly elevated in late pregnancy and during labour, but sexual activity and stress also stimulate its release. In addition to its role in inducing uterine contractions during labour, oxytocin also plays a major role in the process of milk-ejection of the breasts. The trigger for oxytocin secretion is the suckling itself. Activation results in release of oxytocin that acts on myoepithelial cells that lie around the alveoli of mammary glands, triggering contraction (**Figure 56.13**). Approximately 30–60 seconds after suckling starts, milk begins to flow. This whole process is referred to as the 'let-down reflex'.[2] Despite the fact that suckling is a unilateral stimulus, both breasts will start to produce milk. The importance of emotional cues are clear from observations that hearing the baby crying (or even cuddling the baby) provides sufficient emotional signal to the hypothalamus to trigger milk ejection.[2] Oxytocin released during breastfeeding also plays a role in reduction of uterine size after birth by stimulation of contractions.

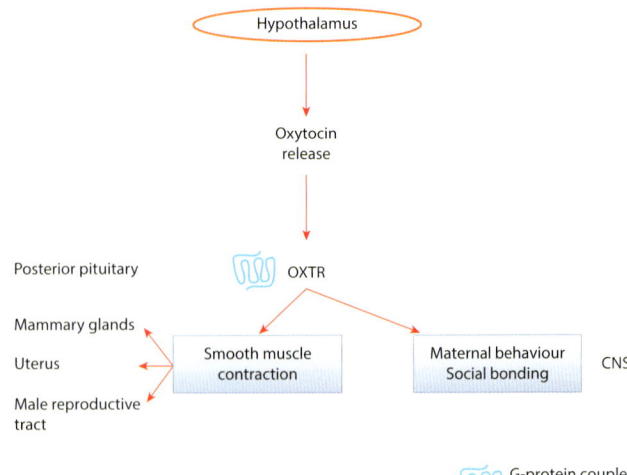

Figure 56.13 Oxytocin effects. Upon hypothalamic stimulation, the posterior pituitary releases oxytocin that binds to its receptor on target smooth muscle cells of the mammary glands and uterus, leading to their contraction. This results in lactation and uterine contractions. It has also been observed that oxytocin in the central nervous system (CNS) plays a role in social bonding and maternal behaviour, and more recently it has been referred to as the 'love hormone'.

Abbreviations: OXTR: oxytocin receptor; CNS: central nervous system.

Extensive research over the past few years has revealed the role of oxytocin in social recognition, pair bonding, maternal behaviour and sexual interaction as well as social anxiety.[39] Oxytocin has gained fame as the 'love hormone', with recent studies implying that it has a determining role in bonding between mothers and their babies,[40, 41] as well as in establishing long-term relationships and falling in love.[42] Recent human studies showed that intra-nasal oxytocin induces increased eye contact and trustful behaviour.[43, 44] CNS effects modulating both the neuronal and behavioural processes associated with alcohol, cocaine and opiate administration in rodents were described,[45, 46] extending possible therapeutic indications to various psychiatric disorders, including drug addiction.[36] A large number of studies have outlined the possible use of intra-nasal oxytocin in behavioural and neural disorders with minimal side effects.[47]

CONCLUSION

The pituitary gland is the central regulator of peripheral hormones. Due to the vicinity of the cells regulating different pathways, abnormalities in the gland can result in a complex pattern of signs and symptoms providing diagnostic and therapeutic challenges.

KEY POINTS

- Pituitary function affects multiple aspects of growth and metabolism.
- Pituitary hormones usually work in tightly controlled feedback loops.
- Both hormone excess and deficiency can lead to complex endocrine disease with multi-system effects.

REFERENCES

1. Blakemore C, Jennett S. Pituitary gland. In: Blakemore C, Jennett S (eds). *The Oxford companion to the body.* Oxford: Oxford University Press; 2001.
2. Guyton AC, Hall JE (eds). *Textbook of medical physiology.* 10th ed. Philadelphia: WB Saunders; 2000.
3. Amar AP, Weiss MH. Pituitary anatomy and physiology. *Neurosurg Clin N Am* 2003; **14**(1): 11–23.
4. Vankelecom H. Non-hormonal cell types in the pituitary candidating for stem cell. *Semin Cell Dev Biol* 2007; **18**(4): 559–70.
5. Nassiri F, Cusimano M, Zuccato JA, et al. Pituitary stem cells: candidates and implications. *Pituitary* 2013; **16**(3): 413–18.
6. Mathioudakis N, Sundaresh R, Larsen A, et al. Expression of the pituitary stem/progenitor marker GFRalpha2 in human pituitary adenomas and normal pituitary. *Pituitary* 2015; **18**(1): 31–41.
7. Raben MS. Growth hormone. 1. Physiologic aspects. *N Engl J Med* 1962; **266**: 31–5.
8. Murray PG, Clayton PE. Endocrine control of growth. *Am J Med Genet C Semin Med Genet* 2013; **163c**(2): 76–85.
9. Hartman ML, Faria AC, Vance ML, et al. Temporal structure of *in vivo* growth hormone secretory events in humans. *Am J Physiol* 1991; **260**(1 Pt 1): E101–10.
10. Scerif M, Goldstone AP, Korbonits M. Ghrelin in obesity and endocrine diseases. *Mol Cell Endocrinol* 2011; **340**(1): 15–25.
11. Kleinau G, Neumann S, Gruters A, et al. Novel insights on thyroid stimulating hormone receptor signal transduction. *Endocr Rev* 2013; **34**(5): 691–724.
12. Zadik Z, de Lacerda L, Kowarski AA. Evaluation of the 6-hour integrated concentration of cortisol as a diagnostic procedure for Cushing's syndrome. *J Clin Endocrinol Metab* 1982; **54**(5): 1072–4.
13. Ghigo E, Aimaretti G, Corneli G. Diagnosis of adult GH deficiency. *Growth Horm IGF Res* 2008; **18**(1): 1–16.
14. Bartke A, Sun LY, Longo V. Somatotropic signaling: trade-offs between growth, reproductive development, and longevity. *Physiol Rev* 2013; **93**(2): 571–98.
15. Baquedano MS, Ciaccio M, Dujovne N, et al. Two novel mutations of the TSH-beta subunit gene underlying congenital central hypothyroidism undetectable in neonatal TSH screening. *J Clin Endocrinol Metab* 2010; **95**(9): E98–103.
16. Nakabayashi K, Matsumi H, Bhalla A, et al. Thyrostimulin, a heterodimer of two new human glycoprotein hormone subunits, activates the thyroid-stimulating hormone receptor. *J Clin Invest* 2002; **109**(11): 1445–52.
17. Levy MJ, Koulouri O, Gurnell M. How to interpret thyroid function tests. *Clin Med* 2013; **13**(3): 282–6.
18. Bizhanova A, Kopp P. Genetics and phenomics of Pendred syndrome. *Mol Cell Endocrinol* 2010; **322**(1–2): 83–90.
19. Ben-Jonathan N, LaPensee CR, LaPensee EW. What can we learn from rodents about prolactin in humans? *Endocr Rev* 2008; **29**(1): 1–41.
20. Freeman ME, Kanyicska B, Lerant A, Nagy G. Prolactin: structure, function, and regulation of secretion. *Physiol Rev* 2000; **80**(4): 1523–631.
21. Ben-Jonathan N, Hugo ER, Brandebourg TD, LaPensee CR. Focus on prolactin as a metabolic hormone. *Trends Endocrinol Metab* 2006; **17**(3): 110–16.
22. Hinuma S, Habata Y, Fujii R, et al. A prolactin-releasing peptide in the brain. *Nature* 1998; **393**(6682): 272–6.
23. Sonigo C, Bouilly J, Carre N, et al. Hyperprolactinemia-induced ovarian acyclicity is reversed by kisspeptin administration. *J Clin Invest* 2012; **122**(10): 3791–5.
24. Mah PM, Webster J. Hyperprolactinemia: etiology, diagnosis, and management. *Semin Reprod Med* 2002; **20**(4): 365–74.
25. Verhelst J, Abs R. Hyperprolactinemia: pathophysiology and management. *Treat Endocrinol* 2003; **2**(1): 23–32.
26. Andrews DW. Pituitary adenomas. *Curr Opin Oncol* 1997; **9**(1): 55–60.
27. Mehta GU, Jane JA Jr. Pituitary tumors. *Curr Opin Neurol* 2012; **25**(6): 751–5.
28. Alama P, Bellver J, Vidal C, Giles J. GnRH analogues in the prevention of ovarian hyperstimulation syndrome. *Int J Endocrinol Metab* 2013; **11**(2): 107–16.
29. Oakley AE, Clifton DK, Steiner RA. Kisspeptin signaling in the brain. *Endocr Rev* 2009; **30**(6): 713–43.
30. Navarro VM, Gottsch ML, Chavkin C, et al. Regulation of gonadotropin-releasing hormone secretion by kisspeptin/dynorphin/neurokinin B neurons in the arcuate nucleus of the mouse. *J Neurosci* 2009; **29**(38): 11859–66.
31. Ubuka T, Son YL, Tobari Y, Tsutsui K. Gonadotropin-inhibitory hormone action in the brain and pituitary. *Front Endocrinol* 2012; **3**: 148.
32. Fechner A, Fong S, McGovern P. A review of Kallmann syndrome: genetics, pathophysiology, and clinical management. *Obstet Gynecol Surv* 2008; **63**(3): 189–94.
33. Molnar AH, Varga C, Janaky T, et al. Biological half-life and organ distribution of [3H]8-arginine vasopressin following administration of vasopressin receptor antagonist OPC-31260. *Regul Pept* 2007; **141**(1–3): 12–18.
34. Raggenbass M. Overview of cellular electrophysiological actions of vasopressin. *Eur J Pharmacol* 2008; **583**(2–3): 243–54.
35. Dale HH. On some physiological actions of ergot. *J Physiol* 1906; **34**(3): 163–206.
36. Carson DS, Guastella AJ, Taylor ER, McGregor IS. A brief history of oxytocin and its role in modulating psychostimulant effects. *J Psychopharmacol* 2013; **27**(3): 231–47.
37. Gimpl G, Fahrenholz F. The oxytocin receptor system: structure, function, and regulation. *Physiol Rev* 2001; **81**(2): 629–83.
38. Rodriguez EM, Blazquez JL, Guerra M. The design of barriers in the hypothalamus allows the median eminence and the arcuate nucleus to enjoy private milieus: the former opens to the portal blood and the latter to the cerebrospinal fluid. *Peptides* 2010; **31**(4): 757–76.
39. Bartz JA, Zaki J, Bolger N, Ochsner KN. Social effects of oxytocin in humans: context and person matter. *Trends Cogn Sci* 2011; **15**(7): 301–9.
40. Nagasawa M, Okabe S, Mogi K, Kikusui T. Oxytocin and mutual communication in mother-infant bonding. *Front Hum Neurosci* 2012; **6**: 31.
41. Tharner A, Luijk MP, Raat H, et al. Breastfeeding and its relation to maternal sensitivity and infant attachment. *J Dev Behav Pediatr* 2012; **33**(5): 396–404.
42. Carter CS, Porges SW. The biochemistry of love: an oxytocin hypothesis. *EMBO Rep* 2013; **14**(1): 12–16.
43. Johansson A, Westberg L, Sandnabba K, et al. Associations between oxytocin receptor gene (OXTR) polymorphisms and self-reported aggressive behavior and anger: interactions with alcohol consumption. *Psychoneuroendocrinology* 2012; **37**(9): 1546–56.
44. Malik AI, Zai CC, Abu Z, et al. The role of oxytocin and oxytocin receptor gene variants in childhood-onset aggression. *Genes Brain Behav* 2012; **11**(5): 545–51.
45. Sarnyai Z. Oxytocin and neuroadaptation to cocaine. *Prog Brain Res* 1998; **119**: 449–66.
46. Kovacs GL, Sarnyai Z, Szabo G. Oxytocin and addiction: a review. *Psychoneuroendocrinology* 1998; **23**(8): 945–62.
47. MacDonald SL, Mulroy L, Wilke DR, Burrell S. PET/CT aids the staging of and radiotherapy planning for early-stage extranodal natural killer/T-cell lymphoma, nasal type: a case series. *Radiat Onc* 2011; **6**: 182.

CHAPTER 57

IMAGING IN HEAD AND NECK ENDOCRINE DISEASE

Steve Colley and Sabena Fareedi

Thyroid gland 643	Pituitary gland 645
Introduction 643	References 649
Parathyroid glands 644	

SEARCH STRATEGY
Data in this chapter may be updated by a PubMed search using the keywords: thyroid, parathyroid, pituitary gland and pituitary tumour.

THYROID GLAND

INTRODUCTION

Ultrasound (US) is the primary imaging modality used to assess size, morphology and pathology of the thyroid gland, and it is the best method for assessing thyroid nodules and possible thyroid cancer. In addition it has the benefit of being able to assess neck lymphadenopathy, and guide appropriate fine-needle aspiration (FNA) for cytological diagnosis.

Since US cannot penetrate bone or air-containing structures, computed tomography (CT) is used to assess the degree of retrosternal extension of thyroid masses. It is also used to image the chest in cases of thyroid malignancy. Magnetic resonance imaging (MRI) is rarely used to assess the thyroid but can occasionally help assess potential tracheal cartilage invasion by cancer.

Positron emission tomography (PET-CT) is sometimes used in the follow-up imaging of thyroid cancer. Thyroid scintigraphy is used less commonly to assess thyroid nodules, with the majority of nuclear isotope scans being therapeutic ^{131}I to treat potential thyroid cancer metastases.

Thyroid nodules and thyroid cancer

Nodules within the thyroid are ubiquitous. Palpable nodules occur in up to 4% but are seen on imaging studies in up to 60–70% of patients, the incidence increasing with age.

US is the best imaging method to assess thyroid nodules. No single US sign has high enough sensitivity or specificity to confirm or exclude malignancy, but a combination of signs or US features can be used in summation to provide an excellent guide to the risk of underlying malignancy. Multiple papers confirm the ability of US to 'risk stratify' nodules and provide an accurate assessment, firstly of whether an FNA is required and secondly which nodule should be sampled.[1,2] Further technology such as US elastography, assessing how firm or compressible a nodule is, have been shown in some studies to assist in this regard.

Features associated with benign nodules[3] are cysts, predominantly cystic nodules with thin septations, cysts with thin peripheral isoechoic tissue, spongiform nodules (microcystic spaces comprising over 50% volume of a nodule), isoechoic well-defined nodules and multiple nodules similar in appearance to isoechoic largely replacing the normal thyroid parenchyma.

Indeterminate or follicular lesions tend to be well defined and iso- to hyperechoic, usually with a thin, low echogenicity halo and often increased internal blood flow. These lesions are usually benign (follicular adenoma), but cytology/biopsy cannot exclude a follicular carcinoma and diagnostic hemithyroidectomy should be considered.

There are a number of US features strongly associated with malignancy: a solid hypoechoic appearance, ill-defined nodule margins, a taller-than-wide shape, and microcalcifications all suggest papillary thyroid cancer and are considered suspicious US features. By using these four characteristics as a guide to FNA of nodules, we can reach a NPV for presence of thyroid cancer of 97%,[4] without undertaking biopsy of the majority of thyroid nodules. If we then consider FNA of well-defined hyperechoic nodules with a peripheral halo (i.e. follicular lesions), our performance is even better. Abnormal neck nodes, either cystic or containing microcalcification, also raise the likelihood of thyroid cancer and usually warrant FNA.

Nodule size and nodule growth have been shown to have poor correlation with underlying thyroid cancer and should not be used as a guide for FNA, but rather the nodule appearances should guide management.

Medullary cancers look very similar to papillary cancers (i.e. solid, hypoechoic, ill-defined), but calcifications are described as more globular in nature. Follicular carcinomas are diagnosed on pathology post excision, not imaging or cytology. Anaplastic cancers, thyroid lymphoma and thyroid metastases from alternate primaries all appear as large, low-echogenicity masses, often with a rapidly progressive history.

Scoring systems, such as the Mayo Clinic Thyroid Ultrasound Chart and the new British Thyroid Association guidelines for the management of thyroid cancer[5] can assist in risk stratifying nodules and improve patient care by reducing unnecessary FNA, speeding up patient pathways and reducing costs.[6]

Benign thyroid disorders

GRAVES' DISEASE

The thyroid gland appears diffusely hyper-reflective on US without nodules. An increase in intrinsic blood flow is seen on Doppler imaging.

HASHIMOTO'S THYROIDITIS

The thyroid is diffusely hypoechoic, often with hyperechoic fibrous bands seen between the areas of affected thyroid. The gland may be of normal size or enlarged. Increased internal blood flow may be seen.

MULTINODULAR GOITRE

The role of imaging in multinodular goitre is to identify the extent of thyroid enlargement (retrosternal extension, superior and inferior extent), tracheal deviation or narrowing, and the presence of any suspicious nodules or masses to suggest whether there may be a thyroid malignancy present.

Ultrasound outperforms CT and MRI in the assessment of the nodules within a goitre. The presence of multiple isoechoic nodules throughout both lobes, with varying degrees of cystic change, is almost certainly due to benign disease and does not represent the pattern of thyroid cancer.

Malignant thyroid disease

Papillary carcinoma is the most common thyroid malignancy. On US, papillary cancer demonstrates four cardinal signs: solid and hypoechoic, ill-defined margins, microcalcifications and a 'taller-than-wide' shape. If none of these four features is present, then the negative predictive value (NPV) for absence of thyroid cancer is in excess of 97%.[4] Papillary cancers may be multifocal and occasionally may be partially cystic; in this setting, it is the appearance of the solid portion of the mass that should be assessed with US.

CT and MRI less reliably show the features of thyroid cancer and rely on extrathyroidal extension or a large ill-defined thyroid mass.

Nodal metastases may be detected by US, CT or MRI. Typically, abnormal nodes from metastatic thyroid cancer show microcalcification or have a propensity for cystic change.

FOLLICULAR CANCER

Unlike papillary cancer, follicular cancer tumours are solitary. Lesions tend to be well defined and iso- to hyperechoic to normal thyroid, with a well-defined peripheral low-echogenicity halo and often prominent internal blood flow.

Metastatic lymph nodes are uncommon. Tumours tend to metastasize to bone and lungs. Tumours tend to take up ^{131}I, and this can be used to treat and follow up metastatic deposits.

ANAPLASTIC THYROID CANCER

Almost exclusively seen in older patients, anaplastic carcinoma has a poor prognosis due to its rapid progression. On US, a large, ill-defined solid low-echogenicity mass with extra thyroidal spread and nodal metastases is typical.

THYROID LYMPHOMA

Extranodal lymphoma of the thyroid may occur following long-standing thyroiditis. Appearances are of a large, hypoechoic mass, which can be indistinguishable from anaplastic carcinoma, requiring core biopsy to differentiate between the two pathologies.

PARATHYROID GLANDS

The parathyroid glands are derived from the third (lower) and fourth (upper) pharyngeal pouches. There are normally four glands, but up to 25% of individuals have more than this. The superior glands are more constant in position, lying posterior to the upper pole, near the recurrent laryngeal nerve (RLN). The lower glands have a more varied position: more commonly glands lie posterior to the lower pole, near the vascular pedicle, but they can vary in location from the level of the hard palate superiorly down to the superior mediastinum.

The role of imaging in hyperparathyroidism is to localize abnormal or hyperfunctioning glands, in order to guide surgical exploration and removal. The major imaging modalities can all be used with varying degrees of success.

Ultrasound

- **Benefits** of US are that it can visualize abnormal parathyroid glands in the region of 10 mm diameter. Abnormal glands appear of low echogenicity compared to adjacent thyroid. Reported sensitivities and specificities vary, but range between 40% and 80%, with specificity up to 98%.[7] US is operator-dependent, but in experienced hands it can outperform nuclear medicine.[8]

- **Limitations** of ultrasound imaging include ectopic glands (ultrasound cannot visualize mediastinal lesions and struggles with tracheaoesophageal lesions) and glands lying posterior to a multinodular goitre.

Nuclear medicine

Nuclear medicine scintigraphy utilizes radioactive substrates that are taken up by both thyroid and parathyroid glands. Technetium (^{99m}Tc) sestamibi is taken up by both thyroid and abnormal parathyroid glands but these have different speeds of washout. Subtraction of the images from one another allows visualization of abnormal parathyroid glands.

- **Benefits** of nuclear medicine are that multiple glands may be visualized in multigland disease, and ectopic glands in the mediastinum may be seen. Reported sensitivity of sestamibi scanning is 70–100%.
- **Disadvantages** include uptake by thyroid nodules/adenoma and poor spatial resolution. The latter has been improved by combining (fusing) the nuclear medicine scan with a low-dose CT study for anatomical and functional detail.

In many centres, the initial investigation may be ultrasound or nuclear medicine, and a combination of the two is a very common method of investigation.

Computed tomography

Contrast enhanced CT is a newer imaging technique for visualization of abnormal parathyroid glands. Adenomas show arterial phase enhancement, with rapid washout of contrast, whereas adjacent lymph nodes show gradual increasing enhancement. Polar feeding vessels may also suggest adenomas.

- **Benefits** include accurate anatomical detail, aiding surgical exploration, and accurate visualization of multigland disease and ectopic glands. Reported sensitivity and specificity appears high, and anatomical information is greater than with US or nuclear medicine techniques.
- **Disadvantages** of CT are radiation doses, as the scan utilizes multiple phases of scanning (typically three or four scans). For this reason, multiphase CT is usually limited to patients with failed surgical exploration or recurrent disease, or where clinical and biochemical suspicion is high and US and nuclear medicine have not provided a potential abnormal gland.

PITUITARY GLAND

The pituitary gland is contained within the sella turcica, a concave depression within the sphenoid bone (basisphenoid). The gland is composed of two lobes, the anterior pituitary or adenohypophysis (AH) and posterior pituitary or neurophypophysis (NH).

The **anterior pituitary** comprises 75–80% of the gland, and it produces somatotropin (growth hormone), prolactin, TSH, FSH, LH and ACTH. The **posterior pituitary** comprises 20–25% of the gland and is an inferior extension of the hypothalamus. The pars nervosa secretes ADH and oxytocin that are both produced by the hypothalamus.[9] The posterior pituitary is subdivided into the large **pars nervosa** and smaller **infundibulum** (pituitary stalk).

Imaging techniques

The best technique for multiplanar imaging of the pituitary gland is high-resolution MRI. A standard pituitary MR imaging study is 3 mm thick coronal and sagittal images pre- and post-contrast. The coronal images are best for simultaneously visualizing the sellar and parasellar structures and the position of the infundibulum in relation to the pituitary gland. The sagittal images demonstrate the midline structures and anterior and posterior extent of any related lesion. Axial T2W images of the brain 5 mm thick aid in excluding any other brain pathology and 3 mm thick coronal T2W images are also acquired to aid in differentiating types of pathology and consistency of any lesion.

ENHANCEMENT PATTERNS

The pituitary gland and infundibulum lack a blood–brain barrier therefore enhance rapidly and intensely after contrast is given.

In patients unable to undergo an MRI study, multislice CT (1 mm) pre- and post-contrast enhancement is an alternative. This can then be reconstructed in coronal and sagittal planes as required.

PRE-OPERATIVE EVALUATION

In those patients suitable for surgery to this region, a pre-operative CT scan is performed to delineate the bony anatomy of the adjacent paranasal sinuses to facilitate a transnasal, endoscopic operative approach.

PITUITARY TUMOURS

Pituitary adenomas constitute 10–15% of all intra-cranial tumours. Small adenomas occur in up to 15% of glands at autopsy and more than 20% of imaging studies. They usually occur in adults and are mostly benign. Tumours less than 1 cm are microadenomas and those greater than 1 cm are macroadenomas (**Figures 57.1** and **57.2**).

Around 25% of pituitary tumours lack hormone activity and are often diagnosed later than hormone-secreting tumours only when they compress adjacent structures (e.g. visual field defects from optic nerve compression or cranial nerve deficits from cavernous sinus invasion) (**Figures 57.3** and **57.4**). Up to 10% of pituitary adenomas invade the cavernous sinus. Clinical signs occur late, as cavernous sinus cranial nerves are lateral to the ICA. An adenoma that extends inferiorly may present as a sphenoid sinus mass.

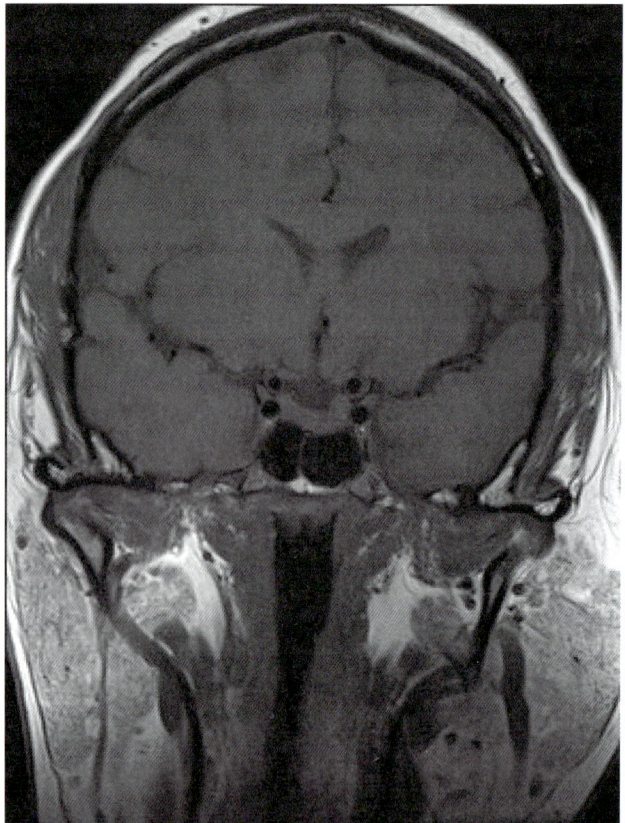

Figure 57.1 Coronal T1W image illustrates a bulky left side of the pituitary gland. There is a slight inferior slope of the sella floor also on the left. The round, dark areas either side of the pituitary gland are due to 'flow voids' which are normally seen due to the cavernous part of the internal carotid artery within the cavernous sinuses.

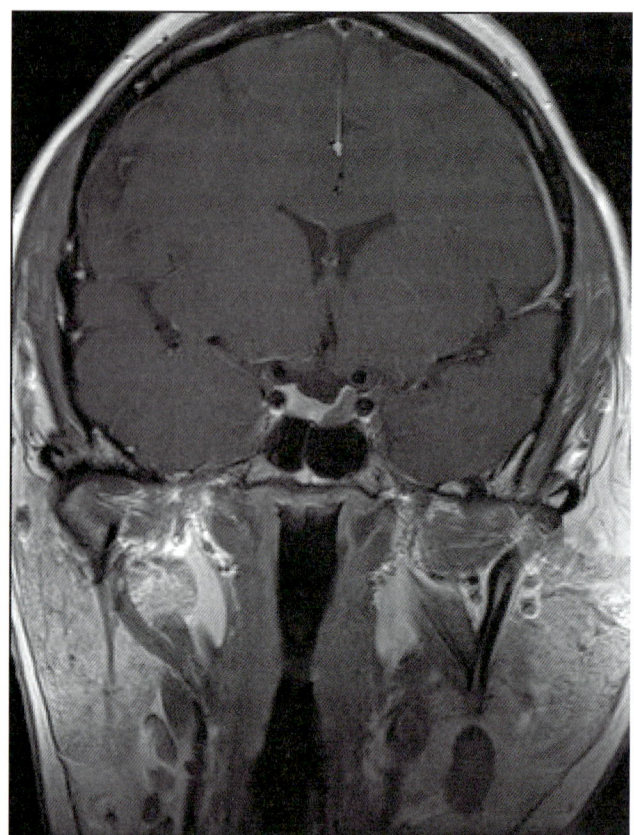

Figure 57.2 Post-contrast coronal T1W image demonstrates the non-enhancing microadenoma within the left side of the pituitary gland. The rest of the pituitary gland enhances normally.

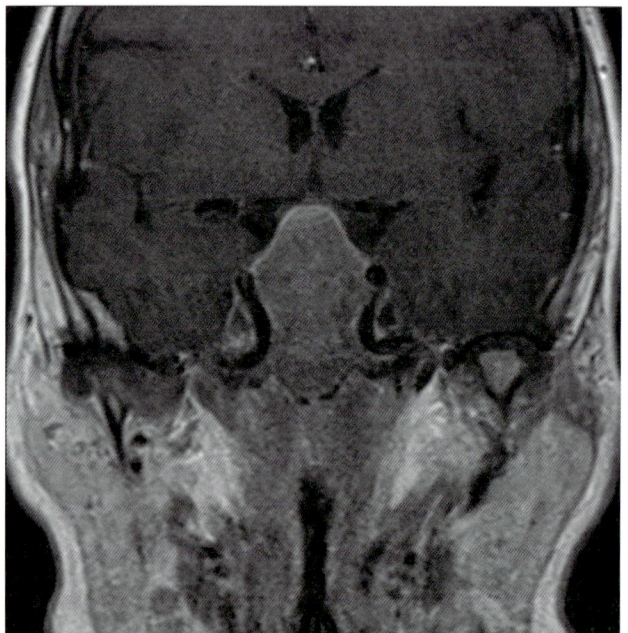

Figure 57.3 Coronal post-contrast image shows a large pituitary macroadenoma. The suprasellar extension causes compression of the optic chiasm in this case. There is also invasion of the adjacent cavernous sinuses.

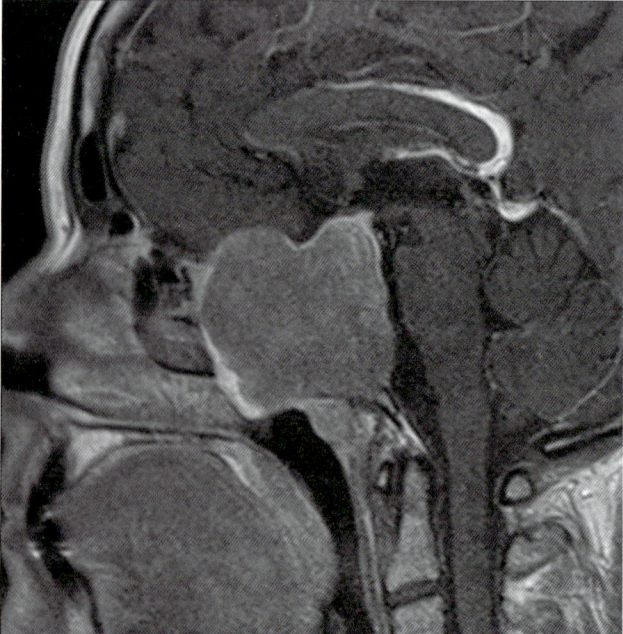

Figure 57.4 Sagittal post-contrast image of the same pituitary macroadenoma shows superior extension up to the optic chiasm and slight posterior extension into the pre-pontine cistern. There is also anterior and inferior extension and inferiorly causing a slight depression of the sella floor.

Most pituitary tumours are sporadic, only 5% being familial. The four inherited familial tumour syndromes are MEN1 (multiple endocrine neoplasia type 1, where pituitary tumours are present in 15–40%), Carney complex, McCune–Albright syndrome and FIPA (familial isolated pituitary adenoma syndrome).[9]

Adenomas originate from the anterior pituitary. The two most common types are prolactinomas and growth hormone (GH)-secreting tumours, which are usually present laterally. TSH, ACTH, LH/FSH-secreting tumours tend to occur in the midline. The most common functioning adenomas are prolactinomas. Clinical symptoms include amenorrhoea, galactorrhoea, infertility and loss of libido or impotence and hence they are more likely to present earlier in premenopausal women than in men and postmenopausal women.

The next most common pituitary tumours produce ACTH and GH. GH-secreting tumours cause gigantism in children and acromegaly in adults. ACTH secretion causes Cushing's disease. **'Dynamic post-contrast' scans** are useful in the investigation of microadenomas caused by suspected Cushing's disease. This utilizes the property of microadenomas having a slower uptake of contrast than the normal pituitary gland. A microadenoma is then visualized as a filling defect (dark) within the rest of the normally enhancing gland. Serial images are acquired of the pituitary gland during intravenous contrast injection to demonstrate the microadenoma. The range of times for optimum detection varies from 30–50 seconds to 1–2 minutes post contrast. Soon after this the contrast within the pituitary gland reduces and the adenoma becomes no longer visible.[10] Cases with known high prolactin levels and a normal-sized gland with or without a filling defect on a normal post-contrast study are treated medically and hence would not require dynamic post-contrast imaging.

Macroadenomas often extend superiorly through the opening of the diaphragm sellae. Cysts and/or foci of haemorrhage are seen in approximately 50% of cases. Most macroadenomas enlarge slowly over years. Imaging features are those of an intrasellar or intra- and suprasellar mass where the pituitary gland cannot be separated from it. Bony CT can show an enlarged sella turcica due to remodelling of the bone. A 'giant' or very large macroadenoma can erode and appear to invade the skull base.

On MRI macroadenomas are usually isointense with cortex and enhance well but heterogeneously with contrast. Tumours that have hyperintense foci on T2W images may be soft or partially necrotic. This knowledge pre-operatively is useful in pre-surgical counselling as a soft tumour can be easily removed compared to a lesion with a more fibrous nature (**Figure 57.5**).

Differential diagnosis

A number of features help to distinguish sellar masses:

- location: is the mass intrasellar, suprasellar, infundibular or a combination of these locations?
- connection: is the mass separate from the pituitary gland or not?
- age of the patient.

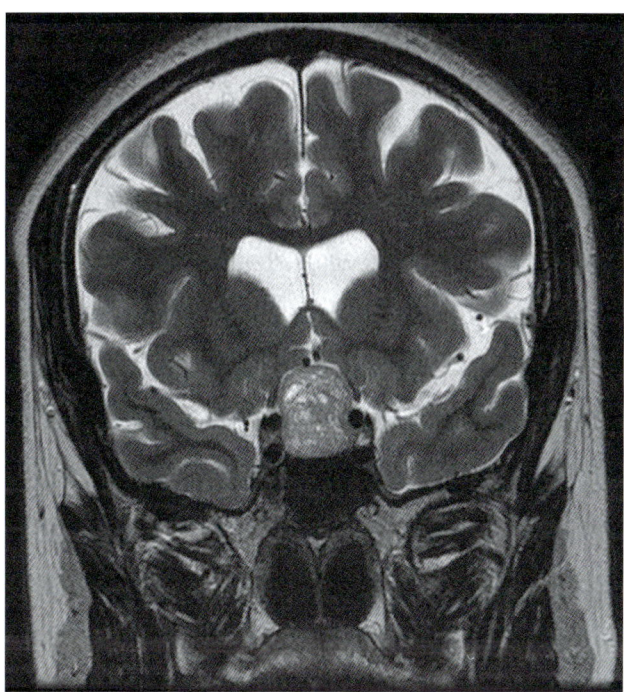

Figure 57.5 Coronal T2W image demonstrates a pituitary macroadenoma with hyperintense foci within it indicating the tumour is 'soft' or partially necrotic. It is extending up to and compressing the optic chiasm which is draped over its superior aspect.

MENINGIOMA

This tumour is rare in children and usually seen as separate from the pituitary gland. Most arise from the undersurface of the diaphragma sella but they can also arise from the walls or floor of the sella. Meningiomas more commonly arise from the parasellar regions and project into the sella turcica.[11] Intrasellar meningiomas are rare.[12]

MRI demonstrates these lesions to be hypointense to isointense to grey matter on T1W and T2W images. They enhance rapidly and avidly and have a 'dural tail'. The most useful feature in allowing differentiation of a sella meningioma from an adenoma is identifying the pituitary gland as separate from the sella mass (Figure 57.6). Also hyperostosis of adjacent bone is seen in 34% of cases. These lesions are benign but can be locally aggressive and recur after incomplete resection. They can encase and eventually occlude the internal carotid artery (ICA). Because most are very vascular tumours, pre-operative embolization is used in some cases to reduce intra-operative blood loss.

METASTASIS

Metastases to the infundibulum and/or pituitary gland are infrequent. They most commonly arise from lung and breast.[13] The posterior pituitary is generally most affected but breast metastases tend to affect the anterior pituitary. It can be difficult to differentiate these lesions from pituitary adenomas. Imaging features that may help to distinguish a pituitary metastasis are: thickening of the infundibulum, loss of high T1W signal from the posterior pituitary,

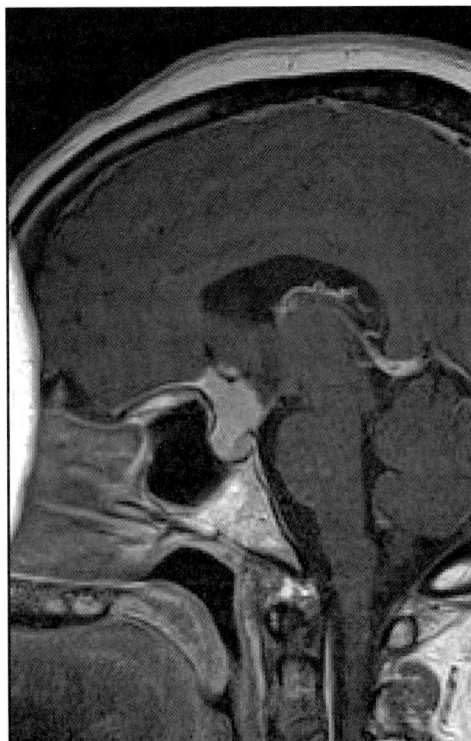

Figure 57.6 Sagittal T1W post-contrast image demonstrates a sella and suprasellar meningioma. The lesion enhances avidly and can be seen separate from the non-enhancing, normal-appearing pituitary gland seen within the posterior aspect of the sella. A 'dural tail' is seen as linear enhancement along the floor of the anterior cranial fossa.

isointense signal on T1W or T2W images, invasion of the cavernous sinus and sclerosis around the sella turcica. These appearances, however, are not specific for pituitary metastasis.

CRANIOPHARYNGIOMA

These tumours arise from epithelial remnants of Rathke's pouch. In children these are the most common suprasellar mass. They have a bimodal age distribution with one peak at 5–10 years of age and another at 50–60 years. Most are suprasellar lesions but a quarter have an intrasellar component. Intrasellar craniopharyngiomas are rare. They can measure from a few millimetres to several centimetres. The large lesions can extend to the anterior and middle cranial fossa (**Figures 57.7** and **57.8**). Two types exist: 90% are adamantinomatous and 10% papillary.

The common type of craniopharyngioma is a multilobulated, mainly cystic suprasellar mass with a solid component. It may contain cysts that are full of viscous 'machinery oil' fluid due to the cholesterol content. Calcification is common and most enhance. The papillary type has a smoother surface and is often solid. Any cysts contain a clear fluid. These tumours rarely calcify. They occur in adults with a peak at 40–44 years. Imaging features are those of a partially calcified, mixed solid and cystic mass. The pituitary can sometimes be seen as separate from the mass.

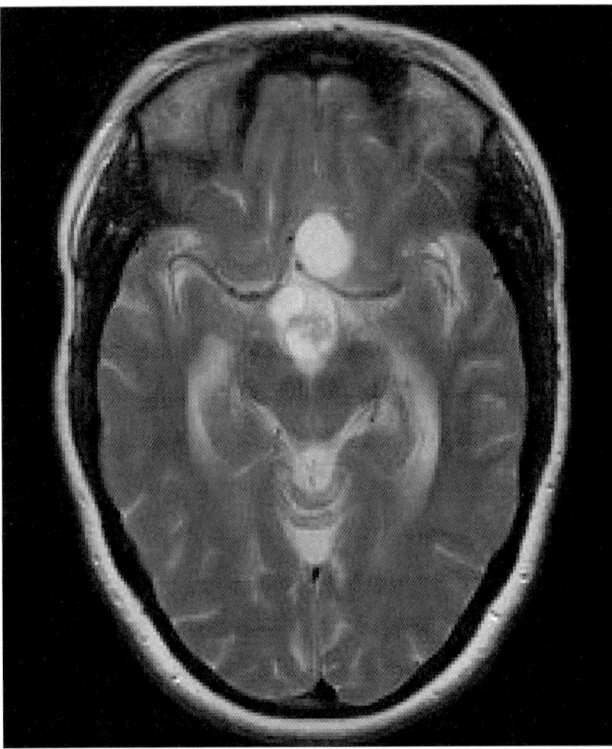

Figure 57.7 Axial T2W image illustrates the high signal intensity cystic components in a suprasellar craniopharyngioma. The posterior aspect of the lesion has some solid material within it which is seen as intermediate signal intensity.

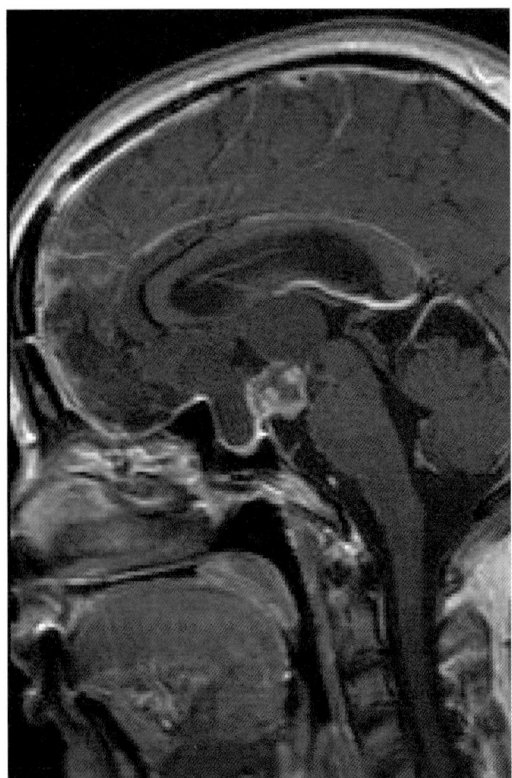

Figure 57.8 Sagittal post-contrast image demonstrates the same lesion as in Figure 57.7. The partially solid, posterior, retrosellar component exhibits patchy enhancement. The anterior and superior cystic components are non-enhancing. A thin rim of pituitary tissue is seen compressed within the sella floor, which is also depressed.

RATHKE CLEFT CYST

Craniopharyngiomas need to be differentiated from Rathke cleft cysts (RCCs). The latter do not calcify, which helps distinguish them. RCCs are a remnant of the embryonic Rathke cleft. Approximately 40% are intrasellar and 60% suprasellar.[9]

If they cause symptoms, patients with an RCC can present with pituitary dysfunction, visual disturbance and headache. MRI signal varies according to the cyst contents, which are mainly mucoid but can be serous.[10] Those which contain mucoid fluid may be indistinguishable from cystic craniopharyngiomas on MRI, with both being hyperintense on T1W and T2W images. They are usually hyperintense on FLAIR imaging. The serous cysts have imaging features of typical benign cysts, that is, low signal (dark) on T1W and high signal (bright) on T2W images. After contrast they have an enhancing rim or 'claw sign' of compressed pituitary gland around the non-enhancing cyst. Around 40–75% of RCCs have an intracystic nodule (**Figures 57.9** and **57. 10**).

NON-ADENOMATOUS PITUITARY TUMOURS

These are rare, WHO grade 1 tumours and are classified as pituicytoma, spindle cell oncocytoma and granular cell tumour.[9] They can also present with visual loss and endocrine disturbance.

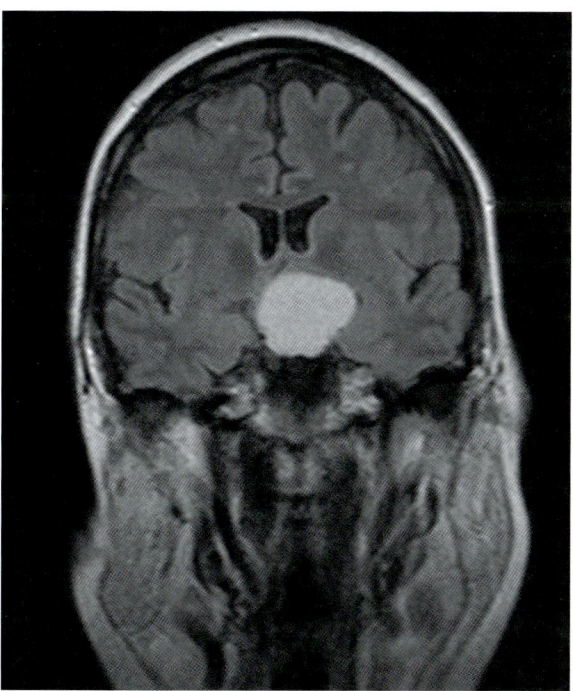

Figure 57.9 Coronal FLAIR image of a Rathke cleft cyst with mucoid fluid within it. This fluid does not 'suppress' like water or CSF on FLAIR imaging and therefore appears hyperintense.

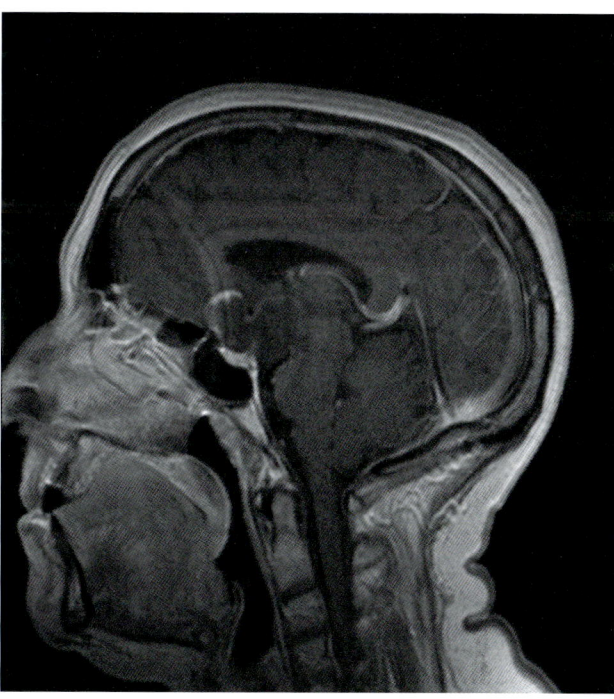

Figure 57.10 Sagittal post-contrast image of a Rathke cleft cyst illustrates the rim-enhancing cystic lesion which has suprasellar and retrosellar extension. There is a normally enhancing pituitary gland within the sella seen separate from the lesion.

KEY POINTS

- Best imaging technique is thin-section multiplanar MRI with a small field of view obtained before and after contrast.
- To distinguish the different types of sellar masses, first consider the location – is the mass intrasellar, suprasellar, infundibular or a combination of these locations?
- Is the mass separate from the pituitary gland or not?
- The age of the patient; as certain lesion are common in adults but not in children.
- Further imaging features of whether the mass is cystic, calcified and its signal intensity on MRI are also helpful.

REFERENCES

1. Hambly NM, Gonen M, Gerst SR, et al. Implementation of evidence-based guidelines for thyroid nodule biopsy. *AJR* 2011; **196**: 655–60.
2. Dominguez JM, Baudrand R, Cerda J, et al. An ultrasound model to discriminate the risk of thyroid cancer. *Acad Radiol* 2011; **18**: 242–5.
3. Kwak JY. Indications for fine needle aspiration in thyroid nodules. *Endocrinol Metab* 2013; **28**: 81–5.
4. Ahn SS, Kim E-K, Kang DR, et al. Biopsy of thyroid nodules: comparison of three sets of guidelines. *AJR* 2010; **194**: 31–7.
5. Perros P, Boelaert K, Colley S, et al. British Thyroid Association guidelines for the management of thyroid cancer. *Clin Endocrinol (Oxf)* 2014; **81** Suppl 1: 1–122.
6. Horvath E, Majlis S, Rossi R, et al. An ultrasonogram reporting system for thyroid nodules stratifying cancer risk for clinical management. *J Clin Endocrinol Metab* 2009; **94**: 1748–51.

7. Chien D, Jacene H. Imaging of the parathyroid glands. *Otolaryngol Clin North Am* 2010; **43**: 399–415.
8. Untch BR, Adam MA, Scheri RP, et al. Surgeon-performed ultrasound is superior to sestamibi scanning to localize parathyroid adenomas in patients with primary hyperparathyroidism. *J Am Coll Surg* 2011; **212**(4): 522–9.
9. Osborn AG. *Osborn's Brain: imaging, pathology and anatomy*. Philadelphia: Amirsys; 2013, pp. 683–724.
10. Atlas SW. *Magnetic resonance imaging of the brain and spine*. 4th ed. Philadelphia: Lippincott Williams and Wilkins; 2008, vol. 2, pp. 1120–91.
11. Satogami N, Miki Y, Koyama T, et al. Normal pituitary stalk: high resolution MR imaging at 3T. *AJNR* 2010; **31**: 355–9.
12. Huang BY, Castillo M. Nonadenomatous tumours of the pituitary and sella turcica. *Top Magn Reson Imaging* 2005; **16**: 289–99.
13. Fassett DR, Couldwell WT. Metastases to the pituitary gland. *Neurosurg Focus* 2004; **16**(4): E8.

CHAPTER 58

THYROID AND PARATHYROID GLAND PATHOLOGY

Ram Moorthy, Sonia Kumar and Adrian T. Warfield

Introduction 651	Parathyroid glands 685
Thyroid gland 651	References 699

SEARCH STRATEGY
Data in this chapter may be updated by a PubMed search using the keywords: benign thyroid disease, thyroid cancer, thyroiditis, benign parathyroid disease, parathyroid cancer, fine needle aspiration cytology and frozen section examination.

INTRODUCTION

The endocrine pathology discussed in this chapter is that affecting the extracranial endocrine system, viz. the thyroid and parathyroid glands found in the anterior triangle of the neck bilaterally. The chapter is not intended to be an encyclopaedic treatise, more a summary overview with selective consideration of clinically important differential diagnoses. Surgical pathology is a visual subject, therefore no apology is offered for the liberal use of illustrations to supplement the text.[1]

THYROID GLAND

The normal thyroid gland

The term 'thyroid gland' was first coined by Thomas Wharton in the 17th century to describe the gland in close proximity to the shield-shaped (scutiform or scutate) thyroid cartilage.[2]

The thyroid gland is the largest of the discrete endocrine organs typically weighing between 15 g and 25 g (roughly 0.4% of body mass), being slightly larger in women,[2] dependent upon age, nutritional and hormonal status. Macroscopically the normal thyroid gland presents a bilobate structure with a reddish-brown colour. The two lobes are connected by a central isthmus. A vestigial, accessory pyramidal lobe is present in 40% of the population.

EMBRYOLOGY

Embryologically, the thyroid gland develops from the median anlage and the two lateral anlagen. The median anlage starts as a thickening of the endodermal epithelium in the foregut between the 1st and 2nd branchial arches at the base of the tongue close to the developing myocardium,[2,3] which in later life constitutes the foramen caecum. The cells proliferate to form the thyroid bud and then a diverticulum, which expands and migrates from the base of tongue to lie anterior to the trachea. The track between the thyroid gland and base of tongue typically disappears by birth. The two lateral anlagen (known as the ultimobranchial bodies) develop from the caudal aspect of the 4th pharyngeal pouch supplemented by migratory neural crest elements and fuse with the median anlage as the thyroid gland descends in the neck. The median anlage forms the thyroid follicular cells and the lateral anlagen form the clear parafollicular cells (C-cells).[4]

CAPSULE

There is no clearly defined anatomical thyroid capsule proper, rather a thin investing fibrous pseudocapsule, which is continuous with the pre-tracheal fascia. This capsule is discontiguous or focally interrupted in approximately 60% of individuals and extracapsular thyroid tissue is present in almost 90% of glands. A variety of pericapsular inclusions, sometimes intra-thyroidal, such as parathyroid tissue, heterotopic thymus, lymph nodes and autonomic paraganglia,

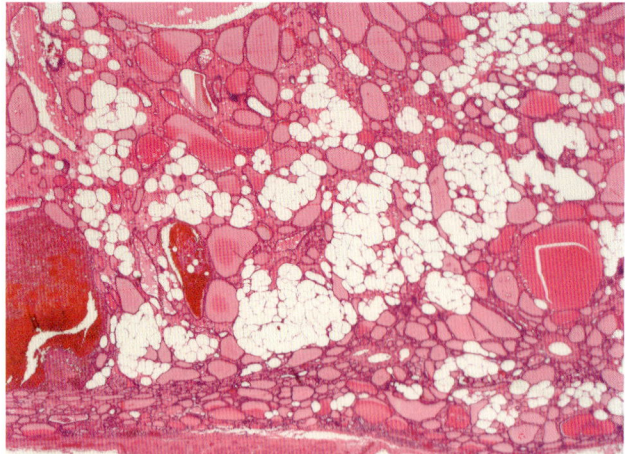

Figure 58.1 Intrathyroidal mature adipocytes intermingled with normofollicular thyroid gland parenchyma. The slender anatomical thyroid gland pseudocapsule is barely discernible at this magnification (*H&E stain, low magnification*).

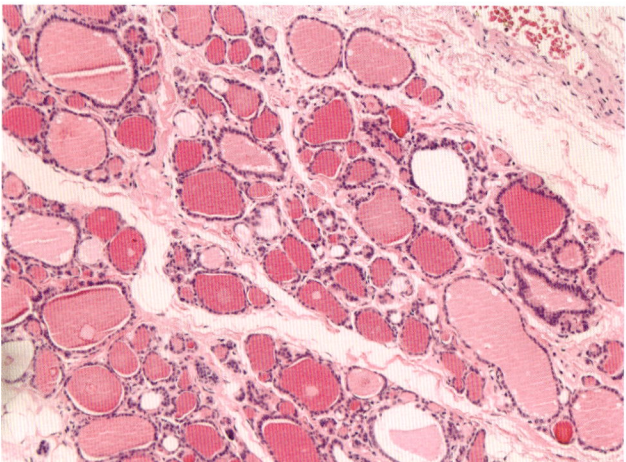

Figure 58.2 Normal thyroid gland demonstrating a lobular architecture with uniform, round/ovoid follicles. The latter contain plentiful stored colloid with fine marginal vacuolation. The parallel linear marks in the colloid ('ripple' or 'wave' effect) are an artefact of microtomy. The C-cell population is typically inconspicuous (*H&E stain, low magnification*).

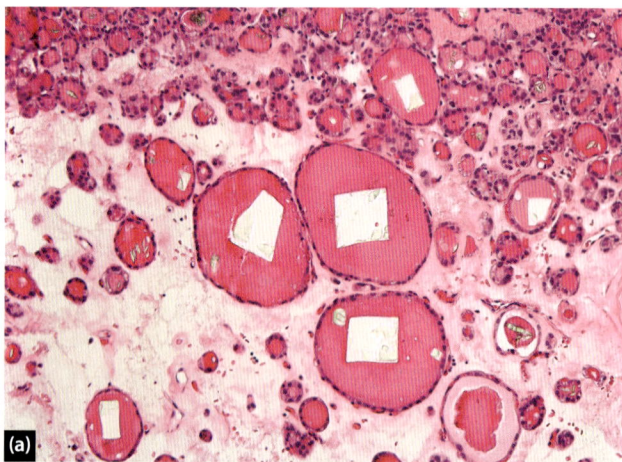

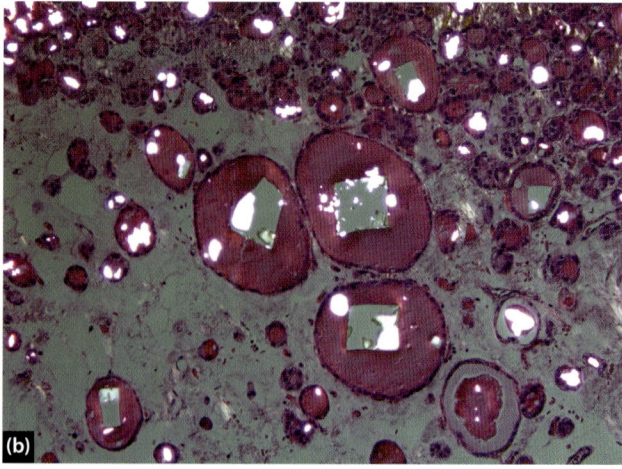

Figure 58.3 Thyroid gland parenchyma with intrafollicular rhomboidal and petaloid oxalate crystals. (a) Viewed under non-polarized brightfield light showing apparent empty geometrical spaces within the stored colloid (*H&E stain, medium magnification*). **(b)** Identical field illuminated by cross-polarized light disclosing many more strongly birefringent crystals against a dark background (*H&E stain, medium magnification*).

are considered normal. Mesenchymal-derived inclusions within the thyroid gland include stromal adipocytic, skeletal muscular and cartilaginous elements[5] (**Figure 58.1**). Awareness of potential comorbid pathological changes in perithyroidal structures is helpful, for example medial calcification of arteries (Monckeberg's sclerosis), which may also occasionally synchronously affect vasculature within the thyroid gland and rarely be encountered in lesional tissue itself.

Breach of this pseudocapsule by tumour constitutes extrathyroidal extension (ETE), defined by infiltration into perithyroidal tissues, typically eliciting inflammatory and/or desmoplastic response. Where discernible grossly to the unaided eye, this is described as macroscopic (or extensive/major/massive/marked). If only appreciable during microscopy, this is designated microscopic (or minimal/minor/limited). This distinction is important prognostically – macroscopic ETE portends a higher recurrence rate and lower disease-free survival than microscopic ETE. Direct infiltration into parathyroid gland is rare but may be arbitrarily regarded as minimal ETE owing to close proximity.

MICROSCOPICAL APPEARANCE

Microscopically, the functional unit of the thyroid gland is the follicle, which in the euthyroid state consists of a monolayer of cuboidal or flattened epithelial cells (thyrocytes) surrounding a central lumen containing stored colloid. The follicles are loosely aggregated into lobules (thyromeres), each containing around 20–50 follicles separated by slender connective tissue septula (**Figure 58.2**). Intracolloidal birefringent oxalate crystals (**Figure 58.3**), brown cytoplasmic lipofuscin ('wear and tear') pigment and haemosiderin pigment are usually of incidental portent, though these may be increased with age and in certain disease states.

The C-cells form a minor cell subpopulation, accounting for less than 10% by number, and are typically concentrated at the junction between the middle and upper thirds of the lateral lobes in a hypothetical central longitudinal axis, corresponding to the planes of medial and lateral anlagen fusion – solid cell nests, C-cell hyperplasia and medullary thyroid carcinoma, therefore, do not ordinarily occur in the isthmus. C-cells are usually larger, more rounded, polyhedral or fusiform in shape, with paler cytoplasm than follicular epithelium.

Solid cell nests

So-called solid cell nests (SCNs) are collections of non-follicular cells, found in approximately 25% of resected thyroid glands, which probably represent remnants of the ultimobranchial apparatus. They are present in greater numbers in infants and children and gradually decline with advancing age. The role of SCNs in the normal structure and function of the thyroid gland is incompletely understood and their biological significance remains a source of controversy and debate. SCNs may harbour minimal properties of a stem cell phenotype with capacity for self-renewal and end differentiation.

SCNs comprise irregularly shaped clusters of interfollicular cells delineated by basal lamina. The dominant cell component (main cell) comprises polygonal to fusiform cells disposed in solid array sometimes with an epidermoid appearance, though generally non-keratinizing and devoid of intercellular bridges (prickles). They less commonly show a glandular morphology and may paradoxically be microcystic, micropapillary and/or mucinous. SCNs co-express cytokeratins, carcinoembryonic antigen (CEA, CD66e), galectin-3 and many pan-neuropeptides such as chromogranin A, synaptophysin and somatostatin, but they are negative for markers of terminal differentiation, viz. thyroglobulin (Tg), thyroid transcription factor-1 (TTF-1) and calcitonin (**Figure 58.4**). They also contain a minor subpopulation of C-cells, which show a partially differentiated immunophenotype. SCNs consistently stain for p63, a homologue of p53, a nuclear transcription factor that induces expression of cytokeratin 5 (CK5) and cytokeratin 14 (CK14). The gene for p63 is universally expressed in basal cells of stratified epithelia and plays a major role in triggering the maturation of these into squamous epithelium.

Solid cell nests are postulated to be precursors of certain thyroid gland neoplasms, notably papillary thyroid carcinoma. They may also play a role in the histogenesis of Hashimoto's thyroiditis, which is also associated with papillary thyroid carcinoma. Papillary thyroid carcinoma and Hashimoto's thyroiditis may therefore be linked in pathogenesis via a common population of pluripotent p63 positive embryonal stem cell remnant progenitors.[6]

Fine-needle aspiration cytology

Fine-needle aspiration cytology (FNAC) is generally recognized as a valuable and cost-effective first-line investigation in the evaluation of a thyroid swelling.[7–10] In experienced hands, FNAC of the thyroid gland is accurate with a sensitivity of 65–98%, a specificity of 72–100%, a false-positive rate of 1–8% and false-negative rate of 1–11%.[7,11] The non-diagnostic or inadequate rate can be as high as 28%[11] but targeting by ultrasound (US) guidance can reduce the incidence of a non-diagnostic FNAC.[12] US guidance is recommended in nodules with a higher chance of non-diagnostic FNAC by simple palpation. These include cystic nodules and smaller or non-palpable lesions.[10] Thus, as a screening test FNAC is highly sensitive, but it lacks specificity: approximately 15–40% of aspirates designated suspect of a follicular neoplasm ultimately prove to be malignant, ergo the remaining 60–85% or so of nodules are benign in the final analysis. Immediate assessment of samples for adequacy at the time of aspiration (rapid on-site evaluation, ROSE) can reduce the rate of unsatisfactory specimens and aid collection of material for ancillary tests.

FNAC is substantially a screening/triage procedure for follicular carcinoma, identifying those patients who require further investigations, and a primary diagnostic test for other thyroid malignancies, principally papillary

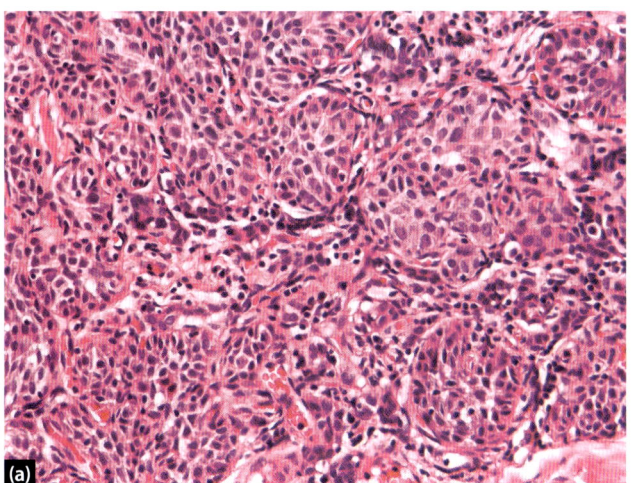
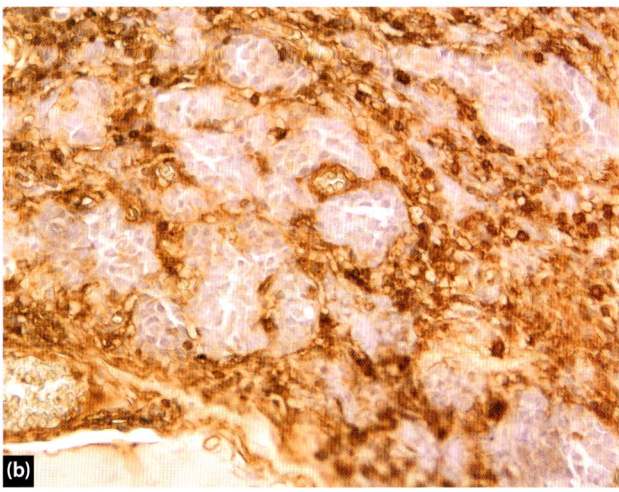

Figure 58.4 Solid cell nests. (a) Ultimobranchial apparatus rests (solid cell nests) disposed as discrete congeries of squamoid (epidermoid) cells without keratinization, discovered incidentally in a thyroidectomy specimen indicated for partially treated Graves' disease (*H&E stain, medium magnification*). **(b)** Such cell rests typically express pan-neuroendocrine immunomarkers but not thyroglobulin and they are thus shown here in negative relief (*thyroglobulin IHC, medium magnification*).

thyroid carcinoma, medullary carcinoma, undifferentiated (anaplastic) carcinoma and lymphoma.

The results of FNAC may reassure that a lesion is benign, triage patients for diagnostic surgery, or provide a definitive diagnosis of selected thyroid malignancies, thereby expediting single-stage therapeutic intervention.[9, 10] There is plentiful experience based upon the traditional wet-fixed and air-dried direct smear methodology, aspirate washings and cyst fluid samples, supplemented by cell concentration techniques, such as centrifugation, filtration and cell blocks. Newer liquid-based technology is favoured by some centres, dependent upon local resources and experience, furthermore handling of FNAC specimens may be influenced by the prospect of ancillary investigations. The success of thyroid FNAC is demonstrably operator-dependent – the cytopathologist can only ever be as good as the quality of the aspiration sample that he or she receives.

Despite acknowledged cytodiagnostic pitfalls, some outlined below, the use of FNAC in the preliminary evaluation of solitary or dominant nodules reduces the use of surgery by approximately one-third, doubles the proportion of malignancies among surgical resections and increases cost-effectiveness. FNAC may be employed in the investigation of suspect lymph nodes and measurement of thyroglobulin in needle wash samples may augment diagnostic accuracy. Molecular studies may also refine the diagnostic process in thyroid FNAC samples. Serious diagnostic delay due to false-negative FNAC is uncommon where there is appropriate clinical follow-up.[13]

Historically, the diagnostic criteria and reporting nomenclature employed internationally have varied somewhat though these have ultimately evolved to broad consensus, aimed at national standardization, stratified for risk of malignancy with corresponding evidence-based recommendations for further patient management.[14] These are epitomized by the North American National Cancer Institute (Bethesda) terminology (2007),[15] Italian (2007, 2014), Australian (2014), Japanese (2013) and British Thyroid Association/Royal College of Pathologists (2002, 2007, 2016) guidelines.[16] The terminology for non-diagnostic, benign, malignant and suspect for malignancy is similar across each of these classifications with minor differences in emphasis for the equivocal/indeterminate category. These schemata and the anticipated rates of malignancy attributed to each diagnostic category are outlined in **Table 58.1**. It is sometimes salutary when deliberating management options during multidisciplinary team conferences to remind participants of the reciprocal likelihood of benignity for each category to maintain a sense of perspective.

The shorthand alpha-numeric diagnostic category codification intrinsic to some of these systems is not intended to supplant a focused narrative cytology report or stymie more comprehensive communication, where appropriate. Additionally, the vernacular habit of grouping together non-diagnostic/unsatisfactory and non-neoplastic/benign aspirates under the rubric of negative reports should be dispelled. As a fundamental principle, it is emphasized that, while the presence of malignant cells is diagnostic, a lack of malignant cells can never be wholly exclusionary – absence of evidence is not *prima facie* evidence of absence.

LIMITATIONS OF FNAC OF THE THYROID GLAND

The follicular-patterned lesion is the most commonly encountered type of thyroid FNAC specimen in clinical practice. Distinction between a hyperplastic (adenomatoid) nodule in a multinodular goitre and a follicular-patterned neoplasm may not always be achievable. The presence of dispersed colloid, monolayered sheets of bland thyrocytes and macrofollicular structures are more typical of hyperplasia. Dense colloid globules, paucity of colloid and microfollicular configuration (**Figure 58.5**) tend to support neoplasia. It is necessary to focus on the predominant cytoarchitectural pattern, rather than a minor subpopulation of microfollicles, with the proviso that this approach is predicated upon adequate cell sampling. The agreed criterion for this is that samples from solid lesions should contain at least six groups of thyroid follicular epithelial cells across all the submitted slides, each composed of at least ten well-visualized epithelial cells. Note that this constitutes a minimum standard, that the degree of diagnostic confidence should increase with higher yield samples and that this threshold does not necessarily preclude a positive diagnosis of malignancy if a lesser quantum of characteristic cells is present.

Reliable discrimination between a benign adenoma and differentiated follicular carcinoma on subjective morphological grounds is now realized to be always difficult, often impossible. While the presence of high cellularity, cell crowding, tri-dimensional (acervate) groups, nucleomegaly, cytonuclear atypia, three or more nucleoli per cell, irregular karyoplasm and necrosis are individually not absolute, in aggregate they tend to favour a diagnosis of malignancy. Follicular variant of papillary thyroid carcinoma (FVPTC) enters the differential diagnosis, where a scrupulous search for its characteristic nuclear morphology is indicated. The diagnosis of non-invasive follicular thyroid neoplasm with papillary-like nuclear features (NIFTP) is not sustainable from SNAC appearances alone. The separation of minimally invasive from widely invasive follicular carcinoma on FNAC, contingent upon extent of extracapsular invasion is obviously untenable *ab initio*.

Oncocytic (oxyphil) cell lesions are problematic on FNAC. Hashimoto's thyroiditis and oncocytic (oxyphil) metaplasia in multinodular hyperplasia are generally separated by conspicuous lymphocytosis in the former (**Figure 58.6**) though the degree of inflammatory cell infiltrate varies with the natural history of the disease and paucilymphocytic variants are described. The cytological distinction between Hürthle cell adenoma and carcinoma is unreliable – benign oncocytic (oxyphil) cells may display extreme pleomorphism and, paradoxically, there is often less cytonuclear variation in Hürthle cell neoplasms. Confident recognition of the rare oncocytic (oxyphil) variant of papillary thyroid carcinoma on FNAC is extremely difficult. The conclusion oncocytic (oxyphil) cell lesion or neoplasm, not otherwise specified, is occasionally the best that can be achieved with a recommendation for excision, as clinically indicated. A solitary thyroid nodule composed of predominantly oncocytes on FNAC merits excision because oncocytic (oxyphil) thyroid neoplasms show on average a 30% malignancy rate based on histology. Moreover, the larger an oncocytic tumour,

TABLE 58.1 Comparison of the BTA/RCPath, Bethesda[16] and other contemporaneous international classification systems for reporting thyroid gland FNAC specimens together with their clinical implications[10, 14]

RCPath	Bethesda	Italian	Australian	Japanese
Thy1 Non-diagnostic for cytological diagnosis Thy 1c Non-diagnostic for cytological diagnosis – cystic lesion	I. Non-diagnostic or unsatisfactory Virtually acellular specimen Other (obscuring blood, clotting artefact, etc.) Cyst fluid only	TIR 1 Non-diagnostic TIR 1c Non-diagnostic cystic	1 Non-diagnostic	1 Inadequate
0–10%	0–10%	Not defined	0–10%	10%
Thy 2 Non-neoplastic Thy 2c Non-neoplastic cystic lesion	II. Benign Consistent with a benign follicular nodule (includes adenomatoid nodule, colloid nodule, etc.) Consistent with lymphocytic (Hashimoto) thyroiditis in the proper clinical context Consistent with granulomatous (subacute) thyroiditis Other	TIR 2 Non-malignant	2 Benign	2 Normal or benign
0–3%	0–3%	<3%	0–3%	<1%
Thy 3a Neoplasm possible, suggesting follicular neoplasm	III. Atypia of undetermined significance or follicular lesion of undetermined significance	TIR 3A Low risk Indeterminate Lesion (LRIL)	3 Indeterminate or follicular lesion of undetermined significance	3 Indeterminate B Others
5–15%	5–15%	<10%	5–15%	40–60%
Thy 3f Neoplasm possible, suggesting follicular neoplasm	IV. Follicular neoplasm or suspicious for a follicular neoplasm Specify if Hürthle cell (oncocytic) type	TIR 3B High risk Indeterminate Lesion (HRIL)	4 Suggestive of a follicular neoplasm	3 Indeterminate A Follicular neoplasm A-1 Favour benign (<15%) A-2 Borderline (15–30%) A-3 Favour malignant (40–60%)
15–30%	15–30%	15–30%	15–30%	
Thy 4 Suspicious of malignancy	V. Suspicious for malignancy Suspicious for papillary carcinoma Suspicious for medullary carcinoma Suspicious for metastatic carcinoma Suspicious for lymphoma Other	TIR 4 Suspicious of malignancy	5 Suspicious of malignancy	4 Malignancy suspected
60–75%	60–75%	60–80%	60–75%	>80%
Thy 5 Malignant	VI. Malignant Papillary thyroid carcinoma Poorly differentiated carcinoma Medullary thyroid carcinoma Undifferentiated (anaplastic) carcinoma Squamous cell carcinoma Carcinoma with mixed features (specify) Metastatic carcinoma Non-Hodgkin lymphoma Other	TIR 5 Malignant	6 Malignant	5 Malignant
97–99%	97–99%	>95%	97–99%	>99%

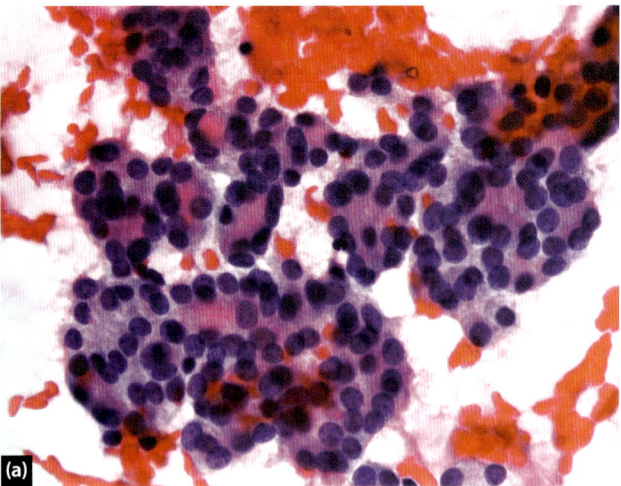
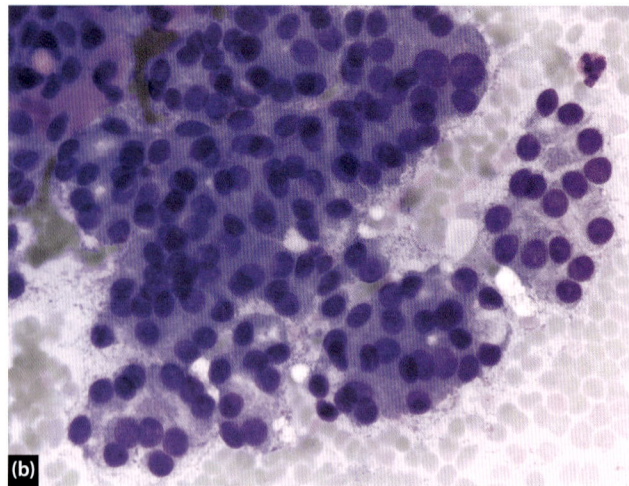

Figure 58.5 FNAC. (a) Cellular FNAC specimen suggestive of a follicular neoplasm. Note several microfollicular structures (defined as 12 or fewer circumferential thyroid epithelial cells, in contrast to macrofollicles composed of 20 or more peripheral cells).[15] Structures of normofollicular configuration are defined within these two extremes (*Pap stain, high magnification*). **(b)** Similar microfollicles seen on its companion air-dried smear. There is sparse colloid in some of the follicles (*MGG stain, high magnification*).

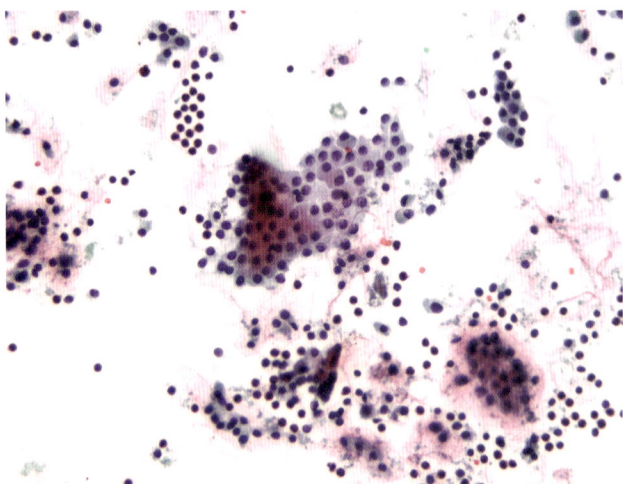

Figure 58.6 FNAC from Hashimoto's thyroiditis. Loosely cohesive, monolayered clusters of mildly pleomorphic oncocytic (oxyphil or Hürthle cell) thyrocytes can be seen admixed with polymorphous small lymphocytes (*Pap stain, medium magnification*).

the greater the likelihood of invasive malignancy: there is a 65–80% chance of malignancy in oncocytic neoplasms exceeding 4 cm maximum dimension.

Aspirates from cystic lesions may not be fully diagnostic, particularly if there is limited or degenerate epithelial sampling. Cysts of any type tend to contain variform inflammatory cells, foam cells, pigmented macrophages and cytolytic debris (**Figure 58.7**). Copious dispersed colloid favours benignity, though in the absence of adequate epithelial cell content the possibility of a cystic neoplasm or cystic degeneration in a neoplasm, of which papillary thyroid carcinoma is paradigmatic, cannot be completely ruled out on FNAC microscopical appearances in isolation since up to 10% of thyroid carcinomas missed on FNAC harbour a cystic component.

The diagnosis of high-grade non-Hodgkin lymphoma is generally straightforward with adequate FNAC material.

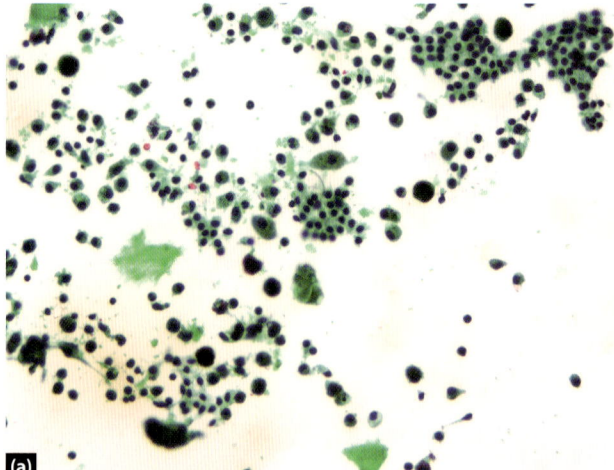
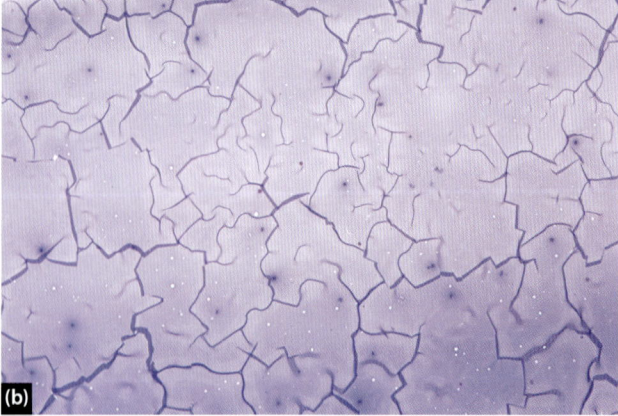

Figure 58.7 Fine-needle aspiration cytology. (a) FNAC from a benign thyroid cyst showing monolayered sheets (honeycomb or frog spawn) of cohesive, isomorphic epithelial cells amidst foam cells and pigmented macrophages with minimal necrolytic debris (*Pap stain, medium magnification*). **(b)** FNAC of the contents of a benign colloid cyst/nodule illustrating abundant, evenly dispersed, tessellated (cracked or 'parched earth') colloid. There is no cell sampling in this field.

Recognition of low-grade non-Hodgkin lymphoma, typically extranodal marginal zone lymphoma ('MALToma'), however, is sometimes fraught, especially if arising in the context of autoimmune thyroiditis where monomorphism of the neoplastic lymphocytes, which triggers the suspicion of neoplasia, is diluted or obscured by reactive lympho-proliferative elements. Histological examination is typically advised, particularly if more definitive subclassification is desired.

FNAC-INDUCED IATROGENIC CHANGE

Although FNAC is popularly considered to be a comparatively atraumatic procedure, the technique is known to induce histological changes, which may modulate or even obscure the underlying pathology and potentially mislead the unwary.

Several studies propose an incidence for FNAC-induced iatrogenic changes of close to 100%.[17] Relevant factors include the nature and size of the target lesion, the calibre of the needle used, the number of passes attempted, the precise FNAC technique employed, how meticulously such effects are sought and the interval between FNAC and excision surgery. The retrospective nature of such audit is prone to underestimate the true frequency.

The resultant secondary damage may broadly be classified into tissue damage and repair effects, tumour and tissue infarction, and epithelial dislodgement/displacement phenomena. The acronym WHAFFT ('worrisome histologic alteration following fine-needle aspiration of the thyroid gland') was originally proposed and has further been divided into acute WHAFFT and chronic WHAFFT.[18]

The tissue damage and repair aspect includes haemorrhage, fibrovascular granulation tissue organization and regenerative/degenerative atypia. Haemorrhagic needle tracks and associated proliferation of fibroblasts/myofibroblasts are typically pericapsular and radiate to the centre of the lesion, perpendicular to the capsule. The influx of inflammatory cells, siderophages, linear fibrosis/hyalinization, cholesterol granulomata, dystrophic mineralization, epithelial metaplasia and epithelial and endothelial atypia may on occasion be so exuberant and kaposiform as to closely mimic a sarcoma (so-called post-FNAC spindle cell nodule) (**Figure 58.8**).

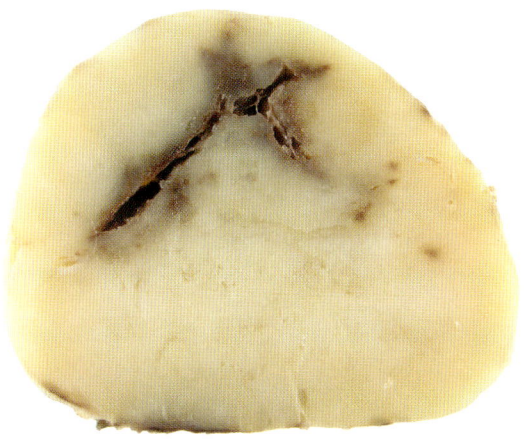
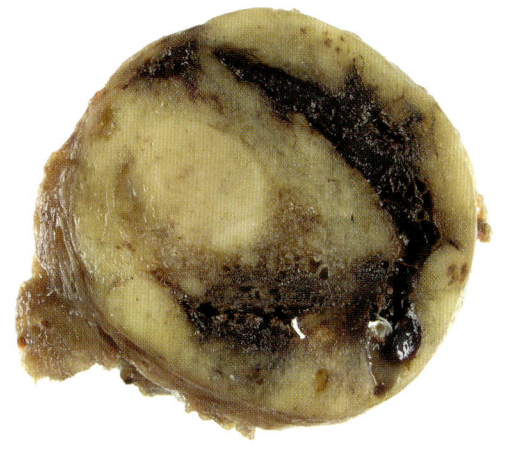
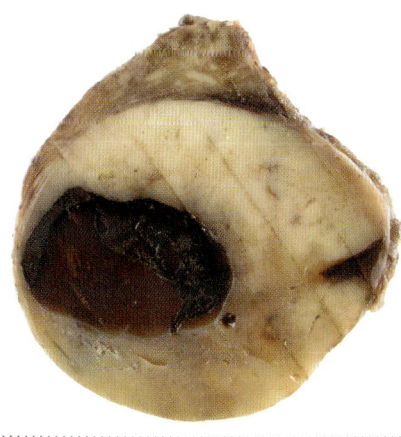
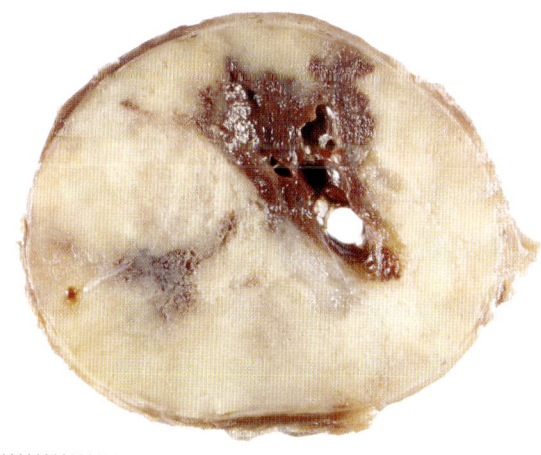

Figure 58.8 FNAC-induced iatrogenic changes. (a) Recent FNAC needle tracks in a follicular neoplasm. The crossed swords ('double skewer') sign indicates that at least two passes of the needle in different directions were conscientiously made by the aspirator. The rectilinear, subcapsular configuration is typical. **(b)** This haemorrhagic recent FNAC needle track, however, appears more curvilinear. **(c)** Circumscribed encysted haematoma post-FNAC. **(d)** Another follicular neoplasm showing post-FNAC linear haemorrhagic infarction with early macrocystic change.

(Continued)

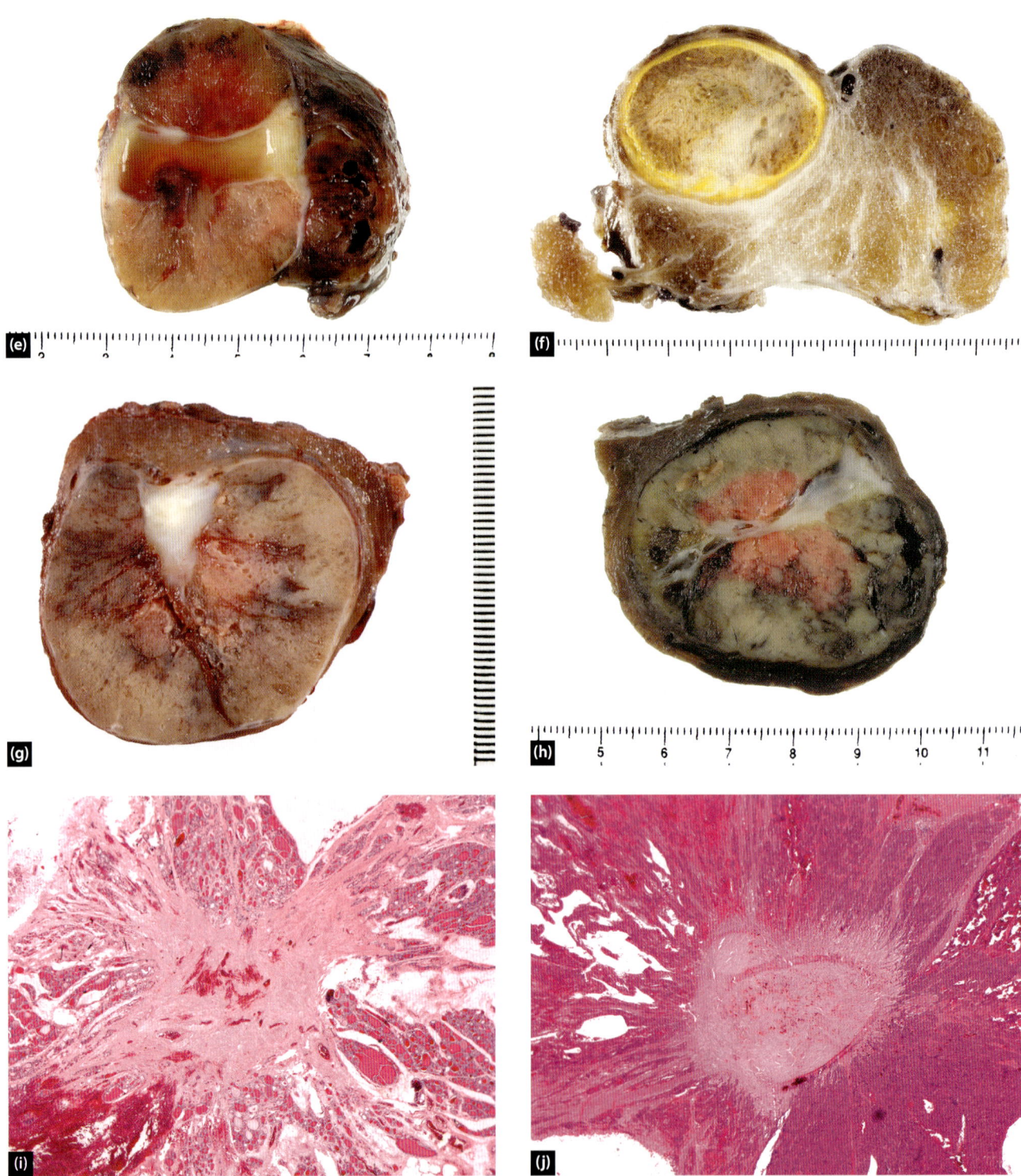

Figure 58.8 (Continued) FNAC-induced iatrogenic changes. (e) Established macrocystic degeneration with localized mural vascular granulation tissue response and limpid, mucoid contents. **(f)** Globally infarcted oncocytic (oxyphil) cell neoplasm, not further sub-classifiable, following FNAC displaying complete yellow ischaemic type necrosis. **(g)** Obvious healing rectilinear FNAC artefact perpendicular to the capsule with a retracted, cuneiform, fibrous pericapsular scar in an otherwise minimally invasive follicular carcinoma. **(h)** Post-FNAC linear fibrous scar traversing an oncocytic (Hürthle cell) neoplasm, contiguous with wedge-shaped, retracted capsular defect. **(i)** Post-FNAC artefact manifest as radial scar-like, central fibroblastic granulation tissue and haemorrhage distorting surrounding lesional parenchyma (*H&E stain, low magnification*). **(j)** Another example of an older post-FNAC radial scar presenting a haemosiderotic, hyalosclerotic nidus with centripetal contracture deformity of lesional architecture (*H&E stain, ultra-low magnification*).

(Continued)

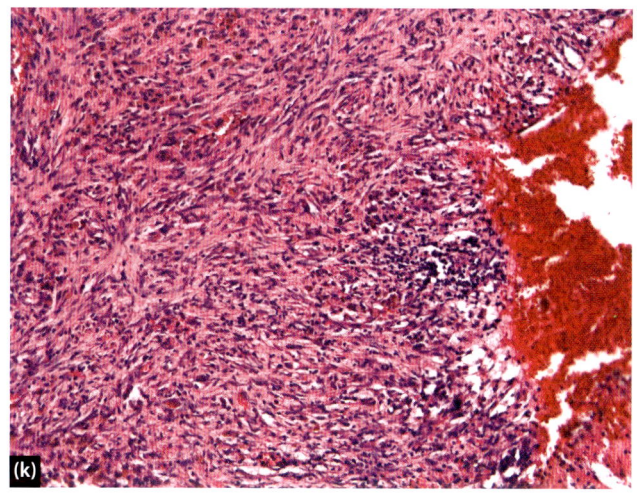

Figure 58.8 (Continued) FNAC-induced iatrogenic changes.
(k) Post-FNAC spindle cell nodule composed of richly vascularized myofibroblastic (kaposiform) stroma bordering encysted haematoma (*H&E stain, medium magnification*).

The thyroid gland is a richly vascularized organ (receiving approximately 2% of total cardiac output) and post-FNAC vascular effects include venous thrombosis, recanalization and papillary endothelial hyperplasia, sometimes to an extent to resemble angiosarcoma (pseudo-angiosarcomatoid). Mitochondrion-rich oncocytic (oxyphil) cell lesions are exquisitely sensitive to ischaemia, and therefore characteristically susceptible to partial or global infarction, either spontaneously or post-FNAC. Where extensive, such infarction may render definitive histological evaluation difficult or impossible and a diagnosis of oncocytic neoplasm, not further specified, may be the best that can be proffered under these circumstances. However, a minor population of better-preserved tissue, the ghost-like outlines of devitalized papillae, necrotic cells or psammoma bodies, together with review of the original FNAC material, may yield some insight into the underlying pathology. Immunocytochemical positivity for certain epitopes persists for a surprising time after infarction – leukocyte common antigen (CD45) and CD20 staining, for example, may reproducibly define lympho-proliferation long after tumour cells have cytolyzed, though antibodies such as carcinoembryonic antigen (CD66e) is more capricious and stains fields of necrotic tissue and abscess cavitation indiscriminately.

Angulated follicles and reparative stromal response, accompanied by nuclear hyperchromasia, fusiform epithelial morphology and squamous metaplasia, may appear infiltrative (pseudo-infiltration), and therefore merit serious consideration of follicular carcinoma, squamous cell carcinoma or muco-epidermoid carcinoma.

Epithelial displacement and/or tumour implantation along FNAC needle tracks into soft tissues or skin does occur, though apart from the uncommon sarcomas such deposits usually disintegrate and viable tumour seeding is rarely of serious clinical importance. Fields of reactive papillary endothelial hyperplasia (Masson's pseudo-tumour) in pericapsular vasculature may closely mimic lymphovascular involvement by papillary thyroid carcinoma. Mechanical tumour cell dislodgement into blood vessels may resemble vascular invasion. Rigorous criteria are recommended, notably the presence of a protruberant connection with the vessel wall, partial or complete endothelialization of the tumour tissue and/or admixture of tumour cells with blood/thrombus, all indicative of a vital response. Opinion is divided as to whether immunostaining (e.g. CD31, CD34 for vascular and D2-40 for lymphatic endothelium) ought to be routinely or selectively utilized. Pericapsular defects in various stages of healing must not be misconstrued as capsular infiltration (pseudo-invasion) or evidence of extrathyroidal extension.

Developmental conditions

Developmental conditions involve the presence of normal thyroid tissue in sites outside the normal thyroid gland (heterotopia or ectopia, hamartoma and choristoma). This includes lingual thyroid, mediastinal thyroid, benign lymph node inclusions, so-called 'lateral aberrant thyroid gland' and sequestrated (parasitic) thyroid nodules. Mature adult cystic teratoma (dermoid cyst) of the ovary may show a preponderance of thyroid tissue (struma ovarii) sometimes with carcinoid elements (strumal carcinoid). The same repertoire of pathological conditions that affect eutopic thyroid gland may also be rarely encountered at these other sites (Figure 58.9).

THYROGLOSSAL TRACT ANOMALIES

Thyroglossal duct remnants persist due to failure of involution of the thyroglossal duct following embryological descent of the thyroid gland. They are the commonest cause of a congenital neck mass and the second most common cause of a cervical mass in childhood.[19]

Thyroglossal duct remnants can occur at almost any site from the base of the tongue to the suprasternal region, predominantly at four locations, namely intralingual, suprahyoid, thyrohyoid and suprasternal[20] (Figure 58.10). Cysts predominate with fewer sinuses and fistulae. Counterintuitively, follicular thyroid tissue is not a prerequisite for diagnosis. Thyroglossal duct carcinoma is rare, estimated as occurring in no more than 1% of thyroglossal duct cysts and, when it supervenes, it is usually a subtype of papillary thyroid carcinoma.

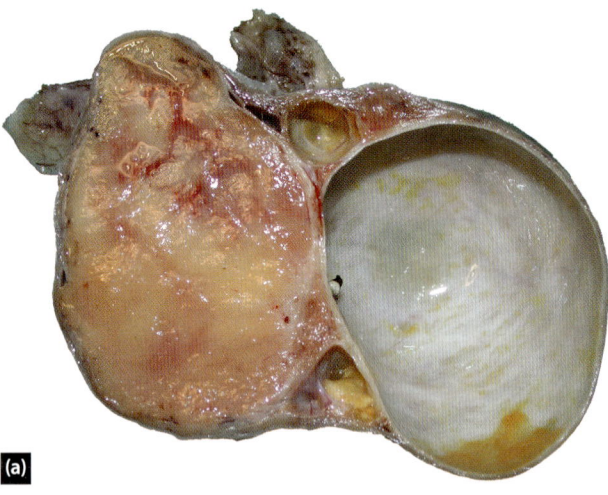

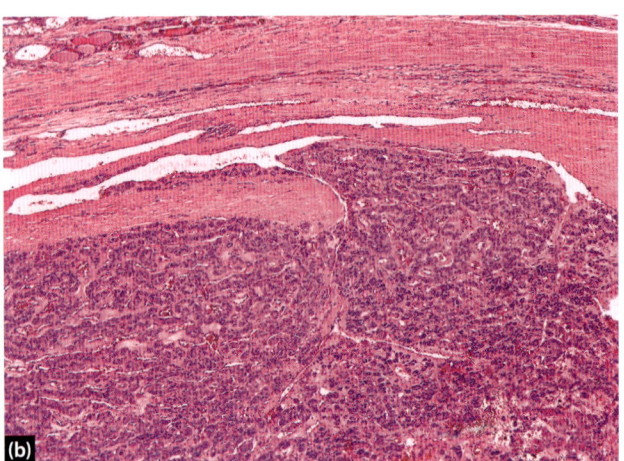
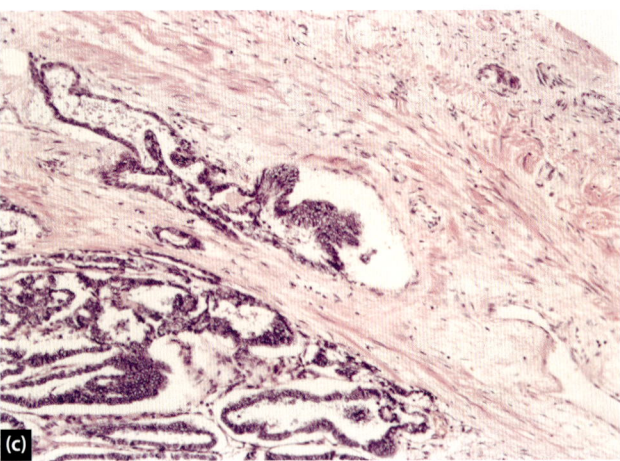

Figure 58.9 Developmental conditions. **(a)** Adult cystic ovarian teratoma (dermoid cyst). The solid component is substantially follicular thyroid tissue with clinically unsuspected fields of minimally invasive (angioinvasive) follicular carcinoma microscopically. **(b)** Minimally invasive follicular carcinoma ex-ovarian teratoma (struma ovarii). The endothelialized tongue-like angioinvasion is identical to that seen in such tumours occurring in eutopic thyroid gland (*H&E stain, medium magnification*). **(c)** Lymphovascular invasion in well-differentiated papillary thyroid carcinoma, classical pattern ex-struma ovarii. Again, this is identical to that occurring in eutopic thyroid gland proper (*H&E stain, medium magnification*).

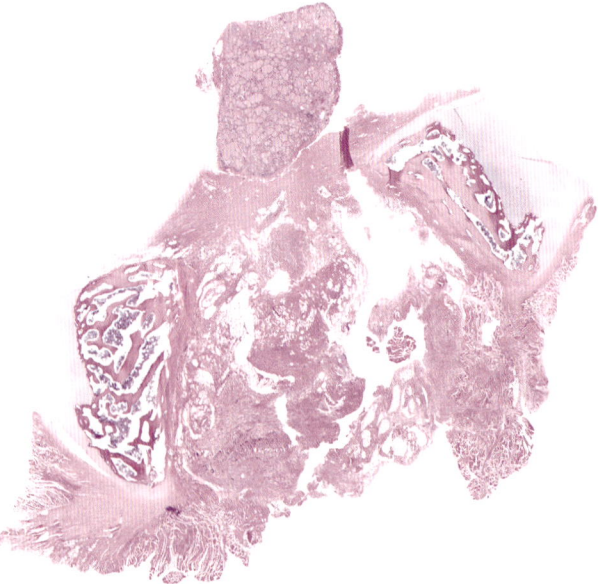

Figure 58.10 Whole mount preparation of a Sistrunk's procedure specimen. It shows hyoid bone, closely associated connective tissue plus a nubbin of normofollicular thyroid tissue representing thyroglossal duct remnants (*H&E stain, ultra-low magnification*).

SQUAMOUS DIFFERENTIATION

The presence of squamous epithelium is not uncommon. It is usually either an acquired, adaptive response (metaplasia) due to inflammation, or related to developmental rests of cells (heteroplasia)[21, 22] though it may also occur in some neoplasms (differentiation) (**Figure 58.11** and **Table 58.2**).

Non-neoplastic squamous epithelium is usually microscopically bland though may sometimes show an alarming degree of reactive/reparative cytonuclear atypia. Benign squamous epithelium generally presents the same immunophenotype as elsewhere, viz. cytokeratins (notably CK5 and CK14), epithelial membrane antigen (EMA) and p63 positivity, usually with thyroglobulin, thyroid transcription factor-1 (TTF-1) and carcinoembryonic antigen (CEA, CD66e) negativity. Malignant squamous differentiation, however, may not conform to this profile and anomalous epitope expression (e.g. CD 56) may be confounding.

ONCOCYTIC CHANGE

Oncocytic (oxyphilic) cells are characterized by swollen, granular, mitochondrion-rich cytoplasm and may occur in both endocrine tissues and non-endocrine organs, including pituitary, parathyroid, thyroid, adrenal, lacrimal and salivary glands, kidney, pancreas, intestine, lung

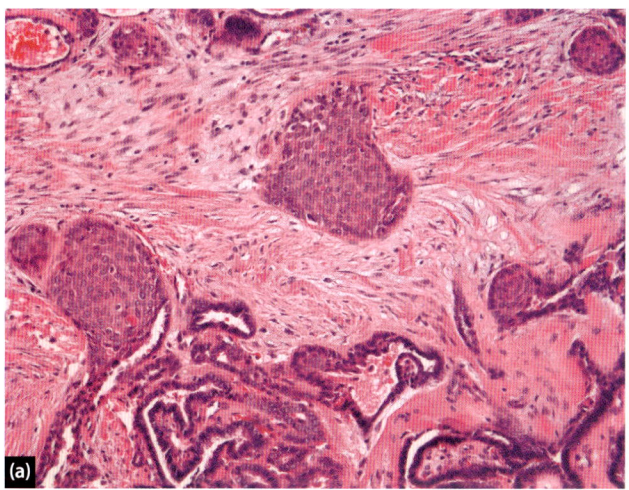 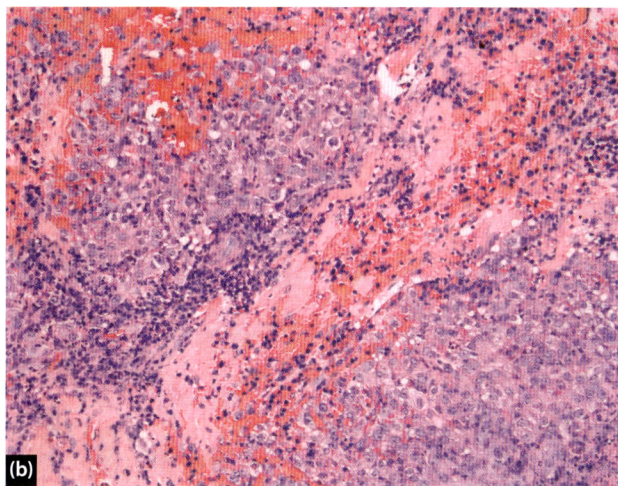

Figure 58.11 Squamous differentiation. (a) Papillary thyroid carcinoma exhibiting isolated areas of squamous differentiation (squamous morulae), which are seen focally in up to 50% of cases. The squamoid cells do not show the typical nuclear features that define PTC (*H&E stain, medium magnification*). (b) Carcinoma with thymus-like elements (CASTLE) showing smooth-contoured lobules of non-keratinizing squamoid epithelial cells demarcated by a central broad fibrous septum, percolated by lymphocytes and plasma cells (*H&E stain, medium magnification*).

TABLE 58.2 Conditions associated with squamous epithelium in the thyroid gland

Non-neoplastic	Neoplastic
Nodular hyperplasia (goitre)	Papillary carcinoma
Chronic lymphocytic thyroiditis and variants	Squamous cell carcinoma, primary or secondary
Hashimoto's thyroiditis	Mucoepidermoid carcinoma, primary or secondary
Following FNAC, core biopsy or contralateral lobectomy	Carcinoma with thymus-like elements (CASTLE)
Developmental solid cell nests and thymic rests	Teratoma

TABLE 58.3 Conditions associated with oncocytic (oxyphilic) epithelium in the thyroid gland[22, 24]

Non-neoplastic	Neoplastic
Hashimoto's thyroiditis	Follicular adenoma
Nodular hyperplasia	Follicular carcinoma
Graves' disease	Papillary thyroid carcinoma
Post-irradiation	Medullary carcinoma
Ageing	Anaplastic carcinoma

and sinonasal tract. The incidence of oncocytic change increases with advancing age and may be extensive at any one site (oncocytosis). When such cells occur in the thyroid, they are termed Hürthle cells (Askanazy cells). It is a purely descriptive term and does not in itself indicate biological potential – oncocytic cells occur in both non neoplastic and neoplastic (benign and malignant) conditions (mitochondriomas) (**Table 58.3**).

Oncocytic metaplasia is believed to occur in response to pathological or physiological stress and the oxygen-sensitive nature of the mitochondria renders the cells unusually susceptible to traumatic/ischaemic injury. There is ongoing debate as to whether such oncocytic transformation is a form of metaplasia or more correctly represents a process of transdifferentiation.[23] The pathogenetic mechanisms underpinning oncocytic change are complex. The genetic events driving oncocytic change involve mutations in mitochondrial DNA and somatic mutations that affect mitochondrial function. Importantly, these changes are largely unrelated to the genetic events that result in proliferation and neoplastic transformation of thyroid follicular epithelial cells.

There is hallmark concomitant nuclear enlargement often with striking nuclear pleomorphism, coarse karyoplasm and conspicuous nucleolation, even in benign oncocytes.

The distinction between oncocytic hyperplasia and neoplasia can be difficult, particularly in the context of thyroiditis. Note that, in autoimmune thyroid disease, oncocytic change is not restricted to Hashimoto's thyroiditis but may also be encountered in long-standing Graves' disease. Oncocytic change occurring in follicular nodules and/or multinodular goitre is conventionally regarded as hyperplastic, whereas clonality studies have demonstrated that many of the larger nodules are in fact monoclonal, thus the biologically correct approach would be to regard these as follicular adenomas.

The mitochondria themselves stain with the phosphotungstic acid haematoxylin (PTAH) method. Positive immunostaining for cytokeratins (notably CK14), vimentin, anti-mitochondrial antibody and weakly for thyroglobulin (TG) is typical. Carcinoembryonic antigen (CEA/CD66e) reactivity is variable. Electron microscopy demonstrates abnormally configured mitochondria (**Figure 58.12**).

Thyroiditis

The various manifestations of thyroiditis are summarized in **Table 58.4**. These may be either non-autoimmune or autoimmune, the latter typified by Hashimoto's thyroiditis and Graves' disease and their variants. Drug-induced thyroiditis is associated with the use of a number of drugs including amiodarone, lithium, interferon-alpha and interleukin-2 (**Figure 58.13**).

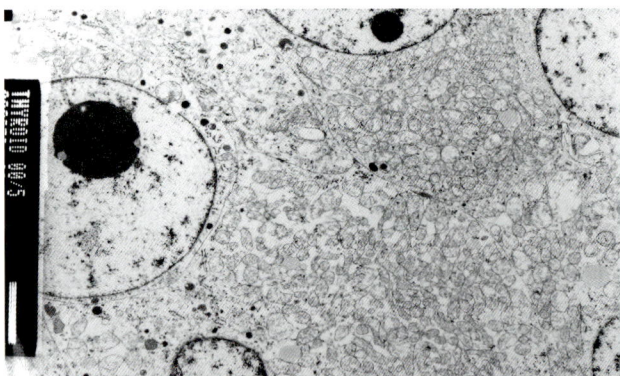

Figure 58.12 Transmission electron micrograph of several tumour cells from a poorly differentiated oncocytic (oxyphil) carcinoma of the thyroid gland. Note the cytoplasmic expansion by scores of swollen mitochondria and paucity of other cell organelles. Two prominent osmiophilic macronucleoli are also plainly seen (*TEM, ultra-high magnification*).

TABLE 58.4 Classification and features of thyroiditis[20, 22]

Characteristics	Hashimoto's thyroiditis (chronic lymphocytic or chronic autoimmune thyroiditis)	*Painless* Postpartum thyroiditis (subacute lymphocytic thyroiditis)	*Painless* Sporadic thyroiditis (subacute lymphocytic thyroiditis)	*Painful* Subacute thyroiditis (de Quervain's, giant-cell, pseudo-granulomatous thyroiditis)	*Suppurative* Thyroiditis (infectious, bacterial, pyogenic thyroiditis)	Riedel's thyroiditis
Age	All ages, peak 30–50	Childbearing age	All ages, peak 30–40	20–60	20–40	30–60
Sex ratio	8–9:1		2:1	5:1	1:1	3–4:1
Cause	Autoimmune	Autoimmune	Autoimmune	Unknown	Infectious	Unknown
Thyroid function	Hypothyroidism	Can be thyrotoxic, hypothyroid or both	Can be thyrotoxic, hypothyroid or both	Can be thyrotoxic, hypothyroid or both	Euthyroid	Euthyroid
TPO status	High	High	High	Low	Absent	Present
ESR	Normal	Normal	Normal	High	High	Normal
Gross pathological features	Symmetrical diffuse enlargement of the thyroid gland Firm consistency, pale colour and multilobulated	Firm to hard, tan white appearance and nodules of varying size	Firm to hard, tan white appearance and nodules of varying size	Firm to hard, tan white appearance and nodules of varying size	Variable appearance including focal or diffuse enlargement and abscess formation Can appear normal	Thyroid replaced by dense, tan-white, firm to hard tissue

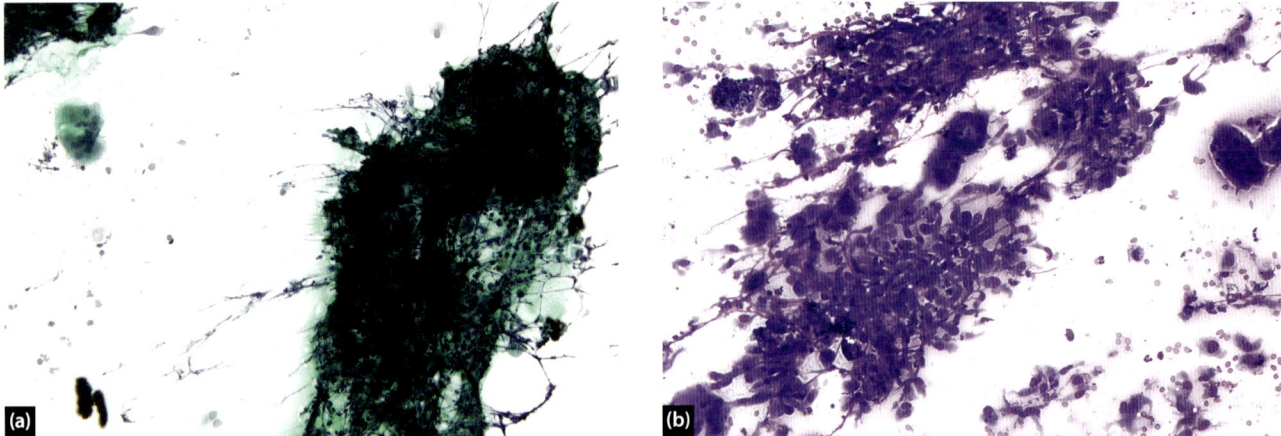

Figure 58.13 Thyroiditis. (a) FNAC sample in granulomatous thyroiditis, suspect of tuberculosis. Part of an epithelioid histiocytic granuloma is shown with characteristic overlapping, tangled, angulated ('hockey sticks') and elongated (smeared or streamed) nucleoplasm plus an adjacent dissociated polykaryocytic giant cell. There is no colloid content and no obvious necrosis (*Pap stain, medium magnification*). **(b)** Complimentary FNAC smear from the same case. Several epithelioid histiocytic granulomata are noted with more numerous plurinucleate giant cells. Again, there is minimal colloid. Care must be taken to discriminate between multi-nucleate giant cells, often of Langhans' type, of mononuclear/macrophage/histiocyte lineage and aspirated intact tri-dimensional thyroid follicles (pseudo-giant cells) (*MGG stain, medium magnification*). *(Continued)*

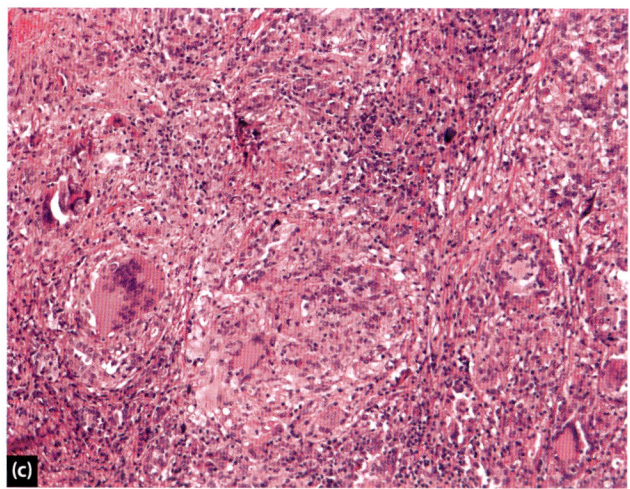
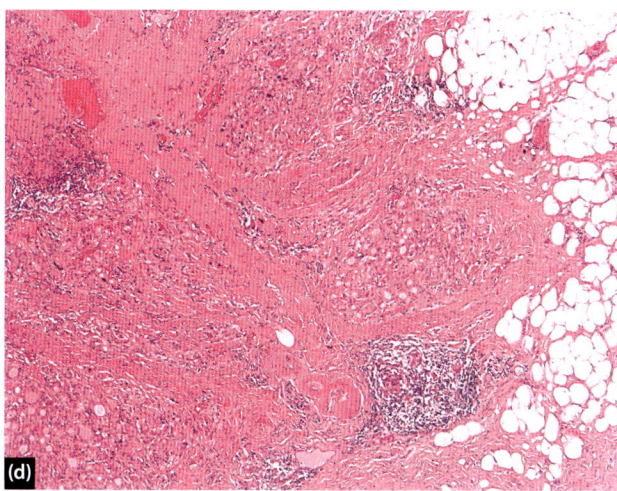
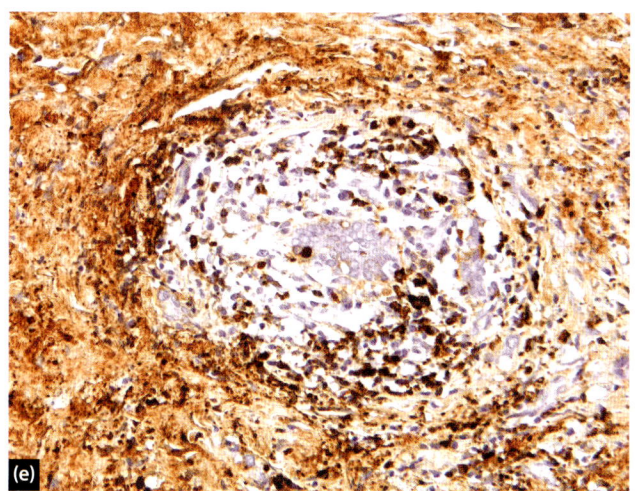

Figure 58.13 (Continued) Thyroiditis. (c) Non-necrotizing granulomatous thyroiditis typical of subacute (De Quervain's) thyroiditis. There is folliculocentric lymphohistiocytic inflammation, loose epithelioid granuloma formation with multinucleate giant cell transformation, follicle destruction and localized colloidophagy. There is little fibrosis in this early phase of the disease (*H&E stain, medium magnification*). **(d)** Riedel's thyroiditis (Riedel's struma, ligneous thyroiditis), acute phase illustrating destructive, non-granulomatous fibroinflammatory tissue percolating beyond thyroid gland pseudocapsule into perithyroidal fat with occasional lymphoid aggregates. Phlebitis and nodular fibro-occlusive vasculopathy were seen throughout this thyroid gland (*H&E stain, low magnification*). **(e)** Replicate section of Riedel's thyroiditis stained for IgG4, highlighting excess numbers of positive plasma cells plus more diffuse background reactivity, presumably of serum origin, supportive of IgG4-related sclerosing disease. Both the IgG4 positive plasma cell count per high-power field and the IgG4:IgG plasma cell ratio were elevated, though not uniformly throughout the specimen (*IgG4 IHC, high magnification*).

Lateral aberrant thyroid tissue

Lateral aberrant thyroid (LAT) tissue or gland describes anomalous deposits of follicular thyroid tissue in the lateral neck. Originally believed to indicate persistent lateral thyroid anlage, the modern view is that the overwhelming majority, but not all, actually represent metastatic follicular thyroid carcinoma or follicular variant of papillary thyroid carcinoma (PTC), the cytonuclear morphology of which may be so deceptively bland as to be virtually indistinguishable from normal or hyperplastic thyroid parenchyma proper.[23]

Pragmatically, any such deposits lateral to the carotid sheath ought to be regarded as metastatic disease until otherwise proven. Those extracapsular deposits medial to the carotid sheath may represent either benign sequestrated (parasitic) thyroid nodules (**Figure 58.14**), which generally recapitulate the appearances in the body of the main gland proper, or metastatic tumour. Benign thyroid tissue inclusions in cervical lymph nodes are rarely encountered and are difficult to confirm with certainty.

Hyperplastic nodules

Historically, multiple nodules as part of multinodular goitre, either incompletely capsulated or unencapsulated, are designated hyperplastic (adenomatoid or cellular colloid) nodules. One or more may predominate, thereby simulating a solitary nodule clinically and/or radiologically (**Figure 58.15**). They do not normally compress the adjacent gland, which oftentimes displays a similar growth pattern. Secondary retrogressive changes frequently present, sometimes extensive, include coarse fibrosclerosis (sometimes resembling a radial scar), cystic degeneration, calcification, infarction, fresh haemorrhage, haemosiderosis, siderophages, foam cells, cholesterol granulomata, endarteritis obliterans and localized inflammation. Squamous, lipocytic, chondroid, osseous and oncocytic (oxyphil) metaplasia are occasionally seen. Simple papillae (papillary hyperplastic nodule) do rarely occur and the papillae tend to radiate towards the centre of the lesion (**Figure 58.16**).[25] Exhaustive efforts to exclude papillary thyroid carcinoma must be pursued under these circumstances.

The concept of thyroid follicular epithelial dysplasia remains theoretical. Up to 70% of hyperplastic nodules are in fact clonal proliferations and can express various markers of malignant follicular-patterned thyroid tumours. However, no morphological, immunohistochemical or molecular study to date has been able to discriminate between adenomatoid nodules, follicular adenoma and follicular carcinoma with absolute sensitivity and specificity.[26]

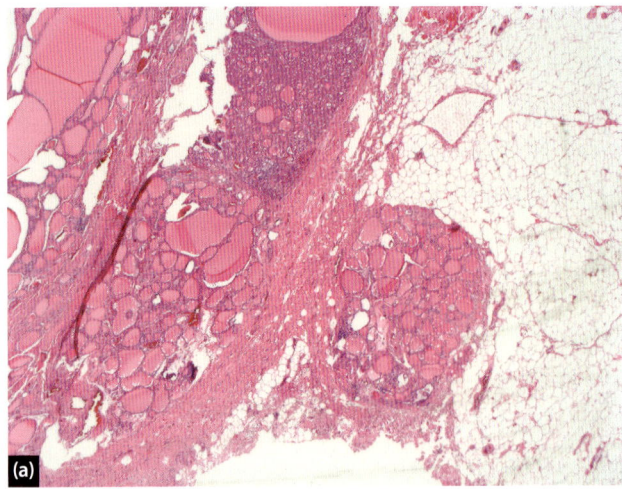
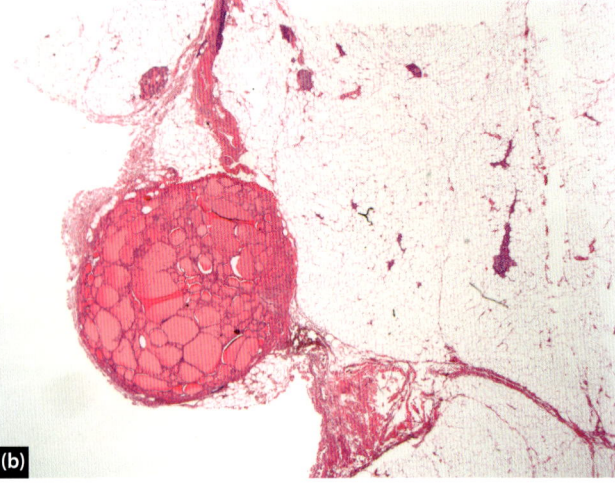

Figure 58.14 Lateral aberrant thyroid tissue. (a) Pericapsular thyroid nodule protruding outside the confines of the anatomical thyroid pseudocapsule, impinging upon perithyroidal fat with an expansile contour. This is the formative stage of sequestration (*H&E stain, low magnification*). **(b)** Extraglandular sequestrated (parasitic) thyroid nodule, completely detached from eutopic thyroid gland proper, but still within the confines of the central neck compartment (*H&E stain, low magnification*).

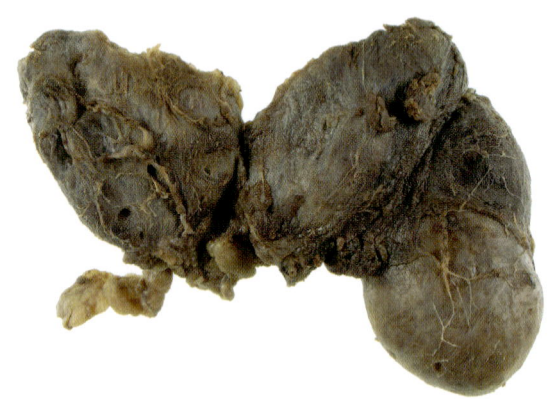

Figure 58.15 Total thyroidectomy specimen showing a protruberant, well-circumscribed, ovoid mass arising from the left lower pole, clinically excised as a solitary thyroid nodule. This proved to be a dominant hyperplastic (adenomatoid) nodule arising in chronic lymphocytic (Hashimoto's) thyroiditis with several smaller intraparenchymal nodules throughout the main body of the gland bilaterally.

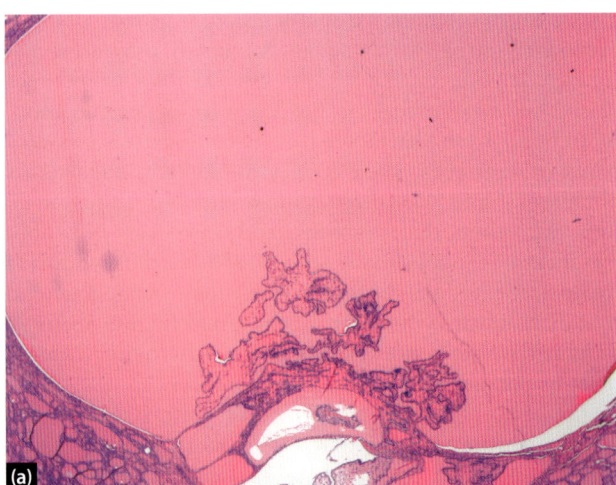
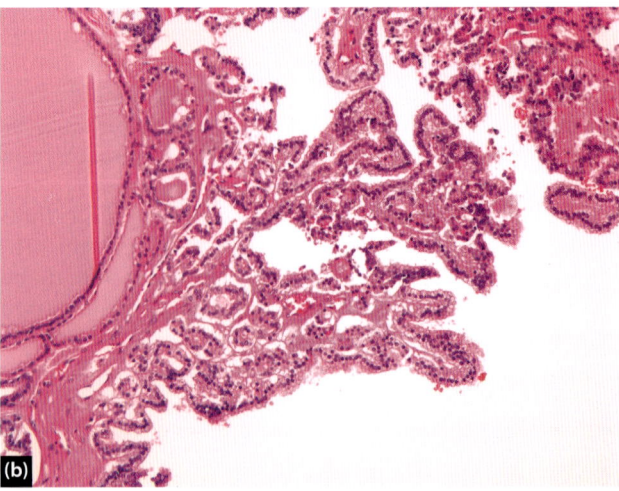

Figure 58.16 Hyperplastic nodules. (a) The edge of a papillary hyperplastic nodule showing localized intracystic mural papillary proliferation immersed in colloid. The papillary projections are simple in contour and tend to project towards the epicentre of the lesion (*H&E stain, low magnification*). **(b)** Part of a different intracystic papillary hyperplastic nodule, also illustrating arborescent centrifugally projecting papillae. The epithelial cells are monolayered, well-polarized and bland. There were no cytonuclear or architectural features to indicate papillary thyroid carcinoma despite a rigorous search (*H&E stain, medium magnification*).

Follicular adenoma

The WHO (4th edition, 2017) classification of tumours of the thyroid gland is reproduced in **Table 58.5**.[27] Follicular adenoma classically occurs as a solitary benign, encapsulated tumour, which shows follicular epithelial differentiation with no evidence of either capsular or vascular invasion and neither architectural nor cytonuclear features of papillary thyroid carcinoma (**Figure 58.17**). It possesses a circumferential, smooth-contoured or gently undulating, slender, fibrous delimiting capsule, usually displaying little variation in thickness – fields of capsular augmentation warrant a conscientious search to exclude a carcinoma, especially if FNAC has not previously been attempted. Surrounding native gland may be compressed and/or atrophic.[8, 22] Internally, there may be a variety of growth patterns, such as normofollicular, microfollicular (foetal), macrofollicular (colloid), solid, trabecular and organoid, though the architecture tends to be fairly uniform within any individual example. Mitoses are few. Degenerative stromal changes, particularly post-FNAC, are identical to multinodular hyperplasia but squamous metaplasia is uncommon and, where present, merits consideration of papillary thyroid carcinoma, follicular variant (FVPTC).

Histological subtypes of adenoma include solid, foetal, oxyphilic (oncocytic), clear cell, signet ring cell (**Figure 58.18**) and lipoadenoma, defined according to the predominant growth pattern (accounting for over 75% of the overall tumour). These, however, do not differ clinically or in biological behaviour from conventional follicular adenoma. There is some commonality in architecture and cytological pattern across the follicular tumours, both adenomas and carcinomata (**Box 58.1**).

Atypical adenoma (follicular tumour of uncertain malignant potential, FT-UMP) is used to describe follicular neoplasms that display some worrisome microscopical features though falling short of unequivocal capsular or vascular infiltration.[28] These include irregularly thickened capsule, partial thickness incursions into, but not completely through, the capsule, hypercellularity, increased mitoses and/or abnormal forms and nuclear atypia (**Figure 58.19**).

TABLE 58.5 WHO classification of tumours of the thyroid gland[35]

Follicular adenoma

Hyalinizing trabecular tumour

Other encapsulated follicular-patterned thyroid tumours
Follicular tumour of uncertain malignant potential
Well-differentiated tumour of uncertain malignant potential
Non-invasive follicular thyroid neoplasm with papillary-like nuclear features

Papillary thyroid carcinoma (PTC)
Papillary carcinoma
Follicular variant of PTC
Encapsulated variant of PTC
Papillary microcarcinoma
Columnar cell variant of PTC
Oncocytic variant of PTC

Follicular thyroid carcinoma (FTC), NOS
FTC, minimally invasive
FTC, encapsulated angioinvasive
FTC, widely invasive

Hürthle (oncocytic) cell tumours
Hürthle cell adenoma
Hürthle cell carcinoma

Poorly differentiated thyroid carcinoma

Anaplastic thyroid carcinoma

Squamous cell carcinoma

Medullary thyroid carcinoma

Mixed medullary and follicular thyroid carcinoma

Mucoepidermoid carcinoma

Sclerosing mucoepidermoid carcinoma with eosinophilla

Mucinous carcinoma

Ectopic thymoma

Spindle epithelial tumour with thymus-like differentiation

Intrathyroid thymic carcinoma

Paraganglioma and mesenchymal/stromal tumours
Paraganglioma
Peripheral nerve sheath tumours (PNSTs)
    Schwannoma
    Malignant PNST
Benign vascular tumours
    Haemangioma
    Cavernous haemangioma
    Lymphangioma
Angiosarcoma
Smooth muscle tumours
    Leiomyoma
    Leiomyosarcoma
Solitary fibrous tumour

Haematolymphoid tumours
Langerhans cell histiocytosis
Rosai-Dorfman disease
Follicular dendritic cell sarcoma
Primary thyroid lymphoma

Germ cell tumours
Benign teratoma (grade 0 or 1)
Immature teratoma (grade 2)
Malignant teratoma (grade 3)

Secondary tumours

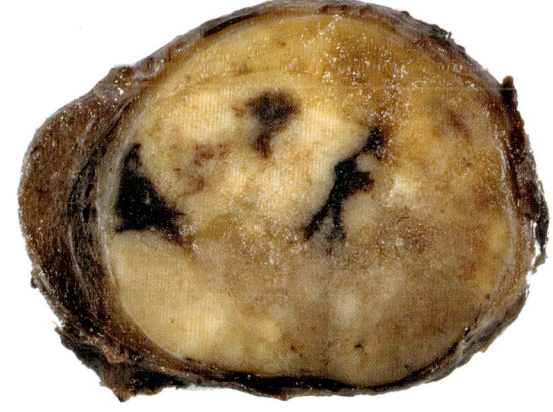

Figure 58.17 The cut surface of a benign follicular adenoma showing a largely solid, fleshy texture with localized cystic change. The perimeter is evenly contoured and the investing capsule is uniformly slender.

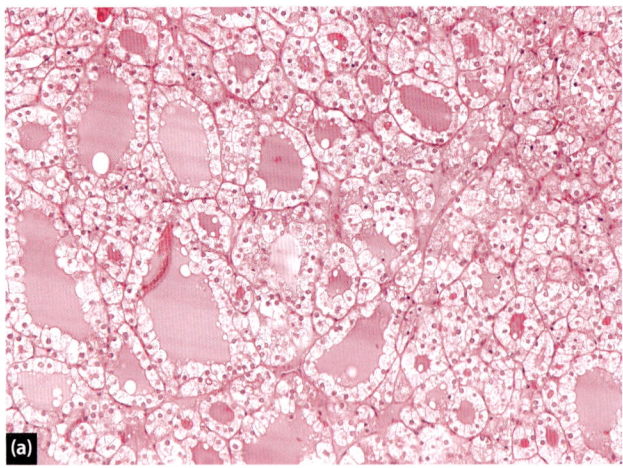 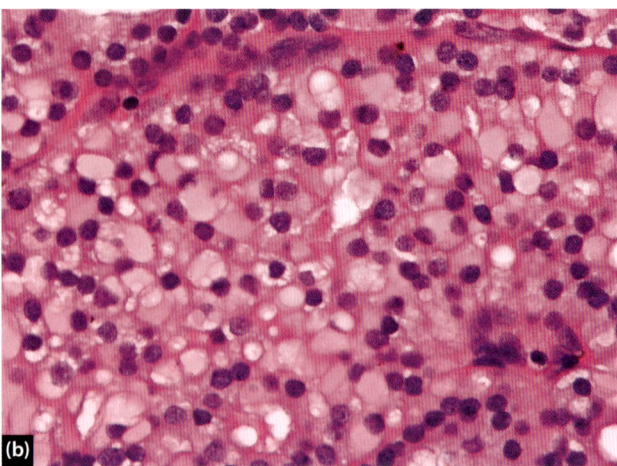

Figure 58.18 Follicular adenoma. (a) Clear cell variant of follicular adenoma. Virtually the entire tumour was composed of colloid filled follicles bounded by thyrocytes possessing abundant faintly reticulated, optically clear cytoplasm (*H&E stain, medium magnification*). **(b)** Signet ring variant of follicular neoplasm. The individual cells are bloated by dense eosinophilic cytoplasm sometimes displacing and/or compressing the nucleus to the cytoplasmic periphery (signet ring appearance) (*H&E stain, high magnification*).

BOX 58.1 Histological variants of follicular neoplasms

- Hyalinizing trabecular adenoma and carcinoma
- Signet ring adenoma and carcinoma
- Mucinous variant
- Clear cell follicular neoplasm (lipid-rich adenoma)
- Follicular adenoma with papillary hyperplasia
- Encapsulated papillary oncocytic neoplasm (follicular adenoma and carcinoma, oncocytic variant with papillary growth)
- Glomeruloid variant
- Meningioma-like tumour of the thyroid
- Follicular neoplasm with lipomatous stroma (adenolipoma/lipoadenoma/thyrolipoma)
- Follicular neoplasm with cartilaginous metaplasia
- Atypical adenoma
- Follicular adenoma with bizarre nuclei
- Hyperfunctioning follicular tumours ('hot nodules')

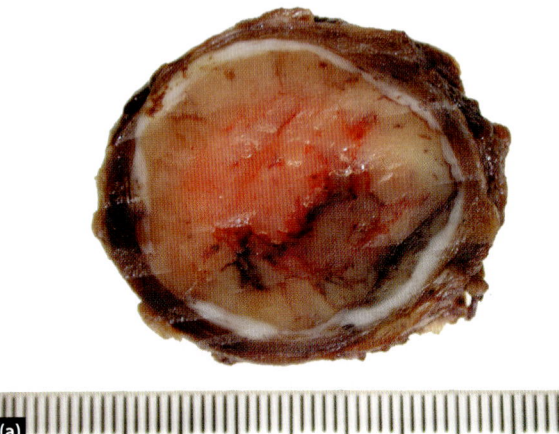 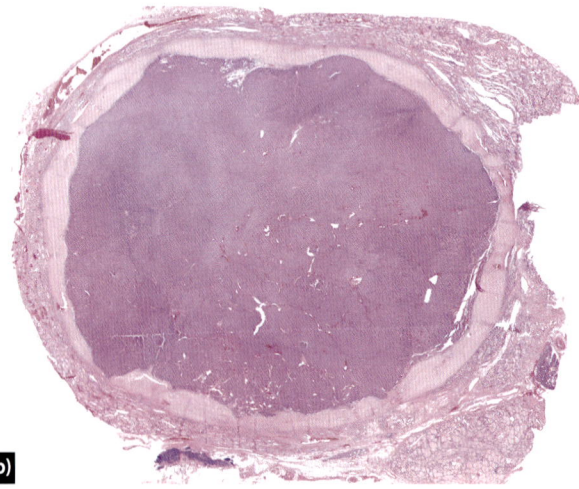

Figure 58.19 Atypical follicular adenoma. (a) A cross-sectional slice through an atypical adenoma (follicular tumour of uncertain malignant potential, FT-UMP). Despite the widespread capsular fibrosis and multiple, irregular, virtually full-thickness internal incursions, at no point can convincing complete transcapsular infiltration be demonstrated. **(b)** Whole mount preparation of the same lesion. Circumferentially, tumour does not invade beyond the original capsular contour (*H&E stain, ultra-low magnification*).

Hyalinizing trabecular tumours

Hyalinizing trabecular tumours (HTTs) are a group of neoplasms originally regarded as adenomas (hyalinizing trabecular adenoma/HTA, paraganglioma-like adenoma of the thyroid/PLAT). It has subsequently transpired that the supposed characteristic organoid growth pattern with interstitial perivascular hyalinization may also be seen focally in nodular hyperplasia plus a number of other benign and malignant thyroid neoplasms, many, though not all, showing histological features of papillary thyroid carcinoma, including *RET/PTC* gene rearrangements. In those examples of pure HTT architecture without papillary carcinomatous morphology

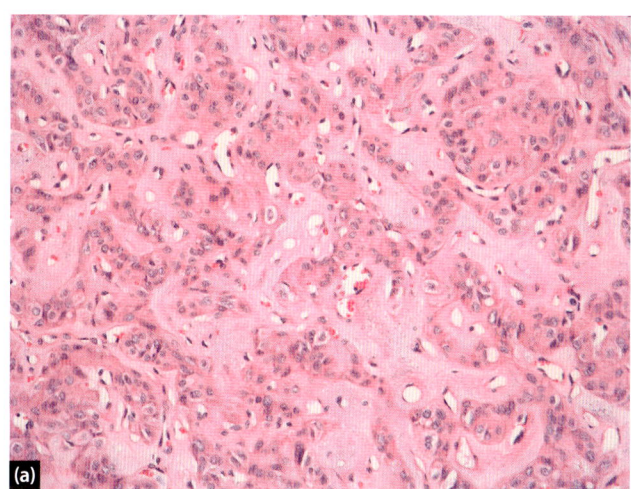
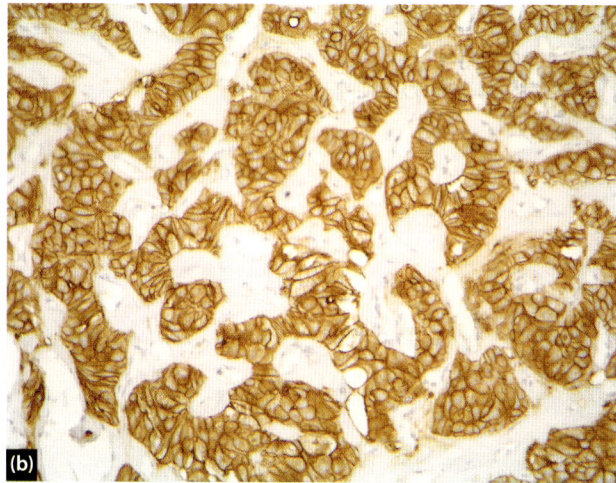

Figure 58.20 Hyalinizing trabecular tumour. (a) Minimally invasive hyalinizing trabecular carcinoma demonstrating the typical organoid nested and trabecular architecture separated by hyalinized interstitium, richly endowed with blood vessels. Elsewhere, this example showed mushrooming transcapsular growth. There are no features to suggest papillary thyroid carcinoma in this neoplasm but there was synchronous classical papillary thyroid carcinoma separately in the specimen (*H&E stain, medium magnification*). **(b)** The same tumour illustrating universal Ki67 (MIB-1) immunoreactivity. Note that this is peculiarly membranous and cytoplasmic in distribution and is antibody clone/manufacturing source dependent. Ki67 is conventionally used as a proliferation marker where, in other circumstances, it stains the nuclei only of those cells in certain phases of the cell cycle (*Ki67 IHC, medium magnification*).

there appears to be a spectrum of biological potential ranging from adenoma to carcinoma, both minimally invasive and widely invasive by conventional criteria.[29] A proportion of such neoplasms exhibit characteristic, peculiar, avid cytoplasmic Ki67 (MIB-1) immunostaining (**Figure 58.20**). Immunopositivity for cytokeratins, thyroglobulin and vimentin generally with negative pan-neuroendocrine marker and calcitonin staining discriminates HTT from paraganglioma proper and medullary thyroid carcinoma.

Follicular carcinoma of the thyroid

Follicular thyroid carcinoma (FTC) is a malignant epithelial tumour arising in both eutopic thyroid gland and/or heterotopic thyroid tissue, showing follicular cell differentiation and bereft of the characteristic features of papillary thyroid carcinoma (PTC). It accounts for 5–15% of all thyroid cancers in iodine-sufficient regions. It spreads via haematogenous routes, preferentially to bone and lung with metastatic disease as a presenting feature in 11% of patients. It is divided into two basic categories defined by the extent of capsular infiltration and/or presence of vascular invasion (**Table 58.6**) and meticulous examination of the tumour capsule and interface with native gland is consequently of paramount importance.

Minimally invasive follicular carcinoma (MIFC) is the common variant and is characterized by microscopical transcapsular invasion and/or pericapsular vascular infiltration.[30] With experience, obvious capsular violation and/or accompanying fibrous capsular thickening may be appreciated in the gross specimen by the unaided eye (**Figure 58.21**), but not more subtle capsular transgression or vascular permeation.

Widely invasive follicular carcinoma (WIFC) is readily identified grossly by infiltrative, destructive or sometimes multinodular growth, the latter separated by fibrous bands, expanding into surrounding native gland. This may be so strikingly obviously nodular as to be mistaken for multinodular hyperplasia by the unwary, particularly if there is no clearly identifiable vestige of pre-existing capsule for reference.

The interpretation of capsular invasion remains somewhat controversial. Most authorities require full-thickness capsular transgression beyond the original lesional contour (capsular invasive MIFC), whereas a dwindling minority of authors accept a given neoplasm as MIFC if it shows only partial-thickness capsular penetration. Full-thickness violation manifests as multiple foci, less commonly a single nidus, of mushrooming herniation bulging into and displacing surrounding native follicles, without infiltrative/permeative growth. Lateral fibrous capsular thickening (buttressing) and neocapsule formation along the advancing tumour to gland interface are paradigmatic,

TABLE 58.6 Classification of follicular thyroid carcinoma[27]

Traditional	AFIP 2015		WHO 2017
Minimally invasive	Minimally invasive	With capsular invasion	Minimally invasive
		With limited vascular invasion (<4 vessels)	Encapsulated angioinvasive
		With extensive vascular invasion (≥4 vessels)	Widely invasive
Widely invasive	Widely invasive		Widely invasive

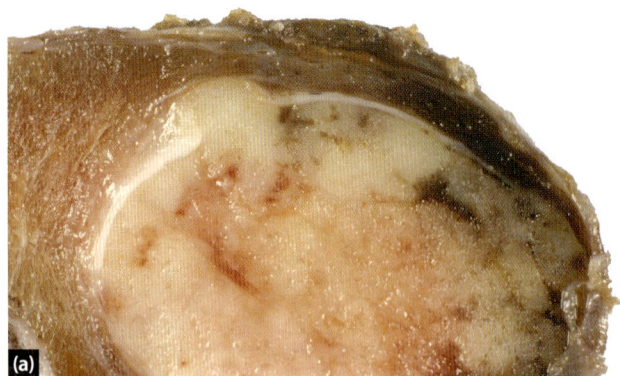
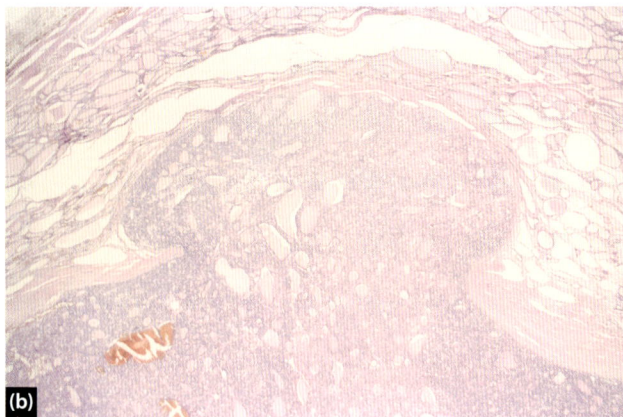

Figure 58.21 **Minimally invasive follicular carcinoma. (a)** Obvious mushrooming, full-thickness, transcapsular herniation qualifying as minimally invasive follicular carcinoma, easily discernible to the unaided eye during dissection. There is slight lateral capsular buttressing but negligible neocapsule formation along the advancing margin in this example. Note that there is no universally endorsed maximum size limit for this phenomenon. **(b)** The same area viewed histologically corroborates streaming impingement into perilesional native gland with no tentacular/permeative infiltration and neither significant host inflammatory nor stromal response (*H&E stain, low magnification*).

but not invariable. Incomplete capsular encroachment includes areas of irregular, serratiform and/or undulating inner capsular contour, perpendicular dentate capsular incursions and horizontally disposed (entrapped) intracapsular follicles, which do not qualify, though they should prompt further detailed scrutiny, as should any unexplained area of capsular expansion. Circumscribed extracapsular (satellite) nodules may represent MIFC visualized outside the plane of connection with the body of the tumour (though such a pedicle may sometimes be impossible to demonstrate) or a sequestrated (parasitic) congerie of benign follicles. Comparison of the cytonuclear features with the main tumour bulk may aid discrimination here. Current recommendation is that, unless there is identifiable connection with the main tumour mass, such satellitosis should not be regarded as definite evidence of capsular violation.

Artefactual capsular puncture, healing and distortion following FNAC should be interpreted with caution and the entry/exit site of normal capsular blood vessels, where there is typically smooth curvilinear capsular interruption, not misconstrued. Well-sampled tumours that fall short of these criteria are termed follicular tumour of uncertain malignant potential (FT-UMP).

There are studies indicating that both the existence and the extent of vascular invasion are of portentous significance. Whilst there is a general consensus as to what defines angioinvasion (grossly encapsulated angioinvasive MIFC), there remains some dissent. The majority opinion is that tumour penetration should be into medium-calibre or large-calibre intracapsular or extracapsular blood vessels and polypoidal intraluminal growth should be endothelialized with/or without thrombus, though not necessarily adherent (**Figure 58.22**). Tumour invasion and obturation of large calibre veins is sometimes a feature, extending beyond the confines of the thyroid gland, in a pattern akin to infiltration of the renal vein/vena cava by clear cell carcinoma of the kidney. A point of attachment of tumour to vessel wall is a prerequisite for some observers. Free-lying nests of tumour cells may represent artefactual dislodgement. Tumour cells occupying capillary-sized intracapsular vessels are of no proven clinical importance and should be discounted. Tumour within intralesional or subcapsular vessels does not qualify. Reactive vascular endothelial hyperplasia may simulate angioinvasion and, when recognized, ought to prompt a rigorous search for vascular invasion proper. Immunostaining for vascular endothelial markers (e.g. CD31, CD34) and lymphatic endothelium (e.g. D2-40) may be helpful in selected instances. Cognizant that absolute discrimination between blood vessel invasion and lymphatic space infiltration may ultimately be impossible, the RCPath defines vascular invasion as involvement of any definite endothelial-lined space and the current College of American Pathologists (CAP) protocol recommends merging the two and reporting under the unifying designation of lymphovascular invasion.[32]

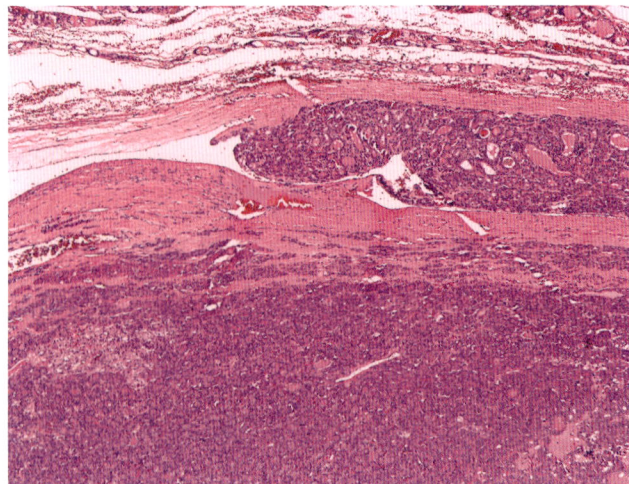

Figure 58.22 **Pericapsular angioinvasion qualifying as encapsulated (angioinvasive) minimally invasive follicular carcinoma.** There is a broad tongue of endothelialized tumour unequivocally protruding into a large-calibre intracapsular vessel (*H&E stain, low magnification*).

Capsular invasive MIFC without lymphovascular invasion portends an extremely low risk of metastasis (less than 1%), justifying the option of a conservative management approach with treatment by lobectomy, acknowledging that there is a small risk of undertreatment in a minority of cases. The term grossly encapsulated angioinvasive follicular carcinoma has been proposed for encapsulated tumours with any foci of lymphovascular invasion, based on the premise that access to even one or a few endothelial-lined vessels confers the capacity for more aggressive behaviour with heightened risk of recurrence, thereby offsetting a designation of minimal invasion. Encapsulated angioinvasive MIFC with limited (minimal) vascular invasion, defined as a few microscopic foci (up to 4 foci) is said to show a low risk of metastasis (approximately 5%). MIFC with more extensive lymphovascular infiltration (defined as 5 or more foci) is said to portend a higher likelihood of metastasis (up to 42%)[33, 34] and the term grossly encapsulated follicular carcinoma with extensive angioinvasion acknowledges this. Specifying a precise threshold for the number of foci of lymphovascular invasion is, however, controversial, not least because a histological section is a two-dimensional representation of a tri-dimensional system and inadvertent replication by counting infiltration potentially into the same vessel visualized in close proximity and/or in a different plane of section is of dubious biological validity and reproducibility.

WIFC is an aggressive neoplasm with a high risk of distant secondaries (29–66%). It displays infiltrative growth within and beyond the anatomical thyroid pseudocapsule proper, sometimes in the form of successive generations of herniating capsular transgression (**Figure 58.23**). Vascular penetration is common and the more widespread it is, the worse the prognosis.

Extrathyroidal extension (ETE) describes involvement of perithyroidal soft tissues by primary thyroid carcinoma. This may be further subdivided into microscopic (minimal/minor/limited) ETE and macroscopic (extensive/major/massive/marked/gross) ETE. As previously noted, the thyroid pseudocapsule is not a discrete anatomical structure, is incomplete or focally absent in a majority of individuals, is additionally fenestrated by lymphovascular channels and contains small nerve radicles. The histological evaluation of minimal ETE into immediate peri-thyroidal soft tissue is consequently subjective, prone to poor reproducibility and, owing to its limited prognostic value, has been expunged from the UICC/TNM (8th edition, 2017) staging schema.[35] Importantly, both adipocytes and skeletal muscle bundles may be normally encountered within the thyroid gland and may also be a component of a variety of pathological thyroid conditions. The identification of a desmoplastic response, adipocytic and/or muscular impingement in close proximity to large-calibre, thick-walled vessels and/or large nerve trunks, on the other hand, may be more helpful, as such would not be expected within the confines of the thyroid gland proper. Extensive ETE is characterized by direct infiltration well beyond the limits of the thyroid gland into anterior strap musculature (sternohyoid M, sternothyroid M, thyrohyoid M and/or omohyoid M), subcutis, neighbouring viscera including larynx, trachea, oesophagus, recurrent laryngeal nerve, carotid artery or mediastinal vasculature. Extensive ETE is invariably obvious, typically identified by the surgeon perioperatively.

The prognosis for those carcinomas with minimal ETE worsens referenced against those without ETE. Similarly, the survival prospects for those suffering carcinomas with extensive ETE are significantly diminished in comparison with minimal ETE.

Gross or microscopic involvement of surgical margins informs the TNM R stage of a tumour and is of prognostic significance. There is no evidence-based definition for the distance required for complete excision, simply that non-neoplastic tissue is interposed between tumour and excision plane. The exercise of measuring the distance of tumour to closest resection margin is therefore somewhat arbitrary.[33, 36] Initial studies suggesting that a microscopically positive posterior margin poses a significantly higher risk of recurrence than a positive anterior margin merits further scrutiny.[33]

Oncocytic (oxyphil) cell tumours

Follicular neoplasms comprising 75% or more oncocytic (oxyphil) cells are designated as such and are subclassified according to the same criteria as their non-oncocytic counterparts based upon morphology, immunohistochemical profiling and molecular markers as oncocytic (oxyphil) adenoma, oncocytic (oxyphil) tumour of uncertain malignant potential, minimally or widely invasive oncocytic (oxyphil) carcinoma (Hürthle cell carcinoma). Oncocytic variants of papillary thyroid carcinoma, poorly differentiated thyroid carcinoma, undifferentiated (anaplastic) carcinoma and medullary thyroid carcinoma are recognized. Focal clear cell change is common in oncocytic tumours and, where this constitutes over 75% of the lesion, it is traditionally designated as clear cell carcinoma. Under such circumstances, it is imperative to exclude metastatic carcinoma (e.g. renal or adrenal),[37] malignant melanoma, intrathyroidal parathyroid gland neoplasms and clear cell variant of medullary thyroid carcinoma.

Grossly, they are usually single nodules (solitary oxyphil follicular tumour, SOFT) (**Figure 58.24**), although they may be multiple (multiple oxyphil follicular tumour, MOFT) and

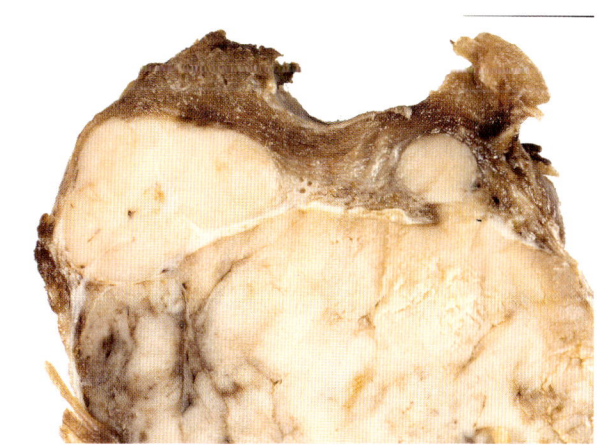

Figure 58.23 The cut surface of a widely invasive follicular carcinoma demonstrating successive generations of capsular transgression to the point where the original lesional capsule becomes almost obscured.

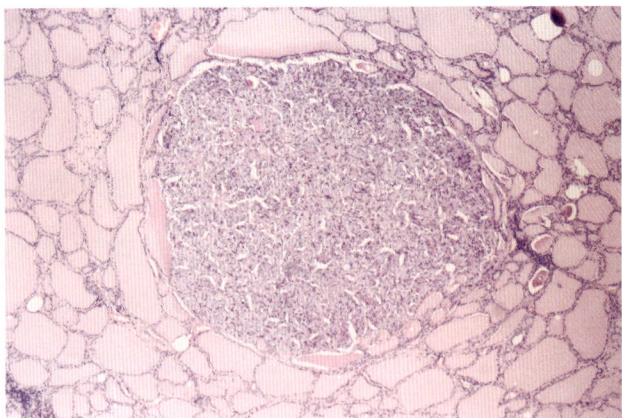

Figure 58.24 A small, benign solitary oncocytic (oxyphil) cell follicular tumour (SOFT), occurring sporadically in a background of chronic lymphocytic (Hashimoto's) thyroiditis. Despite its lack of capsule and occasional rudimentary papillae, there were no diagnostic features to suggest papillary thyroid carcinoma (*H&E stain, low magnification*).

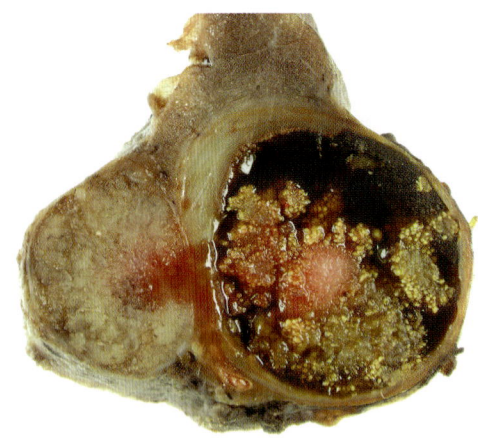

Figure 58.25 The cut surface of a classical papillary thyroid carcinoma illustrating a solid, granular appearance with adjoining encysted elements distended by inspissated colloid. The yellow punctate structures represent psammoma calcification and imparted a gritty texture.

are sometimes associated with Hashimoto's thyroiditis and/or conventional papillary thyroid carcinoma (PTC). A higher proportion of oncocytic (oxyphil) tumours are malignant than other follicular lesions, and when staged comparably there is some experience that they fare worse than their non-oncocytic counterparts, possibly a sequela of their low avidity for radioiodine. The incidence of malignancy in oncocytic (oxyphil) cell neoplasms increases with size, with 17%, 23% and 65% or more associated with maximum dimensions of less than 1 cm, between 1 cm and 4 cm and larger than 4 cm respectively.[38] Most examples are sporadic. Familial examples are rare and may indicate a germline mutation.[39]

Macroscopically they are classically mahogany brown tumours with a propensity for ischaemic infarction, either spontaneously or post-FNAC. They may show numerous histological patterns, including papillary areas, which may morphologically overlap with oncocytic (oxyphil) papillary thyroid carcinoma (PTC). They are typified by cytonuclear atypia and mitoses, though in isolation these do not reproducibly predict biological behaviour.

Oncocytic (oxyphil) parathyroid gland neoplasms should always be considered when evaluating a potential oncocytic (oxyphil) thyroid neoplasm, as they may be indistinguishable by routine orthodox microscopy without recourse to immunostaining.

Papillary thyroid carcinoma

Papillary thyroid carcinoma (PTC) is a malignant epithelial tumour showing follicular cell differentiation with characteristic nuclear features. It accounts for approximately 80% of all thyroid cancer and is also the commonest paediatric thyroid malignancy. In adults it typically occurs between the ages of 20 and 50 years with a female preponderance with less pronounced gender bias in patients over 50 years old. It normally carries an excellent prognosis, especially in younger patients. In areas of adequate dietary iodine, papillary thyroid carcinoma usually presents as a solitary thyroid nodule. In regions of iodine insufficiency multinodular goitre is common and papillary thyroid carcinoma can present as a more prominent or distinctive nodule. It has a propensity for lymphatogenous spread, initially to locoregional lymph nodes.

The potential macroscopical and microscopical manifestations of PTC are protean. Prototypically, it is invasive with irregular outline and either a scirrhous or granular, gritty texture often with multiloculated cystic change and colloid contents (**Figure 58.25**). The encapsulated follicular variant of PTC (EFVPTC, Lindsay tumour) is usually well circumscribed possessing a solid, fleshy cut-surface, closely resembling an adenoma.

The principal defining feature of PTC is its nuclear morphology by light microscopy (**Figure 58.26**), thus the diagnosis of PTC is sustainable even in the absence of invasive growth. Crucially, however, the distinctive appearances may be very localized and, in an appropriate context, the diagnosis may still be entertained in their absence. Ordinarily, there is at least focal nucleomegaly, nuclear crowding and nuclear overlap ('basket of eggs'). Homogenization of karyoplasm ('ground glass' nuclei) with margination of chromatin (likened to the empty-looking, pupil-less eyes of Harold Gray's cartoon strip characters, most famously the waif Little Orphan Annie and her canine companion Sandy) is characteristic, but not pathognomonic. It is not invariable, it is rarely present in FNAC and frozen sections, it may be encountered in other non-neoplastic conditions (notably Hashimoto's thyroiditis, Graves' disease and dyshormonogenetic goitre), it may be simulated by suboptimal tissue fixation (bubbly or pseudo-clear artefact) and is subject to vagaries of inter-observer and intra-observer reproducibility. Longitudinal nuclear grooves ('coffee beans'), nucleolemmal scalloping ('rat bites'), rents and irregularity formed by redundant, folded nuclear membrane and intranuclear cytoplasmic inclusions (pseudo-inclusions) formed by cytoplasmic herniation are typical and may be visualized on both FNAC and frozen section (**Figure 58.27**), but these again are not exclusive and may be mimicked by emptier looking intranuclear bubble artefact (pseudo-pseudo-inclusions,

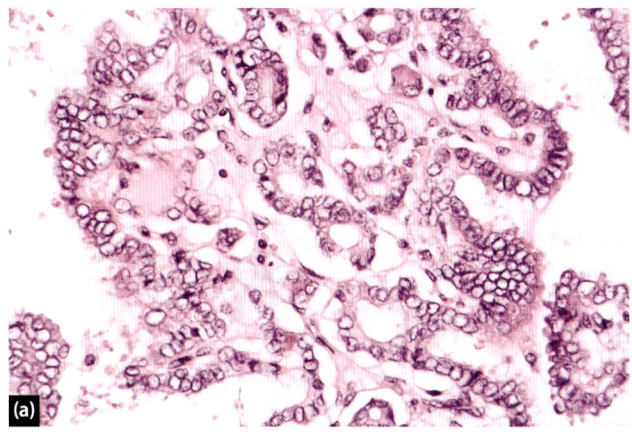
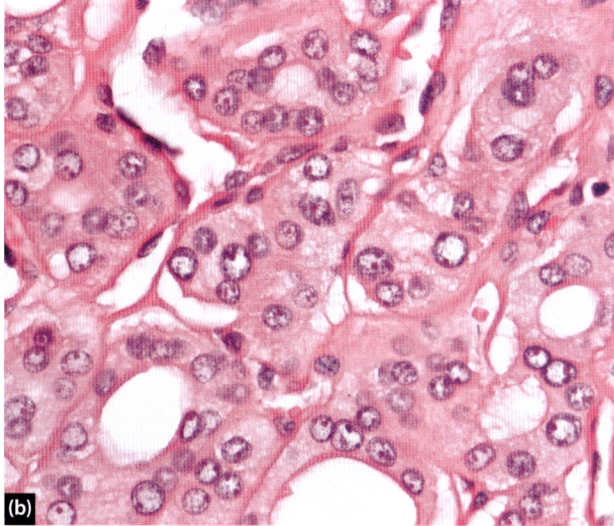
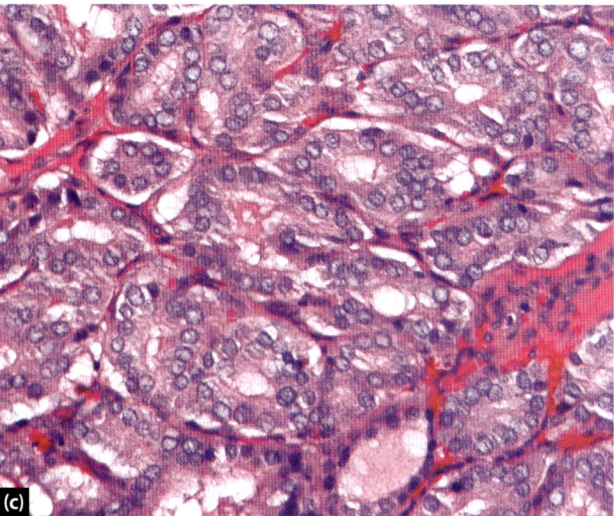

Figure 58.26 Papillary thyroid carcinoma. (a) The characteristic nuclear enlargement, nuclear crowding, nuclear overlap (basket of eggs) and optically clear karyoplasm (Little Orphan Annie eye) of papillary thyroid carcinoma. A few nuclear grooves (coffee beans) and isolated intranuclear cytoplasmic inclusions are also present. **(b)** For comparison, this depicts pseudo-clear (bubbly) nuclear artefact, consequent upon suboptimal tissue fixation and processing. Although there is some anisonucleosis and margination of chromatin, there is no real nuclear crowding or overlap. The nucleoplasm is polyvacuolated with conspicuous nucleolation. Pseudo-inclusions (vacuoles or holes) are numerous, much less densely staining than the thyrocyte cytoplasm and they lack any sharply delimiting nucleolemmal rim. Furthermore, these changes are strikingly zonated, seen towards the centre of a dominant hyperplastic nodule and gradually merged with propitiously preserved follicles more peripherally (*H&E stain, high magnification*). **(c)** Dyshormonogenetic goitre from an adolescent with Pendred's syndrome. Again, there is apparent homogenization of chromatin with plentiful nuclear grooves ('coffee beans'), albeit with evenly disposed nuclei and preponderant follicular-patterned growth. The very comprehensive, bilateral and diffuse distribution of these changes throughout the entire gland with preserved lobular architecture militates against malignancy here, with the proviso that this may be a vexatious differential diagnosis (*H&E stain, high magnification*).

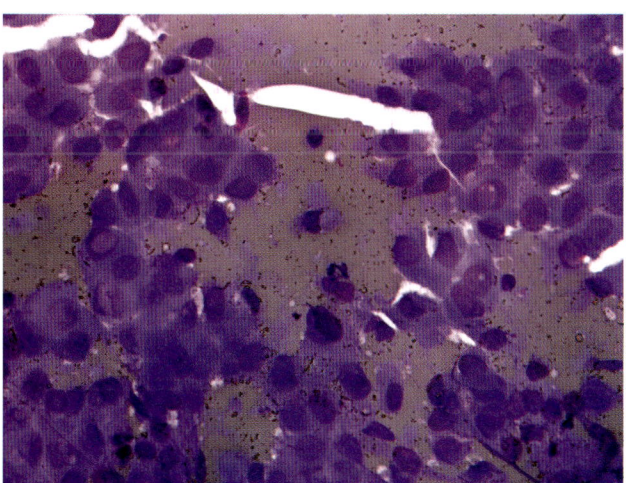

Figure 58.27 FNAC preparation illustrating numerous rounded intranuclear cytoplasmic inclusions and several longitudinal nuclear grooves (coffee beans) in papillary thyroid carcinoma (*MGG stain, high magnification*).

vacuoles, holes). The latter is often unduly widespread and lacks the discrete nuclear membrane rimming of true intranuclear cytoplasmic inclusions in *forme pleine*.

A papillary architecture is typical though by no means universal. The papillae are often well vascularized and complexly arborescent, sometimes oedematous (hydropic), hyalinized, fibrocellular, calcified or micropapillary in configuration (**Figure 58.28**). Follicles are usually present, albeit with an elongated, tortuous or crenated outline ('twisted' follicles) sometimes with rudimentary or abortive papillae and colloid is often more densely hypereosinophilic compared to autochthonous follicles. Intrafollicular multinucleated giant cells of macrophage/histiocyte lineage phagocytosing colloid (colloidophagy) are more often seen in PTC than in other lesions (**Figure 58.29**).

Psammoma bodies (laminated calcospherites) are present in roughly 50% of PTCs histologically, less frequently on FNAC and are virtually pathognomonic. They probably represent mineralized stromal cores and, therefore, must be stromal in location, in contradistinction to calcified, inspissated intrafollicular colloid (psammomatoid calcification or pseudo-psammoma bodies) seen in normality and other

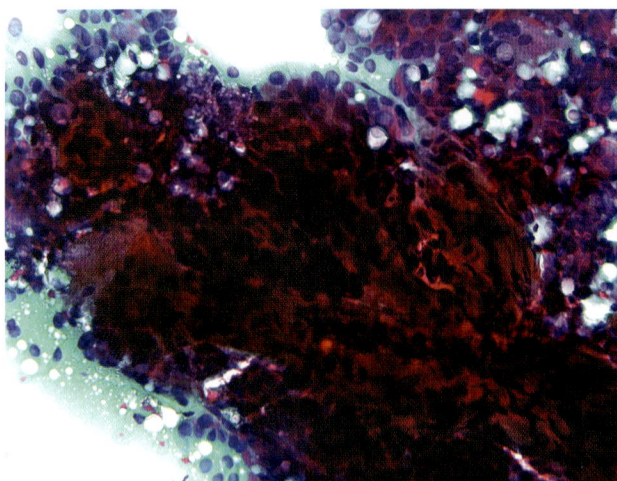

Figure 58.28 FNAC tissue microbiopsy from a papillary thyroid carcinoma. Despite its thickness, obscuring much cytonuclear detail (a few nuclear inclusions and nuclear grooves are nonetheless visible), the branching vascularized fronds are a useful diagnostic feature. Colloid, where present, tends to be globular or in strands ('chewing gum' or stringy colloid) (*Pap stain, medium magnification*).

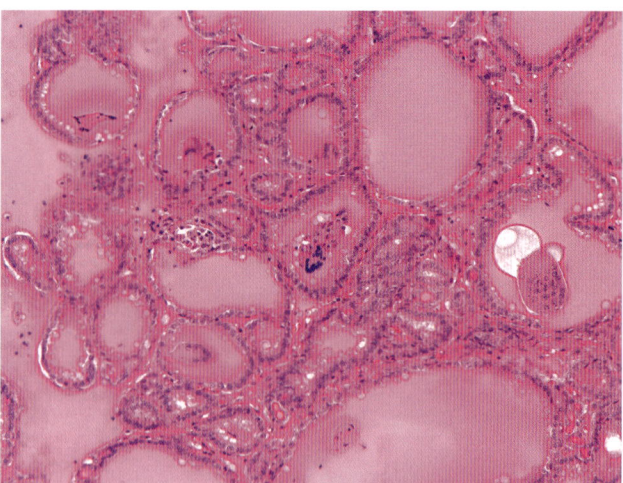

Figure 58.29 Several intrafollicular multinucleate giant cells, of macrophage/monocyte lineage, phagocytosing vacuolated colloid (colloidophagy) in a PTC. This phenomenon is often seen in PTC, but not exclusively so (*H&E stain, high magnification*).

disease states (such as oncocytic tumours) (**Figure 58.30**). Importantly, psammoma bodies may also be seen in other neoplastic and non-neoplastic conditions, both within and outside the thyroid gland. Rarely, psammoma bodies or linear scoring artefact following microtomy provide the only presumptive evidence of regressed or infarcted PTC. Multicentric PTC is common and represents either intrathyroidal lymphatic spread or synchronous primary tumourogenesis with different *RET/PTC* translocations.

Numerous variants of PTC have been described, none mutually exclusive within an individual tumour (**Box 58.2**). A single tumour is classified according to its predominant histological pattern. Most subtypes are of no prognostic significance, although tall cell, diffuse sclerosing, diffuse follicular, solid, trabecular, hobnail/micropapillary and dedifferentiated variants (**Figure 58.31**) are biologically more aggressive in contrast to the encapsulated variant (where conventional infiltrative growth may not be apparent), which portends a highly favourable outcome. Increased mitoses (over two mitoses per ten high-power fields) and tumour necrosis signify worse survival in PTC. PTCs measuring less than 1 cm are associated with an excellent prognosis and the outlook worsens for those tumours exceeding 4 cm. Positive lymph nodal metastasis in PTC is usually an indication for radioactive iodine therapy and the presence of extranodal extension heightens risk of distant metastasis and death. Areas of squamous differentiation (morulae) occur in approximately 50% of cases

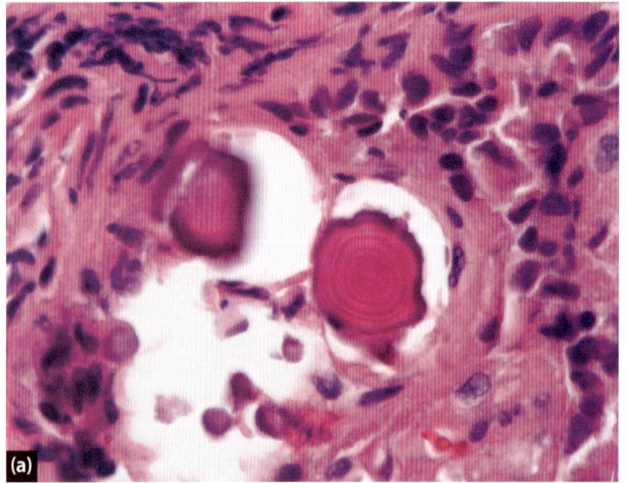
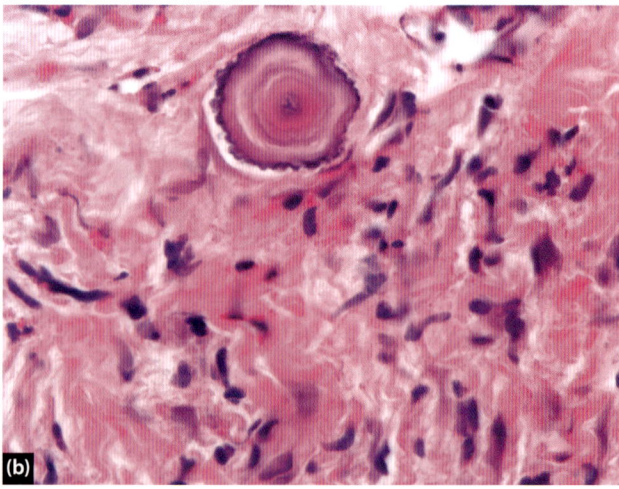

Figure 58.30 Psammoma bodies. (a) Psammoma bodies in papillary thyroid carcinoma. These concentrically laminated concretions are stromal in location. They are often said to represent mineralized tombstones to a mummified cell or papilla, the latter forming the initial nidus for mineral encrustation. They may occasionally be large and complex in configuration. Some of these have splintered during microtomy. Any calcified deposits or other hard objects are prone to dislodgement by the microtome blade and being swept across the tissue section to give parallel linear score artefact (*H&E stain, medium magnification*). **(b)** Psammoma body within fibroblastic interstitium encountered as part of retrogressive change in multinodular hyperplasia. There was no evidence of neoplasia (*H&E stain, high magnification*).

(Continued)

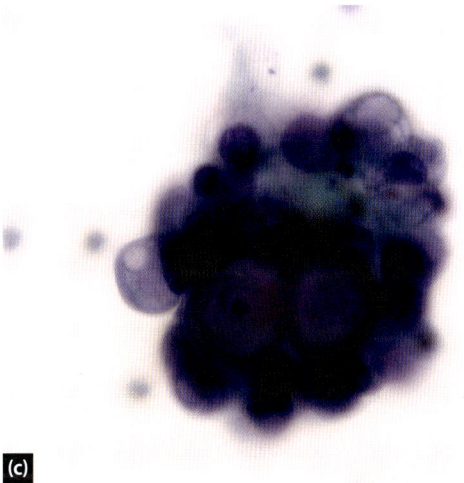 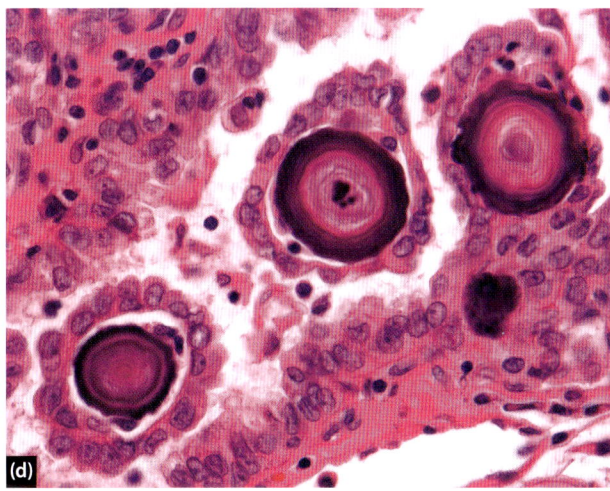

Figure 58.30 (Continued) Psammoma bodies. **(c)** FNAC from a papillary thyroid carcinoma showing two concentrically lamellated psammoma bodies mantled by vacuolated epithelial cells. Psamoma bodies are seen in 40–60% of papillary thyroid carcinomas in histological sections but in only 20% of cases in FNAC specimens[36] (*H&E stain, high magnification*). **(d)** Three psammomatoid spheroliths (concretions or pseudo-psammoma bodies) occupying follicular lumina, again composed of inspissated, partially mineralized intrafollicular colloid in a case of PTC, but also commonly a feature of oncocytic (oxyphil or Hürthle cell) neoplasms (*H&E stain, high magnification*).

BOX 58.2 Histological variants of papillary thyroid carcinoma[22]

Non-invasive follicular tumour with papillary-like nuclei (NIFTP)	Warthin tumour-like variant
Encapsulated follicular variant (EFVPTC)	Hobnail variant
Invasive follicular variant	Solid pattern
Diffuse follicular variant	Diffuse sclerosing pattern
Macrofollicular variant	Trabecular pattern
Classical papillary carcinoma	Cribriform-morular (including familial adenomatous polyposis-associated carcinomas)
Papillary microcarcinoma (papillary microtumour)	Papillary carcinoma with lipomatous stroma
Micropapillary variant.	Variant with exuberant nodular fasciitis-like stroma
Tall cell variant	Variant with spindle cell metaplasia
Columnar cell variant	Adenoid cystic-like variant
Clear cell variant	Angiomatoid variant
Oncocytic (oxyphil/Hürthle cell)	Dedifferentiated variant

Note that fields of squamous differentiation (common), ossification (uncommon) and mucinous differentiation (rare) may be independently encountered.

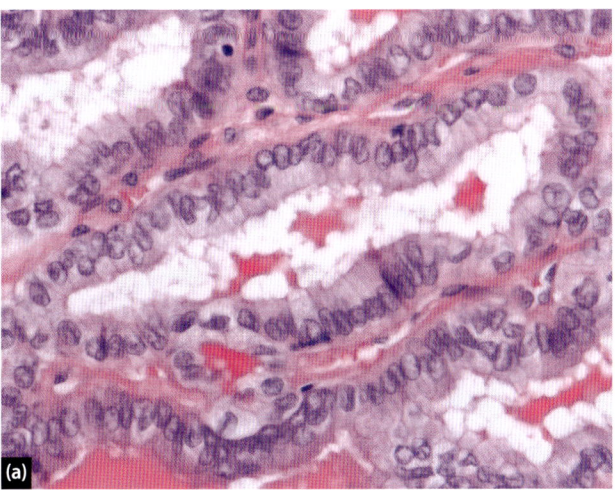 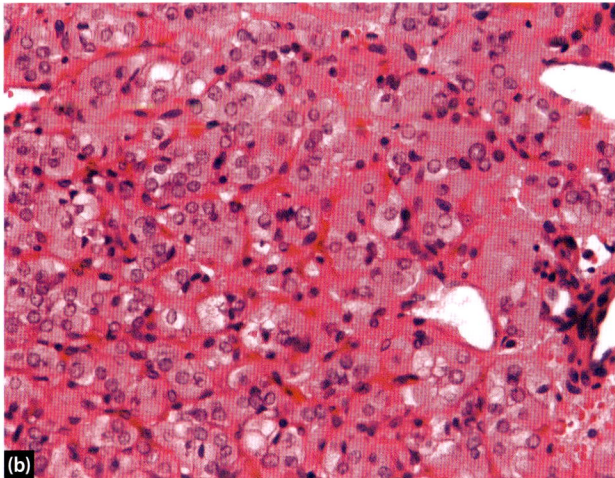

Figure 58.31 PTC variants. **(a)** Tall cell variant of papillary thyroid carcinoma. The cells are columnar, their height being at least three times greater than their width, and they are not hyperstratified, in contradistinction to columnar cell carcinoma (*H&E stain, high magnification*). **(b)** Solid variant of papillary thyroid carcinoma. The small cell nests demonstrate the distinctive nuclear features. This example behaved extremely aggressively (*H&E stain, high magnification*).

(Continued)

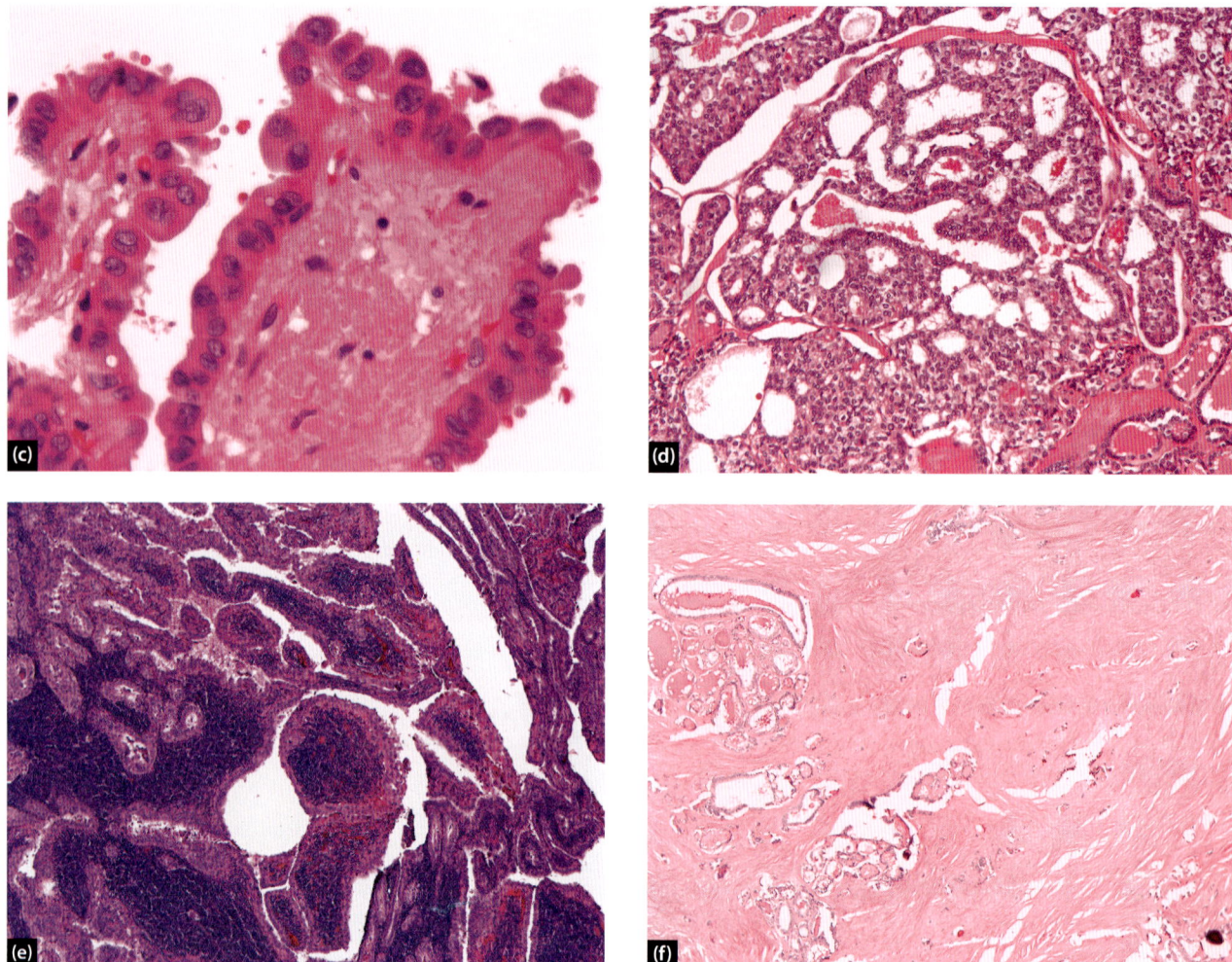

Figure 58.31 (Continued) PTC variants. (c) Hobnail variant of PTC characterized by a significant proportion of the cells showing reverse nuclear polarity with protruberant apical nuclei and/or luminal blebs (snouting) of cytoplasm (*H&E stain, high magnification*). **(d)** Contiguous tubulocribriform arcades of thyrocytes of the pattern seen in cribriform-morular variant PTC (*H&E stain, medium magnification*). **(e)** Papillary thyroid carcinoma, Warthin tumour-like variant, microscopically resembling Warthin's tumour (adenolymphoma) of salivary gland (usually parotid gland) derivation. The epithelium is oncocytic (Hürthle cell) and there is marked reactive lymphocytosis expanding papillary stromal cores (*H&E stain, low magnification*). **(f)** Diffuse sclerosing variant of PTC dominated by dense, acellular, paucivascular sclerohyaline stroma. Psammoma body formation and associated parallel linear microtomy score marks traversing the section are exemplary (*H&E stain, medium magnification*).

and the distinctive PTC nuclear morphology is absent from such areas (**Figure 58.11a**). The WHO definition of tall cells in PTC is merely a preponderance of tumour cells whose height is at least threefold (previously twofold) greater than their width, and this pattern should not be confused with columnar cell carcinoma. Note that there is presently no unanimous agreement on the percentage of tall cell morphology required to define an entire PTC as tall cell variant. The appellation solid variant is reserved for tumours displaying 50% or more solid growth pattern.

PTC stains immunohistochemically for cytokeratins (CKs), thyroglobulin (Tg) and thyroid transcription factor-1 (TTF-1) but not pan-neuroendocrine markers. Areas of squamous differentiation lose their Tg and TTF-1 reactivity. A plethora of markers have been proposed to aid discrimination between follicular variant of PTC and other follicular lesions, notably high molecular weight cytokeratins (HMWCKs), low-molecular weight cytokeratin (cytokeratin 19/CK19), Hector Battifora mesothelial-1 antibody (HBME-1), galectin-3 (GAL-3), neural cell adhesion molecule (NCAM), (CD56), Leu7 (CD57), LeuM1 (CD15), fibronectin-1 (FN-1), platelet-derived growth factor (CD44), p63 protein, trophoblastic cell surface antigen (TROP2), paired box gene 8 (PAX8), Thyroid transcription factor-2 (TTF-2), thyroperoxidase (TPO), BRAF mutation specific antibody and *RET* among others. None, individually or in combination, is entirely sensitive or specific for PTC: they may be capricious even in classical PTC, and a number of inflammatory and other neoplastic conditions may yield ambiguous and/or spurious results. CK19 staining in isolation has a low specificity and low sensitivity. The panel of cytokeratin 19 and HBME-1 has a higher exclusionary power than positive predictive power: if both markers are negative, this militates against a diagnosis of PTC, whereas positivity of either, or both, is supportive but not conclusive (**Figure 58.32**). CD56 is expressed by normal thyrocytes,

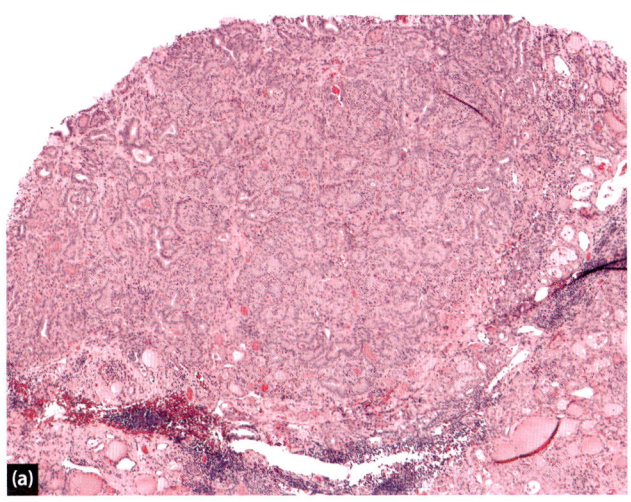
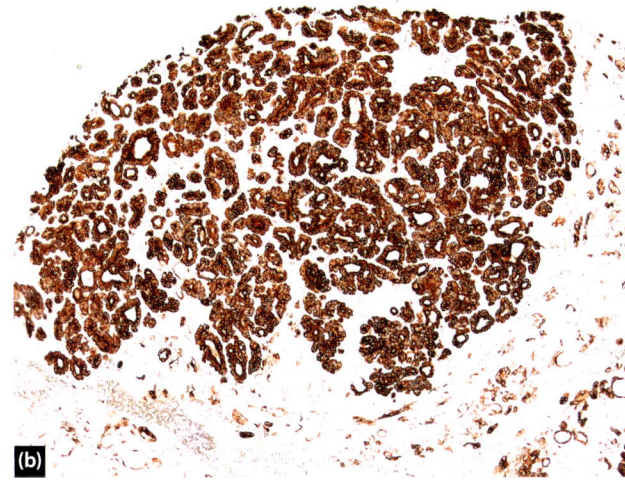
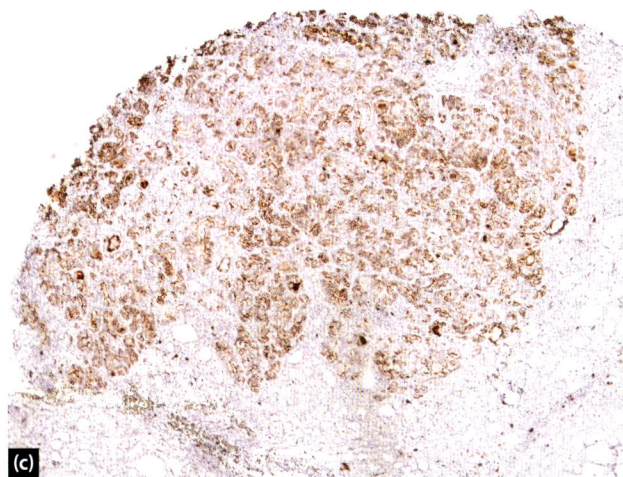

Figure 58.32 PTC staining. (a) Part of an IFVPTC showing follicular architecture (*H&E stain, low magnification*). **(b)** Identical field of IFVPTC showing diffuse avid cytokeratin 19 immunoreactivity (*CK19 IHC, low magnification*). **(c)** The same field of IFVPTC showing moderate positive staining for HBME-1 (*HBME-1 IHC, low magnification*).

benign and malignant follicular lesions but generally not by PTC. Absent, or low, CD56 expression (typically less than 5% or so, confined to the tumour-native tissue interface) in a follicular-patterned neoplasm is claimed to be consistently specific and extremely sensitive for PTC, more so than CK19. In the appropriate context, CD 56 immunonegativity, or loss of CD56 expression in various degrees, is supportive of malignancy and may compliment diagnostic accuracy of PTC when used as a panel in conjunction with CK19, p63 protein and/or HBME-1 antibodies. However, undue reliance should not be placed upon immunostaining in isolation.

Three independent molecular pathways are recognized in the tumourogenesis of PTC with distinct gene expression profiles, namely activation of the proto-oncogene receptor tyrosine (*RET*) kinase, mutation of the gene for B-raf (*BRAF*) and *ras* mutation. *RET* kinase activation consequent upon chromosomal translocation is collectively referred to as *RET/PTC* translocation and occurs in up to 60% of PTCs. *RET/PTC 1* fusion correlates to classical PTC and papillary microcarcinoma. *RET/PTC 3* fusion is seen in tall cell and solid PTC variants plus irradiation-induced tumours. *RET/PTC* expression is not a feature of follicular carcinoma, poorly differentiated carcinoma or undifferentiated (anaplastic) carcinoma. Mutation of the gene for B-raf (*BRAF*) accompanies 29–69 % of PTCs, more prevalent in classical PTC, tall cell, Warthin tumour-like and oncocytic (oxyphil) variants. FVPTC harbours *ras* gene mutations and may show *PAX8/PPARγ* translocation, but rarely *RET/PTC* translocation or *BRAF* mutations, a profile akin to that of follicular adenoma and follicular carcinoma.[4]

Follicular-patterned tumours of uncertain malignant potential

Perhaps the most controversial development relating to thyroid pathology over the past two decades has been the recognition and incorporation into mainstream classification of a group of well-differentiated follicular-patterned neoplasms (intermediate or borderline) that lie morphologically and behaviourally between follicular adenoma and follicular carcinoma/FVPTC – tumours of uncertain malignant potential (atypical adenoma, adenoma with atypia, well-differentiated tumour of uncertain behaviour). Whether these lesions constitute distinct entities, and if so, whether they qualify as carcinoma/neoplasms of low malignant potential has yet to be categorically determined.

Historically, limited follow-up data, compounded by subjective judgement and well recognized poor inter-observer concordance and intra-observer variation has

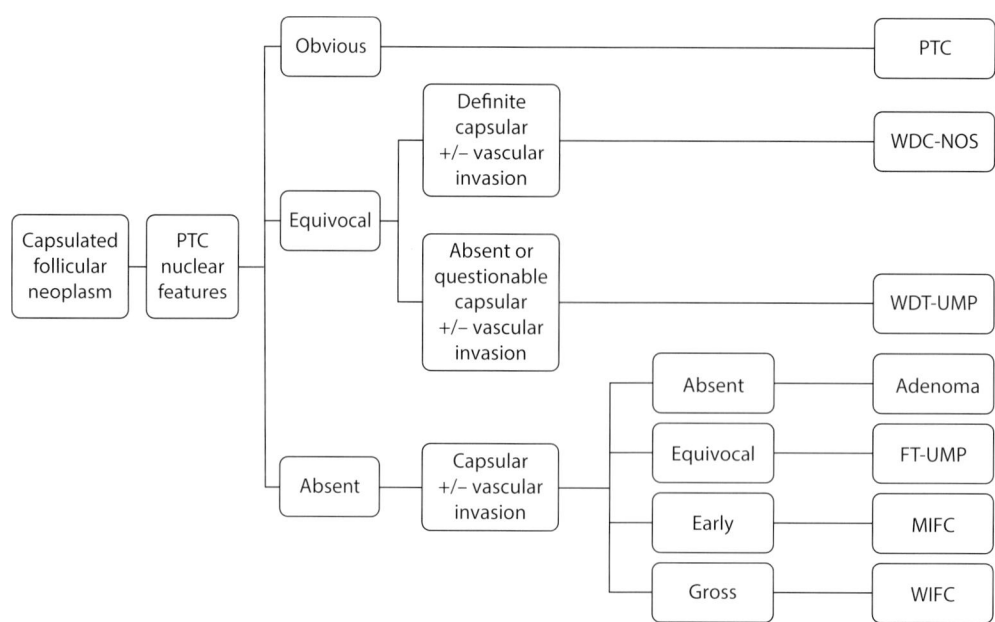

Figure 58.33 Chernobyl Pathologists' Group nosology and diagnostic algorithm for resolution of the differential diagnosis of encapsulated follicular-patterned lesions of the thyroid gland. PTC: papillary thyroid carcinoma; WDC-NOS: well-differentiated carcinoma, not otherwise specified; WDT-UMP: well-differentiated tumour of uncertain malignant potential; FT-UMP: follicular tumour of uncertain malignant potential; MIFC: minimally invasive follicular carcinoma; WIFC: widely invasive follicular carcinoma.

been problematical, prompting recourse to a pragmatic *ipse dixit* diagnosis.[25] Furthermore, RET/PTC expression in some cases of FVPTC shows multicentric rather than diffuse alterations, suggestive of carcinomatous transformation ex-adenoma, though by convention it is recommended that the entire encapsulated lesion is arbitrarily regarded as PTC for staging purposes.[26]

In recognition of these difficulties, the Chernobyl Pathologists' Group proposed alternative nomenclature to accommodate this diagnostic uncertainty and this is summarised in **Figure 58.33**. For more than a decade this provided a more descriptive schema, which could be invoked in the minority of cases where diagnostic equivocation was irresolvable by conventional morphology and the stigma of malignancy was potentially unjustifiable and equally undesired. Until recently, however, this approach was not wholly accepted into mainstream diagnostic practice. The Armed Forces Institute of Pathology (AFIP) fascicle 2015 did embrace this philosophy and adopted the terminology into its classification (**Table 58.7**). Subsequently, the WHO (4th edition, 2017) classification has refined this further (**Table 58.8**).[27]

For encapsulated follicular-patterned tumours indeterminate between follicular adenoma and follicular carcinoma, lacking nuclear features of PTC, where capsular invasion is equivocal, the WHO (4th edition, 2017) classification retains the descriptor *follicular tumour of uncertain malignant potential (FT-UMP)*, but has expanded its scope to include equivocal vascular invasion.[27]

For encapsulated, or well circumscribed, follicular-patterned tumours with well-developed or equivocal nuclear features of PTC, the term *well-differentiated tumour of uncertain malignant potential (WDT-UMP)* was also adopted by the AFIP fascicle 2015. The WHO (4th edition, 2017) classification further recognizes that non-invasive encapsulated FVPTC is associated with an excellent prognosis and possesses molecular features more akin to follicular adenoma/carcinoma than those of conventional PTC – the term *non-invasive follicular thyroid neoplasm with papillary-like nuclear features (NIFTP)* has been introduced to encompass non-invasive encapsulated follicular-patterned tumours previously called encapsulated FVPTC as well as *WDT-UMP*.[27] The designation *WDT-UMP* is reserved in this classification for well-developed or incompletely developed PTC-type nuclei and questionable capsular or vascular invasion.

Where diagnostic distinction between invasive follicular carcinoma and invasive PTC is difficult, the generic

TABLE 58.7 AFIP recommended nomenclature for encapsulated well-differentiated follicular-patterned tumours based on the presence or absence of PTC nuclear features and capsular invasion, AFIP fascicle 2015.[32]

		Capsular invasion		
		Present	Questionable	Absent
Nuclear features of PTC	Present	Follicular variant of PTC		
	Questionable	Well-differentiated carcinoma, NOS	Well-differentiated tumour of uncertain malignant potential	
	Absent	Follicular carcinoma	Follicular tumour of uncertain malignant potential	Follicular adenoma

TABLE 58.8 WHO classification recommended nomenclature for encapsulated follicular-patterned tumours on the basis of presence or absence of PTC nuclear features and capsular or vascular invasion, WHO, 4th edition, 2017.[27]

		Capsular or vascular invasion		
		Present	Questionable	Absent
Nuclear features of PTC	Present	Invasive encapsulated follicular variant of PTC	Well-differentiated tumour of uncertain malignant potential	Non-invasive follicular thyroid neoplasm with papillary-like nuclear features
	Questionable	Well-differentiated carcinoma, NOS		
	Absent	Follicular carcinoma	Follicular tumour of uncertain malignant potential	Follicular adenoma

rubric *well-differentiated thyroid carcinoma, not otherwise specified (WDT-NOS)* may still rarely be employed, though every effort to sub-classify more precisely should be expended.[40]

NON-INVASIVE FOLLICULAR THYROID NEOPLASM WITH PAPILLARY-LIKE NUCLEAR FEATURES

The follicular variant of papillary thyroid carcinoma (FVPTC) is the most prolific variant of PTC, accounting for around 30% of all PTCs. Small variations in outcome (dependent upon the presence/absence of invasion) notwithstanding, the long-term prognosis is near universally excellent, supporting the notion that these tumours are biologically indolent. Discounting the rare diffuse follicular and macrofollicular variants of PTC and encapsulated papillary carcinoma (the latter denoting classical PTC bounded by a thick capsule but with dominant papillary rather than follicular architecture), further subclassification into invasive follicular variant (IFVPTC), encapsulated follicular variant with invasion (EFVPTC) and encapsulated follicular variant without invasion (non-invasive follicular thyroid neoplasm with papillary-like nuclear features, NIFTP), is clinically useful.

In terms of follicular growth and nuclear morphology, IFVPTC is identical to EFVPTC, except that capsulation is typically incomplete and it shows wide infiltration into adjacent parenchyma with commensurate risk of locoregional recurrence and likelihood of metastasis, behaviour more analogous to classical PTC.

Both EFVPTC (which encompasses non-capsulated and incompletely capsulated but circumscribed tumours) and NIFTP are associated with an excellent outcome when managed conservatively, with disease persistence/recurrence rates of 3% and less than 1% in the first 15 years, respectively, such that NIFTP is not now considered a malignant neoplasm. This terminology is intended to encourage more conservative management and to spare the psychological burden of cancer diagnosis for indolent tumours that may be adequately managed by lobectomy or hemi-thyroidectomy alone. This proposed nomenclature and shift in emphasis has been provisionally accepted internationally, justifying inclusion in the revised WHO (4th edition, 2017) classification of thyroid tumours ('blue book').[27]

An algorithm has been proposed along with standards to stringently define this NIFTP subset, stipulating inclusion and exclusion criteria (**Figure 58.34**) supplemented by an objective nuclear scoring schema (**Table 58.9**). There is

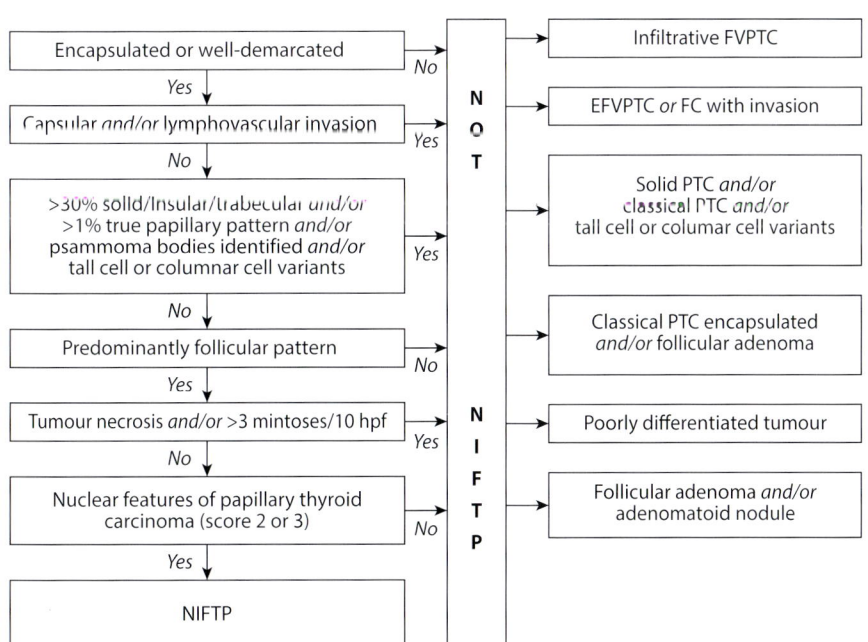

Figure 58.34 Algorithm aiding the subclassification of a follicular-patterned thyroid lesion where NIFTP is a consideration.[38]

TABLE 58.9 Nuclear morphology scoring system intended to enhance reproducibility in the diagnosis of NIFTP[41, 42]

Three-point scoring criteria for the nuclear features of papillary thyroid carcinoma

Nuclear features	Score = 0	Score = 1
1. Size and shape Enlargement, elongation, crowding, overlapping	Absent or only slightly expressed	Present or well-developed (1 point for each feature)
2. Membrane irregularities Irregular contours, grooves, folds, intranuclear cytoplasmic inclusions		
3. Chromatin characteristics Chromatin clearing, margination to the nuclear membranes, glassy nuclei, fine–even delicate chromatin		
Total score: 0 or 1: Not diagnostic		
Total score: 2 or 3: Diagnostic of PTC nuclei		

no prescribed minimum size criterion and the terminology is not fully validated for sub-centimetre or incidentally discovered tumours, indeed it may be challenging to apply the diagnostic criteria to neoplasms measuring less than 0.5 cm. Equally there is no prescribed upper size limit, with the proviso that the collective experience of NIFTP exceeding 4 cm maximum dimension is restricted. Importantly, where possible the entire lesional capsule should be submitted for microscopical scrutiny. Careful fixation and tissue processing are obligatory. A conclusive diagnosis of NIFTP is not feasible on frozen section or FNAC examination.[41]

Major inclusion criteria include sharp demarcation, majority capsulation, dominant follicular growth (less than 1% papillae), less than 30% other architecture (solid, trabecular or insular) and papillary nuclear characteristics (scored for size and shape, membrane irregularity and chromatin characteristics). Minor inclusion features are listed as dark colloid, follicular irregularity and haphazardly scattered microfollicles (sprinkling sign) often displaying artefactual retraction clefts (**Figure 58.35**). Exclusion criteria dictate any capsular or vascular invasion, true papillae (exceeding one percent of the tumour), psammoma bodies, infiltrative interface, coagulative necrosis (excepting ischaemic FNAC injury), increased mitoses (at least 3 per 10 hpf), features of some other aggressive PTC variant (tall cell, columnar cell, cribriform-morular, hobnail/micropapillary, diffuse sclerosing or dedifferentiated) and oncocytic (Hürthle cell) lesions.[42] Lymph node metastasis at presentation is incompatible with a diagnosis of NIFTP, cognizant that central cervical compartment lymph nodal micrometastasis might represent spread from a different occult primary thyroid carcinoma and that heterotopic (ectopic) lymphadenoidal inclusions enter the differential diagnosis.

Papillary thyroid microcarcinoma

Papillary thyroid microcarcinomas (papillary microtumours) are by definition less than 10 mm in diameter, constituting pT1a disease. They may be an incidental finding in thyroid glands removed for other pathology or serendipitously detected on imaging of the thyroid gland (latent carcinoma).[43] Alternatively, they may be found retrospectively in patients presenting with metastatic disease from an initially unsuspected small primary lesion (occult/cryptic/covert carcinoma). Historical subdivision into tumours less

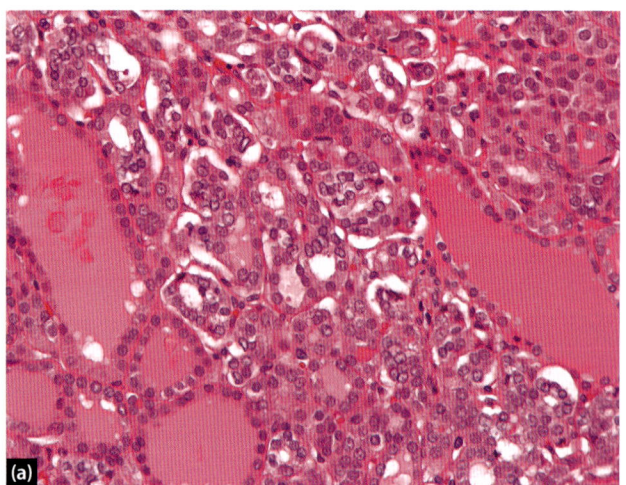 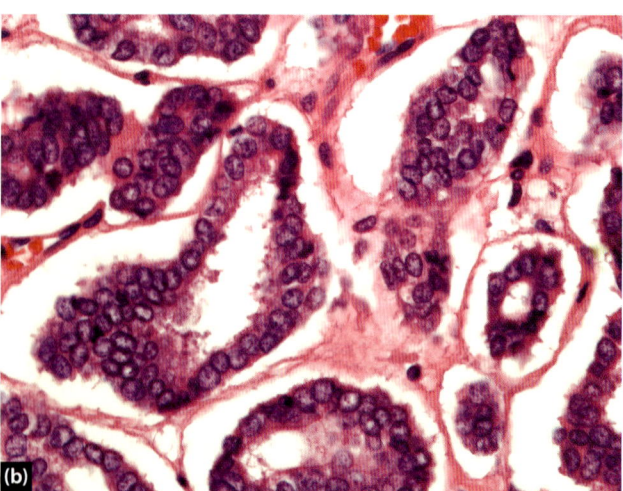

Figure 58.35 Non-invasive follicular thyroid neoplasm with papillary-like nuclear features. (a) A congerie of small follicles displaying PTC nuclear features nested between larger non-descript follicles in NIFTP (sprinkling sign). There is limited artefactual perifollicular clefting (shrinkage artefact) (*H&E stain, medium magnification*). (b) A similar nidus of small follicles displaying PTC nuclear characteristics in NIFTP, albeit with very florid, diffuse follicle-stromal interface retraction artefact (*H&E stain, high magnification*).

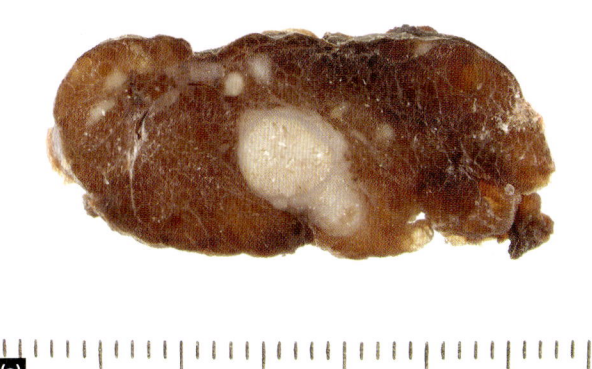
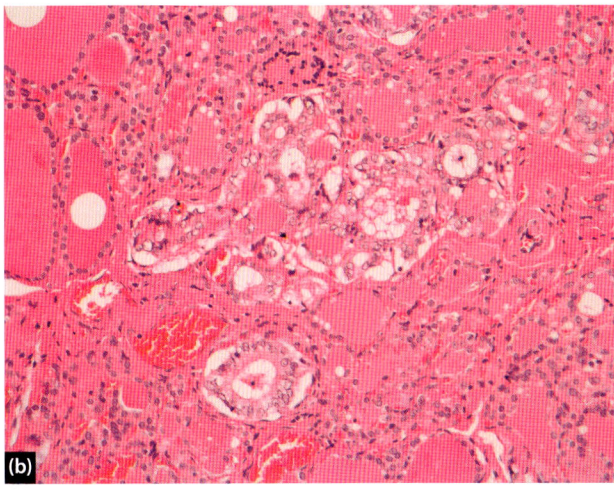

Figure 58.36 Papillary thyroid microcarcinoma. (a) Multicentric papillary thyroid microcarcinoma each deposit measuring less than 10 mm in diameter. These show a sclerotic morphology. (b) Microscopical deposit of papillary microcarcinoma. This is poorly demarcated and is eliciting no stromal or inflammatory response whatsoever. Such foci are readily overlooked on cursory or low-power examination (*H&E stain, medium magnification*).

than 5 mm ('minute') and 5 mm to 10 mm ('tiny') maximum dimension is of no clinical relevance. Occult and latent papillary carcinomas may or may not be microcarcinomas. Follicular and medullary microcarcinomas are independently recognized though less frequently encountered.

Most studies report a prevalence for latent papillary microcarcinomas of around 5% to 10%, but figures as high as 30% or so are acknowledged. Despite their propensity for multifocality in one lobe (23%), bilaterality (17%) and locoregional lymph node metastasis (16%), they almost always pursue an indolent clinical course with excellent prognosis, usually not requiring aggressive intervention.[43] Exceptionally, however, papillary microcarcinomas behave more aggressively and the presence of two or more foci, lymphovascular invasion, extrathyroidal extension and higher risk morphology (e.g. tall cell features) may prompt more comprehensive treatment, despite limited long-term vindication for this. A significant number of sub-centimetre PTCs occurring in children and adolescents harbour extrathyroidal extension and/or distant metastasis, prompting the CAP recommendations to restrict use of the term papillary thyroid microcarcinoma to those over 19 years of age.[33]

Morphologically, papillary microcarcinomas are usually either infiltrative and sclerotic or circumscribed but unencapsulated, located between native follicles without discernible host response (**Figure 58.36**). Such microscopical foci therefore are therefore easily missed on cursory histological screening and are apt to mimic solid cell nests or even heterotopic thymic rests on scanning magnification.

Poorly differentiated thyroid carcinoma

Poorly differentiated carcinoma of the thyroid (PDCAT) encompasses a spectrum of heterogeneous tumours showing limited evidence of follicular cell differentiation associated with biological behaviour intermediate between differentiated (follicular and papillary) thyroid carcinoma and undifferentiated (anaplastic) carcinoma.[44]

Poorly differentiated carcinomas typically arise *de novo*, but they may occur through transformation of differentiated carcinoma (**Figure 58.37**). They may progress to undifferentiated (anaplastic) carcinoma either *ab initio* or after recurrence (**Figure 58.38**).

PDCAT may be defined mainly on the basis of growth pattern. Insular (primordial) carcinoma represents the archetype and is composed of large solid nests (insulae) punctuated by occasional primitive follicles (**Figure 58.39**). Minor elements of classical papillary thyroid carcinoma and/or follicular carcinoma may be recognized. Obversely, an insular growth pattern is by no means exclusive to poorly differentiated carcinoma and important differential diagnoses include medullary thyroid carcinoma, solid variant papillary thyroid carcinoma and undifferentiated (anaplastic) carcinoma.

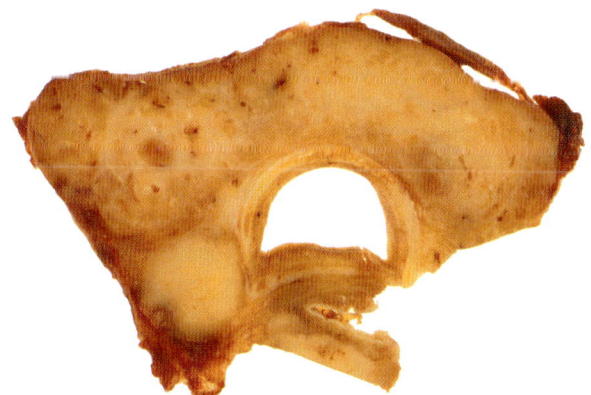

Figure 58.37 Transverse slice through a total laryngopharyngectomy and bilateral radical neck dissection specimen for advanced stage, poorly differentiated thyroid carcinoma. The bulk of the specimen comprises heterogeneous tumour largely enclaving upper trachea and cervical tubular oesophagus. Microscopically this showed intermingled areas of papillary thyroid carcinoma, follicular carcinoma and insular carcinoma with localized squamous differentiation.

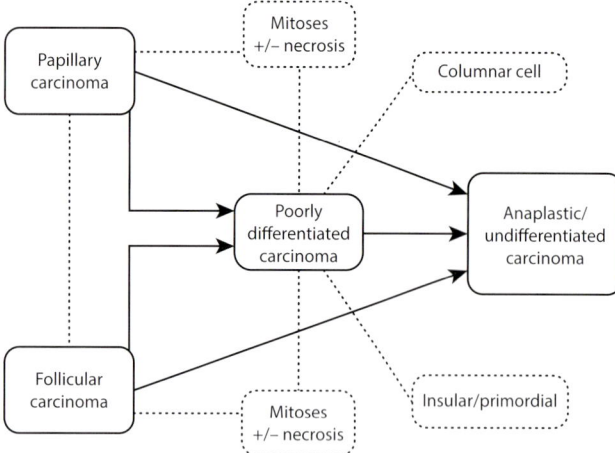

Figure 58.38 Schematic outlining the theoretical developmental relationships between differentiated, poorly differentiated and undifferentiated (anaplastic) thyroid carcinomas.

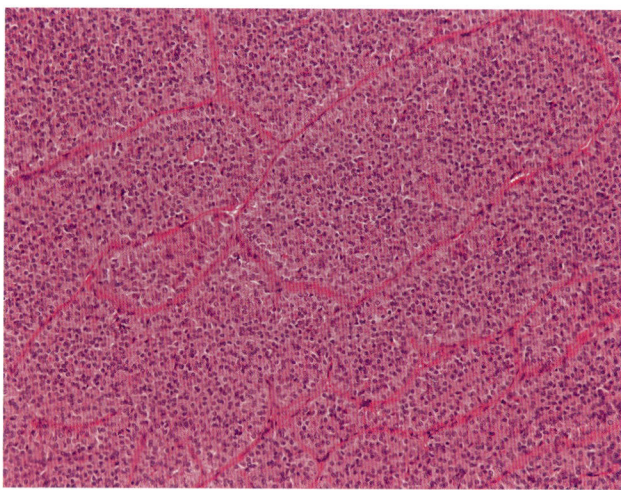

Figure 58.39 Classical poorly differentiated (insular) thyroid carcinoma displaying the characteristic solid tumour cell islands (insulae) separated by narrow fibrovascular septa. There is no hint of follicular or other differentiation here (*H&E stain, medium magnification*).

Alternatively, PDCAT may be specified according to mitotic state (exceeding 5 mitoses per 10 high-power fields ×400) and/or comedo-like tumour necrosis. These portend a survival rate of 60% at 5 years, irrespective of tumour architecture. Furthermore, the combination of solid growth and the presence of at least one of convoluted nuclei, tumour necrosis and/or over 3 mitoses per 10 high-power fields is a powerful predictor of poor outcome. This group constitutes the major cause of radioiodine refractory positron emission tomography (PET)-positive incurable thyroid carcinomas. Some authors propose a so-called 'high-grade carcinoma' of the thyroid as a malignancy in which there are recognizable elements of differentiated thyroid carcinoma but which also show histological and cytological features placing the lesion into a 'high-grade' category. However, this concept has yet to be endorsed in the WHO (4th edition, 2017) classification and most would classify such neoplasms under the rubric of PDCAT.[27]

Confusingly, the term poorly differentiated carcinoma is also applied by some observers to differentiated carcinomas showing a solid, trabecular or scirrhous pattern, to tall cell papillary carcinomas and to columnar cell carcinomas. There are insufficient data to determine whether the spectrum of PDCAT should be widened to incorporate a small subset of tumours that exhibit high-risk pathological and clinical features despite low-grade histomorphology.[49] This lack of consensus may explain conflicting data as to whether a minority component of insular carcinoma in an otherwise differentiated carcinoma is an independent prognostic factor or not and, if so, at what threshold this begins to be a clinically valid observandum. When such poorly differentiated carcinoma comprises the majority of tumour mass (greater than 50%), pragmatically the lesion is best classified as poorly differentiated overall.[36] The response of PDCAT to radio-iodine is generally poor.

Unsurprisingly, the tumour cells demonstrate cytokeratins (CK), thyroglobulin (Tg) and thyroid transcription factor-1 (TTF-1) immunopositivity but negative pan-neuroendocrine markers and calcitonin.

Columnar cell carcinoma

Columnar cell carcinoma is a rare thyroid neoplasm, which once invasive pursues a more aggressive course than other differentiated thyroid carcinomas. Where it remains encapsulated, however, there appears to be little risk of metastasis.[44] There is disagreement as to whether it is best classified as a distinct entity rather than a variant of papillary thyroid carcinoma. There is indeed morphological overlap between columnar cell carcinoma, the cribriform-morular variant of papillary thyroid carcinoma and also so-called FAP-associated thyroid carcinoma, remembering that thyroid carcinomas of conventional pattern also occur in familial adenomatous polyposis (FAP) patients.

This notwithstanding, the typical architecture resembles that of intestinal and endometrioid carcinomas with complex glandular, cribriform and solid growth. The individual cells are tall and columnar but striking nuclear pseudostratification and hyperchromasia enable separation from tall cell variant of papillary thyroid carcinoma (**Figure 58.40**). Immunohistochemically, it is usually CK, Tg and TTF-1 positive.

Undifferentiated (anaplastic) carcinoma

Undifferentiated (anaplastic) carcinoma is a highly malignant tumour typically seen in elderly patients with preponderance in females. It accounts for approximately 2–10% of all malignant thyroid neoplasms,[45] with a predilection for iodine-deficient regions though its overall incidence is declining.[46] Undifferentiated (anaplastic) thyroid carcinoma is usually widely invasive at presentation and inoperable in roughly half of cases. It carries a high mortality and accounts for nearly half of all deaths associated with thyroid malignancy.[8] The overall median survival is 4 months and the 5-year survival rate is less than 10%.

All undifferentiated (anaplastic) thyroid carcinomas are arbitrarily UICC/TNM staged as pT4 due to their anticipated

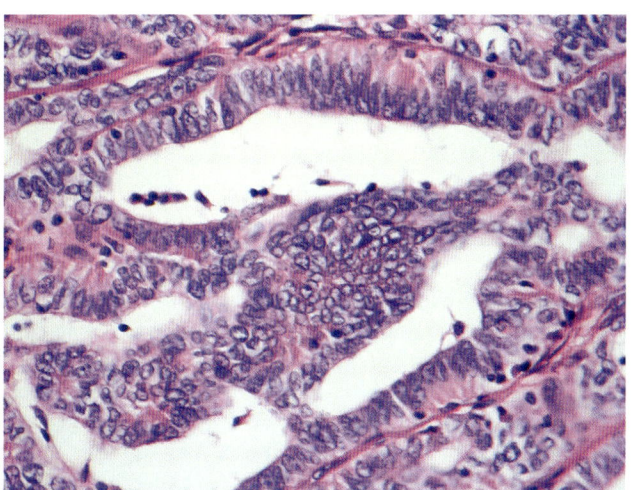

Figure 58.40 Columnar cell carcinoma illustrating the classical, complex glandular growth pattern resembling gastric, colorectal or endometrial adenocarcinoma. The tumour cells are columnar with characteristic nuclear pseudo-stratification (*H&E stain, high magnification*).

aggressive behaviour, classically showing widespread infiltration of surrounding structures, regional lymph node metastases and distant metastasis to any site.[8] Presentation with early, intracapsular anaplastic carcinoma, which is more amenable to surgical extirpation, portends a slightly more favourable outlook but is uncommon. Where there is any focus of anaplasia within a differentiated tumour, the lesion is conventionally classified overall as undifferentiated (anaplastic) carcinoma thereby by default becomes stage T4 disease. Obversely, the presence of better-differentiated elements may mitigate the poor prognosis of undifferentiated (anaplastic) carcinoma to some extent.

Undifferentiated (anaplastic) carcinoma can arise *de novo* but the presence of synchronous better-differentiated carcinomatous elements in over 50% of cases is taken as evidence of de-differentiation of a pre-existing neoplasm.[45] Ergo, there may be a history of long-standing thyroid disease complicated by a recent phase of accelerated growth. The histological features are tremendously variable with two main patterns being pleomorphic epithelioid (giant cell) and spindle cell (sarcomatoid) (**Figure 58.41**). A variety of other microscopical

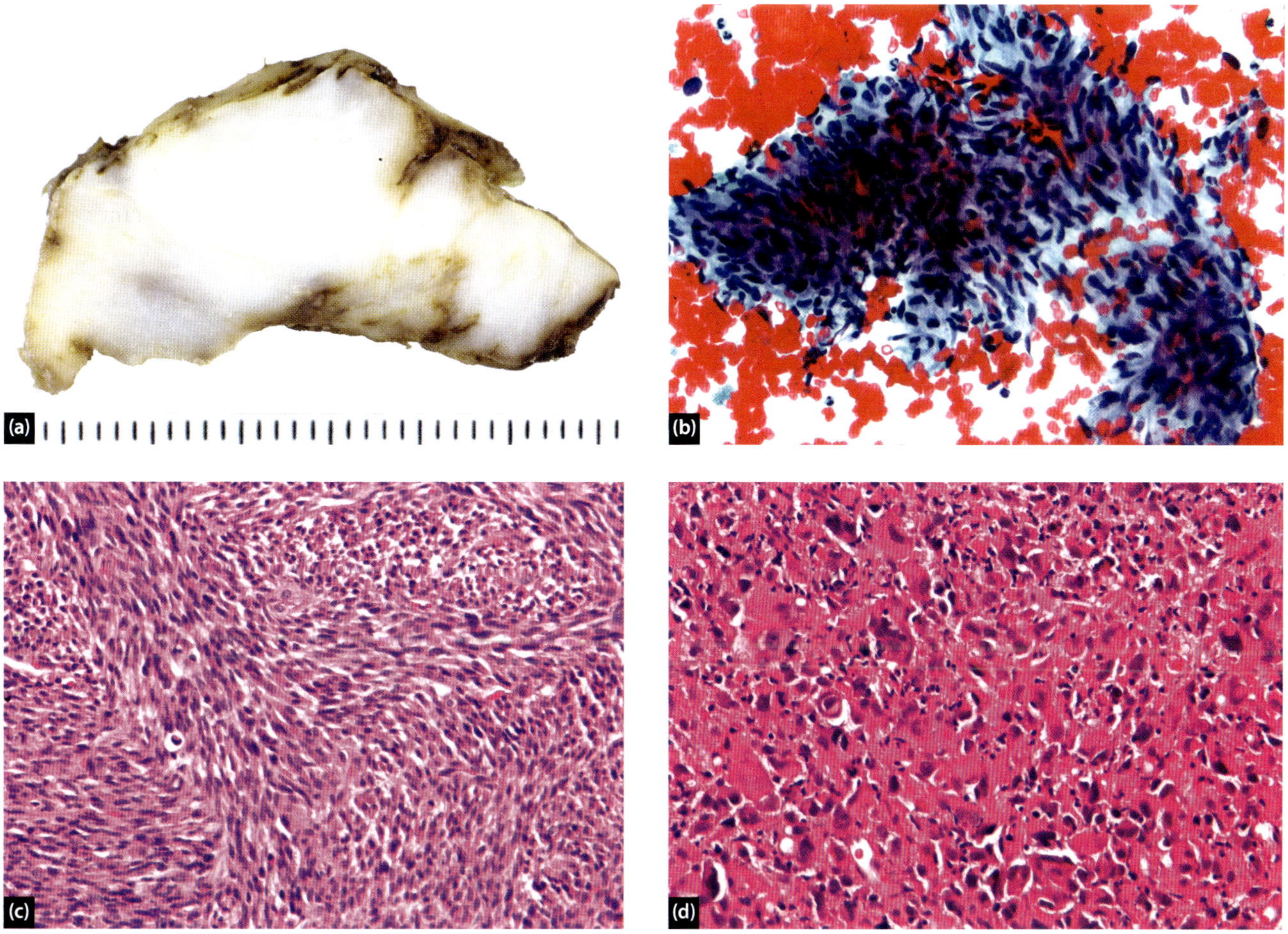

Figure 58.41 Undifferentiated (anaplastic) carcinoma. (a) A cross-sectional slice through a thyroid lobectomy specimen substantially replaced by undifferentiated (anaplastic) thyroid carcinoma. The solid, dense, featureless and infiltrative nature is paradigmatic. **(b)** FNAC specimen from undifferentiated (anaplastic) thyroid carcinoma showing a tri-dimensional, acervate clump of pleomorphic, high-grade malignant spindle cells (*Pap stain, medium magnification*). **(c)** A field of fibrosarcoma-like undifferentiated (anaplastic) thyroid carcinoma composed of fasciculated, malignant fusiform cells (*H&E stain, medium magnification*). **(d)** Undifferentiated (anaplastic) thyroid carcinoma showing highly pleomorphic epithelioid tumour cells with numerous bizarre giant cells and monster cells ('monstrocytes'), some polykaryocytic (*H&E stain, medium magnification*).

TABLE 58.10 Recognized histological variants of undifferentiated (anaplastic) thyroid carcinoma and their mimics. Note that any individual tumour may present a mixture of appearances in any combination or permutation

Pattern	Major differential diagnosis
Epithelioid	Poorly differentiated (insular) carcinoma Papillary carcinoma, solid variant Metastatic carcinoma
Sarcomatoid	Sarcoma proper
Angiomatoid	Angiosarcoma
Osteoclastic	Pleomorphic sarcoma
Rhabdoid	Rhabdomyosarcoma
Lymphoepithelioma-like	CASTLE
Paucicellular/fibrosing	Riedel's thyroiditis
Carcinosarcomatoid	Osteosarcoma Rhabdomyosarcoma
Adenosquamous	Metastatic carcinoma Sclerosing mucoepidermoid with eosinophilocytosis
Squamous cell carcinoma	Metastatic disease Direct extension Papillary thyroid carcinoma CASTLE

patterns are recognized and are renowned for troublesome differential diagnosis (**Table 58.10**). Angiolymphatic penetration is characteristic and a brisk inflammatory response is often encountered.

While the term carcinoma is conventionally applied, compelling proof of epithelial differentiation is not always forthcoming by light microscopy, morphologically or immunophenotypically, and the diagnosis ultimately rests upon an acceptable histological pattern allied to an appropriate clinicoradiological context. Immunohistochemical staining for cytokeratin and vimentin are at least focally positive in around 90% of cases with epithelial membrane antigen reactivity in 50% of examples. Tg, TTF-1, calcitonin and pan-neuroendocrine epitopes are typically negative; diffusion of thyroglobulin from destroyed follicles, however, may give rise to spurious immunopositivity. The thyroid lineage marker PAX 8 is retained in roughly half of all cases and immunopositivity may assist in the exclusion of metastatic giant cell lung cancer, which is generally negative. Endothelial markers (CD31, CD34 and factor VIII) may be focally demonstrated in some tumours presenting an angiosarcomatoid morphology, which may rarely prevail. EDFR, VEGFR and ALK may be expressed with the prospect of targetted protein kinase inhibitor therapy. Occasional cases are completely immunoinert and ultrastructural studies are seldom rewarding. Where appropriate, a haematolymphoid immunopanel should always be considered, particularly on FNAC and needle core biopsies, so as not to overlook high-grade or anaplastic non-Hodgkin lymphoma.

Medullary thyroid carcinoma

Medullary thyroid carcinoma (MTC) is a malignant tumour displaying parafollicular C-cell differentiation,[47] which secretes calcitonin and often a variety of other neuropeptides.[48] It is an uncommon tumour accounting for 5–8% of all thyroid cancers.[50] It may occur sporadically or against a background of an inherited autosomal dominant trait related to a mutation of the *RET* proto-oncogene, which causes multiple endocrine neoplasia (MEN) types 2A or 2B or familial MTC (FMTC).

Sporadic MTC is more common in females and presents at a mean age of 50 years. MEN 2A presents in adolescence or young adults, while MEN 2B presents in infancy or childhood.[8] Sporadic tumours are usually single whereas hereditary tumours are often multicentric and/or bilateral. FMTC arises from C-cell hyperplasia, which is considered a precursor lesion and can be identified histologically with due diligence.

Regional lymph node metastasis and distant lymphatogenous spread are found in 20% and 8% of cases at presentation, respectively. Secondary sites of predilection include lung, liver, adrenal and bone. MEN 2B MTC generally pursues a more aggressive course than MEN 2A MTC, which in turn portends a less favourable prognosis than sporadic MTC, though for those with neoplasms confined to within the thyroid gland, overall long-term survival approaches 95%, and many patients survive for years despite secondary systemic involvement.[4] Micro-MTCs (defined as smaller than 1 cm maximum dimension) detected through screening are associated with a better outcome than those examples over 1 cm.

MTCs may be well demarcated or infiltrative, sometimes encapsulated (**Figure 58.42**). They are commonly located in the middle third of the lateral lobes, where C-cell concentration is greatest. Microscopically, they comprise solid sheets, nests and trabecula of cells separated by slender fibrovascular septa (**Figure 58.43**). A panoply of histological variants is seen, most of no clinical importance other than they may masquerade as other tumours (**Box 58.3**). There is often a mixed pattern in any individual example. There is usually only modest nuclear pleomorphism but necrosis may be a feature. Amyloid protein deposition is present in around 80% of cases (**Figure 58.44**) and may mineralize or elicit a foreign body granulomatous response.

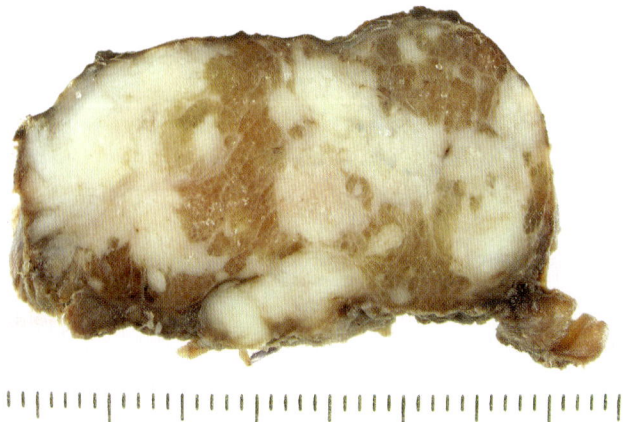

Figure 58.42 The cut surface of multicentric medullary thyroid carcinoma occurring in MEN2B demonstrating widespread effacement of thyroid tissue by infiltrative, solid, white tumour, which abuts and focally violates anatomical thyroid capsule.

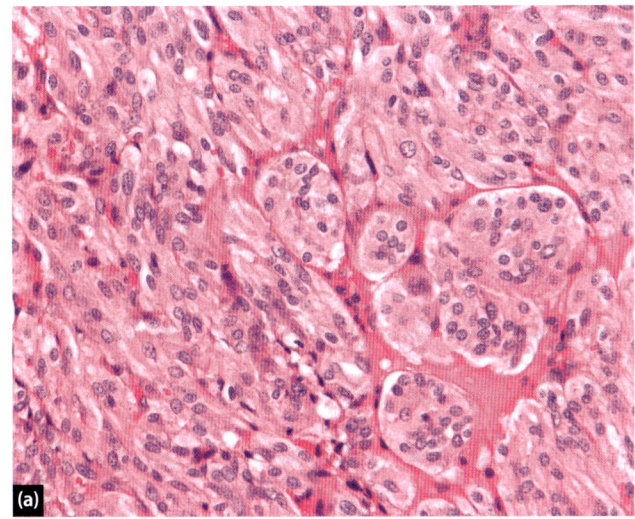
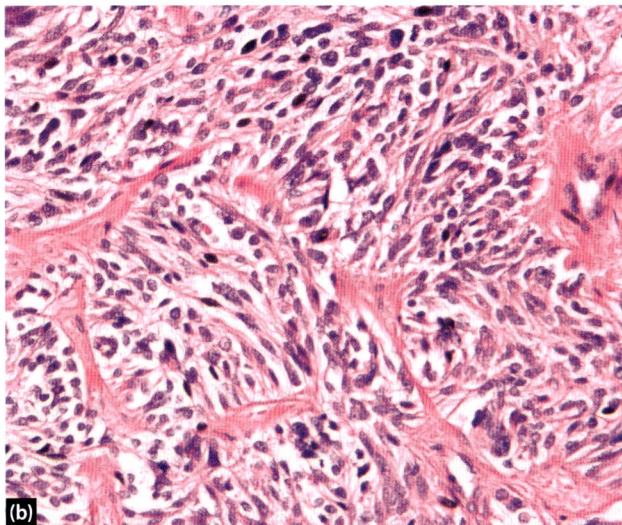

Figure 58.43 Medullary thyroid carcinoma. (a) The typical nested or pseudo-alveolar (Zellballen) architecture of medullary thyroid carcinoma, *type ordinaire*. These tumour cells are largely epithelioid and monotonous (*H&E stain, high magnification*). **(b)** This field shows mild pleomorphism and a more fusiform cell morphology (*H&E stain, high magnification*).

BOX 58.3 Histological variants of MTC

Follicular (glandular/tubular)
Oncocytic (oxyphilic)
Giant cell (anaplastic)
Pigmented
Papillary (pseudo-papillary)
Neuroblastoma-like
Paraganglioma-like
Small cell
Clear cell
Spindle cell
Squamous melanotic
Amphicrine
Angiosarcoma-like (Pseudo-angiosarcomatoid)
Carcinoid-like
Medullary microcarcinoma (latent carcinoma)
Encapsulated ('C-cell adenoma')

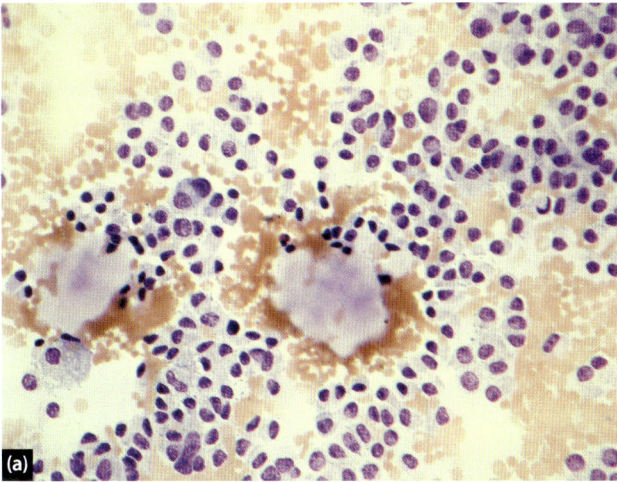
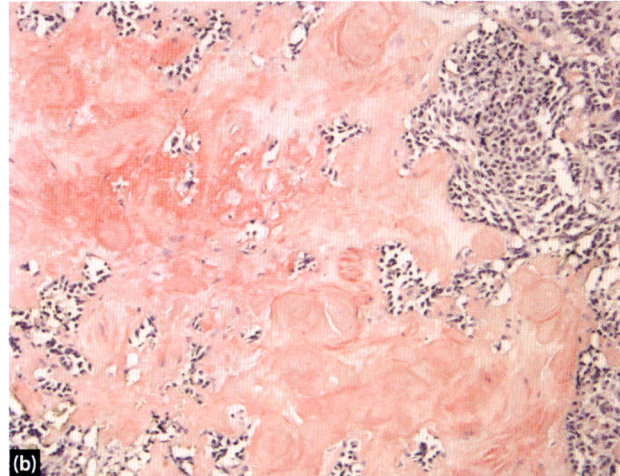
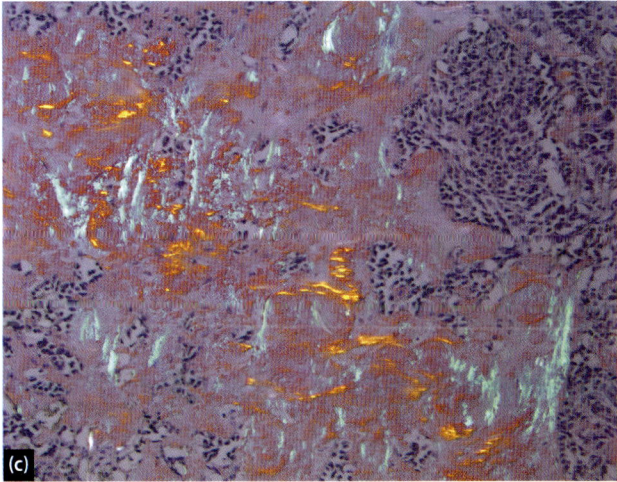

Figure 58.44 MTC. (a) FNAC preparation from medullary thyroid carcinoma, depicting loosely cohesive, moderately pleomorphic, plasmacytoid tumour cells together with several globules of amorphous amyloid protein (*MGG stain, high magnification*). **(b)** Medullary thyroid carcinoma with conspicuous amorphous, dense, pink/red amyloid protein stroma separating groups of tumour cells (*Congo red stain, low magnification*). **(c)** The identical field viewed under high intensity, cross-polarized light corroborates anomalous red/green colouration (sometimes incorrectly termed 'apple green birefringence') highly characteristic of amyloid protein (*Congo red stain, high magnification*).

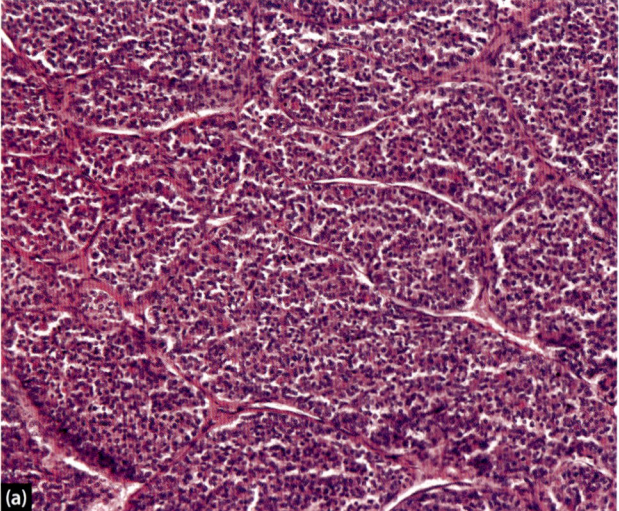
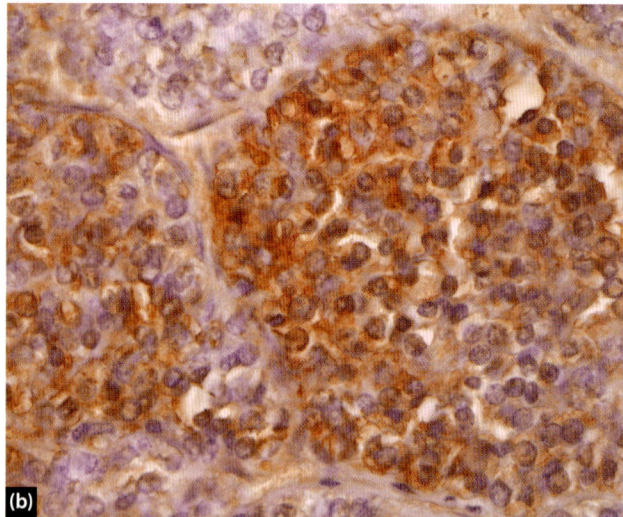

Figure 58.45 Small cell variant MTC. (a) Calcitonin-poor, small cell variant of medullary thyroid carcinoma. Note the insular growth pattern (*H&E stain, intermediate magnification*). **(b)** The same tumour exhibiting carcinoembryonic antigen (CEA, CD66e) positivity. This example was negative for calcitonin and only weakly positive for chromogranin A, reflecting a paucity of intracytoplasmic storage granules, despite raised circulating serum calcitonin levels (*CEA IHC, high magnification*).

The usual immunophenotype is positive for CK, calcitonin, TTF-1, CEA, (CD66e) and pan-neuroendocrine markers. Calcitonin-depleted tumours may behave more aggressively, but almost invariably stain for CEA (**Figure 58.45**). Other neuropeptides may be demonstrated including calcitonin gene-related peptide, somatostatin, ACTH, serotonin, gastrin, bombesin and histaminase amongst others. An S100 protein-positive subpopulation of sustentacular cells is more commonly seen in hereditary cases (**Figure 58.46**), potentially overlapping morphologically with paraganglioma, though paragangliomas (with the rare, anomalous exception of those involving the cauda equina) are cytokeratin negative. It is wise to be aware that neuroendocrine neoplasms other than MTC may sometimes express aberrant calcitonin immunoreactivity, for example laryngeal and bronchopulmonary atypical carcinoid tumours, although the latter are typically immunonegative for CEA (CD66e) and there is more often than not normocalcaemia.

Electron microscopy identifies membrane-bound electron-dense storage granules ranging from 100–300 nm in diameter with augmented rough endoplasmic reticulum and Golgi apparatus (**Figure 58.47**).

C-cell hyperplasia and neoplasia

FMTC develops in a milieu of C-cell hyperplasia and there is no recognized benign C-cell adenoma counterpart. Reactive (physiological) C-cell hyperplasia occurs with advancing age, in thyroiditis, in hyperparathyroidism, in close proximity to other thyroid neoplasms or solid cell nests and in hypergastrinaemia. There is no unanimously accepted definition of nodular (neoplastic, MTC *in situ*)

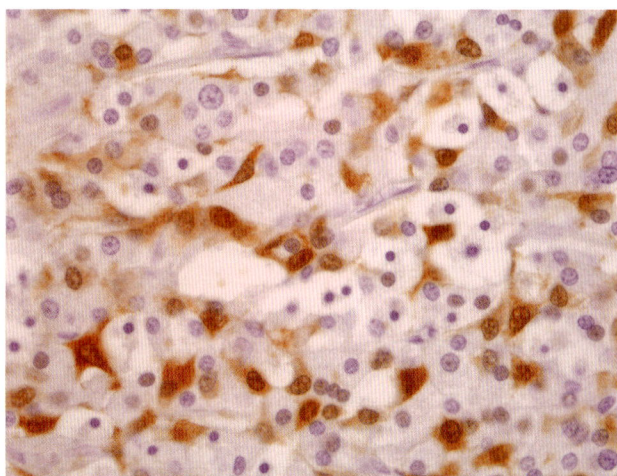

Figure 58.46 Medullary thyroid carcinoma in MEN2 showing typical S100 protein reactive, spindly sustentacular cells mantling small nests of secretory tumour cells (*S100 IHC, high magnification*).

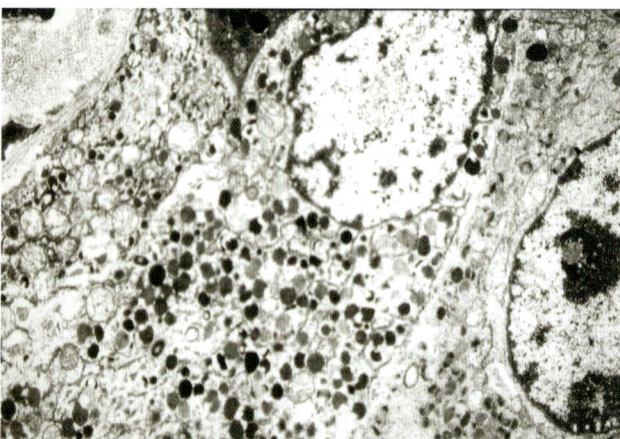

Figure 58.47 Transmission electron micrograph depicting several tumour cells from a medullary thyroid carcinoma, occurring in a child with known MEN2B. Numerous dense, membrane-bound neurosecretory vesicles are present in the cytoplasm (*TEM, ultra-high magnification*).

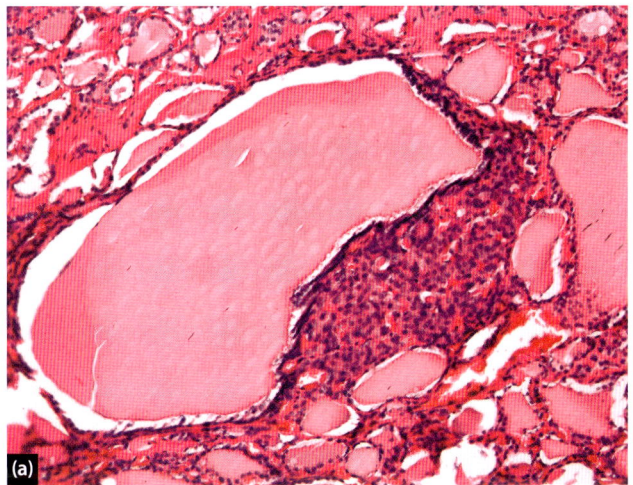
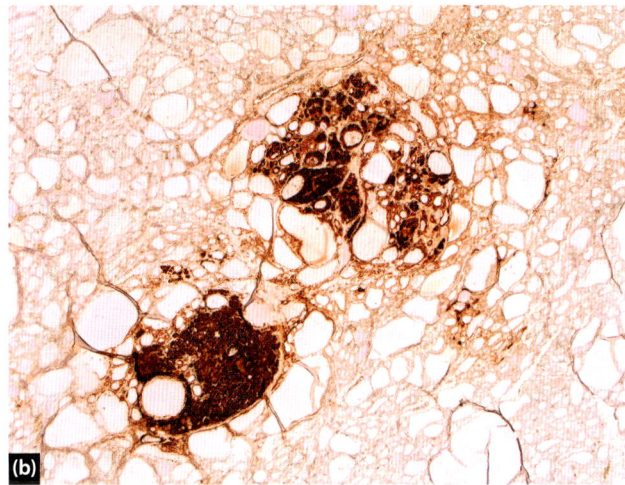

Figure 58.48 C-cell hyperplasia. (a) Early nodular (neoplastic) C-cell hyperplasia in MEN2, readily identified on routine staining. There is expansion of C-cells within the follicular basement membrane but no destructive or infiltrative growth (*H&E stain, medium magnification*). **(b)** More marked and multicentric nodular (neoplastic) C-cell proliferation with follicular obliteration and interstitial expansion. This probably amounts to at least medullary carcinoma *in situ*, if not medullary thyroid microcarcinoma (microtumour) proper (*calcitonin IHC, high magnification*).

C-cell proliferation but over 50 C-cells per ×100 field has been proposed,[51] where there is obliteration of follicular spaces by solid, intrafollicular C-cell growth delimited by basement membrane, as demonstrated by immunostaining for collagen IV (**Figure 58.48**). Once there is violation of basement membrane and/or tumour-derived basal lamina reduplication, that intuitively constitutes MTC proper, although the distinction between medullary microcarcinoma (minute MTC) and intrathyroidal spread of MTC may be impossible.

C-cells cannot be reliably identified by morphology on routine histological slides without recourse to calcitonin or pan-neuroendocrine immunophenotyping. This has, however, assumed less importance with the advent of more sensitive and specific molecular analysis looking for *RET* proto-oncogene germline mutations in the diagnosis of hereditary MTC syndromes.

Tumours displaying joint follicular and C-cell differentiation

The concept of mixed follicular–parafollicular carcinoma (mixed medullary and follicular thyroid carcinoma, MMNFTC) is enigmatic. Collision (combined) tumours include follicular carcinoma plus MTC and papillary carcinoma plus MTC. True follicular–parafollicular carcinoma (differentiated carcinoma of intermediate type) occurring as a genuine hybrid (composite/compound/biphasic) neoplasm is exceptionally rare. Theoretically, the two cell populations may either share origin from a common stem cell or be of dual clonality. The follicular component is sometimes non-neoplastic, thereby raising the possibility of implicated follicles within a slowly growing MTC. False-positive Tg staining may result from passive diffusion out of nearby native follicles or following active pinophagocytosis by tumour cells, rather than endogenous synthesis proper. The conventional ontogenetic explanation proposing different origins for follicular cells and C-cells, however, fails to reconcile the observation of apparent genuine coexpression of both Tg and calcitonin by the same tumour cell.[4]

An appreciation of primary small cell thyroid tumours and allied variants, with or without neuroendocrine features, is however emerging. What was initially described as small cell primary non-neuroendocrine thyroid carcinoma has more recently been redesignated carcinoma of the thyroid with Ewing family tumour elements (CEFTE) on the basis of *EWSR1/FLI1* gene rearrangement studies, and as such may overlap with so-called adamantinoma-like Ewing tumours. Rare examples of non-medullary primary neuroendocrine carcinoma closely resemble small cell neuroendocrine carcinoma of lung, also with absent C-cell differentiation. There is some immunophenotypic overlap between this and non-small cell calcitonin-free medullary carcinomas (calcitonin-negative neuroendocrine tumours of the thyroid). Some authors have postulated that this phenotype is a manifestation of least differentiated tumours of C-cell histogenesis that have lost the capacity to secrete calcitonin but maintain calcitonin gene-related peptide expression, thereby potentially providing a developmental pathway to explain the controversial concept of so-called mixed medullary–follicular/papillary carcinoma.[52]

Other neoplasms and tumour-like lesions

Rare, but distinct forms of primary thyroid carcinoma may morphologically simulate tumours of salivary gland derivation, notably muco-epidermoid carcinoma, muco-epidermoid carcinoma with eosinophilia and secretory carcinoma/mammary secretory analogue carcinoma. There are very many other less common or incredibly rare neoplasms affecting the thyroid gland of epithelial, mesenchymal, haematolymphoid, thymic, parathyroid gland and developmental origin, together with a few tumour-like lesions (**Box 58.4**). The list

> **BOX 58.4** Uncommon or rare tumours and tumour-like lesions described in the thyroid gland
>
> Squamous cell carcinoma
> Mucoepidermoid carcinoma
> Mucoepidermoid carcinoma with eosinophilocytosis
> Mucinous carcinoma
> Spindle cell tumour with thymus-like differentiation (SETTLE)
> Carcinoma showing thymus-like differentiation (CASTLE)
> Malignant lymphomas and leukaemias
> Extramedullary plasmacytoma
> Langerhan's cell histiocytosis
> Angiosarcoma
> Solitary fibrous tumour
> Smooth muscle neoplasms
> Peripheral nerve sheath tumours
> Paraganglioma
> Teratoma
> Fibromatosis
> Granular cell tumour
> Synovial sarcoma
> Haemangiopericytoma
> Lipoma
> Liposarcoma
> Chondrosarcoma
> Osteosarcoma
> Haemangioma
> Lymphangioma
> Rhabdomyoma
> Epithelioid haemangioendothelioma
> Small cell neuroendocrine carcinoma
> IgG4-related sclerosing disease/inflammatory pseudotumour

is not exhaustive and a few may arguably be reclassified differently in the light of modern thinking.

Metastatic tumours

The thyroid gland is commonly affected by metastases either by direct extension from neighbouring structures, haematogenous or lymphatic spread. Local structures include the larynx or lymph nodes and common non-head and neck primary sites include bronchopulmonary, breast, malignant melanoma and renal cell carcinoma (**Figure 58.49**). The latter may occur metachronously following an interval of up to 19 years or be a synchronous presenting feature of the disease.[37]

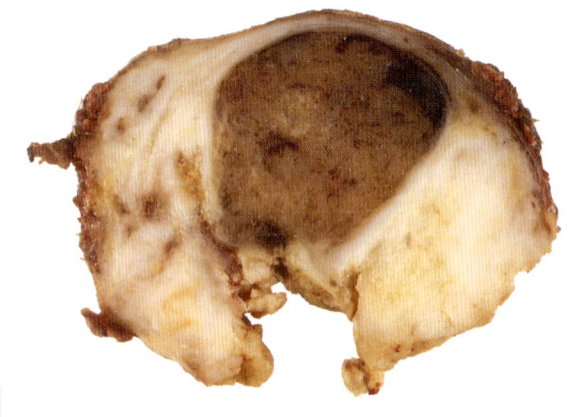

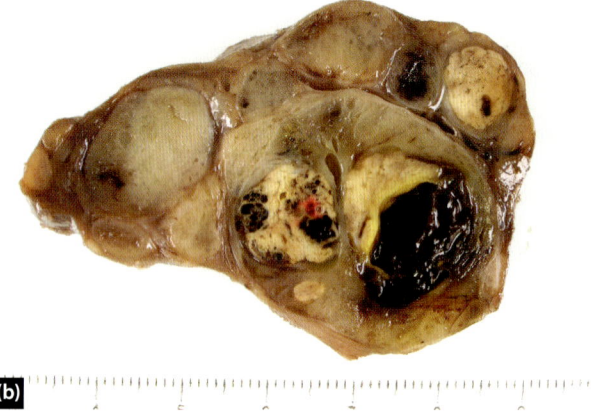

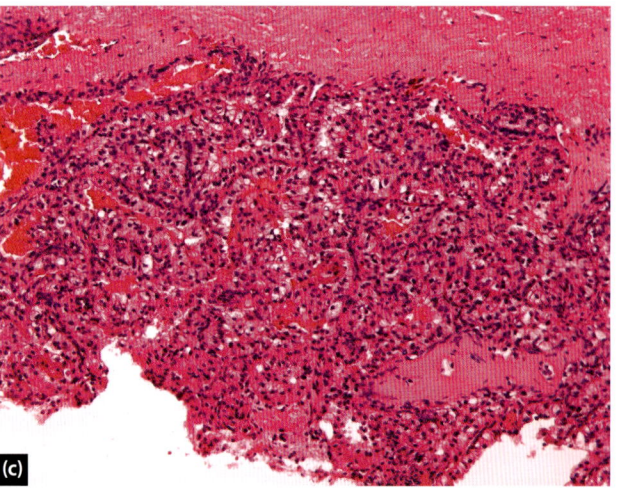

Figure 58.49 Metastatic tumours. (a) Thyroid lobectomy specimen corticated by squamous cell carcinoma, secondary to direct contiguous infiltration from an advanced stage, upper aerodigestive tract primary site. **(b)** Metastatic clear cell renal carcinoma colonizing nodules in a pre-existing hyperplastic multinodular goitre. This was accompanied by characteristic radiological imagery. **(c)** Needle core biopsy of metachronous, metastatic clear cell renal carcinoma presenting as a mass in the thyroid gland some 13 years after nephrectomy for clear cell carcinoma. Its true nature was completely unsuspected clinically – there was no mention of a previous operation in the clinical records. Nonetheless, the pathological findings were unequivocal and the previous kidney specimen was eventually retrieved from the archives of a neighbouring hospital for comparison and review (*H&E stain, medium magnification*).

Intra-operative frozen examination

The use of peri-operative frozen section examination to assist in the diagnosis of thyroid lesions has dwindled in recent years. The widespread adoption of FNAC has enabled broad pre-operative categorization of many lesions, which by their very nature cannot be further refined by frozen section assessment, for example follicular lesion, follicular neoplasm and oncocytic (oxyphil) neoplasm. Frozen section examination on a lesion, definite for malignancy on FNAC, is also unlikely to confer any significant benefit – if the distinction between high-grade lymphoma and undifferentiated (anaplastic) carcinoma has not already been made on FNAC or needle core biopsy, then frozen section is equally unlikely to resolve this. Fleshy, solitary encapsulated lesions are likely to represent follicular adenoma, MIFC, EFVPTC or even MTC, but attempts to comprehensively sample the capsule in the fresh state should be resisted pending tissue fixation with a view to proper paraffin sections in order to obviate artefactual disruption and distortion of the all important peri-capsular tissue planes. The indications for peri-operative frozen section examination of thyroid gland lesions are best agreed by the relevant multidisciplinary team at a local level, taking into consideration local circumstances, individual experience and preferences, together with clinical expectations.[53]

Thyroid cancer staging

The UICC/AJCC TNM classification of malignant tumours is internationally ratified, currently in its 8th edition (2017) (Table 58.11).[54] Most importantly, the definition of T3 has been revised for papillary, follicular and medullary thyroid carcinomas, compared to the 7th edition (2009) and the age threshold for a poor prognosis has been amended from over 45 years to over 55 years.

TABLE 58.11 UICC/TNM 8th edition staging schema for thyroid carcinoma[54, 55]

THYROID GLAND (ICD-o-3 C73.9)[54]

Rules for Classification

The classification applies only to carcinomas. There should be microscopic confirmation of the disease and division of cases by histological type.

The following are the procedures for assessing T, N, and M categories:

T categories	Physical examination, endoscopy, and imaging
N categories	Physical examination and imaging
M categories	Physical examination and imaging

Regional Lymph Nodes

The regional lymph nodes are the cervical and upper/superior mediastinal nodes.

TNM Clinical Classification

T – Primary Tumour*

TX	Primary tumour cannot be assessed
T0	No evidence of primary tumour
T1	Tumour 2 cm or less in greatest dimension, limited to the thyroid
T1a	Tumour 1 cm or less in greatest dimension, limited to the thyroid
T1b	Tumour more than 1 cm but not more than 2 cm in greatest dimension, limited to the thyroid
T2	Tumour more than 2 cm but not more than 4 cm in greatest dimension, limited to the thyroid
T3	Tumour more than 4 cm in greatest dimension, limited to the thyroid with gross extrathyroidal extension invading only strap muscles (sternohyoid, sternothyroid, or omohyoid muscles)
T3a	Tumour more than 4 cm in greatest dimension, limited to the thyroid
T3b	Tumour of any size with gross extrathyroidal extension invading strap muscles (sternohyoid, sternothyroid, or omohyoid muscles)
T4a	Tumour extends beyond the thyroid capsule and invades any of the following: subcutaneous soft tissues, larynx, trachea, oesophagus, recurrent laryngeal nerve
T4b	Tumour invades prevertebral fascia, mediastinal vessels, or encases carotid artery

Note: *Including papillary, follicular, poorly differentiated, Hürthle cell and anaplastic carcinomas.

N – Regional Lymph Nodes

NX	Regional lymph nodes cannot be assessed
N0	No regional lymph node metastasis
N1	Regional lymph node metastasis
N1a	Metastatis in Level VI (pretracheal, paratracheal, and prelaryngeal/Delphian lymph nodes) or upper/superior mediastinum
N1b	Metastasis in other unilateral, bilateral or contralateral cervical (Levels I, II, III, IV or V) or retropharyngeal

(Continued)

TABLE 58.11 (Continued) UICC/TNM 8th edition staging schema for thyroid carcinoma[54, 55]

THYROID GLAND (ICD-o-3 C73.9)[54]

M – Distant Metastasis

M0	No distant metastasis
M1	Distant metastasis

pTNM Pathological Classification

The pT and pN categories correspond to the T and N categories. pM1 denotes distant metastasis microscopically confirmed. Note that pM0 and pMX are not valid categories – the MX category is considered to be inappropriate as clinical assessment can be based on physical examination alone (the use of MX may result in exclusion from staging). The categories M1/pM1 may be further specified employing dedicated codes denoting anatomical site(s) of metastasis, i.e. pulmonary, osseous, hepatic, brain, lymph nodes, bone marrow, pleura, peritoneum, adrenals, skin and others.

pN0   Histological examination of a selective neck dissection specimen will ordinarily include 6 or more lymph nodes. If the lymph nodes are negative, but the number ordinarily examined is not met, classify as pN0.

Histopathological Types

The four major histopathological types are:

- Papillary carcinoma (including those with follicular foci)
- Follicular carcinoma (including so-called Hürthle cell carcinoma)
- Medullary carcinoma
- Anaplastic

Stage

Separate stage groupings are recommended for papillary and follicular (differentiated), medullary, and anaplastic (undifferentiated) carcinomas:

Papillary and Follicular* under 55 years

Stage I	Any T	Any N	M0
Stage II	Any T	Any N	M1

Papillary or Follicular 55 years and older

Stage I	T1a, T1b, T2	N0	M0
Stage II	T3	N0	M0
	T1, T2, T3	N1	M0
Stage III	T4a	Any N	M0
Stage IVA	T4b	Any N	M0
Stage IVB	Any T	Any N	M1

Medullary

Stage I	T1a, T1b	N0	M0
Stage II	T2, T3	N0	M0
Stage III	T1, T2, T3	N1a	M0
Stage IVA	T1, T2, T3	N1b	M0
	T4a	Any N	M0
Stage IVB	T4b	Any N	M0
Stage IVC	Any T	Any N	M1

Anaplastic

Stage IVA	T1, T2, T3a	N0	M0
Stage IVB	T1, T2, T3a	N1	M0
Stage IVB	T3b, T4a, T4b	N0, N1	M0
Stage IVC	Any T	Any N	M1

Note: *Including papillary, follicular, poorly differentiated, and Hürthle cell carcinomas.

(Continued)

TABLE 58.11 *(Continued)* UICC/TNM 8th edition staging schema for thyroid carcinoma[54, 55]			
PROGNOSTIC FACTOR GRID – Papillary and Follicular Thyroid Carcinoma[55]			
Prognostic factors for survival in differentiated thyroid carcinoma of follicular cell derivation			
Prognostic factors	**Tumour-related**	**Host-related**	**Environment-related**
Essential	Extrathyroid extension T category M category Post-treatment Thyroglobulin	Age	Residual disease: R0, 1 or 2
Additional	N category Site of metastases BRAFV600E mutation	Gender	Extent of resection Iodine ablation Endemic goitre
New and promising	Molecular profile		
PROGNOSTIC FACTOR GRID – Medullary Cancer[55]			
Prognostic factors	**Tumour-related**	**Host-related**	**Environment-related**
Essential	Pre- and post-operative calcitonin and CEA	Age	Extent of resection
Additional	MEN Germline mutation Calcitonin doubling time		
New and promising	Molecular profile		

PARATHYROID GLANDS

Normal parathyroid glands

Most individuals possess at least two pairs of parathyroid glands (PTG). The cephalad pair are embryologically derived from the 4th branchial cleft and are usually located over the posterior surface of the thyroid gland close to the point of entry of the inferior thyroid artery. The caudad glands are of 3rd branchial pouch origin and typically lie over the lower thyroid gland pole, though they are more variably placed and may be found within the mediastinum or even the pericardium, consequent upon co-migration with the thymus, which is similarly of 3rd branchial pouch ontogeny. Supernumerary or heterotopic (ectopic) glandular tissue may consist of less well-formed, more diffuse cell aggregates within cervical soft tissues (parathyromatosis) often in close proximity to eutopic glands and this pattern also characterizes surgically implanted gland tissue.[5]

The parathyroid glands secrete parathyroid hormone (parathormone, PTH), which elevates serum calcium via direct effects on kidney and bone and indirectly through the intestine. To the unaided eye, the glands are a yellow-brown colour. At operation, brown fat, yellow fat, sequestrated thyroid tissue, thymus, lymph node and autonomic ganglia may all mimic these appearances and these are not infrequently submitted for frozen section examination in lieu of parathyroid gland proper. Microscopically, in the normal state, the glands are lobulated, richly vascularized and composed of nests and/or trabecula of polygonal parenchymal cells, viz. a mixture of chief (principal) cells, water-clear cells and oncocytic (oxyphil) cells, interspersed with adipocytes (**Figures 58.50** and **58.51**). The number, size and composition of the glands, however, are subject to wide normal and abnormal variation (**Table 58.12**) influenced by age, gender, nutritional and hormonal status. With advancing age, congeries of oncocytic (oxyphil) cells are increasingly encountered.

Hyperparathyroidism

Hyperparathyroidism is defined by elevated serum PTH and is the commonest pathological condition affecting the parathyroid glands. It is classified into primary, secondary and tertiary forms dependent upon the identification of a driving stimulus (**Table 58.13**) though the end result is an absolute increase in parenchymal cell mass affecting one or more glands (**Figure 58.52**). Parathyroid proliferative disease (PPD) is a collective term encompassing all histological causes of hyperparathyroidism.

In primary parathyroid gland hyperplasia, all of the parathyroid glands are enlarged, albeit unevenly in some cases. In parathyroid gland adenoma, paradigmatically only a single gland is enlarged, the remaining glands being of normal size or small. This is typically accompanied by marked diminution in intraglandular adipocytes and reduced or absent intracytoplasmic lipid droplets (**Figure 58.53**), though rarely the latter may paradoxically be more abundant in chief cells located between hyperplastic nodules. Additionally, foci of irregularly distributed stromal fat cells may persist, recapitulating a rim of normal glandular tissue which, when juxtaposed to a fat depleted hyperplastic nodule, may lead to erroneous interpretation as an adenoma. The most reliable discrimination between hyperplasia and adenoma is achieved through histological examination of multiple glands augmented by multiple sections through larger glands. If only one parathyroid gland is available for

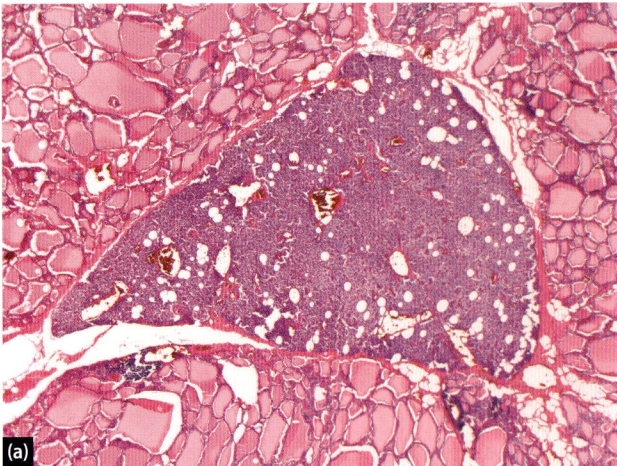
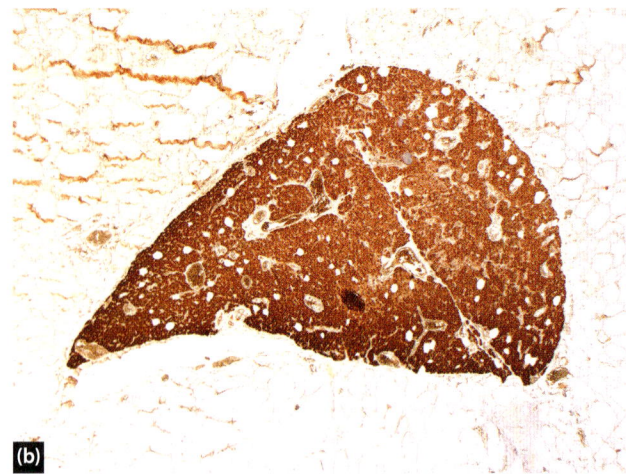

Figure 58.50 Normal parathyroid glands 1. **(a)** An intrathyroidal parathyroid gland presenting a normal vascularized, lobular microarchitecture comprising parenchymal cells interspersed with a normal complement of mature fat cells that are of haphazard distribution and density. Note its clear circumscription and delicate fibrous capsule (*H&E stain, low magnification*). **(b)** A replicate section immunostained with anti-PTH antibody showing intense parenchymal positivity, in sharp contrast to the surrounding negative thyroid gland follicles acting as an internal control (*PTH IHC, low magnification*).

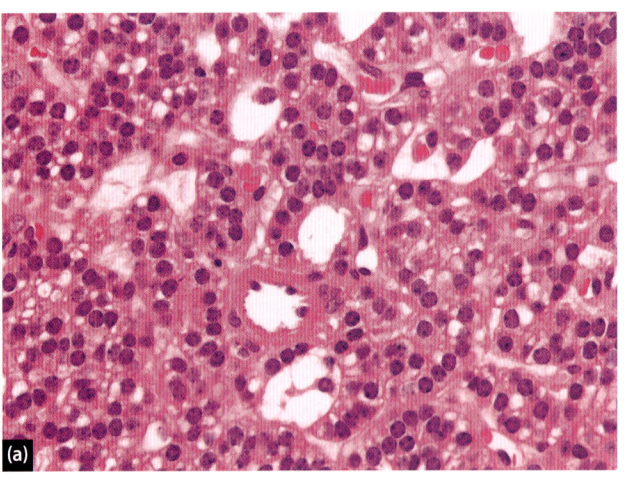
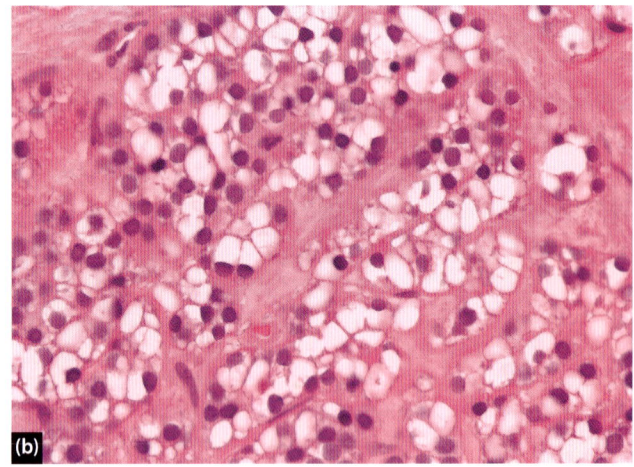
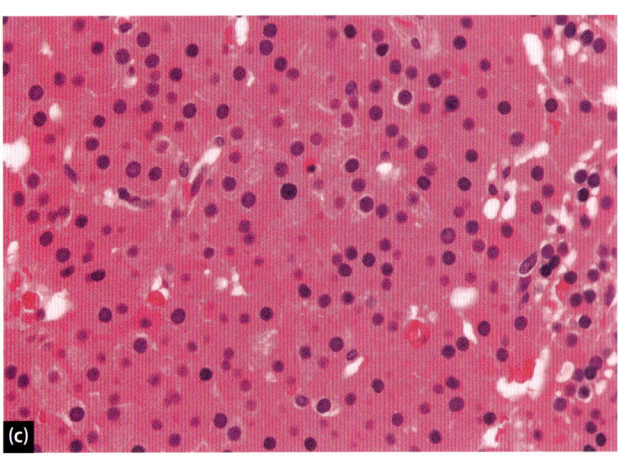

Figure 58.51 Normal parathyroid glands 2. **(a)** Nests and trabecula of isomorphic chief cells forming occasional glandular lumina or so-called microfollicular/pseudofollicular growth pattern (*H&E stain, high magnification*). **(b)** Clusters of water-clear cells displaying their characteristic clear, generally univacuolar cytoplasm with eccentrically displaced nuclei (*H&E stain, high magnification*). **(c)** Nodular sheets of oncocytic (oxyphil) cells illustrating their hallmark, copious, granular and densely eosinophilic cytoplasm, attributable to plentiful mitochondria. A minor degree of random nuclear pleomorphism is often encountered (*H&E stain, high magnification*).

examination and proves to be enlarged and/or hypercellular, definitive pathological distinction between hyperplasia and adenoma cannot always be reliably achieved.

The term lipohyperplasia may be used to designate the extremely rare occurrence of hyperplastic glands with plentiful fat, in which the glands are enlarged albeit with predominant lipocytes and limited parathyrocyte cell content.

Parathyromatosis is a rare cause of persistent or recurrent hyperparathyroidism characterized by multiple nests of hyperfunctioning parathyroid tissue throughout the neck and mediastinum. These may range in size from

TABLE 58.12 Attributes of normal and abnormal parathyroid glands in man[4]

Characteristic	Normal range	Abnormal
Number	Usually 4, but ranges from 1–12	
Size	Length 3–6 mm Width 2–4 mm Depth 0.5–2 mm	>6 mm in any plane
Weight	Each gland approx. 30 mg – the inferior glands are often heavier than the superior ones Total parathyroid gland mass 120 ± 3.5 mg in males 142 ± 5.2 mg in females	Any individual gland >60 mg
% fat	17–50% Male average 20.5% Female average 15.6%	Complete absence or very marked reduction
Intracytoplasmic lipid	Abundant	Absent or sparse

TABLE 58.13 Classification of hyperparathyroidism

Type	Definition	Causes	Pathological changes
Primary	Overproduction of PTH due to intrinsic abnormality of one or more glands causing elevated serum calcium with depressed serum phosphate	PTG adenoma 85% PTG carcinoma 1% PTG hyperplasia 14% • Sporadic • MEN 1 • MEN 2 • Familial isolated hyperparathyroidism • Familial hypocalcuric hypercalcaemia	Adenoma or carcinoma changes Chief cell hyperplasia Reduced or absent intra-parenchymal fat Diffuse or nodular changes
Secondary	Compensatory hyperplasia of parathyroid glands due to decreased serum calcium, usually resulting in normocalcaemia	Chronic renal failure Malabsorption Vitamin D deficiency Renal tubular acidosis	Hyperplasia of all glands May be indistinguishable from primary hyperparathyroidism Multinodular or diffuse
Tertiary	Autonomous parathyroid gland hyper-function following secondary hyperparathyroidism	Any cause of secondary hyperparathyroidism	Very similar to secondary hyperparathyroidism though glands are typically larger and multinodular May rarely be associated with adenoma or carcinoma

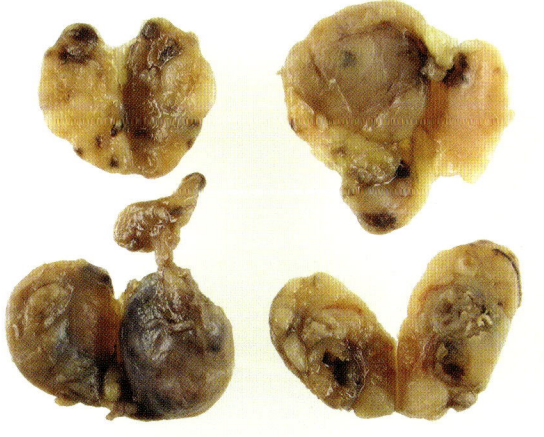

Figure 58.52 Left and right upper and lower parathyroid glands in quadriglandular hyperplasia of secondary hyperparathyroidism following renal transplantation. These each weighed between 0.5 g and 1.2 g and were incised bivalvate peri-operatively to disclose the variegated, multinodular cut surfaces seen here to be irregular, both within and between glands. The lower glands are often asymmetrically larger than the upper glands.

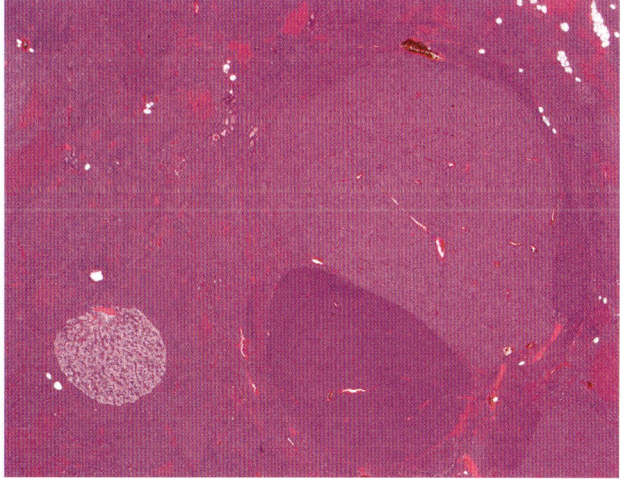

Figure 58.53 A hyperplastic gland in hyperparathyroidism, secondary to chronic renal disease, displaying hypercellularity with hugely reduced stromal fat cell content. The multinodular appearance is due to proliferation of groups of cells with different cytological features, mostly chief cells here with, unevenly distributed, water-clear cell and oxyphil cell nodules (*H&E stain, ultra-low magnification*).

microscopical congeries of cells within skeletal muscle and fat to larger soft yellow/white nodules visible to the unaided eye. Primary parathyromatosisis is associated with the MEN syndromes, most commonly MEN 1. Secondary parathyromatosis occurs as a sequela of surgical exploration of the neck, supposedly due to inadvertent contamination of the operative field following spillage (seeding) of cells. It may mimic invasive carcinoma to the unwary.

Only primary and tertiary hyperparathyroidism are associated with hypercalcaemia and its attendant systemic sequelae, but all three forms may manifest with bone disease. Aberrant PTH-related peptide secretion may occur as a paraneoplastic phenomenon (humoral hypercalcaemia of malignancy) in some malignant neoplasms, notably squamous cell carcinoma of primary bronchopulmonary, upper aerodigestive tract and female genital tract origin, sometimes with renal cell carcinoma. Approximately 50% of metastatic prostatic adenocarcinoma deposits evince anomalous PTH immunopositivity, cross-reacting with PTH-related protein, which may prove to be a source of differential diagnostic confusion. Hypercalcaemia directly related to the osteolytic effects of bone metastasis, independent of PTH-related protein, may occur in mammary carcinoma and haematological malignancies. Lithium therapy prescribed for psychiatric disorders may induce a form of primary hyperparathyroidism, which abates on cessation of the drug, though parathyroidectomy may still be indicated.

Parathyroid gland adenoma

The WHO (4th edition, 2017) classification of parathyroid gland tumours is reproduced in **Table 58.14**.[27] Parathyroid gland adenoma is the predominant cause of primary hyperparathyroidism. It may occur spontaneously or within the context of various syndromes. Irradiation of the neck is a potential risk factor with a latency/interval period in the order of 30–40 years. Excision of the abnormal gland is curative and results in normalization of biochemical indices and increased bone mineral density. Up to 10% of patients relapse, sometimes after an interval of many years. Adenomas are not usually palpable clinically, unless cystic, and rarely cause compressive symptoms. Haemorrhagic infarction, either post-FNAC or spontaneously, complicated by haematoma, may result in an acutely painful neck lump.

The morphological spectrum of parathyroid adenomas occurring in supernumerary glands and in heterotopic sites such as mediastinum, thyroid gland or oesophagus is identical to that in eutopic locations. However, not only may they lead to unsuccessful cervical exploration, they may mimic thyroid gland adenomas or medullary thyroid carcinoma histologically.

Double adenomas may rarely occur (responsible for between 1.7% and 12% of cases of primary hyperparathyroidism) and are usually bilateral. All of the patients are symptomatic and show a higher PTH level and tumour weight compared to solitary adenoma and parathyroid gland hyperplasia. Distinction from asymmetrical parathyroid gland hyperplasia, particularly in the context of MEN, is extremely difficult. The diagnosis is therefore only considered conclusive when follow-up after removal of two abnormal glands shows no recurrence. Gene profiling studies indicate that multiple gland neoplasia represents a distinct molecular entity.

Parathyroid gland adenomas occur more frequently in the lower parathyroid glands. The mean weight is 0.55 g but tumours weighing as much as 53 g are recorded and, generally, the more severe the hypercalcaemia, the bulkier the adenoma. Macroscopically, parathyroid gland adenomas are well marginated, soft and vary from yellow-red to orange-brown in colour (**Figure 58.54**), more blue tinged if toluidine blue has been used as an aid to peri-operative

TABLE 58.14 WHO classification of tumours of the parathyroid glands[35]
Parathyroid carcinoma
Parathyroid adenoma
Secondary, mesenchymal and other tumour

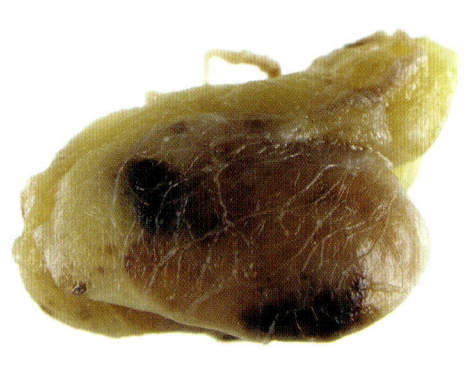 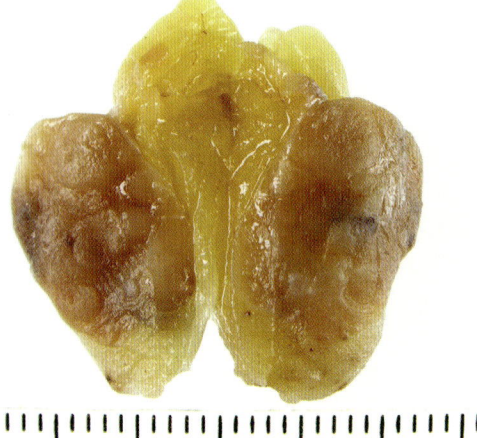

Figure 58.54 **(a)** The external surface of a parathyroid gland adenoma, weighing 1.2 g in primary hyperparathyroidism, demonstrating a delicate capsule with ramifying surface blood vessels. **(b)** When transected, its variegated, multinodular texture is very similar to a hyperplastic gland, though in this instance it was the only abnormal gland of those recovered at operation.

localization. The oncocytic (oxyphil) cell variant presents a so-called mahogany brown cut surface, characteristic of such mitochondria-rich tumours at many sites. Secondary haemorrhage and/or cystic change (**Figure 58.55**) may be encountered, either spontaneously occurring or post-FNAC. The remaining, uninvolved parathyroid glands should be normal or reduced in size.

Microscopically, parathyroid gland adenomas are circumscribed and may be lobulated or nodular. They are hypercellular and substantially or completely bereft of intraglandular adipocytes, with the exception of lipoadenoma. An attenuated, part-circumferential mantle of normal or compressed parathyroid gland tissue is identified in 50% or so of cases, dependent upon the planes of section examined (**Figure 58.56**), often near the vascular hilum of the gland, with the caveat that a compressed tissue rim is occasionally encountered around hyperplastic nodules.

The tumour cells may be disposed in solid sheets, cords, acini, follicle-like and/or microcystic configuration. Glandular structures may contain eosinophilic colloid-like secretions (pseudo-follicular growth). These are dPAS-positive but immunonegative for thyroglobulin. Intrafollicular or interstitial amyloid protein may rarely be deposited.

Most adenomas are composed of chief (principal) cells, though oncocytic (oxyphil) cells and/or water-clear cells are often present, either dispersed or in nodular aggregates. The chief cells of an adenoma are usually larger than their non-neoplastic counterparts present in the uninvolved rim of parathyroid tissue, where present, and in the remaining, non-neoplastic glands. They also typically possess less intracellular fat than the uninvolved tissue and the other suppressed glands. Mitoses usually number less than 1 per 10 high-power fields without abnormal forms. There may be random nuclear pleomorphism and/or multinucleation

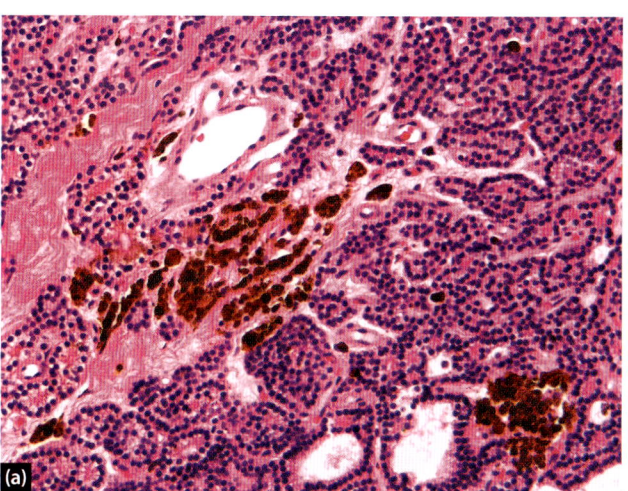
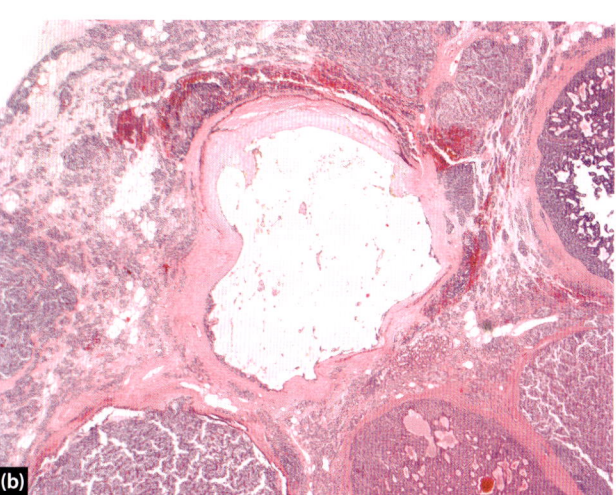

Figure 58.55 (a) This adenoma shows scattered collections of interstitial siderophages containing phagocytosed, coarsely granular, golden brown haemosiderin pigment, indicative of antecedent haemorrhage (*H&E stain, intermediate magnification*). **(b)** Another example displays focal cystic change with accompanying fibrocollagenous scar tissue plus part-circumferential, dystrophic, mural calcification (*H&E stain, low magnification*).

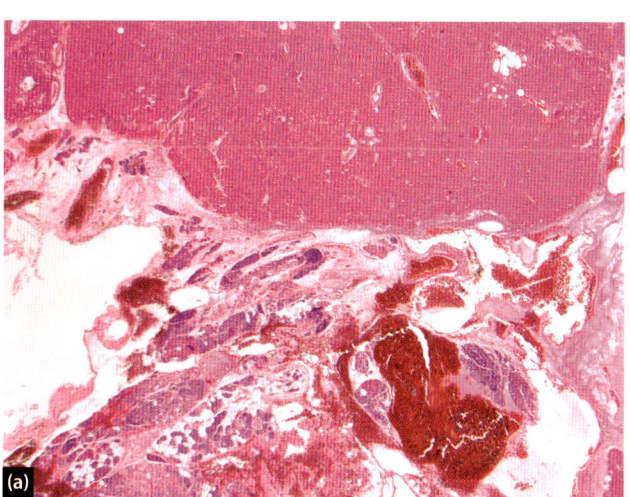
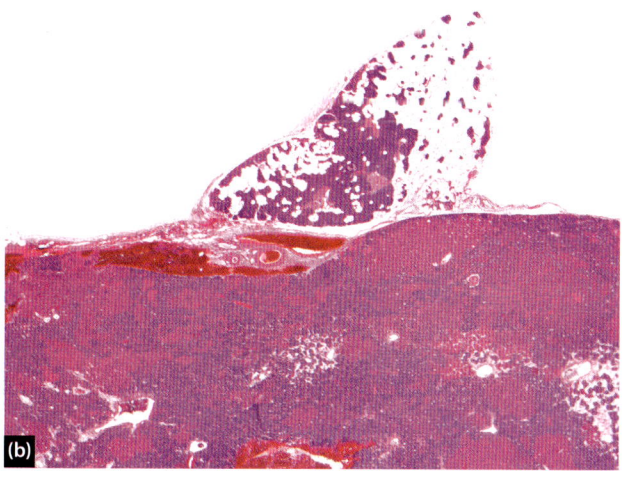

Figure 58.56 (a) View of the edge of a parathyroid gland adenoma. Note its sharp demarcation, hypercellularity and absence of intratumoural lipocytes. There is a peripheral nubbin of attenuated-looking parathyroid glandular tissue with preserved intraglandular fat cells for comparison (*H&E stain, ultra-low magnification*). **(b)** Perimeter of another parathyroid gland adenoma depicting extrinsic atrophic looking parathyroid gland remnant with juxtaposed vascular hilus (*H&E stain, ultra-low magnification*).

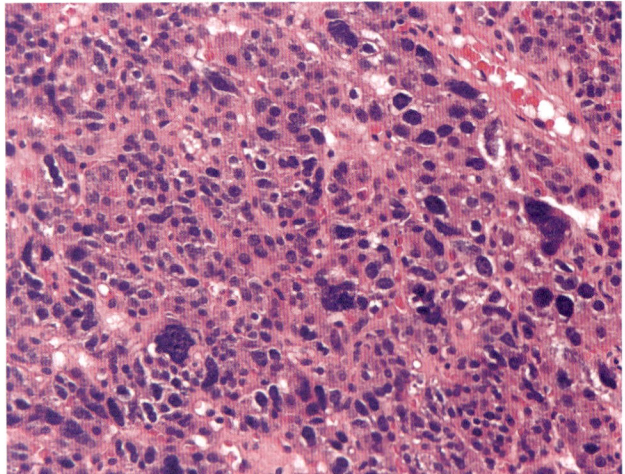

Figure 58.57 The presence of bizarre giant cell transformation (monster cells), some polykaryocytic, possessing enlarged hyperchromatic nuclei, albeit without mitoses or other worrisome features, against a background of bland-looking cells should not be taken as evidence of malignancy (*H&E stain, medium magnification*).

sometimes with bizarre, hyperchromatic giant cells (**Figure 58.57**), though in the absence of other indicators of potential malignancy these should not be misconstrued as evidence portending aggressive behaviour. Flow cytometry is of limited assistance in discriminating between parathyroid gland adenoma and carcinoma because aneuploidy is found in up to 25% of histologically and clinically benign tumours.

VARIANTS OF PARATHYROID GLAND ADENOMA

In addition to their fundamental cytological and architectural patterns, parathyrocyte proliferations, including adenomata, are susceptible to a host of engrafted secondary phenomena, mostly retrogressive, none entirely specific diagnostically. These include inflammation, infarction, haemorrhage, haemosiderosis, Gamna–Gandy nodulosis, hydrops, necrosis, hypervascularity and peliosis-like (pseudo-angiomatoid/telangiectatic) change, microcystic and macrocystic degeneration, fibrosis/hyalinosis, lipometaplasia, metaplastic ossification, mineralization and pseudo-invasion (**Figure 58.58**). These may occur *de novo* or in response to trauma, such as FNAC. The following histological subtypes, however, are recognized.

- **Cystic adenoma** may be cystic *ab initio* or secondarily as a consequence of subsiding haematoma post-infarction. Morphologically, it may mimic a benign simple parathyroid cyst but should not be confused with adenoma *type ordinaire* displaying a minority cystic growth pattern.
- **Lipoadenoma (parathyroid hamartoma)** is a very rare occurrence showing admixture of parenchymal cells with copious mature adipocytes and/or brown fat cells, the fat content variably accounting for 20–90% of the tumour (**Figure 58.59**). There may be accompanying inflammation, mineralization and mucomyxoid change (myxoid lipoadenoma) and, where dominant, the term myxoadenoma is sometimes invoked.[56] Distinction should be drawn diagnostically between lipoadenoma, benign lipoma thymolipoma and lipohyperplasia. Approximately 50% of lipoadenomas are associated with hypercalcaemia. The uninvolved parathyroid glands are normal.
- **Papillary variant** is rare and apt to be mistaken for papillary thyroid carcinoma.
- **Water-clear adenoma** is substantially or wholly composed of water-clear cells. The histological differential diagnosis includes adenoma composed of hydropic and/or vacuolated chief cells (rather than ultrastructurally distinct water-clear cells proper) and water-clear cell

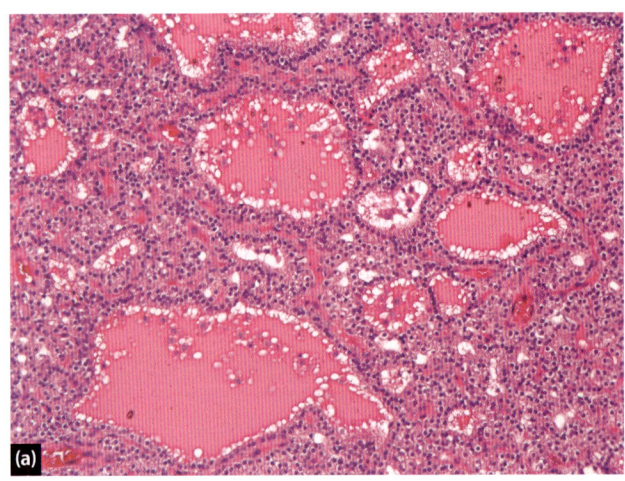
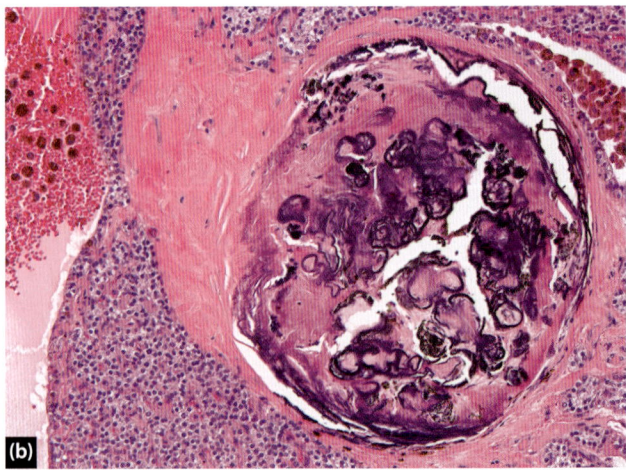

Figure 58.58 (a) Pseudo-follicular growth in a parathyroid adenoma closely resembling normofollicular and macrofollicular thyroid gland follicles with stored colloid-like secretions, even mimicry of marginal vacuoles (*H&E stain, medium magnification*).
(b) Parathyroid gland adenoma showing sequelae of prior haemorrhage, i.e. localized haemosiderosis with adjacent Gamna-Gandy body. These fibrosiderotic nodules consist of degenerate elastin fibres encrusted with iron and calcium salts upon a hyalinized background. They are by no means exclusive to either haemoglobinopathies or the spleen and may occasionally be encountered in tumours at other sites, for example cardiac myxoma (*H&E stain, medium magnification*).

(Continued)

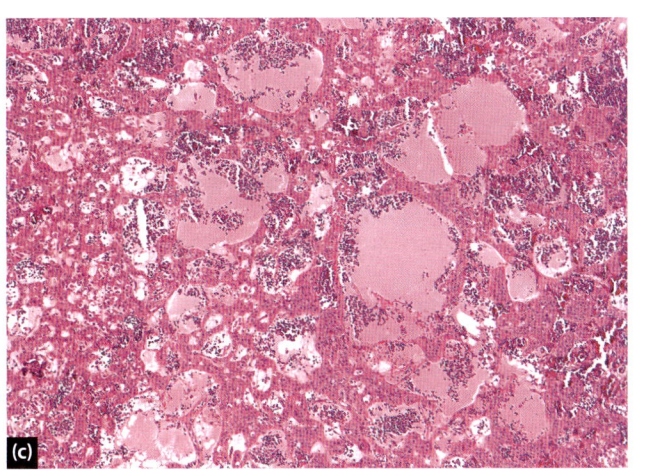
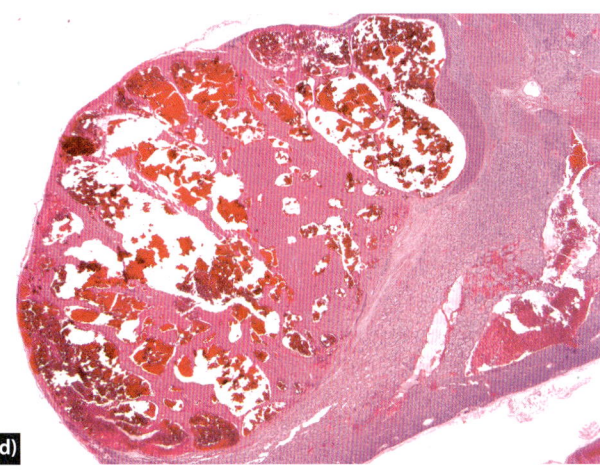

Figure 58.58 (Continued) **(c)** Parathyroid adenoma showing a conspicuous field of spongiform microectatic cisternae filled with erythrocytes, resembling so-called peliosis (pseudoangiomatoid change) more commonly encountered in the liver, spleen and lymph nodes. Its significance at this site is unknown but it should not be mistaken for a vascular malformation, haemangioma or vascular tumour (*H&E stain, low magnification*). **(d)** Another parathyroid adenoma exhibiting circumscribed pseudoangiomatoid growth (*H&E stain, ultra-low magnification*).

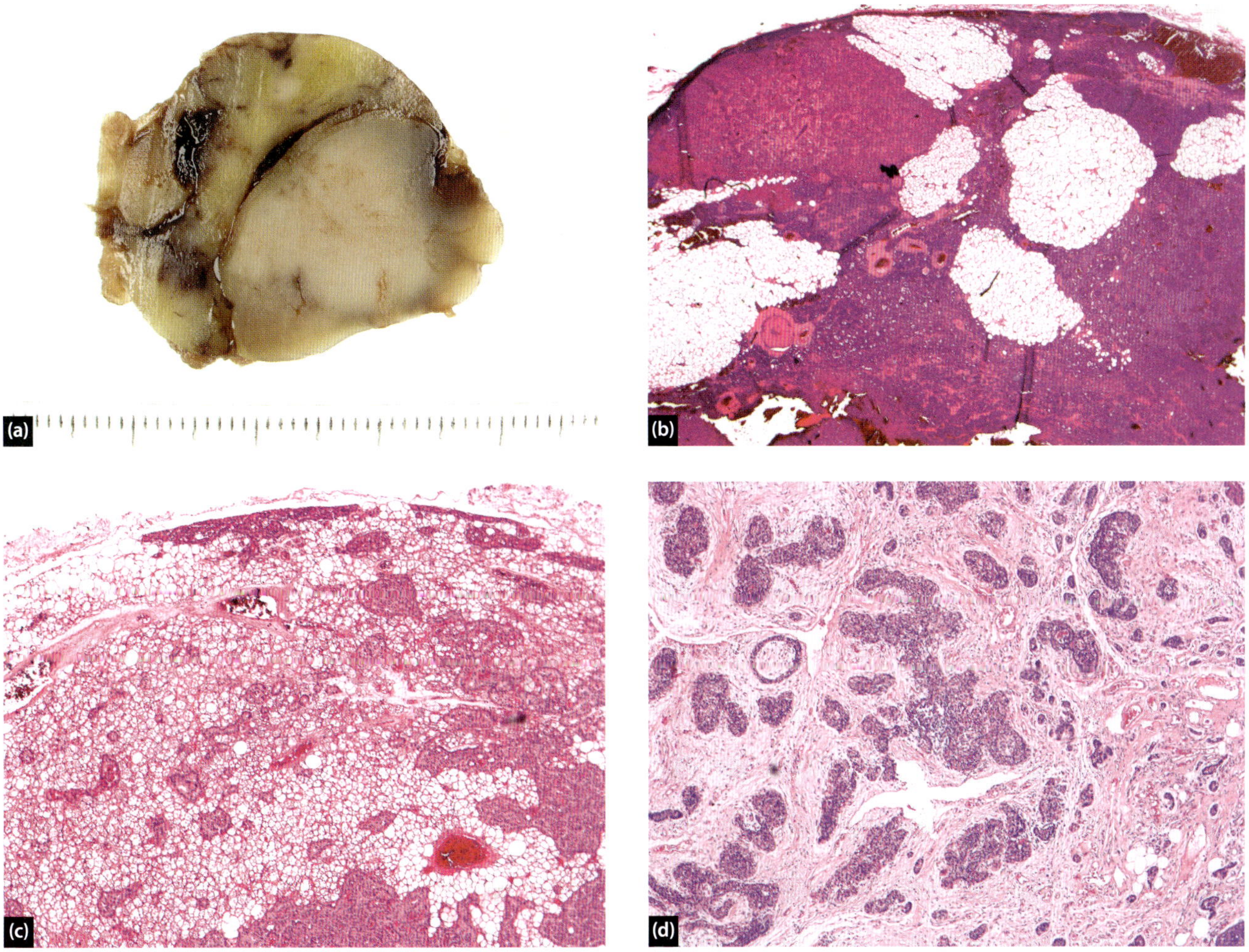

Figure 58.59 **(a)** The cut-surface of a parathyroid gland lipoadenoma illustrating its multinodular architecture comprising solid parenchymal elements interspersed with yellow fat. **(b)** The same lesion histologically confirms solid paratyhyrocyte nodules intimately admixed with mature lipocytes (white fat cells), all within the confines of the delimiting capsule (*H&E stain, low magnification*). **(c)** The pericapsular region of a different lipoadenoma showing similar features, albeit with brown fat cells predominant (*H&E stain, low magnification*). **(d)** Myxoid lipoadenoma comprising prominent loose mucomyxomatous interstitium enclaving discrete islands and sheets of parathyroid cells. A minority cluster of mature adipocytes is evident within the right lower quadrant of this particular field and these provide a clue to the diagnosis (*H&E stain, medium magnification*).

hyperplasia. It may be mistaken for a clear cell neoplasm of the thyroid gland, including metastasis, and paraganglioma.

- **Follicular variant** shows a predominant pseudofollicular (acinar) architecture often with intraglandular secretions and may be misinterpreted as a follicular-patterned thyroid neoplasm.
- **Oxyphil adenoma (oncocytic adenoma)** is comprehensively composed (at least 90% of the cell population) of mitochondria-rich oncocytic (oxyphil) cells and may or may not be functional. It must be distinguished from nodular oxyphilic cell change with advancing age and, when intrathyroidal, from oxyphil (Hürthle) cell neoplasms of the thyroid gland. Commensurate nuclear pleomorphism with polykaryocytosis and bizarre giant cell transformation (monster cells) often feature and, in isolation, should not be overinterpreted as evidence suggestive of malignancy.
- **Microadenoma** is defined as a single lesion of less than 6 mm maximum dimension, weighing no more than 0.1 g, occurring in an otherwise grossly normal parathyroid gland. It may present as an unencapsulated micronodule wholly or partially within the substance of the gland, as a hypercellular proliferation affecting an entire gland or as an area of hypercellular growth showing poor demarcation from juxtaposed normal glandular parenchyma. Demonstration of these may be surgically and pathologically challenging.
- **Parathyroid adenoma with prominent lymphocytic infiltrate** is an unusual histological phenomenon, not necessarily associated with autoimmune response. There may, or may not, be background chronic lymphocytic parathyroiditis of adjacent remnant parathyroid tissue, where glandular destruction may be seen, at least focally. Caution must be exercised to exclude lymphoma.[56] Very rarely parathyroid gland adenoma may present with granulomatous infiltration, not associated with sarcoidosis, underlying infection or other primary granulomatous conditions, themselves associated with hypercalcaemia independent of parathyroid gland disease (**Figure 58.60**).
- **Atypical parathyroid gland adenoma** (*parathyroid neoplasm of uncertain malignant potential*) is a descriptive term attributed to a parathyroid gland tumour that displays equivocal, worrisome, borderline or suspicious features of parathyroid carcinoma, though falls short of fulfilling the first-order criteria for a confident designation of malignancy. This rubric acknowledges the limitations of predicting the behaviour of an individual tumour based upon conventional histomorphological assessment (it is the pathologist who is uncertain, not the tumour) and it is not proffered as a distinct clinicopathological entity. Only a small minority of such atypical adenomas are expected to recur and/or metastasize and the rank importance of second-order criteria in quantifying this small risk of more aggressive behaviour has yet to be established.

Atypical parathyroid gland adenomas are generally indistinguishable from adenoma of usual type by the unaided eye (**Figure 58.61**). The commonest microscopical features, ranked according to frequency, however, include intracapsular entrapment (87%), intratumoural fibrosis (75%), haemosiderosis (58%), cyst formation (50%), mitoses (25%) and peritumoural fibrosis (25%). The Ki67 proliferative index typically lies intermediate between adenoma and frank carcinoma. The value of ploidy studies in predicting local recurrence is based upon small studies. Nonetheless, the use of this terminology serves to highlight those patients who merit closer surveillance, such as regular serum calcium measurements, while avoiding the stigma of a firm label of malignancy, wholly unjustified in most cases.[4]

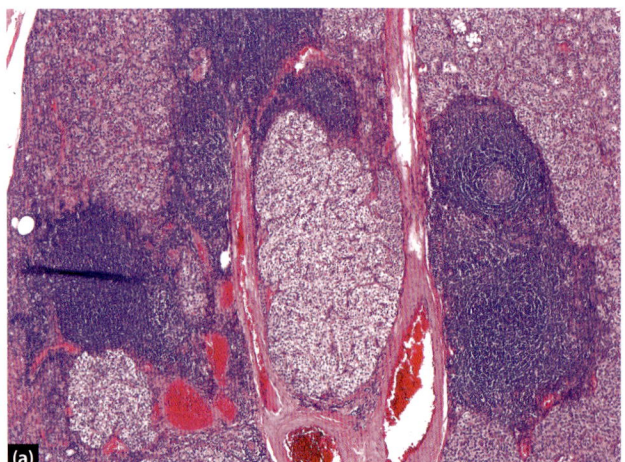
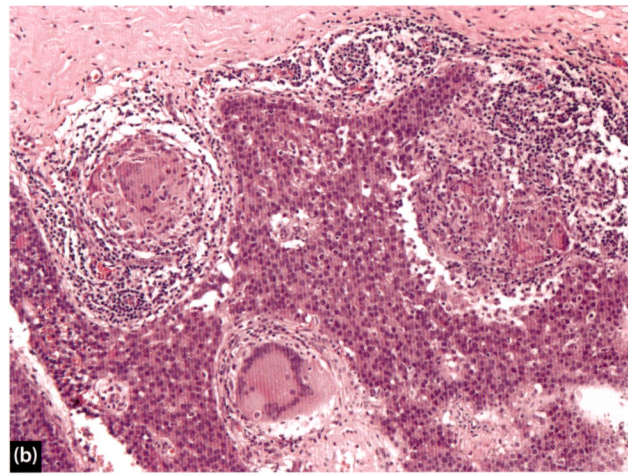

Figure 58.60 **(a)** Parathyroid adenoma variant with prominent lymphocytic infiltrate, demonstrating sheets of chief cells and nodules of water-clear cells intimately associated with a population of lymphocytes and mature plasma cells. Two lymphoid follicles, one with reactive germinal centre formation, are present (*H&E stain, low magnification*). **(b)** Parathyroid adenoma associated with non-necrotizing granulomatous inflammation. Three sharply circumscribed epithelioid histiocytic granulomata, each containing multinucleate giant cells, one of Langhans' type, are visible. This is a rare occurrence and should prompt efforts to exclude comorbid systemic granulomatous disease (*H&E stain, medium magnification*).

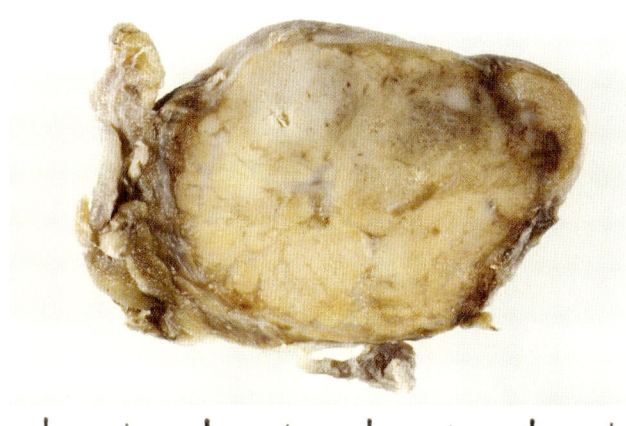

Figure 58.61 This atypical parathyroid gland adenoma is macroscopically indistinguishable from adenoma *type ordinaire*. The cut surface displays subtle capsular irregularity and localised fibrous thickening. First-order criteria of malignancy were absent.

Immunohistochemistry is occasionally valuable in the differential diagnosis between parathyroid gland adenoma and other neoplasms, notably of the thyroid gland, and it also has a role in differentiating between atypical adenoma and parathyroid carcinoma. Parathyrocytes are cytokeratin-positive and stain for many pan-neuroendocrine markers, both membrane-bound peptide products, such as PTH, chromogranin A and synaptophysin, and cytosol epitopes including neuron-specific enolase. Chief cells show nuclear immunoreactivity for thyroid transcription factor-1. Reciprocal negative staining for thyroglobulin may also be helpful. Typically, nuclear parafibromin immunoreactivity is globally or focally lost in parathyroid carcinoma. Atypical adenomata expressing parafibromin are said to behave as adenomata, in contradistinction to those with loss of immunopositivity, which portend a heightened risk of recurrence. Immunostaining for anti-mitochondrial antibody highlights oncocytic (oxyphil) differentiation, but in itself it does not discriminate between oncocytic parathyroid gland tissue and oncocytic change in other tissues. Staining for fat on frozen section is seldom of diagnostic help.

Molecular genetic studies by X-linked restriction fragment length polymorphism provide evidence for monoclonality in many parathyroid gland adenomas. Tumour-specific DNA alterations are present in the PTH gene in some cases. A minority of cases demonstrate pericentric inversion of chromosome 11, which causes translocation of the cyclin D1 gene with the PTH gene resulting in overexpression of cyclin D1 and cell proliferation. Cyclin D1 expression is identified by immunohistochemistry more frequently than this cyclin D1 gene rearrangement, suggesting that other molecular factors are operant in cyclin D1 deregulation. Cyclin D1 is also common in parathyroid hyperplasia and parathyroid carcinoma.

The germline mutation underlying MEN 1 is associated with some sporadic parathyroid gland adenomas. The *RET* proto-oncogene germline mutation underlying MEN 2 does not appear to be involved in the genesis of sporadic parathyroid gland adenomas. Other chromosomal abnormalities are detected by comparative genomic hybridization and fluorescence *in situ* hybridization (FISH) techniques.

Parathyroid carcinoma

This is defined as a malignant neoplasm of parathyroid parenchymal cells and is responsible for approximately 0.5–2% of all cases of primary hyperparathyroidism, though some series report as high as 5%. It occurs most frequently in the fifth and sixth decades (i.e. roughly a decade younger than adenomas) with no gender predilection. Most patients are severely hypercalcaemic with active bone and renal disease at presentation, they tend to suffer worse symptoms attributable to this compared to those with adenoma and there is more often a palpable neck mass, though this presentation is by no means invariable. Initial designation as adenoma may be revised at a later time following recurrence and/or metastasis.[57]

Parathyroid carcinoma tends to invade local structures, is slow-growing and metastasizes late. Complete surgical excision at first operation affords the best opportunity for cure, though this relies upon early recognition of its malignant nature, which cannot always be achieved. Following surgery, approximately 30% of patients suffer local recurrence, usually within 3–5 years. Roughly 30% develop metastasis, typically late in its course, generally to regional lymph nodes (30%), lungs (40%), liver (10%) and bone. Survival is 60–85% and 40–70% at 5 years and 10 years respectively with an average survival following recurrence of 7–8 years. Non-functioning examples may behave more aggressively than functioning ones. Death is usually attributable to the metabolic complications of hypercalcaemia rather than overwhelming tumour burden. Repeated surgery may palliate and adjuvant radiotherapy has a limited role. The response to chemotherapy is poor. The hypercalcaemia may become refractory to medical management and specialist anti-PTH immunotherapy has proven beneficial in very severe cases (**Figure 58.62**), occasionally eliciting a direct anti-tumour effect.[58]

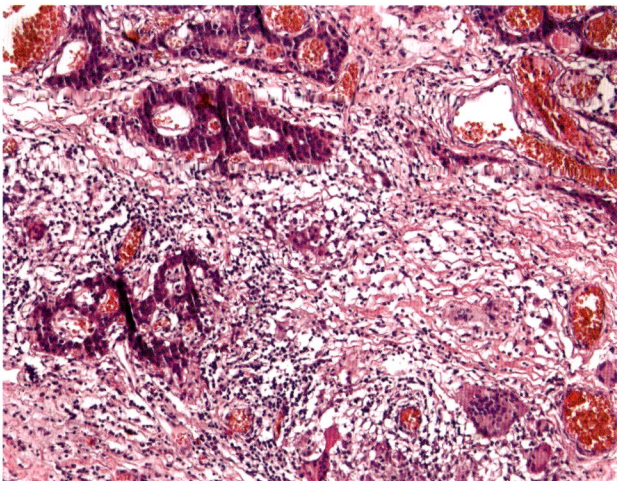

Figure 58.62 Metastatic parathyroid carcinoma in the lung, following anti-PTH immunotherapy for refractory, severe hypercalcaemia. Note the vigorous granulomatous inflammatory response, secondary to Freund's complete adjuvant, which was used to intensify the immune response, closely associated with the nests of residual tumour cells (H&E stain, medium magnification).

The tumour size is generally larger than that of parathyroid gland adenoma with an average weight between 6.7 g and 12 g, although smaller tumours are being identified earlier in recent times. It may be encapsulated or obviously infiltrative. There may be a soft, brown appearance indistinguishable from adenoma, or a firm, grey-white texture. Troublesome intra-operative dissection, owing to adherence to contiguous structures, should alert the perceptive surgeon to a possibility of malignancy.

Microscopically, parathyroid carcinomas may be deceptively bland or overtly malignant and anything in between. It is the biological behaviour, however, which ultimately defines parathyroid carcinoma. In rare cases, there may be no histomorphological clues to indicate potential aggressiveness. Nonetheless, first-order morphological criteria of malignancy (absolute criteria) include invasion into adjacent tissues and/or histologically documented metastasis. When these are absent or inconclusive, a combination of second-order facultative features (features associated with malignancy), each in themselves not fully diagnostic, are invoked (Table 58.15).

The capsule is often thickened and is classically contiguous with broad internal fibrous septula, dividing the tumour into irregular nodular compartments. (This must be differentiated from scarring in an adenoma, secondary to spontaneous infarction, FNAC or previous surgery.) Invasion beyond the delimiting capsule (Figure 58.63) may or may not be obvious (and can be mimicked by pseudo-infiltration, sequestration/benign entrapment and/or implantation of benign tissue following rupture of a parathyroid adenoma capsule). Fibrosis and haemosiderin deposition may be encountered in hyperplasia, degenerate adenomas and carcinomas. Pericapsular vascular invasion (Figure 58.64) is virtually diagnostic of malignancy (though artefactual dislodgement of cells simulating tumour embolus must be considered) but is present in only 10–15% of cases. Perineural infiltration is also diagnostic of malignancy but is also an uncommon finding. There may be a variety of growth patterns and a trabecular or rosettoid architecture favours malignancy (but it is not common and not entirely specific). Diffuse growth of isomorphic cells with elevated nucleus–cytoplasmic ratio is

TABLE 58.15 Microscopical criteria for the diagnosis parathyroid carcinoma[53]

First-order criteria	Second-order criteria

Presence of either or both of the following:
1. Invasion into surrounding tissues
  • Thyroid
  • Oesophagus
  • Nerves
  • Connective tissue
2. Histologically documented locoregional or distant metastasis
	In the absence of first-order criteria, at least two or more of the following:
	• Capsular invasion
	• Vascular invasion
	• Mitoses >5 per 10 hpf
	• Broad intralesional fibrous septa with division into nodules
	• Coagulative-type necrosis
	• Diffuse growth with elevated nucleus to cytoplasmic ratio
	• Diffuse cellular atypia
	• Abundant macronucleoli

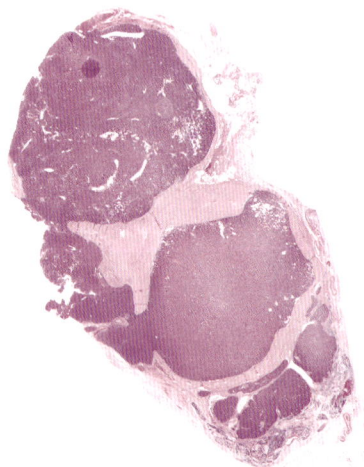 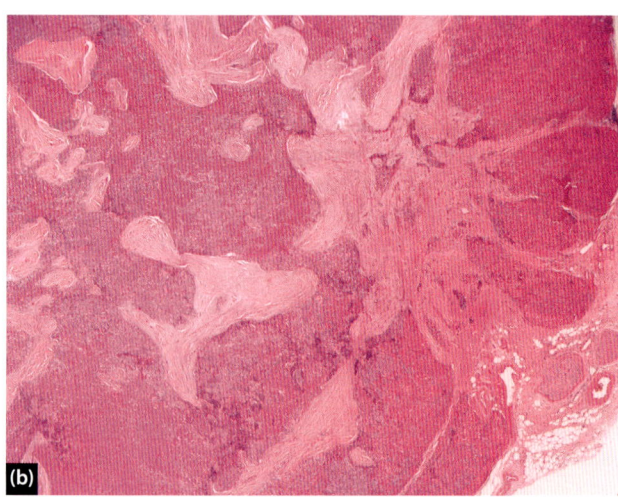

Figure 58.63 (a) Whole mount preparation of an oncocytic parathyroid carcinoma in a patient with MEN2 demonstrating irregular, thick fibrous capsulation contiguous with conspicuous internal fibrous septa. This gland was adherent to surrounding structures at operation and dissected out with some difficulty (H&E stain, ultra-low magnification). (b) The edge of another parathyroid carcinoma depicting an irregular, thick peripheral capsule, together with coarse intratumoural fibrous bands separating the expansile tumour nodules. This presents a broad advancing margin with surrounding soft tissues, rather than direct tentacular, permeative infiltration (H&E stain, low magnification).

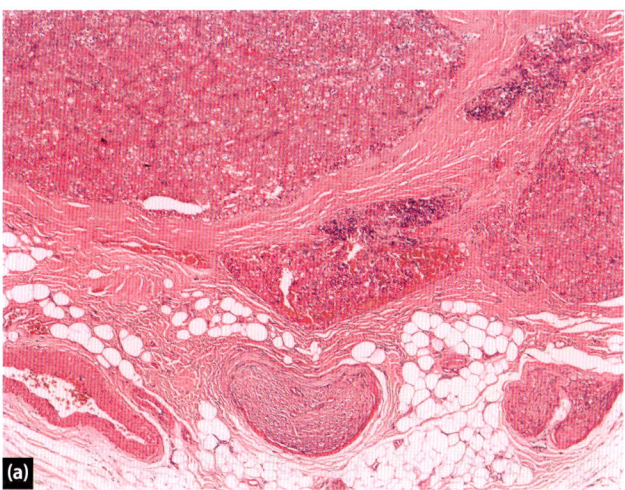
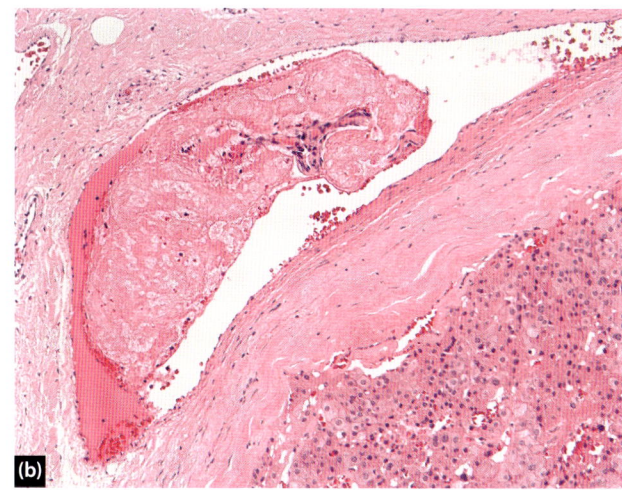

Figure 58.64 **(a)** A pericapsular neurovascular bundle showing endothelialized intravascular tumour invasion characteristic of parathyroid carcinoma (*H&E stain, medium magnification*). **(b)** Angioinvasion of a medium-calibre blood vessel at the perimeter of a parathyroid carcinoma, exemplified by parathyrocytes enveloped in endoluminal fibrin clot (*H&E stain, high magnification*).

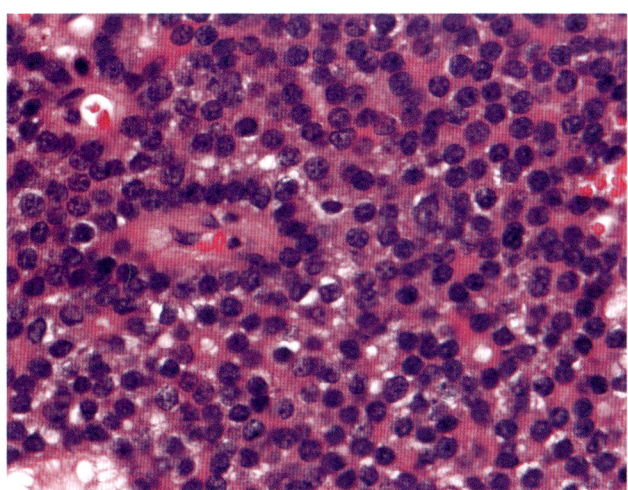

Figure 58.65 Parathyroid carcinoma composed of monotonous tumour cells showing raised nucleus-cytoplasmic ratio, nuclear hyperchromasia, coarse chromatin, macronucleolation and focal multinucleolation. A solitary mitosoid body is present towards the upper left-hand corner (*H&E stain, high magnification*).

a tocsin (**Figure 58.65**), as is generalized nuclear pleomorphism (in contrast to focal, random cytonuclear atypia). Macronucleolation may be conspicuous. Areas of coagulative necrosis may be seen (and should not be mistaken for ischaemic damage or haemorrhage). The interpretation of mitoses has proven controversial: mitoses are present in both hyperplasia and adenoma, though generally below 1 mitosis per 10 high-power fields (obversely, mitotic figures may be completely absent in some metastasizing carcinomas and care must be taken to distinguish mitoses in endothelial and other stromal elements from those in tumour cells). The presence of very many mitoses and/or abnormal forms, however, is usually taken as presumptive evidence of malignant potential. The proposed UICC/AJCC TNM staging classification[35] for parathyroid carcinomas is given in **Table 58.16**. T staging predicated upon size criteria has also been proposed.[59]

The immunohistochemical proliferation marker Ki67 (MIB-1) is slightly higher in parathyroid carcinoma than adenoma, though there is overlap, with a proliferative index greater than 5% suggestive of malignancy. Ki67 may also help in discriminating genuine mitotic figures from pyknotic nuclei (mitosoid bodies) in equivocal cases. An immunopanel comprising Ki67 in combination with galectin-3, parafibromin and PGP9.5 augments both specificity and sensitivity, compared to a single marker. Alternative studies, including retinoblastoma protein, cyclin D1, bcl-2, adenomatous polyposis coli antibody and p27 immunostaining, are presently of limited diagnostic and/or prognostic utility. Cytokeratin 14 (CK14) immunoreactivity has been reported as positive in oncocytic (oxyphil) adenomas but never in oncocytic carcinomas.

An increased incidence of parathyroid carcinoma is reported in some hereditary hyperparathyroidism syndromes. Familial hyperparathyroidism represents a clinically and genetically heterogeneous group of disorders that includes multiple endocrine neoplasia type 1 (MEN 1), multiple endocrine neoplasia type 2 (MEN 2), familial hypocalciuric hypercalcaemia (FHH), hyperparathyroidism-jaw tumour (HPT-JT) syndrome and familial isolated hyperparathyroidism (FIHP). Parathyroid carcinoma is seen in 10–15% of the autosomal dominant HPT-JT syndrome but it is exceptionally rare in MEN 1 and MEN 2. Early studies of FIHP suggested an increased risk of parathyroid carcinoma, but the inclusion of some patients with HPT-JT syndrome casts doubt upon this conclusion. There are no reported cases of parathyroid carcinoma with FHH.

TABLE 58.16 Proposed TNM staging schema for parathyroid carcinoma

T – Primary Tumour

TX	Primary tumour cannot be assessed
T0	No evidence of primary tumour
Tis	Atypical parathyroid neoplasm (neoplasm of uncertain malignant potential)
T1	Localized to the parathyroid gland with extension limited to soft tissue
T2	Direct invasion into the thyroid gland
T3	Direct invasion into laryngeal nerve, oesophagus, trachea, skeletal muscle, adjacent lymph nodes, or thymus
T4	Direct invasion into major blood vessels or spine

N – Regional Lymph Nodes

NX	Regional lymph nodes cannot be assessed
N0	No regional lymph node metastasis
N1	Regional lymph node metastasis
N1a	Metastasis to Level VI (pretracheal, paratracheal, and prelaryngeal/Delphian lymph nodes) or upper/superior mediastinal lymph nodes
N1b	Metastasis to unilateral, bilateral or contralateral cervical (Levels I, II, III, IV, or V) or retropharyngeal nodes

M – Distant Metastasis

M0	No distant metastasis
M1	Distant metastasis

Stage

There are not enough data to propose a formal staging system at this time.

Source: Adapted from AJCC Cancer Staging Manual, 8th edition, 2017. Note that there are insufficient data to enable stage group stratification.[35]

Other parathyroid gland tumours

Paraganglioma may rarely occur at this site. Tumour-like lesions, which may on occasion enter the differential diagnosis, include parathyroid cysts, branchiogenic cysts and amyloidosis. Secondary neoplasms may be the result of direct extension from adjacent structures, such as larynx or thyroid, or from distant metastatic disease, most commonly of primary mammary, haematolymphoid, renal, malignant melanoma or bronchopulmonary derivation. Despite their close proximity, metastasis to parathyroid gland from a primary thyroid carcinoma is uncommon (**Figure 58.66**).

Frozen section examination

Intra-operative frozen section examination of parathyroid gland tissue in cases of hyperparathyroidism is intended to establish the nature of the excised tissue and ascertain whether it is normal or abnormal. Without knowledge of the status of the remaining glands, a more definitive diagnosis of hyperplasia or adenoma (very rarely carcinoma) cannot always be proffered. Incisional biopsies render the task more difficult, as do freezing (ice crystal) artefact, other technical constraints and sampling error. The process is inevitably subject to inter-observer variation. Some workers advocate routine lipid stains as an adjunct to assessing intracytoplasmic fat; others do not. Oncocytic (oxyphil) cells, however, contain minimal lipid and occasional non-oncocytic hyperplastic and adenomatous parathyrocytes may retain significant lipid content. This notwithstanding, the overall accuracy of frozen section evaluation is surprisingly high and demonstrates good concordance with subsequent paraffin sections in experienced hands (**Figure 58.67**). The frozen section diagnosis of parathyroid carcinoma is understandably seldom sustainable, although alerting the surgeon to the possibility may alter pre-operative management should there be other suspect features.

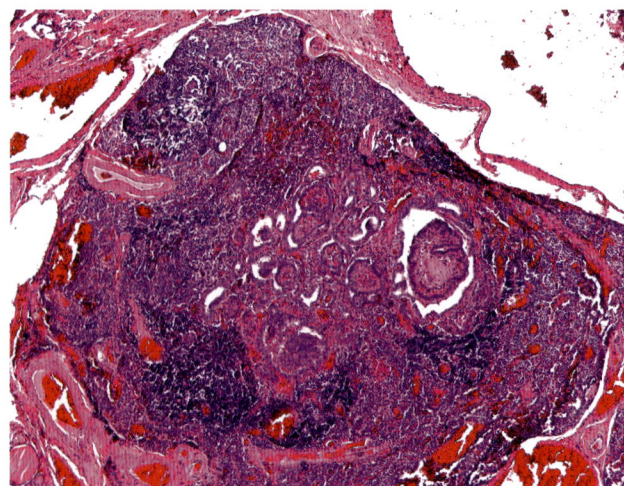

Figure 58.66 Parathyroid gland of normal size, albeit with diminished fat content, containing an intracapsular deposit of metastatic papillary thyroid carcinoma. There was no contiguity with similar tumour elsewhere in the neck (*H&E stain, low magnification*).

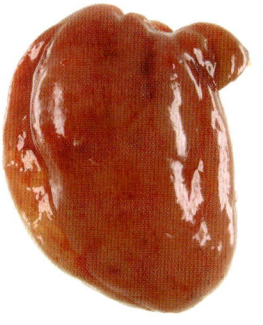
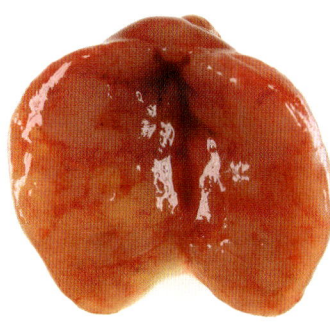
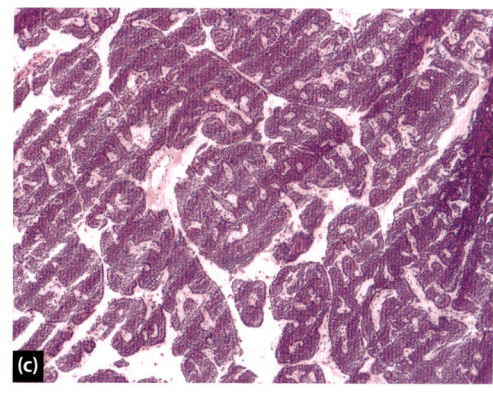

Figure 58.67 (a) The external surface of a fresh parathyroid gland nodule, weighing 1.8 g, sent for intra-operative frozen section examination – see Figure 58.54 for comparison with the appearances of a similar fixed specimen. (b) The same nodule bivalved in the unfixed state to demonstrate ill-defined parenchymal multinodularity. (c) Frozen section histology confirms hypercellular parathyroid gland tissue devoid of intraglandular fat. The entire consultation was completed in less than 5 minutes following receipt of the specimen in the laboratory. The linear striations and folds/rents in the section are artefactual. Without knowledge of the status of the remaining parathyroid glands, this could represent either an adenoma or hyperplasia. This notwithstanding, the findings supported the clinical impression of an adenoma. Subsequent paraffin sections on routinely processed tissue served as a quality audit (*H&E stain, medium magnification*).

Based on the premise that most primary hyperparathyroidism is due to single gland disease, there is sound rationale for unilateral neck exploration to remove the adenoma and visualize and/or biopsy any ipsilateral gland(s). Furthermore, advances in pre-operative localization techniques now facilitate targeted minimally invasive parathyroidectomy (MIP), variously through a mini incision, video-assisted surgery or endoscopic operation alone. Intra-operative frozen section or cytology examination merely confirms tissue nature rather than functional status. Intra-operative quick assay of intact parathyroid hormone (IOQPTH) can be undertaken prior to and post removal of a gland – a significant reduction in parathormone concentration predicts extirpation of abnormally functioning tissue, indicative of cure. Radioguided parathyroidectomy is guided by pre-operative radionucleide injection and radioguidance is helpful in second-look parathyroidectomy. MIP is, however, unsuitable in individuals with discordant imaging and/or comorbid thyroid disease.

KEY POINTS

- Accurate and timely pathological tumour subtyping, tumour grading and tumour staging underpin subsequent effective clinical management of thyroid gland and parathyroid gland neoplasia.
- Morphology remains the gold standard of histocytological diagnosis, increasingly facilitated, but not yet supplanted, by advances in ultrastructural, immunohistochemical, molecular and genetic understanding of normality and disease states.
- Advancement in diagnostic pathology has traditionally evolved along heuristic lines, assimilating observational studies with careful clinico-pathologico-radiological and treatment outcome correlation at population and individual case study levels. This has enabled recognition of new entities and clinically relevant reclassification and/or subclassification of existing conditions with time.
- There is a new era of pathological, clinical and molecular integration informing our understanding of thyroid disease and enabling patient management and clinical treatment decisions to be guided by evidentially based risk stratification with de-escalation of therapy in differentiated thyroid carcinoma.
- The apparently limited repertoire of thyroid gland disease belies its subtlety, masking some of the most highly contentious fields in any area of current surgical pathology.
- Fine needle aspiration cytology (FNAC) of the thyroid gland is a generally accepted first-line investigation for triage of solitary thyroid nodules, is helpful in evaluating diffuse, non-toxic goitre, aids the diagnosis of clinically suspected malignancy and potentially discriminates between treatable lymphomas and poor prognosis undifferentiated (anaplastic) carcinoma.
- Papillary thyroid carcinoma in its numerous guises accounts for approximately 80% of all thyroid malignancies. It generally portends an excellent prognosis, particularly in younger patients, modulated by both patient-specific and tumour-specific variables.
- The capsule of any follicular-patterned neoplasm should be comprehensively sampled specifically searching for both capsular and lymphovascular microinvasion.
- Oncocytic (oxyphil, Hürthle cell) change is a cellular adaptive process occurring in a wide variety of non-neoplastic and neoplastic conditions. It is subject to its own molecular basis, independent to that of any underlying tumour.
- There remain a number of unresolved issues in the histopathological diagnosis of thyroid carcinomas. Large clinicopathological studies subject to long-term follow up are still required with anticipation that many of these controversial areas will be ultimately resolved with evidential basis.
- The role of ancillary immunohistochemical, molecular and genetic studies in the determination of malignancy of the thyroid gland is evolving and has yet to be fully realized in routine diagnostic practice.
- All patients newly diagnosed with medullary thyroid carcinoma should be offered genetic testing given its association with multiple endocrine neoplasia syndromes.
- The value of peri-operative frozen section examination of thyroid gland lesions is disputed amongst pathologists and surgeons. The indications for such are best agreed by the local multi-disciplinary team according to local circumstances, preferences and experience.
- Parathyroid carcinoma is rare, slow growing and metastasizes late in its natural history. The diagnosis is predicated upon clinical, biochemical, imaging and pathological criteria.

REFERENCES

1. Moorthy R, Warfield AT. Thyroid and parathyroid gland pathology. In: Watkinson JC, Gilbert RW (eds). *Stell & Maran's textbook of head and neck surgery and oncology*. London: Hodder Arnold; 2012, pp. 328–66.
2. McGlashan J. The thyroid gland: anatomy and physiology. In: Gleeson MB, et al. (eds). *Scott-Brown's otorhinolaryngology, head and neck surgery*. London: Hodder Arnold; 2008, pp.314–27.
3. De Felice M, Di Lauro R. Thyroid development and its disorders: genetics and molecular mechanisms. *Endocr Rev* 2004; **25**(5): 722–46.
4. Chan JKC. Tumours of the thyroid and parathyroid glands. In: Fletcher CDM (ed.). *Diagnostic Histopathology of Tumours*. Oxford: Elsevier; 2013, pp. 1177–293.
5. Wenig BH, Heffess CS, Adair CF. *Atlas of endocrine pathology*. Philadelphia: WB Saunders; 1999.
6. Akhtar MS, Scognamiglio T. Solid nest cells: role in thyroid disease. *Adv Anat Pathol* 2007; **14**(2): 141–2.
7. Gharib H, Goellner JR. Fine-needle aspiration biopsy of the thyroid: an appraisal. *Ann Intern Med* 1993; **118**(4): 282–9.
8. DeLellis RA. *Pathology and genetics of tumours of endocrine organs*. Lyons: IARC Press; 2004.
9. Perros P, Colley S, Boelaert K, et al. Guidelines for the management of thyroid cancer. *Clin Endocrinol (Oxf)* 2014; **81** Suppl 1: 1–122.
10. Haugen BR, Alexander EK, Bible KC, et al. 2015 American Thyroid Association management guidelines for adult patients with thyroid nodules and differentiated thyroid cancer: The American Thyroid Association Guidelines Task Force on Thyroid Nodules and Differentiated Thyroid Cancer. *Thyroid* 2016; **26**(1): 1.
11. Carr S, Visvanathan V, Hossain T, et al. How good are we at fine needle aspiration cytology? *J Laryngol Otol* 2010; **124**(7): 765–6.
12. Carmeci C, Jeffrey RB, McDougall IR, et al. Ultrasound-guided fine-needle aspiration biopsy of thyroid masses. *Thyroid* 1998; **8**(4): 283–9.
13. Buley I. Problems in fine needle aspiration of the thyroid. *Curr Diagn Pathol* 1995; **2**(1): 23–31.
14. Wise O, Howard MR. Thyroid cytology: a review of current international reporting systems and emerging developments. *Cytopathology* 2016; **27**(3): 161–7.
15. Cibas ES, Ali SZ. NCI Thyroid FNA State of the Science Conference. The Bethesda System for Reporting Thyroid Cytopathology. *Am J Clin Pathol* 2009; **132**(5): 658–65.
16. Cross P, CA, Giles T, et al. *Guidance on the reporting of thyroid cytology specimens*. London: Royal College of Pathologists; 2016.
17. Chau YC, Chan JKC. Fine needle aspiration induced changes. *Curr Diagn Pathol* 2003; **9**: 78–88.
18. LiVolsi VA, Merino MJ. Worrisome histologic alterations following fine-needle aspiration of the thyroid (WHAFFT). *Pathol Annu* 1994; **29**(Pt 2): 99–120.
19. Sturgis EM, Miller RH. Thyroglossal duct cysts. *J La State Med Soc* 1993; **145**(11): 459–61.
20. Shahin A, Burroughs FH, Kirby JP, Ali SZ. Thyroglossal duct cyst: a cytopathologic study of 26 cases. *Diagn Cytopathol* 2005; **33**(6): 365–9.
21. Harcourt-Webster JN. Squamous epithelium in the human thyroid gland. *J Clin Pathol* 1966; **19**(4): 384–8.
22. Wenig BH. *Atlas of head and neck pathology*. Philadelphia: Saunder Elsevier; 2008.
23. Watson MG, Birchall JP, Soames JV. Is 'lateral aberrant thyroid' always metastatic tumour? *J Laryngol Otol* 1992; **106**(4): 376–8.
24. Mete O, Asa SL. Oncocytes, oxyphils, Hürthle, and Askanazy cells: morphological and molecular features of oncocytic thyroid nodules. *Endocr Pathol* 2010; **21**(1): 16–24.
25. Rosai J, Kuhn E, Carcangiu ML. Pitfalls in thyroid tumour pathology. *Histopathol* 2006; **49**(2): 107–20.
26. Baloch ZW, LiVolsi, VA. Our approach to follicular-patterned lesions of the thyroid. *J Clin Pathol* 2007; **60**(3): 244–50.
27. Lloyd RV, Osamura RY, Klöppel G, Rosai J (eds). *WHO Classification of Tumours of Endocrine Organs*, 4th Edn. International Agency for Research on Cancer, France, 2017.
28. Williams ED. Guest editorial: Two proposals regarding the terminology of thyroid tumors. *Int J Surg Pathol* 2000; **8**(3): 181–3.
29. LiVolsi VA. Hyalinizing trabecular tumor of the thyroid: adenoma, carcinoma, or neoplasm of uncertain malignant potential? *Am J Surg Pathol* 2000; **24**(12): 1683–4.
30. LiVolsi VA, Baloch ZW. Follicular neoplasms of the thyroid: view, biases, and experiences. *Adv Anat Pathol* 2004; **11**(6): 279–87.
31. Rosai J. DeLellis RA, Carcangiu ML, et al. (eds).Tumours of the thyroid and parathyroid glands. In: *AFIP Atlas of Tumour Pathology*. Series 4, Fascicle 21. Washington DC: American Registry of Pathology Press; 96–98, 2015.
32. Ghossein R, Asa SL, Barne L. *Protocol for the examination of specimens from patients with carcinomas of the thyroid gland*. Washington DC: College of American Pathologists; 2009.
33. Ghossein R. Update to the College of American Pathologists reporting on thyroid carcinomas. *Head Neck Pathol* 2009; **3**(1): 86–93.
34. Xu B, Ghossein RA. Crucial parameters in thyroid carcinoma reporting-challenges, controversies and clinical implications. *Histopathology* 2018; **72**, 32–39.
35. Brierley JD, Gospodarowicz MK, Wittekind C (eds). *TNM classification of malignant tumours*. 8th ed. Oxford: Wiley-Blackwell; 2017.
36. Stephenson TJ, Johnson SJ. *Dataset for thyroid cancer histopathology reports*. London: Royal College of Pathologists; 2014.
37. Wada N, Hirakawa S, Rino Y, et al. Solitary metachronous metastasis to the thyroid from renal clear cell carcinoma 19 years after nephrectomy: report of a case. *Surg Today* 2005; **35**(6): 483–7.
38. Chen H, Nicol TL, Zeiger MA, et al. Hürthle cell neoplasms of the thyroid: are there factors predictive of malignancy? *Ann Surg* 1998; **227**(4): 542–6.
39. Katoh R, Harach HR, Williams ED. Solitary, multiple, and familial oxyphil tumours of the thyroid gland. *J Pathol* 1998; **186**(3): 292–9.
40. Baloch ZW, LiVolsi VA. Follicular-patterned lesions of the thyroid: the bane of the pathologist. *Am J Clin Pathol* 2002; **117**(1): 143–50.
41. Johnson SJ, Stephenson TJ, Poller DN. *NIFTP addendum to Dataset for thyroid cancer histopathology reports*. London: Royal College of Pathologists; 2016.
42. Thompson LDR. Update on follicular variant of papillary thyroid carcinoma with an emphasis on new terminology: noninvasive follicular thyroid neoplasm with papillary-like nuclear features. *Diagn Histopathol* 2016; **22**(5): 171–8.
43. Grodski S, Delbridge L. An update on papillary microcarcinoma. *Curr Opin Oncol* 2009; **21**(1): 1–4.
44. Baloch ZW, LiVolsi VA. Newly described tumours of the thyroid. *Curr Diagn Pathol* 2000; **6**(3): 151–64.
45. Lang BH, Lo CY. Surgical options in undifferentiated thyroid carcinoma. *World J Surg* 2007; **31**(5): 969–77.
46. Hodgson NC, Button J, Solorzano CC. Thyroid cancer: is the incidence still increasing? *Ann Surg Oncol* 2004; **11**(12): 1093–7.
47. Williams ED. Histogenesis of medullary carcinoma of the thyroid. *J Clin Pathol* 1966; **19**(2): 114–18.
48. Bussolati G Foster GV, Clark MB, Pearse AG. Immunofluorescent localisation of calcitonin in medullary (C cell) thyroid carcinoma, using antibody to the pure porcine hormone. *Virchows Arch B Cell Pathol* 1969; **2**(1): 234–8.
49. Baloch ZW, Li Volsi VA. Special types of thyroid carcinoma. *Histopathology* 2018; **72**: 40–52.
50. Pacini F, Castagna MG, Cipri C, Schlumberger M. Medullary thyroid carcinoma. *Clin Oncol (R Coll Radiol)* 2010; **22**(6): 475–85.
51. McNicol AM. The role of the pathologist. In: Mazaferri ELH, Mallick C, Kendall-Taylor P (eds). *Practical management of thyroid cancer. A multidisciplinary approach*. Springer-Verlag: London; 2006.
52. Eloy C. Newly described thyroid tumours and variants. *Diagn Histopathol* 2016; **22**(5): 179–83.

53. Anderson CE, McLaren KM. Best practice in thyroid pathology. *J Clin Pathol* 2003; **56**(6): 401–5.
54. O'Sullivan B, Brierley JD, D'Cruz AK, et al. *UICC manual of clinical oncology*. 9th ed. Oxford: Wiley-Blackwell; 2015.
55. Nanji SS, Roth SI. A parathyroid myxoadenoma observed grossly. *Endocr Pathol* 2007; **18**(1): 53–5.
56. DeLellis RA. Parathyroid carcinoma: an overview. *Adv Anat Pathol* 2005; **12**(2): 53–61.
57. Betea D, Bradwell AR, Harvey TC, et al. Hormonal and biochemical normalization and tumor shrinkage induced by anti-parathyroid hormone immunotherapy in a patient with metastatic parathyroid carcinoma. *J Clin Endocrinol Metab* 2004; **89**(7): 3413–20.
58. Johnson SJ, Stephenson TJ. *Dataset for parathyroid cancer histopathology reports*. London: Royal College of Pathologists; 2016.

Thyroid disease

CHAPTER 59

CLINICAL EVALUATION OF THE THYROID PATIENT

Andrew Coatesworth and Sebastian Wallis

Introduction	705	Miscellaneous others	706
Functional disorders	705	References	707
Structural disorders	706		

SEARCH STRATEGY

Data in this chapter may be updated by on a PubMed search using the keywords: hypothyroidism, hyperthyroidism, Grave's disease, thyrotoxicosis and thyroid nodule.

This chapter succinctly covers the various clinical presentations of differing thyroid pathologies. More detail of specific presentations is available in chapters specific to those presentations.

INTRODUCTION

Thyroid disorders are common; serious or sinister problems are rare. They can broadly be divided into disorders of function, and disorders of structure, with a few miscellaneous others.

Thyroid disorders are managed by primary care and endocrine physicians, and endocrine and ENT surgeons.

FUNCTIONAL DISORDERS

Endocrine thyroid disorders affect approximately 2% of the adult population, with a 10:1 female to male ratio. Hypothyroidism is predominantly diagnosed and treated in primary care. Hyperthyroidism is primarily managed by physicians, with a surgical opinion generally being sought in cases where medical treatment has failed. It is therefore rare for a patient with an endocrine disorder to present *de novo* to an ENT clinic in the UK.

Symptoms and signs of hypothyroidism

The majority of patients with an underactive thyroid will have little or no symptoms or signs. The commonest symptoms are fatigue, weight gain with a poor appetite, and feeling cold.[1] Other recognized symptoms are poor concentration and memory, hoarse voice, shortness of breath, abnormal sensation, and a change in menstruation.[1] Constipation and dyspepsia are also recognized.[2] Coma is a rare life-threatening state of extreme hypothyroidism. Untreated congenital hypothyroidism can result in cretinism.

Signs of hypothyroidism are: dry coarse skin, cool extremities, hair loss and bradycardia. Reinke's oedema, myxoedema, delayed tendon reflexes, carpal tunnel syndrome, pleural effusion, ascites and pericardial effusions have all been described, but these are generally rare and late features.[1] Reinke's oedema is far more commonly associated with smoking.

Symptoms and signs of hyperthyroidism

Graves' disease, toxic multinodular goitre and toxic adenoma are the commonest causes of thyrotoxicosis. Overactivity of the thyroid gland can cause a wide range of symptoms. These include: weight loss, often in the presence of an increased appetite; nervousness, anxiety and irritability; sweating, palpitations and tremor; thin skin, thin hair and muscle weakness; gastrointestinal and menstrual disturbance. Eye symptoms are a feature of Graves' disease, with bulging eyes, a staring appearance and diplopia. In severe cases, a thyroid storm may occur with tachydysrhythmia, pyrexia, vomiting, diarrhoea and mental agitation. This is a medical emergency which has a 20–50% mortality even when treated.[3]

Signs of thyrotoxicosis are: agitation, evidence of weight loss, perspiration, tremor, palmer erythema and proximal muscle wasting. Thin skin and thin hair, tachycardia and/or atrial fibrillation can also be found.

Thyroid ophthalmopathy is a feature of Graves' disease, and is strongly associated with smoking. Axial proptosis with lid lag (von Graffe sign), lid retraction (Dalrymple sign), and conjunctival injection (Goldzeiher's sign) can be elicited. Diplopia, particularly on upward gaze in abduction, occurs with increased pressure at the orbital apex. In severe cases optic neuropathy can occur.[3]

Graves' disease can also cause dermopathy, with pre-tibial myxoedema and thyroid acropachy. Pre-tibial myxoedema presents with waxy indurated skin that itches. It can extend onto the dorsum of the foot, and rarely affects other parts of the body.[4] Thyroid acropachy is characterized by soft-tissue swelling of the hands which can be in association with clubbing.[5]

STRUCTURAL DISORDERS

Thyroid nodules are common in adults and may be palpated in 3–7% of cases.[6] If ultrasound is used, the prevalence is nearer 70%.[7] The majority of thyroid nodules are solitary, but they may be part of a multinodular goitre. A focal or diffuse goitre can occur physiologically, and in association with thyroiditis. A first-degree relative with thyroid cancer, and prior exposure to radiation, increase the likelihood of malignancy.[7]

Symptoms and signs of thyroid swellings

The commonest presentation of a thyroid nodule is with an asymptomatic lump. Increasingly referrals are arising as incidental findings from radiological investigations. Pain, rapid increase in size, hoarse voice and the presence of a lateral neck mass are all features that raise concern about a malignant underlying pathology, but the commonest cause for a sudden painful thyroid nodule is bleeding into a pre-existing cyst, and the commonest presentation of a differentiated thyroid cancer is an asymptomatic nodule.[8] Prior exposure to ionizing radiation is a risk factor for developing thyroid cancer. Patients may also have a relevant family history.

With increasing size, goitres can cause compressive symptoms; these are usually at or above the level of the thoracic inlet, causing cervical dysphagia, exertional dyspnoea, inspiratory or biphasic stridor, and venous congestion of the superior vena caval territory.[9]

A thyroid nodule can often be diagnosed when the patient swallows on their way into the clinic room. Berry first described the fascial attachments of the thyroid to the trachea.[10] This means that thyroid swellings elevate with swallowing.

A hard mass that is tender to touch is more likely to indicate malignancy or Riedel's thyroiditis. Associated cervical lymphadenopathy and fixation to surrounding structures are also highly worrisome findings. Tracheal deviation can be elicited by examining the neck from the anterior aspect. The lower extent of a retrosternal goitre cannot be felt when the neck is examined from behind and the patient swallows. Percussion of the anterior chest wall to elicit the lower extent of a retrosternal goitre is largely of historical interest with the emergence of readily available cross-sectional imaging techniques. A large retrosternal goitre can cause venous congestion of the head, neck and upper torso. When venous congestion is impending, it can be elicited by asking the patient to raise both arms until they touch the side of their face, and holding that position for a minute (Pemberton's sign). There may also be cyanosis and respiratory distress induced by this manoeuvre.[9]

Flexible nasendoscopy can reveal a vocal cord palsy, Reinke's oedema, tracheal deviation and, in severe cases, tracheal compression. Direct invasion of the upper aerodigestive tract may also be seen.

MISCELLANEOUS OTHERS

Structural thyroid disorders can arise as part of an underlying systemic disorder.

Medullary thyroid cancer is part of multiple endocrine neoplasia syndrome type 2 (MEN2) in 20% of cases, along with phaeochromocytoma. In those cases not diagnosed through genetic screening, medullary thyroid cancer is the commonest initial manifestation.[11] With MEN2a, parathyroid hyperplasia occurs causing primary hyperparathyroidism. With MEN2b mucosal neurofibromas and Marfanoid features may be evident.

Lymphoma of the thyroid gland can occur in isolation, or as part of wider haematological malignancy. As such, it can be associated with lymphadenopathy in the axilla and groins, and hepatosplenomegally. The patient may also have the 'B' symptoms of lymphoma, with fever, unintentional weight loss, and drenching night sweats.[12]

BEST CLINICAL PRACTICE

- ✓ Clinical evaluation of the thyroid patient starts when the patient enters the clinic room. Features of hormone dysfunction and the presence of a goitre may be apparent before the patient sits down.
- ✓ The history should cover systemic as well as locoregional symptoms, and also elicit any family and past history of relevance, including prior exposure to ionizing radiation.
- ✓ ENT examination covers the upper aerodigestive tract and neck, including flexible nasendoscopy. There are systemic signs of thyroid disease in a minority of cases that are evaluated by the ENT surgeon.

KEY POINTS

- Thyroid disorders are common.
- They are often asymptomatic but can be associated with a diverse range of locoregional and systemic signs and symptoms.
- They are managed by a wide range of clinicians.
- They can broadly be broken down into functional and structural disorders.
- Thyroid nodules are common.
- Rapid growth, pain and hoarseness are worrying symptoms for thyroid cancer. The commonest cause for a rapidly enlarging painful swelling, however, is bleeding into a pre-existing cyst, and the commonest presentation of thyroid cancer is with an asymptomatic nodule.

REFERENCES

1. Jameson JL, Weetman AP. Disorders of the thyroid gland. In: Longo DL, Fauci AS, Kasper DL, et al. (eds). *Harrison's principles of internal medicine*. 18th ed. New York: McGraw-Hill; 2011, Ch. 341.
2. Ebert E. The thyroid and the gut. *J Clin Gastroenterol* 2010; **44**(6): 402–6.
3. Devereaux D, Tewelde SZ. Hyperthyroidism and thyrotoxicosis. *Emerg Med Clin North Am* 2014; **32**(2): 277–92.
4. Schwartz KM, Fatourechi V, Debra DF, et al. Dermopathy of Graves' disease (pretibial myxedema): long-term outcome. *J Clin Endocrinol Metab* 2002; **87**(2): 438–46.
5. Fatourechi V, Ahmed DD, Schwartz KM. Thyroid acropachy: report of 40 patients treated at a single institution in a 26 year period. *J Clin Endocrinol Metab* 2002; **87**(12): 5435–41.
6. Hegedus L, Bonnema SJ, Bennedbaek FN. Management of simple nodular goitre: current status and future perspectives. *Endocr Rev* 2003; **24**: 102–32.
7. Perros P, Buelart K, Colley S, et al. Guidelines for the management of thyroid cancer. *Clin Endocrinol* 2014; **81**(1): 1–122.
8. Nix P, Nicolaides A, Coatesworth AP. Thyroid cancer review 1: presentation and investigation of thyroid cancer. *Int J Clin Pract* 2005; **59**(11): 1340–4.
9. Pemberton HS. Sign of submerged goitre. *Lancet* 1946; **248**: 501.
10. Berry J. (IV-V of the Proceedings of the Anatomical Society). *J Anat Physiol* 1888; **22**.
11. Moline J, Eng C. Multiple endocrine neoplasia type 2: an overview. *Genet Med* 2011; **9**(13): 755–64.
12. Carbone PP, Kaplan HS, Musshoff K, et al. Report of the committee on Hodgkin's disease staging classification. *Cancer Res* 1971; **31**(11): 1860–1.

CHAPTER 60

INVESTIGATION OF THYROID DISEASE

Anthony P. Weetman

Introduction 709
Investigation of thyroid dysfunction 709
Determining the cause of thyroid dysfunction 711

Determining the nature of structural lesions 713
References 714

SEARCH STRATEGY

Data in this chapter may be updated by a PubMed search using the keywords hyperthyroidism, hypothyroidism, thyroid function, thyroid nodule and thyroid cancer, and published guidelines which are cited in the chapter.

INTRODUCTION

Clinical signs and symptoms are inadequate to diagnose the presence of any thyroid disorder. Even sophisticated scoring systems are unable to categorize around 40% of euthyroid individuals,[1] and there is considerable inter-user variation in the findings made from thyroid palpation.[2] The investigation of thyroid disease can be broken down into three sets of tests aimed at: (i) determining whether there is biochemical thyroid dysfunction (i.e. hypothyroidism or thyrotoxicosis); (ii) determining the cause of any thyroid dysfunction and (iii) determining the nature of any structural lesion in the thyroid, most typically nodular thyroid disease. This chapter will not cover the use of fine-needle aspiration biopsy (FNAB) to evaluate thyroid nodules but it is worth recording here that FNAB can also be a useful investigative tool in rare non-neoplastic circumstances, for instance where there is an unexplained diffuse enlargement of the thyroid gland or to obtain material to diagnose acute (suppurative) thyroiditis.

INVESTIGATION OF THYROID DYSFUNCTION

Measurement of thyroid-stimulating hormone

Current sandwich immunoassays, employing two monoclonal thyroid-stimulating hormone (TSH) antibodies to immobilize and identify TSH, are highly reliable and capable of measuring TSH levels as low as 0.01 mU/L, although not all available assays perform equally well.[3] Serum TSH levels show a log-linear relationship to serum free thyroxine (FT4) levels and this makes the TSH the most sensitive test to detect primary dysfunction of the thyroid.[4] A number of factors can affect TSH levels and need to be taken into consideration in interpreting TSH measurements (Box 60.1).

Elevation or suppression of the TSH level, outside the reference range, may be associated with normal levels of

---

BOX 60.1 Factors affecting the measurement of serum TSH levels

Serum FT3 and FT4; TSH is inversely proportional to free thyroid hormone levels

Physiological factors: intra-individual variation is ±0.5 mU/L (and there is an insignificant diurnal variation) but inter-individual variation is greater due to the effects of age, genetic factors and obesity

Pituitary or hypothalamic disease; TSH ↓

First trimester of pregnancy; TSH ↓ due to thyroid-stimulating effects of human chorionic gonadotrophin

Non-thyroid illness, including psychiatric disorders; typically TSH ↓, but depends on phase of illness

Drugs; TSH ↓ by dopamine, somatostatin and high dose glucocorticoids

Assay-specific artefacts, especially interference by heterophilic antibodies

free tri-iodothyronine (FT3) or FT4. These are the biochemically defined states of subclinical hypothyroidism and subclinical thyrotoxicosis[5] and their recognition depends therefore on the cut-off levels used to define the TSH reference range. This is an area that has provoked recent debate, with some data suggesting that the reference range for TSH should be narrowed from around 0.4–4.5 mU/L to 0.4–2.5 mU/L.[6] On balance, however, the arguments for lowering the upper limit of the reference range in iodine-replete populations are insufficient to warrant a change.[7, 8]

Measurement of FT3 and FT4

Over 99% of circulating T3 and T4 is bound to thyroxine-binding globulin, albumin or pre-albumin, and variation in the levels of these binding proteins can thus have a profound impact on measurements of total thyroid hormone levels. To eliminate such artefacts, a number of immunoassays have been devised to measure the concentration of free (active) thyroid hormone, and although these may still give anomalous results in certain circumstances (**Box 60.2**), by and large these assays are robust and reliable.[9] If a serum FT3 or FT4 measurement is unexpectedly abnormal, especially if it is inconsistent with the serum TSH level, more detailed analysis is necessary, including measurement of total thyroid hormone levels.

Measurement of FT3 is particularly indicated in the following circumstances: (i) diagnosis of T3-toxicosis, the earliest stage of overt thyrotoxicosis in which the TSH is suppressed and FT4 is still normal, and (ii) if the patient is taking propylthiouracil or amiodarone, both of which impair the deiodination of T4 to T3 and so give rise to euthyroid elevations of FT4. On the other hand, FT3 measurement is not indicated in the diagnosis of hypothyroidism as FT3 levels are frequently normal until very late in the disease process, despite low FT4 and elevated TSH levels.

Evaluation of the symptomatic patient

Several guidelines have been produced which address the optimal strategy to diagnose thyroid dysfunction.[4, 10–12] Local policy will generally dictate whether TSH alone is used as a first-line test, progressing to measurement of FT4 only if the TSH is abnormal; the drawback of this approach is that rare cases of hypothyroidism and thyrotoxicosis which are secondary to pituitary or hypothalamic disease may be missed.[13] If such an approach of using the TSH level as a screening test is adopted, the limitations of TSH measurement have to be continually borne in mind (**Box 60.1**).[14] In general, however, a normal serum TSH level rules out primary thyroid disease. If the TSH is elevated, the most likely diagnosis is hypothyroidism; other causes are detailed in **Box 60.3**. If the TSH is suppressed, the most likely cause is thyrotoxicosis; other causes are detailed in **Box 60.4**.

Screening for thyroid disease

Given the frequency of thyroid disease in the population, the question arises as to whether population-based screening is worthwhile. At present there seems to be no overall benefit, given that most of the cases identified will have subclinical thyroid dysfunction and the benefits of treating this are not yet clear due to the lack of robust trials.[11, 15]

The occurrence of postpartum thyroid dysfunction in up to 5% of women after pregnancy, and the association between impaired fetal neurological development and untreated maternal hypothyroidism, have suggested there may be a benefit from screening women prior to conception. However, a recent review has indicated that there is insufficient evidence to recommend for or against universal TSH screening at the first trimester visit[16] and in any case there is no evidence that treatment of unrecognized maternal hypothyroidism improves fetal outcome.[17]

BOX 60.2 Factors affecting the measurement of serum FT3 and FT4 levels

Thyroid dysfunction; overt primary or secondary hypothyroidism or thyrotoxicosis

Non-thyroidal illness, including psychiatric disorders; typically ↓ FT3, but ↑ FT3 and ↓ or ↑ FT4 possible

Drugs; non-steroidal anti-inflammatory drugs, furosemide, phenytoin, carbamazepine, heparin may rarely affect some assays; propylthiouracil and amiodarone inhibit deiodinase activity, altering the ratio of FT3 to FT4

Pregnancy; FT3 and FT4↓ by 30% in the last trimester

BOX 60.3 Causes of an elevated TSH

Primary hypothyroidism
- Subclinical (FT3 and FT4 normal)
- Overt (FT4 ↓; FT3 ↓ in 25%)

Non-thyroidal illness (FT3 and FT4 variable), especially during recovery phase

TSH-secreting pituitary tumour (FT3, FT4 ↑)

Rare cases of thyroid hormone resistance (FT3, FT4 ↑)

TSH assay interference (FT3 and FT4 normal)

BOX 60.4 Causes of a suppressed TSH

Primary thyrotoxicosis
- Subclinical (FT3 and FT4 normal)
- Overt (FT3 ↑, FT4 usually ↑)

Secondary hypothyroidism due to pituitary or hypothalamic disease (FT4 ↓, FT3 normal or ↓)

Non-thyroidal illness (FT3 and FT4 normal)

Treatment with dopamine or glucocorticoids (FT3 and FT4 normal)

First trimester of pregnancy (FT3 and FT4 normal)

Hydatidiform mole, choriocarcinoma (FT3 and FT4 ↑)

Activating TSH-receptor mutations (FT3 and FT4 ↑)

There is a stronger case for screening certain high-risk populations for thyroid dysfunction, although formal cost–benefit analysis has not been performed: these include individuals with another associated autoimmune disorder (e.g. Addison's disease, vitiligo, coeliac disease, pernicious anaemia, type 1 diabetes mellitus) or who are taking drugs which may precipitate thyroid dysfunction (e.g. lithium, amiodarone, alpha-interferon, alemtuzumab, sorafenib, sunitinib). The risk of congenital hypothyroidism is around 1 in 3500 births and routine neonatal TSH screening on heel-prick specimens is now well established in all developed countries.[18] Following irradiation of the neck for cancer, including lymphoma, the frequency of hypothyroidism is very high and annual TSH screening is recommended.[19]

Monitoring treatment for thyroid dysfunction

In patients receiving antithyroid drug treatment for hyperthyroidism, persistent suppression of TSH levels may occur during and even after cessation of treatment, which is then associated with a higher risk of relapse.[20] As a result, such treatment is best monitored by measuring serum FT4 levels; in patients taking propylthiouracil which blocks T4 deiodination, FT3 levels may be a more accurate indicator of thyroid status. Thyroid hormone levels can fluctuate rapidly in some patients following radioiodine, with transient episodes of thyrotoxicosis or hypothyroidism during the first 6 months.[21] Routine measurement of serum TSH and FT4 levels should be made around 6 and 12 weeks after first treatment, and then every 3 months until a year after radioiodine. Thereafter annual monitoring is indicated. After subtotal thyroidectomy, serum TSH levels often rise and may indicate either a temporary state in which the thyroid remnant is developing capacity to resume function under TSH stimulation, or permanent hypothyroidism. Recent guidelines recommend near-total or total thyroidectomy for Graves' disease and toxic multinodular goitre, if surgery is chosen as treatment, and in these circumstances levothyroxine is commenced immediately after the operation without the need for further testing.[11]

Monitoring the adequacy of levothyroxine replacement in primary hypothyroidism depends on measurement of serum TSH levels, which provide an integrated estimate of the effect of treatment during the preceding weeks.[12, 22] Measurement of TSH should only be made 2 months after any change in levothyroxine dosage, as the TSH level does not stabilize before then. There is no place for measuring serum FT4 levels in the management of primary hypothyroidism, as TSH provides far more reliable information, but FT4 is the only available method to monitor treatment in secondary hypothyroidism: levothyroxine dosage should be adjusted to give a FT4 level in the upper third of the reference range.[23] Once the dose of levothyroxine is stable, TSH should be measured annually, or prior to conception if a pregnancy is planned between annual tests.

Thyroid function testing in pregnancy

Pregnancy has many effects on thyroid function (Box 60.5). As a result of these changes, it is recommended that trimester-specific reference ranges for TSH and FT4 should be applied during pregnancy; in their absence, the following are recommended for TSH: first trimester 0.1–2.5 mU/L; second trimester 0.2–3.0 mU/L; third trimester 0.3–3.0 mU/L.[16]

BOX 60.5 Effects of pregnancy on thyroid function

Increase in human chorionic gonadotrophin during first trimester, reciprocal ↓TSH and ↑ FT4 (in some cases, this effect may be so large that it may cause transient gestational hyperthyroidism, often associated with hyperemesis gravidarum)

Increase in thyroxine-binding globulin; ↑ in total T3 and T4

Increase in plasma volume; ↑ T3 and T4 pool size

Placental type III deiodinase; ↑ T3 and T4 degradation

Increase in iodine clearance; ↓ in T3 and T4 depending on iodine intake

Serum FT3 and FT4 ↓ by 20–40% during the last trimester but also prone to assay artefacts depending on methodology

TSH-receptor autoantibodies ↓ leading to remission of Graves' disease in second half of pregnancy

DETERMINING THE CAUSE OF THYROID DYSFUNCTION

Thyroid antibodies

The diagnosis in the vast majority of cases of spontaneous hypothyroidism is autoimmune hypothyroidism, and in hyperthyroidism, around 60–80% of cases are due to Graves' disease, caused by TSH-receptor stimulating antibodies. Measurement of serum thyroid antibodies can confirm the aetiology of thyroid dysfunction, but there are two important caveats: (i) thyroid antibodies are found in around 10% of the healthy, euthyroid population, and (ii) measurement of thyroid antibodies is only indicated clinically if it alters management. For instance, if radioiodine is going to be used in a particular hyperthyroid patient, it matters little whether TSH receptor antibodies are positive, whereas it would be futile to consider using a course of antithyroid drug treatment to achieve cure in a hyperthyroid patient unless the diagnosis of Graves' disease is firmly established.

Thyroglobulin (Tg) and thyroid peroxidase (TPO) antibodies were originally measured by immunofluorescence or haemagglutination methods, but more sensitive and reliable immunoassays calibrated against standard sera are now widely used.[24, 25] Almost all patients with autoimmune thyroid disease who have Tg antibodies also have TPO antibodies, but the reverse is much less common,[26] and therefore some laboratories only offer TPO antibody measurement to diagnose autoimmune thyroid disease.

The main indication for the estimation of Tg antibodies is in patients being followed up after treatment for differentiated thyroid cancer. In these individuals, measurement of Tg (see below) is only reliable in the absence of Tg antibodies, especially when immunometric Tg assays are used.[27] There is some evidence that the presence of Tg antibodies, found in 15–20% of such patients, is itself a marker for persistent thyroid tissue and a decline in Tg antibody level over time is a good prognostic sign.[28] On the other hand, the presence of Tg antibodies has been associated with a higher risk of malignancy in patients presenting with a thyroid nodule.[29]

Measurement of the TPO antibodies is helpful in defining the risk of overt hypothyroidism developing in individuals with subclinical hypothyroidism (**Figure 60.1**).[30, 31] If a patient presents with subclinical hypothyroidism, the TSH and FT4 should be repeated after 3 months, since an elevated TSH may simply be the result of a non-thyroidal illness and in these cases the elevation is only transient. In those who have an isolated elevated TSH, or isolated TPO antibodies, the annual risk of progression to overt hypothyroidism is 2% per year, but it is 5% per year if both are present. Those with positive TPO antibodies are also more likely to develop hypothyroidism after amiodarone or alpha-interferon treatment, or with other drugs which affect the immune system.[32, 33]

The availability of new, robust immunoassays for TSH receptor antibodies has improved the diagnosis of Graves' disease, as these have sensitivities of around 95% with nearly 100% specificity.[34] Although this test does not distinguish between those antibodies which stimulate the receptor and those which block it, in practice this distinction is readily made by taking into account the biochemical picture: a patient with thyrotoxicosis and positive TSH-receptor antibodies must have Graves' disease, while those with blocking TSH-receptor antibodies will be hypothyroid. Occasionally patients switch production from one functional type of antibody to the other, with sometimes confusing consequences unless this possibility is recognized.[35]

The two other clinical situations in which measurement of TSH receptor antibodies can be helpful are (i) in predicting the possibility of neonatal Graves' disease by measuring these antibodies in the serum of pregnant women previously treated for Graves' disease[16, 36] and (ii) in the diagnosis of euthyroid Graves' opthalmopathy.[37] Persistently raised TSH receptor antibody levels are an adverse feature for a successful outcome after antithyroid drug treatment for Graves' disease, but the results are not sufficiently sensitive or specific for routine use in individual patients.[38] High levels of TSH-receptor antibodies are an independent risk factor for the development of ophthalmopathy in patients with Graves' disease.[39]

Inflammatory markers

The erythrocyte sedimentation rate (ESR) and C-reactive protein (CRP) measurements are useful in the diagnosis of subacute thyroiditis, although these inflammatory markers may also be raised in acute suppurative thyroiditis and even in occasional patients with Hashimoto's thyroiditis.[40]

Thyroglobulin

The measurement of serum thyroglobulin (Tg), alone or following recombinant TSH stimulation, is most useful in the follow-up of patients with differentiated thyroid cancer.[28, 41] A low serum Tg level before giving radioiodine to ablate any thyroid remnant has 94% negative predictive value for the absence of disease at future follow-up.[42]

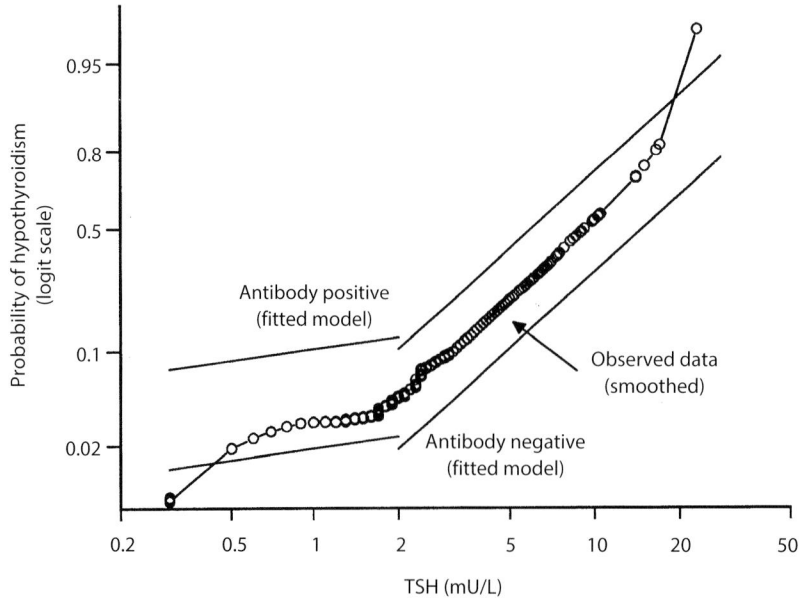

Figure 60.1 Probability of developing overt hypothyroidism in patients with subclinical hypothyroidism. The risks increase in proportion to the initial TSH at the time of diagnosis of subclinical hypothyroidism and the upper line shows the additional risk conferred by having positive thyroid autoantibodies. From Vanderpump et al. The incidence of thyroid disorders in the community – a twenty-year follow-up of the Whickham survey. *Clin Endocrinol* 1995; **43**: 55-69, with permission.

There is no utility in measuring Tg in the initial evaluation of a thyroid nodule. However, there is a role for its measurement in diagnosing factitious thyrotoxicosis, in which the Tg level is low, rather than elevated as in other types of thyrotoxicosis.[43]

DETERMINING THE NATURE OF STRUCTURAL LESIONS

Scintiscanning

The use of radioisotope uptake tests and thyroid scintiscanning has declined markedly in the last two decades with the introduction of better blood tests and thyroid ultrasound. In benign thyroid diseases, ^{99m}Tc is the most frequently used isotope for scanning and is particularly useful (i) to localize congenital anatomical defects of the thyroid,[44] and (ii) to distinguish between thyrotoxicosis caused by destructive thyroiditis (e.g. subacute thyroiditis, postpartum thyroiditis), in which the uptake of isotope is reduced, and hyperthyroidism (e.g. Graves' disease, nodular thyroid disease), in which the uptake is increased (**Figure 60.2**). Radioisotope uptake is also reduced in factitious thyrotoxicosis and in the presence of excessive stable iodine (e.g. after administration of amiodarone or iodine-containing contrast media).

American guidelines for the management of newly presenting thyroid nodules recommend the use of scintiscanning with ^{99m}Tc or I123, for any nodule associated with a subnormal TSH,[41] as a hyperfunctioning nodule is only rarely associated with malignancy. Others take the view that the role of scintiscanning is limited and do not recommend routine use of scintiscanning in the initial evaluation of thyroid nodules.[45] The use of isotope scanning in the management of treated thyroid cancer is considered elsewhere (see Chapters 62 and 66).

Ultrasound

Thyroid ultrasound is now the most cost-effective approach to gaining structural information about the gland and is increasingly being performed by endocrinologists and surgeons, rather than being confined to use by radiologists.[46, 47] Most benign thyroid diseases can be diagnosed by clinical presentation and appropriate blood tests, but colour-flow Doppler ultrasonography has utility in distinguishing between the hyperthyroid (type 1) and destructive (type 2) forms of amiodarone-induced thyrotoxicosis; blood flow is increased in the former and reduced in the latter.[32]

Ultrasound is recommended in the evaluation of all thyroid nodules, including multinodular goitre, as simple palpation is imprecise and insensitive.[41, 48] Features suggestive of malignancy are shown in **Box 60.6** and **Figure 60.3**. It is important to emphasize that ultrasonography is complementary to FNAB in making a diagnosis; for instance, ultrasound is useful in planning the extent of surgery when FNAB is suggestive of carcinoma.[49] Furthermore, the increasing use of thyroid ultrasound has led to the detection of a large number of nodules which previously would have been ignored. The population prevalence for thyroid nodules is around 5% by palpation, but 10% of 25 year olds and 55% of women aged over 70 have nodules on ultrasonography: only a small fraction of these will be malignant.[50] A detailed cost–benefit analysis for the investigation of thyroid nodules found incidentally on neck ultrasound has not been undertaken.

Thyroid ultrasound has an increasingly important role in thyroid cancer follow-up, with the recognition

---

BOX 60.6 Ultrasonographic features suggestive of (a) a malignant thyroid nodule, and (b) a benign thyroid nodule in decreasing order of specificity

- Microcalcification
  - Irregularity of the border of the nodule
  - Increased blood flow in nodule on colour-flow Doppler
  - Hypoechogenicity
  - Absence of a halo
- Diameter less than 1 cm (those less than 0.5 cm do not require further intervention)
  - Simple cyst with no solid component
  - Comet tail sign, due to colloid content
  - Honeycomb appearance

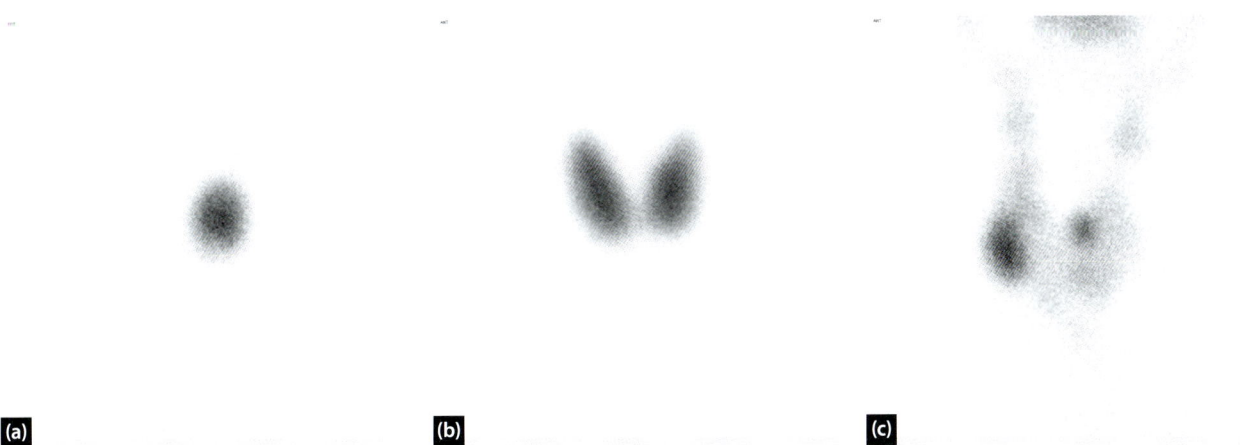

Figure 60.2 Thyroid ^{99m}Tc scintiscans. (a) Toxic adenoma; **(b)** Graves' disease; **(c)** multinodular goitre. Images courtesy of Colleen Brown, Sheffield Teaching Hospitals NHS Foundation Trust.

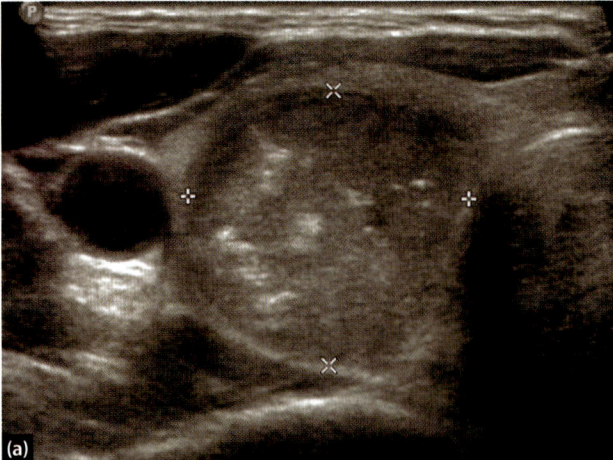 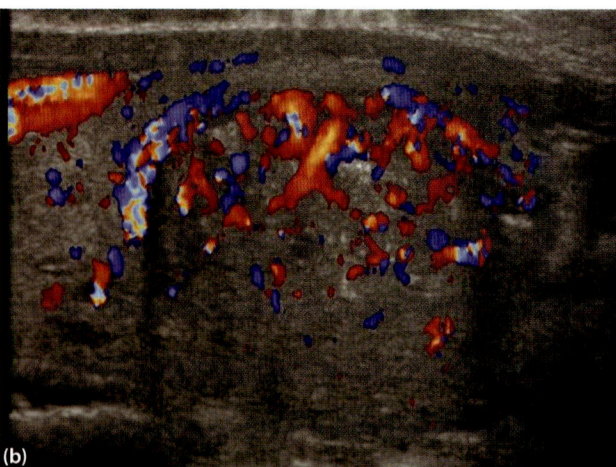

Figure 60.3 Thyroid ultrasound images of papillary carcinoma. **(a)** Microcalcification; **(b)** chaotic vascular pattern on colour-flow Doppler. Images courtesy of Dr Catherine Clout, Sheffield Teaching Hospitals NHS Foundation Trust.

that whole-body scintiscanning has low sensitivity. Measurement of serum Tg and cervical ultrasound is the best current method to detect recurrent disease in low-risk patients.[41, 50] Ultrasound elastography is a technique that assesses nodule consistency by measuring the amount of distortion produced by an external force. Although initial reports have been encouraging, based on the premise that malignant nodules are firm and thus have low elastic strain,[51] other studies have found no improvement over conventional ultrasound, even if the two are combined.[52] This technique is operator-dependent and at present elastography is inadequate to guide management of thyroid nodules.[53]

Other imaging techniques

Computed tomography (CT) and magnetic resonance imaging (MRI) have only an ancillary use to ultrasound in the investigation of thyroid disease.[47] Such scans are useful in the assessment of large goitres to determine whether there is any tracheal compression or substernal extension.[48] In the initial phase of acute thyroiditis, CT scanning is as good as ultrasound at demonstrating the inflammatory process but more accurate with regard to anatomical involvement; barium swallow imaging is superior to both in detecting a pyriform sinus fistula when the acute inflammatory process subsides.[54]

^{18}F-FDG-position emission tomography (PET) has generally been used to localize thyroid cancer recurrence in patients with raised Tg levels but no evidence of disease on whole-body scintiscans. However, its overall impact remains to be defined, and specificity and sensitivity figures are unclear.[41, 55] Non-malignant false-positive results from FDG-PET may be encountered with reactive lymph nodes, suture granulomas and muscle activity. Additional proposed uses for this technique include (i) the initial work-up of patients, although half of patients with indeterminate nodules on fine needle aspiration biopsy and a positive FDG-PET result have benign lesions,[56] (ii) staging and follow-up of invasive Hürthle cell carcinoma, and (iii) categorization of risk in patients with known distant metastases.[41]

KEY POINTS

- Thyroid dysfunction can be diagnosed and managed by simple blood tests: a normal serum TSH level rules out primary thyroid dysfunction.
- Although modern tests for TSH, FT3 and FT4 are robust, occasional artefacts may be encountered, and the possibility of non-thyroid illness as an explanation for abnormal results should always be considered.
- Autoimmune thyroid disease can be diagnosed by the detection of serum TPO antibodies; robust immunoassays for TSH-receptor antibodies make these the test of choice to diagnose Graves' disease.
- Ultrasound has superseded scintiscanning for the structural evaluation of the thyroid and is recommended for the detailed investigation of thyroid nodules.

REFERENCES

1. Zulewski H, Müller B, Exer P, et al. Estimation of tissue hypothyroidism by a new clinical score: evaluation of patients with various grades of hypothyroidism and controls. *J Clin Endocrinol Metab* 1997; 82: 771–6.
2. Jarløv AE, Nygaard B, Hegedüs L, et al. Observer variation in the clinical and laboratory evaluation of patients with thyroid dysfunction and goiter. *Thyroid* 1998; 8: 393–8.
3. Thienpont LM, Van Uytfanghe K, Beastall G, et al. Report of the IFCC Working Group for Standardization of Thyroid Function Tests; part 1: thyroid-stimulating hormone. *Clin Chem* 2010; 56: 902–11.
4. Baloch Z, Carayon P, Conte-Devolx B, et al. Laboratory medicine practice guidelines. Laboratory support for the diagnosis and monitoring of thyroid disease. *Thyroid* 2003; **13**: 3–126.
5. Franklyn JA. The thyroid – too much and too little across the ages: the consequences of subclinical thyroid dysfunction. *Clin Endocrinol* 2013; **78**: 1–8.

6. Wartofsky L, Dickey RA. The evidence for a narrower thyrotropin reference range is compelling. *J Clin Endocrinol Metab* 2005; **90:** 5483–8.
7. Surks MI, Goswami G, Daniels GH. The thyrotropin reference range should remain unchanged. *J Clin Endocrinol Metab* 2005; **90:** 5489–96.
8. Brabant G, Beck-Peccoz P, Jarzab B, et al. Is there a need to redefine the upper normal limit of TSH? *Eur J Endocrinol* 2006; **154:** 633–7.
9. Thienpont LM, Van Uytfanghe K, Beastall G, et al. Report of the IFCC Working Group for Standardization of Thyroid Function Tests; part 2: free thyroxine and free triiodothyronine. *Clin Chem* 2010; **56:** 912–20.
10. Association for Clinical Biochemistry, British Thyroid Association, Thyroid Foundation. UK Guidelines for the Use of Thyroid Function Tests. Available from: http://www.british-thyroid-association.org/current-bta-guidelines.
11. Bahn RS, Burch HB, Cooper DS, et al. Hyperthyroidism and other causes of thyrotoxicosis: management guidelines of the American Thyroid Association and American Association of Clinical Endocrinologists. *Thyroid* 2011; **21:** 593–646.
12. Garber JR, Cobin RH, Gharib H, et al. Clinical practice guidelines for hypothyroidism in adults: co-sponsored by American Association of Clinical Endocrinologists and the American Thyroid Association. *Thyroid* 2012; **22:** 1200–35.
13. Dayan CM. Interpretation of thyroid function tests. *Lancet* 2001; **357:** 619–24.
14. Beckett G, MacKenzie F. Thyroid guidelines – are thyroid-stimulating hormone assays fit for purpose? *Ann Clin Biochem* 2007; **44:** 203–8.
15. Surks MI, Ortiz E, Daniels GH, et al. Subclinical thyroid disease: scientific review and guidelines for diagnosis and management. *J Am Med Assoc* 2004; **291:** 228–38.
16. Stagnaro-Green A, Abalovich M, Alexander E, et al. Guidelines of the American Thyroid Association for the diagnosis and management of thyroid disease during pregnancy and postpartum. *Thyroid* 2011; **21:** 1081–125.
17. Lazarus JH, Bestwick JP, Channon S, et al. Antenatal thyroid screening and childhood cognitive function. *N Engl J Med* 2012; **366:** 493–501.
18. LaFranchi SH. Approach to the diagnosis and treatment of neonatal hypothyroidism. *J Clin Endocrinol Metab* 2011; **96:** 2959–67.
19. Boomsma MJ, Bijl HP, Langendijk JA. Radiation-induced hypothyroidism in head and neck cancer patients: a systematic review. *Radiother Oncol* 2011; **99:** 1–5.
20. Quadbeck B, Hoermann R, Roggenbuck U, et al; Basedow Study Group. Sensitive thyrotropin and thyrotropin-receptor antibody determinations one month after discontinuation of antithyroid drug treatment as predictors of relapse in Graves' disease. *Thyroid* 2005; **15:** 1047–54.
21. Report of a Working Party. Radioiodine in the management of benign thyroid disease. Royal College of Physicians of London. 2007. Available from: https://shop.rcplondon.ac.uk/products/radioiodine-in-the-management-of-benign-thyroid-disease-clincial-guidelines?variant=6637100933
22. Roberts CG, Ladenson PW. Hypothyroidism. *Lancet* 2004; **363:** 793–803.
23. Shimon I, Cohen O, Lubetsky A, Olchovsky D. Thyrotropin suppression by thyroid hormone replacement is correlated with thyroxine level normalization in central hypothyroidism. *Thyroid* 2002; **12:** 823–7.
24. Sinclair D. Clinical and laboratory aspects of thyroid autoantibodies. *Ann Clin Biochem* 2006; **43:** 173–83.
25. Sinclair D. Analytical aspects of thyroid antibodies estimation. *Autoimmunity* 2008; **41:** 46–54.
26. Nordyke RA, Gilbert FI, Jr., Miyamoto LA, Fleury KA. The superiority of antimicrosomal over antithyroglobulin antibodies for detecting Hashimoto's thyroiditis. *Arch Intern Med* 1993; **153:** 862–5.
27. Spencer C, Petrovic I, Fatemi S. Current thyroglobulin autoantibody (TgAb) assays often fail to detect interfering TgAb that can result in the reporting of falsely low/undetectable serum Tg IMA values for patients with differentiated thyroid cancer. *J Clin Endocrinol Metab* 2011; **96:** 1283–91.
28. Spencer CA. Clinical review: clinical utility of thyroglobulin antibody (TgAb) measurements for patients with differentiated thyroid cancers (DTC). *J Clin Endocrinol Metab* 2011; **96:** 3615–27.
29. Kim ES, Lim DJ, Baek KH, et al. Thyroglobulin antibody is associated with increased cancer risk in thyroid nodules. *Thyroid* 2010; **20:** 885–91.
30. Vanderpump MP, Tunbridge WM, French JM, et al. The incidence of thyroid disorders in the community: a twenty-year follow-up of the Whickham Survey. *Clin Endocrinol* 1995; **43:** 55–68.
31. Effraimidis G, Strieder TG, Tijssen JG, Wiersinga WM. Natural history of the transition from euthyroidism to overt autoimmune hypo- or hyperthyroidism: a prospective study. *Eur J Endocrinol* 2011; **164:** 107–13.
32. Martino E, Bartalena L, Bogazzi F, Braverman LE. The effects of amiodarone on the thyroid. *Endocr Rev* 2001; **22:** 240–54.
33. Hamnvik OP, Larsen PR, Marqusee E. Thyroid dysfunction from antineoplastic agents. *J Natl Cancer Inst* 2011; **103:** 1572–87.
34. Ajjan RA, Weetman AP. Techniques to quantify TSH receptor antibodies. *Nat Clin Pract Endocrinol Metab* 2008; **4:** 461–68.
35. McLachlan SM, Rapoport B. Thyrotropin blocking autoantibodies and thyroid stimulating autoantibodies: insight into the pendulum from hypothyroidism to hyperthyroidism or vice versa. *Thyroid* 2013; **23**(1): 14–24.
36. Laurberg P, Bournaud C, Karmisholt J, Orgiazzi J. Management of Graves' hyperthyroidism in pregnancy: focus on both maternal and foetal thyroid function, and caution against surgical thyroidectomy in pregnancy. *Eur J Endocrinol* 2009; **160:** 1–8.
37. Matthews DC, Syed AA. The role of TSH receptor antibodies in the management of Graves' disease. *Eur J Intern Med* 2011; **22:** 213–16.
38. Quadbeck B, Hoermann R, Hahn S, et al. Binding, stimulating and blocking TSH receptor antibodies to the thyrotropin receptor as predictors of relapse of Graves' disease after withdrawal of antithyroid treatment. *Horm Metab Res* 2005; **37:** 745–50.
39. Eckstein AK, Plicht M, Lax H, et al. Thyrotropin receptor autoantibodies are independent risk factors for Graves' ophthalmopathy and help to predict severity and outcome of the disease. *J Clin Endocrinol Metab* 2006; **91:** 3464–70.
40. Samuels MH. Subacute, silent, and post-partum thyroiditis. *Med Clin North Am* 2012; **96:** 223–33.
41. American Thyroid Association (ATA) Guidelines Taskforce on Thyroid Nodules and Differentiated Thyroid Cancer, Cooper DS, Doherty GM, et al. Revised American Thyroid Association management guidelines for patients with thyroid nodules and differentiated thyroid cancer. *Thyroid* 2009; **19:** 1167–214.
42. Webb RC, Howard RS, Stojadinovic A, et al. The utility of serum thyroglobulin measurement at the time of remnant ablation for predicting disease-free status in patients with differentiated thyroid cancer: a meta-analysis involving 3947 patients. *J Clin Endocrinol Metab* 2012; **97:** 2754–63.
43. Bogazzi F, Bartalena L, Scarcello G, et al. The age of patients with thyrotoxicosis factitia in Italy from 1973 to 1996. *J Endocrinol Invest* 1999; **22:** 128–33.
44. Noussios G, Anagnostis P, Goulis DG, et al. Ectopic thyroid tissue: anatomical, clinical, and surgical implications of a rare entity. *Eur J Endocrinol* 2011; **165:** 375–82.
45. Mehanna HM, Jain A, Morton RP, et al. Investigating the thyroid nodule. *BMJ* 2009; **338:** b733.
46. Kangelaris GT, Kim TB, Orloff LA. Role of ultrasound in thyroid disorders. *Otolaryngol Clin North Am* 2010; **43:** 1209–27.
47. Vazquez BJ, Richards ML. Imaging of the thyroid and parathyroid glands. *Surg Clin North Am* 2011; **91:** 15–32.
48. Bahn RS, Castro MR. Approach to the patient with nontoxic multinodular goiter. *J Clin Endocrinol Metab* 2011; **96:** 1202–12.
49. Kwak JY, Kim EK, Kim MJ, et al. The role of ultrasound in thyroid nodules with a cytology reading of "suspicious for papillary thyroid carcinoma". *Thyroid* 2008; **18:** 517–22.
50. Sipos JA. Advances in ultrasound for the diagnosis and management of thyroid cancer. *Thyroid* 2009; **19:** 1363–72.
51. Rago T, Santini F, Scutari M, et al. Elastography: new developments in ultrasound for predicting malignancy in thyroid nodules. *J Clin Endocrinol Metab* 2007; **92:** 2917–22.
52. Moon HJ, Sung JM, Kim EK, et al. Diagnostic performance of gray-scale US and elastography in solid thyroid nodules. *Radiology* 2012; **262:** 1002–13.
53. Carneiro-Pla D. Ultrasound elastography in the evaluation of thyroid nodules for thyroid cancer. *Curr Opin Oncol* 2013; **25:** 1–5.
54. Masuoka H, Miyauchi A, Tomoda C, et al. Imaging studies in sixty patients with acute suppurative thyroiditis. *Thyroid* 2011; **21:** 1075–80.

55. Facey K, Bradbury I, Laking G, Payne E. Overview of the clinical effectiveness of positron emission tomography imaging in selected cancers. *Health Technol Assess* 2007; **11**: xi–267.

56. Vriens D, de Wilt JH, van der Wilt GJ, et al. The role of [18F]-2-fluoro-2-deoxy-d-glucose-positron emission tomography in thyroid nodules with indeterminate fine-needle aspiration biopsy: systematic review and meta-analysis of the literature. *Cancer* 2011; **117**: 4582–94.

CHAPTER 61

BENIGN THYROID DISEASE

Christopher M. Jones and Kristien Boelaert

Introduction 717	Euthyroid glandular enlargement 740
Hyperthyroidism 717	Conclusions 745
Hypothyroidism 733	References 746
Thyroid disease in pregnancy 738	

SEARCH STRATEGY

Data in this chapter may be updated by a Medline search using the keywords: hyperthyroidism, thyrotoxicosis, subclinical hyperthyroidism, Graves' disease, hypothyroidism, myxoedema, subclinical hypothyroidism, thyroiditis, subacute thyroiditis, Hashimoto's thyroiditis, goitre, thyroid nodule and multinodular goitre. Secondary search criteria included thyroid-stimulating hormone, thyroxine, triiodothyronine, antithyroid peroxidase, elastography and fine-needle aspiration cytology. Emphasis has been placed on pathogenesis, diagnosis and treatment with level 1 and 2 evidence reported wherever possible.

INTRODUCTION

Benign thyroid disease is commonly encountered by clinicians. The term encompasses thyroid hormone imbalance, abnormal enlargement of thyroid gland tissue and, less commonly, thyroid tenderness. These abnormalities constitute a significant burden within clinical practice, particularly in relation to the elderly, and often require significant biochemical, immunological, radiological and histological investigations in addition to thorough clinical assessment. Thyroid dysfunction encompasses deficient and excess thyroid hormone production, respectively hypothyroidism and hyperthyroidism, which together affect approximately 2% of women and 0.2% of men.[1] While it is clear that the sequelae of overt thyroid dysfunction affect nearly all body systems and that they are therefore associated with significant morbidity and mortality, the significance of subclinical thyroid dysfunction is yet to be fully elucidated. Enlargement of the thyroid gland, or goitre, whether generalized or focal, augments the burden imposed by thyroid disease and may affect up to 60% of the population, with higher frequencies seen in the elderly and women.[2] Although the majority of cases of thyroid enlargement may be managed conservatively, the need to first exclude malignant aetiology and the more intensive management of these patients pose significant challenges to the clinician.

HYPERTHYROIDISM

Definitions

Hyperthyroidism refers to hyperfunction of the thyroid gland and is defined by reduced levels of thyroid-stimulating hormone (TSH) and raised free T4 (fT4) and free T3 (fT3) concentrations. It leads to thyrotoxicosis, which is the clinical syndrome resulting from a biochemical excess of fT4, fT3 or both. Hence, biochemical tests of thyroid function may identify hyperthyroidism before it becomes clinically apparent, with a rise in fT3 and fall in TSH concentrations typically seen prior to a rise in fT4. **Thyrotoxicosis** may be a consequence of a disorder of the thyroid gland itself, which is referred to as primary disease, or may be secondary to abnormal production of TSH resulting from pathology of the anterior pituitary gland. **Subclinical hyperthyroidism** is diagnosed in patients for whom TSH levels fall below the normal reference range but who have normal fT4 and fT3 concentrations. This must be in the absence of disease of the pituitary or hypothalamus, ingestion of drugs that inhibit TSH secretion or the presence of non-thyroidal illness (**Box 61.1**).

> **BOX 61.1** Key definitions in thyroid hormone excess (hyperthyroidism)
>
> | | |
> |---|---|
> | Hyperthyroidism | *Hyperfunction of the thyroid gland (raised T4 and T3 with suppressed TSH)* |
> | Thyrotoxicosis | *Clinical syndrome resulting from excess thyroid hormones* |
> | Subclinical hyperthyroidism | *Normal T4 and T3 in the presence of low TSH* |

Epidemiology

Hyperthyroidism is approximately ten times more common in women than in men within iodine-replete communities, affecting between 0.5% and 2% of the female population.[3] The Third National Health and Nutrition Examination Survey (NHANES III) reported the prevalence of clinically significant hyperthyroidism to be 2 per 1000, whereas the prevalence in older persons is reported between 0.4% and 2.0%.[4, 5] The reported annual incidence for men and women respectively varies between 0.4–0.8/1000 and 0.1/1000 per year; higher rates are seen in iodine-deficient areas.[6] Unlike for hypothyroidism, there is no documented increase in the probability of the development of overt hyperthyroidism with age.

Subclinical hyperthyroidism is more common and can be readily diagnosed following the introduction of sensitive assays for determining TSH concentrations. The incidence of subclinical hyperthyroidism is reported to increase with age. In a UK survey of 1210 persons aged over 60 years and registered within a single general practice, 6.3% of women and 5.5% of men were identified to have TSH levels below normal.[7] The overall prevalence of low TSH levels in the Colorado study of 25 862 individuals was 2.2%.[8] Of the 13 334 persons enrolled in NHANES III, only 0.8% of randomly selected individuals met criteria for subclinical hyperthyroidism, though this rose to 3% of those aged over 80 years.[4]

Aetiology

There are myriad causes of hyperthyroidism, as summarized in **Table 61.1**, alongside causes of thyrotoxicosis. The most common is Graves' disease, an autoimmune disorder in which antibodies are directed against and stimulate the TSH receptor. Toxic multinodular goitre is commonly seen and features one or more autonomous thyroid hormone-producing nodule(s) that cause thyroid hormone excess. Inflammation of the thyroid may also result in clinically important thyrotoxicosis, in addition to exogenous ingestion of thyroid hormones, the presence of ectopic thyroid tissue or aberrations of thyroidal autonomy. Each carries a specific clinical presentation and requires specific treatment strategies.

Clinical manifestations

Hyperthyroidism may be accompanied by a constellation of signs and symptoms, the breadth of which is attributable to the diversity of action of thyroid hormones. Apathetic or masked thyrotoxicosis may be seen in some patients who fail to develop any symptoms of thyroid excess whatsoever.[9] Older individuals may additionally demonstrate a paucity of symptoms though cardiovascular complaints are seen most frequently; it is therefore appropriate to adopt a low threshold for performing thyroid function testing in older persons.[10] There nevertheless exists a rough correlation between circulating thyroid hormone concentrations and symptom severity. The signs and symptoms of hyperthyroidism are summarized in **Table 61.2**.

SYMPTOMS

The symptoms of thyrotoxicosis result from both β-adrenergic overactivity and the intracellular action of thyroid hormones. Patients may complain of anxiety, poor

TABLE 61.1 Causes and classification of thyrotoxicosis and hyperthyroidism

	Thyrotoxicosis with hyperthyroidism	Thyrotoxicosis without hyperthyroidism
Common	Graves' disease Toxic multinodular goitre Solitary toxic adenoma	Silent (painless) thyroiditis Postpartum thyroiditis Subacute thyroiditis Exogenous thyroid hormone
Uncommon	TSH-secreting pituitary adenoma Iodine intake Radiographic contrast agents Iodine-containing drugs (amiodarone) Pituitary resistance to thyroid hormone Neonatal Graves' disease Hyperemesis gravidarum Struma ovarii Metastatic follicular thyroid carcinoma	Drug-induced thyroiditis (amiodarone, lithium, interferon-α) Acute infectious thyroiditis Radiation thyroiditis Infarction of thyroid adenoma 'Hamburger' thyrotoxicosis

TABLE 61.2 Clinical manifestations of hyperthyroidism

Symptoms	Signs
Weight loss	Sinus tachycardia
Anxiety	Atrial fibrillation
Agitation	Fine tremor
Irritability	Warm moist skin
Palpitation	Palmar erythema
Fatigue and weakness	Onycholysis
Breathlessness	Hair loss
Heat intolerance	Proximal myopathy
Sweating	Muscle wasting
Increased appetite	High output heart failure
Menstrual irregularity	Thyroid bruit
Hair loss	
Brittle nails	

concentration and irritability. They may report insomnia despite extreme fatigue, and a paradoxical fall in weight may be seen in the presence of increased appetite as a consequence of increased basal metabolic rate. Weight loss in conjunction with depression and agitation in this context has previously been termed 'apathetic hyperthyroidism'.

Heat intolerance and increased perspiration are common complaints. Stool frequency is also increased yet frank diarrhoea is rare. Oligomenorrhoea and infertility may occur in women, although amenorrhoea is seen only rarely. Men may report reduced libido and painful gynaecomastia.

SIGNS

Clinical findings include agitation, rapid speech, palmar erythema, the presence of a fine tremor and warm, moist skin. Hair may be fine and thin while sympathetic overactivity and thyroid orbitopathy contribute to lid retraction and lid lag. Examination of the neurological system may reveal a fine tremor of the outstretched hands, hyperreflexia and a proximal myopathy. Sinus tachycardia or atrial fibrillation (AF) is frequently noted on cardiovascular examination. Approximately 15% of older persons with new-onset AF have thyrotoxicosis, while a study of 40 628 patients with hyperthyroidism identified a prevalence of AF of 8.3%.[11] Consequently, new-onset AF warrants an assessment of thyroid status, particularly in older patients among whom AF is seen more commonly and in whom cerebral emboli or worsening cardiac failure may be readily precipitated by its development.[12]

Thyroid enlargement is commonly noted in patients with hyperthyroidism. There may be a single nodule in patients with an autonomously functioning adenoma or a nodular goitre in those with toxic multinodular goitre. A smooth goitre is seen in many patients with Graves' disease although the thyroid is impalpable in 30% of those with Graves' and toxic nodular hyperthyroidism.[3] Other features seen in hyperthyroidism include osteoporosis, signs of hypercalcaemia and shortness of breath. Signs relating to the excess production of thyroid hormones, including the development of goitre, may be less evident among older persons.

In rare instances, established or new-onset hyperthyroidism may present as an acute 'thyroid storm'. This potentially life-threatening condition should be considered in patients with a fever and altered mental state. It commonly comprises psychiatric disturbance such as agitation or psychosis coupled with hyperpyrexia, AF and congestive cardiac failure.[13] Patients may subsequently become comatose. This condition is commonly precipitated by stressors such as infection, surgery or childbirth.

Thyrotoxicosis may also very rarely be associated with periodic paralysis (thyrotoxic periodic paralysis; TPP), particularly among Asian populations and especially in Chinese and Japanese patients aged between 20 and 40 years.[14] Patients typically experience recurrent episodes of transient skeletal muscle weakness which initially affects the lower limbs prior to afflicting the truncal muscles and then all four limbs. Attacks may last 3–72 hours. Severe cases have been accompanied by total paralysis of respiratory, bulbar and ocular muscles. The hallmark of TPP is hypokalaemia, which is thought to result from the action of thyroid hormone on Na^+, K^+-ATPase activity. Treatment with intravenous potassium during an attack may therefore hasten muscle recovery and reduce the potential risk of cardiac arrhythmia. Prophylaxis against further attacks can be achieved using spironolactone or propranolol yet definitive treatment of hyperthyroidism remains the mainstay of management.

Diagnostic evaluation

A history and examination suggestive of thyroid overactivity requires further investigation prior to the initiation of treatment or further investigation. Laboratory investigations used in the workup of suspected thyrotoxicosis are shown in **Table 61.3**. The single most important test is the measurement of serum TSH. If TSH is within normal range, a diagnosis of hyperthyroidism can usually be ruled out. Rare cases in which thyrotoxicosis is caused by a pituitary lesion, such as a TSHoma, or syndromes of thyroid hormone resistance stand as the exception to this rule. In these instances serum TSH may be normal or slightly raised in association with raised fT3 and fT4 concentrations.

In most cases of hyperthyroidism the typical picture is of undetectable serum TSH with elevated serum concentrations of fT4 and fT3. A low TSH and a normal fT4 concentration should prompt fT3 measurement as 10% of cases of thyrotoxicosis are so-called 'T3 toxicosis'. This is most commonly seen in mild cases of toxic nodular hyperthyroidism (either a single autonomous nodule or a multinodular goitre) or early in relapse of Graves' disease. It is important to note that not all laboratories perform T3 assays unless specifically requested.

A low TSH is not specific for thyrotoxicosis. 'Nonthyroidal illness' or treatment with a variety of drugs may lower the TSH below the normal range, although it is still usually detectable in these circumstances. For these reasons it is preferable to measure the TSH in conjunction with serum fT4 and, in specific cases, fT3 as well (**Box 61.2**).

TABLE 61.3 Laboratory investigations in suspected thyrotoxicosis

Laboratory test	Findings	Comment
Thyroid function tests	Elevated free T4 and/or free T3	Unless TSH-secreting pituitary adenoma or thyroid hormone resistance
	Suppressed TSH	
Immunology	Raised TSH-receptor antibodies	Pathognomonic for Graves' disease
	Raised anti-TPO antibodies	Indicative of underlying thyroid autoimmunity
Biochemistry	Elevated alkaline phosphatase	
	Elevated calcium	
Haematology	Normochromic normocytic anaemia	Long-standing cases
	Raised ESR	Subacute thyroiditis

> **BOX 61.2 Key considerations in TSH testing**
>
> Low TSH is not specific for thyrotoxicosis.
> Measurement of serum fT4 should be undertaken if TSH is abnormal.
> A low TSH and normal fT4 may mask T3 toxicosis.

The specific patterns seen in thyroid function tests (TFTs), as depicted in **Table 61.4**, are accompanied by non-specific changes in other laboratory tests. Hypercalcaemia is seen in approximately 10% of patients as a consequence of increased bone turnover and secondary suppression of parathyroid hormone.[15] Levels of alkaline phosphatase may increase and both a raised ESR and normocytic normochromic anaemia seen.

TSH-receptor (TSH-R) antibodies are analysed in the laboratory through binding assays or bioassays.[16] These respectively measure TSH-R levels through respectively quantifying either the degree to which radiolabelled TSH–TSH receptor binding is inhibited by the presence of immunoglobulins, or the effect immunoglobulins have on thyroid cell function. The routine use of TSH-R antibody testing is increasing for the diagnosis of Graves' disease and the presence of these antibodies acts as a specific indicator of the disease. Interestingly, high levels of TSH-R antibodies seen in patients with Graves' disease who are pregnant predict neonatal thyrotoxicosis.[17] The additional presence of thyroid peroxidase (TPO) antibodies is suggestive but not pathognomonic for Graves' disease.

THYROID SCINTIGRAPHY IN THE INVESTIGATION OF THYROTOXICOSIS

In cases in which the aetiology of thyrotoxicosis remains unclear despite history, examination and laboratory investigations, thyroid scintigraphy may be utilized. This technique analyses radioactive iodine uptake by the thyroid gland and can be used to differentiate between 'hot' and 'cold' areas of increased and decreased function respectively. In most hyperthyroid states uptake will be at the higher end of normal or raised and there are specific scintigraphic appearances associated with different conditions (**Figure 61.1**). Uptake is typically low in transient thyroiditis and in iodine-induced hyperthyroidism. Isotope imaging, typically with technetium, can be useful to differentiate between focal uptake in one or more autonomous nodules and diffuse uptake in Graves' disease, but it is less specific than iodide-uptake scans. Radioisotope scanning lacks specificity, with high values also seen in individuals who have a normal thyroid gland in addition to those with iodine deficiency and conditions such as Hashimoto's thyroiditis.

Specific disorders of thyroid hormone excess

GRAVES' DISEASE

In iodine-replete parts of the world, Graves' disease is the most common cause of thyrotoxicosis (**Figure 61.2**). First described in 1835, Graves' disease is a syndrome consisting of hyperthyroidism, moderate diffuse goitre, ophthalmopathy and dermopathy. In many patients, hyperthyroidism and goitre are the only features. It is more common in women than men at a ratio of greater than 5:1. Men are affected later and the disease may be more severe. Its peak incidence is in the twenties and thirties, but the disease can occur at any age, albeit uncommonly before puberty. Graves' disease is both more common and more likely to be complicated by ophthalmopathy in smokers, in whom the risk of Graves' disease is almost doubled.[18]

Pathogenesis

Graves' disease is an autoimmune condition characterized by the presence of circulating IgG oligoclonal autoantibodies directed against the TSH receptor within thyroid tissue (TSHR-Ab). These bind to the extracellular domain of the TSH receptor where they cause activation of intracellular cyclic AMP and thereby mimic the effect of pituitary TSH to stimulate thyroid hormone synthesis and secretion. Increased expression of fibroblast growth factor (FGF) contributes to enlargement of the gland resulting in

TABLE 61.4 Specific patterns of thyroid function tests

Suspected pathology	Specific diagnosis	TSH	T4	T3	TSH response to TRH
Hyperthyroidism	Primary hyperthyroidism	↓	↑	↑	N/A
	T3 toxicosis	↓	↔	↑	N/A
	Subclinical hyperthyroidism	↓	↔	↔	N/A
	TSHoma	↑/↔	↑	↑	N/A
	Amiodarone effect without overt thyroid dysfunction	↔	↑	↓	N/A
Hypothyroidism	Primary hypothyroidism	↑	↓	↓	↑
	Central hypothyroidism	↔/↓	↓	N/↓	↔/↓
	Resistance to thyroid hormone	↔/↑	↑	↑	↑
	Non-thyroidal illness	↔/↓	↔/↓	↓	↔/↓

Note: ↑: increased; ↓: decreased; ↔: normal.

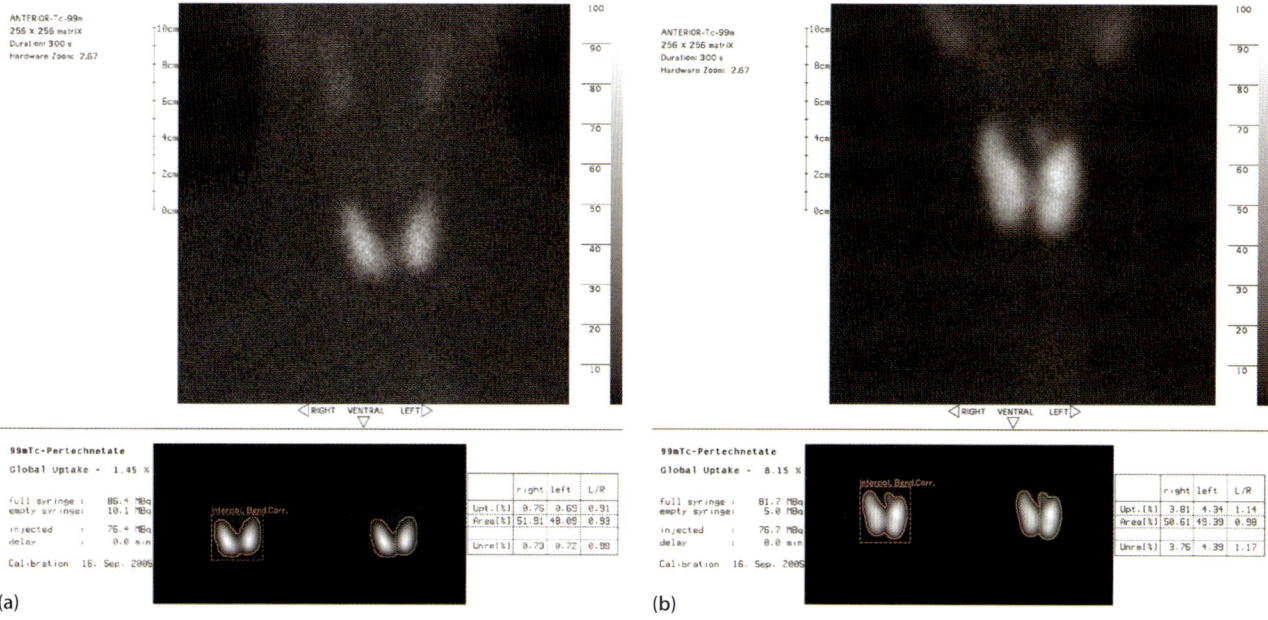

Figure 61.1 Scintigraphic appearances. **(a)** Normal thyroid; **(b)** Graves' disease with pyramidal lobe.

a diffuse swelling. Antibodies which specifically activate phospholipase A_2 are especially goitrogenic.[19]

The expression of CD80 and CD86 by dendritic cells and B cells may trigger Graves' hyperthyroidism by acting to co-stimulate infiltrating T cells.[20] These are targeted against antigens such as the thyrotropin receptor, which is presented to them by thyroid cells that express HLA class II molecules in response to interferon-γ production. The presentation of antigen and molecules such as CD40, CD54 and IL-6 by thyroid cells may later exacerbate the autoimmune process.[21] Cross-reactivity between these thyroidal antigens and antigens in orbital and extra-orbital tissues may explain the close relationship between Graves' disease and both ophthalmopathy and dermopathy. The thyrotopin receptor is additionally expressed in preadipocytes of orbital fibroblasts and has therefore been suggested as a possible cross-reactive antigen.[22,23]

The aetiology of Graves' disease remains unknown. It runs in families and a concordance rate in monozygotic twins of 20% suggests a genetic contribution to its development, albeit with additional contribution from environmental factors responsible for promoting development of the disease. Graves' is well known to be associated with HLA-DR3 and HLA-DQA1*0501 in Caucasians, while HLA-DRB1*0701 is protective.[24] Environmental factors linked with the development of disease include life stress and subsequent activation of specific neuroendocrine pathways, female sex, steroids, smoking, dietary iodine intake and immune modulators such as interferon α.[25-27] Lithium may also promote Graves' hyperthyroidism via its immunologic sequelae.[28] Graves' disease has been associated with other diseases mediated by the immune system, including Type 1 diabetes, vitiligo (**Figure 61.3**), coeliac disease, pernicious anaemia and Addison's disease.

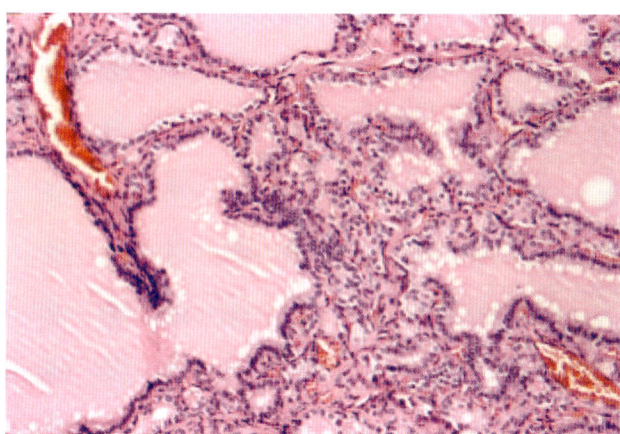

Figure 61.2 Graves' disease. A vascular gland displaying characteristic tortuous, hyperplastic follicles with blunt papillary infolding. The thyrocytes are columnar in outline and there is accentuated marginal vacuolation of stored colloid.

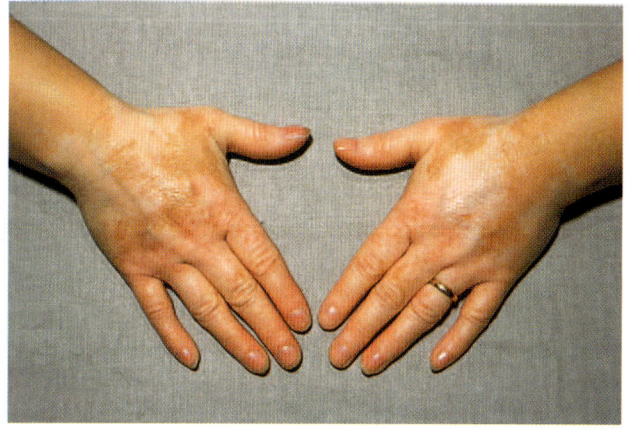

Figure 61.3 Vitiligo in hands of patient with Graves' disease.

Clinical manifestations and natural history

Although Graves' disease can occur rapidly over a few weeks, in most the onset is gradual and insidious. Patients exhibit many of the clinical features discussed above but may in addition have extrathyroidal manifestations such as ophthalmopathy (with exophthalmos and conjunctival oedema) and, rarely, dermopathy and acropachy.

A diffuse goitre is present in the majority of cases but its absence does not rule out Graves' disease, as the thyroid may be of normal size in around 3%.[15–18] The goitre is usually symmetrical, there may be an overlying palpable thrill and a bruit may often be heard. The thrill and bruit result from the increased blood flow to the thyroid.[15–18]

Graves' disease is usually treated with antithyroid medication in the first instance. While adequate therapy is given, the disease may be quiescent, but it can return if compliance diminishes or if drug dosage is inappropriately reduced. As with many autoimmune conditions, Graves' disease is sometimes self-limiting, although this is rare. Around 30% of patients experience lasting remission after treatment with antithyroid drugs.

Extrathyroidal manifestations of Graves' disease

Thyroid eye disease

Ophthalmopathy is common in Graves' disease. It is clinically apparent in approximately 50% of patients and may present prior to the onset of Graves' disease.[18] In 75% of those for whom eye disease is clinically apparent, eye signs appear within a year before or following the diagnosis of hyperthyroidism.[18] Even in the absence of clinical signs, imaging such as MRI has provided evidence of eye involvement in most patients (**Figure 61.4**). Approximately 90% of patients with thyroid eye disease also have Graves' disease.[29] The majority of the remainder have autoimmune hypothyroidism.

The ophthalmopathy seen in Graves' disease is characterized by swelling of the extraocular muscles, proliferation of periorbital fat and late fibrosis leading to muscle tethering.[30] The lesions develop due to an accumulation of glycosaminoglycans and a lymphocytic infiltration of the orbital and retro-orbital tissues. Patients who smoke are more likely to suffer eye disease of greater severity than non-smokers and hypothyroidism is an additional potentially exacerbating factor.[31, 32]

Patients with thyroid eye disease may complain of irritation in the eyes and the feeling of a foreign body. There may be excessive watering, especially in the wind. As the disease progresses, there is sometimes a change in physical appearance with periorbital oedema and/or a staring expression caused by exophthalmos and/or eyelid retraction. Eyelid retraction may give the false impression of proptosis, though both most often coexist. This may be bi- or unilateral and patients can complain of a feeling of pressure behind the eyes. Even in apparent unilateral cases, evidence of bilateral disease may be apparent on imaging. In severe cases the patient cannot close their eyes at night, leading to corneal ulceration and scarring. Apparent nerve palsies are also seen due to infiltration of the extraocular muscles with fat and fibrotic changes.

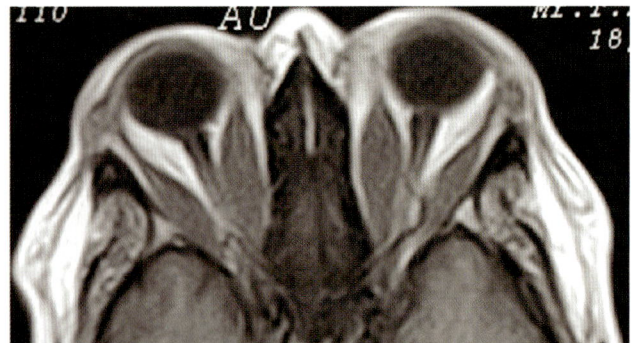
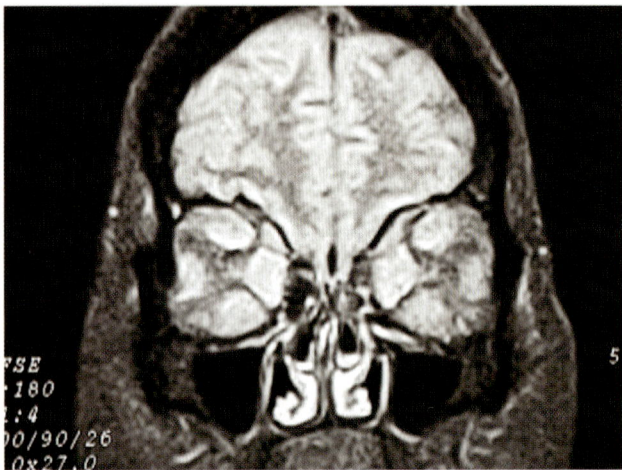

Figure 61.4 Thyroid eye disease. MRI orbits, showing enlarged extraocular muscles.

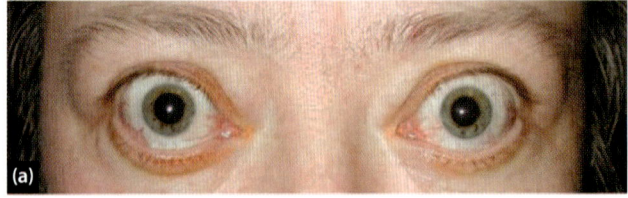
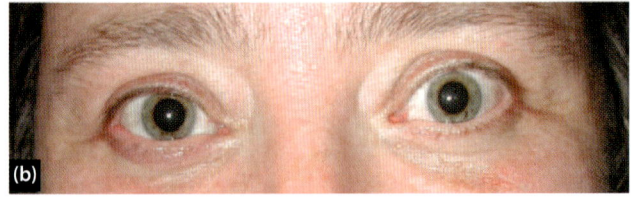

Figure 61.5 Patient with thyroid eye disease and optic neuropathy. (a) Pre-corrective surgery and **(b)** after surgical decompression. Note the upper lid retraction, corneal injection, periorbital fat deposition and proptosis pre-surgery.

Diplopia is noted in a significant proportion of patients and corrective surgery may be required (**Figure 61.5**).[33]

A rapid deterioration in visual acuity and loss of colour vision are ominous signs and may be caused by pressure on the optic nerve by swollen extraocular rectus muscles or sheer stretch of the optic nerve. Urgent treatment is required if permanent visual loss is to be avoided. Patients must also be referred urgently to an ophthalmologist if they develop strabismus or poor eye movement, or corneal ulceration or if their visual acuity is less than 6/18 (**Box 61.3**).[34]

> **BOX 61.3 Urgent referral criteria in thyroid eye disease**
>
> Rapid deterioration in visual acuity
> Ocular nerve palsies
> Unacceptable cosmetic appearance
> Visual acuity of less than 6/18
> Decreased colour vision
> Corneal ulceration

The most frequently seen signs of thyroid eye disease include eyelid retraction and periorbital oedema. Lid lag also occurs frequently and in mild cases arises as a consequence of sympathetic overactivity, whereas in more significant instances is the result of Graves' ophthalmopathy. Exophthalmos is seen in up to a third of patients. Compression of the optic nerve at the apex of the orbit is rare but can result in visual loss.

Thyroid eye disease occurs in two phases: a dynamic phase and a quiescent phase. Unfortunately, even when Graves' ophthalmopathy is well-treated and quiescent, patients do not always achieve a return in physical appearance to their pre-morbid state. Mild to moderate thyroid eye disease often requires no treatment and may improve spontaneously. Local discomfort can be managed with artificial tears and elevation of the head of the bed to reduce oedema. Severe ophthalmopathy requires management in a multidisciplinary team with experienced ophthalmologists. High-dose glucocorticoids as well as other immunosuppressive agents and orbital radiotherapy can be used successfully in early and active disease, which will have beneficial effects in approximately two-thirds of patients.[35, 36] The chimeric anti-CD20 monoclonal antibody Rituximab acts to deplete B-cells and may also be of benefit in thyroid eye disease, though trials are ongoing.[36, 37] Ocular nerve palsies require treatment from an experienced ophthalmologist, either initially or after failure of glucocorticoid treatment.

Dermopathy

This occurs in 1–2% of patients with Graves' disease, almost always accompanied by severe eye disease.[38] Usually occurring over the shins and known as pretibial myxoedema, it may affect other areas of the body.[39] Dermopathy in Graves' disease also occurs at sites of trauma, thereby exhibiting the Koebner phenomenon.

The skin appears raised, oedematous, nodular and discoloured with a pink or brownish tinge (**Figure 61.6**).[40] It is characterized by a florid lymphocytic infiltrate and a build-up of glycosaminoglycans. Although not usually treated, fluorinated steroids may be used topically with occlusive dressings.[39]

Acropachy

This very rare condition occurs in less than 1 per 1000 patients. It presents as clubbing of the fingers with subperiosteal new bone formation seen on plain X-ray films.[41] Acropachy arises from glycosaminoglycan accumulation and is seen in association with dermopathy and ophthalmopathy. There is no treatment.

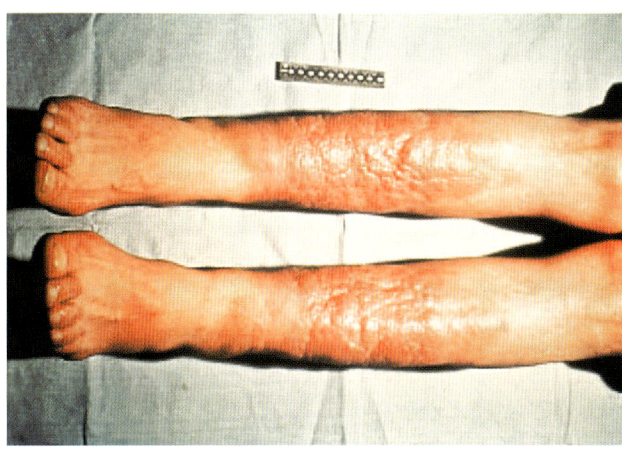

Figure 61.6 Pretibial myxoedema.

Laboratory diagnosis

The routine measurement of TSH-R antibodies for the diagnosis of Graves' disease is increasingly regarded to be both valid and reliable.[16] Anti-TPO antibodies are also commonly measured. Laboratory results otherwise typically identify raised serum fT4 and fT3 with undetectable serum TSH.

> **KEY POINTS**
>
> **GRAVES' DISEASE**
>
> - Graves' disease is the most common cause of thyrotoxicosis in iodine-replete populations.
> - It is more common in women than men.
> - It is an autoimmune condition characterized by the presence of IgG anti-TSH receptor antibodies.
> - Antithyroid peroxidase antibodies are present in 75% of patients.
> - Ophthalmopathy, dermopathy and acropachy are important extrathyroidal manifestations.
> - Antithyroid medication is used in most cases at least initially.

TOXIC MULTINODULAR GOITRE

Nodular thyroid disease predominates in the elderly and surpasses Graves' disease as the most common cause of hyperthyroidism in older persons living within iodine-replete areas.[42] In regions in which iodine is relatively deficient, toxic nodular thyroid disease is the most common cause of hyperthyroidism.[43] A toxic multinodular goitre (MNG) occurs when two or more autonomously functioning thyroid nodules secrete excess thyroid hormone. Its precise cause is not known but may relate to genetic change that occurs within specific nodules and thereby drives clonal expansion.[44] As a consequence of its long natural history, an elderly patient presenting with a toxic MNG may describe the presence of the goitre many years before the thyrotoxicosis develops.[45] Exposure to pharmacological doses of iodine, such as those found in contrast media, may also precipitate hyperthyroidism through the Jod Basedow effect.[46] This is commonly seen in areas of iodine deficiency.

Toxic MNGs are generally observed in an older patient group than those who present with Graves' disease and the degree of thyroid hyperfunction is typically less marked.

For these reasons, the classical clinical symptoms and signs of thyrotoxicosis may not all be present. It is the cardiovascular effects that predominate, including palpitation, AF and other tachyarrhythmias.[47] Patients with toxic MNG may also report the presence of a long-standing goitre. Compressive symptoms are a possible consequence of the presence of a MNG and include dysphagia to solids and dyspnoea that worsen at night.

> **KEY POINTS**
>
> **TOXIC MULTINODULAR GOITRE**
> - This occurs in older patients.
> - Thyroid hyperfunction is less marked than in Graves' disease.
> - Cardiovascular symptoms predominate.
> - Definitive treatment with radioiodine is required.

SOLITARY TOXIC ADENOMAS (PLUMMER'S DISEASE)

A single toxic adenoma is a benign tumour autonomously secreting sufficient thyroid hormone to suppress pituitary TSH secretion. Solitary adenomas tend to grow to at least 3 cm in diameter prior to causing overt hyperthyroidism.[48] They are a rare cause of thyrotoxicosis and account for only around 5% of cases.[48] A mutation in the TSH receptor gene occurs in 20–83% of cases.[49] Several point mutations of this gene have been identified, mostly in the transmembrane domain. These are somatic and result in TSH receptor activation and consequent autonomous thyroid hormone secretion. Other activating mutations have been identified downstream in the stimulatory G protein pathway linked to cyclic AMP production.[50, 51]

Subclinical hyperthyroidism, characterized by below-normal serum TSH and normal serum fT4 and fT3 concentrations, is often evident on biochemical testing.[52] It occurs early in the clinical history of a toxic adenoma as a consequence of negative feedback prompted by TSH receptor activation and the resultant autonomous production of thyroid hormones.[53] Patients with a toxic adenoma are often younger than those with a toxic MNG, and present in the fourth or fifth decade. There may be a history of a slowly enlarging neck mass and many will have a palpable nodule. The autonomously functioning tissue may nevertheless be diffuse and a palpable nodule will not therefore be apparent in all patients. The level of thyroid hyperfunction is less than that seen in Graves' disease and signs may thus be less florid.[52] Radionuclide scanning may be utilized to distinguish a solitary toxic adenoma from toxic MNG and Graves' disease. It typically demonstrates a focus of isotope accumulation with no other visible areas of uptake.

Management of hyperthyroidism

The initial approach to the hyperthyroid patient is to minimize symptoms (often with a beta-adrenergic blocking drug) and to reduce the synthesis of thyroid hormones. Overt hyperthyroidism necessitates effective therapy in all cases in order to reduce the risk of psychological, cardiovascular and skeletal sequelae. The principles of management are summarized in **Box 61.4**.

> **BOX 61.4 Principles of management of hyperthyroidism**
>
> Minimize symptoms (e.g. with the use of a beta-adrenergic blocking drug)
> Treat hyperthyroidism to reduce risk of psychological, cardiovascular and skeletal sequelae:
>
> - Thionamides
> - Radioiodine
> - Surgical resection

Three modalities of treatment exist: drug therapy, radioiodine treatment and surgery. Their relative indications, advantages and disadvantages are summarized in **Table 61.5**. It has been demonstrated that each of the three treatment modalities is as effective at reducing thyroid hormone concentration, with similar improvements seen in quality of life and patient satisfaction following their use.[54–56] Treatment selection therefore depends on the underlying aetiology, the preference of the clinician and patient factors. Service considerations often also play a role in determining treatment choice and include cost, local restrictions on the use of radioisotopes and the availability of a skilled surgical team.

Standard practice in Europe has been to favour antithyroid medication in patients under 40 years of age, with surgery reserved for patients who relapse.[57] In contrast, radioiodine therapy is not restricted to use in older patients within the USA and antithyroid drug regimens are consequently not commonplace. Radioiodine is considered first-line therapy in Graves' disease and toxic multinodular goitres yet its use, which is commonly associated with hypothyroidism, is not without controversy.[2, 32]

A long-term increase in all-cause and vascular mortality after treatment of hyperthyroidism with radioiodine has for instance been described, though this is probably due to an underlying diagnosis of thyrotoxicosis rather than a consequence of radioiodine therapy itself.[58] Induction of hypothyroidism after radioiodine treatment reduces this risk, perhaps because hypothyroidism is the best marker of reversal of adverse tissue effects. Fears about the development of cancer after radioiodine have not been realized, although Graves' hyperthyroidism itself might be associated with a slight increase in the absolute risk of thyroid cancer.[59–61]

There is consequently a lack of consensus regarding appropriate thyroid hormone replacement in patients rendered hypothyroid by radioiodine, and some evidence to suggest that antithyroid drugs may be safely used longer term for the management of relapsing and remitting hyperthyroidism.

PHARMACOLOGICAL MANAGEMENT

The thionamides (carbimazole, its active metabolite methimazole [not available in the UK] and propylthiouracil) are the most effective antithyroid drugs and represent the mainstay of drug treatment of thyrotoxicosis.[57]

TABLE 61.5 Specific indications, advantages and disadvantages of treatment modalities used in the management of thyrotoxicosis

	Treatment modality		
	Antithyroid drugs	Radioactive iodine	Surgery
Indications			
Graves' disease	✓	✓	✓
Toxic nodular hyperthyroidism		✓	✓
Pregnancy	✓		✓
Children	✓		✓
Significant ophthalmopathy	✓		✓
Advantages			
Definitive treatment		✓	✓
Non-invasive	✓	✓	
Outpatient therapy	✓	✓	
Low cost	✓	✓	
No exposure to radiation	✓		✓
Low risk of hypothyroidism	✓		
Relief of compressive symptoms		✓	✓
Histological diagnosis			✓
Disadvantages			
Permanent hypothyroidism		✓	✓
Worsening ophthalmopathy		✓	
Frequent follow-up	✓	✓	
Invasive			✓
Expensive			✓
Specifics	Low cure rates	Slow cure	Risk of hypocalcaemia
		Radiation thyroiditis risk	Scar
		Need to defer pregnancy	Surgical complications
		Radiation protection required	

They act by blocking the synthesis of T4 and T3 early in their biosynthetic pathway by disrupting the organification and oxidation of iodide through inhibition of the thyroperoxidase enzyme. Propylthiouracil (PTU) additionally acts to inhibit the conversion of T4 to T3 but this is not thought to be of clinical relevance. Thionamides have also been associated with a possible immunomodulatory effect, although this is of doubtful clinical significance given that most patients relapse following drug withdrawal.[62] Carbimazole can be dosed as a once-daily preparation in order to improve compliance and results in fewer adverse effects than propylthiouracil.[63] It is therefore generally given in preference, with propylthiouracil reserved for use in pregnancy, women attempting to conceive or patients who have developed an adverse reaction (other than agranulocytosis) to carbimazole or methimazole.[64]

Dosage

All patients with hyperthyroidism require specialist referral and patients should be commenced on antithyroid drug treatment while they await further clinical review.[65] Carbimazole is available as 5 mg and 20 mg tablets and is usually given in a starting dose of 20–30 mg per day in a single dose. Treatment should usually begin at 30 mg in cases of severe disease (fT3 and fT4 levels more than twice the upper limit of the normal reference range). Propylthiouracil is given in divided doses, with a dose of 200 mg approximately equivalent to 20 mg carbimazole. Patients begin to feel an improvement at 10–14 days and fT4 and fT3 values return to normal levels over 4–6 weeks.

Side effects

Side effects are seen in 1–5% of patients taking thionamides and can occur with both carbimazole and PTU (**Table 61.6**). The most common side effect is pruritic rash, which can usually be managed conservatively. Occasionally, the rash necessitates a change from one drug to the other and cross-reactivity in this context is not typically a problem. Other relatively minor side effects include fever, urticaria and arthralgia.[57,66]

TABLE 61.6 Side effects of thionamides	
Severity	Side effects
Mild	Pruritic rash
	Fever
	Urticaria
	Arthralgia
Serious	ANCA-associated vasculitis
	Hepatitis
	Liver failure
	Agranulocytosis
A fever and sore throat in a patient taking thionamides requires measurement of full blood count.	

More serious side effects are rare and include development of an antineutrophil cytoplasmic antibody (ANCA)-associated vasculitis (typically associated with PTU) and hepatitis.[67, 68] Agranulocytosis is a serious side effect and occurs in 0.2–0.5% of patients.[67] This typically occurs in the first few weeks of treatment but may occur at any point during antithyroid drug therapy since it is an idiosyncratic reaction. It is more common in patients taking high doses. For this reason it is essential that all patients are warned (preferably in writing) of the risk of agranulocytosis and that clear instructions are given to present urgently for a full blood count if they develop a fever or sore throat. The agranulocytosis is usually transient and resolves after thionamide withdrawal.

PTU can also result in fulminant hepatic failure, which can necessitate liver transplantation or lead to death. PTU-related acute liver failure occurs in an estimated 1 in 10 000 adults, although it is more commonly seen in children.[69] The US Food and Drug Administration has consequently issued a warning relating to the use of PTU, and its first-line use in adults and children is now not recommended unless the patient is in the first trimester of pregnancy, if side effects are reported with carbimazole or methimazole therapy, if radioiodine or surgery is not an option or in some instances of life-threatening thyrotoxicosis.[70]

The development of agranulocytosis, hepatitis or vasculitis is an absolute contraindication to the further use of thionamides.

Graves' disease

In cases of Graves' disease patients may be offered a full course of thionamide therapy in the hope of inducing remission. Treatment should be offered for a period of 12–18 months as shorter courses are associated with higher rates of relapse.[71, 72] Treatment duration is agreed with the patient at the outset, but at any point medication may be stopped if definitive therapy is preferred. Serum fT4 should be measured regularly, ideally every 4–6 weeks initially, then 8–12 weekly once control is achieved. Drug doses are titrated according to the serum concentration of fT4. Serum TSH may remain suppressed in the medium to long term in patients with Graves' disease due to delayed recovery of thyrotrophs. Most patients require a maintenance dose of 5–10 mg carbimazole and 50–100 mg PTU. Poor compliance should be suspected if larger doses are required.

Treatment efficacy

Remission rates with this regimen are less than 50%, but they may be higher in the elderly.[55–73] Relapse usually occurs within 3–6 months of thionamide withdrawal, in which case patients should be offered definitive treatment. Efforts to risk-stratify patients for their likelihood of relapse using markers such as goitre size, thyroid suppressibility, HLA status, the presence of TSH-receptor antibody and TSH response to thyrotropin-releasing hormone have been unsuccessful.

On a population basis, increased likelihood of remission is most strongly associated with age and sex.[73] Remission occurs in approximately 20% of men, compared to 40% of women, in addition to 33% of those less than 40 years of age compared to 48% of those aged over 40. A small goitre or one that shrinks during therapy also appears related to an increased risk of remission.[74] Once remission is achieved, cure is likely if the patient remains euthyroid for 6 months, although a slowly increasing proportion relapses with length of time of follow-up. Ninety per cent of relapses occur within 3 years. Table 61.7 summarizes poor prognostic factors for relapse of medically treated Graves' disease.

Block and replace

Although most clinicians use thionamides alone to treat Graves' disease, some prefer the 'block and replace' regimen. This uses thionamides to block endogenous hormone production completely with hypothyroidism avoided in the long term by supplementing with exogenous thyroxine. The dose of thyroxine is then adjusted to maintain serum TSH within the lower reference range. Advocates of this regime suggest that it requires less monitoring and leads to better compliance. Remission rates are not, however, improved by standard block and replace therapy and there is no substantial evidence for any advantage of this regime.[75, 76] There is clear evidence of increased adverse effects, some of which are serious and are related to the higher doses of thionamides required.[75] This regimen is also contraindicated in pregnancy because thionamides cross the placenta more easily than T4, leading to the potential for foetal goitre and hypothyroidism.

Toxic multinodular goitre and toxic adenoma

Thionamides may be used in the short term in order to induce euthyroidism in patients with nodular disease but do not lead to remission or cure of thyrotoxicosis in

TABLE 61.7 Poor prognostic factors for relapse of medically treated Graves' disease	
Factor type	Prognostic factor
Demographic	Male gender
	Age < 40 years
Clinical history	Repeated episodes of relapse
	Presence of a large goitre
Biochemical	Severe biochemical disease
	Greatly increased T3:T4 ratio
	High levels of TSH receptor antibodies

this context. Definitive treatment with radioiodine or surgery is therefore required. As the thyrotoxicosis is usually biochemically less severe than Graves' disease, the starting dose of thionamides may be smaller. If surgery or radioiodine is not appropriate, thionamides can be continued indefinitely.

Adjuncts to antithyroid drugs

Beta-adrenergic blockers are useful adjuncts to thionamides in the management of thyroid hormone excess. They act promptly to reduce symptoms such as tremor, palpitations and tachycardia. Their use is cautioned in the elderly where heart failure may be present. The most commonly used beta-adrenergic blocker is propranolol. Thyrotoxicosis may result in accelerated clearance of propanolol and higher doses of this drug may therefore be required.

Patients who develop AF are at risk of embolic complications. Anticoagulation with warfarin or a novel oral anticoagulant (NOAC) such as rivaroxaban or apixaban should therefore be considered, in accordance with the patient's CHA_2DS_2-VASc score and the specific licence of the NOAC. There have been no controlled trials of the use of anticoagulants in thyrotoxic AF but overwhelming evidence for their efficacy in other settings argues in favour of their use for as long as there are not clear contraindications. There is also no evidence for or against the preferential use of NOACs in this context. Approximately half of those with thyrotoxic AF will revert spontaneously to sinus rhythm and this typically occurs within 3 months of the initiation of antithyroid therapy. For those who remain in AF, joint cardiological management involving specific therapy to restore sinus rhythm may be considered when the patient is euthyroid. Chemical or electrical cardioversion is more likely to restore sinus rhythm in those whose AF is of short duration and in those who have no underlying heart disease.[77]

RADIOIODINE

Radioiodine is increasingly used both as first-line therapy in Graves' disease, for toxic multinodular goitre and in patients with Graves' disease for whom initial treatment with a course of thionamides has failed (Box 61.5).[32] It may also be used to induce shrinkage of benign goitres and in the management of autonomous thyroid nodules.[2] Permanent hypothyroidism results in most patients treated with radioiodine, though this may occur many years later. The incidence of hypothyroidism is dose-dependent.[78]

Administration

Radioiodine is administered orally as sodium ^{131}I in capsule form and can be given in the outpatient department. It is incorporated into thyroid tissue and acts principally through the emission of beta rays with a range of 0.5–2 mm. These penetrate into tissue and result in high absorbed doses of radiation within thyroid tissue while sparing the surrounding anatomy. Lasting thyroid tissue damage results but usually lags with maximum thyroid ablation occurring over 6 weeks to 4 months. Scintigraphic imaging may be employed following the administration of radioiodine as a result of emitted gamma rays in order to determine its distribution within thyroid tissue and to support dosimetry.

BOX 61.5 Radioiodine treatment

Used in toxic multinodular goitres and Graves' disease
Administered orally as a sodium ^{131}I capsule
Thyroid tissue damage results from emission of beta rays
Pre-treatment with thionamides and symptomatic relief usually required
Side effects include radiation thyroiditis and exacerbation of ophthalmopathy
Long-term safety is proven but hypothyroidism is common
Contraindicated in pregnancy, women who are breastfeeding and children

---

There is no national consensus regarding the most appropriate dose of radioiodine. The Royal College of Physicians of London recommend that the dose used should be enough to achieve euthyroidism with an acceptable risk of the subsequent development of hypothyroidism. Most centres will administer a fixed dose of 400–600 MBq, which is large enough to induce cure in the majority of patients.[79] Some centres give larger doses to men and those with large goitres in whom it is suggested that relative radioiodine resistance may be found. Larger doses may be preferable in the elderly, especially those with concomitant heart disease, to be certain of rapid resolution of hyperthyroidism.[80]

Many investigators have attempted to determine a method for calculating a radioiodine dose sufficient to cure hyperthyroidism without resulting in hypothyroidism. Postulated methods have involved assessment of the target volume mass, calculations of likely isotope uptake and assessment of isotope turnover.[81] These have not, however, been supported by prospective studies and it has been shown that the use of a calculated dose carries no advantages over a fixed dose in terms of outcome, but results in extra cost and inconvenience for the patient as a consequence of the planning required.

National radiation protection policies exist and include measures to avoid contamination of the home or workplace with radioiodine. They include avoidance of close contact with small children, avoiding sharing utensils and the recommendation to sleep alone.

Pre-treatment with antithyroid medication

Symptom relief may be achieved by beta-adrenergic blocking agents used peritherapeutically in patients undergoing radioiodine administration with coexistent AF. Pre-treatment with thionamides (preferably with carbimazole) should be administered unless the hyperthyroidism is very mild and radioiodine administered once biochemical euthyroidism is restored. This is because it may take 3–4 months for radioiodine to induce euthyroidism whereas thionamides act much more quickly.

There may be a temporary exacerbation of hyperthyroidism as the radiation damage causes follicular destruction and 'dumping' of preformed thyroid hormone into the circulation.[82] Thionamides may therefore be restarted temporarily following radioiodine administration in order to reduce the risk of radiation-related thyroiditis causing an exacerbation of hyperthyroidism, particularly in the elderly and those with cardiac disease.[83]

There is evidence to suggest that use of methimazole and PTU during radioiodine therapy impacts on radioiodine kinetics within the thyroid gland. Whichever thionamide is used, it should thus be discontinued 1 week before radiodiodine administration in order to reduce the risk of negative impacts on therapeutic outcomes.[84, 85] Most clinicians advise restarting thionamides after radioiodine administration, particularly in those with severe disease or who tolerate hyperthyroidism poorly. The antithyroid drug can then be tailed off according to measurements of serum fT4 concentration. In instances in which thionamide therapy is continued during radioiodine administration, success rates are reported to fall from over 90% to under 50%.

Follow-up

In the short term, clinical assessment of the patient should be carried out every 4–6 weeks. In addition to serum TSH, serum fT4 concentration should be measured. Measurement of TSH concentration alone may be misleading as it may be suppressed for many months after treatment and does not necessarily imply that relapse is imminent, especially if the patient is clinically euthyroid and the serum T4 concentration is normal. If biochemical hyperthyroidism persists after a 6-month period, it is likely that a second (and rarely a third) dose of radioiodine will be required. Hypothyroidism commonly results in these patients.

All patients who have received radioiodine require long-term biochemical follow-up. Effectively achieved with a computerized recall system, this is essential as the incidence of hypothyroidism is significant many years after treatment with radioiodine and, eventually, up to 90% may become hypothyroid. Annual measurement of serum TSH is appropriate.

Efficacy

Dependent on the administered dose, 50–70% of patients achieve euthyroidism and shrinkage of goitre around 2 months after therapy.[32] Around 15–20% of patients require a second dose 6–12 months after their initial treatment. A small proportion of patients require a third dose. Those treated with low-dose radioiodine, males, those with severe hyperthyroidism and those with a medium to large goitre are less likely to be cured after a single dose of radioiodine.[86]

Side effects and safety

Many patients are concerned about the concept of radiation treatment and perceive that there may be an increased risk of subsequent cancer. Radioiodine has been used for many years, with well-established efficacy. In terms of cancer, long-term safety has been well demonstrated.[32, 87, 88] The thyroid appears more sensitive to the effects of radiation in children and adolescents. Consequently, most paediatricians would avoid radioiodine in these cases.

Patients who have received radioiodine therapy may notice a sore throat or neck tenderness. This reflects radiation thyroiditis and is thought to occur in around 1% of cases. Symptoms are usually mild and transient. As a result of thyroid ablation, the main side effect of radioiodine treatment is hypothyroidism, although the percentage of patients who develop this during the first year varies according to the dose of radioiodine used. The risk of hypothyroidism with a dose of 600 MBq is around 60%. After the first year, the annual incidence is around 2–3% and seems to be dose-independent.

Radioiodine may worsen moderate to severe ophthalmopathy, particularly in smokers.[31, 89] Adjunctive administration of corticosteroids may ameliorate or even prevent the development of ophthalmopathy.[22] Most physicians delay administration of radioiodine until moderate or severe eye disease has been stable for 12 months. Those with mild eye disease are given radioiodine alongside a course of steroid prophylaxis.[22]

Contraindications

Pregnancy is an absolute contraindication to the use of radioiodine due to the risk of ablating foetal thyroid tissue. A pregnancy test is therefore necessary prior to administration of radioiodine and effective contraception required for 4–6 months after treatment in order to allow for resolution of the effects of transient gonadal radiation. Inadvertent pregnancies require close monitoring, although there is little evidence to suggest that birth defects are increased as a result of exposure to radioiodine during pregnancy. Exposure in early pregnancy is nevertheless associated with a theoretical potential late cancer risk due to foetal irradiation, and exposure after 14 weeks may result in thyroid ablation.

Radioiodine is also contraindicated in women who are lactating, in young children because of fears of increased risk of developing subsequent thyroid carcinoma, and in those who are unable to understand or comply with local radiation protection measures.

Use of radioiodine is associated with worsening of Graves' ophthalmopathy and its use is therefore relatively contraindicated in this group.[90] Radioiodine should not be used in patients with active thyroid eye disease, whereas steroid prophylaxis is recommended for patients with clinically apparent but stable eye disease.[91] Prophylactic steroid treatment is otherwise not recommended for patients who do not have evidence of thyroid eye disease because of the low absolute risk of developing eye disease after receiving radioiodine.[92] Routine steroid prophylaxis has, however, been recommended by consensus statement for smokers given radioiodine treatment, even in the absence of established eye disease, in light of this group's increased risk of complications with radioiodine.[93]

Specific applications of radioiodine

Graves' disease

Radioiodine is increasingly regarded as the treatment of choice in Graves' disease. In certain groups of patients, such as young women or those with mild disease, a course of thionamide therapy may be appropriate in an attempt to induce remission. However, in general radioiodine is considered first line, especially in those whom antithyroid medication is unlikely to result in a cure, such as young men.

Some clinicians target the therapeutic ideal of euthyroidism in patients with Graves' disease by using low-dose radioiodine. There are, however, a number of problems with this approach. Firstly, Graves' may recur in the thyroid remnant, resulting in recurrent hyperthyroidism. This uncontrolled hyperthyroidism results in a permanent reduction in bone density. Secondly, subclinical hyperthyroidism is a risk factor for AF. Many clinicians give radioiodine in a dose large enough to attain euthyroidism in the majority and to avoid recurrence, with a consequent greater risk of hypothyroidism. A dose of 4–600 MBq results in euthyroidism in 90% of cases but at the expense of around 70% hypothyroidism over 20 years.

Nodular thyroid disease

Radioiodine is an effective and definitive treatment option in toxic nodular thyroid disease. It can be used as first-line treatment in those who have mild biochemical hyperthyroidism and who tolerate it well. In the elderly, pre-treatment with a thionamide is necessary to rapidly relieve hyperthyroidism prior to administration of radioiodine.

Radioiodine is effective in achieving euthyroidism and, in those with autonomously functioning nodules, hypothyroidism is less common. The autonomously functioning nodule causes TSH suppression, which, in turn, suppresses surrounding thyroid tissue so that radioiodine is then preferentially taken up into the nodule with sparing of the rest of the gland. Radioiodine may also cause shrinking of nodular goitres with a reduction in thyroid size of 45% after 2 years.

Although around 90% are cured, those with large goitres or with severe hyperthyroidism may not achieve a cure with a single dose of radioiodine and a subsequent dose may be necessary after 6 months' treatment with antithyroid medication.

SURGERY

Although most experts agree that surgery has little part to play in the routine management of thyrotoxicosis, there are instances where partial or subtotal thyroidectomy may be regarded to be a safe and effective treatment for thyroid overactivity.

Indications for surgery

Indications for surgery are summarized within **Table 61.8** and include patient preference, the presence of a cosmetically unacceptable goitre, severe ophthalmopathy, uncontrolled disease, poor response to antithyroid drugs and presence of a coexisting potentially malignant lesion.

TABLE 61.8 Indications for surgery

Indication	Notes
Patient factors	
Patient fear/rejection of radioiodine	
Radioiodine contraindicated	Pregnancy, breastfeeding mothers
Pregnancy with side effect to thionamides	
Pregnancy with severe uncontrolled disease	Radioiodine contraindicated
Clinical features	
Additional non-functioning nodule	If carcinoma cannot be excluded
Cosmetically unacceptable goitre	Radioiodine causes only slow shrinkage of goitre
Severe uncontrolled ophthalmopathy	Radioiodine may worsen ophthalmopathy
Local compressive symptoms	

Preparation

Thyroid surgery may result in the liberation of preformed thyroid hormone, which can lead to 'thyroid storm'. This rare, potentially life-threatening condition carries a mortality of up to 50% and is described in **Table 61.9**. Thorough preparation is required in order to avoid post-operative thyroid storm and significant cardiovascular complications.

Antithyroid drugs are routinely used prior to operative intervention in order to restore euthyroidism. Pre-operative beta-adrenergic blockade may be required if euthyroidism has not been effectively achieved prior to surgery or if a patient is unable to take antithyroid medication due to serious side effects. Use of beta-adrenergic blockers may confer additional technical advantages for the surgeon by decreasing gland vascularity.

Lugol's iodine had traditionally been used in patients awaiting surgery in an effort to reduce iodide uptake and therefore inhibit thyroid hormone release, as well as reducing the vascularity of the thyroid gland. It is now avoided due both to the unpredictable response to its administration and to its potential for exacerbating, rather than improving, thyrotoxicosis.

Complications

Complications of thyroidectomy are relatively unusual, as there is universal agreement that those who perform such surgery should be experienced and perform it frequently.[94, 95] In order of importance, potential complications include bleeding, recurrent laryngeal nerve injury, hypocalcaemia secondary to parathyroid hypofunction or hungry bone disease, infection, thyroid storm, keloid formation and seroma (**Box 61.6**).

Bleeding into the operative site may result in airway compromise due to the development of a haematoma. Immediate clot evacuation and ligation of bleeding vessels

TABLE 61.9 Features and management of extremes of thyroid dysfunction, myxoedema coma and thyroid storm

	Predisposing factors	Features/signs	Treatment General measures	Specific measures
Myxoedema coma	Occurs in elderly patients with hypothyroidism who: • have withdrawn thyroxine • have a severe concomitant illness • are inactive, immobile or live in unheated accommodation	Coma Hypothermia Bradycardia Hyponatraemia Hypoglycaemia Hypotension	*Ideally HDU/ITU* Treat precipitating illness with antibiotics if necessary Slow rewarming (0.5 °C/h) Warm humidified oxygen or ventilation if necessary Monitor and treat arrhythmias Correct hypotension and electrolyte imbalance	T4 300–500 µg via NG tube, then 50–100 µg daily If no improvement T3 10 µg i.v. 8-hourly or 25 µg orally Hydrocortisone 50–100 mg 6–8-hourly unless hypocortisolism excluded
Thyroid storm	Develops in hyperthyroid patients with acute infection who: • are postpartum • have undergone thyroid or non-thyroid surgery • reactive iodine containing contrast agents • withdraw antithyroid medication	*Rare but life-threatening condition, significant mortality (up to 50%)* Severe signs of hyperthyroidism Fever/hyperpyrexia Alteration in mental state Tachycardia/tachyarrhythmia Vomiting and diarrhoea Multi-organ failure – cardiac failure, hepatic congestion with hyperbilirubinaemia and jaundice, dehydration and renal failure	*Best carried out in ITU* Cooling, fluid balance, antibiotics, respiratory support if necessary Correction of electrolyte imbalance Standard antiarrhythmic therapy Anticoagulation if in atrial fibrillation Chlorpromazine if agitated	PTU 300 mg 6-hourly via NG tube (PTU blocks T4 to T3 conversion) Potassium iodide 60 mg 6-hourly via NG tube (inhibits thyroid hormone release; start 6 hours after PTU. Propanolol 160–180 mg in divided doses or by infusion to block adrenergic manifestations Prednisolone 60 mg o.d. may also stop T4 to T3 conversion Plasmapheresis may be necessary in refractory cases

BOX 61.6 Complications of surgical thyroid resection

- Bleeding
- Recurrent laryngeal nerve injury
- Hypocalcaemia
- Infection
- Thyroid storm
- Keloid formation
- Seroma

is therefore required. Damage to the recurrent laryngeal nerve is also possible and vocal cords should be checked prior to surgery. Unilateral damage causing some hoarseness usually improves after a few weeks. Bilateral damage is rare but serious, as stridor develops soon after extubation. The ensuing airway obstruction necessitates a tracheostomy.

Damage to the parathyroid glands can occur and may be transient. It can follow a direct insult or an interruption of blood flow to the glands. The frequency and severity of damage increases with the extent of thyroid surgery and also correlates with the incidence of post-operative hypothyroidism. Transient hypocalcaemia may be seen post-operatively and the patient may be symptomatic with signs of neuromuscular excitability such as Chvostek's sign, Trousseau's sign and carpopedal spasm. Hypocalcaemia typically occurs 1–7 days post-surgery and repeated measurement of serum calcium concentration during this period is therefore mandatory, as is close clinical monitoring of the patient for relevant signs. Mild hypoparathyroidism is managed with oral calcium supplementation but more severe cases require intravenous calcium gluconate.

Effective pre-operative preparation means thyroid storm is now exceedingly rare. It should be managed in the intensive care setting with oxygen, cooling, sedation, PTU and the use of intravenous beta-adrenergic blockers and steroids. Aspirin may exacerbate the condition by causing an increase in free thyroid hormone levels and should be avoided.

Thyroid function in the post-operative setting

The relative degree of thyroid function following thyroidectomy depends on the volume of the thyroid remnant preserved. Thyroid function in the immediate post-operative period should include measurement of fT3, fT4 and TSH. Approximately 20% of patients who are initially hypothyroid will be euthyroid within 3–6 months of surgery. Permanent hypothyroidism tends to become apparent in the first 2 years after surgery. The rate of post-operative hypothyroidism is reported to be in the range of 2–48%, with recurrent hyperthyroidism seen in 0–15% of patients. Measurement of fT3 and fT4 may be necessary in patients who have been managed for post-operative hypothyroidism because their clinical state may not be accurately reflected by serum TSH.

Specific applications of surgery

Graves' disease
In most large centres the surgical treatment of choice in Graves' disease is a total thyroidectomy. In expert hands the recurrence rate with this procedure is less than 4% but at the expense of hypothyroidism, such that patients leave hospital taking levothyroxine therapy.

Nodular thyroid disease
Toxic nodular hyperthyroidism may be treated by thyroid lobectomy or excision of a single hot nodule. The adenomas are often easy to excise and there is very little risk of either recurrence or post-operative hypothyroidism. For patients with a toxic MNG, surgery is appropriate for those with compressive symptoms, such as dysphagia and upper airway obstruction, and for those with a cosmetically unacceptable goitre. Radioiodine may cause shrinkage of the gland and may be preferable in the high-risk patient, although the rate of shrinkage is relatively slow.

> **KEY POINTS**
>
> **THYROTOXICOSIS**
>
> *Clinical features*
> - Classical symptoms may not be present in the elderly.
>
> *Investigations*
> - Measure fT4, TSH and thyroid autoantibodies in suspected hyperthyroidism. fT3 and ESR may be useful.
> - Ultrasound and nuclear medicine scans should be reserved for specialist use.
> - Hyperthyroidism due to thyroiditis is often self-limiting. Treat with NSAIDs +/− beta blockers.
>
> *Treatment*
> - Initial management should consist of antithyroid drugs +/− beta blockers and endocrine referral.
> - Thionamides: warn patients of side effects. 'Block and replace' or titration regimes may be used.
> - Radioiodine: safe and effective. This is the first-line treatment in the elderly and those with cardiac dysfunction.
> - Surgery: used in toxic multinodular goitre, compressive symptoms, Graves' disease, eye disease.

Subclinical hyperthyroidism

Subclinical hyperthyroidism is essentially a biochemical diagnosis, though it is increasingly associated with a number of potential complications. Its detection relies on sensitive assays of TSH and it is therefore only in recent years that our understanding of this condition has widened.

AETIOLOGY

The biochemical finding of low TSH with normal fT4 and fT3 may result from an exogenous source, as a consequence of treatment with thyroxine or a raft of other drugs, or from an endogenous pathology. These include nodular thyroid disease, undetected early Graves' disease or non-thyroidal illness. Exogenous subclinical hyperthyroidism is by the far the largest group with over 20% of patients taking thyroxine having low TSH values on at least one occasion.[8, 96]

COMPLICATIONS

Long-term survival appears to be affected by suppressed TSH, contributing to an increased mortality due to cardiovascular causes.[97] The transience of TSH reduction in patients with illness or drug therapy suggests that for these individuals subclinical hyperthyroidism is likely to be of little consequence. Potential complications of subclinical hyperthyroidism are therefore likely confined to those in whom TSH suppression reflects a minor degree of thyroid hormone excess.

A specific complication associated with subclinical hyperthyroidism is that of AF, with those aged over 60 years who have an undetectable TSH harbouring a threefold increase in relative risk.[98] Subclinical disease is also associated with reductions in bone mineral density and increased fracture risk, especially in postmenopausal women.[99, 100]

MANAGEMENT

The management of subclinical hyperthyroidism remains both complex and controversial. The prevailing consensus is that in those with persistent TSH suppression and evidence for underlying thyroid disease antithyroid treatment is warranted, particularly if the subclinical hyperthyroidism is associated with cardiac disease or AF.[101, 102] As these patients are usually elderly, radioiodine is the treatment of choice unless contraindications exist. There does, however, remain a paucity of evidence for a beneficial effect of this therapy in this setting and the results of relevant randomized controlled trials are awaited.

Practically, it is prudent to repeat TFTs on a 6-monthly basis in those who have endogenous subclinical hyperthyroidism where AF and osteoporosis may have been exacerbated by excess thyroid hormone treatment.[102]

> **KEY POINTS**
>
> **SUBCLINICAL HYPERTHYROIDISM**
>
> *Aetiology*
> - Some causes are related to thyroid disease and its management: thyroxine therapy, previous Graves' hyperthyroidism, Graves' ophthalmopathy, nodular goitre.
> - Other causes relate to non-thyroidal illness: any significant illness, therapy with drugs such as glucocorticoids, iodine-containing compounds, pregnancy.
>
> *Investigations*
> - Findings show low TSH with normal fT4 and fT3.
>
> *Complications*
> - AF
> - Osteoporosis
>
> *Management*
> - Antithyroid treatment may be warranted

Thyrotoxicosis in the absence of hyperthyroidism

Perhaps confusingly, thyrotoxicosis may present in the absence of hyperthyroidism. In these instances thyrotoxicosis results from thyroid hormone excess originating either from the thyroid gland as a consequence of a destructive lesion or from a source outside the thyroid. The absence of hyperthyroidism refers to thyrotoxicosis occurring despite there being no increased synthesis of thyroid hormones in the thyroid gland. Consequently, a low uptake of radioiodine is seen on scintigraphy.

DESTRUCTIVE THYROIDITIS

Thyroiditis refers to any inflammatory condition of the thyroid. It may be associated with transient thyrotoxicosis during its acute phase as a consequence of disruption to the normal architecture of the thyroid gland, which results in the release of T4 and T3 from the colloid.

Classification of thyroiditis

The classification of thyroiditis is confusing but may be divided into those processes in which pain and tenderness develop, and those that do not have pain as a predominant feature (**Table 61.10**). Generally, the former rarely result in permanent hypothyroidism but the latter often do. Subacute, painless and postpartum thyroiditis are generally associated with only mild thyrotoxicosis which lasts only a few weeks as a consequence of the restoration of normal thyroid architecture.

Subacute granulomatous/De Quervain's thryoiditis

Clinical features

De Quervain's, giant cell or subacute thyroiditis is an uncommon cause of transient thyrotoxicosis. The typical patient is female and aged between 40 and 60 years.[103] Presentation is with pain in the region of the thyroid, often (but not always) associated with swelling. This is associated with systemic symptoms such as fever, dysphagia and malaise. The pain is a striking feature, may radiate to the ear and is worse on turning the head. On examination there is often swelling of either thyroid lobe, which may be extremely painful to palpate. Signs of thyrotoxicosis may be present, such as tachycardia, tremor and irritability. There may also be fever. It can take 8 weeks for pain to resolve and a complete resolution is seen in 6 months.

Investigations

Laboratory tests show raised inflammatory markers, such as erythrocyte sedimentation rate (ESR) and C-reactive protein (CRP), and there may be a normocytic normochromic anaemia.[104] Thyroid scintigraphy with ^{99m}Tc or $^{121/131}$I shows a complete absence of uptake, although this can also occur with thyrotoxicosis factitia and iodine-induced hyperthyroidism. Histology is characteristic and lends the condition its name, with multinucleate giant cells surrounding a central core of colloid. Initial TFTs show thyrotoxicosis with a suppressed TSH and an elevated serum fT4. This reflects destruction of the thyroid follicles by the inflammatory process and release of pre-formed thyroid hormone.

Clinical course

At 12–16 weeks there may be a hypothyroid phase during which the damaged tissue is unable to generate thyroid hormone. Most patients do not require treatment with thyroxine and most are ultimately euthyroid. Rarely, hypothyroidism may be permanent. Initially, thyroid autoantibodies may be positive but again this is often transient although some retain thyroid autoimmunity for life. The course of subacute thyroiditis is shown in **Figure 61.7**.

Management

Treatment is supportive. Non-steroidal anti-inflammatory drugs such as aspirin and indomethacin are effective analgesics, while beta-adrenergic blockers are useful if symptomatic in the thyrotoxic phase. Rarely, the severity may necessitate high-dose oral corticosteroids

TABLE 61.10 Classification of thyroiditis		
Pain and tenderness	Diagnosis	Subcategories
Yes	Subacute granulomatous thyroiditis	De Quervain's Giant cell thyroiditis
	Infectious thyroiditis	
	Radioiodine-induced thyroiditis	
No	Subacute lymphocytic thyroiditis (silent)	Postpartum thyroiditis Drug-induced thyroiditis
	Chronic lymphocytic thyroiditis	Hashimoto's thyroiditis Postpartum thyroiditis
	Fibrous thyroiditis (Riedel's thyroiditis)	
	Amiodarone-induced thyroiditis	

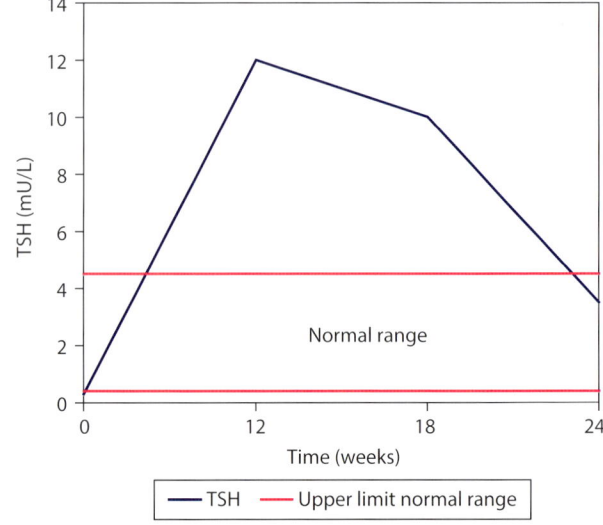

Figure 61.7 Typical course of subacute thyroiditis.

(e.g. prednisolone 30–40 mg daily) which are extremely effective in reducing the pain and swelling but must be withdrawn slowly over some months if the condition is not to recur.[105]

Aetiology

The female preponderance, seasonal incidence, geographical aggregation and raised inflammatory markers have led to a hypothesis of a viral aetiology.[106] Mumps virus, Coxsackie, influenza and adenoviruses have been implicated in the development of the disease although a viral role in the pathogenesis remains obscure.

Silent/painless thyroiditis

Painless thyroiditis can occur in the early stages of autoimmune thyroiditis. This may lead to mild biochemical hyperthyroidism and occasionally to symptomatic thyrotoxicosis. The thyrotoxicosis is generally mild and raised markers of inflammation are rarely found, in contrast to subacute thyroiditis. The thyroid is enlarged in approximately half of all patients and is not painful. Fine-needle aspirate reveals the changes associated with Hashimoto's disease and includes extensive lymphocytic infiltrate with plasma cells rather than multinucleate giant cells. Thyroid autoantibodies are often positive.

The duration of the thyrotoxic phase is around 8 weeks and symptomatic treatment with beta-adrenergic blockers may be required. There then follows a hypothyroid phase that can last for more than 6 months. In most patients, euthyroidism is eventually restored but permanent hypothyroidism is almost certain to develop over time.

Radiation-induced thyroiditis

Administration of large doses of radioiodine may result within 2 weeks in thyroiditis. There is usually a requirement only for simple analgesia and this condition tends to self-resolve within 2 weeks of its onset. Significant pain or swelling may necessitate the use of oral glucocorticoid therapy.

Iodine-induced thyrotoxicosis

Iodide-induced thyrotoxicosis (IIT) results from genetic change that leads to autonomous thyroid hormone production within sufficient numbers of thyrocytes to cause hyperthyroidism in the presence of an increased supply of iodine. This 'Jod Basedow' effect is often seen in patients with toxic MNGs in areas of iodine deficiency. It may also occur in the absence of pre-existing thyroid disease and generally resolves within 6 months. Iodine-containing contrast agents are a common source of excess iodine and confer a 0.3% risk of IIT within iodine-deficient areas.[107]

Amiodarone-induced thyrotoxicosis

Use of amiodarone may result in thyrotoxicosis by one of two ways. In patients with pre-existing thyroid disease, the high iodine content of amiodarone may induce thyrotoxicosis.[108] This is termed amiodarone-induced thyrotoxicosis (AIT) type 1. AIT type 2 arises when a destructive thyroiditis occurs as a consequence of the cytotoxic effect of amiodarone and its metabolite, desethylamiodarone. AIT is prevalent in iodine-deficient areas whereas in areas which are iodine-replete, amiodarone-induced hypothyroidism (AIH) predominates.

Withdrawal of amiodarone may result in an improvement for patients with both AIT type 1 and AIT type 2. Oral corticosteroid therapy may restore euthyroidism in those with AIT type 2 while thionamides are effective in AIT type 1. Antithyroid drugs may be given with potassium perchlorate, which inhibits thyroidal iodide uptake and consequently increases sensitivity to thionamide action.

HYPOTHYROIDISM

Definitions

Hypothyroidism refers to the insufficient production and secretion of thyroid hormones from the thyroid gland. It may occur due to a disturbance within the thyroid gland itself (**primary hypothyroidism**) or within the hypothalamic–pituitary–thyroid axis (**secondary hypothyroidism**).[109] The term **myxoedema** is not synonymous with hypothyroidism and refers to the accumulation of glycosaminoglycans occurring in severe hypothyroidism. These hydrophilic substances are deposited within the dermis, leading to induration of the skin and the characteristic facial features of hypothyroidism. The term **hypothyroxinaemia** may be used to refer to low serum fT4 concentrations in the presence of normal levels of TSH (**Box 61.7**).

BOX 61.7 Key definitions in thyroid hormone deficiency (hypothyroidism)

Hypothyroidism	Insufficient production and secretion of thyroid hormone
Primary hypothyroidism	Pathology of the thyroid gland itself
Secondary hypothyroidism	Pathology of the hypothalamic–pituitary–thyroid axis
Myxoedema	Accumulation of glycosaminoglycans in the dermis
Hypothyroxinaemia	Low serum fT4 concentrations in the presence of normal TSH concentrations

---

Epidemiology

Like hyperthyroidism and other autoimmune conditions, hypothyroidism is more common in women, amongst whom its prevalence is estimated at 2%.[1] This compares to 0.2% of men.[1] Incidence peaks in the 40–50 years age group so that prevalence in women aged over 65 rises to 5–10%.[97] Juvenile hypothyroidism is nevertheless not uncommon. Neonatal hypothyroidism, which if untreated results in severe intellectual impairment, occurs in around 1 in 4000 births and is routinely screened for in the postnatal period in the UK.[110]

Aetiology

The causes of hypothyroidism are outlined in **Table 61.11**. The most common cause in areas replete with iodine is chronic autoimmune hypothyroidism, otherwise termed Hashimoto's thyroiditis.[111, 112] Hypothyroidism may also be an iatrogenic phenomenon, resulting either from thyroidectomy, use of radioiodine therapy or external beam irradiation of the neck.[32, 112, 113] Worldwide, the most common cause of hypothyroidism is iodine deficiency.[114]

Clinical manifestations

Insufficiency of thyroid hormone affects almost every organ system in the body. The effects of hypothyroidism can be broadly categorized into those relating to the generalized slowing of all metabolic processes and those resulting from the tissue accumulation of glycosaminoglycans, as summarized in **Table 61.12**. Among other features, the slowing of metabolic processes results in fatigue, cold intolerance and weight gain. Characteristic features of hypothyroidism such as coarse dry skin, hair loss and doughy peripheral oedema relate to glycosaminoglycan accumulation. A low threshold for thyroid function testing is necessary, given that few patients have all signs and symptoms of hypothyroidism. There is, however, no consensus for routine screening of thyroid function.

SYMPTOMS

The onset of symptoms may be insidious and go unrecognized, such that severe myxoedema may result. The typical patient complains of lethargy and fatigue, and these complaints, plus the accompanying apathy and listlessness, mean that the ability to work is impaired. There may be a slow increase of weight despite a reduction in appetite and constipation is a common feature. Cold intolerance is typical with the patient wearing multiple layers of clothes at initial consultation.

Menstrual periods may be heavy and a desired conception elusive. Myopathy may cause difficulty in walking upstairs or rising from a chair, and numbness and paraesthesia in the hands may develop as carpal tunnel syndrome results from peripheral oedema. Occasionally, neuropsychiatric complications may result and 'myxoedema madness', though now largely confined to historical literature, was previously described.

SIGNS

There may be a husky voice incorrectly attributed to laryngitis but which actually results from oedema of the vocal cords. Women may complain of dry coarse hair and brittle nails. Peripheral and facial oedema is also seen, as is bradycardia, the presence of a goitre and slow-relaxing tendon reflexes. The rare but life-threatening condition of

TABLE 61.11 Causes of hypothyroidism

Primary			Secondary	
Associated with goitre (TSH raised, T4 low)	Not associated with goitre (TSH raised, T4 low)	Self-limiting	Hypothalamic (TSH low, T4 low)	Pituitary (TSH low, T4 low)
Hashimoto's thyroiditis (chronic thyroiditis)	Atrophic thyroiditis	Transient thyroiditis; e.g. subacute or silent	Congenital; e.g. lack of TRSH	Congenital; e.g. lack of TSH
Iodine deficiency (affects 800 million worldwide)	Iatrogenic; e.g. radioiodine, surgery, neck irradiation	Postpartum thyroiditis	Infiltrative; e.g. sarcoidosis, tuberculosis, primary or metastatic malignancy	Panhypopituitarism; e.g. pituitary tumour, cranial irradiation, infection, inflammation
Inherited defects of biosynthesis	Congenital anomaly; e.g. thyroid agenesis	Iatrogenic; e.g. overtreatment with antithyroid medication		
Maternal transmission; e.g. antithyroid agents	Drug-induced; e.g. amiodarone, lithium, iodides, phenylbutazone		Infective; e.g. encephalitis	

TABLE 61.12 Manifestations of hypothyroidism

	Clinical manifestations					
	General	Skin	Gastrointestinal	Cardiovascular	Reproductive	Neurological
Symptoms	Weakness/fatigue	Coarse, dry skin	Decreased appetite	Peripheral oedema	Menorrhagia	Slow/hoarse speech
	Decreased appetite	Pale skin/flush (peaches and cream)	Weight gain		Ovulatory failure	Intellectual impairment
	Weight gain		Constipation		Galactorrhoea	
	Coarse facial features	Loss/drying of hair				Carpal tunnel syndrome
	Cold intolerance					Neuropsychiatric problems
	Peripheral oedema					
Signs	Characteristic facial features	Pale, cool skin		Bradycardia		Slow-relaxing tendon reflexes
	Goitre	Peripheral/facial oedema				Hoarse voice

myxoedema coma can occur in hypothyroidism, particularly in older patients, and can be precipitated by infection, trauma or cold.

Diagnostic evaluation

Thyroid function testing may help support clinical suspicion of hypothyroidism. Low serum fT4 concentration is the hallmark of reduced thyroid function.[115] This is usually associated with a raised TSH concentration, though this may be normal or low in secondary hypothyroidism. Concentrations of fT3 tend to be decreased but may be normal. Microsomal antibodies may be significantly raised in cases of autoimmune hypothyroidism. Other non-specific changes are seen, including a normochromic normocytic anaemia and an atherogenic lipid profile consisting of raised serum levels of cholesterol, triglycerides and low-density lipoprotein (LDL) in addition to lowered high-density lipoprotein (HDL). Reduced negative feedback from thyroid hormones and a consequent excess of thyrotropin-releasing hormone stimulates excess production of prolactin from the anterior pituitary gland so that serum levels may be raised. Laboratory investigations and findings are summarized in **Table 61.13**.

Ultrasound evaluation of the thyroid may provide support in determining the cause of hypothyroidism although should not be performed routinely. Low echogenicity and gross inhomogeneity are seen in autoimmune thyroiditis. Use of colour-flow Doppler may identify greater vascularity in autoimmune thyroiditis than in the atrophic variant of the disease. The identification of nodular tissue should raise suspicion of coexisting adenomas or malignancy.

Specific conditions associated with hypothyroidism

CHRONIC AUTOIMMUNE HYPOTHYROIDISM (HASHIMOTO'S THYROIDITIS)

Seen in 3.5 per 1000 women per year and fewer than 1 per 1000 men per year, this condition is in many respects the archetypal autoimmune disease.[116] In addition to occurring more commonly in females, it runs in families where Graves' disease may feature along with other autoimmune conditions, such as vitiligo, pernicious anaemia, rheumatoid arthritis and type 1 diabetes mellitus.[112] It is more common in older women yet it can occur in infants as young as 2 years of age and it is the major cause of hypothyroidism in children.

The pathogenesis of this condition is well understood.[117] Histology reveals diffuse lymphocytic infiltration of the thyroid gland and the presence of circulating thyroid autoantibodies, reflecting the direct cellular injury induced by cytotoxic T-cells and the role of humoral factors.

Although patients have high circulating antibodies to thyroid microsomes and to thyroglobulin, these are not thought to have functional activity. Histologically, the gland is infiltrated with lymphocytes and areas of follicular destruction and fibrosis may be evident.[117] Enlarged epithelial cells with oxyphilic changes in the cytoplasm and Askenazy cells are commonly found in this condition (**Figure 61.8**).

Initially, the thyroid hypofunction may be subclinical, but it may become overt with a rate of developing hypothyroidism of around 5% per year. A slowly growing goitre may have been found on examination or noted by the patient or a family member.

The typical goitre is moderate in size and smooth. Although both lobes are affected, the gland may appear asymmetrical. The presence of the goitre may predate the development of overt hypothyroidism and, generally, the goitre remains static or may decrease in size. Some patients present without a palpable goitre and are said to have atrophic autoimmune thyroiditis, which is thought to represent the end point of Hashimoto's thyroiditis.[111]

IATROGENIC HYPOTHYROIDISM

This may be seen as a consequence of surgery, treatment with radioactive iodine or external beam radiotherapy, such as that used in the management of head

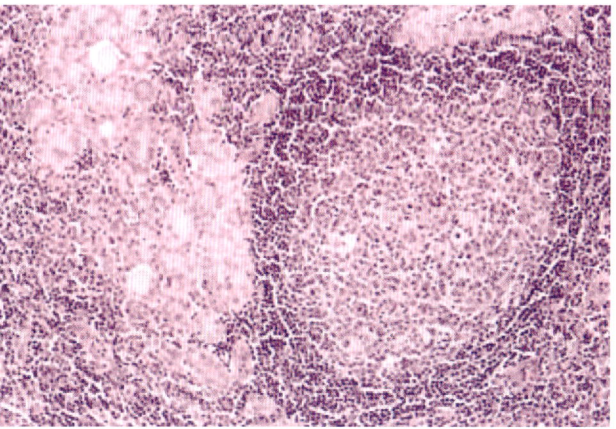

Figure 61.8 Histology of Hashimoto's thyroiditis. There is a dense interstitial lymphocytic infiltrate, with secondary germinal centre formation, enveloping small colloid-depleted follicles. These are lined with plump cuboidal oxyphil (Askanazy or Hürthle) cells possessing characteristic copious pink granular cytoplasm.

TABLE 61.13 Laboratory investigations in suspected hypothyroidism			
		Results in hypothyroidism	
Investigation		Primary	Central
Thyroid function	TSH	↑	↓/↔
	fT4	↓	↓
	fT3	↓/↔	↓/↔
Immunology		Positive thyroid microsomal autoantibodies	
Biochemistry		Raised serum cholesterol, triglycerides, LDL Lowered HDL	
Endocrine		Raised serum prolactin	
Haematology		Normochromic normocytic anaemia	

and neck malignancy. Hypothyroidism may occasionally result from overtreatment of hyperthyroidism with antithyroid medication, but with close monitoring this is not common.

Thyroidectomy

Hypothyroidism would become evident in all patients who have undergone total thyroidectomy at around 2–4 weeks without treatment. Thyroid hormone replacement should therefore be commenced in these patients prior to their discharge from hospital. Subtotal thyroidectomy may also result in hypothyroidism, with most patients becoming so within a year.

Radioiodine therapy

The majority of patients treated with 400–600 MBq of radioiodine will develop hypothyroidism.[18, 113] This may be transient, resulting from radiation thyroiditis some 4–6 weeks after treatment, or permanent. Sustained hypothyroidism may not ensue until months or even years after therapy.

External beam neck irradiation

Radiotherapy given to the neck may result in both hypothyroidism and an increased risk of thyroid malignancy, especially in children and adolescents.[113]

For patients who have had more than 25 Gy there may be a slow-onset dose-dependent development of hypothyroidism. Such patients should be carefully monitored for both the hypothyroidism, which can initially be subclinical, and for nodular thyroid disease which may herald a thyroid malignancy.

Tyrosine kinase inhibitor therapy

Small molecular tyrosine kinase inhibitors (TKIs) are used across a spectrum of disorders and have been associated with thyroid dysfunction.[118, 119] The vascular endothelial growth factor receptor (VEGFR) disruptor sunitinib has, for instance, been linked to both hypothyroidism and thyrotoxicosis. Other TKIs have also been implicated in thyroid dysfunction including Imatinib, which targets the Philadelphia chromosome in chronic myeloid leukaemia, and motesanib, which is used in differentiated thyroid carcinoma.[120]

IODINE DEFICIENCY

Iodine deficiency remains the most common cause of hypothyroidism and goitre worldwide.[43, 114] Iodine is present in the body in only minute amounts and must therefore be sourced from the diet. When iodine requirements are not met, thyroid hormone synthesis is impaired and goitre follows due to increased secretion of TSH, which is released to maximize utilization of available iodine and acts to stimulate the thyroid. Goitres may be present from young adulthood and can become sufficiently large to cause obstructive symptoms. Other iodine deficiency disorders include mental retardation and neonatal cretinism, a combination of intellectual impairment, ataxia, coarse facies and deaf mutism. This has a substantial effect on mental development.[121]

It is estimated that iodine intake is insufficient in 36.5% of school-age children and 35.2% of the general population worldwide. South-east Asia, Africa and the Western Pacific are the most affected by iodine deficiency whereas the addition of iodine to salt in the USA and, to a lesser extent Europe, results in sufficient dietary intake of iodine for the majority of the population. Mild-to-moderate iodine deficiency is nevertheless recognized in the United Kingdom, where salt iodization is not commonplace.[43] Diets high in goitrogens, such as cassava and some soya beans, can exacerbate complications of iodine deficiency.

NEONATAL HYPOTHYROIDISM

This is routinely screened for during the postnatal period in iodine replete regions.[109] It may be caused by inherited defects in thyroid hormone synthesis, transplacental transmission of anti-TSH antibodies causing transient neonatal thyroid underactivity or thyroid gland agenesis and dysgenesis.

CENTRAL HYPOTHYROIDISM

Lack of hypothalamic thyrotropin-releasing hormone or pituitary TSH may lead to hypothyroidism, although central hypothyroidism accounts for less than 1% of all cases of hypothyroidism. The commonest cause is a tumour in the hypothalamic or pituitary region and the surgery or radiotherapy used to treat them.[122] Such central causes may be distinguished from primary hypothyroidism by a normal or low-serum TSH concentration that is inappropriate given a low serum fT3 and fT4 concentration. Approximately a third of patients with central hypothyroidism display marginal elevation of TSH, which is bio-inactive.

Patients with a pituitary adenoma may have other features of hypopituitarism, such as hypogonadism and hypoadrenalism. These may mask the symptoms of thyroid hormone deficiency. Patients with central hypothyroidism should be referred for specialist consultation.

Management of hypothyroidism

Levothyroxine is the drug of choice for the treatment of hypothyroidism.[123, 124] It is absorbed from the upper small bowel with approximately 80% efficiency and is a pro-hormone which is deiodinated in peripheral tissues to the active hormone T3. T3 has a tenfold higher affinity than T4 for thyroid hormone receptors. Treatment is provided with the aim of returning the patient to a euthyroid state both clinically as judged from symptoms, and biochemically as judged from serum TSH estimations.

ADMINISTRATION OF LEVOTHYROXINE

At 7 days, the half-life of levothyroxine is long enough to allow for daily or even weekly dosing if compliance is an issue. The average daily dose is around 125 μg but variation exists and typical doses required to achieve euthyroidism range between 100 µg and 150 µg. In those less than 50 years of age with no evidence of ischaemic heart disease, a moderate dose (1.6 mcg/kg or typically 100 µg) may be started immediately. In older patients, or those with known cardiac disease, a starting dose of 25 µg is prudent due to the risk of exacerbating or precipitating cardiac disease as a consequence of the rise in cardiac output associated with initiation of therapy. Increments of 25 µg can be added every 4–6 weeks until TSH concentrations are within the normal range.

Due to the long half-life of thyroxine, 4–6 weeks should elapse before measuring TSH concentration after initiating therapy or after dose adjustment. Once stable, serum TSH needs to be checked on an annual basis to ensure ongoing compliance.[109]

SPECIFIC CONSIDERATIONS WHEN PRESCRIBING THYROXINE

Central hypothyroidism

In those with central hypothyroidism, it is imperative that hypoadrenalism be excluded before initiating thyroxine therapy. An adrenal crisis may be precipitated if hypoadrenalism is not treated before thyroxine therapy is commenced. In central hypothyroidism, the serum TSH concentration is of no value in monitoring therapy, thus dose adjustments should be made on serum fT4 and fT3 concentrations alone, aiming to keep serum fT4 in the upper half of the reference range.

Elderly patients

Thyroxine therapy should be started at a dose of 25–50 µg daily and increased every 4 weeks until stable. Overtreatment, resulting in a suppressed TSH concentration, should be avoided due to the risk of precipitating AF.

Pregnant women

Women need more thyroid hormone during pregnancy and those with pre-existing hypothyroidism cannot increase T4 and T3 secretion in the same manner as women who do not have hypothyroidism. Hypothyroid women need around 40% more thyroxine in pregnancy and the dosage should be increased upon finding of a positive pregnancy test. Thyroid function tests should be monitored using pregnancy and gestation specific reference ranges preferentially. Repeat measurements should be undertaken 4-weekly during the first trimester and once per trimester thereafter. Most international guidelines recommend treating with levothyroxine to keep serum TSH below 2.5 mIU/L prior to and during pregnancy.[124–126]

T3 THERAPY

A minority of patients feel that their symptoms of hypothyroidism are not controlled on thyroxine therapy despite normal concentrations of TSH and T4. Some choose to take T3 in addition to or instead of thyroxine, although due to its rapid absorption and short half-life it must be taken three times a day and fluctuations in thyroid hormone levels exist. Current national and international guidance does not recommend the use of T3 monotherapy or T3/T4 combination therapy in the management of hypothyroidism based on the lack of evidence supporting these treatment strategies.[127, 128] Similarly, the use of desiccated thyroid extract is not advisable.[129]

> **KEY POINTS**
>
> **HYPOTHYROIDISM**
>
> *Clinical features*
> - Manifestations presented are those of the slowing of metabolic processes and tissue accumulation of glycosaminoglycans.
>
> *Investigations*
> - Low serum T4 and raised TSH is seen in primary hypothyroidism.
> - Low serum T4 with normal or suppressed TSH are seen in central hypothyroidism.
> - A pro-atherogenic lipid profile and a normochromic normocytic anaemia are seen in chronic disease.
>
> *Treatment*
> - Levothyroxine is the drug treatment of choice.
> - A lower starting dose may be required in older patients.
> - There is no evidence to suggest an advantage from T3 therapy.

Subclinical hypothyroidism

Subclinical hypothyroidism is a biochemical diagnosis made where a raised TSH is seen in conjunction with a normal fT4 concentration.

EPIDEMIOLOGY

It is common, affecting 7–8% of women and 2–4% of men. The prevalence rises with age to approximately 15% in women over 60.[130] It is also more common in those with other autoimmune conditions.

AETIOLOGY

Subclinical hypothyroidism may be endogenous or iatrogenic, resulting from either previous radioiodine treatment or surgical resection of the thyroid gland. Around 60% of women with subclinical hypothyroidism have positive antibodies to thyroid peroxidase.[131] Prospective studies have confirmed that those with both positive thyroid autoantibodies and elevated TSH concentrations are at risk of developing overt hypothyroidism at a rate of around 5% per year, although this figure is likely to be greater in older patients.

MANAGEMENT

Given the potential risks to bone and cardiovascular health of overtreatment with thyroxine, there remains controversy as to who should be treated and at what point.

Recent guidelines have highlighted evidence linking raised TSH and cholesterol but otherwise state that data for a clear benefit to treatment are lacking. Many clinicians would opt to treat in the presence of symptoms and serum TSH concentration of greater than 10 mU/L as well as positive antibodies, as a result of the high risk of progression to overt hypothyroidism. For asymptomatic patients with a modestly raised TSH (below 10 mU/L) or with a low or negative titre of microsomal antibodies, retest on a 6-monthly basis is advised.[132]

> **KEY POINTS**
>
> **SUBCLINICAL HYPOTHYROIDISM**
>
> Aetiology
>
> - This is an autoimmune condition.
> - It is iatrogenic: previous radioiodine treatment, surgical resection.
>
> Investigations
>
> - Raised TSH with normal fT4 and fT3 is seen.
>
> Complications
>
> - These are unclear.
> - There is a possible association between raised TSH and cholesterol.
>
> Management
>
> - Best practice is unclear: treat if serum TSH >10 mIU/L or during pregnancy.

THYROID DISEASE IN PREGNANCY

Thyroid dysfunction is relatively common in pregnancy, during which both overt and subclinical disease are associated with adverse outcomes.[125] Foetal development is dependent on maternal thyroid hormone delivered via the transplacental route until around 18 weeks of gestation, although maternal thyroid hormone transfer continues up to delivery. Thyroid hormones are known to influence foetal size and the maturation of tissues, in addition to uteroplacental development. The foetal brain additionally responds to thyroid hormones from 5 weeks of gestation. Euthyroidism is therefore essential throughout pregnancy in order to minimize risk to the foetus.

Physiological changes to the thyroid axis during pregnancy have been extensively described previously.[133] Maternal TSH is seen to decline during the first trimester but resolves to pre-pregnancy levels by the end of gestation. Maternal fT4 concentrations decline throughout pregnancy. Gestation-specific ranges, which are both population- and age-specific, should therefore be used by the clinician caring for a pregnant patient with thyroid disease.

Hyperthyroid states in pregnancy

The immunological changes associated with pregnancy and delivery can affect thyroid status in different ways. Those with pre-existing disease may find symptoms are aggravated or ameliorated at different times during the pregnancy.

Postpartum, around 5–10% of women develop thyroid dysfunction. The risk is higher in those who have positive thyroid antibodies, Type 1 diabetes mellitus (25%), a family history of thyroid disease or another coexisting autoimmune condition.[125] Of those who develop postpartum thyroid dysfunction, around one-third have postpartum thyroiditis. The remainder may present with either Graves' disease or Hashimoto's thyroiditis. In those with biochemical and clinical thyrotoxicosis developing later than 3–6 months postpartum, Graves' disease is more likely, and in these cases the hyperthyroidism will be sustained.[125]

Radioisotope uptake measurements are the investigation of choice and can help to distinguish between postpartum thyroiditis and Graves' disease. The distinction is important, as treatment choices differ according to the aetiology of thyroid dysfunction. Those with postpartum thyroiditis will show reduced uptake on scintigraphic scanning whereas those with Graves' disease will show elevated uptake. Breastfeeding should be avoided for 24 hours if ^{99m}Tc is used.

POSTPARTUM THYROIDITIS

This commonly presents with symptoms of thyrotoxicosis at around 12 weeks post delivery, followed by a period of hypothyroidism at around 3–6 months. Histologically, there is a destructive thyroiditis with a florid lymphocytic infiltrate seen at around 16 weeks in those who are antibody-positive. In some women, only the hypothyroid phase is evident and eventually there will be a return to a euthyroid state. Patients may be managed symptomatically with propranolol during the thyrotoxic phase if necessary. Treatment of the hypothyroid phase may be needed in around a third of women and T4 may be necessary for up to 12 months.[134]

Long term, patients who have experienced postpartum thyroiditis are at risk of further episodes in subsequent pregnancies. About 25% of women will develop permanent hypothyroidism, and recurrent postpartum thyroiditis is seen in up to 80% of subsequent pregnancies. Specialist monitoring and annual monitoring of TFTs are essential.

HYPEREMESIS GRAVIDARUM

Transient thyrotoxicosis may be seen in hyperemesis gravidarum. It is likely to arise as a consequence of the shared alpha subunit of beta-HCG and TSH, with high levels of HCG in hyperemesis gravidarum causing stimulation of the TSH receptor. Around 60% of women with hyperemesis gravidarum have a raised serum fT4 concentration with a suppressed serum TSH. Management is supportive and antithyroid medication should be avoided.

Thyrotoxicosis resulting from hyperemesis gravidarum may be distinguished from that occurring as a consequence of Graves' disease by a negative family history, a lack of any other autoimmune illness and negative thyroid antibodies (anti-TSH-receptor antibodies in particular). Physical signs typically associated with Graves' disease, such as a diffuse goitre, will also be absent.

GRAVES' DISEASE

This accounts for around 90% of cases of thyrotoxicosis observed in pregnancy and around 1 in every 500 women are affected.[134] Graves' disease may contribute to menstrual irregularities, difficulties in conception and an increased rate of miscarriage. In those who do conceive, the recognition and effective management of Graves' is crucial given that untreated hyperthyroidism is associated with miscarriage, premature labour, low birthweight and pre-eclampsia.

Graves' disease may rarely develop *de novo* in pregnancy but diagnosis may be delayed as signs and symptoms may be wrongly attributed to physiological changes occurring in pregnancy, such as increased metabolic rate, increased cardiac output, heat intolerance and mood changes. Other symptoms may include hyperemesis gravidarum, muscle fatigue and, occasionally, cardiovascular problems such as pregnancy-induced hypertension or high output cardiac failure.

Treatment of thyrotoxicosis in pregnancy seeks to achieve rapid biochemical euthyroidism while alleviating symptoms.[92, 125, 126] Specific beta-adrenergic blocking agents may be used as adjuncts but the mainstay of treatment is antithyroid medication. Radioiodine cannot be used as it is contraindicated in pregnancy. Propylthiouracil is preferred to carbimazole in the first trimester as it is associated with fewer teratogenic effects. If antithyroid drugs are continued during the second and third trimester, carbimazole remains the drug of choice in view of fears of liver function abnormalities with propylthiouracil treatment. Antithyroid drugs are excreted in breast milk and babies from mothers taking doses of carbimazole of 20 mg daily or more while breastfeeding should have 4-weekly thyroid function testing.

The presence of circulating anti-TSH-receptor antibodies in pregnancy may result in foetal thyrotoxicosis due to transplacental transfer. Current guidance recommends the determination of TSH-receptor antibody concentrations at 20 weeks' gestation and close monitoring of those with significantly raised levels.[125, 135]

Joint management with the endocrinologist, obstetrician and paediatrician is important as there is a risk of foetal and neonatal thyrotoxicosis indicated by low birthweight, irritability and tachycardia.

Hypothyroid states in pregnancy

Overt hypothyroidism is associated with both anovulation and first trimester abortion. It is therefore unlikely to present at conception or during early pregnancy though it is seen in approximately 0.2–1% of women during the first trimester. If untreated during pregnancy, hypothyroidism confers a two- to threefold increased risk of spontaneous miscarriage, pregnancy-induced hypertension and pre-eclampsia, low birthweight (which is largely a consequence of prematurity) and perinatal mortality. There is additional data to link maternal hypothyroidism with an increased incidence of neurodevelopmental defects.[135]

OVERT HYPOTHYROIDISM

Pre-conception thyroid hormone replacement may offer protection against early pregnancy hypothyroidism. During pregnancy the requirement for thyroid hormone increases due to weight gain, transfer of T4 to the foetus and raised concentrations of thyroxin binding globulin. Gastrointestinal absorption is also known to decrease. An increased dose of thyroxine may be required as early as 4 weeks' gestation. Treatment should target the prevention of hypothyroidism and it is important patients are counselled prior to or during early pregnancy in order to ensure compliance with therapy. It is prudent to counsel women to double their dose of thyroxine on 2 days each week should they have a positive pregnancy test, given that a routine antenatal visit does not occur until 10–12 weeks of gestation.

Between 40% and 70% of patients will require further dose adjustment even following this empirical dose increase. Most clinicians would measure TFTs around 4–6 weeks' gestation, 4 weeks after any increase in dose of T4 and at least once per trimester. Levothyroxine dosage can be reduced to pre-pregnancy levels 2 weeks after delivery with TFTs reviewed after 6 weeks in order to ensure adequate thyroid hormone replacement. Dose adjustment of levothyroxine should be based on serum TSH as it demonstrates less inter-individual variation than fT4 concentrations. Some authors do, however, advocate the use of fT4 concentrations in light of the key role of T4 in determining foetal brain development. Ingestion of iron supplementation and antacid for gastroesophageal reflux may affect thyroxine absorption and further complicate dosing.

Obstetricians advocate managing pregnancies complicated by hypothyroidism as high risk. As such, aspirin is advised for pre-eclampsia prophylaxis in addition to uterine artery Doppler studies to screen for malplacentation. Routine observations should be undertaken frequently to assess for pre-eclampsia.

SUBCLINICAL HYPOTHYROIDISM

Rates of subclinical hypothyroidism in pregnancy are dependent on the iodine status of the population.[136] A recent meta-analysis of studies which included subclinically hypothyroid populations demonstrated a significant increase in risk of pregnancy loss (including miscarriages, stillbirths and perinatal deaths), pre-term delivery (OR 1.3; 95% CI 1.05–1.60), placental abruption (OR 2.16; 95% CI: 1.15–4.06) and breech presentation at term.[137] Raised serum TSH is also associated with breech presentation, reduced external cephalic version success rate and an increased incidence of neurodevelopmental defects.[138–141]

There is a paucity of evidence relating to the management of subclinical hypothyroidism either during pregnancy or in those attempting to conceive. Interestingly, treatment of subclinical hypothyroidism favours increased live birth rates in subjects undergoing assisted conception. Many endocrine professional bodies advocate the use of levothyroxine therapy, ideally prior to conception, given that the risk ratio is highly favourable with the potential risk of hyperthyroidism minimized by regular monitoring of thyroid function. Recent ATA guidelines support treatment only in TPO antibody-positive women but are relatively undecided on the merits of treatment in TPO antibody-negative disease. The American Congress of Obstetricians and Gynecologists does not endorse recommendations for the treatment of subclinical hypothyroidism in pregnancy.

> **KEY POINTS**
>
> **THYROID DISEASE IN PREGNANCY**
>
> - Joint management with an endocrinologist, obstetrician and a paediatrician is important.
> - Hyperemesis may be associated with thyrotoxicosis.
> - Graves' disease should be managed with pregnancy – propylthiouracil is preferable to carbimazole.
> - TSH should be maintained at <2.5 mLU/L in hypothyroid women.
> - Postpartum thyroiditis is common.

EUTHYROID GLANDULAR ENLARGEMENT

Classification

The term 'goitre' refers to a thyroid gland which exceeds the upper limit defined for normal volume. This may simply be described as 18 mL for women and 25 mL for men but assessment of thyroid size should also respect age-specific criteria for normal values. Thyroid enlargement may be diffuse or may result from the presence of one or multiple thyroid nodules. It may additionally occur in the context of euthyroidism, hypothyroidism or hyperthyroidism. This section will review the enlargement of the thyroid gland which commonly occurs in the absence of aberrant hormone concentrations.

Epidemiology

Enlargement of the thyroid gland is common. The Wickham Survey identified the presence of a palpable goitre in 15% of persons within an iodine-replete region and a visible goitre in 7%, supported by data from the US Framingham study that identified a 5–10% lifetime risk of developing a thyroid nodule.[6, 142] The prevalence of goitre is closely related to dietary intake of iodine. This is such that, while 35.9% of the 3941 participants without known thyroid disease in the Study of Health in Pomerania had a goitre in its first phase, goitre was significantly rarer in the 5-year follow-up as iodine intake increased.[143, 144]

The advent of high-resolution ultrasound has led to reported rates of goitre of between 19% and 67% in imaged individuals, even if the gland is normal on palpation. Higher frequencies have been noted in women and the elderly.[2]

Aetiology

Thyroid enlargement occurring in the absence of thyroid hormone excess or deficiency may be diffuse or nodular. The potential for malignancy is of concern, although thyroid cancer remains rare and accounts for only 1% of all new malignant disease.[145] Papillary and follicular thyroid cancers are together termed differentiated thyroid cancers and represent 72–85% and 10–20% of thyroid cancers respectively.[146] The remainder comprise of follicular (10–20%), medullary (1.7–35%), anaplastic (<1%) and other carcinomas (1–4%). Benign and malignant causes of nodular thyroid enlargement are summarized in **Table 61.14**.

Risk factors for the development of thyroid cancer include exposure to head and neck irradiation in infancy and childhood.[147] Increased rates of childhood papillary cancer have been noted in Belarus and Ukraine and are thought to reflect the Chernobyl nuclear reactor accident.[148]

Women are disproportionately affected by thyroid cancer with data suggesting a prevalence of 1.5%, which compares to 0.5% for men. Conversely, the presence of a thyroid nodule in a man is more likely to represent an underlying carcinoma.[2, 149] This is explained by the equal rates of thyroid carcinoma for men and women despite a 5–10 times greater prevalence of nodular thyroid disease in females. Those at the extremes of age are also at most risk of harbouring thyroid cancer.[149]

Survival rates are favourable with percentage cancer deaths of 0.21% and 0.3% for men and women respectively.[150] The incidence of thyroid cancer is rising rapidly and this is, at least in part, due to increased detection of

TABLE 61.14 Causes of nodular thyroid enlargement

| | Malignant | |
Benign	Follicular or C-cell origin	Malignancy of other origin
Follicular adenoma	Papillary carcinoma	Thyroid lymphoma
Hürthle cell adenoma	Follicular carcinoma	Malignancy metastatic to the thyroid
Colloid cyst	Hürthle cell carcinoma	
Simple/haemorrhagic cyst	Medullary thyroid carcinoma	
Lymphocytic thyroiditis	Anaplastic carcinoma	
Granulomatous thyroiditis		
Infectious processes		

incidental thyroid cancers.[150] Clinicians must increasingly respond to the challenge of identifying the minority of patients with thyroid cancer who require surgical intervention and additional therapies.

Clinical manifestations

Goitre development is asymptomatic in the majority of cases but is often visible once thyroid volume exceeds 40 mL. Patients may note that they have changed their collar size or stopped wearing necklaces. As many as 30–85% of patients are reported to develop mechanical compression of the trachea and/or the oesophagus but the majority remain asymptomatic.[151] In those who do develop obstructive sequelae, the location of the goitre may predict symptomatology. Retrosternal goitres often result in dysphagia, for example, whereas retrotracheal goitres are more commonly associated with dyspnoea.

Diagnostic evaluation

History and physical examination are key to the evaluation of suspected goitre and may suggest thyroid carcinoma in some instances.[149] History should focus on the presence of mechanical symptoms, the temporal nature of thyroid enlargement, the presence of risk factors for malignancy such as previous head and neck irradiation, and family history relevant to a potential hereditary cancer syndrome.

The neck and upper thorax must be assessed on examination and palpation undertaken to determine goitre size and the presence of nodularity. The presence of signs suggestive of excess or insufficient thyroid hormone should be noted, as should evidence of mechanical compression.[151]

Features which strongly suggest the presence of thyroid carcinoma include rapid enlargement during hormonal therapy, vocal cord paralysis, ipsilateral lymphadenopathy and the presence of a hard, fixed nodule (Table 61.15).[2, 149] These are, however, absent in the vast majority of cases and thyroid enlargement as a consequence of malignancy is indistinguishable from enlargement of benign aetiology in many cases. There is in addition considerable inter- and intra-observer variation regarding assessment of the size and morphology of the thyroid. A potential consequence is the increase in the use of ultrasound imaging to assess for and characterize thyroid nodularity.

Investigations in thyroid enlargement

LABORATORY INVESTIGATIONS

Recent guidelines published by both the American Thyroid Association (ATA) and the British Thyroid Association (BTA) advocate determination of the serum TSH concentration during the initial evaluation of a patient with a thyroid nodule.[152, 153] Thyroid function tests must also be utilized to exclude thyroid dysfunction. Raised TSH should result in assessment of fT4 to identify either subclinical or overt hypothyroidism. Similarly, measurement of fT3 and fT4 should be undertaken in the presence of a suppressed TSH in order to delineate overt from subclinical hyperthyroidism or T3 toxicosis.

However, while virtually all patients with thyroid carcinoma are euthyroid, TSH may be suppressed in cases of malignancy. Interestingly, TSH concentration is increasingly recognized as an independent risk factor for thyroid malignancy. In a study of 1500 patients investigated with fine-needle aspiration cytology (FNAC) following presentation with thyroid enlargement, an increased odds ratio for malignancy was noted in those with serum TSH >0.9 mU/L.[154] Subsequent analysis of 843 patients undergoing resection of likely thyroid malignancy confirmed an increased likelihood of thyroid cancer with higher serum TSH concentration.[155] Levels of serum TSH were also found to be greater in patients with advanced malignancy (stage III/IV disease) compared with those with stage I or II disease.[156]

Serum levels of thyroglobulin are influenced by the size of a thyroid gland and factors such as iodine intake. Routine assessment of serum thyroglobulin is therefore not recommended for the initial evaluation of thyroid nodules by both the ATA and the BTA as it is neither a sensitive nor a specific diagnostic test in this context.[152, 153] Serum thyroglobulin measurements either under TSH suppression or stimulated do, however, remain the gold-standard tumour marker in patients with proven thyroid cancer.

There remains considerable controversy over the measurement of other potential serum markers of thyroid malignancy. Antithyroid peroxidase measurements are, for instance, undertaken by more than half of clinicians, yet they are found in approximately 10% of the general population and may reflect a coexistent autoimmunity rather than directly relate to the thyroid nodule.[2] The immunometric calcitonin assay is a sensitive marker for

TABLE 61.15 Elements suggestive of thyroid carcinoma in a patient's clinical workup		
History	Clinical examination	Imaging
Family history	Hard, fixed nodule	Hypoechogenicity
Male	Vocal cord paralysis	Solid nodule
Extremes of age	Ipsilateral lymphadenopathy	Microcalcification
Head and neck irradiation in infancy/childhood		Irregular margins
Previous radiation exposure		Increased intranodular flow
Compressive symptoms		Increased anterior–posterior dimension
Nodular enlargement during hormonal therapy		Invasion
		Lymphadenopathy

detection of medullary thyroid cancer, albeit with a high false-positive rate as a consequence of heterophilic antibodies. Calcitonin levels of greater than 10 pg/mL are very sensitive for the detection of medullary thyroid cancer and should elicit further investigation.[157] Despite evidence to suggest that use of calcitonin is cost-effective and a useful tool in the evaluation of thyroid nodules, its use is not widely recognized in the US and is more commonplace within Europe.[158]

DIAGNOSTIC IMAGING

The imaging modality used in the assessment of thyroid enlargement is at least partly dependent on the clinical scenario. There is a growing array of options for the clinician, including ultrasonography, scintigraphy, computed tomography (CT) scanning, magnetic resonance (MR) imaging and, most recently, positron emission tomography (PET).

Ultrasound

The most widely used imaging modality in the detection and evaluation of thyroid nodules is ultrasonography, which is now recommended routinely in the assessment of goitre by BTA, ETA and ATA guidelines.[152, 153] This non-invasive technique has the capacity to detect non-palpable nodules, in addition to permitting estimation of the size of goitres and nodules and allowing accurate guidance of fine-needle aspiration biopsy (FNAB).

A number of specific ultrasonographic changes are associated with malignancy, including hypoechogenicity, solid nodules, microcalcifications, irregular margins, increased intranodular flow, increased ratio of anterior/posterior dimensions in transverse and longitudinal views (more tall than wide), the presence of invasion or evidence of regional lymphadenopathy.

There are several retrospective case series that have together indicated a role for ultrasound imaging in reliably detecting malignancy.[159, 160] Consequently, radiologists may use a US (U) grading system (U1–U5) to predict malignancy and guide clinicians in deciding whether biopsy of a thyroid nodule is required.[152] The U classification system is depicted in **Table 61.16**. Ultrasound findings that represent a benign nodule (U1–U2) are regarded as not requiring FNAB unless the patient has a high risk of malignancy. Those that are equivocal (U3) or show a higher risk of malignancy (U4–U5) should lead to cytological assessment via FNAB.

Elastography may also be utilized and typically identifies diminished compressibility in malignant thyroid nodules.[161] Interestingly, neither the number of nodules nor their size is predictive of malignancy. The presence of multiple suspect ultrasonographic findings confers an 83–99% sensitivity and 56–85% specificity for thyroid malignancy.[161, 162] This high sensitivity may result in unnecessary investigations and intervention for clinically insignificant nodules. The low specificity continues to render ultrasound assessment of thyroid nodules inferior to FNAB for the diagnosis of malignancy.

TABLE 61.16 Ultrasound (U) classification of thyroid nodules

U classification	Nodule type	Ultrasound characteristics
U1	Normal	
U2	Benign	Vascularity, egg shell calcification, cystic change, iso-echoic or mildly hyper-echoic
U3	Indeterminate/ equivocal	Homogenous, hyper-echoic, equivocal echogenic foci, mixed or central vascularity, solid or halo
U4	Suspicious	Solid, hypo-echoic, peripheral calcification, lobulated outline
U5	Malignant	Solid, hypo-echoic, lobulated outline, intranodular vascularity, taller > wide, lymphadenopathy

Thyroid scintigraphy

Scintigraphy is of little value in the differentiation between benign and malignant nodular disease due both to its poor sensitivity and specificity. While this technique permits differentiation between 'hot' (functional) and 'cold' (non-functional) nodules, most malignant nodules trap isotope less well than normal thyroid tissue and thus appear cold, yet the risk of malignancy in cold nodules is nevertheless as high as 8–25%.[163] Both the BTA and the ATA have published guidelines stating that scintigraphy has no role in the routine management of the thyroid nodule.[152, 153]

Other imaging modalities

Use of CT and MRI provides high-resolution three-dimensional imaging of the thyroid gland but affords no advantage over thyroid ultrasound for the detailed assessment of thyroid architecture. They additionally afford little value in the differentiation between benign and malignant lesions.[164] The use of 2-deoxy-2-fluoro-D glucose (FDG-PET) has met with promise but is limited by both cost and availability. For patients with large goitres, flow volume loop assessment may be helpful.[151]

Suspicious nodules are now not uncommonly identified incidentally during FDG-PET imaging undertaken for a separate indication.[165] Effective workup of patients with incidentally identified focal hypermetabolic thyroid lesions on FDG-PET imaging is crucial, with approximately one-third of identified lesions likely to be malignant.[166]

FINE-NEEDLE ASPIRATION BIOPSY

FNAB is the gold-standard investigation in the evaluation of patients presenting with thyroid enlargement and provides both direct and specific information about the pathology of nodules.[152, 153] This inexpensive and easy-to-learn technique carries a low complication rate and is the preferred diagnostic tool by the majority of thyroidologists. It remains the investigation of choice in the evaluation of thyroid nodules as advocated in new ATA guidance.[167]

Current BTA guidance recommends a combination of US and cytological findings in the diagnosis of thyroid cancer.[152] The BTA and ATA have additionally provided guidance for the classification of cytological aspirates, as summarized in **Table 61.17**.

In summary, under BTA guidance nodules with seemingly benign US characteristics in patients of usual or low risk of thyroid cancer can be discharged from follow-up with no requirement for routine follow-up ultrasound. In instances of benign (Thy2) cytology and benign ultrasound findings there is again no requirement for follow-up ultrasound. Repeat FNAB is, however, required if US findings are suspicious and the initial FNA result is Thy1, or if the previous FNAB result is Thy2.

Cystic lesions which repeatedly yield non-diagnostic aspirates require close observation and, particularly in if the nodule is solid, may necessitate surgical intervention. Surgery may also be offered to patients with benign cytology who belong to a high clinical risk group or who have pressure symptoms or rapid nodular growth.

Indeterminate cytology results are common and are reported in 15–30% of FNA specimens. Gender, nodule size and cytological features such as the presence of atypia may improve diagnostic accuracy but overall predictive values remain low. The use of molecular markers in refining the diagnosis of thyroid cancer is a rapidly expanding field and gene expression classifiers and mutation analysis panels are regularly in some US centres.[168] However, there is as yet insufficient evidence to recommend the routine use of molecular markers in the diagnosis of thyroid cancer.[152]

The risk of malignancy is similar in those with multiple thyroid nodules compared with those presenting with a single nodule. Since sonographic characteristics are superior to nodule size in identifying malignancy current ATA and BTA guidance recommends diagnostic ultrasound in those with multinodular thyroids. Fine-needle aspiration should be undertaken in those with suspicious features. If none of the nodules has a suspicious appearance, the likelihood of malignancy is low and it is reasonable to aspirate the largest nodule only.

TABLE 61.17 Cytological classification of fine-needle aspirates and action required

ATA classification (Bethesda System)

Diagnostic category	Cytological diagnosis	Management
I	Non-diagnostic	Repeat US-guided FNA
II	Benign	Clinical follow-up
III	Atypia/follicular lesion of undetermined significance	Repeat FNA
IV	Suspicious	Surgical hemithyroidectomy
V	Suspicious	Near-total thyroidectomy / surgical hemithyroidectomy
VI	Malignant	Near-total hemithyroidectomy

BTA classification (RCPath Thy System)

Diagnostic category	Cytological diagnosis	Management
Thy1	Non-diagnostic	US assessment +/− repeat FNAB
Thy2	Non-neoplastic	Correlate with clinical / US findings
Thy3	Neoplasm possible	
	Thy3a – Atypia (uncategorized)	Further US +/− repeat FNAB
	Thy3f – Atypia (possible follicular neoplasm)	Diagnostic hemithyroidectomy
Thy4	Suspicious of malignancy	Diagnostic hemithyroidectomy
Thy5	Diagnostic of malignancy	Surgical resection

> **KEY POINTS**
>
> **THYROID ENLARGEMENT**
>
> **AETIOLOGY**
>
> - Benign causes include follicular and Hürthle cell adenoma, colloid cyst, infectious processes and thyroiditis.
> - Malignant causes include papillary, follicular, Hürthle cell, and anaplastic or medullary thyroid carcinoma.
> - Malignancies may be metastatic to the thyroid.
>
> *Clinical features suggesting carcinoma in a patient with thyroid enlargement*
>
> - Clinical history: rapid tumour growth, vocal cord paralysis, male sex, age <20 or >60 years, history of head or neck irradiation, presence of compressive symptoms, family history of multiple endocrine neoplasia or medullary thyroid carcinoma.
> - Examination: firm nodules, fixation to adjacent structures, regional lymphadenopathy.
>
> *Investigations*
>
> - High-resolution ultrasound is the diagnostic imaging modality of choice.
> - Fine-needle aspiration biopsy is required for cytological assessment.
>
> *Management*
>
> - Cytological diagnosis of Thy1 and Thy2 will require at least one repeat.
> - Cytological diagnosis of Thy3, Thy4 or Thy5 will likely necessitate surgical intervention.

Medical management of nodular thyroid disease

NON-TOXIC MULTINODULAR GOITRE

Surgery is the treatment of choice where there is evidence of moderate to severe compressive symptoms, where FNAC of a dominant nodule is suspicious of malignant or where the patient prefers surgery for cosmetic reasons.

Radioiodine therapy

Medical treatment of goitre previously involved the use of suppressive thyroid hormone but this is now considered outdated.[169] Use of suppressive therapy necessitates acceptance of a state of subclinical hyperthyroidism and consequent increased risk of reduced bone mineral density and cardiovascular disease.[97] Its discontinuation often also results in the resumption of growth of thyroid nodules or goitres. Contemporary management therefore typically utilizes the administration of radioactive iodine in cases in which a patient has refused surgery or if age, frailty or comorbidities preclude operative intervention.

Reduction in goitre size may be as significant as 60% and may continue for years after treatment, although most shrinkage occurs soon after treatment. Favourable outcomes are more likely in patients with small goitres who are young, have a shorter history of goitre and who receive higher doses of radioiodine.

Approximately 75% of those with the largest goitres will achieve relief from dyspnoea, accompanied by a reported 36% increase in the cross-sectional area of the trachea.[170] These patients may require large doses of radioiodine and may require hospitalization and isolation as a requirement of radiation protection legislation. Alternatively, therapy may be fractionated over a course of a few months.

The use of radioiodine is not, however, without side effects. Hypothyroidism commonly results from its use and is more likely if multiple doses of radioiodine are administered. The prevalence varies according to the amount of radiation exposure, with figures quoted ranging between 8% and 40% at 1–2 years.[2] While uncommon, radiation thyroiditis may occur in 3–13% of patients and causes neck pain and tenderness. Graves' hyperthyroidism associated with the development of TSH receptor antibodies occurs in up to 5% of patients and is usually transient.

Goitre size may transiently increase following the administration of radioiodine. Some concern has been voiced previously that this might contribute to a deterioration in respiratory function in those with tracheal compression. This fear is not well substantiated within the literature with studies demonstrating only a small decrease in tracheal cross-sectional area after therapy with no increase in upper airways obstruction. The use of prednisolone peri- and post-radioiodine to minimize risks of tracheal compression has been advocated but there is no evidence base for this practice.

Recombinant TSH may be employed as an adjunct to radioiodine therapy.[171] Its use in this setting is aimed towards increasing the stimulus for radioiodine uptake into a goitre so as to maximize the effect per dose ratio. Preliminary data relating to the use of this adjuvant treatment are encouraging but evidence for efficacy in volume reduction is not yet available. Consequently, recombinant TSH is not widely used at present.[172]

SOLITARY NON-TOXIC NODULE

Treatment of a solitary toxic nodule is similar to the management of multinodular goitre.[173] Surgery remains the treatment option of choice in cases of suspected malignancy and for cosmetic effect. Suppressive therapy with thyroid hormones is not recommended for solitary nodules for reasons outlined previously in this chapter.

Radioiodine therapy

Nodules which take up iodine (hot nodules) may be managed with radioiodine. This simple treatment is safe and cost-effective for this purpose, with a single dose delivering a thyroid volume reduction of up to 40%. Hypothyroidism is seen in approximately 10% of patients at 5 years post-radioiodine, although its frequency is higher in those with pre-existing thyroid autoimmunity.

Aspiration

Approximately 10–15% of solitary thyroid nodules are cystic. Many will resolve over time and small cysts of less than 3 mL volume are managed with a conservative expectant approach. Larger cysts should be aspirated with FNAB performed on any residual nodule. Surgery may be considered in these cases as around 10% of large lesions may harbour thyroid cancer. Recurrence rates following aspiration are poor and may be as high as 80%.

THYROID INCIDENTALOMAS

This area of thyroid disease has gained growing importance as a consequence of the increasing recognition of previously unrecognizable thyroid nodules through various imaging modalities. Usually measuring less than 1.5 cm, these incidentalomas are often diagnosed during evaluation for non-diagnostic neck disorders and pose a management quandary for clinicians.[152, 153]

The Society of Radiologists in Ultrasound recently released a consensus statement which stipulated that highly suspicious ultrasonographic features, such as microcalcifications, should prompt a biopsy in nodules 1 cm or larger, other suspicious features such as solid consistency should prompt biopsy at 1.5 cm or larger and less suspicious appearances such as mixed solid and cystic consistency should be considered only if nodules measure 2 cm or larger.[159] These guidelines have, however, met with controversy as patients undergoing surgery for papillary cancers as small as <1.5 cm have been identified to have distant metastasis.[174] The revised British Thyroid Association Guidelines on the management of thyroid cancer do not take size into consideration when evaluating incidentalomas and suggest FNAB of nodules that are indeterminate or suspicious on ultrasound (U3–U5 categories).[152]

An alternative approach may be to observe small nodules, in the absence of features of malignancy, and to proceed to FNAB for larger or rapidly growing incidentalomas and those with features suggestive of malignancy, such as irregular margins and increased intranodular flow. Most will require US-guided FNAB as they will be impalpable, and mixed radiological and clinical follow-up is advocated.

CONCLUSIONS

Thyroid dysfunction is common, affecting more than 2% of the population and is usually caused by autoimmune disease. Thyrotoxicosis is most commonly caused by Graves' disease, with other important causes including toxic nodular hyperthyroidism and thyroiditis. The mainstays of treatment of thyrotoxicosis—namely, antithyroid drugs, radioiodine, and surgery—have not changed for more than 60 years, although the evidence base directing treatment choices and modes of administration is improving. Importantly, there is a rapidly increasing evidence base that mild or subclinical hyperthyroidism is associated with serious consequences, especially cardiovascular effects and osteoporosis.

Worldwide iodine deficiency is the most common cause of hypothyroidism, although in developed countries this is usually caused by Hashimoto's thyroiditis, another autoimmune disease. A number of definitive treatment modalities for hyperthyroidism result in permanent hypothyroidism. Levothyroxine mono-therapy remains the standard of care for patients with hypothyroidism. Significant controversy continues to surround the long-term consequences and need for thyroid hormone replacement therapy in mild subclinical hypothyroidism. The management of thyroid dysfunction in pregnancy requires a coordinated multidisciplinary approach involving endocrinologists and obstetricians.

Thyroid enlargement and nodules affect up to 50% of the population and the challenge is to identify patients harbouring malignancy from the large majority who have benign disease. When thyroid dysfunction is excluded, the use of high-resolution ultrasound and fine-needle aspiration cytology are the most important diagnostic tools in this setting. A multidisciplinary approach involving thyroid surgeons, radiologists, nuclear physicists and endocrinologists are crucial for optimal management approaches in patients presenting with thyroid gland enlargement. If the presence of malignancy is excluded, often a conservative approach can be adopted. Treatment of suspected thyroid cancer usually involves surgery, whereas a conservative approach is usually adopted in those with benign thyroid enlargement. If there is significant compression, surgery or administration of radioiodine to shrink the goitre may be indicated.

FUTURE RESEARCH

Hyperthyroidism
- Investigation of novel and safe ways to modulate the underlying disease process in Graves' disease including immunological and other biological agents
- Further evaluation of the mechanisms of and risk factors for the development of severe side effects of the antithyroid drugs
- Determination of the long-term outcomes following treatment and their dependence on the treatment modalities employed
- Prospective randomized controlled trials assessing the indications for and outcomes following treatment of subclinical hyperthyroidism

Hypothyroidism
- Development of superior biomarkers of euthyroidism to supplement serum TSH measurements

- Mechanistic research on serum triiodothyronine levels, including effects of age and disease status, relationship with tissue concentrations, as well as potential therapeutic targeting
- Long-term outcome clinical trials testing combination therapy with T3/T4 or thyroid extracts
- Development of thyroid hormone analogs with a favourable benefit to risk profile
- Prospective randomized trials assessing the indications for and outcomes following treatment of subclinical hypothyroidism

Nodules
- Refinement of long-term follow-up strategies in patients with benign nodular thyroid disease
- Improvements in diagnostic accuracy of fine-needle aspiration cytology of thyroid nodules
- Identification of useful molecular markers diagnostic of thyroid malignancy
- Investigation of the role of elastography in the diagnosis of thyroid nodules

KEY POINTS
- Both overt and subclinical thyroid dysfunction are of clinical importance.
- Classical symptoms of thyrotoxicosis may not be present in the elderly.
- Levothyroxine is the mainstay of treatment in hypothyroidism with inconclusive evidence to indicate an advantage from T3 therapy.
- Thyroid disease in pregnancy requires a specialist-driven multidisciplinary approach.
- Thyroid cancer is rare but must be considered in cases of euthyroid glandular enlargement.
- High-resolution ultrasound, with or without fine-needle aspiration cytology, is used first-line in the investigation of euthyroid goitre.

REFERENCES

1. Tunbridge WM, Evered DC, Hall R, et al. The spectrum of thyroid disease in a community: the Whickham survey. *Clin Endocrinol* 1977; **7**(6): 481–93.
2. Hegedüs L, Bonnema SJ, Bennedbaek FN. Management of simple nodular goiter: current status and future perspectives. *Endocr Rev* 2003; **24**(1): 102–32.
3. Vanderpump MPJ. The epidemiology of thyroid disease. *Br Med Bull* 2011; **99**(1): 39–51.
4. Hollowell JG, Staehling NW, Flanders WD, et al. Serum TSH, T(4), and thyroid antibodies in the United States population (1988 to 1994): National Health and Nutrition Examination Survey (NHANES III). *J Clin Endocrinol Metab* 2002; **87**(2): 489–99.
5. Golden SH, Robinson KA, Saldanha I, et al. Clinical review: Prevalence and incidence of endocrine and metabolic disorders in the United States: a comprehensive review. *J Clin Endocrinol Metab* 2009; **94**(6): 1853–78.
6. Vanderpump MP, Tunbridge WM, French JM, et al. The incidence of thyroid disorders in the community: a twenty-year follow-up of the Whickham Survey. *Clin Endocrinol* 1995; **43**(1): 55–68.
7. Parle JV, Franklyn JA, Cross KW, et al. Prevalence and follow-up of abnormal thyrotrophin (TSH) concentrations in the elderly in the United Kingdom. *Clin Endocrinol* 1991; **34**(1): 77–83.
8. Canaris GJ, Manowitz NR, Mayor G, Ridgway EC. The Colorado thyroid disease prevalence study. *Arch Intern Med* 2000; **160**(4): 526–34.
9. Lahey FF. Non-activated (apathetic) type of hyperthyroidism. *N Engl J Med* 1931; **204**: 747–8.
10. Boelaert K, Torlinska B, Holder RL, Franklyn JA. Older subjects with hyperthyroidism present with a paucity of symptoms and signs: a large cross-sectional study. *J Clin Endocrinol Metab* 2010; **95**(6): 2715–26.
11. Frost L, Vestergaard P, Mosekilde L. Hyperthyroidism and risk of atrial fibrillation or flutter: a population-based study. *Arch Intern Med* 2004; **164**(15): 1675–8.
12. Trivalle C, Doucet J, Chassagne P, et al. Differences in the signs and symptoms of hyperthyroidism in older and younger patients. *J Am Geriatr Soc* 1996; **44**(1): 50–3.
13. Hampton J. Thyroid gland disorder emergencies: thyroid storm and myxedema coma. *AACN Adv Crit Care* 2013; **24**(3): 325–32.
14. Vijayakumar A, Ashwath G, Thimmappa D. Thyrotoxic periodic paralysis: clinical challenges. *J Thyroid Res* 2014; 2014: 649502.
15. Cooper DS. Hyperthyroidism. *Lancet* 2003; **362**(9382): 459–68.
16. Tozzoli R, Bagnasco M, Giavarina D, Bizzaro N. TSH receptor autoantibody immunoassay in patients with Graves' disease: improvement of diagnostic accuracy over different generations of methods. Systematic review and meta-analysis. *Autoimmun Rev* 2012; **12**(2): 107–13.
17. Wilson R, Fraser WD, Gray CE, et al. Thyrotropin receptor antibodies associated with post-operative relapse of thyrotoxicosis in a pregnancy complicated by neonatal thyrotoxicosis. *Scott Med J* 1990; **35**(1): 21–2.
18. Weetman AP. Graves' disease. *N Engl J Med* 2000; **343**(17): 1236–48.
19. Di Cerbo A, Di Paola R, Menzaghi C, et al. Graves' immunoglobulins activate phospholipase A2 by recognizing specific epitopes on thyrotropin receptor. *J Clin Endocrinol Metab* 1999; **84**(9): 3283–92.
20. Wiersinga WM. Thyroid autoimmunity. *Endocr Dev* 2014; **26**: 139–57.
21. Anderson MS. Update in endocrine autoimmunity. *J Clin Endocrinol Metab* 2008; **93**(10): 3663–70.
22. Wiersinga WM, Prummel MF. Pathogenesis of Graves' ophthalmopathy: current understanding. *J Clin Endocrinol Metab* 2001; **86**(2): 501–3.
23. Bahn RS. Thyrotropin receptor expression in orbital adipose/connective tissues from patients with thyroid-associated ophthalmopathy. *Thyroid* 2002; **12**(3): 193–5.
24. Tomer Y, Davies TF. Searching for the autoimmune thyroid disease susceptibility genes: from gene mapping to gene function. *Endocr Rev* 2003; **24**(5): 694–717.
25. Matos-Santos A, Nobre EL, Costa JG, et al. Relationship between the number and impact of stressful life events and the onset of Graves' disease and toxic nodular goitre. *Clin Endocrinol* 2001; **55**(1): 15–19.
26. Vestergaard P, Rejnmark L, Weeke J, et al. Smoking as a risk factor for Graves' disease, toxic nodular goiter, and autoimmune hypothyroidism. *Thyroid* 2002; **12**(1): 69–75.
27. Wong V, Fu AX-L, George J, Cheung NW. Thyrotoxicosis induced by alpha-interferon therapy in chronic viral hepatitis. *Clin Endocrinol* 2002; **56**(6): 793–8.
28. Thompson CJ, Baylis PH. Asymptomatic Graves' disease during lithium therapy. *Postgrad Med J* 1986; **62**(726): 295–6.
29. Villadolid MC, Yokoyama N, Izumi M, et al. Untreated Graves' disease patients without clinical ophthalmopathy demonstrate a high frequency of extraocular muscle (EOM) enlargement by magnetic resonance. *J Clin Endocrinol Metab* 1995; **80**(9): 2830–3.
30. Bartalena L, Fatourechi V. Extrathyroidal manifestations of Graves' disease: a 2014 update. *J Endocrinol Invest* 2014; **37**(8): 691–700.
31. Wiersinga WM. Smoking and thyroid. *Clin Endocrinol* 2013; **79**(2): 145–51.
32. Weetman AP. Radioiodine treatment for benign thyroid diseases. *Clin Endocrinol* 2007; **66**(6): 757–64.
33. Laurberg P, Berman DC, Pedersen IB, et al. Double vision is a major manifestation in moderate to severe graves' orbitopathy, but it correlates negatively with inflammatory signs and proptosis. *J Clin Endocrinol Metab* 2015; **100**(5): 2098–105.
34. Perros P, Dayan CM, Dickinson AJ, et al. Management of patients with Graves' orbitopathy: initial assessment, management outside specialised centres and referral pathways. *Clin Med* 2015; **15**(2): 173–8.
35. Bartalena L, Marcocci C, Pinchera A. Treating severe Graves' ophthalmopathy. *Baillieres Clin Endocrinol Metab* 1997; **11**(3): 521–36.
36. Fatourechi V. Medical management of extrathyroidal manifestation of graves disease. *Endocr Pract* 2014; **20**(12): 1333–44.
37. Salvi M, Vannucchi G, Currò N, et al. Efficacy of B-cell targeted therapy with rituximab in patients with active moderate to severe Graves' orbitopathy: a randomized controlled study. *J Clin Endocrinol Metab* 2015; **100**(2): 422–31.
38. Fatourechi V, Bartley GB, Eghbali-Fatourechi GZ, et al. Graves' dermopathy and acropachy are markers of severe Graves' ophthalmopathy. *Thyroid* 2003; **13**(12): 1141–4.
39. Schwartz KM, Fatourechi V, Ahmed DDF, Pond GR. Dermopathy of Graves' disease (pretibial myxedema): long-term outcome. *J Clin Endocrinol Metab* 2002; **87**(2): 438–46.
40. Cheng S-P, Liu C-L. Images in clinical medicine: dermopathy of Graves' disease. *N Engl J Med* 2005; **352**(9): 918.
41. Vanhoenacker FM, Pelckmans MC, De Beuckeleer LH, et al. Thyroid acropachy: correlation of imaging and pathology. *Eur Radiol* 2001; **11**(6): 1058–62.
42. Morganti S, Ceda GP, Saccani M, et al. Thyroid disease in the elderly: sex-related differences in clinical expression. *J Endocrinol Invest* 2005; **28**(11 Suppl Proceedings): 101–4.
43. Zimmermann MB, Boelaert K. Iodine deficiency and thyroid disorders. *Lancet Diabetes Endocrinol* 2015; **3**(4): 286–95.
44. Tonacchera M, Agretti P, Chiovato L, et al. Activating thyrotropin receptor mutations are present in nonadenomatous hyperfunctioning nodules of toxic or autonomous multinodular goiter. *J Clin Endocrinol Metab* 2000; **85**(6): 2270–4.
45. Vitti P, Rago T, Tonacchera M, Pinchera A. Toxic multinodular goiter in the elderly. *J Endocrinol Invest* 2002; **25**(10 Suppl): 16–18.
46. Roti E, Uberti ED. Iodine excess and hyperthyroidism. *Thyroid* 2001; **11**(5): 493–500.
47. Klein I, Danzi S. Thyroid disease and the heart. *Circulation* 2007; **116**(15): 1725–35.
48. Hamburger JI. Solitary autonomously functioning thyroid lesions. *Am J Med* 1975; **58**(6): 740–8.
49. Tonacchera M, Chiovato L, Pinchera A, et al. Hyperfunctioning thyroid nodules in toxic multinodular goiter share activating thyrotropin receptor mutations with solitary toxic adenoma. *J Clin Endocrinol Metab* 1998; **83**(2): 492–8.
50. Kleinau G, Neumann S, Grüters A, et al. Novel insights on thyroid-stimulating hormone receptor signal transduction. *Endocr Rev* 2013; **34**(5): 691–724.
51. Spiegel AM. Mutations in G proteins and G protein-coupled receptors in endocrine disease. *J Clin Endocrinol Metab* 1996; **81**(7): 2434–42.
52. Burch HB, Shakir F, Fitzsimmons TR, et al. Diagnosis and management of the autonomously functioning thyroid nodule: the Walter Reed Army Medical Center experience, 1975–1996. *Thyroid* 1998; **8**(10): 871–80.
53. Van Sande J, Parma J, Tonacchera M, et al. Somatic and germline mutations of the TSH receptor gene in thyroid diseases. *J Clin Endocrinol Metab* 1995; **80**(9): 2577–85.

54. Abraham-Nordling M, Törring O, Hamberger B, et al. Graves' disease: a long-term quality-of-life follow up of patients randomized to treatment with antithyroid drugs, radioiodine, or surgery. *Thyroid* 2005; **15**(11): 1279–86.
55. Törring O, Tallstedt L, Wallin G, et al. Graves' hyperthyroidism: treatment with antithyroid drugs, surgery, or radioiodine – a prospective, randomized study. Thyroid Study Group. *J Clin Endocrinol Metab* 1996; **81**(8): 2986–93.
56. Ljunggren JG, Törring O, Wallin G, et al. Quality of life aspects and costs in treatment of Graves' hyperthyroidism with antithyroid drugs, surgery, or radioiodine: results from a prospective, randomized study. *Thyroid* 1998; **8**(8): 653–9.
57. Franklyn JA, Boelaert K. Thyrotoxicosis. *Lancet* 2012; **379**(9821): 1155–66.
58. Boelaert K, Maisonneuve P, Torlinska B, Franklyn JA. Comparison of mortality in hyperthyroidism during periods of treatment with thionamides and after radioiodine. *J Clin Endocrinol Metab* 2013; **98**(5): 1869–82.
59. Read CH, Tansey MJ, Menda Y. A 36-year retrospective analysis of the efficacy and safety of radioactive iodine in treating young Graves' patients. *J Clin Endocrinol Metab* 2004; **89**(9): 4229–33.
60. Ron E, Doody MM, Becker DV, et al. Cancer mortality following treatment for adult hyperthyroidism. Cooperative Thyrotoxicosis Therapy Follow-up Study Group. *JAMA* 1998; **280**(4): 347–55.
61. Essi R, Saara M, Pia J, et al. Cancer incidence and mortality in patients treated with RAI or thyroidectomy for hyperthyroidism: a nation-wide cohort study with a long-term follow-up. *J Clin Endocrinol Metab* 2015; jc20151874.
62. Humar M, Dohrmann H, Stein P, et al. Thionamides inhibit the transcription factor nuclear factor-kappaB by suppression of Rac1 and inhibitor of kappaB kinase alpha. *J Pharmacol Exp Ther* 2008; **324**(3): 1037–44.
63. Nicholas WC, Fischer RG, Stevenson RA, Bass JD. Single daily dose of methimazole compared to every 8 hours propylthiouracil in the treatment of hyperthyroidism. *South Med J* 1995; **88**(9): 973–6.
64. Bahn RS, Burch HS, Cooper DS, et al. The role of propylthiouracil in the management of Graves' disease in adults: report of a meeting jointly sponsored by the American Thyroid Association and the Food and Drug Administration. *Thyroid* 2009; **19**(7): 673–4.
65. Vanderpump MP, Ahlquist JA, Franklyn JA, Clayton RN. Consensus statement for good practice and audit measures in the management of hypothyroidism and hyperthyroidism. The Research Unit of the Royal College of Physicians of London, the Endocrinology and Diabetes Committee of the Royal College of Physicians o. *BMJ* 1996; **313**(7056): 539–44.
66. Hedley AJ, Young RE, Jones SJ, et al. Antithyroid drugs in the treatment of hyperthyroidism of Graves' disease: long-term follow-up of 434 patients. Scottish Automated Follow-Up Register Group. *Clin Endocrinol* 1989; **31**(2): 209–18.
67. Tajiri J, Noguchi S. Antithyroid drug-induced agranulocytosis: special reference to normal white blood cell count agranulocytosis. *Thyroid* 2004; **14**(6): 459–62.
68. Gunton JE, Stiel J, Clifton-Bligh P, et al. Prevalence of positive anti-neutrophil cytoplasmic antibody (ANCA) in patients receiving anti-thyroid medication. *Eur J Endocrinol* 2000; **142**(6): 587.
69. Heidari R, Niknahad H, Jamshidzadeh A, et al. An overview on the proposed mechanisms of antithyroid drugs-induced liver injury. *Adv Pharm Bull* 2015; **5**(1): 1–11.
70. US Food and Drug Administration. Postmarket drug safety information for patients and providers. *FDA drug safety communication: new boxed warning on severe liver injury with propylthiouracil*. Available from: http://www.fda.gov/Drugs/DrugSafety/PostmarketDrugSafetyInformationforPatientsandProviders/ucm209023.htm [Accessed June 22, 2017].
71. Allannic H, Fauchet R, Orgiazzi J, et al. Antithyroid drugs and Graves' disease: a prospective randomized evaluation of the efficacy of treatment duration. *J Clin Endocrinol Metab* 1990; **70**(3): 675–9.
72. Maugendre D, Gatel A, Campion L, et al. Antithyroid drugs and Graves' disease – prospective randomized assessment of long-term treatment. *Clin Endocrinol* 1999; **50**(1): 127–32.
73. Allahabadia A, Daykin J, Holder RL, et al. Age and gender predict the outcome of treatment for Graves' hyperthyroidism. *J Clin Endocrinol Metab* 2000; **85**(3): 1038–42.
74. Laurberg P, Buchholtz Hansen PE, et al. Goitre size and outcome of medical treatment of Graves' disease. *Acta Endocrinol* 1986; **111**(1): 39–43.
75. Abraham P, Avenell A, Watson WA, et al. Antithyroid drug regimen for treating Graves' hyperthyroidism. *Cochrane Database Syst Rev* 2005; (2): CD003420.
76. Vaidya B, Wright A, Shuttleworth J, et al. Block & replace regime versus titration regime of antithyroid drugs for the treatment of Graves' disease: a retrospective observational study. *Clin Endocrinol* 2014; **81**(4): 610–13.
77. Lubitz SA, Yin X, Rienstra M, Schnabel RB, et al. Long-term outcomes of secondary atrial fibrillation in the community: the Framingham Heart Study. *Circulation* 2015; **131**(19): 1648–55.
78. Allahabadia A, Daykin J, Sheppard MC, et al. Radioiodine treatment of hyperthyroidism: prognostic factors for outcome. *J Clin Endocrinol Metab* 2001; **86**(8): 3611–17.
79. Vaidya B, Williams GR, Abraham P, Pearce SHS. Radioiodine treatment for benign thyroid diseases: results of a nationwide survey of UK endocrinologists. *Clin Endocrinol* 2008; **68**(5): 814–20.
80. Ross DS. Radioiodine therapy for hyperthyroidism. *N Engl J Med* 2011; **364**(6): 542–50.
81. Bockisch A, Jamitzky T, Derwanz R, Biersack HJ. Optimized dose planning of radioiodine therapy of benign thyroidal diseases. *J Nucl Med* 1993; **34**(10): 1632–8.
82. Tamagna EI, Levine GA, Hershman JM. Thyroid-hormone concentrations after radioiodine therapy for hyperthyroidism. *J Nucl Med* 1979; **20**(5): 387–91.
83. Imseis RE, Vanmiddlesworth L, Massie JD, et al. Pretreatment with propylthiouracil but not methimazole reduces the therapeutic efficacy of iodine-131 in hyperthyroidism. *J Clin Endocrinol Metab* 1998; **83**(2): 685–7.
84. Koroscil TM. Thionamides alter the efficacy of radioiodine treatment in patients with Graves' disease. *South Med J* 1995; **88**(8): 831–6.
85. Sabri O, Zimny M, Schulz G, et al. Success rate of radioiodine therapy in Graves' disease: the influence of thyrostatic medication. *J Clin Endocrinol Metab* 1999; **84**(4): 1229–33.
86. Isgoren S, Daglioz Gorur G, Demir H, Berk F. Radioiodine therapy in Graves' disease: is it possible to predict outcome before therapy? *Nucl Med Commun* 2012; **33**(8): 859–63.
87. Franklyn JA, Maisonneuve P, Sheppard M, et al. Cancer incidence and mortality after radioiodine treatment for hyperthyroidism: a population-based cohort study. *Lancet* 1999; **353**(9170): 2111–15.
88. Hall P, Lundell G, Holm LE. Mortality in patients treated for hyperthyroidism with iodine-131. *Acta Endocrinol* 1993; **128**(3): 230–4.
89. Nwatsock JF, Taieb D, Tessonnier L, et al. Radioiodine thyroid ablation in Graves' hyperthyroidism: merits and pitfalls. *World J Nucl Med* 2012; **11**(1): 7–11.
90. Royal College of Physicians. *Radioiodine in the management of benign thyroid disease: clinical guidelines. Report of a Working Party 2007.* Available at: https://shop.rcplondon.ac.uk/products/radioiodine-in-the-management-of-benign-thyroid-disease-clincial-guidelines?variant=6637100933 [Accessed June 22, 2017].
91. Acharya SH, Avenell A, Philip S, et al. Radioiodine therapy (RAI) for Graves' disease (GD) and the effect on ophthalmopathy: a systematic review. *Clin Endocrinol* 2008; **69**(6): 943–50.
92. Bahn Chair RS, Burch HB, Cooper DS, et al. Hyperthyroidism and other causes of thyrotoxicosis: management guidelines of the American Thyroid Association and American Association of Clinical Endocrinologists. *Thyroid* 2011; **21**(6): 593–646.
93. Bartalena L, Baldeschi L, Dickinson AJ, et al. Consensus statement of the European group on Graves' orbitopathy (EUGOGO) on management of Graves' orbitopathy. *Thyroid* 2008; **18**(3): 333–46.
94. Alsanea O, Clark OH. Treatment of Graves' disease: the advantages of surgery. *Endocrinol Metab Clin North Am* 2000; **29**(2): 321–37.
95. Sosa JA, Bowman HM, Tielsch JM, et al. The importance of surgeon experience for clinical and economic outcomes from thyroidectomy. *Ann Surg* 1998; **228**(3): 320–30.
96. Parle J V, Franklyn JA, Cross KW, et al. Thyroxine prescription in the community: serum thyroid stimulating hormone level assays as an indicator of undertreatment or overtreatment. *Br J Gen Pract* 1993; **43**(368): 107–9.
97. Parle J V, Maisonneuve P, Sheppard MC, et al. Prediction of all-cause and cardiovascular mortality in elderly people from one low serum thyrotropin result: a 10-year cohort study. *Lancet* 2001; **358**(9285): 861–5.

98. Sawin CT, Geller A, Wolf PA, et al. Low serum thyrotropin concentrations as a risk factor for atrial fibrillation in older persons. *N Engl J Med* 1994; **331**(19): 1249–52.
99. Faber J, Galløe AM. Changes in bone mass during prolonged subclinical hyperthyroidism due to L-thyroxine treatment: a meta-analysis. *Eur J Endocrinol* 1994; **130**(4): 350–6.
100. Uzzan B, Campos J, Cucherat M, et al. Effects on bone mass of long-term treatment with thyroid hormones: a meta-analysis. *J Clin Endocrinol Metab* 1996; **81**(12): 4278–89.
101. Fatourechi V. Adverse effects of subclinical hyperthyroidism. *Lancet* 2001; **358**(9285): 856–7.
102. Surks MI, Ortiz E, Daniels GH, et al. Subclinical thyroid disease: scientific review and guidelines for diagnosis and management. *JAMA* 2004; **291**(2): 228–38.
103. Fatourechi V, Aniszewski JP, Fatourechi GZE, et al. Clinical features and outcome of subacute thyroiditis in an incidence cohort: Olmsted County, Minnesota, study. *J Clin Endocrinol Metab* 2003; **88**(5): 2100–5.
104. Pearce EN, Bogazzi F, Martino E, et al. The prevalence of elevated serum C-reactive protein levels in inflammatory and noninflammatory thyroid disease. *Thyroid* 2003; **13**(7): 643–8.
105. Volpé R. The management of subacute (De Quervain's) thyroiditis. *Thyroid* 1993; **3**(3): 253–5.
106. Desailloud R, Hober D. Viruses and thyroiditis: an update. *Virol J* 2009; **6**: 5.
107. Reinhardt W, Luster M, Rudorff KH, et al. Effect of small doses of iodine on thyroid function in patients with Hashimoto's thyroiditis residing in an area of mild iodine deficiency. *Eur J Endocrinol* 1998; **139**(1): 23–8.
108. Bogazzi F, Tomisti L, Bartalena L, et al. Amiodarone and the thyroid: a 2012 update. *J Endocrinol Invest* 2012; **35**(3): 340–8.
109. Roberts CGP, Ladenson PW. Hypothyroidism. *Lancet* 2004; **363**(9411): 793–803.
110. Vanderpump MPJ, Tunbridge WMG. Epidemiology and prevention of clinical and subclinical hypothyroidism. *Thyroid* 2002; **12**(10): 839–47.
111. Zimmerman RS, Brennan MD, McConahey WM, et al. Hashimoto's thyroiditis: an uncommon cause of painful thyroid unresponsive to corticosteroid therapy. *Ann Intern Med* 1986; **104**(3): 355–7.
112. Neufeld M, Maclaren NK, Blizzard RM. Two types of autoimmune Addison's disease associated with different polyglandular autoimmune (PGA) syndromes. *Medicine (Baltimore)* 1981; **60**(5): 355–62.
113. Hancock SL, Cox RS, McDougall IR. Thyroid diseases after treatment of Hodgkin's disease. *N Engl J Med* 1991; **325**(9): 599–605.
114. Delange F, de Benoist B, Pretell E, Dunn JT. Iodine deficiency in the world: where do we stand at the turn of the century? *Thyroid* 2001; **11**(5): 437–47.
115. Devdhar M, Ousman YH, Burman KD. Hypothyroidism. *Endocrinol Metab Clin North Am* 2007; **36**(3): 595–615, v.
116. Caturegli P, De Remigis A, Rose NR. Hashimoto thyroiditis: clinical and diagnostic criteria. *Autoimmun Rev* 2014; **13**(4–5): 391–7.
117. Pyzik A, Grywalska E, Matyjaszek-Matuszek B, Roliński J. Immune disorders in Hashimoto's thyroiditis: what do we know so far? *J Immunol Res* 2015; **2015**: 979167.
118. Nearchou A, Valachis A, Lind P, et al. Acquired hypothyroidism as a predictive marker of outcome in patients with metastatic renal cell carcinoma treated with tyrosine kinase inhibitors: a literature-based meta-analysis. *Clin Genitourin Cancer* 2015; **13**(4): 280–6.
119. Abdel-Rahman O, Fouad M. Risk of thyroid dysfunction in patients with solid tumors treated with VEGF receptor tyrosine kinase inhibitors: a critical literature review and meta analysis. *Expert Rev Anticancer Ther* 2014; **14**(9): 1063–73.
120. Fallahi P, Ferrari SM, Vita R, et al. Thyroid dysfunctions induced by tyrosine kinase inhibitors. *Expert Opin Drug Saf* 2014; **13**(6): 723–33.
121. Bougma K, Aboud FE, Harding KB, Marquis GS. Iodine and mental development of children 5 years old and under: a systematic review and meta-analysis. *Nutrients* 2013; **5**(4): 1384–416.
122. Rose SR. Cranial irradiation and central hypothyroidism. *Trends Endocrinol Metab* 2001; **12**(3): 97–104.
123. Toft AD. Thyroxine therapy. *N Engl J Med* 1994; **331**(3): 174–80.
124. Okosieme O, Gilbert J, Abraham P, et al. Management of primary hypothyroidism: statement by the British Thyroid Association Executive Committee. *Clin Endocrinol* 2016; **84**(6): 799–808.
125. Chan S, Boelaert K. Optimal management of hypothyroidism, hypothyroxinaemia and euthyroid TPO antibody positivity preconception and in pregnancy. *Clin Endocrinol* 2015; **82**(3): 313–26.
126. De Groot L, Abalovich M, Alexander EK, et al. Management of thyroid dysfunction during pregnancy and postpartum: an Endocrine Society clinical practice guideline. *J Clin Endocrinol Metab* 2012; **97**(8): 2543–65.
127. Bunevicius R, Kazanavicius G, Zalinkevicius R, Prange AJ. Effects of thyroxine as compared with thyroxine plus triiodothyronine in patients with hypothyroidism. *N Engl J Med* 1999; **340**(6): 424–9.
128. Walsh JP, Ward LC, Burke V, et al. Small changes in thyroxine dosage do not produce measurable changes in hypothyroid symptoms, well-being, or quality of life: results of a double-blind, randomized clinical trial. *J Clin Endocrinol Metab* 2006; **91**(7): 2624–30.
129. Clyde PW, Harari AE, Getka EJ, Shakir KMM. Combined levothyroxine plus liothyronine compared with levothyroxine alone in primary hypothyroidism: a randomized controlled trial. *JAMA* 2003; **290**(22): 2952–8.
130. Boelaert K, Franklyn JA. Thyroid hormone in health and disease. *J Endocrinol* 2005; **187**(1): 1–15.
131. Rosenthal MJ, Hunt WC, Garry PJ, Goodwin JS. Thyroid failure in the elderly. Microsomal antibodies as discriminant for therapy. *JAMA* 1987; **258**(2): 209–13.
132. Biondi B. Natural history, diagnosis and management of subclinical thyroid dysfunction. *Best Pract Res Clin Endocrinol Metab* 2012; **26**(4): 431–46.
133. Sack J. Thyroid function in pregnancy: maternal-fetal relationship in health and disease. *Pediatr Endocrinol Rev* 2003; **1 Suppl 2**: 170–6; discussion 176.
134. Cooper DS, Laurberg P. Hyperthyroidism in pregnancy. *Lancet Diabetes Endocrinol* 2013; **1**(3): 238–49.
135. Stagnaro-Green A, Abalovich M, Alexander E, et al. Guidelines of the American Thyroid Association for the diagnosis and management of thyroid disease during pregnancy and postpartum. *Thyroid* 2011; **21**(10): 1081–125.
136. Lazarus J, Brown RS, Daumerie C, et al. 2014 European Thyroid Association guidelines for the management of subclinical hypothyroidism in pregnancy and in children. *Eur Thyroid J* 2014; **3**(2): 76–94.
137. Velkeniers B, Van Meerhaeghe A, Poppe K, et al. Levothyroxine treatment and pregnancy outcome in women with subclinical hypothyroidism undergoing assisted reproduction technologies: systematic review and meta-analysis of RCTs. *Hum Reprod Update* 2013; **19**(3): 251–8.
138. Haddow JE, Palomaki GE, Allan WC, et al. Maternal thyroid deficiency during pregnancy and subsequent neuropsychological development of the child. *N Engl J Med* 1999; **341**(8): 549–55.
139. Pop VJ, de Vries E, van Baar AL, et al. Maternal thyroid peroxidase antibodies during pregnancy: a marker of impaired child development? *J Clin Endocrinol Metab* 1995; **80**(12): 3561–6.
140. Pop VJ, Kuijpens JL, van Baar AL, et al. Low maternal free thyroxine concentrations during early pregnancy are associated with impaired psychomotor development in infancy. *Clin Endocrinol* 1999; **50**(2): 149–55.
141. Pop VJ, Brouwers EP, Vader HL, et al. Maternal hypothyroxinaemia during early pregnancy and subsequent child development: a 3-year follow-up study. *Clin Endocrinol* 2003; **59**(3): 282–8.
142. Vander JB, Gaston EA, Dawber TR. The significance of nontoxic thyroid nodules. Final report of a 15-year study of the incidence of thyroid malignancy. *Ann Intern Med* 1968; **69**(3): 537–40.
143. Völzke H, Lüdemann J, Robinson DM, et al. The prevalence of undiagnosed thyroid disorders in a previously iodine-deficient area. *Thyroid* 2003; **13**(8): 803–10.
144. Völzke H, Ittermann T, Albers M, et al. Five-year change in morphological and functional alterations of the thyroid gland: the study of health in Pomerania. *Thyroid* 2012; **22**(7): 737–46.
145. Sherman SI. Thyroid carcinoma. *Lancet* 2003; **361**(9356): 501–11.
146. Schneider AB, Ron E. Carcinoma of the follicular epithelium: epidemiology and pathogenesis. In: Braverman LE, Utiger RD (eds). *The thyroid: a fundamental and clinical text*. 9th ed. Philadelphia: Lippincott, Williams & Wilkins; 2005, pp. 889–906.
147. Marcello MA, Malandrino P, Almeida JFM, et al. The influence of the environment on the development of thyroid tumors: a new appraisal. *Endocr Relat Cancer* 2014; **21**(5): T235–54.
148. Nagataki S, Takamura N. A review of the Fukushima nuclear reactor accident: radiation effects on the thyroid and strategies for prevention. *Curr Opin Endocrinol Diabetes Obes* 2014; **21**(5): 384–93.

149. Hegedüs L. Clinical practice: the thyroid nodule. *N Engl J Med* 2004; **351**(17): 1764–71.
150. La Vecchia C, Malvezzi M, Bosetti C, et al. Thyroid cancer mortality and incidence: a global overview. *Int J Cancer* 2015; **136**(9): 2187–95.
151. Gittoes NJ, Miller MR, Daykin J, et al. Upper airways obstruction in 153 consecutive patients presenting with thyroid enlargement. *BMJ* 1996; **312**(7029): 484.
152. Perros P, Boelaert K, Colley S, et al. Guidelines for the management of thyroid cancer. *Clin Endocrinol* 2014; **81** Suppl 1: 1–122.
153. Cooper DS, Doherty GM, Haugen BR, et al. Revised American Thyroid Association management guidelines for patients with thyroid nodules and differentiated thyroid cancer. *Thyroid* 2009; **19**(11): 1167–214.
154. Boelaert K, Horacek J, Holder RL, et al. Serum thyrotropin concentration as a novel predictor of malignancy in thyroid nodules investigated by fine-needle aspiration. *J Clin Endocrinol Metab* 2006; **91**(11): 4295–301.
155. Haymart MR, Repplinger DJ, Leverson GE, et al. Higher serum thyroid-stimulating hormone level in thyroid nodule patients is associated with greater risks of differentiated thyroid cancer and advanced tumor stage. *J Clin Endocrinol Metab* 2008; **93**(3): 809–14.
156. McLeod DSA, Watters KF, Carpenter AD, et al. Thyrotropin and thyroid cancer diagnosis: a systematic review and dose-response meta-analysis. *J Clin Endocrinol Metab* 2012; **97**(8): 2682–92.
157. Grogan RH, Mitmaker EJ, Clark OH. The evolution of biomarkers in thyroid cancer: from mass screening to a personalized biosignature. *Cancers (Basel)* 2010; **2**(2): 885–912.
158. Bennedbaek FN, Perrild H, Hegedüs L. Diagnosis and treatment of the solitary thyroid nodule: results of a European survey. *Clin Endocrinol* 1999; **50**(3): 357–63.
159. Frates MC, Benson CB, Charboneau JW, et al. Management of thyroid nodules detected at US: Society of Radiologists in ultrasound consensus conference statement. *Radiology* 2005; **237**(3): 794–800.
160. Lee YH, Kim DW, In HS, et al. Differentiation between benign and malignant solid thyroid nodules using an US classification system. *Korean J Radiol* 2011; **12**(5): 559–67.
161. Rago T, Santini F, Scutari M, et al. Elastography: new developments in ultrasound for predicting malignancy in thyroid nodules. *J Clin Endocrinol Metab* 2007; **92**(8): 2917–22.
162. Bojunga J, Herrmann E, Meyer G, et al. Real-time elastography for the differentiation of benign and malignant thyroid nodules: a meta-analysis. *Thyroid* 2010; **20**(10): 1145–50.
163. Agrawal K, Esmail AAH, Gnanasegaran G, et al. Pitfalls and limitations of radionuclide imaging in endocrinology. *Semin Nucl Med* 2015; **45**(5): 440–57.
164. Hoang JK, Branstetter BF, Gafton AR, et al. Imaging of thyroid carcinoma with CT and MRI: approaches to common scenarios. *Cancer Imaging* 2013; **13**: 128–39.
165. Agrawal K, Weaver J, Ngu R, Krishnamurthy Mohan H. Clinical significance of patterns of incidental thyroid uptake at (18)F-FDG PET/CT. *Clin Radiol* 2015; **70**(5): 536–43.
166. Shie P, Cardarelli R, Sprawls K, et al. Systematic review: prevalence of malignant incidental thyroid nodules identified on fluorine-18 fluorodeoxyglucose positron emission tomography. *Nucl Med Commun* 2009; **30**(9): 742–8.
167. Haugen BR, Alexander EK, Bible KC, et al. 2015 American Thyroid Association management guidelines for adult patients with thyroid nodules and differentiated thyroid cancer: The American Thyroid Association Guidelines Task Force on Thyroid Nodules and Differentiated Thyroid Cancer. *Thyroid* 2016; **26**(1): 1–133.
168. Bernet V, Hupart KH, Parangi S, Woeber KA. AACE/ACE disease state commentary: molecular diagnostic testing of thyroid nodules with indeterminate cytopathology. *Endocr Pract* 2014; **20**(4): 360–3.
169. Gharib H. Changing concepts in the diagnosis and management of thyroid nodules. *Endocrinol Metab Clin North Am* 1997; **26**(4): 777–800.
170. Huysmans DA, Hermus AR, Corstens FH, et al. Large, compressive goiters treated with radioiodine. *Ann Intern Med* 1994; **121**(10): 757–62.
171. Huysmans DA, Nieuwlaat WA, Erdtsieck RJ, et al. Administration of a single low dose of recombinant human thyrotropin significantly enhances thyroid radioiodide uptake in nontoxic nodular goiter. *J Clin Endocrinol Metab* 2000; **85**(10): 3592–6.
172. Bonnema SJ, Hegedüs L. Radioiodine therapy in benign thyroid diseases: effects, side effects, and factors affecting therapeutic outcome. *Endocr Rev* 2012; **33**(6): 920–80.
173. Lawrence W, Kaplan BJ. Diagnosis and management of patients with thyroid nodules. *J Surg Oncol* 2002; **80**(3): 157–70.
174. Baskin HJ, Duick DS. The endocrinologists' view of ultrasound guidelines for fine-needle aspiration. *Thyroid* 2006; **16**(3): 207–8.

CHAPTER 62

MANAGEMENT OF DIFFERENTIATED THYROID CANCER

Hisham M. Mehanna, Kristien Boelaert and Neil Sharma

Introduction 751	Assessment of the outcomes of treatment 754
Investigations 751	Follow-up 754
Treatment 752	References 756

SEARCH STRATEGY

Data in this chapter may be updated by a Medline search using the keywords: thyroid, cancer, carcinoma, management, radioiodine, as well as published guidelines from the British and American Thyroid Associations. Reference lists for selected papers were examined for further sources.

INTRODUCTION

The prognosis of differentiated thyroid cancer (DTC) is excellent for most patients. Patients with Stage I–Stage III disease have a 10-year survival rate of over 98%,[1] but the survival rate drops dramatically for patients with Stage IV disease, especially when gross local invasion or distant metastases are present in patients older than 45 years.

The management of DTC is mainly surgical, with adjuvant radioiodine ablation followed by TSH suppression in some cases. In the past almost all patients received similar treatment with a combination of all three therapeutic modalities. Over the past 5–10 years, however, a more personalized approach to treatment has been introduced. This tailors the specific treatment that a patient receives according to their individual requirements and risk of recurrence. The type and size of their tumour and the presence or absence of aggressive features such as lymph node metastases or aggressive histological features mainly determine stratified treatment. This change in treatment paradigms has also recently extended to the stratification of risk of recurrence following the completion of treatment, leading to variable follow-up requirements.

INVESTIGATIONS

The investigation of a patient with suspected thyroid cancer[1,2] has been covered appropriately in Chapter 59.

Briefly, this includes a detailed clinical history, which should in particular elicit a family history of thyroid cancer, previous neck irradiation and a history of Hashimoto's disease (predisposing to lymphoma). The diagnosis will have been obtained using a combination of high-resolution ultrasound scan (USS) and fine-needle aspiration cytology in most cases. Once thyroid cancer is diagnosed, ideally the extent of the disease should be further staged to assess tumour size, invasion of important central structures such as trachea and oesophagus, and the presence of nodal metastases and/or distant metastases (**Table 62.1**). This is undertaken using a combination of ultrasound of the neck, CT and/or MRI.

Use of iodinated contrast for CT scanning will impose some restrictions on the use of ablative radioiodine within 2 months of the scan due to the high concentration of iodinated contrast taken up by the thyroid, which may diminish the effectiveness of radioiodine.[1,2] However, this is usually not a problem because the treatment period will include surgery and recovery from this in the first instance and in view of more recent evidence indicating that the clearance period for iodine in both thyroidectomized and euthyroid patients is only 4 weeks.[3] Importantly, subjects requiring radioiodine ablation are frequently intermediate-risk patients, in whom a small delay in this treatment will have little effect on outcome. Those patients with more aggressive thyroid cancer tend to have non-iodine avid disease or iodine-refractory disease in which case a

TABLE 62.1 TNM classification of thyroid cancer[38]

Primary tumour	
Tx	Primary tumour cannot be assessed
T0	No evidence of primary tumour
T1	Tumour ≤2 cm in greatest dimension limited to the thyroid
T1a	Tumour ≤1 cm, limited to the thyroid
T1b	Tumour >1 cm but ≤2 cm in greatest dimension, limited to the thyroid
T2	Tumour >2 cm but ≤4 cm in greatest dimension, limited to the thyroid
T3	Tumour > 4 cm limited to the thyroid, or gross extrathyroidal extension invading only strap muscles
T3a	Tumour > 4 cm limited to the thyroid
T3b	Gross extrathyroidal extension invading only strap muscles (sternohyoid, sternothyroid, thyrohyoid, or omohyoid muscles) from a tumour of any size
T4a	Tumour of any size extending beyond the thyroid capsule to invade subcutaneous soft tissues, larynx, trachea, oesophagus or recurrent laryngeal nerve
T4b	Tumour invades prevertebral fascia or encases carotid artery or mediastinal vessels
Regional lymph nodes (cervical or upper mediastinal)	
Nx	Regional lymph nodes cannot be assessed
N0	No regional lymph node metastasis
N1	Regional lymph node metastasis
N1a	Metastases to Level 6/7 nodes unilateral or bilateral
N1b	Metastases to unilateral, bilateral or contralateral cervical (Levels 1, 2, 3, 4 or 5) or retropharyngeal nodes
Distant metastases	
M0	No distant metastases
M1	Distant metastases
Residual tumour	
RX	Cannot assess presence of residual primary tumour
R0	No residual primary tumour
R1	Microscopic residual primary tumour
R2	Macroscopic residual primary tumour

Note: TNM: tumour, node, metastasis.

delay in receiving radioiodine ablation is significant only in that it can increase time to other adjuvant modalities such as external beam radiotherapy.

TREATMENT

Over the past decade, a more evidenced-based approach to treatment and follow-up has been espoused by both the American Thyroid Association[2] and the British Thyroid Association.[1] This has resulted in the concept of treatment planning tailored to patients' individual needs. The introduction of personalized medicine has also extended to the need for and duration of TSH suppression as well as to follow-up strategies. Where there is no evidence or conflicting evidence, an open and frank approach with the patient is now recommended so that a full discussion of the potential benefits and risks of adjuvant treatment can be undertaken, leading to shared decision-making.

An assessment of both patient and tumour factors before and after surgery helps determine the extent of the thyroidectomy, the need for neck dissection, the need for radioiodine ablation and the requirement for post-treatment TSH suppression. In addition, the intensity of follow-up the patient requires can be predicted.

Extent of thyroidectomy

Thyroidectomy is the mainstay of treatment for thyroid cancers. In recent years there has been a move towards the more conservative hemithyroidectomy rather than total thyroidectomy. This has coincided with a decrease in the indications for radioiodine ablation. Generally speaking, for DTC, a total thyroidectomy is recommended for patients with tumours >4 cm in size and for patients with tumours where there is multifocal disease, bilateral disease, extrathyroidal spread or confirmed nodal or distant metastases. Additional factors that may warrant bilateral surgery are older age (>55 years), a history of radiation exposure, familial differentiated thyroid cancer, adverse histopathological features and potential difficulties with follow-up.[4]

The evidence for doing a total thyroidectomy rather than a hemithyroidectomy for patients with low-risk papillary thyroid cancer (PTC) of <4 cm with no poor prognostic features is equivocal and conflicting. Careful review of the data indicates that, while there is a decreased risk of recurrence with total thyroidectomy, and while in the long term this may be a more cost-effective approach, the difference is small when compared with more limited surgery.[5–7] In these cases one should have a discussion with the patient regarding the benefits and risks of total thyroidectomy vs. hemithyroidectomy.

Patients with follicular thyroid cancer associated with any of the above poor prognostic features should be advised to undergo a total thyroidectomy.

If tumour is found during the operation to be encasing the recurrent laryngeal nerve (RLN), the clinician should aim to preserve the nerve if it was functioning preoperatively. This may mean a small amount of disease is left on the nerve but this is acceptable in view of the functional detriments of vocal cord palsy, the gain in quality of life and, importantly, the fact that there is no survival benefit to be gained from nerve sacrifice.[8]

Pre-operatively, one should assess the trachea and the oesophagus radiologically, to identify the need for partial tracheal or oesophageal resection in order to achieve macroscopic tumour clearance. This is important because, unlike for RLN involvement, residual disease left at these sites leads to a significant decrease in survival.[9] Furthermore, careful pre-operative assessment allows determination of the need for input from a cardiothoracic surgeon.

Treatment of papillary thyroid microcarcinoma

Papillary thyroid microcarcinoma (PTMC) is defined as a tumour no greater than 1 cm in maximum diameter. In general this has an excellent prognosis with almost no mortality. A recent meta-analysis,[10] however, indicated that there are at least two types of PTMC those found incidentally during histological evaluation postoperatively and those that are identified pre-operatively, either incidentally during radiological investigation or because they caused symptoms. Those patients who are diagnosed incidentally on histology have no mortality and almost no recurrence risk and therefore can be considered as cured and can be discharged to their GP. They should, however, undergo annual thyroid function test monitoring since hemithyroidectomy carries a medium- to long-term risk of hypothyroidism.

Those patients with lesions that were identified radiologically may have a slightly higher risk of recurrence. If there are no poor prognostic features (such as aggressive histology, extracapsular spread or lymph node metastasis), these patients can be followed up for 5 years in the same manner as patients with low-risk DTC and then be discharged to a lower-intensity setting. Any patient who has PTMC with aggressive features should be managed in the same way as a patient with non-low risk papillary thyroid cancer.

Neck dissection

There is no evidence of benefit from doing a prophylactic lateral neck dissection in patients with no overt lateral neck disease.[2] The evidence for potential benefits from prophylactic central neck dissection is unclear and conflicting, with some studies indicating improved outcomes[10, 11] while others do not.[12] In addition, some studies show no additional complications from central neck dissection, whereas others have shown that there is considerable added morbidity.[13–16] There is a suggestion, however, that central neck dissection may be of benefit in tumours >4 cm in size and in tumours with extrathyroidal extension, but the evidence is unclear. Prophylactic central neck dissection is not recommended in patients who have low-risk disease, or have tumours <4 cm in size with classical PTC and no extrathyroidal extension.

Once surgery is completed, TSH suppression should be undertaken with either thyroxine T4 (2 mcg/kg) or with Liothyronine (20 mcg t.d.s.) until the histopathology is available, and a decision can be made as to the need for adjuvant treatment.

Radioiodine ablation

Of all the treatments for thyroid cancer, the practice of radioiodine ablation has undergone the most radical change in recent years. The evidence of the American Thyroid Association Guidelines in 2009 heralded personalized evaluation and decision-making for radioiodine ablation, a decision that should be made at the multidisciplinary team discussion following surgical resection. For radioiodine ablation to be effective, a total thyroidectomy is required, and therefore patients who have had a hemithyroidectomy require a completion thyroidectomy prior to consideration of this treatment.

The benefits of radioiodine ablation have to be weighed carefully against the potential side effects. Positive effects include the possibility of improved survival, reduced recurrence and better monitoring with thyroglobulin in the long term. The downsides, however, include the inconvenience of being in an isolation ward and the requirement not to come into contact with adults and children for 14–25 days following radioiodine ablation. For younger female patients, the implications on pregnancy and breastfeeding must also be considered. Amenorrhoea/oligomenorrhea may occur for 4–10 months following radioiodine ablation, as the gonadal tissue is exposed to radiation via blood and excretion in urine and faeces. Current recommendations are to defer pregnancy for 6 months (BTA guidelines[1]) or 6–12 months (ATA guidelines[2]) following radioiodine treatment. Breastfeeding should be discontinued at least 8 weeks prior to radioiodine administration to prevent excessive uptake by lactating breast tissue.[1] Male patients are advised to defer fathering a child for 4 months following treatment.[1]

Patients also sometimes complain of dryness of the mouth, swelling of the submandibular glands and feeling tired soon after the treatment. Xerostomia can increase with time. Finally, sperm banking is often offered to men, as infertility is possible.

Patients in whom radioiodine is indicated include those patients with tumours >4 cm or with gross extrathyroidal spread or distant metastasis. These patients will receive an ablative dose of radioiodine followed by a treatment dose. Patients for whom radioiodine is not indicated include those who have unifocal or multifocal tumours <1 cm in size which are histologically classed as papillary or follicular variant, or minimally invasive follicular cancer, with no angioinvasion or extension outside the thyroid capsule.

The difficulty arises in the group of patients who have intermediate features, as data regarding the benefits of radioiodine ablation are sparse. These include patients with tumours 1–4 cm in size. Those patients who have poorer prognostic features could be offered radioiodine ablation. The poor prognostic features include aggressive histology (tall cell or poorly differentiated or diffuse sclerosing PTC), widely invasive follicular thyroid cancer, extracapsular invasion, multiple involved lymph nodes or a high ratio of involved to non-involved nodes and large size of individual nodes that are involved.

Recently, two large randomized controlled trials (RCTs) have shown that a lower dose of 1.1 Mbq is as effective as a higher dose of 3.7 Gbq. The lower dose, however, had fewer side effects.[17, 18] Patients have to be prepared for radioiodine ablation by either recombinant TSH injection 5 days before treatment or by Levothyroxine withdrawal, which is more prolonged and has greater side effects. An iodine scan is undertaken 2–10 days after the treatment. This allows assessment of radioiodine uptake and whether uptake has occurred in areas outside the neck.

High treatment doses of radioiodine are recommended in patients who have gross residual disease or distant metastases. These patients may require repeat treatments every 6–12 months, especially those with disease not amenable to surgery.

Further details on radioiodine treatment are provided in Chapter 66.

External beam radiotherapy

Patients with gross evidence of local tumour invasion at surgery are candidates for external beam radiotherapy (EBRT), as are those with residual or recurrent tumour that is non-radioiodine avid. Intensity-modulated radiotherapy (IMRT) is the method of choice as it reduces damage to other surrounding tissues[19] and reduces toxicity. There is no clear-cut evidence as to the best timing of EBRT in relation to radioiodine remnant ablation. Detailed information on EBRT is provided in Chapter 66.

ASSESSMENT OF THE OUTCOMES OF TREATMENT

The post-radioiodine scan, carried out between 2 and 10 days after ablation, helps assess the uptake of radioiodine in the thyroid bed, as well as the extent of residual and metastatic disease. However, the main evaluation of success of treatment occurs 9–12 months afterwards. Evidence suggests that stimulated thyroglobulin measurements provide the most sensitive method of detecting recurrent or residual disease. Stimulated thyroglobulin should be undertaken along with high-definition ultrasound of the neck and thyroid gland. Together these are more accurate than undertaking a whole-body radioiodine scan.[20, 21]

An injection of recombinant TSH 9–12 months after surgery with a measurement of the thyroglobulin and thyroglobulin autoantibodies following this enables an assessment of disease activity. Stimulated thyroglobulin can also be undertaken using thyroxine withdrawal, but this causes more symptoms and takes more time.[22–24] A stimulated thyroglobulin of <0.5 mcg/L after TSH stimulation has been shown to predict disease-free status with 98–99% accuracy. A stimulated thyroglobulin of >2 mcg/L is highly predictive of persistent disease.[20, 25–28] It should be noted, however, that stimulated thyroglobulin can only be used in the absence of thyroglobulin antibodies and is most sensitive in patients who have had both total thyroidectomy and radioiodine ablation. Conversely, it can predict absence of recurrence with 95–99% accuracy.[29, 30]

An unstimulated thyroglobulin of <0.1 mcg/L in the absence of thyroglobulin antibodies and a negative USS has a very high negative predictive value in low-risk patients and can be used as a cost-effective alternative to stimulated thyroglobulin.[31–33]

CT scanning should be used only if the measurement of serum thyroglobulin is unreliable or when the post-radioiodine ablation scan shows uptake beyond the neck.

FOLLOW-UP

Dynamic risk stratification produces three groups (**Table 62.2**): those with an excellent response, those with persistent disease, and those with equivocal or indeterminate response to treatment. Patients with an excellent response are defined as those who have had surgery and radioiodine ablation and in whom the stimulated thyroglobulin is <1 mcg/L, with a negative USS. Patients who have an excellent response can undergo a less stringent follow-up regimen with annual thyroglobulin assessments. Their TSH should be maintained in the low-normal range at 0.3–2.0 mU/L (**Table 62.3**). If they are disease-free after 5 years, consideration can be given to following them up in a less intensive setting, such as a nurse-led clinic.[2, 34–37] It should be noted that the appearance of thyroglobulin antibodies when they were previously absent, or their gradual rise, may indicate evidence of recurrent disease.

Patients with an incomplete response include those with a stimulated thyroglobulin >10 mcg/L or a

TABLE 62.2 Dynamic risk stratification following treatment for thyroid cancer[1]

Response	Criteria	Risk stratification	Follow-up
Excellent	*All of the following:* Suppressed and stimulated Tg <1 mcg/L Neck USS without evidence of disease Cross-sectional and/or nuclear medicine imaging negative (if performed)	High	6-monthly for first year Annually thereafter
Indeterminate	*Any of the following:* Suppressed Tg <1 mcg/L and stimulated Tg ≥1 and <10 mcg/L Neck USS with non-specific changes or stable sub-1 cm nodes Cross-sectional and/or nuclear medicine imaging with non-specific changes, not completely normal	Intermediate	More frequently depending on individual need
Incomplete	*Any of the following:* Suppressed Tg ≥1 mcg/L or stimulated Tg ≥10 mcg/L Rising Tg values Persistent or newly identified disease on cross-sectional and/or nuclear medicine imaging	Low	Investigate and more frequently depending on individual need

TABLE 62.3 Grading of TSH suppression[1]

Response	TSH suppression (mU/L)
Excellent	0.3–2.0
Indeterminate	0.1–0.5 (for 5–10 years)
Incomplete	<0.1 (indefinitely)

rising thyroglobulin concentration. They may have a neck USS that shows recurrence. If their ultrasound is normal, then they require a CT scan or MRI. In these patients where cross-sectional imaging is negative, a PET-CT scan should be undertaken. If this is still negative, then a ^{131}I scan should be undertaken. If there is evidence of surgically resectable disease in these patients, that should be undertaken. If there is no surgically resectable disease, then further radioiodine therapy can be offered. These patients should then have TSH suppression (<0.1 mU/L) indefinitely and should undergo close follow-up.

Patients with an indeterminate or equivocal response (stimulated thyroglobulin 1–10 mcg/L with non-specific changes on neck ultrasound) should be kept under close review with serial thyroglobulin measurements and ultrasound scans to attempt to detect recurrence at an earlier stage. The TSH should be maintained in the range 0.1–0.5 mU/L for at least 5–10 years.

BEST CLINICAL PRACTICE

- ✓ For appropriately selected low-risk patients, hemithyroidectomy may be appropriate surgical management.
- ✓ A small amount of disease may be left on a functioning recurrent laryngeal nerve without compromising survival.
- ✓ Prophylactic central neck dissection should be reserved for high-risk patients.
- ✓ Lateral neck dissection should only be undertaken in patients with overt lateral neck disease.
- ✓ Dynamic risk stratification should be undertaken for all patients who have had total thyroidectomy and radioiodine ablation to guide their follow-up and further management.
- ✓ Radioiodine ablation is indicated for high-risk cases and some selected intermediate-risk cases.

FUTURE RESEARCH

- ➤ Molecular profiling of tumours as an aid to risk stratification
- ➤ Methods of identifying high-risk radioiodine-resistant tumours early to escalate treatment and reduce recurrence
- ➤ The role of the immune response in thyroid cancer and how this may influence lateral neck dissection

KEY POINTS

- Differentiated thyroid cancer is rare but has a rising global incidence.
- Thyroid cancer remains a predominantly surgical disease.
- Personalized treatment based on the patient's individual disease and recurrence risks is now the mainstay.
- Management of all patients with thyroid cancer should be discussed in the context of a multidisciplinary team.

REFERENCES

1. Perros P, Boelaert K, Colley S, et al. Guidelines for the management of thyroid cancer. *Clin Endocrinol (Oxf)* 2014; **81** Suppl 1(s1): 1–122.
2. American Thyroid Association (ATA) Guidelines Taskforce on Thyroid Nodules and Differentiated Thyroid Cancer, Cooper DS, et al. Revised American Thyroid Association management guidelines for patients with thyroid nodules and differentiated thyroid cancer. *Thyroid* 2009; **19**(11): 1167–214.
3. Ho JD, Tsang JF, Scoggan KA, Leslie WD. Urinary iodine clearance following iodinated contrast administration: a comparison of euthyroid and postthyroidectomy subjects. *J Thyroid Res* 2014; **2014**(6): 580569.
4. Haugen BR, Alexander EK, Bible KC, et al. 2015 American Thyroid Association management guidelines for adult patients with thyroid nodules and differentiated thyroid cancer. *Thyroid* 2016; **26**(1): 1–133.
5. Nixon IJ, Ganly I, Patel SG, et al. Thyroid lobectomy for treatment of well differentiated intrathyroid malignancy. *Surgery* 2012; **151**(4): 571–9.
6. Hay ID, Grant CS, Taylor WF, McConahey WM. Ipsilateral lobectomy versus bilateral lobar resection in papillary thyroid carcinoma: a retrospective analysis of surgical outcome using a novel prognostic scoring system. *Surgery* 1987; **102**(6): 1088–95.
7. Mendelsohn AH, Elashoff DA, Abemayor E, St John MA. Surgery for papillary thyroid carcinoma: is lobectomy enough? *Arch Otolaryngol Head Neck Surg* 2010; **136**(11): 1055–61.
8. Lang BH-H, Lo C-Y, Wong KP, Wan KY. Should an involved but functioning recurrent laryngeal nerve be shaved or resected in a locally advanced papillary thyroid carcinoma? *Ann Surg Oncol* 2013; **20**(9): 2951–7.
9. McCaffrey JC. Aerodigestive tract invasion by well-differentiated thyroid carcinoma: diagnosis, management, prognosis, and biology. *Laryngoscope* 2006; **116**(1): 1–11.
10. Mehanna H, Al-Maqbili T, Carter B, et al. Differences in the recurrence and mortality outcomes rates of incidental and nonincidental papillary thyroid microcarcinoma: a systematic review and meta-analysis of 21 329 person-years of follow-up. *J Clin Endocrinol Metab* 2014; **99**(8): 2834–43.
11. Lang BH-H, Ng S-H, Lau LLH, et al. A systematic review and meta-analysis of prophylactic central neck dissection on short-term locoregional recurrence in papillary thyroid carcinoma after total thyroidectomy. *Thyroid* 2013; **23**(9): 1087–98.
12. Wang TS, Cheung K, Farrokhyar F, et al. A meta-analysis of the effect of prophylactic central compartment neck dissection on locoregional recurrence rates in patients with papillary thyroid cancer. *Ann Surg Oncol* 2013; **20**(11): 3477–83.
13. Tisell LE, Nilsson B, Mölne J, et al. Improved survival of patients with papillary thyroid cancer after surgical microdissection. *World J Surg* 1996; **20**(7): 854–9.
14. Sywak M, Cornford L, Roach P, et al. Routine ipsilateral level VI lymphadenectomy reduces postoperative thyroglobulin levels in papillary thyroid cancer. *Surgery* 2006; **140**(6): 1000–5; discussion 1005–7.
15. Roh J-L, Park J-Y, Park CI. Total thyroidectomy plus neck dissection in differentiated papillary thyroid carcinoma patients: pattern of nodal metastasis, morbidity, recurrence, and postoperative levels of serum parathyroid hormone. *Ann Surg* 2007; **245**(4): 604–10.
16. Lee YS, Kim SW, Kim SW, et al. Extent of routine central lymph node dissection with small papillary thyroid carcinoma. *World J Surg* 2007; **31**(10): 1954–9.
17. Mallick U, Harmer C, Yap B, et al. Ablation with low-dose radioiodine and thyrotropin alfa in thyroid cancer. *N Engl J Med* 2012; **366**(18): 1674–85.
18. Schlumberger M, Catargi B, Borget I, et al. Strategies of radioiodine ablation in patients with low-risk thyroid cancer. *N Engl J Med* 2012; **366**(18): 1663–73.
19. Nutting CM, Convery DJ, Cosgrove VP, et al. Improvements in target coverage and reduced spinal cord irradiation using intensity-modulated radiotherapy (IMRT) in patients with carcinoma of the thyroid gland. *Radiother Oncol* 2001; **60**(2): 173–80.
20. Mazzaferri EL, Kloos RT. Is diagnostic iodine-131 scanning with recombinant human TSH useful in the follow-up of differentiated thyroid cancer after thyroid ablation? *J Clin Endocrinol Metab* 2002; **87**(4): 1490–8.
21. Rosario PW, Furtado M de S, Campos Mineiro Filho AF, et al. Value of diagnostic radioiodine whole-body scanning after initial therapy in patients with differentiated thyroid cancer at intermediate and high risk for recurrence. *Thyroid* 2012; **22**(11): 1165–9.
22. Lee J, Yun MJ, Nam KH, et al. Quality of life and effectiveness comparisons of thyroxine withdrawal, triiodothyronine withdrawal, and recombinant thyroid-stimulating hormone administration for low-dose radioiodine remnant ablation of differentiated thyroid carcinoma. *Thyroid* 2010; **20**(2): 173–9.
23. Borget I, Corone C, Nocaudie M, et al. Sick leave for follow-up control in thyroid cancer patients: comparison between stimulation with Thyrogen and thyroid hormone withdrawal. *Eur J Endocrinol* 2007; **156**(5): 531–8.
24. Mernagh P, Suebwongpat A, Silverberg J, Weston A. Cost-effectiveness of using recombinant human thyroid-stimulating hormone before radioiodine ablation for thyroid cancer: the Canadian perspective. *Value Health* 2010; **13**(2): 180–7.
25. Mazzaferri EL, Robbins RJ, Spencer CA, et al. A consensus report of the role of serum thyroglobulin as a monitoring method for low-risk patients with papillary thyroid carcinoma. *J Clin Endocrinol Metab* 2003; **88**(4): 1433–41.
26. David A, Blotta A, Bondanelli M, et al. Serum thyroglobulin concentrations and (131)I whole-body scan results in patients with differentiated thyroid carcinoma after administration of recombinant human thyroid-stimulating hormone. *J Nucl Med* 2001; **42**(10): 1470–5.
27. Haugen BR, Ridgway EC, McLaughlin BA, McDermott MT. Clinical comparison of whole-body radioiodine scan and serum thyroglobulin after stimulation with recombinant human thyrotropin. *Thyroid* 2002; **12**(1): 37–43.
28. Lima N, Cavaliere H, Tomimori E, et al. Prognostic value of serial serum thyroglobulin determinations after total thyroidectomy for differentiated thyroid cancer. *J Endocrinol Invest* 2002; **25**(2): 110–15.
29. Kloos RT, Mazzaferri EL. A single recombinant human thyrotropin-stimulated serum thyroglobulin measurement predicts differentiated thyroid carcinoma metastases three to five years later. *J Clin Endocrinol Metab* 2005; **90**(9): 5047–57.
30. Castagna MG, Brilli L, Pilli T, et al. Limited value of repeat recombinant human thyrotropin (rhTSH)-stimulated thyroglobulin testing in differentiated thyroid carcinoma patients with previous negative rhTSH-stimulated thyroglobulin and undetectable basal serum thyroglobulin levels. *J Clin Endocrinol Metab* 2008; **93**(1): 76–81.
31. Smallridge RC, Meek SE, Morgan MA, et al. Monitoring thyroglobulin in a sensitive immunoassay has comparable sensitivity to recombinant human TSH-stimulated thyroglobulin in follow-up of thyroid cancer patients. *J Clin Endocrinol Metab* 2007; **92**(1): 82–7.
32. Iervasi A, Iervasi G, Ferdeghini M, et al. Clinical relevance of highly sensitive Tg assay in monitoring patients treated for differentiated thyroid cancer. *Clin Endocrinol (Oxf)* 2007; **67**(3): 434–41.
33. Malandrino P, Latina A, Marescalco S, et al. Risk-adapted management of differentiated thyroid cancer assessed by a sensitive measurement of basal serum thyroglobulin. *J Clin Endocrinol Metab* 2011; **96**(6): 1703–9.
34. Jonklaas J, Sarlis NJ, Litofsky D, et al. Outcomes of patients with differentiated thyroid carcinoma following initial therapy. *Thyroid* 2006; **16**(12): 1229–42.
35. Hovens GC, Stokkel MP, Kievit J, et al. Associations of serum thyrotropin concentrations with recurrence and death in differentiated thyroid cancer. *J Clin Endocrinol Metab* 2007; **92**(7): 2610–15.
36. Pujol P, Daures JP, Nsakala N, et al. Degree of thyrotropin suppression as a prognostic determinant in differentiated thyroid cancer. *J Clin Endocrinol Metab* 1996; **81**(12): 4318–23.
37. Pacini F, Castagna MG, Brilli L, et al. Thyroid cancer: ESMO clinical practice guidelines for diagnosis, treatment and follow-up. *Ann Oncol* 2012; **23**(suppl 7): 110–19.
38. O'Sullivan B, Brierley JD, D'Cruz AK, et al. *UICC manual of clinical oncology*. 9th ed. Oxford: Wiley-Blackwell; 2015.

MANAGEMENT OF MEDULLARY THYROID CANCER

Barney Harrison

Incidence 757	Follow-up 761
Pathology 757	Persistent/recurrent hypercalcitonaemia and recurrent MTC 761
Hereditary MTC 758	Localization of persistent/recurrent MTC 762
Clinical features of sporadic and hereditary MTC 758	Outcome and prognosis 762
Diagnosis of MTC 759	Non-surgical treatment of MTC 762
Pre-operative investigations 759	Prophylactic surgery for hereditary MTC 762
Surgery for MTC 760	References 763

SEARCH STRATEGY

Data in this chapter may be updated by a PubMed search using the keywords: medullary thyroid cancer, MEN2, calcitonin and thyroidectomy.

INCIDENCE

Medullary thyroid cancer/carcinoma (MTC) is diagnosed in approximately 1000 people each year in the United States and 25–50 people per year in the UK and it is responsible for 5–10% of paediatric thyroid cancers. In patients with nodular thyroid disease screened for MTC the prevalence is reported as 0.4%–1.8% (see below).

PATHOLOGY

MTC arises from C-cells located in the middle and upper third of the thyroid gland, adjacent to or within thyroid follicles, between the follicular cell basement membrane and the surface epithelium. C-cells are of neural crest origin and produce calcitonin, calcitonin gene-related peptide (CGRP) and carcinoembryonic antigen (CEA).

The physiological role of calcitonin is unclear. In patients with metastatic medullary thyroid cancer, in whom calcitonin levels are grossly elevated, and after total thyroidectomy for benign disease when levels are low, no derangement of calcium homeostasis is apparent.

C-cell hyperplasia

C-cell hyperplasia (CCH) is defined as a multifocal (diffuse or nodular) quantitative increase in C-cells. Two types of CCH are described:

- **neoplastic:** typically nodular and diffuse and indistinguishable from invasive MTC cells
- **reactive/physiological:** typically diffuse, associated with hypercalcaemia, hyperparathyroidism, chronic lymphocytic thyroiditis and follicular thyroid tumours.

Medullary thyroid cancer

MACROSCOPIC

Sporadic tumours are usually solitary (90%) and unilateral. In familial disease, MTC is usually bilateral and multifocal.

CYTOLOGY

Cell morphology is variable, oval/round/spindle-shaped cells may be seen in clusters or as single cells with pleomorphic nuclei and eosinophilic cytoplasm. Eosinophilic extracellular material is amyloid.

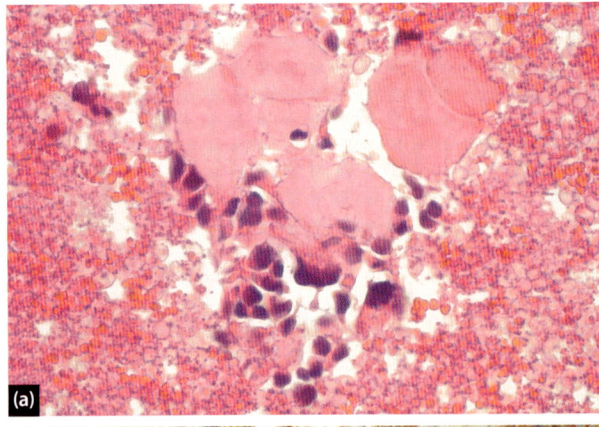
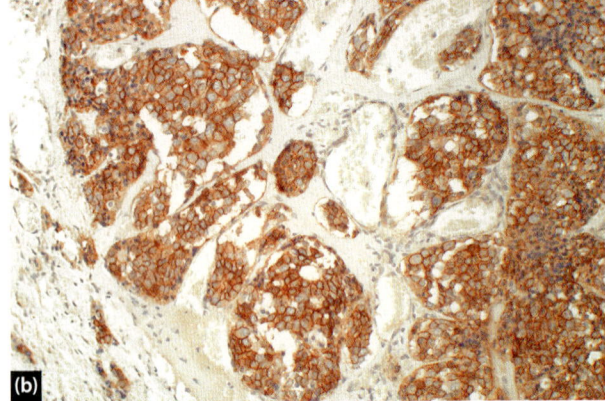

Figure 63.1 (a) MTC cytology from fine needle aspiration (b) MTC histology showing strongly positive immunohistochemical staining for calcitonin.

HISTOPATHOLOGY

Variants of classical MTC include papillary, follicular, squamous and oncocytic subtypes. Amyloid is seen in 80% of tumours on immunohistochemistry, and tumour cells stain positive for calcitonin (**Figure 63.1**), CEA and chromogranin A. Thyroglobulin staining is negative.

MTC is staged as described in the *AJCC Cancer Staging Manual*.[1]

HEREDITARY MTC

Genetically determined disease accounts for 25% of MTC cases. The three main clinical variants are all inherited as autosomal dominant disorders with age-related penetrance and variable expression:

- multiple endocrine neoplasia type 2A (MEN 2A): >50% of cases
- multiple endocrine neoplasia type 2B (MEN 2B): 5% of cases
- familial medullary thyroid cancer (FMTC).

The prevalence is estimated at 1 in 30 000. MTC is expressed in almost all patients and is usually the first manifestation of the syndrome; the age at onset can be roughly predicted according to the genotype.

Gain of function germline and somatic mutations of the *RET* proto-oncogene (chromosome 10q11.2) are implicated in the pathogenesis of MTC. *RET* encodes a plasma membrane-bound receptor tyrosine kinase that is expressed by thyroid C-cells, cells of the adrenal medulla, autonomic nerve ganglia, colonic ganglia and parathyroid cells.

Germline mutations associated with MEN 2/FMTC are found in 7 of the *RET* gene's 21 exons. The codon mutations correlate with the MTC phenotype.[2]

The extracellular, codon 634 mutation (found in 85% of MEN 2A cases) induces a dimerization of the RET receptor which leads to abnormal cell growth, differentiation defects and cellular transformation. The intracellular, codon 918 mutation found in 95% of cases of MEN 2B is associated with receptor activation in the absence of receptor dimerization by alteration of kinase substrate specificity.

Somatic mutations of *RET*, usually at codon 918, are found in approximately 25% of sporadic MTC and linked with poorer prognosis.

CLINICAL FEATURES OF SPORADIC AND HEREDITARY MTC

Sporadic MTC presents usually in the fourth to sixth decade, MEN2A typically presents in the second or third decades, MEN2B in the first and second decades, and FMTC in the fourth and fifth decades. The sex ratio is almost equal.

A thyroid mass is normally the first indication of disease (>75%), cervical lymphadenopathy is a presenting feature in approximately 40–50% of patients. Around 10% of patients will have distant metastases, and symptoms include diarrhoea (the specific cause of which is unknown), flushing and bone pain. Rarely (<1%), ACTH/CRH production by MTC causes Cushing's syndrome[3] and is associated with poor prognosis.

Phaeochromocytoma is most frequently associated with *RET* codon mutations 634 and 918,[4] occurs in 50% of MEN 2 patients most commonly in the third and fourth decades and may be the presenting feature of MEN 2 in up to 25% of cases.

In patients with MEN 2A, hyperparathyroidism occurs in 20–30% of individuals with *RET* 634 mutations. The hypercalcaemia is often mild. Asymmetric parathyroid gland enlargement is likely and resection of only enlarged glands is recommended.[5]

Rare variants of MEN 2A with specific *RET* mutations are associated with Hirschsprung's disease and cutaneous lichen amyloidosis (brownish plaques of multiple tiny papules, usually in the interscapular area).

In FMTC, the age at onset of MTC is later than is seen in MEN 2A and MEN 2B; the phenotype is less aggressive. MEN 2B has a specific phenotype that may be apparent in infancy and progresses as the patient ages. There is a typical facial appearance with enlarged lips (**Figure 63.2**). Mucosal ganglioneuromas arise in the digestive tract – associated with abdominal distension, megacolon, constipation and diarrhoea. In infants, the colonic manifestations of MEN 2B may be confused with Hirschsprung's disease. Ganglioneuromas are seen on the conjunctivae, lips and tongue (**Figure 63.3**).

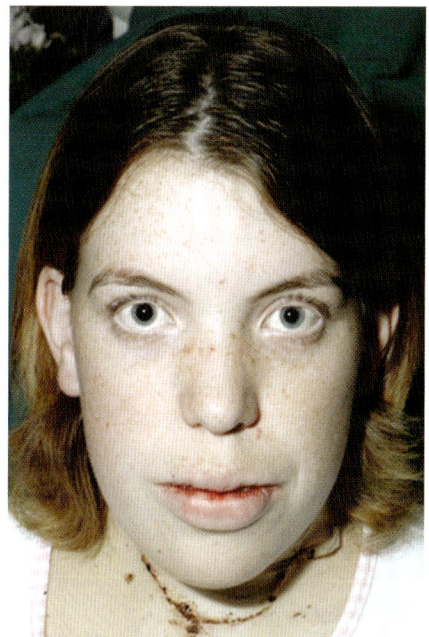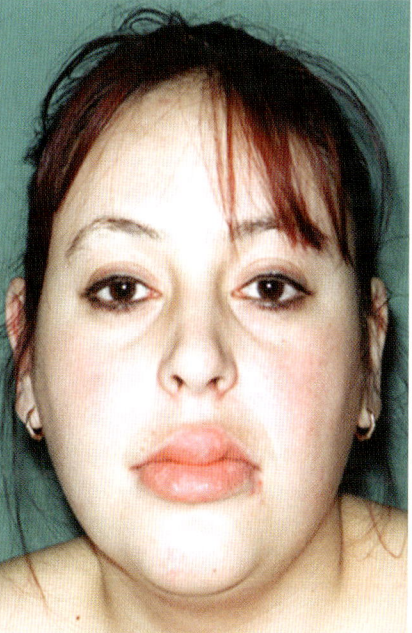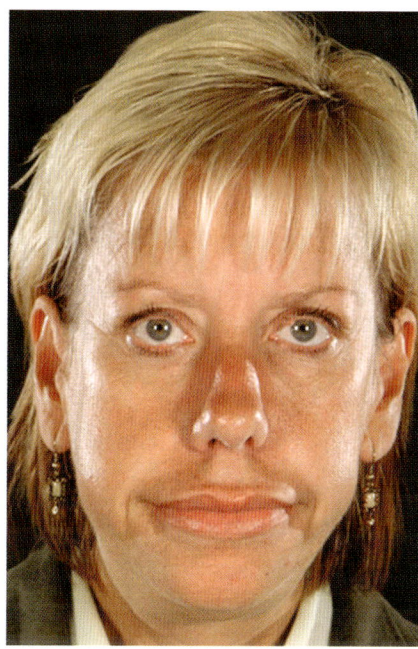

Figure 63.2 Typical facial phenotype of three unrelated MEN 2B patients.

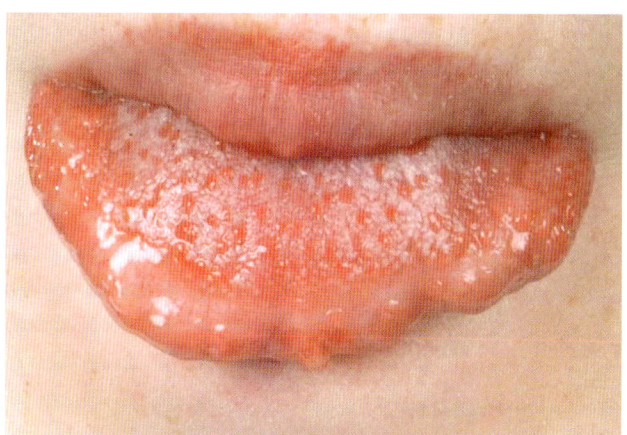

Figure 63.3 Tongue of an 11-year-old MEN 2B patient showing typical ganglioneuromas.

Other manifestations include skeletal abnormalities such as Marfanoid habitus, joint laxity, pes cavus and pectus excavatum, and markedly thickened corneal nerves. Around 95% of patients have a mutation at codon 918, and 75% of patients are the index case (i.e. *de novo* mutations).

DIAGNOSIS OF MTC

The diagnosis of MTC in most cases will result from the investigation of patients who present with a thyroid or lymph node mass. Fine-needle aspiration cytology (FNAC) will result in a diagnosis in 50% of cases,[6] and the additional use of calcitonin assay of the fine-needle aspirate has high sensitivity and specificity for MTC diagnosis.[7] When necessary, targeted core needle biopsy avoids the need for open biopsy.

Routine measurement of basal calcitonin in patients presenting with nodular thyroid disease is recommended by some, to identify otherwise undetected MTC and lead to the potential benefit of better outcome. Basal hypercalcitonaemia will be evident in at least 1.5% of screened individuals but approximately 60% of those with a high basal calcitonin do not have MTC. The positive predictive value of an abnormal basal calcitonin greater than 100 pg/mL is 100%.[8] Recommendations on the use of routine calcitonin screening in patients with nodular thyroid disease in recent draft guidelines of the American Thyroid Association[9] and British Thyroid Association[2] (against) are at variance with European Thyroid Association guideline recommendations (in favour).[10]

PRE-OPERATIVE INVESTIGATIONS

Calcitonin

Serum calcitonin is a sensitive and accurate marker of MTC. False-positive serum calcitonin levels are recorded in patients with autoimmune thyroid disease, hypercalcaemia, foregut-derived neuroendocrine tumours and renal failure. Normal basal calcitonin levels are higher in neonates and children than adults.[11] MTC with normal basal serum calcitonin is described in less than 1% of patients, more often in those with advanced disease.[12]

Basal calcitonin should be measured in all MTC patients prior to surgery. The level of calcitonin is a good indicator of disease extent. Lymph node involvement may be found in patients with calcitonin as low as 10–40 pg/mL; distant metastasis and extra-thyroidal growth can occur with calcitonin levels of 150–400 pg/mL.[13]

In patients with potentially false-positive basal calcitonin levels, or when there is uncertainty about the histological diagnosis, a calcium stimulation test should be performed.[14] Basal calcitonin levels that are false positives (i.e. not MTC) do not respond significantly to calcium stimulation.

Urinary or plasma catecholamines / metanephrines

Biochemical testing for phaeochromocytoma (24-hour urine, or plasma for metanephrines and normetanephrines) is mandatory prior to surgery in all patients with a diagnosis of MTC. Phaeochromocytoma should be treated before the thyroid disease. Annual biochemical screening for phaeochromocytoma is warranted from the age of 11 years in carriers of *RET* codon mutations 918 and 634, and from the age of 16 in the remainder.[15]

Calcium

A serum calcium level should be obtained from all patients prior to surgery. Hypercalcaemia and high or inappropriate serum PTH will indicate the need for careful assessment of the parathyroid glands at the time of thyroidectomy and excision of enlarged glands. Age of commencement of screening for primary hyperparathyroidism is recommended as for phaeochromocytoma.[15]

RET mutation analysis

RET mutation analysis should be performed in all patients diagnosed with MTC. Your 'sporadic' patient may represent the index case of a previously undiagnosed MEN kindred. The prevalence of a germline *RET* mutation in patients with apparently sporadic MTC is reported as 7%.[16]

DNA-based testing will identify mutations in more than 95% of individuals with MEN 2A and MEN 2B and in about 85% of individuals with FMTC. When a patient with MTC is identified as carrying a *RET* mutation, genetic screening should be offered to first-degree relatives. Family members identified as gene-positive can be offered therapeutic, risk reduction or prophylactic surgery for MTC (see below).

Ultrasound

Neck ultrasound performed as a part of thyroid workup or to guide FNA can identify bilateral and or multiple thyroid lesions – suggestive of genetically determined disease, and enlarged or abnormal lymph nodes.

CT/MRI scanning

Cross-sectional imaging of the neck and mediastinum is required to identify tracheal/oesophageal invasion and mediastinal lymphadenopathy (**Figure 63.4**).

Systemic staging to include lungs, liver and axial skeleton (including bone scintigraphy) is appropriate in patients with extensive neck disease, symptoms of metastatic disease or a calcitonin >500 pg/mL.[17] Positive findings may restrict the extent of neck surgery.

Pre-operative laryngoscopy is essential in patients with proven or suspected MTC.

Staging

For staging of MTC, please refer to Chapter 58.

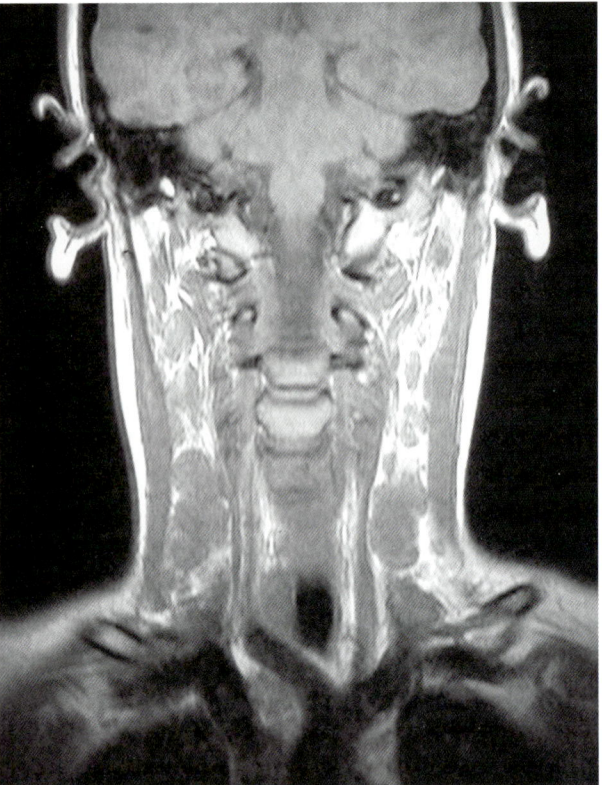

Figure 63.4 Magnetic resonance image showing bilateral cervical and infrabrachiocephalic lymphadenopathy in a 17-year-old MEN 2B patient following previous thyroidectomy.

SURGERY FOR MTC

The aims of surgery in patients with MTC are to remove all disease in the neck, produce biochemical and clinical cure and minimize the risk of locoregional relapse that might compromise the airway, oesophagus or recurrent laryngeal nerves. This requires total thyroidectomy and lymph node dissection in most patients. Surgery should be performed with the intention to preserve the recurrent laryngeal nerves, superior laryngeal nerves and parathyroid function.

Rationale for lymph node dissection in MTC

Node metastases are common (>75%) in patients with palpable MTC[18] and occur early in the disease. Lymph node involvement may be found when the basal calcitonin level is only minimally above the normal range:[13] the frequency can be predicted by tumour size and ranges from 17% (pT1) to 100% (pT4).[19] Node metastases in sporadic medullary microcarcinoma (1 cm diameter or less) have been reported to occur in 43% of patients.[20]

Ipsilateral lateral neck nodes may be involved in over 80% of cases and contralateral lateral nodes in over 50%.[21] The frequency of ipsilateral and contralateral lateral compartment node involvement reflects the degree of central compartment node positivity.[21] Skip metastases (negative central and positive lateral or mediastinal compartments) are found in approximately 20% of patients. Mediastinal node disease is more likely to occur in patients with positive cervical nodes and extra-thyroidal extension; contralateral cervical or mediastinal lymph node involvement predicts an increased risk of distant metastases.[22]

The normal recommendation for the treatment of MTC is total thyroidectomy, although sporadic disease is usually unilateral and unifocal (80%). Total thyroidectomy and compartment-orientated node dissection is associated with improved survival and a reduced risk of recurrence.[23] Biochemical cure can be obtained in 95–100% of patients without lymph node metastases, and in 32–45% of patients with lymph node metastases.[24, 25] When fewer than 10 lymph nodes are involved, an undetectable calcitonin level is observed in 57% of patients.[25]

A reasonable approach to the primary surgical treatment of MTC without distant metastases includes the following:

- Clinically evident MTC: a minimum of total thyroidectomy and central neck lymph node dissection (levels VI-VII). Therapeutic selective lateral neck dissection should be performed if there is clinical or radiological evidence of nodal disease. Ipsilateral prophylactic selective lateral neck dissection (levels IIa–Vb) is advised if central neck nodes are involved as there is a high risk of lateral neck node disease. In the absence of overt central neck node disease, histological confirmation of node metastasis by intra-operative frozen section should be performed prior to prophylactic lateral neck dissection. Alternatively, a two-stage procedure may be performed. As biochemical cure is unlikely when node metastases are present in more than two lymph node compartments,[26] prophylactic bilateral lateral neck dissection is not recommended.
- Incidental MTC >1 cm diagnosed at hemithyroidectomy with elevated post-operative basal calcitonin: treat as above.
- Incidental micro MTC <5 mm (*RET*-ve) and normal post-operative basal calcitonin: completion thyroidectomy is not required.
- MTC >5 mm in diameter when the post-operative basal calcitonin is elevated, or when the basal calcitonin is normal and stimulated calcitonin levels are elevated: total thyroidectomy and central neck dissection.
- After previous surgery and five or fewer lymph nodes removed with calcitonin <1000 pg/mL: central and ipsilateral lateral neck node dissection as above should be considered.
- When pre-operative imaging identifies infrabrachicephalic mediastinal nodal disease and no evidence of distant metastases: mediastinal lymphadenectomy (via a trans-sternal approach) should be performed.

Patients with known distant metastases at diagnosis should be considered for total thyroidectomy and central neck lymph node dissection, and/or resection of enlarged mediastinal nodes to prevent subsequent compromise of the airway, recurrent laryngeal nerves and oesophagus. Survival may be prolonged in patients with disseminated disease.

FOLLOW-UP

Thyroid function and serum calcium should be monitored post-operatively, the former in conjunction with replacement doses of thyroxine to maintain normal TSH levels. After surgery, measurement of calcitonin levels should be delayed as the post-operative fall in levels may be delayed for up to 3 months.[27] All patients with MTC require life-long review, and regular monitoring of calcitonin and CEA. Patients with MEN 2 require multidisciplinary follow-up (endocrinology/oncology/surgery) to diagnose, treat and monitor the other components of their syndrome.

PERSISTENT/RECURRENT HYPERCALCITONAEMIA AND RECURRENT MTC

Historically, patients have undergone less than optimal initial surgery, approximately 50% of patients having less than treatment guidelines recommend. Surgical treatment that is compliant with recognized guidelines is said to result in fewer reoperations and more biochemical cure.[28]

Residual/recurrent disease is diagnosed on the basis of clinical symptoms, signs or an elevated/rising calcitonin or CEA. Locoregional and distant metastases from MTC occur preferentially within the first 5 years.

When a patient presents with persistent or recurrent hypercalcitonaemia, there are three key issues for the surgeon:

- Was the initial surgery less that that recommended according to best practice?
- Is the source of calcitonin in the neck (residual thyroid or lymph nodes) or mediastinum and amenable to further surgery?
- Will further surgery result in cure or improved survival?

The fundamental issue is whether residual disease lies within the neck and is remediable by surgery. Reoperation in selected patients can result in normalization of calcitonin in up to 44% of cases. Biochemical cure is most likely to occur in those patients who have previously undergone inadequate first-time surgery and have serum calcitonin ≤1000 pg/ml or five or fewer nodes removed at previous surgery.[29]

Radiographic evidence of recurrent disease is unlikely when the calcitonin level is at or below 250 pg/mL.[23] In the 'absence' of metastases and when first-time neck surgery was less than adequate, reoperation should be considered for what is persistent disease. This will usually require compartment-orientated cervical node dissection. When localization studies identify recurrent locoregional disease after appropriate first-time surgery, reoperative surgery should also be performed. The presence of distant disease should not in isolation preclude surgery. The aim of surgery is not only to cure or significantly reduce disease bulk or symptoms but also to relieve or prevent future compression of the airway and oesophagus as well as involvement of the brachial plexus or recurrent laryngeal nerves.

LOCALIZATION OF PERSISTENT/RECURRENT MTC

Diagnostic imaging studies in patients with persistent/recurrent hypercalcitonaemia are used to identify surgically remediable locoregional disease that may put the patient at risk of airway or oesophageal compression. They also provide baseline criteria to facilitate entry of patients into clinical trials, and measurement of responses to systemic therapy.

In patients with elevated calcitonin levels following thyroidectomy, metastases are best detected when serum calcitonin levels are greater than 800 pg/mL. The most efficient detection of metastatic MTC consists of neck ultrasound, chest CT, liver MRI, bone scintigraphy and axial skeleton MRI.[30] FDG PET/CT identifies residual/recurrent MTC in patients with progressive disease and suggests poor survival. F-DOPA PET/CT more accurately assesses the extent of residual MTC[31] with sensitivity of 80%,[32] but access to this latter scan is limited in the UK.

OUTCOME AND PROGNOSIS

Reported survival rates at 10 years range from 56%[33] to 96%[24] respectively. More than 50% of patients with sporadic MTC will die of their disease. Biochemical cure following surgery is associated with 97.7% survival at 10 years;[34] disease-specific survival for patients with micro MTC is reported as 96% at 10 years.[35] Children with medullary carcinoma thyroid have 5-year survival rates of 95%. Patients with advanced disease have a median survival of 8 years,[36] and a third of patients with systemic symptoms die within 5 years.[37]

When post-thyroidectomy calcitonin/CEA levels are raised, measurement of doubling times at 6-month intervals predicts outcome. Post-treatment calcitonin/CEA doubling times of less than 1 year[38] or more than 2 years[39] correlate with worse and better outcomes respectively.

NON-SURGICAL TREATMENT OF MTC

Adjuvant radiotherapy

Adjuvant radiotherapy has been found to be independently associated with a decreased survival although its use is inevitably confined to those patients with a worse prognosis. External beam radiotherapy is reported to reduce local relapse in high-risk patients and in those presenting with more advanced disease. It has not been shown to produce a survival benefit. It should be considered in those patients at high risk of locoregional recurrence.

Targeted biological therapy

The rationale for the use of tyrosine kinase inhibitors arises from the knowledge that nearly all patients with genetically determined MTC and approximately 50% of patients with sporadic MTC have germline or somatic *RET* mutations respectively. *RET* encodes a receptor for tyrosine kinase. Clinical benefit from treatment of patients with symptomatic progressive/metastatic MTC with Vandetanib and Cabozantinib is seen in more than half the patients, but toxicity is considerable and side effects common.[40]

Diarrhoea can be an extremely distressing symptom of widespread metastatic MTC and is often resistant to treatment with antimotility drugs. Somatostatin analogues may reduce symptoms, and chemoembolization of liver metastases may be effective.[41]

PROPHYLACTIC SURGERY FOR HEREDITARY MTC

Children and adolescents identified by *RET* screening to be at risk for the development of medullary thyroid cancer can be treated with prophylactic thyroidectomy before developing the disease. The timing of the intervention **and** the extent of surgery should be based on the affected codon, the age of the patient and the calcitonin level. Gene carriers with serum calcitonin less than 60 pg/mL who have undergone surgery appear to have intra-thyroidal MTC without evidence of nodal spread.[42]

The timing of thyroidectomy

Children with *RET* codon 918, 883, mutations (MEN 2B) have the **highest** risk from aggressive MTC – neoplastic transformation of C-cells occurs in the first year of life. Prophylactic thyroidectomy should be performed within the first year of life, preferably in the first 6 months.

Children with a *RET* codon 634 mutation have a **high** risk for MTC – neoplastic transformation of C-cells occurs in the first decade. Prophylactic thyroidectomy should be performed at 5 years of age, or earlier if the calcitonin level is elevated above 40 pg/mL.[13]

Children with other *RET* codon mutations are now recommended to undergo 6-monthly clinical examination, and measurement of serum calcitonin around the age of 5 years. With parents involved in decision-making, thyroidectomy may be delayed until later in childhood or the teenage years if calcitonin levels do not rise above the normal range. Although some national guidelines recommend the use of neck ultrasound in assessment of at-risk patients, it appears to be ineffective in identifying MTC in this patient group.[43]

The need for and timing of lymph node surgery

In ideal circumstances, risk reduction surgery – total thyroidectomy – should be performed before the onset of MTC thereby reducing the need for lymph node dissection, which is associated in children with an increased risk of hypoparathyroidism and recurrent laryngeal nerve injury. In reality, cases often manifest when it is likely or evident that MTC is already present and occult lymph node metastasis may have occurred.

It has been suggested that children from known kindred with highest-risk mutations (918, 883) should be considered for lymph node dissection at the time of prophylactic thyroidectomy in the first year of life. Because the risk of post-operative hypoparathyroidism is so high in these children, if parathyroid glands cannot be identified or preserved at surgery, it may be appropriate to avoid node dissection.

Children with MEN 2A with a mutation of codon 634 should undergo central neck dissection at the time of prophylactic thyroidectomy if the calcitonin level is greater than 40 pg/ml or when there is evidence of node metastasis on imaging.

Results of 'prophylactic' surgery

Previously reported outcomes of 'prophylactic' surgery should be interpreted with the knowledge that MTC was often present at the time of surgery; the intervention would have been better termed 'risk reduction' or indeed therapeutic. Until 2005 only 15% of the 275 reported 'prophylactic' thyroidectomies performed on *RET* 634 children were carried out before the age of 5.[44] Studies of outcome from **risk reduction** surgery in young patients up to the age of 21 years confirm that biochemical cure is possible and sustained at follow-up in the majority of individuals, but the highest chance of 'cure' results when age-appropriate prophylactic surgery is performed on individuals **at risk** of MTC.[45]

KEY POINTS

- Care for adult and paediatric MTC patients should be provided in a tertiary centre and treated according to the recommendations of the specialist MDT.
- All patients with MTC should be offered *RET* gene mutation analysis. If the patient is confirmed to have genetically determined disease, first-degree relatives should be offered genetic screening.
- Risk reduction/prophylactic surgery should be offered to gene carriers prior to the onset of malignant disease.
- All patients with proven or suspected MTC must have undergone biochemical testing to exclude phaeochromocytoma prior to neck surgery.
- Patients with MTC and an elevated basal calcitonin should undergo a minimum of total thyroidectomy and central neck lymph node dissection.

REFERENCES

1. Edge SB, Compton CC. The American Joint Committee on Cancer: the 7th edition of the AJCC cancer staging manual and the future of TNM. *Ann Surg Oncol* 2010; **17**(6): 1471–4.
2. Perros P, Boelaert K, Colley S, et al. Guidelines for the management of thyroid cancer. *Clin Endocrinol (Oxf)* 2014; **81**(Suppl 1): 1–122.
3. Nella AA, Lodish MB, Fox E, et al. Vandetanib successfully controls medullary thyroid cancer-related Cushing syndrome in an adolescent patient. *J Clin Endocrinol Metab* 2014; **99**(9): 3055–9.
4. Machens A, Brauckhoff M, Holzhausen HJ, et al. Codon-specific development of pheochromocytoma in multiple endocrine neoplasia type 2. *J Clin Endocrinol Metab* 2005; **90**(7): 3999–4003.
5. Kraimps JL, Denizot A, Carnaille B, et al. Primary hyperparathyroidism in multiple endocrine neoplasia type IIa: retrospective French multicentric study. Groupe d'Etude des Tumeurs a Calcitonine (GETC, French Calcitonin Tumors Study Group), French Association of Endocrine Surgeons. *World J Surg* 1996; **20**(7): 808–12; discussion 12–13.
6. Trimboli P, Treglia G, Guidobaldi L, et al. Detection rate of FNA cytology in medullary thyroid carcinoma: a meta-analysis. *Clin Endocrinol (Oxf)* 2015; **82**(2): 280–5.
7. Trimboli P, Cremonini N, Ceriani L, et al. Calcitonin measurement in aspiration needle washout fluids has higher sensitivity than cytology in detecting medullary thyroid carcinoma: a retrospective multicentre study. *Clin Endocrinol (Oxf)* 2014; **80**(1): 135–40.
8. Costante G, Durante C, Francis Z, et al. Determination of calcitonin levels in C-cell disease: clinical interest and potential pitfalls. *Nat Clin Pract Endocrinol Metab* 2009; **5**(1): 35–44.
9. Wells SA, Asa SL, Dralle H, et al. Revised American Thyroid Association Guidelines for the Management of Medullary Thyroid Carcinoma. *American Thyroid Association* 2015; **25**(6): 567–610.
10. Elisei R, Romei C. Calcitonin estimation in patients with nodular goiter and its significance for early detection of MTC: European comments to the guidelines of the American Thyroid Association. *Thyroid Res* 2013; **6**(Suppl 1): S2.
11. Verga U, Morpurgo PS, Vaghi I, et al. Normal range of calcitonin in children measured by a chemiluminescent two-site immunometric assay. *Horm Res* 2006; **66**(1): 17–20.
12. Frank-Raue K, Machens A, Leidig-Bruckner G, et al. Prevalence and clinical spectrum of nonsecretory medullary thyroid carcinoma in a series of 839 patients with sporadic medullary thyroid carcinoma. *Thyroid* 2013; **23**(3): 294–300.
13. Machens A, Schneyer U, Holzhausen HJ, Dralle H. Prospects of remission in medullary thyroid carcinoma according to basal calcitonin level. *J Clin Endocrinol Metab* 2005; **90**(4): 2029–34.
14. Mian C, Perrino M, Colombo C, et al. Refining calcium test for the diagnosis of medullary thyroid cancer: cutoffs, procedures, and safety. *J Clin Endocrinol Metab* 2014; **99**(5): 1656–64.
15. Machens A, Lorenz K, Dralle H. Peak incidence of pheochromocytoma and primary hyperparathyroidism in multiple endocrine neoplasia 2: need for age-adjusted biochemical screening. *J Clin Endocrinol Metab* 2013; **98**(2): E336–45.
16. Elisei R, Romei C, Cosci B, et al. RET genetic screening in patients with medullary thyroid cancer and their relatives: experience with 807 individuals at one center. *J Clin Endocrinol Metab* 2007; **92**(12): 4725–9.
17. Machens A, Dralle H. Biomarker-based risk stratification for previously untreated medullary thyroid cancer. *J Clin Endocrinol Metab* 2010; **95**(6): 2655–63.
18. Moley JF, DeBenedetti MK. Patterns of nodal metastases in palpable medullary thyroid carcinoma: recommendations for extent of node dissection. *Ann Surg* 1999; **229**(6): 880–7; discussion 7–8.
19. Ukkat J, Gimm O, Brauckhoff M, et al. Single center experience in primary surgery for medullary thyroid carcinoma. *World J Surg* 2004; **28**(12):1271–4.
20. Machens A, Dralle H. Biological relevance of medullary thyroid microcarcinoma. *J Clin Endocrinol Metab* 2012; **97**(5): 1547–53.
21. Machens A, Hauptmann S, Dralle H. Prediction of lateral lymph node metastases in medullary thyroid cancer. *Br J Surg* 2008; **95**(5): 586–91.
22. Machens A, Holzhausen HJ, Dralle H. Contralateral cervical and mediastinal lymph node metastasis in medullary thyroid cancer: systemic disease? *Surgery* 2006; **139**(1): 28–32.

23. Yen TW, Shapiro SE, Gagel RF, et al. Medullary thyroid carcinoma: results of a standardized surgical approach in a contemporary series of 80 consecutive patients. *Surgery* 2003; **134**(6): 890–9; discussion 899–901.
24. Ito Y, Miyauchi A, Yabuta T, et al. Alternative surgical strategies and favorable outcomes in patients with medullary thyroid carcinoma in Japan: experience of a single institution. *World J Surg* 2009; **33**(1): 58–66.
25. Scollo C, Baudin E, Travagli JP, et al. Rationale for central and bilateral lymph node dissection in sporadic and hereditary medullary thyroid cancer. *J Clin Endocrinol Metab* 2003; **88**(5): 2070–5.
26. Machens A, Gimm O, Ukkat J, et al. Improved prediction of calcitonin normalization in medullary thyroid carcinoma patients by quantitative lymph node analysis. *Cancer* 2000; **88**(8): 1909–15.
27. Fugazzola L, Pinchera A, Luchetti F, et al. Disappearance rate of serum calcitonin after total thyroidectomy for medullary thyroid carcinoma. *Int J Biol Markers* 1994; **9**(1): 21–4.
28. Verbeek HH, Meijer JA, Zandee WT, et al. Fewer cancer reoperations for medullary thyroid cancer after initial surgery according to ATA guidelines. *Ann Surg Oncol* 2015; **22**(4): 1207–13.
29. Machens A, Dralle H. Benefit-risk balance of reoperation for persistent medullary thyroid cancer. *Ann Surg* 2013; **257**(4): 751–7.
30. Giraudet AL, Vanel D, Leboulleux S, et al. Imaging medullary thyroid carcinoma with persistent elevated calcitonin levels. *J Clin Endocrinol Metab* 2007; **92**(11): 4185–90.
31. Verbeek HH, Plukker JT, Koopmans KP, et al. Clinical relevance of 18F-FDG PET and 18F-DOPA PET in recurrent medullary thyroid carcinoma. *J Nucl Med* 2012; **53**(12): 1863–71.
32. Beheshti M, Pocher S, Vali R, et al. The value of 18F-DOPA PET-CT in patients with medullary thyroid carcinoma: comparison with 18F-FDG PET-CT. *Eur Radiol* 2009; **19**(6): 1425–34.
33. Hyer SL, Vini L, A'Hern R, Harmer C. Medullary thyroid cancer: multivariate analysis of prognostic factors influencing survival. *Eur J Surg Oncol* 2000; **26**(7): 686–90.
34. Modigliani E, Cohen R, Campos JM, et al. Prognostic factors for survival and for biochemical cure in medullary thyroid carcinoma: results in 899 patients. The GETC Study Group. Groupe d'etude des tumeurs a calcitonine. *Clin Endocrinol (Oxf)* 1998; **48**(3): 265–73.
35. Kazaure HS, Roman SA, Sosa JA. Medullary thyroid microcarcinoma: a population-level analysis of 310 patients. *Cancer* 2012; **118**(3): 620–7.
36. Chen H, Roberts JR, Ball DW, et al. Effective long-term palliation of symptomatic, incurable metastatic medullary thyroid cancer by operative resection. *Ann Surg* 1998; **227**(6): 887–95.
37. Kebebew E, Ituarte PH, Siperstein AE, et al. Medullary thyroid carcinoma: clinical characteristics, treatment, prognostic factors, and a comparison of staging systems. *Cancer* 2000; **88**(5): 1139–48.
38. Meijer JA, le Cessie S, van den Hout WB, et al. Calcitonin and carcinoembryonic antigen doubling times as prognostic factors in medullary thyroid carcinoma: a structured meta-analysis. *Clin Endocrinol (Oxf)* 2010; **72**(4): 534–42.
39. Laure Giraudet A, Al Ghulzan A, Auperin A, et al. Progression of medullary thyroid carcinoma: assessment with calcitonin and carcinoembryonic antigen doubling times. *Eur J Endocrinol* 2008; **158**(2): 239–46.
40. Klein Hesselink EN, Steenvoorden D, Kapiteijn E, et al. Therapy of endocrine disease: response and toxicity of small-molecule tyrosine kinase inhibitors in patients with thyroid carcinoma: systematic review and meta-analysis. *Eur J Endocrinol* 2015; **172**(5): R215–25.
41. Fromigue J, De Baere T, Baudin E, et al. Chemoembolization for liver metastases from medullary thyroid carcinoma. *J Clin Endocrinol Metab* 2006; **91**(7): 2496–9.
42. Elisei R, Romei C, Renzini G, et al. The timing of total thyroidectomy in *RET* gene mutation carriers could be personalized and safely planned on the basis of serum calcitonin: 18 years experience at one single center. *J Clin Endocrinol Metab* 2012; **97**(2): 426–35.
43. Morris LF, Waguespack SG, Edeiken-Monroe BS, et al. Ultrasonography should not guide the timing of thyroidectomy in pediatric patients diagnosed with multiple endocrine neoplasia syndrome 2A through genetic screening. *Ann Surg Oncol* 2013; **20**(1): 53–9.
44. Piolat C, Dyon JF, Sturm N, et al. Very early prophylactic thyroid surgery for infants with a mutation of the *RET* proto-oncogene at codon 634: evaluation of the implementation of international guidelines for MEN type 2 in a single centre. *Clin Endocrinol (Oxf)* 2006; **65**(1): 118–24.
45. Shepet K, Alhefdhi A, Lai N, et al. Hereditary medullary thyroid cancer: age-appropriate thyroidectomy improves disease-free survival. *Ann Surg Oncol* 2013; **20**(5): 1451–5.

MANAGEMENT OF ANAPLASTIC THYROID CANCER/LYMPHOMA

James D. Brierley and Richard W. Tsang

Introduction 765	Lymphomas 768
Anaplastic thyroid cancer 765	References 771

SEARCH STRATEGY

Data in this chapter may be updated by a PubMed search using the keywords: anaplastic thyroid cancer and thyroid lymphoma.

INTRODUCTION

Apart from both being malignancies of the thyroid gland, the other similarity between anaplastic thyroid cancer and thyroid lymphoma is that for the majority of cases the role of surgery is limited to diagnosis and maintaining an airway. The majority of anaplastic thyroid cancer is advanced at presentation, either locally or distantly or both, and complete resection is rarely possible. In the majority of thyroid lymphomas with the exception of limited stage IE mucosa-associated lymphoid tissue (MALT) surgery is not curative and radiation with or without chemotherapy is the optimal treatment.

ANAPLASTIC THYROID CANCER

Anaplastic thyroid carcinoma (ATC) is at the extreme end of a continuum of dedifferentiation of follicular adenomas and differentiated thyroid cancer (DTC). In contrast to DTC, however, it occurs in older patients (median age 65). The female:male ratio (3:2) still is in favour of female patients but it is relatively more common than DTC in men. Unlike DTC and thyroid lymphoma it is a highly fatal cancer with a median survival of only 3–5 months. Given the appalling survival after diagnosis of the majority of patients with ATC, it is essential in any discussion of treatment that the potential risks and side effects of any treatment are discussed along with a discussion of best supportive care. Fortunately, ATC is rare in the US, accounting for less than 2% of all thyroid cancers.[1–2]

Patients usually present with rapid onset of locoregional symptoms in the background of a pre-existing thyroid goitre or mass. In a large review of over 3000 patients an enlarging neck mass occurred in 86%, also change in voice, swallowing and breathing in about a third of patients for each symptom.[1] Local pain was less common (approximately 15%). Extrathyroid extension is usual, local invasion occurring in up to 90% of cases and distant metastases are identified at presentation in 30–50%. Although the lung is the commonest site of metastasis (35%), metastases can occur in any part of the body. Given the aggressive nature of ATC, the UICC/AJCC staging is unique in that all patients are staged as stage IV: Stage IVa (confined to the thyroid), stage IVb (extrathyroid extension) and stage IVc (distant metastastic disease).[3] Along with extent of local invasion and presence of metastases, male gender, age above 60 and size of the primary (>5–7 cm) are associated with poorer survival.[2, 4, 5]

Imaging for staging should consist of CT head and neck, chest and abdomen and, when available, fluorine-18-labelled deoxyglucose positron emission tomography (FDG-PET) to assess local and distant disease. USS and MRI of the neck and a bone scan may also be of value.[6] As a third of patients have a change in voice at presentation, assessment of vocal cord function, airway adequacy and intral-uminal extension of tumour into the trachea, preferably by fibre-optic endoscopy, is essential. Once initial investigations are complete, stage of the tumour has been assessed and potential surgical resectability has been determined, the options of treatment which require a multidisciplinary approach with surgical, medical oncology, and radiation oncology opinions along with best supporting care can be discussed with the patient and family.[7]

The morphological appearance of ATC can be very varied but spindle cells are the commonest, and giant cells and cells with squamoid differentiation can also occur. All, however, have numerous and often atypical mitoses.[8] Extensive necrosis, sometimes with inflammatory infiltrates, is common. The pathogenesis from differentiated thyroid cancer is shown in that 20% or more can coexist with areas of DTC. Surgical resection with negative margins and consequently survival is more likely in cases where ATC is only a small component.[9] A fine-needle aspiration may be diagnostic but often a core biopsy is required.

Treatment

See **Figure 64.1**.

SURGERY FOR POTENTIALLY RESECTABLE LOCOREGIONAL DISEASE

No more than 10% of patients have ATC confined to the thyroid; of these, ATC may be found incidentally.[9] In the majority of other patients, an assessment by an experienced surgeon is essential to assess whether a resection with either negative (R0) or microscopic margins (R1) is possible. In the recent guidelines on the management of ATC by the American Thyroid Association it was clearly stated that: 'Gross tumor resection, not debulking, is the goal of surgery.'[7] If the tumour is resectable, a total or near-total thyroidectomy with central and lateral lymph node dissection should probably be performed. Survival for patients with an R0 or R1 resection can result in long-term survival. However, it is important to balance the aggressiveness of the surgery with the quality of life and prognosis of a patient with ATC. An R0 or R1 resection should be performed only if surgical morbidity is minimal. Ablative surgery such as a total laryngectomy should be avoided.[7, 10] A tracheostomy, however, may be required if the patient is in acute airway distress or stridor.

ADJUVANT THERAPY

Following a successful resection, adjuvant therapy should be considered along the lines described below for unresectable ATC. Although there are no randomized controlled studies in the management of ATC, two population-based studies support the use of multimodality therapy and suggest that survival is improved. A large Surveillance, Epidemiology, and End Results (SEER)-based study of 516 patients found in a multivariate analysis that surgery combined with external beam radiotherapy (EBRT) was an independent predictor of survival.[11] In a smaller study from British Columbia, survival was better in patients who had more extensive surgery and had high-dose radiation with or without chemotherapy.[12] That these were population-based studies is important: a number of single institutional studies also support the use of multimodality therapy compared to mono therapy but they are all subject to bias as there is always an element of case selection with patients with less extensive disease, young age and better performance status potentially receiving more aggressive therapy.[9, 13-17]

The role of additional therapy after resection of an incidental ATC is uncertain. The ATA working group did not come to a consensus on whether to advise additional therapy in this situation. The role for neoadjuvant therapy for patients with unresectable disease is also uncertain. Although there have been a few reports recommending neoadjuvant therapy, the majority of patients remain unresectable. Rather than planned neoadjuvant therapy, the ATA guidelines recommend combined modality therapy for unresectable disease and, if the disease response is durable and distant metastases do not develop, then consideration of surgical resection.[7, 18-20]

UNRESECTABLE LOCOREGIONAL DISEASE

Data on outcome when a resection is not possible are mainly from single institutional reports and again subject to case selection bias, but patients with good performance status with no evidence of metastatic disease appear to have a better outcome following high-dose radiation with or without chemotherapy.[14] A response rate of 80% to radiation alone has been reported with suggestion of a dose response with higher doses resulting in a trend to improved survival but not tumour response.[21] To overcome the rapid growth rate of ATC and potential for tumour cell repopulation after radiation has commenced, the radiation may be hyperfractionated and accelerated with two fractions given a day, so that the overall treatment time is reduced. In addition, chemotherapy may be given concurrently in an attempt at radiation sensitization.[22] The most frequently prescribed chemotherapy agent in the past was doxorubicin. In a multimodality approach combining mostly doxorubicin with hyperfractionated radiation, a local control rate of 60% has been reported, but the 2-year survival rate was only 9%.[23] In contrast, the Mayo Clinic experience found no benefit in median survival, although more survived to 1 year (23%) when chemotherapy + radiation was compared with radiation alone (10%).[24]

Several more recent reports of other agents that are better established as head and neck cancer radiosensitization (cisplatin and taxanes) have suggested encouraging results with concurrent chemoradiation. In a report on 6 patients treated with intensity-modulated radiation therapy (IMRT) and docetaxel all patients had at least a partial response and 4 had a complete response.[25] In another report on 10 patients, 5 were alive and free from disease at 32 months with a median survival of 60 months. However, due to either metastatic disease or patient preference, only 10 out of 25 patients with ATC were treated on the protocol.[26] In a report of hyperfractionated radiation without chemotherapy the median survival was greater than with conventional therapy (13.6 vs 10.3 months).²² In contrast in another study, however, a hyperfractionated accelerated protocol with larger fraction size, no survival advantage was reported but there was significant toxicity.²⁷

Typical radiation doses would be hyperfractionated 60–70 Gy in 40–45 fractions over 4–5 weeks or daily fractions such as 60–70 Gy in 30–35 fractions.

Most of the newer studies combining radiation and chemotherapy utilize IMRT. With this technique it is possible to generate concave dose distributions and narrow margined dose gradients so that normal structures can be spared while complex volumes are treated.[17, 28, 29] Despite modern radiation techniques, the toxicity from hyperfractionated radiation or concurrent chemoradiation can be significant and enteral nutrition with a feeding tube and growth factor support may be required, especially if large tumour volumes are treated. There has been no comparison of altered fractionation alone

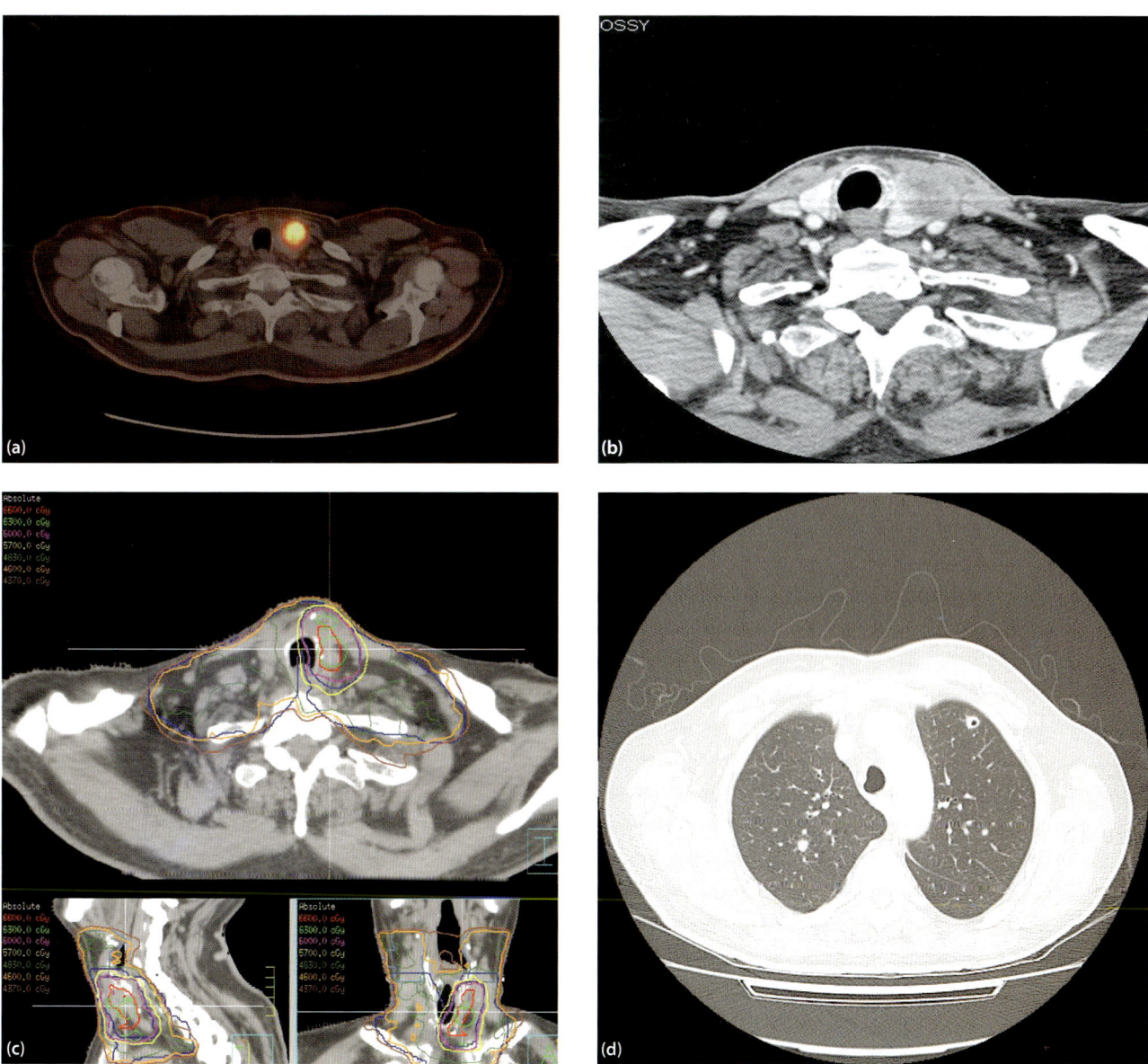

Figure 64.1 Anaplastic thyroid cancer. A 68-year-old man who had a long-standing history of a thyroid nodule that had increased in size. Fine-needle aspiration showed large and spindle cells and necrosis diagnostic of anaplastic thyroid. **(a)** Axial CT scans of his head and neck showed a 4 cm mass. There was no evidence of local invasion or lymph node involvement. **(b)** A PET scan showed uptake at the site of the lesion and nowhere else. He underwent surgical resection. Pathology revealed a 4 cm widely invasive anaplastic thyroid carcinoma. The tumour arose from a well-differentiated papillary carcinoma showing tall cell change but 70% of the total tumour volume was anaplastic carcinoma. There was extensive perineural invasion, and focal angioinvasion. The tumour infiltrated extrathyroidal skeletal muscle. **(c)** He received post-operative radiation therapy using an IMRT technique: 60 Gy in 40 fractions twice daily over 4 weeks was given to the post-operative site and concurrent 44 Gy in 40 fractions to the rest of the thyroid bed and adjacent nodal areas. **(d)** Within 2 months of completing his radiation he developed lung metastases which have progressed on paclitaxel.

compared to chemoradiation with standard or hyperfractionated radiation and the potential benefits remain unanswered especially when more aggressive therapy is associated with increased toxicity.[30]

There is no consensus whether there is any benefit in high-dose radiation with or without concurrent chemotherapy in patients with limited metastatic disease and otherwise good performance status, but it has been recommended in selected highly motivated patients.[7, 31] For patients of poor performance status who decline or who would not tolerate high-dose radiation, low-dose radiation may be of palliative benefit in controlling pain and possibly obstructive symptoms.[21] As noted earlier, radiation can result in an 80% response rate and, although higher doses of radiation resulted in improved survival, the response rate was no better. Palliative doses such as 20 Gy in five fractions (which may be repeated 4–6 weeks later) or 30 Gy in ten fractions may be of benefit in these patients.

METASTATIC DISEASE

In the presence of metastatic ATC, life expectancy is poor and therefore maintaining a good quality of life for as long as possible is imperative. Short 1–2-week courses of radiation as described above may control local symptoms. Unfortunately, ATC is not a chemosensitive disease and the response rates to systemic therapy are generally poor and short-lived. Currently, of the available chemotherapeutic agents the taxanes (paclitaxel or docetaxel), doxorubicin and cisplatin have the greatest clinical effect. Docetaxel (60 mg/m^2 i.v. every 3 weeks) can stabilize disease for a time and rarely results in a complete response.[25] There are several small reports on the use of molecular targeted agents. Antimicrotubular agents and kinase inhibitors occasionally result in a partial response or stable disease but more research is required.[2, 7, 32] Palliative radiation may be required for bone and lung metastases.[33]

KEY POINTS

ANAPLASTIC THYROID CARCINOMA

- Uncommon
- Poor survival (median 3–5 months)
- Best if incidental or R0 resection possible
- Often disseminated at diagnosis
- The role of surgery is for:
  - diagnosis
  - secure airway
  - resect to R0 or R1 if possible
- Local regional control important
- Multimodality treatment: surgery, radiation, chemotherapy
- Not chemosensitive but taxanes and molecular targeted agents show some promise
- Quality of life and palliative care are important
- Treatment guidelines:
  - American Thyroid Association – comprehensive
  - National Comprehensive Cancer Network – limited
  - European Thyroid Association – very limited

LYMPHOMAS

The management of non-Hodgkin lymphoma (NHL) in the thyroid gland is primarily influenced by the acuteness of the presentation, histology and the Ann Arbor stage.[6] A thyroid presentation occurs in only 1–2% of all patients diagnosed with lymphoma, and these are usually in stage IE (when the thyroid gland alone is involved) or stage IIE (when the cervical or superior mediastinum lymph nodes are involved additionally). The 'E' designations indicate that an extranodal organ (the thyroid gland) is involved as a primary site. The principle role for surgery is to establish the diagnosis of lymphoma[34] and to ensure a stable airway since thyroid lymphomas often present with a bulky mass with significant compression of the upper aerodigestive tract. A tracheostomy (temporary) may sometimes be necessary for tracheal lumen compromise if the patient presents with stridor. While fine-needle aspirate (FNA) may suggest lymphoma, it may be inadequate for subtyping the histology, in which case either core-needle biopsy or an open biopsy will be required. Optimal pathology interpretation involves immunophenotypic and sometimes special molecular studies, which can be done on cytology specimens if there is good cell yield. Special fixative and fresh tissue are necessary and therefore specific protocols for tissue retrieval and processing are required. If the FNA biopsy is diagnostic and able to subtype the lymphoma accurately, the therapeutic role of surgery is limited[34] as most patients are treated with chemotherapy, radiation therapy, or a combination of the two. In most cases a philosophy of functional preservation is followed. The need for the use of chemotherapy and/or radiation therapy is generally not diminished following surgical excision of lymphoma, except in the case of MALT lymphoma where a thyroidectomy if performed may be considered curative if there has been a complete excision.[35] However, aggressive surgical approaches that compromise function, including neck dissection and cosmesis, should be avoided.

Staging investigations should include CT scans of neck, chest, abdomen and pelvis and a FDG-PET scan. Thyroid scintigraphy tests with radioactive iodine or ^{99m}Tc are generally unhelpful. Blood work including complete blood count, lactate dehydrogenase (LDH) (which as a tumour marker for lymphoma usually correlates with the disease burden), liver function tests and creatinine should be done. A bone marrow aspirate and biopsy is standard. Approximately 90% will be found to have localized (stage IE or stage IIE) disease.[36] Advanced stages (stages III–IV) of lymphoma where there is documented lymphoma outside the thyroid gland and cervical lymph nodes are treated primarily with chemotherapy and will not be discussed further here. In these situations the thyroid involvement is considered secondary spread as part of disseminated lymphoma. For stage I–II presentations in the thyroid, the curative treatment approach involves radiation alone, or combined modality therapy with chemotherapy followed by consolidation radiation.

Indolent lymphoma

The most common indolent lymphomas in the thyroid are **MALT lymphomas** (also known as extranodal marginal zone lymphomas), with **follicular lymphomas** being second most common;[36, 37] both are radiation-sensitive diseases. MALT lymphomas present with localized (stage IE–IIE) disease in 90% of cases,[38, 39, 41] involving the thyroid gland as a nodule or mass, occasionally diffusely enlarging the thyroid gland, usually non-bulky (<5 cm). It is almost always associated with pre-existing Hashimoto's thyroiditis and occasionally other autoimmune diseases which are predisposing conditions to the development of MALT lymphomas.[41] Cervical lymph nodes are involved in 20–30% of cases. Females are more commonly affected than males with a ratio of 3:1.[36]

Stage I and stage II MALT or follicular lymphomas of the thyroid gland are treated with involved-site radiation therapy (RT), covering the thyroid site and the immediate drainage lymph node regions (zones 3, 4, 5 and 6). If a total thyroidectomy was performed and the MALT lymphoma was localized within the thyroid gland and has been completely excised, no further therapy may be required and the patient should be carefully followed.[35] Local treatment is therefore highly successful, resulting in an excellent local control rate exceeding 95% and long-term disease-free survival of >90% for MALT lymphoma,[38, 39, 41, 42] and 50–60% for follicular lymphoma.[44, 45] Because of exquisite radiation sensitivity, low to moderate doses (24–30 Gy, fractionated over 2–4 weeks) has been the standard approach.

Aggressive histology lymphoma

Thyroid lymphoma with aggressive histology is the most common, accounting for 65–70% of cases.[36, 37, 45] It usually presents with a rapidly enlarging mass, sometimes growing to 10 cm or even larger when diagnosed. It can arise *de novo* or from pre-existing indolent lymphoma or Hashimoto's thyroiditis, recognized as histological transformation to aggressive disease with a poorer prognosis. There is a female predominance with typical presenting age of over 65 years.[37, 46] Cervical lymph nodes are commonly involved (20–50%).[45, 46] The most frequent histology is diffuse large B-cell lymphoma (DLBCL)[37] (**Figure 64.2**) for which standard therapy has been well established based on phase III clinical trials. Other types of aggressive lymphomas (e.g. T-cell lymphomas) rarely present in the thyroid and the management is based on a similar philosophy of treatment with combined modality therapy (CMT) and functional preservation.

Despite a presentation at an early stage (IE–IIE), the recognition of the high risk for occult systemic disease mandates the use of systemic immunochemotherapy to achieve the best cure rates.[37, 45, 46] Patients are treated with CMT, typically the CHOP-R regimen (cyclophosphamide, doxorubicin, vincristine, prednisone and rituximab), with chemotherapy first for 3–6 cycles, followed by moderate dose radiation (30–40 Gy) 3–6 weeks later. In general, a cure rate ranging from 70–85% is achieved, depending on age, tumour burden and other prognostic factors such as performance status and LDH level.[46, 47] For the typical B-cell lymphomas, the addition of immunotherapy with anti-CD20 antibody (rituximab) in combination with chemotherapy improves the clinical outcome compared with CHOP alone[48–50] and is considered the standard approach. Because of the moderate radiation doses required (30–40 Gy), short-term toxicity is mild and serious long-term toxicity is rare, particularly with IMRT, with improved ability to further reduce the dose to uninvolved normal tissues. For stage IE patients treated with CMT, the radiation volume can be limited to the primary thyroid disease site, without intentional coverage of the drainage lymph nodes. For stage IIE patients, the coverage should include the thyroid site and the immediate drainage lymph node regions (typically bilateral zones 3, 4, 5 and 6).

Toxicity of treatment

When chemotherapy is required, the principle toxicities depend on the drugs used. For the CHOP-R regimen, the most common toxicities include nausea and vomiting, fatigue, alopecia, mucositis, myelosuppression, increased risk of infections and bleeding, neuropathy (vincristine), infusion-related reactions (rituximab) and prednisone-related side effects. More serious toxicities, such as cardiac failure, are fortunately rare. Standard management protocols including use of pre-medication, cardiac ejection fraction assessment and monitoring, and use of growth factor support minimizes these risks.

The toxicities of radiation therapy are moderate and significantly less severe than for treatments given for thyroid cancer, due to the lower total dose required for lymphoma. Short-term toxicity is mild and serious long-term toxicity is rare in virtually all head and neck tissues irradiated in the lower neck area. Xerostomia is not expected since the treated volume is generally below the level of the salivary glands. There is a significant risk of radiation-induced hypothyroidism (30% risk for a dose of 30–40 Gy).

770 Section 2: Head and Neck Endocrine Surgery

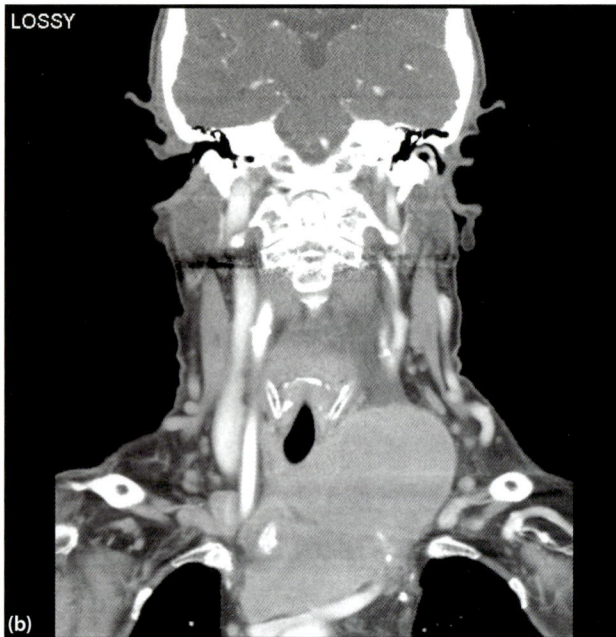

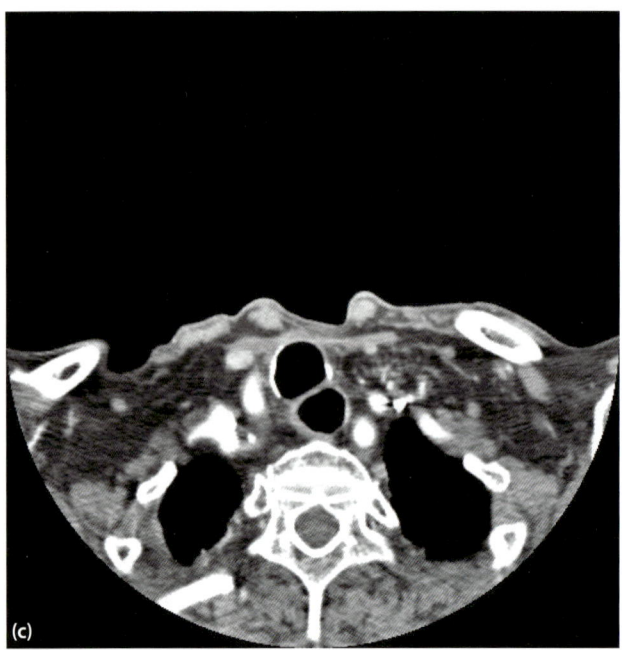

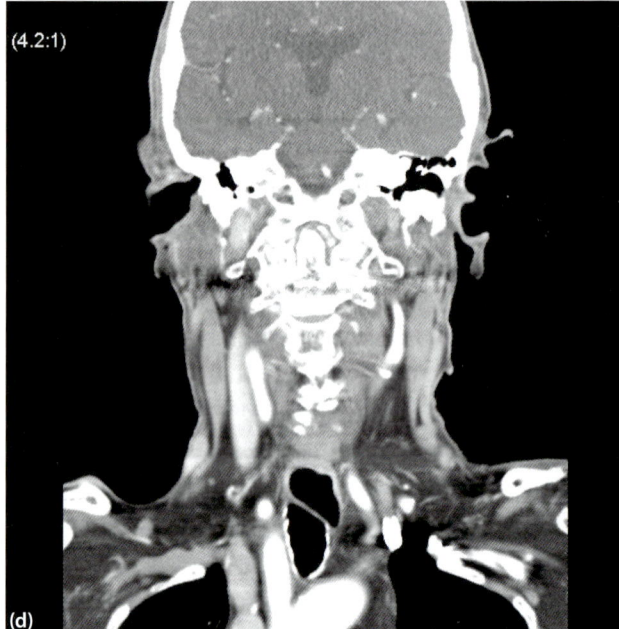

Figure 64.2 Lymphoma. An 82-year-old woman with a rapidly enlarging thyroid mass, with biopsy (right hemithyroidectomy) showing diffuse large B-cell lymphoma. There was significant residual disease involving the left lobe of the gland, right paratracheal area, and also lymphadenopathy in the left neck. Stage IIAE. Pre-treatment CT scans: **(a)** axial; **(b)** coronal. Treatment was with combined chemotherapy and radiation (CHOP-R × 6 cycles and 35 Gy) with curative intent. There was complete resolution of the disease 2 years post therapy. Post-treatment CT scans: **(c)** axial; **(d)** coronal.

KEY POINTS

Primary thyroid lymphomas

- Uncommon
- Usually localized
- The role of surgery is for:
  - diagnosis
  - secure airway
- Almost always B-cell lymphomas
- The MALT-type lymphoma has a high cure rate (>90%) with local therapy (surgery or radiation)
- Diffuse large B-cell lymphoma requires combined chemotherapy and radiation with long-term cure in 75% of patients

REFERENCES

1. Smallridge RC. Approach to the patient with anaplastic thyroid carcinoma. *J Clin Endocrinol Metab* 2012; **97**(8): 2566–72.
2. Smallridge RC, Copland JA. Anaplastic thyroid carcinoma: pathogenesis and emerging therapies. *Clin Oncol* 2010; **22**(6): 486–97.
3. Brierley JD, Gospodarowicz MK, Wittekind C, (eds). *TNM Classification of Malignant Tumours* 8th edn. New York: Wiley Blackwell, 2016.
4. Kim TY, Kim KW, Jung TS, et al. Prognostic factors for Korean patients with anaplastic thyroid carcinoma. *Head Neck* 2007; **29**(8): 765–72.
5. Brierley JD, Asa SL. Thyroid cancer. In: Gospodarowicz MK, O'Sullivan B, Sobin LH (eds). *Prognostic factors in cancer*. Hoboken, NJ: John Wiley; 2006.
6. Sobin LH, Gospodartowicz MK, Wittekind C (eds). *TNM classification of malignant tumours*. 7th ed. Oxford: Wiley-Blackwell (in affiliation with UICC); 2009.
7. Smallridge RC, Ain KB, Asa SL, et al. American thyroid association guidelines for management of patients with anaplastic thyroid cancer. *Thyroid* 2012; **22**(11): 1104–39.
8. Yoshida A, Kamma H, Asaga T, et al. Proliferative activity in thyroid tumors. *Cancer* 1992; **69**(10): 2548–52.
9. Haigh PI, Ituarte PH, Wu HS, et al. Completely resected anaplastic thyroid carcinoma combined with adjuvant chemotherapy and irradiation is associated with prolonged survival. *Cancer* 2001; **91**(12): 2335–42.
10. Ito K, Hanamura T, Murayama K, et al. Multimodality therapeutic outcomes in anaplastic thyroid carcinoma: improved survival in subgroups of patients with localized primary tumors. *Head Neck* 2012; **34**(2): 230–7.
11. Kebebew E, Greenspan FS, Clark OH, et al. Anaplastic thyroid carcinoma: treatment outcome and prognostic factors. *Cancer* 2005; **103**(7): 1330–5.
12. Goutsouliak V, Hay JH. Anaplastic thyroid cancer in British Columbia 1985–1999: a population-based study. *Clin Oncol* 2005; **17**(2): 75–8.
13. Swaak-Kragten AT, de Wilt JH, Schmitz PI, et al. Multimodality treatment for anaplastic thyroid carcinoma: treatment outcome in 75 patients. *Radiother Oncol* 2009; **92**(1): 100–4.
14. Pierie JP, Muzikansky A, Gaz RD, et al. The effect of surgery and radiotherapy on outcome of anaplastic thyroid carcinoma. *Ann Surg Oncol* 2002; **9**(1): 57–64.
15. De Crevoisier R, Baudin E, Bachelot A, et al. Combined treatment of anaplastic thyroid carcinoma with surgery, chemotherapy, and hyperfractionated accelerated external radiotherapy. *Int J Radiat Oncol Biol Phys* 2004; **60**(4): 1137–43.
16. Schlumberger M, Parmentier C, Delisle MJ, et al. Combination therapy for anaplastic giant cell thyroid carcinoma. *Cancer* 1991; **67**(3): 564–6.
17. Bhatia A, Rao A, Ang KK, et al. Anaplastic thyroid cancer: clinical outcomes with conformal radiotherapy. *Head Neck* 2010; **32**(7): 829–36.
18. Brignardello E, Gallo M, Baldi I, et al. Anaplastic thyroid carcinoma: clinical outcome of 30 consecutive patients referred to a single institution in the past 5 years. *Eur J Endocrinol* 2007; **156**(4): 425–30.
19. Besic N, Hocevar M, Zgajnar J, et al. Prognostic factors in anaplastic carcinoma of the thyroid: a multivariate survival analysis of 188 patients. *Langenbecks Arch Surg* 2005; **390**(3): 203–8.
20. Tan RK, Finley RK 3rd, Driscoll D, et al. Anaplastic carcinoma of the thyroid: a 24-year experience. *Head Neck* 1995; **17**(1): 41–7; discussion 7–8.
21. Junor E, Paul J, Reed N. Anaplastic thyroid carcinoma: 91 patients treated by surgery and radiotherapy. *Eur J Surg* 1992; **18**: 83–8.
22. Wang Y, Tsang R, Asa S, et al. Clinical outcome of anaplastic thyroid carcinoma treated with radiotherapy of once- and twice-daily fractionation regimens. *Cancer* 2006; **107**(8): 1786–92.
23. Tennvall J, Lundell G, Wahlberg P, et al. Anaplastic thyroid carcinoma: three protocols combining doxorubicin, hyperfractionated radiotherapy and surgery. *Br J Cancer* 2002; **86**(12): 1848–53.
24. McIver B, Hay ID, Giuffrida DF, et al. Anaplastic thyroid carcinoma: a 50-year experience at a single institution. *Surgery* 2001; **130**(6): 1028–34.
25. Troch M, Koperek O, Scheuba C, et al. High efficacy of concomitant treatment of undifferentiated (anaplastic) thyroid cancer with radiation and docetaxel. *J Clin Endocrinol Metab* 2010; **95**(9): E54–7.
26. Foote RL, Molina JR, Kasperbauer JL, et al. Enhanced survival in locoregionally confined anaplastic thyroid carcinoma: a single-institution experience using aggressive multimodal therapy. *Thyroid* 2011; **21**(1): 25–30.
27. Dandekar P, Harmer C, Barbachano Y, et al. Hyperfractionated accelerated radiotherapy (HART) for anaplastic thyroid carcinoma: toxicity and survival analysis. *Int J Radiat Oncol Biol Phys* 2009; **74**(2): 518–21.
28. Nutting CM, Convery DJ, Cosgrove VP, et al. Improvements in target coverage and reduced spinal cord irradiation using intensity-modulated radiotherapy (IMRT) in patients with carcinoma of the thyroid gland. *Radiother Oncol* 2001; **60**(2): 173–80.
29. Brierley J, Rumble R, Warde P, Panel IIE. *The role of IMRT in thyroid cancers*. Toronto, ON: Cancer Care Ontario; 2010.
30. Brierley JD. Update on external beam radiation therapy in thyroid cancer. *J Clin Endocrinol Metab* 2011; **96**(8): 2289–95.
31. Levendag PC, De Porre PM, van Putten WL. Anaplastic carcinoma of the thyroid gland treated by radiation therapy. *Int J Radiat Oncol Biol Phys* 1993; **26**(1): 125–8.
32. Bible KC, Foote RL, Smallridge RC. Toward improved outcomes in patients with anaplastic thyroid cancer. *Oncology* 2012; **26**(4): 398, 401, 406.
33. Brierley JD, Tsang RW. External beam radiation therapy for thyroid cancer. *Endocrinol Metab Clin North Am* 2008; **37**(2): 497–509, xi.
34. Meyer-Rochow GY, Sywak MS, Reeve TS, et al. Surgical trends in the management of thyroid lymphoma. *Eur J Surg Oncol* 2008; **34**(5): 576–80.
35. Thieblemont C, Mayer A, Dumontet C, et al. Primary thyroid lymphoma is a heterogeneous disease. *J Clin Endocrinol Metab* 2002; **87**(1): 105–11.
36. Graff-Baker A, Roman SA, Thomas DC, et al. Prognosis of primary thyroid lymphoma: demographic, clinical, and pathologic predictors of survival in 1,408 cases. *Surgery* 2009; **146**(6): 1105–15.
37. Alzouebi M, Goepel JR, Horsman JM, Hancock BW. Primary thyroid lymphoma: the 40 year experience of a UK lymphoma treatment centre. *Int J Oncol* 2012; **40**(6): 2075–80.
38. Zucca E, Conconi A, Pedrinis E, et al. Nongastric marginal zone B-cell lymphoma of mucosa-associated lymphoid tissue. *Blood* 2003; **101**(7): 2489–95.
39. Tsang RW, Gospodarowicz MK, Pintilie M, et al. Localized mucosa-associated lymphoid tissue lymphoma treated with radiation therapy has excellent clinical outcome. *J Clin Oncol* 2003; **21**(22): 4157–64.
40. Bible KC, Smallridge RC, Morris JC, et al. Development of a multidisciplinary, multicampus subspecialty practice in endocrine cancers. *J Oncol Pract* 2012; **8**(3 Suppl): e1s–5s.
41. Oh SY, Kim WS, Kim JS, et al. Primary thyroid marginal zone B-cell lymphoma of the mucosa-associated lymphoid tissue type: clinical manifestation and outcome of a rare disease: consortium for improving survival of lymphoma study. *Acta Haematol* 2012; **127**(2): 100–4.
42. Goda JS, Gospodarowicz M, Pintilie M, et al. Long-term outcome in localized extranodal mucosa-associated lymphoid tissue lymphomas treated with radiotherapy. *Cancer* 2010; **116**(16): 3815–24.
43. Sampson E, Brierley JD, Le LW, et al. Clinical management and outcome of papillary and follicular (differentiated) thyroid cancer presenting with distant metastasis at diagnosis. *Cancer* 2007; **110**(7): 1451–6.
44. Clarke A, Tsang R, Sun A, et al. Stage I–II follicular lymphoma: long-term outcomes. *Radiother Oncol* 2010; **96**(2): S60.
45. Onal C, Li YX, Miller RC, et al. Treatment results and prognostic factors in primary thyroid lymphoma patients: a rare cancer network study. *Ann Oncol* 2011; **22**(1): 156–64.
46. Mian M, Gaidano G, Conconi A, et al. High response rate and improvement of long-term survival with combined treatment modalities in patients with poor-risk primary thyroid diffuse large B-cell lymphoma: an International Extranodal Lymphoma Study Group and Intergruppo Italiano Linfomi study. *Leuk Lymphoma* 2011; **52**(5): 823–32.
47. Lopez-Guillermo A, Colomo L, Jimenez M, et al. Diffuse large B-cell lymphoma: clinicobiological characterization and outcome according to the nodal or extranodal primary origin. *J Clin Oncol* 2005; **23**(12): 2797–804.

48. Pfreundschuh M, Trumper L, Osterborg A, et al. CHOP-like chemotherapy plus rituximab versus CHOP-like chemotherapy alone in young patients with good-prognosis diffuse large-B-cell lymphoma: a randomised controlled trial by the MabThera International Trial (MInT) Group. *Lancet Oncol* 2006; 7(5): 379–91.
49. Coiffier B, Lepage E, Briere J, et al. CHOP chemotherapy plus rituximab compared with CHOP alone in elderly patients with diffuse large-B-cell lymphoma. *N Engl J Med* 2002; 346(4): 235–42.
50. Pfreundschuh M, Schubert J, Ziepert M, et al. Six versus eight cycles of bi-weekly CHOP-14 with or without rituximab in elderly patients with aggressive CD20+ B-cell lymphomas: a randomised controlled trial (RICOVER-60). *Lancet Oncol* 2008; 9(2): 105–16.

CHAPTER 65

MANAGEMENT OF LOCOREGIONALLY RECURRENT DIFFERENTIATED THYROID CANCER

Iain J. Nixon and Ashok R. Shaha

Introduction 773	Complications of treatments 776
Risk group stratification 773	Practical tips in the management of recurrent thyroid cancer 776
Definition of recurrence in differentiated thyroid cancer 774	Conclusion 777
Management of recurrence 775	References 777
Evaluation of thyroglobulin level 776	

SEARCH STRATEGY

Data in this chapter may be updated by a PubMed search using the keywords: thyroid cancer, recurrence, papillary thyroid cancer and follicular thyroid cancer.

INTRODUCTION

As differentiated thyroid cancer (DTC) becomes increasingly common, so does the challenge of managing patients with post-treatment evidence of recurrent disease. The appropriate management of such patients requires an understanding of the biology of DTC and the concept of recurrence versus persistent disease. Clinicians must also recognize the high potential for morbidity from salvage therapy and balance that against the benefit likely to be gained by their patients. In this chapter we will discuss recurrent DTC and outline an approach to management of this complex problem. The discussion will be limited to the surgical management of locoregional recurrence as systemic therapies for disseminated disease are discussed elsewhere.

RISK GROUP STRATIFICATION

Initial risk stratification systems for differentiated thyroid cancer focused on mortality.[1–3] Using these systems, patients can be classified as low, intermediate or high risk of death from disease. However, the majority of patients will fall into the low- and intermediate-risk groups with few fatalities. In 2009 the American Thyroid Association (ATA) recognized the importance of risk group stratification in recurrence prediction.[4] They published a system which again stratified patients in to low, intermediate and high risk of recurrence (**Table 65.1**).

Initial disease extent and the extent of primary surgical resection are important predictors of locoregional recurrence.[5] Those patients with advanced local disease or bulky nodal metastases have higher rates of recurrence than those with smaller lesions. Patients who have gross disease following surgery are clearly at high risk of disease progression.

Specific factors associated with locoregional recurrence include macroscopic extrathyroid extension, multiple or large volume nodal metastases, locally invasive disease and aggressive histological subtypes (insular, tall cell or poorly differentiated carcinoma). Other factors which can also predict poor outcome include advanced age, the presence of *BRAF* mutations and Tg doubling time.

A recent publication from the ATA recognized the importance of the status of the neck in predicting locoregional recurrence.[6] This work, which summarized the

TABLE 65.1 American Thyroid Association risk of recurrence stratification							
	Regional metastases	Distant metastases	Extrathyroid extension	Surgical resection	Aggressive pathology	RAI uptake outside thyroid bed	
Low risk	Absent	Absent	Absent	Complete	Absent	Absent	Only low risk if all are true
Intermediate risk	Present	Absent	Microscopic	Complete	Present	Present	Intermediate or high risk if any are true
High risk		Present	Macroscopic	Incomplete			

TABLE 65.2 Level of risk associated with specific nodal metastatic features in papillary thyroid cancer (adapted from Randolph et al[6])		
	Descriptor	Locoregional recurrence rate
Clinically N0 (cN0)	All patients	6%
	Young patients*	0%
	Older patients *	9%
Clinical N1 (cN1)	All patients	13–30%
	All patients*	19–42%
Pathological N1 (pN1)	All patients	7–14%
	All patients*	13%
Specific pN1 descriptors	<5 positive lymph nodes	3%
	>5 positive lymph nodes	19%
	>10 positive lymph nodes	21%
	Extranodal extension	15%

* Denotes that papillary micro carcinomas were excluded from these cohorts.

available literature at the time, demonstrated the importance of size and number of nodal metastases as well as the significance of extranodal extension (Table 65.2).

DEFINITION OF RECURRENCE IN DIFFERENTIATED THYROID CANCER

The approach to managing DTC has become increasingly standardized over the past 50 years.[4, 7–11] Recognition of the relatively indolent biology of the disease and the role of therapy has led to well-defined international treatment guidelines. However, over the same time period a significant change has taken place in relation to recurrent disease.

In the mid-20th century, clinicians followed their patients with clinical examination including palpation of the neck and visualization of the larynx. Investigations including chest X-rays would soon be surpassed by more advanced imaging including computed tomography (CT) scanning, magnetic resonance imaging (MRI) and ultrasound. Further progress with ever-improving imaging, particularly with the widespread adoption of high-resolution ultrasound, allowed clinicians to subject the central and lateral neck to increasing levels of scrutiny following initial therapy.

During the same period the introduction of serum thyroglobulin (Tg) measurement allowed a biochemical assessment of residual or recurrent tissue of thyroid origin. Improvements in the sensitivity of Tg assays have now allowed the detection of recurrence which is of such small volume that even the most advanced imaging systems cannot identify structural disease. In addition to measuring Tg in patients' serum, when structurally suspicious nodal disease is targeted for biopsy, cytology can be supported with thyroglobulin measurements in fine-needle aspiration biopsy specimens in order to confirm metastatic thyroid cancer.[12]

While our ability to identify biochemical and structural evidence of recurrent disease has improved, so too has our understanding of the biology of DTC. The majority of patients with DTC will have papillary thyroid cancer (PTC). This malignancy has a behaviour which does not conform to that of other head and neck malignancies. Groups who routinely dissect the regional lymph nodes in PTC report high rates (up to 40%) of histologically demonstrable metastatic lymph nodes, despite a lack of pre-operatively identifiable disease.[13] The more scrutiny such nodal dissections are subjected to, the higher the rate of demonstrable metastasis, with one group showing over 50% of nodal specimens to contain evidence of thyroid tissue in resected lymph node specimens by immunohistochemistry when conventional staining showed no evidence of thyroid cells.[14]

Unlike squamous cell carcinoma, however, where the presence of regional lymph node metastases is associated with a halving of survival, the impact of subclinical metastases in PTC has little impact on survival.[6] Indeed, the impact on recurrence has also be questioned.[15,16] So small is the perceived impact of occult nodal disease that no major international guideline now supports prophylactic lateral neck dissection in DTC and the tide is turning away from prophylactic central neck dissection also except in high-risk patients.[7,17]

In understanding recurrent DTC, therefore, the clinician must appreciate some critical distinctions. Structural recurrence which can be suspected based on clinical examination or imaging studies and supported by cytological sampling must be distinguished from biochemical recurrence alone. In addition, when disease is identified following initial therapy, a distinction must be drawn between likely persistent disease in the nodes of an untreated neck and truly recurrent disease which presents within the previously operated field. It should also be recognized that, when unresectable disease is identified either pre-operatively or following surgical exploration, progression of disease in that site presents another separate challenge for the disease management team.

Most recurrences are now detected by biochemical evaluation and/or ultrasound screening. Following initial therapy, a rising Tg tends to be an indication of recurrence which is generally in the lymph nodes of the neck. Although cross-sectional imaging and radioactive iodine (RAI) scans can be used to detect structural recurrence, ultrasound is usually the most convenient modality to assess the regional lymphatics. Positron emission tomography (PET) scanning can be useful, particularly for de-differentiating cancers which lose their radioactive iodine avidity. Such PET-positive, RAI-negative disease is more aggressive and associated with poor outcome. An outline for considering recurrent thyroid cancer is provided in Table 65.3.

MANAGEMENT OF RECURRENCE

The goals of managing recurrent disease in thyroid cancer should be considered prior to embarking on a course of management. The ultimate goals include removing recurrent disease and preventing further recurrence.[18] When considering these aims, one must also consider the goal of minimizing morbidity and negatively affecting a patient's quality of life. Indeed, if the decision is made to observe potentially recurrent disease, the goal of management is to prevent disease progression, with a particular focus on invasion of critical structures during follow-up.

Disease recurrence in the central neck may involve the nodal tissue, the thyroid bed or both. Local, thyroid bed recurrence is rare but, when it occurs, the anatomical location of disease presents a significant challenge in terms of surgical resection. Involvement of the recurrent laryngeal nerve (RLN) may be a presenting feature of the recurrence, and invasion of the larynx or trachea should be suspected based upon the relationship between the airway and the site of disease. Airway involvement can be categorized as by Shin et al. into tumour adherent to the perichondrium (stage 1), invading cartilage (stage 2), involving submucosa (stage 3) or involving mucosa (stage 4) (**Figure 65.1**).[19]

Pre-operative assessment of the airway is critical in managing thyroid cancer recurrence, particularly with regard to assessment of the function of the RLNs. If a tumour involves the oesophagus, unlike in primary disease where a plane can often be dissected between muscle and mucosa, scarring may require full-thickness oesophageal resection which will then mandate appropriate reconstruction with free tissue transfer or gastric pull-up. Following surgery, external beam radiotherapy should be considered as an adjunct as it has been shown to improve rates of local control in patients demonstrating gross extrathyroidal extension.[20-23]

A contrast should be made between visceral and nodal recurrence in the neck. Isolated nodal recurrence which does not involve the laryngopharyngeal complex should be carefully assessed prior to deciding to operate. Again the function of the RLNs, the size of the lesion and its

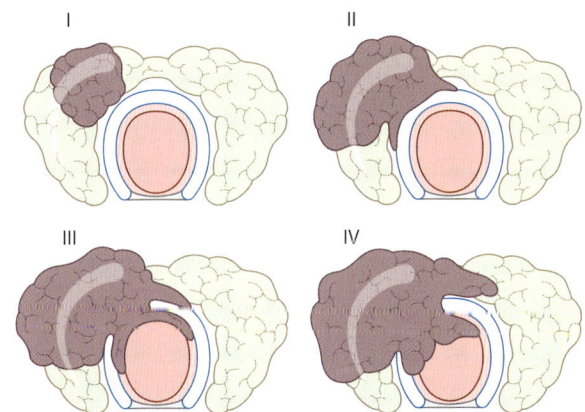

Figure 65.1 Shin classification of airway involvement with thyroid cancer.

TABLE 65.3 Types of differentiated thyroid cancer recurrence				
Central compartment			**Lateral neck**	**Distant**
Thyroid bed	Central compartment lymph nodes	Levels I–V	Retropharyngeal and parapharyngeal nodes	Pulmonary > non-pulmonary metastases
Recurrence involving visceral structures	(Levels VI and VII)			

precise anatomical location should be determined. Small-volume nodal tissue which is distant from the nerve and airway may be safely followed. In contrast, rapidly enlarging nodes or disease in close proximity to the central neck viscera should be treated more aggressively in order to prevent extension into vital structures.

A compartment-orientated approach to a previously unoperated nodal field harbouring recurrence includes a level II–V selective neck dissection for lateral neck disease and levels VI–VII for central neck disease. However, for recurrence within an operated field, such an approach is likely to be associated with high morbidity and a more targeted approach may be reasonable.

Evidence relating to oncological outcomes following surgical therapy for recurrent DTC suggests that a significant number of patients can be 'cured'. However, the literature is difficult to interpret due to differences in definitions of cure (biochemical versus structural), the inclusion of patients of various risk groups in different studies and the differences in duration of follow-up. Nonetheless, groups report success rates of 25–90% of appropriately selected patients.[24–30]

For example, research from MD Anderson Cancer Center, USA, found that, of 210 patients with recurrent or persistent PTC who underwent comprehensive central compartment dissection, 71% of pre-operatively Tg positive had no evidence of post-operative disease and 66% had no measurable Tg at last follow-up (median 7.25 years). Those patients who did suffer recurrence were able to be surgically salvaged giving an overall 98% central compartment control rate and 10-year disease-specific survival of 99% for young patients and 78% for older patients. In this surgical series from a tertiary referral cancer centre the rate of hypoparathyroidism was 1% and new RLN palsy was encountered in 2%.[27]

A group from Ohio State University reported outcomes of 95 patients with recurrent or persistent PTC. They found that 27% of patients achieved a biochemical complete response following lymphadenectomy and 42% achieved a stimulated Tg of <2.0 ng/mL. Even those who did not achieve a complete response did have a significant reduction in Tg following initial and, if required, subsequent surgeries. None of these patients developed distant metastases or died of disease.[28]

It should be noted, though, that the senior authors of such publications are experienced, high-volume surgeons often working in tertiary referral centres. Such outcomes are unlikely to be achieved in less experienced hands.

Traditional surgical therapy has been the standard of care for structural disease following initial therapy in DTC. However, some groups have adopted an alternative approach including both ethanol and radiofrequency ablation of small-volume recurrences with apparently high rates of success. Although not widely practised, these treatment modalities are particularly attractive for low-risk patients with small nodes in a site amenable to a percutaneous approach.[31–34]

EVALUATION OF THYROGLOBULIN LEVEL

The introduction of routine Tg monitoring following treatment for DTC has resulted in a paradigm shift in such patients' management. Small-volume recurrences can now be identified prior to the development of structural disease. The identification of a rising Tg should prompt further imaging. In most circumstances, persistent disease is in the neck and ultrasonography will be the initial imaging modality of choice. If significant structural disease is encountered, surgical excision should be recommended.

If small-volume (<8 mm) suspicious nodes are identified, clinicians should proceed with caution. When one study observed 166 low-risk patients with abnormal lateral neck nodes, only 20% of patients demonstrated progression and 14% regressed.[35] Assessment of the potential disease extent and relationship to critical structures should guide further management in this situation. Small-volume nodes which are distant from the RLN may safely be monitored without the need for biopsy or intervention. If a decision is made to pursue such small-volume disease, even in experienced hands, identification of the nodes in question can be challenging and techniques such as charcoal tattooing and intra-operative ultrasound should be considered to aid localization.

When a rising Tg is encountered in the absence of any evidence of structural disease on imaging, surgery is not indicated. The role of RAI in this situation is controversial with some advocating empirical treatment in an attempt to address occult micrometastases. In general, however, this approach is not supported.[36]

COMPLICATIONS OF TREATMENTS

Rates of complication in the setting of revision surgery, particularly in a previously operated field, are higher than those following initial therapy.[37] Although common complications include injury to the RLN and temporary or permanent hypoparathyroidism when re-entering the central neck, revision lateral neck surgery is also associated with high rates of injury to the accessory nerve, the lower division of the facial nerve or the sympathetic trunk. Due to the relatively high rates of complication, the disease management team must develop a balanced approach and incorporate what they consider the best surgical intervention to control disease while minimizing rates of complication.

PRACTICAL TIPS IN THE MANAGEMENT OF RECURRENT THYROID CANCER

The management of recurrent thyroid cancer is complex and surgical intervention may be difficult due to involvement or proximity of the structures in the central compartment. Thorough evaluation with cross-sectional imaging is very important. The decision about tracheal shave versus sleeve-resection of the trachea will directly depend on the tracheal involvement by recurrent tumour. A majority of the tumours can be easily shaved off the trachea, unless there is a direct submucosal or intra-luminal extension of the disease. The surgeon should be prepared to make these complex decisions intra-operatively for the best oncologic resection of the recurrent tumour.

The nodal recurrence in the central compartment and at level IV may be also a complex surgical undertaking, primarily related to complications of nerve injury and hypoparathyroidism. The operating surgeon should evaluate the extent of the disease and be prepared to manage the patient with a multidisciplinary approach. These patients will require lifetime follow-up.

A sub-centimetre recurrent tumour may be difficult to find and may present a higher risk of injuring the nerve. Generally these patients are secondary references to a cancer centre and involvement of the surgeon, endocrinologist and the multidisciplinary team is very critical. Patients should be warned of the complications of the surgical procedure and the appropriate decision-making should be undertaken for the best form of treatment. Patients should be informed that the thyroglobulin level may not be normalized after the surgery, or they may recur in the future, either in the same neck, quadrilateral neck or in the superior mediastinum. It is very important to have a best understanding with the patient, their family and the treating physicians. The first principal of surgery should be maintained – *Primum non nocere* – first do no harm.

CONCLUSION

Patients with recurrent differentiated thyroid cancer truly require multidisciplinary team management. Not only a surgeon and endocrinologist but nuclear medicine physician, radiologist, pathologist, cytologist and even oncologist must collaborate for optimal evaluation and overall control of disease. By balancing the risks of treatment against the chance of successful outcome, the disease management team must consider options from observation through limited resection to aggressive surgical therapy on a case-by-case basis.

KEY POINTS

- Recurrent thyroid cancer may be biochemical or structural.
- Careful assessment of recurrence should include cross-sectional imaging and endoscopy.
- Small volume nodal recurrence in areas without critical structures may be suitable for observation.
- Large-volume recurrence in high-risk areas (around the recurrent laryngeal nerve for example) should be managed surgically.
- The potential complications of revision surgery should be carefully weighed against the potential benefits on an individual patient basis.

REFERENCES

1. Byar DP, Green SB, Dor P, et al. A prognostic index for thyroid carcinoma. A study of the EORTC Thyroid Cancer Cooperative Group. *Eur J Cancer* 1979; **15**(8): 1033–41.
2. Hay ID, Bergstralh EJ, Goellner JR, et al. Predicting outcome in papillary thyroid carcinoma: development of a reliable prognostic scoring system in a cohort of 1779 patients surgically treated at one institution during 1940 through 1989. *Surgery* 1993; **114**(6): 1050–7; discussion 7–8.
3. Shaha AR, Shah JP, Loree TR. Risk group stratification and prognostic factors in papillary carcinoma of thyroid. *Ann Surg Oncol* 1996; **3**(6): 534–8.
4. Cooper DS, Doherty GM, Haugen BR, et al. Revised American Thyroid Association management guidelines for patients with thyroid nodules and differentiated thyroid cancer. *Thyroid* 2009; **19**(11): 1167–214.
5. Shah JP, Loree TR, Dharker D, et al. Prognostic factors in differentiated carcinoma of the thyroid gland. *Am J Surg* 1992; **164**(6): 658–61.
6. Randolph G, Duh QY, Heller KS, et al. The prognostic significance of nodal metastases from papillary thyroid carcinoma can be stratified based on the size and number of metastatic lymph nodes, as well as the presence of extranodal extension. ATA Surgical Affairs Committee's Taskforce on Thyroid Cancer Nodal Surgery. *Thyroid* 2012 Aug 10. PubMed PMID: 22881837.
7. Perros P, Boelaert K, Colley S, et al. Guidelines for the management of thyroid cancer. *Clin Endocrinol* 2014; **81** Suppl 1: 1–122.
8. Singer PA, Cooper DS, Daniels GH, et al. Treatment guidelines for patients with thyroid nodules and well-differentiated thyroid cancer. American Thyroid Association. *Arch Intern Med* 1996; **156**(19): 2165–72.
9. Watkinson JC. The British Thyroid Association guidelines for the management of thyroid cancer in adults. *Nucl Med Commun* 2004; **25**(9): 897–900.
10. British Thyroid Association, Royal College of Physicians. *Guidelines for the management of thyroid cancer* (Perros P, ed.) 2nd ed. Report of the Thyroid Cancer Guidelines Update Group. London: Royal College of Physicians; 2007.
11. Dottorini ME, Mansi L. P. Perros (ed.), British Thyroid Association, Royal College of Physicians. Guidelines for the management of thyroid cancer 2nd edition. Report of the Thyroid Cancer Guidelines Update Group. *Eur J Nucl Med Mol Imaging* 2008; **35**(6): 1218–19.
12. Uruno T, Miyauchi A, Shimizu K, et al. Usefulness of thyroglobulin measurement in fine-needle aspiration biopsy specimens for diagnosing cervical lymph node metastasis in patients with papillary thyroid cancer. *World J Surg* 2005; **29**(4): 483–5.
13. Hartl DM, Leboulleux S, Al Ghuzlan A, et al. Optimization of staging of the neck with prophylactic central and lateral neck dissection for papillary thyroid carcinoma. *Ann Surg* 2012; **255**(4): 777–83.
14. Qubain SW, Nakano S, Baba M, et al. Distribution of lymph node micrometastasis in pN0 well-differentiated thyroid carcinoma. *Surgery* 2002; **131**(3): 249–56.
15. Nixon IJ, Ganly I, Patel SG, et al. Observation of clinically negative central compartment lymph nodes in papillary thyroid carcinoma. *Surgery* 2013; **154**(6): 1166–72; discussion 72–3.
16. Monchik JM, Simon CJ, Caragacianu DL, et al. Does failure to perform prophylactic level VI node dissection leave persistent disease detectable by ultrasonography in patients with low-risk papillary carcinoma of the thyroid? *Surgery* 2009; **146**(6): 1182–7.
17. Haugen BRM, Alexander EK, Bible KC, et al. 2015 American Thyroid Association Management Guidelines for Adult Patients

with Thyroid Nodules and Differentiated Thyroid Cancer. *Thyroid* 2015 Oct 14. PubMed PMID: 26462967.
18. Urken ML, Milas M, Randolph GW, et al. A review of the management of recurrent and persistent metastatic lymph nodes in well differentiated thyroid cancer: a multifactorial decision making guide created for the Thyroid Cancer Care Collaborative. *Head Neck* 2014 Jan 17. PubMed PMID: 24436291.
19. Shin DH, Mark EJ, Suen HC, Grillo HC. Pathologic staging of papillary carcinoma of the thyroid with airway invasion based on the anatomic manner of extension to the trachea: a clinicopathologic study based on 22 patients who underwent thyroidectomy and airway resection. *Hum Pathol* 1993; **24**(8): 866–70.
20. Rosenbluth BD, Serrano V, Happersett L, et al. Intensity-modulated radiation therapy for the treatment of nonanaplastic thyroid cancer. *Int J Radiat Oncol Biol Phys* 2005; **63**(5): 1419–26.
21. Terezakis SA, Lee KS, Ghossein RA, et al. Role of external beam radiotherapy in patients with advanced or recurrent nonanaplastic thyroid cancer: Memorial Sloan-kettering Cancer Center experience. *Int J Radiat Oncol Biol Phys* 2009; **73**(3): 795–801.
22. Kim TH, Chung KW, Lee YJ, et al. The effect of external beam radiotherapy volume on locoregional control in patients with locoregionally advanced or recurrent nonanaplastic thyroid cancer. *Radiat Oncol* 2010; **5**: 69.
23. Schwartz DL, Lobo MJ, Ang KK, et al. Postoperative external beam radiotherapy for differentiated thyroid cancer: outcomes and morbidity with conformal treatment. *Int J Radiat Oncol Biol Phys* 2009; **74**(4): 1083–91.
24. Shah MD, Harris LD, Nassif RG, et al. Efficacy and safety of central compartment neck dissection for recurrent thyroid carcinoma. *Arch Otolaryngol Head Neck Surg* 2012; **138**(1): 33–7.
25. Farrag TY, Agrawal N, Sheth S, et al. Algorithm for safe and effective reoperative thyroid bed surgery for recurrent/persistent papillary thyroid carcinoma. *Head Neck* 2007; **29**(12): 1069–74.
26. Clayman GL, Shellenberger TD, Ginsberg LE, et al. Approach and safety of comprehensive central compartment dissection in patients with recurrent papillary thyroid carcinoma. *Head Neck* 2009; **31**(9): 1152–63.
27. Clayman GL, Agarwal G, Edeiken BS, et al. Long-term outcome of comprehensive central compartment dissection in patients with recurrent/persistent papillary thyroid carcinoma. *Thyroid* 2011; **21**(12): 1309–16.
28. Al-Saif O, Farrar WB, Bloomston M, et al. Long-term efficacy of lymph node reoperation for persistent papillary thyroid cancer. *J Clin Endocrinol Metab* 2010; **95**(5): 2187–94.
29. Yim JH, Kim WB, Kim EY, et al. The outcomes of first reoperation for locoregionally recurrent/persistent papillary thyroid carcinoma in patients who initially underwent total thyroidectomy and remnant ablation. *J Clin Endocrinol Metab* 2011; **96**(7): 2049–56.
30. Onkendi EO, McKenzie TJ, Richards ML, et al. Reoperative experience with papillary thyroid cancer. *World J Surg* 2014; **38**(3): 645–52.
31. Hay ID, Charboneau JW. The coming of age of ultrasound-guided percutaneous ethanol ablation of selected neck nodal metastases in well-differentiated thyroid carcinoma. *J Clin Endocrinol Metab* 2011; **96**(9): 2717–20.
32. Hay ID, Lee RA, Davidge-Pitts C, et al. Long-term outcome of ultrasound-guided percutaneous ethanol ablation of selected "recurrent" neck nodal metastases in 25 patients with TNM stages III or IVA papillary thyroid carcinoma previously treated by surgery and 131I therapy. *Surgery* 2013; **154**(6): 1448–54; discussion 54–5.
33. Lee SJ, Jung SL, Kim BS, et al. Radiofrequency ablation to treat locoregional recurrence of well-differentiated thyroid carcinoma. *Korean J Radiol* 2014; **15**(6): 817–26.
34. Kim JH, Yoo WS, Park YJ, et al. Efficacy and safety of radiofrequency ablation for treatment of locally recurrent thyroid cancers smaller than 2 cm. *Radiology* 2015; **276**(3): 909–18.
35. Robenshtok E, Fish S, Bach A, et al. Suspicious cervical lymph nodes detected after thyroidectomy for papillary thyroid cancer usually remain stable over years in properly selected patients. *J Clin Endocrinol Metab* 2012 Aug; **97**(8): 2706–13.
36. Sabra MM, Grewal RK, Tala H, et al. Clinical outcomes following empiric radioiodine therapy in patients with structurally identifiable metastatic follicular cell-derived thyroid carcinoma with negative diagnostic but positive post-therapy ^{131}I whole-body scans. *Thyroid* 2012; **22**(9): 877–83.
37. Chadwick D, Kinsman R, Walton P. *The British Association of Endocrine & Thyroid Surgeons Fourth National Audit Report*. Henley-on-Thames, Oxfordshire: Dendrite Clinical Systems Ltd; 2012.

CHAPTER 66

NON-SURGICAL MANAGEMENT OF THYROID CANCER

Laura Moss

Differentiated thyroid cancer..779
Medullary thyroid carcinoma...786
Metastatic medullary thyroid cancer 787
Anaplastic thyroid cancer..788
References 789

SEARCH STRATEGY

Data in this chapter may be updated by a PubMed search using the keywords: radioactive iodine, risk stratification, thyroglobulin, radiation protection and targeted therapy.

DIFFERENTIATED THYROID CANCER

There is limited prospective randomized controlled data relating to the management of differentiated thyroid cancer (DTC) as it is an uncommon disease with a long natural history. Many areas of thyroid cancer management remain controversial, including the indications for ablation using radioactive iodine (RAI, also called radioiodine), the optimal administered activity of radioiodine, the degree and duration of thyroid-stimulating hormone (TSH) suppression, as well as indications for external beam radiotherapy and optimal timing for initiation of targeted therapies for the treatment of metastatic disease. The recommendations in this chapter reflect common UK practice and advice from the British Thyroid Association (BTA) and American Thyroid Association (ATA) guidelines.[1,2]

^{131}I treatment

Normal thyroid gland tissue and differentiated thyroid cancer can concentrate iodine from the circulation and ^{131}I (an unsealed radionuclide of iodine) is taken up in the same way as stable iodine in the diet.

In practice, it is very difficult to achieve complete surgical ablation of the thyroid gland and some residual tissue, known as the thyroid remnant, is inevitably present. As a rule, normal thyroid tissue within the remnant will preferentially take up the iodine compared to thyroid cancer tissue. Hence, if a large remnant is present post-operatively, the post-ablation whole-body radioiodine scan cannot be relied upon to exclude the presence of residual malignancy either locally in the neck or at distant sites as the iodine may be seen in the remnant only. Only when this remnant of normal thyroid tissue is ablated can you reliably expect to see any significant radioiodine uptake in regional and distant sites of differentiated thyroid cancer.

RADIOIODINE REMNANT ABLATION

Radioiodine uptake is usually seen in the thyroid bed following a total or near-total thyroidectomy. ^{131}I destruction of this residual tissue is called radioiodine remnant ablation (RRA).

RRA aids the detection and earlier treatment of persistent/metastatic disease by destroying normal thyroid tissue; it may destroy microscopic foci of cancer in the thyroid remnant, and aids interpretation of serum thyroglobulin (Tg) measurements during follow-up. Remnant ablation may reduce local recurrence and increase survival,[3,4] although not all reported series support these findings.[5-8]

It is important to individualize patient management and to use radioiodine selectively by allocating patients to a risk category post-operatively (**Table 66.1**).

TABLE 66.1 Post-operative risk stratification for risk of recurrence of DTC[1]

Category of risk	Patient characteristics
Low risk	No local or distant metastases
	All macroscopic tumour has been resected, i.e. R0 or R1 resection
	No tumour invasion of locoregional tissues or structures
	The tumour does not have aggressive histology (tall cell, or columnar cell PTC, diffuse sclerosing PTC, poorly differentiated elements) or angioinvasion
Immediate risk	Microscopic invasion of tumour into the perithyroidal soft tissues (T3) at initial surgery
	Cervical lymph node metastases (N1a or N1b)
	Tumour with aggressive histology (tall cell, or columnar cell PTC, diffuse sclerosing PTC, poorly differentiated elements) or angioinvasion
High risk	Extrathyroidal invasion
	Incomplete macroscopic tumour resection (R2 resection)
	Distant metastases (M1)

The following is the British Thyroid Association's guidance on the indications for ^{131}I ablation.[1]

- **No indication for ^{131}I ablation**
  These patients are at low risk of recurrence or cancer-specific mortality.
  o Tumour <1 cm unifocal or multifocal, and on histology classical papillary or follicular variant or follicular minimally invasive without angioinvasion and no invasion of thyroid capsule.
- **Definite indications for ^{131}I ablation**
  o Tumour >4 cm.
  o Any tumour size with gross extrathyroidal extension (pT4).
  o Distant metastases present.
- **Uncertain indications for ^{131}I ablation**
  Patients in this category may or may not derive a benefit from ablation. Factors that may influence the decision on whether to proceed include:
  o large tumour size
  o extrathyroidal extension
  o presence of unfavourable histological cell type (tall cell, or columnar cell papillary thyroid cancer (PTC), diffuse sclerosing PTC, poorly differentiated elements)
  o widely invasive histology
  o multiple metastatic lymph nodes
  o resected metastatic lymph nodes large in size, high ratio of positive to negative nodes, extracapsular nodal involvement.

HIGH VERSUS LOW ADMINISTERED ACTIVITY OF ^{131}I FOR REMNANT ABLATION

Administered activities of ^{131}I of 1.1 GBq or 3.7 GBq show similar rates of successful remnant ablation,[10–13] although there is a trend towards higher success rates with higher administered activities.

Results from two large multicentre randomized trials[14, 15] have shown that 1.1 GBq of ^{131}I was as effective as 3.7 GBq in ablating the thyroid remnant, while adverse events were fewer in the 1.1 GBq group. In these studies all patients had undergone total thyroidectomy and had an R0 (no microscopic residual disease) resection. Most patients were staged pT1 N0 and pT2 N0. One of the trials[14] included patients with pT3 tumours, and patients with N1 disease, who were ablated successfully with 1.1 GBq. A recent meta-analysis found no difference in efficacy between 1.1 GBq and 3.7 GBq.[16]

^{131}I ADMINISTRATION PROCEDURE

Those prescribing radionuclide therapies in the UK must hold an appropriate Administration of Radioactive Substances Advisory Committee (ARSAC) certificate and the treatment must be given in appropriately designed areas.

Radioiodine is administered orally. Although it is available in liquid or capsule formulations, the latter is the preferred format as it is easier and safer to handle.

For successful remnant ablation to be achieved, the TSH level prior to the isotope administration must be elevated to >25–30 mU/L. This stimulates the sodium iodide symporter (membrane protein involved in active transport) and hence radioiodine uptake into thyrocytes. This can be achieved in two ways.

- **Recombinant human TSH injections (rhTSH, Thyrogen™):** These can be administered as an exogenous source of TSH and allow the patient to continue with thyroid hormones throughout the radioisotope treatment period. The benefit with using rhTSH is the avoidance of potential significant physical and psychological symptoms of hypothyroidism resulting from thyroid hormone withdrawal.[17, 18]
- **Thyroid hormone withdrawal:** If the period between surgery and RRA is expected to be longer than 4 weeks, patients should be commenced on thyroid hormone replacement. If liothyronine is commenced (usual dose 20 mcg tds), this should be withdrawn 14 days prior to radioactive iodine treatment. If levothyroxine is used, it should be substituted with liothyronine starting 28 days prior to radioactive iodine treatment and this is then stopped for the last 14 days prior to treatment. By swapping the thyroid hormones in this way, it is possible to reduce the length of time that the patient is rendered hypothyroid. If ^{131}I ablation can be performed approximately 4 weeks after surgery, there may be no need for thyroid hormone supplementation to be commenced in the immediate post-operative period but this might be associated with the development of unnecessary hypothyroid symptoms.

The decision whether a patient should receive ^{131}I remnant ablation after thyroid hormone withdrawal (THW) or after rhTSH injections depends on the current licensed indications of use for rhTSH, the patient's comorbidities and the local availability of rhTSH injections.

The current licensed indications for rhTSH (Thyrogen™) use are as follows:

- With serum Tg testing with or without radioiodine imaging for the detection of thyroid remnants and well-differentiated thyroid cancer in post-thyroidectomy patients maintained on thyroid hormone suppression therapy (THST). Low-risk patients with well-differentiated thyroid carcinoma who have undetectable serum Tg levels on THST and no rhTSH-stimulated increase of Tg levels may be followed up by assaying rhTSH-stimulated Tg levels.
- For pre-therapeutic stimulation in combination with a range of 1.1–3.7 GBq radioiodine for ablation of thyroid tissue remnants in patients who have undergone a near-total or total thyroidectomy for well-differentiated thyroid cancer and who do not have evidence of distant metastatic thyroid cancer.

Patient factors that would warrant rhTSH use in preference to THW include hypopituitarism, functional metastases causing TSH suppression, severe ischaemic heart disease, previous history of psychiatric disturbance precipitated by hypothyroidism, advanced disease and frailty.

Injections of rhTSH (0.9 mg) are given by deep i.m. injection into the buttock on days 1 and 2 with radioiodine being administered on day 3.

Possible rhTSH side effects include flu-like myalgia, mild nausea and headache. There is also the possibility of stimulating thyroid remnant tissue and metastases, resulting in local symptoms, and consideration should be given to prophylactic corticosteroids before use if residual neck disease or metastases are known to be present.

Serum Tg should be measured immediately prior to ^{131}I administration if THW preparation is undertaken or ideally on day 5 if rhTSH is used and local facilities are set up to handle radioactive samples.

Patients with pT1-2, N0 with R0 resection should receive 1.1 GBq. For patients with pT3 and/or N1 disease, the final choice of ^{131}I activity should be decided by the MDT on an individual case basis, taking all prognostic factors into consideration.

^{131}I therapy doses are usually in the range 3.7–5.5 GBq. Whole-body radioiodine scans are performed 2–10 days after giving radioiodine for ablation or therapy to determine the sites of radioiodine uptake and are more sensitive than diagnostic whole-body scans due to the higher administered activity of radiation used. The addition of SPECT CT to planar gamma camera imaging allows more precise anatomical localization of any iodine uptake demonstrated. The timing of the scan will depend on the administered activity of ^{131}I, the method of patient preparation (rhTSH versus thyroid hormone withdrawal) and the clinician's choice of the residual activity at which to image the patient.

Physiological ^{131}I uptake is seen in salivary tissue, genitourinary tract, gastrointestinal tract and sinuses.

Hürthle cell lesions are generally poorly responsive to radioiodine treatment and in particular distant metastases are often resistant to radioiodine therapy.

A pre-ablation radioisotope scan is not routinely indicated, but it may be used to demonstrate the size of thyroid remnant. If a large remnant is seen, consideration of further surgery may be warranted. If further surgery is not appropriate, it may influence the activity of radioiodine that is administered and prompt the prescription of pre-medication with corticosteroids prior to RAI to limit radiation thyroiditis symptoms.

If a preablation scan is performed, a low administered activity of ^{99m}Tc pertechnate or ^{123}I are preferred to ^{131}I as they reduce the risk of stunning,[19, 20] which is the term used for the reduction in uptake of the ^{131}I therapy dose as a result of the pre-treatment diagnostic dose.

Thyroid hormones can be started 1–3 days after radioiodine administration if the patient has been withdrawn from hormones. If the patient has been given rhTSH, they can stay on thyroxine throughout the procedure.

Prior to radioiodine administration, the total body iodine pool should be reduced. A low daily intake of iodine can increase the effective radiation dose achieved with ^{131}I in the regions of interest.[21–23] There is little consensus on the degree and the duration of dietary iodine restriction, but duration of the diet is often 1–2 weeks.

Other sources of excess iodine (e.g. iodinated i.v. contrast and amiodarone) should be eliminated before proceeding with ^{131}I administration.

^{131}I TOXICITY

- Neck discomfort and swelling may be caused by an inflammatory response in the remnant, residual tumour or involved cervical lymph nodes. This is most likely to be seen when there is a large thyroid remnant present. Discomfort is usually adequately treated with simple analgesics. If the patient has only had a debulking procedure and gross residual thyroid tissue is present, prophylactic corticosteroids are advisable to minimize the pain and swelling associated with the inflammatory response and can be started just prior to RAI administration.
- Patients may experience an altered sense of taste, and nausea (although vomiting is uncommon and prophylactic antiemetics are not routinely indicated).
- Sialadenitis arises due to physiological uptake of ^{131}I and subsequent excretion from salivary tissue. This can be reduced by encouraging patients to drink liberal quantities of fluids. In the long term, it is possible for intermittent parotid swelling, which may be tender, to develop. This can often be managed by parotid duct massage and the use of post-meal sialogogues if there is no evidence of duct stenosis or calculus.
- Lacrimal gland dysfunction.
- Radiation cystitis. The risk may be reduced by maintaining a high fluid intake following radioiodine administration and during the isolation period.
- Gastritis.
- Bleeding/oedema in metastases.

- Bone marrow suppression. This reaches its peak 4–6 weeks after treatment. It is more likely in those patients who have extensive skeletal metastases or who have received prior external beam radiotherapy or chemotherapy.
- Gonadal tissue is exposed to radiation from radioiodine in the blood, urine and faeces.
- **Male fertility:** a temporary rise in follicle-stimulating hormone (FSH) and a reduction in sperm count may be seen. High cumulative doses (e.g. >14 GBq) may reduce fertility, and consideration should be given to sperm storage in high-risk cases where multiple therapeutic doses of ^{131}I are expected.[24]
- **Female fertility:** no significant difference in fertility rate, birth weights or prematurity rates have been documented. Temporary alterations in the menstrual cycle may last for 4–10 months in about a quarter of female patients. Increased risk of miscarriage may persist for up to 1 year following ^{131}I ablation/therapy.[25–29] The risk of impaired fertility may be reduced by maintaining a high fluid intake following radioiodine administration and for the duration of the isolation period. This is in order to dilute the urine and therefore reduce concentration of radioactive iodine in the bladder and hence exposure of gonadal tissues.
- If the patient has undergone thyroid hormone withdrawal, constipation is a common symptom of the hypothyroid state so laxatives may help in reducing radiation exposure to gonadal tissue.
- If miliary pulmonary metastases are present, the patient may be at risk of developing pulmonary fibrosis especially if a high cumulative activity of radioiodine is administered. Consideration of pulmonary function test monitoring and corticosteroids immediately before and during treatment may reduce this risk. The data available are, however, fairly limited.[30]
- An increased risk of leukaemia and second cancers in organs that concentrate ^{131}I (salivary gland, breast, bladder, colon) is seen, with the risk being highest with high cumulative activities of radioiodine, i.e. greater than 18.5 GBq, and after external beam radiotherapy. The risk of leukaemia is lower than reported in earlier series due to deliberate attempts to limit the total body dose and to increase the interval between radioiodine administrations, whereas the risk of second solid malignancy might be higher than previously thought.[31, 32]
- Good hydration, frequent micturition and regular bowel activity will help reduce the level of whole-body radiation.

Consideration should be given to the use of high-dose corticosteroids before radioiodine if there is bulky neck disease or metastatic disease.

RADIATION PROTECTION ISSUES

Before the administration of ^{131}I, pregnancy and lactation must be excluded. Following the administration of ^{131}I, pregnancy must be avoided for 6 months and male patients must avoid fathering a child for 4 months.[33]

During the patient's stay in the isolation room, visiting of family and friends must be restricted to non-pregnant adults. Visiting options vary between centres but often entail no direct entry into the patient's room, with visitors needing to stay in a designated area outside the room.

The patient's clothing must be washed separately on their return home, unless it is heavily soiled, when storage on the hospital site or disposal may be needed. The method of transport home may be determined by the patient's residual activity. For example, short-distance travel in a private family vehicle, unoccupied by children, may allow discharge home with a higher residual activity than a longer journey via public transport where exposure to other members of the public, particularly children, may occur. Once at home, the patient must double-flush the toilet, use separate cutlery and crockery, sleep alone, and restrict the time with and extend the distance between them and their contacts. The duration of the restrictions is individualized for each patient and is longer for prolonged and close contact with children and pregnant women than with non-pregnant adults. Timing of a patient's return to work will depend on the type of work undertaken, the work environment and the surrounding work personnel involved. The patient will be given dates on discharge home which advise how long radiation protection restrictions need to be followed for adults and a second longer date for children and pregnant (or potentially pregnant) women

TSH LEVEL

Following total thyroidectomy, thyroxine is required both to replace thyroid hormones no longer produced endogenously and to suppress TSH levels. The dosage tends therefore to be larger than that used for replacement purposes following thyroidectomy for a benign aetiology.

Thyroxine in these larger doses prevents the pituitary from being stimulated to produce TSH and hence prevents stimulation of any remaining thyroid tissue, whether normal or malignant, with the intention of reducing the risk of recurrence, tumour progression and death.

The degree of suppression has not been tested in prospective studies and, due to concerns regarding the effects of prolonged suprapenhysiological thyroxine doses in low-risk cases, there has been a recent move to relax the degree of TSH suppression in low-risk cases, aiming for a TSH within the lower part of the normal range.

The BTA Guidelines 2014 recommend the following:[1]

- Patients who have not received RRA do not require TSH suppression and the serum TSH should be maintained in the low–normal range.
- Following initial treatment with total thyroidectomy and RRA, and before evaluation of the patient's response to treatment after 9–12 months, TSH should be suppressed to below 0.1 mU/L in all patients.
- In patients with an excellent response to treatment for thyroid cancer, the serum TSH should be maintained in the low–normal range.

- In patients who have an indeterminate response, it is recommended that the goal of TSH suppressive therapy be adjusted to maintain serum TSH concentrations between 0.1 mU/L and 0.5 mU/L for 5–10 years.
- In patients with an incomplete response to treatment for thyroid cancer, the serum TSH should be suppressed below 0.1 mU/L indefinitely in the absence of specific contraindications.

When TSH is being suppressed, the free T4 (fT4) level is often seen to be above the upper limit of the normal range. Moderate elevation does not commonly result in symptoms or signs of 'hyperthyroidism'.

Thyroxine is taken once daily, usually in the morning, and on an empty stomach. A number of medications can interfere with the absorption of thyroxine, so it is advisable to leave a 2-hour gap between taking thyroxine and other medications, such as calcium supplements, antacids, iron and multivitamins.

THYROGLOBULIN

Thyroglobulin is a glycosylated protein which is a key substrate for biosynthesis and storage of thyroid hormones. It is secreted by normal and cancerous thyroid cells and its release is TSH-dependent. The diagnostic sensitivity of Tg is increased when the TSH level is elevated. The Tg level may be undetectable in 20% of cases in the presence of isolated lymph node metastases if it is measured while the patient is on TSH suppression therapy. The serum Tg level is more sensitive than ^{131}I whole-body scan (WBS) in detecting recurrent or metastatic disease.

Thyroglobulin autoantibodies (TgAb) interfere with the ability to accurately measure and follow Tg trends. The prevalence of thyroglobulin antibodies is higher in patients with differentiated thyroid cancer (DTC) than in the general population (up to 25% versus 10%).[34] There is evidence that measuring TgAb levels and trends is of value in monitoring patients with thyroid cancer if the Tg cannot be relied upon in the presence of the autoantibodies; a rising trend in TgAb levels may indicate disease relapse in a patient.[35–39]

In order to interpret the serum Tg level, it is necessary to know the TSH level and TgAb level.

Serum thyroglobulin is not useful as a diagnostic test pre-operatively because Tg is a product of normal thyroid tissue and can be markedly elevated by inflammatory thyroid diseases. It is therefore not specifically a serum tumour marker; however, if elevated in a patient who has previously been rendered athyroid by surgery and radioiodine ablation, it may indicate recurrent or metastatic differentiated tumour.

A serum Tg which starts rising over time while on suppressive thyroxine therapy is highly suggestive of tumour recurrence and needs further investigation. There is no need to measure Tg under TSH stimulation if the basal serum Tg is already detectable.[40–45]

FOLLOW-UP

There is some variation in practice relating to the timing and modalities used for assessing success of thyroid remnant ablation. Whole-body radionuclide imaging has largely been superseded by neck ultrasound and stimulated Tg assessment in many centres. Cervical ultrasound is a sensitive method for detection of residual disease in the thyroid bed or cervical lymph nodes. It is essential for the ultrasound to be performed by a highly skilled operator with knowledge of thyroid cancer behaviour and not as a routine investigation by a general ultrasonographer.

Diagnostic ^{131}I or ^{123}I scans can, however, provide useful information on the effectiveness of ablation and the need for further ^{131}I if uptake was seen outside the neck on the post-ablation whole-body scan and can be considered for patients with thyroglobulin antibodies.

A follow-up neck ultrasound scan and stimulated Tg should ideally be performed 9–12 months following ablation.[1] The results from these two investigations will be used to allocate patients to a treatment response group. This process is 'dynamic risk stratification' (Table 66.2).[46–48]

For low-risk cases, if initial follow-up serum Tg is undetectable under TSH stimulation conditions, subsequent long-term follow-up Tg assessments can be performed under TSH suppression conditions.[49]

If the follow-up neck ultrasound scan and stimulated Tg are within normal limits, the patient is kept on clinical follow-up with Tg monitoring. If the scan or the Tg is abnormal, a decision needs to be made on further management. This may be surgery if localized disease is identified in the thyroid bed or cervical lymph nodes or ^{131}I therapy. The usual administered activity of ^{131}I in this setting is 5.5 GBq[1] and this too will be followed up with repeat imaging and Tg assessment to assess response.

TABLE 66.2 Dynamic risk stratification: definitions of response to initial therapy of DTC (9–12 months after total thyroidectomy with R0 resection and subsequent RRA) (Adapted from American Thyroid Association[46, 47])

Excellent response	Indeterminate response	Incomplete response
All of the following are present: • Suppressed and stimulated Tg <1 µg/L • Neck ultrasound without evidence of disease • Cross-sectional and/or nuclear medicine imaging negative	Any of the following are present: • Suppressed Tg <1 µg/L and stimulated Tg ≥1 and <10 µg/L • Neck ultrasound with non-specific changes or stable subcentimetre lymph nodes • Cross-sectional and/or nuclear medicine imaging with non-specific changes, although not completely normal	Any of the following are present: • Suppressed Tg ≥1 µg/L or stimulated Tg ≥10 µg/L • Rising Tg values • Persistent or newly identified disease on cross-sectional and/or nuclear medicine imaging

The TSH stimulated Tg level may remain detectable at low levels after ^{131}I ablation. This could represent residual/recurrent cancer but in the majority of cases represents thyroid remnant. An expectant policy in low-risk cases is recommended with repeat TSH-stimulated Tg assessment at 6–12 month intervals. In many cases, repeat assessments will reveal a gradual decline in stimulated Tg to the point of no detection, when routine follow-up should then be commenced.

Thyroglobulin-positive, imaging negative disease

This is a not uncommon scenario seen in the follow-up of patients with differentiated thyroid cancer and there is uncertainty regarding optimal management.

When Tg is detectable, additional investigations aiming to localize the disease recurrence and offer specific therapy (in particular, surgical resection of the disease wherever possible) are indicated.

A possible imaging strategy is as follows:

1. Neck ultrasound/MRI of neck and mediastinum – the thyroid bed, cervical and mediastinal nodes are the most common sites of recurrence for PTC. *If negative:*
2. CT lungs – to look for micronodular lung metastases. Remember the potential for iodinated intravenous contrast to inhibit subsequent radioiodine uptake. *If negative:*
3. ^{99m}Tc isotope bone scan. MRI spine is more sensitive and may be considered if the bone scan is equivocal and the patient has localized symptoms. *If negative, consider proceeding with:*
4. ^{18}FDG-PET/CT imaging. TSH stimulation prior to positron emission tomography (PET) imaging has shown increased sensitivity in some studies.[50, 51] Patients with positive FDG-PET imaging have a reduced 3-year survival compared with those who are FDG-PET scan-negative. If PET imaging is positive, ^{131}I imaging is typically negative and the patient is radioiodine refractory. This is often referred to as the 'flip flop' phenomenon.

If imaging fails to identify sites of disease, there are two main approaches:

- continued monitoring until repeat imaging demonstrates recurrent disease or the patient becomes symptomatic
- empirical ^{131}I therapy.[52, 53]

The decision on whether to proceed with an empirical dose of ^{131}I needs to be made, bearing in mind the risk category of the patient and the rate of Tg rise. It is uncertain whether empirical ^{131}I treatment is beneficial in patients with raised serum Tg, compared to active surveillance. There is no evidence from randomized controlled trials for or against empirical ^{131}I. Proponents argue that a high proportion of patients will have positive post-therapy scans and/or thyroglobulin response and some may achieve cure. Opponents argue that some of these patients have minimal disease and hence radioiodine is unlikely to improve survival and that treatment is associated with acute toxicity. A meta-analysis showed that 50% of post-therapy scans will be positive and of these positive cases 60% will also show a fall in Tg.

Recurrent or metastatic disease

Between 5% and 20% of patients with papillary thyroid cancer relapse in the thyroid bed or cervical nodes, and surgery is the treatment of choice for such locoregional recurrence. Ideally, complete resection is recommended but, if this is not feasible, debulking is beneficial as this will facilitate greater radioiodine uptake in a smaller volume of disease. Distant metastases develop in 10–20% with pulmonary and bone accounting for the majority. If the patient has radioiodine-avid disease, repeated doses of radioiodine are indicated provided there is evidence of symptomatic, radiological or biochemical response.

Remission can be achieved in about two-thirds of patients with neck recurrence and one-third of those with distant metastases. Remission is more likely when a limited tumour burden is present.[54, 55]

Prognosis depends on the distribution and number of metastatic sites, tumour burden (microscopic foci are more likely to respond) and age at the time of diagnosis of metastases.[56, 57] If tumour takes up ^{131}I, then long-term survival is possible. The preferred treatment is repeated doses of ^{131}I with administered activities ranging between 3.7 GBq and 5.5 GBq at 6–12-month intervals.

Fixed administered activities of ^{131}I are generally used, but dosimetrically calculated activities are used in some centres.[58] There is no maximum limit to the cumulative administered activity of ^{131}I that can be used in the treatment of a patient with persistent disease. Normal bone marrow function is needed and reductions in the administered activity are required in the presence of renal impairment.

Extensive bony metastases are generally not curable by ^{131}I alone. For solitary or a limited number of bone metastases, external beam radiotherapy, resection or embolization with or without post-operative external beam irradiation may be associated with increased survival. Other potential treatments include thermal ablation and cement injection.

External beam radiotherapy

The use and role of radiotherapy in differentiated thyroid cancer is debated due to conflicting results in published series. There are no randomized controlled trials and the retrospective reviews often extend over several decades, resulting in considerable variation in extent of surgery and accuracy of staging investigations. Problems with selection bias are also encountered, as well as inappropriately short follow-up for a disease with a long natural history.

The published data are also often lacking with regards to the radiotherapy techniques and doses used, the acute and late toxicity and study end points. The long natural history of the disease means that drawing conclusions from any treatment intervention is difficult.[59–61]

External beam radiotherapy (EBRT) is infrequently used but the main indications are:

- gross local invasion with significant gross macroscopic residual
- residual or recurrent neck disease that fails to concentrate iodine and that is not amenable to surgery
- palliation of inoperable metastatic disease.

The area treated (target volume) generally includes the thyroid bed (in particular the tracheo-oesophageal groove) and draining lymph nodes (perithyroidal lymph nodes in the central compartment, paratracheal, pretracheal, superior mediastinum and cervical lymph nodes) in papillary and oncocytic follicular (Hürthle cell) cancers. Draining lymph nodes do not need to be irradiated in non-oncocytic follicular thyroid cancer unless there is confirmed nodal involvement.

Technical difficulties arise due to the irregular shape of the areas requiring treatment and their proximity to the spinal cord, which is more sensitive to the effects of radiotherapy than tumour tissue and is therefore a dose-limiting structure. Without careful attention to radiotherapy planning and delivery, the patient is at risk of radiation myelopathy. The anatomical relationship between the target area and the spinal cord makes it difficult to deliver a homogenous dose to the areas at risk with conventional radiotherapy techniques.

Intensity-modulated radiotherapy (IMRT) allows a better radiation dose distribution to the tumour while reducing the dose to radiosensitive organs close to the target areas.

During radiotherapy the patient is treated supine. Due to the proximity of the area for treatment to critical structures and the need to deliver treatment accurately and precisely over a number of weeks, an immobilization shell is required to keep the patient in a reproducible position.

The most common acute toxicities seen with external beam radiotherapy in this situation are mucositis with associated odynophagia, skin erythema, skin desquamation and laryngitis. If level I and II cervical lymph node areas need irradiating, taste changes, xerostomia and accelerated dental decay and a small risk of osteoradionecrosis of the mandible can arise.

It is possible that radiotherapy may reduce the uptake of radioiodine into residual thyroid tissue and therefore consideration should be given to administering radioiodine therapy before external beam radiotherapy. However, in practice, there may be a significant delay before the patient can be admitted to the isolation room for RRA and for some patients it may be advisable to proceed with external beam radiotherapy rather than delay both treatment modalities.

Targeted therapies

The principal indication for targeted treatments is progressive, symptomatic disease, refractory to conventional treatments. Efficacy for increased progression-free survival (PFS), but not overall survival, has been demonstrated for several agents. The agents demonstrating the most activity and clinical benefit to date are sorafenib and lenvatinib. A randomized phase 3 trial of sorafenib versus placebo resulted in a PFS benefit of 5 months for patients on sorafenib over those on placebo (10.8 versus 5.8 months; $p < 0.0001$).[62] Studies continue to evaluate the role of molecular profiling in determination of the most appropriate targeted agent.

Targeted therapy agents are administered orally and have a different toxicity profile compared to conventional chemotherapy. The common toxicities are:

- hypertension
- hand–foot skin reaction (palmar–plantar erythrodysaesthesia) and rash
- diarrhoea, constitutional symptoms such as anorexia and weight loss
- cardiac ischaemia
- increased risk of bleeding
- alopecia.

These agents should only be prescribed by a specialist and patients need to be closely observed especially during the initial weeks of therapy in order to detect early signs of toxicity. There is a high incidence of toxicity which will require treatment breaks and dose reductions.

Targeted therapy is a rapidly evolving area and information on current clinical trial activity can be found at the websites listed in 'Key points' below.

Chemotherapy

There are no data to support the use of adjuvant chemotherapy in the management of differentiated thyroid cancer and it is also not routinely used in the management of locally recurrent or metastatic disease. Its use has largely been superseded by targeted therapies. Published studies of chemotherapy have usually only included small numbers of patients and have often had a mixture of histological tumour types within the study population.

Doxorubicin is the most extensively studied agent in advanced thyroid cancer and the most frequently used drug, with a partial response rate of approximately 20–30% reported.[64–66] There is no clear evidence, however, that its use increases survival. Doxorubicin in combination with cisplatin has demonstrated a higher response rate but with additional toxicity and no improvement in outcome.

Childhood

Thyroid nodules are more likely to be malignant in children. Papillary carcinoma is the most common differentiated thyroid cancer seen, with 30–40% being multifocal; 40–90% of patients are found to have involved cervical nodes at initial surgery.

Differentiated thyroid cancer tends to behave more aggressively in children younger than 10 years of age and the chance of recurrence is also higher.[67–70]

^{131}I ablation is generally indicated for all children and adolescents with differentiated thyroid cancers >1 cm following total thyroidectomy, and selective neck dissection is recommended for children with positive nodes. The dynamic risk stratification model has not been specifically validated in the setting of paediatric differentiated thyroid cancer but the same general principles should be considered when deciding on the pros and cons of radioiodine remnant ablation.

At presentation, 10–20% have lung metastases, while bone metastases are rare (<1%). Fewer than 10% will die as a result of their disease.

Management of differentiated thyroid cancer during pregnancy

If differentiated thyroid cancer is diagnosed during pregnancy, it is essential to consider the risk to both mother and foetus of both the cancer treatment options and the continuation of the pregnancy. Thyroid cancer discovered during pregnancy does not behave more aggressively than that diagnosed in a similar aged group of non-pregnant women. Women of childbearing age with thyroid cancer generally have an excellent prognosis, similar to that of non-pregnant women.

Thyroidectomy in the first trimester of pregnancy is associated with a very high risk of miscarriage, but it may be performed safely in the second trimester. Alternatively, surgery can be deferred until after the baby is delivered provided the patient is monitored and the thyroid cancer lesion remains stable. Suppressive doses of thyroxine are safe in pregnancy and may be considered until surgery is possible. The dosage of thyroxine will need to be increased during pregnancy.[71] Termination of pregnancy is rarely indicated.

It is advisable to stop breastfeeding at least 8 weeks and preferably 8 weeks prior to ^{131}I.

Follow-up

Frequency and type of follow-up depends on an individual's risk of recurrence.[1]

Patients who have undergone hemithyroidectomy for a low-risk cancer do not require TSH suppression.

Once the thyroid remnant has been ablated and following dynamic risk stratification the frequency of attendance will be decided in each case individually:

- Patients with excellent response should be followed 6-monthly for the first year, and annually thereafter.
- Patients with indeterminate or incomplete response should be followed up more frequently depending on individual need.

Follow-up should be lifelong for the following reasons:

- The disease has a long natural history.
- Late recurrences can occur, which can be successfully treated with a view to cure or long-term survival.
- The consequences of supraphysiological levothyroxine replacement (such as atrial fibrillation and osteoporosis) need monitoring, especially as the patient ages.
- Late side effects of ^{131}I treatment may develop.

Clinical trials

A list of websites where information on current clinical trials can be found is given in 'Key points' below.

MEDULLARY THYROID CARCINOMA

Surgery is the main modality of treatment for this disease and monitoring of serum calcitonin post-operatively is important in establishing whether biochemical control has been achieved.[72, 73] The calcitonin level of many patients, however, remains elevated after surgery and it is frequently difficult to locate the site of residual disease and determine whether it is local or at a distant site. Blood samples taken for calcitonin must be immediately stored in ice since rapid degradation occurs at room temperature and may give falsely low results. Carcinoembryonic antigen (CEA) is also commonly raised and can similarly be used to monitor progress and response to therapeutic intervention.

It is presumed that rendering a patient calcitonin-negative will give them an improved chance of long-term survival and cure. Many patients with a raised calcitonin level remain well with an excellent performance status for many years, whereas others become symptomatic over a much shorter interval. In a retrospective review of 65 patients,[74] calcitonin doubling time during follow-up was a significant predictor of survival in both univariate and multivariate analyses. A calcitonin doubling time greater than 2 years was associated with long-term survival, whereas patients with a doubling time of less than 6 months all died as a result of their medullary thyroid cancer. An online calcitonin and CEA doubling-time calculator can be found on the American Thyroid Association website (https://www.thyroid.org).

External beam radiotherapy

Due to a lack of prospective studies, the role of adjuvant radiotherapy to the thyroid bed and cervical nodes remains uncertain.[75–77] It is difficult to compare published series due to considerable differences in radiotherapy dose fractionation and eligibility criteria, and the relative rarity of the disease means that recruitment has been over very long periods of time. Reported series also often fail to report the associated toxicity and impact on quality of life of any treatment intervention.

Radiotherapy may be indicated in the following situations:

- post-operatively, when the disease was locally advanced at presentation and a macroscopic clearance has not been achieved
- multiple involved lymph nodes, especially if extracapsular spread is present
- bulky inoperable tumours
- palliation of distant metastases (e.g. bone).

Routine adjuvant radiotherapy in the post-operative setting has not been shown to improve survival.

METASTATIC MEDULLARY THYROID CANCER

Many patients' survival can be measured in years and, even in the presence of significant disease bulk, quality of life can often be good.

Distant metastases frequently involve the liver, lungs and the skeleton and may first come to light when the serum calcitonin level rises significantly. Occasionally, the first sign of the development of distant metastases may be when the patient starts to experience diarrhoea as a result of excess peptide release or symptoms related to excess hormone production. As well as experiencing frequent loose bowel actions often with urgency, wheezing and flushing are also possible. Cushing's syndrome may also rarely occur. These symptoms may respond to somatostatin analogue therapy (e.g. octreotide). Chemotherapy is rarely helpful and has largely been superseded by targeted therapies.

There is no curative treatment option. Treatment interventions are therefore usually reserved until the patient becomes symptomatic and/or develops significant radiological progression with accelerated calcitonin doubling times rather than at first presentation of asymptomatic radiologically diagnosed metastases or raised tumour markers.

Unlabelled somatostatin analogue therapy for diarrhoea

Diarrhoea can be a challenging symptom for some patients and, in the first instance, is usually managed with loperamide and/or codeine. If these agents fail, consideration can be given to the use of somatostatin analogue agents.

Somatostatin receptors can be found on medullary thyroid cancer cells and therefore blocking these receptors can result in a decrease in the amount of peptide and calcitonin released. However, a significant decrease in tumour mass is not seen and the aim of treatment is an improvement in symptoms – diarrhoea and flushing and quality of life. Unfortunately, any recorded benefits often seem to be short-lived.

If a patient responds favourably to a twice or three times daily subcutaneous administration of octreotide, a synthetic somatostatin analogue, with a reduction in diarrhoea frequency or severity, then they can be commenced on a monthly depot preparation. With prolonged use, there is a risk of tachyphylaxis developing with loss of symptomatic benefit. However, if symptom control deteriorates, it is important to consider if disease progression is the cause before attributing the change to tachyphylaxis. Octreotide and lanreotide have a different spectrum of somatostatin receptor blockade. Side effects of the somatostatin analogues include gastrointestinal disturbances, such as anorexia, nausea, vomiting, abdominal pain, flatulence, diarrhoea and steatorrhoea, and rarely with long-term use gallstones may occur. Abnormalities of glucose metabolism may also occur. Local reactions at the site of administration may be seen and rotation of the injection site is recommended.

Targeted radiolabelled therapies

Once metastatic disease has been established, imaging with ^{123}I metaiodobenzylguanidine (mIBG) or ^{111}In octreotide may demonstrate selective uptake at sites of known tumour relapse, thereby opening up the possibility of using similar agents as targeted radiolabelled therapies.

As medullary thyroid cancer is not derived from follicular cells, it does not accumulate radioiodine.

METAIODOBENZYLGUANIDINE (mIBG) THERAPY

Metaiodobenzylguanidine is a guanethidine derivative, structurally similar to noradrenaline. It is transported into neuroendocrine tumour cells by monoamine transport proteins and may be useful as a therapy in a small number of cases.

Approximately 30–40% of medullary thyroid cancers concentrate ^{131}I-mIBG, but histological tumour characteristics that reliably predict isotope uptake and hence suitability for therapy have not yet been defined.

Prior to treatment, care must be taken to prevent the use of drugs that may interfere with the uptake and retention of mIBG. The following are some examples, but not an exhaustive list: tricyclic antidepressants, phenothiazines, calcium channel blockers, salbutamol and opioids. Administered activities of ^{131}I-mIBG vary and treatment is often given at 2–3-month intervals for three cycles, depending on the patient's tolerance and the benefits observed.

The treatment is given in an isotope isolation room by intravenous infusion usually over a 1–2 hour period through a lead-shielded infusion system. Frequent blood pressure monitoring is required during the infusion and for a period of time afterwards, as unstable blood pressure can result. In practice, this is usually managed by slowing or interrupting the infusion, but in the case of a hypertensive crisis, intravenous alpha and beta blockers such as phentolamine boluses and an esmolol infusion may be required. These drugs should be prescribed in advance and should be available at the time of the mIBG administration.

Prophylactic antiemetics, such as ondansetron, are indicated prior to the infusion and should be continued for 72 hours afterwards. It is advisable to insert two cannulae to allow simultaneous i.v. fluids to be given to ensure good hydration in case the patient is unable to take adequate fluids orally as a result of nausea. It is possible that the patient may experience diarrhoea, wheezing and flushing related to peptide and hormone release from the tumour. The patient remains in the isolation room for several days and will follow similar radiation protection procedures as described above under 'Differentiated thyroid cancer'.

Whole-body gamma camera imaging is performed preferably with SPECT CT just before the patient is discharged home to demonstrate the distribution and intensity of isotope uptake.

A full blood count (FBC) should be checked weekly for 6 weeks afterwards as myelosuppression, particularly thrombocytopenia, can occur. This is more likely if there is widespread bone marrow involvement or if the patient has received chemotherapy.

Response to treatment can be assessed in terms of symptom improvement, decreasing calcitonin levels or tumour regression on imaging. It is the former, however, which tends to dictate management decisions. Up to 60% of patients may derive symptom benefit and 30–80% may achieve disease stabilization. However, these data are derived from small series.[78–80] mIBG is traditionally reserved until patients become symptomatic from metastatic disease and it is unknown whether its use earlier in the natural history of the disease may be beneficial.

RADIOLABELLED SOMATOSTATIN ANALOGUE THERAPY

Somatostatin receptor imaging is reported to have a sensitivity of 50–70% in localizing medullary thyroid tumour.[81, 82]

Somatostatin analogues bound to ^{90}Yttrium or ^{177}Lutetium can therefore be used as therapy in those patients who demonstrate sufficient somatostatin analogue uptake within sites of tumour when compared to background physiological uptake. A subjective benefit may be seen after one or two treatments and this may be associated with a reduction in calcitonin/CEA and tumour stabilization. It is important to realize that a formal radiological assessment of response can be misleading. Often, overall tumour size remains static on cross-sectional imaging, even in the presence of significant radioisotope uptake, symptomatic response and biochemical response. Toxicity includes myelosuppression and nephrotoxicity. Pre-treatment with an amino acid infusion reduces binding of the somatostatin analogue to the renal tubules and hence reduces renal damage.

Other targeted therapies

Various vascular endothelial growth factors (VEGFs) and VEGF receptors (VEGFRs) are often overexpressed in MTC, both in tumour cells and in the supporting vascular endothelium.

Two agents are now licensed for the treatment of symptomatic inoperable locally advanced or metastatic medullary thyroid cancer:

- vandetanib[83–85] (Caprelsa™) which targets *RET*, epidermal growth factor receptors (EGFRs) and VEGFR
- cabozantinib[86] (Cometriq™) which targets *RET*, c-Met and VEGFR.

These agents have shown the potential to provide high rates of disease control (partial response and stable disease) with durable responses and a highly statistically significant improvement in PFS. These treatments are given orally on a daily basis for as long as tumour control persists.

Common acute toxicities include:

- photosensitivity
- palmar plantar syndrome, rash
- prolonged QTc interval and risk of sudden death
- hypertension
- fatigue, reduced appetite, diarrhoea, nausea, vomiting
- corneal deposits
- proteinuria, nephrolithiasis.

Short-term toxicity can be significant and often requires dose reductions or treatment withdrawal. Treatment should only be initiated by a specialist and close monitoring is required. Long-term toxicity needs to be investigated further and includes concerns over the potential for skin malignancy to develop.

Chemotherapy

This is rarely used now that targeted therapies have become available but it might rarely be considered for rapidly progressive and symptomatic metastatic disease.

There are no randomized controlled trials and no significant survival benefit has ever been demonstrated.

As medullary thyroid cancer is a neuroendocrine tumour (NET), chemotherapy regimens with activity in other NETs, such as carcinoids, have been suggested, such as 5-fluorouracil and streptozocin.

Clinical trials

A list of websites where information on current clinical trials can be found is given in 'Key points' below.

ANAPLASTIC THYROID CANCER

Patients with anaplastic thyroid cancer (ATC) have a very poor prognosis, with the median survival being 6 months from symptom onset.[87–89]

External beam radiotherapy

This tumour is the least radiosensitive of the thyroid tumours. Tumour response tends to be partial even with high doses and the majority of patients still die as a result of locally progressive disease. It is also very important to appreciate that patients may spend a very significant proportion of their remaining lives undergoing treatment and recovering from its significant toxicity.

Attempts have been made to improve response to treatment by intensifying the radiotherapy regimen by hyperfractionation (delivering more than the standard one fraction of radiotherapy per day) or by shortening the time period over which it is delivered (accelerated radiotherapy) and combining this with chemotherapy.[90–93] This intensification has in some series resulted in improved response rates but at the cost of increased toxicity and no increase in overall survival.[94]

Chemotherapy

There is no definitive evidence to demonstrate prolonged survival or improved quality of life for ATC patients treated with systemic therapy. Tumour regression can, however, be induced in some patients. Risks and potential benefits must be carefully considered in each case. The agents with the greatest clinical activity in metastatic ATC are the taxanes (paclitaxel or docetaxe), the anthracycline doxorubicin, and the platins (carboplatin and cisplatin).

Fosbretabulin, a prodrug of the antimicrotuble-disrupting agent combretastatin was assessed in the randomized phase II functional assessment of cancer therapy (FACT) trial. Unfortunately, the study closed prematurely due to slow patient recruitment but stable disease was seen in 27% with a median survival of 4.7 months and 23% of patients surviving 1 year.[95]

Clinical trials

A list of websites where information on current clinical trials can be found is given in 'Key points' below.

KEY POINTS

- Decisions on radioiodine remnant ablation should be individualized taking into account both patient and tumour factors.
- Administered activity of radioiodine in the ablation setting is dependent on the risk category.
- Recombinant human TSH should be used where possible in the radioiodine ablation setting to avoid hypothyroidism and reduced quality of life caused by thyroid hormone withdrawal.
- Degree and duration of long-term TSH suppression depends on the dynamic risk stratification outcome.
- Metastatic thyroid cancer may be low volume, slowly progressive and asymptomatic in many cases and an active surveillance approach is appropriate during this time.
- Information on current clinical trials can be found at the following websites:
  - https://www.ukctg.nihr.ac.uk/
  - https://www.clinicaltrials.gov/
  - https://www.cancer.gov/
  - https://www.centerwatch.com/
  - https://www.thyroid.org/

REFERENCES

1. Perros P (ed.). British Thyroid Association, Royal College of Physicians. Guidelines for the management of thyroid cancer, 3rd ed. Report of the Thyroid Cancer Guidelines Update Group. London: Royal College of Physicians; 2014.
2. Cooper DS, Doherty GM, Haugen BR, et al. Revised American Thyroid Association management guidelines for patients with thyroid nodules and differentiated thyroid cancer. *Thyroid* 2009; **19**: 1167–214.
3. Sawka A, Thephamongkhol K, Brouwers M, et al. Clinical review 170: a systematic review and meta analysis of the effectiveness of radioactive iodine remnant ablation for well differentiated thyroid cancer. *J Clin Endocrinol Metab* 2004; **89**: 3668–76.
4. Samaan N, Schultz P, Hickey R, et al. The results of various modalities of treatment of well differentiated thyroid carcinomas: a retrospective review of 1599 patients. *J Clin Endocrinol Metab* 1992; **75**: 714–20.
5. Hay I, Thompson G, Grant C, et al. Papillary thyroid carcinoma managed at the Mayo Clinic during six decades (1940–1999): temporal trends in initial therapy and long term outcome in 2444 consecutively treated patients. *World J Surg* 2002; **26**: 879–85.
6. Sanders L, Cady B. Differentiated thyroid cancer: reexamination of risk groups and outcome of treatment. *Arch Surg* 1998; **133**: 419–25.
7. Kim S, Wei J, Braverman J, Brams D. Predicting outcome and directing therapy for papillary thyroid carcinoma. *Arch Surg* 2004; **139**: 390–4.
8. Sugitani I, Fujimoto Y. Symptomatic versus asymptomatic papillary thyroid microcarcinoma: a retrospective analysis of surgical outcome and prognostic factors. *Endocr J* 1999; **46**: 209–16.
9. Tuttle RM, Tala H, Shah J, et al. Estimating risk of recurrence in differentiated thyroid cancer after total thyroidectomy and radioactive iodine remnant ablation: using response to therapy variables to modify the initial risk estimates predicted by the new American Thyroid Association staging system. *Thyroid* 2010; **20**: 1341–9.
10. Rosario P, Reis J, Barroso A, et al. Efficacy of low and high I^{131} doses for thyroid remnant ablation in patients with differentiated thyroid carcinoma based on post operative cervical uptake. *Nucl Med Commun* 2004; **25**: 1077–81.
11. Bal C, Padhy A, Jana S, et al. Prospective randomized clinical trial to evaluate the optimal dose of I^{131} for remnant ablation in patients with differentiated thyroid carcinoma. *Cancer* 1996; **77**: 2574–80.
12. Creutzig H. High or low dose radioiodine ablation of thyroid remnants? *Eur J Nucl Med* 1987; **12**: 500–2.
13. Johansen K, Woodhouse N, Odugbesan O. Comparison of 1073 MBq and 3700 MBq iodine 131 in postoperative ablation of residual thyroid tissue in patients with differentiated thyroid cancer. *J Nucl Med* 1991; **32**: 252–4.
14. Mallick U, Harmer C, Yap B, et al. Ablation with low-dose radioiodine and thyrotropin alfa in thyroid cancer. *N Engl J Med* 2012; **366**(18): 1674–85.
15. Schlumberger M, Catargi B, Borget I, et al. Strategies of radioiodine ablation in patients with low-risk thyroid cancer. *N Engl J Med* 2012; **366**: 1663–73.
16. Cheng W, Ma C, Fu H, et al. Low or high-dose radioiodine remnant ablation for differentiated thyroid carcinoma: a meta-analysis. *J Clin Endocrinol Metab* 2013; **98**: 1353–60.
17. Robbins R, Larson S, Sinha N, et al. A retrospective review of the effectiveness of recombinant human TSH as a preparation for radioiodine thyroid remnant ablation. *J Nucl Med* 2002; **43**: 1482–8.
18. Pacini F, Ladenson P, Schlumberger M, et al. Radioiodine ablation of thyroid remnants after preparation with recombinant human thyrotropin in differentiated thyroid carcinoma: results of an international, randomized, controlled study. *J Clin Endocrinol Metab* 2006; **91**: 926–32.
19. Leger FA, Izembart M, Dagousset F, et al. Decreased uptake of therapeutic doses of iodine 131 after 185 MBq iodine 131 diagnostic imaging for thyroid remnants in differentiated thyroid carcinoma. *Eur J Nucl Med* 1998; **25**: 242–6.

20. Park H, Park Y, Jhow X. Detection of thyroid remnant/metastases with stunning: an ongoing dilemma. *Thyroid* 1997; 7: 277–80.
21. Maxon H, Boehringer T, Drilling J. Low iodine diet in I 131 ablation of thyroid remnants. *Clin Nucl Med* 1983; 8: 123–6.
22. Pluijmen M, Eustatia-Rutten C, Goslings B, et al. Effects of low-iodide diet on postsurgical radioiodide ablation therapy in patients with differentiated thyroid carcinoma. *Clin Endocrinol* 2003; 58: 428–35.
23. Maxon H. Quantitative radioiodine therapy in the treatment of differentiated thyroid cancer. *Q J Nucl Med* 1999; 43: 313–23.
24. Krassas G, Pontikides N. Gonadal effect of radiation from ^{131}I in male patients with thyroid carcinoma. *Arch Androl* 2005; 51: 171–5.
25. Schlumberger M, De Vathaire F, Ceccarelli C, et al. Exposure to radioiodine (I^{131}) for scintigraphy or therapy does not preclude pregnancy in thyroid cancer patients. *J Nucl Med* 1996; 37: 606–12.
26. Ayala C, Navarro E, Rodriguez J, et al. Conception after I^{131} therapy for differentiated thyroid cancer. *Thyroid* 1998; 8: 1009–11.
27. Dottorinin M, Lomuscio G, Mazzucchelli L, et al. Assessment of female fertility and carcinogenesis after iodine I^{131} therapy for differentiated thyroid carcinoma. *J Nucl Med* 1995; 36: 21–7.
28. Bal C, Kumar A, Tripathi M, et al. High dose radioiodine treatment for differentiated thyroid carcinoma is not associated with changes in female fertility or any genetic risk to the offspring. *Int J Radiat Oncol Biol Phys* 2005; 63: 449–55.
29. Vini L, Hyer S, Al-Saadi A, et al. Prognosis for fertility and ovarian function after treatment with radioiodine for thyroid cancer. *Postgrad Med J* 2002; 78: 92–3.
30. Rall J, Alpers J, Lewallen C, et al. Radiation pneumonitis and fibrosis: a complication of radioiodine treatment of pulmonary metastases from cancer of the thyroid. *J Clin Endocrinol Metab* 1957; 17: 1263–76.
31. Rubino C, de Vathaire F, Dottorinin M, et al. Second primary malignancies in thyroid cancer patients. *Br J Cancer* 2003; 89: 1638–44.
32. Sawka AM, Thabane L, Parlea L, et al. Second primary malignancy risk after radioactive iodine treatment for thyroid cancer: a systematic review and meta-analysis. *Thyroid* 2009; 19: 451–7.
33. Administration of Radioactive Substances Advisory Committee. *ARSAC notes for guidance on the clinical administration of radiopharmaceuticals and use of sealed radioactive sources*. Didcot, UK: ARSAC; 2006 (updated 2014).
34. Spencer C, Takeuchi M, Kazarosyan M, et al. Serum thyroglobulin autoantibodies: prevalence, influence on serum thyroglobulin measurement, and prognostic significance in patients with differentiated thyroid carcinoma. *J Clin Endocrinol Metab* 1998; 83: 1121–7.
35. Chiovato L, Latrofa F, Braverman L, et al. Disappearance of humoral thyroid autoimmunity after complete removal of thyroid antigens. *Ann Intern Med* 2003; 139: 346–51.
36. Tsushima Y, Miyauchi A, Ito Y, et al. Prognostic significance of changes in serum thyroglobulin antibody levels of pre- and post-total thyroidectomy in thyroglobulin antibody-positive papillary thyroid carcinoma patients. *Endocr J* 2013; 60(7): 871–6.
37. Gorges R, Maniecki M, Jentzen W, et al. Development and clinical impact of thyroglobulin antibodies in patients with differentiated thyroid carcinoma during the first 3 years after thyroidectomy. *Eur J Endocrinol* 2005; 153: 49–55.
38. Kim WG, Yoon JH, Kim WB, et al. Change of serum antithyroglobulin antibody levels is useful for prediction of clinical recurrence in thyroglobulin-negative patients with differentiated thyroid carcinoma. *J Clin Endocrinol Metab* 2008; 93: 4683–9.
39. Spencer CA. Clinical review: Clinical utility of thyroglobulin antibody (TgAb) measurements for patients with differentiated thyroid cancers (DTC). *J Clin Endocrinol Metab* 2011; 96: 3615–27.
40. Smallridge RC, Meek SE, Morgan MA, et al. Monitoring thyroglobulin in a sensitive iummunoassay has comparable sensitivity to recombinant human TSH-stimulated thyroglobulin in follow-up of thyroid cancer patients. *J Clin Endocrinol Metab* 2007; 92: 82–7.
41. Iervasi A, Iervasi G Ferdeghini M, et al. Clinical relevance of highly sensitive Tg assay in monitoring patients treated for differentiated thyroid cancer. *Clin Endocrinol* 2007; 67: 434–41.
42. Malandrino P, Latina A, Marescalco S, et al. Risk adapted management of differentiated thyroid cancer assessed by a sensitive measurement of basal serum thyroglobulin. *J Clin Endocrinol Metab* 2011; 96:1703–9.
43. Chindris AM, Diehl NN, Crook JE, et al. Undetectable sensitive serum thyroglobulin (<0.1 ng/ml) in 163 patients with follicular cell-derived thyroid cancer: results of rhTSH stimulation and neck ultrasonography and long-term biochemical and clinical follow-up. *J Clin Endocrinol Metab* 2012; 97: 2714–23.
44. Spencer C, Fatemi S, Singer P, et al. Serum basal thyroglobulin measured by a second-generation assay correlates with the recombinant human thyrotropin-stimulated thyroglobulin response in patients treated for differentiated thyroid cancer. *Thyroid* 2010; 20: 587–95.
45. Castaga MG, Tala Jury HP, Cipri C, et al. The use of ultrasensitive thyroglobulin assays reduces but does not abolish the need for TSH stimulation in patients with differentiated thyroid carcinoma. *J Endocrinol Invest* 2011; 34: 219–23.
46. Tuttle RM, Tala H, Shah J, et al. Estimating risk of recurrence in differentiated thyroid cancer after total thyroidectomy and radioactive iodine remnant ablation: using response to therapy variables to modify the initial risk estimates predicted by the new American Thyroid Association staging system. *Thyroid* 2010; 20: 1341–9.
47. Pitoia F, Bueno F, Urciuoli C, et al. Outcomes of patients with differentiated thyroid cancer risk: stratified according to the American Thyroid Association and Latin American Thyroid Society risk of recurrence classification systems. *Thyroid* 2013; 23: 1401–7.
48. Castagna MG, Maino F, Cipri C, et al. Delayed risk stratification, to include the response to initial treatment (surgery and radioiodine ablation), has better outcome predictivity in differentiated thyroid cancer patients. *Eur J Endocrinol* 2011; 165: 441–6.
49. Mazzaferri E, Robbins R, Spencer C, et al. A consensus report of the role of serum thyroglobulin as a monitoring method for low risk patients with papillary thyroid carcinoma. *J Clin Endocrinol Metab* 2003; 88: 1433–41.
50. van Tol K, Jager P, Piers D, et al. Better yield of 18 fluorodeoxyglucose positron emission tomography in patients with metastatic differentiated thyroid cancer during thyrotropin stimulation. *Thyroid* 2002; 12: 381–7.
51. Petrich T, Borner A, Otto D, et al. Influence of rhTSH on 18 fluorodeoxyglucose uptake by differentiated thyroid cancer. *Eur J Nucl Med Mol Imaging* 2002; 29: 641–7.
52. Ma C, Xie J, Kuang A. Is empiric I^{131} therapy justified for patients with positive Tg and negative I^{131} whole body scanning results? *J Nucl Med* 2005; 46: 1164–70.
53. van Tol K, Jager P, de Vries E, et al. Outcome in patients with differentiated thyroid cancer with negative diagnostic whole body scanning and detectable stimulated thyroglobulin. *Eur J Endocrinol* 2003; 148: 589–96.
54. Leeper R. The effect of I^{131} therapy on survival of patients with metastatic papillary or follicular thyroid carcinoma. *J Clin Endocrinol Metab* 1973; 36: 1143–52.
55. Bernier M, Leenhardt L, Hoang C, et al. Survival and therapeutic modalities in patients with bone metastases of differentiated thyroid carcinomas. *J Clin Endocrinol Metab* 2001; 86: 1568–73.
56. Schlumberger M, Mancusi F, De Vathaire F, et al. Radioactive iodine treatment and external radiotherapy for lung and bone metastases from thyroid carcinoma. *J Nucl Med* 1996; 37: 598–605.
57. Maxon H, Thomas S, Samaratunga R. Dosimetric considerations in the radioiodine treatment of macrometastases and micrometastases from differentiated thyroid cancer. *Thyroid* 1997; 7: 183–7.
58. Van Nostrand D, Atkins F, Yeganeh F, et al. Dosimetrically determined doses of radioiodine for the treatment of metastatic thyroid carcinoma. *Thyroid* 2002; 12: 121–34.
59. Schwartz DL, Lobo MJ, Ang KK, et al. Postoperative external beam radiotherapy for differentiated thyroid cancer: outcomes and morbidity with conformal treatment. *Int J Radiat Oncol Biol Phys* 2009; 74: 1083–91.
60. Terezakis SA, Lee KS, Ghossein RA, et al. Role of external beam radiotherapy in patients with advanced or recurrent nonanaplastic thyroid cancer: memorial Sloan–Kettering Cancer Center experience. *Int J Radiat Oncol Biol Phys* 2009; 73(3): 795–801.
61. Sia MA, Tsang RW, Panzarella T, et al. Differentiated thyroid cancer with extra-thyroidal extension: prognosis and the role of external beam radiotherapy. *J Thyroid Res* 2010 May 6; 2010:183461.
62. Brose M, Nutting C, Jarzab B, et al. Sorafenib in locally advanced or metastatic patients with radioactive iodine-refractory differentiated thyroid cancer: the phase III DECISION trial. *J Clin Oncol* 2013: 31(suppl, abstr 4).

63. Ho AL, Grewal RK, Leboeuf R, et al. Selumetinib-enhanced radioiodine uptake in advanced thyroid cancer. *N Engl J Med* 2013; **368**: 623–32.
64. Ahuja S, Ernst H. Chemotherapy of thyroid carcinoma. *J Endocrinol Invest* 1987; **10**: 303–10.
65. Shimaoka K, Schoenfeld D, Dewys W, et al. A randomized trial of doxorubicin versus doxorubicin plus cisplatin in patients with advanced thyroid cancer. *Cancer* 1985; **56**: 2155–60.
66. Williams S, Birch R, Einhorn L. Phase II evaluation of doxorubicin plus cisplatin in advance thyroid cancer: a Southeastern Cancer Study Group Trial. *Cancer Treat Rep* 1986; **70**: 405–7.
67. Rivkees SA, Mazzaferri EL, Verburg FA, et al. The treatment of differentiated thyroid cancer in children: emphasis on surgical approach and radioactive iodine therapy. *Endocr Rev* 2011; **32**: 798–826.
68. Hay ID, Gonzalez-Losada T, Reinalda MS, et al. Long-term outcome in 215 children and adolescents with papillary thyroid cancer treated during 1940 through 2008. *World J Surg* 2010; **34**: 1192–202.
69. Pawelczak M, David R, Franklin B, et al. Outcomes of children and adolescents with well-differentiated thyroid carcinoma and pulmonary metastases following 131I treatment: a systematic review. *Thyroid* 2010; **20**: 1095–101.
70. A Multi-Disciplinary Consensus Statement of Best Practice from a Working Group Convened Under the Auspices of the BSPED and UKCCSG (rare tumour working groups). *Paediatric endocrine tumours. A multi-disciplinary consensus statement of best practice.* 2005. Available from: https://www.bsped.org.uk/clinical/docs/RareEndocrineTumour_final.pdf
71. Mandel S, Larsen P, Seely E, Brent G. Increased need for thyroxine during pregnancy in women with primary hypothyroidism. *N Engl J Med* 1990; **323**: 91–6.
72. The American Thyroid Association Guidelines Task Force, Kloos RT, Eng C, et al. *Thyroid* 2009; **19**(6): 565–612.
73. Van Heerden J, Grant C, Grarib H, et al. Long-term course of patients with persistent hypercalcitonaemia after apparent curative primary surgery for medullary thyroid carcinoma. *Ann Surg* 1990; **212**: 395–401.
74. Barbet J, Campion L, Kraeber-Bodéré F, Chatal JF. GTE Study Group. Prognostic impact of serum calcitonin and carcinoembryonic antigen doubling-times in patients with medullary thyroid carcinoma. *J Clin Endocrinol Metab* 2005; **90**: 6077–84.
75. Brierly J, Tsang RWS, Gospodaowicz M, et al. Medullary thyroid cancer: analysis of survival and prognostic factors and the role of radiation therapy in local control. *Thyroid* 1996; **6**: 305–10.
76. Schwartz D, Rana V, Shaw S, et al. Postoperative radiotherapy for advanced medullary thyroid cancer: local disease control in the modern era. *Head Neck* 2008; **30**: 883–8.
77. Fife K, Bower M, Harmer C. Medullary thyroid cancer: the role of radiotherapy in local control. *Eur J Surg Oncol* 1996; **22**: 588–91.
78. Troncone L, Rufini V, Maussier M, et al. The role of I^{131}mIBG in the treatment of medullary thyroid carcinoma: results in five cases. *J Nucl Biol Med* 1991; **35**: 327–31.
79. Schwartz C, Delisle M. Results of I^{131} metaiodobenzylguanidine therapy administered to two patients with medullary carcinoma of the thyroid. *J Nucl Biol Med* 1991; **35**: 332–3.
80. Hoefnagel C, Delprat C, Valdes Olmos R. Role of [^{131}I]metaiodobenzylguanidine therapy in medullary thyroid carcinoma. *J Nucl Biol Med* 1991; **35**: 334–6.
81. Kwekkeboom D, Reubi J, Lamberts S. *In vivo* somatostatin receptor imaging in medullary thyroid carcinoma. *J Clin Endocrinol Metab* 1993; **76**: 1413–17.
82. Tisell L, Ahlman H, Wängberg B, et al. Somatostatin receptor scintigraphy in medullary thyroid carcinoma. *Br J Surg* 1997; **84**: 543–7.
83. Leboulleux S, Bastholt L, Krause TM, et al. Vandetanib in locally advanced or metastatic differentiated thyroid cancer: a randomized, double-blind phase II trial. *Ann Oncol* 2010; **21**(Suppl 8): viii 315 (abstr 1008PD).
84. Wells SA Jr, Gosnell JE, Gagel RF, et al. Vandetanib for the treatment of patients with locally advanced or metastatic hereditary medullary thyroid cancer. *J Clin Oncol* 2010; **28**(5): 767–72.
85. Wells SA Jr, Robinson BG, Gagel RF, et al. Vandetanib in patients with locally advanced or metastatic medullary thyroid cancer: a randomized, double-blind phase III trial. *J Clin Oncol* 2012; **30**(2): 134–41.
86. Viola D, Cappagli V, Elisei R. Cabozantinib (XL184) for the treatment of locally advanced or metastatic progressive medullary thyroid cancer. *Future Oncol* 2013; **9**(8): 1083–92.
87. Neff RL, Farrar WB, Kloos RT, Burman KD. Anaplastic thyroid cancer. *Endocrinol Metab Clin North Am* 2008; **37**: 525–38.
88. Smallridge RC, Copland JA. Anaplastic thyroid carcinoma: pathogenesis and emerging therapies. *Clin Oncol* 2010; **22**: 486–97.
89. Smallridge RC, Ain KB, Asa SL, et al. American Thyroid Association guidelines for management of patients with anaplastic thyroid cancer. *Thyroid* 2012; **22**(11): 1104–39.
90. Tennvall J, Lundell G, Hallsquist A, et al. Combined doxorubicin, hyperfractionated radiotherapy and surgery in anaplastic thyroid carcinoma: report on two protocols. *Cancer* 1994; **15**: 1348–54.
91. Tennvall J, Lundell G, Wahlberg P, et al. Anaplastic thyroid carcinoma: three protocols combining doxorubicin, hyperfractionated radiotherapy and surgery. *Br J Cancer* 2002; **86**: 1848–53.
92. De Crevoisier R, Baudin E, Bachelot A, et al. Combined treatment of anaplastic thyroid carcinoma with surgery, chemotherapy, and hyperfractionated accelerated external radiotherapy. *Int J Radiat Oncol Biol Phys* 2004; **60**: 1137–43.
93. Haigh P, Ituarte P, Wu H, et al. Completely resected anaplastic thyroid carcinoma combined with adjuvant chemotherapy and irradiation is associated with prolonged survival. *Cancer* 2001; **91**: 2335–42.
94. Mitchell G, Huddart R, Harmer C. Phase II evaluation of high dose accelerated radiotherapy for anaplastic thyroid carcinoma. *Radiother Oncol* 1999; **50**: 33–8.
95. Sosa JA, Balkissoon J, Lu SP, et al. Thyroidectomy followed by fosbretabulin (CA4P) combination regimen appears to suggest improvement in patient survival in anaplastic thyroid cancer. *Surgery* 2012; **152**(6): 1078–87.
96. Miller T, Dalhberg S, Cassady J, et al. Chemotherapy alone compared with chemotherapy plus radiotherapy for localized intermediate- and high-grade non-Hodgkin's lymphoma. *N Engl J Med* 1998; **339**: 21–6.
97. Matsuzuka F, Miyauchi A, Katayama S, et al. Clinical aspects of primary thyroid lymphoma: diagnosis and treatment based on our experience of 119 cases. *Thyroid* 1993; **3**: 93–9.

Thyroid surgery

CHAPTER 67

THYROIDECTOMY

Ricard Simo, Iain J. Nixon and Ralph P. Tufano

History of thyroidectomy 793	Consent 795
Surgical concepts 794	Pre-operative considerations 795
Indications and extent of surgery 794	Surgical technique for standard thyroidectomy ... 795
Surgery for benign disease 794	Post-operative care 802
'Diagnostic' surgery 795	References 803
Surgery for malignant disease 795	

SEARCH STRATEGY

Data in this chapter may be updated by a PubMed search using the keywords: thyroidectomy, thyroid surgery, thyroid lobectomy, total thyroidectomyt, recurrent laryngeal nerve, thyroid cancer.

There is lack of substantive high-level evidence due to the intrinsic nature of the chapter. In most areas the evidence is at most level 2.

HISTORY OF THYROIDECTOMY

The first recorded thyroidectomy was attributed to Abdul Kasan Kelebis Abis in Baghdad in AD 500. The first in Europe was performed in Spain by another Arabic physician Abu Al-Qasim (El-Zahra 936–1013) and its record published in his book *Al-Tasrif* in AD 952.

In 1646 the first thyroidectomy using scalpels was performed. However the patient, a 10-year-old, died and the surgeon was imprisoned. During the subsequent two centuries surgery for the thyroid gland was hazardous due to the inability to adequately control bleeding, and the lack of antisepsis and anaesthesia. Most patients died and this surgery was extremely unpopular and even condemned by prominent physicians and surgeons. The mortality rate from thyroid surgery by 1850 was about 40%.

During the first part of the 19th century advances were made in the understanding of the function of the thyroid gland and the role of iodine. Two Swiss physicians, Johan Straub and Francious Coindet, recommended the use of iodine to reduce the size and vascularity of goitres before surgery was undertaken.

The second half of the century saw two crucial developments that helped to usher in a new era of thyroid surgery: the discovery of anaesthesia and the introduction of antisepsis by Joseph Lister meant that surgery became much safer. These developments coincided with the arrival of Theodor Kocher and Albert Theodor Billroth.

Albert Theodor Billroth (1829–1894), one of the most prominent surgeons of his time, reduced his thyroidectomy mortality rate from 40% to 8% thanks to anaesthesia and antisepsis. However, thyroid surgery will always be associated with Theodor Kocher (1841–1917). While he was Chair of Surgery in Bern, he performed more than 5000 thyroidectomies. He was extremely meticulous and paid close attention to haemostasis. He was the first surgeon to systematically ligate the inferior thyroid artery, which reduced significantly the risk of haemorrhage. His mortality rate plummeted from 12.6% in 1870 to 0.2% in 1898. He introduced the collar incision, preserved the strap muscles whenever possible and pioneered anaesthesia and antisepsis for thyroid surgery. However, by removing the entire thyroid gland, many patients were left severely hypothyroid and Kocher described this as *chachexia struma priva*. This prompted him to study the physiology, pathology and surgery of the thyroid gland in great detail, which in 1909 earned him the Nobel Prize. It was from then on that he was acknowledged as the 'father of modern thyroid surgery'.

William S. Halsted (1852–1922) brought the Kocher surgical philosophy to the USA. He also introduced antisepsis and developed a new set of haemostats, which together with his meticulous technique made thyroid surgery very safe. Halsted also introduced the first residency programme at the John Hopkins Hospital in Baltimore where he was made Professor of Surgery. From this programme, many famous future thyroid surgeons were trained including Charles Horace Mayo, Frank Lahey and George Crile.

Further refinements to thyroid surgery were introduced by Thomas Peel Dunhill, Jan Mikuliz, Wolfler, Eugene Gley and Harold Floss who first introduced the use of motion pictures to teach thyroid surgery.

Thyroidectomy is now a common procedure with rates increasing year-on-year.[1] In contrast to early results, complications related to thyroidectomy are now uncommon, with the highest volume surgeons reporting the lowest risk of morbidity.[2]

Despite all of these developments, the principles of Kocher's surgical philosophy with meticulous surgical technique and exemplary attention to detail continue to serve as the cornerstone of thyroid surgery.[3, 4]

SURGICAL CONCEPTS

- **Total lobectomy (TL):** the removal of the one lobe, often performed with a thyroid isthmusectomy.
- **Thyroid isthmusectomy (TI):** the excision of the thyroid isthmus, often with the pyramidal lobe of the gland, a procedure that should be reserved for nodules in the isthmus which measure no more than 4 cm in diameter and do not encroach significantly on either lobe.
- **Subtotal thyroidectomy (ST):** the bilateral excision of more than one half of the thyroid gland on each side together with the isthmus. This technique is currently not recommended.
- **Near-total thyroidectomy or Dunhill's thyroidectomy (NTT):** the excision of 90% of the gland, leaving a small remnant of tissue on one side at the level of the Berry's ligament.
- **Total thyroidectomy (TT):** the excision of the entire thyroid gland.

Partial lobectomy, subtotal lobectomy and nodulectomy are confusing terms and are best avoided.

INDICATIONS AND EXTENT OF SURGERY

Thyroidectomy is a benchmark procedure for surgeons, and a thorough understanding of the indications for surgery results in the ability to select the most appropriate primary operation, which is critical to maintaining excellent outcomes. When selecting an appropriate thyroid procedure, the surgeon must first consider whether the surgery is for benign disease, malignancy or diagnostic purposes.

Excision of a nodule from the thyroid gland or 'nodulectomy' has been abandoned. The reasons for this include the bloody nature of the operation itself, but more importantly the high rates of recurrence of benign or malignant disease following surgery. Not only are recurrence rates high, but re-operative surgery for recurrence typically involves unacceptably high risks to both the recurrent laryngeal nerve (RLN) and the parathyroid glands. In addition, for malignant disease, unacceptable oncological outcomes have been associated with less than total thyroid lobectomy.

For most purposes, then, the complete removal of one entire thyroid lobe should be considered the minimum thyroid surgery performed by the modern surgeon.[5]

SURGERY FOR BENIGN DISEASE

Patients without evidence of malignancy may be considered for surgery either due to benign nodular thyroid disease causing compression or cosmetic concerns, or in the setting of hyperthyroidism.

Non-toxic multinodular goitres

In the event that nodular disease has resulted in compression of the trachea or oesophagus, surgical decompression should be considered. Pre-operative assessment is crucial. The surgeon must not only consider the site of compression, but the entire gland, as some patients will have bilateral multinodular disease.[6]

In patients with a single nodule which has enlarged sufficiently to cause compression, TL alone may be sufficient to relieve symptoms, while preventing the need for contralateral tracheoesophageal groove dissection, and therefore eliminating the chance of permanent hypoparathyroidism and bilateral vocal cord palsy. Post-surgical surveillance of the remaining thyroid remnant will be required, as will regular thyroid function tests as up to a third of patients will develop hypothyroidism during long-term follow-up.[7] The need for later thyroid hormone replacement is more common in those with a raised pre-operative thyroid-stimulating hormone level or thyroiditis.[8]

For those patients with bilateral multinodular goitre (MNG), TT is the operation of choice.[9] This removes all nodules and minimizes the chance of recurrence.

ST should only be considered in healthcare settings where an adequate supply of exogenous thyroid hormone cannot be ensured, and functioning thyroid tissue is preserved to maintain endocrine function.

Thyrotoxicosis

The choice of surgery for patients with hyperthyroidism will be related to the pre-operative findings in the gland as a whole. Analysis suggests that surgery for Graves' disease is successful, with total thyroidectomy the preferred option.[10]

For those patients with an autonomously functioning solitary nodule, TL alone may suffice. For those patients with multinodular disease or global glandular dysfunction (e.g. Graves' disease), TT should be recommended. Such an approach again reduces the chance of recurrent hyperthyroidism, and the need for reoperative surgery. Patients considered for such surgery must understand that they will require lifelong hormone supplementation.

'DIAGNOSTIC' SURGERY

This term is controversial but just under 30% of patients investigated for thyroid malignancy will have an indeterminate pre-operative diagnosis.[11] In this setting, each patient should be considered on an individual basis.

Those patients with uninodular disease, which would be adequately treated with TL alone in the setting of malignancy, should undergo TL.[12, 13] Those with multinodular disease should be considered for TT for ipsilateral diagnostic purposes and also to prevent the need for lifelong serial assessment of contralateral nodules.

Patients who have uninodular disease but are likely to require completion thyroidectomy in the event of a malignant diagnosis can be offered either diagnostic TL with completion thyroidectomy as a staged procedure, TT up front, or TL with on-table frozen section analysis with immediate completion if malignancy is confirmed.

Each approach has advantages and disadvantages. Clinicians must assess each case, including the clinical, biochemical, ultrasonographic and cytological features in order to make an individualized decision. A number of statistical models are available to assist in predicting the risk of malignancy within an individual thyroid nodule, which can be used in the clinical setting to aid decision-making and informed consent.[14]

SURGERY FOR MALIGNANT DISEASE

Many patients who undergo surgery for thyroid nodules do so with a biopsy-proven malignant lesion.[15]

For patients with T3 and above differentiated thyroid cancers (DTC), medullary carcinoma of the thyroid, poorly differentiated thyroid cancer, multinodular glands, multifocal cancer, evidence of extrathyroidal extension or overt nodal metastases, the majority of authors agree that TT is the procedure of choice.[16–20]

Patients with disease limited to the isthmus may have a T1 lesion[21] but for the majority of patients with uninodular DTC, without extra thyroid extension or metastases, TL results in oncological outcomes equal to TT.[22, 23]

When considering the extent of surgery for thyroid cancer, the surgeon, endocrinologist, nuclear medicine physician and patient must all agree to the proposed treatment plan. Bear in mind that it is rare for a patient with DTC to die of disease following appropriate primary therapy, so a balance between maximizing outcome while minimizing morbidity must be achieved in every case.

CONSENT

The consent for thyroidectomy should include the explanation of the procedure, its rationale and the options of alternative treatments relevant to the condition. The potential complications should be discussed and should include the risks of general anaesthesia, scarring, infection, haemorrhage, injury to the external branch of the superior laryngeal nerve (EBSLN) and to the RLN, hypocalcaemia and hypothyroidism. In cases of large retrosternal goitre or invasive thyroid carcinoma, the risks of airway obstruction with the potential need for tracheostomy should also be discussed. If extensive intrathoracic goitre requires sternal split or lateral thoracotomy, all relevant complications such as injury to pleura and pneumothorax, pneumonia, and injury to phrenic nerves and the pericardium should be discussed.[8, 24, 25]

PRE-OPERATIVE CONSIDERATIONS

1. Evidence of clinical examination, cytological or histopathological analysis and adequate imaging should be available.
2. Laryngeal examination and pre-operative voice assessment with fibre-optic laryngoscopy should be performed on all patients.[26]
3. Patients should be euthyroid; in thyrotoxic patients adequate precautions should be taken to avoid the possibility of a thyroid storm.
4. Patients should be adequately consented.
5. Patients undergoing general anaesthesia should have a north-facing endotracheal tube so it does not interfere with the surgical field.
6. Local anaesthetic should be considered to help haemostasis while raising the flaps and to aid analgesia in the post-operative period.
7. Neuromonitoring and surgical aids such as loops, microscope, fine bipolar forceps, ligaclips and energy devices should be encouraged to facilitate surgery.
8. Mild hypotensive anaesthesia should be used but reversed before the procedure is completed.

SURGICAL TECHNIQUE FOR STANDARD THYROIDECTOMY

Position The patient should be in a supine position, with a soft shoulder support and a soft head ring to allow maximum extension of the neck and aid stabilization of the head during surgery (**Figure 67.1**).

Incision and incision planning

The classical Kocher collar incision consists of a transverse cervical incision in a skin crease placed halfway between the cricoid cartilage and the sternal notch. There is no one-size-fits-all rule for the incision placement, but the following aspects should be considered (**Figure 67.2**).

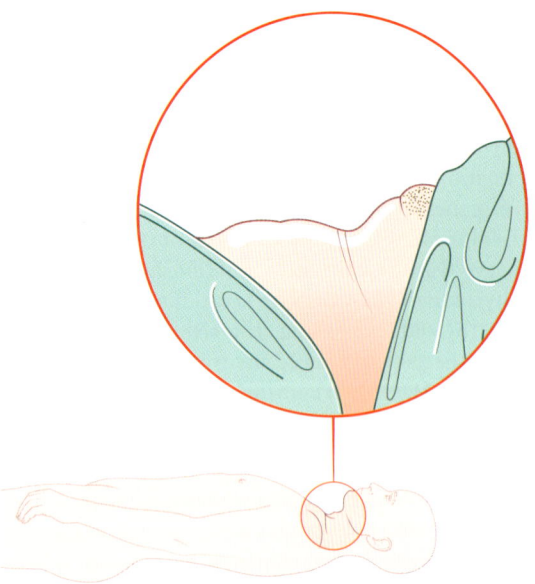

Figure 67.1 Position of patient undergoing thyroidectomy, demonstrating the supine posture with neck extension.

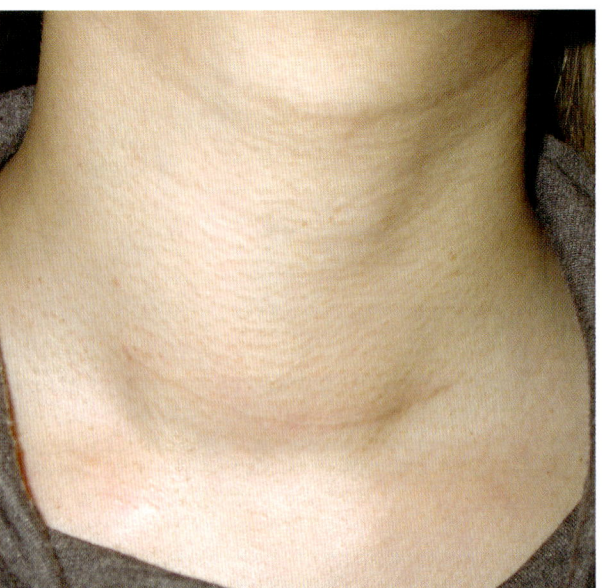

Figure 67.2 Typical Kocher incision 6 months after thyroidectomy.

- **Access:** The incision must be of adequate length to provide sufficient access to the superior, inferior and lateral aspects of the thyroid to ensure a safe dissection. Many surgeons prefer an incision as small as 3 cm and use retraction to move the incision in relation to the gland, exposing the areas of interest in sequence.
- **Cosmesis:** To avoid unnecessary attention drawn to the wound, it should be symmetrical across the midline. By placing the incision in a deep skin crease, the end result will be excellent, and in many cases this will outweigh the need for a small incision: it may be more cosmetically appealing to make a longer incision placed in a skin crease than a short incision between creases.
- **Secondary movement:** When planning the incision, breast size should be considered. In women with large breasts, significant inferior movement of the scar will occur over time. In this case, placing an incision higher in the neck will prevent the scar from migrating to an unsightly position in the presternal area.
- **Future procedures:** Particularly in high-risk patients with extrathyroid extension, for example, the surgeon should bear in mind the possibility that future access to the central and lateral neck may be required. An incision above the level of the cricoid cartilage can easily be extended along a skin crease to the level of the trapezius in order to access all levels of the neck if required at a later date. The modified extended Kocher incision is particularly helpful in this setting.[27]

Approach

Following the skin incision the tissues should be divided through the subcutaneous fat and the platysma. Traditionally, flaps are raised in the immediate subplatysmal plane up to a level above the thyroid cartilage and down to the suprasternal notch. The anterior jugular

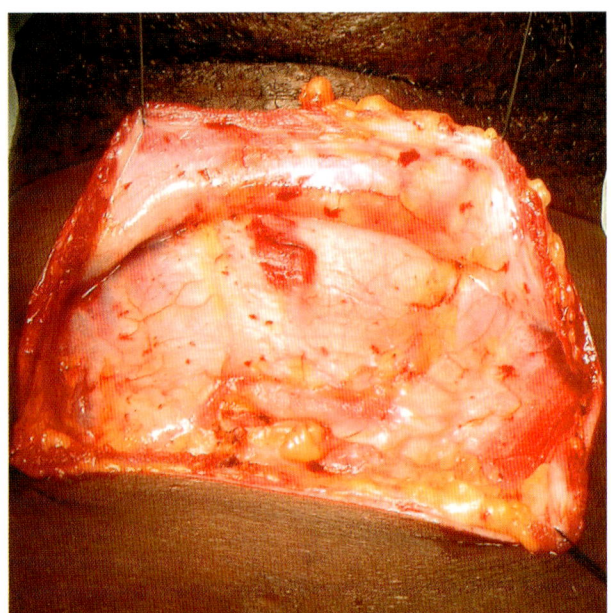

Figure 67.3 Subplatysmal flaps elevated.

veins should be identified and protected during this dissection as damage to these vessels during the early dissection can result in significant post-operative haemorrhage. The extent of dissection should be tailored to the gland in question. The exposure required for a small atrophic gland will be significantly less than for a retrosternal goitre (**Figure 67.3**).

When an extensive dissection is required, flaps should be raised over the sternomastoids, and indeed the muscle can be dissected from its fascial envelope to improve access to the lateral aspect of the gland. The most inferior tendinous insertions of the sternomastoid muscles are connected by ligamentous fibres which can be divided to improve access to an intrathoracic goitre.

Incision of the cervical fascia

The investing cervical fascia is then incised in the midline and opened to the level of the thyroid cartilage and to the level of the sternal notch. Care should be taken to identify any communicating vessels crossing the midline (**Figure 67.4**).

Thyroid isthmus (TI)

The TI is identified once the cervical investing fascia has been opened. In cases of performing a TL only, it can be divided early to help the mobilization of the gland or can be dealt with at the end of the procedure. The timing of the division will depend on the experience of the surgeon.

Division of the strap muscles

This is often necessary, especially in cases of large glands. This allows access and better visualization of the vascular pedicles, particularly the superior pedicles. Either the sternothyroid and/or the sternohyoid muscles can be divided. They should be divided in the upper third as this will prevent injury to the ansa cervicalis, which enters the muscles in their inferior aspect (**Figure 67.5**).

Dissection proceeds on one side initially. The sternohyoid should be separated from the sternothyroid and the medial aspect of the carotid sheath, with the ansa cervicalis identified laterally.

Lateral retraction of the sternohyoid muscle allows access to the sternothyroid muscle. This should again be grasped with atraumatic forceps. Medial traction on the thyroid gland allows dissection of the muscle from the surface of the gland. Attention should be paid to this plane, which is elevated close to the muscle. Evidence of extrathyroid extension at this point should alert the surgeon to the advanced local stage and will alter the approach to the gland. If extrathyroid extension into the straps is evident, the muscle should be excised by dividing above and below the gland.

Identification and division of the vascular pedicles

This is an essential step in thyroidectomy. Individual vessels should be carefully dissected, identified, ligated and divided. This is best done with a curved dissector such as a Lahey or a Mixter dissector. This will allow adequate haemostasis, reducing the risk of post-operative haemorrhage, and will reduce the risk of injury to the superior laryngeal nerve and of leaving large glandular remnants that invariably exist between the vessels.

The superior pole

Management of the superior pole is critical to achieving total removal of the thyroid lobe. Great care should be taken to identify and control the multiple vessels, which fan out from the superior pedicle to insert on the gland.

Traditional descriptions of identifying the superior thyroid artery and dividing distant to the gland should be discouraged as they increase the potential for damage to the EBSLN as it crosses to innervate the cricothyroid muscle. Instead, these vessels should be taken close to the gland, ensuring that the entire superior pole is dissected (**Figure 67.6**).

Some authors now consider identification of the EBSLN mandatory in all procedures. Most, however, prefer to take care to stay close to the gland rather than exploring the area to formally identify the nerve.

Having started the mobilization, the next step is identification of the superior parathyroid gland (PTG). This will be found adjacent to the posterior capsule of

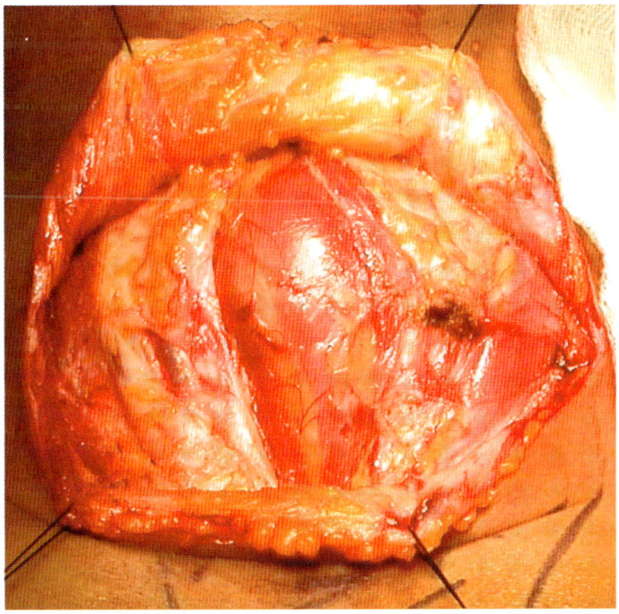

Figure 67.4 Incision cervical fascia, demonstrating the exposure of the thyroid isthmus.

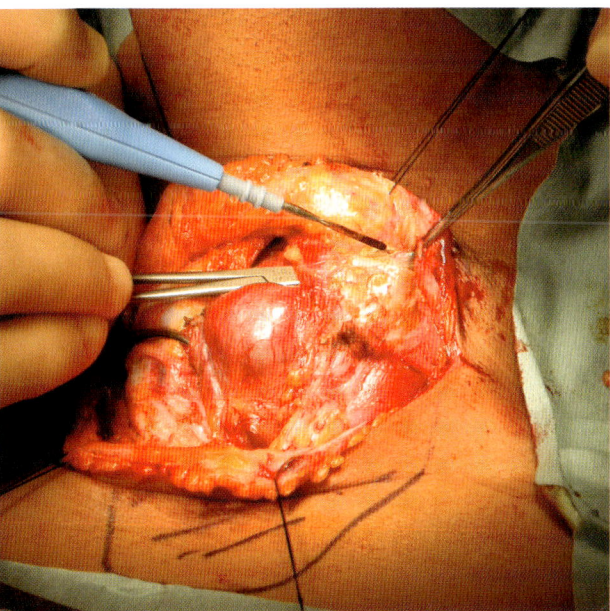

Figure 67.5 Division of the strap muscles using monopolar cutting diathermy.

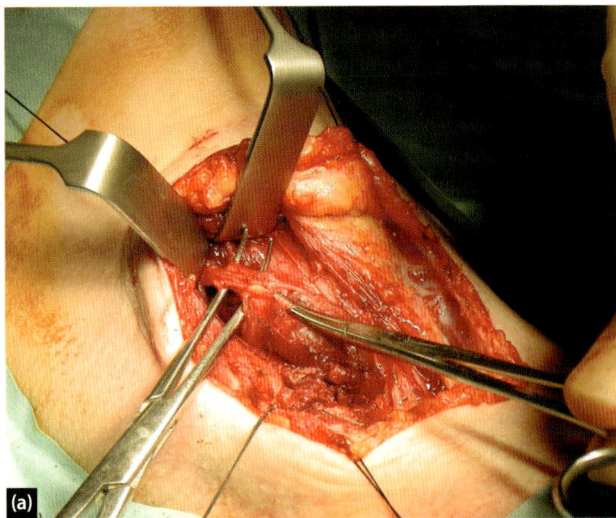 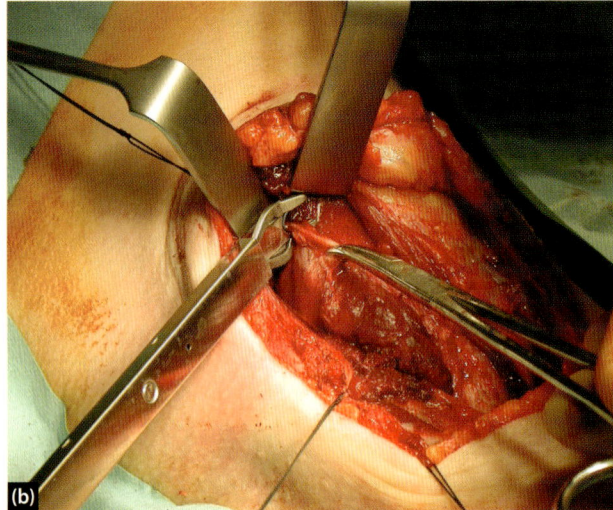

Figure 67.6 Identification, dissection and division of the superior vascular pedicle vessels.

the superior pole. The blood supply must be maintained, and the gland dissected off the thyroid in order to maintain function.

The lateral aspect

With the superior pole mobilized, attention can be turned to the lateral aspect of the gland. The surface of the gland is identified and dissected from the strap muscles. The dissection is done using a combination of sharp and blunt dissection to expose the whole length of the gland. At the lateral aspect of the gland the middle thyroid veins are ligated and divided to allow delivery of the gland and access to the paratracheal areas.

The fascia surrounding the gland is dissected and the thyroid is slowly mobilized, allowing visualization of the tracheosophageal groove (**Figure 67.7**).

The inferior pole

With the superior and medial aspects of the gland mobilized, attention can be turned to the inferior pole.

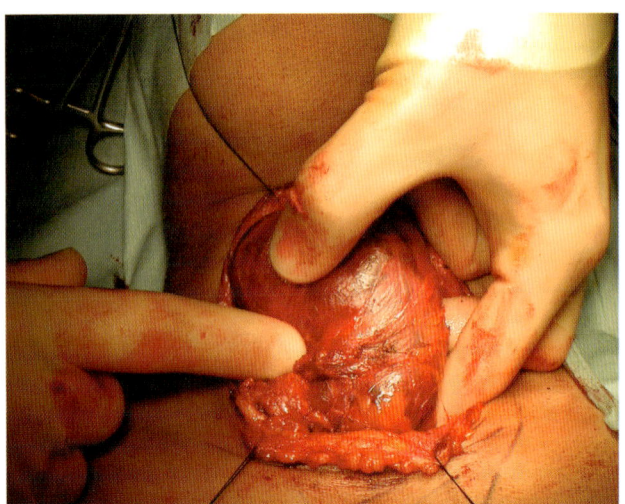

Figure 67.7 Mobilization of the lateral aspect of the gland.

By identifying the trachea, a safe plane of dissection can be developed which allows the inferior pole to be dissected from the trachea without jeopardizing the RLN.

External branch superior laryngeal nerve

The EBSLN should be identified whenever possible during the dissection of the superior pole.[28–30] This is done at the sternothyrolaryngeal or Joll's triangle, which is delineated by the superior thyroid pedicle and upper lobe of the gland, the cricothyroid muscle and the lower edge of the thyroid cartilage (**Figure 67.8**).

Recurrent laryngeal nerve

The position of the RLN varies depending on the side, as previously described in the anatomy section. Although most RLNs are single, up to 30% of nerves can branch before entering the larynx and this may lead to higher risk of injury (**Figure 67.9**).[31, 32]

- **Lateral approach:** The nerve is usually identified in the Beahrs triangle in the lower lateral part the neck. This triangle is defined by the inferior thyroid artery superiorly, the trachea medially and the common carotid artery laterally. This is safest way of identifying the recurrent laryngeal nerve (**Figure 67.10**).[33]
- **Superior approach:** The nerve can be identified at the level of the cricothyroid junction at its entry into the larynx. This approach can be very useful in cancer patients with extensive nodal disease, reoperative surgery, when other approaches have failed and when considering a non-recurrent laryngeal nerve. Once the nerve is identified, it should be dissected in a caudal direction, tunnelling the tissue surrounding the nerve with a mosquito fine-tip dissector (toboggan technique). The tissue above the tunnel is then diathermized with bipolar diathermy and divided (Figure 67.11).[33]

67: THYROIDECTOMY 799

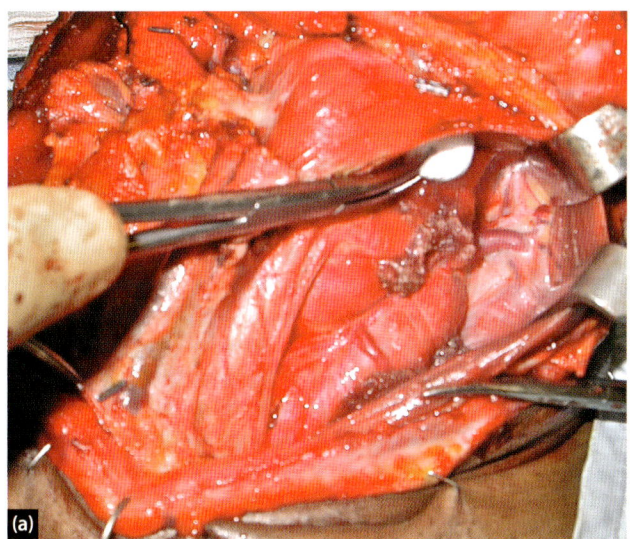

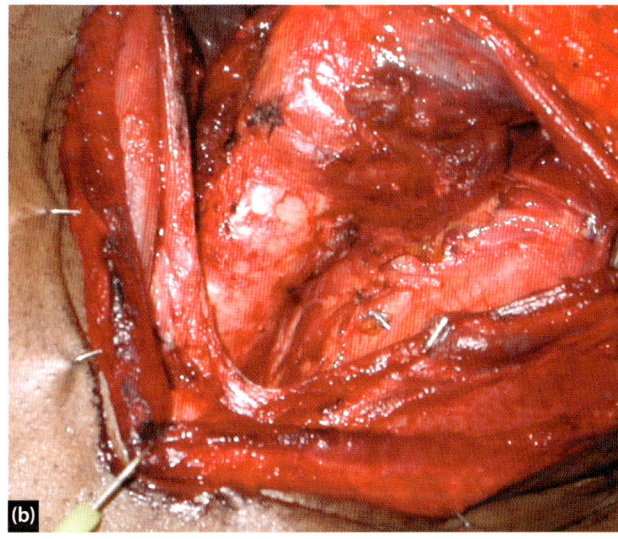

Figure 67.8 Identification of the SLN in the Joll's triangle.

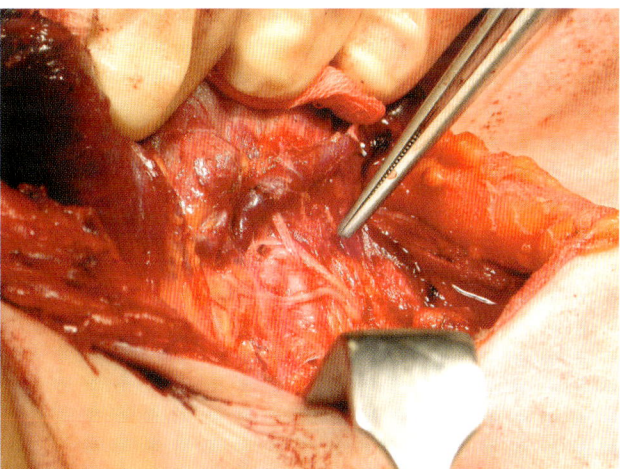

Figure 67.9 RLN demonstrating two extralaryngeal branches.

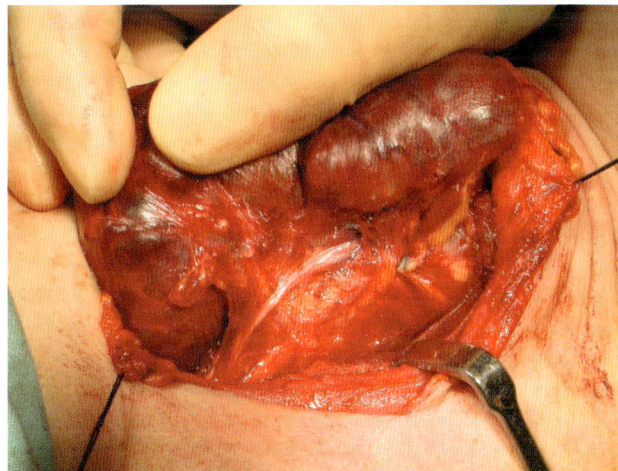

Figure 67.10 Identification of the RLN using a standard lateral approach.

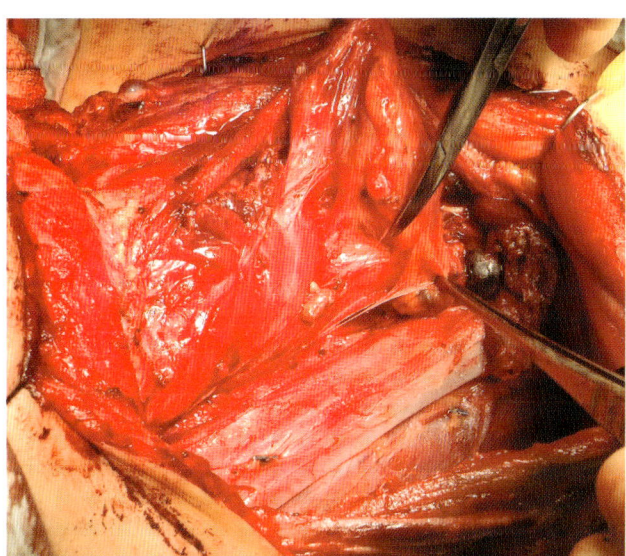

Figure 67.11 Identification of the RLN at the cricothyroid joint using a superior approach.

- **Inferior approach:** In large goitres or in revision surgery, an inferior approach can be used. This allows identification of the nerve in a virgin site (**Figure 67.12**).[33]

In every thyroidectomy, an attempt should be made to identify the nerve. Without this attention to detail, injury rates can be unacceptably high. Having identified the nerve, there is no need for it to be traced for any great distance. With experience, the surgeon will come to recognize the importance of the relationship between Berry's ligament and the nerve. In patients with a low Berry's ligament, which sits posterior on the trachea, the nerve will be in close proximity to the gland at this crucial point. In these cases the nerve must be carefully traced and the gland mobilized off the nerve. When Berry's ligament is high, the nerve is often quite laterally placed in comparison, and minimal dissection will be required. This minimizes the chance of inadvertent injury.

Around 2% of RLNs are non-recurrent and this is almost always present on the right. Pre-operative imaging

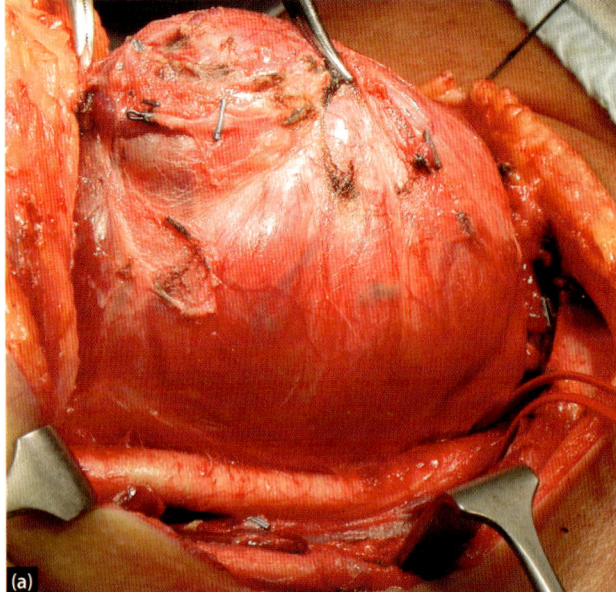
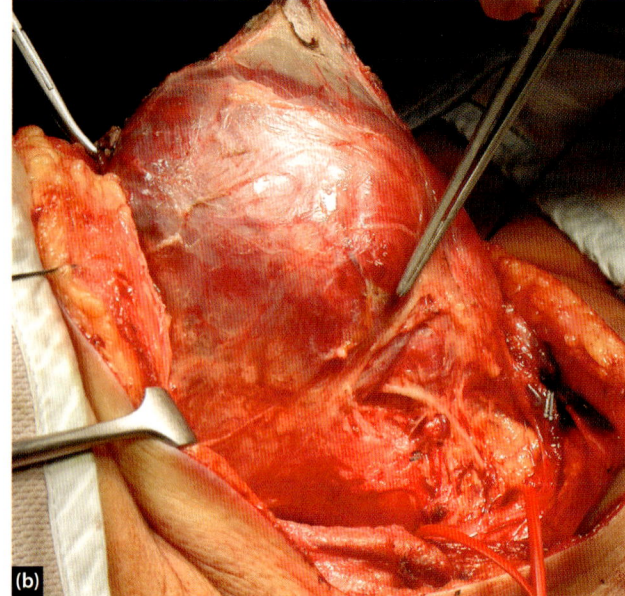

Figure 67.12 Identification of the RLN at the apex of the Beahrs triangle using an inferior approach.

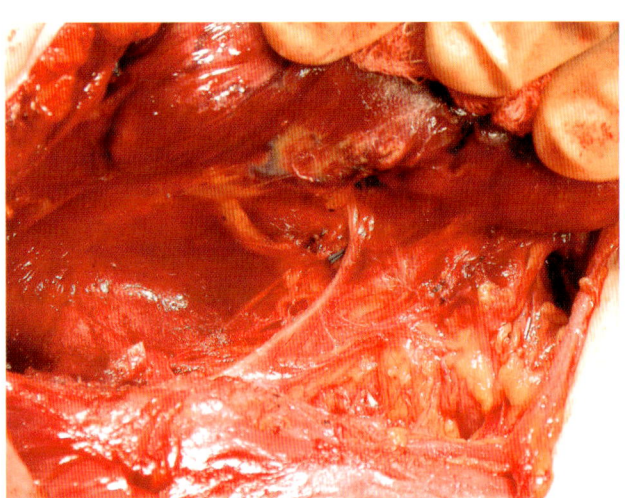

Figure 67.13 Non-RLN arising directly from the right vagus nerve.

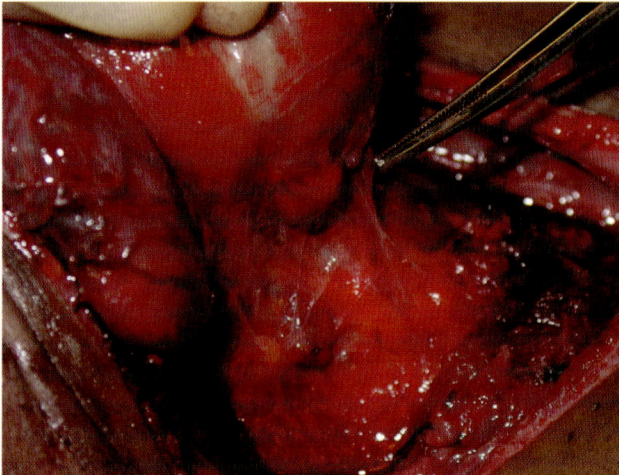

Figure 67.14 Typical position of the parathyroid glands once the right thyroid lobe has been mobilized, demonstrating the superior parathyroid gland in a superior-lateral position and the inferior parathyroid gland in an anterior-inferior position with the RLN crossing from a caudal to cranial position.

which identifies situs inversus, or more commonly a retroesophageal subclavian artery, may raise the index of suspicion. If the RLN cannot be identified in the traditional position, the surgeon must consider the possibility of a non-recurrent nerve. This structure will be running inferomedially from the vagus nerve and will be wide in comparison to a normal RLN (**Figure 67.13**).

RLN MONITORING

Recent technological advances have allowed surgeons to assess the integrity of the recurrent laryngeal nerve during thyroidectomy. Proponents of these techniques highlight the potential reduction in rates of iatrogenic injury and find the nerve monitor useful in the training of junior surgeons. Those who oppose the routine use of nerve monitors cite increases in operative time and cost as well as the lack of clear evidence of overall patient benefit. The topic remains controversial, and it is covered in detail elsewhere.

Management of the parathyroid glands

The parathyroid glands should be identified whenever possible. The position of the glands can be variable and 25% of the glands may not be in the position that the surgeon expects them to be (**Figure 67.14**). When the thyroid gland has been mobilized, the superior parathyroid gland should fall in a posterior position from the nerve and the inferior parathyroid gland in an anterior one. Once identified, the tissue handling needs to be very precise and delicate so the glands can be dissected with their blood supply preserved.

The superior glands are relatively uniform in their position. The inferior glands are traditionally described as ventral to the RLN in the region of the inferior thyroid artery. However, it is not uncommon for these glands to be aberrant in position, and lie somewhere between the level of the cricoid to the thymus. Traditionally, 1% of parathyroids have been considered to be intrathyroidal, although with careful scrutiny of resected thyroid tissue this may be an underestimate.

Parathyroid glands rely on their blood supply to function, and it is critical that their nutrient vessels are preserved. The glands should be gently dissected from the thyroid, taking care not to cause traction or diathermy injury to their blood supply. In the event that a parathyroid is excised, or is considered non-viable, a sample should be sent for frozen section analysis and, on confirmation, the gland should be divided into around 12 pieces for implantation into a muscle. Often the sternomastoid muscle is used due to its convenience, although this view has recently been challenged.[34]

Berry's ligament

At this level the recurrent laryngeal nerve is at greatest risk. The ligament is dissected using fine and judicious bipolar diathermy. The blades of the bipolar should be resting on the thyroid gland and away from the nerve. Once the diathermy has been performed, the ligament is divided with a size 15 blade scalpel. This provides the best accuracy and reduces the risk of injury. It is important to note that the ligament is often very vascular and its thickness variable. It is therefore often necessary to dissect and divide the ligament in several steps until the perichondrium of the trachea is reached (**Figure 67.15**).

Pyramidal lobe

The pyramidal lobe should always be identified, dissected and excised together with the thyroidectomy specimen.

Having delivered the thyroid from Berry's ligament, the gland should be dissected off the anterior tracheal wall towards the midline. Great care should be taken at this point to identify any pyramidal tissue. If this is left behind, it will be evident on post-operative imaging and may result in the need for adjuvant RAI, or sampling to exclude the possibility of local recurrence. The pyramidal lobe tends to be a central structure, although it is not always immediately in the midline. It extends in the direction of the thyroglossal tract towards the hyoid, and should be divided as superiorly as possible (**Figure 67.16**).

Closure

1. **Wound wash.** Once the thyroidectomy is completed, the wound is washed with water or normal saline. Iodine-based solutions are best avoided, especially when performing surgery for thyroid cancer, as this may interfere with subsequent radioiodine ablation.
2. **Haemostasis.** Haemostasis is essential. To check for any bleeding points, the wound must be clean of clots. When this has been done, a Valsalva manoeuvre should be used at least twice to check for any bleeding.

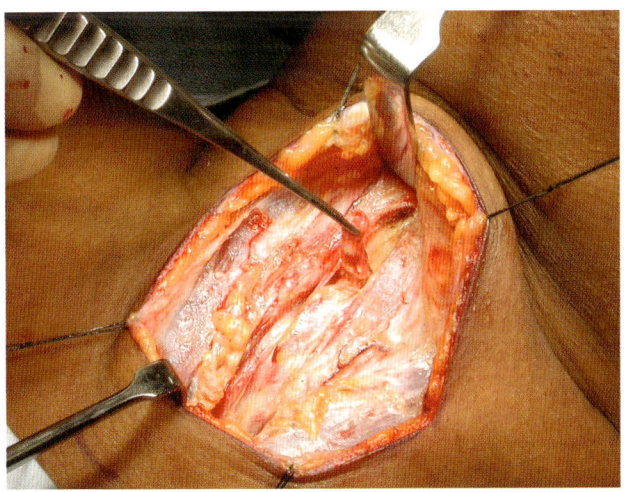

Figure 67.16 Dissection of the pyramidal lobe.

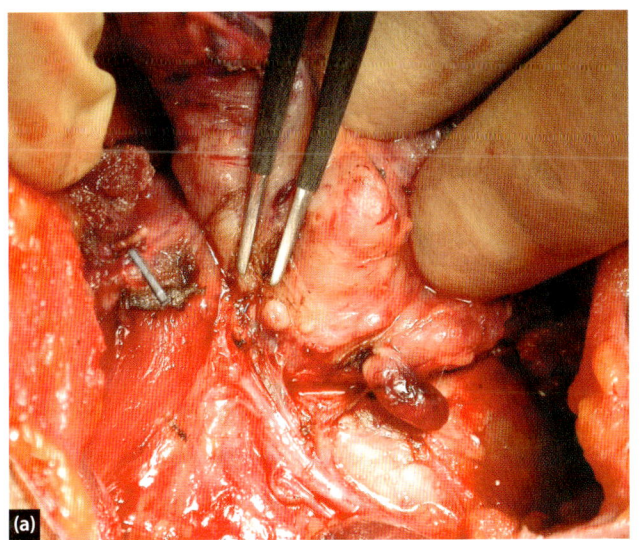
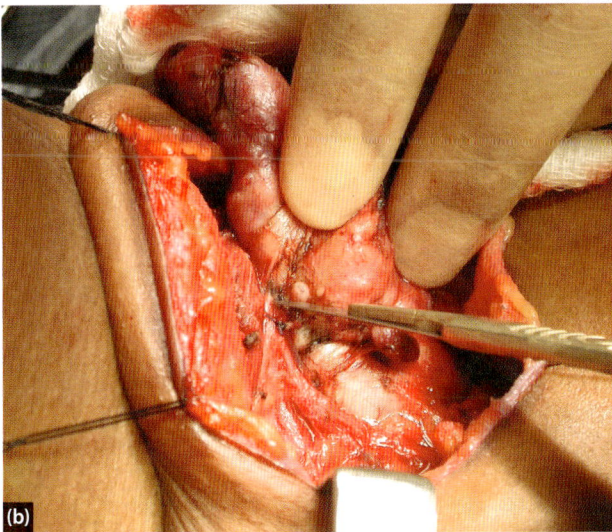

Figure 67.15 Management of the Berry's ligament using careful bipolar coagulation of the fine vessels followed by division of the ligament with a size 15 scalpel.

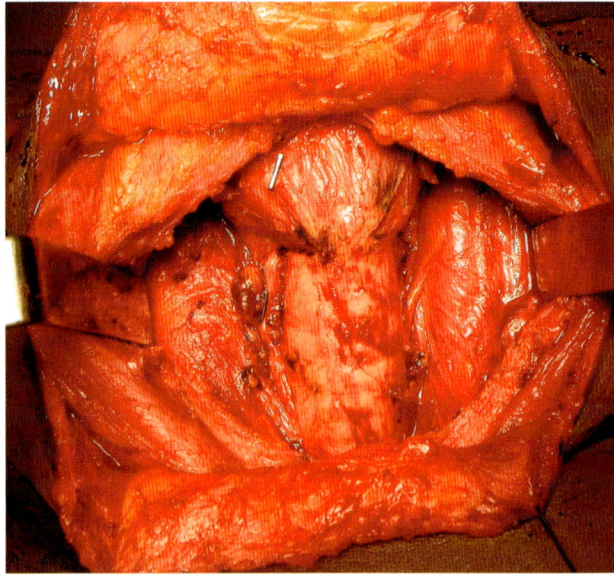

Figure 67.17 Post-operative appearance of a thyroid bed after total thyroidectomy, demonstrating the trachea, larynx, RLNs and parathyroid gland.

3. **Check the RLNs and parathyroid glands.** Once haemostasis is completed, the RLNs and the parathyroid glands should be checked to ensure that they are intact anatomically. If neuromonitoring is used, an EMG signal should be obtained and recorded (**Figures 67.17** and **67.18**).
4. **Drainage.** The need for drains should be considered on an individual patient basis. Many prospective, randomized trials have shown that drains do not reduce haematomas or seroma rates. Despite this, some units use suction drains, particularly when a significant dissection has resulted in a large dead space or the patient uses anticoagulation.[35]
5. **Subcutaneous tissues and skin closure.** The wound is closed in layers. The strap muscles should be approximated with an absorbable suture. Many surgeons now advocate only one suture to prevent trachea–cutaneous adhesion, while maintaining a connection between the deep central neck and the more superficial planes. The theory is that this may prevent the development of high lymphovascular pressure in the perilaryngeal tissue in the event of a hematoma, thereby reducing the risk of airway oedema and respiratory obstruction.

The platysma should then be re-approximated using an absorbable suture. The skin should then be closed with meticulous attention to detail to optimize wound healing. The technique (interrupted nylon, staples, subcuticular sutures, skin glue, etc.) is less important than the need to be precise and treat the skin edges with respect. The ideal closure will allow easy reopening in the event of haematoma.

POST-OPERATIVE CARE

- **Position.** Patients should be nursed head up in a 45 degree position for the first 4 hours before they can start mobilizing.
- **Venous thromboembolism (VTE) prophylaxis.** Patients undergoing thyroid surgery should have adequate VTE prophylaxis. As a general rule, anticoagulant VTE prophylactic agents should be commenced 24 hours from the procedure and continued until the patient is discharged.
- **Nursing.** Patients should be monitored in an adequate post-operative care facility or ward. An adequate pathway of monitoring and enhanced recovery should be instigated in all units dealing with thyroid surgery. Suture or staple removal forceps should be available at the bedside.
- **Steroid therapy.** The use of intravenous steroid therapy in the first 24 hours is a valuable adjunct to analgesia as an antiemetic and in one randomized controlled trial has shown to reduce the rate of RLN neuropraxia.[36]
- **Antibiotic prophylaxis.** This is not usually necessary. In complex cases with extensive dissection, ETE involving the airway structures or lateral neck dissection, prophylactic antibiotics up to three doses in 24 hours should be considered.
- **Analgesia.** Adequate analgesia is imperative. Opiates are preferred to non-steroidal analgesics to minimize the risk of post-operative bleeding.
- **Resume oral intake.** Patients can resume oral intake as soon as they are fully awake and have a normal diet 4 hours from completion of the procedure.
- **Mobilization.** Early mobilization should be encouraged.
- **Drain removal.** Monitoring of drainage volume should be every 8 hours. If the volume is less than 20 mL at 24 hours or 10 mL at 8 hours, the drain may be removed.
- **Removal of sutures or staples** – most surgeons use either staples or subcuticular sutures. Staples can be removed as early as 36 hours from completion of the procedure, and edges reinforced with Steri-Strip™ tapes for 7–10 days. This will ensure adequate healing and optimal cosmesis.
- **Calcium management.** This is addressed in Chapter 79 on the prevention and management of complications.
- **Post-operative vocal cord check.** A post-operative vocal cord check should be done as soon as possible after the surgery if RLN injury is suspected. If there is no suspicion of RLN injury, a post-operative vocal cord check can be done in the first post-operative appointment.[26]

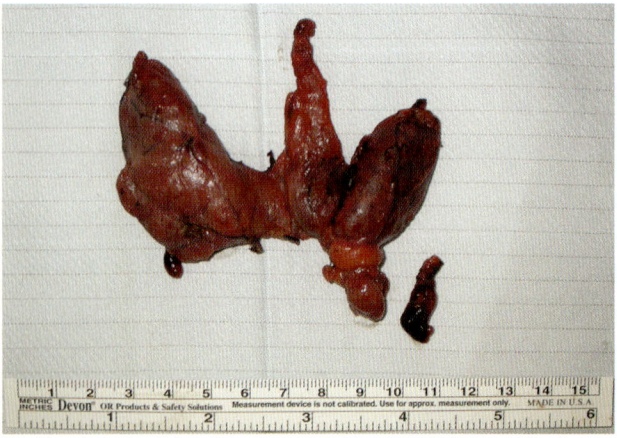

Figure 67.18 Specimen of a total thyroidectomy for thyroid cancer.

KEY EVIDENCE

- Essential pre-operative investigations for thyroid surgery include clinical examination, thyroid function test, thyroid antibodies, ultrasound-guided FNAC, pre-operative voice assessment with fibre-optic laryngoscopy and, for established malignancy, appropriate cross-sectional imaging investigations.
- Thyroid lobectomy is the minimum procedure acceptable except for those nodules located in the isthmus or pyramidal lobe.
- During thyroidectomy the recurrent laryngeal nerves and parathyroid glands should be identified and preserved unless there is pre-operative evidence of involvement with locally invasive thyroid cancer.

KEY POINTS

- Evidence of clinical examination, FNAC, core needle biopsy and adequate imaging USS, CT or MRI should be available.
- Laryngeal examination and pre-operative voice assessment with fibre-optic laryngoscopy should be performed in all patients undergoing thyroid surgery.
- Patients should be euthyroid or in cases of thyrotoxicosis in which the thyroid function is abnormal adequate precautions should be taken to avoid the possibility of a thyroid storm.
- Patients should be adequately consented.
- Patient undergoing general anaesthesia should have a north-facing endotracheal tube so it does not interfere with the surgical field.
- Local anaesthetic should be considered pre-operatively to help haemostasis while raising the flaps and to aid analgesia in the post-operative period.
- Nerve monitoring should be used whenever possible.
- Surgical aids such as loops, microscope, fine bipolar forceps, ligaclips and harmonic knives are very useful and should be encouraged to facilitate surgery.
- Mild hypotensive anaesthesia should be used but reversed before the procedure is completed.
- Adequate incision and approach should be employed for the extent of the procedure.
- Surgery is the mainstay of thyroid cancer treatment and total thyroidectomy should be performed in the majority of patients.
- Level VI selective or central compartment neck dissection should be performed whenever indicated.
- Careful tissue handling is paramount as the thyroid gland is one of the most vascular glands in the body.
- The RLN should always be identified and preserved.
- The EBSLN should be identified whenever possible. This may only be possible in up to 60% of cases due to the position of the nerve in relation to the superior thyroid pedicle.
- Parathyroid glands should be identified and preserved whenever possible. If, however, a parathyroid gland is removed during surgery or its blood supply is lost, frozen section should be used to confirm the nature of the tissue and, if positive, the gland should be reimplanted in a pocket made in the sternocleidomastoid muscle.

REFERENCES

1. Loyo M, Tufano RP, Gourin CG. National trends in thyroid surgery and the effect of volume on short-term outcomes. *Laryngoscope* 2013; **123**(8): 2056–63.
2. Kandil E, Noureldine SI, Abbas A, Tufano RP. The impact of surgical volume on patient outcomes following thyroid surgery. *Surgery* 2013; **154**(6): 1346–52; discussion 52–3.
3. Terris DJ, Gourin GC. *Thyroid and parathyroid diseases: Medical and surgical Management*. New York: Thieme; 2009.
4. Watkinson JC. Fifteen years' experience in thyroid surgery. *Ann R Coll Surg Engl* 2010; **92**(7): 541–7.
5. Caragacianu D, Kamani D, Randolph GW. Intraoperative monitoring: normative range associated with normal postoperative glottic function. *Laryngoscope* 2013; **123**(12): 3026–31.
6. Mehanna H. Diagnosis and management of thyroid nodules. *Journal of ENT Masterclass* 2008; **1**(1): 98–102.
7. De Carlucci D Jr, Tavares MR, Obara MT, et al. Thyroid function after unilateral total lobectomy: risk factors for postoperative hypothyroidism. *Arch Otolaryngol Head Neck Surg* 2008; **134**(10): 1076–9.
8. Kandil E, Krishnan B, Noureldine SI, et al. Hemithyroidectomy: a meta-analysis of postoperative need for hormone replacement and complications. *ORL J Otorhinolaryngol Relat Spec* 2013; **75**(1): 6–17.
9. Barczynski M, Konturek A, Hubalewska-Dydejczyk A, et al. Five-year follow-up of a randomized clinical trial of total thyroidectomy versus Dunhill operation versus bilateral subtotal thyroidectomy for multinodular nontoxic goiter. *World J Surg* 2010; **34**(6): 1203–13.
10. Genovese BM, Noureldine SI, Gleeson EM, et al. What is the best definitive treatment for Graves' disease? A systematic review of the existing literature. *Ann Surg Oncol* 2013; **20**(2): 660–7.
11. Alexander EK, Kennedy GC, Baloch ZW, et al. Preoperative diagnosis of benign thyroid nodules with indeterminate cytology. *N Engl J Med* 2012; **367**(8): 705–15.
12. Watkinson JC. The British Thyroid Association guidelines for the management of thyroid cancer in adults. *Nucl Med Commun* 2004; **25**(9): 897–900.
13. Cooper DS, Doherty GM, Haugen BR, et al. Revised American Thyroid Association management guidelines for patients with thyroid nodules and differentiated thyroid cancer. *Thyroid* 2009; **19**(11): 1167–214.
14. Nixon IJ, Ganly I, Hann LE, et al. Nomogram for selecting thyroid nodules for ultrasound-guided fine-needle aspiration biopsy based on a quantification of risk of malignancy. *Head Neck* 2013; **35**(7): 1022–5.
15. Aschebrook-Kilfoy B, Ward MH, Sabra MM, Devesa SS. Thyroid cancer incidence patterns in the United States by histologic type, 1992–2006. *Thyroid* 2011; **21**(2): 125–34.
16. Sturniolo G, Bonanno L, Gagliano E, et al. Surgical therapy of medullary thyroid carcinoma. *Chir Ital* 2007; **59**(6): 781–7.
17. Pelizzo MR, Boschin IM, Bernante P, et al. Natural history, diagnosis, treatment and outcome of medullary thyroid cancer: 37 years' experience on 157 patients. *Eur J Surg Oncol* 2007; **33**(4): 493–7.
18. Kloos RT, Eng C, Evans DB, et al. Medullary thyroid cancer: management guidelines of the American Thyroid Association. *Thyroid* 2009; **19**(6): 565–612.
19. Nixon IJ, Whitcher M, Palmer FL, et al. The impact of distant metastases at presentation on prognosis in patients with differentiated carcinoma of the thyroid gland. *Thyroid* 2012; **22**(9): 884–9.
20. McCaffrey TV, Bergstralh EJ, Hay ID. Locally invasive papillary thyroid carcinoma: 1940–1990. *Head Neck* 1994; **16**(2): 165–72.
21. Nixon IJ, Palmer FL, Whitcher MM, et al. Thyroid isthmusectomy for well-differentiated thyroid cancer. *Ann Surg Oncol* 2011; **18**(3): 767–70.

22. Nixon IJ, Ganly I, Patel SG, et al. Thyroid lobectomy for treatment of well differentiated intrathyroid malignancy. *Surgery* 2012; **151**(4): 571–9.
23. Mendelsohn AH, Elashoff DA, Abemayor E, St John MA. Surgery for papillary thyroid carcinoma: is lobectomy enough? *Arch Otolaryngol Head Neck Surg* 2010; **136**(11): 1055–61.
24. Hekkenberg RJ, Irish JC, Rotstein LE, et al. Informed consent in head and neck surgery: how much do patients actually remember? *J Otolaryngol* 1997; **26**(3): 155–9.
25. Chan Y, Irish JC, Wood SJ, et al. Patient education and informed consent in head and neck surgery. *Arch Otolaryngol Head Neck Surg* 2002; **128**(11): 1269–74.
26. Jeannon JP, Orabi AA, Bruch GA, et al. Diagnosis of recurrent laryngeal nerve palsy after thyroidectomy: a systematic review. *Int J Clin Pract* 2009; **63**(4): 624–9.
27. Simo R, Nixon I, Tysome JR, et al. Modified extended Kocher incision for total thyroidectomy with lateral compartment neck dissection – a critical appraisal of surgical access and cosmesis in 31 patients. *Clin Otolaryngol* 2012; **37**(5): 395–8.
28. Cernea CR, Ferraz AR, Furlani J, et al. Identification of the external branch of the superior laryngeal nerve during thyroidectomy. *Am J Surg* 1992; **164**(6): 634–9.
29. Aina EN, Hisham AN. External laryngeal nerve in thyroid surgery: recognition and surgical implications. *Aust NZ J Surg* 2001; **71**(4): 212–14.
30. Pagedar NA, Freeman JL. Identification of the external branch of the superior laryngeal nerve during thyroidectomy. *Arch Otolaryngol Head Neck Surg* 2009; **135**(4): 360–2.
31. Sancho JJ, Pascual-Damieta M, Pereira JA, et al. Risk factors for transient vocal cord palsy after thyroidectomy. *Br J Surg* 2008; **95**(8): 961–7.
32. Barczynski M, Nowak W, Sancho JJ, Sitges-Serra A. The motor fibers of the recurrent laryngeal nerves are located in the anterior extralaryngeal branch. *Ann Surg* 2010; **251**(4): 773–4; author reply 4–5.
33. Randolph GW, Kobler JB, Wilkins J. Recurrent laryngeal nerve identification and assessment during thyroid surgery: laryngeal palpation. *World J Surg* 2004; **28**(8): 755–60.
34. Lorente-Poch L, Sancho JJ, Ruiz S, Sitges-Serra A. Importance of in situ preservation of parathyroid glands during total thyroidectomy. *Br J Surg* 2015; **102**(4): 359–67.
35. Sanabria A, Carvalho AL, Silver CE, et al. Routine drainage after thyroid surgery: a meta-analysis. *J Surg Oncol* 2007; **96**(3): 273–80.
36. Schietroma M, Cecilia EM, Carlei F, et al. Dexamethasone for the prevention of recurrent laryngeal nerve palsy and other complications after thyroid surgery: a randomized double-blind placebo-controlled trial. *JAMA Otolaryngol Head Neck Surg* 2013; **139**(5): 471–8.

CHAPTER 68

SURGERY FOR LOCALLY ADVANCED AND NODAL DISEASE

Joel Anthony Smith and John C. Watkinson

Introduction 805	Surgery for recurrent disease: Locoregional recurrence 809
Advanced thyroid cancer..805	Surgery for distant disease 809
Extrathyroidal spread..805	References 810

SEARCH STRATEGY

Data in this chapter may be updated by a PubMed search using the keywords: well-differentiated thyroid cancer, advanced thyroid cancer, extrathyroidal spread, nodal disease, laryngotracheal invasion, oesophageal invasion and recurrent laryngeal nerve invasion.

Key evidence has come from the British Thyroid Association guidelines for the management of well-differentiated thyroid cancer, the American Thyroid Association guidelines for the management of well-differentiated thyroid cancer and the American Head and Neck Society Consensus statement.

INTRODUCTION

In the majority of cases, differentiated thyroid cancer (DTC) carries an excellent prognosis and behaves in an indolent manner.[1-3] However, in advanced disease, including direct spread beyond the thyroid capsule or extranodal spread, surgical management is challenging with higher associated morbidity and mortality.[1,4] Surgery is well accepted as the primary modality of treatment of both primary and recurrent DTC although adjunctive therapies play an important role.[3,5] Awareness of poor prognostic features pre-, intra- and post-operatively can aid in appropriate surgical planning and decision-making and there is a move towards patient-specific risk stratification in management strategy.[4] Treatment planning should be patient-centred and be made within the context of a multidisciplinary team setting (MDT).[3] When treating patients with advanced thyroid cancer, decision-making is the most important part of management, as often a balance must be struck between achieving clear margins and the potential morbidity of surgical intervention. Patients with residual thyroid cancer may survive for many years and be minimally symptomatic. As such, in DTC, leaving microscopic and sometimes macroscopic disease behind to preserve function may be the most appropriate course of action.

ADVANCED THYROID CANCER

Surgical management of advanced thyroid cancer includes:

- direct disease extension beyond the thyroid capsule (extrathyroidal spread)
- recurrent or residual disease in the thyroid bed and neck
- extracapsular nodal disease
- surgery for distant metastasis.

EXTRATHYROIDAL SPREAD

Spread of disease beyond the thyroid capsule into surrounding tissues represents a poor prognostic sign with significant potential for increased post-operative morbidity and early mortality.[6] Extrathyroidal extension (ETE) can be present at some level in up to 25% of patients and occurs in papillary and follicular disease with equal frequency although papillary thyroid cancer has a much greater incidence and is therefore more likely to be encountered.[2,6-10] Extrathyroidal spread can range from minimal extension into surrounding strap muscles and fat (T3) to invasion of the laryngobronchial tree and prevertebral muscles (T4a/b).

Extrathyroidal spread occurs most commonly in those with other risk factors for adverse prognosis.[9, 11-12]

Residual and unrecognized disease is likely to represent the most common manifestation leading to local recurrence and macroscopic disease clearance is associated with higher survival.[2, 13] As such, early recognition of extrathyroidal spread with appropriate pre-operative planning is likely to minimize the risk of inadvertently leaving residual disease. Patient factors that increase the risk of extracapsular spread mirror the risk factors for detecting malignancy in a thyroid nodule and include extremes of age at presentation, size of primary tumour (>4 cm), advanced nodal disease or clinical evidence of distant metastases.[8-9, 11] Presentation with features of upper aerodigestive tract invasion including voice change, recurrent laryngeal nerve palsy, stridor and dysphagia should alert the surgeon to the need for careful clinical assessment of the aerodigestive tract including flexible laryngoscopy to assess vocal fold function as a well as bronchoscopy and oesophagoscopy if directed clinically.[14] In addition, patients with suspected aerodigestive tract invasion should have analysis of pre-operative imaging by a radiologist with a special interest in head and neck radiology, preferably within the context of the MDT such that surgery can be planned with the patient fully informed.

Histological factors that should alert the surgeon to a higher risk of ETE include poorly differentiated and unencapsulated histological subtypes associated with more aggressive disease such as diffuse sclerosing, solid and tall cell types.[9]

Once identified pre-operatively, management planning should be discussed in detail with the patient such that the appropriate resection boundaries and the morbidity associated with obtaining completely clear margins can be adequately understood.[3] The operative skills, experience and repertoire of the surgeon are important factors when obtaining clear surgical margins in patients with cancer spread beyond the thyroid capsule.[14-16]

Involvement of non-vital structures around the thyroid bed

The greatest chance of cure is obtained through macroscopic removal of disease with clear margins. This is the case primarily and for residual or recurrent disease where there is direct spread from the thyroid gland. Predicting extrathyroidal spread is important but not always possible and subtle involvement of local structures are often not identified on imaging.[2] If extrathyroidal spread involves the strap muscles or surrounding lympho-fatty tissue where en-bloc excision leads to little added morbidity, it is generally accepted that these structures should be excised as far as the disease progresses.[3, 17]

Involvement of the recurrent laryngeal nerve

In locally advanced thyroid cancer, the recurrent laryngeal nerve (RLN) can be involved to a greater or lesser extent in up to 60% of cases by direct cancer spread from the gland or by paratracheal lymph nodes.[6] RLN involvement can range from tumour abutting the nerve to partial or total encasement and direct invasion.[18] Evidence that nerve and functional voice preservation can be achieved without compromising local recurrence has led many to adopt a nerve-preserving technique, although large-scale trial data supporting this are not available.[17-19] Further, some studies suggest RLN function can return after tumour has been peeled off the nerve, even when extensively dissected.[20] RLN involvement, in the presence of a still-functioning nerve, is not usually possible to predict on radiological grounds. Most patients with RLN involvement or encasement have no predictive features. Where a pre-existing, ipsilateral cord palsy exists in the context of an encased nerve, most would advocate nerve excision.[17] In a functional ipsilateral vocal cord, with solitary RLN involvement, some would advocate removal as the balance of morbidity from a unilateral RLN palsy may outweigh the risk of leaving disease behind. Others, however, would aim to preserve the nerve while removing macroscopic disease on the basis that adjuvant treatment would be employed to reduce the risk of local recurrence.[17-19] Decisions such as these should be patient-specific. Where both RLNs are involved and functional pre-operatively, a more difficult decision has to be made, but most would advocate RLN preservation to avoid tracheostomy. The British Thyroid Association (BTA) recommends leaving one or both nerves in situ regardless of macroscopic disease and relying on non-surgical post-operative treatment modalities to achieve local control.[3] In addition, RLN monitoring is widely used in thyroid surgery and may aid intra-operative decision-making regarding nerve preservation.[21] This may be particularly helpful in the presence of an apparently functional nerve where nerve signal has been lost.[22] There is debate, however, on the ability of intra-operative nerve monitoring to predict voice outcome following thyroid surgery and large-scale prospective studies are needed to evaluate this further.[23, 24]

Where resection of the recurrent laryngeal nerve is anticipated, such as in the context of a pre-existing vocal fold paralysis, there is some evidence albeit from small studies that primary re-anastamosis of the RLN may improve voice outcome.[25] Such repair may involve end-to-end or cable graft repair. The skills of the operating surgeon may be a factor in whether this is achievable and donor nerve morbidity must be taken into account.

Involvement of the trachea and larynx

Oesophageal and pharyngeal involvement is rare in isolation, and normally occurs in association with involvement of the laryngobronchial tree.[2] When disease recurs, it is most likely to do so locally (70%).[26] Up to 50% of death from DCT is from direct invasion of the airway. The prognosis for those with locoregional recurrence is better than those with distal disease, however, and where locoregional control can be achieved, death is more likely from distant metastasis.[27] Treatment should therefore be directed towards macroscopic, local disease clearance.

Again, where resection is being considered, patient and tumour factors should be at the forefront of the decision-making process. Whether tumour breaches the inner lumen of the airway is the key to surgical planning and all patients with suspected airway invasion should undergo thorough pre-operative evaluation. Clinically, laryngoscopy and bronchoscopy should be performed if luminal spread is suspected. Imaging in the form of contrast-enhanced CT is specific if not particularly sensitive in detecting both tracheal and laryngeal invasion and MRI may add further information regarding laryngeal cartilage invasion.[28] Depending on the skills of the surgeon, the extent of resection may mandate involvement of other specialities or onward referral to tertiary care.

Where macroscopic disease invades the outer layers of the laryngobronchial tree, most agree it is acceptable to shave cartilage as far as macroscopic disease is seen and treat post-operatively with ^{131}I and/or external beam radiotherapy (ERBT).[29, 30] In tracheal invasion, local control rates as high as 95% have been reported when adopting such strategies, even with high rates of microscopically involved margins.[31] It is likely that post-surgical, adjuvant treatment reduces recurrence and improves survival in these circumstances.[29, 32] Where macroscopic disease excision necessitates entering the lumen of the airway, formal resection and reconstruction should be considered.[29, 33] Although this is likely to increase surgical morbidity from anastomotic breakdown, laryngotracheal stenosis and tracheostomy dependence, revision surgery for residual or recurrent disease is likely to be very challenging and carry significantly higher morbidity.[34–36] Options for segmental tracheal and laryngeal resection can be seen in **Figures 68.1–68.4**.[37]

As with tracheal involvement, where the outer layers of the larynx are involved, macroscopic resection of disease with preservation of the larynx is likely to achieve good rates of local control. Where disease spreads through the cartilage, consideration of partial or total laryngectomy should be made as leaving behind macroscopic disease is associated with a high risk of recurrence, regardless of post-operative treatment, and salvage surgery is again likely to involve high morbidity.[17] Often laryngeal preservation can be achieved, however, with good functional and local outcomes.[38] Again decisions should be made

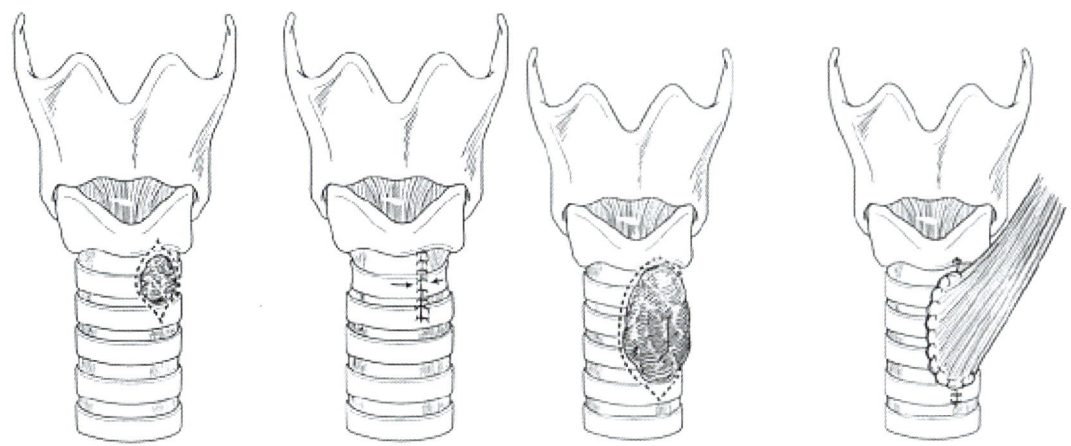

Figure 68.1 Options for tracheal resection and repair. A small defect can be closed primarily and a larger defect reconstructed with a local muscle flap.

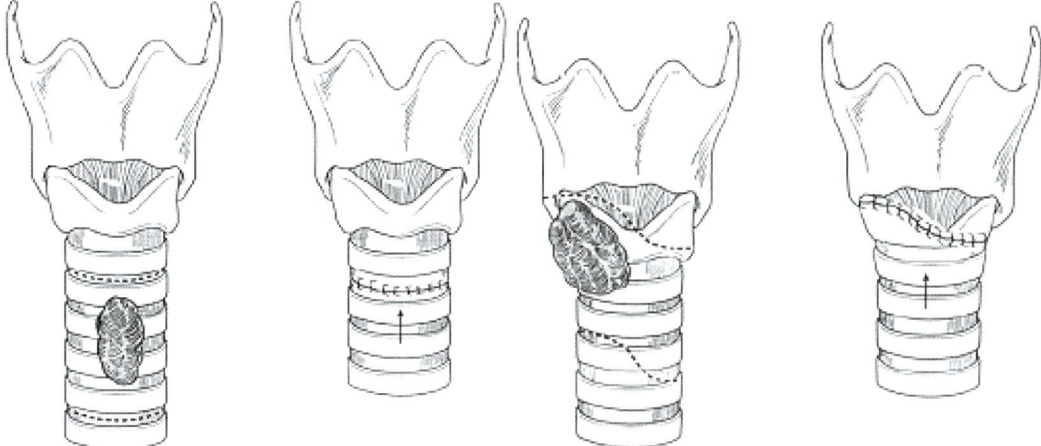

Figure 68.2 Segmental tracheal resection – with an end-to-end primary anastomosis and a stepped closure involving partial resection of the cricoid cartilage.

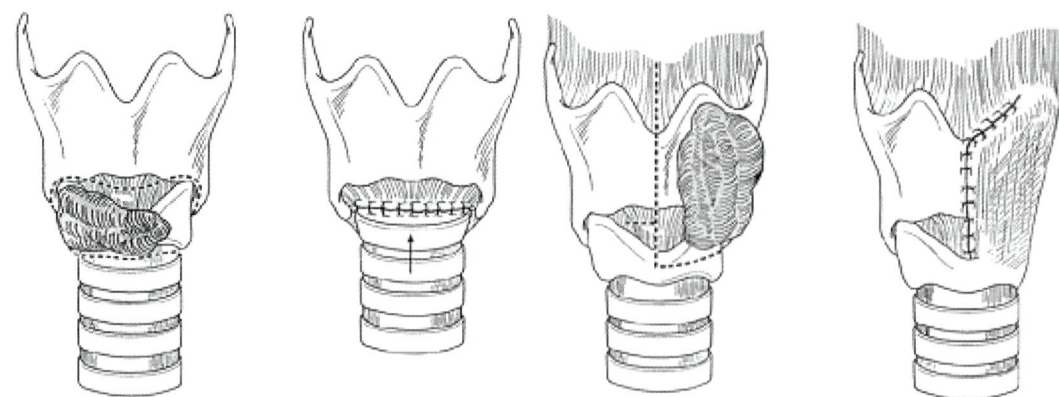

Figure 68.3 Total cricoid resection – with trachea to cricothyroid membrane anastomosis and vertical hemilaryngectomy.

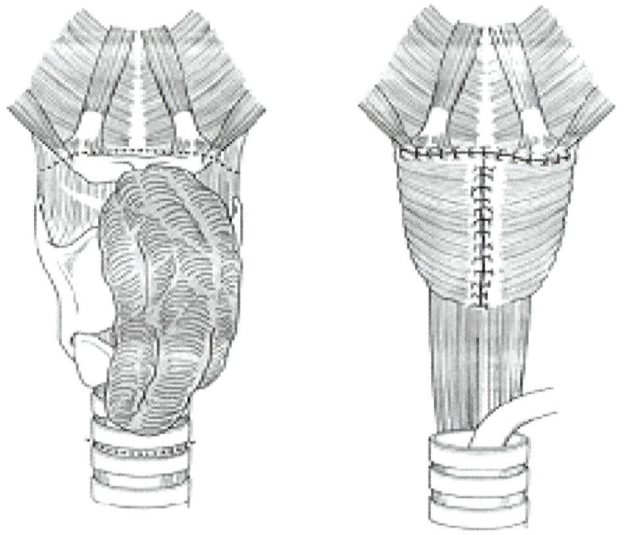

Figure 68.4 Total laryngectomy – for advanced disease extending across the midline.

with the patient at the centre of the discussion and including surgeons with the appropriate skill mix to complete the procedure.[39]

Involvement of the pharynx and oesophagus

Pharyngeal and oesophageal invasion are rare in thyroid cancer and most commonly occur from direct primary tumour extension rather than extranodal disease in the central compartment.[36] A history of true dysphagia should prompt a thorough evaluation of the aerodigestive tract although in most cases involvement is asymptomatic. This is in part because intra-luminal involvement is rare with extension most frequently involving the muscularis layer in isolation without submucosal or mucosal spread.[10] As such, endoscopic examination of the pharynx and oesophagus is often not predictive. As involvement is most likely due to direct spread, the position of the primary within the thyroid may give an important clue to the presence of invasion. MRI scanning is both sensitive and specific at predicting invasion and should be performed whenever invasion is suspected.[40]

Surgery to the pharynx and oesophagus will be dictated by the extent of involvement but should follow the principals of macroscopic disease resection. Where the lumen is breached, segmental resection is required which may be repairable by layered closure or by direct reanastomosis.[17] More extensive defects may require myofascial or myocutaneous reconstruction from pedicled local flaps, free microvascular tissue transfer or gastric pull-up procedures.

Involvement of the vascular compartment

Although rare, vascular involvement occurs and every effort should be made to recognize involvement in the pre-operative phase.[41] Both the internal jugular vein (IJV) and common carotid artery can be involved by direct primary tumour spread although IJV compression and thrombosis is more commonly caused by extensive nodal disease.[42] Again, it is patients with high risk features who are more likely to present with vascular involvement. Clinical signs of arterial involvement are often minimal but major venous involvement should be suspected in the presence of facial flushing, oedema, venous congestion and unexplained headaches or vascular events. Where vascular involvement is suspected, extensive pre-operative evaluation should be performed as there is significant potential for morbidity and mortality if the IJV and or carotid has to be resected.[17] Imaging should be directed towards assessment of resectability and, if so, what structures would need repair. Combination imaging including ultrasound Doppler, MRI, MRA and CT angiography may be sufficient to evaluate intra-luminal involvement and distinguish thrombus from intra-luminal tumour.[42] Formal angiography may be required, however, in particular to assess the arterial supply to the circle of Willis if arterial resection is contemplated.

Ipsilateral IJV involvement can be resected with no recourse to reconstruction of the venous system. There is consensus, however, that in bilateral IJV resection, reconstruction with autologous vein graft should be considered, due to the significant morbidity associated with bilateral IJV excision.[17, 43] Most authors consider a completely encased carotid to be akin to inoperable disease although cases of carotid resection and are reported.[42]

Encasement up to 270 degrees is usually amenable to resection assuming the artery itself is not directly invaded. Where an attempt to resect disease that is advanced to that extent is being considered, careful consideration of the surgical morbidity and the likelihood of improving survival should be undertaken.

SURGERY FOR RECURRENT DISEASE: LOCOREGIONAL RECURRENCE

As with primary disease, recurrent disease should be managed surgically where possible and with curative intent.[13, 3] Local disease recurrence is most often seen in the thyroid bed with the central and lateral neck compartment less commonly affected. Patients with high-risk features are more likely to die from their disease and as such the case for surgical intervention for recurrent local disease is more clear cut.[3] In those with low-volume or low-risk disease, however, close clinical observation may be a better strategy.[3] Consideration should be paid to the position of the recurrence prior to any attempt at surgical excision as well as ^{131}I uptake status. Patients with locoregional recurrence have a better prognosis than those with distant disease, a reflection of the fact that recurrent disease is most likely enlarging residual disease rather than loss of disease control and that all modalities of treatment are still available. Where resection is undertaken, a complete clearance of the central compartment should be performed with invasion into local structures managed as previously discussed.[17]

Where disease recurs in the lymphatics, the central and lateral compartments are most commonly affected and disease can be confined to the nodes themselves or spread extranodally into the free tissue spaces of the neck. Where nodal compartments are macroscopically affected, the aim should be to clear all affected levels in their entirety, avoiding 'berry picking' at all times. In the lateral compartment clearing levels IIa to IV with level Vb if affected is considered the treatment of choice.[1] Where extranodal extension affects other structures such as the vascular compartment or neural structures, consideration of the balance between morbidity and increased survival should be made on a case-by-case basis.

Where nodal disease recurs in previously dissected nodal levels, a comprehensive dissection of the lateral neck should be considered in patients with high-risk disease. In previously operated levels, this may involve excision of the residual node, affected local structures and and scar tissue only. Again, a watchful waiting strategy may be adopted for those with low-risk recurrent disease.[3] Non-surgical treatments should be explored with ^{131}I uptake status as well as the possibility of EBRT for patients not amenable to surgery.

SURGERY FOR DISTANT DISEASE

Distant metastatic spread carries a poor prognosis, in part a representation of the disease process itself and in part due to the limitation of treatment modalities available, particularly surgery.[44] Distant spread is most common to the lung followed by bone, soft tissues and brain.[45] Although metastasis reduces life expectancy by 50%, the disease can progress slowly and may be relatively asymptomatic.[44] For many patients with distant metastases, including to mediastinum and lung, surgery is not considered an option and an assessment should be made as to whether metastases uptake iodine.[3] In these situations ^{131}I may be the treatment of choice with or without EBRT. For isolated or limited bony metastases in accessible places where morbidity is low, surgery may be considered, especially as ^{131}I is relatively ineffective at treating these lesions.[46] Selection should be on a case-by-case basis and multimodal treatment considered. Pain, weight-bearing positions, risk to neuronal structures and risk of other treatment modalities such as EBRT should be considered prior to or instead of surgery. Surgery may be considered first-line treatment for isolated cerebral metastases in patients with good performance status as greater long-term survival has been demonstrated.[3, 47, 48] Surgery for cerebral metastasis should be considered regardless of ^{131}I uptake and a decision made in conjunction with a neurosurgical team.

FUTURE RESEARCH

- Imaging modalities for the detection of early recurrence or residual disease
- Centralization of data and patients with advanced disease for the purpose of audit and research
- Randomized trials in the surgical management of locoregional recurrence and distant disease
- Biomarkers to predict subtypes more likely to recur
- Surgical technology to aid in monitoring intra-operative nerve function

KEY POINTS

- Where possible, individual patient and tumour factors (risk stratification) should be included in decision-making.
- Management should be patient-centred and made within the context of the MDT with consideration of non-surgical treatment where appropriate.
- Assessment and anticipation of advanced disease allows management decisions to be made in advance of surgery.
- Microscopic residual disease may not adversely affect long-term survival.
- A balance must be struck between extent of planned excision and associated morbidity, particularly when there is involvement of the upper aerodigestive tract.

REFERENCES

1. Cooper DS, Doherty GM, Haugen BR, et al. Revised American Thyroid Association management guidelines for patients with thyroid nodules and differentiated thyroid cancer. *Thyroid* 2009; 19(11): 1167–214.
2. Watkinson J, Gilbert RW (eds). *Stell & Maran's textbook of head and neck surgery and oncology*. 5th ed. Boca Raton, FL: CRC Press; 2012. Available from: http://www.crcpress.com/product/isbn/9780340929162
3. Perros P, Boelaert K, Colley S, et al. Guidelines for the management of thyroid cancer. *Clin Endocrinol (Oxf)* 2014; 81 Suppl 1: 1–122.
4. Shaha AR. Recurrent differentiated thyroid cancer. *Endocr Pract* 2012; 18(4): 600–3.
5. Sipos JA, Shah MH. Thyroid cancer: emerging role for targeted therapies. *Ther Adv Med Oncol* 2010; 2(1): 3–16.
6. Hay ID, Thompson GB, Grant CS, et al. Papillary thyroid carcinoma managed at the Mayo Clinic during six decades (1940–1999): temporal trends in initial therapy and long-term outcome in 2444 consecutively treated patients. *World J Surg* 2002; 26(8): 879–85.
7. Thyroid Cancer Treatment (PDQ®) [Internet]. National Cancer Institute. Available from: http://www.cancer.gov/cancertopics/pdq/treatment/thyroid/HealthProfessional/page3
8. Andersen PE, Kinsella J, Loree TR, et al. Differentiated carcinoma of the thyroid with extrathyroidal extension. *Am J Surg* 1995; 170(5): 467–70.
9. Ortiz S, Rodríguez JM, Soria T, et al. Extrathyroid spread in papillary carcinoma of the thyroid: clinicopathological and prognostic study. *Otolaryngol Head Neck Surg* 2001; 124(3): 261–5.
10. McCaffrey TV, Bergstralh EJ, Hay ID. Locally invasive papillary thyroid carcinoma: 1940–1990. *Head Neck* 1994; 16(2): 165–72.
11. Segal K, Shpitzer T, Hazan A, et al. Invasive well-differentiated thyroid carcinoma: effect of treatment modalities on outcome. *Otolaryngol Head Neck Surg* 2006; 134(5): 819–22.
12. Shaha AR. TNM classification of thyroid carcinoma. *World J Surg* 2007; 31(5): 879–87.
13. Tsang RW, Brierley JD, Simpson WJ, et al. The effects of surgery, radioiodine, and external radiation therapy on the clinical outcome of patients with differentiated thyroid carcinoma. *Cancer* 1998; 82(2): 375–88.
14. The British Association of Endocrine & Thyroid Surgeons. *Fourth National Audit Report 2012* [Internet]. Available from: http://www.baets.org.uk/wp-content/uploads/2013/05/4th-National-Audit.pdf
15. Smith JA, Watkinson JC, Shaha A. Who should perform thyroid surgery? United Kingdom (UK) and United States (US) perspectives with recommendations. *Eur Arch Otorhinolaryngol* 2012; 269(1): 1–4.
16. McHenry CR. Patient volumes and complications in thyroid surgery. *Br J Surg* 2002; 89(7): 821–3.
17. Shindo ML, Caruana SM, Kandil E, et al. Management of invasive well-differentiated thyroid cancer: an American Head and Neck Society consensus statement. AHNS consensus statement. *Head Neck* 2014; 36(10): 1379–90.
18. Nishida T, Nakao K, Hamaji M, et al. Preservation of recurrent laryngeal nerve invaded by differentiated thyroid cancer. *Ann Surg* 1997; 226(1): 85–91.
19. Falk SA, McCaffrey TV. Management of the recurrent laryngeal nerve in suspected and proven thyroid cancer. *Otolaryngol Head Neck Surg* 1995; 113(1): 42–8.
20. Chiang F-Y, Lu I-C, Tsai C-J, et al. Does extensive dissection of recurrent laryngeal nerve during thyroid operation increase the risk of nerve injury? Evidence from the application of intraoperative neuromonitoring. *Am J Otolaryngol* 2011; 32(6): 499–503.
21. Randolph GW, Dralle H, Group with the IIMS, et al. Electrophysiologic recurrent laryngeal nerve monitoring during thyroid and parathyroid surgery: international standards guideline statement. *Laryngoscope* 2011; 121(S1): S1–16.
22. Dralle H, Sekulla C, Lorenz K, et al. Loss of the nerve monitoring signal during bilateral thyroid surgery. *Br J Surg* 2012; 99(8): 1089–95.
23. Smith J, Douglas J, Smith B, et al. Assessment of recurrent laryngeal nerve function during thyroid surgery. *Ann R Coll Surg Engl* 2014; 96(2): 130–5.
24. Pisanu A, Porceddu G, Podda M, et al. Systematic review with meta-analysis of studies comparing intraoperative neuromonitoring of recurrent laryngeal nerves versus visualization alone during thyroidectomy. *J Surg Res* 2014; 188(1): 152–61.
25. Yumoto E, Sanuki T, Kumai Y. Immediate recurrent laryngeal nerve reconstruction and vocal outcome. *Laryngoscope* 2006; 116(9): 1657–61.
26. Mazzaferri EL, Kloos RT. Clinical review 128: Current approaches to primary therapy for papillary and follicular thyroid cancer. *J Clin Endocrinol Metab* 2001; 86(4): 1447–63.
27. Czaja JM, McCaffrey TV. The surgical management of laryngotracheal invasion by well-differentiated papillary thyroid carcinoma. *Arch Otolaryngol Head Neck Surg* 1997; 123(5): 484–90.
28. Seo YL, Yoon DY, Lim KJ, et al. Locally advanced thyroid cancer: can CT help in prediction of extrathyroidal invasion to adjacent structures? *Am J Roentgenol* 2010; 195(3): W240–4.
29. McCaffrey JC. Aerodigestive tract invasion by well-differentiated thyroid carcinoma: diagnosis, management, prognosis, and biology. *Laryngoscope* 2006; 116(1): 1–11.
30. Bayles SW, Kingdom TT, Carlson GW. Management of thyroid carcinoma invading the aerodigestive tract. *Laryngoscope* 1998; 108(9): 1402–7.
31. Tsukahara K, Sugitani I, Kawabata K. Surgical management of tracheal shaving for papillary thyroid carcinoma with tracheal invasion. *Acta Otolaryngol* 2009; 129(12): 1498–502.
32. Su SY, Milas ZL, Bhatt N, et al. Well-differentiated thyroid cancer with aerodigestive tract invasion: long-term control and functional outcomes. *Head Neck* 2016; 38(1): 72–8.
33. Honings J, Stephen AE, Marres HA, Gaissert HA. The management of thyroid carcinoma invading the larynx or trachea. *Laryngoscope* 2010; 120(4): 682–9.
34. Ozaki O, Sugino K, Mimura T, Ito K. Surgery for patients with thyroid carcinoma invading the trachea: circumferential sleeve resection followed by end-to-end anastomosis. *Surgery* 1995; 117(3): 268–71.
35. Musholt TJ, Musholt PB, Behrend M, et al. Invasive differentiated thyroid carcinoma: tracheal resection and reconstruction procedures in the hands of the endocrine surgeon. *Surgery* 1999; 126(6): 1078–88.
36. Machens A, Hinze R, Dralle H. Surgery on the cervicovisceral axis for invasive thyroid cancer. *Langenbecks Arch Surg* 2001; 386(5): 318–23.
37. Prinz RA, Rossi HL, Kim AW. Difficult problems in thyroid surgery. *Curr Probl Surg* 2002; 39(1): 5–91.
38. Moritani S. Surgical management of laryngeal invasion by papillary thyroid carcinoma: a retrospective analysis. *Thyroid* 2015; 25(5): 528–33.
39. Kim KH, Sung M-W, Chang K-H, Kang B-S. Therapeutic dilemmas in the management of thyroid cancer with laryngotracheal involvement. *Otolaryngol Head Neck Surg* 2000; 122(5): 763–7.
40. Wang J, Takashima S, Matsushita T, et al. Esophageal invasion by thyroid carcinomas: prediction using magnetic resonance imaging. *J Comput Assist Tomogr* 2003; 27(1): 18–25.
41. Kebebew E, Clark OH. Locally advanced differentiated thyroid cancer. *Surg Oncol* 2003; 12(2): 91–9.
42. Lee YS, Chung WY, Chang H-S, Park CS. Treatment of locally advanced thyroid cancer invading the great vessels using a Y-shaped graft bypass. *Interact Cardiovasc Thorac Surg* 2010; 10(6): 1039–41.
43. Kamizono K, Ejima M, Taura M, Masuda M. Internal jugular vein reconstruction: application of conventional type A and novel type K methods. *J Laryngol Otol* 2011; 125(06): 643–8.
44. Schlumberger M, Baudin E, Travagli JP. [Papillary and follicular cancers of the thyroid.] *Presse Med* 1998; 27(29): 1479–81.
45. Muresan MM, Olivier P, Leclère J, et al. Bone metastases from differentiated thyroid carcinoma. *Endocr Relat Cancer* 2008; 15(1): 37–49.
46. Wexler JA. Approach to the thyroid cancer patient with bone metastases. *J Clin Endocrinol Metab* 2011; 96(8): 2296–307.
47. Henriques de Figueiredo B, Godbert Y, Soubeyran I, et al. Brain metastases from thyroid carcinoma: a retrospective study of 21 patients. *Thyroid* 2014; 24(2): 270–6.
48. Tsuda K, Tsurushima H, Takano S, et al. Brain metastasis from papillary thyroid carcinomas. *Mol Clin Oncol* 2013; 1(5): 817–19.

CHAPTER 69

MINIMALLY INVASIVE AND ROBOTIC THYROID SURGERY

Neil S. Tolley

Introduction 811
Minimally invasive thyroidectomy 811
Scarless in the neck techniques 813
Robotic-assisted thyroidectomy (RAT) 813
Conclusion 817
References 817

SEARCH STRATEGY

Data in this chapter may be updated by a PubMed search using the keywords: robotic thyroidectomy, minimal invasive thyroid surgery (MIVAT).

INTRODUCTION

The principles for safe thyroid surgery were laid down by Kocher at the beginning of the 20th century. Until recently there has been little change to the technique he described, an approach to thyroidectomy that conferred him Nobel laureate in 1909. His incision is still eponymously used although this rarely reflects the incision that he performed.

The site of incision and scar is often a significant focus of patient anxiety when considering surgery. Studies have revealed that 71% of patients surveyed in a thyroid clinic would prefer not to have a neck scar given a choice, a view independent of sex and skin colour. Furthermore, validated scar assessments reveal that professionals rate the aesthetics of a scar more favourably when compared to patients.[1]

Until further advances in medical research permit an incision that is truly scarless, techniques will continue to evolve to minimize scarring. This will facilitate safe surgery through a smaller and cosmetically more desirable incision or for the incision to be placed at a site where the scar is unobtrusive and invisible.

MINIMALLY INVASIVE THYROIDECTOMY

Technological developments of the endoscope and energy sealing devices provided essential prerequisites to develop small incision thyroidectomy techniques. These are known by several euphemisms: minimally invasive video-assisted thyroidectomy (MIVAT) or Miccoli technique, minimally invasive thyroidectomy (MIT), endoscopic-assisted thyroidectomy (EAT) and, finally, the Henry technique. Endoscopic-assisted thyroidectomy more accurately describes these techniques in practice.

Paolo Miccoli in Pisa and Jean-François Henry in Marseille largely pioneered the techniques of minimal invasive thyroidectomy.

Miccoli technique

Miccoli described the open method (gas-less), where a 2–3 cm midline incision facilitates endoscopic dissection of the superior pole and its delivery into the neck. Dissection of the lower pole and completion thyroidectomy is then done in a conventional manner once the thyroid is delivered through the incision. It has the disadvantage of requiring both two competent assistants and video stacks. Nonetheless, it avoids the potential complications of insufflation and it is possible to perform a total thyroidectomy through a single incision.

Excellent visualization of structures such as the recurrent, external laryngeal nerves and the parathyroids is obtained. Its limitation, as in all minimal invasive techniques, is the size and nature of the lesion for which the technique is suitable. This equates to approximately 8% of a UK surgeon's practice.[1] Volume outcome data would indicate that only surgeons with a large thyroid practice would have sufficient numbers to hone and maintain the skills required to adopt this technique both safely and

811

responsibly. A steep learning curve exists requiring over 50 cases before a surgeon obtains expert status.[2] This on a background where 86% of the British Association of Endocrine and Thyroid Surgeons (BAETS) membership perform fewer than 50 thyroidectomies a year[3] is indicative of why few surgeons have adopted this technique in the UK.

MIVAT permits solitary nodules of 3 cm to be safely removed. Highly experienced and skilled surgeons in the technique have extended its application to selected Graves' and cancer patients. It is wise to avoid its use in patients with a history of thyroiditis, cancer or previous surgery. It is recommended that total thyroid lobe volume should not exceed 20 mL with nodules up to 3 cm being suitable, equating to a volume of 14 mL.

In the author's experience, if the small incision necessitates excessive traction (which it does), this can predispose to hyperpigmentation and hypertrophy of the scar. This is clearly undesirable given the reason for using this technique in the first place. Long-term cosmetic analysis of scars is therefore essential for adequate evaluation of minimally invasive techniques. **Figure 69.1** shows the Miccoli instrumentation.

Henry technique

Virtually synchronous to the advent of Miccoli's technique was the insufflation method largely pioneered by Jean-François Henry in Marseille. This relies on the creation of three lateral ports along the anterior border of sternomastoid, two 3 mm ports for instrumentation and a 1 cm port for introduction of the insufflator endoscope. CO_2 at a pressure of 8 mmHg facilitates working space and achieves a bloodless field in which to dissect. It requires an assistant to hold and manipulate the endoscope while dissection proceeds with the other port instruments.

Dissection takes places completely within the neck and delivery of the thyroid lobe once completed is through the endoscope port. Indications for the technique replicate that of Miccoli. A total thyroidectomy is not possible by this method. Technically it is much more challenging than the Miccoli method and, while lending itself very well to parathyroidectomy, it has not been widely adopted for thyroid surgery. **Figure 69.2** shows the Henry instrumentation.

Minimally invasive thyroidectomy – the evidence base

There have been many peer-reviewed publications and even meta-analyses on minimally invasive thyroidectomy. The meta-analysis of Radford contained only five studies with a low degree of freedom and study heterogeneity. It also included a series from Miccoli, the pioneer of the technique. The analysis of 318 patients concluded that complications were no higher and supported superior cosmetic outcomes at the expense of operative time. Scar cosmesis was studied in the early post-operative period only and validated scar assessment methods were not used.[4]

The literature gives clear guidance on the indications, methodology, safety and learning curves. It has been less clear on volume outcome metrics. The latter will assume greater prominence with the advent of revalidation and surgical outcomes being placed in the public domain. Long-term prospective cohort studies comparing conventional and MIT are regrettably lacking. However, a personal communication with JFH has suggested there may be little or no difference in scar satisfaction after 18 months once full healing has taken place.

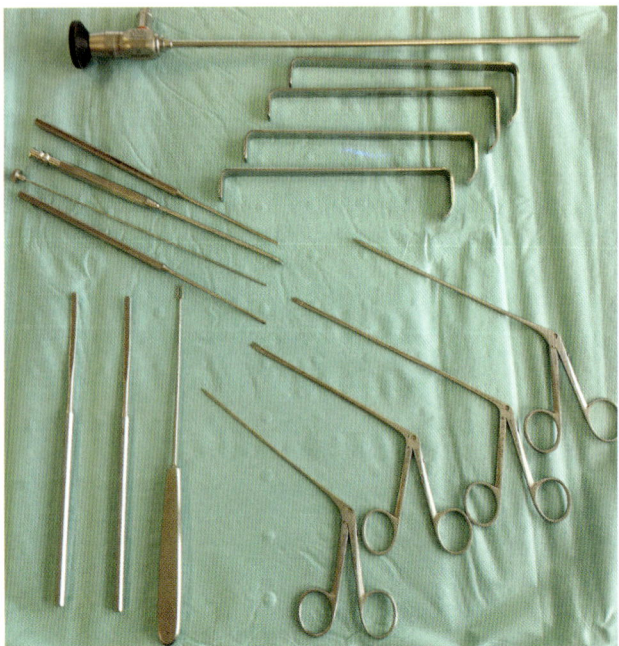

Figure 69.1 The Miccoli range of instruments (gas-less) technique inclusive of suction dissectors, spatulas and specially designed retractors. A 30 degree 4 mm endoscope is used.

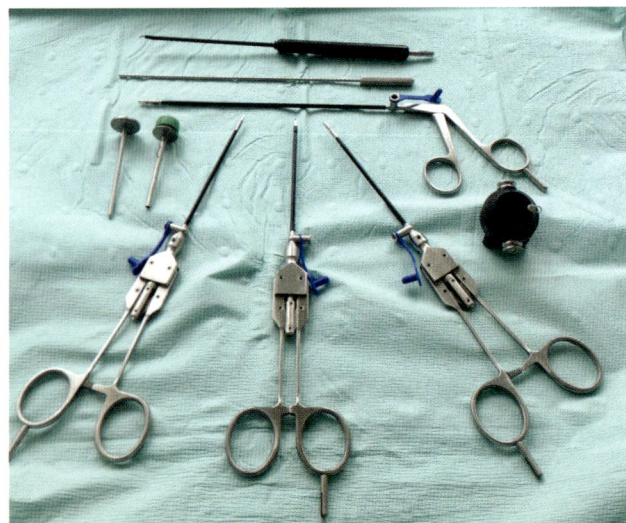

Figure 69.2 The range of instruments available for the Henry (gas) technique. Three ports are used and operative space is created by CO_2 insufflation.

Despite these reservations there is nonetheless a patient demand for this procedure. In the highly skilled such as Miccoli and Henry with high volume practices there is undoubtedly a niche for this technique. It is particularly attractive to those patients who have a tendency to hypertrophic scarring and possible keloid, although in the author's experience true keloid is very rare in thyroidectomy scars. However, because of the technical difficulty of achieving competency, steep learning curves and a regular supply of suitable cases, a large volume thyroid practice is essential. For this reason very few centres in the UK perform truly minimally invasive thyroidectomy.

SCARLESS IN THE NECK TECHNIQUES

Despite advances conferred by minimally invasive techniques they nonetheless have the disadvantage of leaving a scar in the neck. Although other endoscopic techniques have been employed, including a facelift approach,[5] the desire to avoid an incision in the head and neck has led to infraclavicular innovations. It is important that emphasis is placed on scarless in the neck rather than minimally invasive because the latter would not be an accurate description of any infraclavicular method.

Transaxillary and breast techniques were pioneered in the Far East particularly by Japanese and Korean surgeons. The cultural desire to avoid a scar in the neck from the negative feng shui in having a horizontal scar in the neck (denoting death) has been a significant driving force behind these innovations. Although technically demanding, the published literature shows that lobectomy or total thyroidectomy can be achieved safely.[6] These techniques are known as the axillo-bilateral-breast approach (ABBA) and bilateral axillo-breast approach (BABA) respectively.

There is not surprisingly a steep learning curve and a requirement to have a competent assistant working with 2D operative view in a confined operative space. Both gasless and insufflation techniques have been used, the latter potentially being complicated by hypercarbia, which can be a serious sequela of insufflation techniques.[7]

With the introduction of the da Vinci telerobot in the late 1990s, the next logical iteration was for this new technology to be used for thyroidectomy.

ROBOTIC-ASSISTED THYROIDECTOMY (RAT)

NASA had long considered the dilemma that would arise if an astronaut became ill in space. The concept of remote or 'tele' robotics was therefore spawned. The Ministry of Defence also declared an interest in developing the concept of bringing surgical expertise to the front line without placing the surgeon in danger. Patents for the technology were ultimately acquired and a system for commercial use developed by Intuitive (Sunnyvale, California).

The da Vinci telerobotic technology makes remote operating a reality with the feasibility of transatlantic surgery being published by Marescaux and colleagues in 2001.[8]

In head and neck surgery, pioneering work in the USA by Weinstein and colleagues in Philadelphia has led to robotics becoming the gold standard for the treatment of oropharyngeal tumours. In the UK, adoption has been frustratingly slow but this will change and a bright future is predicted for telerobotics in this domain of head and neck surgery.

The da Vinci system has also been used for both thyroid[9] and parathyroid[10] surgery. Lobe and colleagues published a lobectomy using the da Vinci with insufflation in 2005.[11] The present transaxillary technique, however, has been pioneered by Chung and other Korean surgeons.[6, 9, 12, 13] In 2013, Korean surgeons had experience in excess of 3000 patients. For reasons to be elaborated upon later, establishment of RAT has been tardy elsewhere in the world.

Chung and colleagues working at the Yonsei University in Seoul have published data on feasibility and learning curves supporting a superior cosmetic outcome and better post-operative swallow.[14, 15] They have also published data supporting its safe use in patients with papillary thyroid cancer. Noteworthy is that the mean size of tumour excised was only 8 mm and therefore fits into a microcarcinoma category.[16] Further studies are required before conclusions can be made with regard to safety in treating thyroid cancer.

A recent meta-analysis[17] supports its safety compared with conventional thyroidectomy (CT). Complications including cord palsy and hypocalcaemia rates were shown to be no different in this analysis. This study, however, has a low degree of freedom and high heterogeneity. There was also a heavy weighting of publications from pioneering units in Korea. Further prospective cohort studies are required before general conclusions can be made about the safety of RAT. There is inherent publication bias as complications of RAT tend not to get published.

Da Vinci telerobotics system

The da Vinci is a master–slave robot that has undergone five iterations from Standard, Xi to SP machines. The system consists of three components: the surgeon console, cart and video stack containing camera control units (charge-coupled devices, CCDs) and other hardware. As a master–slave device, movements of the robotic arms are controlled by the surgeon sitting remotely in the console.

The surgical cart engages with the patient through a process termed 'docking'. The cart has four arms, one holding an endoscopic camera with other arms being used for surgical instruments. In practice this equates to instruments in the right and left hands with fourth arm instrumentation serving as a surgical retractor or assistant.

Endoscopes are 8 mm or 12 mm and, unlike standard endoscopes that give a 2D view, images seen with the da Vinci are in 3D. This is brought about by the endoscope casing containing two endoscopes thereby replicating a truly 3D surgical experience. This gives the surgeon a depth of field dimension to the operative field. The endoscope can be moved to alter magnification and also moved in various planes to avoid line of sight conflicts that accompany standard endoscopic methods.

Movement of instruments within the hand of a surgeon are restricted by anatomical limitations brought about by evolution. The human hand is able to adduct, abduct, supinate, pronate, flex and extend through a defined range of movements. This limitation is apparent during standard suturing and it limits what a surgeon can achieve in confined spaces where visualization is limited. These anatomical restrictions are overcome by the Endowristed capability of robotic instrumentation.

Robotic instruments are capable of moving through an arc of 270 degrees in both clockwise and anticlockwise directions. Clever algorithms within the system are finally able to remove natural human tremor, a process termed 'tremor-filtration'. Finally, motion-scaling permits the range of movement of instruments in the operative field to be scaled so that movements of the hands at the console can lead to smaller or larger movements at the patient interface. In essence this gives the surgeon 7 degrees of freedom and confers a capability of being equally dextrous with dominant and non-dominant hands.

The CCDs are able to transmit images of each endoscope to the right or left eyes when seen through the viewing binoculars. This replicates a truly 3D surgical experience. The Si has a screen resolution of 1080, a 30% improvement in quality compared to 720 in the S and 480 in the standard machines.

Fine control of the instrument jaws is brought about by movement of thumb with index and middle fingers that are inserted through the rings of the hand control, as shown in **Figure 69.3**.

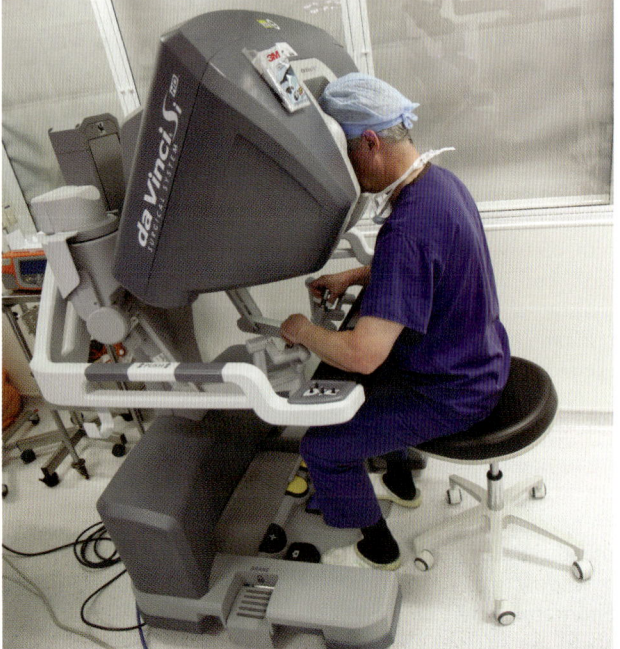

Figure 69.3 The operating surgeon at the console controlling the robotic arms and instruments by the hand cradle.

Infrared sensors in the console stop any movement of the robotic instruments once the surgeon moves his head from the console as a safety measure. The development of dual consoles, bolt-on simulators and telestration aid both training and proctorship of robotic surgery.

Ethical considerations

The da Vinci is now routinely used for hemithyroidectomy, lobectomy, total thyroidectomy and level VI central compartment dissection. More recently, applications have extended to lateral compartment neck dissection through the axillary approach.[18]

A review of published literature from South East Asia shows that the majority of patients undergoing robotic surgery have had relatively small nodules, with the mean size of cancerous nodule removed 8 mm. Although median nodule size would have been more appropriate, it is clear that surgery is being undertaken on patients with small volume pathology. This has been confirmed by personal communication from several surgeons who have visited Korea.

A different healthcare system in association with screening of the thyroid, a variance in reimbursement tariff for robotic compared to conventional approaches (by a factor of five) combined with a national psyche for avoiding a neck scar have combined to create the perfect environment for advancing robotic thyroid surgery in Korea.

Ethical, safety and economic factors need to be considered before the introduction of new technology and surgical techniques. Surgeons practise in an environment of scrutiny with a medicolegal dimension that appears insatiable. However, without the adoption of innovation, advances which improve patient care will be stifled. The history of surgery abounds with examples of innovations that were initially resisted – some quite vehemently – anaesthesia, antisepsis, caps, gowns, gloves and even 'keyhole' surgical techniques to name but few. The environment in which RAT takes place in the Far East may not necessarily translate to a western European population. The body habitués of patients, cultural perception to neck scars and the health system in which doctors operate are very different.

The author received training in robotic surgery in 2007 before publication of RAT. To innovate and learn RAT unassisted has been a long and arduous journey involving cadaveric dissection in Paris, Strasbourg and Geneva. Furthermore, ethical permission was sought and finally granted after two submissions. Funding for prospective evaluation studies was obtained for the initial 50 patients. Obtaining recognition from private companies to recognize robotic head and neck surgery was another hurdle that had to be negotiated for fee-paying patients. Finally, peer perception of RAT had to be negotiated and addressed as we all work in an environment where to be considered maverick and an outlier confers professional risk.

There are thyroid-specific and generic considerations for RAT. My personal view is that RAT is suitable for hemithyroidectomy of nodules or nodular pathology of up to 6 cm and a total thyroidectomy, provided the

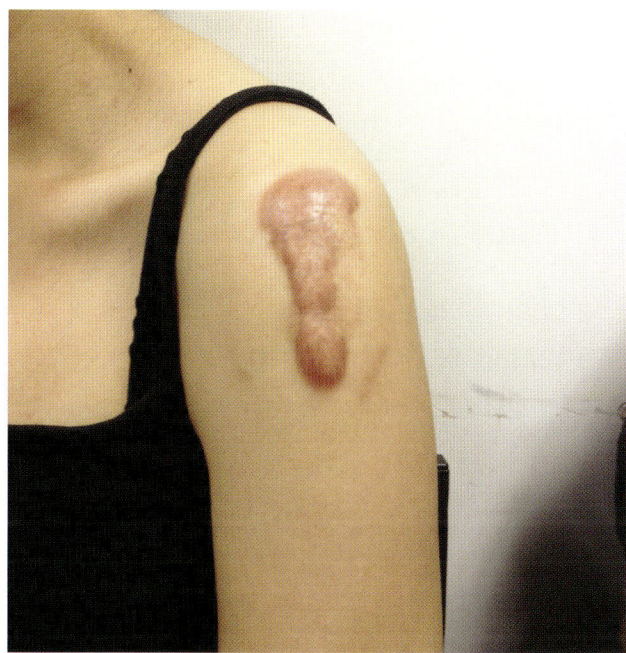

Figure 69.4 Keloid scarring on the upper arm following vaccination – a patient typically who may have valid reasons for avoiding a visible neck scar.

contralateral lobe is 'near' normal. I would counsel avoidance for cancer other than for microcarcinoma in the young and for Graves' disease. It is an attractive option for patients having a history of hypertrophic scarring (**Figure 69.4**) or those simply expressing a personal preference to avoid neck scarring. The approach should be avoided in obese patients with a BMI over 30, those with degenerative shoulder pathology and those with other significant comorbidity placing them in an ASA category greater than 2. The ideal patient, therefore, would be a thin, narrow-chested female with a thyroid nodule of up to 4 cm. Nodules of greater than 4 cm can be removed but are technically more challenging. Large cystic nodules can also be made suitable by aspiration at the time of surgery.

Consent

As for all surgery, informed consent should take place. It is my opinion that all consent but particularly RAT should be performed by the consultant. The literature supports that RAT is as safe as conventional surgery with the same risk of bleeding, infection, vocal cord palsy and parathyroid dysfunction. RAT, however, has the additional rare potential complication of brachial plexus dysfunction. The operation achieves the objective of translocation of an incision from neck to axilla at the expense of an increased operative time. The inpatient stay and time off work are identical.

Reservation of RAT regarding airway obstruction from a bleed is often a concern quite reasonably raised. It may come as a surprise that airway obstruction will not occur following a bleed from RAT simply because the potential space for a bleed to disseminate is so capacious compared to conventional thyroidectomy. In this respect it is safer than CT, although this would not be a cogent argument for the routine introduction of RAT.

Operative set-up

PRE-OPERATIVE CONSIDERATIONS

Teamwork is essential in the pre-operative preparation of the patient. On the arm of the side of surgery no identification bracelet, lines, blood pressure cuffs or ECG leads must be placed. I routinely use laryngeal nerve monitoring.

It is very important to mark the 5–6 cm axillary incision while the patient is awake, with the back of the patient's hand touching the central portion of the forehead, a position which I describe as an extended salute (**Figure 69.5**). In my experience this is the only technique that successfully identifies the best site for the incision. Otherwise, part of the incision can migrate to the upper arm or onto the anterolateral chest wall. I often extend the incision superiorly in a curvilinear fashion so it sits in a natural crease, which reduces tension and a tendency towards a hypertrophic and pigmented scarring. The axilla is not an environment well suited for healing because of its damp anaerobic nature but, with experience and correct planning, the incision heals well and becomes invisible (**Figure 69.6**).

At induction the patient is routinely given i.v. Augmentin and 4 mg Dexamethasone.

THEATRE SET-UP

Prior to transfer of the patient to the operating table it is important that all three components of the da Vinci are appropriately positioned. The cart is placed on the opposite side of the operating table (**Figure 69.7**) and is draped

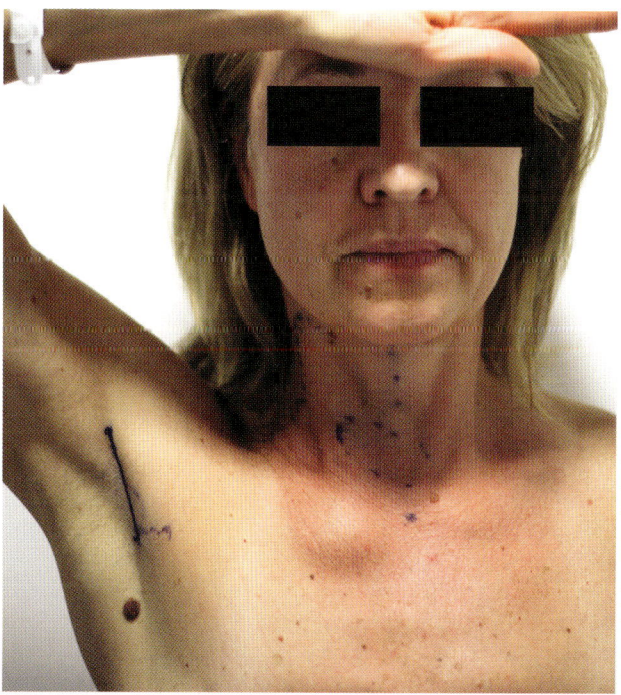

Figure 69.5 Marking of the incision immediately prior to surgery. This is of fundamental importance and is a vital component of pre-operative planning.

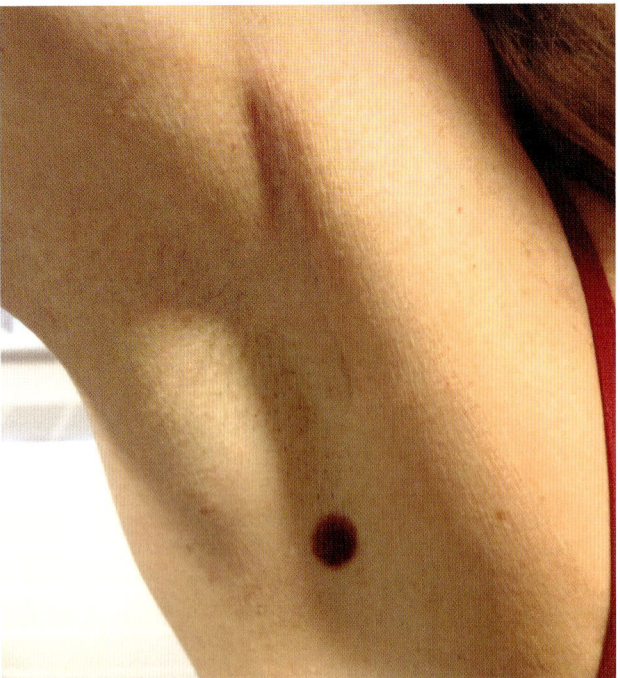

Figure 69.6 The same patient as in Figure 69.5, showing the axillary scar 9 months following surgery.

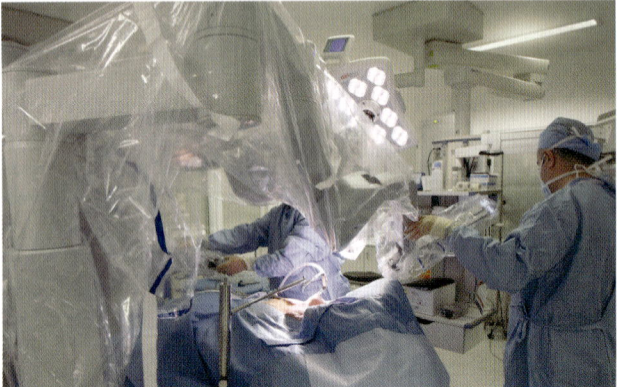

Figure 69.7 The cart is docked at right angles to the operating table, on the opposite side to the incision.

and correctly positioned before the patient is moved onto the operating table, thereby being ready for docking.

Contrary to CT, a shoulder roll is not placed under the shoulders as this has a tendency to overextend the neck and move the superior pole away from the robotic instruments. I place the patient's head and shoulders under a pillow so that there is adequate and comfortable support in a subtle 'sniffing the morning air' position. The head of the table is then dropped by about 20 degrees to widen the angle between the arm and the chest.

A special arm rest supports the arm, which is abducted and flexed with the forearm pronated so that the back of the hand rests on the central portion of the forehead. I stabilize this position with a Velcro coin attached to the hand and forehead. This movement has the effect of elevating and externally rotating the clavicle to that the distance between the incision site and thyroid gland is shortened.

The positioning of the arm in this way is a modification to Chung's method where the arm is fully extended over the head. This puts the brachial plexus at risk and should never be used in my opinion. I have had no problems since I modified Chung's method of arm positioning.

Once completed, the incision site is infiltrated with 2% Xylocaine and 1:200 000 adrenaline. Skin preparation and draping then take place while the surgeon scrubs.

The operation

PREPARATION OF THE ROBOTIC FIELD

The area to be dissected extends from the thyroid cartilage to sternal notch in a subcutaneous plane. The superior and inferior extent of the axillary incision is level with the thyroid and sternal notches respectively. An imaginary line in a horizontal plane connects the two with the area to be dissected being trapezoid-shaped.

Dissection extends medially in the subfascial and subcutaneous planes above pectoralis major and over the clavicle. The natural dehiscence between the sternal and clavicular heads of the sternomastoid is entered to get to the plane of the strap muscles. Dissection then extends under the strap muscles to access the thyroid gland. The surgical planes are then developed as in a standard CT. The lower insertion of the sternothyroid into the back of the manubrium and first rib is divided as is its superior attachment to the thyroid cartilage; this allows full access to superior pole structures. I routinely divide the omohyoid muscle as it extends over the internal jugular vein. Once the strap muscles have been separated off the thyroid gland to approximately a third of the contralateral thyroid lobe, dissection is complete. A modified retractor is then inserted (Chung, Kuppersmith, Modena or Imperial) and the robot docked.

DOCKING

The cart is docked at right angles to the operating table (**Figure 69.7**). All four arms can be placed through a single axillary incision or the fourth arm can be inserted through a periareolar incision. The last incision has little morbidity and the scar is invisible once it has healed.

The 30 degree down 12 mm stereoscopic endoscope is placed at an angle of 220 degrees and is inserted low laterally, extending high and upwards medially towards the thyroid gland. The fourth arm can then be placed under the endoscope, which functions as the assistant. Finally, the first and third arms, which carry the instruments for dissection and haemostasis, are positioned. The fourth assistant arm holds the 8 mm Prograsp, while the first and third arms hold a combination of 5 mm Maryland, Debakey and Harmonic shears.

THE PROCEDURE

It is my preference to identify the recurrent laryngeal nerve and parathyroid glands first by using Maryland and Debakey forceps. Once these have been clearly defined, I then swap the Debakey for the Harmonic shears. The shears use old CS14 harmonic technology that will seal and transect vessels of up to 3 mm, which is adequate for RAT. As with all energy sealing devices, care must be taken when using this instrument close to the nerve.

Standard technique is to divide the superior pole vessels, identify the external branch of the superior laryngeal nerve then dissect the thyroid off the trachea and divide the isthmus as in a standard lobectomy. For a total thyroidectomy the approach is to divide the superior pole vessels first then dissect the thyroid off the trachea to help mobilize the remaining lobe. The inferior pole vessels and middle thyroid vein are then divided before identification and careful dissection of the nerve off the thyroid gland. This part of the operation often involves repositioning of the retractor, which has a tendency to slip. If a subtotal thyroidectomy is to be avoided, the contralateral thyroid lobe is required to be near normal in my opinion.

As in all thyroid surgery, haemostasis should be meticulous and a reversed Valsalva in the presence of normotension must be adhered to before closure. As in conventional surgery, I do not insert a drain and have found this to be unproblematic.

Closure of the incision is with 4-0 subcuticular Vicryl Rapide and Dermabond. An anterior chest wall compression dressing is applied overnight and patients are advised to wear a sports bra or vest for 2 weeks to provide light compression to the anterior chest wall. I routinely give antibiotics for 7 days. Follow-up is at 2 weeks, then 3, 6, 12 and 18 months as all patients are in a prospective study for long-term RAT evaluation.

CONCLUSION

RAT is an exciting technological development in thyroidectomy. It is here to stay but presently will have niche indications. It is not for every surgeon, hospital or patient in its present state of technological development.

Economically it is difficult to justify and lack of competition in the robotic market is hindering the expansion of robotic surgery. Training, proctorship and credentialing are factors of vital and fundamental importance to guarantee safety.

The use of RAT is technically challenging with a steep learning curve. It is still in an evaluation phase and incorporation of patients into long-term studies will assist this process. Robotic technology must be used sensibly, responsibly and ethically to ensure patient safety.

KEY POINTS

- The evidence base for minimal invasive and scarless in the neck techniques for thyroid surgery are outlines.
- This is an evolving field that will witness the indications, applications and approach for remote thyroid surgery change with advances in robotic technology.

REFERENCES

1. Presentation at the Annual BAETS Meeting, October 2012, Cardiff.
2. Del Rio P, Sommaruga L, Cataldo S, et al. Minimally invasive video-assisted thyroidectomy: the learning curve. *Eur Sur Res* 2008; **41**: 33–6.
3. 1st BAES Audit, 2003.
4. Radford PD, Ferguson MS, McGill JC, et al. Meta-analysis of video-assisted minimal invasive thyroidectomy. *Laryngoscope* 2011; **121**: 1675–81.
5. Terris, DJ, Singer MC, Seybt MW. Robotic facelift thyroidectomy: II. Clinical feasibility and safety. *Laryngoscope* 2011; **121**: 1636–41.
6. Tae K, Ji YB, Jeong JH, et al. Robotic thyroidectomy by a gasless unilateral axillo-breast or axillary approach: our early experiences. *Surg Endosc* 2011; **25**(1): 221–8.
7. Gottlieb A, Sprung J, Zheng X-M, Gagner M. Massive subcutaneous emphysema and hypercarbia in a patient during endoscopic transcervical parathyroidectomy using carbon dioxide insufflation. *Anaesth Analg* 1997; **84**: 1154–6.
8. Marescaux J, Leroy J, Gagner M, et al. Transatlantic robot-assisted telesurgery. *Nature* 2001; **413**: 379–80.
9. Lee KE, Rao J, Youn Y-K. Endoscopic thyroidectomy with the da Vinci robot system using the bilateral axillary breast approach (BABA) technique: our initial experience. *Surg Laparosc Endosc Percutan Tech* 2009; **19**: 71–5.
10. Tolley N, Arora A, Palazzo F, et al. Robotic-assisted parathyroidectomy: a feasibility study. *Otolaryngol Head Neck Surg* 2011; **144**: 859–66.
11. Lobe TE, Wright SK, Irish MS. Novel uses of surgical robotics in head and neck surgery. *J Laparoendosc Adv Surg Tech A* 2005; **15**(6): 647–52.
12. Kang SW, Jeong JJ, Yun JS, et al. Robotic-assisted endoscopic surgery for thyroid cancer: experience with the first 100 patients. *Surg Endosc* 2009; **23**: 2399–406.
13. Ryu HR, Kang SW, Lee HL, et al. Feasibility and safety of a new robotic thyroidectomy through a gasless, transaxillary single incision approach. *J Am Coll Surg* 2010; **211**(3): e13–19.
14. Lee J, Nah KY, Kim RM, et al. Differences in postoperative outcomes, function, and cosmesis: open versus robotic thyroidectomy. *Surg Endosc* 2010; **24**: 3186–94.
15. Lee J, Jun JH, Nam KH, et al. The learning curve for robotic thyroidectomy: a multicentre study. *Annal Surg Oncol* 2010; **18**: 226–32.
16. Lee J, Yun JH, Nam KH, et al. Perioperative clinical outcomes after robotic thyroidectomy for papillary thyroid cancer: a multicentre study. *Surg Endosc* 2011; **25**: 906–12.
17. Jackson NR, Yao L, Tufano RP, Kandil EH. Safety of robotic thyroidectomy approaches: meta-analysis and systematic review. *Head Neck* 2014; **36**(1): 137–43.
18. Kim CH, Chang JW, Choi EC, et al. Robotically assisted selective neck dissection in parotid gland cancer: a preliminary report. *Laryngoscope* 2013; **123**: 646–50.

SURGERY FOR THE ENLARGED THYROID

Neeraj Sethi, Josh Lodhia and R. James A. England

Introduction 819	Management 821
Terminology 819	Non-surgical management 821
Aetiology 819	Surgery 822
Clinical presentation 820	References 825
Investigations 820	

SEARCH STRATEGY

Data in this chapter may be updated by a Medline search using the keywords: goiter, goitre, retrosternal, thyroidectomy, mediastinal, thyroid, intrathoracic. There are no randomized controlled trials comparing treatments for the enlarged thyroid. Evidence to support statements made in the chapter are level 2b at best.

INTRODUCTION

The term 'goitre' derives its etymological origins from the Latin 'gutter' meaning throat.[1] Today goitre can be used to describe any thyroid considered to be larger than normal. Prior to widespread salt iodination, Gerber found the average thyroid weight in women over 50 years was 80–90 g and in men 55–75 g.[2] The same study found 30 years after salt iodination the average thyroid weight reduced by approximately half. Pankow et al. reported that the average weight of thyroids in men aged 20–29 years was 16.4 g and 14.4 g for women, suggesting that subjects spending their entire life under the influence of iodinated salt are likely to have a smaller thyroid.[3] The upper limit of the normal thyroid gland in the iodine-replete population is considered to be 20 g.[4,5]

In 1994, the World Health Organization (WHO) defined goitre as any palpably enlarged thyroid.[6] A number of geographically different radiographical studies in iodine-replete regions found the upper limit of the impalpable thyroid to be approximately 15 cm^3 in men and 12 cm^3 in women.[7–9]

In this chapter we discuss the clinical and radiological assessment and management of the enlarged thyroid. This includes both retrosternal goitre and goitre without intra-thoracic extension.

TERMINOLOGY

The Swiss anatomist Haller first described the finding of a thyroid with intra-thoracic extension in 1749.[10] The first report describing removal of such a thyroid was by Klein in 1820.[11] Intra-thoracic, secondary intra-thoracic, substernal and cervicomediastinal are all terms that have been used synonymously with retrosternal. Up to ten definitions for these are found in the literature with the most commonly used being either (i) any goitre which extends below the thoracic inlet (with the patient in the surgical position) or (ii) any goitre where more than 50% of the gland is below the thoracic inlet.[12–21] Primary intra-thoracic goitre is a distinct entity and describes a thyroid mass that originates from ectopic thyroid tissue in the mediastinum, rather than from cervical thyroid tissue.[22]

Large goitres without intra-thoracic extension comprise a group without a clear definition in terms of volume or weight. One study of 813 goitres divided patient groups by weight of gland after thyroidectomy and defined the huge goitre as heavier than 400 g.[23]

AETIOLOGY

Crile attributed goitre with intra-thoracic extension to neck musculature obstructing extra-thoracic growth and directing the goitre downwards.[14] In 1934, Lahey and Swinton discussed the potential role of negative intra-thoracic pressure and downward traction from swallowing.[24] These goitres tend to extend into the anterior mediastinum with only 10–15% growing into the posterior mediastinum.[25] The majority of these tend to be right-sided due to the great vessels impeding extension into the left thorax.[26] Primary intra-thoracic goitre is due to an abnormality of embryologic migration. A key point is that goitres with intra-thoracic extension still derive their blood supply from the superior and inferior thyroid arteries, while primary intra-thoracic goitre is supplied by intra-thoracic vessels.[27, 28]

In accordance with the variation in terminology describing goitre with intra-thoracic extension, the incidence described in the literature varies from 0.2–45%.[16, 29] Using one of the most common definitions (where the majority of the goitre lies below the thoracic inlet) the incidence is up to 20%.[16, 25, 30] Primary intra-thoracic goitre represents less than 1% of all goitres and up to 12% of all mediastinal tumours.[31]

CLINICAL PRESENTATION

In goitre without intra-thoracic extension, the most common presenting symptom is an anterior neck mass. Compressive symptoms (dysphagia, cough, dyspnea, wheeze, stridor) occur in up to 17% of patients and are associated with increasing size of goitre.[32–34] In benign disease recurrent laryngeal nerve palsy at presentation is rare (0.7%).[35]

The goitre with intra-thoracic extension often presents without any palpable, or a barely palpable, neck mass with the majority of the thyroid bulk being in the chest.[1, 36] Approximately 40% of these can be asymptomatic. The most common presenting symptoms are secondary to airway compression, with acute distress occurring in up to 20%, followed by dysphagia.[16, 37, 38] Less common presentations include superior vena cava syndrome (venous distention of neck and chest wall, dyspnoea, facial oedema, upper limb oedema, plethora, cyanosis, papilloedema, cough, confusion), which can also lead to the development of downward oesophageal varices.[39–42] Pemberton's sign (facial congestion and cyanosis while elevating both arms) indicates increased thoracic inlet pressure due to a retrosternal mass.[43] Horner's syndrome due to direct compression of the sympathetic chain, chylothorax due to thoracic duct compression and transient ischaemic attacks secondary to thyrocervical steal have also been reported.[44–46]

Primary intra-thoracic goitre presents either as an incidental finding or with compressive symptoms similar to goitre with intra-thoracic extension.[28, 31]

INVESTIGATIONS

Biochemical assessment of thyroid function is necessary for management of all goitres. The majority are euthyroid, particularly goitres with intra-thoracic extension (80%).[1, 16, 39, 47] Up to 30% may have suppressed serum TSH levels without raised thyroid hormone levels (subclinical thyrotoxicosis).[48]

Ultrasound is highly sensitive and specific for evaluating morphology and measuring volume of accessible, extra-thoracic goitre.[49, 50] It cannot evaluate intra-thoracic goitre, except as an occasional adjunct in transluminal endobronchial fine-needle aspiration to aid pre-operative diagnosis of posterior mediastinal goitre.[51] CT remains the best imaging modality when evaluating the extent of intra-thoracic extension. As a basic rule, if it is not possible to palpate the distal extent of a thyroid goitre, a CT scan is necessary to assess its intra-thoracic extent.

CT allows assessment of the full inferior extent of the intra-thoracic goitre, as well as the shape and position of the goitre in terms of the mediastinal compartment.[52] A number of studies have examined CT findings as predictors of whether a thoracic approach is needed. Although CT is not a definitive predictor, it is more likely a sternotomy will be required if the goitre extends below the level of the aortic arch or there is evidence of extra-thyroid extension suggesting malignancy.[52–55] The risk of malignancy in goitres with intra-thoracic extension has been reported to be up to 11%.[39, 56] Factors that increase the likelihood of requiring a lateral thoracotomy are a goitre extending into the posterior mediastinum or a primary intrathoracic goitre that is primarily right-sided.[52]

Scintigraphy plays no role in the pre-operative evaluation of the biochemically euthyroid patient.[57] Indeed, intra-thoracic goitres often demonstrate limited iodine avidity despite their size (**Figures 70.1–70.4**).

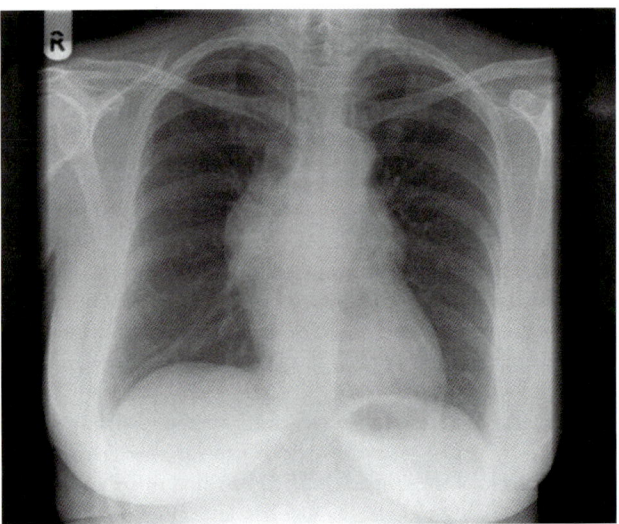

Figure 70.1 Incidental plain chest X-ray abnormality suggesting a mediastinal mass due to primary intra-thoracic goitre.

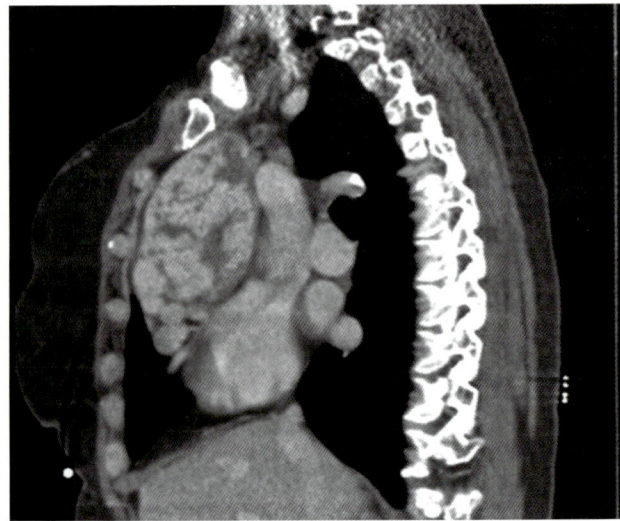

Figure 70.2 Confirmation of the mass as a likely primary intrathoracic goitre on parasagittal MR image.

70: SURGERY FOR THE ENLARGED THYROID

loops characterized by plateaus of flow during both forced inspiration and expiration.[59] However, studies have found that flow volume loop results correlate poorly with goitre weight, extent of tracheal narrowing or patient-reported symptoms.[60–63]

MANAGEMENT

When assessing the need for thyroidectomy in a patient with an enlarged thyroid and particularly retrosternal goitre, two questions need to be asked. First, will the patient benefit from the procedure and second are the surgical risks outweighed by the potential surgical benfits? The American Thyroid Association guidelines suggest that in the absence of lower airway disease, a patient will gain from retrosternal thyroidectomy from a respiratory perspective if the trachea is compressed by 35% or greater on axial CT imaging preoperatively.[64, 65] However, the American literature shows us that patients with retrosternal goitre are older, have more comorbidities, and a 73% increased risk of death during admission.[66]

In addition, patients undergoing sternotomy have a 25% risk of respiratory complications compared to a 2% risk for those who undergo a cervical approach only and the risk of deep sternal infection is cited as 1–5%, with sternal dehiscence carrying a 50% mortality rate.

A significant body of thyroid surgeons will cite the risk of spontaneous intragoitre haemorrhage leading to acute respiratory embarrassment as a reason to perform retrosternal thyroidectomy. However, Hsu tells us that in a retrospective group of patients presenting to the intensive care unit of Singapore General Hospital over a 15 year period with acute respiratory distress caused by mediastinal mass, only 1 of 19 was due to retrosternal goitre and this patient made a full recovery following surgery whilst admitted.[67] Perhaps therefore this risk, although real, is over exaggerated.

When assessing patients with retrosternal goitre therefore, it is important to remember that the majority comprise an older more frail patient subgroup.

NON-SURGICAL MANAGEMENT

No intervention

In the asymptomatic, euthyroid, benign goitre without intra-thoracic extension a conservative approach is appropriate.[68] A Scandinavian study followed up 261 patients with euthyroid goitre over 10 years.[69] Of these patients 21.8% required surgery due to worsening symptoms, 1.9% were diagnosed with carcinoma over the 10-year period and 5% developed thyrotoxicosis. Three patients died of their disease (two after developing anaplastic carcinoma and one with aggressive papillary carcinoma).

An operative approach is advocated by some as the only option to avoid the risks associated with bleeding or continued growth.[39, 70, 71] One of the largest series of thyroidectomies published included 1153 goitres with intra-thoracic extension or primary intra-thoracic goitre.

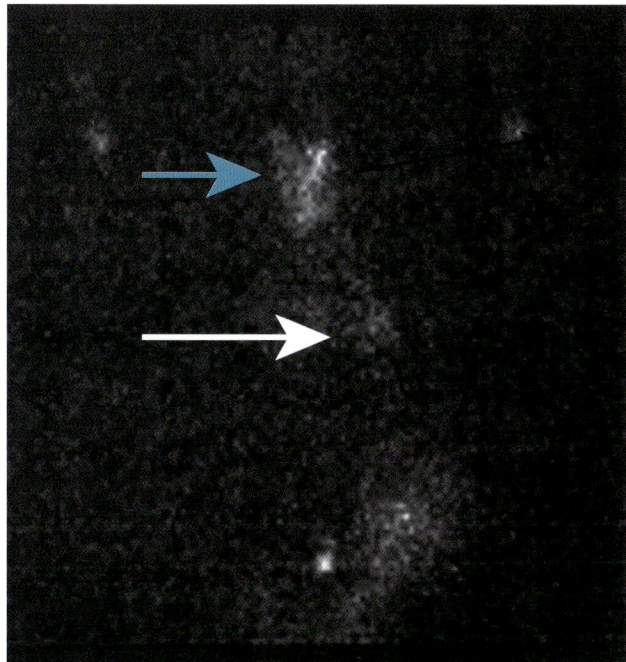

Figure 70.3 ^{123}I image demonstrating reduced iodine avidity often demonstrated by primary intrathoracic goitre (blue arrow demonstrates thyroid uptake in the neck; white arrow demonstrates uptake in the intrathoracic portion).

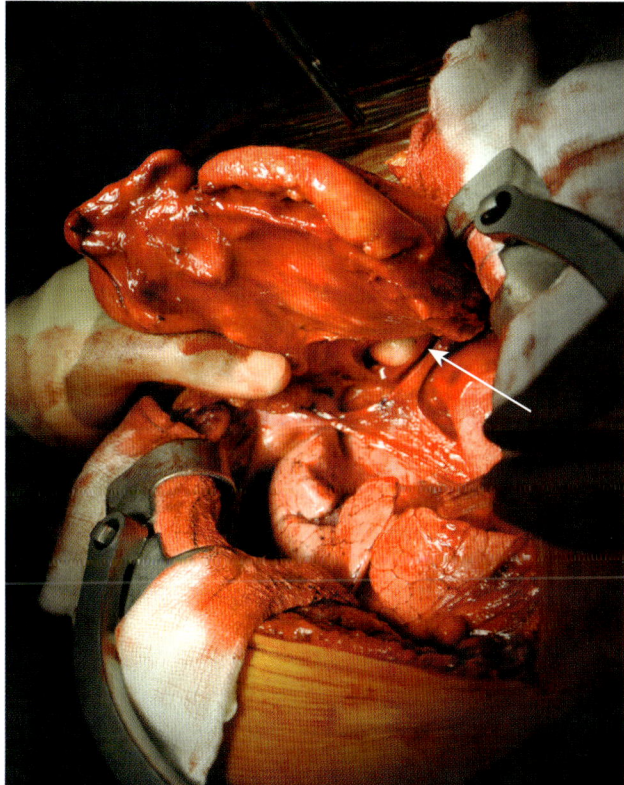

Figure 70.4 Removing the intra-thoracic goitre from the chest cavity preserving the innominate vein (arrow).

Objective assessment of respiratory compromise secondary to retrosternal goitre is difficult. The most common test performed is flow loop spirometry.[58] Obstruction secondary to goitre theoretically produces flow volume

This found that they were at a higher risk of post-operative complications compared to goitres without intra-thoracic extension.[72]

Radioiodine therapy

In symptomatic patients who refuse or are unfit for surgery, radioiodine (^{131}I) therapy remains an option. This has been used in the treatment of hyperthyroidism for over six decades.[73] Conventional ^{131}I has been shown to reduce non-toxic goitre size by approximately 30–45% after 1–2 years in around 80% of patients.[74–77] The effect does diminish with increasing goitre size and approximately 10% of goitres will continue to grow.[74] In a small series conventional ^{131}I does appear to have the same effect on the intra-thoracic portion of goitres as the extra-thoracic portion.[78] Goitres causing compressive symptoms should not be considered for ^{131}I as it can induce an acute increase in size.[73] Other adverse effects of ^{131}I include radiation-induced thyroiditis, transient hyperthyroidism and long-term hypothyroidism (up to 58%).[73] The long-term risk of thyroidal or extra-thyroidal malignancy does not appear significant but is not definitively known.[79–82] Recombinant human TSH-augmented ^{131}I has been demonstrated to improve radioiodine uptake and increase volume reduction by 33–56% compared to conventional ^{131}I therapy.[83–85]

SURGERY

Anaesthetic considerations

Traditionally, the two primary anaesthetic concerns related to massive goitre were intubation difficulty and problems extubating due to tracheomalacia. A number of series have been published detailing the rate of difficulty intubating and/or the need for tracheostomy in patients with goitre.[86, 87] These suggest that the majority of patients with huge goitres with or without intra-thoracic extension can be intubated successfully using i.v. induction or awake fibreoptic intubation. In a report from an endemic goitre region, the rate of tracheostomy was not increased in goitres weighing >400g compared to those <400g.[23] As might be expected, there is a significant increase in the proportion of difficult intubations in huge goitres. Tracheomalacia is also reported to be a rare occurrence in iodine-replete regions (<1%) though it may be more common in endemic goitre regions (up to 33%) in the huge goitre with or without intra-thoracic extension.[23, 86, 88, 89] Treatment options for this include prolonged intubation, placement of supporting sutures, tracheal stenting and tracheostomy.[23, 42]

Another concern is sudden, post-induction cardiorespiratory collapse, which has been described in patients with mediastinal masses.[90] Cardiopulmonary bypass is the necessary option in this situation. The risk of requiring this may be more common in posterior mediastinal goitre and in those with extremely low tracheal compression where prophylactic tracheostomy is not beneficial.[91, 92]

Surgical considerations

The patient is consented ideally prior to the day of surgery. The aims of the operation should have been clarified by the operating surgeon and understood by both parties. Any imaging performed should be available in theatre. The important things to note on imaging are whether the thyroid extends into the posterior mediastinum, whether it extends behind the oesophagus and whether it extends between the trachea and oesophagus. Other significant factors include evidence of extra-thyroidal extension, and evidence of oesophageal or tracheal invasion. Careful study of the CT scan is necessary as tracheal invasion may be subtle but may make goitre delivery extremely difficult (**Figures 70.5** and **70.6**).

With retrosternal disease the likely necessity for cardiothoracic input should be identified pre-operatively. The overwhelming majority of retrosternal goitres are deliverable through a collar incision. However, it is foolhardy to perform such procedures in units where

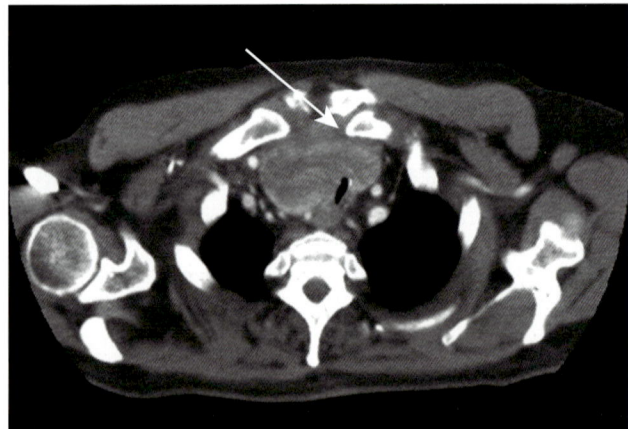

Figure 70.5 Axial CT scan of the chest demonstrating early invasion of the tracheal wall (arrowed) from a poorly differentiated thyroid cancer in the 10 o'clock position.

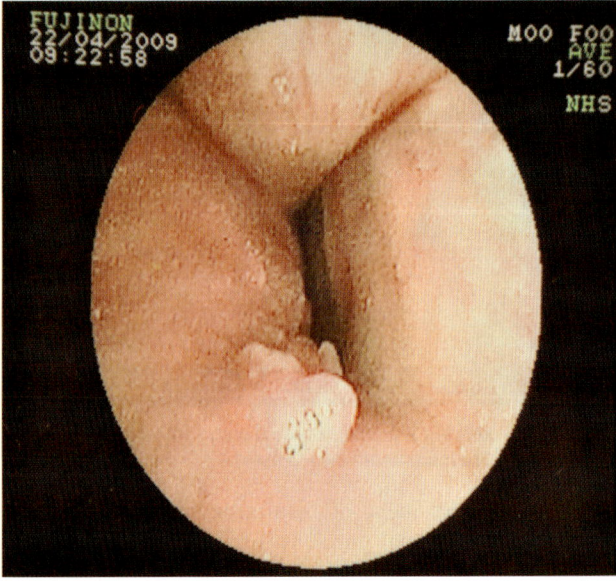

Figure 70.6 Tracheoscopic confirmation of the CT findings.

cardiothoracic expertise is not available. Cardiothoracic input is necessary in primary intrathoracic goitre and occasionally in malignant thyroid disease where the tumour has extended beyond the boundaries of the thyroid within the chest. In the latter instance the benefit of resection should be carefully discussed with the patient pre-operatively because often the patient has comorbidities and the procedure is palliative rather than curative, so a careful risk–benefit analysis should be considered. Rarely, thoracic access is necessary due to patient proportion. A short, obese patient may provide limited access through the neck to the thyroid. The majority of these patients have incidental retrosternal glands, which begs the question: just because the thyroid is retrosternal, will its removal confer significant benefit to the patient?

Extension of the goitre to the level of the carina has previously predicted the need for sternotomy.[13, 14] Thyroid weight greater than 800 g has also been linked with the need for an extra-cervical approach, but this is a post-operative finding.[13, 15] The choice of which extra-cervical approach to take depends on whether access to either hemithorax or mediastinum is required.

In the infrequent situation where greater exposure is required, the option for a partial upper median sternotomy, anterior thoracotomy in the second or third space or video-assisted thoracoscopic approach may be sought. Given that the majority of thyroid masses lie anterior to the innominate vein, a median sternotomy or partial upper median sternotomy provides ideal exposure to the mass and bilaterally towards the pleura. In posterior mediastinal goitre a lateral thoracotomy may be considered. If there is asymmetry to the retrosternal extension, entering via the side with the majority of the mass is appropriate, although the aortic arch can limit access on the left, especially if there is suggested involvement of posterior mediastinal structures such as the trachea. In this situation a right-sided posterolateral thoracotomy is the incisional choice. In the rare situation that there is lateral extension into the upper thorax, a Dartevelle approach (**Figure 70.7**) would provide better control of the subclavian vessels, though this may limit exposure in the neck. Additionally, the use of video-assisted thoracoscopic surgery (VATS) has aided the excision of retrosternal goitres.

The patient is positioned 30° semi-supine with the right side slightly elevated. A double lumen tube allows for lung isolation. The possible approaches include a lateral camera position with medial utility ports allowing for retraction and dissection, or a subxiphoid camera position which can allow for visualization of both hemithoracic cavities. This approach provides good visualization from below and of the phrenic nerves, internal mammary vessels and great vessels. The mass is removed through the cervical incision. The subxiphoid approach limits visualization of the posterior mediastinum as the pericardium lies in the way.

Surgical procedure

A collar incision is made, normally extended to the membranous insertion of the sternomastoid muscles. A superior subplatysmal flap is raised and the flap extended laterally beyond the bodies of the sternomastoid muscles. In virtually every case, once the linea alba is divided to gain access to the thyroid isthmus, the strap muscles are divided. This is best performed superiorly as innervation of the straps is from inferior to superior.

The key to successful delivery of the retrosternal gland is to achieve mobility without excessive blood loss. A plane is therefore developed laterally between the thyroid lobe and the carotid sheath which may lie lateral to the cervical component of the gland, or anterior or posterior to the gland. An anteriorly placed carotid does not preclude thoracic delivery as lateral retraction will still enable delivery in the majority of cases. While the surgeon develops the plane, keeping on the gland surface, it is possible to assess the initial intra-thoracic extent of the gland, and indeed sometimes reach a finger to the inferior extent of the gland.

The next step is to devascularize the lobe. The superior thyroid pedicle is identified in the normal manner, retracted laterally from the cricothyroid muscle, to minimize risk of damage to the external branch of the superior laryngeal nerve, and divided vessel by vessel. The superior vessels are generally far larger in retrosternal glands so there is an increased need for ties or Ligaclips®. Once the pedicle is ligated, the mobility of the lobe is increased. Further blunt dissection laterally improves mobility further. This can be facilitated by placing a gauze swab on the lobe and digitally retracting the lobe out of the chest, the swab reducing slippage. A finger gently slid down the lobe into the mediastinum will give an indication of the extent of intrathoracic extension. Using these manoeuvres, the lobe can often simply be delivered from the chest. This becomes more difficult if the thyroid is particularly firm or if the central isthmic portion of the gland is enlarged pushing the trachea away from the manubrium as this reduces the potential of swinging the enlarged lobe in a superiomedial direction during extra-thoracic passage. In this circumstance it is often useful to palpate for the plane between the trachea and the lobe below the isthmus so that retraction from the chest can be performed both medially and laterally on the lobe.

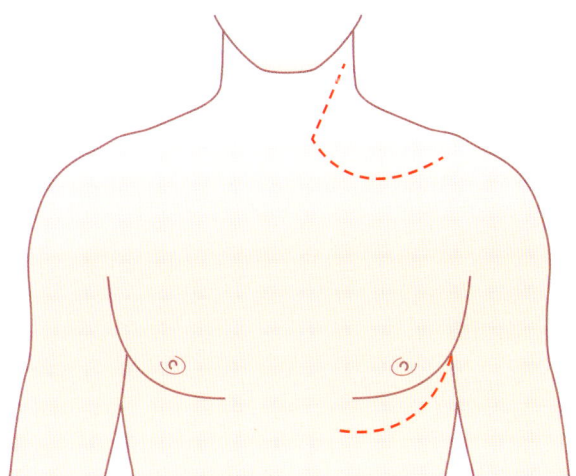

Figure 70.7 Dartvelle approach.

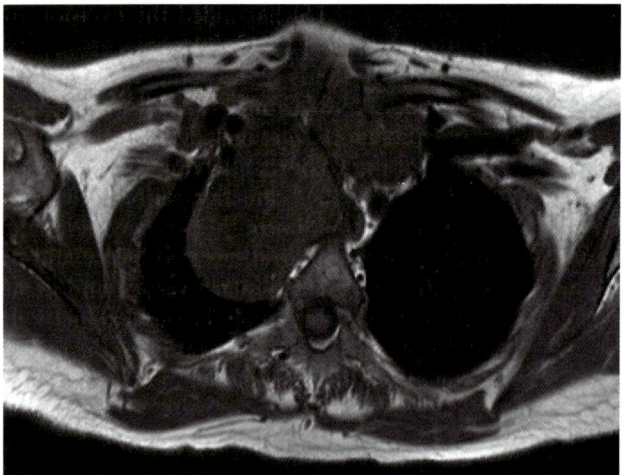

Figure 70.8 Axial MR demonstrating huge goitre with right posterior mediastinal component.

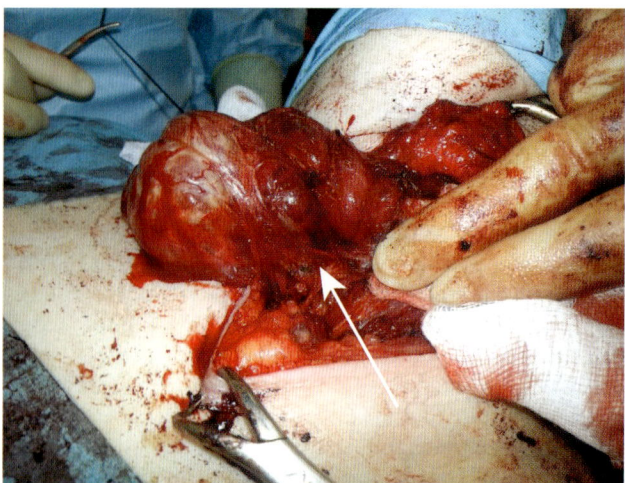

Figure 70.9 Delivery of right posterior mediastinal goitre through a cervical incision. The recurrent laryngeal nerve lies anterior to the goitre (arrow).

The search for the recurrent laryngeal nerve is generally performed once the lobe has been delivered from the chest as the nerve will lie deep to the lobe. However, in posterior mediastinal goitre this is not always the case and the nerve can lie anterior to the retrosternal portion. In this instance, therefore, the nerve needs identifying prior to lobe delivery (**Figures 70.8** and **70.9**). Continuous vagal nerve monitoring if available is a great advantage in such cases.

On completion of the operation the strap muscles are restored and often a drain is inserted to reduce the risk of haematoma formation in the mediastinal space.

In a study comparing morbidity of surgery for goitres with and without intra-thoracic extension Pieracci, Fahey and others found that those with intra-thoracic extension experienced significantly higher rates of recurrent laryngeal nerve injury (2.1%), post-operative bleeding (2.2%) and deep-vein thrombosis (0.5%).[68, 93–95] Multiple series suggest there is not necessarily a higher risk of permanent post-operative hypoparathyroidism following surgery for goitres with intra-thoracic extension.[68, 94, 96] Increasing size or weight of thyroid alone does not appear to be associated with an increased risk of intra-operative surgical complications.[23, 97–99]

KEY POINTS

- Surgery is performed on the enlarged thyroid to relieve obstructive symptoms, to manage thyroid overactivity, and to manage thyroid cancer or suspicious goitres.
- Pre-operatively the goitre should be assessed for function and extension. If the distal extent cannot be manually palpated, or if the goitre is an incidental intra-thoracic or retrosternal presentation, three-dimensional imaging should be obtained pre-operatively.
- Pre-operatively, the surgeon needs to know the extent of thyroid extension, whether the trachea or bronchi are compressed, and the relationship of the gland to the retro-oesophagus, and retropharyngotracheal area, beware the gland passing between the trachea and oesophagus. A significant isthmic retrosternal goitre is harder to deliver through the neck, and a patient's thoracic proportions should be considered.
- Surgeons should carefully assess imaging, paying particular attention to the integrity of the tracheal wall as tracheal invasion may be subtle.
- Surgery on large goitres, particularly with retrosternal extension, should involve an experienced thyroid anaesthetist.
- The thyroid will be deliverable through a collar incision in virtually every case but, if there is evidence of extra-thyroidal extension or primary intra-thoracic goitre, cardiothoracics should be alerted.
- When performing retrosternal thyroid surgery, the first part of the operation involves mobilizing the portion of the gland in the neck to facilitate thoracic delivery. During this phase it is not normally necessary to look for the nerve (except in posterior mediastinal presentation). Delivery is simplified by splitting the straps, dividing the isthmus, dealing with the upper pole, and digital dissection often both medial and lateral to the thoracic component at the level of the thoracic inlet.
- Retrosternal thyroid surgery should only be performed in a centre with cardiothoracic availability.
- In posterior mediastinal goitre be vigilant for the recurrent laryngeal nerve passing anterior to the thoracic portion of the goitre.
- When dissecting in the presumed tracheo-oesophageal groove, it is often worth inserting an oesophageal bougie to accurately locate the oesophagus and avoid mucosal transgression.
- Tracheomalacia is vanishingly rare in a first world economy but, if encountered, it will normally respond to extended intubation post-operatively.

REFERENCES

1. Newman E, Shaha AR. Substernal goiter. *J Surg Oncol* 1995; **60**(3): 207–12.
2. Gerber D. Thyroid weights and iodized salt prophylaxis: a comparative study from autopsy material from the Institute of Pathology, University of Zurich. *Schweiz Med Wochenschr* 1980; **110**(52): 2010–17.
3. Pankow BG, Michalak J, McGee MK. Adult human thyroid weight. *Health Phys* 1985; **49**(6): 1097–103.
4. Langer P. Minireview: discussion about the limit between normal thyroid goiter. *Endocr Regul* 1999; **33**(1): 39–45.
5. Langer P. Normal thyroid size versus goiter: postmortem thyroid weight and ultrasonographic volumetry versus physical examination. *Endocrinol Exp* 1989; **23**(2): 67–76.
6. WHO/UNICEF/ICCIDD. *Indicators for assessing iodine deficiency disorders and their control through salt iodination.* WHO, Editor 1994, WHO: Geneva.
7. Yokoyama N, Nagayama Y, Kakezono F, et al. Determination of the volume of the thyroid gland by a high resolutional ultrasonis scanner. *J Nucl Med* 1986; **27**: 1475–79.
8. Berghout A, Wiersinga WM, Smits NJ, Touber JL. The value of thyroid volume measured by ultrasonography in the diagnosis of goitre. *Clin Endocrinol* 1988; **28**: 409–14.
9. Gutekunst R, Smolarek H, Hasenpusch U, et al. Goitre epidemiology: thyroid volume, iodine excretion, thyroglobulin and thyrotropin in Germany and Sweden. *Acta Endocrinologica (Copenh)* 1986; **112**: 494–501.
10. Haller A. *Disputationes anatomica selectae 1749.* Gottingen: Vandenhoek.
11. Klein F. Veber die Austrotting verschiedener geschwulste, besonders jener der Ohrsperscheldruse und der Schiddruse; Aussachalung der Schilddruse. *J Chir Augenlleilk* 1820; **12**: 106–13.
12. Ríos A, Rodríguez JM, Balsalobre MD, et al. The value of various definitions of intrathoracic goiter for predicting intra-operative and postoperative complications. *Surgery* 2010; **147**(2): 233–8.
13. Wong CK, Wheeler MH. Thyroid nodules: rational management. *World J Surg* 2000; **24**(8): 934–41.
14. Crile G. Intrathoracic goiter. *Cleve Clin Q* 1939; **6**: 313–22.
15. Goldenberg IS, Lindskog GE. Differential diagnosis, pathology, and treatment of substernal goiter. *J Am Med Assoc* 1957; **163**(7): 527–9.
16. Katlic MR, Grillo HC, Wang CA. Substernal goiter. Analysis of 80 patients from Massachusetts General Hospital. *Am J Surg* 1985; **149**(2): 283–7.
17. Modlin IM. Surgical triumvirate of Theodor Kocher, Harvey Cushing, and William Halsted. *World J Surg* 1998; **22**(1): 103–13.
18. Sancho JJ, Kraimps JL, Sanchez-Blanco JM, et al. Increased mortality and morbidity associated with thyroidectomy for intrathoracic goiters reaching the carina tracheae. *Arch Surg* 2006; **141**(1): 82–5.
19. Torre G, Borgonovo G, Amato A, et al. Surgical management of substernal goiter: analysis of 237 patients. *Am Surg* 1995; **61**(9): 826–31.
20. Lahey FH. Diagnosis and management of intrathoracic goiter. *JAMA* 1920; **75**: 163–6.
21. deSouza FM, Smith PE. Retrosternal goiter. *J Otolaryngol* 1983; **12**(6): 393–6.
22. Falor WH, Kelly TR, Krabill WS. Intrathoracic goiter. *Ann Surg* 1955; **142**(2): 238–47.
23. Agarwal A, Agarwal S, Tewari P, et al. Clinicopathological profile, airway management, and outcome in huge multinodular goiters: an institutional experience from an endemic goiter region. *World J Surg* 2012; **36**(4): 755–60.
24. Lahey F, Swinton NW. Intrathoracic goitre. *Sur Gynaecol Obstet* 1934; **59**: 627–37.
25. Mack E. Management of patients with substernal goiters. *Surg Clin North Am* 1995; **75**(3): 377–94.
26. Buckley JA, Stark P. Intrathoracic mediastinal thyroid goiter: imaging manifestations. *AJR Am J Roentgenol* 1999; **173**(2): 471–5.
27. Rives JD. Mediastinal aberrant goiter. *Ann Surg* 1947; **126**(5): 797–810.
28. Hall TS, Caslowitz P, Popper C, Smith GW. Substernal goiter versus intrathoracic aberrant thyroid: a critical difference. *Ann Thorac Surg* 1988; **46**(6): 684–5.
29. Singh B, Lucente FE, Shaha AR. Substernal goiter: a clinical review. *Am J Otolaryngol* 1994; **15**(6): 409–16.
30. Madjar S, Weissberg D. Retrosternal goiter. *Chest* 1995; **108**(1): 78–82.
31. Foroulis CN, Rammos KS, Sileli MN, Papakonstantinou C. Primary intrathoracic goiter: a rare and potentially serious entity. *Thyroid* 2009; **19**(3): 213–18.
32. Shaha AR, Burnett C, Alfonso A, Jaffe BM. Goiters and airway problems. *Am J Surg* 1989; **158**(4): 378–80; discussion 380–1.
33. Alfonso A, Christoudias G, Amaruddin Q, et al. Tracheal or esophageal compression due to benign thyroid disease. *Am J Surg* 1981; **142**(3): 350–4.
34. Sabaretnam M, Mishra A, Chand G, et al. Assessment of swallowing function impairment in patients with benign goiters and impact of thyroidectomy: a case control study. *World J Surg* 2012; **36**(6): 1293–9.
35. Holl-Allen RT. Laryngeal nerve paralysis and benign thyroid disease. *Arch Otolaryngol* 1967; **85**(3): 335–7.
36. White ML, Doherty GM, Gauger PG. Evidence-based surgical management of substernal goiter. *World J Surg* 2008; **32**(7): 1285–300.
37. Landerholm K, Järhult J. Should asymptomatic retrosternal goitre be left untreated? A prospective single-centre study. *Scand J Surg* 2015; **104**(2): 92–5.
38. Shaha AR, Alfonso AE, Jaffe BM, Operative treatment of substernal goiters. *Head Neck* 1989; **11**(4): 325–30.
39. Vadasz P, Kotsis L. Surgical aspects of 175 mediastinal goiters. *Eur J Cardiothorac Surg* 1998; **14**(4): 393–7.
40. Gomes MN, Hufnagel CA. Superior vena cava obstruction: a review of the literature and report of 2 cases due to benign intrathoracic tumors. *Ann Thorac Surg* 1975; **20**(3): 344–59.
41. Barber PV, Edwards JD, Enoch BA, et al. Retrosternal goitre presenting as bleeding oesophageal varices. *Br Med J* 1976; **1**(6009): 564.
42. Anders HJ. Compression syndromes caused by substernal goitres. *Postgrad Med J* 1998; **74**(872): 327–9.
43. Pemberton HS. Sign of submerged goitre. *Lancet* 1946; **248**(6423): 509.
44. Delgado C, Martin M, de la Portilla F. Retrosternal goiter associated with chylothorax. *Chest* 1994; **106**(6): 1924–5.
45. Lowry SR, Shinton RA, Jamieson G, Manché A. Benign multinodular goitre and reversible Horner's syndrome. *Br Med J (Clin Res Ed)* 1988; **296**(6621): 529–30.
46. Gadisseux P, Minette P, Trigaux JP, Michel L. Cerebrovascular circulation "steal" syndrome secondary to a voluminous retrotracheal goiter. *Int Surg* 1986; **71**(2): 107–9.
47. Vanderpump MP, Tunbridge WM, French JM, et al. The incidence of thyroid disorders in the community: a twenty-year follow-up of the Whickham Survey. *Clin Endocrinol (Oxf)* 1995; **43**(1): 55–68.
48. Fast S, Bonnema SJ, Hegedüs L. The majority of Danish nontoxic goitre patients are ineligible for Levothyroxine suppressive therapy. *Clin Endocrinol (Oxf)* 2008; **69**(4): 653–8.
49. Brito JP, Gionfriddo MR, Al Nofal A, et al. The accuracy of thyroid nodule ultrasound to predict thyroid cancer: systematic review and meta-analysis. *J Clin Endocrinol Metab* 2014; **99**(4): 1253–63.
50. Sheth S. Role of ultrasonography in thyroid disease. *Otolaryngol Clin North Am* 2010; **43**(2): 239–55, vii.
51. Jeebun V, Natu S, Harrison R. Diagnosis of a posterior mediastinal goitre via endobronchial ultrasound-guided transbronchial needle aspiration. *Eur Respir J* 2009; **34**(3): 773–5.
52. Qureishi A, Garas G, Tolley N, et al. Can pre-operative computed tomography predict the need for a thoracic approach for removal of retrosternal goitre? *Int J Surg* 2013; **11**(3): 203–8.
53. Grainger J, Saravanappa N, D'Souza A, et al. The surgical approach to retrosternal goiters: the role of computerized tomography. *Otolaryngol Head Neck Surg* 2005; **132**(6): 849–51.
54. Rugiu MG, Piemonte M. Surgical approach to retrosternal goitre: do we still need sternotomy? *Acta Otorhinolaryngol Ital* 2009; **29**(6): 331–8.
55. Kilic D, Findikcioglu A, Ekici Y, et al. When is transthoracic approach indicated in retrosternal goiters? *Ann Thorac Cardiovasc Surg* 2011; **17**(3): 250–3.
56. Nervi M, Iacconi P, Spinelli C, et al. Thyroid carcinoma in intrathoracic goiter. *Langenbecks Arch Surg* 1998; **383**(5): 337–9.
57. Tindall H, Griffiths AP, Penn ND. Is the current use of thyroid scintigraphy rational? *Postgrad Med J* 1987; **63**(744): 869–71.
58. Thusoo TK, Gupta U, Kochhar K, Hira HS. Upper airway obstruction in patients with goiter studies by flow volume loops and effect of thyroidectomy. *World J Surg* 2000; **24**(12): 1570–2.
59. Parker MJ. Interpreting spirometry: the basics. *Otolaryngol Clin North Am* 2014; **47**(1): 39–53.
60. Menon SK, Jagtap VS, Sarathi V, et al. Prevalence of upper airway obstruction in patients with apparently asymptomatic

euthyroid multi nodular goitre. *Indian J Endocrinol Metab* 2011; **15**(Suppl 2): S127–31.
61. Albareda M, Viguera J, Santiveri C, et al. Upper airway obstruction in patients with endothoracic goiter enlargement: no relationship between flow-volume loops and radiological tests. *Eur J Endocrinol* 2010; **163**(4): 665–9.
62. Geraghty JG, Coveney EC, Kiernan M, O'Higgins NJ, et al. Flow volume loops in patients with goiters. *Ann Surg* 1992; **215**(1): 83–6.
63. Jauregui R, Lilker ES, Bayley A. Upper airway obstruction in euthyroid goiter. *JAMA* 1977; **238**(20): 2163–6.
64. Stang MT, Armstrong MJ, Ogilvie JB, et al. Positional dyspnea and tracheal compression as indicators for goiter resection. *Arch Surg* 2012; **147**: 621–6.
65. Chen AY, Bernet VJ, Carty SE, Davies TF, et al. American Thyroid Association statement on optimal surgical management of goiter. *Thyroid* 2014; **24**(2): 181–9.
66. Moten AS, Thibault DP, Willis AW, Willis AL. Demographics, disparities and outcomes in substernal goiters in the United States. *Am J Surg* 2016; **211**: 703–09.
67. Hsu AL. Critical airway obstruction by mediastinal masses in the intensive care unit. *Anaesth Int Care* 2013; **41**(4): 543–8.
68. Gharib H, Papini E, Garber JR, et al. American Association of Clinical Endocrinologists and Associazione Medici Endocrinologi medical guidelines for clinical practice for the diagnosis and management of thyroid nodules. *Endocr Pract* 2006; **12**(1): 63–102.
69. Winbladh A, Jarhult J. Fate of the non-operated, non-toxic goitre in a defined population. *Br J Surg* 2008; **95**(3): 338–43.
70. Testini M, Nacchiero M, Miniello S, et al. Management of retrosternal goiters: experience of a surgical unit. *Int Surg* 2005; **90**(2): 61–5.
71. Hardy RG, Bliss RD, Lennard TW, et al. Management of retrosternal goitres. *Ann R Coll Surg Engl* 2009; **91**(1): 8–11.
72. Pieracci FM, Fahey TJ 3rd. Substernal thyroidectomy is associated with increased morbidity and mortality as compared with conventional cervical thyroidectomy. *J Am Coll Surg* 2007; **205**(1): 1–7.
73. Fast S, Nielsen VE, Bonnema SJ, Hegedüs L. Time to reconsider nonsurgical therapy of benign non-toxic multinodular goitre: focus on recombinant human TSH augmented radioiodine therapy. *Eur J Endocrinol* 2009; **160**(4): 517–28.
74. Le Moli R, Wesche MF, Tiel-Van Buul MM, Wiersinga WM. Determinants of longterm outcome of radioiodine therapy of sporadic non-toxic goitre. *Clin Endocrinol (Oxf)* 1999; **50**(6): 783–9.
75. Kay TW, d'Emden MC, Andrews JT, Martin FI. Treatment of non-toxic multinodular goiter with radioactive iodine. *Am J Med* 1988; **84**(1): 19–22.
76. Huysmans DA, Hermus AR, Corstens FH, et al. Large, compressive goiters treated with radioiodine. *Ann Intern Med* 1994; **121**(10): 757–62.
77. Nygaard B, Hegedüs L, Gervil M, et al. Radioiodine treatment of multinodular non-toxic goitre. *BMJ* 1993; **307**(6908): 828–32.
78. Bonnema SJ, Knudsen DU, Bertelsen H, et al. Does radioiodine therapy have an equal effect on substernal and cervical goiter volumes? Evaluation by magnetic resonance imaging. *Thyroid* 2002; **12**(4): 313–17.
79. Ron E, Doody MM, Becker DV, et al. Cancer mortality following treatment for adult hyperthyroidism. Cooperative Thyrotoxicosis Therapy Follow-up Study Group. *JAMA* 1998; **280**(4): 347–55.
80. Metso S, Auvinen A, Huhtala H, et al. Increased cancer incidence after radioiodine treatment for hyperthyroidism. *Cancer* 2007; **109**(10): 1972–9.
81. Metso S, Jaatinen P, Huhtala H, et al. Increased cardiovascular and cancer mortality after radioiodine treatment for hyperthyroidism. *J Clin Endocrinol Metab* 2007; **92**(6): 2190–6.
82. Angusti T, Codegone A, Pellerito R, Favero A. Thyroid cancer prevalence after radioiodine treatment of hyperthyroidism. *J Nucl Med* 2000; **41**(6): 1006–9.
83. Bonnema SJ, Nielsen VE, Boel-Jørgensen H, et al. Improvement of goiter volume reduction after 0.3 mg recombinant human thyrotropin-stimulated radioiodine therapy in patients with a very large goiter: a double-blinded, randomized trial. *J Clin Endocrinol Metab* 2007; **92**(9): 3424–8.
84. Nielsen VE, Bonnema SJ, Boel-Jørgensen H, et al. Stimulation with 0.3-mg recombinant human thyrotropin prior to iodine 131 therapy to improve the size reduction of benign nontoxic nodular goiter: a prospective randomized double-blind trial. *Arch Intern Med* 2006; **166**(14): 1476–82.
85. Silva MN, Rubió IG, Romão R, et al. Administration of a single dose of recombinant human thyrotrophin enhances the efficacy of radioiodine treatment of large compressive multinodular goitres. *Clin Endocrinol (Oxf)* 2004; **60**(3): 300–8.
86. Bennett AM, Hashmi SM, Premachandra DJ, Wright MM. The myth of tracheomalacia and difficult intubation in cases of retrosternal goitre. *J Laryngol Otol* 2004; **118**(10): 778–80.
87. Dempsey GA, Snell JA, Coathup R, Jones TM. Anaesthesia for massive retrosternal thyroidectomy in a tertiary referral centre. *Br J Anaesth* 2013; **111**(4): 594–9.
88. Abdel Rahim AA, Ahmed ME, Hassan MA. Respiratory complications after thyroidectomy and the need for tracheostomy in patients with a large goitre. *Br J Surg* 1999; **86**(1): 88–90.
89. Findlay JM, Sadler GP, Bridge H, Mihai R. Post-thyroidectomy tracheomalacia: minimal risk despite significant tracheal compression. *Br J Anaesth* 2011; **106**(6): 903–6.
90. Bittar D. Respiratory obstruction associated with induction of general anesthesia in a patient with mediastinal Hodgkin's disease. *Anesth Analg* 1975; **54**(3): 399–403.
91. Wang G, Lin S, Yang L, et al. Surgical management of tracheal compression caused by mediastinal goiter: is extracorporeal circulation requisite? *J Thorac Dis* 2009; **1**(1): 48–50.
92. Lalwani P, Chawla R, Kumar M, et al. Posterior mediastinal mass: do we need to worry much? *Ann Card Anaesth* 2013; **16**(4): 289–92.
93. Raffaelli M, De Crea C, Ronti S, et al. Substernal goiters: incidence, surgical approach, and complications in a tertiary care referral center. *Head Neck* 2011; **33**(10): 1420–5.
94. Hedayati N, McHenry CR. The clinical presentation and operative management of nodular and diffuse substernal thyroid disease. *Am Surg* 2002; **68**(3): 245–51; discussion 251–2.
95. Erbil Y, Bozbora A, Barbaros U, et al. Surgical management of substernal goiters: clinical experience of 170 cases. *Surg Today* 2004; **34**(9): 732–6.
96. Hsu B, Reeve TS, Guinea AI, et al. Recurrent substernal nodular goiter: incidence and management. *Surgery* 1996; **120**(6): 1072–5.
97. McHenry CR, Piotrowski JJ. Thyroidectomy in patients with marked thyroid enlargement: airway management, morbidity, and outcome. *Am Surg* 1994; **60**(8): 586–91.
98. Gardiner KR, Russell CF. Thyroidectomy for large multinodular colloid goitre. *J R Coll Surg Edinb* 1995; **40**(6): 367–70.
99. Mishra A, Agarwal A, Agarwal G, Mishra SK. Total thyroidectomy for benign thyroid disorders in an endemic region. *World J Surg* 2001; **25**(3): 307–10.

Parathyroid disease

CHAPTER 71

CLINICAL EVALUATION OF HYPERCALCAEMIA

Mo Aye and Thozhukat Sathyapalan

Introduction 827	Laboratory evaluation 828
Interpretation of serum calcium 827	References 832
Clinical evaluation... 828	

SEARCH STRATEGY

Data in this chapter may be updated by a PubMed search using the keywords: hypercalcaemia, parathyroid hormone, primary hyperparathyroidism, familial hypocalciuric hypercalcaemia and hypercalcaemia of malignancy.

INTRODUCTION

Since the advent of the automated serum biochemistry analyser in the 1970s, mild to moderate hypercalcaemia has become a common incidental finding in clinical practice. Very high serum calcium (more than 3 mmol/L, 12 mg/dL), however, remains uncommon. Whenever hypercalcaemia is confirmed, a definitive diagnosis needs to be established. Primary hyperparathyroidism (PHPT) and malignancy are the two commonest causes of hypercalcaemia and account for more than 90% of cases.[1] Initial evaluation should be directed at distinguishing between the two.

INTERPRETATION OF SERUM CALCIUM

Before any further investigation, it is essential to make sure that the apparent hypercalcaemia is not a false-positive laboratory test result. Biologically relevant hypercalcaemia is due to an elevated ionized ('free') calcium concentration. Most standard laboratories measure total calcium rather than ionized calcium. Up to 45% of serum calcium is bound to protein, principally albumin. Increased protein binding can result in apparent elevation in serum total calcium concentration without any rise in the ionized calcium.

This phenomenon is called 'pseudohypercalcaemia'. It may occur in those with hyperalbuminaemia from severe dehydration. Rarely, calcium-binding paraproteins in multiple myeloma present with pseudohypercalcaemia. Conversely, when albumin is low as in chronic illness, severe malnutrition or liver disease, serum total calcium may appear to be falsely low although ionized calcium is normal. If a laboratory is able to measure ionized calcium reliably, it would be preferable to measure it directly in clinical situations where serum albumin may be high or low.

Most laboratories will correct measured serum total calcium with respect to albumin, assuming normal albumin to be 40 g/L:

$$[Ca]_{adjusted} = [Ca]_{total} + \{0.02 \times (40 g/L - [Alb]_{serum})\}$$

where:

$[Ca]_{adjusted}$: adjusted serum calcium, in mmol/L

$[Ca]_{total}$: measured serum total calcium, in mmol/L

$[Alb]_{serum}$: measured serum albumin concentration, in g/L.

With US units measuring calcium in mg/dL and albumin in g/dL, the correction formula is:

$$[Ca]_{adjusted} = [Ca]_{total} + \{0.8 \times (4 g/dL - [Alb]_{serum})\}$$

A single, unexpected serum calcium reading should be repeated to confirm the diagnosis. If hypercalcaemia is detected in association with dehydration, calcium should be retested after correction of dehydration. Where cumulative results are available, previous calcium results should be reviewed to see if hypercalcaemia is acute or chronic. Chronic, stable, asymptomatic hypercalcaemia is likely to be benign, the commonest cause being PHPT. Familial hypocalciuric hypercalcaemia (FHH), an inherited condition characterized by a loss of function mutation of the calcium-sensing receptor (CaSR), may also present as chronic asymptomatic hypercalcaemia.

The degree of hypercalcaemia also may be useful diagnostically. Primary hyperparathyroidism usually presents with borderline or mild hypercalcaemia (serum calcium concentration often below 2.75 mmol/L, 11 mg/dL). Values above 3.25 mmol/L (13 mg/dL) are unusual in primary hyperparathyroidism, although they do occur, and are more common in patients with malignancy-associated hypercalcaemia.

CLINICAL EVALUATION

Mild to moderate hypercalcaemia is usually asymptomatic. Signs and symptoms of hypercalcaemia are non-specific and similar regardless of the cause. These include constitutional symptoms such as weakness, lethargy, intellectual weariness and depression.[2] Very severe hypercalcaemia both contributes to and is exacerbated by dehydration. Additional features should be sought in the clinical presentation to help uncover the underlying cause of hypercalcaemia.

An adult with asymptomatic hypercalcaemia probably has PHPT. Clinical features which favour this diagnosis include chronicity, modest elevation in serum calcium levels, slow or no progression of hypercalcaemia over time, normal physical examination and lack of obvious alternative diagnoses. Established end-organ damage such as osteoporotic fragility fractures, declining renal function and kidney stones may be surrogate features of chronicity and their presence may provide some reassurance that the underlying cause of hypercalcaemia is not neoplastic.

PHPT typically occurs in middle-aged or older women. A finding of high calcium in a patient outside this demographic group should prompt consideration of causes other than PHPT. Younger patients with hypercalcaemia may have a familial cause. Parathyroid cancer should be suspected in young men presenting with PTH-driven hypercalcaemia.

Although hypercalcaemia can be the first manifestation of malignancy, in most patients with malignancy-associated hypercalcaemia, the disease is not occult. Typically, features of underlying disease would have brought the patient to medical attention; hypercalcaemia is detected as an additional finding during further investigations. Rapidly progressive or very high serum calcium concentrations should raise concerns about malignancy. Breast, lung, colon and prostate cancers are the commonest solid organ tumours with skeletal metastases.[3]

TABLE 71.1 Causes of hypercalcaemia

Parathyroid hormone dependent

I. Primary hyperparathyroidism
   a. Solitary or multiple adenomas
   b. Parathyroid hyperplasia
   c. Parathyroid cancer
II. Tertiary hyperparathyroidism (end-stage renal failure)
III. Ectopic PTH secretion (very rare)
IV. Multiple endocrine neoplasia – MEN 1 and 2a
V. Inactivating mutations in CaSR or G proteins: familial hypocalciuric hypercalcaemia (FHH)
VI. Lithium therapy (alteration in CaSR function)

Parathyroid hormone independent

I. Neoplastic
   a. Osteolytic skeletal metastases
   b. Multiple myeloma
   c. Paraneoplastic syndrome (PTHrP mediated)
II. Chronic granulomatous disease (e.g. sarcoidosis)
III. Endocrine disorders
   a. Hyperthyroidism
   b. Acromegaly
   c. Hypoadrenalism
IV. Medications
   a. Thiazide diuretics
   b. Hypervitaminosis A or D
   c. Theophylline
   d. Teriparatide (human recombinant PTH 1-34)
V. Excessive calcium intake
   a. Milk-alkali syndrome
   b. Total parenteral nutrition
VI. Miscellaneous
   a. Immobilization
   b. Metaphyseal chondrodysplasia
   c. Congenital lactase deficiency

Clinical evaluation should include an enquiry about weight loss, change in bowel habit, examination of the respiratory system, breast examination in women and prostate examination in men. Multiple myeloma may present with hypercalcaemia alone.

Dietary calcium intake and medications (prescription and non-prescription drugs, herbal preparations, calcium and vitamin supplements) are important to diagnose drug-induced hypercalcaemia (**Table 71.1**). If possible, any medication that may be causing hypercalcaemia should be discontinued. With the exception of vitamin D excess, hypercalcaemia is generally mild in drug-induced hypercalcaemia. Diagnoses are not mutually exclusive. It is possible for thiazide diuretics to accentuate or unmask mild or incipient PHPT.

LABORATORY EVALUATION

Once hypercalcaemia has been confirmed, the next step should be to determine whether this elevation is PTH-driven. PTH mediates hypercalcaemia both in PHPT and FHH. All other causes of hypercalcaemia suppress PTH (**Table 71.2**).

TABLE 71.2 Differential diagnosis of hypercalcaemia

Condition	Total adjusted serum calcium	Ionized serum calcium	Phosphate	Parathyroid hormone (PTH)	Urinary calcium excretion	Vitamin D	Comments
Pseudohypercalcaemia	↑	⇔	⇔	⇔	⇔	⇔	May occur in presence of calcium-binding proteins other than albumin (e.g. in myeloma)
Primary hyperparathyroidism (PHPT)	↑	↑	⇔ or ↓	↑ or high-normal	High-normal or ↑	⇔ or ↓	Usually mild to moderate. More common in postmenopausal women. May be hereditary, e.g. MEN 1 and 2a
Familial hypocalciuric hypercalcaemia (FHH)	↑	↑	⇔ or ↓	↑	Ca:creatinine excretion ratio <0.01	⇔	Autosomal dominant. Usually presents with asymptomatic hypercalcaemia
Osteolytic skeletal metastases	↑↑	↑↑	⇔ or ↑	↓↓	↑ but routine measurement not needed	⇔	May present with very high calcium level, often over a short duration. Clinical features of primary solid organ tumour usually predominates
Multiple myeloma	↑	↑	⇔ or ↑	↓	⇔ or ↑	⇔	Hypercalcaemia may be the first presenting clinical feature. Usually has normal alkaline phosphatase
Paraneoplastic syndrome	↑	↑	⇔ or ↑	↓	⇔ or ↑	⇔	Raised PTHrP. Features of malignancy may predominate
Vitamin D excess (oral ingestion, granulomatous disease, lymphoma)	↑	↑	↑ or ⇔	↓	⇔ or ↑	⇔ or ↑	1,25-DHCC raised in granulomatous disease and lymphoma

Serum parathyroid hormone (PTH)

ELEVATED OR MID- TO HIGH-NORMAL PTH

Hypercalcaemia with elevated PTH is likely to be PTH-driven. Elevated PTH in the setting of hypercalcaemia is most likely to be due to PHPT.[4] For reasons which are not clear, PHPT also appears to be more common in cancer patients than in the general population.[5,6] PTH should still be measured even in patients with known malignancy who present with elevated calcium. Confirmation of PHPT in this situation could obviate a psychologically distressing and ultimately futile search for metastatic or paraneoplastic disease.

Parathyroid hormone levels should be interpreted in context. Physiologically, once hypercalcaemia is established, production of PTH from the parathyroid glands should be switched off. A PTH level within the upper half of the reference range despite hypercalcaemia is 'inappropriately elevated'; this picture is still consistent with PTH-driven hypercalcaemia and hence with the diagnosis of PHPT. It should also be noted that PTH levels rise with age. In a younger individual (age <45 years), the normative range is lower and narrower. PHPT in a young individual may show a PTH value that is within normal range for the population.[7]

However, with a PTH level within the upper end of the normative range, other diagnoses such as FHH should also be considered. PTH levels may be influenced by pre-analytic factors related to collection, storage and transit.[8] PTH should be repeated when the test results appear equivocal.

In chronic kidney disease, there is complex interplay of regulatory hormones (PTH, calcitriol and fibroblast growth factor 23 (FGF-23)). The characteristic biochemical picture is elevated PTH in response to high phosphate, low calcitriol (1,25 dihydroxycholecalciferol), with or without low serum calcium. Hypercalcaemia is relatively rare until relatively later stages of chronic kidney disease (estimated glomerular filtration rate <30 mL/min/1.73 m^2 BSA). Hypercalcaemia in this situation may occur as a progression of compensatory ('appropriate') parathyroid hyperplasia to an autonomous overactivity of parathyroid glands. This is known as tertiary hyperparathyroidism. The diagnosis is relatively straightforward since the emerging trend would be well documented in a patient with progressive renal decline; most patients who develop tertiary hyperparathyroidism also have end-stage renal failure. Hypercalcaemia may be absent in those patients if they are on haemodialysis.

Hypercalcaemia may also be seen patients with adynamic bone disease, a form of chronic kidney disease mineral bone disorder (CKD-MBD) characterized by low bone turnover. In such patients, calcium elevation results from failure of the bone to take up calcium after an oral calcium load, such as calcium carbonate to treat hyperphosphataemia.[9] PTH in adynamic bone disease is only modestly elevated, typically (<11 pmol/L, 110 pg/mL) and may appear disproportionately low relative to the degree of renal dysfunction.

Following renal transplantation, the parathyroid hyperplasia subsides over a period of months to years. Sometimes, hypercalcaemia develops after successful renal transplantation as calcitriol production is restored before parathyroid hyperplasia has subsided completely.

SUPPRESSED PTH

PTH-independent causes should be considered if the PTH is low or within the lower half of the reference range. Serum intact PTH levels below 2.2 pmol/L (20 pg/mL) are highly suggestive of a non-PTH related cause.

Malignancy should be suspected if the hypercalcaemia is of short duration and especially if the calcium level is very high (>3 mmol/L). More often than not, the primary tumour is a solid organ tumour and the patient may present with clinical features attributable to the primary cancer. Hypercalcaemia may arise from direct lytic metastases from non-small cell lung cancer, breast cancer, renal cell carcinoma and gastrointestinal tumours. Skeletal symptoms such as bone pain and pathological fractures may be present. It is recognized, however, that hypercalcaemia and the extent of skeletal metastases are poorly correlated.[10]

In the absence of overt skeletal metastases, humoral hypercalcaemia of malignancy may arise from the action of tumour-derived humoral factors, such as PTH-related protein (PTHrP). PTHrP-related hypercalcaemia has been described in association with solid organ tumours, particularly squamous cell carcinoma of the lung and skin, head and neck tumours and renal cell carcinoma. PTHrP does not react with PTH assays. Humoral hypercalcaemia is accompanied by suppressed PTH levels on standard second- and third-generation PTH assays. Measurement of PTHrP is seldom justified in clinical practice as the underlying malignancy should be self-evident. Levels of PTH and 1,25DHCC are both suppressed appropriately.[11]

Hypercalcaemia occurs in as many as 30% of patients with multiple myeloma.[10] Anaemia, bicytopenia or pancytopenia may be accompanied by reversal of albumin–globulin ratio and impaired renal function. Alkaline phosphatase usually remains normal as osteoclastic bone resorption in myeloma is not accompanied by osteoblastic attempts at bone formation. A number of cytokines have been implicated, including tumour necrosis factor α (TNF-α), transforming growth factor β (TGF-β), interleukin-1 and leukaemia inhibitory factor. In the past, these humoral agents were collectively covered under a generic term 'osteoclast activating factor'. Elevated PTHrP has also been described in myeloma patients.

24-hour urinary calcium and urine calcium/creatinine excretion ratio

Urinary calcium should be measured routinely in suspected PHPT. The 2013 Fourth International Workshop consensus criteria lists calcium excretion of more than 10 mmol/day (400 mg/day) as one of the criteria for considering surgery in asymptomatic PHPT.

Familial hypocalciuric hypercalcaemia is rare in the general population but it is clinically important because the biochemical picture is indistinguishable from PHPT except for hypocalciuria.[12] The 24-hour urinary calcium is typically less than 5 mmol/day (200 mg/day) in FHH. Calculating urinary calcium/creatinine (Ca/Cr) excretion ratio is preferable to simply measuring 24-hour urinary calcium for excluding FHH. The ratio is calculated using paired serum and urinary calcium and creatinine samples, using the following formula:

$$\text{Ca/Cr excretion ratio} = \frac{\text{Urine calcium}\left(\frac{\text{mmol/L}}{\text{L}}\right) \times \text{Plasma creatinine}\left(\frac{\mu\text{mol/L}}{1000}\right)}{\text{Plasma calcium}\left(\frac{\text{mmol/L}}{\text{L}}\right) \times \text{Urine creatinine}\left(\frac{\text{mmol}}{\text{L}}\right)}$$

The Ca/Cr excretion ratio is less than 0.01 in approximately 80% of patients with FHH. In PHPT, the Ca/Cr excretion ratio is typically greater than 0.02.

When evaluating patients with apparent hypocalciuria, other factors which may cause hypocalciuria should also be considered and eliminated. These include vitamin D deficiency (<30 nmol/L, <12 ng/mL), very low calcium intake, treatment with thiazide drugs and lithium therapy.

In FHH, there may be a family history of hypercalcaemia as FHH follows an autosomal dominant pattern of inheritance. Patients with FHH have few, if any, symptoms. Hypercalcaemia tends to be modest. PTH itself may be high-normal or just modestly elevated. Serum magnesium levels may also be raised. Hypocalciuric hypercalcaemia may be acquired as an autoimmune disorder and may be associated with antithyroid, antigliadin or antiendomyseal antibodies.

Vitamin D metabolites

Except in cases of obvious humoral hypercalcaemia of malignancy, serum vitamin D should be performed routinely in non-PTH dependent hypercalcaemia. An elevated 25-hydroxycholecalciferol [25(OH)D] is indicative of excessive ingestion of vitamin D. There is no agreement on the level of 25(OH)D at which hypercalcaemia typically occurs. Many experts define vitamin D intoxication as a value greater than 375 nmol/L (150 ng/mL).[13]

Parathyroid hormone catalyses the conversion of 25(OH)D to 1,25 dihydroxycholecalciferol (1,25-DHCC). With long-standing PHPT, it is common for the substrate 25(OH)D to become depleted. Serum calcium may drift lower with coexisting vitamin D deficiency with the true extent of hypercalcaemia being revealed only after vitamin D deficiency has been corrected.

Measurement of 1,25-DHCC is not required routinely but should be considered if the cause of hypercalcaemia is unclear. Extra-renal conversion of 25(OH)D to 1,25-DHCC occurs in granulomatous diseases and in lymphoma. A chest X-ray to look for malignancy or sarcoidosis may be helpful. Most patients with sarcoidosis or lymphoma generally have clinically evident pulmonary and extrapulmonary manifestations. In the absence of such clinical involvement, a thorough search for occult pulmonary, renal, hepatic, ocular and bone marrow granulomas is indicated.

PTH-independent hypercalcaemia associated with normal or low vitamin D metabolites may result from unsuspected stimulation of bone resorption (as in multiple myeloma, thyrotoxicosis, prolonged immobility, hypervitaminosis A), or unrecognized high calcium intake especially in the face of milk-alkali syndrome.

Serum phosphate

Parathyroid hormone is phosphaturic. A low phosphate level may occur in PHPT and in PTHrP-driven humoral hypercalcaemia. Vitamin D increases reabsorption of phosphate from renal tubules. Hypercalcaemia which occurs in association with vitamin D excess or in granulomatous diseases is associated with high or high-normal phosphate levels. Phosphate levels are variable in FHH.

Diagnostic imaging

Evidence of osteitis fibrosa on a bone film is very specific for primary hyperparathyroidism but is only seen in about 5% of cases. Radiographs of the skeleton are no longer recommended in view of the rarity of radiologically detectable bone disease. There is no role for high-resolution neck ultrasound, computed tomography or technetium ^{99m}Tc sestamibi (MIBI) scintigraphy in routine evaluation of suspected PHPT. These tests are useful only for pre-operative localization of confirmed disease.

Tests of other endocrine diseases

In most situations, hypercalcaemia occurring in association with other endocrine diseases is an ancillary finding. The clinical presentation is usually dominated by signs and symptoms of the underlying endocrine condition.

THYROID FUNCTION TESTS

Mild hypercalcaemia occurs in 15–20% of patients with thyrotoxicosis.[14] Hypercalcaemia persisting after control of thyrotoxicosis should be evaluated on its own merits, as there may be concomitant hyperparathyroidism.

EVALUATION OF ADRENAL FUNCTION

Hypercalcaemia is an occasional finding in adrenal insufficiency.[15] Possible contributory factors are: increased bone resorption, ECF volume contraction, haemoconcentration and increased proximal tubular reabsorption of calcium. Cortisol administration reverses hypercalcaemia within days. Again, persistence of hypercalcaemia despite treatment should prompt evaluation. Hypercalcaemia has also been described in central hypoadrenalism due to hypophysitis.[16]

EXCLUSION OF PHAEOCHROMOCYTOMA

PHPT occurs as part of multiple endocrine neoplasia (MEN 2a). Rarely, hypercalcaemia can be a feature of phaeochromocytoma itself due to humoral production of PTHrP.

Miscellaneous conditions

Other less common causes of hypercalcaemia due to increased bone resorption include Paget's disease of the bone, especially if the patient is immobilized, administration of oestrogen or a selective-oestrogen receptor modifier (SERM) to patients with breast cancer who have extensive skeletal metastases[17] and hypervitaminosis A (ingestion of more than 50 000 IU daily).[18] Retinoic acid causes a dose-dependent increase in bone resorption, resulting in overall incidence of hypercalcaemia of approximately 30%.[19, 20] Theophylline toxicity has been associated with mild hypercalcaemia.[21] In Jansen-type metaphyseal chondrodysplasia, a rare form of dwarfism, mutations in PTH or PTHrP receptor genes result in continuous activation of the receptor even with low PTH levels of PTH secretion.[22] The clinical picture is that of asymptomatic but significant hypercalcaemia with low phosphate and normal or low PTH.

KEY POINTS

- Primary hyperparathyroidism and malignancy are the two commonest causes of hypercalcaemia.
- Once hypercalcaemia is confirmed, the next step is to determine whether this elevation is parathyroid hormone driven by measuring parathyroid hormone.
- Parathyroid hormone levels will be raised or inappropriately normal in primary hyperparathyroidism and suppressed in malignancy related hypercalcaemia.
- In patients with familial hypocalciuric hypercalcaemia the urine calcium creatinine excretion ratio is typically less than 0.01.

REFERENCES

1. Lafferty FW. Differential diagnosis of hypercalcemia. *J Bone Miner Res* 1991; **6** Suppl 2: S51–9; discussion S61.
2. Silverberg SJ. Non-classical target organs in primary hyperparathyroidism. *J Bone Miner Res* 2003; **17**(Suppl 2): N117–25.
3. Stewart AF. Clinical practice. Hypercalcemia associated with cancer. *N Eng J Med* 2005; **352**(4): 373–9.
4. Endres DB, Villanueva R, Sharp CF Jr, Singer FR. Immunochemiluminometric and immunoradiometric determinations of intact and total immunoreactive parathyrin: performance in the differential diagnosis of hypercalcemia and hypoparathyroidism. *Clin Chem* 1991; **37**(2): 162–8.
5. Fierabracci P, Pinchera A, Miccoli P, et al. Increased prevalence of primary hyperparathyroidism in treated breast cancer. *J Endocrinol Invest* 2001; **24**(5): 315–20.
6. Burtis WJ, Wu TL, Insogna KL, Stewart AF. Humoral hypercalcemia of malignancy. *Ann Intern Med* 1988; **108**(3): 454–7.
7. Silverberg SJ, Bilezikian JP. Primary hyperparathyroidism. In: Jameson JL, De Groot LJ, de Krester DM, et al. (eds). *Endocrinology: Adult and pediatric*. 7th ed. Philadelphia: Elsevier Saunders; 2015, vol. 1, pp. 1105–24.
8. Hanon EA, Sturgeon CM, Lamb EJ. Sampling and storage conditions influencing the measurement of parathyroid hormone in blood samples: a systematic review. *Clin Chem Lab Med* 2013; **51**(10): 1925–41.
9. Meric F, Yap P, Bia MJ. Etiology of hypercalcemia in hemodialysis patients on calcium carbonate therapy. *Am J Kidney Dis* 1990; **16**(5): 459–64.
10. Ray DW. Ectopic hormone syndromes. In: Jameson JL, De Groot LJ, de Krester DM, et al. (eds). *Endocrinology: Adult and pediatric*. 7th ed. Philadelphia: Elsevier Saunders; 2015, p. 2628.
11. Schilling T, Pecherstorfer M, Blind E, et al. Parathyroid hormone-related protein (PTHrP) does not regulate 1,25-dihydroxyvitamin D serum levels in hypercalcemia of malignancy. *J Clin Endocrinol Metab* 1993; **76**(3): 801–3.
12. Hinnie J. Familial benign hypocalciuric hypercalcaemia. *Scott Med J* 2011; **56**(1): 36–8.
13. Holick MF. Vitamin D Deficiency. *N Engl J Med* 2007; **357**(3): 266–81.
14. Iqbal AA, Burgess EH, Gallina DL, et al. Hypercalcemia in hyperthyroidism: patterns of serum calcium, parathyroid hormone, and 1,25-dihydroxyvitamin D3 levels during management of thyrotoxicosis. *Endocr Pract* 2003; **9**(6): 517–21.
15. Montoli A, Colussi G, Minetti L. Hypercalcaemia in Addison's disease: calciotropic hormone profile and bone histology. *J Intern Med* 1992; **232**(6): 535–40.
16. Vasikaran SD, Tallis GA, Braund WJ. Secondary hypoadrenalism presenting with hypercalcaemia. *Clin Endocrinol (Oxf)* 1994; **41**(2): 261–4.
17. Legha SS, Powell K, Buzdar AU, Blumenschein GR. Tamoxifen-induced hypercalcemia in breast cancer. *Cancer* 1981; **47**(12): 2803–6.
18. Bhalla K, Ennis DM, Ennis ED. Hypercalcemia caused by iatrogenic hypervitaminosis A. *J Am Diet Assoc* 2005; **105**(1): 119–21.
19. Villablanca JG, Khan AA, Avramis VI, Reynolds CP. Hypercalcemia: a dose-limiting toxicity associated with 13-cis-retinoic acid. *Am J Pediatr Hematol Oncol* 1993; **15**(4): 410–15.
20. Akiyama H, Nakamura N, Nagasaka S, et al. Hypercalcaemia due to all-trans retinoic acid. *Lancet* 1992; **339**(8788): 308–9.
21. Jacobs TP, Bilezikian JP. Clinical review: rare causes of hypercalcemia. *J Clin Endocrinol Metab* 2005; **90**(11): 6316–22.
22. Schipani E, Langman CB, Parfitt AM, et al. Constitutively activated receptors for parathyroid hormone and parathyroid hormone-related peptide in Jansen's metaphyseal chondrodysplasia. *N Engl J Med* 1996; **335**(10): 708–14.

CHAPTER 72

INVESTIGATION OF HYPERPARATHYROIDISM

M. Shahed Quraishi

Introduction 833	Complex clinical settings 839
Non-invasive localization studies 833	References 840
Invasive localization techniques 838	

SEARCH STRATEGY

Data in this chapter may be updated by a Medline search using the keywords: hyperparathyroidism, localization, invasive, non-invasive, imaging, intra-operative and sestamibi.

INTRODUCTION

Primary hyperparathyroidism (PHPT) is the commonest cause of hypercalcaemia in the outpatient population. Over the last decade the advent of improved pre-operative imaging, intra-operative PTH monitoring (IOPTH) techniques and radioguided surgery has resulted in the development of various techniques of 'minimal access parathyroidectomy'. These have succeeded the classic 'four-gland bilateral exploration', with better outcomes.[1,2] Primary hyperparathyroidism is usually caused by a solitary adenoma (80–85%), hyperplasia (10–15%), double adenoma (2–5%) or parathyroid carcinoma (<1%).[3]

Pre-operative localization studies are useful in determining the appropriate surgical technique and approach; they should not be used as a diagnostic tool or as a factor to decide the need to operate and should be ordered only after a decision has been made to operate. Information gained contributes to reduced surgical time, reduced hospital stay, less risk of permanent hypoparathyroidism and use of local/regional anaesthesia.[4]

Several modalities can be used to image the parathyroid gland and can be categorized into:

- **non-invasive studies:** radiology/sonography-based imaging, nuclear medicine imaging
- **invasive techniques:** selective venous sampling (SVS), parathyroid arteriography, fine-needle aspiration.

NON-INVASIVE LOCALIZATION STUDIES

Ultrasonography

The neck is scanned with the patient in the supine position and head slightly extended to simulate the position during surgery. Usually sonography is performed with a 10 MHz or a higher transducer to provide gray scale and colour Doppler imaging in the transverse and longitudinal planes. Ultrasound (US) provides detailed anatomical information of the gland and structures adjacent to it. Techniques can be utilized to aid identification of enlarged parathyroid glands, which include rotating the neck away from the side being examined, gentle compression of the neck and asking the patient to swallow during the scanning.

The results are highly operator-dependent with sensitivity and specificity of US imaging in the ranges 51–96% and 90–98% respectively.[4-6] The sensitivity of glands >500 mg is 86% compared with 75% for glands <500 mg.[7] Factors that reduce the sensitivity of US are a background of concomitant multinodular thyroid, parathyroid hyperplasia and multiple adenomas. There seems to be no difference in US detection of adenomas due to serum calcium and PTH values.[8]

Attention is focused on the area posterior and inferior to the thyroid gland, medial to the carotid sheath and the tracheo-oesophageal grove. The superior parathyroid glands are less commonly ectopic as compared to the inferior pair. Up to 20% of PAs are found at ectopic sites. The usual sites are the retro-oesophageal, retro- or paratracheal, superior mediastinum, within the carotid sheath, thymus tissue and adjacent to the hyoid bone. Scanning should be extended to the retromandibular area superiorly down to the clavicle/suprasternal notch if not found in the usual sites.

The classic enlarged parathyroid adenoma is greater than 1 cm and typically a homogeneously hypoechoic, ovoid, well-marginated, extrathyroidal solid lesion with a fat or connective tissue plane separating it from the thyroid gland. Parathyroid adenomas are typically highly vascular lesions, which on colour Doppler sonography reveal a peripheral vascular arc arising from a vascular pedicle on the superior or inferior pole of the adenoma (**Figure 72.1**). The main supply is from a branch of the inferior or superior thyroid artery. In comparison, normal lymph nodes have a central echogenic fatty hilum surrounded by hypoechogenic cortex with small hilar vessels and are typically kidney-shaped.

Larger adenomas may be multilobed, pear-shaped or complex with cystic/solid components. Other structures in the vicinity which may mimic PA are the oesophagus and the longus colli muscle. They are recognized on US imaging by identifying the striated muscles, position and their elongated structures. Parathyroid carcinomas may show cystic degeneration, calcification, heterogeneity with local invasion and local lymphadenopathy. Intra-thyroidal adenomas (**Figure 72.2**) may mimic thyroid nodules whereas thyroid nodules may appear like parathyroid adenomas (**Figure 72.3**). In Hashimoto's thyroiditis central compartment lymphadenopathy may make it difficult to identify parathyroid adenomas due to similar features.[9]

US-guided fine-needle aspiration and rapid PTH assay can help differentiate an adenoma from a lymph node, and it is utilized especially to evaluate patients before revision surgery.[10] If all four parathyroid glands are enlarged on ultrasound, the diagnosis may be PT hyperplasia; the glands may appear asymmetrically enlarged and individual hyperplastic glands may be difficult to distinguish from an adenoma. The advantages and disadvantages of US scanning are listed in **Table 72.1**.

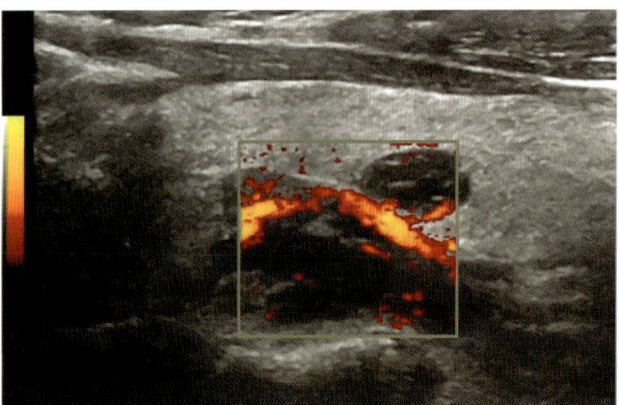

Figure 72.1 Colour Doppler sonography reveals a peripheral vascular arc arising from a vascular pedicle on adenoma.

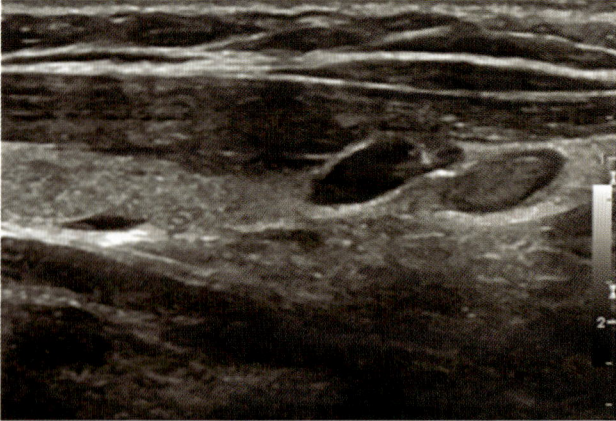

Figure 72.2 Intrathyroidal adenoma.

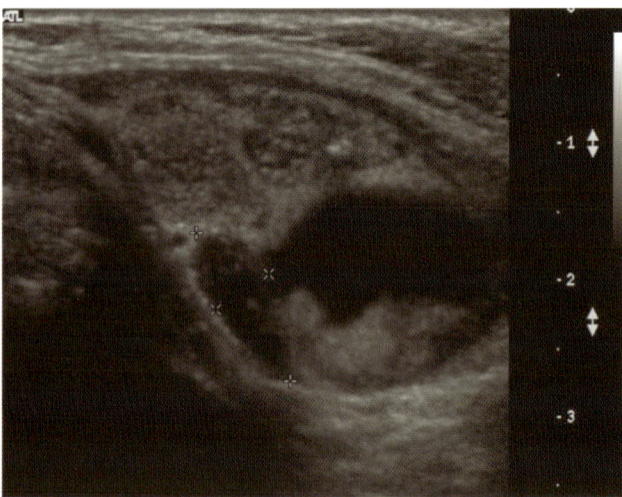

Figure 72.3 Multinodular goitre with parathyroid adenoma.

TABLE 72.1 Ultrasonography for parathyroid adenomas

Advantages	Pitfalls
Inexpensive	Operator-dependent
No radiation exposure	Ectopic or intra-thyroid adenomas missed
Non-invasive	
Helpful in fine-needle biopsy	Limited value in retro-oesophageal, paratracheal and mediastinal adenomas
	Difficult to differentiate between small adenomas and lymph nodes

For best results and interpretation of parathyroid sonography, well-trained and experienced personnel with a specialist interest are essential and lead to successful localization of the parathyroid adenomas in the surgical field.

Imaging using radioactive tracers

SESTAMIBI SCINTIGRAPHY

^{99m}Tc sestamibi was originally used for diagnostic cardiology and was accidentally found to be concentrating in parathyroid adenoma tissue.[11]

TABLE 72.2 Predictive factors for sestamibi scan

Positive	Negative
High oxyphil content (>20%)	Thyroid nodules
Vitamin D deficiency	Multigland disease
High PTH levels	Adenomas <600 mg
High calcium levels	Calcium channel blockers

Sestamibi diffuses passively through cell membranes and accumulates almost exclusively in mitochondria. High mitochondria content in oxyphilic cells in parathyroid adenomas is considered to be the reason for the excessive tissue uptake in PHPT.[12] A meta-analysis of 35 ultrasound and 14 sestamibi-SPECT studies had a pooled sensitivity of 76.1% and 78.9% respectively.[13]

Factors influencing sestamibi imaging include the following and are summarized in **Table 72.2**:

- **Calcium:** A higher calcium level is more likely to be observed in patients with positive sestamibi scans. In a study of 102 patients, a positive sestamibi scan was found in over 95% of patients with calcium over 11.3 mg/dL.[14] Other studies suggested that the severity of hyperparathyroidism has an influence on sestamibi scans, with positive scans in 64% of asymptomatic patients, in 83% with nephrolithiasis and in 100% of patients with severe bone involvement.[15]
- **PTH:** A high PTH level was directly related to the uptake ratio and positive scans, with almost 100% sensitivity when the PTH levels exceed 200 pg/mL.[16] This was not replicated by others[17] and PTH levels do not allow selection of candidates for pre-operative scanning.[18]
- **Vitamin D deficiency:** In a study of 421 patients with low cholecalciferol levels, positive scans were more likely in those who were vitamin D-deficient than in those with normal vitamin D.[19]
- **Calcium channel blockers:** The use of these interferes with the sestamibi uptake by parathyroid cells and reduces the sensitivity of ^{99m}Tc-MIBI parathyroid SPECT.[20]
- **Oxyphil content:** Adenomas with >20% oxyphil cell content are associated with a positive scan while small adenomas (<600 mg) and low oxyphil cells (<20%) are likely to give negative results.[21]
- **Multigland disease:** In a study of 123 patients, none of the 15 patients with multigland disease were identified pre-operatively. It is a major shortcoming of sestamibi scanning in identifying multigland disease.[22]
- **Thyroid disease:** In the presence of thyroid nodules, the sensitivity of sestamibi scanning is low (92% vs 53%).[23] However, a large retrospective study did not find any difference.[24]

Sestamibi scintigraphy is the imaging of choice for pre-operative localization of parathyroid adenomas. ^{99m}Tc sestamibi is taken up by the mitochondria of the salivary, thyroid and parathyroid tissue. In parathyroid adenomas the mitochondria-rich oxyphil cells retain the radiotracer for longer than in thyroid tissue.[25] It is a functional scan and provides limited anatomical details.

The patient should be positioned as on the operating table with a sandbag under the shoulders under the gamma camera. Dual phase planer images are taken 10 minutes after injection of ^{99m}Tc sestamibi and again 2 hours later to identify a focus of retained radiotracer consistent with a hyperfunctioning parathyroid gland. It is better at picking up mediastinal ectopic glands not identified in ultrasound imaging (**Figure 72.4**). It is also used to identify adenomas during radioguided surgery. The combination of sestamibi scans with 3-dimensional (SPECT) imaging, fusion with

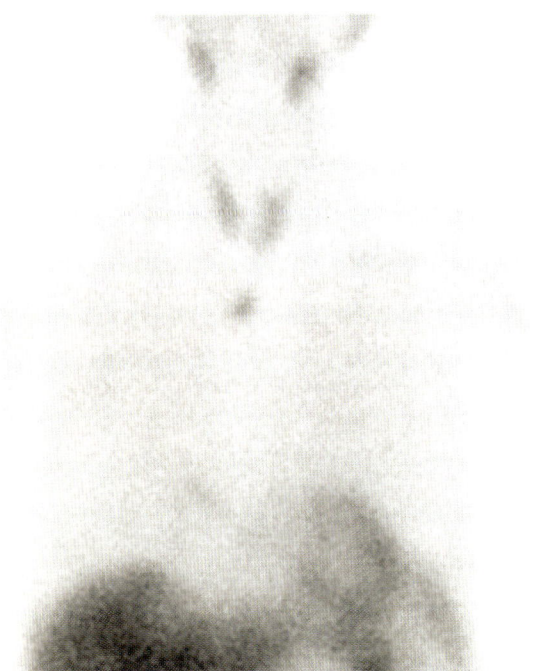 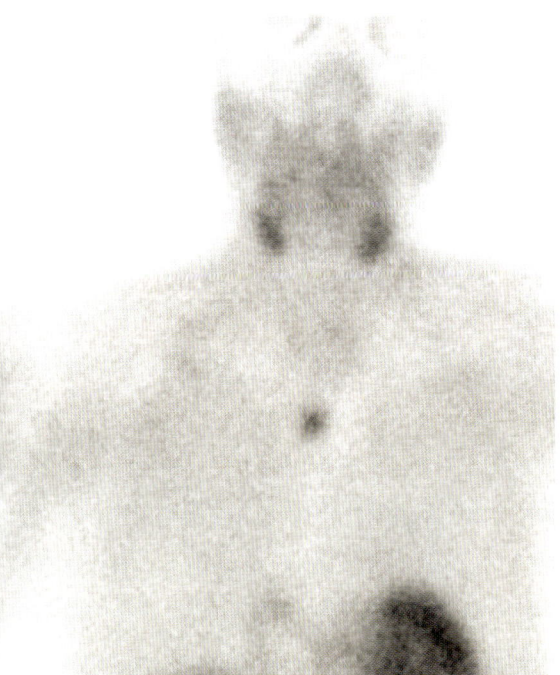

Figure 72.4 Sestamibi scan showing ectopic parathyroid in the mediastinum.

computed tomography (MIBI-SPECT-CT) and thyroid subtraction scans helps obtain better results.

SPECT

Sestamibi–single-photon emission computed tomography (SPECT-MIBI) provides multidimensional higher-resolution images, which helps to detect glands deep in the neck and improves detection of ectopic glands, hence aiding focused surgical techniques. Various studies have shown that SPECT (92–98%) improves the sensitivity of abnormal parathyroid gland in comparison to sestamibi scintigraphy (71–79%).[26, 27] Its sensitivity to identify multigland disease is, however, limited (**Figure 72.5**).

SPECT-CT FUSION

The addition of an integrated SPECT-CT scanner combines the gamma camera with a multidetector CT (**Figure 72.6**). The SPECT provides the functional information while the CT provides the anatomical information which facilitates surgical exploration.[28] A study using SPECT-CT revealed the exact position of the abnormal gland in 102 out of 116 patients (88%), while CT or SPECT-MIBI alone was predictive in 65% and 55% respectively.[29]

SUBTRACTION THYROID SCAN

Dual isotope subtraction scintigraphy is useful in identifying abnormal parathyroid glands in the presence of thyroid pathology. The patient is given a radiotracer which accumulates in thyroid and parathyroid (sestamibi) followed by a thyroid-specific radiotracer (radioiodine ^{123}I or technetium pertechnetate (^{99m}Tc pertechnetate).[30]

After taking images of both radiotracers, computer software is used to subtract the thyroid element from the combined thyroid parathyroid (sestamibi) image, revealing the parathyroid area (**Figure 72.7**). The limitation of this technique is that the image quality can be compromised due to motion artefact.

COMPUTED TOMOGRAPHY (CT)

Axial contrast-enhanced fine cuts (2.5–3 mm) through the neck will help localize PAs in 46–87% of cases,[31, 32] allowing accurate imaging for focused surgical techniques. This modality is available in most hospitals but it is a costly procedure with exposure to radiation. On routine use, studies have not found any advantage over ultrasound in identifying abnormal parathyroid glands. It is helpful in identifying ectopic glands in the mediastinum or

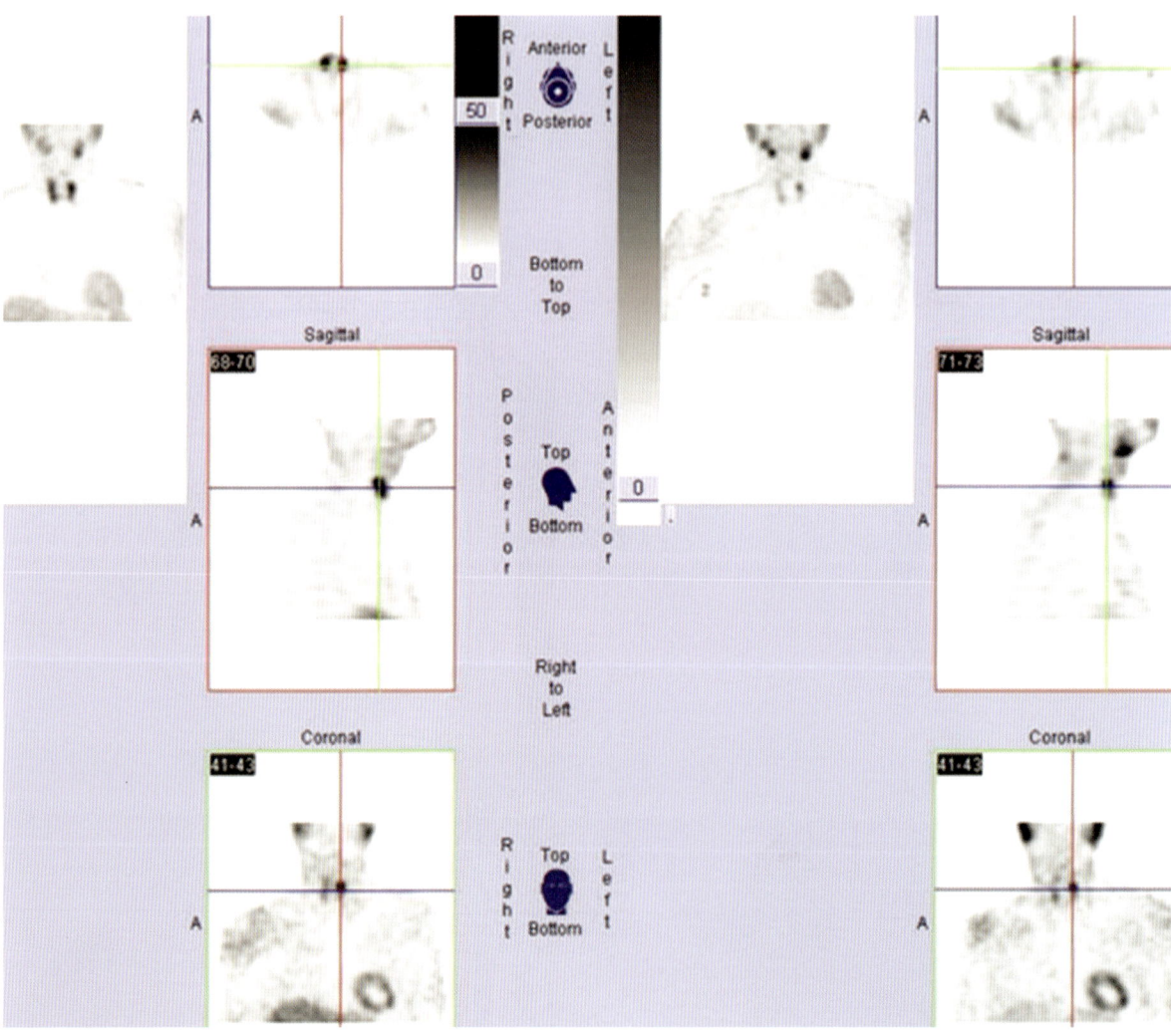

Figure 72.5 SPECT-MIBI.

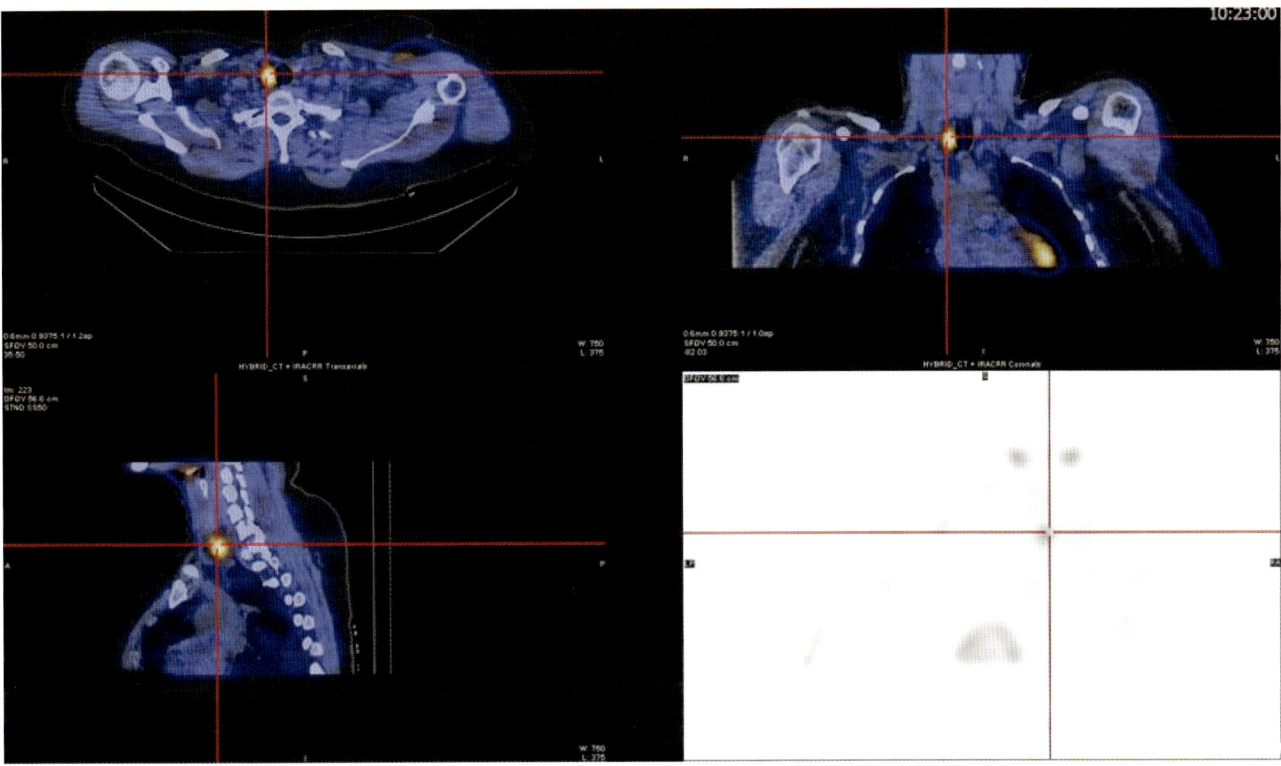

Figure 72.6 MIBI-SPECT-CT.

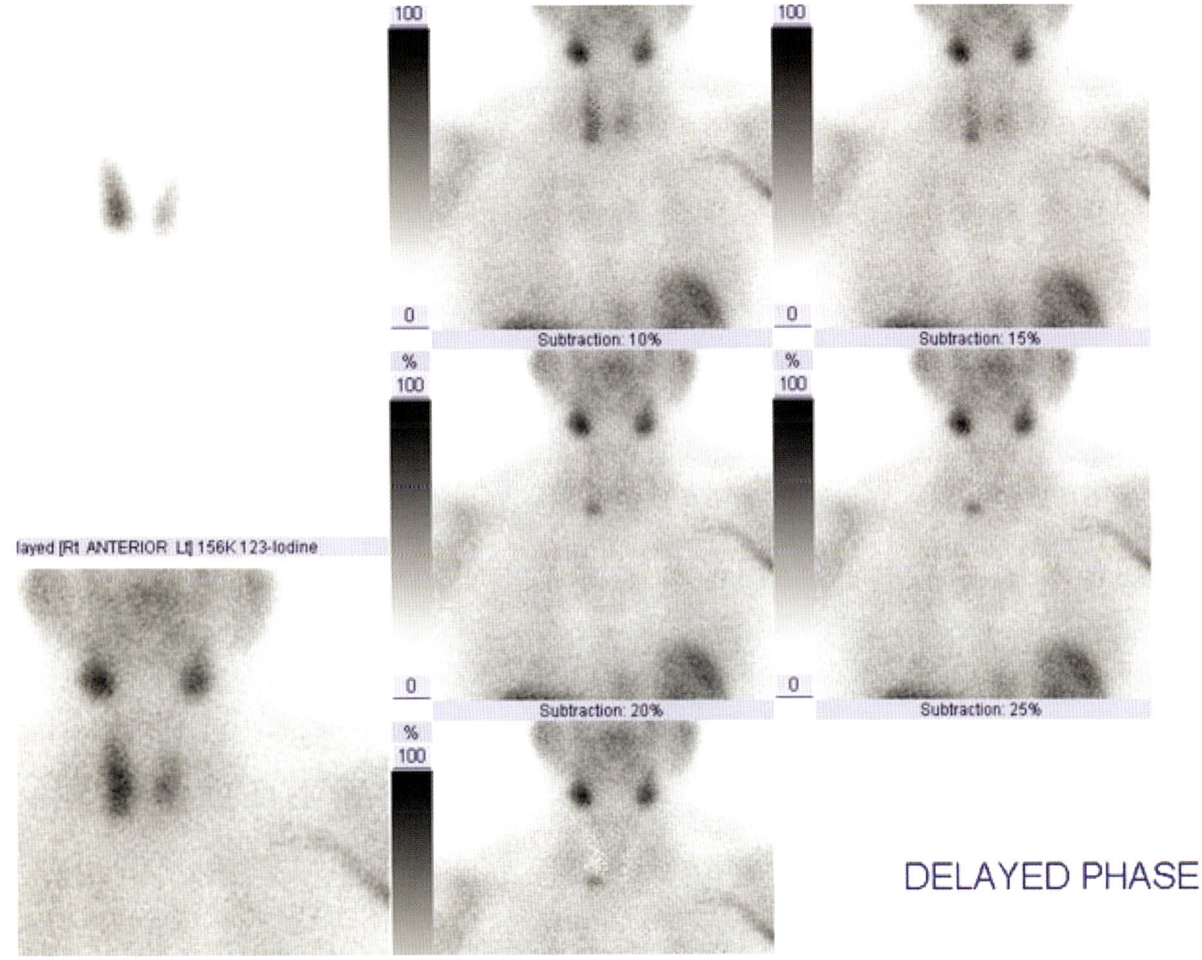

Figure 72.7 Dual isotope: Sestamibi/iodine 123, subtraction study.

trachea-oesophageal groove, especially in patients with a prior failed neck exploration and distorted tissue planes.[33]

Four-dimensional computed tomography (4D-CT) techniques utilize the characteristic of rapid contrast uptake and washout of parathyroid adenomas. The name is derived from an added dimension from the rapid changes of perfusion of contrast over time to 3D-CT. It provides both anatomical and functional data about the abnormal parathyroid glands. The image protocol for 4D-CT scans initially consists of an unenhanced scan followed by an intravenous bolus of non-ionic contrast (2 mL/kg with a maximum of 120 mL at 4 mL/second). Triple-phase 1.5 mm axial scans are repeated from the angle of the mandible to the carina at 30, 60 and 90 seconds after the administration of contrast.

Information from 4D-CT helps to localize ectopic glands (in the deep neck, mediastinum or laterally within the carotid sheath) or intra-thyroid parathyroid adenomas. Prior to the intravenous administration of contrast material, parathyroid adenomas demonstrate attenuation similar to that of muscle. Parathyroid adenomas tend to be hypervascular structures with variable contrast enhancement and early washout. A hypervascular soft-tissue mass near the expected location of the parathyroid glands is considered to represent a parathyroid adenoma (**Figure 72.8**). Ectopic glands may be seen, most commonly within the mediastinum. This helps to improve pre-operative planning in revision surgery in a scarred field with poor tissue planes and thus reduces operative morbidity.[34–36]

MAGNETIC RESONANCE IMAGING (MRI)

This modality is less commonly used than ultrasound and sestamibi scans for pre-operative localization but is still useful for evaluation of abnormal parathyroid glands due to its excellent anatomic detail. For revision surgery, it provides a non-invasive, radiation-free modality to localize abnormal parathyroid tissue. The reported sensitivity of MRI for abnormal parathyroid tissue ranges from 74% to 88%[37, 38] and images are not degraded by streak artefacts from surgical clips or previous surgery. However, compared to CT scans, MRI appears especially useful in detecting ectopic mediastinal glands, with sensitivities exceeding 80%.[39] Parathyroid adenomas are identified as soft-tissue masses in the expected location of the parathyroid glands. The most common tissue characteristics are intermediate to low T1-weighted images and high signal intensity on T2-weighted images.[40] The accuracy of MRI imaging of parathyroid disease is reduced in concomitant thyroid disease, which is present in up to 40% of patients with hyperparathyroidism.[41]

POSITRON EMISSION TOMOGRAPHY AND CT (PET-CT)

Studies of FDG-PET do not confirm that it is as good an imaging technique as MIBI and ultrasound for abnormal parathyroid glands.[42] In patients with initial diagnosis of hyperparathyroidism, the sensitivity of PET-CT for detection and localization of parathyroid adenomas is not as promising as previously thought.[43] While performance was better in secondary hyperparathyroidism, we believe that PET-CT cannot be recommended for PHPT localization although it may be useful for patients in whom other imaging modalities have failed to find the abnormal parathyroid gland.[44]

INVASIVE LOCALIZATION TECHNIQUES

Selective venous sampling

Selective venous sampling (SVS) is the most common invasive modality used for parathyroid localization and the accuracy is much better than large venous sampling. In patients with suspected residual parathyroid adenomas after unsuccessful surgery or in those where non-invasive methods are negative or conflicting, invasive localization techniques may be helpful. In these situations, SVS has a sensitivity of 75% compared to sestamibi (65%) or ultrasound (50%).[45] A 1.5–2-fold increase in PTH levels allows for identification of side (left vs. right) and region (cervical vs. thoracic). False positive results in SVS can be attributed to post-operative changes in venous flow due to ligatures or scarring.

Factors that need to considered with SVS include costs, expertise, radiation exposure and risks such as haematoma at catheter site, adverse reactions to contrast material and vascular accidents. With intact PTH assays, the sensitivity of SVS has been reported as high as 98%[46] and can be considered as the gold standard in patients with persistent or recurrent hyperparathyroidism and unhelpful non-invasive localization techniques.

Parathyroid arteriography

Selective arteriography was performed to localize adenomas in the past when other non-invasive techniques were not available, with varying results. Due to the risk of central venous system complications associated with this technique, it is rarely used. There may be limited benefit in post-operative patients with altered venous or fascial anatomy due to surgical sequelae.

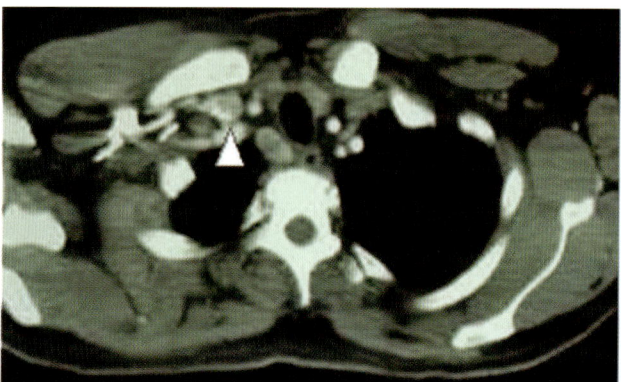

Figure 72.8 4D CT scan. (Courtesy: Dr F. Riffat.)

Fine-needle aspiration

For revision surgery, CT or ultrasound-guided fine-needle aspiration (FNA) can be helpful in distinguishing parathyroid from non-parathyroid tissue.[47, 48] Testing the sample for PTH levels is more sensitive than cytology as thyroid follicular cells may look similar to parathyroid tissue.

COMPLEX CLINICAL SETTINGS

Localization techniques in multigland disease patients such as multiple endocrine neoplasia (MEN) type 1, familial HPT, secondary or tertiary hyperparathyroidism are less accurate. Often the dominant hyperactive parathyroid(s) is prominent and other less active ones may be suppressed in the background. **Figure 72.9** shows the parathyroid localization flow charts for surgery in hyperparathyroidism used at the University of California, San Francisco.[49]

In a systematic review of more than 20 000 cases of solitary adenomas (SA), multiple gland hyperplasia disease (MGHD) and double adenomas (DA), ^{99m}Tc-sestamibi and ultrasound were 88.44% and 78.55% sensitive, respectively, for SA, 44.46% and 34.86% for MGHD, and 29.95% and 16.20% for DA.[50]

In minimal access parathyroidectomy one of the challenges is to identify the posteriorly placed superior adenoma. This not uncommonly placed in the trachea–oesophageal groove, retro-oesophageal area or adherent to the lateral oesophageal wall. It may erroneously be interpreted as an inferior gland in planar sestamibi scans but better identified in SPECT scans. Standard 10 Mhz ultrasound probes may give negative results in these cases due to poor penetration in glands placed in a deep plane.[51]

Hyperparathyroidism in pregnancy could limit the choices of imaging modalities. The first choice would be to try ultrasonography alone and consider surgery only in severe hyperparathyroidism with renal and/or bony complications. Ultrasound-guided FNA with PTH aspiration directly from the gland may be useful for confirmation.[52] If the need for further imaging is necessary, MRI and low-dose sestamibi with radiation shielding to the embryo may help.[53, 54] Mild or moderate presentations are best deferred until pregnancy is over.

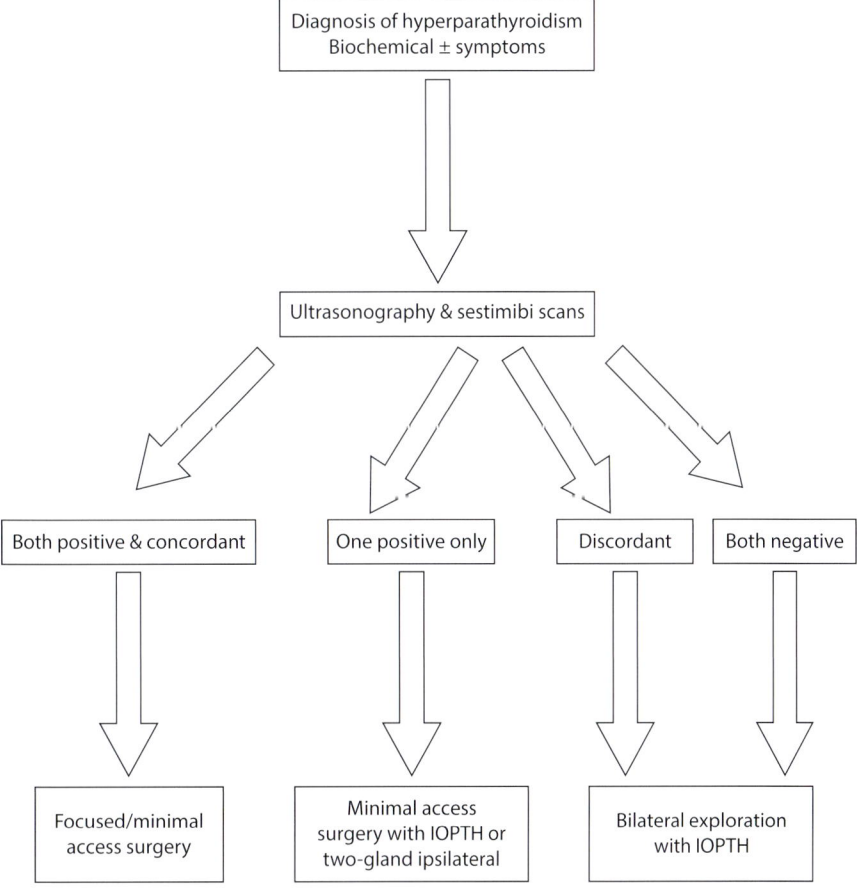

Figure 72.9 Parathyroid localization flow charts for **(a)** first-time surgery used at the University of California, San Francisco. (Modified from Randolph GW. *Surgery of the thyroid and parathyroid glands*, Figures 57.9 and 57.10.)[49]   *(Continued)*

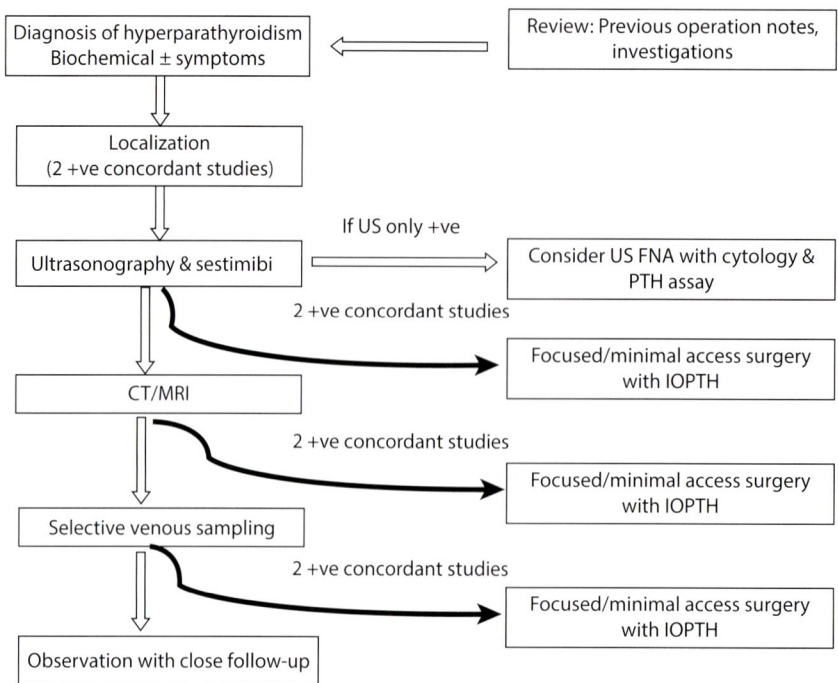

Figure 72.9 (Continued) Parathyroid localization flow charts for **(b)** revision surgery in hyperparathyroidism used at the University of California, San Francisco. (Modified from Randolph GW. *Surgery of the thyroid and parathyroid glands*, Figures 57.9 and 57.10.)[49]

> **KEY POINTS**
>
> - Minimal access, minimally invasive parathyroidectomy is now producing cure rates equal to the traditional four-gland bilateral exploration.
> - This requires good localization studies, and non-invasive techniques such as ultrasound with sestamibi scans are quite often adequate to give satisfactory information to perform a focused surgical procedure as a day case.
> - Invasive techniques are best reserved for revision surgery and negative imaging studies.
> - The final choice of the pre-operative localization studies depends on local expertise, choice and final surgical outcomes.

REFERENCES

1. Greene AB, Butler RS, McIntyre S, et al. National trends in parathyroid surgery from 1998 to 2008: a decade of change. *J Am Coll Surg* 2009; **209**(3): 332–43.
2. Udelsman R, Lin Z, Donovan P. The superiority of minimally invasive parathyroidectomy based on 1,650 consecutive patients with primary hyperparathyroidism. *Ann Surg* 2011; **253**(3): 585–91.
3. Fraker DL, Harsono H, Lewis R. Minimally invasive parathyroidectomy: benefits and requirements of localization, diagnosis, and intraoperative PTH monitoring. Long-term results. *World J Surg* 2009; **33**(11): 2256–65.
4. Kelly CW, Eng CY, Quraishi SM. Open mini-incision parathyroidectomy for solitary parathyroid adenoma. *Eur Arch Otorhinolaryngol* 2014; **271**(3): 555–60.
5. Gritzmann N, Koischwitz D, Rettenbacher T. Sonography of the thyroid and parathyroid glands. *Radiol Clin North Am* 2000; **38**: 1131–45.
6. Abboud B, Sleilaty G, Rabaa L, et al. Ultrasonography: highly accurate technique for preoperative localization of parathyroid adenoma. *Laryngoscope* 2008; **118**(9): 1574–8.
7. Soon PS, Delbridge LW, Sywak MS, et al. Surgeon performed ultrasound facilitates minimally invasive parathyroidectomy by the focused lateral mini-incision approach. *World J Surg* 2008; **32**(5): 766–71.
8. Erbil Y, Barbaros U, Tukenmez M, et al. Impact of adenoma weight and ectopic location of parathyroid adenoma on localization and study results. *World J Surg* 2008; **32**(4): 566–71.
9. Kamaya A, Quon A, Jeffrey RB. Sonography of the abnormal parathyroid gland. *Ultrasound Q* 2006; **22**(4): 253–64.
10. Maser C, Donovan P, Santos F, et al. Sonographically guided fine needle aspiration with rapid parathyroid hormone assay. *Ann Surg Oncol* 2006; **13**(12): 1690–5.
11. Coakley AJ, Kettle AG, Wells CP. et al. 99Tcm sestamibi: a new agent for parathyroid imaging. *Nucl Med Commun* 1989; **10**(11): 791–4.
12. Hetrakul N, Civelek AC, Stagg CA, et al. In vitro accumulation of technetium-99m-sestamibi in human parathyroid mitochondria. *Surgery* 2001; **130**(6): 1011–18.
13. Cheung K, Wang TS, Farrokhyar F, et al. A meta-analysis of preoperative localisation techniques for patients with primary hyperparathyroidism. *Ann Surg Oncol* 2012; **19**: 577–83.
14. Parikshak M, Castillo ED, Conrad MF, et al. Impact of hypercalcaemia and parathyroid hormone level on the sensitivity of preoperative sestamibi scanning for primary hyperparathyroidism. *Am Surg* 2003; **69**(5): 393–8.
15. Bandeira FA, Oliveira RI, Griz LH, et al. Differences in accuracy of ^{99m}Tc-sestamibi scanning between severe and mild forms of primary hyperparathyroidism. *J Nucl Med Technol* 2008; **36**(1): 30–5.
16. Hung GU, Wang SJ, Lin WY. Tc-99m MIBI parathyroid scintigraphy and intact parathyroid hormone levels in hyperparathyroidism. *Clin Nucl Med* **28**: 180–5.
17. Mihai R, Gleeson F, Buley ID, et al. Negative imaging studies for primary hyperparathyroidism are unavoidable: correlation of sestamibi and high-resolution ultrasound scanning with histological analysis in 150 patients. *World J Surg* 2006; **30**: 697–704.

18. Siegal A, Alvarado M, Barth RJ Jr, et al. Parameters in the prediction of the sensitivity of parathyroid scanning. *Clin Nucl Med* 2006; **31**: 679–82.
19. Kandil E, Tufaro AP, Carson KA, et al. Correlation of plasma 25-hydroxyvitamin D levels with severity of primary hyperparathyroidism and likelihood of parathyroid adenoma localization on sestamibi scan. *Arch Otolaryngol Head Neck Surg* 2008; **134**: 1071–5.
20. Friedman K, Somervell H, Patel P, et al. Effect of calcium blockers on the sensitivity of preoperative 99mTc-MIBI SPECT for hyperparathyroidism. *Surgery* 2004; **136**: 1199–204.
21. Erbil Y, Kapran Y, Issever H, et al. The positive effect of adenoma weight and oxyphil cell count on preoperative localization with 99mTc-sestamibi scanning for primary hyperparathyroidism. *Am J Surg* 2008; **195**: 34–9.
22. Katz SC, Wang GJ, Kramer EL, et al. Limitations of technetium 99m sestamibi scintigraphic localization for primary hyperparathyroidism associated with multiglandular disease. *Am Surg* 2003; **69**: 170–5.
23. Sukan A, Reyhan M, Aydin M, et al. Preoperative evaluation of hyperparathyroidism: the role of dual-phase parathyroid scintigraphy and ultrasound imaging. *Ann Nucl Med* 2008; **22**: 123–31.
24. Siperston A, Berber E, Barbosa GF, et al. Predicting the success of limited exploration for primary hyperparathyroidism using ultrasound, sestamibi, and intraoperative parathyroid hormone: analysis of 1158 cases. *Ann Surg* 2008; **248**: 420–8.
25. Palestro CJ, Tomas MB, Tronco GG. Radionuclide imaging of the parathyroid glands. *Semin Nucl Med* 2005; **35**(4): 266–76.
26. Civelek AC, Ozalp E, Donovan P, et al. Prospective evaluation of delayed technetium-99m sestamibi SPECT scintigraphy for preoperative localization of primary hyperparathyroidism. *Surgery* 2002; **131**(2): 149–57.
27. Nichols KJ, Tomas MB, Tronco GG. Preoperative parathyroid scintigraphic lesion localization: accuracy of various types of readings. *Radiology* 2008; **248**(1): 221–32.
28. Sharma J, Mazzaglia P, Milas M, et al. Radionuclotide imaging for hyperparathyroidism (HPT): which is the best technetium-99m sestamibi modality? *Surgery* 2006; **140**(4): 856–63.
29. Prommegger R, Wimmer G, Profanter C, et al. Virtual neck exploration: a new method for localizing abnormal parathyroid glands. *Ann Surg* 2009; **250**(5): 761–5.
30. Leslie WD, Dupont JO, Bybel B, et al. Parathyroid 99mTc-sestamibi scintigraphy: dual tracer subtraction is superior to double-phase washout. *Eur J Nuc Med Mol Imaging* 2002; **29**(12): 1566–70.
31. Johnson NA, Tublin ME, Ogilvie JB. Parathyroid imaging: technique and role in the preoperative evaluation of primary hyperparathyroidism. *Am J Roentgenol* 2007; **188**(6): 1706–15.
32. Gross ND, Weissman JL, Veenker E, et al. The diagnostic utility of computed tomography for preoperative localization in surgery for hyperparathyroidism. *Laryngoscope* 2004; **114**: 227–31.
33. Spieth ME, Gough J, Kasner DL. Role of US with supplemental CT for localization of parathyroid adenomas. *Radiology* 2002; **223**(3): 878–9.
34. Rogers SE, Hunter GJ, Hamberg LM, et al. Improved preoperative planning for directed parathyroidectomy with 4-dimensional computed tomography. *Surgery* 2006; **140**: 932–40.
35. Mortenson MM, Evans DB, Lee JE, et al. Parathyroid exploration in the reoperative neck: improved preoperative localization with 4D-computed tomography. *J Am Coll Surg* 2008; **206**(5): 888–96.
36. Beland MD, Mayo-Smith WW, Grand DJ, et al. Dynamic MDCT for localization of occult parathyroid adenomas in 26 patients with primary hyperparathyroidism. *Am J Roentgenol* 2011; **196**(1): 61–5.
37. Wakamatsu H, Noguchi S, Yamashita H, et al. Parathyroid scintigraphy with 99mTc-MIBI and 123I subtraction: a comparison with magnetic resonance imaging and ultrasonography. *Nucl Med Commun* 2003; **24**(7): 755–62.
38. Lopez Hanninen E, Vogl TJ, Steinmuller T, et al. Preoperative contrast-enhanced MRI of the parathyroid glands in hyperparathyroidism. *Invest Radiol* 2000; **35**(7): 426–30.
39. Ruf J, Lopez Hanninen E, Steinmuller T, et al. Preoperative localization of parathyroid glands: use of MRI, scintigraphy and image fusion. *Nuklearmedizin* 2004; **43**(3): 85–90.
40. Stevens SK, Chang JM, Clark OH, et al. Detection of abnormal parathyroid glands in postoperative patients with recurrent hyperparathyroidism: sensitivity of MR imaging. *Am J Roentgenol* 1993; **160**(3): 607–12.
41. Lee VS, Spritzer CE. MR imaging of abnormal parathyroid glands. *Am J Roentgenol* 1998; **170**(4): 1097–103.
42. Neumann DR, Esselstyn CB, MacIntyre WJ, et al. Comparison of FDG-PET and sestamibi-SPECT in primary hyperparathyroidism. *J Nucl Med* 1996; **37**(11): 1809–15.
43. Herrmann K, Takei T, Kanegae K, et al. Clinical value and limitations of [11c]-methionine PET for detection and localization of suspected parathyroid adenomas. *Mol Imaging Biol* 2009; **11**(5): 356–63.
44. Grassetto G, Alavi A, Rubello D. PET and parathyroid. *PET Clin* 2007; **2**(3): 385–93.
45. Jones JJ, Brunaud L, Dowd CF, et al. Accuracy of selective venous sampling for intact parathyroid hormone in difficult patients with recurrent or persistent hyperparathyroidism. *Surgery* 2002; **132**(6): 944–50.
46. Mihai R, Simon D, Hellman P. Imaging for primary hyperparathyroidism: an evidence-based analysis. *Langenbecks Arch Surg* 2009; **394**(5): 765–84.
47. Doppman JL, Krudy AG, Marx SJ, et al. Aspiration of enlarged parathyroid glands for parathyroid hormone assay. *Radiology* 1983; **148**(1): 31–5.
48. Gooding GA, Clark OH, Stark DD, et al Parathyroid aspiration biopsy under ultrasound guidance in the postoperative hyperparathyroid patient. *Radiology* 1985; **155**(1): 193–6.
49. Randolph GW. *Surgery of the thyroid and parathyroid glands.* 2nd ed. Toronto: Elsevier; 2013, Figures 57.9 and 57.10.
50. Ruda JM, Hollenbeak CS, Stack BC. A systematic review of the diagnosis and treatment of primary hyperparathyroidism from 1995 to 2003. *Otolaryngol Head Neck Surg* 2005; **132**(3): 359–72.
51. Harari A, Mitmaker EJ, Grogan RH, et al. Primary hyperparathyroidism patients with positive pre-operative sestamibi scan and negative ultrasound are more likely to have posteriorly located upper gland adenomas (PLUGs). *Ann Surg Oncol* 2011; **18**(6): 1717–22.
52. Pothiwala P, Levine SN. Parathyroid surgery in pregnancy: review of the literature and localization by aspiration for parathyroid hormone levels. *J Perinatol* 2009; **29**(12): 779–84.
53. McMullen TP, Learoyd DL, Williams DC. Hyperparathyroidism in pregnancy: options for localization and surgical therapy. *World J Surg* 2010; **34**(8): 181–16.
54. Steenvoorde P, Pauwels EK, Harding LK, et al. Diagnostic nuclear medicine and risk for the fetus. *Eur J Nucl Med* 1998; **25**(2): 193–9.

CHAPTER 73

MANAGEMENT OF HYPERPARATHYROIDISM

Neil J.L. Gittoes and John Ayuk

Classification of hyperparathyroidism............843	Is asymptomatic PHPT benign?...............844
Introduction to primary hyperparathyroidism......843	Medical management of PHPT without surgery......847
Changing clinical presentation of PHPT............843	Conclusion 847
What are the indications for parathyroidectomy?........844	References 848
Asymptomatic PHPT 844	

SEARCH STRATEGY

Data in this chapter may be updated by a Medline search using the keywords: hypercalcaemia, parathyroidectomy, primary hyperparathyroidism, cinacalcet. Further relevant articles were obtained by manual screening of the reference lists of selected papers and contemporary textbooks.

CLASSIFICATION OF HYPERPARATHYROIDISM

Hyperparathyroidism literally means excess secretion of parathyroid hormone (PTH). In isolation, the term 'hyperparathyroidism' is of little value in informing clinical practice. For instance, hyperparathyroidism may occur as the result of autonomous hypersecretion of PTH causing hypercalcaemia; conversely physiologically appropriate hypersecretion of PTH may be seen in conditions where hypocalcaemia prevails. Thus the classification of hyperparathyroidism into primary, secondary and tertiary allows an aetiology-based approach to management. Typical biochemical features of primary, secondary and tertiary hyperparathyroidism are shown in Table 73.1.

Depending on specific underlying causes of secondary and susceptibility to tertiary, specific biochemical features will differ. This chapter will focus on the management of primary hyperparathyroidism (PHPT). Because secondary hyperparathyroidism (SHPT) has underlying medical causes, management of the range of conditions causing SHPT (e.g. vitamin D deficiency and chronic renal impairment) is beyond the scope of this chapter.

INTRODUCTION TO PRIMARY HYPERPARATHYROIDISM

PHPT represents a biochemical syndrome of inappropriate or unregulated hypersecretion of parathyroid hormone (PTH) by one or more of the four parathyroid glands in the absence of a recognized stimulus, leading to hypercalcaemia. Most cases are sporadic and caused by a single parathyroid adenoma (85–95%) or multigland disease (5–10%), with parathyroid carcinoma accounting for <1%.[1]

CHANGING CLINICAL PRESENTATION OF PHPT

PHPT was previously considered a relatively rare disorder, with clinical manifestations dominated by renal and/or bone disease. However, in modern times the diagnosis is most frequently recognized coincidentally on biochemical testing in patients evaluated for unrelated complaints. The annual incidence of PHPT is around 20 cases per 100 000, although the prevalence does vary depending on the populations studied and detection methods used.[2, 3]

TABLE 73.1 Biochemical features of primary, secondary and tertiary hyperparathyroidism

	Primary	Secondary	Tertiary
PTH	↑/↑↑	↑↑	↑↑↑
Calcium	↑	↓	↑/↑↑
Phosphate	↓/→	↓ – vitamin D deficiency ↑ – renal failure	↓/↑
Alkaline phosphatase	→/↑	→/↑	↑
Notes		Biochemistry differs according to underlying cause	

Classical skeletal complications (osteitis fibrosa cystica) are present in less than 5% of newly presenting patients and the incidence of renal stones has fallen to around 15–20%.[4] The latter, however, is still the most common complication of PHPT. More diffuse calcification may also be seen in the renal parenchyma (nephrocalcinosis) in association with hypercalciuria and a decline in renal function may be seen with long-standing PHPT.

Neuromuscular manifestations tend to be vague and include fatigue and subjective weakness, as opposed to a definable myopathy. Reduction in neurocognitive function that sometimes ameliorates following successful parathyroidectomy has been described.[5] Psychological and psychiatric symptoms are not in isolation regarded as indications for parathyroidectomy, however.[6]

Peptic ulcer disease and pancreatitis are associations of classical primary hyperparathyroidism. Pancreatitis is rarely seen nowadays because most PHPT is 'mild'. Peptic ulcer disease may be seen in patients who have PHPT in association with multiple endocrine neoplasia syndrome type 1 (MEN-1). Cardiovascular risk is increased in PHPT, particularly with respect to increased vascular stiffness.[7] There is an increased incidence of hypertension with PHPT, although the underlying mechanisms are not fully understood. Results of a number of recent studies suggest parathyroidectomy in hypertensive patients reduces systolic and diastolic blood pressure.[8,9]

WHAT ARE THE INDICATIONS FOR PARATHYROIDECTOMY?

Parathyroidectomy is the only curative treatment for PHPT, with first-time cure rates exceeding 95% of cases.[10] In symptomatic patients or those with evidence of end-organ disease, such as low bone mineral density (BMD) or kidney stones, cohort studies have demonstrated that after successful parathyroidectomy BMD improves substantially and the incidence of kidney stones declines; cognitive function may improve and cardiovascular disease rates and premature death also appear to decrease.[11–14] For these reasons, if no contraindications exist, all patients with symptomatic PHPT or in whom there is evidence of end-organ disease should receive parathyroidectomy.

ASYMPTOMATIC PHPT

The clinical profile of PHPT has shifted from a symptomatic disorder with hypercalcaemia-related symptoms, kidney stones and overt bone disease to a symptomatically more mild condition, and there remains controversy concerning surgical intervention in patients with no clear clinical features. Some clinicians believe 'asymptomatic' patients with no complications can be managed non-surgically, while others believe virtually all patients with biochemical evidence of PHPT, irrespective of how mild, should undergo parathyroidectomy as there may be 'insidious' elements to chronic mild PHPT.[15]

IS ASYMPTOMATIC PHPT BENIGN?

Consequences of untreated asymptomatic PHPT

Developing robust clinical guidelines for the management of asymptomatic PHPT requires a clear understanding of the natural history of the disease. However, large-scale high-quality data in this area are lacking. A prospective study published in 1999 reported no significant change in serum calcium concentration, urinary calcium excretion and BMD after 10 years in 52 patients with asymptomatic PHPT who did not undergo parathyroidectomy.[16] The same group published 15-years follow-up data in the same cohort of patients, reporting a small but significant increase in serum calcium concentration compared to baseline, along with a 10% decline in BMD at one or more sites, although lumbar spine BMD remained unchanged.[17] In addition, there was progression of PHPT in 37% of patients over the 15 years of observation, to the point that criteria for surgery were met.

In a recent well-characterized cohort of 904 untreated patients with mild PHPT (median follow-up 4.7 years), serum calcium did not rise in the group but there was a significant rise in PTH concentration over the follow-up duration.[18] There was progression of PHPT in 121 patients (13%) and 26 (3%) underwent parathyroidectomy for progressive disease during the follow-up period. Baseline age (higher) and PTH concentration were markers for disease progression.[18]

Impact of asymptomatic PHPT on BMD and fracture risk

A small number of studies have prospectively examined bone density changes in treated and untreated asymptomatic PHPT. Studies have generally been short term over 1–2 years. A meta-analysis of such studies has shown small but significant loss of bone density in untreated PHPT, ranging from 0.6% to 1.0% per year.[19] Following parathyroidectomy, there was a rise in bone density, broadly similar to that observed in patients with mild PHPT who did not undergo parathyroidectomy but who were treated with antiresorptive medical therapies.[19]

In a randomized controlled trial of parathyroidectomy versus observation, 28 patients followed up without surgery were found to have a loss of BMD at the femoral neck (−0.4% per year) and total hip (−0.6% per year), but not at the spine or forearm.[20] In 25 patients managed surgically, following parathyroidectomy there was an increase in BMD of the spine, femoral neck, total hip and forearm. Similar findings were reported in two randomized controlled trials comprising 191 patients[21] and 50 patients[22] with asymptomatic PHPT randomized to surgery or observation. The trial of 191 patients reported a significant increase in BMD compared to baseline at the lumbar spine following surgery, with a similar trend at the femoral neck.[21] BMD remained stable in the observation group. At 1 year, the second trial observed a statistically significant change in lumbar spine and total hip BMD between the parathyroidectomy and observation groups.[22] There was no difference in distal radius BMD between the two groups.

In the prospective study of the natural history of asymptomatic PHPT over 15 years, a 10% decline in BMD at one or more sites was observed in patients managed without surgery, although lumbar spine BMD remained unchanged.[17] In patients who underwent parathyroidectomy, there was post-surgical improvement in BMD at all sites (lumbar spine, femoral neck and distal radius). BMD increased and remained above the 10% line for 15 years after surgery.

There are no controlled studies on the risk of fracture in asymptomatic PHPT patients. However, cohort and population studies suggest that fracture risk is increased up to 10 years before diagnosis and treatment of PHPT (relative risk up to 1.8), suggesting fracture risk may be increased in undiagnosed, asymptomatic PHPT patients.[13, 23] The impact of surgery on this potential increased fracture risk remains unclear.

Impact of asymptomatic PHPT on cardiovascular morbidity and mortality

Population and cohort studies have demonstrated that both serum calcium and PTH are independent risk factors for coronary artery disease in subjects *without* PHPT.[24, 25] A number of studies suggest patients with moderate to severe PHPT may have an increased risk of coronary artery disease that appears to decrease after successful parathyroidectomy.[26, 27] However, a small randomized study of 49 patients with mild PHPT demonstrated no significant differences in echocardiographic features at 2 years in untreated and parathyroidectomy patients.[28]

Increased peripheral vascular resistance is an independent marker of cardiovascular risk. A small number of studies have reported increased vascular stiffness in patients with mild PHPT.[29, 30] One study demonstrated that 15% of the variance in the difference between the second and first systolic peaks in the pressure waveform of the radial artery was uniquely accounted for by the presence of PHPT.[30] Interestingly there was a strong positive correlation between PTH and arterial stiffness and PHPT was a stronger predictor of arterial stiffness than traditional risk factors such as age, smoking and hypertension. This suggests that mild asymptomatic PHPT may represent a prominent risk factor for arterial stiffness, which in turn is a predictor of early cardiovascular pathology. The effect of successful parathyroidectomy on arterial stiffness is unknown.

A matched cohort study, using hospital episode statistics and mortality data, demonstrated that patients with mild PHPT had significantly worse cardiovascular outcomes, in terms of mortality and non-fatal events.[18] The risk of other comorbidities was also increased. These adverse outcomes were subsequently shown to be linked to high baseline PTH concentration but not baseline calcium.[31]

Mild PHPT and risk of malignancy

An almost twofold increased incidence of malignant tumours has been reported in patients with PHPT compared with matched controls.[32, 33] However, bias may be present due to a number of factors: some patients may have endocrine tumour syndromes that have PHPT as a feature; in addition, an underlying malignancy is often a prompt for biochemical testing during which incidental PHPT might be detected, and patients with hypercalcaemia detected unexpectedly are likely to undergo detailed assessments for underlying malignancy.[34] Long-term follow-up of patients with mild PHPT has also demonstrated a significant increased risk of malignancy compared to controls (hazard ratio and cardiac index: HR 2.18, CI 1.80–2.65).[35]

Impact of asymptomatic PHPT on neurocognitive function/quality of life

Neurological and neuropsychiatric symptoms have been described in classical PHPT,[36, 37] but it is less clear to what extent they are present (and are reversible) in milder forms of PHPT seen commonly today. Neurological and neuropsychiatric symptoms are especially difficult to define and investigate in mild PHPT. Some studies have demonstrated improvements in quality of life (QOL),[38–40] but others have not.[41, 42] Potential reasons for the inconsistent results include the observational nature of many of the studies, small sample sizes, the inclusion of subjects with symptomatic hyperparathyroidism, lack of appropriate control groups and testing at short intervals after parathyroidectomy.[6]

A number of randomized studies of surgery versus observation have been conducted in patients with mild PHPT that addressed aspects of neuropsychiatric function. In 53 patients randomized to surgery or observation, QOL scores measured using the SF-36 general health survey showed significant decline in five of the nine domains (social functioning, physical problem, emotional problem, energy and health perception) in patients followed up without surgery, but in only one of the nine domains (physical function) in the patients who had parathyroidectomy.[20]

These findings suggest a modest measurable benefit of parathyroidectomy in social and emotional role function. Psychological function as assessed by the Symptom Checklist-90 (SCL-90) scale did not change significantly in either group, except for a decline in anxiety and phobia in patients who had surgery in comparison with those who did not. More recently, in a cohort of 191 patients with mild PHPT randomized to medical observation or surgery, significantly lower QOL and more psychological symptoms were found compared with age- and sex-matched healthy subjects.[21] Both groups were similar at baseline, and no clinically significant changes in these parameters were seen during the 2-year observation period. Another randomized controlled trial of surgery versus observation in 50 patients assessed QOL and psychosocial well-being using Short Form health survey SF-36 and SCL-90 at baseline and after 1 year of follow-up.[22] A modest but significant beneficial effect on QOL (bodily pain, general health, vitality and mental health) was observed in the parathyroidectomy group compared with observation group. One study demonstrated increased anxiety and depression at baseline that did respond positively to parathyroidectomy.[43]

Overall, the findings of these studies are inconsistent and the available data remain incomplete on the precise nature and reversibility of neuropsychological symptoms following surgery for mild PHPT. However, some of the data support a modest beneficial effect of parathyroidectomy on QOL and psychological functioning.[6, 43]

Impact of asymptomatic PHPT on survival

A number of large population-based cohort studies have demonstrated that patients with PHPT appear to be at risk of premature death,[44, 45] with a 50% increase in mortality, predominantly due to cardiovascular disease. However, these data were not specifically derived from asymptomatic patients. A study that examined outcome in an unselected cohort of patients with predominantly uncomplicated, asymptomatic PHPT[46] found overall survival was not reduced, compared to age- and gender-matched controls. Although patients in the highest quartile of serum calcium levels had significantly worse survival than patients in the three lower quartiles, even in this group, compared to age- and gender-matched controls, there was only a trend towards reduced survival in the patients who did not undergo surgery. Based on these data, the authors concluded that the current practice of observing patients with uncomplicated mild PHPT does not compromise survival. However, a recent matched cohort study from Scotland found all-cause mortality was increased in patients with mild primary hyperparathyroidism, demonstrating a hazard ratio of 2.24 (CI 1.99–2.51), incorporating an increase in cardiovascular deaths (HR 2.67 [CI 2.21–3.23]) and cancer deaths (2.69 [CI 2.16–3.56]).[35] Cumulative survival was not linked to baseline calcium, but higher PTH concentrations at baseline did predict worse survival outcome.[31]

Thresholds for surgery in asymptomatic PHPT

Parathyroidectomy is the only cure for PHPT and should be recommended in all patients with symptomatic PHPT or evidence of end-organ damage such as low BMD or kidney stones. However, considerable controversy exists regarding the need for surgery in asymptomatic patients.[47] Emerging data on the natural history of asymptomatic PHPT have demonstrated that the chronic course of the disease may not be as benign as once considered.[15] A small but significant fall in BMD over many years, particularly at sites rich in cortical bone, can also be anticipated after 15 years of observation.[17] In addition, a number of randomized controlled trials of parathyroidectomy versus observation in patients with asymptomatic PHPT have demonstrated improvements in BMD, neurocognitive function and QOL.[20–22] Recent epidemiological data on adverse long-term outcomes in patients with mild untreated PHPT have caused a drift towards a lower threshold for parathyroidectomy. The National Institutes of Health (NIH) have developed consensus guidelines, most recently updated in 2009,[48] giving specific indications for when surgery is recommended in patients with asymptomatic PHPT (**Box 73.1**).

BOX 73.1 National Institutes of Health consensus guidelines for surgery in asymptomatic PHPT

- Age < 50
- Serum calcium > 0.25 mmol/L above upper limit of normal
- Renal
   A. Creatinine clearance < 60 c/min
   B. 24-h urine for calcium > 400 mg/d (> 10 mmol/d)
   C. Presence of nephrolithiasis or nephrocalcinosis by X-ray, ultrasound, or CT
- Bone mineral density (by DXA):
   A. BMD by DXA: T-score < –2.5 at lumbar spine, total hip, femoral neck, or distal 1/3 radius
   B. Vertebral fracture by X-ray, CT, MRI, or VFA
- Medical follow-up undesired or impractical

(Adapted from Bilezikian 2014)

The consensus guidelines also recommend a structured conservative follow-up protocol for patients who do not fulfil the guidelines for surgery (**Box 73.2**) and advice regarding hydration status and symptom recognition. It is in this situation that the potential benefits of a permanent cure need to be balanced against the risks of surgery. A particular concern is that mild disease will progress to disease fulfilling surgical criteria at a time when the patient's fitness for surgery has decreased.

BOX 73.2 Monitoring protocol for patients with asymptomatic PHPT (eGFR: estimated glomerular filtration rate)

Serum calcium annually
   eGFR, annually; serum creatinine, annually. If renal stones suspected, 24-h biochemical stone profile, renal imaging by X-ray, ultrasound, or CT
   Every 1–2 years (3 sites), X-ray or VFA of spine if clinically indicated (e.g., height loss, back pain)

(Adapted from Bilezikian 2014)

These guidelines do not overtly encompass the most recent epidemiological data and, on balance, making an individualized assessment of pros and cons of parathyroidectomy in individual patients is the authors' preferred stance.[34]

MEDICAL MANAGEMENT OF PHPT WITHOUT SURGERY

Although surgery is the only cure for PHPT, medical treatments can be considered for patients who do not fulfil criteria for surgery or those who are unsuitable for or decline surgery. Bisphosphonates and hormone replacement therapy (HRT) are treatment options for those individuals with PHPT for whom the primary goal is skeletal protection, while the calcimimetic cinacalcet effectively lowers serum calcium and PTH levels in PHPT; however, there is a dearth of data demonstrating positive end-organ outcomes.[49]

Intravenous and oral bisphosphonates may cause a transient reduction in serum calcium, but these are not effective in maintaining lower serum calcium levels in patients with PHPT in the long term.[3] However, they can prove useful in managing the bone disease associated with PHPT. Alendronate is the most extensively studied bisphosphonate in PHPT and has been shown to significantly increase BMD in the lumbar spine and femoral neck in patients treated for up to 2 years.[3, 50, 51] The findings of these studies suggest that bisphosphonates, in particular alendronate, may be useful in the treatment of bone disease associated with PHPT when parathyroidectomy is not recommended or possible. However, there are no data demonstrating that BMD changes reflect a reduced fracture risk. In one meta-analysis there was a similar positive effect on BMD with bisphosphonates compared to parathyroidectomy in patients with mild PHPT.[19] Quantitatively similar effects have also been demonstrated with HRT.[19]

Extracellular ionized calcium regulates PTH secretion via the calcium-sensing receptor (CaSR). Stimulation of the CaSR results in inhibition of PTH gene transcription, reduced PTH secretion and reduced parathyroid cell proliferation. Cinacalcet is an orally active calcimimetic, which acts by modifying the CaSR, causing downstream (calcium-like) effects without having true calcium effects peripherally. By mimicking the action of extracellular calcium on the CaSR, cinacalcet blocks PTH secretion. Studies in humans have demonstrated that cinacalcet lowers PTH levels and improves calcium/phosphate homeostasis in patients with primary and secondary hyperparathyroidism.[52, 53] A double-blind, randomized, placebo-controlled study reported normalization of serum calcium in 73% of patients treated with cinacalcet, compared with 5% of placebo-treated patients.[53] PTH decreased by 7.6% in the cinacalcet group, but increased by 7.7% in the placebo group. There were no significant differences in 24-hour urinary calcium levels between the cinacalcet- and placebo-treated patients. Hip and forearm BMD were in the osteopaenic range and remained unchanged throughout the study in both groups. An open-label extension of this study was recently reported, in which 45 subjects from both groups were treated with 30 mg or 50 mg of cinacalcet twice daily for up to 4.5 years.[49] Cinacalcet normalized serum calcium in all patients, and maintained eucalcaemia for the duration of the study. Plasma PTH levels reduced substantially, especially in the latter years, but did not normalize. Mean BMD remained in the normal range (Z-scores of −1 to +1) for the length of the study, with no improvements in BMD observed when expressed as mean change from parent study baseline at the spine, wrist, femoral neck and total femur. A review of studies on the use of cinacalcet in PHPT has confirmed these findings, reporting that cinacalcet effectively lowers serum calcium and PTH levels but does not alter bone turnover or increase BMD.[54]

Despite cinacalcet's beneficial effects on serum calcium and PTH levels in patients with PHPT, there are no data supporting beneficial effects on hard clinical endpoints of fractures (or changes in bone density), kidney stones or cardiovascular disease. QOL has been assessed in a study of 17 patients with persistent PHPT after parathyroidectomy or with contraindications to parathyroidectomy that were treated with cinacalcet;[55] using the SF-36 and Medical Outcomes Study (MOS) Cognitive Functioning scales, the authors found that cinacalcet treatment was associated with improved functional status and well-being in patients with intractable PHPT. The improvements in the Physical Component Summary and Mental Component Summary scores were comparable with the improvements observed in patients with PHPT following parathyroidectomy. This was a small trial, and the results need corroborating in larger studies. In 2008 cinacalcet was approved by the European Commission for the treatment of hypercalcaemia in patients with PHPT for whom parathyroidectomy is indicated on the basis of serum calcium levels but in whom parathyroidectomy is not clinically appropriate or is contraindicated. However, its high cost and lack of data showing improvements in BMD mean that cinacalcet cannot presently be advocated as an alternative to parathyroidectomy.

CONCLUSION

Parathyroidectomy offers the only potential cure for PHPT and should be recommended in all patients with symptomatic PHPT or with evidence of end-organ damage, where there is no obvious contraindication. However, considerable controversy exists regarding the need for surgery in asymptomatic patients. Recently published guidelines have outlined criteria for surgery in the management of asymptomatic PHPT, recommending structured follow-up for patients who do not fulfil these criteria. However, emerging data on the natural history of asymptomatic PHPT have demonstrated that the chronic course of the disease may not be as benign as once considered, with significantly worse cardiovascular outcomes in terms of mortality and non-fatal events, as well as significantly increased risk of malignancy. This has led some clinicians to propose that virtually all patients with biochemical evidence of PHPT, irrespective of how mild, should undergo parathyroidectomy.

Presently there is no alternative medical therapy to parathyroidectomy that has proven efficacy in managing all aspects of PHPT. Alendronate has beneficial effects on BMD but has not been shown to reduce fracture risk or significantly lower serum calcium, while cinacalcet normalizes serum calcium but does not alter BMD.

Despite the high success rate, low morbidity and convenience of modern parathyroidectomy, patients need to be assessed on a case-by-case basis and important clinical considerations need to be balanced to determine whether parathyroidectomy is the best option for individual patients with mild asymptomatic PHPT (**Box 73.3**).

BOX 73.3 Factors influencing management of patients with mild PHPT

Favours conservative management	Favours parathyroidectomy
Old age	Young age
Short life expectancy	Long life expectancy
High operative risk	Low operative risk
Patient preference	Patient preference
Initial low fracture risk	Risk of worsening bone disease
	Risk of worsening renal function
	Neuropsychiatric features
	Cardiovascular risk*
	High baseline PTH*

(Adapted from Gittoes & Cooper 2010[34] and incorporating more recent data* from Yu et al. 2011[35])

KEY POINTS

- PHPT is caused by inappropriate/unregulated hypersecretion of parathyroid hormone by one or more of the four parathyroid glands.
- The clinical profile of PHPT has shifted to a symptomatically more mild condition.
- Skeletal complications, renal stones, neuromuscular manifestations, peptic ulcer disease and pancreatitis are now rarely seen in the context of PHPT.
- Parathyroidectomy is the only curative treatment for PHPT, and if no contraindications exist should be performed in all patients with symptoms or end-organ disease.
- Medical treatments can improve bone mineral density and normalize serum calcium, but have not been shown to improve long-term outcomes.
- Asymptomatic PHPT may have clinical sequelae, and specific indications exist for when surgery is recommended.
- Structured follow up is required for patients with asymptomatic PHPT who do not fulfil criteria for surgery.

REFERENCES

1. Sitges-Serra A, Bergenfelz A. Clinical update: sporadic primary hyperparathyroidism. *Lancet* 2007; **370**: 468–70.
2. Wermers RA, Khosla S, Atkinson EJ, et al. Incidence of primary hyperparathyroidism in Rochester, Minnesota, 1993–2001: an update on the changing epidemiology of the disease. *J Bone Miner Res* 2006; **21**: 171–7.
3. Fraser WD. Hyperparathyroidism. *Lancet* 2009; **374**: 145–58.
4. Silverberg SJ, Shane E, Jacobs TP, et al. Nephrolithiasis and bone involvement in primary hyperparathyroidism. *Am J Med* 1990; **89**: 327–34.
5. Roman SA, Sosa JA, Pietrzak RH, et al. The effects of serum calcium and parathyroid hormone changes on psychological and cognitive function in patients undergoing parathyroidectomy for primary hyperparathyroidism. *Ann Surg* 2011; **253**: 131–7.
6. Silverberg SJ, Lewiecki EM, Mosekilde L, et al. Presentation of asymptomatic primary hyperparathyroidism: proceedings of the third international workshop. *J Clin Endocrinol Metab* 2009; **94**: 351–65.
7. Walker MD, Silverberg SJ. Cardiovascular aspects of primary hyperparathyroidism. *J Endocrinol Invest* 2008; **31**: 925–31.
8. Broulik PD, Broulikova A, Adamek S, et al. Improvement of hypertension after parathyroidectomy of patients suffering from primary hyperparathyroidism. *Int J Endocrinol* 2011; **2011**: article ID 309068.
9. Schiffl H, Lang SM. Hypertension secondary to PHPT: cause or coincidence? *Int J Endocrinol* 2011; **2011**: article ID 974647.
10. Udelsman R. Six hundred fifty-six consecutive explorations for primary hyperparathyroidism. *Ann Surg* 2002; **235**: 665–70.
11. Udelsman R, Pasieka JL, Sturgeon C, et al. Surgery for asymptomatic primary hyperparathyroidism: proceedings of the third international workshop. *J Clin Endocrinol Metab* 2009; **94**: 366–72.
12. Mollerup CL, Vestergaard P, Frokjaer VG, et al. Risk of renal stone events in primary hyperparathyroidism before and after parathyroid surgery: controlled retrospective follow up study. *BMJ* 2002; **325**: 807.
13. Vestergaard P, Mollerup CL, Frokjaer VG, et al. Cohort study of risk of fracture before and after surgery for primary hyperparathyroidism. *BMJ* 2000; **321**: 598–602.
14. Khosla S, Melton LJ, III, Wermers RA, et al. Primary hyperparathyroidism and the risk of fracture: a population-based study. *J Bone Miner Res* 1999; **14**: 1700–7.
15. Macfarlane DP, Yu N, Donnan PT, Leese GP. Should 'mild primary hyperparathyroidism' be reclassified as 'insidious': is it time to reconsider? *Clin Endocrinol* 2011; **75**: 730–7.
16. Silverberg SJ, Shane E, Jacobs TP, et al. A 10-year prospective study of primary hyperparathyroidism with or without parathyroid surgery. *N Engl J Med* 1999; **341**: 1249–55.
17. Rubin MR, Bilezikian JP, McMahon DJ, et al. The natural history of primary hyperparathyroidism with or without parathyroid surgery after 15 years. *J Clin Endocrinol Metab* 2008; **93**: 3462–70.
18. Yu N, Leese GP, Smith D, Donnan PT. The natural history of treated and untreated primary hyperparathyroidism: the parathyroid epidemiology and audit research study. *QJM* 2011; **104**: 513–21.
19. Sankaran S, Gamble G, Bolland M, et al. Skeletal effects of interventions in mild primary hyperparathyroidism: a meta-analysis. *J Clin Endocrinol Metab* 2010; **95**: 1653–62.
20. Rao DS, Phillips ER, Divine GW, Talpos GB. Randomized controlled clinical trial of surgery versus no surgery in patients with mild asymptomatic primary hyperparathyroidism. *J Clin Endocrinol Metab* 2004; **89**: 5415–22.
21. Bollerslev J, Jansson S, Mollerup CL, et al. Medical observation, compared with parathyroidectomy, for asymptomatic primary hyperparathyroidism: a prospective, randomized trial. *J Clin Endocrinol Metab* 2007; **92**: 1687–92.

22. Ambrogini E, Cetani F, Cianferotti L, et al. Surgery or surveillance for mild asymptomatic primary hyperparathyroidism: a prospective, randomized clinical trial. *J Clin Endocrinol Metab* 2007; **92**: 3114–21.
23. Vestergaard P, Mosekilde L. Fractures in patients with primary hyperparathyroidism: nationwide follow-up study of 1201 patients. *World J Surg* 2003; **27**: 343–9.
24. Lind L, Skarfors E, Berglund L, et al. Serum calcium: a new, independent, prospective risk factor for myocardial infarction in middle-aged men followed for 18 years. *J Clin Epidemiol* 1997; **50**: 967–73.
25. Kamycheva E, Sundsfjord J, Jorde R. Serum parathyroid hormone levels predict coronary heart disease: the Tromso Study. *Eur J Cardiovasc Prev Rehabil* 2004; **11**: 69–74.
26. Vestergaard P, Mollerup CL, Frokjaer VG, et al. Cardiovascular events before and after surgery for primary hyperparathyroidism. *World J Surg* 2003; **27**: 216–22.
27. Nilsson IL, Aberg J, Rastad J, Lind L. Maintained normalization of cardiovascular dysfunction 5 years after parathyroidectomy in primary hyperparathyroidism. *Surgery* 2005; **137**: 632–8.
28. Persson A, Bollerslev J, Rosen T, et al. Effect of surgery on cardiac structure and function in mild primary hyperparathyroidism. *Clin Endocrinol* 2011; **74**: 174–80.
29. Smith JC, Page MD, John R, et al. Augmentation of central arterial pressure in mild primary hyperparathyroidism. *J Clin Endocrinol Metab* 2000; **85**: 3515–19.
30. Rubin MR, Maurer MS, McMahon DJ, et al. Arterial stiffness in mild primary hyperparathyroidism. *J Clin Endocrinol Metab* 2005; **90**: 3326–30.
31. Yu N, Leese GP, Donnan PT. What predicts adverse outcomes in untreated primary hyperparathyroidism? The Parathyroid Epidemiology and Audit Research Study (PEARS). *Clin Endocrinol* 2013; **79**: 27–34.
32. Wajngot A, Werner S, Granberg PO, Lindvall N. Occurrence of pituitary adenomas and other neoplastic diseases in primary hyperparathyroidism. *Surg Gynecol Obstet* 1980; **151**: 401–3.
33. Farr HW, Fahey TJ Jr, Nash AG, Farr CM. Primary hyperparathyroidism and cancer. *Am J Surg* 1973; **126**: 539–43.
34. Gittoes NJ, Cooper MS. Primary hyperparathyroidism: is mild disease worth treating? *Clin Med* 2010; **10**: 45–9.
35. Yu N, Donnan PT, Leese GP. A record linkage study of outcomes in patients with mild primary hyperparathyroidism: the Parathyroid Epidemiology and Audit Research Study (PEARS). *Clin Endocrinol* 2011; **75**: 169–76.
36. Fitz TE, Hallman BL. Mental changes associated with hyperparathyroidism; report of two cases. *AMA Arch Intern Med* 1952; **89**: 547–51.
37. Coker LH, Rorie K, Cantley L, et al. Primary hyperparathyroidism, cognition, and health-related quality of life. *Ann Surg* 2005; **242**: 642–50.
38. Pasieka JL, Parsons LL, Demeure MJ, et al. Patient-based surgical outcome tool demonstrating alleviation of symptoms following parathyroidectomy in patients with primary hyperparathyroidism. *World J Surg* 2002; **26**: 942–9.
39. Sheldon DG, Lee FT, Neil NJ, Ryan JA Jr. Surgical treatment of hyperparathyroidism improves health-related quality of life. *Arch Surg* 2002; **137**: 1022–6.
40. Quiros RM, Alef MJ, Wilhelm SM, et al. Health-related quality of life in hyperparathyroidism measurably improves after parathyroidectomy. *Surgery* 2003; **134**: 675–81.
41. Brown GG, Preisman RC, Kleerekoper M. Neurobehavioral symptoms in mild primary hyperparathyroidism: related to hypercalcemia but not improved by parathyroidectomy. *Henry Ford Hosp Med J* 1987; **35**: 211–15.
42. Chiang CY, Andrewes DG, Anderson D, et al. A controlled, prospective study of neuropsychological outcomes post parathyroidectomy in primary hyperparathyroid patients. *Clin Endocrinol* 2005; **62**: 99–104.
43. Walker MD, McMahon DJ, Inabnet WB, et al. Neuropsychological features in primary hyperparathyroidism: a prospective study. *J Clin Endocrinol Metab* 2009; **94**: 1951–8.
44. Palmer M, Adami HO, Bergstrom R, et al. Mortality after surgery for primary hyperparathyroidism: a follow-up of 441 patients operated on from 1956 to 1979. *Surgery* 1987; **102**: 1–7.
45. Hedback G, Oden A. Increased risk of death from primary hyperparathyroidism: an update. *Eur J Clin Invest* 1998; **28**: 271–6.
46. Wermers RA, Khosla S, Atkinson EJ, et al. Survival after the diagnosis of hyperparathyroidism: a population-based study. *Am J Med* 1998; **104**: 115–22.
47. Silverberg SJ, Bilezikian JP, Bone HG, et al. Therapeutic controversies in primary hyperparathyroidism. *J Clin Endocrinol Metab* 1999; **84**: 2275–85.
48. Bilezikian JP, Brandi ML, Eastell R, et al. Guidelines for the management of asymptomatic primary hyperparathyroidism: summary statement from the Fourth International Workshop. Consensus Statement. *J Clin Endocrinol Metab* 2014; **99**(10): 3561–9.
49. Peacock M, Bolognese MA, Borofsky M, et al. Cinacalcet treatment of primary hyperparathyroidism: biochemical and bone densitometric outcomes in a five-year study. *J Clin Endocrinol Metab* 2009; **94**: 4860–7.
50. Parker CR, Blackwell PJ, Fairbairn KJ, Hosking DJ. Alendronate in the treatment of primary hyperparathyroid-related osteoporosis: a 2-year study. *J Clin Endocrinol Metab* 2002; **87**: 4482–9.
51. Chow CC, Chan WB, Li JK, et al. Oral alendronate increases bone mineral density in postmenopausal women with primary hyperparathyroidism. *J Clin Endocrinol Metab* 2003; **88**: 581–7.
52. Block GA, Martin KJ, de Francisco AL, et al. Cinacalcet for secondary hyperparathyroidism in patients receiving hemodialysis. *N Engl J Med* 2004; **350**: 1516–25.
53. Peacock M. Clinical effects of calcimimetics in hyperparathyroidism. *J Musculoskelet Neuronal Interact* 2004; **4**: 414–15.
54. Khan A, Grey A, Shoback D. Medical management of asymptomatic primary hyperparathyroidism: proceedings of the third international workshop. *J Clin Endocrinol Metab* 2009; **94**: 373–81.
55. Marcocci C, Chanson P, Shoback D, et al. Cinacalcet reduces serum calcium concentrations in patients with intractable primary hyperparathyroidism. *J Clin Endocrinol Metab* 2009; **94**: 2766–72.

CHAPTER 74

MANAGEMENT OF PERSISTENT AND RECURRENT HYPERPARATHYROIDISM

David M. Scott-Coombes

Introduction 851	Steps to success 852
Definitions 851	The future 854
Incidence 851	References 855
Reasons for failure 851	

SEARCH STRATEGY

Data in this chapter may be updated by a PubMed search using the keywords: recurrent, persistent, hyperparathyroidism and re-operation and localization.

'The second hardest decision in surgery is when to operate; the hardest decision is when to reoperate.'

Dr Claude H. Organ Jr, MD (1926–2005)

INTRODUCTION

Patients requiring reoperative surgery pose a significant clinical challenge for a number of reasons. Someone has already failed to cure the hyperparathyroidism, suggesting that this case is not 'straightforward'. That 'someone' could be a very good parathyroid surgeon – you or me. This heightens the likelihood of it being difficult and, if you were the surgeon who failed in the first place, it is challenging to encourage the patient to maintain their faith in you. Furthermore, the operative field is going to be more treacherous and so one needs all the help one can get to minimize complications and maximize success. When faced with this clinical challenge, it is wise to have a predetermined strategy.[1]

DEFINITIONS

Persistent hyperparathyroidism (HPT) is defined as the development of hypercalcaemia within 6 months of the first parathyroid operation, whereas hypercalcaemia presenting after an interval of 6 months is termed recurrent HPT.

It is important to understand this distinction because it will give clues to help derive a successful outcome at the next operation, see **Boxes 74.1** and **74.2**.

INCIDENCE

How common is failure? Percentages for bilateral neck exploration and targeted surgery are the same in published data and national disease registries, with a failure rate in the order of 5%.[2]

REASONS FOR FAILURE

In two landmark publications investigating the reasons for failed parathyroidectomy from California (*n* = 102)[3] and Uppsala, Sweden (*n* = 69),[4] the percentage of distribution between persistent and recurrent disease is remarkably similar. Most (76%) reoperative surgery is for persistent disease. The main causes for failure are shown in **Table 74.1**. While cause of the majority of the failures were classified as 'ectopia', most ectopic tumours were in the neck in the classically recognized locations such as paraoesophageal and intrathymic.

Recurrent disease is very rare. In the Uppsala series it accounted for only 13 cases over 20 years. Most patients had hyperplasia and nearly all of them (89%) were diagnosed to have multiple endocrine neoplasia type 1 (MEN 1).

> **BOX 74.1 Clue number 1**
>
> Persistent HPT is a consequence of inadequate first-time surgery whereas recurrent HPT is a result of the underlying disease process.

> **BOX 74.2 Clue number 2**
>
> If no gland or a normal gland was excised at the original operation, then it is highly likely that the patient has single gland disease (Table 74.2).[13]

TABLE 74.1 Causes of failure in first-time parathyroidectomy[3]

Cause	%	Number
Tumour in ectopic position	53	54
Incomplete resection of multiple abnormal glands	37	38
Tumour in normal position (missed at previous operation)	7	7
Re-growth of partially resected tumour	3	3

TABLE 74.2 The outcome at the first operation is a guide to the underlying pathology[13]

First operation	Underlying pathology	(%)
No gland or normal gland excised	SGD	84
	MGD	11
	Unknown	5
Pathological gland excised	MGD	90
	Regrowth of partially resected adenoma	10

SGD, single gland disease; MGD, multiple gland disease.

Sporadic adenoma as a cause of recurrent disease was exceptionally rare in this series. Of the four cases, one had seeding at the time of the first operation, one recurred at 2 years after a partial resection and only two true second adenomas presented at 8 and 16 years after the first parathyroidectomy.

Another important factor contributing to success at the first operation is the experience of the surgeon. Preventable operative failures are more common in low volume (fewer than 50 cases per year) hospitals.[5]

MEN 1

Recurrent HPT is an inevitable outcome of surgery, even when performed to the highest standard, in patients with MEN 1.[6] There are a number of surgical options for patients with MEN-HPT (see Chapter 77) with recurrence rates reported to vary from 11% at 6 years[7] to 63% at 10 years.[8] National Registry data such as those from Scandinavia and the United Kingdom paint a worse picture than the published data, with persistent hypercalcaemia rates of 25% reported in Scandinavia and 17% in the UK.[9, 10]

STEPS TO SUCCESS

Step 1: Confirm the diagnosis

The clinician should start at the beginning in terms of establishing a biochemical diagnosis of HPT (see Chapter 72). Particular attention should be given to ensuring that there is no evidence of renal insufficiency, vitamin D deficiency, and familial hypercalcaemic hypocalciuria or paraneoplastic hypercalcaemia.

Step 2: Does the patient need further surgery?

Reoperation should only be considered if the patient has symptomatic hypercalcaemia or when there is evidence of progressive disease (nephrolithiasis or bone disease). The decision about whether to operate is determined by balancing the severity of the disease with the risks of surgery. The main complications of reoperative parathyroidectomy are hypoparathyroidism and recurrent laryngeal nerve injury. Both of these are more common in redo surgery. Hypoparathyroidism (2–20%)[11] is more common due to the increased rate of multiple gland disease and the fact that normal glands may have been removed at the first operation. RLN injury is more common (up to 6%)[4, 12] owing to the scarred operative field.

In addition, unlike first-time surgery, the decision to reoperate may be influenced by a successful localization result that would both facilitate a targeted approach and increase the likelihood of a successful outcome.

Step 3: Research

There is a need to thoroughly sift through all the evidence from the previous attempt to cure the patient. You might have to be prepared to be cynical about the operation note – is what was written an accurate reflection of what was done? If possible, a conversation with the previous surgeon may be helpful, more so if it was in the recent past. The aim is to try to identify clues that describe the boundaries of the previous exploration in order to establish the region(s) where scar tissue will be worst.

In the histopathology report, if parathyroid glands were removed, were they normal or abnormal? Take note not only of the histology but also the weight of the resected specimen.

Review all of the previous localization studies. It is worth while viewing the images **yourself** as sometimes a surgeon will be prepared to place more emphasis than the radiologist on an indeterminate finding.

Step 4: Localization

Parathyroid localization (see Chapter 72) is an essential step in reoperative surgery. The goal is to be able to perform a limited operative procedure targeted according to the localization results in order to minimize risk to both recurrent laryngeal nerves. As stated, it may be that a decision about whether to proceed with surgery is taken once the results of the localization are known.

^{99m}Tc sestamibi (MIBI) scintigraphy and ultrasound are requested first. Non-invasive localization studies have become more successful in recent times compared with 20 years ago.[14] MIBI can be complemented with SPECT-CT coregistration to provide a three-dimensional image. Any lesions identified on ultrasound can be considered for aspiration for PTH. If these modalities are positive, it is reasonable to proceed to surgery.[13] Cross-sectional imaging with MRI or CT would be the next mode of imaging. Four-dimensional computed tomography is an emerging technique that explores the changes in perfusion of contrast over time to provide a new 'dimension'. Results have been promising for reoperative parathyroidectomy.[15]

As each localization studies fails, so the available procedures become more invasive. Angiography either by digital subtraction or conventional methods is the next technique to consider. In expert hands impressive results can be achieved.[16] However, these invasive studies can be associated with significant morbidity.[17] Selective venous sampling (SVS) of all patent superior, middle and inferior thyroid, thymic, brachiocephalic and vertebral veins (as well as a peripheral sample) attempts to 'regionalize' the tumour rather than precisely locate it. A gradient of at least twofold is considered significant.[18] Ligation of veins at the time of the first operation can lead to anomalous venous draining and give misleading results. Many Units use SVS in combination with angiography.

The Uppsala group has published the impact of localization on their practice.[19] Few patients underwent surgery before 1980. Between 1980 and 1990 localization was undertaken in one-third of patients, more between 1990 and 2000 (75%) and in all patients after 2000. Localization has had a profound impact on the ability to perform a targeted approach; 66% underwent bilateral neck exploration between 1962 and 1989, whereas since 1990 no fewer than 73% underwent a unilateral neck exploration.

Step 5: Surgery

PREPARATION

Reoperative parathyroid surgery is a difficult procedure and should be undertaken only by surgeons experienced in this field. The surgeon should be familiar with the anatomical variants that are a consequence of either embryology or migration of a pathological gland. Vocal cord examination by nasoendoscopy is mandatory. The patient must be thoroughly consented to the risk of complications including permanent and temporary nerve injury, haematoma/return to theatre as well as failure to find the abnormal gland(s).

OPERATION

The surgical strategy is influenced by the clues from previous surgery and the outcome of the localization studies (Table 74.3). It is advisable to set aside plenty of time in theatre to undertake the case and make sure that you have good assistance. The site of the surgical incision should be through the previous incision. Consider asking your radiologist to place a mark on the skin over the site of the presumed adenoma or perform an ultrasound in the operating room yourself. Obviously, if the localization places the gland in the mediastinum, then midline sternotomy, thoracotomy or thoracoscopy should be considered, especially if the tumour does not appear to be intra-thymic such that a cervical approach is contraindicated.

TABLE 74.3 Surgical strategy in reoperative parathyroidectomy

Expected pathology	Strategy
Solitary abnormal gland	Focused approach
Multiple glands	Bilateral approach
Carcinoma/parathyromatosis	En-bloc resection

The surgical approach to the deeper structures in the neck will be influenced by the previous operation and the localization result. For example, if the first-time operation was unilateral (targeted/minimally invasive) and the localization study identifies the gland to the contralateral side, a traditional midline approach will suffice. But if the previous operation was a bilateral exploration and/or the localization result is ipsilateral to the previous operation, then a lateral approach should be adopted. This is achieved by dissecting between the lateral edge of the sternohyoid (strap) muscle and the medial edge of the sternocleidomastoid muscle. In this area the tendon of omohyoid is encountered and divided. Immediately deep to this tendon is the middle thyroid vein (if not already divided) as it drains into the internal jugular vein. The carotid sheath is carefully retracted laterally and the tracheo-oesophageal groove is explored. The intention is to identify the recurrent laryngeal nerve (RLN) in previously unexplored territory and this is most likely to be in a caudal direction. Consideration should be given towards using the nerve monitor. A positional statement by the European Society of Endocrine Surgeons on modern techniques in parathyroid surgery did not recommend the routine use of neuromonitoring in first-time neck exploration but stated that it may be of value in reoperative surgery.[20]

Once the RLN has been located, a careful search for the abnormal gland is made. For the inferior gland, incise the strap lateral to the midline and follow the surface of the thyroid towards the thyrothymic ligament. For the superior gland, the intersection of the RLN with the inferior thyroid artery is the key area to start looking (see Chapter 77). Intra-operative ultrasound scanning (IOUS) has been reported to be helpful in identifying abnormal glands (normal glands are not identified) and results in shorter operative time in the hands of enthusiasts.[14] If an abnormal gland cannot be located, blind thyroid lobectomy should not be undertaken owing to the rarity of the intra-thyroidal adenoma,[21] unless confirmed by IOUS.[14]

Once a gland has been located and excised, both frozen section and intra-operative PTH (ioPTH) assay will provide clues to success. The key information from the pathologist is to confirm that the excised tissue is 'parathyroid'. Localization tells you where to start and ioPTH tells you when to stop! While the literature is not unanimous, most evidence is that ioPTH helps to decide when the operation can be terminated and is an accurate predictor of cure.[19, 22] There is no real evidence, however, that it increases the success rate.

POST-OPERATION

As with all parathyroid surgery, the patient should be closely monitored for the development of a wound haematoma. Results from the UK national audit suggest that the rate of haematoma in redo parathyroidectomy more than doubles compared with first-time surgery (1.2% vs 0.5%).[10] Attention is also given towards the complications of RLN injury and hypocalcaemia. Post-operative nasoendoscopy should be undertaken routinely. The rate of permanent hypoparathyroidism (see Step 2) is between 5% and 11% in most series.[12, 14] A protocol for managing this complication should be written and available in the medical record. A suggested algorithm is shown in **Table 74.4**.

The serum calcium will provide biochemical evidence of surgical success. In expert centres success rates of over 95% are reported.[3, 19]

THE FUTURE

There are two reasons why some surgeons fear that reoperative surgery may become more common.

1. **Focused surgery** – does it lead to higher failure rates? The increased success of pre-operative parathyroid localization and the widespread adoption of ioPTH assay has led to an explosion in the use of a focused approach to first-time parathyroidectomy.[23] Critics of this approach are concerned that ioPTH is inaccurate in determining complete excision among patients with multiple gland disease.[24, 25] In a recent review of 845 cases of focused parathyroidectomy using ioPTH, with a failure rate of 2.9%, the main cause of operative failure was the inability of the surgeon to find the abnormal gland, not the failure to diagnose multiglandular disease.[26] In other words, the most common cause of failed parathyroidectomy remains the surgeon, and experience counts.[27]

2. **Mild disease.** A study that looked at outcomes in patients with double negative parathyroid localization found an alarmingly high rate of persistent hyperparathyroidism (13.3%).[28] It is telling that the median weight of adenoma was small (350 mg). Parathyroid localization is less reliable with smaller tumours[29] although ioPTH assay remains a valuable tool in patients with milder HPT.[30] Either the threshold for parathyroidectomy is being set too low or the wrong surgeon is undertaking this surgery.

TABLE 74.4 Algorithm for managing hypocalcaemia

Corrected plasma calcium mmol/L (mg/dL)	Symptomatic	Asymptomatic
>2.15 (8.6)	Milk	nil
2.00–2.15 (8.0–8.5)	Calcichew 1 g b.d.	nil
1.90–2.00 (7.6–8.4)	Calcichew 1 g t.d.s. 1-alfacalcidol 1 μg o.d.	Calcichew 1 g t.d.s.
1.80–1.90 (7.2–7.5)	Calcichew 1 g t.d.s. 1-alfacalcidol 1 μg b.d.	Calcichew 1 g t.d.s. 1-alfacalcidol 1 μg b.d.
<1.80 (<7.2)	Tetany: 10–30 mL i.v. calcium gluconate over 10–15 min*	Calcichew 1 g t.d.s. 1-alfacalcidol 1 μg t.d.s.

b.d., twice daily; t.d.s., three times per day; i.v., intravenous
* The cannula must be carefully sited to avoid extravasation.

KEY POINTS

- Reoperative parathyroidectomy is a challenging situation.
- The steps to success include careful pre-operative research and a skilled operative technique.
- Localization is mandatory and should be successful prior to contemplating a reoperation. ioPTH assay and neuromonitoring may be useful tools.
- There is a case for centralizing these cases in expert centres but, as with most other aspects of surgery; it is better to get it right the first time.

REFERENCES

1. Bartsch DK, Rothmund M. Reoperative surgery for primary hyperparathyroidism. *Brit J Surg* 2009; **96**: 699–701.
2. Allendorf J, DiGeorgi M, Spanknebel K, et al. 1112 consecutive bilateral neck explorations for primary hyperparathyroidism. *World J Surg* 2007; **31**: 2075–80.
3. Shen W, Duren M, Morita E, et al. Reoperation for persistent or recurrent primary hyperparathyroidism. *Arch Surg* 1996; **131**: 861–9.
4. Akerstrom G, Rudberg C, Grimelius L, et al. Causes of failed primary exploration and technical aspects of re-operation in primary hyperparathyroidism. *World J Surg* 1992; **16**: 562–9.
5. Chen H, Wang TS, Ywen TWF, et al. Operative failures after parathyroidectomy for hyperparathyroidism. *Ann Surg* 2010; **252**: 691–5.
6. Goudet P, Cougard P, Vergès B, et al. Hyperparathyroidism in multiple endocrine neoplasia type I: surgical trends and results of a 256-patient series from Groupe D'etude des Néoplasies Endocriniennes Multiples Study Group. *World J Surg* 2001; **25**: 886–90.
7. Arnalsteen LC, Alesina PF, Quiereux JL, et al. Long-term results of less than total parathyroidectomy for hyperparathyroidism in multiple endocrine neoplasia type 1. *Surgery* 2002; **132**: 1119–25.
8. Elaraj DM, Skarulis MC, Libutti SK, et al. Utility of rapid intraoperative parathyroid hormone assay to predict severe postoperative hypocalemia after reoperation for hyperparathyroidism. *Surgery* 2003; **134**: 858–64.
9. Bergenfelz AOJ, Jansson SKG, Wallin KG, et al. Impact of modern techniques on short-term outcome after surgery for primary hyperparathyroidism: a multicenter study comprising 2,708 patients. *Langenbecks Arch Surg* 2009; **394**: 851–60.
10. Chadwick D, Kinsman R, Walton P. The British Association of Endocrine and Thyroid Surgeons fourth national audit report 2012, ISBN 978-0-9568154-3-9. Available from: www.baets.org.uk/audit.
11. Karakas E, Zieleke A, Dietz C, Rothmund M. Reoperations for primary hyperparathyroidism. *Chirurg* 2005; **76**: 207–16.
12. Jaskowiak N, Norton JA, Alexander HR, et al. A prospective trial evaluating a standard approach to reoperation for missed parathyroid adenoma. *Ann Surg* 1996; **224**: 308–21.
13. Yen TW, Wang TS, Doffek KM, et al. Reoperative parathyroidectomy: an algorithm for imaging and monitoring of intraoperative parathyroid hormone levels that results in a successful focused approach. *Surgery* 2008; **144**: 611–19.
14. Powell AC, Alexander HR, Chang R, et al. Reoperation for parathyroid adenoma: a contemporary experience. *Surgery* 2009; **146**: 1144–55.
15. Mortenson MM, Evans DB, Lee JE, et al. Parathyroid exploration in the reoperative neck: improved preoperative localisation with 4D-computed tomography. *J Am Coll Surg* 2008; **206**: 888–95.
16. Miller DL, Chang R, Doppman JL, et al. Localisation of parathyroid adenomas: superselective arterial DSA versus superselective conventional angiography. *Radiology* 1989; **170**: 1003–6.
17. Wells SA, Debendetti MK, Doherty GM. Recurrent or persistent hyperparathyroidism. *J Bone Miner Res* 2002; **17** suppl 2: N158–62.
18. Sugg SL, Fraker DL, Alexander HR, et al. Prospective evaluation of selective venous sampling for parathyroid hormone concentration in patients undergoing reoperations for primary hyperparathyroidism. *Surgery* 1993; **114**: 1004–10.
19. Hessman O, Stalberg P, Sundin A, et al. High success rate of parathyroid reoperation may be achieved with improved localisation diagnosis. *World J Surg* 2008; **32**: 774–81.
20. Bergenfelz AO, Hellman P, Harrison B, et al. Positional statement of the European Society of Endocrine Surgeons (ESES) on modern techniques in pHPT surgery. *Langenbecks Arch Surg* 2009; **394**: 761–4.
21. Libutti SK, Bartlett DL, Jaskowiak NT, et al. The role of thyroid resection during a reoperation for persistent or recurrent hyperparathyroidism. *Surgery* 1997; **122**: 1183–7.
22. Richards ML, Thompson GB, Farley DR, et al. Reoperative parathyroidectomy in 228 patients during the era of minimal-access surgery and intra-operative parathyroid hormone monitoring. *Am J Surg* 2008; **196**: 937–43.
23. Udelsman R. Six hundred and fifty six consecutive explorations for primary hyperparathyroidism. *Ann Surg* 2002; **235**: 665–72.
24. Siperstein A, Berber E, Mackey R, et al. Prospective evaluation of sestamibi scan, ultrasonography, and rapid PTH to predict the success of limited exploration for sporadic primary hyperparathyroidism. *Surgery* 2004; **136**: 872–80.
25. Clerici T, Brandle M, Lange J, et al. Impact of intraoperative parathyroid hormone monitoring on the prediction of multiglandular parathyroid disease. *World J Surg* 2004; **28**: 182–92.
26. Lew JI, Rivera M, Irvin GL, et al. Operative failure in the era of focused parathyroidectomy. *Arch Surg* 2010; **145**: 628–33.
27. Chen H, Wang TS, Ywen TWF, et al. Operative failures after parathyroidectomy for hyperparathyroidism. *Ann Surg* 2010; **252**: 691–5.
28. Bergenfelz AO, Wallin G, Jansson S, et al. Results of surgery for sporadic primary hyperparathyroidism in patients with preoperatively negative sestamibi scanning and ultrasound. *Langenbecks Arch Surg* 2011; **396**: 83–90.
29. Mihai R, Gleeson F, Buley ID, et al. Negative imaging studies for primary hyperparathyroidism are unavoidable: correlation of sestamibi and high-resolution ultrasound scanning with histological analysis in 150 patients. *World J Surg* 2006; **30**: 697–704.
30. Hathaway TD, Jones G, Stechman M, et al. The value of intraoperative PTH measurements in patients with mild primary hyperparathyroidism. *Langenbecks Arch Surg* 2013; **398**: 723–7.

CHAPTER 75

MANAGEMENT OF PARATHYROID CANCER

Pamela Howson and Mark Sywak

Introduction 857	Histopathology and diagnosis 860
Incidence and natural history 857	Medical therapy 861
Aetiology and molecular pathways 858	Prognosis 861
Clinical presentation 858	References 862
Operative findings and surgery 859	

SEARCH STRATEGY

Data in this chapter may be updated by a PubMed search using the keywords: parathyroid and cancer, hypercalcaemia, parathyroid and tumour.

INTRODUCTION

Parathyroid carcinoma (PAC) is a rare cause of primary hyperparathyroidism which presents with clinical manifestations of severe hypercalcaemia. It was first described in 1904 by Swiss surgeon Fritz de Quervain who reported a non-functioning metastatic PAC, and Sainton and Millot were the first to describe a functioning metastatic PAC in 1933. Around 90% of PACs are functional and may present with a palpable neck mass which invades locally. Skeletal and renal complications are commonly present at presentation. Surgery remains the only effective treatment for primary tumours where en bloc resection is key. Medical therapies are critical for controlling hypercalcaemia. Germ-line DNA testing for the *HRPT2* mutation should be considered for patients who present with PAC.

INCIDENCE AND NATURAL HISTORY

PAC is a very rare malignancy accounting for less than 1% of cases of primary hyperparathyroidism in Europe and the United States, and up to 5% in Japan.[1-3] According to the Surveillance, Epidemiology and End Results cancer registry data, the annual incidence is 5.73 per 10 000 million. This represents a prevalence of 0.005% of all cancers.[4]

PAC occurs equally in males and females, unlike parathyroid adenomas, which have a female preponderance (3–4:1).[2] PACs present mostly in the fourth to fifth decades of life, which is a decade earlier than their benign counterpart. However, the age of diagnosis is in the range of 23–90 years old. There is no racial predisposition in PAC, whereas benign parathyroid tumours more commonly occur in the Western population.

PAC generally runs a slow but progressive course. Less than 8% of patients have lymph node or distant metastases at initial presentation. The mean time to recurrence is generally within 2–5 years of operation and takes the form of locoregional or cervical node involvement (30%), lung metastases (40%), liver secondaries (10%), or bone or brain deposits. Failure of treatment can result in death from hypercalcaemic-related end-organ damage within 14 months. In general, however, PAC tends to have a relatively indolent course because of the tumour's low malignant potential, with a 5-year survival of 86% and a 10-year survival of 35–79%.[2,4,5] A significant proportion of patients (25%) will be diagnosed with PAC after initial surgical treatment following review of histopathology or after developing metastatic disease.

AETIOLOGY AND MOLECULAR PATHWAYS

The pathogenesis of PAC is poorly understood with few known environmental or genetic causative agents. Animal models show that parathyroid glands are histologically resistant to X-ray damage at doses less than 5 Gy, but doses of 5–25 Gy cause oedema and hyperaemia, and higher doses cause severe damage with hyperplasia, cyst and adenoma formation and carcinoma.[6] Head and neck irradiation has been associated with the development of PAC.[7]

PAC has also been reported in patients with secondary and tertiary hyperparathyroidism.[8] End-stage renal failure can promote clonal expansion of cells within the parathyroid hyperplasia that progresses to parathyroid carcinoma. Chronic hypercalcaemia alone in the setting of renal failure has been postulated as a possible trigger for the development of PAC,[9] although the association is weak. An increased risk of PAC has also been associated with multiple endocrine neoplasia type 1 (MEN 1) and with autosomal dominant familial isolated hyperparathyroidism, which is due to mutations in the tumour suppressor genes *MEN1* and *CDC73* or the calcium-sensing receptor (*CaSR*) gene, resulting in the formation of one or more parathyroid adenomas.[2]

Interestingly, several oncogenes and tumour suppressor genes have been linked to PAC. Cyclin D1 or *PRAD1* (parathyroid adenoma 1) is an oncogene involved in cell cycle regulation and is located on chromosome 11q13.[10] It is overexpressed in 91% of PAC specimens and up to 61% of benign parathyroid tumours,[11] but the exact mechanism of carcinogenesis remains unclear. PAC also lacks the retinoblastoma tumour suppressor gene on chromosome 13.[12, 13] Retinoblastoma protein prevents excessive cell growth by inhibiting cell cycle progression, and hence its absence results in dysregulation of cell growth.

The *HRPT2* gene, which encodes the parafibromin protein, has attracted much attention in PAC. Most of the data on the genetics involved in this rare disease are derived from studying inherited disorders of primary hyperparathyroidism such as hereditary hyperparathyroidism-jaw tumour syndrome (HPT-JT). HPT-JT is an autosomal dominant disease characterized by fibromas of the maxilla and mandible and tumours of the parathyroid. In this condition 30% of the parathyroid tumours are PACs.[2] HPT-JT is associated with an inactivating germ-line mutation of the *HRPT2* gene on chromosome 1q25-q32. This is a tumour suppressor gene encoding the protein parafibromin which has anti-proliferative properties. However, it is also defective in sporadic PAC,[14] and parafibromin expression is decreased or absent in PAC, which may have significant implications for diagnosis and management. Kim and colleagues[15] showed that the loss of parafibromin expression was 94.4% specific for the diagnosis of PAC, and recurrences and metastases only occurred in cases with a loss of parafibromin. Moreover, it has been found that *HRPT2* gene mutation results in the upregulation of up to four proteins including histone H1 and H2, E-cadherin and amyloid BA4 precursor protein (APP).[16] Histone proteins are involved in gene repair mechanisms. E-cadherin is involved in cell–cell adhesion, and loss of function contributes to tumorigenesis by increased proliferation, invasion and metastasis. Its upregulation is indicative of the cell's loss of function in cell adhesion. APP is a functional neuronal receptor but its upregulation in PAC is of uncertain significance. Staining for these proteins provides a diagnostic marker for PAC.

CLINICAL PRESENTATION

To treat PAC effectively, the clinician should have a high index of suspicion prior to initial surgery so that an appropriate operative approach may be undertaken. This requires an awareness of the differences in presentation between primary hyperparathyroidism due to benign disease and cancer. Patients with PAC are typically younger than those with benign causes of hyperparathyroidism (fourth to fifth decades).[17] PAC occurs equally in both genders. Since 90% of PAC are functioning tumours, most manifest with symptoms similar to benign hyperparathyroidism, namely weakness, fatigue, anxiety and depression, bone pain, renal stones, abdominal pain, peptic ulcer disease and pancreatitis. However, bone disease and renal involvement are far more common in parathyroid malignancy, occurring in up to 80–90% of patients with PAC[18, 19] and the presence of both is strongly predictive of malignancy. Bone disease includes bone pain, osteopenia, osteoporosis, pathological fractures, osteitis fibrosa cystica, 'salt and pepper' skull and subperiosteal bone resorption. Renal involvement includes ureteric calculi, nephrocalcinosis or renal impairment. Acute pancreatitis, peptic ulceration and hypercalcaemic crisis occur in 12–18% of patients with PAC. These symptoms usually occur before local invasion by the tumour.

Around 50–70% of patients with PAC present with a palpable neck mass.[2, 20] This is extremely uncommon in benign disease, and can be associated with evidence of local invasion including recurrent laryngeal nerve palsy and dysphagia. Non-functioning tumours do not present with symptoms of hypercalcaemia and therefore are more likely to present with a palpable neck mass.

Serum calcium and parathyroid hormone are elevated in PAC, but the average calcium is much higher in PAC than in benign causes of hyperparathyroidism.[2, 18] Most patients with parathyroid adenomas have serum calcium levels within 1 mg/dL above the upper limit of normal; patients with PAC have serum calcium in excess of 3.5 mmol/L (14 mg/dL) and serum parathyroid hormone levels 10–15-fold greater than the normal range. A parathyroid hormone level 10 times the upper limit of normal carries a positive predictive value of 81% for PAC.[21]

Imaging of PAC differs to that for parathyroid adenomas due to a greater emphasis on the detection of locoregional tumour infiltration and distant metastasis. Neck ultrasound is a non-invasive and sensitive study for the detection of enlarged parathyroid glands. PAC are typically large (>15 mm), hypoechoic, lobulated, irregular lesions.[22]

Ultrasound has been shown to have a high accuracy in detecting parathyroid lesions 1 cm or larger.[23] Infiltration and calcification seen on ultrasound have a high positive predictive value for identifying parathyroid malignancy.[24] A meta-analysis of pre-operative localization techniques found that ultrasound had a sensitivity of 76% and a positive predictive value (PPV) of 93%.[25] Ultrasound can also be used to guide fine-needle aspiration (FNA) biopsy of neck lymphadenopathy, but FNA of the primary lesion should be avoided to prevent disruption of the primary tumour.[26] FNA is not useful in distinguishing benign from malignant parathyroid disease.[2]

^{99m}TC sestamibi scintigraphy is useful for localizing primary, recurrent and metastatic disease and to confirm ultrasonographic localization. The radiolabelled isotope has a particular affinity for parathyroid mitochondria.[20] It cannot, however, discriminate benign from malignant disease. Sestamibi has a high sensitivity of 79% and a PPV of 91% and continues to be the most useful imaging modality in benign and malignant causes of hyperparathyroidism.[25]

Four-dimensional computed tomography (4D CT) is increasingly used for parathyroid localization in hyperparathyroidism, particularly when ultrasound and sestamibi imaging are negative or indeterminate (**Figure 75.1**). It has a sensitivity and specificity of 82% and 92% respectively for the localization of parathyroid adenomas.[27, 28] Parathyroid glands have unique angiographic and perfusion characteristics[29] including a 'blush' following intra-arterial contrast used to distinguish abnormal parathyroid tissue. 4D CT uses non-contrast imaging to differentiate thyroid from parathyroid tissue, as well as an early post-contrast phase to determine a hypervascular gland, and a delayed post-contrast scan to detect altered enhancement or abnormal contrast retention.[30] However, 4D CT delivers a significant radiation dose despite dose reduction techniques (20–40 mGy per phase of imaging) and no study has elucidated its importance in PAC diagnosis or localization. Its use may be supported in determining infiltration pre-operatively if PAC is suspected and in reoperative surgery.

In circumstances of recurrence, ^{18}F-FDG PET CT has been used to detect locoregional recurrence or distant metastases.[31] MRI may also be useful for mediastinal recurrence.[32]

OPERATIVE FINDINGS AND SURGERY

Surgical resection is the main therapeutic modality for PAC, even in the presence of metastatic disease. Treatment of hypercalcaemia and correction of renal dysfunction is often necessary prior to surgical intervention. Hydration with saline, correction of electrolyte imbalance, diuretics and bisphosphonates are useful to optimize the patient's condition prior to surgery.

PAC can be difficult to diagnose intra-operatively but usually appears as a large, firm, grey-white mass with adherence to adjacent tissue and is often greater than 3 cm in maximal diameter (**Figure 75.2**). Parathyroid adenomas, in contrast, are smaller, softer and are reddish-brown or tan in colour.[3, 33] En bloc resection involves carefully removing the parathyroid lesion and resecting all adherent tissues with grossly clear margins. This will typically involve ipsilateral thyroid lobectomy and the adjacent level 6 lymphatic component. This approach frequently requires autotransplantation of the ipsilateral parathyroid gland where it appears macroscopically normal as well as cervical thymectomy. It is important not to rupture the capsule, as this increases the risk of seeding and recurrence.[34] PAC can also involve the overlying strap muscles, trachea, oesophagus and recurrent laryngeal nerve. In order to provide the best chance of cure these structures may require en bloc resection.[34, 35] Recurrent laryngeal nerve involvement is suspected pre-operatively if the patient has a hoarse voice and warrants resection in cases where its function is lost due to tumour infiltration or where it is involved circumferentially by malignancy. Sacrifice of a normally functioning nerve is generally not

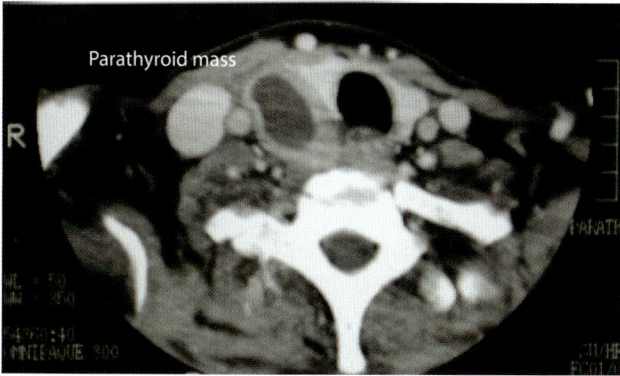

Figure 75.1 Neck CT axial image depicting large right parathyroid mass that proved to be a PAC causing tracheal deviation.

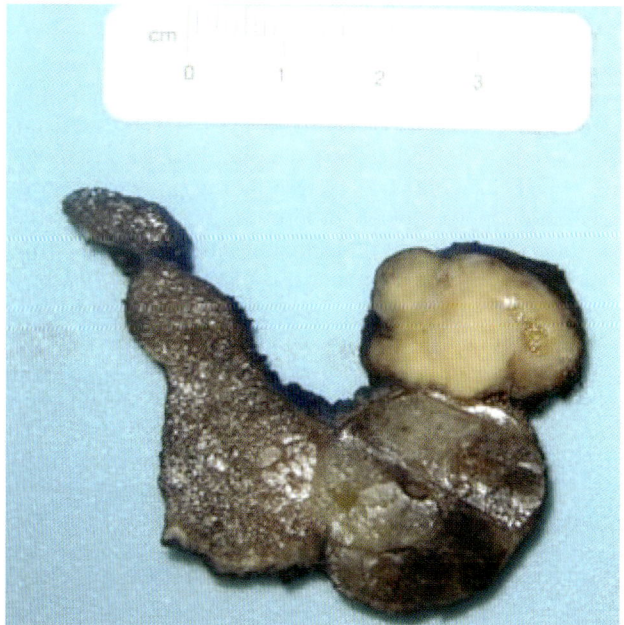

Figure 75.2 Resection specimen of parathyroid carcinoma removed en bloc with adjacent thyroid tissue. The parathyroid carcinoma is adherent to the thyroid. (Photo courtesy of Prof Anthony Gill, Dept of Anatomical Pathology, Royal North Shore Hospital, Sydney Australia.)

required unless its preservation results in gross residual tumour remaining in the thyroid bed. Lymph node involvement is uncommon, occurring in only up to 8% of patients, and as a result comprehensive lymphadenectomy is usually not necessary except in the local area, level 6. Prophylactic modified radical neck dissection does not improve survival and is not typically performed at the primary surgical procedure. It may be of greater utility in reoperative cases.

In at least 25% of initial presentations PAC is diagnosed after primary surgery on histopathology or with the development of distant metastases.[36] In patients with PAC who undergo routine parathyroidectomy because cancer is not suspected, 50% or more will develop local recurrence.[7, 33] The mean time for recurrence in this population is 41 months and the mean disease-free survival time is 62 months.[7] Conversely, if detected before or during operation, then local recurrence rates are 10–33% and long-term survival improves significantly.[7]

The main issue of controversy is the management of PAC diagnosed after initial surgery on histology. O'Neill and colleagues[37] found that subsequent unilateral hemithyroidectomy and lymphadenectomy did not reveal any residual disease and therefore further radical surgery may not be warranted. This is supported by Fujimoto and colleagues[38] who recommended post-operative follow-up at 3-month intervals for PAC that had minimal invasion and low malignant potential as these tumours did not necessarily locally recur. Alternatively, it has been suggested that aggressive histopathological features of extensive capsular and vascular spread should prompt re-exploration and completion of resection.[39]

After initial resection, all patients require immediate monitoring and lifelong surveillance. In the early post-operative period, temporary hypocalcaemia may occur due to secondary uptake of calcium into bones (hungry bone syndrome) which requires treatment with supplemental calcium and vitamin D. PTH levels should also be checked post-operatively to ensure curative resection. Thereafter, PTH and corrected serum calcium are monitored every 3 months.[32] If these increase, sites of recurrence should be evaluated with sestamibi scintigraphy and anatomical imaging. If these imaging studies are inconclusive, selective venous catheterization and PTH measurement are recommended to regionalize the recurrence.[40]

Recurrence is most often locoregional and occurs within 2–3 years of the initial operation.[19, 34] For recurrent locoregional disease, cervical and/or mediastinal re-exploration with wide resection including thymectomy are indicated.[32, 34] Pre-operative vocal cord examination should be performed prior to reoperative surgery.[34] A reoperative neck is challenging due to scar tissue and distorted anatomical planes, but various techniques have been described to aid in re-resection. These include injection of methylene blue dye, which is selectively taken up by parathyroid tissue,[41, 42] or intravenous injection of technetium-99m 1 hour pre-operatively and subsequent use of the gamma probe intra-operatively to localize the recurrence.[43] The low incidence of PAC makes evaluation of these modalities difficult, but extrapolation of the experience with benign parathyroid disease suggests that methylene blue dye and the gamma probe offer little advantage to the experienced parathyroid surgeon. Intra-operative PTH testing, however, is useful in confirming resection of the target lesion.[43, 44]

Even for distant PAC metastasis, resection is advocated to provide palliative control of hypercalcaemia, which can be debilitating and life-threatening. Where possible, even small metastatic deposits should be considered for resection. The most common sites of distant metastatic PAC spread are to the lungs, liver and bone, and up to 30% of patients already have metastases at initial presentation.[45, 46] Radical resections which have provided symptomatic relief include liver or pulmonary wedge resections, bone and cerebral metastasis resections, and oesophageal resection with gastric transposition.[47–51]

HRPT2 germ-line DNA testing should be considered for patients presenting with apparently sporadic PAC. It is unclear whether genetic testing should be offered to at-risk relatives, but monitoring serum calcium levels offers a simple alternative to definitive DNA diagnosis.[14]

HISTOPATHOLOGY AND DIAGNOSIS

Schantz and Castleman[52] developed a set of criteria for the histopathologic diagnosis of PAC in 1973. These included the presence of a fibrous capsule or fibrous trabeculae, rosette-like cellular architecture, presence of mitotic figures, and capsular or vascular invasion. Stojadinovic and colleagues[53] added the presence of adjacent skeletal muscle invasion by tumour. This study found capsular and vascular invasion in 92% and 81% of PAC specimens respectively, and 19% had perineural invasion. However, the histological criteria are often equivocal and hence the World Health Organization (WHO) defined PAC in 2004 as those parathyroid lesions displaying vascular invasion, perineural space invasion, capsular penetration with growth into adjacent tissues and/or metastases (Figure 75.3).[54] While the presence of fibrosis is common, it was not consistent and not considered pathognomonic of PAC, and the trabecular growth only occurs in a minority of cases, with rosette formation a rare finding. In addition, the presence of coagulative necrosis, macronucleoli and mitotic activity greater than 5 mitoses per 50 high-power field is a diagnostic pathologic triad that reflects a high risk of malignant versus benign behaviour. A proliferation marker ki-67 greater than 5% is suggestive of malignancy.

There is generally no accepted staging system for PAC. Tumours tend to be classified as localized when confined to the parathyroid and local soft tissues or metastatic when distant metastases occur.

Since not all PACs exhibit the above diagnostic histopathologic criteria, markers have been sought to distinguish benign from malignant tumours. These include immuno-histochemistry markers for ki-67, bcl2, cyclin D1, Rb, CaSR, although false negatives with these arose owing to the rarity of PAC.[55] The HRPT2 tumour suppressor gene encodes the protein parafibromin. As mentioned previously, parafibromin is involved in apoptosis, inhibits G1 to S phase

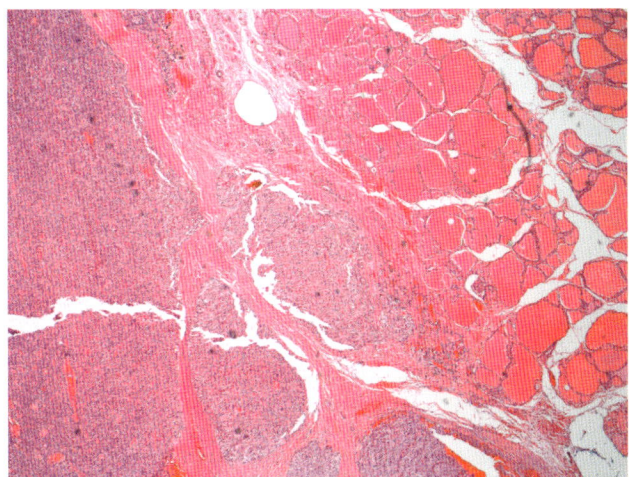

Figure 75.3 Histological section of parathyroid carcinoma invading into adjacent thyroid tissue. The presence of unequivocal invasive growth is the basis of the WHO 2004 criteria for the diagnosis of parathyroid carcinoma (*H&E, original magnification ×100*). (Photo courtesy of Prof Anthony Gill, Dept of Anatomical Pathology, Royal North Shore Hospital, Sydney Australia.)

of the cell cycle, regulates the wingless type (Wnt) pathway, and regulates growth factor expression.[56] Loss of the protein parafibromin will therefore increase cellular proliferation. It has been found that 77% of all PAC harbour mutations in the *HRPT2* gene[14, 57] in contrast to benign adenomata where the mutation is demonstrated in less than 1%.[58] Demonstration of the *HRPT2* mutation is therefore relatively specific for PAC. Tumours with inactivation of *HRPT2* will show loss of parafibromin staining on immunohistochemistry.[55, 59] The absence of nuclear staining for parafibromin is diagnostic of PAC or an HPT-JT-related tumour and is a useful adjunct to the traditional histological criteria for malignancy.[56] Another molecular marker called protein gene product (PGP 9.5) is used to complement parafibromin in the immunohistochemistry process, and this is upregulated in the majority of PAC.[55]

MEDICAL THERAPY

Hypercalcaemia

Medical control of hypercalcaemia is important preoperatively and also in cases of inoperable PAC. Hypercalcaemic crisis is a medical emergency and requires prompt intervention.[34] Aggressive fluid resuscitation with isotonic saline is required as patients become severely dehydrated due to nephrogenic diabetes insipidus and associated nausea and vomiting. Loop diuretics such as frusemide increase urinary calcium excretion and are effective once the patient is euvolaemic. Bisphosphonates (e.g. pamidronate, clodronate, etidronate) inhibit osteoclast-mediated bone resorption and cause apoptosis of osteoclasts and are critical in reducing serum calcium in PAC.[60] Intravenous pamidronate is infused slowly at a dosage of 60–90 mg and decreases calcium in 2–4 days.[2]

The effect has a duration of 1–3 weeks but efficacy reduces with time.

Calcimimetic agents (e.g. cinacalcet) increase the sensitivity of parathyroid cells to the suppressive effects of high extracellular calcium by binding to calcium-sensing receptors on parathyroid cells.[2, 60] Cinacalcet is an oral agent given 30–60 mg daily with a rapid onset of action that reduces calcium within 48 hours and is generally well tolerated.

Other useful agents in PAC include calcitonin and plicamycin. Calcitonin inhibits osteoclast bone resorption and increases urinary excretion of calcium. Calcitonin can be used in conjunction with corticosteroids, which in isolation are useful in reducing hypercalcaemia.[61] Plicamycin is an antineoplastic antibiotic that transiently inhibits bone resorption but has toxic effects on the liver, kidneys and bone marrow. Gallium nitrate, octreotide and haemodialysis can also be used to reduce hypercalcaemia.[2, 34, 62]

Chemotherapy

Chemotherapeutic agents do not offer significant benefit to patients with PAC. There is no standard chemotherapy regime for PAC as there are no randomized trials to support its use. Several case studies involving the use of dacarbazine, fluorouracil, cyclophosphamide, methotrexate and doxorubicin[63, 64] have shown some success.

Radiotherapy

PAC has historically been considered radioresistant.[7, 34] However, the Mayo Clinic reports disease-free survival of 60 months in four patients who received post-operative radiotherapy[65] and this is supported by the MD Anderson experience of a lower local recurrence rate from 77% to 17% with adjuvant radiation.[35] Other case reports support findings that PAC may be a radiosensitive tumour.[66, 67] Given the lack of strong evidence for the routine use of external beam radiotherapy in PAC, it seems prudent to incorporate it when surgical options have been exhausted.

PROGNOSIS

PAC is generally a slow-growing cancer and the median overall survival is 14.3 years but can range from 1 month to more than 20 years.[4, 46, 68] Overall survival ranges from 85% at 5 years to 35–79% at 10 years.[2] As there is no widely accepted adjuvant therapy, complete surgical resection remains the mainstay of cure for both primary and recurrent disease.[40] En bloc resection results in 10–30% local recurrence and 90% long-term survival rates; incomplete resection results in a 50% recurrence rate and a mortality rate of 46%.[7] Other negative prognostic indicators include lymph node or distant metastases and non-functioning tumours. Tumour size is not a prognostic indicator.[46, 68] There is currently no prognostic staging system. Mortality from functional PAC is due to end-organ failure (e.g. renal failure) from uncontrolled hypercalcaemia.[39, 40]

Overall, PAC is a rare, slowly progressive malignancy, which requires medical control of hypercalcaemia, surgical resection and long-term follow-up. It is best managed in a multidisciplinary setting with clinicians experienced in the management of parathyroid disease. Expert histological assessment is critical as is an understanding of the genetic associations this rare cancer exhibits.

> **KEY POINTS**
>
> - Parathyroid cancer is a rare cause of primary hyperparathyroidism and typically presents with marked hypercalcaemia with corrected serum calcium greater than 14 mg/dL or 3.5 mmol/L.
> - Parathyroid cancers typically present in the fourth to fifth decades of life and are distributed equally between males and females.
> - Pre-operative treatment requires correction of metabolic and electrolyte disturbances with saline hydration, loop diuretics, bisphosphonates and calcimimetics.
> - Surgery is the mainstay of treatment and the only curative modality.
> - The surgical approach should incorporate four-gland parathyroid exploration with en-bloc resection of the tumour and involved structures to achieve complete removal.
> - Mutations of the *HRPT2* tumour suppressor gene are strongly associated with the hyperparathyroidism-jaw tumour syndrome and parathyroid cancers.
> - Parathyroid cancer is generally a slowly progressive malignancy with a 10-year disease-specific survival of 49–77%.
> - Immunohistochemical staining for parafibromin and PGP 9.5 are useful adjuncts to histological diagnosis of parathyroid cancer.

REFERENCES

1. Brown S, O Neill C, Suliburk J, et al. Parathyroid carcinoma: increasing incidence and changing presentation. *ANZ J Surg* 2011; **81**(7-8): 528–32.
2. Mohebati A, Shaha A, Shah J. Parathyroid carcinoma: challenges in diagnosis and treatment. *Haematol Oncol Clin N Am* 2012; **26**: 1221–38.
3. Dudney W, Bodenner D, Stack B Jr. Parathyroid carcinoma. *Otolaryngol Clin N Am* 2010; **43**: 441–53.
4. Hundahl SA, Fleming ID, Fremgen AM, Menck HR. Two hundred eighty-six cases of parathyroid carcinoma treated in the US between 1985–1995: a National Cancer Data Base Report. The American College of Surgeons Commission on Cancer and the American Cancer Society. *Cancer* 1999; **86**: 538.
5. Lee PK, Jarosek SL, Virnig BA, et al. Trends in the incidence and treatment of parathyroid cancer in the United States. *Cancer* 2007; **109**: 1736.
6. Upton AC. *Health effects of exposure to low levels of ionizing radiation: BEIR V*. Washington DC: National Academy Press; 1990.
7. Koea JB, Shaw J. Parathyroid cancer: biology and management. *Surg Oncol* 1999; **8**: 155–65.
8. Khan MW, Worcester EM, Straus 2nd FH, et al. Parathyroid carcinoma in secondary and tertiary hyperparathyroidism. *J Am Coll Surg* 2004; **199**(2): 312–19.
9. Kameyama K, Takami H. DNA cytofluorometric analysis using HP/DAPI double staining of parathyroid carcinoma arising in a patient with chronic renal failure and secondary hyperparathyroidism. *Oncol Rep* 1999; **6**:1345.
10. Arnold A, Kim HG, Gaz RD, et al. Molecular cloning and chromosomal mapping of DNA rearranged with the parathyroid hormone gene in a parathyroid adenoma. *J Clin Invest* 1989; **83**(6): 2034–40.
11. Vasef MA, Brynes RK, Sturm M, et al. Expression of cyclin D1 in parathyroid carcinoma, adenoma and hyperplasias: a paraffin immunohistochemical study. *Mod Pathol* 1999; **12**(4): 412–16.
12. Cryns VL, Thor A, Xu HJ, et al. Loss of the retinoblastoma tumour suppressor gene in parathyroid carcinoma. *N Engl J Med* 1994; **330**(11): 757–61.
13. Subramaniam P, Wilkinson S, Shepherd JJ. Inactivation of retinoblastoma gene in malignant parathyroid growths: a candidate genetic trigger? *ANZ J Surg* 1995; **65**(10): 714–16.
14. Shattuck TM, Valimaki S, Obara T, et al. Somatic and germline mutations of the HRPT2 gene in sporadic parathyroid carcinoma. *N Engl J Med* 2003; **349**: 1722.
15. Kim HK, Oh YL, Kim SH, et al. Parafibromin immunohistochemical staining to differentiate parathyroid carcinoma from parathyroid adenoma. *Head Neck* 2012; **34**(2): 201–6.
16. Haven CJ, Howell VM, Eilers PH, et al. Gene expression of parathyroid tumours: molecular subclassification and identification of the potential malignant phenotype. *Cancer Res* 2004; **64**: 7405–11.
17. Sandelin K, Farnebo F. Parathyroid carcinoma. In: Doherty GM, Skogseid B (eds). *Surgical endocrinology*. Philadelphia: Lippincott Williams & Wilkins; 2001, pp. 189–93.
18. DeLellis RA. Parathyroid carcinoma. *Adv Anat Pathol* 2005; **12**(2): 53–61.
19. Obara T, Okamoto T, Kanbe M, Ilhara M. Functioning parathyroid carcinoma: clinicopathologic features and rational treatment. *Semin Surg Oncol* 1997; **13**(2): 134–41.
20. Rodgers SE, Perrier ND. Parathyroid carcinoma. *Curr Opin Oncol* 2006; **18**(1): 16–22.
21. Schaapveld M, Jorna FH, Aben KK, et al. Incidence and prognosis of parathyroid gland carcinoma: a population-based study in the Netherlands estimating the preoperative diagnosis. *Am J Surg* 2011; **202**(5): 590–7.
22. Sharretts JM, Kebebew E, Simonds WF. Parathyroid cancer. *Semin Oncol* 2010; **37**(6): 580–90.
23. Reeder S, Desser T, Weigel R, et al. Sonography in primary hyperparathyroidism: a review with emphasis on scanning techniques. *J Ultrasound Med* 2002; **21**: 539–52.
24. Sidhu PS, Talat N, Patel P, et al. Ultrasound features of malignancy in the preoperative diagnosis of parathyroid cancer: a retrospective analysis of parathyroid tumours larger than 15 mm. *Eur Radiol* 2011; **21**(9): 1865–73.
25. Cheung K, Wang T, Farrokhyar F, et al. A meta-analysis of preoperative localisation techniques for patients with primary hyperparathyroidism. *Ann Surg Oncol* 2012; **19**(2): 577–83.
26. Spinelli C, Bonadio AG, Berti P, et al. Cutaneous spreading of parathyroid carcinoma after fine needle aspiration cytology. *J Endocrinol Invest* 2000; **23**(4): 255–7.
27. Rodgers SE, Hunter GJ, Hamberg LM, et al. Improved preoperative planning for directed parathyroidectomy with 4-dimensional computed tomography. *Surgery* 2006; **140**(6): 932–40.
28. Beland MD, Mayo-Smith W, Grand DJ, et al. Dynamic MDCT for localisation of occult parathyroid adenomas in 26 patients with primary hyperparathyroidism. *AJR Am J Roentgenol* 2011; **196**: 61–5.
29. Muller DL, Doppman JL. Parathyroid angiography. *Ann Intern Med* 1987; **107**: 942–3.
30. Chazen JL, Gupta A, Dunning A, Phillips CD. Diagnostic accuracy of 4D CT for parathyroid adenomas and hyperplasia. *Am J Neuroradiol* 2012; **33**: 429–33.
31. Gardner CJ, Wieshmann H, Gosney J, et al. Localization of metastatic parathyroid carcinoma by 18F FDG-PET scanning. *J Clin Endocrinol Metab* 2010; **95**(11): 4844–5.
32. Rawat N, Khetan N, Williams DW, Baxter JN. Parathyroid carcinoma. *Br J Surg* 2005; **92**: 1345–53.
33. Wang CA, Gaz RD. Natural history of parathyroid carcinoma: diagnosis, treatment and results. *Am J Surg* 1985; **149**(4): 522–7.

34. Wei CH, Harari A. Parathyroid carcinoma: update and guidelines for management. *Curr Treat Options Oncol* 2012; **13**: 11–23.
35. Clayman GL, Gonzalez HE, El-naggar A, Vassilopoulou-Sellin R. Parathyroid carcinoma: evaluation and interdisciplinary management. *Cancer* 2004; **100**(5): 900–5.
36. Obara T, Fujimoto Y. Diagnosis and treatment of patients with PTC: an update and review. *World J Surg* 1991; **15**: 738–44.
37. O'Neill CJ, Chan C, Symons J, et al. Parathyroid carcinoma encountered after minimally invasive focused parathyroidectomy may not require further radical surgery. *World J Surg* 2011; **35**(1): 147–53.
38. Fujimoto Y, Obara T, Ito Y, et al. Localisation and surgical resection of metastatic parathyroid carcinoma. *World J Surg* 1986; **10**: 539–47.
39. Shane E. Clinical review 122: parathyroid carcinoma. *J Clin Endocrinol Metab* 2001; **86**: 485–93.
40. Kebebew E, Arici C, Duh QY, Clark O. Localisation and reoperation results for persistent and recurrent parathyroid carcinoma. *Arch Surg* 2001; **136**(8): 878–85.
41. Ghandran M, Deftos LJ, Stuenkel CA, et al. Thymic parathyroid carcinoma and postoperative hungry bone syndrome. *Endocr Pract* 2003; **9**(2): 152–6.
42. Schell SR, Dudley NE. Clinical outcomes and fiscal consequences of bilateral neck exploration for primary idiopathic hyperparathyroidism without preoperative radionuclide imaging or minimally invasive techniques. *Surgery* 2003; **133**(1): 32–9.
43. Placzkowski K, Christian R, Chen H. Radioguided parathyroidectomy for recurrent parathyroid cancer. *Clin Nucl Med* 2007; **32**(5): 358–60.
44. Sharma J, Milas M, Berber E, et al. Value of intraoperative parathyroid hormone monitoring. *Ann Surg Oncol* 2008; **15**(2): 493–8.
45. Kebebew E. Parathyroid carcinoma. *Curr Treat Options Oncol* 2001; **2**(4): 347–54.
46. Busaidy NL, Jimenez C, Habra MA, et al. Parathyroid carcinoma: a 22-year experience. *Head Neck* 2004; **26**(8): 716–26.
47. Dotzenrath C, Goretzki PE, Sarbia M, et al. Parathyroid carcinoma: problems in diagnosis and the need for radical surgery even in recurrent disease. *Eur J Surg Oncol* 2001; **27**(4): 383–9.
48. Yoshida S. Intracranial metastatic parathyroid carcinoma: case report. *Surg Neurol* 2006; **65**(1): 81–3.
49. Hundley JC, Albertson DA, Bradley RF, Levine EA. Resection of pulmonary metastasis from parathyroid carcinoma. *Am Surg* 2003; **69**(9): 779–83.
50. Van Haaren ER, Kievit J, Huysmans HA, van de Velde CJ. Successful resection of hepatic and pulmonary metastases in a patient with parathyroid carcinoma. *Jpn J Clin Oncol* 1996; **26**(2): 99–102.
51. Koyano H, Shishiba Y, Shimizu T, et al. Successful treatment by surgical removal of bone metastasis producing PTH: new approach to the management of metastatic parathyroid carcinoma. *Intern Med* 1994; **33**(11): 697–702.
52. Schantz A, Castleman B. Parathyroid carcinoma: a study of 70 cases. *Cancer* 1973; **31**: 600–5.
53. Stojadinovic A, Hoos A, Nissan A, et al. Parathyroid neoplasms: clinical, histopathological and tissue microarray based molecular analysis. *Hum Pathol* 2003; **34**: 54–64.
54. Bondeson L, Grimelius L, DeLellis RA, et al. Parathyroid carcinoma. In: DeLellis RA, Lloyd RV, Heitz PU, Eng C (eds). *World Health Organization classification of tumours. Pathology & genetics: Tumours of endocrine organs.* Lyon: IARC Press; 2004.
55. Lim S, Elston MS, Gill AJ, et al. Metastatic parathyroid carcinoma initially misdiagnosed as parathyroid adenoma: the role of parafibromin in increasing diagnostic accuracy. *Internl Med J* 2011; **41**(9): 695–9.
56. Juhlin CC, Hoog A. Parafibromin as a diagnostic instrument for PTC – lone ranger or part of the posse? *Int J Endocrinol* 2010; 1–5.
57. Howell VM, Haren CJ, Kahnoski K, et al. HRPT2 mutations are associated with malignancy in sporadic parathyroid tumours. *J Med Genet* 2003; **40**: 657–63.
58. Krebs LJ, Shattuck TM, Arnold A. HRPT2 mutational analysis of typical sporadic parathyroid adenomas. *J Clin Endocrinol Metab* 2005; **90**: 5015–17.
59. Gill AJ, Clarkson A, Gimm O, et al. Loss of nuclear expression of parafibromin distinguishes parathyroid carcinomas and hyperparathyroidism-jaw tumor (HPT-JT) syndrome-related adenomas from sporadic parathyroid adenomas and hyperplasias. *Am J Surg Pathol* 2006; **30**(9): 1140–9.
60. Strewler GJ. Medical approaches to primary hyperparathyroidism. *Endocrinol Metab Clin N Am* 2000; **29**(3): 523–39.
61. Au WY. Calcitonin treatment of hypercalcaemia due to parathyroid carcinoma. Synergistic effect of prednisone on long term treatment of hypercalcaemia. *Arch Intern Med* 1975; **135**(12): 1594–7.
62. Warrell RP, Israel R, Frisone M, et al. Gallium nitrate for acute treatment of cancer-related hypercalcaemia: a randomized, double-blind comparison to calcitonin. *Ann Intern Med* 1988; **108**(5): 669–74.
63. Bukowski RM, Sheeler L, Cunningham J, Esselstyn C. Successful combination chemotherapy for metastatic parathyroid carcinoma. *Arch Intern Med* 1984; **144**(2): 399–400.
64. Chahinian AP. Chemotherapy for metastatic parathyroid carcinoma. *Arch Intern Med* 1984; **144**(9): 1889.
65. Munson ND, Foote RL, Northcutt RC, et al. Parathyroid carcinoma: is there a role for adjuvant radiation therapy? *Cancer* 2003; **98**: 2378–84.
66. Rasmuson T, Kristoffersson A, Boquist L. Positive effect of radiotherapy and surgery on hormonally active pulmonary metastases of primary parathyroid carcinoma. *Eur J Endocrinol* 2000; **143**(6): 749–54.
67. Selvan B, Paul MJ, Seshadri MS, et al. High index of clinical suspicion with optimal surgical techniques and adjuvant radiotherapy is critical to reduce locoregional disease progression in PTC. *Am J Clin Oncol* 2013; **36**(1): 64–9.
68. Harari A, Waring A, Fernandez-Ranvier G, et al. PTC: a 43-year outcome and survival analysis. *J Clin Endocrinol Metab* 2011; **96**(12): 3679–86.

Parathyroid surgery

CHAPTER 76

BILATERAL PARATHYROID EXPLORATION

R. James A. England and Nick McIvor

Introduction 865
When to perform bilateral parathyroid exploration 865
The operation of bilateral parathyroid exploration..........868
References 871

SEARCH STRATEGY

Data in this chapter may be updated by a PubMed search using the keywords: bilateral exploration, four-gland exploration and parathyroid.

INTRODUCTION

Primary hyperparathyroidism (HPT) is only curable surgically. It is a common endocrine condition with approximately 100 000 new cases diagnosed annually in the United States.[1] Traditionally, the operative procedure of choice involves a search for all four parathyroid glands and the selective removal of any gland(s) judged enlarged by visual inspection. The principles of bilateral parathyroid exploration (BPE) have remained unchanged since their first description by Felix Mandl in 1926.[2]

More recently, improved localization techniques and the use of intra-operative parathyroid hormone level monitoring have led to a shift away from BPE towards more focused surgery, the often-labelled minimally invasive parathyroidectomy (MIP). This procedure enables ambulatory parathyroidectomy and parathyroidectomy under sedation or local anaesthesia. However, most parathyroid surgeons agree that MIP is only feasible for single-gland disease.

The traditional four gland exploration is therefore mainly for patients with suspected multigland disease, negative imaging and patients undergoing revision surgery. The significant incidence of such patients demands that a parathyroid surgeon has the ability to perform the traditional operation.

This chapter discusses the situations in which BPE is generally the preferred surgical option and the operative steps of BPE.

WHEN TO PERFORM BILATERAL PARATHYROID EXPLORATION

Cases where bilateral parathyroid exploration may be performed fall into four broad groups:

- suspected multigland disease
- parathyroid cancer
- failed pre-operative localization
- failed MIP.

Suspected multigland disease

Approximately 15% of primary HPT patients and all those with secondary HPT have multigland disease. Those with primary HPT having multigland disease include those with double adenoma, non-familial hyperplasia, and familial HPT.

PRIMARY HPT – DOUBLE ADENOMA / PRIMARY HYPERPLASIA

There is some debate as to whether double adenoma is a distinct entity. Some argue that double adenomas are rare and the distinction between adenoma and asymmetrical hyperplasia is difficult pathologically.[3] Hyperplasia can be localized within a gland and asymmetrical between glands.

It is not surprising therefore that there is poor correlation between surgeons and pathologists and even among pathologists themselves when interpreting hyperfunctioning glands.[4]

Clonal studies confirm that adenomas are monoclonal whereas hyperplastic glands and normal glands are polyclonal.[5] However, the likelihood of monoclonal growth occurring simultaneously in two separate glands should be low. Increased proliferative activity is reported in normal glands of some double adenoma patients, suggesting adenomas may arise in a background of hyperplasia.[6] Furthermore, clonal studies have confirmed monoclonal growth occurring within hyperplastic glands in both primary hyperplasia and renal hyperparathyroidism.[6–8] Thus the concept of double adenoma is supportable albeit probably in a setting of asymmetrical hyperplasia. The question remains as to how long a patient should be observed after removal of double adenomas to exclude the possibility of recurrence and/or diagnosis of hyperplasia. An interval of 5 years has been recommended.[3]

In primary HPT, therefore, the surgeon needs to know that double adenoma/primary hyperplasia exists, that imaging is unreliable in this situation,[9, 10] and that a small proportion of patients undergoing MIP will require BPE.

PRIMARY HPT – FAMILIAL

Familial HPT comprises approximately 10–20% of all HPT presentations is discussed further in other chapters.

The hereditary syndromes, most frequently caused by mutations within specific genes, include multiple endocrine neoplasia (MEN) familial HPT and non-MEN familial HPT. MEN HPT occurs in MEN 1 and MEN 2A. Non-MEN HPT includes familial hypocalciuric hypercalcaemia (FHH) and neonatal severe hyperparathyroidism caused by heterozygous and homozygous calcium-sensing receptor gene mutations respectively. Also included is familial isolated HPT for which no specific genetic mutation has thus far been identified, and hyperparathyroidism-jaw tumour syndrome (HPT-JT).[11]

A familial syndrome should be suspected in young patients (teens, 20s), those with a family history of HPT, and those with a previous history or family history of medullary carcinoma, phaeochromocytoma, insulinoma, carcinoid or pituitary tumour. Familial syndromes exist in an autosomal dominant pattern.

Traditional BPE is the procedure of choice in most of these patients with the exception of FHH, which requires no treatment.

MEN familial HPT

MEN 1 HPT MEN 1 is relatively rare, occurring in approximately 1 in 30 000 people. The *MEN1* gene, identified in 1997, is the only gene known to be associated with the syndrome.[12] Primary hyperparathyroidism is the most common clinical manifestation of multiple endocrine neoplasia type 1.[2] It represents approximately 2–4% of all PHPT, making it the most common form of inherited HPT.

Clinically evident disease is present in 95% of carriers by 25 years of age, with all being affected by 50.[13] The severity of the condition mandates surgery is performed in most cases but the type of procedure performed varies. The aim of surgery has to be to control HPT, minimize HPT recurrence and avoid hypoparathyroidism. Because of the genetic nature of the condition, removal of only enlarged glands at surgery is not practised because recurrence rates are too high.

Currently, two surgical approaches tend to be practised: subtotal parathyroidectomy removing at least 3–3.5 glands, and total parathyroidectomy with autotransplantation. In both procedures transcervical thymectomy is advised as the thymus often contains ectopic and/or supernumerary parathyroid glands and may develop thymic carcinoids.[14]

Subtotal parathyroidectomy generally involves the removal of the three largest glands and part of the fourth, maintaining approximately 50 g of parathyroid tissue. In 20% of cases all four glands cannot be found and in this situation a three-gland parathyroidectomy is performed. Large series with long-term follow-up are sparse, but persistent HPT rates range from 0% to 33%, recurrence rates from 0% to 51% and hypoparathyroidism rates from 0% to 27%.[15–19]

Total parathyroidectomy aims to remove all functioning parathyroid tissue. Hypoparathyroidism is then avoided by reimplantation of approximately 50 mg of autologous parathyroid tissue harvested from the most macroscopically normal of the parathyroid glands removed.

The optimum surgical approach is debatable. A cohort study from the Netherlands concluded that the most effective surgical approach involved subtotal parathyroidectomy (SPTX) with bilateral transcervical thymectomy. This was because persistence/recurrence was statistically more frequent when thymectomy was not performed, but permanent hypoparathyroidism was much more likely following total parathyroidectomy (TPTX). However, due to the rarity of the condition, a sample size of 73 patients undergoing a variety of surgical procedures in a non-randomized fashion makes it hard to draw firm conclusions.[20] The conclusions obtained correlated with those from a previous meta-analysis searching Medline, Embase and Cochrane from 1966 to 2008 which resulted in the analysis of 12 studies comparing SPTX with TPTX. The analysis concluded that <SPTX (defined as <three gland resection) should not be preformed because of the high risk of persistent and recurrent disease. Also TPTX carried too high a risk of permanent hypoparathyroidism (67%). Once again, more caution should be observed, no RCTs were found and all data was retrospective. In addition, follow-up periods varied and the study group was from the same institution as the more recent Netherlands study.[21]

MEN 2A HPT The MEN 2A subtype constitutes 70–80% of cases of MEN 2. In MEN 2A the overriding concern is to manage medullary thyroid cancer (MTC) in a timely fashion, ideally operating on the patient prior to malignant transformation, but after diagnosis or exclusion of phaeochromocytoma. MEN 2A hyperparathyroidism occurs in approximately 20–30% of MEN 2A patients and is generally mild or asymptomatic.[22] In the majority of cases, hyperplasia occurs prior to adenoma formation although at surgery a single adenoma may be found.[23] It tends to occur in the third decade of life, but generally before the age of 39.[24] Although hyperparathyroidism is associated with various *RET* codon mutations, it tends to occur primarily in association with the exon 11 codon 634 mutation, which accounts for 85% of patients with MEN 2A.[25]

Recommended surgery depends on whether the neck has previously been operated on as is frequently the case to manage/avoid medullary thyroid cancer. In the unoperated neck with diagnosed PHPT in MEN 2A, ATA guidelines suggest removal of either enlarged glands only, a 3–3.5-gland parathyroidectomy (subtotal) or total parathyroidectomy, all with forearm autograft. For patients who develop PHPT after thyroid surgery it is recommended that parathyroid surgery is directed by pre-operative imaging, again with forearm autograft unless a functioning graft already exists. Patients are controlled medically if there is a high risk of surgical mortality, recurrent disease after previous surgeries or limited life expectancy. All recommendations are grade C.[26] It is felt that the optimal surgical intervention should be individualized as the condition is mild and, indeed, often asymptomatic, and most series have significant numbers of permanent hyper- and permanent hypoparathyroid patients.[27,28]

Non-MEN familial HPT

Severe neonatal hyperparathyroidism This is a very rare but life-threatening disease in neonates demanding urgent management. Total parathyroidectomy via BPE following medical stabilization with biphosphonate therapy is usually required within the first few months of life. The morbidity of permanent hypoparathyroidism has encouraged surgeons to autotransplant parathyroid tissue, with variable success.[29]

Hyperparathyroidism-jaw tumour syndrome HPT-JT is a rare autosomal dominant familial cancer syndrome. The condition comprises primary HPT, ossifying tumours of the maxilla and mandible and less commonly renal cysts and/or uterine tumours.[30] HPT is the commonest feature of this disease. In affected individuals HPT occurs in approximately 80% of cases. The HPT occurs at a young age (mean 32 years), and it has a high incidence of severe hypercalcaemia and 15% malignancy rate. Treatment comprises a protocol similar to the management of MEN 2A, where only macroscopically enlarged glands are removed, although all glands should be found and assessed because of the high cancer rate. Some advocate total parathyroidectomy to negate the cancer risk.[31] If a likely cancer diagnosis is made at surgery, then en bloc resection of tumour, ipsilateral thyroid lobe and adjacent involved tissue is performed.

SECONDARY/TERTIARY HPT

Parathyroid surgery in renal failure

With decreasing renal function there is an associated decrease in renal 1-alpha hydroxylase activity, with a resultant drop in calcitriol or vitamin D3 synthesis. This in turn decreases the stimulation of the vitamin D receptor on parathyroid cells, causing an increased production of PTH and secondary HPT.[32] This leads to extraskeletal calcification and cardiac disease, causing an increased risk of cardiovascular morbidity and mortality. Indeed, dialysis patients on multivariant analysis have a 30 times greater risk of cardiovascular mortality than the general population.[33]

Renal failure patients are treated to normalize biochemical parameters, minimize bone disease and prevent extraskeletal calcium deposition. Nephrologists use serum calcium, phosphate, vitamin D and PTH levels as surrogate markers of disease severity. Treatment involves replacing serum vitamin D and restricting phosphate in the diet; vitamin D replacement in renal failure patients has been shown to reduce the risk of mortality, particularly cardiac related mortality.[34] If phosphate restriction proves insufficiently effective, phosphate binders such as calcium acetate and aluminium hydroxide are prescribed. In addition, calcimimetic agents such as cinecalcet may be used. Its implementation has led to a reduction in fracture risk, hospitalization rates for cardiovascular disease and requirement of parathyroid surgery.[35]

The need for parathyroidectomy in renal hyperparathyroidism has fallen due to improved medical control, a retrospective US survey reporting a 30% decline in the 1990s.[36] Currently, 1–2% of these patients will undergo surgery annually, with 10% ultimately requiring parathyroidectomy.[37] The cut-off point for deciding on a surgical option is not well established. The National Kidney Foundation Kidney Disease Quality Outcomes Initiative (KDOQI) suggest that patients with PTH >800 pg/mL associated with hypercalcaemia and/or hyperphosphataemia, despite medical therapy, should be offered parathyroidectomy.[38] Uncontrolled renal HPT results in morbidity classically from pruritus, the severity of which has been directly correlated to intact PTH levels,[39] bone pain, fractures or calciphylaxis and increased mortality rates.[40] In addition, a survival benefit has been demonstrated in renal failure patients undergoing parathyroidectomy.[41]

The optimal operative strategy for these patients is debatable. The main options include total parathyroidectomy versus subtotal parathyroidectomy (a 3.5-gland parathyroidectomy), with or without autotransplantation. In addition, the practice of simultaneous transcervical thymectomy varies.

A recent international survey assessing surgical practice in the management of renal hyperparathyroidism primarily within Europe obtained analysable results from 86 different surgeons performing renal parathyroidectomy.[42] The survey suggests that 20.9% of respondents operated without any pre-operative imaging. When used, the most popular imaging modalities are ultrasound (36%) and sestamibi

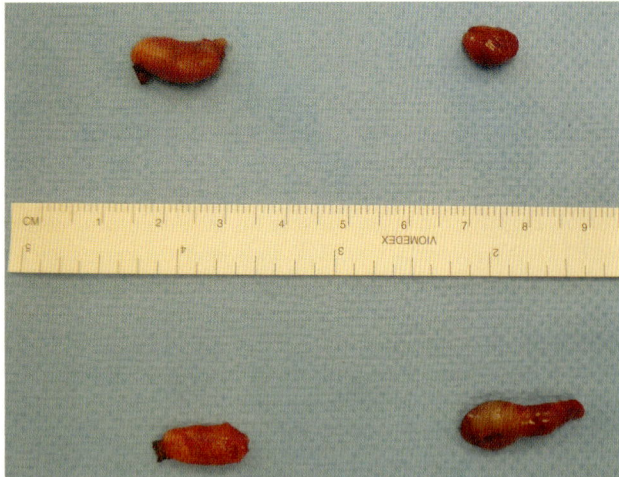

Figure 76.1 Four-gland parathyroidectomy specimen during renal parathyroidectomy in secondary hyperparathyroidism.

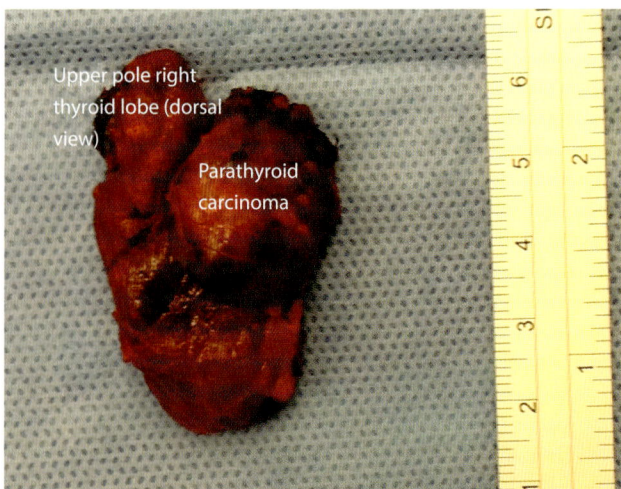

Figure 76.2 Right superior parathyroid carcinoma removed en bloc with right thyroid lobe.

scintigraphy (9.3%), with both in combination in 33.7%. Respondents reported that 98.8% perform subtotal or total parathyroidectomy, with or without immediate autotransplantation (**Figure 76.1**). In addition, 74.4% routinely perform transcervical thymectomy with 25.6% prepared to perform a transsternal exploration during initial surgery.

In the study, the practice of autotransplantation (AT) is extremely variable: 40.7% perform immediate AT while 36% do not. Smaller percentages tailor their practice to ioPTH results or dialysis techniques. The forearm is the implantation site of choice in 72.7% and the sternocleidomastoid in 16.4%. Graft function is assessed with serum PTH monitoring from grafted versus non-grafted forearms in 62.9% of cases, with 13.6% ($n = 5$) performing a temporary implantectomy ('Casanova test') and one using sestamibi scintigraphy (2.6%).

Parathyroid cancer

Parathyroid cancer is the cause of primary hyperparathyroidism in approximately 1% of cases. In advanced cases it has a high morbidity and mortality rate, mortality usually caused by intractable hypercalcaemia. If parathyroid cancer is suspected either pre-operatively or intra-operatively, the most likely way of achieving cure is through thorough surgical resection of the tumour and any involved surrounding tissue; the only appropriate surgical option is therefore BPE.

The involved parathyroid gland tends to invade immediately surrounding tissues including ipsilateral thyroid lobe, recurrent laryngeal nerve and ipsilateral strap muscles. If these structures are involved clinically, most surgeons advocate en bloc resection, avoiding breach of the tumour capsule to minimize risk of tumour seeding, with ipsilateral level 6 clearance if there is evidence of nodal involvement (**Figure 76.2**). Failure to perform en bloc resection or to clear the ipsilateral neck at revision surgery carries a significantly higher risk for local recurrence and death.[43, 44] Because of failure to make a correct clinical diagnosis at the time of first surgery and/or different management beliefs, en bloc resection only occurs in approximately 12% of cases with up to 86% of patients having inadequate resection at first surgery.[45, 46]

Failed pre-operative localization

Pre-operative sestamibi localization is negative in up to 20% of PHPT patients. This is reported to occur with increased incidence in multigland disease (32%). In a recent analysis of over 2600 patients with PHPT at a single institution, a curative operation was performed in 90.4 % with a negative MIBI compared to 97.5 % with localization ($P < 0.001$).

4D-CT is an emerging technique that uses high-resolution CT images, multiplanar reformats and perfusion characteristics to identify abnormal parathyroid glands in patients with hyperparathyroidism. 4D-CT correctly identifies unilateral vs bilateral disease in 90% of patients, potentially reducing the need for BPE.[47]

Failed MIP

MIP may require conversion to BPE when there is failure to find a pre-operatively imaged gland or failure of ioPTH to drop to below 50% baseline at 10 minutes after adenoma excision, suggesting multigland disease.

This is especially significant in double adenoma. In a dual institution study of patients undergoing bilateral exploration, the ioPTH incorrectly indicated success after removal of the first adenoma in 55% of cases of double adenoma.[48] In comparison between the two groups, the authors found that the second adenoma was significantly smaller than the first in the false positive group ($p = 0.03$).

THE OPERATION OF BILATERAL PARATHYROID EXPLORATION

The patient is ideally consented before the day of surgery. The surgeon reviews the diagnosis, the indications for surgery and any imaging performed. The aims of the operation are defined. The incidence of adverse events should be cited according to the surgeon's audited data. Specific risks include surgical failure and disease recurrence, recurrent laryngeal nerve damage and post-operative haematoma. The option of no surgery with its risks and consequences is discussed to enable an informed decision.

On the day of surgery, the neck is marked for level of incision by sitting the patient in a neutral position looking straight ahead. A surgical marker places a line at the bony soft-tissue junction at the level of the sternoclavicular joints.

The procedure is normally performed under general anaesthesia. The patient is intubated with a north-facing armoured endotracheal tube. The patient is placed in a supine position with 30 degrees of head elevation. Where possible, the neck is extended using a sandbag placed under the shoulders with the head stabilized on a headring.

The surgical field is prepared and draped. An incision of approximately 5 cm is made through skin and platysma. To optimize access, a subplatysmal flap is raised to approximately 1 cm above the cricoid cartilage and laterally superficial to the sternomastoid muscles. An inferior flap does not enhance surgical access. The strap muscles are separated at the linea alba. Occasionally, the linea alba is hard to identify as the muscle bodies are closely approximated. In this situation, the strap muscles are followed inferiorly towards the sternal notch as the muscles diverge caudally.

The plane between the deep straps and the thyroid lobe is developed from medial to lateral. The thyroid lobe is partially delivered from deep to the straps by lateral retraction of the ipsilateral strap muscles while the thyroid lobe is digitally retracted medially by the surgeon with a single layer of surgical gauze between the lobe and the middle finger. Fibrous bands are separated by the action of opening the surgical scissors in a medial to lateral direction. Bands that fail to divide are normally small blood vessels under tension which require bipolar diathermy. Once the lobe is adequately mobilized, a suture may be placed through the lobe in a cephalocaudal direction to enable the assistant to retract the thyroid out of the operative field. Simultaneously, the strap muscles and carotid sheath are retracted laterally so that the area directly surrounding the dorsal thyroid and tracheo-oesophageal gutter may be explored. A dry surgical field is vital as bleeding causes tissue discoloration and may create problems with parathyroid identification, especially with normal suppressed glands. Rinsing the wound with saline may help.

A successful search for the parathyroid glands requires a thorough knowledge of their surgical anatomy and embryology. The surgeon should understand the positions of parathyroid ectopia, which are mandated both embryologically and by the effects of increasing gland mass and deglutition.

The search should proceed in a methodical way. Ideally, no gland should be removed until all are visualized, but in a significant number of cases only one adenomatous gland and two suppressed/normal glands are found. In this situation it is acceptable to remove the enlarged gland, note the position of the identified normal glands and record the identity of the missing gland.

The superior gland is the more constant in position and generally lies on the posterior surface of the thyroid gland within 1 cm of the cricothyroid joint and posterior to the recurrent laryngeal nerve. As the thyroid lobe is retracted out of the neck and onto the trachea, its relationship with the nerve is inverted so the nerve lies deep to the superior parathyroid (**Figure 76.3**). An enlarged superior gland often works its way into a retropharyngeal/retro-oesophageal position by the combined actions of swallowing and gravity. It is found by identifying the inferior thyroid artery laterally, the recurrent laryngeal nerve inferomedially and entering the retropharyngeal space by mosquito dissection above the artery. Gentle soft-tissue dissection will identify the gland, which can be drawn out by gentle traction on its pedicle (**Figure 76.4**). If no gland is evident, the retropharyngeal compartment and the posteriomedial surface of the superior thyroid pole should be explored, the latter often requiring full mobilization of the pole by division of the superior vascular pedicle.

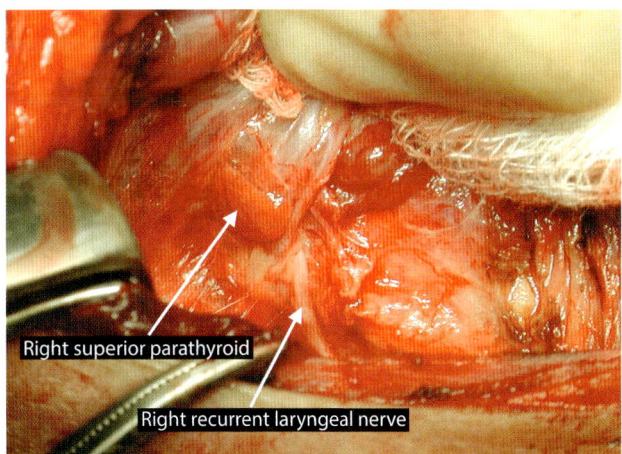

Figure 76.3 Demonstrating the inverted relationship between the right superior parathyroid and the right recurrent laryngeal nerve when the right thyroid lobe is retracted onto the trachea.

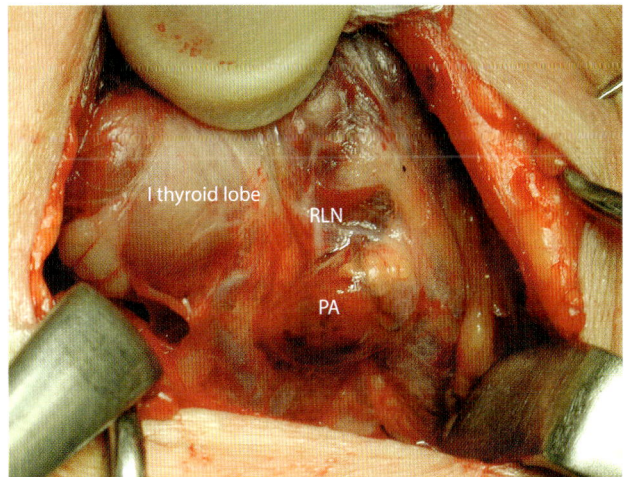

Figure 76.4 Left thyroid lobe retracted medially and enlarged left superior parathyroid adenoma (PA), having been delivered from the retro-oesophageal gutter, lying on top of the left recurrent laryngeal nerve (RLN).

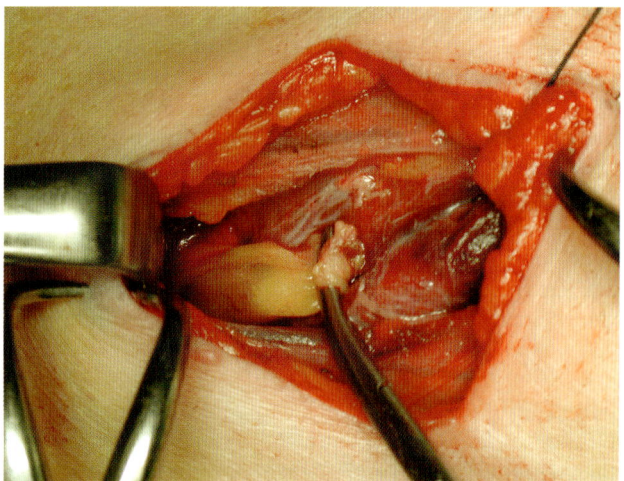

Figure 76.5 Left thymic remnant being delivered from the mediastinum and containing an ectopic inferior parathyroid adenoma.

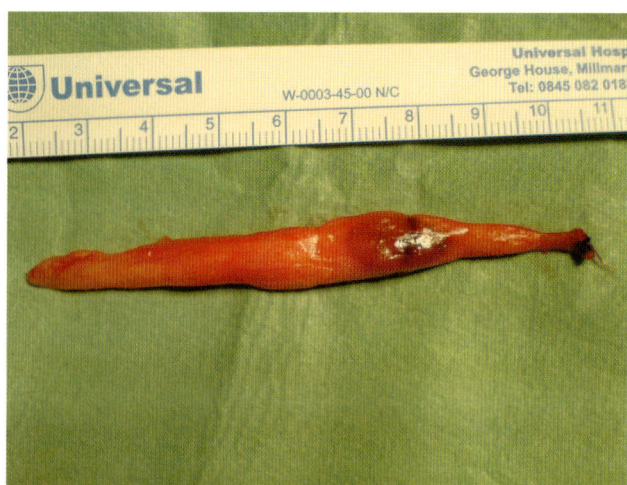

Figure 76.6 Delivered thymic remnant containing ectopic adenoma.

The inferior gland is typically found near or within the thyrothymic tract, extending from the lower pole into the superior mediastinum, and it usually lies in a plane anterior to the nerve. Again, fascia is carefully dissected from the inferior pole out towards the recurrent laryngeal nerve. Progressive dissection into the thyrothymic tract will usually identify the gland. Further search for the inferior gland by delivery of the thymus into the neck is required only if an adenoma has not been identified on either side of the neck. This is to avoid devascularizing a normal but suppressed gland. If no gland has been found, the lower pole itself should be carefully inspected as a gland can often be found deep to the fascia compressed onto the thyroid.

Thymic delivery is effected by dissection inferiorly, anterior to the carotid artery, but medial to the recurrent nerve and lateral to the trachea at the level of the clavicle. The thymus continues as an extension of the thyrothymic tract and may be delivered from the chest by gentle and progressive traction on its capsule (**Figures 76.5** and **76.6**).

Surgical failure necessitates a thorough review of all dissected areas with documentation of clearly identified parathyroids and those missing. A 'second look' often identifies parathyroids which have changed colour due to devascularization or bruising.

If a superior gland, which is of 4th branchial arch origin, is missing, then inspection behind the hyoid, larynx, pharynx and within the carotid sheath at inferior thyroid artery level is performed. The possibility of an intra-thyroidal gland must be considered, best identified with ultrasound. Hemithyroidectomy is performed only if there are good grounds for suspecting an intra-thyroidal adenoma. If an inferior gland is missing, the carotid sheath is explored from the level of the superior thyroid artery down to the sternoclavicular joint.

Failure after such a meticulous and sequential operation occurs in a small minority of patients. The possibility of an incorrect diagnosis must be considered. The surgeon must accept that the gland may be beyond the dissected field and that further imaging studies are required. Accurate operative documentation is essential. Before closing, blood may be taken for PTH assay from the upper IJV and lower IJV on each side as this may help narrow the subsequent search by suggesting the area of the rogue gland. Further surgery is then dictated by the severity of the hyperparathyroidism, positive imaging and patient consent.

KEY POINTS

- Bilateral parathyroid exploration (BPE) is normally reserved for multigland disease, familial disease, cases with negative imaging and revision surgery.
- When performing BPE, the surgeon should be aware of the embryology of the parathyroid glands and hence the most likely positions of ectopia for a missing gland.
- In 80% of cases, a gland on one side is symmetrical with that on the other, so finding the corresponding contralateral gland may aid the search for a missing gland.
- The dissection should be as bloodless as possible to avoid discoloration of surrounding tissues, which makes parathyroid identification difficult, particularly when glands are suppressed.
- The commonest position of an ectopic superior gland is retro-oesophageal, and an inferior intra-thymic.

REFERENCES

1. Arnalsteen LC, Alesina PF, Quiereux JL, et al. Long-term results of less than total parathyroidectomy for hyperparathyroidism in multiple endocrine neoplasia type 1. *Surgery* 2002; **132**(6): 1119–24; discussion 1124–5.
2. Mandl F. Klinisches und experimentelles zur Frage der lokalisierten und generalisierten Ostitis fibrosa. *Arch Klin chir* 1926, **143**: 245.
3. Baloch, ZW, LiVolsi VA. Editorial: Double adenoma of the parathyroid gland does the entity exist? *Arch Pathol Lab Med* 2001; **125**:178–9.
4. Saxe AW, Baier R, Tesluk H, Tureson W. The role of the pathologist in the surgical treatment of hyperparathyroidism. *Surg Gynecol Obstet* 1985; **161**: 101–5.
5. Arnold A, Staunton CE, Kim HG, et al. Monoclonality and abnormal parathyroid hormone genes in parathyroid adenomas. *N Engl J Med* 1988; **318**: 658–62.
6. Larian B, Sassan Alavi S, Roesler J, et al. The role of hyperplasia in multiple parathyroid adenomas. *Head Neck* 2001; **23**(2): 134–9.
7. Arnold A, Brown MF, Urena P, et al. Monoclonality of parathyroid tumors in chronic renal failure and in primary parathyroid hyperplasia. *J Clin Invest* 1995; **95**: 2047–53.
8. Shan L, Kakudo K, Nakamura M, et al. Clonality of the parathyroid nodules with uremic parathyroid hyperplasia. *Pathol Oncol Res* 1997; **3**(3): 198–203.
9. Dy BM, Richards ML, Vazquez BJ, et al. Primary hyperparathyroidism and negative Tc99 sestamibi imaging: to operate or not? *Ann Surg Oncol* 2012; **19**: 2272–6.
10. Norton KS, Johnson LW, Griffen FD, et al. The sestamibi scan as a preoperative screen tool. *Am Surg* 2002; **68**: 812–15.
11. Sharretts JM, Kebebew E, Simonds WF. Parathyroid cancer. *Semin Oncol* 2010; **37**(6): 580–90.
12. Chandrasekharappa SC, Guru SC, Manickam P, et al. Positional cloning of the gene for multiple endocrine neoplasia type 1. *Science* 1997; **276**(5311): 404–7.
13. Giusti F, Tonelli F, Brandi M. Primary hyperparathyroidism in multiple endocrine neoplasia type 1: when to perform surgery? *Clinics Sao Paolo* 2012; **67**(S1): 141–4.
14. Tonelli F, Giudici F, Cavalli T, Brandi M. Surgical approach in patients with hyperparathyroidism in multiple endocrine neoplasia type 1: total versus partial parathyroidectomy. *Clinics Sao Paolo* 2012; **67**(S1): 155–160.
15. Hubbard JGH, Sebag F, Maweja S, Henry JF. Subtotal parathyroidectomy as an adequate treatment for primary hyperparathyroidism in multiple endocrine neoplasia type 1. *Arch Surg* 2006; **141**(3): 235–9.
16. Prinz RA, Gamvros OP, Sellu D, Lynn JA. Subtotal parathyroidectomy for primary chief cell hyperplasia of multiple endocrine neoplasia type 1 syndrome. *Surgery* 1981; **193**(1): 26–9.
17. Elaraj DM, Skarulis MC, Libutti SK, et al. Results of initial operation for hyperparathyroidism in patients with multiple endocrine neoplasia type 1. *Surgery* 2003; **134**(6): 858–65.
18. Hellman P, Skogseid B, Oberg K, et al. Primary reoperative parathyroid operations in hyperparathyroidism of multiple endocrine neoplasia type 1. *Surgery* 1998; **124**(6): 993–9.
19. Hellman P, Skogseid B, Oberg K, et al. Findings and long-term results of parathyroid surgery in multiple endocrine neoplasia type 1. *World J Surg* 1992; **16**(4): 718–25.
20. Pieterman CR, van Hulsteijn LT, den Heijer M, et al. Primary hyperparathyroidism in MEN 1 patients: a cohort study with long-term follow-up on preferred surgical procedure and the relation with genotype. *Ann Surg* 2012; **255**(6): 1171–8.
21. Schreinemakers JMJ, Pieterman CRC, Scholten A, et al. The optimal surgical treatment for primary hyperparathyroidism in MEN 1 patients: a systematic review. *World J Surg* 2011; **35**: 1993–2005.
22. Eng C, Clayton D, Schuffenecker I, et al. The relationship between specific RET proto-oncogene mutations and disease phenotype in multiple endocrine neoplasia type 2. International RET mutation consortium analysis. *JAMA* 1996; **276**: 1575–9.
23. Alevizaki M. Management of hyperparathyroidism (PHP) in MEN 2 syndromes in Europe. *Thyroid Res* 2013; **6** supp 1: S10.
24. Schuffenecker I, Virally-Monod M, Brohet R, et al. Risk and penetrance of primary hyperparathyroidism in multiple endocrine neoplasia type 2A families with mutations at codon 634 of the RET proto-oncogene. Groupe D'etude des tumeurs a Calcitonine. *J Clin Endocrinol Metab* 1998; **83**: 487–91.
25. Raue F, Frank-Raue K. Genotype-phenotype relationship in multiple endocrine neoplasia type 2. Implications for clinical management. *Hormones (Athens)* 2009; **8**: 23–8.
26. Kloos RT, Eng C, Evans DB, et al. Medullary thyroid cancer: management guidelines of the American Thyroid Association. *Thyroid* 2009; **19**(6): 565–612.
27. Kraimps JL, Denizot A, Caranaille B, et al. Primary hyperparathyroidism in multiple endocrine neoplasia type IIa: retrospective French multicentric study. Group d'Etude des Tumeurs a Calcitonine (GETC, French Calcitonin Tumours Study Group), French Association of Endocrine Surgeons. *World J Surg* 1996; **20**: 808–12.
28. Herfarth KK, Bartsch D, Doherty GM, et al. Surgical management of hyperparathyroidism in patients with multiple endocrine neoplasia type 2A. *Surgery* 1996; **120**: 966–73.
29. Al-Shanafey S, Al-Hosaini R, Al-Ashwal A, Al-Rabeeah A. Surgical management of severe neonatal hyperparathyroidism: one center's experience. *J Ped Surg* 2010; **45**: 714–17.
30. Sharrets JM, Simonds WF. Clinical and molecular genetics of parathyroid neoplasms. *Best Pract Res Clin Endocrinol Metab* 2010; **24**(3): 491–502.
31. Carling T, Udelsman R. Parathyroid surgery in familial hyperparathyroid disorders. *J Int Med* 2005; **257**(1): 27–37.
32. Tomasello S. Secondary hyperparathyroidism and chronic kidney disease. *Diabetes Spectr* 2008; **21**: 19–25.
33. Block GA, Klassen PS, Lazarus JM, et al. Mineral metabolism, mortality, and morbidity in maintenance hemodialysis. *J Am Soc Nephrol* 2004; **15**: 2208–18.
34. Duranton F, Rodriguez-Ortiz ME, Duny Y, et al. Vitamin D treatment and mortality in chronic kidney disease: a systematic review and meta-analysis. *Am J Nephrol* 2013; **37**(3): 239–48.
35. Moe SM, Chertow GM, Coburn JW, et al. Achieving NKF-K/DOQI bone metabolism and disease treatment goals with cinacalcet HCl. *Kidney Int* 2005; **67**(2): 760–71.
36. Kestenbaum B, Seliger SL, Dillen DL, et al. Parathyroidectomy rates among United States dialysis patients: 1990–1999. *Kidney Int* 2004; **65**: 282–8.
37. Triponez F, Clark OH, Vanrenthergem Y, Evenepoel P. Surgical treatment of persistant hyperparathyroidism after renal transplantation. *Ann Surg* 2008; **248**: 18–30.
38. National Kidney Foundation K/DOQI clinical practice guidelines for bone metabolism and disease in chronic kidney disease. *Am J Kidney Dis* 2003; **42**(3): 1–201.
39. Makhlough A, Emadi N, Sedighi O, et al. Relationship between serum intact parathyroid hormone and pruritus in hemodialysis patients. *Iran J Kidney Dis* 2013; **7**: 42–6.
40. Costa-Hong V, Jorgetti V, Gowdak LHW, et al. Parathyroidectomy reduces cardiovascular events and mortality in renal hyperparathyroidism. *Surgery* 2007; **5**: 699–703.
41. Sharma J, Raggi P, Kutner N, et al. Improved long-term survival of dialysis patients after near-total parathyroidectomy. *J Am Coll Surg* 2012; **214**(4): 400–7.
42. Riss P, Asari R, Scheuba C, Niederle B. Current trends in surgery for renal hyperparathyroidism (RHPT): an international survey. *Langenbecks Arch Surg* 2013; **398**: 121–30.
43. Talat N, Schulte KM. Clinical presentation, staging and long-term evolution of parathyroid cancer. *Ann Surg Oncol* 2010; **17**(8): 2156–74.
44. Kebebew E, Arici C, Duh QY, Clark OH. Localization and reoperation results for persistent and recurrent parathyroid carcinoma. *Arch Surg* 2001; **136**: 878–85.
45. Lee PK, Jarosek SL, Virnig BA, et al. Trends in the incidence and treatment of parathyroid cancer in the United States. *Cancer* 2007; **109**: 1736–41.
46. Hundahl SA, Fleming ID, Fremgen AM, Menck HR. Two hundred eighty-six cases of parathyroid cancer treated in the US between 1985-1995: a National Cancer Data Base Report. The American College of Surgeons Commission on Cancer and the American Cancer Society. *Cancer* 1999; **86**: 538–44.
47. Kelly HR, Hamberg LM, Hunter GJ. 4D-CT for preoperative localization of abnormal parathyroid glands in patients with hyperparathyroidism: accuracy and ability to stratify patients by unilateral versus bilateral disease in surgery-naive and re-exploration patients. *AJNR* 2014; **35**: 176–81.
48. Gauger PG, Agarwal G, England BG, et al. Intraoperative parathyroid hormone monitoring fails to detect double parathyroid adenomas: a 2-institution experience. *Surgery* 2001; **130**(6): 1005–10.

CHAPTER 77

MINIMALLY INVASIVE PARATHYROIDECTOMY

Parameswaran Rajeev and Gregory P. Sadler

Introduction 873	Operative steps 875
Surgical anatomy of the parathyroid glands 873	Complications 876
Investigations for parathyroid disease 874	Post-operative care 876
Pre-operative imaging 874	References 876
Indications for MIP 875	

SEARCH STRATEGY

Data in this chapter may be updated by a PubMed search using the keywords: parathyroidectomy, hyperparathyroidism and imaging.

INTRODUCTION

The surgical management of primary hyperparathyroidism has evolved from open neck exploration to minimally invasive surgery since the first successful parathyroidectomy was performed by Felix Mandl in Vienna in 1925. Minimally invasive parathyroidectomy (MIP) is now the treatment of choice for patients with sporadic hyperparathyroidism, with a parathyroid tumour localized by pre-operative imaging. The success of the technique is attributable to the improvements in pre-operative localization with sestamibi scanning and high-resolution neck ultrasound. This chapter describes the indications and technique of MIP in the management of sporadic primary hyperparathyroidism.

Primary hyperparathyroidism (HPT) is a common medical problem and is the most frequent cause of hypercalcaemia in the outpatient setting. The incidence of the disease has increased over the last decade worldwide,[1, 2] with the disease being more prevalent in women and with advancing age.[3, 4] Primary HPT is caused by a solitary adenoma in 80–85%, hyperplasia in 15–20%, usually in familial syndromes,[5] and carcinoma in less than 1% of cases.[6] Surgical extirpation of the gland is the mainstay of treatment in this condition.

Bilateral neck exploration has been considered the gold standard in the surgical management of primary parathyroid disease. However, with the emergence of improved pre-operative parathyroid localization with high-resolution ultrasound scan, sestamibi and SPECT scans, the technique of MIP has evolved.[7–9] The operation is performed under local anaesthesia (superficial cervical block) and intravenous sedation[10, 11] or general anaesthesia.[12]

The success of the procedure has been demonstrated in numerous studies with or without intra-operative PTH assay.[9, 10, 12, 13] The advantages of performing minimally invasive parathyroid surgery have been shown to be lower cost,[14] shorter operating time,[15, 16] shorter stay in hospital[12, 16] and improved cosmesis and patient satisfaction.[17] Technically, the operation is performed with a small incision measuring 2–3 cm on the neck and excludes the extrathyroidal approaches via the axilla or chest wall.

Surgical anatomy of the parathyroid glands

The success of parathyroid surgery must lie in the ability of the surgeon to know a parathyroid gland when he sees it, to know the distribution of the glands, where they hide, and also to be delicate enough in technique to be able to make use of this knowledge.

Edward D. Churchill (1931)[18]

This statement should fundamentally apply to all surgeons practising parathyroid surgery, more so in minimally invasive surgery. A thorough understanding of the embryology and anatomy is essential before performing the technique of MIP.

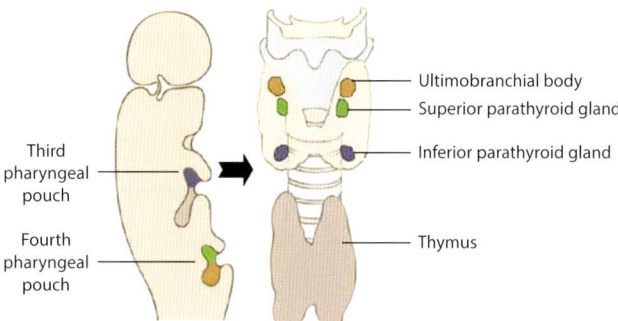

Figure 77.1 Diagram of normal pharyngeal organ development.
The superior parathyroid glands and ultimobrachil body derive from the fourth pharyngeal pouch. The inferior glands originate from the third pharyngeal pouch along with the thymus. Reproduced with permission from Chen H, Senda T, Emura S, Kubo K. An update on the structure of the parathyroid gland. *Open Anat J* 2013; **5**: 1–9.[19]

Parathyroid glands are usually four in number and usually lie on the posterior surface of the thyroid gland, each with its own connective tissue capsule. The glands develop from the third and fourth pharyngeal pouches in the fifth week and descend to join the thyroid gland by about the seventh week of development. The inferior parathyroid gland arises from the superiorly located third pouch and the superior from the inferiorly located fourth pouch, as shown in **Figure 77.1**. This anatomical positioning of the parathyroid is linked to the development of the thymus. The thymus originates from the caudal portion of the third pharyngeal pouch and as it descends into the thorax, the inferior parathyroid usually accompanies it. The inferior parathyroid detaches from the thymus during the migration and takes its position on the posterior surface of the thyroid gland. Occasionally the inferior parathyroid moves with the thymus into the thorax and rests in an ectopic position.

The anatomical landmark that helps the surgeon in identifying the parathyroid gland intra-operatively is the inferior thyroid artery. The superior parathyroid glands are usually located within a circumscribed area about 2.5 cm above the intersection of the recurrent laryngeal nerve (RLN) with the inferior thyroid artery and the inferior glands located about the same distance below it. However, both the glands may be located outside the normal position and this is more commonly seen with the inferior parathyroid glands. Variations in the position of the superior glands include the upper thyroid pole in the posterior aspect of the neck, the retropharyngeal or retro-oesophageal space or rarely intra-thyroidally.[20, 21]

The inferior parathyroid glands have a wider distribution and may be located anterior, inferior or lateral to the inferior thyroid pole besides its conventional position. They may be seen in eutopic positions in the neck close to the thyrothymic ligament or within the cervical portion of the thymus or carotid sheath and, rarely, intra-thyroidally. They may also be located ectopically in the anterior mediastinum or in the aortopulmonary window.[20, 21]

It is not uncommon to confuse fat, accessory thyroid nodules or even lymph nodes with parathyroid glands.

The parathyroid glands are usually vascular and bleed or bruise easily, unlike fat or thyroid tissue.[21] The glands are softer than thyroid tissue and lymph nodes. A simple technique to differentiate parathyroid from non-parathyroid tissue is to apply gentle pressure with a fine surgical instrument to the parathyroid glands; they appear to move inside their own capsule unlike non-parathyroid tissue.

INVESTIGATIONS FOR PARATHYROID DISEASE

The most important aspect in the use of minimally invasive parathyroid surgery is to establish the correct diagnosis and localize the disease accurately. Primary HPT can be differentiated from other forms of hypercalcaemia by careful history, physical examination and laboratory investigations. The disease has evolved from the classical symptomatic to asymptomatic form. Most patients today present with abnormal biochemistry results and do not have any manifestations of the disease.

The presence of the disease is confirmed biochemically with elevated calcium and parathyroid hormone levels, in the presence of normal renal function. It is important to measure vitamin D levels as the disease is characterized by low plasma levels of 25-hydroxyvitamin D and high plasma levels of 1,25-dihydroxyvitamin D. An autosomal dominant condition that mimics primary HPT is benign familial hypocalciuric hypercalcaemia (FHH), and this is excluded by measuring 24-hour urinary calcium excretion.

PRE-OPERATIVE IMAGING

The only localizing study indicated in a patient with untreated primary HPTH is to localize an experienced parathyroid surgeon.

J.L. Doppman[22]

For many years until the development of MIP, the role of pre-operative imaging was considered to be less important than the skill of the surgeon. Imaging in parathyroid disease has evolved over the last 60–70 years, with significant improvement in pre-operative localization. For MIP, it is essential to have a 'road map' of the anatomical location of the parathyroid gland and this is usually achieved by non-invasive modalities in the form of ultrasound and sestamibi scan, computed tomography (CT) and magnetic resonance imaging (MRI)[22] (**Figure 77.2**).[22] The invasive modalities are usually reserved for re-operative parathyroid surgery.

Imaging with sestamibi is the first-line investigation using the single-radioisotope technetium-99m (^{99m}Tc) sestamibi followed by high-resolution ultrasound scan. Recent studies have shown the combination of sestamibi with SPECT to be superior to single modality imaging [23, 24] and effective in detecting posterior glands.

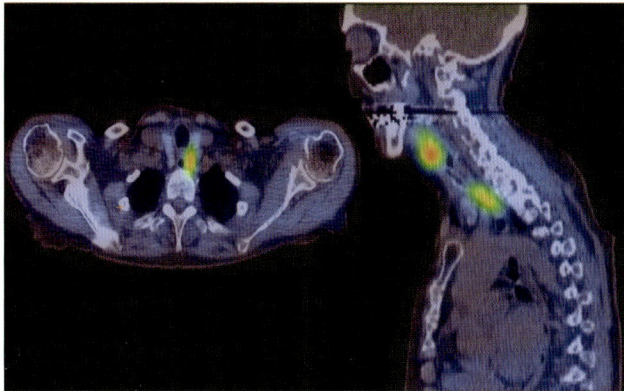

Figure 77.2 Sestamibi/CT functional overlay showing a left superior parathyroid adenoma. The tumour has dropped in the retro-oesophageal position and is not viewable on ultrasound scanning.

Ultrasound scanning (USS) has a complementary role to sestamibi and is useful in assessing the anatomy of the neck. It can easily differentiate parathyroid glands from thyroid nodules, which may be seen in up to 40% of patients. However, USS is operator-dependent and may miss smaller and deeper glands.

Where the scans are discordant, the current practice is to perform a CT or MRI scan for further confirmation of the adenoma. As a single modality, CT and MRI are of little use in localizing parathyroid adenomata for a minimally invasive approach. Their role is more in localizing ectopic disease or in the context of re-operative surgery.

INDICATIONS FOR MIP

The indications for MIP are no different from the conventional cervical exploration – symptomatic or asymptomatic patients fulfilling the established NIH criteria.[25] The technique is reserved for patients with uniglandular disease with concordant scans. Where there is discordance, absent imaging or negative scans MIP should not be performed. A scoring model for uniglandular disease has been developed by Kebebew et al[26] and includes: single site on sestamibi scan, single site on ultrasound, concordant localization, serum calcium >1 mg/dL above the upper normal limit, and PTH twice the upper limit of normal. The predictive value of the scoring system is 100% and therefore patients with a score of more than 3 should be offered MIP. Conditions that make patients unsuitable for MIP are listed in Box 77.1.

BOX 77.1 Contradictions to MIP

Multiglandular disease
Family history of MEN or familial hyperparathyroidism
History of irradiation
Previous neck surgery
Chronic renal insufficiency
Lithium therapy

OPERATIVE STEPS

Preparation and incision

The surgery may be performed under general anaesthesia or local anaesthesia with intravenous sedation (LA+IVS). All patients have a superficial cervical block with 20 mL of 0.25% Marcaine infiltrated on the involved side. Patients have an ultrasound scan on the morning of the surgery with pre-operative skin marking, and the image acts as the 'road map' to the adenoma (Figure 77.3). The patient is positioned on the table supine with slight neck extension by placing a gel pad or pillow behind the shoulder blades. The patient's head is supported in a gel donut and hyperextension is thereby prevented. The table is tilted 30 degrees in a reverse Trendelenburg position. The surgical site is prepped and sterile-draped from the chin to the sternal notch.

The skin incision is made according to the position of the adenoma that is pre-operatively marked by ultrasound. Either a medial or a focused lateral approach may be used to remove the adenoma. The medial approach is more suitable for a superficial inferior adenoma whereas the lateral approach is useful in picking a posterior inferior or a superior adenoma. We routinely use the focused lateral approach for superior and inferior adenomas. A 2–2.5 cm incision is placed along the skin crease overlying the medial border of the sternocleidomastoid muscle corresponding to the position of the parathyroid adenoma (Figure 77.3).

Once the skin incision is made, the platysma is divided gently by electrocautery and the subplatysmal plane is developed using blunt scissors. The medial edge of the sternocleidomastoid muscle is identified and the fascia divided superiorly and inferiorly. Any small vessel encountered is cauterized. The sternocleidomastoid muscle is retracted laterally and the lateral edge of the strap muscles is exposed. The plane below the muscles is entered and the strap muscles are retracted medially to expose the thyroid. By this technique, of medial retraction of straps and lateral retraction of the jugular vein underlying the sternocleidomastoid, most parathyroid glands are identified in the neck.

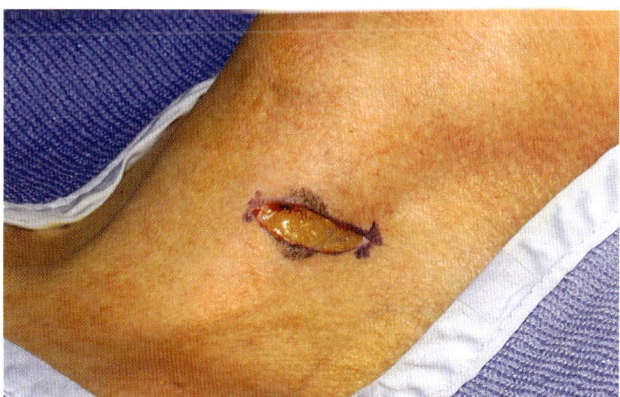

Figure 77.3 Incision for MIP, positioned over medial border of left sternomastoid (20 mm).

Exposure of the inferior parathyroid adenoma

The inferior parathyroid glands are usually seen at the inferior pole of the ipsilateral thyroid lobe or in or around the thyrothymic ligament. The adenomas are usually seen anterior to the RLN and inferior to the inferior thyroid artery. Once the plane between the straps and sternocleidomastoid is exposed, the thyroid is retracted medially and anteriorly. Using blunt artery forceps the parathyroid is circumferentially dissected free from the thyroid and the gland is gently lifted using vascular forceps, taking care not to fracture the parathyroid. Tributaries to the gland are clamped with a small haemostat and ligated. The gland is then excised and sent for histological evaluation. Adenomas located in the thyrothymic ligament or even in the thymus can be removed by this approach.

Exposure of the superior parathyroid adenoma

The superior adenoma is usually located in an area above the intersection of the inferior thyroid artery with the RLN, posteriorly in the retropharyngeal or in the retro-oesophageal space. The thyroid gland is retracted medially and the inferior thyroid artery is identified along with the RLN. In the case of large adenomas the artery may need dividing, as they lie usually posteriorly. Once the adenoma is identified, the dissection is performed in the avascular plane posterolaterally and, using the vascular forceps, the gland is gently mobilized, taking care not to injure the RLN. The pedicle, located posteromedially, is identified, clipped and divided. If the adenoma cannot be located in the positions described, one may need to consider that the adenoma may be intra-thyroidal. In this scenario, a decision for open-neck exploration is advised.

Once the adenoma is excised and haemostasis achieved, the wound is irrigated. The platysma and the skin are closed with subcuticular Vicryl Rapide, and Steristrips or glue applied to the wound.

Confirmation of cure

Most centres recommend the use of intra-operative PTH (IOPTH) levels to ensure that the adenoma is resected and also to assess cure. When this is achieved, the PTH levels fall to 50% of the pre-operative value at 10 minutes and this is predictive of cure in 98% of cases.[27]

COMPLICATIONS

The complications of MIP are rare in the best of hands and in centres of excellence. They are listed in **Box 77.2**.

BOX 77.2 Complications of MIP

Recurrent laryngeal nerve palsy
Bleeding
Hypoparathyroidism (rare)
Persistent disease
Failure to cure

POST-OPERATIVE CARE

Patients are routinely prescribed analgesia and calcium supplementation on discharge. On discharge, irrespective of symptoms of hypocalcaemia and patients are generally advised to take calcium for a minimum of 24–48 hours post excision. While most of these cases are performed as day cases, patients are monitored for a minimum of 4–6 hours for any signs of haematoma. A patient leaflet on wound care is provided on discharge. Patients are reviewed in clinic at 4–6 weeks post-surgery, and calcium and PTH levels are checked to confirm cure.

KEY POINTS

- Confirm diagnosis of PHPT.
- Perform localization studies.
- Concordant studies: consider MIP.
- Ensure adequate exposure to perform operation safely.
- Establish protocol to manage post-operative hypocalcaemia and bleeding.

REFERENCES

1. Abood A, Vestergaard P. Increasing incidence of primary hyperparathyroidism in Denmark. *Dan Med J* 2013; 60(2): A4567.
2. Yu N, Donnan PT, Murphy MJ, Leese GP. Epidemiology of primary hyperparathyroidism in Tayside, Scotland, UK. *Clin Endocrinol (Oxf)* 2009; 71(4): 485–93.
3. Minisola S. Primary hyperparathyroidism is one of the three most frequent endocrine disorders, typically diagnosed in the years following menopause and with advancing age. *J Endocrinol Invest* 2012; 35(7 Suppl): 1.
4. Fraser WD. Hyperparathyroidism. *Lancet* 2009; 374(9684): 145–58.
5. Brandi ML, Gagel RF, Angeli A, et al. Guidelines for diagnosis and therapy of MEN type 1 and type 2. *J Clin Endocrinol Metab* 2001; 86(12): 5658–71.
6. Clayman GL, Gonzalez HE, El-Naggar A, Vassilopoulou-Sellin R. Parathyroid carcinoma: evaluation and interdisciplinary management. *Cancer* 2004; 100(5): 900–5.
7. Sackett WR, Barraclough B, Reeve TS, Delbridge LW. Worldwide trends in the surgical treatment of primary hyperparathyroidism in the era of minimally invasive parathyroidectomy. *Arch Surg* 2002; 137(9): 1055–9.
8. Udelsman R, Donovan PI, Sokoll LJ. One hundred consecutive minimally invasive parathyroid explorations. *Ann Surg* 2000; 232(3): 331–9.
9. Grant CS, Thompson G, Farley D, van Heerden J. Primary hyperparathyroidism surgical management since the introduction of minimally invasive parathyroidectomy: Mayo Clinic experience. *Arch Surg* 2005; 140(5): 472–8; discussion 8–9.

10. Rajeev P, Stechman MJ, Kirk H, et al. Safety and efficacy of minimally invasive parathyroidectomy (MIP) under local anaesthesia without intra-operative PTH measurement. *Int J Surg* 2013; **11**(3): 275–7.
11. Norman J, Chheda H, Farrell C. Minimally invasive parathyroidectomy for primary hyperparathyroidism: decreasing operative time and potential complications while improving cosmetic results. *Am Surg* 1998; **64**(5): 391–5; discussion 5–6.
12. Mihai R, Palazzo FF, Gleeson FV, Sadler GP. Minimally invasive parathyroidectomy without intraoperative parathyroid hormone monitoring in patients with primary hyperparathyroidism. *Br J Surg* 2007; **94**(1): 42–7.
13. Agarwal G, Barakate MS, Robinson B, et al. Intraoperative quick parathyroid hormone versus same-day parathyroid hormone testing for minimally invasive parathyroidectomy: a cost-effectiveness study. *Surgery* 2001; **130**(6): 963–70.
14. Goldstein RE, Blevins L, Delbeke D, Martin WH. Effect of minimally invasive radioguided parathyroidectomy on efficacy, length of stay, and costs in the management of primary hyperparathyroidism. *Ann Surg* 2000; **231**(5): 732–42.
15. Palazzo FF, Sadler GP. Minimally invasive parathyroidectomy. *Br Med J* 2004; **328**(7444): 849–50.
16. Udelsman R. Surgery in primary hyperparathyroidism: the patient without previous neck surgery. *J Bone Miner Res* 2002; **17**(Suppl 2): N126–32.
17. Burkey SH, Van Heerden JA, Farley DR, et al. Will directed parathyroidectomy utilizing the gamma probe or intraoperative parathyroid hormone assay replace bilateral cervical exploration as the preferred operation for primary hyperparathyroidism? *World J Surg* 2002; **26**(8): 914–20.
18. Cope O. The study of hyperparathyroidism at the Massachusetts General Hospital. *N Engl J Med* 1966; **274**(21): 1174–82.
19. Chen H, Senda T, Emura S, Kubo K. An update on the structure of the parathyroid gland. *TOANATJ* 2013; **5**: 1–9.
20. Noussios G, Anagnostis P, Natsis K. Ectopic parathyroid glands and their anatomical, clinical and surgical implications. *Exp Clin Endocrinol Diabetes* 2012; **120**(10): 604–10.
21. Thompson NW, Eckhauser FE, Harness JK. The anatomy of primary hyperparathyroidism. *Surgery* 1982; **92**(5): 814–21.
22. Treglia G, Trimboli P, Huellner M, Giovanella L. Imaging in primary hyperparathyroidism: focus on the evidence-based diagnostic performance of different methods. *Minerva Endocrinol* 2017, June 23.
23. Melton GB, Somervell H, Friedman KP, et al. Interpretation of 99mTc sestamibi parathyroid SPECT scan is improved when read by the surgeon and nuclear medicine physician together. *Nucl Med Commun* 2005; **26**(7): 633–8.
24. Eslamy HK, Ziessman HA. Parathyroid scintigraphy in patients with primary hyperparathyroidism: 99mTc sestamibi SPECT and SPECT/CT. *Radiographics* 2008; **28**(5): 1461–76.
25. Udelsman R, Pasieka JL, Sturgeon C, et al. Surgery for asymptomatic primary hyperparathyroidism: proceedings of the third international workshop. *J Clin Endocrinol Metab* 2009; **94**(2): 366–72.
26. Kebebew E, Hwang J, Reiff E, et al. Predictors of single-gland vs multigland parathyroid disease in primary hyperparathyroidism: a simple and accurate scoring model. *Arch Surg* 2006; **141**(8): 777–82; discussion 82.
27. Carneiro DM, Irvin GL 3rd. New point-of-care intraoperative parathyroid hormone assay for intraoperative guidance in parathyroidectomy. *World J Surg* 2002; **26**(8): 1074–7.

CHAPTER 78

SURGICAL FAILURE AND REOPERATIVE SURGERY

Schelto Kruijff and Leigh Delbridge

Background 879	Review: Results and post-operative complications 884
Investigation of persistent or recurrent disease (the three 'R's)..... 882	Summary 884
Conservative options 883	References 885
Surgical approach 883	

SEARCH STRATEGY

Data in this chapter may be updated by a PubMed search using the keywords: parathyroid and reoperative parathyroid surgery.

BACKGROUND

General introduction

Primary hyperparathyroidism (PHPT) is a disease characterized by elevated serum calcium and parathyroid hormone (PTH) levels. It is a common disorder although multiple factors can influence its incidence such as regional influences, nutritional status, the availability of routine biochemical screening, sex (incidence higher in females), previous irradiation and age. Where the average incidence is 4.3/1000 in the United States, in women aged between 55 and 75 years the incidence can rise up to 21/1000.[1] It is most frequently caused by a single benign adenoma and is associated with a range of symptoms. The parathyroid glands play a key role in regulating the calcium homeostasis through an interaction between PTH, serum ionized calcium and vitamin D with the gastrointestinal tract, kidney and skin. Calcium is the single most potent activator of PTH release and, when its levels decrease, the calcium-sensing receptor (CaSR), situated on the parathyroid chief cells, is activated and stimulates the release of PTH.[2]

Historically, patients with hyperparathyroidism would present with advanced clinical features such as fractures, skeletal deformities, 'brown tumours', renal calculi and even kidney failure. After the discovery of the PTH and the introduction of routine biochemical screening with the autoanalyzer in the 1970s, a significant change took place such that most patients were diagnosed at an earlier stage, with an associated dramatic increase in presentations for surgery.

Historical perspective on surgical management

The only cure for PHPT is to surgically remove the hyperfunctioning parathyroid adenoma or adenomata (in the case of multigland disease) or to reduce the bulk of parathyroid tissue in patients with hyperplasia. The historical evolution of surgery for PHPT, as well as the surgical strategies after operative failure, can be considered in three distinct phases. The first phase was the 'learning curve'. While the first documented removal of a parathyroid adenoma by Bland-Sutton in 1910 was successful, he was certainly not aware of the pre-operative diagnosis.[3] Most of the early documented intentional parathyroid procedures in the 1920s were associated with failure for a variety of reasons that may still plague parathyroid surgeons today. In Vienna in 1925, Hirsch undertook a four-gland parathyroid exploration which turned out to be negative with no tumour found. The patient was subsequently diagnosed with fibrous dysplasia, which was the wrong diagnosis. Also in Vienna in 1925, Mandl performed the first initially successful intentional parathyroidectomy, although a number of years later the patient developed recurrent disease and died.[4] In 1927, Churchill performed a total of seven parathyroid explorations on the same patient before finally removing a large mediastinal adenoma. Unfortunately, his patient died post-operatively of renal failure, albeit cured of his hyperparathyroidism.[5]

The second phase was the open four-gland exploration approach. With an increasing understanding of parathyroid anatomy and embryology over subsequent decades, open four-gland parathyroid exploration became the gold standard procedure for patients with hyperparathyroidism, providing cure rates in experienced hands of over 95% with minimal complications. In that phase, failure in the 5% of patients was largely related either to surgery being performed by an inexperienced surgeon, or to the presence of an ectopic parathyroid adenoma, usually located in a mediastinal position. Multigland disease was readily managed since all four parathyroid glands were routinely identified and any large glands removed.

The third and current phase of minimally invasive parathyroidectomy (MIP) was ushered in with the report of the first endoscopic parathyroidectomy by Gagner in 1996.[6] The initial techniques employed endoscopic assistance, but it soon became clear that a more direct approach via a 2 cm open mini-incision (either central or lateral) was feasible and much more direct.[7] The perceived advantages with a minimally invasive approach were patients with less post-operative pain, smaller scar and shorter hospital stay, and MIP has now become standard of care, with reported cure rates of over 95%, at least in the short term.[7] Unlike open four-gland parathyroid exploration, the most common cause of failure in MIP is the presence of multigland disease. Up to 15% of patients have historically been reported to have multigland disease present, which represents the number who, in theory, require more than one gland excised to achieve normocalcaemia.[8] However, with the advent of MIP, aiming at a pre-operatively identified parathyroid abnormality, a much higher frequency of solitary adenomas of 96% was found.[8] The extent of the pre-operative workup influences the number of observed solitary adenomas. Lee came to a supporting conclusion comparing the presence of multigland disease before and after the introduction of MIP and found that the incidence of multiple enlarged glands being removed dropped from 15% to 4%, although there was no documented change in the incidence of surgical failure. These findings indicate that many enlarged glands in patients with multigland disease do not contribute to hypercalcaemia.[9]

Numerous techniques have been introduced to minimize the risk of failure during MIP. The most widely utilized is the intra-operative measurement of serum PTH levels (IOPTH) first introduced by Irvin.[10] Many authors claim this reduces the risk of failure, although there are no convincing data to support this proposal. IOPTH works best when not required, when a single localized adenoma is removed at MIP, but it fails most often when most needed, especially in the presence of multigland disease. Therefore, we recommend IOPTH is not utilized, rather emphasis is placed upon high-quality concordant imaging for localization, providing a success rate of 98% as documented in our last published series of over 100 successive cases.[11] If a single abnormal gland cannot be localized, then open parathyroidectomy is still offered.

While short-term failure is no higher in patients having a MIP, there is increasing concern that long-term recurrence may be rising. For example, after having performed more than 17 000 parathyroid operations having, Norman has recently abandoned the unilateral MIP claiming that the procedure carries a 10-year recurrence rate of 4–6%.[12] He recommends that the only way to achieve 10-year cure rates of over 95% is to examine all four parathyroid glands.[12] The group claims that no diagnostic tool such as intra-operative PTH (IOPTH) is able to confirm with enough certainty that all the abnormal glands have been removed. They also argue that several studies have shown that 20% of patients have more than one abnormal, enlarged gland, and in 16% an initial IOPTH drop after removing one enlarged gland will still require the removal of additional tumours.[12–14] As previously noted, in general, the experience is that high-quality imaging, with appropriate selection for MIP based upon concordant localization studies (4D CT, sestamibi scan and ultrasound), is the most appropriate means of minimizing initial parathyroidectomy failure to around 2% (**Figure 78.1**). When that inevitably occurs, reoperative parathyroidectomy can still be undertaken (by experienced surgeons) with very high success rates and minimal complications (**Figure 78.2a,b**).[15]

Anatomy and embryology of difficult locations

The parathyroid glands are small tan brown organs which arise from the dorsal aspect of the pharyngeal pouch in the fifth week and descend in the direction of the caudal thyroid gland. They are soft, weigh 35–55 mg, and measure 2–7 mm in length.[15] Multiple shapes, ranging from leaf to bean form, are found.[16] Adenomas are usually oval, red-brown masses that can replace the normal parathyroid gland, although haemorrhagic and cystic lesions can also be seen. An adenoma can weigh anywhere from 50 mg to several grams. On histologic examination, parathyroid chief cells will be seen clustered around capillary networks.[16] Localization studies may help the surgeon locate any pathological glands; success in parathyroid surgery, however, is mainly based upon a thorough knowledge of

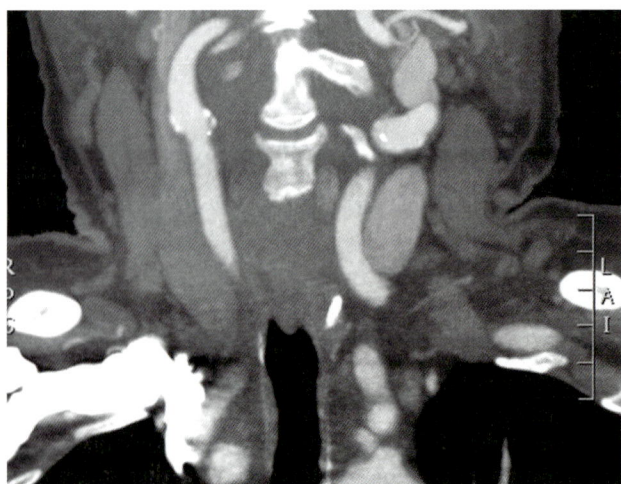

Figure 78.1 4D CT scan showing a left retropharyngeal undescended superior adenoma.

LOCATION OF THE SUPERIOR PARATHYROID GLANDS (PIV)

The superior glands arise from the dorsal wing of the fourth pharyngeal pouch and descend in a caudal direction with the thyroid gland itself. Most superior parathyroid glands (PIVs) are located immediately adjacent to inferior cornu of the thyroid cartilage, close to the recurrent nerve, cranial to the branch of the inferior artery nerve. Exposure of the posterior aspect of the thyroid lobe is made by displacing the gland inwards and retracting the jugular–carotid bundle outwards. After this simple exposure, the superior glands are then found immediately superior to the junction of the recurrent laryngeal nerve and the inferior thyroid artery.[17]

These glands are closely associated with the recurrent nerve and so, when mobilizing them, especially with a minimal invasive approach, identification and dissection of the nerve are of vital importance. However, when the superior gland is abnormal, it tends to migrate posteriorly and downwards. Therefore, when it is not in immediate contact with the thyroid, it should be sought lateral to or behind the oesophagus, bearing in mind that the lower a superior descended gland travels the more posterior it becomes.

The origin of the pedicle is usually at the upper third of the thyroid lobe and can be located by simple traction on the pedicle. The superior parathyroid gland can also be situated just under the perithyroidal sheath, close to the posterior aspect of the lobe. Quite often a flattened parathyroid adenoma is located at the posterior aspect of the upper pole of the thyroid lobe which may easily be missed when one does not know where to look for it.

LOCATION OF THE INFERIOR PARATHYROID GLANDS (PIII)

Because of a longer descent, the inferior parathyroid glands (PIIIs) have a much higher variability in location when compared with the superior parathyroid glands; the inferior parathyroid glands arise from the dorsal aspect of the third pharyngeal pouch and, following the development of the thymus, they descend in a caudal-medial direction. Over 40% are situated at the posterior aspect of the thyroid lobe from the inferior thyroid artery to the lower pole of the lobe and along the thyrothymic ligament. PIII is very rarely situated posteriorly and becomes more anterior the lower it descends. Quite often these glands are located at the posterior aspect of the lower pole of the lobe, situated anterior to the recurrent nerve. The thyrothymic ligament is a common location for a gland and it can be situated at the thymic upper pole. It is important to remember that, in 80% of patients, the location of the inferior and superior parathyroid glands is symmetrical when compared with the glands on the contralateral side of the neck.[18]

Definitions of failure – persistent disease vs. recurrent disease

Persistent hyperparathyroidism is defined as the presence of an elevated serum calcium and inappropriately elevated

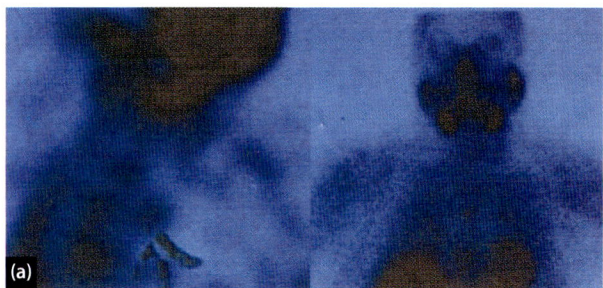
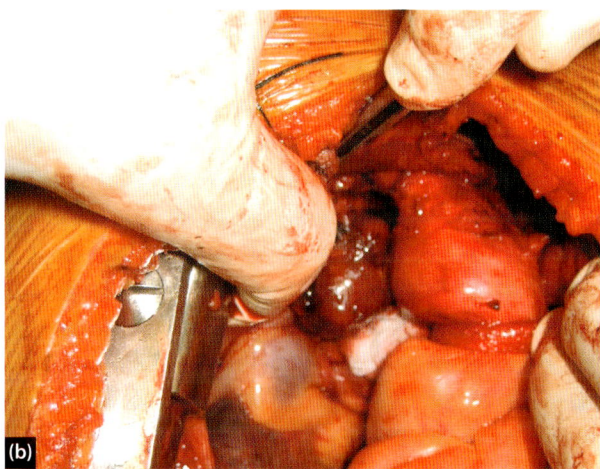

Figure 78.2 (a) Sestamibi scan of fifth ectopic adenoma in aorta pulmonary window. (b) Operative photo of removal of right inferior parathyroid adenoma in aorta pulmonary window.

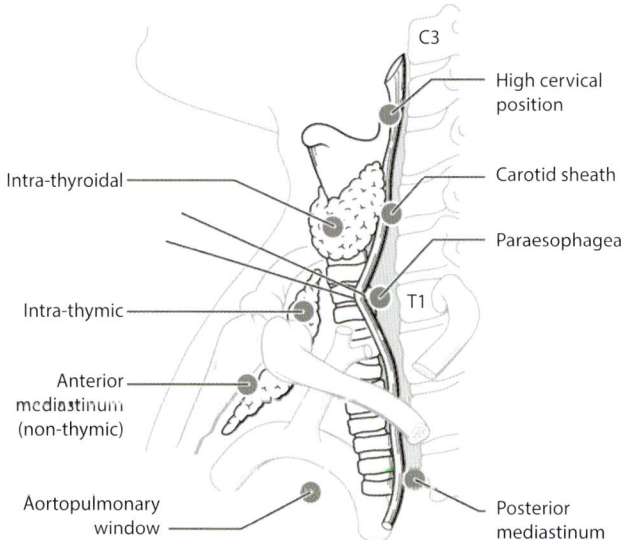

Figure 78.3 Common ectopic locations of missed parathyroid adenomas leading to surgical failure.

the anatomy and a thorough understanding of the embryology of the glands (**Figure 78.3**).

The first procedure is the golden opportunity to cure the patient. Reoperative surgery for failure is almost always a more challenging procedure due to loss of normal anatomical planes, as well as the presence of scarring and fibrosis that may obscure the classic appearance of both normal and abnormal parathyroid glands that experienced surgeons rely on.

or non-suppressed serum PTH within 6 months of the initial surgical procedure; recurrent hyperparathyroidism is defined as the same biochemical scenario developing after at least 6 months of hypercalcaemia. Persistent PHPT (80–90%) is much more common than recurrent (10–20%) PHPT. While this definition is somewhat arbitrary, it acts to separate out those patients with multigland disease in whom hypercalcaemia appears subsequent to an initial successful operation, presumably since the second adenoma was present but inactive at the time of initial surgery. Even in the most experienced hands, persistent hyperparathyroidism following failure at initial surgery for PHPT will never reach zero although centres with a high turnover of cases should achieve an initial success rate of 95–98%.[13]

As noted, there is a conceptual difference between failure following an open parathyroidectomy, where this is largely due to either surgical inexperience or ectopic location, and failure after MIP, where this is largely due the presence of multigland disease in the neck that has not been identified on pre-operative localization studies. Recurrent hyperparathyroidism due to multigland disease may even develop after several years, often being associated with a familial disorder; in contrast, the development of a second adenoma is very rare and mostly seen in patients who have had previous irradiation.[19] Parathyroid carcinoma should also be considered in the differential diagnosis of failure and in some situations a recurrence corrects an original misdiagnosis for an atypical adenoma. Local recurrence can be a parathyroid carcinoma, although this can also be seen after capsular rupture of benign lesions (parathyromatosis).

INVESTIGATION OF PERSISTENT OR RECURRENT DISEASE (THE THREE 'R'S)

Before undertaking any second exploration in the neck for recurrent primary hyperparathyroidism it is of vital importance to understand fully the causes for the failure of the initial operation. The workup before any reoperative exploration should consist of 'the three R's'; **reconfirm** the diagnosis, **review** the operative and pathology reports, and **repeat** the imaging.

Reconfirm the diagnosis and reassess the patient

The diagnosis of PHPT can only be made again if other causes of hypercalcaemia are excluded. In the first place serum analysis and 24-hour urine should be repeated to look for raised PTH and calcium to confirm the diagnosis of PHPT. Elevated PTH with normal calcium can occur in up to 30% post-op due to hungry bone syndrome (secondary response to bone remineralization), low vitamin D levels, impaired renal hydroxylation of vitamin D-25 or decreased peripheral PTH sensitivity or an impaired renal function. Elevated calcium in the presence of suppressed PTH suggests a misdiagnosis such as bone metastases. A modestly elevated serum calcium and serum PTH can be seen in familial hypocalciuric hypercalcaemia (FHH), which mimics PHPT and is a well-recognized cause of failure in an index case. It is of crucial importance to assess a family history properly to be able to exclude FHH because the disorder is not cured by parathyroidectomy. FHH is caused by various mutations in the gene coding for the CaSR. The CaSR responds to serum calcium and mediates feedback inhibition of PTH release. A loss-of-function mutation results in a rising of the calcium threshold that triggers reduction of PTH secretion. Serum concentration of calcium is thus maintained at higher levels since more calcium is needed to trigger negative feedback. This results in hypercalcaemia, and since more calcium is sequestered in the serum, this often results in hypocalciuria.[20] FHH is excluded by demonstration of a 24-hour urinary calcium/creatinine ratio greater than 2%. A family history of PHPT should be sought in order to exclude not only FHH but also other familial endocrinopathies such as MEN 1 and MEN 2A.

Review the operative and pathology reports

It is important to consider factors that might have made the previous surgery difficult such as a very short neck, a coexisting multinodular goitre, or a poorly placed incision, in order to be able to form an operative strategy. It is then vital to obtain and review the operative and pathology reports to determine which parathyroid glands have already been identified or removed. Issues such as who performed the procedure (experience), what kind of procedure was performed (MIP or four-gland exploration) and what was removed (parathyroid normal or abnormal; fat; nodes) all need to be identified. In addition, more detailed information, such as the position of glands identified and/or removed and the time that was spent exploring the neck looking for sites of ectopic parathyroid to be explored, should be documented. Is there anything abnormal to be noted in the report such as thyroid nodules or lymph nodes that might have formed distracting conditions during surgery and the pathology reports should be assessed thoroughly?

Repeat the imaging

A reoperative procedure for PHPT without a positive localization study will most likely lead to a second failed procedure and is a potential recipe for disaster. Localization studies are mandatory although there is no consensus as to which provide the best information. Because the specificity and sensitivity for each method vary greatly, combined localization studies, commencing with the least invasive, are generally recommended.[21]

Our own recently published series showed that 4D CT had an accuracy of 91% in reoperative cases and is significantly more accurate than either sestamibi or ultrasound.[22] In another study it was reported that imaging before reoperation with sestamibi has a 59% identification rate, ultrasound 36%, CT 41% and selective venous sampling 78%.[15] Non-invasive imaging studies (ultrasound, sestamibi, 4D CT) are the studies of first choice, with invasive procedures such as venous sampling and arteriography used only if non-invasive studies are inconclusive or conflicting. In evaluating venous sampling it is important to realize that the study does not image the abnormal parathyroid gland but rather provides information to the surgeon regarding the region where the parathyroid is located.[23] Sometimes image-guided fine-needle aspiration (FNA) with biochemical assessment of the diluted aspirate (not cytological examination) may help distinguish a parathyroid tumour from other structures. A recent report demonstrated that fewer patients now undergo invasive studies (56% versus 73%), which was attributed to improvements in imaging technology.[24] The anatomical diagnosis should ideally be established by a concordance of the results of at least two investigations. When used together, imaging techniques correctly identify abnormal glands in nearly 95% of cases.[25]

CONSERVATIVE OPTIONS

Although parathyroid surgery forms the only definite cure for PHPT, the risks and benefits of surgery need to be appropriately considered and discussed with the patient. When there is an urgent need to treat hypercalcaemia or surgery is contraindicated, or the patient decides against it, non-surgical alternatives are available.

For acute treatment of severe hypercalcaemia, intravenous saline solution loop, diuresis and bisphosphonates are recommended.[26] Subcutaneous calcitonin is also an option, but its efficacy is limited to the first 2 days. Cinacalcet is a calcimimetic drug and lowers PTH secretion by enhancing receptor sensitivity to extracellular calcium. Normocalcaemia can be achieved after 1 day of treatment, the response to cinacalcet can be persistent and it is generally well tolerated.[30] The drug has been shown to be effective in reducing or normalizing serum calcium levels in several groups of patients with PHPT, including patients with mild to moderate PHPT, parathyroid carcinoma, and in PHPT as a part of MEN type 1.[27] Cinacalcet at low dosages is well tolerated, but side effects are more frequent and severe when relatively high doses are needed to control hypercalcaemia. The most common adverse events are nausea, vomiting and paresthesias.[26] Cinacalcet may be of benefit in a wide spectrum of PHPT, offering a novel therapeutic option for the control of hypercalcaemia in PHPT patients who are not able to undergo parathyroidectomy. To what extent the reduction of serum calcium translates into a clinical benefit, particularly in patients with mild to moderate hypercalcaemia, is currently unknown.[28]

SURGICAL APPROACH

In a reoperative situation, a focused exploration is the goal, aiming to locate only the abnormal gland and remove it without disturbing normal glands, mostly positioned in scar tissue and easily damaged or devascularized. There is almost no role for a blind open four-gland exploration in the reoperative situation.

Operative strategy for previous failed open parathyroidectomy

If localization studies have provided a lateralization or a more specific regionalization, a focused re-exploration on the side of localization is performed. If the patient had a standard anterior approach through a cervical incision at the first operation, the same skin incision is used, followed by a lateral approach, in the plane lateral to the strap muscles and medial to the sternocleidomastoid muscle (SCM), rather than the standard approach between the strap muscles. This approach is preferred to avoid heavily scarred planes from the previous anterior neck exploration.

The dissection begins from the medial aspect of the SCM muscle, finding the plane medial to the internal jugular vein then continuing that down to the pre-vertebral fascia, which is often virgin, unscarred tissue. The thyroid lobe can then be identified. The recurrent laryngeal nerve should be identified at this stage using the inferior approach as described for reoperative thyroid surgery.[29] The nerve is located in the trachea-oesophageal groove below the plane of initial surgery and tracing it upwards. As the carotid sheath is retracted to the lateral side, the neck is explored superiorly to the level of the hyoid bone, inferiorly to the brachiocephalic vessels and posteriorly in the trachea-oesophageal plane.[29] Common missed positions of the inferior parathyroid are the inferior and posterior surface of the thyroid gland beneath a thin layer of the capsule, the thyrothymic ligament and the thymus tissue situated in the anterosuperior mediastinum. A parathymus (a parathyroid gland that remained undescended during embryological development) may leave an inferior gland, as high as the mandibular angle. An inferior adenoma positioned here is thus located more superior than the superior parathyroid gland.

During the thorough search along the embryological descent of the gland itself, we dissect towards the superior mediastinum and on the way open and explore the carotid sheath, removing a major portion of the thymus. For the search of the superior parathyroid, the superior pole vessels should then be ligated to facilitate exposure of the superior-posterior side of the thyroid and the tracheaoesophageal groove can be explored by entering this area immediately posterior to the inferior thyroid artery. The technique of palpating the posterosuperior mediastinum digitally can be used to exclude large adenomas that might have been missed in the initial operation. This superior adenoma would thus be situated inferior to the inferior parathyroid gland (PIII).[30, 31]

If the above strategy fails to locate any abnormal parathyroid tissue despite imaging having demonstrated a possible candidate lesion on that side, the contralateral side should not be blindly explored at the time. Bilateral reoperative surgery after a previous bilateral exploration has the potential to lead to bilateral recurrent laryngeal nerve palsy and tracheostomy. Under these circumstances, surgery for the contralateral side should be deferred and reconsidered after further imaging.

Operative strategy for previous failed MIP

Minimal invasive unilateral exploration has now become the procedure of first choice for most first-time parathyroid procedures. In a reoperative situation after a unilateral-focused operation for the first operation, the approach should depend upon the initial incision placement and operative approach. For an adenoma localized to the same side as the initial procedure, if a lateral mini-incision approach was initially utilized, an anterior cervical approach should be considered instead of the lateral approach extending the scar to a classic Kocher incision. However, if a midline mini-incision or videoscopic approach was utilized initially, then a lateral approach second time around is preferable. Should the adenoma be localized to the contralateral side to the initial operation, a lateral mini-incision approach on that side is entirely appropriate.

Mediastinal exploration

Most mediastinal adenomas are located in the posterior mediastinum or in the anterior mediastinum just superior to the aortic arch and can usually be explored from the same cervical approach. Previous extensive cervical surgery (particularly if a cervical thymectomy had been attempted and the thymic tissue was disrupted) may prevent a cervical delivery and necessitate a median sternotomy. Likewise, a large adenoma lying below the aortic arch may not be deliverable and may require a sternotomy. An adenoma located deep in the middle mediastinal window requires a thoracotomy. Confident localization must be obtained before the surgeon proceeds to mediastinal exploration (**Figure 78.2a,b**). There is absolutely no role for blind mediastinal clearance in the futile hope of retrieving or devascularizing a non-localized tumour.

REVIEW: RESULTS AND POST-OPERATIVE COMPLICATIONS

Results

For patients with persistent or recurrent hyperparathyroidism, pre-operative localization studies and a focused surgical approach can result in a 95% success rate with a minimum of complications.[32] However, management of persistent or recurrent hypercalcaemia after failed initial surgery remains one of the greatest challenges in endocrine surgery. Neither the cure rates nor the complication rates of reoperative surgery have changed significantly over the last few decades despite the revolutionary development of imaging.

Although multigland disease is still the most important cause for primary failure, Thompson demonstrated that 40% of missed abnormal glands reside in a normal anatomical position.[33] Despite the success rates for reoperative surgery varying from 82% to 98%, the fact that most missed adenomas are located in abnormal anatomical positions challenges all surgeons to strive for a primary cure to prevent a patient having to face the risks of reoperation.[30]

The rates of persistent hyperparathyroidism after surgery vary considerably around the world, with some centres reporting rates as high as 24% and other centres in Europe and Australia rates as low as 2–3%. This, of course, may simply reflect referral pattern in these countries where most primary operations are performed by experienced endocrine surgeons.[32, 33] However, Lew reported a failure rate for reoperative parathyroid surgery of 2.9%, of which most failures (76%) were due to failure of the surgeon to locate the abnormal gland.[34, 35] Only 24% of missed adenomas in this study were caused by multigland disease.[35] Their group also concluded that the surgeon's judgement and experience are paramount, especially in these cases.

Complications

The most significant complication of reoperative parathyroid surgery is a recurrent laryngeal nerve injury, resulting in vocal cord paralysis. Despite the difficulty of dissecting in scarred tissue planes, the permanent nerve injury rate is exceptionally low in most published series, ranging from 0.4% to 4%, and the rates of permanent hypocalcaemia in reoperative parathyroid surgery have been reported to be in the range of 5–11% in the most recent series.[36–40] The use of intra-operative nerve monitoring was studied recently by comparing nerve injury rates. Since there was only one unintentional nerve injury in each group, the authors concluded that, although monitoring can be performed safely, it does not decrease the injury rate.[41] Careful dissection and visualization of the nerve remain the best protection against injury. However, if the surgeon decides to use intra-operative nerve monitoring, employing it routinely in these cases is more effective to gain more experience with the technique and to be able to make best use of it in the reoperative setting.

Permanent hypocalcaemia is the other significant complication of reoperative parathyroid surgery, where the normal glands may have been damaged, biopsied, or all three normal glands may even have been excised during the first operation.

SUMMARY

Patients with recurrent or persistent PHPT present a challenge, even for the experienced parathyroid surgeon. It is crucial to reconfirm the diagnosis, consider the risks and benefits of the reoperation, and review the operative notes and pathology reports and the results of localization tests. The success rates are high in the hands of an experienced surgeon who has excellent knowledge of the embryology and anatomy of the parathyroid glands. The complication rate of recurrent laryngeal nerve injury and permanent hypocalcaemia is acceptable but considerably higher than during initial parathyroid operations. Most missed adenomas seem to be located in a normal anatomical position, which challenges all parathyroid surgeons to strive for a primary cure in the first operation and to prevent a patient needing to face the risks of reoperation.

> **KEY POINTS**
>
> - The only cure for PHPT is to surgically remove the hyperfunctioning parathyroid adenoma or adenomata.
> - Unlike open four-gland parathyroid exploration, the most common cause of failure in MIP is the presence of multi-gland disease.
> - High-quality imaging, with appropriate selection for MIP based upon concordant localization studies (4D CT, sestamibi scan and ultrasound), is the most appropriate means of minimizing initial parathyroidectomy failure.
> - Persistent PHPT (80–90%) is much more common than recurrent (10–20%) PHPT.
> - The workup before any reoperative exploration should consist of 'the three R's'; reconfirm the diagnosis, review the operative and pathology reports, and repeat the imaging.
> - In a reoperative situation, a focused exploration is the goal, aiming to locate only the abnormal gland and remove it without disturbing normal glands.
> - The most significant complications of reoperative parathyroid surgery are recurrent laryngeal nerve injury and permanent hypoparathyroidism.
> - The success rates are high in the hands of an experienced surgeon who has excellent knowledge of the embryology and anatomy of the parathyroid glands.
> - Most missed adenomas seem to be located in a normal anatomical position, which challenges all parathyroid surgeons to strive for a primary cure in the first operation and to prevent a patient having to face the risks of reoperation.

REFERENCES

1. Adami S, Marcocci C, Gatti D. Epidemiology of primary hyperparathyroidism in Europe. *J Bone Miner Res* 2002; 17: N18–23.
2. Heath H, Hodgson SF, Kennedy MA. Primary hyperparathyroidism: incidence, morbidity, and potential economic impact in a community. *N Engl J Med* 1980; 302: 189–93.
3. Delbridge LW, Palazzo FF. First parathyroid surgeon: Sir John Bland-Sutton and the parathyroid. *ANZ J Surg* 2007; 77: 1058–61.
4. Mandl F. Therapeutischer Versuch bei Ostitis fibrosa generalisata mittels Exstirpation eines Epithelkörperchentumors. *Wien Klin Wochenschr* 1925; 50: 1343–4.
5. Welbourn RB, Friesen SR, Johnston IDA, Sellwood RA. *The history of endocrine surgery*. New York: Praeger; 1990.
6. Gagner M. Endoscopic subtotal parathyroidectomy in patients with primary hyperparathyroidism. *Br J Surg* 1996; 83: 875.
7. Pang T, Stalberg P, Sidhu S, et al. Minimally invasive parathyroidectomy using the lateral focused mini-incision technique without intraoperative parathyroid hormone monitoring. *Br J Surg* 2007; 94: 315–19.
8. Twigt BA, Vollebregt AM, van Dalen T, et al. Shifting incidence of solitary adenomas in the era of minimally invasive parathyroidectomy: a multi-institutional study. *Ann Surg Oncol* 2011; 18: 1041–6.
9. Lee NC, Norton JA. Multiple-gland disease in primary hyperparathyroidism: a function of operative approach? *Arch Surg* 2002; 137: 896–9.
10. Carneiro-Pla DM, Solorzano CC, Lew JI, et al. Long-term outcome of patients with intraoperative parathyroid level remaining above the normal range during parathyroidectomy. *Surgery* 2008; 144: 989–93.
11. Agarwal G, Barraclough BH, Robinson BG, et al. Minimally invasive parathyroidectomy using the 'focused' lateral approach. I. Results of the first 100 consecutive cases. *ANZ J Surg* 2002; 72: 100–4.
12. Norman J, Lopez J, Politz D. Abandoning unilateral parathyroidectomy: why we reversed our position after 15 000 parathyroid operations. *J Am Coll Surg* 2012; 214: 260–9.
13. Norman J, Chheda H, Farrell C. Minimally invasive parathyroidectomy: reducing operative time and potential complications while decreasing potential complications. *Am Surg* 1998; 5: 391–6.
14. Siperstein A, Berber E, Barbosa GF, et al. Predicting the success of limited exploration for primary hyperparathyroidism using ultrasound, sestamibi, and intraoperative parathyroid hormone: analysis of 1158 cases. *Ann Surg* 2008; 248: 420–8.
15. Liew V, Gough IR, Nolan G, Fryar B. Re-operation for hyperparathyroidism. *ANZ J Surg* 2004; 74: 732–40.
16. LiVolsi VA, Hamilton R. Intraoperative assessment of parathyroid gland pathology: a common view from the surgeon and the pathologist. *Am J Clin Pathol* 1994; 102: 365–73.
17. Wang C-A. The anatomic basis of parathyroid surgery. *Ann Surg* 1976; 183: 271–5.
18. Silberfein EJ, Bao R, Lopez A, et al. Reoperative parathyroidectomy: location of missed glands based on a contemporary nomenclature system. *Arch Surg* 2010; 145: 1065–8.
19. Ippilito P, Palazzo F, Sebag F, et al. Long-term follow-up after parathyroidectomy for radiation-induced hyperparathyroidism. *Surgery* 2007; 142: 819–22.
20. Heath H III. Familial benign hypercalcaemia from clinical description to molecular genetics. *West J Med* 1994; 164: 554–62.
21. Mitchel BK, Merrel RC, Kinder BK. Localization studies in patients with hyperparathyroidism. *Surg Clin North Am* 1993; 31: 991–1015.
22. Brown SJ, Lee JC, Christie J, et al. Four-dimensional computed tomography for parathyroid localization: a new imaging modality. *ANZ J Surg* 2015; 85(6): 483–7.
23. Feingold DL, Alexander HR, Chen CC, et al. Ultrasound and sestamibi scan as the only preoperative imaging tests in reoperation for parathyroid adenomas. *Surgery* 2000; 128: 1103–10.
24. Sugg SL, Franker DL, Alexander HL, et al. Prospective evaluation of selective venous sampling for parathyroid hormone concentration in patients undergoing re-operations for primary hyperparathyroidism. *Surgery* 1993; 114: 1004–10.
25. Wadstrom C, Zedenius J, Guinea A, et al. Re-operative surgery for recurrent or persistent primary hyperparathyroidism. *Aust N Z J Surg* 1998; 68(2): 103–7.
26. Jacobs L, Samson MM, Verhaar HJ, Koek HL. Therapeutic challenges in elderly patients with symptomatic hypercalcaemia caused by primary hyperparathyroidism. *Neth J Med* 2012; 70: 35–8.
27. Farford B, Presutti RJ, Moraghan TJ. Nonsurgical management of primary hyperparathyroidism. *Mayo Clin Proc* 2007; 82: 351–5.
28. Saxe AW, Brennan M.F. Strategy and technique of re-operative parathyroid surgery. *Surgery* 1981; 89: 417–23.
29. Prichard R, Delbridge L. Reoperation for benign disease. In: Randolph GW (ed). *Surgery of the thyroid and parathyroid glands*. 2nd edn. Philadelphia: Elsevier, 2013.
30. Norton JA, Shawker TH, Jones BL, et al. Intraoperative ultrasound and re-operative parathyroid surgery: an initial evaluation. *World J Surg* 1986; 10: 631–9.

31. Libutti SK, Bartlett DL, Jaskowiak NT, et al. The role of thyroid resection during a reoperation for persistent or recurrent hyperparathyroidism. *Surgery* 1997; **122**: 1183–7.
32. Shen W, Duren M, Morita E, et al. Reoperation for persistent or recurrent primary hyperparathyroidism. *Arch Surg* 1996; **131**: 861–9.
33. Thompson GB, Grant CS, Perrier ND, et al. Re-operative parathyroid surgery in the era of Sestamibi scanning and intraoperative parathyroid hormone monitoring. *Arch Surg* 1999; **134**: 699–704.
34. Heerden van JA. Lessons learned. *Surgery* 1997; **122**(6): 979–88.
35. Lew JI, Rivera M, Irvin GL, Solozano CC. Operative failure in the era of focussed parathyroidectomy. *Arch Surg* 2010; **145**; 628–33.
36. Udelsman R, Lin Z, Donovan P. The superiority of minimally invasive parathyroidectomy based on 1650 consecutive patients with primary hyperparathyroidism. *Ann Surg* 2011; **253**(3): 585–91.
37. Brennan MF, Marx KJ, Doppman J, et al. Results of reoperation for persistent and recurrent hyperparathyroidism. *Ann Surg* 1991; **194**: 671–6.
38. Cheung PS, Borgstrom A, Thompson NW. Strategy in re-operative surgery for hyperparathyroidism. *Arch Surg* 1989; **124**: 676–80.
39. Jaskowiak N, Norton JA, Alexander HR, et al. A prospective trial evaluating a standard approach to reoperation for missed parathyroid adenoma. *Ann Surg* 1996; **224**: 308–20.
40. Powell AC, Alexander HR, Chang R, et al. Reoperation for parathyroid adenoma: a contemporary experience. *Surgery* 2009; **146**: 1144–55.
41. Yarbrough DE, Thompson GB, Kasperbauer JL, et al. Intraoperative electromyographic monitoring of the recurrent laryngeal nerve in re-operative thyroid and parathyroid surgery. *Surgery* 2004; **136**: 1107–15.

COMPLICATIONS OF THYROID AND PARATHYROID SURGERY AND HOW TO AVOID THEM

Erin A. Felger, Dipti Kamani and Gregory W. Randolph

Introduction 887	Aerodigestive injury 889
Seroma 887	Hypothyroidism 889
Infection 887	Hyperthyroidism 890
Haematoma 888	Airway concerns 890
Recurrent laryngeal nerve injury 888	Hypertrophic or keloid scar 890
Injury to the external branch of the superior laryngeal nerve 888	References 891
Hypoparathyroidism 889	

SEARCH STRATEGY

Data in this chapter may be updated by a PubMed search using the keywords: thyroid surgery, complications, haematoma, recurrent laryngeal nerve injury, oesophageal injury, tracheal injury, airway complications, hypoparathyroidism, hypothyroidism and thyroid storm. The evidence in this chapter is mainly levels 3 and 4. The clinical recommendations are mainly B and C.

INTRODUCTION

Complications in thyroid and parathyroid surgery are uncommon but significant when they occur. Averting the complications should begin pre-operatively with an assessment of risk factors for potential complications and a thorough discussion with the patient outlining the risk factors, treatment approaches and outcomes. Sound anatomical knowledge and meticulous surgical technique aid in minimizing complication risk. Post-operatively, close observation of the patient is the key to identifying and managing problems early and successfully, leading to a better overall outcome.

SEROMA

The incidence of seroma formation is low, occurring in 1–7% of cases. Seromas are more likely to occur after surgery for a large goitre or a total thyroidectomy. Post-operative neck swelling should be taken seriously and monitored for rapid enlargement or tenderness. In most cases, seromas are managed conservatively with observation and by reassuring the patient.[1] When seromas are painful or lead to tightness, aspiration of the fluid using sterile technique eases the patient's discomfort but may need to be repeated several times before reaccumulation of the fluid stops. Placing a drain into the dead space left after the surgery may also be helpful. If there is a concern of infection, the aspirated fluid should be sent for culture and antibiotics should be started. In the majority of patients, seromas resolve over 6–8 weeks with watchful waiting.[1]

INFECTION

Infection of the surgical site is quite rare in thyroid and parathyroid surgery, occurring in less than 1% in most cases series. These surgeries are considered clean by the Centers for Disease Control and the National Safety Network criteria for wound classification and do not require peri-operative antibiotics.[2] In certain instances, using a peri-operative antibiotic selectively may be reasonable given a patient's risk factors for potential infection.

Intra-operatively, if there is a break in sterility or another source of contamination such as entry into the aerodigestive tract is identified, then antibiotics are warranted. Superficial wound infections are treated with local wound care and oral antibiotics. Deep wound infections are more serious: they require incision and drainage with wound culture, placement of a drain in addition to i.v. antibiotics and investigation for the source, which is often a missed aerodigestive injury.[3, 4] Cervical infections after thyroid and parathyroid surgery should never be underestimated and should be treated definitively and swiftly to prevent mortality from this complication.[5]

HAEMATOMA

Minimizing the risk of post-operative haematoma begins pre-operatively by identifying risk factors for each patient that contribute to an increased likelihood of a post-operative haematoma. Several articles have defined significant risk factors including male gender, older age, smoking, large thyroid, benign pathology, antiplatelet/anticoagulation therapy and Graves' disease.[6, 7] Obtaining a good history is important; hypertension and taking herbal supplements such as fish oil increase the risk of bleeding and potential haematoma formation.[8] Following surgery, hypertension, vomiting and excessive coughing or sneezing can induce haematoma formation.[8, 9]

Maintaining meticulous haemostasis intra-operatively, particularly at the end of the case, is essential. There are several thermal haemostatic instruments that can be used including monopolar cautery, bipolar cautery and vessel-sealing devices, none of which confers better haemostasis over another. Many surgeons utilize the Valsalva manoeuvre to identify and control any potential areas of bleeding prior to closure.[1] Drains do not decrease the rate of post-operative haematoma; in fact one study shows that a drain is a risk factor for haematoma. Drains should be used very selectively in this setting and, because they increase the risk of infection, antibiotics should be administered while the drain is in place.[10-13] Haemostatic agents may be used in the thyroid bed but they have not been shown to decrease the rate of haematoma. Most haematomas occur within the first 6-12 hours after surgery. However, a small percentage of haematomas form greater than 24 hours after surgery and up to 1-2 weeks afterwards.[6, 14] Haematomas can be superficial (above the strap muscles) or deep (below the strap muscles). As the haematoma expands, it causes venous and lymphatic congestion which exacerbates laryngopharyngeal oedema leading to eventual airway compromise. Decompressing and evacuating the clot is the first and most important manoeuvre in order to help alleviate airway narrowing. While the patient is awake, the incision is released and the strap muscles are incised to release pressure from the haematoma.[15] Securing the airway is paramount; placement of an endotracheal tube when necessary is preferred. If this is not possible, then an emergency tracheostomy may be needed. The patient is then returned expeditiously to the operating theatre for haematoma evacuation, identification and control of the bleeding source. After achieving complete haemostasis, the wound is closed again.[1, 15] Most patients who return to the operating room for haematoma evacuation recover well from this second procedure and are discharged the day after surgery.

RECURRENT LARYNGEAL NERVE INJURY

In the pre-operative setting, a thorough history and physical examination should be performed to identify any concurrent factors such as significant smoking history, lung cancer or reflux disease, affecting the voice quality of the patient. Pre-operative laryngoscopy should be performed on all patients to document baseline vocal cord function.[16, 17]

Intra-operative direct visualization of the recurrent laryngeal nerve (RLN) lowers the rates of temporary and permanent RLN injury rates and is considered the gold standard.[18-21] Intra-operative neural monitoring (IONM) is an important complement to visualization of the nerve. IONM have shown a trend towards lower RLN injury rates but statistical proof is lacking in part due to lack of adequate statistical powering of most studies. IONM aids in mapping the RLN, in assessing nerve function, and in identification of an injured nerve segment.[16, 22, 23] Having real-time monitoring allows the surgeon to change the technique or the amount of retraction that is causing harmful impact on the RLN.[16] When injury is suspected, identification of the injured segment, assessment of the injury and the possibility of repair should be explored. The RLN injury should be managed appropriately at the time of identification.[24, 25]

An analysis of 27 articles, reviewing more than 25 000 patients undergoing thyroidectomy, found the average post-operative vocal cord paralysis (VCP) rate was 9.8% and ranged from 0% to 18.6%.[26] Post-operative laryngoscopy should be performed to reliably document post-operative glottic function and for early identification of VCP to initiate appropriate management.[16] There are multiple methods for restoring voice quality in patients who have vocal cord dysfunction. In the first 3 months, cordal injections can enhance contact between the vocal cords and improve swallowing, voice and cough. If the injury is permanent, procedures like thyroplasty and medialization laryngoplasty can be performed.[27] These methods rely on placement of a structural implant to reapproximate the injured cord with the normal cord. Finally, reinnervation is another option that can be accomplished by mobilizing a functioning nerve, typically the ansa cervicalis to the distal RLN stump. It may take several months to regain voice function after this procedure.[27]

INJURY TO THE EXTERNAL BRANCH OF THE SUPERIOR LARYNGEAL NERVE

IONM can be very helpful in intra-operative identification of the external branch of the superior laryngeal nerve (EBSLN), as up to 20% of EBSLN are subfacial and visually unidentifiable.[28] A precise surgical technique with careful superior pole dissection and ligation of the superior pole vessels on the gland itself is important.[29, 30] Understanding the anatomical variations of the EBSLN course is the best guide for protecting the nerve. With monitoring there is a standardized approach to identification and dissection of the EBSLN.[31]

Post-operatively, the surgeon should inquire about voice strength, pitch and fatigue. If the patient has any of these complaints, EBSLN injury should be suspected and a formal voice evaluation with videostroboscopy as well as speech therapy should be performed.[29]

HYPOPARATHYROIDISM

For patients with thyroid cancer, substernal goitre, Graves' disease and reoperation, hypoparathyroidism is a significant concern. Pre-operative Vitamin D, serum calcium and PTH evaluations are helpful in establishing a baseline for calcium homeostasis prior to surgery. If the vitamin D is low, replacement before surgery is helpful in order to decrease risk of symptomatic hypocalcemia secondary to lack of calcium absorption.[32]

Meticulous dissection with preservation of the parathyroid glands and their blood supply is required to avert hypoparathyroidism.[33] The standard method for preserving the parathyroid glands and their blood supply is capsular dissection. The glands are mobilized and reflected away from the thyroid gland while keeping their blood supply intact.[20, 21, 24] Disruption of parathyroid gland vascularity is the most common reason for post-operative hypoparathyroidism. If a parathyroid gland seems non-viable after surgical dissection, a portion may be sent for frozen section to confirm parathyroid tissue and the remainder can be autotransplanted into the sternocleidomastoid muscle.[35] Inadvertent removal of one or more parathyroid glands with the thyroid can also cause hypoparathyroidism.[36]

Post-operatively, serum calcium levels can be checked to determine the need for calcium supplementation. Some surgeons give post-operative calcium supplementation to all patients. Hypoparathyroidism can be temporary, less than 6 months post-surgery (8–30%) or permanent, more than 6 months post-surgery (1.7–3.5%).[19, 32] In the acute setting with serum calcium levels less than 1.75 mmol/L, i.v. calcium gluconate is administered to alleviate symptoms which can include paraesthesia, muscle cramps and spasms, twitching, tetany, seizures and cardiopulmonary dysfunction. If serum calcium is at least 2 mmol/L, then it is treated with oral calcium carbonate and vitamin D. For patients with a history of gastric bypass surgery or reflux disease, calcium citrate is used instead of calcium carbonate because it is better absorbed in these patients.[37] The starting dose of calcium is usually 500–1000 mg three times a day with upward titration if symptoms persist. For vitamin D administration, the most active form, 1,25-dihydroxy D3 (calcitriol), is used with a starting dose of 0.25 μg each day. Ionized calcium, phosphorous, PTH and vitamin D should be checked at regular intervals if the patient is not improving. The goal is to maintain a low-normal serum calcium with normal phosphorous levels and low urinary calcium excretion.[32] For patients with permanent hypoparathyroidism, maintaining calcium and phosphorous levels is more difficult and requires routine monitoring and changes to supplementation as needed. Urine calcium levels tend to increase over time and lead to renal insufficiency. Osteoporosis is also a concern for these patients because their bone resorption is decreased.[32] A new treatment option is recombinant PTH (rhPTH), an injectable synthetic human PTH administered subcutaneously once or twice a day.[38] It has been shown to maintain serum calcium levels, decrease phosphorous levels and decrease or eliminate the need for vitamin D supplementation. From a physiological standpoint, there is improved bone turnover and a decreased urinary calcium level.[38, 39]

AERODIGESTIVE INJURY

In patients with known thyroid cancer with a concern for tracheal or oesophageal invasion, a thorough workup including imaging and endoscopy should be completed pre-operatively. This is helpful for surgical planning and for avoidance of aerodigestive injury.

During surgery, inadvertent entry into the oesophagus or trachea is uncommon but, when it occurs, it is usually secondary to adherent tumour or lymph nodes.

Tracheal injuries can be small or large. Small injuries can be repaired primarily with absorbable sutures.[40] If primary closure is not possible, segmental tracheal resection may be performed or a tracheostomy tube placed. Oesophageal repair includes debridement of the tissues edges with two-layer closure of the mucosa and muscle separately. A strap muscle may be used to buttress the repair. A closed drainage system is placed, antibiotics and parenteral nutrition are started and the patient is kept nil by mouth for 7–10 days when a contrast swallow is done to check for a leak.[40–42] If there is no leak, a soft diet is introduced. Long-term complications from a leak include stricture and fistula, both of which require further workup and treatment.[42]

HYPOTHYROIDISM

Surgical hypothyroidism should be a point of pre-operative discussion for any patient undergoing thyroid surgery. Typically, the starting dose for levothyroxine is 1.6–1.8 mcg/kg/day and is titrated based on thyroid function tests thereafter. Patients with thyroid cancer may need a higher dose in order to suppress growth of cancer cells.[43]

For patients who have undergone lobectomy, there is a 15–50% risk of abnormal thyroid function after surgery with the need for levothyroxine. Hashimoto's disease, higher TSH or lower free T4 or a smaller remaining lobe increase the likelihood of requiring T4 supplementation.[44, 45]

Bloods should be checked 6–8 weeks after surgery because the half-life of levothyroxine is 7 days and it takes about this period of time to reach a steady level.[43, 46, 47]

HYPERTHYROIDISM

Patients with hyperthyroidism secondary to Graves' disease and less often toxic multinodular goitre or a toxic nodule are at risk for development of thyroid storm throughout the disease course. Usually an external source such as infection, surgery, trauma or increased iodine intake is the inciting factor for thyroid storm.[48] Multiple systems are affected in thyroid storm – cardiopulmonary, thermoregulatory, metabolism, neurological and gastrointestinal. It is quite rare to develop this extreme form of thyrotoxicosis but when it occurs, early recognition and prompt supportive treatment are essential for survival.[48] Pre-operatively the surgeon needs to discuss with the patient the risks of thyroid storm and the importance of compliance with medication up to the day of surgery. Thyroid function tests should be checked regularly prior to surgery to ensure that free T4 and free T3 levels remain within an acceptable range. If free T4 is above 20 pmol/L and the free T3 remains high, surgery is postponed until those levels decrease appropriately.[48]

In the operating theatre, a shift in vital signs alerts anaesthesia to the possibility of thyroid storm. Tachycardia, dysrhythmia (usually atrial fibrillation), high fever and respiratory changes are the most common symptoms.[48] Cooling the patient, administering a beta blocker and hydrocortisone are initiated to mitigate the associated symptoms. Concurrently, antithyroidal medication, PTU or carbimazole is also started to stop synthesis of new hormone and to prevent peripheral conversion of T4 to T3. Of note, most anaesthetists give a dose of Dantrolene in this situation because the symptoms of malignant hyperthermia and thyroid storm are difficult to differentiate.[48] Post-operatively, patients with thyroid storm need close monitoring and continuation of supportive care until thyroid hormone levels normalize and the patient is no longer symptomatic.

AIRWAY CONCERNS

Determining potential airway risk pre-operatively is the best way to minimize airway complications both during intubation and post-operatively. Recognizing patients who are at higher risk because of their disease extent, by a thorough pre-operative assessment recognizing shortness of breath, dysphagia and hoarseness helps guide anaesthesia and surgical planning.[49, 50] Patients with large goitres, substernal goitres and invasive cancers have a higher risk of airway complications. If there is concern for a substernal component or tracheal narrowing, neck and chest CT scan should be performed.[50] Anaesthetics should be consulted early in the workup of these patients so that a joint anaesthetic–surgical plan can be developed pre-operatively. In some instances, a planned tracheostomy may be considered if there is significant tracheal narrowing, a long-standing goitre or thyroid cancer. On the day of surgery, anaesthesia and surgery jointly decide the best approach based on the patient's pre-operative findings.[49, 51] Options include induction and traditional intubation or use of a glidoscope, awake fibreoptic intubation or planned tracheostomy. At the completion of the surgery, the surgeon and anaesthetist should discuss the likelihood of success with extubation.[51] The majority of patients can be safely extubated and will experience improvement in airway symptoms. Some patients may need prolonged intubation if there is concern for tracheomalacia, which is rare. In other cases, a tracheostomy may be done at the end of the surgery, because of intra-operative detection of significant tracheal narrowing or bilateral RLN injury.[1, 52] Any patient who has a difficult airway or airway complications at the time of surgery should be counselled in the post-operative setting about these difficulties and instructed to convey this information prior to future surgeries.

HYPERTROPHIC OR KELOID SCAR

During the pre-operative visit, a thorough history of prior operations and scar formation is key to having the best possible outcome for the surgical scar. All old scars should be examined for healing issues. In a patient with known keloid formation, a surgical as well as post-surgical plan is developed. The skin should be marked in the holding area just prior to surgery while the patient is still awake in order to find the most natural skin crease for the incision. In theatre, less is more for closing these incisions including use of suture and manipulation of the tissues. Steroid injections can also be employed prior to skin closure.[1] A tension-free closure also helps minimize scarring. Close follow-up for hypertrophy or keloid formation post-operatively and early plastic surgery or dermatology consultation are important so that advanced options for scar treatment can be explored in a timely manner. Post-operatively patients should be educated about sun exposure and use of sunscreen on the incision as well as use of over-the-counter scar care products to aid in minimizing scar formation.[1]

BEST CLINICAL PRACTICE

✓ Pre-operatively, a thorough history, physical examination and laryngoscopy can help identify risk factors that can increase the likelihood of intra-operative and post-operative complications and also provide the opportunity to discuss post-operative expectations with the patient.
✓ Intra-operatively a sound anatomical knowledge, meticulous surgery, avoidance of harmful manoeuvres and use of complementary technology such as nerve monitoring can help avert complications.
✓ Post-operative active surveillance for complications, especially in high-risk patients, and early identification with appropriate management of complications are of paramount importance.

KEY POINTS

- The post-operative course starts in the pre-operative setting with a detailed discussion about surgery, risks and benefits.
- Knowledge of the anatomy and excellent surgical technique are essential for positive outcomes.
- Early recognition of complications with applicable treatment offers better outcomes.

REFERENCES

1. Randolph G. *Surgery of the thyroid and parathyroid glands.* 2nd ed. Philadelphia: W.B. Saunders; 2012.
2. Jarvis WR. Benchmarking for prevention: the Centers for Disease Control and Prevention's National Nosocomial Infections Surveillance (NNIS) system experience. *Infection* 2003; **31** Suppl 2: 44–8.
3. Johnson JT, Wagner RL. Infection following uncontaminated head and neck surgery. *Arch Otolaryngol Head Neck Surg* 1987; **113**(4): 368–9.
4. Tabet JC, Johnson JT. Wound infection in head and neck surgery: prophylaxis, etiology and management. *J Otolaryngol* 1990; **19**(3): 197–200.
5. Elfenbein DM, Schneider DF, Chen H, Sippel RS. Surgical site infection after thyroidectomy: a rare but significant complication. *J Surg Res* 2014; **190**(1): 170–6.
6. Campbell MJ, McCoy KL, Shen WT, et al. A multi-institutional international study of risk factors for hematoma after thyroidectomy. *Surgery* 2013; **154**(6): 1283–9; discussion 1289–91.
7. Morton RP, Mak V, Moss D, et al. Risk of bleeding after thyroid surgery: matched pairs analysis. *J Laryngol Otol* 2012; **126**(3): 285–8.
8. Morton RP, Vandal AC. Postoperative systolic blood pressure as a risk factor for haematoma following thyroid surgery. *Clin Otolaryngol* 2015; **40**(5): 462–7.
9. Bononi, M, Amore Bonapasta S, Vari A, et al. Incidence and circumstances of cervical hematoma complicating thyroidectomy and its relationship to postoperative vomiting. *Head Neck* 2010; **32**(9): 1173–7.
10. Lee SW, Choi EC, Lee YM, et al. Is lack of placement of drains after thyroidectomy with central neck dissection safe? A prospective, randomized study. *Laryngoscope* 2006; **116**(9): 1632–5.
11. Kennedy SA, Irvine RA, Westerberg BD, Zhang H. Meta-analysis: prophylactic drainage and bleeding complications in thyroid surgery. *J Otolaryngol Head Neck Surg* 2008; **37**(6): 768–73.
12. Suslu N, Vural S, Oncel M, et al. Is the insertion of drains after uncomplicated thyroid surgery always necessary? *Surg Today* 2006; **36**(3): 215–18.
13. Woods RS, Woods JF, Duignan ES, Timon C. Systematic review and meta-analysis of wound drains after thyroid surgery. *Br J Surg* 2014; **101**(5): 446–56.
14. Liu J, Li Z, Liu S, et al. Risk factors for and occurrence of postoperative cervical hematoma after thyroid surgery: a single-institution study based on 5156 cases from the past 2 years. *Head Neck* 2016; **38**(2): 216–19.
15. Dixon JL, Snyder SK, Lairmore TC, et al. A novel method for the management of post-thyroidectomy or parathyroidectomy hematoma: a single-institution experience after over 4,000 central neck operations. *World J Surg* 2014; **38**(6): 1262–7.
16. Randolph GW, Dralle H, International Intraoperative Monitoring Study Group, et al. Electrophysiologic recurrent laryngeal nerve monitoring during thyroid and parathyroid surgery: international standards guideline statement. *Laryngoscope* 2011; **121** Suppl 1: S1–16.
17. Wang CC, Wang CP, Tsai TL, et al. The basis of preoperative vocal fold paralysis in a series of patients undergoing thyroid surgery: the preponderance of benign thyroid disease. *Thyroid* 2011; **21**(8): 867–72.
18. Thompson NW, Olsen WR, Hoffman GL, The continuing development of the technique of thyroidectomy. *Surgery* 1973; **73**(6): 913–27.
19. Rosato L, Avenia N, Bernante P, et al. Complications of thyroid surgery: analysis of a multicentric study on 14,934 patients operated on in Italy over 5 years. *World J Surg* 2004; **28**(3): 271–6.
20. Delbridge L, Reeve TS, Khadra M, Poole AG. Total thyroidectomy: the technique of capsular dissection. *Aust N Z J Surg* 1992; **62**(2): 96–9.
21. Bliss RD, Gauger PG, Delbridge LW, Surgeon's approach to the thyroid gland: surgical anatomy and the importance of technique. *World J Surg* 2000; **24**(8): 891–7.
22. Kandil E, Mohamed SE, Deniwar A, et al. Electrophysiologic identification and monitoring of the external branch of superior laryngeal nerve during thyroidectomy. *Laryngoscope* 2015; **125**(8): 1996–2000.
23. Jatzko GR, Lisborg PH, Müller MG, Wette VM. Recurrent nerve palsy after thyroid operations: principal nerve identification and a literature review. *Surgery* 1994; **115**(2): 139–44.
24. Chiang FY, Wang LF, Huang YF, et al. Recurrent laryngeal nerve palsy after thyroidectomy with routine identification of the recurrent laryngeal nerve. *Surgery* 2005; **137**(3): 342–7.
25. Calo PG, Pisano G, Medas F, et al. Identification alone versus intraoperative neuromonitoring of the recurrent laryngeal nerve during thyroid surgery: experience of 2034 consecutive patients. *J Otolaryngol Head Neck Surg* 2014; **43**: 16.
26. Jeannon JP, Orabi AA, Bruch GA, et al. Diagnosis of recurrent laryngeal nerve palsy after thyroidectomy: a systematic review. *Int J Clin Pract* 2009; **63**(4): 624–9.
27. Misono S, Merati AL, Evidence-based practice: evaluation and management of unilateral vocal fold paralysis. *Otolaryngol Clin North Am* 2012; **45**(5): 1083–108.
28. Lennquist S, Cahlin C, Smeds S. The superior laryngeal nerve in thyroid surgery. *Surgery* 1987; **102**(6): 999–1008.
29. Orestes MI, Chhetri DK. Superior laryngeal nerve injury: effects, clinical findings, prognosis, and management options. *Curr Opin Otolaryngol Head Neck Surg* 2014; **22**(6): 439–43.
30. Morton RP, Whitfield P, Al-Ali S. Anatomical and surgical considerations of the external branch of the superior laryngeal nerve: a systematic review. *Clin Otolaryngol* 2006; **31**(5): 368–74.
31. Barczynski M, Randolph GW, Cernea CR, et al. External branch of the superior laryngeal nerve monitoring during thyroid and parathyroid surgery: International Neural Monitoring Study Group standards guideline statement. *Laryngoscope* 2013; **123** Suppl 4: S1–14.
32. Walker Harris V, Jan De Beur S. Postoperative hypoparathyroidism: medical and surgical therapeutic options. *Thyroid* 2009; **19**(9): 967–73.
33. Shaha AR, Jaffe BM. Parathyroid preservation during thyroid surgery. *Am J Otolaryngol* 1998; **19**(2): 113–17.
34. Park I, Rhu J, Woo JW, et al. Preserving parathyroid gland vasculature to reduce post-thyroidectomy hypocalcemia. *World J Surg* 2016; **40**(6): 1382–9.
35. Shaha AR, Burnett C, Jaffe BM. Parathyroid autotransplantation during thyroid surgery. *J Surg Oncol* 1991; **46**(1): 21–4.
36. Page C, Strunski V. Parathyroid risk in total thyroidectomy for bilateral, benign, multinodular goitre: report of 351 surgical cases. *J Laryngol Otol* 2007; **121**(3): 237–41.
37. Antakia R, Edafe O, Uttley L, Balasubramanian SP. Effectiveness of preventative and other surgical measures on hypocalcemia following bilateral thyroid surgery: a systematic review and meta-analysis. *Thyroid* 2015; **25**(1): 95–106.
38. Clarke BL, Kay Berg J, Fox J, et al. Pharmacokinetics and pharmacodynamics of subcutaneous recombinant parathyroid hormone (1–84) in patients with hypoparathyroidism: an open-label, single-dose, phase I study. *Clin Ther* 2014; **36**(5): 722–36.
39. Rubin MR, Cusano NE, Fan WW, et al. Therapy of hypoparathyroidism with PTH(1–84): A prospective six year investigation of efficacy and safety. *J Clin Endocrinol Metab* 2016; **101**(7): 2742–50.
40. Gupta NM, Kaman L. Personal management of 57 consecutive patients with esophageal perforation. *Am J Surg* 2004; **187**(1): 58–63.
41. Vogel SB, Rout WR, Martin TD, Abbitt PL. Esophageal perforation in adults: aggressive, conservative treatment lowers morbidity and mortality. *Ann Surg* 2005; **241**(6): 1016–21; discussion 1021–3.
42. Wu JT, Mattox KL, Wall MJ Jr. Esophageal perforations: new perspectives and treatment paradigms. *J Trauma* 2007; **63**(5): 1173–84.
43. Jonklaas J, Bianco AC, Bauer AJ, et al. Guidelines for the treatment of hypothyroidism: prepared by the American Thyroid Association task force on thyroid hormone replacement. *Thyroid* 2014; **24**(12): 1670–751.
44. McHenry CR, Slusarczyk SJ, Hypothyroidisim following hemithyroidectomy: incidence, risk factors, and management. *Surgery* 2000; **128**(6): 994–8.
45. Morris LF, Iupe IM, Edeiken-Monroe BS, et al. Pre-operative ultrasound identification of thyroiditis helps predict the need for thyroid hormone replacement after thyroid lobectomy. *Endocr Pract* 2013; **19**(6): 1015–20.
46. Stoll SJ, Pitt SC, Liu J, et al. Thyroid hormone replacement after thyroid lobectomy. *Surgery* 2009; **146**(4): 554–8; discussion 558–60.
47. De Carlucci D Jr, Tavares MR, Obara MT, et al. Thyroid function after unilateral total lobectomy: risk factors for postoperative hypothyroidism. *Arch Otolaryngol Head Neck Surg* 2008; **134**(10): 1076–9.
48. Nayak B, Burman K. Thyrotoxicosis and thyroid storm. *Endocrinol Metab Clin North Am* 2006; **35**(4): 663–86, vii.
49. Shen WT, Kebebew E, Duh QY, Clark OH. Predictors of airway complications after thyroidectomy for substernal goiter. *Arch Surg* 2004; **139**(6): 656–9; discussion 659–60.
50. Singh B, Lucente FE, Shaha AR. Substernal goiter: a clinical review. *Am J Otolaryngol* 1994; **15**(6): 409–16.
51. Bouaggad A, Nejmi SE, Bouderka MA, Abbassi O. Prediction of difficult tracheal intubation in thyroid surgery. *Anesth Analg* 2004; **99**(2): 603–6, table of contents.
52. Abdel Rahim AA, Ahmed ME, Hassan MA. Respiratory complications after thyroidectomy and the need for tracheostomy in patients with a large goitre. *Br J Surg* 1999; **86**(1): 88–90.

CHAPTER 80

THYROID AND PARATHYROID SURGERY: AUDIT AND OUTCOMES

David Chadwick

Introduction 893	Other uses of audit data 896
Outcomes: Establishing the magnitude of risk 893	Conclusion 897
Outcomes: Comparison between providers 896	References 897

SEARCH STRATEGY

Data in this chapter may be updated by a PubMed search using the keywords: thyroidectomy, parathyroidectomy, complications, hypocalcaemia, laryngeal nerve palsy and outcomes.

INTRODUCTION

Surgery of the thyroid and parathyroid glands is generally considered very safe. Mortality is minimal, so relevant outcomes relate mainly to the avoidance of specific surgical complications. These are reasonably well defined, and their incidence may depend to a large extent upon the operative skill of the surgeon, thereby providing an ideal opportunity for clinical audit.

OUTCOMES: ESTABLISHING THE MAGNITUDE OF RISK

Accurate knowledge of the frequency of surgical complications may be considered important for many reasons. These include: assistance in patient counselling and consent for surgery; use in surgical decision-making in selection of patients for surgery; identification of risk factors which influence complication rates, particularly if these can be modified to improve results; and provision of benchmarking data by which surgeons can be compared, with the aim of improving surgical performance.

The principal complications to be addressed, related to thyroid and parathyroid surgery, are the following:

- **Post-operative bleeding,** particularly that which requires re-exploration of the neck/evacuation of a haematoma, to protect the airway.
- **Hypocalcaemia,** secondary to the disturbance of parathyroid function. This may occur in the early post-operative phase, usually during the index admission, and may or may not require treatment. In a proportion of these cases, hypocalcaemia will be transient, as parathyroid glands recover their function, but a smaller proportion may progress to permanent hypoparathyroidism.
- **Recurrent laryngeal nerve (RLN) injury,** leading to vocal cord paralysis. As with hypocalcaemia, this may be transient, with recovery of function occurring over a variable time period, or permanent.
- **Persistent hypercalcaemia,** in surgery for primary hyperparathyroidism, where this outcome represents a failure to cure the disease.

Other complications exist, but estimates of their incidence are highly unreliable, due to considerable variation in their definition, perceived impact, detection strategies and geographical factors. For example:

- severe wound infection is rare, and the definitions of milder infection vary widely between studies
- evidence of superior laryngeal nerve injury may be subtle, and frequently is not actively sought
- some complications are simply extremely rare and also influenced by the nature of the presenting disease (e.g. tracheomalacia, chyle leak).

For this reason, the remaining discussion will focus on the principal complications of bleeding, hypocalcaemia and recurrent laryngeal nerve injury.

Estimates of the rates of these complications may derive from individual (often retrospective) case series reported in the medical literature or from large-scale prospective audits/registries designed to measure these outcomes.

Interpretation of the data from retrospective case series is prone to several difficulties. First, there may be issues of case selection bias. Even within a consecutive series, the rationale for the selected time period of study is often not stated, and clusters of complications either side of this time interval can significantly affect results, particularly in smaller series. Many publications do not explicitly record the degree of missing data, nor cases excluded from analysis or lost to follow-up.

Second, studies often vary greatly in the definitions of relevant complications, and in the strategy for their detection. This is particularly relevant for hypocalcaemia and recurrent laryngeal nerve palsy (RLNP). Calcium levels may be uniformly measured after surgery, but hypocalcaemia may be defined in several ways: for example, any result below the local reference range; a result below various other biochemical thresholds; the presence or absence of hypocalcaemic symptoms; the requirement for treatment with calcium and/or vitamin D supplements; or combinations of these variables. Such differences in definitions may result in widely disparate estimates of hypocalcaemia rate, even when applied to the same group of patients.[1] Early hypocalcaemia may also be avoided by the use of prophylactic calcium/vitamin D supplements, and protocols vary greatly between surgeons in this regard.

Likewise, the diagnosis of post-operative RLNP is dependent on the incidence and timing of post-operative laryngeal examination.[2–4] Voice changes after thyroidectomy are commoner than documented RLNP, but vocal cord palsy may also be asymptomatic and is often transient. Many surgeons do not routinely arrange post-operative laryngeal examination, and the available methods for performing such examinations differ in their accuracy. It is clear that routine laryngeal examination reveals much higher rates of RLNP than where vocal cord function is assessed solely on the basis of vocal symptoms and that the earlier in the post-operative course such examination occurs, the higher will be the rate of (at least transient) RLNP.[3,4] For these reasons, rates of RLNP are extremely difficult to compare across retrospective case series.

For both hypocalcaemia and RLNP, the point at which the complication is described as 'permanent' is also variable. Recovery may occur beyond 12 months post-operatively, but data on very long-term follow-up are harder to obtain, and may be incomplete. Results at 6 months may represent a reasonable compromise, but this approach risks overestimation of truly permanent outcomes.

Third, results may be affected by variation in case mix, which is often poorly described. Relevant variables might include, for instance, re-operative versus first-time surgery, indication for surgery (e.g. malignant versus benign), and extent of thyroidectomy and of concomitant central compartment lymphadenectomy.

Fourth, there may be use of 'inappropriate denominators'. For instance, the rate of hypocalcaemia within a series of thyroidectomies will be influenced by the proportion of cases having bilateral surgery, as hypoparathyroidism will not usually result from unilateral dissection. The overall rate of hypocalcaemia will therefore be artificially low if unilateral lobectomies are included in the denominator. This is often inadequately described in published series. Similar considerations apply to recurrent laryngeal nerve injury, where the rate of RLNP per patient may differ significantly for a given rate per nerve at risk, because bilateral surgery carries twice the risk of injury to one or other nerve.

Finally, retrospective series are prone to publication bias, reflecting individuals' tendency only to publish 'good' results. Genuinely excellent outcomes might thus be reported from some highly specialized centres and represent an aspirational target, but these may not reflect more general, routine practice.

Regarding persistent hypercalcaemia after surgery for primary hyperparathyroidism (HPT), additional considerations apply in interpreting the available literature. Although historical series[5,6] report cure rates of over 97%, there has been a resurgence of interest in recent years in performing targeted surgery, following localization studies such as sestamibi and ultrasound scanning. Such surgery may be performed via a mini-incision open method or by various endoscopic techniques. Recent case series, frequently reporting only targeted surgery, are therefore restricted to a subgroup of patients, with obvious abnormalities on imaging, who may potentially have larger adenomas and therefore be 'easier' to cure. Conversely, the limitations of pre-operative imaging in excluding multigland disease may reduce the cure rate in a proportion of targeted cases, while those with entirely negative imaging are possibly the most difficult to cure, in turn affecting the results of bilateral exploration.[7] Individual units' or surgeons' results may therefore be dependent not only on the quality of the surgery but on referral practices and case selection, and they can be reliably compared only if information on all their operated HPT cases is made available.

Despite these concerns, some estimate of risk can be made, and **Table 80.1** summarizes recent results from larger case series.

Prospective audits and registries may partly avoid some of these problems, as they may be able to apply more consistent definitions of relevant outcomes, remain contemporaneous and potentially collect uniform information on case mix and other factors which might influence outcomes. They also have the potential to study much larger numbers of patients than would be feasible in most single centres, thereby increasing the precision of any risk estimates.

The best-established national registries examining global results of thyroid and parathyroid surgery are the Scandinavian Quality Register[21] and the UK-wide Audit of the British Association of Endocrine and Thyroid Surgeons (BAETS).[22]

The Scandinavian Quality Register[21] was established in 2004 and receives data on thyroid, parathyroid and adrenal surgery, submitted from multiple centres across Sweden (and Denmark). Coverage is high, with participating units accounting for over 90% of the cases currently being performed in Sweden, and with a full spectrum of thyroid pathology being represented.

The BAETS National Audit[22] was initiated in 2000 and currently receives data on thyroid, parathyroid, adrenal and endocrine pancreatic surgery from BAETS members, via a standardized electronic pro forma. The distribution of pathology represented is similar to that of the Scandinavian Registry, although coverage within the UK is lower, at about 35% of thyroid cases (estimated from English Hospital Episode Statistics).

Results from both registries have been published in national reports[21, 22] and, as is apparent in Table 80.1, show rates of complications generally higher than the best results previously reported in the medical literature.

It is likely, therefore, that they represent a more realistic assessment of the true rate of complications in routine practice, for the reasons alluded to above.

Even within large, specifically designed registries, however, difficulties remain in providing reliable estimates of risk. These include the following:

- **Data entry issues.** Registries and large prospective audits are dependent on entry of data by external agents, such as by hospital coding departments or individual members of a host specialty association. Such data may therefore be liable to incomplete case acquisition,

TABLE 80.1 Summary rates of complications in recent large case series and national registries

	Reference	Re-exploration for haemorrhage	Early RLNP	Permanent RLNP	Early hypocalcaemia*	Late/permanent hypocalcaemia*
Single centres	Burkey et al[8] (n = 13817) (Thyroid and parathyroid)	0.3%				
	Rosenbaum et al[9] (n = 1050) (Thyroid and parathyroid)	0.6%				
	Promberger et al[10] (n = 30142)	1.7%				
	Leyre et al[11] (n = 6830)	1.0%				
	Lee et al[12] (n = 2636)		0.7%	0.2%	35.3%	0.4%
	Efremidou et al[13] (n = 932)	0.2%	1.3%	0.3%	7.3%	0.3%
	Karamanakos et al[14] (n = 2043)	1.3%	1.7%	0.9%	27.8%	4.8%
	Hermann et al[15] † (n = 16443)		5.1%	1.4%		
	Erbil et al[16] † (n = 3250)		1.8%	0.3%	6.6%	0.3%
	Tartaglia et al[17] (n = 1636)	1.2%	1.9%	0.9%		0.8%
Multicentre studies and National Registries	Godballe et al[18] (n = 5490)	4.2%				
	Duclos et al[19] † (n = 3574)			2.1%		2.7%
	Baldassarre et al[20] (n = 119567)				9.0%	
	Scandinavian Quality Register[21] Thyroid (n = 13975) Parathyroid (n = 6113)	2.0% 0.5%	3.0% 3.0%	1.1% 0.3%	16%	3.0%
	BAETS Audit Thyroid[22] (n = 26222) Parathyroid (n = 11923)	1.1% 0.4%		1.0%	22.7%	6.3% 2.5%
		Persistent hypercalcaemia (all primary HPT)				
	Scandinavian Quality Registry[21] Parathyroid			5.9%		
	BAETS Audit[22] Parathyroid			4.9%		

* Bilateral resections only
† Routine post-operative laryngoscopy

variations in how the definitions of index complications are applied, incorrect coding and data transposition errors.
- **Data quality issues,** in particular the possibility of duplicate entries, and the rates of missing data.[22] The latter are particularly liable to affect estimates of risk, as it is feasible that poorer outcomes may be more frequent within the cohort whose data on that outcome are missing.
- **Choice of a suitable period of analysis,** balancing the need to provide the most contemporaneous data against the advantages of greater patient numbers which might be provided by a longer time period of study. Comparisons between individual units' or surgeons' results may be especially prone to misinterpretation in this regard, due to the greater random variation existing around point estimates of risk with small patient numbers.

These considerations aside, it is likely that national registries provide the most realistic estimates of risk for the purposes of consent and provision of benchmarking data.

OUTCOMES: COMPARISON BETWEEN PROVIDERS

A natural use of audit and registry data is to compare surgical performance between surgeons or hospitals. This may be useful for individual surgeons, to reassure themselves that their practice is satisfactory, or to identify areas where performance might be improved, and so enhance the quality of care. Such considerations may also contribute significantly to surgeons' appraisal processes and, in the UK, to revalidation with professional regulatory bodies (General Medical Council). With appropriate refinement, such data may also assist patients and service commissioners in selecting hospitals or surgeons.

This issue has recently gained increasing attention in the UK, with the introduction of NHS England's Consultant Outcomes Publication process,[23] through which individual surgeons' outcomes for various subspecialty procedures have been made available in the public domain. For thyroid surgery, this was first made publically available in 2013, using data derived from the BAETS audit, via a web-based portal. These data have been updated annually since 2013.[24]

In addition to the above-mentioned problems, further difficulties exist in using audit data for this purpose, particularly issues of random variation and case mix.

Even when the overall risk of a surgical complication is known, the exact number of events observed in any given series of operations will be subject to some random variation. Statistical methods can help identify when the observed variation is within that expected by chance, and traditionally confidence intervals are calculated, outlining the limits beyond which chance is less likely to explain the observed variation. Selection of appropriate confidence limits, however, is difficult. Set too widely, they risk designation of all surgeons as 'within control limits', and so miss those whose performance may in fact be lower than average. Set too tightly, they risk inappropriate identification of surgeons as 'outliers', with the potential for damage to reputation and career.

With any operation, the risk of certain complications occurring may also be affected by case mix, for example variation in patient characteristics, such as age or comorbidity, or in surgical complexity. Surgeons taking on more complex cases might be expected to have a higher complication rate, even if their performance is no worse than the average.

In some surgical fields, the factors affecting results are well defined, allowing for risk adjustment, to allow for case mix. In endocrine surgery, however, there are no established, validated models for this purpose.

For thyroidectomy, factors identified from individual case series as potential confounders include:

- patient age and gender[10, 18, 25]
- extent of thyroid resection (lobectomy versus subtotal versus total thyroidectomy)[10, 14, 16, 18, 25]
- re-operative versus first-time surgery[10, 14, 16, 25, 26]
- malignant versus benign disease[14, 18, 26]
- Graves' disease versus other benign diseases[14]
- central neck dissection, in addition to thyroidectomy[27, 28]
- goitre size and retrosternal versus cervical goitre[29, 30]
- surgeon caseload/experience[19, 31, 32]

As mentioned above, however, it is difficult to combine the results from these disparate studies into a unified mathematical model of risk-adjustment, and it is likely that only analyses from prospective registries will have the power and consistency of definition of relevant variables to do this. A preliminary, multivariate analysis from the BAETS dataset[33] has been a first step towards this, generating estimates of odds ratios for those factors most strongly affecting certain complications, namely:

- for bleeding: extent of thyroidectomy and patient age
- for early hypocalcaemia: Graves' disease, age, gender and level 6 node dissection
- for late hypocalcaemia: cancer diagnosis and particularly level 6 node dissection.

It must also be recognized that risk-adjustment models can only make allowance for those variables included within the original dataset, and that other, unrecorded, factors may influence results, for instance patient comorbidity or ethnicity[34, 35] or thyroid volume.[30]

There remains an urgent need to explore this issue further, if accurate comparison is to be made between surgeons, on the basis of registry data.

OTHER USES OF AUDIT DATA

Published registry data[21, 22] also provide interesting insights into:

- use and accuracy of pre-operative investigations, such as fine-needle aspiration cytology (FNAC)

- trends over time in the management of certain conditions, e.g. the gradual replacement of subtotal by total thyroidectomy for most benign conditions, or the increasing trend to perform pre-operative localization studies in first-time primary hyperparathyroidism
- management and staging of thyroid cancer, particularly variations in the extent of 'prophylactic' lymph node surgery
- rare diseases, including medullary thyroid cancer and parathyroid cancer
- trends in the use of technological innovations, such as a slow increase in intra-operative laryngeal nerve monitoring, more rapid increase in the use of vessel sealing devices, such as the Harmonic scalpel or Ligasure, and decreasing use of intra-operative PTH monitoring during parathyroidectomy.

CONCLUSION

Surgeons are coming under increasing scrutiny and they need to demonstrate that their outcomes are acceptable, for their own satisfaction in addition to meeting the needs of patients, commissioners and regulatory bodies. This is particularly pertinent to thyroid and parathyroid surgery, as outcomes are clearly under the direct influence of the operating surgeon, and publication of these outcomes is already occurring in the public domain.

Estimation of complication rates from published case series is highly problematic. Participation in national registries contributes to more accurate analysis of outcomes, and is recommended to all surgeons with an interest in thyroid and parathyroid surgery.

KEY POINTS

- Assessment of complication rates of thyroid and parathyroid surgery from published data is prone to many limitations.
- Large case series and national registries suggest the following range of risk estimates:
  - Re-operation for bleeding 0.2–4.2%.
  - Early/transient recurrent laryngeal nerve palsy 0.7–5.1%.
  - Persistent recurrent laryngeal nerve palsy 0.2–1.0%.
  - Persistent hypocalcaemia (bilateral thyroid resection) 0.3–6.3%.
- There is a need for validated risk-adjustment models to be developed, if outcomes are to be accurately compared between healthcare providers.

REFERENCES

1. Mehanna HM, Jain A, Randeva H, et al. Postoperative hypocalcemia: the difference a definition makes. *Head Neck* 2010; **32**: 279–83.
2. Dionigi G, Boni L, Rovera F, et al. Postoperative laryngoscopy in thyroid surgery: proper timing to detect recurrent laryngeal nerve injury. *Langenbecks Arch Surg* 2010; **395**: 327–31.
3. Mihai R, Randolph GW. Thyroid surgery, voice and the laryngeal examination. Time for increased awareness and accurate evaluation. *World J Endocr Surg* 2009; **1**: 1–5.
4. Jeannon J-P, Orabi AA, Bruch GA, et al. Diagnosis of recurrent laryngeal nerve palsy after thyroidectomy: a systematic review. *Int J Clin Pract* 2009; **63**: 624–9.
5. Mortier P-E, Mozzon MM, Fouquet OP, et al. Unilateral surgery for hyperparathyroidism: indications, limits and late results. New philosophy or expensive selection without improvement of surgical results? *World J Surg* 2004; **28**: 1298–304.
6. van Heerden JA, Grant CS. Surgical treatment of primary hyperparathyroidism: an institutional perspective. *World J Surg* 1991; **15**: 688–92.
7. Bagul A, Patel HP, Chadwick D, et al. Primary hyperparathyroidism: an analysis of failure of parathyroidectomy. *World J Surg* 2014; **38**: 534–41.
8. Burkey SH, van Heerden JA, Thompson GB, et al. Re-exploration for symptomatic hematomas after cervical exploration. *Surgery* 2001; **130**: 914–20.
9. Rosenbaum MA, Haridas M, McHenry CR. Life-threatening neck hematoma complicating thyroid and parathyroid surgery. *Am J Surg* 2008; **195**: 333–43.
10. Promberger R, Ott J, Kober F, et al. Risk factors for postoperative bleeding after thyroid surgery. *Br J Surg* 2012; **99**: 373–9.
11. Leyre P, Desurmont T, Lacoste L, et al. 2008. Does the risk of compressive hematoma after thyroidectomy authorize 1-day surgery? *Langenbecks Arch Surg* 2008; **393**: 733–7.
12. Lee YS, Nam K-H, Chung WY, et al. Postoperative complications of thyroid cancer in a single center experience. *J Korean Med Sci* 2010; **25**: 541–5.
13. Efremidou EI, Papageorgiou MS, Liratzopoulos N, Manolas KJ. The efficacy and safety of total thyroidectomy in the management of benign thyroid disease: a review of 932 cases. *Canadian J Surg* 2009; **52**: 39–44.
14. Karamanakos SN, Markou KB, Panagopoulos K, et al. Complications and risk factors related to the extent of surgery in thyroidectomy: results from 2,043 procedures. *Hormones* 2010; **9**: 318–25.
15. Hermann M, Alk G, Roka R, et al. Laryngeal nerve injury in surgery for benign thyroid diseases: effect of nerve dissection and impact of individual surgeon in more than 27,000 nerves at risk. *Ann Surg* 2002; **235**: 261–8.
16. Erbil Y, Barbaros U, Issever H. et al. Predictive factors for recurrent laryngeal nerve palsy and hypoparathyroidism after thyroid surgery. *Clin Otolaryngol* 2006; **32**: 32–7.
17. Tartaglia F, Sgueglia M, Muhaya A. et al. Complications in total thyroidectomy: our experience and a number of considerations. *Chirurgia Italiana* 2003; **55**: 499–510.
18. Godballe C, Madsen AR, Pedersen HB et al. Post-thyroidectomy hemorrhage: a national study of patients treated at the Danish departments of ENT Head and Neck surgery. *Eur Arch Otorhinolaryngol* 2009; **266**: 1945–52.
19. Duclos A, Peix J-L, Colin C, et al. Influence of experience on performance of individual surgeons in thyroid surgery: prospective cross sectional multicentre study. *Br Med J* 2012; **344**: d8041.
20. Baldassarre RL, Chang DC, Brumund KT, Bouvet M. Predictors of hypocalcemia after thyroidectomy: results from the nationwide inpatient sample. *ISRN Surgery* 2012 Article ID 838614.
21. Nordenström E. Scandinavian quality register for thyroid, parathyroid and adrenal surgery. Annual Report 2012. Malmö, Sweden.
22. Chadwick D, Kinsman R, Walton P. Fifth National Audit Report, British Association of Endocrine and Thyroid Surgeons. Henley-on-Thames: Dendrite Clinical Systems Ltd., 2017. ISBN 978-0-9929942-004 Available at www.baets.org.uk [last accessed 4 Nov 2017]
23. Healthcare Quality Improvement Partnership; Clinical Outcomes Publication. www.hqip.org.uk/national-programmes/clinical-outcomes-publicaiton/ [last accessed 4 Nov 2017]
24. Surgeon-specific outcome reports for endocrine surgery 2013. http://baets.e-dendrite.com/ [accessed 23 Jan 2018].
25. Sousa Ade A, Salles JM, Soares JM, et al. Predictor factors for post-thyroidectomy hypocalcaemia. *Rev Col Bras Cir* 2012; **39**(6): 476–82.

26. Hayward NJ, Grodski S, Yeung M, et al. Recurrent laryngeal nerve injury in thyroid surgery: a review. *ANZ J Surg* 2013; **83**: 15–21.
27. Chisholm EJ, Kulinskaya E, Tolley NS. Systematic review and meta-analysis of the adverse effects of thyroidectomy combined with central neck dissection as compared with thyroidectomy alone. *Laryngoscope* 2009; **119**: 1135–9.
28. Sitges-Serra A, Ruiz S, Girvent M, et al. Outcome of protracted hypoparathyroidism after total thyroidectomy. *Br J Surg* 2010; **97**: 1687–95.
29. Pieracci FM, Fahey TJ. Substernal thyroidectomy is associated with increased morbidity and mortality as compared with conventional cervical thyroidectomy. *J Am Coll Surg* 2007; **205**: 1–7.
30. Karabeyoglu M, Unal B, Dirican A, et al. The relation between preoperative ultrasonographic thyroid volume analysis and thyroidectomy complications. *Endocr Regul* 2009; **43**: 83–7.
31. Gonzalez-Sanchez C, Franch-Arcas G, Gomez-Alonso A. Morbidity following thyroid surgery: does surgeon volume matter? *Langenbecks Arch Surg* 2013; **398**: 419–22.
32. Sosa JA, Bowman H, Tielsch JM, et al. The importance of surgeon experience for clinical and economic outcomes from thyroidectomy. *Ann Surg* 1998; **228**: 320–30.
33. Chadwick D, Kinsman R, Walton P. Fourth National Audit Report, British Association of Endocrine and Thyroid Surgeon. Henley-on-Thames: Dendrite Clinical Systems Ltd., 2012. ISBN 987-0-9568154-3-9
34. Radowsky JS, Helou LB, Howard RS, et al. Racial disparities in voice outcomes after thyroid and parathyroid surgery. *Surgery* 2013; **153**: 103–10.
35. Schlosser K, Maschuw K, Hassan I, et al. Are diabetic patients at a greater risk to develop a vocal fold palsy during thyroid surgery than nondiabetic patients? *Surgery* 2008; **143**: 352–8.

CHAPTER 81

MEDICOLEGAL ASPECTS OF HEAD AND NECK ENDOCRINE SURGERY

Barney Harrison

Introduction 899	When things go wrong 900
The law 899	A claim arises 901
The likelihood and facts around litigation and thyroid surgery 899	References 902
Consent to surgery 900	

SEARCH STRATEGY

Data in this chapter may be updated by a PubMed search using the keywords: thyroid, thyroidectomy, litigation, malpractice, informed consent and medicolegal.

INTRODUCTION

England and Wales have among the highest level of personal injury damages awards in the world, with an increasing frequency of claims. In England, the number of surgery claims received by the National Health Service Litigation Authority (NHSLA), which manages negligence and other claims against the NHS on behalf of its member organizations, rose by 66% from 2009 to 2013 with General Surgery representing 33.8% and Others – including ENT – 2.5%. Since 2011 the annual payments made by the NHSLA in respect of clinical negligence have exceeded a billion pounds per year.

Clinical negligence claims in 2013/14 were 11 945 compared with 10 129 in 2012/13. In 2013/14, 44% of clinical negligence claims were resolved without a payment and 79% of the small number of cases that were decided in court (historically less than 5%) were successfully defended at trial.

THE LAW

A successful claim of medical negligence is required to prove that:

- the treatment received fell below the reasonable/accepted standard of competence that a patient had a right to expect – **breach of duty of care**
- the patient suffered an injury or loss – **damage**
- it is more likely than not that the injury would not have occurred or been less severe if appropriate treatment had been given, i.e. there is a link between the breach of duty and the injury – **causation**.

The claim must be brought within a specific time after the injury – **period of limitation.**

Successful damages awards will reflect two elements:

- pain, suffering 'loss of amenity'
- financial loss and extra expenses caused by the injury.

THE LIKELIHOOD AND FACTS AROUND LITIGATION AND THYROID SURGERY

Legal systems around the world differ but, in general, cases that arise from medical negligence that end up in court are civil prosecutions. In relation to thyroid surgery the studies described below provide some insight into the likelihood and outcome of claims or prosecutions reaching court subsequent to thyroid surgery.

Europe

From England, the NHSLA recorded 17 claims related to thyroidectomy and vocal cord dysfunction between 1995 and 2005.[1]

A German report[2] reviewed outcomes of 75 thyroidectomy-related malpractice claims in which expert opinion was provided by a single 'witness' over a 15-year period. Unilateral vocal cord palsy was the cause of the action in 28%, bilateral vocal cord palsy in 29%, hypoparathyroidism (all patients requiring calcium and vitamin D) alone in 13%. In 37% of the cases more than one major complication occurred. The claimant was successful in 77% of bilateral RLN palsies, 24% of unilateral palsy and 25% in post-operative hypoparathyroidism.

A prior German study[3] found that between 1975 and 1998 thyroidectomy represented 1% of litigation cases. A successful claim was more likely if a second operation was necessary, if the goal of the operation had been missed, or if any kind of complication was followed by a fault in post-operative care.

USA

Three studies are based on data from the Physicians Insurers Association of America said to represent 60% of privately insured physicians in the United States and 25% of malpractice claims.

Over a 24-year period, approximately 2 585 000 thyroidectomies were performed. The authors[4] estimated from their study that 5.9 claims are filed per 10 000 thyroid operations. Of thyroidectomy-related claims, 11% went to trial and a third (2 per 10 000) resulted in an indemnity payment.

Between 1986 and 2007, 112 closed claims (claims made irrespective of whether dismissed, settled or went to trial) were identified involving iatrogenic vocal cord palsy.[5] Of these, 42% resulted from thyroid and parathyroid surgery. Failure to recognize the complication and consent issues were responsible for 36% and 19% of the claims respectively.

A review of 315 closed malpractice claims related to otolaryngology–head and neck surgery between 1978 and 2007 found that nerve injuries accounted for 20.3% of claims including the accessory (5.4%) and recurrent laryngeal nerve (3.5.%); 5.1% of claims related to thyroidectomy.[6]

Two studies from the USA have assessed thyroid-related claims that went to court, the cases identified by review of legal databases.

Of 30 thyroid-related post-verdict cases (1987–2000), 33% were associated with surgical complications.[7] In respect of nine RLN injuries, the claim related to lack of informed consent in seven cases. In six of eight cancer-related cases, the claim related to delayed diagnosis.

The second study identified 33 cases that went to court in relation to alleged negligence associated with thyroid surgery between 1989 and 2009.[8] Of these, 46% involved RLN injury (five bilateral, five unilateral, five unspecified), and 6% delayed diagnosis. The majority of the seven claims where the outcome favoured the plaintiff were filed because of a lack of informed consent.

Finally, a review of 81 spinal accessory nerve injury claims that went to trial (1985–2007) found that the causative procedure was lymph node biopsy (68%), and neck dissections in only 5%. Lack of informed consent and failure to diagnose the injury were the basis of the allegation in 21% and 20% respectively.[9]

CONSENT TO SURGERY

The importance of adequate informed consent prior to an intervention cannot be overstated, most importantly for best patient care and, secondly, as indicated above, your avoidance of undesired consequence if a claim of negligence is submitted.

In the UK, the General Medical Council document *Consent: patients and doctors making decisions together*[10] includes imperatives (as an overriding duty) with regard to providing information on diagnostic uncertainty, options for treatment, the potential benefits and risks. In addition the document recommends that it is your duty to ensure patients understand information and how this can be enhanced.

Further clarification on who may obtain consent, what should be discussed and how it should be recorded is provided in *Good surgical practice* published by The Royal College of Surgeons (2014).[11]

Risks will usually be 'side effects, complications, failure of an intervention to achieve the desired aim'. Additional information in the form of information leaflets can be useful, and is recommended, but should not be considered as a replacement for a thorough discussion with the patient.[12]

Historically if a claim for litigation arose in the UK, a legal test (*Bolam*) was applied to determine whether the conduct of a doctor could be supported by a responsible body of medical opinion. In the *Sidaway* judgment that followed it was for doctors to decide how much to inform a patient of the risks of a treatment. Since early 2015, following a judgment in the Supreme Court (*Montgomery* v. *Lanarkshire Health Board*), this no longer applies to the law on consent. It is now required that a doctor takes 'reasonable care to ensure that the patient is aware of any material risks involved in any recommended treatment and of any reasonable alternative or variant treatments'. A material risk is one to which a reasonable person would be likely to attach significance, i.e. a risk that might alter the particular patient's decision.

WHEN THINGS GO WRONG

In the UK, since 2014, NHS providers have been required to comply with a duty of candour. It places a legal duty on hospitals and other providers to inform and apologize to patients, or their families if there have been mistakes in their care that led to death, severe or moderate harm. The duty of candour legislation applies to all Care Quality Commission registered providers since 2015. This contractual statutory requirement is, of course, in addition to the ethical duty of a doctor to inform patients and their families when an incident has occurred.

Good surgical practice[11] emphasizes the requirement to inform patients as soon as possible of any harm that has occurred, to apologize and to offer reassurance.

A useful overview of the background and threshold levels at which disclosure should be applied can be found via the RCS website.[13]

A CLAIM ARISES...

The plaintiff's/defendant's solicitors will instruct an expert witness to provide a report on possible breach of duty and/or condition and prognosis. An expert witness should provide, from knowledge and experience, an independent and balanced opinion **for the court** (not the instructing lawyers) on the facts of a case, an explanation of 'technical' issues, a view on what is considered 'reasonable', and matters of causation (symptoms or condition) that have arisen as a result of damage.

Some of the typical issues on which an expert witness may be asked to provide an opinion in a thyroid/parathyroid medical negligence claim are discussed below with current relevant 'evidence'.

IMPACT OF A DELAY IN CANCER DIAGNOSIS

For patients with differentiated or medullary thyroid cancer there are staging and prognostic scoring symptoms that allow an opinion on outcome from the time of actual diagnosis. The expert, in relation to the impact of delay, is unlikely to be able to state (as is often asked) what might have been the prognosis at a previous point in time. The evidence base on the clinical significance of any delay in the diagnosis of thyroid cancer is very limited.

A study using data from the Korean Central Cancer Registry[14] assessed the impact of delay from thyroid cancer diagnosis to first curative treatment and found the small number of deaths in these patients precluded precise estimates. The lowest mortality was observed for patients who had surgery between 1 and 4 weeks after diagnosis but there was no clear pattern of increased risk found with delay of up to 12 weeks in thyroid cancer.

In a study cohort of 1355 patients with DTC,[15] factors influencing the prognosis of patients who died found that cancer mortality was 4% in patients who underwent initial therapy within a year, compared with 10% in the others. The 'delay' group had twice the cancer mortality at 30 years (6% compared to 13%).

In contrast, a study including 47 patients with a delayed diagnosis of differentiated thyroid cancer as a consequence of initial benign cytology – median delay 52 months; range 13–205 months – found no difference in 5-year disease-free survival when compared with a historical cohort of patients treated with 'immediate' surgery.[16]

FAILURE TO PERFORM A SECOND FNA OF A SUSPICIOUS THYROID NODULE

False negative thyroid FNA rates of <3%–10.2%[17, 18] are reported in patients subsequently confirmed as having thyroid cancer. As suspicious features on ultrasound are reported in 90% of patients with thyroid cancer **and** false negative FNA,[17] inadequate cytology (Thy1) or benign cytology (Thy2) in association with sonographic features of concern indicates at the very least a need for further FNA as recommended in the British Thyroid Association Guidelines.[19]

RECURRENT LARYNGEAL NERVE PALSY AND INTRA-OPERATIVE NERVE MONITORING

Risk factors for vocal cord palsy include Graves' disease, post-operative bleed, retrosternal, malignant, recurrent benign and malignant goitre, no identification of the recurrent laryngeal nerve.[20–23]

At thyroidectomy, intermittent intra-operative nerve monitoring (IONM) is useful for identification of the recurrent nerve and its branches, but loss of signal in at least one in three cases is not associated with post-operative nerve dysfunction. The limitation of intermittent IONM is that injury to the nerve from whatever cause is identified after the event. Implicit in its use is that IONM is carried out in the recommended manner.[24]

There are two key issues in the context of litigation.

- There is a lack of evidence that intermittent IONM is associated with a decrease in the risk of permanent vocal cord palsy at first time[25–28] and reoperative thyroidectomy.[28] Temporary nerve dysfunction in both operative scenarios appears to be reduced with IONM use.[25, 29]
- If nerve monitoring is used, what is the appropriate next step if there is loss of signal on the first side of a bilateral thyroid procedure? Continue with the second side or abandon the operation and await laryngoscopy? The risk of bilateral vocal cord palsy at thyroidectomy is variously reported as 1 to >3 per thousand cases.[30, 31] The next step will clearly depend upon the indication for surgery (benign vs malignant disease), the experience of the surgical team, the nature of the signal loss and familiarity with the technicalities of IONM. Two studies from the same unit[32, 33] propose staged thyroidectomy in this worrying scenario; both have limitations that affect the interpretation of their results.

The natural evolution from intermittent to continuous IONM and evolving technology may help resolve the limitations associated with its use.

APPROPRIATENESS OF AN INPATIENT STAY OF LESS THAN 24 HOURS AFTER THYROIDECTOMY IN THE CONTEXT OF NECK HAEMATOMA/HYPOCALCAEMIA

The instructing solicitors might enquire as to the safety of a less than 24 hour inpatient stay for a patient who developed neck haematoma after day-case surgery.

Risk factors for post-operative bleeding include reoperative surgery and bilateral procedures. Life-threatening neck haematoma that requires reoperation will occur in 0.6–2.1% of cases.[31, 34–37] Although most will occur within 6 hours of surgery, 20–37% will occur after 6–24 hours and 0–10% after 24 hours.[35, 36, 38]

An assessment of parathyroid function after completion or total thyroidectomy is mandatory. National specialist databases record post-operative hypocalcaemia rates of 21% (British Association of Endocrine and Thyroid Surgeons) after total thyroidectomy for MNG and, from Scandinavia, 6.4% patients required i.v. calcium after bilateral thyroidectomy.[34]

Post-operative measurement of serum calcium/PTH and/or routine calcium supplementation is used to identify and minimize risks of significant hypocalcaemia. Be aware that in patients who become hypocalcaemic, the lowest level of serum calcium is on or after the second post-operative day.[39,40] If a patient is discharged too soon, they may develop severe untreated hypocalcaemia.

EXPERIENCE OF THE SURGEON

There are an increasing number of publications to support the concept that high-volume thyroid surgeons have better patient outcomes than low-volume surgeons. This is reported for post-operative neck haematoma,[41,42] hypocalcaemia,[42,43] adequacy of thyroidectomy in patients with thyroid cancer[44] and RLN palsy.[22,42,43] There is, however, little consistency in what constitutes a high-, intermediate- or low- volume surgeon (Table 81.1).

Surgeon experience is particularly important in relation to paediatric cases.[45] Children whose thyroidectomy or parathyroidectomy was performed by a low-volume surgeon (<30 endocrine cervical per year) had more endocrine complications than those whose operation was performed by a high-volume surgeon (11% compared to 5.6%). Sosa[46] reported complication rates after thyroidectomy/parathyroidectomy in 1199 patients 17 years old or younger. Children had significantly higher endocrine-specific complication rates than adults after parathyroidectomy and thyroidectomy. Even when thyroidectomy is performed by high-volume surgeons, 7% of patients will require intravenous calcium[47] and post-operative hypocalcaemia is reported in 34% of children <10 years of age.[48]

TABLE 81.1 Variation in classifications of thyroid surgeon operative volumes

Author	Year	Low volume	Intermediate volume	High volume
Sosa[49]	1998	1–9 per year		>100 per year
Tuggle[45]	2008			>30 per year
Kandil[42]	2013	<10 in 10 years	10–99 in 10 years	≥100 in 10 years
Loyo[43]	2013	≤9 per year	9–23 per year	>23 per year
Dehal[41]	2014	<10 in 10 years	10–99 in 10 years	≥100 in 10 years
Adkisson[44]	2014	–		≥30 per year
Landerholm[50]	2014	–	<50 per year	–

KEY POINTS

- Ensure that thyroid function and serum calcium are normal prior to and after surgery. This is your responsibility unless someone else has agreed to take over these aspects of care.
- Ensure at the very least that the content and legibility of your clinical record, the consent form and the operation note would stand up to scrutiny by an 'expert' third party.
- The contents of an operation note should include that indicated in *Good surgical practice*. It would seem entirely appropriate and necessary in the context of thyroid/parathyroid surgery (for your potential benefit in a claim) to record findings related to the parathyroid glands and their preservation as well as the recurrent laryngeal nerves.
- Ensure that for complex patients (e.g. the non-compliant thyrotoxic patient) there is adequate peri-operative support from endocrinology colleagues.
- Post-operative laryngoscopy should be performed in a patient with post-operative voice symptoms.
- The defence of a claim will depend upon your statement of:
  - what you did – were you the appropriate surgeon?
  - why you did it – what were the indications for operation?
  - what your notes say
  - how you managed the complication(s).
- Be reassured that complications are not necessarily due to error.

REFERENCES

1. Mihai RR, Randolph GW. Thyroid surgery, voice and the laryngeal examination: time for increased awareness and accurate evaluation. *World J Endocr Surg* 2009; **1**(1): 1–5.
2. Dralle H, Lorenz K, Machens A. Verdicts on malpractice claims after thyroid surgery: emerging trends and future directions. *Head Neck* 2012; **34**(11): 1591–6.
3. Schulte KM, Roher HD. Medico-legal aspects of thyroid surgery. *Chirurg* 1999; **70**(10): 1131–8.
4. Singer MC, Iverson KC, Terris DJ. Thyroidectomy-related malpractice claims. *Otolaryngol Head Neck Surg* 2012; **146**(3): 358–61.
5. Shaw GY, Pierce E. Malpractice litigation involving iatrogenic surgical vocal fold paralysis: a closed-claims review with recommendations for prevention and management. *Ann Otol Rhinol Laryngol* 2009; **118**(1): 6–12.
6. Simonsen AR, Duncavage JA, Becker SS. Malpractice in head and neck surgery: a review of cases. *Otolaryngol Head Neck Surg* 2012; **147**(1): 69–73.

7. Lydiatt DD. Medical malpractice and the thyroid gland. *Head Neck* 2003; **25**(6): 429–31.
8. Abadin SS, Kaplan EL, Angelos P. Malpractice litigation after thyroid surgery: the role of recurrent laryngeal nerve injuries, 1989–2009. *Surgery* 2010; **148**(4): 718–22; discussion 22–3.
9. Morris LG, Ziff DJ, Delacure MD. Malpractice litigation after surgical injury of the spinal accessory nerve: an evidence-based analysis. *Arch Otolaryngol Head Neck Surg* 2008; **134**(1): 102–7.
10. General Medical Council. *Consent: patients and doctors making decisions together.* 2008. Available from: http://www.gmc-uk.org/guidance/ethical_guidance/consent_guidance_index.asp [Accessed July 19, 2017].
11. Royal College of Surgeons of England. *Good surgical practice.* 2014. http://www.rcseng.ac.uk/surgeons/surgical-standards/professionalism-surgery/gsp [Accessed July 19, 2017].
12. Anderson OA, Wearne IM. Informed consent for elective surgery: what is best practice? *J R Soc Med* 2007; **100**(2): 97–100.
13. Royal College of Surgeons of England. https://www.rcseng.ac.uk
14. Shin DW, Cho J, Kim SY, et al. Delay to curative surgery greater than 12 weeks is associated with increased mortality in patients with colorectal and breast cancer but not lung or thyroid cancer. *Ann Surg Oncol* 2013; **20**(8): 2468–76.
15. Mazzaferri EL, Jhiang SM. Long-term impact of initial surgical and medical therapy on papillary and follicular thyroid cancer. *Am J Med* 1994; **97**(5): 418–28.
16. Amit M, Rudnicki Y, Binenbaum Y, et al. Defining the outcome of patients with delayed diagnosis of differentiated thyroid cancer. *Laryngoscope* 2014; **124**(12): 2837–40.
17. Kwak JY, Kim EK, Kim HJ, et al. How to combine ultrasound and cytological information in decision making about thyroid nodules. *Eur Radiol* 2009; **19**(8): 1923–31.
18. Chernyavsky VS, Shanker BA, Davidov T, et al. Is one benign fine needle aspiration enough? *Ann Surg Oncol* 2012; **19**(5): 1472–6.
19. Perros P, Boelaert K, Colley S, et al. Guidelines for the management of thyroid cancer. *Clin Endocrinol (Oxf)* 2014; **81** Suppl 1: 1–122.
20. Chiang FY, Wang LF, Huang YF, et al. Recurrent laryngeal nerve palsy after thyroidectomy with routine identification of the recurrent laryngeal nerve. *Surgery* 2005; **137**(3): 342–7.
21. Dralle H, Sekulla C, Haerting J, et al. Risk factors of paralysis and functional outcome after recurrent laryngeal nerve monitoring in thyroid surgery. *Surgery* 2004; **136**(6): 1310–22.
22. Enomoto K, Uchino S, Watanabe S, et al. Recurrent laryngeal nerve palsy during surgery for benign thyroid diseases: risk factors and outcome analysis. *Surgery* 2014; **155**(3): 522–8.
23. Lo CY, Kwok KF, Yuen PW. A prospective evaluation of recurrent laryngeal nerve paralysis during thyroidectomy. *Arch Surg* 2000; **135**(2): 204–7.
24. Randolph GW, Dralle H, Abdullah H, et al. Electrophysiologic recurrent laryngeal nerve monitoring during thyroid and parathyroid surgery: international standards guideline statement. *Laryngoscope* 2011; **121** Suppl 1: S1–16.
25. Barczynski M, Konturek A, Cichon S. Randomized clinical trial of visualization versus neuromonitoring of recurrent laryngeal nerves during thyroidectomy. *Br J Surg* 2009; **96**(3): 240–6.
26. Cavicchi O, Caliceti U, Fernandez IJ, et al. Laryngeal neuromonitoring and neurostimulation versus neurostimulation alone in thyroid surgery: a randomized clinical trial. *Head Neck* 2012; **34**(2): 141–5.
27. Higgins TS, Gupta R, Ketcham AS, et al. Recurrent laryngeal nerve monitoring versus identification alone on post-thyroidectomy true vocal fold palsy: a meta-analysis. *Laryngoscope* 2011; **121**(5): 1009–17.
28. Pisanu A, Porceddu G, Podda M, et al. Systematic review with meta-analysis of studies comparing intraoperative neuromonitoring of recurrent laryngeal nerves versus visualization alone during thyroidectomy. *J Surg Res* 2014; **188**(1): 152–61.
29. Barczynski M, Konturek A, Pragacz K, et al. Intraoperative nerve monitoring can reduce prevalence of recurrent laryngeal nerve injury in thyroid reoperations: results of a retrospective cohort study. *World J Surg* 2014; **38**(3): 599–606.
30. Sarkis LM, Zaidi N, Norlen O, et al. Bilateral recurrent laryngeal nerve injury in a specialized thyroid surgery unit: would routine intraoperative neuromonitoring alter outcomes? *ANZ J Surg* 2017; **87**(5): 364–7.
31. Vashishta R, Mahalingam-Dhingra A, Lander L, et al. Thyroidectomy outcomes: a national perspective. *Otolaryngol Head Neck Surg* 2012; **147**(6): 1027–34.
32. Goretzki PE, Schwarz K, Brinkmann J, et al. The impact of intraoperative neuromonitoring (IONM) on surgical strategy in bilateral thyroid diseases: is it worth the effort? *World J Surg* 2010; **34**(6): 1274–84.
33. Melin M, Schwarz K, Lammers BJ, Goretzki PE. IONM-guided goiter surgery leading to two-stage thyroidectomy: indication and results. *Langenbecks Arch Surg* 2013; **398**(3): 411–18.
34. Bergenfelz A, Jansson S, Kristoffersson A, et al. Complications to thyroid surgery: results as reported in a database from a multicenter audit comprising 3,660 patients. *Langenbecks Arch Surg* 2008; **393**(5): 667–73.
35. Lang BH, Yih PC, Lo CY. A review of risk factors and timing for postoperative hematoma after thyroidectomy: is outpatient thyroidectomy really safe? *World J Surg* 2012; **36**(10): 2497–502.
36. Leyre P, Desurmont T, Lacoste L, et al. Does the risk of compressive hematoma after thyroidectomy authorize 1-day surgery? *Langenbecks Arch Surg* 2008; **393**(5): 733–7.
37. Rosenbaum MA, Haridas M, McHenry CR. Life-threatening neck hematoma complicating thyroid and parathyroid surgery. *Am J Surg* 2008; **195**(3): 339–43; discussion 43.
38. Promberger R, Ott J, Kober F, et al. Risk factors for postoperative bleeding after thyroid surgery. *Br J Surg* 2012; **99**(3): 373–9.
39. Pattou F, Combemale F, Fabre S, et al. Hypocalcemia following thyroid surgery: incidence and prediction of outcome. *World J Surg* 1998; **22**(7): 718–24.
40. Sperlongano P, Sperlongano S, Foroni F, et al. Postoperative hypocalcemia: assessment timing. *Int J Surg* 2014; **12** Suppl 1: S95–7.
41. Dehal A, Abbas A, Al-Tememi M, et al. Impact of surgeon volume on incidence of neck hematoma after thyroid and parathyroid surgery: ten years' analysis of nationwide in-patient sample database. *Am Surg* 2014; **80**(10): 948–52.
42. Kandil E, Noureldine SI, Abbas A, Tufano RP. The impact of surgical volume on patient outcomes following thyroid surgery. *Surgery* 2013; **154**(6): 1346–52; discussion 52–3.
43. Loyo M, Tufano RP, Gourin CG. National trends in thyroid surgery and the effect of volume on short-term outcomes. *Laryngoscope* 2013; **123**(8): 2056–63.
44. Adkisson CD, Howell GM, McCoy KL, et al. Surgeon volume and adequacy of thyroidectomy for differentiated thyroid cancer. *Surgery* 2014; **156**(6): 1453–59; discussion 60.
45. Tuggle CT, Roman SA, Wang TS, et al. Pediatric endocrine surgery: who is operating on our children? *Surgery* 2008; **144**(6): 869–77; discussion 77.
46. Sosa JA, Tuggle CT, Wang TS, et al. Clinical and economic outcomes of thyroid and parathyroid surgery in children. *J Clin Endocrinol Metab* 2008; **93**(8): 3058–65.
47. Chen Y, Masiakos PT, Gaz RD, et al. Pediatric thyroidectomy in a high volume thyroid surgery center: risk factors for postoperative hypocalcemia. *J Pediatr Surg* 2015; **50**(8): 1316–19.
48. Kundel A, Thompson GB, Richards ML, et al. Pediatric endocrine surgery: a 20-year experience at the Mayo Clinic. *J Clin Endocrinol Metab* 2014; **99**(2): 399–406.
49. Sosa JA, Bowman HM, Tielsch JM, et al. The importance of surgeon experience for clinical and economic outcomes from thyroidectomy. *Ann Surg* 1998; **228**(3): 320–30.
50. Landerholm K, Wasner AM, Jarhult J. Incidence and risk factors for injuries to the recurrent laryngeal nerve during neck surgery in the moderate-volume setting. *Langenbecks Arch Surg* 2014; **399**(4): 509–15.

Pituitary disease

CHAPTER 82

CLINICAL EVALUATION OF THE PITUITARY PATIENT

Sean Carrie, John Hill and Andrew James

Introduction 905	Neuro-ophthalmological features of pituitary disease 910
Clinical manifestations of hormone deficiency 905	Conclusions 913
Clinical manifestations of excess hormone secretion 906	References 913

SEARCH STRATEGY AND EVIDENCE BASE

Data in this chapter may be updated by a Medline search using the keywords pituitary disease and pituitary adenoma and focusing on clinical features and ophthalmological assessment. The evidence in the chapter is mainly levels 3 and 4 but also with some level 2 evidence.

INTRODUCTION

The commonest lesion arising in the pituitary gland is a pituitary adenoma.[1] The clinical manifestations of pituitary adenomata may relate to their endocrine effects of hormone deficiency, hormone excess or a combination of both.[2] In addition there may be a physical effect related to a space-occupying lesion. Occasionally the presentation may be acute with infarction into a previously undiagnosed pituitary adenoma. Increasingly, with the widespread use of sophisticated imaging techniques, lesions within the pituitary gland may be identified before they become symptomatic, the so-called 'pituitary incidentaloma'.[3]

CLINICAL MANIFESTATIONS OF HORMONE DEFICIENCY

The syndrome of pituitary hyposecretion occurs when the mass effect of a lesion within the pituitary gland compresses the normal tissue leading to a reduction or absence of the normal secretion of pituitary hormones. This resulting hypopituitarism (**Figure 82.1**) affects the reproductive system most commonly.[4] Typically, women experience oligomenorrhoea or amenorrhoea with associated infertility; men commonly experience symptoms of hypogonadism, with increasing loss of libido and erectile dysfunction and associated infertility. There is a characteristic delayed onset of puberty in those adolescents affected.

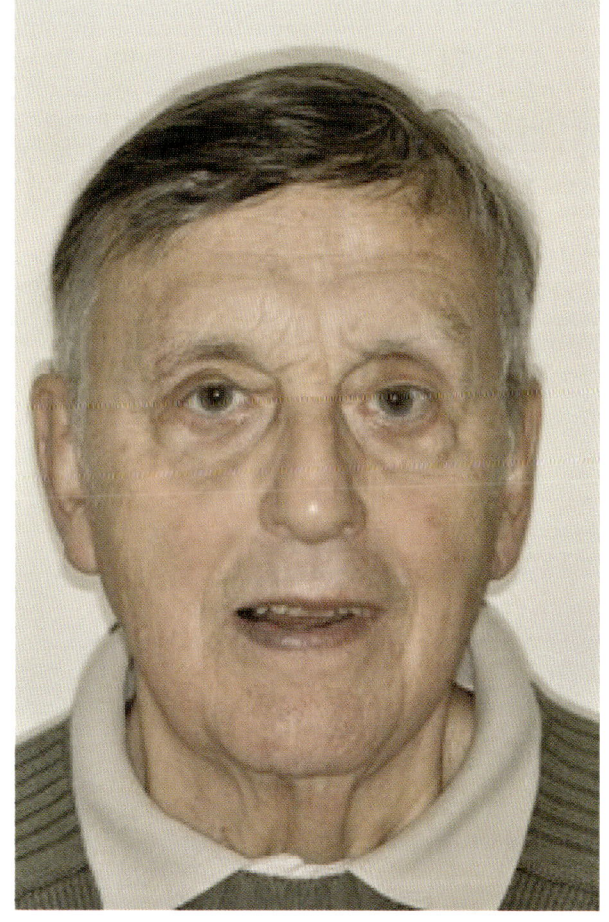

Figure 82.1 Hypopituitarism.

A specific effect of growth hormone hyposecretion in children and adolescents may result in reduced growth velocity and short stature. Thyrotropin (TSH) deficiency leads to mild hypothyroidism with low but not absent levels of circulating T4 and T3. The thyroid is capable of low-grade autonomous secretion of thyroid hormones so symptomatically and biochemically central hypothyroidism is not as profound as primary thyroid failure. It is, however, often missed due to 'TSH-only' screening policies in primary care when a TSH can be normal but inappropriately so for the low levels of circulating T4 and T3.

Adrenocorticotropic hormone (ACTH) deficiency results in symptoms of lethargy, postural hypotension and electrolyte disturbance (hyponatraemia) but, again, this may not become manifest until the patient with a pituitary adenoma is placed under physiological stress with an intercurrent infection or illness and is unable to mount an appropriate cortisol stress response. Varying degrees and combinations of hormone insufficiency may be manifest in a patient with a pituitary adenoma and invariably present with insidious onset.

Prolactin (PRL) is a pituitary hormone related to the lactation response, with its own functional suppressive effect on pituitary luteinizing hormone (LH) and follicle-stimulating hormone (FSH), which constitutes nature's own 'natural contraceptive'. It is under tonic inhibition from hypothalamic dopamine delivered down the pituitary stalk. As a result, anything interrupting the secretion of dopamine can cause an ambient rise in PRL, commonly between 1000 mU/L and 5000 mU/L (NR < 450), often referred to as 'stalk hyperprolactinaemia'.[5] PRL is therefore the last hormone to become deficient in the presence of a pituitary lesion. Clinically hypoprolactinaemia is significant only if it occurs in the postpartum period as part of Sheehan's syndrome. This is a vascular problem and not usually related to the presence of a pituitary adenoma.

Diabetes insipidus is a deficiency of one of the posterior lobe pituitary hormones, arginine vasopressin (AVP), previously known as antidiuretic hormone (ADH). Diabetes insipidus is much rarer at presentation in patients with pituitary adenomas whatever their size and, if present, alternative diagnoses, such as craniopharyngiomas, germinomas, metastases or inflammatory pituitary lesions (sarcoidosis, Generalized Polyangiitis, Langerhans cell histiocytosis) should be considered. Of course, surgical intervention is a recognized cause of diabetes insipidus which may be just transient or permanent following transphenoidal or transcranial surgery. The clinical effects of pituitary deficiency are shown in **Table 82.1**.

Pituitary hormones can be given pharmacologically (e.g. GH, AVP (DDAVP), LH (HCG) or FSH) or the end-organ hormone can be replaced (e.g. hydrocortisone, thyroxine, testosterone, oestrogen/progesterone) to ensure homeostasis titrated to normal physiological and clinical function.

CLINICAL MANIFESTATIONS OF EXCESS HORMONE SECRETION

Excessive hormone secretion by a pituitary adenoma produces several classical clinical syndromes (**Table 82.2**).

Prolactinoma

The commonest type of secreting pituitary adenoma is the prolactinoma, accounting for approximately 40% of adenomas.[1] Prolactin is a peptide hormone that stimulates mammary tissue to produce milk. The hormone also counteracts the effects of dopamine, which is thought to be responsible for sexual arousal. This antagonist effect of PRL is thought to cause reduced libido and impotence.

Until the 1970s surgery was the mainstay of treatment for prolactinoma but, following the introduction of the dopamine 2 receptor agonist Bromocriptine, the majority of prolactinomas are now treated medically. Bromocriptine has a significant side effect profile in certain patients (nausea, nasal stuffiness, postural hypotension) and hence newer dopamine agonists such as

TABLE 82.1 Pituitary hormone deficiency: modes of presentation

Hormone deficiency	Presentation
Hypogonadism (LH/FSH)	Amenorrhoea Infertility Erectile dysfunction Loss of libido
Hypoadrenalism (ACTH) (hypocorticosteroidism)	Malaise Hypotension Hypoglycaemia Hyponatraemia
Hypothyroidism (central (TSH))	Tiredness, lethargy, dry hair, dry skin
Growth hormone deficiency	Lethargy, reduced exercise capacity, central adiposity, reduced muscle mass, premature coronary artery disease, reduced bone density and short stature
AVP (ADH) deficiency	Diabetes insipidus (polyuria/polydipsia) Hypernatraemia Dehydration/coma

TABLE 82.2 Excess pituitary hormone secretion

Hormone in excess	Clinical manifestation
Prolactin (prolactinoma or stalk compression)	Galactorrhoea Amenorrhoea infertility and loss of libido
Growth hormone	Acromegaly
ACTH	Pituitary-dependent Cushing's disease
TSH (TSHoma)	Central thyrotoxicosis (rare)
FSH/LH (gonadotrophinoma)	Macrogonadism (extremely rare)

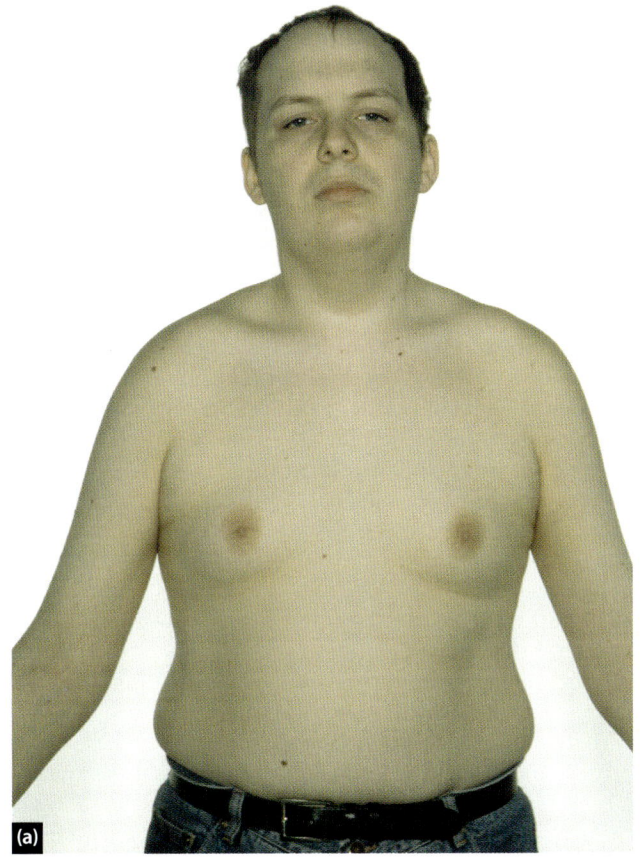 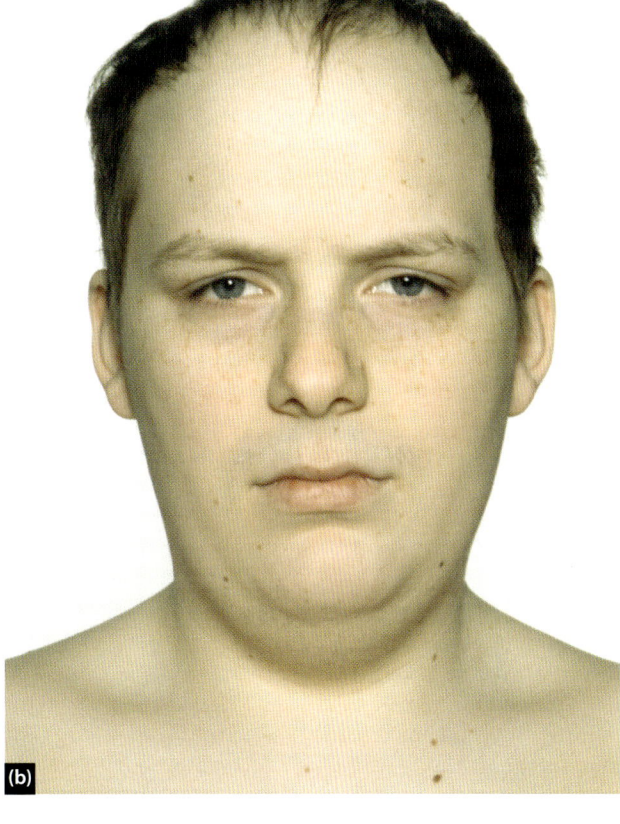

Figure 82.2 Clinical features of hyperprolactinaemia.

Quinagolide (non-ergot) and Cabergoline have become useful alternative drugs in the management of prolactinomas. Dopamine agonists will reduce PRL levels whatever the cause but in addition will cause significant tumour shrinkage and involution in true prolactinomas – often diagnostically so. Non-shrinkage of a pituitary lesion (on serial MRI) despite a good suppression of PRL means that the lesion is unlikely to be a true prolactinoma and the elevated PRL is due to 'stalk hyperprolactinaemia'. This may change management towards a more surgical approach.

Recent concern has been raised about the potential for Cabergoline to cause cardiac valvulopathy with long-term high-dose use.[6] The most recent analyses, however, reassure us that this is unlikely to occur in prolactinoma patients in the doses we use in endocrine practice.[7]

CLINICAL FEATURES

See **Figure 82.2** and **Table 82.3**.

The presenting features of a prolactinoma are related to hyperprolactinaemia, the mass effect of the tumour and other associated endocrine insufficiencies or more rarely pituitary apoplexy.

HYPERPROLACTINAEMIA

The features of hyperprolactinaemia in females and males are shown in **Table 82.3**. Osteoporosis occurs in both males and females as a result of oestrogen and testosterone deficiency, and bone density should be assessed appropriately as part of the initial and long-term management strategy.

TABLE 82.3 Clinical features of prolactinoma/hyperprolactinaemia

Patient gender	Clinical features
Female	Galactorrhoea
	Loss of libido
	Infertility
	Irregular menses
	Osteoporosis
Male	Loss of libido
	Gynaecomastia
	Infertility
	Osteoporosis

The tumour may present with features related to that of an expanding mass within the pituitary fossa, reduction in visual fields and/or acuity as a result of pressure on the under surface of the optic chiasm, or more rarely with involvement of cranial nerves within the cavernous sinuses (III, IV, VI). Headache may be present and is considered to be related to stretching of the overlying dura. Very large prolactinomas may present with hydrocephalus and deterioration in cortical brain function with lateral extension resulting in temporal lobe symptoms which usually resolve with surgical resection or more commonly dopamine agonist-induced tumour involution.

DIFFERENTIAL DIAGNOSIS OF HYPERPROLACTINAEMIA

Hyperprolactinaemia is also associated with conditions other than pituitary adenomas (Table 82.4). In particular 'stalk compression' of the hypothalamic pituitary pathway by any form of mass lesion in the pituitary fossa may interrupt dopamine inhibition of prolactin-secreting cells resulting in hyperprolactinaemia as previously mentioned.

Acromegaly

Acromegaly is a disorder of adults as a consequence of the overproduction of growth hormone which results in significant changes to the patient's appearance over considerable time. If growth hormone excess occurs before fusion of the epiphyses in adolescence, the condition is known as pituitary gigantism.

The commonest underlying cause of acromegaly is that of a spontaneously occurring pituitary adenoma, although rarely it may be a result of a genetic syndrome such as multiple endocrine neoplasia type I (MEN I – along with parathyroid and pancreatic endocrine tumours), GSP mutations, McCune–Albright syndrome[8] or more recently familial acromegaly due to mutation in the aryl hydrocarbon receptor protein.[9]

Pituitary tumours occasionally co-secrete other hormones such as growth hormone and prolactin (somato-mamotroph adenomas) occasionally with the additional secretion of TSH causing central hyperthyroidism. Co-secretion of prolactin often indicates a co-responsivity to the suppressive effects of dopamine agonists.

INCIDENCE

Acromegaly has an incidence of 3–4 per million per year with an incidence in the general population of approximately 60 cases per year. This condition affects all races and both sexes with patients typically presenting between the ages of 40 and 50 years.[10]

CLINICAL FEATURES

Acromegaly has an insidious onset with features of bone and soft-tissue overgrowth. The initial features include changes in shoe size, ring size and coarsening of facial features (Figure 82.3). However, symptom onset is non-specific with sweating, lassitude and musculoskeletal pain resulting in a concomitant delay of diagnosis. The mean time to diagnosis is 8 years with a range of 6–10 years.[11]

Table 82.5 includes the features commonly associated with a diagnosis of acromegaly. Consideration of these should prompt further investigation.

Acromegaly is recognized as causing reduction in life expectancy by up to 10 years in those untreated.[11] Suppression of growth hormone levels to < 1 µg/L and normalization of IgF1 (age and sex adjusted), returns the death rate to that expected of the normal background population.[12] The increase in mortality is related to duration of symptoms prior to diagnosis, disease duration, increasing age and presence of complications at diagnosis.[13]

Reduction in morbidity and mortality relies upon prompt diagnosis and early investigation and treatment. General practitioners and primary care physicians should be alert to the possibility of agromegaly in patients presenting with coarse features, excess sweating, increased ring or shoe size and sleep apnoea,[14] resistant hypertension unresponsive to three or more agents and/or difficult-to-control diabetes.

Cushing's disease

Cushing's syndrome is the term applied to a wide group of disorders with symptoms and signs due to chronic exposure to excess glucocorticoid, irrespective of the underlying cause. The commonest cause is exogenous steroid treatment.

Cushing's disease is the term applied to Cushing's syndrome of pituitary origin (pituitary-dependent adrenal hyperplasia). The disease was described by Harvey Cushing in 1932 as pituitary basophilism.

Table 82.6 shows the causes of endogenous Cushing's syndrome and their approximate frequency.

AETIOLOGY

Cushing's disease often presents with non-specific symptoms which may be slowly progressive and therefore missed as a developing condition in primary care. The mean time to diagnosis after the first presenting symptom is 6 years.[15] Chances to diagnose are often missed in clinical consultations. Cushing's disease mimics common conditions such as obesity, poorly controlled diabetes and hypertension and consideration may not be given to its possibility by the treating doctor.

TABLE 82.4 Differential diagnosis of hyperprolactinaemia

Underlying cause	Differential diagnosis
Physiological	Pregnancy Breastfeeding Mental stress
Drugs	Drugs antagonizing the effects of dopamine including major tranquilizers (phenothiazines and haloperidol) Metoclopromide Domperidone and methyldopa and the combined oral contraceptive pill
Diseases	Chronic renal failure Hypothyroidism Bronchogenic carcinoma Sarcoidosis Idiopathic

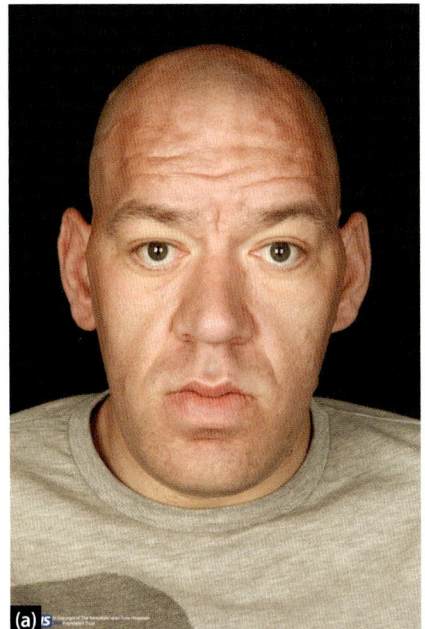
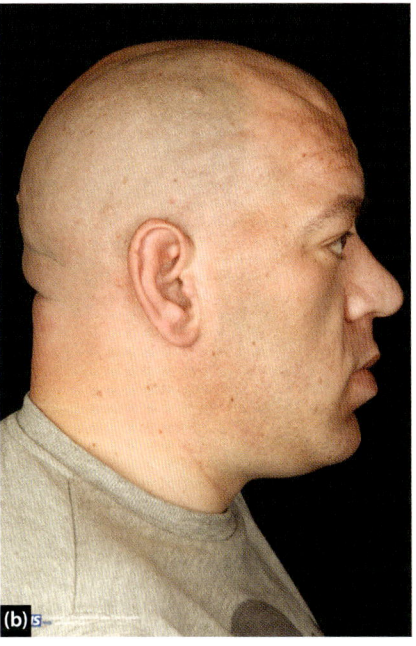
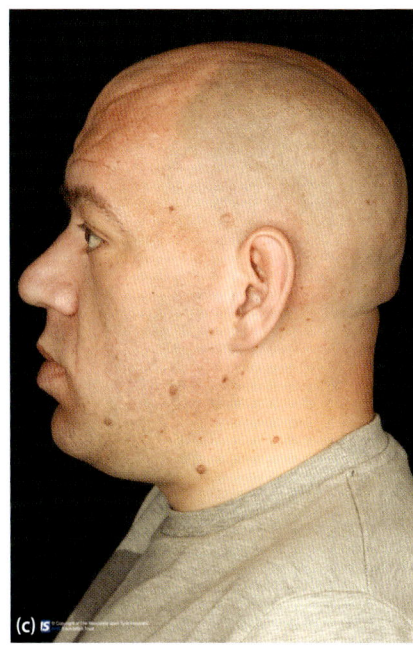
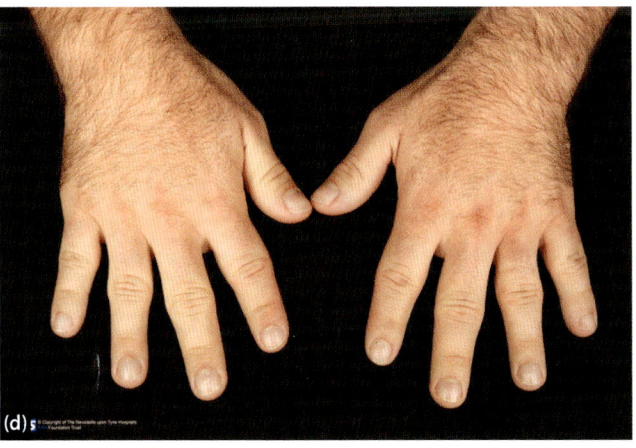
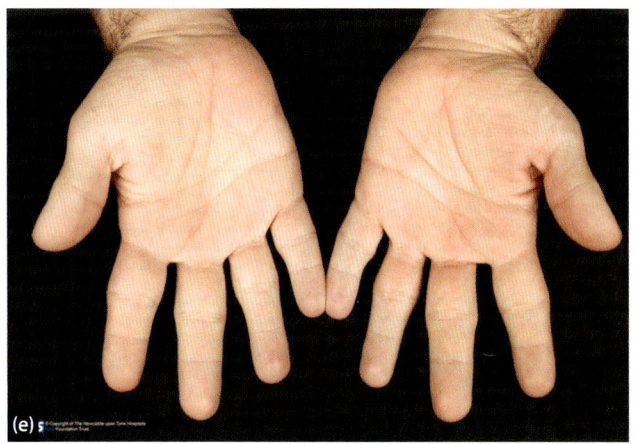

Figure 82.3 Clinical features of acromegaly.

TABLE 82.5 Features commonly associated with acromegaly	
Disorder type	**Feature(s)**
Musculoskeletal	Macroglosia, enlargement of lips, hands and feet Prominent brow Prognathism, interdental separation Skeletal abnormalities – degenerative osteoarthritis Carpal tunnel syndrome and hearing loss
Cardiovascular	Hypertension Cardiomyopathy Arrhythmias Heart failure
Respiratory	Obstructive sleep apnoea
Metabolic	Diabetes mellitus Excess sweating
Gastrointestinal	Colonic polyps

TABLE 82.6 Aetiology of Cushing's Syndrome		
Cause of Cushing's Syndrome	**F:M**	**%**
ACTH-dependent[a]		
Cushing's disease	3.5:1[b]	70
Ectopic ACTH syndrome	1:1	10
Unknown source of ACTH[c]	5:1	5
ACTH-independent	4:1	10
Adrenal adenoma	1:1	5
Adrenal carcinoma		<2
Other causes (PPNAD, AIMAH, McCune-Albright)		

Note: PPNAD primary pigmented nodular adrenal disease, AIMAH ACTH-independent massive adrenal hyperplasia.

[a] In women 9:1 ratio of Cushing's disease to ectopic ACTH
[b] Male preponderance in children
[c] Patients may ultimately prove to have Cushing's disease, ectopic CRH <1% of all cases of ACTH-dependent disease

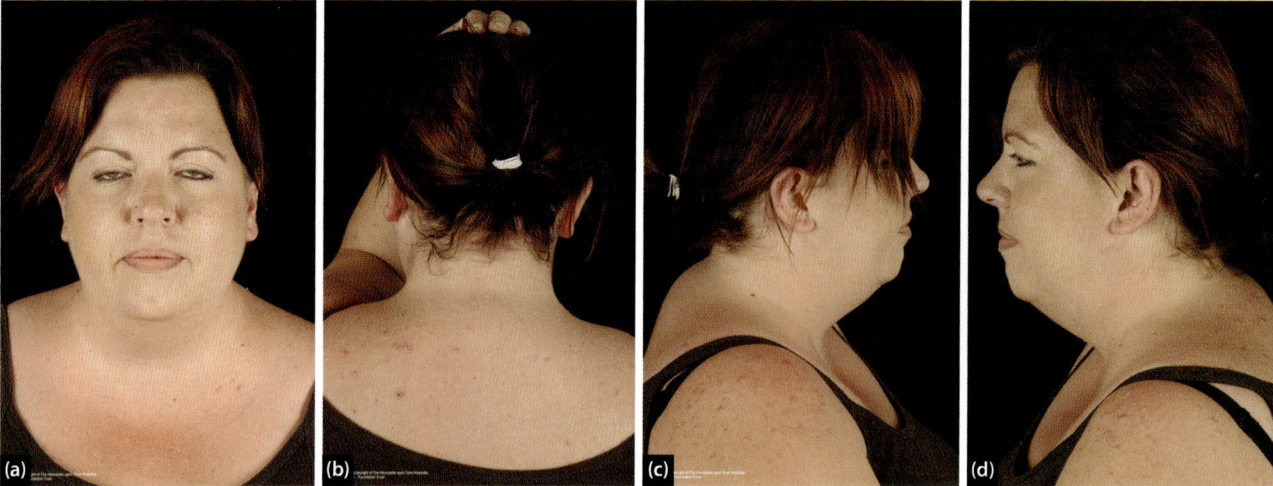

Figure 82.4 Clinical features of Cushing's disease.

Untreated, Cushing's disease is associated with a 50% mortality rate at 5 years, commonly as a result of cardiovascular complications.[16] Significant morbidity results from irreversible organ damage over a prolonged period.

CLINICAL FEATURES OF CORTISOL OVERPRODUCTION

The features of excess cortisol exposure are well described – the typical central obesity, plethora and spontaneous purpura (**Figure 82.4**). However, it is important to realize that certain features are of more diagnostic value than others (**Table 82.7**).[17]

It is important to assess the use of exogenous glucocorticoid and in particular the use of inhalers and skin creams. Several photographs of the patient's appearance over a period of months to years may also indicate the developing changes in appearance associated with Cushing's disease.

TABLE 82.7 Clinical value of symptoms and signs of Cushing's disease	
Clinical diagnostic value	Symptoms and signs
High	Skin atrophy Proximal myopathy and wasting Bruising Childhood growth arrest Osteoporosis
Medium	Oedema Striae Moon face Facial hirsuitism Labile mood
Non-specific	Buffalo hump Hypertension Diabetes mellitus Plethora Acne

NEURO-OPHTHAIMOLOGICAL FEATURES OF PITUITARY DISEASE

The relationship between the optic chiasm and pituitary gland is intimate with lesions expanding superiorly out of the pituitary fossa impacting on the chiasm.

Afferent visual pathway

The optic nerves transverse the orbit and pass through the optic canal where their dural sheath fuses to the wall of the canal. In up to 4% of patients the optic nerves may be dehiscent of bone as they traverse the lateral wall of the sphenoid sinuses.[18] The intra-cranial portion of the optic nerve passes superiorly and medially to form the optic chiasm. Chiasm is named after the Greek letter chi but in life more closely resembles the letter H. Within the chiasm 50% of the axons within each optic nerve decussate to run in the opposite optic tract to the centres higher in the brain.

The location of the chiasm relative to the pituitary gland varies. In the vast majority it lies directly above the pituitary fossa but in a minority of patients it may either be anterior (pre-fixed), or posterior to the pituitary (post-fixed) above the dorsum sellae. On average[19] it lies approximately 10 mm above the pituitary gland, although in a minority (14%) it may be as little as 2 mm above it.

Efferent pathways

Within the cavernous sinus on either side of the pituitary fossa lie the cranial nerves responsible for eye movements and papillary responses to light. **Figure 82.5** shows the relationship of the oculomotor, trochlear and abducens nerves within the cavernous sinuses. The oculomotor is the nerve most frequently involved by pituitary adenoma expansion. Also within the cavernous sinuses lie the ophthalmic and maxillary divisions of the trigeminal nerve.

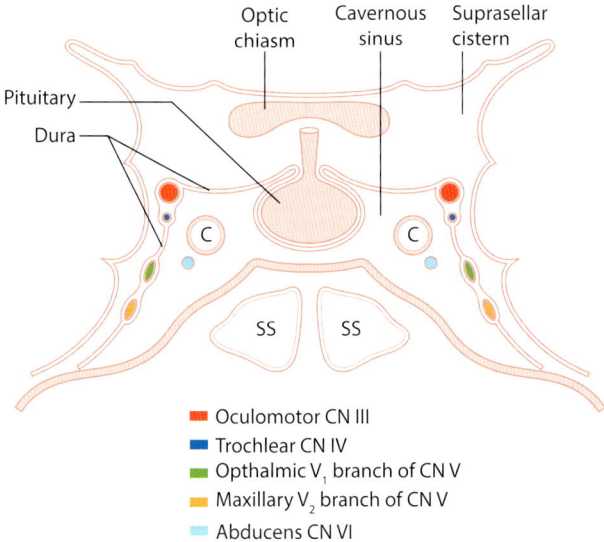

Figure 82.5 Cavernous sinus.

Ophthalmic presentations related to pituitary disease

The classic presentation of an expanding non-functioning pituitary tumour is a bitemporal hemianopia caused by compression of the axons within the chiasm (**Figure 82.6**).

Typically a superior quadrantanopia occurs initially as the axons subserving the temporal visual fields are involved initially by the pituitary compression from below. It should be noted that visual acuity can also be affected. In addition, pituitary tumours do not always respect the midline and can give an asymmetrical visual field defect. A pre- and post-fixed chiasm would produce variable hemianopias, an important consideration when assessing the visual fields.

Clinically patients may not be aware of selective visual field loss, although with progression symptoms may become apparent, for example failing to notice the edges of a doorway when walking through it and bumping into it. Prolonged compression of the optic fibres results in atrophy of the optic disc noted on fundoscopy. More severe or generalized atrophy is associated with a poorer prognosis to visual recovery.[20]

Formal assessment of visual fields should be undertaken by a specialist technician to minimize operator dependency and ensure accuracy. Static perimetry techniques (Goldman visual field assessment) have largely been replaced by kinetic perimetry. The Humphrey visual field analyser (**Figure 82.7**) consists of a bowl-shaped background of set luminescence. The patient fixates on a central target and presses a button when a light stimulus in the periphery is perceived. Testing takes up to 30 minutes for both eyes and is largely automated, reducing margins for error.

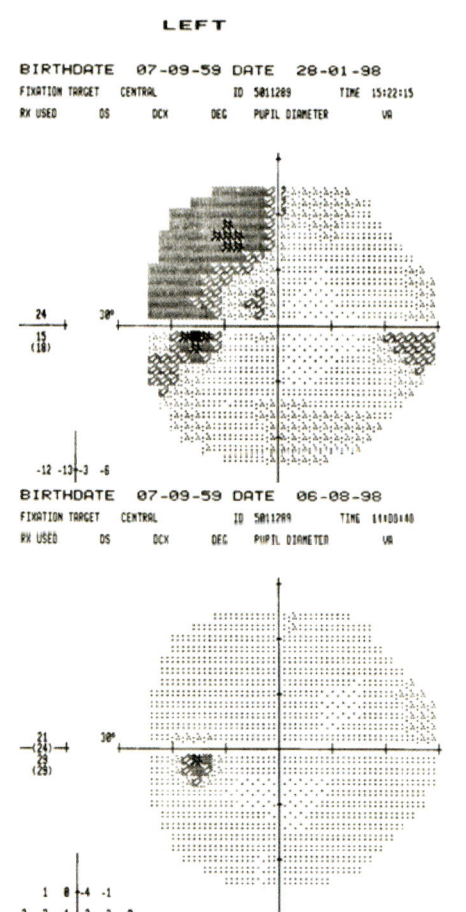
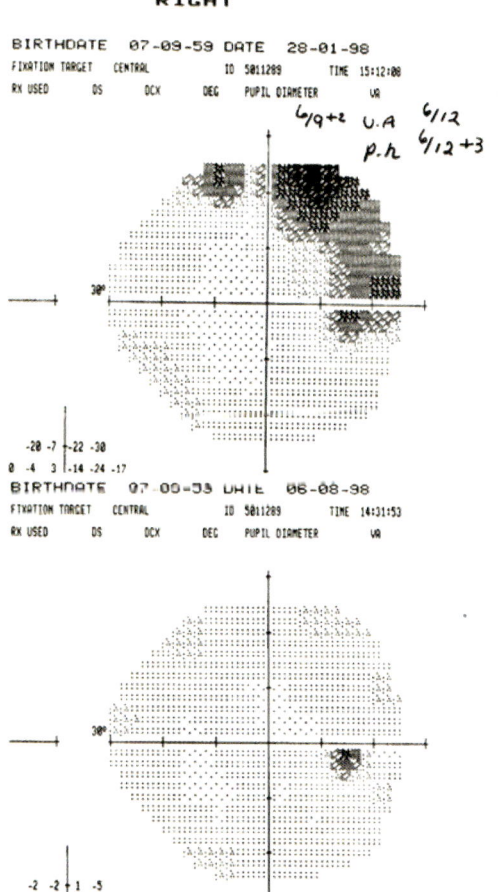

Figure 82.6 Bitemporal hemianopia.

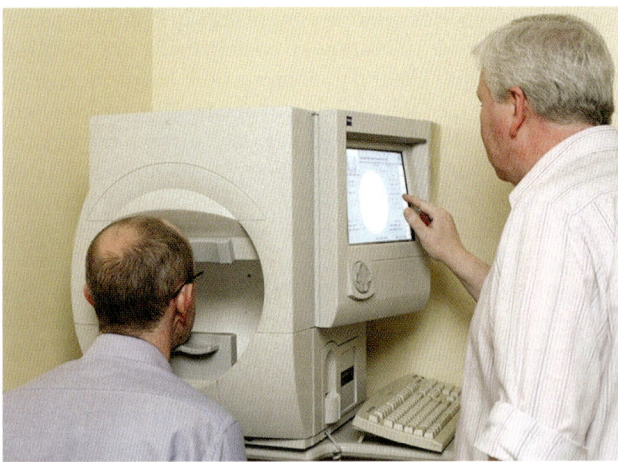

Figure 82.7 The Humphrey visual field analyser.

Motor nerve involvement

Pituitary tumours also have a tendency to compress or invade the cavernous sinus as they expand. In the majority of cases this involvement is asymptomatic but pituitary apoplexy characteristically presents with severe headache and, on occasion, acute oculomotor nerve palsies and hemianopias with loss of acuity. However, all cranial nerves within the cavernous sinus may be involved with palsies potentially affecting III, IV and VI. There is a consequent diplopia and reduced range of ocular movement. Involvement of the sympathetic fibres may result in a Horner's syndrome and facial sensation may be disturbed by involvement of the ophthalmic and maxillary divisions of the trigeminal nerve. Visual field disturbances are much more common than those of ocular motor nerves but in each case formal assessment, documentation and management should be undertaken by a specialist neuro-ophthalmologist.

Vision following surgical decompression

All large series demonstrate a majority of patients experience visual improvement following surgery to macroadenomas with optic apparatus involvement. A study of 67 patients undergoing resection of adenomas compressing the visual pathway reported 88% showing improvement of visual function, despite half of those having significant optic atrophy.[21] Another study demonstrated normalization in 35% of eyes and improvement in 60%.[20] In keeping with most studies the duration and severity of visual field involvement directly affects prognosis for visual recovery. Recovery of vision can be equally dramatic with medical management of a macroprolactinoma with dopamine agonists. Radiotherapy treatment alone is rarely if ever used in this situation as it can pose an additional threat to the optic apparatus. Surgical debulking is invariably recommended prior to adjuvant radiotherapy.

TSHomas

Pituitary thyrotrophin-secreting adenomas (TSHomas) are extremely rare tumours causing hyperthyroidism by chronic stimulation of a normal thyroid gland. In the past 50 years approximately 50 cases have been reported in literature.[22]

Patients present with signs and symptoms of hyperthyroidism, commonly thyrotoxicosis and a goitre with a vascular bruit. The characteristics of this condition are centrally driven thyrotoxicosis with high levels of thyroid hormones in the presence of detectable and invariably elevated TSH and alpha subunit levels.

Gonadotrophinoma

These tumours are often indistinguishable from other non-functioning pituitary adenomas as they are usually 'silent' and not associated with excess secretion of LH and FSH. Therefore, they are usually detected upon histological analysis following operative intervention for a clinically and biochemically non-functioning pituitary macroadenoma.

Non-functioning adenomas

A systematic review of pituitary adenomas in 2004 reported an estimated prevalence of 16% in the population.[1] Non-functioning adenomas are the most common subgroup requiring surgical intervention.

Occasionally, apparently functionless pituitary adenomas will stain for ACTH in the absence of biochemical or clinical cortisol excess. It is important to note this category of pituitary adenoma, the so-called 'silent corticotrophinoma', as they are more prone to physical recurrence and require more assiduous post-decompressive surveillance and early recourse to external beam radiotherapy (EBRT) is often indicated.

True null cell adenomas are rare, accounting for less than 10% of non-functioning adenomas biopsied and examined histologically.

Non-functioning adenomas commonly present as expanding pituitary lesions (visual disturbance), as hypopituitarism or as lesions found incidentally on CT or MRI of the brain. The clinical manifestations of hypopituitarism and stalk compression have already been discussed.

These patients with non-functioning adenomas should be assessed for the loss of visual fields and visual acuity, as well as an assessment of pituitary hormone status. Management may involve serial MR imaging for small asymptomatic lesions, or a combination of surgery or radiotherapy for symptomatic lesions.

Pituitary apoplexy

This is an uncommon but well-described clinical presentation found in a small minority of pituitary adenomas.[23] It occurs as a result of either haemorrhage into or infarction of a pituitary adenoma and may be the presenting feature of a previously undiagnosed tumour.[24] The typical features are of a sudden severe headache mimicking subarachnoid haemorrhage, which may be associated with a deterioration in visual acuity or visual fields. Subsequently an acute loss of pituitary hormones may produce acute adrenal insufficiency or diabetes insipidus or the so-called 'triple response' of transient diabetes insipidus rapidly followed by a period of syndrome of inappropriate antidiuretic hormone (SIADH) and hyponatraemia due to disordered AVP leakage with ultimate exhaustion of AVP stores and a return to diabetes insipidus.[25] It is important to recognize this phenomenon acutely and in the post-operative period as it requires close monitoring of serum and urine electrolytes/osmolalities and fastidious attention to fluid balance, fluid type and the timely use of fluid restriction or DDAVP® administration dependent on which phase the patient is going through.

Larger tumours are more prone to bleeding and more rapidly growing lesions may be at a high risk of apoplexy.[23] Initially, aggressive medical management is appropriate with high dose steroids both to replace the acute adrenal insufficiency and to provide anti-inflammatory effect if visual disturbance is minimal, provided there is close observation of the patient. Deterioration in symptoms or lack of spontaneous improvement indicates the need for surgical intervention.[26]

CONCLUSIONS

Lesions within the pituitary fossa generally present either with disturbance of pituitary hormone function or as a result of a mass lesion extending outside the pituitary fossa. Mass lesions most commonly result in deficiencies in the patient's visual field or more rarely with cranial nerve palsies.

All lesions within the sellar or parasellar areas require a comprehensive endocrine evaluation and, if there is a lesion approximating the optic chiasm or apparatus a specialist opthalmological assessment should also be made.

Endocrine assessment should continue in the post-treatment phase in order that any hormone deficiencies are corrected.

KEY POINTS

- All lesions involving the pituitary fossa should undergo a formal endocrinology assessment.
- The commonest secreting adenoma is a prolactinoma, the majority of which are managed medically.
- Untreated, acromegaly and Cushing's Disease are life shortening conditions.
- Macroadenomas may not produce a classical bitemporal field defect.
- Pituitary apoplexy is an emergency and may require surgical intervention.

REFERENCES

1. Ezzat S, Asa SL, Couldwell WT, et al. The prevalence of pituitary adenomas: a systematic review. *Cancer* 2004; **101**(3): 613–19.
2. Nussey S, Whitehead S. *Endocrinology: An integrated approach*. Oxford: BIOS Scientific Publishers; 2001.
3. Freda PU, Beckers AM, Katznelson L. Pituitary incidentaloma: an endocrine society clinical practice guideline. *J Clin Endocrinol Metab* 2011 Apr; **96**(4): 894–904.
4. Ferrante E, Ferraoni M, Castrinano T, et al. Non functioning pituitary adenoma database: a useful resource to improve the clinical management of pituitary tumours. *Eur J Endocrinol* 2006; **155**: 823–9.
5. Weiss M. Pituitary tumours: an endocrinological and neurosurgical challenge. *Clin Neurosurg* 2003; **25**: 1–6.
6. Schade R, Andersohn F, Suissa S. Dopamine agonists and the risk of cardiac-valve regurgitation. *N Eng J Med* 2007; **356**(1): 29–38.
7. Bogazzi F, Buralli S, Manett, L, et al. Treatment with low doses of cabergoline is not associated with increased prevalence of cardiac valve regurgitation in patients with hyperprolactinaemia. *Int J Clin Prac* 2008; **62**(12): 1864–9.
8. Galland F, Kamenicky P, Affres H, et al. McCune-Albright syndrome and acromegaly: effects of hypothalamopituitary radiotherapy and/or pegvisomant in somatostatin analog-resistant patients. *J Clin Endocrinol Metab* 2006; **91**(12): 4957–61.
9. Korbonits M, Storr H, Agith V, et al. Familial pituitary adenomas: who should be tested for AIP mutations? *Clin Endocrinol* 2012; **77**(3): 351–6.
10. Daly AF, Rixhon M, Adam C, et al. High prevalence of pituitary adenomas: a cross-sectional study in the province of Liege, Belgium. *J Clin Endocrinol Metab* 2006; **91**(10): 4769–75.
11. Holdaway IM, Rajasoorya RC, Gamble GD. Factors influencing mortality in acromegaly. *J Clin Endocrinol Metab* 2004; **89**: 667–74.
12. Giustina A, Barkan A, Casanueva FF, et al. Criteria for cure of acromegaly: a consensus statement. *J Clin Endocrinol Metab* 2000; **85**: 526–9.
13. Beauregard C, Truong U, Hardy J, et al. Long-term outcome and mortality after transsphenoidal adenomectomy for acromegaly. *Clin Endocrinol* 2003; **58**: 86–91.
14. Watson NF, Vitiello MV. Management of obstructive sleep apnoea in acromegaly. *Sleep Med* 2007; **8**: 539–40.
15. Psaras T, Milian M, Hatterman V, et al. Demographic factors and the presence of comorbidities do not promote early detection of Cushing's disease and acromegaly. *Exp Clin Endocrinol Diabetes* 2011; **119**(1): 21–5.
16. Plotz CM, Knowlton AI, Ragan C. The natural history of Cushing's syndrome. *Am J Med* 1952; **13**: 597–614.
17. Ross EJ, Linch DC. Cushing's syndrome – killing disease: discriminatory value of signs and symptoms aiding early diagnosis. *Lancet* 1982; **2**: 646–9.
18. Perlmutter D, Rhoton AL Jr. Microsurgical anatomy of the anterior cerebral – anterior communicating – recurrent artery complex. *J Neurosurg* 1976; **45**: 259–72.
19. Renn WH, Rhoton AL Jr. Microsurgical anatomy of the sellar region. *J Neurosurg* 1975; **43**: 288–98.
20. Gnanalingham KK, Bhattacharjee, Pennington R, et al. The time course of visual field recovery following transsphenoidal surgery for pituitary adenomas: predictive factors for a good outcome. *J Neurol Neurosurg Psychiatry* 2005; **76**: 415–19.
21. Powell M. Recovery of vision following transsphenoidal surgery for pituitary adenomas. *Br J Neurosurg* 1995: **9**: 367–73.
22. Beck-Peccoz P, Persani L. TSH-producing adenomas. In: Jameson JL, De Groot LJ (eds). *Endocrinology: Adult and pediatric*, 6th ed. Philadelphia: Saunders; 2010, vol. 1, pp. 324–31.
23. Randeva HS, Schoebel J, Byrne J, et al. Classical pituitary apoplexy: clinical features, management and outcome. *Clin Endocrinol* 1999; **51**: 181–8.
24. Semple PL, Jane JA Jr, Laws ER Jr. Clinical relevance of precipitating factors in pituitary apoplexy. *Neurosurgery* 2007; **61**, 956–61, discussion 961–2.
25. Rajasekaran S, Vanderpump M, Baldeweg S, et al. UK guidelines for the management of pituitary apoplexy. *Clin Endocrinol* 2011; **74**(1): 9–20.
26. Gruber A, Clayton J, Kumar S, et al. Pituitary apoplexy: retrospective review of 30 patients – is surgical intervention always necessary? *Br J Neurosurg* 2006; **20**: 379–85.

CHAPTER 83

INVESTIGATION OF PITUITARY DISEASE

Thozhukat Sathyapalan and Stephen L. Atkin

Introduction 915
Investigating anterior pituitary dysfunction 915
Investigating posterior pituitary dysfunction 919
References 920

SEARCH STRATEGY

The information in this chapter is taken from standard UK endocrinology clinical practice. It reflects expert opinion (level 4 evidence) with regard to endocrinology tests currently performed in the UK.

Data in this chapter may be updated by a Medline search using the keywords: prolactin, IGF-1, ACTH stimulation test, dexamethasone suppression test, pituitary function testing, SIADH, diabetes insipidus, Cushing's disease, acromegaly, pituitary adenoma and hypopituitarism.

INTRODUCTION

The pituitary gland lies in the sella turcica which is situated in the middle cranial fossa at the base of the brain. It is linked functionally to the hypothalamus by the pituitary stalk. The anterior pituitary secretes growth hormone (GH), thyrotropin or thyroid-stimulating hormone (TSH), corticotropin or adrenocorticotropic hormone (ACTH), follicle-stimulating hormone (FSH) and luteinizing hormone (LH), all of which are under positive stimulatory control, and prolactin (PRL) which is under the inhibitory control of dopamine. The posterior lobe releases arginine vasopressin (AVP, also called antidiuretic hormone) and oxytocin.

INVESTIGATING ANTERIOR PITUITARY DYSFUNCTION

The anterior pituitary hormonal secretion is regulated by hypothalamic releasing and inhibitory factors delivered via portal capillaries, and by negative feedback inhibition of the respective hormones secreted by the target endocrine glands such as the thyroid gland and adrenal cortex.

The presentation of anterior pituitary disease, most commonly associated with a structural lesion, may result from:

- local mass effects – causing headache, visual field defects and ocular nerve palsies
- pituitary hormone deficiencies – producing wide-ranging effects as a result of single or multiple deficiencies, with GH and gonadotropins (LH and FSH) usually affected first, followed much later by ACTH and TSH
- pituitary hormone hypersecretion – usually arising as a consequence of neoplastic proliferation of particular cell types within the gland.[1, 2]

Investigation includes:

- tests for hormone hyper- or hyposecretion, by measuring TSH and thyroxine, FSH/LH and testosterone or oestradiol and prolactin – dynamic testing is required for the ACTH/cortisol axis and determination of GH deficiency or excess
- imaging – MRI is the modality of choice for radiological assessment
- neuro-ophthalmological evaluation, including assessment of visual acuity and visual fields.[3]

Investigating anterior pituitary hormonal hypersecretion

Pituitary masses may present with a typical clinical syndrome resulting from hypersecretion of one or more anterior pituitary hormones. Alternatively, they may present through compression of surrounding structures such as the optic chiasm or the adjacent normal pituitary, causing hypopituitarism. Functional pituitary tumours can produce a complex picture of combined hormonal excess and/ or deficiencies.

LABORATORY INVESTIGATION

The presenting clinical features of functional pituitary adenomas (e.g. acromegaly, Cushing's syndrome) guide the laboratory studies. However, for a sellar mass with no obvious clinical features of hormone excess, laboratory studies are geared towards determining the nature of the tumour and assessing the possible presence of hypopituitarism. When a pituitary adenoma is found incidentally on MRI scan, the initial hormonal evaluation will be guided by the history and clinical examination to look for signs of hormone excess including: (i) prolactin; (ii) insulin-like growth factor-1 (IGF-I); (iii) 24-hour urinary free cortisol and/or overnight oral dexamethasone (1 mg) suppression test; (iv) α-subunit, FSH and LH; and (v) thyroid function tests (free T4 and TSH). Additional hormonal evaluation may be indicated based on the results of these tests (Table 83.1). Pending more detailed assessment of hypopituitarism, 8 a.m. cortisol and testosterone levels, and thyroid function tests usually identify patients with pituitary hormone deficiencies that require hormone replacement before further testing or surgery.[4]

Diagnosis of hyperprolactinaemia

Basal morning PRL levels should be measured to assess hypersecretion. It may be necessary to measure prolactin levels on different occasions when clinical suspicion is high. Since prolactin may be elevated as a stress response in a random sample, cannulated prolactin levels with samples taken through a cannula at 60-minute intervals after insertion to reduce this stress response can be helpful.[5] In patients with markedly elevated PRL levels (>2000 mU/L), results may be falsely lowered because of assay artefacts (the high-dose hook effect); sample dilution is required to measure these high values accurately, but it is rare with modern assays. Falsely elevated values may be caused by aggregated forms of circulating PRL, which are biologically inactive (macroprolactinemia).[6] Hypothyroidism should be excluded by measuring serum TSH and T4 levels.

Diagnosis of acromegaly

Age- and gender-matched serum IGF-I levels are elevated in acromegaly. Consequently, an IGF-I level provides a useful laboratory screening measure when clinical features raise the possibility of acromegaly. Due to the pulsatility of GH secretion, measurement of a single random GH level is not useful for the diagnosis or exclusion of acromegaly and does not correlate with disease severity. The diagnosis of acromegaly is confirmed by demonstrating the failure of GH suppression to <1 µg/L within 1–2 hours after a 75 g oral glucose load.[7] PRL is elevated in approximately a quarter of patients with acromegaly. Thyroid function, gonadotropins and sex steroids may be reduced because of tumour mass effects. Since most patients will undergo surgery with glucocorticoid coverage, tests for ACTH reserve in asymptomatic patients could be deferred until after surgery.[8]

Diagnosis of Cushing's disease

The diagnosis of Cushing's syndrome is based on laboratory documentation of endogenous hypercortisolism.[9] Measurement of 24-hour urine free cortisol is often used as the screening test, ideally two collections with measurement of creatinine that should not differ by more than 10% to indicate adequacy of collection. Alternatively, the failure to suppress plasma cortisol after an overnight 1 mg dexamethasone suppression test can be used to identify patients with hypercortisolism. However, this test has a false positive rate of 2% in the normal population, 13% in obese subjects and 23% in hospital inpatients and is not favoured by many clinicians. A low-dose dexamethasone suppression test is also used to confirm hypercortisolemia, which has a higher sensitivity of 98% for screening Cushing's syndrome. This is done by administering 0.5 mg of dexamethasone 6 hourly for 48 hours at 9 a.m., 3 p.m., 9 p.m. and 3 a.m., and should lead to complete suppression of cortisol to <50 nmol/L in normal subjects with serum cortisol measurement at baseline and 48 hours. As nadir levels of cortisol occur at night, elevated midnight samples of cortisol are suggestive of Cushing's syndrome and this test will require admission to hospital. More recently, however,

TABLE 83.1 Baseline tests to evaluate pituitary hormone hypersecretion

Disorder	Tests	Comments
Acromegaly	Serum IGF-I	Interpret IGF-I relative to age- and gender-matched controls
	Oral glucose tolerance test with GH obtained at 0, 60 and 120 min	Normal subjects should suppress growth hormone to <1 µg/L
Prolactinoma	Serum prolactin	Prolactin levels can be higher in patients who take medications including antidepressants, antipsychotics and antiemetics as well as some over-the-counter medications and homeopathic remedies MRI of the pituitary if prolactin significantly elevated (<2000 mU/L)
Cushing's disease	24-hour urinary free cortisol	Ensure urine collection is total and accurate ideally with 2 × 24-hour samples with measurement of creatinine that should not differ by more than 10%
	Dexamethasone (1 mg) at 11 p.m. and plasma cortisol measured at 8 a.m.	Normal subjects suppress to <1.8 µg/dL (< 50 nmol/L)
	ACTH assay	Distinguishes adrenal adenoma (ACTH suppressed) from ectopic ACTH or Cushing's disease (ACTH normal or elevated) after biochemical confirmation of hypercortisolemia

midnight salivary free measurements have been used which are simpler. Basal plasma ACTH levels often distinguish patients with ACTH-independent (adrenal or exogenous glucocorticoid) from those with ACTH-dependent (pituitary, ectopic ACTH) Cushing's syndrome.[10] Mean basal ACTH levels are about eightfold higher in patients with ectopic ACTH secretion compared to those with pituitary ACTH-secreting adenomas. However, extensive overlap of ACTH levels between these two disorders (ectopic ACTH versus pituitary ACTH-secreting adenoma) precludes using ACTH to make the distinction.[11]

If the investigations are highly suggestive of pituitary Cushing's disease, then pituitary MRI with gadolinium enhancement is undertaken but it is often not sensitive enough to detect small (<2 mm) pituitary ACTH-secreting adenomas. In this case, bilateral inferior petrosal sinus ACTH sampling before and after corticotropin-releasing hormone (CRH) administration may be required to distinguish a pituitary lesion from ectopic ACTH-secreting tumours that may have similar clinical and biochemical characteristics.[12] Simultaneous assessment of ACTH concentrations in each inferior petrosal vein and in the peripheral circulation provides a strategy for confirming and localizing pituitary ACTH production. Sampling is performed at baseline and 2, 5 and 10 min after intravenous bovine CRH (1 µg/kg) injection. An increased ratio (>2) of inferior petrosal to peripheral vein ACTH confirms pituitary Cushing's syndrome. After CRH injection, peak petrosal-to-peripheral ACTH ratios of ≥3 confirm the presence of a pituitary ACTH-secreting tumour when there is unequivocal endogenous hypercortisolemia. The sensitivity of this test is >95%, with rare false-negative results encountered in patients with aberrant venous drainage. Petrosal sinus catheterizations are technically difficult, and about 0.05% of patients develop neurovascular complications.

Most ACTH-secreting pituitary tumours are <5 mm in diameter, and about half are undetectable by sensitive MRI. The high prevalence of incidental pituitary microadenomas diminishes the ability to distinguish ACTH-secreting pituitary tumours accurately by MRI.

Diagnosis of TSH-secreting adenomas

TSH-producing macroadenomas are rare but are often large and locally invasive when they occur. Patients usually present with thyroid goitre and hyperthyroidism, reflecting overproduction of TSH. Diagnosis is based on demonstrating elevated serum free T4 levels, inappropriately normal or high TSH secretion, and MRI evidence of a pituitary adenoma.[13] The commonest cause of elevated FT4 and normal or high TSH is failure to comply with treatment for hypothyroidism and taking thyroxine supplementation a few days prior to thyroid function tests. It is, however, also important to exclude other causes of inappropriate TSH secretion, such as resistance to thyroid hormone, an autosomal dominant disorder caused by mutations in the thyroid hormone β receptor and resistance to thyrotropin.[14] The presence of a pituitary mass and elevated α-subunit levels are suggestive of a TSH-secreting tumour.

Diagnosis of non-functioning and gonadotropin-secreting pituitary adenomas

Clinically non-functioning tumours often present with optic chiasm pressure and other symptoms of local expansion or may be incidentally discovered on an MRI performed for another indication.[15] Menstrual disturbances or ovarian hyperstimulation rarely occur in women with large tumours that produce FSH and LH. More commonly, adenoma compression of the pituitary stalk or surrounding pituitary tissue leads to attenuated LH and features of hypogonadism. PRL levels are usually slightly increased due to stalk compression. Most non-functioning tumours respond poorly to medical treatment, but these can be given an empirical treatment with a dopamine agonist, unless decompression of the chiasm is warranted if prolactin levels are raised.

Free α-subunit levels may be elevated in 10–15% of patients with non-functioning tumours. In female patients, peri- or postmenopausal basal FSH concentrations are difficult to distinguish from tumour-derived FSH elevation.

Testosterone levels are usually low, despite the normal or increased LH level, perhaps reflecting reduced LH bioactivity or the loss of normal LH pulsatility. Because this pattern of hormone levels is also seen in primary gonadal failure and with ageing, the finding of increased gonadotropins alone is insufficient for the diagnosis of a gonadotropin-secreting tumour. For non-functioning and gonadotropin-secreting tumours, the diagnosis usually rests on immunohistochemical analyses of resected tumour tissue, as the mass effects of these tumours usually necessitate resection.[16] Although acromegaly or Cushing's syndrome usually present with unique clinical features, clinically unapparent somatotroph or corticotroph adenomas can be excluded by a normal IGF-I value and normal 24-hour urinary free cortisol levels.

MAGNETIC RESONANCE IMAGING

Sagittal and coronal T1-weighted magnetic resonance imaging (MRI), before and after administration of gadolinium, allows precise visualization of the pituitary gland with clear delineation of the surrounding structures. Adenoma density is usually lower than that of surrounding normal tissue on T1-weighted imaging, and the signal intensity increases with T2-weighted images. The high phospholipid content of the posterior pituitary results in a 'pituitary bright spot'.

Sellar masses are commonly encountered as incidental findings on MRI, and most of these are incidentalomas. In the absence of hormone hypersecretion, these small lesions can be safely monitored by MRI, which is performed annually and then less often if there is no evidence of growth. Resection may be considered for incidentally discovered macroadenomas, as about one-third become invasive or cause local pressure effects. If hormone hypersecretion is evident, specific therapies are indicated. When larger masses (>1 cm) are encountered, they should also be distinguished from non-adenomatous lesions including meningiomas (associated with bony hyperostosis), craniopharyngiomas (usually calcified and hypodense) and gliomas (hyperdense on T2-weighted images).

OPHTHALMOLOGICAL EVALUATION

Visual field assessment that uses perimetry techniques should be performed on all patients with sellar mass lesions that abut the optic chiasm. Bitemporal hemianopia or superior bitemporal defects are classically observed, reflecting the location of these tracts within the inferior and posterior part of the chiasm. Homonymous cuts reflect postchiasmal lesions and monocular field cuts prechiasmal lesions.

HISTOLOGICAL EVALUATION

Immunohistochemical staining of pituitary tumour specimens obtained at transsphenoidal surgery confirms clinical and laboratory studies and provides a histological diagnosis when hormone studies are equivocal and in cases of clinically non-functioning tumours.

Investigating anterior pituitary hormonal hyposecretion (hypopituitarism)

The clinical manifestations of hypopituitarism depend on which hormones are lost and the extent of the hormone deficiency. Biochemical diagnosis of pituitary insufficiency is made by demonstrating low levels of trophic hormones in the setting of low target hormone levels (**Table 83.2**).[1] For example, low free thyroxine in the setting of a low

TABLE 83.2 Tests of pituitary sufficiency: dynamic pituitary hormonal testing

Hormone	Test	Blood samples	Interpretation
Growth hormone[19]	Insulin tolerance test: Regular insulin (0.05–0.15 U/kg i.v.)	–30, 0, 30, 60, 120 min for glucose and GH	Glucose <40 mg/dL (2 mmol/L); GH should be >3 µg/L (5 mU/L)
	Glucagon stimulation test: 0.5–1.5 mg of glucagon i.m.	0, 30, 60, 90, 120, 150, 180, 210, 240 min for GH	Peak GH should be >3 µg/L (5 mU/L)
	GHRH test: 1 µg/kg i.v.	0, 15, 30, 45, 60, 120 min for GH	Normal response is GH >3 µg/L (5 mU/L)
	L-arginine test: 30 g i.v. over 30 min	0, 30, 60, 120 min for GH	Normal response is GH >3 µg/L (5 mU/L)
	L-dopa test: 500 mg p.o.	0, 30, 60, 120 min for GH	Normal response is GH >3 µg/L (5 mU/L)
ACTH	Insulin tolerance test:[18] Regular insulin (0.05–0.15 U/kg i.v.)	–30, 0, 30, 60, 120 min for glucose and GH	Glucose <40 mg/dL (2 mmol/L); cortisol should increase by >7 µg/dL (180 nmol/L) or to >20 µg/dL (550 nmol/L)
	Glucagon stimulation test: 0.5–1.5 mg of glucagon i.m.	0, 30, 60, 90, 120, 150, 180, 210, 240 min for cortisol	Cortisol should increase by >7 µg/dL (180 nmol/L) or to >20 µg/dL (550 nmol/L)
	CRH test: 1 µg/kg CRH i.v. at 8 a.m.	0, 15, 30, 60, 120 min for ACTH and cortisol	Basal ACTH increases two- to fourfold and peaks at 20–100 pg/mL
	Metyrapone test:[20] Metyrapone (30 mg/kg) at midnight	Plasma 11-deoxycortisol and cortisol at 8 a.m.; ACTH can also be measured	Plasma cortisol should be <4 µg/dL to ensure an adequate response. Normal response is 11-deoxycortisol >7.5 µg/dL or or ACTH >75 pg/mL
	Standard ACTH stimulation test: ACTH 1-24 (Cosyntropin), 0.25 mg i.m. or i.v.	0, 30, 60 min for cortisol and aldosterone	Normal response is cortisol >21 µg/dL and aldosterone response of >4 ng/dL above baseline
	Low-dose ACTH test: ACTH 1-24 (Cosyntropin), 1 µg i.v.	0, 30, 60 min for cortisol	Cortisol should be >21 µg/dL
	3-day ACTH stimulation test consists of 0.25 mg ACTH 1-24 given i.v. over 8 hours each day	0 and 72 hours for cortisol	Cortisol should be >21 µg/dL
TSH	Basal thyroid function tests: T4, T3, TSH	Basal tests	Low free thyroid hormone levels in the setting of TSH levels that are not appropriately increased
	TRH test: 200–500 µg i.v.: 0, 20, 60 min for TSH and PRL		TSH should increase by >5 mU/L unless thyroid hormone levels are increased. Evoked prolactin response indicates lactotrope integrity
LH, FSH	Basal LH, FSH, testosterone, oestrogen		Basal LH and FSH should be increased in postmenopausal women. Low testosterone levels in the setting of low LH and FSH
	GnRH test: GnRH (100 µg) i.v.	0, 30, 60 min for LH and FSH	In most adults, LH should increase by 10 IU/L and FSH by 2 IU/L. Normal responses are variable
Multiple hormones	Combined anterior pituitary test: GHRH (1 µg/kg), CRH (1 µg/kg), (or insulin stress test or glucagon stimulation test), GnRH (100 µg), TRH (200 µg) are given i.v.	–30, 0, 15, 30, 60, 90, 120 min for GH, ACTH, cortisol, LH, FSH and TSH	Combined or individual release hormone responses must be elevated in the context of basal target gland hormone values and may not be uniformly diagnostic

or inappropriately normal TSH level suggests secondary hypothyroidism. Similarly, a low testosterone level without elevation of gonadotropins suggests hypogonadotropic hypogonadism.

Provocative tests may be required to assess pituitary reserve.[17] GH responses to insulin-induced hypoglycaemia, arginine, l-dopa, growth hormone-releasing hormone (GHRH) or growth hormone-releasing peptides (GHRPs) can be used to assess GH reserve. Corticotropin-releasing hormone (CRH) administration induces ACTH release, and administration of synthetic ACTH (cosyntropin – Cortrosyn) evokes adrenal cortisol release as an indirect indicator of pituitary ACTH reserve.

ACTH reserve is most reliably assessed during insulin-induced hypoglycaemia.[18] However, this test should be performed cautiously in patients with suspected adrenal insufficiency because of enhanced susceptibility to hypoglycaemia and hypotension. Insulin-induced hypoglycaemia is contraindicated in patients with active coronary artery disease or seizure disorders. The glucagon stimulation test is also used for dynamic pituitary function testing and can be used safely when insulin is contraindicated.

INVESTIGATING POSTERIOR PITUITARY DYSFUNCTION

The neurohypophysis, or posterior pituitary gland, is formed by axons that originate in large cell bodies in the supraoptic and paraventricular nuclei of the hypothalamus. It produces two hormones: (i) arginine vasopressin (AVP), also known as antidiuretic hormone; and (ii) oxytocin. AVP acts on the renal tubules to reduce water loss by concentrating the urine. Oxytocin stimulates postpartum milk letdown in response to suckling.

AVP deficiency causes diabetes insipidus (DI), characterized by the production of large amounts of dilute urine. Excessive or inappropriate AVP production predisposes to hyponatremia if water intake is not reduced in parallel with urine output.

Deficiency of AVP secretion: diabetes insipidus

Decreased secretion or action of AVP causes diabetes insipidus and is characterized by the production of abnormally large volumes of dilute urine. The 24-hour urine volume is >50 mL/kg body weight and the osmolarity is <300 mOsmol/L. The polyuria produces symptoms of urinary frequency, enuresis, and/or nocturia, which may disturb sleep and cause mild daytime fatigue or somnolence. It is also associated with thirst and a commensurate increase in fluid intake (polydipsia). Clinical signs of dehydration are uncommon unless fluid intake is impaired.

INVESTIGATION

When clinically suspected, a 24-hour urine should be collected on an *ad libitum* fluid intake to confirm polyuria.

If the volume exceeds 50 mL/kg per day, polyuria is present. If the osmolarity is >300 mOsmol/L, the polyuria is due to a solute diuresis and the patient should be evaluated for glucosuria or other less common causes of excessive solute excretion. However, if the 24-hour urine osmolarity is <300 mOsmol/L, the patient has a water diuresis and should be evaluated further to determine which type of DI is present.

Except in the rare patient who is clearly dehydrated under basal conditions of *ad libitum* fluid intake, the evaluation should begin with a fluid deprivation test. The test should be started in the morning and water balance should be monitored closely, with hourly measurements of body weight, plasma osmolarity and/or sodium concentration, and urine volume and osmolarity.

If fluid deprivation does not result in urine concentration (osmolarity >300 mOsmol/L, specific gravity >1.010) before body weight decreases by 5% or plasma osmolarity/sodium exceeds the upper limit of normal, the patient has severe pituitary or severe nephrogenic DI. These disorders can usually be distinguished by administering desmopressin (DDAVP, 0.03 μg/kg s.c. or i.v.) and repeating the measurement of urine osmolarity 1–2 hours later. An increase of >50% indicates severe pituitary DI, whereas a smaller or absent response is strongly suggestive of nephrogenic DI.

The differential diagnosis of DI may also be facilitated by MRI of the pituitary and hypothalamus. In most healthy adults and children, the posterior pituitary emits a hyperintense signal in T1-weighted midsagittal images. This 'bright spot' is almost always present in patients with primary polydipsia but is invariably absent or abnormally small in patients with pituitary DI. It is usually also small or absent in nephrogenic DI, presumably because of high secretion and turnover of vasopressin. A normal bright spot virtually excludes pituitary DI, is unlikely in nephrogenic DI, and strongly suggests primary polydipsia.

Excess AVP secretion: syndrome of inappropriate ADH secretion

Excessive secretion or action of AVP results in the production of decreased volumes of more highly concentrated urine. If not accompanied by a commensurate reduction in fluid intake or an increase in insensible loss, the reduction in urine output results in excess water retention with expansion and dilution of all body fluids. In some patients, excessive intake results from inappropriate thirst. If the hyponatremia develops gradually or has been present for more than a few days, it may be largely asymptomatic. However, if it develops acutely, it is almost always accompanied by symptoms and signs of water intoxication that may include mild headache, confusion, anorexia, nausea, vomiting, coma and convulsions, and it could be lethal.

AETIOLOGY

Hyponatremia and impaired urinary dilution can be caused by a primary defect in the regulation of AVP secretion or action or can be secondary to a recognized non-osmotic stimulus such as hypovolemia, hypotension, nausea or glucocorticoid deficiency. The primary forms are generally referred to as syndromes of inappropriate ADH secretion (SIADHs). They have many different causes, including ectopic production of AVP by lung cancer or other neoplasms; eutopic release by various diseases or drugs; and exogenous administration of AVP, desmopressin or large doses of oxytocin.

SIADH is a diagnosis of exclusion that can usually be accomplished with routine historic, physical and laboratory information. In a patient with hyponatremia, the possibility of simple dilution caused by an osmotically driven shift of water from the intracellular to the extracellular space should be excluded by measuring plasma glucose and/or plasma osmolarity. Normal results of liver function tests, lipids and glucose concentration exclude rare causes of artifactual pseudohyponatraemia (hyperproteinaemia and hyperlipidaemia) or hyperosmolar hyponatraemia, where water moves from the intracellular to the extracellular compartment (in severe hyperglycaemia).

SIADH needs to be confirmed by results of paired serum and urine samples: serum hyposmolality must be <275 mOsm/kg (normal range: 275–295 mOsm/kg), and urine osmolality >100 mOsm/kg and sodium ≥30 mmol/L, in the absence of hypovolaemia, hypervolaemia, adrenal or thyroid dysfunction and use of diuretics.[21, 22] Paired serum and spot urine samples need to be sent for osmolality and sodium to confirm both hyponatraemia and SIADH. Serum osmolality measurement is not necessary when there is an obvious contributory cause. It can confirm true hyponatraemia (<275 mOsmol/kg) and rules out the rarer hyperosmolar hyponatraemia and pseudohyponatraemia (serum osmolality ≥275 mmol/L).[23]

Urine osmolality (normal range 300–900 mOsm/kg) is needed to confirm SIADH but it also helps in differentiating it from two other conditions. By definition, SIADH is an incomplete suppression of antidiuretic hormone (urine osmolality >100 mOsm/kg); a spot urinary osmolality <100 mOsm/kg indicates appropriate complete suppression. Complete suppression of antidiuretic hormone is seen in psychogenic polydipsia (history of mental illness) and malnutrition (history of heavy alcohol consumption).[24]

Urinary sodium concentration is helpful when the cause of hyponatraemia is not apparent from the history and examination or when SIADH is suspected. In euvolaemic hyponatraemia (including SIADH), the urinary sodium is ≥30 mmol/L.[22, 25] Hypervolaemic hyponatraemia should be apparent clinically; because of the reduced effective circulating volume, the kidney concentrates the urine (>100 mOsm/kg) and conserves sodium (<30 mmol/L; but it can be higher when the patient is taking diuretics).[22] The clues to hypovolaemia in the history include obvious fluid loss (through diuretics, for example) or third space fluid loss, when fluid with high sodium content is sequestered in a body space, as occurs in burns patients. The urinary sodium concentration in all hypovolaemic hyponatraemia is <30 mmol/L except when the kidney is the site of the loss, for example with diuretic use, salt-losing nephropathy, or mineralocorticoid deficiency.[26]

When the fluid status is difficult to determine clinically, low serum concentrations of urea and uric acid indicate SIADH, and a raised concentration of urea is more likely to reflect hypovolaemia.[24]

> **KEY POINTS**
>
> - Pituitary adenomas can cause local mass effects as well as hyper- or hyposecretion of pituitary hormones.
> - Magnetic resonance imaging of the pituitary is the modality of choice for imaging pituitary pathology.
> - Visual field assessment using perimetry techniques should be performed on all patients with sella mass lesions that abut the optic chiasm.
> - The initial hormonal evaluation of a pituitary adenoma will be guided by the history and clinical examination for evidence of hormone insufficiency or excess.
> - Biochemical diagnosis of pituitary insufficiency is made by demonstrating low levels of trophic hormones in the setting of low target hormone levels. Provocative tests may be required to assess pituitary reserve.
> - Dynamic pituitary function testing is required for testing the integrity of the ACTH/cortisol axis and determination of GH deficiency or excess.
> - Water deprivation testing can be useful for the diagnosis of diabetes insipidus.

REFERENCES

1. Gsponer J, De Tribolet N, Deruaz JP, et al. Diagnosis, treatment, and outcome of pituitary tumors and other abnormal intrasellar masses: retrospective analysis of 353 patients. *Medicine (Baltimore)* 1999; **78**: 236–69.
2. Herman V, Fagin J, Gonsky R, et al. Clonal origin of pituitary adenomas. *J Clin Endocrinol Metab* 1990; **71**: 1427–33.
3. Levy A. Pituitary disease: presentation, diagnosis, and management. *J Neurol Neurosurg Psychiatry* 2004; **75** Suppl 3: iii47–52.
4. Lissett CA, Shalet SM. Management of pituitary tumours: strategy for investigation and follow-up. *Horm Res* 2000; **53** Suppl 3: 65–70.
5. Melmed S, Casanueva FF, Hoffman AR, et al. Diagnosis and treatment of hyperprolactinemia: an Endocrine Society clinical practice guideline. *J Clin Endocrinol Metab* 2011; **96**: 273–88.
6. Leslie H, Courtney CH, Bell PM, et al. Laboratory and clinical experience in 55 patients with macroprolactinemia identified by a simple polyethylene glycol precipitation method. *J Clin Endocrinol Metab* 2001; **86**: 2743–6.
7. Rosario PW. Frequency of acromegaly in adults with diabetes or glucose intolerance and estimated prevalence in the general population. *Pituitary* 2011; **14**: 217–21.
8. Ribeiro-Oliveira A Jr, Barkan A. The changing face of acromegaly: advances in diagnosis and treatment. *Nat Rev Endocrinol* 2012; **8**: 605–11.
9. Invitti C, Pecori Giraldi F, de Martin M, Cavagnini F. Diagnosis and management of Cushing's syndrome: results of an Italian multicentre study. Study Group of the Italian Society of Endocrinology on the Pathophysiology of the Hypothalamic–Pituitary–Adrenal Axis. *J Clin Endocrinol Metab* 1999; **84**: 440–8.
10. Feek CM, Marante DJ, Edwards CR. The hypothalamic–pituitary–adrenal axis. *Clin Endocrinol Metab* 1983; **12**: 597–618.

11. Nieman LK, Biller BM, Findling JW, et al. The diagnosis of Cushing's syndrome: an Endocrine Society Clinical Practice Guideline. *J Clin Endocrinol Metab* 2008; **93**: 1526–40.
12. Booth GL, Redelmeier DA, Grosman H, et al. Improved diagnostic accuracy of inferior petrosal sinus sampling over imaging for localizing pituitary pathology in patients with Cushing's disease. *J Clin Endocrinol Metab* 1998; **83**: 2291–5.
13. Beck-Peccoz P, Persani L, Mannavola D, Campi I. Pituitary tumours: TSH-secreting adenomas. *Best Pract Res Clin Endocrinol Metab* 2009; **23**: 597–606.
14. Refetoff S. Resistance to thyrotropin. *J Endocrinol Invest* 2003; **26**: 770–9.
15. Ruiz M, Rajatanavin R, Young RA, et al. Familial dysalbuminemic hyperthyroxinemia: a syndrome that can be confused with thyrotoxicosis. *N Engl J Med* 1982; **306**: 635–9.
16. Molitch ME. Nonfunctioning pituitary tumors and pituitary incidentalomas. *Endocrinol Metab Clin North Am* 2008; **37**: 151–71, xi.
17. Lamberton RP, Jackson IM. Investigation of hypothalamic-pituitary disease. *Clin Endocrinol Metab* 1983; **12**: 509–34.
18. Landon J, Greenwood FC, Stamp TC, Wynn V. The plasma sugar, free fatty acid, cortisol, and growth hormone response to insulin, and the comparison of this procedure with other tests of pituitary and adrenal function. II. In patients with hypothalamic or pituitary dysfunction or anorexia nervosa. *J Clin Invest* 1966; **45**: 437–49.
19. Hartman ML, Crowe BJ, Biller BM, et al. Which patients do not require a GH stimulation test for the diagnosis of adult GH deficiency? *J Clin Endocrinol Metab* 2002; **87**: 477–85.
20. Spark RF. Simplified assessment of pituitary-adrenal reserve: measurement of serum 11-deoxycortisol and cortisol after metyrapone. *Ann Intern Med* 1971; **75**: 717–23.
21. Ellison DH, Berl T. Clinical practice: the syndrome of inappropriate antidiuresis. *N Engl J Med* 2007; **356**: 2064–72.
22. Verbalis JG, Goldsmith SR, Greenberg A, et al. Hyponatremia treatment guidelines 2007: expert panel recommendations. *Am J Med* 2007; **120**: S1–21.
23. Adrogue HJ, Madias NE. Hyponatremia. *N Engl J Med* 2000; **342**: 1581–9.
24. Milionis HJ, Liamis GL, Elisaf MS. The hyponatremic patient: a systematic approach to laboratory diagnosis. *CMAJ* 2002; **166**: 1056–62.
25. Zenenberg RD, Carluccio AL, Merlin MA. Hyponatremia: evaluation and management. *Hosp Pract* 1995; **38**: 89–96.
26. Schrier RW. Body water homeostasis: clinical disorders of urinary dilution and concentration. *J Am Soc Nephrol* 2006; **17**: 1820–32.

CHAPTER 84

PRIMARY PITUITARY DISEASE

Christopher M. Jones and John Ayuk

Introduction 923	Pituitary adenomas 930
The spectrum of pituitary disease 925	Pituitary carcinoma 937
Congenital primary hypopituitarism 925	Familial pituitary tumour syndromes 937
Acquired primary hypopituitarism 926	Post-operative pituitary function 937
Empty sella syndrome 929	References 938

SEARCH STRATEGY

Data in this chapter may be updated by a Medline search using the keywords: pituitary, adenohypophysis, neurohypophysis, adenoma, macroadenoma, non-functioning adenoma, prolactin, prolactinoma, growth hormone, acromegaly, adrenocorticotrophic hormone, Cushing's disease, Cushing's syndrome, thyroid-stimulating hormone and gonadotrophins. Secondary search criteria included epidemiology, aetiology, management and pathogenesis. Particular focus has been placed on the epidemiology, aetiology and management of key disorders of the pituitary with level 1 and 2 evidence reported wherever possible.

INTRODUCTION

Disease of the pituitary gland may result in a broad spectrum of clinical phenotypes.[1,2] This is perhaps unsurprising given the function of the pituitary as the 'conductor of the endocrine orchestra'. Consisting of both an anterior and a posterior portion, respectively termed the adenohypophysis and the neurohypophysis, the pituitary lies immediately below the hypothalamus.

Anterior pituitary (adenohypophysis)

FUNCTION

The anterior pituitary secretes thyroid-stimulating hormone (TSH), adrenocorticotrophic hormone (ACTH), growth hormone (GH), prolactin (PRL) and the gonadotrophins follicle-stimulating hormone (FSH) and luteinizing hormone (LH) (**Table 84.1**). Their secretion is subject to marked clinical rhythms and varies widely between the different hormones. Gonadotrophin release is, for instance, well recognized to follow a 28-day cycle in women, where it is critical for ovulation and implantation. ACTH follows a circadian rhythm and normal GH secretion is pulsatile, with more pulses secreted during sleep. Knowledge of these fluctuations is important, both for the recognition that isolated measurement of pituitary hormones or their downstream mediators may be misleading and because loss of a recognizable rhythm may indicate disease, such as in Cushing's disease. Interestingly, seasonal rhythms are known to impact on pituitary hormone synthesis in other species but are unlikely to be of significance in humans.

ANATOMY

The anterior portion of the pituitary may be divided into three constituent parts. The largest of these is the pars anterior, which constitutes approximately 80% of gland volume.[3] A smaller contribution to pituitary mass is made by the pars intermedia, which is well developed in the foetus, and the pars tuberalis, which forms from an upward extension of the anterior wall of the gland and wraps around the lower end of the pituitary stalk.[3]

FUNCTION AND FEEDBACK

Secretion of hormones from the pituitary gland is controlled by the hypothalamus. For the hypophysiotrophic cells of the anterior gland, this regulation is derived by

TABLE 84.1 Principle pituitary hormones and their regulators, secreting cell and action

	Pituitary hormone	Abbreviation	Secreting cell	Downstream target	+ve feedback	−ve feedback	Effects
Anterior pituitary	Adrenocorticotrophic hormone	ACTH	Corticotrophs	Adrenal gland	CRH	Cortisol	Corticosteroid secretion
	Growth hormone	GH	Somatotrophs	Liver Adipose tissue	GHRH	IGF-1 Somatostatin	Growth Modulation of lipid/carbohydrate metabolism (effects modulated by insulin-like growth factor 1; IGF-1)
	Luteinizing hormone	LH	Gonadotrophs	Gonads	GnRH Ostrogen	Sex steroids Inhibin (FSH)	Reproductive system development Gametogenesis
	Follicle-stimulating hormone	FSH					
	Prolactin	PRL	Lactotrophs	Breast	TRH	Dopamine	Lactation
	Thyroid-stimulating hormone	TSH	Thyrotrophs	Thyroid	TRH	T4 and T3	Thyroid hormone (T4 and T3) synthesis and release
Posterior pituitary	Oxytocin		Supraoptic and paraventricular nuclei (hypothalamus)	Myoepithelial cells (uterine) Prefrontal cortex	Cervix stretch Suckling		Supports lactation Uterine contraction Emotional bonding
	Antidiuretic hormone	ADH		Liver Kidney Brain Vasculature	Reduced plasma volume/osmolality Angiotensin II Cholecystokinin	Atrial natriuretic peptide	Regulate water retention Induce vasoconstriction

Note: CRH: corticotrophin-releasing hormone; GHRH: growth hormone-releasing hormone; GnRH: gonadotrophin-releasing hormone; TRH: thyrotrophin-releasing hormone; IGF-1: insulin-like growth factor 1; T4: thyroxine; T3: triiodothyronine.

neural stimuli and feedback from circulating hormones, whether these are secreted by the anterior pituitary itself (such as growth hormone (GH)) or a target organ (such as thyroxine). Active hormones influence pituitary hormone production both by directly exerting feedback on anterior pituitary cells and, more significantly, by inducing the synthesis of neurohormones by hypophysiotrophic neurons, which are then transported down their axons and released into the pituitary portal circulation, from where they are carried to target cells in the anterior pituitary.

These neurohormones will have either a stimulatory or an inhibitor effect on the cells of the anterior pituitary gland. Stimulatory neurohormones include gonadotrophin-releasing hormone (GnRH), thyrotrophin-releasing hormone (TRH), corticotrophin-releasing factor (CRF) and GH-releasing hormone (GHRH). The inhibitory neurohormones include somatostatin, which inhibits the release of GH, and dopamine, which inhibits prolactin release.

PITUITARY GLAND VASCULATURE AS IT RELATES TO TESTS FOR NORMAL FUNCTION

The pituitary gland arterial blood supply derives from the superior and inferior hypophyseal arteries, both of which are branches of the internal carotid artery. The superior hypophyseal arteries supply a plexus which is closely associated with the median eminence of the hypothalamus and the axons of the hypophysiotrophic neurons within the hypothalamus. These vessels then form a pituitary portal circulation, which runs down the pituitary stalk into sinusoids in the anterior pituitary. The venous drainage of the gland is into the cavernous sinuses. These are venous lakes, which contain the last part of the internal carotid arteries, and cranial nerves III, IV, V and VI. They are connected across the midline by a variable array of intercavernous connecting veins and they drain into the superior and inferior petrosal sinuses. The venous connections are of importance when considering inferior petrosal sinus sampling as a method of locating secreting adenomas.

Posterior pituitary (neurohypophysis)

The posterior pituitary sits in continuity with the hypothalamus and secretes oxytocin and antidiuretic hormone (ADH, otherwise known as vasopressin).[3] These are released from the axons of supraoptic and paraventricular neurons that run through the pituitary stalk from the hypothalamus. Granules of oxytocin and ADH are stored at the distal end of these axons and are released into the systemic circulation when stimulated to do so.

> **KEY POINTS**
>
> **PITUITARY GLAND STRUCTURE, FEEDBACK AND FUNCTION**
>
> **Structure**
> - The pituitary gland is formed of both an anterior portion (itself split into three constituent parts) and a posterior portion.
> - Pituitary venous drainage is into the cavernous sinuses.
>
> **Feedback**
> - Release of pituitary hormones is governed by hypothalamic input and systemic feedback.
>
> **Function**
> - The pituitary gland is the 'conductor of the endocrine orchestra' – responsible for coordinating metabolism, growth and reproduction.

THE SPECTRUM OF PITUITARY DISEASE

There are a wide range of pathologies of the pituitary gland, the clinical manifestations of which reflect the complexity of a diverse organ formed of two constituent parts and various different cell types. Broadly, anterior pituitary diseases include congenital hypopituitarism and isolated growth hormone deficiencies, in addition to the development of functioning and non-functioning pituitary adenomas. This chapter will focus on clinical presentations arising from the development of anterior pituitary adenomas. Disease of the posterior pituitary tends to be acquired and will also be discussed, albeit in less detail.

CONGENITAL PRIMARY HYPOPITUITARISM

A large number of genes have now been associated with congenital hypopituitarism. Mutations seen in genes encoding specific cell types or hormone subunits generally give rise to isolated pituitary hormone deficiencies; mutations in genes responsible for early pituitary development result in combined hypopituitarism. A complete outline of congenital hypopituitarism is beyond the scope of this chapter but key disorders and – where known – their underlying genetic aetiology are discussed.

Congenital combined pituitary hormone deficiency

Recessive mutations of the chromosome 5q gene *PROP1* underlie the majority of cases of combined pituitary hormone deficiency, accounting for approximately 50% of familial cases.[4] The deficiency in hormone production resulting from mutations of *PROP1* is variable but generally accounts for growth hormone, TSH and prolactin deficiency. More significant deficiency of these same hormones occurs with mutations of the chromosome 3p gene *POU1F1*, though TSH deficiency may present later in childhood and is in some instances preserved.[5]

Combined pituitary hormone deficiency may also arise as part of a syndrome, as is the case in septo-optic dysplasia, Rieger's syndrome and holoprosencephaly.[6] Septo-optic dysplasia carries an incidence of approximately 1:10000 and both sporadic and familial cases have been described with *HESX1*, *SOX2* and *SOX3* implicated in the pathogenesis of this disorder.[7] Hypoplasia of both the pituitary and optic nerve is seen as a consequence, in addition to defects of the midline forebrain. This commonly results in neurological defects. Visual impairment and variable endocrine deficiencies – the most common of which are isolated GH deficiency and combined TSH and ACTH deficiency – are also seen.

Reduced levels of GH have also been noted in the autosomal dominant condition Rieger's syndrome, which encompasses a constellation of craniofacial and eye abnormalities. Conversely, holoprosencephaly is more commonly associated with posterior hormone deficiency and diabetes insipidus. Mutations in the sonic hedgehog (SHH) pathway are thought to result in this condition, which is characterized by a failure of the prosencephalon (the embryonic forebrain) to develop into two hemispheres.[8]

> **KEY POINTS**
>
> **CONGENITAL COMBINED PITUITARY HORMONE DEFICIENCY**
>
> - This may occur as part of a syndrome or independent of non-pituitary clinical features.
> - Mutations in *PROP1* and *POU1F1* are responsible for most non-syndromic cases.
> - Syndromic causes include septo-optic dysplasia, holoprosencephaly and Rieger's syndrome.

Congenital isolated pituitary hormone deficiency

Congenital isolated hormone deficiencies are rare but both familial and sporadic cases of specific anterior and posterior pituitary hormone deficiencies have been reported.

ISOLATED GONADOTROPHIN DEFICIENCY (HYPOGONADOTROPHIC HYPOGONADISM)

One of the most fascinating forms of isolated hormone deficiency is that of isolated GnRH-deficiency (IGD). This may be sporadic or of X-linked, autosomal dominant or autosomal recessive inheritance.[9] It is characterized by hypogonadism, which itself results from LH and FSH deficiency and is thus alternatively termed hypogonadotrophic hypogonadism (HH).

IGD may occur alone or in association with a loss of sense of smell (anosmia). Kallmann syndrome refers to the association of anosmia with IGD. This accounts for approximately 60% of subjects with IGD and affects approximately 1:10 000 males and 1:40 000 females.[10] Around three quarters of patients with Kallmann syndrome exhibit olfactory bulb agenesis on neuroimaging.[11]

Patients with IGD may present early in life or during adulthood. When present at birth, IGD is associated with the development of a micropenis and cryptorchidism.[9] Later in life patients with IGD demonstrate evidence of hypogonadism, the most notable clinical consequence of which is limited development of secondary sexual characteristics. 'Scratch and sniff' tests can be used to formally test for anosmia. Treatment is targeted towards both stimulating gametogenesis with pulsatile GnRH or combined gonadotrophins and inducing secondary sexual characteristics with gonadal steroids. A number of causative genes have been mapped for Kallmann syndrome and normosmic IGD,[12] as summarized in Box 84.1.

ISOLATED GH DEFICIENCY

Congenital deficiency of GH occurs in every 1:4000–1:10 000 births and may have a familial component.[13] Four distinct forms have been characterized. In type IA congenital isolated GH deficiency large homozygous mutations in the GH-encoding *GH1* gene result in exceptionally low levels of GH, even on provocation. Antibodies are generated against GH on treatment so that the adult's final height is low. Smaller mutations in either *GH1* or *GHRH* are seen in type IB isolated GH deficiency, in which a similar but milder GH deficiency is seen.

Congenital isolated GH deficiency type II is an autosomal dominant disorder in which patients present with short stature.[14] It is now recognized that this condition arises as a result of a splice site mutation in intron 3 of the *GH1* gene. This produces a mutant 17.5 kDa molecule containing a deletion between amino acids 32 and 71 (the Del32-71-GH deletion), which has a dominant negative effect and prevents secretion of wild-type GH. As a consequence, supplementation with GH is generally an effective treatment for this condition.

BOX 84.1 Isolated GnRH deficiency (IGD)-associated genes. These account for approximately 50% of all cases of IGD

Kallmann syndrome	Kallmann syndrome and normosmic IGD
KAL1	KAL1
Normosmic IGD	FGFR1
KISS1	PROKR2
KISS1R (GPR54)	PROK2
TAC3	CHD7
TACR3	FGF8
GNRHR	
GNRH1	

Type III isolated GH deficiency is X-linked and may be associated with agammaglobulinaemia. Its pathogenesis is yet to be fully elucidated.[15]

> **KEY POINTS**
>
> **CONGENITAL ISOLATED GROWTH HORMONE DEFICIENCY**
>
> **Type Ia**
> - Autosomal recessive
> - GH undetectable
> - Anti-GH antibodies raised against exogenous GH
>
> **Type Ib**
> - Autosomal recessive
> - GH low but no anti-GH antibodies raised
>
> **Type II**
> - Autosomal dominant
> - Short stature – effectively managed with GH replacement
>
> **Type III**
> - X-linked
> - Associated with agammaglobulinaemia
> - Causative gene not yet known

ISOLATED TSH DEFICIENCY (CENTRAL HYPOTHYROIDISM)

Central hypothyroidism describes underactivity of the thyroid gland resulting from insufficient TSH stimulation. It is rare, affecting around 1:50 000 live births, and both sporadic and familial cases have been described.[16] There are existing programmes already in place to screen for hypothyroidism, such as the 'blood spot' test used within the UK NHS. In the absence of this, infants may present with non-specific symptoms and failure to thrive. In cases of established central hypothyroidism, hormonal assays reveal low free thyroxine (fT4) with inappropriately normal or low TSH levels.

ISOLATED ACTH DEFICIENCY

ACTH deficiency is generally associated with other pituitary hormone deficiencies and isolated ACTH deficiency is vanishingly rare, with only a few cases reported to date. Symptoms may vary from failure to thrive to signs of acute adrenal insufficiency.[17]

ACQUIRED PRIMARY HYPOPITUITARISM

Aetiology

Hypopituitarism may arise in later life through a variety of aetiologies which include tumour growth, radiotherapy, pituitary infarction, pituitary gland infiltration, trauma and infection.[18] These are summarized in Table 84.2.

TABLE 84.2 Causes of acquired hypopituitarism

Category	Examples
Neoplasia	Non-functioning pituitary adenomas Functioning pituitary adenomas Parapituitary tumours Craniopharyngioma Meningioma Metastatic deposits Chordoma Glioma
Iatrogenic	Radiotherapy Pituitary Cranial Nasopharyngeal Surgery (see Trauma)
Systemic disease	Sarcoidosis Haemochromatosis Langerhans cell histiocytosis Granulomatosis with polyangiitis (Wegener's disease) Lymphocytic hypophysitis
Infection	Tuberculosis Pituitary abscess
Vascular	Subarachnoid haemorrhage Pituitary apoplexy Sheehan's syndrome
Trauma	Traumatic brain injury Direct pituitary trauma (e.g. surgery)

PITUITARY APOPLEXY AND SHEEHAN'S SYNDROME

Overview

Pituitary apoplexy refers to a medical emergency in which infarction of the pituitary gland occurs due to haemorrhage or ischaemia. Predisposing factors include radiotherapy, coagulation disorders, the use of anticoagulants and a reduction in intra-cranial pressure.[19] Pituitary infarction due to postpartum haemorrhage has also been described and is termed Sheehan's syndrome.[20]

Clinical assessment

Pituitary apoplexy should be considered in all patients presenting with a sudden onset headache, vomiting, visual impairment, meningism and reduced consciousness. This constellation of symptoms may be accompanied by second, third, fourth and/or sixth cranial nerve palsies.

Patients with pituitary tumours should be considered at risk of apoplexy and should be provided with information regarding relevant signs and symptoms. In those who are not known to harbour pituitary adenomas, a detailed history is required to identify symptoms of pituitary dysfunction.[19] Subsequent clinical examination should focus on the cranial nerves and visual fields for confrontation. More formal assessment of the visual fields can be undertaken using the Humphrey visual field analyser or Goldmann perimeter and can be undertaken once the patient is clinically stable.

Endocrine workup

In all patients suspected to have pituitary apoplexy, blood samples should be sent to assess electrolytes, renal function, liver function, full blood count and clotting. Assessment of anterior pituitary hormones and their downstream mediators is also required and should include cortisol, fT4, prolactin, TSH, IGF1, GH, LH, FSH and gonadotrophins.[21]

Diagnostic imaging

An urgent MRI or dedicated pituitary CT should be performed in patients with suspected apoplexy.[21] High signal will be seen on both T1- and T2-weighted MRI images.

Management

The first priority in managing a patient with pituitary apoplexy is to ensure haemodynamic stability. Empirical steroid therapy is used in patients who are haemodynamically unstable, demonstrate reduced visual acuity or who have a reduced consciousness level. It is recommended that a 100–200 mg bolus of hydrocortisone is used as initial therapy, followed by either continuous intravenous infusion of hydrocortisone or 6-hourly intra-muscular injections.[21]

In patients who are not haemodynamically unstable, steroid treatment is considered in those for whom 9 a.m. serum cortisol is less than 550 nmol/L. Patients with mild, stable or improving symptoms can be managed conservatively; in cases with severe or progressive visual impairment or altered mental state, early surgery provides the optimal chance for neurological recovery. The decision on whether to proceed to surgery must be taken by a multi-disciplinary team with appropriate expertise in endocrinology, ophthalmology and neurosurgery. If conservative management is elected for and a new visual deficit arises, decompressive surgery should be reconsidered.

> **KEY POINTS**
>
> **PITUITARY APOPLEXY**
>
> - Pituitary apoplexy is a medical emergency in which infarction of the pituitary gland occurs.
> - It should be considered in all patients with sudden onset headache, meningism, reduced consciousness and visual impairment.
> - Pituitary hormones should be assayed.
> - Urgent MRI or focused pituitary CT should be undertaken in all patients suspected of pituitary apoplexy.
> - Use empirical steroid therapy if the patient is haemodynamically unstable.
> - Early surgery may support recovery in patients with severe or progressive symptoms.

LYMPHOCYTIC HYPOPHYSITIS

This rare chronic inflammatory condition of the pituitary most commonly presents in late pregnancy or in the first postpartum year.[22] It is considered to be autoimmune in origin and antipituitary antibodies have been implicated in its pathogenesis. A lymphoplasmacytic infiltrate is seen and causes variable destruction, oedema and fibrosis of the pituitary parenchyma with resultant mass effects and hypopituitarism. Corticosteroids may play a role in the management of this condition but its natural history is yet to be determined. Spontaneous recovery has been reported.

Investigations

Biochemical and imaging tests used in cases of suspected hypopituitarism are complex and discussed in Chapter 83. Briefly, these investigations are employed both to identify and determine the extent of hormone deficiency, and to elucidate the cause of the hormone deficiency. Biochemical analyses to identify hypopituitarism include both the assessment of basal hormone levels and dynamic testing. Additional investigations such as angiotensin-converting enzyme (ACE), ferritin, hCG and aFP may be required to identify an underlying cause for the hypopituitarism, and imaging with MRI is mandatory. In some instances biopsy may be required to determine the aetiology of an underactive pituitary gland.

Anterior pituitary hormone replacement

Table 84.3 summarizes the clinical features associated with adult-onset anterior pituitary hormone deficiency.

GROWTH HORMONE DEFICIENCY AND REPLACEMENT

Clinical features of GH deficiency

Adult-onset growth hormone deficiency occurs in 1/10 000 persons. It is specifically associated with a triad of poorer skeletal health, increased cardiovascular risk and impaired quality of life (QOL).[18, 23] Patients with GH deficiency most frequently report reductions in their energy and vitality, and manifest greater emotional liability, impaired socioeconomic performance and poorer relationship-building than matched control subjects.[24]

TABLE 84.3 Clinical features associated with adult-onset anterior pituitary hormone deficiency

Hormone deficiency	Symptoms and signs
Gonadotrophins (LH and FSH)	Male: Loss of secondary sexual hair, erectile dysfunction, testicular atrophy
	Female: Anovulatory cycles, oligomenorrhoea, amenorrhoea
Prolactin	Inability to lactate
Growth hormone	Poor skeletal health, increased cardiovascular risk, impaired quality of life
ACTH	Addisonian features without hyperpigmentation
TSH	Weight gain, cold insensitivity, constipation, dry skin, hair loss, fatigue
ADH	Polyuria, polydipsia

Given the vital role of GH in lipid, protein and carbohydrate metabolism, it is perhaps unsurprising that GH deficiency is associated with increased cardiovascular risk. This is specifically conferred by a cacophony of changes that include increased central fat deposition, decreased lean mass, increased total and low-density lipoprotein cholesterol, increased triglycerides, a reduction in insulin sensitivity and hypertension.[25] Endothelial dysfunction has also been reported, as has an increase in inflammatory markers, the development of microvascular abnormalities and changes in cardiac size and function.[26]

A reduction in bone turnover is a further consequence of GH deficiency and bone mineral density falls as a consequence. There are in addition reports of a resultant increase in the risk of radiologically diagnosed vertebral fractures and clinically identified non-vertebral fractures. GH deficiency is also seen to negatively impact on exercise capacity, renal function and the maintenance of healthy skin.[25]

Rationale for GH replacement

There is no evidence to date to conclude that GH replacement eliminates the excess mortality seen in instances of GH deficiency and the degree to which GH replacement should be administered remains controversial.[25, 27] In many countries universal replacement is provided to all patients with deficiency in order to counter the deleterious clinical features outlined above. For a number of European countries, however, GH replacement is provided only to those with impaired QOL or reduced bone mass. Guidelines published by the UK National Institute for Health and Care Excellence (NICE) in 2003 restrict GH to patients with severe GH deficiency (GH < 9 mU/L) and impairment of QOL (defined as a QOL–Assessment of Growth Hormone Deficiency in Adults (AGHDA) score of greater than or equal to 11).[28]

Treatment and monitoring

In paediatrics GH is generally administered at a dose based on each patient's body weight and surface area. A similar approach in adults resulted in a number of side effects, including significant fluid retention, and this dosing strategy is consequently not commonly used. Management of adult GH deficiency instead relies on dose titration.[25] Respective starting doses of 0.2 mg/day and 0.3 mg/day are recommended for males and females, though this dose should be reduced to 0.1 mg/day in older patients. Serial IGF-1 measurements are then used to monitor GH replacement with a target of the middle-upper end of the age-matched IGF-1 range. In the steady state IGF-1 levels should be repeated at least annually. Repeat measurements are nevertheless required 6 weeks after each dose change. Close monitoring of markers of HbA1c, lipids and bone mineral density are also required during treatment with GH.

GH replacement cannot be continued in cases of active malignancy, in patients with idiopathic intra-cranial hypertension and in patients with proliferative retinopathy as a consequence of diabetes mellitus.

> **KEY POINTS**
>
> **ISOLATED GH DEFICIENCY**
>
> - Isolated GH deficiency is associated with poor skeletal health, impaired quality of life and increased cardiovascular disease.
> - There is no absolute evidence for a reduction in mortality following GH replacement.
> - Guidelines differ. Current UK NICE guidelines advocate treatment if quality of life is impaired.
> - Dose titration is required to establish the correct GH regime.
> - GH replacement may be contraindicated in certain circumstances.

THYROID-STIMULATING HORMONE DEFICIENCY AND REPLACEMENT

Once-daily thyroxine is sufficient for hormone replacement in central thyroid hormone deficiency.[29] Given that TSH is deficient, it cannot be used to identify the optimal replacement dose. This should instead be estimated based on clinical assessment and measurement of circulating (free) thyroid hormone levels, which are conventionally recommended to be in the middle or upper part of the albeit rather broad normal range. It is important that fT4 levels are taken prior to ingestion of thyroxine on the day of sampling.

GONADOTROPHIN DEFICIENCY AND REPLACEMENT

Oestrogen and testosterone replacement are respectively the usual method of sex hormone replacement for males and females with gonadotrophin deficiency. Gonadal steroid replacement will not, however, induce fertility. Patients who are seeking to conceive must therefore receive gonadotrophin therapy.[23]

Therapy in males

Testosterone replacement is required by males with gonadotrophin deficiency both to relieve the symptoms of hypogonadism (such as a reduction in libido) and to counter the long-term consequences of hypogonadism (such as osteoporosis). A link between testosterone deficiency and cardiovascular disease has been postulated but is far from proven. When given as replacement, testosterone may be administered via the transdermal route as a gel or patch, as an intra-muscular depot or as oral therapy. Patient preference, pharmacokinetics, treatment burden and cost should be considered in choosing between administration routes when initiating testosterone therapy.

The Endocrine Society has published guidelines for the management of adult men receiving testosterone therapy.[30] These advise that patients are evaluated within 3–6 months of treatment initiation in order to assess both response to treatment and the presence of adverse effects. Serum testosterone levels should be monitored at 3–6 months after treatment initiation and kept within the mid-normal range.

Baseline assessment and regular reassessment of haematocrit is required as excess androgen replacement is known to cause polycythaemia. Bone mineral density assessment is also advised within 2 years of testosterone replacement initiation in patients with osteoporosis or previous low trauma fracture. Prostate-specific antigen (PSA) levels also require regular monitoring in patients for whom initial levels exceed 0.6 ng/mL. The adverse sequelae of testosterone replacement remain uncertain and further research is required to conclude whether there is any association with increased prostate volume and a greater burden of cardiovascular disease.

Induction of spermatogenesis can occur with both gonadotrophin injections and subcutaneous pulsatile infusions of GnRH. Patients should be aware that this induction of spermatogenesis takes at least 3 months and may require over a year of therapy.

Therapy in females

Oestrogen is required by women of premenopausal age and may be administered as oral or transdermal therapy. The risks postulated for the use of hormone replacement therapy (HRT) in postmenopausal women are not thought to apply to the premenopausal setting.

Gonadotrophin injections and subcutaneous pulsatile infusions of GnRH are successful treatments for both hypothalamic gonadotrophin deficiency and primary pituitary disease. Ultrasound monitoring is required to assess ovarian response.

ACTH DEFICIENCY AND REPLACEMENT

Glucocorticoids are generally required in instances of ACTH deficiency. Strategies for effective glucocorticoid replacement are discussed elsewhere in this book and apply to this setting.

EMPTY SELLA SYNDROME

Empty sella syndrome (ESS) refers to a rare condition in which the sella turcica – a saddle-shaped depression of the sphenoid bone that forms the pituitary fossa in which the pituitary gland ordinarily sits – appears on radiological imaging to be partially or completely filled with cerebrospinal fluid.[31] This occurs as a consequence of the herniation of the suprasellar subarachnoid space into the intrasellar space, with resultant compression of the pituitary gland. Both primary and secondary forms of ESS have been described.

In primary ESS weakness of the diaphragma sella or increased intra-cranial pressure is thought to promote arachnoid membrane herniation. This most commonly occurs in obese women and both hypertension and headache are common concomitant features. Hypopituitarism is uncommon and management is supportive. ESS is considered to be secondary in instances in which it follows pituitary radiation, surgery, infection or infarction. Clinical findings in cases of secondary ESS commonly include visual abnormalities and symptoms reflecting loss of pituitary function.

PITUITARY ADENOMAS

Benign tumours arise within the pituitary gland and have been recognized in as many as one in four persons in post-mortem and radiological studies. Only a small proportion of these are clinically apparent. These result in considerable morbidity both as a consequence of the production of excess pituitary hormone and through mass effect from compression of surrounding structures.

> **BOX 84.2** Key molecular mechanisms implicated in pituitary tumour pathogenesis
>
> Oncogene activation: e.g. GNAS, CCND1, HMGA2, FGFR4 and H-Ras
>
> Tumour suppressor gene inactivation: e.g. AIP, MEN1, PPKAR1A, Rb and BRG1
>
> Cyclin mutation: e.g. the CCNB2 cyclin and CDKN2A cyclin-dependent kinase inhibitor
>
> Securin overexpression: PTTG has been found to be overexpressed in pituitary tumours

Definitions

Pituitary adenomas are benign neoplasms which do not typically metastasize and which may be categorized into those that produce hormones and those that fail to efficiently secrete their gene product.[32] These are respectively termed 'functioning' and 'non-functioning'. Functioning adenomas may arise from any one (or more) of the anterior pituitary cell types and are commonly categorized by their cytodifferentiation. While the majority produce a single hormone, 1–30% express more than one hormone and are described as plurihormonal.

Pituitary tumours are additionally classified by size, with those exceeding 1 cm in diameter termed macroadenomas and those less than 1 cm in diameter referred to as microadenomas.

Pathophysiology

There has been considerable interest in pituitary tumourigenesis and a number of potential subcellular therapeutic targets have been delineated.[33] Our understanding of the development of pituitary adenomas nevertheless remains incomplete. A number of mechanisms have been implicated in pituitary tumourigenesis, including tissue plasticity and the dysregulation of both transcription and the cell cycle through a number of specific tumour-initiating and tumour-promoting factors.

Although no single initiating factor has been identified as pathognomonic for pituitary adenoma pathogenesis, these tumours are monoclonal and intrinsic molecular events are thus thought to lead to pituitary tumourigenesis. These early events are recognized to include epigenetic changes and increasing pituitary chromosome instability. Despite this, pituitary adenomas are invariably benign and their mitotic activity remains at relatively low frequency with key mutations found in common malignancies (such as p53 mutations) only rarely found. Proliferative restraint may be conferred by mechanisms required to ensure the tissue plasticity required by the pituitary gland to maintain physiological homeostasis. **Box 84.2** summarizes key molecular mechanisms implicated in pituitary tumour pathogenesis.

An understanding of the growth of pituitary adenomas is also important for delineating symptoms relating to their mass effect. Extension of pituitary adenomas outside of the pituitary fossa may occur in a superior, inferior or lateral direction (**Table 84.4**).

Investigations

BIOCHEMISTRY

Biochemical evaluation of pituitary function involves both direct assessment of hormone levels and dynamic testing. This is discussed in more detail below.

IMAGING

Imaging of the pituitary is covered in more detail in Chapter 83. In summary, imaging may be used to identify both intrinsic and extrinsic pituitary abnormalities in suspected adenomas (**Figures 84.1–84.4**).[34, 35]

The identification of an intrinsic lesion within a normal-sized pituitary in a patient with clinical features of a functioning adenoma may, however, be misleading because there is a significant background prevalence of asymptomatic pituitary adenomas in the general population. Concluding in a systematic review published in 2004, Ezzat and colleagues, for instance, identified an overall prevalence of pituitary adenomas of 16.7% (14.4% in autopsy studies and 22.5% in radiological studies).[36]

TABLE 84.4 Extrinsic pituitary adenoma spread		
Direction of extrinsic pituitary spread	Expected symptoms	Notes
Superior, into the suprasellar cistern	Visual field defects: superior temporal quadrantanopia, bitemporal hemianopia	Most common direction of spread
Lateral, into the cavernous sinus	Usually asymptomatic	
Inferior, into the sphenoid sinus	Usually asymptomatic. Possibility of CSF rhinorrhoea or meningitis	May result in a connection between the CSF spaces and the nose

84: PRIMARY PITUITARY DISEASE

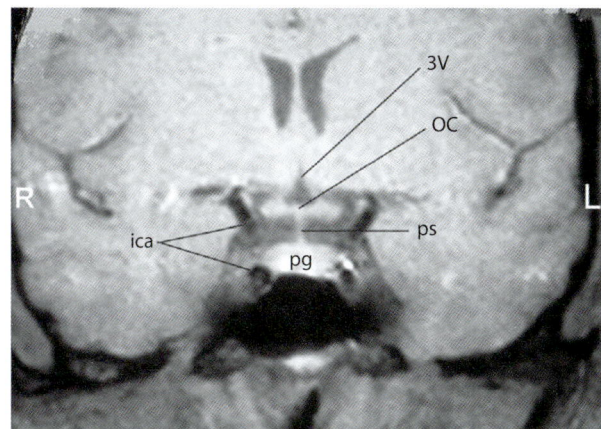

Figure 84.1 Normal pituitary gland. 3V, third ventricle; ica, internal carotid artery; oc, optic chiasm; pg, pituitary gland; ps, pituitary stalk; ss, sphenoid sinus.

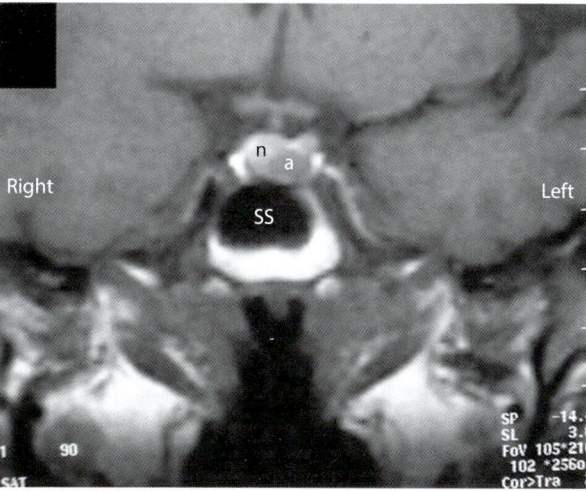

Figure 84.2 T1-weighted MR scan without contrast showing a left-sided microadenoma as a hypointense area. a, adenoma; n, normal pituitary; ss, sphenoid sinus.

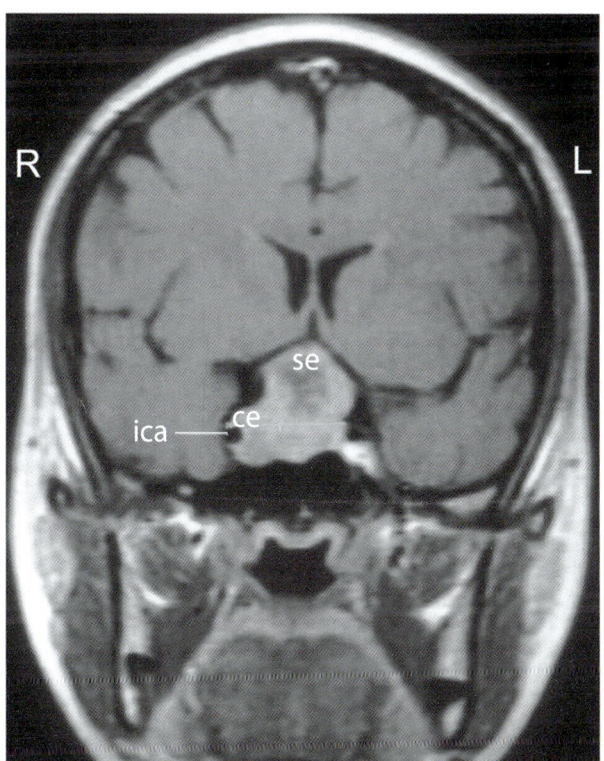

Figure 84.3 Macroadenoma of the pituitary with suprasellar extension and extension into the right cavernous sinus. ce, cavernous sinus extension; ica, internal carotid artery; se, suprasellar extension.

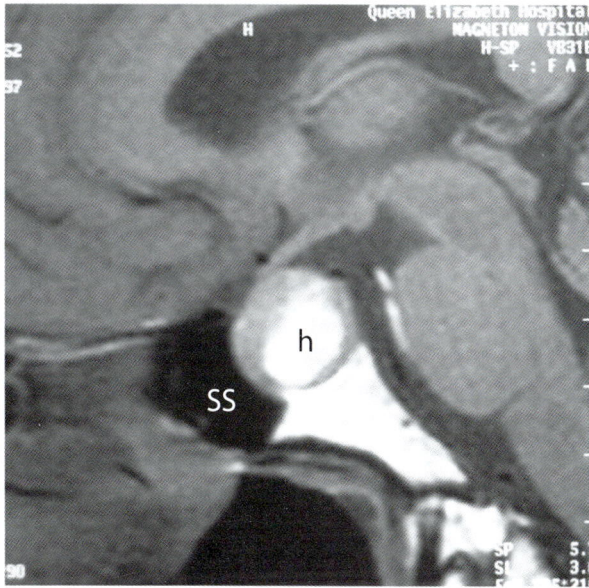

Figure 84.4 Sagittal T1-weighted MRI showing haemorrhage into a macroadenoma. H, area of haemorrhage; ss, sphenoid sinus.

A more recent review authored by Karavitaki in 2012 reported a prevalence of 78–94 cases/100000 inhabitants.[37] It is also apparent that small functioning adenomas may not be visible on imaging.

Imaging is also used to provide information on invasion or displacement of adjacent structures if a tumour extends out of the pituitary fossa (termed an extrinsic pituitary abnormality).

VISUAL FIELD ASSESSMENT

Pituitary tumours result in visual field defects in some, but not all, patients.[38] When present, the typical visual field abnormality is a bitemporal superior quadrantanopia or hemianopia, but this will depend on the position of the optic chiasm in relation to the pituitary. The earliest detectable abnormality is loss of perception of a red target.

In most cases the visual field impairment is reversible if detected and treated early. It is thus imperative that all patients with pituitary tumours who complain of visual disturbance are referred for an ophthalmologist's opinion and visual field testing. Similarly, visual field assessment is vital pre- and post-operatively in patients with a macroadenoma that abuts the optic nerves or chiasm, even if there are no ocular symptoms.[38]

Functioning pituitary adenomas

PROLACTINOMA

Prolactin

Human prolactin is a protein consisting of 199 amino acids. It has similarities with GH and, though its predominant and most active form is a monomer, it also circulates as a dimer and polymer. Serum assessment of prolactin level is a reliable measure of this hormone and is used for both the diagnosis of prolactinoma and to monitor the effect of treatment. Circulating levels are higher in women than in men.

Prolactin regulation occurs via neural and feedback pathways to the hypothalamus and anterior pituitary. Inhibitory factors – PIF – and releasing factors are involved in the control of prolactin release. The main PIF is dopamine. Around 12–28% of cells in the normal anterior lobe produce prolactin. The control of secretion is complex and a wide range of factors and conditions influence prolactin secretion.

The main site of action of prolactin is the mammary gland where it acts to prepare for milk production and to maintain it.

Prolactin excess

Physiologically high levels of prolactin are to be expected during pregnancy and lactation. Pathological causes of hyperprolactinaemia include autonomous secretion of prolactin by a pituitary prolactinoma and loss of PIF from the hypothalamus. Levels of prolactin may be very high in prolactinomas and can exceed 10 000 mU/L. It is important to note that non-functioning adenomas may cause a moderate rise in prolactin levels of up to approximately 2000 mU/L.[39] This is likely a consequence of a loss of PIF due to stalk compression by the adenoma. Prolactin may also be elevated in GH-secreting adenomas as it can be produced in excess along with GH.[39]

Clinical features Physiological and pathological hyperprolactinaemia provide negative feedback on the hypothalamo-pituitary axis and suppress the release of GnRH. Clinical sequelae of hyperprolactinaemia include galactorrhoea. Amenorrhoea may also occur in women as a consequence of reduced gonadotrophins.[39, 40] Men are usually relatively asymptomatic but low gonadotrophin levels may reduce the secretion of testosterone, causing loss of libido.[40] Importantly, prolactinomas may cause few symptoms and no pituitary macroadenoma should be assumed to be non-functioning unless serum prolactin is less than 2000 mU/L.

Management Dopamine agonists, such as bromocriptine and cabergoline, are the first-line treatment for prolactinomas.[40, 41] Serum prolactin levels can be used to monitor their effect, as can neuroimaging. It is expected that prolactin levels will fall and that the tumour will shrink with dopamine agonist therapy but neither is guaranteed. Surgery or radiotherapy may be used in patients intolerant of or resistant to dopamine agonist therapy, and serum prolactin levels would again be used to monitor the result of either of these interventions.[42]

> **KEY POINTS**
>
> **PROLACTINOMA**
>
> - Prolactin has an important role in preparing for lactation.
> - Prolactin is physiologically raised during lactation and in pregnancy.
> - Mild hyperprolactinaemia may occur in stress, with use of antidopaminergic drugs and in pituitary stalk compression.
> - Prolactinomas can cause very high levels of prolactin and may result in galactarrhoea or amenorrhoea.
> - Dopamine agonists are first-line treatment.

SOMATOTROPH ADENOMAS (SOMATOTROPHINOMAS)

Growth hormone

Also known as somatotrophin, GH is a single-chain 191 amino acid protein synthesized by somatotrophic cells, which contribute approximately half of the cells of the anterior pituitary. GH acts either directly on cells when it binds to GH receptors, or indirectly when it triggers the production of insulin-like growth factors (IGFs), which are mainly synthesized in the liver. IGF-1 is the most important of the IGFs and its mean concentration reflects that of GH over time. Concentrations of both GH and IGF-1 can be measured in serum but, because normal secretion of GH is pulsatile and the hormone has a short half-life in circulation, unlike IGF-1 which has a long half-life, the concentration of IGF-1 is a very useful indicator of mean GH output.

The pulsatile release of GH means that the volume secreted may be varied by the frequency or the amplitude of its pulses. When considering the diurnal rhythm, output is highest during slow-wave sleep. Over a lifetime, output is highest during adolescence and decreases with age. A random GH is normally less than 5.5 mU/L.

GH is anabolic and stimulates protein synthesis. It is essential for normal growth and protein metabolism. It also induces lipolysis and is secreted during hypoglycaemia, raising energy from body stores. Conversely, hyperglycaemia suppresses GH output. GH is also known to antagonize insulin, which is why acromegaly (excess of GH) may induce the onset of diabetes mellitus or make it worse.

Growth hormone excess: acromegaly

Excess GH results from the development of a functioning somatotroph adenoma.[43] If this occurs prior to closure of the epiphyseal plate, the result is gigantism. Excess GH after epiphyseal plate closure is referred to as acromegaly.

Clinical features The clinical features that characterize acromegaly derive largely from GH/IGF-1 excess but may also reflect excess prolactin, given that it is co-secreted in approximately 30% of tumours.[44] Common signs and

TABLE 84.5 An overview of the symptoms, signs and complications of acromegaly

Symptoms	Signs	Complications
• Sweating • Arthralgia • Headaches • Increased shoe size • Increased hand size • Preoccupation with appearance can result from physical changes	• Musculoskeletal • Enlargement of the hands and feet • Myopathy • Osteoarthritis • Deepening of the voice • Coarsening of the facial features • Jaw growth and macroglossia • Obstructive sleep apnoea commonly seen • Soft-tissue swelling • Carpal tunnel may result	• Metabolic syndrome • Hypertension • Insulin resistance • Ischaemic heart disease • Cerebrovascular disease • Congestive cardiac failure • Visual field defects • Obstructive sleep apnoea • Colonic polyp formation

symptoms of acromegaly are summarized in **Table 84.5**, as are the complications of this condition.

Diagnosis Random estimation of serum GH levels is unreliable as a consequence of its pulsatile release. Current Endocrine Society guidelines propose measurement of the downstream GH mediator IGF-1 in patients with features or conditions typically associated with acromegaly and in patients with a pituitary mass.[45] Acromegaly should subsequently be confirmed by identification of a lack of GH suppression to less than 1 µg/L in the presence of hyperglycaemia following on oral glucose load.[44] It is important to measure other pituitary hormones in view of potential pan-hypopituitarism. Serum calcium is also worth assessing as hypercalciuria may result from the stimulation of renal 1α-hydroxylase by GH. MRI demonstrates a pituitary tumour in 98% of cases following biochemical diagnosis.

It is important to screen for conditions associated with acromegaly following diagnosis. This should include evaluation for hypertension, multinodular thyroid enlargement, diabetes mellitus, osteoarthritis, sleep apnoea and cardiovascular disease. Patients should also be screened for colonic neoplasia.

Management First-line treatment for most patients is transsphenoidal surgery.[46] Endoscopic approaches are increasingly employed to improve the success of this procedure, recurrence rates for which currently stand at 6% at 5 years.[47] Specific complications of surgical intervention include hypopituitarism, transient mild syndrome of inappropriate antidiuretic hormone (SIADH – see 'Postoperative pituitary function' below) and CSF leak. Surgery should be considered even in those patients for whom cure is not expected (such as in the case of large invasive macroadenomas), because it improves cure rate with medical management.[48]

Radiotherapy is rarely used as a primary treatment for somatotroph adenomas but may be employed if transsphenoidal surgery is unsuccessful.[49,50] GH levels fall slowly after radiotherapy and may not return to normal for many years after treatment, meaning that adjunctive medical treatment is usually required and must be monitored at least annually. Side effects of radiation treatment include a risk of hypopituitarism and an approximate 2% increase in the incidence of second tumours within the radiation field. Newer approaches to radiation therapy include intensity-modulated radiotherapy (IMRT) and stereotactic radiosurgery (SRS).[51]

Three broad classes of drugs are used in the medical management of acromegaly.[50] Long-acting somatostatin analogues suppress GH secretion in approximately two thirds of patients with acromegaly, with symptomatic improvement common. Tumour volume reduction is seen in a significant proportion of patients managed with somatostatin analogues.[52,53] Side effects include colic, diarrhoea and the development of gallstones.

Dopamine agonists also lower GH and IGF-1 levels but do not usually return these hormones to normal levels. Cabergoline is known to be more effective than bromocriptine and restores IGF-1 to normal in approximately one third of acromegalic patients.[54] Finally, for those patients who do not respond to somatostain analogues, pegvisomant is indicated. This acts by inhibiting GH receptor functional dimerization. IGF-1 should be used to monitor response to this therapy and has been reported to return to normal in more than 90% of patients.[55,56]

> **KEY POINTS**
>
> **FUNCTIONING SOMATROTROPH ADENOMA**
>
> - Acromegaly results from GH excess occurring after closure of the epiphyseal plate.
> - Profound changes in physical appearance occur in untreated GH excess.
> - Failure to suppress GH during a 75 g oral glucose tolerant test and elevated IGF-1 confirm the diagnosis of acromegaly.
> - Transsphenoidal surgery is first-line therapy.
> - There are long-term consequences to GH excess, including the metabolic syndrome and increased risk of colonic polyposis.

CORTICOTROPH ADENOMAS (CORTICOTROPHINOMAS)

ACTH

ACTH is a 39 amino acid peptide. It is derived from a large precursor protein which is found in the corticotrophic cells of the anterior and intermediate lobes of the pituitary, in some neuronal cell groups, in peripheral chromaffin cells and some immune cells. In the anterior pituitary, 6–10% of cells are corticotrophs.

ACTH usually has a short circulating half-life and it is more usual to assay plasma cortisol levels and 24-hour urinary free cortisol production to screen patients for Cushing's syndrome. Both can be reliably measured. In normal subjects, plasma cortisol levels are highest in the morning and lowest at night. In Cushing's syndrome, this rhythm is absent and both plasma cortisol and urinary free cortisol levels are elevated.

Normal ACTH output is regulated by CRF and vasopressin. These two potentiate each other, but CRF output is suppressed by high circulating levels of glucocorticoids, whereas vasopressin is not. ACTH acts mainly on the adrenal cortex which secretes glucocorticoids, mineralocorticoids and androgens.

ACTH excess: Cushing's syndrome and Cushing's disease

Clinical features These are outlined in **Table 84.6**. They may gradually worsen over a period of years prior to a formal diagnosis being established.

Diagnosis Establishing a diagnosis of Cushing's syndrome is complex as a consequence of the diurnal rhythm of cortisol release. Endocrine Society guidelines advise testing for Cushing's syndrome in patients with early-onset features such as osteoporosis and hypertension, and patients with progressive symptoms typical of Cushing's syndrome. The first aim in investigating Cushing's syndrome is to confirm elevated cortisol. The underlying cause must then be clarified.

Is this Cushing's syndrome? Circulating glucocorticoid levels and 24-hour urinary free cortisol can be measured by routine laboratory assays. Investigations commonly employed to screen for excess cortisol secretion are outlined in **Table 84.7**. Two late-night salivary cortisol measurements may also be used for initial testing.

Physiological causes of hypercortisolism should be ruled out prior to confirming Cushing's syndrome. These include alcohol dependence, morbid obesity, poorly controlled diabetes mellitus, physical stress and pregnancy.

TABLE 84.6 Symptoms and signs of Cushing's syndrome

Symptoms	Signs
Mood disturbance	Change in facial appearance – 'moon facies'
Impairment of short-term memory	Development of striae
Loss of libido	Hirsutism
Irregular menstrual cycles	Easy bruising
	Weight gain & centripetal fat distribution
	Proximal myopathy
	Hypertension
	Osteoporosis/osteopenia
	Impaired glucose tolerance

TABLE 84.7 Investigations used to screen for Cushing's syndrome[57]

Test	Comments
24-hour urinary free cortisol	This is a useful screening test but should not be used in isolation for diagnosis because of a significant false negative rate.
Circulating glucocorticoid levels	Levels are measured by routine laboratory assays. Normal plasma cortisol levels are subject to large diurnal variation and the precise levels will depend on the laboratory used. In our institution, University Hospitals Birmingham NHS Foundation Trust, Birmingham, UK, normal levels are 180–550 nmol/L at 09:00 and <130 nmol/L at 00:00. Loss of diurnal rhythm is a feature of Cushing's syndrome.
Overnight dexamethasone suppression test	Dexamethasone is administered at midnight and serum cortisol assayed at 09:00. Plasma cortisol is effectively suppressed in normal subjects but not in patients with autonomous ACTH secretion.

What is the underlying cause? Once cortisol excess has been confirmed, its aetiology must be identified in order to differentiate Cushing's disease from Cushing's syndrome.[57, 58] This must be defined if treatment is to be appropriate and effective. Raised cortisol levels may be a consequence of excess production from the adrenal glands themselves, as in an adrenal adenoma or carcinoma, or due to excessive stimulation of the adrenal cortex by overproduction of ACTH, secreted from the pituitary or an ectopic source. The commonest cause of Cushing's syndrome is excess ACTH from the pituitary (70%), termed Cushing's disease.

The following investigations and results are used to determine the underlying cause of Cushing's syndrome:

- **ACTH:** If the source of excess glucocorticoids is adrenal, the plasma ACTH level will be suppressed.
- **Hypokalaemic alkalosis:** This is a feature of Cushing's syndrome due to ectopic ACTH, but not of Cushing's disease.
- **The high-dose dexamethasone suppression test:** This is used to differentiate between a pituitary source and an ectopic source of ACTH. While there are several variations of this test, the broad approach of this investigation is to exploit the differential sensitivity of feedback with increasing doses of dexamethasone between different causes of ACTH-dependent Cushing's syndrome. At low doses of 0.5 mg four times a day, for instance, the powerful glucocorticoid dexamethasone will suppress secretion of ACTH in normal subjects but not in subjects with autonomous ACTH secretion. However, pituitary secretion of excess ACTH is not totally autonomous, and so high doses of dexamethasone (2 mg four times a day) will suppress ACTH output from the pituitary. Conversely, ectopic sources of ACTH are more autonomous and suppression will not occur with either low- or high-dose dexamethasone.

TABLE 84.8 The dexamethasone suppression test			
	Normal	Pituitary Cushing's	Ectopic Cushing's
Low-dose dexamethasone	Suppression of plasma cortisol and UFC	No effect	No effect
High-dose dexamethasone	Suppression of plasma cortisol and UFC	Suppression of plasma cortisol and UFC	No effect

A common approach to this test is to administer 2 mg dexamethasone orally every 6 hours for 48 hours. Serum cortisol is assessed prior to and following the administration of dexamethasone. Unfortunately, this test is not invariably accurate because 10–20% of ACTH-secreting pituitary adenomas do not suppress on high dose whereas 50% of ACTH-secreting bronchial carcinoid tumours show some suppression on high dose. It is therefore important to have additional evidence of a pituitary adenoma before concluding that the cause of Cushing's syndrome is a pituitary adenoma as opposed to an ectopic source of ACTH. This test is summarized in **Table 84.8**.

- **CRF test:** If CRF is administered, ACTH levels will rise in normal subjects. This response is exaggerated in Cushing's disease but is typically absent if the source of ACTH is ectopic. However, once again this test is not foolproof. Up to 10% of pituitary adenomas do not respond to infused CRF as would be expected and a few ectopic ACTH-producing tumours do respond by secreting more ACTH.
- **Metyrapone test:** This is a sensitive test of ACTH reserve but is now used less frequently given the wide availability of ACTH assays. Briefly, metyrapone blocks glucocorticoid metabolism and should therefore result in a rise in ACTH. This response is usually exaggerated in Cushing's disease, but not if the source of ACTH is ectopic.[59]
- **Inferior petrosal sinus sampling:** This is an invasive test used to define the source of excess ACTH, usually in instances in which pituitary MRI is normal or equivocal.[60] Given that Cushing's disease results from a microadenoma in more than 90% of cases, it is postulated that MRI identifies a causative lesion in only one third to two thirds of cases.[61] Inferior petrosal sinus sampling is regarded as the 'gold standard' for the diagnosis of Cushing's disease.[62] It may also predict adenoma lateralization, although it is usually accurate in only two thirds of patients, and holds out the prospect of localizing the source of ACTH within the pituitary itself.

This is an invasive technique, requiring cannulation of both inferior petrosal sinuses under radiographic control via the femoral vein. With the catheters in place, samples can be taken for hormonal assay. After baseline samples are taken to assay the pituitary hormone levels from each side, CRF is administered intravenously and further samples are taken to measure the effect on pituitary hormone output. High levels of ACTH in blood obtained from IPSS are strongly indicative of a pituitary source of ACTH. A differential between the levels of ACTH in the IPS and peripheral sample is further evidence of a pituitary source. If this is combined with a CRF test, a rise in the ACTH levels can be demonstrated with CRF. This raises the sensitivity of the test to 95%. Although there are large venous connections between the cavernous sinuses, the venous blood between the two may not mix very much.[63] If there is a marked difference in the ACTH levels between the two sides, without a similar asymmetry in the levels of the other pituitary hormones (prolactin, GH, FSH, LH), tumours can be localized by this technique.

Management This section refers only to the management of Cushing's disease. The first-line approach in most instances is selective adenomectomy via transsphenoidal surgery. Delayed normalization of cortisol levels following this procedure is not uncommon and complications of surgery are high as a consequence of patients' poor preoperative performance status.[64] Up to 25% of patients will develop a recurrent adenoma.[65]

Second-line treatment generally involves the use of radiotherapy.[64] Control of cortisol levels will not occur for a number of years (mean period of 2 years) and may induce hypopituitarism.

Medical management of Cushing's disease is often required during radiotherapy to control cortisol levels. Medical therapy is also indicated in instances in which surgery fails to control cortisol output or to treat acute, potentially life-threatening disease complications such as opportunistic infections, psychosis and severe hypertension.[66] Approaches include pituitary-directed treatments such as somatostatin analogues, administration of adrenal blocking drugs including mitotane and ketoconazole, and in a proportion of patients use of glucocorticoid antagonists such as mifepristone. Combination therapy is often required.

Bilateral adrenalectomy was previously favoured as the treatment of choice for Cushing's disease and may still be indicated if pituitary surgery, radiotherapy and medical treatment fail to control cortisol levels.[67] A laparoscopic approach can be used to reduce morbidity. An important complication of bilateral adrenalectomy is Nelson's syndrome.[68] This describes the rapid enlargement of a pituitary lesion as a consequence of the loss of negative feedback from high cortisol levels following adrenalectomy. It presents with visual and ocular effects, in addition to hyperpigmentation as a consequence of high circulating levels of ACTH. Prophylactic radiotherapy can be used to minimize the risk of this complication.

> **KEY POINTS**
>
> **CORTICOTROPH ADENOMA**
>
> - Cushing's disease results from a functioning corticotroph adenoma.
> - Hypercortisolaemia results in mood disturbance, loss of libido, change in facial appearance, proximal myopathy, weakened skin, easy bruising and a raft of other signs.
> - Investigations into suspected Cushing's syndrome should first identify hypercortisolaemia and subsequently locate the source of the hypercortisolaemia.
> - Inferior petrosal sinus sampling is essential when there is doubt about the origin of ACTH-dependent Cushing's syndrome.

TSHOMA

TSH

TSH induces release of both T4 and, to a lesser extent, T3. Most T4 is converted to T3 within the peripheries. In cases of primary hyperthyroidism, negative feedback from fT4 and fT3 results in inhibition of TSH release.

TSH excess

TSH secreting adenomas are rare and represent only a very small percentage of functioning adenomas.[69, 70]

Clinical features Patients may present with features of hyperthyroidism but on investigation for this will be identified to have inappropriately normal or elevated TSH levels.

Establishing a diagnosis Thyroid function tests are a key first-line investigation. If a TSHoma is suspected following thyroid function testing, an MR scan of the pituitary gland should be undertaken. Tumours may be micro- or macroadenomas.

Management Surgical excision, radiotherapy and medical treatment are all options for the management of TSHomas. These tumours respond well to somatostatin analogues.[69] They can, however, be more aggressive than standard pituitary adenomas and long-term biochemical and imaging follow-up is therefore appropriate. Radiotherapy can be considered if surgical cure is not possible.

GONADOTROPHINOMAS

These seldom present as functioning tumours. The diagnosis of a gonadotrophinoma is usually made on immunohistochemical analysis of non-functioning adenoma tissue following surgery.

FSHOMA

FSH

FSH is secreted by the gonadotrophin cells of the anterior pituitary and shares an alpha-subunit with LH, TSH and HCG. The specific actions of FSH, conferred by its beta-subunit, include stimulating germ-cell maturation, initiation of follicular growth in females and regulation of androgen-binding production from Sertoli cells in males. FSH secretion is enhanced by activin and reduced by inhibin.

FSH excess

FSH-secreting adenomas are seen more commonly in men and premenopausal women but are nevertheless rare.

Clinical features FSH-secreting pituitary adenomas are usually asymptomatic. Clinical features in male patients generally relate to tumour mass effect and the development of hypogonadism. An association between FSHoma and macroorchidism has also been reported, particularly in prepubertal males.[71] Development of an FSHoma in a premenopausal woman can result in ovarian hyperstimulation syndrome. This manifests as abdominal bloating secondary to increased ovarian size or the accumulation of ascites. FSH-secreting adenomas arising in postmenopausal women are invariably asymptomatic and present a significant diagnostic challenge.

Establishing a diagnosis Measurement of FSH is key in women.[72] In premenopausal women, elevated serum oestradiol with inappropriately high FSH is indicative of an FSHoma. LH is usually normal or suppressed, differentiating the clinical picture from that of polycystic ovarian syndrome. In postmenopausal women, a raised FSH may represent an FSHoma and warrants further investigation, with a higher index of suspicion confirmed by concomitant suppression of LH. Pituitary MRI is required to assess for a macroadenoma and this may often be the first-line investigation in men, who generally present with mass effect, though FSH should also be assessed.[72] Ultrasonography may additionally be employed in premenopausal women and in men in order to respectively identify ovarian cysts and macroorchidism.

Management Management requires multidisciplinary team input. Options include watchful waiting, surgery and radiotherapy.[73] Medical therapy is not generally effective for gonadotroph adenomas.

Non-functioning pituitary adenomas

These do not present with overt hormone excess and are instead characterized by the consequence of a space-occupying lesion spreading out of the pituitary fossa. They may be associated with partial or complete hypopituitarism. This classically involves a progressive loss of pituitary hormone secretion with gonadotrophins (LH and FSH) affected first, followed by GH, TSH and ACTH. Children may present with cessation of growth or delayed puberty.[74]

Diagnosis of non-functioning adenomas relies on both neuroimaging and the biochemical assessment of pituitary function. Prolactin should also be assessed but may be elevated in non-functioning pituitary adenomas. It is essential both that any hormone deficiency is corrected and that asymptomatic functioning adenomas are identified, particularly in the case of prolactinomas as medical management may render surgery unnecessary.

PITUITARY CARCINOMA

Pituitary carcinoma accounts for less than 0.1% of all tumours and is most commonly ACTH- or prolactin-secreting, though a significant proportion are non-functioning.[75] These tumours are more likely to be p53 positive. By definition, pituitary carcinomas feature evidence of metastatic disease. Metastases are more likely to be systemic (to liver, bone, lungs and the lymphatic system) than craniospinal. Mass effects predominate and surgery forms the mainstay of management. There is some evidence for the use of chemotherapy but data from controlled trials are lacking. Favourable responses have been reported with use of the alkylating agent Temozolomide.[76] Palliation may otherwise be afforded through medical management with dopamine agonists for malignant prolactinomas, and from the use of radiotherapy. Prognosis is poor and most patients die within a year.[75]

FAMILIAL PITUITARY TUMOUR SYNDROMES

Familial pituitary tumours are rare and account for less than 1 in 20 pituitary adenomas. They are nevertheless recognized to occur as part of multiple endocrine neoplasia type 1 (MEN 1), multiple endocrine neoplasia type 4 (MEN 4), Carney complex and familial isolated pituitary adenomas.

Multiple endocrine neoplasia type 1

MEN 1, alternatively known as Wermer's syndrome, is characterized by dermal tumours (including lipomas, lentiginosis and angiofibromas) in addition to tumours of the parathyroid, pancreas and pituitary. This occurs as a result of mutations in the *MEN1* gene and genetic analysis is recommended in patients with a strong family history and recurrent neoplasia in the organ distribution described above.[77]

Multiple endocrine neoplasia type 4

MEN 4 has only recently been described and occurs as a consequence of mutations in the *CDKN1B* tumour susceptibility gene.[78] The number of patients with MEN 4 remains low and there are consequently not yet guidelines in place for the management of patients with MEN 4.

Pituitary adenomas are the second most common tumour type occurring in patients with *CDKN1B* mutations.[77]

Carney complex

Pituitary adenomas are seen in approximately one in five patients with this rare autosomal dominant condition.[79] Other tumours seen include myxomas of the breast, skin and heart, in addition to adrenal testicular and thyroid tumours.

Familial isolated pituitary adenomas

Familial isolated pituitary adenomas (FIPAs) represent 2% of all pituitary adenomas.[80] Around one in five cases of FIPA are thought to result from mutations of the aryl hydrocarbon receptor-interacting protein (AIP) gene, which causes pituitary adenoma predisposition of variable penetrance. Gigantism is a particular feature of AIP mutations and germline *AIP* mutations have been shown to correlate with the development of large pituitary adenomas.

POST-OPERATIVE PITUITARY FUNCTION

In functioning adenomas, successful surgery should correct the excess hormone secreted by the adenoma. It may, however, additionally render the patient deficient in other pituitary hormones and is unlikely to restore hormone levels which were deficient pre-operatively.

Hormone assays are used to assess the results of treatment. In microadenomas a resolution of the hormonal excess and persistently normal or low levels of that hormone indicate a cure and are a more accurate method of assessing the results of treatment than imaging. It is essential to test for all the pituitary hormones because the patient may develop a deficiency of any of them. If the pituitary is irradiated, the onset of hypopituitarism may be gradual. Lifelong follow-up is important, as recurrence or hypopituitarism can occur years later.

Patients should be advised that they may experience headaches following their procedure, that they must double their hydrocortisone dose if they are unwell and that they should not discontinue their medication without prior discussion with a health professional. Importantly, patients should also be advised not to drive following surgery until their vision is reassessed and to avoid sporting activities for 6–12 weeks.

FUTURE RESEARCH

There are a number of promising areas of future research in pituitary disease. Advances in genetically engineered mouse models and DNA sequencing technology may provide insight into mechanisms underlying tumour pathogenesis and invasiveness, leading to personalized genetic characterization and tailored treatments.

Chemokines (signalling proteins secreted by cells) have been identified as novel regulators of normal and tumour pituitary cell function; studies targeting chemokine networks may reveal novel therapeutic approaches for managing pituitary tumours.[81]

The role of tyrosine nitration in pituitary disease has also been studied; elucidation of mechanisms and biological functions of tyrosine nitration in pituitary tumourigenesis could potentially provide biomarker targets for novel pharmacological agents.[82]

KEY POINTS

- The pituitary gland plays an important role in regulating reproduction, metabolism and growth.
- Production of pituitary hormones is subject to marked cyclical rhythms, necessitating dynamic testing to diagnose some pituitary hormone excesses or deficiencies.
- Hypopituitarism may be congenital or acquired, and may feature isolated or combined hormone deficiencies.
- Benign pituitary adenomas are common, though many do not present clinically. They may be functioning or non-functioning.
- In functioning adenomas, clinical characteristics are determined by the effects of the excess hormone.
- Extrinsic growth of a pituitary adenoma can result in visual field impairment, or rarely CSF rhinorrhoea and meningitis.
- Management of post-operative pituitary hormone deficiencies requires specialist multidisciplinary team input led by an experienced endocrinologist.

References

1. Schneider HJ, Aimaretti G, Kreitschmann-Andermahr I, et al. Hypopituitarism. *Lancet* 2007; 369(9571): 1461–70.
2. Lamberts SW, de Herder WW, van der Lely AJ. Pituitary insufficiency. *Lancet* 1998; 352(9122): 127–34.
3. Amar AP, Weiss MH. Pituitary anatomy and physiology. *Neurosurg Clin N Am* 2003; 14(1): 11–23.
4. Castinetti F, Reynaud R, Saveanu A, et al. Genetic causes of combined pituitary hormone deficiencies in humans. *Ann Endocrinol* 2012; 73(2): 53–5.
5. Turton JPG, Reynaud R, Mehta A, et al. Novel mutations within the POU1F1 gene associated with variable combined pituitary hormone deficiency. *J Clin Endocrinol Metab* 2005; 90(8): 4762–70.
6. Bancalari RE, Gregory LC, McCabe MJ, Dattani MT. Pituitary gland development: an update. *Endocr Dev* 2012; 23: 1–15.
7. McCabe MJ, Alatzoglou KS, Dattani MT. Septo-optic dysplasia and other midline defects: the role of transcription factors: HESX1 and beyond. *Best Pract Res Clin Endocrinol Metab* 2011; 25(1): 115–24.
8. Choudhry Z, Rikani AA, Choudhry AM, et al. Sonic hedgehog signalling pathway: a complex network. *Ann Neurosci* 2014; 21(1): 28–31.
9. Buck C, Balasubramanian R, Crowley WF Jr. Isolated gonadotropin-releasing hormone (GnRH) deficiency. In: Pagon RA, Adam MP, Ardinger HH, et al. *GeneReviews* [Internet]. Seattle: University of Washington; 2013–2016.
10. Bouloux P-M, Hu Y, MacColl G. Recent advances in the pathogenesis of Kallmann's syndrome. *Prog Brain Res* 2002; 141: 79–83.
11. Zaghouani H, Slim I, Zina N Ben, et al. Kallmann syndrome: MRI findings. *Indian J Endocrinol Metab* 2013; 17(Suppl 1): S142–5.
12. Layman LC. Clinical genetic testing for Kallmann syndrome. *J Clin Endocrinol Metab* 2013; 98(5): 1860–2.
13. Alatzoglou KS, Webb EA, Le Tissier P, Dattani MT. Isolated growth hormone deficiency (GHD) in childhood and adolescence: recent advances. *Endocr Rev* 2014; 35(3): 376–432.
14. Alatzoglou KS, Kular D, Dattani MT. Autosomal dominant growth hormone deficiency (Type II). *Pediatr Endocrinol Rev* 2015; 12(4): 347–55.
15. Duriez B, Duquesnoy P, Dastot F, et al. An exon-skipping mutation in the btk gene of a patient with X-linked agammaglobulinemia and isolated growth hormone deficiency. *FEBS Lett* 1994; 346(2–3): 165–70.
16. Schoenmakers N, Alatzoglou KS, Chatterjee VK, Dattani M. Recent advances in central congenital hypothyroidism. *J Endocrinol* 2015; 227(3): R51–71.
17. Harano Y, Kitano A, Akiyama Y, et al. A case of isolated adrenocorticotropic hormone deficiency: a rare but possible cause of hypercalcemia. *Int Med Case Rep J* 2015; 8: 77–9.
18. Toogood AA, Stewart PM. Hypopituitarism: clinical features, diagnosis, and management. *Endocrinol Metab Clin North Am* 2008; 37(1): 235–61.
19. Oldfield EH, Merrill MJ. Apoplexy of pituitary adenomas: the perfect storm. *J Neurosurg* 2015; 122(6): 1444–9.
20. Errarhay S, Kamaoui I, Bouchikhi C, et al. Sheehan's syndrome: a case report and literature review. *Libyan J Med* 2009; 4(2): 81–2.
21. Rajasekaran S, Vanderpump M, Baldeweg S, et al. UK guidelines for the management of pituitary apoplexy. *Clin Endocrinol (Oxf)* 2011; 74(1): 9–20.
22. Foyouzi N. Lymphocytic adenohypophysitis. *Obstet Gynecol Surv* 2011; 66(2): 109–13.
23. Capatina C, Wass JAH. Hypopituitarism. *Endocrinol Metab Clin North Am* 2015; 44(1): 127–41.
24. Carroll P V, Christ ER, Bengtsson BA, et al. Growth hormone deficiency in adulthood and the effects of growth hormone replacement: a review. Growth Hormone Research Society Scientific Committee. *J Clin Endocrinol Metab* 1998; 83(2): 382–95.
25. van Bunderen CC, van Varsseveld NC, Erfurth EM, et al. Efficacy and safety of growth hormone treatment in adults with growth hormone deficiency: a systematic review of studies on morbidity. *Clin Endocrinol (Oxf)* 2014; 81(1): 1–14.
26. Miljic D, Miljic P, Doknic M, et al. Growth hormone replacement normalizes impaired fibrinolysis: new insights into endothelial dysfunction in patients with hypopituitarism and growth hormone deficiency. *Growth Horm IGF Res* 2013; 23(6): 243–8.
27. Molitch ME, Clemmons DR, Malozowski S, et al. Evaluation and treatment of adult growth hormone deficiency: an Endocrine Society Clinical Practice Guideline. *J Clin Endocrinol Metab* 2011; 96(6): 1587–609.
28. NICE. Human growth hormone (somatropin) in adults with growth hormone deficiency. *Technology Appraisal Guide TA64*. 2003.
29. Persani L. Central hypothyroidism: pathogenic, diagnostic, and therapeutic challenges. *J Clin Endocrinol Metab* 2012; 97(9): 3068–78.
30. Bhasin S, Cunningham GR, Hayes FJ, et al. Testosterone therapy in men with androgen deficiency syndromes: an Endocrine Society Clinical Practice Guideline. *J Clin Endocrinol Metab* 2010; 95(6): 2536–59.
31. Lenz AM, Root AW. Empty sella syndrome. *Pediatr Endocrinol Rev* 2012; 9(4): 710–15.
32. Fernandez A, Karavitaki N, Wass JAH. Prevalence of pituitary adenomas: a community-based, cross-sectional study in Banbury (Oxfordshire, UK). *Clin Endocrinol (Oxf)* 2010; 72(3): 377–82.
33. Melmed S. Pituitary tumors. *Endocrinol Metab Clin North Am* 2015; 44(1): 1–9.
34. Patronas NJ, Liu C-Y. State of art imaging of the pituitary tumors. *J Neurooncol* 2013; 117(3): 395–405.
35. Ouyang T, Rothfus WE, Ng JM, Challinor SM. Imaging of the pituitary. *Radiol Clin North Am* 2011; 49(3): 549–71.
36. Ezzat S, Asa SL, Couldwell WT, et al. The prevalence of pituitary adenomas: a systematic review. *Cancer* 2004; 101(3): 613–19.
37. Karavitaki N. Prevalence and incidence of pituitary adenomas. *Ann Endocrinol (Paris)* 2012; 73(2): 79–80.
38. Dhasmana R, Nagpal RC, Sharma R, et al. Visual fields at presentation and after trans-sphenoidal resection of pituitary adenomas. *J Ophthalmic Vis Res* 2011; 6(3): 187–91.
39. Glezer A, Bronstein MD. Prolactinomas. *Endocrinol Metab Clin North Am* 2015; 44(1): 71–8.
40. Rogers A, Karavitaki N, Wass JAH. Diagnosis and management of prolactinomas and non-functioning pituitary adenomas. *Br Med J* 2014; 349: g5390.
41. Melmed S, Casanueva FF, Hoffman AR, et al. Diagnosis and treatment of hyperprolactinemia: an Endocrine Society Clinical Practice Guideline. *J Clin Endocrinol Metab* 2011; 96(2): 273–88.
42. Barber TM, Kenkre J, Garnett C, et al. Recurrence of hyperprolactinaemia following discontinuation of dopamine agonist therapy in patients with prolactinoma occurs commonly especially in macroprolactinoma. *Clin Endocrinol (Oxf)* 2011; 75(6): 819–24.

43. Chanson P, Salenave S, Kamenicky P, et al. Pituitary tumours: acromegaly. *Best Pract Res Clin Endocrinol Metab* 2009; **23**(5): 555–74.
44. Andersen M. Management of endocrine disease: GH excess: diagnosis and medical therapy. *Eur J Endocrinol* 2014; **170**(1): R31–41.
45. Katznelson L, Laws ER, Melmed S, et al. Acromegaly: an Endocrine Society Clinical Practice Guideline. *J Clin Endocrinol Metab* 2014; **99**(11): 3933–51.
46. Giustina A, Chanson P, Kleinberg D, et al. Expert consensus document: a consensus on the medical treatment of acromegaly. *Nat Rev Endocrinol* 2014; **10**(4): 243–8.
47. Lobo B, Heng A, Barkhoudarian G, et al. The expanding role of the endonasal endoscopic approach in pituitary and skull base surgery: a 2014 perspective. *Surg Neurol Int* 2015; **6**: 82.
48. Karavitaki N, Turner HE, Adams CBT, et al. Surgical debulking of pituitary macroadenomas causing acromegaly improves control by lanreotide. *Clin Endocrinol (Oxf)* 2008; **68**(6): 970–5.
49. Jenkins PJ, Bates P, Carson MN, et al. Conventional pituitary irradiation is effective in lowering serum growth hormone and insulin-like growth factor-I in patients with acromegaly. *J Clin Endocrinol Metab* 2006; **91**(4): 1239–45.
50. Katznelson L. Approach to the patient with persistent acromegaly after pituitary surgery. *J Clin Endocrinol Metab* 2010; **95**(9): 4114–23.
51. Abu Dabrh AM, Asi N, Farah WH, et al. Radiotherapy versus radiosurgery in treating patients with acromegaly: a systematic review and meta-analysis. *Endocr Pract* 2015; **21**(8): 943–56.
52. Colao A, Auriemma RS, Pivonello R. The effects of somatostatin analogue therapy on pituitary tumor volume in patients with acromegaly. *Pituitary* 2016; **19**(2): 210–21.
53. Giustina A, Mazziotti G, Torri V, et al. Meta-analysis on the effects of octreotide on tumour mass in acromegaly. *PLoS One* 2012; **7**(5): e36411.
54. Sandret L, Maison P, Chanson P. Place of cabergoline in acromegaly: a meta-analysis. *J Clin Endocrinol Metab* 2011; **96**(5): 1327–35.
55. Neggers SJCMM, Franck SE, de Rooij FWM, et al. Long-term efficacy and safety of pegvisomant in combination with long-acting somatostatin analogs in acromegaly. *J Clin Endocrinol Metab* 2014; **99**(10): 3644–52.
56. van der Lely AJ, Hutson RK, Trainer PJ, et al. Long-term treatment of acromegaly with pegvisomant, a growth hormone receptor antagonist. *Lancet* 2001; **358**(9295): 1754–9.
57. Nieman LK, Biller BMK, Findling JW, et al. The diagnosis of Cushing's syndrome: an Endocrine Society Clinical Practice Guideline. *J Clin Endocrinol Metab* 2008; **93**(5): 1526–40.
58. Guignat L, Bertherat J. The diagnosis of Cushing's syndrome: an Endocrine Society Clinical Practice Guideline: commentary from a European perspective. *Eur J Endocrinol* 2010; **163**(1): 9–13.
59. Morris DG, Grossman AB. Dynamic tests in the diagnosis and differential diagnosis of Cushing's syndrome. *J Endocrinol Invest* 2003; **26**(7 Suppl): 64–73.
60. Deipolyi A, Karaosmanoglu A, Habito C, et al. The role of bilateral inferior petrosal sinus sampling in the diagnostic evaluation of Cushing's disease. *Diagn Interv Radiol* 2011; **18**(1): 132–8.
61. Testa RM, Albiger N, Occhi G, et al. The usefulness of combined biochemical tests in the diagnosis of Cushing's disease with negative pituitary magnetic resonance imaging. *Eur J Endocrinol* 2007; **156**(2): 241–8.
62. Deipolyi A, Bailin A, Hirsch JA, et al. Bilateral inferior petrosal sinus sampling: experience in 327 patients. *J Neurointerv Surg* 2016 Feb 15. pii: neurintsurg-2015-012164 [Epub ahead of print].
63. Oldfield EH, Girton ME, Doppman JL. Absence of Intercavernous venous mixing: evidence supporting lateralization of pituitary microadenomas by venous sampling. *J Clin Endocrinol Metab* 1985; **61**(4): 644–7.
64. Nieman LK, Biller BMK, Findling JW, et al. Treatment of Cushing's syndrome: an Endocrine Society Clinical Practice Guideline. *J Clin Endocrinol Metab* 2015; **100**(8): 2807–31.
65. Patil CG, Prevedello DM, Lad SP, et al. Late recurrences of Cushing's disease after initial successful transsphenoidal surgery. *J Clin Endocrinol Metab* 2008; **93**(2): 358–62.
66. Feelders RA, Hofland LJ. Medical treatment of Cushing's disease. *J Clin Endocrinol Metab* 2013; **98**(2): 425–38.
67. Wong A, Eloy JA, Liu JK. The role of bilateral adrenalectomy in the treatment of refractory Cushing's disease. *Neurosurg Focus* 2015; **38**(2): E9.
68. Patel J, Eloy JA, Liu JK. Nelson's syndrome: a review of the clinical manifestations, pathophysiology, and treatment strategies. *Neurosurg Focus* 2015; **38**(2): E14.
69. Beck-Peccoz P, Persani L. Medical management of thyrotropin-secreting pituitary adenomas. *Pituitary* 2002; **5**(2): 83–8.
70. Beck-Peccoz P, Persani L, Mantovani S, et al. Thyrotropin-secreting pituitary adenomas. *Metabolism* 1996; **45**(8 Suppl 1): 75–9.
71. Sargın G, Unubol M, Güney E, et al. Macroorchidism in a patient with FSH-secreting pituitary macroadenoma. *Turkish J Endocrinol Metab* 2012; **16**(4): 95–8.
72. Borgato S, Persani L, Romoli R, et al. Serum FSH bioactivity and inhibin levels in patients with gonadotropin secreting and nonfunctioning pituitary adenomas. *J Endocrinol Invest* 1998; **21**(6): 372–9.
73. Gandhi CD, Post KD. Gonadotropin-secreting and nonsecreting pituitary adenomas. In: Kufe DW, Pollock RE, Weichselbaum RR, et al. *Holland-Frei Cancer Medicine.* 6th ed. BC Decker; 2003.
74. Fernández-Balsells MM, Murad MH, Barwise A, et al. Natural history of nonfunctioning pituitary adenomas and incidentalomas: a systematic review and metaanalysis. *J Clin Endocrinol Metab* 2011; **96**(4): 905–12.
75. Kaltsas GA, Nomikos P, Kontogeorgos G, et al. Clinical review: diagnosis and management of pituitary carcinomas. *J Clin Endocrinol Metab* 2005; **90**(5): 3089–99.
76. Ortiz LD, Syro LV, Scheithauer BW, et al. Temozolomide in aggressive pituitary adenomas and carcinomas. *Clinics (Sao Paulo)* 2012; **76** Suppl 1: 119–23.
77. Thakker RV. Multiple endocrine neoplasia type 1 (MEN1) and type 4 (MEN4). *Mol Cell Endocrinol* 2014; **386**(1–2): 2–15.
78. Lee M, Pellegata NS. Multiple endocrine neoplasia type 4. *Front Horm Res* 2013; **41**: 63–78.
79. Correa R, Salpea P, Stratakis CA. Carney complex: an update. *Eur J Endocrinol* 2015; **173**(4): M85–97.
80. Daly AF, Beckers A. Familial isolated pituitary adenomas (FIPA) and mutations in the aryl hydrocarbon receptor interacting protein (AIP) gene. *Endocrinol Metab Clin North Am* 2015; **44**(1): 19–25.
81. Grizzi F, Borroni EM, Vacchini A, et al. Pituitary adenoma and the chemokine network: a systemic view. *Front Endocrinol (Lausanne)* 2015; **6**: 141.
82. Zhan X, Wang X, Cheng T. Human pituitary adenoma proteomics: new progresses and perspectives. *Front Endocrinol (Lausanne)* 2016; **7**: 54.

CHAPTER 85

SURGICAL MANAGEMENT OF RECURRENT PITUITARY TUMOURS

Mihir R. Patel, Leo F.S. Ditzel Filho, Daniel M. Prevedello, Bradley A. Otto and Ricardo L. Carrau

Incidence of recurrent pituitary tumours 941	Reconstruction options 945
Pre-operative evaluation 941	Post-operative management 948
Intra-operative imaging navigation and positioning 942	Conclusion 948
Technical pearls for tumour removal 944	References 949

SEARCH STRATEGY

Data in this chapter may be updated by a PubMed search using the keywords: pituitary tumours, pituitary surgery, revision pituitary surgery, recurrent pituitary tumours and functional pituitary adenomas.

INCIDENCE OF RECURRENT PITUITARY TUMOURS

Recurrence of pituitary adenomas after traditional microsurgical removal is not uncommon. In the relevant literature, recurrence rates for pituitary adenomas vary between 7% and 21%.[1] Similarly, it is clear that regrowth after incomplete tumour removal is a very likely event, being reported in 39–75% of cases.[2-9] Risk factors for recurrence include incomplete resection at the initial surgery, frank invasion of the cavernous sinus, tumour type and strong expression of pituitary tumour transforming gene.[10-12] Gross total removal rates after endoscopic endonasal approach (EEA) removal of primary non-recurrent pituitary adenomas have been reported to be high, in the range of 77–96%.[13-16] In a meta-analysis of endoscopic surgery for pituitary adenomas, Tabaee and colleagues reported the overall gross total resection rate to be 78%.[17] The main factor limiting total resection was frank invasion of the cavernous sinus.[17]

Cavallo et al. noted a recurrence rate of 9% (59 of 635) of pituitary adenomas. After retrospectively analysing the patients who recur, they noticed that at primary surgery 38.9% of them (23 of 59 patients) had a lesion with negative predictive factors, such as a cavernous sinus invasion, high labelling index or young age at diagnosis.[18]

Surgery for recurrent tumours is indicated in the presence of mass effect or systemic effects of persistent hormonal hypersecretion, as observed in Cushing's disease and acromegaly/gigantism. Small recurrences confined to the lateral cavernous sinus region must be considered for radiation treatment.

PRE-OPERATIVE EVALUATION

In addition to the necessary clinical and diagnostic information used to indicate revision surgery, additional information should be sought in order to improve the safety and efficiency of subsequent surgery. Accordingly, the aims of the pre-operative evaluation are:

- to identify sequelae of the previous procedure that may hinder the efficient creation of a sinonasal corridor (e.g. significant sinonasal scarring or the presence of a foreign body used for the previous reconstruction)
- to develop an understanding of the reconstructive options available
- to identify any contraindications to surgery, such as active, untreated infection
- to identify sequelae of the previous procedure that may increase the risk of subsequent procedures (e.g. pseudoaneurysm).

Office-based nasal endoscopy is useful to guide the surgical planning, particularly in the setting of revision surgery. This allows the surgeon to assess the sinonasal cavity for surgical approach and reconstructive options, as well as to rule out sinonasal sequelae and the presence of infection. First, nasal endoscopy provides the surgeon with the necessary information to determine what form of reconstruction was performed prior to the revision (i.e. free graft or nasoseptal flap, NSF). Furthermore, careful inspection of a potential NSF will guide reconstructive options, in the event that a large cerebrospinal fluid (CSF) leak requiring vascular reconstruction occurs during the surgery. During the conventional transseptal approach with a microscope, there is risk of septal perforation or compromise of the sphenopalatine artery (SPA) or posterior septal artery, which supply the nasoseptal flap (Hadad-Bassagasteguy flap).[19] Therefore, in patients who have been operated on in this fashion previously, alternative flaps or other techniques will need to be considered in the event that a vascularized reconstruction is necessary (see 'Reconstruction options' below).

Meticulous radiological assessment is crucial when planning a revision pituitary surgery, particularly when dealing with recurrent functional microadenomas. Dedicated magnetic resonance imaging (MRI) of the sellar and parasellar regions can demonstrate tumour location, status of the medial cavernous sinus wall, distance of the lesion to the optic apparatus, signs of stalk deviation and degree of scarring tissue the surgeon may expect to find.

Any patient who underwent a previous transsphenoidal procedure must be considered for a vascular study in order to evaluate the internal carotid arteries (ICAs). It is very important to rule out the presence of pseudoaneurysm from previous cavernous sinus manipulation particularly if the same skull base team did not perform the original surgery. Furthermore, imaging such as computed tomography angiography (CTA) can be very helpful in ruling out previous vascular complications and can be used in the image guidance system localizing the ICAs, which may be completely exposed out of their canal due to the previous surgery. The CTA is also useful in determining the presence of buttress materials left during the previous procedure.

Complete endocrine evaluation is always necessary before any pituitary procedure in order to establish the patient's baseline and to rule out or confirm pre-operative hormonal deficits. This evaluation includes assessment of the following hormones:

- prolactin
- growth hormone (GH)
- insulin-like growth factor 1 (IGF-1)
- cortisol
- adrenocorticotrophic hormone (ACTH)
- thyroid-stimulating hormone (TSH)
- free triiodothyronine (T3)
- total thyroxine (T4)
- testosterone
- luteinizing hormone (LH)
- follicle-stimulating hormone (FSH).

Patients with hypopituitarism require appropriate replacement to avoid peri-operative complications, particularly if their cortisol levels are found to be low. Conversely, if cortisol levels are normal, the patients do not receive a steroid stress dose during anaesthetic induction to prevent confusion in the immediate post-operative lab values. Diabetes insipidus (DI) must be ruled out and addressed properly when present; the anaesthesiology and post-operative care teams must be aware of this condition and maintain the use of desmopressin when it is detected before surgery.

Patients with tumours causing compression of the optic apparatus must also be evaluated by ophthalmology. As with the endocrine assessment, this seeks to establish a baseline for post-operative comparison. If the patient has no objective visual deficit but the original tumour presented with optic compression, the ophthalmological evaluation is also required.

INTRA-OPERATIVE IMAGING NAVIGATION AND POSITIONING

In the setting of revision surgery, pre-operative imaging plays a critical role; this is in part due to the close relationship to important orbital and intra-cranial structures. Transsphenoidal approaches to the sella demand a high degree of surgical precision and an accurate understanding of the pertinent anatomical relationships.[20] This task can be challenging in patients with altered anatomy and poor anatomical landmarks, frequent in those patients who have had previous surgery or who have disease invading or engulfing the surrounding structures.[21, 22]

Both osseous and neurovascular structures may serve as important landmarks during transsphenoidal approaches to the sella. Hence, both computed tomography (CT) and MRI have their advantages and disadvantages: CT scans are generally optimal for identifying bone integrity and bony landmarks, while MRI is more suited for soft-tissue differentiation. The CT can also provide additional surface points during surgery and thus increase navigation accuracy.

The authors find that intra-operative navigation is especially useful during revision surgery, where normal anatomical structures may be distorted and, as mentioned above, there is a need to rule out previous vascular complications.[23, 24] In this setting, we resort to MRI navigation with the intent to better define the interface of tumour and normal anatomy fused with CTA, which can demonstrate more clearly the bony formation and changes caused by the previous procedure and the vascular structures. Ideally, fusion of the two modalities allows for discrimination of the tumour not only with surrounding soft tissue but also with the ICA and other vessels for more complex tumours, such as the relationship with the basilar artery and anterior circulation. That said, the surgeon often finds the tumour/gland interface to be misleading and must rely on direct observation during dissection to achieve optimal resection rates. These tumours may expand superiorly to the suprasellar space, laterally to the cavernous sinus or inferiorly to the clivus. Information regarding key anatomical landmarks can be provided by the intra-operative image guidance system and are valuable in order to achieve safe tumour removal.[25]

Prior to setting up the intra-operative navigation system, the surgical team must decide if there is a need to fix the head of the patient. The authors typically use a three-pin Mayfield head clamp when there is cavernous sinus invasion (because electromyographic monitoring precludes the use of paralytics) or if there is more than 180 degrees of internal carotid encasement.[26] In cases where intra-operative monitoring is not necessary, the patient's head rests on a horseshoe head holder (**Figure 85.1a**). In these cases, a mask attached to a transmitter is placed on the face of the patient (**Figure 85.1b**) covered by clear drapes during the entire procedure, which is tracked by the optic system and allows dynamic image guidance (**Figure 85.1c,d**).

Finally, the authors always prepare the abdomen and the lateral thigh for a potential fat or fascia lata graft respectively (or in a high-risk patient, for the possibility of harvesting muscle to patch an injured artery) (**Figure 85.1e**).

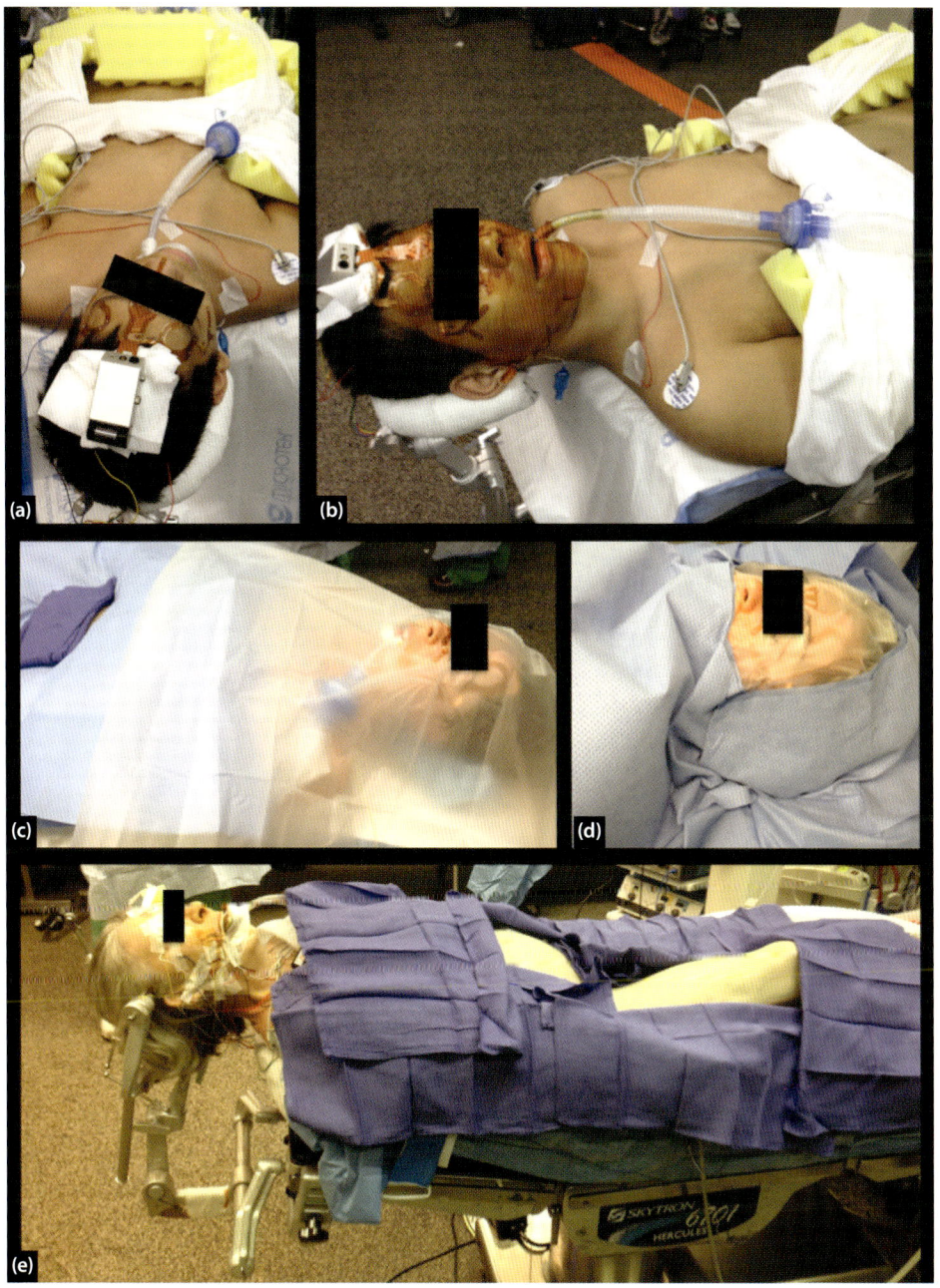

Figure 85.1 Patient and image guidance positioning. (a,b) The patient is supine with the head slightly tilted to the right, resting on a horseshoe head holder. The navigation mask and transmitter are placed on the patient's face; the abdomen has been prepared. **(c,d)** The patient's face is covered with transparent sterile drapes and surrounded by standard drapes. **(e)** In this case both the abdomen and thigh were prepped; the head is secured on a Mayfield head holder and the navigation transmitter is attached to it.

TECHNICAL PEARLS FOR TUMOUR REMOVAL

Recurrent tumours must first be distinguished between secreting or non-secreting; this classification carries implications during the procedure itself regarding the goals of surgery (total resection versus debulking). Appropriate workup is performed as outlined in previous chapters to establish the endocrine profile of the lesion. Functional tumours, such as those seen in the setting of Cushing's disease, acromegaly/gigantism and hyperprolactinemia, on average have a higher recurrence rate than non-functional tumours (15–30% versus 10% respectively).[27]

The first and foremost surgical pearl is to maximize the exposure of the sphenoid sinus and sella. A recent study demonstrated that the lack of exposure during initial tumour removal was a significant cause for recurrence.[28] For this reason, the sphenoid keel must be completely removed or drilled down to expose the sphenoid floor; this manoeuvre provides the necessary working angle for the cranial to caudal exposure. Removing all bony septations within the sphenoid sinus maximizes horizontal exposure, thus, providing access from lateral wall to lateral wall with clear visualization of the lateral opticocarotid recesses (LOCR), when is present (**Figure 85.2a**). We favour the use of a high-speed drill for the removal of septations in lieu of rongeurs because the drill provides more control. These inter- and intra-sinus septations often end on a dehiscent ICA and their removal with a blunt forcep or rongeur may fracture the ICA canal and lacerate the vessel.[29]

When drilling down the face of the sella, enough bone must be removed as to expose the 'four blues'.[30] These represent the walls of the cavernous sinus laterally and the intercavernous sinuses superior and inferiorly (**Figure 85.2b**). The authors typically drill the face of the sella until its wall is very thin, and then use a Kerrison rongeur as a dissector to separate and then lift the bone off the dura, avoiding the urge to bite the bone with the rongeur. This technique helps to avoid an inadvertent internal carotid injury as well as tears in the cavernous sinus wall. Bone that does not fracture with a gentle pull from the Kerrison rongeur indicates the need for further drilling. In addition, drilling of the sellar floor and the surrounding bone provides the ability to retract the internal carotid artery laterally and the use of a cotton tip applicator[31] to manipulate the tumour from below.

Once the bone is satisfactorily removed, one frequently encounters the material that was previously used for reconstruction; most often this is a fat graft that turns into dense scar. Typically, fat becomes too fibrous to remove with a two-suction technique; thus, the authors typically use dissectors and true-cutting instruments to separate and remove the fibrosis. During this phase of dissection, CTA-based image guidance is helpful to define those areas of the ICA that became dehiscent from previous exposures. If there is bone protecting the ICA, sharp dissection can be used to separate the tissues safely.

Once the dura of the sella is well exposed, a feather blade (Mizuho; Tokyo, Japan) is used to make the incision, usually starting in the centre of the sella and carrying it down vertically. The dura is separated from the underlying gland or tumour with a ball probe, avoiding separating the two layers of dura. The incision is then extended laterally towards the cavernous sinus using 45° angled microscissors, both superior and inferiorly. The superior cuts must be performed parallel to the sphenoid floor, so as to avoid violation of the arachnoid membrane of the diaphragm sellae and a subsequent CSF leak. A dissecting instrument is then used to explore the tumour and identify landmarks, including the medial wall of the cavernous sinus and the diaphragm sellae. The use of navigation and endonasal acoustic Doppler sonography probes (Mizuho; Tokyo, Japan), to confirm intra-operative anatomy, is prudent in all revision cases.[32]

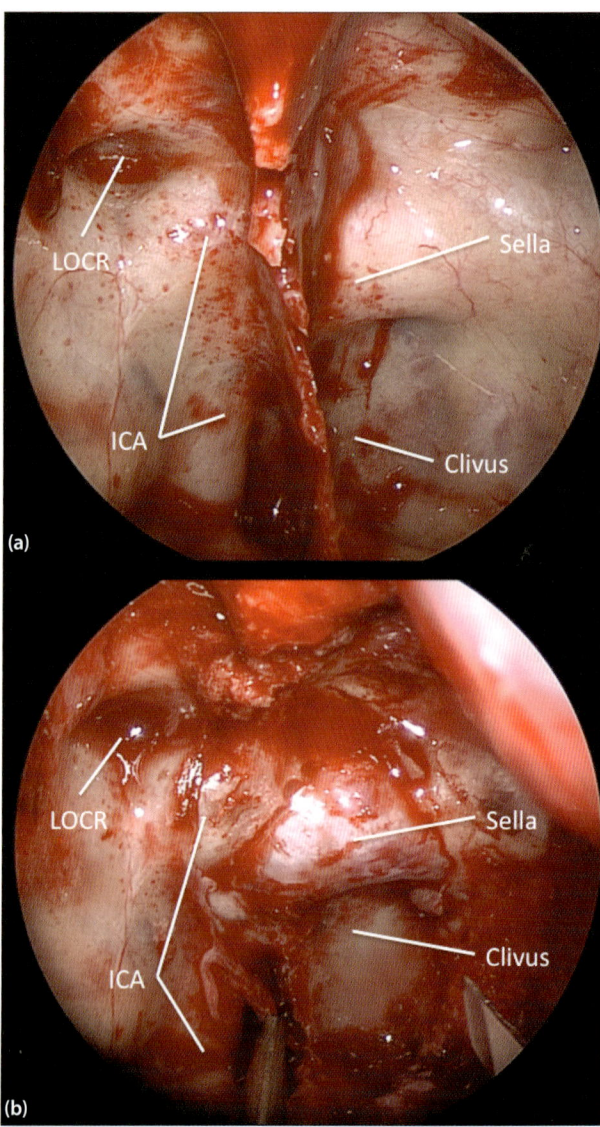

Figure 85.2 Exposure for resection of a pituitary microadenoma. (a) The sphenoid sinus has been entered; observe the bony landmarks and the relation between the septation and the right ICA. **(b)** The face of the sella has been removed, from ICA to ICA and from superior to inferior intercavernous sinuses. Note the proximity between the ICAs, narrowing the operative corridor. ICA, internal carotid artery; LOCR, lateral opticocarotid recess.

Tumour consistency dictates the instrumentation choices. Tumours that are soft are dissected and debrided using a two-suction technique. More fibrous tumours require the use of microscissors or a side-cutting power instrument (Myriad, NICO Corporation; Indianapolis, Indiana). The authors find that the ultrasonic aspirators currently available are aggressive and may inadvertently draw neurovascular structures into the instrument.

If a solid or extremely fibrous tumour is encountered but it is not invading the cavernous sinus, an extracapsular dissection is attempted, provided that the lesion is of reasonable size. Extracapsular dissection is safer than powered instrumentation and the surgeon can define the landmarks and planes for dissection while freeing the tumour from the surrounding structures. It is crucial to find the compressed pituitary gland early during this dissection in order to avoid extracapsular resection of the gland along with the tumour and consequent panhypopituitarism. The dissection must take place between the pituitary gland and tumour interface. If the lesion is very large, it can be debulked before these manoeuvres are employed.

A cotton tip applicator is a practical and relatively atraumatic retractor that decreases the risk of damaging the arachnoid membrane and producing a CSF leak while retracting the descending diaphragma sellae. More importantly, this manoeuvre greatly assists in identifying the tumour–gland interface, exposing the plane of dissection.[31, 33]

RECONSTRUCTION OPTIONS

Rescue flap

A rescue flap is elevated in most patients undergoing an endoscopic endonasal resection of a pituitary adenoma.[34] In this setting, the rescue flap allows the mobilization of the pedicle from the face of the sphenoid, therefore allowing for a wide sphenoid opening without compromising the blood supply to the nasoseptal flap. The rescue flap technique avoids the donor site morbidity associated with a nasoseptal flap.[35] A rescue flap harvest begins by incising the mucosa over the rostrum of the sphenoid sinus from the lateral wall of the nose at the level of the sphenoid ostium, carrying the incision over the sphenoid rostrum, and then anteriorly into the nasal septum mucosa (for approximately one third to half of the septum following the sagittal plane). Recently, the authors have incorporated an additional inferior incision as a modification to the original description, to increase the pedicle inferior mobility.[36] At the end of tumour resection, if a nasoseptal flap is not needed, absorbable packing reapproximates the pedicle to the bony rostrum.

Endoscopic reconstruction with free tissue grafts

Free tissue grafts are commonly used to reconstruct skull base defects after an EEA for a recurrent pituitary adenoma. Typically, they are used to reconstruct small to moderate (i.e. less than 1 cm), low-flow CSF leaks; however, in revision cases, there may not be a middle turbinate from which to harvest a graft if an EEA was performed at the time of primary resection. In this scenario, a variety of techniques such as a 'bath plug' repair or inlay–onlay strategy with acellular dermis or fascia lata may be employed. Regardless of which reconstructive tissues are employed, a multilayer technique and complete defect coverage are critical to achieve a dependable reconstruction.

First, a subdural or epidural inlay graft of collagen matrix (Duragen, Integra Life Sciences) or fascia lata is placed; this helps to stop (or at least reduce) the flow of CSF and decrease the dead space. Collagen matrix is pliable and soft, thus allowing for its safe manipulation around neurovascular structures. This subdural or epidural graft should extend beyond the dural margins, ideally 5–10 mm in all directions. If the graft is placed in the subdural space, a subsequent inlay graft of acellular dermis or fascia lata is placed in the epidural space (between the dura and the skull base). Occasionally, the bony edges are not adequate to support an inlay graft; the graft is then placed extracranially as an onlay (on the nasal side of the defect). It is critical that the edges of the defect are meticulously denuded of mucosa to allow for revascularization of the graft and to avoid mucocele formation.

Once the in- and onlay grafts are in place, a free tissue graft is applied if one is available. Healing of free mucosal grafts (i.e. take) is excellent; however, they are limited by size and the fact that they can only be used as onlay grafts. If a mucosal graft is not available, the reconstruction is bolstered with a free fat graft, typically harvested from the abdomen, or a free fascial graft, which can be fascia lata or temporalis fascia. The final layer consists of non-adherent packing such as absorbable gelatin sponge squares and expandable sponge packing or the balloon of a Foley catheter to further bolster the reconstruction. Any nasal packing is removed 3–5 days after the procedure.

Nasoseptal flap takedown

Increasingly, we have encountered patients who have had prior NSF placement for reconstruction. Although the authors generally do not use a nasoseptal flap for the reconstruction of a CSF leak associated with pituitary surgery (since the success rate with free tissue grafts is excellent), they do try to reuse the flap in patients who have had one previously. This manoeuvre has been termed 'the nasoseptal flap takedown technique'.[37]

The edges of the flap and the nasal mucosa can usually be clearly defined; however, the longer the period after the first surgery, the more difficult this delineation becomes. Once this interface is identified, the edges of the flap can be followed down to its pedicle (usually found overlying the pterygoid wedge). This pedicle must be preserved during the second surgery. The edges of the flap are mobilized centripetally using the sharp end of a Cottle elevator, thus exposing the underlying bony edges of the prior surgical defect. The nasoseptal flap is then elevated in a distal to proximal fashion towards the pedicle. Any soft-tissue structure that was exposed as part of the primary operation will heal and adhere to the undersurface of the flap (periosteal side) and therefore commonly requires a two-surgeon, four-hand sharp dissection. The pedicle is then mobilized from the underlying bony pterygoid wedge, and the flap is stored in the nasopharynx. Once the extirpative portion of the case is complete, the flap is repositioned over the defect.

There are some specific limitations of the nasoseptal flap takedown that do not apply to primary nasoseptal flap skull base reconstructions: its shape is defined by the healing process over the defect (as it heals and contracts, the flap conforms and moulds itself to the defect); it is less pliable and will retain the shape of the previous defect; it tends to migrate out of the nasopharynx into the surgical field due to increased stiffness and fibrosis. These must be kept in mind when the takedown is performed.

A case illustration of a 45-year-old female who presented with a recurrent adenoma is shown in **Figures 85.3** and **85.4**.

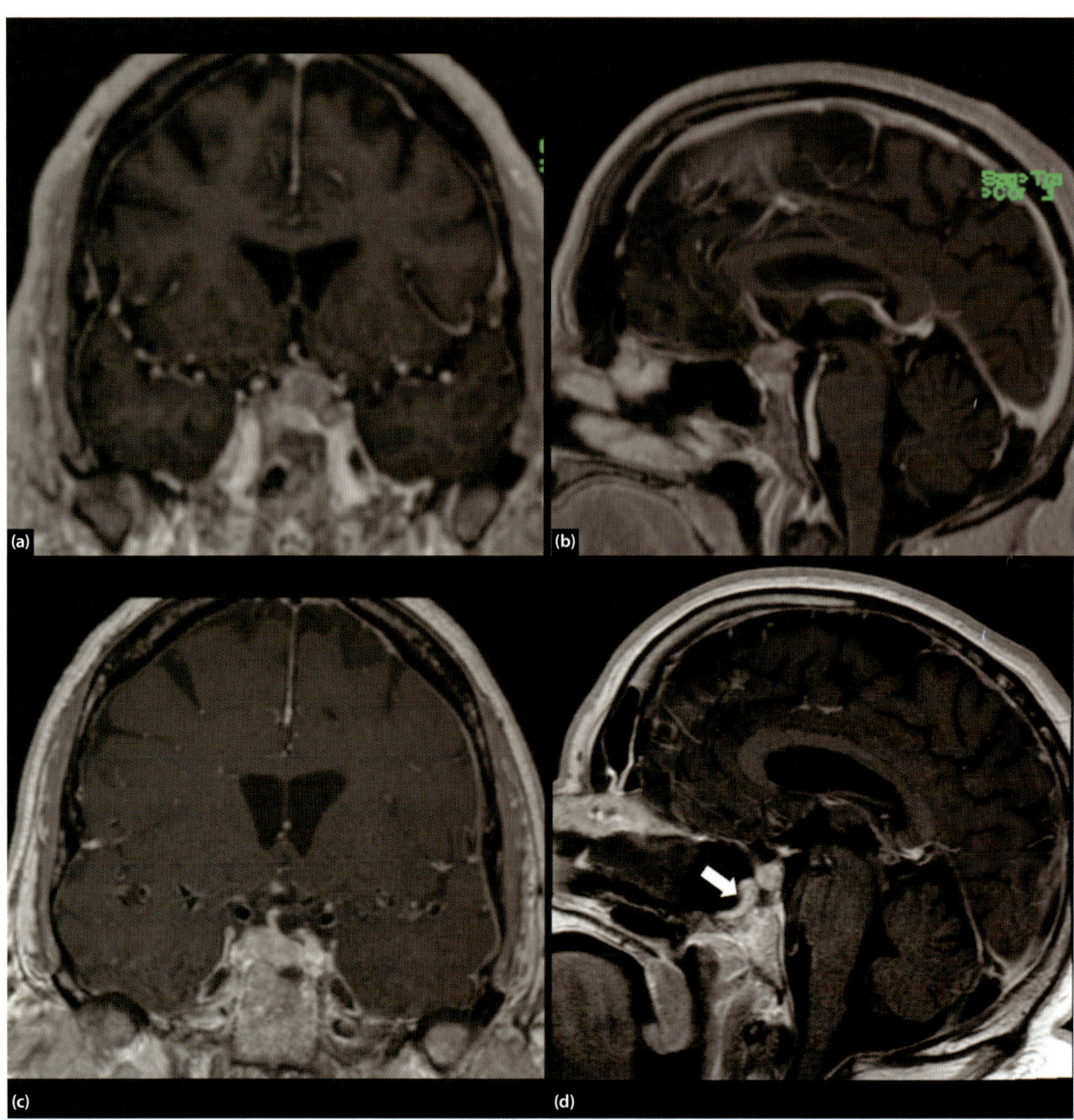

Figure 85.3 Case illustration 1. This 45-year-old female presented with a recurrent adenoma expanding into the suprasellar space and abutting the optic chiasm; her initial surgery was performed endonasally elsewhere. Pre-operative coronal **(a)** and sagittal **(b)** contrast T1-weighted MR imaging reveals the tumour on the superior left portion of the sella; the gland is seen inferiorly and to the right. Note the relation of the lesion to the optic chiasm. Post-operative coronal **(c)** and sagittal **(d)** contrast T1-weighted MR imaging confirms a thorough resection of the tumour with decompression of the optic apparatus; note the enhancing nasoseptal flap (white arrow).

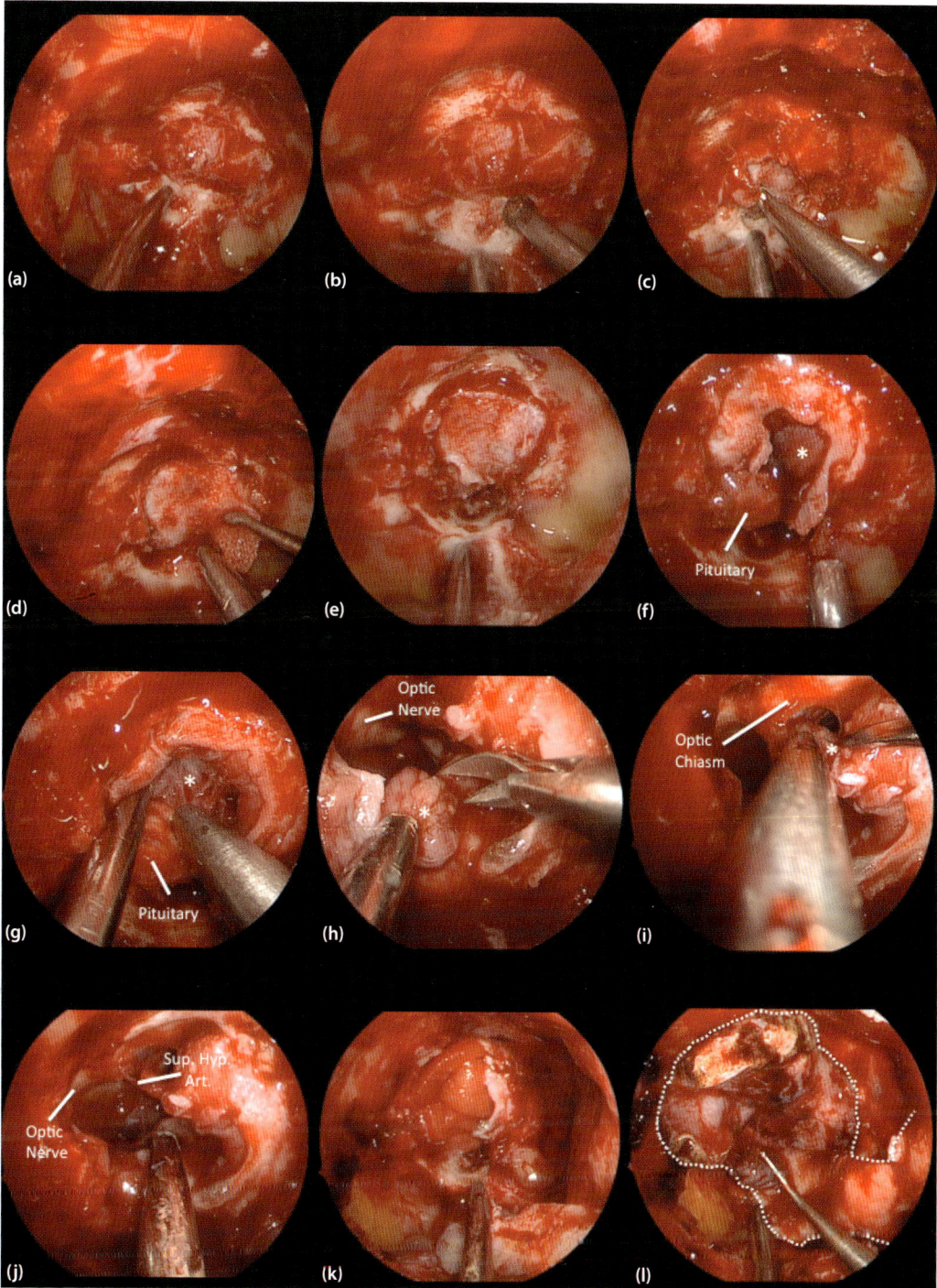

Figure 85.4 Case illustration 2. Stepwise depiction of the case illustration surgery shown in Figure 85.3. **(a)** Sphenoid sinus exposure; note the poor definition of the surgical landmarks. **(b)** The sellar bony opening is expanded with the use of a high-speed drill. **(c)** Scar tissue is displaced by blunt dissection and rongeur removal. **(d)** The Cottle dissector is used to elevate the buttress material employed in the previous surgery from the underlying dural replacement. **(e)** The sella is outlined, from ICA to ICA and from superior to inferior intercavernous sinuses. Note the dural replacement. **(f)** The dura has been opened and the pituitary gland and tumour (*) are visible. **(g)** The double-suction technique is employed to debulk the lesion (*). **(h)** Sharp dissection enables safe removal of the tumour (*) from the optic apparatus. **(i)** The last tumour remnants (*) are separated from the optic chiasm with a fine dissector. **(j)** Final view after tumour removal, prior to reconstruction; the right superior hypophyseal artery (Sup. hyp. art) has been preserved. **(k)** The dural defect is plugged with a collagen matrix replacement. **(l)** A left nasoseptal flap, raised during the approach, is applied over the defect (dotted line). Observe the pedicle arising from the left sphenopalatine foramen.

POST-OPERATIVE MANAGEMENT

All patients submitted to an endonasal endoscopic resection for a recurrent pituitary tumour are sent to an intermediate care unit after surgery where specific monitoring for DI and hypotension secondary to acute hypocortisolism can take place. If the patient is already on desmopressin and/or steroid replacement pre-operatively, these are maintained and rigorous electrolyte surveillance is performed. If pituitary function is normal before surgery, patients are monitored clinically and with prolactin and cortisol serum levels the morning after the procedure. If hypocortisolism is detected, steroid replacement is instated. If new onset DI is observed and the patient is awake and coherent, oral fluid replacement with water is encouraged. If sodium levels remain stable after the initial 48 post-operative hours, it is likely that the posterior gland recovers function and there will be no permanent DI. Otherwise, if desmopressin is initiated, the patient must be challenged by the endocrinologist with increasingly lower doses to determine whether function is still present or is permanently gone.

Patients with Cushing's disease are observed more closely, with ACTH levels checked during and after surgery and cortisol sampling every 6 hours for the initial post-operative 48 hours. This period of time is usually sufficient to determine whether steroid levels will drop enough to cause symptoms ('crashing'). If cortisol levels drop below 5 mcg/dL, steroid replacement is initiated regardless of the patient's clinical status.

Patients with acromegaly or gigantism do not require specific measures other than cortisol and prolactin sampling the morning after surgery. Long-term remission is assessed with GH and IGF-1 levels, typically in an endocrinology clinic within the first 6 weeks after the operation.

Whether and which nasal packing is necessary is determined by the reconstructive technique. As previously mentioned, packing is kept in place for the initial 3–5 days after the procedure. For the first 24 hours, the same antibiotics given during anaesthetic induction (typically cefepime and vancomycin, when needed) are maintained. An oral broad-spectrum antibiotic is used after that for as long as the packing is in.

All patients are seen at the otolaryngology clinic within the first week of discharge; the nasal packing is removed and endoscopy is used to assess healing and debridement of crusting. The degree of crusting will ultimately determine the frequency of visits the patient must endure during the recovery period for nasal hygiene.

CONCLUSION

In summary, recurrent pituitary adenomas are an excellent indication for an endoscopic endonasal approach. The wide-field visualization afforded by the endoscope allows a superior level of safety where the surgeons can observe the key sphenoid landmarks. As with any reoperation, there is a need for adequate preparation before the procedure and adequate planning for surgical resection and reconstruction. Intra-operative image guidance plays a crucial role in avoiding complications, particularly of the vascular kind.

KEY POINTS

Pre-operative management and planning

- Meticulous radiological investigation with head CTA and pituitary MRI is required.
- Assess pituitary function.
- Assess visual function.
- Conduct endonasal evaluation with office endoscopy (rule out infection, assess reconstruction options).

Image guidance

- Fusion between CTA and MRI increases accuracy.
- CT bone window can be used to provide additional reference points.

Intra-operative management

- Bone removal and exposure are paramount to adequate tumour resection.
- Image guidance and acoustic Doppler sonography help to avoid vascular injuries.

Skull base reconstruction

- The rescue flap minimizes nasal morbidity while securing the flap pedicle.
- Free tissue grafting is effective for the majority of CSF leaks after pituitary surgery.

Post-operative management

- Endocrine function and electrolyte levels must be closely monitored.
- Clinic visits are key to preventing excessive crusting and infection.

REFERENCES

1. Alahmadi H, Dehdashti AR, Gentili F. Endoscopic endonasal surgery in recurrent and residual pituitary adenomas after microscopic resection. *World Neurosurg* 2012; 77(3-4): 540–7.
2. Baskin DS, Boggan JE, Wilson CB. Transsphenoidal microsurgical removal of growth hormone-secreting pituitary adenomas: a review of 137 cases. *J Neurosurg* 1982; **56**: 634–41.
3. Laws ER Jr, Fode NC, Redmond MJ. Transsphenoidal surgery following unsuccessful prior therapy: an assessment of benefits and risks in 158 patients. *J Neurosurg* 1985; **63**: 823–9.
4. Laws ER, Kern EB. Complications of transsphenoidal surgery. In: Laws ER, Randall RV, Kern EB, Abboud CF (eds). *Management of pituitary adenomas and related lesions with emphasis on transsphenoidal microsurgery*. New York: Appleton-Century-Crofts; 1982, pp. 329–46.
5. Benveniste RJ, King WA, Walsh J, et al. Repeated transsphenoidal surgery to treat recurrent or residual pituitary adenoma. *J Neurosurg* 2005; **102**: 1004–12.
6. Chang EF, Sughrue ME, Zada G, et al. Long-term outcome following repeat transsphenoidal surgery for recurrent endocrine-inactive pituitary adenomas. *Pituitary* 2010; **13**: 223–9.
7. Ciric I, Ragin A, Baumgartner C, Pierce D. Complications of transsphenoidal surgery: results of a national survey, review of the literature, and personal experience. *Neurosurgery* 1997; **40**: 225–36, discussion 236-7.
8. D'Haens J, Van Rompaey K, Stadnik T, et al. Fully endoscopic transsphenoidal surgery for functioning pituitary adenomas: a retrospective comparison with traditional transsphenoidal microsurgery in the same institution. *Surg Neurol* 2009; **72**: 336–40.
9. Laws ERJ. Transsphenoidal surgery. In: Apuzzo MLJ (ed.). *Brain surgery: Complications avoidance and management*. New York: Churchill Livingstone; 1993, pp. 357–62.
10. Hofmann BM, Hlavac M, Martinez R, et al. Long-term results after microsurgery for Cushing's disease: experience with 426 primary operations over 35 years. *J Neurosurg* 2008; **108**: 9–18.
11. Chang EF, Zada G, Kim S, et al. Long-term recurrence and mortality after surgery and adjuvant radiotherapy for nonfunctional pituitary adenomas. *J Neurosurg* 2008; **108**: 736-45.
12. Filippella M, Galland F, Kujas M, et al. Pituitary tumour transforming gene (PTTG) expression correlates with the proliferative activity and recurrence status of pituitary adenomas: a clinical and immunohistochemical study. *Clin Endocrinol (Oxf)* 2006; **65**: 536–43.
13. Prevedello DM, Doglietto F, Jane JA Jr, et al. History of endoscopic skull base surgery: its evolution and current reality. *J Neurosurg* 2007; **107**: 206–13.
14. Frank G, Pasquini E, Farneti G, et al. The endoscopic versus the traditional approach in pituitary surgery. *Neuroendocrinology* 2006; **83**: 240–8.
15. Kabil MS, Eby JB, Shahinian HK. Fully endoscopic endonasal vs. transseptal transsphenoidal pituitary surgery. *Minim Invas Neurosurg* 2005; **48**: 348–54.
16. Dehdashti AR, Ganna A, Karabatsou K, Gentili F. Pure endoscopic endonasal approach for pituitary adenomas: early surgical results in 200 and comparison with previous microsurgical series. *Neurosurgery* 2008; **62**: 1006–15.
17. Tabaee A, Anand VK, Barrón Y, et al. Endoscopic pituitary surgery: a systematic review and meta-analysis. *J Neurosurg* 2009; **111**(3): 545-54.
18. Cavallo LM, Solari D, Tasiou A, et al. Endoscopic endonasal transsphenoidal removal of recurrent and regrowing pituitary adenomas: experience on a 59-patient series. *World Neurosurg* 2013; 80(3–4): 342–50.
19. Hadad G, Bassagasteguy L, Carrau RL, et al. A novel reconstructive technique after endoscopic expanded endonasal approaches: vascular pedicle nasoseptal flap. *Laryngoscope* 2006; **116**(10): 1882–6.
20. de Lara D, Ditzel Filho LF, Prevedello DM, et al. Application of image guidance in pituitary surgery. *Surg Neurol Int* 2012; 3(Suppl 2): S73–8.
21. Kuroki A, Kayama T. Endoscopic approach to the pituitary lesions: contemporary method and review of the literature. *Biomed Pharmacother* 2002; 56 Suppl 1: 158s–64s.
22. Metson R, Gliklich RE, Cosenza M. A comparison of image guidance systems for sinus surgery. *Laryngoscope* 1998; **108**: 1164–70.
23. Asthagiri AR, Laws ER Jr, Jane JA Jr. Image guidance in pituitary surgery. *Front Horm Res* 2006; **34**: 46–63.
24. Gong J, Mohr G, Vezina JL. Endoscopic pituitary surgery with and without image guidance: an experimental comparison. *Surg Neurol* 2007; **67**: 572–8, discussion 578.
25. Wiltfang J, Rupprecht S, Ganslandt O, et al. Intraoperative image-guided surgery of the lateral and anterior skull base in patients with tumors or trauma. *Skull Base* 2003; **13**: 21–9.
26. Thirumala PD, Kassasm AB, Habeych M, et al. Somatosensory evoked potential monitoring during endoscopic endonasal approach to skull base surgery: analysis of observed changes. *Neurosurgery* 2011; **69**: ons64–76.
27. Charalampaki P, Ayyad A, Kockro RA, Perneczky A. Surgical complications after endoscopic transsphenoidal pituitary surgery. *J Clin Neurosci* 2009; **16**(6): 786–9.
28. Mattozo CA, Dusick JR, Esposito F, et al. Suboptimal sphenoid and sellar exposure: a consistent finding in patients treated with repeat transsphenoidal surgery for residual endocrine-inactive macroadenomas. *Neurosurgery* 2006; **58**(5): 857–65.
29. Gardner PA, Tormenti MJ, Pant H, et al. Carotid artery injury during endoscopic endonasal skull base surgery: incidence and outcomes. *Neurosurgery* 2013; **73**(2 Suppl Operative): ons261–9; discussion ons269–70.
30. Kassam AB, Prevedello DM, Carrau RL, et al. Endoscopic endonasal skull base surgery: analysis of complications in the authors' initial 800 patients: a review. *J Neurosurg* 2011; **114**(6): 1544-68.
31. Prevedello DM, Kassam AB, Gardner P, et al. 'Q-tip' retractor in endoscopic cranial base surgery. *Neurosurgery* 2010; **66**(2): 363–6; discussion 366-7.
32. Pinheiro-Neto CD, Carrau RL, Prevedello DM, et al. Use of acoustic Doppler sonography to ascertain the feasibility of the pedicled nasoseptal flap after prior bilateral sphenoidotomy. *Laryngoscope* 2010; **120**(9): 1798–801.
33. Prevedello DM, Ebner FH, de Lara D, et al. Extracapsular dissection technique with the Cotton Swab for pituitary adenomas through an endoscopic endonasal approach: how I do it. *Acta Neurochir (Wien)* 2013; **155**(9): 1629–32.
34. Rivera-Serrano CM, Snyderman CH, Gardner P, et al. Nasoseptal 'rescue' flap: a novel modification of the nasoseptal flap technique for pituitary surgery. *Laryngoscope* 2011; **121**(5): 990–3.
35. Rawal RB, Kimple AJ, Dugar DR, Zanation AM. Minimizing morbidity in endoscopic pituitary surgery outcomes of the novel nasoseptal rescue flap technique. *Otolaryngol Head Neck Surg* 2012; **147**(3): 434–7.
36. Otto BA, Bowe SN, Carrau RL, et al. Transsphenoidal approach with nasoseptal flap pedicle transposition: modified rescue flap technique. *Laryngoscope* 2013; **123**(12): 2976–9.
37. Zanation AM, Carrau RL, Snyderman CH, et al. Nasoseptal flap takedown and reuse in revision endoscopic skull base reconstruction. *Laryngoscope* 2011; **121**(1): 42–6.

CHAPTER 86

ADJUVANT TREATMENT OF PITUITARY DISEASE

Andy Levy

Overview of pituitary adenomas ... 951	Thyrotroph adenoma ... 955
Primary treatment ... 951	Pituitary carcinomas ... 955
Why is adjuvant treatment needed? ... 952	Endocrinologically inactive adenomas and gonadotrophinomas ... 955
Prolactinoma ... 952	Craniopharyngioma ... 955
Somatotrophinoma ... 952	References ... 955
Corticotrophinoma ... 954	

SEARCH STRATEGY

Data in this chapter may be updated by a PubMed search using the keywords: adjuvant treatments for pituitary tumours.

OVERVIEW OF PITUITARY ADENOMAS

The incidence of clinically overt pituitary adenomas is around 15–20 per million per year. Fifty to sixty percent are microadenomas and these, by definition, regain trophic stability after a period of deregulated post-induction growth. A further proportion of pituitary macroadenomas grow slowly or not at all and may not require intervention if bioactive hormone secretion is not a feature. Overall, approximately one third of pituitary adenomas require surgical intervention at least once, and as their prevalence is relatively high – 2.5 cases per 10 000 – pituitary adenomas constitute the third most common intra-cranial tumour requiring neurosurgical intervention. Occult pituitary adenomas are more common still, with histological evidence of pituitary adenomas at the time of death from unrelated causes in 11–14% of the population.[1, 2]

Approximately 50% of newly diagnosed pituitary adenomas are prolactinomas. Endocrinologically inactive adenomas account for 30%, somatotrophinomas for 15–20%, corticotroph adenomas for 5–10% and thyrotroph adenomas for less than 1%.[3] Limited dural invasion is fairly typical in all macroadenomas and slow expansion over a period of years expected. Aggressive expansion, requiring repeated surgery and adjuvant treatment is atypical, and frank metastatic spread is exceptionally rare.[4]

Non-specific symptoms

Headaches typically associated with pituitary adenomas are non-specific, variable in their characteristics and insidious in onset. They can mimic classical migraine, tension headaches, sinusitis and various causes of facial pain. Analgesics, tricyclic antidepressants at low dose, verapamil and beta-blockers can sometimes be helpful, as can a trial of withdrawing dopamine analogues if possible (e.g. bromocriptine). Headaches caused by haemorrhage that originates within a pituitary mass (pituitary apoplexy) or haemorrhage following pituitary infarction (e.g. in some cases of Sheehan's syndrome) are characteristic of meningeal irritation and tend to start abruptly. Headaches can be cured by transsphenoidal surgery or precipitated by the same.

PRIMARY TREATMENT

With the exception of prolactinomas, first-line treatment for pituitary adenomas that hypersecrete or cause mass effects remains transsphenoidal decompression. This remains the case if the lesion extends into the suprasellar cistern although, if the diaphragma is substantially intact, a pterional or subfrontal approach is sometimes preferred. Outcomes depend critically on the skill of the operator, but even the most gifted and experienced surgeons are rarely able to fully excise a pituitary macroadenoma.

Meningitis and damage to visual apparatus or vascular structures is rare with standard or endoscopic surgery, but longer-term problems of hypopituitarism, impaired olfaction or gustation and a tendency to sinusitis if the nasal septum is damaged or displaced are more common. Endoscopic transsphenoidal surgery requires more generous access and has a higher risk of CSF leakage.

WHY IS ADJUVANT TREATMENT NEEDED?

Most clinically significant pituitary disease results from sporadic pituitary adenoma formation. Complete excision of a pituitary adenoma of any description is far from a universal surgical outcome. Approximately 30% of non-functioning pituitary macroadenomas increase in size to some extent within 5–10 years of the original surgical intervention[5] and micro-invasion of surrounding structures is common.[6] Certainly for endocrinologically inactive macroadenomas the aim of primary surgical intervention is debulking rather than attempted complete excision as this addresses immediate issues of space occupation and seems in many cases to discourage remnant growth. Even in optimistic series, clinically significant residual tumour tissue is present in at least 20% of cases.[7] After surgery for tumour recurrence, almost 40% of patients experience a sustained remission,[8] yet up to 60% of functioning pituitary macroadenomas remain biochemically active after primary treatment[9, 10] and, particularly for these, adjuvant treatment may be required.

Recognition of the benign nature of the vast majority of pituitary adenomas, technical advances in transsphenoidal surgery, particularly more effective and comfortable ways to close the bony deficit in the pituitary fossa and sphenoid, nagging concerns about potential long-term side effects of radiotherapy and improved screening with the ready availability of high-quality (and X irradiation-free) MRI has made watchful waiting the norm.

If the adenoma extends laterally into a cavernous sinus, proximal to the carotid syphon and cranial nerves without any danger of impingement on the optic apparatus, other treatments are likely to be first line.

PROLACTINOMA

A dopaminergic drug, typically cabergoline (0.25–1 mg once or twice a week) or bromocriptine (2.5–10 mg daily) is first-line treatment for prolactinomas. Although dopamine agonists are not teratogenic, current best practice at the time of writing, with no clear rationale, is to stop dopamine analogues when pregnancy is confirmed. Symptomatic tumour regrowth during pregnancy is unusual. The convenience and excellent side-effect profile of the long-acting, ergot-derived D2 agonist cabergoline made it the preferred treatment in most cases until 2007 when (along with pergolide) an association with valvular heart disease was described[11, 12] At the low doses used for prolactinoma rather than Parkinson's disease, the same association has not been demonstrated in pituitary disease[13, 14] and echocardiographic screening is not generally considered necessary.

Microprolactinoma

Where drug treatment is not first-line owing to side effects or costs, microadenomectomy in symptomatic premenopausal women may be curative if a suitably skilled and experienced surgeon is available. If fertility is not required and galactorrhoea is not an issue, oestrogen replacement may be a satisfactory alternative to a dopamine agonist. Postmenopausally, it may be perfectly appropriate to offer no specific treatment other than reassurance. Microprolactinomas occasionally spontaneously resolve (about 7% overall, increasing to almost one third after a pregnancy) but change little in size in response to dopamine analogues.

Macroprolactinoma

It is rare for surgical decompression alone to bring prolactin output from a macroprolactinoma into a range when no further treatment is required. Biopsy is rarely required to confirm the diagnosis, but very occasionally surprisingly large prolactinomas release very modest amounts of prolactin and are mistaken for endocrinologically inactive macroadenomas that are assumed to be restricting portal dopamine flow by compressing the pituitary stalk. Surgery may be appropriate, however, if the patient's compliance with tablet treatment is poor or if the patient is intolerant of dopamine analogues, usually because of psychoses or intractable nausea and dysphoria. Prolactinomas are rarely resistant to dopamine analogues but occasionally response times are relatively prolonged.

Unless accompanied by haemorrhage and altered blood or cystic degeneration, 90% of macroprolactinomas can be expected to shrink with dopamine analogue treatment,[15] to the extent that, if the sphenoid bone has been eroded, a CSF leak may result. A small proportion of macroprolactinomas involute completely after long-term dopamine analogue treatment and treatment can be cautiously withdrawn without tumour recurrence.

The second generation alkylating chemotherapeutic agent temozolomide, related to the imidazotetrazines used primarily for grade IV astrocytomas (i.e. glioblastoma multiforme) and sometimes for oligodendrogliomas, has been used successfully for exceptionally rare and resistant cases of malignant pituitary adenomas including a case of malignant (i.e. metastatic) prolactinoma.[16] Anecdotally, a useful effect of temozolomide has been reported in approximately two thirds of 16 pituitary carcinomas and 30 aggressive pituitary adenoma cases.[17]

SOMATOTROPHINOMA

Even in the hands of experienced surgeons, primary transsphenoidal decompression of somatotroph adenomas in isolation has only a 50:50 chance of achieving immediate and longer-term biochemical remission. At least one third of post-operative patients have persistent disease despite additional medical therapy.[18] Even if the GH response to a glucose load meets the current criterion of 'cure', i.e. GH suppression to <1 mcg/L after a 75 g oral glucose load, a further post-operative cohort continues to experience subtle symptoms that significantly impair quality of life, associated with a normal or only modestly elevated IGF1. Persistent disease is associated with an approximately fourfold increased risk of colorectal carcinoma and with widespread arthralgia and arthritis, impaired glucose tolerance, hypertension, carpal tunnel syndrome, sweating, obstructive sleep apnoea and dysmorphophobia, all of which contribute to a 30% increase in all-cause mortality[19] and all of which need individual and specific management irrespective of ongoing pituitary function or dysfunction.

Somatostatin analogues

Evidence for a beneficial effect of somatostatin analogue treatment before pituitary surgery is inconsistent and unconvincing. In the event that surgery and sometimes repeated pituitary surgery does not secure remission, or when surgery is inappropriate owing to comorbidity, infirmity, technical difficulty (i.e. tumour remnants are out of reach) or because it does not concord with the patient's wishes, long-acting somatostatin analogues are typically the adjuvant treatment of first choice. Somatostatin analogues are reasonably well tolerated, although they produce variable abdominal cramping and bloating that diminishes over time but may recur for a short time after each injection. Accumulation of biliary sludge resulting from reduction in gallbladder motility is rarely a problem. A modest degree of remnant tumour shrinkage (typically by about one third volume (10–50%) in a third to a half of cases[20-22] probably results from a reduction in the size of individual somatotroph cells and hence in overall tumour size rather than an absolute reduction in somatotroph cell numbers. Circulating growth hormone and IGF1 levels drop fairly rapidly into the reference range in about 50% of cases, and typically the efficacy of treatment becomes more pronounced over time such that, after about 5 years, most patients have circulating GH levels within the 'normal range'. Doses are titrated up if control is not achieved after several months' treatment, but over time it may be possible to reduce the dose or increase the dosing interval further.[23] Long-term treatment has significant economic costs and can over time become irksome for patients for whom uncomfortable and socially disruptive injections are a life sentence. For many patients who are not put into remission by initial surgery, somatostatin analogues are used until such time as fractionated radiotherapy takes effect.

Newer long-acting and broad spectrum somatostatin receptor ligand with high affinity to receptor subtypes 1,2,3 and 5 (pasireotide) and chimeric somatostatin and dopamine receptor agonists – dopastatins[24] (BIM-23A760[25]) – have yet to show any particular advantage in terms of comfort or control.[26]

Growth hormone receptor antagonists

Pegvisomant is a growth hormone (GH) antagonist with a half-life of greater than 70 hours delivered as a daily or weekly subcutaneous bolus.[27, 28] It interferes with growth hormone signalling and by so doing produces a high rate of normalization of insulin-like growth factor 1 in patients with somatotroph adenomas, including those in whom somatostatin analogues alone are insufficient to gain control of hormone secretion.[29, 30] Used in isolation, reduced feedback inhibition results in a concurrent increase in circulating growth hormone levels by about 75%. Concerns that tumour growth may accelerate if pegvisomant is used in patients without concurrent somatostatin analogues or prior radiotherapy have not been substantiated, at least during the first 3 years of treatment,[31] although increases have been reported in around 2% of cases.[32] The prohibitive costs of these analogues and side effects, particularly liver function abnormalities that affect approximately 25% of patients, albeit transient, mean that its place in acromegaly management alone and in combination with somatostatin analogues has yet to be established.[33]

Dopamine receptor agonists

Cabergoline, a second-generation long-acting dopamine agonist, reduces GH to within the reference range in a quarter to a third of patients with acromegaly[34, 35] and reduced IGF1 to within the reference range in one third,[36] an effect that is additive to that of somatostatin analogues[36] and independent of prolactin levels.[37] Despite these data, controversy persists, with groups reporting no effect of cabergoline but efficacy with quinagolide,[38] and others contending that bromocriptine has no effect and cabergoline only modest efficacy in fewer than 10% of patients as an adjunct to treatment with somatostatin analogues.[19]

Conventional fractionated radiotherapy

Radiotherapy is no longer an automatic adjunct to pituitary tumour surgery owing to the ease and safety of follow-up with MRI and computerized visual fields, and the expectation that remnant growth will be minimal and predictable. Nevertheless, it remains a useful and safe but relatively slow-acting treatment in selected patients in whom progression of unresectable tumour or excess hormone secretion persists.[39] In patients who have yet to complete their families the significant ongoing risk of hypopituitarism over the first 8–10 years is a further contraindication, given the expense of ovulation induction and restoration of male fertility using exogenous gonadotrophins.[40] External beam radiotherapy is remarkably safe, but long-term effects of external beam radiotherapy on cerebral vasculature and on the induction of secondary brain tumours within the radiation field, which amounts to a 2–4% risk at 20 years, is a more significant concern in young patients.[41, 42]

Early side effects of radiotherapy are generally limited to tiredness during the latter stages of treatment and for several weeks after treatment, and occasionally headaches and transient loss of a small amount of scalp hair, particularly with the older linear accelerator protocols using just three trans-cerebral windows.

Stereotactic radiosurgery

Stereotactic or gamma knife radiosurgery for acromegaly allows radiotherapy to be delivered in one rather exhausting and uncomfortable day for the patient rather than fractionated over several weeks. Somatotrophinomas are not the pituitary adenoma subtype most amenable to Gamma knife radiosurgery owing to their size when they tend to come to treatment.[43] In patients who for the most part have already failed conventional treatment with surgery, conventional fractionated stereotactic radiotherapy and drugs, local tumour control is typically achieved in 37–100% and hormonal control in 17–82% within 2–3 years. New pituitary hormone deficiency occurs in 33–40% of patients over this time[44–48] but otherwise side effects are minimal.[49]

CORTICOTROPHINOMA

Corticotroph adenomas are typically microadenomas at diagnosis and extension beyond the confines of the sella is unusual. Nevertheless, even in the most optimistic published series, pituitary surgery alone fails to induce remission in Cushing's disease in 10–30% of cases and as many as 10% of patients are still obviously affected in the long term. If surgical remission is achieved, there remains a significant, persistent and unpredictable tendency to relapse that affects almost one third of patients by 10 years.

Depending on the clinical circumstances, disease that clearly persists immediately after attempted transsphenoidal microadenomectomy may be addressed by a further, more radical transsphenoidal clearance often within hours or days of the first approach. If preservation of pituitary function, in particular fertility, is a priority and no obvious microadenomatous remnants are visible on pituitary imaging, laparoscopic bilateral adrenalectomy rather than pituitary radiotherapy or a further transsphenoidal approach may be preferred. Nelson's syndrome, disinhibition of corticotroph remnant growth following bilateral adrenalectomy owing to reduced glucocorticoid feedback, is rare, particularly so if very little corticotroph adenoma tissue is present in the fossa, and there is no established rationale for prophylactic pituitary radiotherapy in these circumstances. Although lifelong treatment with glucocorticoids and mineralocorticoids is required, cure is immediate and the morbidity of the procedure itself low.

Many different groups of drugs have been proposed as useful in Cushing's disease, including metyrapone, mitotane, ketoconazole, etomidate, aminoglutethimide, trilostane, mifepristone, sodium valproate, dopamine D2 agonists, reserpine, serotonin antagonists, somatostatin receptor agonists, Bexarotene (a retinoid targeted to retinoid X receptors), the NF-kappaB inhibitor parthenolide, PPAR-gamma receptor ligands and Lapatinib, a tyrosine kinase inhibitor that interrupts the human epidermal growth factor receptor 2 (HER2) pathway.

In practical terms metyrapone, a steroid 11β-hydroxylase inhibitor that has been available in Europe for the last 50 years (500 mg–4 g daily in divided doses) is a reliable, reversible inhibitor of adrenal cortisol synthesis and secretion. It is sometimes used to improve overall metabolic and tissue status prior to transsphenoidal surgery or occasionally to help determine whether more invasive treatment of mild hypercortisolaemia is likely to yield symptomatic benefit. Metyrapone is also exploited as an interim adjunctive therapy while waiting for pituitary radiotherapy to reduce corticotroph function or as sole treatment in the longer term if patients are unable or unwilling to tolerate surgery, as its effects are not subject to tachyphylaxis. The drug should not be used in pregnancy or during lactation, but otherwise significant side effects are few, other than gastrointestinal upset and mild hirsutism.[50] Even if hypocortisolaemia is avoided, the effects of a rapid fall in circulating cortisol levels to within normal limits may for some patients result in depressed mood, arthralgia and in the slightly longer term by disappointment that weight loss is not sustained and that dyslipidaemia, hypertension and impaired glucose tolerance may continue to need specific treatment. Failure of the phenotype to completely regress even after full biochemical remission contributes to a significantly reduced quality of life in the long term and demoralizing recognition that, despite biochemical remission, the perceived pre-morbid 'self' may be very slow to re-emerge.

Ketoconazole, an imidazole derivative used to treat mycoses by inhibiting fungal sterol synthesis, is also used when physical treatments such as transsphenoidal surgery are inappropriate or have failed or the effects of radiotherapy are awaited. Although unlicensed for this indication in the UK, ketoconazole is believed to be effective in reducing circulating cortisol levels in up to 70% of cases – an endpoint that does not equate with remission.[51]

Mitotane is a hepatotoxic, neurotoxic and teratogenic adrenal cytotoxic agent that is highly persistent in the body and generally reserved for unresectable, metastatic or relapsed adrenal cortical carcinoma. It has been used in Cushing's disease (i.e. pituitary-dependent Cushing's syndrome) as first- or second-line treatment[52] but is slow to induce remission, not well tolerated, requires monthly plasma level monitoring and, even if effective in the short term, does not prevent recurrence of the disease in most patients over a median of 13 months.[52]

Etomidate is an intravenous inducing agent that at sub-anaesthetic doses (0.1 mg/kg per hour) powerfully inhibits adrenal 11β-hydroxylase.[53] It has a very rapid onset of action and can be easily titrated against circulating cortisol levels in a high dependency setting.[54] For patients in whom metyrapone or ketoconazole is ineffective in controlling severe hypercortisolaemia, etomidate as a continual infusion is uniquely effective and can be used to rapidly suppress otherwise intractable neuropsychiatric symptoms and give tissues time to recover from high-level cortisol exposure prior to bilateral adrenalectomy.

Centrally acting drugs such as sodium valproate, cabergoline and cyproheptadine are rarely effective. The broad spectrum somatostatin receptor agonist pasireotide shows only partial efficacy in a minority of patients and is associated with significant side effects such as impaired glucose tolerance and frank diabetes[55] in the majority. Mifepristone, a synthetic steroid inhibitor of progesterone receptors used as an emergency contraceptive, is also a powerful type 2 glucocorticoid receptor antagonist. It is approved by the FDA as a therapy to diminish the metabolic effects of hypercortisolaemia in Cushing's syndrome.

Even in remission, patients with a history of corticotroph adenoma have an increased standardized mortality ratio compared to age-matched controls.

THYROTROPH ADENOMA

Debulking transsphenoidal adenomectomy is the primary treatment of choice for thyrotroph adenomas. Even if primary surgical treatment restores euthyroidism in this rare secretory subtype (which accounts for less than 1% of pituitary tumours coming to surgery), external beam radiotherapy to the pituitary bed is often strongly considered as early adjuvant treatment as thyrotroph adenomas have a particular propensity to recur and as, if they do, the presence of thyrotoxicosis, which would be a significant additional surgical risk, can only be directly controlled at the expense of further disinhibition of thyrotroph function. Somatostatin analogues are effective in suppressing thyrotrophin release but tumours typically escape control over time.

PITUITARY CARCINOMAS

The limited dural invasion often seen in pituitary adenomas explains the occasional persistence of symptoms of excess hormone secretion even in the presence of an apparently empty sella. Pituitary carcinoma presenting as metastatic pituitary disease, however, is fortunately rare, constituting less than 0.2% of pituitary adenomas.[56] Over the last 50 years fewer than 150 have been reported in the literature, 36% of which were prolactinomas and 30% corticotroph adenomas.[57] The correlation between behavioural characteristics and mitotic markers such as $p53$ mutation and Ki-67 is too weak to allow pre-emptive treatment and the diagnosis only becomes apparent when repeated imaging discloses aggressive trophic characteristics and metastatic spread. In addition to debulking and radiotherapy, the orally active second-generation alkylating agent temozolomide has been used in cases of aggressive pituitary adenomas and pituitary carcinomas having previously been reserved for malignant glioma. In a recent series of 44 patients, three cycles of treatment (200 mg/m^2 daily for 5 days every 28 days) produced a response rate of around one third of patients, with reduction in tumour volume, or more typically, reduction in the rate of tumour progression. It is of some interest that, at the time of writing, several patients who have received ipilimumab, a cytotoxic T-lymphocyte-associated antigen 4 (CTLA-4) monoclonal antibody used to treat metastatic melanoma, have rapidly developed anterior pituitary failure presumably of autoimmune origin. Whether this could be used in extremis in pituitary carcinoma has not yet been explored.[58]

ENDOCRINOLOGICALLY INACTIVE ADENOMAS AND GONADOTROPHINOMAS

No specific management options are available after surgery and radiotherapy, although agents such as dopamine analogues have been tried. *In vitro*, the dopamine–somatostatin chimeric compound BIM-23A760 has been shown to have very modest antiproliferative actions,[59] but any medical therapy for endocrinologically inactive pituitary adenomas is a triumph of optimism over evidence. Endocrinologically inactive pituitary adenomas are sensitive to radiotherapy and trophic stasis or tumour shrinkage after a medium of 12.5 Gy delivered by stereotactic radiosurgery (gamma knife) controls tumour size in at least 90% of patients, with reduced risks of secondary tumour induction and cerebral vasculopathy compared to standard fractionated radiotherapy.[60, 61]

CRANIOPHARYNGIOMA

At one time craniopharyngioma was thought to be relatively radioresistant, and some centres withhold radiotherapy after primary surgery pending an evaluation of further growth even when initial decompression has been relatively modest.[62] Aggressive attempts to resect craniopharyngioma are associated with significant morbidity, and experimental therapies such as intracystic P32, bleomycin or yttrium-90 have not gained acceptance.[63, 64]

> **KEY POINTS**
> - Surgical outcomes of pituitary adenoma treatment continue to depend very heavily on the innate skill of specialist surgeons.
> - In adults, LINAC remains a very effective and safe treatment that reduces significant craniopharyngioma and pituitary tumour space occupying-recurrence 5-fold.
> - A significant minority of non-cystic macroprolactinomas involute completely after prolonged dopamine agonist treatment.
> - In acromegaly, quality of life depends primarily on attention to the management of obstructive sleep apnoea, arthritis, orthodontic problems, dysmorphophobia and cardiovascular risks.
> - Metyrapone is a reliable and safe inhibitor of adrenal cortisol synthesis and secretion in the medium if not long term.

REFERENCES

1. Molitch ME. Pituitary incidentalomas. *Endocrinol Metab Clin North Am* 1997; **26**: 725–40.
2. Ezzat S, Asa SL, Couldwell WT, et al. The prevalence of pituitary adenomas: a systematic review. *Cancer* 2004; **101**(3): 613–19.
3. Lindholm J, Juul S, Jørgensen JO, et al. Incidence and late prognosis of Cushing's syndrome: a population-based study. *J Clin Endocrinol Metab* 2001; **86**(1): 117–23.
4. Levy A. Molecular and trophic mechanisms of tumorigenesis. *Endocrinol Metab Clin North Am* 2008; **37**(1): 23–50.
5. Chanson P, Brochier S. Non-functioning pituitary adenoma. *J Endocrinol Invest* 2005; **28**(11 Suppl International): 93–9.
6. Pegolo G, Buckwalter JG, Weiss MH, Hinton DR. Pituitary adenomas: correlation of the cytologic appearance with biologic behavior. *Acta Cytol* 1995; **39**(5): 887–92.
7. Meij BP, Lopes MB, Ellegalla DB, et al. The long-term significance of microscopic dural invasion in 354 patients with pituitary adenomas treated with transsphenoidal surgery. *J Neurosurg* 2002; **96**(2): 195–208.
8. Benveniste RJ, King WA, Walsh J, et al. Repeated transsphenoidal surgery to treat recurrent or residual pituitary adenoma. *J Neurosurg* 2005; **102**(6): 1004–12.
9. Jenkins D, O'Brien I, Johnson A, et al. The Birmingham pituitary database: auditing the outcome of the treatment of acromegaly. *Clin Endocrinol (Oxf)* 1995; **43**(5): 517–22.
10. Prevedello DM, Pouratian N, Sherman J, et al. Management of Cushing's disease: outcome in patients with microadenoma detected on pituitary magnetic resonance imaging. *J Neurosurg* 2008; **109**(4): 751–9.
11. Schade R, Andersohn F, Suissa S, et al. Dopamine agonists and the risk of cardiac-valve regurgitation. *N Engl J Med* 2007; **356**: 29–38.
12. Zanettini R, Antonini A, Gatto G, et al. Valvular heart disease and the use of dopamine agonists for Parkinson's disease. *N Engl J Med* 2007; **356**: 39–46.
13. Bogazzi F, Buralli S, Manetti L, et al. Treatment with low doses of cabergoline is not associated with increased prevalence of cardiac valve regurgitation in patients with hyperprolactinaemia. *Int J Clin Practice* 2008; **62**(12): 1864–9.
14. Wakil A, Rigby AS, Clark AL, et al. Low dose cabergoline for hyperprolactinaemia is not associated with clinically significant valvular heart disease. *Eur J Endocrinol* 2008; **159**: R11–R14.
15. Bevan JS, Webster J, Burke CW, Scanlon MF. Dopamine agonists and pituitary tumor shrinkage. *Endocr Rev* 1992; **13**(2): 220–40.
16. Byrne S, Karapetis C, Vrodos N. A novel use of temozolomide in a patient with malignant prolactinoma. *J Clin Neurosci* 2009; **16**(12): 1694–6.
17. Ortiz LD, Syro LV, Scheithauer BW, et al. Temozolomide in aggressive pituitary adenomas and carcinomas. *Clinics* 2012; **67**(S1): 119–23.
18. Arosio M, Reimondo G, Malchiodi E, et al. Predictors of morbidity and mortality in acromegaly, an Italian survey. *Eur J Endocrinol* 2012; **167**(2): 189–98.
19. Melmed S, Colao A, Barkan A, et al. Guidelines for acromegaly management: an update. *J Clin Endocrinol Metab* 2009; **94**: 1509–17.
20. Bevan JS. The anti-tumoral effects of somatostatin analog therapy in acromegaly. *J Clin Endocrinol Metab* 2005; **90**: 1856–63.
21. Melmed S, Sternberg R, Cook D, et al. A critical analysis of pituitary tumor shrinkage during primary medical therapy in acromegaly. *J Clin Endocrinol Metab* 2005; **90**: 4405–10.
22. Giustina A, Mazziotti G, Torri V, et al. Meta-analysis on the effects of octreotide on tumor mass in acromegaly. *PLoS One* 2012; **7**(5): e36411.
23. Colao A, Auriemma RS, Galdiero M, et al. Effects of initial therapy for five years with somatostatin analogs for acromegaly on growth hormone and insulin-like growth factor-1 levels, tumor shrinkage, and cardiovascular disease: a prospective study. *J Clin Endocrinol Metab* 2009; **94**(10): 3746–56.
24. Jaquet P, Gunz G, Saveanu A, et al. BIM-23A760, a chimeric molecule directed towards somatostatin and dopamine receptors, vs universal somatostatin receptors ligands in GH-secreting pituitary adenomas partial responders to octreotide. *J Endocrinol Invest* 2005; **28**(11 Suppl International): 21–7.
25. Kumar SS, Ayuk J, Murray RD. Current therapy and drug pipeline for the treatment of patients with acromegaly. *Adv Ther* 2009; **26**(4): 383–403.
26. Petersenn, S., J. Schopohl, Barkan A, et al. Pasireotide (SOM230) demonstrates efficacy and safety in patients with acromegaly: a randomized, multicenter, phase II trial. *J Clin Endocrinol Metab* 2010; **95**(6): 2781–9.
27. Feenstra J, de Herder W, ten Have SM, et al. Combined therapy with somatostatin analogues and weekly pegvisomant in active acromegaly. *Lancet* 2005; **365**(9471): 1620.
28. Higham CE, Thomas JD, Bidlingmaier M, et al. Successful use of weekly pegvisomant administration in patients with acromegaly. *Eur J Endocrinol* 2009; **161**: 21–5.
29. Colao A, Pivonello R, Auriemma RS, et al. Efficacy of 12-month treatment with the GH receptor antagonist pegvisomant in patients with acromegaly resistant to long-term, high-dose somatostatin analog treatment: effect on IGF-I levels, tumor mass, hypertension and glucose tolerance. *Eur J Endocrinol* 2006; **154**: 467–77.
30. Plöckinger U. Medical therapy of acromegaly. *Int J Endocrinol* 2012; **2012**: 268957.
31. Jimenez C, Burman P, Abs R, et al. Follow-up of pituitary tumor volume in patients with acromegaly treated with pegvisomant in clinical trials. *Eur J Endocrinol* 2008; **159**: 517–23.
32. van der Lely AJ, Biller BMK, Brue T, et al. Long-term safety of pegvisomant in patients with acromegaly: comprehensive review of 1288 subjects in ACROSTUDY. *J Clin Endocrinol Metab* 2012; **97**(5): 1589–97.
33. Moore DJ, Yaser A, Connock MJ, Bayliss S. Clinical effectiveness and cost-effectiveness of pegvisomant for the treatment of acromegaly: a systematic review and economic evaluation. *BMC Endocr Disord* 2009; **9**: 20.
34. Abs R, Verhelst J, Maiter D, et al. Cabergoline in the treatment of acromegaly: a study in 64 patients. *J Clin Endocrinol Metab* 1998; **83**(2): 374–8.
35. Moyes VJ, Metcalfe KA, Drake WM. Clinical use of cabergoline as primary and adjunctive treatment for acromegaly. *Eur J Endocrinol* 2008; **159**(5): 541–5.
36. Sandret L, Maison P, Chanson P. Place of cabergoline in acromegaly: a meta-analysis. *J Clin Endocrinol Metab* 2011; **96**(5): 1327–35.
37. Cozzi R, Attanasio R, Lodrini S, Lasio G. Cabergoline addition to depot somatostatin analogues in resistant acromegalic patients: efficacy and lack of predictive value of prolactin status. *Clin Endocrinol (Oxf)* 2004; **61**(2): 209–15.
38. Colao A, Ferone D, Marzullo P, et al. Effect of different dopaminergic agents in the treatment of acromegaly. *J Clin Endocrinol Metab* 1997; **82**(2): 518–23.
39. Schalin-Jäntti C, Valanne L, Tenhunen M, et al. Outcome of fractionated stereotactic radiotherapy in patients with pituitary adenomas resistant to conventional treatments: a 5.25-year follow-up study. *Clin Endocrinol (Oxf)* 2010; **73**(1): 72–7.
40. Plowman PN. Pituitary adenoma radiotherapy: when, who and how? *Clin Endocrinol (Oxf)* 2001; **51**(3): 265–71.
41. McCord MW, Buatti JM, Fennell EM, et al. Radiotherapy for pituitary adenoma: long-term outcome and sequelae. *Int J Radiat Oncol Biol Phys* 1997; **39**(2): 437–44.
42. Erfurth EM, Hagmar L. Cerebrovascular disease in patients with pituitary tumors. *Trends Endocrinol Metab* 2005; **16**(7): 334–42.
43. Kobayashi T. Long-term results of stereotactic gamma knife radiosurgery for pituitary adenomas. Specific strategies for different types of adenoma. *Prof Neurol Surg* 2009; **22**: 77–95.
44. Pamir MN, Kilic T, Belirgen M, et al. Pituitary adenomas treated with gamma knife radiosurgery: volumetric analysis of 100 cases with minimum 3 year follow-up. *Neurosurgery* 2007; **61**(2): 270–80.
45. Jagannathan J, Sheehan JP, Pouratian N, et al. Gamma knife radiosurgery for acromegaly: outcomes after failed transsphenoidal surgery. *Neurosurgery* 2008; **62**(6): 1262–9.
46. Swords FM, Monson JP, Besser GM, et al. Gamma knife radiosurgery: a safe and effective salvage treatment for pituitary tumours not controlled despite conventional radiotherapy. *Eur J Endocrinol* 2009; **161**(6): 819–28.
47. Stapleton CJ, Liu CY, Weiss MH. The role of stereotactic radiosurgery in the multi-modal management of growth hormone-secreting pituitary adenomas. *Neurosurg Focus* 2010; **29**(4): E11.
48. Liu X, Kano H, Kondziolka D, et al. Gamma knife radiosurgery for clinically persistent acromegaly. *J Neurooncol* 2012; **109**(1): 71–9.
49. Wilson PJ, De-Loyde KJ, Williams JR, Smee RI. A single centre's experience of stereotactic radiosurgery and radiotherapy

49. for non-functioning pituitary adenomas with the Linear Accelerator (Linac). *J Clin Neurosci* 2012; **19**(3): 370–4.
50. Jeffcoate WJ, Rees LH, Tomlin S, et al. Metyrapone in long-term management of Cushings' disease. *Br Med J* 1977; **2**(6081): 215–17.
51. Nieman LK. Medical therapy of Cushing's disease. *Pituitary* 2002; **5**(2): 77–82.
52. Baudry C, Coste J, Bou Khalil R, et al. Efficiency and tolerance of mitotane in Cushing's disease in 76 patients from a single centre. *Eur J Endocrinol* 2012; **167**(4): 473–81.
53. Schulte HM, Benker G, Reinwein D, et al. Infusion of low dose etomidate: correction of hypercortisolemia in patients with Cushing's syndrome and dose-response relationship in normal subjects. *J Clin Endocrinol Metab* 1990; **70**(5): 1426–30.
54. Drake WM, Perry LA, Hinds CJ, et al. Emergency and prolonged use of intravenous etomidate to control hypercortisolemia in a patient with Cushing's syndrome and peritonitis. *J Clin Endocrinol Metab* 1998; **83**(10): 3542–4.
55. Colao A, Petersenn S, Newell-Price J, et al. A 12-month phase 3 study of pasireotide in Cushing's disease. *N Eng J Med* 2012; **366**(10): 914–24.
56. Roncaroli F, Scheithauer BW, Young WF, et al. Silent corticotroph carcinoma of the adenohypophysis: a report of five cases. *Am J Surg Pathol* 2003; **27**(4): 477–86.
57. Dudziak K, Honegger J, Bornemann A, et al. Pituitary carcinoma with malignant growth from first presentation and fulminant clinical course: case report and review of the literature. *J Clin Endocrinol Metab* 2011; **96**(9): 2665–9.
58. Min L, Vaidya A, Becker C. Association of ipilimumab therapy for advanced melanoma with secondary adrenal insufficiency: a case series. *Endocr Pract* 2012; **18**(3): 351–5.
59. Peverelli E, Olgiati L, Locatelli M, et al. The dopamine-somatostatin chimeric compound BIM-23A760 exerts antiproliferative and cytotoxic effects in human non-functioning pituitary tumors by activating ERK1/2 and p38 pathways. *Cancer Lett* 2010; **288**(2): 170–6.
60. Thorén M, Höybye C, Grenbäck E, et al. The role of gamma knife radiosurgery in the management of pituitary adenomas. *J Neurooncol* 2001; **54**(2): 197–203.
61. Sheehan JP, Niranjan A, Sheehan JM, et al. Stereotactic radiosurgery for pituitary adenomas: an intermediate review of its safety, efficacy, and role in the neurosurgical treatment armamentarium. *J Neurosurg* 2005; **102**(4): 678–91.
62. Van Effenterre R, Boch AL. Craniopharyngioma in adults and children: a study of 122 surgical cases. *J Neurosurg* 2002; **97**(1): 3–11.
63. Wisoff JH. Craniopharyngioma. *J Neurosurg Pediatr* 2008; **1**(2): 124–5.
64. Di Mambro A, Giuliani C, Ammannati F, et al. A single-institution restrospective experience of brachytherapy in the treatment of pituitary tumors: transsphenoidal approach combined with (192) Ir-afterloading catheters. *J Endocrinol Invest* 2010; **33**(7): 455–60.

Section 3
Rhinology

87	Anatomy of the nose and paranasal sinuses 961		103	Nasal septum and nasal valve 1135
88	Outpatient assessment 977		104	Nasal septal perforations 1149
89	Physiology of the nose and paranasal sinuses 983		105	Management of the enlarged turbinates 1157
90	Measurement of the nasal airway 991		106	Epistaxis 1169
91	Allergic rhinitis 999		107	Nasal and facial fractures 1183
92	Non-allergic perennial rhinitis 1011		108	CSF leaks 1203
93	Occupational rhinitis 1017		109	Granulomatous conditions of the nose 1211
94	Rhinosinusitis: Definitions, classification and diagnosis 1025		110	Abnormalities of smell 1227
			111	Disorders of the orbit 1243
95	Nasal polyposis 1037		112	Diagnosis and management of facial pain 1253
96	Fungal rhinosinusitis 1047		113	Juvenile angiofibroma 1265
97	Medical management for rhinosinusitis 1059		114	Endoscopic management of sinonasal tumours 1269
98	Surgical management of rhinosinusitis 1071		115	Surgical management of pituitary and parasellar diseases 1281
99	The frontal sinus 1081			
100	Mucoceles of the paranasal sinuses 1107		116	Extended anterior skull base approaches 1289
101	Complications of rhinosinusitis 1113		117	Imaging in rhinology 1305
102	The relationship between the upper and lower respiratory tract 1125			

ANATOMY OF THE NOSE AND PARANASAL SINUSES

Dustin M. Dalgorf and Richard J. Harvey

Introduction 961	Paranasal sinuses 969
Development of the nose and paranasal sinus 961	Developmental and functional anatomy of the paranasal sinuses....... 972
External nose..964	Conclusion..976
Nasal septum 966	References 976

SEARCH STRATEGY

Data in this chapter may be updated by a PubMed and Medline search using the following keywords: paranasal sinuses, maxillary sinus, ethmoid sinus, frontal sinus, nasal cavity, nasal bone, nasal cartilages, nasal mucosa, nasal septum and turbinates. Evidence presented in this chapter is Levels 3 and 4 while recommendations are Grace C.

INTRODUCTION

This chapter outlines the embryological development of the nose and paranasal sinuses, neurovascular and anatomical structures of the external nose, nasal cavity and nasal septum. A surgically relevant approach to the paranasal sinus anatomy is discussed with a focus on fixed anatomical landmarks and the concept of the horizontal and vertical components of the paranasal surgical box. The anatomical descriptions and surgically relevant anatomical concepts are based on standard text, peer reviewed journals referenced in the bibliography and the author's personal experience.

DEVELOPMENT OF THE NOSE AND PARANASAL SINUS

Traditional teaching of paranasal sinus anatomy focused on embryological development and pathways of pneumatization with limited clinical application. These descriptions are included for completeness but the emphasis in this chapter is on the surgically relevant anatomy

External nose and nasal cavity

The nose develops from a number of mesenchymal processes around the primitive mouth during the fourth week of gestation. Collections of neural crest cells undergo proliferation and form the nasal placodes. Sinking of the nasal placodes leads to formation of the nasal pits which further deepen to form the nasal sac. Adjacent mesoderm cells proliferate to give rise to the medial and lateral nasal prominences of the frontonasal process which surround the nasal pit and sac to eventually become the nares (**Figure 87.1**).

The maxillary processes grow anteriorly and medially to fuse with the medial nasal prominences and frontonasal process to close off the nasal pits and form separate nasal cavities. The primitive nasal cavity and mouth are initially separated by the bucconasal membrane. This membrane gradually thins as the nasal sacs extend posteriorly and

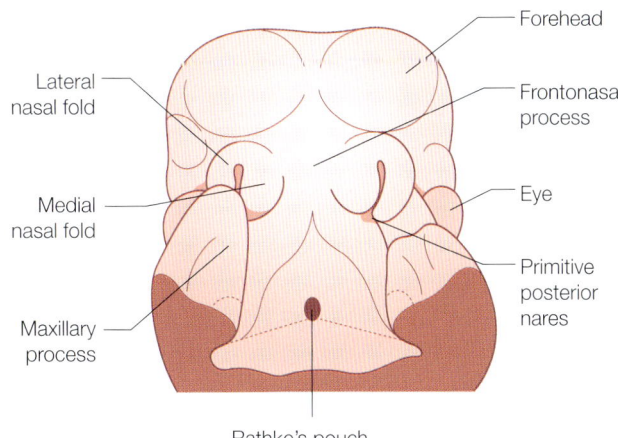

Figure 87.1 Embryological development of the primitive nose and palate during fusion of the maxillary process to the lateral and medial nasal prominences.

> **BOX 87.1**
>
> Failure of the bucconasal membrane to break down during embryological development results in choanal atresia

eventually breaks down to form the choanae. Failure of this membrane to break down results in choanal atresia.

The frontal and maxillary processes fuse to give origin to the lateral two thirds of the upper lip, superior alveolar ridges and palatal shelves. The medial nasal prominences fuse with the maxillary process to form the philtrum and medial crus of the lower lateral cartilages. The lateral nasal prominences form the nasal bones, upper lateral cartilages and lateral crus of the lower lateral cartilages.

Palate and nasal septum

The septum develops from the posterior midline growth of the frontonasal process in the root of the oral cavity and extends posteriorly to the opening of Rathke's pouch. The primitive or primary palate begins to form anteriorly with fusion of the maxillary and frontonasal processes. As the nasal cavities enlarge, the palatal processes, derived from lateral maxillary mesoderm, grow medially towards each other and the nasal septum. Initially, the palatal processes are vertically oriented and lateral to the tongue (**Figure 87.2**). Further growth of the jaw and oral cavity enables the palatal processes to migrate medially towards the midline and fuse (**Figure 87.3**). The fusion begins along the posterior margin of the primitive palate and progresses from anterior to posterior to form the secondary palate. Partial notching of the posterior hard palate represents an incomplete fusion of the secondary palate and may indicate a submucus cleft. A midline dehiscence in the fusion of the primary and secondary palate forms the incisive foramen.

Maxillary sinus

The maxillary sinus is the first sinus to appear between the 7th and 10th weeks of gestation. The maxillary sinus appears as a shallow groove expanding from the primitive ethmoidal infundibulum into the mass of the maxilla. Expansion and absorption results in a small sinus cavity present at birth. Rapid growth of this cavity occurs during childhood until age seven followed by gradual enlargement, reaching its final size by age 17–18 years. Growth may continue beyond this period with extensive pneumatization involving the entire hard palate (**Figure 87.4**).

Any disruption or abnormality in the development of the maxillary sinus may result in maxillary sinus aplasia or hypoplasia. Maxillary sinus hypoplasia is present in up to 10% of CT scans.[1] Radiographic diagnostic criteria for maxillary hypoplasia include: (1) enlargement of the vertical orbit, (2) lateral position of the infraorbital

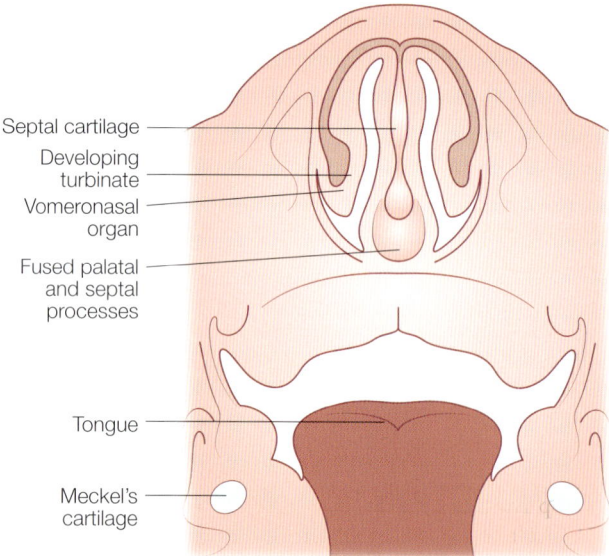

Figure 87.3 Section through the developing palate of a 48 mm human foetus. With further growth of the oral cavity to accommodate the tongue, the palatal shelves are able to migrate medially into a horizontal position and begin to fuse in an anterior to posterior direction.

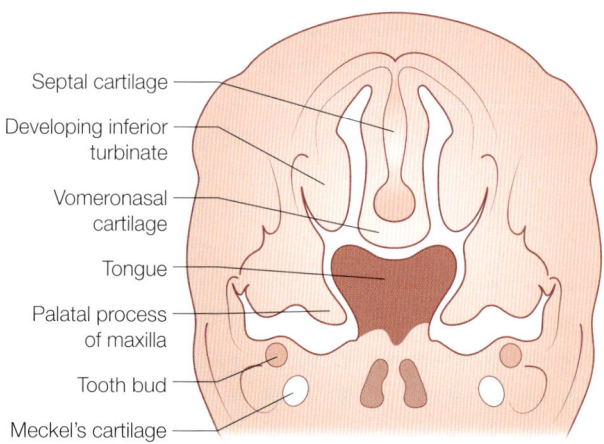

Figure 87.2 Section through the developing palate of a 20 mm human foetus. The palatal shelves are positioned vertically due to occupation of this space by the tongue.

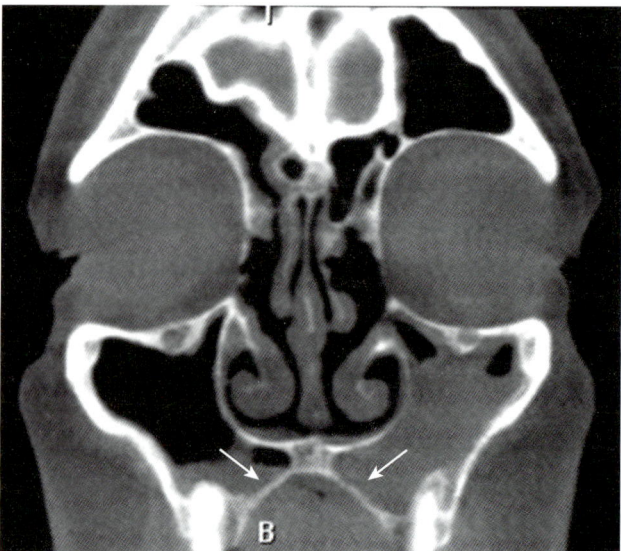

Figure 87.4 Coronal CT of extensive maxillary sinus penumatization into the hard palate (arrows) with evidence of maxillary sinus dysfunction (left greater than right).

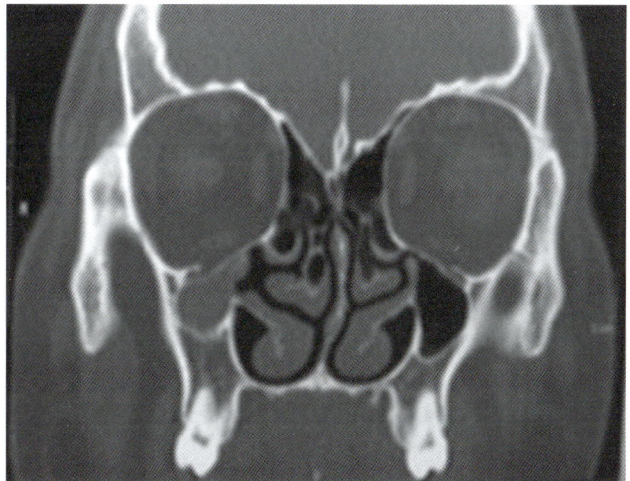

Figure 87.5 Coronal CT demonstrating maxillary sinus hypoplasia on the right side and maxillary sinus atelectasis on the left side.

neurovascular canal, (3) elevated canine fossa, (4) enlargement of superior orbital fissure and (5) enlargement of pterygopalatine fissure (**Figure 87.5**).[2]

Ethmoid sinus

During the 9th and 10th weeks of gestation, a series of folds called ethmoturbinals that are separated from each other by corresponding grooves appear in the lateral wall of the nasal capsule. Fusion of these folds leads to the development of crests, each with an ascending and descending portion. All permanent ethmoidal structures are present at birth and develop from these crests and the furrows between them. As a result, acute sinusitis in children often involves the ethmoid cavity which can extend laterally through the lamina papyracea causing orbital complications.

> **BOX 87.2**
>
> The ethmoid structures are present at birth and acute sinusitis involving this cavity can extend laterally and result in orbital complications.

Understanding the basic embryology of the four or five ethmoturbinals defines a series of lamella that must be removed in order to pass from the anterior of the sinonasal cavity to the sphenoid sinus. In order from anterior to posterior, these lamella include: FIRST: agger nasi (ascending portion) and uncinate process (descending portion), SECOND: bulla ethmoidalis, THIRD: basal lamella of the middle turbinate, FOURTH: superior turbinate and FIFTH: supreme turbinate if present.

Sphenoid sinus

The sphenoid sinus begins to develop in the twelfth week of gestation as an evagination from the sphenoethmoidal recess. A small sphenoid sinus is present at birth with progressive enlargement starting at age three during pneumatization of the sphenoid bone. Three pneumatization patterns have been described with reference to the sella turcica.[3] These pneumatization patterns are important for surgical planning of transphenoid approaches to pituitary tumours. These include sellar (90%), pre-sellar (9%) and conchal (1%) type pneumatization patterns (**Figure 87.6**). The sellar type is most common and describes sphenoid pneumatization posterior to the sella turcica. The presellar type describes sphenoid pneumatization up to the anterior sella and the conchal type describes a shallow bowl with minimal sphenoid pneumatization and trabecular bone between the sinus and sella. The sphenoid sinuses can also pneumatize laterally into the pterygoid root resulting in the presence of a lateral sphenoid recess (**Figure 87.7**). This pneumatization pattern results in exposure of the neurovascular structures surrounding the sphenoid sinus.

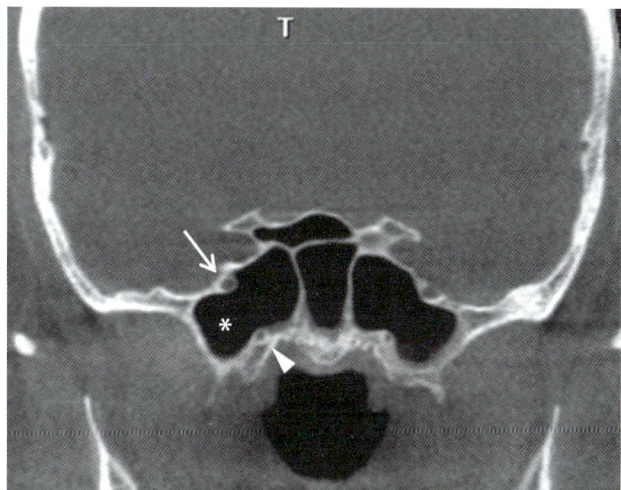

Figure 87.7 Coronal CT of sphenoid sinus. Lateral sphenoid recess (asterisk), maxillary division of trigeminal nerve (arrow), vidian nerve (arrow head).

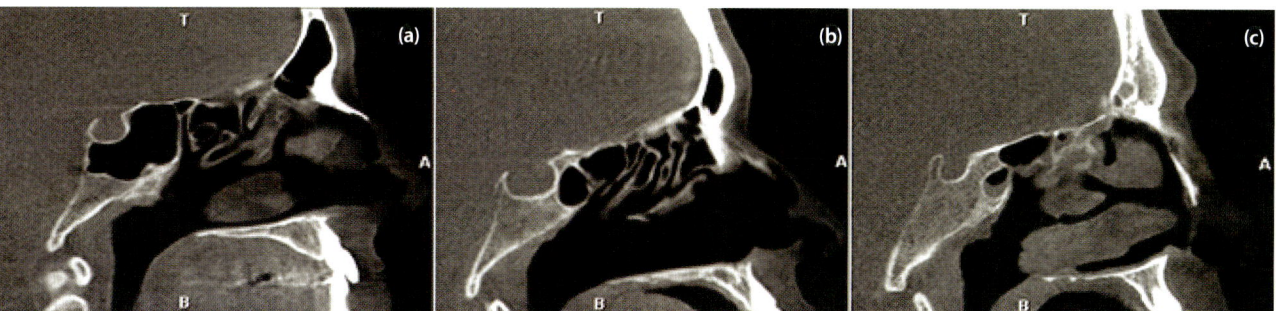

Figure 87.6 Sphenoid sinus pneumatization patterns. Midline sagittal CT indicating the **(a)** sellar **(b)** pre-sellar and **(c)** conchal types of sphenoid sinus pneumatization patterns.

The lateral recess pneumatization pathway occurs between the second trigeminal division and the vidian nerve.

> **BOX 87.3**
>
> The three different sphenoid sinus pneumatization patterns are described with reference to the sella turcica and include: sellar (90%), pre-sellar (9%) and conchal (1%) type. These pneumatization patterns are important for surgical planning of transphenoid approaches to pituitary tumours.

Frontal sinus

The frontal sinus is the most variable sinus in terms of size and shape. Pneumatization of the frontal bone begins during the 16th week of gestation originating from the anterior ethmoid complex. At birth, the frontal sinuses appear only as a small blind pocket that is difficult to distinguish from the anterior ethmoid air cells on imaging. With gradual pneumatization, the frontal sinuses are seen in most radiological studies by the age of 8 years. Significant frontal pneumatization does not occur until early adolescence and continues until 18 years of age. Although still developing, the relative proportions of the frontal sinus have reached adult ratios by age 10–12 years and just prior to the second growth spurt.

EXTERNAL NOSE

Skin and muscles of the external nose

The thickness of the skin and soft tissues of the nasal bridge vary according to individual skin type and anatomical location. Over the dorsum and sides of the nose, the nasal skin is thin and loosely adherent to the underlying framework. The nasal skin becomes thicker and more adherent towards the nasal tip and alar cartilages where it contains numerous sebaceous glands. The elasticity and mobility of the skin over the nose also varies according to the quality of the collagen fibers anchoring the skin to the underlying structures.

The extension of the facial SMAS (subcutaneous musculoaponeurotic system) layer continues over the nose as numerous muscles of the external nose which function to compress, dilate, depress or elevate the nostrils and nasal tip. These muscles are all supplied by branches of the facial nerve. The nasal elevators include the procerus, levator labii-superioris alaeque nasi, and anomalous nasi muscles. The depressors include the alar nasalis and depressor septi nasi muscles. Compressor muscles include the transverse nasalis and compressor narium minor. The dilator naris anterior muscle acts as a minor dilator.

The subcutaneous tissue of the nose is made up of four layers: superficial fatty, fibromuscular, deep fatty and periosteal layers. The superficial fatty layer is directly connected to the dermis. The fibromuscular layer comprises the nasal SMAS. The deep fatty layer lies deep to the SMAS and contains the neurovascular system. The deepest layer is the periosteum and perichondrium. During external approach rhinoplasty, dissection deep to the third layer minimizes post-operative scarring and retraction because the neurovascular and SMAS structures are preserved.

> **BOX 87.4**
>
> Dissection deep to the third layer of the nose (deep fatty layer) minimizes post-operative scarring and retraction because the neurovascular and SMAS structures are preserved.

Vestibule

The nasal vestibule is the anterior most aspect of the nasal cavity and serves as the entry point from the external nares into the nasal cavity. The vestibule is demarcated by the limen nasi located at the caudal border of the lower lateral cartilage. The limen nasi is the location where the marginal incision is made during external approach rhinoplasty. It is lined by keratinizing stratified squamous epithelium, and coarse hairs called vibrissae, sebaceous glands and sweat glands. A layer of mucous typically covers the outer surface of the vibrissae which functions to filter airborne particles during inspiration. It is important to note that only a small part of the alar rim is composed of cartilage from the lateral crus, the majority is composed of fibrofatty tissue.

Nasal cartilages

While much focus is placed on the internal septal and turbinate anatomy, the anterior third of the nasal passage has a critical functional role and can greatly influence nasal airflow. The nasal cartilages consist of hyaline cartilage that attach to the bones of the anterior nasal aperture to form the skeletal framework of the external nose. These cartilages include the upper and lower lateral cartilages, septum and sesamoid complex.

The lower lateral cartilage is divided into medial, intermediate and lateral crus that form the natural arch of the nasal ala. The upper lateral cartilages are trapezoid shaped cartilages that attach to the dorsal septum in the midline, nasal bones cranially at the rhinion and lower lateral cartilages caudally via the scroll area.

The relationship and architecture of these cartilages form the external and internal nasal valves which are critical to nasal airflow. The external nasal valve is comprised of the septum medially, alar rim (lateral crus, sesamoid complex and fibrofatty tissue) laterally and nasal sill inferiorly (**Figure 87.8**). Anatomical abnormalities or compromise in the structural integrity of these components can cause external valve narrowing, stenosis or dynamic valve collapse that is exacerbated during inspiration.

The internal nasal valve, in normal development, is the narrowest portion of the nasal cavity and is bounded by the septum medially, caudal edge of the upper lateral cartilage and head of the inferior turbinate laterally and nasal floor inferiorly (**Figure 87.8**). The apex of the internal nasal valve is approximately 10–15 degrees in Caucasians and wider in non-Caucasian populations. Changes in the relationship of any structure within this space can cause symptoms of nasal obstruction.

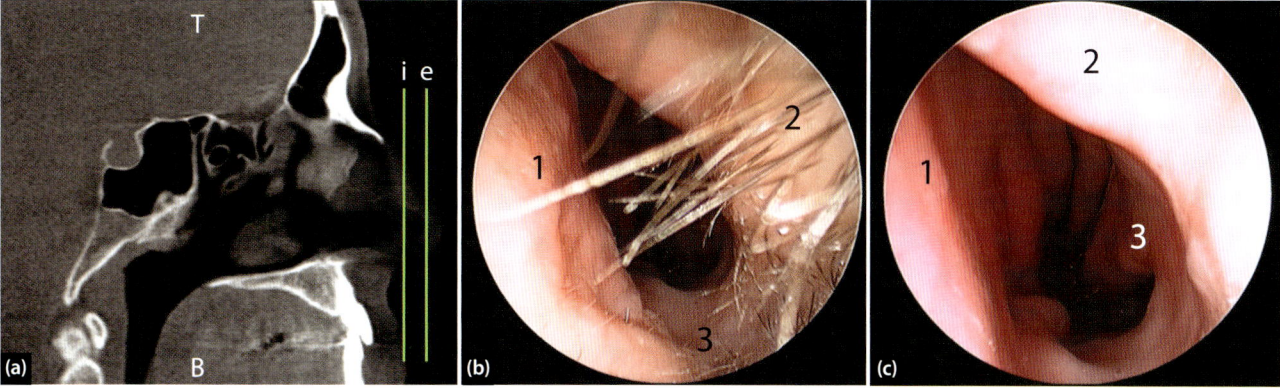

Figure 87.8 Nasal valves (a) Midline sagittal CT scan with green line indicating the relative positions of the external (e) and internal (i) nasal valves. (b) Endoscopic view of the left external nasal valve including (1) septum (2) alar rim (comprised of lower lateral crus, sesamoid complex and fibrofatty tissue) and (3) nasal sill. (c) Endoscopic view of the left internal nasal valve including (1) septum (2) caudal edge of upper lateral cartilage and (3) head of inferior turbinate.

BOX 87.5

The structures of the external and internal nasal valve are critical to nasal airflow with the internal nasal valve representing the narrowest portion of the nasal cavity. The internal nasal valve is bounded by the septum medially, caudal edge of the upper lateral cartilage and head of the inferior turbinate laterally and nasal floor inferiorly.

KEY POINTS

- The upper lip and nose are considered the danger area of the face because infections in this region may be transmitted in a retrograde fashion through a valveless venous system to the cavernous sinus.

Blood supply

Arterial supply to the external nose has both external and internal carotid artery contributions. Branches of the facial artery supply the alar region and include the angular and superior labial arteries. The angular artery and its lateral nasal branch supply the nasal side wall and ala. The superior labial artery gives rise to a columellar branch that supplies the nasal sill and columella and a septal branch that supplies the anterior nasal septum. The ophthalmic artery gives rises to a dorsal nasal branch which anastomoses with the lateral nasal branch of the angular artery to supply the dorsum and nasal side wall. The nasal dorsum and nasal side wall also receive vascular supply from the external nasal branch of the anterior ethmoid artery and infraorbital artery respectively. There are rich anastomoses between these vessels on each side and between right and left sides of the nose.

The venous networks do not parallel the arterial supply but correspond to territories termed arteriovenous units. The frontomedian area drains to the facial vein and the orbitopalpebral area drains to the ophthalmic vein. The facial vein originates as the angular vein located at the inner canthus. The angular vein forms as the confluence of the supratrochlear and supraorbital veins. The upper lip and nose are considered the danger area of the face because infections in this region may be transmitted in a retrograde fashion intracranially to the cavernous sinus. This phenomenon can occur because the facial vein communicates through a valveless venous system with the cavernous sinus via the ophthalmic vein.

Nerve supply

A working knowledge of the neural supply to the external nose has clinical value when performing a nerve block to this region during procedures such as rhinoplasty or closed reduction of nasal fractures (**Figure 87.9**). The supratrochlear and infratrochlear branches of the ophthalmic nerve supply the skin of the nasal root, bridge and upper portion of the side wall of the nose. The infraorbital branch of the maxillary nerve supplies the remaining skin of the nasal side wall. The external nasal branch of the anterior ethmoid nerve exits between the nasal bone and upper lateral cartilage to supply the skin over the dorsum and nasal tip.

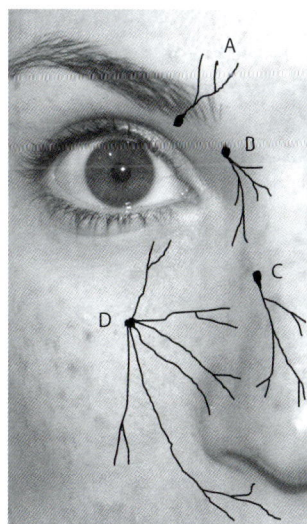

Figure 87.9 External nasal innervation (A) supratrochlear nerve (B) infratrochlear nerve (C) anterior ethmoid nerve (D) infraorbital nerve.

Lymphatic drainage

The lymphatic drainage of the external nose is directed towards the submandibular, submental and facial nodes. Drainage of the external nose is often bilateral and drainage to the parotid region may be possible.

Nasal cavity

The nasal cavity extends from the external nares to the posterior choanae, where it becomes continuous with the nasopharynx. The nasal cavity is divided into two passage ways by the nasal septum. Each side consists of a floor, roof, lateral and medial (septum) wall. The nasal floor is concave from side to side, flat anteroposteriorly and horizontally oriented. The anterior three-quarters are comprised of the palatine process of the maxilla and the posterior one-quarter by the horizontal process of the palatine bone. Approximately 12 mm behind the anterior aspect of the nasal floor is a slight depression which corresponds to the incisive canal. The incisive canal contains terminal branches of the nasopalatine nerve and greater palatine artery. The roof of the nasal cavity is formed by the skull base and slopes downward anteroposteriorly. This is important to recognize during endoscopic sinus surgery as dissection progresses posteriorly towards the sphenoid sinus.

The superior aspect of the nasal cavity including the superior septum, superior turbinate and upper aspect of the middle turbinate is lined by olfactory epithelium. With the exception of the vestibule, the remainder of the nasal cavity is lined by respiratory epithelium. The respiratory epithelium of the nasal cavity is continuous with the mucosal lining of the entire upper and lower airway system.

BOX 87.6

Three different types of epithelium within the nasal cavity consist of squamous (nasal vestibule), olfactory (superior septum, superior turbinate and upper aspect of the middle turbinate) and respiratory (remainder of nasal cavity) epithelium.

Nerve supply

Innervation of the nasal mucosa includes both autonomic and sensory components. The autonomic nervous system regulates the degree of vascular tone, turbinate congestion and nasal secretions present in the nose. Nasal secretion is regulated by the parasympathetic nervous system. Presynaptic parasympathetic fibers travel along the vidian nerve (contribution from the greater superficial petrosal (parasympathetic) and deep petrosal (sympathetic) nerves) and synapse within the sphenopalatine ganglion to innervate the nasal mucosa via postsynaptic fibers. Vascular tone and turbinate congestion is regulated by the sympathetic nervous system. Post-synaptic sympathetic fibers pass through the sphenopalatine ganglion and terminate in the nasal mucosa. The ophthalmic and maxillary divisions of the trigeminal nerve provide the sensory innervation to the nasal mucosa. Trigeminal nerve fibers also pass through the sphenopalatine ganglion and transmit sensations of pain, temperature and touch. The lateral wall of the nose and turbinates are supplied by the posterolateral nasal nerves from V2 arising from the sphenopalatine foramen and the ethmoidal nerves arising from V1. Although an artery supplies the inferior turbinate posteriorly, the neural innervation is from the lateral wall nerves continuing caudally.

BOX 87.7

The parasympathetic nerve regulates nasal secretions, sympathetic nerve regulates vascular tone and turbinate congestion, and the trigeminal nerve controls nasal cavity sensation.

NASAL SEPTUM

The nasal septum serves many functions, including separation of the nasal airway into two nasal cavities, support of the nasal dorsum, and maintenance of the nasal tip and forms part of the nasal valves. Deviation of the nasal septum can lead to significant nasal airway obstruction and cosmetic deformity. The nasal septum consists of a bony, cartilaginous and membranous portion (**Figure 87.10**).

The bony portion is comprised of the perpendicular plate of the ethmoid bone, vomer, maxillary crest and palatine bone (**Figure 87.10**). The perpendicular plate of the ethmoid forms the upper one-third of the nasal septum. It is continuous superiorly with the cribriform plate and crista galli and abuts a variable amount of the nasal and frontal bones. Posteriorly the perpendicular plate articulates with the sphenoid crest, posteroinferiorly with the vomer and anteroinferiorly with the septal cartilage. The vomer forms the posterior and inferior nasal septum and articulates by its two alae with the sphenoid rostrum creating the vomerovaginal canals through which the pharyngeal branches of the maxillary artery travel. The inferior border of the vomer articulates with the nasal crest formed by the maxillary and palatine bones. The anterior border articulates with the septal cartilage and the posterior edge of the vomer forms the posterior free edge of the septum.

The cartilaginous portion of the nasal septum is composed of the septal or quadrilateral cartilage (**Figure 87.10**). The quadrilateral cartilage is bound firmly by collagenous fibers to the nasal bones, perpendicular plate of the ethmoid and vomer. The septal cartilage is continuous with the upper lateral cartilages towards the bridge of the nose. A projection of the septal cartilage called the sphenoidal process or septal tail extends posteriorly between the vomer and perpendicular plate of the ethmoid. The septal tail can serve as an additional source of cartilage to harvest especially during revision rhinoplasty. The inferior attachment sits within the nasal crest of the maxilla and is bound by looser connective tissue creating a pseudoarthrosis. This joint allows mobility of the septal cartilage base during flexion thereby reducing the risk of fracture or dislocation with trauma. The membranous septum is a segment of connective tissue between the caudal portion of the septal cartilage and columella.

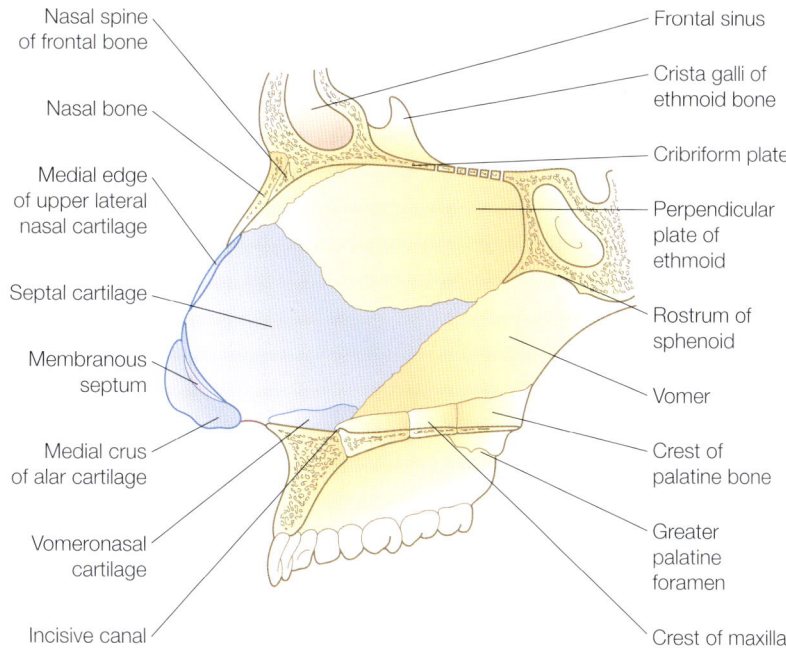

Figure 87.10 The cartilaginous and bony components of the nasal septum.

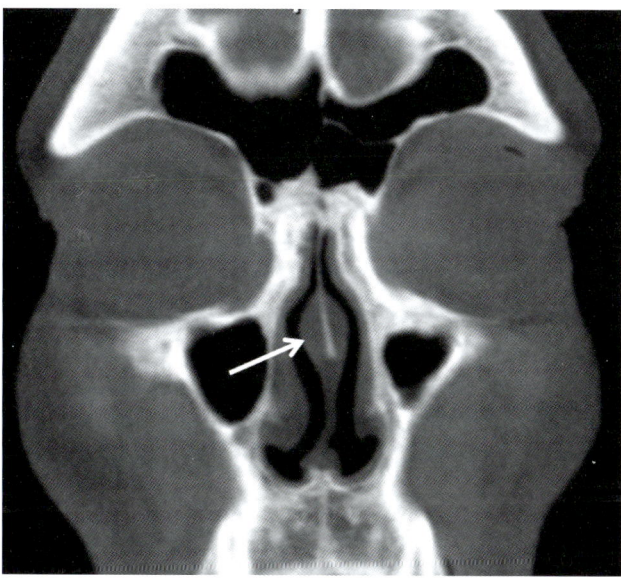

Figure 87.11 Coronal CT of septal swell body (arrow).

The nasal septal swell body is a widened region of the anterior nasal septum located anterior to the middle turbinate at the internal nasal valve (**Figure 87.11**).[4] Histological analysis of this tissue demonstrates an increased amount of venous sinusoids and fewer glandular elements compared to adjacent septal mucosa.[4] The high proportion of venous sinusoids suggests the capacity to alter nasal airflow in a similar manner to the inferior turbinates.

Blood supply of the nasal septum

Both the external and internal carotid arteries contribute to the vascular supply of the nasal septum (**Figure 87.12**). The external carotid artery branches supplying the septum include the sphenopalatine and greater palatine arteries (branches of the internal maxillary artery). The sphenopalatine artery supplies the posteroinferior septum by a branch called the posterior septal artery. The posterior septal artery is the basis of the nasoseptal mucosal flap which is the workhorse for endoscopic skull base reconstruction. The greater palatine artery enters the nasal cavity through the incisive canal to supply the anteroinferior portion of the septum. The septal branch of the superior labial artery (branch of the facial artery) contributes to the vascular supply of the caudal septum and columella. The internal carotid artery branches supplying the septum include the anterior and posterior ethmoid arteries (branches of the ophthalmic artery). The anterosuperior and posterosuperior portions of the nasal septum receive vascular supply from the anterior and posterior ethmoid arteries respectively.

The anterior ethmoid artery, posterior septal artery and septal branch of superior labial artery contribute to Kisselbach's plexus which is located along the anterior nasal septum at Little's area (**Figure 87.12**). This region is formed by the anastomosis of these arteries which terminate as a rich vascular bed of long capillary loops. Kisselbach's plexus is the most common location of epistaxis due to its rich vascular supply and susceptibility to injury from such factors as turbulent airflow and digital trauma.

BOX 87.8

Kisselbach's plexus is the most common location of epistaxis due to its rich vascular supply (confluence of the anterior ethmoid, posterior septal and septal branch of superior labial arteries) and susceptibility to injury from turbulent airflow and digital trauma.

The venous system drains via the sphenopalatine vessels into the pterygoid plexus posteriorly and into the facial

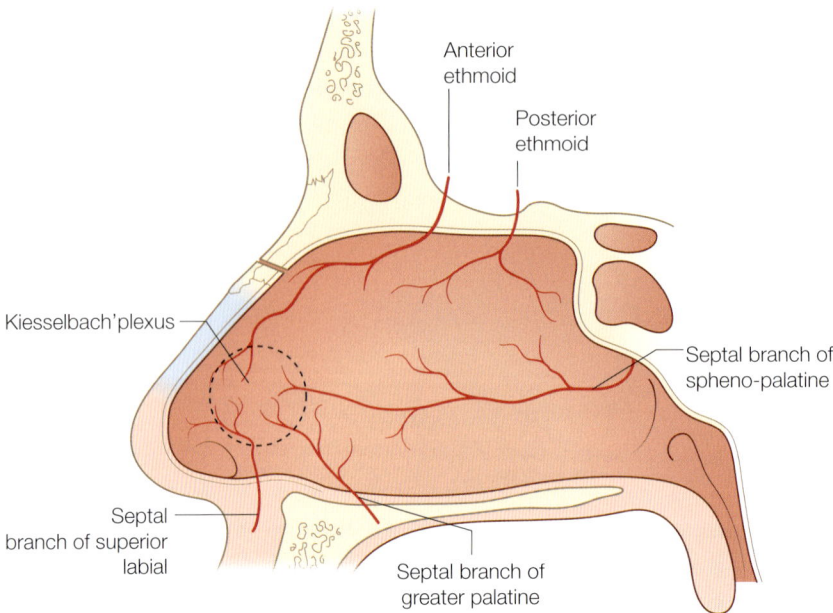

Figure 87.12 Vascular supply of the nasal septum.

veins anteriorly. Superiorly, the ethmoidal veins communicate with the superior ophthalmic system and there may be direct intracranial connections through the foramen caecum into the superior sagittal sinus.

Lateral nasal wall and turbinates

The inferior, middle and superior turbinates are internal structures found along the lateral nasal wall. The middle and superior turbinates arise from extensions of the ethmoid bones whereas the inferior turbinate is an embryologically independent osseus structure. The space between the lateral nasal wall and inferior, middle and superior turbinates is called the inferior, middle and superior meatus respectively. Each meatus is associated with the connection between a specific anatomical structure and the nasal cavity along a series of well-defined drainage pathways. The lacrimal duct drains into the inferior meatus approximately 1 cm posterior to the head of the inferior turbinate. Although not considered a true valve, the opening of the nasolacrimal duct is called Hasner's valve which is formed by small folds of mucosa. The middle meatus forms the common drainage pathway of the maxillary, anterior ethmoid and frontal sinus into the nasal cavity. The superior meatus forms the common drainage pathway of the posterior ethmoid air cells.

Turbinates are structures filled with vascular channels and venous sinusoids which serve to warm and humidify air and modify nasal airflow resistance. The turbinates continuously dilate and constrict under sympathetic control in response to environmental conditions. A process occurs every 0.5–3 hours in a normal physiological phenomenon known as the 'nasal cycle' resulting in alternating congestion and decongestion of the nasal cavities. Turbinate hypertrophy is a common cause of nasal obstruction in which the turbinates are either chronically congested or hypertrophied due to allergic or non-allergic triggers as part of an inflammatory rhinitis conditions.

> **BOX 87.9**
>
> The nasal turbinates continuously dilate and constrict every 0.5–3 hours in a normal physiological phenomenon known as the 'nasal cycle'.

Blood supply of the lateral nasal wall

Both the internal and external carotid arteries supply the lateral nasal wall. The sphenopalatine artery contributes the majority of the arterial supply to the turbinates and lateral nasal wall (**Figure 87.13**). It enters through the sphenopalatine foramen which lies just inferior to the horizontal attachment of the middle turbinate. The sphenopalatine foramen is formed by the sphenopalatine notch of the palatine bone in articulation with the sphenoid bone. The crista ethmoidalis is a small crest of the perpendicular plate of the palatine bone located anterior to sphenopalatine foramen and serves as a consistent and reliable landmark to identify this vessel during endoscopic dissection.[5] The sphenopalatine artery commonly branches lateral to the crista ethmoidalis with many variations in the branching pattern. In one cadaver study, 97% of specimens had two or more branches of the sphenopalatine artery medial to the crista ethmoidalis.[6] It is critical that the surgeon is aware of these variations and controls all branches to ensure successful endoscopic ligation of the sphenopalatine artery for epistaxis. If more proximal vascular control is required, the internal maxillary artery can be ligated in the pterygopalatine or infratemporal fossa by removal of the posterior wall of the maxillary sinus.

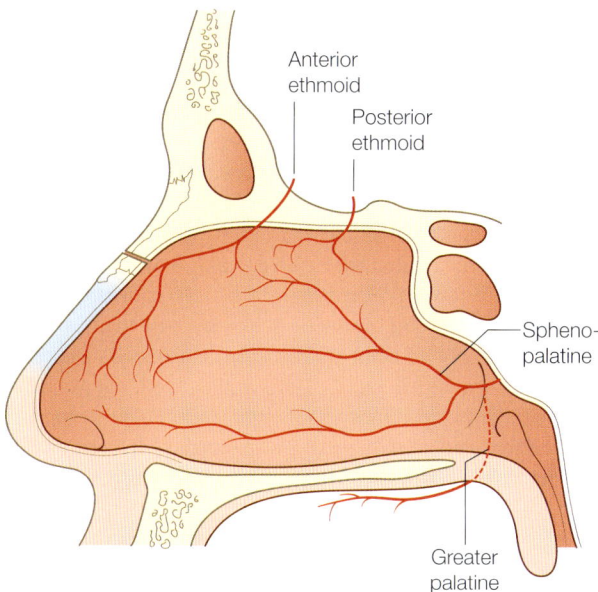

Figure 87.13 Vascular supply of lateral nasal wall.

BOX 87.10

The crista ethmoidalis is a small crest of the perpendicular plate of the palatine bone located anterior to sphenopalatine foramen and serves as a consistent and reliable landmark to identify the sphenopalatine artery during endoscopic dissection. There are often two or more branches of the sphenopalatine artery medial to the crista ethmoidalis.

A small area along the anterior aspect of the lateral nasal wall is supplied by a branch of the facial artery. The inferior part of the lateral nasal wall adjacent to the palate is supplied by the greater palatine artery. The internal carotid artery contribution is via the anterior and posterior ethmoid arteries (branches of the ophthalmic artery) which supply the superior lateral wall. The anterior ethmoid artery traverses three compartments of the head during its course from the orbit to the olfactory fossa and into the nasal cavity. After branching from the ophthalmic artery in the orbit, the anterior ethmoid artery passes between the superior oblique and medial rectus muscles through the anterior ethmoid foramen. This portion is easily identified on pre-operative coronal CT imaging. The anterior ethmoid artery travels through the ethmoid cavity obliquely in a posterior to anterior direction either within the bone of the skull base or a mucosal mesentery. The artery traverses intra-cranially into the olfactory fossa through the lateral lamella of the lamina cribrosa. After entering the intra-cranial cavity, it gives off anterior meningeal branches before re-entering the nasal cavity through the cribroethmoidal foramen. Within the nasal cavity, it divides into the anterior and posterior nasal arteries. The anterior and posterior nasal arteries each give rise to lateral and medial branches that supply the lateral nasal wall and nasal septum respectively.

The anterior ethmoid artery is more difficult to access surgically, with only 20% of arteries found within a mesentery that can be successful clipped via a transnasal approach.[7] Endoscopic removal of the lamina papyracea allows identification of the anterior and posterior ethmoid arteries between the periobita and skull base. Alternatively, an external approach via a modified Lynch incision can be used. There is considerable overlap between the internal and external carotid arterial systems on each side and between sides of the nasal cavity which can complicate attempts at arterial ligation in the management of epistaxis.

BOX 87.11

The anterior ethmoid artery is more difficult to access endoscopically as it is only found within a mesentery that can be ligated in a small portion of cases. An external approach using a modified Lynch incision is often the preferred method of ligation.

PARANASAL SINUSES

Anatomy of the paranasal sinuses can be divided into anatomy that has surgical relevance and descriptions that are academic in nature.

Surgical anatomy of the paranasal sinuses

Traditional descriptions of paranasal sinus anatomy focus on pneumatization patterns of air cells with corresponding clefts and spaces. Such descriptions are academic and have little clinical relevance to modern endoscopic sinus surgery. Although an understanding of sinonasal anatomy is critical to ensure safe and complete endoscopic sinus surgery, the concept of pneumatization pathways and development is highly variable and often distorted by disease or prior surgery. Endoscopic sinus surgery is an exercise of anatomical dissection around fixed anatomical landmarks. Akin to traditional mastoid surgery, the sinus surgeon must identify certain key anatomical landmarks in order to delineate the limits of dissection. These landmarks must be based on fixed anatomical structures rather than variable anatomy that can be distorted or absent from disease processes or prior surgery. The goal of surgery is to identify these landmarks early during the procedure in order to provide orientation for the remainder of the operation. These consistent anatomical landmarks include: (1) the maxillary sinus, (2) the orbit from the maxillary sinus roof / orbital floor and medial orbital wall (lamina papyracea) and (3) skull base identified posteriorly by the sphenoid sinus. These defined anatomical limits establish the boundaries of the paranasal surgical box including the horizontal and vertical components of this box.[8] The concept of the paranasal surgical box forms the basic framework of endoscopic sinus surgery (**Figure 87.14**).

The boundaries of the horizontal portion of the paranasal surgical box include the middle turbinate medially,

970 Section 3: Rhinology

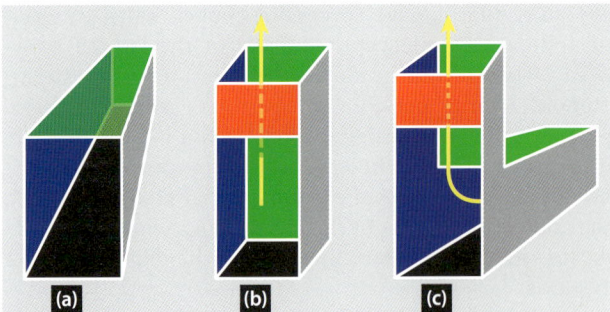

Figure 87.14 Schematic diagram of the right paranasal surgical box. **(a)** Horizontal component of the right surgical box with limits of dissection including medial orbital wall (blue), middle turbinate (grey), skull base (green), sphenoid sinus (yellow). **(b)** Vertical component of the right surgical box with limits of dissection including medial orbital wall (blue), middle turbinate (grey), skull base (green), anterior nasal beak (red). **(c)** Combined schematic diagram of the horizontal and vertical components of the paranasal surgical box.

medial orbital wall (lamina papyracea) laterally, floor of nose inferiorly and skull base superiorly (**Figure 87.15**).[8] The boundaries of the vertical portion of the paranasal surgical box include the middle turbinate and intersinus septum medially, lamina papyracea laterally, nasofrontal beak anteriorly and skull base posteriorly (**Figure 87.16**).[8]

Upon completion of the maxillary antrostomy (or any maxillary sinus opening), identification of the maxillary sinus roof/orbital floor exhibits the first key anatomical landmark (**Figure 87.17**). This landmark first provides the location of the orbit and then provides a safe working distance from the skull base during identification of the sphenoid sinus whether via the natural ostium or not (**Figure 87.18**).[9, 10] Although conceptually the floor of orbit should be below the skull base, anatomical studies have demonstrated that the maxillary sinus roof / orbital floor was below the level of the skull base (lowest portion of the cribriform plate) in 100% of cases with an mean distance of 10.1 ± 2.7 mm.[9] This landmark was also found to be below the level of the sphenoid planum in 100% of cases with a mean distance of 11.0 ± 3.7 mm and located at approximately 50% the height of the sphenoid.[9] As a surgical rule, staying below or at the level of the maxillary sinus roof / orbital floor as dissection proceeds posterior will avoid the skull base. Although a well-pneumatized maxillary sinus reduces the height of the posterior ethmoid cavity and may lead to poor surgical trajectory and skull base injury this surgical rule still applies.

The ethmoid bulla is attached to the medial orbital wall (lamina papyracea) laterally. With the orbital floor on view, removal of the ethmoid bulla enables identification of second key anatomical landmark (**Figure 87.19**). Identification of where the floor turns vertically to become the medial orbital wall enables safe exposure of the entire orbital axis and delineation of the lateral boundary of the paranasal surgical box (**Figure 87.19**).

The third key landmark is the sphenoid sinus/posterior skull base (**Figure 87.20**). The maxillary sinus roof/orbital floor landmark is used as a reference to mark the level of the sphenoid ostium. Any dissection medial to the orbital axis and below or at the level of the orbital floor will allow safe entry into the sphenoid. While structures such as the superior turbinate are incredibly useful in defining the medial boundary of dissection for the ethmoid cavity, this

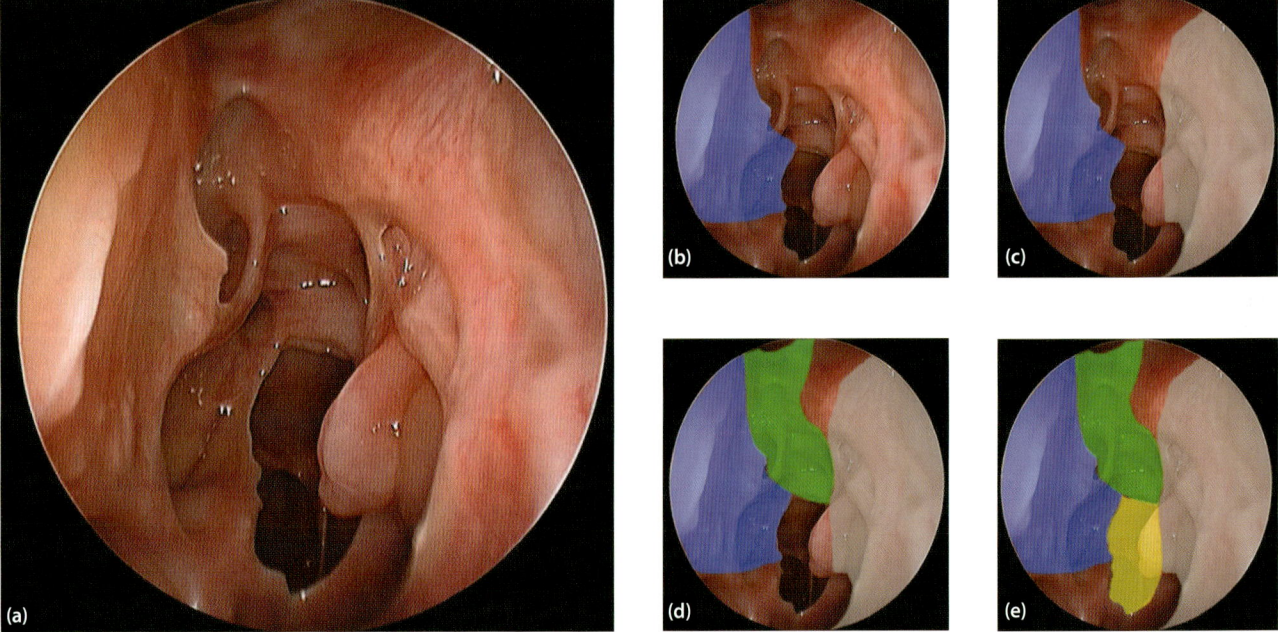

Figure 87.15 (a) Endoscopic view of the right horizontal component of the paranasal sinus surgical box with the medial, lateral, superior and inferior limits of dissection visible with a single position of the endoscope. The lateral, medial and superior boundaries of the horizontal surgical box are indicated as **(b)** medial orbital wall (blue) **(c)** middle turbinate (grey) **(d)** skull base (green) respectively. **(e)** Sphenoid sinus (yellow) serves as an important landmark to identify the skull base at its most posterior position.

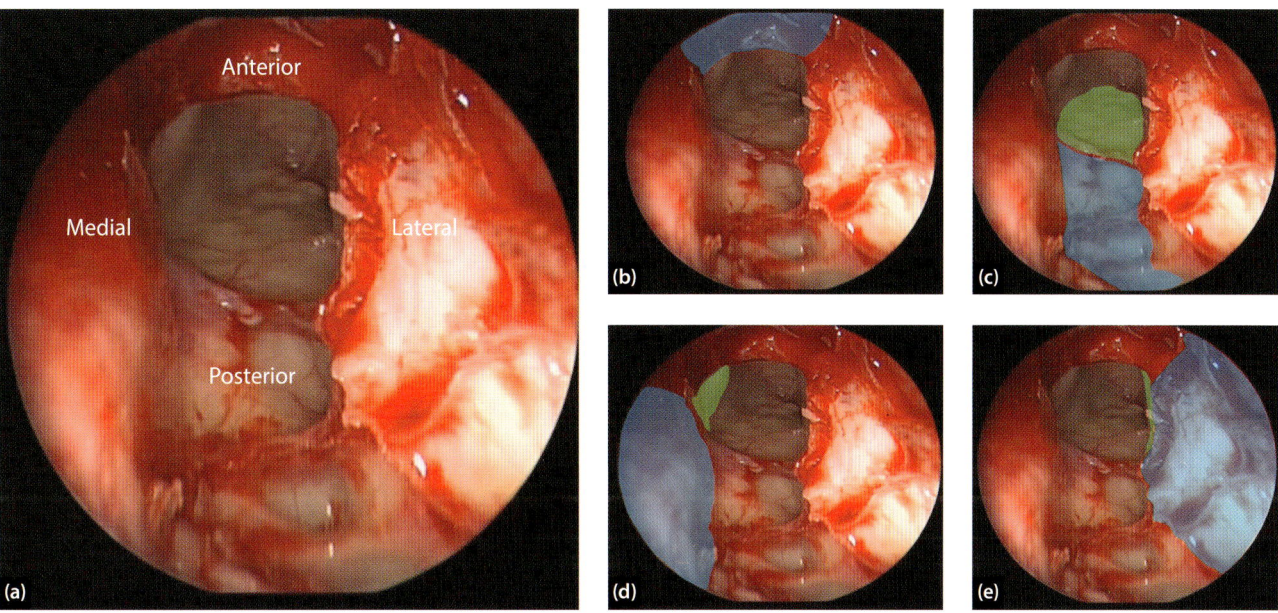

Figure 87.16 (a) Endoscopic view of the left vertical component of the paranasal sinus surgical box with anterior, posterior, medial and lateral limits of dissection visible with a single position of the endoscope. The anterior, posterior, medial and lateral boundaries of the vertical surgical box are indicated as **(b)** nasal beak (blue) **(c)** skull base (blue) and posterior table of frontal sinus (green) **(d)** middle turbinate (blue) and frontal intersinus septum (green) **(e)** medial orbital wall (blue) and supraorbital roof (green) respectively.

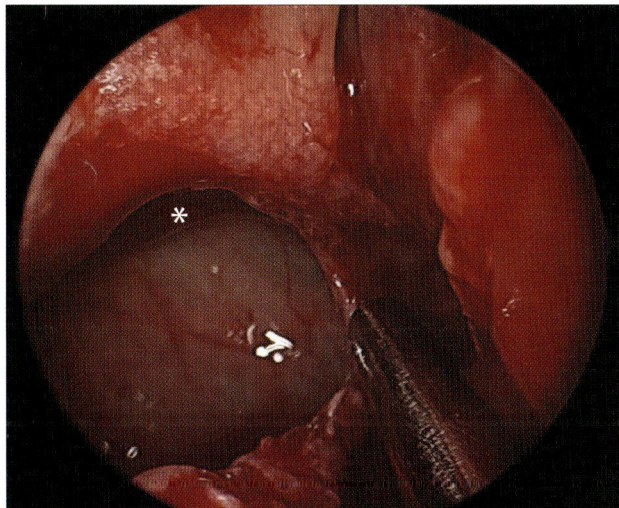

Figure 87.17 Maxillary sinus roof/orbital floor landmark. Endoscopic view of right maxillary sinus antrostomy. Asterisk indicates the position of the right maxillary sinus roof/orbital floor which serves as the first surgical landmark during endoscopic sinus surgery.

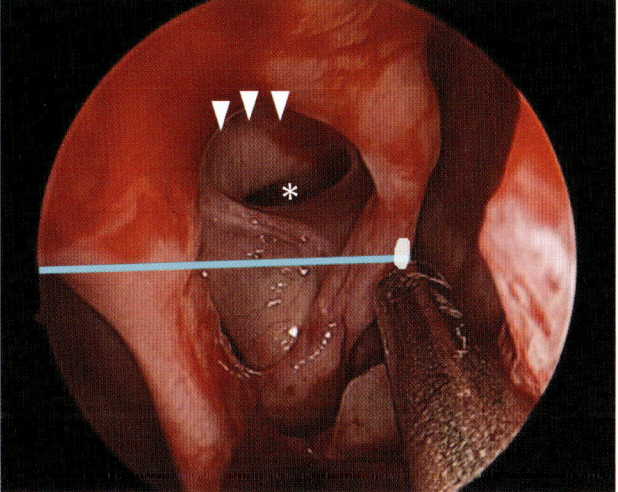

Figure 87.18 Endoscopic view of right maxillary sinus antrostomy after removal of anterior ethmoid cells and basal lamella. Line indicates the horizontal relationship between the maxillary sinus roof / orbital floor landmark and position of the sphenoid ostium. White oval indicates the relative position of the sphenoid ostium. Application of this landmark will ensure safe and easy identification of the sphenoid sinus and avoids mistaking a posterior ethmoid cell or Onodi cell (asterisk) for the true sphenoid sinus. Note that within the Onodi cell is the presence of an exposed optic nerve (arrow heads).

structure cannot be relied upon as it is often removed by pathology or previous surgery. Opening of the sphenoid ostium and removal of the anterior sphenoid wall enables clear visualization of the posterior skull base. The skull base slopes downwards from anterior to posterior, thus, the posterior skull base is at its lowest height within the horizontal portion of paranasal surgical box at the level of the sphenoid sinus (**Figure 87.20**). The sphenoid can be widely opened laterally as the orbital axis (and thus the lateral limit) is previously identified. Once the posterior skull base is identified, all four limits of dissection of the horizontal portion of the paranasal surgical box are defined (**Figures 87.14** and **87.15**) and all cells within the confines of these boundaries must be removed.

Performing a complete dissection of the horizontal portion of the paranasal surgical box serves to define the limits of dissection for the vertical portion of the box (**Figures 87.14** and **87.16**). The limits of dissection that

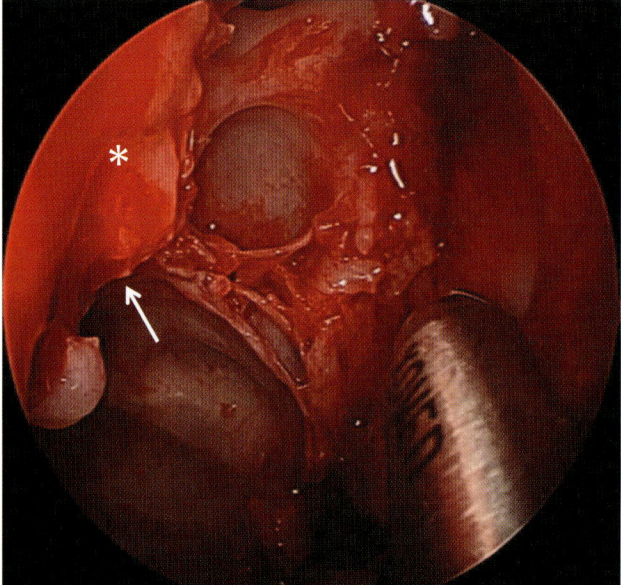

Figure 87.19 Endoscopic view of right anterior ethmoid sinus cavity. The position of the right medial orbital wall (asterisk) is identified after removal of the ethmoid bulla. The transition from the orbital floor to the medial orbital wall is clearly delineated (arrow).

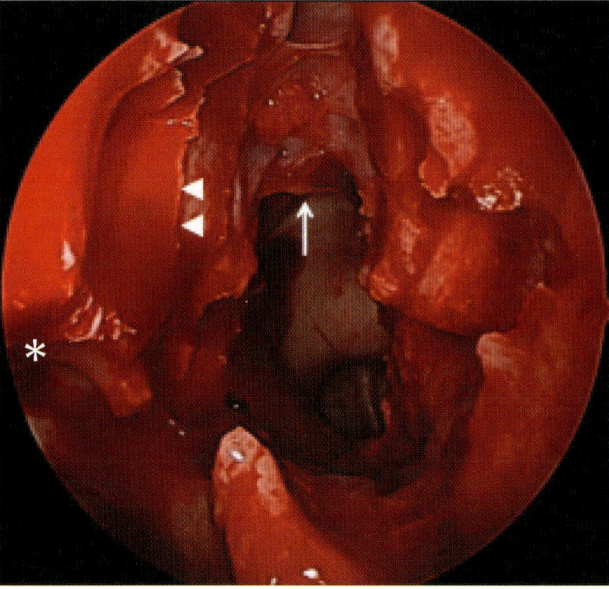

Figure 87.20 Endoscopic view of right sphenoid sinus cavity. The position of the posterior skull base (arrow) is identified after removal of the anterior wall of the sphenoid sinus. The positions of the orbital floor (asterisk) and medial orbital wall (arrow heads) landmarks are visible with a single position of the endoscope.

BOX 87.12

- Endoscopic sinus surgery is based on the identification of key fixed anatomical landmarks including the orbital floor, medial orbital wall, sphenoid sinus and posterior skull base.
- These landmarks help to define the anatomical limits of dissection during surgery and establish the boundaries of the paranasal surgical box including the horizontal and vertical components of this box.
- The horizontal component of the paranasal surgical box includes the medial orbital wall laterally, middle turbinate medially and skull base posteriorly. These limits are extended superiorly to define the boundaries of the vertical component of the paranasal surgical box which includes the middle turbinate and intersinus septum medially, lamina papyracea laterally, nasofrontal beak anteriorly and skull base posteriorly.

DEVELOPMENTAL AND FUNCTIONAL ANATOMY OF THE PARANASAL SINUSES

The paranasal sinuses are paired structures lined by ciliated pseudostratified columnar respiratory epithelium identical to that in the lower airway. The cilia beat in a coordinated fashion to carry the mucous blanket which traps particles from the sinus into the nose through a series of well-defined pathways. The paranasal sinuses are divided into anterior, posterior and sphenoid compartments that serve as functional units based on these drainage pathways. The anterior functional unit is comprised of the maxillary, anterior ethmoid and frontal sinuses. These sinuses drain into the nose through the osteomatal complex in the middle meatus. The posterior functional unit is comprised of the posterior ethmoid sinus and drains into the nose through the superior meatus. The sphenoid functional unit is comprised of the sphenoid sinus and drains through the sphenoethmoid recess located medial and posterior to the superior turbinate. Although the anterior and posterior ethmoid cavities share a common name, they are completely separate functional entities with different drainage pathways and embryologic origins.

The concept of the sinonasal compartment or functional unit has clinical relevance during endoscopic sinus surgery. Once a compartment is entered with surgical instrumentation, all diseased mucosal cells within the compartment must be completely dissected in order to remove obstructive phenomenon, avoid leaving behind disconnected cells from the surgical cavity, prevent mucocele formation, re-establish post-surgical mucociliary function that is free of recirculation effects, and enable maximal delivery of topical therapy. The ultimate goal of surgery (whether limited or extensive) is the creation of a new functional sinus cavity.

are defined during the complete sphenoethmoidectomy include the medial orbital wall laterally, middle turbinate medially and skull base posteriorly. These limits are extended superiorly to define the boundaries of the vertical portion of the surgical box and all cells within the confines of these boundaries are removed (**Figure 87.14**).

Anterior functional unit

> **BOX 87.13 Uncinate process and maxillary sinus**
>
> - The uncinate process is a sickle-shaped bone which attaches inferiorly to the inferior turbinate and palatine bone and anterosuperiorly to the lacrimal bone.
> - The posterosuperior attachment will be discussed later along with the frontal sinus.
> - The true maxillary ostial opening is covered by the uncinate process and cannot be viewed endoscopically in a sinus cavity that has not been previously opened surgically.
> - The uncinate, together with a fold of mucosa called the anterior and posterior fontanelle cover the opening to the maxillary sinus. Accessory ostia may be present in the fontanelle that can be mistaken for the true maxillary ostium.
> - Failure to correctly identify the true ostia and connect it with the common sinus cavity may result in a phenomenon known as mucous recirculation. During recirculation, mucous is directed towards the natural opening along the mucociliary drainage pathway and re-enters the sinus through the accessory ostium.

ETHMOID BULLA

The ethmoid bulla is the largest and most consistent anterior ethmoid air cell. It attaches to the lamina papyracea laterally and has variable attachments to the skull base and basal lamella creating a series of clefts and spaces within the middle meatus that are well described, but have little clinical significance. The reader is referred to the consensus document produced by the Anatomic Terminology Group for a detailed description of anatomic terminology and nomenclature.[11] A variant of normal anatomy in this region is called a Haller cell. A Haller cell is an infraorbital anterior ethmoid cell that pneumatizes into the maxillary sinus and may cause obstruction of the maxillary sinus ostium. Complete removal of the ethmoid bulla is critical to define the medial orbital wall as a landmark.

MIDDLE TURBINATE

The complex shape of the middle turbinate is divided into three segments according to the sagittal, coronal and axial planes to which it is oriented. The sagittal segment attaches to the skull base at the lateral lamella. The coronal segment creates the basal lamella which separates the anterior ethmoid (those cells draining in the middle meatus) and posterior ethmoid (draining via the superior meatus) cavities. There is no natural connection between these two cavities. This partition is often not smooth due to posterior projections of the anterior ethmoid air cells and anterior projections of the posterior ethmoid air cells. The safe working distance from the skull base established by the maxillary sinus roof/orbital floor is used as a reference point to proceed through the basal lamella and enter the posterior ethmoid cavity.[9] The axial segment of the middle turbinate attaches to the lateral nasal wall and is the entry point of a terminal branch of the sphenopalatine artery.

FRONTAL SINUS

The vertical portion of the paranasal surgical box defines the anatomical limits of dissection of the frontal recess. The boundaries of the vertical portion of the paranasal surgical box include the intersinus septum and middle turbinate medially, lamina papyracea laterally, nasofrontal beak anteriorly and skull base posteriorly (**Figures 87.14** and **87.16**). Successful identification of these anatomical limits of the surgical box and removal of all cells within its confines ensures complete dissection of the frontal recess. To define the limits of the vertical portion of the paranasal surgical box, one must consider the various cells that may encroach on this space from the anterior, posterior, medial and lateral directions.

Agger nasi, posterosuperior uncinate process and frontal ethmoid cells

Anterior structures encroaching on the frontal recess include the agger nasi, lateral uncinate process and frontal cells (**Figure 87.21**). The agger nasi is the anterior-most ethmoid air cell and its medial border is formed by the uncinate process.[12] The degree of pneumatization of the agger nasi influences the position of the superior uncinate process and thickness of the bony nasofrontal beak.

The uncinate process can insert into the medial orbital wall, skull base or middle turbinate. Recent studies have demonstrated that the uncinate has multiple attachments in more than 50% of cases rather than a single attachment pattern (**Figure 87.22**).[12,13] Classic teaching that describes three distinct attachments of the uncinate process which determines the direction of the frontal sinus drainage pathway is neither surgically relevant nor accurate (**Figure 87.22**). The uncinate process inserts onto the medial orbital wall in 85% of cases.[13] Thus, the frontal recess drainage pathway is medial to the uncinate process in 85% of cases. An uncinate process with an isolated attachment to either the skull base or middle turbinate (without attachment to the medial orbital wall) occurs in only 15% of cases.[13] This attachment pattern leads to a surgically obvious frontal drainage pathway located lateral to the uncinate process that is easily identified at the time of surgery. The surgical rule holds true that the frontal recess is medial to the remnant uncinate process or 'vertical bar' in 85% of cases[14] with the other uncinate attachments representing easy surgical arrangements.

> **BOX 87.14**
>
> The uncinate process inserts onto the medial orbital wall in 85% of cases resulting in a frontal recess drainage pathway that is medial to the uncinate.

Frontal cells represent cells of the first ethmoturbinal that pneumatize above the agger nasi towards the frontal sinus. According to the Kuhn classification, a type 1 frontal cell is a single frontal ethmoidal cell above the agger nasi and below the frontal sinus floor, type 2 is a tier of

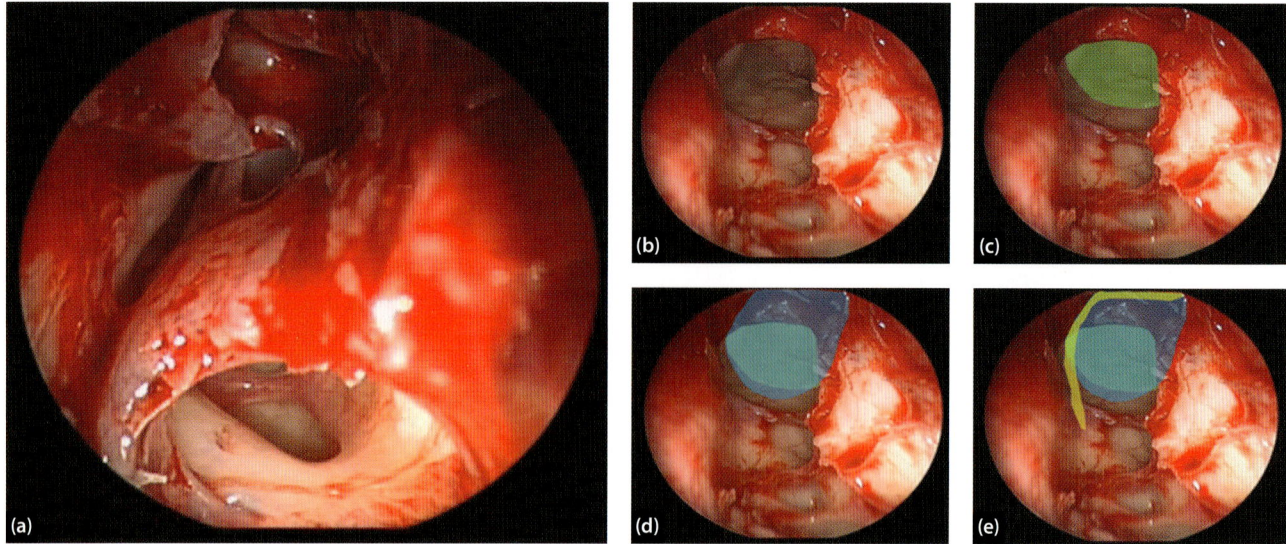

Figure 87.21 Anterior structures encroaching on the frontal recess depicted by a series of onlay diagrams. (a) Left frontal recess with all cells intact prior to surgical dissection, **(b)** left Draf 2A frontal sinusotomy with removal of all cells encroaching on the frontal recess. The relative positions of the anterior cells are superimposed including: **(c)** frontal cells (green), **(d)** agger nasi (blue), **(e)** superior uncinate process (yellow).

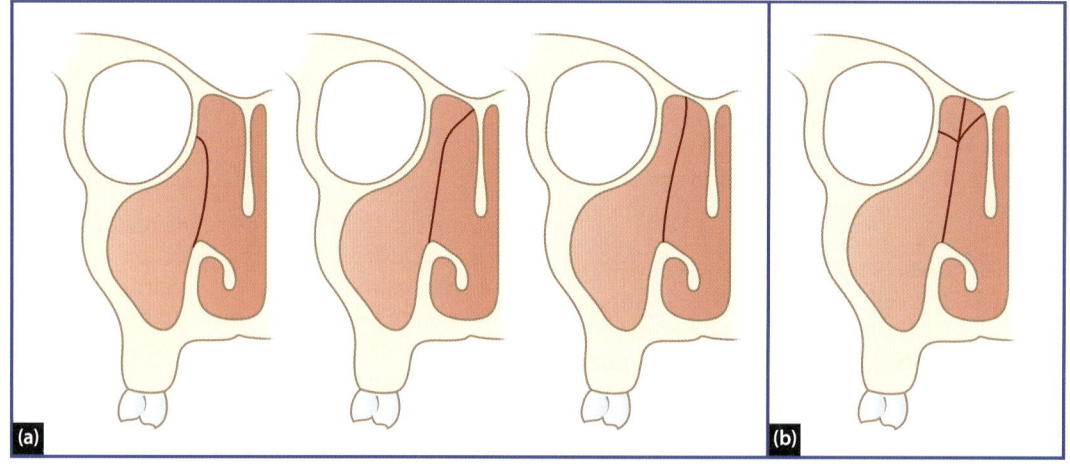

Figure 87.22 Schematic diagram of the uncinate process with different arrangements of its superior attachment. (a) Classic teaching describes 3 distinct attachments to the medial orbital wall, middle turbinate and skull base respectively which determines the direction of the frontal sinus drainage pathway. This description is not accurate. **(b)** The uncinate process has multiple attachments in greater than 50% of cases rather than a single attachment.

cells above the agger nasi, type 3 is a cell pneumatizing into the floor of the frontal sinus and type 4 is an isolated frontal ethmoid cell within the frontal sinus. Using multiplanar reconstructed imaging, Wormald further modified this classification to more accurately describe type 3 cells as frontal ethmoidal cells that fill less than 50% of the frontal sinus and type 4 cells as filling greater than 50% of the frontal sinus.[15] These classifications of frontal cells are primarily to ensure that the surgeon's view of a large frontal recess cell lumen will not be mistaken for the true frontal sinus. Identification of these frontal cells on preoperative imaging prevents false assumption of completion sinusotomy (see Chapter 99 on the frontal sinus).

Supraorbital ethmoid and suprabulla cells

Posterior structures encroaching on the frontal recess include supraorbital ethmoid cells, suprabulla cells and the ethmoid bulla (**Figure 87.23**). Supraorbital ethmoid cells are anterior ethmoid air cells that extend superiorly and laterally over the orbital roof.[16] These cells are recognized on imaging giving the appearance of a septated frontal sinus on coronal view and a cell located posterior and lateral to the frontal sinus on axial view.[16] Supraorbital ethmoid cells have three clinically significant features relevant to the frontal recess: (1) they can cause obstruction of the frontal recess, (2) they can be falsely mistaken for the true frontal sinus leading to incomplete surgical dissection and (3) they are associated with a low position of the anterior ethmoid artery within a mesentery because these cells pneumatize downward from the skull base behind the artery.[17] The supraorbital ethmoid cell also creates a very narrow orbitocranial cleft posteriorly that can be very challenging to operate within.[18] Suprabulla or frontal bulla cells are pneumatized extensions above

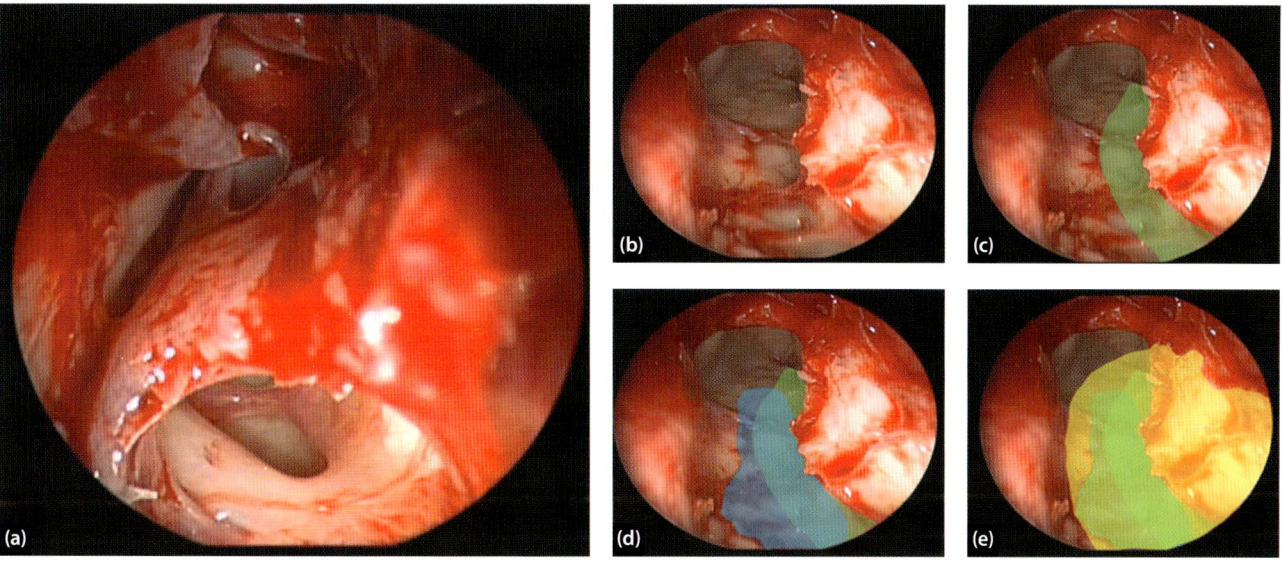

Figure 87.23 Posterior structures encroaching on the frontal recess depicted by a series of onlay diagrams. (a) Left frontal recess with all cells intact prior to surgical dissection, (b) left Draf 2A frontal sinusotomy with removal of all cells encroaching on the frontal recess. The relative positions of the posterior cells are superimposed including: (c) supraorbital ethmoid cell (green), (d) suprabulla cell (blue), (e) ethmoid bulla (yellow).

the ethmoid bulla up the skull base and on the posterior table of the frontal sinus. These cells can become quite large and mistaken for either the skull base or posterior table of the frontal sinus. Failure to recognize these cells on pre-operative imaging will also result in incomplete surgical dissection of the frontal recess.

BOX 87.15

- Supraorbital ethmoid cells have significant features relevant to the frontal recess as the can: (1) cause obstruction of the frontal recess, (2) be falsely mistaken for the true frontal sinus leading to incomplete surgical dissection and (3) be associated with a low position of the anterior ethmoid artery within a mesentery placing this artery at risk of injury during surgery.
- Suprabulla cells pneumatize up the skull base and failure to recognize these cells pre-operatively will result in incomplete surgical dissection of the frontal recess.

Medial structures encroaching on the frontal recess include intersinus septal cells and medially inserting uncinate process. Intersinus septal cells represent pneumatization of the frontal sinus septum. Lateral encroaching structures include frontal cells, agger nasi and a lateral uncinate process attachment.

Posterior functional unit

The posterior functional unit is comprised of the posterior ethmoid air cells with drainage into the superior meatus. A variant of normal anatomy in this region is a lateral and posterior pneumatization of a posterior ethmoid cell called an Onodi cell (**Figure 87.18**). Onodi cells pneumatize over the optic nerve exposing this critical structure to injury during surgery. These cells can also be mistaken for the true sphenoid sinus leading to incomplete surgery. Application of the maxillary sinus roof/orbital floor landmark identifies the level of the sphenoid ostium and enables complete dissection of the sphenoid sinus.

BOX 87.16

Onodi cells pneumatize over the optic nerve placing the optic nerve at risk for injury during surgery. An Onodi cell can be identified on the coronal view CT sinus as giving the appearance of a horizontal septation within the sphenoid sinus.

Sphenoid functional unit

The sphenoid functional unit is comprised of the sphenoid sinus which drains into the sphenoethmoid recess. Identification of the sphenoid sinus enables the surgeon to determine the level of the posterior skull base at its lowest position. The sphenoethmoid recess is the space between the superior meatus and septum. The supreme turbinate may be seen here. The sphenoid ostium opens behind the superior turbinate and is neither medial nor lateral to it.[19] Complete removal of the anterior sphenoid wall laterally enables the surgeon to identify the medial orbital wall at its posterior position. The main structures associated with the sphenoid sinus include the optic nerve, carotid artery and sella turcica where the pituitary gland is located. The pneumatization pattern of the sphenoid sinus can be variable. The different types include sellar (90%), pre-sellar (9%) and conchal (1%) pneumatization patterns (**Figure 87.6**). The sellar type describes sphenoid pneumatization posterior to the sella turcica. The pre-sellar type describes sphenoid pneumatization up to the anterior sella and the conchal type describes a shallow bowl with minimal sphenoid pneumatization and trabecular bone between the sinus and sella. The sphenoid sinuses can also pneumatize laterally into the pterygoid root resulting in the presence of a lateral sphenoid recess (**Figure 87.7**).

CONCLUSION

The paranasal sinuses represent some of the most variable human anatomy. An understanding of the developmental and functional anatomy is critical to understand patterns of disease and pathophysiological events in the sinuses. However, it is an understanding of the anatomical boundaries of paranasal sinuses that are critical for the surgeon to avoid major complications. Ensuring the ostia are incorporated into the common surgical cavity provides the basis for a functional post-surgical cavity rather than discreet identification of their location.

BEST CLINICAL PRACTICE

- ✓ The paranasal sinuses represent some of the most variable in human anatomy.
- ✓ Although a knowledge of the developmental and functional anatomy is critical to understand patterns of disease and pathophysiological events in the sinuses, they are often of limited assistance during surgery.
- ✓ The anatomical boundaries of the paranasal sinuses are critical for the surgeon to avoid major complications. Variable clefts, pneumatization patterns and features that are easily distorted by pathology and prior surgery are not good guides for a surgeon.
- ✓ Ensuring complete surgical dissection with ostia incorporated into the common surgical cavity provides the basis for creating a new functional neo-sinus cavity post-operatively.

FUTURE RESEARCH

➤ Understanding the epithelial dysfunction with intrinsic mucosal inflammation, local microbial colonization and mucociliary dysfunction as the contributing factors in patients with chronic sinus inflammation is still evolving.

KEY POINTS

- Identify key fixed anatomical landmarks to delineate the limits of dissection of the paranasal sinus surgical cavity (box) for safe and complete endoscopic sinus surgery.
- The main structures are the orbit and skull base. These are defined by (1) maxillary sinus roof (orbital floor) (2) medial orbital wall (3) sphenoid sinus roof (skull base) and (4) the lateral sphenoid wall (orbital apex).
- Paranasal sinuses are divided into anterior, posterior and sphenoid compartments that serve as functional units based on mucociliary drainage pathways.
- Once a compartment is surgically entered, all mucosal cells within the compartment must be completely dissected to create a new functional neo-sinus cavity.

REFERENCES

1. Bolger WE, Woodruff WW Jr., Morehead J, et al. Maxillary sinus hypoplasia: classification and description of associated uncinate process hypoplasia. *Otolaryngol Head Neck Surg* 1990; **103**(5 (Pt 1)): 759–65.
2. Geraghty JJ, Dolan KD. Computed tomography of the hypoplastic maxillary sinus. *Ann Otol Rhinol Laryngol* 1989; **98**(11): 916–18.
3. Hammer G, Radberg C. The sphenoidal sinus: an anatomical and roentgenologic study with reference to transsphenoid hypophysectomy. *Acta Radiol* 1961; **56**: 401–22.
4. Costa DJ, Sanford T, Janney C, et al. Radiographic and anatomic characterization of the nasal septal swell body. *Arch Otolaryngol Head Neck Surg* 2010; **136**(11): 1107–10.
5. Bolger WE, Borgie RC, Melder P. The role of the crista ethmoidalis in endoscopic sphenopalatine artery ligation. *Am J Rhinol* 1999; **13**(2): 81–6.
6. Simmen DB, Raghavan U, Briner HR, et al. The anatomy of the sphenopalatine artery for the endoscopic sinus surgeon. *Am J Rhinol* 2006; **20**(5): 502–5.
7. Floreani SR, Nair SB, Switajewski MC, et al. Endoscopic anterior ethmoidal artery ligation: a cadaver study. *Laryngoscope* 2006; **116**(7): 1263–7.
8. Dalgorf DM, Harvey RJ. Chapter 1: Sinonasal anatomy and function. *Am J Rhinol Allergy* 2013; **27** Suppl 1: 3–6.
9. Harvey RJ, Shelton W, Timperley D, et al. Using fixed anatomical landmarks in endoscopic skull base surgery. *Am J Rhinol Allergy* 2010; **24**(4): 301–5.
10. Casiano RR. A stepwise surgical technique using the medial orbital floor as the key landmark in performing endoscopic sinus surgery. *Laryngoscope* 2001; **111**(6): 964–74.
11. Stammberger HR, Kennedy DW, Anatomic Terminology Group. Paranasal sinuses: anatomic terminology and nomenclature. *Ann Otol Rhinol Laryngol Suppl* 1995; **167**: 7–16.
12. Wormald PJ. The agger nasi cell: the key to understanding the anatomy of the frontal recess. *Otolaryngol Head Neck Surg* 2003; **129**(5): 497–507.
13. Zhang L, Han D, Ge W, et al. Anatomical and computed tomographic analysis of the interaction between the uncinate process and the agger nasi cell. *Acta Otolaryngol* 2006; **126**(8): 845–52.
14. Stamm A, Nogueira JF, Americo RR, et al. Frontal sinus approach: the 'vertical bar' concept. *Clin Otolaryngol* 2009; **34**(4): 407–8.
15. Kew J, Rees GL, Close D, et al. Multiplanar reconstructed computed tomography images improves depiction and understanding of the anatomy of the frontal sinus and recess. *Am J Rhinol* 2002; **16**(2): 119–23.
16. Owen RG, Jr., Kuhn FA. Supraorbital ethmoid cell. *Otolaryngol Head Neck Surg* 1997; **116**(2): 254–61.
17. Otto KJ, DelGaudio JM. Operative findings in the frontal recess at time of revision surgery. *Am J Otolaryngol* 2010; **31**(3): 175–80.
18. Harvey RJ, Gallagher RM, Sacks R. Extended endoscopic techniques for sinonasal resections. *Otolaryngol Clin North Am* 2010; **43**(3): 613–38.
19. Millar DA, Orlandi RR. The sphenoid sinus natural ostium is consistently medial to the superior turbinate. *Am J Rhinol* 2006; **20**(2): 180–1.

CHAPTER 88

OUTPATIENT ASSESSMENT

Martyn L. Barnes and Paul S. White

Introduction 977	Examination 978
History taking 977	References 982
Patient reported outcome measures (PROMs) 978	

SEARCH STRATEGY

Data in this chapter may be updated by PubMed MeSH searches using the following keywords: otolaryngology, diagnosis, nose and outpatients, as well as selected subheadings e.g. 'otolaryngology/diagnosis'[Majr]. Several thousand articles were identified, almost all too specific in context to guide this short overview chapter. Notable exceptions are cited. See also the future research comments.

INTRODUCTION

Rhinology is an increasingly broad sub-speciality in which outpatient assessment is adjusted to suit each individual case. This chapter explores basic rhinologic history taking, clinical examination, nasendoscopy and the use of patient reported outcome measures (PROMs). Interpretation and use of more specialist assessments such as rhinometry, facial pain and lacrimal testing are described in their respective chapters. Investigations are described in their respective chapters, for example 'Measurement of the Nasal Airway' and 'Radiological imaging in rhinology and skull base surgery'.

The aim of an outpatient assessment is to reach a diagnosis in order to guide management. In many patients this may be clear from the history alone.

HISTORY TAKING

This is best initiated by characterizing the index nasal symptom(s), noting duration, periodicity, nocturnal variation, seasonal effects, laterality, association with trauma or prior surgery, and whether there are any alleviating or provoking factors. The enquiry should cover the presence of nasal obstruction or congestion, facial pain, hyposmia, anosmia, rhinorrhoea and post-nasal discharge. Secondary symptoms such as sneezing, itch, epiphora, taste disturbance and dry mouth should be elicited where appropriate. Understanding the symptoms and their associations is not only useful diagnostically, but also helps to create a picture of the level of quality-of-life impairment suffered. The character of any nasal discharge can give clues to an acutely infective (mucopurulent) versus chronic rhinosinusitis or inflammatory origin. Increasing unilateral nasal obstruction associated with epistaxis (often minor) or facial pain and swelling suggests neoplasia and indicates the need for urgent assessment.

It is important to enquire about allergies, hay-fever, exposure to animal dander, asthma (or more general respiratory symptoms), and aspirin hypersensitivity. A previous history of nasal trauma may suggest nasal obstruction resulting from septal fracture or dislocation causing obstruction or failure of support to the internal nasal valve. Surgical procedures such as rhinoplasty, alar base reduction, and cleft palate surgery may all be associated with similar restrictive changes on the nasal airway.

Many systemic diseases have nasal manifestations. Granulomatosis with polyangiitis (previously Wegener's granulomatosis) is a systemic vasculitis in which nasal obstruction is associated with diffuse crusting of the nasal mucosa. Other conditions such sarcoidosis, Churg-Strauss vasculitis and Bechet's syndrome have a similar presentation. Cocaine abuse and habitual nose picking can cause septal crusting, septal perforation, and saddle deformity all of which have the potential to cause nasal impairments. Immunodeficiencies and ciliary defects are also commonly associated with nasal pathology.

A history of cigarette smoking is relevant as it may potentiate allergic rhinitis, and vasomotor rhinitis is sometimes seen as a cause of nasal obstruction during smoking cessation.

The psychological aspects of the history are important to address. Many rhinologic symptoms relate to stress, anxiety, and psychosomatic manifestations. Directed enquiry into work and home situations will often elicit a patient's own concerns to this end.

Previous and current therapeutic trials of medication and their efficacy should be recorded. Many drugs exacerbate nasal symptoms, especially common are those with anti-muscarinic effects, such as anti-prostatic medications, anti-epileptics, antidepressants, antipsychotics, antihistamines, and drugs for Parkinson's. Non-steroidal anti-inflammatory drugs (NSAIDs) such as aspirin and ibuprofen in patients who have Samter's triad (nasal polyposis, asthma and NSAID intolerance) can trigger non-infective rhinitis and rhinosinusitis. Nasal obstruction associated with vasomotor rhinitis is a side effect of a number of drugs, including antihypertensives (such as beta blockers and calcium channel blockers), sedatives, phenothiazines, antidepressants, oral contraceptives and drugs used to treat erectile dysfunction. Overuse of sympathomimetic decongestant nasal sprays can cause rhinitis medicamentosa.

PATIENT REPORTED OUTCOME MEASURES (PROMs)

Contemporary practice should include the evaluation of the full-patient presentation. This process is simplified by the routine use of PROMs – questionnaires that aim to capture and quantify the bulk of symptomatology and disease impact. These should be supplemented and validated by direct questioning and inviting patients to discuss other ways in which they have been affected. When patients complete forms prior to the appointment, the administrative burden is minimized and the exercise will add to the efficiency and efficacy of the history taking process. Capture of these data (ideally digital) should facilitate research, audit, and service evaluation.

The following are selected examples of the more prevalent and well-validated patient reported outcome measures that may be useful in a rhinology clinic (**Table 88.1**).

EXAMINATION

Nasal Structure / Aesthetics

A full facial aesthetic assessment should be performed in patients with external deformity or cosmetic concerns. Examination of the external nose should begin with careful inspection and palpation of the nasal bones and alar cartilages. The detail should include an evaluation of skin type, skin scars, soft-tissue envelope thickness, integrity of the upper and lower lateral cartilages, nasal tip support, tip configuration, nares shape and integrity of the external and internal nasal valves. These factors can offer useful information on the more subtle causes of nasal dysfunction such as nasal valve insufficiency. Abnormalities of relevance to function as well as cosmesis include saddle deformity, septal deviation and deficiencies of the upper or lower lateral cartilages.

Functional assessment / anterior rhinoscopy

Nasal patency is assessed through anterior rhinoscopy – examination of the anterior nose using a Thudicum's speculum and head light illumination. First the patient is asked to breathe normally through their nose, noting any difficulty or noise. A thumb is used to gently occlude each nostril in turn and assess unilateral patency, remembering that many normal subjects are unable to breathe comfortably through a single nasal airway.

The degree of alar margin or 'external nasal valve' collapse is observed on normal and on forced inspiration, again noting that some dynamic narrowing is normal. The inferior turbinates should be evaluated for congestion, mucosal thickening and the presence of exudate.

TABLE 88.1 Select examples of the more prevalent and well-validated patient reported outcome measures that may be useful in a rhinology clinic

Instrument	Domain Focus	PubMed Citations	Licensing
Sinonasal Outcomes Test (SNOT-22)[2]	Sinonasal	59	See wustl.edu website.[3] Contact Jay Piccirillo (+1-314-362-8641)
Glasgow Benefit Inventory (GBI)[4]	Change in Generic QoL (Benefit)[a]	129	Free for non-commercial use. Contact maa@ihr.gla.ac.uk
Rhinasthma[5]	The Unified Airway	17	No details provided. Contact canonica@unige.it
Rhinoconjunctivitis Quality of Life Questionnaire (RQLQ)[6]	Allergic Rhinitis	140	No details provided. Contact jill@qoltech.co.uk
SF-36[7]	Generic QoL	12K+	See Qualitymetricwebsite.[8] Contact info@qualitymetric.com

[a] As a benefit inventory, the GBI can be used on a single occasion (e.g., at post-operative follow-up) in order to assess the effects of an intervention – a significant administrative advantage. The Sinosasal Outcome Test-22 Questionnaire version 4 is the domain (rhinology) specific instrument recommended by the Clinical Audit and Practice Advisory Group of ENT-UK[1] based on a PubMed search conducted on July 2013 PubMed citations prior to 2009 publications.

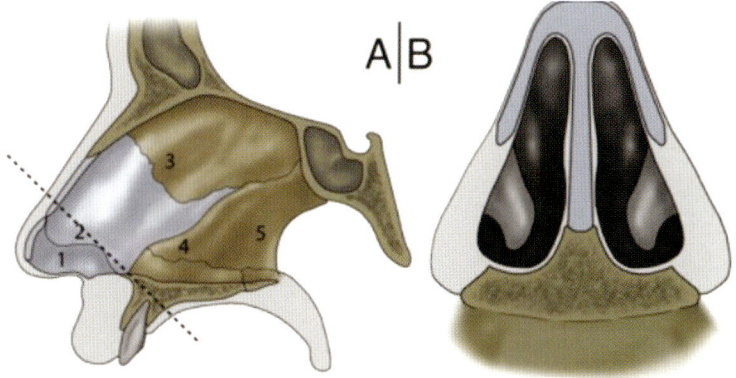

Figure 88.1 Cottle's areas of the nasal septum and the internal nasal valve region (dotted line). Deviations of the nasal septum can be classified by location and by severity. Locations include, 1 – Caudal septum, 2 – Internal nasal valve, 3 – High mid septum, 4 – Low mid septum, 5 – Posterior septum. Severity is graded 0 – No deviation, 1 – Minimal, 2 – Less than 50% lateralized, 3 – More than 50% lateralized, 4 – Fully lateralized (mucosal contact with lateral wall). This figure is released by SurgTech Ltd. (see www.SurgTech.net). They are available free of charge for anyone to use with certain provisos (see www.surgtech.net/terms). http://www.surgtech.net/Rhino/Exam/

The area between the inferior turbinate head, upper lateral cartilage and the nasal septum is the narrowest part of each nasal airway, termed the 'internal nasal valve' (**Figure 88.1**). The cross-sectional area of this space should be assessed at rest, on normal and forced inspiration. Any restriction may be due to septal deformity, turbinate engorgement or internal valve collapse. The latter may be static or dynamic due to upper lateral cartilage deformity or weakness respectively. Static internal nasal valve collapse is associated with an acute 'valve angle' at the junction of the septal and upper lateral cartilages (less than 15°). Poor septal support can also result in a shallow valve height, with nasal restriction despite an even more obtuse angle (more than 15°). Septal obstruction elsewhere in the nose can be classified and graded as shown in **Figure 88.1**.

Simple tests such as the peak nasal inspiratory flow, nasal vapour condensation, or nasal valve splinting tests can be helpful adjuncts to confirm the clinical evaluation of nasal patency (**Figure 88.2**).

Cottle's manoeuvre (testing for improvement in nasal patency with lateral traction on the alar) tends to improve all nasal airways and is not advocated as a usefully discriminant test. Other clinical tests can be helpful – internal

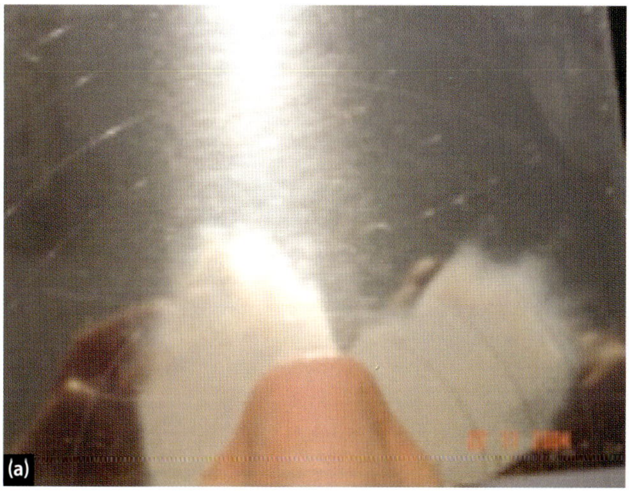

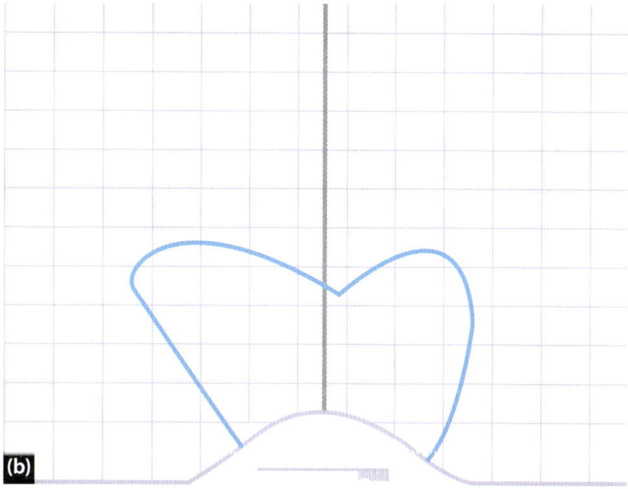

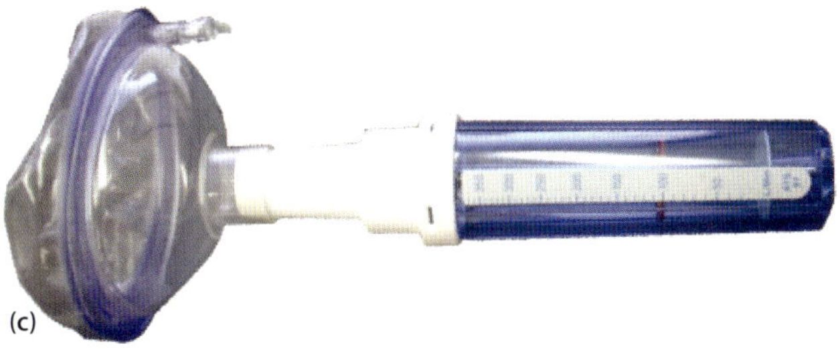

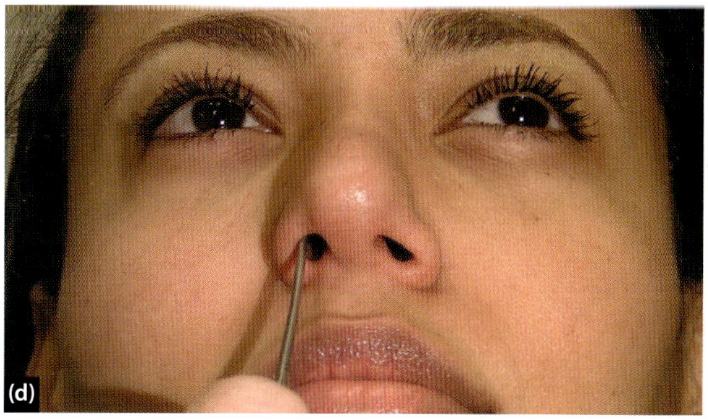

Figure 88.2 Nasal patency tests. (a,b) A vapour condensation test can be performed with a metal tongue depressor or a Glatzel calibrated mirror and gives a ready reckoning of relative flow. **(c)** A peak nasal inspiratory flow (PNIF) meter can evaluate overall nasal patency (normally more than 100 Lmin^{-1} in an adult). **(d)** Splinting tests on the external and internal nasal valve can confirm anatomical deficiencies.

TABLE 88.2 Nasendoscopy Technique
First Pass – Front to back
The endoscope is passed along the nasal floor, visualizing the septum and inferior turbinate.
In the post-nasal space, the eustachian cushion and orifice, and the fossa of Rosenmüller are seen. Any mucopurulent post-nasal drainage can be noted.
On withdrawal, the inferior meatus and, where possible, Hasner's valve are inspected.
Second Pass – Medial to the middle turbinate
Passing the endoscope medial to the middle turbinate, the sphenoethmoid recess, superior turbinate, and slit-like opening of the sphenoid ostium are visualized.
The olfactory cleft is seen more anteriorly.
Head repositioning may be required, and an angled endoscope is recommended.
Third Pass – The middle meatus
Retracting, rotating the view laterally, and rolling the endoscope into the middle meatus will medialize the turbinate to expose any middle meatal mucopurulence accessory ostia or other pathology.
The hiatus semi-lunaris, bounded by the uncinate and ethmoid bulla can be seen, as well as the membranous fontanelles and any associated accessory ostia.
An angled endoscope is recommended.

valve collapse may respond to a trial of *Breathe-Right®* strips®. Similarly, nasal vestibule stents such as France's alar dilators®, AirMax Nasal splints®, or Max-Air Sinuscones® can have a positive effect on both valve areas.

Nasendoscopy

This is a necessary investigation for all patients referred for a specialist investigation of nasal or paranasal sinus disease. It is best performed after the application of decongestant (often combined with a local anaesthetic).The effect of the vasoconstriction on the turbinate mucosa will give a useful indication of the reversibility of any congestion. Endoscopic evaluation using a three-pass technique (**Table 88.2**) should enable visualization of the inferior meatus, middle meatus, superior meatus, spheno-ethmoidal recess, olfactory cleft, septal areas, and the nasopharynx. Narrow diameter (2.5–3.0 mm) angled endoscopes (30–45°) confer greater opportunity to look around corners into each narrow nasal meatus. Patient confidence is enhanced by initiating the examination with passes though the more patent parts of the airway, for example, on the side opposite to any septal deviation. Conditions causing severe obstruction of the anterior airway such as a dramatic septal deviation or large polyps may preclude endoscopy beyond this level, but the clinical relevance will be obvious. Examples of the endoscopic anatomy, and common pathologic and findings are provided in **Figures 88.3** and **88.4**.

Endoscopic nasal biopsy

Any nasal masses should be evaluated for colour, consistency, vascularity and origin. Bilateral nasal polyps need not be biopsied unless the mucosal appearance is unusual, however, it is a sensible precaution to obtain histopathology in all primary polypectomy cases. Other endonasal masses can often be biopsied in a clinic situation, but the possibility of a vascular nature (e.g. juvenile angiofibroma) or meningo(encephalo)coele must be considered based on the appearance, location and apparent margins. In such cases, a CT with contrast or MRI scan may prevent significant complications. If a biopsy is still required, it may be best performed in the operating theatre. In all cases, preparations should be made to address any epistaxis following biopsy.

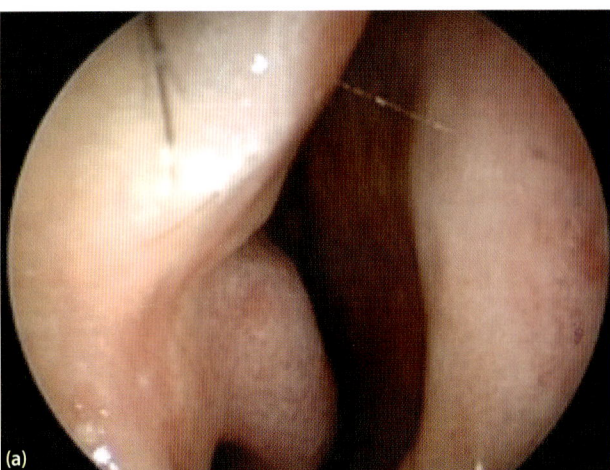
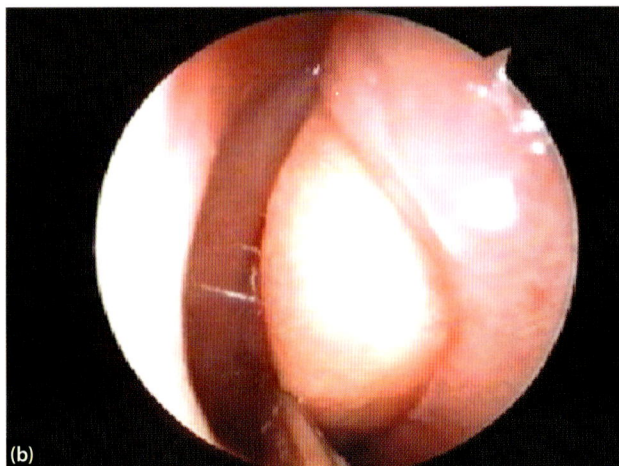

Figure 88.3 Stills of endoscopic anatomical findings. (a) Endoscopic view of the right internal nasal valve. (b) Endoscopic view of right middle meatus.
(Continued)

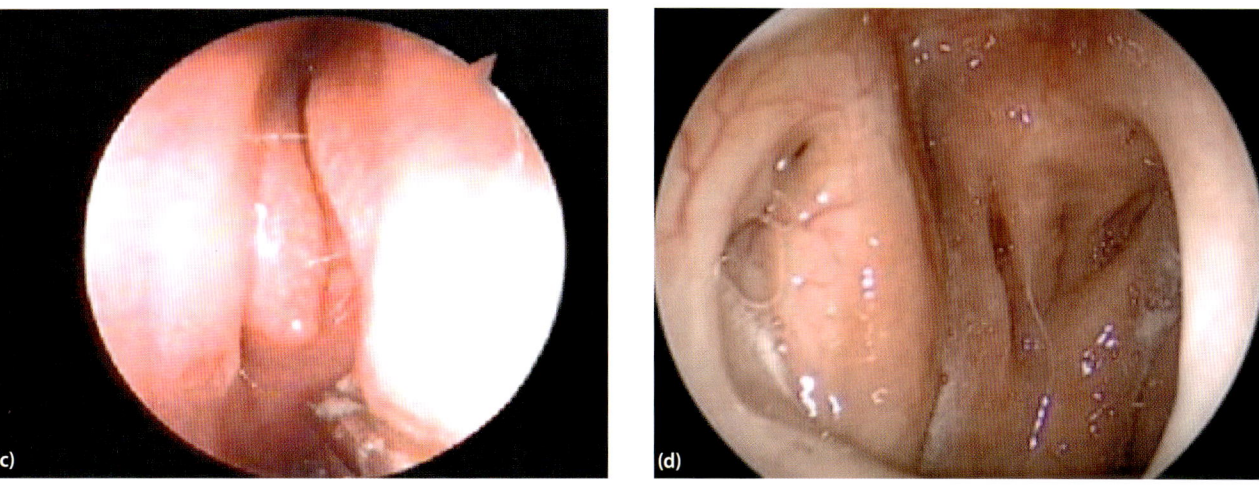

Figure 88.3 (Continued) Stills of endoscopic anatomical findings. (c) Endoscopic view of right middle meatus, showing the uncinate process, hiatus semilunaris and ethmoidal bulla. **(d)** Endoscopic view of the right side of the nasopharynx.

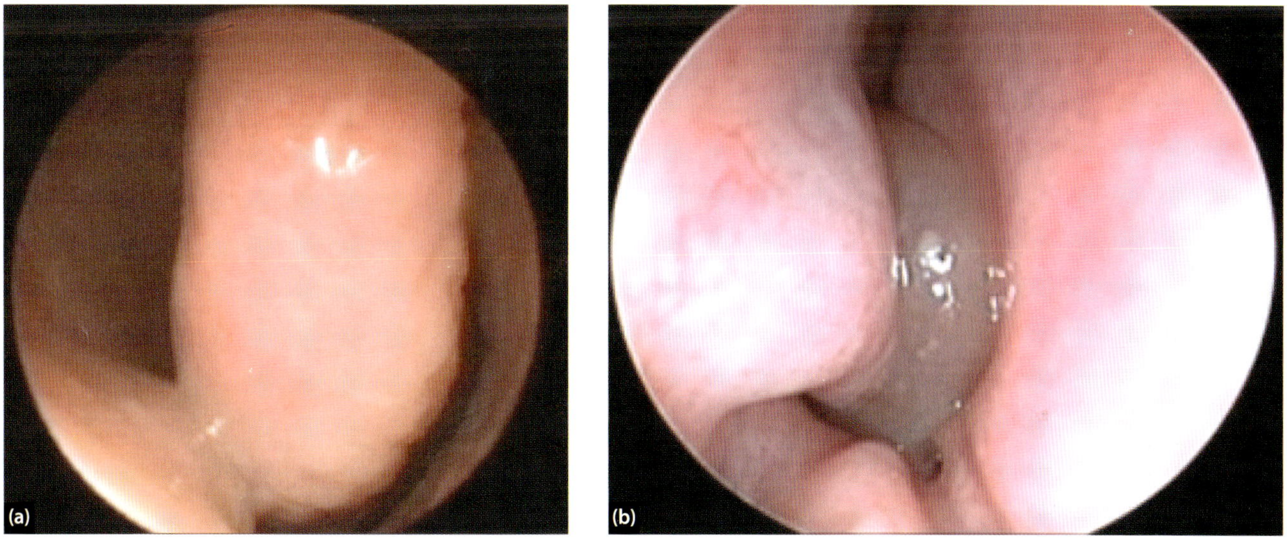

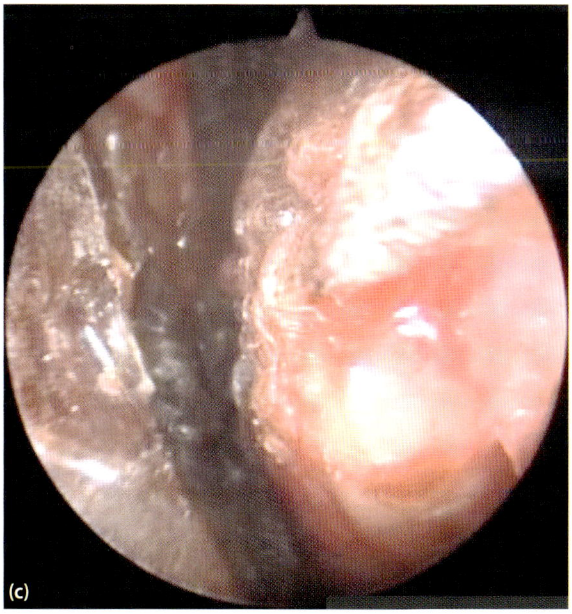

Figure 88.4 Stills of common endoscopic pathological findings. (a) Left inferior turbinate hypertrophy in allergic rhinitis. **(b)** Right nasal polyp. **(c)** Severe crusting of the right inferior turbinate and septum in granulomatosis with polangitis.

BEST CLINICAL PRACTICE

✓ Systematic approach to history and examination based on presenting concerns.
✓ Appropriate PROMs used to record presentation and clinical progress - patient completed.
✓ Formally recorded benefits for surgery and other interventions.

FUTURE RESEARCH

➤ Rarely do we formally study our greatest tool – the medical history and examination.
➤ In the future, the coming together of medical informatics, the electronic patient record, patient reported outcome measures, and innovative (largely patient led) data collection techniques applied to routine clinical practice will bring together a wealth of data we currently fail to recognize and interpret. This will give us greater opportunities to improve our understanding of the patient symptom journey, diagnostic implications, and the effect our interventions truly have on this. It may also trivialize clinician involvement. Such changes seem some way off yet – a good start would be a 'Rhinology' MeSH term.

KEY POINTS

- Well-developed skills in clinical history and examination are key to efficiently arriving at the correct diagnosis and implementing appropriate management in all our patients.
- PROMs have become an integral component of patient assessment.
- Nasal endoscopy is a necessary investigation for all patients referred for a specialist rhinologic assessment.

REFERENCES

1. Clinical outcome: Approved ENT-UK CAPAG (clinical audit and practice advisory group) patient reported outcome measures (proms); Available from: https://entuk.org/professionals/clinical_outcomes. Accessed 24 August 2017.
2. Hopkins C, Gillett S, Slack R, et al. Psychometric validity of the 22-item sino-nasal outcome test. *Clin Otolaryngol* 2009, Oct; **34**(5): 447–54.
3. Otolaryngology outcomes; Available from: http://otooutcomes.wustl.edu/research/forms/. Accessed 24 August 2017.
4. Robinson K, Gatehouse S, Browning GG. Measuring patient benefit from otorhinolaryngological surgery and therapy. *Ann Otol Rhinol Laryngol* 1996; **105**(6): 415–22.
5. Baiardini I, Pasquali M, Giardini A, et al. Rhinasthma: a new specific QoL questionnaire for patients with rhinitis and asthma. *Allergy* 2003; **58**(4): 289–94.
6. Juniper EF, Guyatt GH. Development and testing of a new measure of health status for clinical trials in rhinoconjunctivitis. *Clin Exp Allergy* 1991; **21**(1): 77–83.
7. Ware JE, Sherbourne CD. The MOS 36-item short-form health survey (SF-36). I. Conceptual framework and item selection. *Med Care* 1992; **30**(6): 473–83.
8. The SF-36v2 health survey from QualityMetric Inc. Acquired by optum, a unitedhealth group company in march 2010; Available from: http://www.qualitymetric.com/WhatWeDo/SFHealthSurveys/SF36v2HealthSurvey/tabid/185/Default.aspx. Accessed 24 August 2017.

CHAPTER 89

PHYSIOLOGY OF THE NOSE AND PARANASAL SINUSES

Tira Galm and Shahzada K. Ahmed

Introduction 983	Nasal aerodynamics 986
The role of paranasal sinuses 984	Nasal cycle 986
Nasal blood flow 984	Nasal resistance 986
Nasal mucosal vessel capacitance 984	Nasal function 987
Autonomic nervous system 984	Defence mechanisms of the nasal mucosa 988
Epithelium-ciliary function 985	Effect of pregnancy on the nose 988
Effect of smoking on the nose 986	References 989

SEARCH STRATEGY

Data in this chapter may be updated by a PubMed and Medline search using the following keywords: nasal obstruction, nasal mucosa, nasal blood flow, nasal cycle, nasal cilia, olfaction, nasal valve and autonomic nervous system.

INTRODUCTION

To understand the pathological process affecting the nose and the paranasal sinuses, it is important to have an understanding of the normal physiological functions of the nose.

The nose is a complex organ that forms an important part of the face and has multiple functions. Anatomically, the nose may be considered to have an external and internal component. The internal component forms the nasal cavities. The external component is prominent, pyramidal with an apex at the tip whose base is attached to the forehead. The nose projects downward with two perforated apertures, the nostrils, which are separated by the columella. The external nose is made up of cartilaginous and bony parts. The cartilaginous part consists of lower lateral cartilages and upper lateral cartilages both of which are in pairs. Fibrous tissue connects the cartilages. The internal nose is divided by the nasal septum into left and right chambers. The entrance of the internal nose: the nasal vestibule is lined by skin, and it contains appendages. The rest of the nasal entry is lined by respiratory mucosa and olfactory epithelium. Each cavity consists of a floor, roof, lateral and medial walls.[1]

The principal physiological function of the nose is to humidify and warm inspired air, as well as to remove noxious particles from the air, thus protecting the delicate distal lower respiratory tract. The nose also serves as a sense organ, housing the olfactory apparatus that allows individuals to smell substances for pleasure and defence purposes. These functions are highly dependent on the anatomical structure of the nose. The vomeronasal organ (VNO) is the peripheral sensory organ of the accessory olfactory system and is located either at the base of the nasal septum in humans or in the roof of the mouth in most amphibians, reptiles and mammals. The VNO role is to detect pheromones and other chemical signals that initiate innate behavioural response between individuals of the same species. These chemical communications facilitate social interactions such as sexual relationships.

The nasal mucosa is the first part of the airways to come in contact with the external environment, with an adult inspiring up to an estimated 10 000 litres of air daily. The nasal mucosa is very vascular containing arterioles, arteriovenous anastomoses and venous sinusoids, with a large surface area of 150 cm^2.[2] During normal breathing the nose contributes up to 50% of the resistance of the entire airway, with any change in this resistance playing a significant role to the total respiratory function.[3] These vital properties allow the nasal airway to play an important role in the normal homeostasis of the body.

THE ROLE OF PARANASAL SINUSES

The paranasal sinuses are air filled cavities found in the maxilla, sphenoid, ethmoid and frontal bones. They develop from an outgrowth of the nasal cavity, and hence pathology affecting the nose also affects the paranasal sinuses. Development of the paranasal sinuses vary, with ethmoid and maxillary sinuses being present at birth and the frontal sinuses developing by the age of six, however they can also be absent. The degree of development of the sphenoid sinus differs considerably.

The physiological role of the paranasal sinuses is uncertain, but a number of possible functions have been suggested.

This includes the following:

- Providing a physical buffer against injury to the face
- Vocal resonance
- Reduction of skull weight
- Humidification
- Heat insulation
- Air conditioning

NASAL BLOOD FLOW

Nasal blood flow plays a crucial part in the normal physiological function of the nose.

It can be determined using temperature change, colour change, photoelectric plethysmography, and laser Doppler techniques (**Figure 89.1**). There can be various combinations of blood flow based on the balance between arteriovenous shunting, arterial airflow as well as venous pooling. The main clinical variations include hyperaemia, reduced arterial perfusion and ischemia. Arteries and arterioles cause resistance while venules and sinusoids give capacitance. The nose has an abundant blood supply, from branches of both the internal and external carotid arteries. A rich vascular bed composed of predominantly arteriovenous anastomosis and venous sinusoids supply the nasal mucosa. The venous sinuses form the erectile tissue that is located on the anterior nasal septum and the inferior turbinates. They have the ability to expand and shrink, which has an impact on the nasal resistance and nasal airflow.[4] Animal studies have shown that venous pressure has a greater impact on the nasal airway resistance, with nasal resistance increasing by 1.2–1.3% per mmHg of venous pressure increase.[5]

NASAL MUCOSAL VESSEL CAPACITANCE

Two main mechanisms, the hydrostatic pressure of blood and the autonomic nervous system influence nasal mucosal vessel capacitance. The change in hydrostatic pressure affects the filling pressure of vessels, where increase in pressure expands the venous sinusoids. The autonomic nervous system controls the activity of smooth muscle found in the walls of the arteriovenous anastomoses leading to changes in nasal blood flow. Other factors which also influence nasal blood flow include medication, temperature and humidity.[6]

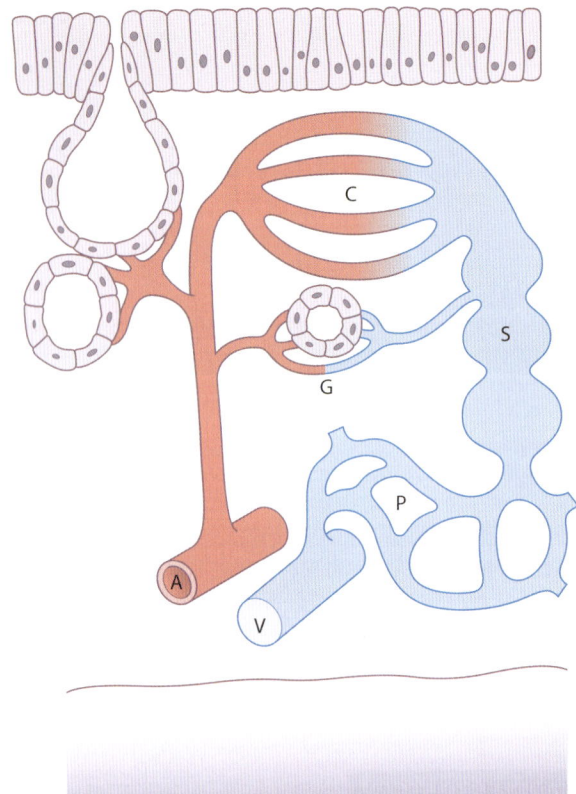

Figure 89.1 Schematic representation of the blood supply of the turbinates. A, arteriole; V, venule; C, capillaries; G, interstitial glands; P, venous plexus; S, venous sinusoids.

AUTONOMIC NERVOUS SYSTEM

The nose is innervated by parasympathetic and sympathetic fibres, which have a profound impact on nasal physiological function. The parasympathetic fibres originate in the midbrain, with the post-ganglionic fibres travelling in the maxillary branch of the trigeminal nerve and providing secretomotor supply to the mucous glands in the nasal mucosa. The primary neurotransmitters are acetylcholine, which induces serous secretion and vasoactive intestinal peptide which causes vasodilation of the blood vessels of the nasal mucosa. The sympathetic innervation to the nose starts from the thoracic spinal nerves, with pre-ganglionic fibres synapsing in the cervical sympathetic ganglion. The post-ganglionic fibres travel alongside the internal carotid artery. Sympathetic fibres predominantly innervate smooth muscle in the walls of arterioles and sinusoids. The primary neurotransmitter is noradrenalin, which has the opposite effect on the nose, causing a reduction in secretomotor activity of mucous glands and causing vasoconstriction of the blood vessels. Drugs may mimic the effects of sympathetic and

TABLE 89.1 Drugs acting on the nasal mucosa		
Drug Group	Mode of action	Example
Sympathomimetics and their antagonists	Compounds act on alpha 1 receptors and cause vasoconstriction	Adrenalin and noradrenaline analogues
		Cocaine blocks uptake of noradrenalin in nerve endings. Also acts as a local anaesthetic
		Drugs used for hypertension such as beta-blockers
Parasympathomimetics and their antagonists	Compounds act to cause vasodilation and increase nasal secretions	Pilocarpine causes vasodilation and watery secretions
		Ipratropium bromide blocks muscarinic receptors, thus preventing acetycholine from binding
Antihistamines	Predominantly block H^1 receptors. Histamine is found mainly in mast cells and causes vasodilation and increases plasma leaking from capillaries	Antihistamines
Local anaesthetics	Inhibit Na channel influx therefore reduce the rate of depolarization/repolarization.	Lignocaine

parasympathetic nerve supply. Table 89.1 gives an overview of drugs frequently used and their mode of action on the nose.

EPITHELIUM-CILIARY FUNCTION

There are three types of epithelium in the nose. First, there is squamous also referred to as the transitional epithelium that consists of the vibrissae, sweat glands, and nasal vestibule (sebaceous glands). Second, there is the pseudostratified columnar epithelium that covers two-thirds of the posterior nasal cavity. This epithelium contains ciliated as well as non-ciliated columnar cells, basal cells as well as mucin secreting goblet cells. The nasal epithelium is located on the lamina propria and basement membrane, which are served by capillaries that facilitate fluid flow through to the nasal mucosa. Finally, there is the olfactory neuroepithelium that forms the superomedial portion of the superior turbinate, nasal root and superior septum. There are various types of cells in the olfactory epithelium but the more common are Bowman glands and ducts, bipolar receptor cells, sustentacular cells and microvillar cells. Cilia are located on the surface cells of the respiratory tract. Their role is to push mucus backwards towards the nasopharynx.

The ultrastructure of all cilia remains the same; however, nasal cilia are somewhat short. The surface membrane of a cilium encloses an organized ultrastructure. The nine outer-paired microtubules enclose a single inner pair of microtubules. The outer pairs of microtubules are linked to one another by nexins and to the inner pair of microtubules by central spokes. In addition, outer pairs of microtubules have both outer and inner dynein arms that are made up of an ATPase. There are two layers of nasal mucus film, the lower layer that is more watery and cilia move freely, and the upper viscous layer. Importantly, there are small hooks on the tips of the cilia to facilitate their movements once they enter the viscous layer.

At body temperature, cilia beat frequency ranges from 7 to 16 Hz. The frequency usually remains constant when the temperatures are between 32 and 40 °C. The cilia can beat rapidly in a propulsive stroke or slowly during the recovery phase. Notably, the propulsive period is characterized by the cilium straightening while the tip points to the viscous layer. The recovery phase sees the cilium bending over in the aqueous layer. During this process, adenosine triphosphate (ATP) is converted to adenosine diphosphate (ADP) using the enzyme ATPase that is found at the dynein arms. This magnesium ion (Mg^{2+}) dependent reaction produces energy. Motion occurs whenever there is sliding of the outer pair microtubules against one another. The mitochondria located near the cell surface next to cilia's basal bodies generate the ATP.[7]

Metachronous movement of cilia propels the mucus blanket backwards, thus only those (cilia) that are at right angle to the direction of the flow form the phase. Cilia that are in the flow-direction are out of phase until the cycle completes. From the front of the nose, mucus flows posteriorly. Thereafter, mucus from the sinuses and from the lateral wall joins together with most passing through the middle meatus. The majority of mucus then passes around the Eustachian orifice before it is swallowed.

The nose is a constantly changing environment where slight fluctuations can affect the function of cilia. Dry conditions stop ciliary action and at temperatures below 10 °C and temperatures above 45 °C, ciliary movement stops. Isotonic saline preserve the activity of cilia, however, if the solutions are 5% above and 2% below the normal isotonic saline conditions, paralysis occurs. Likewise, potassium ions do not affect ciliary function except when the levels become non-physiological.[8] Furthermore, cilia can beat above pH 6.4 as well as function in a slightly alkaline medium of up to pH 8.5 for a prolonged period. Infections in the upper respiratory tract can cause damage to the epithelium and the function of cilia also deteriorate with age.[9]

EFFECT OF SMOKING ON THE NOSE

Tobacco contains hundreds of noxious chemicals and when smoked can irritate the lining of the nose resulting in increased nasal secretions and congestion caused by impairment of mucociliary clearance. Smoking causes a reduction in the number of cilia and change in mucous viscosity. Studies have shown that eight hours after exposure to tobacco smoke the efficiency of mucociliary clearance had reduced, with heavier smokers having more marked impact.[10]

NASAL AERODYNAMICS

Knowledge of the aerodynamic behaviour of the nasal airway provides an aid to the decision-making process of medical and surgical management of pathological processes affecting the nose.

At rest the normal inspiratory flow rate in an adult ranges between 5 L/min to 12 L/min and has a pressure change of 50 Pa between the nostrils and the nasopharynx. During exercise the flow rate increases with a correspondent drop in pressure, where the flow rate can increase to as much as 150 L/min.[11]

Fluid dynamic experiments of the nose (**Figure 89.2**) have shown that nasal flow is laminar as it enters the nasal vestibule, with no mixing of the different air layers at low velocity.

The velocity of the air increases as it passes through the nasal valve, the narrowest site of the upper respiratory tract. At this point turbulent flow is observed in the nasal cavity, with different air layers swirling together. The change from laminar to turbulent flow is paramount as it allows the velocity of the air to reduce, thus allowing prolonged contact of inspired air with the nasal mucosa and therefore allowing the nose to perform its vital functions.

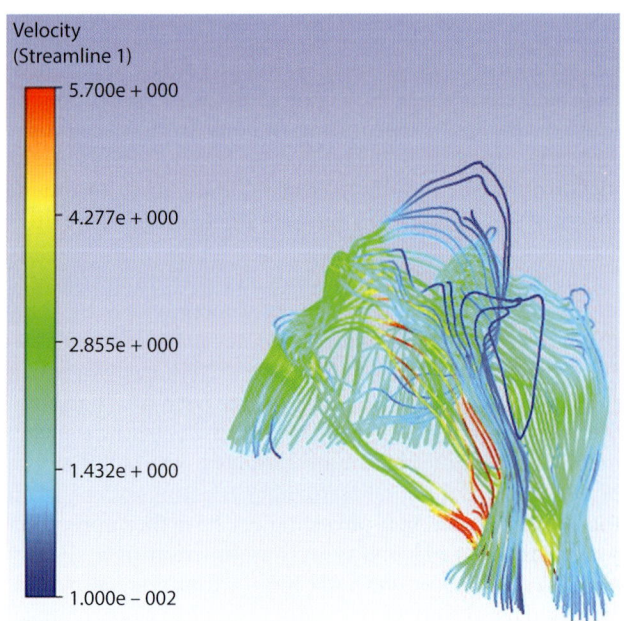

Figure 89.2 Velocity streamlines.

Septal deviation and turbinate hypertrophy can cause a reduction in the cross-sectional area of the nasal mucosa and thus also affect nasal function.[12, 13]

NASAL CYCLE

The nasal cycle is a well-recognized physiological activity whereby each side of the nose alternates the phases of congestion and decongestion.[14] Vascular activity produces the changes, especially the volume of blood in capacitance vessels (venous sinusoids). The changes are cyclical and occur every 4 to 12 hours with the changes being constant for each person. The nasal cycle can be demonstrated in up to 80% of adults, however, it is not easy to demonstrate in children.[15]

The physiological significance of the nasal cycle is not clear. However, resistance and airflow leads to increased cyclical secretions in the side that is experiencing the greatest flow. Several factors affect the nasal cycle; these include exercise, pregnancy, hormones, infections, allergy, fear, emotions and sexual activity. The autonomic nervous system regulates many of the changes. Notably, vagal over activity can lead to congestion while high levels of CO_2 present in inspired air that is produced as a result of rebreathing may reduce the nasal resistance. Hyperventilation reverses the situation.[16] Nasal congestion may also occur due to drugs that block the action of the noradrenaline. Antihistamines also produce anticholinergic effects that can halt parasympathetic activity. This results in increased sympathetic tone that improves the nasal airway. Hormonal changes seen in puberty also affect the nasal mucosa.

NASAL RESISTANCE

Nasal resistance plays a crucial role in preventing the collapse of the lower respiratory tract, notably the lungs, with nasal resistance contributing up to 50% of the total airway resistance. As nasal airway resistance is increased, it causes an increase in negative intra-thoracic pressure and in turn enhances pulmonary ventilation. Mathematically, resistance of nasal airflow is equal to the pressure of the nasal flow divided by flow rate. Nasal air flow is affected by the radius of the nose. Based on laminar flow equations, a decrease in the nasal radius can cause a four-fold decrease in nasal air flow (see Chapter 90, Measurement of the nasal airway). The presence of laminar and turbulent flow in the nasal passageway is vital to the physiology of air exchange. Nasal airway resistance is achieved through three key components. These include the nasal vestibule, the nasal valve and the inferior turbinates.

Nasal vestibule

The nasal vestibule is composed of a compliant wall that can collapse in response to the negative pressure caused by inspiration thus increasing nasal resistance. A flow of 30 L/min is the limiting rate during inspiration at which nasal airway collapse occurs at the nasal

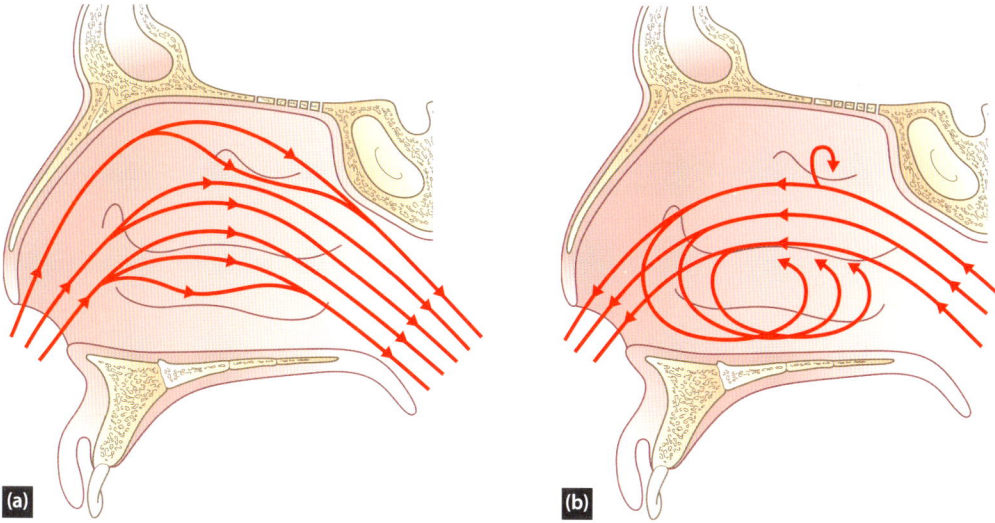

Figure 89.3 (a) The direction of inspiratory airflow. **(b)** The direction of expiratory airflow.

vestibule (**Figure 89.3a**). However, this airway collapse can be prevented by activation of the ala nasi muscle during inspiration. Contraction of this muscle results in a change of the shape of the vestibule which leads to a reduction in air flow turbulence without affecting the cross-sectional area. Paralysis of ala nasi, as seen in facial nerve palsy, causes the nasal vestibule to collapse during inspiration and hence increase nasal resistance. During exercise the ala nasi muscle contracts, which increases the radius of the nasal cavity and hence reduces nasal resistance.[17]

Expiration has the opposite effect, as the positive pressure within the vestibule increases the radius of the nose and in turn improves nasal airflow (**Figure 89.3b**).

Internal nasal valve

This is the narrowest part of the nasal airway and helps to direct the airflow upward and backward across the anterior part of the inferior turbinate. It is found approximately 2 cm posterior to the anterior nares and has a cross-sectional area between 55–83 mm^2. The size of the inferior turbinate (an erectile tissue) and position of the nasal septum determines the dimensions of nasal valve.

The nasal valve is bound superiorly by the caudal end of upper lateral cartilages and septum medially. The inferior boundary is the nasal floor, laterally is the bony piriform aperture with the adjacent fibrofatty tissue and posteriorly is the head of the inferior turbinate. The nasal valve makes a significant contribution to upper airway resistance and produces the most turbulent airflow.[12] During quiet respiration, the velocity of the anterior valve ranges from 12 to 18 m/sec. The nasal valve is often referred as the internal nasal valve. Therefore any change in the size of the inferior turbinate and deviation of the septum at this level has an impact on the nasal valve. The nasal valve plays a key role clinically, and the treatment of the components that make up the nasal valve area can have a marked impact on nasal airway resistance.

The Cottle maneuver is used to assess the narrowing of the nasal valve area at rest. The test is conducted by lateralizing the soft tissue and the nasal vestibule. It is considered positive if it improves nasal airflow. Swelling of the inferior turbinate has a profound effect on nasal resistance. Consequently, treatments that aim to reduce the size of the inferior turbinate have a significant effect on the nasal resistance as opposed to that of the nasal surgery that removes septal spurs.

Inferior turbinate

The turbinates of the nose can swell and recede, thereby reducing the dimensions of the nasal cavity contributing to nasal airway resistance. The inferior turbinates are part of the nasal valve area and they help the change of laminar inspired air into turbulent flow. The large surface area and extensive blood supply of the inferior turbinate increases the interaction of inspired air with nasal mucosa which enables the nose to carry out its functions more effectively.[18]

Pathological processes causing enlargement of the inferior turbinate by only a small incremental increase of 1–2 mm have been shown to lead to a significant reduction in the nasal airflow velocity down to 0.42 m/s when compared to 0.89 m/s in the normal healthy nose.[19]

NASAL FUNCTION

The nose has various physiological functions. Respiratory functions include heat exchange, filtration, humidification, nasal neurovascular reflexes and voice modification. Olfaction functions are stimulus pathways and there is trigeminal input.

Heat exchange

The temperature of inspired air can range from −50 to 50°C. Since various racial groups live in different environments, the nose has evolved to suit different local conditions.

Filtration

The turbinates organize the pattern of airflow, enabling the nose to exhale all of the inspired air to the airstream. This happens fairly slowly around and along the ciliated turbinates. In the process, heat and energy is emitted into the inspired airstreams thereby saturating the airborne particles as well as micro-organisms. Eventually, the particles and micro-organisms become heavier, sinking into the mucosal layer where they are processed using enzymes and immune system cells.

Olfaction

Sense of smell plays an important role in protection from danger, such as fire. It is also central in forming positive and negative memories affecting individual psychological wellbeing, socialization and interpersonal relationships, with dysfunction leading to a poor quality of life (see Chapter 110. Abnormalities of Smell).

DEFENCE MECHANISMS OF THE NASAL MUCOSA

The nose has a role in protective mechanisms to prevent noxious substances entering the lower respiratory tract. This defence mechanism can be divided into mechanical and immunological defence.

Mechanical defence

The nose is able to protect the lower airway by removing particles of approximately 30 μm or upward such as pollen in inspired air. The velocity of the inspired air drops significantly after the nasal valve. As turbulence increases, so does the deposition of particles. Particles with irregular shapes resist change to the greatest extent because they have a larger surface area. Vibrissae only stop the largest particles. Mucociliary flow is the main mechanical defence of the nasal mucosa because it physically cleans inspired air. The mucociliary transport system is made up of cilia of the respiratory epithelium as well as a mucous blanket. The latter consists of a deeper layer where ciliary motion occurs as well as a superficial thicker gel layer. Viscoelastic properties enable it to trap larger particles. This mechanical defence is predominant and expels filtered particles and debris into the nasopharynx and oropharynx as well as elimination through sneezing and coughing.[20]

Immunological defence

Mucus consists of compounds that are able to neutralize antigens through innate mechanisms, learned, and adaptive immunological responses. Immunoglobulin A (IgA) and immunoglobulin E (IgE) are found on the surface, and they act whenever the mucosa is breached. In most cases, bacterial allergens are destroyed, but there are other viruses and bacteria that require the activation of the cell-mediated immune responses. IgA is the main immunoglobulin in secretions and has distinctive characteristics. IgA has two subgroups, namely IgA_1 and IgA_2. IgA_1, with a monomeric structure, is frequent in serum while IgA_2, with a dimer structure, is common in nasal secretions.[21] Immunoglobulin A constitutes 70% of the total proteins in nasal secretions.

EFFECT OF PREGNANCY ON THE NOSE

Pregnancy induced rhinitis (PIR) is a common problem, and has an incidence of around 22%. PIR has been defined as nasal congestion that is not present before pregnancy, but manifests itself in the second or third trimester, lasting 6 or more weeks with no known allergic cause, which then resolves completely within 2 weeks of delivery.[22] The cause of PIR is still under debate as is the impact of pregnancy hormones on the nasal mucosa. Studies have shown that during pregnancy there is a decrease in mucociliary clearance and increase in nasal resistance, with oestrogen having possible role in inducing histamine receptors on epithelial cells.[23, 24]

> **BEST CLINICAL PRACTICE**
>
> ✓ Pregnancy induced rhinitis (PIR) is a common problem, and has an incidence of around 22%.
> ✓ PIR has been defined as nasal congestion that is not present before pregnancy, but manifests itself in the 2nd or 3rd trimester, lasting 6 or more weeks with no known allergic cause, which then resolves completely within 2 weeks of delivery.[22]

> **FUTURE RESEARCH**
>
> ▶ Nasal morbidity, unlike in disorders affecting the other senses, is difficult to quantify, yet conditions such as sinusitis are chronic and affect a significant percentage of the population.
> ▶ Continued basic science research is desperately needed that may lead to a better understanding of the physiology of nasal function to ultimately help in better treating common nasal complaints.

> **KEY POINTS**
>
> - The principal physiological function of the nose is to
>   - humidify and warm inspired air
>   - remove noxious particles from the air
>   - also serves as a sense organ
> - The nose has an abundant blood supply, from branches of both the internal and external carotid arteries.
> - The venous sinuses form the erectile tissue that is located on the anterior nasal septum and the inferior turbinates.
> - Smoking causes a reduction in the number of cilia and change in mucous viscosity.
> - The nasal cycle is a well-recognized physiological activity whereby each side of the nose alternates the phases of congestion and decongestion.[14]
> - Nasal resistance plays a crucial role in preventing the collapse of the lower respiratory tract, notably the lungs, with nasal resistance contributing up to 50% of the total airway resistance.

REFERENCES

1. Jones N. The nose and paranasal sinuses: physiology and anatomy. *Adv Drug Deliv Rev* 2001; **51**(1–3): 5–19.
2. Patou J, De Smedt H, van Cauwenberge P, et al. Pathophysiology of nasal obstruction and meta-analysis of early and late effects of levocetirizine. *Clin Exp Allergy* 2006; **36**(8): 972–81.
3. Hilberg O. Objective measurement of nasal airway dimensions using acoustic rhinometry: methodological and clinical aspects. *Allergy* 2002; **57** Suppl 70: 5–39.
4. Holmberg K, Bake B, Pipkorn U. Nasal mucosal blood flow after intranasal allergen challenge. *J Allergy Clin Immunol* 1988; **81**(3): 541–7.
5. Lung MA, Wang JC. Nasal airway response to mucosal perfusion and outflow resistance in the dog and rat. *Acta Otolaryngol* 1987; **104**(5-6): 526–32.
6. Tsai KK, Yen CF, Chu YH, et al. Using dynamic analysis of Laser-Doppler blood flowmetry to measure nasal mucosa bloody flow in postural changes. *Rhinology* 2012; **50**(4): 376–80.
7. Robson AM, Smallman LA, Drake-Lee AB. Factors affecting ciliary function in vitro: a preliminary study. *Clin Otolaryngol Allied Sci* 1992; **17**(2): 125–9.
8. Ho JC, Chan KN, Hu WH, et al. The effect of aging on nasal mucociliary clearance, beat frequency, and ultrastructure of respiratory cilia. *Am J Respir Crit Care Med* 2001; **163**(4): 983–8.
9. Cauna N. Electron microscopy of the nasal vascular bed and its nerve supply. *Ann Otol Rhinol Laryngol* 1970; **79**(3): 443–50.
10. Proenca M, Fagundes Xavier R, et al. Immediate and short term effects of smoking on nasal mucociliary clearance in smokers. *Rev Port Pneumol* 2011; **17**(4): 172–6.
11. Chen XB, Lee HP, Chong VF, et al. Impact of inferior turbinate hypertrophy on the aerodynamic pattern and physiological functions of the turbulent airflow: a CFD simulation model. *Rhinology* 2010; **48**(2): 163–8.
12. Bridger GP, Proctor DF. Maximum nasal inspiratory flow and nasal resistance. *Ann Otol Rhinol Laryngol* 1970; **79**(3): 481–8.
13. Mlynski G, Grutzenmacher S, Plontke S, et al. Correlation of nasal morphology and respiratory function. *Rhinology* 2001; **39**(4): 197–201.
14. Soane RJ, Carney AS, Jones NS, et al. The effect of the nasal cycle on mucociliary clearance. *Clin Otolaryngol Allied Sci* 2001; **26**(1): 9–15.
15. Van Cauwenberge PB, Deleye L. Nasal cycle in children. *Arch Otolaryngol* 1984; **110**(2): 108–10.
16. Series F, Cormier Y, Desmeules M, et al. Influence of respiratory drive on upper airway resistance in normal men. *J Appl Physiol* 1989; **66**(3): 1242–9.
17. Hol MK, Huizing EH. Treatment of inferior turbinate pathology: a review and critical evaluation of the different techniques. *Rhinology* 2000; **38**(4): 157–66.
18. Lee HP, Poh HJ, Chong FH, et al. Changes of airflow pattern in inferior turbinate hypertrophy: a computational fluid dynamics model. *Am J Rhinol Allergy* 2009; **23**(2): 153–8.
19. Huang ZL, Ong KL, Goh SY, et al. Assessment of nasal cycle by acoustic rhinometry and rhinomanometry. *Otolaryngol Head Neck Surg* 2003; **128**(4): 510–16.
20. Pilette C, Ouadrhiri Y, Godding V, et al. Lung mucosal immunity: immunoglobulin-A revisited. *Eur Resp J* 2001; **18**(3): 571–88.
21. Kerr MA. The structure and function of human IgA. *Biochem J* 1990; **271**(2): 285–96.
22. Ellegard EK. The etiology and management of pregnancy rhinitis. *Am J Respir Med* 2003; **2**(6): 469–75.
23. Philpott CM, El-Alami M, Murty GE. The effect of the steroid sex hormones on the nasal airway during the normal menstrual cycle. *Clin Otolaryngol Allied Sci* 2004; **29**(2): 138–42.
24. Armengot M, Basterra J, Marco J. Nasal mucociliary function during the menstrual cycle in healthy women. *Rev Laryngol Otol Rhinol* 1990; **111**(2): 107–9.

CHAPTER 90

MEASUREMENT OF THE NASAL AIRWAY

Ron Eccles

Introduction 991	Subjective measurements 994
Rhinomanometry 991	Measurement of the nasal airway by the rhinologist 995
Acoustic rhinometry 994	References 997
Peak nasal flow 994	

SEARCH STRATEGY

Data in this chapter may be updated by a PubMed search using the keywords: rhinomanometry, acoustic rhinometry, nasal peak inspiratory flow and human. The data were supplemented by further searches and use of a personal database. The evidence in this chapter is not aimed at any specific treatments, only methods to measure the patency of the nasal airway, and based on a range of studies that include randomized clinical trials of Level 1 evidence.

INTRODUCTION

Nasal obstruction is one of the most common complaints presenting to ENT surgeons, but treatment is usually initiated without any objective measurement of nasal airflow or nasal patency. Pneumologists have access to useful normal ranges for lung function, whereas rhinologists have not established generally accepted ranges for normal nasal patency.

Establishing a normal range of nasal patency is confounded by several factors related to nasal physiology. First, the nose is directly exposed to the external environment and acts as an air conditioner to protect the lungs from infection and variations in environmental conditions, whereas the lungs operate as part of the internal environment at a constant temperature of 37°C in a sterile environment. Second, the nose is subject to spontaneous changes in nasal patency associated with the 'nasal cycle', with spontaneous congestion and decongestion of the large veins found in the nasal epithelium.[1] The direct exposure of the nose to the external environment and the spontaneous changes in nasal patency associated with the nasal cycle make normal or 'physiological' nasal patency unstable and difficult to define.[2]

'Anatomical' nasal patency is the nasal patency measured after decongestion of the nasal blood vessels by application of a topical nasal decongestant or by standard exercise. Anatomical nasal patency is a useful measure for the nasal surgeon as it is determined solely by the hard tissues of the nose such as cartilage and bone.[3]

Measures of nasal obstruction usually involve measurement of nasal airflow or an assessment of the cross sectional area of the airway. The nasal airway can be considered as a simple tube, and measurement of the airflow through the tube and its driving pressure, by means of rhinomanometry, can provide a measure of nasal patency. The prime factor determining nasal patency is the cross sectional area of the nasal airway and this can be measured by means of acoustic rhinometry. Rhinomanometry provides a functional measure of nasal patency, whereas acoustic rhinometry provides an anatomical measurement of cross sectional area or nasal volume. Rhinomanometry and acoustic rhinometry are the major techniques used for measuring the nasal airway but other techniques such as measurement of nasal peak inspiratory flow can also provide useful measures of nasal patency.

This section will discuss the most commonly used measurements of nasal patency and their relevance to research and clinical practice in rhinology.

RHINOMANOMETRY

Rhinomanometry normally provides a measure of nasal resistance to airflow and measures of nasal patency in units of nasal airflow may be further calculated from this parameter. Nasal resistance to air flow is calculated from two measurements: nasal airflow and trans-nasal pressure.[4] Both these parameters are measured by means of differential pressure transducers (manometers) and this is why the study of nasal pressure and flow is termed 'rhinomanometry', since manometry involves the measurement of pressure. Nasal airflow can be measured by means of a flow head that usually consists of a mesh resistance inside a tube. The pressure difference across the mesh generated by airflow through the tube is used to measure airflow. Trans-nasal pressure can be measured by relating the pressure at the posterior nares to that at the entrance of the nostril, which will normally be atmospheric pressure or nasal mask pressure.

Active rhinomanometry involves the generation of nasal airflow and pressure with normal breathing. Passive rhinomanometry involves the generation of nasal airflow and pressure from an external source, such as a fan or pump, to drive air through the nose.

Active rhinomanometry can be divided into anterior and posterior methods according to the location of the pressure-sensing tube. In active anterior rhinomanometry, the pressure-sensing tube is normally taped to one nasal passage. The sealed nasal passage acts as an extension of the pressure-sensing tube to measure pressure in the posterior nares. With this method, nasal airflow is measured from one nostril at a time and the pressure-sensing tube is moved from one side of the nose to the other. Therefore, nasal resistance is determined separately for each nasal passage and the total resistance is then calculated by summing the values as shown in the formulae below.

In active posterior rhinomanometry as shown in **Figure 90.1**, the pressure-sensing tube is held in the mouth and detects the posterior nares pressure when the soft palate allows an airway to the mouth.

Total nasal airflow can be measured from both nasal passages simultaneously. The right and left nasal airflows can be measured separately by taping off one nostril at a time. Total nasal resistance can be determined directly from the total nasal airflow and trans-nasal pressure with this method. A disadvantage of this method, when compared with the anterior method, is that not all subjects can obtain an airway around the soft palate into the mouth. With some training of subjects it is possible to obtain satisfactory results from about 90% of subjects.

Passive rhinomanometry involves the direction of an external flow of air through the nose and out of the mouth. The method may involve either measurement of a driving pressure at a constant flow or measurement of the flow at a constant pressure. Passive rhinomanometry is particularly useful if it is necessary to separate the upper and lower airways for experimental work.

Active anterior rhinomanometry, using surgical tape to seal a pressure-sensing tube into the nasal passage, is one of the most commonly used methods for clinical determination of nasal resistance and it is recommended by standardization committees,[5, 6] but posterior rhinomanometry has been used successfully in clinical trials on nasal surgery and nasal decongestants.[7–9]

Nasal airway resistance can also be measured by use of a head-out body plethysmograph (displacement type) and with this method the flow head is located on the side of the body-box and the pressure-sensing tube is passed along the floor of the nasal cavity. This method has the advantage that the nose is unimpeded by any mask.[10]

When making measurements of nasal airway resistance it is important to take several measurements with repositioning of the mask between measurements. This is to control for air leaks around the mask that are a common source of error. A single measurement of nasal airway resistance is unreliable and a standard operating procedure should be implemented to prevent investigator bias when gathering data.[4]

Nasal resistance to air flow may be calculated from the following equation:

$$R = \frac{\delta P}{V}$$

R = resistance to air flow/cm H_2O/litre per second or Pa/cm^3 per second
δP = trans-nasal pressure, in cm H_2O or Pa
V = nasal air flow, in litre/s or cm^3/s

This equation is a compromise that has been generally accepted by rhinologists and it does not take into consideration the separate components of laminar and turbulent air flow.[5,6]

A plot of the dynamic relations of trans-nasal pressure and flow on an x/y plotter shows a curvilinear relationship for the $\frac{\delta P}{V}$ plot. Nasal airflow increases with increase of trans-nasal pressure, but at higher pressures there is a limitation of flow due to the increased frictional effects of turbulent airflow. The flow-limiting effect of nasal alar collapse is only apparent during rapid or close to maximum inspiratory manoeuvres.

The curvilinear relationship between trans-nasal pressure and flow means that one cannot simply determine

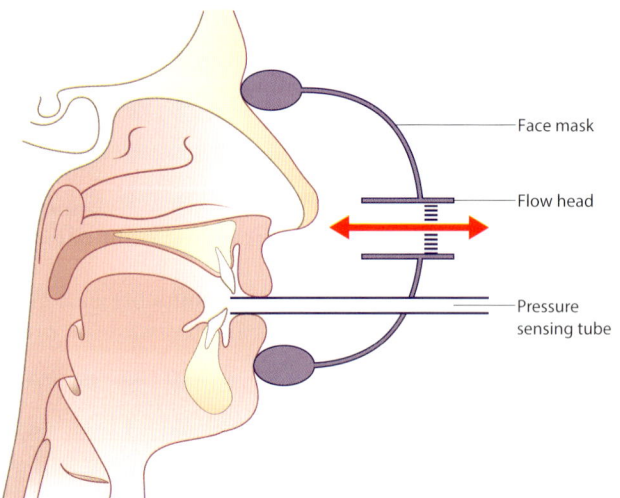

Figure 90.1 The technique of posterior rhinomanometry. This involves a pressure-sensing tube in the mouth that detects the changes in pressure in the posterior nares, and a flow head to measure nasal airflow.

nasal resistance from the slope of the graph, as would be the case with a straight-line relationship. The slope of the $\frac{\delta P}{V}$ plot varies along its length and, therefore, it is not possible to describe the whole curve with a single numerical value for resistance. It is, however, possible to define the resistance at any given sample point along the curve and this has been the solution recommended for a standardized measurement of nasal resistance.[5,6]

The positive or negative pressure at the posterior nares results in airflow through both nasal passages. The right and left nasal airflows are normally asymmetrical due to the nasal cycle and therefore a single pressure value may relate to two different airflows. It is, therefore, sensible to standardize nasal resistance by measuring both nasal airflows at the same sample pressure point rather than by measuring trans-nasal pressures at the same sample flow point.

Unilateral nasal airflow measured at a sample pressure point of 150 Pa and bilateral nasal airflow measured at 75 Pa are recommended.[5] Other parameters may be calculated from the pressure flow curve but these are not in general use and are not generally accepted.[6] The Asian population cannot always achieve the higher sample pressure of 150 Pa during normal quiet breathing, and the lower sample pressures of 100 and 50 Pa, respectively, are generally accepted for nasal resistance measurements in Japan.

The lower nasal pressures in the Asian population compared to Caucasians is due to smaller body size and smaller lung volume.

Total nasal resistance to air flow can be either determined directly using the posterior method of rhinomanometry or it can be calculated by combining the two separate values of nasal resistance for the two nasal passages as shown in the formula below:

$$\frac{1}{R(total)} = \frac{1}{r(left)} + \frac{1}{r(right)}$$

The reciprocal of total resistance is equal to the sum of the reciprocals of left and right resistance.

When quoting values for total nasal resistance it should be stated whether the value was obtained by measurement of total nasal air flow using posterior rhinomanometry, or whether the air flows of the nasal passages have been measured separately.

Normal nasal airflow

As discussed above, nasal patency in health is unstable and may be even more variable in disease, therefore it is difficult to give any normal range. The variability in nasal patency is especially marked for unilateral patency as it is normal for one nasal passage to be obstructed and the other quite patent as a normal phase of the nasal cycle. However, total nasal patency is more stable because of the reciprocal relationship between the two nasal passages.[1]

In adult subjects free from signs of nasal disease mean total resistance has been reported to be around 0.23 Pa cm^3 s with a range of 0.15–0.39 Pa cm^3 s.[11] As a routine screening procedure in our laboratory we normally consider a total nasal resistance to airflow of 0.3 Pa cm^3 s as an upper limit of the normal range. Cole considers any total airway resistance greater than 0.25 Pa cm^3 s as obstructed.[10] Nasal resistance is at a maximum in the infant at around 1.2 Pa cm^3 s,[12-13] declines to the adult value at around 16–18 years of age and then shows only a slow decline with increasing age.[14] In a study on healthy male volunteers a relationship between age and nasal resistance was reported, with resistance declining with increasing age from 0.6 Pa cm^3 s (age 5–12 years) to 0.29 Pa cm^3 s (age 13–19 years) and 0.22 Pa cm^3 s (age >20 years) in males.[15] The relationship between age and nasal resistance was similar in females but in general nasal resistance was lower in females than males.[15]

If the nose is decongested by exercise or application of a topical decongestant then this eliminates any physiological variation in resistance and allows one to investigate the anatomical factors influencing resistance. Studies by Broms[16] have provided a table of predictive values for height and nasal resistance in the decongested nose that are useful in assessing the extent of any deviation from normality in patients with nasal skeletal stenosis.

Total nasal resistance gives an overall measure of nasal function but it is a very crude measurement, as it provides no information about the separate nasal passages. Rhinologists have a dilemma when assessing nasal function as the nose consists of two separate dynamic airways. However, it is not very informative to quote the mean of unilateral resistance when measured over several hours because this mean value will have a large standard deviation due to the instability of unilateral resistance. The range of unilateral nasal airway resistance in a group of healthy volunteers when recorded over a 6–8 hour period has been shown to vary from 0.36 to 1.36 Pa cm^3 s[17] and 0.28–0.63 Pa cm^3 s.[18] This indicates that there is often almost a fourfold change in unilateral resistance associated with the spontaneous congestion and decongestion of the nasal venous sinuses.

One way to overcome the dilemma of spontaneous changes in unilateral nasal resistance is to decongest the nose prior to assessment. This solution is of use to the surgeon whose main interest may be in assessing the extent of any nasal anatomical problem,[16] however one study reports that nasal patency after decongestion is not always reproducible over several months in healthy subjects[19] but it is reported to be stable over shorter periods of 12 hours.[4] However, decongestion of the nose is of no use in studying nasal physiology and pathophysiology as it is the spontaneous changes in unilateral resistance that are of interest to the physiologist and clinician. One solution is to quantify the extremes of unilateral resistance or the amplitude of the unilateral changes in resistance that occur over a period of several hours. This approach has been used to determine the unilateral changes in resistance and to assess the efficacy of nasal surgery.[7] The disadvantage of unilateral nasal measurements is that in order to assess the amplitude of changes in unilateral nasal resistance it is necessary to make measurements over several hours. The advantage of unilateral measurements are that they give a comprehensive assessment of the dynamic nose rather than the crude snap shot that is provided by a single measure of total resistance.

ACOUSTIC RHINOMETRY

Acoustic rhinometry has been developed from methods previously used to measure lower respiratory tract resistance. The method consists of generating an acoustic pulse from a spark source or speaker and the sound pulse is transmitted along a tube into the nose. The sound pulse is reflected back from inside the nose according to changes in the local acoustic impedance which are related to the cross sectional area of the nasal cavity. The reflected sound is detected by a microphone, which transmits the sound signal to an amplifier and computer system for processing into an area distance graph.

The cross sectional area measurements obtained with acoustic rhinometry correlate very well with area measurements made by computed tomography scans, and nasal airway resistance measured by rhinomanometry, but the accuracy of acoustic rhinometry is unreliable in the posterior part of the nose, especially when the nasal passage is congested.[20]

Acoustic rhinometry is also subject to artefacts caused by noise and breathing.[21] The volume of the nasal cavity (e.g. between 2 and 5 cm depth into the nose) can be calculated from the cross sectional areas across a measured distance into the nose, and nasal volumes are often used to study the effects of medical and surgical treatments.

A major advantage of the technique of acoustic rhinometry is that it provides a measure of nasal cross sectional area and volume along the length of the nasal passage, unlike rhinomanometry that is limited to measuring the effects of the narrowest point of the nasal airway on nasal airflow. Technical specifications for standard operating procedures for acoustic rhinometry have been standardized as regards the accuracy and repeatability of measurements and the acquisition of data.[22]

Normal values for acoustic rhinometry

Normal values for acoustic rhinometry have the same limitations described above for rhinomanometry, due to the spontaneous changes in nasal patency associated with the nasal cycle. The normal adult value for minimum cross sectional area for a nasal passage is quoted as 0.7 cm^2 with a range of $0.3–1.2 \text{ cm}^2$ and this increases on decongestion to 0.9 cm^2 with a range of $0.5–1.3 \text{ cm}^2$.[23]

The volume of the nasal cavity, between 2 and 5 cm depth into the nasal passage, has been reported to be 3.71 cm^3 (3.58–3.84) in school children aged 9–11 years and 5.44 cm^3 (5.21–5.67) in adults, after decongestion.[24]

The diagnostic value of acoustic rhinometry has been investigated by Lenders and Pirsig (1990), who could distinguish various deviations of nasal structure, such as valve stenosis, septal deviation, turbinate hypertrophy and tumour masses.[25]

The accuracy of acoustic rhinometry like rhinomanometry is dependent on the interface between the equipment and the nose. For example, the cross sectional area of the nasal vestibule is susceptible to distortion if a tube is inserted into the nose. Mispositioning of the nasal tube and air leaks are just as likely to give spurious measurements with acoustic rhinometry as face mask leaks with rhinomanometry, but with care the technique of acoustic rhinometry provides reproducible data.

PEAK NASAL FLOW

The peak inspiratory or expiratory airflow through the nose associated with maximal respiratory effort can be used as a measure of nasal conductance. The measurement is effort dependent and is less sensitive than rhinomanometry or acoustic rhinometry in determining small changes in conductance.[26] Expiratory measurements are likely to cause expulsion of nasal secretions into the measuring instrument, and inspiratory flow measurements are likely to cause nasal alar collapse and flow limitation. Simple peak flow instruments such as the Wright, mini-Wright, and Youlten flow meters are often used to measure peak nasal inspiratory flow (PNIF) with the use of a face mask. However, the use of more sensitive spirometers can improve the accuracy and reproducibility of nasal measurements,[27] and reliable measurements can be made with standard pulmonary spirometry equipment.[28] Measurement of PNIF may be useful for the assessment of large changes in nasal conductance such as those associated with nasal challenge and nasal decongestion,[29] and for this type of work the measurement of PNIF compares well with rhinomanometry for the assessment of nasal patency.

Normal values for peak nasal inspiratory flow

Normal values for PNIF have been reported in both adults[30] and children aged 6–11.[31] Normal values for PNIF in a healthy adult Caucasian population have been described as related to age, sex and height with PNIF declining with age and being greater in males than females.[30] Mean PNIF in adult males was 143 L/min, and 122 L/min in females.[30]

SUBJECTIVE MEASUREMENTS

Nasal sensations are important in the study of nasal disease, as it is the patient's perception of nasal sensations (symptoms) that is of primary concern to the patient. However, the clinician in the assessment and treatment of nasal disease is mainly concerned with restoring normal nasal function to the nasal airway by reducing nasal obstruction by medical or surgical means. The clinician has various objective measures of nasal function such as rhinomanometry and acoustic rhinometry but the problem is that these objective measures of nasal function do not always correlate with the patient's own assessment of nasal sensations such as the sensation of nasal airflow.[32]

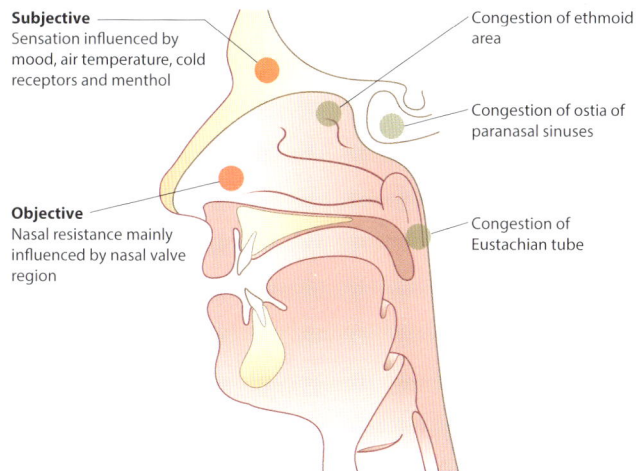

Figure 90.2 Factors that influence the patient's perception of nasal airflow and relationship to objective and subjective measures of nasal obstruction. *Objective measurements* are mainly determined by the cross sectional area of the nasal valve region at the tip of the inferior turbinate. *Subjective measurements* are influenced by the stimulation of cold receptors in the airway and the patient's perception of obstruction may be influenced by menthol and mood. Congestion in the ethmoid area, ostia of paranasal sinuses and Eustachian tube cause a perception of congestion and pressure that is unrelated to any change in nasal airway resistance as these areas are distant from the nasal valve.

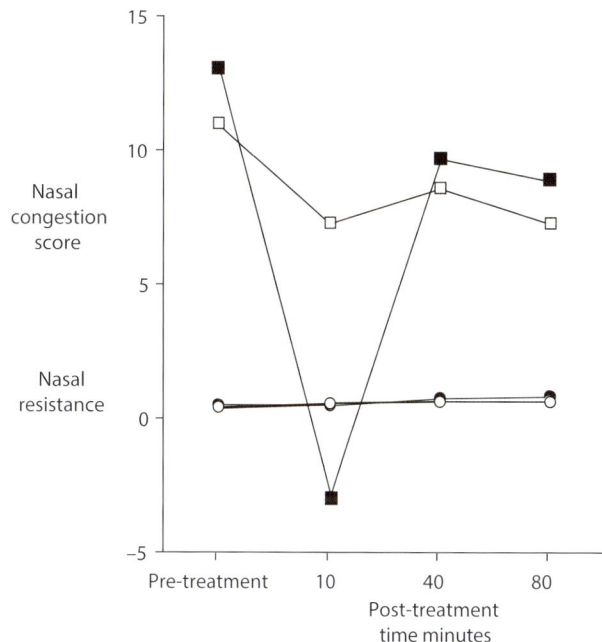

Figure 90.3 The effects of ingestion of an 11 mg l-menthol lozenge on subjective sensation of nasal congestion and nasal resistance to airflow in human volunteers with common cold. The subjective sensation of nasal congestion, measured on a 100mm visual analogue scale, was significantly reduced 10 min. after ingestion of the lozenge but nasal airway resistance as measured by rhinomanometry was unaffected. Shaded symbols represent the values for the menthol treated group and the open symbols represent the mean values for the placebo treated group.[34]

The reason for the lack of correlation between the perception of nasal airflow and nasal resistance as measured by rhinomanometry may be because the resistance to nasal airflow is primarily determined by the nasal valve area, whereas the symptoms of nasal obstruction may be influenced by other areas of the nose as well as the nasal valve area, as illustrated in **Figure 90.2**.

Congestion in the ethmoid region may cause contact of ethmoid surfaces and a sensation of pressure and obstruction that would have little or no effect on nasal airway resistance. Similarly, pressure changes in the middle ear and paranasal sinuses may cause a sensation of nasal obstruction and pressure without any effect on nasal airway resistance. Another factor that may explain the lack of correlation between objective and subjective measures of nasal obstruction is that the nasal airway consists of two parallel airways and the total nasal conductance may be near normal even if one nasal passage is completely obstructed. Subjects with nasal obstruction associated with acute upper respiratory tract infection have a total nasal airway resistance that is close to normal yet they still complain of nasal obstruction because one nasal passage may be severely congested whilst the other is patent.[17] Objective and subjective unilateral measures of nasal obstruction have been shown to have a much better correlation than combined bilateral measures for the two nasal passages indicating that the nose should be assessed as two separate organs rather than a single combined airway.[33]

Studies on the effects of menthol on nasal sensation of airflow clearly demonstrate the lack of any correlation between objective measures of nasal airway resistance and subjective measures of airflow.[34] In patients with nasal obstruction associated with common cold, ingestion of a menthol lozenge causes a great improvement in the sensation of nasal airflow without any change in nasal airway resistance, as shown in **Figure 90.3**. This is because the menthol vapour causes an increase in the sensitivity of cold receptors that detect nasal airflow, and a perception of nasal decongestion, without any objective change in nasal resistance.

Subjective scores of nasal symptoms provide the main outcome criteria for clinical trials on new treatments for rhinitis yet our knowledge of the factors influencing the perception of symptoms is still very superficial.

MEASUREMENT OF THE NASAL AIRWAY BY THE RHINOLOGIST

The rhinologist may be interested in measuring the patency of the nasal airway for two reasons: first to assess the severity of any nasal obstruction and select patients for medical and/or surgical treatment and second to assess the efficacy of any treatment in increasing nasal airflow. There is a large literature on the assessment of medical and surgical treatments aimed at improving nasal airflow and only two examples will be given here to demonstrate the usefulness of rhinomanometry in assessing patient response to surgical or medical treatments of nasal obstruction.

The efficacy of nasal surgery as a treatment for chronic nasal obstruction was demonstrated by measuring changes

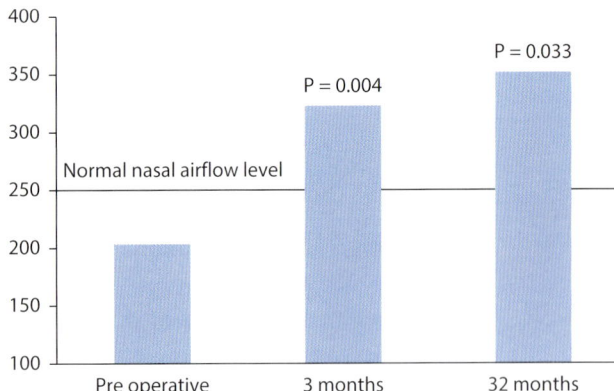

Figure 90.4 The effect of Coblation inferior turbinate surgery on total nasal conductance of airflow pre-operatively, at 3 months and 32 months follow-up. The Y axis is nasal airflow patency cm^3 sec as measured by posterior rhinomanometry. The line represents normal level of airflow in health in health. P values relate to comparison with preoperative airflow.[35]

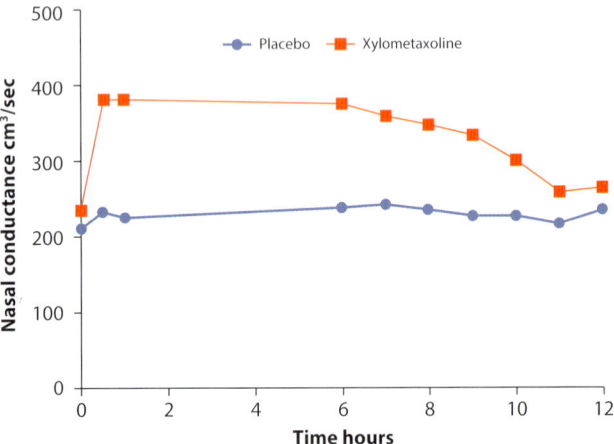

Figure 90.5 Effects of xylometazoline and placebo nasal sprays on nasal conductance in subjects with nasal congestion associated with common cold. The figure demonstrates the reproducibility of the mean nasal conductance measurements over a 12 hour period in the placebo treatment group (n = 29). The sensitivity of rhinomanometry is demonstrated by the significant increase in mean nasal conductance over 10 hours after treatment with xylometazoline (n = 32).[9]

in nasal airflow by posterior rhinomanometry before and after Coblation inferior turbinate reduction surgery at 3 and 32 months post-operatively as illustrated in **Figure 90.4**. The mean baseline nasal conductance was 248.6 cm^3/s (range 2.5–614.8), which improved significantly (p = 0.033) to 342.1 cm^3/s (range 166.7–500) at 32 months post-operatively.[35]

The efficacy of medical treatment of acute nasal obstruction associated with common cold was demonstrated by measuring changes in nasal airflow before and after treatment with a topical nasal decongestant, xylometazoline as illustrated in **Figure 90.5**. The decongestant effect of xylometazoline was significantly greater than placebo, as shown by the nasal conductance at 1 hour (384.23 versus 226.42 cm^3/s; p < or = 0.0001).[9]

BEST CLINICAL PRACTICE

✓ Nasal surgery for the treatment of nasal obstruction should be guided by objective measurement of nasal airway patency pre- and post-operatively

FUTURE RESEARCH

➤ The major deficiency in our knowledge concerning measurement of the nasal airway is that there is no generally accepted standard measurement to assess the degree of obstruction of the nasal airway.

➤ Rhinomanometry is generally accepted as the 'gold standard' for the assessment of nasal obstruction but this technique is only available in research centres and is not generally used in the clinic. Even when rhinomanometry is used, there is a choice between various techniques such as anterior and posterior, and various sample pressures (75 Pa for posterior, and 150 Pa for anterior) that make it difficult to compare results from different laboratories.

➤ Standardization of rhinomanometry was attempted in 1984[5] but little progress has been made since then. The new recommendations for standardization of rhinomanometry and acoustic rhinometry add little more than mathematical modelling to the older standardization recommendations.[6]

➤ The introduction of acoustic rhinometry was initially proclaimed as a method that would replace rhinomanometry but this has not taken place as the technique is not quicker or more reproducible than rhinomanometry.

➤ A major problem in measuring the nasal airway is the lack of any generally accepted reference tables for nasal patency related to age, height, sex and race etc. and future research is needed to provide some reference values for the rhinologist for each of the methods described above.[2]

➤ Measurements of the nasal airway will be restricted to research laboratories unless a cheap and portable instrument is developed for use in the clinical setting and some progress has been made in establishing the use of the much cheaper and easily used peak flow meter to measure nasal obstruction in adults and children.[30–31]

KEY POINTS

- Objective and subjective measurements of nasal conductance do not correlate well for bilateral measures but do correlate for unilateral measures
- The spontaneous changes in unilateral nasal resistance associated with the nasal cycle cause great variability in physiological nasal airflow
- Subjective measurements are important as they relate directly to symptoms
- Decongestion of the nose eliminates the effects of the nasal cycle and allows the measurement of anatomical nasal airflow
- Acoustic rhinometry provides anatomical rather than functional measurements of the nasal airway
- Rhinomanometry is generally accepted as the 'gold standard' for measurement of nasal airway resistance
- Acoustic rhinometry and rhinomanometry in their current forms have not found a routine place in the day to day assessment of patients in the rhinology clinic.

REFERENCES

1. Eccles R. Nasal airflow in health and disease. *Acta Oto-laryngol* 2000; **120**(5): 580–95.
2. Moore M, Eccles R. Normal nasal patency: problems in obtaining standard reference values for the surgeon. *J Laryngol Otol* 2012; **126**(6): 563–9.
3. Broms P, Johnson B, Malm L. Rhinomanometry. IV. A pre- and postoperative evaluation in functional septoplasty. *Acta Oto-laryngol* 1982; **94**(5-6): 523–9.
4. Eccles R. A guide to practical aspects of measurement of human nasal airflow by rhinomanometry. *Rhinology* 2011; **49**(1): 2–10.
5. Clement PAR. Committee report on standardisation of rhinomanometry. *Rhinology* 1984; **22**: 151–5.
6. Clement PA, Gordts F. Consensus report on acoustic rhinometry and rhinomanometry. *Rhinology* 2005; **43**(3): 169–79.
7. Quine SM, Aitken PM, Eccles R. Effect of submucosal diathermy to the inferior turbinates on unilateral and total nasal airflow in patients with rhinitis. *Acta Oto-laryngol* 1999; **119**(8): 911–15.
8. Farmer SE, Quine SM, Eccles R. Efficacy of inferior turbinate coblation for treatment of nasal obstruction. *J Laryngol Otol* 2009; **123**(3): 309–14.
9. Eccles R, Eriksson M, Garreffa S, et al. The nasal decongestant effect of xylometazoline in the common cold. *Am J Rhinol* 2008; **22**(5): 491–6.
10. Cole P. Acoustic rhinometry and rhinomanometry. *Rhinol Suppl.* 2000; **16**: 29–34.
11. Morris S, Jawad M, Eccles R. Relationships between vital capacity, height and nasal airway resistance in asymptomatic volunteers. *Rhinology* 1992; **30**: 259–64.
12. Polgar G, Kong GP. The nasal resistance of newborn infants. *J Ped* 1965; **67**: 557–67.
13. Stocks J, Godfrey S. Nasal resistance during infancy. *Respir Physiol* 1978; **34**: 233–46.
14. Syaballo NC, Bundgaard A, Entholm P, et al. Measurement and regulation of nasal airflow resistance in man. *Rhinology* 1986; **24**: 87–101.
15. Vig PS, Zajac DJ. Age and gender effects on nasal respiratory function in normal subjects. *Cleft Palate Craniofac J* 1993; **30**: 279–84.
16. Broms P. Rhinomanometry. III Procedures and criteria for distinction between skeletal stenosis and mucosal swelling. *Acta Oto-laryngol* 1982; **94**(3-4): 361–70.
17. Eccles R. A role for the nasal cycle in respiratory defense. *Eu Respir J* 1996; **9**(2): 371–6.
18. Flanagan P, Eccles R. Spontaneous changes of unilateral nasal airflow in man: a re-examination of the 'nasal cycle'. *Acta Oto-laryngol* 1997; **117**(4): 590–5.
19. Thulesius H. *Rhinomanometry in clinical use: A tool in the septoplasty decision making process* 2012. Published Thesis. Department of Otorhinolaryngology, Lund University.
20. Tomkinson A, Eccles R. The identification of the potential limitations of acoustic rhinometery using computer-generated, 3-dimensional reconstructions of simple-models. *Am J Rhinol* 1996; **10**(2): 77–82.
21. Tomkinson A, Eccles R. Errors arising in cross-sectional area estimation by acoustic rhinometry produced by breathing during measurement. *Rhinology* 1995; **33**(3): 138–40.
22. Hilberg O, Pedersen OF. Acoustic rhinometry: recommendations for technical specifications and standard operating procedures. *Rhinol Suppl* 2000; **16**: 3–17.
23. Grymer LF, Hilberg O, Pedersen OF, et al. Acoustic rhinometry: values from adults with subjective normal nasal patency. *Rhinology* 1991; **29**: 35–47.
24. Straszek SP, Schlünssen V, Sigsgaard T, et al. Reference values for acoustic rhinometry in decongested school children and adults: the most sensitive measurement for change in nasal patency. *Rhinology* 2007; **45**(1): 36–9.
25. Lenders H, Pirsig W. Diagnostic value of acoustic rhinometry: patients with allergic and vasomotor rhinitis compared with normal controls. *Rhinology* 1990; **28**: 5–16.
26. Clarke RW, Jones AS. The limitations of peak nasal flow measurement. *Clin Otolaryngol* 1994; **19**(6): 502–4.
27. Harar RP, Kalan A, Kenyon GS. Assessing the reproducibility of nasal spirometry parameters in the measurement of nasal patency. *Rhinology* 2001; **39**(4): 211–14.
28. Goyal M, Verma NS, Goel A, et al. Nasal spirometery. *Indian J Physiol Pharmacol* 2010; **54**(3): 271–6.
29. Holmström M, Scadding GK, Lund VJ, et al. Assessment of nasal obstruction: a comparison between rhinomanometry and nasal inspiratory peak flow. *Rhinology* 1990; **28**(3): 191–6.
30. Ottaviano G, Scadding GK, Coles S, et al. Peak nasal inspiratory flow: normal range in adult population. *Rhinology* 2006; **44**(1): 32–5.
31. van Spronsen E, Ebbens FA, Fokkens WJ. Normal peak nasal inspiratory flow rate values in healthy children aged 6 to 11 years in the Netherlands. *Rhinology* 2012; **50**(1): 22–5.
32. Quine S, Eccles R. Nasal resistance from laboratory to clinic. *Curr Opin Otolaryngol Head Neck Surg* 1999; **7**: 20–5.
33. Clarke JD, Hopkins ML, Eccles R. Evidence for correlation of objective and subjective measures of nasal airflow in patients with common cold. *Clin Otolaryngol* 2005; **30**(1): 35–8.
34. Eccles R, Jawad MS, Morris S. The effects of oral administration of menthol on nasal resistance to airflow and nasal sensation of airflow in subjects suffering from nasal congestion associated with the common cold. *J Pharm Pharmacol* 1990; **42**: 652–4.
35. Leong SC, Farmer S, Eccles R. Coblation inferior turbinate reduction: a long-term follow up with subjective and objective assessment. *Rhinology* 2010; **48**(3): 108–12.

CHAPTER 91

ALLERGIC RHINITIS

Quentin Gardiner

Introduction 999	Diagnosis 1002
Definition 999	Treatment 1002
Prevalence 1000	Children with rhinitis 1007
Natural history 1001	Pregnancy 1008
Presentation 1001	References 1009
Examination 1001	

SEARCH STRATEGY

Data and recommendations in this chapter are taken from the ARIA 2008 update and 2010 revision, and may be updated by a Medline search using the keywords: allergic rhinitis, allergic rhinosinusitis and allergic rhinoconjunctivitis linked with aetiology, presentation, epidemiology, prevalence, allergen avoidance, treatment, immunotherapy, children, pregnancy and surgery.

INTRODUCTION

Allergic rhinitis is characterized by inflammatory changes in the nasal mucosa caused by exposure to inhaled allergens. It is a common disease, affecting between 0.8 and 39.7% of the world population[1] (depending on location) with prevalence in Western Europe of 23%. It causes significant disability and is often poorly managed. There may be co-morbidities with other organs being involved, commonly the eyes causing allergic conjunctivitis and the lungs with allergic asthma. Indeed, these diseases are increasingly considered to be a single entity, with a spectrum of respiratory allergic response, termed the unified allergic airway. They have a common epidemiology, pathophysiology, and in many cases, treatment approach.

Allergic rhinitis and allergic rhinoconjunctivitis are caused by an inflammatory response to an allergen to which the patient has already been exposed. In this abnormal response the individual has produced allergen specific immunoglobulin E (IgE) which binds to mast cell surface receptors. Subsequent allergen exposure causes this receptor/IgE complex to trigger mast cell degranulation with the release of preformed mediators. This inflammatory mediator release includes not only histamine, but also other granule contents (serine proteases, heparin), and newly synthesized eicosanoid mediators (leukotriene C4, prostaglandin D2, thromboxane and PAF).

For further details please see Chapter 14, 'Allergy: basic mechanisms and tests'.

These inflammatory mediators cause the classic symptoms of allergic rhinitis: nerve irritation causing sneezing and itching, loss of mucosal integrity causing rhinorrhoea and vascular engorgement causing block. Histamine drives the majority of acute nasal symptoms such as sneezing and itching with leukotrienes and prostaglandins being involved in longer term symptoms such as block.

DEFINITION

Rhinitis is defined clinically as having two or more symptoms of anterior or posterior rhinorrhoea, sneezing, nasal blockage and/or itching of the nose during two or more consecutive days for more than one hour on most days.[2]

Allergic rhinitis is diagnosed when these symptoms are caused by allergen exposure leading to an IgE mediated reaction. Allergic rhinitis is subdivided into intermittent (IAR) or persistent (PER) disease and the severity into mild or moderate/severe (**Figure 91.1**).

These definitions are not interchangeable with the terms seasonal and perennial and were introduced to relate the patient's symptoms, rather than an allergen, to a diagnosis.[4] In one large study of people with allergic

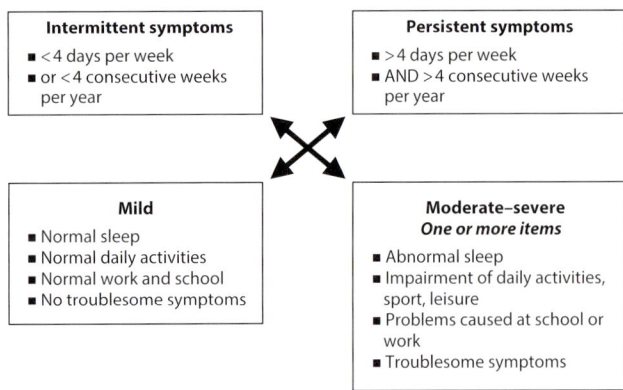

Figure 91.1 **Classification of allergic rhinitis.** Reproduced with permission.[3]

rhinitis, 10% were classified as having mild intermittent rhinitis, 14% mild persistent rhinitis, 17% moderate/severe intermittent rhinitis and 59% moderate/severe persistent rhinitis; therefore approximately 75% of patients will be diagnosed as having a persistent rhinitis and 25% intermittent.[5] Whether the disease is classified as mild or moderate/severe depends on the effect on the patient's social life[6, 7] work/school[8–10] and sleep.[11] Sleep disturbance is common in patients with moderate/severe allergic rhinitis[12] and may lead to daytime sleepiness.[13] This is also linked to problems with learning at school[14] and examination success in children[15] and time off work and loss of productivity in adults.[16]

Patients with non-allergic rhinitis may have similar symptoms[17] which are discussed in other chapters – infectious rhinitis, occupational rhinitis, drug-induced rhinitis, hormonal rhinitis, irritant rhinitis, tobacco mucositis, persistent non-allergic rhinitis with eosinophilia (NARES) and idiopathic (vasomotor) rhinitis. The diagnosis of an allergic rhinitis is made by correlating the allergic symptoms and history with diagnostic tests demonstrating allergen-specific IgE, whether by skin prick testing or by measuring specific IgE levels in the blood (RAST).

PREVALENCE

The prevalence of allergic rhinitis varies widely around the world. The International Study on Asthma and Allergy in Childhood (ISAAC 1)[1] and its follow-up (ISAAC 3)[18] showed the prevalence of rhinoconjunctivitis to vary between 0.8% and 39.7% in different populations (**Figure 91.2**).

Countries with a low prevalence of asthma (<5%) such as Indonesia, Romania and Greece had a low prevalence of allergic rhinitis. Conversely, countries with a high prevalence of asthma (>30%) such as the United Kingdom, Australia and New Zealand had a high prevalence of rhinitis (15–20%).

There has been a steep increase in the prevalence of allergic rhinitis over the last 40 years,[19, 20] though this may now be slowing.[21] The reasons for this increase are uncertain. Children who live on farms and have contact with livestock are less likely to develop allergic rhinitis than their urban peers[22, 23] suggesting a possible protective effect of microbial exposure. Larger family size, more frequent infections and unhygienic contact may all be protective – the hygiene hypothesis.[24] This suggests

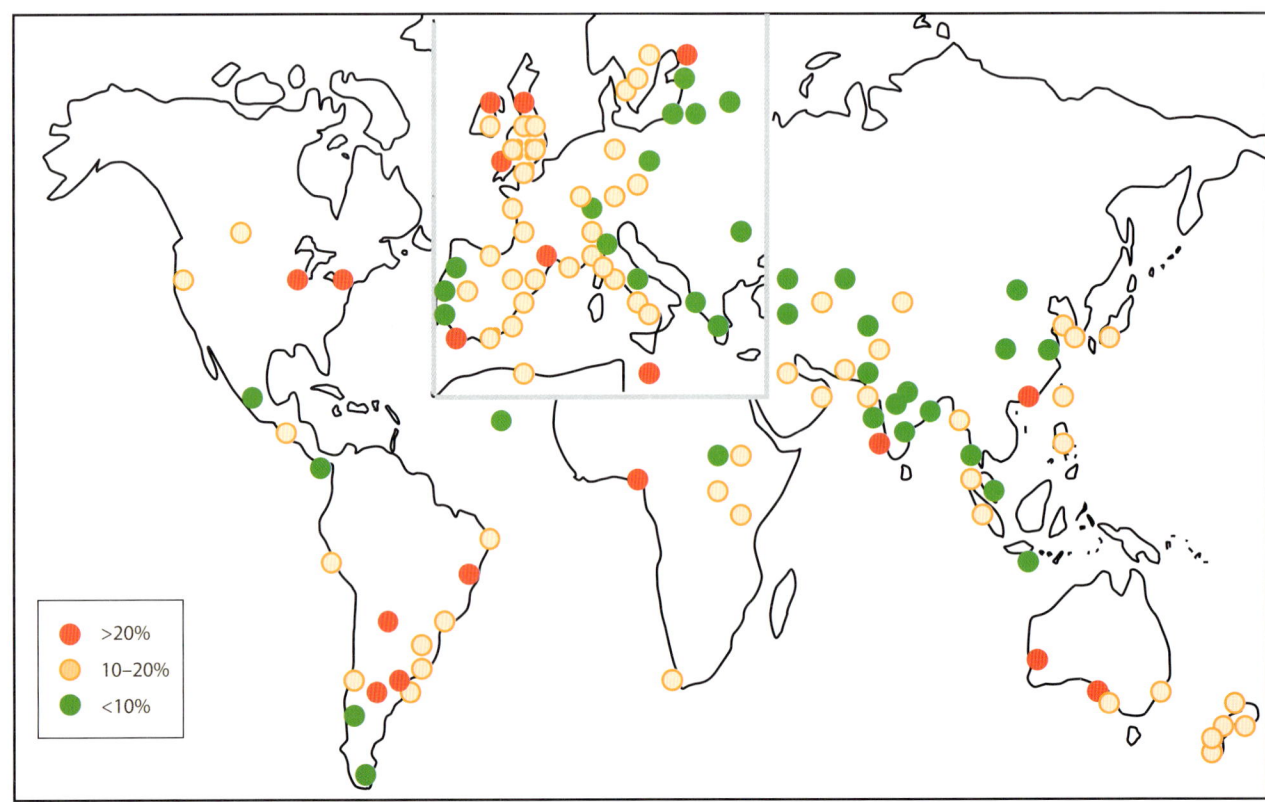

Figure 91.2 **Prevalence of allergic rhinitis worldwide, 13–14 year olds.** Reproduced with permission.[1]

that reduced exposure to infective agents reduces the Th1 response and leads to an overdrive of the Th2 immune response leading to excessive production of IgE and consequent atopy. There are however some uncertainties about this concept.[25] Chronic parasitic disease (for example with worms) is also protective, possibly because of the production of blocking antibodies (IgG4).[26] Eradication of worm infestation increases skin reactivity to aeroallergens.[27]

All these reasons suggest that an urbanized, Western lifestyle promotes the development of allergic disease. The link with helminth infection may also point the way to future treatment options.

NATURAL HISTORY

Genetic factors are certainly involved in the aetiology of allergic rhinitis. Having parents who are atopic may increase the risk of a child having an allergic disease by 3–6 times.[28] Exposure to an allergen is also required before sensitivity develops therefore environmental factors are also important. Pollen-induced allergic rhinitis is uncommon before the age of 2 years suggesting that exposure over two seasons is required for sensitization.[29] The 'atopic march'[30] in children refers to the sequential development of allergic diseases, often starting in infants with atopic eczema then the development of allergic rhinitis and finally allergic asthma.[31] Several studies have shown that adult-onset asthma is more likely to occur in patients with allergic rhinitis than in those without, usually increasing the risk by a factor of three,[32] though whether allergic rhinitis is an earlier manifestation of allergic disease in patients who will go on to develop asthma or whether the nasal disease itself causes asthma is unclear. Remission of symptoms may occur over time. One study showed that although the overall prevalence of allergic rhinitis increased from 12.4% in 1992 to 15% in 2000 in keeping with the worldwide increase, 23.1% of patients who had allergic rhinitis in 1992 no longer had symptoms in 2000.[33] Symptoms of rhinitis generally become less severe with age and skin prick testing shows less reactivity in the elderly.[34]

KEY POINTS

- Allergic rhinitis is an IgE mediated disease
- In Western societies it is common (>20%)
- It is often associated with other allergic diseases such as allergic conjunctivitis and asthma
- It may have significant negative effects on sleep, work and study
- Patients with allergic parents are more likely to be allergic
- Lack of helminth infection may be important in development of disease
- Allergic disease is often less severe in the elderly

PRESENTATION

Most patients will be referred from general practice with two or more symptoms of anterior or posterior rhinorrhoea, sneezing, nasal blockage and/or itching of the nose. Young children may simply present with block. Other complaints such as itchy eyes, pharyngeal itch, hearing loss due to otitis media with effusion, atopic eczema, asthma, loss of smell, chronic cough, snoring, fatigue, sore throat and halitosis may occur.[35, 36] Unilateral symptoms, mucopurulent rhinorrhoea, thick post-nasal discharge, epistaxis, pain and anosmia are not usually associated with allergic rhinitis and should prompt further investigation.

The history is crucial. When symptoms started, how long they last and when they occur will allow determination of likely long-term atopy, whether the problem is persistent or intermittent and the possible allergens. Ask direct questions regarding symptoms suggestive of asthma such as wheeze or cough. A family history of atopy is important as it makes the diagnosis of allergy more likely.

Symptoms of rhinitis, conjunctivitis, cough and wheeze during the summer months suggest grass pollen sensitivity; waking with a blocked nose might be linked to house dust mites in the bed. The main presenting symptoms and their severity should be determined. Does the nasal block cause problems with sleep or work?

Ask about the character of the nasal discharge. A coloured discharge suggests infection whereas the discharge is usually clear in allergy. Does the block switch from side to side? This is common in patients with mucosal inflammation and less likely with anatomical abnormalities alone such as septal deviation.

More direct questions should be asked regarding endocrine problems that may cause rhinitis (hypothyroidism) and medication (the combined oral contraceptive pill may cause congestion). Specific questions may be helpful in patients with seasonal symptoms. Tree pollen allergy (birch particularly) may be associated with oral allergy syndrome which causes swelling or tingling of the lips when eating uncooked fruits and vegetables such as potatoes, carrots, cherries, celery, apples, pears, plums, peaches, parsnip, kiwi, hazelnuts and apricots and is found in approximately half the patients with birch pollen sensitivity.[37] It may also be reported with other pollen sensitivities.

EXAMINATION

A general examination of the patient may reveal other signs of atopic disease such as eczema or allergic conjunctivitis and sometimes an allergic crease may be seen on the patient's nose.

Examination of the nose should always be performed, if only to exclude causes other than allergy. Anterior rhinoscopy will allow an assessment to be made of the colour and state of the nasal mucosa and to see whether it is swollen and causing obstruction. It may be oedematous, blue or pale in colour and covered in thin mucus, but this is not always the case. In children a blocked nose with normal nasal mucosa may suggest adenoid enlargement. Endoscopic examination will allow polyps and other nasal disease to be excluded. In severe or atypical presentations (especially in the presence of cartilage or mucosal loss, cosmetic changes, systemic illness or refractory bleeding) exclusion of other inflammatory or neoplastic diseases is important.

A history suggesting asthma such as wheeze or night-time cough may necessitate examination of the chest or referral to a respiratory physician.

DIAGNOSIS

For many patients, a clear history that fits with allergic rhinitis and a corresponding nasal examination will allow a diagnosis to be made confidently, though in specialist practice skin prick tests will normally be carried out as part of the standard workup. If there is diagnostic uncertainty, or if the consequences of a possible allergy are important (such as a pet allergy), then allergy testing should be performed. This will normally be either a skin prick test (SPT)[38] or measurement of specific IgE in the blood (often referred to as radioallergosorbent testing or RAST[39] (see Chapter 14).

Skin prick testing is usually the preferred option as it allows the patient to see the results directly and gives time for patient education about avoidance measures if required.

The method of skin prick testing involves the use of a small lancet to introduce an allergen into the skin. If the patient is sensitized to the allergen then IgE sensitized mast cells will degranulate and cause a wheal and flare reaction in the skin. Negative (saline) and positive (histamine) controls are also used to rule out dermographism and non–reactivity respectively. If the negative control shows a reaction or the positive control shows no reaction then blood IgE levels should be measured. If an oral antihistamine has been taken in the preceding 7–10 days then the positive control may not react. A positive reaction is noted by a wheal size 2 mm or greater than the negative control. In the United Kingdom the main four allergens that should be tested for are grass pollen, house dust mite, cat and dog but the prevalence of sensitivities varies around the world with cockroach sensitivity common in tropical countries. Patients with particular exposure can have various other allergens tested depending on their history (for example exposure to horses or moulds). It should be noted that a positive skin test shows atopy but it does not necessarily mean that the patient has a clinically relevant reaction to that allergen. The reaction has to be correlated with the patient's symptoms. Approximately 25% of adults have a positive reaction on skin prick testing but only 10–15% are symptomatic (though some patients with positive tests will go on to develop allergic disease in the future).[40]

RAST testing is usually reserved for patients who require a diagnosis but where SPTs are unavailable or inappropriate. A blood sample is taken and radio- or enzyme-labelled anti-IgE is added to the serum. A positive result is shown by an IgE level of 0.35 kU/l or greater. As for SPTs, a positive result may not necessarily be clinically relevant.

Nasal allergen challenge is the gold standard of allergy diagnosis but it is infrequently required or available. It may be useful where the history is suggestive of a particular allergen being responsible for symptoms but the skin prick tests are negative. An allergen is applied to the nasal mucosa, or the patient exposed to an airborne allergen, and subjective measurements made (symptom scores) as well as objective measurements (sneeze count, peak nasal inspiratory flow, rhinomanometry, pulmonary peak flow, etc.).[41] This method of testing can also be used in patients suspected of having salicylate intolerance using lysine aspirin applied to the nose and is a possible substitute for an oral salicylate challenge. Nasal challenge testing is complex and has the risk of inducing anaphylaxis and is therefore is used only in specialist centres.

Various other methods of determining sensitivity are also described including the measurement of inflammatory mediators such as histamine, PGD2, leukotrienes, kinins and tryptase in blood or nasal secretions, nasal cytology and histology and measurement of nitric oxide in exhaled air.[42] None of these methods are generally used in clinical practice.

Symptoms of asthma may indicate the need for respiratory assessment with pulmonary function tests and reversibility with a bronchodilator.

> **KEY POINTS**
>
> - The history and symptoms are crucial in diagnosis.
> - The timing of symptoms will often lead to diagnosing the allergy.
> - Nasal examination is mainly to exclude other causes.
> - In severe or atypical presentations (especially in the presence of cartilage or mucosal loss, cosmetic changes, systemic illness or refractory bleeding) exclusion of other inflammatory or neoplastic diseases is important.
> - Ask about asthma symptoms (wheeze and cough).
> - Skin prick testing is useful particularly in persistent allergic rhinitis where the cause may not be clear.

TREATMENT

- The prevention of allergic rhinitis
- Methods of reducing allergen exposure
- Pharmacological treatment of allergic rhinitis (see also Chapter 28)
- Immunotherapy for allergic rhinitis
- Surgical treatment
- Complementary therapies

The prevention of allergic rhinitis

Various areas have been examined to determine if sensitization can be reduced in infancy – no definite triggers have been found but recommendations have been made on the available evidence. It has been advised that children should breastfeed for at least the first three months after birth,[43] that there is no benefit in having a reduced antigen diet for the mother in pregnancy and during lactation[44] and that parents should not smoke in pregnancy or near children, although no definite link with allergy has been found.[45] There was also limited evidence of benefit in reducing exposure to house dust mite but no benefit in not exposing children to furry pets.[46]

REDUCING ALLERGEN EXPOSURE

As the clinical effects of allergic rhinitis are caused by allergens it would seem logical that reduced exposure would benefit symptoms. The major allergens to be found indoors are house dust mite, cat, dog and other furry animals, cockroach and moulds. Outdoors the main allergens are airborne pollens which vary during the year and depend on local conditions. In Europe tree pollen is found during the spring, grass and weed pollens during the summer and various mould spores during the summer and autumn. In North America ragweed sensitivity is a common problem but this is not found in Europe. Tropical areas will have less seasonal variation.

METHODS TO ACHIEVE ALLERGEN REDUCTION

House dust mite allergen reduction aims to reduce the amount of mite allergens in the home:

- Wash bedding regularly (every 1–2 weeks) at 55–60°C to kill mites (washing with cold water removes 90% of mite allergens; washing at 55–60°C kills mites)
- Wash pillows and duvets in hot water (55–60°C) and encase pillows and mattresses with protective coverings that have a pore size of 6 μm or less
- Sufficient ventilation of dwellings to decrease humidity; aim to reduce indoor relative humidity to below 50% and avoid damp housing conditions.

Reproduced with permission of the WHO.[47]

ADDITIONAL STRATEGIES

- Use a good quality vacuum cleaner (if possible, one fitted with a HEPA filter)
- Use a damp duster when dusting and cleaning surfaces
- Replace wall to wall carpets with linoleum or wooden floors which can be wiped clean
- Remove/reduce curtains and soft furnishings in the bedroom
- Replace fabric-covered seating with leather or vinyl
- Remove soft toys from the bedroom; wash them at 55–60°C or freeze them (in a kitchen deep-freezer) to kill house dust mites
- Exposure of mattresses, rugs and carpets to direct strong sunlight (for more than 3 hours) kills mites and can be used in appropriate regions.

Pollen avoidance provides mechanical barriers to pollen contact.

- Keep windows closed at peak pollen times
- Wear glasses or sunglasses to help prevent pollens entering the eyes
- Consider wearing a mask over nose and mouth to prevent inhalation of pollens at peak time
- Use air-conditioning where possible
- Install car pollen filters where possible

Pet allergen avoidance reduces the amount of pet allergen indoors.

- If possible, find another home for the pet and do not introduce new animals into the home. If the pet is not removed from the home then:
  o Exclude pets from bedrooms and if possible keep pets outdoors
  o Vacuum carpets, mattresses and upholstery regularly
  o Change clothes before going to school or work if you have had contact with any animal (e.g. horse/cat/dog).

Cockroach allergen avoidance involves removing the cockroaches, eliminating the places and conditions in which they can live and removing all allergens.

- Eradicate cockroaches with appropriate insecticidal bait
- Seal cracks in floors and ceilings
- Enclose all food
- Do not store waste in the home
- Scrub floors with water and detergent to remove allergens.

Mould allergen avoidance aims to prevent mould from growing and mould spores from becoming airborne during mould removal.

- Use dehumidifiers in the home if relative humidity is consistently high (above 50%)
- Ensure heating, ventilation or air-conditioning systems are properly maintained
- Use 5% ammonia solution to remove mould from bathrooms and other contaminated surfaces
- Replace carpets with hard flooring and replace wallpaper with paint
- Repair indoor water damage immediately.

Unfortunately despite these measures it is very difficult to achieve significant allergen reduction or elimination and clinical benefit from these strategies has been limited. For example a study looking at the results of using impermeable covers on mattresses and pillows demonstrated a reduction in dust mite allergen to 30% of the initial level, but found no evidence of clinical benefit.[48]

Table 91.1[49] summarizes the evidence of efficacy for some of these measures. Although the evidence base for recommending allergen reduction is poor it may nevertheless benefit some patients and a trial of avoidance may be useful.

Food allergy

It is very unusual for food allergy to cause isolated nasal symptoms, although the nose may be involved in more generalized systemic reactions. Foods such as peanuts, nuts, shellfish, fish and fruits such as strawberry may be involved. Milk and egg allergy is more common in younger children but usually resolves by 4–6 years old.

TABLE 91.1 Effect on allergen levels and evidence of clinical benefit

Measure	Evidence of effect on allergen levels	Evidence of clinical benefit
House dust mites		
Encase bedding in impermeable covers	Some	None (adults): evidence A Some (children): evidence B
Wash bedding on a hot cycle (55–60 °C)	Some	None: evidence A
Replace carpets with hard flooring	Some	None: evidence A
Acaricides and/or tannic acid	Weak	None: evidence A
Minimize objects that accumulate dust	None	None: evidence B
Vacuum cleaners with integral HEPA filter and double-thickness bags	Weak	None: evidence B
Remove, hot wash or freeze soft toys	None	None: evidence B
Pets		
Remove cat/dog from the home	Weak	None: evidence B
Keep pet from main living areas/bedrooms	Weak	None: evidence B
HEPA-filter air cleaners	Some	None: evidence B
Wash pet	Weak	None: evidence B
Replace carpets with hard flooring	None	None: evidence B
Vacuum cleaners with integral HEPA filter and double-thickness bags	None	None: evidence B

Reproduced with permission.[49]

Skin prick testing or IgE levels can confirm a true allergy but may give false positive results, therefore should be targeted at specific allergens rather than having a screening role. Avoidance of allergenic foods may be difficult (particularly in the case of peanut allergen which may be found in many processed foods) and suitable substitutes must be found to avoid dietary insufficiency and consequent malnutrition.

True food allergy should not be confused with oral allergy syndrome where there is cross-reactivity with a pollen allergen and which is relatively common.

Pharmacological treatment of allergic rhinitis

The basic summary of recommendations for treatment according to the ARIA guidelines[50] are shown in **Figure 91.3**.

The effects of the various medications used are summarized in **Table 91.2**.

The most widely used and effective medications to treat allergic rhinitis are oral or topical antihistamines and topical nasal steroids.

It should be stressed that these medications aim to achieve improved symptom control and are not a cure for allergy. They generally need to be taken for as long as there is allergen exposure causing symptoms. Symptom control is better for patients with intermittent allergic rhinitis if they start treatment prior to exposure to the allergen to which they are sensitized. For example, patients with grass pollen allergy should be advised to start treatment a month before the pollen season starts to try to avoid the development of symptoms and nasal inflammation and to stop treatment at the end of the season.

In keeping with the idea of the unified allergic airway, treatment for asthma may also be required, whether this be long-term or to manage wheeze only during the peak pollen season (peak seasonal wheeze). Treatment of the nose with topical steroids reduces asthma symptoms[51] and treatment of the lungs may reduce nasal symptoms[52] therefore symptom control will be better if both nose and lungs are assessed and treated together in symptomatic patients.

ANTIHISTAMINES

The symptoms of running, sneezing and nasal and eye itching are histamine driven and antihistamines are the first-line treatment for these symptoms in patients who have no problem with nasal obstruction. They have little effect on nasal blockage.[53] The older first-generation antihistamines (chlorphenamine, diphenhydramine) are rarely used now due to their sedative effects, though ketotifen may still have a role with some additional effect as a mast cell stabilizer. Second generation oral antihistamines such as loratadine and cetirizine are non-sedating, safe for long-term use and can be used for children. They have a rapid onset of action (usually less than an hour) and will give symptom reduction on a once daily dosing. Antihistamines give better symptomatic control when used regularly rather than on an as required basis.[54] Topical antihistamines (for example azelastine) may be used intranasally to achieve rapid symptom control and can be combined with a topical nasal steroid. It has the disadvantages of having a bitter taste that some patients

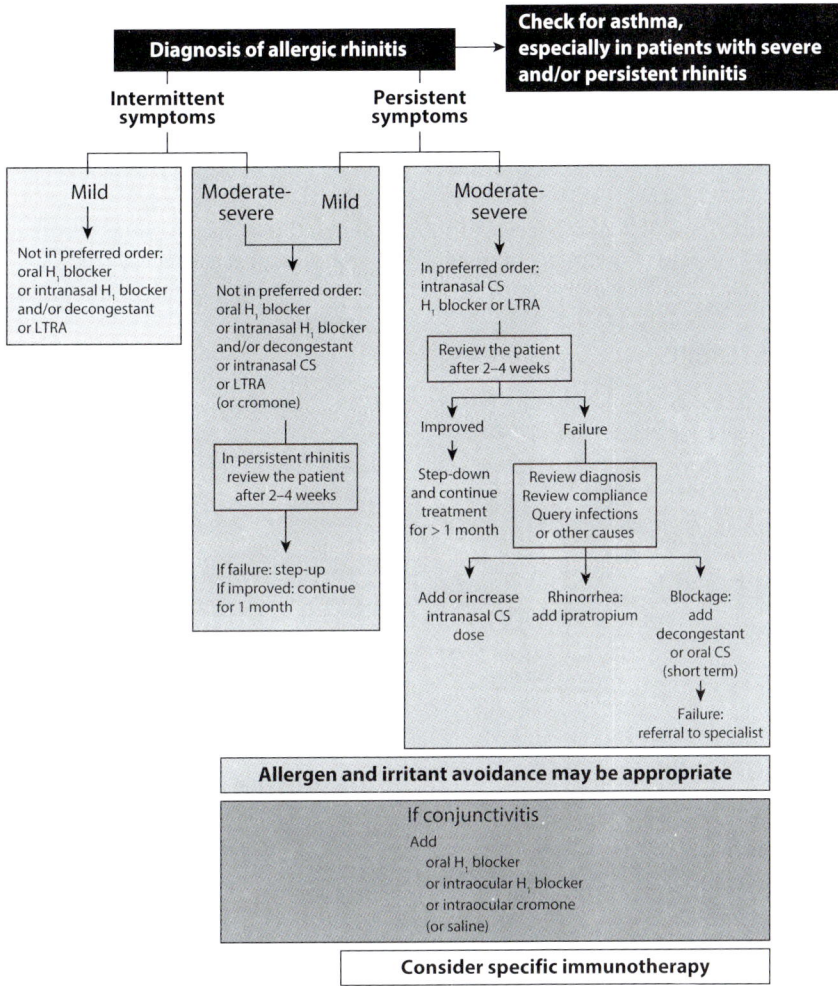

Figure 91.3 Allergic rhinitis management (algorithm of the ARIA update recommendations 2008). Reproduced with permission.[50]

TABLE 91.2 Pharmacological treatments and their effects in allergic rhinitis

	Itch/sneezing	Discharge	Blockage	Impaired smell
Sodium cromoglicate	+	+	+/−	−
Oral antihistamines	+++	++	+/−	−
Ipratropium bromide	−	+++	−	−
Topical decongestants	−	−	+++	−
Topical corticosteroids	+++	+++	++	+
Oral corticosteroids	+++	+++	+++	++
Antileukotrienes	−	++	+	+/−

dislike and needs twice daily dosing. Azelastine eyedrops may also be useful in reducing ocular symptoms.

Antihistamines alone may control symptoms adequately in some patients though many will require the addition of a topical nasal steroid.

INTRANASAL GLUCOCORTICOSTEROIDS

Glucocorticosteroids are the most effective treatment for allergic rhinoconjunctivitis.[55] Topical use in the form of a spray or drops is preferred to oral use to reduce side effects, although occasionally oral steroids may be useful. Intra-nasal application allows a high concentration of the active drug to be delivered to the nasal mucosa with minimal systemic absorption. The drugs reduce all symptoms of allergic rhinitis and ocular symptoms and are the first-line treatment of choice in patients who complain of nasal block.[56] As steroids have an effect on the production of pro-inflammatory mediators within the cell nucleus their effect is slow to occur and long lasting. Most steroids will not have an appreciable effect on symptoms for several hours or days and it can take two weeks for full benefit to be noticed. Patients should be warned of this as some will give up on treatment if it does not work rapidly.

Side effects of intra-nasal steroids are few but include epistaxis. This may be caused by incorrect use of the spray delivery system causing trauma as there is no evidence of nasal mucosal atrophy even with long-term use.[57] The systemic bioavailability of these drugs is low. Minor growth retardation has been noted in children treated with intra-nasal beclometasone[58] but this has not been shown with fluticasone[59] or mometasone.[60] These drugs are generally relatively cheap and in many countries can be bought without prescription.

SYSTEMIC GLUCOCORTICOSTEROIDS

Oral steroids may occasionally be useful in patients with severe symptoms to allow reduction of mucosal swelling and subsequent use of topical medication or to cover a short period when symptom control is particularly bad. Prednisolone 20–40 mg/day is normally sufficient[61] but oral steroids may cause serious side effects so their use should be considered carefully and length of treatment be kept as short as possible. For this reason depot injectable steroids, while effective at symptom control, are not recommended as once injected their effects cannot be stopped.[62]

LEUKOTRIENE RECEPTOR ANTAGONISTS (LTRAS)

Cysteinyl leukotrienes are a family of eicosanoid inflammatory mediators (LTC4, LTD4 and LTE4) produced in leukocytes, mast cells, eosinophils, basophils and macrophages by the oxidation of arachidonic acid by the enzyme arachidonate 5-lipoxygenase. Their effects are to cause bronchoconstriction, increase vascular permeability and attract inflammatory cells and as such are involved in the processes underlying asthma and allergic rhinitis.[63] In the UK montelukast (a leukotriene receptor antagonist) is licensed for the treatment of allergic rhinitis associated with asthma. In studies it was found to be as effective as loratadine in reducing nasal symptoms but less effective than a topical nasal steroid.[64] Combined use of cetirizine and montelukast was shown not to improve symptom control above each drug individually in one study[65] but to be more effective when combined in another.[66] There is a significant variation in responsiveness to LTRAs and a closely monitored trial of treatment may be useful in some patients. It now has a place in the updated ARIA treatment guidelines (**Figure 91.3**).

SODIUM CROMOGLICATE

Sodium cromoglicate nasal spray has modest effects on rhinitis symptoms but must be used four times daily, which limits compliance.[67] It has no side effects and can be used on young children.[4] Cromoglicate eye drops can be effective against ocular itching.[68]

DECONGESTANTS

Topical (e.g. xylometazoline) and systemic decongestants (e.g. pseudoepedrine) are available and have a place in allergic rhinitis management. The topical decongestants are more effective and have a more rapid onset of action. They reduce nasal obstruction and may allow access of a topical steroid into an otherwise obstructed nose. The disadvantage is of rebound vasodilation when their use is stopped leading to a worsening of symptoms and of rhinitis medicamentosa with longer term use. A maximum length of treatment of 7–10 days therefore is advised. Systemic decongestants may also have side effects such as insomnia, tachycardia and tremor.[4]

IPRATROPIUM

Topical ipratropium bromide spray is effective at controlling watery rhinorrhoea and can be a useful addition to a topical steroid if rhinorrhoea is not being well controlled.[69] Side effects are infrequent but include prostatic symptoms and worsening of glaucoma.[4]

NASAL DOUCHING

Saline nasal douches may help with symptom control[70] and can physically remove an allergen from the nasal mucosa. If pollen levels are high regular douching may be of benefit.

Immunotherapy

Immunotherapy (sometimes called desensitization) is a method of inducing tolerance to an allergen and therefore reducing unwanted symptoms. It can reduce the symptoms of allergic rhinitis, offer long-lasting reduction of symptoms (even when treatment has stopped) and can prevent the progression of allergic disease.[71] It involves repeated exposure of the patient to the allergen usually, but not always, with a gradual increase in allergen dose. It can be given subcutaneously by injection (SCIT) or sublingually in drops or tablets (SLIT). Studies have shown similar efficacy for SCIT and SLIT.[72] It is effective in reducing symptoms in adults and older children[71] though the results are less clear for children under five.[73] There are several guidelines regarding the selection of patients and treatment protocols, one of which is published by the British Society for Allergy and Clinical Immunology.[74]

Immunotherapy use in the UK is limited but it is widely used elsewhere. Patients considered are those who have severe symptoms but whose response to standard medical treatment has been unsatisfactory, or those patients who have unacceptable side effects from their medication.

This group may be larger than generally supposed with up to 40% of patients in UK general practice stating that symptom control of their rhinitis was poor.[75] The diagnosis of an IgE mediated response should be confirmed by skin prick tests or measurement of IgE levels before treatment and correlated with the patient's history to ensure the correct allergen is used. The main allergens used in Europe are for the main causes of allergic rhinitis – house dust mite, grass pollen, cat, dog and tree pollen. These extracts are all available in standardized doses. Treatment is usually continued over a 3-year period to achieve a long lasting tolerance after treatment has stopped.[76]

Recent exposure of the nose to allergen may lead to asymptomatic eosinophil infiltration and a pro-inflammatory mucosal environment – a concept known as priming. Such changes are likely to be reflected in the bone marrow also, with an increased production of allergy-associated cellular and biochemical mediators which are effective systemically. This can cause a patient who has specific IgE to an allergen but no clinical allergy to be 'primed' and who will subsequently react clinically to an allergen to which they would not normally react.[77] For example a patient with IgE to dog and grass pollen may not normally have an allergic response to either but if exposed to dog will then show an allergic response to grass pollen later in the season. This explains why immunotherapy treatment for one allergen may have a beneficial effect for others.

EFFICACY

With good patient selection immunotherapy can be very effective. In a study of patients with grass pollen sensitivity treated with SCIT, over the peak pollen season mean symptom and medication scores were 32% and 41% lower respectively than those in a placebo group,[78] and these results or better have been replicated in many other studies.[79] Immunotherapy for older children with allergic rhinitis also reduces the risk of developing allergic asthma later in life[80] and of developing new allergies.[81]

PROCEDURE AND SIDE EFFECTS

With SCIT there is usually an updosing phase of between 2 and 4 months when the dose of allergen is gradually increased to the maintenance dose. This maintenance dose is then injected every 4–6 weeks for a 3-year period. SLIT may be updosed or, in some treatment protocols, the patient starts with the maximum dose and continues with this daily for 3 years. Giving the patient a product to which they are known to be sensitized carries the risk of side effects. These are usually transient redness and itching around an injection site, or oral itching, and can be reduced by pre-treatment with an oral antihistamine. Very occasionally patients may suffer a generalized reaction such as urticaria, bronchoconstriction or anaphylaxis and resuscitation facilities with adrenaline must be available.[71] Almost all reactions will occur within 30 minutes of treatment therefore patients should be observed for an hour after injection. SLIT should be taken under medical supervision for the first dose but can then be taken by the patient at home if they do not react severely.

ANTI-IgE ANTIBODY (OMALIZUMAB)

Omalizumab is a monoclonal antibody that binds to circulating IgE preventing it from binding to mast cells and causing degranulation.[82] Omalizumab reduces all nasal symptoms and improves asthma control[83] but has the risk of causing anaphylaxis and is expensive. It is administered by monthly injection. Currently it is recommended only for patients with severe allergic asthma with or without rhinitis symptoms.

Surgery

Surgery cannot cure allergy but can give relief of nasal blockage if other methods fail. Reduction of submucosal fibrotic tissue on the inferior turbinates that has developed due to long-standing inflammatory changes may improve the airway and allow access for topical nasal steroids.[84] If the nose remains congested even after the application of a decongestant in clinic then surgery should be considered as the mucosal swelling may be fixed. Polypoidal mucosa may also be found in some patients with severe allergic rhinitis and occasionally this needs to be removed.

Complementary treatments

Trials of homeopathy, acupuncture and herbal remedies have not shown any evidence of beneficial effect in allergic rhinitis[85] but many patients use them and are satisfied with the results.

> **KEY POINTS**
>
> - Although allergen avoidance seems logical there is minimal evidence of beneficial effect.
> - Food allergies do not present with isolated allergic rhinitis.
> - Antihistamines and topical nasal steroids are the main treatments for allergic rhinitis.
> - Antihistamines work better if used regularly rather than on demand.
> - Leukotriene receptor antagonists may be useful.
> - Immunotherapy is highly effective but access to treatment is limited.
> - Reduction surgery to the inferior turbinates may be of use occasionally.

CHILDREN WITH RHINITIS

Allergic rhinitis is the most prevalent allergic disease in children[86] and can have significant effects on the child's quality of life. It may exacerbate other allergic disease such as asthma.[87] Younger children may get frequent episodes of acute infective rhinitis in a year and it can be difficult to differentiate these from allergy. If the episodes last more than 2 weeks and are associated with other allergic symptoms such as itching then allergy should be considered. In children with nasal obstruction but healthy nasal mucosa and clear anterior nares then adenoidal hypertrophy may be present.[88]

Skin prick testing may be performed on young children, though some will not tolerate it. It can be done on the skin of the back rather than the forearm if the child is afraid of the lancet.

The treatment algorithm is similar to that for adults but it may be more difficult to get a child to use a nasal spray. As many of these children also have asthma, however, they may be used to using an inhaler. Oral non-sedating antihistamines are the standard first-line treatment but a trial of a leukotriene receptor antagonist should also be considered if a nasal spray is not tolerated or if the steroid load is excessive. Fluticasone (from 4 years old) and mometasone and triamcinolone (from 6 years old) have low systemic bioavailability and are the steroids of choice.[89] As with adults depot steroids are not recommended. Growth should be monitored if the child is already using steroids (such as an inhaled steroid for asthma or steroid creams for eczema) although there is no evidence of an effect on the hypothalamic-pituitary-adrenal axis with normal doses.[90] Beclometasone has been associated with growth retardation and is not recommended for children.[58] SCIT is generally not recommended for children under 5 years, though SLIT may be used increasingly in the future. Its efficacy in young children is, however, still uncertain.[73, 91]

PREGNANCY

Rhinitis of pregnancy is relatively common and probably caused by high levels of oestrogen. It may occur in women without any past history of rhinitis, allergic or otherwise. Symptoms of allergic rhinitis may also be exacerbated during pregnancy, probably by the same cause. Although topical nasal steroids with low bioavailability are relatively safe, hypertonic saline douches or occasional use of topical decongestants may be preferable. The condition is self-limiting and resolves rapidly following childbirth.

BEST CLINICAL PRACTICE

- ✓ Advice to reduce allergen exposure in high-risk families has not been shown to be effective in reducing prevalence of allergy.
- ✓ Avoidance of parental smoking during pregnancy and childhood is probably important, though evidence is lacking.
- ✓ Breastfeeding is recommended.
- ✓ Although allergen avoidance is desirable, it is frequently expensive, time-consuming, impracticable or, in the case of pollens, not feasible.
- ✓ Recent trials and a meta-analysis have failed to demonstrate efficacy of house dust mite avoidance or reduction methods in adult patients with persistent rhinitis and asthma.
- ✓ Patients with allergic rhinitis and /or asthma who are sensitive to cats and dogs should be advised to remove the animals, not replace them, or at a minimum keep them out of the bedroom.
- ✓ Food allergy almost never causes isolated nasal symptoms.
- ✓ Antihistamines all rapidly relieve itching and sneezing but have minimal effect on block.
- ✓ Antihistamines appear to be more effective if used regularly.
- ✓ Topical glucocorticoids are the most effective treatment for rhinitis, especially if started prior to allergen exposure.
- ✓ There is no difference in efficacy between the various topical glucocorticoid preparations, but fluticasone and mometasone have the lowest systemic bioavailability and therefore should be considered in paediatric practice or patients having inhaled or cutaneous steroids.
- ✓ Specific immunotherapy is highly effective and may prevent development of future allergic disease.

FUTURE RESEARCH

- ➤ Should allergen avoidance methods be used by parents to prevent the development of allergy in children? What effect does this have?
- ➤ Should occupational allergen avoidance methods be used?
- ➤ Should patients with allergic rhinitis and/or conjunctivitis use antihistamines, glucocorticosteroids, antileukotrienes, cromones, decongestants or ipratropium bromide? What is the relative effect of these medications? Can decongestants be used long term if used with a nasal steroid? For what period and how regularly should they be used?
- ➤ Should allergen specific immunotherapy be used in patients with allergic rhinitis? What is the effect of subcutaneous and sublingual specific immunotherapy?
- ➤ Do complementary and alternative treatments for allergic rhinitis have an effect?
- ➤ Should medications for allergic rhinitis be used in patients with concomitant asthma for the treatment of symptoms of asthma?
- ➤ What is the role of helminths in the development of allergic disease?

KEY POINTS

- Allergic rhinitis is best considered in the context of the unified allergic airway, or even as a systemic disease.
- Diagnosis is based on the symptomatic presentation, exposure and evidence of allergen sensitization.
- The disease has a strong association with asthma and an underestimated prevalence, cost and impact on quality of life.
- The mainstay of contemporary treatment are avoidance of allergen, oral or topical antihistamines and topical corticosteroids, but immunotherapy has a re-emerging role.

REFERENCES

1. Strachan D, Sibbald B, Weiland S et al. Worldwide variations in prevalence of symptoms of allergic rhinoconjunctivitis in children: the International Study of Asthma and Allergies in Childhood (ISAAC). *Pediatr Allergy Immunol* 1997; 8: 161–76.
2. International rhinitis management working group. International Consensus Report on diagnosis and Management of Rhinitis. *Allergy* 1994; 49: S1–34.
3. Scadding GK, Durham SR, Mirakian R, et al. BSACI guidelines for the management of allergic and non-allergic rhinitis. *Clin Exp Allergy* 2008; 38: 19–42.
4. Bousquet J, Van Cauwenberge P, Khaltaev N. Allergic rhinitis and its impact on asthma. *J Allergy Clin Immunol* 2001; 108: S147–334.
5. Bousquet J, Annesi-Maesano I, Carat F, et al. Characteristics of intermittent and persistent allergic rhinitis: DREAMS study group. *Clin Exp Allergy* 2005; 35(6): 728–32.
6. Dykewicz MS, Fineman S. Executive summary of joint task force practice parameters on diagnosis and management of rhinitis. *Ann Allergy Asthma Immunol* 1998; 81: 463–8.
7. Leynaert B, Neukirch C, Liard R, et al. Quality of life in allergic rhinitis and asthma: a population-based study of young adults. *Am J Respir Crit Care Med* 2000; 162: 1391–6.
8. Blaiss MS. Allergic rhinitis and impairment issues in schoolchildren: a consensus report. *Curr Med Res Opin* 2004; 20(12): 1937–52.
9. Vuurman EF, van-Veggel LM, Uiterwijk MM, et al. Seasonal allergic rhinitis and antihistamine effects on children's learning. *Ann Allergy* 1993; 71(2): 121–6.
10. Simons FE. Learning impairment and allergic rhinitis. *Allergy Asthma Proc* 1996; 17(4): 185–9.
11. Young T, Finn L, Kim H. Nasal obstruction as a risk factor for sleep–disordered breathing. The University of Wisconsin Sleep and Respiratory Research Group. *J Allergy Clin Immunol* 1997; 99(2): S757–62.
12. Leger D, Annesi-Maesano I, Carat F, et al. Allergic rhinitis and its consequences on quality of sleep: an unexplored area. *Arch Intern Med* 2006; 166(16): 1744–8.
13. Stuck BA, Czajkowski J, Hagner AE, et al. Changes in daytime sleepiness, quality of life, and objective sleep patterns in seasonal allergic rhinitis: a controlled clinical trial. *J Allergy Clin Immunol.* 2004; 113(4): 663–8.
14. Sundberg R, Toren K, Hoglund D, et al. Nasal symptoms are associated with school performance in adolescents. *J Adolesc Health* 2007; 40(6): 581–3.
15. Walker S, Khan–Wasti S, Fletcher M, et al. Seasonal allergic rhinitis is associated with a detrimental effect on examination performance in United Kingdom teenagers: case-control study. *J Allergy Clin Immunol* 2007; 120: 381–7.
16. Lamb CE, Ratner PH, Johnson CE, et al. Economic impact of workplace productivity losses due to allergic rhinitis compared with select medical conditions in the United States from an employer perspective. *Curr Med Res Opin* 2006; 22: 1203–10.
17. Molgaard E, Thomsen SF, Lund T, et al. Differences between allergic and nonallergic rhinitis in a large sample of adolescents and adults. *Allergy* 2007; 62(9): 1033–7.
18. Asher MI, Montefort S, Bjorksten B, et al. Worldwide time trends in the prevalence of symptoms of asthma, allergic rhinoconjunctivitis, and eczema in childhood: ISAAC Phases One and Three repeat multicountry cross-sectional surveys. *Lancet* 2006; 368: 733–43.
19. Linneberg A, Nielsen NH, Madsen F, et al. Increasing prevalence of allergic rhinitis symptoms in an adult Danish population. *Allergy* 1999; 54(11): 1194–8.
20. Butland BK, Strachan DP, Lewis S, et al. Investigation into the increase in hay fever and eczema at age 16 observed between the 1958 and 1970 British birth cohorts. *BMJ* 1997; 315: 717–21.
21. von Hertzen L, Haahtela T. Signs of reversing trends in prevalence of asthma. *Allergy* 2005; 60(3): 283–92.
22. Leynaert B, Neukirch C, Jarvis D, et al. Does living on a farm during childhood protect against asthma, allergic rhinitis, and atopy in adulthood? *Am J Respir Crit Care Med* 2001; 164: 1829–34.
23. Kilpelainen M, Terho EO, Helenius H, Koskenvuo M. Childhood farm environment and asthma and sensitization in young adulthood. *Allergy* 2002; 57(12): 1130–5.
24. Strachan DP. Hay fever, hygiene, and household size. *BMJ* 1989; 299(6710): 1259–60.
25. Platts-Mills TA, Erwin E, Heymann P, et al. Is the hygiene hypothesis still a viable explanation for the increased prevalence of asthma? *Allergy* 2005; 60: S25–31.
26. Hussain R, Poindexter RW, Ottesen EA. Control of allergic reactivity in human filariasis: predominant localization of blocking antibody to the IgG4 subclass. *J Immunol* 1992; 148(9): 2731–7.
27. van den Biggelaar AH, Rodrigues LC, van Ree R, et al. Long-term treatment of intestinal helminths increases mite skin-test reactivity in Gabonese schoolchildren. *J Infect Dis* 2004; 189(5): 892–900.
28. Burke W, Fesinmeyer M, Reed K. Family history as a predictor of asthma risk. *Am J Prev Med* 2003; 24: 160–9.
29. Kulig M, Klettke U, Wahn V, et al. Development of seasonal allergic rhinitis during the first 7 years of life. *J Allergy Clin Immunol* 2000; 106(5): 832–9.
30. Hahn EL, Bacharier LB. The atopic march: the pattern of allergic disease development in childhood. *Immunol Allergy Clin North Am* 2005; 25(2): 231–46.
31. Gustafsson D, Sjoberg O, Foucard T. Development of allergies and asthma in infants and young children with atopic dermatitis: a prospective follow-up to 7 years of age. *Allergy* 2000; 55(3): 240–5.
32. Bodtger U, Poulsen LK, Linneberg A. Rhinitis symptoms and IgE sensitization as risk factors for development of later allergic rhinitis in adults. *Allergy* 2006; 61(6): 712–16.
33. Nihlen U, Greiff L, Montnemery P, et al. Incidence and remission of self-reported allergic rhinitis symptoms in adults. *Allergy* 2006; 61(11): 1299–304.
34. Simola M, Holopainene E, Malmberg H. Changes in skin and nasal sensitivity to allergens and the course of rhinitis: a long-term follow-up study. *Ann Allergy Asthma Immunol* 1999; 82(2): 152–6.
35. Hadley JA, Schaefer SD. Clinical evaluation of rhinosinusitis: history and physical examination. *Otolaryngol Head Neck Surg* 1997; 117: S8–11.
36. Doty RL, Mishra A. Olfaction and its alteration by nasal obstruction, rhinitis, and rhinosinusitis. *Laryngoscope* 2001; 111(3): 409–23.
37. Skypala IJ, Calderon MA, Leeds AR, et al. Development and validation of a structured questionnaire for the diagnosis of oral allergy syndrome in subjects with seasonal allergic rhinitis during the UK birch pollen season. *Clin Exp Allergy* 2011; 41(7): 1001–11.
38. Pepys J. Skin testing. *Br J Hosp Med* 1975; 14: 412.
39. Wide L, Bennich H, Johansson SG. Diagnosis of allergy by an in-vitro test for allergen antibodies. *Lancet* 1967; 2(7526): 1105–7.
40. Kerkhof M, Droste JH, de Monchy JG, et al. Distribution of total serum IgE and specific IgE to common aeroallergens by sex and age, and their relationship to each other in a random sample of the Dutch general population aged 20–70 years. Dutch ECRHS Group, European Community Respiratory Health Study. *Allergy* 1996; 51(11): 770–6.
41. Andersson M, Greiff L, Svensson C, et al. Various methods for testing nasal responses in vivo: a critical review. *Acta Otolaryngol* 1995; 115: 705–13.
42. Olin AC, Alving K, Toren K. Exhaled nitric oxide: relation to sensitization and respiratory symptoms. *Clin Exp Allergy* 2004; 34(2): 221–6.
43. Muraro A, Dreborg S, Halken S, et al. Dietary prevention of allergic diseases in infants and small children. Part III: Critical review of published peer-reviewed observational and interventional studies and final recommendations. *Pediatr Allergy Immunol* 2004; 15(4): 291–307.
44. Kramer MS, Kakuma R. Maternal dietary antigen avoidance during pregnancy or lactation, or both, for preventing or treating atopic disease in the child. *Cochrane Database Syst Rev* 2012; Iss 9. Art No CD000133.
45. Strachan DP, Cook DG. Health effects of passive smoking: parental smoking and allergic sensitisation in children. *Thorax* 1998; 53(2): 117–23.
46. Halmerbauer G, Gartner C, Schierl M, et al. Study on the Prevention of Allergy in Children in Europe (SPACE): allergic sensitization at 1 year of age in a controlled trial of allergen avoidance from birth. *Pediatr Allergy Immunol* 2003; 14(1): 10–17.
47. World Health Organization. Prevention of allergy and allergic asthma; 2003. http://whqlibdoc.who.int/hq/2003/WHO_NMH_MNC_CRA_03.2.pdf. [Accessed 30 June 17]
48. Terreehorst I, Hak E, Oosting AJ, et al. Evaluation of impermeable covers for bedding in patients with allergic rhinitis. *N Engl J Med* 2003; 349(3): 237–46.

49. Custovic A, Wijk RG. The effectiveness of measures to change the indoor environment in the treatment of allergic rhinitis and asthma: ARIA update (in collaboration with GA(2)LEN). *Allergy* 2005; **60**(9): 1112–15.
50. Bousquet J Khaltaev N, Cruz AA et al. Allergic Rhinitis and its Impact on Asthma (ARIA) 2008 update (in collaboration with the World Health Organization, GA(2)LEN and AllerGen). *Allergy* 2008; **63**: S8–160.
51. Corren J, Adinoff AD, Buchmeier AD, et al. Nasal beclomethasone prevents the seasonal increase in bronchial responsiveness in patients with allergic rhinitis and asthma. *J Allergy Clin Immunol* 1992; **90**(2): 250–6.
52. Grieff L, Andersson M, Svensson C, et al. Effects of orally inhaled budesonide in seasonal allergic rhinitis. *Eur Resp Journal* 1998; **11**(6): 1268–73.
53. Simons FE. Advances in H1-antihistamines. *N Engl J Med* 2004; **351**(21): 2203–17.
54. Ciprandi G, Passalacqua G, Mincarini M, et al. Continuous versus on demand treatment with cetirizine for allergic rhinitis. *Ann Allergy Asthma Immunol* 1997; **79**: 507–11.
55. Weiner JM, Abramson MJ, Puy RM. Intranasal corticosteroids versus oral H1 receptor antagonists in allergic rhinitis: systematic review of randomised controlled trials. *BMJ* 1998; **317**(7173): 1624–9.
56. Bhatia S, Baroody FM, deTineo M, et al. Increased nasal airflow with budesonide compared with desloratadine during the allergy season. *Arch Otolaryngol Head Neck Surg* 2005; **131**(3): 223–8.
57. Laliberte F, Laliberte MF, Lecart S, et al. Clinical and pathologic methods to assess the long-term safety of nasal corticosteroids. French Triamcinolone Acetonide Study Group. *Allergy* 2000; **55**(8): 718–22.
58. Skoner D, Rachelefsky G, Meltzer E, et al. Detection of growth suppression in children during treatment with intranasal belcomethasone dipropionate. *Pediatrics* 2000; **105**: E23.
59. Allen DB, Meltzer EO, Lemanske RF, Jr., et al. No growth suppression in children treated with the maximum recommended dose of fluticasone propionate aqueous nasal spray for one year. *Allergy Asthma Proc* 2002; **23**(6): 407–13.
60. Schenkel EJ, Skoner DP, Bronsky EA, et al. Absence of growth retardation in children with perennial allergic rhinitis after one year of treatment with mometasone furoate aqueous nasal spray. *Pediatrics* 2000; **105**(2): E22.
61. Plaut M, Valentine MD. Clinical practice: allergic rhinitis. *N Engl J Med* 2005 Nov 3; **353**(18): 1934–44.
62. Bousquet J. Primum non nocere. *Prim Care Respir J* 2005; **14**(3): 122–3.
63. Dahlen S-E, Bjork J, Hedqvist P, et al. Leukotrienes promote plasma leakage and leukocyte adhesion in postcapillary venules: in vivo effects with relevance to the acute inflammatory response. *PNAS* 1981; **78**(6): 3887–91.
64. Pullerts T, Praks L, Skoogh BE, et al. Randomized placebo-controlled study comparing a leukotriene receptor antagonist and a nasal glucocorticoid in seasonal allergic rhinitis. *Am J Respir Crit Care Med* 1999: **159**: 1814–18.
65. Nayak AS, Philip G, Lu S, et al. Montelukast Fall investigator group. Efficacy and tolerability of montelukast alone or in combination with loratadine in seasonal allergic rhinitis: a muticenter, randomised, double-blind, placebo-controlled clinical trial. *Ann Allergy Asthma Immunol* 2002: **88**: 562–600.
66. Meltzer E, Malmstrom K, Lu S, et al. Concomitant montelukast and loratadine as treatment for seasonal allergic rhinitis: placebo-controlled clinical trial. *J Allergy Clin Immunol* 2000; **105**: 917–22.
67. Meltzer E. Efficacy and patient satisfaction with cromolyn sodium nasal solution in the treatment of seasonal allergic rhinitis: a placebo-controlled study. *Clin Ther* 2002; **24**(6): 942–52.
68. Owen CG, Shah A, Henshaw K, et al. Topical treatments for seasonal allergic conjunctivitis: systematic review and meta-analysis of efficacy and effectiveness. *Br J Gen Pract* 2004: **54**: 451–6.
69. Dockhorn R, Aaronson D, Bronsky E, et al. Ipratropium bromide nasal spray 0.03% and beclomethasone nasal spray alone and in combination for the treatment of rhinorrhea in perennial rhinitis. *Ann Allergy Asthma Immunol* 1999; **82**: 349–59.
70. Taccariello M, Parikh A, Darby Y, Scadding G. Nasal douching as a valuable adjunct in the management of chronic rhinosinusitis. *Rhinology* 1999; **37**(1): 29–32.
71. Bousquet J, Lockey R, Malling H. WHO Position Paper. Allergen Immunotherapy: therapeutic vaccines for allergic diseases. *Allergy* 1998; **53**, suppl 54.
72. Wilson DR, Lima MT, Durham SR. Sublingual immunotherapy for allergic rhinitis: systematic review and meta-analysis. *Allergy* 2005; **60**(1): 4–12.
73. Marseglia GL, Incorvaia C, La Rosa M, et al. Sublingual immunotherapy in children: facts and needs. *Ital J Pediatr* 2009 23; **35**(1): 31.
74. Frew AJ. Injection immunotherapy. British Society for Allergy and Clinical Immunology Working Party. *BMJ* 1993; **307**: 919–23.
75. White P, Smith H, Baker N, et al. Symptom control in patients with hay fever in UK general practice: how well are we doing and is there a need for allergen immunotherapy? *Clin Exp Allergy* 1998; **28**: 266–70.
76. Durham SR, Walker SM, Varga EM, et al. Long-term clinical efficacy of grass-pollen immunotherapy. *N Engl J Med* 1999; **341**: 468–75.
77. Bousquet J, Vignola AM, Campbell AM, et al. Pathophysiology of allergic rhinitis *Int Arch Allergy Immunol* 1996; **110**(3): 207–18.
78. Frew AJ, Powell RJ, Corrigan CJ, et al. Efficacy and safety of specific immunotherapy with SQ allergen extract in treatment-resistant seasonal allergic rhinoconjunctivitis. *J Allergy Clin Immunol* 2006; **117**: 319–25.
79. Walker SM, Pajno GB, Lima MT, et al. Grass pollen immunotherapy for seasonal rhinitis and asthma: a randomized, controlled trial. *J Allergy Clin Immunol* 2001; **107**: 87–93.
80. Moller C, Dreborg S, Ferdousi HA, et al. Pollen immunotherapy reduces the development of asthma in children with seasonal rhinoconjunctivitis (the PAT-study). *J Allergy Clin Immunol* 2002; **109**: 251–6.
81. Des Roches A, Paradis L, Menardo JL, et al. Immunotherapy with a standardized *Dermatophagoides pteronyssinus* extract. VI. Specific immunotherapy prevents the onset of new sensitizations in children. *J Allergy Clin Immunol* 1997; **99**(4): 450–3.
82. Holgate S, Casale T, Wenzel S, et al. The anti-inflammatory effects of omalizumab confirm the central role of IgE in allergic inflammation. *J Allergy Clin Immunol* 2005; **115**(3): 459–65.
83. Vignola AM, Humbert M, Bousquet J, et al. Efficacy and tolerability of anti-immunoglobulin E therapy with omalizumab in patients with concomitant allergic asthma and persistent allergic rhinitis: SOLAR. *Allergy* 2004; **59**(7): 709–17.
84. Mori S, Fujieda S, Igarashi M, et al. Submucous turbinectomy decreases not only nasal stiffness but also sneezing and rhinorrhea in patients with perennial allergic rhinitis. *Clin Exp Allergy* 1999; **29**(11): 1542–8.
85. Passalacqua G, Bousquet PJ, Carlsen KH, et al. ARIA update: Systematic review of complementary and alternative medicine for rhinitis and asthma. *J Allergy Clin Immunol* 2006; **117**(5): 1054–62.
86. Selnes A, Nystad W, Bolle R, et al. Diverging prevalence trends of atopic disorders in Norwegian children: results from three cross-sectional studies. *Allergy* 2005; **60**(7): 894–9.
87. Gelfand EW. Pediatric allergic rhinitis: factors affecting treatment choice. *Ear Nose Throat J* 2005; **84**(3): 163–8.
88. Hellings PW, Fokkens WJ. Allergic rhinitis and its impact on otorhinolaryngology. *Allergy* 2006; **61**(6): 656–64.
89. Daley-Yates PT, Richards DH. Relationship between systemic corticosteroid exposure and growth velocity: development and validation. *Clin Ther* 2004; **26**(11): 1905–19.
90. Sheth KK, Cook CK, Philpot EE, et al. Concurrent use of intranasal and orally inhaled fluticasone propionate does not affect hypothalamic-pituitary-adrenal-axis function. *Allergy Asthma Proc* 2004; **25**: 115–20.
91. Roder E, Berger MY, de Groot H, et al. Immunotherapy in children and adolescents with allergic rhinoconjunctivitis: a systematic review. *Pediatr Allergy Immunol* 2008; **19**(3): 197–207.

CHAPTER 92

NON-ALLERGIC PERENNIAL RHINITIS

Jameel Muzaffar and Shahzada K. Ahmed

Introduction 1011	Drug-induced rhinitis 1013
Pathophysiological considerations................ 1012	Other forms of rhinitis 1013
Types of non-allergic rhinitis 1012	Conclusion 1015
Hormonal rhinitis 1013	References 1016

SEARCH STRATEGY

Data in this chapter may be updated by a Medline and Embase searches using the keywords: rhinitis, vasomotor rhinitis, non-allergic rhinitis, NANIPER, occupational rhinitis, drug-induced rhinitis, NARES, drug therapy and surgery.

INTRODUCTION

Although rhinitis is a cause of widespread morbidity, medical treatment costs, reduced work productivity and lost school days, the disease is often trivialized. Non-infectious rhinitis can broadly be subdivided into two subclasses, allergic and non-allergic rhinitis, depending predominantly on whether or not an allergic aetiology is implicated. Whilst allergic rhinitis has been extensively investigated and the underlying mechanisms are relatively well understood, there is comparatively little information on non-allergic rhinitis. The term 'non-allergic rhinitis' is commonly applied to a diagnosis of any nasal condition in which the symptoms are identical to those seen in allergic rhinitis but an allergic aetiology has been excluded. These non-allergic aetiologic entities can broadly be classified as:

- idiopathic rhinitis (also referred to as vasomotor rhinitis, or non-allergic non-infectious perennial rhinitis (NANIPER));
- non-allergic occupational rhinitis;
- hormonal rhinitis;
- drug-induced rhinitis; and
- other forms (non-allergic rhinitis with eosinophilia syndrome (NARES), rhinitis due to physical and chemical factors, food-induced rhinitis, emotion-induced rhinitis, atrophic rhinitis).[1,2]

Unlike allergic rhinitis there are no specific diagnostic tests for non-allergic rhinitis, and diagnosis is made on the basis of rhinitis symptoms in the absence of identifiable allergy (by allergy testing), structural abnormality, immune deficiency, sinus disease or other causes.

Ninety-five percent of normal subjects without rhinitis complaints have been shown to sneeze up to four times a day and to blow their noses up to four times a day, as an average over 2 weeks.[3] This would suggest that five or more sneezes and/or nose blowing per day may possibly be indicative of nasal disease. Whilst it is difficult to readily diagnose non-allergic rhinitis, it has been suggested that in patients with perennial non-allergic rhinitis this condition persists for greater than 9 months each year and produces two or more symptoms, including hypersecretion, blockage, sneezing and post-nasal drip.

Although there are some studies of the prevalence of non-allergic rhinitis amongst the rhinitic population, large variations (ranging from around 20 to 50%) have been reported,[4,5] presumably due to difficulties in definition and diagnosis of the disease. It is evident that the incidence of positive skin tests to inhalant allergens is far greater than the incidence of rhinitis symptoms in large cross-sectional epidemiological studies. This also implies that rhinitis symptoms in a patient with a positive skin test are not necessarily caused by the allergen, suggesting that the contribution of non-allergic rhinitis to the total number of rhinitis patients may be substantially greater than hitherto estimated. A survey of nearly 1000 rhinitis patients seen in 18 allergy clinics in the USA showed that 23% of the patients had pure non-allergic rhinitis and, importantly, 34% of the patients were diagnosed with 'mixed' rhinitis (a combination of allergic and non-allergic rhinitis),[6,7] a group not considered in the other studies. Furthermore, both non-allergic and mixed rhinitis occur more frequently in adults than in children, may be more common in females and are more likely to be perennial than seasonal. More recently, the survey was extended to include more than 22 000 practitioners, each of whom contributed ten patients with rhinitis to the survey. The interim results of the survey indicated that as many as 70% of these patients have mixed rhinitis, with only 9% having the non-allergic rhinitis component alone.

PATHOPHYSIOLOGICAL CONSIDERATIONS

Non-allergic rhinitis, allergic rhinitis and post-infectious rhinitis have nasal hyper-reactivity to various stimuli (for example odours, position, temperature, histamine, etc.) in common, which consequently does not allow differentiation between allergic and non-allergic causes. Unlike patients from some subgroups of non-allergic rhinitis (particularly drug-induced, hormone-induced and NARES) and patients with allergic rhinitis for whom the aetiology is well defined, the aetiology and pathophysiology for the majority of patients with non-allergic non-infectious rhinitis are largely unknown. Although the term 'vasomotor' implies increased neuronal efferent traffic to the blood vessels supplying the nasal mucosa, this has never been proved.[1] Some mechanistic studies have suggested that the functional abnormality in NANIPER may be associated with an imbalance between the sympathetic and parasympathetic nervous systems, which leads to an imbalance in neuronal control of the end organs in the nose.[8] Indeed, nasal provocation with capsaicin, which specifically stimulates afferent nerve fibres, has been shown to result in a dose-dependent leukocyte influx, albumin leakage and glandular secretion in patients with allergic rhinitis[9] and to be efficacious in the treatment of NANIPER.[10] However, reports on the underlying mechanisms are conflicting. Whilst some studies have suggested that capsaicin induces neurogenic inflammation in patients with allergic rhinitis, possibly as a consequence of abnormal nociceptor function, this has been shown not to be the case in NANIPER.[11] Forced expiration through the nose has been found to significantly increase nasal airway resistance, but not mucous production or sneezing, within the first minute in NANIPER patients and not in non-rhinitic controls, suggesting that mechanical stimulation may also be an important mechanism in NANIPER patients.[12] However, in view of the fact that sympathetic stimulation leads to vasoconstriction and parasympathetic stimulation leads to nasal congestion, it is likely that the imbalance is biased towards parasympathetic stimulation since rhinorrhoea is the predominant complaint in this condition.[8]

Review of the limited data available for idiopathic rhinitis, which comprises the largest group of patients with non-allergic rhinitis, has indicated that several pathologic mechanisms, including non-IgE-mediated inflammatory responses, C-fibre stimulation, parasympathetic hyper-reactivity and/or sympathetic hyporeactivity, and glandular hyper-reactivity, might play a role in these patients.[13] However, it is not clear whether these mechanisms operate separately or in combination in the same patient, and whether these mechanisms may be caused by different aetiological entities.

Some attempts have been made to develop diagnostic tools for this condition. Assessment of skin reactivity to a variety of vasomotor agents, including Papaverine, Methacholine, Histamine and Compound 48/40, has demonstrated that the frequency of pathological skin reactivity to Papaverine, but not the other three agents, is significantly increased in patients with perennial non-allergic rhinitis, compared with healthy subjects.[14] This suggests that Papaverine-induced skin reactivity may be a useful diagnostic tool for non-allergic rhinitis. A dose–response study has shown that histamine-induced total nasal resistance follows a model exponential curve, suggesting that it may be possible to classify non-specific nasal hyper-reactivity in allergic and non-allergic subjects as a function of the regression b coefficient of the empirical equation used in reactivity classes.[15] Methacholine tests may be able to differentiate idiopathic rhinitis subjects from controls, but only in those suffering from rhinorrhoea as the main symptom. Recently, cold dry air (CDA) challenge has been suggested to differentiate best between controls and idiopathic rhinitis patients.[13] However, none of these tests is suitable to differentiate the non-allergic idiopathic from other forms of rhinitis, nor has any been demonstrated to be superior to a simple case history.

TYPES OF NON-ALLERGIC RHINITIS

Idiopathic rhinitis

Idiopathic rhinitis is characterized primarily by symptoms of nasal blockage, rhinorrhoea and sneezing, although the prevalence of sneezing, conjunctival symptoms and pruritis is lower than that in allergic rhinitis. Although the subjects have traditionally been classified as either 'runners' (those with predominantly rhinorrhoea) or 'blockers' (those with predominantly nasal congestion and blockage), many patients suffer from more than one type of these symptoms, therefore making it difficult to subdivide the patients into these groups. The aetiology is unknown in most cases and the disease is thought to be triggered mainly by irritants and changes in atmospheric conditions.[16] Among patients with chronic symptoms, the percentage with a non-allergic aetiology increases progressively with age and reaches >60% beyond the age of 50 years, therefore suggesting that functional abnormality in this condition may be associated with the ageing process in the nasal mucosa.[16]

Non-allergic occupational rhinitis

Occupational rhinitis, as the term implies, may be defined as rhinitis caused by exposure to airborne agents present in the work place. These agents elicit predominantly sneezing, nasal discharge and/or blockage and may act via both immunologic (IgE-mediated) and non-immunologic mechanisms. The non-immunologic triggers are often irritant or toxic small molecular weight compounds such as aldehydes, isocyanates, aircraft fuel and jet stream exhaust, solvents, etc.,[1, 8, 17] or may be physical (long-term exposure to cold air). Whilst the specific mechanisms underlying the effects of these irritants and toxic agents have not been fully elucidated, it is possible that damage and/or stimulation of the epithelial cells and neurons by the irritants may lead to proinflammatory mediators and neuromediators, which may predispose the nasal mucosa to inflammation and infection, subsequently resulting in the symptoms of rhinitis. Indeed, a study investigating the effect of airborne exposure to the non-allergenic microbial agents endotoxin and beta(1,3)-glucan in compost workers has reported that concentrations of total cells (predominantly neutrophils), myeloperoxidase (MPO), IL-8, nitric oxide (NO) and albumin were significantly higher in compost workers than in controls.[18] Similarly, occupational exposure to vanadium pentoxide, a constituent of fuel oil ash and a known respiratory irritant, has been shown to significantly increase the number of polymorphonuclear cells in nasal lavage of boilermakers.[19]

HORMONAL RHINITIS

Hormonal rhinitis is often associated with pregnancy in particular, although puberty is also known to induce the symptoms of rhinitis.[1, 8] A large multicentre study has indicated that the cumulative incidence of pregnancy rhinitis was 22%, and in women who were smokers this was significantly increased with a relative risk enhancement of 69%.[20] Neither asthma nor rhinitis were, apparently, risk factors for pregnancy rhinitis. In contrast, only 2% of patients with non-allergic rhinitis may be afflicted by rhinitis due to hypothyroidism or acromegaly.[21]

Oestrogens cause vascular engorgement, not only in the female genital tract, but also in the nose, leading to nasal obstruction and/or nasal hypersecretion. Beta-oestradiol and progesterone have been shown to increase the expression of histamine H_1 receptors on human nasal epithelial cells and mucosal microvascular endothelial cells,[22] and to induce eosinophil migration and/or degranulation, in marked contrast to testosterone, which decreases eosinophil activation and viability.[23] Compared with pregnancy rhinitis, the evidence linking hypothyroidism with nasal pathology is sparse, and the reported increase in nasal secretion associated with thyroid disease is anecdotal.[1]

DRUG-INDUCED RHINITIS

Several commonly employed medications, such as aspirin, other non-steroidal antiinflammatory drugs (NSAIDs), beta-blockers, angiotensin-converting enzyme (ACE) inhibitors, methyldopa, oral contraceptives, psychotropic agents and nasal topical decongestants (Oxymetazoline, Naphazoline, Xylometazoline) may induce symptoms of rhinitis when they are administered either topically or systemically. The symptoms may be either predictable, as would be the case for known side effects of particular drugs, or unpredictable, based on individual hypersensitivity to certain drugs, in particular aspirin, which commonly exacerbates rhinitis and asthma. However, intolerance to aspirin and/or NSAIDs predominantly produces rhinorrhoea, which may be either isolated or part of a complex involving hyperplastic rhinosinusitis, nasal polyps and asthma.[1] In contrast, intolerance to ACE inhibitors, methyldopa or oral contraceptives, which is less common than aspirin intolerance, leads predominantly to nasal blockage.[1] Whilst persistent overuse of the topical nasal vasoconstrictors also leads to nasal decongestion by a mechanism involving a rebound effect following withdrawal of these drugs, excessive use of these agents may also lead to nasal hyper-reactivity and hypertrophy of the nasal mucosa, a condition known as 'rhinitis medicamentosa'.[1, 8]

OTHER FORMS OF RHINITIS

NARES

The term NARES was originally introduced by Mullarkey and colleagues, who characterized the condition on the basis of a presence of greater than 20% eosinophils in nasal smears of symptomatic patients with perennial sneezing attacks, a profuse watery rhinorrhoea, nasal pruritis, incomplete nasal obstruction and occasional loss of smell.[1, 4, 7, 8] In addition to these symptoms, a marked feature of the disease is the lack of evidence of allergy, as indicated by negative skin prick tests and/or absence of serum IgE antibodies to specific allergens.

The prevalence of NARES has been shown to range between 13 and 33% in patients with non-allergic rhinitis.[21, 24] Although the specific aetiology of NARES is not clear, in view of the features shared by this syndrome and the triad (nasal polyposis, intrinsic asthma and intolerance to aspirin) and because NARES patients frequently develop nasal polyps and asthma later on in life, it has been suggested that NARES may be an early expression of the triad.[24] Indeed, in approximately 50% of NARES patients without a history of respiratory symptoms, bronchial responsiveness is associated with an increase in the number of sputum eosinophils, but not with an increase in the number of nasal eosinophils.[25] Some investigators have suggested that NARES is a variant of vasomotor rhinitis, and referred to the condition as 'perennial intrinsic rhinitis'.

Rhinitis due to physical and chemical factors

Nasal symptoms similar to those of rhinitis can be induced by physical and chemical factors in individuals with sensitized nasal mucous membranes.[2] Cold, dry air has been shown to lead to a condition known as skier's nose, in which rhinorrhoea features prominently. Exposure to chemicals, particularly air pollutants derived from cigarette smoke and liquid petroleum fuels, have also been shown to directly exacerbate symptoms of rhinitis in non-allergic individuals,[2] although their effects have generally been extensively investigated and well documented in the lower airways of allergic individuals.[26] Little information is available on the acute or chronic effects of air pollutants on the nasal mucosa.

Food-induced rhinitis

Few studies have documented that certain foods and alcoholic beverages can induce non-allergic rhinitis, although the underlying mechanisms are largely unknown. Hot and spicy foods, in particular, which contain capsaicin, lead to a watery rhinorrhoea termed 'gustatory rhinitis', probably as a result of the capsaicin stimulating the sensory nerves to release neuropeptides and tachykinins.[1, 2] In contrast, alcoholic beverages are thought to induce symptoms as a result of vasodilation. Dyes and preservatives, as well as sulphites, appear to play a role in a very few cases, whereas some foods may contain clinically relevant concentrations of histamine or other biogenic amines.

Emotionally induced rhinitis

Although not studied extensively, emotional factors such as stress and sexual arousal have been documented to affect the nose, likely as a result of autonomic stimulation.[2, 27] In patients suffering from post-coital rhinitis, anxiety appears to be a predominant feature, which leads to worsening of their disease.[27]

Atrophic rhinitis

Primary atrophic rhinitis is a condition that occurs predominantly in women and is characterized by progressive atrophy of the nasal mucosa and underlying bone of the turbinates.[1, 2] This leads to the formation of thick crusts, which leave a constant foul smell (ozaena) in the nose.[1, 2] Furthermore, the nasal cavities are enlarged and there is the sensation of nasal congestion. Although the precise aetiology of this condition is not clear, it has been suggested that this may be a result of infection with *Klebsiella ozaenae* and other bacteria. However, primary atrophic rhinitis is distinct from secondary atrophic rhinitis, which develops directly as a result of granulomatous nasal infections, chronic rhinosinusitis, excessive nasal surgery, trauma and irradiation.

Differential diagnosis

Allergic rhinitis is the major disease to differentiate from non-allergic rhinitis and may be excluded by appropriate allergy tests. However, the possibility of a local IgE production within the nasal mucosa may account for some cases where skin prick tests or IgE antibodies to common allergens are not positive. Several other conditions, including polyps, sinusitis, congenital and acquired anatomical abnormalities (e.g. nasal septal deviation, adenoid hypertrophy, hypertrophy of nasal turbinates, choanal atresia), benign and malignant tumours, granulomas, ciliary defects and cerebrospinal rhinorrhoea,[1, 2] are known to mimic symptoms of non-allergic non-infectious rhinitis and therefore have to be excluded by careful examination in order to make the correct diagnosis. Anatomical nasal abnormalities block the flow of nasal secretions and lead to rhinorrhoea, post-nasal drip and nasal blockage. In children, congenital choanal atresia can lead to reduced nasal airflow, resulting in nasal blockage. Tumours are not very common in the nasal passages, but when established and growing rapidly they often lead to unilateral nasal obstruction, bleeding and pain. Rhinorrhoea and nasal congestion, in the absence of pruritus, are also characteristic features of nasal mastocytosis, an extremely rare condition, in which eosinophils are absent and tests for IgE-mediated disease are negative.

Diagnosis as a step-wise approach

In daily clinical practice, the diagnosis of non-allergic rhinitis and its subgroups is mainly based on a thorough case history, followed by the step-wise exclusion of possible differential diagnoses, as follows.

If the case history is suggestive of clinically relevant non-infectious rhinitis:

- check possible stimuli, severity and duration of disease;
- check drug use (systemic and topical), exposure at work place, hormonal status (pregnancy, hypothyroidism, acromegaly) and involvement of other organs (asthma, hormonal status);
- exclude other nasal disease (rigid nasal endoscopy);
- exclude allergy: skin prick test, serum IgE-antibodies to the most frequent inhalant allergens, and ultimately nasal provocation testing in selected cases;
- exclude chronic rhinosinusitis (nasoendoscopy +/− computed tomography (CT) scan);
- perform nasal cytology (eosinophilia), and if shown to be positive then perform oral Aspirin challenge.

Therapy for non-allergic perennial rhinitis

First, an evaluation of the severity of the disease should be performed to confirm the need for therapy, in connection with counselling on how to avoid non-specific stimuli. In case of drug-induced, food-induced or occupational rhinitis, specific avoidance measures are employed as first-line therapy.

Several treatments (pharmaceutical, non-conventional and surgery) have been employed for idiopathic non-allergic rhinitis.[28] Intra-nasal anticholinergics (Ipratropium Bromide) may be useful in patients with nasal secretion as the predominant symptom, whereas nasal decongestants should be avoided or limited to 10 days. Topical steroids and antihistamines are the two main classes of drugs employed, of which only Fluticasone Propionate, Budesonide, Beclomethasone and Azelastine, respectively, have been approved by the Food and Drug Administration (FDA). Azelastine nasal spray has been found to be more effective than placebo for control of rhinorrhoea, post-nasal drip, sneezing and nasal congestion in most patients, although its effect on nasal congestion was rather marginal.[29] The efficacy of intra-nasal steroids in patients with vasomotor rhinitis has been inconsistent. Furthermore, whilst the topical nasal steroids are more frequently used for treatment of more severe symptoms, they are mostly useful in patients in whom an inflammatory pathogenesis is a prominent feature of their disease, for example NARES. Recent evidence suggests that in patients who do not respond to treatment with nasal steroids, treatment with non-conventional therapies such as silver nitrate, botulin toxin and particularly intra-nasal capsaicin may be beneficial. Studies in patients suffering from NANIPER have demonstrated that intra-nasal capsaicin leads to a significant and long-term reduction in clinical VAS scores, compared with placebo.[10] In another study, treatment once daily for 5 weeks with intranasal capsaicin was also shown to significantly improve all symptoms and produce a larger vascular response throughout a 6-month follow-up period in patients suffering from severe chronic non-allergic rhinitis with nasal vasoconstrictor abuse.[30] In cases where nasal obstruction is resistant to medical treatment and if the inferior turbinate is hyperplastic, surgical intervention to reduce the size of the turbinate by various procedures has been shown to be useful. Endoscopic transnasal vidian neurectomies have also been performed by excision, diathermy and cryotherapy, and have produced results with varying degrees and duration of success.[31-33]

Recent interest in intranasal capsaicin prompted a Cochrane Review that included 302 patients with idiopathic non-allergic rhinitis.[34] Whilst the quality was judged to be low to moderate there was sufficient evidence that capsaicin was superior to both placebo and Budesonide. Studies were of variable follow-up ranging from 4 to 38 weeks. Given the limited treatment options for non-allergic rhinitis and good safety profile[35] Capsaicin represents a reasonable therapeutic choice.

Small scale non-powered studies have shown therapeutic potential for intra-nasal Botulinum toxin for non-allergic rhinitis.[36-38] Symptoms of nasal obstruction, discharge, sneezing and itching all improved, though the duration of improvement was limited to 2–3 months.

CONCLUSION

Despite increasing evidence for the various forms of non-allergic rhinitis, many of these conditions are often underrated and trivialized, primarily due to the paucity of information on the causative factors, the underlying mechanisms and/or the absence of specific diagnostic tests. Furthermore, there are differences in opinion amongst clinicians and researchers regarding classification of disease and in conditions such as occupational rhinitis, in particular, the situation is further compounded as a consequence of legal and financial compensatory implications, for both employers and employees alike. To date, no specific diagnostic test is available, and clinical diagnosis is based on case history and exclusion of other disease. Despite these difficulties, however, recent evidence suggests that relevant diagnostic tools and specific information regarding the mechanisms underlying some of these conditions is more forthcoming and should therefore lead to a better overall understanding and management of these conditions in the future.

BEST CLINICAL PRACTICE

✓ Wherever possible, the treatment should take into account the aforementioned subgroups of non-allergic perennial rhinitis.
✓ In idiopathic rhinitis, antihistamines and topical steroids are the two main classes of drugs for treatment. Topical steroids are to be preferred if an inflammatory pathogenesis is suggested.
✓ Intra-nasal capsaicin is supported by a better evidence base than intra-nasal Botulinum toxin but both treatments remain outside widespread clinical use.
✓ Surgery is an option in patients with persistent nasal obstruction not improved by medication.

FUTURE RESEARCH

➤ There is a marked lack of diagnostic tools/procedures for determining each type of these conditions.
➤ There is a marked lack of controlled trials for determining diagnosis.
➤ Epidemiological studies on prevalence of different types of non-allergic rhinitis are required.
➤ Research on mechanisms underlying these conditions is needed.

KEY POINTS

- Approximately half of rhinitis patients may suffer from non-allergic rhinitis.
- There are no specific diagnostic tests for non-allergic rhinitis.
- A thorough case history is the best diagnostic tool available and should focus on drug intake, work exposure and hormonal status to subdivide the condition into subgroups.
- As the symptoms are quite non-specific, the differential diagnoses have to be excluded.

REFERENCES

1. *Dykewicz MS, Fineman S, Skoner DP, et al. Diagnosis and management of rhinitis: complete guidelines of the Joint Task Force on Practice Parameter in Allergy, Asthma and Immunology. American Academy of Allergy, Asthma, and Immunology. *Ann Allergy Asthma Immunol* 1998; **81**: 478–518.
2. *Bousquet J, van Cauwenberge P, Khaltaev N, the ARIA Workshop Group. Allergic rhinitis and its impact on asthma – ARIA Workshop Report. *J Allergy Clin Immunol* 2001; **108**: S147–333.
3. Hansen B, Mygind N. How often do normal persons sneeze and blow the nose? *Rhinology* 2002; **40**: 10–12.
4. Mullarkey MF, Hill JS, Webb DR. Allergic and nonallergic rhinitis: their characterization with attention to the meaning of nasal eosinophilia. *J Allergy and Clin Immunol* 1980; **65**: 122–6.
5. Jessen M, Janzon L. Prevalence of nonallergic nasal complaints in urban and a rural population in Sweden. *Allergy* 1989; **44**: 582–7.
6. Data presented at the National Allergy Advisory Council Meeting (NAAC). The broad spectrum of rhinitis: etiology, diagnosis and advances in treatment. St. Thomas, US Virgin Islands, Oct 16, 1999.
7. Settipane RA, Lieberman P. Update on nonallergic rhinitis. *Ann Allergy Asthma Immunol*. 2001; **86**: 494–507.
8. *van Cauwenberge PB, Wang D-Y, Ingels KJAO, et al. Rhinitis: the spectrum of the disease. In: Busse WW, Holgate ST (eds). *Asthma and rhinitis*. 2nd ed. Oxford: Blackwell Science; 2000, pp. 6–13.
9. Sanico A, Atsuta S, Proud D, et al. Dose-dependent effects of capsaicin nasal challenge: in vivo evidence of human airway neurogenic inflammation. *J Allergy Clin Immunol* 1997; **100**: 632–41.
10. Blom HM, van Rijswijk JB, Garrelds IM, et al. Intranasal capsaicin is efficacious in nonallergic, non-infectious perennial rhinitis: a placebo-controlled study. *Clin Exp Allergy* 1997; **27**: 796–801.
11. Blom HM, Severijnen LA, van Rijswijk JB, Mulder PGH, Gerth van Wijk R, Fokkens WJ. The long-term effects of capsaicin aqueous spray on the nasal mucosa. *Clin Exp Allergy* 1998; **28**: 1351–8.
12. Braat JPM, Fokkens WJ, Mulder PG, et al. Forced expiration through the nose is a stimulus for NANIPER but not for controls. *Rhinology* 2000; **38**: 172–6.
13. *Fokkens WJ. Thoughts on the pathophysiology of nonallergic rhinitis. *Curr Allergy Asthma Rep* 2002; **2**: 203–9.
14. Milosevic DN, Janosevic LJB, Janosevic SB. Intradermal tests with vasomotor agents in perennial nonallergic rhinitis. *Acta Otorhinolaryngol Belg* 2000; **54**: 465–71.
15. Zambetti G, Moresi M, Romeo R, et al. Non-specific nasal provocation test with histamine: analysis of the dose-response curve. *Rhinology* 1999; **37**: 168–74.
16. *Sanico A, Togias A. Noninfectious, nonallergic rhinitis (NINAR): considerations on possible mechanisms. *Am J Rhinology* 1998; **12**: 65–72.
17. Tunnicliffe WS, O'Hickey SP, Fletcher TJ, et al. Pulmonary function and respiratory symptoms in a population of airport workers. *Occup Environ Med* 1999; **56**: 118–23.
18. Douwes J, Wouters I, Dubbeld H, et al. Upper airway inflammation assessed by nasal lavage in compost workers: a relation with bio-aerosol exposure. *Am J Ind Med* 2000; **37**: 459–68.
19. Hauser R, Elreedy S, Hoppin JA, et al. Upper airway response in workers exposed to fuel oil ash: nasal lavage analysis. *Occup Environ Med* 1995; **52**: 353–8.
20. Ellegard E, Hellgren M, Toren K, et al. The incidence of pregnancy rhinitis. *Gynecol Obstet Invest* 2000; **49**: 98–101.
21. Settipane GA, Klein DE. Non allergic rhinitis: demography of eosinophils in nasal smear, blood total eosinophil counts and IgE levels. *N Engl Reg Allergy Proc* 1985; **6**: 363–6.
22. Hamano N, Terada N, Maesako K, et al. Expression of histamine receptors in nasal epithelial cells and endothelial cells: the effects of sex hormones. *Int Arch Allergy Immunol* 1998; **115**: 220–7.
23. Hamano N, Terada N, Maesako K, et al. Effect of sex hormones on eosinophilic inflammation in nasal mucosa. *Allergy Asthma Proc* 1998; **19**: 263–9.
24. Moneret-Vautrin DA, Hsieh H, Wayoff M, et al. Nonallergic rhinitis with eosinophilia syndrome a precursor of the triad: nasal polyposis, intrinsic asthma, and intolerance to aspirin. *Ann Allergy* 1990; **64**: 513–18.
25. Leone C, Teodoro C, Pelucchi A, et al. Bronchial responsiveness and airway inflammation in patients with nonallergic rhinitis with eosinophilia syndrome. *J Allergy Clin Immunol* 1997; **100**: 775–80.
26. Devalia JL, Rusznak C, Wang J, et al. Air pollutants and respiratory hypersensitivity. *Toxicol Lett* 1996; **86**: 169–76.
27. Shah A, Sircar M. Postcoital asthma and rhinitis. *Chest* 1991; **100**: 1039–41.
28. Lieberman P. Treatment update: nonallergic rhinitis. *Allergy Asthma Proc* 2001; **22**: 199–202.
29. Banov CH, Lieberman P. Efficacy of azelastine nasal spray in the treatment of vasomotor (perennial nonallergic) rhinitis. *Ann Allergy Asthma Immunol* 2001; **86**: 28–35.
30. Lacroix JS, Buvelot JM, Polla BS, Lundberg JM. Improvement of symptoms of nonallergic chronic rhinitis by local treatment with capsaicin. *Clin Exp Allergy* 1991; **21**: 595–600.
31. Tan G, Ma Y, Li H, et al. Long-term results of bilateral endoscopic vidian neurectomy in the management of moderate to severe persistent allergic rhinitis. *Arch Otolaryngol Head Neck Surg* 2012; **138**: 492–7.
32. Ma Y, Tan G, Zhao Z, et al. Therapeutic effectiveness of endoscopic vidian neurectomy for the treatment of vasomotor rhinitis. *Acta Otolaryngol* 2014; **134**: 260–7.
33. Jang TY, Kim YH, Shin SH. Long-term effectiveness and safety of endoscopic vidian neurectomy for the treatment of intractable rhinitis. *Clin Exp Otorhinolaryngol* 2010; **3**: 212–6.
34. Gevorgyan A, Segboer C, Gorissen R, et al. Capsaicin for non-allergic rhinitis. *Cochrane Database Syst Rev Library* 2015; **14**:
35. Van Rijswijk JB, Boeke EL, Keizer JM, et al. Intranasal Capsaicin reduces nasal hyperreactivity in idiopathic rhinitis: a double-blind randomised application regimen study. *Allergy* 2003; **58**: 754–1.
36. Özcan C, Vayisoglu Y, Doğu O, Görür K. The effect of intranasal injection of botulinum toxin A on the symptoms of vasomotor rhinitis. *Am J Otolaryngol* 2006; **27**(5): 314–18.
37. Sapci T, Yazici S, Evcimik MF, et al. Investigation of the effects of intranasal botulinum toxin type A and ipratropium bromide nasal spray on nasal hypersecretion in idiopathic rhinitis without eosinophilia. *Rhinology* 2008; **46**(1): 45–51.
38. Rohrbach S, Junghans K, Köhler S, Laskawi R. Minimally invasive application of botulinum toxin A in patients with idiopathic rhinitis. *Head Face Med* 2009; **5**(1): 18.

CHAPTER 93

OCCUPATIONAL RHINITIS

Hesham Saleh

Introduction	1017
Risk factors	1018
Pathogenesis	1018
High risk occupations	1018
Effects of air pollution	1021
Sick building syndrome	1021
Diagnosis	1021
Management	1022
References	1023

SEARCH STRATEGY

Data in this chapter may be updated by a Medline search and an Embase search using the key words: rhinitis, occupational rhinitis, rhinitis and occupation, air pollutants and occupational, occupational disease, occupational accident, occupational allergy, occupational exposure, occupational hazard, occupational health, occupational medicine, occupational safety, work environment, industrial medicine, industry, industry and industrial phenomena, work and disability.

INTRODUCTION

Occupational rhinitis (OR) is an inflammatory disease of the nose, which is characterized by intermittent or persistent symptoms (i.e. nasal congestion, sneezing, rhinorrhoea, itching), and/or variable nasal airflow limitation and/or hypersecretion arising out of causes and conditions attributable to a particular work environment and not to stimuli encountered outside the workplace.[1] Symptoms usually manifest in weekdays and abate during weekends and holidays. When exposure has been prolonged the condition may become irreversible and symptoms persist.[2,3] OR frequently coexists with asthma and conjunctivitis, and it has been documented that occupational rhinitis precedes the development of occupational asthma especially when high molecular weight compounds (HMW) are involved (see below).[1,3,4] Occupational rhinitis is commoner than occupational asthma and most reports show that it tends to occur two to four times more frequently.[1,3,5]

The prevalence of occupational rhinitis is unknown. Studies have dealt primarily with occupational asthma with less work on rhinitis. It has been estimated that 2–5% of all patients with asthma in the United States have work-induced asthma.[1] It is possible that the incidence of occupational rhinitis is underestimated due to failure to diagnose and because, unlike asthma, it is not a life-threatening condition. Workers may be reluctant to report symptoms for this reason as well as for fear of job loss, loss of seniority, or fear of repercussions from co-workers.[1] A variety of cross-sectional studies of populations from diverse occupations exist but, because of the different methodologies used, interpretation of data is difficult. Furthermore, data from epidemiological studies are lacking. Information from the Finnish Institute of Health showed that 20% of all cases of rhinitis were occupational in origin.[7] The same study also showed that the number of cases more than doubled between 1987 and 1991. Another study, utilizing the Finnish Register, showed that the incidence of occupational rhinitis is higher in men than women (60% and 40% respectively). Also a gender difference exists for the age at which occupational rhinitis develops. Men have the highest incidence at the age range of 25–29 years, after which the incidence gradually declines. In women, the incidence of occupational rhinitis gradually increases and peaks between 40 and 44 years of age.[4] It has been suggested that this difference is related to the fact that men and women are engaged in different jobs and hence exposed to different kinds of causative agents.[8]

More than 200 chemicals and organic dusts have been implicated as a cause of occupational rhinitis and asthma.[1] The pathological effects of these are either due to an allergic reaction or irritation of the nasal mucosa. Well-documented causative agents include laboratory animals such as rats, mice and guinea pigs, grains (bakers), storage mite (agricultural workers), wood dust, particularly hard wood such as western red cedar (furniture manufacturers), guar gum (workers in the food processing and carpet industry), *Bacillus subtilis* enzymes (detergent manufacturing workers), persulphate salts (hairdressers), latex and chemicals such as acid anhydrides, isocyanates, platinum salts, glues and solvents.[1, 3, 6] Symptoms may develop after a latency period of 2 months to 18 years in the case of allergic occupational rhinitis.[1, 6] This observation does not apply to irritant occupational rhinitis which can develop on immediate exposure.

RISK FACTORS

Risk factors for developing occupational rhinitis include exposure (intensity and duration), atopy and smoking.[6] Most reports on exposure have focused on intensity, and associations have been confirmed in laboratory animal workers, wool textile mill workers and bakery workers amongst others.[3] Duration of exposure has seldom been studied. Other studies have shown an association between atopy and specific sensitization to high molecular weight agents in grain elevators, fish and seafood workers, bakers, workers exposed to latex, coffee and others. Although smoking is known to induce the release of inflammatory mediators and to cause mucosal changes, its impact on occupational rhinitis is yet to be shown. The current evidence on this matter is still inconclusive as some studies show higher risk of occupational rhinitis in smokers and some do not.[3, 6, 9]

PATHOGENESIS

The nose is the first portal of entry to the respiratory tract and is exposed to a constant stream of air. Materials that accompany the air stream tend to impact on the mucus surface as a function of their aerodynamic equivalent diameter (AED).[10] Approximately 80% of those that have an AED of more than 9 μm, 50% of those with 2–9 μm AED and 40% of material with less than 2 μm stick to the nasal wall. Highly soluble materials such as ammonia, sulphur dioxide, and formaldehyde also deposit in the upper airway. Smaller particles and less water-soluble gases generally pass to the lower airways.[8] According to the nature of the offending agent, occupational rhinitis may be allergic or irritant.

Allergic occupational rhinitis

Allergic occupational particles may trigger an IgE-mediated (Type 1) immune response. A late-phase response may also develop 4–6 hours after the initial reaction.[8] The causative agents are classified into high molecular weight compounds (HMWC), such as animal and vegetable proteins, and low molecular weight compounds (LMWC), such as isocyanates and anhydrides. IgE dependant mechanisms, that can be assessed through skin prick test and specific IgE levels have been demonstrated with most high molecular weight compounds (HMWC).[3, 8] Low molecular weight compounds (LMWC) can also produce specific IgE antibodies by acting as a hapten to form hapten-protein conjugate. However, an IgE-mediated mechanism has been elicited only rarely with LMWC. **Table 93.1** shows a number of HMWC and **Table 93.2** shows LMWC implicated in allergic occupational rhinitis with the related occupations.[1, 3, 6]

Irritant occupational rhinitis

Non-allergic, irritant chemicals may trigger the release of substance P and other inflammatory mediators from sensory C-fibres after binding to chemoreceptors on their surface.[11, 12] This sequence, known as neurogenic inflammation, leads to vasodilatation, oedema, and other manifestations of inflammation. The patients complain of burning, stinging or painful sensation in the nasal passages in addition to nasal congestion and rhinorrhoea.[1] Delayed response does not occur in cases of irritant rhinitis.[8] Existing evidence shows the release of substance P in the nose with exposures to nicotine, capsaicin, ether, and formaldehyde. Chronic irritant rhinitis requires protracted exposure to one or more irritating chemicals. However, in reactive upper airways dysfunction syndrome (RUDS) rhinitis results from an acute exposure to high concentrations of a respiratory irritant, and persists after the exposure.[12] Table 93.3 shows a number of agents implicated in irritant occupational rhinitis with the related occupations.[1, 6]

Corrosive reactions may also occur due to excessive concentrations of irritating and soluble chemical gases. Substances implicated in causing corrosion are ammonia, hypochloric acid, vinyl chloride, organic sulphur containing compounds, acrylamide, cyanide, nitriles and organophosphoside compounds.[1] Disorders of olfaction may occur a result of rhinitis or as a direct effect of irritants on the olfactory receptors and their central connections.[13] Anosmia and hyposmia have been reported after single high-dose exposure to sulphuric acid, hydrogen selenide, phosphorus oxychloride and a mixture of pepper and cresol.[8] Other case reports of olfactory disorders present workers chronically exposed to low levels of chemicals such as benzene, benzol, cadmium, carbon disulphide, ethyl acetate, formaldehyde, hydrazine, menthol, solvents, and oil of peppermint.[8, 14] However, olfactory disorders in occupational rhinitis are otherwise under-investigated.

Similar to other patients with allergic and non-allergic rhinitis, patients with occupational rhinitis may manifest nasal hyperreactivity to non-specific environmental agents such as changes in temperature and humidity, exposure to tobacco smoke and strong odours.[1] The prevalence of this entity is, however, unknown.

HIGH RISK OCCUPATIONS

Data from the Finnish Register of Occupational Diseases identified furriers, who are exposed to different kinds of animal epithelium, as the highest risk group for developing occupational rhinitis. Livestock breeders and bakers were the occupations following in rank.[4] Other commonly

TABLE 93.1 High molecular weight compounds (HMWC) causing allergic occupational rhinitis

High molecular weight compounds	Occupation
Animal proteins (rats, mice, guinea pigs, rabbits, hamsters)	Laboratory animal workers, pet shop owners, veterinarians, farmers
Other animal derived allergens (pig)	Swine confinement workers
Grain dust	Grain elevators
Flour, alpha amylase	Bakery workers
Bacillus subtilis	Detergent workers
Enzymes (papain, trypsin, pancreatic extracts, lactase)	Pharmaceuticals
Wool	Wool textile workers
Insects (locust, fruit fly)	Laboratory workers
Arthropods	Laboratory workers
Mites (storage, red spider)	Bakers, farmers, grain elevators, food processors
Mould spores	Librarians
Latex	Healthcare workers
Guar gum/vegetable gum	Food processors, carpet workers, printing
Green coffee bean	Coffee production
Tea	Tea workers
Dried fruits	Dried fruit workers
Tobacco leaf	Tobacco workers
Cayenne peppers	Hot pepper workers
Pollens	Gardeners, greenhouse workers
Sunflower pollen	Bakers, agricultural workers
Soybean dust	Farmers, food processors
Saffron flower	Saffron workers
Cocoa	Packers
Garlic	Food workers
Milk proteins (alpha Lactalbumin, casein)	Chocolate manufacturing, tannery
Fish, prawn, crab	Food processors
Bird proteins	Poultry breeders, farmers
Raw poultry	Food processors
Cow dander	Dairy farms

TABLE 93.2 Low molecular weight compounds (LMWC) causing allergic occupational rhinitis

Low molecular weight compounds	Occupation
Diisocyanates (toluene diisocyanates, diphenyl-methan diisocyanates)	Painters, urethane mould workers
Anhydrides (trimellitic anhydride, methyl tetrahydrophtalic anhydride, pyrotomellitic anhydride)	Epoxy resin production, plastics, electric condenser workers, chemical workers
Wood dust (western red cedar, several other woods)	Furniture making, carpentry
Colophony	Electronics, welders
Metals (platinum, nickel, chromium)	Platinum refinery, metal processing or plating
Drugs (psyllium, senna, spiramycin)	Healthcare workers, bulk laxatives factory workers, pharmaceuticals
Chemicals (reactive dyes, carmine, polyamide, polyester, para-amide)	Reactive dye product producers, synthetic fibre workers
Cotton	Farmers, cotton mill workers
Persulphates	Persulphage product manufacturers, hairdressers
Solvents and organic dust	Shoe manufacturing
Azo dyes	Textile dying
Chlorine	Pulp and paper production

TABLE 93.3 Causative agents of irritant occupational rhinitis

Irritant substance	Occupation
Ammonia, nitrogen dioxide, hydrogen sulphide	Agricultural workers
Smoke	Firefighters
Cooking vapour	Food service workers
Glutaraldehyde, formaldehyde	Healthcare workers
Inorganic acid vapours	Laboratory workers
Sulphur dioxide	Power plant, oil refinery workers
Solvent vapours	Printers, painters
Zinc chloride smoke	Military personnel
Chloride, chlorine dioxide, hydrogen sulphide	Pulp mill workers
Oxides of nitrogen, ozone, diesel exhaust	Traffic wardens, lorry drivers, railroad workers
Asphalt vapours, polycyclic aromatic hydrocarbons	Roofers, pavers
Metallic oxide fumes	Welders
Talc	Pharmaceutical workers, cosmetic manufacturers

reported occupations include farmers, food-processing workers, wood workers, detergents manufacturers, animal laboratory workers, hairdressers and healthcare workers.

Bakers

A large number of cross-sectional studies show that work-related symptoms of rhinitis and sensitization are common among bakery workers. Work-related rhinitis has been shown in 18% to 29% of workers and specific sensitization in 10% to 38%.[3] The offending agents are wheat and cereal flours, cereal amylases, fungal amylases, storage mites contaminating wheat flour and others such as baking additives.

Farmers

The prevalence of occupational rhinitis in farmers is unknown. However, a variety of agricultural exposures have been associated with rhinitis. These include grain farming and handling, livestock breeding, feed manufacture and handling, dairy farming, tea farming, cotton, flax, and hemp processing and organophosphorous pesticides.[15] Storage mites, present in storage hay have been described as a cause of barn allergy. A number of reports on grain elevator workers showed prevalence of sensitization in 9% to 28%.[3]

Food processing workers

It has been suggested that the food industry accounts for the largest number of cases of occupational rhinitis.[3] Cases of occupational rhinitis due to guar gum are well documented. It is obtained from the seeds of the tree *Cyamopsis tetragonoloba*, and used as a food additive as well as a laxative and a colour fixing agent in the carpet industry. The prevalence of symptoms in workers is, however, less well documented. Symptoms related to other plant-related allergens such as soybean, coffee bean, garlic, cinnamon and hot peppers have also been reported.[1] Occupational rhinitis has also been correlated to fish and seafood proteins. Prevalence of symptoms of 5% to 25% in fish factory workers has been reported.[3]

Wood manufacturers

Hard woods, often of tropical origin, are well-known factors in causing work-related symptoms. Plicatic acid, found in western red cedar, has been suggested as the causative agent of rhinitis in carpenters and furniture manufacturing workers.[3, 16] Symptom prevalence figures are less well documented. Oak, beech and pine have also been implicated.[16] Soft woods, used in joiner shops, have been less reported than hard woods in relation to rhinitis.[16]

Detergent manufacturers

Biological enzymes are used extensively in the detergent industry as well as pharmaceutical and food industries. *Bacillus subtilis* enzymes and lactase have been commonly implicated in occupational rhinitis.[1, 3, 6] Prevalence rates of occupational rhinitis from 7% to 16% have been reported in workers. Specific sensitization ranged from 22% to 52%.[3]

Animal laboratory workers

Laboratory workers are one of the groups most commonly affected with occupational rhinitis.[1] It has been suggested that proteins from virtually any mammalian species may induce an allergic response in human beings.[1] Rats are the most commonly implicated but mice, guinea pigs, rabbits and hamsters are also known to cause occupational rhinitis.[1, 3] Immunological substances implicated include saliva, urine, dander and serum. Previous reports demonstrate symptom prevalence of 10% to 33% and specific

IgE antibodies to animal protein in 6% to 46% of workers. Recent evidence suggests a trend towards a progressive decline in the prevalence, which may be due to the reduction of exposure since the early 1980s.[3, 17]

Healthcare workers

Concern has been raised about latex allergy in healthcare workers and patients due to the extensive use of latex gloves. Rubber latex is a naturally occurring cytoplasmic exudate obtained from the tree *Hevea brasiliensis*.[18] It is used extensively in the manufacture of surgical gloves and other medical devices (drains, bag and valve masks, mouth gags and bandages are some examples).[19] Aerosolized particles of latex proteins are carried in the cornstarch used to powder the gloves and may remain airborne for hours.[19, 20] Significant quantities of airborne latex have been measured in areas using powdered latex gloves.[20] These proteins have been implicated in causing rhinitis, asthma and anaphylaxis.[18–20] Exposed personnel may also develop contact dermatitis as a reaction to the chemical accelerators and preservatives that are added to latex to improve its physical property.[19] Anaphylaxis most often affects patients during open surgery due to mucosal absorption, and has been reported in those who have had multiple surgical procedures and in patients with spina bifida.[18] However, anaphylactic reactions were also reported during gloving and inhaling latex in the workplace.[18] Healthcare workers with regular latex exposure have been reported to have symptom prevalence rates of 3% to 17%.[21] Specific skin tests have been shown to be positive in 5% to 20% in contrast to prevalence in the general population of less than 1%.[18]

Other substances that may cause occupational rhinitis in healthcare workers include formaldehyde and drugs such as psyllium, senna and spiramycin.[3] Formaldehyde is also used widely in industry in addition to its use as a sterilizing agent in medicine. It is toxic at high doses and can induce irritant reaction. It is also been suggested that it can act as a hapten and cause an IgE mediated reaction.[22]

Other occupations

Workers reported to have occupational rhinitis in other occupations have been referred to in **Tables 93.1–93.3**.

EFFECTS OF AIR POLLUTION

In the first half of the 20th century dramatic episodes of severe pollution, caused by sulphur dioxide (SO_2) derived from coal combustion, occurred in the Western world. Regulations to decrease the use of coal in homes and industry were set and other fuels like petrol and gas substituted coal. The by-products of petrol consumption in transport and industry, however, have replaced the decline of coal-associated pollution. Exhaust fumes consist of oxides of nitrogen, namely nitric oxide (NO) and nitric dioxide (NO_2), ozone (O_3), particulate matter (PM) and volatile organic compounds (VOCs).[23] Much of the research done on pollution has been on its effects on the lower airway. However, epidemiological studies suggest an association between pollution and rhinitis.[9] Laboratory studies have shown that exposures to NOx, O_3 and diesel exhaust particles result in the release of inflammatory mediators in the nasal mucosa.[24] A link between high levels of environmental pollutants and increased prevalence of allergy has also been suggested.[9] Whether this would have an impact on allergic occupational rhinitis remains to be examined.

Certain occupations such as traffic wardens, railroad workers and lorry drivers may be exposed to high levels of pollution that result in high prevalence of symptoms of rhinitis.[25]

SICK BUILDING SYNDROME

Sick building syndrome (SBS) is described as the high prevalence of eye, nose and throat irritation, fatigue and headache among office workers temporally associated with time at work and characterized by an absence of abnormal physical findings and laboratory results.[8] It is a diagnosis of exclusion as multiple causative agents have been implicated. More than 300 volatile organic compounds (VOCs) were identified as indoor pollutants causing SBS. They originate from building materials, combustion fumes, cleaning compounds, paints and stains in addition to tobacco smoke. It has been suggested that workers in buildings with mechanical ventilation and air conditioning have a higher risk of SBS symptoms than workers in naturally ventilated buildings.[26, 27]

DIAGNOSIS

Diagnosing occupational rhinitis can be difficult. A combination of history, examination and investigation will aid the diagnosis. Nasal provocation test (NPT) with the suspected agent is particularly central to secure the diagnosis.

History

The patients present with a variable number of symptoms including nasal obstruction, anterior rhinorrhoea, postnasal discharge, crusting, disturbed sense of smell and taste and epistaxis.[2] A detailed history of the patient's complaint in addition to occupational history is essential to aid the diagnosis. Development of symptoms during the working week with improvement at weekends and holidays provide the clue for diagnosis. However, history in itself is not sufficient for diagnosis and could be feigned by workers claiming compensation. The history can be further compounded by the presence of symptoms of rhinitis due to atopy in allergic patients. In patients with protracted exposure, the symptoms may continue during absence from work further complicating matters.[1] The difference in presentation between allergic and irritant occupational rhinitis should be also borne in mind. In allergic patients, rhinitis may take longer to develop and may be manifested by a delayed response a few hours after exposure. On the other hand, patients with irritant rhinitis may develop the symptoms instantly on exposure and do not have a delayed response.[1] A history of eye, throat, skin and chest symptoms should be elicited. It is important to enquire about smoking and drug history including over-the-counter decongestants, substance abuse and other drugs known to cause nasal symptoms such as aspirin, alpha-blockers, beta-blockers, antidepressants and ACE inhibitors. Enquiries should be made on history of atopy in the patient and first-degree relatives.[1,2] An enquiry about problems of the sense of smell and taste should also be made.

A detailed occupational history includes the patient's account of a typical working day, the nature of chemicals, duration and intensity of daily exposure and use of protective masks.[8] A substance information sheet or an engineer's report may also be required particularly in medico-legal cases. Other work factors such as type and efficiency of ventilation, history of accidents and spills, and effects on co-workers should also be considered.[2,6] A site visit has been recommended if the history of work conditions is unhelpful.[1]

Examination

The physical findings in occupational rhinitis are non-specific. Nasal examination should include description of mucosal changes, nature of secretions, crusting, epistaxis, ulceration and perforation. These are particularly important in medico-legal cases.[1] Crusting and epistaxis are commoner in irritant rhinitis. Eye inspection for conjunctivitis and oral cavity/oropharynx examination for ulceration should also be done. Chest examination for signs of asthma is important as well as inspection for dermatitis, which occurs in latex allergy.

Investigations

The skin prick test is useful in allergic occupational rhinitis for most HMW and some LMW agents. It is also be helpful in diagnosing suspected atopy. However, sensitization to an occupational agent is not sufficient to diagnose occupational rhinitis, because it only indicates an immunological response and not necessarily a clinical syndrome.[3] Skin prick tests have been used extensively in cross-sectional studies to assess sensitization to a specific agent. Sensitivity and specificity have been evaluated with differing results.[3] Measuring serum specific IgE has also been used in a number of studies. The sensitivity and specificity is probably less than that of the skin prick test but a combination of both tests may enhance sensitivity and specificity.[1]

A secure diagnosis cannot be made without a nasal provocation test (NPT).[1,6] This is more conclusive when performed in controlled conditions in the laboratory with known agents. Carefully graded exposure to increasing doses of the suspected agent in specialized ventilated environmental chambers is the best method. Difficulties arise when dealing with unknown or multiple agents.[3] On these occasions a workplace provocation test may be an option.[1,3] Unfortunately, no standardized method for nasal provocation is yet recommended and the test is time consuming. The test must be accompanied by an objective measure of the nasal response such as acoustic rhinometry or rhinomanometry.[4,28] Nasal inspiratory flow rate measurement (NIPF) is also useful with nasal provocation. It can be also be used by the patient to measure fluctuations of the nasal airway during the working week.[3] Other measures such as collecting nasal lavage for analysis of cells and inflammatory markers and brush biopsies have been used with nasal provocation. They are generally more suitable for research situations and have been used extensively in various trials.[3] Exhaled nitric oxide measurement has also been used in clinical trials but not in routine clinical practice.[29]

When an olfactory disorder is suspected and in medico-legal cases, olfaction should be tested using one of the commercially available tests such the University of Pennsylvania Smell Identification Test (UPSIT).[2]

MANAGEMENT

The best management approach for occupational rhinitis is prevention. In established cases avoidance methods should be instituted and medical therapy may be tried. Immunotherapy may have a part to play in treating severe cases of allergic occupational rhinitis.

Prevention

Primary prevention in the workplace may be effective and should always be considered.[1] Environmental control measures are undertaken by recognizing potentially sensitizing allergens and controlling the point source of any mucosal irritant. Enclosing previously open operations and automating hand operations should be considered. Masks, gloves and protective clothing should be used and ventilation improved.[1,6] It has been suggested that applicants for high-risk jobs should be screened for atopy by history taking and skin prick test. However, this has not been shown to be efficient, particularly when the marker of susceptibility (e.g. atopy) is prevalent in the general population.[1]

In workers with established diagnosis certain avoidance measures may be effective. For example, laboratory workers who become sensitive to rats generally react to rat urinary protein rather than epithelium. It has been suggested that it may be possible for them to perform surgery on rats, if the cage containing the rats – which is soaked with urine – is kept out of the laboratory. In healthcare workers sensitive to latex the use of powder-free gloves by all co-workers has been shown to reduce symptoms and allow allergic patients to continue their work.[18] Non-latex gloves are available and may be used as an alternative for sensitive individuals. In some occupations where preventive measures are ineffective, relocation of the worker or even changing jobs may be recommended.

Medical therapy

Medical therapy of occupational rhinitis is similar to that of non-occupational allergic rhinitis and should be instituted according to evidence-based guidelines.[30] Antihistamines, sodium cromoglycate, topical corticosteroids, anticholinergic spray and saline douches have all been used.[1, 6] Systemic steroids have also been suggested in severe cases. Treatment may be most effective in allergic occupational rhinitis.[1] However, no studies on the efficacy of these medications in occupational rhinitis are available at present. The choice of agent is often based on trial and error according to efficacy and frequency of side effects. Sedating antihistamines affect work productivity adversely and second-generation antihistamines are preferred. Patients may use them regularly when they have chronic symptoms or periodically before an expected exposure to an allergen.[1]

Immunotherapy

Studies have reported some improvement in symptoms during immunotherapy with purified rodent proteins, wheat flour extracts, and natural rubber latex.[31] Fear of severe reactions with continued exposure to the offending antigen at the same time of the administration of immunotherapy have precluded its use.[1] Furthermore, many of the offending antigens are not available for treatment. However, where alternative jobs are not a consideration, the risks of treatment should be balanced against the benefits.[1]

FUTURE RESEARCH

- Epidemiological studies are required to detect incidence and prevalence in various populations.
- Longitudinal studies should be conducted to document the natural history of the condition.
- The impact of occupational rhinitis on the quality of life of affected workers needs to be studied.
- Characterization of the clinical features and pathophysiology of non-allergic occupational rhinitis.
- More studies of the role of atopy and smoking in the development of occupational rhinitis are needed.
- The agreed diagnostic test, nasal provocation, should be standardized and other tests such as exhaled nitric oxide measurements should be further investigated.
- Randomized controlled trials should be designed to identify the best possible therapy.

KEY POINTS

- The prevalence of occupational rhinitis in the general population is still unknown.
- Occupational rhinitis is either allergic or irritant.
- Occupational rhinitis frequently coexists with asthma and conjunctivitis.
- Exposure, atopy and smoking are risk factors.
- History of work-related symptoms with improvement in weekends and holidays is typical.
- Nasal provocation is the main diagnostic test.
- Prevention is the best approach.
- Medical therapy is similar to that for other types of rhinitis.

REFERENCES

1. EAACI Task Force on Occupational Rhinitis, Moscato G, Vandenplas O, Gerth Van Wijk R. et al. Occupational rhinitis. *Allergy* 2008; **63**(8): 969–80.
2. Drake-Lee A, Ruckley R, Parker A. Occupational rhinitis: a poorly diagnosed condition. *J Laryngol Otol* 2002; **116**: 580–5.
3. Siracusa A, Desrosiers M, Marabini A. Epidemiology of occupational rhinitis: prevalence, aetiology and determinants. *Clin Exp Allergy* 2000; **30**: 1519–34.
4. Hytonen M, Kanerva L, Malmberg H, et al. The risk of occupational rhinitis. *Int Arch Occup Environ Health* 1997; **69**(6): 487–90.
5. Ameille J, Hamelin K, Andujar P, et al. Occupational asthma and occupational rhinitis: the united airways disease model revisited. *Occup Environ Med* 2013; **70**(7): 471–5.
6. Sublett JW, Bernstein DI. Occupational rhinitis. *Immunol Allergy Clin North Am* 2011; **31**(4): 787–96.
7. Kanerva L, Vaheri E. Occupational allergic rhinitis in Finland. *Int Arch Occup Environ Health* 1993; **64**: 565–8.
8. Epling CA. Upper respiratory problems. *Occup Environ Med* 2000; **27**(4): 997–1007.
9. Higgins TS, Reh DD. Environmental pollutants and allergic rhinitis. *Curr Opin Otolaryngol Head Neck Surg* 2012; **20**(3): 209–14.
10. Andersen I, Lundqvist GR, Proctor DF, et al. Human response to controlled levels of inert dust. *Am Rev Respir Dis* 1979; **119**: 619–27.
11. Keh SM, P Facer, K Simpson, et al. Increased nerve fiber expression of sensory sodium channels nav1.7, nav1.8, and nav1.9 in rhinitis. *Laryngoscope* 2008; **118**(4): 573–9.
12. Meggs WJ. RADS and RUDS – The toxin induction of asthma and rhinitis. *Clin Toxicol* 1994; **32**(5): 487–501.
13. Castano R, Trudeau C, Castellanos L, et al. Prospective outcome assessment of occupational rhinitis after removal from exposure. *J Occup Environ Med* 2013; **55**(5): 579–85.
14. Emmett EA. Parosmia and hyposmia induced by solvent exposure. *Brit J Int Med* 1976; **33**: 196–8.
15. Schenker MB, Christiani D, Cormier Y, et al. Respiratory health hazards in agriculture *Am J Resp Crit Care Med* 1998; **158**: S1–S76.
16. De Zotti R, Gubian F. Asthma and rhinitis in wooding workers. *Allergy Asthma Proc* 1996; **17**(4): 199–203.
17. Folletti I, Forcina A, Marabini A, et al. Have the prevalence and incidence of occupational asthma and rhinitis because of laboratory animals declined in the last 25 years? *Allergy* 2008; **63**(7): 834–41.
18. Sussman GL, Beezhold DH. Latex allergy: a clinical perspective. *J Long-Term Eff Med Implants* 1994; **4**(2&3): 95–101.

19. Deacock S. Latex allergy. *CPD Bull Immunol Allergy* 2001; **2**(1): 8–11.
20. Swanson MC, Buback ME, Hunt LW, et al. Quantification of occupational latex aeroallergens in a medical center. *J Allergy Clin Immunol* 1994; **94**: 445–51.
21. Charous B, Hamilton R, Yunginger J. Occupational latex exposure: characteristics of contact and systemic reactions in 47 workers. *J Allergy Clin Immunol* 1994; **94**: 12–18.
22. Bousquet J, Michel FB. Allergy to formaldehyde and ethylene oxide. *Clin Rev Allergy* 1991; **9**: 357–70.
23. Saleh HA, Lund VJ. The nose as a target of air pollution. *Eur Resp Mon* 2001; **18**(6): 143–52.
24. Bascom R, Naclerio RM, Fitzgerald TK, et al. Effect of ozone inhalation on the response to nasal challenge with antigen of allergic subjects. *Am Rev Resp Dis* 1990; **142**(3): 594–601.
25. Wnogsurakiat P, Maranetra KN, Nana A, et al. Respiratory symptoms and pulmonary function of traffic policemen in Thonburi. *J Med Assoc Thailand* 1999; **82**(5): 435–43.
26. Clerico DM. Sources and effects of indoor air pollution, including sick building syndrome. *Curr Opin Otolaryngol Head Neck Surg* 1996; **4**(1): 44–49.
27. Mendell MJ, Lei-Gomez Q, Mirer AG, et al. Risk factors in heating, ventilating, and air-conditioning systems for occupant symptoms in US office buildings: the US EPA BASE study. *Indoor Air* 2008; **18**(4): 301–16
28. Zerah-Lancer F, Pichon B, Pairon JC, et al. Usefulness of nasal provocation tests in occupational rhinitis. *Rhinology* 2009; **47**(4): 432–7.
29. Baatjies R, Jeebhay MF. Sensitisation to cereal flour allergens is a major determinant of elevated exhaled nitric oxide in bakers. *Occup Environ Med* 2013; **70**(5): 310–16.
30. Brozek JL, Bousquet J, Baena-Cagnani CE, et al. Allergic rhinitis and its impact on asthma (ARIA) guidelines: 2010 revision. *J Allergy Clin Immunol* 2010; **126**(3): 466–76.
31. Sastre J, Quirce S. Immunotherapy: an option in the management of occupational asthma? *Curr Opin Allergy Clin Immunol* 2006; **6**: 96–100.

CHAPTER 94

RHINOSINUSITIS: DEFINITIONS, CLASSIFICATION AND DIAGNOSIS

Carl Philpott

Rhinosinusitis and rhinitis definitions 1025	Chronic rhinosinusitis 1028
Epidemiology and socioeconomic impact 1026	Systemic conditions causing rhinosinusitis 1032
Diagnostic aids 1027	References 1034
Acute rhinosinusitis 1027	

SEARCH STRATEGY

Data in this chapter may be updated by a Medline search using the keywords: rhinosinusitis, rhinitis, sinusitis, classification and differential diagnosis and by reference to the European position paper on rhinosinusitis and nasal polyps.

RHINOSINUSITIS AND RHINITIS DEFINITIONS

The European position paper on rhinosinusitis and nasal polyps (EPOS) has now defined rhinosinusitis as a diagnosis made on clinical grounds based on the presence of characteristic symptoms, combined with objective evidence of mucosal inflammation (Table 94.1).[1]

This has been widely accepted internationally, although alternative classifications and guidelines have been produced, such as by the American Academy of Otorhinolaryngologists/Head & Neck Surgeons (AAOHNSF) Rhinosinusitis Task Force Committee.[2] The most recent international guidelines have supported the EPOS definition, confirming the need for objective evidence to confirm the symptom profile (ICORS).[3] The defining symptoms and signs listed in the EPOS 2012 document apply to both adults and children and can be further qualified in terms of severity by use of a visual analogue score for the question 'how troublesome are your symptoms of rhinosinusitis?' (Table 94.2). In practice, the severity is often defined by individual responses on Patient Reported Outcome Measures (PROMs) such as the SNOT-22 with recent consensus statements considering minimum scores for surgical candidates.[4]

Rhinosinusitis can then be further defined as acute or chronic based on duration of symptoms: acute being less than 12 weeks duration and chronic being greater.[1,5] Within acute rhinosinusitis (ARS), further distinctions can be made on a timeline basis such that a common cold

TABLE 94.1 Clinical definition of rhinosinusitis[1]

Diagnostic criteria for rhinosinusitis	Symptoms should be correlated by either endoscopic and/or radiological findings
Primary symptoms (requires at least one to be present, but if both present it is sufficient to make diagnosis on the basis of symptoms)	Nasal blockage/obstruction/congestion Nasal discharge (anterior/posterior)
Additional symptoms (may also be present and at least one is needed if only one of the primary symptoms is present)	Facial pain/pressure Olfactory dysfunction Hyposmia/anosmia
Duration	>10 days, <3 months = acute >3 months = chronic
Endoscopy (any of these)	Nasal polyps Mucopurulent discharge (middle meatus) Oedema/mucosal obstruction in middle meatus
CT scan findings (as well as or instead of endoscopic findings)	Mucosal changes within the ostiomeatal complex and/or sinuses

TABLE 92.2 Visual Analogue Scores (VAS) for rhinosinusitis symptoms[1]

Severity	VAS scale (10 cm line)
Mild	0il
Moderate	4od
Severe	8eve

1025

> **BOX 94.1 Additional symptoms or signs for acute bacterial rhinosinusitis[1]**
>
> **At least three of the following should be present:**
> - Discoloured discharge (unilateral predominance)
> - Severe local pain (unilateral predominance)
> - Fever (>38°C)
> - Elevated ESR/CRP
> - 'Double-sickening' – deterioration after initial milder phase of illness

(acute viral rhinosinusitis) will last for less than 10 days and acute post-viral rhinosinusitis will last between 100 days and 12 weeks in duration. ARS is considered to be bacterial (ABRS) if at least three of the symptoms in **Box 94.1** exist.[1]

For a diagnosis of recurrent acute rhinosinusitis, there must be symptom-free episodes between the clinical events. Chronic rhinosinusitis (CRS) is phenotypically divided into those cases with polyps (CRSwNPs) and those without (CRSsNPs) based on endoscopic findings. This division has also been broadly based up the pathophysiological themes within these two main subgroups which is discussed further below. Allergic fungal rhinosinusitis (AFRS)[6–8] is a smaller subgroup, believed to represent 10% of those with CRSwNPs, and is discussed in Chapter 96. A proportion of patients with CRSwNPs also fall into a unique subset, characterized by coexistent asthma and aspirin sensitivity known as Samter's triad or aspirin exacerbated respiratory disease (AERD).[8] AERD is believed to account for approximately 15% of CRSwNPs, classically manifest by severe nasal and/or respiratory symptoms following ingestion of salicylates, and there may be considerable overlap with AFRS-like cases.[9]

Finally, in all cases of CRS, some patients may experience acute exacerbations with worsening of symptoms for short periods, which may be triggered by viral URTIs.

Despite all the above definitions, there remain areas of uncertainty as not all patients adhere to the diagnostic symptoms and in primary care settings, diagnosis is often based on symptoms alone as the equipment to perform suitable nasal examinations is lacking. Rhinosinusitis should be distinguishable from rhinitis but inevitably there will be overlap. Rhinitis can broadly be categorized into allergic and non-allergic types, with the former now defined as persistent or intermittent according to the WHO committee Allergic Rhinitis In Asthma (ARIA) (**Figure 94.1**).[10, 11] Rhinitis is defined as the presence of at least two of the following: nasal blockage, rhinorrhoea (clear), sneezing or itching. Other varieties of rhinitis is discussed further in Chapters 91–93. Clinicians need to also be mindful that systemic diseases can manifest themselves in the nose, as is discussed further below.

EPIDEMIOLOGY AND SOCIOECONOMIC IMPACT

ARS is a very common condition and based on the current literature, prevalence rates vary from 6 to 15% with a prevalence of recurrent ARS estimated at 0.035%.[1] In a 3-year case-control study of the Dutch population, van Gageldonk-Lafeber estimated that annually, 900 000 individual patients consulted their primary care physician for acute respiratory tract infection.[12] This high volume of patients then receives a variable response from medical practitioners in terms of treatment.[13–15] Given that the proportion of bacterial causes amongst all ARS is believed to be as little as 0.5–2.0%,[16] this results in over-prescribing of antibiotics as found by a Danish study, where diagnostic certainty was found to be 70% based on symptoms and limited examination and where penicillin V was the preferred agent of choice.[17] German healthcare data over 1 year showed that 6.3 million separate diagnoses of ARS were made and in conjunction with this 8.5 million prescriptions were provided.[18]

CRS represents a significant disease burden worldwide, affecting at least 11% of the population[19] and consequently carrying with it a substantial economic burden to healthcare systems, to patients and to the economy from loss of productivity in the workplace.[18, 19] In fact 'sinusitis' was cited as one of the top ten most costly physical health conditions to American businesses in 1999,[20] as it has an increasing incidence in middle age with a significant socio-economic impact and impairment of quality of life.[21, 22] As a disease entity in the UK its prevalence is greater than ischaemic heart disease (3.7%), diabetes (4%), chronic obstructive pulmonary disease (1.5%), heart failure (<1%) and stroke (<1%) and equivalent to that of peripheral vascular disease, arthritis and back pain, several of which have been shown to have a lesser impact on patients' quality of life than CRS.[23] Patients with CRS also have a 5–17% prevalence of asthma as shown by a recent European study. This figure is higher in secondary care cohorts.[22, 25]

In the EPOS 2012 document stated: 'The overview of the currently available literature illustrates the paucity of accurate information on the epidemiology of CRSsNPs and CRSwNPs, especially in European countries, and highlights the need for large-scale epidemiologic research exploring their prevalence and incidence.'[1] A recent UK study has shown that CRS affects the social spectrum equally and that poor socioeconomic status does not

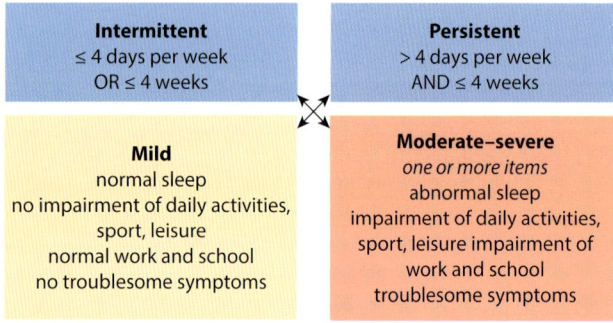

Figure 94.1 ARIA classification.[9]

appear to be a risk factor for CRS,[22] but there remains a need for larger scale studies that may also examine the natural history of the disease.

There are about 2.7 million outpatient consultations for ENT disorders per year in England and Wales and sinonasal disease is thought to account for at least 120,000 visits per year).[26] Failure of medical treatment usually leads to an operation being offered with over 40,000 nose and sinus operations performed per year in England and Wales;[26] based on current tariffs this is an estimated £30 million spent each year. Furthermore, in patients who undergo surgery, the UK Sinonasal audit revealed a surgical revision rate of up to 20% within 5 years[27] and also a ten to fifteen fold variation in surgical practice around the UK;[28] the cost of this revision surgery is estimated at £15 million per year.[25]

There are no published estimates of cost of healthcare and productivity losses for patients with CRS in the UK. Previoius findings from the USA estimate that patients with CRS spend more than $500 each year on healthcare and miss an average of 5.67 workdays per year versus 3.74 days per year for patients without CRS,[29] suggesting a significant disease burden on both the healthcare system and on individuals that is equal to or exceeds that for diseases that are thought to be more serious. An earlier study found that the overall yearly economic cost was $1500 per patient[30] and that estimated healthcare expenditures attributable to CRS and common comorbidities were close to $5.78 billion in 1996 excluding out-of-pocket expenditures or time off work for patients. Bringing this up to date, yearly estimated costs for CRS in the USA now exceed $60 billion.[31, 32] Another USA study concluded that the direct costs associated with CRS are higher than the background costs due to increased clinic visits and prescriptions, as well as significant productivity losses.[33] Surgical treatment for CRS certainly appears to influence drug costs,[34, 35] but this may depend on the level of intervention. There is also increasing evidence that earlier surgical intervention may reduce the prevalance of late onset asthma.[36]

DIAGNOSTIC AIDS

As stated above, EPOS 2012 has included the need for endoscopic or radiological findings to confirm the evidence from a patient's history and the flow diagrams within the EPOS document can be used to guide clinicians as to when to implement the latter. Thus rigid nasal endoscopy and CT scanning of the sinuses are at the present time the gold standard investigations for CRS. Endoscopy allows the clinician to assess the nose for the presence of polyps, mucopus discharge or middle meatal oedema. Furthermore the endoscope can be used to accurately sample any mucopus for microbiological analysis.[37] In cases of suspected allergic or eosinophilic fungal/mucinous rhinosinusitis, a fungal smear and culture should be requested, although diagnostic yield from such samples can be hugely variable depending on local laboratory resources and techniques.[33] CT scanning should be considered mandatory for all cases where surgical intervention is planned.[28]

There are a number of adjuncts beyond endoscopy, radiology and microbiology that may aid diagnosis or perhaps the differential diagnosis, although they may also give more specific information about the aetiology or presence of concurrent disease and predict response to treatment. These include:[38]

- Allergy testing – skin prick testing or RAST
- Nasal brushings for cytology
- Nasal biopsy for exclusion of neoplasia, to look for granulomas/vasculitides or to examine for evidence of eosinophilia and fungal hyphae
- Blood tests – full blood count (serum eosinophilia), ANCA (Wegener's granulomatosis), ACE (sarcoidosis)
- Olfactory testing:
  ○ Psychophysical (threshold (quantitative) and iscrimination/identification (qualitative))
  ○ Olfactory event-related potentials (OERPs) (objective)
- Physiological testing
  ○ Peak inspiratory nasal flow
  ○ Rhinomanometry
  ○ Acoustic rhinometry
  ○ Mucociliary clearance (saccharin test)
- Ciliary function testing
  ○ Ciliary beat frequency
  ○ Ciliary beat pattern analysis
  ○ Electron microscopy
- Patient reported outcome measures/symptom scores – these include the Sinonasal Outcome Text (SNOT),[39] Rhinosinusitis Outcome Measure (RSOM-31),[40] Chronic Sinusitis Survey (CSS),[41] and other validated questionnaires.

ACUTE RHINOSINUSITIS

ARS is a very common condition that is predominantly managed in primary care and hence rarely seen by hospital specialists unless complications occur. As stated above, the primary cause of ARS is viruses[34] and only 0.5–2.0% of patients are believed to develop ABRS. Current EPOS guidelines for primary care therefore suggest the use of symptomatic relief, nasal douching and decongestants with consideration given to the use of topical steroids depending on severity. Cases with the features listed in **Box 94.1** or where duration has been greater than 10 days are more likely to benefit from antibiotics. Predisposing factors to ARS include anatomical factors (e.g. Haller/infra-orbital ethmoid cells, conchae bullosa), allergy, smoking and poor mental health. Whilst there is evidence in some of these factors to support the contrary, both anatomical and allergy factors have a reasonable weight of evidence in the literature.[1]

The viruses most commonly implicated in ARS include rhinoviruses (50%), influenza and parainfluenza viruses, adenovirus, respiratory syncytial virus and enterovirus.[42] If bacteria do become implicated the organisms most commonly see are *S. pneumoniae* (27%), *H. influenzae* (44%), *M. catarrhalis* (14%) with other organisms sometimes seen including *S. pyogenes* and *S. aureus*. The proportion of these organisms has changed in recent years with vaccination schemes.[43] Pathophysiological mechanisms relating to viral agents include cell invasion of the respiratory epithelium leading to inflammatory changes including mechanical changes, epithelial damage and activation of humoral and cellular defences. In bacterial cases, this is largely a superinfection following an initial viral insult where epithelial disruption has already occurred and there has been an associated decrease in ciliated cells and increase in goblet cells which eventually cause sinus ostial obstruction. The accumulating mucus causes an initial increase in the intra-sinus pressure followed quickly by negative pressure due to the lack of ventilation. This then sets up a vicious cycle of further congestion, mucus retention, impaired gas exchange and pH balance and largely prevents clearance of inflammatory products and debris leading to an ideal medium for bacteria to flourish.

Most cases will be self-limiting with complications of ARS exceedingly rare; an estimated 2–4 cases per million of the population per year. This was perhaps thought to be due to the high rate of antibiotic use but there is evidence to suggest that in cases where complications have occurred, this has not been prevented by prior use of oral antibiotics.[44] Complications of ARS can be subdivided into orbital (60–75%), intra-cranial (15–20%) and osseous (5–10%) (Table 94.3). In orbital cellulitis, 90% are secondary to ABRS. A national survey in the UK found 78 cases of complications relating to ABRS over a 1-year period.[44] A review of the literature on complications shows that the mortality rate varies between 2 and 19%.

CHRONIC RHINOSINUSITIS

Please refer to Figure 94.2.

At the present time CRS is largely subcategorized into cases with polyps (CRSwNPs) and cases without polyps (CRSsNPs). The clinical definition has been outlined above but relates to a heterogeneous group of patients that fall loosely within one of these two subgroups.[1] The reason for this coarse subcategorization is the apparent themes within the pathophysiology of these two groups. CRSwNPs is characterized by an intense oedematous stroma in the sinonasal epithelium, with albumin deposition, pseudocyst formation and subepithelial/perivascular inflammatory cell infiltration. It appears to be associated with a typical T-helper 2 cell (TH$_2$) skewed eosinophilic inflammation, with high interleukin (IL-5) and eosinophil cationic protein (ECP) concentrations in the polyps. By comparison, CRSsNPs is characterized by fibrosis, basement membrane thickening, goblet cell hyperplasia, subepithelial oedema,

TABLE 94.3 Complications of ABRS

Orbital	Intra-cranial	Osseous
Pre-septal cellulitis	Subdural empyema	Pott's puffy tumour (subperiosteal abscess of frontal sinus)
Orbital cellulitis	Meningitis/encephalitis	Maxillary osteomyelitis (in infancy)
Subperiosteal abscess	Intra-cerebral abscess	
Orbital abscess	Epidural abscess	
	Superior sagittal sinus thrombosis	
Cavernous sinus thrombosis		

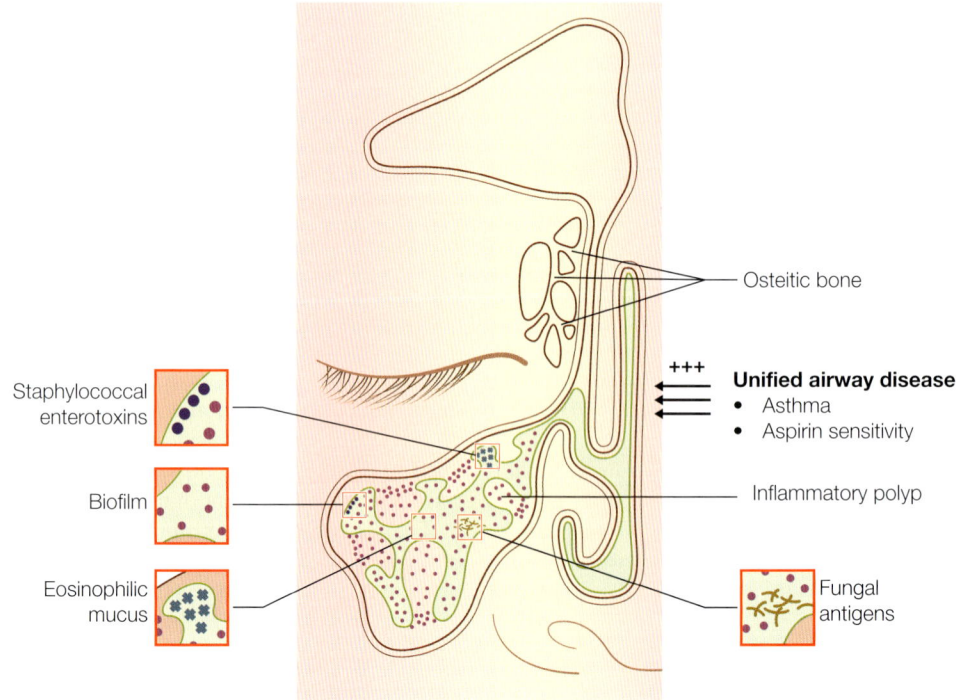

Figure 94.2 Aetiological mechanisms proposed for CRS.

and mononuclear cell infiltration. It exhibits a T-helper 1 cell (TH$_1$) milieu, with increased levels of interferon gamma (IFN-γ) in inflamed sinus mucosa and low ECP/myeloperoxidase ratios.[45] This basic division into the two subgroups does however represent a gross oversimplification of a heterogeneous disease. These categories can therefore be further divided as discussed below (**Tables 94.4** and **94.7**). The various aetiological mechanisms that have been proposed for CRS are summarized in **Figure 94.2**.

Polypoidal chronic rhinosinusitis

It is important that 'nasal polyposis' is not considered a diagnosis, merely a description of a pathological endpoint of sinonasal disease, hence why the term chronic rhinosinusitis with nasal polyposis is used to denote the most common manifestation of polyps; other examples of nasal polyps will include antrochoanal polyps and reactive polyps such as may be seen around other inflammatory focus such as a fungal ball or inverted papilloma. The clinician finding nasal polyps inside the nose should always ask why they have formed, although the answer may not always be readily apparent. The classifications below provide a useful framework around which to base the potential aetiology of nasal polyps.

LOCALIZED NASAL POLYPOSIS (CRSWNPS – LOCALIZED)

Please refer to **Figure 94.3**. A unilateral nasal polyp should always be viewed with suspicion, especially in older patients and in anyone exposed to wood dust. It may represent a benign entity such as an antro-choanal polyp or be part of a tumour such as an inverted papilloma or sinonasal malignancy. A unilateral polyp may occur as a result of a prior inflammatory event, predisposing to sinus ostia obstruction, hypoxia and subsequent bacterial infection. Microbiology sampling in clinic should be performed if appropriate but computed tomography and biopsy of the polyp are indicated in order to decide on the medical and surgical treatment strategy to pursue. Caution should be advised with performing a biopsy of any polyp that arises superiorly within the nose, or from the back of the nose in a juvenile male patient.

DIFFUSE NASAL POLYPOSIS (CRSwNP – DIFFUSE)

A number of recognized mechanisms appear to have a role in polyp formation, although this is by no means fully understood and there may well be crossover between them. These include bacterial (super-antigen response), fungal sensitization, and atopy. These may be associated with biofilm formation or frank eosinophilia, both exacerbating and propagating the inflammatory process. When severe bilateral nasal polyposis is present with aspirin sensitivity and asthma, the possibility of AERD and hence salicylate desensitization therapy should be considered. CT scanning will further elucidate a pansinus opacification typical of AFRS/AERD (**Figure 94.4**), (double density signs) or show less marked disease consistent with atopy and superantigen cases. In cases of suspected AFRS/AERD, thick granular

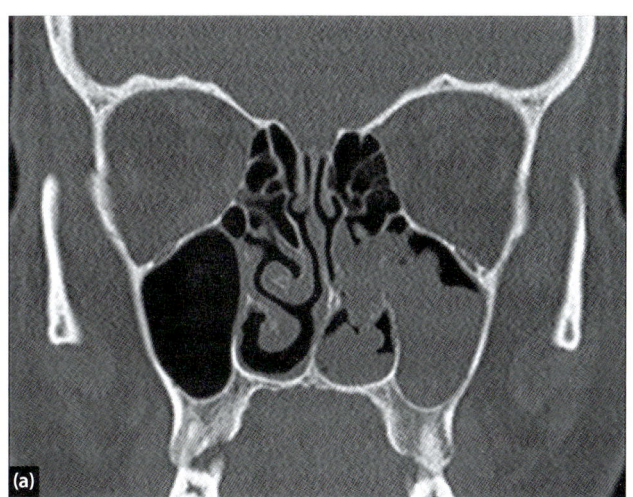

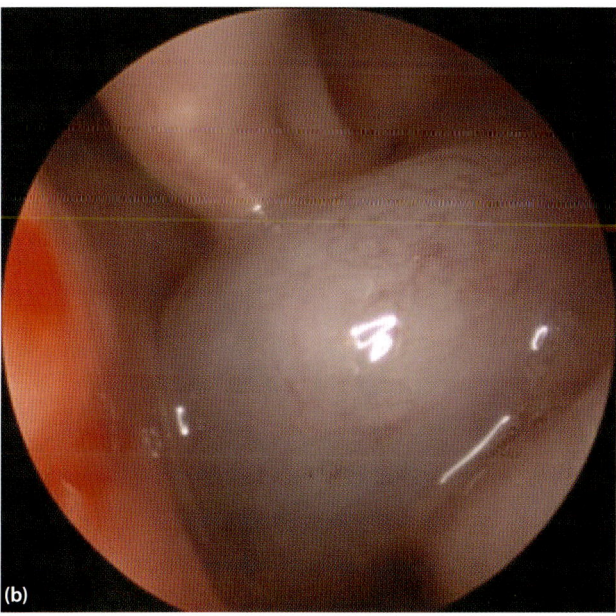

Figure 94.3 (a) Radiological and (b) endoscopic appearance of an antro-choanal polyp.

TABLE 94.4 Classification for the finding of nasal polyps

Polypoid CRS

Localized	Reactive polyp(s)	Inflammatory
		Neoplastic
Diffuse (CRSwNPs)	Host	Anatomical e.g. poor OMC function, aspirin sensitivity (AERD)
		Atopy
	External agent	Staphylococcus superantigen
	Combined host/external agent interaction	Allergic fungal rhinosinusitis and its related derivatives
Systemic	Cystic fibrosis, Churg/EMRSexternal	

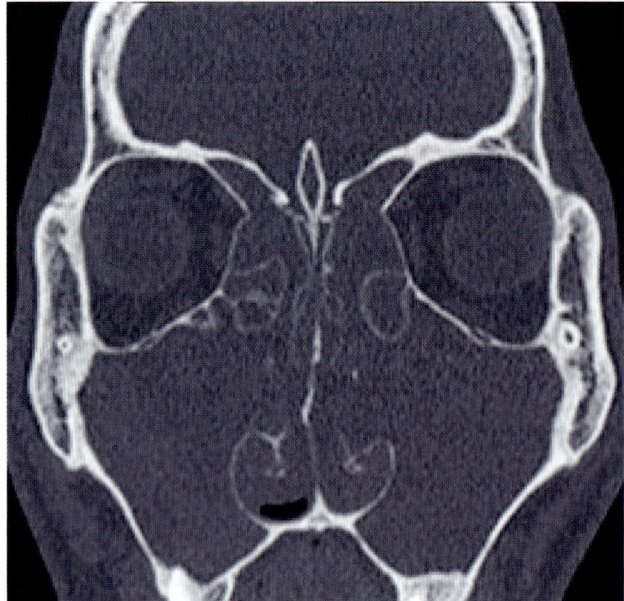

Figure 94.4 Pan-sinus opacification consistent with AFRS and AERD cases.

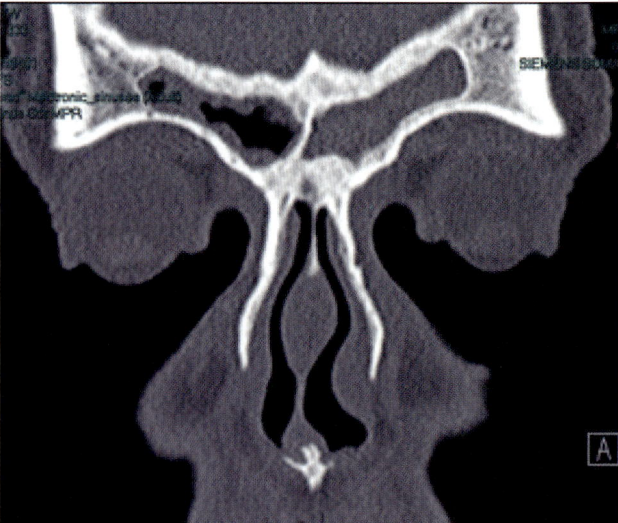

Figure 94.5 CRSwNPs with marked osteitis.

(eosinophilic) mucin will usually be found at initial presentation, during surgery or sometimes in the post-operative period. Less viscous mucus will perhaps suggest bacterial superantigen aetiology.

Bacterial superantigens, fungal antigens and allergic allergens have all been suggested as mechanisms driving T-cell activation, IgE and IL5 production resulting in subsequent tissue eosinophilia. Lack of consistency in studies suggests that each of these pathogens cannot be solely responsible, and the pathogenesis is likely to represent a multifactorial interaction. Also Asian studies have identified a predominantly TH_1 cell and TH_{17} pattern within polyp tissue[46] and in cystic fibrosis, patients exhibit a neutrophilia.[45] These observations highlight the apparently heterogenous nature of biochemical pathways that ultimately result in the clinical phenotype of CRSwNPs.

Furthermore some cases show polyps confined to the OMC on CT scanning indicating poor OMC function perhaps with narrowing features such as Haller cells. All cases should have appropriate mucus samples sent for routine and/or fungal cultures with fungal smears in the latter case. Both gram positive and negative bacteria have been cultured from the nasal cavity of CRSwNPs patients, the latter of which are rarely cultured from healthy subjects.[47-49] However, it is uncertain as to whether identification of a specific bacterium represents infection, or simply colonization. Data on biofilms in CRSwNPs is lacking but some recent evidence suggests up to 75% of cases may elicit biofilm;[50] clearly further evidence is needed to confirm this.

The super-antigen hypothesis proposes that non-invasive *S. aureus* in the nasal mucosa of CRS patients secretes exotoxins, which produce a localized eosinophilic inflammatory response as studies have shown exotoxin, specific super-antigen IgE, eosinophils and markers of eosinophilic inflammation are higher in cases of CRSwNPs compared to CRSsNPs.[51, 52] To counter this hypothesis is the evidence that there are differing levels of *S. aureus* (65%), superantigen-specific IgE (50%) and T-cell changes (33%)[53, 54] suggesting that the superantigens may have a role in some cases of CRSwNPs patients, but not all. Tissue eosinophilia can be a useful marker of severity and may help predict severity in these patients.[55]

Much of the evidence around fungal hypotheses is muddied by the difficulties in proving fungal organisms are present and with studies that do not carefully select cases more likely to represent fungal aetiology leading to the conclusion that fungi are mere bystanders and antifungals do not work.[56] Studies have demonstrated a high frequency of both fungi and eosinphilic mucin in CRS patients compared to control subjects suggesting a unique, T-cell driven hypersensitivity to fungi, independent of IgE mediated/atopic pathways.[57] This is supported with evidence that peripheral blood mononuclear cells and eosinophils of CRS patients react to Alternaria fungal extracts, in contrast to controls.[47] However a T-cell receptor mediated hypersensitivity response to fungal antigen has yet to be definitively elucidated and it is possible that a non-specific protease-based reaction to Alternaria is occurring.

The role and significance of osteitis in CRS is currently unclear, although may explain why some cases are resistant to standard oral treatment regimens. In CRSwNPs, osteitis may act as a marker of severity and has been shown to occur significantly more often in revision cases[58, 59] (Figure 94.5).

NASAL POLYPOSIS SECONDARY TO SYSTEMIC DISEASE

Two main systemic conditions should be considered in the presence of diffuse nasal polyposis: Churg-Strauss Syndrome (CSS) and cystic fibrosis (CF). Up to 76% of CSS cases demonstrate nasal polyps and ANCA positivity should alert the clinician to the underlying vasculitis characterized by necrotizing inflammation of the vessel wall, particularly of small arteries, arterioles, capillaries and venules.[60] Although newborn screening for CF will pick up most cases, any doubt in a child presenting with diffuse nasal polyposis in conjunction with total opacification of the sinuses as well as hypoplastic sinuses (typically frontal and sphenoid), should be followed up with a sweat test. Nasal endoscopy demonstrates polyp formation in up to 45% of adults with cystic fibrosis (CF), although most will show radiological evidence of disease.[61] Polyps from children with CF have a significantly lower eosinophil count than patients with 'typical' adult onset CRSwNPs.[62] However, there have also been studies to demonstrate significant overlap in eosinophil concentrations between groups.[63] Absent mucociliary clearance exhibited in primary ciliary dyskinesia results in recurrent bacterial infections and CRSwNPs in approximately 40% of patients.[64]

NON-POLYPOIDAL CHRONIC RHINOSINUSITIS (CRSsNPS)

It is worth noting here that some cases of CRSsNPs may be classified as CRSwNPs due to polypoid change around obstructed sinus ostia, rather than representing more diffuse polyps seen in other cases of CRSwNPs. Careful consideration of the relevant treatment paradigms should therefore be given in conjunction with relevant radiological findings. However, it is also likely, given the insidious nature of CRS, that some cases appear as CRSsNPs at first presentation but eventually develop nasal polyposis.

Localized CRSsNP (isolated sinus disease and odontogenic disease)

Anatomical variation may predispose a patient to isolated inflammation in only one of the sinuses (**Figure 94.6**) as a post-obstructive phenomenon.

Infundibular opacification has been shown to be associated with maxillary sinus disease in approximately three-quarters of cases in a series of 100 prospectively evaluated CT scans,[65] suggesting that anatomic variants such as infra-orbital ethmoid cells, concha bullosa, and narrow nasal cavity secondary to deviated nasal septum correlated with mucosal thickening, particularly in the maxillary sinus (**Figure 94.7**).

Preceding events may include an allergic or viral exacerbation, leading to obstruction of the sinus ostia, with secondary bacterial infection. Depending on the attachment of the uncinate process, some cases may also involve the frontal and anterior ethmoid sinuses on that same side and endoscopy typically reveals a bulging uncinate process where the infection appears to be 'walled-off' in the anterior sinuses. Microbiology sampling of mucopus should be performed in conjunction with surgical drainage and aeration as medical therapy typically fails but these patients tend not to need any sustained post-operative medical treatment. In approximately 10% of these cases the cause will be odontogenic.[66] Therefore, all unilateral cases should include an oral examination and a careful review of the maxillary sinus floor on the CT scan to look for signs of an oro-antral fistula.[67] Involvement of oral maxillofacial colleagues will be beneficial at an early stage where odontogenic aetiology is suspected to enable optimization of management.[68]

DIFFUSE NON-POLYPOIDAL CRSsNP

CRSsNPs is histologically characterized by fibrosis, goblet cell hyperplasia, basement membrane thickening, subepithelial oedema and mononuclear cell infiltration (**Figure 94.8**).

It accounts for about 45% of the cases seen in secondary care[22] but presents a lower surgical burden than CRSwNPs.[25, 55] Remodelling is a dynamic process in both health and disease that balances extra-cellular matrix (ECM) production and degradation, which is regulated by diverse mediators among which TGF-β takes a central role. Indeed, the up-regulation of the TGF-β signalling pathway in patients with CRSsNP and its down-regulation in patients with CRSwNPs on the protein level are reflected by oedema formation and a lack of collagen production in patients with CRSwNPs and excessive collagen deposition associated with

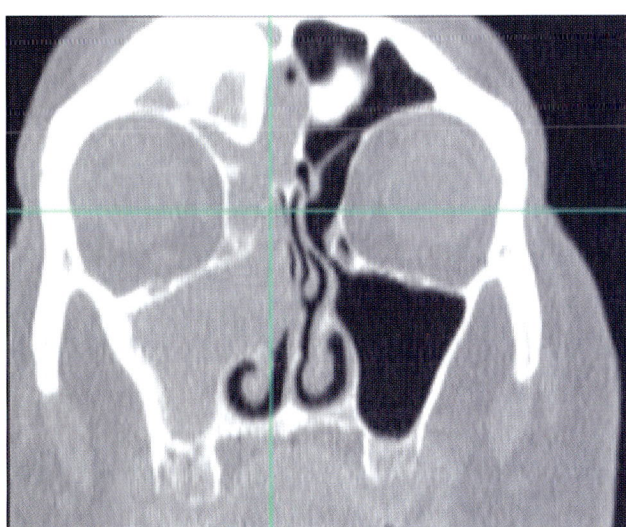

Figure 94.6 Localized CRSsNPs.

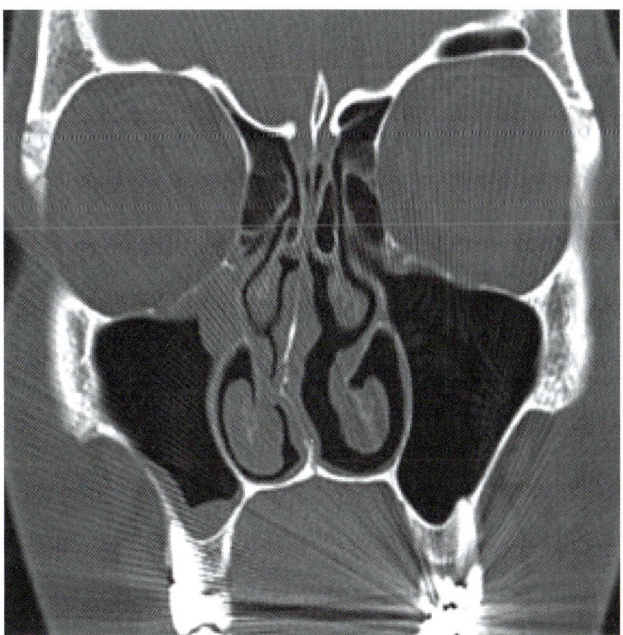

Figure 94.7 Infundibular disease due to anatomical narrowing.

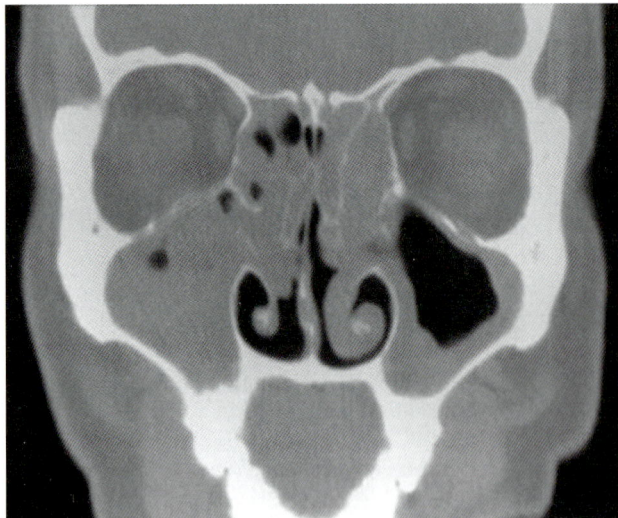

Figure 94.8 Coronal CT image demonstrating diffuse pansinusitis and mucosal thickening, indicative of severe CRSsNPs.

fibrosis in patients with CRSsNPs.[56] CRSsNPs is also distinct from CRSwNPs immunologically, characterized by a TH_1 milieu with increased levels of IFN-γ in the inflamed sinus mucosa and low ECP/myeloperoxidase ratios.

Much like CRSwNPs, bacterial colonization of the paranasal sinuses in CRSsNPs has a similarly uncertain significance.[69] While identifiable bacteria are comparable between the two subtypes,[47–49, 69, 70] *S. aureus* colonization appears to be more statistically significant in patients with CRSwNPs (63.6%) compared to controls, which is not apparent in CRSsNPs patients (27.3%),[52] however, the organism is identified as the most common pathogen in CRS patients as a whole, especially post-operatively.[71] This former observation has thus largely rejected the superantigen hypothesis in CRSsNPs. Conversely, reports on biofilms are more abundant in CRSsNPs patients, with detection rates ranging from 28.6 to 100%.[72–76] Multiple bacterial species have been identified, including *P. aeruginosa*, *S. aureus*, *S. pneumonia*, *H. influenza* and *M. catarrhalis*. Again, their overall relevance in the context of disease pathogenesis remains incompletely defined, but biofilms are thought to be at least partially responsible for a subset of recalcitrant CRSsNPs cases. The same can be said for the clinical significance of fungal pathogens isolated from CRSsNPs patients.

The significance of OMC obstruction in the context of CRSsNP is more clear-cut than the polypoidal variant. In the latter, OMC obstruction may be a 'barometer' of overall disease burden, in that increasing Lund-Mackay scoring is associated with OMC involvement overall.[77]

SYSTEMIC CONDITIONS CAUSING RHINOSINUSITIS

The systemic conditions likely to manifest with nasal polyps have been discussed above in the section on CRSwNPs. This section will therefore focus on other systemic conditions that give rise to CRS or should perhaps be considered as a differential diagnosis for CRS.[78,79] Granulomatous diseases to consider include granulomatosis with polyangiitis (GPA) formerly known as Wegener's Granulomatosis and sarcoidosis.[80] Clues to the diagnosis may be derived from blood tests including Anti-nuclear cytoplasmic antibody (ANCA) and angiotensin converting syndrome (ACE) which if elevated may need corroboration with tissue biopsy and other imaging. These conditions typically manifest with intranasal crusting and the former can be locally destructive with erosion of sinus lamellae and septal cartilage, the latter giving rise to a characteristic saddle-nose deformity. Ciliary dyskinesias represent another group of disorders that will manifest with rhinosinusitis.[81] Primary ciliary dyskinesia is often associated with situs inversus and known in this circumstance as Kartagener's syndrome. Patients often present in adolescence and may have a prior history of otitis media with effusion; they may also suffer with bronchiectasis.[82] Ciliary dyskinesias will show delayed mucociliary clearance times and require investigation at specialist centres, of which there are three in the UK.[83] Clear rhinorrhoea, especially unilaterally, should always prompt investigation for a CSF leak, initiated by collecting nasal fluid to test for β-2 transferrin. Tumours will typically present with unilateral symptoms such as blockage or bleeding but inverted papillomas may sometimes be found amongst bilateral CRSwNPs, hence it is important to send material for histology during any surgery to remove polyps, especially the first time, if there is any index of suspicion. Tumours may also present when they cause secondary infection by sinus ostial occlusion.

Rhinosinusitis may also be a presenting or secondary feature of patients with immunodeficiencies (e.g. HIV[84]) or who are immunocompromised by systemic treatment for other disorders (e.g receiving immunosuppressive drugs for organ transplantation). In those cases, patients require endoscopic retrieval of mucopus where possible, as unusual organisms may be found.[85] Immunodeficiency should always be considered a possibility in patients who appear not to respond to standard medical and surgical care for CRS[86, 87] and in cases of recurrent ARS. Common variable immune deficiency (CVID), selective IgA deficiency, IgG subclass deficiency, and specific antibody deficiency are all possible immunodeficiencies that can be detected in cases of CRS.[88] Refractory cases of CRS have been shown to have low IgG in 18%, low IgA in 17% and low IgM in 5%[89] with both IgA and IgG deficiencies postulated as potential contributory factors for patients failing medical therapy for CRS.[90] In children, where a higher index of suspicion accompanies the onset of CRS, IgG_3 subclass deficiency has been reported in association with the presence of nasal polyposis.[91] Another study looking at 245 CRS patients failing prolonged antibiotic therapy found that about 8% had an IgG deficiency[92] with IgG_3 deficiency being implicated as the most common Ig deficiency in the wider group of patients with CRS[93] and IgG_2 in cases of recurrent ARS.[94] Certainly there is a role for screening for immunodeficiency in CRS patients refractory to standard treatment.[88, 95]

A list of differential diagnosis and key diagnostic features is found in **Table 94.5**. This is by no means exhaustive but does provide a guide to other conditions that should be considered.

TABLE 94.5 Systemic conditions causing rhinosinusitis or possible differential diagnosis

Congenital	Cystic fibrosis	Abnormal sweat test CFTR gene mutation on chromosome 7
	Primary ciliary dyskinesia	Abnormal mucociliary clearance and cilial ultrastructure
	Primary immunodeficiencies (CVID, SCID, hypo/dys–gammaglobulinaemias)	Low/absent antibodies
Infectious/inflammatory	HIV	Positive ELISA for HIV
	Sarcoidosis	Elevated ACE CXR signs (hilar lymphadenopathy)
	Tuberculosis	Acid-fast bacilli Mantoux test positive
	Granulomatosis with polyangitis (Wegener's)	cANCA positive Leukocytoclastic vasculitis on biopsy
	Eosinophilic granulomatosis with polyangitis (Churg-Strauss Syndrome)	pANCA positive
Neoplastic	Haematological malignancies	Abnormal FBC/bone marrow
	Sinonasal malignancies	Biopsy positive Radiological changes
Iatrogenic	Atrophic rhinitis	Excessive crusting following radical nasal surgery
	Chemotherapy/immunosuppression	Relevant drug history
Metabolic	Malnutrition	Low BMI

FUTURE RESEARCH

➤ The EPOS paper[1] and more recently the European Forum for Research and Education in Allergy and Airway Disease (EUFOREA)[96] have carefully detailed where future research efforts need to be directed and hence the tables below summarize this.

➤ There is clearly much work to be done, above all, in understanding the complexities of this heterogeneous disease and perhaps in the future separating patients out into distinct groups based on cytokine profiling, allowing personalized medical treatment for individual patients.[97]

➤ Through the characterization of CRS phenotype subsets, well-defined endotype groups should become distinguishable.

➤ Continual identification of specific disease subgroups, genetic changes and biomarkers as directed by good epidemiological studies will be valuable undertakings for future research, particularly in the context of implementing novel treatment strategies and the overall prognosis of the condition.

BOX 94.2 EPOS 2012 Aetiological Research Priorities

Future research should consider the role of:

- Socioeconomic status
- Severity staging with respect to QoL
- Prognostic symptoms in primary care
- Endotyping and phenotyping – including how to assess this and the impact upon management and outcomes
- Osteitis (long-term study and RCT of treatment options)
- Purulence in assessing response to treatment
- Childhood events, smoking and AR as risk factors
- Psychological, neurological, GORD risk factors
- Genetic profiling on susceptibility to disease and therapeutic response
- CRSsNPs pathophysiology

Future research should further investigate:

- Olfactory disorders, headache, facial pain
- The development of new classifications based on endotypes and phenotypes
- Better understanding of inflammatory pathways including TGF-β, T-cells, dendritic cells, microbiomes and search for new and clinically applicable biomarkers
- The pathogenesis of 'allergic' fungal rhinosinusitis and AERD.
- Understanding of the link between CRSwNPs and lower airway disease.
- The natural history of CRS and epidemiology studies.

BOX 94.3 EPOS[1] and EUFOREA[96] research priorities for CRS management

- Improve professional education and efficient dissemination of evidence-based guidelines to optimize outcomes and reduce referral rates to secondary care.
- Conduct a large prospective placebo controlled study of long-term antibiotic treatment in a well-defined CRS population, exploring effects on the patient's quality of life, immune system, microbiota of the airway as well as the health economic impact.
- Seek better local therapies for immunomodulation.
- Conduct an RCT on oral steroids versus surgery on the long-term outcomes of CRSwNPs.
- Conduct an RCT studying the effects of oral corticosteroids on olfactory function in CRSwNP.
- Conduct multicentre RCTs on surgery versus no treatment for patients with CRSwNPs to establish the natural course of disease.
- Conduct RCTs on minimal versus more extensive endoscopic sinus surgery.
- Investigate the effect of early surgical intervention on CRSwNPs to see if it alters the course of the disease.
- Better tools for the diagnosis and differential diagnosis of facial pain in assessment of rhinosinusitis symptoms and examination in CRS.
- To establish whether treatment of CRS affects outcomes of comorbid lower airways disease (eg asthma, COPD)
- To undertake further RCTs studying the effects of surgery and medical treatment on the lower airways (lung function/QoL/symptoms) in CRSwNP and concomittant asthma.
- Demonstrate whether the relative frequency of different symptoms and signs in CRSwNPs and CRSsNPs predict a differential response to different therapies.
- Cost effectiveness of biological treatment versus surgery.
- Socioeconomic impact of implementation of phenotyping and endotyping into care pathways.

KEY POINTS

- Rhinosinusitis is a common disease with CRS affecting an estimated 10% of the population worldwide.
- Most ARS is not bacterial and requires symptomatic relief only.
- CRS is a heterogeneous disease with differing phenotypes and endotypes; the latter have yet to be clearly determined.
- CRS presents a significant burden on healthcare resources but guidelines exist for its medical and surgical management.
- Where other clues are present, consideration must be given to other systemic causes for sinonasal disease.
- Due to the relative paucity of evidence, more clinical trials are needed to determine the most effective treatment strategies for the various forms of CRS.

REFERENCES

1. Fokkens WJ, Lund VJ, Mullol J, et al. European position paper on rhinosinusitis and nasal polyps 2012. *Rhinol Suppl* 2012; (**23**):3 p preceding table of contents, 1–298.
2. Rosenfeld RM, Piccirillo JF, Chandrasekhar SS, et al. Clinical practice guideline (update): adult sinusitis. *Otolaryngol Head Neck Surg* 2015; **152**(2 Suppl): S1–S39.
3. Ferguson BJ. Definitions of fungal rhinosinusitis. *Otolaryngol Clin North Am* 2000; **33**(2): 227–35.
4. Bent JP, 3rd, Kuhn FA. Diagnosis of allergic fungal sinusitis. *Otolaryngol Head Neck Surg* 1994; **111**(5): 580–8.
5. Chan Y, Kuhn FA. An update on the classifications, diagnosis, and treatment of rhinosinusitis. *Curr Opin Otolaryngol Head Neck Surg* 2009; **17**(3): 204–8.
6. Chakrabarti A, Denning DW, Ferguson BJ, et al. Fungal rhinosinusitis: a categorization and definitional schema addressing current controversies. *Laryngoscope* 2009; **119**(9): 1809–18.
7. Simon RA, Dazy KM, Waldram JD. Aspirin-exacerbated respiratory disease: characteristics and management strategies. *Expert Rev Clin Immunol* 2015; **11**(7): 805–17.
8. Ferguson BJ. Eosinophilic mucin rhinosinusitis: a distinct clinicopathological entity. *Laryngoscope* 2000; **110**(5 Pt 1): 799–813.
9. Bachert C, van Cauwenberge P. The WHO ARIA (allergic rhinitis and its impact on asthma) initiative. *Chem Immunol Allergy* 2003; **82**: 119–26.
10. van Gageldonk-Lafeber AB, Heijnen ML, Bartelds AI, et al. A case-control study of acute respiratory tract infection in general practice patients in The Netherlands. *Clin Infect Dis* 2005; **41**(4): 490–7.
11. Trinh N, Ngo HH. Practice variations in the management of sinusitis. *J Otolaryngol* 2000; **29**(4): 211–7.
12. Smith SS, Kern RC, Chandra RK, et al. Variations in antibiotic prescribing of acute rhinosinusitis in United States ambulatory settings. *Otolaryngol Head Neck Surg* 2013; **148**(5): 852–9.
13. Wang DY, Wardani RS, Singh K, et al. A survey on the management of acute rhinosinusitis among Asian physicians. *Rhinology* 2011; **49**(3): 264–71.
14. Revai K, Dobbs LA, Nair S, et al. Incidence of acute otitis media and sinusitis complicating upper respiratory tract infection: the effect of age. *Pediatrics* 2007; **119**(6): e1408–12.
15. Hansen JG. Management of acute rhinosinusitis in Danish general practice: a survey. *Clin Epidemiol* 2011; **3**: 213–6.
16. Bachert C, Hormann K, Mosges R, et al. An update on the diagnosis and treatment of sinusitis and nasal polyposis. *Allergy* 2003; **58**(3): 176–91.
17. Hastan D, Fokkens WJ, Bachert C, et al. Chronic rhinosinusitis in Europe—an underestimated disease. A GA(2)LEN study. *Allergy* 2011; **66**(9): 1216–23.
18. Bhattacharyya N. Contemporary assessment of the disease burden of sinusitis. *Am J Rhinol Allergy* 2009; **23**(4): 392–5.
19. Erskine SE, Verkerk MM, Notley C, et al. Chronic rhinosinusitis: patient experiences of primary and secondary care – a qualitative study. *Clin Otolaryngol* 2015; **41**: 8–14.
20. Goetzel RZ, Hawkins K, Ozminkowski RJ, et al. The health and productivity cost burden of the 'top 10' physical and mental health conditions affecting six large U.S. employers in 1999. *J Occup Environ Med* 2003; **45**(1): 5–14.
21. Gliklich RE, Metson R. The health impact of chronic sinusitis in patients seeking otolaryngologic care. *Otolaryngol Head Neck Surg* 1995; **113**(1): 104–9.
22. Jarvis D, Newson R, Lotvall J, et al. Asthma in adults and its association with chronic rhinosinusitis: the GA2LEN survey in Europe. *Allergy* 2012; **67**(1): 91–8.
23. Gulliford MC, Dregan A, Moore MV, Ashworth M, Staa T, McCann G, et al. Continued high rates of antibiotic prescribing to adults with respiratory tract infection: survey of 568 UK general practices. *BMJ* 2014; **4**(10): e006245.
24. Hospital Episode Statistics: Department of Health, 2013.
25. Hopkins C, Slack R, Lund V, et al. Long-term outcomes from the English national comparative audit of surgery for nasal polyposis and chronic rhinosinusitis. *Laryngoscope* 2009; **119**(12): 2459–65.
26. Hopkins C, McCombe A, Philpott C, et al. Commissioning Guide: Rhinosinusitis: ENT UK/Royal College of Surgeons of England, 2013.

27. Philpott C, Hopkins C, Erskine S, et al. The burden of revision sinonasal surgery in the UK–data from the Chronic Rhinosinusitis Epidemiology Study (CRES): a cross-sectional study. *BMJ open* 2015; **5**(4): e006680.
28. Bhattacharyya N. The economic burden and symptom manifestations of chronic rhinosinusitis. *Am J Rhinol* 2003; **17**(1): 27–32.
29. Ray NF, Baraniuk JN, Thamer M, et al. Healthcare expenditures for sinusitis in 1996: contributions of asthma, rhinitis, and other airway disorders. *J Allergy Clin Immunol* 1999; **103**(3 Pt 1): 408–14.
30. Bhattacharyya N. Incremental health care utilization and expenditures for chronic rhinosinusitis in the United States. *Ann Otol Rhinol Laryngol* 2011; **120**(7): 423–7.
31. Anand VK. Epidemiology and economic impact of rhinosinusitis. *Ann Otol Rhinol Laryngol Suppl* 2004; **193**: 3–5.
32. Gliklich RE, Metson R. Economic implications of chronic sinusitis. *Otolaryngol Head Neck Surg* 1998; **118**(3 Pt 1): 344–9.
33. Vogan JC, Bolger WE, Keyes AS. Endoscopically guided sinonasal cultures: a direct comparison with maxillary sinus aspirate cultures. *Otolaryngol Head Neck Surg* 2000; **122**(3): 370–3.
34. Heikkinen T, Jarvinen A. The common cold. *Lancet* 2003; **361**(9351): 51–9.
35. Brook I, Gober AE. Frequency of recovery of pathogens from the nasopharynx of children with acute maxillary sinusitis before and after the introduction of vaccination with the 7–valent pneumococcal vaccine. *Int J Pediatr Otorhinolaryngol* 2007; **71**(4): 575–9.
36. Babar-Craig H, Gupta Y, Lund VJ. British Rhinological Society audit of the role of antibiotics in complications of acute rhinosinusitis: a national prospective audit. *Rhinology* 2010; **48**(3): 344–7.
37. Van Zele T, Claeys S, Gevaert P, et al. Differentiation of chronic sinus diseases by measurement of inflammatory mediators. *Allergy* 2006; **61**(11): 1280–9.
38. Zhang N, Van Zele T, Perez–Novo C, et al. Different types of T–effector cells orchestrate mucosal inflammation in chronic sinus disease. *J Allergy Clin Immunol* 2008; **122**(5): 961–8.
39. Doyle PW, Woodham JD. Evaluation of the microbiology of chronic ethmoid sinusitis. *J Clin Microbiol* 1991; **29**(11): 2396–400.
40. Gordts F, Halewyck S, Pierard D, et al. Microbiology of the middle meatus: a comparison between normal adults and children. *J Laryngol Otol* 2000; **114**(3): 184–8.
41. Hsu J, Lanza DC, Kennedy DW. Antimicrobial resistance in bacterial chronic sinusitis. *Am J Rhinol* 1998; **12**(4): 243–8.
42. Tatar EC, Tatar I, Ocal B, et al. Prevalence of biofilms and their response to medical treatment in chronic rhinosinusitis without polyps. *Otolaryngol Head Neck Surg* 2012; **146**(4): 669–75.
43. Seiberling KA, Conley DB, Tripathi A, et al. Superantigens and chronic rhinosinusitis: detection of staphylococcal exotoxins in nasal polyps. *Laryngoscope* 2005; **115**(9): 1580–5.
44. Van Zele T, Gevaert P, Watelet JB, et al. Staphylococcus aureus colonization and IgE antibody formation to enterotoxins is increased in nasal polyposis. *J Allergy Clin Immunol* 2004; **114**(4): 981–3.
45. Conley DB, Tripathi A, Seiberling KA, et al. Superantigens and chronic rhinosinusitis: skewing of T–cell receptor V beta–distributions in polyp–derived CD4+ and CD8+ T cells. *Am J Rhinol* 2006; **20**(5): 534–9.
46. Sacks PLt, Harvey RJ, Rimmer J, et al. Antifungal therapy in the treatment of chronic rhinosinusitis: a meta–analysis. *Am J Rhinol Allergy* 2012; **26**(2): 141–7.
47. Shin SH, Ponikau JU, Sherris DA, et al. Chronic rhinosinusitis: an enhanced immune response to ubiquitous airborne fungi. *J Allergy Clin Immunol* 2004; **114**(6): 1369–75.
48. Telmesani LM, Al–Shawarby M. Osteitis in chronic rhinosinusitis with nasal polyps: a comparative study between primary and recurrent cases. *Eur Arch Otorhinolaryngol* 2010; **267**(5): 721–4.
49. Bacciu A, Bacciu S, Mercante G, et al. Ear, nose and throat manifestations of Churg–Strauss syndrome. *Acta Otolaryngol* 2006; **126**(5): 503–9.
50. Brihaye P, Clement PA, Dab I, et al. Pathological changes of the lateral nasal wall in patients with cystic fibrosis (mucoviscidosis). *Int J Pediatr Otorhinolaryngol* 1994; **28**(2–3): 141–7.
51. Henderson WR, Jr., Chi EY. Degranulation of cystic fibrosis nasal polyp mast cells. *J Pathol* 1992; **166**(4): 395–404.
52. Rowe–Jones JM, Shembekar M, Trendell–Smith N, et al. Polypoidal rhinosinusitis in cystic fibrosis: a clinical and histopathological study. *Clin Otolaryngol Allied Sci* 1997; **22**(2): 167–71.
53. Pedersen M, Mygind N. Rhinitis, sinusitis and otitis media in Kartagener's syndrome (primary ciliary dyskinesia). *Clin Otolaryngol Allied Sci* 1982; **7**(6): 373–80.
54. Yousem DM, Kennedy DW, Rosenberg S. Ostiomeatal complex risk factors for sinusitis: CT evaluation. *J Otolaryngol* 1991; **20**(6): 419–24.
55. Dykewicz MS, Hamilos DL. Rhinitis and sinusitis. *J Allergy Clin Immunol* 2010; **125**(2 Suppl 2): S103–15.
56. Van Bruaene N, Derycke L, Perez–Novo CA, et al. TGF–beta signaling and collagen deposition in chronic rhinosinusitis. *J Allergy Clin Immunol* 2009 **124**(2): 253–9, 59 e1–2.
57. Hoyt WH, 3rd. Bacterial patterns found in surgery patients with chronic sinusitis. *J Am Osteopathic Assoc* 1992; **92**(2): 205, 09–12.
58. Schlosser RJ, London SD, Gwaltney JM, Jr, et al. Microbiology of chronic frontal sinusitis. *Laryngoscope* 2001; **111**(8): 1330–2.
59. Genoway KA, Philpott CM, Javer AR. Pathogen yield and antimicrobial resistance patterns of chronic rhinosinusitis patients presenting to a tertiary rhinology centre. *J Otolaryngol Head Neck Surg* 2011; **40**(3): 232–7.
60. Ferguson BJ, Stolz DB. Demonstration of biofilm in human bacterial chronic rhinosinusitis. *Am J Rhinol* 2005; **19**(5): 452–7.
61. Prince AA, Steiger JD, Khalid AN, et al. Prevalence of biofilm–forming bacteria in chronic rhinosinusitis. *Am J Rhinol* 2008; **22**(3): 239–45.
62. Psaltis AJ, Weitzel EK, Ha KR, et al. The effect of bacterial biofilms on post–sinus surgical outcomes. *Am J Rhinol* 2008; **22**(1): 1–6.
63. Ramadan HH, Sanclement JA, Thomas JG. Chronic rhinosinusitis and biofilms. *Otolaryngol Head Neck Surg* 2005; **132**(3): 414–7.
64. Sanderson AR, Leid JG, Hunsaker D. Bacterial biofilms on the sinus mucosa of human subjects with chronic rhinosinusitis. *Laryngoscope* 2006; **116**(7): 1121–6.
65. Leung RM, Kern RC, Conley DB, et al. Osteomeatal complex obstruction is not associated with adjacent sinus disease in chronic rhinosinusitis with polyps. *Am J Rhinol Allergy* 2011; **25**(6): 401–3.
66. Ryan MW. Diseases associated with chronic rhinosinusitis: what is the significance? *Curr Opin Otolaryngol Head Neck Surg* 2008; **16**(3): 231–6.
67. Wang X, Cutting GR. Chronic rhinosinusitis. *Advances in oto-rhino-laryngology* 2011; **70**: 114–21.
68. Tami TA. Granulomatous diseases and chronic rhinosinusitis. *Otolaryngologic clinics of North America* 2005; **38**(6): 1267–78, x.
69. Garg A, Wadher R, Gulati SP, et al. Primary ciliary dyskinesia—an underdiagnosed entity. *J Assoc Physicians India* 2010; **58**: 704–6.
70. Philpott CM, McKiernan DC. Bronchiectasis and sino–nasal disease: a review. *J Laryngol Otol* 2008; **122**(1): 11–5.
71. Bush A, Cole P, Hariri M, et al. Primary ciliary dyskinesia: diagnosis and standards of care. *Eur Respir J* 1998; **12**(4): 982–8.
72. Miziara ID, Araujo Filho BC, et al. Chronic rhinosinusitis in HIV–infected patients: radiological and clinical evaluation. *Braz J Otorhinolaryngol* 2005; **71**(5): 604–8.
73. Franzen C, Muller A, Salzberger B, et al. Chronic rhinosinusitis in patients with AIDS: potential role of microsporidia. *Aids* 1996; **10**(6): 687–8.
74. Alqudah M, Graham SM, Ballas ZK. High prevalence of humoral immunodeficiency patients with refractory chronic rhinosinusitis. *Am J Rhinol Allergy* 2010; **24**(6): 409–12.
75. Woodbury K, Ferguson BJ. Recalcitrant chronic rhinosinusitis: investigation and management. *Curr Opin Otolaryngol Head Neck Surg* 2011; **19**(1): 1–5.
76. Ocampo CJ, Peters AT. Antibody deficiency in chronic rhinosinusitis: epidemiology and burden of illness. *Am J Rhinol Allergy* 2013; **27**(1): 34–8.
77. Chee L, Graham SM, Carothers DG, et al. Immune dysfunction in refractory sinusitis in a tertiary care setting. *Laryngoscope* 2001; **111**(2): 233–5.
78. Carr TF, Koterba AP, Chandra R, et al. Characterization of specific antibody deficiency in adults with medically refractory chronic rhinosinusitis. *Am J Rhinol Allergy* 2011; **25**(4): 241–4.
79. Chinratanapisit S, Tunsuriyawong P, Vichyanond P, et al. Chronic rhinosinusitis and recurrent nasal polyps in two children with IgG subclass deficiency and review of the literature. *J Med Assoc Thai* 2005; **88** Suppl 8: S251–8.
80. May A, Zielen S, von Ilberg C, et al. Immunoglobulin deficiency and determination of pneumococcal antibody titers in patients with therapy–refractory recurrent rhinosinusitis. *Eur Arch Otorhinolaryngol* 1999; **256**(9): 445–9.
81. Scadding GK, Lund VJ, Darby YC, et al. IgG subclass levels in chronic rhinosinusitis. *Rhinology* 1994; **32**(1):15–9.
82. Silk H, Geha RS. Asthma, recurrent infections and IgG2 deficiency. *Ann Allergy* 1988; **60**(2): 134–6.
83. Bernatowska E, Mikoluc B, Krzeski A, et al. Chronic rhinosinusitis in primary antibody immunodeficient patients. *Int J Pediatr Otorhinolaryngol* 2006; **70**(9): 1587–92.

CHAPTER 95

NASAL POLYPOSIS

Louise Melia

Introduction 1037	Diagnosis 1041
Incidence and prevalance 1038	Classification 1042
Clinical presentation 1038	Management 1042
Pathogenesis 1038	Summary 1043
Associated diseases 1039	References 1044

SEARCH STRATEGY

Data in this chapter may be updated by a Medline search using the keywords: nasal polyps, chronic rhinosinusitis with nasal polyps, cystic fibrosis, asthma, aspirin exacerbated respiratory disease, eosinophilic granulomatosis with polyangiitis, Young's syndrome, intranasal corticosteroids, systemic corticosteroids and endoscopic sinus surgery.

INTRODUCTION

Nasal polyps represent the end stage local manifestation of chronic inflammatory disease of the sinonasal tract. The condition is a distinct subgroup of chronic rhinosinusitis, chronic rhinosinusitis with polyps (CRSwNP). Despite the prevalence of polyps, the long history of recognition and extensive research and literature, their aetiology remains elusive and poorly understood. In the last few decades numerous studies have tried to determine the exact pathogenesis of this disease and although many have shown factors thought to be related and associated, none have come to a definitive conclusion about causation. CRSwNP can significantly affect quality of life, and places significant financial burden on society, directly as a result of outpatient appointments, prescriptions, investigations and hospitalization, and indirectly as a result of missed work days and decreased productivity at work. Despite adequate treatment CRSwNP runs a chronic and recurrent course. Nasal polyps continue to be a challenge for rhinologists treating patients with this chronic disease and for those searching for a cause.

Definition

Nasal polyps are best thought of as 'chronic rhinosinusitis with nasal polyps' (CRSwNP), and European guidelines define these conditions clinically as:

- inflammation of the nose and paranasal sinuses associated with two or more symptoms, one of which should be nasal blockage/obstruction/congestion or nasal discharge:
  o +/− facial pain/pressure
  o reduction or loss of smell

and either

- endoscopic evidence of
  o polyps and/or
  o mucopurulent discharge from the middle meatus or oedema, mucosal obstruction primarily in the middle meatus

and/or

- CT changes:
  o mucosal changes within the osteomeatal complex and/or sinuses[1]

Morphologically nasal polyps are oedematous grape-like protrusions most often originating in the upper part of the nose around the osteomeatal complex on the lateral wall. The surface epithelium tends to be smooth and consists of pale translucent tissue which distinguishes them from the more vascular mucosa of the nasal cavity. Polyps can vary widely in size and should be considered a bilateral condition. Rare cases of unilateral polyps should only be diagnosed once all other more likely pathologies have been reliably excluded.

INCIDENCE AND PREVALANCE

The annual incidence of CRSwNP is between 1 and 20 per 1000 population.[2] This incidence declines after 60 years of age. In the normal population the prevalence is between 1 and 4% in adults and 0.1% in children. Nasal polyps are more common in males (2–4:1). There is no racial predilection. Certain systemic diseases, as mentioned below, carry a much higher incidence of nasal polyps.

CLINICAL PRESENTATION

Clinical presentation is variable and depends on the extent of polyp disease. Small polyps may not produce symptoms and may be identified incidentally during rhinoscopic examination, whilst larger polyps may cause significant symptoms. In general, patients with nasal polyps will present with various symptoms that have generally persisted over months to years, progressing from mild nasal congestion with a watery rhinorrhoea to a persistent nasal obstruction associated with hyposmia or anosmia, as well as a thicker post nasal discharge and very occasionally headaches. Epistaxis is not associated with benign polyps and may suggest a more serious pathology in the nasal cavities. Massive polyps or a single large polyp that obstructs the nasal cavities or nasopharynx can cause chronic mouth breathing and obstructive sleep symptoms. Rarely, proptosis, hypertelorism and diplopia can result from alterations in the craniofacial structure. Generally, because of their slow-growing nature, massive polyposis does not cause neurological symptoms or pain, even if they extend into the intracranial cavity (**Figure 95.1**).

PATHOGENESIS

Polyps arise in the presence of inflammation that may be initiated by a number of factors, resulting in dysregulated interaction between the sinus epithelium and the lymphoid system.[3] Histologically, they consist of loose connective tissue, inflammatory cells and fluid, and are usually covered by pseudostratified, columnar, ciliated epithelium (**Figure 95.2**). Polyps form when oedematous connective tissue stroma ruptures and herniates through the basement membrane.[4]

Despite a growing body of evidence that bacteria, fungi, allergens, and superantigens play a prominent role in the pathophysiology of nasal polyps the exact cause remains unknown.

In the last decade, research has revealed unique cytokine and cellular inflammatory profiles that may contribute

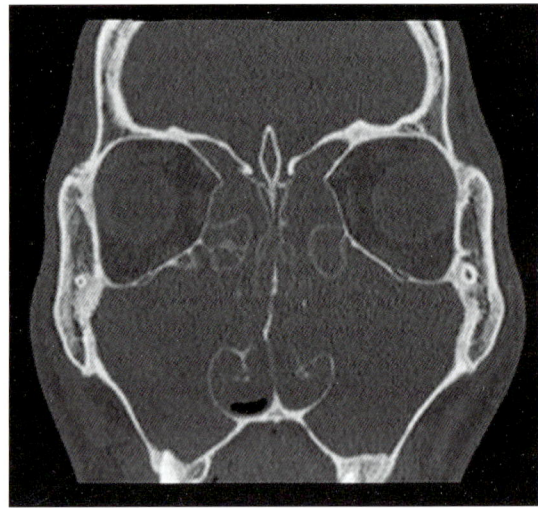

Figure 95.1 Coronal CT image showing complete opacification of sinuses secondary to nasal polyps.

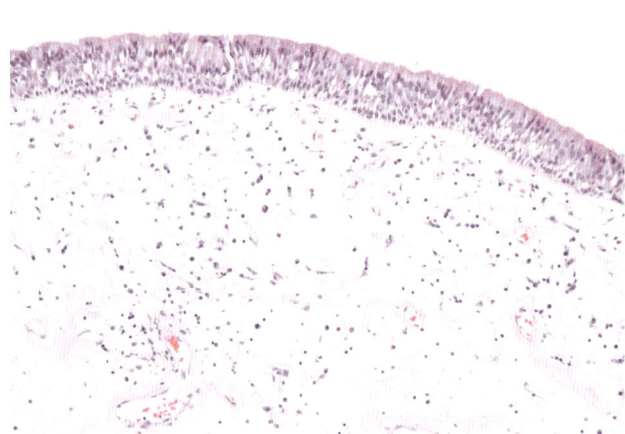
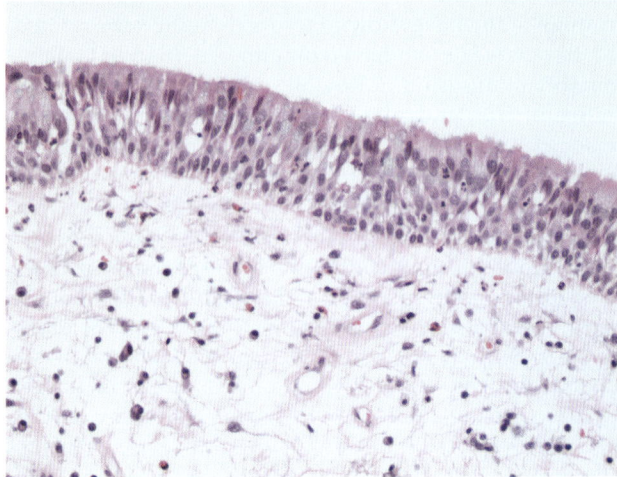

Figure 95.2 Photomicrographs of a simple inflammatory nasal polyp (magnifications of X250 and X400).

to nasal polyps. Approximately 80% of nasal polyps in Western countries are characterized by a robust T-helper 2 response, eosinophilic infiltration[5, 6] decreased T regulatory function,[6] and an abundance of IL-5 cytokine.[7, 8]

Allergy

It is not yet completely clear whether there is an increased risk for the development of nasal polyps in allergic patients, and the evidence in the literature is conflicting. Only 0.4–4.5% of patients with allergic rhinitis have nasal polyps,[9–11] which is similar to the normal population. However, nasal polyps have been shown in 25.6% of patients with allergy compared to 3.9% in a control population.[12] The prevalence of allergy in patients with nasal polyps has been shown to vary from 10%[13] to 64%.[14] Elevated levels of immunoglobulin E (IgE) and positive skin tests to inhalant allergens have been determined in the majority of patients with nasal polyps[10, 15] and association has been found between levels of both total and specific IgE and eosinophilic infiltration in nasal polyps. In patients with nasal polyps however the total serum IgE levels are only partially correlated to local tissue IgE levels and local eosinophilic inflammation.[16] The highly increased local tissue IgE levels in nasal polyps are often polyclonal and independent of total serum IgE levels or allergy skin prick test responses[17] and it has recently been demonstrated that mucosal polyclonal IgE is functional by inducing mast cell degranulation independent of serum IgE levels.[18]

Bacteria

A link between bacterial colonization and nasal polyps has been postulated, but remains unproven. Examination of microbial organisms in the nasal cavity has revealed the presence of a diverse flora, consisting mostly of aerobic and anaerobic bacteria. These include gram-negative organisms such as *Moraxella catarrhalis*, *Haemophilus influenzae*, *Prevotella* species, *Enterobacter* species, and *Pseudomonas* species.[19, 20] Gram-positive organisms include streptococci, coagulase-negative staphylococci, and *Staphylococcus aureus*.[21] It is believed that the main species involved in the exacerbation of nasal polyps is *Staphylococcus aureus* which harbours genes coding for enterotoxins.[16, 22–25]

In one study, 42.5% of *Staphylococcus aureus* strains isolated from nasal polyp patients and controls harboured at least one classic enterotoxin gene.[26] The secreted toxins coded for by these genes behave as superantigens, which, unlike conventional antigens, do not need processing.[23–28] Superantigens induce the activation of numerous T-cell clones and a massive secretion of cytokines, and therefore have the ability to activate as much as 20% of the body's T cells, compared with only 0.001–0.0001% for regular antigens.[29, 30] In CRSwNP this is characterized by an increased eosinophilic inflammation and formation of IgE antibodies.[31] The formation of bacterial biofilms on the sinus mucosa has also been suggested to be responsible for chronic rhinosinusitis.[32, 33] Biofilms are bacteria enclosed within a self-developed matrix of polysaccharides which renders the bacteria inaccessible to antimicrobial agents. Clinically, cases of nasal polyps with the presence of biofilms may be associated with a more severe form of the disease and worse postoperative outcome.[34, 35]

ASSOCIATED DISEASES

The prevalence of CRSwNP is around 7% in patients with asthma, compared to 4% of the general population,[36] and increases to 30–60% in patients with aspirin exacerbated respiratory disease (AERD).[37] Chronic inflammation and allergic fungal sinusitis have also been considered to be potential risk factors for nasal polyps, and the association between genetic variations and chronic rhinosinusitis suggests that genetic polymorphisms could be related to nasal polyps development.[38, 39]

Asthma

The link between the upper and lower airways has been reported since the beginning of 1800s, with both being lined by the same pseudostratified ciliated columnar epithelium. In patients with nasal polyps 30–71% have been shown to have asthma,[10, 40] and there is a direct association between asthma severity and the presence of nasal polyps.[41] Of patients with late-onset asthma, 10–15% develop nasal polyps, with patients generally developing asthma first, then polyps within 9–13 years. This occurs faster in patients with aspirin-induced asthma, about 2 years from the onset of symptoms.[42] Asthma and nasal polyps share the same basic features of eosinophilia, mucus cell hyperplasia, oedema, thickened basal membrane and increased pro-inflammatory mediators, for example cysteine leukotrienes.[43–45]

The relationship between upper and lower airway pathology is further corroborated by the improvement in lower airway disease that is observed when nasal polyps are effectively treated.[46]

Aspirin-exacerbated respiratory disease (AERD, *Samter's Triad*)

The combination of bronchial asthma, nasal polyposis and aspirin sensitivity is also well described in the otolaryngology literature. It was first described by Wimal in 1922 and then formally recognized as a triad of clinical manifestations by *Samter* et al. in 1967.[47] Its prevalence is reported to be as high as 0.3% in the general population and between 5 and 10% of the adult asthmatic population.[48] The prevalence of patients with nasal polyps, asthma and aspirin sensitivity increases over 40 years of age, and these patients are normally non-atopic. The currently accepted pathophysiology behind aspirin sensitivity syndrome lies in the inhibition of cycle-oxygenase in the arachidonic acid pathway. By blocking cycle-oxygenase, the arachidonic acid is shunted into lipoxygenase and there is an increased production of leukotrienes. The subsequent decreased prostaglandin E2 leads to mast cell instability with release of histamine. The combination of increased histamine release and increased leukotriene causes increased vascular permeability, leakage from the vascular system and oedema. It is thought that this cycle of inflammation and oedema results in the formation of polyps.[49] The nasal polyps associated with AERD/*Samter's* Triad are often very extensive, with significantly higher radiological CT scores than non-AERD patients with nasal polyps.[48] They can be difficult to treat and have a higher rate of recurrence. One cohort study of 549 patients with nasal polyposis found the polyp-free rates at 5 years following FESS for failed medical treatment to be 84% for control patients, 55% for patients with asthma and 10% for patients with AERD. At 10 years these rates dropped to 78% and 45% for the control patients and the patients with asthma. 100% of those with AERD had already recurred.[50]

Allergic fungal rhinosinusitis

Allergic fungal rhinosinusitis (AFRS) was first reported in 1976.[51] It is a type 1 hypersensitivity reaction to fungal antigens in which patients usually present with unilateral or bilateral nasal polyps. Approximately 80% of patients with fungal sinusitis have nasal polyps.[36] Theories on pathogenesis include hypersensitivity and T-cell mediated reactions as well as a humoral immune response. Treatment is largely surgical, with a strong role for oral corticosteroids and an emerging role for immunotherapy. Antifungals, both systemic and topical, currently have a limited role in treatment, although this area needs further study.[52] In 1994, Bent and Kuhn published their diagnostic criteria centred on the histologic, radiographic, and immunologic characteristics of the disease (**Table 95.1**).[53] Patients must meet all the major criteria for diagnosis, while the minor criteria serve to support the diagnosis and describe individual patients but are not used to make a diagnosis. The major criteria include a history of type I hypersensitivity by history, skin testing, or *in vitro* testing; nasal polyposis; characteristic computed tomography (CT) scan findings with soft tissue differential densities; the presence of eosinophilic mucin without fungal invasion into the sinus tissue; and a positive fungal stain of sinus contents removed at the time of surgery. The minor criteria include a history of asthma, unilateral predominance of disease, radiographic evidence of bone erosion, fungal cultures, presence of Charcot-Leyden crystals in surgical specimens, and serum eosinophilia. A wide variety of fungi have been isolated from the sinuses of patients with chronic rhinosinusitis and as fungal detection techniques improve, so does the sensitivity to detect them, with some studies demonstrating fungal presence in almost 100% of patients, both controls and CRS patients.[54] Therefore the only features that appear to be unique to AFRS are type 1 hypersensitivity and the characteristic CT findings.

Cystic fibrosis

Cystic fibrosis (CF) is an autosomal recessive disorder caused by mutations of a gene on chromosome 7. The gene prevalence is approximately 1:25 in the Caucasian population and it currently affects 9000 people in the UK.[55] CF patients have thick, tenacious mucus secondary to a mutation in the CF transmembrane conductance regulator chloride channel that affects mucociliary transport.[56] Although the majority of CF patients do not report sinonasal symptoms, CRS is prevalent,[57] with nasal polyps present in up to 86% of patients.[58] In CF CRS, inflammation is neutrophil driven with IL-8 being the primary cytokine.[59, 60] Sinus cultures typically grow *Staphlococcus aureus* or *Pseudomonas aeruginosa*.[61, 62] Examination of CF patients with nasal polyps usually reveals bilateral polyposis with thick rhinorrhoea and facial deformities such as hypertelorism.[63] In addition to nasal polyps, CT scan findings include hypoplasia of the frontal or sphenoid sinuses as well as demineralization and medial displacement of the uncinate process.[59, 64-67]

Mucocele formation is not uncommon in CF, and therefore the presence of mucoceles in a child should raise suspicion for CF.[68, 69]

Primary ciliary dyskinesia

Primary ciliary dyskinesia (PCD) is a rare autosomal recessive disease in which abnormal or absent beating of cilia hinders normal mucociliary clearance. The commonest presentations are in the upper and/or lower respiratory tracts, with mucus retention and recurrent infection leading to nasal polyposis and/or bronchiectasis.[70] Kartagener's syndrome is a clinical variant of PCD and is a triad of chronic sinusitis, bronchiectasis and situs inversus. Twenty-seven per cent of patients with Kartagener's syndrome have nasal polyps (**Figure 95.3**).[36]

Young's syndrome

Young's syndrome is a rare disease consisting of three components: obstructive azoospermia, bronchiectasis and sinus disease. Although it is a recognized cause of male infertility and is well known in the field of infertility,[71] the exact nature and natural history of the sinus disease component is not widely understood. The prevalence of Young's syndrome remains unknown. In the 1980s, the syndrome was reported to affect one in 500 males and was described as being more common than cystic fibrosis.[72] However, in the last 20 years only a handful of case reports have been published on this syndrome.[73-75] A reduction in the use of mercury in Europe and the USA has been cited as a potential reason for this decline. Mercury exposure in

TABLE 95.1 Bent and Kuhn Classfication of Allergic fungal rhinosinusitis[53]

Major	Minor
Type I Hypersensitivity	Asthma
Nasal polyposis	Unilateral disease
Characteristic CT findings	Bone erosion
Eosinophilic mucin without invasion	Fungal cultures
Positive fungal stain	Charcot-Leyden crystals
	Serum eosinophilia

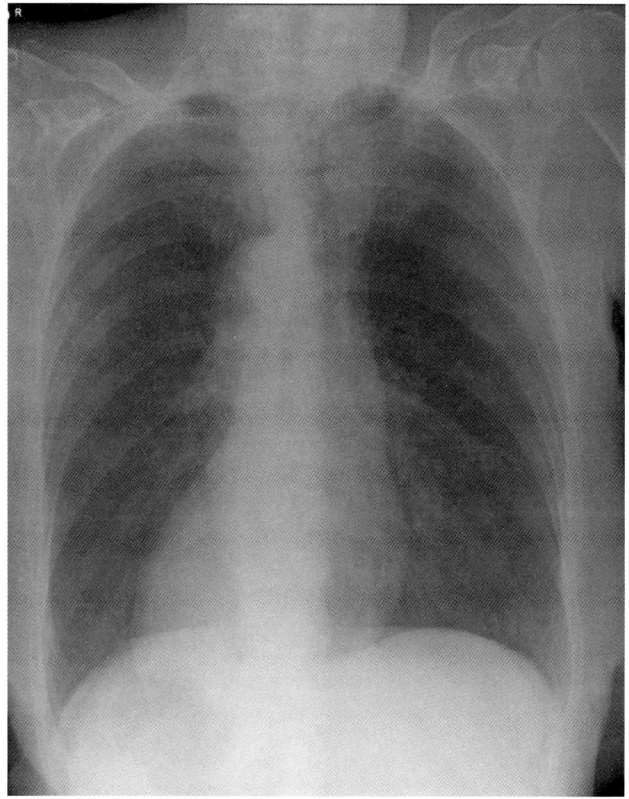

Figure 95.3 Chest radiograph showing dextrocardia.

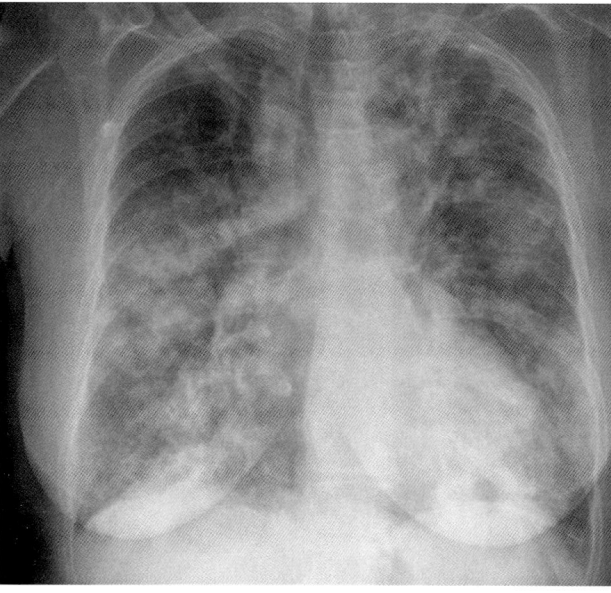

Figure 95.4 Chest radiograph showing pulmonary infiltrates.

childhood is likely to be the only aetiological factor identifiable in Young's syndrome, with a history of mercury intoxication seen in 10% of Young's syndrome patients in one series.[76] Mercury inhibits enzymes containing sulphydryl by reacting with thiols to form mercaptides. Mercaptides are thought to inhibit glycolysis, which is necessary for the normal function and energy supply of sperm and cilia.[77]

EGPA (Churg Strauss)

Previously known as Churg Strauss syndrome, this entity has now been recognized by the 2012 revised nomenclature for vasculitides as eosinophilic granulomatosis with Polyangiitis (EGPA). It is a systemic small-vessel vasculitis associated with asthma and eosinophilia, and is traditionally described to evolve through a prodromic, allergic phase characterized by asthma and rhinosinusitis, an eosinophilic phase hallmarked by peripheral eosinophilia and organ involvement, and a vasculitic phase with clinical manifestations due to small-vessel vasculitis.[78] These phases partially overlap and may not appear in such a defined order, although asthma and rhinosinusitis only rarely arise after the vasculitic manifestations.[79] Criteria for classification from the American College of Rheumatology[80] consist of the following:

- asthma
- eosinophilia of >10% in peripheral blood
- paranasal sinusitis
- pulmonary infiltrates, sometimes transient
- histologic evidence of vasculitis with extravascular eosinophils
- mononeuritis multiplex or polyneuropathy
- if ≥4 criteria are present, sensitivity is 85%, and specificity is 99.7%.

The typical case that should raise suspicion of EGPA is that of a patient with adult-onset asthma and a history of rhinosinusitis, who develops pronounced eosinophilia and lung infiltrates. Eosinophilia may occur in straightforward asthmatic patients but is usually mild (<10%); likewise, lung infiltrates due to bronchial plugging by mucus and superimposed infection may complicate asthma, but they are uncommon. Nasal polyps affect approximately 50% of patients with EGPA and consistently recur after surgery in patients not receiving immunosuppressive therapy (**Figure 95.4**).[81]

Genetics

Despite many previous attempts to explain disease pathogenesis, the exact genetic mechanisms underlying the development of nasal polyps remain unclear. Suggestion for a potential genetic basis to nasal polyps is afforded by degree of inheritability suggested from family and twin studies as well as the existence of chronic rhinosinusitis and nasal polyps in simple mendelian diseases. Associations between chronic rhinosinusitis and polymorphisms in over 30 genes have been published, however, studies of monozygotic twins have not shown both siblings to always develop polyps, indicating that environmental factors are also likely to play a role in the development of nasal polyps.[82–85]

DIAGNOSIS

Anterior rhinoscopy is the first step to diagnosis, but is inadequate alone and cannot exclude polyps. Rod Lens nasendoscopy after topical decongestant is needed for diagnosis, as well as identifying discharge, crusting or scarring secondary to previous surgery. Plain sinus radiographs are insensitive[86–88] and should not be used to diagnose polyps. CT scanning with coronal sections is the investigation of choice for assessing the extent of the disease and detailing the anatomy before surgery.[89–91] Magnetic resonance imaging may be helpful to differentiate from tumour, or if intracranial extension of disease is suspected. History for features of systemic disease should be taken, including lower airway symptoms, and tests for factors associated with nasal polyps can be performed. The effects of treatment on nasal obstruction and polyp masses can be documented objectively via nasal inspiratory peak flow,[92] rhinomanometry,[93] acoustic rhinometry,[94] olfactory tests and symptom scoring (**Figure 95.5**).[95]

CLASSIFICATION

Endoscopic and CT-based staging systems are used to determine the extent of disease within the nose and sinuses, and facilitate both medical communication and evaluation of therapeutic responses. The clinical staging system and endoscopic scoring systems are based on the assumption that the polyp grows from the middle meatus down towards the floor of the nose (**Table 95.2**).[96, 97] The radiological staging system includes all sinuses and the osteomeatal complex bilaterally. Various radiological staging systems have been described. The Lund–Mackay system gives a score of 0–2 depending on the absence, partial or complete opacification of each sinus system and of the osteomeatal complex on computed tomography scanning. A maximum score of 12 per side can be achieved (**Table 95.3**).[98] The Lund-Mackay score increases with increasing grade of polyposis.

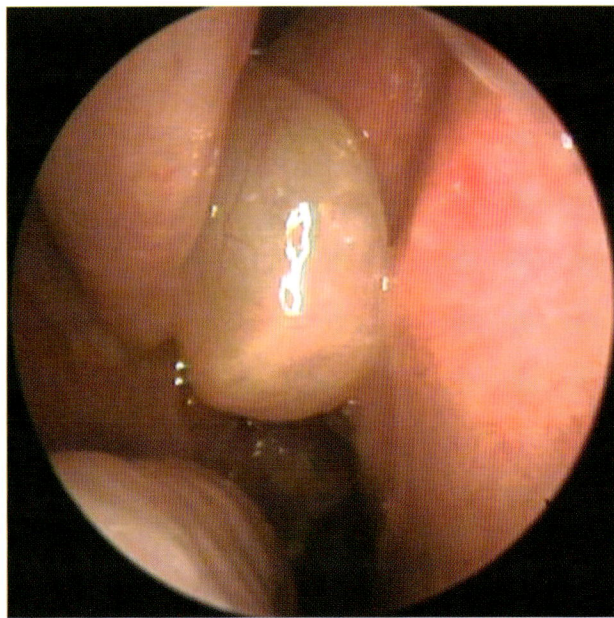

Figure 95.5 Endoscopic view of a nasal polyp.

MANAGEMENT

Treatment aims to eliminate symptoms and nasal polyps, re-establish nasal breathing and olfaction, prevent recurrence and improve patients' quality of life. Treatment can be divided into medical and surgical.

Medical

All patients should have a trial of medical therapy first, unless histology is required. Medical treatment consists mainly of topical and systemic corticosteroids, which are thought to affect eosinophil function directly by reducing both eosinophil viability and activation,[99] and indirectly by reducing the secretion of haemotactic cytokines by nasal mucosa and polyp epithelial cells.[100] Intranasal corticosteroids (INCS) have been shown to be more effective than placebo at improving nasal airflow, reducing polyp size and decreasing rate of recurrence.[1] The effect on sense of smell is poor when compared to systemic steroids, which may be due to the sprays being unable to reach the olfactory mucosa because of oedema. Nasal drops are more effective than sprays and have a significant positive effect on sense of smell, however, they are relatively potent topical steroids, and may be used initially, although not for longer than 2 months at one time unless under specialist supervision, or for longer than 4 months in one

TABLE 95.2 Endoscopic staging of nasal polyps[96]	
Polyp	0 = absence of polyp 1 = polyps in middle meatus only 2 = beyond middle meatus
Oedema	0 = absent 1 = mild 2 = severe
Discharge	0 = no discharge 1 = clear, thin discharge 2 = thick, purulent discharge
Scarring	0 = absent 1 = mild 2 = severe
Crusting	0 = absent 1 = mild 2 = severe

TABLE 95.3 Radiological staging of CRS[99]		
Paranasal sinuses	Right	Left
Maxillary 0,1,2		
Anterior ethmoid 0,1,2		
Posterior ethmoid 0,1,2		
Sphenoid 0,1,2		
Osteomeatal complex 0*, 2*		
Total points to each side		

0 = no abnormalities, 1 = partial opacification, 2 = complete opacification
0* = not occluded, 2* = occluded

12-month period, as they can be absorbed systemically. Larger polyps may require systemic corticosteroids,[101] for example prednisolone 0.5 mg/kg each morning for 5–10 days. Maintenance therapy with topical corticosteroid spray is recommended as these may have lower bioavailability than drops and are less likely to be administered incorrectly.

It is recommended that patients are started on sprays, drops or systemic steroids depending on their initial presentation and examination findings. On review, a decision can be made whether to continue with medical treatment, request further investigations or consider surgical intervention.[1] Antihistamines only help if allergy is present,[102] and leukotriene inhibitors may help patients with coexisting asthma and/or aspirin sensitivity.[103–105]

Common side effects of intranasal corticosteroids include local irritation and epistaxis. Potential adverse events related to the administration of intranasal corticosteroids are effects on growth, ocular effects, effects on bone and effects on the hypothalamic pituitary-adrenal axis. Cases of adrenal suppression and Cushing's syndrome from systemic absorption have been reported, but are rare.[106] Measurement of salivary cortisol is a useful, non-invasive and economical test for monitoring patients using intranasal corticosteroids.[107] There is evidence that a 3-month course of a macrolide antibiotic can help nasal polyps.[108] Macrolides have been shown to increase mucociliary transport, reduce goblet cell secretion and cause accelerated apoptosis of neutrophils, all of which would reduce the symptoms of chronic inflammation. However, acute cardiac toxicity is an increasingly recognized potential adverse effect of antimicrobial drug treatment and several agents of the macrolide class of antibiotics are known to interfere with the delayed rectifier potassium current, which results in accumulation of potassium ions in cardiac myocytes and thereby delays cardiac repolarization. Evident on an electrocardiogram as a prolongation of the QT interval, this mechanism is thought to underlie an increase in the risk of torsade de pointes, a potentially fatal arrhythmia, with macrolides. A recently published large cohort study has found a significantly increased risk of cardiac death associated with clarithromycin. No increased risk was seen with roxithromycin.[109] Nasal douching provides symptomatic benefit, and should be used with sterilized or distilled water to avoid contamination.

Surgical

Surgical management is considered for patients who have failed to respond to maximal medical treatment and for those with complications.

Functional endoscopic sinus surgery aims to improve sinus ventilation and drainage as well as removing polyps. The extent of surgery varies with the extent of disease, the surgeon's individual practice and available technology. Functional endoscopic sinus surgery has been used for many years to treat sino-nasal conditions and permits a better view of the surgical field, allowing more precise clearance of the inflammatory change than conventional surgery. It may be associated with fewer complications and lower recurrence rates.[110, 111]

Patients being treated for polyp disease derive the greatest benefit from functional endoscopic sinus surgery, and those whose main preoperative symptom is nasal obstruction or headache report higher benefit. Coexistent asthma, allergic rhinitis or aspirin intolerance does not decrease the benefit of sinus surgery in patients with polyps.

Postoperatively, patients should be treated with nasal douching and intranasal or systemic corticosteroids, and compliance with this treatment will influence the long term efficacy of surgery. There is good evidence that postoperative use of topical nasal steroids reduce the rate of polyp recurrence.[112]

SUMMARY

Nasal polyps are a chronic disease of the upper respiratory tract that form as an end result of severe inflammation in the nose and paranasal sinuses and are considered to be a subgroup of chronic rhinosinusitis. Although not life-threatening, they can cause severe symptoms with a significant impact on quality of life. Nasal polyps arise in patients with chronic inflammation resulting from many different pathologies and why certain patients develop polyps remains unknown. Extensive research has resulted in a greater understanding of this disease, with evidence that bacteria, fungi, allergens, and superantigens play a prominent role in the pathophysiology of nasal polyps. However the exact cause remains elusive. The annual incidence of nasal polyps is between 1 and 20 per 1000 population. Certain systemic diseases are associated with a much higher incidence of CRSwNP with a prevalence of around 7% in patients with asthma and up to 30–60% in patients with aspirin exacerbated respiratory disease.

Anterior rhinoscopy is the first step to diagnosis, but cannot exclude polyps. Rigid nasendoscopy after is required for diagnosis. CT scanning with coronal sections is the investigation of choice for assessing the extent of the disease and detailing the anatomy before surgery.

A combined treatment strategy involving both medical and surgical management is recommended for long-term control because of the chronic and recurrent nature of the disease, with treatment aiming to eliminate nasal polyps and rhinitic symptoms, re-establish nasal breathing and olfaction, prevent recurrence and improve patients' quality of life. Medical treatment consists mainly of intranasal

> **BEST CLINICAL PRACTICE**
>
> ✓ Initial medical treatment with topical intranasal corticosteroids
> ✓ Clinical review allows adjustment of medical therapy, planning of further investigations and reduces need for surgery
> ✓ Consider surgery in patients who have failed to respond to maximal medical therapy
> ✓ Unilateral nasal polyps are tumours until proved otherwise

and systemic corticosteroids, thought to affect eosinophil function by reducing both eosinophil viability and activation, and by reducing the secretion of chemotactic cytokines. This improves nasal airflow, reduces polyp size and decreases the rate of recurrence. Surgical management should be reserved for patients who have failed to respond to maximal medical treatment.

> **KEY POINTS**
>
> - Nasal polyps can cause severe symptoms and can have a significant impact on quality of life.
> - Although known to be associated with chronic inflammation the exact aetiology remains elusive.
> - Nasal polyps are associated with many chronic conditions including asthma, aspirin exacerbated respiratory disease and cystic fibrosis.
> - Nasal polyps can be easily diagnosed with anterior rhinoscopy and nasendoscopy.
> - Combined medical and surgical treatment is recommended for long-term control of symptoms.
> - Unilateral nasal polyps should be treated as suspected malignancy until biopsy proves otherwise.

REFERENCES

1. Fokkens WJ, Lund VJ, Mullol J, et al. EPOS: European position paper on rhinosinusitis and nasal polyps 2012. A summary for otorhinolaryngologists. *Rhinology* 2012; **50**: 1–12.
2. Johansson L, Akerlund A, Holmberg K, et al. Prevalence of nasal polyps in adults. *Ann Otol Rhinol Laryngol* 2003; **112**(7): 625–9.
3. Chaaban MR, Walsh EM, Woodworth BA. Epidemiology and differential diagnosis of nasal polyps. *Am J Rhinol Allergy* 2013; **27**: 473–8.
4. Berger G, Kattan A, Bernheim J, Ophir D. Polypoid mucosa with eosinophilia and glandular hyperplasia in chronic sinusitis: a histopathological and immunohistochemical study. *Laryngoscope* 2002; **112**(4): 738–45.
5. Zhang N, Van Zele T, Perez-Novo C, et al. Different types of T-effector cells orchestrate mucosal inflammation in chronic sinus disease. *J Allergy Clin Immunol* 2008; **122**: 961–8.
6. Van Zele T, Claeys S, Gevaert P, et al. Differentiation of chronic sinus diseases by measurement of inflammatory mediators. *Allergy* 2006; **61**: 1280–9.
7. Jiang XD, Li GY, Li L, et al. The characterisation of IL-17A expression in patients with chronic rhinosinusitis with nasal polyps. *Am J Rhinol Allergy* 2011; 25: e171–5.
8. Wen W, Liu W, Zhang L, et al. Increased neutrophilia in nasal polyps reduces the response to oral corticosteroid therapy. *J Allergy Clin Immunol* 2012; **129**: 1522–8.
9. Caplin I, Haynes JT, Spahn J. Are nasal polyps an allergic phenomenon? *Ann Allergy* 1971; **29**(12): 631–4.
10. Settipane GA, Chafee FH. Nasal polyps in asthma and rhinitis: a review of 6,037 patients. *J Allergy Clin Immunol* 1977; **59**(1): 17–21.
11. Bunnag C, Pacharee P, Vipulakom P, Siriyananda C. A study of allergic factor in nasal polyp patients. *Ann Allergy* 1983; **50**(2): 126–32.
12. Kern R. Allergy: a constant factor in the etiology of so-called mucous nasal polyps. *J Allergy* 1993; **4**: 483.
13. Delaney JC. Aspirin idiosyncrasy in patients admitted for nasal polypectomy. *Clin Otolaryngol* 1976; **1**(1): 27–30.
14. English G. Nasal polyposis. In: English GM, (ed). *Otolarygology*. Harper and Row, Philadelphia: 1985, pp. 1–30.
15. Slavin RG. Allergy is not a significant cause of nasal polyps. *Arch Otolaryngol Head Neck Surg* 1992; **118**: 771.
16. Bachert C, Gevaert P, Holtappels G, et al. Total and specific IgE in nasal polyps is related to local eosinophilic inflammation. *J Allergy Clin Immunol* 2001; **107**(4): 607–14.
17. Van Zele T, Gevaert P, Watelet JB, et al. Staphylococcus aureus colonization and IgE antibody formation to enterotoxins is increased in nasal polyposis. *J Allergy Clin Immunol* 2004; **114**: 981–3.
18. Zhang N, Holtappels G, Gevaert P, et al. Mucosal tissue polyclonal IgE is functional in response to allergen and SEB. *Allergy* 2011; **66**: 141–8.
19. Brook I, Frazier EH. Bacteriology of chronic maxillary sinusitis associated with nasal polyposis. *J Med Microbiol* 2005; **54**(6): 595–7.
20. Hashemi M, Sadeghi MM, Omrani MR, Torabi MA. Microbiology and antimicrobial resistance in chronic resistant rhinosinusitis with or without polyp after functional endoscopic sinus surgery. *J Res Med Sci* 2005; **10**(3): 167–71.
21. Araujo E, Palombini BC, Cantarelli V, et al. Microbiology of middle meatus in chronic rhinosinusitis. *Am J Rhinol* 2003; **17**(1): 9–15.
22. Bachert C, van Zele T, Gevaert P, et al. Superantigens and nasal polyps. *Curr Allergy Asthma Rep* 2003; **3**(6): 523–31.
23. Conley DB, Tripathi A, Seiberling KA, et al. Superantigens and chronic rhinosinusitis II: analysis of T-cell receptor V beta domains in nasal polyps. *Am J Rhinol* 2006; **20**(4): 451–5.
24. Tripathi A, Kern R, Conley DB, et al. Staphylococcal exotoxins and nasal polyposis: analysis of systemic and local responses. *Am J Rhinol* 2005; **19**(4): 327–33.
25. Bernstein JM, Ballow M, Schlievert PM, et al. A superantigen hypothesis for the pathogenesis of chronic hyperplastic sinusitis with massive nasal polyposis. *Am J Rhinol* 2003; **17**(6): 321–6.
26. Van Zele T, Vaneechoutte M, Holtappels G, et al. Detection of enterotoxin DNA in Staphylococcus aureus strains obtained from the middle meatus in controls and nasal polyp patients. *Am J Rhinol* 2008; **22**(3): 223–7.
27. Van Cauwenberge P, Gevaert P, Van Hoecke H, et al. New insights into the pathology of nasal polyposis: the role of superantigens and IgE. *Verb K Acad Geneeskd Belg* 2005; **67**(1): 5–28.
28. Seiberling KA, Conley DB, Tripathi A, et al. Superantigens and chronic rhinosinusitis: Detection of staphylococcal exotoxins in nasal polyps. *Laryngoscope* 2005; **115**(9): 1580–5.
29. Al-Daccak R, Mehindate K, Damdoumi F, et al. Staphylococcal enterotoxin D is a promiscuous superantigen offering multiple modes of interactions with the MHC class II receptors. *J Immunol* 1998; **160**(1): 225–32.
30. Herman A, Kappler JW, Marrack P, Pullen AM. Superantigens: mechanism of T-cell stimulation and role in immune responses. *Annu Rev Immunol* 1991; **9**: 745–72.
31. Bachert C, Zhang N, Holtappels G, et al. Presence of IL-5 protein and IgE antibodies to staphylococcal enterotoxins in nasal polyps is associated with comorbid asthma. *J Allergy Clin Immunol* 2010; **126**(5): 962–8, 8 e1–6.
32. Sanclement JA, Webster P, Thomas J, Ramadan HH. Bacterial biofilms in surgical specimens of patients with chronic rhinosinusitis. *Laryngoscope* 2005; **115**(4): 578–82.
33. Sanderson AR, Leid JG, Hunsaker D. Bacterial biofilms on the sinus mucosa of human subjects with chronic rhinosinusitis. *Laryngoscope* 2006; **116**(7): 1121–6.
34. Sun Y, Zhou B, Wang C, et al. Clinical and histopathologic features of Biofilm associated chronic rhinosinusitis with nasal polyps in Chinese patients. *Chin Med J* 2012; **125**(6): 1104–9.
35. Cohen M, Kofonow J, Nayak JV, et al. Biofilms in chronic rhinosinusitis: a review. *Am J Rhinol Allergy* 2009; **23**(3): 255–60.
36. Hedman J, Kaprio J, Poussa T, Nieminen MM. Prevalence of asthma, aspirin intolerance, nasal polyposis and chronic obstructive pulmonary disease in a population-based study. *Int J Epidemiol* 1999; **28**(4): 717–22.
37. Picado C. Aspirin intolerance and nasal polyposis. *Curr Allergy Asthma Rep* 2002; **2**: 488–93.

38. Castano R, Bosse Y, Endam LM, et al. Evidence of association of interleukin-1 receptor-like 1 gene polymorphisms with chronic rhinosinusitis. *Am J Rhinol Allergy* 2009; **23**: 377–84.
39. Kilty SJ, Bosse Y, Cormier C, et al. Polymorphisms in the SERPINA1 (Alpha-1-Antitrypsin) gene are associated with severe chronic rhinosinusitis unresponsive to medical therapy. *Am J Rhinol Allergy* 2010; **24**: e49.
40. Larsen K. The clinical relationship of nasal polyps to asthma. *Allergy Proc* 1996; **17**(5): 243–9.
41. Fasano MB. Combined airways: impact of upper airways on lower airway. *Curr Opin Otolaryngol Head Neck Surg* 2010; **18**: 15–20.
42. Szczeklik A, Nizankowska E, Duplaga M. Natural history of aspirin-induced asthma. AIANE Investigators. European Networkon Aspirin-Induced Asthma. *Eur Respir J* 2000; **16**(3): 432–6.
43. Bachert C, Gevaert P, Holtappels G, et al. Nasal polyposis: from cytokines to growth. *Am J Rhinol* 2000; **14**: 279–90.
44. Poynter ME, Cloots R, van Woerkom T, et al. NF-kappa B activation in airways modulates allergic inflammation but not hyperresponsiveness. *J Immunol* 2004; **173**: 7003–9.
45. McGee HS, Agrawal DK. Naturally occurring and inducible T-regulatory cells modulating immune resonse in allergic asthma. *Am J Resp Crit Care* 2009; **180**: 211–25.
46. Mattos JL, Woodard CR, Payne SC. Trends in common rhinologic illnesses: analysis of U.S. healthcare surveys 1995–2007. *Int Forum Allergy Rhinol* 2011; **1**: 3–12.
47. Knight A. Desensitization to aspirin in aspirin-sensitive patients with rhino-sinusitis and asthma: a review. *J Otolaryngol* 1989; **18**(4): 165–7.
48. McMains KC, Kountakis SE. Medical and surgical considerations in patients with Samter's Triad. *Am J Rhinol* 2006; **20**(6): 573–6.
49. Chen BS, Virant FS, Parikh SR, Manning SC. Aspirin sensitivity syndrome (Samter's Triad): an unrecognized disorder in children with nasal polyposis International *J Pediatr Otorhinolaryngol* 2013; **77**(2): 281–3.
50. Mendelsohn D, Jeremic G, Wright ED, Rotenberg BW. Revision rates after endoscopic sinus surgery: a recurrence analysis *Ann Otol Rhinol Laryngol* 2011; **120**(3): 162–6.
51. Arikan OK, Unal B, Kazkayasi M, Koc C. The analysis of anterior skull base from two different perspectives: coronal and reconstructed sagittal computed tomography. *Rhinology* 2005; **43**(2): 115–20.
52. Safirstein B. Allergic bronchopulmonary aspergillosis with obstruction of the upper respiratory tract. *Chest* 1976; **70**: 788–90.
53. Glass D, Amedee RG. Allergic fungal rhinosinusitis: a review. *Ochsner J* 2011; **11**(3): 271–5.
54. Bent JP, 3rd, Kuhn FA. Diagnosis of allergic fungal sinusitis. *Otolaryngol Head Neck Surg* 1994; **111**(5): 580–8.
55. Cystic Fibrosis Trust. www.cysticfibrosis.org.uk [Accessed 29 Jan 2018]
56. Ponikau JU, Sherris DA, Kern EB, et al. The diagnosis and incidence of allergic fungal sinusitis. *Mayo Clinic Proc* 1999; **74**(9): 877–84.
57. Riordan JR, Rommens JM, Kerem B, et al. Identification of the cystic fibrosis gene: cloning and characterization of complementary DNA. *Science* 1989; **245**: 1066–73.
58. Tandon R, Derkay C. Contemporary management of rhinosinusitis and cystic fibrosis. *Curr Opin Otolaryngol Head Neck Surg* 2003; **11**: 41–4.
59. Ryan MW. Diseases associated with chronic rhinosinusitis: what is the significance? *Curr Opin Otolaryngol Head Neck Surg* 2008; **16**: 231–6.
60. Gentile VG, Isaacson G. Patterns of sinusitis in cystic fibrosis. *Laryngoscope* 1996; **106**: 1005–9.
61. Scapa VI, Ramakrishnan VR, Kingdom TT. Upregulation of Bcl-2 in nasal polyps from patients with cystic fibrosis. *Int Forum Allergy Rhinol* 2013; **3**(3): 199–203.
62. Shapiro ED, Milmoe GJ, Wald ER, et al. Bacteriology of the maxillary sinuses in patients with cystic fibrosis. *J Infect Dis* 1982; **146**: 589–93.
63. Digoya GP, Dunna JD, Stonera JA, et al. Bacteriology of the paranasal sinuses in pediatric cystic fibrosis patients. *Int J Pediatr Otorhinolaryngol* 2012; **76**(7): 934–8.
64. Hui Y, Gaffney R, Crysdale WS. Sinusitis in patients with cystic fibrosis. *Eur Arch Otorhinolaryngol* 1995; **252**: 191–6.
65. Ledesma-Medina J, Osman MZ, Girdany BR. Abnormal paranasal sinuses in patients with cystic fibrosis of the pancreas: radiological findings. *Pediatr Radiol* 1980; **9**: 61–4.
66. Neely JG, Harrison GM, Jerger JF, et al. The otolaryngologic aspects of cystic fibrosis. *Trans Am Acad Ophthalmol Otolaryngol* 1972; **76**: 313–24.
67. Woodworth BA, Ahn C, Flume PA, Schlosser RJ. The delta F508 mutation in cystic fibrosis and impact on sinus development. *Am J Rhinol* 2007; **21**: 122–7.
68. Seifert CM, Harvey RJ, Mathews JW, et al. Temporal bone pneumatisation and its relationship to paranasal sinus development in cystic fibrosis. *Rhinology* 2010; **48**: 233–8.
69. Guttenplan MD, Wetmore RF. Paranasal sinus mucocele in cystic fibrosis. *Clin Pediatr (Phila)* 1989; **28**: 429–30.
70. Tunkel DE, Naclerio RM, Baroody FM, Rosenstein BJ. Bilateral maxillary sinus mucoceles in an infant with cystic fibrosis. *Otolaryngol Head Neck Surg* 1994; **111**: 116–20.
71. Bush A, Cole P, Hariri M, et al. Primary ciliary dyskinesia: diagnosis and standards of care. *Eur Respir J* 1998; **12**: 982–8.
72. Arya AK, Beer HL, Benton J, et al. Does Young's syndrome exist? *J Laryngol Otol* 2009; **123**: 477–81.
73. Handelsman DJ, Conway AJ, Boylan LM, Turtle JR. Young's syndrome: obstructive azoospermia and chronic sinopulmonary infections. *N Engl J Med* 1984; **310**: 3–9.
74. Armengot M, Juan G, Carda C, et al. Young's syndrome: a further cause of chronic rhinosinusitis. *Rhinology* 1996; **34**: 35.
75. Hasegawa A, Ohe M, Yamazaki K, et al. A rare case of Young's syndrome in Japan. *Intern Med* 1994; **33**: 649–53.
76. Shiraishi K, Ono N, Eguchi S, et al. Young's syndrome associated with situs inversus totalis. *Arch Androl* 2004; **50**: 169–72.
77. Hendry WF, Levison DA, Parkinson MC, et al. Testicular obstruction: clinicopathological studies. *Ann R Coll Surg Engl* 1990; **72**: 396–407.
78. Brown JR, Kulkarni MV. A review of the toxicity and metabolism of mercury and its compounds. *Med Serv J Can* 1967; **23**: 786–808.
79. Vaglio A, Casazza I, Grasselli C, et al. Churg–Strauss syndrome. *Kidney Int* 2009; **76**: 1006–11.
80. Noth I, Strek ME, Leff AR. Churg–Strauss syndrome. *Lancet* 2003; **361**: 587–94.
81. Masi AT, Hunder GG, Lie JT, et al. The American College of Rheumatology 1990 criteria for the classification of Churg-Strauss syndrome (allergic granulomatosis and angiitis). *Arthritis Rheum* 1990; **33**: 1094–100.
82. Vaglio A, Buzio C, Zwerina J. Eosinophilic granulomatosis with polyangiitis (Churg–Strauss): state of the art. *Allergy* 2013; **68**: 261–73.
83. Rugina M, Serrano E, Klossek JM, et al. Epidemiological and clinical aspects of nasal polyposis in France; the ORLI group experience. *Rhinology* 2002; **40**(2): 75–9.
84. Alexiou A, Sourtzi P, Dimakopoulo K, et al. Nasal polyps: heredity, allergies, and environmental and occupational exposure. *J Otolaryngol Head Neck Surg* 2011; **40**(1): 58–63.
85. Mfuna-Endam L, Zhang Y, Desrosiers MY. Genetics of rhinosinusitis. *Curr Allergy Asthma Rep* 2011; **11**(3): 236–46.
86. Lockey RF, Rucknagel DL, Vanselow NA. Familial occurrence of asthma, nasal polyps and aspirin intolerance. *Ann Intern Med* 1973; **78**(1): 57–63.
87. Jonas I, Mann W. Misleading x-ray diagnosis due to maxillary sinus asymmetries (author's transl). *Laryngol Rhinol Otol (Stuttg)* 1976; **55**(11): 905–13.
88. McAlister WH, Lusk R, Muntz HR. Comparison of plain radiographs and coronal CT scans in infants and children with recurrent sinusitis. *Am J Roentgenol* 1989; **153**(6): 1259–64.
89. Iinuma T, Hirota Y, Kase Y. Radio-opacity of the paranasal sinuses: conventional views and CT. *Rhinology* 1994; **32**(3): 134–6.
90. Erdem C, Erdem T, Miman MC, Ozturan O. A radiological anatomic study of the cribriform plate compared with constant structures. *Rhinology* 2004; **42**(4): 225–9.
91. Arikan OK, Unal B, Kazkayasi M, Koc C. The analysis of anterior skull base from two different perspectives: coronal and reconstructed sagittal computed tomography. *Rhinology* 2005; **43**(2): 115–20.
92. Kazkayasi M, Karadeniz Y, Arikan OK. Anatomic variations of the sphenoid sinus on computed tomography. *Rhinology* 2005; **43**(2): 109–14.
93. Ottaviano G, Scadding GK, Coles S, Lund VJ. Peak nasal inspiratory flow; normal range in adult population. *Rhinology* 2006; **44**(1): 32–5.
94. Lund VJ, Scadding GK. Objective assessment of endoscopic sinus surgery in the management of chronic rhinosinusitis: an update. *J Laryngol Otol* 1994; **108**(9): 749–53.
95. Ragab SM, Lund VJ, Scadding G. Evaluation of the medical and surgical treatment of chronic rhinosinusitis: a prospective, randomised, controlled trial. *Laryngoscope* 2004; **114**(5): 923–30.

96. Koo Ng NK, Young D, McGarry GW. Reversible nasal airway obstruction: does change in nasal peak inspiratory flow following decongestion predict response to topical steroids in chronic rhinosinusitis patients? *J Laryngol Otol* 2012; 126(12): 1238–40.
97. Lund VJ, Kennedy DW. Quantification for staging sinusitis. In: Kennedy DW. International Conference on Sinus Disease: Terminology, Staging, Therapy. *Ann Otol Rhinol Laryngol* 1995; **104**(Suppl 167): 17–21.
98. Johansson L, Akerlund A, Holmberg K, et al. Evaluation of methods for endoscopic staging of nasal polyposis. *Acta Otolaryngol* 2000; **120**(1): 72–6.
98. Lund VJ, Mackay IS. Staging in rhinosinusitus. *Rhinology* 1993; **31**(4): 183–4.
100. Xaubet A, Mullol J, Lopez E, et al. Comparison of the role of nasal polyp and normal nasal mucosal epithelial cells on in vitro eosinophil survival: mediation by GM-CSF and inhibition by dexamethasone. *Clin Exp Allergy* 1994; **24**(4): 307–17.
101. Mullol J, Xaubet A, Gaya A, et al. Cytokine gene expression and release from epithelial cells: a comparison study between healthy nasal mucosa and nasal polyps. *Clin Exp Allergy* 1995; **25**(7): 607–15.
102. Benitez P, Alobid I, de Haro J, et al. A short course of oral prednisone followed by intranasal budesonide is an effective treatment of severe nasal polyps. *Laryngoscope* 2006; **116**(5): 770–5.
103. Bernstein JM, Gorfien J, Noble B. Role of allergy in nasal polyposis: a review. *Otolaryngol Head Neck Surg* 1995; **113**(6): 724–32.
104. Blomqvist EH, Lundblad L, Anggard A, et al. A randomized controlled study evaluating medical treatment versus surgical treatment in addition to medical treatment of nasal polyposis. *J Allergy Clin Immunol* 2001; **107**(2): 224–8.
105. Bachert C, Hormann K, Mosges R, et al. An update on the diagnosis and treatment of sinusitis and nasal polyposis. *Allergy* 2003; **58**: 176–91.
106. Gevaert P, Lang-Loidolt D, Lackner A, et al. Nasal IL-5 levels determine the response to ant-IL-5 treatment in patients with nasal polyps. *J Allergy Clin Immunol* 2006; **118**: 1133–41.
107. Bateman ND, Fahy C, Woolford TJ. Nasal polyps: still more questions than answers. *J Laryngol Otol* 2003; **117**(1): 1–9.
108. Patel RS, Wallace AM, Hinnie J, McGarry GW. Preliminary results of a pilot study investigating the potential of salivary cortisol measurements to detect occult adrenal suppression secondary to steroid nose drops. *Clin Otolaryngol Allied Sci* 2001; **26**(3): 231–4.
109. Cervin A. The anti-inflammatory effect of erythromycin and its derivatives, with special reference to nasal polyposis and chronic sinusitis. *Acta Otolaryngologica* 2001; **121**: 83–92.
110. Svanström H, Pasternak B, Hviid A. Use of clarithromycin and roxithromycin and risk of cardiac death: cohort study. *BMJ* 2014; **349**: g4930.
111. Lund VJ. Evidence-based surgery in chronic rhinosinusitis. *Acta Otolaryngol* 2001; **121**(1): 5–9.
112. Khalil HS, Nunez DA. Functional endoscopic sinus surgery for chronic rhinosinusitis. 2006; *Cochrane Database Syst Rev* 3: CD004458.
113. Mehanna H, Mills J, Kelly B, McGarry GW. Benefit from endoscopic sinus surgery. *Ann Otol Rhinol Laryngol* 1996; **105**: 415–22.

FUNGAL RHINOSINUSITIS

Eng Cern Gan and Amin R. Javer

Introduction 1047	*Invasive FRS* *1055*
Non-invasive FRS *1047*	Acute (fulminant) invasive FRS 1055
Saprophytic fungal infection 1047	Granulomatous invasive FRS 1056
Fungal ball 1048	Chronic invasive FRS 1056
Fungus-related eosinophilic FRS including allergic fungal rhinosinusitis (AFRS) 1048	Conclusion 1057
	References 1057

SEARCH STRATEGY

Data in this chapter may be updated by a PubMed and Medline search using the following keywords: fungal rhinosinusitis, fungal ball, mycetoma, allergic fungal rhinosinusitis, invasive fungal rhinosinusitis.

INTRODUCTION

Fungal rhinosinusitis (FRS) can be categorized into two broad groups; invasive and non-invasive.[1] This is based on the presence or absence of fungus in the tissue (mucosa, blood vessel or bone) respectively.[2]

NON-INVASIVE FRS

SAPROPHYTIC FUNGAL INFECTION

Saprophytic fungal infection refers to visible fungal colonization of mucus crusts seen within the nose and paranasal sinuses on nasoendoscopy (**Figure 96.1**).[3, 4] These patients are usually asymptomatic or may present with a foul smelling odour.[2] The proposed mechanism is dysfunction in mucociliary transportation from surgery leading to crust formation. The crust then acts as a platform for growth of fungal spores.[3] It has been suggested that saprophytic fungal infections may be precursors to fungal balls if left untreated.[3] Endoscopic cleaning of the infected crust with or without continued self-irrigation with saline is usually the only treatment required.[3]

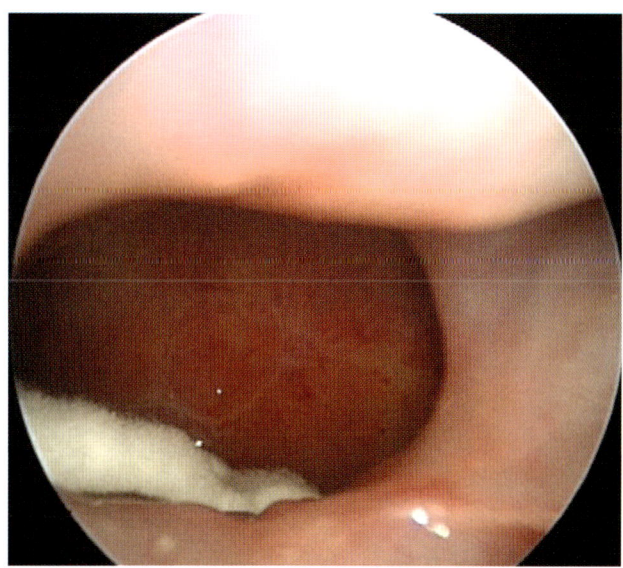

Figure 96.1 Saprophytic fungal infection where visible fungus is seen growing on mucosal crust.

FUNGAL BALL

A fungal ball is a dense accumulation of extramucosal fungal hyphae, usually within one sinus, most commonly the maxillary sinus.[2] Although the most common organism in a fungal ball is *Aspergillus*, the cultures are often negative and other fungal species have also been identified.[2] Fungal balls are seen more commonly in immunocompetent, middle-aged and elderly females, often with a history of previous dental procedure, especially dental fillings.[2]

The diagnosis of fungal ball is based on the following features: radiological findings of sinus opacification often with areas of hyperattenuation, cheesy or clay-like debris within the sinus (**Figure 96.2a and 96.2b**), accumulation of fungal hyphae without evidence of tissue fungal invasion seen microscopically, non-specific chronic inflammation of the sinus and the absence of eosinophil predominance, granuloma or allergic mucin.[1]

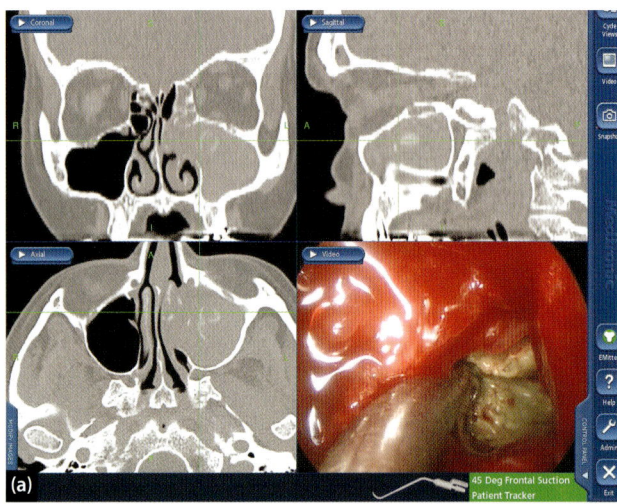

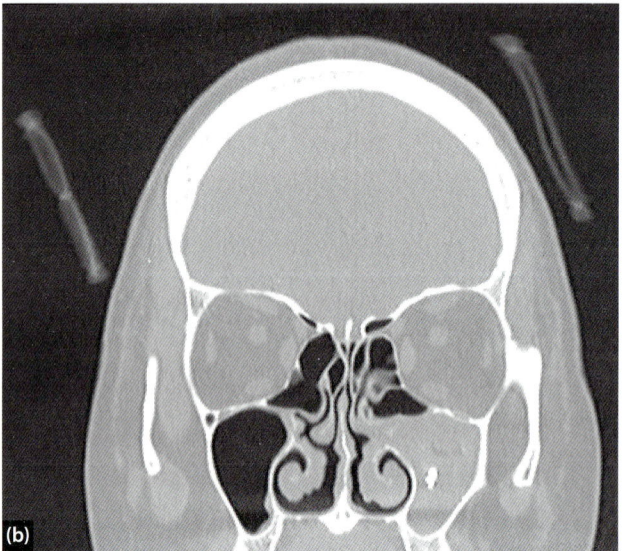

Figure 96.2(a–b) (a) Image guidance system (IGS) CT images of a left maxillary sinus fungal ball showing areas of hyperattenuation. (b) A centrally located calcification within a completely opacified left maxillary sinus from a fungal ball. The calcification is due to metabolic deposits of calcium within the fungal concretions.

The management involves a wide opening of the involved sinus and complete removal of the fungal debris. Examination of the involved sinuses with angled scopes is crucial to ensure complete surgical extirpation. Subsequent regular surveillance in the clinic is necessary. Oral or topical antifungals are not necessary.

FUNGUS-RELATED EOSINOPHILIC FRS INCLUDING ALLERGIC FUNGAL RHINOSINUSITIS (AFRS)

Introduction

AFRS is a non-invasive fungal sinusitis resulting from an allergic and immunologic response to the presence of extramucosal fungal hyphae in the sinuses. It was first recognized as an upper airway manifestation of allergic bronchopulmonary aspergillosis (ABPA) in the 1970s.[5] Although *Aspergillus* was the presumed pathogen in the first few early case series, subsequent case series showed that dematiaceous fungi such as *Bipolaris*, *Curvularis* and *Alternaria* were more common.[6]

Epidemiology

The prevalence of FRS amongst chronic rhinosinusitis (CRS) patients who undergo surgery is between 12 and 47%.[7, 8] Of this, AFRS is the most common form, accounting for between 56 and 72% of patients with FRS.[7, 8] The typical AFRS patients are young immunocompetent adults.[9] The mean age at presentation is between 21 and 33 years old.[10] There is a higher male to female ratio of between 1.5 and 2.6 to 1.[10] Wise et al. found that AFRS patients also have a lower socioeconomic status and a higher African American ratio compared to CRS patients.[10]

Pathophysiology

Although it has been over 30 years since AFRS was first described, the underlying pathophysiology remains unknown and controversial. A number of popular theories have evolved. Manning et al. proposed a mechanism derived from the ABPA model.[11] Based on studies demonstrating raised fungal-specific IgE antibodies and IgG antibodies in AFRS patients, it is believed that an atopic host exposed to fungi resulted in antigenic stimulation by a combination of Gell and Coombs type I and type III hypersensitivity.[11, 12]

While the immunologic theory proposed by Manning et al. is supported in the literature, it fails to explain the unilateral or asymmetric nature of AFRS, the persistence of a raised IgE level after prolonged fungal immunotherapy and the failure of a rise in specific IgG levels resulting from the formation of IgG-blocking antibodies following fungal immunotherapy.[13] An alternative theory was later proposed by Panikou et al.[14] Their landmark but non-peer-reviewed paper stated that fungi were present in the nasal secretions of 96% (202 patients) of consecutive CRS patients and 100% (14 patients) of healthy volunteers with no sinus disease. Elevated total and specific IgE levels were not prevalent amongst the AFRS patients and not significantly different to that of the control group. Hence, they rejected the role of an IgE-mediated reaction in the pathogenesis of AFRS. Rather, eosinophilic chemotaxis in response to extramucosal fungi was the hallmark of the inflammatory reaction in AFRS. The term **eosinophilic fungal rhinosinusitis** (EFRS) was introduced. Similarly, the term **eosinophilic mucin** was suggested as a replacement for **allergic mucin** to emphasize the importance of eosinophils in the pathophysiology of AFRS. However, the eosinophilic theory does not explain the triggering factor for eosinophil chemotaxis.

In 2000, Ferguson performed a literature review and concluded that there may be two different disease processes in play: allergic and non-allergic fungal rhinosinusitis.[15] The term **eosinophilic mucin rhinosinusitis** (EMRS) was used to describe non-allergic fungal sinusitis. These patients were felt to have histological features similar to AFRS but without the presence of fungus. The underlying mechanism was believed to be a systemic dysregulation of immunologic controls resulting in upper and lower airway eosinophilia. By recognizing EMRS and AFRS as two separate entities with a similar phenotypic endpoint, the treatment strategies for these patients can be formulated according to their pathogenesis. Antifungal agents and fungal immunotherapy should theoretically benefit only AFRS and not EMRS patients.[15]

Diagnostic criteria

In 1994, Bent and Kuhn described a diagnostic criteria for AFRS based on 15 consecutive AFRS patients.[16] They found 11 important clinical features, 5 of which were present in all 15 patients. These 5 features were termed major criteria and the remaining 6 features as minor criteria. All 5 major criteria were necessary to define AFRS while the minor criteria were considered supporting features (Box 96.1). These criteria set the benchmark for diagnosis of AFRS for many years with minor variations proposed over the years.

There exists a subgroup of patients who do not meet all five major criteria but behave like AFRS patients and respond to AFRS treatment strategies (previously known as **atypical AFRS**). We have therefore adopted the Bent and Kuhn criteria with minor modifications to be more inclusive. An elevated IgE level is not always present in all AFRS patients and may fluctuate within the normal range as the disease stage changes.[9, 17] We currently utilize the following five major criteria to diagnose patients with AFRS (Box 96.2).

BOX 96.2 St Paul's Sinus Center Diagnostic Criteria for AFRS

Major criteria
- Immunocompetent patient
- Presence of nasal polyposis
- Characteristic CT findings
- Presence of allergic mucin
- Positive fungal cultures or the presence of fungal hyphae on fungal staining

Clinical presentation

Although there are no pathognomonic symptoms for AFRS, clinical suspicion should be high when one encounters a young patient with uni- or bi-lateral nasal polyposis with thick, sticky yellow/green mucus, characteristic double density sign on CT and who responds to oral steroids. Often, the symptoms are subtle and similar to that of chronic sinusitis with nasal polyposis.[18] On nasoendoscopy, inspissatted thick yellow or brown peanut-butter like mucus may be seen among the polyps (Figure 96.3a–c).

Investigation

IMMUNOLOGIC TEST

Patients with AFRS have an elevated IgE level. In a long term follow-up of AFRS patients by Marple et al. the total IgE levels were found to be between 50 and >1000 IU/ml. The average total IgE level was about 550 IU/mL. Because of the wide range of total serum IgE levels in AFRS patients, it is not useful as a screening tool.[19] However, total serum IgE level may be useful in monitoring clinical activity in the management of AFRS.[17] An *in-vivo* (skin prick) or *in-vitro* (RAST) test can be utilized to demonstrate fungal specific IgE as a diagnostic criteria for AFRS.[20, 21]

IMAGING – COMPUTED TOMOGRAPHY (CT) AND MAGNETIC RESONANT IMAGING (MRI) SCANS

AFRS patients have typical features that are present on an unenhanced CT and enhanced MRI scans of the paranasal sinuses (Box 96.3).[22, 23]

CT without contrast is the imaging of choice in suspect patients. The focal or diffuse areas of hyperintensity seen on CT are due to calcium and manganese deposits in the necrotic debri of the fungus and allergic mucin.[22] This results in a 'double density' or rail-track sign, (Figure 96.4). The optimum setting in the bone protocol

BOX 96.1 Bent and Kuhn Diagnostic Criteria for AFRS

Major criteria	Minor criteria
• Evidence of type I IgE–mediated hypersensitivity • Nasal polyposis • Characteristic CT findings • Eosinophilic mucus • Positive fungal smear	• Asthma • Unilateral predominance • Radiographic bone erosion • Fungal culture • Charcot-Leyden crystals • Serum eosinophilia

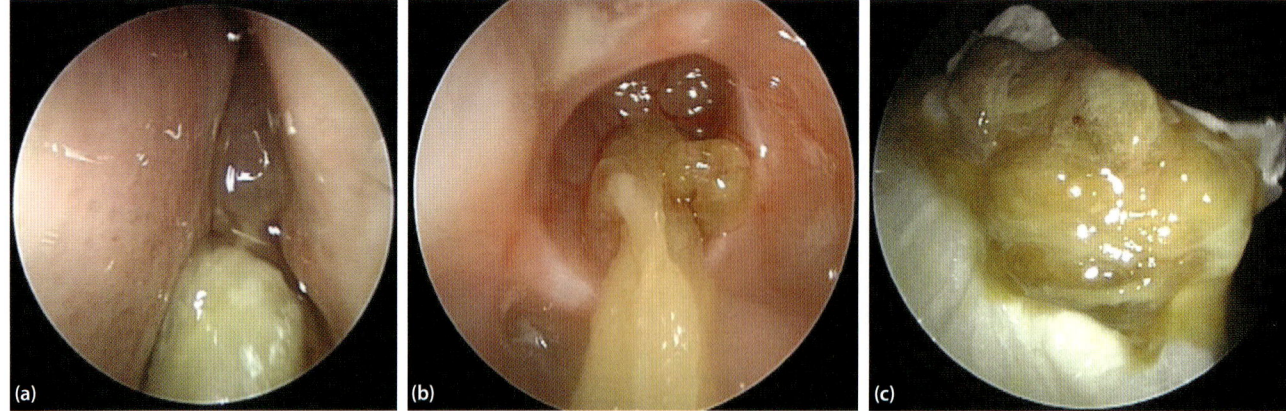

Figure 96.3(a–c) Clinical appearance of AFRS. **(a)** Nasoendoscopic picture of the left nasal cavity of an AFRS patient with allergic mucin covering a nasal polyp. **(b)** Allergic mucin is being suctioned out from the left sphenoid sinus. **(c)** Gross appearance of allergic mucin.

BOX 96.3 Characteristic findings of AFRS on CT and MRI scans of the paranasal sinuses

CT features	MRI features
• Heterogenous signal intensities within the paranasal sinuses filled with allergic mucin ('double density sign') • Expansion of the paranasal sinuses/nasal cavity • Unilateral or asymmetric disease load • Bony erosion	• T1 weighted images – central areas of hypointensity with peripheral enhancement • T2 weighted images – central areas of hypointensity or signal void with peripheral enhancement

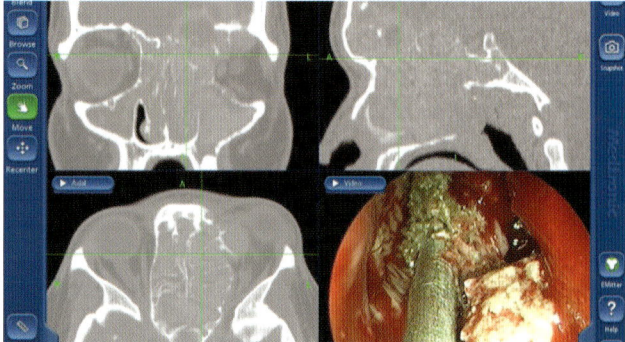

Figure 96.4 IGS CT images of a patient with extensive AFRS. There is a large erosion of the left skull base with intra-cranial extension as well as erosion of the left lamina papyracea. There is complete opacification of all sinuses with heterogeneity in signal intensity that is most obvious in the left maxillary sinus ('double density' sign).

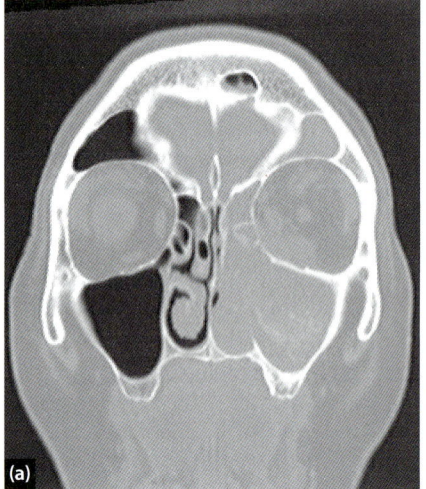 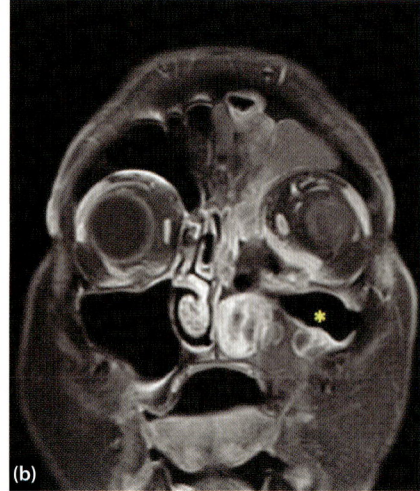 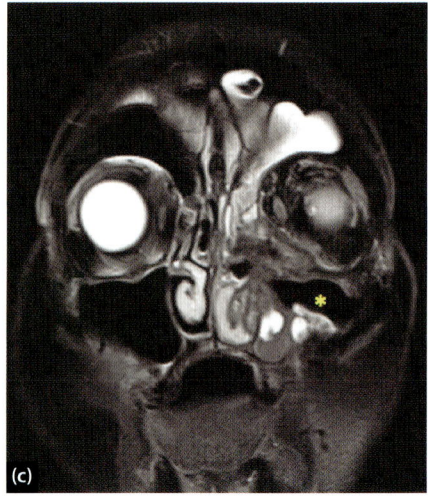

Figure 96.5(a–c) Radiographic imaging of a patient with chronic invasive fungal rhinosinusitis with fungal concretions in the left maxillary sinus. **(a)** Coronal cut of a CT scan showed complete opacification of the left maxillary sinus with areas of hyperattenuation, suggestive of fungal concretions. **(b & c)** Coronal cut of a T1–weighted MRI **(b)** and T2–weighted image **(c)** of the same patient showing a signal void (asterisk) from the fungal concretions in the left maxillary sinus. The signal void is due to heavy metals (iron, magnesium and manganese) within the fungal concretions.

to accentuate this sign is a window width of ~2000 House unit (HU) and centred at ~−250/−200.[24]

MRI of the paranasal sinus with intra-venous gadolinium contrast can be considered when the diagnosis of AFRS is uncertain or if there are concerns with rare intra-cranial or intra-orbital complications. The protein content and viscosity of the secretion will determine the signal intensity seen on MRI. In fungal infections, the consistency of the secretion usually results in a low intensity on T1 and a much lower intensity to signal void on T2 (**Figure 96.5**a–c).[22] This is due to higher concentration of iron and manganese as well as calcium deposits within the fungal concretions.[23]

HISTOLOGY

The hallmark of AFRS is the presence of allergic mucin. Grossly, it is thick, tenacious and highly viscous in consistency.[18] Hence, the terms 'peanut butter' and 'axle-grease' are often used to describe the characteristic appearance of the mucus. Histologically, allergic mucin consists of an eosinophilic mucin with necrotic eosinophils, inflammatory cells, Charcot-Leyden crystals (the by-product of eosinophil) and fungal hyphae (**Figure 96.6**a).[25] As fungal hyphae are infrequent and scattered within allergic mucin, their detection is difficult unless specific stains with a silver stain such as Grocott's or Gomori's methamine silver (GMS) stain are performed (**Figure 96.6**b).[18]

FUNGAL CULTURE

A positive fungal culture provides supporting evidence in the diagnosis of AFRS. However, its absence does not exclude the diagnosis of AFRS. The presence of a positive fungal culture in AFRS patients ranged from 49 to 100%, depending on the culture method used.[6, 12, 14, 26, 27] In our institution, positive fungal cultures were obtained in 64% of AFRS patients using a modified Mayo Clinic fungal culture technique. Likewise, a positive fungal culture does not confirm the diagnosis of AFRS. The histological identification of allergic mucin is still the most reliable marker for the diagnosis of AFRS.[18]

Management

Once a diagnosis of AFRS has been established, patients are enrolled into a committed long-term management program with regular and long-term follow-up considered critical to the success of the treatment. A combination of surgery with a comprehensive post-operative medical regimen to keep the disease under control is almost always required.[28]

SURGICAL TREATMENT

Unlike the management of classical CRS, surgery is usually the first line treatment in the management of AFRS. Meticulous and complete endoscopic sinus surgery is the gold standard for the surgical extirpation of polypoid disease and allergic mucin in an attempt to restore ventilation and drainage of the sinuses.[9] Removal of allergic mucin and fungal debris eliminates the antigenic factor that incites the disease in an atopic host. Surgery also provides wide access for surveillance, clinical debridement and application of topical medication. In our center, functional endoscopic sinus surgery (FESS) for AFRS patients is routinely carried out with image-guidance system (IGS). We feel that the use of IGS allows complete removal of diseased cells in the sinuses and minimizes the risk of complications from distorted anatomy.

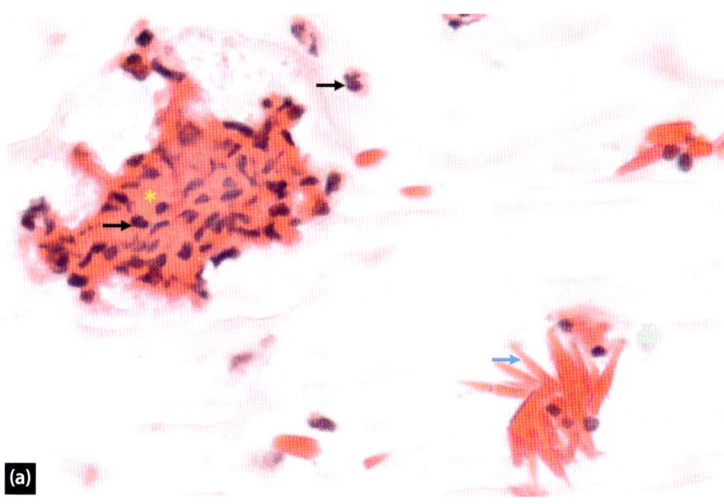
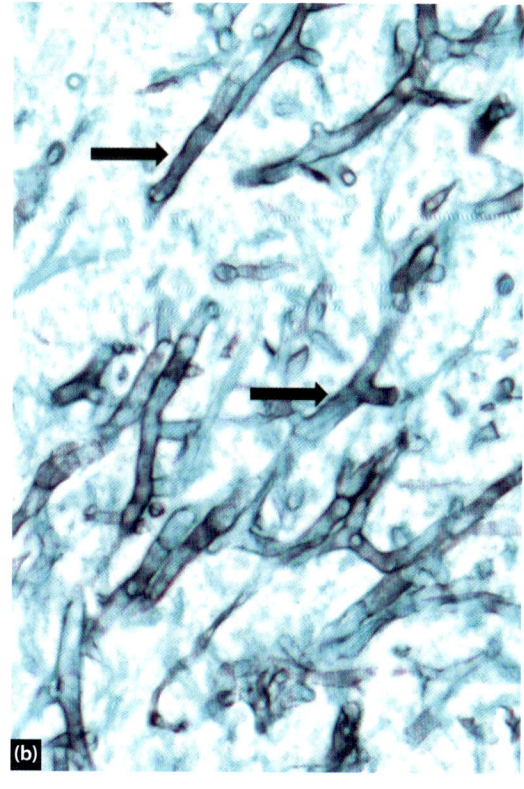

Figure 96.6(a–b) Histology of allergic mucin and fungal hyphae. (a) H&E stain of allergic mucin showing eosinophils (black arrows), eosinophil aggregate (yellow asterisk) and Charcot-Leyden crystals (blue arrow) on a mucinous background. **(b)** Fungal hyphae (black arrows) with 45° branching and septation typical of *Aspergillus sp*. (GSM stain). Slides are courtesy of Dr Blair Walker, Department of Pathology and Laboratory Medicine, University of British Columbia, Vancouver, Canada.

ENDOSCOPIC STAGING OF MUCOSAL DISEASE POST-SURGERY

Regular follow-up and accurate documentation of the sinonasal mucosa of AFRS patients after surgery is critical to monitor disease status and response to adjunctive medical treatments. Kupferberg et al. devised a 4-stage system for endoscopic follow-up in these patients post-surgery (Table 96.1).[30] However, the Kupferberg staging system lacks sensitivity, often resulting in patients remaining in the same endoscopic stage despite having improved symptomatically and endoscopically. In 2010, Philpott et al. introduced a new endoscopic staging system for AFRS. The Philpott-Javer system[30] is a validated mucosal staging system that was derived from modifications made to the Kupferberg system. Such a system is much more sensitive and allows for much better tracking of disease control post-operatively (**Figure 96.7**).

TABLE 96.1 Kupferberg post-operative endoscopic staging system for AFRS

Stage	Endoscopic finding
I	Normal mucosa
II	Mucosal oedema/allergic mucin
III	Polypoid oedema/allergic mucin
IV	Sinus polyps and fungal debris

Medical treatment

SYSTEMIC MEDICATIONS

I. Corticosteroids

Oral steroids are useful in the perioperative period of patients with AFRS. In the pre-operative period, a short course of coritcosteroids reduce intra-operative bleeding

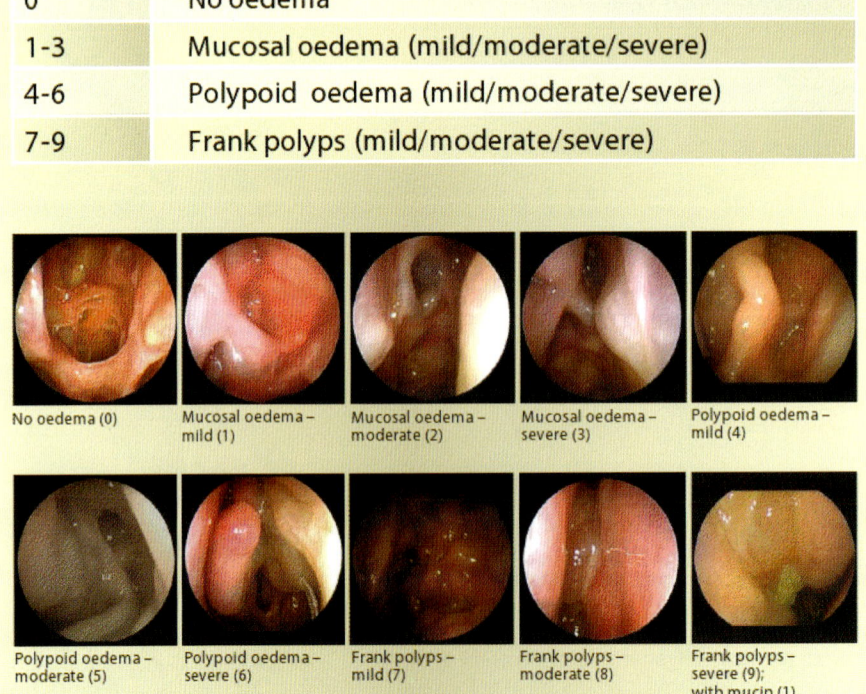

Figure 96.7 A clinic poster for the Philpott-Javer endoscopic staging system for AFRS.

and size of the polyps.[13] In a prospective comparative study by Landsberg et al, AFRS patients who received oral steroids pre-operatively showed greater radiologic and endoscopic improvement compared to CRSwNP patients.[31]

In the post-operative period, the corticosteroids regimen was initially derived from the protocol used in treatment of ABPA.[32] In a 4-year follow-up study of 11 AFRS patients by Kuhn and Javer, a reduction in IgE and mucosal disease post-operatively were seen in patients who were on steroids. They found that in order to prevent recurrence, a minimum of 6 months of normal sinus mucosa while on steroids is necessary before steroids can be slowly discontinued.[17] A 6-month post-operative regimen of tapering corticosteroid therapy was proposed by Kuhn and Javer, including the use of high-dose intra-nasal corticosteroids.[29]

Systemic steroids, although beneficial in the perioperative period, are not without adverse side effects. Although long-term oral corticosteroid may be necessary in some patients, its use should be judicious and limited to short courses in the perioperative period and in acute exacerbations of AFRS to suppress growth of recurrent polyps.[33]

II. Antifungals

Oral antifungals are considered a viable treatment option for patients with recalcitrant AFRS. They are also used as a steroid-sparing medication, allowing some patients to be weaned off from long-term oral corticosteroid therapy.[34] Early reports by Bent and Kuhn on the efficacy of oral antifungals in AFRS patients showed mixed to poor results.[35] However, subsequent retrospective case series showed that oral itraconazole (200–400 mg daily) has potential benefits as a steroid sparing alternative and in prolonging time to disease recurrence.[34, 36, 37] Oral itraconazole is associated with risk of elevated liver enzymes, congestive heart failure, nausea, rash, headache, malaise, fatigue and oedema (Janseen Pharmaceutica, Beerse, Belgium). Asymptomatic transaminitis is not uncommon (4–19%)[34, 36] and cessation of treatment is usually sufficient for the elevated liver enzymes to revert back to normal. It appears that a subset of AFRS patients seem to respond to antifungals. Future RCTs are needed to identify the ideal candidate and to assess the efficacy, safety and optimal dosage and regime for oral antifungals in the treatment of AFRS.

TOPICAL MEDICATION

I. Corticosteroid

Topical corticosteroids are used as standard treatment for patients with AFRS. They are most effective in the post-operative period when open sinus cavities and middle meati allow access to the paranasal sinuses. The benefit of topical over systemic steroid lies in the ability of topical steroid to achieve the highest drug concentration in the target tissue (sinonasal mucosa) without the undesirable systemic side effects.[38] Although studies on the efficacy of intra-nasal steroids in AFRS patients are lacking, their benefits have been well established in CRS patients with nasal polyposis.[39] An evidence-based review with recommendations based on Grade A evidence by Rudmik et al. provided a strong recommendation for the use of standard topical nasal steroids for the management of CRS.[40] Standard topical nasal steroids are metered-dose topical steroid solutions that have been approved for use in the nasal cavity by the U.S. Food and Drug Administration (FDA). These include metered-dose nasal sprays such as mometasone furoate, fluticasone propionate, fluticasone furoate, budesonide, beclomethasone dipropionate monohydrate, ciclesonide, flumisolide and triamcinolone acetonide.[40]

The use of budesonide administered as drops, atomized sprays or through low volume saline rinses have gained popularity in the treatment of AFRS patients. These are 'non-standard' topical nasal steroids and are not FDA approved for application in the nasal cavity. Other 'off-label' non-standard topical steroids that have been used in the sinonasal cavity include low-volume solutions such as intra-nasal dexamethasone ophthalmic drops (0.1%), prednisolone ophthalmic drops (1%) and ciprofloxacin/dexamethasone otic drops (0.3/0.15).[40] Non-standard topical nasals steroids have the advantage of delivering higher volume and/or high concentration of steroids into the sinonasal cavity. In the treatment of post-operative refractory CRS patients, topical budesonide (Pulmicort Respules) via the Mucosal Atomization Device (MAD; Wolfe-Tory Medical, Salt Lake City, UT) resulted in improvements in both physician and patient global assessments and also reduction in the use of oral prednisolone (**Figure 96.8**).[41]

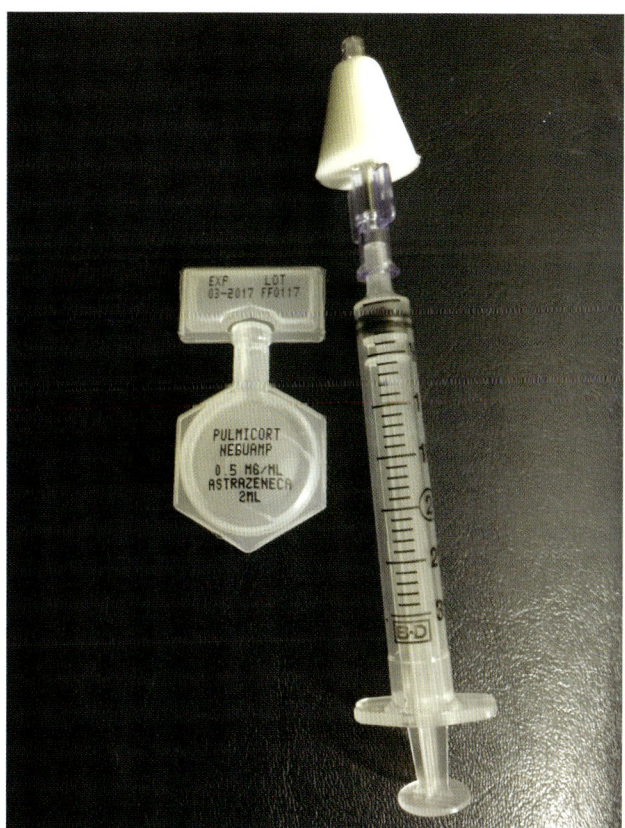

Figure 96.8 Pulmicort nebule and the MAD syringe.

The main concern of non-standard topical nasal steroids sprays is systemic absorption resulting in unwanted systemic side effects. In post-surgical CRS patients, Sachanandani et al. demonstrated that budesonide nasal irrigation (2.5 mg of budesonide diluted in 5 ml of normal saline in each nasal cavity) for 30 days improved clinical symptoms of CRS without hypothalamic-pituitary-adrenal (HPA) axis suppression.[42] A prospective study was conducted in our centre to determine if application of high dose budesonide (1 mg of Pulmicort Respules twice a day) via the MAD over 2 months causes HPA suppression and results in an increase in plasma cortisol and detection of plasma budesonide. The result of the ten patients subjected to high dose budesonide delivered via the MAD did not show any evidence of HPA suppression nor any elevation of plasma cortisol or presence of plasma budesonide.[43] Hence, the use of topical budesonide delivered via the MAD looks promising as an effective and safe adjunct in the treatment of AFRS.

At our centre, AFRS patients are instructed to use budesonide rinses (2 ml of 0.5 mg/ml Pulmicort Respules in every 60 ml of normal saline) in the immediate post-operative period. After 3 weeks post-operatively, the budesonide is delivered through a MAD (1 ml in each nostril). Patients are taught to apply the spray in the Mygind position (**Figure 96.9**). We favour the Mygind position as it is supported by our recently completed study on post-FESS cadaveric heads. Our study showed superior distribution of fluorescein within the ethmoid and frontal sinuses and the frontal recess when the head was placed in the lateral-head-back (LHB) position compared to the vertex-to-floor (VTF).[44]

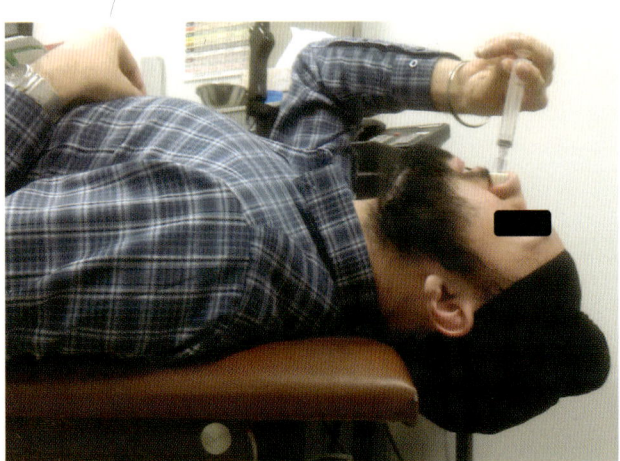

Figure 96.9 Application of Pulmicort through the MAD in the Mygind position.

II. Antifungals

In CRS, topical antifungals have been deemed ineffective in a number of meta-analyses and systemic reviews.[40, 45–48] As AFRS is a different disease entity resulting from an immunologic hyperreaction to extramucosal fungus,[11, 12] topical antifungals should hypothetically reduce the immunologic reaction of an atopic host by decreasing the antigenic load. In a RCT of 50 AFRS patients by Khalil et al., the fluconazole nasal spray arm had the best recurrence rate (10%) followed by combined oral itraconazole and topical fluconazole (14.3%), fluconazole nasal irrigation (28.6%), oral itraconazole alone (66.7%) and control (75%).[49] Although results from this RCT appeared promising, larger RCTs will be required to establish the role of topical antifungals in the management of AFRS.

III. Immunotherapy (IT)

In ABPA, IT has been avoided due to the possibility of an immune complex-mediated reaction developing from the IgG produced by IT.[50] As opposed to ABPA, the fungal antigenic stimulus can be removed surgically in AFRS patients. Surgical removal of fungal debris and allergic mucin in AFRS patients has also been shown to decrease allergen-specific IgE levels for fungal antigen.[11] Hence, it can be argued that fungal IT after surgery may potentially provide benefit rather than harm in the management of AFRS.[50]

A literature review by Hall and deShazo in 2012 revealed ten studies on fungal IT in AFRS patients.[50] In most studies, there were improvements in clinical outcomes. No major systemic reactions, nor evidence of worsening of disease in patients treated with fungal IT were reported. The only side effects reported were minor local reaction. Although the results of fungal IT appeared promising, the lack of RCT warrants better-designed research to establish the efficacy and safety of fungal IT in the treatment of AFRS.

Adjunctive treatment

MANUKA HONEY

Manuka (*Leptospermum scoparium*) honey from New Zealand is the most therapeutically potent honey.[51] It has been shown to be active against a broad spectrum of gram-positive and gram-negative bacteria.[52] The principal active ingredient responsible for the antibacterial property in Manuka honey is methylglyoxal (MGO).[53] MGO is present in Manuka honey at a concentration of up to 100-fold that of conventional honey.[53] In an *in vitro* study by Alandejani et al., Manuka honey at a concentration of 33% v/v was shown to be effective in eradicating methicillin-susceptible *Staphylococcus aureus* (MSSA), methicillin-resistant *Staphylococcus aureus* (MRSA) and *Pseudomonas aeruginosa* (PA) biofilms.[54] In fact, conditions that rapidly induced antibiotic resistance did not cause bacterial resistance to honey.[55]

At St Paul's Sinus Centre, our early experience with Manuka honey irrigation (**Figure 96.10**) in AFRS patients refractory to surgery and post-operative oral and intra-nasal steroids showed a partial response to Manuka honey with 21% of patients showing mucosal improvement after treatment with Manuka honey irrigation in one nostril.[56] It appears that there is a subgroup of AFRS patients who do respond well to Manuka honey irrigation. In our recently completed RCT (unpublished) comparing post-FESS patients treated with either Manuka honey or saline solution for 3 months, we found a cytokine signature of up-regulated interleukin (IL)-1b, IL-4, IL-6 and

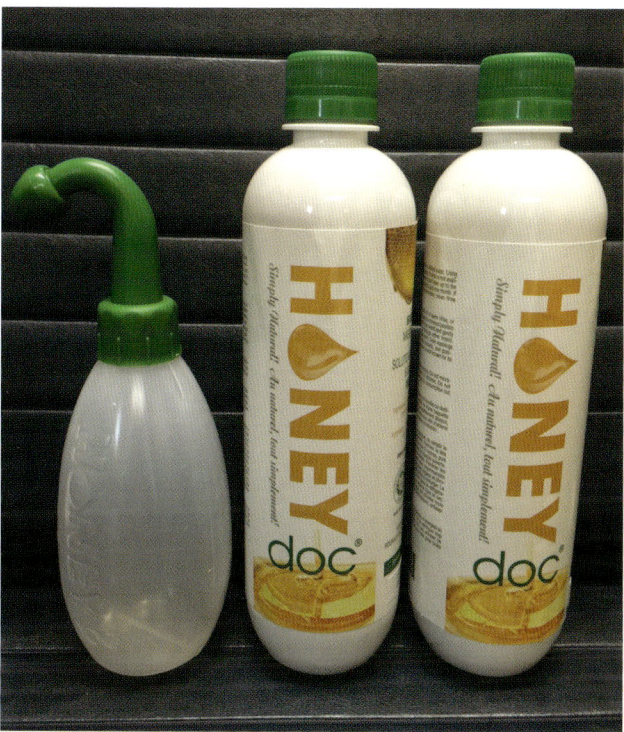

Figure 96.10 Manuka honey preparation and the power rinse bottle for sinus irrigation.

IL-12 in the sinonasal mucosa of patients who responded to Manuka honey treatment. This preliminary result looks promising and larger studies to confirm the result of this study will be warranted.

Future treatment strategy

ANTI-IMMUNOGLOBULIN E (IGE) THERAPY

Omalizumab (Xolair) is a humanized monoclonal anti-IgE antibody that has been used as an adjuvant treatment in severe atopic asthma, allergic rhinitis and CRS with nasal polyposis.[57, 58] In the only randomized double-blind placebo-controlled trial on omalizumab therapy on nasal polyps and asthma patients, Gevaert et al. demonstrated that there was significant improvement in total nasal endoscopic polyp scores, CT findings, airway symptoms and quality of life scores after 16 weeks of omalizumab treatment.[59] These improvements were seen irrespective of the presence of allergy. Omalizumab therapy has also been shown to be effective in ABPA patients.[60] Given the pathophysiological similarity between ABPA and AFRS, the use of omalizumab in AFRS patients should be explored. At our centre, seven patients with refractory AFRS and raised IgE levels with moderate or severe asthma underwent subcutaneous omalizumab injections (mean number of injections = 7.57; mean dosage = 287 mg; mean follow-up period = 9.7 months). They had improved sinonasal symptoms and endoscopic scores and were less dependent on corticosteroid and antifungal treatments.[61] We are excited about the outcome of this study which we hope will pave the way for a double blind RCT to determine the efficacy of this drug.

INVASIVE FRS

ACUTE (FULMINANT) INVASIVE FRS

Acute or fulminant invasive FRS is a life-threatening disease present usually in immunocompromised patients with impaired neutrophilic response. These patients include those with uncontrolled diabetes mellitus, acquired immunodeficiency syndrome (AIDS), iatrogenic immunosuppression, organ transplantation and haematological malignancies.[62] This condition is characterized by the presence of hyphal invasion of sinus tissue and a time course of less than 4 weeks.[3, 4] Histological features include mycotic infiltration of blood vessels, vasculitis with thrombosis, tissue infarction, haemorrhage and acute neutrophilic infiltrate.[1] *Aspergillus* species and the fungi in the order of mucorale (e.g. *Rhizopus*, *Rhizomucor* and *Mucor*) are the most commonly implicated species.[1]

The inability to mount a host response to invasive fungal disease in immunocompromised patients can make the diagnosis of this disease entity difficult, especially in the early stages.[63] Although common reported clinical symptoms include fever, cough, crusting of the nasal mucosa, epistaxis and headaches,[1] a high index of suspicion of this disease entity should be present in any immunosuppressed patients with localizing sinonasal symptoms. Often, fever of unknown origin that has failed to respond to 48 hours of broad-spectrum intravenous antibioitcs may be the initial presenting symptom.[64]

In the early stages, nasoendoscopic findings may be as subtle as the presenting symptoms. Alteration in mucosal appearance such as a discoloration, granulation and ulceration are the most consistent physical findings.[65] There are no pathognomonic features for invasive FRS on imaging and a CT scan is the initial radiologic investigation of choice (**Figure 96.11**). Compared to AFRS, invasive FRS tends to have more focal bony erosions, lacks expansion of the sinuses, has more limited sinus disease and has more disease outside of the sinuses than within when there is intra-orbital or intra-cranial extension.[73]

Without early treatment, rapid progression of disease with 50–80% mortality rates from intra-orbital and intra cranial complications have been reported.[64] Improvement of the host immune response is paramount for survival. Surgery is necessary to halt or slow progression of the disease (allowing time for bone marrow recovery), to reduce fungal load and to provide a tissue culture.[64]

Prior to definitive identification of the causative fungi, empirical treatment with intravenous amphotericin B, a broad-spectrum antifungal agent, has been recommended.[66] Once a causative fungal species has been identified, the use of the triazoles (fluconazole, itraconazole and variconazole) can be considered.[63, 66] The triazoles are effective in the treatment of invasive FRS without the associated nephrotoxicity seen in standard amphotericin B.[66] However, the triazoles lack effectiveness against the *Mucorales* species and their presence should be ruled out before its use is considered.[1, 63]

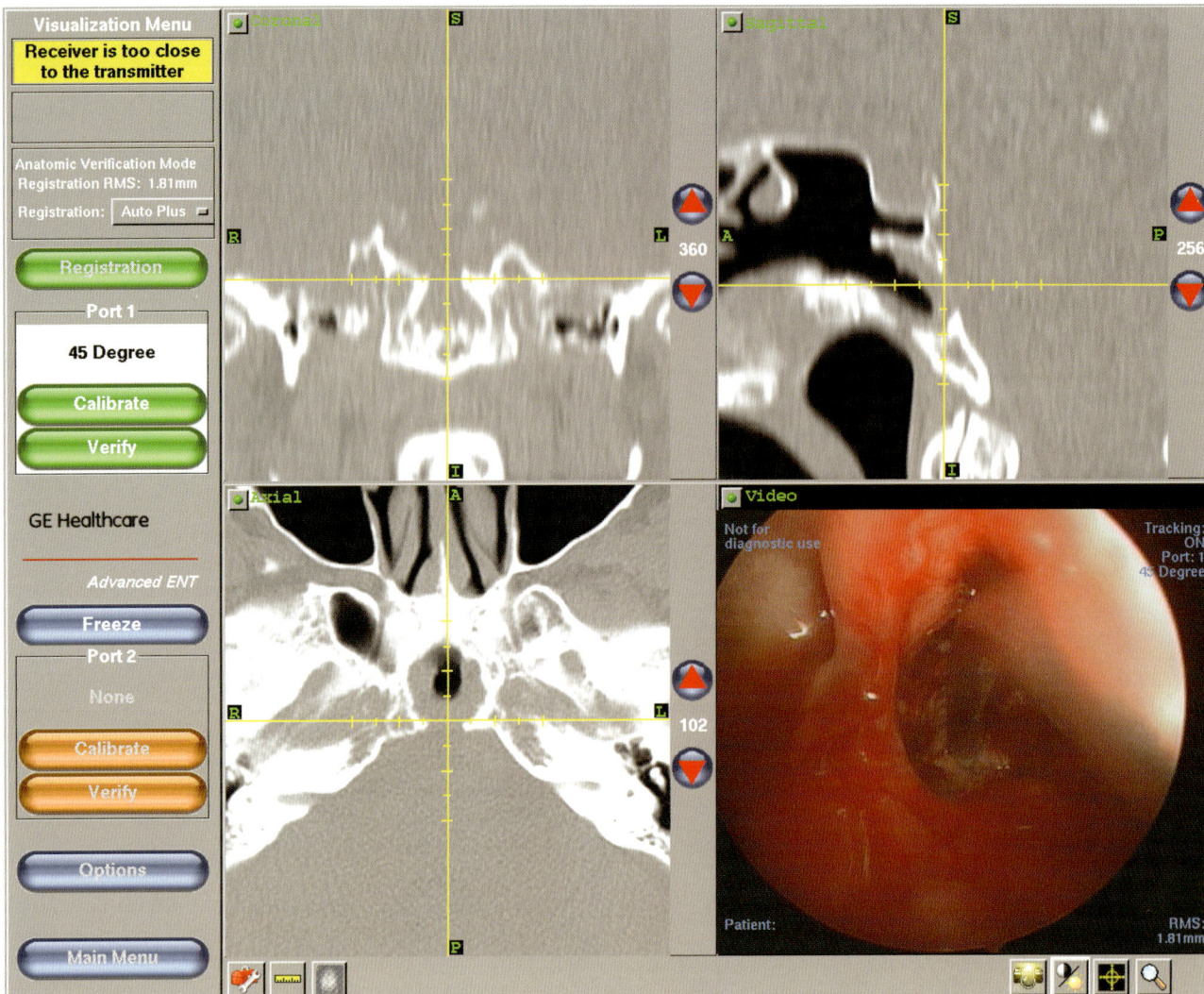

Figures 96.11 Intra-operative IGS images of the sphenoid sinus of a patient with invasive FRS. The fungal disease has eroded the infero-posterior wall of the sphenoid sinus (which is formed by a pneumatized clivus).

GRANULOMATOUS INVASIVE FRS

This disease entity is defined by invasive fungal infection lasting more than 12 weeks.[4] It is usually of gradual onset and is seen more commonly in Sudan, India, Pakistan and Saudi Arabia.[1] The causative agent is almost exclusively *Aspergillus flavus*.[1] Patients are typically immunocompetent and the predominant clinical features include proptosis with an enlarging mass in the cheek, nose, paranasal sinus and orbit.[1,63] CT findings are not different to that of chronic invasive FRS although they have a tendency for multiple sinus involvement.[67] The distinguishing feature from chronic invasive FRS is histological findings of fungal tissue invasion and a granulomatous reaction with considerable fibrosis. This is evident from the presence of non-caseating granulomas with foreign body or Langerhans-type giant cells, occasional vasculitis and sparse hyphae.[1,4,63] Treatment includes complete surgical removal and antifungal agents.

CHRONIC INVASIVE FRS

Chronic invasive FRS is a slowly destructive disease with a time-course of more than 12 weeks duration. Patients are usually immunocompetent or have subtle abnormalities in the immune system from diabetes mellitus, chronic low dose corticosteroid use and AIDS.[4,63] The most common fungi implicated is *Aspergillus fumigatus*.[4] The clinical picture of chronic invasive FRS is similar to that of granulomatous invasive FRS. The ethmoid and sphenoid sinuses are most commonly involved.[4] On histology, chronic invasive FRS demonstrates invasion of fungi into the sinonasal mucosa with a dense accumulation of fungal hyphae, occasional vascular invasion, and chronic or sparse inflammatory reaction.[1,4] There is no difference in the prognosis or the management of both chronic invasive and granulomatous invasive FRS.[4] For the occasional patients with invasive FRS with a time line between 4 and 12 weeks, the term subacute invasive FRS has been recommended.[4]

CONCLUSION

In summary, FRS is an uncommon but important part of the disease spectrum of CRS. Although there are certain clues from clinical and radiological findings, histology is key in distinguishing the different subtypes of FRS. Obtaining the correct diagnosis is crucial as each disease entity differs in the optimal management strategy. Antifungal agents are usually not required in the management of non-invasive FRS but are part of the first line treatment in invasive FRS.

BEST CLINICAL PRACTICE

- ✓ In the management of AFRS, endoscopic sinus surgery is required to decrease antigenic stimulation from the fungus; drain and ventilate the paranasal sinuses; and provide access to the surgeon for clinical surveillance, debridement and application of topical medication.
- ✓ Post-operative oral steroids and standard topical nasal steroids are recommended to maintain a healthy sinus cavity in the medical management of AFRS.
- ✓ Non-standard topical nasal steroid (e.g. budesonide), oral antifungals and immunotherapy are options in cases of refractory AFRS.

FUTURE RESEARCH

- ➤ There is insufficient evidence for the use of topical antifungals in the management of AFRS or invasive FR and more research in this area is required
- ➤ Omalizumab therapy may be a potential treatment option for the management of refractory AFS. The safety and effectiveness of this treatment modality should be explored in randomized controlled trials

KEY POINTS

- FR is categorized into non-invasive and invasive groups depending on the absence or presence of fungus within the sinonasal tissue respectively.
- AFRS is the most common type of FR.
- In medically fit patients with FR, endoscopic sinus surgery is indicated to remove fungal load and ventilate the involved paranasal sinuses.
- Intravenous antifungal agents and reversal of the immunocompromised status of the host are paramount in the management of invasive FR.

REFERENCES

1. deShazo RD, Chapin K, Swain RE. Fungal sinusitis. *N Eng J Med* 1997; **337**: 254–9.
2. Grosjean P, Weber R. Fungus balls of the paranasal sinuses: a review. *Eur Arch Otorhinolaryngol* 2007; **264**: 461–70.
3. Ferguson BJ. Definitions of fungal rhinosinusitis. *Otolaryngol Clin North Am* 2000; **33**: 227–35.
4. Chakrabarti A, Denning DW, Ferguson BJ, et al. Fungal rhinosinusitis: a categorization and definitional schema addressing current controversies. *Laryngoscope* 2009; **119**: 1809–18.
5. Safirstein BH. Allergic bronchopulmonary aspergillosis with obstruction of the upper respiratory tract. *Chest* 1976; **70**: 788–90.
6. Manning SC, Schaefer SD, Close LG, et al. Culture-positive allergic fungal sinusitis. *Arch Otolaryngol Head Neck Surg* 1991; **117**: 174–8.
7. Granville L, Chirala M, Cernoch P, et al. Fungal sinusitis: histological spectrum and correlation with culture. *Hum Pathol* 2004; **35**: 474–81.
8. Das A, Bal A, Chakrabarti A, et al. Spectrum of fungal rhinosinusitis; histopathologist's perspective. *Histopathology* 2009; **54**: 854–9.
9. Kuhn FA, Javer AR. Allergic fungal rhinosinusitis: perioperative management, prevention of recurrence, and role of steroids and antifungal agents. *Otolaryngol Clin North Am* 2000; **33**: 419–33.
10. Wise SK, Ghegan MD, Gorham E, et al. Socioeconomic factors in the diagnosis of allergic fungal rhinosinusitis. *Otolaryngol Head Neck Surg* 2008; **138**: 38–42.
11. Manning SC, Mabry RL, Schaefer SD, et al. Evidence of IgE-mediated hypersensitivity in allergic fungal sinusitis. *Laryngoscope* 1993; **103**: 717–21.
12. Manning SC, Holman M. Further evidence for allergic pathophysiology in allergic fungal sinusitis. *Laryngoscope* 1998; **108**: 1485–96.
13. Marple BF. Allergic fungal rhinosinusitis: current theories and management strategies. *Laryngoscope* 2001; **111**: 1006–19.
14. Panikou JU, Sherris DA, Kern EB, et al. The diagnosis and incidence of allergic fungal sinusitis. *Mayo Clin Proc* 1999; **74**: 877–84.
15. Ferguson BJ. Eosinophilic mucin rhinosinusitis: a distinct clinicopathological entity. *Laryngoscope* 2000; **110**: 799–813.
16. Bent JP, Kuhn FA. Diagnosis of allergic fungal sinusitis. *Otolaryngol Head Neck Surg* 1994; **111**: 580–8.
17. Kuhn FA, Javer AR. Allergic fungal sinusitis: a four year follow up. *Am J Rhinol* 2000; **14**: 149–56.
18. Marple BF. Allergic fungal rhinosinusitis: a review of clinical manifestation and current treatment strategies. *Med Mycol* 2006; **44**: S277–84.
19. Marple B, Newcomer M, Schwade N, et al. Natural history of allergic fungal rhinosinusitis: a 4- to 10-year follow-up. *Otolaryngol Head Neck Surg* 2002; **127**: 361–6.
20. Mabry RL, Manning S. Radioallergosorbent microscreen and total immunoglobulin E in allergic fungal sinusitis. *Otolaryngol Head Neck Surg* 1995; **113**: 721–3.
21. Mabry RL, Marple BF, Mabry CS. Mold testing by RAST and skin test methods in patients with allergic fungal sinusitis. *Otolaryngol Head Neck Surg* 1999; **121**: 252–4.
22. Manning SC, Merkel M, Kriesel K, et al. Computed tomography and magnetic resonance diagnosis of allergic fungal sinusitis. *Laryngoscope* 1997; **107**: 170–6.

23. Reddy CE, Gupta AK, Singh P, et al. Imaging of granulomatous and chronic invasive fungal sinusitis: comparison with allergic fungal sinusitis. *Otolaryngol Head Neck Surg* 2010; **143**: 294–300.
24. Lund VJ, Lloyd G, Savy L, et al. Fungal rhinosinusitis. *J Laryngol Otol* 2000; **114**: 76–80.
25. Meltzer EO, Hamilos DL, Hadley JA, et al. Rhinosinusitis: establishing definitions for clinical research and patient care. *Otolaryngol Head Neck Surg* 2004; **131**: S1–62.
26. Cody DT II, Neel HB III, Ferreiro JA, et al. Allergic fungal sinusitis: the Mayo Clinic experience. *Laryngoscope* 1994; **104**: 1074–9.
27. Javer AR, Genoway KA, Gervais M, et al. Fungal cultures in patients with allergic fungal rhinosinusitis: improving the recovery of potential fungal pathogens in the Canadian laboratory. *J Otolaryngol* 2007; **36**: 1–5.
28. Gan EC, Thamboo A, Rudmik L et al. Medical management of allergic fungal rhinosinusitis following endoscopic sinus surgery: an evidence-based review and recommendations. *Int Forum Allergy Rhinol* 2014; **4**: 702–15.
29. Kuhn FA, Javer AR. Allergic fungal rhinosinusitis: our experience. *Arch Otolaryngol Head Neck Surg* 1998; **124**: 1179–80.
30. Philpott CM, Clark A, Javer AR. Allergic fungal rhinosinusitis: a new staging system. *Rhinology* 2011; **49**: 318–23.
31. Landsberg R, Segev Y, DeRowe A, et al. Systemic corticosteroids for allergic fungal rhinosinusitis and chronic rhinosinusitis with nasal polyposis: a comparative study. *Otolaryngol Head Neck Surg* 2007; **136**: 252–7.
32. Waxman JE, Spector JG, Sale SR, et al. Allergic aspergillus sinusitis: concepts in diagnosis and treatment of a new clinical entity. *Laryngoscope* 1987; **97**: 261–6.
33. Ryan MW. Allergic fungal rhinosinusitis. *Otolaryngol Clin North Am* 2011; **44**: 697–710.
34. Seiberling K, Wormald PJ. The role of itraconazole in recalcitrant fungal sinusitis. *Am J Rhinol Allergy* 2009; **23**: 303–6.
35. Bent JP, Kuhn FA. Antifungal activity against allergic fungal sinusitis oragnisms. *Laryngoscope* 1996; **106**: 1331–4.
36. Chan KO, Genoway KA, Javer AR. Effectiveness of itraconazole in the management of refractory allergic fungal rhinosinusitis. *J Otolaryngol Head Neck Surg* 2008; **37**: 870–4.
37. Rains BM III, Mineck CW. Treatment of allergic fungal sinusitis with high-dose itraconazole *Am J Rhinol* 2003; **17**: 1–8.
38. Benninger MS, Ahmad N, Marple BF. The safety of intranasal steroids. *Otolaryngol Head Neck Surg* 2003; **129**: 739–50.
39. Rudmik L, Schlosser RJ, Smith TL, et al. Impact of topical nasal steroid therapy on symptoms of nasal polyposis: a meta-analysis. *Laryngoscope* 2012; **122**: 1431–7.
40. Rudmik L, Hoy M, Schlosser RJ et al. Topical therapies in the management of chronic rhinosinusitis: an evidence-based review with recommendations. *Int Forum Allergy Rhinol* 2013; **3**: 281–98.
41. Kanowitz SJ, Batra PS, Citardi MJ. Topical budesonide via mucosal atomization device in refractory postoperative chronic rhinosinusitis. *Otolaryngol Head Neck Surg* 2008; **139**: 131–6.
42. Sachanandani NS, Piccirillo JF, Kramper MA, et al. The effect of nasally administered budesonide respules on adrenal cortex function in patients with chronic rhinosinusitis. *Arch Otolaryngol Head Neck Surg* 2009; **135**: 303–7.
43. Thamboo A, Manji J, Szeitz A, et al. The safety and efficacy of short-term budesonide delivered via mucosal atomization device for chronic rhinosinusitis without nasal polyposis. *Int Forum Allergy Rhinol* 2014; **4**: 397–402.
44. Habib AR, Thamboo A, Manji J, et al. The effect of head position on the distribution of topical nasal medication using the Mucosal Atomization Device: a cadaver study. *Int Forum Allergy Rhinol* 2013; **3**: 958–62.
45. Isaacs S, Fakhri S, Luong A, et al. A meta-analysis of topical amphotericin B for the treatment of chronic rhinosinusitis. *Int Forum Allergy Rhinol* 2011; **1**: 250–4.
46. Sacks PL, Harvey RJ, Rimmer J, et al. Topical and systemic antifungal therapy for the symptomatic treatment of chronic rhinosinusitis. *Cochrane Database Syst Rev* 2011; (8): CD008263.
47. Sacks PLt, Harvey RJ, Rimmer J, et al. Antifungal therapy in the treatment of chronic rhinosinusitis: a meta-analysis. *Am J Rhinol Allergy* 2012; **26**: 141–7.
48. Huang A, Govindaraj S. Topical therapy in the management of chronic rhinosinusitis. *Curr Opin Otolaryngol Head Neck Surg* 2013; **21**: 31–8.
49. Khalil Y, Tharwat A, Abdou AG, et al. The role of antifungal therapy in the prevention of recurrent allergic fungal rhinosinusitis after functional endoscopic sinus surgery: a randomized, controlled study. *Ear Nose Throat J* 2011; **90**: E1–7.
50. Hall AG, DeShazo RD. Immunotherapy for allergic fungal sinusitis. *Curr Opin Clin Immunol* 2012; **12**: 629–34.
51. Molan PC. The role of honey in the management of wounds. *J Wound Care* 1999; **8**: 415–18.
52. Lusby PE, Coombes AL, Wilkinson JM. Bactericidal activity of different honey against pathogenic bacteria. *Arch Med Res* 2005; **36**: 464–7.
53. Mavric E, Wittmann S, Barth G, et al. Identification and quantification of methylglyoxal as the dominant antibacterial constituent of Manuka (*Leptospermum scoparium*) honeys from New Zealand. *Mol Nutr Food Res* 2008; **52**: 483–9.
54. Alandejani T, Marsan J, Ferris W, et al. Effectiveness of honey on Staphylococcus aureus and Pseudomonas aeruginosa biofilms. *Otolaryngol Head Neck Surg* 2009; **141**: 114–18.
55. Blair SE, Cokcetin NN, Harry EJ, et al. The unusual antibacterial activity of medical-grade Leptospermum honey: antibacterial spectrum, resistance and transcriptome analysis. *Eur J Clin Microbiol Infect Dis* 2009; **28**: 1199–208.
56. Thamboo A, Philpott C, Javer A, et al. Single-blind study of manuka honey in allergic fungal rhinosinusitis. *J Otolaryngol Head Neck Surg* 2011; **40**: 238–43.
57. Holgate S, Buhl R, Bousquet J, et al. The use of omalizumab in the treatment of severe allergic asthma: a clinical experience update. *Respir Med* 2009; **103**: 1098–113.
58. Casale T, Condemi J, LaForce C, et al. Effect of omalizumab on symptoms of seasonal allergic rhinitis: a randomized controlled trial. *JAMA* 2001; **286**: 2956–67.
59. Gevaert P, Van Zele T, Blomme K, et al. Omalizumab is effective in allergic and nonallergic patients with nasal polyps and asthma. *J Allergy Clin Immunol* 2013: **131**: 110–16.
60. Tille-Leblond I, Germaud P, Leroyer C, et al. Allergic bronchopulmonary aspergillosis and omalizumab. *Allergy* 2011; **66**: 1254–6.
61. Gan EC, Habib AR, Rajwani A, et al. Omalizumab therapy for refractory allergic fungal rhinosinusitis patients with moderate or severe asthma. *Am J Otolaryngol* 2015; **36**: 672–7.
62. deShazo RD. Fungal sinusitis. *Am J Med Sci* 1998; **316**: 39–44.
63. Thompson GR, 3rd, Patterson TF. Fungal disease of the nose and paranasal sinuses. *J Allergy Clin Immunol* 2012; **129**: 321–6.
64. Gillespie MB, O'Malley BW. An algorithmic approach to the diagnosis and management of invasive fungal rhinosinusitis in the immunocompromised patient. *Otolaryngol Clin North Am* 2000; **33**: 323–34.
65. Gillespie MB, O'Malley BW, Francis HW. An approach to fulminant invasive fungal rhinosinusitis in the immunocompromised host. *Arch Otolaryngol Head Neck Surg* 1998; **124**: 520–6.
66. Luna B, Drew RH, Perfect JR. Agents for treatment of invasive fungal infections. *Otolaryngol Clin North Am* 2000; **33**: 277–99.
67. Challa S, Uppin SG, Hanumanthu S et al. Fungal rhinosinusitis: a clinicopathological study from South India. *Eur Arch Otorhinolaryngol* 2010; **267**: 1239–45.

CHAPTER 97

MEDICAL MANAGEMENT FOR RHINOSINUSITIS

Claire Hopkins

Medical management of acute rhinosinusitis 1059	Treatment aimed at reducing microbial load 1063
Introduction 1059	Treatment aimed at improvement in mucociliary clearance 1064
Reduction of infective load 1059	Assessment of the response to medical treatment 1065
Differentiating bacterial from viral ARS 1060	When does a medical therapy only approach fail? 1066
Medical management of chronic rhinosinusitis 1061	Medical treatment post-surgery 1067
Introduction 1061	Summary 1068
Overview of the pathophysiology of CRS 1061	References 1068
Treatment targeting intrinsic mucosal inflammation ... 1061	

SEARCH STRATEGY

The author consulted the suite of Cochrane reviews on chronic rhinosinusitis (www.cochrane.org/news/suite-cochrane-reviews-chronic-rhinosinusitis) to underpin the recommendations in this chapter.

MEDICAL MANAGEMENT OF ACUTE RHINOSINUSITIS

INTRODUCTION

Acute rhinosinusitis is common, affecting 6–15% of the population each year. The vast majority of cases are viral, with bacterial infection estimated in less than 2% of cases; however there is significant overlap, with viral infection triggering inflammatory changes that facilitate secondary bacterial infection. Most cases resolve spontaneously within 10 days, and the incidence of complications is very low. Medical treatment may be antimicrobial or anti-inflammatory, with an aim of reducing the infective and inflammatory load to both reduce the severity and duration of illness, to prevent recurrence and complications, or reducing symptom severity alone.

REDUCTION OF INFECTIVE LOAD

Inappropriate antibiotic use is a significant threat to public health in terms of increasing resistance, yet antibiotics are prescribed in over 80% of outpatient visits in the United States for acute rhinosinusitis (ARS),[5] and ARS is the fifth most common indication for antibiotic treatment.

Although the majority of ARS is viral, antibiotics are often both expected by patients and prescribed by physicians.[1–4]

The majority of studies and meta-analyses have shown little benefit from antibiotics in most patients with ARS.[5–8] The most recent systematic review, published by the Cochrane Collaboration in 2012, included 10 trials with a total of 2450 adult participants.[9] Irrespective of antibiotic usage, 47% of participants were cured after one week and 71% after 14 days. Five more participants per 100 had shortened time to cure between 7 and 14 days if they received antibiotics instead of placebo (number needed to treat = 18). Purulent secretion resolved faster with antibiotics (odds ratio (OR) 1.58 (95% CI 1.13 to 2.22)), (NNT = 11, three trials). However, 27% of the participants who received antibiotics and 15% of those who received placebo experienced adverse events (OR 2.10) (number needed to treat to harm NNTH = 8, seven trials). Therefore, while there was a small beneficial clinical effect with antibiotics, there was also an increased risk of adverse effect.

While there are limitations with the evidence (there is often marked heterogeneity of patients, different diagnostic criteria applied, and most studies conducted in subspecialty clinics, rather than primary care), current evidence supports restricting antibiotic usage in uncomplicated ARS.

DIFFERENTIATING BACTERIAL FROM VIRAL ARS

If those with bacterial infection can be identified, a more selective approach to antibiotic prescribing may be applied. The gold-standard for confirmation is a positive bacterial culture from a maxillary sinus aspirate. However, this requires specialist care, and incurs patient morbidity. Endoscopically guided middle-meatal cultures have been shown to have good specificity but lower sensitivity when compared with direct aspiration. Symptomatic selection alone is unreliable, unilateral facial pain and nasal purulence have a positive predictive value of 40% and 50% only for positive bacterial culture. When a combination of 3 out of 4 of nasal purulence, purulence in the post-nasal space, high fever (>39C) and raised ESR are used, specificity may be increased to 80%.

Choice of antibiotic if indicated

Where a decision to treat with antibiotics has been made, due to the presence of complications or in severe infection, the choice can be based on culture results, or local resistance to common classes. A Cochrane review comparing different classes of antibiotics found no significant difference between penicillins or non-penicillins (cephalosporins, macrolides) or between non-penicillins and amoxicillin-clavulate. Prolonged courses (10–14 days) do not significantly increase cure rates, thus a short course of narrow-spectrum agents may reduce the risk of increasing antibiotic resistance.

Role of treatment in preventing complications

The incidence of complications of ARS is low. Of those cases of complicated ARS reported to a UK audit, 50% had received antecedent antibiotic treatment. When comparing the prevalence of complicated ARS is countries with widely differing rates of antibiotic prescribing, there seems to be little difference; in the Netherlands, with the lowest rates of antibiotic usage, the prevalence is reported at 3 per million population per annum while in the US it is 2.7–4.3 per million. Thus antibiotic usage does not seem to prevent the development of complications.

Reduction of inflammation

Studies of topical glucocorticoids have demonstrated some benefit for the relief of symptoms in both viral and bacterial ARS. A meta-analysis of three studies, with ARS diagnosed by symptoms and confirmed by radiologic or endoscopic studies, found that adult participants receiving INCS were more likely to have resolution or improvement of symptoms than those receiving placebo (73% versus 66.4%; risk ratio (RR) 1.11).[10] Higher doses of INCS had a stronger effect on improvement or complete relief of symptoms. When used as an adjunct to antibiotic therapy in the treatment of ABRS, a meta-analysis of placebo-controlled trials suggests that 15 patients would need to be treated with intra-nasal glucocorticoids to improve clinical symptoms in one patient.[11] As the risk of adverse events with short-term usage INCS is low, INCS can be recommended in ARS.

Similarly, meta-analysis supports a role for systemic steroid treatment as adjunctive treatment.[12] Four RCTs with a total of 1008 adult participants met our inclusion criteria. Acute sinusitis was defined clinically in all studies, with radiological confirmation in three. All participants received oral antibiotics and were assigned to either oral corticosteroids or the control (placebo in three trials and non-steroidal anti-inflammatory drugs in one). In all trials, participants treated with oral corticosteroids were more likely to have short-term resolution or improvement of symptoms than those receiving the control treatment: at Days 3 to 7, risk ratio (RR) 1.4; risk difference (RD) 20% and at Days 4 to 10 or 12, RR 1.3, RD 18%. An analysis of the three trials with placebo as a control treatment showed similar results but with a lesser effect size: Days 3 to 6: RR 1.2, RD 12% and Days 4 to 10 or 12: RR 1.1, RD 10%.

Symptomatic improvement

There is limited evidence to suggest that nasal decongestants may have a small beneficial clinical effect in reducing nasal congestion, but not overall duration of ARS.

There is little evidence that saline therapies assist in symptom relief. Low-volume saline sprays may assist in mucus and crusting but there is evidence that high-volume irrigations are poorly tolerated in the setting of acute inflammation and are currently not recommended.[13] A randomized study comparing hypertonic with isotonic saline found no difference between groups in terms of severity or duration of symptoms, but higher adverse events (local discomfort) associated with hypertonic saline.

Medical management in complicated ARS

The management of complications of ARS will often require surgical intervention to address the complication itself, but will also require ongoing medical management to treat the underlying sinus infection. Where possible, choice of antibiotic should be culture directed, and are usually be given intravenously, followed by an oral course on discharge. There are no randomized trials of the medical management of complicated ARS; however, in many published case series, decongestants are given. There is little evidence regarding the use of systemic steroids in such cases, but they are often given to reduce cerebral oedema associated with intra-cranial complications, and are likely to be more beneficial than detrimental.

Prevention of ARS

There is a growing body of evidence identifying allergic rhinitis as a predisposing factor for ARS. It would be reasonable to assume that optimal medical management of

AR may reduce the risk of ARS, but there are no studies to confirm or refute this. A recent systematic review found only a weak association between laryngeal reflux and ARS. Therefore, there does not appear to be any role for antireflux medication. One study has evaluated the benefit of INCS at the onset of symptoms of a common cold in reducing the risk of developing post-viral rhinosinusitis, and found no benefit.

MEDICAL MANAGEMENT OF CHRONIC RHINOSINUSITIS

INTRODUCTION

'The treatment of chronic rhinosinusitis is primarily medical, with surgery reserved for those who fail a trial of maximal medical therapy', is a commonly quoted approach in the management of CRS. However, what maximal medical therapy entails, and how to define those who fail to respond is perhaps more controversial than it may appear. This chapter hopes to address this and summarize current evidence.

OVERVIEW OF THE PATHOPHYSIOLOGY OF CRS

Chronic rhinosinusitis is a heterogenous group of several phenotypes, and is likely to represent the end-point of multiple aetiologies, rather than a single disease process. In some cases, sinonasal disease is a manifestation of systemic disease; examples include vasculitides, cystic fibrosis, sarcoidosis and cilial motility disorders. Medical treatment in these groups is usually directed at systemic disease management, where possible. CRS may also occur as a direct result of focal abnormalities; a foreign body, fungal ball, odontogenic infection or very rarely, an anatomical obstruction. Medical management plays no significant role in first-line management in this group, and treatment is usually surgical correction of the focal abnormality. Medical treatment may be required to facilitate normalization of the sinonasal mucosa post-operatively. These groups of *secondary* CRS will not be considered further in this section.

Primary CRS refers to the vast majority of patients that present to otolaryngologists with unexplained inflammation of the upper airway. It is common to find lower airway disease as part of a broader respiratory condition but not as a result of systemic disease. In these patients, with *primary* CRS, there is an interaction of intrinsic mucosal inflammation, local microbial community and mucociliary dysfunction, with each factor being of varying importance in individual patients.[14] Considerations of these three factors will help direct medical therapy in these patients; the aim will be to reduce inflammation, reduce bacterial load and optimize ciliary function by removing mucus. Chronic rhinosinusitis may be subcategorized by the endoscopic assessment of the middle meatus, if necessary after decongestant; polyps presenting to the middle meatus or nasal cavity is defined as *CRS with polyps* (CRSwNP), CRS *sine (without) polyps* (CRSsNP) is used when no polyps are visible on endoscopy, accepting that there may be polypoid change within the sinuses. While there is increasing recognition that CRSwNP and CRSsNP are opposing ends of a spectrum, there remains overlap between the conditions, and many studies to date have not separated according to phenotype. It is acknowledged that there is a move away from phenotyping the disease, and greater endotyping of the mucosal condition is anticipated.[15–16] Greater distinction occurs when separating the eosinophil dominated (or Th2 skewed) CRS group. This better defines the inflammatory process and often referred to as eosinophilic CRS (eCRS). However, little distinction occurs in routine clinical practice beyond phenotype. Therefore this review will combine both groups, but will highlight where medical therapies differ in efficacy.

TREATMENT TARGETING INTRINSIC MUCOSAL INFLAMMATION

Mucosal inflammation is the defining feature of CRS; it may be intrinsic, as in those with asthma and aspirin sensitivity, or occur as a result of local infection or environmental exposure. Glucocorticoids have formed the mainstay of medical therapy for CRS, while long-term macrolides, doxycycline and other novel approaches also target the inflammatory pathway.

Intra-nasal corticosteroids

There are many studies supporting the role of topical corticosteroids. For CRSwNP, 40 studies (3624 patients) met the inclusion criteria for a recent Cochrane review.[17] The primary outcomes were sino-nasal symptoms, polyp size and polyp recurrence after surgery. When compared to placebo, topical corticosteroids improved overall symptom scores (standardized mean difference (SMD) −0.46; $P < 0.00001$; seven trials, $n = 445$) and had a higher proportion of patients whose symptoms improved (responders) (risk ratio (RR) 1.71, $P = 0.0002$, four trials, $n = 234$). Topical corticosteroids also decreased the polyp score (SMD −0.73; $P < 0.00001$; three trials, $n = 237$) and had a greater proportion of patients with a reduction in polyp size (responders) (RR 2.09; $P < 0.00001$; eight trials, $n = 785$) when compared to placebo. Topical corticosteroids also prevented polyp recurrence after surgery (RR 0.59; $P = 0.0004$; six trials, $n = 437$). However, there is a significant amount of heterogeneity in the included studies. Some of these showed very little or no benefit. Subgroup analyses by sinus surgery status helps to explain this heterogeneity, revealing a greater benefit in reduction of polyp score when topical steroid was administered in patient groups who had undergone previous sinus surgery (SMD −1.19) compared to patients who had never had surgery (SMD −0.13; $P < 0.00001$). There was no difference between groups in terms of adverse events. In CRSsNP, the number of studies available smaller, and the risk of bias greater, but a beneficial effect for INCS is found; ten studies (590 patients) met the inclusion criteria for meta-analysis.[18] The primary outcome was sino-nasal symptoms. When compared to placebo, topical steroid improved symptom scores (SMD −0.37; P = 0.002; five trials, n = 286) and had a greater proportion of responders (risk ratio 1.69; P = 0.002; four trials, n = 263). Even with a limited number of studies, heterogeneity was present and subgroup analyses of patients who had received sinus surgery versus those who had not was not significant (P = 0.35). However, only the sinus surgery group had a positive effect on meta-analysis. Subgroup analyses by topical delivery method revealed more benefit when steroid was administered directly to the sinuses than with simple nasal delivery (P = 0.04). There were no differences between groups for quality of life and adverse events.

Intra-nasal corticosteroids have an excellent safety profile, with the systemic bioavailability for second-generation compounds (mometasone and fluticasone) less than 1%[12] There is a low incidence of adverse events, with nasal irritation and epistaxis the most common, and are safe for long-term use. Studies show no evidence of nasal mucosal atrophy with long-term use,[19] or growth retardation in the paediatric population.[20] Patient education regarding delivery techniques and the need for compliance is essential (**Figure 97.1**).

In summary, INCS are beneficial in CRSwNP and CRSsNP, and the risk of adverse events low. However, the effect size is often very small and penetration into previously unoperated sinuses is limited, and there may be a greater response to topical therapy after surgery, utilizing direct delivery to the sinuses.

Systemic corticosteroids

In contrast, there is a relative paucity of comparative data for the efficacy of systemic corticosteroids. In CRSsNP, there are no RCTs, or studies evaluating systemic steroids alone: instead all case series supporting the use of systemic steroids combine therapy with antibiotics and INCS, and are at best level 4 or 5.[21-22] In CRSwNP, three trials (166 patients) were suitable for inclusion in systematic review,[23] and showed a short-term benefit of a short (2- to 4-week) course of oral steroids of variable doses and duration when compared to placebo. There was an objective reduction of polyp size and a subjective improvement of nasal symptoms and quality of life. There was no report of significant adverse effects of treatment with a short course of steroids. Therefore, for short periods, when the risk of adverse event is small, systemic steroids can be recommended for the treatment of CRSwNP. There are no studies to inform us as to the optimum interval between repeated courses of systemic steroids, and use should be weighed up against potential adverse events and discussed with individual patients. However, deriving a plan from best evidence may suggest that a course should last at least as long as the life-span of a tissue eosinophil, have a total or maximal dose below that reported in most case series of serious adverse event from systemic steroid and be infrequent enough to protect against long-term risks of osteoporosis and posterior subcapsular cataract formation. This is further discussed later in this chapter.

Immunomodulatory antibiotics

Long-term macrolide antibiotics are used for their anti-inflammatory effects, based on their efficacy in lower airways disease. They target markers including IL-8, IL-4, IFNγ and TNFα, and have a predominant effect on neutrophil-mediated inflammation. Open label studies have demonstrated improvement in symptoms. There are two prospective randomized controlled trials, one published after a Cochrane review on the topic. The first study included only CRSsNP and showed a significant effect of roxithromycin on symptom scores and IL-8 levels, with greater efficacy in patients with normal IgE levels. A subsequent study has found no effect; however this study included both CRSwNP and CRSsNP, and therefore it is likely that this study included more patients with elevated IgE than the first.[24]

Long-term use of macrolide antibiotics is associated with increasing levels of macrolide resistance, and gastrointestinal side effects are relatively common. Therefore use should be directed at those patients most likely to benefit (i.e. CRSsNP, normal IgE levels), and further studies are required.[25]

Doxycycline has been investigated for a potential anti-inflammatory role. In a PCRCT, a 20-day course of doxycycline was shown to reduce levels of myeloperoxidase,

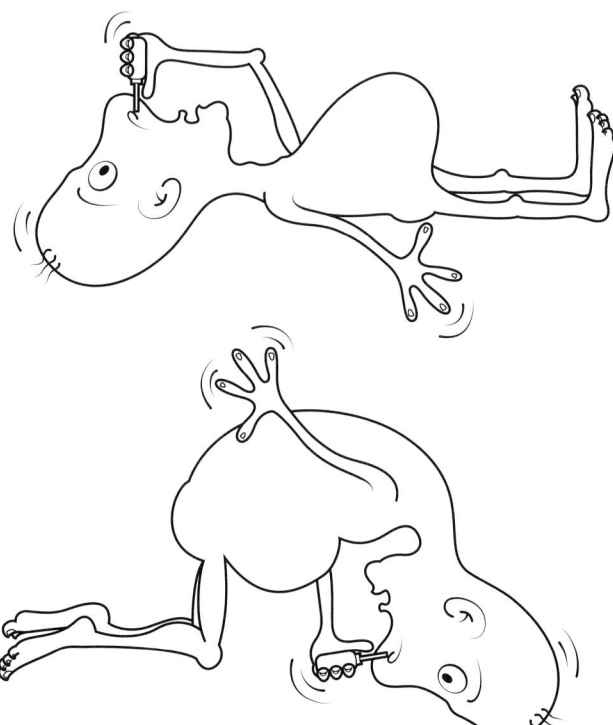

Figure 97.1 Correct application for nasal drops. **(a)** Head back position. **(b)** Head down position.

eosinophil cationic protein, matrix metalloproteinase-9 in CRSwNP patients, and had a moderate and sustained effect on polyp size over a 12-week period.[26] The clinical impact of this effect, while present at 90 days, is likely to be of minimal clinical benefit. The difference between corticosteroid and the doxycycline was dramatic, but simple withdrawal of the corticosteroid at 20 days prevents sustained benefit. Doxycycline may be an adjunct in the eCRS subgroup while macrolides may assist in the non-eCRS patient.

Leukotriene receptor antagonists

Montelukast, a leukotriene receptor antagonist has been investigated in studies primarily as an adjunct to steroid treatment inpatients with CRSwNP and asthma. There is one positive single-blinded placebo controlled cross-over study with methodological problems, that shows benefit over placebo, while three other randomized trials were negative for change in polyp scores, although there were some benefits on some symptoms including sneezing and facial pain.[27] Most studies found greater benefit in patients with associated nasal allergy. There is the definite possibility of leukotriene receptor antagonists assisting with concomitant allergic rhinitis symptom control in these patients and may be the mechanism of effect as many of these patients have both conditions. This is also the basis of some benefit seen and reported by studies on immunotherapy and CRS.[28]

Novel immunoregulation

Direct targeting of the inflammatory pathway is possible using monoclonal antibodies. In two recent small PCRCTs, omalizumab (anti-IgE) has been shown to significantly reduce both symptom scores and polyp size,[29] and mepolizumab (anti-IL-5) has a significant effect on polyp size.[30] High cost, risk of anaphylaxis and need for subcutaneous injection are limiting factors in widespread application of such treatments at present. Many other anticytokine and antichemokine agents have been trialled in asthma and lower airway disease.[31] The respiratory epithelium is likely to co-ordinate the inflammatory process in eCRS with many mediators enacting a pro-inflammatory response.[32] It is highly likely that 'downstream' inhibition of a single agent may be suboptimal as redundancy of inflammatory pathways is present, and while one may be inhibited, others may persist. This is likely to explain why some of these medications have an effect but are not a panacea of treatment.

Aspirin desensitization

Aspirin sensitivity is usually associated with nasal polyposis and asthma (Samter's triad). Patients often have extensive polyposis, with high rates of recurrence after both medical and surgical treatment. Immune tolerance may be achieved and maintained by regular administration of aspirin, either orally or intra-nasally.

Tolerance is achieved by giving incrementally increasing dosages of oral aspirin until several hundred milligrams per day are tolerated. Used in this fashion, there is evidence of significant improvement in many parameters affecting both nose and chest, and has been found to be beneficial in patients with Samter's triad,[33–34] but comes with a significant risk of gastrointestinal side effects. More recently, doses as low as 100 mg have been used, and a placebo controlled randomized trial has shown a reduction in polyp recurrence in trial patients.[35] In the event of polyp recurrence requiring surgical intervention, oral aspirin is normally discontinued, and therefore desensitization must be repeated.

Lysine aspirin, a soluble from, is used for diagnosis of aspirin sensitivity by nasal or bronchial challenge and topical nasal desensitization. In a double-blind, placebo-controlled crossover study, topical lysine aspirin was associated with a reduction on cysteinyl leukotriene receptors, however, there was no significant clinical effect.[36]

TREATMENT AIMED AT REDUCING MICROBIAL LOAD

Treatment aimed at reducing microbial load or eradicating pathogens from the sinuses assumes that these play a role in causing or propagating CRS. Bacteria may play a role in acute infective exacerbations. Bacterial capsules and exotoxin may trigger an inflammatory response, while superantigens (predominantly Staphylococcal) and fungi may induce eosinophilic inflammation. The organisms isolated from patients with CRS differ from those in ARS, with *Staphylococcus aureus*, *S. epidermidis*, and anaerobic and Gram-negative bacteria predominating. Some, such as *S. epidermidis* are likely to be innocent colonizers. Polymicrobia is common. *S. aureus* may be isolated in up to 50% of CRSwNP, and MRSA is being increasingly grown, with more than 40% *S. aureus* cultures in the US now resistant to methicillin. Anaerobes are identified in 14–93% cultures, and may be involved in acute exacerbations.

Culture directed short-term antibiotics may be of use during acute exacerbations of CRS, but there are no studies evaluating effect on short courses on long-term symptom control. Long-term macrolides are discussed above, and are used predominantly for an anti-inflammatory effect.

Doxycycline has been compared with oral steroids in a placebo-controlled RCT in CRSwNP, and was found to have a moderate, but more sustained effect when compared with methylprednisolone. While doxycycline reduced post-nasal drip, it had no effect on nasal congestion, anosmia or rhinorrhea. Therefore it may be considered as an adjunct in treatment of CRSwNP but needs further evaluation.

While topical antibiotics have been shown to reduce bacterial colonization in animal studies, there is no evidence in the current literature that topical antibiotics are beneficial in the treatment of CRS. There have been three placebo-controlled RCTs, two in patients without previous surgery, one in difficult to treat CRS.[37] In all three there was no additional benefit of topical antibiotic compared to the placebo arm of nasal irrigation alone.

Even more recent trials of mupirocin, as an antistaphylococcal, delivered post-surgically in large volume irrigation, demonstrated little effect on patient outcomes. They are not therefore currently recommended.

Biofilms, both bacterial and fungal, have been demonstrated within the sinuses of patients with CRS, and their presence is associated with more severe disease and recalcitrance to surgical therapy. Systemic antibiotics are relatively ineffective against biofilms; topical antibiotics and surfactants may be more beneficial, but are likely to penetrate the sinuses only after surgery, and therefore will play a limited role in the treatment of the pre-operative patient with CRS.

The role of antifungal agents in the treatment of CRS has caused much controversy since the Mayo clinic made a patent application for the topical application of antifungals in patients with CRS in the late 1990s. However, the encouraging results of open label studies have not been repeated in randomized trials. A Cochrane meta-analysis identified 5 PCRCTs evaluating topical treatment, and one comparing systemic treatment with placebo.[38] Symptomatic response rates were better, and adverse event rate was lower in the placebo arm in all studies. These studies were conducted on groups of patients with CRSwNP (2), CRSsNP (1), and a mixed group of both (2 without previous surgery, 1 with). Therefore in any of these patients there is no evidence to support the use of antifungals. There are no randomized trials assessing antifungal agents in the treatment of selected patients with allergic fungal sinusitis, except for one PCRCT demonstrating reduced recurrence rates up to 9 months after surgery in patients treated with topical fluconazole when compared with itraconazole of placebo.[39]

TREATMENT AIMED AT IMPROVEMENT IN MUCOCILIARY CLEARANCE

Normal mucociliary clearance is dependent upon both ciliary function and the mucus blanket. Saline irrigation can improve mucociliary clearance by the removal of mucus, infected crusts and pro-inflammatory agents. Eight studies were eligible for inclusion in a Cochrane meta-analysis in 2007,[40] which demonstrated benefit from saline irrigation both when used as sole modality treatment and as an adjunct, albeit less efficacious than intranasal steroid. Large volume irrigation appears to have a greater impact on mucus management than simple sprays on RCT.[41] A subsequent RCT published in 2012 found hypertonic saline irrigations and saline spray alone had a comparable response rate to patients treated with hypertonic saline irrigation and INCS.[42] Studies directly comparing isotonic and hypertonic saline have not reported symptomatic outcomes, but suggest some benefit of hypertonic saline in terms of radiological improvement, at the cost of higher rates of local adverse effects. One small cross-over randomized trial demonstrated greater effectiveness of saline irrigation with xylitol compared with saline alone.[43]

As irrigation is generally well tolerated, it can be recommended for use in patients with CRS. As with other topical treatments, patients should be instructed on correct techniques for irrigation (**Figure 97.2**).

Mucoactive agents

Amphiphatic molecules possess the ability to be soluble in both water and organic solutions. They form the basis of surfactants. This effects both the solution and remaining molecular load behaviour at air–surface interfaces.[44] Pulmonary surfactant greatly improves the efficiency of mucociliary clearance by reducing adhesiveness of mucus to the respiratory epithelium. Acute respiratory distress of the newborn is the case example of the requirement of such agents in respiratory function. Surfactants can have both mucoactive properties and antimicrobial properties. Chemical surfactants can interfere with microbial cell membrane permeability and cause membrane disruption. These agents are often classified as cationic, anionic or zwitterioninc (possessing non-adjacent positive and negative charges) based on the charge of the hydrophilic domain present in these molecules. Cationic surfactants possess the most antimicrobial properties but are also the most irritating.[45]

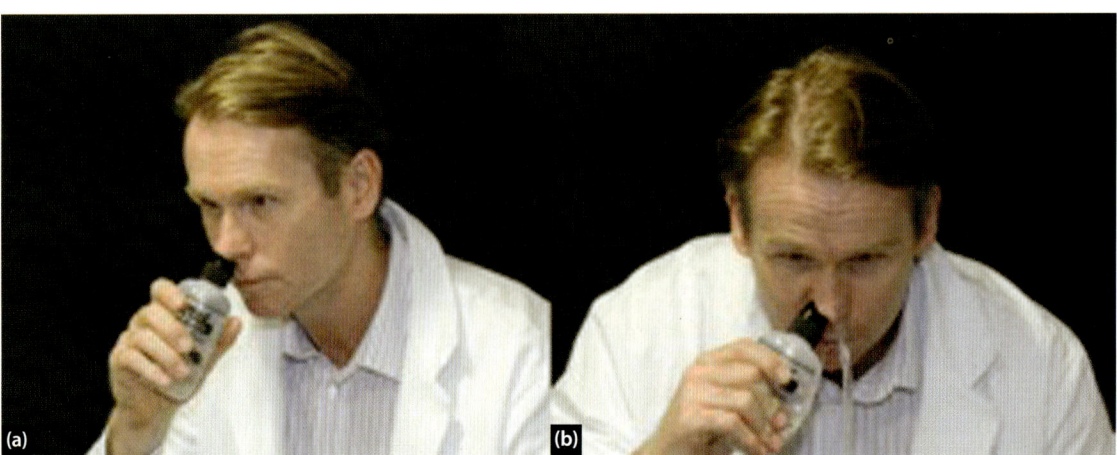

Figure 97.2 Technique for nasal irrigation.

Commercial agents such as detergents, soil wetting agents, paints, antifogging solutions and ski wax are all examples of surfactants. The combination of PEG-80 sorbitan laurate, cocamidopropyl betaine and sodium trideceth sulfate (Johnson & Johnson Baby Shampoo®) has been shown to have both antibiofilm forming properties at 1% solution and clinical efficacy in managing refractory CRS patients.[45] Surfactants may not be a direct therapy for aggressive polypoid mucosal change that is dominated by inflammatory Th2 response but they are useful for treating crusting, thick mucus and chronic bacterial mucosal colonization.

Delivery of medical therapy

Cadaveric studies have documented poor penetration of topical therapies into the sinuses, particularly the frontal and sphenoid sinuses.[46] ESS can improve delivery, but only if ostial enlargement and the extent of surgery are sufficient to do so; the minimum ostial size is 4 mm to achieve maxillary sinus penetration, and retention of the uncinate in minimally invasive techniques is likely to act as a barrier to penetration.[47] Therefore, in the pre-operative state, topical therapies reach only the nasal cavity, potentially treating nasal polyps, oedema at the ostiomeatal complex and any associated turbinate hypertrophy. In order to treat the sinus mucosa, systemic therapy must be employed. In the post-operative state, topical therapy plays a greater role in managing disease control. Studies in humans support the data from these studies with less than 0.1% of solution making the maxillary sinus.[48]

The delivery device is important, with aerosol sprays achieving poor penetration beyond the anterior third of the nose. The most effective delivery devices are the positive pressure, high-volume irrigation bottles or Neti pots, which can penetrate all sinuses in a post-operative patient following wide sinus surgery or frontosphenoethmoidectomy (**Figure 97.3**).[49]

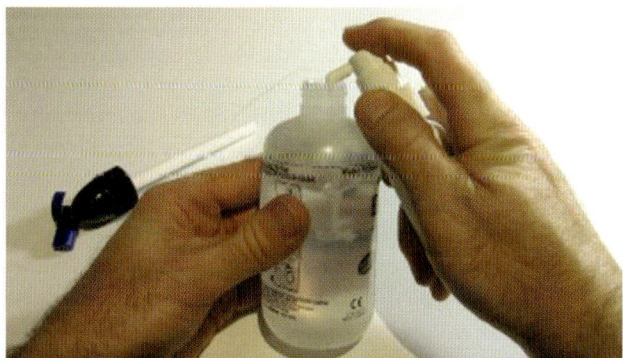

Figure 97.3 Combining local topical corticosteroid into a delivery device (such as an irrigation bottle with a volume > 100ml) makes an enormous difference to the distribution of local therapy. When combined with a wide post-surgical cavity, the ability to control the sinus mucosa is vastly different than simple nasal sprays and without prior surgery. This shift in transitioning a patient from relying on systemic medication to delivery treatment to the sinuses to a local-based therapy has dramatically changed the outcomes for patients with chronic conditions.

ASSESSMENT OF THE RESPONSE TO MEDICAL TREATMENT

As the aim of treatment for CRS is to reduce the symptom load and impact on quality of life, these subjective symptoms need to be quantified to allow repeated measures in order to evaluate response to therapy. There are several validated disease specific quality of life measures for use in CRS. Knowledge of scores in the normal population and the minimum clinical important difference facilitates detecting improvement (**Table 97.1**). Alternatively a VAS scale may be used.

Response to treatment should be considered as relief of the symptoms of CRS to the point that they are no longer present or bothersome.[13] If this is maintained, with or without ongoing medical therapy, then disease can be considered as controlled. This concept of disease control is well defined for asthma, but has been largely neglected in CRS until the recent EPOS guideline (**Table 97.2**); however, the proposed table needs to be data driven. Recent publication has suggested a refinement of this to focus on nasal obstruction, endoscopic evidence of oedema and mucus production and systemic medication use as either corticosteroid or antibiotics.[50] A proposed NOSE system was proposed (Nasal Obstruction, Systemic Medication, Endoscopy).

Control of disease is both to prevent infective exacerbations and control baseline symptoms. 'Normal' mucosa on endoscopy is the reference point but even this is not associated with 'no' nasal symptoms as many will have rhinitis reactions to account for some disease burden.

Usually 4–8 weeks should be allowed before considering treatment to have failed in patients with established CRS. If there has been improvement but incomplete resolution, a further period of ongoing medical treatment is recommended, although this is rarely with systemic corticosteroids. Persistent evidence on either endoscopy or CT of active mucosal inflammation is associated with

TABLE 97.1 Summary of outcome instruments and their key properties

Instrument	Items/ Domains	MID	Normal	Completion time (min)
Adult Acute Rhinosinusitis				
SNOT-16	16/1			5
Adult Chronic Rhinosinusitis				
RSOM-31	31/7			20
SNOT-16	16/1			5
SNOT-20	20/1			5–10
SNOT-22	22/1	8.9	7	5
RSDI	20/1	10.4		5
Rhinoqol	17/3			5–10
CSS	6/2	9.8		5
FNQ	12/1			<5
SNAQ-11	11/1			<5

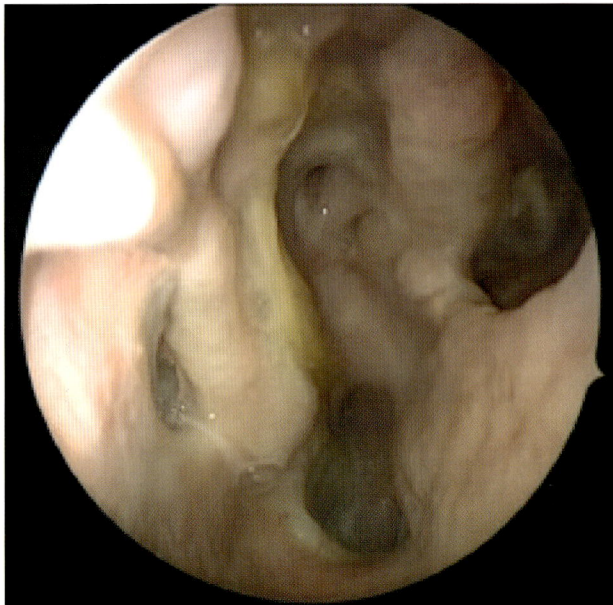

Figure 97.4 Poorly controlled CRS requiring ongoing medical treatment and likely revision surgery.

TABLE 97.2

	Controlled	Partly controlled	Uncontrolled
Blockage	-	Present	3 or more
Rhinorrhoea		Mucopurulent	
Facial pain		Present	
Smell		Impaired	
Sleep		Disturbed	
Nasendoscopy		Diseased	
Systemic medication		Required in last 3 months	

a high rate of relapse even in the asymptomatic patient (**Figure 97.4**).[51] Where patients are asymptomatic, treatment can be withdrawn in the presence of normal endoscopy and or CT. Where endoscopy remains abnormal, the patient should continue with saline irrigation and intranasal corticosteroid and counselled on the potential need for future therapy.

Where there has been no response, the history and examination findings should be reviewed to ensure both the correct diagnosis, and to exclude symptom amplifiers that may be less amenable to standard treatment – for example, coexisting depression may lead to higher levels of symptoms for a given disease burden. Secondary CRS should be considered, and assessment of the full respiratory system undertaken, including testing for secondary eosinophilic disorders, vasculatides and immunodeficiencies where appropriate. Smoking cessation should be strongly encouraged. If there is no response, and surgical treatment is being considered, a CT scan should be performed, even with positive endoscopy, as an aid to surgery and exclusion of other diagnoses (fungal ball, AFS, neoplasia) if not already performed.

Any patient with unilateral polypoid disease, where there is a suspicion of malignancy, the presence of associated neurological or orbital symptoms or atypical features should not be considered for a trial of maximum medical therapy. They require urgent radiological imaging, followed by surgery and histological examination where indicated.

WHEN DOES A MEDICAL THERAPY ONLY APPROACH FAIL?

The question of when to be more aggressive in therapy for CRS is a common question. The dictum of a trial of conservative medical therapy before surgery in every case is false. Both fungal ball and AFS are examples where initial surgery is required. Especially in CRSwNP, there is little basis to the concept of either medical or surgical treatment alone, as combined therapy is critical to control disease.[52] Thus, what is being achieved from intervening surgically? There will be CRSsNP patients in whom the mucosal oedema, basement membrane thickening and fibrosis are causing ostial occlusions, which cannot be resolved medically and are leading to persistent disease. However, this concept is not true for CRSwNP, eCRS or eosinophilic subtypes.[53, 54] Simply operating to 'unblock' or 'ventilate' the sinus is not an endpoint supported by evidence. Access for topical therapies is critical as a goal of surgery for CRS patients, and thus allows a patient to switch from relying on systemic therapies to local treatments.[52]

Failure is defined by patient-focused outcomes rather than evidence of mucosal inflammation. Those patients who have a high symptom burden despite treatment, or go on to have infective exacerbations, are failures. The benefits of repeated courses of systemic treatment need to be weighed against the risk of adverse events. We would consider the need for more than two courses of systemic treatment per year indications that medical-only treatment has failed. Greater frequency may expose patients to deleterious effects of systemic corticosteroid use.[55] Each course is recommended for 14–21 days as this best equates to the lifespan of a tissue eosinophil.[56] An accumulative dose less than 290–1000 mg is recommended, with a maximum of 30–40 mg daily, as this is the range in which significant complications and medicolegal complaints occurred.[57] Those patients that fail to derive sufficient benefit from pre-surgical medical treatment and fulfil the diagnostic criteria for CRS, in whom an alternative diagnosis is not found, and who have confirmation of mucosal disease on CT, should be considered for surgery.

Patients with complete nasal obstruction due to nasal polyps, where there has been no reduction in size following initial medical treatment, are unlikely to be able to achieve access to topical treatment. In the van Zele study,[26] symptomatic improvement was maximal shortly after completing prednisolone, and the benefit had significantly waned by 12 weeks. It may be worth considering surgical intervention at an earlier point in such patients.

MEDICAL TREATMENT POST-SURGERY

Allowing a transition to effective local or topical therapy is a critical role for surgical intervention. With this aim, surgery is often complete, wide and designed to remodel the paranasal sinus to a common cavity that can be managed. Hypersecretory mucus can be easily removed and anti-inflammatory therapy effective delivered.[52] This is especially true for CRSwNP, where local ostial obstruction is unlikely to play a major role in the perpetuation of the disease process.[53, 54]

Although nasal polyps or the presence of asthma might identify these inflammatory patients, they are still often missed. A structured histopathology of sinus tissue using defined criteria for eosinophilic CRS or greater than 10 eosinophils per high power field (>10 per hpf) will reveal an additional 20% of CRSsNP to be classified as eCRS (**Figures 97.5, 97.6**).[58] The diagnosis of eCRS has prognostic implications. eCRS is associated with greater clinical and radiological severity,[58, 59] higher risk of asthma[59] and higher risk of polyp recurrence when compared to non-eCRS.[60] Serum eosinophilia, while associated with eCRS and predictive of asthma,[59] is not predictive of the localized inflammatory processes[61] and was less sensitive for eCRS.[58] Surgery provides an ideal opportunity to make this disease distinction.

Corticosteroid irrigations are the mainstay of topical anti-inflammatory therapy post-ESS.[52–62] They are delivered in large-volume positive pressure saline irrigations. These treatments are often mislabelled as 'high dose' or 'high concentration' but neither of these is true. The delivered steroid dose is mostly in a more diluted form than

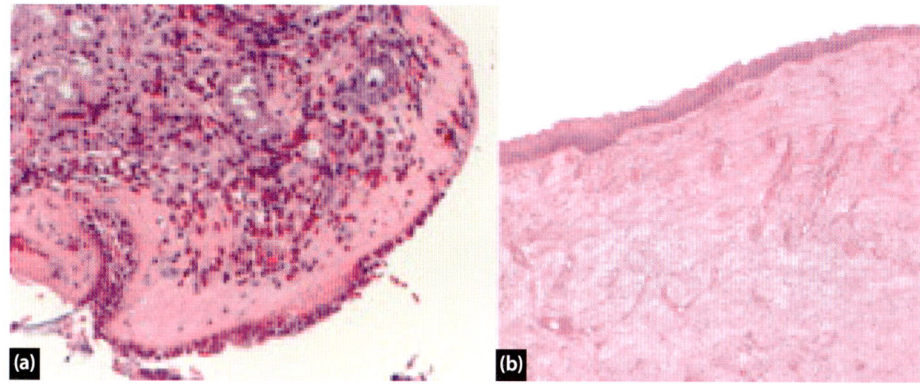

Figure 97.5 (a) Tissue eosinophilia is a marker of more severe disease and generally corticosteroid sensitive. **(b)** Significant subepithelial fibrosis is a feature of long-term tissue remodelling and likely portends a poor prognosis similar to studies on tissue remodelling and in asthma.

Chronic Rhinosinusitis Histopathology Report	
Tissue	
Overall degree of inflammation	Absent / mild / moderate / severe
Eosinophil count	<10 / 10–100 / >100 per hpf
Neutrophil infiltrate	Absent / focal / < 20 / > 20 per hpf
Inflammatory predominance	Lymphocytic / lymphoplasmocytic / lymphohistiocytic / neutrophilic / eosinophilic/ other
Basement membrane thickening	<7.5 µm / 7.15–15 µm / >15 µm
Sub-epithelial oedema	Absent / mild / moderate / severe
Hyperplastic / papillary change	Absent / present
Mucosal ulceration	Absent / present
Squamous metaplasia	Absent / present
Fibrosis	Absent / partial / extensive
Mucin	
Fungal elements	Absent / present
Charcot-Leyden Crystals	Absent / present
Eosinophil aggregates	Absent / present

Figure 97.6 An example of routine efforts to improve histopathologic profiling in CRS during routine clinical care. The structured outline provides simple information on eosinophilic inflammatory activity, eosinophil activation (aggregates and Charcot-Leyden crystals), neutrophilic infiltrate and tissue remodelling (squamous metaplasia, fibrosis and basement thickening). Simple algorithms such as corticosteroids for eosinophilic disease and potential macrolide therapy for neutrophilic predominant patients are possible with just a little pathologic assessment.

simple sprays and the total residual delivered is usually less than 5% making the exposure to the patient less than simple spray therapy.[63] They are effective since they actually deliver the pharmaceutical to the sinus mucosa. Studies have shown no effect on serum cortisol,[64] urinary cortisol or the adrenocorticotropin hormone stimulation test.[65]

SUMMARY

Medical therapy is the mainstay of management for rhinosinusitis.

For acute infections, antibiotics are rarely required and treatment is largely supportive, except in the presence of complications.

For chronic disease, reducing mucosal inflammation is a cornerstone of treatment. Intra-nasal corticosteroids are the first line of treatment. Systemic steroids, immune-modulatory drugs and novel monoclonal antibodies may be used in carefully selected cases. Antibiotics may be of benefit in acute infective exacerbations. Endoscopic sinus surgery plays an adjunctive role in facilitating delivery of topical medications when standard delivery approaches have failed.

KEY POINTS

- Medical therapy should have a 3-way goal of reducing inflammatory load, normalizing microbial community and restoration of mucocillary function.
- Medical therapy to the paranasal sinus is primarily via the systemic route in the unoperated patient.
- Systemic corticosteroid is effective, but use is usually limited to 2 courses a year, of 2–3 weeks duration and often less than 30–40mg maximal daily dose as a reducing course.
- There is little evidence of ostial obstruction as a cause of CRSwNP or the eosinophilic subgroup.
- Surgery, while potentially curative for some, is more commonly utilized to enable long-term local or topical therapy to control disease.
- Corticosteroid irrigations are a common effective delivery mechanism in the post-surgical patient. Their use is similar to that of a prophylactic inhaler for asthma patients.

REFERENCES

1. Stafford C. The clinician's view of sinusitis. *Head Neck Surg* 1990; 103: 870–5.
2. Williamson IG, Rumsby K, Benge S, et al. Antibiotics and topical nasal steroid for treatment of acute maxillary sinusitis: a randomized controlled trial. *JAMA* 2007; 298(21): 2487–96.
3. Hickner JM, Bartlett JG, Besser RE, et al. Principles of appropriate antibiotic use for acute rhinosinusitis in adults: background. *Ann Intern Med* 2001; 134(6): 498–505.
4. Rosenfeld RM, Andes D, Bhattacharyya N, et al. Clinical practice guideline: adult sinusitis. *Otolaryngol Head Neck Surg* 2007; 137(3 Suppl): S1–31.
5. de Ferranti SD, Ioannidis JP, Lau J, et al. Are amoxicillin and folate inhibitors as effective as other antibiotics for acute sinusitis? A meta-analysis. *BMJ* 1998; 317(7159): 632–7.
6. Arroll B. Non-antibiotic treatments for upper-respiratory tract infections (common cold). *Respir Med* 2005; 99(12): 1477–84.
7. Falagas ME, Giannopoulou KP, Vardakas KZ, et al. Comparison of antibiotics with placebo for treatment of acute sinusitis: a meta-analysis of randomised controlled trials. *Lancet Infect Dis* 2008; 8(9): 543–52.
8. Ahovuo-Saloranta A, Borisenko OV, Kovanen N, et al. Antibiotics for acute maxillary sinusitis. *Cochrane Database Syst Rev* 2008; 2: CD000243.
9. Lemiengre MB, van Driel ML, Merenstein D, et al. Antibiotics for clinically diagnosed acute rhinosinusitis in adults. *Cochrane Database Syst Rev* 2012; 10: CD006089.
10. Zalmanovici A, Yaphe J. Intranasal steroids for acute sinusitis. *Cochrane Database Syst Rev* 2009; 4: CD005149.
11. Chow AW, Benninger MS, Brook I, et al. IDSA clinical practice guideline for acute bacterial rhinosinusitis in children and adults. *Clin Infect Dis* 2012; 54(8): e72–e112.
12. Sastre J, Mosges R. Local and systemic safety of intranasal corticosteroids. *J Investig Allergol Clin Immunol* 2012; 22(1): 1–12.
13. Fokkens WJ, Lund VJ, Mullol J, et al. European Position Paper on Rhinosinusitis and Nasal Polyps 2012. *Rhinol* Suppl 2012; 23: 3 p preceding table of contents, 1–298.
14. Timperley D, Schlosser RJ, Harvey RJ. Chronic rhinosinusitis: an education and treatment model. *Otolaryngol Head Neck Surg* 2010; 143(5 Suppl 3): S3–8.
15. Lam M, Hull L, McLachlan R, et al. Clinical severity and epithelial endotypes in chronic rhinosinusitis. *Int Forum Allergy Rhinol* 2013; 3(2): 121–8.
16. Snidvongs K, Lam M, Sacks R, et al. Structured histopathology profiling of chronic rhinosinusitis in routine practice. *Int Forum Allergy Rhinol* 2012; 2(5): 376–85.
17. Kalish L, Snidvongs K, Sivasubramaniam R, et al. Topical steroids for nasal polyps. *Cochrane Database Syst Rev* 2012; 12: CD006549.
18. Snidvongs K, Kalish L, Sacks R, Craig JC, Harvey RJ. Topical steroid for chronic rhinosinusitis without polyps. *Cochrane Database Syst Rev* 2011; 8: CD009274.
19. Klossek JM, Laliberte F, Laliberte MF, et al. Local safety of intranasal triamcinolone acetonide: clinical and histological aspects of nasal mucosa in the long-term treatment of perennial allergic rhinitis. *Rhinology* 2001; 39(1): 17–22.
20. Moller C, Ahlstrom H, Henricson KA, et al. Safety of nasal budesonide in the long-term treatment of children with perennial rhinitis. *Clin Exp Allergy* 2003; 33(6): 816–22.
21. Lal D, Hwang PH. Oral corticosteroid therapy in chronic rhinosinusitis without polyposis: a systematic review. *Int Forum Allergy Rhinol* 2011; 1(2): 136–43.
22. Howard BE, Lal D. Oral steroid therapy in chronic rhinosinusitis with and without nasal polyposis. *Curr Allergy Asthma Rep* 2013; 13(2): 236–43.
23. Martinez-Devesa P, Patiar S. Oral steroids for nasal polyps. *Cochrane Database Syst Rev* 2011; 7: CD005232.
24. Videler WJ, Badia L, Harvey RJ, et al. Lack of efficacy of long-term, low-dose azithromycin in chronic rhinosinusitis: a randomized controlled trial. *Allergy* 2011; 66(11): 1457–68.
25. Harvey RJ, Wallwork BD, Lund VJ. Anti-inflammatory effects of macrolides: applications in chronic rhinosinusitis. *Immunol Allergy Clin North Am* 2009; 29(4): 689–703.
26. Van Zele T, Gevaert P, Holtappels G, et al. Oral steroids and doxycycline: two different approaches to treat nasal polyps. *J Allergy Clin Immunol* 2010; 125(5): 1069–76 e4.
27. Stewart RA, Ram B, Hamilton G, et al. Montelukast as an adjunct to oral and inhaled steroid therapy in chronic nasal polyposis. *Otolaryngol Head Neck Surg* 2008; 139(5): 682–7.
28. Nathan RA, Santilli J, Rockwell W, Glassheim J. Effectiveness of immunotherapy for recurring sinusitis associated with allergic rhinitis as assessed by the Sinusitis Outcomes Questionnaire. *Ann Allergy Asthma Immunol* 2004; 92(6): 668–72.

29. Gevaert P, Calus L, Van Zele T, et al. Omalizumab is effective in allergic and nonallergic patients with nasal polyps and asthma. *J Allergy Clin Immunol* 2013; **131**(1): 110–6 e1.
30. Gevaert P, Van Bruaene N, Cattaert T, et al. Mepolizumab, a humanized anti-IL-5 mAb, as a treatment option for severe nasal polyposis. *J Allergy Clin Immunol* 2011; **128**(5): 989–95 e1–8.
31. Pease JE, Horuk R. Chemokine receptor antagonists: Part 1. *Expert Opin Ther Pat* 2009; **19**(1): 39–58.
32. Coffman RL. Origins of the T(H)1–T(H)2 model: a personal perspective. *Nat Immunol* 2006; **7**(6): 539–41.
33. Zeiss CR, Lockey RF. Refractory period to aspirin in a patient with aspirin-induced asthma. *J Allergy Clin Immunol* 1976; **57**(5): 440–8.
34. Berges-Gimeno MP, Simon RA, Stevenson DD. Long-term treatment with aspirin desensitization in asthmatic patients with aspirin-exacerbated respiratory disease. *J Allergy Clin Immunol* 2003; **111**(1): 180–6.
35. Fruth K, Pogorzelski B, Schmidtmann I, et al. Low-dose aspirin desensitization in individuals with aspirin-exacerbated respiratory disease. *Allergy* 2013; **68**(5): 659–65.
36. Parikh AA, Scadding GK. Intranasal lysine-aspirin in aspirin-sensitive nasal polyposis: a controlled trial. *Laryngoscope* 2005; **115**(8): 1385–90.
37. Lim M, Citardi MJ, Leong JL. Topical antimicrobials in the management of chronic rhinosinusitis: a systematic review. *Am J Rhinol* 2008; **22**(4): 381–9.
38. Sacks PL, Harvey RJ, Rimmer J, et al. Topical and systemic antifungal therapy for the symptomatic treatment of chronic rhinosinusitis. *Cochrane Database Syst Rev* 2011; **8**: CD008263.
39. Khalil Y, Tharwat A, Abdou AG, et al. The role of antifungal therapy in the prevention of recurrent allergic fungal rhinosinusitis after functional endoscopic sinus surgery: a randomized, controlled study. *Ear Nose Throat J* 2011; **90**(8): E1–7.
40. Harvey R, Hannan SA, Badia L, Scadding G. Nasal saline irrigations for the symptoms of chronic rhinosinusitis. *Cochrane Database Syst Rev* 2007; **3**: CD006394.
41. Pynnonen MA, Mukerji SS, Kim HM, et al. Nasal saline for chronic sinonasal symptoms: a randomized controlled trial. *Arch Otolaryngol Head Neck Surg* 2007; **133**(11): 1115–20.
42. Friedman M, Hamilton C, Samuelson CG, et al. Dead Sea salt irrigations vs saline irrigations with nasal steroids for symptomatic treatment of chronic rhinosinusitis: a randomized, prospective double-blind study. *Int Forum Allergy Rhinol* 2012; **2**(3): 252–7.
43. Weissman JD, Fernandez F, Hwang PH. Xylitol nasal irrigation in the management of chronic rhinosinusitis: a pilot study. *Laryngoscope* 2011; **121**(11): 2468–72.
44. Van Hamme JD, Singh A, Ward OP. Physiological aspects. Part 1 in a series of papers devoted to surfactants in microbiology and biotechnology. *Biotechnol Adv* 2006; **24**(6): 604–20.
45. Chiu AG, Palmer JN, Woodworth BA, et al. Baby shampoo nasal irrigations for the symptomatic postfunctional endoscopic sinus surgery patient. *Am J Rhinol* 2008; **22**: 34–7.
46. Harvey RJ, Lund VJ. Biofilms and chronic rhinosinusitis: systematic review of evidence, current concepts and directions for research. *Rhinology* 2007; **45**(1): 3–13.
47. Grobler A, Weitzel EK, Buele A, et al. Pre- and postoperative sinus penetration of nasal irrigation. *Laryngoscope* 2008; **118**(11): 2078–81.
48. Snidvongs K, Chaowanapanja P, Aeumjaturapat S, et al. Does nasal irrigation enter paranasal sinuses in chronic rhinosinusitis? *Am J Rhinol* 2008; **22**(5): 483–6.
49. Harvey RJ, Goddard JC, Wise SK, Schlosser RJ. Effects of endoscopic sinus surgery and delivery device on cadaver sinus irrigation. *Otolaryngol Head Neck Surg* 2008; **139**(1): 137–42.
50. Snidvongs K, Heller G, Sacks R, Harvey RJ. Validation of EPOS 2012 disease control assessment in chronic rhinosinusitis. *Otolaryngol Head Neck Surg* 2013; **149**(2): 136–7.
51. Baguley C, Brownlow A, Yeung K, et al. The fate of chronic rhinosinusitis sufferers after maximal medical therapy. *Int Forum Allergy Rhinol* 2014; **4**: 525–532.
52. Chin D, Harvey RJ. Nasal polyposis: an inflammatory condition requiring effective anti-inflammatory treatment. *Curr Opin Otolaryngol Head Neck Surg* 2013; **21**(1): 23–30.
53. Snidvongs K, Chin D, Sacks R, et al. Eosinophilic rhinosinusitis is not a disease of ostiomeatal occlusion. *Laryngoscope* 2013; **123**(5): 1070–4.
54. Leung RM, Kern RC, Conley DB, et al. Osteomeatal complex obstruction is not associated with adjacent sinus disease in chronic rhinosinusitis with polyps. *Am J Rhinol Allergy* 2011; **25**(6): 401–3.
55. Bonfils P, Halimi P, Malinvaud D. Adrenal suppression and osteoporosis after treatment of nasal polyposis. *Acta Otolaryngol* 2006; **126**(11): 1195–200.
56. Bachert C. Evidence-based management of nasal polyposis by intranasal corticosteroids: from the cause to the clinic. *Int Arch Allergy Immunol* 2011; **155**(4): 309–21.
57. Howard BE, Lal D. Oral steroid therapy in chronic rhinosinusitis with and without nasal polyposis. *Curr Allergy Asthma Rep* 2013; **13**(2): 236–43.
58. Snidvongs K, Lam M, Sacks R, et al. Structured histopathology profiling of chronic rhinosinusitis in routine practice. *Int Forum Allergy Rhinol* 2012; **2**: 376–385.
59. Sakuma Y, Ishitoya J, Komatsu M, et al. New clinical diagnostic criteria for eosinophilic chronic rhinosinusitis. *Auris Nasus Larynx* 2011; **38**(5): 583–8.
60. Soler ZM, Sauer D, Mace J, Smith TL. Impact of mucosal eosinophilia and nasal polyposis on quality-of-life outcomes after sinus surgery. *Otolaryngol Head Neck Surg* 2010; **142**(1): 64–71.
61. Hu Y, Cao PP, Liang GT, et al. Diagnostic significance of blood eosinophil count in eosinophilic chronic rhinosinusitis with nasal polyps in Chinese adults. *Laryngoscope* 2012; **122**(3): 498–503.
62. Snidvongs K, Pratt E, Chin D, et al. Corticosteroid nasal irrigations after endoscopic sinus surgery in the management of chronic rhinosinusitis. *Int Forum Allergy Rhinol* 2012; **2**(5): 415–21.
63. Harvey RJ, Debnath N, Srubiski A, et al. Fluid residuals and drug exposure in nasal irrigation. *Otolaryngol Head Neck Surg* 2009; **141**(6): 757–61.
64. Welch KC, Thaler ER, Doghramji LL, et al. The effects of serum and urinary cortisol levels of topical intranasal irrigations with budesonide added to saline in patients with recurrent polyposis after endoscopic sinus surgery. *Am J Rhinol Allergy* 2010; **24**(1): 26–8.
65. Bhalla RK, Payton K, Wright ED. Safety of budesonide in saline sinonasal irrigations in the management of chronic rhinosinusitis with polyposis: lack of significant adrenal suppression. *J Otolaryngol Head Neck Surg* 2008; **37**(6): 821–5.

CHAPTER 98

SURGICAL MANAGEMENT OF RHINOSINUSITIS

A. Simon Carney and Raymond Sacks

Introduction 1071	Evidence based surgery for chronic rhinosinusitis 1077
Diagnosis.. 1071	Rhinosinusitis in children 1078
Surgical options... 1072	Conclusions 1078
Surgical procedures... 1072	References 1079
Surgical complications 1076	

SEARCH STRATEGY

Data in this chapter may be updated by a Medline search using the following keywords: rhinosinusitis, sinusitis and surgery, restricted to English language and abstract publication. A secondary literature review of reference lists from keynote papers and relevant book chapters was also undertaken.

INTRODUCTION

As the mucosa of the paranasal sinuses are in direct continuity with that of the nasal cavity, the term 'rhinosinusitis' has now been recognized as the correct description of a disease defined as: 'inflammation of the nose and the paranasal sinuses characterized by two or more symptoms, one of which should be either nasal blockage/obstruction/congestion or nasal discharge (anterior/posterior nasal drip): +/− facial pain/pressure +/− reduction or sense of smell'.[1]

Rhinosinusitis of less than 12 weeks with complete resolution of symptoms is termed acute rhinosinusitis (ARS) with chronic rhinosinusitis (CRS) developing at or after 12 weeks of symptoms without complete resolution.[1]

There are many exacerbating factors, which can cause or influence the severity of rhinosinusitis. These include (but are not restricted to): asthma, aspirin exacerbated respiratory disease (AERD), cystic fibrosis and immunodeficiency.[1-4]

A comprehensive history of surgery for the management of rhinosinusitis is beyond the scope of this chapter; however, it is fair to say that the advent of antibiotics and the rigid endoscope have both completely revolutionized the indications and surgical techniques for operative management of rhinosinusitis.[5]

The aetiological causes of both ARS and CRS remain controversial, incompletely understood and subject to continued speculation.[6] It is becoming increasingly apparent that surgical indications and techniques for the management of rhinosinusitis depend, to a greater or lesser degree, on the belief by the individual surgeon or local surgical community in these various aetiological theories. For example, in countries where osteo-meatal complex (OMC) obstruction is seen as paramount for disease causation, simple middle meatal antrostomy and anterior ethmoidectomy ('mini-FESS') may be considered as standard of care; whereas, in countries where surgery is predominantly seen as optimizing the environment for the application of topical medical therapies, a more complete fronto-spheno-ethmoidectomy ('full-house FESS') is deemed as a more appropriate primary procedure.[7, 8]

With new technological developments, minimally invasive options such as balloon sinus dilatation are now available[9] and yet at the other end of the spectrum, extensive 'nasalization' of all the paranasal sinuses is now possible using high powered drills, haemostatic agents and computer navigation systems.[10]

In this chapter, we will examine the literature surrounding this complex area and attempt to present it in an evidence-based manner.

DIAGNOSIS

The diagnosis of both ARS and CRS depends on an accurate history and clinical examination of the patient. Whilst nasal endoscopy and CT scanning are critical in confirming the diagnosis, these are usually only available through an ENT specialist or allergist. CRS is subdivided into disease with nasal polyps (CRSwNP) and without (CRSsNP).[1] Bilateral nasal polyps are required for a diagnosis of CRSwNP.[1] It can further be subdivided by histological phenotypes such as eosinophilic or neutrophilic CRS, which is now recognized to influence both the medical (both pre- and post-operative) and surgical management of the patient.[11]

In the specialist setting, rigid nasal endoscopy can be used to visualize the osteo-meatal complex in patients. It can also aid the collection of sinus secretions for microbiological analysis.[1] Whilst the presence of pus, erythema and oedema can be valuable positive findings, endoscopic findings remain extremely subjective and there is little evidence they alter outcomes.[1, 12–14]

Radiology

Due to the poor resolution, high false positive and false negative results, plain sinus x-rays are no longer recommended for the investigation of either ARS or CRS.[1] The advance in CT scanning technology has meant it is now possible for high resolution CT images to be rapidly obtained with a very small radiation dose. CT scans should ideally be reconstructed into three planes (coronal, axial and para-sagittal).[15] The use of laptop-based computer programs such as OsiriX, and the routine availability of images on CD-ROM, has now made further manipulation of CT images possible on an individual patient basis.[16]

SURGICAL OPTIONS

Indications for surgery

ACUTE RHINOSINUSITIS

Medical management remains the mainstay for ARS with antibiotic therapy being reserved for patients with severe disease, especially with the presence of high fever or severe (unilateral) facial pain.[1] In rare cases, ARS may progress to complications involving the orbit, the cranium or frontal bone. Where sub-periosteal and intra-orbital abscess, epidural or subdural abscesses, meningitis and/or intra-cranial sinus thrombosis, surgical options may then enter the management algorithm.[17] A good principle is that where the ARS complication is managed medically (e.g. meningitis), the ARS may be managed medically as well; whereas when a complication is to be managed surgically (e.g. orbital or intra-cranial abscess, Pott's puffy tumour), then simultaneous surgical drainage of the affected sinuses should be considered.[18]

CHRONIC RHINOSINUSITIS

There is a huge amount of evidence on the medical management of CRSwNP and also CRSsNP.[19] Well produced guidelines such as the EPOS2012 document[1] have concluded that topical steroids and nasal irrigation should be tried by primary care physicians for at least 4 weeks before considering a referral to an ENT specialist. If the diagnosis is clinically confirmed and maximal medical therapy has not improved symptoms, a CT scan is then indicated. The CT findings not only enable assessment of the presence of residual disease that could be addressed by surgery but also provide the surgeon with the ability to recognize the presence of anatomical risk factors for the development of CRS and to facilitate surgical planning. There are multiple factors which need to be considered before a decision to undertake surgery is reached;[20] these include i) patient factors; such as general cardio-respiratory health, anticoagulation treatment and social factors, ii) facility factors; such as access to (and the availability of) appropriately trained personnel and acceptable equipment levels for the type of surgery being considered and iii) economic factors; which include cost both to the individual and to the relevant healthcare system.

Appropriate informed consent must be obtained from all patients when considering surgery and this consent must include an honest discussion of the natural history of their condition,[21] the risks and sequelae of surgical complications,[22] the potential for recurrent disease,[23] the usual need for ongoing medical management and always the option of continuing non-surgical management.[24]

SURGICAL PROCEDURES

Anaesthesia for sinus surgery

Although it is entirely possible to do most forms of endoscopic sinus surgery under local anaesthetic, it is common practice for patients to have a general anaesthetic in many Western countries.[1, 25] Whilst the use of laryngeal mask anaesthesia has not yet been universally accepted, it is the authors' view that, unless there are significant increased risks of laryngeal soiling (significant laryngopharyngeal reflux, obesity or other medical factors), laryngeal mask anaesthesia is generally preferred over endotracheal intubation.[26] The use of volatile inhalation agents has declined and with the increasing availability of short acting opiates such as Remifentanil, many surgeons prefer total intravenous anaesthesia (TIVA). With TIVA there is a very small but real risk of awake anaesthesia and therefore the use of bispectoral index (BIS) monitoring is recommended to avoid this potentially serious medicolegal complication. The evidence regarding TIVA and an improved surgical field remains controversial.[27] Whilst some authors claim that there is significant benefit from TIVA,[28] the use of sevoflurane (at low concentration only) and remifentanil combined probably provides just as good a surgical field and avoids the need for BIS monitoring. Mean arterial blood pressure (MAP) is determined by the following equation: MAP = heart rate (HR) x stroke volume (SV) x systemic vascular resistance (SVR). In order to optimize the surgical field, hypotensive anaesthesia is desirable. Our evidence-based recommendation is to maintain a systolic MAP of approximately 90 mmHg, which is best achieved by maintaining the HR at approximately 60 beats per minute.[25, 27, 28] Volatile agents, which achieve hypotension by reducing SVR, can paradoxically cause a deterioration of the surgical field due to vasodilatation of the nasal microvasculature. Further discussion on anaesthesia for sinus surgery can be found in several good review articles.[25, 29, 30]

Surgical position

There is good evidence that the surgical field is optimized by placing the patient in the reverse Trendelenberg position.[31] Many surgeons remain concerned about the effect of head elevation and its potential reduction in cerebral blood flow (CBF) and oxygenation. Whilst physiological studies have confirmed that CBF does vary with head elevation, the cerebral perfusion pressure remains constant at elevations of between 0 and 30°.[31]

Intranasal preparation

There is evidence that transpalatal injection of the greater palatine canal decreases intra-operative blood loss during sinus surgery[32] but despite the evidence, the technique has failed to break through it into routine clinical practice. This may be due to the fact that whilst head elevation has been demonstrated to produce a 38.3% reduction in nasal blood flow, injection of the greater palatine canal only produces a reduction of 4.7%.[31, 32]

Topical decongestion in the form of cocaine and adrenaline, +/– sodium bicarbonate ('Moffat's solution') soaked on neuro-patties, ribbon gauze or pledgets remains most commonly used[33] although a randomized controlled trial has shown that the use of co-phenylcaine (ENT Technologies, Victoria, Australia) which is a combination of lignocaine 5% and phenylephrine 0.5%, is just as effective.[34] There are many legal restrictions on the use of cocaine and in many countries it is simply not possible for ENT surgeons to use cocaine and other alternatives are therefore required. Oxymetazoline alone is utilized in many centres with effective results.[35] Local anaesthetic infiltration of the middle turbinate, nasal septum and frontal process of the maxilla is then commonly performed. 1–2 mls of 1% lignocaine with 1 in 80 000 adrenaline is typically utilized.[35] It is always important to be aware of the total dose of cocaine, lignocaine or other local anaesthetics that are given both topically and intra-mucosally. Toxic reactions from overdose have been reported and the use of adrenaline will frequently cause a rise in heart rate with a corresponding temporary deterioration in the operative field (which may be greater than the gained benefit of the vasoconstrictor effect). Rather than immediately proceeding to surgery, it is therefore preferable to allow a period of time for topical and injected vasoconstrictors to establish their local effect, whilst allowing their systemic effect to dissipate.

Functional endoscopic sinus surgery (FESS) for rhinosinusitis

GENERAL PRINCIPLES

Recent CT scans of the patient's sinuses are mandatory and should be available to the surgeon throughout the operation.[36] If scans are available in traditional x-ray film format, these can be placed on a mobile viewing box adjacent to the surgeon. It is increasingly common for images to be provided in electronic format (DICOM-viewers). In this case, a large plasma screen TV or monitor can be placed adjacent to the surgeon and multiple images displayed on the screen simultaneously. It is important that a member of the theatre team is computer skilled to change the displayed images, if required. It is difficult for a surgeon to remember the multiple anatomical nuances of each individual patient and without the presence of images during surgery, increased complications may occur. If intra-operative image navigation is available, some surgeons regard this as an adequate replacement for the above but it is the personal preference of the authors to have standard images available at all times, in case of equipment failure or poor registration of the image navigation system.

EYE PREPARATION

Traditionally, the eyes have been left open with lubrication but many surgeons now accept limited or even complete taping of the eye, still allowing rapid access to the globe but providing for better corneal protection. There have been several medicolegal cases whereby corneal abrasions have resulted in successful lawsuits.[37]

SURGICAL TECHNIQUES[36, 38]

i) Uncinectomy

The free edge of the boomerang-shaped uncinate process can be identified in most cases by the use of a Freer's elevator. The use of a sickle knife on the interior portion of the uncinate is to be discouraged as orbital penetration can easily occur.[37] Either adult or paediatric back-biting forceps are readily available which allow for safer uncinate incision (Figure 98.1).

Superiorly on the uncinate process, the orbit is relatively more protected by the hard bone of the frontal process of the maxilla.[36] A sickle knife can be used safely in this area although a back-biter remains an acceptable alternative. The uncinate process can then be removed using

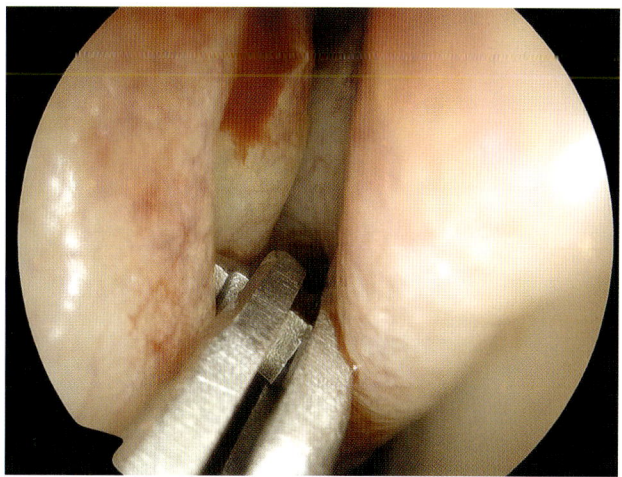

Figure 98.1 A paediatric back-biting forcep is used to perform the inferior uncinectomy incision.

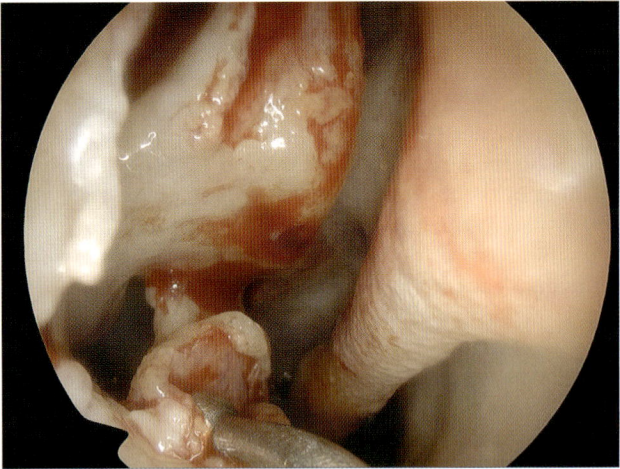

Figure 98.2 Dissecting out the bone of the horizontal process of the uncinate.

angled through-biting forceps or can be dislocated forward using a double right-angled ball probe and then cautiously removed with the microdebrider or through-biting forceps. Any rough edges can be removed using a 2 mm Kerrison's punch.[38] It is always important to then address the horizontal part of the uncinate which extends inferior to the natural ostium of the maxillary sinus. The bone of the horizontal portion can be dissected free from the mucosa (**Figure 98.2**) and the natural ostium can simply be stretched open with an angled probe or sucker, without removing any mucosa. For more advanced disease (or in revision cases), it may be necessary to remove mucosa to create a large middle meatal antrostomy.

ii) Removal of the ethmoidal bulla

The natural ostium of the ethmoidal bulla sits postero-medial to the anterior face. The ostium can be located by several methods; a double right angled ball probe or 45° antral curette can then be used to fracture the anterior face forwards (**Figure 98.3**). A microdebrider can then be used to remove the bulla, aiming for complete removal of partitions between the lamina papyracea and the middle turbinate. When removing the bulla superiorly, it is important to recognize the location of the anterior ethmoidal artery. Although commonly located in the supra-bullar recess, on rare occasions, the artery can sit within the anterior wall of the bulla and be damaged by inadvertent use of the microdebrider in this area. If present, other anterior ethmoidal cells can be removed in a similar manner. The use of through-biting instruments is preferred to standard Blakesley-Wells forceps as the latter can tear mucosa and leave exposed bone in the final sinus cavity.

iii) Posterior ethmoidectomy

The ground lamella of the middle turbinate defines the junction between the anterior and posterior ethmoid sinuses. After reference to the CT scan, the ground lamella should be perforated in the infero-medial quadrant. This avoids inadvertent injury to the skull base or lamina papyracea. Once the posterior ethmoid is opened, the roof of the maxillary sinus can be used as a guide to the superior limit of dissection within the posterior ethmoid. Anatomical studies have shown that the antral roof will always be below the skull base and allow for safe passage to the sphenoid sinus.[38, 39] A microdebrider, Kerrison's punch or through-biting instruments can be used to remove the partitions between the posterior ethmoid cells. Care should be taken in the posterior ethmoid as the optic nerve may traverse through an Onodi cell and the surgeon should always be aware of their exact surgical location at all times.

iv) Sphenoidotomy

The natural sphenoid ostium is located in the sphenoethmoidal recess, medial to the superior turbinate and at the height of the antral roof. It is not always possible to pass an endoscope medial to the superior turbinate to identify the ostium and part of the middle turbinate can be resected with a back-biting forceps, entering the superior meatus and locating the forward projection of the superior turbinate from within the posterior ethmoid cavity. The inferior third of the superior turbinate can then be resected in order to gain access to the sphenoethmoidal recess. If the sphenoid ostium can still not be located using this method, an artificial opening to the sphenoid can be made through the posterior ethmoid and then extended medially to incorporate the natural sphenoid ostium. Again, if accessing the sphenoid through the posterior ethmoid cavity, perforating the ground lamella of the superior turbinate should always be done in the infero-medial portion to avoid accidental injury to the skullbase.

v) Frontal sinus surgery

The Agger nasi cell is key to all approaches to the frontal recess.[36] In a small percentage of patients it may be absent but it is a good landmark in the vast majority of cases. Using a Kerrison's punch in the axilla of the middle turbinate (**Figure 98.4**), the anterior portion of the Agger nasi can be removed.[38]

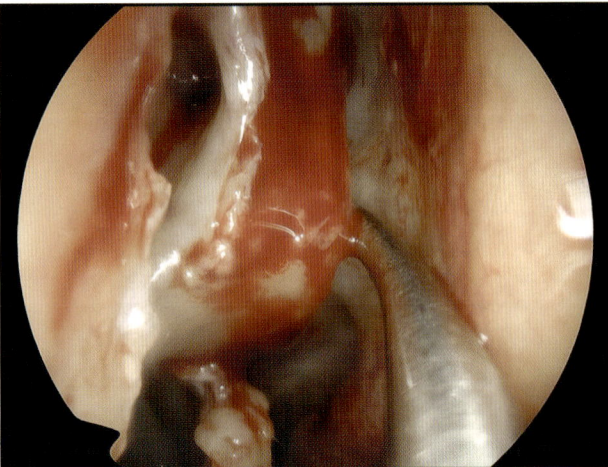

Figure 98.3 A double right-angle ball probe is inserted into the natural ostium of the bulla ethmoidalis (medial) then the anterior face is fractured anteriorly.

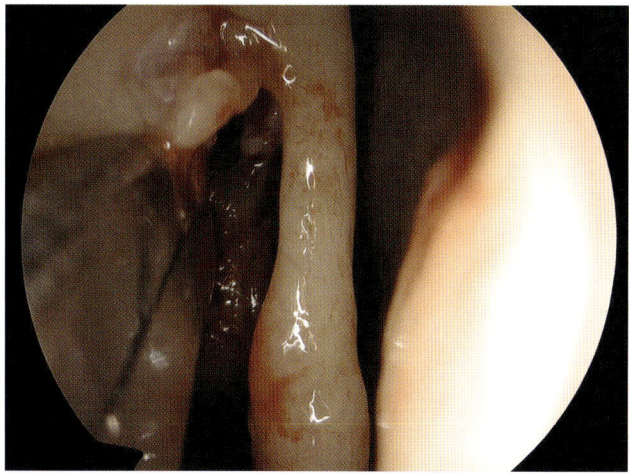

Figure 98.4 A 2 mm 450 forward-angled Kerrison's punch is used to raise the axilla of the middle turbinate and improve access to the Agger nasi and the frontal recess.

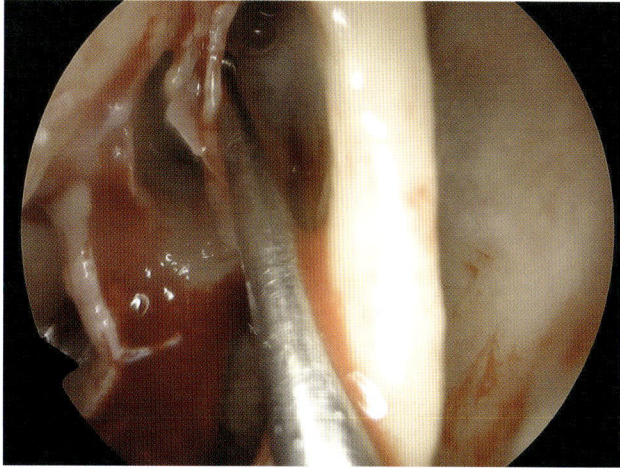

Figure 98.5 Exposure of the frontal recess by removing the posterior wall and roof of the Agger nasi cell.

Curettes and angled instruments can then be used to remove the posterior wall and roof of the Agger nasi to expose the frontal recess (**Figure 98.5**).

Although mucosal flaps have been advocated for this approach,[36] the authors no longer regularly utilize axillary flaps as adhesions can easily be prevented using other methods and regular post-operative review. Once the Agger nasi has been removed, any remaining fronto-ethmoidal cells can be removed using through-biting instruments, curettes or angled microdebrider blades. Care must be taken to avoid a circumferential injury to the mucosa in this area as this will undoubtedly result in stenosis of the frontal recess and recurrent frontal sinusitis. When dissecting the frontal recess, the position of the anterior ethmoidal artery needs to be identified and maintained in the surgeon's mind at all times. Any inter-sinus septal cells or supraorbital ethmoid cells may also need to be addressed and these generally require the use of angled endoscopes and curved microdebrider blades. Advanced frontal instrumentation such as a giraffe forceps or 3.5 mm Hosemann punch (**Figure 98.6**) may greatly facilitate surgery in this area.[38]

POST-OPERATIVE MANAGEMENT

It is critical to see patients regularly in the immediate post-operative period. Although surgeons routinely perform debridement of the sinus cavity in several countries, there is controversy as to whether this is absolutely necessary. Randomized controlled trials have shown no difference in outcomes between patients who receive regular toilet of their sinus cavities versus those that do not.[40]

Most surgeons routinely use high volume saline irrigations to clean the nose of mucopus, blood clot and other tissue.[1] Although the choice of solution is largely an individual one, a recent randomized controlled trial demonstrated improved outcomes using Ringer's lactate solution, when compared to either isotonic or hypotonic saline solution.[41] However, the cost of pre-made irrigation sachets needs to be offset against any potential benefit. There is no evidence that the use of prophylactic

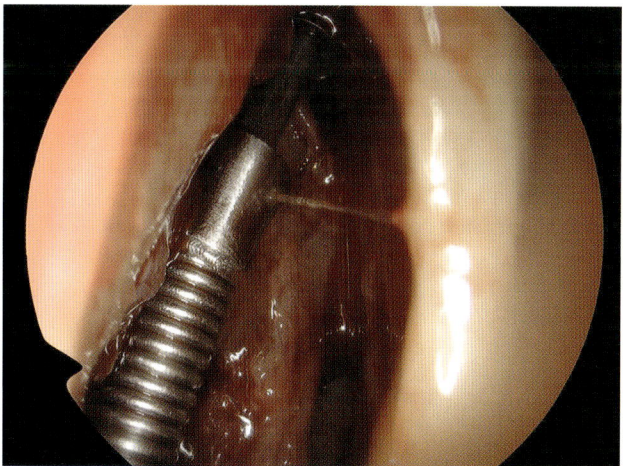

Figure 98.6 Use of a Hosemann punch to facilitate removal of Kuhn cells in the frontal recess. It is critical to avoid circumferential mucosal injury in this location.

post-operative antibiotics improves outcomes following routine endoscopic sinus surgery.[1] If mucopus is found at the time of surgery, a swab should be taken and targeted antibiotic treatment should then be prescribed. Institutional guidelines may now prevent the surgeons from prescribing routine prophylactic antibiotics unless infection is identified at the time of surgery. In the case of severe disease (and usually in most cases of CRSwNP) a 10 day course of oral Prednisolone can be given. It is the authors' practice to use 25 mg prednisolone daily for 10 days without tapering. However, individual surgeons will have their own preferred steroid regimes. It is important to remember that eosinophils can last up to 3 weeks in the tissues and if there is extensive eosinophilic disease (usually in the case of CRSwNP), it may be logical to use an extended course of steroids for 3 weeks or longer.[38] In this case, the steroid dose will need to be tapered off to avoid an Addisonian crisis. It is the authors' practice to see patients 7–10 days following surgery then weekly if there are any concerns or fortnightly if not. At 6 weeks, one would expect the sinus cavity to be fully healed and at that stage, routine nasal steroids and less frequent irrigations can be continued until review at 3 months. It is important to emphasize to patients with severe disease that they may need to be on topical steroid sprays or irrigations for some time (and in some cases, e.g. eosinophilic CRS, for an indefinite period) to prevent recurrence of their nasal polyps.

SURGICAL COMPLICATIONS

In the hands of experienced clinicians, reported complications are rare. Analysis of the literature reveals a range of significant complications between 0.3 and 22.4% (median 7.0%).[22] Although the majority of these are minor and do not result in any adverse outcome to the patient, damage to the orbit or skull-base can be severe and result in significant morbidity and mortality. Excessive bleeding and poor visualization of the operative field is associated with an increase in complication rates. When a bloody field is encountered, if this cannot be controlled, it is always safer to abandon the procedure and plan elective second stage surgery. Continuing with surgery without proper visualization can result in a catastrophic outcome. A recent meta-analysis from Australia has demonstrated that the use of intra-operative image guidance does significantly reduce the incidence of complications.[42] Such equipment however is costly and in the UK and Australia, surgeons would not routinely use intra-operative image guidance for primary, uncomplicated sinus surgery.

Avoiding complications

A proper pre-operative history will identify if the patient is taking significant medication (e.g. warfarin, clopidogrel or aspirin). There are many other drugs and homeopathic preparations that can also effect bleeding. NSAID's, fish oil and vitamin preparations are amongst those often missed. Correct interpretation of the CT scans will alert the surgeon to any presence of any high risk anatomical features which might increase the chance of damage to the orbit or cribriform plate. Dehiscence of the lamina papyracea, angulation of the vertical lamella of the cribriform plate and congenital defects in the skull base and over the carotid artery can all be identified pre-operatively.

HAEMORRHAGE

Knowledge of the anatomical location of the major branches of the sphenopalatine artery and anterior ethmoidal artery will prevent injury in the first instance. Aggressive resection of the horizontal part of the middle turbinate and extending the sphenoid ostium inferiorly will damage two of the major branches of the SPA. Identification and avoidance of the anterior ethmoidal artery should be performed in all cases where the bulla is elevated up to the skull base or the frontal recess is dissected. Small bleeding vessels can usually be controlled with topical vasoconstrictors (1 in 80 000 adrenaline, with or without cocaine). Larger vessels can be controlled with dedicated suction bipolar diathermy. Caution must be used if monopolar diathermy is considered as heat dissipation can damage surrounding structures, including the optic nerve.[43] In cases of diffuse mucosal bleeding, topical haemostats such as Surgiflo or Floseal can be utilized to good effect. Very rarely, formal ligation of the SPA[36] or exploration of the orbit for clipping of the anterior ethmoidal artery may be required. Direct bipolar diathermy of the anterior ethmoid artery is rarely required and may be problematical, owing to the presence of varying degrees of bone thickness over the artery.

ORBITAL INJURY

The orbit can be damaged with the first incision of a sickle knife through the inferior portion of the uncinate process (**Figure 98.7**). Other high risks areas are when performing a middle meatal antrostomy where there is a long thin infundibulum. If orbital fat is exposed, it is essential that the surgeon recognizes this immediately. No repair of the defect is usually necessary and the eye should be routinely checked to identify any intra-orbital haemorrhage. Any proptosis should be regarded as significant and decompression of the orbit by removing the lamina papyracea and incising the orbital periosteum may be required, with or without a lateral canthotomy and/or cantholysis.[36]

If a surgeon fails to recognize they have exposed orbital fat and continues manipulation in this area, damage to the medial rectus or other ocular muscle can occur. The use of the microdebrider has been associated with an increased risk of damage to the medial rectus muscle. If damage to the ocular muscles is suspected, an ophthalmological opinion should be obtained although there is usually little that can be done to repair a transected muscle and late oculoplastic surgery may never restore normal movement to the damaged eye.[37]

OPTIC NERVE INJURY

The optic nerve can be damaged due to intra-orbital haematoma (see above) or direct injury from within the

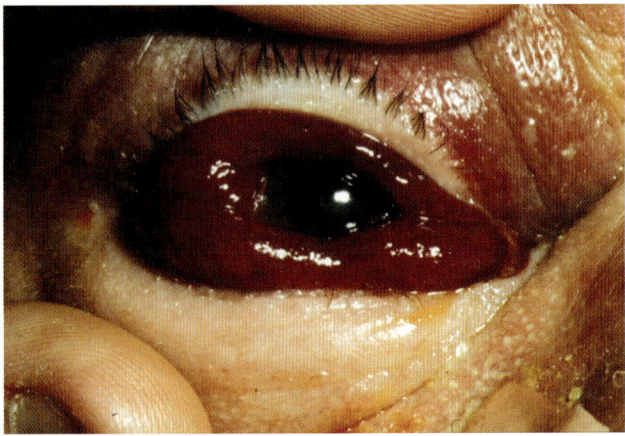

Figure 98.7 An orbital haematoma caused by a breach of the lamina papyracia during sinus surgery.

posterior ethmoid or sphenoid. It is most at risk if the optic nerve is on a mesentery within an Onodi cell. If injury to the optic nerve is suspected during a surgical procedure, steroids should be given and an urgent ophthalmological consultation should be obtained as soon as possible.

CSF LEAK

If the skull base is damaged during sinus surgery, a CSF leak can be created (**Figure 98.8**). The estimated prevalence of this is 0.5% of sinus surgical cases.[37] The area at greatest risk is surrounding the vertical lamella of the cribriform plate. If this lamella is at an angle (rather than vertical) it is more easily damaged, especially with angled instruments or microdebrider blades. Again, a bloody surgical field increases the risks of CSF leak.

Often a CSF leak can be identified immediately and can be repaired without any long-term morbidity to the patient. Repair of CSF leaks has been covered elsewhere in this book but options include fat plugs, artificial materials or homografts with or without covering mucosal grafts. The use of fibrin glue has greatly facilitated the closure of CSF leaks.

CAROTID ARTERY INJURY

The internal carotid artery can be damaged during sphenoid surgery, especially if there is a bony dehiscence over the artery. Pre-operative identification of such a dehiscence will reduce the chance of such complications arising. A carotid injury can be catastrophic and devastating. It can be extremely difficult to manage due to the high volume of exuding blood, which will obscure the operative field. The anaesthetist must commence immediate haemostatic resuscitation and the sphenoid packed. Although direct carotid artery repair (with either a J-suture or muscle pack) has been advocated,[44] placement of an endovascular stent is an effective alternate treatment option.

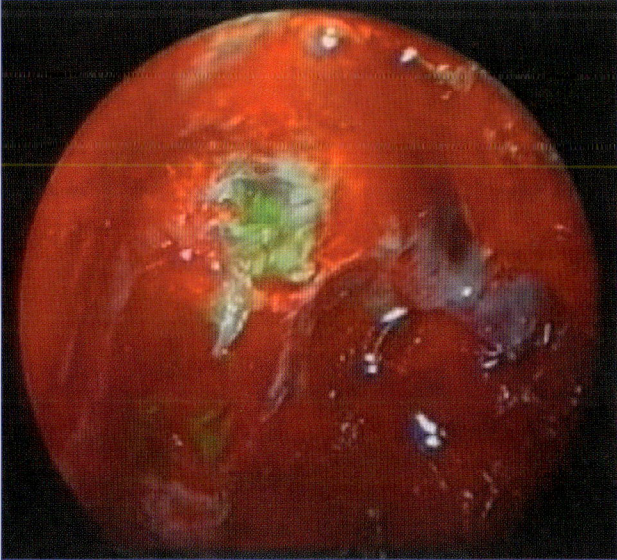

Figure 98.8 Iatrogenic CSF leak caused by damage to the skull base during FESS.

EVIDENCE BASED SURGERY FOR CHRONIC RHINOSINUSITIS

Whilst most surgeons would feel that sinus surgery benefits the vast majority of their patients, critical analysis of the literature reveals that this is not always the case. Owing to the phenomenon of cognitive dissonance,[45] surgeons will always be reminded of their successes and psychologically repress their failures. There have been few randomized controlled trials (RCT) looking at surgery for chronic rhinosinusitis. The Cochrane collaboration continues to update its analysis of evidence behind surgery for CRS and have only found six RCT's in this area and excluded three of them.[46] One trial compared twelve patients undergoing endoscopic middle meatal antrostomy with seventeen patients undergoing inferior meatal antrostomy. The trial showed no difference between the groups but was poorly powered and poorly designed.[47] A second study looked at patients undergoing FESS versus antibiotics and again found no difference between the two groups.[48] The third and best study randomized ninety patients to medical treatment (long-term antibiotics, intra-nasal corticosteroids and saline irrigations) or FESS. Whilst both treatments had significant benefit to the patients, there was no significant difference between the medical and surgical arm.[49]

In patients with CRSwNP, thirty-one patients were randomized to receive FESS on one side after oral and topical steroids. Whilst surgery provided additional benefit in some patient symptom scores, there was no difference in post-operative smell between the two groups.[50] The RCT evidence does demonstrate more benefit for patients with CRSwNP than CRSsNP.[51] Other non-RCT data provides more support for surgery, especially in patients who have failed medical management.[51] The Royal College of Surgeons of England performed the national comparative audit of surgery for nasal polyposis and chronic rhinosinusitis in 2000. This audit looked at over 3000 patients and found that patients with CRSwNP did better following surgery than patients with CRSsNP. Three point six percent had revision surgery within 12 months and 11.8% within 36 months.[52] A 5-year follow-up study published in 2009[53] revealed that 19% of patients had undergone revision sinus surgery during a 5-year post-operative period. Revision rate was 21% in patients with CRSwNP compared to 15% with CRSsNP.

Recently, studies have evaluated the implications of tissue eosinophilia on post-operative outcome. Eosinophilic CRS has been shown to be of greater clinical severity as well as having a higher recurrence of disease following surgery.[54] One recent study also showed that 'full-house' FESS with post-operative steroid irrigations significantly reduces the risk of recurrence in CRSwNP.[55]

Whilst several clinical factors have been shown to decrease baseline quality of life (QOL) scores (including; asthma, ASA status, depression, and female gender), few of these factors appear to correlate with poorer outcomes post-operatively.[56] Asthma and ASA status have been demonstrated to influence clinical outcome post-ESS.[57] One trial showed that patients with asthma or higher ASA generally had worse endoscopy scores post-operatively but showed greater symptom improvement than those without asthma.[58] Depression, whilst having no effect on objective measures, demonstrated greater degrees of improvement on QOL scores.[59] Patients who had undergone previous FESS had worse post-operative endoscopy scores although their degree of symptom improvement was similar to that seen in primary surgical patients.[60] Although contrary to established conceptions, neither smoking nor allergy has been shown to affect post-surgical outcomes following FESS.

These QOL studies have been reviewed well in several published articles.[60]

In conclusion, although there is little RCT evidence to demonstrate the benefit of FESS over medical treatment, there is a large amount of level 2 and level 3 data demonstrating that FESS is safe and produces significant symptom and QOL improvement for patients with both CRSwNP and CRSsNP.

Balloon sinuplasty

Balloon dilatation of either the maxillary, frontal and/or the sphenoid sinus ostia is an alternative technique that is increasingly being performed, especially in North America. It is a highly controversial topic and yet there is a large amount of evidence that balloon dilatation can maintain patency of the sinus ostia with 80.5% patency at 6 months, 85.1% at 1 year and 91.6% at 2 years.[61] However, cadaveric studies have shown that, when the maxillary sinus 'ostium' is dilated, the true ostium may be missed and a false ostium created in the posterior fontanelle. These findings have been confirmed by a clinical study performed in Austria.[9] There are significant health care costs with the disposable balloons used for most sinus dilatations, although reusable balloons are now entering the marketplace, which should reduce costs in the future. Small RCTs have shown balloon dilatation to be non-inferior to FESS[62] and a non-randomized trial has shown balloon dilatation to produce lower sinonasal outcome test (SNOT-20) scores compared to conventional FESS at three months.[63] Larger and more robust trials are certainly required to establish which patients should be treated with this new treatment modality and at what stage during their disease progression.[64]

RHINOSINUSITIS IN CHILDREN

The management of children with rhinosinusitis remains controversial. There is a large body of evidence to support the use of adenoidectomy alone as a first-line treatment and to reserve any form of endoscopic sinus surgery for rare and resistant cases.[1] In a meta-analysis and systematic review of adenoidectomy in paediatric CRS, 50–80% of children with CRS improved following adenoidectomy alone.[65] Whilst there does not appear to be any evidence that endoscopic sinus surgery produces any deleterious effects on mid-facial growth, it is widely accepted that conservative treatment should be pursued with all medical management options exhausted before surgery is considered in this patient age group.[1] There may be a role for surgery in patients with cystic fibrosis and immune deficiencies to provide better access for topical irrigations and medications to control their disease although fortunately, such cases remain in the minority treated by most paediatric rhinologists.

CONCLUSIONS

The advent of endoscopic sinus surgery has largely replaced external approaches to the sinuses with some exceptions relating to disease involving the lateral frontal sinus or pre-maxilla. Outcomes of FESS surgery in patients with CRSwNP and CRSsNP remain excellent where medical management has failed, however there is little evidence for endoscopic sinus surgery over medical management as a primary treatment. When significant extra-sinus complications are associated with ARS, and surgical intervention is indicated, most cases can be managed endoscopically. It should always be remembered that FESS does carry a risk of significant and severe complications and rare mortality. Good patient selection, meticulous operative technique and post-operative care remain critical to optimize patient outcomes.

> **FUTURE RESEARCH**
>
> ➤ Better evidence about the best treatment regimes for 'maximal medical therapy' prior to consideration of FESS is required.
> ➤ The relative benefits of aggressive 'full-house' FESS versus conservative 'mini-FESS' need to be ascertained.
> ➤ Balloon sinus dilatation remains an intervention where further clinical trials would clarify its role in current management algorithms.
> ➤ More research is necessary to provide an adequate evidence-basis for post-FESS medical management regimes.

> **KEY POINTS**
>
> - FESS is an effective technique for patients with both CRSwNP and CRSsNP when medical management has failed.
> - Revision rates for FESS are generally between 10–20% over a 5-year period, more so in patients with CRSwNP.
> - Good pre-operative planning, surgical technique and post-operative follow-up have been demonstrated to produce optimal outcomes.
> - FESS has been demonstrated to improve the effective medical management of patients with eosinophilic CRS.
> - CRS remains a mucosal disease and ongoing medical management is typically required to prevent recurrent symptoms despite adequate FESS.

REFERENCES

1. Fokkens WJ, Lund VJ, Mullol J, et al. European Position Paper on Rhinosinusitis and Nasal Polyps 2012. *Rhinol Suppl* 2012; **23**: 1–298.
2. Settipane RA, Peters AT, Chandra R. Chapter 4: Chronic rhinosinusitis. *Am J Rhinol Allergy* 2013; **27** Suppl 1: S11–15.
3. Settipane RA, Peters AT, Chiu AG. Chapter 6: Nasal polyps. *Am J Rhinol Allergy* 2013; **27** Suppl 1: S20–5.
4. Hanna BC, Wormald PJ. Gastroesophageal reflux and chronic rhinosinusitis. *Curr Opin Otolaryngol Head Neck Surg* 2012; **20**(1):15–18.
5. Smith TL, Kern R, Palmer JN, et al. Medical therapy vs surgery for chronic rhinosinusitis: a prospective, multi-institutional study with 1-year follow-up. *Int Forum Allergy Rhinol* 2013; **3**: 4–9.
6. Snidvongs K, Chin D, Sacks R, et al. Eosinophilic rhinosinusitis is not a disease of ostiomeatal occlusion. *Laryngoscope* 2013; **123**: 1070–4.
7. Bassiouni A, Naidoo Y, Wormald PJ. When FESS fails: the inflammatory load hypothesis in refractory chronic rhinosinusitis. *Laryngoscope* 2012; **122**: 460–6.
8. Harvey RJ, Psaltis A, Schlosser RJ, et al. Current concepts in topical therapy for chronic sinonasal disease. *J Otolaryngol Head Neck Surg* 2010; **39**: 217–31.
9. Tomazic PV, Stammberger H, Braun H, et al. Feasibility of balloon sinuplasty in patients with chronic rhinosinusitis: the Graz experience. *Rhinology* 2013; **51**: 120–7.
10. Pynnonen MA, Davis MM. Extent of sinus surgery, 2000 to 2009: a population-based study. *Laryngoscope* 2014; **124**: 820–5.
11. Lam M, Hull L, McLachlan R, et al. Clinical severity and epithelial endotypes in chronic rhinosinusitis. *Int Forum Allergy Rhinol* 2013; **3**: 121–8.
12. Marseglia GL, Pagella F, Klersy C, et al. The 10-day mark is a good way to diagnose not only acute rhinosinusitis but also adenoiditis, as confirmed by endoscopy. *Int J Ped Otorhinolaryngol* 2007; **71**: 581–3.
13. Hsu J, Pacheco JA, Stevens WW, et al. Accuracy of phenotyping chronic rhinosinusitis in the electronic health record. *Am J Rhinol Allergy* 2014; **28**: 140–4.
14. Esposito S, Marchisio P, Tenconi R, et al. Diagnosis of acute rhinosinusitis. *Ped Allergy Immunol* 2012; **23** Suppl 22: 17–19.
15. Kew J, Rees GL, Close D, et al. Multiplanar reconstructed computed tomography images improves depiction and understanding of the anatomy of the frontal sinus and recess. *Am J Rhinol* 2002; **16**: 119–23.
16. Shamshuddin S, Matthews HR. Use of OsiriX in developing a digital radiology teaching library. *Clin Radiol* 2014; **69**: e373–80.
17. Hansen FS, Hoffmans R, Georgalas C, et al. Complications of acute rhinosinusitis in The Netherlands. *Fam Pract* 2012; **29**: 147–53.
18. Desrosiers M, Evans GA, Keith PK, et al. Canadian clinical practice guidelines for acute and chronic rhinosinusitis. *Allergy Asthma Clin Immunol* 2011; **7**: 2.
19. Orlandi RR, Smith TL, Marple BF, et al. Update on evidence-based reviews with recommendations in adult chronic rhinosinusitis. *Int Forum Allergy Rhinol* 2014; **4** Suppl 1: S1–S15.
20. Higgins TS, Lane AP. Chapter 12: Surgery for sinonasal disease. *Am J Rhinol Allergy* 2013; **27** Suppl 1: S42–4.
21. Snidvongs K, Heller GZ, Sacks R, et al. Validity of European position paper on rhinosinusitis disease control assessment and modifications in chronic rhinosinusitis. *Otolaryngol Head Neck Surg* 2014; **150**: 479–86.
22. Krings JG, Kallogjeri D, Wineland A, Nepple KG, Piccirillo JF, Getz AE. Complications of primary and revision functional endoscopic sinus surgery for chronic rhinosinusitis. *Laryngoscope* 2014; **124**: 838–45.
23. Mendelsohn D, Jeremic G, Wright ED, et al. Revision rates after endoscopic sinus surgery: a recurrence analysis. *Ann Otol Rhinol Laryngol* 2011; **120**: 162–6.
24. Baguley C, Brownlow A, Yeung K, et al. The fate of chronic rhinosinusitis sufferers after maximal medical therapy. *Int Forum Allergy Rhinol* 2014; **4**(7): 525–32.
25. Amorocho MR, Sordillo A. Anesthesia for functional endoscopic sinus surgery: a review. *Anesthesiol Clin* 2010; **28**(3): 497–504.
26. Atef A, Fawaz A. Comparison of laryngeal mask with endotracheal tube for anesthesia in endoscopic sinus surgery. *Am J Rhinol* 2008; **22**(6): 653–7.
27. DeConde AS, Thompson CF, Wu EC, et al. Systematic review and meta-analysis of total intravenous anesthesia and endoscopic sinus surgery. *Int Forum Allergy Rhinol* 2013; **3**(10): 848–54.
28. Wormald PJ, van Renen G, Perks J, et al. The effect of the total intravenous anesthesia compared with inhalational anesthesia on the surgical field during endoscopic sinus surgery. *Am J Rhinol* 2005; **19**(5): 514–20.
29. Baker AR, Baker AB. Anaesthesia for endoscopic sinus surgery. *Acta Anaesthesiol Scand* 2010; **54**(7): 795–803.
30. Danielsen A, Gravningsbraten R, Olofsson J. Anaesthesia in endoscopic sinus surgery. *Eur Arch Otorhinolaryngol* 2003; **260**(9): 481–6.
31. Amedee RG. The relationship between hypotension, cerebral flow, and the surgical field during endoscopic sinus surgery. *Am J Rhinol Allergy* 2015; **29**(1): 83.
32. Valdes CJ, Al Badaai Y, Bogado M, et al. Does pterygopalatine canal injection with local anaesthetic and adrenaline decrease bleeding during functional endoscopic sinus surgery? *J Laryngol Otol* 2014; **128**(9): 814–17.
33. Valdes CJ, Bogado M, Rammal A, et al. Topical cocaine vs adrenaline in endoscopic sinus surgery: a blinded randomized controlled study. *Int Forum Allergy Rhinol* 2014; **4**(8): 646–50.
34. Douglas R, Hawke L, Wormald PJ. Topical anaesthesia before nasendoscopy: a randomized controlled trial of co-phenylcaine compared with lignocaine. *Clin Otolaryngol* 2006; **31**(1): 33–5.
35. Rodriguez Valiente A, Roldan Fidalgo A, et al. Bleeding control in endoscopic sinus surgery: a systematic review of the literature. *Rhinology* 2013; **51**(4): 298–305.
36. Wormald PJ. *Endoscopic Sinus Surgery*. 3rd ed. New York: Thieme; 2013.
37. Cottrill E, Becker SS, DeLaurentis D. Pearls and pitfalls: medico-legal considerations for sinus surgery. *Curr Opin Otolaryngol Head Neck Surg* 2014; **22**(1): 75–9.
38. Schlosser RJ, Harvey RJ. *Endoscopic sinus surgery: Optimizing outcomes and avoiding failures*. San Diego: Plural; 2012.
39. Dalgorf DM, Harvey RJ. Chapter 1: Sinonasal anatomy and function. *Am J Rhinol Allergy* 2013; **27** Suppl 1: S3–6.
40. Green R, Banigo A, Hathorn I. Postoperative nasal debridement following functional endoscopic sinus surgery, a systematic review of the literature. *Clin Otolaryngol* 2015; **40**(1): 2–8.
41. Low TH, Woods CM, Ullah S, Carney AS. A double-blind randomized controlled trial of normal saline, lactated Ringer's, and hypertonic saline nasal irrigation solution after endoscopic sinus surgery. *Am J Rhinol Allergy* 2014; **28**(3): 225–31.
42. Dalgorf DM, Sacks R, Wormald PJ, et al. Image-guided surgery influences perioperative morbidity from endoscopic sinus surgery: a systematic review and meta-analysis. *Otolaryngol Head Neck Surg* 2013; **149**(1): 17–29.
43. Asaka D, Nakayama T, Hama T, et al. Risk factors for complications of endoscopic sinus surgery for chronic rhinosinusitis. *Am J Rhinol Allergy* 2012; **26**(1): 61–4.
44. Valentine R, Wormald PJ. Carotid artery injury after endonasal surgery. *Otolaryngol Clin North Am* 2011; **44**(5): 1059–79.
45. Homer JJ, Sheard CE, Jones NS. Cognitive dissonance, the placebo effect and the evaluation of surgical results. *Clin Otolaryngol Allied Sci* 2000; **25**(3): 195–9.
46. Khalil HS, Nunez DA. Functional endoscopic sinus surgery for chronic rhinosinusitis. *Cochrane Database Syst Rev* 2006(3): CD004458.
47. Fairley JW. A prospective randomized controlled trial of functional endoscopic sinus surgery: endoscopic middle meatal antrostomy versus conventional inferior meatal antrostomy. Interim results. *Clin Otolaryngol* 1994; **19**: 267.
48. Hartog B, van Benthem PP, Prins LC, et al. Efficacy of sinus irrigation versus sinus irrigation followed by functional endoscopic sinus surgery. *Ann Otol Rhinol Laryngol* 1997; **106**(9): 759–66.
49. Ragab SM, Lund VJ, Scadding G. Evaluation of the medical and surgical treatment of chronic rhinosinusitis: a prospective, randomised, controlled trial. *Laryngoscope* 2004; **114**(5): 923–30.
50. Blomqvist EH, Lundblad L, Bergstedt H, et al. A randomized prospective study comparing medical and medical-surgical treatment of nasal polyposis by CT. *Acta Otolaryngol* 2009; **129**(5): 545–9.
51. Georgalas C, Cornet M, Adriaensen G, et al. Evidence-based surgery for chronic rhinosinusitis with and without nasal polyps. *Curr Allergy Asthma Rep* 2014; **14**(4): 427.
52. Hopkins C, Browne JP, Slack R, et al. The national comparative audit of surgery for nasal polyposis and chronic rhinosinusitis. *Clin Otolaryngol* 2006; **31**(5): 390–8.
53. Hopkins C, Slack R, Lund V, et al. Long-term outcomes from the English national comparative audit of surgery for nasal polyposis and chronic rhinosinusitis. *Laryngoscope* 2009; **119**(12): 2459–65.

54. Snidvongs K, McLachlan R, Chin D, et al. Osteitic bone: a surrogate marker of eosinophilia in chronic rhinosinusitis. *Rhinology* 2012; **50**(3): 299–305.
55. Snidvongs K, Pratt E, Chin D, et al. Corticosteroid nasal irrigations after endoscopic sinus surgery in the management of chronic rhinosinusitis. *Int Forum Allergy Rhinol* 2012; **2**(5): 415–21.
56. Goldstein GH, Kennedy DW. Long-term successes of various sinus surgeries: a comprehensive analysis. *Curr Allergy Asthma Rep* 2013; **13**(2): 244–9.
57. Vashishta R, Soler ZM, Nguyen SA, et al. A systematic review and meta-analysis of asthma outcomes following endoscopic sinus surgery for chronic rhinosinusitis. *Int Forum Allergy Rhinol* 2013; **3**(10): 788–94.
58. Nakamura H, Kawasaki M, Higuchi Y, et al. Effects of sinus surgery on asthma in aspirin triad patients. *Acta OtoLaryngol* 1999; **119**(5): 592–8.
59. Litvack JR, Mace J, Smith TL. Role of depression in outcomes of endoscopic sinus surgery. *Otolaryngol Head Neck Surg* 2011; **144**(3): 446–51.
60. Soler ZM, Smith TL. Quality of life outcomes after functional endoscopic sinus surgery. *Otolaryngol Clin North Am* 2010; **43**(3): 605–12.
61. Weiss RL, Church CA, Kuhn FA, et al. Long-term outcome analysis of balloon catheter sinusotomy: two-year follow-up. *Otolaryngol Head Neck Surg* 2008; **139**(3 Suppl 3): S38–46.
62. Cutler J, Bikhazi N, Light J, Truitt T, Schwartz M, Investigators RS. Standalone balloon dilation versus sinus surgery for chronic rhinosinusitis: a prospective, multicenter, randomized, controlled trial. *Am J Rhinol Allergy* 2013; **27**(5): 416–22.
63. Friedman M, Schalch P, Lin HC, et al. Functional endoscopic dilatation of the sinuses: patient satisfaction, postoperative pain, and cost. *Am J Rhinol* 2008; **22**(2): 204–9.
64. Batra PS. Evidence-based practice: balloon catheter dilation in rhinology. *Otolaryngol Clin North Am* 2012; **45**(5): 993–1004.
65. Brietzke SE, Brigger MT. Adenoidectomy outcomes in pediatric rhinosinusitis: a meta-analysis. *Int J Ped Otorhinol* 2008; **72**(10): 1541–5.

CHAPTER 99

THE FRONTAL SINUS

Salil Nair

Introduction	1081	Osteomas	1099
Anatomy	1081	Malignant tumours involving the frontal sinus	1103
The frontal recess	1081	Other conditions	1103
Congenital frontobasal malformations	1086	Aetiology	1103
Inflammatory conditions of the frontal sinus	1087	Clinical features and investigations	1103
Frontal sinus surgery	1089	Management	1103
Tumours	1098	References	1104
Benign tumours	1098		

SEARCH STRATEGY

Data in this chapter may be updated by a Medline search (as well as PubMed) using the following keywords: frontal sinus, Draf, Lothrop, frontal sinus drill out, osteoplastic flap, osteoma focusing on anatomy, diagnosis, outcomes, management and surgical strategy. The evidence in this chapter is mainly levels 3/4 with some level 2 evidence. The clinical recommendations are predominantly B and C.

INTRODUCTION

The frontal sinus is arguably the most complex of the paranasal sinuses. It demonstrates great variability in size and septation and is rarely symmetrical. In up to 5% of the population this sinus is absent or rudimentary.[1]

ANATOMY

An overview of the anatomy of the paranasal sinuses is covered in Chapter 87. This section refers specifically to the complex anatomy of the frontal recess and frontal sinus.

The frontal sinus ostium drains into an hourglass shaped space termed the frontal recess. Previously, this was incorrectly termed the frontonasal duct but it is not a tubular structure. The frontal recess is a three-dimensional space which communicates with the ethmoidal infundibulum within the middle meatus. In essence the ventilation and drainage of both the maxillary and frontal sinuses pass through narrow complex clefts and spaces before they reach the middle meatus. These clefts and spaces are part of the anterior ethmoid air cells. A normal healthy frontal sinus is therefore dependent on the health of the anterior ethmoids.

Only in the frontal sinus is mucus actively transported inwardly. This is along the frontal intersinus septum, laterally along the roof and back medially along the floor. Less than 60% exits the sinus in any given circuit. Hence, there is a significant recirculation of mucus.[2]

THE FRONTAL RECESS

The frontal recess is bound anteriorly by the agger nasi and the frontal process of the maxilla, the frontal beak. The thickness of the frontal beak depends on the pneumatization of the agger nasi and the presence of frontoethmoidal cells. In general, but not invariably, the greater the number of cells and pneumatization present the smaller the beak and the wider the frontal ostium.[3] The medial border of the frontal recess is the superior attachment of the middle turbinate, the lateral lamella of the cribriform plate, the height and angle of which can vary considerably. The lateral and posterior boundaries are formed by the lamina papyracea and the upward continuation of the anterior face of the bulla, respectively. If the bulla lamella is absent superiorly, a suprabulla space will communicate directly with the frontal recess. In this situation the anterior ethmoidal artery is not protected by the bulla lamella and may be at risk during dissection of the frontal recess. The anterior ethmoidal artery, traversing the skull base

1081

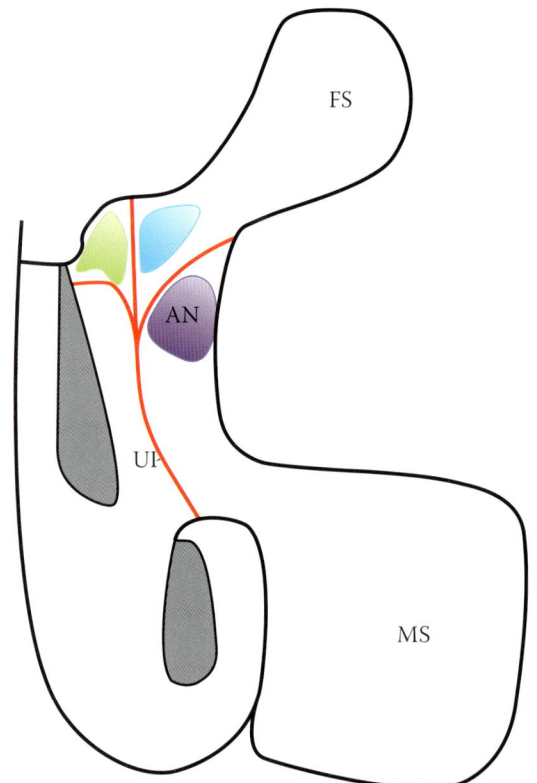

Figure 99.1 Attachments of the uncinate process (UP). Note the presence of frontal ethmoidal cells may alter the attachment of the uncinate process to the skull base, middle turbinate or a combination of these (AN, Agger nasi; FS, Frontal sinus; MS, Maxillary sinus).

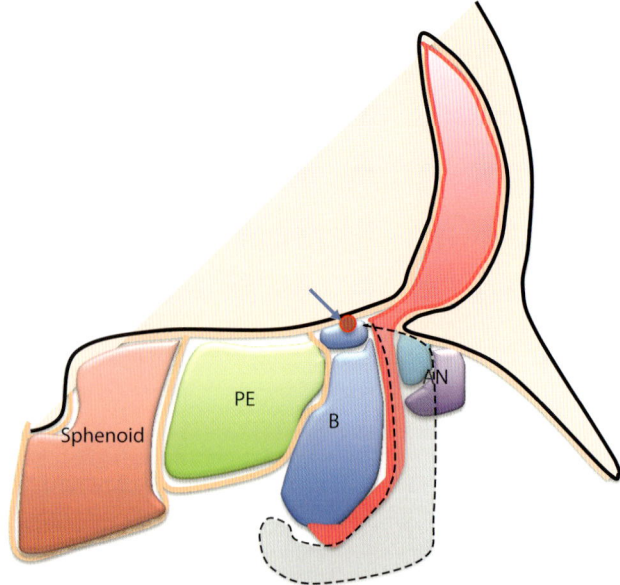

Figure 99.2 The lateral nasal wall. The uncinate process is outlined in a black dotted line. Note its relationship with the agger nasi (AN), B (bulla) and PE (posterior ethmoid). Arrow highlights the anterior ethmoidal artery.

from laterally posteriorly to medially anteriorly, is more likely to lie in a mesentery when the olfactory fossa depth is greater than 4 mm.[4] Superiorly, the frontal recess communicates with the frontal sinus but posterior to this, the roof is formed by the fovea ethmoidalis.

Both the agger nasi and uncinate process are key structures in understanding the frontal recess. The agger nasi cell is present in over 90% of patients.[5] The crescent shaped uncinate process attaches inferiorly to the inferior turbinate but superiorly it can attach to the lamina papyracea (33%), skull base (10%) or middle turbinate and a combination of these (57%) (**Figure 99.1**). When present, the medial, posterior and even superior walls of the agger nasi cell are often attached or intimately related to the superior aspect of the uncinate process (**Figure 99.2**).[6]

There are many complex anatomical variations within the frontal recess. Building a three-dimensional image of the various cells is crucial to understanding the anatomy and safe dissection in this area. This has been elegantly described by Wormald et al. in numerous articles and texts.[3, 7, 8]

The simplest configuration within the frontal recess is the presence of an agger nasi cell only. In this instance the uncinate process, curving around the agger cell, would most likely attach directly to the lamina papyracea. Following an uncinectomy and viewed from below, the superior cut end of the uncinate resembles 'a vertical bar'. Access to the frontal sinus is medial to the vertical bar.[9]

Accessory cells in the frontal recess

The array of cells within the frontal recess can be complex and confusing. In an attempt to provide clarity, Bent and Kuhn proposed an early classification of these cells.[10] This has since been modified.[3] The most recent classification describes the various cells as anterior or posterior, and medial or lateral, with respect to the frontal recess.[11]

Frontal ethmoidal cells are frequently present and classified 1 to 4 (**Table 99.1**). These are anterior ethmoidal cells that are in contact with the frontal process of the maxilla, the anterior limit of the frontal recess. They sit above the agger nasi cell and are described by their number and degree of extension into the frontal sinus. Recently, a more simplified classification has been proposed. The IFAC (International Frontal Sinus Anatomy Classification), primarily describes these accessory cells based on their location and relationship with the agger nasi and ethmoid bulla.[12] Anterior cells are termed supra agger cells and if extending into the frontal sinus are called supra agger frontal cells (SAF). Supra bulla cells are posterior cells and similarly if these extend into the frontal sinus are called supra bulla frontal (SBF) cells. When multiple or large they can obstruct ventilation of the frontal sinus (**Figure 99.3**). Being able to *read* the configuration of these cells, and how it affects the outflow tract is an important step in dissecting the frontal recess. In general, frontal ethmoidal cells tend to push the frontal sinus drainage pathway either posteriorly and/or medially (**Figure 99.4**).

In order to build a three-dimensional understanding of the frontal recess, CT images in the coronal, axial and parasagittal planes are required. In **Figure 99.5** the coronal CT image depicts bilateral frontal cells (**a**). If one merely looked at image (**b**), the frontal ethmoidal cell on the left

TABLE 99.1 Classification of frontal sinus and recess cells

Cell type	Description	Significance	Best CT view
Anterior*			
Agger nasi	A cell that sits anterior to, or directly above to the origin of the middle turbinate	Push the drainage pathway of the frontal sinus medial, posterior or posteromedially	Coronal, Sagittal
Frontal ethmoidal	Anterior lateral ethmoid cells above the agger nasi cell (in contact with the frontal process of the maxilla)		
Type 1/SAC	Single cell above the agger nasi cell – supra agger cell (SAC)	Tend to push the drainage pathway posteriorly	
Type 2/SAC	Tier of cells above the agger nasi cell		
Type 3/SAFC	A frontal cell that pneumatizes into the frontal sinus – supra agger frontal cell (SAFC)		
Type 4/SAFC	A frontal cell that pneumatizes into the frontal sinus and extends by more than 50% of the vertical height of the sinus (**Figure 99.6**)	Removal of these cells will often require an extended frontal sinus procedure	
Posterior*			
Supra bulla	Cell above the bulla not pneumatizing into the frontal sinus	May contain the anterior ethmoid artery	Sagittal
Frontal bulla or supra bulla frontal cell (SBFC)	A cell pneumatizing forward from the bulla or suprabulla space. These 'crawl' along the skull base. Posterior wall of the cell is the skull base.	They tend to push the frontal sinus drainage pathway anteriorly	Coronal, Axial
Supraorbital ethmoid	Pneumatization of the orbital plate of the frontal bone. Posterior wall is the skull base	Give the impression that one has entered the frontal sinus. They open posterior and lateral to the frontal ostium. Associated with anterior ethmoid artery in a mesentery	
Medial*			
Intersinus or frontal septal	Cell based medially in the anterior ethmoid region or pneumatizing the interfrontal sinus septum	Tend to push the drainage pathway laterally	Coronal, Axial

* Refers to EPOS anatomical terminology classification.[11] Supra agger frontal cell (SAFC), based on the IAFC (International Frontal Sinus Anatomy Classification), is an anterior lateral ethmoidal cell that extends into the frontal sinus (T3 cell) whereas a large SAFC can significantly pneumatize into the frontal sinus (T4 cell).[12]

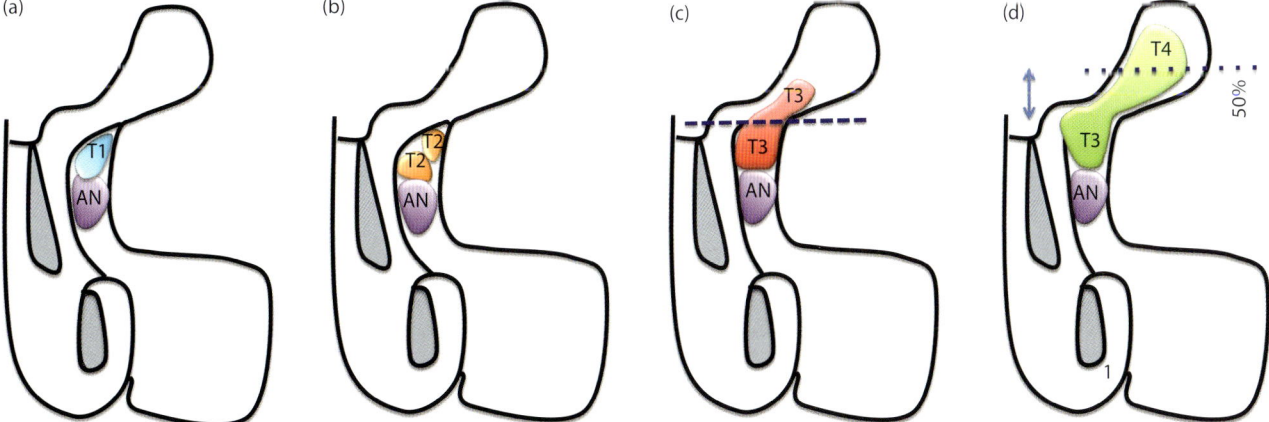

Figure 99.3 Frontal ethmoidal cells. A type 1 or Supra Agger cell (SAC), a single cell sitting above the aggger nasi **(a)**. Multiple supra cells, but not entering the frontal sinus **(b)**. Any cell extending beyond the floor of the frontal sinus (hashed line) is at least a type 3 cell or supra agger frontal cell (SAFC) **(c)**. In **(d)** a cell extending beyond 50% of the height of the sinus (dotted line), is termed a type 4 cell or large SAFC.

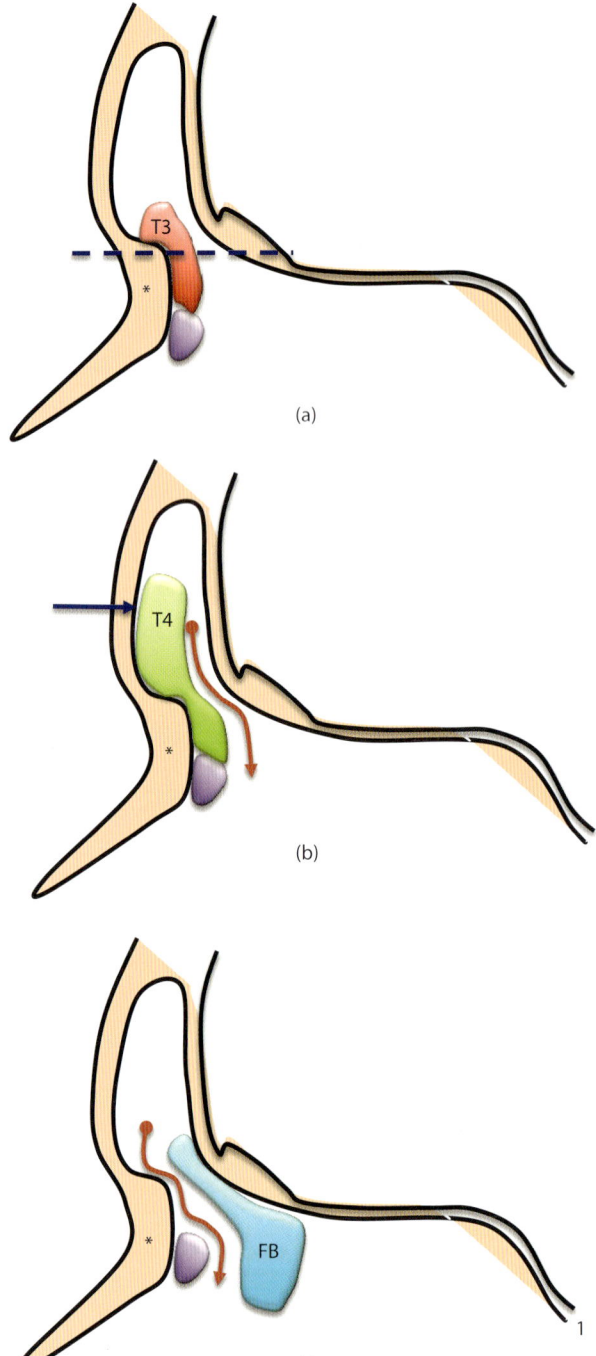

Figure 99.4 Parasagittal views. In **(a)**, a type 3, or small supra agger frontal (SAF) cell pushes above the floor of the frontal sinus (dotted line). In **(b)** a type 4, or large supra agger frontal (SAF) cell extends above 50% of the height (solid arrow) of the frontal sinus. In **(c)** a frontal bulla (FB), or supra bulla frontal (SBF) cell pneumatizes forward from the bulla. It is not in contact with the frontal process of the maxilla or frontal beak (*). The red arrows indicate the drainage pathway of the frontal sinus, which is anterior to the frontal bulla cell and posterior to the frontal ethmoidal cell.

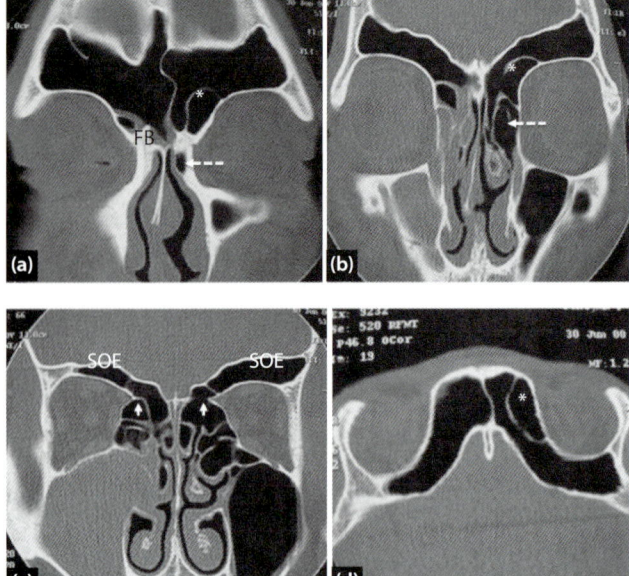

Figure 99.5 In the coronal CT scans **(a)** and **(b)**, the frontal beak (FB), agger nasi cell (dotted arrow) and type 3 cell can be seen (*). Pneumatization of the orbital plate of the frontal bone, the supraorbital ethmoids (SOE), produces a curious 'double lamina' effect of the orbital roof. The anterior ethmoidal artery (solid arrow) is seen traversing the space in a mesentery **(c)**. Axial image identifying the type 3 cell within the frontal sinus **(d)**.

extending superiorly into the frontal sinus, thus making this a type 3 cell. The drainage pathway is best studied in the axial images, and in this case is medial to the type 3 cell (d). It is through these pathways that one can dissect the frontal recess and remove obstructing cells.

Type 4 cells are rarely isolated within the frontal sinus and usually pneumatize from the frontal recess. They can be extensive (**Figure 99.6**) and cause disease by direct obstruction of the outflow tract or be diseased themselves. In most instances, it is not possible to completely remove these cells via a standard frontal sinus approach and an extended procedure such as a modified endoscopic Lothrop may be required.

In approximately 65% of Caucasian patients, the orbital plate of the frontal bone can be extensively pneumatized, resulting in supraorbital ethmoid cells (SOEC) (**Figure 99.5c**). An ethnic variation does exist with the incidence being much lower in east Asia.[13] SOEC can present a number of surgical challenges. Firstly, the anterior ethmoidal artery is more likely to be present in a mesentery and hence susceptible to injury.[4] Secondly, a greater proportion of the orbit and skull base are exposed within the surgical field. Finally, it is easy to mistake the opening of the supraorbital cells as that of the frontal sinus. The former tends to open more posteriorly and laterally.

Cells can pneumatize forward from the bulla itself (frontal bulla cells) or above the bulla (suprabulla cells). These 'crawl' along the skull base and if large enough can push the frontal sinus drainage pathway anteriorly (**Figure 99.4**). Large frontal bulla cells can appear as isolated cells within the frontal sinus and be mistaken for a type 4 cell on a coronal CT scan image. They are readily

side would have been identified incorrectly as a type 1 cell sitting above the agger nasi cell. However, 'walking' forwards through the images one can identify the same cell

99: THE FRONTAL SINUS

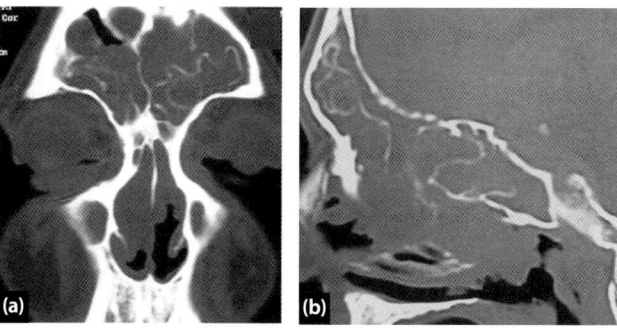

Figure 99.6 Extensive bilateral type 4 cells (a) coronal view and (b) parasagital.

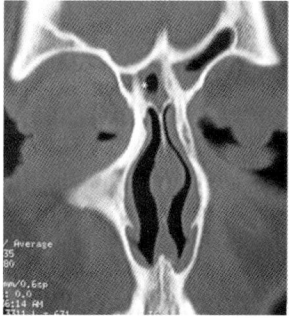
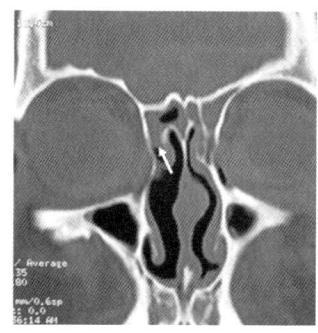

Figure 99.8 Interfrontal sinus septal cells (*). Drainage pathway (solid arrow).

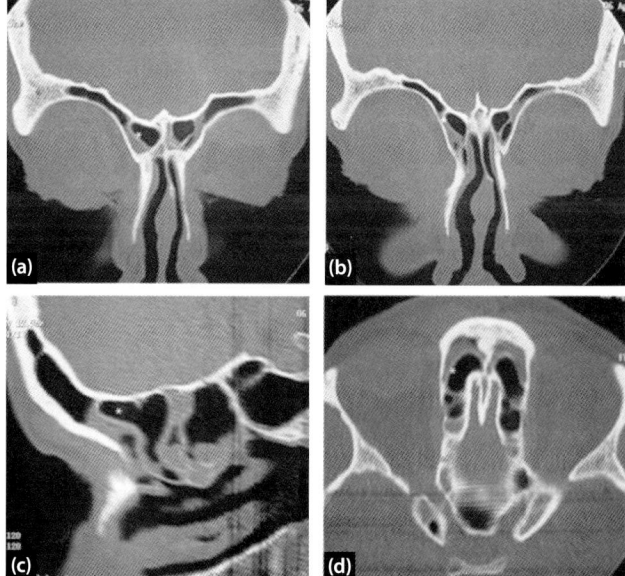

Figure 99.7 Frontal bulla cells. (a) CT image shows cells within the frontal sinus (*). These cells are present in the frontal recess and closely applied to the skull base (b). The parasagittal view confirms forward pneumatisation of the bulla (c). Note the mucosal thickening and frontal sinus drainage pathway anterior to the frontal bulla cells (d).

distinguished from frontal ethmoidal cells as they are not in contact with the frontal process of the maxilla or the frontal beak. Instead they hug the skull base and are best identified on the axial and parasagittal CT sections (**Figure 99.7**). On coronal CT images supraorbital ethmoid cells are found lateral to the frontal sinus, whereas frontal bulla cells are medially placed.

As the name indicates, frontal intersinus septal cells arise from the frontal sinus septum. These tend to push the drainage pathway laterally and ultimately drain into the frontal recess on that side (**Figure 99.8**). According to the most recent classification proposed by the EPOS (European position paper) group, an intersinus septal cell is therefore a medial frontoethmoidal cell.[11]

Diagnosis

A carefully taken clinical history is indispensible. This is particularly important with frontal sinus symptoms where often a diagnosis of headache has been mislabelled as frontal sinusitis. Sinus headaches are uncommon. An excellent review on the subject by Jones explains that the vast majority of people presenting with symmetrical frontal headache have a tension type headache. Unilateral, episodic headaches are vascular in origin.[14] The headache history is important to try and characterize the symptoms and exclude frontal sinusitis.

A history of facial trauma, previous sinonasal surgery and comorbidities such as asthma and aspirin sensitivity are relevant.

Most patients would undergo a full otorhinolaryngological examination. Rarely inspection of the forehead might reveal a swelling which may or may not be tender. Painful percussion is suggestive of acute frontal sinusitis or even osteomyelitis, so called Pott's puffy tumour. A painless swelling may indicate a mucocoele.

Endoscopy

Although anterior rhinoscopy is routinely performed, the accepted gold standard is nasal endoscopy. Traditionally, 4 mm rigid endoscopes have been used to examine the nose. However, smaller 3 mm endoscopes provide very similar optics and tend to be better tolerated by most patients. Narrower 2.7 mm and 1.9 mm endoscopes are available but compromise image quality and are less robust. Despite the use of narrow endoscopes, access to the middle meatus may be difficult. In patients who have had previous surgery an angled endoscope (30° or 45°) is useful in examining the frontal recess. In addition, a flexible nasendoscope can be navigated into the frontal sinus for inspection purposes.

Imaging

Plain sinus X-rays are inadequate for the routine diagnosis and management of frontal sinus disease. They are useful in providing a template of the frontal sinus when considering an osteoplastic flap procedure. The recommended view is an occipitofrontal sinus plain X-ray.

Ultrasonography is not routinely used for imaging of the paranasal sinuses. Scintigraphy is useful in diagnosing osteomyelitis of the frontal bone. It is helpful in assessing the extent of disease and for follow-up purposes.

COMPUTER ASSISTED TOMOGRAPHY (CT)

Clinical history and nasal endoscopy are essential in managing patients with frontal sinus symptoms but this must be complemented by imaging. CT is the first choice of radiological imaging for sinus disease and is essential for planning surgery. In pre-operative planning, coronal sinus images are most frequently used due to better correlation of radiological and clinical findings during surgery. However, studies have demonstrated that parasagittal views are very helpful in not only identifying the complex cells within the frontal sinus but also the drainage pathways.[15, 16] Ideally, CT images should be available in coronal, axial and parasagittal planes. Although Zinreich et al.[17] proposed a protocol for CT imaging of the sinuses, most institutions will have developed their own preferred technique. Current low dose spiral and multidetector CT scanners are able to acquire images quickly and reformat axial images into coronal and parasagittal planes. The need to acquire direct coronal images is no longer necessary and the effective dose of paranasal sinus CT can be reduced to the order of a chest radiograph.[18] Advantages of axial scanning include improved patient comfort during scanning and avoidance of dental artifacts. Furthermore, raw data from thin section axial scanning can be used for intra-operative computer assisted navigation, if available. Excellent detail can be achieved with contiguous axial cuts of 0.6 mm thickness. A satisfactory compromise might be to use thin-collimation contiguous, 1 mm thickness axial slices. Scan should be reconstructed in the axial, coronal and sagittal planes using both soft-tissue and high resolution algorithm bone windows with a reconstruction thickness of 3 mm or less.[19] The standard bone window/level settings range between 1500–2000/300 Hounsfield units (HU) and 450/50 HU for soft tissue windows. Many centres have access to picture archiving and communication systems (PACS), which allow the end user to easily alter the window settings. This is particularly helpful in fungal ball and chronic fungal sinus disease, where soft tissue window settings may demonstrate double densities associated with calcification and eosinophillic mucin, respectively.

MAGNETIC RESONANCE IMAGING (MRI)

MRI offers excellent soft tissue detail but no bony definition. It is very useful in differentiating tumour from retained secretions. Tumours tend to enhance with T1-weighted gadolinium enhanced scans while fluids do not. Mucus and secretions tend to avidly enhance on T2-weighted images. MRI is very helpful in assessing the dual interfaces between the nasal cavity, and the orbit and the intra-cranial cavity.[20] Enhancement of the lamina papyracea or dura may indicate tumour involvement. Indeed, dural thickening of greater than 2 mm, loss of the hypointense zone and nodular enhancement are highly predictive of dural invasion by malignancy.[21] MRI is particularly useful in assessing patients with ongoing symptoms, who have previously undergone an osteoplastic flap with obliteration. The scans can helpfully distinguish mucocole formation from fat necrosis and infection.[22, 23]

It is recommended that in cases of unilateral sinus disease, both CT and MRI are routinely performed. The two imaging modalities are complementary in diagnosing tumours such as inverted papilloma and fungal disease. The characteristic appearances of fungal disease are an iso- or hypo-attenuated signal on T1-weighted images and a signal void on T2-weighted images.[24]

CONGENITAL FRONTOBASAL MALFORMATIONS

Nasal dermoids, cysts and fistulae

Rarely, the frontal sinus can be involved in congenital abnormalities of the skull base. This may be secondary to craniofacial dysostosis or persistence of embryonic remnants. Congenital midline nasal lesions include nasal dermoids, encephaloceles and gliomas. The nasal dermoid is the least rare of these, and is an uncommon midline developmental anomaly. Unlike other craniofacial dermoids, these lesions can present as a cyst, a sinus or a fistula (**Figure 99.9a**) and may have an intra-cranial extension (**Figure 99.9b**).[25] The incidence is estimated at between 1 : 20,000 and 1 : 40,000 live births.[26] These fistulas may extend from the skin to the frontal bone, leading to pressure atrophy and narrowing of a frontal sinus if it is developed. Progressive enlargement of the nasal dermoid can cause local infection, meningitis and brain abscesses.

Typically, nasal dermoids present as a midline mass anywhere from the base of the columella, along the dorsum to the glabellar region. They are non-compressible and can discharge sebaceous material.[27]

Pathogenesis

Sessions[25] was the first to coin the term *nasal dermal sinus cyst* to include all the lesions containing ectoderm and mesoderm located in the nose. Briefly, as the neuroectodermal tract recedes, dermal attachments can be drawn in along its course. As the dura mater recedes from the prenasal space it may pull nasal ectoderm upward and inward to form a sinus or a cyst.[28]

Imaging

Imaging is a critical component in the evaluation of nasal dermoids given the associated risk of intra-cranial extension. CT and MRI provide complementary information. For CT, fine cut multiplanar, contrast enhanced imaging is optimal. On CT imaging, the presence of a widened foramen caecum and bifid crista galli do not necessarily indicate intra-cranial extension. However, a normal foramen caecum and crista galli rule out intra-cranial disease.[28]

Surgery

The following principles are important when considering the ideal surgical approach: permit access to a midline cyst

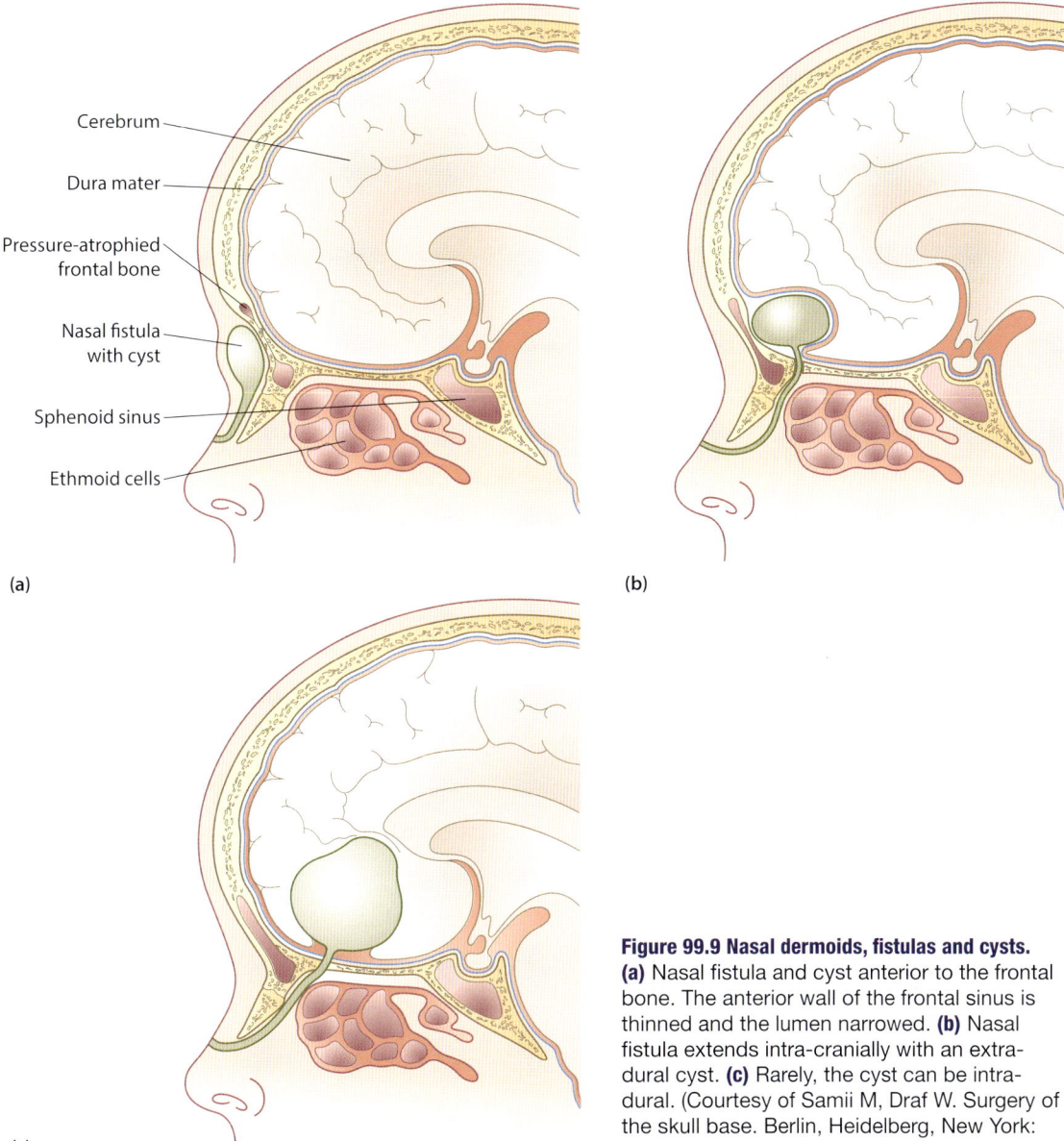

Figure 99.9 Nasal dermoids, fistulas and cysts.
(a) Nasal fistula and cyst anterior to the frontal bone. The anterior wall of the frontal sinus is thinned and the lumen narrowed. **(b)** Nasal fistula extends intra-cranially with an extra-dural cyst. **(c)** Rarely, the cyst can be intra-dural. (Courtesy of Samii M, Draf W. Surgery of the skull base. Berlin, Heidelberg, New York: Springer; 1989.)[123]

and allow access for medial and lateral osteotomies; allow access to the skull base; facilitate reconstruction of any resulting nasal deformity and finally have a cosmetically acceptable scar.[27] The midline vertical approach is commonly used for extra-cranial lesions although some favour an external rhinoplasty approach for better cosmesis. The latter can be combined with a direct excision if necessary.[29] When there is evidence of intra-cranial extension, a combined approach with the neurosurgical team is recommended. Endoscope assisted excision of extra-cranial dermoids using bilateral intercartilagenous incisions have been described. Recent publications have suggested that it may be feasible to endoscopically access some intra-cranial dermoids.[30]

Although the recurrences following surgery are low, they can occur many years later. Long-term follow-up is therefore essential.

INFLAMMATORY CONDITIONS OF THE FRONTAL SINUS

Acute frontal sinusitis

Acute rhinosinusitis (ARS) is sudden in onset and often follows an upper respiratory tract infection (URTI). It is defined as an increase in symptoms after 5 days or persistent symptoms after 10 days with less than 12 weeks duration. It is estimated that only 0.5% to 2% of viral URTI are complicated by bacterial infection, although the true incidence is unknown due to the difficulty in clinically distinguishing bacterial from viral infections. The prevalence rates for ARS vary from 6% to 12%.[31]

Acute frontal sinusitis occurs as part of a generalized acute rhinosinusitis. In most cases ARS resolves without complication or the need for antibiotic treatment.

Mild symptoms are effectively managed with intra-nasal corticosteroid monotherapy or in conjunction with antibiotics (see Chapter 97, 'Medical Therapy for Rhinosinusitis'). Although topical nasal decongestants are often used, there is little evidence to suggest any effect in relieving ostial oedema. However, they may provide symptomatic relief of nasal congestion. Isotonic and hypertonic saline nasal douches are effective in alleviating symptoms.[31]

Extrasinus complications of acute frontal sinusitis are relatively rare in the current antibiotic era. Nonetheless, in some patients acute frontal sinusitis may become complicated. This is most commonly seen in young adolescent men.[32, 33] The frontal sinus is the most common sinus associated with intra-cranial infection. Clinically, patients may present with a persistent severe headache, frontal or periorbital swelling, altered mental status or meningeal signs. The possible complications are outlined in **Table 99.2**.

The general management of the complications of rhinosinusitis are discussed elsewhere (see Chapter 101, 'Complications of Rhinosinusitis'). If culture results are unavailable, antibiotic therapy should target the common organisms which include *H. Influenzae, S. pneumonia, S. pyogenes* and *alpha haemolytic streptococci*.[34] Despite antibiotic therapy, there is not an insignificant incidence of morbidity and occasionally mortality estimated between 5% and 15%.[35]

CT is the imaging modality of choice. Multiplanar imaging of the brain, orbit and sinuses with contrast enhancement is necessary as the incidence of concomitant complications is significant. In one study, approximately 24% of patients aged 7 or older attending theatre for surgical intervention of an orbital complication also had an intra-cranial complication.[36] Evidence of intra-cranial or orbital involvement requires a multidisciplinary approach.

As mentioned above the surgical management is covered elsewhere. In brief, neurosurgical complications may require a craniotomy. Traditionally, the frontal sinus can be trephined and irrigated via a small infrabrow approach and the placement of a drain. An alternative approach has been described which involves performing a 'mini' frontal sinus trephine.[37] The disadvantage of this method is the difficulty in establishing irrigation via the small trephine port. Orbital abscesses not responding to maximal medical therapy require surgical drainage. A classical Lynch-Howarth approach is favoured.

Increasingly, orbital complications such as subperiosteal abscesses and acute complicated frontal sinusitis are being managed endoscopically. In the acutely infected state, dissection of the frontal recess can be very challenging and requires a significant level of advanced endoscopic skills. However, the role of endoscopic frontal sinus surgery in the initial management of intra-cranial complications of sinusitis remains unclear. In a recent 6 year retrospective review of 23 patients, ESS did not appear to influence the need for neurosurgical intervention, even with lesions less than 1 cm.[38]

Chronic frontal sinusitis

Although much work has improved our understanding, the aetiology and pathogenesis of chronic rhinosinusitis (CRS) is still described as multifactorial. The bacteriology of CRS differs from that of ARS with a higher prevalence of anaerobic organisms. Chronic rhinosinusitis with (CRSwNP) or without (CRSsNP) may cause obstruction of the frontal sinus outflow tract and lead to chronic frontal sinusitis. The current mainstay of treatment for CRS involves medical therapy.[31] The majority of patients respond to a combination of antibiotics, nasal irrigations, intra-nasal and if necessary oral steroids therapy. The optimal management is discussed in Chapter XX (The management of CRS). However, despite maximal medical therapy some patients may have persistent symptoms. As in CRS, the diagnosis of frontal sinusitis is based on symptoms (frontal pressure or headache), clinical findings and CT imaging. In these patients, surgical intervention may be necessary. However, despite surgery a proportion of patients may continue to suffer with frontal sinus symptoms and develop recalcitrant chronic frontal sinus disease. This may be related to persistent disease or scarring and stenosis secondary to surgery.

The frontal recess is a complex space and anatomical variations, inflammation and scarring may play an important role in the aetiology of chronic frontal sinusitis. The relative contribution of each of these factors to chronic frontal sinusitis requiring surgical intervention has not been well quantified. A number of retrospective studies have examined the impact of accessory cells within the frontal recess and the development of frontal sinusitis. One study has reported that the presence of suprabulla cells, supraorbital ethmoid cells, frontal bulla cells and recessus terminalis was significantly associated with frontal sinusitis.[39] In another study, the prevalence of frontal sinus mucosal thickening was increased in patients with type 3 and 4 frontal ethmoidal cells.[40] Other studies suggest that although scarring, retained agger and frontal cells may contribute to anatomical obstruction, the ongoing mucosal inflammation is the most important factor leading to frontal sinusitis.[41–44]

TABLE 99.2 Complications of acute frontal sinusitis

Local (frontal sinus)	Orbital	Intra-cranial
Mucocele Pyocele Osteomyelitis (Potts puffy tumour)	Orbital cellulitis (including subperiosteal, intra-orbital abscess)	Meningitis Epidural abscess Subdural empyema Intra-cerebral abscess Superior sagittal sinus thrombosis Cavernous sinus thrombosis

FRONTAL SINUS SURGERY

Despite advances in medical and surgical therapy, chronic frontal sinusitis remains a difficult disease to manage. Over the years, the surgical management of frontal sinus disease has evolved from open obliterative procedures to endoscopic mucosal sparing techniques. Although extensive and complex frontal sinus pathology can be managed endoscopically there remains a definitive role for open procedures such as the osteoplastic flap.

There are no simple guidelines for the management of chronic frontal sinusitis. Prior to considering any surgery it is wise to review the clinical history, imaging and indications. Underlying conditions such as diabetes, immune disorders and aspirin exacerbated respiratory diseases need to be identified.[45]

In the past, treatment of chronic frontal sinusitis was directed towards the sinus itself. However, contemporary management is based on the understanding that the problem most often involves the drainage pathway, the frontal recess rather than the sinus. The principles of surgery are to relieve obstruction that may lead to inflammatory changes. Mucosal preservation is important as mucosa regenerating over bare bone lacks effective cilia.[46]

There is much debate regarding the philosophies of managing the frontal sinus in CRS. These range from minimal invasive sinus techniques (MIST) where following an uncinectomy transitional spaces are opened, to addressing an obstructed frontal recess irrespective of patient symptoms.[7, 47] Most rhinologists would agree that the best surgical approach to the frontal sinus is a graduated one (Table 99.3).

Numerous descriptions and approaches to the frontal sinus have been described. Not only is this confusing but it makes it difficult to draw meaningful comparisons from the published literature. The most widely accepted classification is that described by Draf and his colleagues although this has waned in popularity, as it too can be open to interpretation.[48] The classification describes increasingly aggressive approaches to the frontal sinus. The general rule would be to choose the least invasive approach to achieve the desired outcome. In some cases, the least invasive may necessarily be quite extensive. The surgery needs to be tailored to the individual needs of each patient and depends on various factors such as previous surgery and extent of disease.

The choice of surgical procedure used to manage recurrent frontal sinus disease will depend on a number of factors outlined in Table 99.4. The surgeon needs to take into account the extent and completeness of the previous surgery, the anatomy of the frontal sinus and the overall burden of disease. An assessment of the surgical complexity based on the anatomy alone is available in Table 99.5.

In an attempt to better define the extent of surgery to the frontal recess and sinus, an international panel of

TABLE 99.3 Graduated approach to frontal sinus surgery

Graduated approach to frontal sinus surgery	
No exploration	No disease
Balloon sinuplasty	May have a role in certain situations with limited disease
Draf type I (frontal sinusotomy), ethmoidectomy*	Removing cells within the frontal recess, following an FESS
Draf type IIa and b*	Remove cells extending into the frontal sinus and resect bone between the lamina papyracea and middle turbinate (a) or nasal septum (b)
Draf type III, modified endoscopic Lothrop (MEL), Frontal sinus drillout*	Resection of the floor of the frontal sinus, superior nasal septum and interfrontal sinus septum
Osteoplastic flap + MEL Osteoplastic flap with obliteration	Above and below approach Removal of all mucosa within the sinus and obliteration with fat
Riedel's procedure	Removal of the anterior table of the frontal sinus
Cranialization	Removal of sinus mucosa and the posterior table of the frontal sinus

* A frontal sinus mini trephine may be used as an adjunct to these procedures.

TABLE 99.4 Factors influencing the surgical approach

	Considerations	Surgical options
Patient	Compliance issues and significant comorbidities	Simple FESS with minimal manipulation of the frontal recess
	Asthma, aspirin sensitivity	Comprehensive clearance of frontal recess If recurrent disease see below
Anatomy	Preserved landmarks, minimal previous surgery, no complex cells	Draf type I procedure
	Poor landmarks, osteoneogenesis, multiple revision procedures, thick frontal beak, complex frontal cells	Draf type (modified endoscopic Lothrop)
Pathology	Chronic frontal sinusitis with or without polyps. No previous surgery	Draf type I procedure
	Recurrent disease, ASA with polyps, eosinophillic mucin CRS, tumours, lateral mucoceles. Recalcitrant	Draf type (modified endoscopic Lothrop)
	Complicated frontal sinusitis with erosion of the posterior table, anterior table osteitis, tumours extending laterally	Draf III or an osteoplastic flap approach. Combined approach

TABLE 99.5 The International classification of complexity of frontal sinus surgery

	Wide AP diameter (≥10 mm)	Narrow AP diameter (9–6 mm)	Very narrow AP diameter (≤5mm)
Cells below ostium (AN, SAC, SBC)	Less complex (Grade 1)	Moderate complexity (Grade 2)	High complexity (Grade 3)
Cells encroaching into the ostium (SAFC, SBFC, SOEC, FSC)	Moderate complexity (Grade 2)	High complexity (Grade 3)	Highest complexity (Grade 4)
Cells extending significantly into the frontal sinus (SAFC, SBFC, SOEC, FSC)	High complexity (Grade 3)	Highest complexity (Grade 4)	Highest complexity (Grade 4)

AP refers to the frontal ostium anterior-posterior (AP) diameter as measured from the frontal beak to the skull base at its narrowest distance on the parasagittal CT scan. Classification of the cells is in accordance to the International Frontal Sinus Classification[12]: AN (Agger Nasi), FSC (frontal septal cell), SAC (supra agger cell), SAFC (supra agger frontal cell), SBC (supra bulla cell), SBFC (supra bulla frontal cell), SOEC (supra-orbital ethmoid cell). Data from Wormald PJ, Bassiouni A, Callejas CA, et al. The International Classification of the radiological Complexity (ICC) of frontal recess and frontal sinus. *Int Forum Allergy Rhinol.* 2016.[123]

TABLE 99.6 Extent of frontal sinus surgery (EFSS). A comparison between the Draf frontal sinus surgery classification and a new proposed international classification of extent of frontal sinus surgery

Draf classification[124]	International classification of the extent of EFSS[12]	Tissue/Bone removal
	0 – No bone or tissue removal. Balloon dilatation	No Tissue removal
Draf 1 – Ethmoidectomy and removal of cells below the frontal sinus	1 – Removal of cells in the frontal recess not directly obstructing the frontal ostium	Removal of cells
	2 – Removal of cells obstructing the ostium but not extending through the ostium	
Draf 2a – Enlargement of the frontal ostium between the lamina papyracea (LP) and the middle turbinate (MT)	3 – Removal of cells extending through the frontal ostium (no widening of the frontal ostium)	
	4 – Removal of cells extending through the frontal ostium with enlargement of the ostium (bone removal, usually frontal beak)	Removal of bone
Draf 2b – Enlargement of the frontal ostium from the LP and the nasal septum	5 – Enlargement of the frontal ostium from the LP to the nasal septum	
Draf 3 – Bilateral enlargement of the frontal ostia, resection of the superior nasal septum, floor of the frontal sinus and inter-sinus septum	6 – Bilateral enlargement of the frontal ostia into a common ostium, with resection of the superior nasal septum, inter-sinus septum and floor of the frontal sinus	

experts have proposed a new classification (**Table 99.6**). The aim is to standardize terminology and provide a framework which should allow better comparison of surgical outcomes.[12]

No frontal recess exploration

Unfortunately, it is not uncommon for frontal sinus obstruction to occur as a result of surgery.[41, 43] In the absence of positive CT scan findings and clinical symptoms the frontal sinus or recess should not be explored. Unnecessary instrumentation in a healthy recess can result in mucosal injury and adhesion formation.[49]

Balloon sinuplasty

Introduced in 2006, balloon sinuplasty is proposed to be a minimally invasive approach to the management of CRS involving the frontal sinus. The technique introduces a balloon over a guide wire, which may be illuminated, to confirm its position in the frontal sinus. Once in place, spanning the ostium, the balloon is dilated with a controlled inflation device. In theory, this gently enlarges the ostium by effecting microfactures of the surrounding bone and compressing the soft tissue. Soft tissue injury is suggested to be minimal but the rate of synechia formation is reportedly at least equal to that seen with conventional endoscopic sinus surgery (ESS). Complications include inability to cannulate the sinus, and CSF leak.[50, 51] Although it is a safe and well tolerated procedure, the evidence in support of its use as an alternative to standard ESS techniques is limited.[31, 52, 53] In many instances balloon dilation is combined with ESS and is termed a hybrid procedure.

Draf type I (ethmoidectomy and frontal sinusotomy)

This is the commonest primary procedure performed for chronic frontal sinusitis and in many cases is sufficient.[54] As the least invasive procedure the aim is to clear obstructing disease **inferior** to the level of the frontal ostium – the frontal recess. The key step is performing a complete ethmoidectomy. This includes removal of any anterosuperior ethmoid cells, the agger nasi and uncinate process (**Figure 99.10**). This approach is best limited to when there

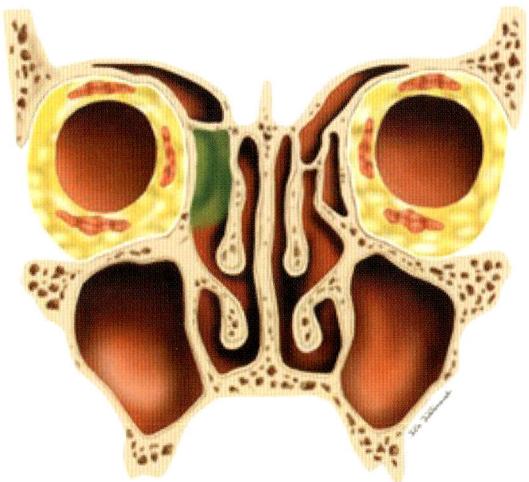

Figure 99.10 A Draf type I frontal sinusotomy with removal of the agger and anterior ethmoid cells in the frontal recess cells.

is only minor pathology in the frontal sinus. It may not be sufficient in cases where the patient suffers from significant nasal polyposis associated with aspirin intolerance and asthma.

Draf type II frontal sinusotomy

Where a more conservative surgical approach has failed an extended frontal sinus procedure may be required. In a Draf type II approach, cells extending into the frontal sinus are removed (**Figure 99.11**). If the frontal ostium is widened from the lamina papyracea to the middle turbinate this is called a type IIa approach. This may be possible by using a Kerrison or Hajek-Kofler punch. Extending this opening beyond the middle turbinate to the nasal septum is a type IIb approach. This involves removing the anterior end of the middle turbinate and drilling the floor of the sinus to the midline. The indications for a Draf type IIb are limited but may be used to address unilateral frontal ostium osteoneogenesis, inverted papilloma, osteomas or medially placed frontal mucoceles. A recent study has suggested using a Draf type IIb approach for addressing contralateral inaccessible frontal sinus disease. Although short-term patency was good, larger patient numbers and longer follow-up data are required before this can be recommended.[55]

Draf type III (modified endoscopic lothrop)

Also known as a median drainage procedure or frontal sinus drill-out, the operation was first described by Lothrop in 1914 as an external procedure.[56] Draf described an intranasal microscopic approach while others described a similar endoscopic technique.[57, 58] The modified endoscopic Lothrop procedure (MELP) has recently gained popularity as a minimally invasive alternative to frontal sinus obliteration. The possible indications for a MELP are highlighted in **Table 99.7**.

The procedure consists of creating a large common drainage pathway for the paired frontal sinuses by resecting the upper nasal septum, the frontal intersinus septum

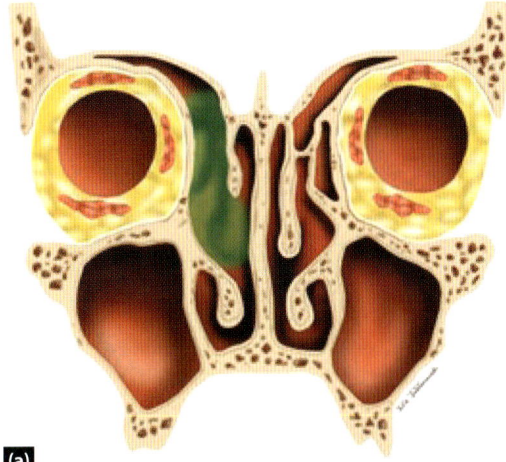

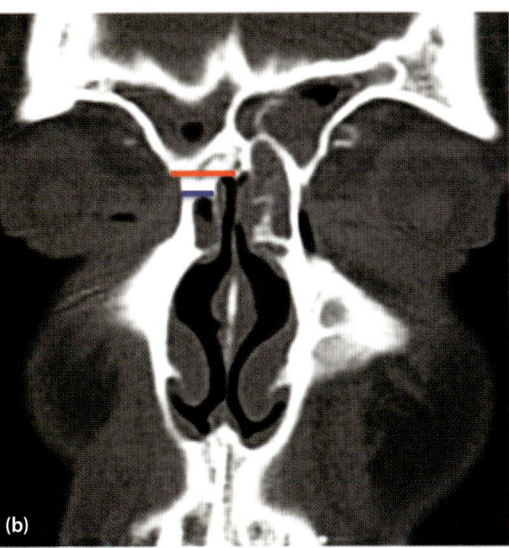

Figure 99.11 The Draf type II, with removal of cells extending into the frontal sinus (a). The coronal CT highlights the extent of bone removal (b). Type IIa involves widening of the ostium from the lamina papyracea to the middle turbinate (blue line) and IIb extending this to the nasal septum (red line).

and the floor of both frontal sinuses (**Figure 99.12**). The procedure is technically demanding as useful landmarks are often absent and the operative field is narrow. A septectomy performed early allows the surgeon to work more freely in the narrow confines. The use of frontal mini trephines helps with early identification of the frontal ostium and hence the posterior limit of dissection. The use of computer assisted navigation may improve efficacy and safety but is no substitute for sound surgical training and anatomical knowledge.[59]

Drilling commences from one frontal recess and proceeds across the midline to the contralateral recess. A small area of skin is often exposed bilaterally just above the axilla of the middle turbinate and demarcates the lateral extent of dissection. To obtain the maximum possible opening it is necessary to drill down the anterior projection of the skull base. In order to do this safely, it is helpful to identify the first olfactory neurons, which are found by peeling back the mucosa between the middle turbinate and the nasal septum. The fibres can be seen to arise just posterior to a linear groove through a small bony opening. When this is performed on both sides the so-called 'frontal T' results (**Figure 99.13**). The long limb corresponds to the posterior aspect of the septectomy (the perpendicular plate of the ethmoid) and the horizontal limbs to the posterior margin of the frontal sinus floor resection. A summary of the essential steps of the procedure is outlined in **Box 99.1**.

In certain situations when access to the frontal sinus is blocked (osteoma or osteoneogenesis) or the anatomy is grossly distorted, one can use a midline approach. Rather than drilling from lateral to medial a transeptal approach can be used. This involves finding the 'frontal T' early and drilling immediately superiorly to enter the floor of the frontal sinus in the midline. This is relatively safe as one is drilling away from the skull base. Drilling then proceeds from medial to lateral in an 'inside to outside' fashion.

Complications of the MELP include injury to the skin and nasal bones, orbital injury, damage to the skull base and CSF leak.

Reasons for failure of frontal recess and sinus surgery

Despite careful pre-operative planning and maximum medical therapy, surgery in the frontal recess can fail. The commonest causes for failure include.

TABLE 99.7 Utility of the modified endoscopic Lothrop procedure (MELP)

Potential indications for a MELP	
Chronic frontal sinusitis	Refractory to previous endoscopic surgery
CRS with nasal polyps, asthma, aspirin exacerbated respiratory disease	Controversial, but may be indicated as a primary procedure
Allergic fungal disease	Includes eosinophilic mucin CRS, fungal sinusitis
Mucoceles	Large frontal mucoceles, even those extending beyond the mid-pupillary line[22]
Salvage osteoplastic flap	'unobliteration' of the frontal sinus[23]
Frontal osteoma	Grade I and II. Less suitable for grade III and IV with significant posterior table erosion and lateral extension[111]
Inverted papilloma	Extending into the frontal sinus. May require an accessory port in to the sinus[72]
Frontal sinus trauma	Closure of CSF leaks
Cranionasal resection	As part of a skull base resection for anterior cranial fossa tumours
Alternative to OPF with obliteration	Preservation of a functioning sinus, able to survey for recurrent disease, improved cosmesis, decreased morbidity, shorter hospital admission, lower cost[125]

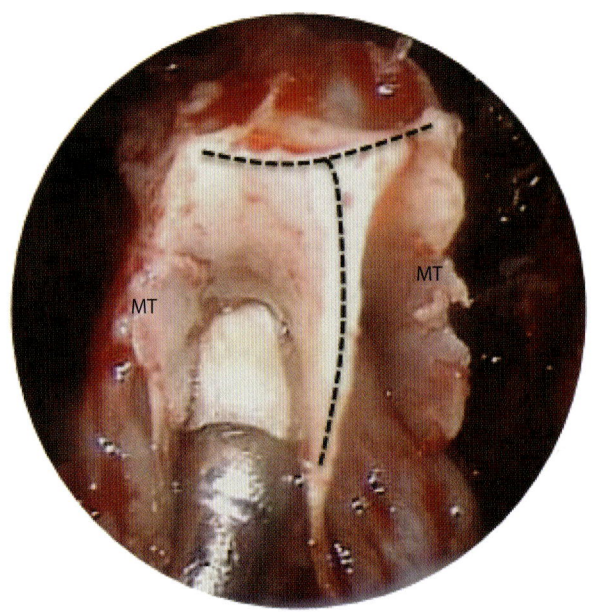

Figure 99.13 The 'frontal T'. An intra-operative view with the olive tip suction on the first olfactory neuron. The vertical limb of the dotted line is the posterior margin of the septectomy (perpendicular ethmoid plate). Horizontal limb is the posterior margin of the frontal ostium and joins the two amputated ends of the middle turbinate (MT).

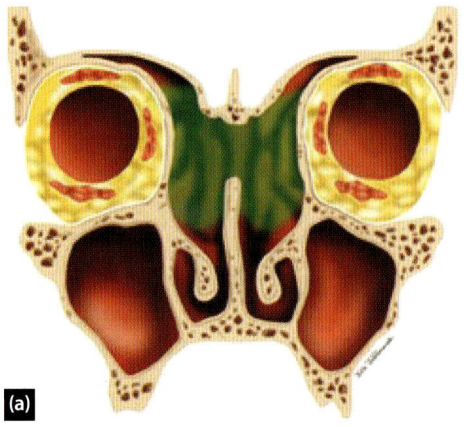
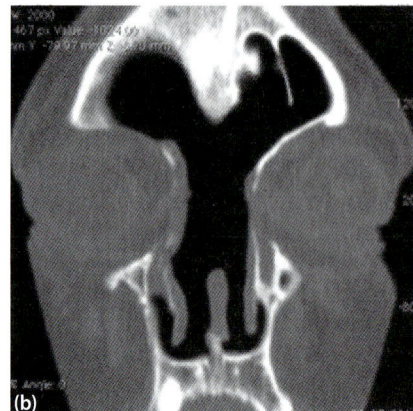
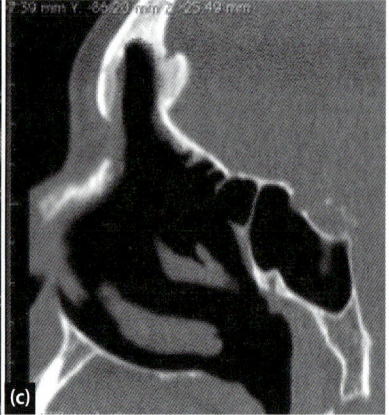

Figure 99.12 The Draf type III or modified Lothrop. Note the widening of the frontal ostium from lamina to lamina **(a)**, the reduction of the frontal intersinus septum **(b)** and the beak **(c)**.

> **BOX 99.1** Summary of operative steps for the MELP
>
> **ESSENTIAL STEPS OF A MODIFIED ENDOSCOPIC LOTHROP (DRAF TYPE III) PROCEDURE**
> 1. Complete sphenoethmoidectomy
> 2. Clear frontal recess and identify frontal ostium. Frontal mini trephines may be required. If no access consider midline, trans-septal approach
> 3. Create septal window. At least 2 × 2 cm. Posterior limit is anterior end of middle turbinate. Inferior limit, to allow visualization of contralateral middle turbinate axilla. Superiorly to the nasal vault
> 4. Trim anterior end of middle turbinate to skull base.
> 5. Dissect mucosa posteriorly between middle turbinate and nasal septum to identify first olfactory neuron
> 6. Drilling commences in an anterior, superior and lateral direction from the frontal ostium through the axilla of the middle turbinate. Small area of skin may be exposed laterally.
> 7. As drilling extends superiorly, it is easier to drill from the contralateral side via the septal window
> 8. Reduce frontal intersinus septum and frontal beak to join the two sides together
> 9. Try to preserve mucosa over posterior aspect of frontal ostium
> 10. Lower bone over anterior projection of the skull base to primary olfactory neuron

ONGOING MUCOSAL DISEASE

Persistent or recurrent nasal polyps frequently obstruct the sinuses. Patients with eosinophilic CRS presenting with polyps fare less well. Similarly patients with asthma and nasal polyps are likely to require revision surgery.[60]

INCOMPLETE DISSECTION WITH RETAINED UNCINATE PROCESS AND RESIDUAL CELLS IN THE FRONTAL RECESS

This can impede drainage and exacerbate ongoing mucosal inflammation.[40, 61]

LATERALIZATION OF THE MIDDLE TURBINATE

Whether partial resection of the middle turbinate predisposes to frontal sinusitis is unclear. However, the incidence of lateralized middle turbinates in revision surgery is high (36–78%).[61, 62] The frontal sinus rescue procedure was described to address frontal recess stenosis secondary to middle turbinate lateralization. Mucosa is dissected from the turbinate and the stump trimmed back to the skull base. The medial mucosa is discarded and the lateral mucosa from the sinus is draped over the denuded stump.[63]

SCARRING AND SYNECHIA

Meticulous attention to detail can help to minimize unnecessary trauma and subsequent scarring. However, synechia and scarring are very common findings in revision frontal sinus surgery but may not always be symptomatic.[60, 62]

OSTEONEOGENESIS

Failure to preserve mucosa results in scarring and osteoneogenesis.[64] The incidence of osteoneogenesis is higher in patients that have undergone sinus surgery. It may occur secondary to a combination of factors such as persistent mucosal inflammation, ongoing infection and surgical trauma. The ongoing osteitis promotes mucosal inflammation and oedema and may contribute to frontal recess stenosis.[65]

Outcomes for endoscopic frontal sinus surgery

Although trials providing high level of evidence are not available, there are a number of well organized prospective studies that have shown endoscopic sinus surgery (ESS) is safe and effective in managing patients with CRS (with and without polyps) when medical therapy has failed.[31] The evidence of effectiveness for various frontal sinus procedures is less well documented.

Most studies define success as objective endoscopic evidence of frontal sinus patency. Subjectively however, despite a patent recess some patients will continue to complain of ongoing symptoms.[66] This mismatch between patient reported outcome measures and clinical or radiological findings poses a challenge in both selecting the ideal candidate for frontal sinus surgery and reporting results. A recent review of the literature has identified at best, level 3 evidence in support of the clinical efficacy of frontal sinus surgery, the main issues being the relative short follow-up periods and the different surgical techniques performed for various indications.[67] Early patency rates of 90% at 12 months, falling to 68% after 72 months, have been reported.[60] Others report a 90% patency rate in non-eosinophilic CRS, dropping to 85% in eosinophilic CRS, over an average follow-up period of 46 months.[68] A recent study with a shorter follow-up reported a high overall ostial patency rate of 92% with symptom resolution in 78% which was unaffected by asthma, EMCRS and smoking when assessed individually but additive when combined together.[69]

There has been much comparison in the literature between the osteoplastic flap procedure (OPF) with obliteration and the MELP. The OPF with obliteration has a reported success rate as high as 93% at 8 years but is not without complications (see 'The osteoplastic flap procedure' below).[70] A systematic review and meta-analysis of the safety and efficacy of the MELP reports an overall patency rate of 95.9%. An overall failure rate of 13.9% is quoted with 80% of those failing undergoing a revision MELP and the remainder an osteoplastic frontal sinus obliteration.

The osteoplastic flap procedure

The OPF procedure was developed to manage chronic frontal sinus disease refractory to procedures such as the external frontoethmoidectomy, which were associated with high failure rates.[71] Obliteration with fat was introduced later and popularized by Goodale and Montgomery. Although the OPF with fat obliteration is reported to be the gold standard treatment with success rates over 90% it does have a long-term failure rate of up to 25%.[72] In addition, it is associated with significant morbidity. These include CSF leaks, persistent forehead numbness, severe headaches without evidence of recurrent disease, frontal bossing, supraorbital neuralgia, mucocele formation, donor site complications after abdominal fat harvesting and difficulties with post-operative surveillance.[70, 73, 74] In a graduated approach to frontal sinus surgery some might consider this the final step, as the frontal sinus is rendered non-functional. Others would argue that it is a safe and effective procedure in carefully selected patients.

Without question, the OPF approach offers unparalleled access to the frontal sinus and is indicated when wide exposure is necessary (**Table 99.8**). However, the role of frontal sinus obliteration for the surgical treatment of frontal sinus abnormalities is much more controversial.[71, 75–77] In a large series, based in a tertiary setting performing over 700 frontal sinus procedures in a 3-year period, less than 2% of cases were managed by an OPF with obliteration.[78] In the current endoscopic era, the indications for obliteration are dwindling. The ability to tackle pathology from above via an OPF approach and simultaneously endoscopically restore ventilation from below has offered an alternative to obliteration. Traditionally, obliteration was suggested for fractures of the anterior table of the frontal sinus involving the outflow tract. Currently however, one might consider repairing the fracture, monitoring with imaging and perhaps endoscopically intervening at a later stage if necessary.[79]

Without obliteration

An OPF can be performed through a number of approaches. Coronal, brow and mid forehead incisions have all been used to expose the anterior table of the frontal sinus. Zigzag coronal incisions are better camouflaged in male pattern baldness. A combination of local anaesthesia (Lignocaine 1%), vasoconstrictors (adrenaline 1:1000), steroid (Adcortyl 5 mg) and Hylase (1,500 iu) aid dissection and minimize bleeding. An incision is made down to the periosteum. Using a combination of blunt and sharp dissection the scalp flap is elevated to the supraorbital ridge and over the root of the nose. The flap is pulled caudally on both sides, leaving behind the periosteum and the bone, thus preserving the supraorbital and supratrochlear vascular nerve bundles. The next step is to precisely define the extent of frontal sinus pneumatization. Conventionally, a 6-foot Caldwell view (occipitofrontal view) X-ray was used as a template to mark out the margin of the frontal sinus. CT-generated frontal sinus templates are virtually identical to the Caldwell radiograph-derived templates and may obviate the need for additional imaging.[80] As an alternative, transillumination can be used to outline the extent of the sinus. When available, surgical navigation has been shown to be more accurate and may reduce the risk of inadvertent intra-cranial entry.[81] Others have developed 3D models of the frontal sinus using pre-operative CT data from which an accurate template is produced (**Figure 99.14**).[82]

The periosteum is incised 1.5 cm outside the frontal sinus margin (or template) and elevated to the margin of the sinus where an osteotomy is performed. An alternative is to entirely elevate the pericranium with the skin flap.[83] An oscillating saw angled at 30° towards the frontal sinus provides an opening with a large surface area for easier fixation of the bone lid. The bony incision is carried to the supraorbital ridge on both sides. When opening the frontal sinus bilaterally, the intersinus septum must be separated from the anterior frontal sinus wall with an angled chisel. The fracture and elevation of the bony lid is undertaken

TABLE 99.8 Relative indications for an osteoplastic flap procedure. (*) May consider frontal sinus obliteration

Possible scenarios	Pathology
Wide exposure of the frontal sinus necessary and endoscopically inaccessible anatomy	Large osteomas Inverted papilloma with significant lateral extension Malignant tumours Far lateral mucoceles in a well-pneumatized sinus
Failed endoscopic procedures for chronic frontal sinusitis	Where maximal medical therapy and MELPs have failed (*)
Extensive frontal bone osteomyelitis	Unresponsive to medical therapy and ESS
Extensive neo-osteogenesis of the frontal recess	May occur secondary to failed endoscopic sinus surgery, facial fractures, frontal bone osteomyelitis (*)
Diseased small underdeveloped sinuses	Anterior-posterior distance less than 8 mm making a MELP difficult (*)
Frontal sinus fractures	Anterior and posterior table fractures, CSF leaks and those involving the frontal sinus outflow tract

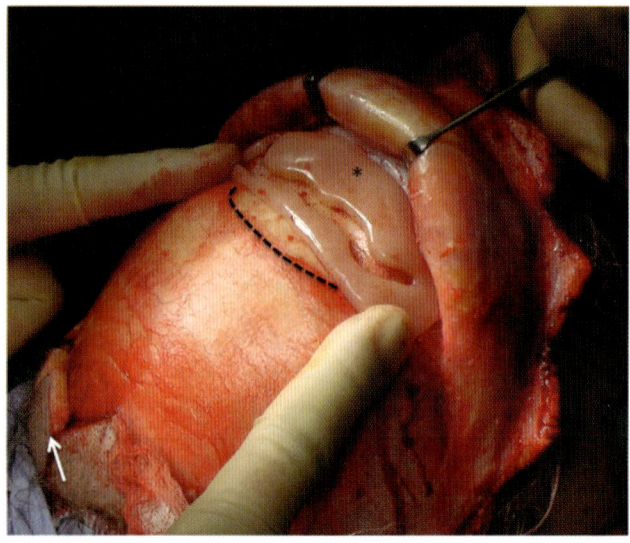

Figure 99.14 Marking out the osteotomy incision during an osteoplastic flap procedure. The template shown (*) was created from a 3D model and provides a guide for the bony osteotomy. Note the cute edge of the periosteum approximately 1.5 cm posterior to the incision site (dotted line) and the zigzag coronal skin incision (white arrow). (Courtesy of Mr A Sama.)

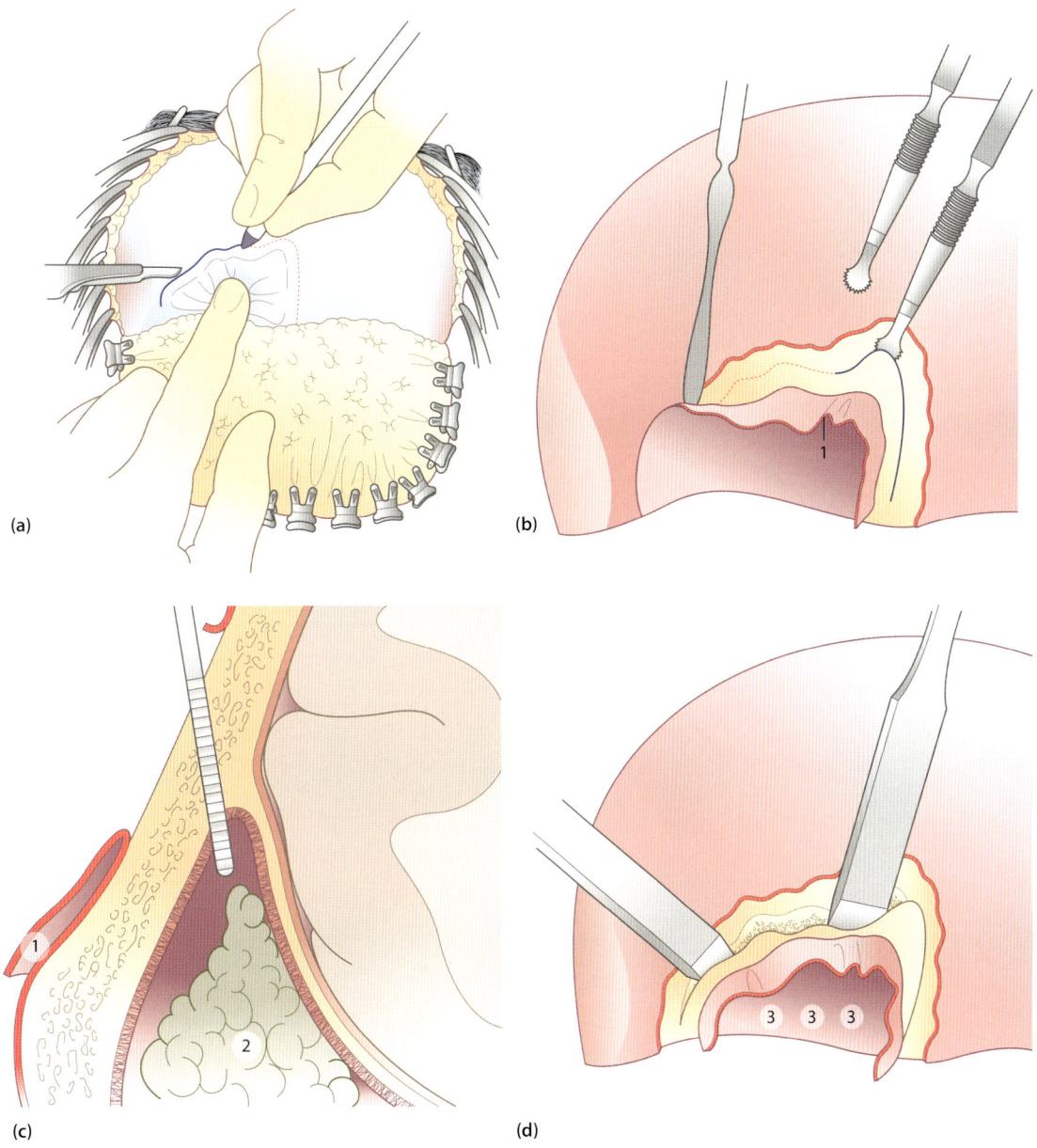

Figure 99.15 Technique of the osteoplastic frontal sinus operation. (a) The periosteal incision is marked approximately 1.5 cm outside the template. (b) The periosteum is elevated just beyond the osteotomy site. The bone flap is created with a drill/saw corresponding to the limits of the frontal sinus. (c) An oblique incision through the bone enlarges the area for replacement of the bony flap. (d) Elevation of the frontal sinus anterior wall with two broad chisels. This ends in a fracture of the frontal sinus floor just posteriorly of the supraorbital ridge. (1: periosteum, 2: pathology, 3: drill holes for fixation.) *(Continued).*

with a wide osteotome. Ideally the bone lid hinges on the periosteal flap, although in practice this is rarely possible. The pathology is now accessible (**Figure 99.15**).[84]

On completion, the bone lid is replaced and the periosteum is sutured. Often the periosteum may not be intact and the bone lid will need securing with mini plates. The scalp wound is closed over a closed-suction drain.

With obliteration

If obliteration is being considered, its success depends on the complete removal of all mucous membrane elements. The use of a diamond burr on the inner cortex of the sinus helps to exenterate mucosal invaginations and promotes neovascularization. The frontal ostium is plugged with fascia, or oxidized cellulose (Surgicell®, Ethicon, Inc., Somerville, NJ).[49] Obliteration is usually performed with fat harvested from the abdomen but alternatives include a vascularized pericranial flap, cancellous bone, muscle and alloplastic material. Monitoring the sinus post-obliteration is an issue. MRI is most useful but it can be difficult to distinguish fat necrosis from mucocele formation and recurrent disease.[75]

Above and below approaches

Endonasal procedures may be combined with external procedures such as an osteoplastic flap or trephine

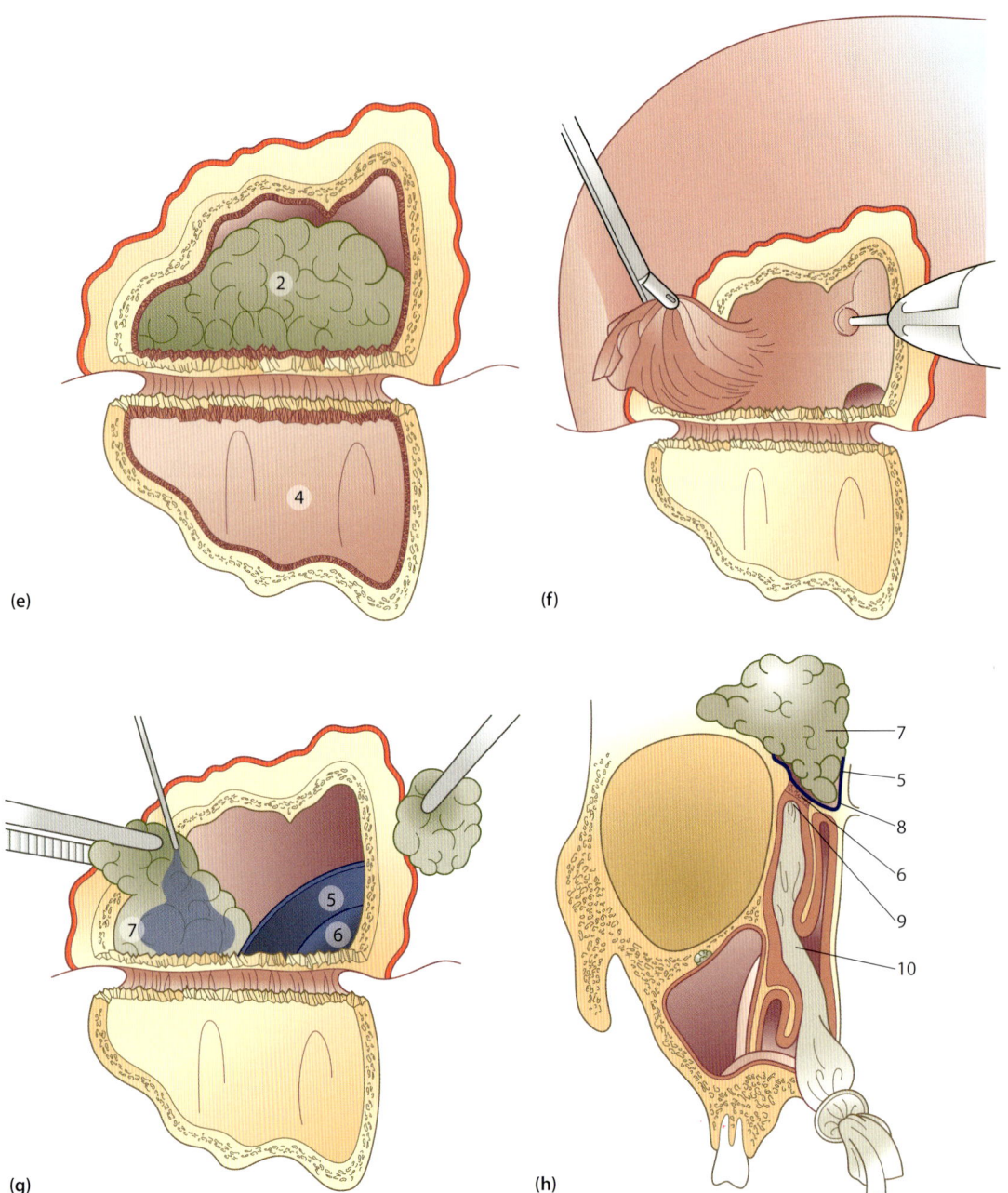

Figure 99.15 (Continued) Technique of the osteoplastic frontal sinus operation. (e) Appearances after down fracturing of anterior wall of frontal sinus. **(f)** The mucosa is completely removed and using the operation microscope, the internal table drilled with the burr. **(g)** After blockage of the ostium, frontal sinus drainage by inverting the mucosa, covering the cartilage with preserved fascia or galea-periosteum and fixing with fibrin glue, the frontal sinus is filled with pieces of fat. These are made to cohere with fibrin glue. Finally, the bony flap is replaced and closure of the wound begins. **(h)** Situation at the end of the operation: (1) Elevated galea-periosteum; (2) pathologically altered mucosa frontal sinus; (3) drill holes; (4) bony flap hinged on periosteum (anterior wall of the frontal sinus); (5) preserved fascia; (6) cartilage; (7) transplanted fat with fibrin glue; (8) fibrin glue; (9) resorbable sponge; (10) rubber finger packs. (Redrawn from Draf W. Surgical treatment of the inflammatory diseases of the paranasal sinuses: indication, surgical technique, risks, mismanagement, and complications, revision surgery (Reproduced with permission from Die chirurgische Behandlung entzuendlicher Erkrankungen der Nasennebenhoehlen: Indikation, Operationsverfahren, Gefahren, Fehler und Komplikationen, Revisionschirurgie). *Arch Otorhinolaryngol* 1982; **235**: 133–205 (Kongressbericht 1982).

(see 'Frontal sinus trephination' below). This combined approach has meant that where some sinuses would have been obliterated in the past it may not be necessary to do so now. The approach may be used when pathology in the frontal sinus outflow tract cannot adequately or safely be addressed by an endonasal approach alone. A MELP can be combined with a frontal trephine or OPF to remove tumours such as inverted papilloma with lateral attachments. The obvious advantage of this is to retain a functioning sinus that is endoscopically accessible and can be monitored by imaging. Medially based osteomas, neo-osteogenesis of the frontal recess, posterior table CSF leaks and encephaloceles can be managed by the 'above and below' approach.[46, 75–78]

Frontal sinus trephination

Trephination of the frontal sinus is a procedure that is normally performed in cases of complicated acute frontal sinusitis not responding to medical management, but it can have a role in chronic frontal sinus disease.[85]

In the acute setting, a small incision (1–1.5 cm) is made below the medial eyebrow and supraorbital rim down through the periosteum. The periosteum is elevated and a drill is used to make a small window at the junction of the floor and anterior wall of the frontal sinus. The sinus is irrigated and a drain placed *in situ*.

A modified frontal trephine technique, the mini trephine (Medtronic, Jacksonville), is useful during surgery for chronic frontal sinus disease. The landmarks are identified in **Figure 99.16**. The use of fluorescein stained saline to irrigate the trephine can aid in dissection of the frontal recess pathway. One must always aspirate prior to irrigation and be cautious when a dehiscence of the orbit is present. Indications include any situation where the frontal sinus outflow tract is difficult to detect, for irrigation of the sinus intra- and post-operatively and as an adjunct to more complex frontal sinus procedures. A pre-operative CT scan to define the depth and extent of pneumatization of the frontal sinus is essential. Complications such as intracranial penetration with CSF leak, periorbital trauma and incision related infection have been reported.[86–88]

External frontoethmoidectomy

This historical procedure, which was associated with a high failure and complication rate, has been replaced by endoscopic approaches to the frontal sinus.[84] The operation was conceptually flawed as it was designed to remove the bony support of the frontal recess. As a result scarring and fibrosis obstructed the outflow tract. It was performed via an external, slightly curved incision (Lynch) made halfway between the nasal dorsum and the medial canthus. The indications for a Lynch incision today are to externally access the anterior ethmoidal artery, in the drainage of periorbital abscesses and if extended superolaterally, to trephine the floor of the frontal sinus.

Cranialization of the frontal sinus

Frontal sinus cranialization for refractory chronic frontal sinusitis is rarely performed. Cranialization has a role in procedures requiring a craniotomy. Performed in conjunction with the neurosurgeons, the commonest indicaton is for extensive fractures of the frontal sinus, particularly the posterior table. Other indications include tumours and osteomyelitis.

Using a coronal incision a midfrontobasal craniotomy can be used.[89] The posterior wall and floor of the sinus are removed. Mucosa of the frontal sinus outflow tract is inverted into the nasal cavity and sealed with fascia or a strip of pericranium and fibrin glue. The success of the procedure relies on meticulous removal of the entire frontal sinus mucosa and drilling the sinus with a diamond burr. Dead space between the anterior wall and dura can be filled with fat or a vascularized pericranial flap.[90] Complications include dural injury with CSF leak, bone flap necrosis, frontal lobe trauma and intra-cranial mucocele formation.

Riedel's procedure

Riedel's procedure involves removing the floor, anterior wall of the frontal sinus and its entire mucosal lining.

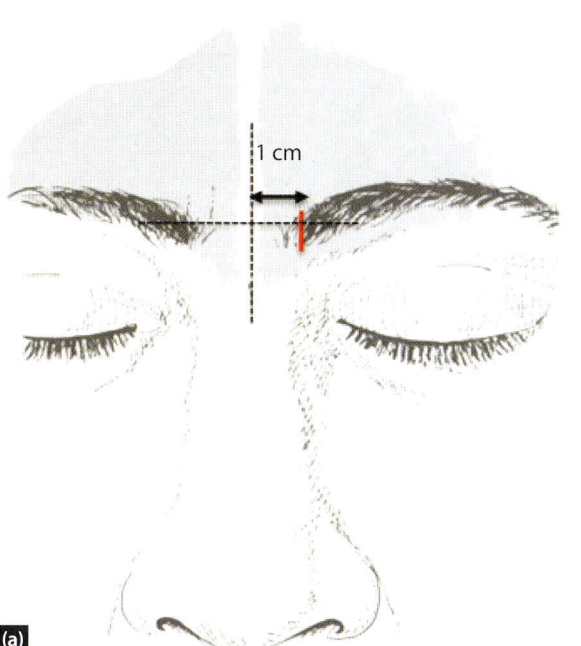
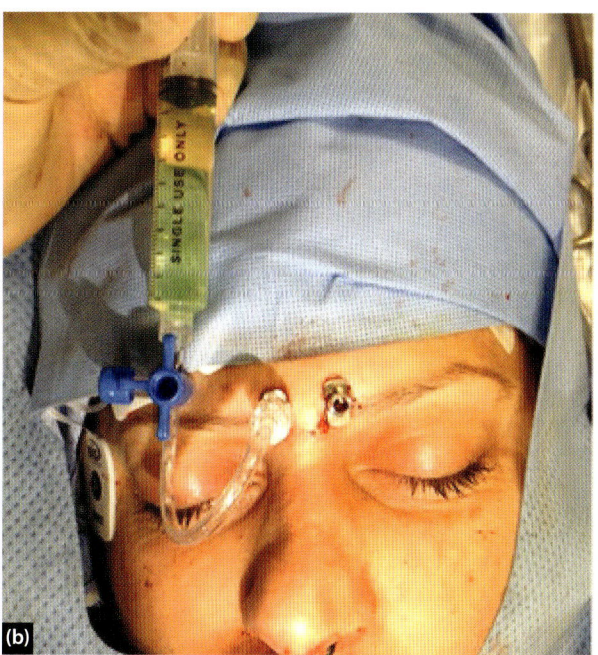

Figure 99.16 (a) Frontal mini-trephine landmarks. The incision can be hidden in the medial aspect of the eyebrow or if necessary in a vertical crease. However, given the possible anatomical variations, careful evaluation of the imaging is essential in every case to avoid inadvertent injury and to help select the safest distance from the midline for frontal sinus trephination.[87] **(b)** Fluorescein tinted saline is injected via the trephine during a MELP.

Although it is rarely performed, it does have a role in a small proportion of patients where frontal sinus drainage cannot be established and frontal sinus obliteration has failed. These include patients who have osteomyelitis or tumours involving the anterior wall of the frontal sinus. The main criticism of the procedure is the cosmetic defect, which can be reduced by chamfering the supraorbital ridge and smoothing out the margin of the sinus to a gentle curve. As the mucosa within the sinus is removed recurrent complications are uncommon.[91]

TUMOURS

Sixty percent of sinonasal tumours arise in the maxillary sinus, 20% arise in the nasal cavity, 5% in the ethmoid sinuses, and only 3% in the sphenoid and frontal sinuses. Fifty-five percent of sinonasal malignancies are carcinomas, squamous cell carcinomas being the commonest. Tumours of the ethmoid sinus and superior nasal vault are usually adenocarcinomas.[92] As it is with chronic frontal sinus disease, tumours of the frontal sinus present a significant challenge in diagnosis and management. Although tumours originating within the frontal sinus are rare, extension into the sinus is not.

Imaging

The aim of imaging is to provide reliable information on the nature of the tumour (benign vs. malignant), map its extent and point of origin, and distinguish concomitant inflammatory reactions. MRI best achieves this. Multiparametric MRI imaging, using a combination of apparent diffusion coefficient and time-signal intensity curve techniques, may help differentiate benign and malignant sinonasal diseases.[93]

CT is often requested as the initial investigation for sinonasal symptoms and it provides useful bony detail particularly in fibro-osseous lesions.

General principles of tumour surgery of the frontal sinus

Ideally, it is preferable to remove a frontal sinus tumour using the most minimally invasive technique. Tumour characteristics (benign or malignant), site, involvement of adjacent structures (dura and orbit), and local expertise determine the surgical approach. Management decisions should be made within a multidisciplinary team including head and neck surgeons and neurosurgery when appropriate. As with chronic frontal sinus disease a stepwise approach is recommended:

- Endonasal (including modified Lothrop procedures)
- Osteoplastic flap (bi-coronal incision, mid forehead, brow)
- Above and below (endoscopic and frontal craniotomy)
- Subcranial, subfrontal and transcranial.

The midfacial degloving approach provides excellent access to bony structures of the midface and posterior parts of the anterior skull base but less satisfactory access to the frontal sinus. Generally, with OPF approaches for tumour removal, frontal sinus obliteration should be considered a contraindication given the inability to detect subsequent tumour recurrence.

Endoscopic considerations

When considering an endoscopic approach, experience in dealing with inflammatory diseases and endonasal duraplasty is mandatory. The endoscopic modified Lothrop procedure (MELP) provides excellent access to the frontal sinus when managing chronic frontal sinus disease but its utility in tumour disease has some limitations. In tumour surgery it is necessary not only to visualize the site of the lesion but also to instrument that area with curettes and drills. The degree of the frontal sinus pneumatization is an important factor. The better the pneumatization, the wider the radius of action of the instrument. The following general guidelines for operating on tumours of the frontal sinus are useful:

1. Lesions not extending beyond a sagittal plane through the lamina papyracea are accessible endoscopically. Lesions extending beyond this may be accessible depending on the anterior-posterior dimension of the floor of the frontal sinus and the intercanthal distance.[94]
2. Tumours arising from the medial quarter of the orbital plate of the frontal sinus may be accessible via a MELP alone or with the aid of an external trephine. (**Figure 99.17**).
3. Lesions originating in the lower third of the posterior wall of the frontal sinus are usually accessible via an endoscopic approach.
4. In general, tumours arising from the anterior wall of the frontal sinus are difficult to access endoscopically.[84] Those arising low down may be accessible via a MELP.
5. A narrow anterior-posterior dimension of the floor of the frontal sinus (<10 mm) can limit endoscopic access and favour open or combined approaches.[95]
6. Superior reach within the sinus may not be possible in well pneumatized sinuses.[96]
7. The junction of the anterior and posterior wall in the most lateral part of the frontal sinus may be too narrow to admit a drill. Similarly, supraorbital ethmoid cells may limit lateral access for tumour removal.[97]

BENIGN TUMOURS

Inverted papilloma

Inverted papilloma (IP) are relatively uncommon benign epithelial tumours of the nasal cavity. They are locally aggressive, have a tendency to recur and are associated with malignancy. Histologically, the tumour is characterized by epithelium inverting into the stroma with a distinct and intact basement membrane. Human papilloma virus has been implicated in the pathogenesis. Viral DNA has been found in the adjacent normal appearing

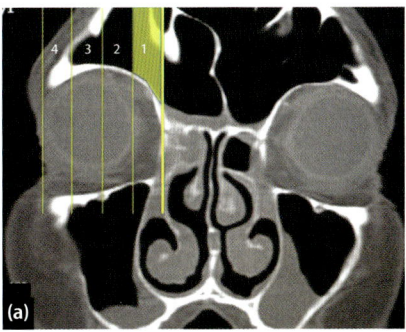 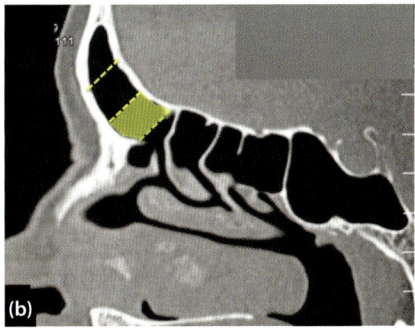 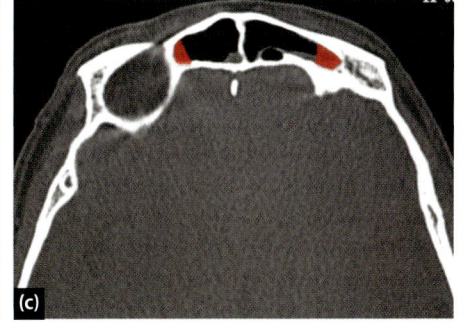

Figure 99.17 (a) Coronal CT demonstrating orbital zones. Zone 1: medial quarter of the orbit (yellow highlight); Zone 2: outer margin of Zone 1 to the midorbital point; Zone 3: laterally from midorbital point to halfway between the midorbital point and the lateral aspect of the orbit; Zone 4: the lateral-most quarter. (Modified with permission.)[97] (b). Parasagittal CT scan. Lesions which originate from the lower third (yellow area) of the posterior or anterior wall of the frontal sinus may be accessible endoscopically.[84] (c) Axial CT scan. The lateral junction of the anterior and posterior walls may be inaccessible due to their narrowness (red area).

tissue and may account for the associated recurrence rates although in many cases this is due to residual disease. The incidence of IP in normal bilateral nasal polyps is rare (<1%). As multiple sites within the paranasal sinus may be involved, localization of the origin is not always easy. The commonest sites of origin are the ethmoid region (48%), lateral nasal wall and maxillary sinus (28%) with the frontal sinus accounting for only 2.5%.[98] Bilateral frontal sinus involvement is not uncommon (16%).[99]

Although CT is the primary mode of imaging, MRI is complementary and recommended. Particularly in the frontal sinus when tumour can obstruct the outflow tract, MRI is very useful in distinguishing mucus from papilloma. Focal hyperostosis on CT imaging is a common finding in patients with IP but may be helpful in identifying the site of origin.[100, 101]

Surgical strategy

The success of surgery is dependent on defining the extent of disease, identifying the site of tumour origin and attachments and fully extirpating all affected tissue. This includes removal of the underlying mucoperiosteum and burring the bone. Within the frontal sinus, the narrow confines and proximity to the anterior skull base and orbit makes this a challenge. This is reflected by the higher recurrence rates (22%) than would be expected for endoscopic management of IP in other locations (3%).[99]

The OPF procedure offers a wide exposure of the frontal sinus, and has traditionally been the preferred approach. The modified Lothrop procedure combined with angled instruments and endoscopes offers similar access and is a valid alternative.[102] Generally, tumours originating medially or from the lower third of the posterior wall of the frontal sinus can be accessed by a frontal sinusotomy or Draf type II approach. Those arising laterally or along the anterior wall will require an extended endoscopic approach or an OPF. A summary of the suggested surgical strategy can be found in **Table 99.9**.

Extended approaches such as a MELP can be augmented by an external trephine, which can provide an additional port for instruments or endoscopes. The relative accessibility is highlighted in **Figure 99.17**.

TABLE 99.9 Suggested surgical strategy for frontal sinus inverted papilloma

Site of origin within the frontal sinus	Surgical approach options
Unifocal, attached to MW or lower AW/PW. Multifocal as above	Draf type IIa/b MELP
Unifocal or multifocal, attached to superior AW, superior PW or LW	OPF, MELP possibly with external trephine
Lateral to midpoint of orbit	OPF, MELP with external trephine

Anterior wall: AW; posterior wall: PW; medial wall: MW; lateral wall: LW; osteoplastic flap: OPF; endoscopic modified Lothrop procedure: MELP.[102]

A recent systematic review suggests that more aggressive primary approaches may facilitate better disease control.[99] Patients should be followed up for a minimum of 3 years. Where tumour removal was performed via a MELP, direct surveillance can be performed. When this is not possible an MRI is recommended.[103]

Fibro-osseous lesions

Fibrous dysplasia, ossifying fibroma and osteoma are a group of benign bony abnormalities that can affect the paranasal sinuses. They lie along a continuum from least to the most bony content.[104]

OSTEOMAS

Osteomas are the most common benign tumour of the paranasal sinuses, with a prevalence of 3%. These slow growing tumours occur most often in the ethmoid followed by the frontal sinuses.[105] There are three main theories regarding the aetiology of osteomas: developmental, traumatic and infectious. The developmental theory suggests that reactivation of embryonic stem cells leads to uncontrolled bone formation. The traumatic and infectious theories propose an inflammatory process as the initiating factor for bony tumour formation.[103] Histologically 3 types are found: ivory or compact, mature or cancellous and mixed. Their attachment may be broad based or occasionally via a stalk.

CT imaging is the investigation of choice with osteomas appearing as homogenous, dense, well-circumscribed lesions. MRI is recommended when extra sinus involvement is suspected.

Most osteomas are asymptomatic. The commonest reported clinical symptoms are headache or a sensation of pressure. However, these symptoms may be non-sinogenic and one must be cautious in attributing them to the presence of an osteoma.[14]

Surgical strategy

Small asymptomatic osteomas do not require surgery. Conservative management with watchful waiting and interval imaging is recommended.[106] The following guidelines are useful indicators for surgery:

- Symptomatic patients (chronic rhinosinusitis and mucoceles secondary to obstruction, facial deformity, orbital or neurological complications)
- Tumours occupying more than 50% of the frontal sinus
- Continued growth on serial CT imaging
- Tumours obstructing the frontal recess
- Tumours extending outwith the paranasal sinuses (orbital and intra-cranial)

Surgical approaches can be classified as external, endoscopic or a combination of both (above and below). The osteoplastic flap approach with or without fat obliteration has been the gold standard as it provides excellent access and visualization (**Figure 99.18a–c**) but it is not without morbidity (see above). Recently, there has been a trend towards an entirely endoscopic approach such as a Draf IIb (**Figure 99.19a–c**) or modified endoscopic Lothrop procedure (MELP/Draf III).

When combined with an OPF procedure, the MELP aims to maintain long-term patency of the frontal neo-ostium by avoiding obliteration. There is some debate as to the limits of the endoscopic approach. Some of these limitations are discussed above under 'Endoscopic considerations'. Other important factors include the extent of intra-cranial extension, significant orbital involvement and erosion of the posterior or anterior wall of the frontal sinus.[95, 107] A grading system for osteomas is outlined in **Table 99.10**. Conventionally mostly grade I and II tumours were removed endonasally. With the advances in endoscopic instrumentation and surgical skill, many grade III and grade IV can be managed endoscopically.[108–110] Tumours extending beyond a vertical plane through the lamina papyracea are accessible endoscopically. However, access to tumours arising lateral to the midpoint of the orbit may be limited.[97] Tumours extending through the anterior table of the frontal sinus are best managed by an external approach. Although large osteomas filling the sinus may be managed endoscopically, the operative duration is likely to be much shorter via an open approach. Clearly, the surgical strategy needs to be based on the individual's anatomy. Variables such as the degree of frontal sinus pneumatization, interorbital width (distance between both lamina papyracea) and A-P dimension of the floor of the frontal sinus are important considerations in determining the most appropriate approach.[94, 111]

Gardner's syndrome

The syndrome consists of a triad of multiple osteomas, colorectal polyps, skeletal abnormalities and supernumerary teeth. The disease is autosomal dominant and carries a 100% risk of malignant transformation of the colonic polyps by the age of 40. Patients usually present in their second decade with rectal bleeding, pain and diarrhoea. As early diagnosis is important, all patients presenting with frontal sinus osteomas should have a thorough systemic enquiry.[104]

Fibrous dysplasia

Fibrous dysplasia (FD) is a slow growing, tumour-like lesion of bone. It occurs when normal cancellous bone is replaced by abnormal fibrous tissue. The fibrous tissue replaces the spongiosa and fills the medullary cavity with poorly calcified trabeculae (**Figure 99.20**). This genetic disease is a result of a mutation in the *GNAS1* gene located on chromosome 20q13, which normally codes for the alpha subunit of the stimulatory G-protein.[112, 113]

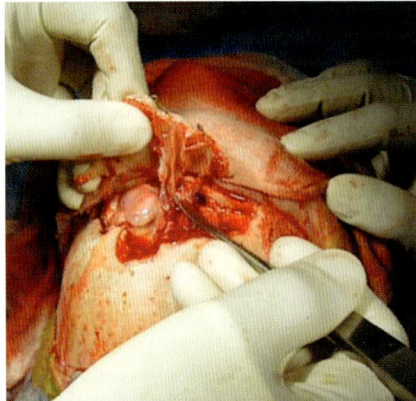 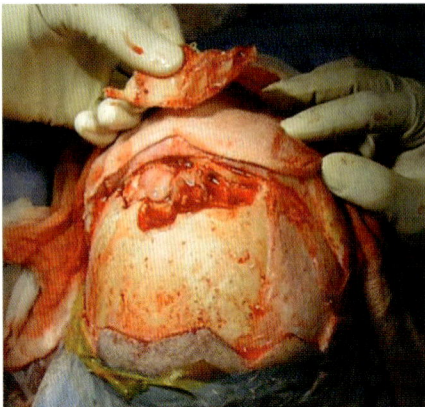 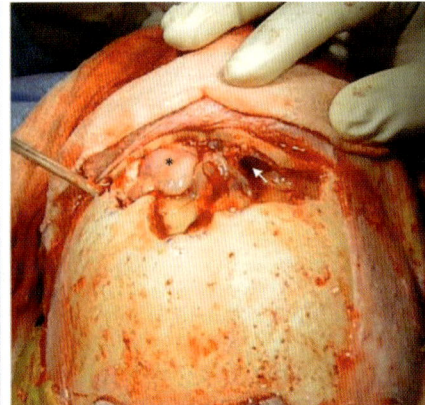

Figure 99.18 Osteoplastic approach for the removal of a large frontal sinus osteoma. Elevation of the bone flap **(a)** and **(b)** reveals the osteoma (*) filling the left frontal sinus **(c)**; the right frontal sinus outflow tract is indicated with a white arrow.

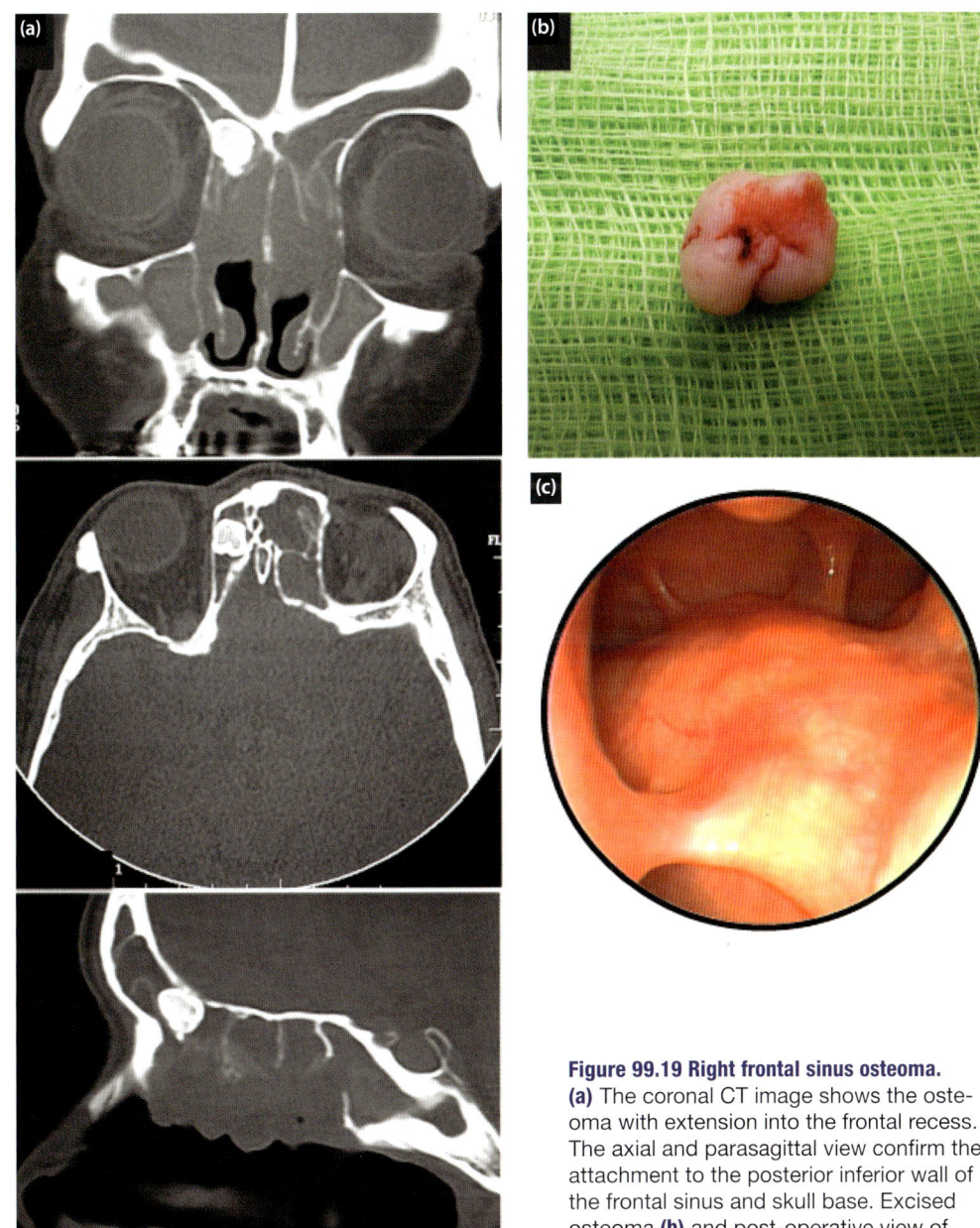

Figure 99.19 Right frontal sinus osteoma.
(a) The coronal CT image shows the osteoma with extension into the frontal recess. The axial and parasagittal view confirm the attachment to the posterior inferior wall of the frontal sinus and skull base. Excised osteoma **(b)** and post-operative view of right frontal sinus following Draf IIb procedure **(c)**.

TABLE 99.10 Frontal sinus osteoma grading system. The grading system highlights three variables: The location of attachment of the base, the relationship of the lesion to a virtual sagittal plane through the lamina papyracea and the A-P width of the frontal recess

Grade	Description
I	Base of attachment is posterior–inferior along the frontal recess.
	Tumour is medial to a virtual sagittal plane through the lamina papyracea.
	Anterior–posterior diameter of the lesion is less than 75% of the anterior–posterior dimension of the frontal recess.
II	Base of attachment is posterior–inferior along the frontal recess.
	Tumour is medial to a virtual sagittal plane through the lamina papyracea.
	Anterior–posterior diameter of the lesion is greater than 75% of the anterior–posterior dimension of the frontal recess.
III	Base of attachment is anterior or superiorly located within the frontal sinus AND/OR
	Tumour extends lateral to a virtual sagittal plane through the lamina papyracea.
IV	Tumour fills the entire frontal sinus.

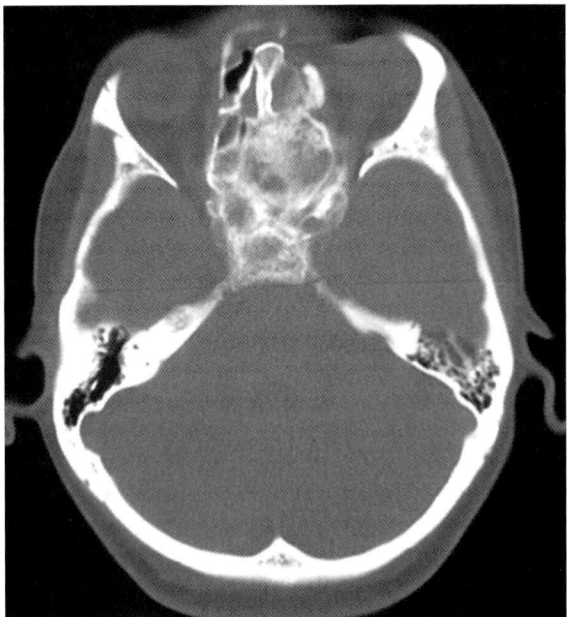

Figure 99.20 Extensive fibrous dysplasia (FD) involving the ethmoid and sphenoid sinus. The patient had previously undergone surgery for FD involving the left frontal sinus.

Most cases (75%) are diagnosed before the age of 30 and tend to stabilize after the patient reaches skeletal maturity.[104, 114] Two forms are present:

- Monostotic (80%) – Craniofacial involvement occurs in up to 25% of cases with the maxilla and mandible most commonly affected. Although monostotic FD in the long bones does not cross the joint line, it can cross bony sutures in the maxillofacial skeleton.
- Polyostotic (20%) – various areas of the skeleton can be affected with craniofacial involvement present in 40% to 50% of cases. Polyostotic FD, endocrine hyperfunction (such as precocious puberty and/or hyperthyroidism) and café-au-lait spots are components of McCune-Albright syndrome. This rare condition primarily affects females.

FD has a low rate of malignant transformation occurring in 0.5% of polyostotic forms and in 4% of lesions with McCune-Albright syndrome.

Patients with the monostotic form are frequently asymptomatic, often diagnosed incidentally. Polyostotic FD can present early with manifestations of bone pain and deformity. Both variants can lead to symptoms of vascular or neurological compression. Craniofacial disease can present as headaches or facial asymmetry. Sphenoid and frontal sinus FD may lead to optic nerve compression and mucocele formation respectively.

CT and MRI are helpful in establishing the diagnosis but if there is any doubt a biopsy is recommended. On CT imaging, lesions appear fairly homogenous with a 'ground glass' appearance. As the lesion scleroses, 'cotton wool' areas appear. MRI helps evaluate the soft tissue component and can distinguish it from other lesions such as meningiomas and bone cysts. FD tends to display an intermediate signal on T1-weighted images and is hypointense on T2-weighted images.[104]

Surgical strategy

Most studies recommend conservative management. Medical treatment is limited to symptomatic relief. Bisphosphonates are useful in reducing the incidence of fractures and bone pain. Asymptomatic patients with monostotic FD can be observed. Endoscopic sinus surgery can provide symptomatic relief by improving sinus drainage pathways.[115] In more severe cases and those with cosmetic deformity, local controlled resection and recontouring may be feasible depending on symptoms and location. Paranasal sinus lesions causing sinusitis or optic nerve compression may be managed endoscopically, ideally with the aid of computer assisted navigation.[84, 103] The rate of malignant transformation to an osteosarcoma is low, at 0.5%, but any painful, rapidly growing lesion should raise suspicion. There is no role for radiotherapy in treating FD.[115]

Ossifying fibroma

The nomenclature surrounding ossifying fibroma (OF) is diverse and confusing. Broadly, OF can be classified into 3 categories:[116]

1. Ossifying fibroma
2. Cemento-ossifying fibroma (COF)
3. Aggressive psammomatoid ossifying fibroma (APOF) or juvenile-aggressive OF.

These benign tumours can have differing biologic behaviour. Histologically, lesions consist of 2 main components: fibrous stroma and bone elements. APOF lesions consist of irregular bony spicules within a cellular fibrous stroma. Classically, this resembles cementum or calcified 'psammomatoid bodies'. COF lesions have similar histologic features with cementum-like material present throughout the lesion.

Clinically, lesions are often asymptomatic but can present with proptosis, diplopia, epiphora, facial swelling, nasal obstruction, epistaxis and headaches. Endoscopically they appear as smooth mucosally covered masses. This locally destructive tumour occurs most commonly in the facial skeleton affecting the mandible in 75% of cases. When arising outside the mandible, OFs appear to affect the ethmoid and maxillary sinuses most frequently. Similarly, APOFs most commonly affect the ethmoid sinus followed by the maxillary sinus, orbit and frontal sinus. Multiple sinus involvement is not uncommon. COF most commonly present in the maxillary and ethmoid sinus and rarely in the frontal and sphenoid sinus.[116]

All three variants display similar features on CT. Sharply circumscribed round lesions with an eggshell rim and central radiolucency are typical of OF. APOF and COF have a thicker bony rim and a central ground glass appearance. MRI features are similar to fibrous dysplasia with a low to intermediate signal on T1-weighted imaging and variable intensity on T2-weighted imaging. An endoscopic biopsy may be required to confirm the diagnosis.

Treatment strategy

If OF is suspected on imaging, a biopsy is recommended to confirm the diagnosis. For paranasal sinus disease this may be achieved endoscopically. The role of biopsy is to exclude malignant pathology such as sarcoma. Ideally, treatment should be complete surgical excision but this is dependent on the site and symptoms. Evidence would suggest that a more conservative approach might be acceptable where there are little or no symptoms.[115, 117] Surgical resection may be achieved by an endoscopic approach, with more extensive disease requiring a combined approach including craniofacial resection. Recurrence rates for APOF, COF and OF are low.[103, 104, 117]

MALIGNANT TUMOURS INVOLVING THE FRONTAL SINUS

Primary malignant tumours of the frontal sinus are very rare. Squamous cell carcinoma is the commonest tumour, affecting the maxillary sinus in up to 30% and the frontal sinus in less than 1%. Other primary tumours include adenocarcinomas and non-epithelial malignancies such as lymphomas. Mostly the frontal sinus becomes involved by direct extension of tumour from adjacent sites. Metastasis of malignant tumours to the frontal sinus is rare. Along with tissue biopsies, CT and multiparametric MRI are helpful in establishing the diagnosis, extent of disease and in particular orbital and dural involvement.[118]

The comprehensive management of sinonasal malignancy is covered elsewhere in this book. However, the principles of surgery are twofold: complete resection of the tumour by the least invasive approach. It would appear that more important than 'en bloc' resection is to achieve negative tumour resection margins.[103]

Malignant tumours of the nasal cavity and other paranasal sinuses, which have not led to major bone destruction and are just reaching the frontal sinus, may be operated on via the endonasal route.

More extensive tumours of this type, or primary malignant frontal sinus tumours, may be approached by the subcranial technique, according to Raveh et al.[119] through a coronal incision, without shaving the hair, sometimes in combination with midfacial degloving, if the lower sinuses are involved. The subcranial approach also allows management of malignancies with skull base or even intradural involvement.

To summarize, there is a stepladder of three surgical techniques: (1) endonasal; (2) midfacial degloving; (3) subcranial approach,[119] which has proved to be very efficient when dealing with malignant tumours of the nasal cavity and the paranasal sinuses, including the frontal sinus and the anterior skull base. The great advantage of all these approaches is the avoidance of visible scars, a fact much appreciated by the patients. The lateral rhinotomy is generally reserved if exenteration of the orbit is needed simultaneously.

OTHER CONDITIONS

Frontal pneumosinus dilatans

Pneumosinus dilatans refers to an abnormally large aerated sinus. This uncommon condition can affect all the paranasal sinuses but has a predilection for the frontal sinus. When associated with the frontal sinus, aeration extends beyond the normal margin of the frontal bone. Characteristically, the walls of the sinus are of normal thickness and there is no evidence of erosion. It is unlike a pneumocele where the aerated sinus is associated with a thinning of its wall and this can be focal or generalized.[120]

AETIOLOGY

A number of theories have been put forward but the pathophysiology remains poorly understood. These theories include: (a) mucocoele growth and spontaneous rupture, (b) a one-way valve mechanism, (c) hormonal influences affecting bone resorption and (d) congenital defects.[121] The mechanism most favoured is that of a one-way valve.

CLINICAL FEATURES AND INVESTIGATIONS

The condition usually presents between the 2nd and 4th decade and has a male preponderance. Most patients are asymptomatic but bony expansion can result in frontal bossing. Less common pressure-related symptoms include diplopia, headache or intra-cranial symptoms.

Pneumosinus dilatans has been shown to be associated with a number of pathological conditions such as planum meningiomas, arachnoid cysts, fibrous dysplasia, acromegaly and prolonged cerebrospinal fluid shunting. Recently, an association with congenital polyosteotic fibrous dysplasia (McCune Albright syndrome) has been reported.[121]

CT imaging is the investigation of choice.

MANAGEMENT

It is important to address any pathology within the sinus or obstructing ventilation of the sinus. If this cannot be achieved endoscopically then an open approach may be required. In patients with functioning ostia the cosmetic deformity is the main issue. This can be corrected by direct, full thickness, resection of horizontal bone strips of the anterior wall of the sinus. Plating of the bone fragments is not required if the galea-periosteum remains attached.[122]

BEST CLINICAL PRACTICE

- ✓ Trial of optimum medical therapy prior to any surgical intervention is important.
- ✓ Recording of outcome data is essential.
- ✓ Post-operative care should include regular saline douches and debridement as necessary.
- ✓ Mucosal preservation during surgery is important. The use of pedicled flaps in more extensive surgery such as the modified Lothrop aids healing and reduces post-operative crusting.
- ✓ The modified Lothrop procedure aims to provide maximal ventilation and facilitate removal of eosinophilic mucin and osteitic bone.
- ✓ Consider more extensive surgery in the following scenarios:
  - ✓ AERD is associated with higher incidence of frontal neo-ostium stenosis.
  - ✓ Asthma (associated with a higher rate of surgical revision).
  - ✓ CRSwNP revision rate higher.
  - ✓ Osteoneogenesis.
  - ✓ Greater burden of disease, Lund McKay score > 16.
  - ✓ Frontal ostium opening on anteroposterior dimension (sagittal CT view) < 4mm.

FUTURE RESEARCH

- ➤ Which patient groups might benefit from more extensive primary frontal sinus surgery?
- ➤ Method of targeted delivery of local steroid and antibiotic therapy within the frontal sinus.
- ➤ Effect of alternative therapies on chronic sinus disease.

KEY POINTS

- The anatomy of the frontal recess is variable and complex. A detailed knowledge of the anatomy is vital when operating within this area.
- One should approach this area with caution. Meticulous attention to detail and careful dissection is key.
- An *all or nothing* approach is suggested.
- It is important to address any disease in the frontal recess/sinus when managing patients with Chronic Rhinosinusitis. Failure of surgery can often be attributed to unaddressed disease within the frontal recess and sinus.
- Incomplete or inadequate surgery in the frontal recess can lead to iatrogenic disease and persistence of symptoms.
- The greater the disease burden as noted by the preoperative Lund-McKay (LM) CT score, the more extensive the surgery required.
- The incidence of more extensive frontal sinus surgery is higher in patients with Asthma and AERD (Aspirin exacerbated respiratory disease)
- Patients with frontal sinus disease may not have *specific* frontal sinus symptoms
- Headache as the predominant symptom without any other significant symptoms of sinusitis is unlikely to be sinogenic in origin.

REFERENCES

1. Lang J. *Clinical anatomy of the nose, nasal cavity and paranasal sinuses.* Stuttgart: Thieme; 1989.
2. Stammberger H. *Functional endoscopic sinus surgery: the messerklinger technique.* Philadelphia: BC Decker; 1991.
3. Wormald P.-J Anatomy of the frontal recess and frontal sinus. In: *Endoscopic sinus surgery: anatomy, three-dimensional reconstruction and surgical technique.* 2nd ed. New York: Thieme; 2008, pp. 43–81.
4. Floreani SR, Nair SB, Switajewski MC, et al. Endoscopic anterior ethmoidal artery ligation: a cadaver study. *Laryngoscope* 2006; **116**(7): 1263–7.
5. Bolger WE, Butzin CA, Parsons DS. Paranasal sinus bony anatomic variations and mucosal abnormalities: CT analysis for endoscopic sinus surgery. *Laryngoscope* 1991; **101**(1 Pt 1): 56–64.
6. Zhang L, Han D, Ge W, et al. Anatomical and computed tomographic analysis of the interaction between the uncinate process and the agger nasi cell. *Acta Otolaryngol* 2006; **126**(8): 845–52.
7. Wormald P-J. Surgery of the frontal recess and frontal sinus. *Rhinology* 2005; **43**(2): 82–5.
8. Wormald P-J. The agger nasi cell: the key to understanding the anatomy of the frontal recess. *Otolaryngol Head Neck Surg* 2003; **129**(5): 497–507.
9. Stamm A, Nogueira JF, Americo RR, et al. Frontal sinus approach: the 'vertical bar' concept. *Clin Otolaryngol* 2009; **34**(4): 407–8.
10. Bent JP, Cuilty-Siller C, Kuhn FA. The frontal cell as a cause of frontal sinus obstruction. *Am J Rhinol* 1994; **8**(4): 185–91.
11. Lund VJ, Stammberger H, Fokkens WJ, et al. European position paper on the anatomical terminology of the internal nose and paranasal sinuses. *Rhinol Suppl* 2014; **24**: 1–34.
12. Wormald P-J, Hoseman, W, Callejas C, et al. The International Frontal Sinus Anatomy Classification (IFAC) and Classification of the Extent of Endoscopic Frontal Sinus Surgery (EFSS). *Int Forum Allergy Rhinol* 2016; **6**(7): 677–96.
13. Cho JH, Citardi MJ, Lee WT, et al. Comparison of frontal pneumatization patterns between Koreans and Caucasians. *Otolaryngol Head Neck Surg* 2006; **135**(5): 780–6.
14. Jones NS. Sinus headaches: avoiding over- and mis-diagnosis. *Expert Rev Neurother* 2009; **9**(4): 439–44.
15. Kew J, Rees GL, Close D, et al. Multiplanar reconstructed computed tomography images improves depiction and understanding of the anatomy of the frontal sinus and recess. *Am J Rhinol* 2002; **16**(2): 119–23.
16. Reitzen SD, Wang EY, Butros SR, et al. Three-dimensional reconstruction based on computed tomography images of the frontal sinus drainage pathway. *J Laryngol Otol* 2010; **124**(3): 291–6.
17. Zinreich SJ, Kennedy DW, Rosenbaum AE, et al. Paranasal sinuses: CT imaging requirements for endoscopic surgery. *Radiology* 1987; **163**(3): 769–75.
18. Dammann F. Imaging of paranasal sinuses today. *Radiologe* 2007; **47**(7): 576, 578–83.
19. Huang BY, Lloyd KM, DelGaudio JM, et al. Failed endoscopic sinus surgery: spectrum of CT findings in the frontal recess. *Radiographics* 2009; **29**(1): 177–95.
20. Loevner LA, Sonners AI. Imaging of neoplasms of the paranasal sinuses. *Neuroimaging Clin N Am* 2004; **14**(4): 625–46.
21. McIntyre JB, Perez C, Penta M, et al. Patterns of dural involvement in sinonasal tumors: prospective correlation of magnetic resonance imaging and histopathologic findings. *Int Forum Allergy Rhinol* 2012; **2**(4): 336–41.
22. Wormald P-J, Ananda A, Nair S. The modified endoscopic Lothrop procedure in the treatment of complicated chronic frontal sinusitis. *Clin Otolaryngol Allied Sci* 2003; **28**(3): 215–20.

23. Wormald P-J, Ananda A, Nair S. Modified endoscopic lothrop as a salvage for the failed osteoplastic flap with obliteration. *Laryngoscope* 2003; **113**(11): 1988–92.
24. Ryan MW, Marple BF. Allergic fungal rhinosinusitis: diagnosis and management. *Curr Opin Otolaryngol Head Neck Surg* 2007; **15**(1): 18–22.
25. Sessions RB. Nasal dermal sinuses: new concepts and explanations. *Laryngoscope* 1982; **92**(8 Pt 2 Suppl 29): 1–28.
26. Hughes GB, Sharpino G, Hunt W, et al. Management of the congenital midline nasal mass: a review. *Head Neck Surg* 1980; **2**(3): 222–33.
27. Zapata S, Kearns DB. Nasal dermoids. *Curr Opin Otolaryngol Head Neck Surg* 2006; **14**(6): 406–11.
28. Rahbar R, Shah P, Mulliken JB, et al. The presentation and management of nasal dermoid: a 30-year experience. *Arch Otolaryngol Head Neck Surg* 2003; **129**(4): 464–71.
29. Blake WE, Chow CW, Holmes AD, et al. Nasal dermoid sinus cysts: a retrospective review and discussion of investigation and management. *Ann Plast Surg* 2006; **57**(5): 535–40.
30. Pinheiro-Neto CD, Snyderman CH, Fernandez-Miranda J, et al. Endoscopic endonasal surgery for nasal dermoids. *Otolaryngol Clin North Am* 2011; **44**(4): 981–7, ix.
31. Fokkens WJ, Lund VJ, Mullol J, et al. European position paper on rhinosinusitis and nasal polyps 2012. *Rhinol Suppl.* 2012; (23): 3 p preceding table of contents, 1–298.
32. Wenig BL, Goldstein MN, Abramson AL. Frontal sinusitis and its intracranial complications. *Int J Pediatr Otorhinolaryngol* 1983; **5**(3): 285–302.
33. Lebovics RS, Moisa, II, Ruben RJ. Sex predilection in patients with acute frontal sinusitis. *Ear Nose Throat J* 1989; **68**(6): 433–4, 7.
34. Maccabee M, Hwang PH. Medical therapy of acute and chronic frontal rhinosinusitis. *Otolaryngol Clin North Am* 2001; **34**(1): 41–7.
35. Lang EE, Curran AJ, Patil N, et al. Intracranial complications of acute frontal sinusitis. *Clin Otolaryngol Allied Sci* 2001; **26**(6): 452–7.
36. Herrmann BW, Forsen JW, Jr. Simultaneous intracranial and orbital complications of acute rhinosinusitis in children. *Int J Pediatr Otorhinolaryngol* 2004; **68**(5): 619–25.
37. McIntosh DL, Mahadevan M. Frontal sinus mini-trephination for acute sinusitis complicated by intracranial infection. *Int J Pediatr Otorhinolaryngol* 2007; **71**(10): 1573–7.
38. DelGaudio JM, Evans SH, Sobol SE, et al. Intracranial complications of sinusitis: what is the role of endoscopic sinus surgery in the acute setting. *Am J Otolaryngol* 2010; **31**(1): 25–8.
39. Lien CF, Weng HH, Chang YC, et al. Computed tomographic analysis of frontal recess anatomy and its effect on the development of frontal sinusitis. *Laryngoscope* 2010; **120**(12): 2521–7.
40. Meyer TK, Kocak M, Smith MM, et al. Coronal computed tomography analysis of frontal cells. *Am J Rhinol* 2003; **17**(3): 163–8.
41. Otto KJ, DelGaudio JM. Operative findings in the frontal recess at time of revision surgery. *Am J Otolaryngol* 2010; **31**(3): 175–80.
42. DelGaudio JM, Hudgins PA, Venkatraman G, et al. Multiplanar computed tomographic analysis of frontal recess cells: effect on frontal isthmus size and frontal sinusitis. *Arch Otolaryngol Head Neck Surg* 2005; **131**(3): 230–5.
43. Han JK, Ghanem T, Lee B, et al. Various causes for frontal sinus obstruction. *Am J Otolaryngol* 2009; **30**(2): 80–2.
44. Bradley DT, Kountakis SE. The role of agger nasi air cells in patients requiring revision endoscopic frontal sinus surgery. *Otolaryngol Head Neck Surg* 2004; **131**(4): 525–7.
45. Gross CW. Surgical treatments for symptomatic chronic frontal sinusitis. *Arch Otolaryngol Head Neck Surg* 2000; **126**(1): 101–2.
46. Kuhn FA. An integrated approach to frontal sinus surgery. *Otolaryngol Clin North Am* 2006; **39**(3): 437–61, viii.
47. Catalano PJ. Minimally invasive sinus technique: what is it? Should we consider it? *Curr Opin Otolaryngol Head Neck Surg* 2004; **12**(1): 34–7.
48. Draf W, Weber R, Keerl R, et al. Current aspects of frontal sinus surgery. I: Endonasal frontal sinus drainage in inflammatory diseases of the paranasal sinuses. *HNO* 1995; **43**(6): 352–7.
49. Metson R, Sindwani R. Endoscopic surgery for frontal sinusitis: a graduated approach. *Otolaryngol Clin North Am* 2004; **37**(2): 411–22.
50. Tomazic PV, Stammberger H, Koele W, et al. Ethmoid roof CSF-leak following frontal sinus balloon sinuplasty. *Rhinology* 2010; **48**(2): 247–50.
51. Andrews JN, Weitzel EK, Eller R, et al. Unsuccessful frontal balloon sinuplasty for recurrent sinus barotrauma. *Aviat Space Environ Med* 2010; **81**(5): 514–16.
52. Plaza G, Eisenberg G, Montojo J, et al. Balloon dilation of the frontal recess: a randomized clinical trial. *Ann Otol Rhinol Laryngol* 2011; **120**(8): 511–18.
53. Ahmed J, Pal S, Hopkins C, et al. Functional endoscopic balloon dilation of sinus ostia for chronic rhinosinusitis. *Cochrane Database Syst Rev* 2011; **7**: CD008515.
54. Becker SS, Han JK, Nguyen TA, et al. Initial surgical treatment for chronic frontal sinusitis: a pilot study. *Ann Otol Rhinol Laryngol* 2007; **116**(4): 286–9.
55. Eloy JA, Friedel ME, Kuperan AB, et al. Modified mini-Lothrop/extended Draf IIB procedure for contralateral frontal sinus disease: a case series. *Int Forum Allergy Rhinol* 2012; **2**(4): 321–4.
56. Lothrop HA. XIV. Frontal sinus suppuration: the establishment of permanent nasal drainage; the closure of external fistulae; epidermization of sinus. *Ann Surg* 1914; **59**(6): 937–57.
57. Draf W. Endonasal micro-endoscopic frontal sinus surgery: the Fulda concept. *Oper Tech Otolaryngol Head Neck Surg* 1991; **2**: 234–40.
58. Gross WE, Gross CW, Becker D, et al. Modified transnasal endoscopic Lothrop procedure as an alternative to frontal sinus obliteration. *Otolaryngol Head Neck Surg* 1995; **113**(4): 427–34.
59. Sindwani R, Metson R. Image-guided frontal sinus surgery. *Otolaryngol Clin North Am* 2005; **38**(3): 461–71.
60. Friedman M, Bliznikas D, Vidyasagar R, et al. Long-term results after endoscopic sinus surgery involving frontal recess dissection. *Laryngoscope* 2006; **116**(4): 573–9.
61. Chiu AG, Vaughan WC. Revision endoscopic frontal sinus surgery with surgical navigation. *Otolaryngol Head Neck Surg* 2004; **130**(3): 312–18.
62. Musy PY, Kountakis SE. Anatomic findings in patients undergoing revision endoscopic sinus surgery. *Am J Otolaryngol* 2004; **25**(6): 418–22.
63. Kuhn FA, Javer AR, Nagpal K, et al. The frontal sinus rescue procedure: early experience and three-year follow-up. *Am J Rhinol* 2000; **14**(4): 211–16.
64. Ling FT, Kountakis SE. Important clinical symptoms in patients undergoing functional endoscopic sinus surgery for chronic rhinosinusitis. *Laryngoscope* 2007; **117**(6): 1090–3.
65. Lee JT, Kennedy DW, Palmer JN, et al. The incidence of concurrent osteitis in patients with chronic rhinosinusitis: a clinicopathological study. *Am J Rhinol* 2006; **20**(3): 278–82.
66. Chiu AG. Frontal sinus surgery: its evolution, present standard of care, and recommendations for current use. *Ann Otol Rhinol Laryngol Suppl* 2006; **196**: 13–19.
67. Silverman JB, Prasittivatechakool K, Busaba NY. An evidence-based review of endoscopic frontal sinus surgery. *Am J Rhinol Allergy* 2009; **23**(6): e59–62.
68. Chan Y, Melroy CT, Kuhn CA, et al. Long-term frontal sinus patency after endoscopic frontal sinusotomy. *Laryngoscope* 2009; **119**(6): 1229–32.
69. Naidoo Y, Wen D, Bassiouni A, et al. Long-term results after primary frontal sinus surgery. *Int Forum Allergy Rhinol* 2012; **2**(3): 185–90.
70. Hardy JM, Montgomery WW. Osteoplastic frontal sinusotomy: an analysis of 250 operations. *Ann Otol Rhinol Laryngol* 1976; **85**(4 Pt 1): 523–32.
71. Silverman JB, Gray ST, Busaba NY. Role of osteoplastic frontal sinus obliteration in the era of endoscopic sinus surgery. *Int J Otolaryngol* 2012; 2012: 501896.
72. Wormald PJ. Salvage frontal sinus surgery: the endoscopic modified Lothrop procedure. *Laryngoscope* 2003; **113**(2): 276–83.
73. Weber R, Draf W, Keerl R, et al. Osteoplastic frontal sinus surgery with fat obliteration: technique and long-term results using magnetic resonance imaging in 82 operations. *Laryngoscope* 2000; **110**(6): 1037–44.
74. Ulualp SO, Carlson TK, Toohill RJ. Osteoplastic flap versus modified endoscopic Lothrop procedure in patients with frontal sinus disease. *Am J Rhinol* 2000; **14**(1): 21–6.
75. Sillers MJ. Frontal sinus obliteration: an operation for the archives or modern armamentarium. *Arch Otolaryngol Head Neck Surg* 2005; **131**(6): 529–31.
76. Lanza DC. Frontal sinus obliteration is rarely indicated. *Arch Otolaryngol Head Neck Surg* 2005; **131**(6): 531–2.
77. Soyka MB, Annen A, Holzmann D. Where endoscopy fails: indications and experience with the frontal sinus fat obliteration. *Rhinology.* 2009; **47**(2): 136–40.
78. Hahn S, Palmer JN, Purkey MT, et al. Indications for external frontal sinus procedures for inflammatory sinus disease. *Am J Rhinol Allergy* 2009; **23**(3): 342–7.
79. Davis WE. Growing obsolescence of the frontal sinus obliteration procedure. *Arch Otolaryngol Head Neck Surg* 2005; **131**(6): 532–3.

80. Fewins JL, Otto PM, Otto RA. Computed tomography-generated templates: a new approach to frontal sinus osteoplastic flap surgery. *Am J Rhinol* 2004; **18**(5): 285–9; discussion 289–90.
81. Melroy CT, Dubin MG, Hardy SM, Senior BA. Analysis of methods to assess frontal sinus extent in osteoplastic flap surgery: transillumination versus 6-ft Caldwell versus image guidance. *Am J Rhinol* 2006; **20**(1): 77–83.
82. Daniel M, Watson J, Hoskison E, et al. Frontal sinus models and onlay templates in osteoplastic flap surgery. *J Laryngol Otol* 2011; **125**(1): 82–5.
83. Al-Qudah M, Graham SM. Modified osteoplastic flap approach for frontal sinus disease. *Ann Otol Rhinol Laryngol* 2012; **121**(3): 192–6.
84. Draf W. The frontal sinus. In: Gleeson M, (ed). *Scott-Brown's Otorhinolaryngology, head and neck surgery.* 7th ed. London: Hodder Arnold; 2009, pp. 1507–20.
85. Gallagher RM, Gross CW. The role of mini-trephination in the management of frontal sinusitis. *Am J Rhinol* 1999; **13**(4): 289–93.
86. Bartley J, Eagleton N, Rosser P, et al. Superior oblique muscle palsy after frontal sinus mini-trephine. *Am J Otolaryngol* 2012; **33**(1): 181–3.
87. Lee AS, Schaitkin BM, Gillman GS. Evaluating the safety of frontal sinus trephination. *Laryngoscope* 2010; **120**(3): 639–42.
88. Seiberling K, Jardeleza C, Wormald PJ. Minitrephination of the frontal sinus: indications and uses in today's era of sinus surgery. *Am J Rhinol Allergy* 2009; **23**(2): 229–31.
89. van Dijk JM, Wagemakers M, Korsten-Meijer AG, et al. Cranialization of the frontal sinus-the final remedy for refractory chronic frontal sinusitis. *J Neurosurg* 2012; **116**(3): 531–5.
90. Donath A, Sindwani R. Frontal sinus cranialization using the pericranial flap: an added layer of protection. *Laryngoscope* 2006; **116**(9): 1585–8.
91. Raghavan U, Jones NS. The place of Riedel's procedure in contemporary sinus surgery. *J Laryngol Otol* 2004; **118**(9): 700–5.
92. Lango MN, Topham NS, Perlis CS, et al. Surgery in the multimodality treatment of sinonasal malignancies. *Curr Probl Cancer* 2010; **34**(5): 304–21.
93. Sasaki M, Sumi M, Eida S, et al. Multiparametric MR imaging of sinonasal diseases: time-signal intensity curve- and apparent diffusion coefficient-based differentiation between benign and malignant lesions. *Am J Neuroradiol* 2011; **32**(11): 2154–9.
94. Georgalas C, Goudakos J, Fokkens WJ. Osteoma of the skull base and sinuses. *Otolaryngol Clin North Am* 2011; **44**(4): 875–90, vii.
95. Castelnuovo P, Giovannetti F, Bignami M, et al. Open surgery versus endoscopic surgery in benign neoplasm involving the frontal sinus. *J Craniofac Surg* 2009; **20**(1): 180–3.
96. Becker SS, Bomeli SR, Gross CW, et al. Limits of endoscopic visualization and instrumentation in the frontal sinus. *Otolaryngol Head Neck Surg* 2006; **135**(6): 917–21.
97. Timperley DG, Banks C, Robinson D, et al. Lateral frontal sinus access in endoscopic skull-base surgery. *Int Forum Allergy Rhinol* 2011; **1**(4): 290–5.
98. Lawson W, Patel ZM. The evolution of management for inverted papilloma: an analysis of 200 cases. *Otolaryngol Head Neck Surg* 2009; **140**(3): 330–5.
99. Walgama E, Ahn C, Batra PS. Surgical management of frontal sinus inverted papilloma: a systematic review. *Laryngoscope* 2012; **122**(6): 1205–9.
100. Al Badaai Y, Chankowsky J, Mah M, et al. Radiological localization of Schneiderian papilloma. *Int Forum Allergy Rhinol* 2011; **1**(6): 488–91.
101. Bhalla RK, Wright ED. Predicting the site of attachment of sinonasal inverted papilloma. *Rhinology* 2009; **47**(4): 345–8.
102. Yoon BN, Batra PS, Citardi MJ, et al. Frontal sinus inverted papilloma: surgical strategy based on the site of attachment. *Am J Rhinol Allergy* 2009; **23**(3): 337–41.
103. Lund VJ, Stammberger H, Nicolai P, et al. European position paper on endoscopic management of tumours of the nose, paranasal sinuses and skull base. *Rhinol Suppl* 2010; **22**: 1–143.
104. Eller R, Sillers M. Common fibro-osseous lesions of the paranasal sinuses. *Otolaryngol Clin North Am* 2006; **39**(3): 585–600, x.
105. Erdogan N, Demir U, Songu M, et al. A prospective study of paranasal sinus osteomas in 1,889 cases: changing patterns of localization. *Laryngoscope* 2009; **119**(12): 2355–9.
106. Seiden AM, el Hefny YI. Endoscopic trephination for the removal of frontal sinus osteoma. *Otolaryngol Head Neck Surg* 1995; **112**(4): 607–11.
107. Bignami M, Dallan I, Terranova P, et al. Frontal sinus osteomas: the window of endonasal endoscopic approach. *Rhinology* 2007; **45**(4): 315–20.
108. Ledderose GJ, Betz CS, Stelter K, et al. Surgical management of osteomas of the frontal recess and sinus: extending the limits of the endoscopic approach. *Eur Arch Otorhinolaryngol* 2011; **268**(4): 525–32.
109. Seiberling K, Floreani S, Robinson S, et al. Endoscopic management of frontal sinus osteomas revisited. *Am J Rhinol Allergy* 2009; **23**(3): 331–6.
110. Sieskiewicz A, Lyson T, Piszczatowski B, et al. Endoscopic treatment of adversely located osteomas of the frontal sinus. *Ann Otol Rhinol Laryngol* 2012; **121**(8): 503–9.
111. Rokade A, Sama A. Update on management of frontal sinus osteomas. *Curr Opin Otolaryngol Head Neck Surg* 2012; **20**(1): 40–4.
112. Lietman SA, Schwindinger WF, Levine MA. Genetic and molecular aspects of McCune-Albright syndrome. *PER* 2007; **4** Suppl 4: 380–5.
113. Schwindinger WF, Francomano CA, Levine MA. Identification of a mutation in the gene encoding the alpha subunit of the stimulatory G protein of adenylyl cyclase in McCune-Albright syndrome. *Proc Natl Acad Sci USA* 1992; **89**(11): 5152–6.
114. Rojas R, Palacios E, Kaplan J, et al. Fibrous dysplasia of the frontal sinus. *Ear Nose Throat J* 2004; **83**(1): 14–15.
115. Ooi EH, Glicksman JT, Vescan AD, et al. An alternative management approach to paranasal sinus fibro-osseous lesions. *Int Forum Allergy Rhinol* 2011; **1**(1): 55–63.
116. Manes RP, Ryan MW, Batra PS, et al. Ossifying fibroma of the nose and paranasal sinuses. *Int Forum Allergy Rhinol* 2013; **3**(2): 161–8.
117. Suarez-Soto A, Baquero-Ruiz de la Hermosa MC, Minguez-Martinez I, et al. Management of fibro-osseous lesions of the craniofacial area: presentation of 19 cases and review of the literature. *Med Oral Patol Oral Cir Bucal* 2013; **18**(3): e479–85.
118. Sasaki M, Sumi M, Kaneko KI, et al. Multiparametric MR imaging for differentiating between benign and malignant thyroid nodules: initial experience in 23 patients. *J Magn Reson Imaging* 2013; **38**: 64–71.
119. Raveh J, Turk JB, Ladrach K, et al. Extended anterior subcranial approach for skull base tumors: long-term results. *J Neurosurg* 1995; **82**: 1002–10.
120. Nowlin TP 4th, Hall DJ, Purdom EB, et al. Pneumosinus dilatans. *Ear Nose Throat J* 2007; **86**(5): 290–1.
121. Walker JL, Jones NS. Pneumosinus dilatans of the frontal sinuses: two cases and a discussion of its aetiology. *J Laryngol Otol* 2002; **116**(5): 382–5.
122. Draf W. Endonasal micro-endoscopic surgery of tumours: state of the art and long term results. In: Fahlbusch R, Buchfelder M, (eds). *The centre of the skull base.* Reinbeck: Einhorn Verlag; 2000, pp. 78–82.
123. Samii M, Draf W. *Surgery of the skull base.* Berlin, Heidelberg, New York: Springer, 1989.
124. Wormald P-J, Bassiouni A, Callejas CA, et al. The International Classification of the Radiological Complexity (ICC) of frontal recess and frontal sinus. *Int Forum Allergy Rhinol* 2017; **7**(4): 332–7.
125. Weber R, Draf W, Kratzsch B, et al. Modern concepts of frontal sinus surgery. *Laryngoscope* 2001; **111**(1): 49–54.
126. Gross CW, Zachmann GC, Becker DG, et al. Follow-up of University of Virginia experience with the modified Lothrop procedure. *Am J Rhinol* 1997; **11**(1): 49–54.

CHAPTER 100

MUCOCELES OF THE PARANASAL SINUSES

Darlene E. Lubbe

Definition	1107	Clinical features	1108
Site of development	1107	Surgical management	1110
Aetiology	1108	Complications	1111
Pathogenesis	1108	References	1111

SEARCH STRATEGY

A PubMed search was conducted to support the data in this chapter using the Medical Subject Headings (MeSH) paranasal, maxillary, frontal, ethmoid, sphenoid sinus and mucocele. The chapter will focus on the etiology and surgical management of mucoceles. The evidence in this chapter is mainly level 2b.

DEFINITION

A mucocele is an epithelium-lined mucus-filled sac within one of the paranasal sinuses with expansion of the sinus cavity and remodelling of the sinus walls. It forms secondary to obstruction of the outflow tract of the involved sinus together with an inflammatory process within the sinus.[1] It is lined by pseudostratified or low-columnar epithelium in contradistinction to a cyst that has a distinct separate membrane. Where bony erosion has taken place, the mucocele's epithelium is often fused with dura or orbital periosteum.

SITE OF DEVELOPMENT

The frontal, ethmoid, maxillary and sphenoid sinuses are involved in descending order of frequency (**Table 100.1**).[2] Frontal sinus mucoceles are probably more common because of the complex and narrow drainage pathway of the frontal sinus that is easily obstructed.[2-3] Mucoceles can form in any other aerated structure such as a concha bullosa of the middle (**Figure 100.1**) or superior turbinate. Obstruction of the nasolacrimal duct can also cause a lacrimal sac mucocele/dacryocele.

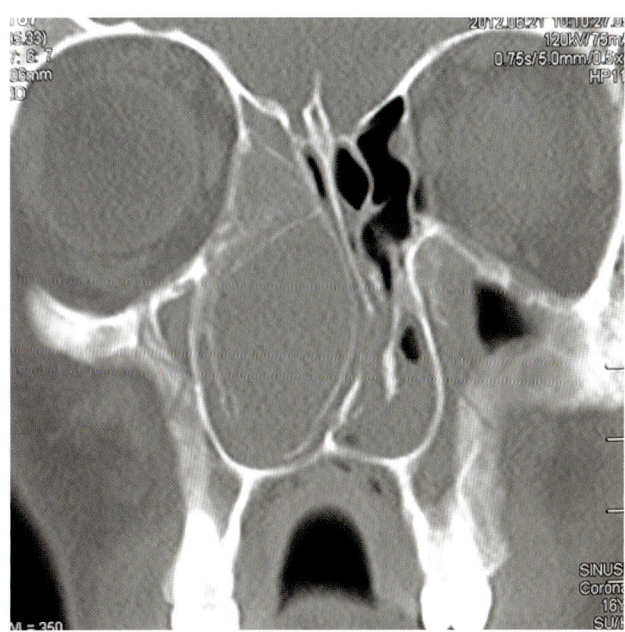

Figure 100.1 Mucocele within a concha bullosa.

TABLE 100.1 Aetiopathogenesis of mucoceles						
Series	Number of cases	Prior sinus surgery	Prior trauma	Spontaneous	CRS without surgery	Tumours
Bockmühl et al.[2]	255	66%	14%	17%	2%	1%
Devars du Mayne et al.[7]	68	75%		15%	7%	
Khong et al.[5]	28	86%	7%			
Nakanishi et al.[6]	24	87.5%		12.5%		
Lund et al.[1]	48			92%	2%	

AETIOLOGY

Sinus surgery is now the leading cause (66–86%)[4–6] of mucocele formation following surgery mostly for chronic sinusitis and nasal polyposis.[2, 7] The interval between surgery and subsequent mucocele formation can range between 1 and 19 years and depends on the location of the mucocele, with frontal and sphenoid mucoceles developing earlier than maxillary sinus mucoceles. Surgery in the region of the frontal recess during functional endoscopic sinus surgery can cause circumferential injury to the frontal sinus outflow tract with subsequent stenosis and mucocele formation. External fronto-ethmoidectomy/Lynch-Howarth operation is a leading cause of mucoceles because of loss of lateral bony support of the frontal recess which causes herniation of the periorbital tissue into the frontal sinus outflow tract. In a large series by Bockmühl et al, 78% of mucoceles following sinus surgery was associated with the Lynch-Howarth and/or Caldwell-Luc operations versus 1.5% after endonasal surgery.[2]

A significant incidence of mucoceles has been reported following endoscopic repair of skull-base fractures in children. In one study 50% of patients developed mucoceles after repair of skull-base defects with a middle turbinate overlay patch.[8] Only 10–14% of mucoceles are secondary to trauma and 15–17% develop spontaneously; the mean interval between head injury and mucocele formation is 9 years.[7] Any benign or malignant tumour can lead to mucocele formation but the incidence in the literature is low and ranges from 1% to 5% (Table 100.2).

PATHOGENESIS

It is thought that in order for a mucocele to form two factors are essential: an obstructed sinus outflow tract and an inflammatory process within the sinus. Osteolytic cytokine-IL-1 and tumour necrosis factor are present within the epithelial lining of mucoceles; it has been postulated that this cytokine may be the responsible for the bony erosion in expanding mucoceles.[1]

CLINICAL FEATURES

Bony erosion leads to expansion of the sac beyond the sinus cavity into the cranial cavity or orbit. Symptoms depend on the sinus involved. A visible mass is often seen on the forehead (Figure 100.2a and b), medial canthus or in the gingivobuccal sulcus or cheek. Ophthalmologic symptoms are more common than rhinological and neurological symptoms.[9] The most common ophthalmologic complaints are periorbital swelling, pain and exophthalmos (Figure 100.3). Displacement of the orbital contents can lead to limited ocular mobility, visual disturbance and diplopia.[4, 9] Optic neuropathy has been reported in up to 18% of patients who present with ophthalmologic symptoms and is due to direct compression of the optic nerve in the posterior ethmoid and sphenoid sinuses.[9] A mucocele within a concha bullosa may present with nasal obstruction and/or secondary sinusitis. Epiphora and a cystic swelling in the medial canthus suggest the presence of a dacryocele.

Radiology

Computed tomography (CT) findings suggestive of a mucocele are a homogeneous, isodense lesion within an expanded sinus with bony remodelling of the sinus walls (Figures 100.2c and 3). Contrast enhancement only occurs with a pyocele. A bony defect of the lamina papyracea and/or superomedial part of the orbital rim is often seen in fronto-ethmoidal mucoceles.[10] The globe may be displaced laterally and/or inferiorly with evidence of proptosis on axial images. The sac can cause erosion of the posterior table of the frontal sinus and compression of the intracranial contents. It can be difficult to differentiate maxillary sinus mucoceles from other benign or malignant lesions.

TABLE 100.2 Site of involvement							
Series	No. of mucoceles	Frontal	Fronto-ethmoidal	Ethmoid	Spheno-ethmoid	Sphenoid	Maxillary
Lee et al[4, 10]	82	45%		28%		18%	9%
Bockmühl et al[2]	290	43%	8%	14%		10%	25%
Har-El et al[11]	108		61%	16%	6%	11%	6%

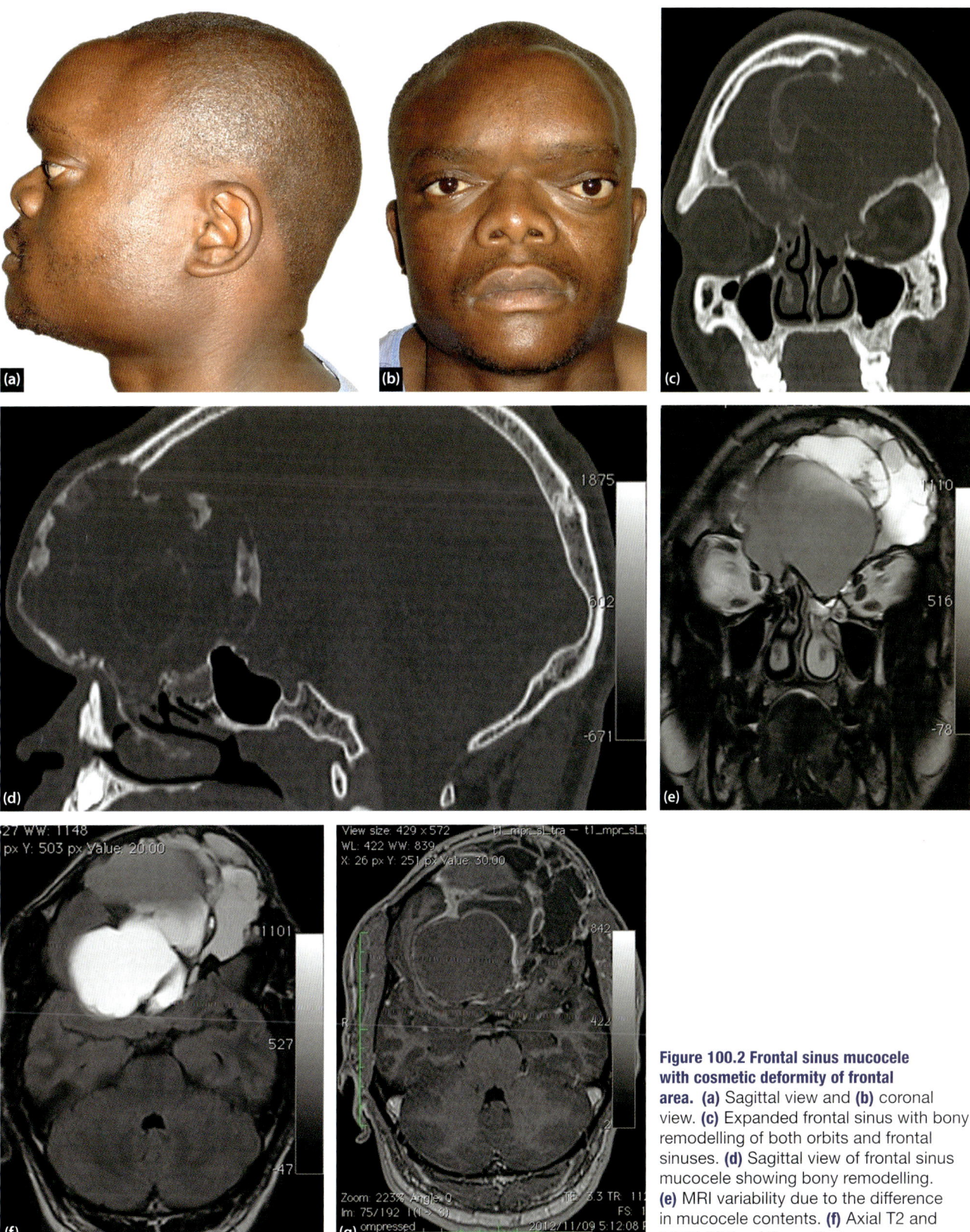

Figure 100.2 Frontal sinus mucocele with cosmetic deformity of frontal area. (a) Sagittal view and (b) coronal view. (c) Expanded frontal sinus with bony remodelling of both orbits and frontal sinuses. (d) Sagittal view of frontal sinus mucocele showing bony remodelling. (e) MRI variability due to the difference in mucocele contents. (f) Axial T2 and (g) T1 MRIs of the patient.

Magnetic resonance imaging (MRI) should be considered in cases of significant bony erosion of the posterior table of the fontal sinus or the orbital lamina papyracea, in order to delineate the mucocele from adjacent soft tissue e.g. cerebral tissue. It should also be recognized that MRI can be misleading due to the variability of mucocele content (Figures 100.2e and 2f). Mucoceles generally have a high-water content and are hyperintense on T1; pyoceles have higher protein content and greater variability of signal intensity on both T1- and T2-weighted images (Figure 100.2e to 2g).

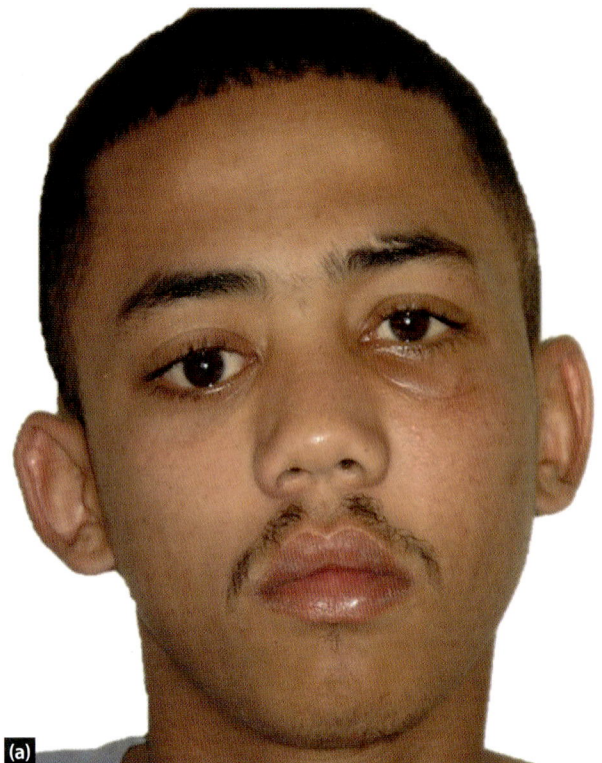 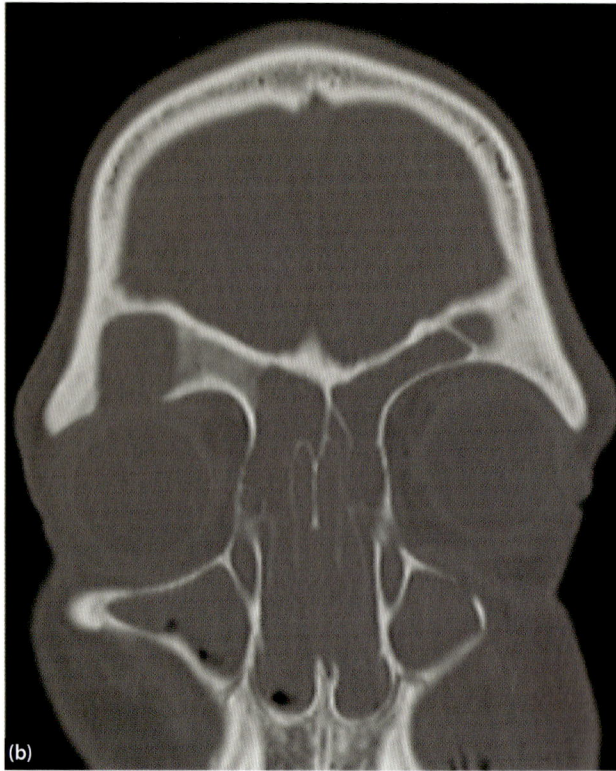

Figure 100.3 (a) Displacement of the left eye secondary to a frontal sinus mucocele. (b) Coronal CT scan of the patient.

Differential diagnosis

1. Benign or malignant tumours
2. Allergic fungal sinusitis/Other fungal disease
3. Cholesterol granuloma (rare).

SURGICAL MANAGEMENT

Treatment is to widely marsupialize the sac to provide permanent ventilation and sinus drainage and to relieve pressure on vital structures. Cosmetic deformities often settle with time as bony remodelling takes place.[11]

Fronto-ethmoidal mucoceles

Wide marsupialization is essential whether by endoscopic and/or open technique. Endoscopic surgery with wide marsupialization/nasalization is the first line of treatment for simple mucoceles but a modified endoscopic Lothrop procedure (MELP) is often required for more complex frontal sinus mucoceles.[5, 11] Good results have been reported with endoscopic techniques with recurrence rates ranging from 0 to 25%.[7, 11] The MELP is especially useful where there is loss of lateral support in the frontal recess due to bony erosion/previous removal of the superior aspect of the lamina papyracea. Combined approaches are often required for laterally located mucoceles as thick bony septations might not allow for endoscopic techniques alone (**Figure 100.3b**). Whilst the Lynch-Howarth approach can be used to access laterally located frontal sinus mucoceles and to assist with the drilling down of bony septations, the approach is associated with risk of long-term frontal outflow obstruction. An osteoplastic frontal flap in combination with a MELP may be required for those mucoceles lying far laterally in the frontal sinus. Transorbital neuroendoscopic surgery (TONES) – and specifically the superior eyelid approach – allows for an alternative, less invasive approach to address pathology of the lateral frontal sinus. Stenting remains controversial; most authors do not advocate the use of stents to maintain patency except in smaller unilateral marsupializations.[6, 11, 12] If a stent is placed, it is important that it is loose fitting to prevent circumferential pressure necrosis that could eventually lead to stenosis.

Obliteration of the frontal sinus has a high success rate (93%) but a major complication rate in excess of 20%.[12] A contraindication to frontal sinus obliteration is extensive erosion of the posterior table of the sinus due to the inability to remove the normal respiratory epithelium on dura.[12] Obliteration has, therefore, largely fallen out of favour.

Maxillary sinus mucoceles

It is important to allow for wide drainage of the maxillary sinus into the nasal cavity; a wide middle meatal antrostomy will usually suffice. A partial medial maxillectomy with preservation of the lacrimal system may be required to gain access to laterally located mucoceles.[11] The Caldwell-Luc approach is only offered in centres where endoscopic surgery is not an option.

Sphenoid sinus mucoceles

A wide sphenoidotomy and intra-nasal marsupialization are all that is required for sphenoid sinus mucoceles.

No attempt is made to remove the lateral sphenoid sinus mucosa as bony erosion place the internal carotid artery or optic nerve at risk of injury.

Other mucoceles

Mucoceles that have formed within a concha bullosa require resection of the lateral aspect of the concha bullosa. Dacryoceles are managed by endoscopic dacryocystorhinostomy.

COMPLICATIONS

Great care needs to be taken when decompressing a large, tense frontal mucocele that displaces the frontal lobe of the brain (**Figure 100.2c and d**) as sudden expansion of the cranial contents can disrupt the dural vessels and cause a subdural haematoma, or disrupt the dura and cause a cerebrospinal fluid (CSF) leak. Close post-operative monitoring is therefore essential in such patients. Because recurrence can occur decades later, long-term follow-up is required.

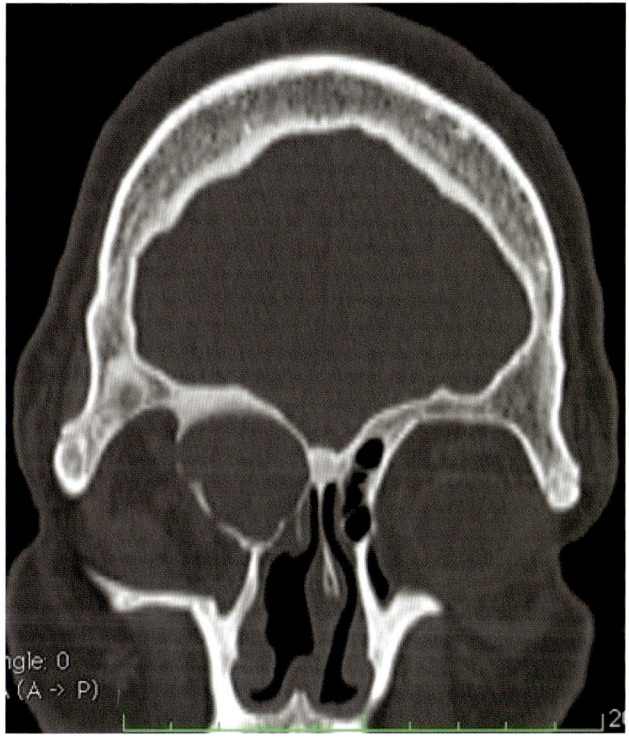

Figure 100.4 Homogeneous, isodense lesion within an expanded ethmoid sinus with bony remodelling of the sinus walls.

BEST CLINICAL PRACTICE

- ✓ CT is the imaging modality of choice and must be performed pre-operatively.
- ✓ Wide endoscopic marsupialization is the first line treatment for simple mucoceles.
- ✓ MELP is a good alternative to obliteration procedures.
- ✓ Combined approaches may be required with laterally located frontal sinus mucoceles.
- ✓ Long-term follow up is required to assess the need for further surgery to correct cosmetic deformities and to ensure patency of the marsupialized sac

FUTURE RESEARCH

- ➤ The pathogenesis of idiopathic mucoceles needs to be further investigated to ascertain if factors exist that make certain people more susceptible to mucoceles.
- ➤ Although cosmetic deformities can settle with time as bony remodelling takes place, no studies have been done to assess the long-term cosmetic outcome with marsupialization alone.

KEY POINTS

- Sinus surgery is now the leading cause of mucoceles.
- Wide marsupialization is required for all mucoceles.
- Bony remodelling can take place after surgery and cosmetic deformities will improve with time.

REFERENCES

1. Lund VJ, Henderson B, Song Y. Involvement of cytokines and vascular adhesion receptors in the pathology of fronto-ethmoidal mucocoeles. *Acta Otolaryngol* 1993; **113**(4): 540–6.
2. Bockmühl U, Kratzsch B, Benda K, Draf W. Surgery for paranasal sinus mucocoeles: efficacy of endonasal micro-endoscopic management and long-term results of 185 patients. *Rhinology* 2006; **44**(1): 62–7.
3. Lund V. Anatomical considerations in the aetiology of fronto-ethmoidal mucoceles. *Rhinology.* 1987; **25**(2): 83–8.
4. Lee T-J, Li S-P, Fu C-H, et al. Extensive paranasal sinus mucoceles: a 15-year review of 82 cases. *Am J Otolaryngol* Elsevier Inc.; 2009 [cited 2013 Mar 31]; **30**(4): 234–8.
5. Khong JJ, Malhotra R, Selva D, Wormald PJ. Efficacy of endoscopic sinus surgery for paranasal sinus mucocele including modified endoscopic Lothrop procedure for frontal sinus mucocele. *J Laryngol Otol* CUP; 2004; **118**(5): 352–6.

6. Nakanishi M, Haruna S, Wada K, et al. Outcomes of frontal mucocele marsupialization: endonasal and external approaches. *Am J Rhinol* 2004; **18**(4): 247–52.
7. Devars du Mayne M, Moya-Plana a, Malinvaud D, et al. Sinus mucocele: natural history and long-term recurrence rate. *Eur Annal Otorhinolaryngol Head Neck Dis* 2012 [cited 2013 Mar 21]; **129**(3): 125–30.
8. Verillaud B, Genty E, Leboulanger N, et al. Mucocele after transnasal endoscopic repair of traumatic anterior skull base fistula in children. *Int J Pediatr Otorhinolaryngol* 2011 [cited 2013 Mar 24]; **75**(9): 1137–42.
9. Kim Y-S, Kim K, Lee J-G, et al. Paranasal sinus mucoceles with ophthalmologic manifestations: a 17-year review of 96 cases. *Am J Rhinol Allergy* 2013 [cited 2013 Mar 28]; **25**(4): 272–5.
10. Lee T-J, Li S-P, Fu C-H, et al. Extensive paranasal sinus mucoceles: a 15-year review of 82 cases. *Am J Otolaryngol* Elsevier Inc.; 2009; **30**(4): 234–8.
11. Har-El G. Endoscopic management of 108 sinus mucoceles. *Laryngoscope* 2001 [cited 2013 Apr 7]; **111**(12): 2131–4.
12. Anderson P, Sindwani R. Safety and efficacy of the endoscopic modified Lothrop procedure: a systematic review and meta-analysis. *Laryngoscope* 2009 [cited 2013 Mar 17]; **119**(9): 1828–33.

CHAPTER 101

COMPLICATIONS OF RHINOSINUSITIS

Stephen Ball and Sean Carrie

Definition 1113	Intracranial complications 1120
Epidemiology 1113	Clinical presentation 1120
Classification 1113	Investigations 1120
Clinical presentation 1114	Treatment 1120
Orbital complications 1114	Bony complications 1122
Examination 1116	Chronic complications 1123
Investigations 1116	Acknowledgements 1123
Treatment 1118	References 1123

SEARCH STRATEGY

Data in this chapter may be updated by a Medline search along with BMJ evidence using the keywords: rhinosinusitis, complications, orbital cellulitis, intra-cranial, cavernous sinus thrombosis and Pott's puffy tumour.

DEFINITION

Complications of rhinosinusitis result from progression of acute or chronic infection beyond the paranasal sinuses, potentially causing significant morbidity from either local or distant spread.

EPIDEMIOLOGY

Epidemiological studies estimate an incidence of three complications from rhinosinusitis per million population per year; approximately one in every 12,000 acute rhinosinusitis episodes,[1] although this probably underestimates the disease burden. Most complications tend to occur in children and young adults, who typically experience six to eight upper respiratory infections per year.[2] Rhinosinusitis occurs in 5–10% of these infections[3] with the majority of complications originating from frontal and ethmoid sinus infections. Complications of rhinosinusitis are more accentuated in children and adolescents because of their thinner, more porous bony septa and sinus walls, open suture lines and larger vascular foramina.

CLASSIFICATION

Complications of rhinosinusitis are generally classified as orbital, intra-cranial, bony or chronic.

Complications may be caused by either local progression or distant spread via the bloodstream. Local progression is typically through areas where the surrounding bone is thin such as the porous lamina papyracea, where there is a direct anatomical connection[6,7] or through osteitic bone. Direct routes of spread occur through neurovascular foramina such as the infraorbital canal, or via the valveless diploeic veins of Breschet of the frontal, ethmoid and sphenoid bones. The venous drainage of the sinus mucosa is via these diploeic veins,[8] which communicate with the dural venous plexus, the absence of valves facilitates retrograde spread of infection. Local complications of rhinosinusitis can be specific for the individual sinus groups and may best be discussed relating to their presumed anatomical sinus of origin. However, isolated sinus infections are rare and usually simultaneous infection is present in more than one sinus group.

Frontal

Anterior spread of acute frontal sinusitis through the outer table of the skull may cause a boggy subperiosteal abscess and osteomyelitis. This condition is commonly referred to as Pott's puffy tumour, following its description by Sir Percival Pott in 1760.[9] Posterior spread of infection can cause acute intracranial complications such as subdural empyema, meningitis, cerebritis and intracranial abscess. Subdural empyema is the most common intracranial complication of sinusitis, and the most common cause of subdural empyema is frontal sinusitis.[5] Spread of infection inferiorly can lead to orbital cellulitis.

Ethmoid

Orbital cellulitis is by far the most frequent acute complication of ethmoid sinusitis. It can vary in degree and severity and is typically graded with the Chandler classification.[10] This clinically useful classification (**Table 101.1** and **Figure 101.2**) also helps to guide the overall management of the patient although its lack of sensitivity and specificity means it has been superseded by the current availability of CT scanning. It is also important to note that orbital cellulitis can present at any stage of the Chandler classification and the disease does not necessarily progress in a chronological order i.e. a stage 2 can progress directly to stage 5 bypassing the steps in between and so on.

Maxillary

Isolated maxillary rhinosinusitis rarely gives rise to acute complications. Acute cheek swelling usually results from complications of dental disease, though there may be an associated secondary maxillary rhinosinusitis.

Sphenoid

Isolated sphenoid sinusitis is rare, but complications can result in meningitis[12] or cavernous sinus thrombosis by direct spread.[13] In cavernous sinus thrombosis infection may spread through veins from the paranasal sinuses and orbit to the cavernous sinuses as thrombophlebitis or by septic emboli. Bacteria themselves are pro-thrombotic, the thrombus provides good conditions for growth and bacteria within the thrombus are shielded by the outer layers from antibiotics which they can later re-infect.[14] In cases arising from acute sinusitis the sphenoid and ethmoid sinuses are the most common source.[14] Intracranial complications can also occur following a skull base fracture through the sphenoid sinus.

CLINICAL PRESENTATION

Any of the complications described above may present with a good history or obvious signs of preceding rhinosinusitis. However, it is not uncommon for the rhinosinusitis itself to be 'occult' or asymptomatic. In children it is more likely that there will be no prior history of rhinosinusitis, with the complication often being the first presentation.

ORBITAL COMPLICATIONS

It is estimated that 3% of sinusitis cases will progress to orbital cellulitis[7] with 60–85% of orbital cellulitis cases being secondary to sinusitis.[15, 16] The remainder are caused by processes such as dacryocystitis or facial infection.[16] In the pre-antibiotic era death or blindness occurred in up to 20% of patients.[7]

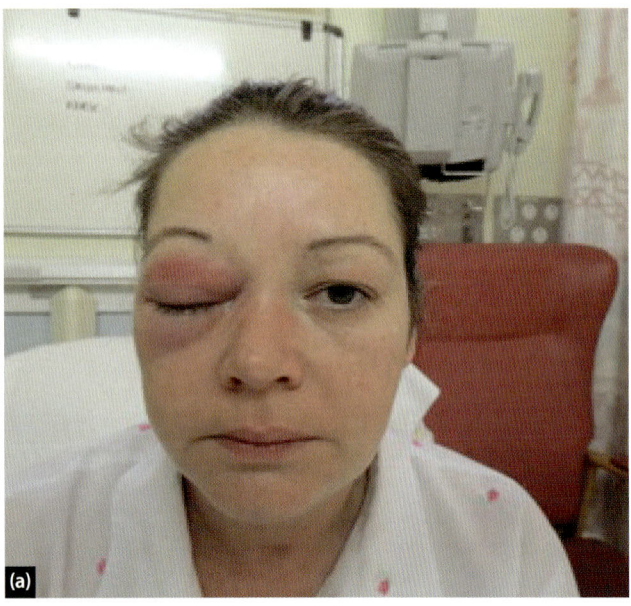 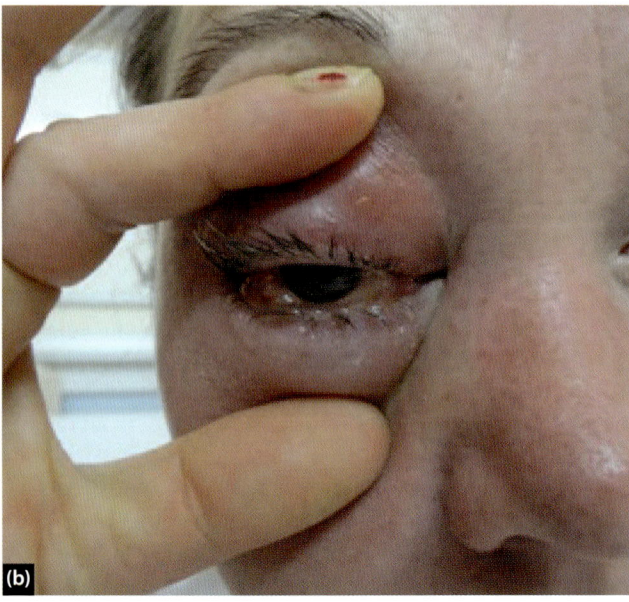

Figure 101.1 Right orbital cellulitis, Chandler classification stage 2; postseptal cellulitis. It is important to open the eyelids to fully examine the eye & vision. Here we see chemosis typical of orbital cellulitis, there was no visual defect, diplopia or relative afferent pupillary defect.

101: COMPLICATIONS OF RHINOSINUSITIS

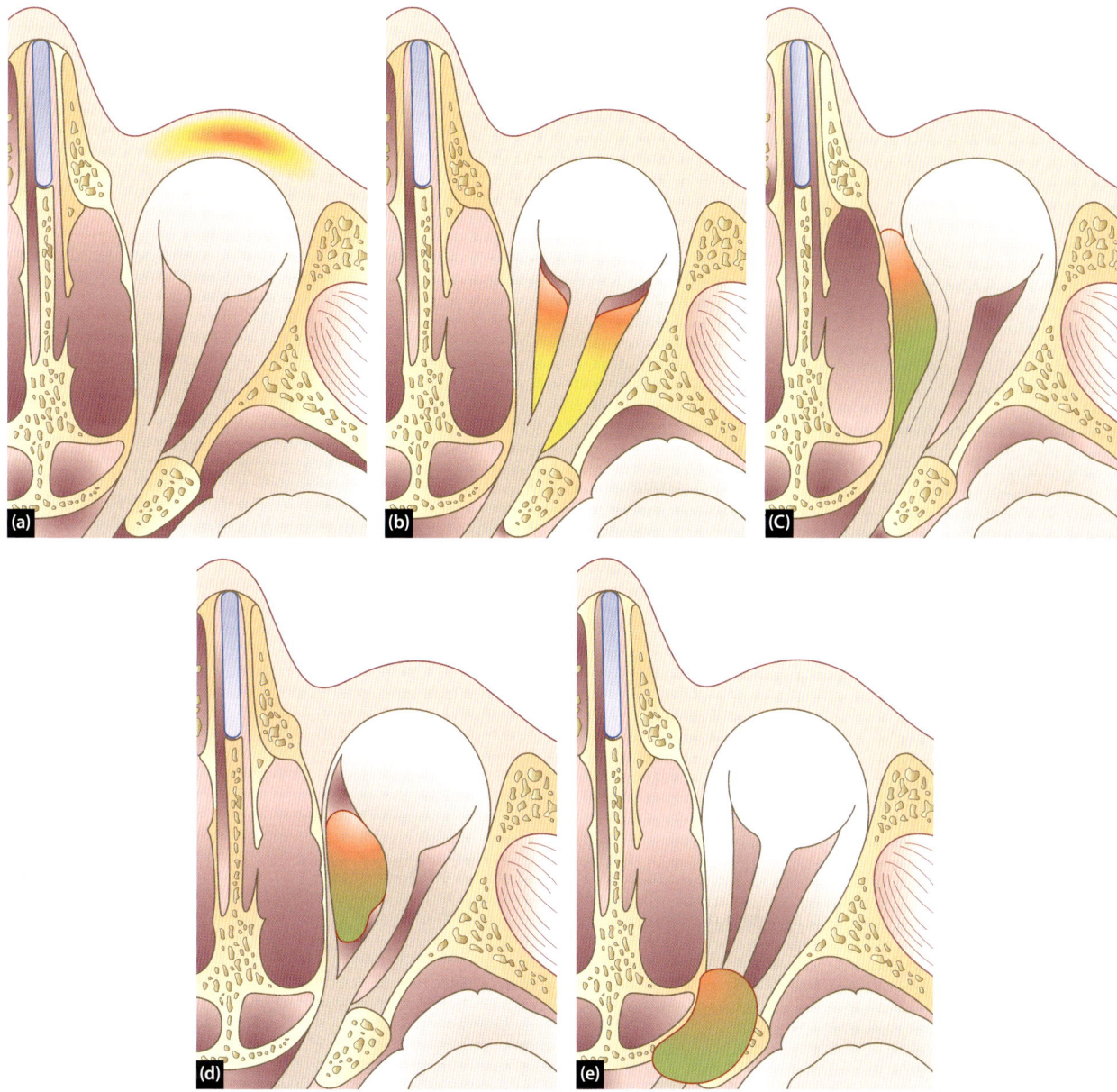

Figure 101.2 Various orbital complications on axial projection: (a) preseptal inflammation; **(b)** orbital cellulitis; **(c)** orbital cellulitis with subperiosteal (extra periosteal) abscess, **(d)** orbital cellulitis with intra-periosteal abscess; **(e)** cavernous sinus thrombosis. Red and yellow shading indicate inflammation/cellulitis, and green shading indicates pus. Redrawn from [11], with permission.

TABLE 101.1 Complications of rhinosinusitis, figures in brackets indicate relative frequency			
Orbital[4]	**Intracranial**[5]	**Bony**	**Chronic**
Preseptal cellulitis (50%)	Sub dural empyema (38%)	Osteomyelitis & Pott's puffy tumour	Mucocele & pyocele
Postseptal cellulitis or orbital cellulitis without abscess (35%)	Intracranial abscess (30%)		
Subperiosteal abscess (15%)	Extradural abscess (23%)		
Orbital abscess (<1%)	Meningitis (2%)		
Cavernous sinus thrombosis	Cavernous or sagittal sinus thrombosis (2%)		

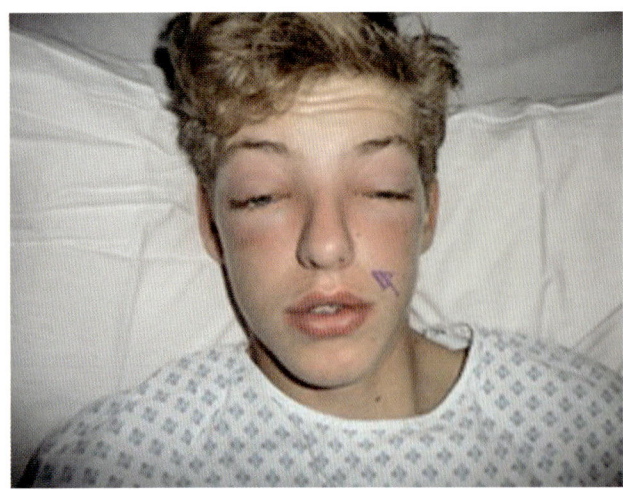

Figure 101.3 Pre-operative clinical photograph from an adolescent male with cavernous sinus thrombosis secondary to rhinosinusitis. Note the bilateral periorbital signs of oedema, cellulits and subtle left VIth cranial nerve palsy.

The onset is noted by swelling around the eye. Oedema results from congestion of veins draining the eyelid and can be present when the infection is still confined to the sinus. Cellulitis from untreated sinusitis represents stage 1 of the disease with local spread of inflammatory elements to the lid. Postseptal cellulitis (stage 2) is confined to the orbit but has extended through the orbital septum, potentially with intraconal involvement. Patients will have eyelid swelling, chemosis and proptosis, potentially with impaired extraocular muscle function and diplopia (**Figure 101.1**). Postseptal cellulitis typically results from transmitted pressure from the sinus to orbital veins with leakage of inflammatory elements into the orbit. It is difficult to clinically differentiate postseptal cellulitis from subperiosteal abscess (stage 3), CT scanning is mandatory here and reflects the fact that the classification system pre-dates the ready availability of scanning.

Orbital cellulitis is far more common in children (50% under 6 years)[17] and young adults (76–85% under 20 years).[18, 19] Visual problems are a late sign, but may be present if the problem is stage 2 (postseptal cellulitis) or beyond. Specific enquiries should be made regarding diplopia, visual acuity and colour vision; signs which indicate compromised optic nerve function. At stage 5 (cavernous sinus thrombosis) signs of chemosis, periorbital oedema, proptosis, progressive opthalmoplegia, visual impairment and symptoms including headache and trigeminal parasthesia will be present (**Figure 101.3**).[20] In the case of orbital infection, cavernous sinus thrombosis will result from septic thrombophlebitis of the superior ophthalmic vein. Initially signs may be unilateral; bilateral disease propagates via the intercavernous sinuses.[21] Published mortality from cavernous sinus thrombosis is high at between 14% and 79% and up to half of patients experience morbidity including residual cranial nerve palsies and blindness.[14, 21] Animal experiments have demonstrated that visual loss may be irreversible if retinal ischaemic time exceeds 100 minutes.[22] Superiorly located orbital subperiosteal abscesses with severe frontoethmoiditis may indicate an increased potential for intracranial suppuration and should be aggressively evaluated.[23]

EXAMINATION

Clinical endoscopic examination of the nose should be performed to help determine the site and extent of disease. In the case of orbital cellulitis, a formal assessment of the degree of chemosis, range of eye movements, degree of proptosis, relative afferent pupillary defect, visual acuity (using a Snellen chart), colour vision (using Ishihara plates) and inspection of the optic disc should be made. This should ideally be carried out by an ophthalmologist. This assessment should be repeated at least twice daily and where there is increasing concern, 4–6 hourly monitoring of the full range of eye movements, visual acuity and colour vision should be undertaken with regular temperature and pulse measurements. For intracranial complications a full neurological examination should be completed. The possibility of occult intracranial complications should always be considered, even in a patient with a normal neurological examination. If intracranial complications are found, neurosurgical opinion is required. Multidisciplinary involvement is important but leadership of care should be clear and preferably by an experienced ENT surgeon.

INVESTIGATIONS

Rhinosinusitis can cause complications in different sites simultaneously. In one series the frequency of developing both intracranial and orbital complications was 5.4%, which rose to 13–24% for those who required surgical intervention to drain orbital disease.[23] Investigations should therefore be used to confirm the diagnosis, extent and any occult complications.

Radiological

There is currently a wide range of techniques available for imaging the paranasal sinuses and surrounding structures. The aim of these investigations is to:

- confirm the diagnosis of the complication
- define the extent and site of the complication
- help plan treatment including surgical approach
- confirm that there is no other covert complication present
- Monitor the response to treatment.

Contrast enhanced computed tomography (CT) is advised as first-line imaging because of its superiority in demonstrating bony anatomy and pathology of the orbit and sinuses with its speed and ease of examination. MRI provides outstanding soft tissue detail without radiation

TABLE 101.2 Chandler stages				
Stage 1	**Stage 2**	**Stage 3**	**Stage 4**	**Stage 5**
Preseptal cellulitis	Postseptal cellulitis or orbital cellulitis without abscess	Subperiosteal abscess	Orbital abscess	Cavernous sinus thrombosis/abscess
Inflammation does not extend beyond the orbital septum (where the medial orbital periosteal reflection attaches to the medial eyelid at the tarsal plate).	Inflammation extends into the tissues of the orbit.	There is abscess formation deep to the periosteum of the orbital bones, typically at the lamina papyracea from ethmoid sinusitis.	There is abscess formation within the orbit which has breached the periosteum.	The inflammatory process has extended into the cavernous sinus which thromboses and may progress to abscess formation.

exposure. It should be noted that CT scanning may miss up to 50% of early stage intracranial complications. A low threshold for MR imaging is advised if there is any clinical suspicion of intracranial involvement.

The diagnosis of the complication should be apparent from the clinical appearance. If there is full ocular movement and normal colour vision, no immediate radiological investigation is indicated unless there is concern about intracranial pathology. Imaging should be undertaken to confirm the presence and site of suspected abscess prior to surgical drainage. Plain X-rays have no role as they are unable to define anything but the grossest orbital abnormalities. The investigation of choice is high-resolution triplanar axial, coronal and sagittal CT scanning. This will give the greatest chance of picking up small abnormalities, which may be missed with uniplanar scans. Although magnetic resonance imaging (MRI) will define abnormalities in the orbit, there is no evidence that it is more accurate than CT[24] and the lack of bone definition for planning surgery makes it of limited value for first-line imaging. Ultrasound also will not demonstrate surgical anatomy and has high false positive and negative rates.[24, 25]

Radiological findings

It is important to be familiar with the interpretation and analysis of triplanar imaging when managing patients with complications of rhinosinusitis as it aids the planning of surgical intervention. We would recommend, where possible, jointly reviewing the imaging with an experienced radiologist. Below are some of the common signs to look out for each stage of the Chandler classification.

1. **Preseptal cellulitis** – eyelid swelling and thickening of the preseptal tissues with possible posterolateral extension to the temporal fossa. Importantly, CT will not distinguish between oedema, preseptal cellulitis and allergy.
2. **Postseptal cellulitis** – the findings as above often with induration of the extraconal, intraconal and retrobulbar fat without abscess.
3. **Subperiosteal abscess** – CT scans show a typical lenticular rim-enhancing collection adjacent to the lamina papyracea with a fat plane between it and the displaced medial rectus muscle (**Figure 101.4**). Lateral deviation and proptosis of the globe may be visible on

TABLE 101.3 Risk factors for simultaneous orbital and intra-cranial complications[23]
Risk factors for intracranial infection in children admitted for orbital complications of acute rhinosinusitis[23]
Male
Age 7 years and older
Failure to improve after appropriate therapy
Changes in neurologic status
Frontal sinus opacification on CT
Superior or lateral position of orbital abscess
Need for surgical intervention to drain orbital abscess

axial images. Sightthreatening complications of optic neuritis or optic nerve ischemia may also be present without radiological signs. Subperiosteal abscess secondary to frontal sinusitis typically forms an abscess superiorly with anteroinferior globe displacement.[16]

4. **Orbital abscess** – Scans may show multiple rim-enhancing orbital abscesses with surrounding cellulitis and a resultant proptosis.
5. **Cavernous sinus thrombosis** – It is important to note that in the early stages CT scans appear normal. CT and MR venography are complementary in the diagnosis of cavernous sinus thrombosis.[27] There may also be thickening and increased signal intensity in the extraocular muscles in T2-weighted MRI.[28]

Haematological investigations

The place of haematological investigations is three-fold:

1. to help identify any serious underlying disease process such as a haematological malignancy;
2. aid in assessment of fitness for surgery;
3. monitor the patient's response to treatment.

Other investigations

- Blood cultures
- Sinonasal/abscess pus culture ideally from initial nasal endoscopy

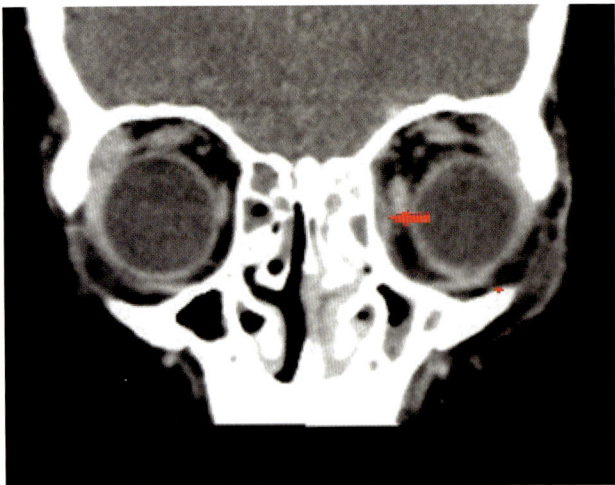

Figure 101.4 Coronal CT scan showing left maxillary and ethmoid sinusitis with associated medial orbital subperiosteal abscess (red arrow) and displacement of the globe.

- Urinalysis for diabetes mellitus, potentially causing immunocompromised
- Clinical observations. The simple regular monitoring of temperature should not be forgotten, any persisting infection may result in sustained or 'spiking' pyrexia requiring further clinical and radiological investigation.

TREATMENT

Medical

Almost all patients with complications of rhinosinusitis require admission for observation and treatment. Unless an abscess is demonstrated by radiological or other investigation, non-surgical management of rhinosinusitis complications is normally first choice. The exception is when vision is affected by pressure on the optic nerve from surrounding inflammation without abscess formation.

The aim of medical management is to control and eliminate both the disease process of the complication and of the primary rhinosinusitis. Antibiotics form the mainstay of medical treatment, but expert opinion suggests decongestant medications such as xylometazoline aids the resolution of acute rhinosinusitis by reducing mucosal oedema, although the evidence is inconclusive.[26] Selection of antibiotics is typically made on clinical grounds prior to identification of any organism or before culture-specific sensitivities are known. Broad-spectrum antibiotics are advised for severe complications of sinusitis to cover the likely organisms including *S. pneumonia*, *S. anginosus* and other *Streptococcus* species, *H. influenzae*, *S. aureus*, *Moraxella catarrhalis* and anaerobic bacteria (*Prevotella*, *Porphyromonas*, *Fusobacterium* and *Peptostreptococcus* species).[19, 29–31]

Polymicrobial and anaerobic isolates are more common in patients older than 15 years of age and in patients with intracranial complications.[29, 32] *Streptococcus anginosus* species represent some of the most frequently cultured organisms from either orbital or intracranial complications and have a tendency towards abscess formation.[33, 34] Complications, especially intracranial, are often one-off events due to highly pathogenic organisms. There will be marked local variation in causative organisms and sensitivities, therefore liaison with microbiology colleagues is recommended. An initial regime of intravenous cephalosporin with metronidazole would be an appropriate first choice until case-specific cultures and sensitivities are known. In patients with antibiotic sensitivities, other appropriate antibiotics should be selected in accordance with local microbiology policies.

The evidence base for systemic corticosteroid use is lacking in complications of rhinosinusitis. The risk of direct pressure from inflammation may possibly be reduced though this needs to be balanced against the immunosuppressive action and side effects of the steroids. In general, the use of systemic steroids is not recommended unless there is evidence of pituitary insufficiency in cavernous sinus thrombosis.

In the absence of abscess formation or reduction in visual signs medical management should initially be implemented for the first 24 hours, with frequent monitoring as described previously (**Figure 101.5**). If there is no significant clinical improvement in the first 24 hours of medical treatment, surgical intervention should be considered. Also, if at any point there is any clinical deterioration, urgent repeat imaging with a view to emergency surgical intervention is likely to be required. For orbital complications, intravenous antibiotic administration should continue until clinical improvement is well established and only then should oral medications be substituted. Evidence for how long oral antibiotics should be continued is limited, though 14 days of culture directed antibiotics is often appropriate. In the early stages of cerebritis, appropriate antibiotic administration can prevent intracerebral abscess formation.[35] Once a brain abscess has formed, surgical drainage combined with a prolonged antibiotic course of 4–8 weeks is recommended.[29]

CAVERNOUS SINUS THROMBOSIS

Prolonged broad-spectrum antibiotics must be given for at least 2 weeks beyond clinical resolution as bacteria sequestered within the thrombus may not be killed until the dural sinuses have started to recanalize.[14] Relapse and recurrence of meningeal and ocular signs have been reported up to 6 weeks after recovery and cessation of antibiotics[14] and follow-up for at least 6 months is advised.[26] Surgery is indicated only to drain any non-draining sinus infection or abscess collection.[14] There remains no consensus for the use of anticoagulation; proponents suggest that anticoagulants prevent thrombus propagation and have anti-inflammatory properties.[36, 37] Those against hypothesize that thrombus formation walls off infection and prevents its spread, with anticoagulants increasing the risk of intracranial bleeding in an already inflammatory environment. If anticoagulation is to be used rapidly reversible agents such as unfractionated heparin infusion should initially be used[14] aiming for an activated partial thromboplastin time (APTT) between 1.5–2,[38] switching to low-molecular weight heparins once the condition has improved.

Surgical

The surgical treatment of patients with complications of rhinosinusitis can be divided into procedures necessary to manage the complication and surgery for the rhinosinusitis. Often these are performed at the same time and may involve joint working with neurosurgeons in the case of intracranial suppuration.

The surgery required for acute complications of rhinosinusitis is often similar to that used for managing chronic rhinosinusitis. The principles of draining any pus and establishing ventilation of the sinuses remain. Where complications have arisen from acute rhinosinusitis it is likely that the operative field will be inflamed and very haemorrhagic, potentially making endoscopic surgery much more difficult than in the presence of chronic rhinosinusitis alone.

Knowledge of the likely sinus origin of the orbital complication is important in planning any surgical treatment. In ethmoid sinusitis orbital abscesses are typically medial to the globe, and in frontal sinusitis abscesses often form more superiorly within the orbit. A relatively large study of 240 patients identified patients with proptosis but normal eye movements and visual acuity are likely to require surgery, whereas infections with cellulitis alone are likely to settle with medical management.[18] Adolescent patients also appear more likely to develop complications requiring surgical intervention.[32]

The debate about the best approach to drain orbital collections remains a current controversy. Advocates of endoscopic surgery suggest that endoscopic ethmoidectomy with removal of the lamina papyracea and pernasal drainage of the orbital abscess is appropriate. The advantages of an endoscopic approach include avoiding facial scarring, ventilating the sinuses endonasally by operating on the osteomeatal complex, less post-operative orbital oedema, a shorter hospital stay and the absence of possible wound complications such as stitch abscesses.[39] More traditional external orbitotomy also has its proponents, and unless the surgeon is very familiar with endoscopic sinus surgery, it is more appropriate to use an external approach. If performing endonasal drainage the surgeon must be prepared to convert to external drainage if required and it is advised that patients and relatives are appropriately consented prospectively for both approaches. The external approach is also advised for abscesses that are not situated medially within the orbit adjacent to the lamina papyracea. The external approach uses a conventional Lynch–Howarth approach for an external ethmoidectomy, allowing an assistant to help keep the operative field clear whilst the subperiosteal abscess is drained. Occasionally, the orbital abscess will lie away from the lamina papyracea, especially if associated with frontal rhinosinusitis. As the abscess may lie in the roof of the orbit or further laterally, it is essential to obtain a CT scan preoperatively to define the position of any orbital collection and plan surgical treatment. Drainage of the abscess can be maintained with surgical drains either into the nasal cavity fixing to the septum or externally through the medial canthal incision. The evidence for performing concurrent surgical ethmoidectomy at the same time as draining the abscess is limited, as opposed to relying on medical treatment to deal with the rhinosinusitis and only draining the

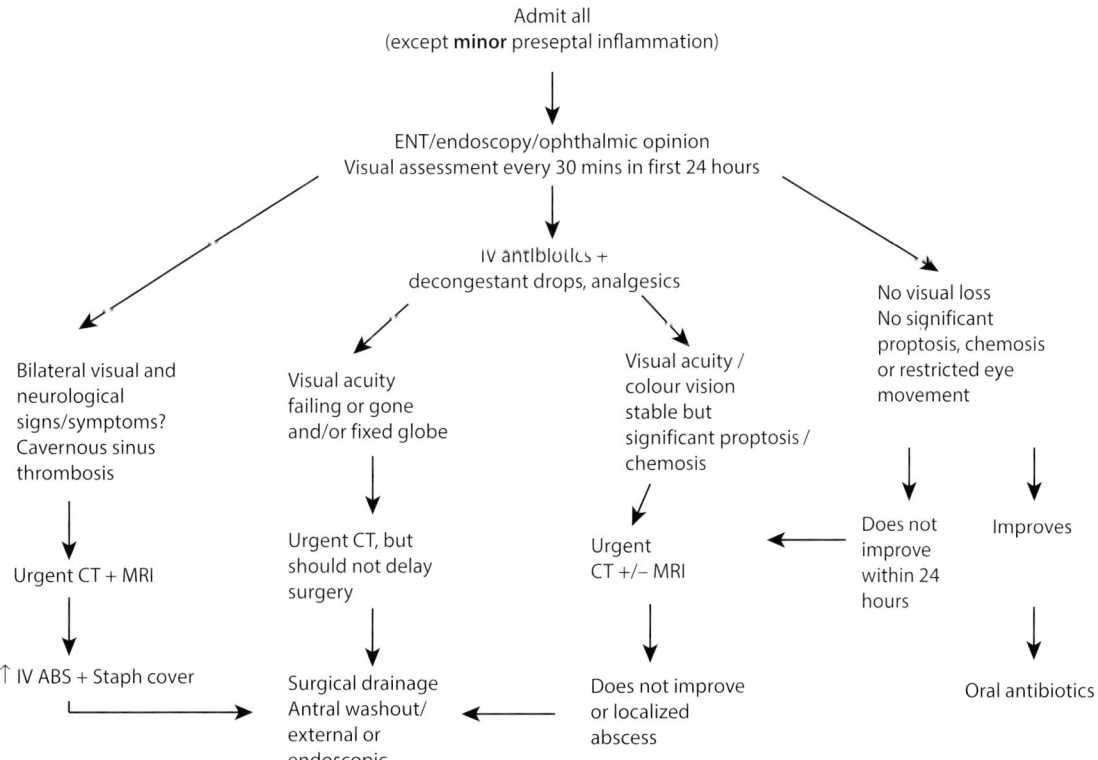

Figure 101.5 Management algorithm for orbital complications.

orbital collection surgically. However, the authors would advocate undertaking a maxillary washout or antrostomy and limited ethmoidectomy to allow all areas of pus to be drained. There are some early reports regarding possible medical management of carefully selected patients with small medial subperiosteal abscesses,[40] though at present we would advocate draining any orbital collection surgically with concurrent medical management.

Prognosis of orbital complications

If prompt treatment is carried out with adequate monitoring of patients, the prognosis for the return of normal vision is excellent. However, there is a small but significant risk of diplopia following surgery.[41] Provided the patient's presentation is not delayed and there is effective teamworking with ophthalmologists, paediatricians where appropriate, and otorhinolaryngologists ensuring prompt surgical intervention if non-surgical management fails, full recovery of eye function should occur.

INTRACRANIAL COMPLICATIONS

Brain abscess

Brain abscess can occur as a complication of either local or distant spread. The frontal sinuses are the most common source followed by the ethmoid, sphenoid and maxillary sinuses.[23] Haematogenous spread is the most likely mechanism of distant spread. It is estimated that 40–60% of brain abscesses arise from paranasal sinus infections.[42] The total reported incidence of intracranial complications from acute rhinosinusitis is between 3% and 17% of hospitalized sinusitis patients.[42, 43]

Subdural empyema

Subdural empyema is one of the commonest intracranial complications of rhinosinusitis, typically from haematogenous spread.[5] The brain is clearly more exposed as the infection is beyond the protective dura mater and allows the possibility of thrombosis of the dense network of veins in this space. Serious neurological injury can occur if not treated rapidly and aggressively with combined medical treatment and neurosurgical drainage to decompress the brain and evacuate the empyema. Subdural empyemas present with meningeal irritation and neurological signs such as seizures or focal deficits.

Extradural empyema

Extradural empyemas tend to be less symptomatic as the brain is protected by the dura mater. The signs are less marked and specific and are often only present when the collection reaches a size to cause mass effect.

Brain infarction

Cerebral ischaemia and infarction are rare vascular complications of sinusitis from either dural venous thrombosis secondary to adjacent empyema, or cavernous carotid artery occlusion.[28]

CLINICAL PRESENTATION

Early symptoms are often non-specific such as headache, fever, seizure, drowsiness, diplopia (VIth cranial nerve palsy) eye pain and nausea.[5] There may not be a preceding history of acute rhinosinusitis and clinical examination will not always identify suppuration from the paranasal sinuses. Adolescent and young adult males are more commonly affected which may be due to the vascularity of the diploeic system in this age group.[23] Frontal lobe abscesses are the most common intracranial abscess location. There may be specific neurological symptoms if there is a well-defined intracranial abscess including acute pain and possible loss of consciousness associated with meningitis. Some authors advocate scanning all patients with acute frontal rhinosinusitis or orbital cellulitis to exclude such serious complications, which may initially be clinically 'silent'.[13, 42]

INVESTIGATIONS

MRI scanning has been shown to be superior to CT in the diagnosis of intracranial complications and is the investigation of choice for the diagnosis of suspected intracranial extension.[24] The example in **Figure 101.6** demonstrates the presence of a small subdural frontal abscess apparent on MR imaging but not visualized by a contrast enhanced CT scan.

As soon as an intracranial complication is detected, joint management of the case with neurological or neurosurgical colleagues is mandatory. If possible, surgery to drain affected paranasal sinuses should be undertaken synchronously with any neurosurgical operative intervention. If synchronous paranasal sinus surgery is to be undertaken, CT scanning is desirable to demonstrate the bony anatomy of the paranasal sinuses, provided any delay incurred in scanning is compatible with the patient's clinical condition. Intracranial complications may be relatively silent and a high index of suspicion should be maintained (**Figure 101.7**). Intracranial complications may also develop after the initial presentation and any change in neurological status should merit consideration for repeat imaging.

TREATMENT

For medical treatment see earlier in the chapter. The surgical treatment of intracranial complications will inevitably involve neurosurgical expertise. As far as the otorhinolaryngologist is concerned, discussion needs to take place as to whether the sinus surgery will be done at the same time as any neurosurgical procedure. There is unfortunately little evidence to help decide whether these should be done as separate procedures but, as with orbital cellulitis, it is the authors' practice to undertake the surgery for the complication at the same time as for the underlying rhinosinusitis. Intracranial complications are most likely to arise

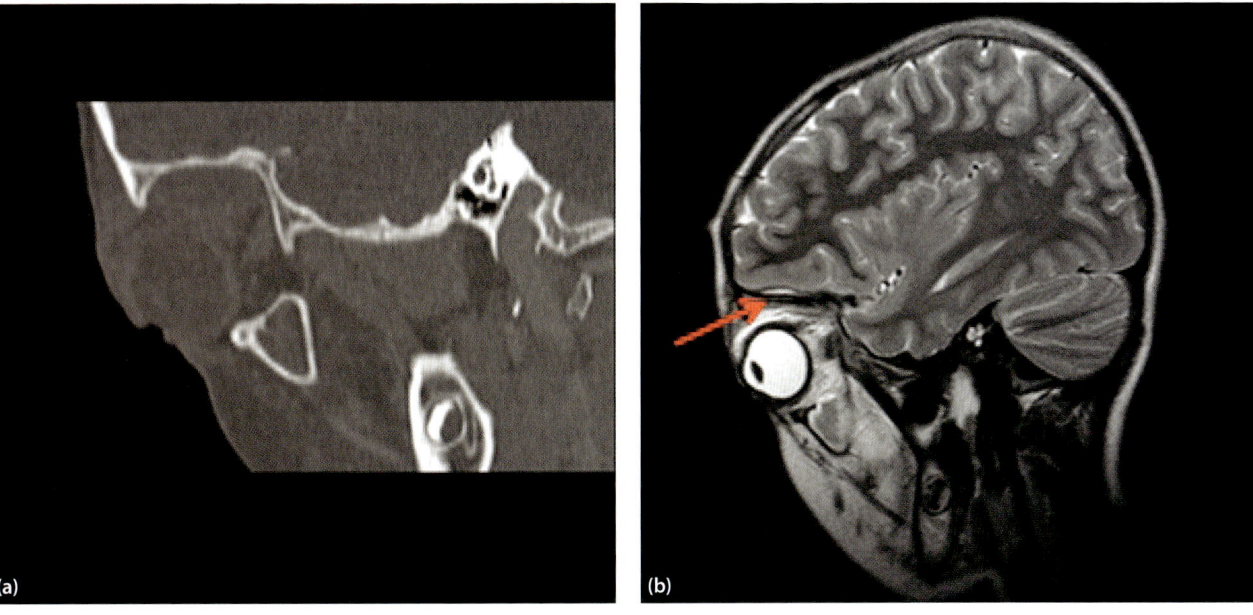

Figure 101.6 Contrast enhanced sagittal CT scan of a child with acute sinusitis and headache. (a) No intracranial pathology was identified to account for the symptoms. An MRI scan of the same child (b) highlighted a small subdural frontal abscess (arrow illustrates pathology).

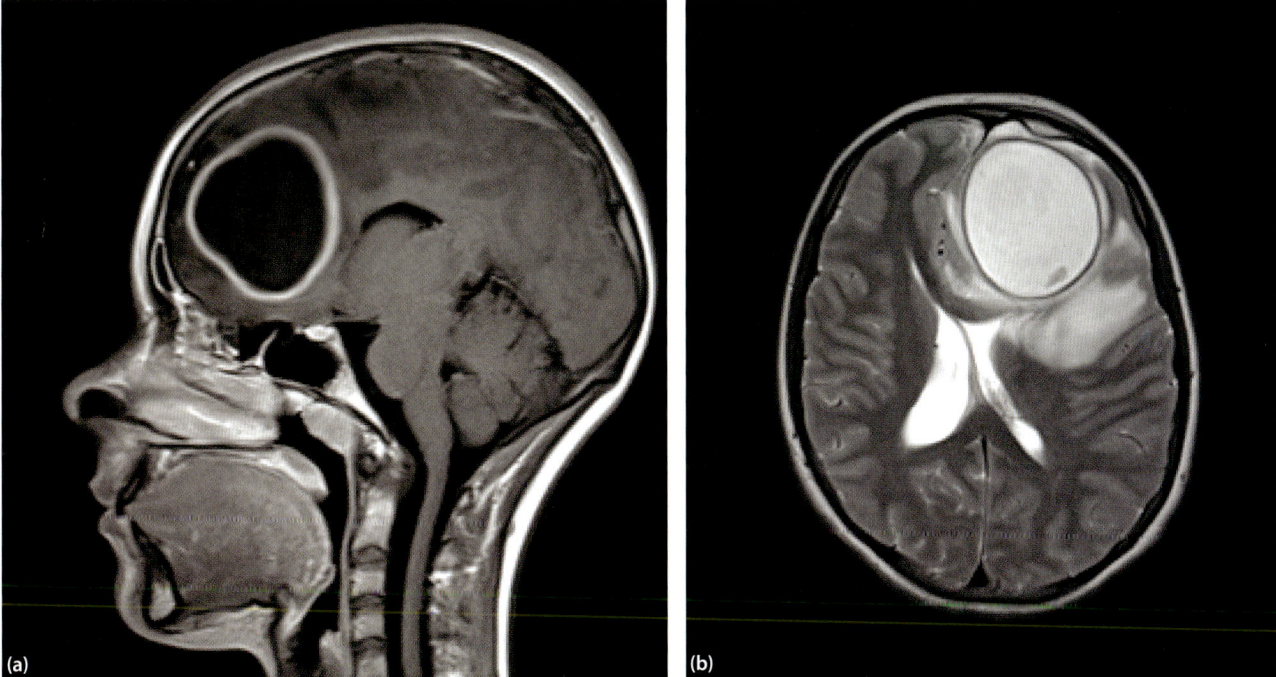

Figure 101.7 MRI images of a large frontal intracerebral abscess secondary to rhinosinusitis.

from frontal rhinosinusitis as opposed to the remaining paranasal sinuses, and endoscopic frontal surgery is likely to be challenging and potentially dangerous. In the acute setting, it is better to undertake a temporary frontal drainage procedure concomitantly with surgery for the intracranial condition. A frontal sinus trephine procedure with placement of an external drain is most commonly used, although endoscopic balloon sinuplasty has been used to drain acute frontal sinus collections pernasally[44] and may become more popular in future. Any definitive frontal sinus surgical procedure can be deferred until the patient has fully recovered from treatment of the complication.[45]

Prognosis from intracranial complications

The increased availability of scanning has no doubt led to earlier diagnosis and better outcomes.[46] Published mortality rates vary between 0 and 25%[5, 30] Unsurprisingly, mortality varies according to the specific complication and increases with age and decreased level of consciousness on presentation.[31, 42] Persistent morbidity such as hemiparesis, epilepsy, altered cognitive function and cranial nerve palsies are reported in between 11% and 40% of cases.[5, 30, 43] Early recognition of complications and multidisciplinary treatment is essential for the best possible outcome.

BONY COMPLICATIONS

Pott's puffy tumour

In the 18th century Percival Pott described the case of a patient with a pericranial abscess related to trauma. The area, he noted, was 'swollen and puffy'. The term Pott's puffy tumour is now used to describe a subperiosteal cellulitis or abscess of the frontal bone associated with frontal oeteomyelitis and presenting with headache, swelling and, on occasion, a discharging frontal fistula (Figure 101.8). The infection can spread posteriorly giving rise to intracranial sepsis either by erosion of the posterior table or more likely by septic thrombophlebitis via the diploeic veins.[47] The reported rate of coexistent intracranial complications is high between 29% and 60%, though not all are present on initial imaging[47, 48] which suggests prompt cross-sectional imaging and treatment are paramount. Both Gallagher and Jones[48, 49] noted a preponderance of Streptococcus anginosus infection in series of such patients, where positive cultures were obtained.

Management requires drainage of pus from the frontal sinuses, achieved either endoscopically or conventionally through a frontal sinus trephination via an incision in the superomedial aspect of the orbit. In the absence of a subperiosteal or intracranial abscess, further surgery may not be necessary acutely. Prolonged antibiotic therapy, ideally culture-directed, for 6–8 weeks covering both aerobic and anaerobic organisms is recommended by the authors. Once the acute phase has subsided the patient should be re-evaluated to determine if a frontal sinus drainage procedure is required for long-term management. This can be undertaken endoscopically or externally through an osteoplastic frontal flap, or in combination (see Chapter 99 Frontal Sinus). However, as these infections rarely recur, in general, patients can be reassured this an unlikely occurrence.

A limited subperiosteal abscess may be drained through a Lynch Howarth brow incision. However, this does not allow adequate inspection of the frontal bone to assess for necrotic bone. An alternative is to perform a spectacle incision providing good exposure to the frontal sinus but resulting in a scar, which may not be acceptable cosmetically. A bicoronal scalp incision and flap provides excellent access to assess the whole frontal sinus enabling removal of diseased bone. This procedure is of such significant complexity that the inexperienced rhinologist should not undertake it.

Associated intracranial complications necessitate prompt neurosurgical intervention. This is typically performed through a bifrontal craniotomy enabling drainage of intracranial pus and removal of necrotic bone.[50] Complete removal of the posterior table will require frontal sinus cranialization. Extensive osteomyelitis of the anterior table may necessitate a Riedel's procedure[51] with removal of the anterior wall and floor of the frontal sinus allowing the forehead skin to collapse onto the posterior table. Whilst this causes a significant cosmetic

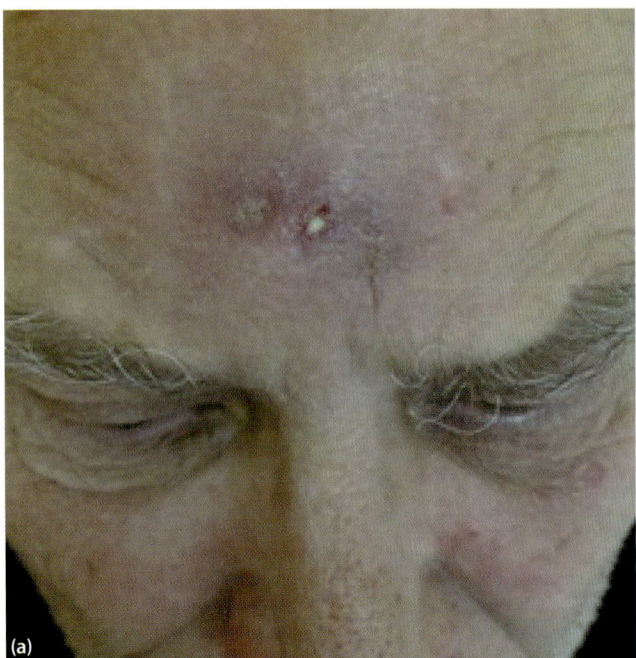 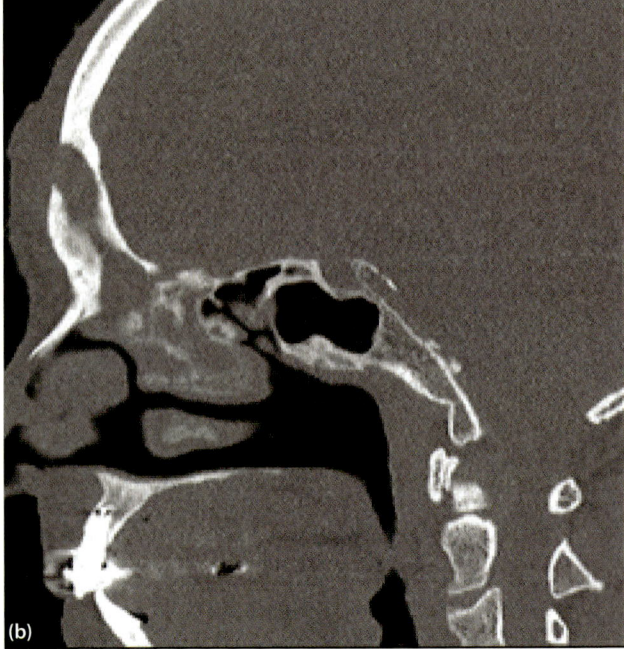

Figure 101.8 Clinical photograph (a) & sagittal CT scan (b) through the frontal sinus showing Pott's puffy tumour; a discharging fronto-cutaneous fistula from the subperiosteal collection, frontal sinusitis with osteomyelitis and bone erosion of the anterior frontal sinus wall.

deformity, reconstruction with split calvarial bone or alloplastic materials can be undertaken at a later stage when all infection has resolved.[52]

CHRONIC COMPLICATIONS

Chronic complications of rhinosinusitis usually result from chronic rhinosinusitis. As with acute complications, the nature of the complication depends on the particular sinus or group of sinuses involved. Mucoceles are chronic, slowly expanding lesions in any of the sinuses that may result in bony erosion and can extend beyond the sinus (see Chapter 100, Mucoceles). It is unusual for chronic rhinosinusitis to cause orbital cellulitis or intracranial complications unless there is an infective exacerbation.

ACKNOWLEDGEMENTS

We would like to acknowledge the previous work of Mr Robert Slack and Mr Richard Sim. This is an updated and revised chapter based initially on their work from the seventh edition. Additional acknowledgement must be made to Professor Nick Jones for his helpful advice and critical reading of the manuscript.

FUTURE RESEARCH

➤ There is continued controversy as to whether surgery for orbital abscess complications is best undertaken endoscopically or externally. The availability of local expertise often determines the preferred approach, though it may be possible for carefully designed clinical trials to provide more evidence.

➤ The numbers of patients presenting with complications of rhinosinusitis is relatively small, the symptoms can be varied and the time required to begin treatment is very short. This makes it very difficult to design studies that would result in level 1 or 2 evidence. Consequently the evidence presented here is mostly based on retrospective case series data.

➤ There is also little information to suggest why some individuals should develop complicated sinus disease when similar organisms are isolated from patients with uncomplicated disease. Bony sinus anomalies that narrow anatomically important areas such as the osteomeatal unit (OMU) which may predispose to sinusitis are seen with similar frequency in children, adults[49] and asymptomatic individuals making their significance unclear.[50] However, when specific measurements of OMU calibre are made, no significant difference between children and adults exists implicating additional mucosal immune mechanisms which require further investigation.[51]

BEST CLINICAL PRACTICE

✓ Careful, repeated clinical observations with a low threshold for repeat imaging if there is deterioration in clinical condition.
✓ Radiological investigations of choice are CT with MRI for suspected intracranial pathology.
✓ Broad-spectrum antibiotics with streptococcal and anaerobic cover form the mainstay of medical treatment.
✓ Surgical treatment is normally required for resolution in patients with abscess formation.
✓ Cultured *Staphylococcus aureus* should not be dismissed as a contaminant.
✓ A multidisciplinary approach is essential to ensure optimal outcome.

KEY POINTS

• The major complications of rhinosinusitis are orbital and intracranial infections, of which orbital complications are the more common.
• The incidence of complications is greatest in children and young adults.
• The speed of initiating treatment and confirming the diagnosis can greatly reduce the morbidity and extent of intervention required.
• Multidisciplinary care involving ENT surgeons with ophthalmology, paediatric and neurology/neurosurgical input as required is a standard of care

REFERENCES

1. Hansen FS, et al. Complications of acute rhinosinusitis in The Netherlands. *Fam Pract* 2012; **29**(2): 147–53.
2. Gwaltney JM, Jr, Sydnor A, Jr, Sande MA. Etiology and antimicrobial treatment of acute sinusitis. *Ann Otol Rhinol Laryngol Suppl*, 1981; **90**(3 Pt 3): 68–71.
3. Wald ER. Sinusitis in children. *N Engl J Med* 1992; **326**(5): 319–23.
4. Ryan JT, et al. Management of pediatric orbital cellulitis in patients with radiographic findings of subperiosteal abscess. *Otolaryngol Head Neck Surg* 2009; **140**(6): 907–11.
5. Jones NS, et al. The intracranial complications of rhinosinusitis: can they be prevented? *Laryngoscope* 2002; **112**(1): 59–63.
6. Arjmand EM, Lusk RP, Muntz HR. Pediatric sinusitis and subperiosteal orbital abscess formation: diagnosis and treatment. *Otolaryngol Head Neck Surg* 1993; **109**(5): 886–94.

7. Som PMC, Curtin HD. *Head and neck imaging*. St. Louis: Mosby; 2011.
8. Gupta M, et al. Pott's puffy tumour in a pre-adolescent child: the youngest reported in the post-antibiotic era. *Int J Pediatr Otorhinolaryngol* 2004; **68**(3): 373–8.
9. Pott P. *The chirurgical works of Percival Pott F.R.S.* Vol. 1. 1808, London, UK: Woods and Innes.
10. Chandler JR, Langenbrunner DJ, Stevens ER, The pathogenesis of orbital complications in acute sinusitis. *Laryngoscope* 1970. **80**(9): 1414–28.
11. Lusk RP. *Pediatric sinusitis*. New York: Raven Press; 1992.
12. Lusk RP, McAlister B, el Fouley A, Anatomic variation in pediatric chronic sinusitis: a CT study. *Otolaryngol Clin North Am* 1996; **29**(1): 75–91.
13. Lew D, et al. Sphenoid sinusitis: a review of 30 cases. *N Engl J Med* 1983; **309**(19): 1149–54.
14. Bhatia K, Jones NS. Septic cavernous sinus thrombosis secondary to sinusitis: are anticoagulants indicated? A review of the literature. *J Laryngol Otol* 2002; **116**(9): 667–76.
15. Zeifer B. Pediatric sinonasal imaging: normal anatomy and inflammatory disease. *Neuroimaging Clin N Am* 2000; **10**(1): 137–59, ix.
16. Pond F, Berkowitz RG. Superolateral subperiosteal orbital abscess complicating sinusitis in a child. *Int J Pediatr Otorhinolaryngol* 1999; **48**(3): 255–8.
17. Hawkins DB, Clark RW. Orbital involvement in acute sinusitis: lessons from 24 childhood patients. *Clin Pediatr (Phila)* 1977; **16**(5): 464–71.
18. Singh B. The management of sinogenic orbital complications. *J Laryngol Otol* 1995; **109**(4): 300–3.
19. Moloney JR, Badham NJ, McRae A. The acute orbit: preseptal (periorbital) cellulitis, subperiosteal abscess and orbital cellulitis due to sinusitis. *J Laryngol Otol Suppl*, 1987; **12**: 1–18.
20. Southwick FS, Richardson EP Jr, Swartz MN. Septic thrombosis of the dural venous sinuses. *Medicine (Baltimore)* 1986; **65**(2): 82–106.
21. Assefa D, et al. Septic cavernous sinus thrombosis following infection of ethmoidal and maxillary sinuses: a case report. *Int J Pediatr Otorhinolaryngol* 1994; **29**(3): 249–55.
22. Hayreh SS, Kolder HE, Weingeist TA. Central retinal artery occlusion and retinal tolerance time. *Ophthalmology* 1980; **87**(1): 75–8.
23. Herrmann BW, Forsen JW Jr. Simultaneous intracranial and orbital complications of acute rhinosinusitis in children. *Int J Pediatr Otorhinolaryngol* 2004; **68**(5): 619–25.
24. Younis RT, Anand VK, Davidson B. The role of computed tomography and magnetic resonance imaging in patients with sinusitis with complications. *Laryngoscope* 2002; **112**(2): 224–9.
25. Varonen H, et al. Acute rhinosinusitis in primary care: a comparison of symptoms, signs, ultrasound, and radiography. *Rhinology* 2003; **41**(1): 37–43.
26. Fokkens WJ, et al. EPOS 2012: European position paper on rhinosinusitis and nasal polyps 2012: a summary for otorhinolaryngologists. *Rhinology* 2012; **50**(1): 1–12.
27. Pinto J, Chaaban M. *Cavernous sinus thrombosis*. British Medical Journal Best Practice, 2013. http://bestpractice.bmj.com/best-practice/monograph/956.html
28. Reid JR. Complications of pediatric paranasal sinusitis. *Pediatr Radiol* 2004; **34**(12): 933–42.
29. Brook I. Microbiology and antimicrobial treatment of orbital and intracranial complications of sinusitis in children and their management. *Int J Pediatr Otorhinolaryngol* 2009; **73**(9): 1183–6.
30. Rosenfeld EA, Rowley AH. Infectious intracranial complications of sinusitis, other than meningitis, in children: 12-year review. *Clin Infect Dis* 1994; **18**(5): 750–4.
31. Singh B, et al. Sinogenic intracranial complications. *J Laryngol Otol* 1995; **109**(10): 945–50.
32. Harris GJ. Subperiosteal abscess of the orbit: age as a factor in the bacteriology and response to treatment. *Ophthalmology* 1994; **101**(3): 585–95.
33. Deutschmann MW, et al. The significance of Streptococcus anginosus group in intracranial complications of pediatric rhinosinusitis. *JAMA Otolaryngol Head Neck Surg* 2013; **139**(2): 157–60.
34. Oxford LE, McClay J. Complications of acute sinusitis in children. *Otolaryngol Head Neck Surg* 2005; **133**(1): 32–7.
35. Boom WH, Tuazon CU. Successful treatment of multiple brain abscesses with antibiotics alone. *Rev Infect Dis* 1985; **7**(2): 189–99.
36. Chaves CJ, Caplan LR. Heparin and oral anticoagulants in the treatment of brain ischemia. *J Neurol Sci* 2000; **173**(1): 3–9.
37. Connor SJ, Grimm MC. Heparin as an anti-inflammatory agent: it's no GAG to forget about chemokines. *Gut* 2001; **48**(5): 738.
38. Levine SR, Twyman RE, Gilman S. The role of anticoagulation in cavernous sinus thrombosis. *Neurology* 1988; **38**(4): 517–22.
39. Migirov L, et al. Endoscopic sinus surgery for medial orbital subperiosteal abscess in children. *J Otolaryngol Head Neck Surg* 2009; **38**(4): 504–8.
40. Coenraad S, Buwalda J. Surgical or medical management of subperiosteal orbital abscess in children: a critical appraisal of the literature. *Rhinology* 2009; **47**(1): 18–23.
41. Swift AC, Charlton G. Sinusitis and the acute orbit in children. *J Laryngol Otol* 1990; **104**(3): 213–16.
42. Johnson DL, et al. Treatment of intracranial abscesses associated with sinusitis in children and adolescents. *J Pediatr* 1988; **113**(1 Pt 1): 15-23.
43. Clayman GL, et al. Intracranial complications of paranasal sinusitis: a combined institutional review. *Laryngoscope* 1991; **101**(3): 234–9.
44. Hopkins C, Noon E, Roberts D. Balloon sinuplasty in acute frontal sinusitis. *Rhinology* 2009; **47**(4): 375–8.
45. Lang EE, et al. Intracranial complications of acute frontal sinusitis. *Clin Otolaryngol Allied Sci* 2001; **26**(6): 452–7.
46. Rosenblum ML, et al. Decreased mortality from brain abscesses since advent of computerized tomography. *J Neurosurg* 1978; **49**(5): 658–68.
47. Jung J, et al. Endoscopic endonasal treatment of a Pott's puffy tumor. *Clin Exp Otorhinolaryngol* 2012; **5**(2): 112–15.
48. Akiyama K, Karaki M, Mori N. Evaluation of adult Pott's puffy tumor: our five cases and 27 literature cases. *Laryngoscope* 2012; **122**(11): 2382–4.
49. April MM, et al. Coronal CT scan abnormalities in children with chronic sinusitis. *Laryngoscope* 1993; **103**(9): 985–90.
50. Coley BD. *Caffey's Pediatric diagnostic imaging*. 12th ed. Philadelphia: Mosby; 2014.
51. Thorp MA, et al. Complicated acute sinusitis and the computed tomography anatomy of the ostiomeatal unit in childhood. *Int J Pediatr Otorhinolaryngol* 1999; **49**(3): 189–95.

CHAPTER 102

THE RELATIONSHIP BETWEEN THE UPPER AND LOWER RESPIRATORY TRACT

Nigel K.F. Koo Ng and Gerald W. McGarry

Introduction 1125	Possible mechanisms of interaction between the upper and lower respiratory tract 1128
Epidemiological relationship between rhinitis and asthma 1125	Management implications 1128
Rhinitis and non-specific bronchial hyperresponsiveness 1126	Quality of life and costs in asthma and rhinitis 1130
Causative agents in rhinitis and asthma 1126	Summary 1130
Rhinitis as a risk factor for asthma 1126	Acknowledgments 1131
Inflammation of the upper and lower respiratory tract in rhinitis, asthma and chronic obstructive pulmonary disease 1127	References 1132

SEARCH STRATEGY

Data in this chapter may be updated by a Medline search using the keywords: rhinitis, allergic rhinitis, sinusitis, nasal polyps, asthma, occupational, chronic obstructive pulmonary disease, hypersensitivity, allergens, bronchial hyperreactivity, nasal mucosa, bronchi, biopsy, nasal provocation tests, bronchial challenge tests, airway remodelling, quality of life, disease management, anti-allergic agents, anti-asthmatic agents, steroids, leukotriene antagonists, anti-IgE antibodies (omalizumab), immunotherapy and nasal surgery.

INTRODUCTION

The close relationship between the upper respiratory tract (nose and paranasal sinuses) and the lower respiratory tract (tracheobronchial tree) is something that is manifestly observed by all practising rhinologists. Whilst it can be observed in a number of rare conditions such as granulomatosis with polyangiitis, this close relationship is most striking in the conditions of asthma, rhinitis and nasal polyposis (**Table 102.1**). The relationship between the upper and lower respiratory tract is so evident in rhinitis and asthma that these conditions may be viewed as ends or parts of a respiratory inflammatory spectrum. Most patients with asthma also have rhinitis[1] and treatment of coexisting rhinitis may improve asthma. The concept of 'one airway, one disease' and the 'unified airway' in which the upper and lower airways act as a whole unit has been proposed, with rhinitis and asthma representing manifestations of the same inflammatory process.[2,3] However, there are also differences between rhinitis and asthma and not all patients with rhinitis have asthma.[4]

EPIDEMIOLOGICAL RELATIONSHIP BETWEEN RHINITIS AND ASTHMA

There is strong epidemiological evidence both from cross-sectional and longitudinal studies that rhinitis and asthma are related. The two conditions often coexist in the same patients, with rhinitis occurring in over 65% of allergic asthma patients and in over 80% of patients with non-allergic asthma.[1] In the Copenhagen Allergy Study,[5] between 40–50% of allergic rhinitis patients had allergic asthma and the risk of allergic asthma was up to 300 times higher in allergic rhinitis patients than those without allergic rhinitis.

It is not only allergic rhinitis however that is associated with asthma; there is also an association between non-allergic rhinitis and asthma. Rhinitis has been shown to be an independent significant risk factor for asthma in both atopic and non-atopic individuals.[6] There is also an association between asthma and chronic rhinosinusitis, irrespective of smoking behaviour.[7] Sixty percent of chronic rhinosinusitis patients have associated lower airway disease (24% asthma, 36% small airway disease).[8]

TABLE 102.1 Examples of disease which affect the upper and lower airways

Asthma
Rhinitis
Chronic rhinosinusitis
Sarcoid
Granulomatosis with polyangiitis
Cystic fibrosis
Ciliary dyskinesias

RHINITIS AND NON-SPECIFIC BRONCHIAL HYPERRESPONSIVENESS

Many patients with allergic rhinitis who do not have asthma symptoms demonstrate bronchial hyperresponsiveness, a key feature of asthma.[9] They showed increased bronchial sensitivity to stimuli such as methacholine (a parasympathomimetic agent) or histamine. In those with seasonal rhinitis and allergy to pollen, the degree and prevalence of bronchial hyperresponsiveness is significantly greater during the pollen season compared to outside this period.[10] Those with perennial rhinitis have a higher risk of bronchial hyperresponsiveness compared to those with seasonal rhinitis.[11, 12]

Patients with allergic rhinitis and bronchial hyperresponsiveness are at greater risk of developing asthma than those with normal bronchial challenges.[13] However, not all patients with allergic rhinitis have increased bronchial hyperresponsiveness and there are large differences in the extent of airway responsiveness exhibited in asthma and rhinitis.

CAUSATIVE AGENTS IN RHINITIS AND ASTHMA

Asthma and rhinitis share many common risk factors. Some of the agents inducing asthma and rhinitis such as allergens and aspirin[14] are well known to affect both the upper and the lower airways. This is compatible with the concept of a 'unified airway', although many studies have shown some differences in the genetic and environmental risk of these two conditions suggesting that there is an element of specificity for each condition.[15]

Bacterial enterotoxins, by acting as a superantigen, may play a role in the development and/or severity of asthma and allergic rhinitis.[16] In a mouse model of allergic asthma, application of *Staphylococcus aureus* enterotoxin B to the nose or to the bronchus each resulted in a more severe bronchial eosinophilic inflammation.[17] It has also been shown that there is increased *Staphylococcus aureus* colonization in the nose and specific IgE antibodies against *Staphylococcus aureus* enterotoxins in patients with nasal polyps.[18]

Upper respiratory tract viral infections, often caused by rhinovirus, are strongly associated with asthma exacerbations in children and adults[19, 20] Experimental induction of upper respiratory tract rhinovirus infection in allergic rhinitis patients has been shown to increase airway hyperreactivity and late asthmatic reactions after allergen challenge.[21] However, rhinovirus also has the ability to infect the lower respiratory tract and induce a pro-inflammatory response, suggesting that rhinovirus-mediated asthma exacerbations may result from a direct lower respiratory tract reaction.[22]

The most common precipitants of occupational asthma can all induce occupational rhinitis. Although rhinitis and asthma are closely related, the relationship in occupational disease is less well known. Occupational rhinitis, however, is often associated with occupational asthma, and this association is significantly greater with high molecular weight agents compared to low molecular weight agents.[22] As patients with occupational rhinitis can often go on to develop occupational asthma, cessation of allergen exposure in occupational allergic rhinitis is important to try to prevent asthma.

RHINITIS AS A RISK FACTOR FOR ASTHMA

There are many studies which support rhinitis as a risk factor for asthma both in children and adults.[6, 23-26] Physician-diagnosed allergic rhinitis in infancy has been shown to be independently associated with doubling the risk of asthma by 11 years old.[27] In another study, allergic rhinitis in childhood was found to be significantly associated with a two- to seven-fold increased risk of asthma in pre-adolescence, adolescence, or adult life.[28] Furthermore, the risk of childhood asthma persisting to middle age was three times higher in children with allergic rhinitis compared to those never having allergic rhinitis.[28]

In adults, a study of college students found that the risk of developing asthma over a 23-year period was significantly higher in those diagnosed with allergic rhinitis compared to those without (10.5% vs. 3.6%).[29] A 15-year prospective study of Finnish twins found that patients with 'allergic rhinitis including hay fever' were more likely to develop asthma by four times if male and six times if female compared to patients without allergic rhinitis.[30] Some have found the prevalence of asthma to be associated to the severity and duration of rhinitis with the highest prevalence in patients with moderate/severe persistent allergic rhinitis[31] whereas others report no correlation between the Allergic Rhinitis and its Impact on Asthma (ARIA) categories of rhinitis and the prevalence of asthma.[32]

Allergic rhinitis usually precedes asthma and the term 'The Allergic March' has been used to describe the progression of allergic nasal disease in the upper airway to the lower airway. It is not clear, however, whether allergic rhinitis causes asthma or whether allergic rhinitis is just an earlier clinical manifestation of allergic disease in atopic patients who would in any case develop asthma. Children with atopic eczema have significantly greater risk of developing asthma and allergic rhinitis than those with non-atopic eczema[33] and it has been suggested that the allergic march may begin even earlier with eczema[34] leading to rhinitis and then asthma.

The increased risk of asthma is not just limited to allergic rhinitis but is also found with non-allergic rhinitis.[15] It has been reported that rhinitis increased the risk of asthma in both atopic and non-atopic patients by about three times.[6] It appears that rhinitis and asthma are not just linked because they share atopy as a common risk factor.

INFLAMMATION OF THE UPPER AND LOWER RESPIRATORY TRACT IN RHINITIS, ASTHMA AND CHRONIC OBSTRUCTIVE PULMONARY DISEASE

Similarities and differences between nasal and bronchial inflammation in asthma and rhinitis

There are many anatomical and physiological similarities between the upper and lower airways. They are both lined by pseudostratified ciliated columnar epithelium on a continuous basement membrane (**Figures 102.1a** and **102.1b**). Throughout the submucosa there are mucous glands, blood vessels, structural cells (fibroblasts), some inflammatory cells (monocytic cells, lymphocytes and mast cells) and nerves. There are also significant differences however, between the upper and lower respiratory tracts. The nasal mucosa is highly vascular with an extensive subepithelial capillary and arterial system and venous cavernous sinusoids. Vascular dilatation can result in increased upper airway resistance and subsequent nasal obstruction. In contrast, bronchoconstriction is due to the contraction of airway smooth muscle which is present from the trachea to the bronchioles, rather than changes in the vasculature.

Inflammation is a key component in the pathogenesis of rhinitis and asthma and studies have shown a similar inflammatory infiltrate (eosinophils, mast cells, T-lymphocytes and cells of the monocytic lineage) involved in the inflammation of the nasal and bronchial mucosa. There also appears to be similar pro-inflammatory mediators (histamine, cysteinyl leukotriene), T-helper 2 (Th2) cytokines (interleukin IL-4, IL-5, IL-13 and granulocyte-macrophage colony-stimulating factor), chemokines (RANTES and eotaxin) and adhesion molecules in the inflammation of the upper and lower airways in rhinitis and asthma. Airway smooth muscle is important in the pathogenesis of asthma not only by causing bronchoconstriction but may also be involved by increased proliferation and the expression and secretion of a variety of proinflammatory mediators and cytokines.[35, 36] In patients with both rhinitis and asthma, the degree of inflammation in the upper and lower airways may be different. Greater eosinophilic inflammation has been found in the bronchi compared to the nose in untreated asthmatic patients with rhinitis.[37] Epithelial shedding and basement membrane thickening are key features of airway remodelling in asthma and have also been found in sinonasal specimens of patients with chronic rhinosinusitis.[38] The extent of epithelial shedding and reticular basement membrane thickening however are greater in the bronchi than in the nose in patients with both asthma and rhinitis.[37]

Nasal and sinus inflammation in asthma and chronic obstructive pulmonary disease

Eosinophilic infiltration of the nasal mucosa has been demonstrated in patients with asthma irrespective of the presence of nasal symptoms,[39] further supporting the hypothesis that asthma and rhinitis are clinical manifestations of the same disease. There is also a strong association between chronic rhinosinusitis and asthma, with a higher

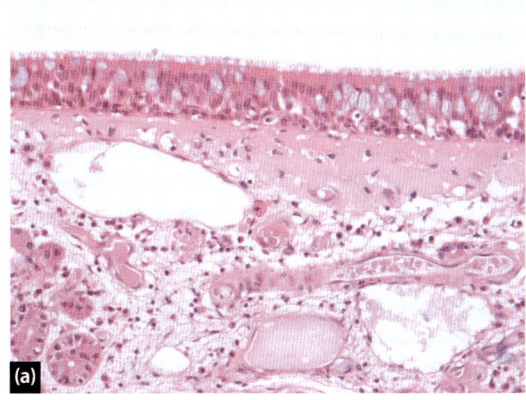 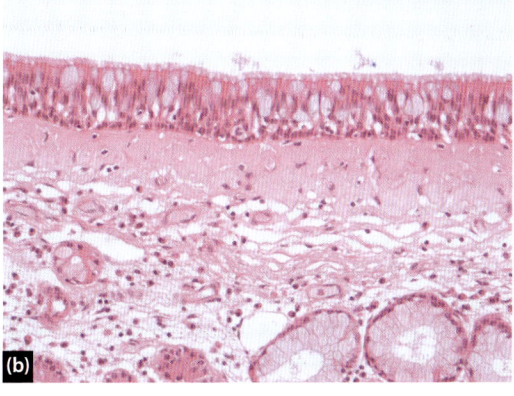

Figure 102.1 **(a)** Photomicrograph of nasal mucosa showing ciliated pseudostratified columnar epithelium on the surface with underlying basement membrane and lamina propria. The lamina propria contains prominent dilated, thin walled vascular channels some of which are filled by red cells or pink, flocculent protein rich material derived from plasma. A few mucosal glands are present towards the left. A light scattering of chronic inflammatory cells is seen in the mucosa. H&Ex200. **(b)** Photomicrograph of lower respiratory mucosa showing ciliated pseudostratified columnar epithelium on the surface with underlying basement membrane and lamina propria. The lamina propria contains a few mucosal glands towards the bottom of the image. No prominent vascular channels are present. A light scattering of chronic inflammatory cells is seen in the mucosa. H&Ex200.

rate of nasal polyps in asthmatic patients compared to non-asthmatics.[40] The triad of aspirin sensitivity, asthma and nasal polyps in aspirin-induced asthma is considered a separate clinical syndrome and found in about 10% to 15% of asthmatics.[41]

Patients with asthma often also have radiological evidence of sinusitis.[42, 43] The frequency of abnormal CT scans has been reported to be similar in patients with mild to moderate asthma (88%) compared to those with severe steroid dependent asthma (100%).[44] However, the extent of sinonasal involvement is greater in the latter, as based on clinical symptoms and CT.

The relationship between the upper and lower airways in patients with COPD has been much less extensively studied than in asthma. Some have found no significant difference in the prevalence of rhinitis in patients with COPD compared to those without[45] and an association between COPD and the upper respiratory tract has not been widely appreciated. There is, however, increasing evidence that upper airway disease may be related to COPD.[46] Some studies have reported increased upper airway symptoms and nasal inflammation in patients with COPD.[47-51] There is a need for further research in this area including the impact of treatment of the upper airway in patients with COPD.[52]

Bronchial inflammation and remodelling in rhinitis

In non-asthmatic patients with allergic rhinitis, there appears to be remodelling in the lower airways similar, although less marked, to that in asthma.[53] Studies of the bronchial mucosa in non-asthmatic allergic rhinitis patients and atopic non-asthmatics have shown an increase in the thickness of the basement membrane and in eosinophils, compared to normal individuals.[54, 55] Natural exposure to pollen in non-asthmatic patients with seasonal allergic rhinitis, results in increased lymphocytes, eosinophils and IL-5 expression in the bronchial mucosa.[56] Nasal allergen challenge in patients with seasonal allergic rhinitis shows increased sputum eosinophils and bronchial responsiveness to methacholine with inflammation of the bronchial and nasal mucosa.[57, 58]

Bronchial challenge of rhinitis patients leads to bronchial and nasal inflammation

In allergic non-asthmatic patients, endobronchial allergen challenge causes bronchial constriction and inflammation, with an increase in inflammatory cells recovered by bronchoalveolar lavage.[59] Endobronchial allergen challenge not only causes bronchial symptoms in non-asthmatic allergic rhinitis patients but also affects the nose, inducing nasal symptoms and inflammation resulting in reduced pulmonary and nasal function.[60] It has been shown that there is an increase in the number of eosinophils in the challenged bronchial mucosa and in the blood. In the nose, there is also an increase in eosinophils as well as eotaxin-positive cells in the nasal lamina propria with enhanced expression of IL-5, after bronchial challenge.[60]

POSSIBLE MECHANISMS OF INTERACTION BETWEEN THE UPPER AND LOWER RESPIRATORY TRACT

The nose plays a crucial role in warming, humidifying and filtering air before it enters the lower airways. Impairment in nasal function can therefore impact on the lower airways. Nasal obstruction can lead to increased oral breathing, reduced filtered air and increased exposure of the lower airways to allergens. Bypassing the nose also results in colder air being delivered to the lower airways, which can also trigger bronchoconstriction in asthmatic patients.[61] Although aspiration of nasal contents can occur in neurologically impaired patients, it is not thought to be responsible for the nasobronchial interaction under normal circumstances.[62]

The upper and lower airways not only interact via their anatomical connection but there may also be neural reflexes and systemic mechanisms.[63] A nasobronchial reflex has been proposed although there has been controversy as to whether it exists with limited evidence to support its presence.[61] A double-blind randomized study of nasal challenges in asthmatic patients with allergic rhinitis and in controls found that methacholine increased lower airway resistance but this could be blunted by pre-medication of phenylephrine to the nasal mucosa.[64] The implication is that the effect was through systemic absorption rather than a nasobronchial reflex. More recently it has been shown that nasal allergen provocation rapidly induces bronchial hyperresponsiveness by substance P binding to the neurokinin 1 receptor with an increased number of substance P-positive pulmonary nerves.[65] However, the precise interactions between the upper and lower airways are yet to be fully understood.

There is increasing evidence that the upper and lower airways are connected via a systemic route. Following local allergen challenge, there is high and rapid absorption of allergens in the nasal and bronchial vasculature.[66] There is also an increase in eosinophils in the blood and airway tissues as well as bone marrow eosinopoiesis.[58, 60, 67, 68] Increased serum IL-5 levels occurs after allergen exposure[69] and appears to play a critical role in allergic airways eosinophilia and eosinopoiesis in the bone marrow.[61, 70-73] In addition, it has been suggested that there is 'in situ haemopoiesis' with basophils/mast cells and eosinophils accumulating in allergic tissue from in situ growth and differentiation of progenitors, stimulated by soluble haemopoietic factors derived from mucosal cell populations.[74]

MANAGEMENT IMPLICATIONS

As rhinitis and asthma often coexist, a combined approach is recommended to manage the airways. The presence of disease in the lower airways can affect the results of investigations of the upper airways such as peak nasal inspiratory flow (PNIF) (**Figure 102.2a**). Although objective measures of nasal patency are not widely used in routine clinical practice, PNIF is reported to be the best validated technique for the evaluation of nasal flow through the nose[75]

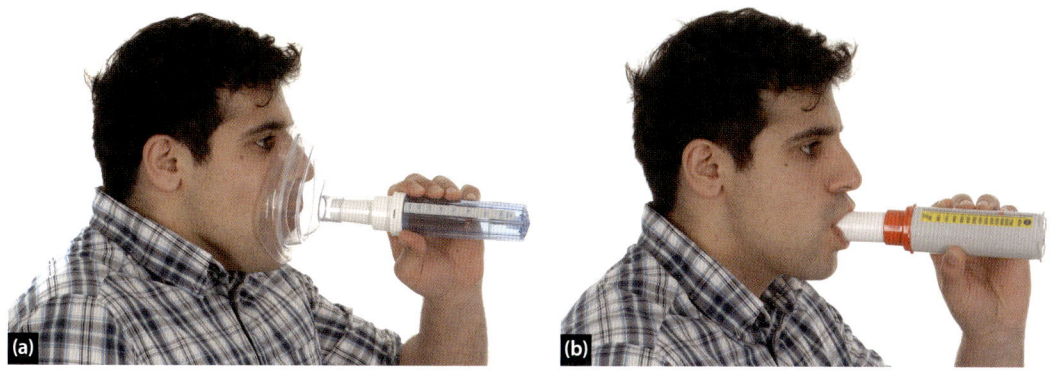

Figure 102.2 (a) Peak nasal inspiratory flow being measured. (b) Peak expiratory flow being measured.

and is quick, simple and cheap to use. It may be particularly helpful in evaluating children and adolescents with allergic rhinitis due to the subjective nature of the clinical information and the possibility that they may underestimate their symptoms.[76] However PNIF is affected by lower airway function[75] and has been reported to positively correlate with peak expiratory flow (PEF) in healthy children and adults (**Figure 102.2b**).[77, 78] PEF has been shown to be predictive of PNIF and low values of PNIF may be reflective of poor lower airway function rather than representing nasal obstruction.[78] Pulmonary function tests (particularly spirometry and PEF), in contrast objective tests of nasal patency are much more commonly used and can be helpful in confirming the diagnosis in asthma.[79]

Treatment of rhinitis may reduce morbidity from asthma and patients with asthma should be assessed for rhinitis and vice versa.[15] A retrospective cohort study of 4 944 patients with both allergic rhinitis and asthma (without any evidence of COPD) found that those treated for allergic rhinitis had a significantly lower rate of asthma-related emergency department visits or hospitalizations compared to those not treated.[80] Another retrospective study of 13 844 patients with asthma found that treatment with intra-nasal steroids of nasal conditions significantly reduces exacerbations of asthma leading to emergency department visits[81] although it has also been reported that there may be bias in such an observational study.[82]

Treatment options for rhinitis and asthma include pharmacological agents, immunotherapy and surgery for chronic rhinosinusitis. Although treatment regimes are well established for each individual condition, optimal management for coexisting rhinitis and asthma is still not agreed. Questions remain as to whether each condition should be treated separately or concurrently and which therapies should be used.[83]

Medical management

Drugs for rhinitis and asthma can be given via local (intra-nasal or inhaled (intra-bronchial)), oral and parenteral routes. Topical glucocorticosteroids to the nose and bronchi are a highly effective treatment for rhinitis and asthma. Intra-nasal glucocorticosteroids administered for rhinitis have been reported to improve asthma symptoms and to reduce asthma exacerbations leading to emergency department visits.[81, 84–87] However, not all studies have shown an improvement in asthma with intra-nasal glucocorticosteroids in patients with rhinitis and asthma.[88, 89]

The effect of inhaled intra-bronchial glucocorticosteroids on the nasal airway has been less well studied. However, one study reported that orally inhaled budesonide in patients with seasonal allergic rhinitis without asthma caused clinically significant anti-inflammatory effects in the whole airway.[90] This included the nasal mucosa which was not directly exposed to the drug with reduced seasonal eosinophilia both in the circulation and in the nose with a reduction in nasal symptoms. Oral glucocorticosteroids are also highly effective in asthma and rhinitis although its long-term use is limited by side effects.

H1-antihistamines are an important part of the treatment for allergic rhinitis. Some studies have also shown an improvement in asthma with oral antihistamines[91–93] although others have not and they are not currently recommended for the treatment of asthma.[94] Anti-leukotrienes have also been found to be effective in improving allergic rhinitis and asthma.[92, 95–101] The clinical response, however, is highly heterogeneous and they are generally considered as second line or add-on treatments.[79, 102, 103]

The anti-immunoglobulin E monoclonal antibody omalizumab has been shown to be a safe and effective additional treatment in moderate to severe asthma in children and adults. By binding with free IgE, it inhibits the release of mediators and production of cytokines from mast cells and it has also been found to be effective in allergic rhinitis. In patients with concomitant allergic asthma and persistent allergic rhinitis, there is a clinically significant improvement in both asthma and rhinitis with omalizumab.[104] The ability to reduce IgE levels irrespective of allergen specificity means that the role of omalizumab in allergic disease is potentially huge; it has also been used in combination with immunotherapy.

Specific Immunotherapy

Immunotherapy is a technique that involves progressive incremental exposure to causative allergens in order to modulate the immune response and achieve clinical tolerance to the allergens. It may be administered via a subcutaneous (SCIT) or a sublingual (SLIT) route and both have been reported to be effective in allergic disease. Serious complications such as anaphylactic reactions are uncommon, although are a major limitation of immunotherapy. SLIT is considered to be much safer than SCIT although less effective.[105]

Immunotherapy is reported to be effective in asthma and allergic rhinitis with improvements in symptoms and medication use.[105-109] However, it has also been highlighted that the quality of reporting of most immunotherapy trials is low[110] and there are many questions about immunotherapy that remain unanswered. Nevertheless, immunotherapy has shown promising results. It appears that immunotherapy in children sensitive to a single allergen can alter the natural history of allergy and prevent development of new sensitizations.[111-113] There is also some evidence, although limited at present, that immunotherapy has the potential to prevent the development of asthma in children with allergic rhinoconjunctivitis.[114-117] There is a need for further research in immunotherapy, which may not only have a therapeutic role but may also prevent and alter the natural course of allergic disease.

Surgical management

In addition to improving nasal symptoms, endoscopic sinus surgery (ESS) may also improve asthma in patients with chronic rhinosinusitis and asthma. Studies have shown improved asthma symptoms and control with a reduction in the use of inhalers, systemic medications and hospital admissions for asthma following ESS in chronic rhinosinusitis patients.[118-125] The positive effect on asthma has also been shown to continue long term following ESS,[126] with an improvement in severity of asthma, frequency of attacks and use of asthma medication, at an average follow-up of 6.5 years after surgery in one study.[127] Benefit in children with asthma and chronic sinusitis following ESS has also been reported, with a significant reduction in hospitalizations for asthma, school days missed and symptom scores in asthma and sinusitis.[128]

Lung function tests following ESS in patients with asthma and chronic rhinosinusitis have shown improvement in some studies[120, 122, 129, 130] whilst others have found no improvement.[119, 128, 131] Some have also not found any significant improvement in asthma following ESS in patients with chronic rhinosinusitis with and without nasal polyps.[132, 133] The reported difference in outcomes may be due to the heterogeneity and relatively small numbers of subjects and also to differences in outcome measures in these studies.[52]

The first randomized prospective study comparing medical and surgical treatment of chronic rhinosinusitis with and without polyps in asthmatic patients found subjective and objective improvements in asthma in both treatment groups.[134] However, overall asthma control was better maintained in the medically treated group and medical treatment was also superior to surgery in the subgroup of patients with nasal polyps.

The presence of asthma has been reported to negatively affect the outcome of ESS on the upper airway.[130, 135] Others, however, have found that asthma only has a negative impact on outcome in those with the most extensive sinonasal disease.[136] Furthermore, some report that asthma does not negatively affect outcome after ESS.[137, 138]

QUALITY OF LIFE AND COSTS IN ASTHMA AND RHINITIS

Asthma and allergic rhinitis results in poorer quality of life, demonstrated by the European Community Respiratory Health Survey,[139] a population-based study of young adults, using the SF-36 questionnaire. They found that patients with both asthma and allergic rhinitis had more physical limitations than patients with only allergic rhinitis, but there was no difference between these two groups for aspects related to social/mental health. Patients with allergic rhinitis but not asthma were more likely to have problems with social activities, daily activities as a result of emotional problems, and poorer mental wellbeing compared to patients with neither asthma nor rhinitis. There were too few patients with asthma without rhinitis to study although it appears that impairment in social life in asthmatics may be related to nasal symptoms.

More recently, however, it has been reported that allergic rhinitis does not seem to further impair health-related quality of life or only has a minor impact in asthmatic patients. Health-related quality of life (based on the SF-36 questionnaire) is markedly reduced in patients with asthma with or without allergic rhinitis, compared to those with allergic rhinitis alone, without any significant difference between those with asthma alone and those with both diseases.[140, 141] Other studies however, have shown that quality of life is worse in patients with asthma and allergic or non-allergic rhinitis compared to those with asthma alone.[142-144]

Rhinitis and asthma are global health problems that cause significant morbidity with loss of productivity and have massive direct and indirect costs. Worldwide, it is estimated that there are 500 million people with allergic rhinitis, 300 million people with asthma and also hundreds of millions of people with non-allergic rhinitis/rhinosinusitis.[79, 145] Although a global problem, there is geographical variation in the prevalence of rhinitis and asthma which tends to be lower in rural communities or low- to middle-income countries compared to Western developed countries.[15] Rhinitis increases asthma costs particularly in children and young adults and those with coexisting asthma and allergic rhinitis have been found to have higher medical care costs by an average of 46% compared to those with asthma alone.[146]

SUMMARY

The upper and lower respiratory tracts are intimately related as demonstrated by the similarities between rhinitis and asthma. Most patients with asthma have coexisting rhinitis whilst many rhinitis patients have asthma and an even greater number demonstrate non-specific bronchial hyperresponsiveness. Rhinitis and asthma are not only linked because they share atopy as a common risk factor; both allergic and non-allergic rhinitis are risk factors for asthma. Inflammation is a key component in the pathogenesis of both rhinitis and asthma and in many respects they appear to be manifestations of the same disease, representing a continuum of disease.

Airway smooth muscle present from the trachea to the bronchioles not only causes bronchoconstriction in asthma but may also be involved by increased proliferation and the expression and secretion of a variety of proinflammatory mediators and cytokines.[35, 36] The difference between rhinitis and asthma may therefore be due to an epithelial-mesenchymal trophic unit[147] in rhinitis whereas in asthma there is an epithelial-mesenchymal-muscular trophic unit. Although the precise interactions between the upper and lower respiratory tracts are not yet fully understood, it is clear that optimal management of patients with rhinitis and asthma requires an integrated upper and lower airway approach.

As rhinitis and asthma often coexist, a combined approach is recommended to investigate and treat the upper and lower airways. Studies strongly support the 1999 World Health Organization workshop 'Allergic rhinitis and its impact on asthma' (ARIA)[1] and the 2008 update,[145] which recommended that:

- Patients with persistent allergic rhinitis should be evaluated for asthma by history, chest examination and, if possible and when necessary, assessment of airflow obstruction before and after bronchodilator;
- History and examination of the upper respiratory tract for allergic rhinitis is performed in patients with asthma;
- Proposal of a strategy combining the treatment of both the upper and lower airway disease in terms of efficacy and safety.

Although there are some recommendations in the treatment of coexisting allergic rhinitis and asthma in the ARIA 2008 update[145] and 2010 revision,[148] further research is required in this area.

ACKNOWLEDGMENTS

Dr Allan McPhaden (Department of Pathology, Southern General Hospital, 1345 Govan Road, Glasgow, G51 4TF) for providing histology images

Craig Richardson and Rosie Smithers (Department of Medical Illustration, Glasgow Royal Infirmary, 84 Castle Street, Glasgow, G4 0SF)

Dr Shuaib Ellahi (photograph model)

BEST CLINICAL PRACTICE

- ✓ H1-antihistamines are effective in rhinitis.
- ✓ Intra-nasal corticosteroids are effective in rhinitis.
- ✓ Intra-nasal corticosteroids are inconstantly effective in asthma.
- ✓ Intra-nasal corticosteroids may reduce asthma exacerbations.
- ✓ Anti-leukotrienes are often effective in rhinitis and asthma.
- ✓ Anti-IgE monoclonal antibody is effective in both rhinitis and asthma.
- ✓ Allergen-specific immunotherapy is effective in both rhinitis and asthma.

FUTURE RESEARCH

- ➤ More prospective studies should assess the relationship between rhinitis and asthma.
- ➤ More studies are needed to assess nasal and bronchial inflammation in patients with asthma and COPD.
- ➤ Nasal remodelling is poorly understood.
- ➤ More studies are needed to understand the mechanisms of interaction between the upper and lower respiratory tract.
- ➤ Further large pivotal clinical trials are needed to assess whether the treatment of one target organ may improve outcome measures of the other target organ and to assess the specific impact of the different pharmacological agents, immunotherapy and surgery on the whole airway.

KEY POINTS

- The close relationship between the upper respiratory tract and the lower respiratory tract is something that is manifestly observed by all practising rhinologists, demonstrated by the similarities between rhinitis and asthma.
- Rhinitis and asthma may be viewed as ends or parts of a respiratory inflammatory spectrum.
- Most patients with asthma also have rhinitis and many patients with rhinitis have asthma.
- Allergy is associated with rhinitis and asthma.
- Allergic and non-allergic rhinitis are risk factors for asthma.
- Asthma and rhinitis share many common risk factors.
- There are many anatomical and physiological similarities between the upper and lower airways although there are also differences.
- There is a similar inflammatory infiltrate in the upper and lower airways in rhinitis and asthma.
- Bronchial challenge of rhinitis patients leads to nasal inflammation. Nasal challenge induces bronchial inflammation.
- The upper and lower airways not only interact via their anatomical connection but there may also be neural reflexes and systemic mechanisms.
- Treatment of rhinitis may reduce morbidity from asthma and patients with asthma should be assessed for rhinitis and vice versa.
- A combined approach is recommended to treat the upper and lower airways in patients with rhinitis and/or asthma.

REFERENCES

1. Bousquet J, Van Cauwenberge P, Khaltaev N, Aria Workshop G. Allergic rhinitis and its impact on asthma. *J Allergy Clin Immunol* 2001; **108**: S147–334.
2. Grossman J. One airway, one disease. *Chest* 1997; **111**: 11S–16S.
3. Togias A. Rhinitis and asthma: evidence for respiratory system integration. *J Allergy Clin Immunol* 2003; **111**: 1171–83; quiz 84.
4. Vignola AM, Bousquet J. Rhinitis and asthma: a continuum of disease? *Clin Exp Allergy* 2001; **31**: 674–7.
5. Linneberg A, Nielsen NH, Madsen F, et al. Secular trends of allergic asthma in Danish adults. The Copenhagen Allergy Study. *Resp Med* 2001; **95**: 258–64.
6. Guerra S, Sherrill DL, Martinez FD, Barbee RA. Rhinitis as an independent risk factor for adult-onset asthma. *J Allergy Clin Immunol* 2002; **109**: 419–25.
7. Jarvis D, Newson R, Lotvall J, et al. Asthma in adults and its association with chronic rhinosinusitis: the GA2LEN survey in Europe. *Allergy* 2012; **67**: 91–8.
8. Ragab A, Clement P, Vincken W. Objective assessment of lower airway involvement in chronic rhinosinusitis. *Am J Rhinol* 2004; **18**: 15–21.
9. Leynaert B, Bousquet J, Neukirch C, et al. Perennial rhinitis: an independent risk factor for asthma in nonatopic subjects: results from the European Community Respiratory Health Survey. *J Allergy Clin Immunol* 1999; **104**: 301–4.
10. Shaaban R, Zureik M, Soussan D, et al. Allergic rhinitis and onset of bronchial hyperresponsiveness: a population-based study. *Am J Resp Crit Care Med* 2007; **176**: 659–66.
11. Riccioni G, Della Vecchia R, Castronuovo M, et al. Bronchial hyperresponsiveness in adults with seasonal and perennial rhinitis: is there a link for asthma and rhinitis? *Int J Immunopathol Pharmacol* 2002; **15**: 69–74.
12. Verdiani P, Di Carlo S, Baronti A. Different prevalence and degree of nonspecific bronchial hyperreactivity between seasonal and perennial rhinitis. *J Allergy Clin Immunol* 1990; **86**: 576–82.
13. Braman SS, Barrows AA, DeCotiis BA, et al. Airway hyperresponsiveness in allergic rhinitis. A risk factor for asthma. *Chest* 1987; **91**: 671–4.
14. Szczeklik A, Stevenson DD. Aspirin-induced asthma: advances in pathogenesis and management. *J Allergy Clin Immunol* 1999; **104**: 5–13.
15. Cruz AA, Popov T, Pawankar R, et al. Common characteristics of upper and lower airways in rhinitis and asthma: ARIA update, in collaboration with GA(2)LEN. *Allergy* 2007; 62 Suppl 84: 1–41.
16. Pastacaldi C, Lewis P, Howarth P. Staphylococci and staphylococcal superantigens in asthma and rhinitis: a systematic review and meta-analysis. *Allergy* 2011; **66**: 549–55.
17. Hellings PW, Hens G, Meyts I, et al. Aggravation of bronchial eosinophilia in mice by nasal and bronchial exposure to Staphylococcus aureus enterotoxin B. *Clin Exp Allergy* 2006; **36**: 1063–71.
18. Van Zele T, Gevaert P, Watelet JB, et al. Staphylococcus aureus colonization and IgE antibody formation to enterotoxins is increased in nasal polyposis. *J Allergy Clin Immunol* 2004; **114**: 981–3.
19. Johnston SL, Pattemore PK, Sanderson G, et al. The relationship between upper respiratory infections and hospital admissions for asthma: a time-trend analysis. *Am J Resp Crit Care Med* 1996; **154**: 654–60.
20. Joao Silva M, Ferraz C, Pissarra S, et al. Role of viruses and atypical bacteria in asthma exacerbations among children in Oporto (Portugal). *Allergologia et Immunopathologia* 2007; **35**: 4–9.
21. Lemanske RF Jr, Dick EC, Swenson CA, et al. Rhinovirus upper respiratory infection increases airway hyperreactivity and late asthmatic reactions. *J Clin Invest* 1989; **83**: 1–10.
22. Papadopoulos NG, Bates PJ, Bardin PG, et al. Rhinoviruses infect the lower airways. *J Infect Dis* 2000; **181**: 1875–84.
23. Ameille J, Hamelin K, Andujar P, et al. Occupational asthma and occupational rhinitis: the united airways disease model revisited. *Occup Environ Med* 2013; 70(7): 471–5.
24. Leynaert B, Neukirch C, Kony S, et al. Association between asthma and rhinitis according to atopic sensitization in a population-based study. *J Allergy Clin Immunol* 2004; **113**: 86–93.
25. Plaschke PP, Janson C, Norrman E, et al. Onset and remission of allergic rhinitis and asthma and the relationship with atopic sensitization and smoking. *Am J Resp Crit Care Med* 2000; **162**: 920–4.
26. Shaaban R, Zureik M, Soussan D, et al. Rhinitis and onset of asthma: a longitudinal population-based study. *Lancet* 2008; **372**: 1049–57.
27. Wright AL, Holberg CJ, Martinez FD, et al. Epidemiology of physician-diagnosed allergic rhinitis in childhood. *Pediatrics* 1994; **94**: 895–901.
28. Burgess JA, Walters EH, Byrnes GB, et al. Childhood allergic rhinitis predicts asthma incidence and persistence to middle age: a longitudinal study. *J Allergy Clin Immunol* 2007; **120**: 863–9.
29. Settipane RJ, Hagy GW, Settipane GA. Long-term risk factors for developing asthma and allergic rhinitis: a 23-year follow-up study of college students. *Allergy Proc* 1994; **15**: 21–5.
30. Huovinen E, Kaprio J, Laitinen LA, Koskenvuo M. Incidence and prevalence of asthma among adult Finnish men and women of the Finnish Twin Cohort from 1975 to 1990, and their relation to hay fever and chronic bronchitis. *Chest* 1999; **115**: 928–36.
31. Bousquet J, Annesi-Maesano I, Carat F, et al. Characteristics of intermittent and persistent allergic rhinitis: DREAMS study group. *Clin Exp Allergy* 2005; **35**: 728–42.
32. Antonicelli L, Micucci C, Voltolini S, et al. Allergic rhinitis and asthma comorbidity: ARIA classification of rhinitis does not correlate with the prevalence of asthma. *Clin Exp Allergy* 2007; **37**: 954–60.
33. Lowe AJ, Hosking CS, Bennett CM, et al. Skin prick test can identify eczematous infants at risk of asthma and allergic rhinitis. *Clin Exp Allergy* 2007; **37**: 1624–31.
34. Dixon AE. Rhinosinusitis and asthma: the missing link. *Curr Opin Pulm Med* 2009; **15**: 19–24.
35. Hirst SJ, Lee TH. Airway smooth muscle as a target of glucocorticoid action in the treatment of asthma. *Am J Resp Crit Care Med* 1998; **158**: S201–6.
36. Chung KF. Airway smooth muscle cells: contributing to and regulating airway mucosal inflammation? *Euro Resp J* 2000; **15**: 961–8.
37. Chanez P, Vignola AM, Vic P, et al. Comparison between nasal and bronchial inflammation in asthmatic and control subjects. *Am J Resp Crit Care Med* 1999; **159**: 588–95.
38. Ponikau JU, Sherris DA, Kephart GM, et al. Features of airway remodeling and eosinophilic inflammation in chronic rhinosinusitis: is the histopathology similar to asthma? *J Allergy Clin Immunol* 2003; **112**: 877–82.
39. Gaga M, Lambrou P, Papageorgiou N, et al. Eosinophils are a feature of upper and lower airway pathology in non-atopic asthma, irrespective of the presence of rhinitis. *Clin Exp Allergy* 2000; **30**: 663–9.
40. Settipane GA, Chafee FH. Nasal polyps in asthma and rhinitis. A review of 6,037 patients. *J Allergy Clin Immunol* 1977; **59**: 17–21.
41. Szczeklik A, Stevenson DD. Aspirin-induced asthma: advances in pathogenesis, diagnosis, and management. *J Allergy Clin Immunol* 2003; **111**: 913–21; quiz 22.
42. ten Brinke A, Grootendorst DC, Schmidt JT, et al. Chronic sinusitis in severe asthma is related to sputum eosinophilia. *J Allergy Clin Immunol* 2002; **109**: 621–6.
43. Matsuno O, Ono E, Takenaka R, et al. Asthma and sinusitis: association and implication. *Int Arch Allergy Immunol* 2008; **147**: 52–8.
44. Bresciani M, Paradis L, Des Roches A, et al. Rhinosinusitis in severe asthma. *J Allergy Clin Immunol* 2001; **107**: 73–80.
45. Sichletidis L, Tsiotsios I, Gavriilidis A, et al. Prevalence of chronic obstructive pulmonary disease and rhinitis in northern Greece. *Respiration* 2005; **72**: 270–7.
46. Hurst JR. Upper airway. 3: Sinonasal involvement in chronic obstructive pulmonary disease. *Thorax* 2010; **65**: 85–90.
47. Montnémery P, Svensson C, Adelroth E, et al. Prevalence of nasal symptoms and their relation to self-reported asthma and chronic bronchitis/emphysema. *Euro Resp J* 2001; **17**: 596–603.
48. van Manen JG, Bindels PJ, Ijzermans CJ, et al. Prevalence of comorbidity in patients with a chronic airway obstruction and controls over the age of 40. *J Clin Epidemiol* 2001; **54**: 287–93.
49. Hurst JR, Wilkinson TM, Donaldson GC, Wedzicha JA. Upper airway symptoms and quality of life in chronic obstructive pulmonary disease (COPD). *Resp Med* 2004; **98**: 767–70.
50. Hens G, Vanaudenaerde BM, Bullens DM, et al. Sinonasal pathology in nonallergic asthma and COPD: 'united airway disease' beyond the scope of allergy. *Allergy* 2008; **63**: 261–7.
51. Roberts NJ, Lloyd-Owen SJ, Rapado F, et al. Relationship between chronic nasal and respiratory symptoms in patients with COPD. *Resp Med* 2003; **97**: 909–14.

52. Fokkens WJ, Lund VJ, Mullol J, et al. European Position Paper on Rhinosinusitis and Nasal Polyps 2012. *Rhinology* Suppl 2012: 3 p. preceding table of contents, 1–298.
53. Chakir J, Laviolette M, Boutet M, et al. Lower airways remodeling in nonasthmatic subjects with allergic rhinitis. *Lab Invest* 1996; 75: 735–44.
54. Braunstahl GJ, Fokkens WJ, Overbeek SE, et al. Mucosal and systemic inflammatory changes in allergic rhinitis and asthma: a comparison between upper and lower airways. *Clin Exp Allergy* 2003; 33: 579–87.
55. Djukanovic R, Lai CK, Wilson JW, et al. Bronchial mucosal manifestations of atopy: a comparison of markers of inflammation between atopic asthmatics, atopic nonasthmatics and healthy controls. *Eur Respir J* 1992; 5: 538–44.
56. Chakir J, Laviolette M, Turcotte H, et al. Cytokine expression in the lower airways of nonasthmatic subjects with allergic rhinitis: influence of natural allergen exposure. *J Allergy Clin Immunol* 2000; 106: 904–10.
57. Bonay M, Neukirch C, Grandsaigne M, et al. Changes in airway inflammation following nasal allergic challenge in patients with seasonal rhinitis. *Allergy* 2006; 61: 111–8.
58. Braunstahl GJ, Overbeek SE, Kleinjan A, et al. Nasal allergen provocation induces adhesion molecule expression and tissue eosinophilia in upper and lower airways. *J Allergy Clin Immunol* 2001; 107: 469–76.
59. Calhoun WJ, Jarjour NN, Gleich GJ, et al. Increased airway inflammation with segmental versus aerosol antigen challenge. The American review of respiratory disease 1993; 147: 1465–71.
60. Braunstahl GJ, Kleinjan A, Overbeek SE, et al. Segmental bronchial provocation induces nasal inflammation in allergic rhinitis patients. *Am J Resp Crit Care Med* 2000; 161: 2051–7.
61. Braunstahl GJ. United airways concept: what does it teach us about systemic inflammation in airways disease? *Proc Am Thorac Soc* 2009; 6: 652–4.
62. Bardin PG, Van Heerden BB, Joubert JR. Absence of pulmonary aspiration of sinus contents in patients with asthma and sinusitis. *J Allergy Clinical Immunol* 1990; 86: 82–8.
63. Hens G, Hellings PW. The nose: gatekeeper and trigger of bronchial disease. *Rhinology* 2006; 44: 179–87.
64. Littell NT, Carlisle CC, Millman RP, Braman SS. Changes in airway resistance following nasal provocation. *Am Rev Resp Dis* 1990; 141: 580–3.
65. Hens G, Raap U, Vanoirbeek J, et al. Selective nasal allergen provocation induces substance P-mediated bronchial hyperresponsiveness. *Am J Resp Cell Mol Biol* 2011; 44: 517–23.
66. Hens G, Bobic S, Reekmans K, et al. Rapid systemic uptake of allergens through the respiratory mucosa. *J Allergy Clin Immunol* 2007; 120: 472–4.
67. Li J, Saito H, Crawford L, et al. Haemopoietic mechanisms in murine allergic upper and lower airway inflammation. *Immunology* 2005; 114: 386–96.
68. Denburg JA, Keith PK. Systemic aspects of chronic rhinosinusitis. *Immunol Allergy Clin North Am* 2004; 24: 87–102.
69. Beeh KM, Beier J, Kornmann O, et al. A single nasal allergen challenge increases induced sputum inflammatory markers in non-asthmatic subjects with seasonal allergic rhinitis: correlation with plasma interleukin-5. *Clin Expl Allergy* 2003; 33: 475–82.
70. Wang J, Palmer K, Lotvall J, et al. Circulating, but not local lung, IL-5 is required for the development of antigen-induced airways eosinophilia. *J Clin Invest* 1998; 102: 1132–41.
71. Saito H, Matsumoto K, Denburg AE, et al. Pathogenesis of murine experimental allergic rhinitis: a study of local and systemic consequences of IL-5 deficiency. *J Immunol* 2002; 168: 3017–23.
72. Denburg JA, Sehmi R, Saito H, et al. Systemic aspects of allergic disease: bone marrow responses. *J Allergy Clin Immunol* 2000; 106: S242–6.
73. Dorman SC, Sehmi R, Gauvreau GM, et al. Kinetics of bone marrow eosinophilopoiesis and associated cytokines after allergen inhalation. *Am J Resp Crit Care Med* 2004; 169: 565–72.
74. Denburg JA, Otsuka H, Ohnisi M, et al. Contribution of basophil/mast cell and eosinophil growth and differentiation to the allergic tissue inflammatory response. *Int Arch Allergy Appl Immunol* 1987; 82: 321–6.
75. Scadding G, Hellings P, Alobid I, et al. Diagnostic tools in Rhinology EAACI position paper. *Clin Transl Allergy* 2011; 1: 2.
76. Gomes Dde L, Camargos PA, Ibiapina Cda C, de Andrade CR. Nasal peak inspiratory flow and clinical score in children and adolescents with allergic rhinitis. *Rhinology* 2008; 46: 276–80.
77. Chaves C, Ibiapina Cda C, de Andrade CR, et al. Correlation between peak nasal inspiratory flow and peak expiratory flow in children and adolescents. *Rhinology* 2012; 50: 381–5.
78. Ottaviano G, Lund VJ, Coles S, et al. Does peak nasal inspiratory flow relate to peak expiratory flow? *Rhinology* 2008; 46: 200–3.
79. From the Global Strategy for Asthma Management and Prevention, Global Initiative for Asthma (GINA) 2012. Available from: http://www.ginasthma.org/. 2012.
80. Crystal-Peters J, Nealusan C, Crown WH, Torres A. Treating allergic rhinitis in patients with comorbid asthma: the risk of asthma related hospitalizations and emergency department visits. *J Allergy Clin Immunol* 2002; 109: 57–62.
81. Adams RJ, Fuhlbrigge AL, Finkelstein JA, Weiss ST. Intranasal steroids and the risk of emergency department visits for asthma. *J Allergy Clin Immunol* 2002; 109: 636–42.
82. Suissa S, Ernst P. Bias in observational study of the effectiveness of nasal corticosteroids in asthma. *J Allergy Clin Immunol* 2005; 115: 714–9.
83. Scadding G, Walker S. Poor asthma control? – then look up the nose. The importance of co-morbid rhinitis in patients with asthma. *Prim Care Resp J* 2012; 21: 222–8.
84. Scichilone N, Arrigo R, Paterno A, et al. The effect of intranasal corticosteroids on asthma control and quality of life in allergic rhinitis with mild asthma. *J Asthma* 2011; 48: 41–7.
85. Stelmach R, do Patrocinio TNM, Ribeiro M, Cukier A. Effect of treating allergic rhinitis with corticosteroids in patients with mild-to-moderate persistent asthma. *Chest* 2005; 128: 3140–7.
86. Reed CE, Marcoux JP, Welsh PW. Effects of topical nasal treatment on asthma symptoms. *J Allergy Clin Immunol* 1988; 81: 1042–7.
87. Lohia S, Schlosser RJ, Soler ZM. Impact of intranasal corticosteroids on asthma outcomes in allergic rhinitis: a meta-analysis. *Allergy* 2013; 68: 569–79.
88. Nathan RA, Yancey SW, Waitkus-Edwards K, et al. Fluticasone propionate nasal spray is superior to montelukast for allergic rhinitis while neither affects overall asthma control. *Chest* 2005; 128: 1910–20.
89. Pedroletti C, Lundahl J, Alving K, Hedlin G. Effect of nasal steroid treatment on airway inflammation determined by exhaled nitric oxide in allergic schoolchildren with perennial rhinitis and asthma. *Pediatr Allergy Immunol* 2008; 19: 219–26.
90. Greiff L, Andersson M, Svensson C, et al. Effects of orally inhaled budesonide in seasonal allergic rhinitis. *Euro Resp J* 1998; 11: 1268–73.
91. Grant JA, Nicodemus CF, Findlay SR, et al. Cetirizine in patients with seasonal rhinitis and concomitant asthma: prospective, randomized, placebo-controlled trial. *J Allergy Clin Immunol* 1995; 95: 923–32.
92. Baena-Cagnani CE, Berger WE, DuBuske LM, et al. Comparative effects of desloratadine versus montelukast on asthma symptoms and use of beta 2-agonists in patients with seasonal allergic rhinitis and asthma. *Int Arch Allergy Immunol* 2003; 130: 307–13.
93. Nathan RA, Finn AF Jr, LaForce C, et al. Comparison of cetirizine-pseudoephedrine and placebo in patients with seasonal allergic rhinitis and concomitant mild-to-moderate asthma: randomized, double-blind study. *Ann Allergy Asthma Immunol* 2006; 97: 389–96.
94. Van Ganse E, Kaufman L, Derde MP, et al. Effects of antihistamines in adult asthma: a meta-analysis of clinical trials. *Euro Resp J* 1997; 10: 2216–24.
95. Nathan RA, Kemp JP, Antileukotriene Working Group. Efficacy of antileukotriene agents in asthma management. *Ann Allergy Asthma Immunol* 2001; 86: 9–17.
96. Philip G, Nayak AS, Berger WE, et al. The effect of montelukast on rhinitis symptoms in patients with asthma and seasonal allergic rhinitis. *Curr Med Res Opin* 2004; 20: 1549–58.
97. Busse WW, Casale TB, Dykewicz MS, et al. Efficacy of montelukast during the allergy season in patients with chronic asthma and seasonal aeroallergen sensitivity. *Ann Allergy Asthma Immunol* 2006; 96: 60–8.
98. Piatti G, Ceriotti L, Cavallaro G, et al. Effects of zafirlukast on bronchial asthma and allergic rhinitis. *Pharmacol Res* 2003; 47: 541–7.
99. Price DB, Swern A, Tozzi CA, et al. Effect of montelukast on lung function in asthma patients with allergic rhinitis: analysis from the COMPACT trial. *Allergy* 2006; 61: 737–42.
100. Virchow JC, Bachert C. Efficacy and safety of montelukast in adults with asthma and allergic rhinitis. *Resp Med* 2006; 100: 1952–9.

101. Kim H, Bouchard J, Renzi PM. The link between allergic rhinitis and asthma: a role for antileukotrienes? *Can Resp J* 2008; **15**: 91–8.
102. Scadding GW, Scadding GK. Recent advances in antileukotriene therapy. *Curr Opin Allergy Clin Immunol* 2010; **10**: 370–6.
103. Scadding GK, Durham SR, Mirakian R, et al. BSACI guidelines for the management of allergic and non-allergic rhinitis. *Clin Exp Allergy* 2008; **38**: 19–42.
104. Vignola AM, Humbert M, Bousquet J, et al. Efficacy and tolerability of anti-immunoglobulin E therapy with omalizumab in patients with concomitant allergic asthma and persistent allergic rhinitis: SOLAR. *Allergy* 2004; **59**: 709–17.
105. Mohapatra SS, Qazi M, Hellermann G. Immunotherapy for allergies and asthma: present and future. *Curr Opin Pharmacol* 2010; **10**: 276–88.
106. Calderon MA, Alves B, Jacobson M, et al. Allergen injection immunotherapy for seasonal allergic rhinitis. *Cochrane Database Syst Rev* 2007: CD001936.
107. Compalati E, Passalacqua G, Bonini M, Canonica GW. The efficacy of sublingual immunotherapy for house dust mites respiratory allergy: results of a GA2LEN meta-analysis. *Allergy* 2009; **64**: 1570–9.
108. Sieber J, Koberlein J, Mosges R. Sublingual immunotherapy in daily medical practice: effectiveness of different treatment schedules – IPD meta-analysis. *Curr Med Res Opin* 2010; **26**: 925–32.
109. Abramson MJ, Puy RM, Weiner JM. Injection allergen immunotherapy for asthma. *Cochrane Database Syst Rev* 2010: CD001186.
110. Bousquet PJ, Calderon MA, Demoly P, et al. The Consolidated Standards of Reporting Trials (CONSORT) Statement applied to allergen-specific immunotherapy with inhalant allergens: a Global Allergy and Asthma European Network (GA(2) LEN) article. *J Allergy Clin Immunol* 2011; **127**: 49–56, 56 e1–11.
111. Des Roches A, Paradis L, Menardo JL, et al. Immunotherapy with a standardized Dermatophagoides pteronyssinus extract. VI. Specific immunotherapy prevents the onset of new sensitizations in children. *J Allergy Clin Immunol* 1997; **9**: 450–3.
112. Pajno GB, Barberio G, De Luca F, et al. Prevention of new sensitizations in asthmatic children monosensitized to house dust mite by specific immunotherapy. A six-year follow-up study. *Clin Exp Allergy* 2001; **31**: 1392–7.
113. Inal A, Altintas DU, Yilmaz M, et al. Prevention of new sensitizations by specific immunotherapy in children with rhinitis and/or asthma monosensitized to house dust mite. *J Invest Allergol Clin Immunol* 2007; **17**: 85–91.
114. Moller C, Dreborg S, Ferdousi HA, et al. Pollen immunotherapy reduces the development of asthma in children with seasonal rhinoconjunctivitis (the PAT-study). *J Allergy Clin Immunol* 2002; **109**: 251–6.
115. Jacobsen L, Niggemann B, Dreborg S, et al. Specific immunotherapy has long-term preventive effect of seasonal and perennial asthma: 10-year follow-up on the PAT study. *Allergy* 2007; **62**: 943–8.
116. Novembre E, Galli E, Landi F, et al. Coseasonal sublingual immunotherapy reduces the development of asthma in children with allergic rhinoconjunctivitis. *J Allergy Clin Immunol* 2004; **114**: 851–7.
117. Hedlin G, van Hage M. The role of immunotherapy in the management of childhood asthma. *Ther Adv Respir Dis* 2012; **6**: 137–46.
118. Nishioka GJ, Cook PR, Davis WE, McKinsey JP. Functional endoscopic sinus surgery in patients with chronic sinusitis and asthma. *Otolaryngol – Head Neck Surg* 1994; **110**: 494–500.
119. Dhong HJ, Jung YS, Chung SK, Choi DC. Effect of endoscopic sinus surgery on asthmatic patients with chronic rhinosinusitis. *Otolaryngol – Head Neck Surg* 2001; **124**: 99–104.
120. Proimos E, Papadakis CE, Chimona TS, et al. The effect of functional endoscopic sinus surgery on patients with asthma and CRS with nasal polyps. *Rhinology* 2010; **48**: 331–8.
121. Dunlop G, Scadding GK, Lund VJ. The effect of endoscopic sinus surgery on asthma: management of patients with chronic rhinosinusitis, nasal polyposis, and asthma. *Am J Rhinol* 1999; **13**: 261–5.
122. Batra PS, Kern RC, Tripathi A, et al. Outcome analysis of endoscopic sinus surgery in patients with nasal polyps and asthma. *Laryngoscope* 2003; **113**: 1703–6.
123. Ehnhage A, Olsson P, Kolbeck KG, et al. Functional endoscopic sinus surgery improved asthma symptoms as well as PEFR and olfaction in patients with nasal polyposis. *Allergy* 2009; **64**: 762–9.
124. Park AH, Lau J, Stankiewicz J, Chow J. The role of functional endoscopic sinus surgery in asthmatic patients. *J Otolaryngol* 1998; **27**: 275–80.
125. Palmer JN, Conley DB, Dong RG, et al. Efficacy of endoscopic sinus surgery in the management of patients with asthma and chronic sinusitis. *Am J Rhinol* 2001; **15**: 49–53.
126. Ehnhage A, Olsson P, Kolbeck KG, et al. One year after endoscopic sinus surgery in polyposis: asthma, olfaction, and quality-of-life outcomes. *Otolaryngol – Head Neck Surg* 2012; **146**: 834–41.
127. Senior BA, Kennedy DW, Tanabodee J, et al. Long-term impact of functional endoscopic sinus surgery on asthma. *Otolaryngol – Head Neck Surg* 1999; **121**: 66–8.
128. Manning SC, Wasserman RL, Silver R, Phillips DL. Results of endoscopic sinus surgery in pediatric patients with chronic sinusitis and asthma. *Arch Otolaryngol – Head Neck Surg* 1994; **120**: 1142–5.
129. Ikeda K, Tanno N, Tamura G, et al. Endoscopic sinus surgery improves pulmonary function in patients with asthma associated with chronic sinusitis. *Ann Otology Rhinol Laryngol* 1999; **108**: 355–9.
130. Dejima K, Hama T, Miyazaki M, et al. A clinical study of endoscopic sinus surgery for sinusitis in patients with bronchial asthma. *Int Arch Allergy Immunol* 2005; **138**: 97–104.
131. Chen FH, Zuo KJ, Guo YB, et al. Long-term results of endoscopic sinus surgery-oriented treatment for chronic rhinosinusitis with asthma. *Laryngoscope* 2014; **24**: 4–8.
132. Goldstein MF, Grundfast SK, Dunsky EH, et al. Effect of functional endoscopic sinus surgery on bronchial asthma outcomes. *Arch Otolaryngol – Head Neck Surg* 1999; **125**: 314–9.
133. Uri N, Cohen-Kerem R, Barzilai G, et al. Functional endoscopic sinus surgery in the treatment of massive polyposis in asthmatic patients. *J Laryngol Otol* 2002; **116**: 185–9.
134. Ragab S, Scadding GK, Lund VJ, Saleh H. Treatment of chronic rhinosinusitis and its effects on asthma. *Euro Resp J* 2006; **28**: 68–74.
135. Dinis PB, Gomes A. Sinusitis and asthma: how do they interrelate in sinus surgery? *Am J Rhinol* 1997; **11**: 421–8.
136. Kennedy DW. Prognostic factors, outcomes and staging in ethmoid sinus surgery. *Laryngoscope* 1992; **102**: 1–18.
137. Mehanna H, Mills J, Kelly B, McGarry GW. Benefit from endoscopic sinus surgery. *Clin Otolaryngol Allied Sci* 2002; **27**: 464–71.
138. Kountakis SE, Bradley DT. Effect of asthma on sinus computed tomography grade and symptom scores in patients undergoing revision functional endoscopic sinus surgery. *Am J Rhinol* 2003; **17**: 215–9.
139. Leynaert B, Neukirch C, Liard R, et al. Quality of life in allergic rhinitis and asthma. A population-based study of young adults. *Am J Resp Crit Care Med* 2000; **162**: 1391–6.
140. Elkholy MM, Khedr MH, Halawa A, Elbaramawy A. Impact of allergic rhinitis on quality of life in patients with bronchial asthma. *Int J Health Sci* 2012; **6**: 194–202.
141. Kalpaklioglu AF, Baccioglu A. Evaluation of quality of life: impact of allergic rhinitis on asthma. *J Invest Allergol Clin Immunol* 2008; **18**: 168–73.
142. Braido F, Baiardini I, Balestracci S, et al. Does asthma control correlate with quality of life related to upper and lower airways? A real life study. *Allergy* 2009; **64**: 937–43.
143. Vandenplas O, Dramaix M, Joos G, et al. The impact of concomitant rhinitis on asthma-related quality of life and asthma control. *Allergy* 2010; **65**: 1290–7.
144. Maio S, Baldacci S, Simoni M, et al. Impact of asthma and comorbid allergic rhinitis on quality of life and control in patients of Italian general practitioners. *J Asthma* 2012; **49**: 854–61.
145. Bousquet J, Khaltaev N, Cruz AA, et al. Allergic Rhinitis and its Impact on Asthma (ARIA) 2008 update (in collaboration with the World Health Organization, GA(2) LEN and AllerGen). *Allergy* 2008; 63 Suppl **86**: 8–160.
146. Yawn BP, Yunginger JW, Wollan PC, et al. Allergic rhinitis in Rochester, Minnesota residents with asthma: frequency and impact on health care charges. *J Allergy Clin Immunol* 1999; **103**: 54–9.
147. Holgate ST, Davies DE, Lackie PM, et al. Epithelial-mesenchymal interactions in the pathogenesis of asthma. *J Allergy Clin Immunol* 2000; **105**: 193–204.
148. Brozek JL, Bousquet J, Baena-Cagnani CE, et al. Allergic Rhinitis and its Impact on Asthma (ARIA) guidelines: 2010 revision. *J Allergy Clin Immunol* 2010; **126**: 466–76.

CHAPTER 103

NASAL SEPTUM AND NASAL VALVE

Shahram Anari and Ravinder Singh Natt

Introduction 1135	*Nasal valve* 1141
Nasal septum 1136	Anatomy 1141
Anatomy 1136	Aetiology 1142
Aetiology 1136	Diagnosis 1142
Diagnosis 1136	Treatment 1143
Treatment 1137	Dressing and splints in nasal airway surgery 1146
Submucosal resection 1137	Complications 1146
Septoplasty 1137	Conclusion 1147
Septoplasty techniques 1139	References 1148
Special septoplasty considerations 1140	

SEARCH STRATEGY

Data in this chapter may be updated by a Medline search using the keywords: septoplasty, rhinoplasty, septorhinoplasty, functional rhinoplasty, nasal valve surgery, turbinate surgery and paediatric.

INTRODUCTION

Nasal breathing is the normal path of respiration in human beings. Nasal airway passage accounts for approximately half of the total airway resistance and this resistance is required for optimal respiratory physiology.[1] Nasal airway patency or its resistance can be measured by objective and subjective tools.

Rhinomanometry measures trans-nasal airflow and pressure during respiration to determine nasal airway resistance. Nasal cycle and mucosal pathology play a part in these measurements and would make the results based on one rhinomanometry reading less reliable or reproducible. Taking objective measurements before and after nasal decongestants can help distinguish between mucosal hypertrophy and structural deformity as the cause of nasal obstruction.[2] Acoustic rhinometry determines the nasal cross-sectional area and nasal volume through the analysis of reflected sound pulses within the nasal cavity but the nasal airflow is not included in this method and therefore the effects of dynamic collapse can be missed. Inaccurate placement of the probes during the measurements can also lead to erroneous results.

Due to the inherent problems with the objective measures, subjective tools are more commonly employed in the clinical and research settings. Visual analogue scale appears to be a simple and adequate tool to measure the nasal patency subjectively. The Nasal Obstruction Symptom Evaluation (NOSE) scale is a validated tool for nasal obstruction in adults. The five domains each score 0 (no symptoms) to 4 (severe symptoms) and the result is multiplied by 5 producing a maximum score of 100.[3]

From a practical point, the current technology cannot accurately determine the level or cause of nasal obstruction; clinical examination remains the mainstay of clinical diagnosis.

The nasal airway is composed of two nasal cavities, each with a medial and a lateral wall as well as a floor. The nasal cavity and its elements are referred to in a three-dimensional structure and we follow the terminology demonstrated in **Figure 103.1** in this chapter.

1. **Medial nasal wall:** This is mainly formed by the nasal septum which in itself is composed of bony, cartilaginous and membranous parts. The columella forms the most caudal part of the medial wall.

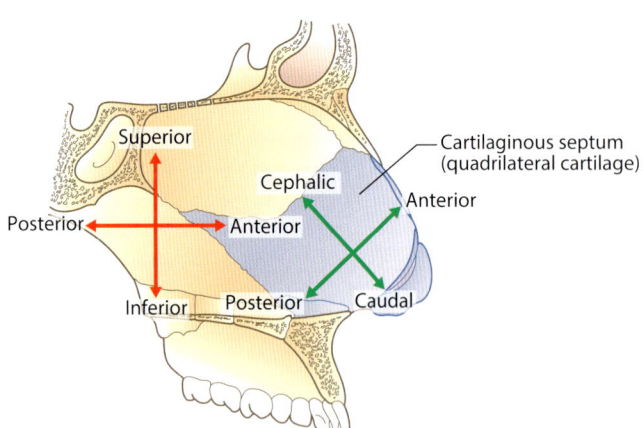

Figure 103.1 Terminology used in nasal and septal orientation. Red arrows refer to the nasal cavity; green arrows refer to the nasal septum.

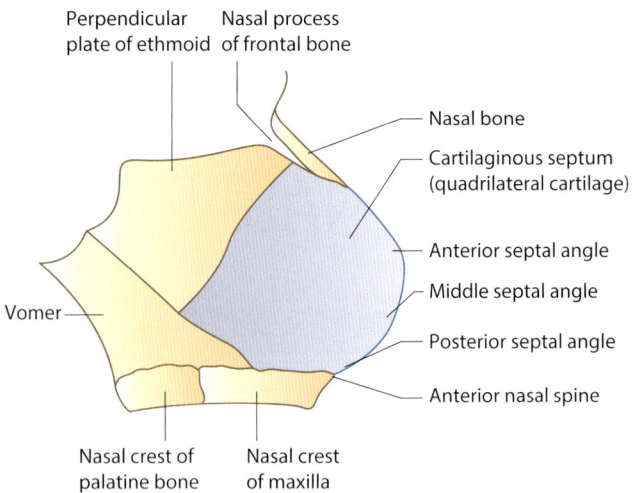

Figure 103. 2 Nasal septal anatomy and its terminology.

2. **Lateral nasal wall:** This is formed by the turbinates, fibrofatty tissue and cartilages (sesamoid cartilages, accessory cartilages, upper lateral cartilage and the lateral crus of the lower lateral cartilage).
3. **Nasal floor:** This wall is formed by the floor of the nasal cavity and the nasal vestibule sill.

The elements involved in the nasal airway could have an adverse effect on the nasal airway patency. These elements are mainly incorporated in the nasal septum and the nasal valve areas and it is essential that they are carefully assessed during clinical examination.

NASAL SEPTUM

ANATOMY

The nasal septum is divided into bony, cartilaginous and membranous parts (from cephalad to caudal). The bony septum is mainly formed by the perpendicular plate of ethmoid and vomer. The palatine bones and maxillary crest form the most posterior parts of the bony septum (**Figure 103.2**). The cartilaginous septum (i.e. quadrilateral cartilage) is not an isolated cartilage and in fact is in unison with the upper lateral cartilages forming one cartilaginous unit.

AETIOLOGY

Nasal obstruction can be caused by septal deflection which can be developmental or secondary to trauma. In some cases, the trauma occurs in childhood and the patient does not necessarily remember the incident.

DIAGNOSIS

An L-shaped strut of septum measuring approximately one centimetre in width is required to support the external nasal skeleton (**Figure 103.3**). Deviation at the nasal septum L-strut needs to be differentiated from the obstruction caused by the rest of the septum, as it will have implications on the management.

Septal examination should include inspection as well as palpation. During inspection, the position of deviation should be mapped in relation to the L-strut. Nasendoscopy will allow inspection of the anatomy in the neutral position and it also allows inspection of the elements that are not visible in anterior rhinoscopy; this at times can reveal adenoid tissue, mucosal abnormalities, nasal polyps or choanal pathology which can cause nasal obstruction.

Nasal airflow can be demonstrated by misting of the examination mirror or metal tongue spatula but this technique needs to be used with caution. Absence or reduction of the misting can be suggestive of a structural blockage but a satisfactory amount of misting does not necessarily indicate a patent nasal airway as perceived by the patient. This will be discussed further in the examination of the nasal valve.

Palpation is used to feel for attachment of the septum to the anterior nasal spine and to feel for fracture lines. In patients who have undergone septal surgery in the past, gentle palpation of the septum with an applicator (e.g. Jobson Horne probe) might indicate the areas deficient of cartilage.

During assessment, a decision is to be made as to whether the septal deflection is the sole cause of nasal obstruction. Nasal valve and mucosal elements need to be taken into consideration. The history of constant nasal obstruction points to an anatomical blockage whereas the intermittent obstruction points to the mucosal elements

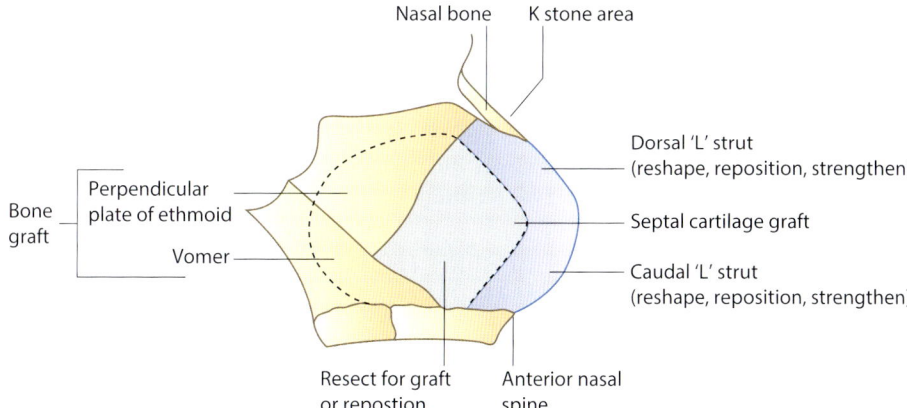

Figure 103.3 Septal cartilaginous L-strut with a minimum 10 mm width is preserved for structural support. The rest of the bony and cartilaginous septum can be used as grafts.

to be at least partially to blame. Significant improvement in nasal obstruction after application of topical nasal decongestants indicates the role of mucosal elements in nasal obstruction. Intermittent nasal obstruction, especially one that changes sides, can be due to nasal cycle. Patients who have had complete nasal obstruction might complain of this phenomenon after their successful nasal airway surgery. If the patient notices obstruction in the lateral decubitus, then the engorgement of turbinates on the dependent side or the collapse of the lateral nasal wall (i.e. nasal valve elements) on the opposite side can be blamed.

TREATMENT

Septal deviation can be present due to the inherent bend of the septal cartilage or as a result of septal tilt due to deviated bony septum. In cases where the septum is inherently straight, the septal tilt may be corrected by addressing the bony attachments; when the cartilage is inherently deformed, special techniques are employed.

Most septal deviations involve the caudal and dorsal L-strut to some degree but in cases where the obstruction does not involve the L-strut, the offending segment can be excised through submucosal resection (SMR).

SUBMUCOSAL RESECTION

In this technique, the L-strut is not addressed therefore a Killian incision for approach would suffice. A Killian incision is placed about 1 cm cephalad from the caudal end of the septum (**Figure 103.4**). At this point the perichondrium is less adherent to the underlying cartilage and the flap can be raised more easily. If the deviation is situated further cephalad, the incision for access can be made close to the offending segment.

The deviated part of the septum is freed from its peripheral cartilaginous and bony attachments. The *in-situ* bony deviation can be in-fractured to put the bony septum in midline or it can be excised conservatively. Bony septum is an invaluable source of graft material for septal reconstruction; therefore the excision should be done conservatively. The harvested septum can then be used as a graft or it can be straightened and reinserted in its place. It can be secured to the remaining septum by sutures to avoid migration; some authors prefer to secure it by inserting bilateral intra-nasal splints.

SEPTOPLASTY

In most cases of septal deviation, the septal L-strut is involved. SMR is not effective in these cases as it cannot address the caudal and dorsal struts. Septoplasty techniques are needed to address these problems and the approach should provide access to the L-strut.

Hemitransfixion incision is designed to provide access to the whole septum including the caudal L-strut. The incision is placed at the caudal edge of the septum. The length of the incision depends on the access required (**Figure 103.4**). If access is required to the whole of caudal arm of the L-strut then a full hemitransfixion is used. However, if access is not required for the most posterior parts of the septum, then a partial hemitransfixion would suffice. If access is required to the floor of the nasal cavity then an extended hemitransfixion incision is used.

Generally, raising the mucosal flap on the concave side would be enough to allow access for excision of septal cartilage and bone, to detach the septal osseocartilaginous junction, to score the concave side and apply other relevant techniques. It also reduces the chance of septal perforation by keeping the opposite mucosa intact. In certain conditions, both mucosal flaps are raised, especially when the surgeon would like to keep the sutures in the mucosal envelope or in cases where access to both sides of the septum is required (e.g. S-shaped septal deformity).

Caudally, the perichondrium is adherent to the septal cartilage and care must be taken to identify the actual plane of dissection at the subperichondrial level. This can be achieved by scoring the area to find the desired plane.

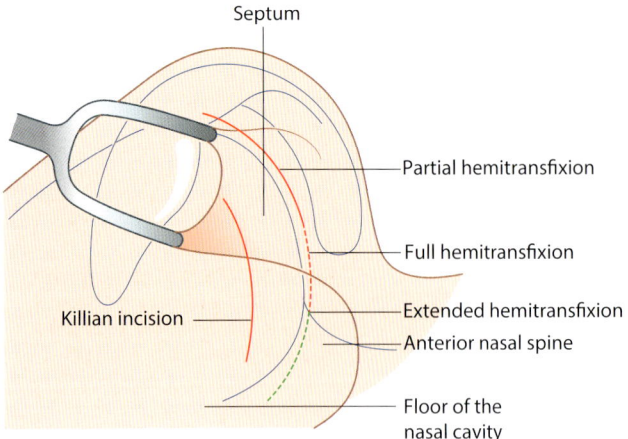

Figure 103.4 Placement of different incisions for approach to the septum.

If the flap is raised at the correct plane, minimal to no bleeding is encountered. The extent of the flap elevation depends on the plan of surgery. The flap can be raised as far cephalically as possible to have access to the perpendicular plate of ethmoid for harvesting bony grafts. Often it is easier to raise the flap anteriorly as far cephalically as possible and then to change direction more posteriorly and raise the flap from cephalic position caudally (i.e. back to front) by the help of a Pennington septum elevator (**Figure 103.5**).

When the bony osseocartilaginous junction between the quadrilateral cartilage and the bony septum is reached, this junction is disarticulated to gain access to the opposite side of the bony septum. Care must be taken not to perforate the mucosa on the other side when raising the mucosal flap from the opposite side of the bony septum. Often the disarticulation is not enough to allow the cartilaginous septum to return to midline and a sliver of bone or cartilage needs to be removed. The excision should be planned carefully to remove the bony or cartilaginous pieces as usable grafts rather than excising them piecemeal. Disarticulation of the quadrilateral cartilage from the maxillary crest is required to allow the septum to move to midline; often a sliver of bone or cartilage needs to be removed. The 1 cm of bony-cartilaginous junction at the L-strut is left undisturbed if possible but often this area requires special attention.

If access is required to the floor of the nasal cavity then an extended hemitransfixion is applied (**Figure 103.4**).

This would allow raising a tunnel underneath the septal spur which reduces the chance of mucosal tear over the spur (**Figure 103.6**). Raising the flap over a spetal spur can be challenging as the perichondrial fibres of the cartilaginous septum and the periosteal fibres of the maxillary crest are interwoven. To reduce the chance of mucosal tear, two techniques can be employed.

BACK TO FRONT TECHNIQUE (CEPHALAD TO CAUDAL)

In this technique, the flap is raised more anteriorly at the caudal septum and raised towards the cephalic position; the direction of dissection is then moved posteriorly and the flap is raised from the cephalic position caudally. This way the plane of dissection is at the correct subperiosteal level initially and then continues at the subperichondrial level reducing the chance of mucosal tear.

FRONT TO BACK TECHNIQUE

In this technique, the mucoperichondrial flap is raised over the quadrilateral cartilage and the bony septum; this constitutes the anterior tunnel over the spur. Then another subperiosteal tunnel is raised posterior to the septal spur which constitutes the posterior tunnel (**Figure 103.6**). The mucosa left attached to the most prominent part of

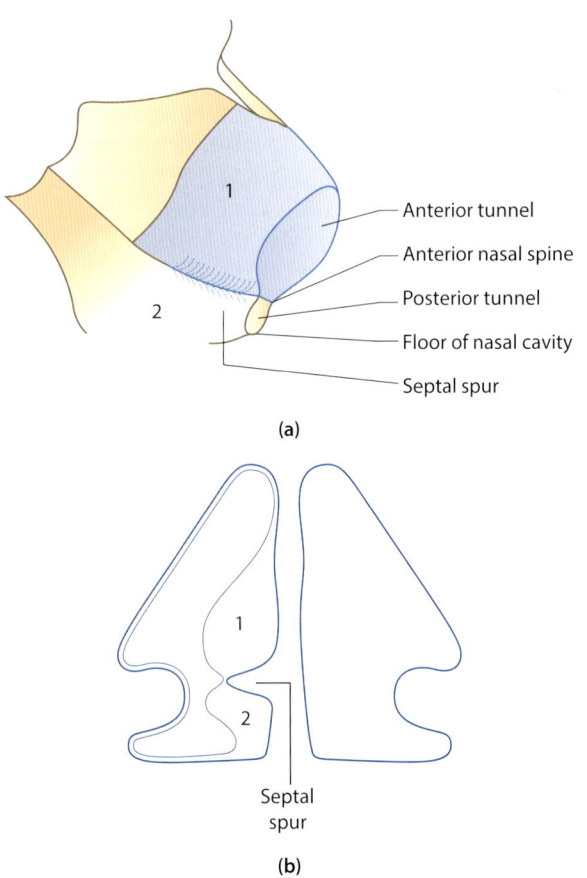

Figure 103.6 Anterior **(1)** and posterior **(2)** tunnels are raised to reduce the chance of mucosal tear over the septal spur.

Pennington Septum Elevator, Double-Ended

Catalog#	Description	Length	Width 1	Width 2
20–246*	Right and left	8-1/4″ (210 mm)	4 mm	4.5 mm

*Miltex® Brand

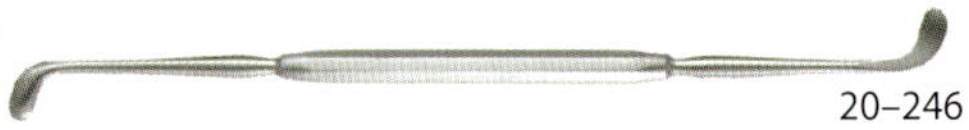

20–246

Figure 103.5 Pennington septum elevator.

spur is then addressed by sharp dissection without the tension of the mucosa on either side.

SEPTOPLASTY TECHNIQUES

In septoplasty, the attention is more on reconstruction rather than excision. The excision alone can be performed as SMR on the body of the septum but deviations of the L-strut require special reconstructive techniques.[4]

The deviated septum can be addressed by 1) Cutting techniques, 2) Grafting techniques, 3) Suturing techniques, and 4) Relocating techniques. The techniques can be used alone or in combination.

The surgical techniques described here are not exhaustive; the techniques and the choice of equipment and sutures are those of the senior author's (SA) who has found them reliable and reproducible.

CUTTING TECHNIQUES

Scoring of the septal cartilage on the concave side allows the septum to become straight, eliminating the deviation. The septum will be kept in position by the scar tissue in grooves created by scoring on the concave side; therefore, the septum should be kept in position, free of any tension until the scar tissue is set in place. This technique is not wholly reliable as under-scoring or over-scoring can result in unsatisfactory results. Also, if the flap is only raised on the concave side, the result of warping might be delayed due to the effects of attached perichondrium on the other side. For these reasons, it will be more predictable if the scored segment is splinted against a batten graft. In S-shaped septal deformities, the scoring needs to be done on the concave segments on both sides; hence the need for raising bilateral mucoperichondrial flaps. If the septum is fractured, the fractured line needs to be weakened by scoring or cutting through to allow the septum to return to midline; in this instance the concomitant grafting technique (splinting) is recommended.

Caudal septal deviation or dislocation is often addressed by excising the excess cartilage at the caudal arm of the L-strut. In the swinging door technique, an appropriate amount of caudal L-strut is excised to allow the septum to return to the midline.[5] The septum then needs to be secured to the midline again; this can be achieved by suturing the septum back to the anterior nasal spine or its periosteum. To apply sutures to the anterior nasal spine, a hole is made in the bone using a strong hypodermic needle or using a drill with a Fissure burr. The septum is then secured in place with 4×0 PDS sutures. Scoring technique is used to correct the convexity but the septum is splinted with a graft in order to avoid unsatisfactory results due to under-scoring or over-scoring (**Figure 103.7**).

Often the deviation at the dorsal L-strut of the quadrilateral cartilage is because of deviation of the bony attachment to the perpendicular plate of ethmoid. In these cases, the osseocartilaginous junction needs to be disarticulated all the way through (and sometimes encroaching into the last 1–1.5 cm). Traditional teaching warns us of septal collapse if this segment is disturbed; however this is simply not true. The quadrilateral cartilage of the septum is attached to the upper lateral cartilages and as long as this attachment and the attachment of the upper lateral cartilages to the nasal bones are intact and the bones are secure and stable, the septum will not collapse. If the bony cartilaginous junction at the dorsal L-strut needs to be disarticulated fully, it should be clearly documented in the operative notes for future operations.

GRAFTING TECHNIQUES

Often the deviated septum can be kept in a straight line if it is splinted against a graft. Both septal cartilage and septal bone (from perpendicular plate of ethmoid or from vomer) can be used for this purpose. The perpendicular plate of ethmoid is stronger and thinner compared to the septal cartilage.[6,7] The technique involves harvesting a suitable piece of perpendicular plate of ethmoid which is then thinned down using a large diamond burr (e.g. 5 mm diamond burr). The graft is then perforated using a Fissure burr and it is splinted against the concave side of the septum (**Figure 103.8**). Care must be taken to position the bony strut a few millimetres from the septal edge so that it is not felt by the patient and it does not cause obstruction for dorsal reconstruction (e.g. spreader grafts). Often the septum is scored to

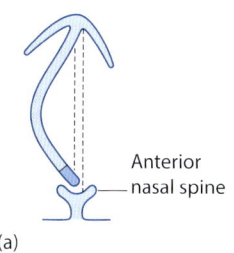
(a) Excess septal length in deviated position

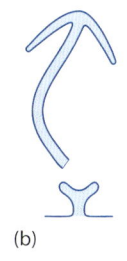
(b) Excess septum excised

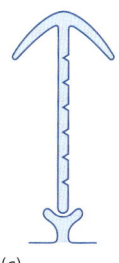
(c) Scoring, straightening and lengthening of the septum

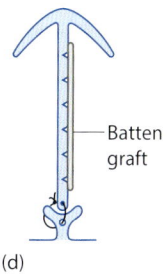
(d) Septum fixed to anterior nasal spine

Figure 103.7 Swinging door technique is a reliable method in dealing with anterior septal deviations: **(a)** Septal convexity to the right has resulted in excess caudal septal length, **(b)** The excess length of the septum is excised, **(c)** The height of septum is restored after scoring of the concave side, **(d)** The weakened septum is splinted against a batten graft and secured to the midline.

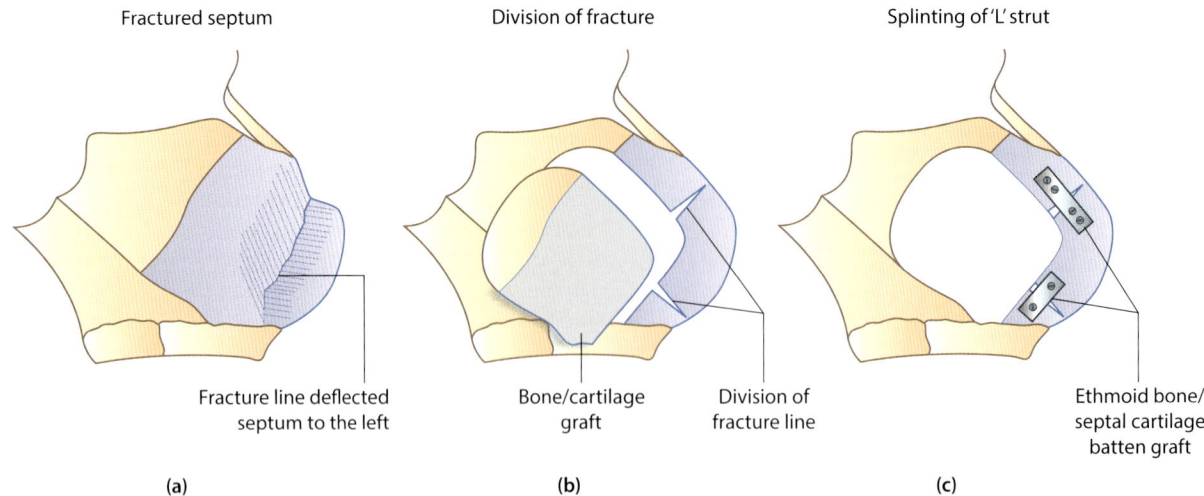

Figure 103.8 Septal bony grafts form the perpendicular plate of ethmoid are used to splint the deviated or fractured parts of the cartilaginous septum: **(a)** Left septal deviation with a vertical fracture line is demonstrated, **(b)** The graft is harvested from the body of septum and the fracture line on the L-strut is cut through and divided, **(c)** The septum is splinted with an ethmoid bone graft.

make it more pliable to conform to the straight ethmoid bone. A fine absorbable or non-absorbable suture is used to secure the graft to the septum (e.g. 5 × 0 PDS®). This technique is more reliable than scoring alone as it eliminates the chance of residual deviation or over-correction due to underscoring or overscoring. A graft made from the septal bone can cause rigidity to the caudal septum; a side effect less noticeable if the batten graft is fashioned from the cartilaginous septum.

The deviation of the dorsal L-strut can be corrected by spreader grafts too. The concave part of the dorsal septum is scored to weaken the septum and to allow it to return to the midline; it is then splinted by spreader grafts and secured in place by sutures (e.g. 5 × 0 PDS®). For this particular technique, external approach provides better access of visualization however spreader grafts can be inserted through endonasal approach too.

SUTURING TECHNIQUES

A mattress suture can be used to control the septal curvature.[8] In this technique, the septum is first scored (preferably underscored) just enough to make it pliable so it can be shaped and kept in shape by fine sutures. The entrance and exit sutures are placed on the convex side and the knot is incrementally tightened until the desired position and shape is achieved. A fine non-absorbable suture (e.g. 5 × 0 Prolene®) is used for this purpose and bilateral mucoperichondrial flaps are raised so that the suture is covered by the septal mucosa.

RELOCATING TECHNIQUES

These techniques are used when the septum is dislocated off the midline and it only requires reinsertion onto the maxillary crest. The septum needs to be secured in its midline position and this is achieved by suturing the septum either onto the periosteum of the anterior nasal spine or to the actual bone by drilling a hole onto it. Fine absorbable or non-absorbable sutures can be used for this purpose. At times other surgical techniques such as scoring and grafting are required to keep the septum in midline.

Often a deviated caudal septum can be improved by door-stop technique where the septal cartilage is dissected free along the maxillary crest and is relocated over the nasal spine which acts as a door stop and secures the caudal septum in a straighter position.[9]

SPECIAL SEPTOPLASTY CONSIDERATIONS

There are special cases related to septoplasty which deserve to be discussed separately.

Endoscopic septoplasty

This technique can be used to improve visualization particularly of more cephalic septal deformities. It also allows minimal access dissection to reach isolated deviated parts of the septum (more relevant in revision cases). Endoscopic septoplasty can be used concomitantly along with sinus surgery. It is also an effective teaching tool.[10]

External approach septoplasty

Most septoplasty techniques can be performed through the endonasal approach; in certain situations especially where the dorsal L-strut deformity is concerned, the external approach septoplasty can improve surgical access. External septorhinoplasty is also favourable in complex septal reconstructive cases such as extracorporeal septoplasty.

Extracorporeal septoplasty

In cases of a severely fractured and deformed septum, the correction and reconstruction can be achieved through an extracorporeal technique.[11] In this method, the septum (both cartilaginous and the bony segment) is excised in one piece as intact as possible. This requires detachment of the cartilaginous septum from upper lateral cartilages and its attachment to the maxillary crest posteriorly. The septum is then measured and a template is made to represent the new septum. Now two different techniques can be employed:

1. **Re-orientation**: The new L-strut is harvested from a straight section of the excised septum and it is re-inserted in place.
2. **Reconstruction**: The septum is reconstructed by a variety of techniques (as described before) and then reinserted in its place. In cases of fractured septum, the fracture line is cut through or weakened to straighten the septum and then the septum is splinted against a graft as previously described. In cases where the septum is broken into many pieces, the segments of septum are splinted against a sheet of thinned down perpendicular plate of ethmoid or a PDS sheet (like a jigsaw puzzle). A fine absorbable or non-absorbable suture (e.g. 5x0 PDS®) is used to secure the pieces of septum to the ethmoid bone graft or the PDS sheet.

The neo-septum is then reinserted into its position. A Fissure burr is used to make a groove onto the maxillary crest for the septum to rest on. A hole is also made onto the anterior nasal spine so that the septum is secured caudally (e.g. 4×0 PDS®). The second point of fixation is to the upper lateral cartilages (e.g. 5×0 Prolene® or PDS). For further security, the neo-septum can be secured to the nasal bones at the K-stone area.

Paediatric septoplasty

There remains controversy about the optimal age and extent of septal surgery in the paediatric population. However, studies have demonstrated that septal surgery performed in children as young as 6 years old provides long-term satisfactory outcomes.[12, 13] Delaying operation on children with deformed nasal skeleton and septal deformities can adversely affect nasal and facial growth and it prolongs patients' suffering from nasal blockage.[12]

Surgeons have addressed septal deformity in children with a range of techniques from closed reduction of septal deviation to the extracorporeal technique through an external approach septorhinoplasty.[12, 14]

The most important aspect of surgery is to resect the cartilage conservatively and to avoid disrupting the endochondral ossification plates if possible. Excision should be kept to minimum and any excised segment should be re-inserted after remodelling.[12]

Evidence from cleft rhinoplasty and septal surgery is used by those advocating surgical intervention in earlier years and justifying more extensive surgery, however, it is wise to avoid over-enthusiastic septal surgery in early years especially if the nasal blockage is unilateral delaying the definitive surgery to later teen years and early adulthood.

NASAL VALVE

The nasal valve is the narrowest portion of the nasal airway. Failure to properly address the nasal valve at primary surgery has been the cause of persistent nasal obstruction in a large proportion of failed septoplasties.[15] The nasal valve is the area caudal to the nasal bones and it is unique in two aspects: 1) It contains the narrowest section of the nasal airway (i.e. internal nasal valve), and 2) It contains a mobile collapsible segment (i.e. lateral nasal wall and its contents).

The nasal valve has traditionally been divided into two 3D-areas: 1) Internal nasal valve, and 2) External nasal valve. This division is arbitrary as in reality there is no clear line between them and they are connected to each other through the lateral nasal wall soft tissues (e.g. at the scroll area).

ANATOMY

The described boundaries of nasal valves have not been consistent in the literature. For the purpose of this chapter, we describe each nasal valve with the following three walls (**Figure 103.9**).

Internal valve

- **Medial wall**: septum
- **Lateral wall**: caudal end of the upper lateral cartilage (ULC), anterior part of the inferior turbinate
- **Nasal floor**: floor of the bony aperture.

External valve

- **Medial wall**: septum, columella
- **Lateral wall**: lateral crus of the lower lateral cartilage (LLC), fibrofatty alar lobule
- **Nasal floor**: nasal sill.

The lateral nasal wall weak triangle contains the sesamoid cartilages and lies between the defined boundaries of the two valves forming part of their lateral walls. There is no universal term for this part of the nasal wall and different terms have been used interchangeably (e.g. weak lateral triangle, external lateral triangle).

Nasal valve angle refers to the angle between the caudal edge of the ULC and the septum, and it is measured at 10–15 degrees in Caucasian Leptorrhine noses (i.e. long narrow noses mostly seen in white individuals as opposed

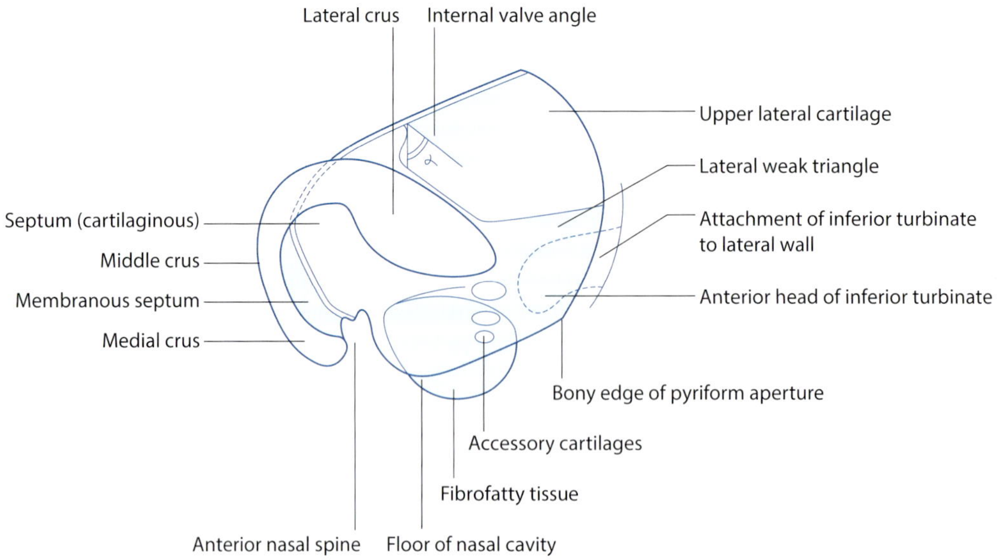

Figure 103.9 The elements incorporated in the nasal valve walls are demonstrated.

to the flat broad Platyrrhine noses seen in the black population). More acute internal nasal valve angles can be associated with nasal blockage and result in dynamic external valve collapse.

AETIOLOGY

The obstruction at the nasal valve can occur due to:

- **Static narrowing**: the nasal airway is narrowed or blocked secondary to deformed anatomy (e.g. congenital, developmental, traumatic or iatrogenic).
- **Dynamic collapse**: in this situation, the nasal airway is patent at rest and in expiration but the lateral wall collapses due to increased intra luminal negative pressure during inspiration. Dynamic collapse follows Poiseuille's principle and the Venturi effect (See Volume 2, Chapter 28) and the surgeon needs to understand the interplay between the nasal airflow, nasal wall resistance and the cross-sectional area of the nasal valve. To address the dynamic collapse, the surgeon needs to increase the cross-sectional area of the nasal airway on the collapsing side and/or strengthen the weakened lateral nasal wall. Also, increasing the airflow on the opposite side will help reduce the excessive flow on the collapsing side, improving the dynamic collapse.

Anatomical narrowing of the nasal valve is caused by the elements in the nasal valve walls.

Medial wall

1. **Septum**: anterior septal deviation or caudal dislocation can narrow the nasal valve area.
2. **Columella**: widened columella is caused by prominent footplates or prominent soft tissue (e.g. depressor septi nasi muscle). Asymmetry, dislocation and deviation of the footplate can narrow the external nasal valve.

Lateral wall

1. **ULC**: anatomical narrowing of the internal valve angle, sequela of lateral osteotomy (e.g. pinched bony nose and medialized ULC).
2. **Lateral crus of LLC**: Its configuration and alignment (e.g. cephalic position) can predispose to nasal obstruction.
3. **Fibrofatty tissue (alar lobule and lateral nasal wall weak triangle)**: Its medialization usually follows weakened or medialized cartilaginous support (e.g. aggressive cephalic trimming, facial palsy).
4. **Inferior turbinate**: Mucosal swelling or bony prominence.

Nasal floor

1. **Soft tissue stenosis**: Developmental or iatrogenic (i.e. secondary to alar base surgery)
2. Bony aperture stenosis is a rare condition but it can be corrected surgically.

DIAGNOSIS

A thorough nasal examination is essential in diagnosing the cause of nasal blockage. Attention to nasal septal deformity as well as the nasal valve area is paramount. In many cases of dynamic external valve collapse, the internal valve is the culprit.

Misting of the examination mirror or a metal tongue spatula on nasal expiration does not equate with a patent nasal airway as it is perceived by the patient. In fact, lack of misting on the spatula test is a more reliable method to demonstrate nasal blockage; in these cases if the lack of misting persists despite adequate decongestion, it confirms static structural obstruction. Misting test relies on nasal expiratory flow and it can therefore miss the dynamic collapse which only occurs on inspiration.

A nasal speculum can be used to examine the anterior nasal cavity; however, the nasal airway and the valve area should be examined by an endoscope to assess the anatomy

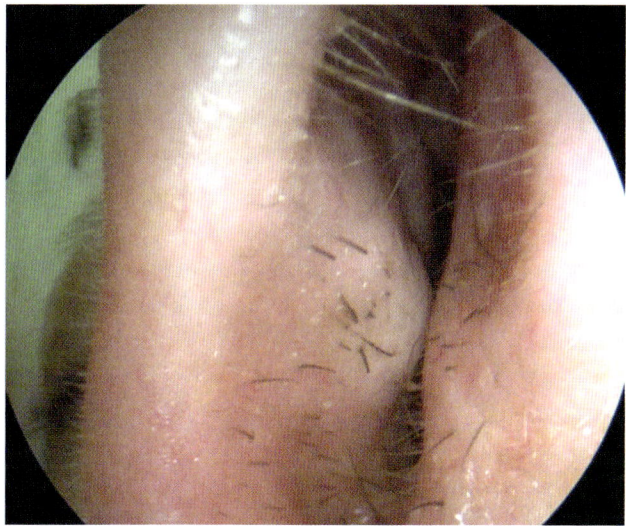

Figure 103.10 **The nasal airway and the nasal valve should be inspected in its neutral position.** Nasal speculum can distort the anatomy and can hide the culprit. (Reprinted with permission from Anari S. Nasal Valve Surgery. *ENT News & Audiology* 2013; **22**(3): 44–6).

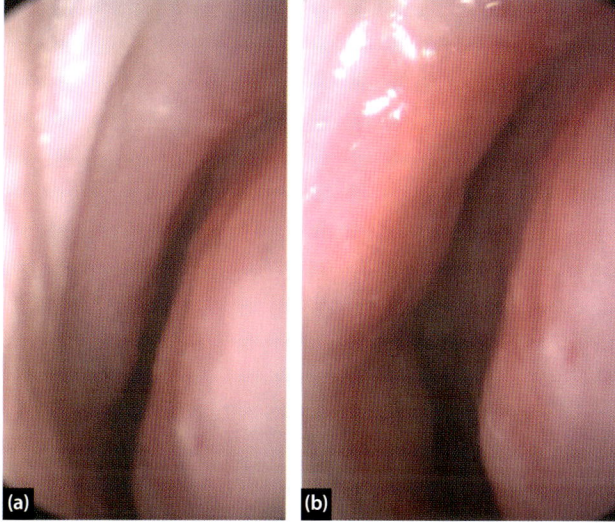

Figure 103.11 **Cottle's manoeuvre is not a specific test for the external valve.** The internal valve is also affected via its attachments to the external valve elements; **(a)** Internal valve angle in resting position, **(b)** Opening of the internal nasal valve angle during Cottle's manoeuvre. (Reprinted with permission from Anari S. Nasal Valve Surgery. *ENT News & Audiology* 2013; **22**(3): 44–6).

in its neutral position. Using a nasal speculum can distort the anatomy and can obscure the culprit (**Figure 103.10**). Nasal airway should be assessed at rest as well as inspiration and expiration; it should also be re-examined after nasal decongestion. Considerable improvement in nasal blockage after decongestion highlights the role of mucosal congestion in nasal obstruction. Treatment of the allergic elements and addressing the inferior turbinates should be part of the management plan in these cases.

Manipulation of the elements on the lateral nasal wall is required to identify the cause of the nasal valve blockage. Cottle's manoeuvre (i.e. gently pulling the cheek laterally) increases the cross-sectional area of the nasal valve however it is not a specific test as it lateralizes elements incorporated in the lateral walls of both the external and the internal nasal valves (**Figure 103.11**). Also, a person with normal nasal airway would generally perceive increased nasal patency with Cottle's manoeuvre. Perhaps a negative Cottle's test is more informative suggesting that the cause of the nasal blockage does not rest in the lateral nasal wall.

A more precise way of examining the lateral nasal wall is by modified Cottle's manoeuvre where a soft-tipped instrument (i.e. Jobson Horne probe) is used to assess the structures internally. The probe can be used to lateralize each element very conservatively to assess patient's perception of nasal patency improvement during inspiration.

TREATMENT

Nasal valve dilators (e.g. Breathe Right® or Nozovent®) (**Figure 103.12**) and nasal steroid medications play a part in the non-surgical management of nasal valve obstruction.

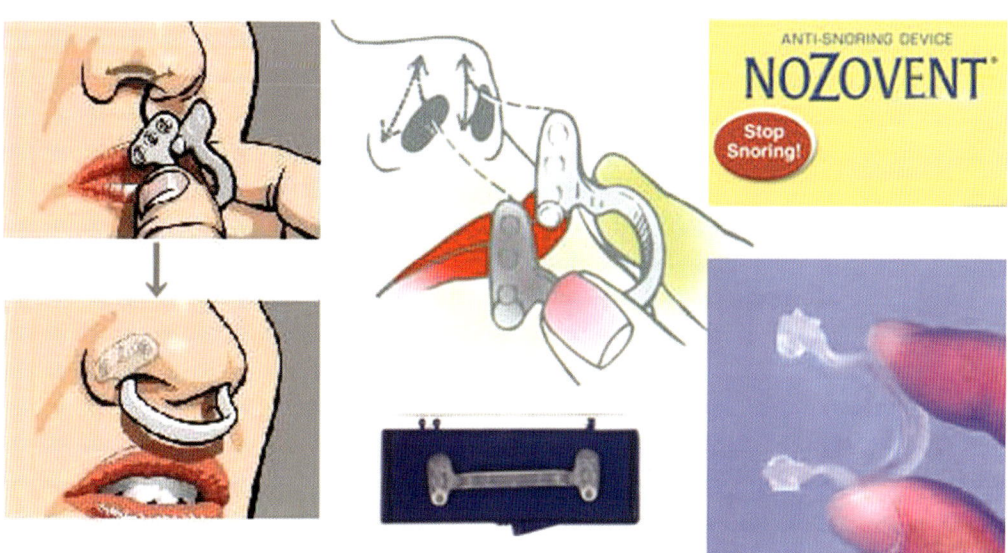

Figure 103.12 Nozovent.

The surgical techniques are divided into: 1) Cutting techniques (incision and excision); 2) Suturing techniques; 3) Grafting techniques; and 4) Relocating techniques.

The following list of surgical techniques is not exhaustive but the senior author has found them to be effective. The techniques are aimed at each of the offending segments.

Septum

The techniques to address the deviated septum have already been described in the previous section of this chapter.

Upper lateral cartilage

CUTTING TECHNIQUES

In cases where the internal nasal valve is narrow, excision of a few millimetres of the caudal ULC can increase the valve angle. This is based on the principle that the angle between the septum and upper lateral cartilage increases when moving cephalad. This can be achieved through external rhinoplasty as well as endonasal approach. If the length of the ULC is reduced, the excess mucosa needs to be trimmed to prevent obstructing the angle.[16]

SUTURING TECHNIQUES

The ULC can be flared using a suture connecting them to each other (**Figure 103.13**). This allows increase in the internal nasal valve angle. The knot needs to be tied incrementally to achieve the beneficial effect but to avoid undesirable aesthetic changes.[17] This technique can be used along with spreader grafts to maximize the benefit.

Suspension sutures can be used to improve the internal valve area (**Figure 103.14**). A non-absorbable suture is used to anchor the ULC to the adjacent bony structures (e.g. orbital rim or frontal process of the maxilla).[18] To improve the efficacy of this technique, the midfacial and nasal soft tissues need to be extensively undermined and the sutures should be placed without tension.

GRAFTING TECHNIQUES

Spreader grafts are used to reconstruct the dorsal 'T' junction between the ULC and septum (**Figure 103.15**). Their use is both for functional and aesthetic purposes although some argue the magnitude of their functional advantage. These grafts can be inserted through the endonasal and external approach.[19]

Butterfly grafts can be taken from the septum or conchal cartilage and they saddle the dorsum to open up the midnasal vault and internal valve. They could have an undesirable aesthetic effect causing the supra-tip fullness. To reduce the supra-tip fullness, a hosting groove can be carved on the septal dorsum.[20]

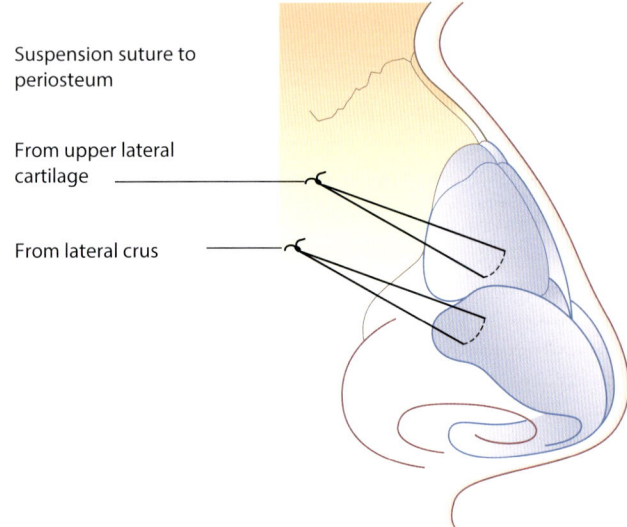

Figure 103.14 Suspension sutures can prevent the collapse of the lateral nasal wall.

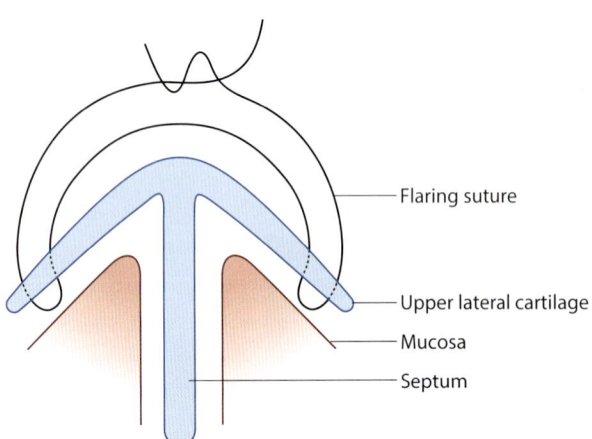

Figure 103.13 Flaring suture is used to splay the upper lateral cartilages and to open up the internal nasal valve angle and the cross sectional area of the internal valve.

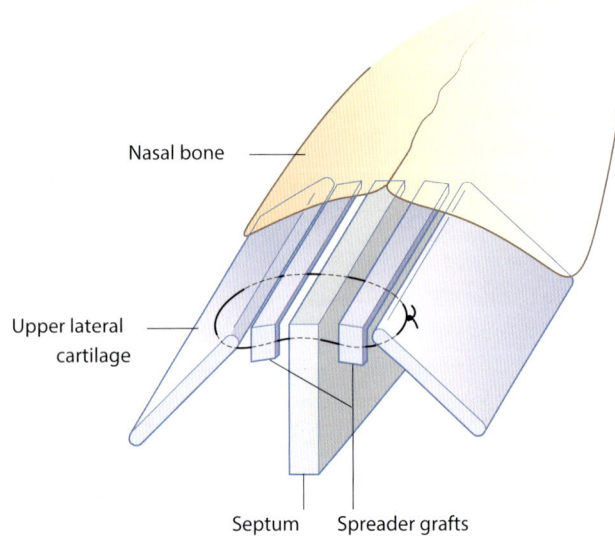

Figure 103.15 Spreader grafts are placed between the upper lateral cartilages and the septum to reconstruct the dorsal septal 'T' segment.

Lateral crus of LLC

CUTTING TECHNIQUES

In cases of nasal tip ptosis (e.g. ageing nose), lateral crus trans-section and overlap (i.e. lateral crural overlay) results in improvement in nasolabial angle and air flow dynamics.[21, 22]

SUTURING TECHNIQUES

Mattress sutures are used to control the lateral crus curvature.[8] Cases of extreme convexity which result in invagination of the crus into the nasal vestibule can be corrected this way (**Figure 103.10**). The domal formation sutures can result in straightening of the lateral crus too.

Spanning sutures have been designed for nasal tip refinement but as they alter the tilt of the lateral crus, they increase support for the nasal side wall too. This is essentially a mattress suture securing the two lateral crura together. This suture is very powerful and it should be used to keep the crura in the desirable position; too much tension on the suture can have adverse effects and could lead to alar retraction.[23]

Alar expansion sutures are essentially mattress sutures designed to splay the lateral crura and improve the valve area. The tension on these sutures should be controlled as they can cause alar retraction.[24]

Lateral crus suspension sutures are used to support the lateral nasal wall (**Figure 103.14**). These are similar in principle and method of execution to suspension sutures used for ULC.[18]

GRAFTING TECHNIQUES

The lateral crus strut graft or alar strut graft is often a septal graft that is secured between the vestibular skin and the defective lateral crus and it may rest over the bony piriform aperture for further stability (**Figure 103.16**).[25] In some cases, a shorter version of the graft (the so-called mini-strut) is inserted underneath the lateral crus to strengthen it and to bring the severely convex or concave lateral crus to a more straightened configuration.

The alar batten graft is usually taken from the septal or conchal cartilage and placed in a subcutaneous pocket over the point of maximum collapse of the lateral nasal wall (**Figure 103.16**). This graft can be positioned cephalad, caudal or on the lateral crus and can extend over the bony piriform aperture for further stability.[26]

Spanning grafts straddle the dorsal septum and they are attached to the lateral crura keeping them in the desired orientation and position. If required, a groove on the dorsal edge of the septum can host the graft preventing supratip fullness.[23]

At times, an extremely convex or concave lateral crus can be completely excised from its bed and reinserted on the opposite side. Also the strip of cephalic trim can be used to splint the remaining lateral crus strip and reduce the excessive curvature; these techniques are described in a variety of names and fashions (e.g. turn-in flap, turn-over grafts, flip-flop grafts etc.).

RELOCATING TECHNIQUES

A cephalically-positioned lateral crus can lead to reduced support for the lateral nasal wall which can lead to external valve collapse. Reorientation of the lateral crus can be achieved by elevating the lateral crus from its original bed and reinserting it into a more caudal and posterior position (**Figure 103.17**). The lateral crus is repositioned on its own or with the added structural support of a strut graft usually taken from septum. This technique has been described both through the endonasal and external approach but the latter is technically less challenging.[27]

Fibrofatty tissue

GRAFTING TECHNIQUES

Non-anatomic grafts (such as alar rim grafts or lateral wall grafts) are used to strengthen the collapsible lateral nasal wall (**Figure 103.16**). The grafts should be carved thin enough to cause little aesthetic disfigurement and yet they need to be strong enough to increase lateral nasal wall strength.

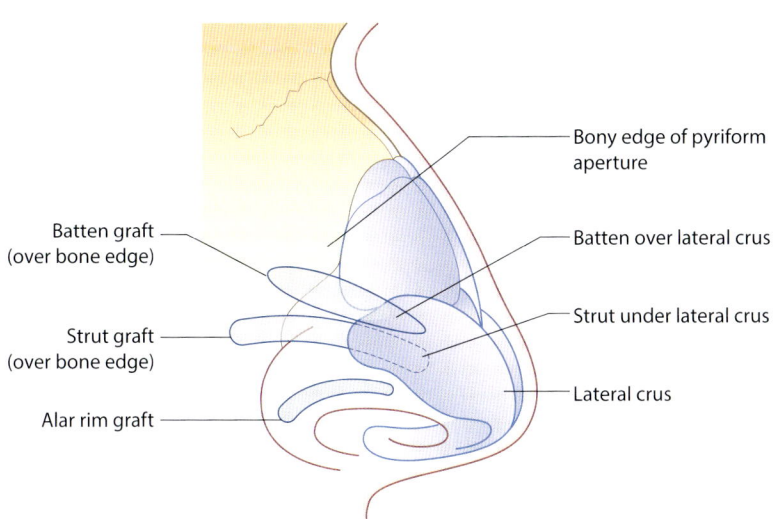

Figure 103.16 Position of alar strut, batten and rim grafts to support the lateral nasal wall from collapse.

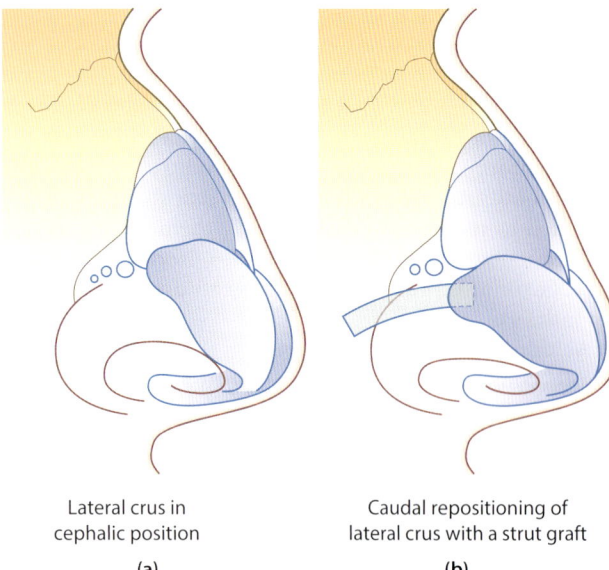

Figure 103.17 Repositioning of the lateral crus: (a) Lateral crus of the lower lateral cartilage is in its cephalic position (i.e. malposition). In this position, there is less support for the lateral nasal wall and the lateral nasal wall is prone to collapse on inspiration, **(b)** the lateral crus is repositioned into its orthotopic position with the help of a lateral crus strut graft. The lateral nasal wall has greater support in this position.

They are usually inserted in tight subcutaneous pockets over the maximum point of nasal wall collapse.

SUTURING TECHNIQUES

Lateral nasal wall suspension sutures are used to improve the narrowing in this segment.[28] Often the sutures are applied to the upper lateral cartilage or the lateral crus of the lower lateral cartilage and as a result the lateral nasal wall lateralizes (**Figure 103.14**). When the sutures are applied to the cartilage rather than the fibrofatty soft tissue, the result seems to last longer.

Inferior turbinates

Inferior turbinate enlargement can be compensatory on the opposite side of nasal obstruction or it can be part of the inflammatory nasal condition (e.g. allergic rhinitis).

The surgical techniques aim to reduce the size of inferior turbinates by reducing the conchal bone or the submucosal expansile venous plexus (See Chapter 105).[29] Cryosurgery, laser cautery, submucous electrocautery, linear mucosal diathermy, microdebridement of the submucosal venous plexus and radiofrequency have been used to address the dynamic mucosal element of the inferior turbinate engorgement. Radiofrequency-assisted turbinate reduction surgery has been suggested to cause minimal disruption to nasal function.[30]

In cases of bony enlargement, the conchal bone is reduced while preserving the mucosa. Turbinate outfracture can improve the nasal airway with minimal trauma to the nasal lining, however the anterior head of the inferior turbinate – which plays an important part in the nasal valve area – is not easily amenable to lateralization.

Nasal sill/vestibule

CUTTING TECHNIQUES

Z-plasty is performed to improve the nasal valve narrowing.[31] This technique is to address the stenosis at the internal valve angle mostly caused by inappropriate septo(rhino)plasty incisions and closure techniques.

GRAFTING TECHNIQUES

Composite skin and cartilage grafts harvested from the pinna concha can be used to improve the stenosis at the internal valve angle or the nasal sill (depending on the source of stenosis).

Columella

Widening of the columella can narrow the nostril size and result in external nasal valve narrowing. Widening of the columella or a protruding footplate can be addressed by excising, relocating or suturing techniques.[32] Grafting techniques (e.g. columella strut graft) can improve the nasal droopy tip and improve nasal airflow dynamics; this is a commonly performed step in treatment of the ageing nose.

DRESSING AND SPLINTS IN NASAL AIRWAY SURGERY

The use of post-operative nasal packing remains a varied practice. Careful dissection and minimal trauma during surgery makes risk of bleeding minimal and obviates the need for nasal packing which would save the patient the discomfort of subsequent nasal pack removal. Septal quilting sutures have demonstrated a greater reduction in post-operative haematoma complications and have improved patient satisfaction in comparison with nasal packing.[33, 34]

Some surgeons use septal splints to prevent adhesions especially when septal mucosal lacerations are present and concomitant turbinate surgery has been performed. Some use septal splints as an extra support for the septum especially when extensive reconstructive surgery has been performed.[35]

Most surgeons protect the outer nasal skeleton after external septoplasty and nasal valve surgery by applying an external splint. Thermoplastic splints or Plaster of Paris can be applied without the need to pinch the nasal skeleton – an action that is best avoided if suturing or grafting techniques of nasal valve surgery have been employed.

COMPLICATIONS

Complications may arise from septal surgery but they are mostly due to poor surgical planning and operative techniques. These include bleeding, infection, saddle deformity, nasal tip depression, septal perforation, adhesion, septal haematoma, septal abscess, sensory changes including upper dental anaesthesia and upper incisors teeth discolouration.[34, 36]

Certain aspects of nasal surgery may not necessarily be considered as complications but more as anticipated side effects; they should be discussed with patients (e.g. rigidity of the septum and nose after certain techniques especially bone grafting techniques; aesthetic changes associated with nasal valve surgery).

CONCLUSION

Septum and nasal valve both play important parts in the nasal airway. The result of nasal airway surgery is dependent on the correct diagnosis and execution of the relevant techniques related to the offending segment of the nasal airway.

The patient must also be informed that almost all of the above nasal valve techniques will result in some aesthetic change to their nose. The option of surgical treatment should be discussed with this side effect in mind. When patients decline major nasal valve surgery which could result in noticeable aesthetic changes, a combination of septal surgery, turbinate surgery and minor nasal valve surgery can achieve comparable results with minimal aesthetic changes.[37]

BEST CLINICAL PRACTICE

- ✓ In most cases of septal deviation, the septal L-strut is involved. SMR is not effective in these cases as it cannot address the caudal and dorsal struts; septoplasty techniques are needed.
- ✓ In certain situations, especially where the dorsal L-strut deformity is concerned, external approach septoplasty can improve surgical access.
- ✓ Certain aspects of nasal surgery may not necessarily be considered as complications but more as anticipated side effects.
- ✓ Nasal valve dilators (e.g. Breathe Right® or Nozovent® (Figure 103.12) and nasal steroid medications play a part in the non-surgical management of nasal valve obstruction.
- ✓ The most important aspect of paediatric septal surgery is to resect the cartilage conservatively and to avoid disrupting the endochondral ossification plates.
- ✓ In cases of severely fractured and deformed septum, the correction and reconstruction can be achieved through an open approach septorhinoplasty with the septum *in situ* or through extracorporeal techniques.[11]

FUTURE RESEARCH

Studies on nasal airway surgery are often observational or retrospective. Variations in the causes of nasal obstruction, the surgical procedures performed and the outcome measures used to measure the change have added to the complexity of analyzing the evidence. It is often impossible to analyze the effects of one particular procedure in a study as often multiple procedures are used simultaneously in nasal airway surgery.

Nasal mucosal swelling, whether in its physiological form (i.e. nasal cycle) or in its pathological form (i.e. rhinitis), adds to the complexity of measuring the effects of surgical intervention. The same problem exists when employing objective measures such as rhinomanometry to measure the effect. There is a need for an objective tool to measure the nasal airway resistance and to identify the level of obstruction taking into account the nasal airflow. This tool should be able to measure nasal flow and resistance during nasal breathing to be able to detect the dynamic elements of nasal obstruction.

The subjective elements of nasal obstruction add to the complexity of analyzing the effects of surgical interventions as the lack of correlation between the subjective and the objective tools have been shown before in the literature.

Like other aspects of surgical practice, it would be very difficult and often unethical to conduct randomized controlled trials to produce the high level evidence for nasal airway surgery.

Future studies on surgical techniques need to have improved designs and their cohort needs to be comparable. Ideally only one surgical procedure needs to be performed so the effect can be measured solely on that particular procedure. Like any surgical study, the operator dependant factors play a part in the results and this needs to be taken into account when designing any study.

Tissue engineering is a rapidly developing field and further advances in this field would be very much welcomed by rhinoplasty surgeons who are always in need of cartilage for nasal support and nasal valve surgery.

KEY EVIDENCE

Several studies demonstrate a consistent benefit for nasal valve repair. Nasal airway surgery benefits are measured by patient-reported outcome measures (PROM) which are more clinically relevant than objective measures.

KEY POINTS

- Nasal airway surgery requires attention to the nasal septum as well as nasal valve areas.
- Correct diagnosis is essential in choosing the correct surgical technique.
- The patient's nasal airway should be examined in the neutral position using an endoscope.
- The nasal expiratory misting test can miss the dynamic elements of nasal obstruction.
- The nasal speculum can distort the anatomy and can hide the culprit.
- Cottle's manoeuvre is not a specific test for the external nasal valve.
- The nasal airway should be examined before and after topical decongestion to assess the effect of mucosal swelling on it.
- Most nasal valve procedures will have an aesthetic effect and the patient should be warned of these prior to the operation.
- Patient-reported outcome measures appear to be more clinically relevant than the objective measures.
- Nasal obstruction can be caused by septal deflection which can be developmental or secondary to trauma.
- In septoplasty, the attention is more on reconstruction rather than excision.
- Complications may arise from septal surgery but they are mostly due to poor surgical planning and operative techniques.
- There remains controversy about the optimal age and extent of septal surgery in the paediatric population.

REFERENCES

1. Sulsenti G, Palma P. Tailored nasal surgery for normalization of nasal resistance. *Facial Plast Surg* 1996; **12**(4): 333–45.
2. André RF, Vuyk HD, Ahmed A, et al. Correlation between subjective and objective evaluation of the nasal airway: a systematic review of the highest level of evidence. *Clin Otolaryngol* 2009; **34**: 518–25.
3. Stewart MG, Witsell DL, Smith TL, et al. Development and validation of the Nasal Obstruction Symptom Evaluation (NOSE) scale. *Otolaryngol Head Neck Surg* 2004; **130**(2): 157–63.
4. Becker DG. Septoplasty and turbinate surgery. *Aesthet Surg J* 2003; **23**(5): 393–403.
5. Wright WK. Principles of nasal septum reconstruction. *Trans Am Acad Ophthalmol Otolaryngol* 1969; **73**(2): 252–5.
6. Foda HM. The role of septal surgery in management of the deviated nose. *Plast Reconstr Surg* 2005; **115**(2): 406–15.
7. Metzinger SE, Boyce RG, Rigby PL, et al. Ethmoid bone sandwich grafting for caudal septal defects. *Arch Otolaryngol Head Neck Surg* 1994; **120**(10): 1121–5.
8. Gruber RP, Nahai F, Bogdan MA, Friedman GD. Changing the convexity and concavity of nasal cartilages and cartilage grafts with horizontal mattress sutures: part II. Clinical results. *Plast Reconstr Surg* 2005; **115**(2): 595–606.
9. Pastorek NJ, Becker DG. Treating the caudal septal deflection. *Arch Facial Plast Surg* 2000; **2**(3): 217–20.
10. Hwang PH, McLaughlin RB, Lanza DC, Kennedy DW. Endoscopic septoplasty: indications, technique, and results. *Otolaryngol Head Neck Surg* 1999; **120**(5): 678–82.
11. Gubisch W. Extracorporeal septoplasty for the markedly deviated septum. *Arch Facial Plast Surg* 2005; **7**(4): 218–26.
12. Lawrence R. Pediatric septoplasy: a review of the literature. *Int J Pediatr Otorhinolaryngol* 2012; **76**(8): 1078–81.
13. Tasca I, Compadretti GC. Nasal growth after pediatric septoplasty at long-term follow-up *Am J Rhinol Allergy* 2011; **25**(1): e7–12
14. Christophel JJ, Gross CW. Pediatric septoplasty. *Otolaryngol Clin North Am* 2009; **42**(2): 287–94.
15. Becker SS, Dobratz EJ, Stowell N, et al. Revision septoplasty: review of sources of persistent nasal obstruction. *Am J Rhinol* 2008; **22**(4): 440–4.
16. Schulte DL, Sherris DA, Kern EB. M-Plasty correction of nasal valve obstruction. *Facial Plast Surg Clin North Am* 1999; **7**(3): 405–9.
17. Park SS. The flaring suture to augment the repair of the dysfunctional nasal valve. *Plast Reconstr Surg* 1998; **101**(4): 1120–2.
18. Roofe SB, Most SP. Placement of a lateral nasal suspension suture via an external rhinoplasty approach. *Arch Facial Plast Surg* 2007; **9**(3): 214–16.
19. Sheen JH. Spreader graft: a method of reconstructing the roof of the middle nasal vault following rhinoplasty. *Plast Reconstr Surg* 1984; **73**(2): 230–9.
20. Clark JM, Cook TA. The 'butterfly' graft in functional secondary rhinoplasty. *Laryngoscope* 2002; **112**(11): 1917–25.
21. Rohrich RJ, Hollier LH. Rhinoplasty with advancing age: characteristics and management. *Clin Plast Surg* 1996; **23**(2): 281–96.
22. Kridel RW, Konior RJ. Controlled nasal tip rotation via the lateral crural overlay technique. *Arch Otolaryngol Head Neck Surg* 1991; **117**(4): 411–15.
23. Tebbetts JB. Shaping and positioning the nasal tip without structural disruption: a new, systematic approach. *Plast Reconstr Surg* 1994; **94**(1): 61–77.
24. Mendelsohn MS, Golchin K. Alar expansion and reinforcement: a new technique to manage nasal valve collapse. *Arch Facial Plast Surg* 2006; **8**(5): 293–9.
25. Gunter JP, Friedman RM. Lateral crural strut graft: technique and clinical applications in rhinoplasty. *Plast Reconstr Surg* 1997; **99**(4): 943–52.
26. Toriumi DM, Josen J, Weinberger M, Tardy ME. Use of alar batten grafts for correction of nasal valve collapse. *Arch Otolaryngol Head Neck Surg* 1997; **123**(8): 802–8.
27. Hamra ST. Repositioning the lateral alar crus. *Plast Reconstr Surg* 1993; **92**(7): 1244–53.
28. Lee DS, Glasgold AI. Correction of nasal valve stenosis with lateral suture suspension. *Arch Facial Plast Surg* 2001; **3**(4): 237–40.
29. Chhabra N, Houser SM. The surgical management of allergic rhinitis. *Otolaryngol Clin North Am* 2011; **44**(3): 779–95.
30. Garzaro M, Landolfo V, Pezzoli M, et al. Radiofrequency volume turbinate reduction versus partial turbinectomy: clinical and histological features. *Am J Rhinol Allergy* 2012; **26**(4): 321–5.
31. Dutton JM, Neidich MJ. Intranasal Z-plasty for internal nasal valve collapse. *Arch Facial Plast Surg* 2008; **10**(3): 164–8.
32. Fischer H, Gubisch W. Nasal valves-importance and surgical procedures. *Facial Plast Surg* 2006; **22**(4): 266–80.
33. Certal V, Silva H, Santos T, et al. Transseptal suturing technique in septoplasty: a systematic review and meta-analysis. *Rhinology* 2012; **50**(3): 236–45.
34. Quinn JG, Bonaparte JP, Kilty SJ. Postoperative management in the prevention of complications after septoplasty: a systematic review. *Laryngoscope* 2013; **123**(6): 1328–33.
35. Jung YG, Hong JW, Eun YG, Kim MG. Objective usefulness of thin silastic septal splints after septal surgery. *Am J Rhinol Allergy* 2011; **25**(3): 182–5.
36. Bloom JD, Kaplan SE, Bleier BS, Goldstein SA. Septoplasty complications: avoidance and management. *Otolaryngol Clin North Am* 2009; **42**(3): 463–81.
37. Anari S, El Badawey MR. Triple-procedure technique in internal nasal valve surgery. *Eur J Plast Surg* 2012; **35**(7): 501–6.

NASAL SEPTAL PERFORATIONS

Charles East and Kevin Kulendra

Introduction 1149	Prevention 1152
Symptomatology 1149	Non-surgical 1152
Clinical assessment 1150	Obturation 1152
Special investigations 1151	Surgical 1152
Prevalence of septal perforations 1151	Surgical repair of septal perforations 1152
Management 1152	References 1155

SEARCH STRATEGY

Data in this chapter may be updated by a Medline search restricted to English papers using the keywords: septum, perforation, and reconstruction from a medline search as well as textbooks of otolaryngology published in English literature and local Audits.

INTRODUCTION

Definition: through and through defect or defects of the nasal septum. The exact prevalence of septal perforations is unknown as many perforations are asymptomatic, but in a general otolaryngology practice the clinician will encounter several patients with septal holes each year. Younger and Blokmanis[1] cite an incidence of just over 1%, which makes the condition relatively common. It must be remembered that racial traditions and fashion dictate that perforations in various parts of the body are a part of normal life and the anterior nasal septum is no exception. The majority of perforations involve the anterior quadrilateral cartilage of the septum. Kuriloff[2] has provided an extensive list of the local and systemic causes (**Table 104.1**). Currently, the most common cause of perforation in the UK is probably local trauma, although in a significant percentage, no clear history exists attracting the label of 'idiopathic'. The trauma is frequently self-induced or iatrogenic following surgery to the nasal septum or nasal instrumentation. Injuries to the cartilagenous skeleton of the nose may result in perforation through a compound fracture of the quadrilateral cartilage in the absence of any external deformity. Recreational drugs, for example crack or cocaine snorted nasally, are becoming increasingly common as a cause of septal necrosis.[3] The prevalence of chronic specific infections producing perforations is small, but there are a significant number of inflammatory conditions which should be excluded, particularly if the history does not give an easy clue to the aetiology.

SYMPTOMATOLOGY

The principle symptoms associated with perforations are crusting, epistaxis and whistling. Other symptoms include a feeling of dryness, emptiness in the nose or a general feeling of discomfort. In a series of 69 septal perforations, Brain[4] showed that 62.4% were completely free from any symptoms. Size and position of the hole had a direct bearing on the presence of symptoms. Anterior perforations and large perforations where the anterior margin is in front of the nasal valve appear to be the most troublesome. This probably relates to the relatively slow mucociliary clearance from the anterior septum, low humidity in the anterior nares compared to controls[5] and the loss of mucosa, all contributing to dryness and crusting. The accumulation of large crusts around the margin of the perforation produces a sensation of blockage. With large stable perforations, patients may feel the nose is empty or complain of 'blockage', even when nasal airflow is greater than average. These features may be due to turbulence of airflow in the nasal vestibule, although there is little evidence to support this. Huge perforations produce a common nasal cavity resulting in rhinolalia and an inability to

TABLE 104.1 Aetiologies of nasal septal perforations				
Traumatic causes	**Surface irritants**	**Infections**	**Neoplastic**	**Inflammatory**
Nasal surgery	Cocaine insufflation	Syphilis	Melanoma	Sarcoidosis
Nose picking	Cocaine adulterants	Typhoid	Adenocarcinoma	Crohn's disease
Septal cauterization (bilateral)	Heroin inhalation	Diptheria	Squamous cell carcinoma	Dermatomyositis
Nasal packing for epistaxis	Decongestant nasal sprays Intra-nasal corticosteroids	Tuberculosis	Metastatic carcinoma	Rheumatoid arthritis
Septal hematoma/abscess	Lime, cement, glass, salt, dust	Rhinoscleroma	Lymphoma	Relapsing polychondritis
Cryosurgery	Tar and pitch	Lepromatous leprosy		Granulomatosis with polyangiitis (GPA)
Intubation (nasogastric/tracheal)	Fumes (chromic/sulfuric acid)	Leishmaniasis		Systemic lupus erythematosus
Desiccation (ozena, deviated septum)	Arsenicals, mercurials	Mucor		
Radiation	Calcium nitrate, cyanide	Rhinosporidiosis		
Stab and gunshot wounds	Phosphorus, sodium carbonate	Alternaria		
Foreign bodies (button batteries)	Copper-smelting fumes	Actinomycosis		
		Aspergillosis		
		Histoplasmosis		
		Cryptococcosis		
		Coccidioidomycosis		
		Paracoccidioidomycosis		
		Candidiasis		

clear secretions.[2] Nasal mucosal cooling is associated with increased sensation of patency but this does not correlate with clinical observation in patients with nasal perforations whose intra-nasal temperature rises after successful closure.[5]

Inflammation in the perforation margin leads to recurrent epistaxes, often triggered when the crust separates or is removed. Epistaxis can be quite significant from the sphenopalatine vessels. Large areas of mucosal deficit, particularly where there is cartilage exposure, prevent normal mucus clearance, contributing to localized infection and more inflammation. The local inflammation in the nose is often perceived as a generalized sense of discomfort, felt internally and over the nasal bridge. Over time, necrosis of septal cartilage will lead to enlargement of the hole in 'active perforations', sometimes to such a size that surgical closure is impossible.

CLINICAL ASSESSMENT

A full history is necessary when investigating septal perforations to cover the wide range of aetiologies. Principally, it is important to identify episodes of nasal trauma, cautery or surgery and, in particular, a history of substance abuse. Though patients may often deny it, aggressive nasal self-toilet with digital trauma or tissues will convert an inflamed mucous membrane to an ischaemic crusty area which ulcerates – the so-called 'pick ulcer'. Continued attempts to remove the crust invariably lead to cartilage exposure, cartilagenous necrosis and subsequent perforation.

An overall assessment of the external and internal nasal skeleton should be made together with nasal endoscopy. Endoscopy is the best method to assess the margins and state of the residual septum. Measurement of the dimensions of the hole is performed by introducing a small paper ruler into the contralateral airway and reading the scale through the hole. Saddle deformities, deviations of the nose or septum, columella retraction and intra-nasal adhesions are commonly seen and may require reconstructive rhinoplasty techniques to correct if surgery is contemplated. Nasal questionnaires using a linear visual analogue scoring system may be used as a measure of symptom severity. Although not essential in routine clinical practice, they do provide subjective assessment for comparing pre- and post-treatment symptoms and are a basic measure of outcome (**Figure 104.1**). Other outcome measures via validated questionnaire have been used to measure patient benefit from surgical repair.[6]

Nasal septal perforation questionnaire

NAME:

Please mark you own score by marking a line at the appropriate point.

0 = No symptoms, 10 = Worst symptoms.

                                                  1   10

1   Crusts/scabs

2   Nose bleeds

3   Whistling

4   Nasal discomfort

Please mark the appropriate point for your symptoms in Questions 5 and 6

5   My nose feels empty   My nose feels blocked

6   Can clear secretions easily   Can't clear secretions at all

Figure 104.1 Nasal septal perforation questionnaire.

SPECIAL INVESTIGATIONS

Because of the wide range of aetiologies for septal perforation, history-taking is crucial. Any signs of inflammation around a perforation, however, should prompt investigation of other anatomical areas in the head and neck, as well as investigations for systemic inflammatory conditions. Nasal perforations may be the first sign of various granulomatous disorders, including Wegener's granulomatosis, and occur with a variety of collagen disorders including relapsing polychondritis, systemic lupus erythematosus (SLE) and dermatomyositis. Of the infective causes, the clinician is guided by the health of the patient, but tuberculosis and syphilis should be excluded. A full blood count, erythrocyte sedimentation rate (ESR), urea and electrolytes, urine analysis, C-ANCA, treponemal investigations, ACE titres and a chest X-ray, together with a nasal swab, provide an adequate baseline. Other symptoms of inflammation in the respiratory tract, for example cough, middle ear effusions, an arthritis or skin rash, should prompt referral to a clinical immunologist.

There is little evidence that extensive investigations for patients with healed, stable and asymptomatic perforations contribute to a change in the management, particularly where the aetiology is clear. Routine biopsy of septal perforations to exclude vasculitis has been suggested,[6, 7] but biopsy rarely reveals anything other than chronic inflammation and is not usually sufficient for a specific diagnosis. Indeed, biopsy may convert an inactive perforation to an 'active state', resulting in significant enlargement of the hole. The role of routine biopsy in idiopathic perforations has recently been questioned. In two retrospective series, septal biopsy was shown to be non-specific for Wegener's and was only of value in those perforations with an irregular margin which were clinically malignant.[8, 9] It is clear that the diagnosis of Wegener's or its reactivation cannot be reliably inferred from biopsy of the nasal septum alone. Practically, therefore, perforations should be biopsied if there is an unexplained aetiology, with persistent inflammation, or if the perforation is irregular. Specimens should be examined for mycobacteria and fungi, and with immunocytochemistry to exclude a neoplasm.[2]

PREVALENCE OF SEPTAL PERFORATIONS

The prevalence of septal perforations following nasal septal surgery shows wide variation and has been reported as between 1.4% and 25%. The prevalence appears higher after submucous resection operations (17–25%) than the more conservative septoplasty procedures (1.4–5%).[10] The use of nasal splints during septal surgery is known to produce a higher incidence of perforation.[11] Splinting is unnecessary in the majority of routine septal surgery unless established adhesions are being treated. Recent retrospective reports[12] have suggested an association between nasal steroid sprays and the development of nasal perforation. It is known that all steroid sprays can cause inflammation over the caudal septum, by direct irritation or their initial vasoconstrictor activity, particularly if there is a septal deviation which takes the brunt of the spray jet. Patients should be directed to use the spray with the opposite hand to the nostril being treated, minimizing the impact on the septum. Any ulceration after starting steroid spray use should be allowed to heal by withdrawing the medication.

MANAGEMENT

The majority of septal perforations are asymptomatic and require no specific treatment.[4] The more anterior the lesion, the more likely it is to cause symptoms. This probably relates to accessibility by the patient to pick at the nose, but may also be related to fast airflow producing drying in the region of the internal nasal valve. The management can be divided into three groups.

PREVENTION

In a series of 50 perforation repairs at the Royal National Throat, Nose and Ear Hospital, 60% had a previous history of septal surgery. Meticulous attention to technique is required in elevating the mucoperichondrial flaps in the correct plane, particularly avoiding overlapping bilateral mucosal tears. Starting the dissection on the easier (usually the concave) side to raise one intact flap first, and using an autograft of cartilage or ethmoid plate to support any tears, is good practice. The mucoperichondrium over large spurs is often very thin, and tears may be inevitable. However, when the spur is removed, there will be a relative excess of mucosa which can be repaired with absorbable sutures. Quilting sutures in the septum after surgery should be tied loosely to allow for postoperative oedema. The authors have seen perforations caused by individual sutures tied tightly in the septum which resulted in ischaemic necrosis. Septal inflammation or ulceration should be treated by withdrawing the source of the irritation and promotion of healing, for example by eradication of pathogenic bacteria, avoidance of aggressive cleaning and use of mucosal protectants (petroleum jelly, sesame seed sprays). Antiseptic silicon barrier creams over 6–8 weeks will stabilize the mucosa in the majority of cases. In recalcitrant inflammation, thin reinforced silastic sheeting can be sutured to cover the caudal septum. If there is a large area of cartilage exposure, however, this still may not be sufficient to prevent progression to perforation. When a septal ulcer heals, the scar produced may leave a persistent area of squamous metaplasia which never reverts to a mucosal surface. Periodic and regular use of barrier creams may be necessary or the regular application of sesame seed oil which has a longer duration of effect than simple saline douching.

NON-SURGICAL

This, essentially, is aimed at reducing the drying effect in the nasal mucosa to alleviate crusts and epistaxis. Alkaline nasal douches, proprietary saline sprays and petroleum-based ointments are commonly used. There are no studies of the effectiveness of this type of regimen, but many patients adopt a twice daily ritual of douching and ointment application. It is usually obvious within 6–8 weeks whether this will be effective in maturing the margins of a perforation.

OBTURATION

The principle of obturation is to cover the inflamed mucosal margin. In 2002, Meyer[13] cited the use of septal obturators in the management of perforations. Inert sheeting (usually silastic) was placed to prevent drying and encourage epithelialization over the cartilage/bony septum to create a mature mucosal edge. Evidence suggests that patients do derive benefit from the use of nasal obturators, but opinion on their usage and effectiveness is divided. Facer and Kern,[14] in a retrospective study of 73 patients, reported 72.8% of obturators remained in place, but 27.4% of buttons were removed or were extruded. Brain[4] described the long-term outcome of 102 patients with medium or large holes (1 cm perforations or larger). He described a good result in 44.4 and 32.4%, respectively. The main benefit from obturation appears to be the control of whistling and epistaxis. Often, crusting and nasal discomfort remain a problem.[6, 15] The feeling of obstruction is improved when crusting is reduced, but the bulk effect of an obturator may increase blockage, particularly in anterior perforations with a narrow nasal valve. Poorly tailored silastic may irritate the mucosa, particularly with anterior holes close to the membranous septum. Patient interference and movement of the mobile membranous septum against the edge of the obturator can lead to granuloma formation. It is often for these reasons that patients request removal of the obturator.

SURGICAL

Enlargement of a nasal septal perforation to prevent whistling was described by Jackson and Coates in 1922,[16] but there is little evidence to support its routine use in clinical practice. One retrospective article of widening of the perforation and posterior edge repair in larger holes (15–50 mm) evaluated the pre- and post-operative symptom scores obtained by a linear visual analogue questionnaire. Benefit was reported for the symptoms of crusting and epistaxis and overall nasal discomfort with a significant reduction in mean scores. This technique appears to offer some value for patients with persistent inflammation who could not retain a nasal obturator and who were deemed unsuitable for surgical repair.

SURGICAL REPAIR OF SEPTAL PERFORATIONS

The plethora of techniques for septal perforation repair described over the years attest to the fact that there is still a challenging technical problem for the nasal surgeon, although reliable surgical techniques with good outcomes have been published in the last 15 years. The variety of repairs may be classified as:

- Free grafts:
  - simple or composite autografts
  - allografts

- Pedicled flaps:
  - local nasal mucosal
  - buccal mucosal
  - composite septal cartilage and mucosa
  - composite skin/cartilage
- Rotation/advancement of mucoperichondrial or mucoperiosteal flaps.

Combinations of techniques have been employed in many small reports. In the larger series of observational outcomes of perforation repairs, two factors emerge that appear to have an important bearing on a successful outcome, to achieve closure in 80–90 % of cases. The first is that there is sufficient residual mucosa in the nasal fossa which can be mobilized and transposed allowing direct suturing of the mucosal defect (**Figure 104.2**).

The second is the routine use of a connective tissue interposition graft to support the repair. Bilateral mucosal flaps with the main blood supply derived from the sphenopalatine vessels form the basis of most techniques. Grafts have been reported using temporalis fascia,[17] mastoid periosteum, cranial periosteum, cartilage (septal, auricular, rib) perichondrium and bone (either locally or from rib or the iliac crest).[18, 19] Small defects can be closed with bipedicled flaps, by making relieving incisions either superiorly or inferiorly.[20] Larger holes up to about 2 cm require larger flaps which are pedicled only posteriorly based on the sphenopalatine vessels, and are effectively transposition/rotation flaps.[1, 20-23] Even if complete bilateral mucoperichondrial suturing of the hole is not possible, the use of a connective tissue graft between the leaves allows for epithelialization on the side of incomplete closure, as long as the flaps are protected from drying out and the reconstruction does not get infected. In the presence of any dehiscence of the sutured mucosal defect, it appears that epithelialization occurs more reliably over fascia than cartilage or bone. Reports using acellular dermal allografts[24, 25] instead of fascia appear to give similar success rates. The allografts are expensive, but it must be remembered that donor site morbidity from fascia is not a major issue and the repair is entirely the patient's own tissue. The use of other collagen xenografts may be an alternative. The primary author has used at least two layers of either temporalis or temporoparietal fascia, if necessary with a sandwich of cartilage as a composite graft where there is little supporting remaining quadrilateral cartilage (**Figure 104.3**), for the last 6 years with a current success rate of 87%.

Auricular cartilage, which is a useful graft, is often curved and care should be taken anterosuperiorly at the internal valve because any excess thickness at this level risks post-operative nasal block, requiring revision surgery. Where this may be a problem, a combined approach by raising an anteriorly based turbinate flap endoscopically either alone or with mobilization of mucosa from the floor and upper nose will often allow a tension free repair of the hole without the need for a cartilage graft between the layers. The patient should be counselled that a second usually minor procedure to divide the pedicle of the flap may be required at about 3 months if restriction of breathing is still present.

The nasal fossa is a contaminated area and therefore antibiotic prophylaxis is important. There are no studies as to the ideal length of the course, but the development of sepsis can have a potentially devastating effect on the residual cartilage producing a saddle deformity. Currently, the authors give a 10-day course and supplement this with topical antibacterial ointment.

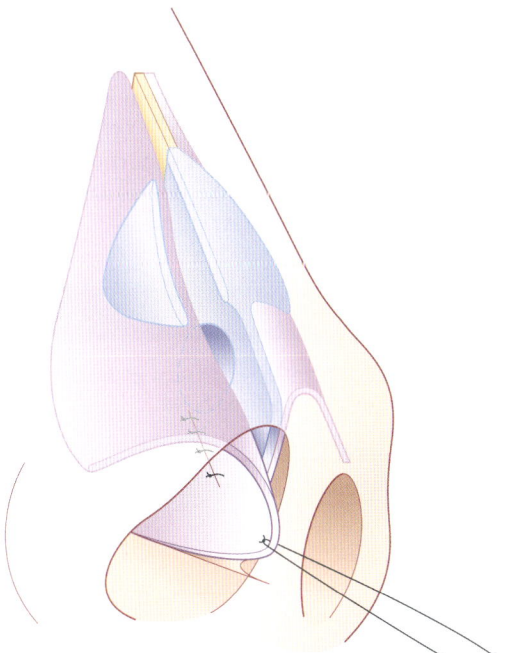

Figure 104.2 Extensive mobilization of the mucosal lining allows a round hole to be closed with sutures in a straight line.

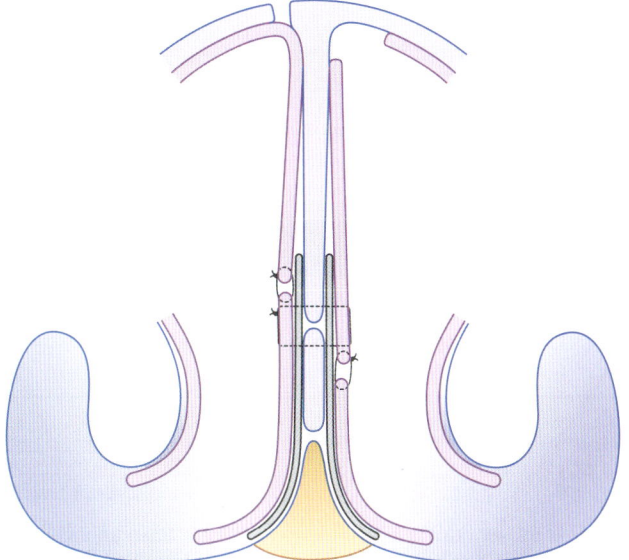

Figure 104.3 Bilateral mucosal flap repair with staggered mucosal rotation/transposition flap closure and connective tissue interposition graft. The fascia should extend to the nasal floor to cover any secondary defect inferiorly.

There is an anatomical limit to the amount of septal mucosa which can be transposed and this is directly inverse to the size of the septal hole. Large perforations (larger than 2.5 cm), particularly with a large vertical dimension as opposed to horizontal linear holes, still pose a problem. However, by extensive undermining along the nasal floor and inferior meatus inferiorly and under the upper lateral cartilage superiorly, substantial flaps may be created. The careful atraumatic elevation of flaps is technically demanding, particularly if the mucoperichondrium is inflamed, atrophic or there is a significant spur of the septum. The surgeon has four options for the approach.

Endonasal[17]

This approach is limited principally by nostril size and position of the hole. Design of the endonasal flaps is critical in this approach due to the limited access. Broad-based elevations via hemitransfixion incisions and bipedicled flaps preserving anterior and posterior blood supplies with horizontal relieving incisions together with interposition grafts should give very good results for small holes (up to 0.5 cm).

Endoscopic

An anterior pedicled turbinate flap is raised to include the mucosa of the medial and inferior surfaces, reflected forwards and sutured to the margins of the septal perforation following submucosal mobilisation.[18] Bilateral flaps provide a more secure repair although if the pedicle remains bulky, a second procedure to divide the attachment may be required. Unilateral septal flaps based on the anterior ethmoid vessels and including mucoperiosteum from the nasal floor can be transposed forward and sutured on one side to the margins of the hole.[19] The opposite side epithelializes over several weeks and disturbance of the valve is minimal.

External rhinoplasty

Approach via a trans columella approach[21] or a columella-philtrum incision: The external approach or its modification by sectioning the columella below the medial crural footplates and connecting to a transfixion and intercartilagenous incisions provides excellent exposure of the septum and lower dorsum, particularly if concomitant rhinoplasty is required and especially when additional grafting is needed to the nasal valve or dorsum. Alar crease incisions only provide limited additional unilateral access and should not be combined with the transcolumella approach because of the risk of ischaemia to the columella flap. It is possible to design larger flaps through this approach and suturing of the mucosal hole is definitely easier than by the endonasal approach. The use of medially based pedicled buccal mucosal flaps have limited use for larger perforations, but are useful to repair secondary deficiencies of the membranous septum when the mucosa has been mobilized to close very anterior holes.

Mid-face degloving approach[26]

This is an extensive dissection of the face which has been employed for very large holes (>2 cm). Used purely as an approach with standard rotation transposition mucosal flaps, it appears to offer little benefit over an external approach for successful closure but with a higher complication rate (vestibular stenosis, 20%). Variation of the technique by employing tissue expansion of the mucosa and skin grafting to the nasal sill appear to improve the success rate and reduce the incidence of nasal vestibular stenosis. Tissue expansion is achieved along the nasal floor using a small (1 × 3 cm) expander over 6–8 weeks with a total volume of 4–7 mL. This technique has the advantage of generating more lining for easier mucosal closure, but the extensive relatively traumatic dissection must be weighed against the degree of benefit to be gained by the patient. Reported success in this series was 18 out of 22 patients with holes from 2 cm to 4 cm diameter.

Although there is evidence of good technical success in surgical repair of the perforated septum for small–medium sized holes, objective evidence of patient benefit following surgical closure is limited. Lindemann et al.[5] have shown improvements in nasal physiology particularly in end-inspiratory humidity and a reduction in symptom scores for epistaxis and nasal dryness.

BEST CLINICAL PRACTICE

✓ Meticulous attention to technique in the execution of septal surgery with adequately supported repair in the event of mucosal tears.

✓ Referral to specialist rhinologist/facial plastic surgeon for repair of small- to medium-sized holes.

FUTURE RESEARCH

➤ More supporting evidence of outcome measures including general health status is needed to confirm the benefits of surgical repair.

➤ Tissue engineering with the possibility to produce cartilage sheets and stable collagen as implants, which are guaranteed free from infection, will remove the need for a donor site.

KEY POINTS

- More than half of perforations are asymptomatic and do not require treatment.
- Trauma is the most common cause of septal perforation.
- Small to medium holes can be closed reliably by surgery.

REFERENCES

1. Younger R, Blokmanis A. Nasal septal perforations. *J Otolaryngol* 1985; **14**: 125–31.
2. Kuriloff DB. Nasal septal perforations and nasal obstruction. *Otolaryngol Clin North Am* 1989; **22**: 333–50.
3. Slavin SA, Goldwyn RM. The cocaine user: the potential problem patient for rhinoplasty. *Plast Reconstr Surg* 1990; **86**: 436–42.
4. Brain D. Septo-rhinoplasty: the closure of septal perforations. *J Otolaryngol* 1980; **94**: 495–505.
5. Lindemann J, Leiacker R, Stehmer V, et al. Intranasal temperature and humidity profile in patients with nasal septal perforation before and after surgical closure. *Clin Otolaryngol* 2001; **26**: 433–7.
6. Toriumi DM, Capelle QM, Chung V. Use of costal perichondrium as an interposition graft for septal perforation closure *JAMA Facial Plast Surg* 2017; **19**: 121–7.
7. Brain D. The nasal septum. In: Scott B (ed.). *Scott-Brown's otolaryngology*. Oxford: Butterworth Heinemann; 1997, pp 4–11.
8. Bridger G. Surgical closure of septal perforations. *Arch Otolaryngol Head Neck Surg* 1986; **112**: 1283–6.
9. Murray A, McGarry GW. The clinical value of septal perforation biopsy. *Clin Otolaryngol* 2000; **25**: 107–9.
10. Diamantopoulos II, Jones NS. The investigation of nasal septal perforations and ulcers. *J Laryngol Otol* 2001; **115**: 541–4.
11. Dommerby H, Rasmussen O, Rosborg J. Long term results of septoplastic operations. *J Otorhinolaryngol Relat Spec* 1985; **47**: 151–7.
12. von Schoenberg M, Robinson P, Ryan R. The morbidity from nasal splints in 105 patients. *Clin Otolaryngol* 1992; **17**: 528–30.
13. Meyer R. *Secondary rhinoplasty including reconstruction of the nose*. 2nd edn. Berlin: Springer; 2002.
14. Facer GW, Kern EB. Nonsurgical closure of nasal septal perforations. *Arch Otolaryngol* 1979; **105**: 6–8.
15. Osma U, Cureoglu S, Akbulut N, et al. The results of septal button insertion in the management of nasal septal perforation. *J Laryngol Otol* 1999; **113**: 823–4.
16. Jackson CL, Coates GM. *Diseases of the throat, nose and ear*. Philadelphia: W. B. Saunders; 1922.
17. Fairbanks DNF. Closure of nasal septal perforations. *Arch Otolaryngol* 1980; **7**: 403–6.
18. Friedman M, Ibrahim H, Ramakrishnan V. Inferior turbinate flap for repair of nasal septal perforation. *Laryngoscope* 2003; **113**(8): 1425–8
19. Castelnuovo P, Ferreli F, Khodaei I, et al. Anterior ethmoid artery septal flap for the management of septal perforation. *Arch Facial Plast Surg* 2011; **13**: 411–14.
20. Goodman WS, Strelzow VV. The surgical closure of nasoseptal perforations. *Laryngoscope* 1982; **92**: 121–4.
21. Kridel RWH, Appling D, Wright WK. Septal perforation closure utilizing the external septorhinoplasty approach. *Arch Otolaryngol* 1986; **112**: 168–72.
22. Schultz-Coulon HJ. Experiences with the bridge-flap technique for the repair of large nasal septal perforations. *Rhinology* 1994; **32**: 25–33.
23. Smith DF, Albathi M, Lee A, et al. Upper lateral cartilage composite flap for closure of complicated septal perforations. *Laryngoscope* 2017; **127**(8): 1767–71.
24. Kridel RWH, Foda H, Lunde KC. Septal perforation repair with acellular human dermal allograft. *Arch Otolaryngol* 1998; **124**: 73–8.
25. Foda H. The one-stage rhinoplasty septal perforation repair. *J Laryngol Otol* 1999; **113**: 728–33.
26. Romo T, Sclafani AP, Falk AN, et al. A graduated approach to the repair of nasal septal perforations. *Plast Reconstr Surg* 1999; **103**: 66–75.

CHAPTER 105

MANAGEMENT OF ENLARGED TURBINATES

Andrew C. Swift and Samuel C. Leong

Management of enlarged turbinates	1157	Complications	1165
Medical treatment for the enlarged inferior turbinate	1160	Outcomes	1165
Surgical management for the enlarged inferior turbinate	1160	Recent research on the inferior turbinate	1166
Mucosal preservation surgery	1162	References	1168
Submucosal techniques requiring specific technology	1162	Links to national guidance documents	1168
Turbinate surgery in specific clinical situations	1164	Cochrane	1168

SEARCH STRATEGY

Data in this chapter may be updated by a search using the keywords: turbinates, nasal surgical procedures, nasal obstruction and nasal procedures.

MANAGEMENT OF ENLARGED TURBINATES

Introduction

The inferior turbinates are dynamic structures that form a crucial part of the normal functional nose. However, they are structures that are relatively easy to access. They have been recognized as a cause of nasal obstruction and therefore subject to numerous operative techniques to either reduce their size or excise them completely.[1] Various surgical techniques of turbinate reduction or destruction have been described since the middle of the 19th century. Despite a declining trend in England (United Kingdom), inferior turbinate reduction surgery remains a commonly performed procedure in ENT practice (**Figure 105.1**). Contemporary otorhinolaryngological literature states that the evidence base for the multitude of techniques for turbinate reduction is weak and that surgeons empirically offer surgery where the predominant symptom is nasal obstruction.[2] In fact, there is currently no ideal surgical procedure and most techniques offer only short-term benefit.[3] Paradoxically, most specialist rhinologists who devote a major part of their practice to conditions of the nose perform surgery to the inferior turbinate infrequently.

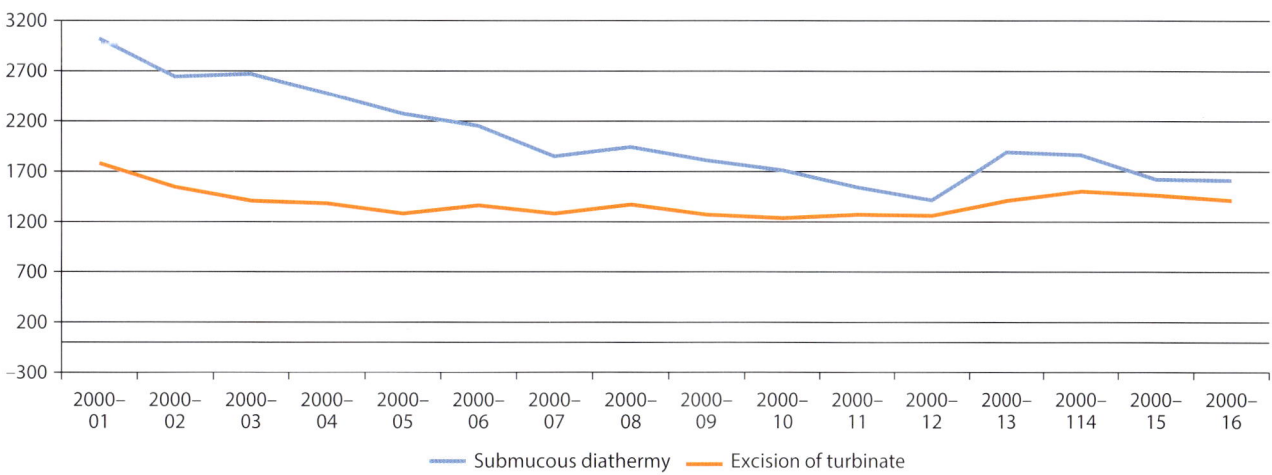

Figure 105.1 Trends in adult turbinate surgery in England from financial year 2000 to 2016. E04.1 = Submucous diathermy to turbinate of nose. E04.2 = Excision of turbinate of nose NEC. (Source: Hosptial Episodes Statistics, http://content.digital.nhs.uk

History of turbinate surgery

Operative techniques to reduce the size of the inferior turbinates have been practiced since 1845. The first technique to be described was electrocautery: at the time this was being used for a wide variety of non-nasal medical complaints, justified by the misconception of nasal reflex neurosis. Hol and Huizing[4] described 13 techniques of interior turbinate reduction up to the present day.

Anatomy of the inferior turbinates

The inferior turbinate consists of a supporting cancellous conchal bone, named after the Greek for scroll, covered by specialized erectile mucosa.[5] The turbinate is attached along the inferolateral aspect of the nasal cavity, extending from the interior nasal valve to just anterior to the Eustachian tube. The conchal bone is firmly attached to the inferomedial surface of maxilla. The adjacent maxilla is very thick anteriorly and becomes thin in the midsection of the nose. The conchal bone is not a completely straight structure but curves superiorly reaching its highest point in the mid nasal cavity. The nasolacrimal duct opens into the superior aspect of the inferior meatus just between the thick anterior bone and the thin section in the mid part of the nose. The entrance of the nasolacrimal duct is protected by Hasner's valve.

From the applied point of view, these anatomical points are important to appreciate: during antral washout the trochar is passed into the inferior meatus below the turbinate to puncture the lateral wall of the nose into the maxillary sinus. The superior part of the attachment of the inferior turbinate is thin in the midsection of the nose and puncture is generally easy.

The blood supply is from the lateral branch of the sphenopalatine artery that enters the posterior aspect of the turbinate. Sensation is supplied by the trigeminal nerve; sympathetic nerves travel along the feeding arterial blood vessels; the parasympathetic supply also travels along the vascular supply but travels along the vidian nerve before entering the nose through the sphenopalatine foramen.

Physiology in health

The inferior turbinate is an important functional component of the normal nose. It warms inspired air and maintains linear rather than turbulent airflow within the nose.[6] The turbinate is covered by a functional ciliated pseudostratified respiratory mucosa that is supported by a lamina propria, below which is a vascular layer rich in venous sinusoids (**Figures 105.2a** and **105.2b**).

The normal inferior turbinate is a dynamic structure that varies in size according to the degree of congestion. The latter is determined by the control of blood flowing through the specialized erectile tissue. This change is governed by the autonomic neural supply: the sympathetic nerves induce reduction of blood flow and a decrease in volume whilst the parasympathetic supply congests the erectile tissue of the turbinate. The degree of congestion varies in a cyclical manner in a healthy nose every few hours and is coordinated so that when one side is congested the other is constricted. This phenomenon is known as the nasal cycle: it can be demonstrated in about 80% of humans but the purpose is unknown.[7]

Definition of an enlarged inferior turbinate

Operations to reduce the size of the inferior turbinate are generally based on the fact that it is enlarged. However, in clinical practice, this is usually a subjective assessment and diagnosis is normally made by exclusion criteria when dealing with the sensation of nasal obstruction. Various terms are used to describe this enlargement and there is a lack of standardization.[8] The various terms include hypertrophic, congested, hyperplastic, and engorged turbinates.

In practice, gross congestion of both inferior turbinates in a patient with severe rhinitis may be obvious. However, it is important to appreciate that congestion may reflect stages of the nasal cycle. It is therefore important to consider the effect of spraying a topical decongestant onto the inferior turbinates before accepting the fact that the inferior turbinates are chronically congested.

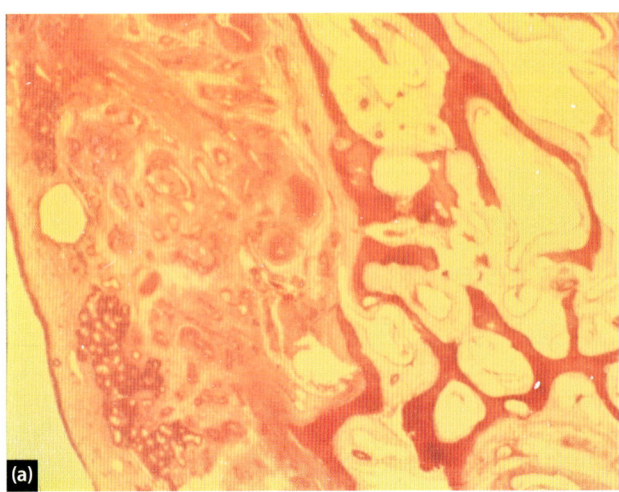 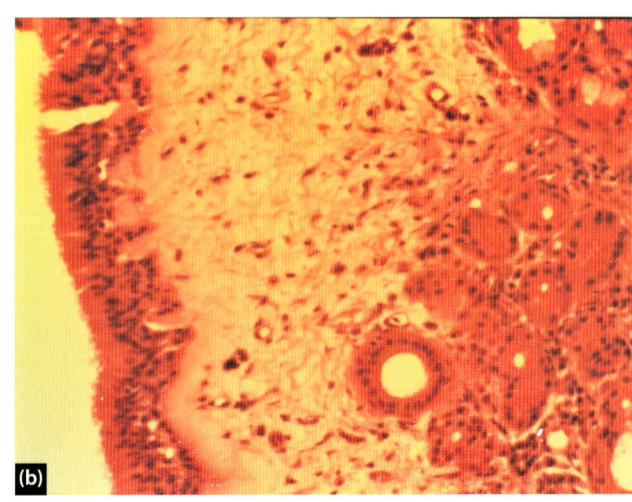

Figure 105.2 Histology IT1 **(a)**; Histology IT2 **(b)**.

Histological studies of bilaterally enlarged inferior turbinates have shown dilated congested venous sinuses, subepithelial inflammatory cell infiltration, fibrosis of the lamina propria, and dilatation of mucous gland ducts.[5] Other changes include an increase in pseudostratified surface epithelium, goblet cells and mucous gland acini. Histology of inferior turbinates from patients with non-allergic perennial and allergic rhinitis has shown degenerative change and fibrosis in the lamina propria in the non-allergic group whereas the allergic turbinates showed gross tissue oedema.[9] In patients with septal deviation and contralateral inferior turbinate enlargement, an additional finding has been a two-fold increase in the bony concha compared to cadaver controls.

It is of note that the medial aspect of the mucosa is thickest in an enlarged turbinate.[10] It has been suggested that surgery should therefore be targeted to the mucosa over the medial aspect of the turbinate and the inferior section that is rich in vascular sinusoids.[11]

Pathogenesis of inferior turbinate enlargement

Whilst assessing a patient with enlarged inferior turbinates, it should be helpful to categorize the enlargement according to a classification proposed by Hol and Huizing.[4, 12] The individual categories are judged according to clinical features as follows:

1. Compensatory hypertrophy
2. Protruded turbinate
3. Hyperplasia of the turbinate head
4. Hyperplasia of the whole turbinate
5. Hyperplasia of the turbinate tail.

Compensatory hypertrophy of the inferior turbinate is seen when the nasal septum is deviated to the opposite side, and the turbinate seems to fill the empty space. **Protrusion** is where the turbinate extends more medially into the nasal cavity than expected. It may be more apparent on the coronal CT images when the conchal bone may be seen to make a less acute angle with the lateral nasal wall. Hyperplasia of the turbinate head and whole length of the turbinate may both occur with chronic rhinitis. Should the head enlarge, the turbinate may enlarge anteriorly and obstruct the nasal valve. Hyperplasia of the posterior end is said to occur in patients with chronic sinusitis and post-nasal discharge.

In patients with rhinitis, the effect of the nasal cycle is accentuated; patients may become aware of the cycling effect on their sensation of nasal obstruction that may become significantly worse whilst in the supine position due to nasal reflexes. In patients with severe forms of rhinitis or significant rhinosinusitis, the inferior turbinates may become chronically enlarged. This effect becomes even more so should the patient self-medicate with xylometazoline to try and decongest the nose.

Sarcoidosis is an unusual disorder that may cause quite severe inferior turbinate enlargement and should be considered if the turbinates do not respond to normal topical treatments for rhinitis.

Clinical features

Patients with enlarged inferior turbinates will invariably present with nasal obstruction. The complete nasal symptom complex together with nasal examination and endoscopy will normally lead to the correct clinical diagnosis of allergic or non-allergic rhinitis or chronic rhinosinusitis. The anterior head of the congested inferior turbinates may appear as a red swelling or be pale and purplish: the latter is typically associated with severe allergic rhinitis (**Figure 105.3**). The swollen anterior end is easily visible on examination of the nose and in primary care this is often mistaken for an inflamed nasal polyp.

Ideally, the nose should be examined before and 10 minutes after mucosal vasoconstriction: chronically congested inferior turbinates normally do not reduce in size but remain large. This is important to note if turbinate surgery is being considered.

Imaging is not normally required unless surgery is being considered for rhinosinusitis. However, when available, helpful information about the turbinates may be demonstrated. CT is the best imaging modality (**Figure 105.4**), although MRI may also yield useful information (**Figure 105.5**).

Physiological evaluation of the inferior turbinates

Nasal obstruction is a subjective symptom that has a complex pathophysiological mechanism that is not yet fully explained.[13] It is not an uncommon phenomenon to find discordance between reported severity of nasal obstruction and clinical findings. It is thus important to measure the degree of obstruction in order to monitor the effects of surgery and audit the effectiveness of medical/surgical intervention. This can be done with a visual

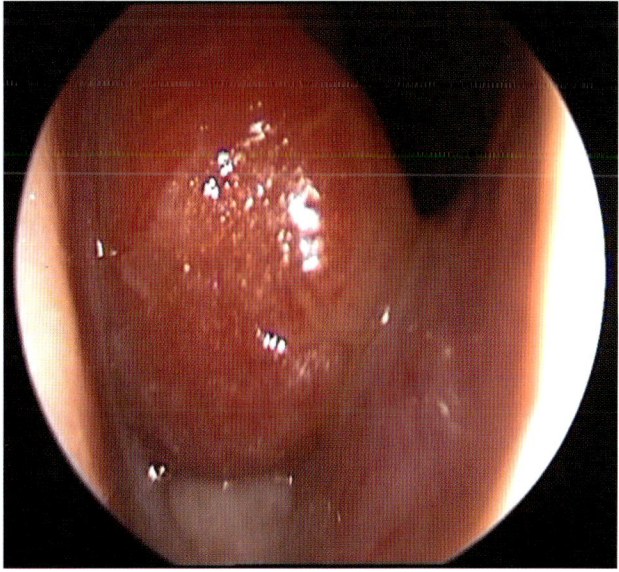

Figure 105.3 Gross enlargement of the right inferior turbinate in allergic rhinitis.

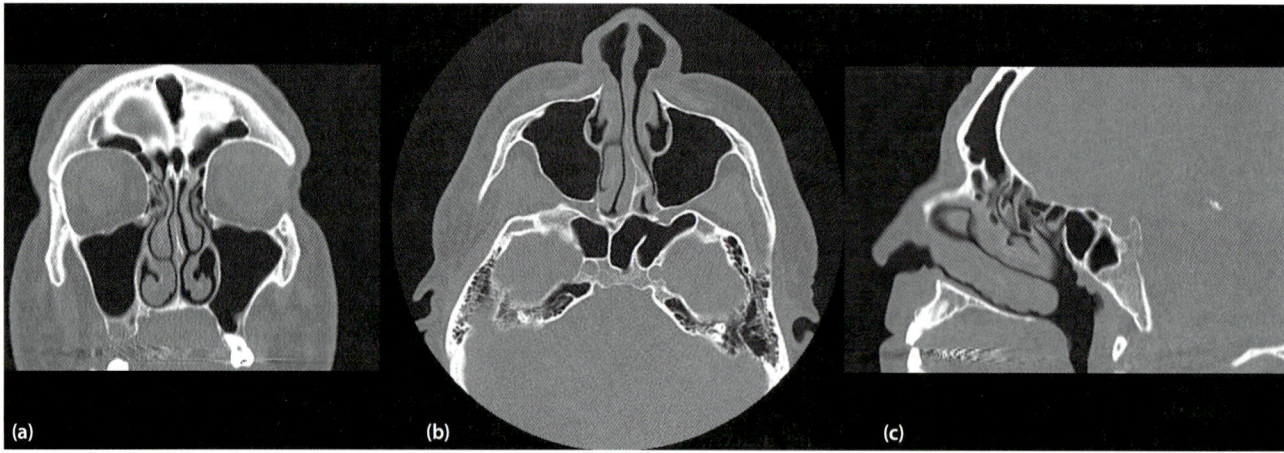

Figure 105.4 Multi-planar CT sinus: enlarged inferior turbinates.

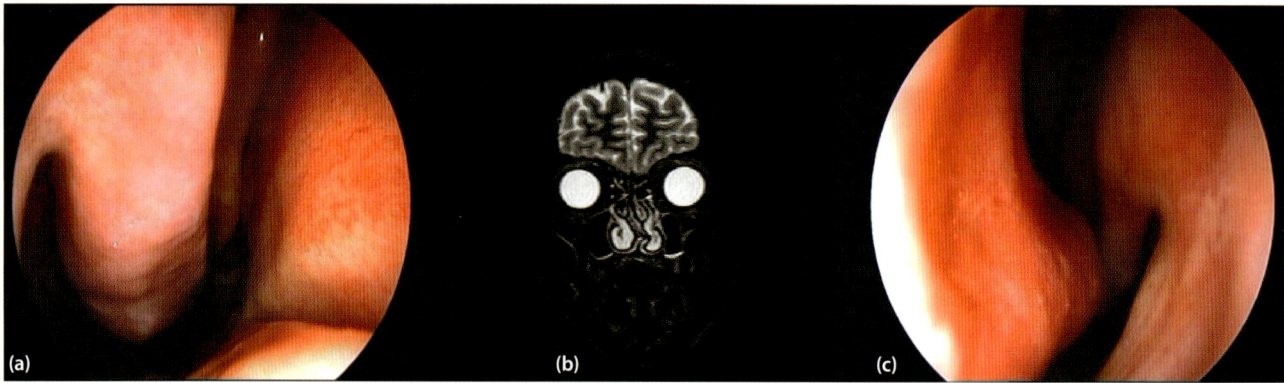

Figure 105.5 Enlarged right inferior turbinate and septal deviation to the left: endoscopic view and MRI appearance.

analogue scale and the 22 question Sino-Nasal Outcome Test (SNOT-22).

A few departments will have access to physiological measuring techniques (**Figure 105.6**) such as acoustic rhinometry, anterior rhinomanometry and rhinospirometry. These tools can demonstrate the degree of obstruction, the difference between each side of the nose and the change with nasal surgery. In the research setting measurements can be obtained before and after vasoconstriction, but in the clinical setting, this is not practical, and mucosal vasoconstriction should be induced in all cases. An overall assessment of the degree of nasal obstruction can also be obtained by measuring the peak nasal inspiratory flow using a specific nasal spirometer.

MEDICAL TREATMENT FOR THE ENLARGED INFERIOR TURBINATE

Firstly, rhinitis medicamentosa due to chronic abuse of vasoconstrictor agents should be sought and excluded. If present, the patient should be counselled on inducing factors and that their nose will become more obstructed until recovery starts to occur.

There is no contention amongst ENT specialists that the first line of treatment for enlarged inferior turbinates is medication. Topical nasal steroids are the mainstay of treatment for both allergic and non-allergic rhinosinusitis.

However, prolonged once/twice daily treatment for at least 3 months is necessary, with reassurance that topical nasal steroids are safe to use every day. Topical steroids are often combined with oral antihistamines, antibiotics and saline in the treatment of chronic rhinosinusitis.[14]

However, should medical intervention fail to provide good control, the option of surgery needs to be considered.

SURGICAL MANAGEMENT FOR THE ENLARGED INFERIOR TURBINATE

Surgery should ideally be restricted to patients with a significant symptomatology in whom operative intervention is likely to be effective. However, this is an area where there may be much diversity in opinion and practice with regard to the management of the inferior turbinate. As previously stated, it is paradoxical that specialist rhinologists operate on the inferior turbinate infrequently, but turbinate surgery is still a common procedure in the generality of the speciality. The explanation for this diversity is that with perceived enlargement of the turbinate it is very tempting to just reduce the size of the turbinate and this will generally result in an improved nasal airway. However, without addressing the driving forces for the condition, it is likely that any beneficial effect from inferior turbinate surgery will be short-lived. On the other hand, if underlying chronic rhinosinusitis is identified and corrected by

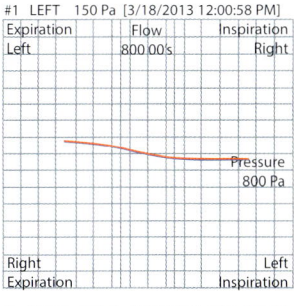

Standard	Inspiration	Expiration
Mean resistance	5.980	4.337
Max deviation	1.444	0.000
Respirations	3	1

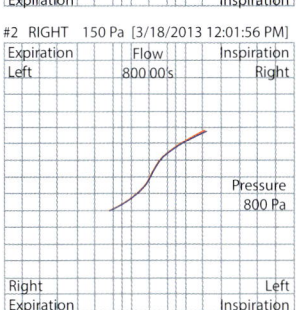

Standard	Inspiration	Expiration
Mean resistance	0.865	0.930
Max deviation	0.053	0.059
Respirations	4	4

(a)

LEFT	Area	Distance
First minimum	0.30	2.07
Second minimum	N/A	N/A
MCA	0.30	2.07
Volume (0-5)	3.44	

RIGHT	Area	Distance
First minimum	0.39	2.07
Second minimum	0.47	3.80
MCA	0.39	2.07
Volume (0-5)	3.16	

(b)

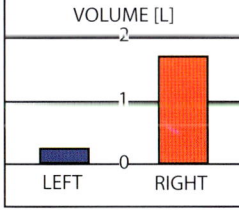

01 S - TEST INSP

	Result
Left volume	0.2473 L
Right volume	−1.0708
NPR	−0.75
Time	10.02 s
Outcome	Y

02 S - TEST INSP

	Result
Left volume	−0.6574 L
Right volume	−1.152 L
NPR	−0.38
Time	10.02 s
Outcome	Y

(c)

Figure 105.6 Nasal physiology. Investigations in a patient with a large left inferior turbinate **(a)** Anterior rhinomanometry showing increased resistance and low flow on the left hand side of the nose. **(b)** Acoustic rhinometry consistent with significant obstruction in anterior nasal cavity. **(c)** Rhinospirometry: partitioning effect shows marked preference for right nasal airway.

endoscopic sinus surgery, with or without septal deformity surgery, the turbinate will often respond in a positive way without the need for turbinate reduction surgery.

As well as the diversity of opinion as to when to operate on the inferior turbinate, there is also a wide range of different operations and techniques, each with their own proponents.

It is not realistic to expect that this situation will ever become standardized, but it may be possible to modify the way that surgeons perceive the inferior turbinate.

Perhaps the most important aspect to consider when operating on the inferior turbinate is to preserve the mucosa and maintain the mucociliary transport.

A simple system of classifying turbinate operations is proposed in **Box 105.1**.

It may be necessary to excise the inferior turbinate for access during tumour surgery such as removal of an angiofibroma or inverted papilloma within the maxillary sinus. Resection may also be necessary in treating malignancy such as adenocarcinoma or melanoma. The inferior turbinate has been utilized as a pedicle graft in the closure of septal perforations or as a free graft source for repairing dural defects in the anterior skull base.

Individual techniques

The authors recommend that ideally inferior turbinate reduction should be restricted to submucosal mucosal preservation techniques where at all possible to minimize the risk of complications. However, acknowledgement is given to the fact that alternative techniques such as mucosal reduction by a microdebrider is safe and effective in experienced hands.

It is also acknowledged that some techniques require specific technology that may be expensive and it is unlikely that any one department will have a choice of all of the possibilities.

All techniques require mucosal vasoconstriction to minimize bleeding during the procedure. Performing the surgery under endoscopic control facilitates precision surgery with minimal collateral damage.

MUCOSAL PRESERVATION SURGERY

The two simplest low-cost techniques are lateralization by outfracture and submucous diathermy.

Lateralization

Lateralization by outfracture can be done by simply using an elevator to mobilize the concha by infracture, and then pushing the whole turbinate laterally. Although this probably results in the least improvement in the airway of the various techniques, it is very low risk, but can often be used as an adjunct to septal surgery or endoscopic sinus surgery to facilitate access to the nose. An alternative that may give a more effective result is to create a submucosal tunnel and outfracture the concha in segments via this tunnel.

Submucosal diathermy

Submucosal diathermy (SMD) is performed by passing an insulated Abbey™ needle along the length of the inferior turbinate in 2–3 different passes, and applying the diathermy at 70 W, as the needle is withdrawn. SMD is monopolar diathermy that generates intense heat at the electrode tip. This causes tissue destruction, inflammation and fibrosis. Initially, the nose is likely to feel more blocked until healing has occurred. There is a risk of extensive tissue destruction following excessive diathermy and the necrotic inferior turbinate will slough and crust over a prolonged period.

Classically, it is said that SMD will only be effective in patients that demonstrate good pre-operative turbinate reduction after applying a topical decongestant. Short-term results are good but this effect is often not maintained in the long term.

SUBMUCOSAL TECHNIQUES REQUIRING SPECIFIC TECHNOLOGY

Turbinate reduction can be achieved very effectively with a mini-microdebrider. A submucosal tunnel is created through a small incision of the anterior end of the turbinate (**Figure 105.7**). The erectile tissue can be reduced over the medial and inferior part of the turbinate by partial resection with a 2 mm diameter oscillating mini-microdebrider blade. Post-operative nasal packing is not necessary. This technique is effective, carries minimal risk, and the microdebrider can be controlled to preserve all of the overlying mucosa.

Submucosal microdebrider reduction has been combined with a procedure to divide the posterior nasal nerve at the sphenopalatine foramen. This procedure is known as functional inferior turbinosurgery (FITS) and aims to interfere with the autonomic control and reduce turbinate sensation.[15]

BOX 105.1 Simple system of classifying turbinate operations

Mucosal preservation surgery
- Lateralization by outfracture
- Mini-microdebrider surgery
- Radiofrequency
- Coblation
- Turbinoplasty
- Submucosal diathermy

Mucosal destructive reduction surgery
- Superficial cautery
- Chemocautery with chromic acid or trichloric acid
- Cryosurgery
- Laser surgery
- Direct microdebrider mucosal reduction

Turbinate excision procedures
- Partial
- Subtotal
- Posterior end

Coblation® techniques utilizes a narrow electrode or wand that creates low temperature plasma of 85 degrees and effectively dissolves tissue and later induces fibrosis. Radiofrequency (RF) has also been used with good effect and utilizes high frequency alternating current to generate heat and ablate tissues.

All of the submucosal techniques allow for precise surgery that can be performed under endoscopic control. Reports suggest the techniques are effective and can be repeated if needed.

Turbinoplasty

This technique is designed to preserve functional mucosa over the surface of the turbinate whilst achieving substantial reduction in the volume of the turbinate. The turbinate is initially in-fractured and an incision made over the anterior head and along the inferior margin (**Figure 105.7**). The mucosa is elevated from both sides of the bony concha. The concha is then resected in varying degrees. The lateral mucosa is removed with a microdebrider and the medial mucosa placed so that it lies laterally and forms a 'neoturbinate'. The anterior end of the turbinate is typically reduced and moved away from the nasal valve by this technique. Support dressings are then placed in the nose.

Mucosal destructive reduction surgery

Some of these procedures will destroy the specialized mucosal surface of the turbinate and may cause long-term crust formation and underlying infection with prolonged healing. It has been suggested that there is very little to justify some of these techniques in modern day surgery.[1]

Turbinate excision techniques

These are much more radical techniques than the techniques described above.

Radical subtotal resection of the turbinate operation includes resection of the mucosa and bony concha along the length of the inferior turbinate (**Figure 105.8**). This operation can be painful and has a much greater chance of damaging the lateral branch of the sphenopalatine artery and cause heavy epistaxis. It also carries long-term risks of crusting and the empty nose syndrome (*vida infra*).

To reduce the risk of significant complications and improve the airway at the region of the nasal valve, the operation of partial resection was devised. The enlarged anterior head and anterior third of the inferior turbinate are excised (**Figure 105.9**). The line of resection is first crushed to limit bleeding. Angled scissors are then used to excise the required section of turbinate. This can be done utilizing a headlight but an endoscope gives greater precision.

Enlargement of the posterior end of the inferior turbinate is occasionally seen. Such cases often have irregular polypoid mucosa over the inferior turbinate and local resection may be appropriate. Historically this was done using a specific snare developed in the days where large posterior ends were seen with the aid of a post-nasal mirror. A more controlled way of doing this now is to use a microdebrider under endoscopic control.

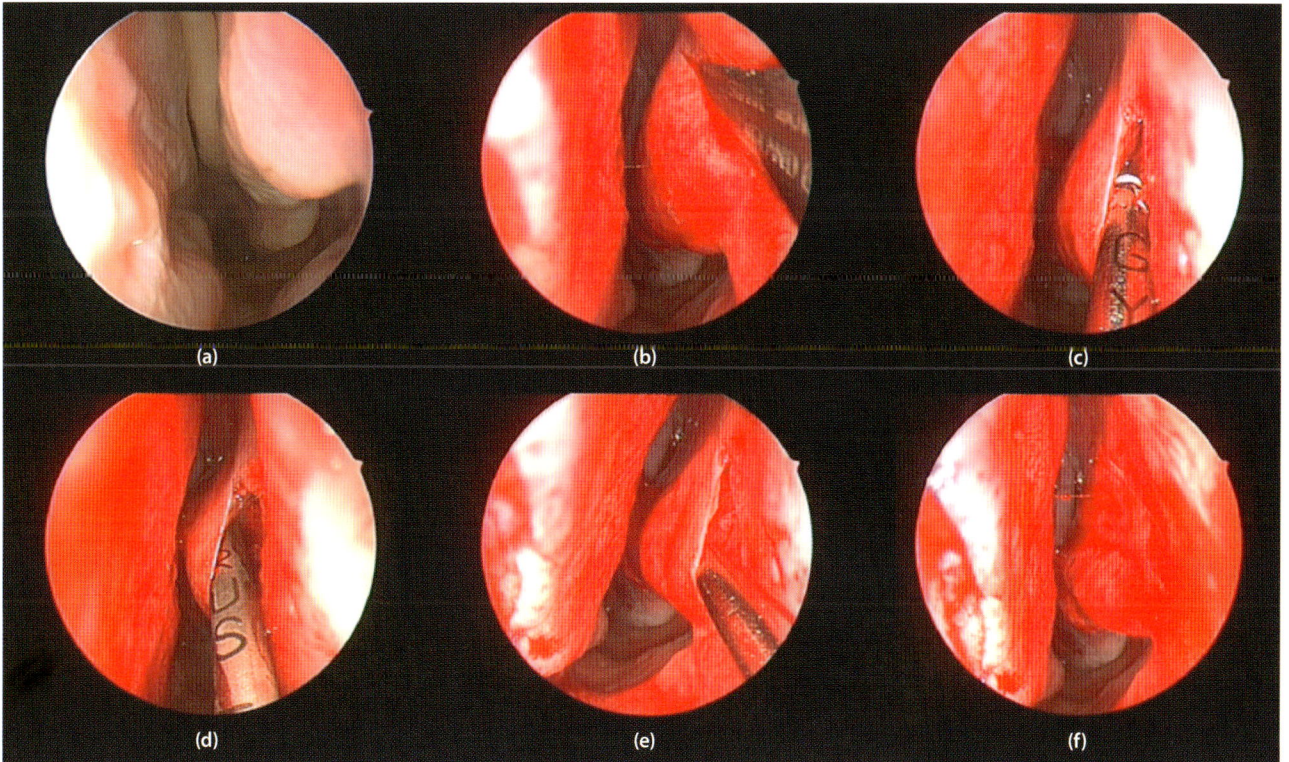

Figure 105.7 Submucosal turbinate reduction with mini-microdebrider blade. (a) Decongested left inferior turbinate **(b)** anterior turbinate incision **(c-e)** submucosal placement of microdebrider blade **(f)** replacement of mucosa against concha.

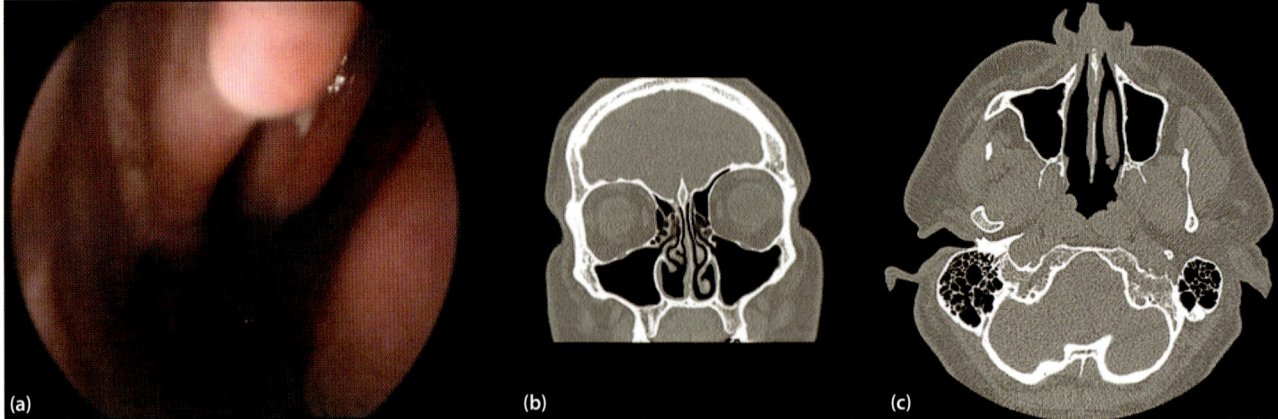

Figure 105.8 Appearance of radical excision of right inferior turbinate: endoscopic view and CT scan images.

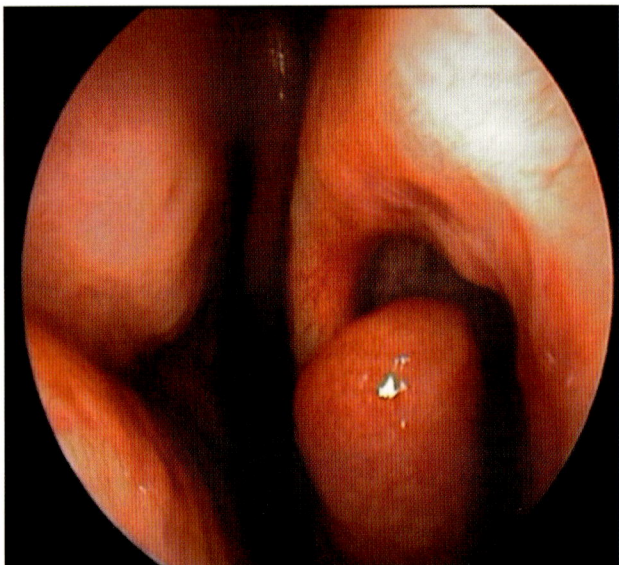

Figure 105.9 Partially resected turbinate.

Laser surgery

Lasers can be used to reduce the size of the inferior turbinate by excision, vaporization or coagulation. They can be used under local anaesthesia as a day-case or office procedure. Several types have laser have been described and their action is dependent on the particular properties of the laser according to the wavelength. Several surgical laser techniques have been described: these vary widely from limited spot applications to the turbinate head through to spot applications, mucosal excision or vaporization of the anterior section or whole length of the turbinate.

The properties of the CO_2 laser favour tissue cutting and vaporization. Normally, a microscope, micromanipulator and angled mirrors to divert the beam onto the turbinate are required. The light energy is absorbed by water causing significant tissue heat to a depth of 4 mm but with limited collateral tissue damage. Long-term benefit and improved results compared to electrocautery have been described.[16]

The neodymium-yttrium aluminium garnet (Nd-YAG), potassium titanyl phosphate (KTP), and argon-ion lasers can all be transmitted down a flexible fibre which makes them suitable to be used under endoscopic control. They are absorbed by haemoglobin and coagulate to a limited depth. The holmium yttrium aluminium garnet (Ho-YAG) is primarily absorbed by water but is able to remove bone as well as soft tissue.[17]

Although reports suggest that laser therapy is effective, the long-term results are in general less certain.[10]

Direct microdebrider mucosal reduction surgery

Direct debridement of the inferior turbinate is utilized as an effective means of relieving nasal obstruction in patients with gross inferior turbinate hypertrophy secondary to allergic or non-allergic chronic rhinitis. The mucosa is debrided down to periosteum along the medial aspect and inferior edge of the anterior two-thirds of the inferior turbinate. Bleeding is minimal as long as the periosteum is undisturbed. Healthy normal mucosa regenerates within 6–12 weeks following surgery and mucociliary clearance problems have not been observed.

TURBINATE SURGERY IN SPECIFIC CLINICAL SITUATIONS

Rhinosinusitis and endoscopic sinus surgery

In most patients undergoing endoscopic sinus surgery for chronic rhinosinusitis, there is no need to perform inferior turbinate surgery. Chronic rhinosinusitis will induce mucosal congestion of the nasal mucosa and inferior turbinates. Following endoscopic sinus surgery and post-operative medication, the degree of mucosal inflammation within the sinuses should significantly improve, with the benefit of reduction in the secondary congestion of the turbinates. Should inferior turbinate surgery still be deemed necessary, the authors would suggest that this is restricted to a mucosal preservation technique of surgery.

Septal deviation

Compensatory enlargement of the inferior turbinate is often observed on the opposite side to a septal deflection. It would therefore seem logical that turbinate reduction surgery would be indicated at the time of septal surgery. Formal study of this dilemma has, however, shown a positive effect from submucous unilateral turbinate reduction as shown by acoustic rhinometry and patient self-assessment at 6 months following surgery.[18]

Histological studies have shown that enlargement of the inferior turbinate on the contralateral side to a septal deviation may be due to an increase in the size of the conchal bone as well as an increase in mucosal thickness.[4] This would favour submucosal conchal resection and turbinoplasty in such cases.

Although these research findings are of interest, not all studies support the concept of simultaneous turbinate reduction and it is of note from clinical experience that most septal corrective surgery is performed without inferior turbinate reduction and patients generally have a satisfactory outcome.[19] The potential risk of bleeding and adhesion formation also needs to be taken into account in deciding on whether to include turbinate reduction with septoplasty.

Septorhinoplasty

Some surgeons will routinely excise the inferior turbinates at the time of doing septorhinoplasty to maximize the chance of improving nasal obstruction. However, this will increase the potential for heavy bleeding post-operatively and is probably not going to result in any significant long-term advantage.

Sleep disordered breathing

There is a cogent argument to maximize the nasal airway in patients with sleep-disordered breathing, particularly when there may be a problem of compliance with CPAP due to nasal obstruction. This is an instance where there may be a tendency for surgeons to be radical in their approach to the inferior turbinate and to excise both turbinates whilst also correcting septal deformity. However, there is a lack of evidence to support a policy of radical excision in this group of patients and a more conservative approach is recommended. Most studies do support mucosal preservation turbinate reduction techniques as an adjunct to septal surgery for snoring, although none have demonstrated significant decrease in the apnoea-hypopnoea index of obstructive sleep apnoea patients.[20]

Inferior turbinate surgery in children

Most children with nasal obstruction have rhinitis or adenoid enlargement. Rhinitis is mostly allergic and generally improves following treatment with anti-allergic medication and allergen avoidance. Should significant nasal obstruction persist and inferior turbinates remain large, there may be a case for turbinate reduction surgery.

Children with sleep disordered breathing and obstructive sleep apnoea may benefit from inferior turbinate surgery.[21] A recent comparison of adenotonsillectomy with and without microdebrider-assisted inferior turbinoplasty has shown improved results in the children who underwent turbinate reduction.[22]

A recent survey of turbinate reduction techniques in the USA showed that 80% of surgeons combined turbinate surgery with another procedure such as adenotonsillectomy, septal surgery and sinus surgery, and the most popular techniques are now the microdebrider and coblation®.[23]

COMPLICATIONS

Inferior turbinate surgery is not without risk and consent for surgery should include a discussion about complications and their subsequent management.

The most immediate significant risk is severe haemorrhage, particularly after turbinate resection.

Procedures that are destructive to the mucosa may be followed by prolonged nasal crust formation that can take several weeks if not months to improve.

Long-term risks include nasal adhesions or synechiae between the turbinate and the septum. Visual change and blindness is rare but has been reported from the use of monopolar diathermy at the posterior end of the turbinate.

The danger of performing radical resection of tissue within the nasal cavities was recognized many years ago as a cause of ozaena and mucosal atrophy. Huizing suggests that too radical turbinectomy should be considered as a 'nasal crime'.[12] Patients undergoing radical resection risk developing chronic infected smelly crusting within the nose. Fortunately, this condition is rarely seen following inferior turbinate reduction surgery in modern otorhinolaryngology.

However, total resection of the inferior turbinate does carry a risk of inducing the 'empty nose syndrome (ENS)' in which the patient complains of nasal obstruction in the absence of an obstructive cause (**Figure 105.9**).[24] The pathophysiology is unclear but probably involves altered nasal receptor sensitivity, associated with humidity and conditioning of inhaled air; neuropsychological factors have also been suspected. Visible dryness or crusting are normally not seen. Should ENS occur after inferior turbinate resection, inserting a submucosal Medpor (Porex Surgical Inc) implant to effectively create a neo-turbinate has recently been described as a successful means of management.[25]

OUTCOMES

Benefit from turbinate surgery would ideally be defined as improvement in both objective and subjective measurements of nasal airflow. Despite overwhelming data supporting the efficacy of turbinate surgery, of 93 studies reporting positive results, most were case series of retrospective reviews: only 14 reported acoustic rhinometry results and 12 had rhinomanometric data[26] (evidence level 4 and 5). There have been few comparative studies and no systematic reviews of outcomes comparing the efficacy of different surgical techniques.[2] Furthermore, there is currently no specific quality of life assessment tool for turbinate reduction surgery.

In the largest randomized study to date, submucous resection and lateralization of the inferior turbinate resulted in sustained long-term improvement in nasal airflow and mucociliary clearance when compared to other surgical techniques (Figure 105.10).[27] Furthermore, over a fifth of patients in this series experienced atrophic rhinitis following radical turbinectomy.

A long-term study on a cohort of 341 patients who had submucous resection of the turbinate reported that 91.3% were symptom free at 10-year follow-up.[28] Rhinomanometric data demonstrated over 90% improvement of nasal airflow compared to the initial baseline and this was sustained at long-term follow-up.

Although newer surgical techniques such as Coblation® and radiofrequency ablation do not have long-term data yet, early results suggest that these techniques appear to offer promising short-term improvement in nasal airflow (Figure 105.11).[29–31] RCT data are unusual but a recent study has shown a definite reduction in turbinate enlargement and subjective improvement in nasal obstruction after bipolar radiofrequency volumetric tissue reduction (RFVTR) compared to placebo at 6–8 weeks.[32]

RECENT RESEARCH ON THE INFERIOR TURBINATE

Computational fluid dynamics (CFD) is a numerical simulation application that enables the visualization of flow factors (velocity, pressure, vector, streamline and vortices) under variation flow conditions and has been used in the aerospace industry and civil engineering. Although computational fluid dynamic studies (CFD) remain an experimental tool in rhinology, CFD has enabled detailed study and understanding of nasal physiology. A three-dimensional nasal cavity is constructed from either MRI or CT scans before CFD simulations are performed by a supercomputer. The physiological effects of modelling septal perforation, deviation and enlarged inferior turbinates have been studied extensively using CFD simulations.[6]

It has been demonstrated that despite a small increment of 1–2 mm in the overall dimensions of the inferior turbinate, a significant change in the air pressure around the nasal valve region occurs: nasal airflow is reduced and there is redistribution of airstreams to the upper parts of the nasal cavity.[33] The resultant negative pressure in the nasopharynx and reduced flow rate have been postulated to adversely affect the function of the surrounding muscles and mobility of the soft palate: the latter are common etiological factors for Eustachian tube dysfunction, snoring and obstructive sleep apnoea.[34]

Although CFD simulations have yet to be performed on actual post-operative cases, it is possible to simulate outcomes following turbinate surgery. Partial turbinectomy, especially when the enlarged turbinate is reduced by a third, result in the return of near-normal airstreams and aerodynamics (Figure 105.12).[35] In contrast, radical turbinectomy causes an alteration of nasal aerodynamics akin to that observed in atrophic rhinitis.[36] Also, excision of the lower third of the inferior turbinate lowers the ability to heat inspired air by 11.7% due primarily to inducing turbulent airflow.

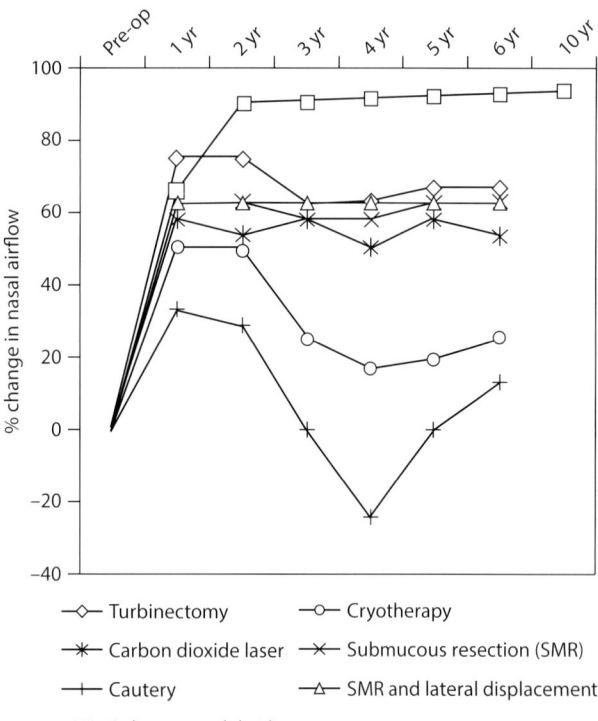

Figure 105.10 A comparison of long-term results between different surgical techniques based on average change in nasal airflow. Data for turbinectomy, carbon dioxide laser, cautery, cryotherapy, SMR and lateral displacement were derived from Passali et al.[27] The submucous debriding data was derived from Yañez and Mora.[28]

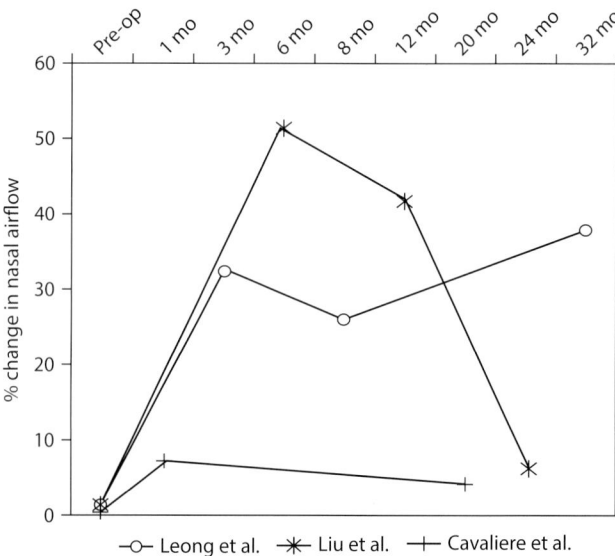

Figure 105.11 Average change in nasal airflow after Coblation® inferior turbinate reduction surgery. Data derived from Leong et al.[29] Liu et al.[30] and Cavaliere et al.[31]

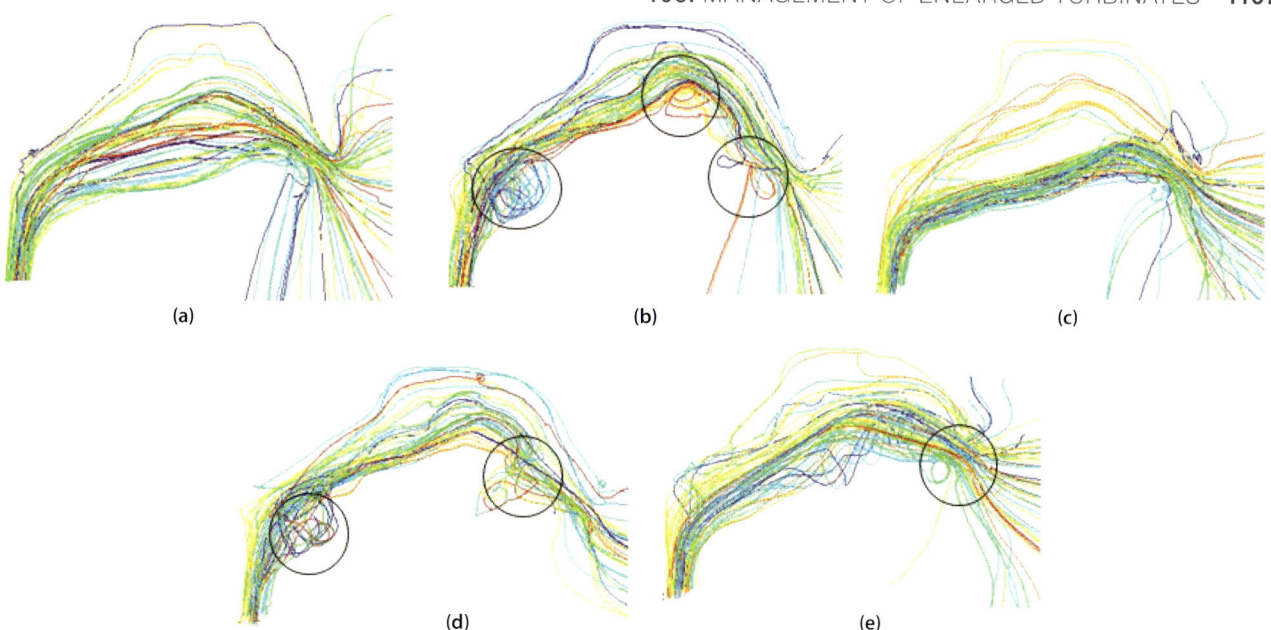

Figure 105.12 Comparison of the velocity streamlines in the nasal cavity with an inspiratory airflow rate of 17.4 L/min. The vortex areas are circled. (a) Healthy nasal cavity. (b) Enlarged inferior turbinates causing nasal obstruction. (c) Lower third of the inferior turbinate excised. (d) Head of the inferior turbinate excised. (e) Radical inferior turbinate resection. (With permission from Prof. D-Y Wang, National University of Singapore.)

BEST CLINICAL PRACTICE

✓ Warn patients and document the risk of nasal crusting postoperatively. Include the possibility of long-term recurrence of nasal obstruction and possible revision surgery in the consent process.
✓ Always seek information about over-the-counter self-medication for the nose and consider the possibility of rhinitis medicamentosa.
✓ Re-examine the inferior turbinates again 10 minutes after applying a topical decongestant to assess the effect of vasoconstriction.
✓ Nasal endoscopy is strongly recommended before listing patients for inferior turbinate surgery.
✓ Consider a sinus CT scan if there is a suspicion of chronic rhinosinusitis in patients with chronically large inferior turbinates.
✓ Inferior turbinate surgery can result in heavy epistaxis. Check patients are not taking anticoagulants and utilize more conservative turbinate reduction techniques in preference to more aggressive techniques.

FUTURE RESEARCH

➤ There is a need for RCTs to compare different techniques of inferior turbinate reduction surgery after failed medical treatment. Comparisons should clearly separate allergic from non-allergic groups and restrict groups to adults or children. Trials should include short and long-term outcome data and review complications as well as clinical effectiveness.
➤ The clinical entity of the 'empty nose syndrome' needs clarification. Aetiology, diagnosis and management issues need to be investigated.

KEY POINTS

- Surgery of the inferior turbinate should be deferred until the patient has undergone an adequate trial of normally-effective medication.
- Large inferior turbinates may reflect an underlying allergic rhinitis. Consider effective conservative management regimes, including allergen identification and prevention, prior to committing to surgery.
- Always consider and exclude co-existent chronic rhinosinusitis prior to operating on enlarged inferior turbinates.
- Great caution should be exercised with regard to turbinate surgery in children. Inferior turbinate surgery is best avoided if at all possible.
- Beware of excessive resection of the inferior turbinates: this can induce chronic crusting and a sense of nasal obstruction.

REFERENCES

1. Clement WA, White PS. Trends in turbinate surgery literature: a 35-year review. *Clin Otolaryngol Allied Sci* 2001; **26**(2): 124–8.
2. Jose J, Coatesworth AP. Inferior turbinate surgery for nasal obstruction in allergic rhinitis after failed medical treatment. *Cochrane Database Syst Rev* 2010; (12): CD005235.
3. Leong SC, Eccles R. Inferior turbinate surgery and nasal airflow: evidence-based management. *Curr Opin Otolaryngol Head Neck Surg* 2010; **18**(1): 54–9.
4. Hol MK, Huizing EH. Treatment of inferior turbinate pathology: a review and critical evaluation of the different techniques. *Rhinology* 2000; **38**(4): 157–66.
5. Farmer SE, Eccles R. Chronic inferior turbinate enlargement and the implications for surgical intervention. *Rhinology* 2006; **44**(4): 234–8.
6. Leong SC, Chen XB, Lee HP, Wang DY. A review of the implications of computational fluid dynamic studies on nasal airflow and physiology. *Rhinology* 2010; **48**(2): 139–45.
7. Hanif J, Jawad SS, Eccles R. The nasal cycle in health and disease. *Clin Otolaryngol Allied Sci* 2000; **25**(6): 461–7.
8. Farmer SE, Eccles R. Chronic inferior turbinate enlargement and the implications for surgical intervention. *Rhinology* 2006; **44**(4): 234–8.
9. Schmidt J, Zalewski P, Olszewski J, Olszewska-Ziaber A. Histopathological verification of clinical indications to partial inferior turbinectomy. *Rhinology* 2001; **39**(3): 147–50.
10. Willatt D. The evidence for reducing inferior turbinates. *Rhinology* 2009; **47**(3): 227–36.
11. Berger G, Gass S, Ophir D. The histopathology of the hypertrophic inferior turbinate. *Arch Otolaryngol Head Neck Surg* 2006; **132**(6): 588–94.
12. Huizing EZ, de Groot JAM. Section 8: Surgery of the Nasal Cavity: Turbinate Surgery. *Functional Reconstructive Nasal Surgery*, 2nd edition, Thieme, Stuttgart, 2003, pp. 276–282.
13. Eccles R. Mechanisms of the symptoms of rhinosinusitis. *Rhinology* 2011; **49**(2): 131–8.
14. Fokkens WJ, Lund VJ, Mullol J, et al. European Position Paper on Rhinosinusitis and Nasal Polyps 2012. *Rhinol Suppl* 2012; **23**: 1–298.
15. Ikeda K, Yokoi H, Saito T, et al. Effect of resection of the posterior nasal nerve on functional and morphological changes in the inferior turbinate mucosa. *Acta Otolaryngol* 2008; **128**(12): 1337–41.
16. Lippert BM, Werner JA. CO_2 laser surgery of hypertrophied inferior turbinates. *Rhinology* 1997; **35**(1): 33–6.
17. Serrano E, Percodani J, Yardeni E, et al. The holmium:YAG laser for treatment of inferior turbinate hypertrophy. *Rhinology* 1998; **36**(2): 77–80.
18. Devseren NO, Ecevit MC, Erdag TK, et al. A randomized clinical study: outcome of submucous resection of compensatory inferior turbinate during septoplasty. *Rhinology* 2011; **49**(1): 53–7.
19. Nunez DA, Bradley PJ. A randomised clinical trial of turbinectomy for compensatory turbinate hypertrophy in patients with anterior septal deviations. *Clin Otolaryngol Allied Sci* 2000; **25**(6): 495–8.
20. Sufioğlu M, Ozmen OA, Kasapoglu F, et al. The efficacy of nasal surgery in obstructive sleep apnea syndrome: a prospective clinical study. *Eur Arch Otorhinolaryngol* 2012; **269**(2): 487–94.
21. Leong SC, Kubba H, White PS. A review of outcomes following inferior turbinate reduction surgery in children for chronic nasal obstruction. *Int J Pediatr Otorhinolaryngol* 2010; **74**(1): 1–6.
22. Cheng PW, Fang KM, Su HW, et al. Improved objective outcomes and quality of life after adenotonsillectomy with inferior turbinatereduction in pediatric obstructive sleep apnea with inferior turbinate hypertrophy. *Laryngoscope* 2012; **122**(12): 2850–4.
23. Jiang ZY, Pereira KD, Friedman NR, et al. Inferior turbinate surgery in children: a survey of practice patterns. *Laryngoscope* 2012; **122**(7): 1620–3.
24. Coste A, Dessi P, Serrano E. Empty nose syndrome. *Eur Ann Otorhinolaryngol Head Neck Dis* 2012; **129**(2): 93–7.
25. Jiang C, Wong F, Chen K, Shi R. Assessment of surgical results in patients with empty nose syndrome using the 25-item Sino-Nasal Outcome Test Evaluation. *JAMA Otolaryngol Head Neck Surg* 2014; **140**(5): 453–8.
26. Batra PS, Seiden AM, Smith TL. Surgical management of adult inferior turbinate hypertrophy: a systematic review of the evidence. *Laryngoscope* 2009; **119**(9): 1819–27.
27. Passàli D, Passàli FM, Damiani V, et al. Treatment of inferior turbinate hypertrophy: a randomized clinical trial. *Ann Otol Rhinol Laryngol* 2003; **112**(8): 683–8.
28. Yañez C, Mora N. Inferior turbinate debriding technique: ten-year results. *Otolaryngol Head Neck Surg* 2008; **138**(2): 170–5.
29. Leong SC, Farmer SE, Eccles R. Coblation® inferior turbinate reduction: a long-term follow-up with subjective and objective assessment. *Rhinology* 2010; **48**(1): 108–12.
30. Liu CM, Tan CD, Lee FP, et al. Microdebrider-assisted versus radiofrequency-assisted inferior turbinoplasty. *Laryngoscope* 2009; **119**(3): 414–18.
31. Cavaliere M, Mottola G, Lemma M. Monopolar and bipolar radiofrequency thermal ablation of inferior turbinates: 20 month follow-up. *Otolaryngol Head Neck Surg* 2007; **137**(2): 256–63.
32. Bran GM, Hünnebeck S, Herr RM, et al. Bipolar radiofrequency volumetric tissue reduction of the inferior turbinates: evaluation of short-term efficacy in a prospective, randomized, single-blinded, placebo-controlled crossover trial. *Eur Arch Otorhinolaryngol* 2013; **270**(2): 595–601.
33. Lee HP, Poh HJ, Chong FH, et al. Changes of airflow pattern in inferior turbinate hypertrophy: a computational fluid dynamics model. *Am J Rhinol Allergy* 2009; **23**(2): 153–8.
34. Chen XB, Leong SC, Lee HP, et al. Aerodynamic effects of inferior turbinate surgery on nasal airflow: a computational fluid dynamics model. *Rhinology* 2010; **48**(4): 394–400.
35. Garcia GJ, Bailie N, Martins DA, et al. Atrophic rhinitis: a CFD study of air conditioning in the nasal cavity. *J Appl Physiol* 2007; **103**(3): 1082–92.
36. Chen XB, Lee HP, Chong VF, et al. Numerical simulation of the effects of inferior turbinate surgery on nasal airway heating capacity. *Am J Rhinol Allergy* 2010; **24**(5): e118–22.

LINKS TO NATIONAL GUIDANCE DOCUMENTS

Radiofrequency tissue reduction for turbinate hypertrophy – guidance (IPG495)
Source: National Institute for Health and Care Excellence – NICE – 25 June 2014, https://www.nice.org.uk/guidance/ipg495

Powered microdebrider turbinoplasty for inferior turbinate hypertrophy – guidance (IPG498)
Source: National Institute for Health and Care Excellence – NICE – 23 July 2014, https://www.nice.org.uk/guidance/ipg498

COCHRANE

1. Surgery to the inferior turbinate (lining of the nose) in order to relieve nose block in allergic rhinitis after failed medical treatment Jose J, Coatesworth AP. *Cochrane Database Syst Rev* 2010; Issue 12. Art. No.: CD005235.DOI: 10.1002/14651858.CD005235.pub2. http://www.cochranelibrary.com

CHAPTER 106

EPISTAXIS

Gerald W. McGarry

Background 1169	Adult primary epistaxis 1174
Surgical anatomy of the nasal vascular system 1169	Secondary epistaxis 1179
Classification of epistaxis 1172	References 1181

SEARCH STRATEGY

Data in this chapter may be updated by multiple searches using the keywords: epistaxis, aetiology, management, treatment and therapies, arterial supply, venous drainage and key clinical areas. Main articles, RCTs and systematic reviews were searched. Results were augmented by a manual search through major references and texts. Many older references are cited because of their quality and value which has stood the test of time. Indeed newer publications frequently, simply repeat (often without acknowledgment) the findings of much earlier works and so in these cases I have used the original publication as the reference.

BACKGROUND

Epistaxis is defined as bleeding from the nose. This simple definition belies the difficulties associated with one of otolaryngology's commonest and most difficult to treat emergencies. The historical literature contains numerous references to epistaxis and its antiquity is reflected in the fact that the simplest treatment for a nose bleed (pinching the ala nasi) is called the Hippocratic technique.

While extensive review of the history of epistaxis is beyond the scope of this book, much of the historical literature remains relevant and students of this subject are advised to review the writings of Morgagni who even predicted nasal endoscopy in 1761![1]

SURGICAL ANATOMY OF THE NASAL VASCULAR SYSTEM

It is vital that the surgeon responsible for managing patients with epistaxis has a sound understanding of the nasal vasculature. The surgical anatomy of this system has in recent years been revisited by those who raise nasal mucosal flaps in skull base surgery and the reader is advised to read some of the articles on that subject to help consolidate understanding of this crucial area.[2]

Arterial supply

The internal and external carotid arteries supply the nose via branches which anastomose extensively within the lateral wall, septum and across the midline. On the anterior septum an arterial plexus was identified as a frequent site of haemorrhage by James Little in 1879 and the same plexus was described one year later by Kiesselbach.[3] As a result of these descriptions, the area most frequently implicated in epistaxis is known as Little's area or Kiesselbach's plexus. In the posterior nasal cavity, the vessels are larger than those in Little's area and can more easily be traced to their external or internal carotid origin.

EXTERNAL CAROTID ARTERY

The external carotid artery supplies the nasal cavity via facial and maxillary branches. The facial artery supplies the most anterior part of the septum (nasal septal rami of superior labial artery), the vestibule (lateral nasal artery) and a small area of the nasal cavity (ascending palatine artery). The maxillary artery supply is via sphenopalatine and greater palatine branches. The greater palatine artery supplies the anteroinferior part of the nasal floor and septum.

The sphenopalatine artery is the most important supply to the nasal cavity. It enters through the sphenopalatine foramen and immediately divides into posterior septal and posterior lateral rami.[4] The posterior lateral division gives the inferior and middle turbinate arteries. These vessels were studied in detail by Burnham in 1935 and his work remains the definitive reference on this subject.[5] Burnham described how the inferior and middle turbinate arteries run in bony tunnels within the turbinates. Shaheen postulated that these bony conduits could reduce the likelihood of the arteries being involved in epistaxis.[6] The posterior septal branch of the sphenopalatine artery runs medially across the face of the sphenoid to the posterior part of the septum then takes an undulating course anteroinferiorly in the muco-perichondrium. Its terminal branches anastomose in Little's area.

INTERNAL CAROTID ARTERY

The internal carotid contributes the anterior and posterior ethmoidal branches of the ophthalmic artery. The anterior ethmoidal artery, after arising in the orbit, runs under the superior oblique muscle to the anterior ethmoidal canal in which it traverses the ethmoid and nasal cavities. It terminates in the region of the ethmoid fovea in a meningeal branch and a larger branch to the nasal roof, olfactory cleft and superior turbinate. The posterior ethmoidal artery is smaller than the anterior ethmoidal artery and is present in only 80% of individuals.[7] Like the anterior vessel, this artery runs medially but this time passes above the superior oblique muscle to enter the posterior ethmoidal foramen situated 5 mm anterior to the optic canal and 10/15 mm behind the anterior ethmoidal foramen. Within its canal, the posterior ethmoidal artery is accompanied by the sphenoethmoidal nerve and a branch of the nasociliary nerve. This vessel also divides into a terminal meningeal branch and a branch to the posterosuperior nasal cavity, olfactory sulcus and sphenoethmoidal recess.

INTERNAL AND EXTERNAL CAROTID TERRITORIES

The nasal cavity is the location of the principal internal-external carotid artery anastomoses in the head and neck. There has been debate over the relative importance of each supply to the nasal cavity. Shaheen showed that the area supplied by the ethmoidal arteries was much smaller than had previously been thought. His findings were supported by observing; sphenopalatine branches to the superior meatus and superior turbinate, the comparatively narrow calibre of the ethmoidal arteries and the fact that the larger of the two ethmoidal arteries, the anterior, is absent in as many as 14% of cadaver dissections.[6] The view that the middle turbinate marks a watershed between internal and external carotid circulations is erroneous as the arteriolar anastomotic network allows varying directions of flow to occur. Compensatory anastomotic flow for example via the facial arteries is thought to explain re-bleeding events which may occur following ligation or embolization.[8]

Venous drainage

The veins follow the arteries within the mucosa. The exception is the periarterial venous cuff surrounding the intra-osseous portions of the inferior and middle turbinate arteries. The veins of the lateral wall drain through the sphenopalatine foramen into the pterygoid venous plexus and to the internal jugular vein. Anteriorly, drainage is via superior labial and greater palatine veins to the facial vein and ultimately the external jugular system. Of particular note clinically is the retro-columellar vein running 2 mm behind and parallel to the columella. This vein is in a particularly superficial area and is a common cause of venous epistaxis in children.

Key clinical areas

WOODRUFF'S PLEXUS

The role of Woodruff's plexus (WP) in epistaxis was at one time frequently discussed, especially in the North American literature.[9, 10] Woodruff (1949) described a plexus of prominent blood vessels lying just inferior to the posterior end of the inferior turbinate (Figure 106.1).[11] He commented on how this plexus was a frequent site of adult epistaxis and described 14 cases of bleeding from this area. Many authors describe WP as a frequent source of so-called 'posterior' epistaxis despite the absence of any numerical evidence to support this. Shaheen in 1967 attempted to study and define WP but was unable to identify the plexus in nasal ethmoidal blocks.[6] A more recent study with endoscopic photography and anatomical micro-dissection confirmed that the plexus does indeed exist but showed it to be a venous plexus and thus very unlikely to be important in epistaxis.[12]

LATERAL WALL OR SEPTAL BLEEDING?

There is general acceptance that overall the vast majority of epistaxis occurs from Little's area but there is debate on the relative importance of various other sites. Some suggest that WP is important and others nominate the septum or other regions of the lateral wall as prime sites. Numerous studies using various methods and examination techniques have produced diverse findings.[10, 13–16] For example, Shaheen failed to find any lateral wall bleeding while Wurman did not report any septal bleeding.[10, 16] Sixty percent of bleeding points identified by el-Simily were septal whereas 62% of those found by Rosnagle were on the lateral wall.[17, 18] In a

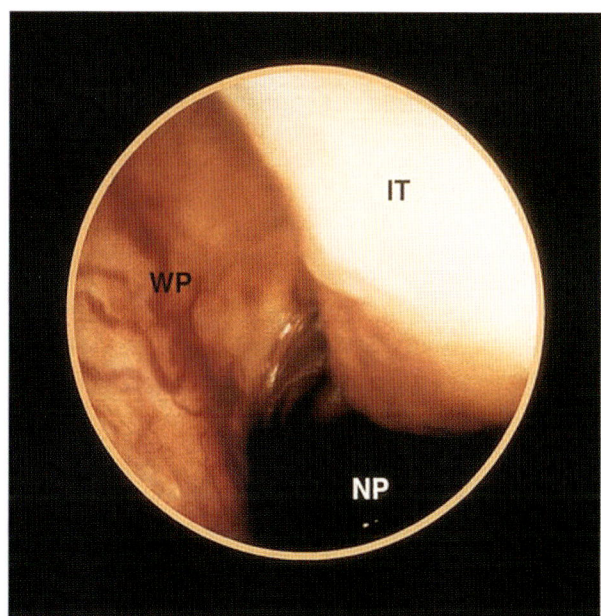

Figure 106.1 Endoscopic photograph of Woodruff's plexus (right). IT: inferior turbinate, WP: Woodruff's plexus, NP: nasopharynx.

study of 50 patients with adult primary *posterior* epistaxis, McGarry identified the bleeding point in 94% (6% not located despite endoscopy), 70% bled from the septum and 24% from the lateral wall. There was no side predilection (50% left nostril and 48% right, 2% bilateral).[19] These findings support the observation that posterior, like anterior, epistaxis is predominantly septal in origin (**Figure 106.2**).

ANTERIOR ETHMOIDAL ARTERY IN ENDOSCOPIC SINUS SURGERY AND IN TRAUMATIC EPISTAXIS

Detailed knowledge of this vessel is essential for surgeons carrying out endoscopic sinus surgery and for those planning its ligation for epistaxis. The artery is frequently encountered in a mesentery just below the skull base between the ethmoid fovea and the lamina papyracea. Inadvertent damage to the mesentery can lead to troublesome bleeding from the artery. Transection of the vessel during sinus surgery can result in retraction of the bleeding end into the orbit with subsequent pressure haematoma and risk of visual loss. In patients with orbito-ethmoidal fractures, severe and often intermittent epistaxis can occur due to damage to this vessel and in such cases open ligation may be the only option to control the bleeding. The vessel can be ligated as a treatment for epistaxis via an external (medial canthal) approach or endoscopically (trans-ethmoidal). The open approach via a medial orbital incision is the most reliable and preferred method and the artery may be clipped, bipolared or ligated without entering the bulbar fascia (**Figures 106.3** and **106.4**).

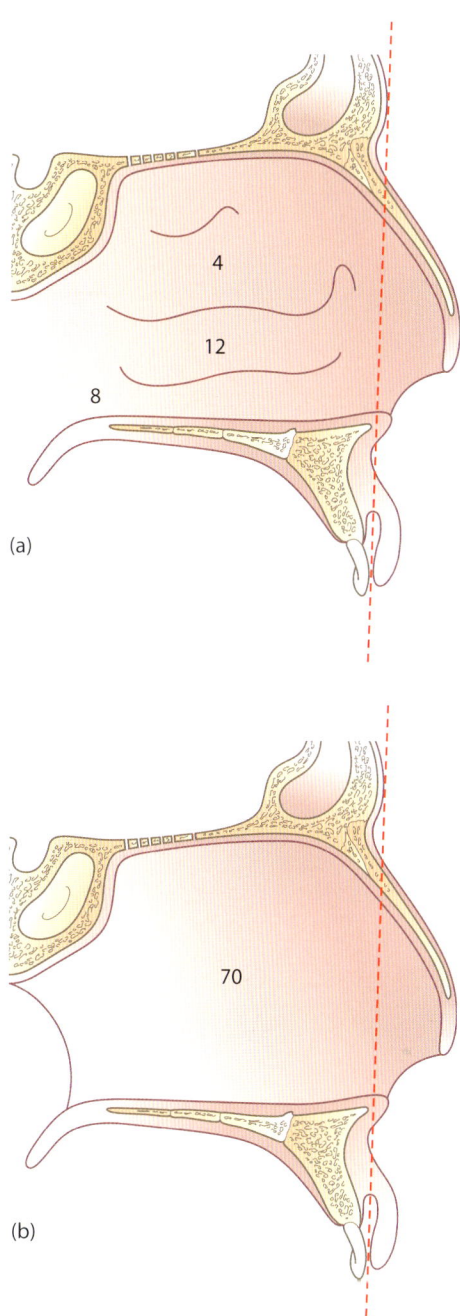

Figure 106.2 Diagram of sites of bleeding in posterior epistaxis. **(a)** lateral nasal wall, **(b)** septum. Numbers are percentages (6% not located).

SURGICAL ANATOMY OF THE SPHENOPALATINE FORAMEN

The sphenopalatine foramen is the portal for the major arterial supply of the nasal cavity. Lateral to the foramen lies the pterygopalatine space. The foramen is formed by a U-shaped notch in the vertical portion of the palatine bone which is closed posterosuperiorly by the sphenoid bone. The foramen transmits the sphenopalatine artery, vein and the nasal palatine nerve (maxillary division of

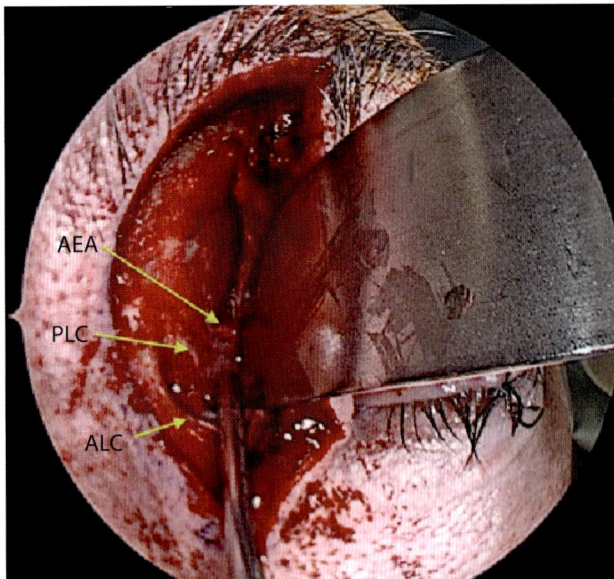

Figure 106.3 Open approach to ligate left anterior ethmoidal artery. ALC: anterior lacrimal crest, PLC: posterior lacrimal crest, AEA: anterior ethmoidal artery.

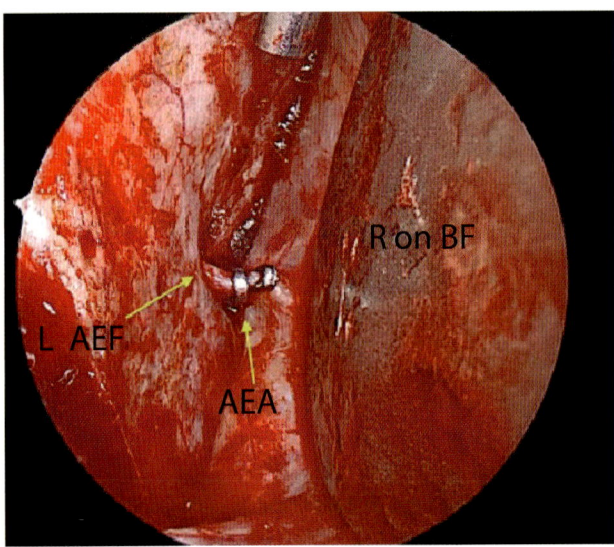

Figure 106.4 Operative field in ligation of anterior ethmoidal artery (left). RonBF: retractor on bulbar fascia, LPEF: lamina papyracea and anterior ethmoidal foramen, AEA: anterior ethmoidal artery with titanium clips applied.

the trigeminal nerve). Clinically this foramen is the key to the procedure of endonasal endoscopic sphenopalatine artery ligation (ESPAL). Surgical localization of the foramen can be difficult. Bolger et al. studied a small bony projection which lies anterior to the foramen in 96% of cases.[20] This landmark is called the crista ethmoidalis and its recognition during surgery may help in finding the foramen. The crista is variable in size but consistent in its position anterior to the artery and so it is a key landmark for the endoscopic surgeon (See **Figure 106.8**).

SURGICAL ANATOMY OF THE BLOOD SUPPLY OF THE INFERIOR TURBINATE

Severe secondary epistaxis is a serious complication of inferior turbinectomy. Understanding the vascular supply of the inferior turbinate may help in both the avoidance and the management of this complication. At its origin, the inferior turbinate artery runs anteroinferiorly in the submucosa where it is vulnerable to damage during radical turbinectomy. On reaching the inferior turbinate, it divides into three parallel branches each of which run in bony tunnels within the substance of the turbinate. These tunnels with their peri-arterial cuff of fibrous tissue and venous elements may prevent the artery constricting following turbinectomy and may predispose to post-operative haemorrhage.[4, 14]

Attempts to control haemorrhage following turbinectomy should be directed towards the posterosuperior aspect of the inferior turbinate where pressure or bipolar to the submucosal segment of the artery should prove effective.

CLASSIFICATION OF EPISTAXIS

Clinical classification

Traditionally, epistaxis has been classified on the basis of presumed aetiology and publications include long lists of factors thought to cause the condition.[21] As most cases are idiopathic and since case-control evidence does not exist for most of the putative aetiological factors, a causation-based classification is inappropriate.

A clinical classification based on the clearly observed patterns of presentation of epistaxis is more useful.

Adult or childhood epistaxis

There is a pronounced bimodal distribution in the age of onset of epistaxis. The condition is common in childhood, becomes less common in early adult life and then peaks in the sixth decade. Thus, while it can occur at any time in life, this variation with age is sufficiently pronounced to classify epistaxis as **childhood** (less than 16 years) or **adult** (greater than 16 years).

Primary or secondary

Between 70% and 80% of all cases of epistaxis are idiopathic, spontaneous bleeds without any proven precipitant or causal factor.[22] This type of bleeding can be classified as **primary** epistaxis. As our understanding of the aetiology advances, the number of cases of true primary epistaxis will decrease but, at present, this definition encompasses the majority of cases.

A small proportion of cases are due to a clear and definite cause such as trauma, surgery or anti-coagulant overdose and can be classified as **secondary** epistaxis. The distinction between primary and secondary epistaxis is

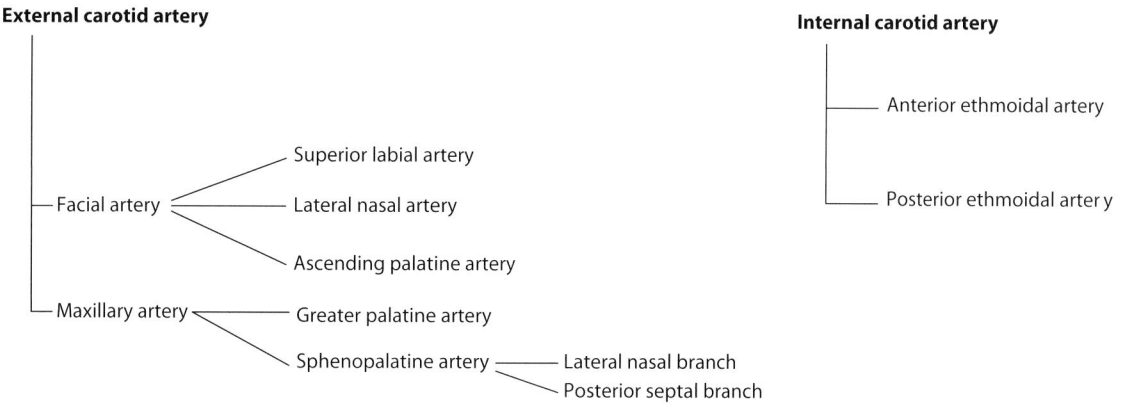

Figure 106.5 Schematic of blood supply to nasal cavity.

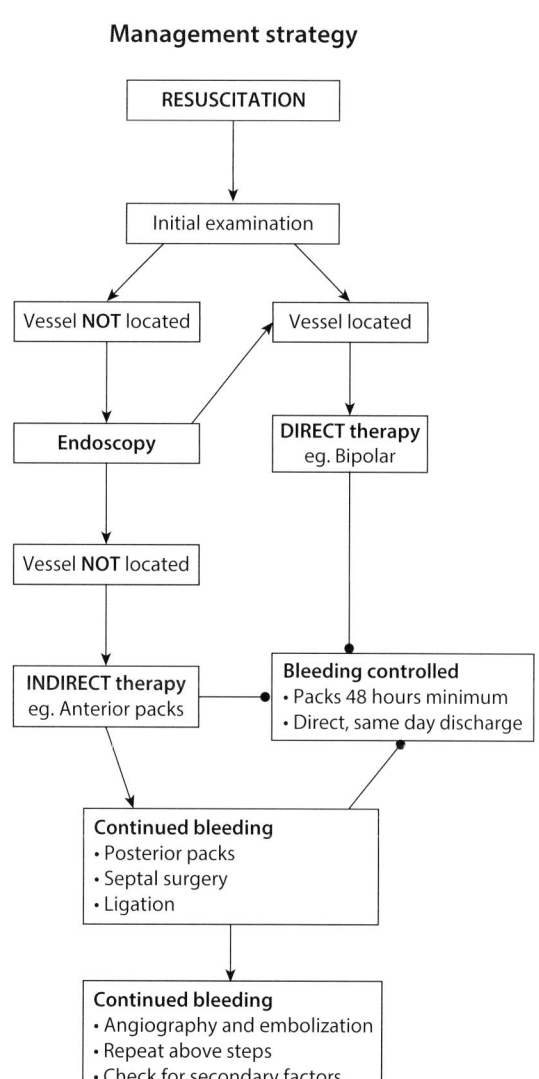

Figure 106.6 Management algorithm.

more than academic as the management of each type is quite different, e.g. techniques used to control primary epistaxis are unlikely to be successful for a secondary epistaxis due to coagulopathy.

Anterior and posterior epistaxis

The terms anterior and posterior epistaxis are frequently used but the definitions are imprecise and inconsistent and really not very useful. Pearson attempted to standardize the term posterior epistaxis as a bleeding point which cannot be located despite examination with a headlight, vasoconstrictors and suction.[9] While this is a clinically useful definition, modern techniques of examination and endoscopy, are likely to see true posterior bleeds moving further and further back! Attempts to define anterior epistaxis as bleeding from Little's area are problematic, due to the lack of a precise definition of Little's area. To standardize the use of the term 'posterior epistaxis' and 'anterior epistaxis', the author proposes that their use be restricted to the following:

- **Anterior epistaxis** – bleeding from a source anterior to the plane of the piriform aperture. This includes bleeding from the anterior septum and rare bleeds from the vestibular skin and mucocutaneous junction. These should be the bleeds where the clinician will easily locate the bleeding point and management should be simple.
- **Posterior epistaxis** – bleeding from a vessel situated posterior to the piriform aperture, i.e. from within the nasal cavity. This allows further subdivision of these posterior or nasal cavity bleeding points into lateral wall, septal and nasal floor bleeding. These are the bleeds that will challenge the clinician the most.

Further descriptive classification based on the severity and frequency of the bleeding can also be used, e.g. whether recurrent (usually minor and non-life-threatening) or acute, severe. It is of interest that for adults at least, the severity of an epistaxis is inversely proportional to its frequency. That is, recurrent primary epistaxis tends to be minor, non-life-threatening and often easily managed whereas acute, severe epistaxis is often a one-time event resulting in hospitalization and carrying a high morbidity.

For the remainder of this chapter, the clinical syndromes of adult epistaxis are discussed. Childhood epistaxis is discussed elsewhere in this textbook (**Table 106.1**).

TABLE 106.1 Classification of epistaxis

- **Primary:** no proven causal factor
- **Secondary:** proven causal factor
- **Childhood:** <16 years
- **Adult:** >16 years
- **Anterior:** bleeding anterior to piriform aperture
- **Posterior:** bleeding point posterior to piriform aperture

ADULT PRIMARY EPISTAXIS

Demography

Adult primary epistaxis is the variant that challenges otolaryngologists the most. The condition can occur at any age but is mainly a disease of the elderly. Between 7% and 14% of adults have epistaxis at some time or other but only 6% of cases are seen by otorhinolaryngologists.[23, 24] The peak presentation is the sixth decade and most large case series reveal a slight male predominance (55 male, 45 female).[15, 25] Most cases are minor, self-limiting or easily managed anterior bleeds but nevertheless a significant number require admission to hospital. The annual rate of admission to otolaryngology units in the northern UK with adult epistaxis is 30 per 100,000 per annum.[26] In Scotland, epistaxis is the commonest reason for adult admission to an ENT ward.[27] Fewer than 10% of hospitalized patients require a general anaesthetic procedure to secure haemostasis.[28] It is not surprising that such a common haemorrhagic condition of elderly patients is associated with significant morbidity and mortality. After head and neck cancer, epistaxis stands out as a prominent cause of mortality in ENT patients.

Aetiology

By definition the aetiology of primary epistaxis is unknown but there are clear suggestions that systemic factors may be important (**Table 106.2**).

CHRONOBIOLOGY

The frequency of admission is greatest in the autumn and winter months.[28, 29] This seasonal variation correlates with fluctuations in environmental temperature and humidity.[30] A chronobiological rhythm is also observed at the circadian level where onset of bleeding and hospital admission show a biphasic pattern with peaks in the morning and late evening.[31, 32] There are strong parallels between the circadian rhythms of primary epistaxis and those observed in subarachnoid haemorrhage.

NON-STEROIDAL ANTI-INFLAMMATORY DRUGS (NSAID)

Adult pattern epistaxis is associated with the use of NSAID. Patients are more likely than controls to consume NSAID. The NSAID used include prescribed and self-administered compounds especially aspirin. The action of non-steroidal anti-inflammatory drugs is mediated via an anti-platelet aggregation effect due to altered platelet membrane physiology.[33–35]

ALCOHOL

Similar aetiological associations to those of NSAID have been found with alcohol. Epistaxis patients are more likely to consume alcohol than matched control patients and are more likely to have consumed alcohol within 24 hours of hospital admission than other emergency admissions. The use of alcohol by epistaxis patients is associated with a prolongation of the bleeding time despite normal platelet counts and coagulation factor activity. Once again, the effects of NSAID and alcohol mirror those reported in subarachnoid haemorrhage.[36, 37]

HYPERTENSION

This has long been considered a cause of epistaxis. However, a number of large studies have failed to show a causal relationship between hypertension and epistaxis.[38] Attempts to correlate epistaxis with secondary effects of hypertension or with the severity of hypertension have proved inconclusive.[39] Even if not causal, elevated blood pressure is observed in almost all epistaxis admissions. This apparent hypertension in acute admissions may be a result of anxiety associated with hospital admission and the invasive techniques used to control the bleeding.

SEPTAL ABNORMALITIES

Septal abnormalities are common and depending on the definition used between 1% and 80% of the population have a significant deviation.[40] Given such a high prevalence, the perceived association between epistaxis and septal abnormalities could be coincidence. One study found an association between septal deviation and *recurrent* epistaxis in young subjects.[41] There is no clear case control evidence of an association between septal abnormalities and adult epistaxis.

Management

In order to be effective the management of adult epistaxis should follow an incremental sequence of interventions (**Figure 106.6**). The theoretical ideal treatment requires identification of the bleeding point and direct control of the bleeding, at source. First, the patient must be resuscitated, bleeding slowed, the nasal cavity examined and a treatment plan established.

RESUSCITATION

Given the high prevalence of coexistent cardiovascular disease, prompt and effective resuscitation is required. Sixty-five percent of cases are referred from an accident and emergency department and thus many will already have had some form of therapy.[28] First aid by pinching the ala nasi (the Hippocratic technique) is supported by the frequency with which the anterior part of the septum

TABLE 106.2 Summary of aetiological evidence of adult primary epistaxis

- **Weather:** proven association
- **NSAID:** proven association
- **Alcohol:** proven association
- **Hypertension:** no association
- **Septal deviation:** no association

is the source of bleeding. Otorhinolaryngologists should ensure medical students, nurses and other team members are fully aware of the precise technique for compression of the nostrils. In one study of Accident and Emergency staff, only 43% of trained medical and nursing staff could correctly demonstrate the Hippocratic technique.[42] Recent surveys of junior doctors show that nothing much has changed and there is still poor understanding of initial management of epistaxis![43] History and examination will help in assessing the amount of blood lost. In all but the most minor of bleeds intravenous access is established and baseline blood estimations are taken. A detailed history should be taken, looking for predisposing factors. Routine coagulation studies in the absence of a positive history are not indicated.[15, 44]

ASSESSMENT

The patient should be assessed in a semi-recumbent position and nursing assistance is mandatory. Everyone involved should wear protective visors and clothing as blood aerosol contamination is common, especially when inserting nasal packing.[45] Basic equipment includes: couch or reclining chair, headlight, suction, vasoconstrictor solutions (lignocaine and pseudoephedrine solution has now widely superseded cocaine solutions) and a selection of packs, tampons and cautery apparatus. All specialist ENT units should also have access to rod lens nasal endoscopy equipment and bipolar electrodiathermy.

DIRECT OR INDIRECT THERAPIES

Treatment may be divided into direct (bleeding point specific therapies) or indirect treatments. Indirect treatments are those that do not require identification of the bleeding point. Direct treatments are logically and theoretically superior and, therefore, a committed search for the bleeding vessel should always be undertaken.[9]

DIRECT MANAGEMENT

There has been a slow but steady uptake of direct strategies throughout the UK. Despite this, however, a minority of cases admitted to otolaryngology units in the UK are managed by direct control of the bleeding point.[28] The reluctance to use direct approaches may be due to a perceived difficulty in locating bleeding points, but probably also reflects the fact that over 70% of cases are managed by the most junior members of the specialty.[27] Anterior epistaxis is usually very straightforward to identify and treat and over 90% of cases can be controlled with silver nitrate cautery or bipolar. The use of packing for primary anterior epistaxis is unwarranted and should be strongly discouraged.

Posterior epistaxis can occur from the lateral wall, floor or septum. As previously discussed there is evidence to support the septum as the principal locus. Systematic examination with a headlight will identify most bleeding points. Once identified, bleeding points can be directly controlled with bipolar diathermy, chemical cautery (difficult in posterior bleeds), electro-cautery or direct pressure from miniature targeted packs.[46]

Endoscopic control

Failure to locate the bleeding point on initial examination is an indication for examination with a rod lens endoscope. Endoscopy identifies the source of posterior epistaxis in over 80% of cases.[26, 10, 14, 46] Endoscopy enables targeted haemostasis of the bleeding vessel using insulated hot wire cautery or modern single fibre bipolar electrodes.[26] Success rates for immediate control by endoscopic guidance are consistently reported in the 90% range.[26] Monopolar diathermy should not be used in the nasal cavity as there have been reports of blindness due to current propogation.[47]

Adoption of direct (including endoscopic) management strategies has been shown to facilitate out-patient management and to significantly reduce in-patient stay (**Figure 106.7**).[26]

Indirect therapies

Failure to find the bleeding point is an indication for use of one of numerous traditionally favoured indirect strategies.

Nasal packing

Packing can be anteriorly or posteriorly placed. Anterior packing has been the mainstay of treatment for centuries. Skills required for accurate packing are difficult to acquire and with modern techniques of nasal surgery, less frequently encountered in a surgeon's training.

Ribbon gauze impregnated with petroleum jelly or Bismuth Iodoform Paraffin paste (BIPP) is inserted the entire length of the nasal cavity in attempt to tamponade the bleeding. Once inserted, the packs are left *in situ* for between 24 and 72 hours.[48] Continued or re-bleeding with packs *in situ* is observed in up to 40% of cases.[49] Complications of packing include; sinusitis, septal perforation, alar necrosis, hypoxia and myocardial infarction. Packing is usually considered an indication for antibiotic cover but the evidence base for this is lacking.

Modern and now more frequently used variations on anterior packing include special tampons (Merocel® and Kaltostat®) and balloon catheters (Brighton or Epistat). Balloons and tampons are favoured by non-specialists as first-line therapy but are associated with similar complications and re-bleed rates to packing. If over inflated, balloons will prolapse anteriorly and posteriorly with the risk of hypoxia and alar necrosis.[50] There is no evidence of greater efficacy for packs compared to balloons or tampons.

Persistent bleeding or re-bleeding is an indication for further examination of the nasal cavity and renewed search for the bleeding point. There is no clear, universally agreed definition of failed packing but patients who continue to bleed should proceed to surgical management sooner rather than later. In the author's institution the agreed protocol is that all admitted epistaxis patients should be haemostased within 24 hours of admission. If this has not been achieved a rhinologist should be summoned to review the case. Patients should not be left on a ward with blood oozing from nasal packs or tampons while on-call teams change shift!

Hot water irrigation

Irrigation of the nasal cavity with water at 50°C has been proposed as an alternative to packing. Although this technique has seen little use in the UK, Stangerup reports similar levels of success comparing the hot water technique to anterior packing and balloon tamponade.[49, 51] Up to one third of patients find the technique difficult to tolerate and so use of specialized irrigation catheters is recommended. The exact mechanism of action of this treatment is unclear but may, paradoxically, involve reflex vasodilatation and reduction in nasal lumen dimensions.[52]

Systemic medical therapy

Tranexamic acid and epsilon aminocaproic acid are systemic inhibitors of fibrinolysis. Tranexamic acid has been shown to reduce the severity and risk of re-bleeding in epistaxis at a dose of 1.5 g three times a day. Tranexamic acid does not increase fibrin deposition and so does not increase the risk of thrombosis. Pre-existing thromboembolic disease is a contraindication. At present antifibrinolytics are best reserved as adjuvant therapy in recurrent or refractory cases. There has been a recent increase of interest in this drug and it may become more important in managing secondary bleeds due to novel anticoagulants.[53]

Topical haemostatic agents

Topical thrombin compounds have been marketed for operative field haemostasis in surgery. The use of these compounds in epistaxis is attractive to those looking for a simple fix. Compounds such as Floseal (Baxter Healthcare) have been used and results have been variable with some authors finding no real benefit.[54] In the author's experience these agents can only be considered an additional tool for the management of difficult (especially secondary) bleeds

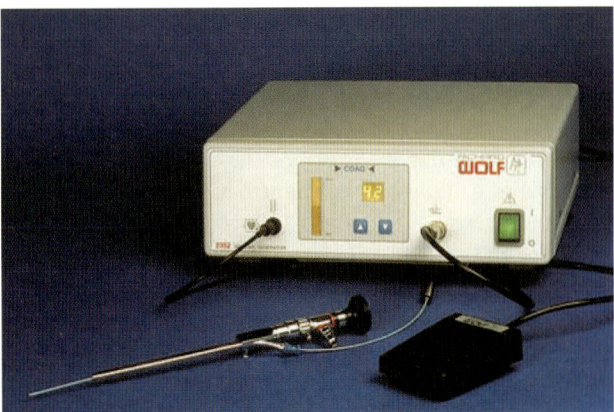

Figure 106.7 Single fibre bipolar unit for direct management of epistaxis.

and should never replace the main aim of identifying and directly treating the source of the bleeding.

Surgical management

If the techniques described above fail, surgical intervention is required. Endoscopic diathermy of the bleeding point under anaesthetic may control the bleeding but if the vessel still cannot be controlled (or even located) indirect surgical therapy is indicated. Surgical management for continued epistaxis consists of:

- Posterior packing
- Ligation techniques
- Septal surgery techniques
- Embolization techniques.

POSTERIOR NASAL PACKS

Posterior packing should be viewed as largely obsolete but in extreme cases or where no specialist rhinologist is available it may be indicated. It can, in extremis, be carried out under local anaesthetic but general anaesthesia is preferable. Nasopharyngeal tamponade is achieved using special gauze packs inserted transorally and positioned by means of tapes passed from the posterior choana to the anterior nares bilaterally. These posterior 'Bellocq' packs are secured against anterior gauze packing. The securing tapes are tied over padding positioned to protect the columella from pressure necrosis. An easier and perhaps kinder alternative is to insert a Foley urethral catheter (size 12 or 14) along the floor of the nasal cavity until the nasopharynx is reached. The Foley catheter is inflated with 15 ml of water, pulled forward to engage in the posterior choana and anterior packing is then inserted. The Foley catheter needs to be secured anteriorly taking care not to cause pressure over the columella. Posterior packing causes considerable pain and may cause hypoxia secondary to soft palate oedema. Sinusitis and middle ear effusions are common. More serious complications include necrosis of the septum and columella. Antibiotics and opiate analgesia are necessary. Once they have been placed, posterior packs should be left in position for a minimum of 48 hours or at least until a rhinological surgeon can attend to the patient.

LIGATION TECHNIQUES

Ligation is reserved for intractable bleeding where the source cannot be located or controlled by the techniques described above. Knowledge of the blood supply of the nasal cavity and the likely sources of epistaxis will inform the choice of ligation technique (**Figure 106.5**).

Ligation should be performed as close as possible to the likely bleeding point thus the hierarchy of ligation is:

- Sphenopalatine artery
- Internal maxillary artery
- External carotid artery
- Anterior /posterior ethmoidal artery.

Endonasal endoscopic sphenopalatine artery ligation (ESPAL)

ESPAL conforms to the ideal of controlling the bleed as close as possible to its nasal source. The sphenopalatine artery is the main supply of the nasal cavity and thus the most logical target for ligation. Modern endoscopic techniques have seen an increase in popularity of this procedure and it has now largely replaced all other ligations as the procedure of choice. The operation has been performed with an operating microscope but much more commonly using modern endoscopic techniques. Under general or local anaesthetic, an incision is made approximately 8 mm anterior to and under cover of the posterior end of the middle turbinate. The incision is carried down to the bone and a mucosal flap is elevated posteriorly until the fibroneurovascular sleeve arising from the sphenopalatine foramen is identified. The foramen can be difficult to identify but its location is signalled by the crista-ethmoidalis.[20] Once the main vessel is identified, it can be ligated using haemostatic clips (**Figure 106.9**) and divided or coagulated using bipolar diathermy (**Figure 106.8**). In some series success rates for this procedure have reached almost 100%.[55] Complications including re-bleeding (anastomoses), infection and nasal adhesions are generally less common than with other procedures.

Internal maxillary artery ligation (IMAL)

This was more frequently used prior to the development of ESPAL procedures. The artery is exposed

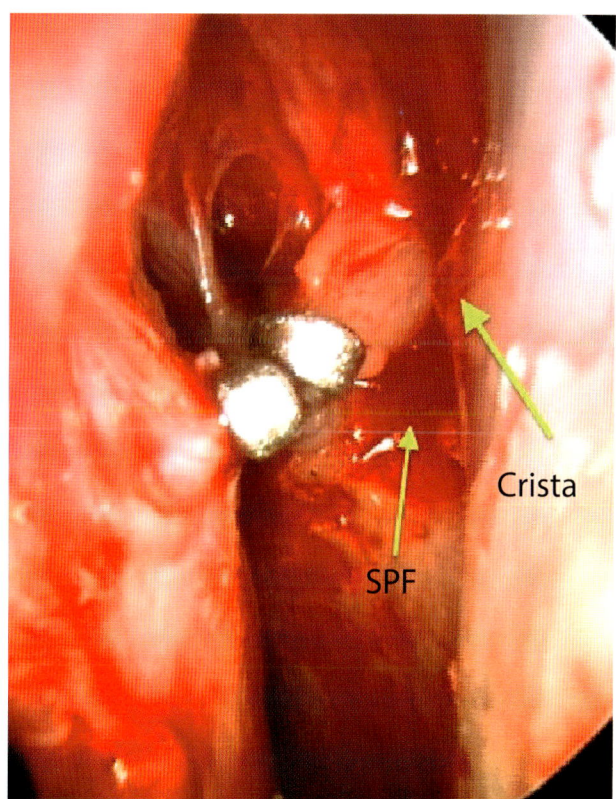

Figure 106.8 Haemostatic clips applied to main trunk of sphenopalatine artery (left) in procedure of ESPAL. Crista: crista ethmoidalis, SPF: sphenopalatine foramen.

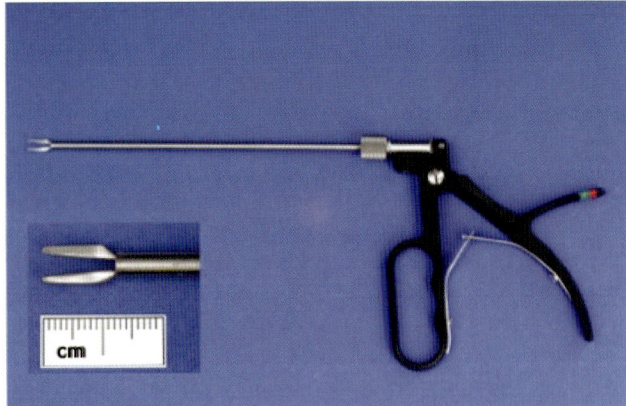

Figure 106.9 Rotatable ligation clip applicators suitable for ESPAL.

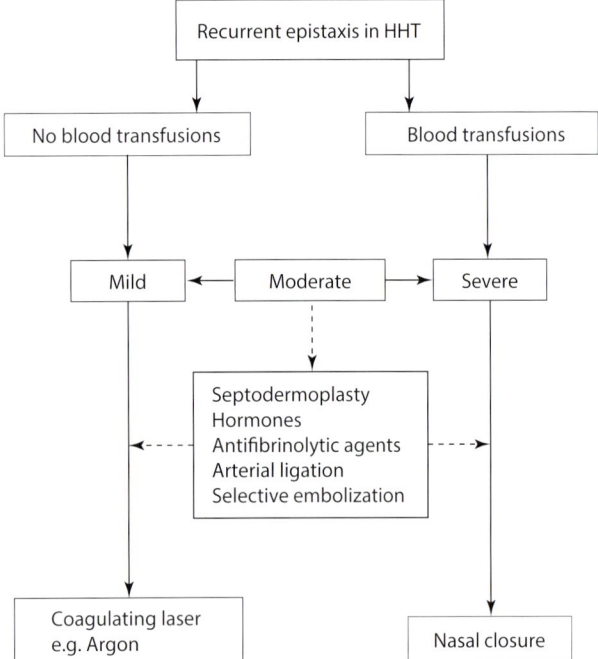

Figure 106.10 The management of HHT. From Lund and Howard, *Am J Rhinol* with permission.[68]

trans-antrally via anterior (sublabial) or combined anterior and medial (endoscopic) techniques. In the traditional sublabial approach an antrostomy is formed taking care to preserve the infra-orbital nerve. The mucosa of the posterior wall of the antrum is then elevated and a window is made through into the pterygopalatine fossa. The branches of the internal maxillary artery are identified pulsating within the fat of the fossa and are carefully dissected out prior to clipping with haemostatic clips. The proximal internal maxillary artery, descending palatine and sphenopalatine branches are all clipped and ideally divided. An endoscopic variation of this technique uses a middle meatus antrostomy as an instrument port with a 4 mm endoscope is inserted through a small canine fossa antrostomy.[56] Trans-antral ligation controls haemorrhage in 89% of cases and is comparable to embolization in both cost and efficacy.[57] Endoscopic trans-antral ligation of the internal maxillary artery can also be carried out via a middle meatus antrostomy and is occasionally required when control of a damaged sphenopalatine artery is lost during ESPAL. Complications include: sinusitis, damage to the infra-orbital nerve, oro-antral fistula, dental damage and anaesthesia and rarely ophthalmoplegia and blindness.

External carotid artery ligation (ECAL)

ECAL represents a step further away from the nasal source of bleeding. Nevertheless, the relative technical ease of this procedure justifies its use in extreme cases and by non-rhinologists. This procedure can be carried out under local or general anaesthetic using either a skin crease incision or a longitudinal incision parallel with the anterior border of the sternomastoid. The carotid bifurcation is identified and the external carotid confirmed, double checked for arterial branches and then ligated in continuity. Some authors advocate anterior and posterior ethmoidal artery ligation as an adjuvant to this procedure. In one study, external carotid artery ligation secured haemostasis in 14 out of 15 patients.[58] Complications include wound infection, haematoma and neurovascular damage.

Anterior/posterior ethmoidal artery ligation (EAL)

Given the minimal contribution of these arteries to the nasal blood supply, their ligation is best reserved as an adjuvant to one of the procedures described above or in cases of confirmed ethmoidal bleeding (e.g. ethmoidal fracture, iatrogenic tear). The arteries are approached by a medial canthal incision which is carried down to the bone of the anterior lacrimal crest. Periosteal elevators are then used to elevate and laterally retract the bulbar fascia. The anterior ethmoidal artery is seen as a fibro-neurovascular mesentry running from the bulbar fascia into the anterior ethmoidal foramen. The vessel is clipped and divided and dissection is continued to identify the posterior artery which is located approximately 12 mm behind. Endoscopic trans-ethmoidal ligation of the anterior ethmoidal artery has been described. The popularity of ligation of these vessels in primary epistaxis possibly reflects the technical ease of the open procedure rather than any logical reason for ligating vessels with such a small contribution to the nasal blood supply (**Figures 106.3** and **106.4**).

SEPTAL SURGERY

When epistaxis originates behind a prominent septal deviation or vomero-palatine spur, septoplasty or submucosal resection (SMR) may be required to access the bleeding point. Some authors have advocated septal surgery as a primary treatment for failed packing. The rationale is that by elevating the mucoperichondrial flap for septoplasty or SMR, the blood supply to the septum is interrupted and haemostasis secured. In one study a strategy involving SMR and re-packing was found to be more effective and economic than ligation in patients who had failed with packing, however, this was prior to widespread adoption of ESPAL techniques.[59]

EMBOLIZATION

Embolization under angiographic guidance has been shown to control severe epistaxis in between 82% and 97% of cases.[57, 60, 61] Under local anaesthetic, transfemoral Seldinger angiography is used to identify the bleeding points and display the nasal circulation. It is essential to exclude arteriovenous malformations, aneurysms and fistulae prior to embolization. Once the bleeding vessel is identified, a fine catheter is passed into the internal maxillary circulation and particles (polyvinyl alcohol, tungsten or steel microcoils) are used to embolize the vessels. The ipsilateral facial artery is also embolized in order to prevent re-circulation. Complications include skin necrosis, paraesthesia, cerebrovascular accident and groin haematomas.

Embolization is of similar efficacy to ligation techniques and, therefore, choice will depend on local expertise, availability and experience. The risks of embolization mean that is should be reserved for failed ligations or where no rhinological surgical expertise is available.

Adult recurrent epistaxis

Recurrent bleeding is more commonly seen in children. When recurrent bleeds occur in adults, secondary epistaxis is most likely. Bleeding is usually minor and troublesome rather than life-threatening and it is uncommon to see bleeding by the time the patient presents. A full and detailed history and examination should identify factors such as aspirin use, liver disease or bleeding from the margins of a septal perforation. Rarely nasal tumours present with recurrent blood-stained discharge which should be distinguished from epistaxis per se. Patients using topical nasal medications (particularly steroid sprays) frequently report minor recurrent bleeds.

If a bleeding point can be identified cautery is used but often no single vessel can be identified and an area of vestibulitis is found. Evidence for the efficacy of topical antiseptic creams is available from paediatric studies and it is likely (but unproven in adults) that chlorhexidine and neomycin creams may reduce the frequency of bleeding. An area of debate is what to do when aspirin being used for cardiovascular prophylaxis is responsible for recurrent bleeds. If there is a history of cardiovascular disease or vascular graft surgery then aspirin should not be discontinued, otherwise temporary cessation of aspirin may be required to allow the recurrent bleeding to settle.

SECONDARY EPISTAXIS

Epistaxis is commonly observed in patients with coagulopathy secondary to liver disease, leukaemia or myelosuppression. In such cases, treatment of the epistaxis demands close liaison with haematologists and physicians. The following causes of secondary epistaxis deserve special mention.

Trauma

Post-traumatic nasal haemorrhage does not conform to the normal pattern of epistaxis and its origin and severity is almost infinitely variable. Persistent bleeding can occur from the ethmoidal arteries following fronto-ethmoidal fracture. In this case the vessels may be lacerated, incompletely divided or even held open by fractures through their bony mesenteries. Severe haemorrhage refractory to packing should be managed by open approach ligation.

Catastrophic bleeding has been reported after head injuries due to delayed rupture of an internal carotid artery pseudo-aneurysm. Thus persistent or unexpectedly severe bleeding even some time after a head injury should be seen as an indication for CT scanning and angiography.[62]

Post-surgical

Bleeding can occur after almost any nasal surgery and is seldom difficult to manage. An exception is the severe haemorrhage which occurs in between 3% and 9% of inferior turbinectomies.[63] As previously discussed bipolar to the main branch of the inferior turbinate artery will usually secure haemostasis. Anterior subtotal turbinectomy may carry a reduced risk of post-operative bleeding.[63]

Iatrogenic damage to the anterior ethmoidal artery during endoscopic sinus surgery should be managed by bipolar of the vessel. Retraction of the vessel into the orbit can give rise to a tension haematoma of the orbit and is a surgical emergency (see elsewhere).

Massive and usually fatal epistaxis can result from damage to the internal carotid artery during posterior ethmoid or sphenoid sinus surgery. The bleeding is usually uncontrollable but packing, angiography and embolization may be tried.

Warfarin

Patients on warfarin constitute between 9% and 17% of epistaxis admissions.[27, 64] Bleeding may be due to overdose or loss of control but can also occur in patients whose INR is within the therapeutic zone. With warfarin, direct therapies seldom work and packing may be required. Bleeding is often from multiple sites and attempts at instrumentation lead to further mucosal damage and bleeding. After resuscitation, anterior packs should be gently inserted and the haematology team consulted. With large areas of bleeding or oozing fibrin glue has been used as a haemostatic dressing.[65] When deciding to reduce, stop or even reverse warfarin, the medical history and the severity of the epistaxis must be considered. If the INR is within the therapeutic range and treatment seems to be controlling the bleeding it may be safe to continue the warfarin.[64]

New oral anticoagulants: TSOACs

New target specific oral anticoagulants such as Rivaroxiban and Dabigataran are seeing increased use throughout the healthcare system. As a result numbers of secondary epistaxis cases in patients on these medications are being seen in our ENT units. Unlike vitamin K antagonists the reversal of these new agents is often difficult to achieve and can be incomplete. Siegal has written a useful paper on the subject.[66]

When dealing with epistaxis in patients on these compounds ENT surgeons are advised to liaise at the earliest opportunity with the local haematology team. In addition to discussing with haematologists about anticoagulant reversal it is important that no steps are taken to stop or reverse agents without first clarifying the indication for the medication. Liaison with cardiologists may be required to avoid catastrophic complications (e.g. stent occlusion) as a result of withholding antiplatelet or anticoagulant medication for what may even after all prove to be a very minor epistaxis.

Hereditary haemorrhagic telangiectasia

Hereditary haemorrhagic telangiectasia (HHT) or Osler-Weber-Rendu disease is an autosomal dominant condition affecting blood vessels in skin, mucous membranes and viscera. Penetrance is variable but reaches 97% by age 50 years and occasional atavistic cases are observed. The genetic abnormality has been located to chromosome 9q (HHT1) and chromosome 12q (HHT2). The classical features are telangiectasia, a-v malformations and aneurysms. Recurrent epistaxis occurs in 93% of cases.[67] Management involves packing, cautery, antifibrinolytics, systemic or topical oestrogens, coagulative lasers, septal dermoplasty, ligation and embolization and as a last resort permanent surgical closure of the nostrils (Young's operation). Laser photocoagulation has become a popular therapy and the NdYAG, Argon and KTP532 lasers have all been used with some success. Large multicentre comparisons of these treatments have not been conducted and due to the relative rarity of the condition this situation is likely to persist. **Figure 106.10** is an algorithm for management of this condition.[68] A recent study showed that the disability produced by Young's operation was more than offset by an improved quality of life due to reduced bleeding. Trials of systemic, topical or locally injectable Bevacizumab have produced conflicting results and at present the efficacy of this drug in HHT is unproven.[69]

Tumours

Nasal tumours seldom present as epistaxis in isolation. More commonly tumours produce blood-stained discharge with other nasal symptoms (unilateral obstruction, pain, swelling). The risk, albeit small, of missing a tumour is another good reason for using nasal endoscopy in epistaxis cases. Juvenile nasopharyngeal angiofibroma (JNA) and haemangiopericytoma (HPC) are rare vascular tumours which can present with recurrent or severe epistaxis in association with nasal obstruction. Treatment of JNA and HPC is mainly surgical but may include pre-operative embolization and are dealt with elsewhere in this textbook.

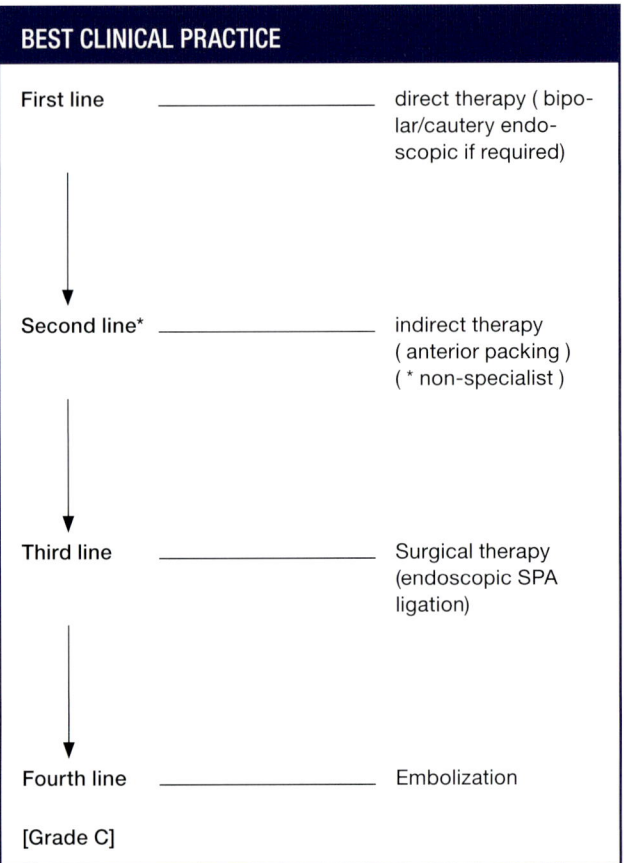

> **BEST CLINICAL PRACTICE**
>
> First line — direct therapy (bipolar/cautery endoscopic if required)
>
> ↓
>
> Second line* — indirect therapy (anterior packing) (* non-specialist)
>
> ↓
>
> Third line — Surgical therapy (endoscopic SPA ligation)
>
> ↓
>
> Fourth line — Embolization
>
> [Grade C]

> **FUTURE RESEARCH**
>
> ➤ Publications still consistently fail to classify epistaxis or define the study population. Thus studies involve heterogenous groups of patients and different types of epistaxis making comparisons difficult. As result level 1 and 2 evidence is scarce.
> ➤ Multicentre comparisons of treatment and management strategies still do not exist.
> ➤ Basic research is required to identify initiating and aetiological factors.

> **KEY POINTS**
>
> - Direct bleeding point specific approaches are superior to indirect nasal packing strategies.
> - Epistaxis secondary to drugs or coagulopathy requires management of the underlying cause.
> - Endoscopic ligation of the sphenopalatine artery is the ligation of choice.
> - The endoscope has revolutionized the treatment of epistaxis.

REFERENCES

1. Morgagni JP. *The seats and causes of diseases*. Vol.1, Alabama: Gryphon Editions Ltd; 1983, pp. 312–54 (first published in 1761).
2. MacArthur FJD, McGarry GW. The arterial supply of the nasal cavity. *Eur Arch Otorhinolaryngol* 2017; **274**(2): 809–15.
3. Mackenzie D. Little's area or the Locus Kiesselbachii. *J Laryngol* 1914; **29**(1): 21–2.
4. Nomina Anatomica 6th ed. Nomina Histologica 3rd ed. and Nomina Embryologica 3rd ed. 1985, A54–A55.
5. Burnham HH. An anatomical investigation of blood vessels of the lateral nasal wall and their relation to turbinates and sinuses. *J Laryngol Otol* 1935; **50**: 569–93.
6. Shaheen OH. Epistaxis in the middle aged and elderly. Thesis for Master of Surgery. London: University of London; 1987.
7. Caliot PH, Plessis JL, Midy D, et al. The intraorbital arrangement of the anterior and posterior ethmoidal foramina. *Surg Radiol Anat* 1995; **17**: 29–33.
8. Lasjaunias P, Marsot-Dupuch K, Doyon D. The radio-anatomical basis of arterial embolisation for epistaxis. *J Neuroradiol* 1979; **6**: 45–53.
9. Pearson BW. Epistaxis: some observations on conservative management. *J Laryngol Otol (Suppl)*, 1983; **8**: 115–19.
10. Wurman LH, Sack JG, Flannery JV, Paulson JO. Selective endoscopic electrocautery for posterior epistaxis. *Laryngoscope* 1988; **98**: 1348–9.
11. Woodruff GH. Cardiovascular epistaxis and the naso-nasopharyngeal plexus. *Laryngoscope* 1949; **15**: 1238–47.
12. Chiu TW, Shaw-Dunn J, McGarry GW. Woodruff's naso-nasopharyngeal plexus: how important is it in posterior epistaxis? *Clin Otolaryngol* 1998; **23**: 272–9.
13. Jackson KR, Jackson RT. Factors associated with active, refractory epistaxis. *Arch Otolaryngol Head Neck Surg* 1988; **114**: 862–5.
14. O'Leary-Stickney K, Makielski K, Weymuller EA. Rigid endoscopy for the control of epistaxis. *Arch Otolaryngol Head Neck Surg* 1992; **118**: 966–7.
15. Padgham N. Epistaxis: anatomical and clinical correlates. *J Laryngol Otol* 1990; **104**: 308–11.
16. Shaheen OH. Arterial epistaxis. *J Laryngol Otol* 1975; **89**: 17–34.
17. el-Silimy O. Endonasal endoscopy and posterior epistaxis. *Rhinology* 1993; **31**: 119–20.
18. Rosnagle RS, Yanagisawa E, Smith HW. Specific vessel ligation for epistaxis & survey of 60 cases. *Laryngoscope* 1973; **83**: 517–25.
19. McGarry GW. MD Thesis. University of Glasgow 1996. Epistaxis.
20. Bolger WE, Borgie RC, Melder P. The role of the crista ethmoidalis in endoscopic sphenopalatine artery ligation. *Am J Rhinol* 1999; **13**(2): 81–6.
21. Maran AGD, Lund VJ. Chapter 2; Section 2.8, Epistaxis. In *Clinical Rhinology*. New York: Thieme; 1990, pp. 101–4.
22. Stell PM. Epistaxis. *Clin Otolaryngol* 1977; **2**: 263–73.
23. Weiss NS. Relation of high blood pressure to headache, epistaxis and selected other symptoms. *N Eng J Med* 1972; **287**(13): 631–3.
24. Lepore ML. Epistaxis. In: Bailey BJ, Johnson JR, Kohut RI, et al. (eds). *Head and Neck Surgery: Otolaryngology*, Vol. 1. Philadelphia, JB Lippincott Company; 1993, pp. 428–46.
25. Juselius H. Epistaxis: a clinical study of 1,724 patients. *J Laryngol Otol* 1974; **88**: 317–27.
26. O'Donnell M, Robertson G, McGarry GW. A new bipolar diathermy probe for the outpatient management of adult acute epistaxis. *Clin Otolaryngol* 1999; **24**: 537–41.
27. Walker TW, MacFarlane TV, McGarry GW. The epidemiology and chronobiology of epistaxis: an investigation of Scottish hospital admissions 1995–2004. *Clin Otolaryngol* 2007; **32**(5): 361–5.
28. Kotecha B, Fowler S, Harkness P, et al. Management of epistaxis: a national survey. *Ann R Coll Surg Eng* 1996; **78**: 444–6.
29. Nunez DA, McClymont LG, Evans RA. Epistaxis: a study of the relationship with weather. *Clin Otolaryngol* 1990; **15**: 49–51.
30. Danielides V, Kontogiannis N, Bartzokas A, et al. The influence of meteorological factors on the frequency of epistaxis. *Clin Otolaryngol* 2002; **27**(2): 84–8.
31. Mehanna H, Robinson K, Gatehouse S, McGarry GW. Otorhinolaryngological Research Society (ORS): a circadian rhythm in adult idiopathic epistaxis? *Clin Otolaryngol* 1998; **23**: 280.
32. Manfredini R, Portaluppi F, Salmi R, et al. Circadian variation in onset of epistaxis: analysis of hospital admissions. *BMJ* 2000; **321**: 1112.
33. Watson MG, Shenoi PM. Drug-induced epistaxis? *J R Soc Med* 1990; **83**: 162–4.
34. McGarry GW. Drug-induced epistaxis? *J R Soc Med* 1990; **83**: 812.
35. Livesey JR, Watson MG, Kelly PJ, Kesteven PJ. Do patients with epistaxis have drug-induced platelet dysfunction? *Clin Otolaryngol* 1995; **20**: 407–10.
36. McGarry GW, Gatehouse S, Hinnie J. Relation between alcohol and nose bleeds. *BMJ* 1994; **309**: 640.
37. McGarry GW, Gatehouse S, Vernham G. Idiopathic epistaxis, haemostasis and alcohol. *Clin Otolaryngol* 1995; **20**: 174–7.
38. Lubianca-Neto JF, Bredemeier M, Carvalhal EF, et al. A study of the association between epistaxis and the severity of hypertension. *Am J Rhinol* 1998; **12**(4): 269–72.
39. Lubianca-Neto JF, Fuchs FD, Facco SR, et al. Is epistaxis evidence of end-organ damage in patients with hypertension? *Laryngoscope* 1999; **109**: 1111–15.
40. Roblin DG, Eccles R. Review: What, if any, is the value of septal surgery? *Clin Otolaryngol* 2002; **27**(2): 77.
41. O'Reilly BJ, Simpson DC, Dharmeratnam R. Recurrent epistaxis and nasal septal deviation in young adults. *Clin Otolaryngol* 1996; **21**: 12–14.
42. McGarry GW, Moulton C. The first aid management of epistaxis by accident and emergency department staff. *Arch Emerg Med* 1993; **10**: 298–300.
43. Fox R, Nash R, Lui ZW, Singh A. Epistaxis management: current understanding amongst junior doctors. *J Laryngol Otol* 2016; **130**(3): 252–5.
44. Smith IM, Ludlam CA, Murray JAM. Haematological indices in elderly patients with epistaxis. *Health Bull (Edinb)* 1988; **46**(5): 277–81.
45. Carney AS, Weir J, Baldwin DL. Contamination with blood during management of epistaxis. *BMJ* 1995; **311**: 1064.
46. McGarry GW. Nasal endoscope in posterior epistaxis: a preliminary evaluation. *J Laryngol Otol* 1991; **105**: 428–31.
47. Vanden Abeele D, Clemens A, Tassignon MJ, van de Heyning PH. Blindness due to electrocoagulation following functional endoscopic sinus surgery. *J Laryngol Otol* 1996; **110**: 261–4.
48. Tan LKS, Calhoun KH. Epistaxis. *Med Clin North Am* 1999; **83**(1): 43–56.
49. Stangerup SE, Dommerby H, Lau T. Hot-water irrigation as a treatment of posterior epistaxis. *Rhinology* 1996; **34**: 18–20.
50. McGarry GW, Aitken D. Intranasal balloon catheters: how do they work? *Clin Otolaryngol* 1991; **16**: 388–92.
51. Stangerup SE, Dommerby H, et al. New modification of hot-water irrigation in the treatment of posterior epistaxis. *Arch Otolaryngol Head Neck Surg* 1999; **125**: 686–90.
52. Stangerup SE, Thomsen HK. Histological changes in the nasal mucosa after hot-water irrigation: an animal experimental study. *Rhinology* 1996; **34**: 14–17.
53. Petruson B. A double-blind study to evaluate the effect of epistaxis with oral administration of the antifibrinolytic drug tranexamic acid (cyclokapron). *Acta Oto-Laryngologica Suppl* 1974; **317**: 57–61.
54. Khan MK, El Badawey MR, Powell J, Idris M. The utility of Floseal haemostatic agent in the management of epistaxis. *J Laryngol Otol* 2015; **129**(4): 353–7.
55. O'Flynn PE, Shadaba A. Management of posterior epistaxis by endoscopic clipping of the sphenopalatine artery. *Clin Otolaryngol* 2000; **25**: 374–7.
56. White PS. Endoscopic ligation of the sphenopalatine artery (ELSA): a preliminary description. *J Laryngol Otol* 1996; **110**: 27–30.
57. Strong EB, Bell DA, Johnson LP, Jacobs JM. Intractable epistaxis: transantral ligation vs. embolization: efficacy review and cost analysis. *Arch Otolaryngol Head Neck Surg* 1995; **113**(6): 674–8.
58. Waldron J, Stafford N. Ligation of the external carotid artery for severe epistaxis. *J Otolaryngol* 1992; **21**(4): 249–51.
59. Cumberworth VL, Narula AA, Bradley PJ. Prospective study of two management strategies for epistaxis. *J R Coll Surg Edinb* 1991; **36**: 259–60.
60. Scaramuzzi N, Walsh RM, Brennan P, Walsh M. Treatment of intractable epistaxis using arterial embolization. *Clin Otolaryngol* 2001; **26**: 307–9.
61. Moreau S, De Rugy MG, Babin E, Courtheoux P, et al. Supraselective embolization in intractable epistaxis: review of 45 cases. *Laryngoscope* 1998; **108**: 887–8.
62. Crow WN, Scott BA, Guinto FC, Jr, et al. Massive epistaxis due to pseudoaneurysm: treated with detachable balloons. *Arch Otolaryngol Head Neck Surg* 1992; **118**: 321–4.

63. Garth RJN, Cox HJ, Thomas MR. Haemorrhage as a complication of inferior turbinectomy: a comparison of anterior and radical trimming. *Clin Otolaryngol* 1995; **20**: 236–8.
64. Srinivasan V, Patel H, John DG, Worsley A. Warfarin and epistaxis: should warfarin always be discontinued? *Clin Otolaryngol* 1997; **22**: 542–4.
65. Walshe P, Harkin C, Murphy S, et al. Rapid communication. The use of fibrin glue in refractory coagulopathic epistaxis. *Clin Otolaryngol* 2001; **26**: 284–5.
66. Siegal DM. Managing TSOACs associated bleeding including an update on pharmacological reversal agents. *J Thromb Thrombolysis* 2015; **39**(3): 395–402.
67. Pau H, Carney AS, Murty GE. Review. Hereditary haemorrhagic telangiectasia (Osler-Weber-Rendu syndrome): otorhinolaryngological manifestations. *Clin Otolaryngol* 2001; **26**: 93–98.
68. Lund VJ, Howard DJ. (A treatment algorithm for the management of epistaxis in hereditary hemorrhagic telangiectasia. *Am J Rhinol* 1999; **13**(4): 319–22.
69. Whitehead KJ, Sautter NB, McWilliams JP, et al. Effect of topical intranasal therapy on epistaxis frequency in patients with hereditary haemorrhagic telangiectasia: a randomized clinical trial. *JAMA* 2016; **316**(9): 943–51.

CHAPTER 107

NASAL AND FACIAL FRACTURES

Dae Kim and Simon Holmes

Nasal Fractures 1183	Aetiology 1189
Introduction 1183	Primary care 1190
Epidemiology and aetiology 1183	Mandibular fractures 1191
Classification and pathophysiology 1183	Fractures of the maxilla 1194
Clinical presentation 1185	Zygomatic complex fractures 1196
Investigations 1185	Orbital floor fractures 1198
Treatment 1186	Naso-orbito-ethmoid complex fractures 1198
Complications 1188	Upper facial third fractures involving the frontal sinus 1199
Facial Fractures 1189	Paediatric facial injuries 1199
Introduction 1189	References 1200

SEARCH STRATEGY

Data in this chapter may be updated by a Medline search using the keywords: nasal fracture, maxillofacial injuries, mandibular fractures, maxillary fractures, orbital floor fractures, nasoethmoid fractures and frontal sinus fractures, focusing on diagnosis, surgery, management and complications.

NASAL FRACTURES

INTRODUCTION

Treatment of nasal fractures was first recorded 5000 years ago during the early Pharonic period in Ancient Egypt. The Edwin Smith papyrus describes repositioning of deviated nasal bones with the fingers or elevators, the insertion of splints and the application of external dressings.[1] Just as then, nasal fractures are still very common. Isolated fractures of the nasal pyramid account for about 40% of all facial fractures. Furthermore, fractures of the nasal bones are often sustained along with other fractures of the facial skeleton. Delays in management can result in significant cosmetic and functional deformity that is often a cause for subsequent medicolegal action. The management of fractures of the nose is an important part of everyday ear, nose and throat (ENT) practice.

EPIDEMIOLOGY AND AETIOLOGY

Relatively little force is required to fracture the nasal bones, as little as 25–75 lb/in.[2] It is perhaps not surprising that young men are twice as likely to sustain a fractured nose as women. Subsequent refracture rates of 5% have been reported.[3] The peak incidence is in the 15–30-year age group when assaults, contact sports and adventurous leisure activities are more common.[4] In childhood, accident-prone toddlers not infrequently fracture their noses as well and these are often of a greenstick nature. Compound and comminuted fractures are more common in the elderly who are prone to falls.

CLASSIFICATION AND PATHOPHYSIOLOGY

Nasal fractures have been classified in a number of ways, for example, by the nature of injury, the extent of deformity and the pattern of the fracture.

Nature of injury

Most fractures result from laterally applied forces (> 66%). In a series reported by Illum et al. fractures following frontal injuries accounted for only 13%.[5] Greater force is required to fracture the nose with a blow directed from the front as the nasal cartilages behave like shock absorbers.

Extent of deformity

A five-point grading system has been developed for the extent of lateral deviation of the nasal pyramid:

- Grade 0: bones perfectly straight
- Grade 1: bones deviated less than half of the width of the bridge of the nose
- Grade 2: bones deviated half to one full width of the bridge of the nose
- Grade 3: bones deviated greater than one full width of the bridge of the nose
- Grade 4: bones almost touching the cheek.

Pattern of fracture

Nasal fractures can also be subdivided into three broad categories that characterize the patterns of damage sustained with increasing force. This classification has some practical utility as each category of fracture requires a different method of treatment.

CLASS 1 FRACTURES

Class 1 fractures are the result of low–moderate degrees of force and hence the extent of deformity is usually not marked. The simplest form of a Class 1 fracture is the depressed nasal bone. The fractured segment usually remains in position due to its inferior attachment to the upper lateral cartilage which provides an element of recoil. The nasal septum is generally not involved.

In the more severe variant, both nasal bones and the septum are fractured. The fracture line runs parallel to the nasomaxillary suture ipsilateral to the side of the applied force to a point approximately two-thirds along the length of the nasal bone, where the bone becomes much thicker. The fracture line then connects across to the contralateral side and runs parallel and just below the dorsum. The cartilaginous septum is fractured approximately 0.5 cm below the dorsum and this aspect of the injury may extend posteriorly into the bony septum, through the perpendicular plate of the ethmoid and skull base. This fracture was first described by Chevallet and bears his name (**Figure 107.1**).

Class 1 fractures tend not to cause gross lateral displacement of the nasal bones and may not even be perceptible. Deformity generally results from a persistently depressed fragment, which is often due to impaction of the flail segment beneath the residual nasal bone. In children, these fractures may be of the 'greenstick' variety and significant nasal deformity may only develop at puberty when nasal growth becomes accentuated.[6]

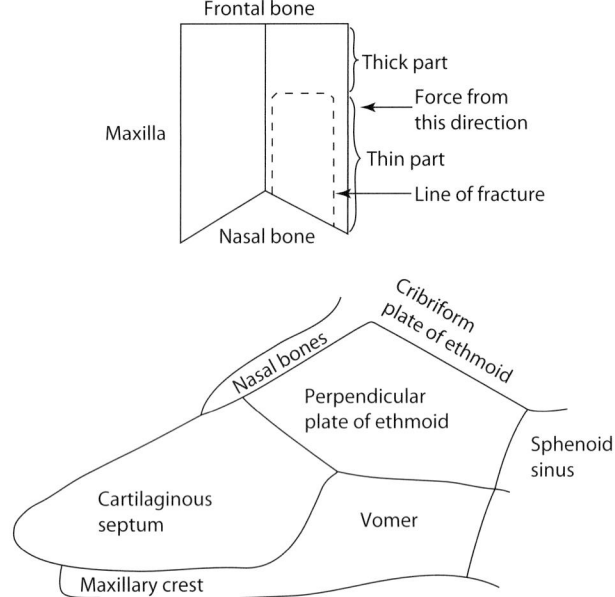

Figure 107.1 The distal part of a nasal bone is half the thickness of the proximal part. When it fractures, the nose is apparently deviated but the impression of deviation is optical (Chevallet fracture). It is important to recognize this injury. The edges of the stable segment can often be palpated. Figure courtesy of AGD Maran.

CLASS 2 FRACTURES

Class 2 fractures are the result of greater force and are often associated with significant cosmetic deformity. In addition to fracturing the nasal bones, the frontal process of the maxilla and septum are also involved. However, the ethmoid labyrinth and adjacent orbital structures remain intact (see Class 3). The pattern of deformity is determined by the direction of the force applied. A frontal impact tends to comminute the nasal bones and cause gross flattening and widening of the dorsum; while a lateral impact produces a high deviation of the nasal skeleton.

What may appear to be a simple dislocation of the quadrangular cartilage from the bony septum is in reality a complex 'C-shaped' fracture that extends from the quadrangular cartilage beneath the nasal tip, posteriorly through to the perpendicular plate of the ethmoid, to the anterior border of the vomer and then forward through the lower part of the perpendicular plate of the ethmoid into the inferior part of the quadrilateral cartilage. This pattern of fracture was first described by Jarjavay and bears his name (**Figure 107.2**).

As a rule of thumb, if the nasal dorsum is deviated laterally greater than half the width of the nose (Grade 2 or greater fracture), then a septal fracture must also be present. Septal fracture-dislocations tend to happen at points of weakness. They are where the quadrangular cartilage inserts into the cartilaginous dorsum, the bony septum and the maxillary crest. Both the nasal bone and septal fractures need to be reduced together in order to achieve a satisfactory cosmetic result.

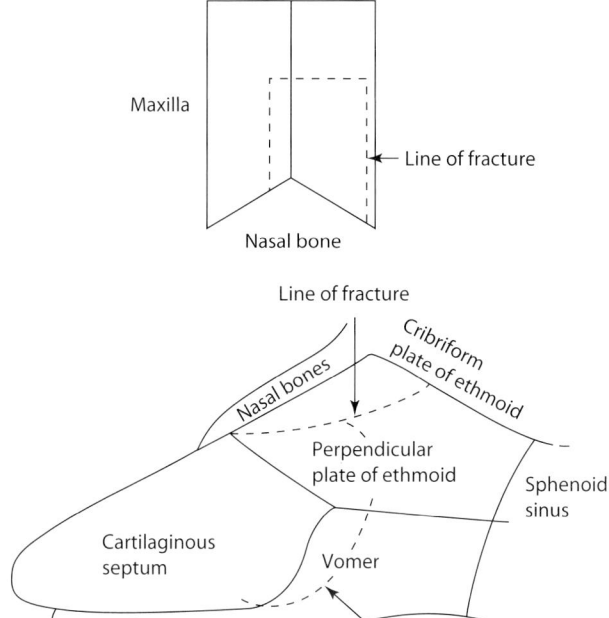

Figure 107.2 A Class 2 nasal fracture involves the thicker proximal portion of the nasal bone. It results in true deviation and also fracture of the perpendicular plate of the ethmoid and quadrilateral cartilage (Jarjavay fracture). Figure courtesy of AGD Maran.

CLASS 3 FRACTURES

Class 3 fractures are the most severe nasal injuries encountered and usually result from high velocity trauma. They are also termed naso-orbito-ethmoid fractures and often have associated fractures of the maxillae. The external buttresses of the nose give way and the ethmoid labyrinth collapses on itself. This causes the perpendicular plate of the ethmoid to rotate and the quadrilateral cartilage to fall backwards. These movements cause a classic, 'pig-like' appearance to the patient, with a foreshortened saddled nose and the nostrils facing more anteriorly, like the snout of a pig. There is also telecanthus, which may be exaggerated further by disruption of the medial canthal ligament from the crest of the lacrimal bone.

Two categories of naso-orbito-ethmoid fractures have been recognized by Raveh.[7] In type I, the anterior skull base, posterior wall of the frontal sinus and optic canal remain intact. In type II, there is disruption of the posterior frontal sinus wall, multiple fractures of the roof of the ethmoid and orbit that may extend posteriorly to the sphenoid and parasellar regions. Multiple dural tears, cerebrospinal fluid leaks (CSF), pneumocranium and cerebral herniation may complicate this type of injury. (The management of this type of nasal fracture is covered later in this Chapter).

CLINICAL PRESENTATION

History

It is prudent to establish how and when the injury was sustained, not only for medicolegal purposes but also because there is a limited period of time during which simple reduction is possible. There will almost certainly be some degree of nasal obstruction associated with the injury, but complete obstruction and persisting pain might indicate the presence of a septal haematoma. Enquiry should be made about any obvious change in the shape of the nose and of previous injuries or past nasal surgery. The patient may have a recent photograph that could be helpful to establish their claim.

Other injuries may also be present and may have been overlooked. Diplopia, visual disturbance and epiphora suggest orbital trauma. Loose teeth, an altered bite or trismus indicate the need for a dental opinion. The onset of watery rhinorrhoea and loss of the sense of smell, though uncommon, signal possible skull base damage and the need for a more detailed evaluation. Finally, it is worth enquiring about their leisure pursuits and any occupational hazards that might influence any decision to correct the deformity.

Key issues to consider when determining history include:

- details of how and when the injury was sustained
- nasal obstruction
- change in appearance
- anosmia; hyposmia; watery rhinorrhoea
- visual disturbance; diplopia; epiphora
- altered bite; loose teeth; trismus
- occupation; leisure pursuits.

Examination

The importance of clear and complete records of the clinical examination cannot be overemphasized. What is and what is not a new injury can be difficult to determine at a later date when litigation is contemplated. Inspect the nose for any external deformity. This may be extremely difficult in the acute situation when swelling may hide an underlying abnormality. A second inspection a few days later may be necessary. Gently palpate the nasal bones for a step deformity and make note of any surgical emphysema that could suggest a more serious injury. Make a detailed record of soft-tissue lacerations. Inspect the nasal cavities and check for the presence of a septal haematoma or deviation. A thorough general ENT/head and neck examination must also be completed.

Key issues to consider when examining a patient include:

- deviation, depression, step deformities
- mobility, crepitus, specific areas of point tenderness
- generalized swelling and specific bruising
- skin and mucosal lacerations
- septal fracture/haematoma/abscess/perforation.

INVESTIGATIONS

Unlike other fractures, nasal X-rays are not required to make the diagnosis or aid subsequent reduction. In a prospective study undertaken by Logan et al., it was concluded that X-rays were not cost effective.[8] Their only possible utility is proof of injury in subsequent litigation. If there is clinical evidence of a more serious facial injury computerized tomography (CT) scan should be acquired. Samples of any watery rhinorrhoea must be collected in those with suspected CSF leak and tested for b2 transferrin.

TREATMENT

The indications for surgical intervention in the acute phase are significant cosmetic deformity and nasal obstruction caused by a septal haematoma. However, a very significant number of patients (up to 80%) do not require any active treatment; many do not have a nasal fracture and, in those that do, the fracture may not be displaced.[4] Soft-tissue swelling can produce the misleading appearance of a deformity which disappears as the swelling subsides. Reassurance is all that these patients may require. Topical vasoconstrictor drops are helpful to alleviate congestion and obstructive symptoms. A reexamination about 5 days later is prudent where there is uncertainty about the need for reduction.

Many patients will have a pre-existing nasal deformity caused by a previous incident. Manipulation of the nose will, at best, only return it to its most recent appearance. Patients that fall into this category may be better advised to consider a formal rhinoplasty when everything has settled down some months later. Others will be at continued risk of further injury because of an occupational hazard, sport or leisure activity. It is better to advise this group of patients to undergo a definitive septorhinoplasty when the risk of further injury no longer exists.

The timing of surgical assessment and subsequent reduction is crucial as there is a narrow window of opportunity to correct the deformity. Failure of referral or timely referral is a common cause of litigation in nasal injuries. Patients should be seen quickly, certainly within the first few days and no later than one week. Patients with a suspected septal haematoma should be seen urgently at the first possible opportunity. The optimal time for clinical assessment is around 4 days, by which time much of the oedema will have subsided and any underlying deformity become apparent. Review at 4 days allows sensible planning for reduction of the fracture on an elective operating list within the next 2 to 3 days, if it is to be reduced under a general anaesthetic. By 7 days, the bony abnormality will be easily palpable and still movable. Further delay makes effective reduction less likely and sometimes impossible without making osteotomies. In children, healing can take place even more quickly and earlier intervention is indicated.

Those patients for whom treatment is considered unnecessary should be given the contact details of the ENT clinic lest deformity become apparent over the ensuing weeks.[4]

Anaesthesia

Reduction of a fractured nose can be performed under local or general anaesthesia. Many studies have shown reduction of nasal fractures under local anaesthesia to be perfectly adequate and acceptable.[9, 10]

Local anaesthesia has several advantages but the injections can be painful and the associated distortion of soft tissues can hinder accurate assessment of the reduction and the literature is divided over the influence on outcomes. In a retrospective analysis of 324 patients, Courtney et al. found a higher number of patients seeking a septorhinoplasty when the initial reduction was performed under local anaesthetic (17.2%) than general anaesthetic (3.2%).[3] On the other hand, Ridder et al. found that there was no significant difference in overall success rate.[11]

Local anaesthetic can be used as a combination of external infiltration with internal application of topical preparations. Lignocaine is injected along the nasomaxillary groove, infraorbital nerve in its foramen and around the infratrochlear nerve. Jones and Nandapalan recently reported the use of topical EMLA (prilocaine and lignocaine) cream or AMETOP (amethocaine) gel to the external nose instead of infiltration.[12] They found less discomfort when the manipulation was carried out using the topical, local anaesthetic preparation compared with local infiltration. They achieved similar cosmetic and functional results.[12] Within the nose, sprays, injections, pastes or packs coated with local anaesthetic are all acceptable, using combinations of cocaine, lignocaine, adrenaline and phenylephrine. The vasoconstrictive element helps to reduce any bleeding associated with mucosal tears from instrumentation during the reduction, but must be used cautiously in hypertensive patients or those with cardiovascular disease.

There are easily identifiable groups of patients who are not suitable for reduction under local anaesthesia. Children and patients with low pain thresholds or significant anxiety states are better admitted for general anaesthesia. Likewise, attempts at reduction of fractures where there has been delay in presentation are better performed under general anaesthetic.

Methods of reduction

Closed techniques for nasal reduction have traditionally been used. The general principle of any fracture reduction is to mobilize the fragments first by increasing and then decreasing the degree of deformity. An initial slight increase in deformity away from the side of the blow to disimpact the fragments, followed by steady movement back towards and often slightly beyond the midline is usually required. Generally, this can be achieved by firm digital pressure. Sometimes instruments are necessary, particularly in those where there has been delay. Various elevators and forceps have been developed specifically for this purpose, such as Freer, Hills and Howarth elevators and Ashe and Walsham forceps (**Figure 107.3**). The instrument is held so that the index finger of the dominant hand is placed along the instrument in the line of the nose. In this way, the depth that the instrument must be inserted into the nasal cavity is easily gauged and inadvertent damage to the orbit avoided (**Figure 107.4**).

All Class 1 and most Class 2 fractures can be reduced with these techniques. In some Class 2 fractures, closed reduction alone may not achieve a satisfactory result as the final position of the nasal dorsum reflects the deformity of the underlying septum.[1, 13–15] At least 50% of

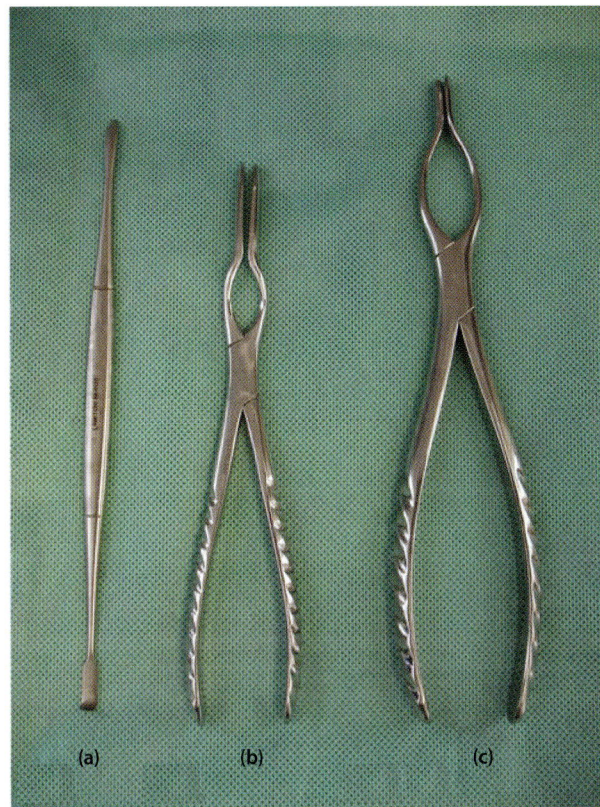

Figure 107.3 Instruments used in nasal fracture manipulation.
(a) Howarth's elevator; **(b)** Ashe's forceps (septum);
(c) Walsham's forceps (nasal bones).

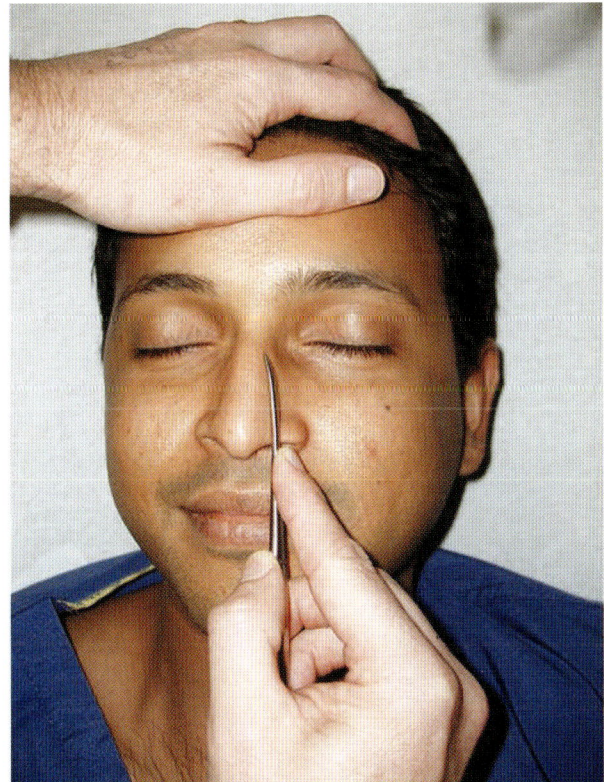

Figure 107.4 Determining depth of insertion of instrument into nasal cavity.

these fractures remain displaced because of overlapping segments of the fractured perpendicular plate of the ethmoid or septal cartilage, which can only be repositioned by open reduction. Occasionally, the bones are fixed, especially if the fracture is old, and osteotomies are necessary to release the fragments before manipulation. These should be performed cautiously to avoid the risk of extension into the orbit or, even worse, intra-cranially.[16]

Splints or packs may be necessary, depending on the stability of the reduction and the surgeon's preference. A splint or plaster applied to the nasal bridge maintains, to some extent, the position of the nasal bones and prevents accidental displacement. Splints are usually kept in place for about 7 days. It is advisable to refrain from contact sports for at least 6 weeks.

Very occasionally, open reduction techniques may be desirable or required to provide optimal results, despite the increased time and effort involved. Verwoerd identified the following indications for open reduction:[15]

- bilateral fractures with dislocation of the nasal dorsum and significant (pre-existent or recent) septal deformity
- infraction of the nasal dorsum
- fractures of the cartilaginous pyramid, with or without dislocation of the upper laterals.

For depressed tip or flail lateral fractures that are unstable despite closed reduction techniques, Kirschner (K) wires can be used. The wire is inserted under fluoroscopic guidance into the depressed fragment as well as neighbouring uninvolved bone (maxilla or frontal bone), and the wires are screwed together externally to maintain the position. The external wire can be covered by dressings or plaster to protect the wires from disruption and the patient from injury. The wires are removed after 2 weeks.

Some authors advocate a more aggressive approach to the treatment of acute nasal fractures which includes some 'rhinoplasty' techniques, such as release of upper lateral cartilages, hump removal and camouflaging cartilage grafts.[17] Incorporation of these more advanced techniques into the management of the fractured nose requires expertise, more instrumentation and more operating time and this may not always be feasible or desirable.

Management of the nasal septum

Septal fracture is often missed and is a major reason for poor functional and cosmetic results. Kim et al. found that 46.9% of nasal fractures have a concomitant septal fracture.[18] If a significant septal fracture-dislocation is present, it is wise to reduce this at the same time as the nasal bones. In fact, a satisfactory reduction of nasal bones is often not possible without improving the position of the septum. An often-quoted aphorism, 'where goes the septum, so does the nose' is not far from the truth.

Septal reduction can sometimes be performed with Ashe's forceps, but often requires a Killian or hemitransfixion incision, elevation of mucosal flaps to expose the cartilage and bone fragments, and replacement and/or removal of cartilaginous and bony fragments, as in a standard septoplasty. Quilting sutures prevent a dead space from forming and a haematoma from collecting.

COMPLICATIONS

Poor cosmetic result

Attempts to reduce deformity are not always successful. Factors which contribute to an unsatisfactory cosmetic result include:

- extent of the injury
- time delay in surgical reduction
- poor surgical technique
- unrecognized and untreated septal fracture
- pre-existing nasal deformity
- post-operative trauma (in recovery room or subsequently)
- scarring and fibrosis.

Unfortunately, it is not uncommon for the shape of the nose to change over time due to subsequent scarring and fibrosis, loss of tip or dorsal support, or hump formation. Some patients inevitably require a septorhinoplasty despite apparent adequate reduction. It is wise to wait at least 6 months after the injury before embarking on septorhinoplasty to allow the fractures to heal, the oedema to settle completely so the underlying nasal skeleton is evident, and for any fibrosis to develop.

Nasal obstruction

Post-operative nasal obstruction is also common and there are many causes that include:

- valve obstruction
- collapse of upper lateral cartilages and depressed nasal bones
- septal deviation
- widened septum (haematoma)
- tip ptosis.

These causes need to be considered and addressed at a subsequent septorhinoplasty.

Epistaxis

Epistaxis at the time of injury may be impressive but is usually relatively brief. Occasionally, fractures involving the nasoethmoidal complex can cause laceration to the anterior ethmoidal artery. This may result in repeated, brisk and significant haemorrhage that only stops once the fracture has been reduced. Very occasionally, prolonged packing or ligation of the artery is required. Bleeding can also be troublesome at the time of reduction, particularly if instruments are used. Preparation of the nose with vasoconstrictive agents helps to minimize this blood loss.

Septal complications

A submucoperichondrial bleed not infrequently complicates nasal fractures. While most septal haematomas are relatively limited, some may strip the mucoperichondrium over an extended area and deprive the underlying cartilage of its source of nutrition. This can lead to cartilage necrosis and ultimately nasal deformity. Septal haematomas present with an acute unilateral or bilateral nasal obstruction and, on inspection, there is a reddish-purple, fluctuant swelling of the caudal septum. A deviated septum can be confused with a septal haematoma. Gentle pressure on the bulging area will ascertain that it is fluctuant if a collection is present. Untreated, an abscess may develop and the patient becomes very unwell with a fluctuating fever and severe facial and cranial pain. Rarely, cavernous sinus thrombosis or other forms of intra-cranial sepsis can ensue.

The haematoma or abscess must be drained as soon as possible. This can be performed under local or general anaesthetic, either by using needle aspiration or preferably an incision. Often the collection will have become organized and so impossible to aspirate. In this situation, a small window of mucoperiostium should be excised ensuring there is no corresponding defect on the contralateral side which could predispose to a perforation. Once drained, quilting sutures from one side through cartilage to the other are inserted to eliminate the dead space. Packs or splints can be used to provide gentle pressure on the septum. The patient must be reexamined within 48 hours to establish that the collection has not recurred. The management of a septal abscess is similar, but with the addition of appropriate antibiotic therapy.

Septal perforations may also develop after nasal fractures, usually as a result of septal haematomas and their surgical treatment. Loss of cartilaginous septal support can also lead to a saddle nose deformity, as well as columellar retraction and a broadened septum.

> **KEY POINTS**
>
> - Nasal fractures are common and awareness of the basic principles of management ensures good outcomes.
> - All significant nasal injuries should be assessed within a few days if there is cosmetic deformity and within 24 hours if nasal obstruction is evident to exclude a septal haematoma.
> - It is important to assess each patient carefully and be vigilant over potential complications.
> - Document all details carefully in case of subsequent litigation.
> - Not all referred patients actually have fractures and even some with fractures do not need surgery.
> - Most cases can be reduced adequately with closed techniques, unless the fractures are complex or a significant septal fracture-dislocation is present.
> - There are no significant differences between the outcomes of local versus general anaesthesia: more important predictors of outcome include pre-existing deformity, severity of injury, delay in assessment and poor surgical technique.
> - Residual cosmetic deformity and nasal obstruction are relatively common complications and it is wise to counsel patients about these from the outset.
> - A formal septorhinoplasty can be performed in cases of poor outcome, best performed at least 6 months after the injury.

> **BEST CLINICAL PRACTICE**
>
> ✓ Prompt medical review within 24–48 hours of all significant nasal injuries, with urgent ENT referral if a septal haematoma or if a Class 3 fracture is present.
> ✓ Exclusion of related injuries to face, orbit, jaws and central nervous system (CNS) at initial assessment and appropriate specialist referral if present.
> ✓ ENT assessment at 4 to 5 days if cosmetic deformity or nasal obstruction are present.
> ✓ Closed reduction at 7 days, or open reduction if more complex.
> ✓ Review 7 days post-operatively with removal of external nasal splint.
> ✓ No contact sports for at least 6 weeks post-operatively.

> **FUTURE RESEARCH**
>
> ➤ More prospective studies are required comparing closed and open reduction techniques.
> ➤ More prospective studies are needed to compare nasal bone reduction with nasal bone reduction and septoplasty.
> ➤ Studies need to be undertaken to determine whether a more aggressive approach to the initial management of nasal fractures (such as open reduction, septoplasty, 'rhinoplasty techniques') will prevent subsequent septorhinoplasty.

FACIAL FRACTURES

INTRODUCTION

Injuries to the face are common and account for 10% of all accident and emergency department attendances. Aesthetically, first impressions of a person in terms of their intellect, ability, trustworthiness and even sexual orientation are influenced by facial appearance. Functionally the facial skeleton provides support to the muscles of facial expression and these in turn act as the sphincter that protects the eyes and make the mouth competent. The facial skeleton holds and supports the eyes in the optimum position for binocular vision and the orbital margins provide additional protection for the globes. Historically the success of facial fracture management was judged entirely on the final dental occlusion. While it is important to ensure that a normal bite is achieved, it is just one of the criteria that define today's standard of care. Equally important is the restoration of both the vertical and transverse facial dimensions. This can be achieved by extended craniofacial bone exposure and the use of rigid and semi-rigid internal fixation. In addition, meticulous attention to the repair of soft tissues injuries ensures the best possible cosmetic result.

> **KEY POINTS**
>
> - Maxillofacial trauma is extremely common. Ten percent of all accident and emergency attendances are related to facial injuries.
> - Immediate assessment of the airway is essential.
> - Most facial fractures are managed by semi-rigid internal fixation through extended subperiosteal exposure of the fracture.
> - Wiring of the jaws is no longer the standard of care.
> - Cerebrospinal fluid (CSF) rhinorrhoea and retrobulbar haematoma should be excluded in all middle-third facial injuries.

AETIOLOGY

Fractures of the nose, mandible and middle third of the face are usually caused by road traffic accidents, physical violence, falls, attempted suicide, and sporting injuries (**Figure 107.5**). Most injuries are low energy and heal predictably. Higher-energy injuries cause gross comminution of the bones and do not heal as well. It is important to ascertain the exact mechanism of injury not only for medicolegal reasons, but also to ensure that an adequate screening examination is undertaken to detect other injuries and so that a prognosis on the likely stability of any repair can be given.

> **KEY POINTS**
>
> - Successful outcome involves restoration of pre-morbid facial proportions, dental occlusion and accurate soft tissue repair.
> - Road traffic accidents, interpersonal violence, attempted suicide and sports injuries are the most common cause of facial fractures.
> - The mechanism of injury will provide insight on the possible degree and extent of the injury and the methods that will be necessary for repair.

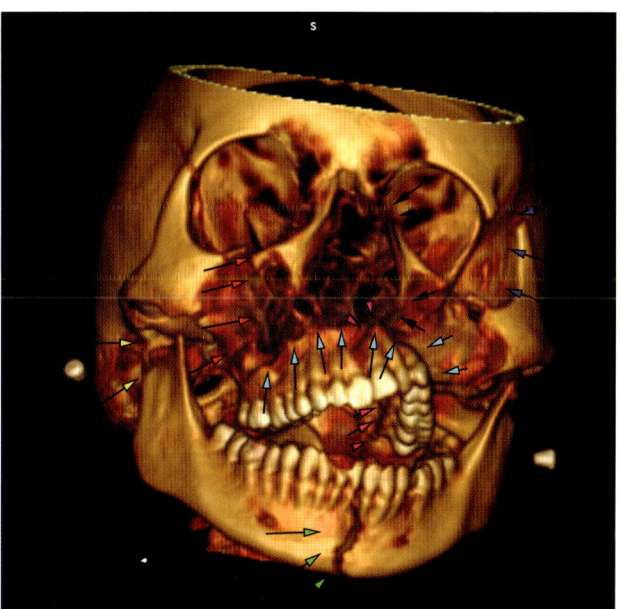

Figure 107.5 A true panfacial fracture. Green arrows – mandibular symphysis : Yellow arrows – right mandibular condyle (left hidden): Red arrows – right Le Fort 2 : Light blue arrows – Le Fort 1.: Dark blue arrows – Le Fort 3 : Black arrows – Naso orbitothmoid : Purple arrows – Parasagittal midline split maxilla.

PRIMARY CARE

The initial survey

Maxillofacial injuries endanger the airway and can cause profuse haemorrhage. Associated neck injuries are common and should always be suspected and excluded. Advanced trauma and life-support protocols dictate that a rapid and accurate primary survey should be undertaken in the following sequence:

1. **Airway.** Evaluate and secure the airway, while maintaining alignment of the neck in case there is an unstable cervical spine injury.
2. **Breathing.** Make sure that there is adequate ventilation.
3. **Circulation.** Control sources of blood loss.
4. **Disability.** Assess the level of consciousness and neurological dysfunction.
5. **Exposure.** Ensure that all other injuries are identified.

The establishment of a safe airway and effective ventilation is essential so that hypoxia and carbon dioxide retention is prevented and the resultant post-traumatic cerebral oedema minimized. Oral or nasal bleeding, posterior displacement of the tongue secondary to mandibular fractures or the result of postero-inferior displacement of the maxilla in middle-third injuries may further compromise the airway. It may be necessary to reduce these fractures immediately and place temporary bridal wires around dentoalveolar segments to increase bony stability. Although the correct surgical procedure for the rapid relief of acute upper airway obstruction is often a cricothyroidotomy, there is occasionally merit in performing an immediate tracheostomy if it can be conducted swiftly and safely. Haemorrhage from facial fractures can be torrential and demands immediate attention. The use of anterior and posterior nasal packs has been abandoned in favour of the epistat (**Figure 107.6**). It is important to remember that any injury to the upper middle third of the face is likely to have shattered the anterior skull base.

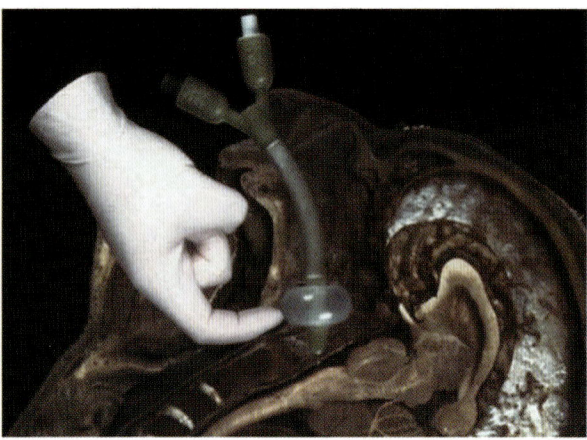

Figure 107.6 Epistat in anatomical model. Palpation of the posterior balloon in the nasopharynx ensures no intra-cranial intubation.

Inadvertent intubation of the anterior cranial fossa through the cribriform plate or medial wall of the orbit is a distinct possibility and should be borne in mind when attempting to pass any tube through the nose. Intense shock should not be attributed to a facial injury until abdominal, pelvic, orthopaedic or thoracic causes have been excluded. Use of the Glasgow Coma Scale will alert the clinician to impending intra-cranial complications. Immediate neurosurgical advice should be obtained if the patient's conscious level deteriorates. CSF rhinorrhea must be suspected in any high-level nasoethmoid or maxillary fractures. This demands prophylactic antibiotic therapy to prevent meningitis. Tetanus prophylaxis should be administered in any non-immune patient.

Principles of primary management

Once the primary survey of the injury has been completed, a secondary survey is carried out to exclude other injuries and to categorize the extent of the facial injury. The soft tissues of the face are carefully scrutinized and any lacerations or cuts noted together with the proximity to relevant anatomical structures including the eyebrows, conjunctival margins, nasal aperture and the vermillion border of the lips. Facial nerve function should be documented and the integrity of the parotid duct assessed. Visual acuity and ocular movements are recorded. Any orbital injury may be complicated by a retrobulbar haemorrhage and retinal detachment, both of which are preventable and treatable causes of permanent blindness.

A full hard-tissue examination is conducted by palpating the orbital margins, zygomatic projection, nasal skeleton and mandibular outline. If conscious, the patient is asked whether their bite is comfortable and if it feels normal, and if there is any numbness. A full dental examination is necessary so that any fractured or missing teeth that may have been inhaled are identified and accounted for. Finally, the dental occlusion and maxillary or mandibular instability is formally assessed and documented.

Radiographic evaluation

All major trauma patients should have chest, cervical spine and pelvic X-rays as soon as possible. The selection of X-rays of the facial skeleton is discussed later, but it is certainly worth including the facial skeleton on any computerized tomography (CT) scan that might be required for a patient with multiple injuries. Early detection of these injuries greatly simplifies their management. The timing of any maxillofacial intervention is controversial. Historically, it was usual to await resolution of any facial swelling before the assessment process began. Patients might wait for 5 to 7 days before surgery was considered. With modern-day techniques, there is a trend to fix facial fractures earlier. This policy avoids the so-called double insult of accidental and surgical trauma. Swelling can be reduced by nursing the patient in the head-up position with ice packs, together with a single dose of dexamethasone. Facial wounds should be cleaned and lacerations closed as soon as possible, if necessary under local anaesthesia.

Any facial fracture that communicates with the oral cavity through the periodontal ligament of teeth should be regarded as compound and parenteral prophylactic antibiotics given.

> **BEST CLINICAL PRACTICE**
>
> ✓ Maxillofacial fractures can endanger the airway.
> ✓ Be aware of associated cervical spine injuries.
> ✓ Consider tracheostomy at the outset in patients with extensive trauma.
> ✓ Close soft tissues injuries as soon as possible.
> ✓ CT scans of the head and facial bones help to define the extent of both facial and cerebral injuries.
> ✓ Do not forget to give tetanus prophylaxis.
> ✓ Exclude cervical spine injuries.
> ✓ Check visual acuity in all patients with middle-third facial injuries lest they have a retrobulbar haemorrhage.

MANDIBULAR FRACTURES

Introduction

The mandible is a parabolic-shaped bone with a complex articulation that consists of paired synovial joints – the temporomandibular joints – and movements that are, in part, guided by the dental occlusion. Satisfactory rehabilitation of the fractured mandible requires accurate reduction, adequate fixation and mobilization. The traditional method of treatment was immobilization of the fracture with intermaxillary fixation (IMF) (**Figure 107.7**). More recently, it has been realized that the advantages of such treatment in terms of cost and simplicity were far outweighed by a number of disadvantages. At the outset, there were always concerns about the airway lest it became compromised by soft-tissue swelling or vomiting. The period of immobilization was uncomfortable and inconvenient for the patient as it imposed dietary restrictions.[19, 20] Furthermore, the use of wires placed the surgeon and nursing staff at risk of needlestick injuries.[21] To make matters worse, the fixation achieved by this method was often inadequate, particularly if the dentition was incomplete or in bad repair (**Figure 107.8**).

The widespread use nowadays of miniplates and extended subperiosteal exposure of the craniofacial skeleton to achieve fixation means that there are now few indications for closed reduction of any facial fracture. In this way, correct anatomy and occlusion is restored.[22, 23] One further and very significant advantage of not using IMF is that in severely injured patients a tracheostomy might be avoided.

Surgical anatomy

The mandible will fracture when subjected to direct and indirect force. Stereotypical fracture configurations are recognized that are determined by the direction and magnitude of the applied force and whether the teeth are in or out of occlusion at the time. Fractures happen at points of potential weakness where the bone is relatively thin (**Figure 107.9**). The angles of the mandible may be weakened by unerupted wisdom teeth, the parasymphysis by the long root of the lower canine and the condylar neck by its slender anatomy. It is also common for the mandible to fracture in more than one place,

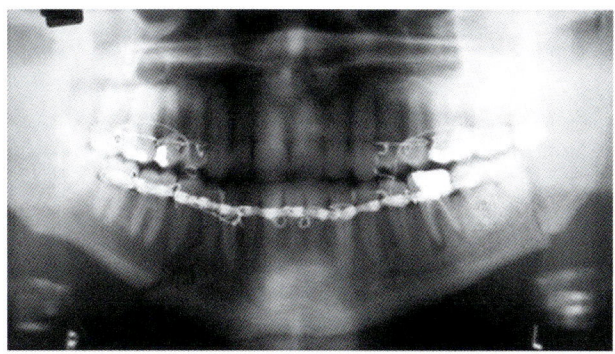

Figure 107.8 This fracture of the angle of the mandible has been managed inappropriately by intermaxillary fixation – the posterior segment of the left mandible is not controlled. The molar tooth in the line of the fracture should be extracted and an alternative form of fixation applied.

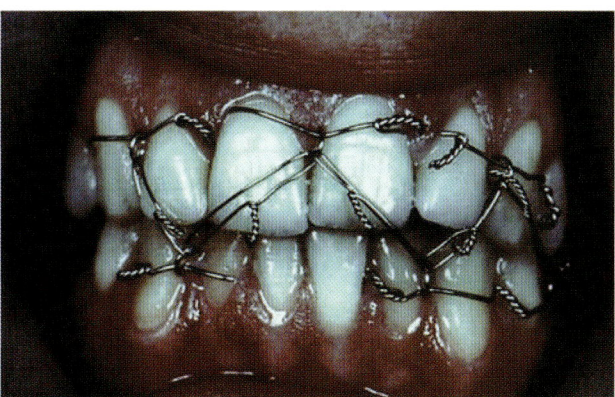

Figure 107.7 Eyelet wires fastened to the dentition and interconnected is the simplest form of intermaxillary fixation.

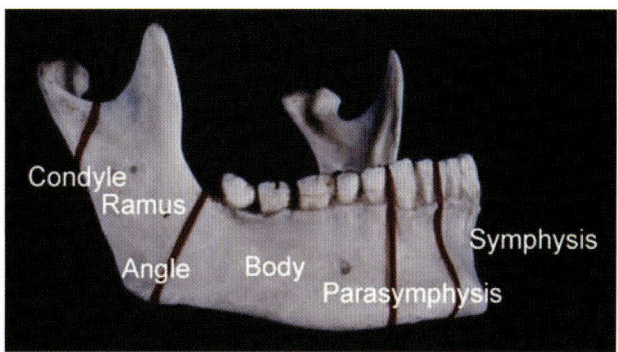

Figure 107.9 Lines of weakness in the mandible that determine the pattern of fractures in the mandible.

for example, the parasymphysis (site of direct violence) and condylar neck (site of indirect violence). It is obviously sensible to look carefully for more than one fracture. Displacement of the fracture depends on a variety of factors, the most important of which are the pull of attached muscles.

Signs and symptoms

The signs and symptoms produced by mandibular fractures are determined by the site of the fracture.

Fractures of the body, angle and symphysis are associated with:

- a step deformity palpable either externally or intraorally
- asymmetry of the lower dental arch and derangement of the occlusion
- pain and paradoxical movement and crepitus on distraction of the fractured segments
- haematomas in the buccal sulcus or floor of the mouth
- blood-stained saliva
- anaesthesia of the lower lip.

Fractures of the condylar neck are associated with:

- tenderness over the temporomandibular joint
- trismus
- deviation of the jaw towards the injured side on opening the mouth
- inability to move the mandible to the side opposite the fracture
- deviation of the jaw to the fractured side at rest with an anterior open bite secondary to gagging of the molar teeth in fracture dislocation
- symmetrical anterior open bite in bilateral fractures of the necks of the condyles.

Closed reduction techniques

As stated previously, the use of IMF plays a much smaller role in modern maxillofacial surgery. Simple mandibular fractures can be held in normal occlusion and plated without much difficulty.[24] Nevertheless, IMF still has a part to play in two groups of patients. First, those with undisplaced fractures and no neural deficits who want to avoid more complex surgery and, second, those with unilateral condylar fractures. In the emergency room, a simple tie wire placed around the teeth either side of a displaced fracture can reduce pain, bleeding from bone ends and make nursing easier in the hours and days before a planned open reduction and internal fixation.

THE INTACT DENTAL ARCH

There are several methods of applying wire to an intact dental arch to provide IMF. Perhaps best known are eyelet wires. This is very simple but is only possible in those situations where there are two adjacent teeth in contact. The main disadvantage is that it is difficult to combine eyelet wires with elastic traction and it can be awkward to thread wire through tight interdental contact points, particularly in an awake patient. A simple and ingenious modification is the Leonard button (**Figure 107.10**), an eyelet wire with a small metal disc instead of a loop.

THE INCOMPLETE DENTAL ARCH

Arch bars

An arch bar is a strip of metal that is wired to each jaw using several individual teeth. The bar may be prefabricated using a model made from a pre-operative dental impression (**Figure 107.11**), or may be made at the time of surgery by adapting a pre-formed pattern. Arch bars can span short gaps within each jaw, but will not cope with large gaps or when there is no posterior tooth. Their main advantage is that they provide a relatively simple means of stabilizing more complex fractures and at the same time provide indirect fixation.

Intermaxillary bone pins

A rapid method of intermaxillary fixation has been described.[25] A mono-cortical screw is placed through the mucosa between the canine and first premolar on each side and jaw. The screws are then wired together or connected with elastic bands. It is important to ensure that

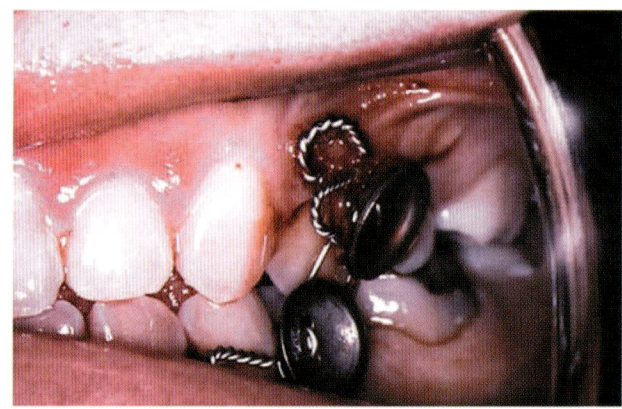

Figure 107.10 **The Leonard button** – a simple device that facilitates intermaxillary fixation by either wire or elastic bands.

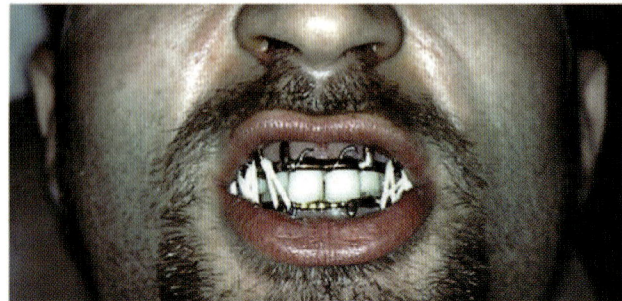

Figure 107.11 **Intermaxillary fixation has been achieved by the use of preformed arch bars connected by elastic bands.**

the path of the screw enters bone and avoids the roots of teeth. These specially designed screws are brittle and care must be exercised when inserting them lest they break.

External fixation

The use of rigid and semi-rigid fixation has diminished the need for external fixation. External fixation is now only indicated for those patients with gross tissue loss as might be seen in the theatre of war and for those with pathological fractures, particularly when the patient is too unwell to undergo extensive surgery. A number of methods have been described and are in current clinical use. By far the simplest is the placement of cortical screws and then connecting them with an external bar made of acrylic. We have found that a mini-Pennig orthopaedic fixator provides an elegant means of stabilizing fractures (**Figure 107.12**), as well as avoiding pin tract problems, and the need for constant tightening and adjustment.

Internal fixation

ACCESS

Intra-oral incisions

Wherever possible, bone plates should be placed through an intra-oral approach. Mucogingival incisions are made so that the resultant flap includes the periosteum. It is essential that a sufficient cuff of mucosa is raised so that the plate is completely covered after closure. Care must be taken to avoid inadvertent damage to the mental nerve in the anterior region.

Extra-oral incisions

External incisions are used for the lower border of the mandible and condylar neck. Lower border plates are ideal when there is gross comminution or tissue loss. They are also preferable in fractures of grossly resorbed edentulous mandibles.[26] In these situations, it is better to use bicortical screws and thicker plates that can provide superior fixation. The incision is made two finger-breadths below the lower border of the mandible in order to avoid damage to the mandibular branch of the facial nerve. The incision is deepened through the platysma muscle and then blunt dissection exposes the lower border of the mandible. Condylar neck fractures are approached through a retromandibular incision while higher condylar neck fractures are better exposed through a pre-auricular incision.[27]

PRINCIPLES OF MANDIBULAR FIXATION

The zones of tension and compression mentioned earlier dictate the ideal position and plate configuration around a fracture site. In simple mandibular fractures, monocortical 2 mm plates provide adequate fixation because of the phenomenon of load sharing between the fracture and the osteosynthesis. In the anterior mandible, two plates are used while posteriorly one plate is usually sufficient[28] and in both situations 6 mm long screws are used. The placement of plates in the region of the mental nerve can be technically demanding (**Figure 107.13**). In complicated fractures where there is gross comminution, tissue loss or infection, a load-bearing osteosynthesis with rigid internal fixation and bicortical screws are required.

CONDYLAR NECK FRACTURES

There is no topic more controversial in maxillofacial trauma than the management of condylar fractures. The 'gold standard' management of most displaced mandibular fractures is reduction and internal fixation. There is just one exception – fractures of the condyle. In the case of condylar fractures, functional adaptation, neuromuscular rehabilitation and altered condylar mechanics may compensate for the deficiencies of IMF in terms of accuracy of reduction. Bilateral displaced condylar neck and high-intra-capsular fractures generally have poor outcomes and are better managed by an open reduction.[29] Several factors determine the best approach to the condyle. These include the position of the fracture, available skin creases, tissue laxity and last but not least, the experience of the operator.

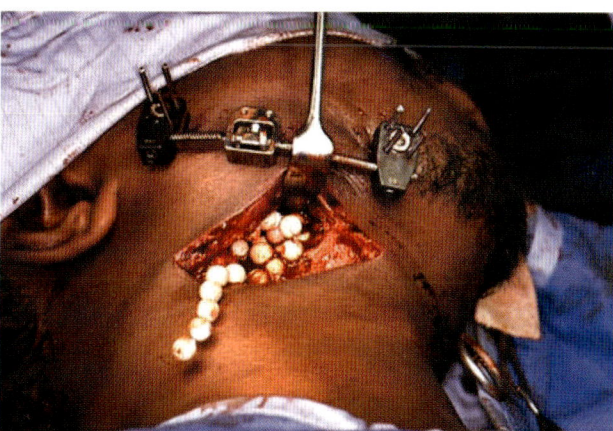

Figure 107.12 A mini-Pennig wrist fixator used to provide external fixation.

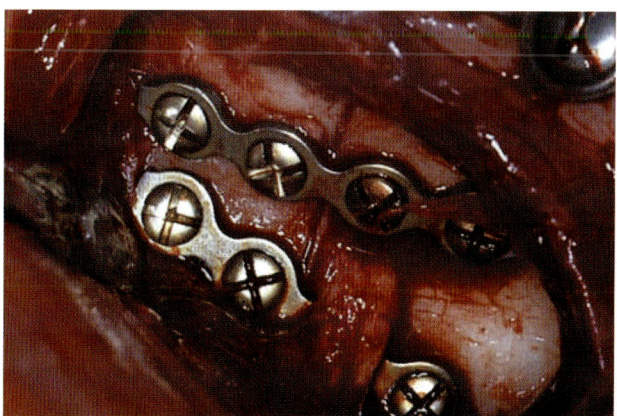

Figure 107.13 Fixation of a fracture in the parasymphyseal region of the mandible using plates. The lower plate has been manipulated beneath the mental nerve.

A retromandibular incision provides the most direct and simple approach to the ramus and subcondylar region, albeit that the surgeon must be careful not to damage the facial nerve. An additional pre-auricular incision can be usefully employed with higher condylar neck fractures. In recent years, there has been enthusiasm for endoscope-assisted repair techniques that are technically difficult to perform but avoid large facial scars.[30, 31] Once exposed, the fracture is reduced and fixed with miniplates.

> **KEY POINTS**
>
> **Mandibular injuries**
>
> - Mandibular injuries are often multiple.
> - IMF following closed reduction is no longer acceptable practice for the majority of mandibular injuries.
> - Most fractures are treated with non-compression miniplates.
> - The management of condylar neck fractures is controversial.
> - Endoscopic techniques may have a role in the management of certain mandibular fractures.
>
> Signs and symptoms of mandibular fractures include:
>
> - bony step deformity;
> - deranged occlusion;
> - pain;
> - sublingual haematoma;
> - blood-stained saliva;
> - mobile teeth in the fracture line;
> - anaesthesia of the lip;
> - trismus.
>
> Signs and symptoms of condylar neck fractures include:
>
> - tenderness over the temporomandibular joint (TMJ);
> - trismus;
> - lateral open bite;
> - anterior open bite.

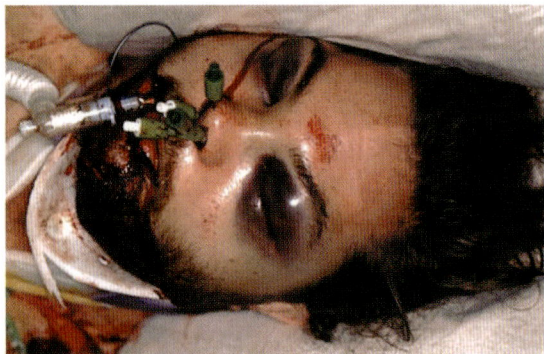

Figure 107.14 Severe multilevel Le Fort fracture with typical 'panda eyes'. An epistat has been inserted to arrest haemorrhage.

FRACTURES OF THE MAXILLA

Introduction

Fractures of the midfacial skeleton can be subdivided into lateral (zygomatic) or central (maxillary, nasal, nasorbito-ethmoid) fractures. The symptoms and signs of maxillary injuries depend on the level of the fracture (**Figures 107.14 and 107.15**). The classical features of a midfacial fracture are circum-orbital ecchymosis (panda facies), facial oedema and emphysema, lengthening of the face and an anterior open bite. Not all of these signs need be present. An infra-orbital nerve sensory deficit is not uncommon in higher fractures and bruising at the junction of the hard and soft palate is frequently present.

Surgical anatomy

The bone of the midfacial region is generally very thin and offers little resistance to anterior and lateral forces.

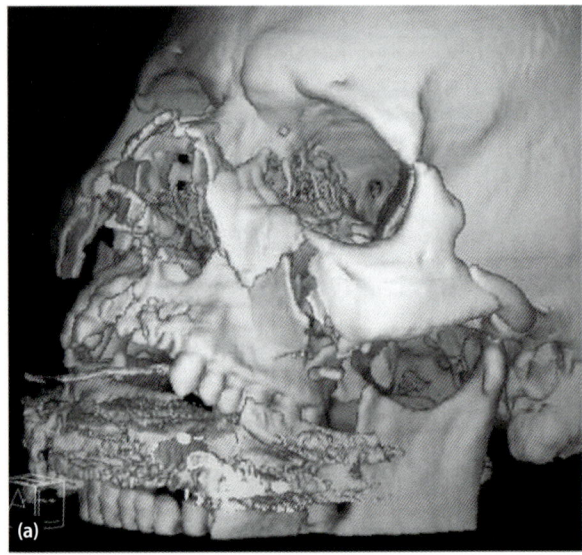

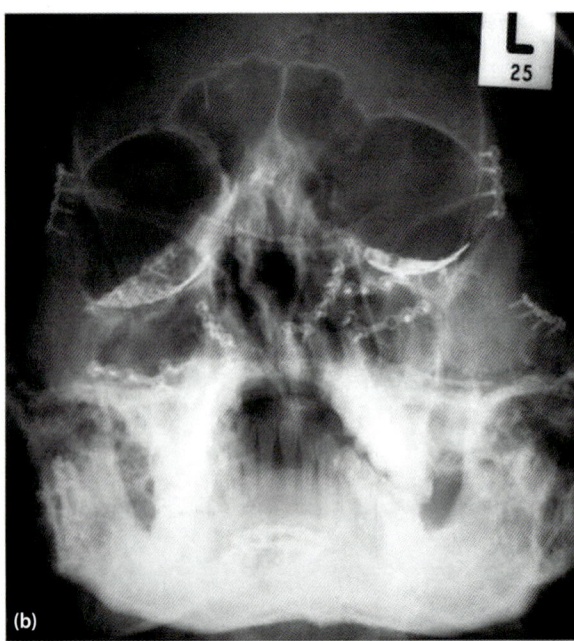

Figure 107.15 (a) 3D CT reconstruction demonstrating vertical, horizonal and transverse disruption to the entire craniofacial skeleton. (b) Post-operative view, note bilateral titanium orbital floor reconstruction.

Le Fort[32] described three levels of midfacial fracture (**Figure 107.16**):

1. **Le Fort 1** This fracture runs above the floor of the nasal cavity, through the nasal septum, maxillary sinuses and inferior parts of the medial and lateral pterygoid plates.
2. **Le Fort 2** This is a fracture which runs from the floor of the maxillary sinuses superiorly to the infraorbital margin and through the zygomaticomaxillary suture. Within the orbit, it passes across the lacrimal bone to the nasion. The infraorbital nerve is often damaged by involvement in this fracture.
3. **Le Fort 3** This represents a disconnection of the facial skeleton from the cranial base. The fracture traverses the medial wall of the orbit to the superior orbital fissure and exits across the greater wing of the sphenoid and zygomatic bone to the zygomaticofrontal suture. Posteriorly, the fracture line runs inferior to the optic foramen, across the lesser wing of the sphenoid to the pterygomaxillary fissure and sphenopalatine foramen. The arch of the zygoma is also broken.

While the Le Fort classification is attractive and accurate for low-energy injuries, in high-energy injuries there are very few instances of pure Le Fort fractures and most configurations involve multiple Le Fort levels,[33] together with zygomatic and nasal/nasoethmoid components. Authors have described thickened areas of bone between the maxilla and skull base which act as buttresses.[34] In essence, these thickened areas of bone provide a strategy for reconstruction[34, 35] and are key areas for osteosynthesis.

Signs and symptoms

Middle third facial fractures produce the following symptoms and signs:

- epistaxis
- circumorbital ecchymosis
- facial oedema
- surgical emphysema
- lengthening of the face
- infraorbital anaesthesia.

Principles of management

EMERGENCY TREATMENT

Midfacial fractures can easily compromise the airway with torrential epistaxes and posterior impaction of the maxilla. The bleeding can be arrested by using epistats or anterior and posterior nasal packs. If retroposition of the maxilla is a problem, it can be pulled forwards using the index and middle finger placed behind the patient's soft palate.

REDUCTION

The maxilla is mobilized by a combination of digital pressure and traction on arch bars or interdental wires. The position of the maxilla is 'eye-balled' with reference to the bony buttresses and dental occlusion. This can be difficult when the bone fragments are comminuted or the dentition is mutilated. Rowe maxillary disimpaction forceps can prove invaluable if the maxilla is impacted.

FIXATION

Modern management of the fractured maxilla parallels that of the mandible.[31] Internal fixation with

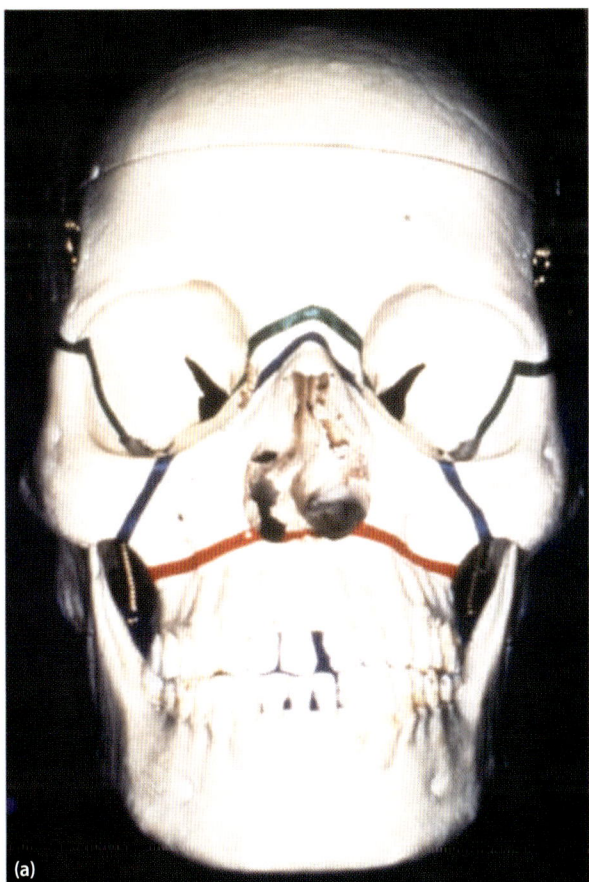

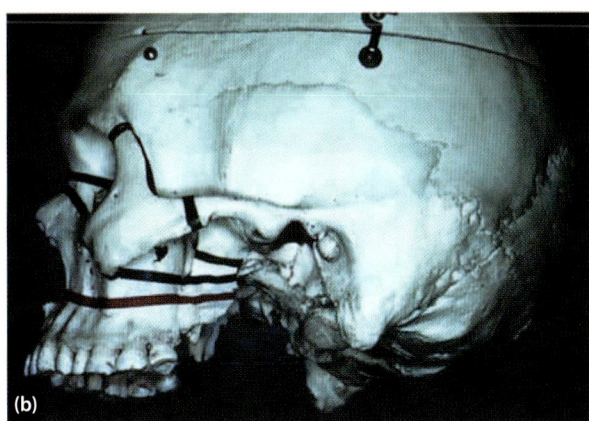

Figure 107.16 **(a)** and **(b)** The Le Fort injuries: red, Le Fort 1; blue, Le Fort 2; green, Le Fort 3.

1.3 or 1.5 mm, low-profile miniplates placed along the buttresses provides very satisfactory stabilization of the fractured segments. Access to fractures of the anterior and lateral maxilla can be achieved through a gingivo-buccal incision ensuring that there is an adequate cuff of unattached mucosa to isolate the plates from the mouth at closure. The posterior limit of the incision should be no further than the first permanent molar to preserve a good blood supply. The buccal fat pad may be avoided by angling the scalpel blade or cutting diathermy at 45° to the gingival cuff. Subperiosteal elevation with preservation of the infraorbital nerve allows reconstruction of the paranasal and zygomatic buttresses. The infraorbital rim needs to be reduced and fixed in Le Fort 2 maxillary fractures, nasomaxillary fractures, zygomatic injuries and orbital floor repairs. A number of skin incisions can be used (**Table 107.1**) all of which have advantages and disadvantages.

> **KEY POINTS**
>
> **Maxillary fractures**
>
> - Maxillary fractures may involve the orbits.
> - They may disrupt the occlusion.
> - Internal fixation has replaced external fixation for the majority of maxillary fractures.
> - Most high-energy maxillary fractures are not pure Le Fort injuries and are also comminuted.
> - Haemorrhage may be arrested with anterior and posterior nasal packs or epistats.

ZYGOMATIC COMPLEX FRACTURES

Surgical anatomy

The body and processes of the zygomatic bone make up the lateral middle third of the facial skeleton. Blows to this part of the face are common and may cause either a depressed fracture of the entire zygomatic bone or a fracture of the zygomatic arch (**Figure 107.17**). These injuries were originally termed 'tripod fracture' because of the disruption of the three commonly recognized articulations:

1. fronto-zygomatic
2. infraorbital rim
3. zygomaticomaxillary buttress.

In fact, there are two further articulations worthy of consideration:

1. zygomatic arch;
2. zygomaticosphenoid.

The lateral middle third of the face provides support and protection for the globe of the eye. Accurate anatomical reduction of such fractures is important for facial appearance, optimum function of the eye, and because of its close proximity to the coronoid process, for opening and closing the mandible.

Signs and symptoms

The lateral aspect of the face is best examined from the front, above and behind the patient. It will be swollen and bruised. A subconjunctival haemorrhage is almost invariably present in fractures of the zygomatic body (**Figure 107.17**). Even if the eyelid is closed by oedema, it is essential that the eye is examined and its acuity recorded. Eye movements may be restricted, particularly in upward gaze if there is an orbital floor dehiscence and blow-out of the orbital contents (**Figure 107.18**). The zygomatic prominence may be difficult to assess initially because of soft tissue swelling but, once this has decreased, reduced projection will become more obvious. A step deformity of the infraorbital margin may be palpable and the frontozygomatic suture may be tender to touch. In arch fractures, there is often a palpable depression and limited mouth opening. Finally, the sensation of the cheek may be altered

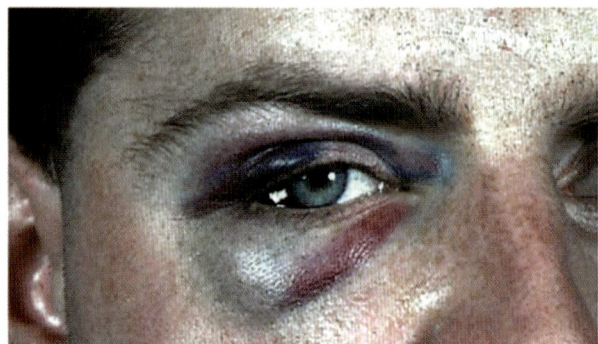

Figure 107.17 Typical appearance of a patient with a fractured zygoma. A slight depression of the cheek is clearly visible and he has a subconjunctival haemorrhage.

TABLE 107.1 Orbital access		
Incision	Advantage	Disadvantage
Transconjunctival	Good exposure, aesthetic	Slight risk of entropion
Transconjunctival with cantholysis	Excellent exposure	Risk of lid malposition
Transconjunctival with transcaruncular extension	Excellent exposure of medial orbit wall	Technically difficult
Lower eyelid	Straightforward to execute	Risk of increased sclera show, ectropion Visible scar
Infraorbital	Rapid, minimal increased scleral show	Poor cosmesis

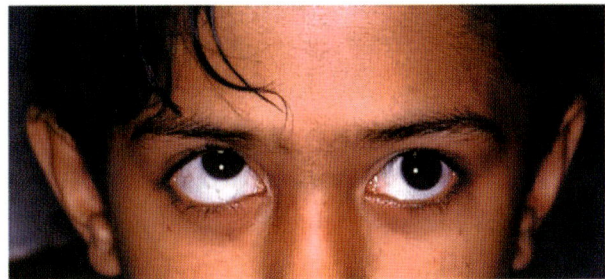

Figure 107.18 Reduced ocular movement and enophthalmos associated with an orbital floor injury.

if there has been damage to either the zygomaticotemporal or zygomaticobuccal nerves.

Imaging

Whilst most fractures are visible on 15 and 30° occipitomental X-rays, CT scanning is increasingly becoming standard of care particularly if there are signs of diminished ocular motility. Hess charting should be obtained in all cases with subjective diplopia.[36]

Management

Minimally displaced fractures may be managed conservatively with a full explanation to the patient and instructions not to blow their nose for a period of 2–3 weeks. It is prudent to review the patient after 10 days when much of the swelling will have resolved to make sure that no active intervention is required. Displaced fractures require reduction with or without fixation. Reduction may be achieved in a number of ways. The precise method will depend on the surgeon's preference and the configuration of the fracture. Each method has its advocates and offers certain advantages over others (**Table 107.2**).

GILLIES TEMPORAL APPROACH

The hair is shaved just anterior to the ear and both infraorbital margins are exposed for comparison. Following infiltration with local anaesthetic and adrenaline solution, a small incision is made down to the superficial temporal fascia. The fascia is then incised and an elevator is passed down on the temporalis muscle so that its tip lies just under the fracture. The bone is then elevated.

POSWILLO HOOK

The point of application of the hook is the intersection of a line drawn vertically from the lateral orbital margin and a horizontal line drawn from the inferior margin of the nose. The hook is inserted through a stab incision and the zygoma lifted back into position.

INTRA-ORAL OR KEEN APPROACH

A mucogingival incision is made in the buccal sulcus in the molar/premolar region. An elevator may be passed behind the zygomatic body to elevate the fracture.

Diastasis at the frontozygomatic suture and high-energy injuries are typically unstable. Closed reduction does not allow examination of the articulations of the zygoma. Minor discrepancies may be missed and only come to light some days later.

In reality, surgical exposure of the relevant articulations together with experience ensures good outcomes for the overwhelming majority of patients. The zygoma may be plated at the frontozygomatic suture, infraorbital margin, zygomatic buttress and zygomatic arch. Wound closure is extremely important. Optimal draping of the soft tissues requires meticulous closure of the periosteum over the plates. Some surgeons 'hitch' the deep tissues to superior tissues to provide further support.[37]

TABLE 107.2 Zygomatic complex fractures – advantages and disadvantages of surgical approaches

Approach	Indication	Advantage	Disadvantage
Gillies	Medially displaced body fractures, zygomatic arch fractures	Elevating site distant from fixation site	Requires skin incision, may be conspicuous in the bald patient
Dingman	Medially displaced body fractures	Uses common skin incision to that of frontozygomatic access	May be difficult to plate frontozygomatic suture and elevate simultaneously. Incision may become stretched
Poswillo hook	Posteriorly displaced fractures. Not arch fractures	Good mechanical advantage, quick, only one suture required	Access point of hook is prominent on the lateral cheek prominence and may be noticeable
Keen	Medially displaced fractures, arch fractures	Avoids cutaneous scars	Does not address displacement at the frontozygomatic suture. Elevation and plating at this site are difficult simultaneously. Theoretical contamination of the fracture site with oral microorganisms
Coronal	Laterally displaced arch fractures	The only approach for this rare fracture	Extensive surgical exposure

Post-operative care

The patient is instructed not to blow their nose and, for the first 12 hours, they should be closely observed for signs or symptoms of a retrobulbar haemorrhage. Increasing pain, proptosis, ophthalmoplegia, diminishing visual acuity and a palpable increase in ocular pressure should alert the attendant to this and indicate the need for urgent exploration and evacuation of any haematoma. Most long-term complications relate to malunited fractures. It is important to realize that early accurate anatomical reduction provides the best results. Secondary reconstruction is difficult because of bony remodelling and fibrosis in the overlying soft tissues.[38, 39]

> **KEY POINTS**
>
> Retrobulbar haemorrhage can involve:
> - decreased visual acuity;
> - diplopia;
> - ophthalmoplegia;
> - proptosis;
> - tense globe;
> - dilated pupil;
> - loss of direct light reflex.

> **BEST CLINICAL PRACTICE**
>
> Management involves:
> - ✓ dexamethasone 4 mg/kg bolus, 2 mg/kg, 6-hourly;
> - ✓ acetazolamide 500 mg i.v.;
> - ✓ mannitol 20%, 200 mL;
> - ✓ finally, remove the sutures and consider surgical decompression by a lateral cathotomy.

ORBITAL FLOOR FRACTURES

Introduction

The form and function of the globe depends on the integrity of the bone and soft tissue of the orbit. Blunt trauma to the globe[40] or adjacent bone can lead to a fracture of the thin bone of the orbital floor.[41]

Signs and symptoms

The cardinal signs of an orbital floor fracture are enophthalmos and hypoglobus (depressed pupillary level). Enophthalmos is most apparent when the contralateral eye is normal. Other signs include supratarsal hollowing, hooding of the eye, narrowing of the palpebral fissure width and an infraorbital nerve deficit. A small fracture of the orbital floor can lead to a trap door phenomenon. If the orbital fat or inferior oblique muscle becomes trapped in the fracture configuration, then interference with muscular function results in diplopia on upward gaze (**Figure 107.18**).

Imaging

CT imaging with axial, coronal and sagittal reformatting provides best standard of care

> **BEST CLINICAL PRACTICE**
>
> **Ophthalmology review**
> - ✓ Assessment of visual acuity is mandatory. Retrobulbar haemorrhage causing loss of sight is a rare occurrence but is treatable and should be sought in every orbital injury.
> - ✓ Hess charting allows comparison of the visual fields of each eye. Post-operative charting can be used to assess the quality of repair.
> - ✓ Hertel exophthalmometry gives an objective analysis of the position of the globe. It has limited value in acute trauma.

Management

Significant orbital floor injury requires exploration and repair. The approach will be determined by the size and position of the blow-out fracture. All soft-tissue components should be mobilized and supported by a graft. Various grafts and materials have been used for this purpose. polydimethylsiloxane (PDS) are readily available and most suited for smaller defects. Titanium alloplasts, either prefabricated or custom-made using CAD-CAM technology are extremely useful especially when there are concomitant zygomatic complex fractures.[42]

NASO-ORBITO-ETHMOID COMPLEX FRACTURES

Definition and classification

Naso-orbito-ethmoid (NOE) fractures involve the anatomical confluence of the nose, orbits and ethmoids. This is a complex area and these injuries are often overlooked. Reconstruction at a later date is extremely difficult. The most useful classification of these injuries was devised by Markowitz et al.[43] who defined them in terms of their attachment to the medial canthal ligaments (**Table 107.3**).

TABLE 107.3 Classification of naso-orbito-ethmoid complex fractures

Classification	
Type I	Single large central fragment bearing the canthal ligaments
Type II	Fragmentation of the central fragment, medial canthal ligaments attached to bone
Type III	Comminution of the central fragment with no bone attached to canthal ligaments

Signs and symptoms

Loss of nasal projection and tipping up of the end of the nose are common features of these injuries (**Figure 107.19**). Splaying of the nasal root and telecanthus indicates gross comminution. There is usually blunting of the canthal angle and movement of the medial canthus can be elicited by displacement of the lateral palpebral ligament.

Management

Type I fractures can be stabilized using miniplates. Surgical access is through a coronal flap, intra-orally and lower eyelid incisions may be required. Type II and III fractures are also repaired with miniplates, but require a transnasal canthopexy to reduce the telecanthus and hold the position of the medial canthal ligaments. This is accomplished by means of plates and/or a wire. The lacrimal integrity should be assessed pre- or peri-operatively and stented primarily if damaged.

UPPER FACIAL THIRD FRACTURES INVOLVING THE FRONTAL SINUS

Fractures involving the frontal sinus may lead to deformity and be complicated by infection. These injuries are classified according to the involvement of the anterior and/or posterior table and whether or not there is damage to the nasofrontal duct.[44] The principal aims of treatment are to leave the patient with a safe and functional sinus and with no cosmetic deformity. Fractures of the anterior table may be treated conservatively if there is no cosmetic deformity, while displaced fractures require reduction and fixation. Fractures of the posterior table demand a neurosurgical opinion and may need an obliterative procedure or cranialization with obliteration of the frontonasal recess and its lining.[45, 46] Persistence of the epithelial lining with inadequate drainage predisposes to mucocoele formation.[47]

Soft tissue injuries

Accurate repair of soft tissue injuries including skin and fascia layers is mandatory for optimum results. Facial wounds should be closed as soon as possible provided they are clean. Meticulous debridement with antiseptic solution is essential. Grit from the roads can tattoo wounds badly and be a real problem and are best removed using a sterile nylon scrubbing brush.

Experience with cutaneous malignancy demonstrates that sizeable areas of tissue loss can be dealt with primarily, so some selective removal of poorly viable wound margins would appear to be sensible. It is crucial to ensure that any underlying bony injury is repaired to enable correct support and soft tissue draping.

The facial nerve and parotid duct are frequently damaged in significant soft-tissue injuries. The facial nerve is easiest to find and repair in the first 48 hours, while the peripheral branches can still be stimulated. Epineural repair provides the patient with the best chance of a good recovery.

Identification and alignment of key landmarks such as the vermillion border of the lip, eyebrow, alar margin of nose, ear and eyelids is essential for a good cosmetic result. Similarly, the use of deep sutures (4/0 vicryl or equivalent) to take tension out of the wound and to avoid dead space together with appropriate skin sutures (5/0 or 6/0 monofilament) produces the best results. Shelved lacerations should be managed by placing sutures with a bigger 'bite' on the more depressed side, and triangular edges by the 'corner stitch' technique. Sutures are best supported by steristrips and removed after 4–7 days. Chloramphenicol eye ointment can be applied to the wound 4 times daily for one week.

The patient should be instructed in wound care and told to avoid direct sunlight on the wound for one year.

PAEDIATRIC FACIAL INJURIES

Fortunately, serious maxillofacial injuries in this age group are uncommon. Minor injuries, particularly soft tissue and dentoalveolar are, however, frequent. The treatment concepts and protocols are similar to adult patients.[48]

Soft tissue injuries

Minor soft-tissue injuries are managed in the same way as adult patients. Consideration should be given to the use of resorbable sutures to avoid unnecessary general anaesthesia for suture removal. Cyanoacrylate glue can be used with care but not in the presence of substantial connective tissue damage.

Injured anterior teeth

Dental injuries to the upper anterior teeth are extremely common, but their management and prognosis is

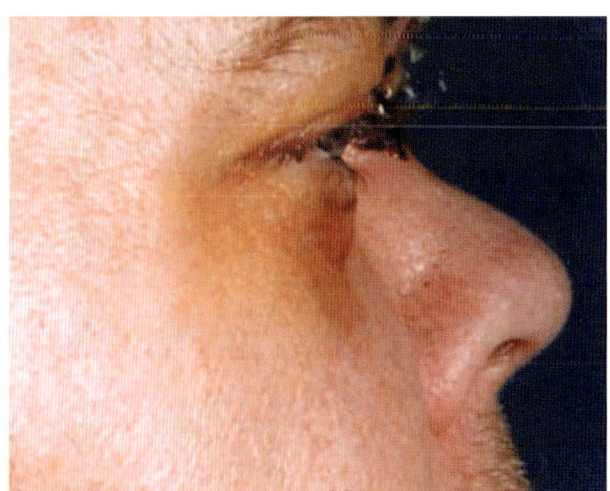

Figure 107.19 Patient with a naso-orbito-ethmoid fracture with typical loss of nasal projection and tilting of the nasal tip.

extremely complex. The optimal treatment protocol is determined by a number of factors that relate to the type of tooth fractured, the presence and level of any root fracture, the vitality of the pulp and the state of development of the root. It is essential that an expert opinion is sought from a maxillofacial surgeon or paedodontist. Fractured teeth can be temporarily repaired, exposed pulps capped with calcium hydroxide based pastes and mobile teeth splinted to adjacent teeth. Anterior permanent teeth that have been avulsed should be reimplanted at the first available opportunity and splinted. If the reimplantation is delayed, the tooth should be kept moist in the mouth of the patient or parent. Alternatively, the tooth could be stored in a glass of milk.

Fractures of the facial bones

As stated previously, the principles of reduction and fixation of facial bone fractures in children are the same as for adults. Plates should be placed using short screws to avoid damaging developing tooth germs and all mandibular metal work removed after 3–6 months so that it does not interfere with growth. Fractures of the condyle are usually treated conservatively as there is an immense capacity for remodelling and any intervention might damage the growth centre.[49] Fronto-naso-ethmoid injuries differ in their fracture pattern because the development of the frontal sinus may not be complete. Any extensive dissection of the medial canthal area may lead to excessive subperiosteal bone formation and therefore repairs in this area should be supported by acrylic buttons in the immediate post-operative phase.[50]

BEST CLINICAL PRACTICE

Paediatric dental injuries

✓ Consider whether the injury might be non-accidental.
✓ Reimplant avulsed teeth as soon as possible.
✓ Use short screws and take care not to damage unerupted teeth.
✓ Remove plates 3–6 months after surgery.
✓ Manage condylar fractures conservatively.

FUTURE RESEARCH

➤ The controversy on the virtues of open and closed management of condylar neck injuries will persist. The management and outcomes of intra-capsular fractures may well become revolutionized by alloplastic materials.

KEY POINTS

Soft tissue injuries

- Accurate repair of soft tissue injuries including skin and fascia layers is mandatory for optimum results.
- It is crucial to ensure that any underlying bony injury is repaired to enable correct support and soft tissue draping.
- Identification and alignment of key landmarks such as the vermillion border of the lip, eyebrow, alar margin of nose, ear and eyelids is essential for a good cosmetic result.

Paediatric Facial Injuries

- Fortunately, serious maxillofacial injuries in this age group are uncommon. Minor injuries, particularly soft tissue and dentoalveolar are, however, frequent.
- The treatment concepts and protocols are similar to adult patients. The principles of reduction and fixation of facial bone fractures in children are the same as for adults.
- Fractures of the condyle are usually treated conservatively as there is an immense capacity for remodelling and any intervention might damage the growth centre.

REFERENCES

1. Murray JAM. Management of septal deviation with nasal fractures. *Facial Plast Surg* 1989; **62**: 88–93.
2. Nahum AM. The biomechanics of maxillofacial trauma. *Clin Plast Surg* 1975; **2**: 59–64.
3. Courtney MJ, Rajapakse Y, Duncan G, Morrissey G. Nasal fracture manipulation: a comparative study of general and local anaesthesia techniques. *Clin Otolaryngol* 2003; **28**: 472–5.
4. Karagama YG, Newton JR, Clayton MGG. Are nasal fractures being referred appropriately from the accident and emergency department to ENT? *Injury* 2004; **35**: 968–71.
5. Illum P, Kristensen S, Jorgensen K, Brahe Pedersen C. Role of fixation in the treatment of nasal fractures. *Clin Otolaryngol* 1983; **8**: 191–5.
6. Persig W, Lehmann I. The influence of trauma on growing septal cartilage. *Rhinology* 1975; **13**: 39–46.
7. Raveh J, Laedrach K, Vuillemin T, Zingg M. Management of combined frontonasoorbital/skull base fractures and telecanthus in 355 cases. *Arch Otolaryngol Head Neck Surg* 1992; **118**: 605–14.
8. Logan M, O'Driscoll K, Masterton J. The utility of nasal bone radiographs in nasal trauma. *Clin Radiol* 1994; **49**: 192.
9. Cook JA, McRae RD, Irving RM, Dowie LN. A randomized comparison of manipulation of the fractured nose under local and general anaesthesia. *Clin Otolaryngol* 1990; **15**: 343–6.
10. Owen GO, Parker AJ, Watson DJ. Fractured-nose reduction under local anaesthesia: is it acceptable to the patient? *Rhinology* 1992; **30**: 89–96.
11. Ridder GJ, Boedeker CC, Fradis M, Schipper J. Technique and timing for closed reduction of nasal fractures: a retrospective study. *Ear Nose Throat J* 2002; **81**: 49–54.
12. Jones T, Nandapalan V. Manipulation of the fractured nose: a comparison of local infiltration anaesthesia and topical local anaesthesia. *Clin Otolaryngol* 1999; **24**: 443–6.
13. Harrison DH. Nasal injuries: their pathogenesis and treatment. *Br J Plast Surg* 1979; **32**: 57–64.
14. Murray JAM, Maran AGD. Open v closed reduction of the fractured nose. *Arch Otolaryngol* 1984; **110**: 797–802.
15. Verwoerd C. Present day treatment of nasal fractures: closed versus open reduction. *Facial Plast Surg* 1992; **8**: 220–3.
16. Fernandes S. Nasal fractures: the taming of the shrewd. *Laryngoscope* 2004; **114**: 587–92.

17. Staffel J. Optimizing treatment of nasal fractures. *Laryngoscope* 2002; **112**: 1709–19.
18. Kim J, Park HS, Yoon, CH, Kim HJ. Analysis of nasal septal fracture combined in nasal bone fracture using CT. *J Korean Soc Plast Reconstr Surg* 1998; **25**: 852–9.
19. Hayter JP, Cawood JI. The functional case for miniplates in maxillofacial surgery. *Int J Oral Maxillofac Surg* 1993; **22**: 91–6.
20. Williams JG, Cawood JI. Effect of intermaxillary fixation on pulmonary function. *Int J Oral Maxillofac Surg* 1990; **19**: 76–8.
21. Pigadas N, Avery CM. Precautions against cross-infection during operations for maxillofacial trauma. *Br J Oral Maxillofac Surg* 2000; **38**: 110–13.
22. Markowitz BL, Manson PN. Panfacial fractures: organization of treatment. *Clin Plast Surg* 1989; **16**: 105–14.
23. Tullio A, Sesenna E. Role of surgical reduction of condylar fractures in the management of panfacial fractures. *Br J Oral Maxillofac Surg* 2000; **38**: 472–6.
24. Fordyce AM, Lalani Z, Songra AK, et al. Intermaxillary fixation is not usually necessary to reduce mandibular fractures. *Br J Oral Maxillofac Surg* 1999; **37**: 52–7.
25. Schneider AM, David LR, DeFranzo AJ, et al. Use of specialized bone screws for intermaxillary fixation. *Ann Plast Surg* 2000; **44**: 154–7.
26. Kunz C, Hammer B, Prein J. Fractures of the edentulous atrophic mandible: fracture management and complications. *Mund-, Kiefer- und Gesichtschirurgie*. 2001; **5**: 227–32.
27. Ellis E, 3rd, Dean J. Rigid fixation of mandibular condyle fractures. *Oral Surg Oral Med Oral Pathol* 1993; **76**: 6–15.
28. Ellis E, 3rd. Treatment methods for fractures of the mandibular angle. *Int J Oral Maxillofac Surg* 1999; **28**: 243–52.
29. Zide MF, Kent JN. Indications for open reduction of mandibular condyle fractures. *J Oral Maxillofac Surg* 1983; **41**: 89–98.
30. Lauer G, Schmelzeisen R. Endoscope-assisted fixation of mandibular condylar process fractures. *J Oral Maxillofac Surg* 1999; **57**: 36–9; discussion 39–40.
31. Lee C, Mueller RV, Lee K, Mathes SJ. Endoscopic subcondylar fracture repair: Functional, aesthetic, and radiographic outcomes. *Plast Reconstr Surg* 1998; **102**: 1434–43; discussion 1444–5.
32. Le Fort R. Etude experimentale sur les fractures de la machoire superieure. *Rev Chirurg* 1901; **23**: 20, 360, 479.
33. Manson PN. Some thoughts on the classification and treatment of Le Fort fractures. *Ann Plast Surg* 1986; **17**: 356–63.
34. Gruss J, MacKinnon SE. Complex maxillary fractures: role of buttress reconstruction and immediate bone grafts. *Plast Reconstr Surg* 1986; **78**: 4.
35. Manson PN, Hooper JE, Su CT. Structural pillars of the facial skeleton: an approached the management of Le Fort fractures. *Plast Reconstr Surg* 1980; **66**: 54–7.
36. Manson PN, Markowitz B, Mirvis S, et al. Toward CT-based facial fracture treatment. *Plast Reconstr Surg* 1990; **85**: 202–12; discussion 213–14.
37. Phillips JH, Gruss JS, Wells MD, Cholet A. Periosteal suspension of the lower eyelid and cheek following subciliary exposure of facial fractures. *Plast Reconstr Surg* 1991; **88**: 145–8.
38. Hammer B, Prein J. Correction of post-traumatic orbital deformities: operative techniques and review of 26 patients. *J Craniomaxillofac Surg* 1995; **23**: 81–90.
39. Freihofer HP. Effectiveness of secondary post-traumatic periorbital reconstruction. *J Craniomaxillofac Surg* 1995; **23**: 143–50.
40. Warwar RE, Bullock JD, Ballal DR, Ballal RD. Mechanisms of orbital floor fractures: a clinical, experimental and theortical study. *Ophthal Plast Reconstr Surg* 2000: **16**: 188–200.
41. Waterhouse N, Lyne J, Urdang M, Garey L. An investigation into the mechanism of orbital blowout fractures. *Br J Plast Surg* 1999; **52**: 607–12.
42. Sugar AW, Kuriakose M, Walshaw ND. Titanium mesh in orbital wall reconstruction. *Int J Oral Maxillofac Surg* 1992; **21**: 140–4.
43. Markowitz B MP, Sargent L, Van der Kolk CA, et al. Management of the medial canthal tendon in nasoethmoid orbitae fractures: the importance of the central fragment in classification and treatment. *Plast Reconstr Surg* 1991; **87**: 843–53.
44. Stanley Jr. RB. Fractures of the frontal sinus. *Clin Plast Surg* 1989; **16**: 115–23.
45. Parhiscar A, Har-El G. Frontal sinus obliteration with the pericranial flap. *Otolaryngol Head Neck Surg* 2001; **124**: 304–7.
46. Mickel TJ RR, Robinson JB. Frontal sinus obliteration: a comparison of fat, muscle, bone, and spontaneous osteoneogenesis in the cat model. *Plast Reconstr Surg* 1995; **95**(3): 586–92.
47. Wallis A, Donald PJ. Frontal sinus fractures: a review of 72 cases. *Laryngoscope* 1988; **98**: 593–8.
48. Kaban LB. Diagnosis and treatment of fractures of the facial bones in children 1943-1993. *J Oral Maxillofac Surg* 1993; **51**: 722–9.
49. Fiefal H, Albert-Deumlich J, Riediger D. Long term follow up of subcondylar fractures in children by electronic computer assisted recording of condylar movements. *Int J Oral Maxillofac Surg* 1992; **21**: 70–6.
50. Ayliffe P, Ward Booth P. Nasoethmoid fractures. In: Ward Booth P, Schendel SA, Hausamen J-E (eds). *Maxillofacial surgery*. Edinburgh: Churchill Livingstone; 1999, pp. 155–6.

CHAPTER 108

CSF LEAKS

Scott M. Graham

Introduction	1203	Imaging for diagnosis of CSF leaks	1207
Head trauma	1204	*Controversies in repair*	1207
Congenital CSF leaks	1204	Intrathecal fluorescein	1207
CSF leaks associated with tumours	1204	Lumbar drains	1208
Spontaneous leaks	1204	Technical aspects of the repair	1208
CSF leaks complicating sinus surgery	1205	Conclusion	1209
Repair of surgically-induced skull base defects	1206	References	1209
Investigation of CSF leaks	1206		

SEARCH STRATEGY

Data in this chapter may be updated by a Medline search using keywords: CSF leak, CSF rhinorrhoea, spontaneous CSF leak, skull base repair and intrathecal fluourescein.

INTRODUCTION

Few procedures reflect the tremendous benefits of endoscopic techniques in quite the same way as the endoscopic closure of CSF leaks. Although the ultimate chance of success may in some measure depend on the aetiology of the leak,[1] remarkable results of 90% success rates at the initial attempt with success rates up to 97% with revision have been published.[1, 2] Despite these impressive figures there continues to be isolated enthusiasm for open approaches in some neurosurgical centres. Some published neurosurgical series have success rates as low as 60% with predictable sequelae from brain retraction and sacrifice of the olfactory nerves, to say nothing of the coronal flap and frontal craniotomy. Recent neurosurgical publications have recommended open approaches in the face of adverse prognostic factors such as prior radiation or elevated intra-cranial pressure.

Although rhinorrhea can be a socially troubling symptom, the principal motivation for repair of CSF leaks is to reduce the risk of meningitis or other intra-cranial complications. The incidence of meningitis in patients with an active CSF leak has been quoted as 10% year on year[3, 4] although a more recent study suggested that the incidence may be as low as 0.3% per year per active leak per person.[5]

Daudia et al. found that in 11 patients with 190 years of active leaks 21 developed meningitis resulting in an overall risk of 19% although most occurred in the first year of the leak.[5]

The repair of a newly diagnosed CSF leak is not an absolute surgical emergency and time can be taken to properly work-up and investigate the patient. During this time the simple advice of telling the patient not to blow their nose or to sneeze 'with their mouth open' and not to use CPAP needs to be reinforced. Nonetheless, because of the risk of meningitis, surgical repair should be performed at the earliest reasonable opportunity. Even today meningitis is associated with a definite mortality rate. Few studies have followed patients with repaired leaks over the long term. A publication from the Mayo Clinic[6] identified recurrence of leaks in a group of 21 patients at an average of 50.8 months after corrective surgery. The longest interval to recurrence in this group of patients was 28 years.

In patients with a history of a CSF leak it is worth checking their pneumococcal antibody titres and recommending vaccination with a 23-valent polysaccharide PNC vaccine or a 7-valent conjugate PNC vaccine if it is low.

In recent years, the spectrum of leaks seen in major centres has changed significantly. Most of the leaks seen today are either 'spontaneous' or what might be termed 'anticipated'. The 'anticipated' category of leaks comprises those seen after anterior skull base or sellar or parasellar tumour resection. In these patients, the bony defect is often substantial and this has required a reappraisal of reconstructive techniques.

While a variety of classification systems of CSF leaks exist, perhaps the most useful is the time-honoured system of classification by aetiology. CSF leaks can be considered as congenital, spontaneous or post-traumatic. Post-traumatic leaks can be further divided into those associated with head trauma, those seen as a complication of sinus surgery and those seen as a part of skull base surgery. A small number of patients with tumours also present with CSF leaks.

HEAD TRAUMA

CSF leaks are quoted as occurring in perhaps 2% of head injuries and 12% to 30% of skull base fractures.[8] Most CSF leaks occur as a result of blunt trauma. They may present as CSF otorrhea, CSF oto-rhinorrhea or CSF rhinorrhea. The conventional viewpoint is that most traumatic CSF leaks will heal with conservative treatment including bedrest. Insertion of a lumbar drain may sometimes be required. It is likely that only the sinus mucosal aspect of the defect closes as the dura does not regenerate. This produces a relatively fragile closure and work by Bernal-Sprekelsen et al.[9] has suggested a substantial continuing risk of meningitis in these patients. The authors suggest that this 'mono-layer of protection' may be eroded by either the pulsatile effect of the brain or by inflammation within the nose.[9] With the widespread availability of endoscopic closure, performed with statistically small risks, this conservative management paradigm might be challenged, changing towards a more active interventionist policy.

Massive head trauma with complex comminuted and displaced fractures of the skull base can be incredibly difficult to treat. Open approaches may be of value for these patients. The decision to proceed with an open approach is sometimes made easier by the presence of intra-cranial injuries requiring attention or significant fractures of the posterior wall of the frontal sinus. Free tissue transfer has been reported as being helpful in carefully selected groups.[10] In massive 'egg-shell' fractures of the sphenoid sinuses, fat obliteration can be considered, leaving the treatment of possible subsequent mucoceles that may develop to a secondary procedure.

CONGENITAL CSF LEAKS

Congenital CSF leaks in association with encephalocele or meningoencephaloceles are uncommon. These are well diagnosed on MRI and this scan is recommended when sinus opacity is demonstrated adjacent to a skull base defect. Brain tissue contained within the encephalocele is invariably non-functioning and can be removed as part of the surgical procedure. Congenital abnormalities of

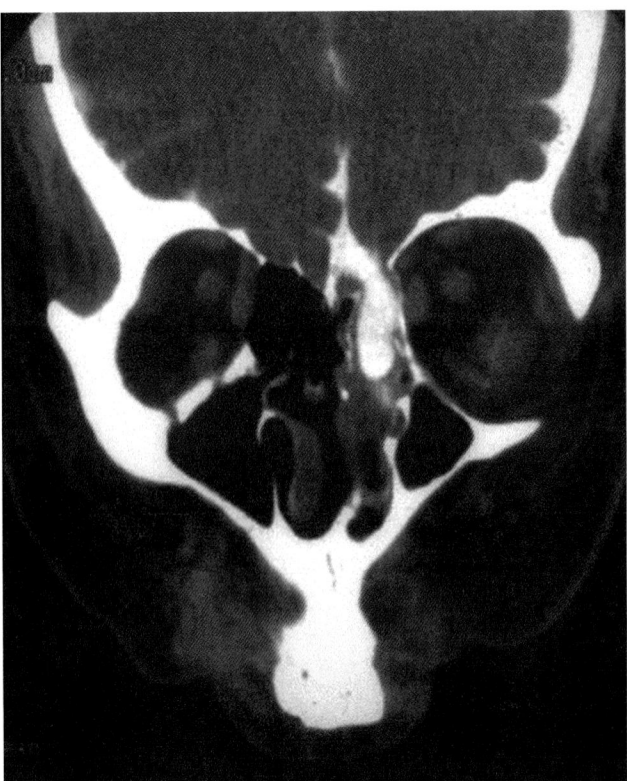

Figure 108.1 Coronal CT scan of meningo – encephalocele medial to and eroding the left middle turbinate.

the inner ear such as the Mondini Dysplasia may present with substantial CSF leaks where the CSF has only briefly transversed the perilymphatic space. Such leaks, in addition to presenting as hearing loss or recurrent meningitis, may also present with CSF otorrhea or CSF oto-rhinorrhea (**Figure 108.1**).

CSF LEAKS ASSOCIATED WITH TUMOURS

Tumours causing substantial erosion of the skull base may present with CSF rhinorrhea. Occasionally where tumour shrinkage occurs, for example during induction chemotherapy, CSF leaks may also occur. The closure of the CSF leak is part of the surgical treatment of the tumour and for the closure to be successful it is important for the margins of the CSF leak to be clear of tumour, particularly in malignant disease. Persisting CSF leaks in the face of residual untreated tumour may present a considerable challenge. A study by Boudreaux and Zins[11] described open treatment of CSF leaks in 14 high-risk patients. Nine of the 14 patients had malignant brain tumours. A success rate of 85% was reported.

SPONTANEOUS LEAKS

A good deal of recent interest has centered on 'spontaneous CSF leaks' sometimes described as 'idiopathic'. The association of spontaneous leaks with middle-aged women with a raised body mass index is now well known. These leaks are thought to represent a variant of benign intra-cranial hypertension.[12] These patients have a generally elevated intra-cranial pressure, this diagnosis being made on lumbar puncture after surgical repair. It is not possible to measure this pre-operatively as the persistent leak reduces the pressure although there may be radiological features of increased intra-cranial pressure such as an empty sella, enlarged ventricles or diffuse erosion of the skull base.[1] When the CSF is actively draining – for example, perhaps at the time of lumbar puncture for fluorescein installation prior to repair, the intra-cranial pressure is often reduced. It is thought that the elevated intra-cranial pressure is due to poor CSF resorption by the arachnoid villi.[12] This increased intra-cranial pressure with associated pulsatile forces produces thinning of bone that is most evident in the weakest areas of the skull base. Herniation of the meninges and brain, often with CSF leakage, most often occurs in the lateral recess of a well pneumatized sphenoid, in the area of the lateral lamella of the cribriform and in the ethmoid roof. These may be multiple sites of weakness of the skull base.

Imaging and diagnosis are similar to other varieties of CSF leaks. In cases of multiple cranial base defects, intrathecal fluorescein can be helpful in localizing the exact location of active leakage. Identification of 'spontaneous' as the likely aetiology of the leak pre-operatively is helpful in counselling the patient.[1] Spontaneous leaks are most likely to recur and the success rates for endoscopic closure are worse than for other aeteologies.[1] In one study, 21% of spontaneous leaks recurred, going up to 46% if there were radiological signs of a raised intra-cranial pressure compared to 2% if the leak was not spontaneous.[1] With spontaneous leaks there can be re-leakage at the site of repair but there can be multiple areas of weakness of the skull base and with untreated underlying elevated intra-cranial pressure other areas may break down and leak.

Areas of substantial skull base dehiscence may benefit from additional reinforcement with a bone or cartilage graft. This is sometimes easier said than done with a thin bony skull base and difficulty in finding a reliable 'edge'. CSF leaks in the lateral recess of well pneumatized sphenoid sinuses may be best approached by the transantral transpterygoid approach described by Bolger.[13] Post-operatively, the elevated intra-cranial pressure may be helped by oral acetazolamide. Selected patients may benefit from shunting. Success with employing a gastric bypass for morbid obesity has also been described.[12]

CSF LEAKS COMPLICATING SINUS SURGERY

A rate of serious complications in the order of 0.5% or less is generally quoted for endoscopic sinus surgery (**Figure 108.2**). CSF leaks diagnosed intra-operatively or post-operatively would be included in this category of serious complications.

A publication by Bachmann et al.[14] looked at the incidence of occult cerebrospinal fluid fistulae during

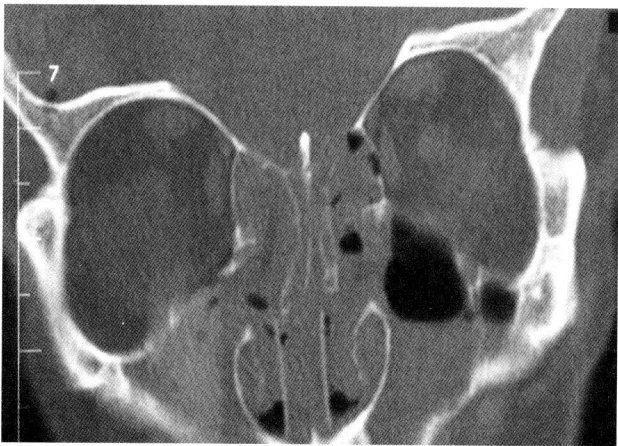

Figure 108.2 Coronal CT scan image revealing left skull base injury, clinically presenting with a CSF leak, complicating endoscopic sinus surgery.

sinus surgery. They found a 3% incidence of occult leaks utilizing the beta-trace protein assay. They had reviewed 69 consecutive patients, 'all-comers', undergoing surgery at the hands of an experienced surgeon in a tertiary referral centre. None of the patients with occult leaks displayed any symptoms or sequelae out to the follow-up period of 6 months. The authors speculated that occult leaks may be more common than previously thought and that small leaks may self-heal. The important caveat to be included with this study is that these patients need to be followed long term to examine the likelihood of delayed meningitis.

Some of the details of CSF leaks complicating sinus surgery are covered in the complications chapter of this book. Image-guided surgery, while indisputably helpful in individual cases, has not reduced the likelihood of complications in large case series. Powered instrumentation, the other great technological advance in sinus surgery in recent times, has changed the scale of complications, making brain parenchymal injury more likely than eminently treatable CSF leaks. With brain parenchymal injuries has come the need to exclude significant intra-cranial adverse vascular events.

As a general rule, CSF leaks complicating sinus surgery, diagnosed intra-operatively should be repaired under the same anaesthetic. Local intra-nasal tissue can be used for the repair with generally good results. The most likely anatomical sites for CSF leaks complicating sinus surgery are the very thin bone of the lateral lamella of the cribriform plate, the area of the anterior skull base where it is weakened by the anterior ethmoid neurovascular bundle and posteriorly where there may be confusion as to the exact anatomical relationship between the last posterior ethmoidal cell and the sphenoid sinus.

In unusual circumstances, a decision can be made not to repair the CSF leak under the same anaesthetic. Where the degree of surgical disorientation is such that attempts at repair might result in further damage such as an orbital or brain parenchymal injury, an argument can be made for referring these patients to specialist centres for closure. The wound can be carefully packed with particular care being exercised during the 'wake-up' from anaesthesia.

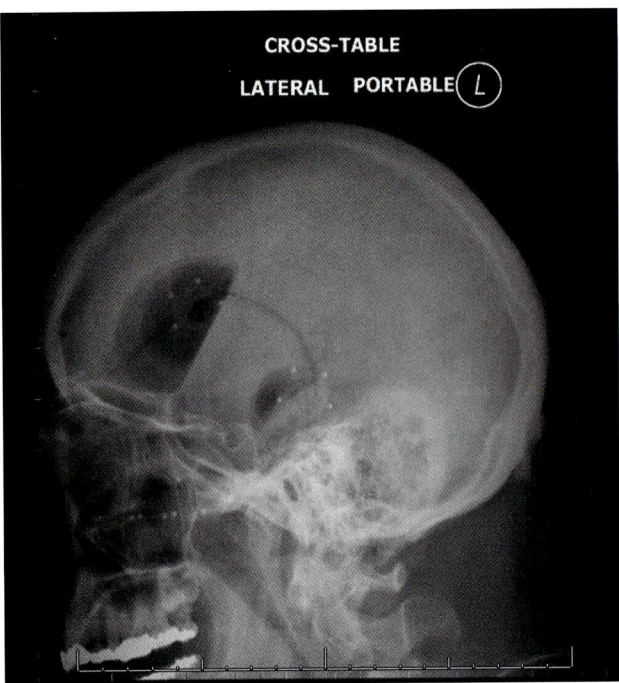

Figure 108.3 Plain skull film demonstrating pneumocephalus complicating the use of positive airway pressure. Permission pending from Kopelovich J, et al. *J Clinical Anesthesia* 2012 Aug; 24(5): 415–18.

It is crucial that the patient does not receive positive pressure mask ventilation after extubation for fear of substantial pneumocephalus developing (**Figure 108.3**).

CSF leaks complicating sinus surgery may also become evident in the post-operative period. Any complaint of clear rhinorrhea post-operatively needs to be taken seriously and investigated vigorously. The appropriate investigation of such leaks will be dealt with later in the chapter.

REPAIR OF SURGICALLY-INDUCED SKULL BASE DEFECTS

Endoscopic approaches to the anterior skull base and sellar and parasellar regions are increasingly employed for the treatment of a variety of pathological processes. Small defects can be repaired in the same way as defects of other aetiologies. For larger defects, free-fat grafts can be successfully employed. More recently, interest has focused on the use of vascularized tissue flaps. The idea of CSF leak repair utilizing vascularized septal or turbinate flaps is not new. Yessenow and McCabe reported excellent success rates utilizing this tissue in transnasal, extracranial, non-endoscopic repair of CSF leaks nearly 30 years ago.[15]

Most reports have focused on posterior septal flaps. The so-called 'Hadad-Bassagasteguy' flap utilizes septal mucoperiosteum and mucoperichondrium based on the nasoseptal artery. Kassam et al.[16] reported its general utility in 75 patients undergoing endonasal endoscopic cranial base surgery. Harvey et al.[17] reported on the experience of two skull-base centres over a 12-month period comprising 30 patients. They related using a variety of flaps including the posterior septal flap as well as inferior turbinate and nasal floor flaps. They emphasized technical aspects relating to the flap including avoiding injudicious initial posterior septectomy, decisions regarding a concomitant hemi-transfixion or Killian septal incision and careful preservation of the flap during surgery. They also emphasized the use of multi-layer skull base reconstruction initially supported by an inflated Foley catheter balloon.[17]

INVESTIGATION OF CSF LEAKS

A story of clear rhinorrhea, sometimes tasting salty and often posturally provoked, with an appropriate antecedent history is clinically suspicious for a CSF leak. Such patients must be investigated vigorously. As compelling as such a history appears, these patients do not always end up having CSF leaks as shown by Bateman and Jones in 9 patients presenting with highly suggestive histories.[18] Further investigation is therefore required. Endoscopic examination of the nose may be unrevealing but is part of the initial work-up.

The next goal is to obtain fluid for testing. Ideally this can be obtained at the office visit, sometimes with postural provocation (**Figure 108.4**). When this is unsuccessful we will sometimes have patients run up stairs in an effort to increase intra-cranial pressure and produce drainage or strain on a closed glottis. If this fails, patients are given vials to take home to catch fluid for testing. In the United States the beta-2-transferrin test is widely available and the most commonly used. A downside of the test is that it may only be performed in certain major centres and thus it may take a few days to get a result. The beta-2-transferrin test provides excellent sensitivity, specificity and positive and negative predictability in the diagnosis of CSF leaks.[19] A concomitant serum value enhances its utility. Occasional false positives have been reported in certain liver diseases or hereditary disorders of protein metabolism. It has been suggested in some European

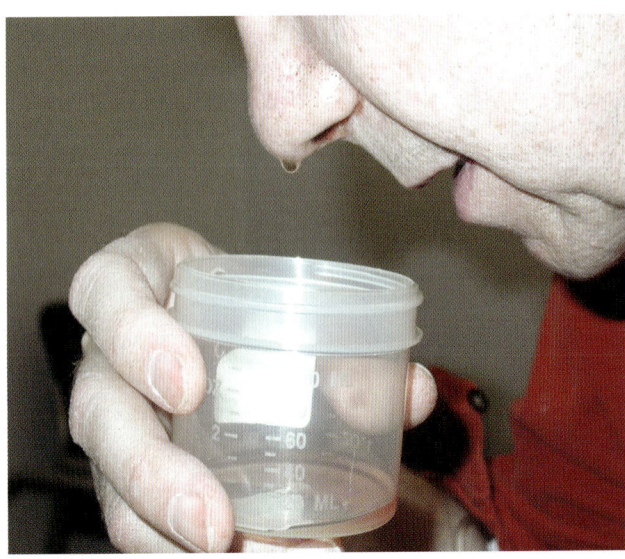

Figure 108.4 Collection of posturally provoked CSF rhinorrhea.

studies that beta-trace protein is an even better test than beta-2-transferin in detecting CSF leaks.[19]

IMAGING FOR DIAGNOSIS OF CSF LEAKS

The clear majority of CSF leaks can be diagnosed using beta-2-transferrin testing and reformatting of ultra-fine cut CT scan images of the sinuses. The coronal scan is most helpful in examining the ethmoid roof but other views are useful in diagnosing leaks at other anatomical sites. These images are most often obtained as part of planning for image-guided surgery. Details of a bony defect may be seen or an area of opacification or an air fluid level in an adjacent sinus. In the situation where there is an opaque sinus adjacent to a skull base defect an MRI scan should be performed to help diagnose a possible encephalocoele or meningocoele. Where a defect is not visualized in the sinuses, a CT examination of the temporal bones should be considered to exclude CSF oto-rhinorrhea in difficult to diagnosis cases.

In some centres MRI cisternography is performed if fine cut CT scans and beta-2-transferrin testing do not provide a diagnosis. A variety of technical modifications of the MRI enhance its ability to detect the area of the leak.[20] More commonly in cases where the diagnosis is unclear, CSF contrast studies are considered (**Figure 108.5**). This may utilize radiographical contrast such as iohexol or alternatively a radio-active tracer. These investigations require the patient to be actively leaking at the time of the study. As they need an intrathecal contrast agent of one sort or another, these tests are associated with a slightly greater risk than non-invasive studies. Radionucleide cisternography involves intrathecal administration of a tracer via a lumbar puncture followed by imaging once the tracer has had an opportunity to make its way to the skull base. Strategically placed nasal pledgets are also used. It is our practice to cut these pledgets into different shapes as this helps to identify their position in the nose after they come out. Radioactive tracers of different half lives can be considered. Localization of CSF leaks by Gadolinium-enhanced MRI cisternography has also been described. Gadolinium is injected into the subarachnoid space. This is an 'off-label' use of gadolinium in the United States and requires a separate consent. Aydin et al.[21] found this technique useful in 43 of 51 patients. No neurological sequelae were seen from the injection.

CONTROVERSIES IN REPAIR

INTRATHECAL FLUORESCEIN

It is my practice to use intrathecal fluorescein as part of the repair of all CSF leaks planned as a discrete procedure. Separate consent is obtained for the intrathecal use of fluorescein as its use via this route is not approved by the FDA. There is at least a theoretical advantage to giving this while the patient is awake and a German publication describes employing intrathecal fluorescein the afternoon before surgery.[22] In this publication, fluorescein is administered without CSF withdrawal to minimize CSF displacement.[22]

As a practical matter in the United States fluorescein is mostly administered in the operating room after induction of general anaesthesia. Our neurosurgical colleagues perform a lumbar puncture and insert a lumbar drain. Ten cc's of the patients CSF is withdrawn and this is mixed with 0.1 cc of 10% fluorescein suitable for injection. The mixture is then re-injected slowly over 10 minutes timed by the clock. The patient is placed slightly head down and sufficient time is allowed for the fluorescein to equilibrate throughout the subarachnoid space. The nose is closely examined with zero degree and angled telescopes and sites of leakage are disclosed by the bright green colour of the fluorescein. Usually the light of the telescope is sufficiently broad spectrum to achieve this – occasionally a blue light filter is helpful. The intrathecal fluorescein is of use, firstly in diagnosing a CSF leak, secondly in disclosing its exact location and thirdly, by its absence, providing evidence of success of the repair (**Figure 108.6**).

Complications of fluorescein's intrathecal use have been reported.[22] The most common complication cited has been seizures but in general this has been associated with use of the wrong formulation of fluorescein, occipital application, a higher than recommended dose or rapid bolus injection. Other complications have been attributed to the simultaneous use of intrathecal radiographical contrast material. Citing these concerns,

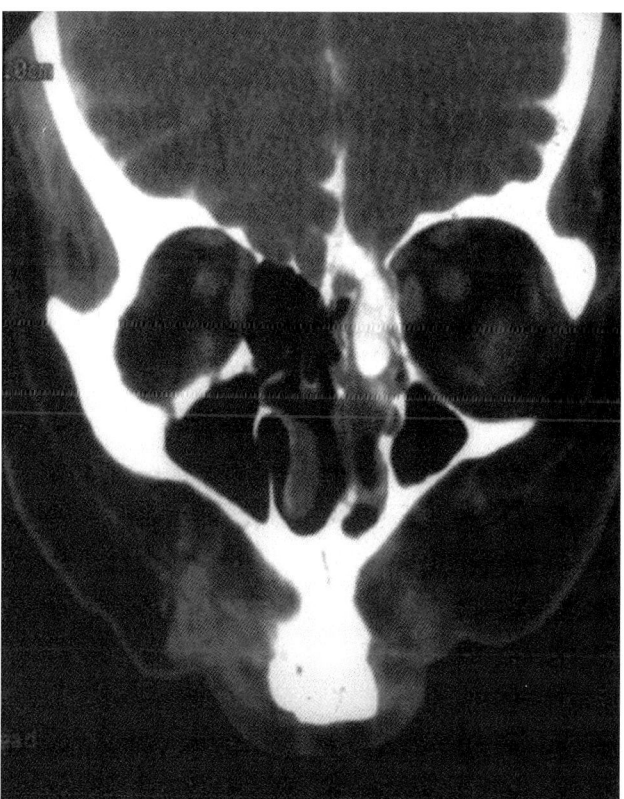

Figure 108.5 Intrathecal contrast CT study revealing left skull base defect.

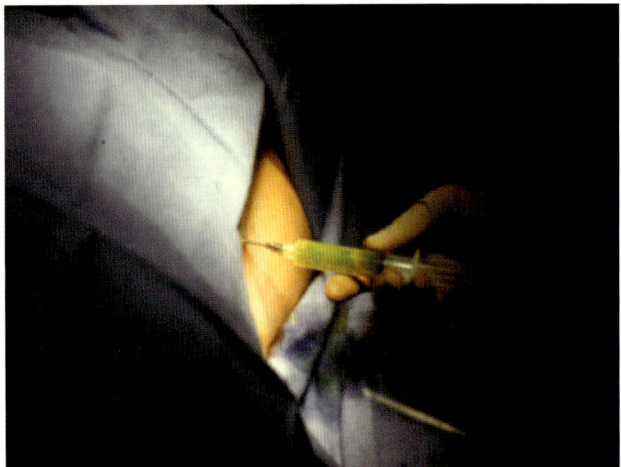

Figure 108.6 Intra-operative slow re-injection of patient's CSF mixed with fluorescein.

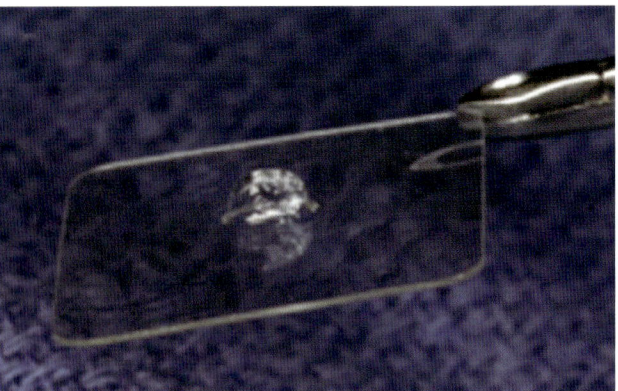

Figure 108.7 Bioabsorbable transparent plate. 'Handle' provides for ease of manipulation. Permission pending from Potter, NJ, et al. *Laryngoscope* 2015; **125**(6): 1313–15.

Zuckerman and Del Gaudio[23] described excellent success rates in 42 CSF leaks repaired without using intrathecal fluorescein or indeed lumbar drains. They relied on high-resolution CT and intra-operative image guidance for leak identification. The use of topical 5% fluorescein applied intra-operatively to the surgical site has also been described.[24] This can also be used as an office-based diagnostic test. The authors recommend skin testing the patient with fluorescein eye drops to rule out allergy the day prior to the procedure.[24]

LUMBAR DRAINS

The routine use of lumbar drains in elective CSF leak repair is controversial. Our practice is to use one when intrathecal fluorescein has been employed. The drain is placed at the time of initial lumbar puncture and then 'closed' and re-opened immediately prior to repair. Lumbar drains can be associated with important complications and their use requires specialist nursing management. In our hospital, patients with lumbar drains are managed on the neurosurgical floor.

We feel that the reduction in intra-cranial pressure afforded by the lumbar drain offers an extra measure of insurance for the repair. Certainly, however, series of successful repair without lumbar drains of selected patients with CSF leaks have been described.[23]

TECHNICAL ASPECTS OF THE REPAIR

Whatever preferences and prejudices a surgeon might have regarding specific aspects of the surgical repair, evidence can be found in the literature to support that view. Successful repair of CSF leaks requires identification of the exact site of leakage. This may require considerable dissection in difficult to find leaks. In contrast to routine endoscopic sinus surgery where mucosal preservation and avoidance of scarring is of paramount importance, in cases of CSF leak repair, scarring incited by mucosal stripping helps form a dense repair. No literature exists favouring one graft material over another and therefore the choice is largely based on surgeon preference, ease of manipulation, cost etc. Likewise no literature exists regarding the use of onlay versus underlay grafts. In general, free grafts have been preferred to vascularized flaps for smaller defects because of technical ease of manipulation and obviation of the potential for contraction with healing. Recent interest in closing large defects associated with skull base surgery has favoured pedicled flaps.[16, 17] While bone or cartilage grafts are helpful in medium-sized defects they have not been used for large repairs or generally in small defects. There is some evidence to support the use of fibrin glue to reinforce the closure. In a pig model, Almeida et al.[25] showed that fibrin glue enhanced closures had superior graft adherence and higher 'burst pressures'. Neurosurgical authors[26] have recommended dural sealants as an adjuvant to surgical repair in high-risk patients. A concern is that these 'sealant' materials may add to the cost of the surgery without significantly improving success rates. Potter et al.[27] have described the use of bio-absorbable plates as part of the surgical repair of CSF leaks in patients with an elevated BMI. Dloughy et al.[27] described young age and elevated BMI as independent variables predictive of post-operative CSF leakage after endoscopic pituitary surgery. Potter et al.[28] recommended use of semirigid bio-absorbable plates as part of the surgical repair of CSF leaks in patients with an elevated BMI, describing a significant reduction in leak rates after pituitary surgery following their use (**Figure 108.7**).

We place a 'break-layer' of Gelfoam® under the area of repair and then place a Merocel® pack. The Gelfoam® isolates the repair from shearing forces when the pack is removed. As mentioned earlier in the chapter, inflated catheter balloons[17] may provide temporary structural support after major skull base repairs.

CONCLUSION

Remarkable progress has been made in the endoscopic treatment of CSF leaks. Advances have occurred both in pre-operative imaging and diagnosis as well as in technical refinements of the surgical closure. Areas of interest in the future might include a better understanding of patients with spontaneous leaks and advances in the reconstruction of significant skull base defects from endo-nasal craniotomies.

KEY POINTS

- Endoscopic repair is treatment of choice.
- Beta-2 transferrin or Beta-trace protein are highly accurate diagnostic tests.
- High-resolution CT scans are needed in all cases.
- Intrathecal fluorescein helps in difficult cases.
- Precise layered closures give best results.

REFERENCES

1. Mirza S, Thaper A, McLelland L, Jones NS. Sinonasal cerebrospinal fluid leaks: management of 97 patients over 10 years. *Laryngoscope* 2005; **115**: 1774–77.
2. Banks CA, Palmer JN, Chiu AG, et al. Endoscopic closure of CSF rhinorrhea: 193 cases over 21 years. *Otolaryngol Head Neck Surg* 2009; **140**: 826–33.
3. Eljamel MS, Foy PM. Non-traumatic CSF fistulae: clinical history and management. *Brit J Neurosurg* 1991; **5**: 275–9.
4. Eljamel MSM. The role of surgery and beta-2-transferrin in the management of cerebrospinal fluid fistula [MD thesis]. Liverpool: University of Liverpool, 1993.
5. Daudia A, Biswas D, Jones NS. The relative risk of meningitis with cerebrospinal fluid rhinorrhoea. *Ann Otol Rhinol Laryngol* 2007; **116**(12) 902–5.
6. Gassner HG, Ponikau JU, Sherris DA, et al. CSF rhinorrhea: 95 consective surgical cases with long term follow-up at the Mayo Clinic. *Am J Rhinol* 1999; **13**: 439–47.
7. Peabody RG, Leino T, Nohynek H, et al. Pneumococcal vaccination policy in Europe. *Euro Surveill* 2005; **10**(9): 174–8.
8. Dalgic A, Okay HO, Gezici AR, et al. An effective and less invasive treatment of post-traumatic cerebrospinal fluid fistula: closed lumbar drainage system. *Minim Invas Neurosurg* 2008; **51**: 154–7.
9. Bernal-Sprekelsen M, Bleda-Vazquez C, Carrau RL. Ascending meningitis secondary to traumatic cerebrospinal fluid leaks. *Am J Rhinol* 2000; **14**: 257–9.
10. Weber SM, Kim J, Delashaw B, et al. Radial forearm free tissue transfer in the management of persistent cerebrospinal fluid leaks. *Laryngoscope* 2005; **115**: 968–72.
11. Boudreaux B, Zins JE. Treatment of cerebrospinal fluid leaks in high risk patients. *J Craniofac Surg* 2009; **20**: 743–7.
12. Wise SK, Schlosser RJ. Evaluation of spontaneous nasal cerebrospinal fluid leaks. *Curr Opin Otolaryngol Head Neck Surg* 2007; **15**: 28–34.
13. Bolger WE, Osenbach R. Endoscopic transpterygoid approach to the lateral sphenoid recess. *Ear Nose Throat J* 1999; **78**: 36–46.
14. Bachmann G, Djenabi V, Jungehülsing M, et al. Incidence of occult cerebrospinal fluid fistula during paranasal sinus surgery. *Arch Otolaryngol Head Neck Surg* 2002; **128**: 1299–302.
15. Yessenow RS, McCabe BF. The osteomucoperiostial flap in repair of cerebrospinal fluid rhinorrhoea: a 20 year experience. *Otolaryngol Head Neck Surg* 1989; **101**: 555–8.
16. Kassam AB, Carrau RL, Snyderman CH, et al. Endoscopic reconstruction of the cranial base using a pedicled nasoseptal flap. *Neurosurgery* **63**(1): Suppl ONS 44-ONS53, 2008.
17. Harvey RJ, Nogueira JF, Schlosser RJ, et al. Closure of large skull base defects after endoscopic transnasal craniotomy. *J Neurosurg* 2009; **111**: 371–9.
18. Bateman N, Jones NS. Rhinorrhoea feigning cerebrospinal fluid leak: nine illustrative cases. *J Laryngol Otol* 2000; **114**: 462–4.
19. Michel O, Bamborschke S, Nekic M, et al. Beta-trace protein (prostaglandin D synthase): a stable and reliable protein in perilymph. *Ger Med Sci* 2005; **3**: 4.
20. Lloyd KM, Del Gaudio JM, Hudgins PA. Imaging of skull base cerebrospinal fluid leaks in adults. *Radiology* 2008; **248**(3): 725–36.
21. Aydin K, Terzibasioglu E, Sencer S, et al. Localization of cerebrospinal fluid leaks by gaddolinium-enhanced magnetic resonance cisternography: a 5-year single center experience. *Neurosurgery* 2008; **62**: 584–9.
22. Keer, R, Weber RK, Draf W, et al. Use of sodium fluorescein solution for detection of CSF fistulas: an analysis of 420 administrations and reported complications in Europe and the United States. *Laryngoscope* 2004; **114**: 266–72.
23. Zuckerman JD, Del Gaudio JM. Utility of pre-operative high resolution CT and intraoperative image guidance in identification of cerebrospinal fluid leaks for endoscopic repair. *Am J Rhinol* 2008; **22**: 151–4.
24. Saafan ME, Ragab SM, Albirmawy OA. Topical intranasal fluorescein: the missing partner in algorithms of cerebrospinal fluid fistula desection. *Laryngoscope* 2006; **116**: 1158–61.
25. de Almeida JR, Ghotme K, Leong L, et al. A new porcine skull base model: fibrin glue improves strength of cerebrospinal fluid leak repairs. *Otolaryngol Head Neck Surg* 2009; **141**: 184–9.
26. Weinstein JS, Liu KC, Delashaw JB, et al. The safety and effectiveness of a dural sealant system for use with non-autologous duraplasty materials. *J Neurosurg* 2010; **112**(2): 428–33.
27. Dloughy BJ, Madhavan K, Clinger JD, et al. Elevated body mass index and risk of postoperative CSF leak following transphenoidal surgery. *J Neurosurg* 2012; **115**(6): 1311–17. Epub 2012 March 23.
28. Potter NJ, Graham SM, Chang EH, Greenlee JD. Bioabsorbable plate cranial base reconstruction. *Laryngoscope* 2015; **125**(6): 1313–15.

CHAPTER 109

GRANULOMATOUS CONDITIONS OF THE NOSE

Joanne Rimmer and Valerie J. Lund

Introduction 1211	Eosinophilic granuloma 1219
Sarcoidosis 1211	Giant cell granuloma 1221
Granulomatosis with polyangiitis (Wegener's) 1214	Cholesterol granuloma 1221
Eosinophilic granulomatosis with polyangiitis (Churg Strauss) 1218	Granulomatous neoplasia – extranodal NK/T-cell lymphoma 1222
Cocaine-induced midline destructive lesion 1219	References 1223

SEARCH STRATEGY

Data in this chapter may be updated by a Medline search using the keywords: granulomatous disease, Wegener's granulomatosis, granulomatosis with polyangiitis, sarcoidosis, Churg Strauss syndrome, cocaine-induced midline destructive lesion, nose and paranasal sinuses. The evidence is mainly levels 2/3 with some level 4 randomized trials. The clinical recommendations are predominantly grades C with some B and D.

INTRODUCTION

A granuloma is an organized collection of macrophages, known as epithelioid cells, which fuse to form multi-nucleated giant cells. This histological configuration is encountered in a number of infective, inflammatory and neoplastic conditions of the nose and sinuses (Table 109.1) and is also seen in various conditions in which vasculitis plays a role. Vasculitis may be primary or secondary and is further classified according to the size of vessel affected (Table 109.2).

Whilst many of these conditions are systemic, they may be limited to the upper respiratory tract or present with otorhinolaryngological symptoms; the ear, nose and throat (ENT) surgeon must therefore maintain a continuous low threshold of suspicion to establish the diagnosis at the earliest opportunity.

SARCOIDOSIS

Sarcoidosis is a systemic granulomatous condition of unknown aetiology which may affect any part of the body, but most frequently involves the lungs and intra-thoracic lymph nodes, in over 90% of cases.[3] It has a global incidence of 6–16 per 100,000 population per annum but there is significant geographical variation, with 64 cases per 100,000 in Scandinavia.[4] It is 10–20 times more common in African-Americans (36.5–81.8 per 100,000) than Caucasians (1.2–19 per 100,000). Besnier first used the term 'lupus pernio' to describe cutaneous lesions in 1889, but it was Boeck who recognized the more generalized nature of the condition 10 years later.[5, 6]

Age and sex

Sarcoidosis is a condition of young adults with a peak onset between the third and fourth decades. It is slightly more common in women than men.[7]

Aetiology

The aetiology of sarcoidosis remains unknown, but theories suggest an immunological response to an unidentified antigen in genetically predisposed individuals.[8] The antigens may be infectious or environmental, and possibilities include mycobacteria, fungi, chemicals such as beryllium and zirconium, pine pollen and peanut dust.[9] There are abnormalities of both the cell-mediated and humoral immune systems.[4] Macrophages and T-cell activation lead to release of cytokines including tumour necrosis factor (TNF), with resultant granuloma formation.[10]

TABLE 109.1 Granulomatous conditions affecting the nose and sinuses

Infective		Inflammatory	Neoplastic
Bacteria			
Tuberculosis	Myobacterium tuberculosis	Sarcoidosis	Extranodal NK/T-cell lymphoma
Leprosy	Myobacterium leprae	Granulomatosis with polyangiitis (Wegener's)	
Rhinoscleroma	Klebsiella rhinoscleromatis	Eosinophilic granulomatosis with polyangiitis (Churg Strauss)	
Syphilis	Treponema pallidum	Cocaine-induced midline destructive lesion	
Actinomycosis	Actinomyces israeli	Giant cell granuloma	
Fungal[a]			
Aspergillus	Asp. fumigatus, flavus, niger	Eosinophilic granuloma	
Zygomycosis	Conidiobolus coronatus	Cholesterol granuloma	
	Rhizopus oryae		
Dematiaceae	Curvularia		
	Alternaria		
	Bipolaris		
Rhinosporidiosis	Rhinosporidiosis seeberi		
Blastomycosis	Blastomyces dermatitidis		
	Cryptococcus neoformans		
Histoplasmosis	Histoplasma capsulatum		
Sporotrichosis	Sporotrichum schenkii		
Coccidioidimycosis	Coccidioides immitis		
Protozoa			
Leishmaniasis	Leishmania spp.		

Source: Modified from reference[1], with permission.
[a]Covered in Chapter 96, Fungal rhinosinusitis.

TABLE 109.2 Primary vasculitis according to vessel size

Large, medium and small blood vessels	Medium and small blood vessels	Small blood vessels	Miscellaneous conditions	Secondary vasculitis
Takayasu arteritis	Polyarteritis nodosa	Microscopic polyangiitis	Buerger's disease	Infection-related vasculitis
Giant cell (temporal) arteritis	Eosinophilic granulomatosis with polyangiitis (Churg Strauss)	Schönlein–Henoch syndrome	Behçet's disease	Serum sickness or drug hypersensitivity-related vasculitis
Granulomatous angiitis of the central nervous system	Granulomatosis with polyangiitis (Wegener's)	Cutaneous leukocytoclastic angiitis	Kawasaki disease	Hypocomplementemic urticarial vasculitis
				Vasculitis associated with rheumatic connective tissue diseases
				Vasculitis associated with other systemic diseases
				Malignancy-related vasculitis
				Post-transplant vasculitis
				Pseudovasculitic syndromes (myxoma, endocarditis, Sneddon syndrome)

Source: Reprinted from reference[2], with permission.

Clinical features

Sarcoidosis is a multisystem disease; the reported distribution of clinical manifestations tends to reflect the bias of the treating physician. It primarily affects the lower respiratory tract but may involve almost any organ or system in the body (Table 109.3). It involves the upper respiratory tract in up to 18% of cases.[11] Sinonasal sarcoid is reported in 1–4%, more frequently than previously realized, and it is generally agreed that nasal manifestations are almost always part of chronic multisystem sarcoid.[12] Nasal symptoms commonly include obstruction, crusting, bleeding or facial pain (Table 109.4). A staging system for sinonasal involvement has been described to help tailor treatment: stage I is reversible involvement of the nose alone; stage II is moderate but potentially reversible disease of the nose and/or limited sinus involvement; and stage III is severe, irreversible and extensive sinonasal disease.[4]

The nasal mucosa often has a rather characteristic granular appearance, sometimes referred to as a 'strawberry skin' because of the tiny pale granulomas against hypertrophic erythematous mucosa. This is generally very friable and there may be ulceration, crusting and adhesions. The anterior nasal septum is most often affected and may perforate, particularly if traumatized by surgery. The nasal bones may be involved by a process similar to the dactylitis seen in the fingers; patients may present with a soft-tissue mass or expansion of the nasal bridge. This may be associated with thickening and purplish discoloration of the overlying skin known as lupus pernio (Figure 109.1), which is a cutaneous manifestation of chronic systemic sarcoid.[3] Facial pain is experienced by one in five patients with nasal sarcoid.[12] There may be hyposmia due to mechanical obstruction of the olfactory cleft by crusting or fibrosis or as a result of direct neuropathy.

Salivary gland enlargement is seen in 5–10% of cases, more rarely associated with facial palsy and uveitis when it is termed uveoparotid fever or Heerfordt's syndrome.[8] The larynx is involved in 1–5% of cases, most commonly the supraglottis (85%), with symptoms of cough, hoarseness, dysphagia and more rarely stridor.[13] Tracheal involvement is rare but bronchial sarcoid is common. Chronic progressive pulmonary fibrosis occurs in 25% of cases of chronic pulmonary sarcoid.[3]

Diagnosis

No test is pathognomonic for sarcoidosis. Diagnosis therefore relies on a combination of clinical features, imaging, histology, biochemical and serological testing and the exclusion of other granulomatous diseases. Previously the most reliable investigation, the Kveim test has been withdrawn in the UK for unproven health and safety reasons.[14] It involved intra-dermal injection of splenic tissue from a patient with sarcoidosis, with biopsy of the resulting skin nodule. The classic histological appearance is that of a non-caseating granuloma with central epithelioid cells

TABLE 109.3 Frequency (%) of clinical involvement of extrapulmonary organs in sarcoidosis

Extrathoracic sites	Percentage
Peripheral nodes	73
Skin	32
Liver	21
Eye	21
Spleen	18
Bone	14
Salivary glands	6
Joints	6
Heart	5
Nervous system	5
Kidneys	4
Nose and mouth	3
Lacrimal glands	3
Skeletal muscle	1
Larynx	1
Stomach and intestine	1
Uterus	1

TABLE 109.4 Incidence (%) of symptoms in patients with nasal sarcoidosis

Symptom	Percentage
Nasal stuffiness and obstruction	88
Crusting	63
Blood-stained discharge	37
Purulent discharge	30
Facial pain	22
Mucoid discharge	15
Anosmia	4

Source: Reproduced with permission from the ©ERS 1988.[12]

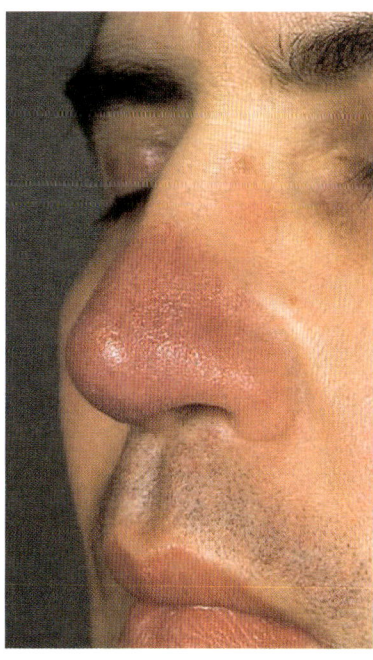

Figure 109.1 Typical appearances of nasal lupus pernio.

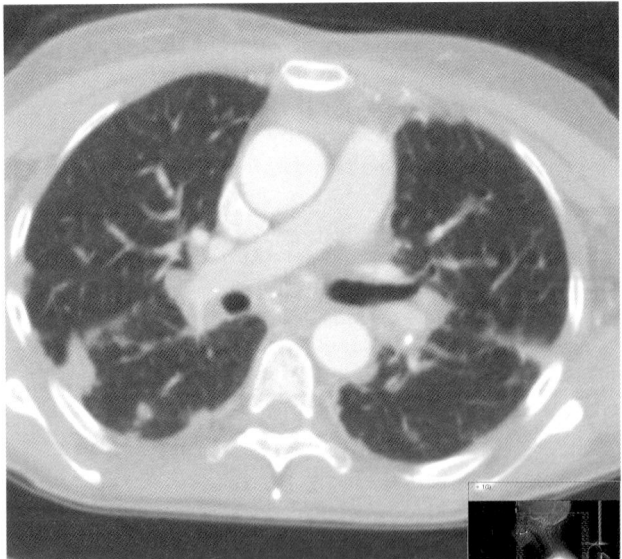

Figure 109.2 Axial CT scan showing typical pulmonary infiltrates in systemic sarcoidosis. (Courtesy of Dr Timothy Beale.)

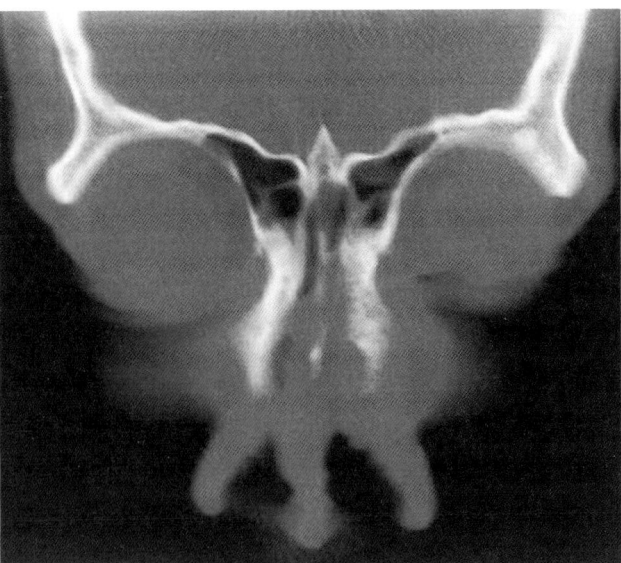

Figure 109.3 Coronal CT scan showing sclerosis and osteolysis of the nasal bones associated with a soft tissue mass in nasal sarcoid.

surrounded by lymphocytes and fibroblasts. Biopsy should target potentially affected tissue such as the lung, skin and lymph nodes; lip biopsy of minor salivary glands can be useful.[8] Biopsy of nasal mucosa is only of use if it appears abnormal, when over 90% of samples are positive; random biopsy of macroscopically normal mucosa is negative in 92%.[12]

Serum angiotensin converting enzyme (ACE) is elevated in up to 85% during active disease, but this is non-specific as it is also elevated in other conditions such as tuberculosis, leprosy and primary biliary cirrhosis.[15] Serum and urinary calcium levels are elevated in approximately 15% of cases.[4]

Imaging of the lower respiratory tract shows varying degrees of pulmonary involvement, which allow staging of the disease (**Figure 109.2**). Stage I is bilateral hilar lymphadenopathy, stage II is hilar lymphadenopathy and pulmonary infiltrates, stage III is pulmonary infiltrates alone and stage IV is pulmonary fibrosis.[16] Bronchoscopy will allow biopsy. Plain X-rays of the nasal bones may show rarefaction or punctate osteolysis in up to one quarter of cases and this, together with soft tissue changes, may also be seen on computerized tomography (CT) scanning (**Figure 109.3**).[17] CT will also demonstrate secondary involvement of the sinuses though will not distinguish between active disease and secondary infection. Bilateral lacrimal gland enlargement may also be seen.

Magnetic resonance imaging (MRI) of the brain may show granulomatous involvement of the basal meninges.

Treatment

Sarcoidosis has a variable clinical course that often correlates with the mode of presentation; an acute onset with arthritis and erythema nodosum is usually self-limiting, whilst a more insidious onset with lupus pernio and sinonasal involvement tends to be more chronic.[18] Up to two-thirds of patients will spontaneously remit, generally those with stage I and II pulmonary disease, while 10–30% follow a chronic course with relapses despite systemic therapy.[19] Some patients require no treatment at all, but international guidelines suggest systemic or intra-lesional steroid treatment for life-threatening disease or if critical organs are involved.[20] Despite a lack of controlled studies, steroids remain the mainstay of treatment for severe disease, with the addition of agents such as methotrexate to reduce the steroid dose if required. Hydroxychloroquine has been used for cutaneous and sinonasal sarcoidosis, although the response rate is less than 50% and there is a risk of ocular toxicity.[21] Lupus pernio may respond dramatically to medical treatment.[22] There has been recent interest in TNF-alpha inhibitors such as infliximab and etanercept.[23]

Nasal symptoms may be helped with topical treatment including intra-nasal steroids, glucose and glycerine drops, and nasal douching. Surgery has a limited role, particularly in the presence of active disease, although endoscopic sinus surgery can be undertaken to remove obstructing lesions or for secondary bacterial infection, with success in selected cases.[24] Septal surgery should be avoided if possible as an increased rate of septal perforation has been reported.[3] Symptomatic laryngeal disease that fails to respond to systemic treatment may be treated with transoral laser and intra-lesional steroid injections.[25]

GRANULOMATOSIS WITH POLYANGIITIS (WEGENER'S)

Granulomatosis with polyangiitis (GPA) is a systemic condition characterized by granulomatous inflammation of the respiratory tract and necrotizing vasculitis affecting small- to medium-sized vessels with focal or proliferative glomerulonephritis.[27] GPA was formerly known as Wegener's granulomatosis, after Wegener's article on rhinogenic granulomatosis in 1939, but has been renamed as part of a move towards a vasculitis terminology based on pathology.[28, 29] GPA classically involves a triad of upper airway, lung and renal disease, but limited or localized forms of the condition have been reported in up to 30% of cases.[30] Thus, the true incidence of the condition is difficult to determine. Whilst up to 1967 only 138 unequivocal cases had been recorded in the literature, the incidence is now estimated to be 10–15 per million per year with a prevalence of up to 5 per 100,000 population in Europe.[30–32]

Age and sex

The mean age at diagnosis is 40–50 years.[33] The age of presentation in our own cohort ranges from 15 to 78 years ($n = 180$ patients), although it has been reported in younger children. Cabral's paediatric series reported a median age at diagnosis of 14.2 years (range 4–17 years).[34] Men and women are equally affected, although in children there appears to be a female preponderance.[34, 35] GPA is predominantly a Caucasian disease (over 90%).[26]

Aetiology

GPA appears to be an autoimmune disease, given its strong association with antineutrophil cytoplasmic antibodies (ANCA). *In vitro* studies have shown that ANCA binds to and activates neutrophils, which then release oxygen radicals, inflammatory cytokines and lytic enzymes and adhere to and kill vascular endothelial cells.[36] ANCA may also induce immune complex formation.[26] In GPA, cytoplasmic ANCA (c-ANCA) are specific for proteinase-3 (PR3), an endogenous peptide. There is evidence that a mimic peptide may be introduced via an exogenous infective agent such as *Staphylococcus aureus*.[36] This theory is supported by the higher rate of chronic nasal *S. aureus* carriage in patients with GPA, in whom it is associated with more frequent relapses.[37]

Clinical features

Any part of the body may be affected and in generalized disease there is often associated general malaise, disproportionate to the clinical findings. Limited forms of the disease are now well recognized; the European Vasculitis Study Group classified GPA as 'localized' (respiratory tract involvement only with no features of systemic vasculitis), 'early systemic' or 'generalized' disease.[38] In the USA, 'limited' GPA refers to systemic non-life threatening disease rather than truly localized forms.[39] Whilst many of these cases may progress to generalized disease, there is some evidence that a subset (approximately 5%) will remain localized.[40] The frequency with which different sites are involved, both at presentation and subsequently, varies with the interest and specialty of the reporting physicians.[41] Duration of symptoms before a diagnosis is made remains highly variable and can be more than one year.[42]

The head and neck is the most common site of involvement at presentation, in 73–93% of cases.[33, 43] The nose and sinuses are involved in more than 80%, with symptoms including nasal obstruction, crusting, discharge and bleeding. In addition, patients may complain of facial pain.[42] Destruction of the intra-nasal structures may follow, including the septum, turbinates and sinuses with formation of a single large cavity. While there is intra-nasal destruction of bone and cartilage in some patients with GPA, leading to septal perforation and a characteristic nasal collapse, there are none of the gross destructive changes of the midfacial skin seen in NK/T-cell lymphomas and basal cell carcinomas.

Approximately one-third of patients develop otitis media with effusion with associated conductive hearing loss due to eustachian tube dysfunction, and more rarely pain and suppuration. Sensorineural hearing loss also occurs in 35%.[43] Facial nerve paralysis has been recorded in 8–10%.[44]

Subglottic or upper tracheal stenosis occurs in 16% of cases, although it is 5 times more common if GPA presents in childhood.[45] It may present as progressive dyspnoea on exertion or as acute airway obstruction. Localized GPA requires exclusion in an adult presenting with an apparently idiopathic subglottic stenosis.[46]

Oral symptoms are rare but ulceration may be seen and 'strawberry' gingival hyperplasia is said to be pathognomonic.[47]

Ocular manifestations, including conjunctivitis, dacryocystitis and episcleritis, occur in approximately 50% of patients at some point.[43] Approximately, 2% develop proptosis from a granulomatous mass within the orbit (**Figure 109.4**). Visual loss occurs in up to 8%, usually from optic nerve ischaemia due to inadequately treated retro-orbital disease.

Necrotizing vasculitis in the lungs causes cough, haemoptysis and pleuritic pain. The pulmonary lesions often cavitate and can usually be seen radiologically. Over 75% of patients develop renal involvement; early treatment is vital since damage is irreversible.[43] Cutaneous manifestations include ulceration and nodules, and both polymyalgia and polyarthritis have been described. Neurological sequelae include meningitis, mononeuritis multiplex and neuropathy of cranial nerves.[26]

Diagnosis

The ANCA test, first described by van der Woude in 1985, has significantly improved the diagnosis of GPA and other vasculitides.[48] There are two main staining patterns: c-ANCA, 90% of which are PR3-ANCA; and perinuclear (p-ANCA), 90% of which are specific for myeloperoxidase (MPO-ANCA).[49] In general, patients with GPA have c-ANCA, whereas p-ANCA tends to occur in other conditions, such as microscopic polyangiitis (MPA) and eosinophilic granulomatosis with polyangiitis (EGPA). Using combined immunofluorescence and enzyme-linked immunosorbent assay techniques, the sensitivity and specificity of c-ANCA are 91% and 99% respectively; the sensitivity falls to 60% with localized disease.[50] C-ANCA is positive

be requested, including a full blood count, erythrocyte sedimentation rate, c-reactive protein, serum urea and creatinine and serum ACE. Urinalysis and chest X-ray should be performed. Tissue biopsy may be helpful in ANCA-negative patents where suspicion remains high, but is nondiagnostic in up to 50% of head and neck specimens.[26] Paranasal sinus biopsies tend to yield more positive results than nasal specimens.[53] The main histological features are granulomatous inflammation, vasculitis and necrosis.

The American College of Rheumatology proposed a clinical classification in 1990 to distinguish GPA (Wegener's) from other vasculitides (Table 109.5).[54] The Chapel Hill Consensus added PR3-ANCA to the definition in 1994.[55]

CT and MRI may show characteristic features (Figure 109.5). In a series of 74 patients, over 90% showed

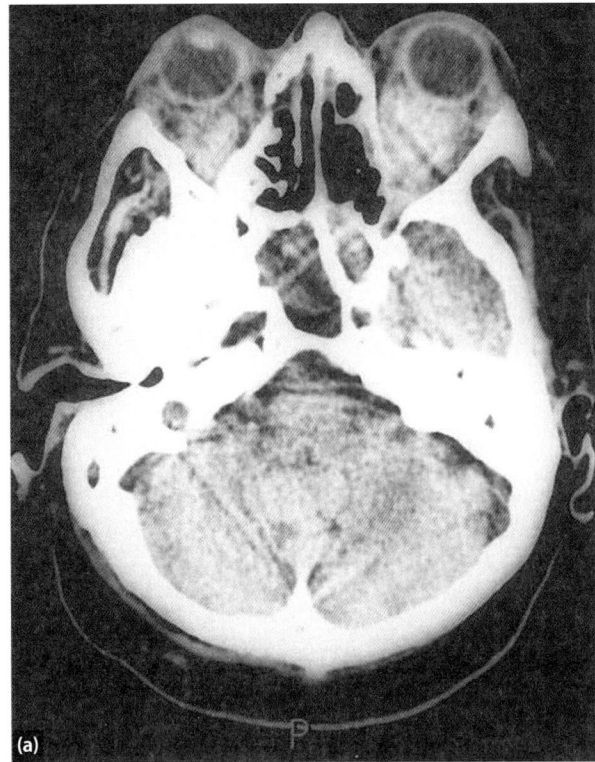
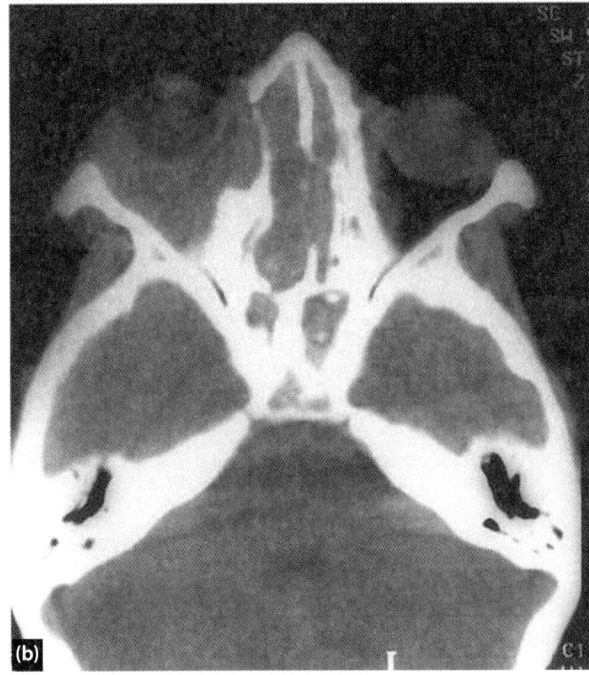

Figure 109.4 (a) and (b) Axial CT scans showing sclerosis and opacification of the nasal cavity associated with widespread infiltration of the orbit in GPA.

in over 90% of patients with generalized active disease and titres have been shown to correlate well with disease activity.[51] However, 10% of patients with GPA have a positive p-ANCA result and up to 20% may be ANCA-negative; in localized disease this figure may rise to 30%.[26] In addition, there may be false-positive c-ANCA results with cocaine abuse.[52] Other blood tests should therefore also

TABLE 109.5 1990 American College of Rheumatology criteria for the classification of Wegener's granulomatosis*

Criteria	Definition
Nasal or oral inflammation	Painful or painless oral ulcers or purulent or bloody nasal discharge
Abnormal chest X-ray	Nodules, fixed infiltrates or cavities
Abnormal urinary sediment	Microscopic haematuria with or without red cell casts
Granulomatous inflammation on biopsy	Histologic changes showing granulomatous inflammation within the wall of an artery or in the peri- or extravascular area (artery or arteriole)

* For classification purposes, a patient shall be said to have Wegener's granulomatosis if he/she has satisfied any two or more of these four criteria. This rule is associated with a sensitivity of 88.2% and a specificity of 92.0%.

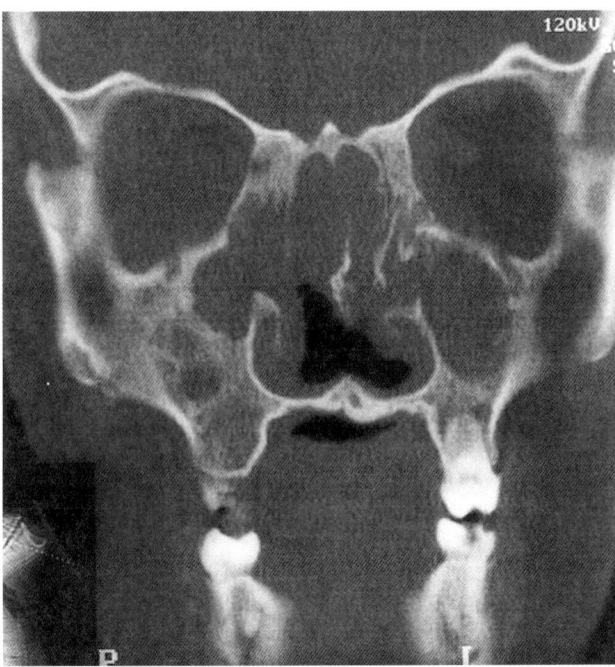

Figure 109.5 Coronal CT showing typical appearances of Wegener's in the nose with septal destruction hyperostosis and opacification of the sinuses together with orbital infiltration.

non-specific mucosal thickening in the nasal cavity or paranasal sinuses, 62% showed evidence of bone destruction and 78% had new bone formation in the walls of the sinus cavities.[56] In addition, the orbit was affected in 37%. Whilst the diagnosis of systemic GPA is made clinically, in a patient without a history of previous sinonasal surgery the combination of bone destruction and new bone formation on CT is virtually diagnostic, especially when accompanied on MRI by a fat signal from the sclerotic sinus wall, so-called 'tramlining'.[57] These findings can be helpful in localized sinonasal GPA, where the clinical diagnosis is uncertain and the c-ANCA test may be negative. Imaging of the chest may show nodules, progressive cavitation or fibrosis. Imaging of the larynx should be considered in any patient with symptoms suggestive of subglottic stenosis.

Treatment

Untreated, GPA is a lethal disease with a mean survival of 5 months.[58] Rapid diagnosis remains of great importance since a fulminating course with a fatal outcome can occur in as little as 48 hours. The introduction of systemic corticosteroid treatment improved mortality rates to 50%.[32] However, it was the combination of oral cyclophosphamide with corticosteroids that improved remission rates to 93%.[59] Despite this, over half of patients will have at least one relapse, and the potential side effects of cyotoxic treatment are not insignificant.[33] Treatment regimes today aim to induce remission and then maintain it, whilst minimizing side effects, and the European Vasculitis Study Group (EUVAS) has undertaken several controlled trials to inform treatment algorithms.[60]

Remission-induction therapy is typically with a combination of high-dose steroids and cyclophosphamide or methotrexate.[26] The usual daily dose of cyclophosphamide is 2 mg/kg, to a maximum of 200 mg per day. There is significant morbidity associated with long-term cyclophosphamide treatment, with side effects including alopecia, haemorrhagic cystitis, opportunistic infections and malignancies; leukaemia and lymphoma are 11 times more likely, and there is a 33 fold increase in the risk of bladder cancer.[61] Strategies to reduce these adverse effects include shorter treatment durations and the use of intermittent 'pulsed' cyclophosphamide. Several randomized trials have shown that pulsed therapy is as effective as oral treatment in achieving remission, but it is associated with a higher relapse rate.[62] Methotrexate, an antimetabolite, has been shown in randomized trials to be an effective alternative to cyclophosphamide in inducing remission in patients with limited and less severe GPA.[63] More recently rituximab, an anti-CD20 monoclonal antibody, has been shown to be as effective as cyclophosphamide in inducing remission.[64] The multicentre randomized double-blind RAVE (Rituximab for ANCA-Associated Vasculitis) trial also suggested that rituximab may be superior in relapsing disease.

High-dose glucocorticoids are an essential part of remission–induction treatment, and prednisolone is initially given at a dose of 0.5–1 mg/kg daily, to a maximum of 80 mg per day; this can then be tapered over the course of several months before stopping completely where possible.[65] Patients may require further courses of glucocorticoids to manage disease exacerbations and relapses. The side effects of long-term systemic therapy are well known, including osteoporosis, diabetes, hypertension, proximal myopathy, weight gain and cataracts.

Remission-maintenance therapy aims to keep GPA quiescent with minimal treatment morbidity. Methotrexate can be used, with similar relapse rates compared to long-term cyclophosphamide treatment.[66] These patients should receive folic acid supplementation to prevent folate deficiency. Azathioprine is an alternative immunosuppressive agent with less morbidity than cyclophosphamide, and a randomized controlled trial showed equivalent remission control.[67] Both methotrexate and azathioprine may be used as monotherapy to maintain remission, but are also given as steroid-sparing agents to reduce the dose of prednisolone required by some patients.

Multiple controlled trials have been undertaken in an effort to try and find less toxic but equally effective immunosuppressive agents. Mycophenolate mofetil, a purine synthesis inhibitor, has shown promise in this area but a large multicentre randomized controlled trial showed a higher relapse rate when compared with azathoprine.[68] Leflunomide, a T-cell inhibitor that targets purine synthesis, appears to be well tolerated and effective in remission maintenance.[69] Deoxyspergualin, an immunomodulatory agent which inhibits lymphocyte differentiation, appears to be effective in maintaining remission and reducing steroid requirements.[70] Tumour necrosis factor antagonists, such as infliximab and etanercept, have shown less promising results. A multicentre placebo-controlled trial of etanercept plus standard therapy showed no benefit compared to placebo.[72]

The possible association between GPA relapses and *S. aureus* infection in the nose prompted trials of long-term antibiotic treatment, namely trimethoprim-sulphamethoxazole (co-trimoxazole), with mixed results. A double-blind placebo-controlled trial showed that relapse rates were reduced compared to controls.[72] However, another randomized trial reported that co-trimoxazole did not maintain remission as effectively as methotrexate.[73]

Whatever treatment is used, patients require regular monitoring for both treatment side effects and disease activity. Serial monitoring of c-ANCA can be useful; it frequently becomes negative when the disease is under control but this is not always the case, particularly in localized forms.

Topical nasal treatment such as douching, intra-nasal steroids and nasal lubricants may be helpful for symptomatic relief of crusting and bleeding. Surgery is generally reserved for cases that are refractory to medical treatment, or for complications of GPA.[26] Endoscopic sinus surgery is rarely helpful in improving symptoms, but may be undertaken in selected cases. Endoscopic dacryocystorhinostomy has been reported to improve epiphora, but should be avoided in active disease.[74] Septal perforation repair is not recommended but the use of a silastic septal button can be beneficial. Augmentation rhinoplasty to correct a saddle-nose deformity should be deferred until the disease has been in remission for at least one year. A series of 13 patients in remission from Wegener's reported a 92% overall success rate from dorsal augmentation without reactivation of disease.[75] Grommets are best avoided if possible, because of the risk of chronic otorrhoea; hearing aids are a better option to treat both conductive and sensorineural hearing loss.[44] It has been said that 50% of patients with subglottic stenosis will require a tracheostomy at some point, but recent studies suggest that conservative treatment may avoid this in most cases. Conservative laser surgery combined with endoluminal balloon dilatation and intra-lesional steroid injection appears to give satisfactory results.[76]

EOSINOPHILIC GRANULOMATOSIS WITH POLYANGIITIS (CHURG STRAUSS)

In 1951, Churg and Strauss described a syndrome of allergic angiitis and granulomatosis, a rare systemic vasculitis which has more recently been named 'eosinophilic granulomatosis with polyangiitis' (EGPA).[77, 78] The Chapel Hill consensus defined it as 'eosinophil-rich and granulomatous inflammation involving the respiratory tract, and necrotizing vasculitis affecting small to medium-sized vessels, associated with asthma and eosinophilia.'[55] It is the rarest of the ANCA-associated vasculitides, with an estimated annual incidence of 0.5–4 per million in Europe, although may be underestimated.[31] However, in asthmatics this incidence rises to 67 per million.[79]

Age and sex

The mean age at diagnosis is 50 years (range 4–75 years).[80] Both male and female preponderances have been reported, but overall there appears to be no significant difference.[79, 81, 82]

Aetiology

The aetiology remains unknown but it may be an autoimmune disease mediated by Th2-cells which activate both eosinophils and neutrophils.[83] Direct eosinophilic infiltration and the release of cationic proteins and cytokines then cause tissue injury.[80] High levels of eosinophils and immunoglobulin E (IgE) in vessels and tissues also suggests a direct role in the development of the vasculitis, possibly an allergic response to an unknown allergen. EGPA has been reported to occur after treatment with the leukotriene receptor antagonist zafirlukast.[84] However, this appears to relate to the unmasking of vasculitis by the reduction in systemic steroid treatment that zafirlukast allowed, rather than be a true causative effect.[85] Other suggested precipitants include vaccination, desensitization therapy and inhalation of various aeroallergens, which all support an allergic aetiology.[86]

Clinical features

Asthma occurs in approximately 99% of patients, and is characteristically late-onset; in 83% of cases it precedes the vasculitis by an average of 8 years.[87] Sinonasal symptoms are present in up to 93%, and have been reported to worsen prior to diagnosis in 28% of patients.[81, 88] Allergic rhinitis and chronic rhinosinusitis with nasal polyps occur in up to 75% of cases.[82] Patients frequently complain of nasal obstruction, rhinorrhoea, anosmia and sneezing, as well as crusting and epistaxis to a lesser degree; nearly half may have undergone previous nasal surgery before the diagnosis is made.[81]

Neurological symptoms are common, with mononeuritis multiplex in up to 76% and peripheral polyneuropathy in approximately one-quarter of cases.[89] Central nervous system involvement is less common, but is the second commonest cause of death.[90]

Cutaneous symptoms including papules and nodules occur in up to 50% of cases. Cardiac involvement is less common but is the major cause of mortality, usually from granulomatous myocarditis.[79]

Three clinical phases of EGPA have been described, although they do not necessarily follow each other consecutively.[90] The first, prodromal, phase may persist for several years, and is characterized by adult-onset asthma and upper respiratory tract inflammation. Phase two is characterized by peripheral eosinophilia, usually with pulmonary infiltrates and eosinophilic gastroenteritis. The third phase is that of the systemic vasculitis, including constitutional symptoms, neurological and cutaneous involvement.[80]

Diagnosis

Diagnosis is based on the typical clinical features with a peripheral eosinophilia of greater than 10% of the white cell differential, plus tissue biopsy. Histology shows necrotizing vasculitis, extravascular necrotizing granulomas and tissue eosinophilia, but it is rare to see all three features on one biopsy.[82] ANCA is positive in 40–75% of cases, typically p-ANCA specific for MPO but occasionally c-ANCA is seen.[80, 86] There is evidence that ANCA modulates the phenotype, with a more vasculitic disease in ANCA-positive patients.[87] The French Vasculitis Study Group series reported significantly more peripheral neuropathy, ENT and renal involvement in patients with a positive p-ANCA, as well as less frequent cardiac pathology.[78] There was a higher relapse rate in ANCA-positive cases but significantly reduced mortality.

Chest X-ray usually shows transient peripheral infiltrates, but pleural effusions are seen in up to 10% of cases.[79] Sinonasal imaging shows non-specific widespread opacification consistent with chronic rhinosinusitis with polyps, and patients are perhaps more likely to develop frontoethmoidal mucocoeles.[61] The American College of Rheumatology clinical criteria for the classification of EGPA includes pulmonary and sinus radiological abnormalities (**Table 109.6**).[91]

Aetiology

Cocaine is the trigger but patients who develop CIMDL appear to be predisposed to produce ANCA. Nearly 90% have a positive p-ANCA against human neutrophil elastase (HNE), which may increase apoptosis and the local inflammatory response to injury.[52]

Clinical features

Patients complain of chronic nasal obstruction and bleeding, with change in shape of the nose and nasal regurgitation as the lesion progresses to destroy the nasal framework and in particular the palate; this is more common than in GPA patients where it occurs only rarely. There are rarely systemic symptoms. Not all patients will admit to cocaine use. Examination confirms a variable degree of destruction of the septum, turbinates, lateral nasal wall and floor (**Figure 109.6**).

Diagnosis

The differential diagnosis includes infections, GPA and neoplasia, and these must be excluded. Whilst the majority of patients with CIMDL will have a positive HNE-ANCA, over 50% of patients will also have a positive PR3-ANCA. This makes differentiation from limited GPA more difficult, but studies have shown no evidence of HNE-ANCA positivity in either normal controls or patients with GPA.[93] Histology is often very similar to that of GPA, with vasculitis and fibrinoid necrosis, so may not be helpful unless it confirms GPA.[52] Urine, blood and hair can be tested for cocaine if necessary.

Treatment

There is no role for immunosuppression, and patients must stop using cocaine to prevent further progression. Conservative treatment includes nasal douching, debridement of necrotic areas and topical or systemic antibiotic therapy. Surgical correction of septal perforation or nasal deformity should not be attempted until the patient has been clear of cocaine for at least 6–12 months.

EOSINOPHILIC GRANULOMA

This is a clonal proliferation of Langerhans cells associated with a heterogeneous inflammatory infiltrate of eosinophils, histiocytes, lymphocytes, plasma cells and neutrophils. It is now regarded as a neoplastic condition with a variable clinical course.[94, 95] It is also considered a manifestation of histiocytosis-X and is sometimes referred to as Langerhans cell histiocytosis or Langerhans granulomatosis.

Age and sex

A wide age range from infancy to over 80 years has been recorded, but about 85% of cases are detected in the first

---

TABLE 109.6 1990 American College of Rheumatology criteria for the classification of Churg Strauss syndrome*

Criteria	Definition
Asthma	History of wheezing or diffuse rales on expiration
Eosinophilia	Eosinophilia >10% on white blood cell differential count
Mononeuropathy or polyneuropathy	Development of mononeuropathy, multiple mononeuropathies, or polyneuropathy
Pulmonary infiltrates, non-fixed	Migratory or transitory pulmonary infiltrates on radiographs
Paranasal sinus abnormality	History of acute or chronic paranasal sinus pain or radiographic opacification of the paranasal sinuses
Extravascular eosinophils	Biopsy including artery, arteriole or venule, showing accumulations of eosinophils in extravascular areas

*For classification purposes, a patient shall be said to have Churg Strauss syndrome if he/she has satisfied any four or more of these six criteria. This rule is associated with a sensitivity of 85% and a specificity of 99.7%.

The differential diagnosis includes parasitic and fungal infections, eosinophilic pneumonia, idiopathic hypereosinophilic syndrome and other vasculitides.

Treatment

Treatment is primarily with high-dose systemic steroids, which are tapered when possible. Those with organ or life-threatening disease, or those requiring persistently high doses of steroids may require treatment with cyclophosphamide to induce remission.[88] Methotrexate has also been used for both induction and maintenance of remission, and azathioprine and mycophenolate mofetil may be helpful as steroid-sparing agents.[79] Interferon-alpha has been successful in treating refractory cases.[92] Overall remission rates are high (91%) but over 25% relapse either within the first 3 months or much later, after 5 years.[86] Survival has improved with the advent of corticosteroid and immunosuppressive treatment, with mortality similar to that of the normal population.[88] Sinonasal symptoms should be treated with topical nasal steroids, douching and endoscopic sinus surgery as required, which may be multiple times.[81]

COCAINE-INDUCED MIDLINE DESTRUCTIVE LESION

Cocaine use via intra-nasal inhalation is known to cause mucosal inflammation. Septal perforation has been reported in approximately 5% of chronic users, but more aggressive midfacial destruction has also been noted.[52] Such cocaine-induced midline destructive lesions (CIMDL) can mimic localized or systemic GPA as well as neoplasia.

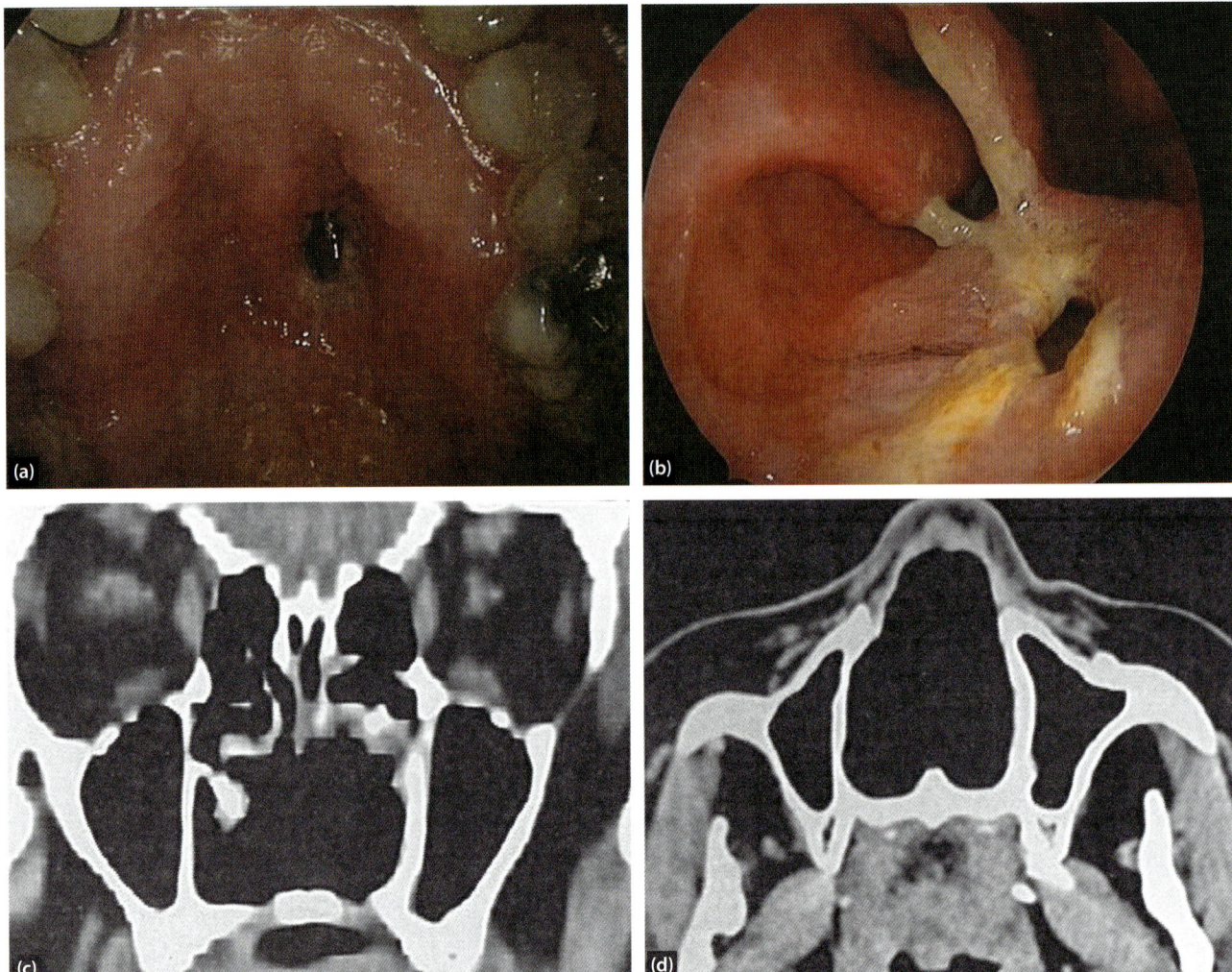

Figure 109.6 Cocaine-induced midline destructive lesions. (a) Oral endoscopy showing a 1cm hard palate perforation with regular margins; **(b)** Nasal endoscopy showing extensive destruction of the nasal septum and inferior turbinate as well as the hard palate perforation; **(c)** Coronal and **(d)** axial CT showing extensive destruction of the septum and turbinates (Courtesy of Dr Matteo Trimachi).

three decades of life; 60% are young children. Males are affected twice as frequently as females.

Clinical features

Whilst all organs may be affected, eosinophilic granuloma predominantly occurs in bones. The skull is a common site of involvement, in particular the temporal, frontal and parietal bones. The usual presentation is a painful swelling of the involved bone, often for many months, associated with cervical lymphadenopathy. Mandibular lesions produce toothache, gum ulceration and loose teeth, whereas involvement of the temporal bone may simulate acute mastoiditis.

Diagnosis

Radiological evaluation shows punched-out bony lesions and radiolucent areas around the teeth. Lesions in the skull often show bevelled margins due to angulated destruction of the cortical bone. Macroscopically, the lesions are soft and yellow or red-brown in colour; biopsy material is best obtained by curettage. Microscopically, the Langerhans cells are mixed with other inflammatory cells. The cytoplasm of the Langerhans cells may be eosinophilic and Charcot–Leyden crystals may be found in ordinary histiocytes. There is intense osteoclastic activity at the periphery of the granuloma due to prostaglandin and cytokine production by the Langerhans cells.[96] During the healing phase of the granuloma, the stroma becomes increasingly fibrotic.

Treatment

Treatment depends on whether or not the eosinophilic granuloma is localized and/or solitary. Solitary, or 'type II disease', is at least five times more common than polyostotic disease. Some solitary lesions will spontaneously regress. With unifocal disease a combination of curettage/excision and radiotherapy is usually curative, provided that no new lesions develop within the first year. A proportion of patients will develop a generalized disease with hepatosplenomegaly, lymphadenopathy, skin lesions and further osseous lesions, so called 'type I disease'.

The course of this can be rapid with a poor prognosis; additional chemotherapy has been advocated in these circumstances. At present, the most effective chemotherapy regime appears to be etoposide and steroids given for periods of 12 months or more dependent on the response.[97] Alpha interferon and bone marrow transplantation have also been used successfully.

GIANT CELL GRANULOMA

Granuloma-like aggregates of giant cells in a fibrovascular stroma characterize this benign condition otherwise referred to as 'giant cell reparative granuloma' or 'giant cell reaction of bone'. It was first described by Jaffe in 1953 in the jaws, although other craniofacial sites have been reported.[98]

Age and sex

These lesions commonly occur in children and young adults, with a female to male preponderance of 2:1.

Clinical features

Pain and swelling over the affected bone are the most common symptoms, but diplopia, hearing loss, vertigo and tinnitus have also been reported. The maxilla and mandible are most commonly affected followed by the sphenoid and temporal bones.[98, 99] Bilateral symmetrical involvement of the jaws by giant cell granulomas is seen in cherubism, a rare inherited childhood condition (Figure 109.7).[100]

Diagnosis

CT shows expansile lytic lesions with a 'soap bubble' centre and well-demarcated edges. Histologically, the granuloma has a cellular fibroblastic stroma containing aggregates of giant cells. These cells are smaller and have fewer nuclei than in a true giant cell tumour. The lesions are benign despite the presence of mitoses, which may cause the inexperienced pathologist difficulties. To add to the confusion, the microscopic appearance of giant cell granulomas is indistinguishable from that of the solid variant of aneurysmal bone cysts. Biochemical investigations (serum calcium, phosphate and alkaline phosphatase) should be undertaken to distinguish it from the brown tumour of hyperparathyroidism.

Treatment

Curettage alone is associated with recurrence in 15% of cases and excision should be undertaken where possible.[99]

CHOLESTEROL GRANULOMA

This is a rare granulomatous foreign body reaction to cholesterol crystals precipitated in the tissues, and has also been referred to as a chocolate cyst or orbital cholesteatoma.

Age and sex

In 6 cases managed by the senior author, the age ranged from 31 to 89 years (mean 59 years) with a male preponderance of 5:1.

Aetiology

It is presumed to result from haemorrhage due to trauma, but there must also be abnormal ventilation and drainage of the involved sinus.[101]

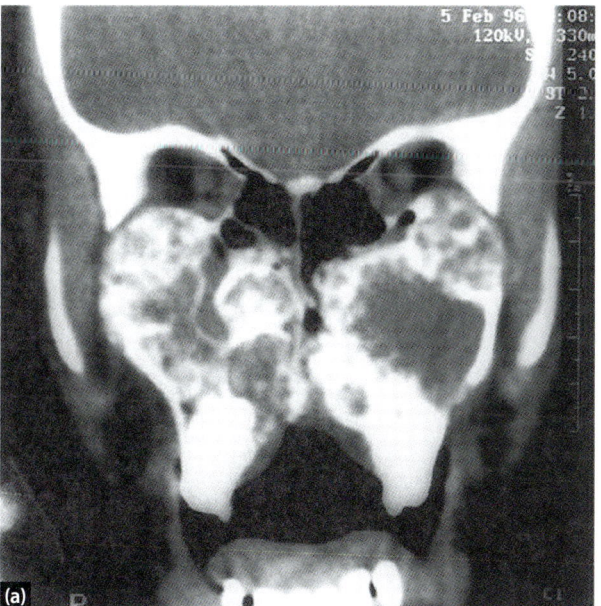
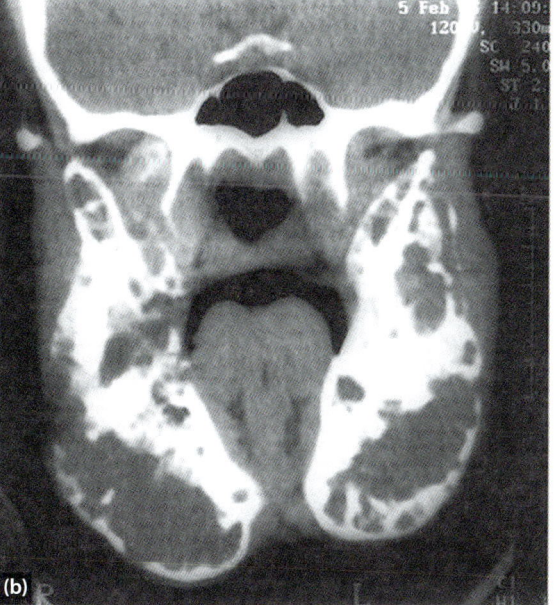

Figure 109.7(a) and (b) Coronal CT scans of upper and lower jaw showing typical appearances of cherubism.

Clinical features

Although more common in the ear, these lesions may affect the maxillary or frontal sinuses, producing bony expansion, cosmetic deformity and displacement of adjacent structures, such as the globe. The differential diagnosis includes a mucocele and a dermoid or epidermoid cyst.

Diagnosis

Typical CT appearances are of a cyst-like expansion of the sinus that does not enhance with contrast. A very high signal is produced on all MRI sequences.

Histologically, it has a characteristic appearance of granulation tissue containing foreign body-type giant cells surrounding clefts created by the cholesterol crystals.[102]

Treatment

Surgical drainage and marsupialization is required, by whichever approach facilitates complete removal of the granulation tissue to prevent recurrence.[103, 104]

GRANULOMATOUS NEOPLASIA – EXTRANODAL NK/T-CELL LYMPHOMA

Many terms, most notably 'midline lethal granuloma', have been used to describe the condition now known to be an extranodal NK/T-cell lymphoma, nasal type (ENKTCL).[105, 106] It is included in this chapter for completeness due to this historical nomenclature. This rare non-Hodgkin's lymphoma (NHL) causes destruction of the midface and was the subject of great pathological debate. Now recognized as a distinct entity by the WHO, it is most common in south-east Asia and South America.[106]

Age and sex

NK/T cell lymphoma may occur at almost any age from the first to the ninth decade, but is most common in the fifth or sixth decades. A male preponderance has been reported.[107]

Aetiology

ENKTCL appears to be caused by the Epstein-Barr virus.[108]

Clinical features

ENKTCL usually arises in the nasal cavity and spreads to involve adjacent structures including the orbits, oral cavity, skin and paranasal sinuses. The intra-nasal granulomatous mass initially causes symptoms of obstruction, discharge and bleeding. Progressive destruction of the nasal skeleton and overlying skin occurs (**Figure 109.8**).

Diagnosis

Early diagnosis is important, as the prognosis for widespread disease is much worse. Good quality representative biopsy material from tissue beneath the slough and crust is essential. Histologically, the infiltrates are polymorphic and atypical cells may to be arranged in a necrotizing angiocentric growth pattern. The tumour consists of neoplastic T-lymphocytes with a significant inflammatory infiltrate.[109] Immunohistochemistry is usually positive for CD56, CD2 and cytoplasmic CD3.[106] Granulomas and giant cells are not present in T-cell lymphomas; thrombosis and necrosis are, however, common findings. Imaging and bone marrow biopsy are also required for staging purposes.

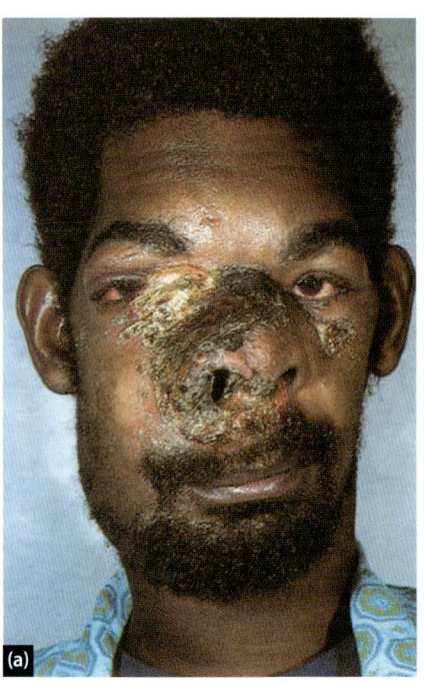
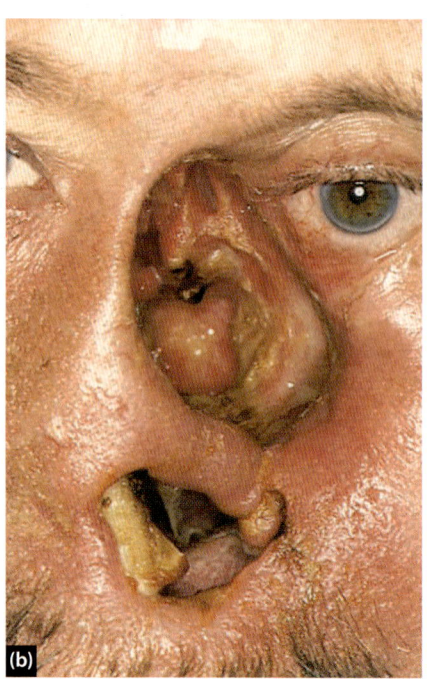

Figure 109.8 ENKTCL affecting the midface with **(a)** early ulceration and **(b)** significant central destruction.

Treatment

This is an aggressive tumour but tends to have a dramatic response to radiotherapy, which is therefore the recommended treatment for localized disease.[110] The role of chemotherapy has not yet been established, but may be given in addition for recurrent or disseminated disease.[111] Local recurrence rates range from 31–67%, with an overall 5-year survival rate of 38–45%.[106]

BEST CLINICAL PRACTICE

- ✓ The sensitivity and specificity of c-ANCA in GPA are 91% and 99% respectively.
- ✓ Pulsed cyclophosphamide therapy is as effective as oral treatment in achieving remission in GPA, but it is associated with a higher relapse rate.
- ✓ Rituximab is as effective as cyclophosphamide in inducing remission in GPA and may be superior in relapsing disease.
- ✓ Methotrexate and azathioprine have shown similar relapse rates compared to long-term cyclophosphamide treatment for GPA.
- ✓ Subglottic stenosis due to granulomatous disease can be satisfactorily treated with conservative laser surgery combined with endoluminal balloon dilatation and intra-lesional steroid injection.

FUTURE RESEARCH

- ➤ The aetiology of these conditions remains obscure and requires further investigation.
- ➤ It is uncertain whether all cases with limited GPA progress to systemic disease or what triggers this progression.
- ➤ The sensitivity of c-ANCA requires refinement, particularly in limited forms of GPA.
- ➤ Further multicentre controlled trials are required to inform treatment with newer, less toxic medications for these rare conditions.

KEY POINTS

- Many patients with systemic granulomatous conditions present first to ENT surgeons. It is important to maintain a low threshold of suspicion in order to make an early diagnosis and avert more severe systemic disease.
- Any patient with blood-stained discharge and crusting in the nose has a granulomatous condition until proven otherwise.
- No one test is completely reliable and a combination of clinical findings combined with diagnostic investigations is required.
- Secondary or tertiary referral may be required to diagnose and manage the condition.
- Management should be multidisciplinary.
- A range of medications is available, of which steroids combined with cytotoxic drugs are the most frequently used.
- Patients on long-term systemic steroids should be monitored for complications.
- Surgery is generally reserved for refractory cases or complications of disease.

REFERENCES

1. Lund VJ. Granulomatous disease and tumours of the nose and paranasal sinuses. In: Kennedy DW, Bolger WE, Zinreich SJ (eds). *Diseases of the sinuses diagnosis and management*. Hamilton: BC Decker; 2001, p. 86.
2. Lie JT. Classification and histopathologic specificity of systemic vaculitis. In: Ansell BM, Bacon PA, Lie TJ, Yazici H (eds). *The vasculitidies*. Springer, Boston, MA; 1996, p. 25.
3. Morgenthau AS, Teirstein AS. Sarcoidosis of the upper and lower airways. *Expert Rev Respir Med* 2011; **5**: 823–33.
4. Krespi YP, Kuriloff DB, Aner M. Sarcoidosis of the sinonasal tract: a new staging system. *Otolaryngol Head Neck Surg* 1995; **112**: 221–7.
5. Besnier E. Lupus pernio de la face. *Ann Dermatol Syphiligr* 1889; **10**: 333–6.
6. Boeck C. Multiple benign sarcoid of the skin. *J Cutan Dis* 1899; **17**: 543–53.
7. Zeitlin JF, Tami TA, Baughman R, Winget D. Nasal and sinus manifestations of sarcoidosis. *Am J Rhinol* 2000; **14**: 157–61.
8. Mrówka-Kata K, Kata D, Lange D, et al. Sarcoidosis and its otolaryngological implications. *Eur Arch Otorhinolaryngol* 2010; **267**: 1507–14.
9. Wright RE, Clairmont AA, Perl JH, Butz WC. Intranasal sarcoidosis. *Laryngoscope* 1974; **84**: 2058–64.
10. Baughman RP, Lower EE, du Bois RM. Sarcoidosis. *Lancet* 2003; **361**: 1111–18.
11. deShazo RD, O'Brien MM, Justice WK, Pitcock J. Diagnostic criteria for sarcoidosis of the sinuses. *J Allergy Clin Immunol* 1999; **103**: 789–95.
12. Wilson R, Lund V, Sweatman M. Upper respiratory tract involvement in sarcoidosis and its management. *Eur Respir J* 1988; **1**: 269–72.
13. Dean CM, Sataloff RT, Hawkshaw MJ, Pribikin E. Laryngeal sarcoidosis. *J Voice* 2002; **16**: 283–8.
14. Du Bois RM, Geddes DM, Mitchell DN. Moratorium on Kveim test. *Lancet* 1993; **342**: 173.
15. Lieberman J. Elevation of serum angiotensin converting enzyme level in sarcoidosis. *Am J Med* 1975; **59**: 365–72.
16. Siltzbach LE, Blaugrund SM. Sarcoidosis of the mucosa of the respiratory tract. *Ann Otol Rhinol Laryngol* 1963; **72**: 923–39.
17. Weiss JA. Sarcoidosis in otolaryngology report of 11 cases. *Laryngoscope* 1960; **70**: 1351–98.
18. Gulati S, Krossnes B, Olofsson J, Danielsen A. Sinonasal involvement in sarcoidosis: a report of seven cases and review of the literature. *Eur Arch Otorhinolaryngol* 2012; **269**: 891–6.
19. Neville E, Walker AN, James DG. Prognostic factors predicting the outcome of sarcoidosis: an analysis of 818 patients. *Q Med J* 1983; **52**: 525–33.

20. Hunninghake GW, Costabel U. ATS/ERS/WASOG statement on sarcoidosis. *Sarcoidosis Vasc Diffuse Lung Dis* 1999; **16**: 149–73.
21. Baughman RP, Costabel U, du Bois RM. Treatment of sarcoidosis. *Clin Chest Med* 2008; **29**: 533–48.
22. Milford CA, Mugliston T, Lund VJ. "Medical rhinoplasty" in nasal sarcoidosis. *Rhinology* 1990; **28**: 137–9.
23. Stagaki E, Mountford WK, Lackland DT, Judson MA. The treatment of lupus pernio: results of 116 treatment courses in 54 patients. *Chest* 2009; **135**: 468–76.
24. Kay DJ, Har-El G. The role of endoscopic sinus surgery in chronic sinonasal sarcoidosis. *Am J Rhinol* 2001; **15**: 249–54.
25. Butler CR, Nouraei SA, Mace AD, et al. Endoscopic airway management of laryngeal sarcoidosis. *Arch Otolaryngol Head Neck Surg* 2010; **136**: 251–5.
26. Erickson VR, Hwang PH. Wegener's granulomatosis: current trends in diagnosis and management. *Curr Opin Otolaryngol Head Neck Surg* 2007; **15**: 170–6.
27. Wegener F. Uber eine eigenartige rhinogene Granulomatose mit besonderer Beteiligung des Arteriensystems und der Nieren. *Beitr Pathol Anat Allg Pathol* 1939; **102**: 36–68.
28. Falk RJ, Gross WL, Guillevin L, et al. Granulomatosis with polyangiitis (Wegener's): an alternative name for Wegener's granulomatosis. *Arthritis Rheum* 2011; **63**: 863–4.
29. McDonald TJ, De Remee RA. Wegener's granulomatosis. *Laryngoscope* 1983; **93**: 220–31.
30. Editorial. Wegener's granulomatosis. *BMJ* 1971; **3**: 446.
31. Lane S, Watts RA, Scott DG. Epidemiology of systemic vasculitis. *Curr Rheumatol Rep* 2005; **7**: 270–5.
32. Gottschlich S, Ambrosch P, Kramkowski D, et al. Head and neck manifestations of Wegener's granulomatosis. *Rhinology* 2006; **44**: 227–33.
33. Reinhold-Keller E, Beuge N, Latza U, et al. An interdisciplinary approach to the care of patients with Wegener's granulomatosis. *Arthritis Rheum* 2000; **43**: 1021–32.
34. Cabral DA, Uribe AG, Benseler S, et al. Classification, presentation, and initial treatment of Wegener's granulomatosis in childhood. *Arthritis Rheum* 2009; **60**: 3413–24.
35. Cotch MF, Hoffman GS, Yerg DE, et al. The epidemiology of Wegener's granulomatosis. *Arthritis Rheum* 1996; **39**: 87–92.
36. Jennette JC, Xiao H, Falk R. Pathogenesis of vascular inflammation by anti-neutrophil cytoplasmic antibodies. *J Am Soc Nephrol* 2006; **17**: 1235–42.
37. Popa ER, Tervaert JW. The relation between Staphylococcus aureus and Wegener's granulomatosis: current knowledge and future directions. *Intern Med* 2003; **42**: 771–80.
38. Rasmussen N, Jayne DRW, Abramowicz D, et al. European therapeutic trials in ANCA-associated systemic vasculitis: disease scoring, consensus regimens and proposed clinical trials. *Clin Exp Immunol* 1995; **101**: 29–34.
39. Stone JH. Limited versus severe Wegener's granulomatosis: baseline data on patients in the Wegener's granulomatosis etanercept trial. *Arthritis Rheum* 2003; **48**: 2299–309.
40. Holle JU, Gross WL, Holl-Ulrich K, et al. Prospective long-term follow-up of patients with localosed Wegener's granulomatosis: does it occur as a persistent disease stage? *Ann Rheum Dis* 2010; **69**: 1934–9.
41. Gubbels SP, Barkhuizen A, Hwang PH. Head and neck manifestations of Wegener's granulomatosis. *Otolaryngol Clin North Am* 2003; **36**: 685–705.
42. Srouji IA, Andrews P, Edwards C, Lund VJ. Patterns of presentation and diagnosis of patients with Wegener's granulomatosis: ENT aspects. *J Laryngol Otol* 2007; **121**: 653–8.
43. Hoffman GS, Kerr GS, Leavitt RY, et al. Wegener granulomatosis: an analysis of 158 patients. *Ann Intern Med* 1992; **116**: 488–98.
44. Takagi D, Nakamaru Y, Maguchi S, et al. Otologic manifestations of Wegener's granulomatosis. *Laryngoscope* 2002; **112**: 1684–90.
45. Lebovics RS, Hoffman GS, Leavitt RY, et al. The management of subglottic stenosis in patients with Wegener's granulomatosis. *Laryngoscope* 1992; **102**: 1341–5.
46. Hoare TJ, Jayne D, Rhys Evans P, et al. Wegener's granulomatosis, subglottic stenosis and antineutrophil cytoplasm antibodies. *J Laryngol Otol* 1989; **103**: 1187–91.
47. Rasmussen N. Management of the ear, nose, and throat manifestations of Wegener's granulomatosis: an otorhinolaryngologist's perspective. *Curr Opin Rheumatol* 2001; **13**: 3–11.
48. van der Woude FJ, Rasmussen N, Lobatto S, et al. Autoantibodies against neutrophils and monocytes: tool for diagnosis and marker of disease activity in Wegener's granulomatosis. *Lancet* 1985; **1**: 425–9.
49. Jennette JC, Falk RJ. Small vessel vasculitis. *N Engl J Med* 1997; **337**: 1512–23.
50. Alam DS, Seth R, Sindwani R, Woodson EA, Rajasekaran K. Upper airway manifestations of granulomatosis with polyangiitis. *Cleve Clin J Med* 2012; **79** Suppl 3: S16–S21.
51. Specks U, Wheatley CL, McDonald TJ, et al. Anticytoplasmic autoantibodies in the diagnosis and follow-up of Wegener's granulomatosis. *Mayo Clin Proc* 1989; **64**: 28–36.
52. Trimarchi M, Bussi M, Sinico RA, et al. Cocaine-induced midline destructive lesions: an autoimmune disease? *Autoimmun Rev* 2013; **12**: 496–500.
53. Devaney KO, Travis WD, Hoffman G, et al. Interpretation of head and neck biopsies in Wegener's granulomatosis: a pathologic study of 126 biopsies in 70 patients. *Am J Surg Pathol* 1990; **14**: 555–64.
54. Leavitt RY, Fauci AS, Bloch DA, et al. The American College of Rheumatology 1990 Criteria for the classification of Wegener's granulomatosis. *Arthritis Rheum* 1990; **33**: 1101–7.
55. Jennette JC, Falk RJ, Andrassy K, et al. Nomenclature of systemic vasculitides: proposal of an international conference. *Arthritis Rheum* 1994; **37**: 187–92.
56. Grindler D, Cannady S, Batra PS. Computed tomography findings in sinonasal Wegener's granulomatosis. *Am J Rhinol Allergy* 2009; **23**: 497–501.
57. Lloyd G, Lund VJ, Beale T, Howard D. Rhinologic changes in Wegener's granulomatosis. *J Laryngol Otol* 2002; **116**: 565–9.
58. Trimarchi M, Sinico RA, Teggi R, et al. Otorhinolaryngological manifestations in granulomatosis with polyangiitis (Wegener's). *Autoimmun Rev* 2013; **12**: 501–5.
59. Fauci AS, Haynes BF, Katz P, Wolff SM. Wegener's granulomatosis: prospective clinical and therapeutic experience with 85 patients for 21 years. *Ann Intern Med* 1983; **98**: 76–85.
60. Holle JU, Dubrau C, Herlyn K, et al. Rituximab for refractory granulomatosis with polyangiitis (Wegener's granulomatosis): comparison of efficacy in granulomatous versus vasculitic manifestations. *Ann Rheum Dis* 2012; **71**: 327–33.
61. Lund VJ, Howard DJ, Wei W. Granulomas and conditions simulating neoplasia In: *Tumours of the Nose, Paranasal Sinuses and Nasopharynx*. Thieme, New York, 2014.
62. Guillevin L, Cordier JF, Lhote F, et al. A prospective, multicenter, randomized trial comparing steroids and pulse cyclophosphamide versus steroids and oral cyclophosphamide in the treatment of generalized Wegener's granulomatosis. *Arthritis Rheum* 1997; **40**: 2187–98.
63. de Groot K, Rasmussen N, Bacon PA, et al. Randomized trial of cyclophosphamide versus methotrexate for induction of remission in early systemic antineutrophil cytoplasmic antibody-associated vasculitis. *Arthritis Rheum* 2005; **52**: 2461–9.
64. Stone JH, Merkel PA, Spiera R, et al. Rituximab versus cyclophosphamide for ANCA-associated vasculitis. *N Engl J Med* 2010; **363**: 221–32.
65. Wung PK, Stone JH. Therapeutics of Wegener's granulomatosis. *Nat Clin Pract Rheumatol* 2006; **2**: 192–200.
66. Reinhold-Keller E, Fink CO, Herlyn K, et al. High rate of renal relapse in 71 patients with Wegener's granulomatosis under maintenance of remission with low-dose methotrexate. *Arthritis Rheum* 2002; **47**: 326–32.
67. Jayne D, Rasmussen N, Andrassy K, et al. A randomized trial of maintenance therapy for vasculitis associated with antineutrophil cytoplasmic autoantibodies. *N Engl J Med* 2003; **349**: 36–44.
68. Hiemstra TF, Walsh M, Mahr A, et al. Mycophenolate mofetil vs azathioprine for remission maintenance in antineutrophil cytoplasmic antibody-associated vasculitis: a randomized controlled trial. *JAMA* 2010; **304**: 2381–8.
69. Metzler C, Fink C, Lamprecht P, et al. Maintenance of remission with leflunomide in Wegener's granulomatosis. *Rheumatology (Oxford)* 2004; **43**: 315–20.
70. Flossman O, Jayne DR. Long-term treatment of relapsing Wegener's granulomatosis with 15-deoxyspergualin. *Rheumatology (Oxford)* 2010; **49**: 556–62.
71. Wegener's Granulomatosis Etanercept Trial (WGET) Research Group. Etanercept plus standard therapy for Wegener's granulomatosis. *N Engl J Med* 2005; **352**: 351–61.
72. Stegeman CA, Tervaert JW, de Jong PE, Kallenberg CG. Trimethoprim-sulfamethoxazole (co-trimoxazole) for the prevention of relapses of Wegener's granulomatosis. Dutch Co-Trimoxazole Wegener Study Group. *N Engl J Med* 1996; **335**: 16–20.

73. de Groot K, Reinhold-Keller E, Tatsis E et al. Therapy for the maintenance of remission in sixty-five patients with generalized Wegener's granulomatosis. Methotrexate versus trimethoprim/sulfamethoxazole. *Arthritis Rheum* 1996; **39**: 2052–61.
74. Eloy P, Leruth E, Bertrand B, Rombaux PH. Successful endonasal dacryocystorhinostomy in a patient with Wegener's granulomatosis. *Clin Ophthalmol* 2009; **3**: 651–6.
75. Congdon D, Sherris DA, Specks U, McDonald T. Long-term follow up of repair of external nasal deformities in patients with Wegener's granulomatosis. *Laryngoscope* 2002; **112**: 731–7.
76. Nouraei SA, Obholzer R, Ind PW, et al. Results of endoscopic surgery and intralesional steroid therapy for airway compromise due to tracheobronchial Wegener's granulomatosis. *Thorax* 2008; **63**: 49–52.
77. Churg J, Strauss I. Allergic granulomatosis, allergic angiitis and periarteritis nodosa. *Am J Pathol* 1951; **27**: 277–301.
78. Comarmond C, Pagnoux C, Khellaf M, et al. Eosinophilic granulomatosis with polyangiitis (Churg-Strauss): clinical characteristics and long-term follow-up of the 383 patients enrolled in the French Vasculitis Study Group cohort. *Arthritis Rheum* 2013; **65**: 270–81.
79. Keogh KA, Specks U. Churg-Strauss syndrome. *Semin Respir Crit Care Med* 2006; **27**: 148–57.
80. Abril A, Calamia KT, Cohen MD. The Churg Strauss syndrome (allergic granulomatous angiitis): review and update. *Semin Arthritis Rheum* 2003; **33**: 106–14.
81. Srouji I, Lund V, Andrews P, Edwards C. Rhinologic symptoms and quality-of-life in patients with Churg-Strauss syndrome vasculitis. *Am J Rhinol* 2008; **22**: 406–9.
82. Bacciu A, Bacciu S, Mercante G, et al. Ear, nose and throat manifestations of Churg-Strauss syndrome. *Acta Otolaryngol* 2006; **126**: 503–9.
83. Kiene M, Csernok E, Muller A, et al. Elevated interleukin-4 and interleukin-13 production by T cell lines from patients with Churg-Strauss syndrome. *Arthritis Rheum* 2001; **44**: 469–73.
84. Wechsler ME, Garpestad E, Flier SR, et al. Pulmonary infiltrates, eosinophilia, and cardiomyopathy following corticosteroid withdrawal in patients with asthma receiving zafirlukast. *JAMA* 1998; **279**: 455–7.
85. Weller PF, Plaut M, Taggart V, Trontell A. The relationship of asthma therapy and Churg-Strauss syndrome: NIH workshop summary report. *J Allergy Clin Immunol* 2001; **108**: 175–83.
86. Guillevin L, Cohen P, Gayraud M, et al. Churg-Strauss syndrome: clinical study and long-term follow-up of 96 patients. *Medicine (Baltimore)* 1999; **78**: 26–37.
87. Keogh KA, Specks U. Churg-Strauss syndrome: clinical presentation, antineutrophil cytoplasmic antibodies, and leukotriene receptor antagonists. *Am J Med* 2003; **115**: 284–90.
88. Moosig F, Bremer JP, Hellmich B, et al. A vasculitis centre based management strategy leads to improved outcome in eosinophilic granulomatosis and polyangiitis (Churg-Strauss, EGPA): monocentric experiences in 150 patients. *Ann Rheum Dis* 2013; **72**(6): 1011–7.
89. Sehgal M, Swanson JW, DeRemee RA, Colby TV. Neurologic manifestations of Churg-Strauss syndrome. *Mayo Clin Proc* 1995; **70**: 337–41.
90. Lanham JG, Elkon KB, Pusey CD, Hughes GR. Systemic vasculitis with asthma and eosinophilia: a clinical approach to the Churg-Strauss syndrome. *Medicine (Baltimore)* 1984; **63**: 65–81.
91. Masi AT, Hunder GG, Lie JT, et al. The American College of Rheumatology 1990 criteria for the classification of Churg-Strauss syndrome (allergic granulomatosis and angiitis). *Arthritis Rheum* 1990; **33**: 1094–100.
92. Tastis E, Schnabel A, Gross WL. Interferon-alpha treatment of four patients with the Churg-Strauss syndrome. *Ann Intern Med* 1998; **129**: 370–4.
93. Wiesner O, Russell KA, Lee AS, et al. Antineutrophil cytoplasmic antibodies reacting with human neutrophil elastase as a diagnostic marker for cocaine-induced midline destructive lesions but not autoimmune vasculitis. *Arthritis Rheum* 2004; **50**: 2954–65.
94. Willman CL. Detection of clonal histiocytes in Langerhans cell histiocytosis: biology and clinical significance. *Br J Cancer Suppl* 1994; **23**: S29–S33.
95. Willman CL, Busque L, Griffiths BB, et al. Langerhans'-cell histiocytosis (histiocytosis X): a clonal proliferative disease. *N Engl J Med* 1994; **331**: 154–60.
96. Gonzalez-Crussi F, Hsueh W, Wiederhold MD. Prostaglandins in histiocytosis X. PG synthesis by histiocytosis-X cells. *Am J Clin Pathol* 1981; **75**: 243–53.
97. Benz-Lemoine E. [Prognostic factors in histiocytosis X]. *Ann Pediatr (Paris)* 1989; **36**: 499–503.
98. Jaffe HL. Giant-cell reparative granuloma, traumatic bone cyst, and fibrous (fibro-osseous) dysplasia of the jawbones. *Oral Surg Oral Med Oral Pathol* 1953; **6**: 159–75.
99. Waldron CA, Shafer WG. The central giant cell reparative granuloma of the jaws: an analysis of 38 cases. *Am J Clin Pathol* 1966; **45**: 437–47.
100. Saleh EA, Taibah AK, Naguib M, et al. Giant cell tumor of the lateral skull base: a case report. *Otolaryngol Head Neck Surg* 1994; **111**: 314–18.
101. Graham J, Michaels L. Cholesterol granuloma of the maxillary antrum. *Clin Otolaryngol Allied Sci* 1978; **3**: 155–60.
102. Butler S, Grossenbacher R. Cholesterol granuloma of the paranasal sinuses. *J Laryngol Otol* 1989; **103**: 776–9.
103. Hellquist H, Lundgren J, Olofsson J. Cholesterol granuloma of the maxillary and frontal sinuses. *ORL J Otorhinolaryngology Relat Spec* 1984; **46**: 153–8.
104. Milton CM, Bickerton RC. A review of maxillary sinus cholesterol granuloma. *Br J Oral Maxillofac Surg* 1986; **24**: 293–9.
105. Michaels L, Gregory MM. Pathology of "non-healing (midline) granuloma". *J Clin Pathol* 1977; **30**: 317–27.
106. Al-Hakeem DA, Fedele S, Carlos R, Porter S. Extranodal NK/T-cell lymphoma, nasal type. *Oral Oncol* 2007; **43**: 4–14.
107. Metgud RS, Doshi JJ, Gaurkhede S, et al. Extranodal NK/T-cell lymphoma, nasal type (angiocentric T-cell lymphoma): a review about the terminology. *J Oral Maxillofac Pathol* 2011; **15**: 96–100.
108. Harabuchi Y, Yamanaka N, Kataura A, et al. Epstein-Barr virus in nasal T-cell lymphomas in patients with lethal midline granuloma. *Lancet* 1990; **335**: 128–30.
109. Hellquist HB. Granulomatous lesions of the nose and sinuses. In: Hellquist HB (ed.). *Pathology of the nose and paranasal sinuses*. London: Butterworths; 1990, pp. 60–81.
110. Koom WS, Chung EJ, Yang WI, et al. Angiocentric T-cell and NK/T-cell lymphomas: radiotherapeutic viewpoints. *Int J Radiat Oncol Biol Phys* 2004; **59**: 1127–37.
111. Isobe K, Uno T, Tamaru J, et al. Extranodal natural killer/T-cell lymphoma, nasal type. *Cancer* 2006; **106**: 609–15.

CHAPTER 110

ABNORMALITIES OF SMELL

Richard L. Doty and Steven M. Bromley

Introduction 1227	Treatment of smell disorders 1238
Anatomy and physiology 1228	Prognosis 1239
Olfactory disorder classification 1230	Acknowledgements 1240
Clinical evaluation of smell function 1231	References 1240
Causes of smell disturbance 1233	

SEARCH STRATEGY

Data in this chapter may be updated by a Medline search using the keywords: olfaction, smell, anosmia, dysosmia, phantosmia, age, odour identification, psychophysics, odour threshold, odour discrimination, presybyosmia, head trauma, olfactory epithelium, olfactory bulb and UPSIT.

INTRODUCTION

The ability to detect environmental chemicals is a primary function of the nose. A proper functioning sense of smell allows a person to discriminate between thousands of largely organic, low-molecular mass, volatile compounds and provides information regarding: (1) the safety of a substance or environment (e.g., spoiled food, leaking natural gas); (2) the aesthetic properties of everyday objects (e.g., rose, dirty laundry); and (3) elements of basic communication (e.g., mother/infant interactions). When combined with gustatory and somatosensory stimuli, the sense of smell determines the flavours of foods and beverages, and aids the process of digestion by triggering normal gastrointestinal secretions. Moreover, the olfactory system contributes significantly to a person's quality of life. Among 750 patients presenting to our centre with largely olfactory problems, more than 68% experienced altered quality of life, 46% described changes in appetite or body weight, and 56% reported influences in daily living or psychological well-being.[1] Loss of smell can result in significant psychological disruption and even generate feelings of physical and social vulnerability and victimization.[2] The importance of smell is also emphasized by the consequences of its loss in those who depend on it for their livelihood (e.g., cooks, homemakers, firefighters, plumbers, wine merchants, chemical plant workers, etc.). Loss of smell can also adversely affect nutrition, especially in the elderly and, importantly, has been associated with longevity. In a recent longitudinal study of over a thousand non-demented older persons, mortality risk was nearly two and a half times higher in those with low than with high odour identification test scores after adjusting for sex, age, education and other variables.[3]

Although otorhinolaryngologists are often the first physicians that patients with smell complaints visit, some patients find themselves making repeated appointments to multiple physicians until their olfactory problem is adequately addressed. Unfortunately, olfactory health is generally disregarded by physicians. This is beside the fact the abnormalities of smell are ubiquitous. There are at least 2.7 million (1.4%) adults in the United States with olfactory dysfunction; presumably similar numbers exist world-wide.[4] Also, most patients who complain of decreased 'taste' function actually have an unrecognized impairment of smell.[1] Diminished 'taste' is typically due to loss of flavour sensations derived from retronasal stimulation of the olfactory receptors, rather than impairment of taste-mediated sensations, per se.[3] Importantly, a patient's lack of olfactory function can be an early sign of a number of serious disease states, including nasopharyngeal carcinoma, Alzheimer's disease, Parkinson's disease, frontal meningiomas, multiple sclerosis, and sinus infections.[5,6] While some patients initially present to their physicians with a frank complaint of smell impairment, others can be completely unaware of their dysfunction, making routine clinical assessments of olfaction imperative.

The necessity of the physician to properly evaluate for abnormalities of smell function is also supported in the medicolegal arena, with claims of accidental and iatrogenic smell disturbance often resulting in substantial financial awards. Routine clinical quantitative measurement of smell function can now be easily performed in the office setting, allowing a physician to:

- validate and characterize a patient's olfactory complaint
- identify patients who might be malingering
- quantify and document known presurgical smell impairment
- longitudinally, follow the course of smell function in the midst of a therapeutic intervention or during recovery from previous loss.

This chapter summarizes important aspects of olfactory anatomy and physiology, describes the common olfactory disorders encountered in clinical practice, and provides current practical techniques for the evaluation and management of smell disturbance.

ANATOMY AND PHYSIOLOGY

The nose: Structure in relation to smell

The human nose contains two independent nasal passages that are dynamic conduits that subserve both respiration and olfaction. The nasal cavities not only warm and humidify inspired air, but they help to eliminate most airborne pathogens and environmental pollutants – a number of which can be toxic to the olfactory system.[7] The olfactory neuroepithelium exists within a small region of nasal mucosa (said to be ~2 cm^2) in the upper recesses of the nasal chambers lining the cribriform plate and sectors of the superior turbinate, middle turbinate, and septum (**Figure 110.1**).[8] The olfactory cleft, an opening of approximately 1 mm wide that sits 7 cm deep to the nostril, harbours the majority of the olfactory neuroepithelium which is difficult to observe even by modern endoscopic techniques.[9] While most of the air stream coming into the nose is shunted through the passages around the inferior and medial turbinates and along the septal wall, only 10–15% of the air reaches the olfactory neuroepithelium.[10] Thus, minor changes in nasal architecture and airflow can result in substantial air-flow blockage to olfactory regions without much impairment in nasal respiratory ability.[7,11] For example, relatively small polyps located in the superior meatus can deflect incoming air currents away from the olfactory cleft, resulting in smell impairment.[11] On the other hand, too patent an airway, as seen with excessive turbinate removal, can improperly shunt air away from the olfactory cleft, resulting in at least some deterioration in olfactory acuity.[12] It is important to remember that while chronic rhinosinusitis can lead to swelling of the mucosa and a mechanical conductive block, there is evidence for local inflammatory toxicity to the olfactory neuroepithelium that may not be alleviated with surgical intervention.[13] A significant amount of retronasal airflow from the nasopharynx occurs during swallowing and

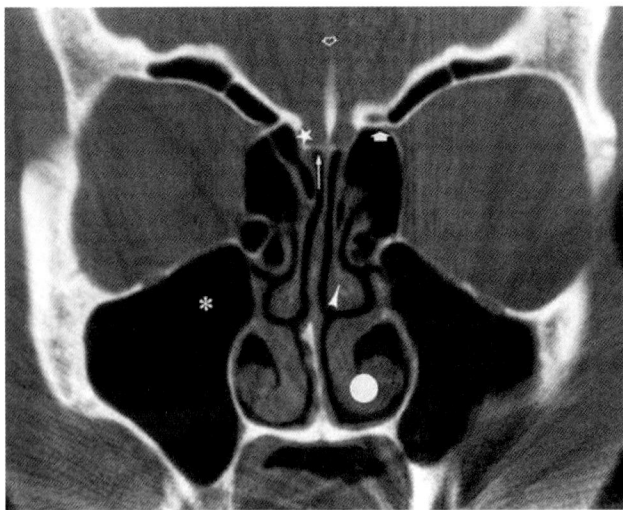

Figure 110.1 CT scan of paranasal sinuses and associated nasal structures. The * is within the right maxillary sinus, below the right eye. The inferior portion of the middle turbinate is indicated by the white arrowhead and the inferior turbinate by the circle. Note the attachment of the middle turbinate to the cribriform above. A short fat white arrow is in the left anterior ethmoid sinus and points to the anterior ethmoidal neurovascular bundle as it emerges from the left orbit and courses along the roof of the ethmoid. The central small open arrow is located in the anterior cranial fossa directly above the bony crista galli. The long thin arrow situated with the olfactory cleft points to the cribriform plate. The five-pointed star in the right olfactory fossa is adjacent to the vertical lamella of the cribriform plate. From: Lanza DC, Clerico DM. Anatomy of the human nasal passages. In: Doty RL (ed) Handbook of olfaction and gestation. New York: Marcel Dekker, 1995, p. 60. Copyright © 1995 by Marcel Dekker, Inc.

deglutition. This retronasal route is vital to the production of flavour from swallowed foods – adding *smell* to both *taste* and *touch*.

The human nasal passage is intermittently affected, at least in some individuals, by the 'nasal cycle'. This cycle, an autonomic ultradian rhythm of periodic alternating side-to-side nasal turbinate engorgement and disengorgement, is said to occur in 80% of the normal population with a cycle frequency ranging from 40 minutes to 4 hours.[7] The nasal cycle itself, which is less frequent in the very young and the very old, does not appear to affect overall olfactory sensitivity in the normal nose; however, intermittent engorgement in the context of a pre-existing structural distortion can result in a noticeable, albeit transient, blockage of a nasal passage (e.g., when turbinate adhesions are present).

Four neural systems within the human nose

Most land mammals have four major specialized neural systems within the left and right sides of the nose:

- The main olfactory system (Cranial Nerve I or CN I).
- The accessory olfactory system (i.e., the vomeronasal system).

- The trigeminal somatosensory system (CN V)
- The nervus terminalis or terminal nerve (CN 0).[14, 15]

While CN I mediates common odour sensations (e.g., vanilla, rose, chocolate), CN V mediates both chemical and non-chemical stimuli in the form of somatosensory sensations (e.g., irritation, burning, cooling, tickling, touch). CN V is also responsible for inducing reflexive responses, such as secretions of mucus and halting of inhalation, that help to prevent or minimize chemically-induced or thermally-induced damage to the linings of the nose and lungs. The vomeronasal system is non-functional in humans; while a rudimentary vomeronasal tube is present on each side of the septum with an opening into the human nose, it has no centrally-projecting nerve and humans do not possess an accessory olfactory bulb, the target of such a nerve. CN 0 was discovered after the other cranial nerves had been named, and consists of a loose plexus of ganglionated nerves that, in most mammals, is in close proximity to the vomeronasal organ and nerve. Its neurons are immunoreactive to the peptide hormone gonadotropin-releasing hormone (GnRH), implying a yet-to-be characterized association with endocrine processes. It has been suggested by some that CN 0 may be a vestige of an ancient nerve whose function was lost or superseded by other parts of the nervous system, although this argument is weak, given that it is so well conserved among a wide range of vertebrates, including humans.

Olfactory neuroepithelium and neural transduction

Before neural transduction can begin, odourants must (a) enter the nose during either active (e.g. sniffing) or passive (e.g., diffusion) processes, (b) pass through the olfactory cleft, and (c) move from the air phase into the largely aqueous phase of the olfactory mucus. During mastication, odourants from the oral cavity actively move into the nasal cavity via the nasal pharynx (retronasal direction). Mucus is important in that it ensures a moist and protective environment for the olfactory neuroepithelium, and aids in dispersing odourants to the olfactory receptors. From the mucus, odourous chemicals either diffuse or are transported by specialized proteins (termed odourant binding proteins) to the receptors.

The olfactory neuroepithelium has an ultrastructure of variable uniformity and, contrary to many textbooks, cannot be discerned reliably from the surrounding respiratory epithelium by the naked eye. It is a pseudostratified columnar epithelium, supported by a highly vascularized lamina propria. Throughout life, islands of respiratory-like epithelial metaplasia appear within the epithelium, presumably as a result of cumulative viral, bacterial, and other insults.[14] In the adult, at least six distinct classes of cells – defined morphologically, biochemically, and functionally – can be identified within the neuroepithelium (**Figure 110.2**).

- The *bipolar sensory receptor neuron* is derived embryologically from the olfactory placode, is of CNS origin, and extends odourant receptor-containing cilia into the mucus.
- The *supporting* or *sustentacular cell* insulates the bipolar receptor cells from one another, regulates mucus production, transports molecules across the epithelium, and detoxifies and degrades odourants.
- The *duct cell of Bowman's glands* secretes most of the mucus within the olfactory receptor region.
- The poorly understood *microvillar cell* is located at the surface of the epithelium and, like the supporting cell, sends tufts of microvilli into the nasal mucus.
- The *horizontal (dark) basal cells*, one of two main classes of stem cells within the basement membrane of the epithelium.
- The *globose (light) basal cells*, a multipotent basal cell that can give rise to neurons and non-neuronal cells, including the horizontal basal cells.[14]

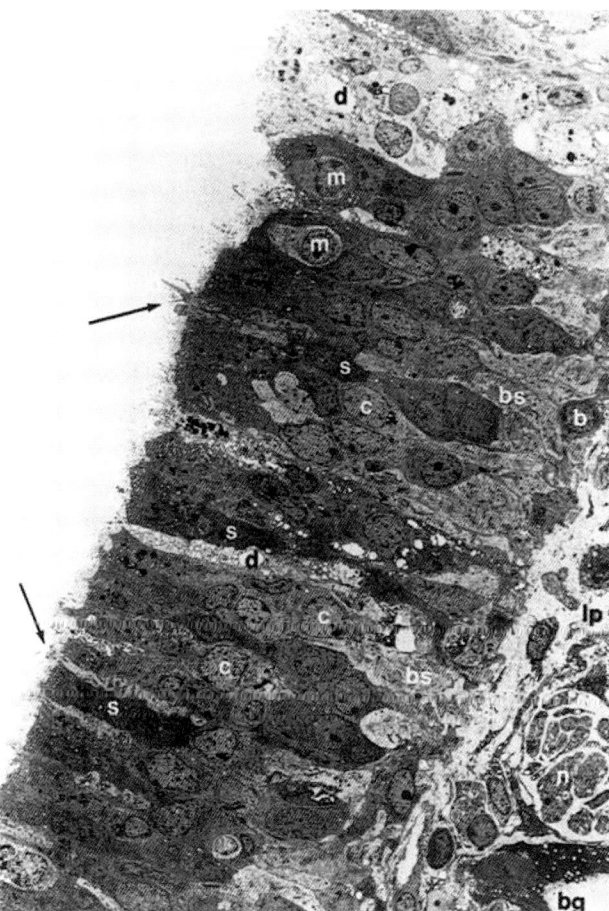

Figure 110.2 Low-power electron micrograph (× 670) of a longitudinal section through a biopsy specimen of human olfactory mucosa taken from the nasal septum. Four cell types are indicated: ciliated olfactory receptors (c), microvillar cells (m), supporting cells (s) and basal cells (b). The arrows point to ciliated olfactory knobs of the bipolar receptor cells. d = degenerating cells; bs = base of the supporting cells; lp = lamina propria; n = nerve bundle; bg = Bowman's gland. Photo courtesy of David T. Moran.

The number of olfactory receptor cells exceeds that of any other sensory system except vision; collectively, the surface area of the cilia is quite large – exceeding 20 cm² in the human.[15] Seven domain transmembrane olfactory receptors, which reflect the expression of the largest known vertebrate gene family (on the order of 1000 genes or pseudogenes, accounting for ~1% of all expressed genes), are found on the 10–30 cilia that project into the nasal mucus from each of these cells.[16] Approximately 6 million receptor cell axons ultimately coalesce into 30–50 fascicles, termed the olfactory fila, which traverse the cribriform plate and pia matter to synapse with second-order neurons within the glomeruli of the olfactory bulb. The olfactory receptor neurons primarily use the neurotransmitter glutamate to excite OB neurons, while dopamine appears to be a necessary modulator of olfactory nerve input.[17] The process of actually transforming the chemical energy of receptor binding into a neural signal – signal transduction – requires a complex cascade of events, some of which involves activation of G proteins (e.g., that of an olfactory-specific subtype, G_{olf}) and various second-messenger enzymes.[18, 19]

It is important to recognize that the olfactory nerve cells, as well as the proximal extraneural spaces, can serve as conduits for the movement of viruses and exogenous agents from the nasal cavity into the brain. This was recognized many years ago as a major route of polio viruses into the brain, leading to programmes to cauterize the olfactory epithelium of school children with zinc sulphate in Toronto and other major cities to avert contracting polio during epidemics. This 'olfactory vector' route has been proposed as a potential explanation for both the olfactory loss and the aetiology of some forms of common neurodegenerative diseases, such as Alzheimer's disease and idiopathic Parkinson's disease,[20] although evidence for this hypothesis in these cases remains largely circumstantial.

The olfactory bulb and central projections

The olfactory bulbs are complex structures located on the ventral surface of the frontal lobes directly over the cribriform plate. The first synapse of the incoming bipolar olfactory receptor cell neurons occurs within spherical structures making up a distinct layer of the bulb – the glomeruli. A given receptor projects to only one glomerulus, and any given glomerulus appears to receive most of its input from a restricted region of the epithelium. The main afferent second-order neurons are termed mitral and tufted cells. A considerable amount of convergence of information occurs at the level of the glomeruli. The mitral and tufted cells, in turn, send collaterals that synapse within the periglomerular and external plexiform layers, resulting in 'reverberating' circuits in which negative and positive feedback occur. The apical dendrites of the mitral and tufted cells are influenced by interneurons and centrifugal fibres, most of which are GABAergic or dopaminergic.[21]

It is generally believed that the olfactory system is unique among sensory systems in that information from the sensory receptors is sent directly, and primarily ipsilaterally, into cortical regions without synapsing in the thalamus. However, some cortical projections from primary to secondary (i.e. orbitofrontal) cortex do ultimately relay through the thalamus, and there are some contralateral projections via the anterior commissure. The latter arise largely from pyramidal cells of the anterior olfactory nucleus (AON; a structure whose cells are primarily in the rostral olfactory peduncle). Higher order brain regions in addition to the AON that are targeted by the mitral and tufted cells of the bulb include (from rostral to caudal):

- The piriform cortex.
- The olfactory tubercle.
- The entorhinal area.
- The amygdaloid cortex (a region contiguous with the underlying amygdala).
- The corticomedial nuclear group of the amygdala.

There is a rich supply of centrifugal fibre projections from sectors of the olfactory cortex and other central structures to the olfactory bulb which modify and control olfactory input.[21, 22] Structures involved in centrifugal activity include the AON, piriform cortex, lateral entorhinal cortex, regions of the amygdala, raphe nuclei, locus ceruleus, and regions of the hypothalamus.[22] Third-order projections occur, in a reciprocal fashion, to numerous regions, including the mediodorsal nucleus of the thalamus, the posterior and medial hypothalamus, the hippocampus, and the orbitofrontal cortex, the latter of which also receives second-order projections. Areas of the cortex that result in smell perception when stimulated include the pre-piriform and intermediate piriform cortices. Lesions of the olfactory system anterior to the olfactory trigone (including the neuroepithelium, fila, bulb, and tract) can result in total lack of smell on the affected side. However, lesions within olfactory structures more posterior to the olfactory trigone do not typically cause complete loss.[22, 23]

OLFACTORY DISORDER CLASSIFICATION

Olfactory disorders are classified according to standard schemata. It is important to differentiate between a patient's chemosensory complaint and the findings of objective testing, which are not always in congruence. *Anosmia* refers to an inability to detect qualitative olfactory sensations (i.e., absence of smell function); *Partial anosmia* defines an ability to perceive some, but not all, odours; *Hyposmia* or *microsmia* refers to decreased sensitivity to odours; *Hyperosmia* reflects increased sensitivity to common odours; *Dysosmia* (sometimes termed cacosmia or parosmia) is distorted or perverted smell perception to odour stimulation; *Phantosmia* is a dysosmic sensation perceived in the absence of an odour stimulus (a.k.a. olfactory hallucination); and *Olfactory agnosia* refers to an inability to recognize an odour sensation, even though olfactory processing, language, and general intellectual functions are essentially intact, as in some stroke patients. Other less commonly used terms include *Heterosmia* – a condition where all odours smell the same, *Presbyosmia* – a decline in smell sense with age, and *Osmophobia* – a dislike or fear of certain smells. Presbyosmia is less specific than the other terms noted above (e.g., it does not distinguish between anosmia and hyposmia) and is laden, by definition, with the notion that it is age *per se* that is causing the age-related deficit. Olfactory dysfunction can be either bilateral or unilateral (sometimes termed binasal or uninasal), and bilateral testing usually reflects the better functioning of the two sides of the nose.

CLINICAL EVALUATION OF SMELL FUNCTION

History

Proper assessment of a patient's smell function requires:

- A detailed clinical history
- Objective quantitative olfactory testing
- A thorough physical examination emphasizing the head and neck with appropriate brain and rhinosinus imaging.

It is important to recognize that patients frequently confuse 'taste problems' with true smell loss, and that many deny any olfactory disturbance until formal testing proves otherwise. Several focused questions can help establish the nature of the olfactory disturbance. Was olfactory functioning previously normal? Does the patient have a problem with smell, taste, or both? What is the timing of onset, duration of impairment, and pattern of occurrence? *Sudden olfactory loss* can be consistent with possible head trauma, ischaemia, infection, or a psychiatric condition. *Gradual loss* may indicate a progressive and obstructive lesion in or around the nasosinus region, particularly if the loss is unilateral. *Intermittent loss* may suggest an inflammatory process in association with nasal and sinus disease. Is the problem seasonal, suggesting an allergic seasonal rhinitis? Is there a history of precipitating antecedent events, such as head trauma, viral upper respiratory infections, chemical or toxin exposures, and nasosinus surgeries? Does the patient have any nasal discharge that is mucous-appearing (e.g., allergy), purulent (e.g., infection), or clear (CSF rhinorrhea after trauma)? Does the patient use drugs of abuse, such as intra-nasal cocaine, ethanol, or tobacco? Each of these substances has been associated with some form of olfactory impairment; for example, chronic alcoholism can result in significant impairment in smell discrimination[24] and cigarette smoking results in a loss of olfactory ability that is proportional to the cumulative smoking dose.[25] Cessation of smoking can result in improvement in olfactory function over time.

It is essential to determine all medications used by the patient since many reportedly cause smell and taste disturbance. For example, smell or taste loss or disturbances are reported in the Physicians' Desk Reference (PDR) as a potential side effect of hundreds of medications.[26] Does the patient have comorbidities that can contribute to smell impairment, such as renal failure, liver disease, hypothyroidism, diabetes, or dementia? Delayed puberty in association with anosmia (with or without midline craniofacial abnormalities, deafness, and renal anomalies) suggests the possibility of Kallmann's syndrome or some variant thereof. Is there a recent history of epistaxis, discharge (clear, purulent or bloody), facial numbness or weakness, nasal obstruction, allergies, headache or irritation (i.e., signs that may have localizing value)? A positive family history suggests a genetic aetiology. A history of headache which can suggest sinusitis, migraine, or intra-cranial tumour should be sought. Are smells present without an obvious stimulus? A simple partial seizure, or aura, may not be obvious and other signs of ictal activity should be explored (e.g. limb shaking, difficulties with speech, unresponsiveness, automatisms, loss of consciousness, and déjà vu). Given the strong relationship of Alzheimer's disease and idiopathic Parkinson's disease to smell impairment, one should also look for memory- and parkinsonism-related complaints in older patients. A physician should also be aware of pending litigation and the possibility of malingering since olfactory loss is a compensatable injury. Malingering is readily detected in most patients by forced-choice olfactory testing. Malingerers frequently perform more poorly than expected on the basis of chance on such tests.[27]

Physical examination and evaluation

Patients complaining of smell disturbance typically require a general assessment of the head and neck and more detailed otolaryngological and neurological examinations. Are there any signs of trauma such as healing wounds, scarring or distorted nasal or skull architecture? Inspection of the nasal passages can begin with a simple nasal forceps examination to view the peripheral nasal cavity for signs of polyps, congestion, deviation of septum, or inflammation. However, this method is limited, and often nasal endoscopy, employing both flexible and rigid scopes, is needed to ensure thorough assessment of the olfactory meatal area. A deviated septum, *per se*, does not imply a smell disturbance since the olfactory cleft can remain patent; however, the additional presence of polyps, masses, adhesions of the turbinates to the septum may adequately obstruct airflow. Rarely, foreign bodies can be present, particularly in the context of a psychiatric disturbance. Nasal mucus membranes must be examined for colour, surface texture, swelling, inflammation, exudate, erosion, ulceration, epithelial metaplasia, and atrophy.

The presence of mucopus above the eustachian tube orifice suggests posterior ethmoid and/or sphenoid sinus disease. However, mucopus below the eustachian tube implies involvement of the osteomeatal complex. A pale mucous membrane suggests allergy, usually as a result of oedema within the lamina propria. Atrophy of the lamina propria is suggested by unusual spaciousness, dryness and crusting, as is seen in atrophic rhinitis. Exposures to environmental or industrial pollutants can result in metaplasia within the epithelium, in addition to swelling, inflammation, exudates, erosion, and ulceration.

The neurological evaluation should focus on cranial nerve function, with particular attention to the optic nerve (CN II), trigeminal nerve (CN V), and the facial nerve (CN VII). Visual acuity, visual field, and optic disc examinations aid in the detection of possible intra-cranial mass lesions resulting in increased intra-cranial pressure (papilloedema) and optic atrophy, especially when considering Foster Kennedy syndrome (described below). General sensation over the face should be done (e.g., cotton, pin-prick, temperature). The nasal tickle, performed by using cotton to tickle the inside of one nostril, is also useful since an asymmetric withdrawal response suggests impairment of trigeminal fibres within the nose. The face should be symmetrical and full strength, with intact taste on the anterior two-thirds of the tongue bilaterally. Signs of frontal lobe injury and memory impairment may also aide in the diagnosis.

Biopsy of the olfactory epithelium is occasionally helpful. However, the interpretation of such biopsies is complicated by sampling issues and the fact that metaplasia of respiratory-like epithelium occurs throughout the olfactory epithelia in persons with no olfactory problems. Some laboratory tests, such as blood serum tests, may also be helpful in evaluating for underlying medical conditions suggested by history and physical examinations, such as infection, nutritional deficiencies (e.g. B6, B12), allergy, diabetes mellitus, and thyroid, liver, and kidney disease.[3] Contrary to many textbooks, there is no proven efficacy of zinc or vitamin A treatments in cases where frank deficiencies are lacking.

Quantitative olfactory testing

Several standardized and practical psychophysical tests have been developed over the last several years, including a number of brief self-administered tests ranging from the 3-item Pocket Smell Test™ to the 40-item University of Pennsylvania Smell Identification Test or UPSIT.[28] The UPSIT is commercially known as the Smell Identification Test™ and is the most widely used olfactory test, having been administered to more than one million patients worldwide (**Figure 110.3**).[29] The UPSIT can be self-administered in 10 to 15 minutes by most patients in the waiting room, and scored in less than one minute by non-medical personnel. Available in more than 30 different languages, this test consists of four booklets containing 10 microencapsulated ('scratch and sniff') odourants apiece. Test results are in terms of a percentile score of a patient's performance relative to age- and sex-matched controls, and olfactory function can be classified on an absolute basis into one of six categories: normosmia, mild microsmia, moderate microsmia, severe microsmia, anosmia, and probable malingering. Since chance performance is 10 out of 40, very low UPSIT scores reflect avoidance, and hence recognition, of the correct answer, allowing for determination of malingering. The reliability of this test is very high (test-retest $r = 0.94$).

Although most olfactory problems are bilateral, and bilateral testing reflects the better functioning side of the nose, in some instances, unilateral testing is warranted.[23] To accurately assess olfaction unilaterally, the naris contralateral to the tested side should be occluded without distorting the patent nasal valve region. Such occlusion not only prevents air from entering the olfactory region from the naris (orthonasal stimulation), but prevents active movement of odour-laden air into the occluded side from the rear of the nasopharynx (retronasal stimulation). An easy way of doing this is to seal the contralateral naris using a piece of Microfoam™ tape (3M Corporation, Minneapolis, MN) cut to fit the naris borders. The patient is instructed to sniff the stimulus normally and to exhale through the mouth.

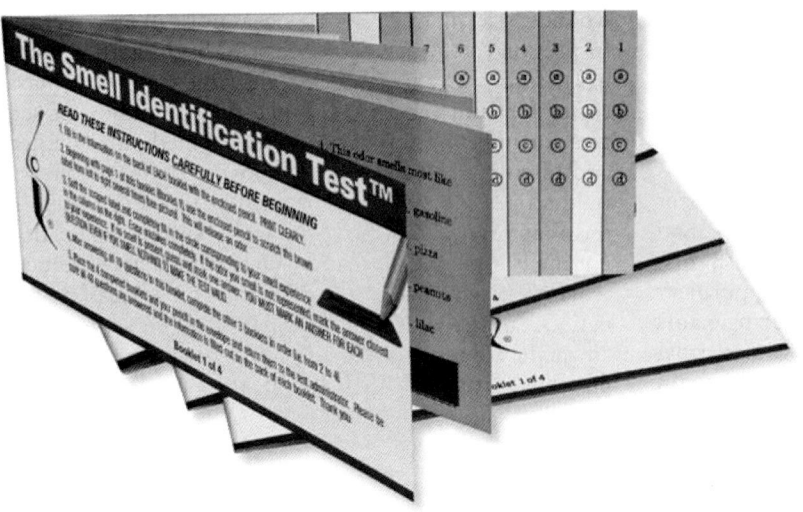

Figure 110.3 The four booklets of the 40-odorant University of Pennsylvania Smell Identification Test (UPSIT; commercially known as the Smell Identification Test™). Each page contains a microencapsulated odorant that is released by means of a pencil tip. This test, which has been administered to ~ 400,000 patients since its development, is the most widely used olfactory test in the world, with English, French, German, and Spanish versions available. The UPSIT is considered to be the "eye chart for the nose." Photo courtesy of Sensonics, Inc., Haddon Hts., NJ 08035 USA. Copyright © 2000 by Sensonics International.

While, in most cases, olfactory dysfunction can be adequately characterized by the UPSIT, some physicians employ, alone or in combination with the UPSIT, a smell threshold test. A commonly employed test employs phenyl ethyl alcohol as the odourant and establishes the threshold employing a staircase procedure.[30] Thresholds determined using this procedure are similar in principle to audiometric thresholds using the von Bekesy procedure. Like the UPSIT, threshold testing can be done either bilaterally or unilaterally.

The recording of olfactory event-related potentials (OERPs) is available in some specialized medical centres as an additional means of assessing the integrity of the olfactory system. Using brain electroencephalography (EEG), the test consists of discerning synchronized brain activity recorded from overall EEG activity following brief presentations of odourants. Unfortunately, OERP testing requires complex, specialized and expensive equipment capable of delivering well-delineated 'square wave' odourant pulses into the nose within the background of continuously flowing warmed and humidified air. Although OERPs can be useful in some cases in detecting malingering, and are generally sensitive to alterations in olfactory function due to a wide range of causes, unlike their visual and auditory counterparts, they are *unable* to discern where in the pathway the anomaly exists that is causing the problem.

Imaging studies

There are multiple ways of medically imaging patients with smell disturbance. Plain radiographs are rarely useful due to an inability to capture details of the osteomeatal complex. Computed tomography (CT), on the other hand, has proven to be the most useful and cost-effective technique to assess sinonasal tract inflammatory disorders, and is superior to magnetic resonance imaging (MRI) in the evaluation of the bony structures (e.g. ethmoid, cribriform plate, olfactory cleft). In particular, coronal CT scans are useful in evaluating paranasal anatomy. MRI is better to evaluate soft tissue, and is the technique of choice to image the olfactory bulbs, tracts, and cortical parenchyma. Positron emission tomography (PET), single-proton emission computed tomography (SPECT), and functional MRI (fMRI) presently have limited usefulness outside of research institutions.

CAUSES OF SMELL DISTURBANCE

There are a number of known aetiologies, many non-mutually exclusive, for olfactory disturbance (Table 110.1). The majority of cases of presumably permanent chronic anosmia or hyposmia are due to prior upper respiratory infections, head trauma, and nasal and paranasal sinus disease – most causes reflecting permanent damage to the olfactory neuroepithelium.[1] **[Level 1 evidence]** Despite extensive evaluations, a substantial proportion remains idiopathic.

TABLE 110.1 Reported agents, diseases, drugs, interventions and other aetiologic categories associated in the medical or toxicologic literature with olfactory dysfunction. Note that categories are not mutually exclusive

Air Pollutants & Industrial Dusts

Acetone	Formaldehyde
Acids (e.g. sulfuric)	Grain
Ashes	Hydrazine
Benzene	Hydrogen selenide
Benzol	Hydrogen sulphide
Butyl acetate	Iron carboxyl
Cadmium	Lead
Carbon disulphide	Nickel
Cement	Nitrous gases
Chalk	Paint solvents
Chlorine	Paper
Chromium	Pepper
Coke/coal	Peppermint oil
Cotton	Phosphorus oxychloride
Cresol	Potash
Ethyl acetate	Silicone dioxide
Ethyl & methyl acrylate	Spices
Flour	Trichloroethylene

Drugs

Adrenal steroids (chronic use)	Propylthiouracil
Amino acids (excess)	Thiouracil
Cysteine	Antivirals
Histidine	Cardiovascular/hypertensives
Analgesics	Gastric medications
Antipyrine	Cimetidine
Anaesthetics, local	Hyperlipoproteinaemia medications
Cocaine HCl	Artovastatin Calcium (Lipitor)
Procaine HCl	
Tetracaine HCl	Cholestyramine
Anticancer agents (e.g., methotrexate)	Clofibrate
Antihistamines (e.g., Chlorpheniramine malate)	Intra-nasal saline solutions with:
	Acetylcholine
	Acetyl, b-methylcholine
Antimicrobials	Menthol
Griseofulvin	Strychnine
Lincomycin	Zinc sulfate
Macrolides	Local Vasoconstrictors
Neomycin	Opiates
Pencillins	Codeine
Streptomycin	Hydromophone HCl
Tetracyclines	Morphine
Tyrothricin	Psychopharmaceuticals (e.g., LSD, psilocybin)
Antirheumatics	
Mercury/gold salts	Sympathomimetics
D-Penicillamine	Amphetamine sulphate
Antithyroids	Fenbutrazate HCl
Methimazole	Phenmetrazine theoclate

Endocrine/Metabolic

Addison's disease	Hypothyroidism
Congenital adreanl hyperplasia	Kallmann's syndrome
Cushing's syndrome	Pregnancy
Diabetes mellitus	Panhypopitutarism
Froelich's syndrome	Pseudohypoparathyroidism
Gigantism	Sjögren's syndrome
Hypergonadotropic hypogonadism	Turner's syndrome

(Continued)

TABLE 110.1 *(Continued)* Reported agents, diseases, drugs, interventions and other aetiologic categories associated in the medical or toxicologic literature with olfactory dysfunction. Note that categories are not mutually exclusive

Infections – Viral/Bacterial

Acquired immunodeficiency syndrome (AIDS)	Fungal
Acute viral rhinitis	Influenza
Bacterial rhinosinusitis	Rickettsial
Bronchiectasis	Microfilarial

Lesions of the nose/Airway blockage

Adenoid hypertrophy	Nasal Polyposis
Allergic rhinitis	Rhinitis medicamentosa
Perennial	Structural abnormality
Seasonal	Deviated septum
Atrophic rhinitis	Weakness of alae nasi
Chronic inflammatory rhinitis	Vasomotor rhinitis
Hypertrophic rhinitis	

Medical Interventions

Adrenalectomy	Influenza vaccination
Anaesthesia	Laryngectomy
Anterior craniotomy	Oophorectomy
Arteriography	Paranasal sinus exenteration
Chemotherapy	Radiation therapy
Frontal lobe resection	Rhinoplasty
Gastrectomy	Temporal lobe resection
Haemodialysis	Thyroidectomy
Hypophysectomy	

Neoplasms – Intra-cranial

Frontal lobe gliomas and other tumours	Paraoptic chiasma tumours
Midline cranial tumours	Aneurysms
Parasagittal meningiomas	Craniopharyngioma
Tumours of the corpus callosum	Pituitary tumours (esp. adenomas)
Olfactory groove/cribriform plate meningiomas	Suprasellar cholesteatoma
	Suprasellar meningioma
Osteomas	Temporal lobe tumours

Neoplasms – Intra-nasal

Neuro-olfactory tumours	Leukemic infiltration
Esthesioepithelioma	Nasopharyngeal tumours with extension
Esthesioneuroblastoma	
Esthesioneurocytoma	Neurofibroma
Esthesioneuroepithelioma	Paranasal tumours with extension
Other benign or malignant nasal tumours	
Adenocarcinoma	Schwannoma

Neoplasms – Extranasal and Extracranial

Breast	Lung
Gastrointestinal tract	Ovary
Laryngeal	Testicular

Neurologic

Amyotrophic Lateral Sclerosis	Familial dysautonomia
Alzheimer's disease	Guam ALS/PD/Dementia
Cerebral abscess (esp. frontal or ethmoidal regions)	Head trauma
	Huntington's disease
Down syndrome	Hydrocephalus

(Continued)

TABLE 110.1 *(Continued)* Reported agents, diseases, drugs, interventions and other aetiologic categories associated in the medical or toxicologic literature with olfactory dysfunction. Note that categories are not mutually exclusive

Neurologic

Korsakoff's psychosis	Syringomyelia
Migraine	Temporal lobe epilepsy
Meningitis	Hamartomas
Multiple sclerosis	Mesial temporal sclerosis
Myesthenia gravis	Scars/previous infarcts
Paget's disease	Vascular insufficiency/anoxia
Parkinson's disease	Small multiple cerebrovascular accidents
Refsum's syndrome	
Restless Leg Syndrome	Subclavian steal syndrome
Syphilis	Transient ischemic attacks

Nutritional/metabolic

Abetalipoproteinemia	Trace metal deficiencies
Chronic alcoholism	Copper
Chronic renal failure	Zinc
Cirrhosis of liver	Whipple's disease
Gout	Vitamin deficiency
Protein calorie malnutrition	Vitamin A
Total parenteral nutrition w/o adequate replacement	Vitamin B6
	Vitamin B12

Pulminary

Chronic obstructive pulminary disease

Psychiatric

Anorexia nervosa (severe stage)	Malingering
	Olfactory reference syndrome
Attention deficit disorder	Schizophrenia
Depressive disorders	Schizotypy
Hysteria	Seasonal affective disorder

In general, loss of olfactory function can be subdivided into two classes: (a) *conductive or transport impairments* from obstruction of the nasal passages (e.g., chronic nasal inflammation, polyposis, etc.); and (b) *sensorineural impairment* from damage to the olfactory neuroepithelium, central tracts, and connections (e.g., viruses, airborne toxins, tumours, seizures, etc.). In some circumstances, it is difficult to classify an olfactory disorder into one of these classes, since blockage of airflow to the receptors and damage to the receptors or other elements of the olfactory neuroepithelium can be simultaneously involved. Chronic rhinosinusitis, for example, can produce damage to the olfactory membrane in addition to blocking airflow, and altered membrane function can, over time, lead to degeneration within the olfactory bulb, a central structure. Although we are currently able to treat many causes of olfactory disturbance due to conductive factors or inflammation of the olfactory epithelium, most olfactory disorders due to sensorineural factors remain untreatable.

In most cases, hyperosmia reflects a patient's heightened response to an odour, rather than an increased ability to smell, *per se*. This problem has been reported in some conditions associated with a change in hormone balance, such as in pregnancy and Addison's disease (adrenal-cortical insufficiency), as well as head trauma, migraine, drug withdrawal, epilepsy (intericatal period), multiple-chemical sensitivity, and psychosis. While hyperosmia is relatively rare, dysosmia is more common. Usually dysosmia reflects dynamic alterations of degeneration or regeneration within the olfactory neuroepithelium over time, and it is not uncommon for patients who eventually develop anosmia to report having experienced weeks of dysosmia preceding the experience of anosmia. Dysosmia implies an olfactory system that is intact at least to some degree, as total smell loss does not typically accompany most cases of dysosmia.[1] Severely debilitating, long-lasting, and intractable chronic dysosmias have been treated by surgical ablation of regions of the olfactory neuroepithelium, or by surgical removal of a diseased olfactory bulb or bulbs.[31] Olfactory hallucinations or phantosmias can occur from a problem anywhere along the olfactory neural pathways, from the nose to the cortex. Sometimes they are associated with ictal epileptiform activity (e.g., simple partial seizures), nasal sinus disease (e.g., infection), and head trauma. If someone believes a smell is present (hallucination) and persistently gives this smell personal reference to outside events, despite contradicting evidence, this patient may suffer from *olfactory reference syndrome* – a depression-related disorder. In some cases, there may be a pathological correlate in the form of right hemispheric lesions.[32] Olfactory agnosia is an extremely rare phenomenon, although it appears to be less commonly investigated than visual and auditory agnosia. It is associated with lesions of the right inferior temporal lobe and often linked to prosopagnosia (agnosia for familiar faces).

The more common disorders or entities associated with olfactory impairment are discussed in more detail below, beginning with the more frequent ones.

Upper respiratory infection

Upper respiratory viruses, such as those associated with the common cold and influenza, are considered the most common aetiology of permanent olfactory loss in man. Other infectious causes that have been reported include hepatitis, herpes simplex encephalitis, and variant Creutzfeldt-Jacob disease. It is not clear what predisposes someone to viral-induced smell dysfunction or the precise mechanisms behind it. Often the smell-affecting respiratory illness is described as being more severe than usual. In a study of olfactory biopsies of 4 patients with anosmia and 11 patients with hyposmia due to a viral illness, Jafek and colleagues[33] noted that patients with anosmia had markedly reduced numbers of receptors and those receptors were abnormal compared to those patients with hyposmia. Given the ability of the olfactory neuron to regenerate, spontaneous recovery of some smell function is theoretically possible over a prolonged period; however, complete recovery is less likely the longer the patient has the loss and is likely inversely related to the degree of dysfunction. In general, it is necessary to exclude other aetiologies prior to making a diagnosis of post-viral anosmia. HIV-infected patients are said to show an early impairment in odour thresholds and a later decline in odour identification and discrimination function which appears to parallel a general reduction in cognitive abilities.[34]

Head trauma

Head trauma often results in smell loss, particularly where rapid acceleration/deceleration of the brain occurs (i.e. coup/contrecoup injury) (**Figure 110.4**). Blunt trauma to the occiput has been found to produce greater olfactory loss than trauma to the front of the head.[35] Following head trauma, the loss of smell is usually, but not always immediate, although it may take a while for the patient to recognize the presence of the dysfunction. In some cases, months can pass before the smell loss is apparent to the patient. Common mechanisms include disruption from shearing forces of the olfactory fila through the sinonasal tract, and direct contusion and ischaemia to the olfactory bulb and frontal and temporal poles. Fracturing of the cribriform plate is not a prerequisite for smell loss. The prevalence of olfactory loss following head trauma is around 15% and, on average, is proportional to the severity of the injury.[35, 36] As would be expected, such prevalence is much higher in patients referred to specialized smell and taste centres for evaluation and treatment. For example, among 268 patients evaluated at our centre who had experienced head trauma, 66.8% had anosmia, 20.5% hyposmia, and 13% had normal smell function. MRI images may reveal damage to the olfactory bulbs, tracts and areas of the temporal and frontal lobes.[36] Animal research shows that intra-cranial haemorrhage and ischaemia can lead to degeneration of the olfactory epithelium without transection of the olfactory nerves.[37] [Level 1 evidence] Iatrogenic trauma, such as surgery, can cause smell impairment and has been seen with such procedures as sinus surgery and laryngectomy.[38]

Nasal and sinus disease

While the olfactory impairment that follows a viral syndrome or head trauma can be classified as *sensorineural*, the dysfunction that results from nasal and sinus disease is usually considered *conductive* – in other words, there is impaired air flow to the olfactory receptors. Theoretically, any inflammatory or obstructive process in the nose can result in a disturbance of smell function, with common examples being allergic rhinitis, rhinosinusitis, nasal polyposis, intra-nasal tumours and previous nasal surgery. In the evaluation of 240 patients with allergic rhinitis, Rydzewski and colleagues found that 21.4% of patients had smell impairment and there was a significant correlation between olfactory thresholds and levels of eosinophils in the blood and nasal discharge.[39] Treatments in the form of surgery (e.g., excision of polyps) or medication (e.g., administration of topical or systemic steroids) may improve olfactory function in some cases; however, complete return is not typical. Thus, while chronic rhinosinusitis

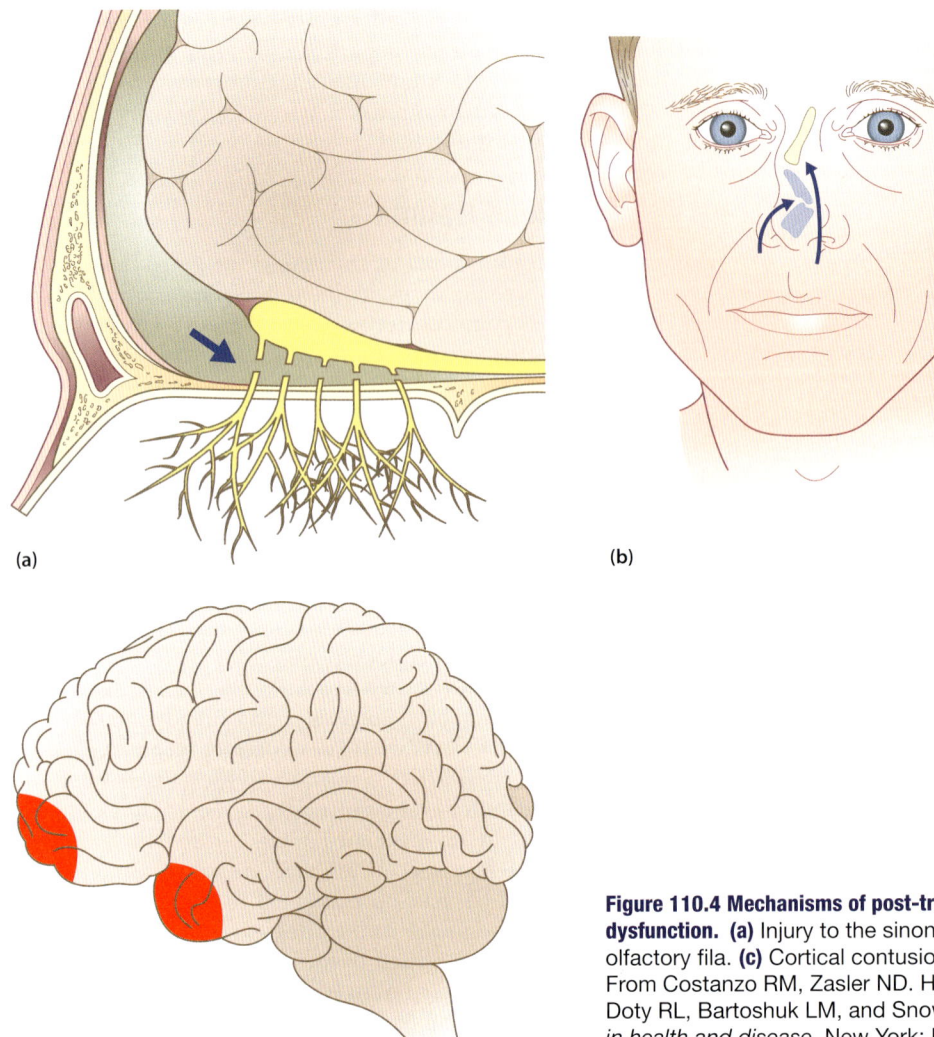

Figure 110.4 Mechanisms of post-traumatic olfactory dysfunction. (a) Injury to the sinonasal tract. **(b)** Tearing of the olfactory fila. **(c)** Cortical contusions and brain hemorrhage. From Costanzo RM, Zasler ND. Head trauma. In: Getchell TV, Doty RL, Bartoshuk LM, and Snow JB Jr (eds) *Smell and taste in health and disease*. New York: Raven Press, 1991, p. 713. Copyright © 1991 by Raven Press, Ltd.

can result in nasal airflow blockage, there is also a component of direct toxicity to olfactory neurons and impaired ciliary motility resulting in abnormal clearance of mucus. These combined factors make any one treatment modality limited. In one study, it was found that systemic steroids can temporarily reverse conductive olfactory impairment in 83% of patients while topical steroids helped in only 25% of patients – making systemic steroids a useful diagnostic tool.[40] The severity of histopathological changes within the olfactory mucosa of patients with chronic rhinosinusitis is positively related to the magnitude of olfactory loss, as measured by the UPSIT.[41] Biopsies from the neuroepithelial region of patients with nasal disease are less likely to yield olfactory-related tissue than biopsies from controls.[42] Anosmic rhinosinusitis patients generally exhibit a more pathological epithelium (e.g., disordered arrangement of cells and increased islands of respiratory epithelium) when compared to non-anosmic patients with rhinosinusitis.[43] Excessive dryness of the nasal mucosa – as seen in atrophic rhinitis, Sjögren's syndrome, and repeated nasal surgery – can cause olfactory dysfunction, since a moist receptor environment aids chemoreception and transduction.

Tumours and mass lesions

A number of tumours in and around the olfactory bulbs or tracts can cause olfactory disturbance. Examples include olfactory groove meningiomas, frontal lobe gliomas, and suprasellar ridge meningiomas arising from the dura of the cribriform plate. Due to the olfactory nerve's close location to the roof and medial wall of the orbit, as well as the optic nerves and tracts, structural lesions affecting smell may also affect vision. Also, olfactory tumours may extend into the frontal lobes resulting in symptoms of dementia and possibly the release of primitive reflexes (e.g., grasping, snout, and glabellar). Mass lesions need not be in the olfactory tracts to cause smell impairment. Ishimaru and colleagues[44] identified two patients with hyposmia from tumours to the right frontal lobe; the hyposmia reversed with craniotomy and tumour resection. Mass lesions around the olfactory region can result in a *Foster-Kennedy syndrome*, which consists of: (a) ipsilateral anosmia, (b) ipsilateral optic atrophy, and (c) contralateral papilledema secondary to raised intra-cranial pressure.[45] *Pseudo Foster-Kennedy syndrome* has been reported in patients with increased intra-cranial pressure who had previous unilateral optic atrophy.[46] Similarly, tumours in central regions of olfactory processing (e.g., mesial temporal lobe) can also potentially affect smell. Headache often accompanies a complaint of smell loss when the aetiology is a mass lesion. Lymphoma has been known to infiltrate into olfactory areas and cause dysfunction. Similarly, granulomatous diseases – such as syphilis, sarcoidosis, SLE, and Wegener's granulomatosis – often result in anosmia. In patients suspected of having a neoplasm, neuroimaging is essential.

Neurodegenerative diseases

Olfactory deficits have been described in a number of neurological disorders (Table 110.1). Importantly, olfactory dysfunction may be the first clinical sign of Alzheimer's disease (AD) and idiopathic Parkinson's disease (PD). Smell testing is useful in identifying persons who have PD, as well as those who either have, or are at risk for having, AD. In PD, bilateral olfactory deficits occur before the onset of most of the classical neurological signs and symptoms and are unrelated to disease stage, use of antiparkinson medications, duration of the illness, and severity of the symptoms, such as tremor, rigidity, bradykinesia or gait disturbance.[5, 6] Measurement of smell function can be useful to distinguish PD among the other disorders that share many non-olfactory symptoms and signs, such as progressive supranuclear palsy, multiple-system atrophy, parkinsonism induced by the proneurotoxin 1-methyl-4-phenyl-1,2,3,6-tetrahydropyridine (MPTP), and essential tremor.[6, 20] In a male patient suspected of PD, based on history and physical who is less than 60 years of age, an UPSIT score of 31 carries a 91% sensitivity and 88% specificity of correctly diagnosing patient suspected of having PD.[6] In a woman suspected of PD, who is less than 60 years old, an UPSIT score of 33 carries a 79% sensitivity and 85% specificity.[6]

With regard to AD, Graves and colleagues[47] found that olfactory dysfunction in the presence of one or more APOE-e4 alleles was associated with a very high risk of subsequent cognitive decline, and smell testing identified persons who came to exhibit later cognitive decline better than did a global cognitive test. Devanand and colleagues[48] found that patients with mild cognitive impairment scored lower on the UPSIT than did the controls, and that patients with low UPSIT scores (<34) were more likely to develop AD than the other patients. When low UPSIT scores were accompanied by a lack of awareness of olfactory deficits on the part of the patients, they found that this predicted the time to development of AD. UPSIT scores from 30 to 35 showed moderate to strong sensitivity and specificity for diagnosis of AD at follow-up. In later life, individuals with Down syndrome show similar clinical and pathological changes to AD patients and have lower performance on a modified UPSIT compared to controls matched on mental age. However, it is not clear whether this is due to AD-related pathology, *per se*, as Down syndrome children as young as 12 years old exhibit smell dysfunction.[49] [Level 1 evidence]

The olfactory loss associated with multiple sclerosis is directly proportional to the number of MS-related demyelinating lesions in central brain regions associated with olfactory processing (e.g., inferior middle temporal lobe and periorbital frontal cortex).[50] [Level 1 evidence] Olfactory function actually increases and decreases as the plaque numbers increase and decrease.[51] Therefore, knowledge of a patient's UPSIT score largely predicts the plaque load in the olfaction-related regions. [Level 1 evidence]

Schizophrenia is associated with significant deficits in olfactory threshold sensitivity and odour identification.[52] [Level 1 evidence] The fact that there is an inverse correlation with UPSIT scores and disease progression suggests that there may be progressive neurodegenerative changes within olfactory-related pathways and smell testing can be used as a marker of disease progression.[52]

Epilepsy and migraine

Olfactory auras, also described as hallucinations, are rare but frequently associated with seizures and headaches. Olfactory auras consist of sudden unexplained sensations of smell that are usually unpleasant (although not always) and are rarely isolated events.[53] In epilepsy, mesial temporal lobe structures involved in the usual processing of odour information – such as the amygdala and hippocampus – have been implicated as the generators of ictal olfactory sensations (simple or complex partial seizures) that often evolve into secondarily generalized seizures.[54] Common aetiologies include mesial temporal sclerosis and tumours.[54] Some cases of epilepsy have been associated with hyperosmia during the inter-ictal period, although most patients with long-standing epilepsy and intractable seizure activity, such as candidates for temporal lobe resection, are hyposmic.[53] The effect of migraine on smell function is less understood. The concept of certain smells provoking or exacerbating a migranous headache – osmophobia – may exist similar to that of photophobia or phonophobia.

Other causes and considerations

Less than 5% of patients who present to a specialized centre for smell and taste disorders have a chemosensory disturbance that can be directly attributed to an exposure of a toxic compound.[1] There are numerous chemical agents that have been reported to affect smell function, including acrylates, cadmium, benzene, formaldehyde, solvents and nickel dust, among others (Table 110.1).[55] Tobacco smoking results in diminished olfactory ability as a function of cumulative smoking dose, and importantly, smoking cessation can result in improvement in olfactory function over time.[25] Medications are also a common cause of smell disturbance and should be considered early, especially in the context of a new drug therapy (Table 110.1).[56]

Several endocrine disorders evidence disorders of smell. For example, Kallmann's syndrome, or hypogonadotropic hypogonadism, is an X-linked or autosomal recessive neuronal migrational disorder associated with anosmia

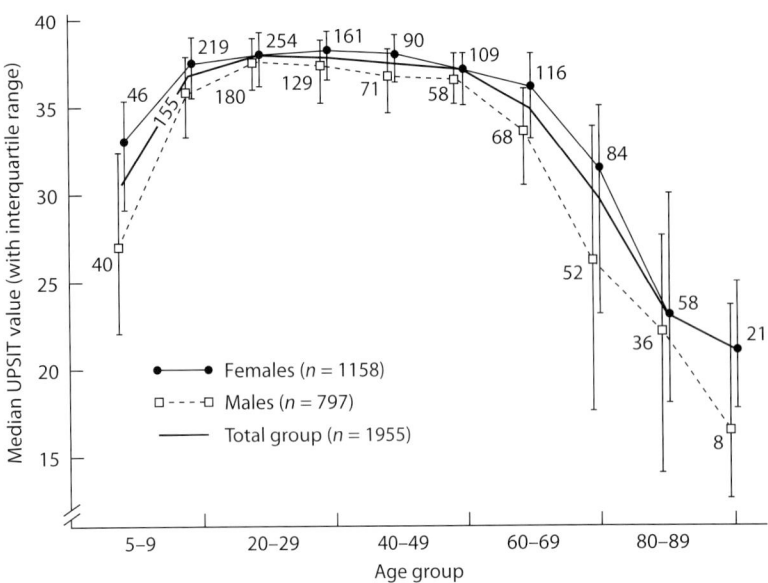

Figure 110.5 **Scores on the University of Pennsylvania Smell Identification Test (UPSIT) as a function of age and gender in a large heterogeneous group of subjects.** Numbers by data points indicate sample sizes. From Doty RL, Shaman P, Applebaum SL, et al. Smell identification ability: changes with age. *Science* 1984; **226**: 1441–3. Copyright © 1984 by the American Association for the Advancement of Science.

(aplasia of the olfactory bulb) and hypogonadism (pituitary involvement). [**Level 1 evidence**] Similarly, patients with septo-optic dysplasia (de Morsier's syndrome) can have hyposmia, visual symptoms, and precocious puberty.

Age-related deficits in smell function are well documented and decreased smell function is present in most elderly patients, including ones who are healthy and taking no medications (**Figure 110.5**).[57] Under the age of 65 years, approximately 1% of the population has major difficulty smelling. Between 65 and 80 years, this increases remarkably, with about half of the population exhibiting at least some decrement in the ability to smell. Over the age of 80, this figure rises to nearly 75%.[54] Despite the association with age, the complaint of smell loss should never be attributed simply to age, as often an accumulation of damage over the years is the culprit and a single event, such as a bad cold, can be the precipitating factor. In general, the age-related changes in smell function are reflected not only in damage to the olfactory receptors but related decreases in number of glomeruli within the olfactory bulb.[58] Whether age-related factors increase the susceptibility of the epithelium to damage from exogenous agents is not clear. What is clear, however, is that smell loss in older persons adversely affects the quality of life. Chemosensory loss has been implicated as a cause – particularly in the elderly – of malnutrition, weight loss, and worsening of a medical illness.

TREATMENT OF SMELL DISORDERS

The most effective treatments available are those for *conductive* anosmia, where there is an obstruction of airflow through the nose to the olfactory neuroepithelium. As noted above, the typical causes of mechanical obstruction include nasal sinus disease, including inflammation, and intra-nasal neoplasms. After diagnosis is confirmed using tools such as nasal endoscopy and CT scanning of the sinuses, the next appropriate course of action may include topical or systemic steroids. Conductive and sensorineural olfactory loss are often distinguishable using a brief course of systemic steroid therapy since patients with conductive impairment often respond positively to the treatment, although long-term systemic steroid therapy is not advised. Topical nasal steroids are often ineffectual in returning smell function because the steroid fails to reach the affected regions in the upper nasal passages. Increased efficacy presumably occurs when the nasal drops or spray are administered in the head-down Moffett's position.[40] Proper allergy management is essential and may require the use of an antihistamine. When a bacterial infection is suspected (e.g., infectious sinusitis), a course of antibiotics should be used. Surgery should be considered for: (1) very large and medically-refractory polyps; or (2) situations where a malignant neoplasm is suspected. Importantly, pre- and post-intervention olfactory testing should be performed to establish intervention efficacy, as well as to screen for subsequent slow relapse that is characteristic of most conductive disorders. In cases where rheumatological granulomatous disease is suspected, such as Wegener's granulomatosis or sarcoidosis, further immunomodulation using agents such as cyclophosphamide or methotrexate may be necessary.

Sensorineural impairment of olfaction is typically more difficult to manage, and the prognosis for patients suffering from long-standing total loss due to upper respiratory illness or head trauma is poor. The majority of patients who recover smell function subsequent to trauma do so within 12 weeks of injury.[35] Patients who quit smoking typically have dose-related improvement in olfactory function and flavour sensation over time.[25] Central lesions, such as CNS tumours that impinge on olfactory bulbs and tracts can often be resected with significant improvement in olfactory function. When epilepsy or migraine is suspected, a course of anti-epileptic or anti-migraine medications might prove beneficial. Medically-refractory epilepsy resulting in olfactory disturbance can be successfully treated with surgery. For example, Chitanondh[59] reported successful treatment of 7 patients with seizure disorder, olfactory hallucinations, and psychiatric problems by stereotactic amygdalotomy, concluding 'stereotactic amygdalotomy has a dramatic effect on olfactory seizures, auras, and hallucinations. It is a safe surgical procedure and can be done without neurological deficit'. In patients with multiple sclerosis, immunomodulatory therapies, including interferon beta and occasional steroids, is the mainstay of treatment. When depression or psychosis is suspected, a course of an anti-depressant and appropriate psychiatric referral may be necessary.

Medications that induce distortions of olfaction can often be discontinued and replaced with other types of medications or modes of therapy. In addition to direct effects on the olfactory system, the side-effects of many medications is to detrimentally dry the nasal mucosa (e.g., anti-cholinergics). Dopaminergic and cholinergic therapies do not improve the olfactory dysfunction seen in Parkinson's disease, and there is no evidence that neuroleptics alter the olfactory loss of patients with schizophrenia. Despite the fact there are advocates for zinc and vitamin therapies, there continues to be no strongly compelling evidence that these therapies work except in cases where frank zinc or vitamin deficiencies exist.

In patients with complete anosmia, supportive measures are necessary to protect them from further harm; thus

- Smoke and carbon monoxide detectors need to be installed and properly working
- When possible, electric appliances should be used instead of gas appliances
- Expiration dates for food products should be scrutinized and old food items checked by someone with normal smell function or discarded
- A balanced diet – particularly in the elderly – must be kept to prevent weight loss and malnutrition. Adding flavour enhancers (e.g., monosodium glutamate, food colouring, chicken or beef stock) to foods can also help with their appeal.

A physician needs to be cognizant of medicolegal ramifications in his or her evaluation and management. In cases of personal injury malingering is not uncommon, and may be distinguished from true anosmia by the pseudo-disappearance of trigeminal function or unusually low UPSIT test scores (i.e., those below chance responding), suggesting active avoidance of the correct answer. When queried on a standardized questionnaire, malingerers were found to minimize factors that might be otherwise associated with their chemosensory complaint. For example, relative to non-malingerers, malingerers reported significantly fewer allergies, dental problems, cigarettes smoked, surgical operations, nasal sinus problems, and use of medications. They also reported significantly more putative symptom-related psychological duress, interference with daily activities, weight loss, decreased appetite, and taste loss. Litigation involvement was found to be higher in malingerers than non-malingerers. Age, sex, education, and length of written symptom descriptions did not differentiate malingerers from non-malingerers.[27]

PROGNOSIS

Spontaneous recovery of function appears to vary depending on the severity of the disturbance. Thus, for patients whose odour identification ability is less severe (e.g., UPSIT scores above 25), prognosis for complete recovery is much better than for those with complete anosmia. In one study, for example, odour identification tests were administered to 542 patients complaining of smell dysfunction on two occasions separated from one another by 3 months to 24 years.[60] The percentage of anosmic and microsmic patients exhibiting statistically significant change in function, as defined by 4 UPSIT points, was 56.72% and 42.86%, respectively. However, only 11.31% of anosmic and 23.31% of microsmic patients regained normal age-related function over time. Age, severity of initial olfactory loss, and the duration of dysfunction at the first test occasion were significant predictors of the amount of change. Interestingly, aetiology, sex, time between the two test administrations, and initial smoking behaviour were not strong predictors.

Given such factors, an important part of management for many patients is to use quantitative olfactory testing and establish the true degree of olfactory loss so that some

---

FUTURE RESEARCH

In general, the medical community needs to become better educated regarding the importance of the chemical senses for the well-being and everyday function of human beings, and to realize that accurate assessment of these senses is critical for (a) establishing the validity of a patient's complaint, (b) distinguishing between complaints of taste and olfactory dysfunction, and (c) monitoring the efficacy of treatment regimens. The basis of the olfactory loss in the earliest stages of a number of neurodegenerative disorders, including Alzheimer's disease and idiopathic Parkinson's disease, needs elucidation, as gene therapy and other therapeutic modes may be of future value in reversing not only the olfactory dysfunction, but other elements of these diseases. There is dire need to establish the mechanisms involved in olfactory cell degeneration and regeneration, as well as in the production of appositional bone growth in the region of the foramina of the cribriform plate, which may be an age-related process. A greater understanding of these and related phenomena, such as the nature of inflammation associated with rhinosinusitis, may ultimately lead to topical or systemic treatments that can mitigate smell dysfunction secondary to damage to the olfactory receptor cells or closure of the foramina of the cribriform plate.

estimate or prognosis can be given. Importantly, age- and sex-related normative data allows one to put into perspective a patient's overall problem. For example, many older patients find it rather therapeutic to know that, while his or her smell function is not what it used to be, it still falls above the average of his or her peer group.

> **KEY POINTS**
>
> - The olfactory system contributes significantly to a person's quality of life.
> - A patient's lack of olfactory function can be an early sign of a number of serious disease states, including nasopharyngeal carcinoma, Alzheimer's disease, Parkinson's disease, frontal meningiomas, multiple sclerosis, and sinus infections.
> - Too patent an airway, as seen with excessive turbinate removal, can improperly shunt air away from the olfactory cleft, resulting in at least some decrement in olfactory acuity.
> - A significant amount of retronasal airflow from the nasopharynx occurs during swallowing and deglutition. This retronasal route is vital to the production of flavour from swallowed foods – adding *smell* to both *taste* and *touch*.
> - Throughout life, islands of respiratory-like epithelial metaplasia appear within the epithelium, presumably as a result of cumulative viral, bacterial, and other insults.
> - The number of olfactory receptor cells exceeds that of any other sensory system except vision; collectively, the surface area of the cilia is quite large – exceeding 20 cm^2 in the human.
> - The olfactory nerve cells, as well as the proximal extraneural spaces, can serve as conduits for the movement of viruses and exogenous agents from the nasal cavity into the brain.
> - It is essential to determine all medications used by the patient since many reportedly cause smell and taste disturbance.
> - Several standardized and practical psychophysical tests have been developed over the last several years, including a number of brief self-administered tests ranging from the 3-item Pocket Smell Test™ to the 40-item University of Pennsylvania Smell Identification Test or UPSIT.
> - The majority of cases of presumably permanent chronic anosmia or hyposmia are due to prior upper respiratory infections, head trauma, and nasal and paranasal sinus disease – most causes reflecting permanent damage to the olfactory neuroepithelium.
> - A number of tumours in and around the olfactory bulbs or tracts can cause olfactory disturbance.
> - Olfactory deficits have been described in a number of neurological disorders. Importantly, olfactory dysfunction may be the first clinical sign of Alzheimer's disease (AD) and idiopathic Parkinson's disease (PD).
> - The olfactory loss associated with multiple sclerosis is directly proportional to the number of MS-related demyelinating lesions in central brain regions associated with olfactory processing (e.g., inferior middle temporal lobe and periorbital frontal cortex).
> - Schizophrenia is associated with significant deficits in olfactory threshold sensitivity and odour identification.
> - Under the age of 65 years, approximately 1% of the population has major difficulty smelling. Between 65 and 80 years, this increases remarkably, with about half of the population exhibiting at least some decrement in the ability to smell. Over the age of 80, this figure rises to nearly 75%.
> - *Sensorineural* impairment of olfaction is typically more difficult to manage, and the prognosis for patients suffering from long-standing total loss due to upper respiratory illness or head trauma is poor.

ACKNOWLEDGEMENTS

This contribution was supported, in part, by the following grants: PO1 DC 00161, RO1 DC 04278, RO1 DC 02974, RO1 AG 17496, and USAMRAA W81XWH-09-1-0467.

REFERENCES

1. Deems DA, Doty RL, Settle RG, et al. Smell and taste disorders: a study of 750 patients from the University of Pennsylvania Smell and Taste Center. *Arch Otolaryngol Head Neck Surg* 1991; **117**: 519–28.
2. Van Toller S. Assessing the impact of anosmia: review of a questionnaire's findings. *Chemical Senses* 1999; **24**: 705–12.
3. Devanand DP, Lee S, Manly J, et al. Olfactory identification deficits and increased mortality in the community. *Ann Neurol* 2015; **78**: 401–11.
4. Hoffman HJ, Ishii EK, Macturk RH. Age-related changes in the prevalence of smell/taste problems among the United States adult population: results of the 1994 disability supplement to the National Health Interview Survey (NHIS). *Ann NY Acad Sci* 1998; **855**: 716–22.
5. Mesholam, RI, Moberg, PJ, Mahr, RN, Doty, RL. Olfaction in neurodegenerative disease: a meta-analysis of olfactory functioning in Alzheimer's and Parkinson's diseases. *Arch Neurol* 1998; **55**: 84–90.
6. Doty RL, Bromley SM, Stern MB. Olfactory testing as an aid in the diagnosis of Parkinson's Disease: development of optimal discrimination criteria. *Neurodegeneration* 1995; **4**: 93–7.
7. Zhao K, Frye RE. Nasal patency and the aerodynamics of nasal airflow in relation to olfactory function. In: Doty RL (ed) *Handbook of olfaction and gustation*. 3rd ed. Hoboken: John Wiley & Sons, 2015, pp. 355–74.
8. Clerico DM, To WC, Lanza DC. Anatomy of the human nasal passages. In: Doty RL (ed). *Handbook of olfaction and gustation*. New York: Marcel Dekker; 2003, pp. 1–16.
9. Moran DT, Jafek B, Rowley JC. The ultrastructure of the human olfactory musoca. In: Laing DG, Doty RL, Breipohl W (eds). *The human sense of smell*. New York: Springer-Verlag; 1991, 3–28.
10. Scherer PW, Hahn II, Mozell MM. The biophysics of nasal airflow. *Otolaryngol Clin North Am* 1989; **22**: 265–78.
11. Leopold DA. The relationship between nasal anatomy and function, *Laryngoscope* 1988; **98**: 1232–8.
12. Schneider RA, Wolf S. Relation to olfactory acuity to nasal membrane function. *J Appl Physiol* 1960; **15**: 914–20.
13. Doty RL, Mishura A. Olfaction and its alteration by nasal obstruction, rhinitis, and rhinosinusitis, *Laryngoscope* 2001; **11**: 409–23.
14. Huard JM, Youngentob SL, Goldstein BL, et al. Adult olfactory epithelium contains mutipotent progenitors that give rise to neurons and non-neural cells. *J Comp Neurol* 1998; **400**, 469–86.

15. Doty RL. Olfaction. *Ann Rev Psychol* 2001; **52**: 423–52.
16. Buck L, Axel R. A novel multigene family may encode odorant receptors: a molecular basis for odor recognition. *Cell* 1991; **65**: 175–87.
17. Berkowicz DA, Trombley PQ. Dopaminergic modulation at the olfactory nerve synapse. *Brain Res* 2000; **855**: 90–9.
18. Firestein S. How the olfactory system makes sense of scents. *Nature* 2001; **413**: 211–18.
19. Shepherd GM, Firestein S. Toward a pharmacology of odor receptors and the processing of odor images. *J Ster Biochem Mol Biol* 1991; **39**: 583–92.
20. Doty, RL. The olfactory vector hypothesis of neurodegenerative disease: is it viable? *Ann Neurol* 2008; **63**: 7–15.
21. Ennis M, Holy TE. Anatomy and neurobiology of the main and accessory olfactory bulbs. In: Doty RL (ed) *Handbook of olfaction and gustation*, 3rd ed. Hoboken: John Wiley and Sons, 2015; pp. 157–82.
22. Gloor P. *The temporal lobe and the limbic system*. New York: Oxford University Press; 1: 273–323.
23. Doty RL, Bromley SM, Moberg PJ, Hummel T. Laterality in human nasal chemoreception. In: S. Christman (ed.), *Cerebral asymmetries in sensory and perceptual processing*. New York: Elsevier Science B.V; 1997, pp. 497–542.
24. Shear PK, Butters N, Jernigan TL, et al. Olfactory loss in alcoholics: correlations with cortical and subcortical MRI indices. *Alcohol* 1992; **9**: 247–55.
25. Frye RE, Schwartz BS, Doty RL. Dose-related effects of cigarette smoking on olfactory function. *JAMA* 1990; **263**: 1233–6.
26. *Physicians' Desk Reference*. 54th ed. Montvale, NJ: Medical Economics Company, Inc., 2000: 1–3355.
27. Doty RL, Crastnopol B. Correlates of chemosensory test malingering. *Laryngoscope* 2010; **8**: 707–11.
28. Doty RL, McKeown DA, Lee WW, Shaman P. A study of the test-retest reliability of ten olfactory tests. *Chem Senses* 1995; **20**: 645–56.
29. Doty RL. *The Smell Identification Test™ administration manual.* 3rd ed. Haddon Hts., NJ: Sensonics, Inc., 1995: pp. 1–57.
30. Doty RL. *The Smell Threshold Test™ administration manual.* Haddon Hts., NJ: Sensonics, Inc., 2000: pp. 1–18.
31. Leopold DA, Loehrl TA, Schwob JE. Long-term follow-up of surgically treated phantosmia. *Arch Otolayngol Head Neck Surg* 2002; **128**: 642–7.
32. Devinsky O, Khan S, Alper K. Olfactory reference syndrome in a patient with partial epilepsy. *Neuropsychiatry Neuropsychol Behav Neurol* 1998; **11**: 103–5.
33. Jafek BW, Hartman D, Eller PM, et al. Postviral olfactory dysfunction. *Am J Rhinol* 1990; **4**: 91–100.
34. Mueller C, Temmel AF, Quint C, et al. Olfactory function in HIV-positive subjects. *Acta Otolaryngol* 2002; **122**: 67–71.
35. Doty RL, Yousem DM, Pham LT, et al. Olfactory dysfunction in patients with head trauma. *Arch Neurol* 1997; **54**: 1131–40.
36. Yousem DM, Geckle RJ, Bilker WB, et al. Posttraumatic olfactory dysfunction: MR and clinical evaluation. *Amer J Neuroradiol* 1996; **17**: 1171–9.
37. Nakashima T, Kimmelman CP, Snow B Jr. Progressive olfactory degeneration due to ischemia. *Surgical Forum* 1983; **34**: 566–8.
38. van Dam FS, Hilgers FJ, Emsbroek G, et al. Deterioration of olfaction and gustation as a consequence of total laryngectomy. *Laryngoscope* 1999; **109**(7 Pt 1): 1150–5.
39. Rydzewski B, Pruszewicz A, Sulkowski WJ. Assessment of smell and taste in patients with allergic rhinitis. *Acta Otolaryngol* 2000; **120**: 323–6.
40. Seiden AM, Duncan HJ. The diagnosis of a conductive olfactory loss. *Laryngoscope* 2001; **111**: 9–14.
41. Kern RC. Chronic sinusitis and anosmia: pathologic changes in the olfactory mucosa. *Laryngoscope* 2000; **110**: 1071–7.
42. Feron F, Perry C, McGrath JJ, Mackay S. New techniques for biopsy and culture of human olfactory epithelial neurons. *Arch Otolaryngol Head Neck Surg* 1998; **124**: 861–6.
43. Lee SH, Lim HH, Lee HM, et al. Olfactory mucosal findings in patients with persistent anosmia after endoscopic sinus surgery. *Ann Otol Rhinol Laryngol* 2000; **109**: 720–5.
44. Ishimaru T, Miwa T, Nomura M, et al. Reversible hyposmia caused by intracranial tumor. *J Laryngol Otol* 1999; **113**: 750–3.
45. Watnick RL, Trobe JD. Bilateral optic nerve compression as a mechanism for the Foster-Kennedy syndrome. *Ophthalmology* 1989; **96**: 1793–8.
46. Schatz NJ, Smith JL. Non tumor causes of the Foster Kennedy syndrome. *J Neurosurg* 1967; **27**: 37–44.
47. Graves AB, Bowen JD, Rajaram L, et al. Impaired olfaction as a marker for cognitive decline: interaction with apolipoprotein E epsilon4 status. *Neurology* 1999; **53**: 1480–7.
48. Devanand DP, Michaels-Marston KS, Liu X, et al. Olfactory deficits in patients with mild cognitive impairment predict Alzheimer's disease at follow-up. *Amer J Psychiat* 2000; **157**: 1399–405.
49. McKeown DA, Doty RL, Perl DP, et al. Olfactory function in young adolescents with Down's syndrome. *J Neurol Neurosurg Psychiat* 1996; **61**: 412–14.
50. Doty RL, Li L, Mannon LJ, Yousem, DM. Olfactory dysfunction in multiple sclerosis. *N Eng J Med* 1997; **336**: 1918–19.
51. Doty RL, Li C, Mannon LJ, Yousem DM. Olfactory dysfunction in multiple sclerosis: relation to longitudinal changes in plaque numbers in central olfactory structures. *Neurology* 1999; **53**: 880–2.
52. Moberg PJ, Doty RL, Turetsky BI, et al. Olfactory identification deficits in schizophrenia: correlation with duration of illness. *Am J Psychiatry* 1997; **154**: 1016–18.
53. West SE, Doty RL. Influence of epilepsy and temporal lobe resection on olfactory function. *Epilepsia* 1995; **36**: 531–42.
54. Acharya V, Acharya J, Luders H. Olfactory epileptic auras. *Neurology* 1998; **51**: 56–61.
55. Doty RL, Hastings L. Neurotoxic exposure and olfactory impairment. *Clin Occupat Environ Med* 2001; **1**: 547–75.
56. Ackerman BH, Kasbekar N. Disturbances of taste and smell induced by drugs. *Pharmacotherapy* 1997; **17**: 482–96.
57. Doty RL, Shaman P, Applebaum SL, et al. Smell identification ability: changes with age. *Science* 1984; **226**: 1441–3.
58. Meisami E, Mikhail L, Baim D, Bhatnagar KP. Human olfactory bulb: aging of glomeruli and mitral cells and a search for the accessory olfactory bulb. *Ann NY Acad Sci* 1998; **855**: 708–15.
59. Chitanondh H. Stereotaxic amygdalotomy in the treatment of olfactory seizures and psychiatric disorders with olfactory hallucination. *Confinia Neurologica* 1966; **27**: 181–96.
60. London B, Nabet B, Fisher AR, et al. Predictors of prognosis in patients with olfactory disturbance. *Ann Neurol* 2008; **63**: 159–66.

CHAPTER 111

DISORDERS OF THE ORBIT

Nithin D. Adappa and James N. Palmer

Introduction 1243	Endoscopic orbital decompression 1247
Relevant surgical anatomy 1243	Optic nerve compression 1248
Endoscopic dacrocystorhinostomy 1245	Conclusion 1251
Thyroid eye disease 1246	References 1251

SEARCH STRATEGY

Data in this chapter may be updated by a Medline search using the keywords: orbital anatomy; nasolacrimal system; epiphora; endoscopic dacrocystorhinostomy; thyroid eye disease; Graves' ophthalmopathy; orbital decompression; optic nerve decompression; silent sinus syndrome; orbital pseudotumor; orbital neoplasm; and orbital tumour. The evidence in this chapter is mainly levels 3 and 4. The clinical recommendations are predominantly B and C.

INTRODUCTION

Given its intimate relationship to the paranasal sinuses, a thorough understanding of the orbit is essential for the otorhinolaryngologist. We are faced with a wide variety of orbital conditions due to the general proximity of the sinonasal cavity as well as the surgical corridor the sinuses provide (**Box 111.1**). The most common conditions include epiphora, thyroid eye disease, optic nerve compression, imploding maxillary sinus, pseudotumor, and orbital neoplasms.

BOX 111.1 Differential diagnosis of orbital pathology

Infectious
- Bacterial
- Fungal

Inflammatory
- Graves' orbitopathy
- Granulomatous disease
- Pseudotumor

Neoplastic
- Benign
  - Fibro-osseous
  - Neural
  - Vascular
- Malignant
  - Lymphoma
  - Epithelial
  - Non-epithelial
  - Metastatic

Traumatic

Other
- Epiphora

RELEVANT SURGICAL ANATOMY

Orbital anatomy

The orbit is a quadrilateral pyramid, with its base facing forwards, laterally and slightly inferiorly (**Figure 111.1**). The orbit contains the globe, extraocular muscles, nerves, vessels and other associated structures including the lacrimal apparatus. The average volume in the adult Caucasian orbit is 30 ml.[1] The orbit receives contribution from 7 distinct bones: maxillary, zygomatic, ethmoid, lacrimal, sphenoid, frontal, and palatine bones all of which make unique contributions to each orbital wall.

Medial wall

The medial wall is most relevant to otorhinolaryngologists due to the proximity of the paranasal sinuses. From an anterior to posterior direction, the boney contribution of anterior lacrimal crest originates at the frontal process of the maxilla. The lacrimal bone makes up the second one half of the lacrimal sac fossa and the posterior lacrimal crest. The lamina papyracea (arising from ethmoid bone) makes up the majority of the medial orbital wall. The paper-thin bone overlies the ethmoid sinuses.[2] The anterior and posterior ethmoid foramina are found in the superior aspect of the orbit along the fronto-ethmoidal suture line. The anterior ethmoid foramen is a useful

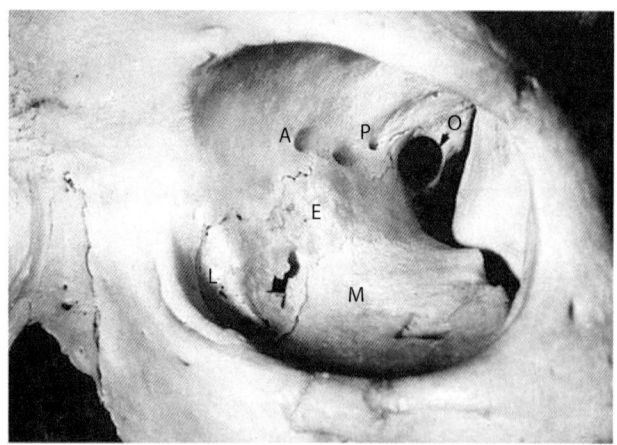

Figure 111.1 The orbit. A, anterior ethmoidal foramen, P, posterior ethmoidal foramen, O, optic canal, E lamina papyracea, M, maxilla, L, lacrimal bone.

landmark and is identified 20–25 mm posterior to the anterior lacrimal crest and the posterior ethmoid foramen is 30–35 mm posterior to the anterior lacrimal crest.[3] The thick bone of the sphenoid body forms the most posterior portion of the medial orbital wall adjoining the optic canal.

Superior wall

The roof of the orbit is formed primarily by the frontal bone.[2] The superior margin has a supraorbital notch or foramen with its respective nerves and vessels.[4] The trochlea is a connective tissue sling anchoring the tendinous portion of the superior oblique muscle to the orbital wall and the trochlear fovea, a small depression lying close to the superomedial orbital margin.[4]

Inferior wall

The floor is formed by the orbital surface of the maxilla, the zygomatic and the palatine bone. At approximately the midpoint of the orbit floor runs the infraorbital groove containing the maxillary division of the trigeminal nerve (V2) leading to the infraorbital foramen. Medial to the infraorbital nerve, the orbital floor is relatively thin and fractures more easily than the lateral aspect.[4]

Lateral wall

The zygomatic process of the frontal bone, the orbital surface of the zygoma and the greater wing of the sphenoid form the lateral wall. These bones join at the zygomaticosphenoid suture line, creating the thickest bony wall. The lateral tendons all attach to the lateral tubercle, which is found 3–4 mm posterior to the lateral orbital rim.[4]

Orbital contents

The orbit is lined by the fibrous periorbita. It is attached to bone at the orbital margin, suture lines, the trochlear fossa, fissures, the lateral tubercle, the anterior lacrimal crest, and perforating vascular foramina. Other than these locations, the periorbita is loosely attached and easily dissected. The globe and other orbital tissue structures are surrounded by orbital fat, which cushions the globe and facilitates in orbital movement. This is further aided by orbital connective tissue septae that slide over each other for smooth movement.[5]

Nasolacrimal system

The nasolacrimal drainage system consists of the superior and inferior canaliculi which feed into the common canaliculus, lacrimal sac and subsequently the nasolacrimal duct.[6] The system begins at the punctum of each eyelid where the canaliculi initially run at 90° to the lid margin for 1–2 mm before running parallel with the lid margin. After 10 mm they join to form the common canaliculus. The common canaliculus angles inferiorly and forward for 3–5 mm before entering the lacrimal sac. The nasolacrimal duct exits from the inferior portion of the lacrimal sac and continues in an inferior direction for approximately 12 mm before entering the nose 10–15 mm behind the anterior end of the inferior turbinate and 16 mm above the floor of the nasal cavity at Hasner's valve. The lacrimal bone that attaches inferiorly with the base of the inferior turbinate forms the posterior wall of the bony canal and the frontal process of the maxilla forms its anterior boundary.

The lacrimal sac is protected in the concavity of the lacrimal fossa of the medial orbital wall. The fossa is formed anteriorly by the harder frontal process of the maxillary bone and posteriorly by the softer lacrimal bone. The frontal process forms the anterior lacrimal crest and the remainder of the anterior portion of the fossa.

Epiphora

Epiphora from nasolacrimal system obstruction is either anatomic (70%) or functional (30%).[7] This includes complete blockages anywhere from the lacrimal punctum to the nasal cavity. Functional obstructions, on the other hand, are a result of either significant narrowing within the lacrimal system that delays normal lacrimal flow or a failure of the lacrimal pumping mechanism. Dacrocystorhinostomy (DCR) is performed to relieve epiphora resulting from an obstruction of the nasolacrimal system.

The majority of nasolacrimal system obstruction is unknown. Idiopathic obstruction is seen more frequently with increasing age and demonstrates a female preponderance. Less common causes include surgical trauma, facial trauma, granulomatous conditions such as Wegener's granulomatosis and sarcoidosis, malignancy, infections, and radiation exposure. It should be noted that while a significant number of patients suffer nasolacrimal injury after FESS (up to 15%), actual obstruction resulting in epiphora is very rare.[8]

ENDOSCOPIC DACROCYSTORHINOSTOMY

Indications

A DCR is indicated when there is a symptomatic distal obstruction of the nasolacrimal duct that is not relieved by probing and syringing. It is not indicated when the obstruction is in the canaliculi or puncti as the endoscopic DCR will not bypass these areas.

Pre-operative evaluation and studies

A thorough history and physical examination is essential to aid in identification of the site of obstruction. The patient should be questioned on history of radiation, neoplasm, midface trauma, systemic diseases, sinonasal disease and ocular conditions.

Syringing and probing the nasolacrimal system can aid in identification of the site of obstruction. Inability to flush through the inferior canaliculus indicates obstruction at the site of the punctum or inferior canaliculus whilst reflux of saline through the other canaliculus indicates a distal obstruction. Probing with a Bowman lacrimal probe also helps identify the level of obstruction. Nasal endoscopy is also useful to exclude anatomic abnormalities that may interfere with an endoscopic approach.

An ophthalmologist will often perform a fluorescein dye disappearance test in the office. Fluorescein is applied to the eye and after 10–15 minutes a bluelight filter is used to attempt to identify fluorescein runoff into the nose. Radiographic tests include a dacryocystogram, which can identify diverticula, stenosis, strictures, dacryoliths or a tumour. Dacryoscintigraphy uses radionucleotide. ^{99m}Tc also may be helpful when identifying for a functional obstruction when there is free flow on a syringe test along with an abnormal fluorescein dye disappearance test. Computed tomography (CT) is generally not indicated unless there is suspicion for neoplastic etiology or history of midface trauma requiring further evaluation.

Surgical procedure

Create a posteriorly based mucosal flap

The initial goal is to expose the lacrimal bone and frontal process of the maxilla. Initially a superior incision should be made horizontally 10 mm above the axilla of the middle turbinate. This incision should extend from 2–3 mm posterior to the axilla and run forwards for approximately 10 mm onto the frontal process of the maxilla. The blade should then be turned vertically and a cut made on the frontal process of the maxilla from the superior incision to just above the insertion of the inferior turbinate. Finally, a cut is made horizontally and the inferior mucosal incision made form the insertion of the uncinate to join the vertical incision.

Elevation of the mucosal flap

Elevation is best accomplished with a suction freer. It is critical to stay on the bone to avoid losing the surgical plane in the transition from the hard bone of the frontal process of the maxilla to the softer lacrimal bone (**Figure 111.2**).

Remove lacrimal bone

A round otologic knife can be used to flake off the lacrimal bone overlying the posterior portion of the lacrimal sac.

Removal of frontal process of the maxilla

This bone is much harder and overlies the anterior aspect of the lacrimal sac. This can be accomplished with a kerrison punch or a DCR drill bur. The sac should be exposes fully by removing all bone up to the mucosal incisions. The sac will form a prominent bulge into the nasal cavity (**Figure 111.3**).

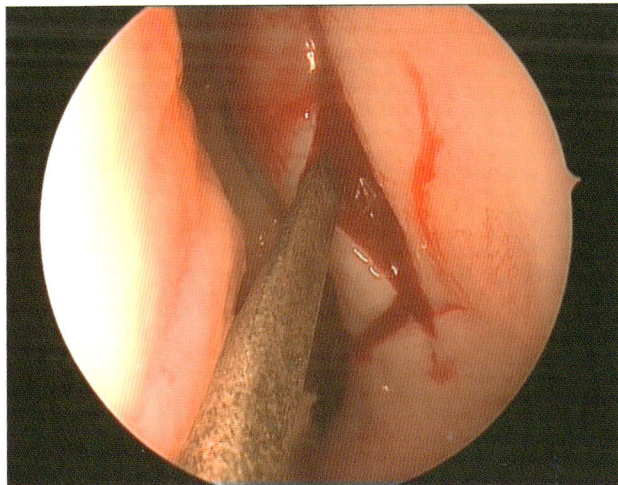

Figure 111.2 Elevation of posteriorly based mucosal flap over left nasolacrimal crest.

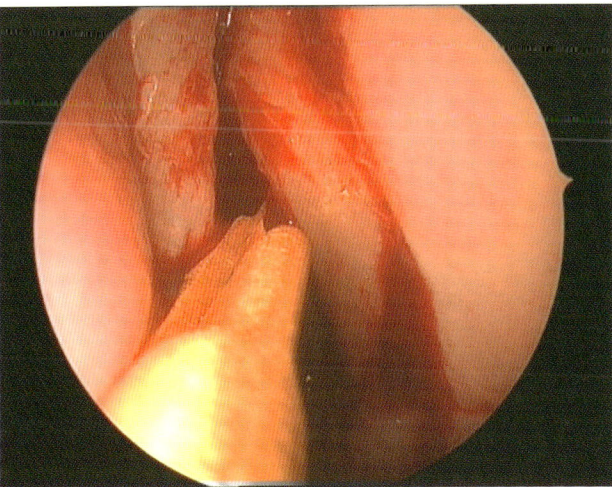

Figure 111.3 Resection of left anterior lacrimal crest with kerrison punch.

Expose the agger nasi cell

By exposing the agger nasi cell, the mucosa of the lacrimal sac will be able to lie against the mucosa of the agger cell, allowing for a wider marsupialization of the lacrimal sac.

Marsupialize the lacrimal sac

Insert a lacrimal probe through the inferior canaliculus (**Figure 111.4**) and tent the lacrimal sac up with the probe. Make a vertical incision with two subsequent horizontal incisions on the superior and inferior portion of the sac to create the widest possible anterior and posterior flaps. Once the sac is marsupialized, it should be lying flat on the lateral nasal wall (**Figure 111.5**).

Reposition the mucosal flap

Cut the mucosal flap so only a superior and inferior limb are present and reapproximate this over the bone at the bone–lacrimal sac junction at both the superior and inferior aspects of the lacrimal sac flaps.

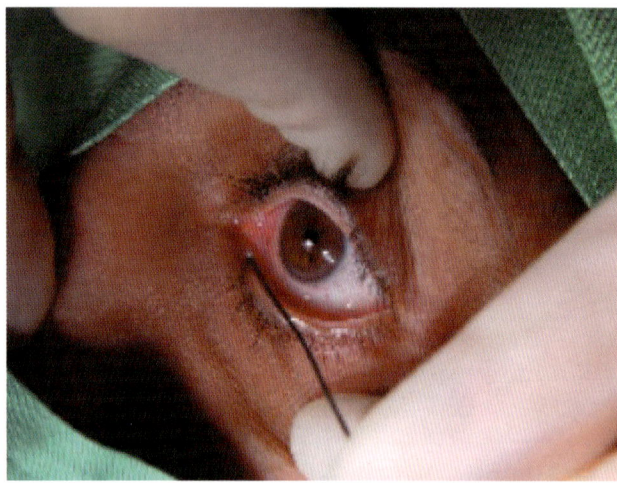

Figure 111.4 Probing of the inferior canaliculus.

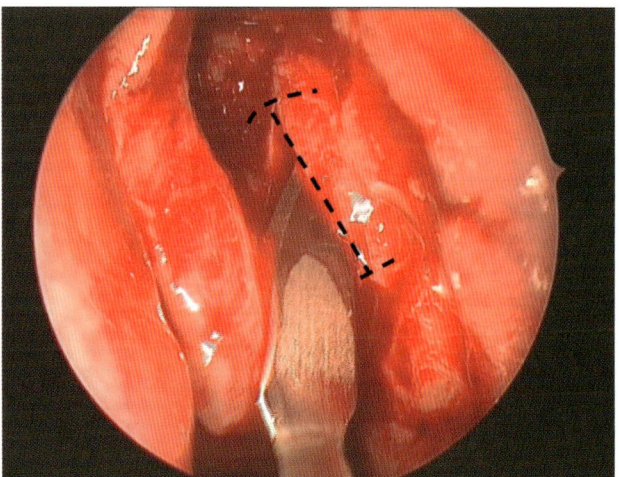

Figure 111.5 Incision of the left lacrimal sac. Then create an anterior and posterior flap, incisions should be made along the dotted lines.

Pass the Crawford silastic tubes

The lacrimal tubes are inserted into the superior and inferior punctae and passed into the nasal cavity. They can be secured by tying the tubes together. Place a small piece of gelfoam along the mucosal flaps to hold them in place.

Post-operative management

Patients are discharged on saline sprays, 7 day course of oral antibiotics, and topical antibiotic eye drops for 2 weeks. Patients are endoscopically evaluated with removal of crusting at 2 weeks. Crawford tubes are removed at 4–6 weeks and the lacrimal system is checked for patency using the fluorescein dye disappearance test.

Complications

Complications demonstrated in endoscopic DCR are similar to those reported in endoscopic sinus surgery including epistaxis, occurring in 2% of patients.[9, 10] Other possible complications of the procedure include obstruction and subsequent rhinosinusitis of the frontal or maxillary sinus, orbital penetration with damage to the extraocular muscles, cerebrospinal fluid leak and orbital haematoma.

THYROID EYE DISEASE

Introduction

Thyroid eye disease (Graves' ophthalmopathy) is an incompletely understood autoimmune disease with infiltration of T lymphocytes and macrophages into the orbital tissue as well as an increased glycosaminoglycan deposition with subsequent enlargement of orbital fat and extraocular muscles.[1, 11, 12] The increased volume in the fixed boney orbit impairs venous drainage resulting in chemosis and periorbital edema. This ultimately leads to increased retrobulbar pressure and enlargement of extraocular muscles potentially leading to loss of vision. The increased volume may result in significant proptosis and possible globe subluxation, exposure keratitis, or corneal ulceration. Approximately 50% of patients who have thyroid eye disease will develop orbital manifestations.[13]

Thyroid eye disease has two phases; an inflammatory phase and a burnt-out phase. The inflammatory phase typically lasts from 6 months to 3 years. During this phase, inflammation, fibrosis, and adipogenesis occur resulting in the changing ocular findings.[14] The burnt-out phase is defined as a period of disease where the ocular findings do not progress during a minimum of 6 months.

Conservative treatment options include eye lubrications, eyelid taping, and patching for the patients with dryness and diplopia, as well as controlling thyroid function. In the inflammatory stage, corticosteroids, immunosuppressants, orbital irradiation, and surgical decompression may also be necessary to improve symptoms and reduce optic nerve compression. Subsequently, in the burnt-out stage, lid surgery, strabismus surgery, and orbital decompression may be required.[14]

ENDOSCOPIC ORBITAL DECOMPRESSION

Indications

Indications for orbital decompression include compressive optic neuropathy, exposure keratitis, diplopia, and cosmesis. Both external and intra-nasal decompression has previously been described. Otorhinolaryngologists typically perform an endoscopic approach only or in conjunction with other approaches.

Pre-operative evaluation and studies

Given the wide variety of procedures possible with varying degrees of decompression, careful discussion with the ophthalmology team is critical for understanding the degree of decompression necessary. In general an endoscopic decompression is indicated for patients with moderate to severe thyroid eye disease. It may be performed in conjunction with an open approach for the orbital floor and lateral wall if further decompression is necessary. The procedure is generally utilized for thyroid orbitopathy but can also be used as a corridor to gain access to orbital tumours, biopsy of indeterminate orbital lesions, or palliative therapy for malignant tumours causing visual symptoms.[15]

A complete ophthalmology examination is necessary prior to the procedure. This includes evaluation of the degree of proptosis, assessment of eye movements and diplopia, measurement of visual acuity, and colour vision. Pre-operative consent must include discussion of risks including permanent double vision and need for strabismus surgery.

A CT scan evaluating the orbits and sinuses is required to review relevant anatomy. Typical findings include a greater than two-fold enlargement of extraocular muscle bodies, sparing the tendinous portions. The medial and inferior rectus muscles are most commonly involved although all muscles may be enlarged (**Figure 111.6**).[16] The surgeon should identify the middle turbinate attachment, location and course of the anterior ethmoid artery, and the presence of an onodi cell as the optic nerve may course through the lateral aspect of the cell.

Surgical procedure

Perform a maxillary antrostomy, complete ethmoidectomy and sphenoidotomy

During sinus surgery, it is important to completely resect the uncinate process. In addition, we advocate resection of the middle turbinate for improved exposure and decreased risk of adhesions. During dissection, special attention should be made to identify all ethmoid cells have been removed along the lamina papyracea. The maxillary antrostomy should be as large as possible to allow for ideal exposure during decompression.

Resection of medial orbital wall bone

The orbital wall should be penetrated in a controlled fashion. Typically a j-curette or Freer elevator can be used. Care should be taken to perform this gently to avoid

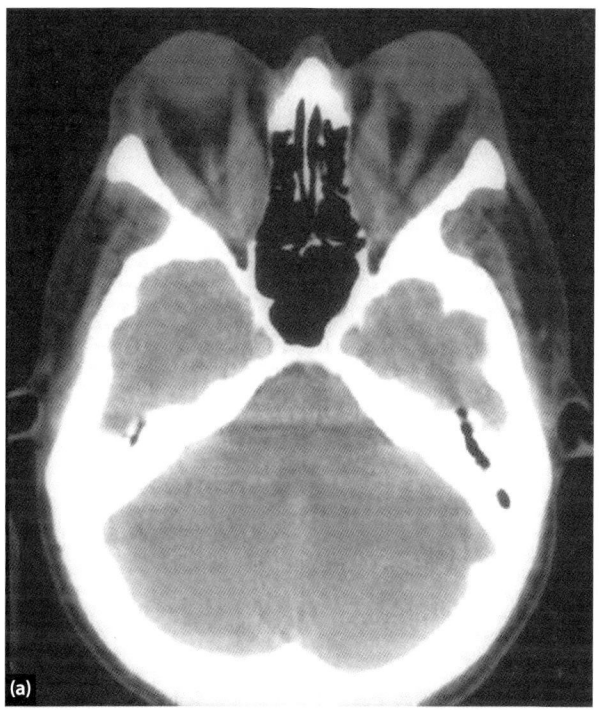

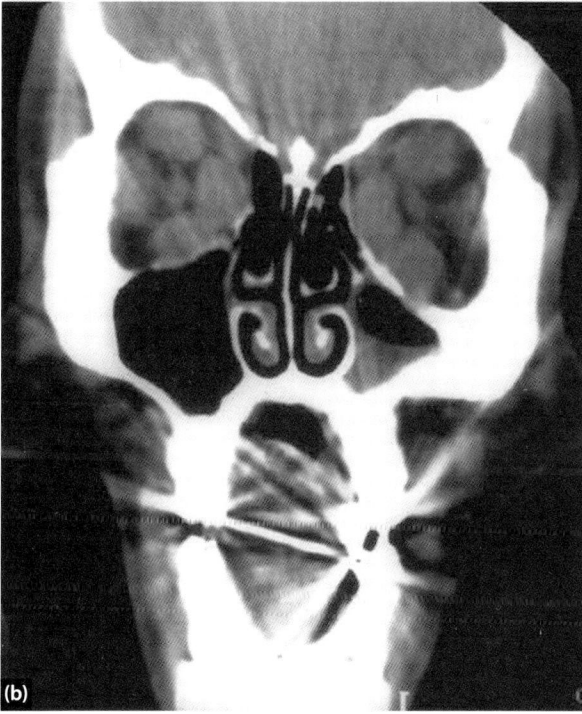

Figure 111.6 (a) Axial and **(b)** coronal CT scans in thyroid eye disease showing the classical 'Coca Cola' bottle sign of auto-decompression (axial) and compression of orbital apex due to enlarged extraocular muscles.

trauma to the periorbita. The fragments can be freed from the periorbita with the j-curette or Freer elevator and subsequently removed with Blakesley forceps. Take care not to penetrate the periorbita at this time as prolapsing fat will make surgery more difficult. All bone should be resected superiorly up to the ethmoid roof, inferiorly to the orbital floor, anteriorly to the maxillary line and posteriorly to the face of the sphenoid sinus. Care should be taken when removing bone superiorly to avoid skull base injury that may produce either a cerebrospinal fluid leak or ethmoidal vessel injury.

Down fracture of the orbital floor

Start by elevating the periorbita off the medial orbital floor. Use a spoon curette to down fracture the medial aspect of the orbital floor. The bone of the orbital floor is significantly thicker than the medial orbital wall and requires increased force. The bone often fractures in one large piece at the infraorbital canal junction. Note that if the down fracturing is not performed bilaterally, there is an increased risk for post-operative diplopia, especially in the horizontal plane.

Incision of periorbita

The incision should begin at the posterior limit of the decompression and follow a posterior to anterior direction to prevent prolapsing orbital fat from obstructing visualization. A series of parallel incisions should be made in this fashion. In patients without optic neuropathy, a fascial sling can be left in place overlying the medial rectus to prevent diplopia.[17] A curved seeker can be used to gently dissect the remaining fibrous bands between fat lobules.

Prolapse of orbital fat into maxillary and ethmoid sinuses

If done completely, a significant amount of fat will prolapse in the sinuses. The eye may be balloted to confirm fat herniation and allow further prolapse.

Post-operative considerations

It is critical prior to extubation and in the immediate post-operative period to have a clear discussion with the anaesthesia team. This potentially will avoid aggressive post-extubation mask ventilation, which can result in orbital subcutaneous emphysema. Expect large amounts of post-operative swelling, oedema, and erythema. Our patients are typically observed overnight and discharged on broad-spectrum antibiotics and instructed to start nasal irrigations. Patients should avoid nose blowing for 2 weeks to prevent subcutaneous emphysema or even prolapse of the globe.

Results

Post-operative diplopia is frequently encountered with 15–63% of post-operative patients reporting new-onset or worsening diplopia.[15, 18–22] In most cases, this is temporary and resolves spontaneously over weeks to months. Strabismus surgery will be considered in 8–10 months following decompression if diplopia persists.

The average ocular recession from endoscopic decompression ranges from 3.2–5.1 mm reduction of proptosis with an inferior and medial wall decompression.[17, 19, 23] Concurrent lateral decompression provides an additional 2 mm of recession.[19] Post-operative deterioration of visual acuity is demonstrated in less than 5% of patients.[24–26]

OPTIC NERVE COMPRESSION

Optic nerve compression is a rare entity requiring decompression. The optic nerve may be decompressed for a number of indications.

Endoscopic optic nerve decompression

Traumatic optic neuropathy is the most common indication for endoscopic or open optic nerve decompression.

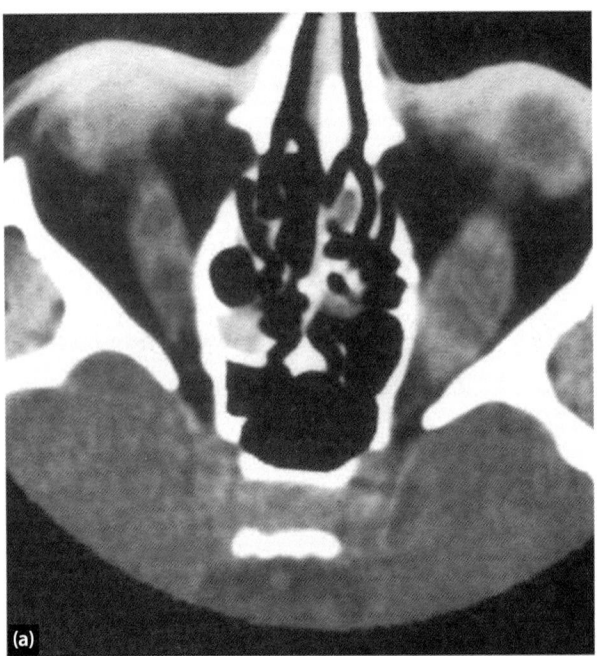
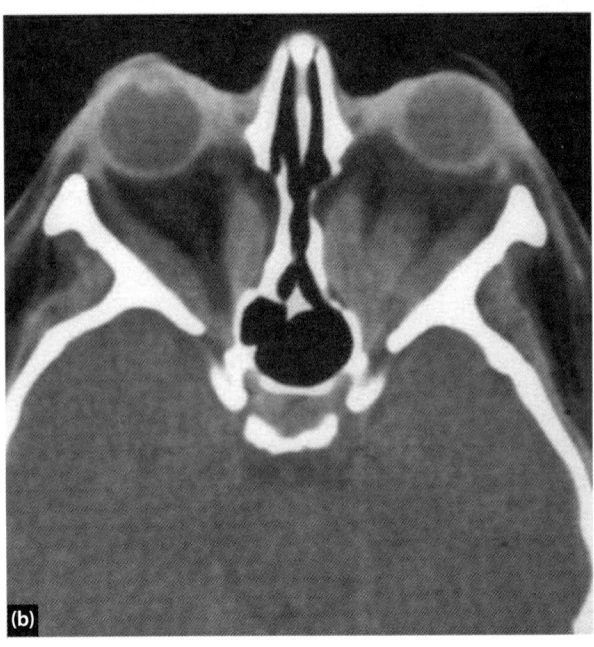

Figure 111.7 (a) Axial and **(b)** coronal CT scans of patient with thyroid eye disease before and after endoscopic decompression.

Unfortunately, success rates are limited for this procedure.[27–30] Traumatic optic neuropathy was initially felt to be secondary to vascular compromise from external compression resulting in injury to the optic nerve. More recent investigation has favoured the theory that manual compression results in a conduction block and focal demyelination leading to compressive optic neuropathy.[31]

Benign or malignant tumours of the skull base can occasionally compress the orbital apex. Meningiomas of the skull base, in particular, produce a hyperostotic reaction with mass effect from the soft tissue component that may directly impact the orbital apex. Benign fibro-osseous lesions or sinonasal tumours can in a similar fashion result in compression of the apex or the optic nerve itself.

Many different approaches have been described for optic nerve decompression including transorbital, transantral, extra-nasal transethmoid, intra-nasal microscopic, and craniotomy approaches. We believe the endonasal approach is superior as it offers a number of advantages over other approaches such as preservation of olfaction, quick recovery period, lack of external scars, and excellent intra-operative visualization. However, the ideal approach should be dictated by the pathology and its location.

PRE-OPERATIVE CONSIDERATIONS AND STUDIES

A thorough ophthalmologic history and physical examination should be performed. A fine cut CT scan of the sinuses and orbit should be evaluated for optic canal compression, fracture, or bone displacement and sinus anatomy for endoscopic considerations. An MRI of the orbits should also be considered for evaluation of the optic nerve and orbital contents.

PROCEDURE

Perform a complete ethmoidectomy and sphenoidotomy

Pay special attention to removing all boney partitions off the lamina papyracea. Additionally, open up the sphenoidotomy maximally, especially laterally. Identify the optic nerve, carotid artery and the opticocarotid recess (**Figure 111.8**). Image guided surgery is ideally employed here.

Fracture the lamina papyracea in posterior ethmoid region

As in orbital decompression, eggshell fracture and remove bone of the lamina in the posterior ethmoids. Again, pay special care not to penetrate the periorbita.

Drill down the bone of the optic strut

Use a diamond drill with copious irrigation to avoid thermal injury to the optic nerve. Drill along the nerve, not across it. As the bone thins, gently flake it away. The amount of decompression depends on the pathology. For cases of traumatic optic neuropathy and thyroid eye disease, the optic nerve should be decompressed for a distance of 1 cm posterior to the face of the sphenoid sinus (**Figure 111.9**).[32] Further decompression of the nerve can

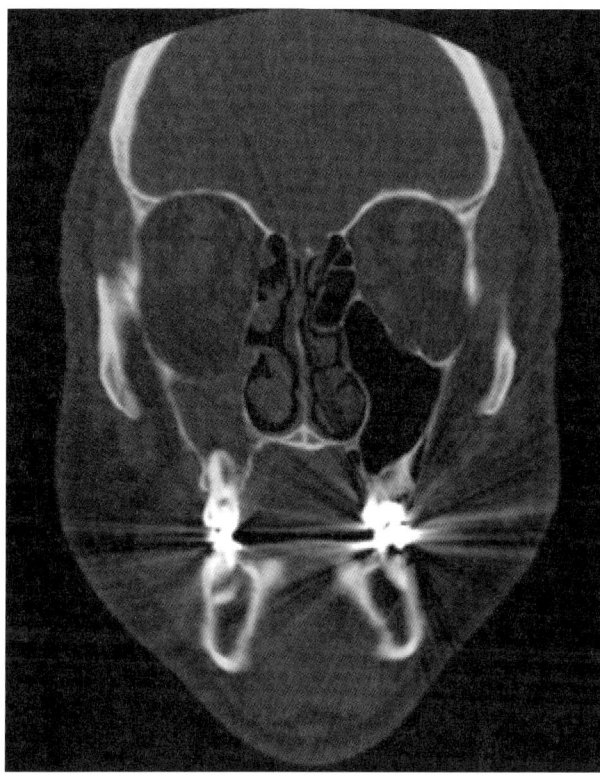

Figure 111.8 Silent sinus syndrome with inferior collapse of orbital floor associated with maxillary sinus outflow obstruction.

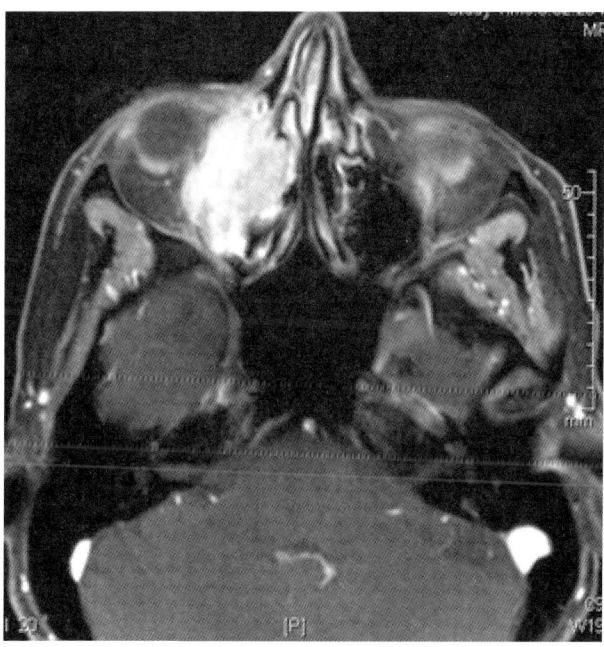

Figure 111.9 Axial T1-weighted post-contrast MRI demonstrating a large infiltrative orbital mass. It was initially reported to be an aggressive malignant neoplasm. Subsequent biopsy demonstrated orbital pseudotumor.

be created with incision of the sheath itself. If this is to be performed, the incision should be in the superomedial quadrant as the ophthalmic artery may lie in the inferiomedial quadrant of the optic nerve sheath in approximately 15% of cases.[33] The incision should be made from a posterior to anterior direction and which includes the release of the tendinous ring of Zinn. Be prepared for a possible CSF leak which can be closed with a mucosal flap.

POST-OPERATIVE CONSIDERATIONS

Close communication with the ophthalmologic team is critical. They will aid in serial eye examination and help guide the generally required high dose oral steroids. Additionally, antibiotics and gentle saline rinses are recommended. To minimize intra-conal pressures, nasal packing is not utilized following the procedure, and the patient should be instructed on avoiding nose blowing and straining post-operatively.

Imploding maxillary sinus

Imploding maxillary sinus or silent sinus syndrome is believed to originate from obstruction of the osteomeatal complex of the paranasal sinuses leading to hypoventilation of the maxillary sinus. This enclosed cavity in certain settings is thought to undergo air resorption, thus creating a suction effect of subatmospheric pressure within the maxillary antrum.[34-36] The development of a pressure vacuum within the sinus, in turn, results in the accumulation of mucous into the antrum, subclinical inflammation and eventual collapse of the maxillary sinus through attenuation of the maxillary bony side walls. The hallmark of the disease is lack of traditional chronic sinusitis symptoms. Instead patients present with enopthalmos, occasionally with double vision as well.

Diagnosis is typically confirmed though CT imaging, demonstrating maxillary atelectasis and decreased height of the orbital floor (**Figure 111.8**). Treatment for imploding maxillary sinusitis is correcting the underlying pressure system of the maxillary sinus. Although historically this was done with a Caldwell-Luc, it is now treated with an endoscopic maxillary antrostomy. Depending on the severity of bone resorption, the patient may also require surgical intervention to restore height to the orbital floor. This can be done as a single procedure or in a staged fashion.

Orbital pseudotumor

Orbital pseudotumor, or idiopathic orbital inflammation, is a diagnosis of exclusion. The exact etiology of this condition is unclear, but it should be in the differential diagnosis of orbital pathology as it comprises 10% of orbital lesions.[37] The clinical signs include proptosis, diplopia, pain, eyelid swelling, ptosis and chemosis. Similar lesions can arise elsewhere in the head and neck including the pterygopalatine and infratemporal fossae.

Pseudotumor presents as a nonspecific orbital mass on CT and/or MRI (**Figure 111.9**).[37] Diagnosis is one of exclusion, most commonly ruling out lymphoma. Most clinicians should have a low threshold for biopsy if the clinical course is not typical of pseudotumor. Histology generally demonstrates polymorphous inflammatory infiltration of T and B cells, plasma cells, eosinophils, neutrophils and a variable degree of fibrous tissue proliferation.[38]

Treatment of orbital pseudotumor is typically medical, most commonly with oral steroids, but is also treated with radiotherapy, chemotherapy or immunosuppression for refractory cases. Surgical intervention is only considered to establish a diagnosis, or for emergent treatment of compressive symptoms as a temporizing measure.

Orbital neoplasms

Orbital neoplasms can broadly be divided into benign and malignant lesions. Otorhinolaryngologists participate as part of a multidisciplinary team in treatment. Benign neoplasms most commonly consist of fibro-osseous lesions, neural lesions, and vascular lesions, while malignant neoplasms are generally divided into epithelial, non-epithelial, lymphoma, and metastatic.

Benign neoplasm

FIBRO-OSSEOUS LESIONS

Benign fibro-osseous lesions affecting the optic nerve and orbit are similar to lesions dealt with in the paranasal sinuses. These lesions are primarily fibrous dysplasia, ossifying fibromas, and osteomas. Fibrous dysplasia is either monostotic or polyostotic fibrous dysplasia (**Figure 111.10**). Asymptomatic lesions are observed with surveillance imaging. Those resulting in orbital or optic nerve compression require surgical intervention. Conversely, ossifying fibromas are aggressive and can be locally destructive, in these cases, early resection

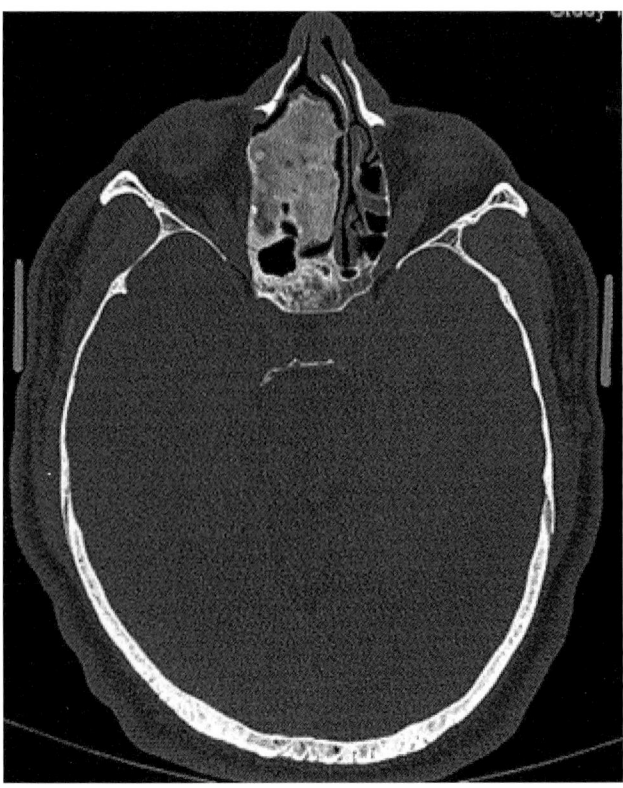

Figure 111.10 Axial CT scan with right-sided fibrous dysplasia with encroachment of the optic nerve.

is recommended. Finally, osteomas are benign, osseous lesions presenting with slow growth. They have an increased incidence along the frontoethmoidal suture line and accordingly may encroach on the orbit. Similar to fibrous dysplasia, if asymptomatic, these can be observed with surveillance imaging.

NEURAL

Neural-derived neoplasms of the orbit and orbital apex most commonly consist of gliomas, neurofibromas, schwannomas, and meningiomas. As with most orbital lesions, presentation is dependent on tumour pathology and position within the orbit. Neurofibromas and schwannomas tend to present more anteriorly within the orbit, and meningiomas and gliomas are often retrobulbar. Optic nerve meningiomas are of special significance as removal or even biopsy of these lesions can cause damage to the blood supply of the optic nerve resulting in visual loss. Typically optic nerve meningiomas are treated conservatively unless the patient develops visual loss.

VASCULAR

Vascular lesions include lymphangioma, orbital varices and arteriovenous malformations. Complete surgical resection for vascular lesions is often not feasible, but orbital apical decompression often may plays a role in management. Non-encapsulated lesions, or lesions that infiltrate critical orbital structures should only be decompressed if they are causing optic neuropathy.

Malignant neoplasms

EPITHELIAL

Primary epithelial tumours of the orbit are very rare. When present, they generally involve the lacrimal gland. Lacrimal gland tumours range from pleomorphic adenoma to aggressive neoplasms such as adenoid cystic and squamous cell carcinoma.[39] Open surgical resection is often the treatment of choice as endoscopic access with clear margins is often challenging.

NON-EPITHELIAL

The most common non-epithelial neoplasm is rhabdomyosarcoma. It typically presents in childhood and should be considered on the differential in any child presenting with progressive proptosis. Other sarcomas such as liposarcoma and leiomyosarcoma, although rare, can present in the orbit.

LYMPHOMA

Lymphoma typically presents as a painless enlarging mass. Surgical intervention, as with lymphoma of other areas, consists of biopsy only. Ultimate treatment depending on tumour type and stage consists of radiation therapy and/or chemotherapy.[39]

METASTATIC

Metastatic neoplasm must be considered in the differential for any orbital lesion. The most common are neuroblastoma, leukaemia, breast carcinoma, lung carcinoma, and prostate carcinoma.

CONCLUSION

Otorhinolaryngologists must have a thorough understanding of the wide variety of pathology that occurs in the orbit due to the close proximity of the paranasal sinuses. This is relevant both in terms of paranasal sinus involvement of orbital lesions as well as treatment corridors through the nose. Most of these lesions are best treated by a multidisciplinary team for optimal outcomes.

KEY POINTS

- A thorough understanding of the orbital anatomy is essential for otorhinolaryngologists given the close proximity to the paranasal sinuses.
- Optimal results in endoscopic DCR require both knowledge the site of obstruction as well as optimal surgical steps to ensure patency.
- Traumatic optic neuropathy is the most common indication for endoscopic optic nerve decompression. Unfortunately, success rates are limited for this procedure.
- There is a wide variety of orbital neoplasms and accurate diagnosis and workup are necessary to identify the correct treatment plan.
- Treatment of orbital pathology requires a close working relationship between ophthalmologists and otorhinolaryngologists.

REFERENCES

1. Gorman CA. Pathogenesis of Graves' ophthalmopathy. *Thyroid* 1994; **4**: 379–83.
2. Moore KL. *Clinically oriented anatomy*. 6th ed: Lippincott Williams & Wilkins; 2010.
3. Rontal E, Rontal M, Guilford FT. Surgical anatomy of the orbit. *Ann Otol Rhinol Laryngol* 1979; **88**: 382–6.
4. Rene C. Update on orbital anatomy. *Eye* 2006; **20**: 1119–29.
5. Koornneef L. New insights in the human orbital connective tissue: result of a new anatomical approach. *Arch Ophthalmol* 1977; **95**: 1269–73.

6. Chastain JB, Sindwani R. Anatomy of the orbit, lacrimal apparatus, and lateral nasal wall. *Otolaryngol Clin North Am* 2006; **39**: 855–64.
7. Wormald PJ, Kew J, Van Hasselt A. Intranasal anatomy of the nasolacrimal sac in endoscopic dacryocystorhinostomy. *Otolaryngol Head Neck Surg* 2000; **123**: 307–10.
8. Bolger WE, Parsons DS, Mair EA, Kuhn FA. Lacrimal drainage system injury in functional endoscopic sinus surgery. Incidence, analysis, and prevention. *Arch Otolaryngol Head Neck Surg* 1992; **118**: 1179–84.
9. Tsirbas A, Wormald PJ. Mechanical endonasal dacryocystorhinostomy with mucosal flaps. *Otolaryngol Clin North Am* 2006; **39**: 1019–36.
10. Wormald PJ. Powered endoscopic dacryocystorhinostomy. *Otolaryngol Clin North Am* 2006; **39**: 539–49.
11. Pletcher SD, Sindwani R, Metson R. Endoscopic orbital and optic nerve decompression. *Otolaryngol Clin North Am* 2006; **39**: 943–58.
12. Weetman AP, Cohen S, Gatter KC, et al. Immunohistochemical analysis of the retrobulbar tissues in Graves' ophthalmopathy. *Clin Exp Immunol* 1989; **75**: 222–7.
13. Eckstein AK, Johnson KT, Thanos M, et al. Current insights into the pathogenesis of Graves' orbitopathy. *Horm Metab Res* 2009; **41**: 456–64.
14. Leung MK, Platt MP, Metson R. Revision endoscopic orbital decompression in the management of Graves' orbitopathy. *Otolaryngol Head Neck Surg* 2009; **141**: 46–51.
15. Metson R, Shore JW, Gliklich RE, Dallow RL. Endoscopic orbital decompression under local anesthesia. *Otolaryngol Head Neck Surg* 1995; **113**: 661–7.
16. Jelks GW, Jelks EB, Ruff G. Clinical and radiographic evaluation of the orbit. *Otolaryngol Clin North Am* 1988; **21**: 13–34.
17. Metson R, Samaha M. Reduction of diplopia following endoscopic orbital decompression: the orbital sling technique. *Laryngoscope* 2002; **112**: 1753–7.
18. Eloy P, Trussart C, Jouzdani E, et al. Transnasal endoscopic orbital decompression and Graves' ophthalmopathy. *Acta Otorhinolaryngol Belg* 2000; **54**: 165–74.
19. Metson R, Dallow RL, Shore JW. Endoscopic orbital decompression. *Laryngoscope* 1994; **104**: 950–7.
20. Michel O, Bresgen K, Russmann W, et al. Endoscopically-controlled endonasal orbital decompression in malignant exophthalmos. *Laryngorhinootologie* 1991; **70**: 656–62.
21. Shepard KG, Levin PS, Terris DJ. Balanced orbital decompression for Graves' ophthalmopathy. *Laryngoscope* 1998; **108**: 1648–53.
22. Wright ED, Davidson J, Codere F, Desrosiers M. Endoscopic orbital decompression with preservation of an inferomedial bony strut: minimization of post-operative diplopia. *J Otolaryngol* 1999; **28**: 252–6.
23. Wee DT, Carney AS, Thorpe M, Wormald PJ. Endoscopic orbital decompression for Graves' ophthalmopathy. *J Laryngol Otol* 2002; **116**: 6–9.
24. Goldberg RA, Shorr N, Cohen MS. The medical orbital strut in the prevention of postdecompression dystopia in dysthyroid ophthalmopathy. *Ophthal Plast Reconstr Surg* 1992; **8**: 32–4.
25. Schaefer SD, Soliemanzadeh P, Della Rocca DA, et al. Endoscopic and transconjunctival orbital decompression for thyroid-related orbital apex compression. *Laryngoscope* 2003; **113**: 508–13.
26. Unal M, Leri F, Konuk O, Hasanreisoglu B. Balanced orbital decompression combined with fat removal in Graves ophthalmopathy: do we really need to remove the third wall? *Ophthal Plast Reconstr Surg* 2003; **19**: 112–18.
27. Kountakis SE, Maillard AA, El-Harazi SM, et al. Endoscopic optic nerve decompression for traumatic blindness. *Otolaryngol Head Neck Surg* 2000; **123**: 34–7.
28. Li KK, Teknos TN, Lai A, et al. Traumatic optic neuropathy: result in 45 consecutive surgically treated patients. *Otolaryngol Head Neck Surg* 1999; **120**: 5–11.
29. Rajiniganth MG, Gupta AK, Gupta A, Bapuraj JR. Traumatic optic neuropathy: visual outcome following combined therapy protocol. *Arch Otolaryngol Head Neck Surg* 2003; **129**: 1203–6.
30. Levin LA, Beck RW, Joseph MP, et al. The treatment of traumatic optic neuropathy: the International Optic Nerve Trauma Study. *Ophthalmology* 1999; **106**: 1268–77.
31. McDonald WI. The symptomatology of tumours of the anterior visual pathways. *Can J Neurol Sci* 1982; **9**: 381–90.
32. Luxenberger W, Stammberger H, Jebeles JA, Walch C. Endoscopic optic nerve decompression: the Graz experience. *Laryngoscope* 1998; **108**: 873–82.
33. Lang J. *Clinical anatomy of the nose, nasal cavity, and paranasal sinuses.* New York: Thieme; 1989.
34. Annino DJ, Jr., Goguen LA. Silent sinus syndrome. *Curr Opin Otolaryngol Head Neck Surg* 2008; **16**: 22–5.
35. Davidson JK, Soparkar CN, Williams JB, Patrinely JR. Negative sinus pressure and normal predisease imaging in silent sinus syndrome. *Arch Ophthalmol* 1999; **117**: 1653–4.
36. Numa WA, Desai U, Gold DR, et al. Silent sinus syndrome: a case presentation and comprehensive review of all 84 reported cases. *Ann Otol Rhinol Laryngol* 2005; **114**: 688–94.
37. Mendenhall WM, Lessner AM. Orbital pseudotumor. *Am J Clin Oncol* 2010; **33**: 304–6.
38. Zurlo A, Sancesario G, Bernardi G, Loasses A. Orbital pseudotumor: case report and literature review. *Tumori* 1999; **85**: 68–70.
39. Robinson D, Wilcsek G, Sacks R. Orbit and orbital apex. *Otolaryngol Clin North Am* 2011; **44**: 903–22.

CHAPTER 112

DIAGNOSIS AND MANAGEMENT OF FACIAL PAIN

Rajiv K. Bhalla and Timothy J. Woolford

Introduction 1253	Dental pain 1259
Background 1253	Other causes of facial pain encountered by the otolaryngologist 1259
Sinogenic facial pain 1254	Persistent idiopathic facial pain (atypical facial pain) 1261
Non-sinogenic facial pain 1255	History taking in facial pain 1261
Neuralgias causing facial pain 1258	References 1263

SEARCH STRATEGY

A systematic search of the available literature was performed using Medline, Embase, Cochrane library and NHS Evidence. Search terms included facial pain, sinusitis, neuropathic pain, migraine, trigeminal autonomic cephalalgia, neuralgia, persistent idiopathic facial pain, referred pain, and medication- or analgesia-dependency headache, focusing primarily on diagnosis and management.

INTRODUCTION

The diagnosis of facial pain is complex, requiring a holistic approach to the patient. Individuals are often convinced or have been convinced, either by reading the internet or by their family doctor, that their facial symptoms have underlying sinus aetiology. Additionally, there may be a strong psychological component to the onset, severity, exacerbation and prolongation of symptoms. These consultations have a propensity to be difficult and are usually time-consuming. However, time invested at an initial consultation is often time well invested, particularly if patients are helped to understand the underlying mechanism of their pain if sinus pathology is not the cause. This chapter examines the presentation and subsequent management to the otolaryngologist of patients with the symptom of facial pain, and includes an extensive discussion on medical and adjuvant therapies currently used to treat diseases that are not isogenic in aetiology.

BACKGROUND

Reaching the correct diagnosis in patients with facial pain is challenging because many patients come with fixed ideas about the cause of their pain. The majority are convinced they have sinusitis, a not unreasonable view because the diagnosis has often been confirmed by their general practitioner or other specialists. A proportion of patients have already undergone unsuccessful nasal or sinus surgery. If all cases of facial pain are assumed to be sinogenic in aetiology, those with other conditions will not receive the correct medical treatment and unfortunately, many patients will continue to be subjected to inappropriate surgery.

The majority of painful stimuli from the face are transmitted to the spinal tract of the brain stem via afferents in the trigeminal nerve. Pain afferents from the VIIIth, IXth and Xth cranial nerves also relay in the spinal tract. Facial pain from deep structures tends to be a dull, poorly localized ache because the afferent nerves innervating them are unmyelinated. Facial skin is supplied by myelinated nerves that produce a sharper pain. Various neurophysiological models have been proposed to explain the nociceptive inputs causing tension headache and migraine, and suggest pathogenesis similar to that of fibromyalgia and irritable bowel syndrome, conditions that frequently coexist. Experimental studies suggest that increased excitability of the central nervous system generated by repetitive and sustained pericranial myofascial input may be partly responsible, along with widespread changes in brain function and connectivity.[1, 2] By extrapolation, facial pain is likely to be caused by central sensitization of the trigeminal nucleus by myofascial, vascular or supraspinal input, with exacerbations or provocation of pain induced by supraspinal inhibition of the trigeminal nucleus by psychological influences.[3] To add to this, surgery, trauma and inflammation may promote nociceptive stimulation of the trigeminal caudal nucleus and initiate pain.

There are many different ways of dividing the subsections in the ensuing descriptive text. However, from the perspective of the otolaryngologist the most important differentiation, perhaps, is between facial symptoms of sinogenic aetiology and those that are not. Hence, the chapter is divided accordingly, with great emphasis on the decision to operate and perhaps more important to avoid surgery. The chapter also furnishes the reader with comprehensive differential diagnoses for the patient that presents with the symptom of facial pain. In truth, the diagnoses, aetiological hypotheses and management options have not changed greatly over the last 10 years. An individual presenting with facial pain represents an extremely common encounter in both specialist rhinology and general otolaryngology out-patient clinics. A thorough grounding in what is and what is not sinus-related, understanding from where this information arises, and starting with a broad and holistic perspective in any new or complex follow-up consultation is of paramount importance to ensure that effective interventions are implemented where indicated, and withheld when they are not.

SINOGENIC FACIAL PAIN

Pain is defined as an unpleasant sensory and emotional experience associated with actual or potential tissue damage, or described in terms of such damage.[4] Unfortunately though, discriminating between *pain* caused by sinusitis and *pain* caused by other pathologies is, perhaps, conceptually too difficult for the large majority of our patients and why, perhaps, we often hear ourselves asking questions such as, 'Describe the pain to me' and, 'What do you mean by pain?'

Pain in sinusitis that is not acute or complicated is probably a misnomer. Enough evidence now exists to suggest that sinusitis per se does not cause *pain* but instead, may be associated with other more vague symptoms. Patients may complain of pressure, fullness or throbbing in the distribution of the paranasal sinuses or at the vertex of the head. Symptoms may be bilateral or unilateral, particularly if individual sinuses are affected by pathology. Examples include pathology such as pyomucocele of the maxillary antrum, or fibrous dysplasia or osteoma of the ethmoid sinus causing secondary obstruction of drainage pathways, or mucocele of the sphenoid sinus (**Figures 112.1** and **112.2**). Exacerbation of these symptoms on bending forwards is not, however, diagnostic or suggestive of rhinosinusitis.[5] Furthermore, symptoms may be acute, recurrent acute (moderated by repeated short courses of antibiotics) or chronic. Associated with these symptoms may be nasal congestion and/or hyposmia, although these symptoms may be difficult for the patient to recall, particularly if the underlying diagnosis is of recurrent acute sinusitis. Clarification often requires some gentle probing. More readily detectable are the endoscopic signs of polyposis and obstruction of outflow drainage pathways, and

mucosal disease (**Figure 112.3**). However, these signs are frequently subtle and may, therefore, be missed. It is also highly relevant that over 80% of patients with endoscopic evidence of purulent secretions have no headache or facial pain.[6] Moreover, if surgery is performed in cases where facial pain is the dominant symptom without firm clinical evidence of rhinosinusitis, not surprisingly, a significant proportion of these patients continue to complain of facial pain post-operatively.[7]

- Management of rhinosinusitis is initially medical, with imaging reserved for failed maximal medical therapy, complications of rhinosinusitis, or suspicion of malignancy.
- Surgery should be targeted, as good correlation between symptoms, signs and radiological findings.

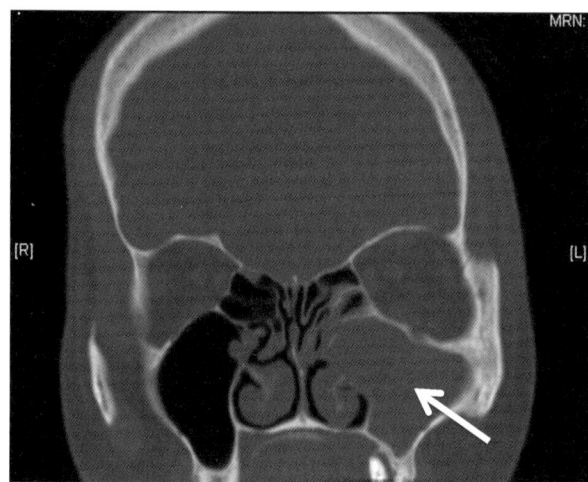

Figure 112.1 Coronal CT image depicting a left antral pyomucocele (arrow).

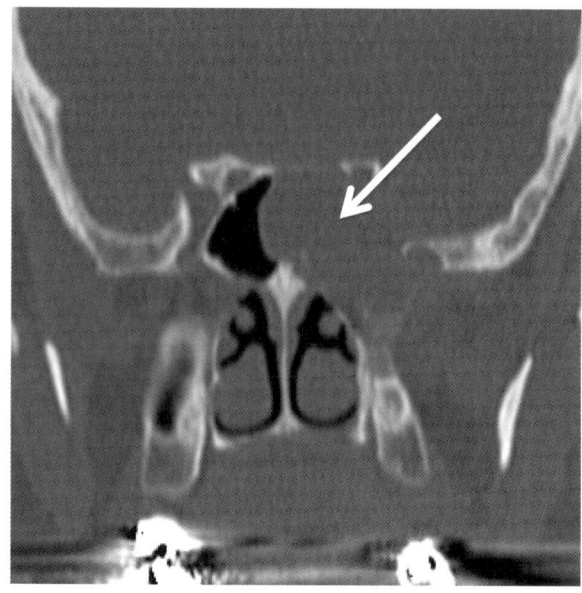

Figure 112.2 Coronal CT image depicting a left sphenoid mucocele (arrow).

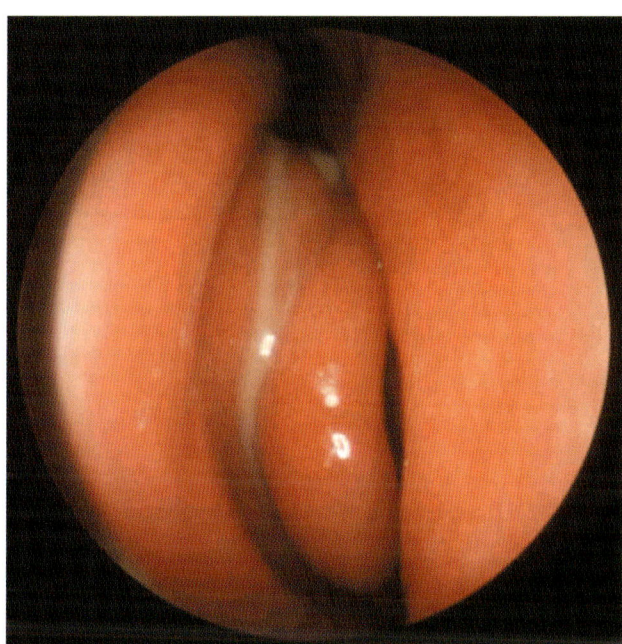

Figure 112.3 Endoscopic digital photograph showing rhinosinusitis with associated purulent discharge in the right middle meatus.

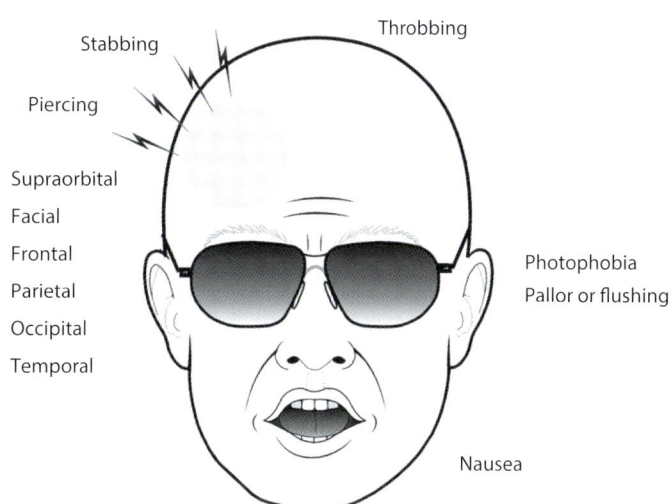

Figure 112.4 The features of migraine.

NON-SINOGENIC FACIAL PAIN

The primary headaches

These are headache disorders not caused by another condition. Each is worth considering in the context of an otolaryngology out-patient setting since they are not infrequently encountered in both specialist rhinology and general situations. Some rhinologists will be very comfortable with the medical management of these headache disorders and will have a thorough understanding of the mechanisms of drug actions and their side effects; some rhinologists will rely heavily on a partnership with a neurologist and/or a colleague with a special interest in pain management. Either approach is acceptable. Not covered in this section are primary headache disorders of the stabbing, cough (precipitated by valsalva), exertional (onset during or immediately after exercise), sexual activity, thunderclap (maximum intensity reached within a minute), hypnic (waking patient from sleep), or new daily-persistent (intractable headache that persists daily for at least 3 months) subtypes.[8] Suspicion should prompt a referral to a neurologist with an interest in headache, for an informed second opinion.

MIGRAINE

Migraine is characterized by recurrent, often unilateral, moderate to severe headaches, which may be associated with a number of symptoms attributable to the autonomic nervous system (**Figure 112.4**). The headache is described as pulsatile or throbbing, and may be severe enough to force the sufferer to bed in a darkened and quiet room as the pain is generally aggravated by physical activity or sensory stimulation. It may last between 2 and 72 hours.

In classical migraine, accounting for 25% of cases, the associated autonomic symptoms may include one or more of nausea, vomiting, photophobia, and phonophobia. Up to one-third of classical migraine sufferers may describe prodromal aura: a transient visual (scintillating scotoma, which is an area of partial alteration in the field of vision that flickers with zigzagging lines resembling fortifications or walls of a castle), sensory (olfaction or taste), or language or motor disturbance (pins-and-needles or numbness), which signals that the headache will soon occur.[9] Common migraine sufferers experience the same throbbing headache and nausea but without the aura associated with classical migraine.

Although previously believed to be a neurovascular disorder, the mechanism for migraine is now believed to be a disorder of the brain itself.[10] Cortical spreading depression is a wave of intense depolarization that starts in the occipital lobe, propagates through the brain and is followed by a period of suppressed activity. Consequent activation of the trigemino-vascular system causes the release of neuropeptides (e.g. calcitonin gene-related peptide, substance P) from peripheral trigeminal nerve endings. It is these neuropeptides that are thought to play a role in causing and maintaining the headache. The pulsating quality of migraine is thought to be caused by a process of peripheral sensitization. The condition runs in families in approximately two-thirds of cases, is more common in women and sufferers may describe triggers, which can be encountered up to 24 hours prior to the onset of an attack.[11–13] Some examples of triggers include stress, hunger, fatigue, hormonal changes, foodstuffs containing tyramine (aged cheeses, smoked fish, cured meats, some types of beer), monosodium glutamate, indoor air quality and lighting, although the evidence base for all of these is poor.

Over 90% of self-diagnosed and doctor-diagnosed sinus headaches meet the International Headache Society criteria for migraines and yet 60% receive an antibiotic prescription.[5] Furthermore, over 40% of migraine sufferers had at least one unilateral nasal symptom of congestion, rhinorrhoea or ocular lacrimation, redness or swelling during an attack, which can confuse the picture somewhat. However, these episodes do not last longer than 72 hours and endoscopic examination during an acute episode yields no evidence of purulent secretion.

> **Main aspects of treatment for acute migraine**
> - Trigger avoidance
> - Acute symptomatic control
> - Pharmacological prevention.

Medications are useful if used early in an attack. For mild to moderate symptoms simple analgesics, such as non-steroidal anti-inflammatory drugs (NSAIDs) or the combination of acetaminophen, acetylsalicylic acid and caffeine, are recommended for initial treatment in acute attacks.[14] Ibuprofen provides effective relief of symptoms in about half of people and diclofenac has also been found to be effective, both prescribed either with or without metoclopramide.[15, 16] Triptans (e.g. sumatriptan, naratriptan, rizatriptan, zolmatriptan) may help individuals with moderate to severe symptoms or those with milder symptoms who do not respond to simple analgesics, and are effective in up to 75%.[14, 17] Most side effects are mild, such as flushing, but they are not recommended for people with cardiovascular disease due to rare cases of myocardial ischaemia.[14] Unfortunately though, they may cause medication-overuse headaches if used for more than 10 days per month. Older medications, such as ergotamine and dihydroergotamine, remain as effective as triptans in the management of acute migraine, are less expensive, and are associated with side effects that are typically benign.[18]

Preventative measures in migraine include medications, nutritional supplements and lifestyle alterations. Prevention is recommended in those that have headaches for more than 2 days a week, cannot tolerate the medications used to treat acute attacks, or those with severe attacks that are not readily controlled. Options for medical prevention include anti-epileptic drugs (e.g. topiramate, sodium valproate), beta-blockers (e.g. propanolol, metoprolol), beta-adrenergic receptor antagonists (e.g. timolol), and antidepressants (e.g. amitriptyline, venlafaxine).[19, 20] It is important, however, to appreciate the side effects and contraindications for each before prescribing. Furthermore, it is often reassuring for patients to know that the doses of antidepressants prescribed to treat headaches and facial pain are somewhat lower than those used in the management of depression.

Botulinum toxin type A, administered intra-muscularly to between 31 and 39 sites around the head and back of the neck, has been found to be useful in those with chronic migraines (15 or more headache days per month of which at least 8 days are with migraines) but not those with episodic ones (0 to 14 headache days per month).[21, 22] The treatment is endorsed by the National Institute for Health and Clinical Excellence.[23] Evidence for effective control of other facial pain conditions using botulinum toxin is scarce, although it has also been used for headaches of tension origin.

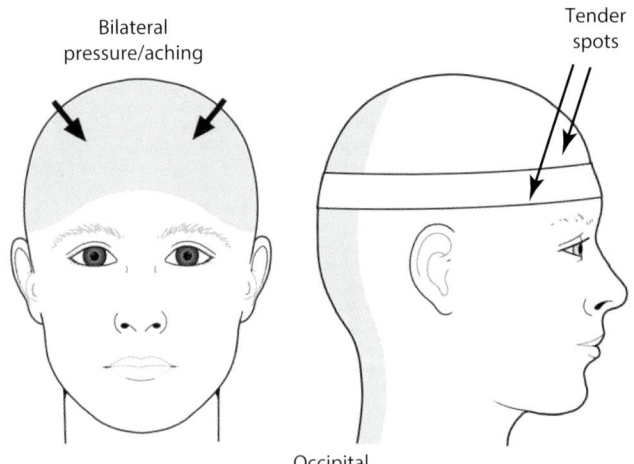

Figure 112.5 The characteristics of tension-type headache.

TENSION-TYPE HEADACHE

This is a headache that can vary in intensity in the same individual, but is usually symmetric and non-pulsatile in nature. The feeling is of tightness, pressure or constriction (vice-like) that may be confined to a small area at the glabella or extend across the whole forehead and into the temporoparietal scalp, often with a tightness or tenderness in the occiput and related trapezius (**Figure 112.5**). There is often some hyperaesthesia of the skin in the area giving the impression to the patient they have sinusitis, and tender trigger points can often be identified in the neck and shoulder areas. Clearly, the aggregate of symptoms suggests an underlying association with stress and tension, but depression and anxiety may also contribute.[3] Furthermore, although many analgesics are being taken, the patients say they offer little relief and, in fact, analgesic-dependent headaches (see below) can complicate the picture. Despite extensive investigation, the underlying pathophysiology remains a matter of speculation, with peripheral muscular and central nervous system components both likely involved. Pericranial myofascial mechanisms are probably of importance in episodic tension-type headache, whereas sensitization of central nociceptive pathways and inadequate endogenous anti-nociceptive circuitry seem to be more relevant in chronic tension-type headache.

Relaxation training, stress management and counselling have been shown to be beneficial in the management of chronic (continuous or last for more than 15 days per month) tension-type headaches although these are, perhaps, therapeutic measures that could be implemented for all non-sinogenic headaches including, for example, temporomandibular joint disorders.[24] Amitriptyline is also effective in the management of tension headache and midfacial segment pain (see below). Dosing begins at 10 mg, taken once daily at night, and increased in increments of 10 mg every 6 weeks until the pain is controlled. Rarely, 50 mg is needed. The main side effect is sedative, which enhances quality of sleep but may cause a 'hangover' effect the following morning. Tolerance to this effect usually develops after a few days. Treatment should be continued for at least 6 weeks before judging its effect, and should be continued for 6 months if it has helped. Alternatively, a triptan may be of value when there is overlap between headaches caused by tension and migraine.

CLUSTER HEADACHE AND OTHER TRIGEMINAL AUTONOMIC CEPHALALGIAS

The trigeminal autonomic cephalalgias are a group of primary headache disorders that include cluster headache, paroxysmal hemicrania, and short-lasting unilateral neuralgiform headache attacks with conjunctival injection and tearing/cranial autonomic features (SUNCT/SUNA).[25] Trigeminal autonomic cephalalgias are generally characterized by relatively short-lasting attacks of severe pain and lateralized associated features including pain, cranial autonomic symptoms and where present, migrainous symptoms, such as photophobia. Key for the otolaryngologist when diagnosing a trigeminal autonomic cephalalgia is the consideration of underlying pituitary or pituitary-region pathology, since the posterior hypothalamus is crucial in the pathophysiology of these headaches.[26] Although the syndromes share much in their pathophysiology and investigation paths, their treatment is distinct, so that accurate differentiation is important for optimal management. Due to the associated autonomic symptoms, there is a great propensity for the presentation to be confused with sinus pathology, causing misdiagnosis and subsequent mismanagement. It is of great value if such patients are managed in conjunction with a neurologist and/or colleague with a special interest in pain management.

Cluster headache

Cluster headaches are excruciating unilateral headaches of extreme intensity affecting the frontal and temporal regions, extending over the cheek and even into the teeth. There is often associated lacrimation, rhinorrhoea and nasal obstruction, symptoms that have led to misdiagnosis of sinusitis. The pain is typically lancinating or boring/drilling in quality, and is located behind the eye or in the temple (**Figure 112.6**). Descriptions range from a red-hot poker inserted into the eye or a spike penetrated from the top of the head, behind one eye, and radiating down the neck. Men are more often affected than women, primarily between the ages of 20 and 50 years. The duration of the common attack ranges from as short as 15 minutes to 3 hours or more with a rapid onset and without preliminary signs that are characteristic of a migraine. 'Side shifting' between cluster periods and bilateral headache have been described.[27] Clusters of headaches often continue for several weeks followed by months or years of remission. The intense pain in cluster headache is caused by dilation of blood vessels creating pressure on the trigeminal nerve. The aetiology of this process is, unfortunately, not fully understood but is, perhaps, due to an abnormality in the hypothalamus. Preventive treatment is always indicated for cluster headaches, to be started at the first sign of a new cluster cycle. Oxygen therapy, triptans, calcium-channel blockers (e.g. verapamil), and systemic corticosteroids have been found to be effective at managing cluster headaches.

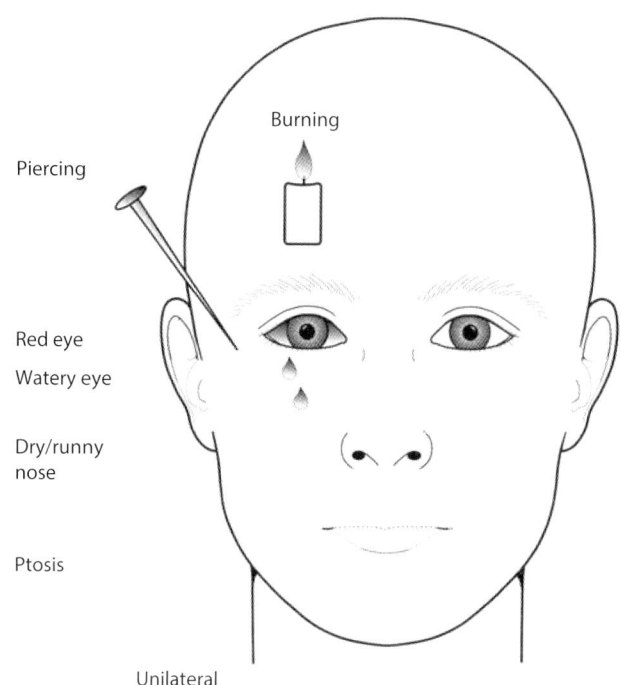

Figure 112.6 The features of cluster headache.

Paroxysmal hemicrania

This is a severe debilitating unilateral headache affecting usually the periorbital and frontotemporal regions, with an average age of onset of 30 to 40 years. Attacks are usually short-lasting, ranging from 2 to 45 minutes, and frequent, happening more than 5 times a day. Trigeminal autonomic symptoms may include nasal congestion, rhinorrhoea and lacrimation, lending itself to diagnostic confusion. The majority of patients with paroxysmal hemicrania respond to indomethacin within 24 hours. In cases where indomethacin fails to work, other drugs that have been suggested include calcium-channel blockers, naproxen, carbamezapine, and sumatriptan.

SUNCT/SUNA

Short-lasting unilateral neuralgiform headache attacks with conjunctival injection and tearing (SUNCT) and short-lasting unilateral neuralgiform attacks with cranial autonomic features (SUNA) have the shortest attack duration and the highest attack frequency. They are typified by severe, brief, unilateral attacks that usually occur in the distribution of the trigeminal nerve. SUNA differs from SUNCT in that autonomic symptoms are less prominent. Possible effective preventive drugs are carbamezapine, lamotrigine, gabapentin, and topiramate. At present, the drug of choice for SUNCT seems to be lamotrigine, whereas SUNA may better respond to gabapentin.[28]

Hemicrania continua

This is also a strictly unilateral headache causing moderately severe pain, without side-shift, with exacerbations that can include cranial autonomic symptoms as part of the phenotype (e.g. conjunctival injection, lacrimation, nasal congestion, rhinorrhoea, ptosis, or miosis). The headache is daily and continuous, without pain-free periods, and lasts for more than 3 months. The condition occurs more often in women and tends to present first in adulthood. Its diagnosis requires response to indomethacin but where side effects are an issue, other treatments may include gabapentin, topiramate, radiofrequency ablation of the supraorbital nerve, nerve blocks or botulinum toxin.

NEURALGIAS CAUSING FACIAL PAIN

Trigeminal neuralgia

Trigeminal neuralgia is characterized by paroxysms of brief but severe pain followed by asymptomatic periods without pain, although a constant dull ache may persist in some patients.[29] The pain is often described as stabbing or lancinating, burning, pressing, crushing, exploding or shooting, and patients may describe a trigger area on the face so sensitive that touching or even air currents may trigger an episode. Individual attacks usually affect one side of the face at a time, lasting from several seconds to a few minutes and may repeat up to hundreds of times throughout the day. The pain also tends to occur in cycles with remissions lasting months or even years. Vascular (arterial and venous) compression of the trigeminal nerve roots has emerged as the likely cause in most cases, with the superior cerebellar artery, the anterior and posterior inferior cerebellar arteries, and the superior petrosal vein including several of its tributaries most often implicated.[30] Such compression can injure the protective myelin sheath of the nerve and cause erratic and hyperactive nerve functioning. Diagnosis should be prompt as the longer a patient suffers with trigeminal neuralgia, the more difficult it may be to reverse the neural pathways responsible for pain. Magnetic resonance imaging should be performed to exclude multiple sclerosis or posterior fossa pathology. The anticonvulsant carbamazepine is the drug of choice for management. Gabapentin, lamotrigine and topiramate are useful as second-line agents. Percutaneous radiofrequency thermo- or chemical rhizotomy of the Gasserian ganglion is a valuable intervention in some cases, whilst stereotactic radiotherapy may offer relief of symptoms for others, although the effectiveness tends to decrease with time. Microvascular decompression produces satisfactory relief of trigeminal neuralgia symptoms in the majority of well-selected cases.

Post-herpetic neuralgia

This is pain following a herpes zoster infection, and is defined as pain recurring or continuing at the site of shingles after the onset of the rash. Up to 50% of elderly patients that have had shingles may develop post-herpetic neuralgia though fortunately, most recover during the first year. Antiviral agents help curtail the pain of acute shingles and they may also reduce the risk of subsequent post-herpetic neuralgia. Various medical treatments may be helpful, particularly carbamazepine or gabapentin with or without a tricyclic antidepressant.[31] However, management of distressing pain in these cases is often the remit of a pain specialist.

Post-surgical/traumatic neuralgia

The external portion of the nose is highly innervated by branches of the ophthalmic and maxillary divisions of the trigeminal nerve including the nasociliary nerve, external nasal nerve, infratrochlear nerve, anterior ethmoidal nerve, and infraorbital nerve. As these nerves are located on the external portion of the nose just deep to the skin, they can be easily traumatized with any impact to the nose, either following trauma or after surgery.[32] The pathophysiology is unclear and may be a central, due to neuroplasticity within the trigeminal nucleus producing spontaneous firing of neurones and reverberating circuits, or a peripheral phenomenon, perhaps due to direct neural damage with fibrosis or neuroma formation, or neural entrapment. Callous formation or post-traumatic focal inflammation may exacerbate the problem.

Removal of prosthetic pressure (e.g. from spectacles), drugs to treat neuropathic pain (amitriptyline, gabapentin, or pregabalin), infiltration with local anaesthetic and corticosteroid, nerve decompression and ultimately, nerve section may offer some symptom relief. These patients often suffer a degree of psychological distress following injury or are dissatisfied with the result of their surgery, and it is not uncommon for symptoms to be exaggerated if associated with ongoing litigation. It should be borne in mind that correction of an aesthetic abnormality is unlikely to alleviate pain and caution should be observed when managing such patients. Furthermore, there is the added risk of worsening the pain syndrome or causing new pain to develop after surgical intervention.

Sluder's neuralgia and 'contact point pain'

The theory that implicates mucosal contact points within the nose as a cause of headache or facial pain has, unfortunately, become firmly entrenched in otolaryngology folklore.[33] The findings have been used by some to support the notion that mucosal contact points within the nasal cavity can cause referred pain, even though the original studies did not describe contact point-induced headache or facial pain. High-quality studies now exist to support the view that the majority of people with contact points experience no facial pain.[34] Although Sluder's description of sphenopalatine ganglion neuralgia described a collective group of neuralgic, motor, sensory and gustatory symptoms and signs including facial pain, he did not actually describe the presence of contact points, which is all the more confusing as to why his theory has been extrapolated by some to include mucosal contact with the lateral nasal wall as a cause for facial pain.[35] Moreover, there is nowhere else in the body where mucosa-to-mucosa contact causes pain. It seems probable that the majority of case series in the literature that describe surgery for anatomical variations (septal spur, concha bullosa, a paradoxically curved middle turbinate, a superior turbinate touching the septum, or a large ethmoid bulla) in patients with facial pain that responded to surgery result from the effect of cognitive dissonance or from surgery altering neuroplasticity within the brainstem sensory nuclear complex.[34] Benefit is more often partial than complete and relatively short-lived. Further prospective, randomized and blinded trials with a minimum follow-up period of 12 months are required to assess the place of contact point surgery.

DENTAL PAIN

Painful teeth

A frequent source of referral to a specialist rhinology clinic is the patient with vague maxillary or piriform aperture pain that has been assessed in an oral or maxillofacial surgery clinic and radiological investigation has identified mucosal thickening in the maxillary antrum. It is important to note that maxillary retention cysts are an extremely common finding in one-third of patients with no sinus complaint. Most will either shrink or remain unchanged over time.[36] Surgery is rarely indicated. True dental pain can often be elicited by percussing the offending tooth, although pain originating from pulp disease may be poorly localized causing misdiagnosis. This pain rarely crosses the midline but radiation to the opposite jaw (e.g. maxilla to mandible) and surrounding structures may further confuse the picture. In contrast, dentino-enamel defects will produce a sharp, well-localized pain often caused by a lost or cracked filling. Once the periodontium is involved the pain becomes localized to the affected tooth, which throbs and is tender to percussion.

Temporomandibular joint disorder

This is not an uncommon presentation in otolaryngology clinics, where muscular hyper- or parafunction may produce acute or chronic pain in the pre- or periauricular areas, deep otalgia, and tenderness in the temporoparietal and cervical regions of the scalp. Clinical findings may include scalloping of the buccal mucosa in cases of bruxism, tenderness in the muscles of mastication or in the temporomandibular joint itself, and smoothed contours of the pre-molar and molar dentition. Other causes include malocclusion, mal-alignment following dental restorative procedures, stress and anger, excessive chewing (e.g. gum), and degenerative joint disease. Treatment includes joint rest, non-steroidal anti-inflammatory analgesia, correction of aetiological factors, and an occlusal splint (e.g. biteguard) worn at night or, sometimes, longer duration can relieve inflammation in a tender joint. Use of a 'one-size-fits-all' splint can worsen symptoms in some people and so these should be custom made. Physiotherapy, temporomandibular joint injection with corticosteroid and local anaesthetic or botulinum toxin, and low-dose amitriptyline may be useful in some resistant cases.

Phantom tooth pain

Patients with unrelenting pain in the teeth, gingival, palatal or alveolar tissues often see multiple dentists and have multiple irreversible procedures performed and still have their pain. Common diagnoses include atypical odontalgia, persistent orodental pain, or if teeth have been extracted, phantom tooth pain.[37] One possibility is that these pain complaints are due to a neuropathic alteration of the trigeminal nerve, but more likely is a diagnosis of persistent idiopathic facial pain (see below). Treatment may include pharmacological medications that suppress nerve activity. The common medications used for atypical odontalgia and phantom tooth pain include gabapentin, tricyclics, topical anaesthetics and opioids.

OTHER CAUSES OF FACIAL PAIN ENCOUNTERED BY THE OTOLARYNGOLOGIST

Mid-facial segment pain

This is a type of tension headache that affects the midface (**Table 112.1** and **Figure 112.7**).[38] The diagnosis can be challenging as patients and their family practitioner are often convinced the symptoms are due to rhinosinusitis. However, dubious endoscopic evidence of rhinosinusitis should prompt the clinician to refute this diagnosis in support of a neurological cause. The mechanism behind tension pain and its management have been described above.

Analgesia-dependency headache or medication-overuse headache

Many headache sufferers, particularly tension-type, midfacial segment pain and migraine, can get into a cycle of taking an excessive amount of analgesics in spite of the fact that they have little effect. Dull, diffuse and band-like headaches, usually starting in the early morning, are suggestive of drug-induced or analgesic-dependent headaches. The drugs most often used are acetaminophen,

TABLE 112.1 Criteria comprising mid-facial segment pain

- A symmetric sensation of pressure or tightness. Some patients may say that their nose feels blocked even though they have no nasal airway obstruction.
- Involves the areas of the nasion, under the bridge of the nose, either side of the nose, the peri- or retro-orbital regions, or across the cheeks. The symptoms of tension-type headache often coexist.
- There may be hyperaesthesia of the skin and soft tissues over the affected area.
- Nasal endoscopy is normal.
- Computerized tomography of the paranasal sinuses is normal (note a third of asymptomatic patients have incidental mucosal changes on CT).
- There are no consistent exacerbating or relieving factors.
- There are no nasal symptoms (note that approximately 20% of most populations have intermittent or persistent allergic rhinitis, which may occur incidentally in this condition).

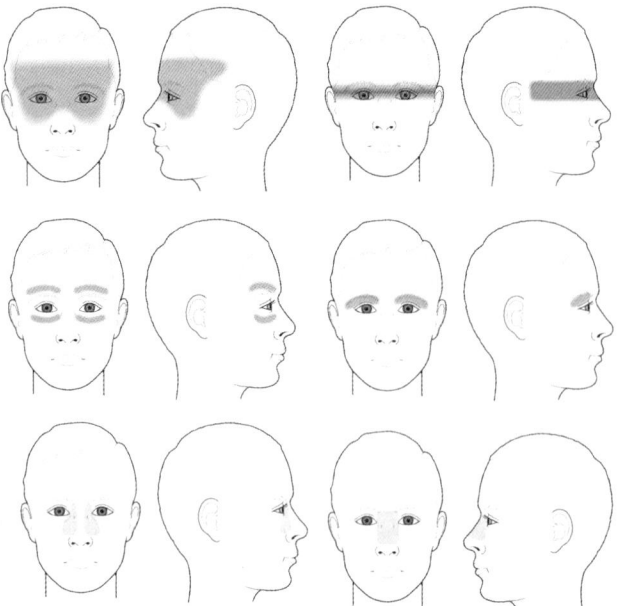

Figure 112.7 Facial map of the patterns of distribution of mid-facial segment pain.

caffeine, non-steroidal anti-inflammatory medications, codeine, ergot alkaloids, and pyrazalone derivatives.[39] On stopping analgesics, headaches disappear or decrease by more than 50% in two-thirds of patients, but withdrawal may be problematic as symptoms can take several weeks to disappear. Positive predictors for successful treatment are migraine as the primary headache, chronic headache lasting less than 10 years, and the regular intake of ergotamine. The underlying mechanisms behind analgesia-dependency headache remain unknown.

Myofascial pain

This is characterized by chronic pain caused by multiple trigger points in the neck, jaw or ear, and is five times more common in post-menopausal women (**Table 112.2**). The condition has many features in common with temporomandibular joint dysfunction, with tender points identifiable in the sternomastoid and trapezius muscles. Aetiological factors include malocclusion and poor deltopectoral posture, but stress and tiredness have a tendency to amplify the symptoms. Chronic myofascial pain may be helped by applying local heat, ultrasound therapy and often massage to relieve trigger point tenderness. Other pharmacological treatments are similar to temporomandibular joint disorders.

TABLE 112.2 Clinical features of a myofascial trigger point

- focal point tenderness
- reproduction of pain on trigger point palpation
- hardening of the muscle upon trigger point palpation
- pseudo-weakness of the involved muscle
- referred pain
- limited range of motion following approximately 5 seconds of sustained trigger point pressure

Cervical spine degenerative disease and cervicogenic headache

Cervicogenic headache is recognized as a referred pain in the head and by muscular association, to the face.[40] Primary sensory afferents from the cervical roots C1 to C3 converge with afferents from the occiput and trigeminal afferents on the same second-order neuron in the upper cervical spine. Consequently, the anatomical structures innervated by the cervical roots C1 to C3 are potential sources of cervicogenic headache. Pain may originate from different muscles and ligaments of the neck, from intervertebral discs and particularly, from the atlanto-occipital, atlanto-axial, and C2/C3 zygapophyseal joints. Treatment may include simple analgesia, physiotherapy, complementary therapies such as acupuncture or massage, cervical epidural corticosteroid injection, local botulinum toxin injection, radiofrequency ablative therapy, and surgery. Severe cases should be managed in conjunction with a spine specialist.

Temporal arteritis

This is an inflammatory vasculitis of the temporal artery. The condition usually presents to the rheumatologist or vascular surgeon but in the rare instance that an affected patient does present to an otolaryngology clinic, it is essential that a prompt diagnosis is made. Delay can, unfortunately, render a patient blind due to disease progression and involvement of the ophthalmic artery. Loss of vision in both eyes may occur very abruptly. Women over 55 years are most commonly affected, presenting with headache, fever, jaw or tongue claudication, and visual disturbance. The temporal area may be tender, with prominence of the temporal arteries, which may be thickened. Diagnosis is confirmed by raised erythrocyte sedimentation rate and a minimum 1 cm length biopsy of the temporal artery, which shows giant cells infiltrating the tissue, intimal hyperplasia and fragmentation of the internal elastic lamina. Unfortunately, a negative biopsy result does not definitely rule out the diagnosis. High-dose corticosteroids (prednisolone 1mg/kg/day) must be started as soon as the diagnosis is suspected, even before biopsy confirmation, if there is a strong clinical suspicion that the condition is present.

Pain caused by tumour

Although tumours rarely present with facial pain, nearly 80% of patients with head and neck cancers experience facial pain related to their tumour or treatment.[41] Constant or progressive dull or gnawing pain, particularly if associated with other suspicious symptoms or neurological signs should alert the clinician. A past history of malignancy may raise the possibility of metachronous tumour or metastasis. A thorough examination of the head, neck and upper aerodigestive tract along with appropriate radiological imaging is mandatory to exclude the possibility of underlying tumour. Occasionally, tumours may have a long natural history of growth, such

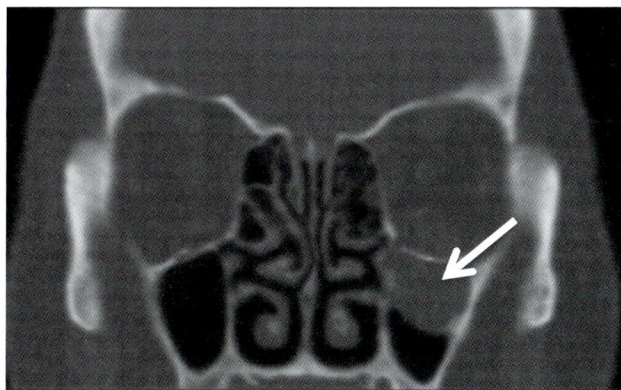

Figure 112.8 Coronal CT image showing a recurrent left infraorbital schwannoma (arrow) causing chronic facial pain.

as a neuroma, and pain may have been present for several years (**Figure 112.8**).

Patients with neoplasia of the paranasal sinuses, benign or malignant, often present with advanced disease. Unilateral nasal obstruction, bloody or discoloured nasal discharge, a proptosed or displaced globe, facial paraesthesia or swelling, and a loose tooth or ill-fitting denture may represent advanced disease. Pain is usually a late feature.

PERSISTENT IDIOPATHIC FACIAL PAIN (ATYPICAL FACIAL PAIN)

This warrants special mention in its own right. A diagnosis of exclusion only, patients are all too easily labelled as suffering *atypical* facial symptoms when actually, a thorough understanding of alternative causes, mechanisms and symptoms, and appropriate management lends itself to a happier outcome for both the patient and attending otolaryngologist. It is described as a persistent facial pain that does not have the classical characteristics of cranial neuralgias and for which there is no obvious cause.[9] The diagnosis is possible if the facial pain is localized, present daily, and throughout all or most of the day and by definition, neurological and physical examination findings in persistent idiopathic facial pain should be normal. Both the incidence and pathophysiology of the condition are unknown, and it is seen primarily in older adults.[42] The pain does not usually stay within the anatomical boundaries of the trigeminal nerve distribution. It may move from one part of the face to another between different consultations and other symptoms, such as 'mucous moving' in the sinuses, are often described. A number of patients have such completely fixed ideas about their condition that they will not be convinced otherwise, whatever the weight of evidence to the contrary.[5] Pain is often disproportionately described in dramatic terms in conjunction with an excess of other unpleasant life events. Many of these patients have a history of other pain syndromes and their extensive records show little progress despite various medications and investigations. They have often undergone previous sinus or dental surgery and may be resentful about their treatment.

Significant psychological disturbance or a history of depression may exist with the suggestion that they are unable to function normally as a result of their pain. Some project a pessimistic view of treatment, almost giving the impression they do not wish to be rid of the pain that plays such a central role in their lives.

The management of such patients is almost always challenging and confrontation is nearly always counterproductive. A good starting point is to reassure the patient that you recognize that they have genuine pain and an empathic consultation with an explanation should be conducted. Drug treatment revolves around a gradual build-up to the higher analgesic and antidepressant levels of amitriptyline (75 to 100 mg) at night. Second-line treatment includes gabapentin and carbamazepine. Patients should sympathetically be made aware that psychological factors may play a role in their condition and referral to a clinical psychologist or psychiatrist may be helpful. Attempts have also been made to further separate idiopathic facial pain syndromes according to topographical criteria. Pain clearly localized in the eye (idiopathic ophthalmodynia) or in the nose (idiopathic rhinalgia) has been described.[43] Whether all such focal syndromes are topographic variants of persistent idiopathic facial pain or independent disorders remains a topic for discussion.

HISTORY TAKING IN FACIAL PAIN

In an effort to draw together the breadth of descriptive text provided in this chapter, an approach to taking a thorough and accurate history is now presented since this is the crux to making a correct diagnosis in a patient that presents with facial pain. It may not be possible to make a correct diagnosis at the first visit, particularly if the patient has seen a number of physicians previously and is emotionally charged. Retaking a history at a subsequent consultation in conjunction with the evidence provided in a symptom diary may further clarify the situation.

In attempting to make a diagnosis, it is helpful to broadly classify symptoms into sinogenic and non-sinogenic in aetiology. Sinus-related symptoms (**Table 112.3**), coupled with endoscopic evidence of disease, should be readily substantiated. Non-sinogenic causes can be broadly classified as primary headache disorders (migraine, tension and cluster), neuralgias, pain caused by tumours, and others (mid-facial segment pain, dental, analgesia-dependency and persistent idiopathic facial pain). It is useful to have a mental algorithm to plan questions and to use these to work through a diagnostic checklist of possible conditions.

- **Where is the pain and does it radiate anywhere?**
  Asking the patient to localize pain can be extremely useful in differentiating sinogenic from other causes of pain, and may differ from information contained in the referral letter. Bilateral facial pain is commonly, although not exclusively, mid-facial segment pain. Migraine, cluster and other trigeminal autonomic headaches, and temporomandibular joint disorders tend to be unilateral. The manner in which the patient outlines

TABLE 112.3 Definitions of headache caused by rhinosinusitis and the diagnosis of rhinosinusitis	
International Headache Society definition of headache due to rhinosinusitis[9]	**European Position Paper on Rhinosinusitis and Nasal Polyps 2012 definition of rhinosinusitis in adults[5] Is it the latest now?**

A. Frontal headache accompanied by pain in one or more regions of the face, ears or teeth and fulfilling criteria C and D
B. Clinical, nasal endoscopic, CT, and/or MRI imaging and/or laboratory evidence of acute or acute-on-chronic rhinosinusitis
C. Headache and facial pain develop simultaneously with onset or acute exacerbation of rhinosinusitis
D. Headache and/or facial pain resolve within 7 days after remission or successful treatment of acute or acute-on-chronic rhinosinusitis
	Rhinosinusitis in adults is defined as:
	• inflammation of the nose and the paranasal sinuses characterized by two or more symptoms, one of which should be either nasal blockage/obstruction/congestion or nasal discharge (anterior/posterior nasal drip):
	  • ± facial pain/pressure
	  • ± reduction or loss of smell
	  • and either
	• endoscopic signs of:
	  • nasal polyps, and/or
	  • mucopurulent discharge primarily from middle meatus and/or
	  • oedema/mucosal obstruction primarily in middle meatus and/or
	• CT changes:
	  • mucosal changes within the ostiomeatal complex and/or sinuses

their pain, and the gestures used, can inform the examiner of the emotional significance of the symptom.

- **Is the pain continuous or intermittent?**
  Sinogenic pain and migraine are unlikely to be continuous or present on a daily basis. Pain of this character is more likely to represent tension headache, mid-facial segment pain, analgesia-dependency headache or atypical facial pain. Constant and predominantly unilateral pain, particularly if it is progressive, may be due to a tumour and this possibility must be considered.

- **What is the character of the pain?**
  Vascular pain tends to be throbbing in nature, with cluster headaches being particularly severe. Mid-facial segment pain, like tension headache, is often described as pressure or band-like pain. Trigeminal neuralgia may cause intense stabbing pain that is initiated by a trigger.

- **What precipitates or is associated with the pain?**
  Sinogenic pain is associated with adverse rhinological symptoms, but should be differentiated from trigeminal autonomic symptoms. Migraine may have preceding aura and is often associated with nausea. Trigger factors, such as certain foods, withdrawal of stress and sleep disruption, are well recognized. Cluster headaches are frequently triggered by alcohol and wake the patient. The pain of temporomandibular joint disorder is exacerbated by chewing, and that of trigeminal neuralgia and myofascial pain is provoked by trigger points.

- **What relieves the pain?**
  Sinogenic facial pain almost always responds to medical treatments such as topical decongestion, either short or long term, and antibiotics. Patients with migraine will retreat to a quiet and darkened room to lie down, which helps them to cope with their symptoms. Although mid-facial segment pain may initially respond to simple analgesics, the benefit is usually short-lived.

- **What effect does the pain have on daily life?**
  Patients with persistent idiopathic facial pain often describe their pain in dramatic detail as severe and unrelenting despite sleeping well and living a relatively normal life. In contrast, some patients with this condition are unable to work and blame the pain for a breakdown in a close relationship. Severe crippling pain that wakes the patient, often a man, is typical of cluster headache.

BEST CLINICAL PRACTICE

- ✓ A careful and meticulous history is key to accurate diagnosis of facial pain, acknowledging that most patients will not have sinogenic pain.
- ✓ Examination must include nasendoscopy to assess the sinus drainage pathways, lateral nasal wall and visible anterior skull base, particularly when the patient is either symptomatic or in pain. A normal endoscopic examination in such circumstances makes the diagnosis of sinogenic pain extremely unlikely.
- ✓ Plain sinus X-rays should not be used. Computed tomography should be reserved for cases of failed maximal medical therapy, complications of rhinosinusitis, or where there is suspicion of malignancy. Non-pathological sinus mucosal thickening is common in asymptomatic patients and management based only on radiological findings, without clinical correlation, will result in unnecessary surgery.
- ✓ Non-sinogenic facial pain should be managed medically, with complementary therapies, using cognitive behavioural therapy and rarely, with surgery if decompression or nerve section is considered. Caution should be observed if consideration is given to offering endoscopic sinus surgery or nasal plastic surgery to manage facial pain.
- ✓ A multidisciplinary approach to managing chronic non-sinogenic facial pain offers the best outcome for the patient.

FUTURE RESEARCH

➤ Neural pathophysiology in rhinosinusitis remains poorly understood.
➤ Neural pathophysiology in non-sinogenic facial pain also remains poorly understood.
➤ Although the psychological aspects of facial pain are well recognized, well-designed epidemiological studies to assess the incidence of anxiety-depressive disorders in patients with facial pain do not exist. Understanding this association may help to drive forward targeted therapy in such individuals.
➤ Future studies should focus on investigation of the source of peripheral nociception, the role of descending pain modulation, and the development of animal models for headache and facial pain to support the pathophysiologic importance of central sensitization in these conditions.

KEY POINTS

- Fundamental to the accurate diagnosis of facial pain is a comprehensive and detailed history.
- Management of patients with chronic facial pain can be time-consuming and complex.
- Facial pain may be exacerbated by an underlying psychological predilection, such as stress, depression or anxiety, or by a litigious motivation.
- Surgery for facial pain is rarely beneficial and may, conversely, either exacerbate or cause de novo pain.
- Rhinosinusitis, unless acute or associated with complications, does not usually cause pain.
- Genuine sinogenic pain may be complicated by non-sinogenic pain of multifactorial aetiology.
- Normal clinical examination and radiology does not usually suggest rhinosinusitis and often does not warrant surgery. Recurrent acute sinusitis moderated by antibiotic therapy may be the exception.
- Incidental sinus mucosal thickening on computed tomography does not automatically indicate that facial pain is sinogenic in aetiology.
- Many headache disorders may have associated trigeminal autonomic symptoms such as lacrimation, nasal congestion and rhinorrhoea.
- Many patients with chronic facial pain that is not sinogenic in aetiology benefit from drugs to manage neuropathic pain.
- It is useful to manage patients with chronic facial pain in a multidisciplinary team with neurology, pain specialty, psychology, oculoplastic and neurosurgical colleagues.

REFERENCES

1. Ashina M. Pathophysiology of tension-type headache: potential drug targets. *CNS Neurol Disord Drug Targets* 2007; 6: 238–9.
2. Charles A. Migraine: a brain state. *Curr Opin Neurol* 2013; [Epub ahead of print].
3. Beghi E, Bussone G, D'Amico D, et al. Headache, anxiety and depressive disorders: the HADAS study. *J Headache Pain* 2010; 11: 141–50.
4. Bonica JJ. The need of a taxonomy. *Pain* 1979; 6: 247–8.
5. European position paper on rhinosinusitis and nasal polyps 2012. *Rhinology* 2012; 50(suppl 23): 5.
6. Clifton NJ, Jones NS. Prevalence of facial pain in 108 consecutive patients with paranasal mucopurulent discharge at endoscopy. *J Laryngol Otol* 2007; 121: 345–8.
7. Kamani T, Jones NS. Evidence based management of a patient with facial pain. *Clin Otolaryngol* 2012; 37: 207–12.
8. Bahra A. Other primary headaches. *Ann Indian Acad Neurol* 2012; 15(suppl 1): S66–71.
9. Headache Classification Subcommittee of the International Headache Society. The international classification of headache disorders, 2nd edition. *Cephalalgia* 2004; 24(suppl 1): 9–160.
10. Kojic Z, Stojanovic D. Pathophysiology of migraine: from molecular to personalized medicine. *Med Pregl* 2013; 66: 53–7.
11. Levy D, Strassman AM, Burstein R. A critical view on the role of migraine triggers in the genesis of migraine pain. *Headache* 2009; 49: 953–7.
12. Martin PR. Behavioural management of migraine headache triggers: learning to cope with triggers. *Curr Pain Headache Rep* 2010; 14: 221–7.
13. Bartleson JD, Cutrer FM. Migraine update: diagnosis and treatment. *Minn Med* 2010; 93: 36–41.
14. Gilmore MB. Treatment of acute migraine headache. *Am Fam Phys* 2011; 83: 271–80.
15. Rabbie R, Derry S, Moore RA, McQuay HJ. Ibuprofen with or without an antiemetic for acute migraine headaches in adults. *Cochrane Database Syst Rev* 2010; 10: CD008039.
16. Derry S, Rabbie R, Moore RA. Diclofenac with or without an antiemetic for acute migraine headaches in adults. *Cochrane Database Syst Rev* 2012; 2: CD008783.
17. Johnston MM, Rapoport AM. Triptans for the management of migraine. *Drugs* 2010; 70: 1505–18.
18. Kelley NE, Tepper DE. Rescue therapy for acute migraine, part 1: triptans, dihydroergotamine, and magnesium. *Headache* 2012; 52: 114–28.
19. Loder E, Burch R, Rizzoli P. The 2012 AHS/AAN guidelines for prevention of episodic migraine: a summary and comparison with other recent clinical practice guidelines. *Headache* 2012; 52: 930–45.
20. Silberstein SD, Holland S, Freitag F, et al. Evidence-based guideline update: pharmacologic treatment for episodic migraine prevention in adults: report of the Quality Standards Subcommittee of the American Academy of Neurology and the American Headache Society. *Neurology* 2012; 78: 1337–45.
21. Katsarava Z, Buse DC, Manack AN, Lipton RB. Defining the differences between episodic migraine and chronic migraine. *Curr Pain Headache Rep* 2012; 16: 86–92.
22. Jackson JL, Kuriyama A, Hayashino Y. Botulinum toxin A for prophylactic treatment of migraine and tension headaches in adults: a meta-analysis. *JAMA* 2012; 307: 1736–45.
23. Botulinum toxin type A for the prevention of headaches in adults with chronic migraine. *NICE technology appraisals* 2012: TA260.
24. Aaseth K, Grande RB, Leiknes KA, et al. Personality traits and psychological distress in persons with chronic tension type headache: the Akershus study of chronic headache. *Acta Neurol Scand* 2011; 124: 375–82.
25. Goadsby PJ, Cittadini E, Cohen AS. Trigeminal autonomic cephalalgias: paroxysmal hemicranias, SUNCT/SUNA, and hemicranias continua. *Semin Neurol* 2010; 30: 186–91.
26. Goadsby PJ. Trigeminal autonomic cephalalgias. *Continuum (Minneap Minn)* 2012; 18: 883–95.
27. Meyer EL, Laurell K, Artto V, et al. Lateralisation in cluster headache: a Nordic multicenter trial. *J Headache Pain* 2009; 10: 259–63.
28. Pareja JA, Alvarez M, Montojo T. SUNCT and SUNA: recognition and treatment. *Curr Treat Options Neurol* 2013; 15: 28–39.
29. Obermann M, Holle D, Katsarava Z. Trigeminal neuralgia and persistent idiopathic facial pain. *Expert Rev Neurother* 2011; 11: 1619–29.

30. Thomas KL, Vilensky JA. The anatomy of vascular compression in trigeminal neuralgia. *Clin Anat* 2013; [Epub ahead of print].
31. Edelsberg JS, Lord C, Oster G. Systematic review and meta-analysis of efficacy, safety, and tolerability data from randomized controlled trials of drugs used to treat post-herpetic neuralgia. *Ann Pharmacother* 2011; **45**: 1483–90.
32. Rozen T. Post-traumatic external nasal pain syndrome (a trigeminal based pain disorder). *Headache* 2009; **49**: 1223–8.
33. McAuliffe AG, Mueller GC, Wolff HG. Experimental studies on headache: pain originating in nasal and paranasal structures. *N Y State J Med* 1950; **50**: 1113–16.
34. Harrison L, Jones NS. Intranasal contact points as a cause of facial pain or headache: a systematic review. *Clin Otolaryngol* 2013; **38**: 8–22.
35. Sluder G. The role of the sphenopalatine (or Meckel's) ganglion in nasal headaches. *N Y Med J* 1908; **87**: 989–90.
36. Wang JH, Jang YJ, Lee BJ. Natural course of retention cysts of the maxillary sinus: long-term follow-up results. *Laryngoscope* 2007; **117**: 341–4.
37. Clark GT. Persistent orodental pain, atypical odontalgia, and phantom tooth pain: when are they neuropathic disorders? *J Calif Dent Assoc* 2006; **34**: 599–609.
38. Jones NS. The prevalence of facial pain and purulent sinusitis. *Curr Opin Otolaryngol Head Neck Surg* 2009; **17**: 38–42.
39. Johnson JL, Hutchinson MR, Williams DB, Rolan P. Medication-overuse headache and opioid-induced hyperalgesia: a review of mechanisms, a neuroimmune hypothesis and a novel approach to treatment. *Cephalalgia* 2013; **33**: 52–64.
40. Becker WJ. Cervicogenic headache: evidence that the neck is a pain generator. *Headache* 2010; **50**: 699–705.
41. Mendelsohn D, Ranjan M, Hawley P, Honey CR. Percutaneous trigeminal rhizotomy for facial pain secondary to head and neck malignancy. *Clin J Pain* 2013; [Epub ahead of print].
42. Cornelissen P, van Kleef M, Mekhail N, et al. Persistent idiopathic facial pain. *Pain Prac* 2009; **9**: 443–8.
43. Pareja JA, Cuadrado ML, Porta-Etessam J, et al. Idiopathic ophthalmodynia and idiopathic rhinalgia: two topographic facial pain syndromes. *Headache* 2010; **50**: 1286–95.

JUVENILE ANGIOFIBROMA

Bernhard Schick

Introduction 1265	Endoscopic resectin: Surgical considerations 1266
Clinical findings 1265	Indication and limitation of endoscopic surgery 1267
Tissue architecture 1266	Acknowledgements 1268
Juvenile angiofibroma and the first branchial arch artery 1266	References 1268

SEARCH STRATEGY

Data in this chapter may be updated by a search on PubMed and Medline which will enable the reader to identify latest information on this condition using the following keywords: nasopharyngeal neoplasms, angiofibroma, adolescent, and child', supplemented by the author's personal bibliography.

INTRODUCTION

Juvenile angiofibroma (JA) is a unique tumour presenting almost exclusively in adolescent males. The tumour is rare, with an incidence of e.g. 0.4 cases per 1 million inhabitants per year in Denmark.[1] A higher incidence has been reported in Southern Europe and even more in Asia. Although tumour biology is still not completely understood, the knowledge about JAs is increasing and the tumour is well-defined clinically. Consideration of the clinical tumour characteristics is of utmost importance in the diagnosis and treatment of JAs.

Therapeutic options for JAs include surgery, radiotherapy and, in rare cases, chemotherapy. Tumour resection is the therapy of choice. Various surgical techniques have been described previously, ranging from endonasal surgery and mid-facial degloving to approaches using skin incisions, e.g. lateral rhinotomy or infratemporal approaches. At the current time, and in the hands of experienced sinonasal surgeons, endoscopic resection has been proven to allow successful treatment of most JAs[2] based on a precise knowledge of the clinical findings.

CLINICAL FINDINGS

The tumour usually arises from the lateral wall of the posterior nasal cavity close to the sphenopalatine foramen and the pterygoid base (**Figure 113.1a**). Due to its early submucosal expansion towards the nasopharynx, it has frequently been termed 'nasopharyngeal angiofibroma'. Due to this location nasal obstruction and nasal bleeding may be symptoms presented by the adolescents. Although the tumour is histopathologically classified as a benign lesion, bony erosions of the pterygoid, the clivus and the sphenoid sinus floor are common hallmarks of JAs. Bony destruction of the sphenoid sinus floor is followed by tumour extension into the sphenoid sinus. Here the tumour may fill the sinus space almost completely without infiltrating the mucosa. Furthermore, the tumour may grow along the central skull base towards the foramen lacerum. In such cases, assessment should be made of the presence, or not, of tumour tissue posterior to the pterygoid plates.

It is important to consider that JAs spread along natural foramina and fissures. Tumour tissue may extend laterally through the sphenopalatine foramen into the pterygopalatine fossa and further into the infratemporal fossa. In this case, a widened sphenopalatine foramen and an anterior displacement of the posterior maxillary sinus wall are typical radiological findings (**Figure 113.1b**).

Finger-like tumour processes may be encountered in the infratemporal fossa. A further lateral extension or tumour growth beyond the maxillary sinus will present as facial swelling. The orbit may be reached via the inferior orbital fissure causing proptosis and/or optic nerve compression with visual disturbance. Intra-cranial tumour spread is observed in advanced stages mainly through the roof of the infratemporal fossa and in some cases via the superior orbital fissure. In cases of intra-cranial tumour growth, JAs are mainly located in the extradural space. Dural infiltration or even brain involvement are rare events.

Blood supply of this highly vascular tumour needs to be evaluated carefully in order to diagnose and treat

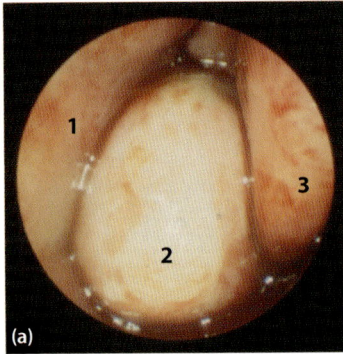 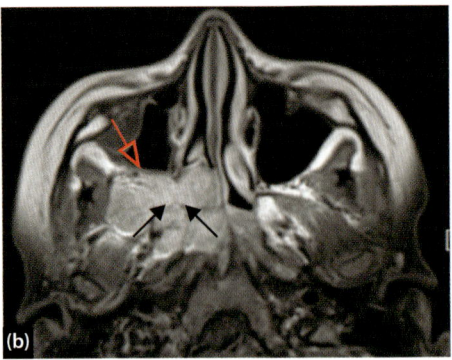 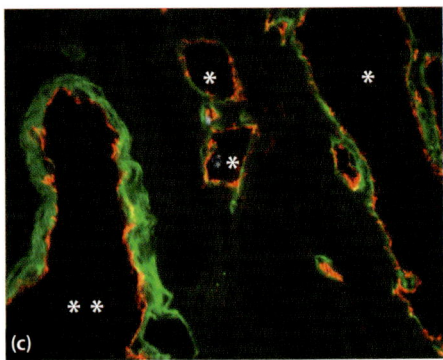

Figure 113.1 (a) Endoscopic view of a juvenile angiofibroma (JA) in the left posterior nasal cavity (1 = nasal septum, 2 = tumour, 3 = inferior turbinate). **(b)** MRI of a juvenile angiofibroma (arrows) after application of contrast medium showing an enlarged sphenopalatine foramen (black arrows) and anterior displacement of the posterior maxillary sinus wall (red arrow). **(c)** Staining of a juvenile angiofibroma (JA) with antibodies against laminin (vascular wall, green) and the endothelial cell marker CD31 (red) demonstrates irregularly shaped vessels lined by endothelial cells only (*) in the vicinity to vessels with a regular vascular wall architechture (**).

JAs successfully. The diagnosis is based on the typical clinical and radiological findings.[3] Tumour biopsy should be avoided due to the risk of severe bleeding. In its early stages, the tumour is supplied by the sphenopalatine and maxillary arteries. In advanced stages, further branches of the external carotid artery (ECA), such as the ascending pharyngeal artery, contribute to tumour blood supply. Besides the internal carotid arteries (ICAs), the vertebral arteries have to be considered as additional feeders, especially in large JAs. In view of this, a careful angiographic evaluation of ipsilateral and contralateral ECAs and ICAs is strongly recommended in all JAs, and should be accompanied by an examination of both vertebral arteries in advanced tumour stages. Pre-operative superselective embolization of this highly vascularized tumour has attracted great attention and is recommended by most authors. Some surgeons do not ask for pre-operative embolization as they close the feeding vessels before tumour removal and have found it wise to detect possible tumour remnants by bleeding, as well as to avoid site effects of embolization e.g. brain infarction. In addition, a cell saver can be used during surgery to avoid allogenic blood donation. As well as defining the tumour feeders in JAs, the vascular tumour architecture deserves special attention, especially as the surgeon is able to reduce blood loss by respecting the unique structure of JAs.

TISSUE ARCHITECTURE

JAs are benign fibrovascular tumours with characteristic irregularly-shaped vessels, which may be lined by endothelial cells only (**Figure 113.1c**) or show an incomplete vascular wall architecture. Therefore, the surgeon is faced with profuse bleeding when opening these non-contractible pathological vessels during dissection of the tumour. The extreme variability in the amount of fibrous tissue and vessel density within JAs is of outstanding importance for the surgeon. The highest density of vessels, in particular those with the characteristic irregular shape, is found below a pseudocapsule at the tumour surface. Thus, the surgeon should always dissect along the pseudocapsule in order to avoid severe bleeding. Towards the centre of the tumour, the amount of fibrous tissue increases, while vessel density decreases. Based on the clinical findings and the specific vascular architecture, JAs have been defined as vascular malformations rather than true neoplasms.[4] Recently published genetic and molecular findings have supported this theory.[5]

JUVENILE ANGIOFIBROMA AND THE FIRST BRANCHIAL ARCH ARTERY

It has been proposed that the tumour origin is based on an incomplete regression of the first branchial arch artery.[6] This theory is especially attractive, as it is able to explain different aspects of JAs:

Firstly, during embryological development, the first branchial arch artery finally recedes close to the pterygoid base and sphenopalatine foramen regions. Secondly, vascular remnants of this artery are incorporated into the sphenopalatine and maxillary arteries themselves. Thus, both the proximity of tumour origin to the sphenopalatine foramen and its main blood supply from the sphenopalatine and maxillary arteries in early stages of JAs can be explained by the 'branchial arch artery' theory. The fact that this embryological vessel is connected to the C4-segment of the ICA deserves special attention in this context: persistent vascular remnants of the first branchial arch artery contacting the ICA are able to account for the observation of a vascular supply from the ICA, despite an anatomical distance between this vessel and the JA. Furthermore, the 'branchial arch artery' theory elucidates the common finding of residual tumour at the pterygoid base and clivus and explains why it is necessary to drill the bone in this specific location in order to remove tumour remnants at the site of origin.[2, 7]

ENDOSCOPIC RESECTIN: SURGICAL CONSIDERATIONS

Endoscopic resection of JAs follows tumour management principles by keeping the specific characteristics of this unique tumour in mind. Basically, the strategy of endoscopic resection takes the following considerations into account:

1. Opening of the maxillary sinus and exposure of its posterior wall are performed early during surgery. The size of the tumour dictates the size of the medial maxillectomy. The bony posterior wall of the maxillary sinus is removed with 'through cutting' punches or drills avoiding trauma to the periosteum in the pterygopalatine fossa before resection of the bone is completed. Following incision of the periosteum, the sphenopalatine and maxillary arteries are identified and clipped or coagulated. Early control of the main feeding vessel is of great value to assist further tumour resection. An alternative in early JAs is to push the tumour gently in a medial direction out of the pterygopalatine and infratemporal fossae and to identify the main feeding vessel by this manoeuvre. In cases where an extended access to the maxillary sinus does not allow exposure of the lateral tumour border within the infratemporal fossa in advanced JAs, the tumour can be pushed medially with a finger placed externally at the lateral border of the maxillary sinus below the jaw.
2. Resection of the posterior nasal septum is advised to widen the access in endoscopic tumour removal and to define tumour margins at the nasal septum.
3. The anterior sphenoid sinus wall is removed in order to expose the tumour within the sphenoid sinus. For this purpose, a bilateral opening of the sphenoid sinus is usually necessary.
4. Finally, the tumour is dissected directly off the pterygoid base and pterygoid canal regions and the clivus. Troublesome venous bleeding from the bone can be managed at this stage with drilling, chemical haemostatic agents or fine endosurgical diathermy.
5. It is of utmost importance to drill at the pterygoid base and the clivus at the end of surgery in order to avoid residual tumour.
6. Endoscopic dissection should always follow the pseudocapsule in order to avoid injury of the tumour at the surface. Finger-like extensions of the tumour can be gently pulled out along the pseudocapsule

INDICATION AND LIMITATION OF ENDOSCOPIC SURGERY

Endoscopic resection of JAs using the nostrils as natural openings is an ideal option to treat the majority of tumours successfully. Nevertheless, the endonasal approach should not be applied in a dogmatic sense. It depends on the personal experience of the surgeon to determine whether endoscopic tumour resection is appropriate in a particular JA. Each surgeon should feel free to convert to an open approach during surgery if the endoscopic resection cannot be performed in a particular situation. From the author's point of view, indications and limitations of endoscopic JA surgery will change for every surgeon with increasing experience in this field.

In general, the endoscopic resection can be used to remove JAs limited to the nasal cavity, the nasopharynx, the sphenoid sinus and the pterygopalatine fossa. With increasing experience, a surgeon might be able to perform an endoscopic resection of JAs which extend into the infratemporal fossa and to the space posterior to the pterygoid plate. With increasing experience, a surgeon will be able to remove tumour tissue from the orbit and the parasellar region in primary surgery. Generally, an endoscopic tumour resection is not recommended in situations of broad skull base infiltration, extensive blood supply from the internal carotid artery, encasement of the internal carotid artery and brain infiltration.[2]

Due to the importance of preserving neurovascular function, the surgeon may be forced to leave residual tumour in areas around the optic nerve, the cavernous sinus, the internal carotid artery and the dura, independent of the surgical approach selected. In cases of revision surgery for residual tumour, the surgeon should be very careful about selecting an endonasal approach, as the limitatons for endocopic approaches are different compared to primary surgery. If the residual tumour is potentially adherent by fibrosis to important neurovascular structures, it may not possible to tease out tumour tissue as one can in primary surgery. Careful radiological follow-up of residual tumour adjacent to delicate neurovascular structures assists in monitoring potential tumour growth. Nicolai has demonstrated that residual tumour does not necessarily expand when assessed on serial MR imaging.[2]

BEST CLINICAL PRACTICE

✓ Tumour biopsy should be avoided due to the risk of severe bleeding.
✓ The surgeon should always dissect along the pseudocapsule in order to avoid severe bleeding.
✓ The endoscopic resection can be used to remove JAs limited to the nasal cavity, the nasopharynx, the sphenoid sinus and the pterygopalatine fossa.
✓ An endoscopic tumour resection is not recommended in situations of broad skull base infiltration, extensive blood supply from the internal carotid artery, encasement of the internal carotid artery and brain infiltration.
✓ Juvenile angiofibromas can be mobilized along the pseudocapsule, but are firmly fixed at the clivus and the pterygoid base.
✓ Dissect strictly along the pseudocapsule and avoid entering the tumour surface, as this will result in severe bleeding due to the high-density of irregularly-shaped vessels at the surface.
✓ Finger-like tumour extensions can be teased out gently in most cases during primary surgery.
✓ Knowledge of the tumour arterial feeders is essential for the surgeon, as these need to be controlled during tumour resection.

- ✓ Always check carefully for tumour extension posterior to the pterygoid plate, as residual tumour can easily be left at this point.
- ✓ Drilling of the pterygoid base and the clivus is of the utmost importance in order to avoid residual tumour at the site of tumour origin.
- ✓ Endoscopic resection has been found to be a valuable alternative to external approaches for the successful management of most juvenile angiofibromas.
- ✓ With increasing experience, endoscopic management allows the surgeon not only to resect small, but also intermediate JAs.

KEY POINTS

- At the current time, and in the hands of experienced sinonasal surgeons, endoscopic resection has been proven to allow successful treatment of most JAs[2] based on a precise knowledge of the clinical findings.
- It is important to consider that JAs spread along natural foramina and fissures.
- The surgeon may be forced to leave residual tumour in areas around the optic nerve, the cavernous sinus, the internal carotid artery and the dura, independent of the surgical approach selected.
- Tumour origin is close to the sphenopalatine foramen and the pterygoid canal; bony destruction at the pterygoid base and the clivus is frequently observed.
- Widening of the sphenoplataine foramen and anterior displacement of the posterior maxillary sinus wall are typical radiological findings.
- Tumour spread takes place along natural foramina and fissures.
- The maxillary/sphenopalatine arteries are the main tumour feeders. However, the surgeon should always bear in mind that further tumour feeders may arise from the internal carotid artery.
- Tumour diagnosis is based on the typical signs on CT, MRI and angiography. A biopsy should not be performed due to the risk of severe bleeding.
- Irregularly-shaped vascular spaces, which may have an endothelial lining only, embedded in a fibrous stroma are the reason for potential profuse tumour bleeding.
- JAs are proposed to be vascular malformations originating from vascular remnants of the first branchial arch.

ACKNOWLEDGEMENTS

The author thanks Julia Dlugaiczyk, MD for a critical reading of the manuscript and valuable suggestions.

REFERENCES

1. Glad H, Vainer B, Buchwald C, et al. Juvenile nasopharyngeal angiofibromas in Denmark 1981–2003: diagnosis, incidence and treatment. *Acta Otolaryngol* 2007; **127**: 292–9.
2. Nicolai P, Schreiber A, Villaret AB. Juvenile angiofibroma: evolution of management. *Int J Ped* 2012; **2012**: 412545.
3. Schick B, Kahle G. Radiological findings in angiofibroma. *Acta Radiol* 2000; **41**: 585–93.
4. Beham A, Beham-Schmid C, Regauer S, et al. "Nasopharyngeal angiofibroma: true neoplasm or vascular malformation?" *Adv Anat Pathol* 2000; **7**: 36–46.
5. Schick B, Wemmert S, Willnecker V, et al. Genome-wide copy number profiling using a 100K SNP array reveals novel disease-related genes BORIS and TSHZ1 in juvenile angiofibroma. *Int J Oncol* 2011; **39**: 1143–51.
6. Schick B, Urbschat S. New aspects of pathogenesis of juvenile angiofibroma. *Hosp Med* 2004; **65**: 269–73.
7. Howard DJ, Lloyd G, Lund V. Recurrence and its avoidance in juvenile angiofibroma. *Laryngoscope* 2001; **111**: 1509–11.

ENDOSCOPIC MANAGEMENT OF SINONASAL TUMOURS

Alkis J. Psaltis and David K. Morrissey

Introduction 1269	Principles of endoscopic management of sinonasal tumours 1273
Evidence base for endoscopic management of sinonasal tumours... 1269	Post-operative care and tumour surveillance 1278
Sinonasal tumour epidemiology 1269	Conclusion 1279
Diagnosis and pre-operative planning 1270	References 1279

SEARCH STRATEGY

This chapter is based on and supported by a detailed search strategy encompassing PubMed, Medline and the Cochrane Library. Searches utilized a combination of keywords associated with the endoscopic management of sinonasal tumours. These keywords included but were not limited to: paranasal sinus, endoscopy, sinonasal tumours, benign sinus lesions, malignant sinus lesions, endoscopic field control, endoscopic access, image guidance, vascular, orbital and intra-cranial extension and injury.

INTRODUCTION

With the advent of the endoscope and its early application to the management of inflammatory sinonasal conditions, surgeons identified significant advantages of endoscopic endonasal surgery over open approaches. Increasing endoscopic experience and advances in instrumentation and imaging technology have led to a natural evolution and expansion of endoscopic endonasal surgery to now commonly include the management of benign and malignant sinonasal tumours. The scope of this chapter is to provide the reader with a general overview of the approach to the endoscopic management of sinonasal tumours. Tumour specific management can be found in other chapters dedicated to the individual pathologies.

EVIDENCE BASE FOR ENDOSCOPIC MANAGEMENT OF SINONASAL TUMOURS

As surgical experience with the endoscopic resection of sinonasal tumours increases, so has the body of evidence supporting its role.[1] Systematic reviews and large case series now support the endoscopic approach as a favourable treatment option for the management of benign tumours, including most cases of sinonasal inverted papilloma,[2-5] juvenile nasal angiofibroma[6-8] and osseous tumours such as osteomas,[9,10] ossifying fibromas[11] and fibrous dysplasia.[12,13]

The application of endonasal endoscopic techniques to the management of malignant sinonasal tumours has been more controversial.[14-16] Early concerns raised included the violation of the oncologic principle of en bloc resection, the ability to deal with vascular complications and the difficulty associated with defect reconstruction. Evidence is now emerging however that refutes such concerns, with large case series showing reduced morbidity,[17] improved vascular control,[18] better quality of life outcomes[19] and equivalent survival outcomes to open approaches. These findings have led to the support of the endoscopic approach for the management of sinonasal tumours by a recently published European Position Paper.[20] Malignant pathologies successfully treated via endoscopic techniques include squamous cell carcinoma, adenoid cystic carcinoma, adenocarcinoma, aesthesioneuroblastoma, sinonasal undifferentiated carcinoma and sinonasal melanoma.[15,17-24]

SINONASAL TUMOUR EPIDEMIOLOGY

Tumours involving the sinonasal cavity are considered rare entities. They can arise from any of the structures comprising the paranasal sinuses or can involve the sinuses by direct extension from adjacent structures. Consequently, these tumours encompass a large and diverse group of lesions (Table 114.1). The most commonly reported benign lesion is a sinonasal osteoma, with a radiological incidence of 1%. Ossifying fibroma, fibrous dysplasia and inverted papilloma are the next most commonly reported

TABLE 114.1 Summary of sinonasal tumours by tissue of origin

Tissue of origin	Benign lesions	Malignant lesions
Epithelial	• Inverted Papilloma • Oncocytic Papilloma • Exophytic Papilloma • Respiratory Epithelial Adenomatoid Hamartoma (REAH) • Salivary Gland Adenomas	• Squamous Cell Carcinoma • Sinonasal Undifferentiated Carcinoma (SNUC) • Lymphoepithelial Carcinoma • Adenocarcinoma • Salivary Gland Carcinomas • Mucoepidermoid • Adenoid Cystic Carcinoma • Acinic cell Carcinoma
Neuroendocrine		• Carcinoid
Soft tissue	• Myxoma • Leiomyoma • Haemangioma • Schwannoma • Meningioma • Neurofibroma • Angiofibroma • Haemangiopericytoma	• Fibrosarcoma • Rhabdomyosarcoma • Angiosarcoma • Malignant Peripheral Nerve Sheath Tumour
Bone and cartilage	• Fibrous Dysplasia • Osteoma • Osteoblastoma • Chondroma • Ameloblastoma	• Chondrosarcoma • Osteosarcoma • Chordoma
Haematological and lymphatic		• Lymphoma • Langerhans cell Histiocytosis
Germ cell tumours	• Dermoid cyst	• Teratoma Sinonasal yolk sac tumour
Neuroectodermal tumours		• Esthesioneuroblastoma

benign lesions of the paranasal sinuses.[20] Sinonasal malignancies are less common with an estimated incidence of 0.5–1/100 000.[25] They account for around 1% of all malignancies and 3–5% of all head and neck cancers.[20, 23] Primary epithelial tumours are the most common type of sinonasal malignant tumour, with squamous cell carcinoma the most common subtype followed by adenoid cystic carcinoma and adenocarcinoma. Of the less common non-epithelial tumours, lymphoma is the most commonly reported tumour.[20]

DIAGNOSIS AND PRE-OPERATIVE PLANNING

Evaluation of sinonasal masses should commence with a complete history and physical examination. In addition to a focused otorhinological examination, a complete cranial nerve assessment should be performed on all these patients. Table 114.2 highlights concerning features that should be looked for on clinical examination.

Endoscopy

Nasal endoscopy forms an integral part of the rhinological assessment. Although large masses may create difficulty with respect to performing a complete endoscopic assessment, it is important to obtain as much information pre-operatively as possible. Documentation of the likely site of origin, as well as involvement or destruction of the septum, lacrimal system, orbit, palate, nasopharynx and skull base is important and may provide useful information regarding the likely pathology, endoscopic resectability and access or approach required. Although biopsy may be performed at the time of endoscopic assessment, we recommend review of the relevant radiological investigation. This may avoid catastrophic complications including torrential bleeding or CSF leak (**Figure 114.1**).

Radiology

Radiological investigations in the form of computed tomography (CT) and magnetic resonance imaging (MRI) are critical in management of sinonasal tumours. Imaging not only helps characterize the tumour and assess the local and regional extension but also aids in the planning of surgery and adjuvant treatments. High resolution CT scans with contrast and slice thickness of 1 mm should be performed in all patients. CT scan permits superior assessment of osseous margins of the skull base and sinus walls which are less effectively demonstrated on MRI. Specific features to assess on CT scan and their clinical implications are shown in **Table 114.3**.

MRI provides inherently superior soft-tissue resolution and multiplanar capabilities, rendering it superior for the assessment of soft-tissue masses and extension of infectious or malignant processes outside the confines of the paranasal sinuses. MRI facilitates the differentiation of retained secretions and haemorrhage from the tumour mass and allows a better appreciation of the tumour margin and its interface with normal tissue and critical structures. MRI of the paranasal sinuses must include

TABLE 114.2 Concerning features on clinical examination

Clinical finding	Reason for concern
Conductive hearing loss/Middle ear effusion	Obstruction/invasion of eustachian tube
Visual change/loss	Optic nerve involvement
Visual field change	Intra-cranial extension, optic chiasm compression
Diplopia/Ophthalmoplegia	Involvement of intra-orbital contents
Pain on eye movement	
Chemosis/Orbital displacement	
Clear rhinorrhea	Dural/Intra-cranial involvement with CSF leak
Facial paraesthesia	Compression/invasion of the maxillary or infraorbital nerve
Loose teeth	Invasion of the alveolar process and dental roots
Dental paraesthesia	
Facial asymmetry	Possible involvement of facial soft tissues
Oronasal or Oroantral fistula	Erosion of the nasal floor or maxillary sinus floor
Palpable cervical nodal disease	Possible metastatic spread
Reduced neck range of motion	Paraspinal muscle involvement

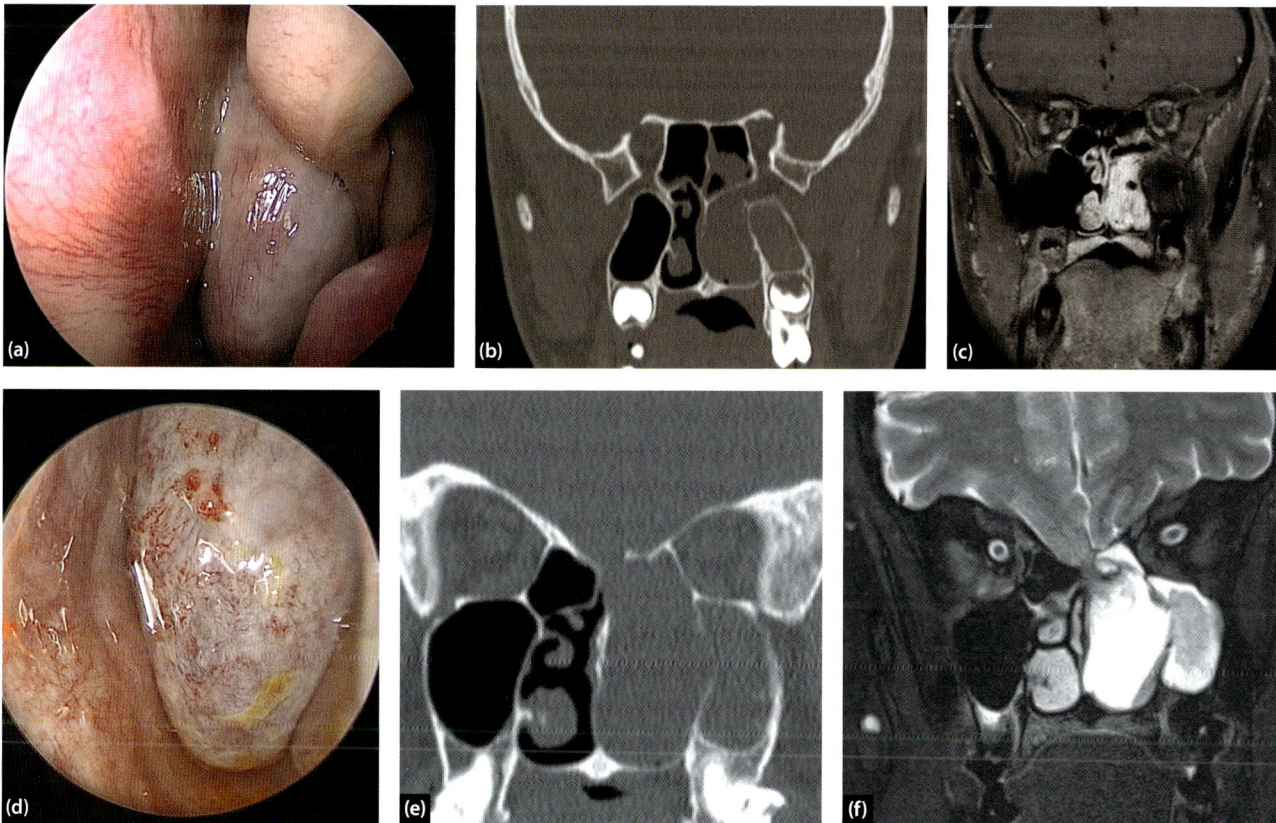

Figure 114.1 Highlights the importance of obtaining imaging prior to the biopsy of a nasal lesion. (a) Endoscopic Image of left juvenile nasal angiofibroma resembling a simple benign nasal polyp in the sphenoethmoidal recess. **(b)** Coronal CT scan of left juvenile nasal angiofibroma showing characteristic expansion of the sphenopalatine foramen and **(c)** an MRI T1 with gadolinium contrast demonstrating the extensive vascularity of the juvenile nasal angiofibroma with the presence of flow voids as well. **(d)** An endoscopic image of a large left sided encephalocele presenting a left sided nasal mass. **(e)** CT and **(f)** MRI coronal images of the left encephalocele showing the clear intra-cranial origin and skull base defect. Although the pathology is suspected from the CT, MRI is needed to confirm the diagnosis prior to surgery.

high resolution (1 mm) T1- and T2-weighted images of the sinonasal cavity, orbit, skull base and the adjacent intra-cranial compartment. Understanding the advantage of each sequence and a systematic approach to the evaluation of the images can be extremely useful to the surgeon in understanding the characteristics of the tumour. The use of gadolinium chelate contrast agents with fat saturation increases the sensitivity of the contrast enhancement, thereby improving the detection of local disease extent and the presence of disease beyond the paranasal sinuses such

TABLE 114.3 Radiological features on CT and their possible implications	
Feature	**Potential clinical implication**
ORBIT	
Breech of lamina papyracea Loss of orbital fat planes Involvement of extra-ocular muscles	May indicate involvement of orbit and the need for orbital exenteration.
SEPTUM	
Erosion of septum	Important implications for surgical access and repair. Lesions crossing midline will require a septectomy and binasal approach. Gross septal involvement may preclude the use of the nasoseptal flap.
SKULL BASE	
Asymmetrical or low lying	Increase risk of inadvertent entry and CSF leak during surgery
Position of anterior ethmoid arteries	Mesentery suspended arteries are at increased risk of injury
Skull base defect	Suggestive of intra-cranial extension of sinonasal pathology or intra-nasal extension of intra-cranial pathology
SPHENOID SINUS	
Extent of pneumatization	Laterally pneumatized sinuses may place the carotid at risk
Onodi cells	May contain optic nerve and be confused with sphenoid sinus
Location of sphenoid septations	Septations may be closely related to carotid artery and optic nerve, requiring great care when removing.
PARANASAL SINUS	
Osteitic changes	Possible site of tumour origin
Widened bony foramina	Perineural invasion of tumour
	Nerve sheath tumour
Tumour calcification	See to varying degrees with aesthesioneuroblastoma, chondroma, chondrosarcoma, osteoma, ossifying fibroma and osteosarcoma
Expansion of paranasal sinus / fossae	Tends to indicate the presence of a mass within the space

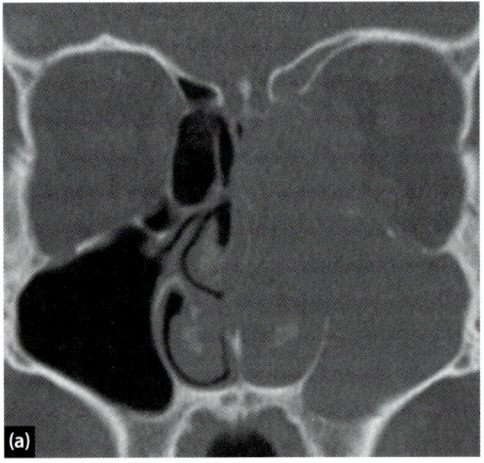
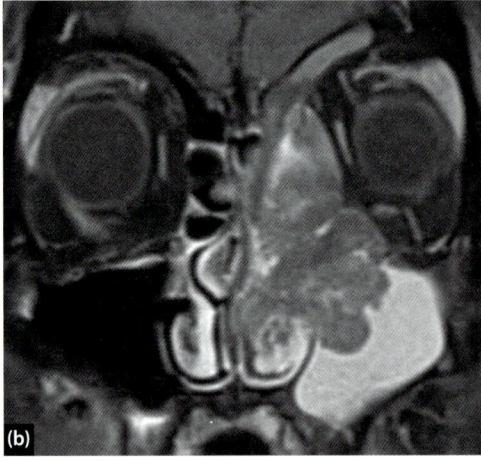

Figure 114.2 Coronal CT and MRI of a sinonasal tumour. Although the CT would suggest involvement of the extra-ocular muscles, the MRI demonstrates clear preservation of the fat plane. The MRI also facilitates a differentiation of tumour from retained secretions seen in the maxillary sinus. These images highlight the importance of obtaining both a CT and MRI for skull base tumours.

as dural involvement or perineural spread. Figure 114.2 demonstrates the complementary features of CT and MRI in the work-up of skull base tumours.

Clinical Positron Emission Tomography (PET) relies on the preferential uptake of 18-fluorodeoxyglucose (18-FDG) by tumour cells that exhibit a higher density of GLUT1 glucose transporters. When combined with CT it can improve tumour localization, although the increased 18-FDG avidity in areas of sinonasal inflammation or infection can confound its utility in the paranasal sinuses.

In the evaluation of these tumours its usefulness is predominantly confined to the detection of distant metastases.

Biopsy

Pre-operative endoscopic-guided biopsies should be taken prior to performing the definitive surgical procedure. Biopsies should typically be performed after reviewing the relevant radiology to exclude vascular lesions or prolapsed meningo-encephaloceles. Whenever possible, multiple deep biopsies from the centre of the tumour should be taken to gain a representative sample and avoid sampling the non-specific and necrotic superficial aspects of the tumour. Tissue should always be sent both fresh, and in formalin fixative, to allow both routine histopathology and flow cytometry. Tumour histopathology will help direct management and intra-operative decision-making.

Multidisciplinary planning meetings

All patients with malignant and complex pathology should be presented to a multidisciplinary team, comprising of surgeons, radiologists, medical and radiation oncologists and allied health professionals. Treatment recommendations made by the team should not only take into account the pathology of the tumour but also the age, health and functional status of the patients, as well as their level of home support. Although complete oncological clearance is the ultimate goal of any treatment, this may not be possible without causing significant morbidity to the patient. Patients and families should be informed of all the different treatment options discussed at tumour board meetings to enable informed consent to be made.

PRINCIPLES OF ENDOSCOPIC MANAGEMENT OF SINONASAL TUMOURS

Case selection

As experience with endoscopic cranial base surgery increases, so have the limits of what is considered endoscopically resectable. Dura, the olfactory bulbs and lamina papyracea can all be safely resected as can the entire anterior cranial base from the cribiform plate to the planum sphenoidale. Transclival approaches allow resection of tumours from the nasopharynx, clivus and the odontoid process, with the inferior limit of endoscopic resectabilty considered the nasopalatine line.[26] Endoscopic medial maxillectomy provides access to the pterygopalatine and infratemporal fossa, while the petrous temporal bone, Meckel's cave and middle cranial fossa can be accessed via the transpterygoid approach. Relative contraindications to an entirely endoscopic approach include the involvement of skin and subcutaneous tissue, the nasolacrimal sac, carotid artery, the anterior table of the frontal sinus and extensive dural and brain involvement (Figure 114.3). Like all forms of surgery, endoscopic endonasal surgery is associated with a steep learning curve. It is recommended that surgeons considering performing oncological surgery first become proficient in the surgical management of sinonasal inflammatory disease, before progressing to benign and eventually malignant tumours. Surgeons should use simpler cases to improve their familiarity with the endoscopic anatomy as well as the ergonomics involved in endoscopic surgery. The latter takes on greater importance when a second surgeon becomes involved.

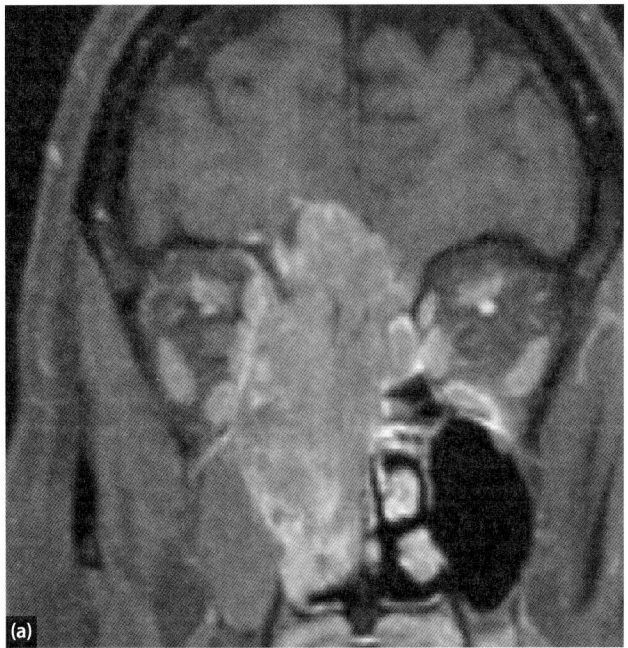
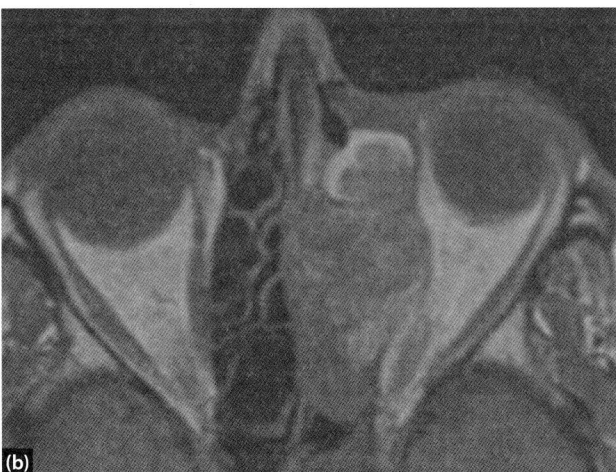
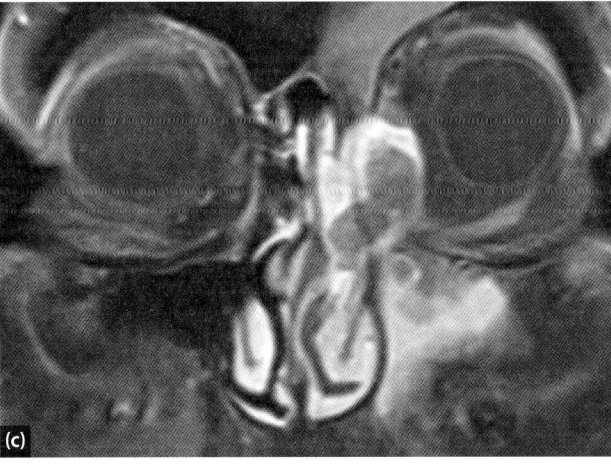

Figure 114.3 Demonstrates relative contraindications to a purely endoscopic resection. (a) shows gross intra-cranial involvement necessitating a combined endoscopic and anterior craniofacial approach; (b) shows frank invasion of the extra-ocular muscles with loss of preservation of the orbital fat planes and (c) shows involvement of the lacrimal apparatus and the anterior soft tissue structures.

Optimizing the surgical field

Poor visualization due to excessive bleeding has been shown to be associated with an increased risk of intra-operative complications.[27–30] Strategies to improve the surgical field include proper patient positioning, regulation of haemodynamic parameters, adequate topicalization and the use of electrocautery. Studies suggest that positioning a patient in 15–20° of reverse Trendelenberg can increase venous drainage without compromising cerebral perfusion. Similarly, the use of total intravenous anaesthesia to maintain a mean arterial blood pressure of approximately 60 mmHg and a pulse rate below 70 bpm has also been shown to decrease surgical bleeding without affecting cerebral blood flow, provided a patient does not have underlying cardiovascular disease. Pre-operative topicalization of the nasal cavity with local anaesthetic infiltration and patties soaked in vasoconstricting agents is also useful as is the intra-operative use of haemostatic agents such as Gelfoam® and Floseal®, along with the use of warm saline irrigations and cautery.[30] Although suction monopolar cautery is extremely useful in tumour debulking, it should be avoided near the skull base and orbit due to the theoretical risk of heat and electrical current transmission to vital structures.

Image guidance technology

Image guidance technology is considered a useful aid when performing endoscopic skull base surgery. It provides the surgeon with enhanced anatomical localization and the current literature suggests that its use may decrease surgical disorientation, improve surgical completeness and potentially lower complication rates.[31, 32] The incorporation of CT/MRI fusion is also thought to provide valuable information with regard to the extent of tumour resection and the clarification of boundaries between the tumour and normal adjacent soft tissues and neurovascular structures.[33]

Principles of oncologic resection

The complete resection of a tumour with as little morbidity as possible is the primary goal of any oncological surgery. Although traditional surgical paradigm dictates that this be performed in an en bloc manner, the anatomical confines of the nasal cavity prevent this for the vast majority of endoscopic tumour resections. Fortunately, despite filling the nasal cavity, many sinonasal tumours have a small, well-defined area of origin or tissue invasion. Provided en bloc excision of this site is performed, ideally with a cuff of normal surrounding tissue, the remainder of the tumour can be selectively debulked down to attachment points, without compromising the completeness of resection or increasing the risk of recurrence.[34]

Surgical access techniques

Prior to debulking the tumour, the initial steps of the procedure are aimed at improving surgical access. The purpose of this is twofold. Firstly it will allow the surgeon more room for instrumentation and improve the vectors needed to approach the peripheral aspects of the tumour and secondly, it will allow early identification of tumour-free zones that can serve as margins or the limits of the resection.

IMPROVING LATERAL ACCESS

Lateral sinonasal tumours, including those involving the maxillary sinus and pterygopalatine or infratemporal fossae have historically proven difficult to access endoscopically. The introduction of angled endoscopes and instrumentation as well as the development of various approaches has meant that many of these tumours can now be resected entirely endoscopically. To access such tumours, surgeons must not only consider the lateral extent of these tumours, but the likely vectors required for instrumentation. Tumours confined to the nasal cavity with no extension beyond the infra-orbital nerve can usually be managed through the ipsilateral nostril, while those extending outside this zone will require additional lateral access. Lateral access can be improved through a transeptal approach often combined with removing varying amounts of the medial maxillary wall.

Transeptal approach

Although various transeptal approaches have been described, they are all variations of the concept of non-opposing septal incisions described by Douglas et al.[35] This procedure allows use of the contralateral nostril for instruments or endoscopes thereby increasing the horizontal plane of access. The additional advantage it confers is that it allows a second surgeon to be involved to provide retraction and additional instrumentation when required. Although septal perforation is a risk of this approach, it can be reduced by preserving rather than resecting septal cartilage, and ensuring that the mucosal incisions on either side of the septum are not opposing (**Figure 114.4**).

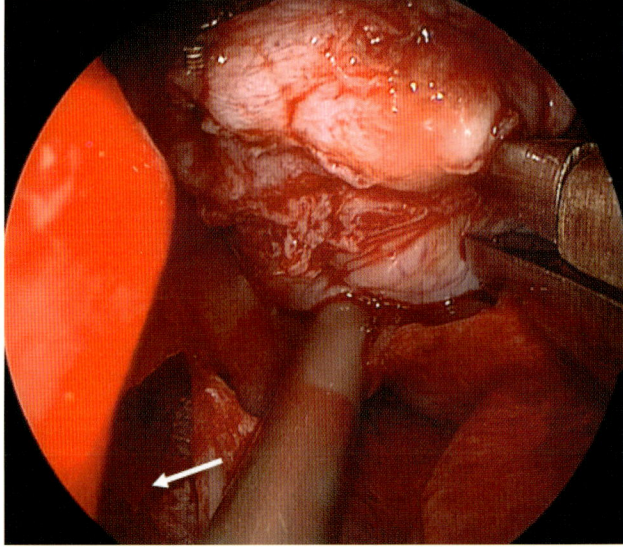

Figure 114.4 This image demonstrates the utility of the trans-septal approach. Here a patient with a Juvenile Nasal Angiofibroma has the mass manipulated via an instrument in the contralateral nostril placed through the transeptal incision (arrow) and the ipsilateral nostril.

Transmaxillary approaches

Surgery for lesions involving the maxillary sinus typically commences by performing a routine uncinectomy to identify the natural maxillary ostium. Depending on the size and location of the tumour, the antrostomy can then be enlarged accordingly. Posteriorly based lesions, including those extending into the pterygopalatine fossa, located medial to the infra-orbital nerve can usually be accessed with a mega-antrostomy. Lesions located lateral to the infra-orbital nerve or those involving the infratemporal fossa require more extensive resection of the medial maxillary wall. A modified medial maxillectomy allows preservation of the lacrimal duct by extending the mega-antrostomy inferiorly below Hasner's valve to the piriform aperture. This approach allows inferiolateral access to the maxillary sinus (**Figure 114.5**).

For more superiorly based lesions, a total medial maxillectomy is needed with transection of the nasolacrimal duct. Although this approach confers an inherent risk of epiphoria, this can be minimized with clean sharp transection of the duct followed by probing and splaying the duct open. The anterolateral area of the maxillary sinus is considered the most difficult to access endoscopically. The pre-lacrimal approach as described by Zhou et al[36] is a modification of the Denker's procedure, that allows direct access to this area, with reduced alar retraction, collapse and risk to the canine root. In this procedure, following reflection of the soft tissues and mucosa of the anterior aspect of the inferior turbinate, osteotomies are used to remove a small buttress of bone at the junction of the antero-medial walls of the maxillary sinus, adjacent to the pre-lacrimal recess, with the nasolacrimal duct visualized and left intact. Through this window, the surgeon has direct access to the entire maxillary sinus including the anterior and lateral walls. Tumours can be carefully removed from these regions and sites of origin/attachment can be directly addressed (**Figure 114.6**).

IMPROVING POSTERIOR ACCESS

Binasal access provides the key to addressing tumours involving the nasopharynx, sphenoid sinus, pituitary fossa and the infratemporal and pterygopalatine fossae. The creation of an adequately sized posterior septectomy affords such access. Through this septal window,

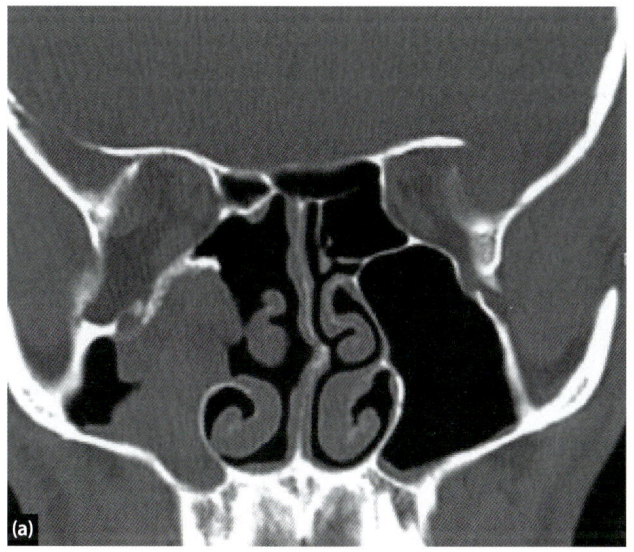

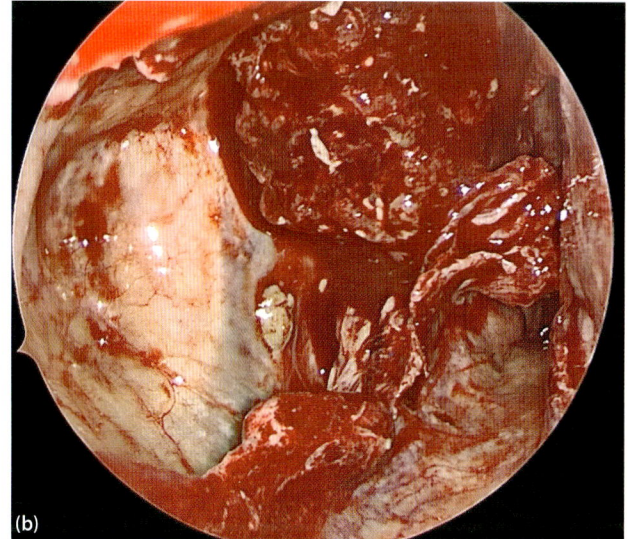

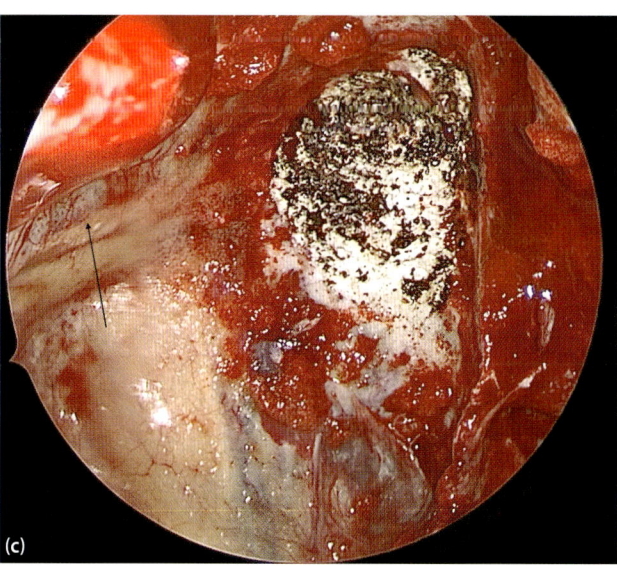

Figure 114.5 **(a)** Coronal CT of the sinuses showing a right maxillary inverted papilloma arising from the roof of the maxillary sinus medial to the infra-orbital nerve. The area of osteitis often indicates the site of origin; **(b and c)** demonstrate the site of origin of the inverted papilloma prior to **(b)** and after **(c)** it has been removed, drilled down and cauterized to reduce the chance of recurrence. The black arrow indicates the infraorbital nerve.

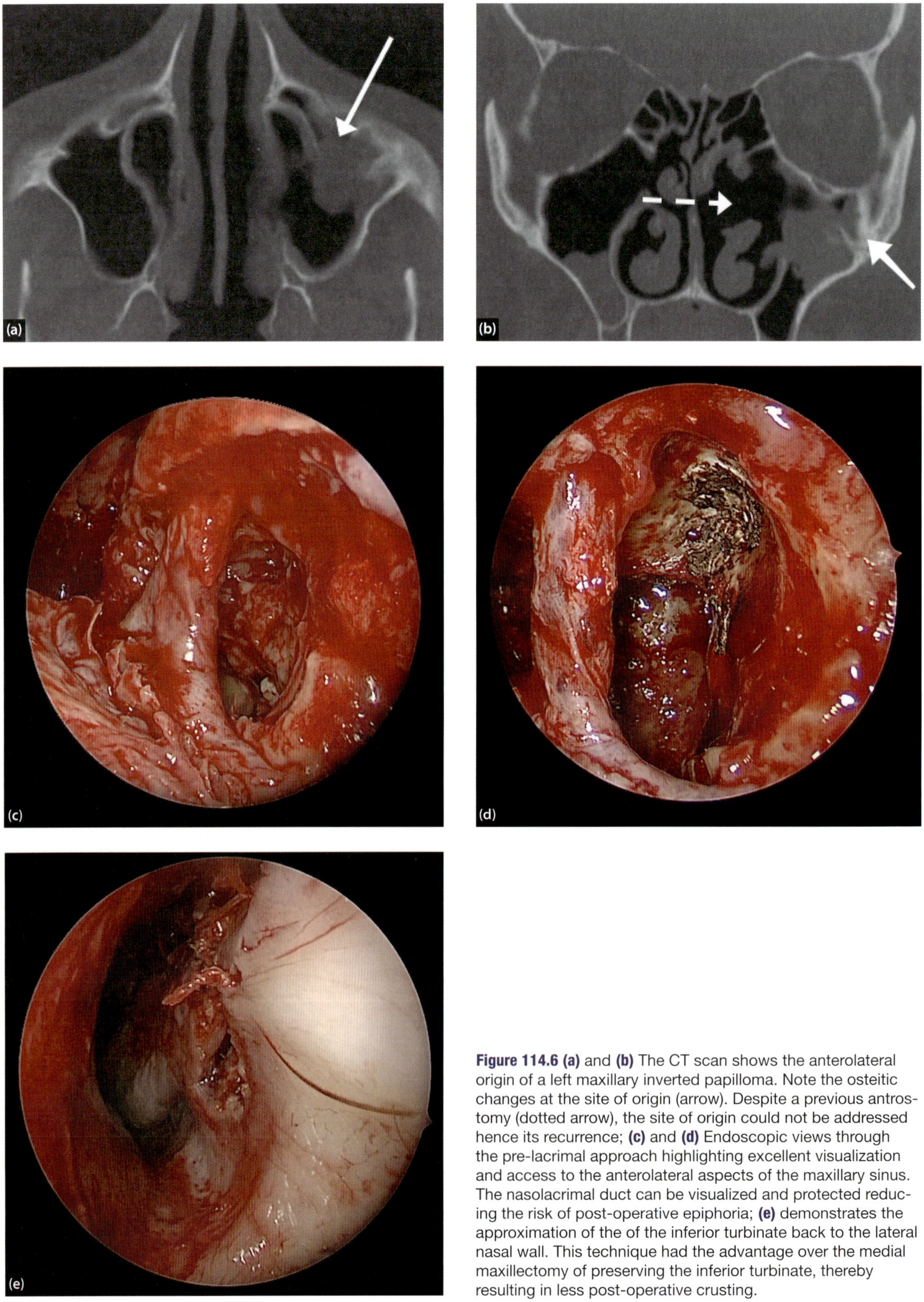

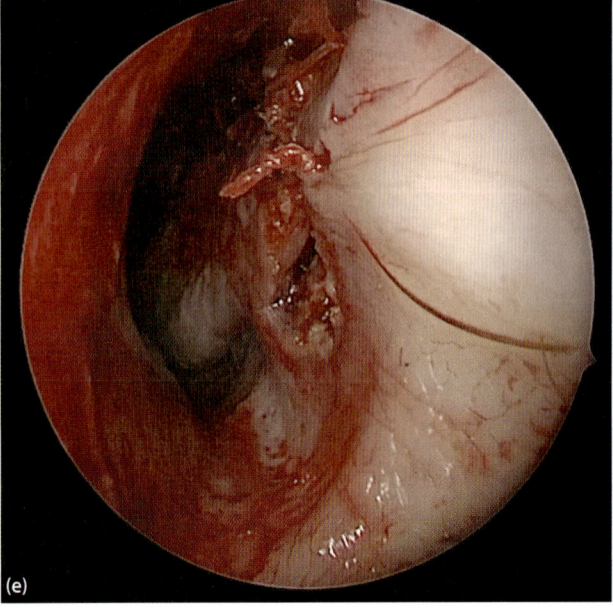

Figure 114.6 (a) and **(b)** The CT scan shows the anterolateral origin of a left maxillary inverted papilloma. Note the osteitic changes at the site of origin (arrow). Despite a previous antrostomy (dotted arrow), the site of origin could not be addressed hence its recurrence; **(c)** and **(d)** Endoscopic views through the pre-lacrimal approach highlighting excellent visualization and access to the anterolateral aspects of the maxillary sinus. The nasolacrimal duct can be visualized and protected reducing the risk of post-operative epiphoria; **(e)** demonstrates the approximation of the of the inferior turbinate back to the lateral nasal wall. This technique had the advantage over the medial maxillectomy of preserving the inferior turbinate, thereby resulting in less post-operative crusting.

a two-surgeon team can utilize an endoscope and up to three surgical instruments to reach the aforementioned posterior regions.

Posterior septectomy

Before performing a posterior septectomy, the surgeon must consider whether a nasoseptal flap will be required for reconstruction. This flap is based on the posterior septal artery, a branch of the sphenopalatine artery, and runs just below the sphenoid ostium to supply the majority of the septal mucosa. If a CSF leak is anticipated, the nasoseptal flap is typically raised before performing the septectomy and then stored either in the nasopharynx or in the maxillary sinus. If a leak is not anticipated, the surgeon must still take care to preserve the pedicle in case a flap may be required later. At this stage, the sphenoid ostia are located on either side and enlarged superiorly to the skull base and laterally to the lamina papyracea. Wide exposure allows visualization of the bony landmarks of the internal carotid artery and optic nerves and avoids inadvertent injury. With this exposure, the surgeon can then perform an appropriately-sized septectomy depending on the access required. For sellar lesions, a limited septectomy may be all that is necessary and this typically involves removing the posterior and inferior aspect of the septum with powered instrumentation or retrograde forceps. The septal window should extend anteriorly enough to enable complete visualization of the entire surgical field and limit contralateral instrument clash. An even larger septectomy will be required for surgery involving the middle cranial fossa, clivus and infratemporal fossae. Where possible, surgeons should attempt to preserve at least 1.5 cm of postero-superior septal mucosa in the region of the olfactory cleft for preservation of smell and taste (**Figure 114.7**). Obviously in the case of malignant tumours, surgical clearance of the tumour takes precedence but patients

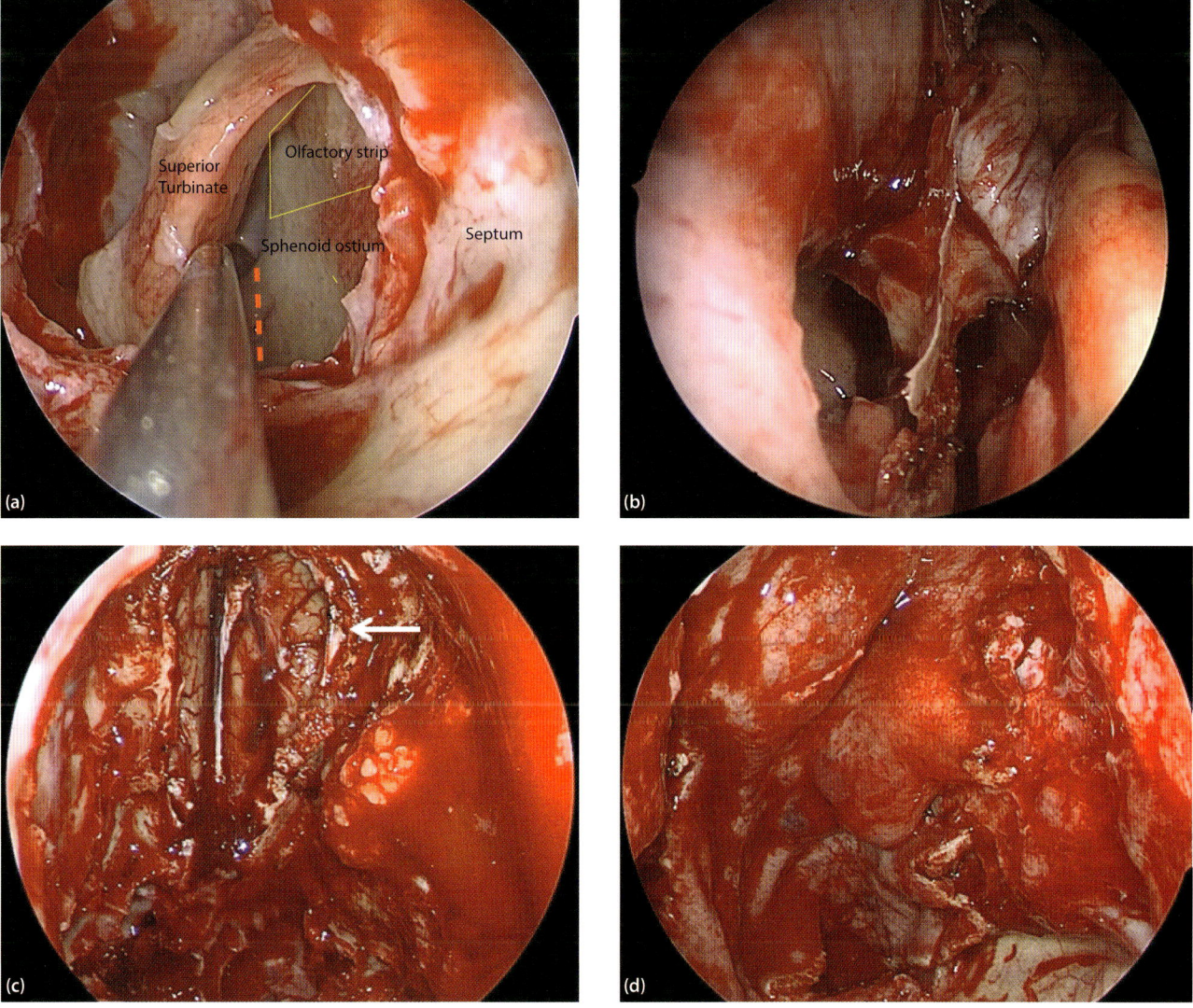

Figure 114.7 (a) Shows an endoscopic view of the nasal cavity and septum via the transethmoid approach. Highlighted in yellow is the olfactory strip that needs to be preserved when harvesting the flap. The red dotted line is the area of the vascular predicle supplying the flap. This should not be violated; **(b)** demonstrates the right nasoseptal flap reflected into the post nasal space. **(c)** shows a skull base defect of the anterior cranial fossa following resection of an aesthesioneuroblastoma. The white arrow represents the edge of the skull base defect and **(d)** shows reconstruction of the defect with a large nasoseptal flap.

should be warned pre-operatively of the possible loss of function of these senses.

IMPROVING SUPERIOR ACCESS

All aspects of the anterior skull base can be accessed endoscopically allowing the complete endoscopic resection of sinonasal tumours with intra-cranial extension. The anterior ethmoid artery provides a useful landmark when planning surgery for these lesions. If the intra-cranial component lies posterior to these vessels, targeted resection of the posterior skull base can usually provide adequate access for tumour removal. If however, the intra-cranial extent of the tumour lies anterior to the level of the anterior ethmoid arteries, an endoscopic modified lothrop procedure (EMLP) will typically be required to access the anterior aspect of the tumour. The EMLP also improves lateral access to lesions within the frontal sinus. Through a superior septectomy, surgeons can use the contralateral nostril to reach lesions well beyond the frontal recess and even beyond the mid-pupillary line. This not only avoids the need for external incisions, but also increases the ease of post-operative surveillance. The surgical site can be directly visualized endoscopically, reducing the need for as frequent imaging.

Tumour resection

Once appropriate access has been created, the tumour can then be debulked in a controlled manner down to its site of attachment. Debulking can be performed using various instruments including powered micro-debriders and radio-frequency ablation wands. Specimen traps should be applied to instruments, so that all of the tumour removed from the patient can be sent for histopathological analysis. Following debulking of the tumour, the site of attachment is usually visualized. The management of this region depends on numerous factors, including the age and functional state of the patient, the histology of the tumour and the location and extent of the attachment. Where possible, attainment of clear surgical margins should be attempted. Frozen sections taken from the margins of the tumour field have been shown to be reliable for ensuring complete resection of most sinonasal tumours, with the exception of mucosal melanoma and adenoid cystic tumours.[37] In addition to these frozen specimens, surgical margin specimens should also be sent in formalin fixative for formal histo-pathological analysis. Careful orientation of specimens and close discussion with the histopathologists should be undertaken for all specimens, to aid in the generation of an accurate histological report and to avoid errors such as the air-tumour interface being erroneously reported as a positive margin.

Whilst the ultimate goal of surgery is a complete oncological resection of the tumour, the nature of the tumour and the characteristics of the individual patient may, on occasion, necessitate a degree of compromise. Benign tumours may be appropriate for sub-total resections with post-operative surveillance where there is significant risk to critical structures or in the elderly frail population. Malignant tumours may also be palliated in this fashion while limiting morbidity from the resection.

Reconstruction

Sinonasal tumour resection may result in a defect in the skull base. If the dura remains intact, and the defect is small, it may be left alone, but large defects and all breaches of the dura should be repaired to avoid meningo-encephalocele formation and ascending meningitis.

Small defects (< 1cm) in the dura mater are typically amenable to a 'Bath Plug' type repair as described by Wormald.[38] Larger defects, however, will usually require multi-layer closure with an underlay of autogenic material such as tensor facia lata harvested from the thigh or dural substitutes (e.g. Duragen®, Integra Life Sciences, Plainsboro, New Jersey USA), followed by an overlay which may be a free-mucosal graft or in most cases a vascularized flap. The most commonly employed vascularized flap is the Hadad nasoseptal flap,[39] described in the previous section, but inferior and middle turbinate flaps have also been successfully used. For very large defects (> 3 cm), reinforcement of the repair site with a rigid buttress of septal cartilage or titanium mesh is also thought necessary, prior to coverage with the mucosal flap, to minimize the risk of encephalocele formation.

Complications of endoscopic techniques

Endoscopic approaches to sinonasal tumours share the minor and major complications seen in endoscopic sinus surgery. Surgeons who wish to perform endoscopic skull base surgery must make themselves familiar with these complications and their management. A thorough understanding of the surgical and radiological anatomy of the sinuses and skull base and the attendance of skull base courses may help to minimize their frequency and severity. Of all the complications, major vascular injury is one of the most serious and anxiety provoking. Through animal wet labs, Valentine and Wormald have developed and evaluated several techniques for controlling such injuries, including the use of the muscle patch.[40] They showed that the application of crushed muscle to the site of a major arterial bleed could primarily control the bleed in all cases while maintaining vascular patency. This led to reduced blood loss and overall improved survival.[41] A follow-up study by the same group highlighted the benefits of surgeons undergoing training in this technique before undertaking complex skull base cases.[41]

POST-OPERATIVE CARE AND TUMOUR SURVEILLANCE

Once the initial perioperative period is complete, the role of the surgeon moves to one of surveillance for recurrence. Surveillance is performed with regular endoscopic examinations and serial imaging. Performance of an early post-operative CT or MRI scan within 3–6 months post-surgery provides a baseline that can be referenced, should the patient develop clinical features suggestive of recurrence.

CONCLUSION

Published data now support the use of endoscopic techniques for the management of appropriately selected benign and malignant tumours of the paranasal sinuses. The decision to undertake such a resection should ultimately be made by a multidisciplinary team that has considered the patient, the pathology in question and the skill set of the endoscopic skull base team. With appropriate training and surgical planning, complications can be minimized and outcomes can become more predictable.

> ### FUTURE RESEARCH
>
> ➤ New technology and increased experience continues to advance the field of endoscopic sinus and skull base surgery. Although still in early development, real-time intra-operative imaging, 3-dimensional endoscopes and remotely controlled robotic instrumentation hold promise in their application to this field. Such technology may one day further improve the safety and oncological results of endoscopic skull base procedures.

> ### KEY POINTS
>
> - The operating surgeon must understand the anatomy of the paranasal sinuses and the nature of the pathology to be managed.
> - A comprehensive history and examination with review of radiology and biopsy specimens will enable a safe and effective plan to be formulated for the endoscopic approach to sinonasal tumours.
> - The surgeon must be aware of the limitations of his or her individual endoscopic skills and the capabilities of the other teams involved to ensure that case selection is appropriate.
> - Endoscopic skills and equipment are rapidly evolving, thus surgeons must remain current in their knowledge and skill development to undertake this complex surgery.

REFERENCES

1. Sciarretta V, Pasquini E, Frank G, et al. Endoscopic treatment of benign tumors of the nose and paranasal sinuses: a report of 33 cases. *Am J Rhinol* 2006; **20**(1): 64–71.
2. Busquets JM, Hwang PH. Endoscopic resection of sinonasal inverted papilloma: a meta-analysis. *Otolaryngol Head Neck Surg* 2006; **134**(3): 476–82.
3. Carta F, Blancal J-P, Verillaud B, et al. Surgical management of inverted papilloma: approaching a new standard for surgery. *Head Neck* 2013; **35**(10): 1415–20.
4. Karkos PD, Fyrmpas G, Carrie SC, Swift AC. Endoscopic versus open surgical interventions for inverted nasal papilloma: a systematic review. *Clin Otolaryngol* 2006; **31**(6): 499–503.
5. Lombardi D, Tomenzoli D, Buttà L, et al. Limitations and complications of endoscopic surgery for treatment for sinonasal inverted papilloma: a reassessment after 212 cases. *Head Neck* 201; **33**(8): 1154–61.
6. Boghani Z, Husain Q, Kanumuri VV, et al. Juvenile nasopharyngeal angiofibroma: a systematic review and comparison of endoscopic, endoscopic-assisted, and open resection in 1047 cases. *Laryngoscope* 2013; **123**(4): 859–69.
7. Huang Y, Liu Z, Wang J, et al. Surgical management of juvenile nasopharyngeal angiofibroma: analysis of 162 cases from 1995 to 2012. *Laryngoscope* 2014; **124**(8): 1942–6.
8. Khoueir N, Nicolas N, Rohayem Z, et al. Exclusive endoscopic resection of juvenile nasopharyngeal angiofibroma: a systematic review of the literature. *Otolaryngol Head Neck Surg* 2014; **150**(3): 350–8.
9. Seiberling K, Floreani S, Robinson S, Wormald P-J. Endoscopic management of frontal sinus osteomas revisited. *Am J Rhinol Allergy* 2009; **23**(3): 331–6.
10. Turri-Zanoni M, Dallan I, Terranova P, et al. Frontoethmoidal and intraorbital osteomas: exploring the limits of the endoscopic approach. *Arch Otolaryngol Head Neck Surg AMA* 2012; **138**(5): 498–504.
11. Wang H, Sun X, Liu Q, et al. Endoscopic resection of sinonasal ossifying fibroma: 31 cases report at an institution. *Eur Arch Otorhinolaryngol* 2014; **271**(11): 2975–82.
12. Amit M, Fliss DM, Gil Z. Fibrous dysplasia of the sphenoid and skull base. *Otolaryngol Clin North Am* 2011; **44**(4): 891–902.
13. Charlett SD, Mackay SG, Sacks R. Endoscopic treatment of fibrous dysplasia confined to the frontal sinus. *Otolaryngol Head Neck Surg* 2007; **136**(4 Suppl): S59–61.
14. Banhiran W, Casiano RR. Endoscopic sinus surgery for benign and malignant nasal and sinus neoplasms. *Curr Opin Otolaryngol Head Neck Surg* 2005; **13**: 50–4.
15. Lund V, Howard DJ, Wei WI. Endoscopic resection of malignant tumors of the nose and sinuses. *Am J Rhinol* 2007; **21**(1): 89–94.
16. Samant S, Kruger E. Cancer of the paranasal sinuses. *Curr Oncol Rep* 2007; **9**(2): 147–51.
17. Vergez S, Mayne du MD, Coste A, et al. Multicenter study to assess endoscopic resection of 159 sinonasal adenocarcinomas. *Ann Surg Oncol* 2014; **21**(4): 1384–90.
18. Nicolai P, Battaglia P, Bignami M, et al. Endoscopic surgery for malignant tumors of the sinonasal tract and adjacent skull base: a 10-year experience. *Am J Rhinol* 2008; **22**(3): 308–16.
19. Su SY, Kupferman ME, DeMonte F, et al. Endoscopic resection of sinonasal cancers. *Curr Oncol Rep* 2014; **16**(2): 369.
20. Lund VJ, Stammberger H, Nicolai P, et al. European position paper on endoscopic management of tumours of the nose, paranasal sinuses and skull base. *Rhinol Suppl* 2010; **22**: 1–143.
21. Luong A, Citardi MJ, Batra PS. Management of sinonasal malignant neoplasms: defining the role of endoscopy. *Am J Rhinol Allergy* 2010; **24**(2): 150–5.
22. Saedi B, Aghili M, Motiee M, et al. Surgical outcomes of malignant sinonasal tumours: open versus endoscopic surgical approaches. *JLO* 2014; **128**(9): 784–90.
23. Swegal W, Koyfman S, Scharpf J, et al. Endoscopic and open surgical approaches to locally advanced sinonasal melanoma: comparing the therapeutic benefits. *JAMA Otolaryngol Head Neck Surg* 2014; **140**(9): 840–5.

24. Tojima I, Ogawa T, Kouzaki H, et al. Endoscopic resection of malignant sinonasal tumours with or without chemotherapy and radiotherapy. *JLO* 2012; **126**(10): 1027–32.
25. Dulguerov P, Jacobsen MS, Allal AS, et al. Nasal and paranasal sinus carcinoma: are we making progress? A series of 220 patients and a systematic review. *Cancer* 2001; **92**(12): 3012–29.
26. de Almeida JR, Zanation AM, Snyderman CH, et al. Defining the nasopalatine line: the limit for endonasal surgery of the spine. *Laryngoscope* 2009; **119**(2): 239–44.
27. Ha TN, van Renen RG, Ludbrook GL, et al. The relationship between hypotension, cerebral flow, and the surgical field during endoscopic sinus surgery. *Laryngoscope* 2014; **124**(10): 2224–30.
28. Nair S, Collins M, Hung P, et al. The effect of beta-blocker premedication on the surgical field during endoscopic sinus surgery. *Laryngoscope* 2004; **114**(6): 1042–6.
29. Wormald PJ, van Renen G, Perks J, et al. The effect of the total intravenous anesthesia compared with inhalational anesthesia on the surgical field during endoscopic sinus surgery. *Am J Rhinol* 2005; **19**(5): 514–20.
30. Gan EC, Alsaleh S, Manji J, et al. Hemostatic effect of hot saline irrigation during functional endoscopic sinus surgery: a randomized controlled trial. *Int Forum Allergy Rhinol* 2014; **4**(11): 877–84.
31. Belier B, Schlosser RJ. Navigation in endoscopic paranasal and skull base surgery. In: Stamm AC (ed.). *Transasal endoscopic skull base and brain surgery*. New York: Thieme; 2011, pp. 64–9.
32. Dalgorf DM, Sacks R, Wormald P-J, et al. Image-guided surgery influences perioperative morbidity from endoscopic sinus surgery: a systematic review and meta-analysis. *Otolaryngol Head Neck Surg* 2013; **149**(1): 17–29.
33. Tabaee A, Schwartz TH, Anand VK. Image guidance in endoscopic skull base surgery. In: Anand VK, Schwartz TH (eds). *Practical endoscopic skull base surgery*. San Diego: Plural Publishing; 2007, pp. 57–69.
34. Wellman BJ, Traynelis VC, McCulloch TM, et al. Midline anterior craniofacial approach for malignancy: results of en bloc versus piecemeal resections. *Skull Base Surg* 1999; **9**(1): 41–6.
35. Douglas R, Wormald P-J. Endoscopic surgery for juvenile nasopharyngeal angiofibroma: where are the limits? *Curr Opin Otolaryngol Head Neck Surg* 2006; **14**(1): 1–5.
36. Zhou B, Han D-M, Cui S-J, et al. Intranasal endoscopic prelacrimal recess approach to maxillary sinus. *Chin Med J* 2013; **126**(7): 1276–80.
37. Chiu AG, Ma Y. Accuracy of intraoperative frozen margins for sinonasal malignancies and its implications for endoscopic resection of sinonasal melanomas. *Int Forum Allergy Rhinol* 2013; **3**(2): 157–60.
38. Wormald PJ, McDonogh M. "Bath-Plug" technique for the endoscopic management of cerebrospinal fluid leaks. *JLO* 1997; **111**: 1042–6.
39. Hadad G, Bassagasteguy L, Carrau RL, et al. A novel reconstructive technique after endoscopic expanded endonasal approaches: vascular pedicle nasoseptal flap. *Laryngoscope* 2006; **116**(10): 1882–6.
40. Valentine R, Wormald P-J. Controlling the surgical field during a large endoscopic vascular injury. *Laryngoscope* 2010; **121**(3): 562–6.
41. Padhye V, Valentine R, Sacks R, et al. Coping with catastrophe: the value of endoscopic vascular injury training. *Int Forum Allergy Rhinol* 2015; **5**(3): 247–52.

CHAPTER 115

SURGICAL MANAGEMENT OF PITUITARY AND PARASELLAR DISEASES

Philip G. Chen and Peter-John Wormald

Introduction	1281	Complications	1287
Pre-operative assessment	1282	Conclusion	1287
Endoscopic transsphenoidal approach to sella	1283	References	1287
Surgical approach for parasellar (carvenous sinus) extension	1286		

SEARCH STRATEGY

Data in this chapter may be updated by a PubMed search using the following keywords: pituitary adenoma, pituitary gland, transsphenoidal pituitary resection, sella, transsellar approach and endoscopic skull base surgery.

INTRODUCTION

History

For years, the surgical approach to the central skull base has been a challenge for surgeons given its relatively inaccessible location. A number of pathologies occur in this region and examples include pituitary adenomas, meningiomas, chordomas, germ cell tumours, and epidermoid cysts.

Sir Victor Horsley is credited with performing the first removal of a pituitary tumour in 1889, using a craniotomy with transfrontal route.[1] Shortly thereafter, Herman Schloffer[2] (1907) utilized a transfacial-transsphenoidal approach to the pituitary fossa, and he was followed by Oskar Hirsch[3] (1909) who used a transnasal transseptal route. Another pioneer of the transnasal route was Harvey Cushing but he eventually abandoned it for open surgery.[2, 4] Pituitary surgery continued to evolve through the 1950s as notable surgeons such as Gerard Guiot realized the merits of the transsphenoidal approach.[5] In the 1960s, James Hardy took advantage of the increasing availability and visualization provided by use of the operative microscope to perform the first microsurgical pituitary surgery via a transsphenoidal route.[6] This became the standard approach for pituitary and sella surgery.

In the early 1990s technological advances in optics, digital cameras, light sources, and monitors afforded surgeons a high-resolution view that was sufficient to safely perform intra-nasal surgery without external incisions. With growing experience in endoscopic sinus surgery, efforts began to expand use of the endoscope to assist in skull base surgery. In 1992, Jankowski published the first description of a fully endoscopic transnasal technique for the pituitary gland.[7]

Microscopic approaches

The transition from open approaches to microscopic was accepted, as there was no brain retraction, decreased wound breakdown, shorter hospitalization, and no scar. The sublabial-transseptal microscopic approach is time tested and has been the standard of care for years. A sublabial incision is made followed by elevation of the septal mucosa off the septal cartilage and bones. The quadrangular cartilage is fractured laterally and bony septum removed followed by removal of the bony sphenoid face. The resulting microscopic view is straight into the sella. A variation is the transseptal approach with a hemitransfixion incision using a self-retaining retractor between the mucosal flaps. While effective, the microscopic view is limited by the speculum with an inability to visualize lateral extension of tumour.

Transition to endoscopic approaches

The use of the rigid endoscope in lieu of the microscope was initially met with resistance by some surgeons. Nonetheless, endoscopic approaches have rapidly gained popularity as experience has grown, and outcomes appear at least as favourable as microscopic approaches.[8, 9] Proponents of an endoscopic transsphenoidal approach to the pituitary and surrounding structures suggest that benefits over microscopic surgery include decreased pain and damage to the nasal mucosa, an improved panoramic view, and good mobility with angled views. Furthermore, there is no external incision or associated numbness which occurs with the sublabial approach. The wide angle provided by the endoscope allows the critical landmarks and tumour to be seen in the same field of view, even in regions which are difficult to see and access (**Figure 115.1**). This is especially helpful when tumour extends beyond the limits of the sella turcica, with an improved ability to remove these tumour extensions and decrease the risk of residual or recurrent diease.[9–11]

Endoscopic surgery of the sellar region requires two surgeons. One surgeon holds the endoscope to provide the second surgeon an optimal view to perform the surgical dissection bimanually. Skilled endoscopic sinus surgeons have a vast experience in the approach to and operating within the sphenoid sinus and can provide fast and efficient access to the sella and skull base. Neurosurgeons with experience in pituitary surgery understand the surgical technique and complexities of operating in this region. Together, these two surgeons form an experienced team that can safely access and remove tumours of the sellar and parasellar regions. These teams should initially gain experience in the endoscopic management of pituitary tumours and learn the nuances of having two to three instruments and an endoscope in the sphenoid simultaneously. This creates challenges for the team in learning how to best prevent the crossing of instruments as well as access to tumour extensions especially in challenging areas. For this learning curve in endoscopic skull base surgery, Snyderman and colleagues described a categorization of cases into five levels of difficulty.[12] With regard to surgery of the sellar and parasellar regions, level II cases have pathology confined to the sella. Level III cases exhibit extrasellar extension but also remain extradural, while intra-dural dissection elevates complexity to level IV out of V.

Pituitary tumours make up the vast majority of endoscopic transsellar surgery,[13] but additional skull base pathologies within the sella turica and parasellar region can be addressed in a similar fashion.[14] Other pathologies include lesions such as Rathke cleft cysts, craniopharyngiomas, fibrous dysplasia, chordomas, chondrosarcomas, epidermoid cysts, and meningiomas.

PRE-OPERATIVE ASSESSMENT

History and physical examination

Prior to embarking upon any surgery, it is critical that the surgeons understand the patient's pathology, extent of disease, neurological deficits, concurrent head and neck disease, and other co-morbites. A comprehensive history should always be obtained with a full head and neck examination. Special attention should be paid to the cranial nerves which pass through the cavernous sinus. Visual status such as acuity, visual fields, and gaze restrictions may be best performed by an ophthalmologist. Inclusion of rigid nasal endoscopy is also warranted to determine whether sinonasal disease or anatomic obstructions are present which would need to be addressed during surgery. Particularly when pituitary tumour surgery is to be performed, an endocrinologist should be involved in the patient's care, and the patient's hormonal status and pituitary function should be determined prior to surgery.

Imaging

Radiographic imaging is critical to preparing for skull base surgery, and details of skull base and sellar region imaging are covered in detail elsewhere in this text. The primary goal of the otolaryngologist is to gain wide transnasal access to the sella (**Figure 115.2**). All patients require

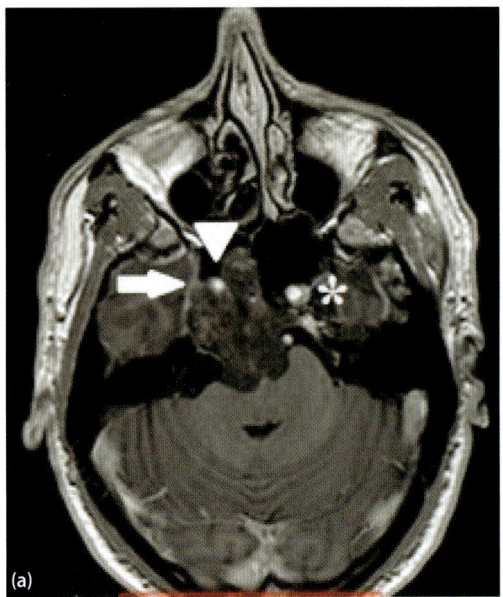
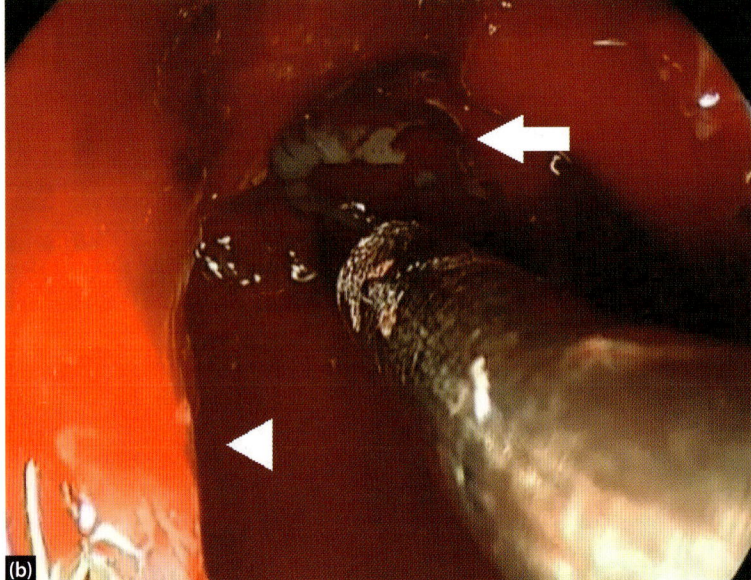

Figure 115.1 (a) MRI chordoma axial labelled. **(b)** Residual tumour.

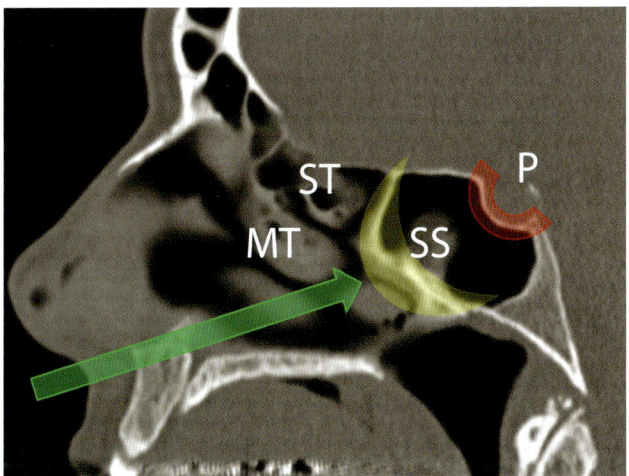

Figure 115.2 CT sella approach.

a computed tomography (CT) scan of the sinuses. Bone windows are helpful to determine presence of tumour invasion or bony remodelling. Further, review of CT scans helps delineate sinonasal disease, septal deviation (which helps with planning of a nasoseptal flap), sinus aeration, access to the sphenoid sinus, and anatomical variations such as Onodi cells, sphenoid intersinus septa, and the course of the carotid artery and optic nerve as well as potential areas of dehiscence (**Figure 115.3**). If there is additional concern about the carotid artery, a CT angiogram is indicated.

In addition to CT, an MRI with image guidance navigation (IGN) protocol should be obtained. This assists with pre-operative planning by differentiating tumour mass from obstructed mucus/fluid. Further, MRI is superior to CT in providing information about tumour morphology and whether dural enhancement or invasion is present. Image guidance is routinely used for all skull base cases, and this practice is widespread at large skull base centres.[15, 16] IGN is never a substitute for thorough understanding of the patient's individual anatomy, but rather should confirm the surgeons' anatomical knowledge. It may be especially helpful for revision cases, challenging anatomy, resident teaching, expanded transsphenoidal approaches, and when extrasellar extension is present.[16] Additional benefits have been reported including improved accuracy, reduced morbidity, and shorter duration of intensive care stays.[17] However, there is associated set-up time and the systems require some practice to become familiar with them. The surgeons must know the limitations of IGN and realize the system is not always accurate.

ENDOSCOPIC TRANSSPHENOIDAL APPROACH TO SELLA

Pre-operative considerations

Optimizing the nasal cavity for an endoscopic approach is an important first objective of the surgery. This includes assessing the CT scan for the need to remove the lateral wall of a concha bullosa or in some cases, the entire

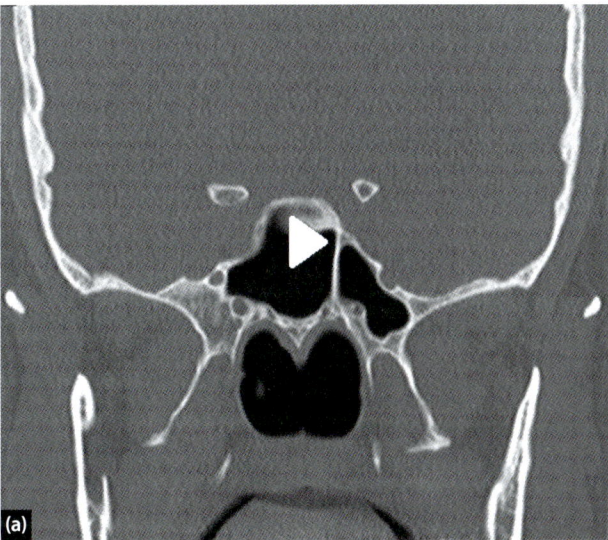

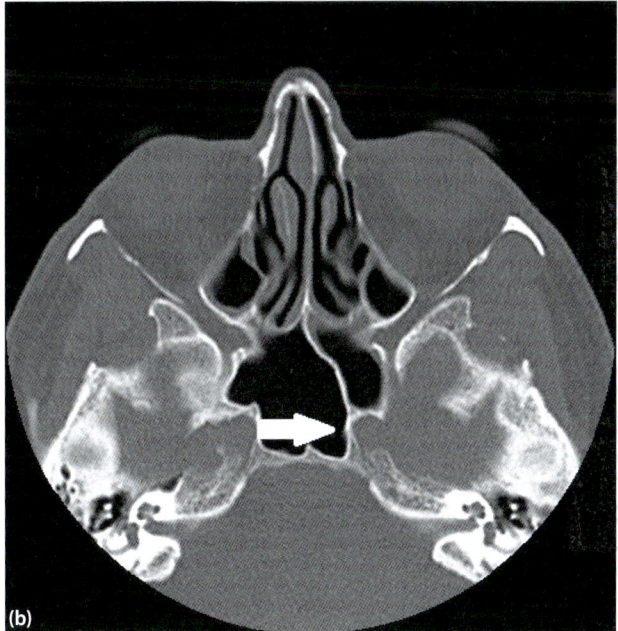

Figure 115.3 (a) CT intersinus septum carotid opt cor. **(b)** CT intersinus-septum carotid artery.

middle turbinate. Septal deviations and need for a septoplasty is evaluated. The transsphenoidal approach can be expanded to transplanum, transclival/transodontoid, and transpterygoid approaches as dictated by the size, type, and extent of the tumour.

The operating theatre is set up for a two-surgeon approach, and usually this is best accomplished by turning the table so that the anaesthetist is at the foot of the patient. The patient should be catheterized for accurate fluid balance management, especially with the risk of diabetes insipitus during pituitary tumour removal. We have found that lumbar drains are not routinely required even if a CSF leak is created during surgery. This prevents the potential complications associated with lumbar drains. Routine broad spectrum prophylactic antibiotic cover is given and the nose is decongested as for sinus surgery with topical and local vasoconstrictive agents. A surgical preparation of abdomen or thigh as a graft donor site is performed. We prepare the abdomen to harvest fat and rectus abdominis fascia in most pituitary tumours, but prepare the right thigh for fat and fascia lata when larger defects are anticipated (craniopharyngiomas, meningiomas, chordomas, etc.). Image guidance is set up usually with a scuba head strap for the electromagnetic IGN system and then the patient is registered.

The head of bed is placed in the reverse Trendelenburg position to decrease venous congestion and bleeding in the operative field. Instruments include the standard sinus and endoscopic skull base instruments, a high-speed drill, bipolar forceps, and an endoscopic ultrasonic aspirator.

Surgical technique

The first step in the surgery is optimizing the nasal cavity. Anatomical obstructions are addressed, such as performing septoplasty and removal of concha bullosa. Eliminating these obstructions improves access and passing of instruments from both sides of the nose. This decreases the risk of striking instruments against the septum which increases bleeding, damages mucosa, and slows surgery. In extended pituitary approaches (substantial opening of the arachnoid mater), a septal flap should be raised.[18] If one is unsure whether a pedicled septal flap will be required, then the vascular pedicle of the flap should be preserved on one side. This is accomplished by placing an incision from the lower edge of the natural ostium of the sphenoid and carrying this incision anterior and horizontal for about 3–4 cm. A suction Freer is used to mobilize this flap to the level of the posterior bony choana (**Figure 115.4**). This will allow the anterior face of the sphenoid to be widely opened while allowing the mobilized mucosa with the posterior nasal artery to be preserved. This ensures that should a septal flap be needed for reconstruction of the skull base or for closure of a large CSF leak, that the flap can still be raised and utilized.

Access to the sella should be created bilaterally to increase the working space for the binasal two-surgeon approach. Wide access yields improve visualization and allows space for the endoscope to be placed out of the way of the suction and dissecting instruments during surgery. The middle corridor of the nasal passage is widened by lateralizing the middle turbinates to expose the sphenoethmoidal recess and superior turbinate. The inferior half of the superior turbinate is removed flush with the face of the sphenoid sinus (**Figure 115.5a**). In many patients, the sphenoid ostium is clearly identified medial to the superior turbinate at the junction of the lower third and upper two-thirds of superior turbinate.[19] If the natural ostium is not visible the blunt end of the 4 mm microdebrider blade can be used to measure 12 mm from the posterior choanae.[20] A blunt Freer elevator is used to palpate the sphenoid face and identify the ostium. Entry with a Freer has a low risk of injuring the critical structures housed within the sphenoid sinus. The sphenoid ostium is widened and the posterior ethmoids opened so the sphenoid ostium can be widened to the lamina papyracea (**Figure 115.5a**). The final size of the sphenoidotomy should be from septum to lamina laterally, and from the roof of sphenoid to the floor of the sphenoid vertically. The Hajek-Koffler and Kerrison punches are ideal to for this purpose. While the bites are aggressive enough to make rapid progress, the biting mechanism minimizes the risk of inadvertently damaging the optic nerve and carotid artery (**Figure 115.5b**). At this point the mucosa of each side of the sphenoid should be elevated from medial to lateral leaving the lateral mucosa still attached to the bone (**Figure 115.5c**). This provides two mucosal flaps that can be used to reconstitute the anterior face of the pituitary fossa at the end of surgery. However, these mucosal flaps are removed if a pedicled septal flap is utilized.

To maximize access and to prevent the posterior edge of the septum being pushed into the endoscope thereby limiting visualization, a posterior septectomy is performed. This can be completed with the microdebrider, scalpel, or large backbiting forceps. If the microdebrider is used, care is taken to protect the pedicle of the septal flap and therefore the septectomy is only performed above the previously mobilized pedicle. Usually about 1–1.5 cm of the posterior edge of the septum is removed (**Figure 115.5d**). Intersinus septations are carefully removed using a rongeur or diamond drill, being conscious that septations frequently veer towards the carotid artery and/or optic nerve (**Figure 115.5f**). Septations are removed flush with the face of the sella. The medial[21] and lateral opticocarotid recesses are identified along with the anterior genu of the carotid arteries and both optic nerves (**Figure 115.5f**). Confirmation of these structures is obtained by using the image guidance suction probe. These limits define the planned bony exposure of the sella and identification reduces the likelihood of damaging them during the bone removal.

In most patients with a pituitary macroadenoma, the sellar face will be soft due to tumour expansion and pressure on the bone. A Freer elevator is used to gently fracture the bone giving an edge for placement of the 2 mm forward biting Kerrison punch. Alternatively, if the bone is hard (often seen with microadenomas), a diamond burr is used to "eggshell" the bone so it can be gently fractured

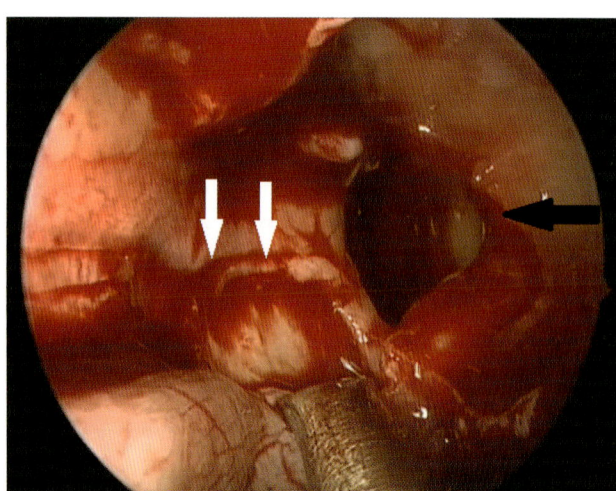

Figure 115.4 Septal flap.

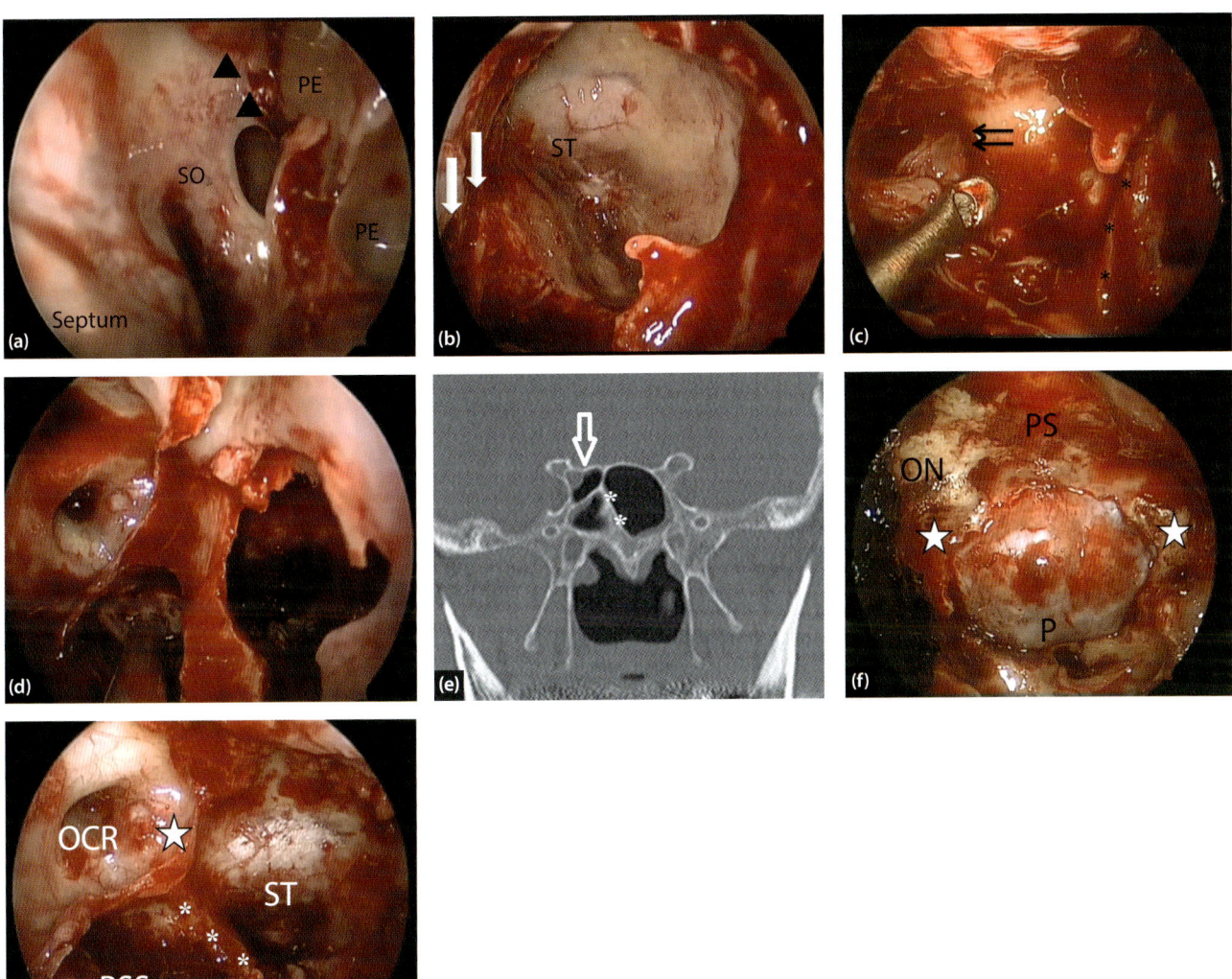

Figure 115.5 **(a)** Sphenoid os. **(b)** Opened sphenoid. **(c)** Sphenoid mucosa. **(d)** Septectomy. **(e)** CT Onodi pituitary. **(f)** Opened sella. **(g)** Onodi.

and removed. The Kerrison punch is used to remove the bone off the dura exposing the underlying dura from one cavernous sinus to the other and from the pituitary fossa floor to just below the tuberculum sella (Figure 115.5f). Once bone removal is complete the surgeon must be able to easily pass instruments below the pituitary fossa and from one sphenoid wall to the other. Creating this large space allows significant freedom of movement for the instruments without the bony walls of the sphenoid limiting access to any part of the sellar or parasellar region.

The dura is opened with a retractable blade or a number 11 blade in a U-shaped incision placed a few millimetres medial to each cavernous sinus and joined at the floor of the sella. This produces a superiorly based U-shaped flap which gives the best possible exposure of the fossa (Figure 115.6a). Cruciate incisions are no longer used as the visualization after such an incision is poor compared to the U-shaped incision.

In patients with macroadenomas the tumour should be immediately apparent and tissue is taken and sent for histology (Figure 115.6b). In patients with microadenomas, the MRI scan and image guidance can be helpful in identifying the tumour. An attempt is made to complete an extracapsular resection of these tumours thereby improving the chances of complete resection. Tumours have varying consistency from soft to firm, and the best instruments for removal will depend on the consistency. They may remain confined to the sella turcica or may extend into the parasellar and suprasellar regions. In cases of parasellar extension, a 30° angled endoscope is very useful to access tumour under vision and appreciate the full extent of the disease. This visualization is paramount to ensuring comprehensive removal, and achieving such views is not possible with microscopic approaches. **Figure 115.1b** is an example of a tumour that has grown laterally and behind the cavernous segment of the carotid artery. This extension would have been impossible to see with the microscope. It has been established that extrasellar extension is a risk factor for persistent disease;[22] thus, we aggressively chase tumour extensions in secreting tumours. However, our philosophy regarding extrasellar extension in cases of non-secreting adenomas is to resect what is relatively easy to remove without putting the patient at undue risk.

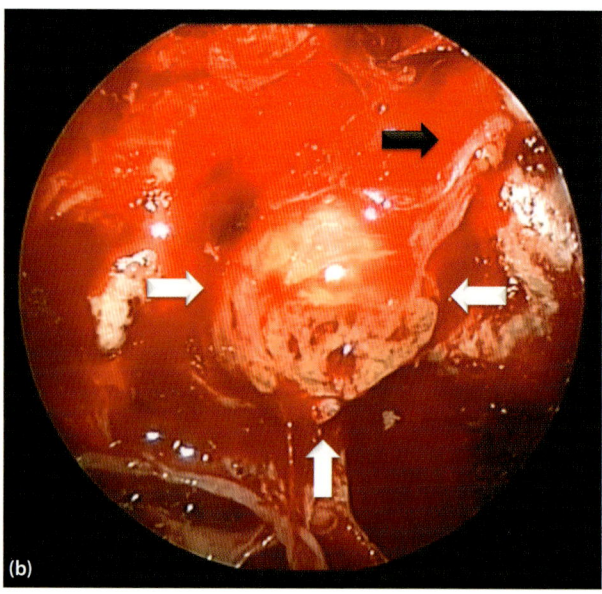

Figure 115.6 (a) Dural incision. (b) Tumour exposed.

After complete tumour removal, haemostasis is ensured using Gelfoam paste (made up of Gelfoam® powder (Pfizer Inc, New York, NY) and saline) and pressure from neuropathies. The pituitary fossa is gently filled with the paste and the dura placed over the paste. The sphenoid mucosal flaps are placed over the dura, secured with Surgicel® (Ethicon, Somerville, NJ) and fixed with a layer of fibrin glue. No packing is placed in the sphenoid sinus.

If a cerebrospinal fluid (CSF) leak is created during tumour removal, the diaphragm sellae defect is identified and a small triangle of fat placed into the defect ensuring cessation of the leak. An additional small piece of fat is placed in the sellar fossa with a layer of fascia over the fat. The dura and sphenoid mucosa are draped over the fascia followed by Surgicel® and fibrin glue. A layer of Gelfoam® is then placed over the glue followed by a ribbon gauze pack soaked in bismuth iodoform paraffin paste (BIPP) or antibiotic ointment. This is removed on day 3 post surgery. For large CSF leaks or in patients who have had an extended approach with a defect in the arachnoid mater, the pedicled septal flap is raised.[18] The fascia (or dural substitute such as DuraGen™ (Integra LifeSciences Corp., Plainsboro, NJ)) is placed as an underlay intra-cranial graft with the pedicled septal flap placed over this graft onto the bone of the defect. The edges of the flap are secured with Surgicel® and fibrin glue and the repair covered with Gelfoam® and the sinus packed with ribbon gauze soaked in BIPP for 3 to 7 days depending on the size of the defect.

SURGICAL APPROACH FOR PARASELLAR (CARVENOUS SINUS) EXTENSION

Parasellar extension beyond the pituitary fossa is initially dealt with as above. In some cases, tumour may extend anterior to the carotid before entering the cavernous sinus (**Figure 115.7a**). As per our philosophy, such tumour extensions are only addressed in secreting tumours as the risks outweigh the benefits in benign non-secreting tumours.

When lateral access is required, bone anterior to the anterior genu of the cavernous carotid artery is very gently removed. It is often safest to perform osteotomies with a 2 mm diamond burr on this bone and then to use a blunt hook to dissect the carotid from this bone before fracturing this bone (osteotomies control the fracture points) and removing it to expose the carotid artery. After complete

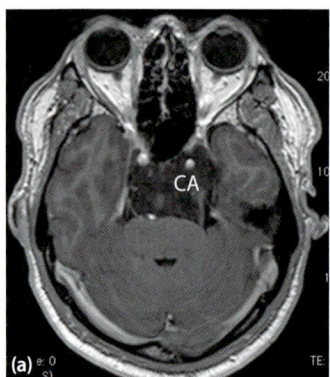
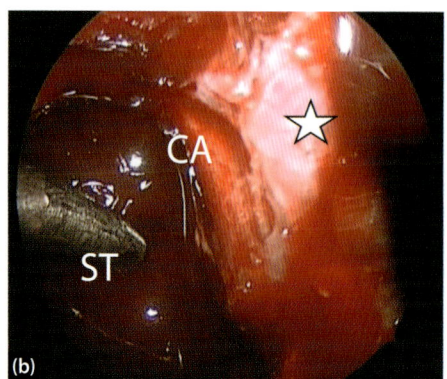
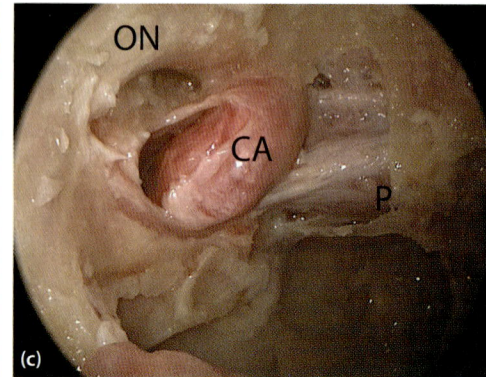

Figure 115.7 (a) MRI tumour encase L carotid. (b) Lateral to carotid intraop. (c) Far lateral approach.

exposure of the anterior genu of the artery, the cavernous sinus can be approached from anterior and lateral to the carotid (**Figures 115.7b** and **115.7c**). Post-tumour removal, the exposed carotid artery should be covered by the pedicled septal flap.

COMPLICATIONS

Delayed complications

The most common complication is CSF leak. Our philosophy is not to limit tumour resection because of fear of creating a CSF leak. We feel that we can successfully deal with any CSF leak at the end of the surgery. However, a post-operative CSF leak is a complication, and while this does occur the accepted rate of post-operative CSF leaks should be less than 5%. We use a multilayer closure including use of fibrin glue and a sphenoid sinus pack to maximally bolster the skull base repair and prevent a post-operative leak. Currently our post-operative CSF leak rate is under 5% with this protocol. Should a post-operative CSF leak occur, the patient is kept on bedrest and a lumbar drain is placed. If, despite these measures, the leak does not cease within 24 hours the patient returns to theatre for a formal closure. Other more common complications include mucosal scarring, hyposmia or anosmia, nasal crusting, and sinusitis.

Immediate complications

Immediate complications other than CSF leak include vision damage and both venous and arterial bleeding. The pre-operative imaging is very useful in preventing devastating complications; therefore, anatomical variations such as an Onodi cell (sphenoethmoidal cell) should be identified pre-operatively (**Figures 115.5e, 115.5f**). The Onodi cell pneumatizes lateral and superior to the sphenoid sinus and the optic nerve often runs within it. Failure to identify this ahead of time places the optic nerve at risk. Similarly, the medial location of the carotid artery (**Figure 115.1a**) or an intersinus septum that attaches to the carotid artery is identified on imaging (**Figures 115.3a** and **115.3b**).

Carotid artery injury is a devastating complication with up to 30% of patients having neurological sequelae and an approximate 20% mortality rate.[23] Carotid injury is one of the most challenging endonasal situations requiring both calmness and skill from both surgeons.[24] Recently, an animal model has been created by our group to provide skull base surgeons with a realistic model where techniques of how to manage high-flow bleeding can be taught and these surgical skills can be practised. This model almost exactly replicates both significant cavernous sinus and carotid artery bleeding.[25] We have used this model to assess the best way to handle such a complication and recommend the use of crushed muscle as a patch on the bleeding vessel as the quickest, safest, and most effective way to handle such a complication.[26]

CONCLUSION

The endoscopic transsphenoidal approach is a safe and effective means to remove many tumours within the sellar and parasellar regions of the central skull base. With improvements in technology, combined with greater surgical experience, the boundaries of safe and effective endoscopic removal of tumours will continually be pushed with the goal of improving patient care.

KEY POINTS

- The endoscopic approach to stellar and parasellar lesions has benefits over the microscopic approach including angled visualization and a dynamic, mobile view. However, this approach requires two surgeons and the image is only in two dimensions.
- An endoscopic skull base surgery team consisting of a neurosurgeon and otolaryngologist should be formed to perform these cases. They should start on easier pathologies before advancing to more difficult cases such as laterally based tumours and those that are adjacent to critical structures.
- Wide nasal access is critical to facilitate visualization and complete tumour removal, which is best accomplished with a binaural approach.
- It is important to salvage the posterior nasal artery so that a nasoseptal flap can be used to cover this defect if a cerebrospinal fluid leak is encountered.

REFERENCES

1. Pollock JR, Akinwunmi J, Scaravilli F, Powell MP. Transcranial surgery for pituitary tumours performed by Sir Victor Horsley. *Neurosurgery* 2003; **52**: 914–25.
2. Schloffer H. Frage der Operationen an der Hypophyse. *Beitr Klin Chir* 1906; **50**: 767–817.
3. Hirsch O. Eine neue methode der endonasalen operation von hypophysentumouren. *Wien Med Wschr* 1909; **59**: 636–7.
4. Cushing H. Surgical experience with pituitary disorders. *JAMA* 1914; **63**: 1515–25.
5. Guiot G, Thibaut B. Excision of pituitary adenomas by transsphenoidal route. *Neurochirurgia (Stuttg)* 1959; **1**: 133–150.
6. Hardy J. Transsphenoidal microsurgery of the normal and pathological pituitary. *Clin Neurosurg* 1969; **16**: 185–217.
7. Jankowski R, Auque, J, Simon C, et al. Endoscopic pituitary tumour surgery. *Laryngoscope* 1992; **102**; 198–202.
8. Higgins TS, Courtemanche C, Karakla D, et al. Analysis of transnasal endoscopic versus transseptal microscopic approach for excision of pituitary tumours. *Am J Rhinol* 2008; **22**: 649–52.
9. Komotar RJ, Starke RM, Raper DM, et al. Endoscopic endonasal compared with microscopic transsphenoidal and open transcranial resection of giant pituitary adenomas. *Pituitary* 2012; **15**: 150–9.
10. Shah S, Hal-El G. Diabetes insipidus after pituitary surgery: incidence after traditional versus endoscopic transphenoidal approaches. *Am J Rhinol* 2001; **15**: 377–9.
11. Cooke R. Experience with the direct transnasal transphenoidal approach to the pituitary fossa. *Br J Neurosurg* 1994; **8**: 193–6.

12. Snyderman C, Kassam A, Carrau R, et al. Acquisition of surgical skills for endonasal skull base surgery: a training program. *Laryngoscope* 2007; **117**: 699–705.
13. Nyquist GG, Anand VK, Brown S, et al. Middle turbinate preservation in endoscopic transsphenoidal surgery of the anterior skull base. *Skull Base* 2010; **20**: 343–7.
14. de Divitiis E, Cappabianca P, Cavallo LM. Endoscopic transsphenoidal approach: adaptability of the procedure to different sellar lesions. *Neurosurgery* 2002; **51**: 699–705; discussion 705–7.
15. Kacker A, Komisar A, Huo J, et al. Transsphenoidal surgery utilizing computer-assisted stereotactic guidance. *Rhinology* 2001; **39**: 207–10.
16. de Lara D, Filho LF, Prevedello DM, et al. Application of image guidance in pituitary surgery. *Surg Neurol Int* 2012; **3**: S73–8.
17. Eliashar R, Sichel JY, Gross M, et al. Image guided navigation system–A new technology for complex endoscopic endonasal surgery. *Postgrad Med J* 2003; **79**: 686–90.
18. Hadad G, Bassagasteguy L, Carrau RL, et al. A novel reconstructive technique after endoscopic expanded endonasal approaches: vascular pedicle nasoseptal flap. *Laryngoscope* 2006; **116**: 1882–6.
19. Orlandi RR, Lanza DC, Bolger WE, et al. The forgotten turbinate: the role of the superior turbinate in endoscopic sinus surgery. *Am J Rhinol* 1999; **13**: 251–9.
20. Kim HU, Kim SS, Kang SS, et al. Surgical anatomy of the natural ostium of the sphenoid sinus. *Laryngoscope* 2001; **111**: 1599–602.
21. Labib MA, Prevedello DM, Fernandez-Miranda JC, et al. The medial opticocarotid recess: an anatomic study of an endoscopic "key landmark" for the ventral cranial base. *Neurosurgery* 2013; **72**(Suppl): 66–76.
22. van Bunderen CC, van Varsseveld NC, Baayen JC, et al. Predictors of endoscopic transsphenoidal surgery outcome in acromegaly: patient and tumour characteristics evaluated by magnetic resonance imaging. *Pituitary* 2013; **16**: 158–67.
23. Laws ER Jr. Vascular complications of transsphenoidal surgery. *Pituitary* 1999; **2**: 163–70.
24. Kassam A, Snyderman CH, Carrau RL, et al. Endoneurosurgical hemostasis techniques: lessons learned from 400 cases. *Neurosurg Focus* 2005; **19**: E7.
25. Valentine R, Wormald PJ. A vascular catastrophe during endonasal surgery: An endoscopic sheep model. *Skull Base* 2011; **21**: 109–14.
26. Valentine R, Boase S, Jervis-Bardy J, et al. The efficacy of hemostatic techniques in the sheep model of carotid artery injury. *Int Forum Allergy Rhinol* 2011; **1**: 118–22.

CHAPTER 116

EXTENDED ANTERIOR SKULL BASE APPROACHES

Carl H. Snyderman, Paul A. Gardner, Juan C. Fernandez-Miranda and Eric W. Wang

Introduction 1289	Outcomes 1301
Classification of approaches 1289	Complications 1302
Indications 1290	References 1303
Surgical techniques 1292	

SEARCH STRATEGY

Data in this chapter may be updated by Medline and PubMed searches using the following keywords: anterior skull base, craniopharyngioma, endoscopic endonasal surgery, meningnioma, nasal dermoid, pituitary adenoma and sinonasal malignancy.

INTRODUCTION

A paradigm shift has occurred in skull base surgery over the last two decades with the introduction of endoscopic techniques for sinus surgery. Endoscopic techniques have been widely adopted for surgery of the pituitary gland and endoscopic endonasal surgery (EES) has been extended to include extrasellar regions of the ventral skull base. EES encompasses parasellar regions for the treatment of sellar pathology that extends to the cavernous sinus and suprasellar area, as well as the anterior cranial base.

The primary principle of EES is not endoscopic visualization but rather utilization of the endonasal corridor to provide optimal access with the least morbidity for the patient. For many tumours that are bounded by the neural and vascular structures of the cranial base, the endonasal corridor allows complete resection while minimizing manipulation of uninvolved cranial nerves, blood vessels, and brain tissue. In comparison to the microscope, the endoscope provides superior visualization with the capability of panoramic views and angled visual pathways. EES is team surgery, requiring the coordination of two specialties to achieve operative goals. Skull base team surgery is a dynamic process that results in enhanced visualization, increased efficiency, and improved communication and problem-solving.

CLASSIFICATION OF APPROACHES

Endonasal approaches to the ventral skull base are classified based on their orientation in sagittal and coronal radiological planes relative to the sphenoid sinus (**Table 116.1**).[1] The sphenoid sinus is the epicenter of endonasal skull base approaches since it is often the starting point for endoscopic skull base experience (pituitary surgery) and it is the location of critical anatomical structures (optic nerves, internal carotid arteries). Sagittal plane surgical modules extend from the frontal sinus to the sella, and from the sella to the upper cervical spine (C1/2). Coronal plane modules extend laterally, in correspondence with each cranial fossa (anterior, middle, and posterior).

The anterior cranial base extends from the sella to the frontal sinus in the midline plane and laterally across the orbital roof. Discrete sagittal plane modules include transfrontal, transcribriform, and transplanum approaches. These can be combined to provide complete access to the anterior cranial fossa for large intra-cranial tumours or excision of sinonasal malignancy that involves the skull base. For example, an endonasal resection of an aesthesioneuroblastoma includes transfrontal (Draf 3 frontal sinusotomy), transcribriform, and transplanum modules. Lateral margins of the anterior cranial base may be extended to the midline of the orbits by removal of the medial orbital roofs.

TABLE 116.1 Classification of endonasal approaches to the skull base

Sagittal plane
Transfrontal
Transcribriform
Transplanum (suprasellar)
Transsellar
Transclival
   Superior: Posterior clinoid
   Middle: Mid-clivus
   Inferior: Foramen magnum
Transodontoid (craniovertebral junction)

Coronal plane
Anterior (anterior cranial fossa)
   Supraorbital
   Transorbital
Middle (middle cranial fossa)
   Medial cavernous sinus
   Medial petrous apex
   Suprapetrous (middle fossa, lateral cavernous sinus)
   Infratemporal skull base
Posterior (posterior cranial fossa)
   Transcondylar
   Infrapetrous
   Parapharyngeal space

INDICATIONS

Pathologic processes may arise from intra-cranial, cranial, or extracranial structures and include a diversity of benign and malignant pathologies (Table 116.2). Isolated transfrontal approaches are primarily performed for inflammatory sinus disease (chronic frontal sinusitis, mucocele) and benign tumours (osteoma). The intracranial component of a nasal dermoid can be removed by following the tract through the foramen cecum, anterior to the crista galli.

Isolated transcribriform approaches are used for meningoencephaloceles that typically involve the lateral lamella of the cribriform. Rarely, tumours may arise from the olfactory nerves (olfactory schwannoma, olfactory hamartoma, aesthesioneuroblastoma). The most common indication for a transcribriform approach is for olfactory meningioma or sinonasal malignancy with skull base involvement. A transcribriform approach is usually combined with transfrontal and transplanum approaches to obtain adequate access and resection margins.

TABLE 116.2 Indications for endoscopic endonasal surgery (by surgical approach)

Transfrontal	chronic sinusitis, mucocele, osteoma, nasal dermoid
Transcribriform	meningoencephalocele, olfactory groove meningioma, olfactory schwannoma, olfactory neuroblastoma, sinonasal malignancy
Transplanum (suprasellar)	Pituitary adenoma, craniopharyngioma, meningioma
Transsellar	Pituitary adenoma, Rathke's cleft cyst, craniopharyngioma
Supraorbital	osteoma, meningioma, sinonasal malignancy

Sellar pathology includes primary pituitary adenomas (functioning and non-functioning) and Rathke's cysts. Large macroadenomas may extend to the suprasellar area and require a combined transsellar-transplanum approach for exposure and removal. A combined approach is also used for craniopharyngiomas and tuberculum meningiomas.

A supraorbital approach augments transcribriform and transplanum approaches by providing access to the roof of the orbit and associated dura. Usual indications for a supraorbital approach include a dural tail for meningiomas and dural margins for sinonasal malignancy.

For patients with sinonasal malignancy, oncological principles can be preserved with EES.[2] The goal of surgery is complete oncological resection with the least morbidity. With such cases, the endoscope is only a surgical tool and resection margins should not be compromised in order to perform an endoscopic resection. Although it is often promoted, en bloc resection is not achievable with an 'open' approach in many patients, due to proximity of the tumour to critical neural and vascular structures and fracturing of the tumour specimen. There is also abundant evidence that en bloc resection is not necessary as long as final resection margins are negative (e.g., inverted papilloma, Moh's surgery for skin cancer, and laser resection of pharyngeal and laryngeal squamous cell carcinoma). For sinonasal malignancy that involves the cribriform plate with risk of intra-cranial extension along olfactory filia to the olfactory bulb, bilateral wide resection of the anterior cranial base is recommended including dura, olfactory bulbs, and olfactory tracts.[3] Potential benefits of endoscopic surgery include better visualization of resection margins with better local control, no transgression of normal tissue planes with risk of tumour seeding, absence of frontal lobe manipulation, and faster recovery with early institution of adjunctive therapies.

A wide variety of sinonasal neoplasms are suitable for EES if properly selected. These include olfactory neuroblastoma (aesthesioneuroblastoma), neuroendocrine carcinoma, sinonasal undifferentiated carcinoma (SNUC), squamous cell carcinoma, adenocarcinoma, adenoid cystic carcinoma, and melanoma. Operability is determined by the biological behaviour of the tumour (diagnosis), stage (extent), and patient factors (age, medical co-morbidities). Surgery is generally preferred as the first treatment option for resectable tumours that do not have a high risk of distant metastases. Brain invasion is not necessarily a sign of inoperability. If a pial or cortical margin of brain tissue can be removed to achieve a negative margin without sacrificing major cerebral vasculature, then the tumour is operable. If there is tumour involvement of cerebral vessels, then the goal of surgery is no longer cure but palliation. Such patients usually receive radiochemotherapy first and surgery is reserved for salvage treatment of residual disease. For tumour with aggressive biological behaviour and increased risk of metastases (SNUC, melanoma), systemic therapy (chemotherapy, immunotherapy) is considered first. Even though the prognosis remains poor for cure of mucosal melanoma, EES is considered for local control.

The endoscope provides additional treatment options in patients with malignancy. In addition to performing a

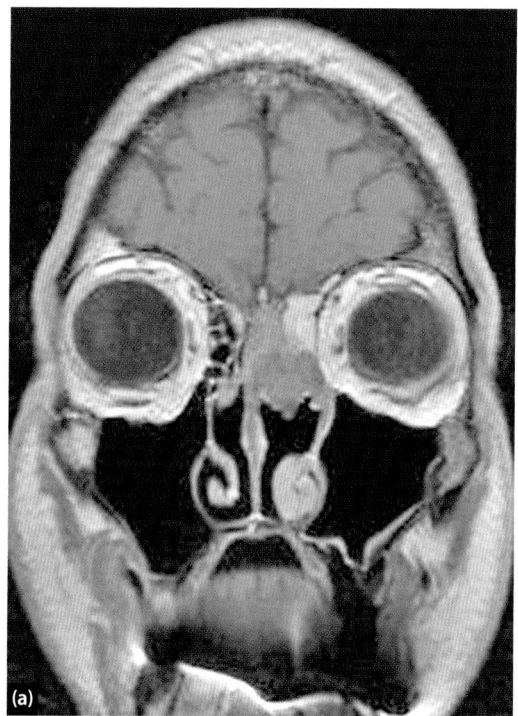
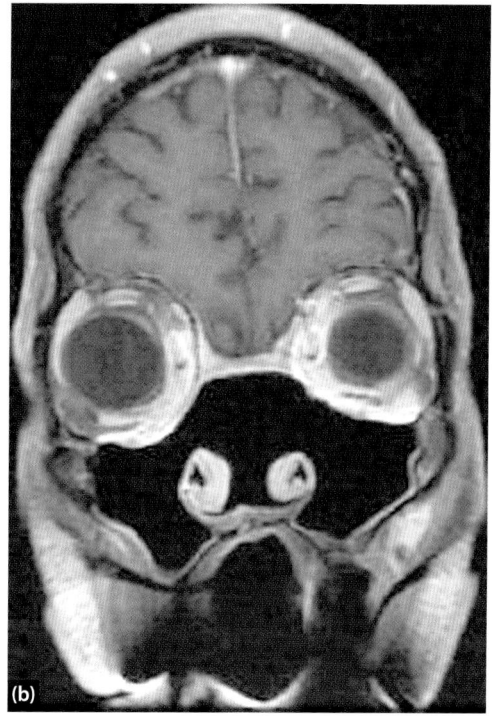

Figure 116.1 Pre-operative (a) and **post-operative (b)** MRI of a complete oncological resection of an adenocarcinoma of the left olfactory cleft with cranial base involvement.

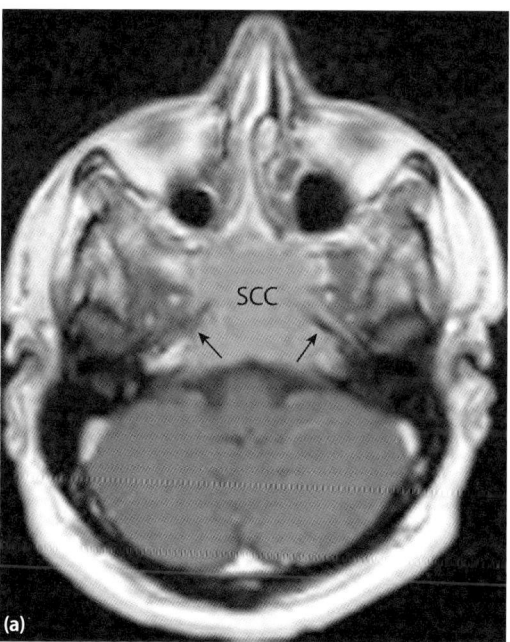
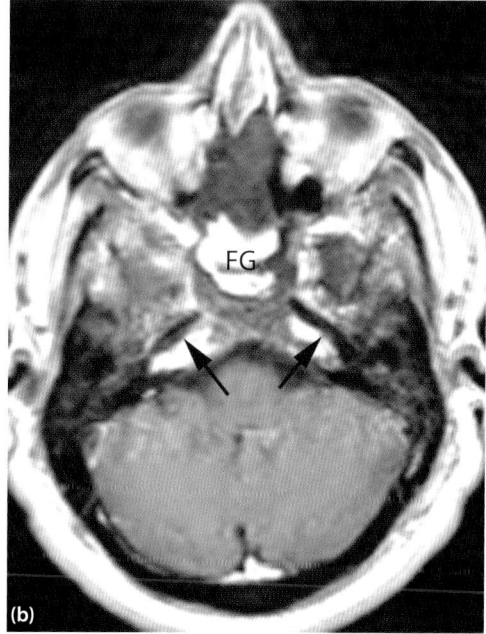

Figure 116.2 Debulking of unresectable squamous cell carcinoma of nasopharynx prior to radiochemotherapy. The patient presented with a VIth nerve palsy that resolved with surgery. **(a)** Pre-operative MRI with tumour encasement of both internal carotid arteries (arrows). **(b)** Post-operative MRI with fat graft (FG) and residual tumour surrounding the internal carotid arteries (arrows). The patient had a complete response to radiochemotherapy and remains disease-free more than 10 years later.

complete oncological resection (**Figure 116.1**), debulking of tumour prior to radiochemotherapy (**Figure 116.2**) may be considered in order to relieve symptoms such as bleeding, infection, pain, or compression (brain, orbit, cranial nerves). In addition, potential benefits of debulking prior to radiotherapy include accurate assessment of tumour margins and areas of invasion, modification of radiation ports to spare uninvolved tissues (optic nerves), and improved therapeutic response. The endonasal approach is ideal for palliation of symptoms in patients with unresectable recurrences (**Figure 116.3**). The morbidity of EES is minimal in such cases and affords the opportunity for multiple outpatient surgeries. Palliative surgery may also be considered for prevention of complications related to continued tumour growth (e.g., visual loss).

Pre-operative planning

The pre-operative evaluation of patients with tumours involving the cranial base starts with a detailed history and thorough physical examination. Presenting symptoms are often minimal and non-specific. Sellar and suprasellar tumours may present with headache, endocrine dysfunction, or visual loss. Intra-nasal tumours may present with

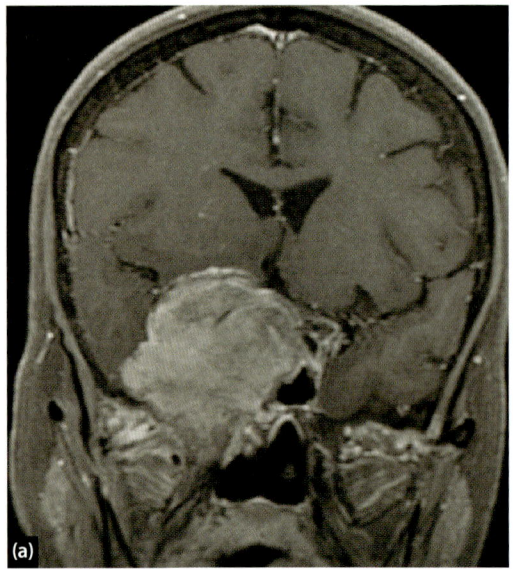 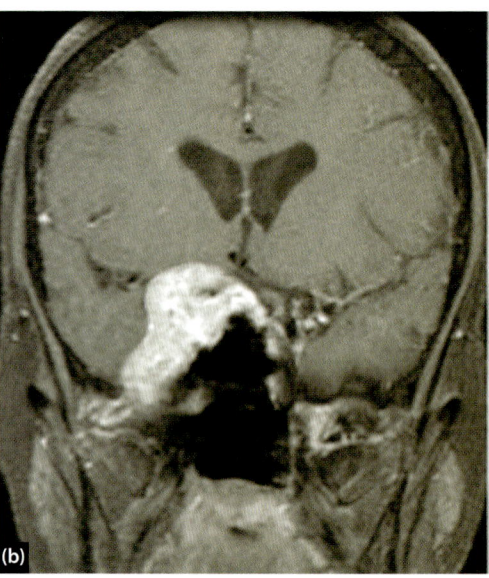

Figure 116.3 (a) Unresectable olfactory neuroblastoma with complete encasement of the right orbital apex and cavernous sinus. **(b)** Palliative EES with limited resection of residual tumour was performed to limit spread of tumour to the uninvolved eye and preserve vision (MRI is 2 years following radiochemotherapy and 1 year following surgery).

nasal obstruction, olfactory loss, epistaxis, or rhinorrhea. Tumours that extend laterally to the orbit may cause diplopia from displacement or invasion of orbital tissues. Intra-cranial tumours are often silent but subtle changes in personality and memory loss may become evident with further questioning.

Physical examination includes nasal endoscopy to assess the location and extent of tumour. Origination medial to the middle turbinate is typical of olfactory neuroblastoma. Coexistent sinus pathology may include infection, mucocele formation, and nasal polyposis. Olfaction may be assessed using available 'scratch and sniff' tests (Sensonics, Inc, Haddon Heights, NJ). Assessment of orbital function includes examination of extraocular motility and visual acuity. Visual field testing can provide evidence of early visual compromise and topographic data (tumour location relative to the chiasm). If there is concern about brain function, neurocognitive testing of executive functions can be performed. Pre-operative testing of visual and brain function is valuable for comparison with postoperative function.

Radiological imaging is essential for proper diagnosis as well as surgical planning. Both computed tomographic (CT) scan and magnetic resonance imaging (MRI) are obtained in many cases due to complementary information. CT is better for demonstrating bone erosion and sinus anatomy and MRI is better for delineating soft-tissue invasion and differentiating tumour from obstructed secretions. Scans are obtained using a skull base format with intra-operative navigation in mind. CT angiography is useful for identification of the internal carotid artery (ICA) or anterior cerebral arteries both pre-operatively and intra-operatively using navigation.

SURGICAL TECHNIQUES

EES is performed in an operative suite that is dedicated to endoscopic procedures. The room is organized around the patient with multiple monitors for viewing endoscopic images. The operative set-up is as shown in **Figure 116.4**. Following induction of anaesthesia, the head is immobilized with 3-point fixation in a Mayfield clamp. This allows precise positioning of the head for endoscopic access and facilitates intra-operative navigation. It also prevents inadvertent movement of the head during periods of critical dissection. The head is extended to increase anterior access and slightly rotated and laterally flexed to align the surgical corridor with the surgeon. Intra-operative navigation is registered and neurophysiological monitoring electrodes are placed. Cortical function (brain ischaemia) is monitored during every case using somatosensory-evoked potentials. If dissection of cranial nerves (III, IV, VI) is anticipated, electromyographic (EMG) monitoring of extraocular muscles is performed.

The nasal mucosal tissues are decongested with pledgets soaked in 0.05% oxymetazoline and the nasal vestibule and midface are prepped with betadine solution. Antiseptic rinses of the nasal cavity are not used due to

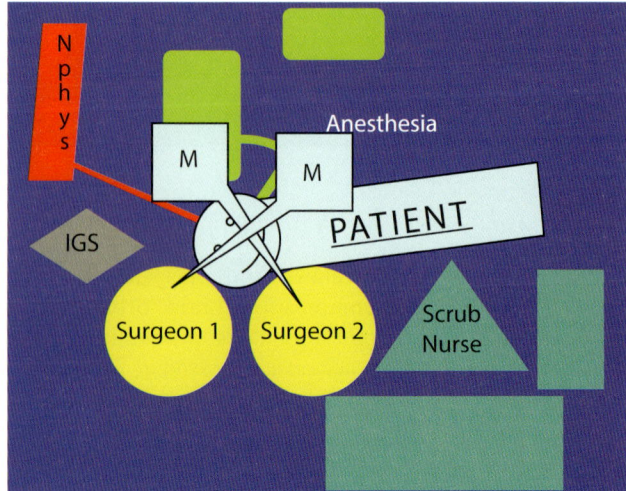

Figure 116.4 Operating room set-up. IGS: image-guidance system; M: monitor; NPhys: neurophysiology.

their deleterious effects on mucociliary function. A third-generation cephalosporin antibiotic is administered intravenously for perioperative prophylaxis.

Standard equipment for endonasal surgery includes a full set of endoscopic sinus surgery instruments including frontal sinus instruments, endoscopic bipolar electrocautery with exchangeable tips, endonasal drill with 4 mm coarse (hybrid) diamond bits, an array of angled Frazier and Fukushima suctions, pistol-grip extended microscissors and fine-tip extended dissectors for microvascular dissection. A nerve stimulator is used to aid identification of cranial nerves and a Doppler probe is used to identify and measure blood flow in major vessels.

Surgical approaches

TRANSFRONTAL APPROACH

The transfrontal approach provides access to the skull base anterior to the cribriform plates. It includes the floor of the frontal sinuses and the foramen cecum and crista galli in the midline. With drilling of the 'beak' of the frontal bone, the majority of the posterior table of the frontal sinus is accessible. Key landmarks and limits of the transfrontal approach are noted in **Table 116.3**.

A Draf 3 frontal sinusotomy is the foundation for the transfrontal approach (**Figure 116.5**). The nasofrontal recess is identified bilaterally by following the uncinate process and opening the anterior ethmoid air cells. The anterior ethmoid artery is identified at the posterior limit of the nasofrontal recess. The anterior tip of the middle turbinate is resected to the first olfactory fibre. The mucosa and periosteum of the olfactory sulcus can be elevated to assist in identification of the anterior margin of the cribriform plate and olfactory fibres. A superior septal window is created between the nasofrontal recesses to provide binarial access and improved angles for instrumentation. With visualization of the frontal sinuses on both sides, the floor of the frontal sinuses is then drilled in a curvilinear fashion anterior to the crista galli. Additional bone is drilled anteriorly in the midline (frontal beak) to increase access superiorly. Intersinus septations are drilled as necessary to provide a wide drainage pathway.

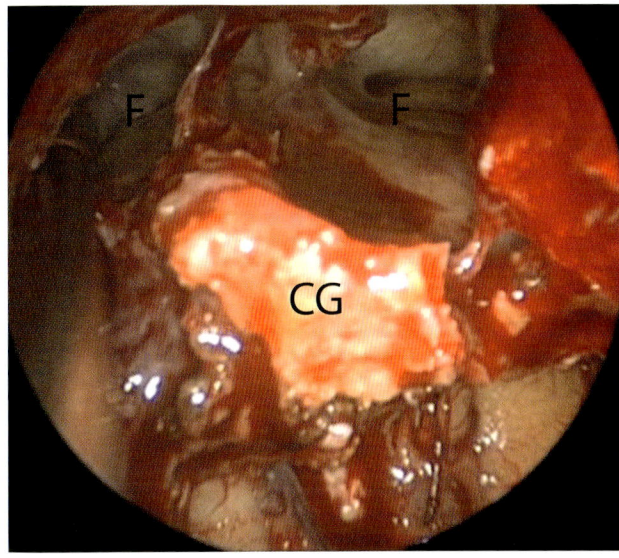

Figure 116.5 Draf 3 frontal sinusotomy for resection of sinonasal malignancy. CG: crista galli; F: frontal cell.

The posterior table of the frontal sinus is thinned with a drill and then elevated with dissecting instruments to expose the dura. The crista galli can be exposed in the midline and partly removed by drilling.

CASE EXAMPLE: NASAL DERMOID
A 5-year-old boy presented with a history of recurrent inflammation of the nasal dorsum despite prior transcutaneous excisions of a dermoid cyst of the nasal dorsum. A well-healed scar of the nasal dorsum was present without active inflammation. Nasal endoscopy revealed swelling of the superior nasal septum. CT and MRI demonstrated swelling of the superior nasal septum with a sinus tract extending through the foramen cecum to a small intra-cranial but extradural collection (**Figure 116.6**). Following frontal sinusotomy, the septal portion of the dermoid cyst was opened and contents were removed. The sinus tract was followed through the skull base by drilling the surrounding bone. The sinus tract was resected to the surface of the dura without a CSF leak. The defect was left open to the nasal cavity to prevent recurrence.

TRANSCRIBRIFORM APPROACH

A transcribriform approach provides access for tumours that arise from the cribriform plate area such as olfactory neuroblastomas and olfactory groove meningiomas. It is also a common site for meningoencephaloceles with spontaneous CSF leaks. A transcribriform approach is often combined with transfrontal and transplanum approaches for complete resection of the anterior cranial base in patients with a sinonasal malignancy. Key landmarks and limits of the transcribriform approach are noted in **Table 116.4**.

A Draf 3 frontal sinusotomy may be necessary to provide access to the anterior limit of the cribriform plates and also avoids problems with post-operative obstruction

TABLE 116.3 Key landmarks and limits of the transfrontal approach

Key landmarks	
	Foramen cecum
	Crista galli
	Frontal sinus
Limits	
	Anterior: anterior table frontal sinus
	Posterior: posterior table frontal sinus
	Medial: crista galli
	Lateral: lacrimal fossa
	Superior: posterior table midpoint

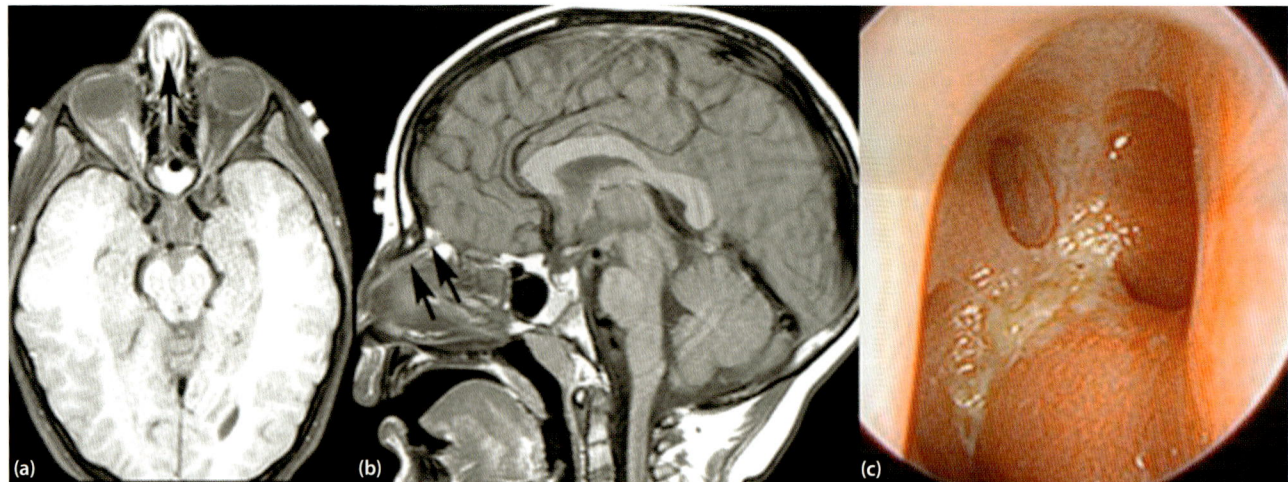

Figure 116.6 Pre-operative axial **(a)** and sagittal **(b)** MRI demonstrate a dermoid cyst extending from the superior nasal septum (arrow) through foramen cecum (arrows) to the surface of the dura. **(c)** Endoscopic view of healed defect of superior septum following surgery.

TABLE 116.4 Key landmarks and limits of the transcribriform approach

Key landmarks	
	Crista galli
	Olfactory filia, olfactory bulbs
	Lateral lamella
Limits	
	Anterior: frontal sinus
	Posterior: planum, posterior ethmoid artery
	Medial: crista galli
	Lateral: orbit

of the frontal sinuses. Bilateral ethmoidectomies are performed and the middle turbinates are resected. It may be necessary to debulk large intra-nasal tumours first in order to delineate the margins of the tumour and expose the area of skull base involvement (**Figure 116.7a**). Devascularization of intra-nasal tumours can be achieved by bipolar electrocautery of the tumour surface and ligation of feeding vessels. The anterior and posterior ethmoidal arteries may be identified where they cross the skull base lateral to the tumour. The paired vessels diverge from each other as they pass medially. The anterior ethmoidal artery is located between the 2nd and 3rd ethmoid lamella just posterior to the nasofrontal recess. Navigation can also be used to locate the artery; it exits the orbit in a coronal plane that is tangential to the posterior surface of the globe. The anterior and posterior ethmoidal arteries are best transected on the orbital side of the skull base. The lamina papyracea is partially removed and the orbital periosteum is dissected from the orbital roof. The periosteum is tethered where the vessels enter the foramina. The vessels are cauterized with bipolar electrocautery prior to transection. It is important to leave a small stump for cauterization so that the vessel does not retract into the orbit and cause a retro-orbital haematoma.

The bone of the skull base is then thinned with the drill and elevated to expose the dura to the margins of resection. If dural margins are important, it is helpful to elevate the dura from the orbital roof; this makes it easier to resect additional dural margins later, if needed. The dura is incised laterally with a retractable sickle knife and the incisions are extended with micro-scissors, taking care to avoid injury to cortical vessels. In the midline anteriorly, it is necessary to detach the dura from the crista galli. The base of the crista galli is removed with the drill prior to dural opening so that the attachment of the falx can be cauterized and cut once the dura is open (**Figure 116.7b**). Transection of the falx is directed posteriorly towards its free edge. This releases the dural specimen anteriorly and the remaining posterior dural cuts can be made. Additional intra-cranial tumour is dissected as needed.

> **CASE EXAMPLE: OLFACTORY SCHWANNOMA**
>
> A 12-year-old male presented with headaches and altered personality. Imaging revealed a large intra-cranial tumour arising from the olfactory area (**Figure 116.8**). A bilateral transcribriform approach was performed with complete intra-dural excision of the tumour. Histological examination confirmed an olfactory schwannoma.

TRANSPLANUM APPROACH

A transplanum approach provides access from the cribriform plates anteriorly to the tuberculum posteriorly (**Figure 116.9**). The planum forms the roof of the sphenoid sinus and is bounded by the optic canals posterolaterally. Most commonly, an isolated transplanum approach is used for access to intra-cranial tumours such as meningiomas. It may be combined with a sellar and suprasellar approach for suprasellar lesions such as pituitary tumours and craniopharyngiomas. Meningiomas that extend into the optic canals can be completely removed by decompressing the optic canals medially out to the optic strut.

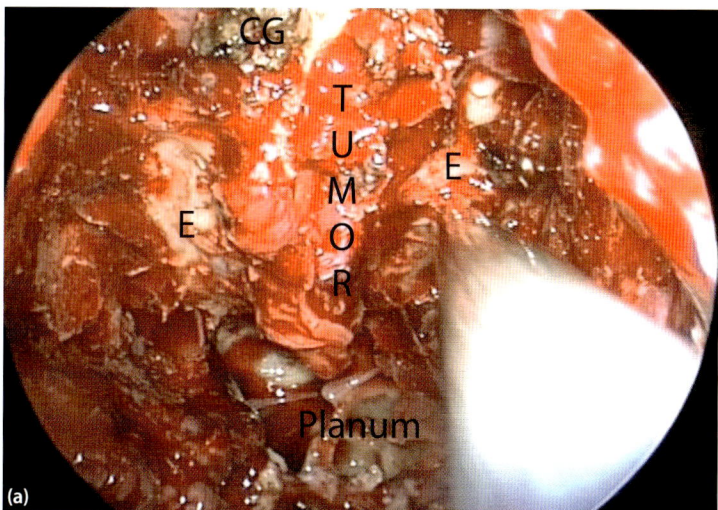
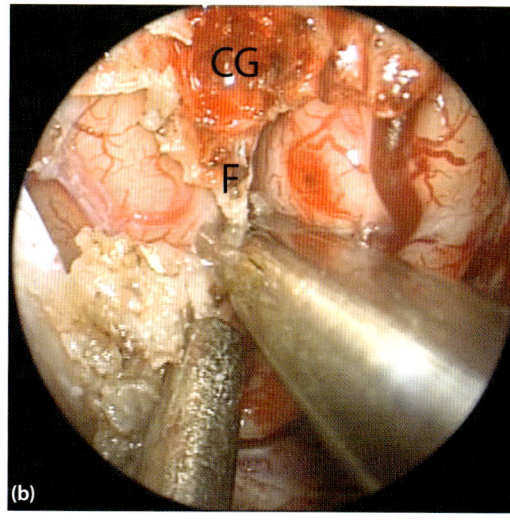

Figure 116.7 (a) The tumour is debulked and surrounding bone landmarks of the skull base are exposed. CG: crista galli; E: ethmoid roof. (b) The falx (F) is transected to release the dural specimen anteriorly. CG: site of crista galli.

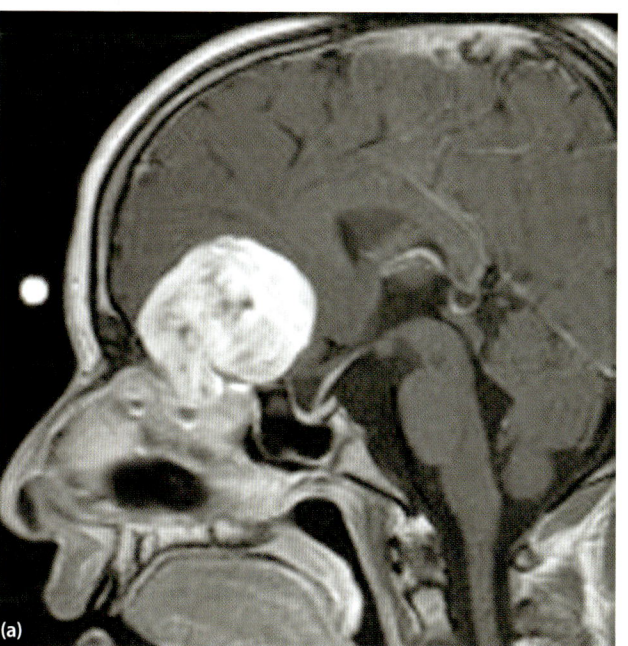
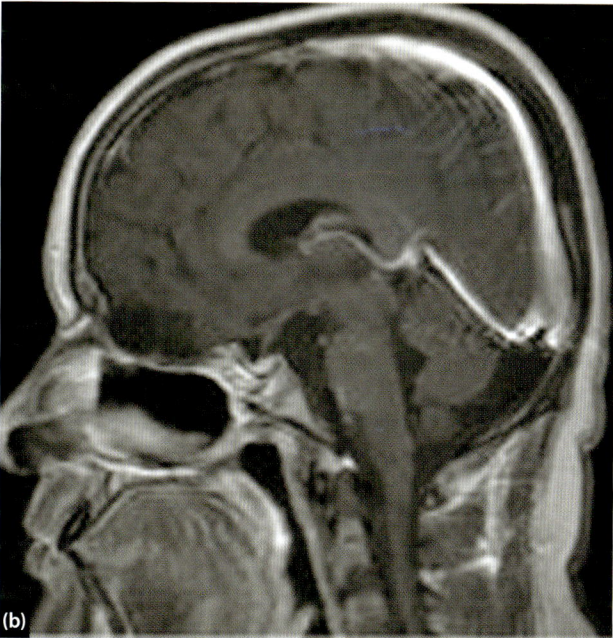

Figure 116.8 Pre-operative (a) and post-operative (b) MRI of olfactory schwannoma in a 12-year-old boy removed using a transcribriform approach.

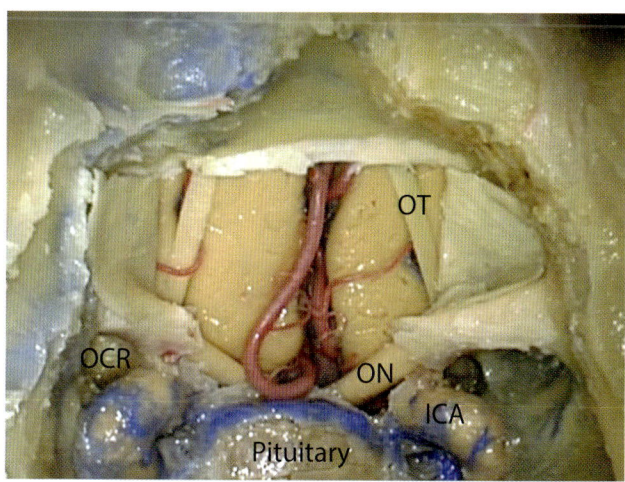

Figure 116.9 **Anatomical dissection of a transplanum approach demonstrating key landmarks.** ICA: internal carotid artery; OCR: optic-carotid recess; ON: optic nerve; OT: optic tract. The transplanum approach is bounded by the cribriform plates anteriorly.

Key landmarks and limits of the transplanum approach are noted in **Table 116.5**.

Bilateral ethmoidectomies and a wide sphenoidotomy are necessary to provide visualization of the planum. The rostrum of the sphenoid is resected to provide binarial access. It is important to avoid aggressive resection of the septal attachment superiorly due to risks of olfactory injury or cerebrospinal fluid leak from the cribriform plates. The sphenoid sinus landmarks are identified and mucosa is stripped from the bone. The posterior ethmoid

TABLE 116.5 Key landmarks and limits of the transplanum approach	
Key landmarks	
	Posterior ethmoid artery
	Olfactory tracts
Limits	
	Anterior: cribriform plate
	Posterior: superior intercavernous sinus
	Posterolateral: optic canals
	Lateral: orbital apex

CASE EXAMPLE: MENINGIOMA

A 45-year-old female presented with headaches and vision loss. MRI revealed a large suprasellar tumour with compression of the optic chiasm and tumour extension into the optic canals (**Figure 116.11**). Gross total excision was achieved using a transplanum approach. The dura of the optic canal was opened medially just above the optic nerve and tumour was dissected without injury to the ophthalmic artery.

arteries are variable in location and diameter but are generally found near the junction of the planum sphenoidale and roof of ethmoid sinus. The foramina are approximately 4–7 mm anterior to the optic canal.

The bone of the planum is outlined with the drill and fragments of bone are dissected from the underlying dura in an anterior to posterior direction. Posteriorly, the optic canals are kept in sight. If tumour dissection from the optic canals is necessary, a 3 mm coarse diamond bit is used to thin the overlying bone. Copious irrigation is used to prevent thermal injury to the optic nerves. The thinned bone is carefully elevated with fine dissectors to avoid compression of the optic nerves. The posterior ethmoid arteries are cauterized and transected on the orbital side of the bone. Excessive bone removal beyond the anterior margin of the tumour should be avoided so that normal brain tissue does not descend and obstruct the view.

The dura is incised with a retractable sickle knife and the incisions are extended with micro-scissors, taking care to avoid injury to cortical vessels. Tumour dissection is performed using standard microsurgical techniques with internal debulking followed by extracapsular dissection. If the dura is incised to the optic canals, care should be taken to identify and preserve the ophthalmic artery, which is often inferior and medial to the optic nerve as it branches from the ICA (**Figure 116.10**).

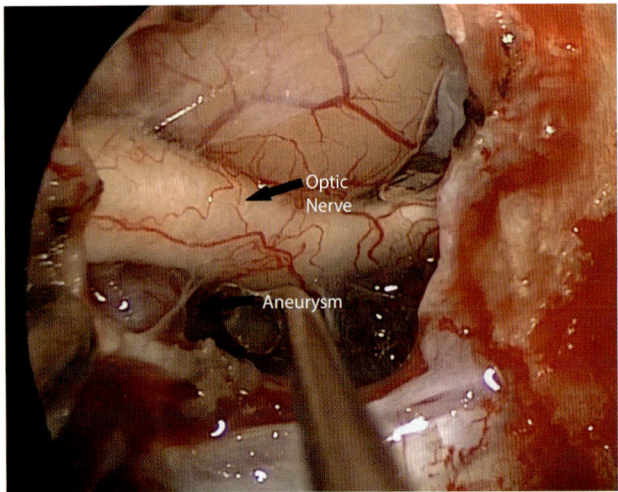

Figure 116.10 Intra-operative view of an aneurysm arising from the right ophthalmic artery.

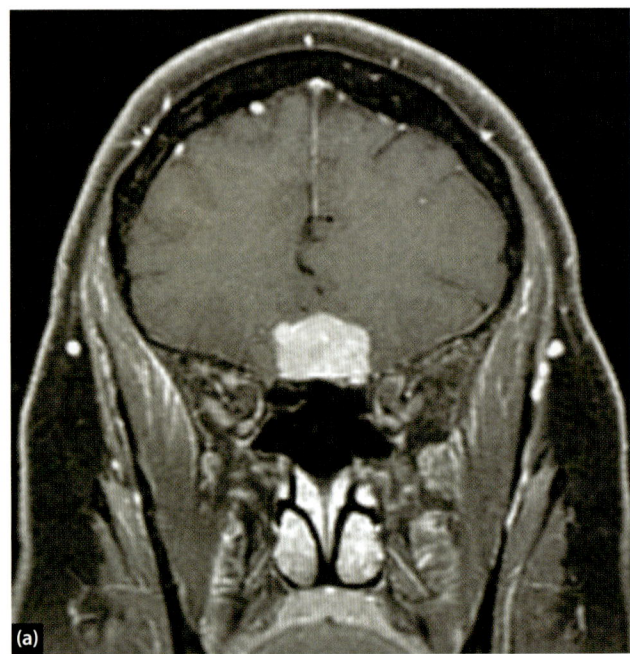

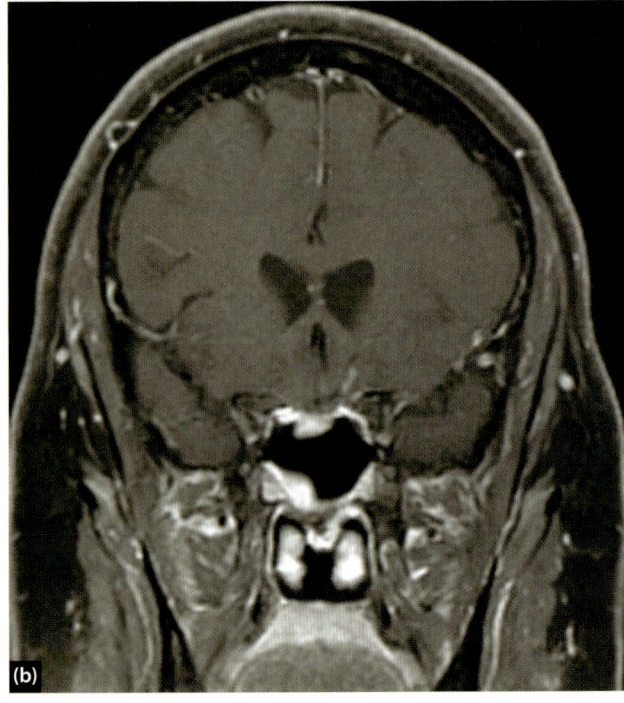

Figure 116.11 Pre-operative **(a)** and post-operative **(b)** MRI of a planum meningioma. GTR was achieved using a transplanum approach with decompression of the optic canals.

SUPRAORBITAL APPROACH

The supraorbital approach is a coronal plane approach that provides access to the orbital roof. The maximal limit of exposure is the mid-sagittal plane of the orbit. This approach is used to remove tumour-involved bone (osteomas, meningioma) and to chase dural margins for sinonasal malignancy or meningiomas. It is often combined with transcribriform or transplanum approaches. The supraorbital approach is bounded anteriorly and posteriorly by the ethmoidal arteries. Key landmarks and limits of the supraorbital approach are noted in **Table 116.6**.

Following a complete sphenoethmoidectomy, the medial wall of the orbit is removed to the level of the skull base. The anterior and posterior ethmoidal arteries are identified and transected following cauterization. Periorbital is then dissected from the orbital roof to the mid-plane of the orbit. Access is greater in the middle and posterior orbit due to the trajectory of the surgical corridor. A binarial approach with a superior septal defect greatly enhances the exposure for instrumentation and minimizes contact of powered instrumentation with the orbital tissues. While the orbital tissues are protected with a suction or retracting instrument, the medial orbital roof is drilled and removed with rongeurs to the margin of resection. Posteriorly, removal of bone can extend to the anterior clinoid and facilitate 270° decompression of the optic canal.

> ### CASE EXAMPLE: SINONASAL MALIGNANCY
>
> A 52-year old man presented with nasal obstruction and a unilateral nasal mass involving the skull base with dural thickening over the medial orbit (**Figure 116.12a**). Biopsy confirmed a diagnosis of undifferentiated carcinoma and resection of the tumour and skull base was performed, including removal of the medial wall of the orbit. The initial dural incision did not provide an adequate resection margin (**Figure 116.12b**) and additional bone was removed from the orbital roof (**Figure 116.12c**) to achieve a negative dural margin.

SUPRASELLAR APPROACH

A suprasellar approach is combined with transsellar and transplanum approaches to gain access to suprasellar pathology. The most common indications include pituitary macroadenomas with suprasellar extension, craniopharyngiomas, and meningiomas. It is bounded by the

TABLE 116.6 Key landmarks and limitations of the supraorbital approach

Key landmarks	
	Anterior and posterior ethmoid arteries
Limits	
	Anterior: frontal sinus
	Posterior: optic canal
	Superolateral: midplane of orbit

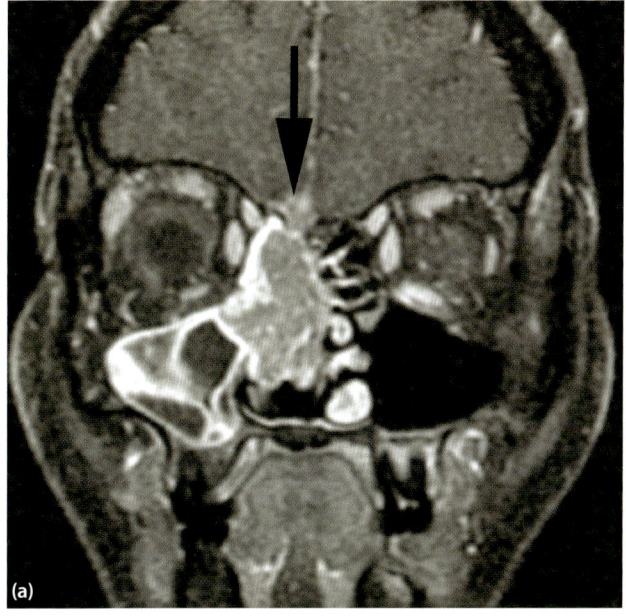

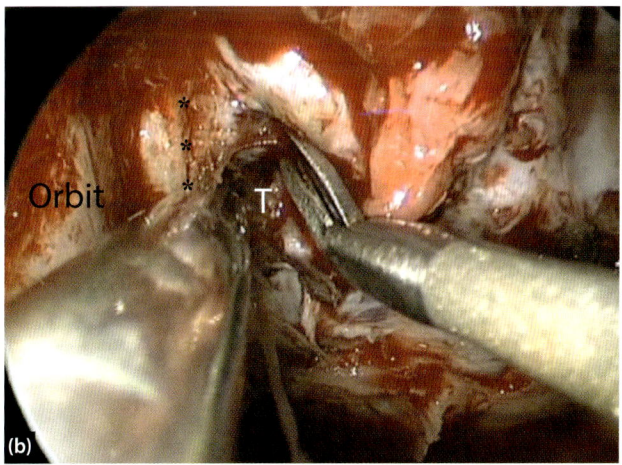

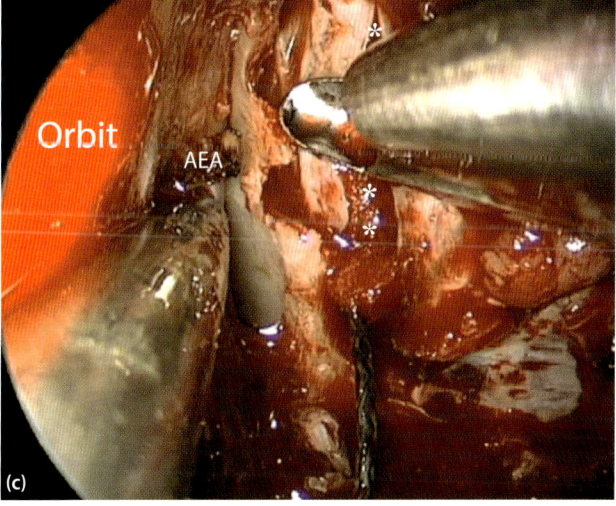

Figure 116.12 **(a)** Pre-operative MRI demonstrating intra-cranial extension of tumour (arrow). **(b)** Intra-operative view of initial dural incision with exposure of tumour (T). The edge of the resected bone is highlighted with asterisks. **(c)** Additional bone is removed from the orbital roof with retraction of orbital contents. The initial dural incision is highlighted with asterisks. AEA: anterior ethmoid artery.

optic chiasm superiorly and pituitary stalk or membrane of Lillequist posteriorly. Key landmarks and limits of the suprasellar approach are noted in **Table 116.7**.

Following a wide sphenoidotomy with opening of posterior ethmoid air cells, the landmarks of the sphenoid sinus are identified (**Figure 116.13**). This includes the sella, optic canals, lateral optic-carotid recess, and parasellar ICA. The medial optic-carotid junction or recess (mOCR) is an important landmark where the ICA courses medially before it passes under the optic nerve. The medial clinoid is a small bony projection below the medial OCR that provides a medial point of attachment of the dural rings next to the anterior genu of the cavernous ICA. In some cases, this can be calcified to form a complete ring around the ICA.

The bone of the sella is first thinned with the drill and removed to the margins of the cavernous sinus superiorly and laterally. Bone rongeurs are used to lift the thinned bone rather than bite the bone due to risk of injury to the ICA, especially at the medial optic-carotid junction. Anteriorly, the bone of the posterior planum is thinned with the drill until dura is exposed. The tuberculum strut (bone between the optic canals) is then disconnected laterally with a drill just medial to the optic canals (**Figure 116.14**). Then the entire tuberculum strut can be dissected free as a single piece of bone.

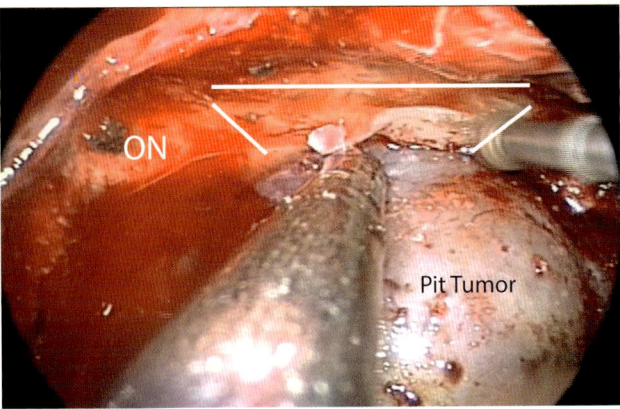

Figure 116.14 The bone cuts (lines) for a suprasellar approach for resection of a pituitary tumour (Pit Tumour) with suprasellar extension are shown. The lateral cuts are made with the drill medial to the optic nerve (ON) canals. Removal of the tuberculum allows descent of the suprasellar component of the tumour.

The dura is then incised above and below the superior intercavernous sinus (SIS). The location of the optic chiasm should be ascertained from pre-operative imaging in case it is prefixed or displaced anteriorly by tumour. The SIS is then cauterized with bipolar electrocautery and transected. Bleeding from the cut edges is controlled with application of Floseal® or Surgifoam®. Dural cuts are extended as necessary to the margins of the tumour.

TABLE 116.7 Key landmarks and limitations of the suprasellar approach

Key landmarks	
	Optic canals
	Tuberculum
	Ophthalmic arteries
Limits	
	Anterior: planum sphenoidale
	Lateral: optic canals, paraclinoidal ICA

CASE EXAMPLE: CRANIOPHARYNGIOMA

A 44-year old man presented with progressive vision loss, headache and fatigue. Imaging showed a heterogeneous, partially cystic suprasellar lesion involving the pituitary stalk and elevating the optic chiasm (**Figure 116.15**). Hormonal evaluation revealed hypogonadism, hypothyroidism and borderline adrenal insufficiency. The patient underwent an endoscopic endonasal suprasellar approach with complete resection of the tumour that was histologically confirmed to be a craniopharyngioma. The tumour extensively involved the pituitary stalk, which was transected as part of complete removal. The patient's vision improved significantly post-operatively and he was treated with oral replacement for panhypopituitarism with the new addition of diabetes insipidus.

Reconstruction (nasoseptal flap, pericranial flap)

Prior to dural reconstruction, it is imperative to have good haemostasis. Bipolar electrocautery is used for bleeding dural edges and small arterioles. Cavernous sinus or venous bleeding can be controlled with application of haemostatic materials such as Surgifoam® or Floseal®. Mild oozing from the surface of the brain or residual tumour can be controlled with copious irrigation of warm saline (40°C).[4] It may take 10 minutes or more of continuous irrigation to confirm that all bleeding is controlled.

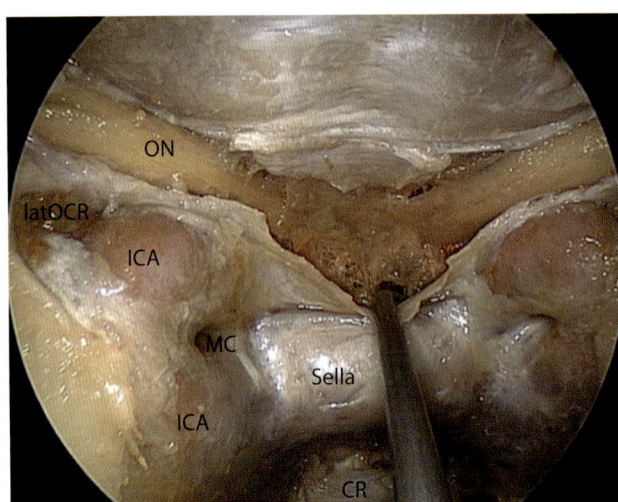

Figure 116.13 Key landmarks of the suprasellar approach. CR: clival recess; ICA: internal carotid artery; latOCR: lateral optic-carotid recess; MC: middle clinoid; ON: optic nerve.

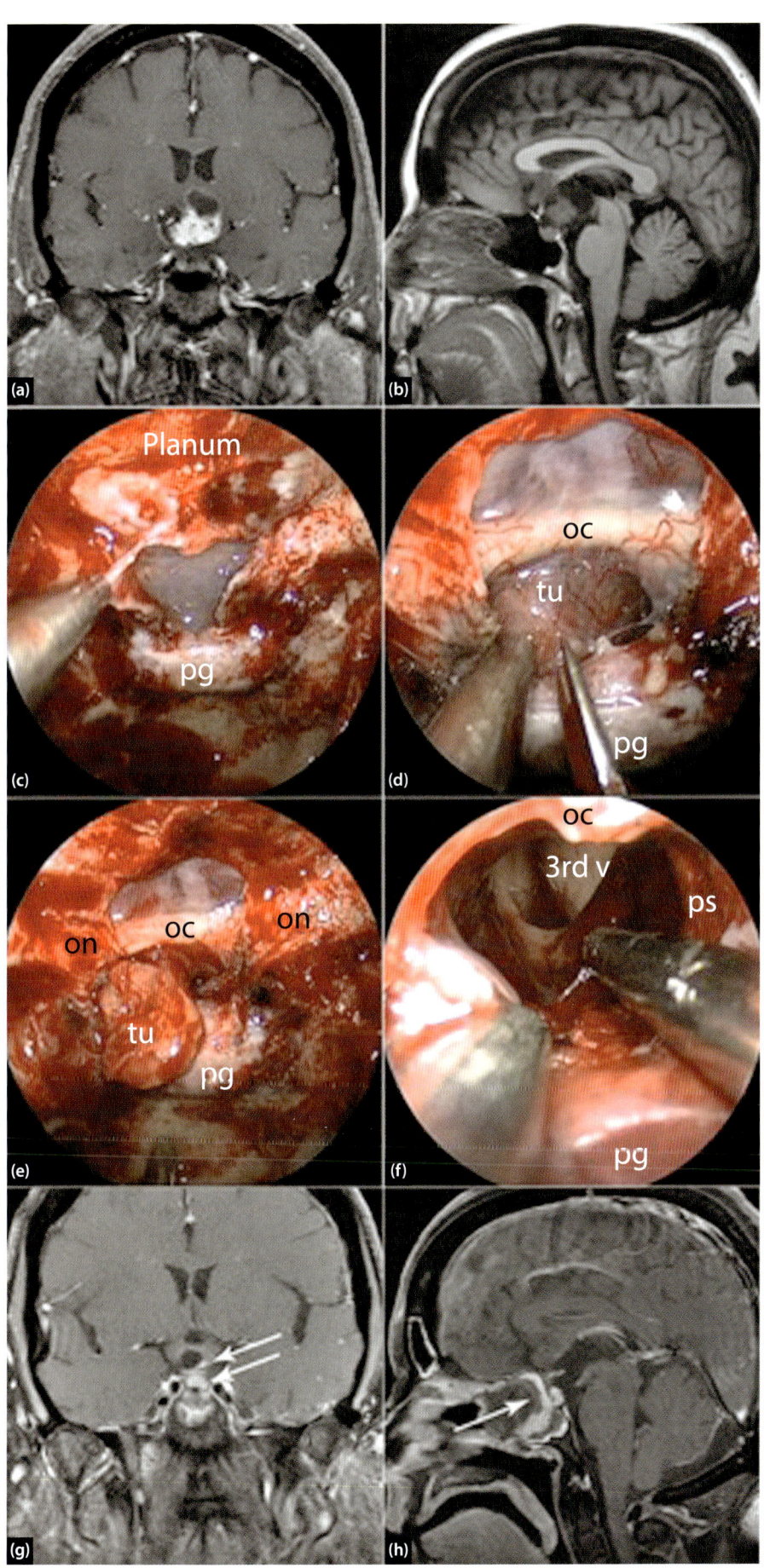

Figure 116.15 Craniopharyngioma. Pre-operative, intra-operative and post-operative images of a suprasellar craniopharyngioma with intraventricular extension that underwent GTR with EES. **(a, b)** Pre-operative MRI demonstrates a mixed solid and cystic suprasellar tumour that invades the floor of the 3rd ventricle. **(c)** Intraoperative view with a 0-degree endoscope after bony resection of the planum, tuberculum and anterior wall of the sella with exposure of the pituitary gland (pg). **(d)** After opening the suprasellar arachnoid, the optic chiasm (oc) is identified and the solid compartment of the tumour (tu) is visualized between the optic chiasm and the pituitary gland (pg). **(e)** The tumour (tu) is dissected and removed from the suprasellar cistern. The dura over the optic nerves (on) remains intact. **(f)** A closer view with the 0-degree endoscope provides direct visualization of the 3rd ventricle (3rd v), the floor of which was eroded by the tumour. Having removed the tumour, the pituitary stalk (ps) is identified with deviation to the left. The optic chiasm (oc) and pituitary gland (pg) remain intact. **(g, h)** Post-operative MRI with contrast confirm GTR of the craniopharyngioma. The pituitary stalk can be seen on the coronal image (upper arrow) deviated to the left, just above the pituitary gland (lower arrow). The linear contrast-enhancing area on the sagittal MRI (arrow) represents the vascularized nasoseptal flap that was used for skull base reconstruction and the enhancing spot behind the flap is the intact pituitary gland.

Reconstruction of dural defects of the anterior cranial base is ideally performed using vascularized tissue.[5] Although small dural defects are effectively repaired using a variety of techniques and materials, the use of vascularized tissue is associated with significantly lower post-operative CSF leak rates for larger defects. Local vascularized flaps include middle turbinate, inferior turbinate, and nasal septal flaps, all of which are based on terminal branches of the sphenopalatine artery. Regional vascularized flaps include pericranial and temporoparietal fascial flaps. Of these, the nasal septal flap and pericranial flap offer the best coverage and are preferred for reconstruction of large defects of the anterior cranial base.

The nasal septal flap[6] is raised at the beginning of the procedure to preserve the vascular pedicle. The superior incision runs parallel to the skull base approximately 1 cm below the skull base. If there are concerns about tumour involvement of the septum, clear margins are assessed by frozen section or reconstruction with a pericranial flap is considered. The inferior incision runs from the posterior choana along the posterior edge of the nasal septum to the junction of the nasal septum and nasal floor. If a wider flap is needed, the nasal floor can be incorporated into the flap. The anterior incision connects the superior and inferior incisions at the junction of the septal mucosa and skin of the nasal vestibule. It is important to include the most anterior-superior septal mucosa that is anterior to the attachments of the middle turbinate in order to harvest a maximal flap. After the flap is elevated from the underlying septal cartilage, it is displaced into the nasopharynx during the remainder of the procedure.

When it is time to repair the dural defect, an inlay fascial graft is placed between the brain and the dura. The septal flap is then transposed to cover the entire defect. All surrounding mucosa should be removed so that the entire flap is in contact with bone or dura. If the flap is not long enough, the reach of the flap can be extended by drilling the sphenoid floor or filling the clival recess with autologous fat grafts. The margins of the repair can also be augmented with onlay fascia grafts placed under the flap or fat grafts placed over the edges of it as needed. The donor site on the anterior nasal septum is covered with a free mucosal graft when available, and Silastic® nasal splints are placed.

An extracranial pericranial flap provides maximal vascularized tissue for reconstruction.[7] After the intradural fascial graft is placed, the flap is harvested using a bicoronal scalp incision. The scalp is elevated to the level of the nasion and supraorbital rims with preservation of the supraorbital neurovascular bundle on one or both sides. The bone at the level of the nasion is then drilled to create a window (approximately 2.0 cm × 0.5 cm) into the nasal cavity that is below the level of the skull base (**Figure 116.16**). The pericranial flap is then dissected from the scalp in a subgaleal plane and passed through the bony defect into the nasal cavity. Rotation of the flap is facilitated by sacrificing the vascular pedicle on one side. Endonasally, the flap is spread out to cover the dural and bony margins of the defect. If possible, the flap pedicle is displaced to one side to prevent obstruction of the drainage

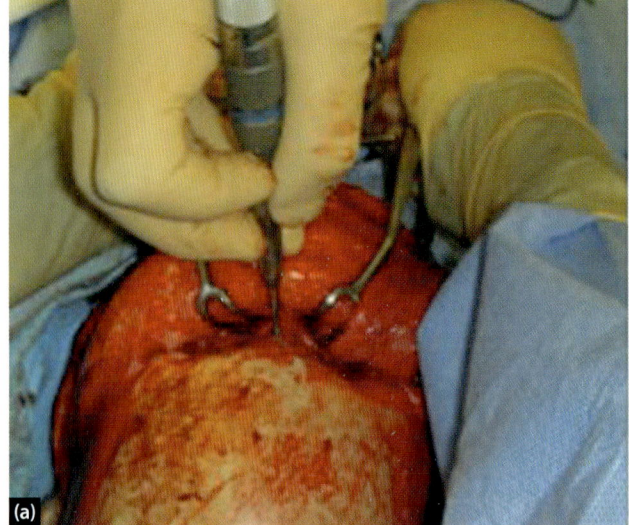

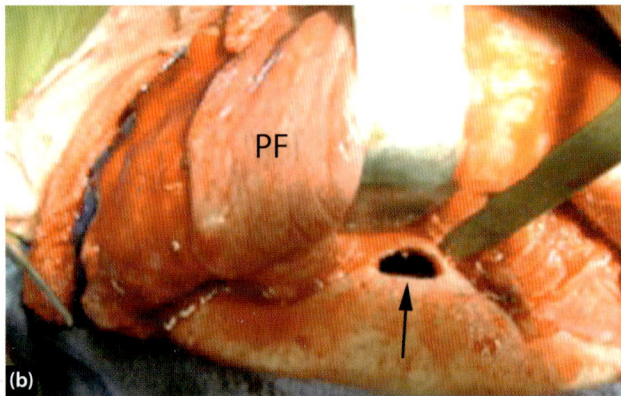

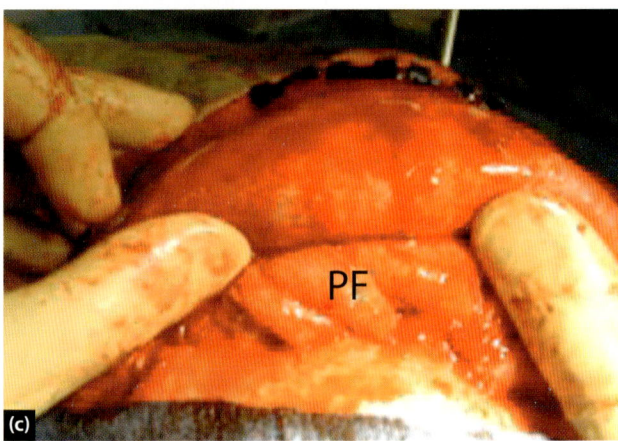

Figure 116.16 An extracranial pericranial flap requires drilling **(a)** of a bone window (arrow) at the nasion that extends from orbit to orbit below the level of the skull base **(b)**. The pericranial flap (PF) is pedicled on one or both supraorbital vessels and passed through the bone window into the nasal cavity **(c)**.

pathway of the Draf 3 frontal sinusotomy. Care should be taken to ensure the proximal flap is in contact with the anterior aspect of the skull base defect or the bone of the posterior table of the frontal sinus.

The reconstructive flap is then covered with layers of Surgicel®, tissue glue, and Gelfoam®. Support of the reconstruction is provided by a Foley catheter inflated with saline or Merocel® tampons. Tampons are preferred for large anterior defects and when the optic nerves are exposed and susceptible to compression.

CASE EXAMPLE: PERICRANIAL FLAP

A 79-year-old female underwent EES for an olfactory neuroblastoma. Because of septal involvement by the tumour, reconstruction of the anterior cranial base defect with a nasoseptal flap was not possible (**Figure 116.17**). An extracranial pericranial flap was harvested using a bicoronal scalp incision and was passed into the nasal cavity inferior to the skull base using a bony window at the level of the nasion and covered the defect widely, including the medial orbits. The post-operative course was not complicated by a CSF leak and sensory and motor function of the frontal scalp was preserved.

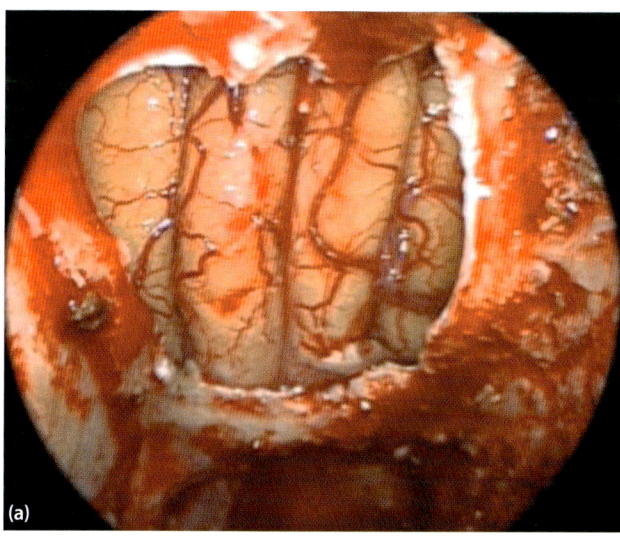

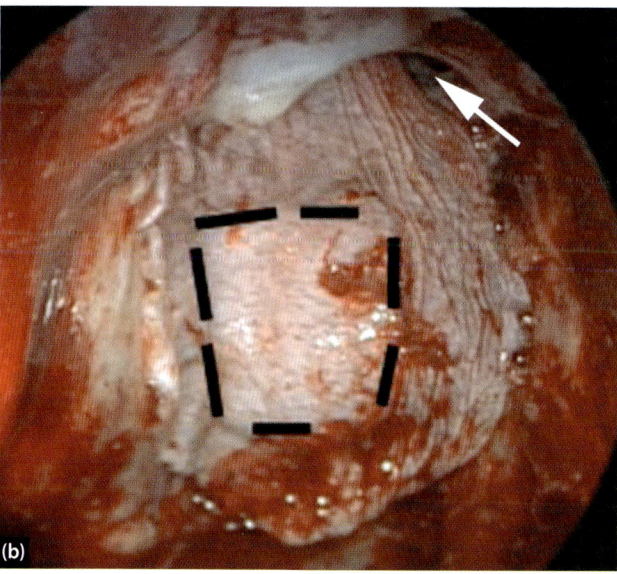

Figure 116.17 A nasoseptal flap was not available for reconstruction of this dural defect. **(a)** Following endoscopic endonasal excision of an aesthesioneuroblastoma. **(b)** An extracranial pericranial flap provided ample coverage of the defect (original dural defect outlined). Note drainage pathway (arrow) for the frontal sinuses to the side of the flap pedicle.

Post-operative care

Patients are monitored for signs of intra-cranial complications and a CT scan of the brain is performed within 8 hours to look for evidence of intra-cranial haemorrhage or tension pneumocephalus. Visual outcomes are assessed if dissection included the optic nerves/chiasm. If a suprasellar approach is performed, patients are also at risk for diabetes insipidus and are managed in conjunction with the endocrinology service. Antibiotic prophylaxis is continued for the duration of nasal packing. After 24 hours, patients can be switched to an oral cephalosporin (Ceftin). Lumbar drainage is used in patients with significant arachnoidal dissection (i.e. high-flow leaks), but there is limited evidence to support this practice.

Nasal packing is removed in 5–7 days; this can be done in the outpatient clinic. Nasal splints are maintained for 1 week if a pericranial flap is used and for 3 weeks if a septal flap is used. This facilitates mucosalization of the septum. Nasal irrigations with saline are performed daily and periodic endoscopic debridement of the nasal cavity is performed until healing is complete.

OUTCOMES

We have successfully treated several nasal dermoids with intra-cranial extension (extradural) through foramen cecum using an endonasal approach. Review of the literature demonstrates minimal data regarding endoscopic endonasal resection of nasal dermoids.[8] The initial experience is positive, however, and suggests that equivalent outcomes can be achieved with these techniques.

Oncological outcomes for sinonasal malignancy are limited. A meta-analysis of 23 studies (361 patients) of treatment for aesthesioneuroblastomas demonstrated a higher published survival rate for endoscopic surgery when compared to open surgery, even when stratifying for year of publication. Although endoscopic series had similar follow up, they had earlier stage (Kadish) disease, suggesting a treatment bias. Data are even more limited for other sinonasal malignancies such as squamous cell carcinoma, adenocarcinoma, and sinonasal undifferentiated carcinoma. Early results suggest that comparable results can be achieved using endoscopic techniques.

The optimal approach for olfactory groove meningiomas remains controversial, but there is a role for EES for debulking large tumours in the elderly and avoiding frontal lobe retraction. In a review of 44 patients who underwent EES for olfactory groove meningiomas (unpublished data), 55% underwent gross total resection, 16% near total and 30% subtotal. In 16 patients, tumours were removed in two stages, both to allow tumour descent/ collapse and as part of the endoscopic learning curve. Overall, the CSF leak rate was nearly 40%, but this decreased throughout the series as reconstructive techniques evolved. As a result, 6.8% of patients suffered post-operative meningitis. As experience improved, the gross total resection rate increased to almost 70% in the last 3 years. No patients had worsening of vision and 64% of those with pre-operative visual impairment improved.

Suprasellar meningiomas often present with visual impairment. In a review of 75 patients with suprasellar meningiomas, visual impairment was the most common presenting symptom in 81%. Following EES, complete resolution or improvement of visual symptoms was seen in 86% of patients with deterioration in only 4% (2 patients). These results compare favourably to the literature for open approaches and suggest that preservation of small vessels of the optic chiasm are better visualized and preserved with EES. Gross total resection (GTR) was achieved in 79%. GTR was limited by large tumours (>3 cm), multi-lobulated tumours, and those with vascular encasement but not by optic canal involvement. CSF leak was the most common complication in 25% of patients but has decreased to 16% since the introduction of the nasoseptal flap for reconstruction.

Craniopharyngiomas are well suited for an endonasal approach. We performed a retrospective review of 64 patients (47 adults, 17 children) with craniopharyngioma who underwent EES.[9] The most common presenting symptom in adults was visual loss (81%); headache was most common in the paediatric population (65%). Resection >95% was achieved in 72% of patients; the resection rate was significantly better in the paediatric population. Of those patients presenting with visual impairment, vision was improved or normalized in 86%. In patients with normal pituitary function (n = 24), new pituitary deficit occurred in 14 (58%). Other than pituitary dysfunction (hypopituitarism and diabetes insipidus), CSF leak was the most common complication (23%) but decreased to 11% following introduction of the nasoseptal flap for reconstruction. Treatment options for recurrent disease (34% of patients) included repeat EES in 55% of recurrences. With the goal of gross total or near total resection, EES can be employed for the treatment of every craniopharyngioma regardless of the location, size and extension (excluding purely intra-ventricular tumours) and can provide acceptable results, comparable to traditional craniotomies. This surgical technique is not limited to adult patients, actually showing higher resection rates in the paediatric population.

In patients undergoing EES of the skull base, excellent QOL scores are noted using the anterior skull base questionnaire.[10] One area of relative deficiency is in specific symptoms, such as olfactory loss. Limited data suggest that QOL is superior to open transcranial approaches for tumours involving the anterior cranial base. Nasal morbidity has been assessed in the endonasal surgical group using the SNOT-22 questionnaire, a validated instrument.[11] The use of a nasoseptal flap for reconstruction had a limited negative impact. As expected, increasing nasal morbidity (decreased QOL) has been noted in the expanded (non-transsellar sagittal plane and coronal plane) surgical modules compared to transsellar surgery.[12]

COMPLICATIONS

Complications may be categorized in multiple ways, by location, type, or time period. Intra-operative complications are rare and depend on the type and extent of pathology and the surgical approach.[13,14] The most serious intra-operative complications are injuries to the optic nerves or carotid arteries. Meticulous surgical technique, familiarity with endoscopic anatomy, and good visualization are key factors in avoiding injury. With a transcribriform approach, the frontopolar vessels are at particular risk and the dura should be initially incised laterally to avoid injury. Visual loss may result from direct trauma to the optic nerves or from loss of vascular supply (branches of superior hypophyseal arteries).

Post-operatively, the most common complication is CSF leak. Potential risk factors include the size and location of the dural defect, patient factors (prior treatment, obesity), reconstructive technique (materials, vascularized flap, packing), and perioperative care (patient activity, lumbar drain, debridement). Most leaks are small and are related to insufficient coverage by the reconstructive tissues. In most cases, endoscopic repair supplemented by a lumbar spinal drain is successful. Intra-cranial infection is rare and is usually associated with a post-operative CSF leak. Prompt repair of CSF leaks and limited use of lumbar spinal drains is encouraged to limit the risk of infection.

Sinonasal complications include sinusitis, epistaxis, synechiae, chronic crusting, cosmetic deformity, and loss of olfaction. Delayed epistaxis is usually due to a branch of the sphenopalatine artery. A saddle-nose deformity can result from loss of septal support. Even if the olfactory nerves are preserved, some loss of olfaction is common and may be due to altered airflow patterns, mucosal oedema and crusting, post-operative irradiation, or direct damage to the olfactory epithelium or olfactory tracts. Fortunately, QOL studies demonstrate that overall sinonasal morbidity is low.

KEY POINTS

- The anterior cranial base from the frontal sinus to the sella and from orbit to orbit is accessible using EES.
- These techniques can be applied to a wide variety of lesions including meningoencephaloceles, benign tumours (nasal dermoids, meningiomas, craniopharyngiomas, pituitary adenomas) and malignant tumours (sinonasal malignancy) with preservation of microsurgical and oncological principles.
- Many of the challenges of endonasal surgery have been solved and large dural defects can be reconstructed effectively using vascularized flaps.
- Oncological and functional outcomes are comparable or superior to other approaches with the potential for decreased morbidity.
- Proper training in endoscopic techniques and adherence to the principles of team surgery is necessary to avoid complications and achieve superior outcomes.

REFERENCES

1. Snyderman CH, Pant H, Carrau RL, et al. Classification of endonasal approaches to the ventral skull base. In: Stamm AC (ed). *Transnasal endoscopic skull base and brain surgery.* New York: Thieme; 2011, pp. 83–91.
2. Snyderman CH, Carrau RL, Kassam AB, et al. Endoscopic skull base surgery: principles of endonasal oncological surgery. *J Surg Oncol* 2008; **97**(8): 658–64.
3. Snyderman CH, Gardner PA. "How much is enough?" Endonasal surgery for olfactory neuroblastoma. *Skull Base* 2010; **20**(5): 309–10.
4. Stangerup SE, Dommerby H, Siim C, et al. New modification of hot-water irrigation in the treatment of posterior epistaxis. *Arch Otolaryngol Head Neck Surg* 1999; **125**(11): 1285.
5. Harvey RJ, Parmar P, Sacks R, Zanation AM. Endoscopic skull base reconstruction of large dural defects: a systematic review of published evidence. *Laryngoscope* 2012; **122**(2): 452–9.
6. Pinheiro-Neto CD, Snyderman CH. Nasoseptal flap. *Adv Otorhinolaryngol* 2013; **74**: 42–55.
7. Patel MR, Shah RN, Snyderman CH, et al. Pericranial flap for endoscopic anterior skull-base reconstruction: clinical outcomes and radioanatomic analysis of preoperative planning. *Neurosurgery* 2010; **66**(3): 506–12; discussion 512.
8. Pinheiro-Neto CD, Snyderman CH, Fernandez-Miranda J, Gardner PA. Endoscopic endonasal surgery for nasal dermoids. *Otolaryngol Clin North Am* 2011; **44**(4): 981–7.
9. Koutourousiou M, Gardner PA, Fernandez-Miranda JC, et al. Endoscopic endonasal surgery for craniopharyngiomas: surgical outcome in 64 patients. *J Neurosurg* 2013; **119**: 1194–207.
10. Cavel O, Abergel A, Margalit N, et al. Quality of life following endoscopic resection of skull base tumors. *J Neurol Surg B Skull Base* 2012; **73**(2): 1121–16.
11. Harrow BR, Batra PS. Sinonasal quality of life outcomes after minimally invasive resection of sinonasal and skull-base tumors. *Int Forum Allergy Rhinol* 2013; **12**(3): 1013–20.
12. Pant H, Bhatki AM, Snyderman CH, et al. Quality of life following endonasal skull base surgery. *Skull Base* 2010; **20**(1): 35–40.
13. Kassam AB, Prevedello DM, Carrau RL, et al. Endoscopic endonasal skull base surgery: analysis of complications in the authors' initial 800 patients. *J Neurosurg* 2011; **114**(6): 1544–68.
14. Snyderman CH, Pant H, Gardner PA, et al. Management of complications of endonasal cranial base surgery. In: Kassam AB, Gardner PA (eds). *Endoscopic approaches to the skull base.* Progress in neurological surgery. 26th ed. Basel: Karger; 2012, pp. 182–90.

CHAPTER 117

IMAGING IN RHINOLOGY

Gregory O'Neill

Introduction	1305	Imaging – new developments	1315
Imaging modalities – technical aspects	1305	Conclusion	1316
Imaging – applications	1307	References	1316

SEARCH STRATEGY
Data in this chapter may be updated by a Medline search using the keywords: sinonasal, paranasal, and diagnostic imaging with cross-referencing from the papers thus identified.

INTRODUCTION

Modern imaging has come to occupy a pivotal role in the pre-/post- (and intra-) operative depiction of patient anatomy and disease localization in the sinonasal region, and can, on occasion, provide insights into pathology. The principal modalities used in sinonasal imaging are CT and MRI, and their role (as outlined in the examples that follow) is frequently complementary. PET-CT, a technique combining anatomical information with metabolic information (by virtue of uptake of the glucose analogue ^{18}F-FDG), is increasingly utilized in head and neck cancer imaging in general (for example, in the investigation of the unknown primary), although its role in sinonasal imaging is still emerging.

Plain film imaging is now largely obsolete (except in the context of trauma or, perhaps on the rare occasion when an AP frontal sinus radiograph may be used in template planning for osteoplastic flap surgery). In one study, comparing plain radiographs and coronal CT scans in a paediatric population with recurrent sinusitis, there was an almost 75% discordance between plain film and CT findings.[1] Plain radiographs are neither necessary nor sufficient to either exclude or confirm sinus disease. This advice may be modified, however, in healthcare systems where access to modern cross-sectional imaging is limited.

IMAGING MODALITIES – TECHNICAL ASPECTS

Computed tomography (CT)

Multi-detector row CT (MDCT) enables a patient to be rapidly scanned in the supine position, resulting in submillimetre slices that can be reformatted, in high resolution, in axial, coronal or sagittal planes.

The main drawback with CT is that it involves ionizing radiation. Radiation dose to the lens of the eye is a specific concern in relation to sinonasal imaging and work has focused on the potential for reducing the dose of radiation whilst still maintaining diagnostically satisfactory images.[2]

With CT, high-attenuation ('white') bone contrasts against low attenuation ('black') air and intermediate ('grey') soft tissue and fluid. In terms of providing contrast between different soft tissues or fluid, intravenous iodinated contrast can be of assistance, to some extent, although MRI is superior and usually to be preferred (particularly in the assessment of neoplastic disease where contrast between tumour and secretions/inflamed mucosa is desirable).

Magnetic resonance imaging (MRI)

Having the advantage of no ionizing radiation and superior soft tissue contrast, the imaging sequences employed usually involve a combination of T1- and T2-weighted images with Gadolinium contrast agents being employed to assess complications of inflammatory disease or to assess spread of neoplasms (particularly to assess perineural tumour spread and dural invasion).

Note that in comparison to CT, no (or very little) contrast is seen on MRI between air and cortical bone (both low signal, or 'black', thus CT more optimally depicts the intricacies of bony anatomy), between cortical bone and fast-flowing blood (for example, between the wall of the sphenoid and the internal carotid artery), or between air and dessicated secretions (both signal voids on T2-weighted images, see below). Thus, there are pros and cons to both CT and MRI and frequently both are needed – particularly in assessing disease involving the skull base.

A particular feature of MR imaging of the paranasal sinuses is the effect that increasing viscosity and protein concentration within secretions has on T1-weighted and T2-weighted images signal intensities – a source of potential confusion. As protein concentration (or viscosity) increases, the signal intensity on T1-weighted images (which for water is low to intermediate) increases and then falls (becomes bright and then dark). For T2-weighted images (starting with bright 'water' signal) there is a gradual decrease in signal intensity[3] (**Figures 117.1 & 117.2**).

At the extreme end of the spectrum, with markedly viscid and dehydrated secretions, a signal void is produced on all imaging sequences.[4] If MRI is the initial investigation then this could be mistaken for air, although a clue to the presence of dessicated secretions may be the finding of expansion of the affected sinus (a mucocele) (**Figure 117.3**). CT will clarify by demonstrating intermediate or high attenuation contents ('grey') within the sinus (as opposed to air which would appear 'black').

Positron-emission tomography/computed tomography (PET-CT)

A technique fusing the anatomical information of CT with metabolic information provided by uptake of the glucose analogue ^{18}F-FDG (fluoro-deoxy-glucose) and predicated on tumour (or inflammatory) tissue having increased metabolism and thus increased glucose uptake in comparison to normal tissue. As indicated, its potential role in sinonasal imaging is gradually being appreciated but we will return to this topic towards the end of this chapter.

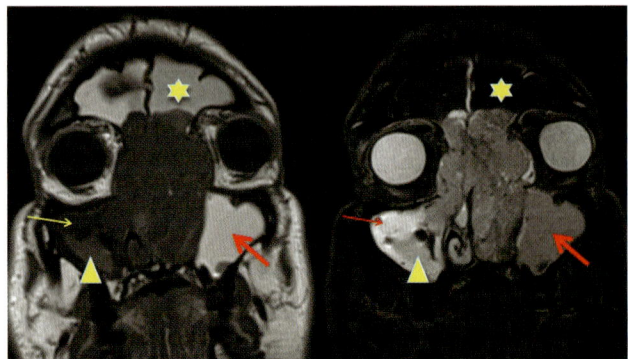

Figure 117.2 MRI of sinus secretions (olfactory neuroblastoma). A large nasal cavity olfactory neuroblastoma causing obstruction of the frontal and maxillary sinuses (T1-weighted image on left, fat-suppressed T2-weighted image on right). Note the differing signal intensities of secretions in the affected sinuses depending on their concentration. Mucosa lining the right maxillary sinus (arrows) is of a similar signal intensity to the aqueous humour (equates to water) in the globe above. Within the right maxillary sinus (arrowheads) the concentration of secretions begins to increase and, as a result, the signal begins to increase on T1-weighted images and decrease on T2-weighted images. Compare with the left maxillary sinus (large arrows) where, as the concentration increases still, the signal on T1-weighted becomes markedly high whilst continuing to reduce (although remaining fairly high) on T2-weighted images. With increasing thickness/concentration of secretions in the frontal sinuses (stars), the signal remains high on T1-weighted images but has now dropped out on T2-weighted images.

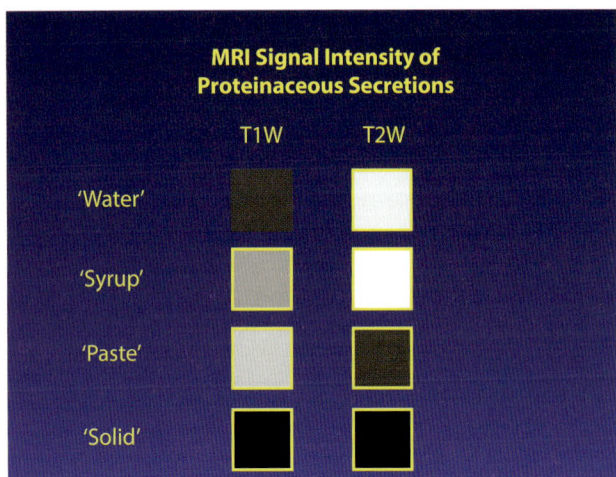

Figure 117.1 MRI of sinus secretions. Note, as the concentration of sinus secretions increases the signal intensity on T1-weighted images goes from intermediate to high to low, whereas on T2-weighted images the signal intensity progressively decreases.

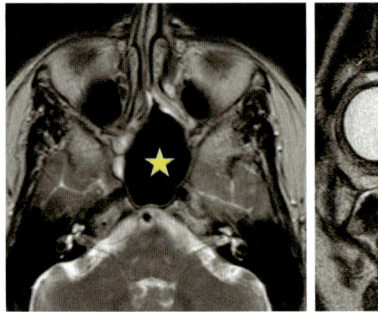 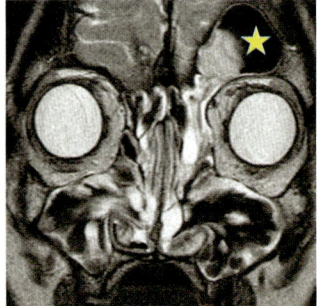

Figure 117.3 Mucoceles containing signal voids. Dessicated secretions can produce a signal void that can be confused for an air-filled sinus, particularly on T2-weighted images. The expansion of the sinus walls hints at a mucocele and in both cases CT confirmed an opacified sinus.

IMAGING – APPLICATIONS

Depicting anatomy

Sinonasal anatomy is subject to tremendous variation and is virtually unique to any one individual such that plain radiographic and, more recently, CT assessment of sinus anatomy are well-recognized techniques for victim identification in forensic investigation.[5]

Some anatomic variants are relevant in terms of potential risk of surgical complications: for example, asymmetry of the anterior skull base (in particular the fovea ethmoidalis) or the presence of an Onodi cell (or sphenoethmoidal cell–a posterior ethmoid cell projecting posteriorly and lateral to, or more commonly above, the sphenoid sinus to be related to the optic nerve).[6]

There are also a number of anatomic variants which have a close relationship to the drainage pathways of the paranasal sinuses. It is controversial as to whether any of these (other than maybe nasal septal deviation) have an aetiologic role in the development of sinusitis.[7] However, an understanding of these variants remains necessary to safe and effective sinus surgery. The reader will be familiar with most anatomic variants including the concha bullosa (pneumatized middle turbinate) and the Haller cell (an air cell located below the ethmoid bulla, inferomedial to the orbit).

More complex are the variants of anatomy occurring in the frontal recess region. This area is of particular concern as this is a difficult area to operate in and as the frontal sinus is an area prone to sinusitis recurrence following FESS.[8]

In understanding frontal recess anatomy, it is useful to start with the basic template of frontal sinus, frontal sinus ostium, frontal sinus drainage pathway, agger nasi cell and ethmoid bulla (**Figure 117.4**). To this template we can consider the various potential frontal recess cells in three groups: medial, anterior and posterior. The medial group consists of the interfrontal sinus septal cell which is best seen on coronal images and easily appreciated as an air cell arising within the interfrontal sinus septum.

The anterior group of frontal cells are classified into types 1 to 4 (**Figure 117.5**).[9] Note that in Kuhn's original classification a type 4 cell is an isolated cell in the frontal sinus. However, Wormald[6] has modified this classification describing both type 3 and 4 cells as frontal cells which pneumatize through the frontal sinus ostium and extend cephalad to a height either less than (type 3) or more than (type 4) 50% of the height of the frontal sinus.

The posterior group consists of the suprabullar cell and the frontal bullar cell, the differentiating characteristic of the latter being that it extends beyond and above the frontal sinus ostium in contradistinction to the former (**Figure 117.6**).

Also belonging to the posterior group, and the hardest cell to illustrate conveniently in a single image (requiring study of both coronal and axial images), is the supraorbital cell.[10] The opening is usually found anterior to the canal for the anterior ethmoidal artery and it extends laterally to pneumatize the orbital plate of the frontal bone, its distinction from the frontal sinus made clear on axial images, where a bony septum can be seen between the two.

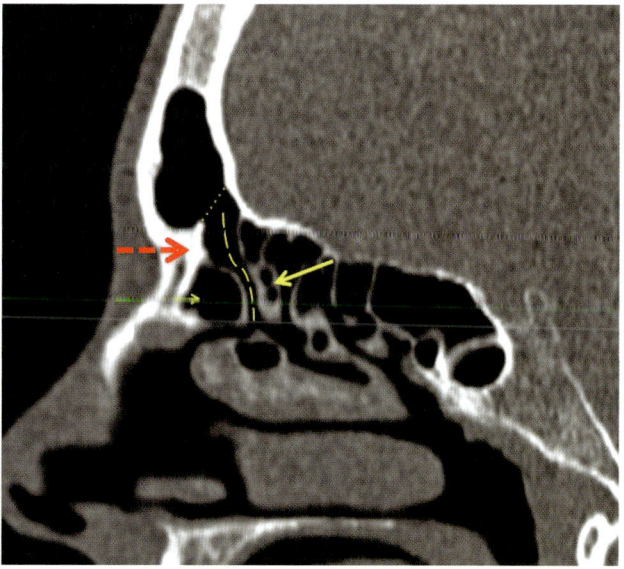

Figure 117.4 Typical frontal recess anatomy as demonstrated in parasagittal section. Frontal sinus ostium (dotted line) runs from frontonasal beak (interrupted arrow) anteriorly to anterior skull base posteriorly. Frontal sinus drainage pathway (dashed line). Note wide superior compartment leading into narrow inferior compartment. Agger nasi cell (small arrow). Ethmoid bulla (large arrow). (Note small suprabullar air cell).

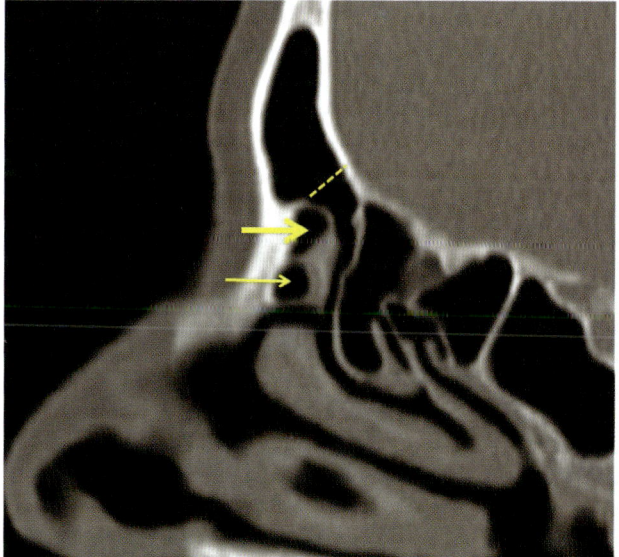

Figure 117.5 Type 1 frontal cell. Type 1 frontal cell (large arrow) sitting above agger nasi cell (small arrow). Note relationship to frontonasal beak. Note the frontal sinus ostium (interrupted line). In a type 2 configuration there are two cells above the agger nasi cell but below the frontal sinus ostium. In type 3 and type 4 configurations a large frontal cell extends through the ostium into the frontal sinus for a variable distance of either <50% (type 3) or >50% (type 4) of the height of the frontal sinus.

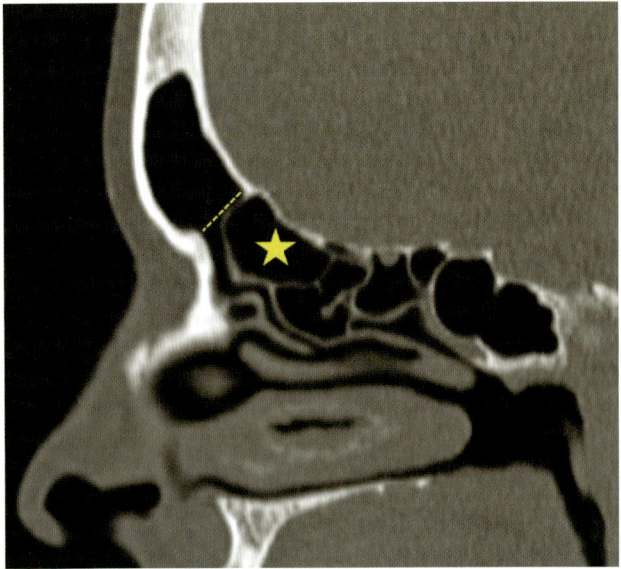

Figure 117.6 Suprabullar cell (star). Note relationship to anterior skull base and frontal sinus ostium (dashed line). A frontal bullar cell extends above the dashed line into the frontal sinus.

Sinus inflammatory disease

INCIDENTAL FINDINGS

Mucosal thickening, fluid-filled sinuses and retention cysts are common findings in asymptomatic patients imaged for other reasons: for example, patients undergoing MRI of the head/brain for neurological symptoms,[11] or of the internal auditory meati,[12] or cone-beam CT for orthodontic patients.[13] It has been said that incidentally found mucosal thickening up to 3 mm is of no clinical significance and that in the ethmoid sinuses 1–2 mm of mucosal thickening occurs in 63% of asymptomatic patients.[14] The concept of an 'incidental' Lund score, with 0–5 considered 'normal', has also been suggested.[15] As regards retention cysts (recognized as dome-shaped, smoothly marginated opacities on CT with high (fluid) signal on T2-weighted MR; **Figure 117.7**), the natural history is that the majority either regress or remain unchanged.[16]

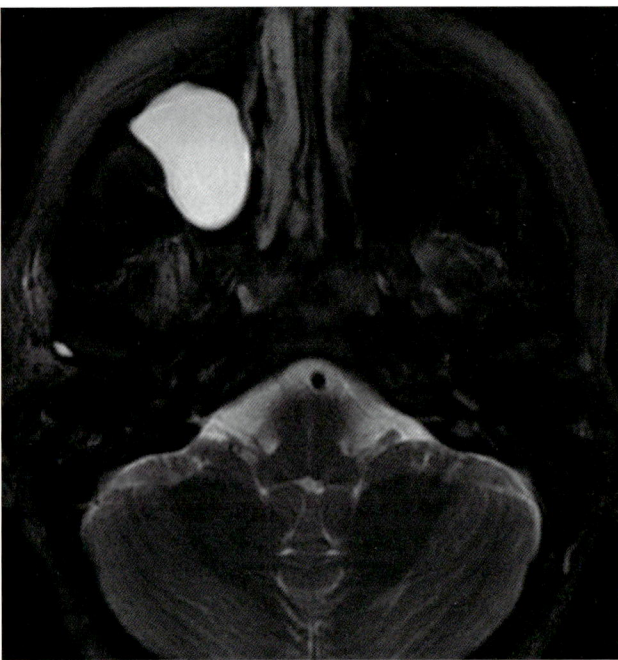

Figure 117.7 Maxillary sinus retention cyst. High signal on T2/fat-saturated images. Typically smooth outlined, 'dome-shaped' lesion.

The relevance of these incidental findings depends on correlation with clinical findings.

RHINOSINUSITIS (TYPICAL)

The diagnosis of rhinosinusitis is largely a clinical/endoscopic one. Whilst a negative CT is useful to rule out rhinosinusitis and provoke the search for an alternative diagnosis (particularly where the predominant symptom is facial pain[17]), the role of CT when sinusitis is diagnosed is largely one of demonstrating the bony anatomy prior to surgery and defining disease extent (**Figure 117.8**). Disease extent can be quantified through the use of one of a number of staging systems of which the Lund-Mackay system[18] is perhaps the best known. CT acquisition is also needed

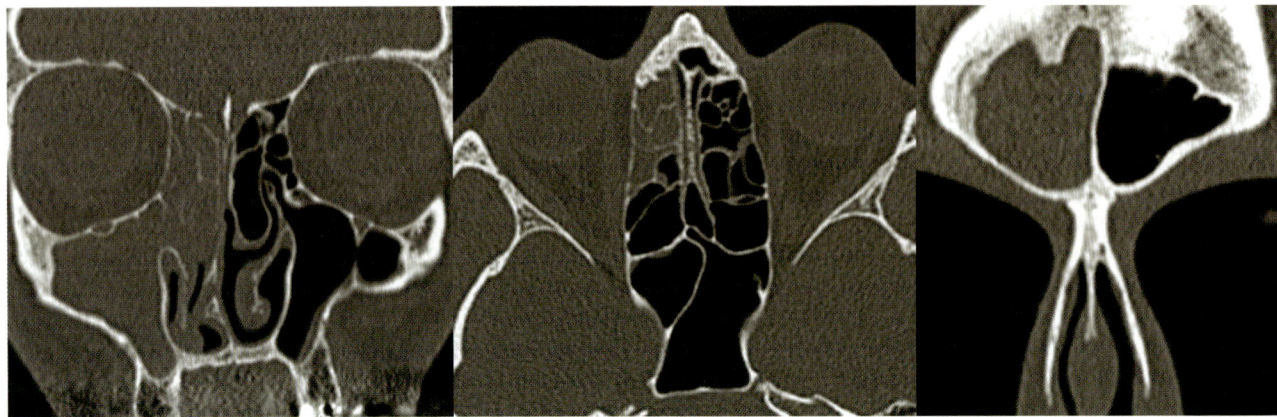

Figure 117.8 Rhinosinusitis. OMU pattern. A case of rhinosinusitis conforming to an ostiomeatal unit pattern of disease involving frontal, maxillary and anterior ethmoid sinuses. Whilst this pattern of disease suggests obstruction at the level of the middle meatus, the CT appearance of the affected sinuses is non-specifically bland.

where the operating surgeon employs a surgical navigation system in theatre.

In terms of diagnostic information, whilst sinus wall sclerosis serves as a pointer to chronicity of disease, the plain CT imaging findings are, for the most part, banal. CT (and MRI) become of more crucial use diagnostically in the investigation of the complications of sinusitis, particularly subperiosteal orbital abscess and intra-cranial infective complications.

FUNGAL SINUSITIS

Fungal sinusitis is a disparate group, with disparate imaging features (**Figure 117.9**), which can be classified into invasive and non-invasive forms:

Invasive (IFS)

Acute invasive fungal sinusitis (AIFS) AIFS usually occurs in immunocompromized patients and is a rapidly progressive, potentially fatal condition. Findings on CT such as bone erosion and mucosal thickening may be subtle.[19] The finding of extrasinus extension (or perisinus soft tissue infiltration)[20] is described as an early and characteristic finding suggesting AIFS (with MR said to be more sensitive in this regard).[21] However, a larger retrospective review[22] found that the commonest early findings on CT in this condition were severe, unilateral, nasal mucosal inflammatory changes (marked mucosal thickening or complete nasal cavity opacification) and that these were found much more frequently, and earlier, than osseous erosion or extra-sinus extension. More recently, the finding on post-contrast MRI of foci of non-enhancement in the nasal cavity (the so-called 'black turbinate' sign – non-enhancing devitalized tissue contrasting with the typical mucosal enhancement normally seen in sinusitis, **Figure 117.9**) has been described in two patients with mucormycosis.[23] In the correct clinical context this finding has the potential to alert the radiologist and surgeon to the correct diagnosis.

Chronic invasive fungal sinusitis (CIFS) Affected patients are usually immunocompetent or have a mild degree of immunocompromise (such as diabetics).

Chronic granulomatous invasive fungal sinusitis (CGIFS) CGIFS usually occurs in Africa (Sudan) or South Asia, is usually caused by *Aspergillus* species, and occurs in immunocompetent individuals. It is considered by some not to be a separate entity but to be a subset of chronic invasive fungal sinusitis.

On CT, chronic (granulomatous) invasive fungal sinusitis tends to display homogeneous soft tissue opacification with no focal hyperdensities (in contrast to allergic fungal sinusitis). Disease tends to be limited in extent or unilateral, sinus expansion is not a feature, focal bony erosion is limited to areas of extra-sinus extension and the burden of disease is often more outwith the sinuses (for example, intra-orbital) than within.[24]

Non-invasive

Allergic fungal sinusitis (AFS) Typically, affected patients are immunocompetent with a history of atopy. A characteristic finding at endoscopy is the presence of so-called 'allergic mucin'.[19]

The typical imaging findings at CT are those of unilateral or bilateral opacification of multiple sinuses, with sinus expansion, bony erosion of the sinus walls, and areas of intra-sinus high attenuation (due to heavy metals, calcium and inspissated secretions).[25]

An important point to note is that whilst AFS is classified as non-invasive (in histopathological terms), advanced disease with sinus expansion and bony erosion can result in extensive intra-cranial and/or intra-orbital 'invasion' with an aggressive appearance on imaging which can mimic malignancy.

Also, it should be noted that the presence of intra-sinus high attenuation is not specific to AFS but can be seen with dessicated secretions in chronic rhinosinusitis. In this case the imaging features of sinus expansion and bony

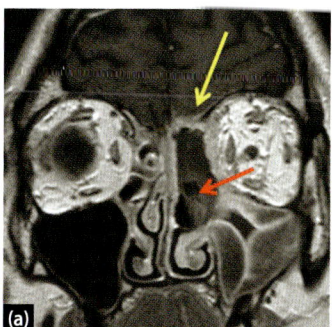 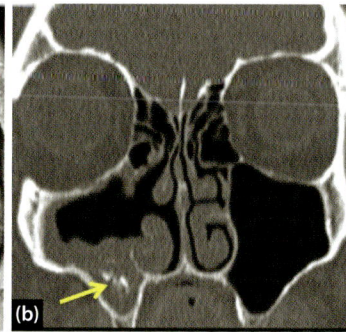 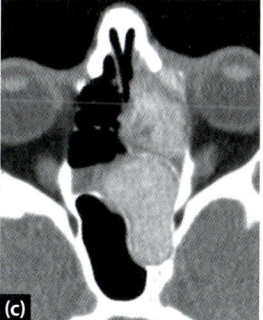 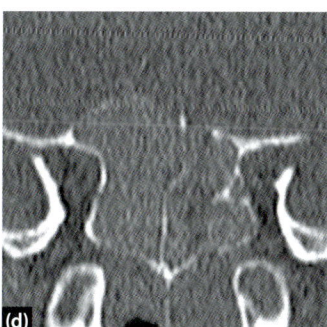

Figure 117.9 Fungal sinusitis. (a) is a case of acute invasive fungal sinusitis (mucormycosis) with cribriform plate extension and dural enhancement as demonstrated on MRI. Note also the non-enhancement of the left middle turbinate and adjacent ethmoid air cells (the so-called 'black turbinate' sign) due to the presence of devitalized tissue. Compare with the normally enhancing right middle turbinate. **(b)** is a case of non-invasive mycetoma or 'fungal ball' on plain CT. The 'ball'-like nature of this condition containing punctate hyperdensities is difficult to appreciate on a non-contrast CT where there is no discrimination with the adjacent inflamed mucosa. **(c)** is a case of allergic fungal sinusitis with the ethmoid sinuses filled with high attenuation material and with expansion of the sinus causing lamina papyracea remodelling. More typically allergic fungal sinusitis is diffuse and bilateral as in **(d)** where there is remodelling of the skull base in the region of the sphenoid. Part **(a)** is reprinted from The Otolaryngologist, Vol **1**(1), Fraser L, McGarry W. Core knowledge and literature review, p. 5. 2006 Copyright with permission from Rila Publications Ltd, London.

thinning point to the former whereas the latter is more characterized by thickening and sclerosis of sinus walls.

The MR appearance is typically low to signal void on T2-weighted image (due to heavy metals and dessicated secretions) and more variable on T1-weighted image.[19]

Fungal ball/ mycetoma A fungus ball is a tangle of fungal hyphae within a sinus, but with no allergic mucin (compare with AFS) and no evidence of submucosal invasion (compare with IFS).[19] Affected individuals tend to be older and immunocompetent.

Typically a single sinus is involved, and on a non-contrast CT, an iso- to hyper-attenuating soft tissue mass is seen, frequently containing punctate or nodular calcifications. In contrast the inflamed mucosa lining the sinus is hypo attenuating on CT, hyper intense on T2-weighted image MRI and demonstrates contrast enhancement.

The fungus ball is low signal on T1-weighted and T2-weighted images as it contains little or no free water. Contained calcifications or heavy metals (iron and manganese)[26] produce a characteristic signal void on T2-weighted image.[27]

Granulomatous inflammation

Covering a range of disorders, this subset is characterized by the common imaging features of nasal septal perforation and destruction of the midline sinonasal skeleton including turbinates and hard palate.

The differential diagnosis for septal perforation and mid-face destruction not only includes the various granulomatous disorders but also neoplasia (for example, squamous cell carcinoma), infection (leprosy, syphilis, tuberculosis, actinomycosis, rhinoscleroma) and cocaine misuse (**Figure 117.10**).

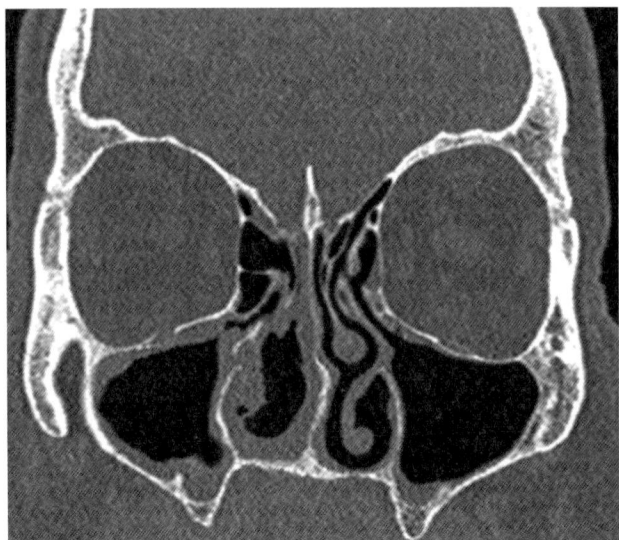

Figure 117.10 Cocaine-induced nasal cavity destruction. Note the mucosal thickening accompanying destruction of the right inferior turbinate and lower aspect of right middle turbinate. Unusually the process is unilateral and the nasal septum is not involved.

Of the granulomatous disorders, Wegener's granulomatosis has a particular propensity for involvement of the nasal cavity and paranasal sinuses.

The early features of the disease may be non-specific (mucosal thickening, sinus opacification) but with disease progression, bony destruction occurs involving nasal septum and turbinates initially. Neo-osteogenesis (to the extent of sinus obliteration) is also a feature on CT, and one which is exacerbated by surgery.[28]

On MRI, as on CT, the early manifestations of sinonasal Wegener's may be non-specific and indistinguishable from sinusitis. In the later stages granulomatous inflammation is depicted as low-signal intensity lesions, best depicted on T2-weighted images. Orbital involvement may occur.[29]

The imaging features of cocaine misuse are similar to Wegener's but at initial presentation the extent of mid-face destruction is usually greater (perhaps reflecting a delay to presentation).[30]

Sarcoidosis shares similar imaging features with other granulomatous disorders, but a feature which is said to be characteristic is the finding of soft tissue nodules on the septum or turbinates.[31]

NK (natural killer cell)/T-cell lymphoma (formerly known as lethal midline granuloma) shows a tendency to spread as a thin sheet of tumour enveloping turbinates and septum[32] and may extend into the nasopharynx[32] or paranasal sinuses.[33] Nodal involvement is not usual. Interestingly, a recent study has shown a majority in their cohort presenting as unilateral nasal cavity disease.[33] However, the imaging findings are not diagnostic and the finding that is most characteristic for this disease is Southeast Asian ethnicity.[32, 33]

Miscellaneous

The imaging features of a miscellaneous group that includes antrochoanal polyp and silent sinus syndrome are virtually diagnostic (**Figure 117.11a** and **117.11b**). In the maxillary sinuses, a possible odontogenic cause of sinusitis (**Figure 117.11c**) should always be considered and one should consider also odontogenic cysts (**Figure 117.11d**) in the differential diagnosis of the 'opacified maxillary sinus'.

Sinonasal neoplasms

It is rare (if ever) that imaging will be able to definitively diagnose a sinonasal lesion without the referring clinician ultimately having to make recourse to biopsy. Conversely, however, the radiologist and clinician must be alert to those occasions when it is mandatory *not* to perform a biopsy (for example highly vascularized tumours, sphenoid sinus internal carotid artery pseudoaneurysm).[34]

But for the most part, the purpose of imaging the sinonasal neoplasm is to delineate the extent of the tumour, both in terms of differentiating tumour from secetions or mucosa (**Figure 117.12**) within the sinonasal compartment (where MRI is of particular use), and in terms of defining extent outwith the sinonasal compartment.

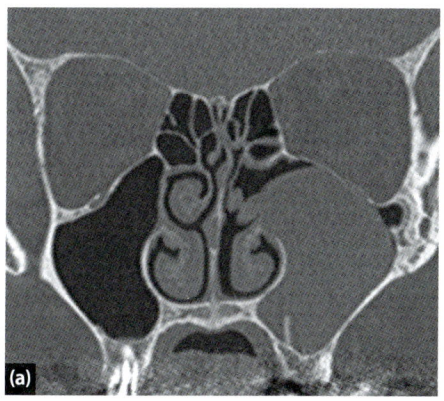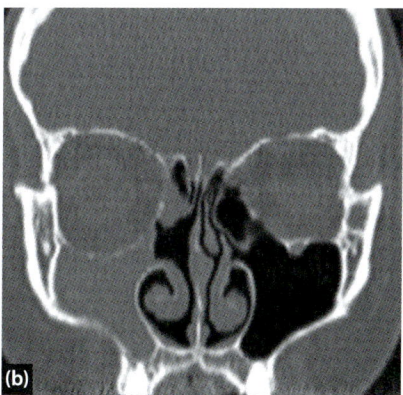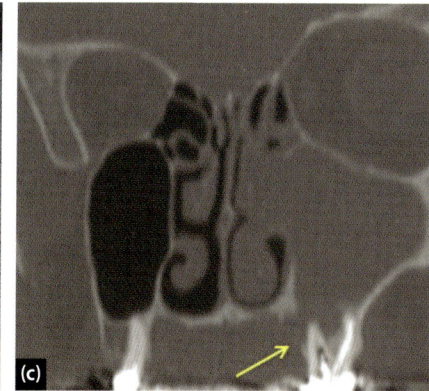

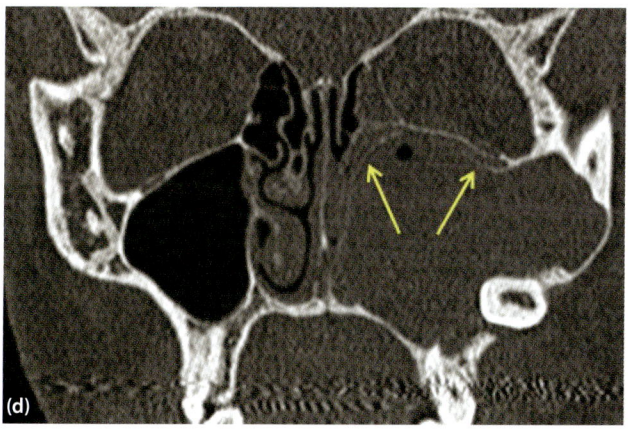

Figure 117.11 Miscellaneous maxillary sinus lesions.
(a) Antrochoanal polyp. **(b)** Silent sinus syndrome (note collapsed walls of right maxillary sinus in this patient with enophthalmos. **(c)** Odontogenic sinusitis (periapical abscess discharging into sinus). **(d)** Dentigerous cyst arising in association with the crown of an unerupted, malpositioned tooth. Note the thin, bony shell of the cyst paralleling the roof and medial wall of the maxillary sinus.

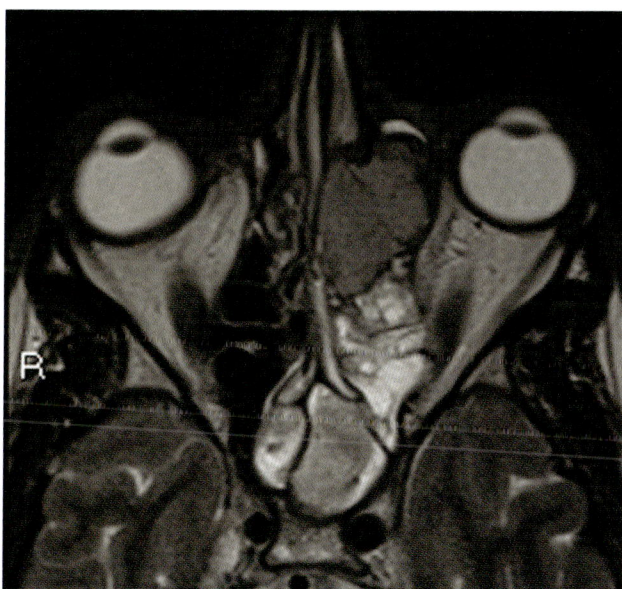

Figure 117.12 Tumour vs. obstructed secretions. MRI sharply defines the extent of this tumour in the anterior ethmoid sinus contrasting with obstructed secretions in the posterior ethmoids and sphenoid.

SPECIFIC TYPES OF NEOPLASMS

Inverting papilloma

A unilateral mass commonly originating in the lateral nasal wall and involving middle meatus and maxillary sinus, although less commonly the site of origin will be the maxillary sinus itself, the anterior ethmoid sinus or, rarely, the sphenoid, frontal or posterior ethmoid sinuses. Though benign, these lesions commonly recur and are associated with squamous cell carcinoma. CT features include internal calcification, and bony erosion or bowing. Focal hyperostosis (**Figure 117.13c**) is a finding which has been said to correlate with the site of origin of this neoplasm – a finding which has potential relevance in planning the extent of surgery needed to achieve extirpation.[35] On MRI a characteristic convoluted, cerebriform pattern (**Figure 117.13a** and **117.13b**) is said to be highly suggestive of this diagnosis, with the concomitant finding of necrosis suggesting a coexistent focus of carcinoma.[36]

Sinonasal carcinoma

These include the common squamous cell carcinoma and the less common adenocarcinoma. Neither have specific imaging characteristics and the purpose of imaging is to define tumour extent.

Adenoid cystic carcinoma is given particular attention because of its poor prognosis, in part because of its propensity for perineural spread. However, this mode of tumour extension will be more frequently encountered in squamous cell cancer simply because the latter is much more common. Thus imaging of all forms of carcinoma must include post-contrast MR sequences with particular care given to examining the cranial nerves (**Figure 117.14**), pterygopalatine fossa, skull base foraminae and the intracranial compartment.

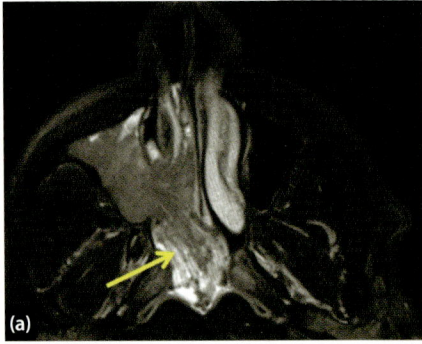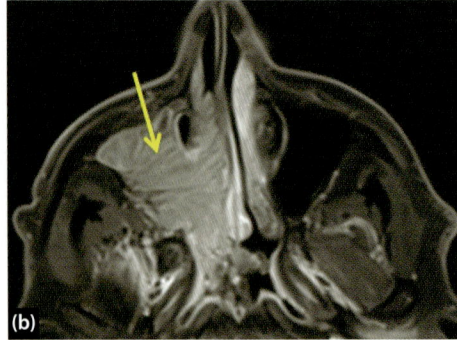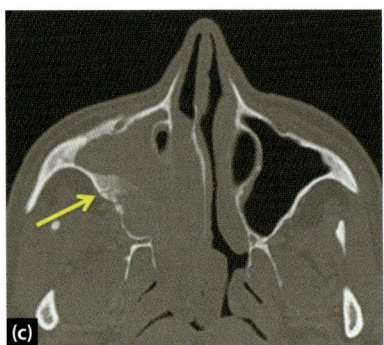

Figure 117.13 Inverted papilloma. Note the striations ('cerebriform' pattern) visible on T2 FS **(a)** and post-contrast **(b)** MRI and the focus of hyperostosis in the lateral wall of the maxillary sinus on CT **(c)** suggesting the site of origin of this growth.

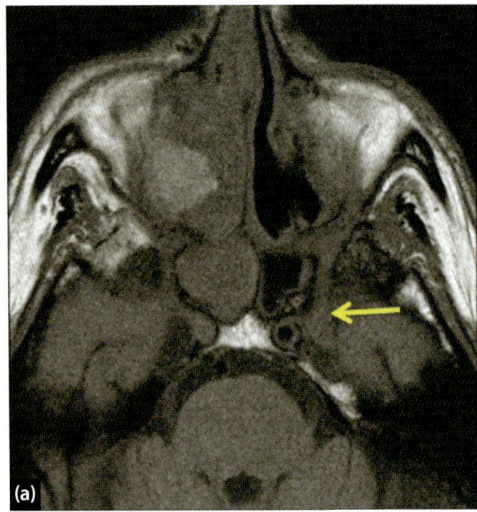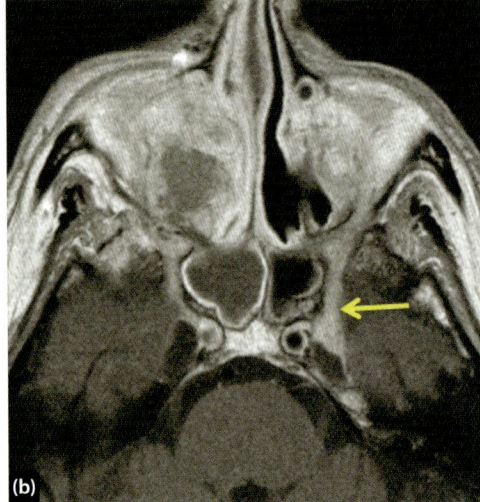

Figure 117.14 Perineural tumour spread (recurrent SCC). Note enhancement of left maxillary nerve (also right). **(a)** Pre-contrast; **(b)** post-contrast.

Sinonasal melanoma

Sinonasal melanoma is infrequent and whilst these lesions may demonstrate high signal on T1-weighted images, presumably because of the paramagnetic effect of melanin[37] or haemorrhage,[38] a number may be amelanotic in which case the imaging features are non-specific.

Bone and cartilage tumours

In contrast to the non-specific imaging features of sinonasal disease in general, imaging (in particular, CT) of lesions arising from bone or cartilage plays a central diagnostic role in concert with pathology.

Benign lesions include osteoma, which can appear as dense cortical bone or ground-glass,[39] and fibro-osseous lesions (fibrous dysplasia or ossifying fibroma). Fibro-osseous lesions are readily recognizable on CT although biopsy may still be required to refine the diagnosis. In contrast, the MRI appearance of fibrous dysplasia can be misleading and may be a trap for the unwary (**Figure 117.15**).

Of the malignant lesions primarily arising from bone, chondrosarcoma is perhaps the most common in the paranasal sinus region and can be suggested on CT by matrix calcification (**Figure 117.16a**) and on MRI by high signal on T2-weighted image (as a result of a high matrix water content) and by curvilinear septal enhancement on post-contrast images (**Figure 117.16b** and **117.16c**).[40, 41]

Vascular lesions

These include haemangioma, haemangiopericytoma, angiomatous polyp and the juvenile nasal angiofibroma (JNA). The clues to the vascular nature of a nasal mass include the finding of flow voids and avid enhancement with contrast (**Figure 117.17**). The location of the lesion is an important feature of the JNA, which characteristically expands the pterygopalatine fossa.

Lymphoma

T cell lymphomas characteristically affect the nasal septum (see above) whilst B cell lymphomas typically arise in the maxillary sinus with an epicenter close to the lateral sinus wall and tumour on either side of the sinus wall.[39]

Neuroendocrine tumours

This is a group of tumours including olfactory neuroblastoma (**Figure 117.2**) and sinonasal undifferentiated carcinoma (SNUC) which tend to arise in the superior nasal fossa but which otherwise frequently have non-specific imaging features.

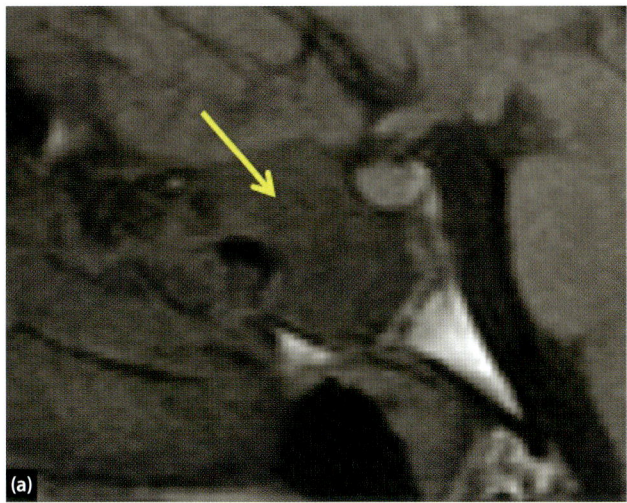
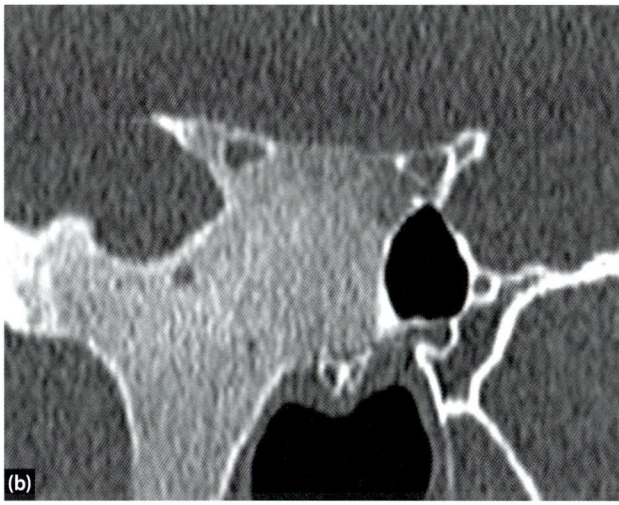

Figure 117.15 **Fibrous dysplasia.** (a) On MRI it is very easy to confuse fibrous dysplasia (in this case involving sphenoid) with tumour. (b) On CT the diagnosis is straightforward.

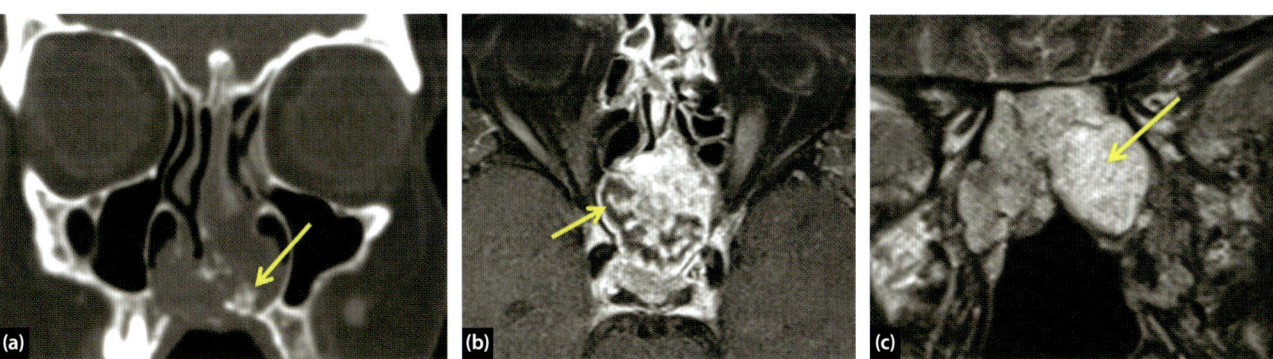

Figure 117.16 **Chondrosarcoma.** (a) Note calcified matrix of a chondrosarcoma of the nasal septum. (b) Internal septal enhancement on post-contrast MRI. (c) High signal on T2-weighted image resulting from high water content of chondroid matrix.

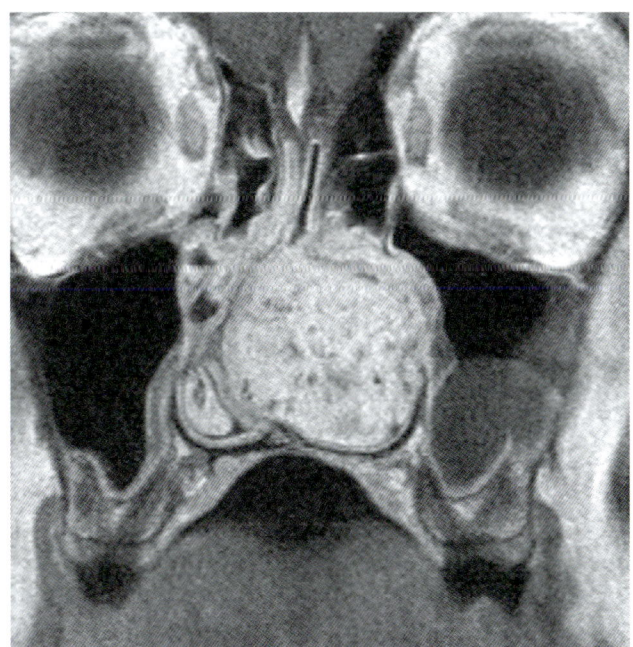

Figure 117.17 **Juvenile angiofibroma.** Note flow voids ('black dots' and curved black lines) within this brightly enhancing tumour indicating that this is a highly vascularized lesion.

Predicting dural invasion

Skull base invasion by (with or without intra-cranial extension of) a sinonasal malignancy has important implications in assessing the feasibility and extent of surgical resection and in deciding between an endoscopic or open approach to the tumour. Whilst CT is important to assess the integrity of the bony skull base owing to the contrast between bone and soft tissue, MRI becomes essential for assessing tumour relationship to dura and brain parenchyma.

Whilst a tumour with clear evidence of intra-cranial extension associated with brain oedema on MRI is generally considered to imply that the tumour has breached the leptomeninges to involve the brain parenchyma (**Figure 117.18**),[42] the use of MRI in predicting earlier degrees of dural invasion has also been studied. Pial enhancement, nodular dural enhancement and dural thickening of more than 5 mm have been found to be predictive of dural invasion. A linear pattern of enhancing dura was more commonly associated with, or interpreted as, reactive inflammation adjacent to tumour.[42] Further, where linear dural enhancement is separated from tumour by a thin hypointense zone this suggests reactive inflammation. In contrast, areas where tumour cannot be

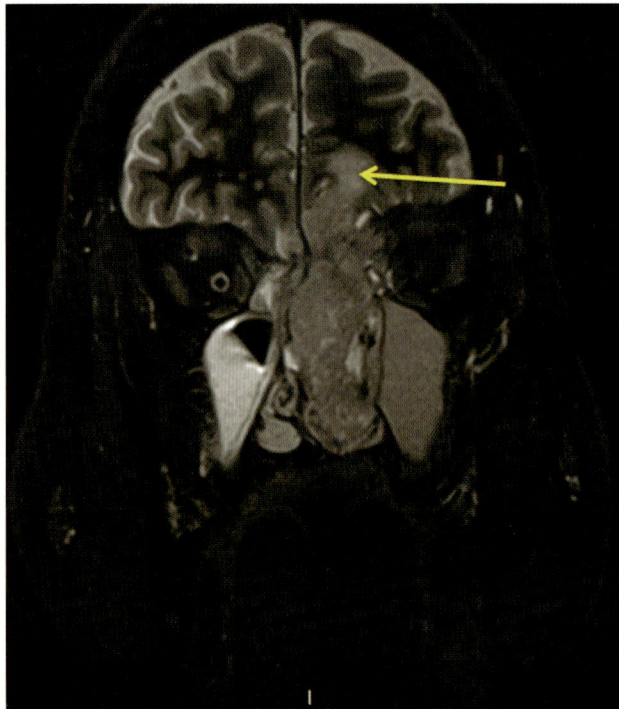

Figure 117.18 Brain parenchymal invasion. Vasogenic oedema in the left frontal lobe implies that this tumour (an olfactory neuroblastoma) has transgressed the dura and is now invading brain.

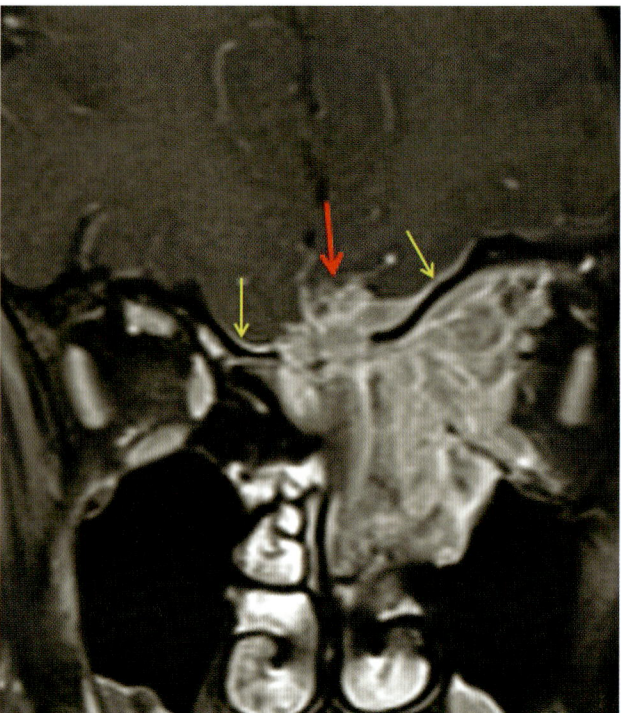

Figure 117.19 Alveolar rhabdomyosarcoma. Note the thin linear dural enhancement (yellow arrows) representing reactive inflammation interrupted by nodular tumour tissue, indistinguishable from enhancing dura. This corresponds to the nodular enhancement described by Eisen[42] or the focal interruption of linear dural enhancement by tumour as described by Ahmadi[43, 44] and is a marker for dural invasion.

visually separated from enhancing dura, or where there is a focal interruption of linear dural enhancement by tumour (**Figure 117.19**), suggest dural invasion.[43, 44]

CSF leaks

CSF rhinorrhoea is most commonly post-traumatic in origin (frequently post-surgical), less commonly non-traumatic (tumours, infection or congenital lesions), and occasionally spontaneous. In most cases, non-contrast CT of the skull base is the only imaging investigation required to identify a skull base defect (**Figure 117.20**).[45]

MRI should be performed in cases where a skull base defect found on CT is associated with opacification in the nasal cavity or sinus below the defect, to exclude an encephalocele or meningoencephalocele (**Figure 117.21**).

More advanced techniques include non-contrast MR cisternography (heavily T2-weighted with fat suppression), which relies on the detection of a continuous, bright CSF column from the subarachnoid space to the nasal cavity or sinus below[46] or, in cases where there remains a diagnostic dilemma, then more invasive cisternography (radionuclide or CT) may be considered.

MR cisternography using intrathecal Gadolinium has been used to detect CSF leaks with reported success,[47] however, its widespread acceptance has been delayed (partly due to a lack of FDA approval) and some have sounded caution regarding the lack of data confirming an absence of neurotoxicity over the long-term.[48]

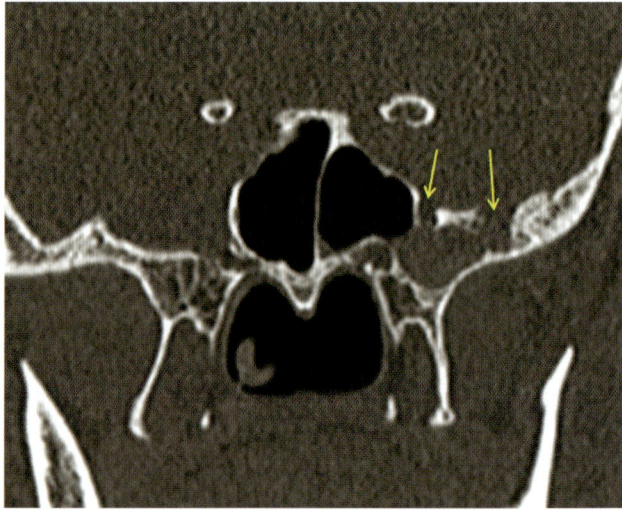

Figure 117.20 Arachnoid granulations. Spontaneous CSF fistula. Arachnoid granulations (yellow arrows) eroding roof of sphenoid sinus with fluid noted in the sinus below. Note extent of lateral pneumatization of the sinus. Non-contrast CT is frequently the only investigation needed to identify the site of a CSF leak.

An alternative to cisternography is the use of intrathecal fluorescein injection coupled with the endoscopic detection of fluorescein-stained CSF leaking through a skull base defect (**Figure 117.22**).

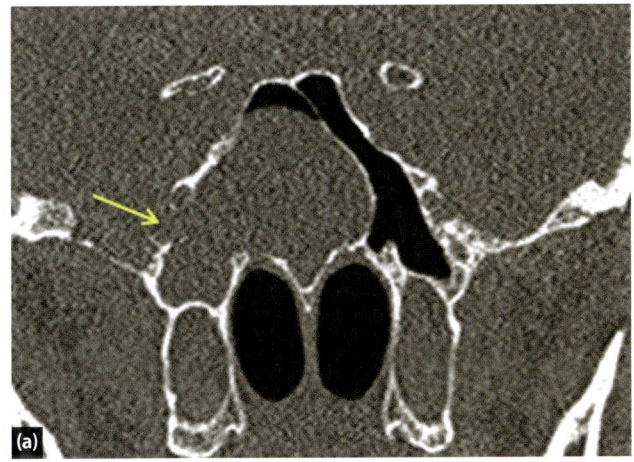
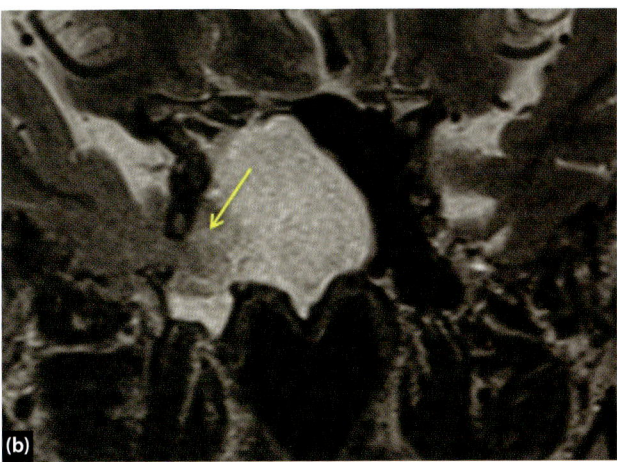

Figure 117.21 Encephalocele. (a) Note the defect in the lateral wall of sphenoid and the contiguous opacification within the sinus on this non-contrast CT. MRI is mandatory subsequent to this. (b) Note herniating brain tissue through the defect. The converse situation, the finding of a sinus 'polyp' or fluid adjacent to the skull base on MRI, may require a subsequent CT to more clearly depict the bony defect.

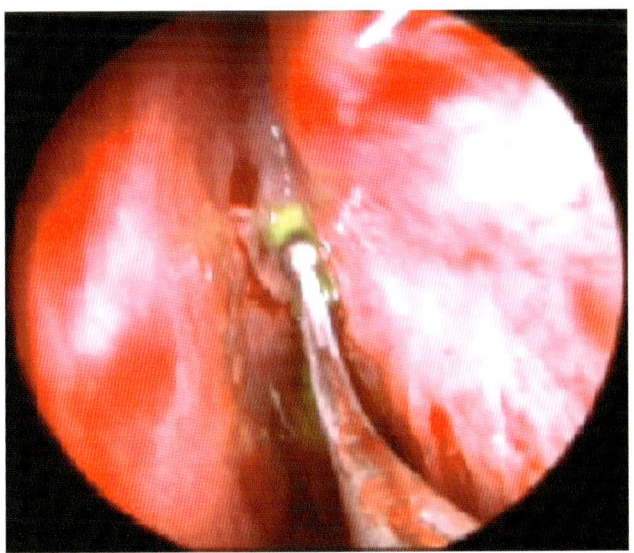

Figure 117.22 Endoscopic detection of CSF leak following intrathecal injection of fluoroscein. Note skull base defect with fluoroscein leakage adjacent to tip of probe. (Courtesy of Gerry McGarry).

IMAGING – NEW DEVELOPMENTS

The roles of PET-CT and DWI (diffusion-weighted imaging) are as yet not clearly defined but are beginning to emerge.

PET-CT

As sinonasal malignancies are rare, and are heterogeneous in terms of pathology, the role of PET-CT has been slow to emerge. Where PET-CT has been used in the staging or re-staging of sinonasal malignancy it has been seen to have a role in altering treatment course, particularly in the detection/exclusion of distant metastases (where consistently high negative predictive values have been demonstrated).[49, 50] However, caution should be exercised regarding the number of false positive studies (24%),[50] which may lead to unnecessary interventions (biopsies), and with regard to the occasional false negative study (for example, in intra-cranial disease where the normal metabolic activity of the brain may obscure disease).

It is unlikely that PET-CT will obviate the need for conventional imaging (in particular, MRI – although PET-MRI has been shown to be feasible), it is being more frequently used as an important adjunct – especially in the settings of advanced disease (where the finding of distant metastases may avoid major, potentially mutilating surgery) and in recurrent disease (where the effects of treatment, residual masses and recurrent disease are difficult to differentiate on conventional imaging).

In the setting of sinonasal papillomas PET-CT has been explored for its potential in identifying co-existent malignancies but with disappointing results.[51]

PET-MRI

This development has so far only been explored in terms of its feasibility but has the potential to improve soft-tissue contrast and reduce radiation exposure compared with PET-CT. Whole body imaging is feasible using this technique although the technique is not widely available and its role remains uncertain.[52]

Diffusion-weighted imaging (DWI)

Essentially, this is an extension of MRI predicated on the degree to which free water molecules diffuse in tissues. In general, the more cellular the tissue the less extracellular space available for water to diffuse. The degree to which diffusion occurs in tissues can then be expressed in terms of the apparent diffusion coefficient (ADC). The more cellular the tissue the lower the ADC and therefore it might be hoped that measuring the ADC of a tumour might help distinguish benign tumours from, usually more cellular, malignancies. Unfortunately, the picture is complicated by factors such as tumour necrosis and the presence of keratin, collagen or debris. A considerable overlap in ADC values has been observed between benign sinonasal tumours and malignancies[53] although other observers report improved differentiation between inflammation, benign lesions and malignancy through the use of ADC mapping (a visual map of ADC values assigned to individual pixels rather than an overall ADC)[54] particularly if interpreted alongside the analysis of time-signal intensity curves generated from dynamic contrast-enhanced MRI (DCE MRI).[55]

Cone beam CT

A low-cost, compact technology used widely in dental practice, as yet the image quality (particularly soft-tissue contrast) does not compare with conventional CT. However, the potential for significant radiation dose-reduction exists and its role in sinonasal imaging could include intra-operative imaging (for example, assessing adequacy of resection).[56]

CONCLUSION

Modern cross-sectional imaging plays a central role in the diagnosis and assessment of sinonasal disease. Whilst MRI and CT are the key imaging modalities it is likely that the use of PET-CT will continue to expand as its role becomes clearer, particularly in the setting of sinonasal malignancy.

This is a complex area, both in terms of the anatomy of the sinonasal region and anterior skull base and in terms of the heterogenous pathologies presenting here. Increasingly therefore, there is a need for increased subspecialization by dedicated head and neck radiologists working closely with head and neck surgeons in the best interests of this patient group.

BEST CLINICAL PRACTICE

- ✓ Radiologists should work closely with clinicians and pathologists in an MDT setting.
- ✓ Radiologists should aim to subspecialize in this challenging area.
- ✓ Audit results.

FUTURE RESEARCH

- ➤ New techniques are being developed in CT to reduce radiation dose whilst maintaining high-quality images.
- ➤ Anticipated developments in cone beam CT are expected to include improved image quality and potentially intra-operative use.
- ➤ The role of Diffusion-weighted MRI is expected to be refined.
- ➤ Advancements in PET MRI are expected.

KEY POINTS

- There is virtually no role for plain radiography in the investigation of sinus disease.
- Radiation to the eyes is a particular concern with CT.
- CT and MRI differ in the contrast demonstrated between different tissues. Thus these two modalities are often complimentary.
- Sinus anatomy is subject to extreme variability between individuals.
- Mucosal thickening, fluid-filled sinuses and retention cysts are common incidental findings.
- In inflammatory disease, imaging is useful to exclude sinusitis as a cause of symptoms, to provide an anatomical roadmap to the surgeon, and to provide diagnostic information.
- In neoplastic disease, the purpose of imaging is to alert the surgeon when not to perform a biopsy and to delineate the extent of the tumour in relation to secretions and inflammation, and spread outwith the sinonasal compartment.
- The role of PET CT is an evolving one but it is of particular use in staging cancer patients with advanced disease and in detecting recurrence.

REFERENCES

1. McAlister WH, Lusk R, Muntz HR. Comparison of plain radiographs and coronal CT scans in infants and children with recurrent sinusitis. *Am J Roentgenol* 1989; **153**: 1259–64.
2. Brem MH, Zamani AA, Riva R, et al. Multidetector CT of the paranasal sinus: potential for radiation dose reduction. *Radiology* 2007; **243**: 847–52.
3. Som PM, Dillon WP, Fullerton GD, et al. Chronically obstructed sinonasal secretions: observations on T1 and T2 shortening. *Radiology* 1989; **172**: 515–20.
4. Dillon WP, Som PM, Fullerton GD. Hypointense MR signal in chronically inspissated sinonasal secretions. *Radiology* 1990; **174**: 73–8.
5. Ruder TD, Kraehenbuehl M, Gotsmy WF, et al. Radiologic identification of disaster victims: a simple and reliable method using CT of the paranasal sinuses. *Eur J Radiol* 2012; **81**: e132–8.
6. Wormald P-J. *Endoscopic Sinus Surgery: Anatomy, Three-dimensional reconstruction, and Surgical Technique*. 2nd ed. New York: Thieme 2008.

7. Jones NS. CT of the paranasal sinuses: a review of the correlation with clinical, surgical and histopathologic findings. *Clin Otolaryngol Allied Sci* 2002; **27**: 11–17.
8. Huang BY, Lloyd KM, DelGaudio JM, et al. Failed endoscopic sinus surgery: spectrum of CT findings in the frontal recess. *Radiographics* 2009; **29**: 177–95.
9. Kuhn FA. Chronic frontal sinusitis: the endoscopic frontal recess approach. *Op Tech Otolaryngol Head Neck Surg* 1996; **7**: 222–9.
10. Owen RG, Kuhn FA. Supraorbital ethmoid cell. *Otolaryngol Head Neck Surg* 1997; **116**: 254–61.
11. Cooke LD, Hadley DM. MRI of the paranasal sinuses: incidental abnormalities and their relationship to symptoms. *J Laryngol Otol* 1991; **105**: 278–81.
12. McNeill E, O'Hara J, Carrie S. The significance of MRI findings for non-rhinological disease. *Clin Otolaryngol* 2006; **31**: 292–6.
13. Pazera P, Bornstein MM, Pazera A, et al. Incidental maxillary sinus findings in orthodontic patients: a radiographic analysis using cone-beam computed tomography. *Orthod Craniofac Res* 2011; **14**: 17–24.
14. Rak KM, Newell JD, Yakes WF, et al. Paranasal sinuses on MR images of the brain: significance of mucosal thickening. *Am J Roentgenol* 1991; **156**: 381–4.
15. Ashraf N, Bhattacharyya N. Determination of the 'incidental' Lund score for the staging of chronic rhinosinusitis. *Otolaryngol Head Neck Surg* 2001; **125**: 483–6.
16. Wang JH, Jang YJ, Lee BJ. Natural course of retention cysts of the maxillary sinus: long-term follow-up results. *Laryngoscope* 2007; **117**: 341–4.
17. West B, Jones NS. Endoscopy-negative, computed tomography-negative facial pain in a nasal clinic. *Laryngoscope* 2001; **111**: 581–6.
18. Lund VJ, Mackay IS. Staging in rhinosinusitis. *Rhinology* 1993; **31**: 183–4.
19. Aribandi M, McCoy VA, Bazan C. Imaging features of invasive and non-invasive fungal sinusitis: a review. *Radiographics* 2007; **27**: 1283–96.
20. Silverman CS, Mancuso AA. Periantral soft-tissue infiltration and its relevance to the early detection of invasive fungal sinusitis: CT and MR findings. *Am J Neuroradiol* 1998; **19**: 321–5.
21. Groppo ER, El-Sayed IH, Aiken AH, et al. Computed tomography and magnetic resonance imaging characteristics of acute invasive fungal sinusitis. *Arch Otolaryngol Head Neck Surg* 2011; **137**: 1005–10.
22. DelGaudio JM, Swain RE, Kingdom TT, et al. Computed tomographic findings in patients with invasive fungal sinusitis. *Arch Otolaryngol Head Neck Surg* 2003; **129**: 236–40.
23. Safder S, Carpenter JS, Roberts TD, et al. The 'black turbinate' sign: an early MR imaging finding of nasal mucormycosis. *Am J Neuroradiol* 2010; **77**: 1–4.
24. Reddy CEE, Gupta AK, Singh P, et al. Imaging of granulomatous and chronic invasive fungal sinusitis: comparison with allergic fungal sinusitis. *Otolaryngol Head Neck Surg* 2010; **143**: 294–300.
25. Mukherji SK, Figureueroa RE, Ginsberg LE, et al. Allergic fungal sinusitis: CT findings. *Radiology* 1998; **207**: 417–22.
26. Zinreich SJ, Kennedy DW, Malat J, et al. Fungal sinusitis: diagnosis with CT and MR imaging. *Radiology* 1988; **169**: 439–44.
27. Seo YJ, Kim J, Kim K, et al. Radiologic characteristics of sinonasal fungus ball: an analysis of 119 cases. *Acta Radiol* 2011; **52**: 790–5.
28. Grindler D, Cannady S, Batra PS. Computed tomography findings in sinonasal Wegener's granulomatosis. *Am J Rhinol Allergy* 2009; **23**: 497–501.
29. Muhle C, Reinhold-Keller E, Richter C, et al. MRI of the nasal cavity, the paranasal sinuses and orbits in Wegener's granulomatosis. *Eur Radiol* 1997; **7**: 566–70.
30. Trimarchi M, Gregorini G, Facchetti F, et al. Cocaine-induced midline destructive lesions. *Autoimmun Rev* 2013; **12**: 496–500.
31. Braun JJ, Imperiale A, Riehm S, et al. Imaging in sinonasal sarcoidosis: CT, MRI, ^{67}Gallium scintigraphy and ^{18}F-FDG PET/CT features. *J Neuroradiol* 2010; **37**: 172–81
32. King AD, Lei KI, Ahuja AT, et al. MR imaging of nasal T-cell/natural killer cell lymphoma. *Am J Roentgenol* 2000; **174**: 209–11.
33. Ou CH, Chen CC, Ling JC, et al. Nasal NK/T cell lymphoma: computed tomography and magnetic resonance imaging findings. *J Chin Med Assoc* 2007; **70**: 207–12.
34. Saket RR, Hetts SW, Tatum JK, et al. CT and MRI findings of sphenoid sinus internal carotid artery pseudoaneurysm: an important and challenging differential diagnosis for a skull base mass. *Clin Radiol* 2012; **67**: 815–20.
35. Lee DK, Chung SK, Dhong HJ, et al. Focal hyperostosis on CT of sinonasal inverted papilloma as a predictor of tumor origin. *Am J Neuroradiol* 2007; **28**: 618–21.
36. Ojiri H, Ujita M, Tada S, et al. Potentially distinctive features of sinonasal inverted papilloma on MR imaging. *Am J Roentgenol* 2000; **175**: 465–8.
37. Yousem DM, Li C, Montone KT, et al. Primary malignant melanoma of the sinonasal cavity: MR imaging evaluation. *Radiographics* 1996; **16**: 1101–10.
38. Kim SS, Han MH, Kim JF, et al. Malignant melanoma of the sinonasal cavity: explanation of magnetic resonance signal intensities with histopathologic characteristics. *Am J Otolaryngol* 2000; **21**: 366–78.
39. Eggesbo HB. Imaging of sinonasal tumours. *Cancer Imaging* 2012; **12**: 136–52.
40. Chen CC, Hsu L, Hecht JL, et al. Bimaxillary chondrosarcoma: clinical, radiologic, and histologic correlation. *Am J Neuroradiol* 2002; **23**: 667–70.
41. Geirnaerdt MJ, Bloem JL, Eulderink F, et al. Cartilaginous tumors: correlation of gadolinium-enhanced MR imaging and histopathologic findings. *Radiology* 1993; **186**: 813–17.
42. Eisen MD, Yousem DM, Montone KT, et al. Use of preoperative MR to predict dural, perineural, and venous sinus invasion of skull base tumours. *Am J Neuroradiol* 1996; **17**: 1937–45.
43. Ahmadi J, Hinton DR, Segall HD, et al. Dural invasion by craniofacial and calvarial neoplasms: MR imaging and histopathologic evaluation. *Radiology* 1993; **188**: 747–9.
44. Ahmadi J, Hinton DR, Segall HD, et al. Surgical implications of magnetic resonance-enhanced dura. *Neurosurgery* 1994; **35**: 370–7.
45. Lloyd KM, Del Gaudio JM, Hudgins PA. Imaging of skull base cerebrospinal fluid leaks in adults. *Radiology* 2008; **248**: 725–36.
46. El Gammal T, Sobol W, Wadlington VR, et al. Cerebrospinal fluid fistula: detection with MR cisternography. *Am J Neuroradiol* 1998; **19**: 627–31.
47. Algin O, Turkbey B. Intrathecal gadolinium-enhanced MR cisternography: a comprehensive review. *Am J Neuroradiol* 2013; **34**: 14–22.
48. Dillon WP. Intrathecal Gadolinium: its time has come? *AM J Neuroradiol* 2008; **29**: 1–4.
49. Wild D, Eyrich GK, Ciernik IF, et al. In-line (18)F- flurodeoxyglucose positron emission tomography with computed tomography (PET/CT) in patients with carcinoma of the sinus/nasal area and orbit. *J Craniomaxillofac Surg* 2006; **34**(1): 9–16.
50. Lamarre ED, Batra PS, Lorenz RR, et al. Role of positron emission tomography in management of sinonasal neoplasms- a single institution's experience. *Am J Otolaryngol* 2012; **33**(3): 289–95.
51. Jeon TY, Kim HJ, Choi JY, et al. 18 F-FDG PET/CT findings of sinonasal inverted papilloma with or without coexistent malignancy: comparison with MR imaging findings in eight patients. *Neuroradiology* 2009; **51**(4): 265–71.
52. Platzek I, Beuthien-Baumann B, Schneider M, et al. PET/MRI in head and neck cancer: initial experience. *Eur J Nucl Med Mol Imaging* 2013; **40**(1): 6–11.
53. White ML, Zhang Y and Robinson RA. Evaluating tumors and tumor-like lesions of the nasal cavity, the paranasal sinuses, and the adjacent skull base with diffusion-weighted MRI. *J Comput Assist Tomogr* 2006; **30**(3): 490–5.
54. Sasaki M, Eida S, Sumi M, et al. Apparent diffusion coefficient mapping for sinonasal diseases: differentiation of benign and malignant lesions. *Am J Neuroradiol* 2011; **32**(6): 1100–6.
55. Sasaki M, Sumi M, Eida S, et al. Multiparametric MR imaging of sinonasal diseases: time-signal intensity curve- and apparent diffusion coefficient-based differentiation between benign and malignant lesions. *Am J Neuroradiol* 2011; **32**(11): 2154–9.
56. Huang BJ, Senior BA and Castillo M. Current trends in sinonasal imaging. *Neuroimag Clin N Am* 2015; **25**(4): 507–25.

INDEX

Note: Page references in *italic* refer to tables or boxes in the text; those underscored refer to figures

A v. Botrill 423
Abciximab 114, 271–2
abducens nerve 617, 910, 911
ABO group 240, *240*
Abortion Act (1991) 405
abscesses
   cerebral 1120–2
   orbital *1028*, 1115, 1117, *1117*
   retropharyngeal 313
   septal 1188
abstracts, critical appraisal 505
ABT-263 (navatoclax) 64
Access to Health Records Act (1990) 417
accessory nerve, injury 447
accidental ingestion 365
acetazolamide 279
acetic acid 276
aciclovir 202, 280
acoustic rhinometry 991, 994, 1135
   artefacts 994
   inferior turbinate enlargement 1161
   methods 994
   normal values 994
acromegaly 630, 908
   adjuvant treatments 952–4
   aetiology 908
   clinical features 908, *909*, 909, 932–3, *933*
   diagnosis 916, *916*, 933
   incidence 908
   management 933
acropachy 723
Actinomyces spp. 192
actinomycin D 43
activated partial thromboplastin time (APTT) 260, *264*, 266
acute invasive fungal rhinosinusitis (AIFR) 209–11
acute myeloid leukaemia (AML) 251
acute otitis media (AOM), systemic antibiotics 277, *278*
acute respiratory distress syndrome (ARDS), management 353–4, *355*
acute rhinosinusitis (ARS) 1027–8
   bacterial 1026, *1026*, 1027–8
   diagnosis 1071–2
   differentiating bacterial from viral 1060
   epidemiology 1026
   frontal sinus 1087–8, *1088*
   indications for surgery 1072
   invasive fungal (AIFR) 209–11
   prevention 1060–1
   treatment
      antibiotics 285–6, 1059, 1060
      antihistamines 287
      complicated ARS 1060
      corticosteroids 283–4, 1060
      decongestants 266
      prevention of complications 1060
      symptomatic improvement 1060
   vaccination 289
   viral 1025–6, 1027
ADAMTS13 268
adaptive immunity 125–6
Addison's disease 638, 1234
adeno-associated virus (AAV), gene vectors 30, *30*, 33
adenocarcinoma, olfactory cleft 1291
adenohypophysis, *see* pituitary gland, anterior
adenoidectomy
   anaesthetic techniques 344–5
   childhood rhinosinusitis 1078
   medical negligence claims 445
adenomas, *see* parathyroid adenoma; pituitary adenomas
adenovirus 197, *197*
   gene therapy vectors 30, *30*, 32–3
adhesion proteins, gene mutations 16–17
adipose stem cells 122
adjustment 475
adrenal insufficiency, hypercalcaemia 831
adrenalectomy, bilateral 935, 954
adrenaline 296, 354
adrenocorticotropic hormone (ACTH) 637–8, 637, 933–4
   deficiency 906, *906*, 928, 929
   excess 638, 908–10, 910, 916–17, 934–5
   inferior petrosal sinus sampling 917, 935
   isolated deficiency 926
   laboratory test 917, *918*
   reserve 919
adverse events
   communication of 384–5
   incidence of 391
aerodynamics, nose 986
aesthesioneuroblastoma 1269, *1272*, 1277
   endonasal endoscopic resection 1289, 1301, 1301
   imaging 1306
afibrinogenaemia *264*, 267
African-Americans, sarcoidosis 1211
AFRS, *see* allergic fungal rhinosinusitis
age/ageing
   and growth hormone levels 633, 634
   and nasal airflow resistance 993
   and skin flap survival 113
   and skin properties 112, *112*
   and smell function 1237–8, 1238
   and wound healing 98
agger nasi 973, 974, 1081, 1082, 1307
   posterior wall and roof removal 1074–5, 1075
aggressive psammomatoid ossifying fibroma 1102–3
agnosia, olfactory 1230–1, 1235
agranulocytosis, propylthiouracil therapy 726
agricultural workers, occupational rhinitis *1019*, 1020

AIDS 230
Aintree catheter 318, 318
air pollutants
   causing smell dysfunction *1233*
   and rhinitis 1013–14, 1021
air-helium mixture 296
airway
   evaluation 310–13, *313*
   gas flow 321, 321
   paediatric anatomy and physiology 361–2
   'shared' 336, 339, 344
   thyroid tumour involvement 806–8, 807–8, 822, 822
   recurrent disease 775, 775
airway compression, intra-thoracic goitre 820
airway devices 336–8, 339
airway management
   critical care 357–8
   laryngeal surgery 347
   laser surgery 339–40, 346
   maxillofacial injuries 1190
   thyroid surgery 890
airway obstruction 321–8
   acute 321, 321
   children 363–4
   chronic 321
   during surgery 337
   evaluation 321–2
   haematological malignancy 252, 254
   jet ventilation 327–8, 327
   low tracheal 326, 327
   management strategy 322
   medical negligence claims 446
   periglottic/glottic 324–5
   subglottic/midtracheal 326
   'supraglottic' 322–4
   tracheostomy under local anaesthesia 325–6
   see also nasal obstruction
airway pressure, measurement 343
airway remodelling, asthma and rhinitis 1127, 1128
airway resistance, nasal 983, 986
airway smooth muscle 1127, 1131
Akt 65–7, 66
ala nasi
   collapse/paralysis 978, 987
   contraction 987
   retraction 435
alar batten graft 1145, 1145
alar expansion sutures 1145
albumin, serum 98
alcohol use, and epistaxis 1174–5
alendronate, primary hyperparathyroidism 847, *848*
1-alfacalcidol 625, 627, *854*
alginate dressings 300

alginates 298
alipogene tiparvovec 29, 30
alkaline phosphatase 830
alkylating agents 299, _299_
allelic deletion 7–9
allergen-specific immunotherapy 143, 147, 215, 1006–7
allergens 137
    avoidance 147, 1003, _1004_
    components and clinical relevance 145, _146_
    inhaled 137, _138_
allergic fungal rhinosinusitis (AFRS) 212–15, 1040, 1048
    adjunctive treatment 1054–5, _1055_
    anti-immunoglobulin E therapy 1055
    classification 1040, _1040_
    clinical presentation 1049
    diagnostic criteria 1049, _1049_
    epidemiology 1048
    imaging 1309–10
    investigation 1049–51
    medical management 215, 1052–5
    nasal polyps 1040
    pathophysiology 1048–9
    post-surgical endoscopic staging 1052, _1052_
    surgical management 214–15, 1051–2
allergic march 1126–7
allergic mucin 1049, 1051, _1051_
allergic reactions, blood transfusion 246
allergic rhinitis 133, 147, 999–1008
    allergen reduction/avoidance 1003, _1004_
    and asthma 142, _143_, 1007, 1125–31
        asthma risk 1126–7
        causative mechanisms 1126
        epidemiology 1007, 1125–6
        management issues 1128–30
        possible mechanisms association 1128
    best clinical practice 1008
    and breastfeeding 1002
    bronchial hyperresponsiveness 1126
    children 1000, 1007–8
    classification 999, _1000_
    diagnosis 1000, 1002
    differentiation from non-allergic disease 1014
    examination 1001–2
    future research 1008
    healthcare costs 1130
    immunotherapy (desensitization) 1006–7
    inferior turbinate enlargement 1159, _1159_
    intermittent _1000_
    local allergic 141–2
    management algorithm _1005_
    nasal polyps 1039
    natural history 1001
    persistent _1000_
    pharmacological treatment 1004–7
    in pregnancy 988, 1008
    presentation 1001
    prevalence 999, 1000–1, _1000_
    quality of life 1130
    role of sensory nerves 141
    smell impairment 1235
    surgery 1007

Allergic Rhinitis and its Impact on Asthma (ARIA) _1005_, 1126, 1131
allergy 133–4
    clinical features of immediate 141, _142_
    current knowledge deficiencies 147
    defined 137
    diagnostic tests 143–6, _147_, 151–2
    effector cells 138–41
    environmental factors 138
    future research 147
    genetics 137–8
    high affinity receptor signalling 141
    mechanisms of tissue damage 133–4, _134_
    mechanisms of treatment 142–3
    and nasal polyps 1039
    'priming' 1007
allografts, demineralized bone matrix (DBM) 120
allopurinol 114
alpha agonists 354
1-alpha hydroxylase 624, 867
Alport syndrome 20
Alternaria spp. 1048
aluminium acetate 276
Alzheimer's disease 1230, 1231, 1237
American Association of Clinical Endocrinologists (AACE) 621–2
American Association of Endocrine Surgeons (AAES) 599
American College of Rheumatology
    criteria for Churg-Strauss syndrome _1219_
    criteria for granulomatosis with polyangiitis _1216_
American Society of Anesthesiologists (ASA)
    difficult airway algorithm _314_
    physical status grading 301, _302_
American Thyroid Association (ATA)
    anaplastic thyroid cancer 766
    retrosternal goitre guidelines 821
    risk of recurrence stratification 773, _774_
    thyroid cancer guidelines 600
    thyroid nodule evaluation 741, 743, _743_, 755
amikacin 223
aminoglycosides
    ototoxicity 20–1, 254
        genetics 20–1, 24
    resistance 225
    site and mode of action 223
amiodarone, inducing thyrotoxicosis 733
amisfostine 217
amitriptyline 1256
amoxicillin, prophylactic 295
amoxicillin/clavulanic acid 285
amphiphatic molecules 1064–5
amphotericin 209, 211, 217, 234, 254, 287
amphotericin B, intravenous 1055
amputations, wound healing 100
amygdalotomy, stereotactic 1238–9
amyloid P, serum 133
amyloid precursor protein (APP) 858
amyloid protein 681, _683_, 693, 758
An organisation with memory 390–1
anaemia
    of chronic disease 255
    haemolytic 255

    iron deficiency 255
    laboratory tests 255
    pernicious 154
    pre-operative management 247
anaerobic bacteria, antimicrobial resistance _225_
anaesthesia
    airway management devices 336–40, _339_
    in airway obstruction 325
    atlanto-axial instability 448
    deaths 319
    ear surgery 347–8, 349
    future research 348–9
    induction
        after securing airway 341
        inhalation 325, 341
        intravenous 340–1
        rapid sequence 341
    informed consent 304
    intra-thoracic goitre 822
    jet ventilation 327–8, _327_, 338
    laryngeal microsurgery 346
    laryngectomy 347
    laser surgery 346
    monitoring 341–3
    nasal fracture reduction 1186
    nasal and sinus surgery 347, 1072–3
    neuromuscular blockade 340, 341
        monitoring 343
    parathyroid surgery 345
    pre-operative visit 304
    premedication 334
    preoxygenation 340
    principles 333–4
    salivary gland surgery 345–6
    temperature management 343
    thyroid surgery 345
    tonsillectomy/adenoidectomy 344–5, 349
    total intravenous 335, 348, 1072, 1274
    triad 333, _334_
    tubeless 338
    variation in patient outcomes 349
anaesthetic agents
    future research 348–9
    inhalation (volatile) 335–6
    inspired/end-tidal sampling 342–3
    intravenous 334–5
anaesthetic reaction testing 152
anaesthetist, discussion with patient 304
anaesthetists' non-technical skills (ANTS) 454
analgesia
    acute post-operative planning 305
    multi-modal 305
    paediatric intensive care 363
    thyroidectomy 802
analgesia-dependency headaches 1259–60
analytical studies 473
anaphylaxis 141
    during surgery 152
    following blood transfusion 245
    latex allergy 1021
anaplastic thyroid cancer _678_, 680–82
    adjuvant therapies 766–8
    chemotherapy 766, 789
    external beam radiotherapy 766–8, 788–9

anaplastic thyroid cancer (*continued*)
   genetics 85–6
   histological variants *682*
   histopathology 680, <u>680–81</u>, 766
   investigations 644, 765
   metastatic disease 768
   presentation 765
   thyroidectomy 766
   ultrasound 644
Andrews v. DPP 422
angioedema
   drug treatment 296, 300
   hereditary 296
angiofibroma, juvenile, *see* juvenile angiofibroma
angiofollicular units 604
angiogenesis
   inhibitors 47–8, <u>47</u>
   stimulators of <u>47</u>
   wound healing 97
angiography, paragangliomas 575, <u>575</u>
angiosome 108, *109*
angiotensin-converting enzyme (ACE) inhibitors, intolerance 1013
angiotensin-converting enzyme (ACE) levels 1214
angular artery 965
angular vein 965
animal laboratory workers 1020–1
anisokaryosis 591
anisotropy 112
Annexin V assay 60–1
anosmia 1230
antenatal diagnosis, neurofibromatosis 2 22
anterior ethmoidal artery 965, 969, 1170
   anatomy 1074, *1075*, 1076, 1081–2, <u>1082</u>, 1171, 1294
   injury 1179, 1188
   ligation 1171, <u>1172</u>, 1178
anterior ethmoidal foramen 1243–4, <u>1244</u>
anterior olfactory nucleus 1230
anthracyclines, cytotoxicity 43
anti-diuretic hormone, *see* arginine vasopressin
anti-leukotrienes, *see* leukotriene receptor antagonists
anti-tuberculous therapy 192
anti-Xa inhibitor 246
antibiotic prophylaxis 295
   septal surgery 1153
antibiotics
   contraindications and precautions 278
   cytotoxic 43, 299, <u>299</u>
   in GPA 1217
   immunomodulatory 1062
   interactions 279
   orbital cellulitis 1118
   otoxicity 20–1, 254, 444–5
   perioperative 295, 300
      thyroid/parathyroid surgery 802, 887–8
   rhinosinusitis 285–6
      acute 1059, 1060
      chronic 1063–4
   systemic in otology 277–9, *278*
   see also antimicrobial resistance; antimicrobials
antibody responses, assessment 150

anticardiolipin antibodies 153, 270
anticholinergics, intra-nasal *1005*, 1006, 1014
anticoagulants 293
   direct (novel) oral (DOACs/NOACs) 246, 270, 271, 1179–80
   heparin 268, 293–4
      low molecular weight (LMWH) 270, 271, 294
      unfractionated 271
   parenteral 271
   warfarin 270–1, 294, <u>294</u>
anticoagulation
   best clinical practice 300
   epistaxis 1179–80
   management of surgical patient 270
   reversal 246, 270, 271
   role of vessel wall 262–3, <u>263</u>
antifibrinolytic drugs 247
antifungal agents 209, 287–8
   chronic rhinosinusitis 1064
   classes 209
   fungal rhinosinusitis 215, 287–8
      acute invasive 1055
      allergic 215, 287, 1053
   in HIV 234
   side effects 1053
   topical nasal 1054
antigen presenting cells (APC) 128, *129*, <u>134</u>, 139–40
antigen recognition 126–9
antigens, tumour cells 160
antihistamines
   in allergic diseases 142–3
   allergic rhinitis 1004–5, *1005*
   asthma 1129
   and nasal mucosa *985*, 986
   occupational rhinitis 1023
   rhinosinusitis 287
   topical intra-nasal 1004–5
   in vertigo 279
antimetabolites 42, <u>43</u>, 299, <u>299</u>
antimicrobial resistance 224
   acquired 225
   challenge of 221
   control of 226
   intrinsic 224, *225*
   mechanisms of 225–6
antimicrobials
   classification 222, *223*
   history of development 221, *222*
   principles of treatment 226–7
   susceptibility testing 222, 224, <u>224</u>
   see also antibiotics, *and* named agents
antineutrophil cytoplasmic antibodies (ANCA) 152, *153*
   Churg-Strauss syndrome 1218
   GPA 1215–16, *1223*
antinuclear antibodies (ANA) 153, *153*
antiphospholipid syndrome 153, 270
antiplatelet agents 271–2, 293
   pre-operative management 303
antisialogogue 323, 334
antithrombin 261
   deficiency 269, *269*, 270
antithyroid drugs 297, 600, 620, 724–7, *725*
   adjuncts 727
   'block and replace' regimen 726

   dosage 725
   efficacy 726
   Graves' disease 726
   monitoring treatment 711
   radioiodine pre-treatment 727–8
   side effects 725–6, *726*
   toxic nodular disease 726–7
antivirals 202–3, 280
   novel 203
antrochoanal polyp 1029, <u>1029</u>, 1310, <u>1311</u>
AP100 (AP50) haemolytic complement test 151
APACHE-II score 352
Apaf-1 63, <u>63</u>
aphthous ulcers, in HIV 233, *235*
Apixaban 271
apoptosis 41
   death receptor pathway 64–5
   definition 59
   in head and neck squamous cell carcinomas 65–7
   identification 60–1, <u>60</u>
   mechanisms of regulation 62–5
   mitochondrial pathway 62–4
   versus necrosis 61, *61*
appraisal, surgeon 375–6
aprepitant 348–9
arachnoid granulations <u>1314</u>
Arcanobacterium haemolyticum 188
arch bars 1192, <u>1192</u>
ARCON 54
ARDS, *see* acute respiratory distress syndrome
ARDSnet RCT 353
L-arginine test *918*
arginine vasopressin (vasopressin/ADH) 614, 637, <u>637</u>, 924
   excess 640, 912–13
   insufficiency 638–9, 906, *906*, 913
   regulation of release 638, <u>639</u>
   structure <u>638</u>
   testing 919–20
arterial stiffness, primary hyperparathyroidism 845
arterial ulcers 101
arteriography, parathyroid 838
Ashcroft v. Mersey Regional Health Authority 411
Ashe's forceps <u>1187</u>
Aspergillus spp. 205, 206–7
   fungal balls 216, 1048
   rhinosinusitis 209–16, *210*, 253–4, 1309
Aspergillus flavus 212, 1056
Aspergillus fumigatus 206, <u>206</u>, 1056
Aspergillus niger 206, <u>207</u>
   otitis externa 209, <u>209</u>
aspirin 272, 293
   pre-operative discontinuation 303
aspirin desensitization 288, 1063
aspirin sensitivity 288, 1013, 1026, 1029, 1039–40
   in asthma 1039, 1128
   chronic rhinosinusitis 1026, <u>1028</u>, 1039–40
   rhinitis 1013
aspirin-exacerbated respiratory disease (AERD) 1026, 1039–40
assault 410, 415, 423

Association of Anaesthetists of Great Britain and Ireland (AAGBI) 302, 303
asthma 140
    and allergic rhinitis 142, *143*, 1007, 1125–31
        common risk factors 1126
        epidemiology 1007, 1125–6
        respiratory inflammation 1127–8
        risk of asthma 1126–7
    cell mechanisms 133
    Churg-Strauss syndrome 1218
    and nasal polyps 1013, 1039, 1127–8
    occupation 1017, 1021
    quality of life and costs 1130
astringents 276
atlanto-axial instability 448
atlanto-occipital movement 312–13
atopic eczema 1126–7
'atopic march' 1001, 1126–7
atopy 133, 134, 137
atrial fibrillation, hyperthyroidism 719, 729, 731
atrophic rhinitis 289, 1014
attenuated familial adenomatous polyposis (AFAP) 89
auditory brainstem responses 528–9
auditory function monitoring 527–9
augmented reality surgery 559–60
auricular cartilage graft 1153
Australia, medical negligence claims 415
autoantibodies 133
    detection 152–4
    liver disease 154
autoimmunity, investigations 152–4
autoinflammatory disease 178
autonomic nervous system, nasal function 984–5, 986
autonomy 398
autophagy 62
autotransplantation (AT), parathyroid tissue 625, 626, 859, 867, 868
awake fibre-optic intubation (AFOI) 322–4, 326
axillary incision, robotic thyroidectomy 815, 815–16
azathioprine, GPA 1217
azelastine 287, 1004–5
    nasal spray 1014–15
azoles 287
    acute invasive fungal rhinosinusitis 211, 1055
    allergic fungal rhinosinusitis 215, 1053, 1054
    oropharyngeal candidiasis 217
    otomycosis 209
    side effects 1053
    topical nasal 1054

B cell signature 161
B cells 125, 127
    activation 127
    CD20+ 161
B-cell lymphomas, thyroid 769, 770
B-RAF mutations 83, 675
    BRAFV600E 83, 85
    thyroid tumours 83, 85
Bacillus spp. 187
Bacillus subtilis enzymes 1018, 1020

bacteria
    anaerobic 191, *191*
    antimicrobial resistance, *see* antimicrobial resistance
    biofilms 185, *185*, 217, 1030, 1039
    culture and identification 181–3
    Gram negative 188–91, *225*
    Gram positive 184–8
    Gram staining 181, 182
bacterial enterotoxins 1126
bacterial lysate preparations 288
bacterial superantigens 1030, 1039, 1126
bacteriophages 203
bad news communication 384, *384*
Bak 62, *62*
bakery workers 1020
balloon sinuplasty 1078, 1090
balloon vessel occlusion 570, *570*, 571, 572
balloons, nasal packing 1176
Barnett v. Chelsea & Kensington Hospital 411
Barret's oesophagus, photodynamic therapy 585
barrier creams, nasal 1152
Basophil Activation Test (BAT) 145–6, 146
basophils 132, 138–9, *140*, 256
bath plug repair, skull base 945, 1278
battery 410, 415, 423
Bax 62–4, *62*, 63
Bcl-2 62, *62*, 63
Beahrs triangle 798, 799
beclomethasone dipropionate 284, 1008
bee allergy *146*
Behçet's disease 176–7
Bell's palsy 201, 232
Belmont Report 399
Bence Jones proteins 154
beneficence 399
benign paroxysmal positional vertigo 443
Bentham, Jeremy 400
benzalkonium chloride 275
benzocaine 295
Bernard Soulier disease 262, 269
Berry's ligament 799, 801, 801
Berwick, Don 393
Berwick report 393, *393*
'best interest' 399
beta agonists 354
beta-2-transferrin test 1206–7
beta-adrenergic blockers, in hyperthyroidism 727, 729
betahistine hydrochloride 279
betamethasone, ear preparations 276
Bethesda classification
    thyroid aspirates 655, *743*
bevacizumab 48, 55, *162*, 1180
bias
    assessment 506
    control of 478–9
    information 475
    minimizing 474–5
    selection 474–5
bilateral parathyroid exploration 865–70
    indications 865–8
    operation 868–70, 869–70
Billroth, Christian Albert Theodor 598, *598*, 793
BIM-23A760 955

Bio-oss 120
bioabsorbable transparent plate 1208, 1208
biofilms 185, *185*
    Candida 217
    chronic rhinosinusitis 1064
    examples in medicine *185*
    Manuka honey treatment 1054
    nasal cavity 1030, 1039
    surfactant treatments 1064–5
biological enzymes, occupational exposure 1018, 1020
biomarkers
    organ dysfunction 359
    parathyroid carcinoma 860–1
    tumour 161, 162–3
biomaterials 119–22
bioreactors 121–2
bioreductive drugs 54–5
biotinidase deficiency 20
bipolar electrocautery
    epistaxis 1176, 1176
    intra-nasal tumours 1294
Bipolaris spp. 1048
bisphosphonates
    parathyroid carcinoma 861
    primary hyperparathyroidism 847
bitemporal hemianopia 911, *911*, 918
bivalirudin 271
'black turbinate' sign 1309
blastomycosis 206
Blau syndrome 179
bleeding disorders 264–5
    blood products and factor replacement 272–3
    coagulation factor disorders 265–7
    information for haematologist 273
    in liver disease 269
    platelet disorders 267–9
    in renal disease 269
    thrombotic disorders 269–72
bleomycin 43
blepharoplasty 438
blinding 471, 478, 504, 513
blood clots, breakdown (fibrinolysis) 263, 263
blood components 243–4, 249–50
blood donation 239, 240, *240*
blood flow, skin vessels 110–11
blood grouping 241, 304
blood groups 240–1, *241*
blood pressure, intra-operative monitoring 342
blood products, in bleeding disorders 272–3
blood sugar, critically ill patient 356
blood tests, basic haematology 254–6
blood transfusion
    alternatives 246–7
    cryoprecipitate 244
    emergency 242–3, 242
    fresh frozen plasma (FFP) 244
    future research 247
    planning for surgery 241, *241*
    platelets 243–4
    red cells 243
    requirement for in ENT 239
    reversal of anticoagulation 246
    safety of 239, *239*
    serious hazards of transfusion (SHOT) 244, 245
    transfusion reactions 244–6

blood vessels, skin 110–11, 110, 111
blow-out fractures 1198
Blyth v. Bloomsbury Health Authority 415
bodily harm 423
body language 383–4
body mass index (BMI), and suitability for day surgery 301–2
Bolam test 410, 410–11, 429, 526, 900
Bolam v. Friern Hospital Management Committee 410–11
Bolitho v. City and Hackney Health Authority 411
bone
　bioengineering 122
　calcium homeostasis 624, 625
　repair 97–8
bone disease
　adynamic 830
　parathyroid carcinoma 858
bone graft materials 119
Brown-Wilkinson, Lord 411
bone marrow 250
bone marrow aspirate (BMA) 121
bone marrow failure syndromes 268
bone marrow suppression, radioiodine therapy 782
bone marrow transplant 256–7
bone metastases
　hypercalcaemia 829
　thyroid cancer 784, 809
bone mineral density (BMD), in primary hyperparathyroidism 844–5, 847, 848
bone morphogenetic protein 7, recombinant human (rhBMP-7) 122
bone morphogenetic proteins (BMPs) 97, 98, 121
Bordatella pertussis 189
Borelia burgdorferi 192
boric acid 209, 276
botulinum toxin 300
　contraindications 296–7
　intra-nasal 1015
　spasmodic dystonia 296–7
　type A in migraine 1256
bougie, gum-elastic 315, 315
Boveri, Theodore 6
bowel preparation 305
Bowman's glands 1229, 1229
brain abscess, complicating rhinosinusitis 1120–2
brain infarction, sinusitis 1120
branchial arch, first artery and juvenile angiofibroma 1266
branchial cyst, FDG PET-CT imaging 551
branchiootorenal syndrome 19
breast cancer 159, 161, 647
breastfeeding, and radioiodine therapy 753–4
Breathe Right® 1143–4, *1147*
Bristol Royal Infirmary Inquiry 391–2, 409
British Association of Day Surgery (BADS) 302
British Association of Endocrine Surgeons (BAES) 599
British Association of Endocrine and Thyroid Surgeons (BAETS) 376, 599, 600
　thyroid/parathyroid surgery audits 894–6, *895*

British Committee for Standards in Haematology (BCSH) 241, 246
British Medical Association (BMA) 397, 405
British Thyroid Association (BTA)
　thyroid cancer guidelines 782–3
　thyroid nodule evaluation 741, 743, *743*
bromhexine 287
bromocriptine 906, 932, 952
bronchial carcinoma, ACTH-secreting 935
bronchial challenge, rhinitis patients 1128
bronchial hyperresponsiveness, allergic rhinitis 1126
broncho-alveolar lavage, children 366
bronchoconstriction 1127
bronchoscopy
　assisted intubation 366
　low tracheal airway obstruction 326
　paediatric intensive care unit 366
broth dilution methods 222, 224
Brown-Wilkinson, Lord 411
budesonide
　allergic fungal rhinosinusitis 1053–4
　croup 364
buffers, in ear preparations 275
bullous pemphigoid 133, 154
Burkitt's lymphoma 160, 201, 250–1
burns 99–100
　dressings 103–4
busulphan 299, 299
butterfly grafts 1144
button batteries, ingestion 447
Byrne v. Boadle 411–12

C cells, *see* parafollicular cells (C cells)
C-cell hyperplasia 684–5, 684, 757
c-Fos, thyroid tumours 84
c-Myc oncogene 84
C-reactive protein 133, 150, 712
c-ret proto-oncogene 87–8
C1 esterase inhibitor protein 296
C3 convertase enzymes 131
cabergoline 907, 932, 933, 952, 953
cabozantinib 762
Cadbury report (1992) 390
cadherin 23 16–17, 20
calcichew 854
calcifediol 298
calcimimetic agents 847, 861, 883
calcitonin 604, 623, 626, 861
　hyperparathyroidism 883
　medullary thyroid cancer 741–2, 759–60, 761, 762
　levels after surgery 786
calcitriol 608, 624, 625, 889
calcium
　serum 604, 608, 624, 827
　after thyroid/parathyroid surgery 298, 345, 625, 730, 854, 889, 902
　'free' ionized 624, 827
　hyperparathyroidism 828, 847
　interpretation 827–8
　medullary thyroid cancer 760
　parathyroid carcinoma 858
　total levels 827
　urinary 829, 830, 1214
calcium homeostasis 298, 624–5, 625
calcium stimulation test 759

calcium supplementation
　parathyroid surgery *854*
　thyroid surgery 889
calcium-sensing receptor (CaSR) 624, 625–6, 828, 847, 858, 879, 882
calcium:creatinine (Ca/Cr) excretion ratio 830
calcofluor white stain 206
Caldwell-Luc procedure 431, 1108, 1250
Calgary–Cambridge model 381
callus formation 98
Calman Report (1993) 372
Canada, prosecution of doctors 422–3
canaliculi 1244
　probing 1246, 1246
cancer, EORTC QLQ-C30 instrument 490
cancer stem cells (CSCs) 72
Candida spp. 205, 207
　biofilms 217
Candida albicans 207, 207
　microscopy 207
　oropharyngeal infections 216–17
Candida dubliniensis 217
Candida glabrata 207, 217
Candida krusei 207, 217
Candida tropicalis 217
candidiasis 207
　diagnosis 207, 207
　oropharyngeal, in HIV 216–17, 233–4, 235, *235*
　pseudomembranous 217
cannula-over-needle devices 320
can't intubate and can't ventilate (CICV) 319
capacity 398, 416
capillary bleeding, ear surgery 348
capnography 342
capsaicin, intra-nasal 1015
carbapenems 223
carbimazole 297, 620, 724–7
　dosage 725
　in pregnancy 739
　radioiodine pre-treatment 727–8
　side effects 725–6
carbon dioxide, end-tidal (ETCO$_2$), monitoring 338, 342
carbon dioxide (CO$_2$), inspired/expired 342
carbon dioxide (CO$_2$) laser 346, 439, 582
carboplatin 42
　ototoxicity 254
carbozantinib 788
carcinoembryonic antigen (CEA) 623, 786
carcinogenesis 7–11
　apoptosis 65–7
　loss of heterozygosity 7–9
　oncogenes 9, 83–4
　telomere shortening 9–10
cardiac output
　intra-operative monitoring 343
　monitors 354, *354*
cardiolipin antibodies 153, 270
cardiovascular disease
　pre-operative assessment 302–3
　risk in primary hyperparathyroidism 844, 845
Care Quality Commission (CQC) 420
Carney complex 647, 937
carotico-optic recess 613

carotid arteries
    cavernous sinus 616–17, <u>617</u>, 944, <u>944</u>
    injury in sinus surgery 1077, 1179
    sphenoid sinus 612–13, <u>612</u>
    see also external carotid artery; internal carotid artery
Carpue, Joseph 107
cartilage, tissue-engineering 71
cartilage scoring technique 435
case presentations
    appraisal of papers 498, *499–500*
    literature searches 497–8, *498*
    portfolio for otorhinolaryngology 496
    preparing discussion 498, *500*
    questions to ask 497
    structuring 496–7, <u>496</u>
case-control studies 477–8
CASH management 321
caspases 59–60, <u>60</u>, 62–3, <u>63</u>
CaSR gene 858
cassava 76
Castleman disease 231
casuistry 396
catecholamines 354, 760
catheters, endovascular 570
cauterization
    epistaxis 447, 1176, <u>1176</u>
    intra-nasal tumours 1294
cavernous sinus
    anatomy 616–17
    cranial nerves 910, <u>911</u>, 912
    endoscopic anatomy 617, <u>617</u>
    pituitary tumour extension 645, <u>646</u>, 1286
        surgical approach 1286–7, <u>1286</u>
cavernous sinus thrombosis *1115*, 1116, 1117, *1117*
    treatment 1118–19
CD4+ T cells
    HIV infection 230, 231
    tumour microenvironment 158
CD8+ T cells 158
CDC73 gene 858
CDH23 gene 17
CDKN1B gene mutations 937
ceftriaxone 189
cefuroxime 300
cell cycle 39–40
    targets for chemotherapy 39, <u>40</u>
cell death
    necrosis 41, 61
    programmed, *see* apoptosis
    radiotherapy 51–2
    terminal differentiation 61
cell division 4
cell salvage <u>242</u>, 247
cell signalling 41
cellulitis, orbital *1028*, 1114–16, <u>1114</u>, *1115*, <u>1115</u>
cemento-ossifying fibroma 1102–3
central venous pressure, intra-operative 343
Centre for Evidence-Based Medicine 504
cephalosporins 223
    antibacterial spectrum *278*
    commonly used *223*
ceramic graft materials 120, *120*
cerebellopontine angle (CPA) surgery, auditory function monitoring 527–9

cerebral metastasis, thyroid cancer 809
cerebrospinal fluid (CSF) leaks 1203–9
    after head trauma 1204
    congenital 1204, <u>1204</u>
    endoscopic closure 1203
    endoscopic detection 1314, <u>1315</u>
    facial fractures 1190
    imaging 1207, <u>1207</u>, 1314, <u>1314–15</u>
    investigation 1206–7
    medical negligence claims 430, 432–3
    nasal fracture 1186
    recurrence 1203
    repair 1206
        controversies 1207–8
        technical aspects 1208
    sinus surgery 1077, <u>1077</u>, 1111, 1205–6
    skull base surgery 1302
    spontaneous 1204–5
    tumour-associated 1204
Certificate of Completion of Training (CCT) 370, 372, 373, <u>373</u>, 376
Certificate of Eligibility for Specialist Registration (CESR) 373, <u>373</u>
cerumenolytics 277, 280
cervical fascia, incision 797, <u>797</u>
cervical lymphadenopathy 251–2
    in HIV 231
    medical negligence 447
cervical smears, misreading 423
ceteris paribus principle 467
cetirizine 287, 1004, 1006
cetuximab 47, 56, 67, 161–2, *162*
CH100 (CH50) haemolytic complement test 151
change scores 486
Chapel Hill Consensus 1216, 1218
charcoal dressings 300
Charcot–Leyden crystals *212*, 213, 1040, *1051*, <u>1067</u>, 1220
charge-coupled devices 813, 814
chemicals
    implicated in occupational rhinitis 1017–18
    and smell disorders *1233*, 1237
chemokines, tumour microenvironment 159–60
chemosensitization 34
chemotherapy
    adjuvant 44
    anaplastic thyroid cancer 766
    CHOP-R regimen 769
    combination 44
    concurrent radiotherapy 44–5, 55, 766–7
    differentiated thyroid cancer 785
    endovascular delivery 572
    future research 48
    in head and neck cancer 44
    medullary thyroid cancer 788
    mucositis 254
    neoadjuvant (induction chemotherapy) 44, 55
    ototoxicity 254
    parathyroid carcinoma 861
    principles of 39
    stridor 254
    targeted therapies 11–12, 45–8, 55–6
    taxanes 789
    thyroid lymphoma 769

chemotherapy agents
    alkylating agents 41, 299, <u>299</u>
    antimetabolites 42, <u>43</u>
    cell cycle specific 41
    cell cycle targets 39, <u>40</u>
    heavy metals 41–2
    novel 45–8
    phase-specific 41
    sites of action 299, <u>299</u>
cherubism 1221, <u>1221</u>
Chester v. Afshar 415
Chevallet fracture 1184, <u>1185</u>
chief cells (principal cells) 608
children
    acute otitis media 201, 277, *278*
    airway anatomy/physiology 361–2
    allergic rhinitis 1000, 1007–8
    'atopic march' 1001
    bacterial tracheitis 364
    differentiated thyroid cancer 785–6
    epiglottitis 325, 364, 446
    facial injuries 1199–200, *1200*
    fluid requirements 362–3, *363*
    foreign body inhalation 364–5
    goitre 76, *76*
    HPV infection 167–8
    immunodeficiency tests 149
    inferior turbinate surgery 1165
    informed consent 416
    nose bleeds 265
    prophylactic thyroidectomy 762–3
    rhinosinusitis management 1078
    septoplasty 1141, *1147*
    viral croup 364
chitosan *120*
chlorambucil 299, <u>299</u>
chlorhexidine gluconate 295
choanal atresia *962*, 1014
cholesteatoma, medical negligence 442–3
cholesterol granuloma 1221–2
¹¹C-choline PET-CT 555
chondrosarcoma 1312, <u>1313</u>
chordoma 927, *1270*
    skull base 1282, <u>1282</u>, 1284
Christmas disease 265
chromophobe cells 613
chromosomes 3–4, *5*
chronic infantile neurologic cutaneous articular syndrome (CINCA) 178
chronic kidney disease
    hypercalcaemia 829–30
    mineral bone disorder (CKD-MBD) 830
chronic lymphocytic leukaemia (CLL) 252, 256
chronic myeloid leukaemia (CML) 251
chronic obstructive pulmonary disease (COPD) 1128
chronic rhinosinusitis (CRS)
    aetiology <u>1028</u>
    in asthma 1127–8
    definitions 283, 1025–6, *1025*
    diagnosis 1027, 1071–2
    eosinophilic 1067, <u>1067</u>
    epidemiology 1026–7
    frontal sinus 1088
    indications for surgery 1072
    management in children 1078

chronic rhinosinusitis (CRS) (continued)
  medical treatment
    antibiotics 285–6, 1063–4
    aspirin desensitization 1063
    assessment of response 1065–6
    corticosteroids 284–5, 1061–2
    delivery methods 1065, 1065
    failure 1066
    immunomodulatory antibiotics 1062–3
    immunoregulation 1063
    leukotriene receptor antagonists 1063
    mucociliary clearance improvement 1064–5
    post-surgery 1067–8
  with nasal polyps (CRSwNP) 284–5, 288, 1026, 1028–31, 1037, 1039, 1061
  pathophysiology 1061
  smell impairment 1234, 1235–6
  surgery 1071–8
    anaesthesia 1072–3
    complications 1076–7
    evidence base 1077–8
    nasal preparation 1073
    post-operative care 1075–6
    techniques 1073–5
  in systemic disease 1032, 1033
  turbinate surgery 1164
  without nasal polyps (CRSsNP) 284, 288, 1026, 1028–9, 1031–2, 1061
Churchill, Edward D. 873
Churg-Strauss syndrome 152, 176, 1030, 1033, 1041, 1218–19
ciclosporin 251
ciliary dyskinesias 1032, 1033, 1040
ciliary function testing 1027
ciliated epithelium, contact endoscopy 589, 589
ciliated pseudostratified columnar epithelium
  inferior turbinates 1158, 1158
  lower respiratory mucosa 1127, 1127
  nasal mucosa 985, 1127, 1127
  paranasal sinuses 972
cinacalcet 847, 861, 883
cinnarizine 279
ciprofloxacin
  antibacterial spectrum 278
  chronic rhinosinusitis 285
  ear drops 276
  systemic 278
circadian variation
  growth hormone 633
  thyroid-stimulating hormone 634
circulatory overload, transfusion-associated (TACO) 245–6
cisplatin 42, 299, 299
  ototoxicity 254
civil law, defined 409
Civil Procedures Rules (1998) 412, 418, 419
cleft lip/palate surgery, paediatric intensive care 365
Client-Oriented Scale of Improvement (COSI) 490
clindamycin 223
clinical audit 391–2
  factors in effective 392
  thyroid and parathyroid surgery 894–7

clinical effectiveness 392
clinical ethics committees 405–6
Clinical Evidence 504, 507
clinical governance
  current issues 393
  definitions 390–1
  domains 390
  historical background 389–90
  and patient safety 392–3
  7 pillars 391–2
  roles of CEO, NHS board and senior management 393
clinical supervisors 374
clinimetric scales 470–1
clinoid process
  anterior 614, 615
  middle 614, 615
  posterior 615
clopidogrel 293
Clostridium difficile 187
clotrimazole 209, 234, 287
  ear drops 276
cluster headaches 1257, 1257
co-phenylcaine 1073
co-triamterzide 279
coagulation
  inhibition 261
  platelet function 261–2, 262
  role of vessel wall 262–3, 263
  screening tests 263–4
coagulation factors 259–61
  disorders 265–7
  recombinant 272
  replacement/blood products 272–3
  von Willebrand factor (vWF) 262
coagulation pathway 259–63, 260
  action of anticoagulants 293–4, 294
Coblation® inferior turbinate surgery 996, 996, 1163, 1166, 1166
cocaine
  causing nasal cavity destruction 1219, 1220, 1310
  and nasal mucosa 985
  nasal preparation 289, 1073
cochlea, stem cell regeneration 71
cochlear implantation
  medical negligence claims 427–8
  parental consent 402–3
cochlear nerve
  direct recordings 529
  injury 527
Cochrane Collaboration 498, 504, 515
Cochrane Database of Systematic Reviews 515
Cochrane Handbook 517
cockroach allergen avoidance 1003
codeine phosphate 296
codons 3
coeliac disease 153–4
Cogan syndrome 177
cohort studies 477
coil embolization 571
cold agglutinins 153
colecalciferol (cholecalciferol) 624, 625
collagen
  scaffolding materials 120
  skin 112
  vocal cord injection 297, 300
  xenografts 120, 1153

collagen matrix grafts 945, 947
collar incision 795–6, 796, 823
collectins 131
colloid fluids 355
colon, microflora 182
colorectal cancer, tumour biomarkers 161
columella 965, 983
  widened 1142, 1146
columella strut graft 1146
columella: philtrum incision 1154
coma, myxoedema 730
Commission for Health Improvement (CHI) 390, 391, 392
common carotid artery, thyroid cancer involvement 808
common cold 197
  efficacy of nasal decongestants 996, 996
common law 410
common variable immune deficiency (CVID) 1032
communication
  adverse incidents 384–5
  closed questions 381
  and compliance 386
  critically ill patient and family 358
  5 Es model 381–3
  'heart sink' encounter 385
  honesty in 404–5
  'illness perspective' 379
  importance for doctors and surgeons 380–1
  issues around loss 385
  learning skills 381
  literature on 381
  medical errors 385
  non-verbal 383–4
  optimization 384
  surgical team 459–60
comparative genomic hybridization (CGH) 6
complaints procedures 413, 420–1
complement
  deficiencies 151
  measurement 151
complement system 126, 130–1, 131
  classical pathway of activation 131
complementary therapies, allergic rhinitis 1007
compliance, and patient communication 386
complications of surgery, informing patients 429–30
component resolved diagnostics (CRD) 145
compound muscle action potentials (CMAP) 525–7
computational fluid dynamics 1166, 1167
computed tomography angiography (CTA) 942
computed tomography (CT)
  cone beam 1316
  four-dimensional (4D) 838, 838, 859, 868, 880, 880, 882–3
  frontal sinus 1082, 1084–5, 1084–5, 1086
  fungal ball 1048, 1309, 1310
  fungal rhinosinusitis 1049, 1050, 1051
  giant cell granuloma 1221
  GPA 1216–17, 1216

computed tomography (CT) (continued)
  inferior turbinate enlargement 1159, 1160
  intra-thoracic goitre 820, 822, 822
  intracranial complications of sinusitis 1120, 1121
  mucoceles 1108, 1109, 1254, 1254
  nasal polyposis 1038, 1042, 1043
  orbital cellulitis 1116–17, 1118
  orbital zones 1098, 1099
  parathyroid adenoma 645, 836, 838, 838, 868
  parathyroid carcinoma 859, 859
  parathyroid glands 645
  radiation exposure 1305
  rhinosinusitis 1308–10, 1308–9
  sarcoidosis 1214, 1214
  sinonasal tumours 1270, 1271–2
  skull base defects 1205, 1207, 1207
  skull base surgery 1282–3, 1283
  smell disorders 1233
  technical aspects 1305
  thyroid cancer 644, 751
  thyroid eye disease 1247, 1247–8
  thyroiditis 714
concha bullosa, mucoceles 1107, 1107, 1108, 1111
condylar fractures 1192, 1193–4
conestat alpha 296
confidence, surgeon 462
confidence intervals 474
Confidential Enquiry into Postoperative Deaths (CEPOD) 306, 326
confidentiality 405, 417
confounding 475
  minimizing 475
congenital adrenal hyperplasia 638
congenital primary hypopituitarism 925–6
Conidiobolus spp. 208
connective tissue disease, autoantibodies 153, *153*
connexin genes 16
consent, *see* informed consent
consequentialism 400–1
conservative treatments, failure to consider 428
Consolidated Standards of Reporting Trials (CONSORT) statement 480
construct validity 485
Consultant Outcomes Publication, NHS England 896
consultant trainers 374
consulting room, seating arrangement 383–4, 384
contact endoscopy 587–93
  application 587–8, 593
  combination with 'narrow band imaging' 588
  development 587–8
  objective 588
  technique 588
  upper aerodigestive tract
    normal patterns 589–90, 589, 590
    pathology 590–3
'contact point pain' 1258–9
continuing professional development 375, *375*, 392
Copenhagen Allergy Study 1125

cophenylcaine 347
Core Outcome Measures in Effectiveness Trials (COMET) 508
Core Surgical Training (CST) programme 373, 373
corona viruses 197
coronary stenting, antiplatelet therapy 303
coroner 417–18
Coroners and Justice Act (2009) 417
corticosteroids
  after thyroidectomy 802
  allergic diseases 142–3, 147
  allergic fungal rhinosinusitis 215, 1052–3
  croup 364
  GPA 1217
  inhaled 1129
  intranasal 283–4, 1005–6
    acute rhinosinusitis 1060
    adverse effects 1006, 1043, 1151
    allergic fungal rhinosinusitis 215, 1053–4
    allergic rhinitis 147, 1005–6, *1005*
    and asthma 1129
    chronic rhinosinusitis 284, 1061–2
    improving delivery 1065, 1065
    nasal polyposis 1042–3
    non-allergic rhinitis 1014–15
    post-sinus surgery 1067–8
  rhinosinusitis 283–5, 1061–2
  and smell dysfunction 1235–6
  sudden sensorineural hearing loss 280
  temporal arteritis 1260
  topical ear preparations 276
  and wound healing 99
corticotrophinomas 916–17, 933–5
  adjuvant treatment 954–5
corticotrophs 613, *631*, 924
corticotrophin-releasing hormone (CRH) 637, 637, 917
corticotrophin-releasing hormone (CRH) test *918*, 935
cortisol
  24-hour urinary *916*, 934, *934*
  overproduction 908–10, *909*
  salivary levels 934
  serum levels 916, *918*
cortisol synthesis 637, 637
Corynebacteria 188
cosmesis, thyroidectomy 796
cosmetic surgery
  facelift 436–8
  laser skin resurfacing 439
  medical negligence claims 436–8
  patient selection 428–9, 437
  rhinoplasty 434–5
Cottle elevator 945, 947
Cottle's manoeuvre 979, 987, 1143, 1143
  modified 1143
cough medicines 296
coumarins 270–1
counter-regulation hypothesis 138
County Court 413
Court of Appeal 410, 411, 416–17, 422, 423
Cowden's disease (multiple hamartoma syndrome) 89
CpG islands 9

cranial nerves
  cavernous sinus 910, 911, 912
  facial pain 1253
  see also individual cranial nerves
craniofacial hypoplasia 65
craniofacial surgery, paediatric intensive care 365
craniofacial syndrome, intubation 366
craniopharyngioma 648, 648, 927, 1290
  adjuvant therapy 955
  endonasal endoscopic surgery 1294, 1297, *1298*, 1299, 1302
Crawford silastic tubes 1246
Crawford v. board of Governors of the Charing Cross Hospital 411
creams, otologic 275
CREST syndrome *153*
Creutzfeldt-Jakob disease, variant 240, 344–5
cribriform plate, fracture 1235
cricoid resection, in thyroid cancer 808
cricothyroid joint 798, 799
cricothyrotomy
  large cannula 320, 320
  needle/small bore cannula 319–20, 319
  surgical 320–1
cricothyrotomy needle 326
criminal law
  defined 409
  offences resulting from medical treatment 421–3
crista ethmoidalis 968, 969, 1172, 1177
criterion validity 485
critical appraisal 498
  abstracts 505
  diagnostic studies 508–11
  formulating questions 506–8
  framework *500*
  importance of 503–4
  levels of evidence 518–21, *519–20*
  methodology of trials 504
  outcomes 507–8
  statistics 506
  systematic reviews 515–21
  therapy studies 512–15
  tips for 504–5
  worksheets *522–4*
critical care 351–9
  admission 352
  cardiovascular support 354
  communication with patient and family 358
  development of 351
  early identification of organ dysfunction 359
  fluid resuscitation 355
  impacts on patients' futures 359
  interface with ENT 356–8
  levels of intensity *351*
  management models 352
  medical staff 352
  mortality 358–9
  multidisciplinary 351–2
  nutritional support 355–6
  renal support 355
  respiratory support 352–4
  scoring systems 352
  types of admission from ENT 356
  see also paediatric intensive care

cross-matching 241, 304
cross-sectional studies 476–7
croup
　　pseudomembranous
　　　　(bacterial tracheitis) 364
　　viral 364
cryoglobulinaemia 153
cryoglobulins 153
cryoprecipitate 244, 272
cryopyrin-associated periodic syndromes (CAPS) 178–9
Cryptococcus neoformans 208
crystalloid fluids 355
Curvularis spp. 1048
Cushing, Harvey 1281
Cushing's disease 638, 647
　　adjuvant therapy 954
　　aetiology 908–9
　　clinical features 910, 910
　　diagnosis 916, 917, 934
　　differentiation from Cushing's syndrome 934–5, 935
　　management 935, 954
　　post-operative care 948
Cushing's syndrome 638, 908
　　cause of endogenous 908
　　diagnosis and investigations 916–17, 934–5, 935
　　medullary thyroid cancer 758
　　topical steroid use 1043
cyclic citrullinated peptide (CCP) antibodies 153
cyclin D1 gene 697, 858
cyclin dependent kinase inhibitors (CDK1) genes 86
cyclizine 279
cyclooxygenase (COX) enzymes 160, 262
　　inhibition 272
cyclophosphamide 299, 299, 1217
cysteinyl leukotrienes 1006
cystic fibrosis (CF)
　　gene therapy 31–3
　　nasal polyposis 1030–1, 1040
cystic fibrosis transmembrane conductance regulator (CFTR) gene 31–2
cystic teratoma, *see* dermoid cysts
cystitis, radiation 781
cytochrome c 62–3, 63
cytogenetics 6
cytokines 120–1
　　allergic rhinitis 1127
　　asthma 1127
　　bone remodelling 121
　　bone/hard tissue healing 98
　　pro-inflammatory 133
　　Th cell secretion 129, 129
　　tumour microenvironment 159–60
　　in wound healing 95, 96
cytomegalovirus (CMV)
　　hearing loss 201
　　in HIV 235
cytopenia 255
cytotoxic T-lymphocyte antigen-4 (CTLA-4) 48
　　monoclonal antibodies 162, 955

Da vinci telerobotics system 813–14, 814
dabigatran 246, 271, 1179–80

dacryocystorhinostomy, endoscopic 1217, 1245–6
dacryoscintigraphy 1245
Dalrymple sign 706
damage-associated molecular pattern molecules (DAMPs) 60
damages (medical negligence claims) 409, 412, 414
　　aid by NHS 414
　　general 409, 412
　　punitive 423
　　special 409, 412
danaparoid 271
dantolene 890
Dartvelle approach (thyroid surgery) 823, 823
Data Protection Act (1997) 417
database searches 497–8, 498, 499
Davies, Dame Sally 221
day surgery
　　ear surgery 348
　　patient suitability 301–2
　　pre-operative assessment 302
DDAVP 266
de Morsier's syndrome 1237
de Quervain's thyroiditis 662, 663, 732, 732
deaf child, ethics of interventions 402–3
deaf culture 403
deafness
　　at birth, negligent causation 439
　　wrongly diagnosed 439–40
death inducing signal complex (DISC) 64
death receptors 64–5
deaths
　　critical care 358–9
　　difficult airway 319, 322, 329
　　prosecutions following 422–3
　　reporting to coroner 417–18
deception 405
decision-making, surgeon 457–8
decongestants 286
　　allergic rhinitis 1005, 1006
　　before nasal airflow assessment 993
　　efficacy in common cold 996, 996
　　pre-surgical 1073, 1292
　　rhinosinusitis 286
deep vein thrombosis (DVT)
　　prophylaxis 294
　　risk factors 269–70, 269
　　treatment 270
deferoxamine-hespan (DFO-H) 114
deiodinases 623
delayed haemolytic transfusion reaction (DHTR) 246
delays in diagnosis
　　cholesteatoma 442
　　dizziness 443
　　hearing disorders 439
　　laryngeal cancer 450
　　malignancy 901
　　meningitis 439, 444
　　skin cancer 436
delays in referral 430–1
delays in treatment
　　cholesteatoma 442
　　nasal trauma 434
delirium, critical care patient 356

demineralized bone matrix (DBM) 120
dendritic cells 126, 126, 139–40
denominator problem 471–2, 471
dental arch, wiring in mandible fractures 1191, 1192, 1192
dental injuries
　　children 1199–200, 1200
　　paediatric surgery 445
dental pain 1259
dentigerous cyst 1310, 1311
deontology 401
Department of Health (UK), antimicrobial resistance 226–7
depth of anaesthesia monitors 343
dermis 108
dermoid cysts
　　nasal, *see* nasal dermoids
　　ovary 607, 659, 660
descriptive studies 474, 475–6
desflurane 335, 336
desmopressin (DDAVP) 266, 919
detergent manufacture 1018, 1020
determinant-occurrence relationships 466
dexamethasone
　　croup 364
　　ear preparations 276
　　lymphomas 252
dexamethasone suppression tests 916, 916
　　high-dose 934–5, 935
　　low-dose 916, 935
dextrocardia 1040, 1041
DFNX3 gene 17–18
di-iodothyronine 620
diabetes insipidus 638–9, 906
　　central 638–9, 906, 913
　　investigations 919
　　nephrogenic 639
　　post-operative monitoring 948
diabetes mellitus
　　and skin flap survival 113
　　wound healing 99, 103
diabetic ulcers 100, 103
diagnostic tests, critical appraisal 509–10, 509
diaphragmatica sella 615
diarrhoea, medullary thyroid cancer 762, 787
diathermy
　　inferior turbinates 429, 1162
　　medical negligence claims 445–6
DIC, *see* disseminated intravascular coagulation
differentiation, terminal 61
difficult airway
　　alternative techniques 315–17
　　best clinical practice 329
　　children 366
　　choice of airway device 339
　　critical care management 357
　　definitions 309–10
　　developments in equipment 349
　　evaluation 310–13
　　extubation 328
　　failed ventilation/emergency cricothyrotomy 319–21
　　follow-up 329
　　future research 330
　　management strategy 314–15, 314

difficult airway (*continued*)
 morbidity/mortality 319, 322, 329
 prediction of difficulty 313–14, *313*
 prevalence 310
 recovery 328–9, *329*
 thyroid/parathyroid surgery 890
Difficult Airway Society (DAS) 309, 314, 329
diffuse large B-cell lymphoma 769, 770
digestive tract, microflora *182*
digital subtraction angiography (DSA), tumour embolization 569, 573, 574
1,25-dihydroxyvitamin D3 624, 625
dimethylsulfoxide (DMSO) 114
Dingman approach *1197*
diphtheria 188
Diploma in Otolaryngology – Head and Neck Surgery (DOHNS) 373
diplopia, after orbital decompression 1248
dipyridamole 293
direct oral anticoagulant agents (DOACs) 246, 271
disc diffusion testing 222, 224
disclosure 404–5
 confidential information 405, 417
 medical errors 405, 900–1
 risks of surgery 415–16, 417, 429
disease-modifying anti-rheumatic drugs (DMARDS) 179–80
disseminated intravascular coagulation (DIC) 267
 causes *267*
 laboratory tests 255
 management 267
distortion product otoacoustic emissions (DPOEs) 254
dizziness 443
 assessment instruments 490
 medical negligence claims 443
Dizziness Handicap Inventory 490
DNA
 amplification 6–7, *7*
 double-stranded (dsDNA) 7, 153, *153*
 fragmentation and identification 5, *5*
 hybridization 6, *6*
 naked 31
 replication 40
 structure and function 3–4
 viruses 196
'do not attempt resuscitation' (DNAR) orders 359
dobutamine 354
docetaxel 43, 766
doctrine of double effect 404
Donaldson, Liam 389–90
L-dopa test *918*
dopamine, pituitary inhibition 932
dopamine agonists 906–7, 932, 933, 952, 953
dopamine antagonists 279
dopastatins 953
Doppler ultrasound, oesophageal *354*
Doppman, J.L. 874
dorsum sellae 614, *615*
double blinding 479
'double density' sign 1049, *1050*
Down syndrome 6, 1237
 atlanto-axial instability 448

doxorubicin 766
doxycycline, anti-inflammatory 1062–3
drainage
 frontal sinus 1088, 1097, 1097, 1121, 1122
 orbital collections 1119–20
 septal haematoma/abscess 1188
 thyroidectomy 802
Dreyfus model skills acquisition 372
Driver and Vehicle Licensing Authority 417
dual isotope subtraction scintigraphy 836, 837
Dunhill, Thomas 598, 599
dural defects, repair 945–6, 947, 1278, 1300
dural grafts 1300
dural substitutes 1286
dusts, organic 1017–18
duty of candour 414, 900–1
Dyazide® 279
dynamic risk stratification, thyroid cancer treatment 754–5, *755*, 783
dysfibrinogenaemia *264*, 267
dyskaryosis 591
dyslipidaemia 735, *735*
dysosmia 1230, 1234–5
dysphonia, rheumatological disorders 174
dysplasia, contact endoscopy 591, 591
dyspnoea, airway obstruction 321

E-cadherin 858
E-test 222, 224, 224
E6/E7 genes 160, 169–70
ear drops 275–7
 use in tympanum perforation 276–7
 wax removal 277, 280
ear sprays 276
ear surgery, anaesthesia 347–8, 349
ear syringing, medical negligence claims 440
EaStER trial 480
echocardiography, cardiac output *354*
ECMO, *see* extracorporeal membrane oxygenation
Edoxaban 271
effect size 473
egg allergy *146*
EGPA, *see* eosinophilic granulomatosis with polyangiitis
Einstein, Albert 581
elastography, thyroid nodules 742
elderly
 epistaxis 1174
 smell dysfunction 1237–8, 1238, 1239
elective surgery
 fasting 306–7
 patient selection 428–9
electrocardiography (ECG)
 intra-operative monitoring 341, 341
 pre-operative 304
electrocochleography 440–1, 528
electroencephalography (EEG) 1233
electrolyte requirements, children 362, *363*
electromyography (EMG)
 facial nerve 343, 345, 346, 525–6
 thyroid/parathyroid surgery 337
electrophoresis 5

electrophysiological monitoring
 auditory function 527–9
 facial nerve 525–7
embolic agents
 liquid 571
 particles 570–1, *571*, 575, 576
embryology
 nose 961–2, *961*
 palate 962, *962*
 parathyroid glands 608, 608, 874, 874, 881, 881
 thyroid gland 605–6, 605, *606*, 651
embryonic stem cells 70
emotionally-induced rhinitis 1014
empathy, patient communication 382–3, 385
empty nose syndrome 1163, 1165
empty sella syndrome 929
empyema
 extradural 1120
 subdural 1120
encephalocele 1204, 1315
end of life 358–9
end-tidal CO_2 338, 342
endobronchial allergen challenge 1128
endocrine disease, causing smell dysfunction *1233*
Endocrine Society
 acromegaly diagnosis 933
 Cushing's syndrome diagnosis 934
 testosterone replacement guidelines 929
endocrine system, negative feedback loops 621, 621, 629, 630
endonasal endoscopic sphenopalatine artery ligation (ESPAL) 1177, 1178
endonasal flaps, septal perforation repair 1154
endoscopes, robotic surgery 813–14
endoscopic endonasal surgery (EES)
 development 1281–2
 nasal preparation 1274, 1292–3
 operative set up 1282, 1283–4, 1292, 1292
 palliative in unresectable tumours 1291, 1292
 pituitary tumours 951–2, 1281–7
 recurrent 941–8
 sinonasal tumours 1274–8
  complications 1278
  evidence base 1269
  optimizing surgical field 1274
  post-operative care 1278–9
  surgical access 1274–8
  tumour resection 1274, 1278
 skull base reconstruction 945–6, 946–7, 1206, 1208, 1278
 tumour debulking 1291, 1291
endoscopic sinus surgery (ESS)
 anaesthesia 1072–3
 and asthma 1130
 children 1078
 chronic rhinosinusitis, post-surgical medical treatment 1067–8
 complications 1076–7, 1205–6, 1205
  carotid artery injury 1077
  CSF leak 1077, 1205–6, 1205
  haemorrhage 1076
  optic nerve injury 975, 1076–7
  orbital injury 1076, 1076

endoscopic sinus surgery (ESS) (continued)
  eye preparation 1073
  image guidance 565, 565
  intra-operative monitoring 432
  intranasal preparation 1073
  key anatomical landmarks 969–72, 970–2, 972
  medical negligence claims 427–8, 429, 432–3, 1073
  post-operative care 432–3, 1075–6
  rhinosinusitis 1072–8
    allergic fungal 1051
    evidence base 1077–8
  surgical position 1073
  video recording 430
  see also functional endoscopic sinus surgery (FESS)
endothelial wall 262–3, 263
endothelin-1 (ET-1) 114
endotracheal tubes 336–7, 337
  laser surgery 339–40, 340
endovascular catheters 570
endovascular embolization 569
  coils and balloons 570, 571
  epistaxis 576–8, 1179
  indications 569–70
  temporary in head and neck surgery 570, 572
  tumours 571–2
    juvenile angiofibroma 576, 577
    meningioma 573–5
    paragangliomas 575–6
endovascular ligation, functional testing 570, 570
energy intake, critical care patient 355
enhanced recovery, day surgery 302
Enhanced Recovery after Head and Neck Cancer Surgery (ERAHNCS) 307
Enhanced Recovery After Surgery (ERAS) 307
enophthalmos, orbital floor injury 1197, 1198
enteral feeding, early post-operative 307
enterobacteriaceae 190, 1039
  examples of species 190
  lactose/non-lactose fermenters 189, 190
enterococci 187
environmental factors
  and allergic disease 138
  goitre formation 76–7, 77
eosinophilia 256
eosinophilic fungal rhinosinusitis 1049
eosinophilic granuloma 927, 1219–21
eosinophilic granulomatosis with polyangiitis (EGPA/Churg-Strauss syndrome) 152, 176, 1030, 1033, 1041, 1218–19
eosinophilic mucin 1049
eosinophilic mucin rhinosinusitis 1049
eosinophils 139, 140
ephedrine nasal drops 286
epidemiology
  analytical studies 473, 476–7
  classical (aetiological) 467
  clinical 467–8
  definition 466
  descriptive studies 474, 475–6
  determinant-occurrence relationships 466

health and public health research 468
as a methodological discipline 466
observational studies 469, 469, 475–6
precision and accuracy 471
research protocol 468
research question 468
results analysis 471–3
'so what' test 468–9
specific conditions
  allergic rhinitis and asthma 1125, 1130
  goitre 740
  Graves' disease 720
  HIV infection 229
  hyperthyroidism 733
  occupational rhinitis 1017
  rhinosinusitis 1026–7
  thyroid cancer 740–1
  thyroid nodules 740
study design
  choosing 474–80
  taxonomy 469, 469
study size 473–4
study subjects 469–70
variables measured 470–1
epidermal growth factor receptor (EGFR) 45–7, 55–6
  antibodies 47, 161, 162
  targeted small molecules 47
epidermis 108
epiglottitis
  anaesthesia 325
  intensive care 364
  medical negligence 446
epilepsy 1237
epiphora 1244
epistat 1190, 1190
epistaxis 265
  adult recurrent 1170, 1179
  aetiology 1174–5
  anterior 1174
  best clinical practice 1180
  cautery 447, 1176, 1176
  classification 1172, 1174
  demography 1174
  direct management 1175–7
  future research 1180
  hereditary haemorrhagic telangiectasia 289, 577, 1178, 1180
  history 1169
  lateral wall or septal bleeding 1170–1
  management algorithm 1173
  medical negligence claims 447
  in nasal fractures 1188
  nasal vascular anatomy 1169–70
  posterior 1170, 1171, 1174
  primary 1172
  primary adult 1174–9
  resuscitation 1175
  secondary 1179–80
  in septal perforation 1150
  surgical management 1177–9
  transarterial embolization 576–8
  traumatic 1179
epithelial-mesenchymal transition (EMT) 72
epithelialization, wounds 96, 103
epithelium
  dysplasia 591, 591

lower airway 1127, 1127
  nasal cavity 966, 985, 1127, 1127
Epstein–Barr virus (EBV) 160, 199, 1222
  and cancers 201, 250–1
Epworth Sleepiness Scales 470–1
equipoise 478
ergocalciferol (vitamin D2) 625
erlotinib 47, 56
erythrocyte sedimentation rate (ESR), thyroid disease 662, 712, 732
erythrocytes, see red blood cells
erythromycin 279
erythropoietin (EPO) 247, 249–50
ETHICAL model 480
ethics
  concepts
    autonomy 398
    consequentialism 400–1
    deontology 401
    justice 400
    non-maleficence 399
    paternalism 399–400
    principles 397
    relativism 396, 397
    rights 400
    welfare, well-being, beneficence 399
  definitions 395–6
  empirical 395
  and law 397, 405
  methods 396–7
  normative 395
  philosophical (analytic) 395
  progress in 395
  and religion 397
  robotic surgery 814–15
ethics of care 396–7
ethinyloestradiol 289
ethmoid air cells 970, 972, 973
ethmoid bone 966
ethmoid bulla 970, 972, 973, 1307
  endoscopy 981
  removal 1074, 1074
ethmoid cell, posterior (Onodi cell) 971, 975, 975
ethmoid foramen
  anterior 1243–4, 1244
  posterior 1243, 1244
ethmoid sinus
  development 963, 963
  tumours 1098
ethmoidal arteries, see anterior ethmoidal artery; posterior ethmoidal artery
ethmoidectomy 1091–2
  bilateral 1295
  posterior 1074
ethmoturbinals 963
ethnicity
  nasal valve anatomy 1141–2
  sarcoidosis 1211
ethylene-vinyl alcohol copolymer (EVAL) 571
etomidate 954
European Community Respiratory Health Survey 1130
European Convention on Human Rights 400, 421
European Forum for Research and Education in Allergy and Airway Disease (EUFOREA) 1033–4

European Organisation for Research and Treatment of Cancer (EORTC) 484, 490
European position paper on rhinosinusitis and nasal polyposis (EPOS) 1025, 1026, *1033–4*, 1065, *1066*, 1072
European Vasculitis Study Group 1215, 1217
European Working Time Directive (EWTD) 372, 392
EuroQol (EQ-5D) 489
event rates 513–14
Evidence-Based Medicine 504
evidence-based medicine (EBM)
   chronic rhinosinusitis 1077–8
   critical appraisal, *see* critical appraisal
   definition 495
   levels of evidence 474, *474*, 480, 518–21, *519–20*
   in medical education 495–500
   minimally-invasive thyroidectomy 812–13
   patient-centred cycle 495, <u>495</u>
   sinonasal tumours 1269
examination under anaesthesia, medical negligence claims 432
exophthalmos
   hyperthyroidism 722, <u>722</u>, 723
   mucoceles 1108, <u>1109</u>
expectorants 296
experimental studies 469, <u>469</u>
expert medical witnesses 413, 418–20
   in clinical negligence 419
   in court 419–20
   duties/responsibilities 418–19
external carotid artery 1169–70, <u>1171</u>
   anastomosis 1170
   ligation in epistaxis 1178
external ear infections
   fungal 208–9
   HIV 232
extracellular matrix (ECM), synthesis in wound healing 96, 97
extracorporeal membrane oxygenation (ECMO) 353–4
   skin flaps 115–16
extractable nuclear antigens (ENA) 153
extranodal NK/T-cell lymphoma (ENKTCL) 1222–3, <u>1222</u>, 1310
extrinsic allergic alveolitis 133
extubation
   difficult airway 328
   nasal surgery 337
   tonsillectomy 344–5
eye care, endoscopic sinus surgery 1073
eye disease
   after eyelid surgery 438
   complicating rhinosinusitis <u>1114</u>, 1116
   in GPA 1215, <u>1216</u>
   hyperthyroidism 706
      conservative treatment 1246
      orbital decompression 1247–8, <u>1247–8</u>
      and radioiodine therapy 728
      symptoms and signs 722–3, <u>722</u>
      urgent referral criteria *723*
   mucoceles 1108, <u>1109–10</u>
   orbital floor injury <u>1197</u>, 1198
   sinonasal tumours *1271*
   see also visual problems

eyelid retraction, thyroid disease 722, <u>722</u>
eyelid surgery 438

face, danger areas 965
face and content validity 485
face mask anaesthesia 336
facelift, potential complications and litigation 436–8
facial appearance, MEN 2B 758, <u>759</u>
facial artery, nasal branch <u>117</u>, 965, 969, 1169
facial fractures 1189–99
   aetiology 1189
   children 1200
   future research *1200*
   mandible 1191–4
   maxilla 1194–6
   naso-orbito-ethmoid complex 1185, 1198–9, <u>1198</u>, <u>1199</u>
   orbital floor 1198
   primary care 1190–1
   soft tissue injuries 1199, *1200*
   upper third/frontal sinus 1199
   zygomatic complex 1196–8
   see also nasal fractures
facial injuries
   paediatric 1199–200, *1200*
   primary care 1190–1
   soft-tissue 1199
   see also facial fractures; nasal fractures
facial nerve monitoring 343, 346, 525–7
   benefits 525–6
   development 525
   difficulties 527
   ear surgery 442
   future research 529
   non-otological procedures 527
   and post-operative outcomes 527
   technique 526–7
facial nerve palsy
   after ear surgery 441–2
   after facelift surgery 437
   ala nasi collapse 987
   in HIV 232
   idiopathic 201
   medical negligence claims 437, 444, 526
   saccus decompression surgery 444
facial pain
   best clinical practice *1262*
   caused by tumours 1260–1
   cervical spine disease 1260
   dental 1259
   diagnosis 1253
   future research *1263*
   history taking 1261–2
   mid-face segment 1259, *1259*, <u>1260</u>
   migraine 1255–6
   myofascial 1260, *1260*
   neuralgias 1258–9
   persistent idiopathic (atypical) 1281
   primary headaches 1255, 1256–7, <u>1256</u>
   sinogenic 1254, <u>1255</u>, 1262, *1262*
   temporal arteritis 1260
facial vein 965
factor V Leiden 269, *269*
factor VII 260, 267
factor VIIa, recombinant (rFVIIa) 265

factor VIII 260, <u>261</u>
   deficiency (haemophilia A) 265
factor VIII bypassing agent (FEIBA) 265, 271
factor IX, deficiency (Christmas disease) 265
factor XI, deficiency 266
factor XII, deficiency 267
factor XIII 259, 267
Fahraeus-Lindqvist effect 111
fallacy of the length-to-width ratio 111, <u>111</u>
familial adenomatous polyposis (FAP) 89
familial cold autoinflammatory syndrome (FCAS) 178
familial hypocalciuric hypercalcaemia (FHH) <u>829</u>, 830, 882
familial isolated hyperparathyroidism (FIHP) 699
familial isolated pituitary adenomas 937
familial Mediterranean fever (FMF) 178
familial medullary thyroid carcinoma (FMTC) 682, 685–6, <u>684</u>, 758–9
familial paragangliomas, genetics 22–4
families
   critically ill patient 358–9
   paediatric intensive care patient 362
farmers 1020
farnesyl transferase inhibitors <u>66</u>, 67
Fas-associated death domain (FADD) 64
Fas-ligand (Fas-L) 64, 128
fasting, elective surgery 306–7
fat grafts 944, 945, 1206, <u>1291</u>, 1300
febrile non-haemolytic transfusion reactions (FNHTR) 246
fellowship programmes 373, <u>373</u>
Fellowship of the Royal College of Surgeons (FRCS(ORL-HNS)) 373, 374–5
fertility
   and radioiodine therapy 782
   Young's syndrome 1040–1
fibrin 260, <u>261</u>
fibrinogen <u>242</u>, 243, 244, 259, <u>260</u>
   defects/deficiency 264, 267
fibrinogen concentrate 273
fibrinolysis, endogenous 263, <u>263</u>
fibrinolytic agents 272
fibro-osseous lesions, orbit 1250–1
fibroblast growth factors (FGF) 122
   skin flap survival 115
   wound healing 95
fibroblasts
   carcinoma-associated 159
   thyroid gland 604
   wound healing 95, 97
fibronectin 97
fibrous dysplasia
   frontal sinus 1100, 1102, <u>1102</u>
   imaging 1312, <u>1313</u>
   orbit 1250, <u>1250</u>
fidaxomycin 187
fine-needle aspiration cytology (FNAC)
   lymphomas 252, 768
   medullary thyroid carcinoma 681, <u>683</u>, 759
   papillary thyroid carcinoma 670–1, <u>671</u>
   parathyroid carcinoma 859
   parathyroid glands 839

fine-needle aspiration cytology (FNAC) (*continued*)
   thyroid gland 653–7, *655*, <u>662–3</u>, 742–3
     iatrogenic changes 657–9, <u>658</u>
     international classification systems 654, *655*, *743*
     limitations 654, 656–7, 901
     lymphoma 768
finite element analysis (FEA) 112
Finnish Institute of Health, occupational rhinitis studies 1017
fissure burr 1141
flexible fibrescopes 316–17
Floseal 1176–7
flow cytometry 252
flow directed catheters 570
flow loop spirometry 313, 321, 821
fluconazole 217, 234
   nasal spray 1054
flucytosine 209, 287
fluid balance, critical care 355
fluid dynamics
   computational 1166, <u>1167</u>
   nose 986, <u>986</u>
fluid requirements, children 362–3, *363*
fluid therapy
   critical care 355
   improving oxygen delivery 357
flumetasone, ear drops 276
fluorescein
   intrathecal 1207–8, 1314, <u>1315</u>
   lacrimal duct patency assessment 1245
fluorescence *in situ* hybridization (FISH) 6
fluorinated nitromidazole compounds, hypoxia imaging 554
5-fluorouracil (5-FU), mechanism of action 42, <u>43</u>, *299*
fluticasone propionate 284
folic acid antagonists 42
follicle stimulating hormone (FSH) <u>636</u>, 637, 906
   excess 912, 917, 936
   measurement *918*, 936
follicular cells 604, <u>604</u>, 605
follicular tumour of uncertain malignant potential (FT-UMP) 665–6
folliculostellate cells 613
fondaparinux 271
food allergy 1003–4
food processing workers 1020
foods, inducing rhinitis 1014
foreign bodies 446–7
   iatrogenic 447
   ingestion 447
   inhaled 364–5, 447
   medical negligence claims 446–7
Forkhead transcription factors 65
Forrest plot 517, <u>518</u>
fosbretabulin 789
fospropofol 348
Foster Kennedy syndrome 1232
foundation training programme 373
fractional cell kill hypothesis 41
fractionation 52–3
fracture risk, primary hyperparathyroidism 844–5, 847
fractures, *see* facial fractures; nasal fractures

Francis Inquiry report 393, 414
free radical scavengers 113–14
free tissue grafts
   development 108
   skull base repair 945
fresh frozen plasma (FFP) 244
   in bleeding disorders 272
   in DIC 267
   reversal of raised INR *271*
frontal bone 1244
   zygomatic process 1244
frontal bulla cells 1084–5, <u>1085</u>
frontal ethmoidal cells 973–5, 1081, *1082*, <u>1082</u>, <u>1083</u>
frontal intersinus septal cells 1085, <u>1085</u>
frontal recess 1081–5, 1307
   accessory cells 1082–5, *1083*, <u>1083–5</u>, 1307, <u>1308</u>
   anatomical variants 1082, 1307
frontal sinus 1081–103
   accessory cells *1083*
   anatomy *972*, 973–5, 1081
   development 964
   endoscopy 1085
   facial fractures involving 1199
   fractures *1094*
   imaging 1085–6
   mucocele 1108–9, <u>1109</u>, 1110, <u>1110</u>
   ostium 1081, 1307, <u>1307–8</u>
   tumours 1098
frontal sinus surgery 1089–98
   benign tumours 1098–1103
   choice of procedure 1089–90, *1089*
   Draf classification *1090*
   Draf type 1 1090–2, <u>1090</u>
   Draf type 2 1091, <u>1091</u>
   Draf type 3 1091–2, *1092*, <u>1092</u>
   external frontoethmoidectomy 1097
   failure 1092–3
   frontal sinus cranialization 1097
   international classification *1090*
   malignant tumours 1103
   medical negligence claims 431
   obliteration 1110
   osteoplastic flap procedure 1093–6, 1100, <u>1100</u>
   outcomes for endoscopic 1093
   pneumosinus dilitans 1103
   Riedel's procedure 1097–8
   trephination 1088, 1097, <u>1097</u>
   complications 431
frontal sinusitis
   acute 1087–8, *1088*
   bony complications 1122–3, <u>1122</u>
   chronic 1088
   intracranial complications 1120–2, <u>1121</u>
frontal 'T' 1092, *1092*
frontobasal malformations, congenital 1086–7, *1087*
frontoethmoidectomy, external 1097
frontonasal beak 1081, <u>1307</u>
full blood count (FBC) 254–5
functional endoscopic sinus surgery (FESS) 214–15, 216
   complications 1076–7, 1205–6, <u>1205</u>
   eye preparation 1073
   nasal polyps 1043
   nasal preparation 289, 1073

   post-operative management 1075–6
   revision rates *1078*
   rhinosinusitis 1073–6
     allergic fungal 1051
     complications 1076–7
     evidence base 1077–8
     post-operative care 1075–6
   surgical position 1073
functional inferior turbinosurgery (FITS) 1162
fungal ball (mycetoma) *210*, 215, 1310
   clinical features 216
   definition 215
   diagnosis/imaging 1048, <u>1048</u>, <u>1309</u>, 1310
   management 216, 1048
   pathogenesis 216
   predisposing factors 215–16
fungal culture 206
fungal hyphae, histology <u>1051</u>
fungal infections
   diagnosis 206, <u>206</u>
   in haematological malignancies 253–4
   in HIV 233, <u>233</u>
   larynx, contact endoscopy 590, <u>590</u>
   otomycosis 208–9
   predisposing factors 208
   see also candidiasis; fungal ball; fungal rhinosinusitis
fungal rhinosinusitis 209–16
   acute invasive 209–11, 253–4, 1055, <u>1056</u>, 1309, <u>1309</u>
   chronic invasive 211–12, 1056, <u>1056</u>
   granulomatous invasive 212, 1056, 1309
   imaging 1309–10, <u>1309</u>
   non-invasive 1047–55
     allergic (AFRS) 212–15, 287, 1026, 1048–55, 1309–10
     fungal ball *210*, 215–16, 1048, <u>1048</u>
     saprophytic 1047, <u>1047</u>
fungal taxonomy 205
fungating wounds, management 300
Fusobacterium spp. 1118
Fusobacterium necrophorum 191

gabapentin 1258
gallium arsenide laser 582
gamma knife surgery, *see* stereotactic radiosurgery
ganciclovir 34
ganglioneuromas 758–9, <u>759</u>
gap junction proteins 16
gape, limitation 311, <u>312</u>
Gardner's syndrome 89, 1100
gastric parietal cell antibodies 154
gastro-oesophageal reflux, anaesthesia in 339
gefitinib 47, 56
gelatin particles 570–1, *571*
gender
   and anaplastic thyroid cancer 765
   and Graves' disease 726
   and occupational rhinitis 1017
   and papillary thyroid carcinoma 669
   and primary hyperparathyroidism 857, 879
   and prolactinoma/hyperprolactinaemia 907, *907*
   and smell function <u>1238</u>

gene, definition 4
gene arrays 11
gene expression 4–5
gene gun 29, 33
gene inactivation 9, 10, 11
gene mapping 10–11
gene methylation, thyroid tumours 85
gene sequencing 9
gene therapy
    clinical trials 29
    compromised skin flap 114–15
    cystic fibrosis 31–2
    definition 29
    delivery 29–30
    future research 35
    head and neck cancer 34–5
    immune modulation 34
    non-viral vectors 30, 31, 33
    restorative 34
    risks of 35
    viral vectors 30–1, 30, 203
gene translocations, thyroid tumours 84
General Medical Council (GMC) 391, 397, 405
    code of Good Medical Practice 305
    consent guidance 416, 900
    Curriculum Advisory Group 370
    ethical guidance 397
    medical negligence complaints 420, 421
    training assessment standards 371
general practitioners (GPs), medical negligence claims 430–1, 439, 440
general surgery, shared responsibility with endocrine/head and neck surgery 599–600
genetic testing
    immune deficiency 151
    MEN1 syndrome 87
    MEN2 syndrome 88, 88
    neurofibromatosis 2 22
genetics
    familial paragangliomas 22–4
    hearing loss 15–21
    neurofibromatosis 2 (NF2) 21–2
genome 3
    mitochondrial 3, 4
    nuclear 4
genotype–phenotype correlation 11
gentamicin 223
    intra-tympanic 279
Gentian Violet 209
GH1 gene mutations 926
ghrelin 632
giant cell granuloma 1221, 1221
gigantism 630
Gillick v. West Norfolk and Wisbech Area Health Authority 416
Gillies, Sir Harold 107, 112
Gillies temporal approach (zygoma fractures) 1197, 1197
Gilligan, Carol 397
gingivitis, in HIV 234, 235
Girard v. Royal Columbian Hospital 412
GJB2 (connexin 26) gene 16
Glanzmann's thromboasthenia 262, 269
Glasgow, OMFS Regional Centre 307
Glasgow Benefit Inventory (GBI) 488–9, 489, 978

Glasgow Hearing Aid Benefit Profile 490
gliomas, orbit 1251
glomus tumours, *see* paragangliomas
glossopharyngeal nerve, blockade 324
glottic irritability 325
gloves, latex 1021
glucagon stimulation test 918
glucocorticoid deficiency, familial 638
glucocorticoids
    circulating levels 934, 934
    exogenous 638
glucose in glycerine solution 289
glucose requirements, children 362–3
glucose tolerance test, oral 916, 916
glutathione (GSH) 54
glycaemic control, critical care 356
glycopeptide antibiotics 223
glycoprotein Ib/V/IX complex 262
glycoprotein IIb/IIIa complex 262
    receptor antagonist (Abciximab) 114, 271–2
glycopyrrolate 323
GNAS1 gene mutations 1100
goitre
    aetiology 76–8
    classification 75, 740, 740
    clinical presentation 706, 741
    definition 75
    diagnostic evaluation 741–3
    epidemiology 740
    Graves' disease 722
    hormonal factors in 79, 79
    intra-thoracic 819
        aetiology 819–20
        assessment for thyroidectomy 821
        clinical presentation 820
        investigations 820–1, 821
        non-surgical management 821–2
        surgery 822–4
    iodine deficiency 78, 78, 79, 736
    malignant potential 740
    management 743–4
    non-toxic multinodular 743–4
        surgery 794
    novel therapies 79
    pathophysiology 78–9, 78
    peri-operative airway concerns 890
    posterior mediastinal 824, 824
    spontaneous haemorrhage 821
    toxic multinodular 718, 723–4
        medical management 725, 726–7
        radioiodine therapy 729
    ultrasound 644
    weight of 819
    WHO definition 819
goitrogens 736
Goldzeiher's sign 706
gonadotrophin deficiency
    adult 928, 929
    isolated 925
gonadotrophin inhibitory hormone (GnIH) 636
gonadotrophin replacement 929
gonadotrophin-releasing hormone (GnRH) 635–6, 636
    isolated deficiency 925–6, 926
gonadotrophin-releasing hormone (GnRH) test 918

gonadotrophinomas 912, 917, 936
gonadotrophs 613, 631, 924
'good for' 399
Good Medical Practice 371, 373, 375
Goodpasture's syndrome 133
Google Scholar 498
GPA, *see* granulomatosis with polyangiitis
GRADE Working Group 474
graft osteoconduction 119
graft osteogenesis 119
graft osteoinduction 119
graft versus host disease (GvHD)
    stem cell transplantation 251, 257
    transfusion-associated (TA-GVHD) 243, 246
grafts
    collagen matrix 945
    nasal valve surgery 1144, 1144, 1145–6
    septal perforation repair 1153
    septoplasty 1139–40, 1140
    skull base reconstruction 945, 1208, 1278
Gram staining 181, 182
granulation tissue 96–7, 101, 103
granulocyte colony stimulating factor (GM-CSF) 159, 160, 249
granulocytes 125
granulomatosis with polyangiitis (GPA) 152, 174, 176, 977, 1214–18
    aetiology 1215
    age and gender 1215
    American College of Rheumatology criteria 1216
    clinical features 1215
    definition 1214–15
    diagnosis 1215–17, 1216, 1223
    failure to investigate 431
    nasal endoscopy 981
    nasal septal perforation 1151, 1215, 1216, 1217–18
    sinonasal 1032, 1033, 1215, 1216, 1217–18, 1310
    treatment 1217–18, 1223
granulomatous disorders 1211, 1212
    best clinical practice 1223
    cholesterol granuloma 1221–2
    classification 1211, 1212
    cocaine-induced midline destruction lesion (CIMDL) 1219, 1220
    eosinophilic granuloma 1219–21
    extranodal NK/T-cell lymphoma 1222–3, 1222, 1310
    future research 1223
    giant cell granuloma 1221, 1221
    GPA 152, 174, 176, 977, 1214–18
    nasal septal perforation 1151
    sarcoidosis 1211–14
granulomatous invasive fungal rhinosinusitis 212, 1056, 1309
grass pollen allergy 146
Graves' disease 621, 661, 720–3
    aetiology 721
    clinical manifestations 719, 722–3, 722, 723
    epidemiology 720
    history of treatment 599
    laboratory diagnosis 723
    medical management 722, 725, 726, 726

Graves' disease (continued)
  pathogenesis 720–1, 721
  in pregnancy 738, 739
  radioiodine therapy 724, 727, 729
  surgical management 731, 794–5
  thyroid antibodies 711–12
  ultrasound 644
Greece 423
growth factors
  in goitre development 79, 79
  tumour microenvironment 159
  in wound healing 95, 97
growth hormone 613, 630–3
  changes through life 633, 634
  deficiency 906, 928
    adult-onset 928, 928
    congenital isolated 926
  excess 630, 647, 908
  laboratory tests 916, 918
  replacement 928
growth hormone antagonists 933, 953
growth hormone receptor (GHR) 630, 631
growth hormone-releasing hormone (GHRH) 632, 632, 918, 919
growth hormone-releasing peptides (GHRPs) 919
guaifensin 233
guar gum 1020

H1N1 virus ('swine 'flu') 198
H5N1 virus ('avian 'flu') 198
Hadad nasoseptal flap 1278
'Hadad-Bassagasteguy' flap 942, 1206, 1278
haematological malignancies 250–1
  aetiologies 250–1
  presentations in ENT 251–3
  treatment 251
  treatment complications 253–4
haematology laboratory
  basic tests 254–6
  management of thrombotic or bleeding patient 273
haematomas
  nasal septum 434, 1186, 1188
  orbit 1076, 1076
  post-operative 888
  tissue compromise 113
haematopoiesis 249–50, 250
haematopoietic stem cell transplantation (HSCT) 251, 253, 254
haematopoietic stem cells (HSC) 70, 249–50
haemodilution, acute normovolaemic 247
haemofiltration 355
haemoglobin (Hb) 255
  blood donor 240
  targets in blood transfusion 243
haemolytic complement tests 151
haemophagocytic lymphohistiocytosis (HLH) 174
haemophilia 265–6
Haemophilus influenzae 189, 233, 1027, 1032, 1039, 1118
Haemophilus influenzae B (Hib) 364
haemorrhage
  after thyroid surgery 888, 893, 895, 901
  after tonsillectomy 345, 349, 445

anaemia 255
  in endoscopic sinus surgery 1076
  facial fractures 1190, 1190
  spontaneous in goitre 821
  transfusion management 242–3, 242
haemostasis
  medication affecting 270–2
  thyroidectomy 797, 801–2
  wound healing 95
haemostatic agents, topical 1176–7
haemostatic clips 1177, 1177
hair cells, stem cell regeneration 71
hairy leukoplakia 201–2, 234, 235
Haller cell 973
hallucinations, olfactory 1230, 1235
halogenated pyrimidines 54
halothane 325, 335
Halsted, William 598, 599, 794
harm principle 398
Hashimoto's thyroiditis 662, 735
  histology 654, 656, 735, 735
  pathogenesis 735
  ultrasound 644
Hasner's valve 968, 1158, 1244
head injuries
  CSF leak 1204
  epistaxis 1179
  smell loss 1235, 1236
head and neck squamous cell carcinoma (HNSCC)
  chemotherapy 44, 45
  genetic changes 65–7
  and HPV infection 170
  immunotherapy 161–2
  photodynamic therapy 585
  recurrence 45
  risk factors 66
  tumour biomarkers 161, 162–3
  tumour escape mechanisms 160
  tumour microenvironment 157–60
head and neck surgery
  enhanced recovery 307
  patient preparation 306
  post-operative ventilation 340
headaches 1255–8
  analgesia-dependency 1259–60
  cervicogenic 1260
  cluster 1257, 1257
  migraine 1255–6, 1255
  pituitary adenomas 951
  pituitary apoplexy 912
  tension-type 1256–7, 1256
health, definitions 399
health promotion 399
Health Service Commissioner 420
health services research 468
Health and Social Care Act (2008) 414
Health Utilities Index (HUI) 486, 487, 489, 491–2
  HUI-II 489, 491
  HUI-III 489, 492
health-related quality of life (HRQoL) 484
healthcare costs
  asthma and allergic rhinitis 1130
  rhinosinusitis 1027
healthcare workers, occupational rhinitis 1021, 1022
hearing aid questionnaires 490

Hearing Handicap Inventory for the Elderly (HHIE) 490
hearing loss
  apoptosis in 59, 64
  failure to diagnose cause 444
  in GPA 1215, 1218
  hereditary 11, 24
    classification 15
    genetics 15–21
    neurofibromatosis 2 20, 21–2
    non-syndromeic 16–18, 19, 24
    syndromic 19–21
  in HIV 232
  medical negligence claims 439–40, 443, 444–5
  noise-induced, medical reports 418
  otosclerosis, treatment 280
  patient communication 385
  patient-reported assessment instruments 490
  post-operative 445
  rheumatological disease 174, 176–7
  virus-associated 199, 200, 201
'heart sink' patients 385
heavy metals, chemotherapy 41–2
Heerfordt's syndrome 1213
Heimlich manoeuvre, children 365
heliox 296, 300, 321
helium-neon laser (He-Ne) 116
hemicrania, paroxysmal 1257
hemicrania continua 1257–8
hemilaryngectomy 347
Henry technique 812, 812
heparin
  adverse effects 268, 294
  low molecular weight 270, 271, 294
  mechanism of action 293–4
  unfractionated 271
heparin-induced thrombocytopenia (HIT) 255–6, 268
hereditary haemorrhagic telangiectasia (HHT/Osler-Weber-Rendu disease) 289, 577, 1178, 1180
hereditary periodic fever syndromes (HPFSs) 178
herpes labialis 234
herpes simplex thymidine kinase (HSV-TK) 34
herpes simplex viruses (HSV) 199
  in HIV 234, 235
  type 1 (HSV-1) 199, 201
  type 2 (HSV-2) 199
herpes zoster infection, neuralgia following 1258
herpes zoster oticus 232, 280
heterosmia 1231
hiatus emilunaris 981
High Court 413
high dependency unit (HDU) 351, 351
high frequency jet ventilation (HFJV) 338
high molecular weight compounds, causing occupational rhinitis 1018, 1019
higher specialty training (HST) 373, 373
highly-active antiretroviral therapy (HAART) 230–1
Hippocratic Oath 393
Hippocratic technique 1175
Hirudo medicinalis 116

histamine 140, 999
histamine H$_2$ receptor antagonists 298
histone proteins 858
histopathology interpretation, medical negligence claims 428
Hodgkin's lymphoma 202, 251
holmium yttrium aluminium garnet (Ho-YAG) laser 1164
holoprosencephaly 925
homocysteine levels 270
honesty, in patient communication 404–5
Hopp v. Lepp 415
hormonal rhinitis 1013
hormone replacement therapy (HRT)
    gonadotrophin deficiency 929
    primary hyperparathyroidism 847
Horner's syndrome, intra-thoracic goitre 820
Horsley, Sir Victor 1281
hospital administration, medical negligence claims 423–4
hospital-acquired infections 450
Hounsfield units 561
house dust mite 147
    allergen reduction 1003, *1004*
House of Lords 399, 410, 411, 415, 422
Howarth's elevator 1187
HRPT2 gene 87, 858, 860–1
Human Genome Mapping Project 9, 10–11
human herpesvirus-8 (HHV-8) 231
human immunodeficiency virus (HIV) 229–30
human immunodeficiency virus (HIV) infection 151
    acute 231
    CD4+ cell counts 230, 231
    cervical lymphadenopathy 231
    epidemiology 229
    Kaposi's sarcoma 231–2
    oropharyngeal candidiasis 216–17, 233–4, 235, *235*
    phases 230
    public health interventions 229
    rhinosinusitis 1032, *1033*
    therapy 230–1
human leucocyte antigens (HLA) 128, 160
human papilloma virus (HPV) 66, 167, 199
    associated pathologies 200, *200*
    and cancer 169–70, *169*, 202
    detection 170
    gene products 167, *168*
    genome 167, *168*
    genotypes 167
    in HIV 234, *234*
    life cycle 167–9, *168*
    p16 163
    transmission 167–8
    vaccines 202
human rights 400, 417
Human Rights Act (1998) 417, 421
Hume, D. 395–6
humoral hypercalcaemia 830, 831
Humphrey visual field analyser 911, *912*
hungry bone syndrome 345
Hunsaker tube 338, 339
Hunter's syndrome 311
Hürthle cell neoplasms 550, 654, 714, 785
Hürthle cells (Askanazy cells) 661, 735

hyalinizing trabecular tumours, thyroid 666, 666
hybridization 6, 6
hydrochlorothiazide 279
hydrogen peroxide 295
hydroxychloroquine 1214
hygiene hypothesis 138
hyper IgD syndrome with periodic fever syndrome 178
hyperbaric oxygen 53, 211
hypercalcaemia
    acute treatment 861, 883
    asymptomatic 828
    causes 828, *828*
    clinical evaluation 828
    diagnostic imaging 831
    differential diagnosis *829*
    familial hypocalciuric (FHH) *829*, 830, 882
    hyperparathyroidism 692, 829–30
        medical management 847
        persistent after surgery 894, *895*
    laboratory evaluation 828–31, *829*
        non-parathyroid endocrine disease 831
        serum calcium 827–8
        serum parathyroid hormone 829–30
        serum phosphate 831
        urinary calcium/Ca: Cr ratio 830
        vitamin d metabolites 830–1
    malignancy-associated 692, 828, *829*, 830, 831
    medullary thyroid cancer 760
    parathyroid carcinoma 858, 861
hypercortisolism 908–10, 916–17
    causes 934
    diagnosis 934–5, *935*
    management 935, 954–5
hyperemesis gravidarum 738–9
hyperfractionation 53
hyperglycaemia, critically ill patient 356
hyperhomocystinaemia 270
hyperkalaemia, heparin therapy 294
hyperosmia 1230, 1234
hyperparathyroidism
    classification 843, *844*
    hereditary syndromes 86, 700, 866–7
        MEN 1 852, 866
        MEN 2A 866–7
        non-MEN 867
    laboratory evaluation 828–31, 829–31, 874
    localization studies 833–9
    persistent 851–4, 881–2
        failure of surgery 851–2, *852*, 854, 882
        investigation 882–3
        reoperation 852–4
    primary, *see* primary hyperparathyroidism
    secondary 345, 691, *691*, 838, 843, *844*, 867–8
    tertiary 691, 828, 829, 843, *844*, 867
hyperparathyroidism with jaw tumours (HPT-JT), genetics 86, 87, 88–9, 700, 858, 867
hyperprolactinaemia 635, 907–8
    diagnosis 916, *916*

differential diagnosis 908, *908*
management 906–7, 932, 952
hypersalivation 444
hypersensitivity 133–5
    type I (immediate) 133, 134, 137, *138*
    type II (cell/membrane reactive) 133, 134, *138*
    type III (immune complex mediated) 133, 134, *138*
    type IV (cell-mediated) 134, 134, *138*
hypertension, and epistaxis 1175
hyperthyroidism 717–33
    aetiology 718, *718*
    clinical manifestations 705–6, 718–19
    definitions 717, *718*
    diagnosis 719–20, *719*, *720*
    epidemiology 718
    eye disease, *see* eye disease, hyperthyroidism
    Graves' disease 720–3
    medical management 297, 724–7, *725*
    pituitary adenoma 912
    in pregnancy 738
    principles of management 724, *724*
    radioiodine therapy 727–9
    solid toxic adenoma (Plummer's disease) 724
    subclinical 717, *718*, 731, *731*
    surgical management 729–31
    toxic multinodular goitre 723–4
hypertrophic scars 102, 433, 815, 890
    medical negligence claims 433
hyperviscosity 253
hypervitaminosis A 831
hypoadrenalism 736, 737, 906, *906*
hypocalcaemia
    after parathyroid surgery 298, 345, 625, 854, 884, 889, 894
    after thyroid surgery 298, 345, 730, 889, 894, *895*, 902
    drugs used 298, 889
hypogonadism 905, *906*
    hypogonadotrophic 925
    hypothalamic 636
hyponatraemia, hypovolaemic 919–20
hypoparathyroidism
    hypocalcaemia management 298, 298, *854*
    post-operative 625, 852, 854, *854*, 889
hypophyseal arteries 614, 614
hypophysis cerebri, *see* pituitary gland
hypophysitis, lymphocytic 927–8
hypopituitarism
    clinical manifestations 905–6, 905
    investigations 918–19, *918*
    post-operative 937
hyposmia 1230
hypotension, controlled in ear surgery 348
hypothalamic–pituitary-adrenal (HPA) axis 619, 621, 637–8, 637
    and corticosteroid therapy 1054
hypothalamus 629, 632, 923, 924
hypothermia, in surgery 343
hypothetical imperative 398
hypothyroidism
    aetiology 734, *734*
    central 736, 737, 906, *906*, 926
    chronic autoimmune, *see* Hashimoto's thyroiditis

hypothyroidism (continued)
    clinical manifestations 705, 734–5
    definitions 733, *733*
    diagnostic tests *720*, 735, *735*, *737*
    effects in adults *620*
    epidemiology 733
    iatrogenic 735–6
        radioiodine therapy 736, 744
        thyroid/parathyroid surgery 889–90
    iodine deficiency 736
    neonatal 712, 736
    in pregnancy 737, 739–40
    subclinical 737–8
        in pregnancy 739–40
        risk of overt hypothyroidism 712, *712*
    treatment 297, 736–7
        pre-operative 626
hypothyroxinaemia 733, *733*
hypoxia inducible factor 1α (HIF-1α) 159
hypoxic cells
    PET tracers detecting 554
    radioresistance 53–4
HYTEC-288 system 145

ibuprofen 1256
icatibant 296
IDEAL Collaboration 480
Ikarian Reefer 418
'illness perspective' 379
illness severity scores 352
I'M SAFE mnemonic 462
image-guided surgery 559–66
    clinical applications 565
    image reconstruction 560–1
    pixels and voxels 561
    recurrent pituitary tumours 942–3, 943
    registration 562–4, 565–6
    skull base surgery 565, 1274, 1283
    surface rendering 561, 562
    surgical planning 565
    tracking 564
    vestibular schwannoma 560
    volume averaging 561
    volume rendering 561–2
imaging 1305–16
    best clinical practice *1316*
    CSF leaks 1314, 1314–15
    diffusion-weighted (DWI) 1315–16
    future research *1316*
    sinonasal anatomy 1307, 1308
    sinonasal tumours 1310–14
    sinus inflammatory disease 1308–10
    see also individual imaging modalities
imatinib 251
imidazoles 287
immediate haemolytic transfusion reactions 244–5
Immulite system 145
immune checkpoint inhibitors 48
immune response
    anti-tumour 160
    cytosolic infectious agents 130, 132
    extra-cellular and vesicular infectious agents 129–32
    stages 126, 126
    tissue damaging 133–4

immune thrombocytopenic purpura (ITP) 255, 267–8
immunity
    adaptive 125–6
    innate 125, 126
immunoassays, allergic disease 145, *145*
ImmunoCAP 145
immunochemotherapy, thyroid lymphoma 769
immunodeficiency
    investigations 149–52, *150*
    presentations in ENT 149, *150*
    primary 149
    rhinosinusitis 1032
    types of pathogens 149, *150*
immunoediting 160
immunoglobulin A (IgA)
    deficiency 154, 1032
    nasal mucosa 988
immunoglobulin E (IgE)
    allergen-specific (sIgE) 137, 138, 999
        measurement 145, 145, 147, 152
    in allergic fungal rhinosinusitis 1049
    anti-IgE antibody therapy 143, 1007, 1055, 1063, 1129
    high affinity receptors (FcεRI) 138–9, 141
    hypersensitivity 140, 141, *142*
    local synthesis 140
    in nasal polyposis 1039
    total levels 152
immunoglobulin G (IgG)
    deficiency 1032
    functional properties *130*
    maternal 130
    subclasses *130*, 150
immunoglobulin G kappa chain (IgGκC) 161
immunoglobulins (Ig) 125
    classes 127, 130, *130*
    effector functions 129–30
    excess 253
    isotype switching 140, 140
    structure 126, *127*
immunological tests 149–54
    autoimmune disease 152–4
    future research 154
    immunodeficiency 149–52
'immunonutrition' 355–6
immunoreceptor tyrosine-based activation motif (ITAM) 141
immunosuppression
    fungal rhinosinusitis 209–11, 253–4, 1055
    haematological cancer therapy 253–4
    rheumatological disease 179
    tumour cells 159
immunotherapy
    allergen-specific 143, 147
        allergic fungal rhinosinusitis 215, 1054
        allergic rhinitis 1006–7
    asthma and rhinitis 1129–30
    cancers 48, 161–2
    occupational rhinitis 1023
in situ hybridization 6, *6*
incidence, definition 467
incompetent adult 398, 416

indoloquinone EO9 54
industrial dusts 1017–18, *1233*
inferior turbinates 987
    anatomy 968, 1158, 1158
    enlargement 987, 1015, 1146, 1157–9, 1158–9, 1159
        clinical features 1159, 1160
        medical management 1160
        pathogenesis 1146, 1159
        in septal deviation 1146, 1165
    evaluation 1159–60, 1161
    functions 987, 988, 1158
    lateralization 1162
    recent research 1166, 1167
    reduction surgery 1146, 1160–7, *1162*
        best clinical practice *1167*
        children 1165
        Cochrane review 1168
        complications 1165, 1179
        future research *1167*
        history 1158
        NICE guidance 1168
        outcomes 1165–6
        rhinosinusitis 1164
        in septal surgery 1165
        in septorhinoplasty 1165
        sleep-disordered breathing 1165
        trends 1157, 1157
    in septal deviation 1165
inflammation 132–3
    asthma and rhinitis 1127
    tumour microenvironment 160
    wounds 96
inflammatory markers, thyroid disease 712
inflammatory mediators 132
    allergic rhinitis 999, 1127
    asthma 1127
influenza virus 195, 198, 198
    antiviral drugs 202–3
information bias 475
informed consent 304–5
    anaesthesia 304
    children 416
    disclosure of risks of surgery 415–16, 417
    incompetent adult 398, 416
    Jehovah's witnesses 416–17
    medical ethics 401–2
    medical negligence and 415–17, 429–30, 900
    planned surgery 304–5
    thyroidectomy 795
    robot-assisted 815
    tonsillectomy 445
infraorbital artery 965
inhalation anaesthesia 325, 341
inhalation anaesthetic agents 335–6
inherited cancer syndromes 87–9
innate immune system 125, 126
inner ear infections 232–3
inpatient stay, thyroidectomy 901
inquests 418
Institute of Medicine (IOM) 389
insulin resistance, and goitre formation 77
insulin therapy, 'intensive' 356
insulin tolerance test *918*, *919*
insulin-like growth factor (IGF), in goitre development 79, *79*

insulin-like growth factor type 1 (IGF-1) 632, 632, 633
   acromegaly diagnosis 933
   in GH replacement 916, 928
integrins 47, 132
intensive care unit (ICU)
   levels of care 351, 351
   paediatric, see paediatric intensive care
intention-to-treat 479, 512–13
intercavernous venous sinuses 615
Intercollegiate Surgical Curriculum Programme (ISCP) assessments 371, 374
interferon gamma (IFN-γ) 129, 129, 139
interferon-alpha/beta (IFN α/β), viral infections 132, 202
interleukin-1 (IL-1) 133
   in wound healing 95
interleukin-4 (IL-4) 129, 129, 143
interleukin-5 (IL-5) 129, 129, 143
   allergic airway diseases 1128
   monoclonal antibody 143, 1063
interleukin-6 (IL-6) 133
interleukin-10 (IL-10) 129, 129
interleukin-12 (12) 139
interleukin-13 (IL-13) 129, 129
interleukin-17 (IL-17) 129, 129
interleukins, tumour microenvironment 159
intermaxillary bone pins 1192–3
intermaxillary fixation (IMF) 1191–3, 1191–2
internal carotid artery 1170, 1173
   anastomosis 1170
   cavernous sinus 944, 944
   injury in sinus surgery 1077, 1179
internal consistency 485–6
internal jugular vein (IJV), thyroid cancer involvement 808–9
internal maxillary artery (IMA)
   embolization 576–7
   ligation 576, 1177–8
International Headache Society 1262
international normalized ratio (INR) 263
   monitoring in anticoagulation 294–5
   reversal of raised 271, 271
International Study on Asthma and Allergy in Children (ISAAC) 1000
interventional neuroradiology (INR) 569
   chemotherapy delivery 572
   future research 578
   indications 569–70, 570
   temporary and permanent large artery occlusions 572
   tools and techniques 570–1
   tumour embolization 571–2
      juvenile angiofibroma 576, 577
      meningioma 573–5
      paragangliomas 575–6
      percutaneous 572
      transarterial 571–2
intra-dermal test (IDT) 144
intra-operative nerve monitoring
   ear surgery 442
   facial nerve 343, 346, 525–7
   thyroid surgery 337, 345, 600, 800, 888–9, 901
intracranial hypertension, benign 1205
intranasal preparation 289, 1073, 1274
intrathecal fluorescein 1207–8, 1314, 1315

intravenous immunoglobulin (IVIg) 267, 273
intrinsic factor antibodies 154
intubating laryngeal mask airway 317, 317
inverted papilloma 1311, 1312
   endoscopic surgery 1275–6
   frontal sinus 1098–9, 1099
involuntary manslaughter 422–3
iodine
   deficiency 76, 76, 622, 736
      epidemiology 736
      goitre formation 78, 78, 79, 736
   excess 622, 723
   intake prior to radioiodine therapy 781
   recommended dietary intake 622
   therapy 297
   and thyroid function 619, 620, 622
ipilimumab 162, 955
ipratropium bromide 289, 985, 1005, 1006, 1014
iron deficiency anaemia 247
irritant chemicals, occupational rhinitis 1018
irritants, respiratory 1013
ischaemia-reperfusion injury, skin flaps 113
ischaemic preconditioning, skin flap 115
isoflavones 77
isoflurane 335
isolated GnRH-deficiency (IGD) 925–6, 926
isolation, radioiodine therapy 782
itraconazole 215, 217, 1053
   side effects 1053

Jansen-type metaphyseal chondrodysplasia 831
Janus kinase 2 (JAK2) 630, 631
Jarjavay fracture 1184, 1185
jaw, receding 311, 311
jaw slide 312
Jehovah's Witnesses 247, 399, 416–17
Jervell and Lange-Nielsen syndrome 20
jet ventilation 327–8, 327, 338
Jobson Horne probe 1143
Jod Basedow effect 723
Joint Committee on Surgical Training (JCST) 371
Joll's triangle 799
jugular veins
   anterior 796
   internal, thyroid cancer involvement 808–9
justice 400
juvenile angiofibroma 1265–8
   arterial supply 1266
   best clinical practice 1267–8
   branchial arch artery theory 1266
   clinical findings 1265–6, 1266
   endoscopic resection 1266–7, 1274, 1274
      indications/limitations 1267
   epidemiology 1265
   imaging 1271, 1312, 1313
   pre-operative embolization 576, 577, 1266
   tissue architecture 1266

Kahneman, Daniel 457
Kallmann's syndrome 636, 926, 926, 1231

Kant, I. 398
Kaposi's sarcoma 231–2, 233
   larynx/pharynx 235
   oral 234, 234, 235
Kartagener's syndrome 1032, 1040, 1041
Kawasaki disease 175–6
Keen intra-oral approach (zygoma fractures) 1197, 1197
keloid scars 102, 815, 890
   medical negligence claims 433
   thyroid/parathyroid surgery 813, 890
Keogh report 393
keratinocytes, wound healing 95, 96
keratosis, vocal cords, contact endoscopy 590–1, 591
Kerrison Rongeur 944
Kerrison's punch 1074–5, 1075
ketoconazole 287
   corticotroph adenomas 954
ketotifen 1004
Kiesselbach's plexus (Little's area) 967, 967, 968, 1169
Killian incision 1137, 1138
KISS-R 636
kisspeptin 636
Klebsiella ozaenae 1014
Knudson's 'two-hit' hypothesis 8
Kocher collar incision 795–6, 796, 811
Kocher, Theodor 598–9, 598, 793, 811
koilocytes 592, 593
Korean Central Cancer Registry 901
Kralj v. McGrath 412
Kupferberg endoscopic staging (AFRS) 1052
Kupffer cells 250
Kveim test 1213

labial artery, superior 965
labour 640
lacrimal bone 1243, 1244, 1244
lacrimal duct 968
lacrimal gland tumours 1251
lacrimal probe 1245, 1246, 1246
lacrimal sac 1244
   marsupialization 1246, 1246
β-lactamases 189, 225
β-lactams 223, 225
lactate dehydrogenase 768
lactation 635, 640, 640
lactotrophs 631, 635, 924
lamellipodia 96
lamina papyracea 970, 1081, 1243, 1244
   breach in sinus surgery 1076, 1076
lamina propria 985, 1127
lamotrigine 1258
Langerhans cell histiocytosis, see eosinophilic granuloma
Langerhans cells 108, 169, 1219, 1220
lanreotide 787
lapatinib 22, 162
Laplace's law 111
Laryngeal Cancer Study Group 44
laryngeal carcinoma
   contact endoscopy 591, 591
   medical negligence claims 450
   PET-CT imaging 548, 548
   photodynamic therapy 585
laryngeal dystonia 296

laryngeal injuries
    children 363
    difficult airway management 329
laryngeal mask airway (LAM) 317–18, 336, <u>336</u>
    intubating 317, <u>317</u>
    intubation via 318, <u>318</u>
laryngeal nerves, *see* recurrent laryngeal nerve; superior laryngeal nerve
laryngeal surgery, children 365–6
laryngectomy
    anaesthesia 347
    Candida biofilms 217
    pre-operative care 306
    thyroid cancer spread 807–8, <u>808</u>
laryngitis
    contact endoscopy 590, <u>590</u>
    medical negligence claims 449–50
laryngopharyngeal injury, children 365
laryngopharyngeal reflux, treatment 298–9
laryngopharyngectomy, poorly differentiated thyroid cancer <u>678</u>
laryngoscope blades 310, 315–17, <u>316</u>
laryngoscopy
    difficult airway 309–10
    prediction of difficult 313–14, *313*
laryngotracheobronchitis, acute viral (croup) 364
larynx
    contact endoscopy 589–93
    cricoid pressure 341
    involvement in thyroid cancer 807–8, <u>808</u>
    optical coherence tomography 535–6, <u>535</u>
    paediatric anatomy 361–2
    papilloma 200, 591–3
    stem cell therapies 71–2
laser capture microdissection (LCM) 7
laser light, nature of 581
laser skin resurfacing 439
laser surgery
    anaesthesia 346
        choice of airway device 339–40
    safety 584
    turbinate reduction 1164
lasers
    applications in ENT 584
    delivery devices 582–3, <u>583</u>
    history of development 581
    micromanipulators 582
    principles of 581–2
    and skin flap survival 116
    tissue interactions 582, 583–4
    types 581–2
Lasting Power of Attorney 398
lateral opticocarotid recess (LOCR) 613, 944, <u>944</u>
latex allergy 306, 1021
Le Fort injuries <u>1194–5</u>, 1195
leadership, surgeon 460–2
leeches, skin flaps 116
legal aid 414
Lemièrre's syndrome 191
lentivirus, gene therapy vectors 30, 31, 33
Leonard button 1192, <u>1192</u>
lethal midline granuloma (extranodal NK/T-cell lymphoma) 1222–3, <u>1222</u>, 1310

leucocytes 249
    digestive 131–2
    inflammatory 132
leucocytosis, neutrophil 256
leucopheresis 253
leucostasis 253
leucotriene receptor antagonists 147
leukaemias 250–1
    aetiology 251
    diagnosis 251, 252
    presentations in ENT 251–3
    risk in radioiodine therapy 782
    treatment 251
leukotriene receptor antagonists 215, 288
    allergic rhinitis 1006, 1129
    asthma 1129
    chronic rhinosinusitis 1063
    and EGPA 1218
levocabastine 287
levothyroxine 297, 736–7
    monitoring of therapy 711
    radioiodine remnant ablation 780
lifestyle changes, reflux oesophagitis 298
lignocaine
    airway topicalization 323–4
    sprays and lozenges 295
    transendoscopic administration 324
likelihood ratio 510, <u>511</u>
Likert scale 486
Lim v. Camden Health Authority 412
limen nasi 964
lincosamides 223
linezolid 223
linkage analysis 10
liothyronine 297, 626
    radioiodine therapy 780
lipoadenoma (parathyroid hamartoma) 694, <u>695</u>
liposomes, gene delivery 33
liposuction 437
5-lipoxygenase (5-LOX) 160
literature, critical appraisal 498, *500*
literature searches 497–8, *498*, <u>499</u>
lithium therapy 692, 721
Little's area 967, *967*, <u>968</u>, 1169
liver disease
    autoimmune 154
    and coagulation 269
Livingstone v. Rawyards Coal Company 412
local allergic rhinitis 141–2
local anaesthesia
    airway 323–4
    nasal fracture reduction 1186
    post-operative 305
local anaesthetics 295
    and nasal mucosa 985
Local Education and Training Boards (LETBs) 370, 374
LOD scores 10
loratadine 287, 1004
loss of heterozygosity (LOH) 7–9, 11
low frequency jet ventilation (LFJV) 338
low molecular weight compounds, causing occupational rhinitis 1018, *1019*
low molecular weight heparins (LMWH) 270, 271, 294
lower respiratory tract, mucosa 1127, <u>1127</u>

lozenges 295
Ludwig's angina <u>321</u>, 322
Lugol's iodine 729
lumbar drains 1208
Lund–Mackay score 1042, *1042*
lung collapse, ventilated child 366
lung disease
    in GPA 1215
    sarcoidosis 1213, 1214, <u>1214</u>
lung injury, transfusion-related acute (TRALI) 245
lupus pernio 1211, 1213, <u>1213</u>, 1214
luteinizing hormone (LH) 636–7, 906, *918*
Lyme disease 192
lymphadenopathy
    cervical, *see* cervical lymphadenopathy
    rheumatological disorders 174
lymphatic system 250
lymphocyte phenotyping (subsets) 150–1
lymphocyte proliferation assays 151
lymphocytes 125, 249, 250
    abnormalities 256
    activation 126
    tumour-infiltrating 158–9, 161, 163
    wound healing 95, 96
lymphocytosis 256
lymphoepithelial cyst 235–6, <u>236</u>
lymphomas 251–3
    diagnosis 252
    and EBV virus 202
    extranodal NK/T-cell 1222–3, <u>1222</u>, 1310
    hypercalcaemia 831
    orbit 1251
    presentations in ENT 251–3
    sinonasal 1312
    T-cell 202, 251, 1310, 1312
    thyroid 644, 656–7, 706, 768–9, <u>770</u>
lymphoproliferative disease, immunological tests 154
Lynch incision 1097
Lynch-Howarth fronto-ethmoidectomy 431, 1110, 1119
lysine-aspirin 288, 1063

MacConkey agar 189, <u>190</u>
McCoy laryngoscope blade 315, <u>316</u>
McCune-Albright syndrome 647, 1102
McGill Pain Questionnaire 491
Macintosh laryngoscope blade 315
macroautophagy 62
macrolide antibiotics 223
    antibacterial spectrum *278*
    commonly used 223
    nasal polyposis 1043
    rhinosinusitis 285–6, 1062
macrophage activation syndromes (MAS) 174
macrophage inhibitory factor (MIF) 159
macrophages 125, 126, <u>126</u>
    wound healing 95, 96
MAGIC syndrome 177
magnetic resonance imaging (MRI)
    cisternography 1207, 1314
    diffusion-weighted 1315–16
    frontal sinus 1086
    frontal sinus tumours 1098
    fungal rhinosinusitis <u>1050</u>, 1051

magnetic resonance imaging (MRI) (*continued*)
  GPA 1216–17
  intracranial complications of sinusitis 1120, 1121
  medullary thyroid cancer 760, 760
  mucoceles 1109, 1109
  paranasal sinuses 1086, 1306, 1306, 1308, 1308
  parathyroid adenomas 838
  PET integration (PET-MRI) 555
  pituitary disease 645–9, 646, 647, 917, 930–1, 931
  sinonasal tumours 1270–2, 1271
  sinus secretions 1306, 1306
  skull base surgery 1283
  technical aspects 1305–6
  thyroid disease 644, 714
    intra-thoracic goitre 820
Mahon v. Osborne 412
major histocompatibility complex (MHC) 128
  class I molecules 128, 128, 132, 160
  class II molecules 128–9, 128
malar augmentation 438
male fertility
  radioiodine therapy 782
  Young's syndrome 1040–1
malignancy
  failures to diagnose 431
  hypercalcaemia 692, 828, *829*, 830, 831
  risk in primary hyperparathyroidism 845
malingering 1231, 1239
Mallampati scoring 312, *313*
malnutrition
  categories 99
  and wound healing 98–9, 99
MALT lymphomas 768, 769
mammalian target of rapamycin (mTOR) 22, 65–7, 66
mammotrophs 613
mandible, lines of weakness 1191, 1191
mandibular fractures 1191–4
  condylar neck 1192, 1193–4
mandibular protrusion 312
mannan-binding lectin (MBL) 131
manslaughter, involuntary 422–3
Manuka honey 1054–5, 1055
mapatumumab 65
Marjolin's ulcer 99
mast cells 132, 133, 134, 138, 139, *140*
  cell membrane stabilizers 147
  degranulation 999
matching 475
matrix 2 ion channel blockers 202
matrix metalloproteinase 2 (MMP-2) 159
mattress sutures, nasal valve surgery 1145
maxilla, fractures 1194–6, 1194
maxillary antrostomy 1247, 1250, 1275
maxillary antrum, pyomucocele 1254, 1254
maxillary artery 1170, 1171
maxillary nerve 965
maxillary sinus
  development 962–3, 962
    fungal ball 1048
    hypoplasia 962–3, 963
    imploding (silent sinus syndrome) 1249, 1250, 1310, 1311

mucoceles 1110
  retention cyst 1308, 1308
  roof (orbital floor) 970, 971, 1244, 1248
maximum surgical blood ordering system (MSBOS) 241, *241*
mean arterial blood pressure (MAP) 1072
mean corpuscular haemoglobin (MCH) 254
mean corpuscular volume (MCV) 254
measles 199
measles, mumps, rubella (MMR) vaccine 199, 439
mecA gene 225
medial maxillectomy 1275
medial opticocarotid recess (MOCR) 613
median thyroid anlage 605
mediastinum
  enlarged thyroid 824, 824
  parathyroid adenoma 884
Medic Alert 329
Medical Devices Agency 584
medical errors
  disclosure 405, 900–1
  discussion with patient 385
  mortality from 389
medical ethics
  acts *versus* omissions 403–4
  changes in focus of 396
  and children 402–3
  and competence 402
  and confidentiality 405
  consultation 405–6
  definitions 395–6
  doctrine of double effect 404
  four principles approach 401
  further study 406
  and informed consent 401–2
  methods 396–7
  official guidance 397, 405–6
  and rationing/resource allocation 404
  and research 403
  and truth-telling/disclosure 404–5
medical negligence
  causation 411
  complaints to NHS Trusts 420–1
  and consent to surgery 415–17, 429–30, 900
  criminal offences 421–3
  damages 409, 414
    general 409, 412
    paid by NHS 414
    punitive 409, 423
    special 409, 412
  legal tort 410–12, 899
  proof of negligence 411–12
  standard of care 410–11
medical negligence claims
  against GPs 430–1, 439, 440
  best clinical practice 451
  coroner's court 417–18
  cosmetic surgery 428–9, 436–8
  difficult airway management 329
  duty of candour 414
  duty of confidentiality 417
  endoscopic sinus surgery 427–8, 429, 1073
  facial nerve injury 526
  failure to consider conservative treatment 428
  funding 414

guidelines 423
head and neck surgery 448–50
histopathology interpretation 428
hospital administration 423–4
interpretation of imaging 427–8
otology and neuro-otology 439–45
paediatric otolaryngology 445–8
patient selection and 428–9
procedures and time limits 412–13
requirements of the law 899
rhinology and facial plastic surgery 430–9
role of medical experts 413, 418–20
settlements 413
skin cancer 436
skin surgery 433
smell dysfunction 1228, 1239
standard of proof 409–10
surgical infection 450
thyroid/parathyroid surgery 899–902
trial and preparation for trial 413–14
tumour recurrence 430
witness statements 413
Medical Outcomes Study (MOS) Cognitive Functioning Scales 847
medical paternalism 399–400, 415
Medical Practitioner's Tribunal Service (MPTS) 420–1
medical records, release in negligence claims 413, 417
Medical Research Council (MRC) 484
medications
  associated with nasal symptoms 978, 1013
  causing smell dysfunction *1233*, 1239
  pre-operative continuation 307
  and wound healing 99
Medline (PubMed) 498
medullary thyroid cancer (MTC) 682–6, 706
  C-cell hyperplasia 684–5, 684, 757
  clinical features 758–9, *759*
  diagnosis 759
  diarrhoea 762, 787
  follow-up 761
  genetics 85, 87–8, 758
  hereditary 682, 684–5, 684, 758
    prophylactic surgery 762–3
  histological variants 681, *681*, 683
  incidence 757
  investigations 759–60
    calcitonin 741–2, 759–60, 761, 762
    calcium 760
    catecholamines/metanephrines 760
    FNAC 681, 683, 759
    imaging 760, 760
    RET mutation analysis 760
    ultrasound 644, 760
  metastatic 681, 787–8
  non-surgical treatment 762, 786–8
    external beam radiotherapy 786–7
    targeted 787–8
  outcome and prognosis 762
  pathology 607, 681–4, 684, 757–8
  recurrent/residual disease 761–2
  sporadic 758
  surgery 760–1
  tumour markers 623
melanoma 551, 1312
Melker Seldinger device 320

Membership of the Royal College of
    Surgeons (MRCS) 373, 373
MEN1 gene 86, 87, 858, 937
Ménière's disease
    management 279
    medical negligence claims 443, 444
MENIN protein 87
meningiomas
    associated with olfactory dysfunction
        1234, 1236
    embolization 573–5
    orbit 1251
    sellar 647
    skull base 1249
    suprasellar 1294–5, 1296, 1296, 1302
        endoscopic endonasal surgery
            1296, 1296
meningitis
    delay in diagnosis 439, 444
    meningococcal 189
meningoencephalocele 1204, 1204
Mental Capacity Act (2005) 416
mentally incompetent patients 416
menthol, effects on nasal sensation 995, 995
mentoplasty 438
mepolizumab 1063
mercaptides 1041
6 mercaptopurine 42, 299
mercury exposure 1040
Merkel cells 108
Merlin protein 21, 22
mesenchymal stem cells (MSC) 70, 97, 121
Met oncogene 84
meta-analysis 497
meta-ethics 395
metabolic syndrome, and goitre
    formation 77
metabolomics 9, 10
metaiodobenzylguanidine (mIBG) therapy
    787–8
metalloproteinases 47, 97
metanephrines 760
metaplasia, upper aerodigestive tract
    mucosa 589
metastases 41
    cancer stem cells 72
    orbit 1251
    parathyroid gland 700, 700
    pituitary 647–8
    skeletal, hypercalcaemia 829
    thyroid cancer, surgery 809
    thyroid gland 684, 686
metformin 77
methacholine tests 1012
methicillin-resistant *Staphylococcus aureus*
    (MRSA) 64, 184–5, 225
    chronic rhinosinusitis 1063
    nasal eradication 289
methimazole 297, 620, 724–5, 726
    use in radioiodine therapy 728
methotrexate 42, 299
    Churg-Strauss syndrome 1219
    GPA 1217
    mechanism of action 42
methyldopa 1013
methylglyoxal 1054
metronidazole 191
    antibacterial spectrum 277, 278

prophylactic 295
as radiosensitizer 54
resistance 225
site and mode of action 223
topical gel 300
metyrapone 954
metyrapone test *918*, 935
Miccoli technique 811–12, 812
miconazole 287
microbiology, basic concepts 181–3
microcalcifications, thyroid cancer 643,
    644, 713, 714
microcolpohysteroscopy 587
microdebrider, sinus surgery 1074
microflora 181, *182*
microRNAs 4, 85
microscopic polyangiitis 152
microsurgery, development 108
microvascular networks, contact endoscopy
    589, 590, 593
mid-face degloving
    frontal sinus tumours 1098, 1103
    juvenile angiofibroma 1265
    septal perforation repair 1154
mid-facial segment pain 1259, *1259*, 1260
midazolam 363
middle ear infections, HIV 232
middle meatus 968, 972, 973
    endoscopy 980, 980–1, 980, 981
middle meatus antrostomy 1178
mifepristone 955
migraine 1237, 1255–6
    clinical features 1255–6, 1255, 1262
    prevention measures 1256
    treatment 1265
Mill, J.S. 398
Milton's theory 111
mini-microdebrider, turbinate reduction
    1162, 1163
mini-Pennig orthopaedic fixator 1193, 1193
minimal invasive sinus techniques
    (MIST) 1089
minimally invasive parathyroidectomy
    (MIP) 839, 840, 865, 873–6, 880
    complications 876, *876*
    contraindications 875
    failed 868, 884
    indications 875
    operative steps 875–6
    post-operative care 876
    pre-operative imaging 874–5, 875
minimally invasive thyroidectomy
    evidence base 812–13
    Henry technique 812, 812
    Miccoli technique 811–12, 812
    scarless in the neck techniques 813
minimally invasive video-assisted
    thyroidectomy (MIVAT) 600
minimum inhibitory concentration (MIC),
    methods of determination 222, 224, 224
misting test (nasal patency) 979, 1136, 1142
mitochondria
    apoptosis pathway 62–4
    genome 3, 4
mitochondrial non-syndromic hearing
    impairment 18, *19*
mitogen-activated protein kinase (MAPK)
    pathway 65, 66, 84

mitomycin C 43, 54
mitosis 40
mitotane 954
mixed lineage kinase domain-like protein
    (MLKL) 61
Modernising Medical Careers (MMC)
    372, 373
modified endoscopic Lothrop procedure
    (MELP) 1091–2, 1092
    essential steps *1093*
    frontal sinus tumours 1098, 1099, 1278
    fronto-ethmoidal mucoceles 1110
    utility *1092*
Moffat's solution 289, 1073
Mohs surgery 436
molecular biology 3–12
    future research 11–12
    methods 5–7
mometasone furoate 284
Monckeberg's sclerosis 652
Mondini dysplasia 20, 1204
mono-iodothyronine 620
monoamine oxidase inhibitors
    (MAOIs) 286
monoclonal antibodies 45
    against EGFR 47
    against tumour antigens 161–2, *162*
    against VEGFR 48, 162
    anti-IgE 143, 1007, 1055, 1063, 1129
    anti-IL-5 143, 1063
    anti-PD1 56
    CD18 114
    chronic rhinosinusitis 1063
    desirable target 45
    rheumatological disease 180
    sources 45
monoclonal gammopathy of uncertain
    significance (MGUS) 154
monocytes 250
    wound healing 95, 96
monocytosis 256
mononuclear phagocyte system 250
montelukast 1006, 1063
Montgomery v. Lanarkshire Health Board
    415–16, 900
Moraxella catarrhalis 189, 233, 1027, 1032,
    1039, 1118
morphine, children 363
moulds 205
    allergen avoidance 1003
mouth opening, limitation 311, 312
mouthwashes 295
MRSA, *see* methicillin-resistant
    Staphylococcus aureus
mucin, allergic 1049, 1051, 1051
Mucle-Wells syndrome 178
mucoactive agents 1064–5
mucoceles 1107–11, 1123
    aetiology and pathogenesis 1108, *1108*
    clinical features 1108, 1109
    complications of surgery 1111
    concha bullosa 1107, 1107, 1108, 1111
    facial pain 1254, 1254
    fronto-ethmoidal 1110, 1111
    imaging 1108–9, 1109
    maxillary sinus 1110
    sphenoid sinus 1110–11, 1254, 1254
    surgical management 1110–11

mucociliary transport
    improving in rhinosinusitis 1064–5
    nasal 985, 988
mucolytics 286–7
mucopolysaccharidosis 311
Mucor spp. 211, 1055
mucormycosis 210, 211, 254, 1309, 1309
mucosa
    nasal 983, 985–6
    olfactory 985, 1228, 1229–30, 1229
    upper aerodigestive tract 588
        contact endoscopy 589–93
Mucosal Atomization Device (MAD)
    1053–4, 1054
mucosal flaps, septal perforation repair
    1153, 1153
mucositis
    chemotherapy 254
    radiation 235
    stem cell transplantation 257
mucus, nasal 985
multiple endocrine neoplasia type 1 (MEN1) 87
    genetics 87
    hyperparathyroidism 852, 866
    parathyroid carcinoma 700
    pituitary tumours 937
multiple endocrine neoplasia type 2
    (MEN2) 87–8
    genetics 87–8, 88, 758
    medullary thyroid cancer 623, 682–3,
        681, 684, 706, 758
    MEN 2A 758, 763, 866–7
    MEN 2B 758–9, 759, 762–3
    parathyroid carcinoma 699
    primary hyperparathyroidism 626, 866–7
multiple endocrine neoplasia type 4
    (MEN4) 937
multiple myeloma 154, 253, 829, 830
multiple sclerosis 1237
mumps (parotitis) 199
mupirocin 289
muscarinics 296
muscle patch, skull base defect 1278
Mustardé technique 435
mustine 299, 299
myasthenia gravis 133, 154
mycetoma, *see* fungal ball
mycobacteria 191–2
    examples of 192
Mycobacterium leprae 192
Mycobacterium tuberculosis 134, 191–2
    in HIV 232
mycophenolate mofetil 1217, 1219
myelodysplastic syndrome (MDS) 268
myelofibrosis 250
myeloma 154, 253, 829, 830
myeloperoxidase 114
Mygind position 1054, 1054
myofascial pain 1260, 1260
myofibroblasts 94
myosins 16
myxoedema 733, 734
    pre-tibial 706, 723, 723
myxoedema coma 534–5, 730

N-butyl-2-cyanoacrylate (NBCA) 571
NAP4 study 322
NARES 1011, 1013, 1015

nasal airflow
    after turbinate reduction surgery
        1166, 1167
    assessment of medical treatments
        995–6, 996
    measurement 991–4
    normal 993
    and smell function 1228, 1234
    subjective measures 994–5, 995
nasal airway patency 991
    'anatomical' 991
    assessment 978–9, 979, 1135, 1136
    improving 979–80
    normal variability 968, 968, 986, 991
nasal airway resistance 983, 986
    calculation 992–3
    total 993
nasal airway surgery
    best clinical practice 1147
    complications 1146–7
    dressings and splints 1146
    future research 1147
    medical negligence claims 431–2
    nasal valves 1141–6
    septoplasty 1137–41
    submucosal resection 1137, 1178–9
    turbinate reduction 1146, 1160–7
nasal allergen challenge 1002
nasal allergen provocation test (NAPT) 142
nasal biopsy
    outpatient assessment 980
    rhinosinusitis 1027
nasal cartilages 964
nasal cavity
    anatomy 966, 1135–6
    bacteria, and nasal polyps 1039
    epithelium 966, 985
    floor 1136
    lateral wall 968–9, 969, 1136
    medial wall 1135
    middle meatus 972, 973, 980, 980–1
    volume 994
nasal cycle 968, 968, 986
    in rhinitis 1159
    and smell 1228
nasal dermoids 1086–7, 1087
    imaging 1086
    intra-cranial extension 1087, 1293, 1294
    pathogenesis 1086
    surgery 1086–7, 1087, 1293, 1294, 1301
nasal discharge 977
nasal douches 1006
    in septal perforation 1152
nasal drops
    administration 289, 290, 1062, 1062
    ephedrine 286
nasal endoscopy 980
    allergic fungal rhinosinusitis 1049, 1050
    allergic rhinitis 981
    anatomical findings 980–1
    biopsy 980
    frontal recess 1085
    GPA 981
    nasal polyps 981, 1041–2
    rhinosinusitis 1027
    sinonasal tumours 1270
    smell dysfunction 1231–2
    three-pass technique 980

nasal fractures 1183–9
    best clinical practice 1189
    class 1 1184
    class 2 1184, 1185
    class 3 1185
    clinical presentation 1185
    complications 1188
    epidemiology and aetiology 1183
    epistaxis 1188
    examination 1185
    future research 1189
    investigations 1185–6
    medical negligence claims 430–1, 434
    treatment 1186–8
nasal inspiratory flow rate
    measurement 1022
nasal irrigation
    epistaxis 1176
    saline 288, 1006, 1060, 1064, 1064
nasal mastocytosis 1014
nasal mucosa 983, 985–6
    comparison with lower respiratory tract
        mucosa 1127, 1127
    defence mechanisms 988
    drugs acting on 984–5, 985, 1013
    effects of smoking 986
    eosinophilic infiltration 1127–8
    examination in smell disorder 1231–2
    mucociliary function 985, 988
        improving 1064–5
    nerve supply 966
    preparation for surgery 289, 1073, 1274,
        1292–3
nasal mucosal vessel capacitance 984
nasal obstruction 991
    after nasal fracture 1188
    effects on lower airway 1128
    evaluation 1159, 1161
    inferior turbinate enlargement 968,
        1159, 1160
    intermittent 1137
    measures of 991
    nasal valves 1142–6
    septal deviation 1136–7
    subjective factors 995, 995
Nasal Obstruction Symptom Evaluation
    (NOSE) scale 1135
nasal obturators 1152
nasal packing
    after nasal airway surgery 1146
    epistaxis 1175, 1176
nasal polypectomy 980, 1043
    post-operative corticosteroids 285
nasal polyposis 1037–44
    associated diseases 1039–41
    in asthma 1013, 1039, 1127–8
    biopsy 980
    chronic rhinosinusitis 284–5, 288, 1026,
        1028–31
    clinical presentation 1038
    definition 1037
    diagnosis 1041–2, 1043
    diffuse 1029–30
    genetics 1041
    imaging 1038, 1042, 1043
    incidence and prevalence 1038, 1043
    medical negligence claims 430
    morphology 1038

nasal polyposis (*continued*)
   non-surgical management 428, 1042–3
   pathogenesis 1038–9, 1038
   secondary to systemic disease 1030–1
   and smell 1228
   staging 1042, *1042*
   surgical management 1043
   unilateral 1029
nasal provocation test 1022
nasal sensations 994–5, 995
nasal septal perforation
   questionnaire 1151
nasal septum
   abnormalities, and epistaxis 1175
   anatomy 966–9, 967, 1136, 1136–7
   blood supply 967, *967*
   cartilaginous (quadrilateral cartilage) 966, 1136, 1136, 1138
   Cottle's area 979
   development 962
   deviation 1136–41
     causes 1136
     diagnosis 1136–7
     inferior turbinate hypertrophy 1146, 1159, 1160
     inferior turbinate reduction 1165
     surgical treatment 1137–41, 1165
   examination 1136
   fractures 1141, 1184, 1185, 1187–8
   haematomas 434, 1186, 1188
   inflammation/ulceration 1152
   perforation
     after nasal fracture 1188
     causes 1149, *1151*, 1220
     differential diagnosis 1310, 1310
     in GPA 1151, 1215, 1216, 1217–18
     non-surgical management 1152
     obturation 1152
     prevalence 1149, 1151
     prevention 1152
     previous septal surgery 1152
     surgical enlargement 1152
     surgical repair 1152–4
   submucosal resection 1137, 1178–9
     medical negligence claims 432
   surgical approach 1137–8
   swell body 967, 967
nasal speculum 1142–3, 1143
nasal sprays 289
   allergic fungal rhinosinusitis 1053–4
   antifungal 1054
   application 289, 289, 1054, 1054
   azelastine 1014–15
   efficacy of delivery 1065
nasal strips 979–80
nasal surgery
   anaesthesia 337, 347
   children 365
nasal symptoms
   history taking 977–8
   in systemic disease 977
nasal tip ptosis, surgery 1145
nasal valve dilators 1143–4, 1143, *1147*
nasal valves 964–5, *965*, 965
   anatomy 1141–2, 1142
   external 964, 965, 978, 1141
   internal 964, 965, 978, 979, 979, 980, 987, 1141

obstruction
   aetiology 1142
   diagnosis 1142–3, 1143
   treatment 1143–6
nasal vestibule 964, 983, 986–7, 987
nasal vestibule stents 980
naseptin 289
naso-orbito-ethmoid fractures 1185, 1198–9, *1198*, 1199
nasobronchial reflex 1128
nasolacrimal duct 968, 1158, 1244
nasolacrimal system 1244
   obstruction 1244
     dacryocystorhinostomy 1245–6, 1245–6
     probing 1245, 1246
nasopharyngeal carcinoma
   and EBV 201
   PET-CT imaging 544, 548
   photodynamic therapy 585
   skull base, endoscopic debulking 1291
nasopharynx, endoscopic view 981
nasoseptal flap 945–6, 946–7, 1277, 1278, 1300
National Cancer Institute of Canada (NCIC) 484
National Clinical Assessment Service (NCAS) 420
National Health and Nutrition Examination Survey, 3rd (NHANES III) 718
National Health Service Litigation Authority (NHSLA) 414, 899
National Health Service (NHS)
   complaints procedures 413, 420–1
   Consultant Outcomes Publication process 896
   failures in patient care 389, 391, 393–4
   medical negligence claims 410, 412–13
   patient and public involvement 391
   see also clinical governance
National Institute for Clinical Excellence (NICE)
   establishment 390, 391, 392
   growth hormone replacement guidelines 928
   medical negligence guidelines 423
   pre-operative tests 303
   and resource allocation 404
   turbinate surgery guidance 1168
National Institutes of Health (NIH), guidelines for asymptomatic PHPT 846
National Justice Compania Naviesa SA v. Prudential Assurance Company Ltd, The Ikarian Reefer 418–19
National Kidney Foundation Disease Quality Outcomes Initiative (KDOQI) 867
National Patient Safety Agency (NPSA) alert, paediatric fluid therapy 363
natural killer (NK) cells 129, 132
near hanging events 363
necessity, doctrine of 416
neck, transillumination 317
neck dissection
   differentiated thyroid cancer 753
   medical negligence claims 447
   medullary thyroid cancer 760–1
   PET-CT imaging 553
   thyroid cancer recurrence 776, 809

necroptosis 61
necrosis 41, 61
   versus apoptosis 61, *61*
necrotic wounds 101, 102
needle cricothyrotomy 319–20, 319
negative feedback loops 621, 621, 629, 630
negligence, proof of 411–12
Neisseria gonorrhoea 189
Neisseria meningitidis 188–9
Nelson, H.L. 398
Nelson, J.L. 398
Nelson's syndrome 638, 935, 954
neodymium yttrium-aluminium-garnet (Nd:YAG) laser 346, 581, 1164
neonatal-onset multi-system inflammatory disease (NOMID) 178
neonate
   fluid and electrolyte requirements 362–3, *363*
   hypothyroidism 736
nerve blocks, airway anaesthesia 324
nerve growth factor 141
Nerve Integrity Monitor (NIM) endotracheal tube 337, 337
nerve monitoring, *see* intra-operative nerve monitoring
Neti pots 1065, 1065
neuralgia
   post-herpetic 1258
   post-surgical/traumatic 1258
   Sluder's 1258–9
   trigeminal 1258
neuraminidase inhibitors 202–3
neuroblastoma, olfactory 1306
neurocognitive function, primary hyperparathyroidism 844, 845–6
neurodegenerative diseases, olfactory deficits 1230, 1231, 1237
neurofibromas, orbit 1251
neurofibromatosis
   differentiation of type I/type II 11
   type 2 (NF2) 20, 21–2, 24
neurogenic inflammation 1018
neurohypophysis, *see* pituitary gland, posterior
neurokinin-1 receptor antagonists 348–9
neurological disease
   delays in diagnosis 450
   smell function *1234*
neuromuscular blockade 340, 341
   measurement 343
neurotransmitters 984
neutropenia 256
neutrophil-endothelial interactions 113–14
neutrophil-to-lymphocyte ratio (NLR) 161
neutrophils 151, 249
   disorders of number 256
   wound healing 95, 96
'never events' 453
The New NHS 389
New Zealand 423
NF2 gene 21–2, 24
NHS Trusts, medical negligence claims 414, 420–1, 423–4
nicotinamide 53–4
nifedipine 114
nilotinib 22
nimorazole 54

nimotuzumab 162, *162*
nitrate 76
nitric oxide 113
nitric oxide synthase, inducible (iNOS) 113
nitro blue tetrazolium (NBT) test 151
nitrogen oxides (NOX) 1021
nitroglycerin (GTN) 114
nitroimidazoles 54, *223*
nitrous oxide, avoidance in ear surgery 348
no reflow phenomenon 113
nodal disease
    thyroid cancer 776, 809
        medullary 760–1
noise-induced hearing loss, medical reports 418
Nolan Committee 389
non-allergic non-infectious perennial rhinitis (NANIPER) 1011, 1012, 1015
non-allergic rhinitis with eosinophilia syndrome (NARES) 1011, 1013, 1015
non-Hodgkin's lymphoma (NHL) 233, 234
    extranodal disease 252
    oropharynx 252
    PET-CT imaging 550, 550
    thyroid 656–7, 768–9
non-maleficence 399
non-nucleoside reverse transcriptase inhibitors (NNRTIs) 230
Non-Religious Ethics 396
non-steroidal anti-inflammatory drugs (NSAIDs)
    antiplatelet action 271–2
    and epistaxis 1174
    migraine 1256
    pre-operative 334
    rhinitis induction 1013
    tonsillectomy 344
    and wound healing 99
non-technical skills for surgeons (NOTSS) 453–63
    aim of 454
    behavioural markers 454
    classification *454*
    communication and teamwork 459–60
    decision-making 457–8
    leadership 460–2
    situational awareness 454–7
non-verbal communication 383–4, *384*
noradrenaline
    cardiovascular support 354
    and nasal function 984, *985*, 986
Northern blotting 6
nose
    aerodynamics 986
    airway resistance 983, 986
    anatomy 983
    blood supply 965, 984, 984, 1169–70, 1173
    development 961–4
    epithelium-ciliary function 985, 988
    examination 978–81
        in allergic rhinitis 1001
        endoscopy, *see* nasal endoscopy
        functional 978–80, 1135
        in occupational rhinitis 1022
        in smell disorders 1231–2
        structure and aesthetics 978
    filtration function 988

foreign bodies 446
fractures, *see* nasal fractures
heat exchange 987–8
lymphatic drainage 966
nerve supply 965, 984–5
olfaction 983, 988
skin and muscles 964
structure/physiology in relation to smell 1228–30
venous drainage 1170
nose blowing 1011
nose deformity
    rhinoplasty 434–5
    saddle 431, 434
NOTCH1 65
NOTCH1 gene 9
Nottingham Health Profile 486, 488
Nozovent® 1143–4, 1143
NTSS, *see* non-technical skills for surgeons
nuclear factor-kappaB (NF-κB) pathway, thyroid tumours 85
nuclear medicine, *see* scintigraphy
nucleoside analogues 209
nucleoside/nucleotide reverse transcriptase inhibitors (NRTIs) 230
nucleotides 3
nucleus: cytoplasm ratio 591, 591
Nurenberg standards 403
null hypothesis 473
numbers needed to treat (NNT) 513, 514
nursing, thyroidectomy 802
nutrition
    critical care patient 355–6
    iodine intake 622
    post-operative 307
    pre-operative 306
    and smell dysfunction 1232, *1234*, 1239
nutritional status, and wound healing 98–9
Nylen, Carl-Olof Siggesson 108
nystatin 209, 217, 234, 287

Obatoclax (Gemin X) 64
obesity
    anaesthesia in 339
    and suitability for day surgery 301–2
observational studies 469, 469, 475–6
obstructive sleep apnoea, anaesthesia in 339, 344
occult tumours, PET-CT studies 543–4, 543
occupational asthma 1126
occupational rhinitis
    allergic 1018, *1019*
    definition 1017
    diagnosis 1021–2
    epidemiology 1017
    future research 1023
    high risk occupations 1018, 1019–21
    immunotherapy 1023
    irritant 1018, *1020*
    medical therapy 1023
    non-allergic 1012–13
    pathogenesis 1018
    prevention 1022
    risk factors 1018
octreotide 787
oculomotor nerve 910, 911
    cavernous sinus 617, 617
    palsies 912

'odds' 472
odds ratio 472, 517
odontogenic cysts 1310, 1311
oesophageal cancer, photodynamic therapy in 585
oesophageal injury
    difficult airway 329
    thyroid/parathyroid surgery 889
oesophagitis
    in HIV 235
    reflux, management 298–9
oesophagus, thyroid cancer involvement 775, 806, 808
17β-oestradiol (E$_2$) 636
oestrogens
    effects on nasal mucosa 1013
    replacement therapy 929
Office for Population Censuses and Surveys (OPCS/Read codes) 306
ointments, otologic 275
olfaction 983, 988
    disorders, *see* smell disorders
olfactory agnosia 1230–1, 1235
olfactory bulbs 1230
olfactory cleft 1228
olfactory event-related potentials 1233
olfactory fila 1230
    tearing 1235, 1236
olfactory nerve 1228–9
olfactory neuroblastoma, *see* aesthesioneuroblastoma
olfactory neuroepithelium 985, 1228, 1229–30, 1229
    biopsy 1232
olfactory receptor cells 1229–30, 1229
olfactory reference syndrome 1235
olfactory schwannoma, endoscopic endonasal surgery 1294, 1295
olfactory testing 1022
    rhinosinusitis 1027
olfactory 'vector route' 1230
omalizumab 143, 1007, 1055, 1063, 1129
oncocytic (oxyphil) cell tumours 669–670, 670
oncocytic (oxyphilic) cells 660–1, *661*
oncogenes 9
    MEN2 syndrome 87–8
    parathyroid carcinoma 858
    thyroid tumours 83–4
oncologic tumour resection 1274
oncolytic virus 35, 203
oncoproteins, HPV E6 and E7 160, 169–70
Onodi cells 971, 975, *975*, 1074, *1272*, 1307
ONYX-015 11–12, 35, 66
operating room set up, endoscopic endonasal surgery 1282, 1283–4, 1292, 1292
ophthalmic artery 965
ophthalmic nerve, cavernous sinus 617
ophthalmic vein 965
optic canal 614, 615
    meningioma 1294–5, 1296, 1296
optic chiasm, effects of pituitary adenomas 910–12, 911
optic nerve
    cavernous sinus 617
    compression 1248–51
        mucoceles 1108
        neoplasms 1250–1

optic nerve (*continued*)
    endoscopic decompression 1248–50
    injury in sinus surgery 975, 1076–7
    sphenoid sinus 612–13
optic neuropathy, traumatic 1248–9
optical coherence tomography 533–7
    clinical studies 536–7
    fourier domain 537
    future research 538
    indications 533–4
    laryngeal imaging 535–6, 535
    long-range 537
    paediatric studies 537
    polarization-sensitive 536
    system operation 534–5
optical frequency domain imaging (OFDI) 537
optical tracking systems 564, 564
oral allergy syndrome 1001
oral cavity
    manifestations of HIV infection 233–5, 235
    microflora *182*
oral contraceptives
    and goitre formation 77
    intolerance 1013
    thrombosis risk 269
oral intake, elective surgery 306–7
oral papillomas *200*, 234
oral T-cell lymphoma 202
orbit
    anatomy 1243–4, 1244
        inferior wall 1244
        lateral wall 1244
        medial wall 970, 972, 1243–4
        superior wall/roof 1244
    complications of rhinosinusitis 1028, *1028*, 1088, 1114–20
    contents 1244
    endoscopic decompression 1247–8, 1248
    GPA involvement 1215, 1216
    injury in sinus surgery 1076
    neoplasms 1250–1
    pseudotumour 1249, 1250
orbital abscess *1028*, 1115, *1117*, *1117*
orbital cellulitis *1028*, 1114–16, 1114, *1115*, 1115
    cavernous sinus thrombosis *1115*, 1116
    Chandler stages 1117, *1117*
    investigations 1116–18
    preseptal *1115*, 1115
    prognosis 1120
    subperiosteal abscess 1115, 1117, 1118
    treatment 1118–20
    visual problems 1116
orbital floor (maxillary sinus roof) 970, 971, 1244
    downfracture 1248
    fractures 1198
orbitofrontal complex 1230
Organ, Dr Claude H Jr. 851
organ dysfunction
    critical care management 352–6
    early identification 359
organochlorides 77
oropharyngeal cancer (OPC), and HPV 170

oropharyngeal candidiasis
    head and neck cancer patients 217
    HIV patients 216–17, 233–4, 235, *235*
oseltamivir 203
Osler-Weber-Rendu disease (hereditary haemorrhagic telangiectasia) 289, 577, 1180
    epistaxis 1178, 1180
osmophobia 1231
ossiculoplasty, medical negligence claims 443
ossifying fibroma
    frontal sinus 1102–3
    imaging 1312, 1313
    orbit 1250–1
osteitis, chronic rhinosinusitis 1030, 1030
osteitis fibrosa cystica 601, 658, 831, 844
osteoblasts 98
osteoclasts 98
osteogenesis 121
osteomas
    frontal sinus 1099–1100, 1100–1, *1101*
    orbit 1251
osteomeatal complex (OMC), obstruction in rhinosinusitis 1071
osteomyelitis, frontal sinus 1122, 1122
osteonecrosis, PET-CT imaging 553
osteoneogenesis, frontal sinus surgery 1093
osteoplastic flap procedure 1093–6
    frontal sinus osteoma 1100, 1100
    indications *1094*
osteoporosis, hyperprolactinaemia 907
otitis externa
    fungal infections 208–9
    malignant 209, 232
    topical preparations 276
otitis media
    acute 201
    chronic suppurative 276
    in GPA 1215, 1218
Otitis Media-6 (OM6) 490
otoacoustic emissions (OAE) 528
otology, medical negligence claims 439–45
otomycosis 208–9
otosclerosis
    medical negligence claims 440–1
    sodium fluoride treatment 280
'otospongiosis-otosclerosis' 280
otosyphilis 232
ototoxicity 59
    aminoglycosides 20–1, 24, 254
    apoptosis in 59, 64
    chemotherapy 254
    medical negligence claims 444–5
out of programme activities (OOPA) 373, 373
outcome variables, analysis 471–2
outcomes research
    patient-based measures 483–4
        acceptability 487
        appropriateness 484–5
        benefits of use 484
        choice of 491–2
        defined 483–4
        disease-specific 489–90
        feasibility 487, 491
        generic 487–9, *487*
        interpretability 487

        precision/sensitivity 486–7
        reliability 485–6
        responsiveness to change 486
        rhinology 491, 978, 1025, 1027, 1065, *1065*
        site-specific 490–1
        validity 485
outpatient assessment, rhinology 977–82
ovary, thyroid tissue (*struma ovarii*) 607, 659
over-the-wire catheters 570
overmatching 475
Owen, Sir Richard 600
oxaliplatin 42
oxazolinidones 223
Oxford Centre for Evidence-Based Medicine, levels of evidence 474, *474*
oxygen analysis, intra-operative 342
oxygen delivery, increasing 354, *354*, 357
oxymetazoline 286, 1073
oxyphil cells 608
oxytocin 614, 640, 640, 924
ozone pollution 1021

p-value 473
p16 65–6, 169–70
p53 65–6
    gene therapy 34, 35
    and HPV 169
    inactivation 9, 10, 11
    thyroid cancer 84
p63 653
pacemakers, pre-operative assessment 303
paclitaxel, mode of action 43
paediatric intensive care 361–7
    bronchoscopy 366
    ENT emergencies 363–5
    evaluation of child 362
    fluid management 362–3, *363*
    major surgery 365–6
Paget's disease of bone 831
pain questionnaires 491
palate, development 962, 962
palatine artery, greater 967, 1170
palatine bones 966, 1136, 1244
palliative care 358–9
pamidronate 861
pancreatitis, primary hyperparathyroidism 844
pancytopenia 252, 255
    causes *255*
panda facies 1194, 1194
Papaverine-induced skin reactivity 1012
papillary thyroid cancer 670–79
    histological variants 673, *673*, 674
    histopathology 671–5, 671–5
    macroscopic appearance 669, 669
    microcarcinoma 678–9, 679, 753
    molecular biology 675
    parathyroid metastasis 700
    recurrence, definition 774–5
    recurrence management 775–8
    recurrence risk 773–4, *774*
    recurrence/metastases 784
    ultrasound 644, 713, 714
papillomas
    laryngeal 200, 591–3
    oral *200*, 234, 234
    see also inverted papilloma

paracetamol 334
parafibromin 88, 858, 860–1
parafollicular cells (C cells) 604, 604, 607, 652–3
  hyperplasia 684–5, 684, 757
paragangliomas (PGs)
  angiography 575, 575
  genetics of familial 22–4
  preoperative embolization 575–6
parainfluenza viruses 199
Parainfluenzae virus type 1 364
paramixoviruses 198–9
paranasal sinuses 984
  anatomy
    developmental and functional 972–6
    surgical 969–72
  benign tumours 1098–103
  development 962–4, 962–3
  fungal disease 209–16, 233
  granulomatous disorders 1032, 1033, 1310
  imaging 1072, 1307–14
    CT 1086
    incidental findings 1308, 1308
    MRI 1086, 1306, 1306, 1308, 1308
    rhinosinusitis 1308–10, 1308–9
  malignancy 1103
  medical negligence claims 431
  mucoceles 1107–11
  physiological role 984
  see also rhinosinusitis; sinonasal tumours, *and individual sinuses*
paranasal surgical box 969–72, 970–2, 972
paraneoplastic syndromes, hypercalcaemia 827, 829
paraproteins 154, 253
parasympathetic nerve 966
parasympathomimetics 985
parathyrocytes 699, 700
parathyroid adenomas 86, 625, 692–7
  asymptomatic 844–7
  atypical 697, 697
  double 692, 833, 839, 865
  ectopic locations 881, 881
  histopathology 692–4, 693–4
  localization 537, 601, 874–5
    arteriography 838
    CT 836, 838, 838, 882–3
    dual isotope subtraction study 836, 837
    failed 868
    fine-needle aspiration 839
    flow charts 839, 839–40
    mediastinal adenoma 884
    MRI 838
    PET-CT 838
    posteriorly placed superior adenoma 839
    in pregnancy 839
    repeat surgery 852–3, 882–3
    selective venous sampling 838
    sestamibi scintigraphy 834–6, 853, 868
    sestamibi/CT 874, 875
    SPECT 836, 836
    SPECT-CT 836, 837
    subtraction thyroid scan 836, 837
    ultrasound 833–4, 834, 875

molecular genetics 86, 697
multigland disease 835, 839, 843, 854, 865, 868
post-operative pituitary function 937
size/weight 854
variants 694–4, 695–6
parathyroid carcinoma 697–700, 833, 857–61
  aetiology and pathogenesis 858
  clinical presentation 858–9
  definition 697
  diagnostic criteria 698, 698
  first described 857
  genetics 86–7
  histopathology 860–1, 861
  hypercalcaemia 858, 861
  imaging 858–9, 859
  incidence and natural history 857
  medical therapy 861
  metastatic 698, 698
  prognosis 861
  recurrence 860
  resection specimen 859
  surgery 859–60, 868
parathyroid glands 689, 688–9
  anatomy 607–8, 873–4, 880–1
    macroscopic 607, 689, 690
    microscopic 607–8, 690–700, 690
  development 608, 608
  embryology 608, 608, 874, 874, 881, 881
  hyperplasia 86, 689–91, 691, 833, 865–6
  imaging 537, 601, 644–5, 833–9
  inferior 874, 874, 881
  injury in thyroidectomy 448, 730, 889
  intra-operative frozen section examination 698, 700
  intra-operative localization 874
  management in thyroidectomy 797–8, 800–1, 800
  normal attributes 689–71, 691
  number, size and position 608, 689, 691
  physiology 623–6
  secondary neoplasms 700, 700
  superior 874, 874, 881
parathyroid hormone (PTH) 298, 298, 345, 607, 623, 624
  first understanding 601
  intra-operative measurement 601, 839–40, 854, 868, 876, 880
  recombinant (rhPTH) 889
  serum levels 829–30, 829
    in hypercalcaemia 829, 830–1
    raised 829–30, 829
    suppressed 829, 830
  and vitamin D 830–1
parathyroid hormone-related protein (PTHrP) 608, 624
  aberrant secretion 692
  hypercalcaemia 830, 831
parathyroid proliferative disease 689
parathyroid surgery 345
  autotransplantation of tissue 625, 626, 867, 868
  bilateral exploration 865–70
  causes of failure 851–2, 852, 854
  complications 887–90, 893
    audits and registers 894–7, 895

hypocalcaemia 345, 625, 854, 884, 894
development 600–1
history 879–80
indications for in PHPT 844, 846, 846
medical management 626
minimally invasive 839, 840, 865, 873–6, 880
  complications 876, 876
  failed 868, 884
  indications 875
  post-operative care 876
  pre-operative imaging 874–5, 875
  surgical steps 875–6
parathyroid carcinoma 859–60
persistent hypercalcaemia 894, 895
persistent hyperparathyroidism 851–2, 852, 881–2
reasons for failure 851–2, 852, 854
in renal failure 867–8, 868
reoperation 852–4
results and complications 854, 884
surgical approach 853–4, 883–4
parathyromatosis 692
parents, consent 416, 445
Parkinson's disease 1230, 1231, 1237, 1239
parotid gland
  lymphoepithelial cysts 235–6, 236
  medical negligence claims 449
  tumours 449
parotitis (mumps) 199, 200
paroxysmal hemicrania 1257
Parry Romberg syndrome 174
pars anterior (pituitary) 611, 611
pars intermedia (pituitary) 611, 611
pars tuberalis 613
partial thromboplastin time (PTT) 260, 264, 264, 267
particulate matter pollution 1021
pasireotide 953
pastilles 295
paternalism 399–400, 415
patient education 383
patient information leaflets 429
patient pathway 301–2
patient preparation for surgery
  assessment 302–3
  consent 304–5
  day surgery 302
  head and neck cancer surgery 306
  investigations 303–4
  nasal/sinus surgery 289, 1073
  nutrition 306
  oral intake 306–7
  post-operative care planning 306
  theatre planning/scheduline 306
  VTE prophylaxis 305–6
patient satisfaction, and surgeon communication 380
patient selection
  elective surgery 428–9
  rhinoplasty 434
patient-reported outcome measures (PROMs) 483–92
  assessment criteria 484–7, 484
  cancer 490
  definition 483–4
  EuroQol (EQ-5D) 489

patient-reported outcome measures (PROMs) (continued)
    Glasgow Benefit Inventory 488–9
    Health Utilities Index (HUI) 489
    hearing 490
    Nottingham Health Profile 488
    otitis media 490
    rhinology 491, 978, 1025, 1027, 1065, 1065
    Short-Form 36-Item Health Survey (SF-36) 488
    Sickness Impact Profile 488
    utility measures 489
    vertigo 490
    voice disorders 491
    WHO-DAS 2 488
pattern-recognition molecules 125
PAX8/PPARG rearrangement 84
peach allergy *146*
peak expiratory flow (PEF) 1129, 1129
peak nasal inspiratory flow (PNIF) 979, 994
    effects of lower airway disease 1128–9, 1129
    normal values 994
peanut allergy *146*
pedicled flaps
    septal perforation repair 1153, 1154
    skull base repair 1206, 1208, 1300–1, 1300
peer-assisted learning 497
pegvisomant 933, 953
Pemberton's sign 820
pemphigus 133, 154
Pendred syndrome 20, 635
pendrin 20, 635
pendrin gene 16
penicillins *223*
    acute rhinosinusitis 285
    antibacterial spectrum *278*
    commonly used *223*
    introduction 221
    resistance 225
Pennington septum elevator 1138
peptic ulcer disease, primary hyperparathyroidism 844
Peptostreptococcus spp. 1118
percentage of glottic opening (POGO) score 309–10
perchlorate 77
perforasomes 109, 109, 110
perforator flaps 109, 110
pericranial flap 1300–1, 1300
periodic paralysis, thyrotoxic 719
periorbita 1244
    incision 1248
personalized medicine 59
pertussis 189
pets, allergen avoidance 1003, *1004*
PFA-100 test 268
PFAPA syndrome 179
phaeochromocytoma 623, 758, 760, 831
phagocytosis 131–2, 250
    apoptotic cells 60
phantom tooth pain 1259
phantosmias 1230, 1235
pharyngeal collapse 336
pharyngo-oesophageal perforation 329

pharynx
    intubation injuries 329
    thyroid cancer involvement 808
Philpott-Javer endoscopic staging (AFRS) 1052, 1052
pholcodine 296
phosphate, serum 831
phosphatidylinositol 3,4,5-triphosphate (PIP3) 65
phosphodiesterase III inhibitor 114
photoablation 582
photochemical reactions 582
photochemotherapy 584
photodynamic therapy (PDT) 584–5
photomechanical effects 582
photosensitizer drugs 582, 584, 585
photothermal reactions 582
Physicians Insurers Association of America 900
PI3K-Akt pathway 65–6, 66, 84–5
PICO acronym 468, 497, 498, 507
pilocarpine 296, 300, *985*
pinna, chondritis 174
pinnaplasty 435–6
    medical negligence claims 535
pituitary adenomas 645, 905, 930–6
    adjuvant treatment 952–5
    cavernous sinus extension 645, 646, 1286
        surgical approach 1286–7, 1286
    corticotrophinomas 916–17, 933–5
        adjuvant treatment 954–5
    definitions 930
    ectopic 851
    extrinsic spread 930, *930*
    familial syndromes 647, 937
    future research 937
    gonadotrophin-secreting 912, 917, 936
    growth hormone secreting (somatotrophinomas) 647, 932–3
        adjuvant treatment 952–4
    histological evaluation 918
    hormone deficiency 905–6
    hormone excess 906–10
    hypothyroidism 736, 737
    imaging 645–7, 646, 917, 930–1, 931
    incidence 951
    macroadenomas 646, 647
    microadenomas 646, 647
    neuro-ophthalmological features 910–12, 911
    non-functioning 912, 917, 936
        treatment 955
    non-specific symptoms 951
    pathogenesis 930, *930*
    prolactinoma 635, 906–8, 952
    recurrence 941
    thyrotrophin-secreting (TSHomas) 912, 917, 936
        adjuvant therapy 955
    visual field loss 911–12, 912, 918, 931
    visual recovery after surgery 912
pituitary apoplexy 912–13
    assessment 927
    management 927
pituitary carcinoma 937
    treatment 955
pituitary fossa
    anatomy 612–13, 613
    endoscopic anatomy 616, 616

pituitary gland
    anatomy 613–14
    anterior (adenohypophysis) 613, 630
        anatomy 923
        cell types 613, 630, *631*, *924*
        hormone replacement 928–9
        hormone secretion 613, 614, 630–8, 923–4, *924*
        investigations of function 915–19, *918*
    blood supply 614, 614, 924
    capsule 614
    embryology 611, 611
    excess hormone secretion 906–10
    first description 629
    gonadal axis 635–7
    hormone deficiency (hypopituitarism) 905–6, 905
        acquired 926–9
        congenital 925–6
        investigation 918–19, *918*
    imaging 645–9
    lymphocytic hypophysitis 927–8
    posterior (neurohypophysis) 613–14, 638, 924
        hormones 638–40
        investigation of dysfunction 919–20
    size 613, 629
pituitary incidentaloma 905, 917
pituitary inhibitory factors 932
pituitary surgery
    history 1281
    primary tumour 951–2, 1281–7
    recurrent tumours 941–8
pituitary tumours
    adenomas, *see* pituitary adenomas
    craniopharyngioma 648, 648
        adjuvant treatment 955
        endonasal endoscopic surgery 1294, 1297, *1298*, 1299, 1302
    metastatic 647–8
    non-adenomatous 649
pixels 561
placebo treatments 479, 512
plasma 249
plasma cells 127, 139
plasma derived factor concentrate 272–3
plasma osmolality 638, 639, 920
plasmapheresis 253
plasmid gene therapy 31
plasmin 263, 263
plasminogen 263, 263
plasminogen activator inhibitor (PAI-1) 263
plasminogen activators (tPA) 263
platelet counts 254–5
    anticoagulation therapy 294, 300
platelet storage pool disorder 269
platelet-derived growth factor (PDGF), wound healing *95*
platelet-rich plasma (PRP) 121
platelets 249
    abnormalities of function 268–9
    disorders of number 255–6, 267–8
    function in blood clotting 261–2, 262
    thresholds in medical/surgical procedures 244, *244*
    transfusion 243–4, 272
    wound healing 95, *95*

platinum-based chemotherapy agents 41–2, 47
pleomorphic adenoma 449
plicamycin 861
plicatic acid 1020
Plummer's disease 724
pneumocephalus 1206, 1206
Pneumocystis jiroveci 232
pneumosinus dilitans, frontal 1103
Poiseuille's law 111
Poiseuille's principle 1142
polio virus 1230
pollen-induced allergic rhinitis 1001
　allergen avoidance 1003
pollutants
　causing smell dysfunction *1233*
　and goitre formation 76–7
　and rhinitis 1013–14, 1021
pollybeak deformity 435
polycystic ovary syndrome 635
polycythaemia 255
polyenes 209
polymerase chain reaction (PCR)
　bacteriological diagnosis 183
　techniques 6–7, 7
polyvinyl alcohol (PVA), embolic particles 570–1
Pope v. St Helen's Theatre 411–12
Porphyromonas spp. 1118
portal hypertension 269
posaconazole 217
positional cloning 10
positive pressure mask ventilation 1206, 1206
positive prick test (PPT) 145
positron emission tomography (PET)
　2-[18F] fluoro-2-deoxy-D-glucose (FDG-PET) 541, 542
　MRI-integrated (PET-MRI) 555, 1315
positron emission tomography (PET)-computed tomography (PET-CT) 541–52, 1306, 1315
　characterization of indeterminate lesions 548–9, 548
　chemotherapy response assessment 549
　CT component 541–2
　FDG radiotracer 541, 542
　FDG uptake and outcomes 549
　limitations/pitfalls 551–2, 552–4, 1315
　non-squamous cell carcinomas 549–50, 549, 550
　normal variants and artefacts 550–1
　occult tumours 543–4
　parathyroid adenoma 838
　PET component 542–3
　radiotherapy planning 549
　radiotracers other than FDG 552–5
　sinonasal malignancy 1272, 1315
　squamous cell carcinoma
　　post-treatment 545–6
　　primary disease 544–5
　　recurrent disease 546–8
　thyroid disease 714, 742
post-herpetic neuralgia 1258
post-operative care
　critical care 356
　endoscopic sinus surgery 432–3, 1075–6

minimally invasive parathyroidectomy 876
　parathyroid surgery 854
　pituitary surgery 948
　skull base surgery 1301
　thyroidectomy 802
post-operative nausea and vomiting (PONV)
　new drugs to minimize 348–9
　tonsillectomy 344
posterior ethmoidal artery
　anatomy 1170, 1173, 1294
　ligation 1178
　skull base surgery 1295–6
posterior ethmoidal foramen 1244
posterior septectomy 1277–8
postseptal cellulitis *1115*, 1115, 1116, 1117, *1117*
Poswillo hook 1197, *1197*
potassium hydroxide (KOH) test 206
potassium titanyl phosphate (KTP) laser 346
Pott's puffy tumour 1122–3, 1122
POU1F1 mutations 925
PRAD1 gene 858
pre-albumin 98
pre-eclampsia 739
pre-operative assessment 302–3
　cardiovascular disease 302–3
　day surgery 302
　investigations 303–4
　respiratory disease 303
pre-operative care
　day of surgery 306–7
　head and neck surgery 306
　venous thromboembolism prophylaxis 294, 305–6
precedent 410
precision, outcome measures 486–7
prednisolone 147, 1006
prednisolone ear drops 276
pregnancy
　hyperparathyroidism 839
　iodine deficiency 76, *76*, 77
　prolactin levels 635
　and radioiodine therapy 753–4
　rhinitis in 988, 1008, 1013
　rubella infection 439
　thrombosis risk 269
　thyroid cancer management 786
　thyroid function 711, *711*, 737, 738–40
　thyroxine therapy 737, 739
premedication 334
　analgesics 334
　sedative 334
preoxygenation 340
presbyosmia 1231
preseptal cellulitis *1028*, *1115*, 1115, 1117, *1117*
pressure ulcers 100–1
　classification 100–1
　management 103
pretibial myxoedema 706, 723, 723
pretracheal fascia 603–4
Pretty, Diane 400
prevalence, definition 467
Prevotella spp. 1039, 1118
primary ciliary dyskinesia 1032, *1032*, 1040

primary hyperparathyroidism (PHPT)
　aetiology 873
　asymptomatic 844–8, *848*
　clinical presentation 843–4
　definition *691*, *844*
　diagnosis 828–31, 874
　familial 86, 700, 866–7
　　MEN 1 852, 866
　　MEN 2A 866–7
　genetics 86, 697
　historical management 879–80
　hypercalcaemia 692, 828
　　acute treatment 883
　　persistent 894, *895*
　incidence 843, 879
　indications for surgery 844, 847, *847*
　medical management 847
　persistent and recurrent 851–4, 881–2
　　investigation 882–3
　　surgical failure 851–2, *852*, 854, 882
　pre-operative localization
　　arteriography 838
　　CT 836, 838, 838
　　dual isotope subtraction study 836, 837
　　failed 868
　　fine-needle aspiration 839
　　flow charts 839, 839–40
　　MRI 838
　　PET-CT 838
　　selective venous sampling 838
　　sestamibi scintigraphy 834–6, 853
　　SPECT-CT 836, 837, 853
　　SPECT/MIBI 836, 836
　　ultrasound 833–4, 834, 875
　skeletal complications 844–5
primum non nocere 393, 399
principles, and ethics 397
principalism 396
PRISMA guidelines 504, 515–16
probability 472
procaspases 63, 63
prochlorperazine 279
prodrugs 34, 54–5
Professional Standards Authority 421
programmed cell death protein 1 (PD-1) 48
prolactin 906
　effects of 635
　excess 635, 906, 916, *916*, 932
　hypothalamic control 633, 635
　role of 630, 636
prolactinoma 635, 647, 906–8, 932
　adjuvant treatment 952
　clinical features 907–8, *907*, 907, 932
　laboratory investigations 916, *916*
　macroprolactinoma 952
　management 906–7, 932, 952
　microprolactinoma 952
PROP1 mutations 925
prophylactic surgery, hereditary MTC 762–3
prophylaxis
　antibiotics 295, 1153
　venous thromboembolism 294, 305–6, 802
propiomelanocortin 637
propofol 323, 334–5
propranolol 626

propylthiouracil (PTU) 620, 724–7
    dosage 725
    in pregnancy 739
    side effects 725–6, 726
prostaglandins (PG) 160
prostate-specific antigen (PSA) 929
protease inhibitors 230–1
protein C 262
    activated 262, 263, <u>263</u>
    deficiency 269, 270
protein gene product (PGP 9.5) 861
protein S 262, 269, 270
proteomics 9, 10
Proteus spp. 190
prothrombin complex concentrate (PCC) 246, 271, *271*, 272
prothrombin (factor II) 259, <u>260</u>, <u>261</u>, 267
prothrombin time (PT) 260, 264
    monitoring in anticoagulation 294–5
    prolonged *264*
proto-oncogenes 9, 83–4
proton pump inhibitors 299
psammoma bodies 672–3, <u>672–3</u>
pseudo-ephedrine 286
pseudohypercalcaemia 827, 829
pseudomembranous candidiasis 217
Pseudomonas spp. 190–1, 1039
Pseudomonas aeruginosa 190, 232, 1032
pseudotumour, orbital <u>1249</u>, 1250
psychiatric disorders, and smell dysfunction *1234*, 1235
psychological aspects, rhinologic symptoms 978
PTEN tumour suppressor 65, 85, 89
public health research 468
public inquiries 391–2
Pulmicort nebule 1053–4, <u>1053–4</u>
pulmonary artery catheter 354, *354*
pulmonary artery wedge pressure 343
pulmonary aspiration of gastric contents 334
pulmonary embolism (PE) 270
pulmonary metastases, thyroid cancer 782
pulse oximetry, intra-operative 342
purine analogues 42
purpura
    immune thrombocytopenic 255, 267–8
    post-transfusion 246
    thrombotic thrombocytopenic 268
pyomucocele 1254, <u>1254</u>
pyramidine analogues 42, <u>43</u>

quadrilateral cartilage 966, 1136, <u>1136</u>, 1138
quality adjusted life years (QALYs) 401
quality of life (QOL)
    asthma and allergic rhinitis 1130
    and critical illness 359
    primary hyperparathyroidism 845–6
    sinus surgery 1077–8
    skull base surgery 1302
quinagolide 907
quinolones 223
    commonly used 223

R v. Bateman 422
R v. Caldwell 422
R v. Lawrence 422

R v. Prentice and Sulliman 422
R v. Sella 423
R v. Seymour 422
R v. Tutton and Tutton 422–3
R v. Yogasakaran 423
Rachels, J. 405
radiation exposure
    CT scanning 1305
    and thyroid cancer 740
radiation mucositis 235
radiation protection, radioiodine therapy 782
Radiation Therapy Oncology Group (RTOG) 91-11 trial 44
radioallergosorbent testing (RAST) 152, 1002, 1049
radiofrequency ablation, turbinate reduction 1163
radioiodine therapy 600, 724
    administration procedures 727, *727*, 780–1
    causing thyroiditis 733
    contraindications 728, 754
    differentiated thyroid cancer 751, 753–4, 779–80
        administration procedure 780–1
        follow-up 783–4, *784*
        high *vs* low activity 780
        thyroglobulin level 783
        TSH level 782–3
    goitre 744
        intra-thoracic 822
    hyperthyroidism 727–9
    indications 725
    patient preparation 754
    post-treatment hypothyroidism 736, 744
    prior iodinated contrast CT scanning 751
    radiation protection 782
    side effects and safety 728, 753–4, 781–2
    solitary thyroid nodule 744
radiological films, reading 427–8
radiosurgery, stereotactic 954, *955*
radiotherapy
    acute-reacting tissues 51–2
    anaplastic thyroid cancer 766–8, 788–9
    bioreductive drugs 54–5
    causing hypothyroidism 736
    concurrent chemotherapy 55
    DNA damage 51
    dose-response curves 52, <u>52</u>
    fractionation 52–3
    hyperfractionated 767–8
    intensity-modulated (IMRT) 766, 785
    late-reacting tissues 52
    medullary thyroid cancer 762, 786–7
    parathyroid carcinoma 861
    planning, FDG PET-CT 549
    radiosensitizers 53–4
    somatotrophinoma 933, 953–4
    targeted 55–6
    thyroid cancer 754, 784–5
Ramsay Hunt syndrome (herpes zoster oticus) 232, 280
random error
    control 469, 471
    sources of 471
random sampling 470

randomization 478, 506, 513
    concealed 513
    inadequate concealment 504, 506
randomized controlled trials (RCTs) 474, 478–80, 497
    critical appraisal 498, *500*, 512–15
    maximizing compliance and follow up 479
    strength of evidence 474
    surgical innovation 480
    systematic reviews 503–4, 515–21
rapid sequence induction 341
Ras 22, <u>66</u>, 67
RAS oncogene 83–4
RASSF1A 85
Rathke's cleft cysts 649, <u>649</u>, 1282, 1290
Rathke's pouch 611, <u>611</u>, 962
rationing 404
Raynaud's syndrome 153
RB tumour suppressor gene 86, 858
reactive oxygen species (ROS) 64, 113
reactive upper airways dysfunction syndrome (RUDS) 1018
Read codes 306
reasoning 396
receptor-interacting serine/threonine-protein kinases 1 and 3 (RIPK1/RIPK3) 61
rectal cancer, PET-CT detection <u>548</u>
recurrent laryngeal nerve (RLN)
    checking in thyroidectomy 802
    injury
        medical negligence claims 448
        parathyroid surgery 852, 884
        thyroid surgery 448, 888, 893, 894, *895*
    intra-operative monitoring 337, 345, 800, 888, 901
    involvement/encasement in thyroid cancer 753, 806
    locating in parathyroid surgery 853, 874, 883
    locating in thyroid surgery 798–800, <u>799–800</u>, 824, <u>824</u>
red blood cells (RBC/erythrocytes) 243, 249, 254
reference manager software 498
referrals, delays in 430–1
reflective equilibrium 396
reflux oesophagitis, treatment 298–9
Refsum disease 20
refusal of medical treatment 416–17
registration 562–4, 565–6
registry data, thyroid/parathyroid surgery 894–7, *895*
Reinke's oedema 705
relapsing polychondritis 177
relative risk 514
relative risk reduction 514
relativism 396, 397
relaxed skin tension lines (RSTL) 112
reliability, outcome measures 485
religion, and ethics 397
remifentanil 323, 335, 1072
remimazolam 348
renal cell carcinoma, thyroid metastases <u>686</u>
renal collecting duct cell, signal transduction 638, <u>639</u>

renal disease
    hypercalcaemia 829–30
    parathyroid carcinoma 858
    and platelet function 269
    secondary hyperparathyroidism 867–8
renal replacement therapy (RRT) 355
reproducibility 485
rescue flap 945
research
    clinical outcomes, see outcomes research
    ethical standards 403
research hypothesis 473
resource allocation 404
respect for autonomy 398
respiratory disease
    pre-operative assessment 303
    upper tract infections 201, 1087, 1126, 1235
    viral 197–9, 1087, 1126
respiratory irritants 1013
respiratory support
    classification 353
    critical care 352–4
    invasive 353
    weaning 353
respiratory syncytial virus (RSV) 198
respiratory tract
    ciliated epithelium 985, 1127, 1127
    microflora 182, 189
restriction endonucleases 5, 5
RET mutations
    children and adolescents 762–3
    hereditary thyroid cancers 85, 758, 760
    MEN2 syndrome 87–8, 758, 760
    phaeochromocytoma 758
RET-PTC gene rearrangements 84, 675
RET-PTC protein 160
retention cysts, sinuses 1308, 1308
reticulocytes 254, 255
retinoblastoma, genetic events 7–8
retinoblastoma protein 169, 700, 858
retinoblastoma tumour suppressor gene 8, 86, 858
retinoic acid 831
retropharyngeal abscess 313
retroviruses 199
    gene therapy vectors 30, 31
revalidation 375–6, 376, 391–2
reverse genetics 10
RFamide-related peptide (RFRP) 636
rhabdomyosarcoma 1251, 1314
rhesus (Rh) antigens 241
rheumatoid arthritis (RA) 133, 134
    airway difficulty 310, 311
    antibodies 153
    presentations 174
rheumatoid factor (RF) 153
rheumatological disease 173–9
    effects of immunosuppression 179
    ENT disease in 173–4, 175–9
    laboratory features 175
    red flags 174–5
    treatments 179–80
Rhinasthma 978
rhinitis
    and air pollution 1013–14, 1021
    allergic, see allergic rhinitis
    atrophic 289, 1014, 1033

definition 999, 1026
drug-induced 1013
due to physical and chemical factors 1013–14
emotionally-induced 1014
food-induced 1014
hormonal 1013
'mixed' 1011–12
non-allergic 1000
    aetiologies 1011
    diagnosis 1012, 1014
    idiopathic 1012
    occupational 1012–13
    symptoms 1011
    treatment 1014–15
non-allergic with eosinophilia syndrome (NARES) 1011, 1013, 1015
non-allergic non-infectious perennial (NANIPER) 1011, 1012, 1015
occupational, see occupational rhinitis
post-infectious 1012
pregnancy-induced 988, 1008, 1013
sick building syndrome 1021
rhinitis medicamentosa 1160
Rhinoconjunctivitis Quality of Life Questionnaire 978
rhinolalia 1149
rhinomanometry 991–3, 996, 1135
    active 992
    inferior turbinate enlargement 1161
    passive 992
    posterior 992, 992
rhinophyma 439
rhinorrhoea
    CSF 1206–7, 1206
        see also cerebrospinal fluid (CSF) leaks
rhinoscopy, anterior 978–9
rhinosinusitis
    acute, see acute rhinosinusitis
    chronic, see chronic rhinosinusitis (CRS)
    complications
        best clinical practice 1123
        bony 1115, 1122–3
        chronic 1123
        classification 1113
        epidemiology 1113
        future research 1123
        intracranial 1115, 1117, 1120–2
        orbital 1028, 1028, 1088, 1114–20
    definition 1262
    delays in referral 431
    diagnosis 1027
    distinction from rhinitis 1026
    epidemiology 1026–7
    ethmoid sinus 1114
    European position paper (EPOS) 1025, 1026, 1033–4, 1072, 1262
    facial pain 1254, 1255, 1262
    frontal sinus 1114
    fungal, see fungal rhinosinusitis
    future research 1033
    imaging 1308–10
    management in children 1078
    maxillary sinus 1114
    medical treatment 286–8
        antibiotics 285–6, 1059, 1060, 1062–4

antifungal agents 215, 287–8, 1053, 1064
antihistamines 287
antileukotrienes 288
corticosteroids 283–5, 1061–2
decongestants 286
ipratropium bromide 289
medications improving immune response 288
mucolytics 286–7
nasal/antral saline irrigation 288, 1006, 1060, 1064
sodium cromoglicate 287
recurrent acute, treatment 285
socioeconomic impact 1027
sphenoid sinus 1114
surgical treatment 1072–8
rhinospirometry 1161
rhinosporidiosis 208, 1150, 1212
rhinoviruses 197, 197
Rhizomucor spp. 1055
Rhizopus spp. 1055
ribavirin 203
Riedel's procedure (frontal sinus) 1097–8, 1122
Riedel's thyroiditis 662, 663, 706
Rieger's syndrome 925
rights 400
risk, definition 391
risk management 391
risk ratio 472–3
risks of surgery, disclosure 415–16, 417, 429
rituximab 161, 769, 1217
rivaroxaban 246, 271, 1179–80
RNA (ribonucleic acid) 4
    messenger (mRNA) 4
    microRNAs 4, 85
    protein production 40
    small interfering (siRNAs) 4
    transfer (tRNA) 4
RNA viruses 196
robotic surgery 560
    advantages 560
    current limitations 560
robotic-assisted thyroidectomy 813–17
    consent 815
    ethical issues 814–15
    operation 816–17
    operative set-up 815–16, 816
    training 814
robotized scanners, laser surgery 583
rocuronium 319, 340, 341
Rogers v. Whitaker 415, 429
rotational thromboelastography (ROTEM) 263
Royal Australasian College of Surgeons 454
Royal College of Nursing, fasting guidelines 307
Royal College of Surgeons of England (RCS)
    audit of sinus surgery 1077
    fellowship (FRCS) 373, 374–5
    Good surgical practice 900–1
    membership (MRCS) 373, 373
Royal Colleges 397, 405
rubella 199, 439
rubivirus 199

saccus decompression surgery 444
Sackett, Professor D 495
saddle nose deformity 431, 434, 435
St Paul's Sinus Centre
  diagnostic criteria for AFRS 1049
  Manuka honey treatment 1054–5, 1055
saline irrigation, nasal
  allergic rhinitis 1006
  application technique 1064, 1064
  rhinosinusitis 288, 1006, 1060, 1064
saliva, artificial 296
salivary gland surgery 345–6
  medical negligence claims 448–9
salivary glands
  involvement in HIV 235–6
  in sarcoidosis 1213
  stones 448–9
  tumours, medical litigation 447, 449
salt, iodinated 819
sample size 473–4
sampling procedures 470
Samter's triad 978, 1026, 1039–40, 1128
Sanders injector 319, 319
saprophytic fungal infections 1047, 1047
sarcoidosis 174, 179, 179, 831, 1033,
    1211–14, 1310
  aetiology 1211
  clinical features 1213, 1213, 1213
  diagnosis 1213–14
  epidemiology 1211
  inferior turbinate enlargement 1159
  nasal 1213, 1214, 1214
  pulmonary 1213, 1214, 1214
  treatment 1214
Savlon 295
scaffolds
  biomaterials 120, 120
  biomimetic 122
scalds 99–100
  dressings 103–4
Scandinavian Quality Register 894–6, 895
scars
  frontal sinus surgery 1093
  keloid/hypertrophic 102, 815, 890
  maturation 97
  medical negligence claims 433
  thyroid/parathyroid surgery 796, 811,
    813, 815, 890
schizophrenia 1237
schwannomas
  causing facial pain 1261, 1261
  olfactory, endoscopic endonasal surgery
    1294, 1295
  orbit 1251
  vestibular 21, 22, 560
Schwartz–Bartter syndrome (SIADH) 640,
    912, 919–20
scintigraphy
  frontal sinus 1085
  parathyroid glands 645
    adenomas 834–6, 835, 836
  thyroid 713, 713
    hyperthyroidism 720, 721
    intra-thoracic goitre 820, 821
    nodules 742
    subacute thyroiditis 732
Scott v. London & St Katherine's
    Docks 411–12

Scottish Intercollegiate Guidelines Network
    (SIGN) 392
search strategies 497–8, 498, 499
seat and desk arrangements 383–4, 384
sedation
  airway obstruction 323
  critical care 356
sedative premedication 334
selectins 132
selection bias 474–5
selective venous sampling (SVS) 838, 853
selective-oestrogen receptor modifiers
    (SERM) 831
selenium 77, 620
self-inflicted disease 401
sella turcica
  anatomy 614–16, 615
  differential diagnosis of masses 647–9
  empty syndrome 929
  endoscopic transsphenoidal approach
    944, 944, 1283–7
semaphorin 3F (SEMA3F) 22
sensitivity 510
sensorineural hearing loss
  drugs used 280
  in HIV 232
  tissue engineering 71
  virus-associated 199, 200, 201
sensory nerves, in allergic disease 141
sepsis 356–7, 357
Sepsis Six 357
septal perforations
  causes 1149, 1150, 1219, 1220
  clinical assessment 1150–1, 1151
  differential diagnosis 1310, 1310
  in granulomatous disorders 1151, 1215,
    1216, 1217–18
  nasal fractures 1188
  non-surgical management 1152
  obturation 1152
  prevalence 1149, 1151
  prevention 1152
  previous septal surgery 1152
  surgical repair 1152–4
  surgical widening 1152
  symptoms 1149–50
septal splints 1146, 1151
septal surgery
  complications 431–2
  perforation repair 1152–4
  septal deviation 1137–41, 1165
septo-optic dysplasia 925
septoplasty 1137–41
  approach 1137–8
  back to front technique 1138
  endoscopic 1140
  in epistaxis management 1178–9
  external approach 1140
  extracorporeal 1141
  front to back technique 1138–9
  paediatric 1141, 1147
  techniques 1139–40
septorhinoplasty
  after nasal fracture 1188
  inferior turbinate excision 1165
  medical negligence claims 434–5
serious hazards of transfusion (SHOT)
    244, 245

serology
  fungal antigens/antibodies 206
  virus specific antibodies 196–7
seroma, after thyroid/parathyroid
    surgery 887
sestamibi scintigraphy, parathyroid
    adenoma 834–6, 835, 853, 868
sestamibi–single-photon emission CT
    (SPECT-MIBI) 836, 836
severe combined immune deficiency
    (SCID) 29
sevoflurane 325, 335, 336, 1072
sex hormone binding globulin (SHBG) 636
sham surgery 444
shared airway 336, 339, 344
Sheehan's syndrome 906, 927, 951
Shipman, Harold 409
Shnitzlers syndrome 179
Short Form 36-Item Health Survey (SF-36)
    487, 488, 492, 846, 978
Shy Drager syndrome, delay in
    diagnosis 450
sialadenitis, radioiodine therapy 781
sick building syndrome 1021
sick euthyroid syndrome 635
sickle cell disease 256
Sickness Impact Profile (SIP) 488, 492
Sidaway v. Board of Governors of the
    Bethlem Royal Hospital 415
signal transducer and activator of
    transcription (STAT) 630, 631
significance level 473
significance test 473
silent sinus syndrome 1249, 1250,
    1310, 1311
silicone barrier creams, nasal 1152
Singer, P. 396
single-photon emission computed
    tomography (SPECT)
  CT fusion 836, 837
  sestamibi scintigraphy fusion 836, 836
sinonasal compartment 972–6
Sinonasal Outcomes Tests 491
  SNOT-16 1065
  SNOT-20 470, 491
  SNOT-22 491, 978, 1025, 1065
sinonasal tumours
  biopsy 1270, 1272–3
  by tissue of origin 1270
  concerning clinical features 1271
  diagnosis and pre-operative planning
    1270–3, 1271–2
  endoscopic management
    case selection 1273, 1273, 1290
    complications 1278
    evidence base for 1269
    image guidance 1274
    optimizing surgical field 1274
    outcomes 1301
    postoperative care 1278–9
    surgical access 1274–8
    tumour resection 1274, 1278
  epidemiology 1269–70
  imaging 1270–2, 1271–2, 1310–14
    CT features and implications 1272
  juvenile angiofibroma 576, 577, 1265–8,
    1312, 1313
  malignant 1270, 1270

sinonasal tumours (continued)
  multidisciplinary management 1273
  skull base 1290, 1293, 1293, 1297, 1297
  see also individual tumours; juvenile angiofibroma
sinonasal undifferentiated carcinoma (SNUC) 1290
sinus secretions, MRI 1306, 1306
sinusitis
  facial pain 1254, 1255
  in HIV infection 233
  medical negligence claims 447–8
  in rheumatological disease 174
  see also rhinosinusitis
situational awareness 454–7
situs inversus 1040, 1041
Sjögren's syndrome 134, 153, 153, 174
skier's nose 1013
skills acquisition, Dreyfus model 372
skin
  anatomy and physiology 108–9, 110
  biomechanics 111–12
  blood flow 109–11
  microflora 182
  vessel biomechanics 110–11
skin biopsies, healing 100
skin cancer, diagnosis and treatment 436
skin closure, thyroidectomy 802
skin disease, hyperthyroidism 723, 723
skin flap surgery
  applied anatomy and physiology 108–10
  history 107–8
skin flaps
  conditioning 115
  design 108
  extracorporeal perfusion 115–16
  laser therapy 116
  leech therapy 116
  management of compromised 112–15
  potential complications 436
  surgical delay 115
skin grafts 100, 436
skin lesions, excision of benign 433
skin prick tests 144, 145, 147, 152
  allergic rhinitis 1002
  occupational rhinitis 1022
skin tension lines, relaxed 112
skin testing, allergic disease 144–5, 144
skull base
  areas of weakness 1205
  congenital malformations 1086–7, 1087
  damage in sinus surgery 1205–6, 1205
    medical negligence claims 430
  defects 1205, 1207, 1207, 1277, 1314, 1314
    CSF leaks 1077, 1205–6, 1205
  fractures 1204
  nasal cavity 966
  and paranasal sinuses 969–72, 970–1
  posterior 970–1, 971, 972
  reconstruction 945–6, 946–7, 1206, 1208, 1278, 1298, 1300–1, 1300–1
    nasoseptal flap 945–6, 946–7, 1277, 1278, 1300
    pericranial flap 1300–1, 1300
    rescue flap 945
  remodelling in fungal sinusitis 1309

tumours 572, 944–5, 944, 1204, 1249, 1313–14, 1314
  imaging 1270–2, 1271–2
skull base surgery
  approaches
    classification 1289, 1290
    supraorbital 1297
    suprasellar 1297–8
    transcribriform 1293–4, 1294, 1294
    transfrontal 1293, 1293
    transplanum 1294–6
    transsphenoidal 1283–6
  complications 1302
  image guidance 565, 1274, 1283
  indications 1290–1, 1290
  nasal preparation 1292–3
  operating room set up 1292, 1292
  outcomes 1301–2
  post-operative care 1301
  pre-operative assessment 1282–3
  pre-operative planning 1291–2
  reconstruction 1298–301, 1300–1
skull base tumours, brain invasion 1290
sleep disturbance, allergic rhinitis 1000
sleep-disordered breathing 1165
sloughy wounds 102
Sluder's neuralgia 1258–9
smell
  importance of 1227
  nasal structure and physiology 1228–30
smell disorders
  causes 1233–5, 1233–4
    head trauma 1235
    neurodegenerative diseases 1230, 1231, 1237, 1239
    sinonasal disease 1234, 1235–6
    tumours and mass lesions 1236–7
    upper respiratory infection 1235
  classification and terms 1230–1
  clinical evaluation 1228, 1231–3
  conductive 1233, 1238
  frequency of 1227
  future research 1239
  imaging studies 1233
  prognosis 1239
  sensorineural 1233–4, 1238–9
  treatment 1238–9
Smell Identification Test ™ 1232–3, 1232
smoking
  and goitre development 77
  and nasal function 977–8, 986
  and olfactory function 1231, 1237
  patient' personal responsibility 400
smooth muscle, airway 1127, 1131
α-smooth muscle actin (α-SMA) 159
sneezing 1011
sodium bicarbonate ear drops 277
sodium cromoglicate 147, 1006, 1023
sodium fluoride 280
sodium iodide symporter (NIS) 78, 619, 622, 640
sodium thiosulphate 254
sodium valproate 955
solicitors, medical negligence claims 413, 414
solutions 295–6

solvent detergent plasma 244
somatomammotrophs 613, 630
somatostatin 632, 632
somatostatin analogues
  medullary thyroid cancer 787, 788
  primary pituitary disease 933, 936, 953, 955
  radiolabelled 788
somatotrophinomas 647, 932–3
  adjuvant treatment 952–4
somatotrophs 613, 630, 631, 924
sonic hedgehog (SHH) pathway mutations 925
sorafenib 22, 785
sore throat, rheumatological disease 174
South Africa, HIV 229
Southern blotting 6
spanning sutures 1145
specificity 509–10
Speech Intelligibility Index 490
Speech, Spatial and Qualities of Hearing Questionnaire 490
sphenoethmoidal nerve 1170
sphenoid functional unit 975–6
sphenoid ostium 970, 971
sphenoid sinus 970–1, 972
  anatomy 612, 612, 970–1, 972, 975–6
  development 963
  intra-sinus septae 612, 944, 1283
    removal 944, 1284, 1285
  invasive fungal rhinosinusitis 1056
  mucoceles 1110–11, 1254, 1254
  pneumatization patterns 612, 963–4, 963, 964, 975–6
  surgical exposure 944, 944, 947
sphenoidal process 966
sphenoidectomy 1074
sphenopalatine artery 967, 968, 968, 1170
  anatomical variants 968
  damage in sinus surgery 1076
  endonasal endoscopic ligation 1177, 1178
  lateral branch 1158
  posterior septal branch 1170
sphenopalatine foramen 1170, 1172–3, 1177
  widened in juvenile angiofibroma 1265, 1266
sphenopalatine ganglion 966
SPIKES framework 384, 384
spindle poisons 43
spirochaetes 192
spirometry 313, 321, 821
spleen 250
splenectomy 257, 267
splinting tests 979
splints, nasal 1146, 1152
spreader grafts 1144, 1144
squamous cell carcinoma
  frontal sinus 1103
  sinonasal 1311, 1312
squamous epithelium
  contact endoscopy 589, 589
  nose 985
staffing 392
stapedotomy 441
stapes, congenital fixation 440
staphylococci 184–5

Staphylococcus aureus 184
    biofilms 185
    chronic rhinosinusitis 1030, 1032
    enterotoxin B 1126
    exotoxins 1030
    flucloxacillin resistance 225
    and GPA aetiology 1215, 1217
    methicillin-resistant, *see* methicillin-resistant *Staphylococcus aureus*
Staphylococcus aureus bacteraemia (SAB) 184
Staphylococcus aureus, and nasal polyps 1039
Staphylococcus lugdunensis 184
staples, thyroidectomy 802
statistics
    critical appraisal 506
    systematic reviews 516
statutes 410
stem cell transplants 251, 253, 254, 257
stem cells
    adipose 122
    adult tissue-specific (somatic) 69–70
    cancer 72
    clinical applications 71–2
    embryonic 70
    haematopoietic 70, 249–50
    induced pluripotent 70
    mesenchymal 70
    methods for tissue/organ generation 70–1
Stenstrom technique 435–6
stenting, fronto-ethmoidal mucocele 1110
stereotactic radiosurgery, pituitary adenomas 954, 955
sternocleidomastoid muscle 875, 883
sternohyoid muscles 797
sternothyroid muscles 797
sternotomy, thyroidectomy 823
Stickler syndrome 19
stomach cancer, PET-CT imaging 548
Storz, Karl 587, 588
strangulation, children 363
strap muscles
    closure 802
    division 797, 797, 823, 853, 875
stratification 475
streptococci 185–7
    α-haemolytic 186–7
    antibiotics 187
    β-haemolytic 186, *186*
Streptococcus anginosus 1118, 1122
Streptococcus pneumoniae 186, 233, 1118
    culture 186
    infections 186–7
    rhinosinusitis 1027, 1032
Streptococcus pyogenes 186
    clinical syndromes *186*
    virulence factors *186*
streptokinase 272
streptomycin 192
stress, surgeon 461–2, *462*
stress assessment, pre-operative 462
stress management 1256
stridor
    airway narrowing 322
    anaesthesia induction 325
    children 363

haematological malignancy
    treatment 254
    management 296, 300
    rheumatological disorders 174
struma ovarii 607, 659, 660
Sub-Saharan Africa, HIV epidemic 229
subarachnoid haemorrhage 1174, 1175
subconjunctival haemorrhage 1196, 1196
subcutaneous immunotherapy (SCIT) 143, 1006, 1007, 1129–30
subcutaneous musculoaponeurotic system (SMAS) 964
subdural empyema 1120–2
subglottic stenosis, granulomatous disease 1215, 1218, *1223*
subgroup analyses 479–80
sublingual immunotherapy (SLIT) 1006, 1007, 1129–30
submandibular gland surgery, medical negligence claims 448–9
submucosal diathermy, inferior turbinates 429, 1162
submucosal resection (SMR), epistaxis 1178–9
subperiosteal abscess
    frontal sinus (Pott's puffy tumour) 1122–3, 1122
    orbit *1028*, 1117, *1117*, 1118
subplatysmal flap 796, *796*
substance P 1128
succinate dehydrogenase (SDH) complex 23
sugammadex 319, 340
sulfamethoxazole 223
sulphatide 114
sulphur dioxide pollution 1021
SUNCT/SUNA 1257
sunitinib 736
superantigens 1030, 1039, 1126
superior intercavernous sinus (SIS) 1298
superior laryngeal nerve
    blockade 324
    external branch identification 798, 799
    external branch injury 888–9
superior vena cava obstruction (SVCO) 252
superoxide dismutase 113–14
Supporting doctors, protecting patients 390
supra agger frontal cells 1082, *1083*, 1083–4
supra bulla frontal cells 1082, *1083*, 1084, 1307, *1308*
supraglottic airway devices (SADs) 336, 336
supraorbital ethmoid cells 1084, 1084, 1307
surface immunoglobulin (sIg) 127, 127
surface rendering 561, 562
surfactants, in rhinosinusitis 1064–5
surgeon experience
    parathyroidectomy 852
    thyroidectomy 902, *902*
surgeon portfolio 375
surgical checklist 453, 463
surgical infections
    medical negligence claims 450
    thyroid/parathyroid surgery 887–8
surgical innovation, clinical trials 480

surgical performance, thyroid/parathyroid surgery 896
surgical simulation 560, 565
surgical training 392
    appraisal and revalidation 375–6, *376*
    assessments 370–1, 374
    Calman Report (1993) 372
    continuing professional development 375, *375*
    curriculum
        aims and objectives 369–70
        assessment 370–1
        resources for delivery 370
        syllabus 370, 376
    delivery 373–5
    evidence-based medicine in 495–500
    evolution in UK 371–2
    future of ENT 376
    GMC standards of assessment 371
    principles 369
    programme evaluation 371
    robotic surgery 814
    structure of UK postgraduate and ENT specialty 373, 373
    time available for 370, 372, *372*, 392
    Unfinished Business (2002) 372
surgical wounds 100
    classification *100*
SurgTech Ltd. 979
Surveillance, Epidemiology, and End Results (SEER) studies, anaplastic thyroid cancer 766
Surviving Sepsis Campaign 356, 357
Sushruta Samhita 107
suspension sutures, lateral nasal wall 1144, 1145
suspensions 296
suspensory ligament of Berry 604
sustenacular cell 1229, 1229
suture marks, litigation 433
suxamethonium 340, 341
swallowing difficulty, rheumatological disease 174
sympathomimetics 286, 985
Symptom Checklist-90 (SCL-90) 846
synchronous malignancies, PET-CT detection 548–9, 548
syndrome of inappropriate antidiuretic hormone (SIADH) 640, 912, 919–20
syndromic hearing impairment, genetics 19–21
synechiae, frontal sinus surgery 1093
synthetic graft materials 120, *120*
syphilis 192
syrups 296
system 1/system 2 thinking 457
systematic error
    control 469, 471
    sources of 471
systematic reviews 497, 503–4, 551
    critical appraisal 516–21
    PRISMA guidelines 504, 515–16
    sources 515
    validity 516
systemic disease
    causing chronic rhinosinusitis 1032, *1033*
    causing nasal polyposis 1030–1
    nasal manifestations 977

systemic lupus erythematosus (SLE) 133, 174, 177–8
   autoantibodies (ANA) 153, *153*
   classification *177*
   diagnostic criteria *178*
   nasal septal perforation 1151
systemic sclerosis *153*, 174, 179

T cells 125, 127–9
   allergic disease 139
   cytotoxic (Tc) 128
   helper (Th) 128, 129, <u>129</u>, 139
   regulatory (T reg) 129, <u>129</u>, 138
   Th17 129
   tumour-infiltrating 158–9, 161
T-cell leukaemia/lymphoma 202, 251, 1312
T-cell receptor (TCR) 127–8
tampons, nasal 1176
Taq polymerase 7
targeted therapies 11–12, 45–8, 55–6
   differentiated thyroid cancers 785
   medullary thyroid cancer 762, 787
   toxicities 785
taxanes 789
taxoids 43
team work 459–69
teeth, painful 1259
telangiectasia, hereditary haemorrhagic (Osler-Weber-Rendu disease) 289, 577, <u>1178</u>, 1180
telomerase 10
telomere, shortening 9–10
temozolomide 952, 955
temperature, intra-operative management 343
temporal arteritis 1260
temporomandibular joint disorder 1259
tension-type headache 1256–7, <u>1256</u>
tentorium cerebelli 615
Terrorism Act (2000) 417
testosterone levels 917
testosterone replacement 929
tetany, hypocalcaemic 298
tetracyclines, resistance 226
tetraiodothyronine, *see* thyroxine
thalassaemia major 250
thalidomide 233
theatre lists 306
theatre team
   communication with 459–60
   surgeon's confidence in 462
theophylline toxicity 831
Thinking Fast and Slow (Kahneman) 457
thiocyanate 76–7
thioguanine 42, <u>299</u>
thionamides 297, 620, 724–7
   adjuncts 727
   'block and replace' regimen 726
   dosage 725
   Graves' disease 726
   indications *725*
   monitoring therapy 711
   in pregnancy 739
   radioiodine pre-treatment 727–8
   side effects 725–6, *726*
   toxic multinodular goitre/toxic adenoma 726–7
   treatment efficacy 726

thiopentone 334–5
throat lozenges/pastilles 295
throat packs 337
thrombin 259, <u>260</u>, <u>261</u>, 262
thrombin inhibitors, direct 246
thrombocytopenia 255, 267–8
    heparin-induced 255–6, 268
    platelet transfusion 243–4
thrombocytosis 255, 268
thromboelastography 263, <u>264</u>
thromboembolism
    acquired causes 270
    management 270, 273
    prophylaxis 294, 305–6
    risk assessment 305
    risk factors 269, *269*
    role of haematology 273
thrombomodulin 262, <u>263</u>
thrombophilia screen 269–70
thrombosis 269–72
    acquired causes 270
    information for haematologist 273
    rare causes 270
    risk factors 269, *269*
    treatment 270
thrombotic thrombocytopenic purpura (TTP) 268
thrush, oral in HIV 233–4, *235*
Thudicum's speculum 978
thymectomy 866
thymidine 3-deoxy-3-¹⁸F-fluorothymidine (FLT) 552
thymoma 154
thymus, embryology 608, 874, *874*
thyroglobulin (Tg) 620, 622, 634–5, 783
    antibodies 711–12, 783
    stimulated 754–5, 783, *783*
    thyroid cancer 712–13, 741, 783–4
      recurrent disease 774–5, 776
thyroglossal duct carcinoma 659
thyroglossal tract 607
    remnants 607, 659
thyroid, cancer 643–4
thyroid adenoma
    follicular adenoma 665–6, *665*, <u>665–6</u>
    solitary toxic (Plummer's disease) 724
thyroid antibodies 711–12
thyroid artery, inferior 874
thyroid bed, cancer recurrence 775, *775*
thyroid cancer
    advanced disease 805
    aetiology 740–1
    airway involvement 806–8, <u>807–8</u>, 822, <u>822</u>
      recurrent disease 775
    columnar cell 680, <u>680</u>
    differentiated
      chemotherapy 785
      childhood 785–6
      external beam radiotherapy 754, 784–5
      follow-up 754–5, 786
      investigations 751
      locoregional recurrence 774–7, 809
      management in pregnancy 786
      metastatic disease 784
      non-surgical treatment 753–4, 779–86

      prognosis 751
      recurrence risk 773–4, *774*
      surgical treatment 752–3
      targeted therapies 785
      thyroglobulin measurement 712–13, 741, 776, 783
      thyroidectomy 752–3, 795
      treatment outcomes assessment 754
    distant metastases 809
    epidemiology 740–1
    extrathyroidal spread 652, 668, 805–9
    FDG PET-CT imaging 549–50, <u>549</u>
    follicular 667–9
      extrathyroidal extension 669
      minimally invasive 667–8, <u>667</u>
      oncocytic cell tumours 669, 670, <u>670</u>
      surgical margins 668
      thyroidectomy 753
      ultrasound 644
      widely invasive 667, 669
    follicular variant 675
    genetics 83–6
    hyalinizing trabecular tumours (HTTs) 666, <u>666</u>
    intra-operative frozen section examination 685
    medullary, *see* medullary thyroid cancer (MTC)
    mixed follicular-parafollicular 684
    neck dissection 753, 776, 809
    nodal disease 776, 809
    non-invasive follicular with papillary-like nuclear features 677–8, <u>677</u>
    oesophagus involvement 775, 806, 808
    papillary, *see* papillary thyroid cancer
    poorly differentiated 679–70, <u>681</u>
    resection specimen <u>802</u>
    residual/unrecognized disease 806
    serum markers 741–2
    staging 685, 687–9, *752*
    thyroidectomy 752–3
    TSH levels 741
    ultrasound 643–4
    undifferentiated, *see* anaplastic thyroid cancer
thyroid eye disease, *see* hyperthyroidism, eye disease
thyroid function tests 709–11
    hypercalcaemia 831
    hyperthyroidism 720, *720*
    hypopituitarism *918*
    hypothyroidism 735, *735*
    peri-operative 889, 890
    population screening 710–11
    pregnancy 711, *711*
    thyroid nodules 741
thyroid gland
    capsule 651–2
    cystic lesions 656, <u>656</u>
    developmental abnormalities 607, 659
    differential diagnosis of follicular-patterned lesions 675, <u>676</u>
    ectopic tissue 607
    embryology 605–6, <u>605</u>, *606*, 651
    enlarged intra-thoracic
      aetiology 819–20
      assessment for surgery 821
      clinical presentation 820

thyroid gland (*continued*)
    investigations 820–1
    non-surgical management 821–2
    surgery 822–4, <u>824</u>
    terminology use 819
euthyroid enlargement 740–5
FNAC 653–7, 655, <u>662–3</u>, 742–3, *743*
    false negatives 901
    iatrogenic changes 657–9, <u>658</u>
    international classification systems 654, *655*, 743, *743*
    limitations 654, 656–7
    thyroid enlargement 742–3, *743*
growth, hormonal factors 79
inferior pole 798
lateral aberrant tissue 663, <u>664</u>
lateral aspect 798, *798*
lymphoma 644, 656–7, 706, 768–9, <u>770</u>
macroscopic anatomy 603–4, 651
metastatic tumours 684, <u>685</u>
microscopic appearance 604, 652–3, <u>652–3</u>
    C cells 652–3
    solid cell nests 653, <u>653</u>
normal anatomical variants 606
oncocytic (oxyphilic) cells 660–1, *661*, 669–670, <u>670</u>
parafollicular cells (C cells) 604, <u>604</u>, 607, 652–3
physiology 619–23
pyramidal lobe 606, 801, <u>801</u>
scintigraphy 713, <u>713</u>
    hyperthyroidism 720, <u>721</u>
    nodular disease 742
    subacute thyroiditis 732
squamous differentiation 660, *661*, <u>661</u>
superior pole 797–8, <u>798</u>
surgical approach 600, 796–7, 823, <u>824</u>
tubercle of Zuckerkandl 606
uncommon/rare neoplasms 684, *684*
vascular pedicle 797, <u>798</u>
weight of normal 619, 651, 819
thyroid hormone withdrawal (THW) 780–1
thyroid hormones 619–20, 633–5
    activity in tissues 623
    drug preparations 297
    feedback control of synthesis 621, <u>621</u>
    release 622
    synthesis 620, <u>621</u>
    and wound healing 99
thyroid incidentalomas 744–5
thyroid isthmus, exposure 797, <u>797</u>
thyroid nodules 663, <u>664</u>, 706
    causes 740
    epidemiology 740
    FNAC 643–4, 742–3, *743*, 901
    hyperplastic 663, <u>664</u>
    medical management 743–5
    presentation 706
    risk of malignancy 713, *713*, 743
    risk stratification 644
    solitary non-toxic 744
    ultrasound 643–4, 713–14, *713*, 742
        classification 742
thyroid peroxidase (TPO) 620, <u>621</u>, 622
    antibodies 622, 711, 720
thyroid storm
    after thyroid surgery 729, *730*, 890

features/signs 705, *730*
treatment *730*
thyroid-stimulating hormone (TSH) 621, <u>621</u>, 633–4, <u>634</u>
causes of elevation/suppression *710*, 912
deficiency 709, *710*, 717, 741, 906, *906*, 928, 929
    isolated (central hypothyroidism) 736, 737, 906, *906*, 926
elevation prior to radioiodine therapy 780–1
excess *710*, 912, 917, 936
follicular cell responses 604
and goitre development 79
hyperthyroidism 719, *719*, 720
hypothyroidism 735, *735*
measurement 709–10, *709*, *918*
normal range 621–2
in pregnancy 711
recombinant (rhTSH) 744, 754, 780–1
    licensed indications 781
in subacute thyroiditis 732, <u>732</u>
subclinical hypothyroidism 737–8
suppression after thyroid cancer treatment 754–5, *755*, 782–3
in thyroid cancer 741
in thyroid nodules 741
thyroid-stimulating hormone receptor (TSH-R) 621
    antibodies 712, 720, 723
thyroidectomy
    airway management 890
    anaplastic thyroid cancer 766
    benign disease 794–5
    complications 729–30, *730*, 887–90, 893
        aerodigestive injury 889
        audits and registers of 894–7, *895*
        bleeding 888, 893
        haematoma 888
        hypocalcaemia 730, 889, 894, 895, 902
        hypoparathyroidism 625, 889
        hypothyroidism 736, 889–90
        infection 887–8
        recurrent laryngeal nerve injury 448, 888, 893, 894, *895*
        revision surgery 776
        superior laryngeal nerve injury 888–9
        and surgeon experience 902, *902*
    development as multidisciplinary specialism 599–600
    'diagnostic' surgery 795
    differentiated thyroid cancer 752–3, 795
    extra-cervical approach 823, <u>824</u>
    haemostasis 797, 801–2
    history 597–9, 619, 793–4
    hyperthyroidism 729–31
    incisions 795–6, <u>796</u>, 823
    informed consent 795
    intra-operative nerve monitoring 337, 345, 600, 888–9, 901
    intra-thoracic goitre 821, 822–4, <u>823</u>, <u>824</u>
    L-thyroxine replacement 626
    length of inpatient stay 901–2
    medical negligence claims 899–902
    minimally invasive 811–13

minimally invasive video-assisted (MIVAT) 600
near-total (Dunhill's) 894
outcomes
    comparison between providers 896
    registry data 894–6, *895*
    and surgeon experience 902, *902*
parathyroid glands
    injury 730, 889
    management 797–8, 800–1, <u>800</u>
perioperative medical management 626, 889
postoperative care 802
postoperative thyroid function 730–1
pre-operative considerations 795
in pregnancy 786
'prophylactic' in hereditary MTC 762–3
recurrent laryngeal nerve preservation 753, 806
robot-assisted 813–17
scarless in the neck techniques 813
scars 796, 811, 813, 815, 890
subtotal 600, 794
surgical outcomes 600
    comparison of providers 896
    national registry data 894–6, *895*
surgical technique 795–802
thyroid isthmusectomy 794
thyroid lobectomy 794
for thyrotoxicosis 794–5
thyroiditis
    destructive 732–3
    drug-induced 661
    FNAC <u>662–3</u>
    Hashimoto's 644, 661, 662, 670, <u>670</u>, 735
    painless sporadic 662
    postpartum 662, 738
    radiation-induced 733
    Riedel's 662, <u>663</u>, 706
    silent/painless 733
    subacute/de Quervain's 662, <u>663</u>, 732, *732*
    suppurative 662
thyromental distance 312, <u>312</u>, *313*
thyrotoxicosis 717, *718*
    in absence of hyperthyroidism 732–3
    aetiology 718, *718*
    amiodarone-induced 733
    clinical manifestations 705–6, 718–19
    diagnostic evaluation 719–20, *720*, 731
    effects/key functions in adults 620
    extent of surgery 794
    eye disease 706
        conservative treatment 1246
        orbital decompression 1247–8, <u>1247–8</u>
        symptoms and signs 722–3, <u>722</u>
        urgent referral criteria 723
    Graves' disease 720–3
    hypercalcaemia 831
    iodine-induced 733
    management before surgery 626
    medical management 724–7, *725*, 731
    periodic paralysis 719
    pituitary thyrotrophin-secreting adenoma 912

thyrotoxicosis (*continued*)
  post-operative 890
  in pregnancy 738–9
  radioiodine therapy 727–9, *727*
  surgical management 729–31
  thyroidectomy 794–5
thyrotrophs 613, *631*
thyrotropin-releasing hormone (TRH) 621, <u>621</u>, 633, <u>634</u>
thyrotropin-releasing hormone (TRH) test *918*
thyroxine (T4) 620, 634–5
  foetal serum 606
  free (fT4)
    hyperthyroidism 719, *719*, *720*
    hypothyroidism 735, *735*
    measurement 710, *710*
thyroxine therapy 297, 736–7
  elderly patients 737
  monitoring 711
  pregnancy 737, 739
  replacement doses 626
thyroxine-binding globulin 622–3, *623*
tidal volume, intra-operative measurement 343
tirapazamine 54–5
tissue engineering 70–2, 122
  applications in otorhinolaryngology 71–2
  bioreactors 121–2
  bone 122
  methods 70–1
  molecular therapy 122
  scaffold biomaterials 120, *120*
tissue expansion 115
tissue inhibitors of metalloproteinases 97
tissue sealants 247
TNM staging, thyroid cancer 685, 687–9, *752*
To Err is Human: Building a safer health system (IOM) 389
tobacco smoking, *see* smoking
tongue base tumour 322, <u>322</u>
tongue resection surgery, PET-CT imaging *552*
tonsillectomy
  anaesthesia 344–5, 349
  antibiotics 295
  epidemiology studies 465–6, 468
  medical negligence claims 445
  PET-CT imaging after *552*
  post-operative bleeding 345, 349, 445
tonsils, asymmetry 252
topical anaesthesia, airway 323–4
topiramate 1258
topoisomerase inhibitors 43–4
tort 410
total intravenous anaesthesia (TIVA) 335, 348, 1072, 1274
TP53 65–6
trachea
  iatrogenic injury 889
  thyroid cancer involvement 806–8, <u>807–8</u>, 822, <u>822</u>
  tissue-engineering 71
tracheal intubation
  'awake' 322–4, 341
  bronchoscopic 366

difficult, *see* difficult airway
fibre-optic 316–17
lighted stylets 317
tracheal ligament, anterior 603–4
tracheal tubes 336–7, <u>337</u>
  laryngeal surgery 347
  laser surgery 339–40, <u>340</u>
tracheitis, bacterial 364
tracheobronchial stent 326, <u>327</u>
tracheomalacia 822, 890
tracheostomy 357–8
  emergency post-extubation 328–9, <u>329</u>
  medical negligence claims 446
  paediatric 365–6
  rapid emergency 326
  under local anaesthesia 325–6
  verification of correct placement 326
Trachlight™ 317
training
  in communication skills 381
  see also surgical training
tramazoline hydrochloride 286
tranexamic acid 247, 266, 1176
tranfusion-associated graft versus host disease (TA-GVHD) 243, 246
transcription 4, 5, <u>40</u>
transferrin, serum 98
transforming growth factor-α (TGF-α) 56
  and goitre 79, *79*
  wound healing 95
transforming growth factor-β (TGF-β) 129, <u>129</u>
  bone healing 97
  chronic rhinosinusitis 1031
  and goitre 79, *79*
  tumour microenvironment 159
  wound healing 95
transfusion reactions 244–6
  acute 244–5, *245*
  delayed 246
transfusion-associated acute lung injury (TRALI) 245
transfusion-associated circulatory overload (TACO) 245–6
translation 4, 5
transoesophageal echocardiography (TOE) 343
transorbital neuroendoscopic surgery (TONES) 1110
transsphenoidal surgery 933, 942, 944, <u>944</u>, 951, 1283–7
trastuzumab 161
trauma, paediatric airway 363, 365
Treacher Collins syndrome 65
tree pollen allergy 1001
trephination
  frontal sinus 1088, 1097, <u>1097</u>
  complications 431
Treponema pallidum 192
triamcinolone 233, 433
Trichophyton mentagrophytes 207
Trichophyton rubrum 207
Trichophyton schoenleinii 207
trigeminal autonomic cephalalgias 1257–8
trigeminal nerve 963, 966, 1158, 1253–4
trigeminal neuralgia 1258
trigeminal somatosensory system 1229

triiodothyronine (T3) 620, 634–5
  free (fT3)
    hyperthyroidism 719, *719*
    hypothyroidism 735, *735*
    measurement 710, *710*
  therapy in hypothyroidism 737
trimethoprim 223
'tripod' fracture 1196
triptans 1256
trisacryl gelatin particles 570–1, *571*, <u>576</u>
trochlear nerve 617, 910, <u>911</u>
truth-telling 404–5
tryptase, serum 141, 152
tubeless surgery 338
tubercle of Zuckerkandl 606
tuberculosis (TB) 134, 191–2, 251, *1033*
  in HIV 232
tuberculum sellae 614, <u>615</u>
tumour associated macrophages (TAM) 158, 159, 160
tumour biology 39–41
tumour biomarkers 161, 162–3
tumour clonogen proliferation 52, 53
tumour debulking 1291, <u>1292</u>
  sinonasal tumours 1278
tumour embolization 571–2, *572*
  chemotherapy delivery 572
  juvenile nasopharyngeal angiofibroma 576, <u>577</u>
  meningioma 573–5
  paraganglioma 575–6
  percutaneous 572
  transarterial 571–2
tumour escape mechanisms 160
tumour growth 40–1
tumour microenvironment 157–60, <u>158</u>
tumour necrosis factor (TNF)
  allergy *139*, *140*
  bone repair 97
  defence mechanisms 128, 133
  sarcoidosis 1211, 1214
  sepsis 356
  tumour microenvironment <u>158</u>, 159–60
tumour necrosis factor (TNF) receptor-associated periodic syndrome (TRAPS) 178
tumour necrosis factor-α (TNF-α)
  antagonists 162, 177, 180
tumour necrosis factor-related apoptosis-inducing ligand (TRAIL) 65
tumour suppressor genes
  parathyroid carcinoma 858, 860–1
  thyroid tumours 84
tumour-associated antigens (TAA) 160
tumour-infiltrating lymphocytes (TIL) 158–9, 161, 163
tumour-specific antigens (TSA) 160
TUNEL assay 60
turbinate surgery 1160–4
  best clinical practice *1167*
  in children 1165
  future research *1167*
  mucosal preservation 1162
  outcomes 1165–6, <u>1167</u>
  in rhinosinusitis 1164–5
  in septal surgery 1165
  in sleep-disordered breathing 1165

turbinate surgery (continued)
    submucosal 429, 1162–4, 1163
    trends in 1157, 1157
turbinates
    anatomy 968
    blood supply 984, 984
    functions 987, 988, 1158
    inferior 987, 1157
        anatomy 1158
        enlargement 987, 1015, 1146,
            1158–9, 1159
        physiology 1158, 1158
    middle 973
        lateralization 1093
    nasal cycle 968, 968, 986, 1158
turbinoplasty 1163, 1163
twin studies, goitre formation 78, 78
tympanic membrane perforation 276–7
tyrosine kinase inhibitors (TKIs) 162,
    251, 736

UK Registry of Endocrine and Thyroid
    Surgery (UKRETS) 376
UK Sinonasal Audit 1027
ulcers
    arterial 101
    diabetic 100, 103
    pressure 100–1, 103
    venous 101
ultimobranchial bodies 605, 605, 607,
    608, 651
ultrasound
    parathyroid glands 644–5, 833–4
        adenoma localization 833–4, 834,
            875
        carcinoma 858–9
    thyroid 643–4, 713–14
        benign disease 713, 713, 742, 742
        cancer diagnosis 643–4
        cancer follow-up 713–14, 783, 783
        intra-thoracic goitre 820
UN Declaration of Human Rights 400
uncinate process 973, 974, 981
    attachments 1082, 1082
    superior attachment 973, 974
uncinectomy 1073–4, 1073–4, 1247
'unified airway' concept 999, 1028,
    1125, 1126
United States (USA), medical negligence
    claims 442, 900
University of Pennsylvania Smell
    Identification Test™ (UPSIT) 1022,
    1232–3, 1232
upper aerodigestive tract
    injury in thyroid/parathyroid
        surgery 889
    microflora 182, 189
    mucosa
        contact endoscopy 589–93
        dysplasia 591, 591
upper airway obstruction, child 363–4
upper respiratory tract infection (URTI)
    disorders of smell 1235
    viral 201, 1126
        frontal sinusitis after 1087–8
uraemia, and platelet function 269
urinary calcium 829, 830
urinary iodine concentration 76, 76

urinary sodium 920
urine
    24-hour cortisol 916, 934, 934
    calcium: creatinine excretion ratio 830
    osmolarity 919, 920
Usher syndrome 20
    type 1D 17
uveoparotid fever 1213

vaccines
    acute rhinosinusitis 289
    Hib infections 364
    inactivated 202
    live attenuated 202
    MMR 199
    therapeutic cancer 162
    viruses 202, 203
validity, outcome measures 485
vanadium pentoxide 1013
vancomycin 223
    resistance 225
vandetanib 788
vapour condensation test 979, 1136, 1142
variant Creutzfeldt-Jakob disease
    240, 344–5
vascular disrupting agents 55
vascular endothelial growth factor receptor
    (VEGFR), monoclonal antibodies
    48, 162
vascular endothelial growth factor
    (VEGF) 122
    gene therapy 114–15
    receptor antagonists 788
    tumour microenvironment 159
    wound healing 95
vascular tumours
    embolization 569–70
    sinonasal 1312, 1313
    see also juvenile angiofibroma
vasculitis 152–3
    Churg-Straus syndrome 152, 176, 1030,
        1033, 1041, 1218–19
    classification 175, 175
    with ENT implications 175–9
    GPA 152, 174, 176, 977, 981, 1032,
        1033, 1214–18
    laboratory diagnosis 152–3, 153
    nasal septal perforation 1151
    temporal arteritis 1260
vasoactive intestinal peptide 984
vasoconstrictor agents, abuse 1160
vasopressin, see arginine vasopressin
vasopressin type 2 receptor (V2R) 639
vasospasm, skin flap 113
vecuronium 319
venous thromboembolism (VTE)
    prophylaxis 294, 305–6
        thyroidectomy 802
    risk assessment 305
    risk factors 269–70, 269
    role of haematology 273
    treatment 270, 273
venous ulcers 101, 103
ventilation
    failed 319–21
    jet techniques 327–8, 327, 338
    post-operative 340
Ventrain device 320, 320

Venturi effect 1142
vertigo
    assessment instruments 490
    management 279
    medical negligence claims 443
Vertigo Handicap Questionnaire 490
vestibular schwannoma 21, 22, 560
vestibulitis (nasal) 289, 447
    treatment 289
video, in endoscopic sinus surgery 430
videolaryngoscopes 315–16
videoscopes 349
vidian nerve 963, 964, 1158
vinblastine, mode of action 43, 299, 299
vinca alkaloids 43, 299, 299
vincristine
    adverse effects 254
    mode of action 43, 299, 299
viral infections
    antiviral drugs 202–3
    haematological malignancies 253
    respiratory 197–9, 1087, 1126
    tumours associated with 160
viral vectors 30–1, 30, 203
Virchow's triad 269
virotherapy 203
virtue ethics 396
viruses
    associated pathologies 200–1, 200
    budding 185
    definition 195
    detection in clinical samples 196–7
    future research 203
    genome 196
    immune response to 132
    life cycle 196, 196
    and malignancy 201–2
    oncolytic 35, 203
    proteins 195–6
viscoelasticity, skin 112
visual analogue scales 486
    nasal patency 1135
    nasal septal perforation 1150, 1151
    rhinosinusitis 1025
visual field assessment 911, 912, 918, 931
visual problems
    after eyelid surgery 438
    orbital cellulitis 1116
    pituitary adenoma 911–12, 911, 918
    sinonasal tumours 1271
    suprasellar meningiomas 1302
vitamin D 298, 298, 624–5, 625
    calcium homeostasis 624–5, 625
    deficiency 625, 830
    excess/toxicosis 829, 830
    serum metabolites 830–1
    supplementation 625, 627, 854, 889
    in renal failure 867
vitamin K
    deficiency 263, 264
    therapy 246, 271, 271
vitiligo, Graves' disease 721, 721
vocal cords
    assessment in ICU patient 358
    collagen injection 297, 300
    contact endoscopy 589, 589, 590
    keratosis 590–1, 591
    optical coherence tomography 535–6

vocal cords (*continued*)
  paralysis
    parathyroid surgery 884
    secondary to chemotherapy 254
    thyroid surgery 888, 901
  rheumatological disease 174
  stem cell therapies 71–2
voice assessment questionnaires 491
Voice Handicap Index 491
voice prosthesis 347
volatile organic compounds (VOCs) 1021
volume averaging 561
volume rendering 561–2
vomer 966, 1136, 1136
vomeronasal system 983, 1229
von Graefe sign 706
von Willebrand disease 266
  management 266, 272–3
von Willebrand factor (vWF) 262, 266
  replacement 272–3
voriconazole 209, 211, 212, 254
voxels 561

Waardenburg syndrome 19, 24
Waldeyer's ring 252
Walsham's forceps 1187
Ward v. James 412
warfarin 270–1
  and epistaxis 1179
  mechanism of action 270–1, 294, 294
  reversal of anticoagulation 246, 271
warts 200
wasp allergy 146
Wegener's granulomatosis, *see* granulomatosis with polyangiitis (GPA)
well-being 399
Wermer's syndrome, *see* multiple endocrine neoplasia type 1 (MEN1)

Western blotting 6
wheat allergy 146
white cell count 253, 254
  and cancer outcomes 161
whooping cough 189
Wilsher v. Essex Area Health Authority 411
Wilson risk sum 313
WNT-β-catenin signalling pathway, thyroid tumours 85
Wolff–Chaikoff effect 622
wood manufacturers 1020
Woodruff's plexus 1170, 1171
working hours, and training 372
workplace-based assessments (WPBA) 370, 371, 374
World Health Assembly 76
World Health Organization (WHO)
  ARIA 1026, 1026, 1131
  definition of health 399
  Disability Assessment Schedule 2.0 (WHO-DAS 2) 488
  iodine deficiency and goitre 76, 76
  surgical checklist 453, 463
wound dressings 102–3
  acute wounds 102
  chronic wounds 102–3
wound healing
  delayed primary (tertiary intention) 94, 94, 104
  diabetic wounds 99, 103
  excessive 102
  impaired 98–9
  phases 94–7, 95
  primary intention 93, 94, 104
  secondary intention 93–4, 94
  superficial (partial-thickness) wounds 94

wound irrigation solutions 295
wounds
  acute 99–100
  assessment 101–2
  chronic 99, 100–1
  contraction 97
  defined 93
  fungating 300
  infection 99, 101, 103
  local anaesthetic infusions 305
  necrotic 101, 102
  surgical 100, 100

X-linked non-syndromic hearing impairment 17–18
X-linked syndromic hearing impairment (Alport syndrome) 20
xenografts
  bone 120
  collagen 120, 1153
xerostomia 234
  radioiodine therapy 754
  treatment 296
xylometazoline 286, 996, 996

yeasts 205
Young's operation 1180
Young's syndrome 1040–1

zafirlukast 1218
zanamivir 202–3
ZFX gene 86
zygomatic bone 1244
zygomatic complex fractures 1196–8, 1196, 1197
zygomatico-sphenoid suture line 1244
Zygomycetes 205